OBSTETRICS

OBSTETRICS

Normal and Problem Pregnancies

Fourth Edition

STEVEN G. GABBE, M.D.
Dean, Vanderbilt University School of Medicine
Professor of Obstetrics and Gynecology
Vanderbilt University Medical Center
Nashville, Tennessee

JENNIFER R. NIEBYL, M.D.
Professor and Head
Department of Obstetrics and Gynecology
University of Iowa College of Medicine
Iowa City, Iowa

JOE LEIGH SIMPSON, M.D.
Ernst W. Bertner Professor and Chairman
Department of Obstetrics and Gynecology
Professor of Molecular and Human Genetics
Baylor College of Medicine
Houston, Texas

Illustrated by
Mikki Senkarik, M.S., A.M.I., and Michael Cooley, A.M.I.

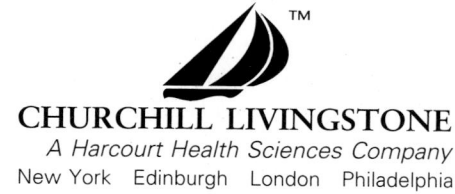

CHURCHILL LIVINGSTONE
A Harcourt Health Sciences Company
New York Edinburgh London Philadelphia

CHURCHILL LIVINGSTONE
A Harcourt Health Sciences Company

The Curtis Center
Independence Square West
Philadelphia, Pennsylvania 19106

Library of Congress Cataloging-in-Publication Data

Obstetrics: normal & problem pregnancies/[edited by] Steven G. Gabbe, Jennifer R.
Niebyl, Joe Leigh Simpson; illustrated by Mikki Senkarik and Michael Cooley.—4th ed.
    p.; cm.
  Includes bibliographical references and index.
  ISBN 0-443-06572-1
    1. Obstetrics. 2. Pregnancy—Complications. I. Title: Normal & problem pregnancies.
II. Title: Normal and problem pregnancies. III. Gabbe, Steven G. IV. Niebyl, Jennifer R.
V. Simpson, Joe Leigh
    [DNLM: 1. Obstetrics. 2. Pregnancy Complications. WQ 100 O165 2002]
  RG524.O3 2002
  618.2—dc21
                                                 00-047461

OBSTETRICS: Normal and Problem Pregnancies   ISBN 0-443-06572-1

Printed in the United States of America.

Last digit is the print number: 9 8 7 6 5 4 3 2 1

To our mentors, during our training at Cornell University Medical College and The New York Hospital: Dr. Irwin R. Merkatz and Dr. John T. Queenan

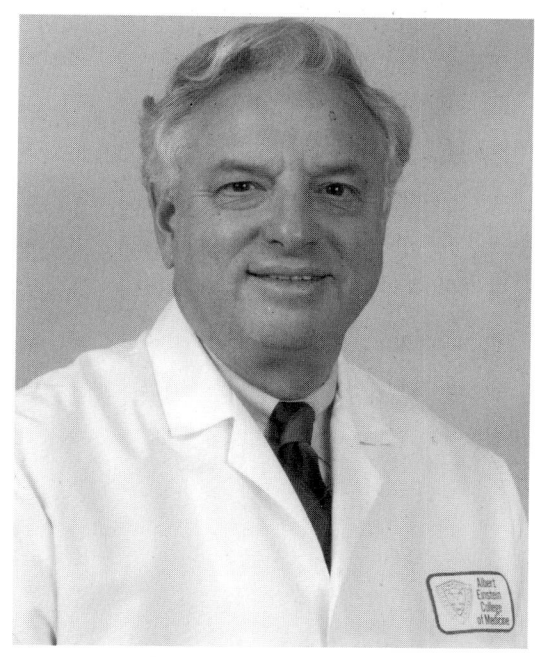

Dr. Irwin R. Merkatz

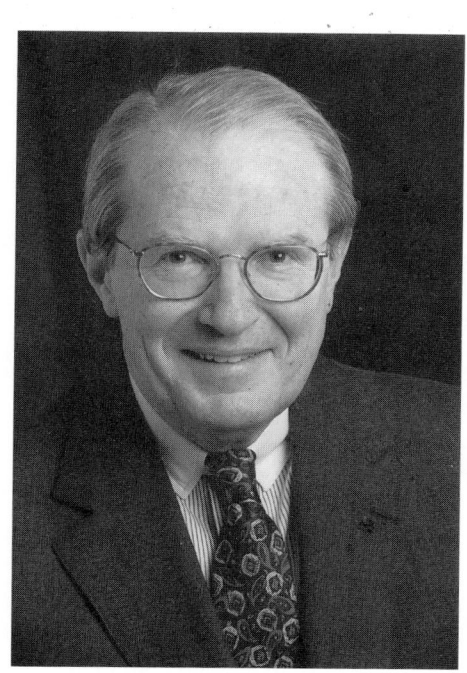

Dr. John T. Queenan

Contributors

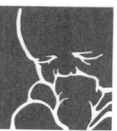

GEORGE J. ANNAS, J.D., M.P.H.
Professor of Health Law, Boston University Schools of Public Health, Medicine, and Law; Cofounder, Global Lawyers and Physicians, Boston, Massachusetts
Legal and Ethical Issues in Obstetric Practice

THOMAS J. BENEDETTI, M.D., M.H.A.
Professor and Director, Division of Perinatal Medicine, Vice-Chair Network Development and Operations, Department of Obstetrics and Gynecology, University of Washington School of Medicine, Seattle, Washington
Obstetric Hemorrhage

RICHARD L. BERKOWITZ, M.D.
Professor and Chairman, Department of Obstetrics, Gynecology, and Reproductive Sciences, Mount Sinai School of Medicine of New York University; Director of Obstetrics and Gynecology, Mount Sinai Hospital, New York, New York
Multiple Gestations

IRA BERNSTEIN, M.D.
Associate Professor, Department of Obstetrics and Gynecology, University of Vermont College of Medicine; Attending Physician, Fletcher Allen Health Care, Burlington, Vermont
Intrauterine Growth Restriction

WATSON A. BOWES, JR., M.D.
Emeritus Professor of Obstetrics and Gynecology, University of North Carolina at Chapel Hill School of Medicine, Chapel Hill, North Carolina
Postpartum Care

D. WARE BRANCH, M.D.
Professor, Department of Obstetrics and Gynecology, University of Utah School of Medicine, Salt Lake City, Utah
Alloimmunization in Pregnancy

JOHN E. BUSTER, M.D.
Professor, Department of Obstetrics and Gynecology, Baylor College of Medicine, Houston, Texas
Endocrinology and Diagnosis of Pregnancy

SANDRA A. CARSON, M.D.
Professor, Department of Obstetrics and Gynecology, Baylor College of Medicine, Houston, Texas
Endocrinology and Diagnosis of Pregnancy

PATRICK M. CATALANO, M.D.
Professor, Department of Reproductive Biology, Case Western Reserve University; Chairman, Department of Obstetrics and Gynecology, MetroHealth Medical Center, Cleveland, Ohio
Diabetes Mellitus

JOHN R.G. CHALLIS, Ph.D.
Professor, Departments of Physiology and Obstetrics and Gynecology, University of Toronto; Scientific Director, Canadian Institutes of Health Research (CIHR), Institute of Human Development, Child and Youth Health, Toronto, Ontario, Canada
Physiology and Endocrinology of Term and Preterm Labor

FRANK A. CHERVENAK, M.D.
Given Foundation Professor and Chairman, Department of Obstetrics and Gynecology, Weill Medical Center of Cornell University; Obstetrician and Gynecologist In-Chief, Department of Obstetrics and Gynecology, New York Presbyterian Hospital, New York, New York
Obstetric Ultrasound: Assessment of Fetal Growth and Anatomy

DAVID H. CHESTNUT, M.D.
Alfred Habeeb Professor and Chairman of Anesthesiology, and Professor of Obstetrics and Gynecology, University of Alabama School of Medicine, Birmingham, Alabama
Obstetric Anesthesia

USHA CHITKARA, M.D.
Professor, Division of Maternal-Fetal Medicine, Department of Gynecology and Obstetrics, Stanford University School of Medicine, Stanford, California
Multiple Gestations

DAVID F. COLOMBO, M.D.
Assistant Professor, Division of Maternal-Fetal
Medicine, Department of Obstetrics and Gynecology,
The Ohio State University College of Medicine,
Columbus, Ohio
Renal Disease

ROY COLVEN, M.D.
Assistant Professor of Medicine, Division of
Dermatology, University of Washington School of
Medicine; Attending Physician, Harborview Medical
Center, Seattle, Washington
Dermatologic Disorders

LARRY J. COPELAND, M.D.
Professor and Chair, Department of Obstetrics and
Gynecology, William Greenville Pace III and Joann
Norris Collins-Pace Chair, The Ohio State University
College of Medicine and Public Health, and James
Cancer Hospital and Solove Research Institute,
Columbus, Ohio
Malignant Diseases and Pregnancy

RICHARD DEPP, M.D.
Professor, Department of Obstetrics
and Gynecology, MCP Hahnemann University School
of Medicine, Philadelphia, Pennsylvania
Cesarean Delivery

MICHAEL Y. DIVON, M.D.
Professor of Obstetrics, Gynecology and Women's
Health, Albert Einstein College of Medicine, Bronx;
Chairman of Obstetrics and Gynecology, Lenox Hill
Hospital, New York, New York
Prolonged Pregnancy

MITCHELL P. DOMBROWSKI, M.D.
Professor, Division of Maternal-Fetal Medicine,
Department of Obstetrics and Gynecology, Wayne State
University School of Medicine, Hutzel Hospital,
Detroit, Michigan
Respiratory Diseases in Pregnancy

MAURICE L. DRUZIN, M.D.
Professor of Gynecology and Obstetrics, Stanford
University School of Medicine; Chief, Division of
Maternal-Fetal Medicine, Director of the Perinatal
Diagnostic Center, Stanford University Medical Center,
Stanford, California
Antepartum Fetal Evaluation

PATRICK DUFF, M.D.
Professor and Residency Program Director, Department
of Obstetrics and Gynecology, University of Florida
College of Medicine, Gainesville, Florida
Maternal and Perinatal Infection

THOMAS R. EASTERLING, M.D.
Associate Professor, Division of Prenatal Medicine,
Department of Obstetrics and Gynecology, University of
Washington School of Medicine, Seattle, Washington
Heart Disease

SHERMAN ELIAS, M.D.
Professor and Head, Department of Obstetrics and
Gynecology, and Professor, Department of Molecular
Genetics, University of Illinois at Chicago; Chief,
Department of Obstetrics and Gynecology, University
of Illinois Hospital, Chicago, Illinois
Legal and Ethical Issues in Obstetric Practice

M. GORE ERVIN, Ph.D.
Professor, Department of Biology, Middle Tennessee
State University, Murfreesboro, Tennessee
Placental and Fetal Physiology

MARK I. EVANS, M.D.
Professor and Chairman of Obstetrics and Gynecology,
Professor of Human Genetics, and Director, Fetal
Therapy Program, MCP Hahnemann University,
Philadelphia, Pennsylvania
Fetal Therapeutic Intervention

ALAN W. FLAKE, M.D.
Associate Professor of Surgery, and Obstetrics and
Gynecology, University of Pennsylvania; Director,
Children's Institute for Surgical Science, Children's
Hospital of Philadelphia, Philadelphia, Pennsylvania
Fetal Therapeutic Intervention

STEVEN G. GABBE, M.D.
Dean, Vanderbilt University School of Medicine,
Professor of Obstetrics and Gynecology, Vanderbilt
University Medical Center, Nashville, Tennessee
*Obstetric Ultrasound: Assessment of Fetal Growth
and Anatomy; Antepartum Fetal Evaluation;
Intrauterine Growth Restriction; Diabetes Mellitus*

THOMAS J. GARITE, M.D.
Professor and Chairman, Department of Obstetrics and
Gynecology, University of California, Irvine, School of
Medicine, Irvine, California
Intrapartum Fetal Evaluation

CHARLES P. GIBBS, M.D.
Professor Emeritus of Anesthesiology, University of
Colorado School of Medicine, Denver, Colorado
Obstetric Anesthesia

MICHAEL C. GORDON, M.D.
Chief of Obstetrics, Wilford Hall United States Air
Force Medical Center, San Antonio, Texas
Maternal Physiology in Pregnancy

MICHAEL R. HARRISON, M.D.
Professor of Surgery and Pediatrics, and Director, The Fetal Treatment Center, Chief, Division of Pediatric Surgery, University of California, San Francisco School of Medicine, San Francisco, California
Fetal Therapeutic Intervention

JOY L. HAWKINS, M.D.
Director of Obstetric Anesthesia and Professor of Anesthesiology, University of Colorado School of Medicine, Denver, Colorado
Obstetric Anesthesia

JAY D. IAMS, M.D.
Frederick P. Zuspan Professor and Director, Division of Maternal-Fetal Medicine, Department of Obstetrics and Gynecology, The Ohio State University College of Medicine and Public Health, Columbus, Ohio
Preterm Birth

MARC JACKSON, M.D.
Associate Professor, Department of Obstetrics and Gynecology, Temple University School of Medicine, Philadelphia; Division of Maternal-Fetal Medicine, Crozer-Chester Medical Center, Upland, Pennsylvania
Alloimmunization in Pregnancy

MARK P. JOHNSON, M.D.
Associate Professor, Departments of Obstetrics and Gynecology, and Surgery, University of Pennsylvania School of Medicine; Director of Obstetrical Services, Center for Fetal Diagnosis and Treatment, Children's Hospital of Philadelphia, Philadelphia, Pennsylvania
Fetal Therapeutic Intervention

TIMOTHY R.B. JOHNSON, M.D.
Bates Professor of the Diseases of Women and Children, Professor and Chair of Obstetrics and Gynecology, Research Scientist, Center for Human Growth and Development, and Professor of Women's Studies, Medical School and College of Literature, Science and the Arts, University of Michigan, Ann Arbor, Michigan
Preconception and Prenatal Care: Part of the Continuum

VERN L. KATZ, M.D.
Clinical Assistant Professor, Department of Obstetrics and Gynecology, University of Oregon School of Medicine, Portland; Director of Perinatal Services, Sacred Heart Medical Center, Eugene, Oregon
Postpartum Care

MARK B. LANDON, M.D.
Professor and Vice Chair, Department of Obstetrics and Gynecology, Division of Maternal-Fetal Medicine, The Ohio State University College of Medicine and Public Health, Columbus, Ohio
Diabetes Mellitus; Gastrointestinal Disease; Malignant Diseases and Pregnancy

SUSAN M. LANNI, M.D.
Assistant Professor of Obstetrics and Gynecology and Maternal Fetal Medicine, Virginia Commonwealth University, Medical College of Virginia Hospitals, Richmond, Virginia
Malpresentations

JACK LUDMIR, M.D.
Professor of Obstetrics and Gynecology, University of Pennsylvania School of Medicine; Chair, Department of Obstetrics and Gynecology, Pennsylvania Hospital, University of Pennsylvania Health System, Philadelphia, Pennsylvania
Surgical Procedures in Pregnancy

STEPHEN J. LYE, Ph.D.
Professor of Obstetrics and Gynaecology, and Physiology, University of Toronto Faculty of Medicine; Head, Program: Development, Samuel Lunenfeld Research Institute; Director, Canadian Institutes of Health Research (CIHR) Group in Fetal Health and Development, Toronto, Ontario, Canada
Physiology and Endocrinology of Term and Preterm Labor

JORGE H. MESTMAN, M.D.
Professor of Medicine and Obstetrics and Gynecology, University of Southern California Keck School of Medicine, Los Angeles, California
Endocrine Diseases in Pregnancy

EDWARD R. NEWTON, M.D.
Professor and Chairman, Department of Obstetrics and Gynecology, Brody School of Medicine, East Carolina University, Greenville, North Carolina
Physiology of Lactation and Breast-Feeding

JENNIFER R. NIEBYL, M.D.
Professor and Head, Department of Obstetrics and Gynecology, University of Iowa College of Medicine, Iowa City, Iowa
Preconception and Prenatal Care: Part of the Continuum; Occupational and Environmental Perspectives of Birth Defects; Drugs in Pregnancy and Lactation

ERROL R. NORWITZ, M.D., Ph.D.
Assistant Professor, Harvard Medical School;
Attending Perinatologist, Division of Maternal-Fetal
Medicine, Department of Obstetrics and Gynecology,
Brigham and Women's Hospital, Boston,
Massachusetts
Labor and Delivery

DONALD NOVAK, M.D.
Professor of Pediatrics and Chief, Section of Pediatric
Gastroenterology, University of Florida College of
Medicine, Gainesville, Florida
Placental and Fetal Physiology

CATHERINE OTTO, M.D.
Professor, Division of Cardiology, Department of
Medicine, University of Washington, Seattle,
Washington
Heart Disease

KATHRYN L. REED, M.D.
Professor, Department of Obstetrics and Gyneology
and Director of Ultrasound and Director of Maternal-
Fetal Medicine, Arizona Health Sciences Center,
Tucson, Arizona
*Antepartum Fetal Evaluation; Intrauterine Growth
Restriction*

JOHN T. REPKE, M.D.
Chris J. and Marie A. Olson Professor of Obstetrics
and Gynecology, and Chairman, Department of
Obstetrics and Gynecology, University of Nebraska
Medical Center, Omaha, Nebraska
Labor and Delivery

JULIAN N. ROBINSON, M.D.
Assistant Professor, and Attending Perinatologist,
Division of Maternal-Fetal Medicine, Department of
Obstetrics and Gynecology, Columbia-Presbyterian
Medical Center, Columbia University, New York,
New York
Labor and Delivery

ADAM A. ROSENBERG, M.D.
Professor of Pediatrics, University of Colorado School
of Medicine; Director of Nurseries, University of
Colorado Hospital, Denver, Colorado
The Neonate

MICHAEL G. ROSS, M.D., M.P.H.
Professor of Obstetrics and Gynecology, Department of
Community Health Sciences, University of California,
Los Angeles, School of Medicine, Los Angeles; Chair,
Department of Obstetrics and Gynecology, Harbor-
University of California, Los Angeles, Medical Center,
Torrance, California
Placental and Fetal Physiology

PHILIP SAMUELS, M.D.
Associate Professor and Director of Residency
Education Program, Department of Obstetrics and
Gynecology, The Ohio State University College of
Medicine and Public Health, Columbus, Ohio
*Renal Disease; Hematologic Complications of
Pregnancy; Collagen Vascular Diseases; Hepatic
Disease; Neurologic Disorders*

JOHN W. SEEDS, M.D.
Professor and Chairman, Department of Obstetrics and
Gynecology, Virginia Commonwealth University, Medical
College of Virginia Hospitals, Richmond, Virginia
Malpresentations

BAHA M. SIBAI, M.D.
Professor and Chairman, Department of Obstetrics and
Gynecology, University of Cincinnati College of
Medicine; Chief of Obstetrics, University Hospital,
Cincinnati, Ohio
Hypertension

JOE LEIGH SIMPSON, M.D.
Ernst W. Bertner Professor and Chairman, Department
of Obstetrics and Gynecology, and Professor of
Molecular and Human Genetics, Baylor College of
Medicine, Houston, Texas
*Occupational and Environmental Perspectives of
Birth Defects; Genetic Counseling and Prenatal
Diagnosis; Fetal Wastage*

ROXANNE STAMBUK, M.D., Ph.D.
Assistant Professor, Division of Dermatology,
University of Southern California Keck School of
Medicine; Attending Physician, Los Angeles County
and University of Southern California Medical Center,
Los Angeles, California
Dermatologic Disorders

PHILLIP G. STUBBLEFIELD, M.D.
Professor and Chairman, Department of Obstetrics and
Gynecology, Boston University School of Medicine;
Director of Obstetrics and Gynecology, Boston Medical
Center, Boston, Massachusetts
Surgical Procedures in Pregnancy

JANICE E. WHITTY, M.D.
Associate Professor, Division of Maternal-Fetal
Medicine, Department of Obstetrics and Gynecology,
Wayne State University School of Medicine, Hutzel
Hospital, Detroit, Michigan
Respiratory Diseases in Pregnancy

Preface to the Fourth Edition

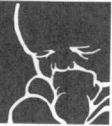

Obstetrics: Normal and Problem Pregnancies was published for the first time in 1986. With this fourth edition, our book thus enters its third decade. During these years, remarkable advances have occurred in some areas of obstetrics, whereas in others progress has been less marked. To provide our readers with the most important and most up-to-date information in our specialty, significant and extensive changes have been made throughout this fourth edition. Three new chapters have been added: Fetal Therapeutic Interventions, Surgical Procedures in Pregnancy, and Endocrine Diseases in Pregnancy. The chapter on Fetal Therapeutic Interventions describes especially exciting advances, both surgical and medical, emphasizing that the fetus as well as the mother is our patient. Other changes in this edition have been made for ease of reading and lucidity. With the exception of cesarean delivery, all surgical procedures in pregnancy were combined in a single chapter, emphasizing common principles of care. A separate chapter on diabetes mellitus complicating pregnancy has been developed, encompassing new information on the pathophysiology, diagnosis, and treatment of this important medical complication. We have replaced the chapter on anatomy with an appendix; readers can quickly access the excellent illustrations provided by Mikki Senkarik.

This fourth edition includes 28 authors who are making their first contributions to our textbook. They represent the vanguard of our specialty; readers will appreciate their expertise in presenting the most recent information in obstetrics. In addition to these new contributors, we want to recognize Drs. George J. Annas, Thomas J. Benedetti, Richard L. Berkowitz, Watson A. Bowes, Jr., D. Ware Branch, John E. Buster, Sherman Elias, Timothy R.B. Johnson, Mark B. Landon, Adam A. Rosenberg, Philip Samuels, John W. Seeds, Baha M. Sibai and Phillip G. Stubblefield. These luminaries have written chapters in every edition of our textbook. We thank them immensely and recognize them as leaders in our specialty.

With the acquisition of Churchill Livingstone by Harcourt Health Sciences Publishing Company, our book has benefited from the energies of a new publishing team, including Judith Fletcher and Ann Ruzycka. Readers will appreciate the more extensive use of color in headings, tables, and other key areas. In addition to the assistance provided by the staff at Harcourt Health Sciences, the editors have had the invaluable editorial and secretarial support of Susan Blewett, Nancy Schaapveld, and Belinda Felder.

This fourth edition of *Obstetrics: Normal and Problem Pregnancies*, like the three preceding it, has been a labor of love. We deliver it to you, our readers, with hopes that you will enjoy it and will find it a valuable resource.

Steven G. Gabbe, M.D.
Jennifer R. Niebyl, M.D.
Joe Leigh Simpson, M.D.

Preface to the First Edition

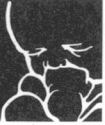

This book is written for a new generation of obstetricians and gynecologists. Today's obstetrician must not only be able to plot and interpret a labor curve and deliver a breech presentation but also must assess fetal heart rate tracings and scalp pH data. While doing so, he or she must also consider the legal and ethical ramifications for these actions. In the past decade, the practice of obstetrics has been altered by a technologic explosion. Antepartum and intrapartum fetal monitoring, diagnostic ultrasound, and a host of advances in prenatal genetic diagnosis have enabled obstetricians to identify and understand some of the most important disease processes. This information has already led to significant improvements in maternal and perinatal outcome. Yet, the practice of obstetrics and the applications of this technology must be built on a firm base of knowledge in anatomy, embryology, physiology, pathology, genetics, and teratology.

Obstetrics: Normal and Problem Pregnancies has been written to meet these needs. The first sections of the book provide the essential foundation for the practice of obstetrics. The reader can then proceed to discussions of the problems encountered in clinical practice and finally progress to the chapters devoted to high-risk obstetrics. Where does the information necessary to be a specialist end and that needed to be a subspecialist begin? This boundary is difficult to define. It is hoped that *Obstetrics: Normal and Problem Pregnancies* will serve as a reference source for the general practice of obstetrics and provide the necessary base of information for those in fellowship programs in maternal–fetal medicine.

The contributors to this book represent the vanguard in their areas of expertise. Each chapter has been written to stand on its own and, in general, can be read in one evening. As editors, we are most indebted to our collaborators for their excellent contributions and their willingness to create a new book with a new approach.

Our book could not have been written without the help of many special people. Toni M. Tracy, Editor-in-Chief at Churchill Livingstone, and Linda Panzarella, Sponsoring Editor, successfully guided us through this enormous but rewarding project. Lynne Herndon got us off to a good start. Mikki Senkarik prepared all of the original artwork for the book and, in doing so, showed her unique artistic skills and understanding. Dr. Gerald Lazarus, Chairman of the Department of Dermatology, Dr. Marshall Mintz of the Department of Radiology, and Dr. James Wheeler of the Department of Pathology, all at the Hospital of the University of Pennsylvania, provided guidance in the selection of illustrations for the chapters on infectious diseases, placental development, and antepartum fetal evaluation. Also, all of us owe so much to the secretarial support provided by Michele Simons and C. Winston Wisehart.

This is the first edition of *Obstetrics: Normal and Problem Pregnancies*. Now a neonate, it has completed its months and years of gestation. Hopefully, it will help those embarking on careers in obstetrics to enjoy the specialty as much as we have. We look forward to hearing comments, both positive and negative, from our readers.

Steven G. Gabbe, M.D.
Jennifer R. Niebyl, M.D.
Joe Leigh Simpson, M.D.

Contents

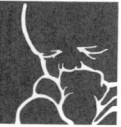

Section 7: LEGAL AND ETHICAL ISSUES IN PERINATOLOGY

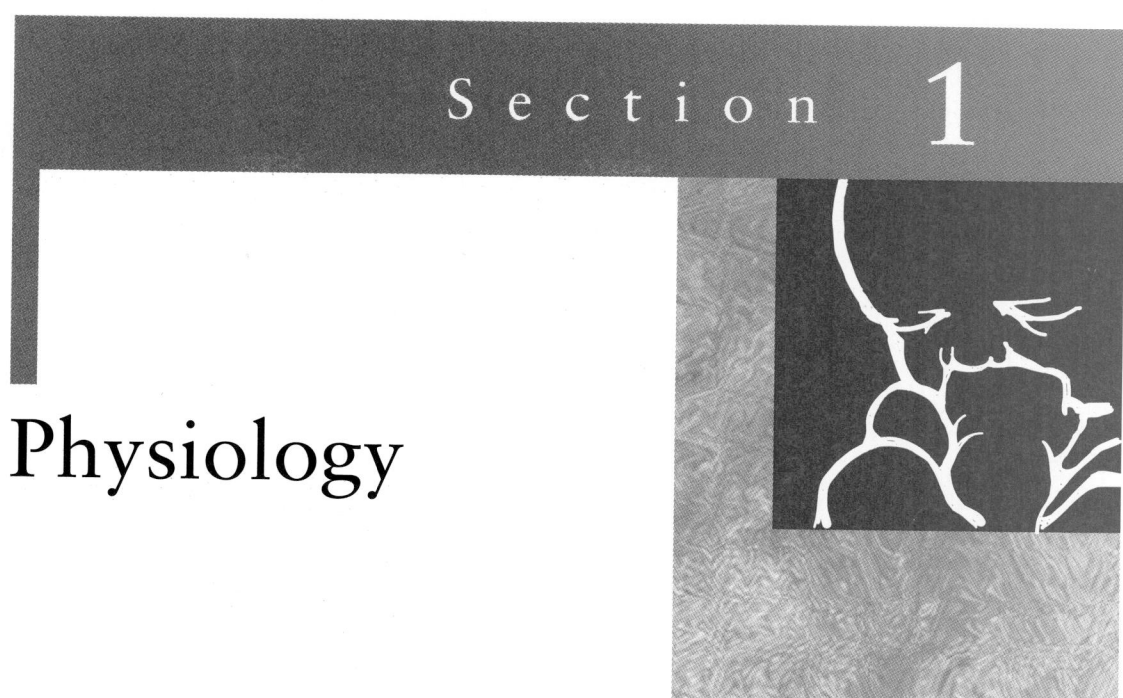

Section 1

Physiology

Chapter 1

Endocrinology and Diagnosis of Pregnancy

JOHN E. BUSTER AND SANDRA A. CARSON

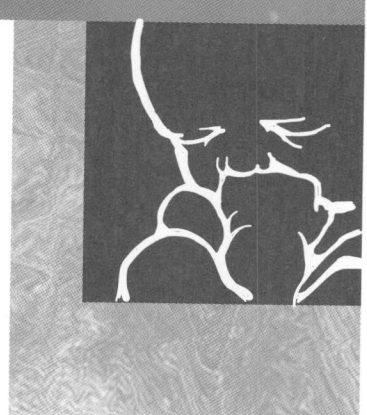

The evolutionary advent of viviparity necessitated changes in the maternal metabolic, hormonal, and immunologic systems. To compensate for the increased and altered demands of an intracorporeal pregnancy, a new organ—the placenta—and a series of proteins specific for and secreted only during pregnancy evolved. These proteins, aided by alterations in the already stimulated steroids, allow invasion of a half-foreign tissue into the maternal system that not only tolerates but actively nourishes and protects the growing fetus. The changes in the hormonal milieu also help to diagnose and monitor pregnancy, and they are the focus of this chapter.

PREGNANCY PROTEINS

Ontogeny of Pregnancy Protein Production

From the moment of conception, proteins are released into the maternal system by the newly formed conceptus, presumably to alter the maternal immune metabolic and hormonal responses to the advancing gestation. The production and secretion of these proteins mirror the demands that each developmental stage of gestation brings.

The Preimplantation Conceptus

Pregnancy proteins are present in the maternal circulation almost at the time of conception. Presumably released from the fertilized ovum after sperm penetration, a platelet-activating factor (PAF)-like substance is evident almost immediately.[1-4] The conceptus remains in the tubal ampulla for approximately 80 hours after follicular rupture, travels through the isthmus for approximately 10 hours, and then enters the uterus as a two- to eight-cell embryo.[5,6] The embryo develops into a blastocyst while freely floating in the endometrial cavity 90 to 150 hours after conception.[6] Although human chorionic gonadotropin (hCG) mRNA is detectable in the blastomeres of six- to eight-cell embryos at 2 days, the hormone is not detectable until 6 days (blastocyst) in culture media.[7-9] Secretion into the maternal serum is limited by the absence of vascular communication.[10] Successful implantation results from a precise orchestration of cytokines and growth factors that bind the foreign embryo to the maternal interface[10] (Fig. 1–1). Only after implantation is completed is hCG detectable in maternal serum, 8 to 11 days after conception.[11-13]

The Implanted Conceptus

Blastomeres destined to form the placenta can be identified as trophectoderm lining the periphery of the blastocyst 5 days after conception (Fig. 1–2). By the tenth day, invading trophoblasts have formed two distinct layers: an inner layer composed of individual, well-defined, and rapidly proliferating cells, the *cytotrophoblasts;* and an outer and thicker layer comprising a continuous mass of cell plasma containing multiple nuclei with indistinct cell borders, the *syncytiotrophoblast* (Figs. 1–3 and 1–4). The syncytiotrophoblasts line the fetal side of the intervillous space opposite the decidualized endometrium on the maternal side (Fig. 1–4).

Cytotrophoblasts stain immunohistochemically for hypothalamic-like peptides: corticotropin-releasing hormone (CRH), gonadotropin-releasing hormone (GnRH), and thyrotropin-releasing hormone (TRH).[14-26] The juxtaposed cytotrophoblasts stain immunohistochemically for corresponding pituitary-like peptides: adrenocorticotropic hormone (ACTH), hCG (analogous to

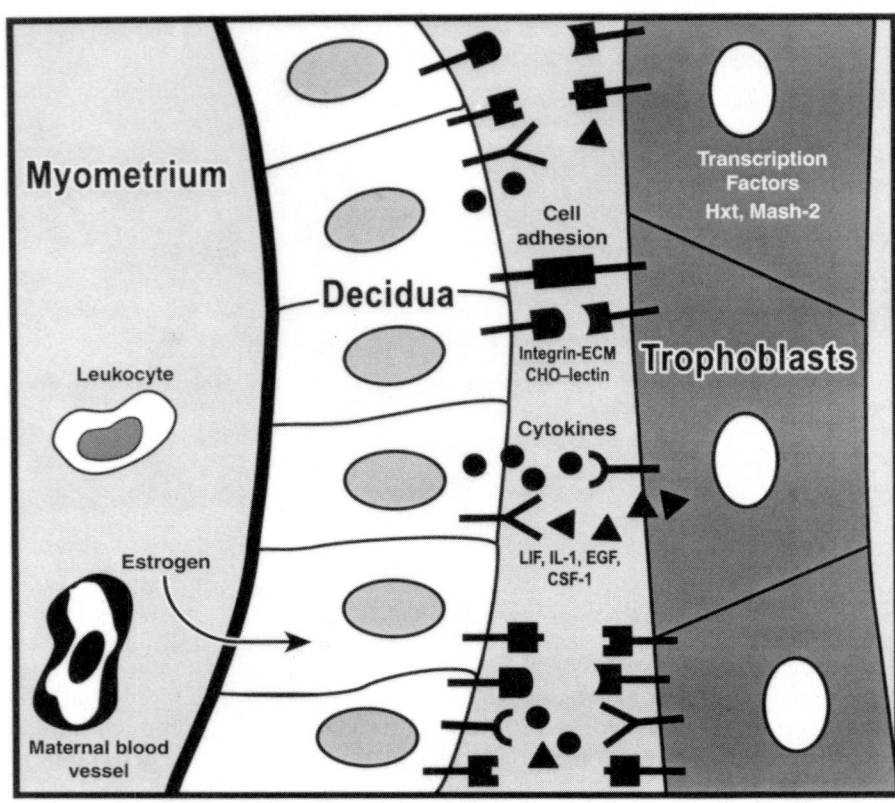

Figure 1–1. Interface between trophoblasts and endometrium at implantation. At approximately day 7 of embryonic life, the blastocyst attaches to the uterine wall. Endometrium clamps around the blastocyst. The uterus is not receptive until the "windows of implantation" are open. Maternal estrogens are believed to induce the endometrial permissiveness needed for blastocyst attachment. Estrogens induce the release of cytokines such as leukemia inhibitory factor (LIF), interleukin-1 (IL-1), epidermal growth factor (EGF), and others. The adhesive mechanisms that regulate embryonic attachment are not well understood but likely involve the interactions of carbohydrates and phospholipids: Cho–lectin, integrin–integrin, and integrin–extracellular matrix (ECM) linkages. (Adapted from Cross JC, Werb Z, Fisher SJ: Implantation and the placenta: key pieces of the development puzzle. Science 266:1508, 1994, with permission.)

pituitary luteinizing hormone [LH]), and human chorionic thyrotropin (hCT). This anatomic arrangement suggests that these two layers mirror the paracrine relationship of the hypothalamic-pituitary axis[14–26] (Table 1–1).

Syncytiotrophoblasts are the principal site of placental steroid and protein hormone biosynthesis. The cells have a large surface area and line the intervillous space, which exposes them directly to the maternal bloodstream without the blood vessel endothelium and basement membrane, which separates them from the fetal circulation. Thus, both cell types are ideal for both hormone secretion and nutrient exchange.[27] This anatomic arrangement also explains why placental proteins are secreted almost exclusively into the maternal circulation in concentrations much higher than those in the fetus.[27]

The syncytiotrophoblast cell layer contains abundant rough endoplasmic reticulum, Golgi complexes, and mitochondria, the subcellular machinery that characterizes hormone syntheses (Fig. 1–4). Prohormones are assembled from amino acids of maternal origin within the rough endoplasmic reticulum of the syncytiotrophoblast. Assembled into early secretory granules in the Golgi complex, these prohormones are transferred across trophoblastic cell membranes as mature granules.

The mature granules then become soluble as circulating hormones in maternal blood passing through the intervillous space[27] (Fig. 1–4).

Decidualized endometrium is a site of maternal steroid and protein biosynthesis that is related directly to the maintenance and protection of the pregnancy from immunologic rejection.

The Mature Placenta

Throughout the second and third trimesters, the placenta adapts its structure to reflect its function. As fetomaternal exchange dominates hormone secretory functions, the relative numbers of trophoblasts decrease.[19] The villi near term (Figs. 1–4 and 1–5) consist largely of fetal capillaries with little or no stroma beyond that required for anatomic integrity. Cytotrophoblasts are sparse, and the remaining syncytium is thin, scarcely visible by light microscopy. In contrast to the early villus, in which the trophoblasts are present in abundance with a continuous basal cytotrophoblast layer and an overlying surface syncytium, the placenta's membranous interface between fetal and maternal circulation is extremely thin.[27] This villous structure facilitates specialized transport of compounds across the fetomaternal interface.[27]

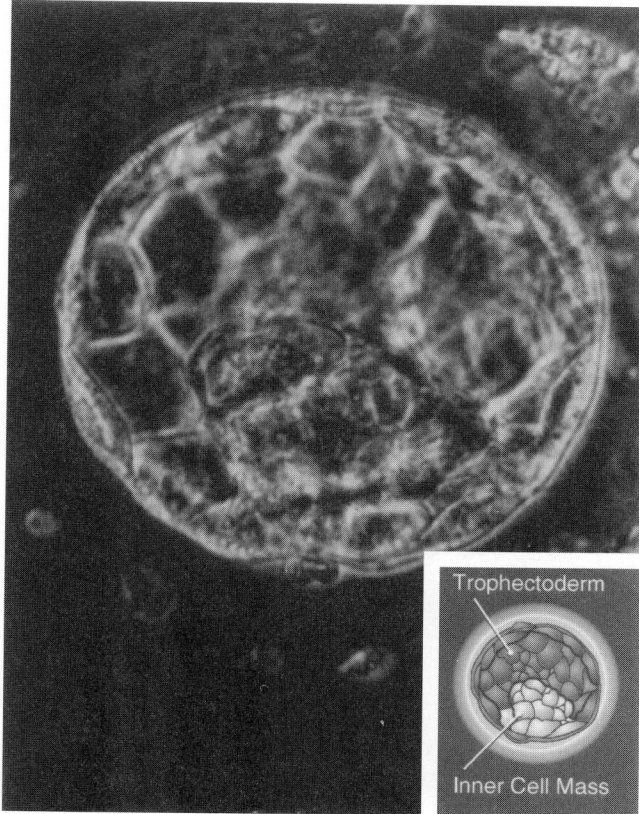

Figure 1–2. The human preimplantation blastocyst. The inner cell mass, the cells destined to form embryonic structure, are seen between 3 and 6 o'clock. Trophectoderm, comprising the remainder, evolves into placenta and membranes. (Adapted from Buster JE, Bustillo M, Rodi LA, et al: Biological and morphologic development of donated human ova recovered by nonsurgical uterine lavage. Am J Obstet Gynecol 153:211, 1985.)

Physiology of Pregnancy Proteins

The sequential appearance is characteristic for each protein, reflecting their various functions unique to pregnancy (Table 1–1).

Early Pregnancy Factor

MOLECULAR STRUCTURE. Early pregnancy factor (EPF) has been purified from human platelets and found to be closely homologous to chaperonin 10 (cpn10), a member of the heat-shock family of proteins.[28] Cpn10 is an intracellular protein that is believed to act together with chaperonin 60 (cpn60) within mitochondria to mediate protein folding.[1,2] EPF, a product of platelet activation and cell proliferation, is secreted into the circulation from cytoplasm by unknown mechanisms. Chaperonin proteins are believed to be highly potent immunosuppressants that assemble immunoglobulins, direct lymphocyte homing, and suppress some autoimmune diseases.[1,2] Although they act intra-

cellularly, they are also expressed on the cell surface.[1,2] One group of investigators reports having purified EPF from human platelets.[29,30] This cpn10 homologue has a molecular mass of 10,843.5 Da.[28] The only assay for EPF is a bioassay, the rosette inhibition test. The rosette inhibition test assesses ability of lymphocytes to bind in vitro and is quantitated by the degree to which rosette formation between lymphocytes and heterologous (sheep) red blood cells is inhibited.[1,2] This bioassay is lengthy, tedious, and imprecise. No radioimmunoassay has been described.

ORIGIN. That EPF is a single molecular substance is not accepted by all investigators.[31–35] EPF is believed to be produced within activated platelets, the maternal ovaries, and other maternal tissues.[1–4] Its release is stimulated by a PAF that is released from the conceptus at fertilization (Fig. 1–6).[3,4] It is believed that sperm entry into the ovum releases PAF, which circulates to other maternal tissues.[3,4] PAF also acts upon the ovum itself to stimulate local EPF release. By blastocyst stage, this local EPF may have endometrial immunosuppressive function.[1,2] Because embryonic EPF probably does not reach the circulation until implantation, removal of the ovaries in experimental animals shortly after conception, but before implantation, produces immediate disappearance of EPF from the circulation.[3,4]

NORMAL VARIATION. Serum EPF is the earliest known marker of fertilization. It is detectable in the circulation within 6 to 24 hours after conception, with maximum levels reached in the early first trimester, diminishing to almost undetectable levels at term[1,2] (Fig. 1–7). In early human studies, EPF was detected after intercourse in 18 of 28 ovulatory cycles, suggesting a fertilization rate of 67 percent. Embryonic loss was high (78 percent), because EPF disappeared from the circulation before the onset of menstruation in 14 of 18 cases.[36] In the remaining four cases, EPF remained detectable beyond 14

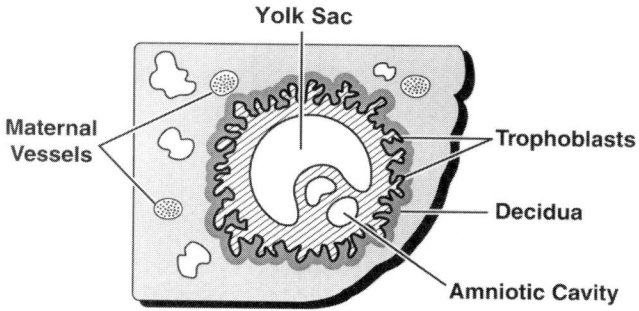

Figure 1–3. Postimplantation embryo and early placental structures. Trophoblasts are seen to invade maternal decidua, which contains blood-filled lacunar spaces. The embryo has evolved as a simple embryonic disk in association with a very large yolk sac and developing amniotic cavity.

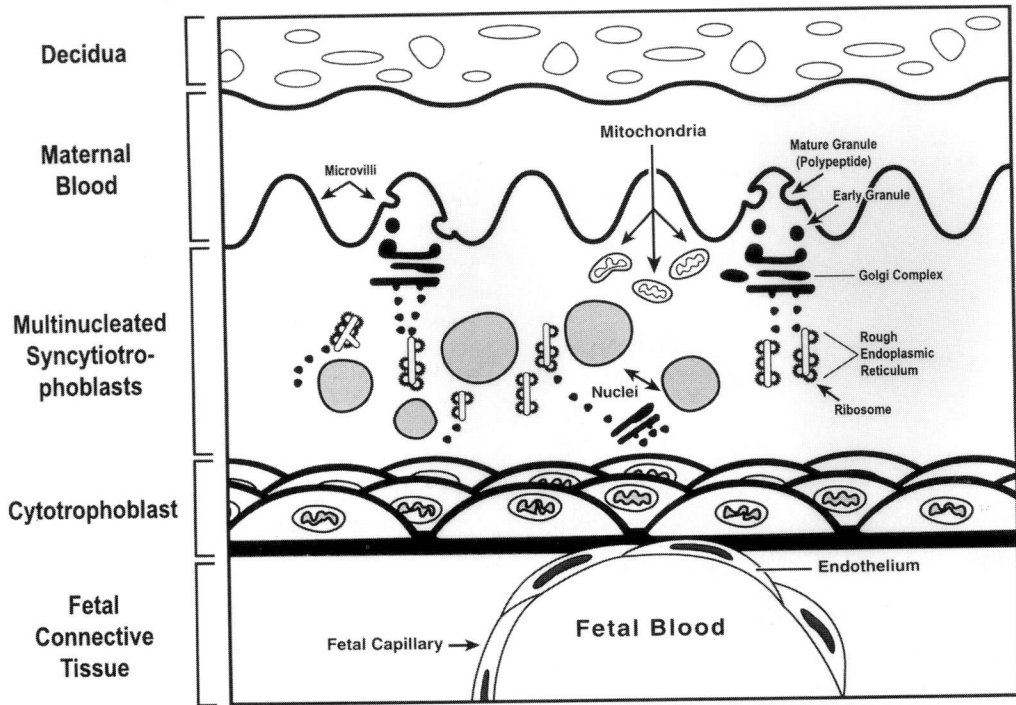

Figure 1–4. The human placenta at term in a cross-sectional electron microscopic view. Syncytiotrophoblasts line the fetal surface of the intervillous space and interact with the maternal blood supply to secrete placental proteins directly into the circulation. Decidua lines maternal surfaces of the intervillous space and secretes its own unique protein hormones into the maternal circulation. (Adapted from Osathanondh R, Tulchinsky D: Placental polypeptide hormones. *In* Tulchinsky D, Ryan KJ [eds]: Maternal-Fetal Endocrinology. Philadelphia, WB Saunders Company, 1980, p 18.)

days with presence of a viable embryo.[36] EPF appears within 48 hours after successful in vitro fertilization and embryo transfer.[1,2] It disappears within 24 hours after reduced abortion and is undetectable in many spontaneous abortions, ectopic pregnancies, and following a complete removal of gestational trophoblastic diseases.[36–43] EPF is detectable in cases of latent trophoblastic disease and disappears when the disease resolves completely.[43]

Inability to detect EPF during pregnancy portends a poor prognosis. Clinical application of EPF measurements is promising but elusive because of difficulties in isolating the molecule and developing practical assays for it.[1–4]

FUNCTION. EPF is believed to prevent rejection of an antigenically alien embryo. Binding to a specific lymphocyte population, it recruits suppressor cells that in turn release soluble suppressor factors that are believed to protect the pregnancy.[1,2,44,45] In its association with dividing cells, EPF also has properties of a growth factor that regulates cell proliferation.[1,2,44,45]

The coding sequence for EPF has a high degree of homology with a sequence for human cpn10.[46] Sequences have been identified in nine locations on eight different chromosomes, suggesting that EPF is a member of a large gene family.[46] EPF-like molecules have also been obtained in culture supernatants from stimulated lymphocytes of pregnant women.[29,30] EPF activity has been confirmed in these supernatants by the rosette inhibition test.[29,30]

Placental Proteins

Placental protein hormone synthesis may be a direct reflection of both trophoblastic mass and intervillous maternal blood flow.[27] Control of their release is poorly understood; one hypothesis suggests that placental hormone production is regulated by negative feedback to maintain a fixed intervillous hormone concentration. An alternative hypothesis suggests the hypothalamic-like placental peptides (CRH, GnRH, TRH, and somatostatin [SRIF]), located in the cytotrophoblasts, stimulate the pituitary-like placental hormones (ACTH, hCG, and hCT) located in the adjacent syncytiotrophoblasts.[14–27] The former hypothesis is only speculative, but does prove a convenient grouping of hormones which, for heuristic reasons, is used in this discussion (Table 1–1).

Table 1–1. CYTOCHEMICAL DISTRIBUTION OF PREGNANCY PROTEINS

Peptide	Abbreviation	Cytotrophoblast	Syncytiotrophoblast	Decidua	References
Hypothalamic-like hormones					
Corticotropin-releasing hormone	CRH	+		+	15,73
Gonadotropin-releasing hormone	GnRH	+			16
Thyrotropin-releasing hormone	TRH	+			17,85
Somatostatin	SRIF	+			26
Pituitary-like hormones					
Adrenocorticotropic hormone	ACTH		+		18,71
Human chorionic gonadotropin	hCG		+		19,22–24
Human chorionic thyrotropin	hCT		?		20
Human placental lactogen	hPL		+		23,24
Growth factors					
Inhibin/activin	N/A		+		73
Transforming growth factor	TGF-β		+		86,108
Insulin-like growth factor 1 & 2	IGF-1; IGF-2		+		83,105
Epidermal growth factor	EGF		+		87,109
Other pregnancy proteins					
Pregnancy-specific β1-glycoprotein	SP1		+		111
Placental protein 5	PP5		+		115
Pregnancy-associated plasma protein-A*	PAPP-A		+		114
Prolactin	PRL			+	25
Relaxin*	N/A			+	103,125,127
IGF-1 binding protein	IGF-1BP, PP12			+	128,132
Placental protein 14	PP14			+	106,131
α-Fetoprotein†	AFP			+	110,134

* Relaxin is secreted principally by the corpus luteum and secondarily from decidua.[131,132]
† AFP is fetal in origin.[134]

PITUITARY-LIKE HORMONES

Human Chorionic Gonadotropin

Molecular Structure. HCG is a glycoprotein with structural similarity to follicle-stimulating hormone (FSH), LH, and thyroid-stimulating hormone (TSH). As are the other glycoprotein hormones, hCG is composed of two nonidentical subunits associated noncovalently[14,47] (Fig. 1–8). The α subunit consists of a 92-amino-acid sequence essentially identical and shared in common with the pituitary glycoprotein hormones (Fig. 1–8). The β subunit, although structurally similar, differs just enough to confer specific biologic activity on the intact (dimer) hormones. The subunits differ primarily at the COOH terminus, where the β subunit of hCG has a 30-amino-acid tailpiece that is not present in the human luteinizing hormone (hLH) β subunit. Assuming an average carbohydrate content of 30 percent, the molecular weight of dimer hCG is approximately 36.7 kDa; the α subunit contributes 14.5 kDa and the β subunit 22.2 kDa.[47] Biologic activity of the hCG molecule is profoundly affected by its carbohydrate content and its resulting tertiary structure (Fig. 1–9).[48–50] Desi-alation of pregnancy hCG renders the molecule biologically inactive.[48]

Origin. HCG mRNA is detectable in blastomeres of six- to eight-cell embryos.[7] After implantation, hormonal hCG is present in the outer syncytial layer.[12,22–24] α-HCG subunits are localized to the cytotrophoblasts with none in the syncytial layer.[19,22]

HCG secretion is related to the mass of the hCG-secreting trophoblastic tissues. Thus, the release of hCG in vivo has been correlated with the respective trophoblast layer widths from weeks 4 through 20 and with placental weights from 20 to 38 weeks.[19] Between 3 and 9 weeks' gestation, rapidly rising hCG coincides with proliferation of immature trophoblastic villi and an extensive syncytial layer.[19] Between 10 and 18 weeks' gestation, declining hCG is associated with a relative reduction in syncytiotrophoblasts and cytotrophoblasts (Fig. 1–5). From 20 weeks to term, a gradual increase in dimer hCG corresponds with a gradual increase in placental weight and villus volume.[19] In summary, rising hCG reflects the histology of a rapidly proliferating and invasive placenta. Falling hCG is associated with a relative reduction in tropho-

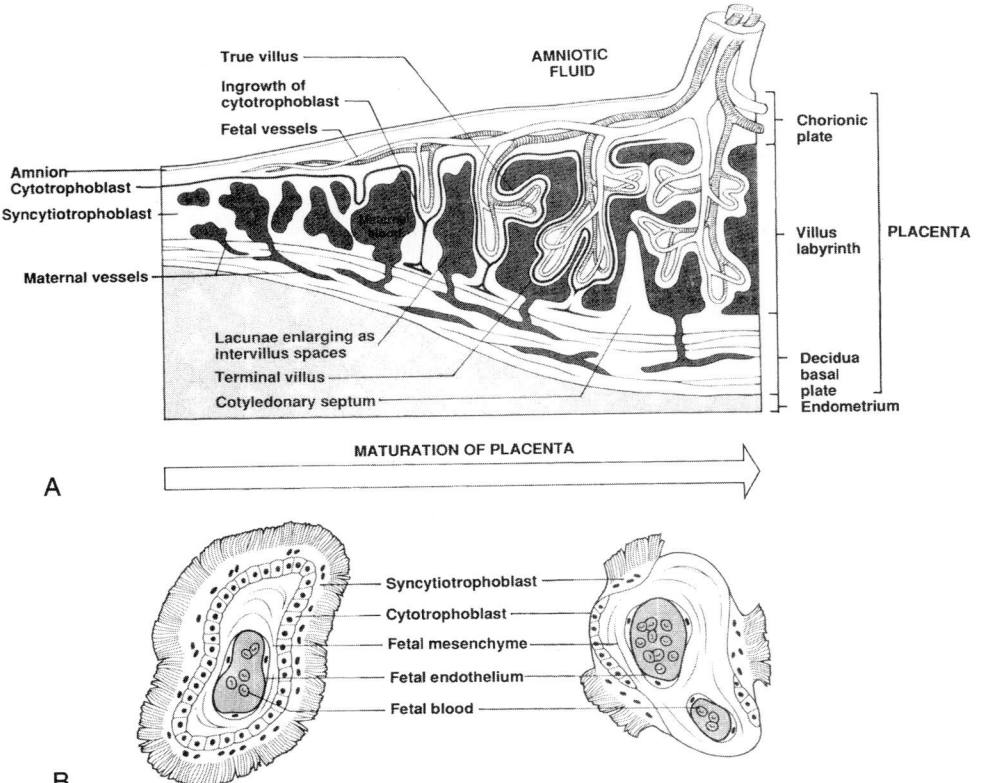

Figure 1–5. *A*, Gross morphology of the human placenta. The effects of advancing gestation on placental morphology evolve from left to right. Placental mass increases and hormonally active and invasive trophoblasts compose a lesser percentage of the total mass as the placenta evolves as an organ of transfer. *B*, Anatomic structure of early and late terminal villi. These transverse sections through terminal villi are from early (*left*) and term (*right*) pregnancy. Cytotrophoblastic cells become infrequent with placental maturity. Increasing fibrin deposits occur by term gestation as placental function adapts more to maternal fetal transfer and relatively less to hormone production. Fetal capillary endothelium is the only structure separating the maternal circulation from the fetal circulation in the mature placenta. (Modified from Williams L, Warwick L: Gray's Anatomy, 36th ed. Philadelphia, WB Saunders Company, 1980, p 125.)

blasts and reflects a morphologic transformation of the placenta into an organ of transfer.[19]

HCG secretion is linked to placental GnRH.[51] In an in vitro trophoblast perfusion system, hCG is released in 11- to 22-minute pulses, where the pulse frequency and amplitude are believed entrained to the release of placental GnRH.[51] HCG production is stimulated by glucocorticoids and suppressed by dehydroepiandrosterone sulfate (DHEA-S).[52] Cyclic adenosine monophosphate (cAMP) analogues augment secretion of hCG and α-hCG in vitro.[51,52] Decidual inhibin and prolactin inhibit hCG production by term human trophoblasts, whereas decidual activin augments it.[47,53]

In a countermechanism, follistatin binds activin and therefore inhibits the stimulatory activity of activin. Other growth factors (insulin-like growth factor 1 [IGF-1], IGF-2, transforming growth factor-β [TGF-β] and epidermal growth factor [EGF]) also impact on gene regulation of the hCG system in the placenta.[54,55]

Although nonpregnancy tissues make hCG, the placenta uniquely glycosylates it (Fig. 1–9).[48–50,56–58] Glycosylation substantially reduces hCG clearance; conse-

quently, the half-life of pregnancy hCG is extended (Fig. 1–9).[48] Thus, nonpregnancy hCG has a very short half-life, as does hLH.[48,59] The DNA sequences of the β-hCG gene and the β-LH gene are close to identical; however, different promoter and transcriptional sites uniquely located upstream in the β-hCG subunit gene, as opposed to β-LH subunit gene, confirm structure as well as regulation.[60] It has been suggested that hCG secretion escapes feedback regulation by the sex steroids, because the β-hCG subunit promoter does not contain steroid hormonal response elements, a phenomenon in contradistinction to FSH and LH.[60–63] The genes that encode for the β subunits of LH, hCG, and TSH are located on chromosome 19q13.3. There are reportedly six genes for the β subunit of hCG as opposed to only one for β-LH. There appears to be a single human gene for the expression of the α subunit. That gene, which also codes for subunits of FSH, LH, and TSH, is located on chromosome 6p21.1 23.[60] Whereas the α subunit gene is expressed in many different cell types, the β subunit genes are restricted in cell type (i.e., β-TSH in thyrotropes, β-FSH in gonadotropes,

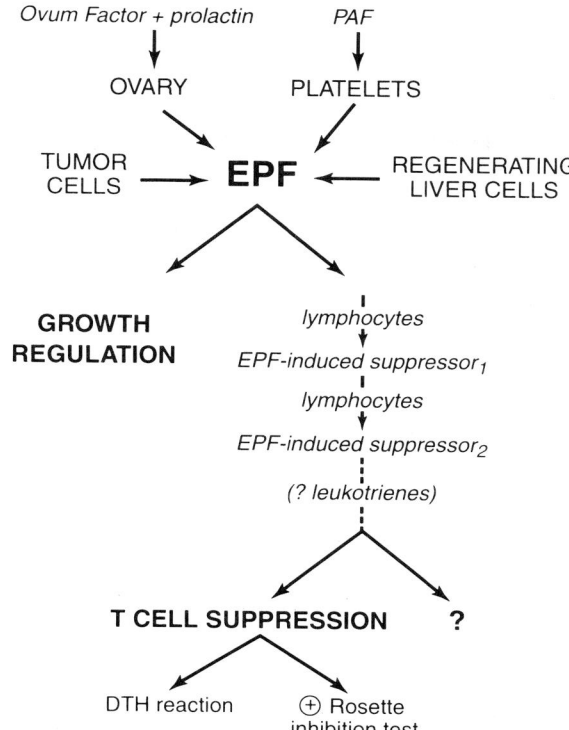

Figure 1–6. Flow chart demonstrating multiple sources of EPF. It is believed to be produced within activated platelets, maternal ovaries, and other maternal tissues. Ovum factor, a form of platelet activating factor, is thought to be released from the conceptus at fertilization, which leads to the above immunologic cascade. DTH, delayed tissue hypersensitivity (Modified from Morton H: Early pregnancy factor: an extracellular chaperonin 10 homologue. Immunol Cell Biol 76: 483, 1998, with permission.)

(Fig. 1–10C). Levels of subunit are very low relative to dimer hCG, approximately 2,000-fold to 150-fold less at 6 and 35 weeks, respectively[19] (Fig. 1–10C).

"Nicked hCG," hCG molecules missing a peptide linkage on the β subunit, increase with advancing gestation in parallel with free α subunits into which it disassociates.[64] A final reduced fragment, the β core fragment, is a product of renal metabolism and is cleared through the kidneys. These are over 30 known hCG isoforms present in maternal blood, with calculating concentrations similar and parallel to the increases observed in hCG in early pregnancy and the decreasing levels seen as pregnancy advances to term.[64]

HCG secretion may be increased in cases of fetal Down syndrome, where up-regulation of hCG occurs as an effect of the extra chromosome 21.[65]

Function. HCG is believed to be the major factor in maintaining the corpus luteum.[66] It stimulates both adrenal and placental steroidogenesis,[67] and it stimulates the fetal testes to secrete increasing amounts of testosterone to induce internal virilization.[68] HCG is immunosuppressive and may be involved in maternal lymphocyte function.[69] Finally, HCG possesses thyrotrophic activity.[70]

Adrenocorticotropin

Molecular Structure and Origin. Placental ACTH is structurally similar to pituitary ACTH. Under paracrine influence of placental CRH from the juxtaposed cyto-

and β-hCG in the placenta).[60–63] HCG may be secreted by maternal tissues including kidneys and pituitary.[56–58] Pituitary secretion of hCG in very small amounts is probably a normal event in healthy postmenopausal women.[58] There are rare case reports of larger amounts being secreted from this source.[56]

Normal Variation. Figure 1–10 depicts maternal levels of dimer hCG, α-hCG subunits, and β-hCG subunits from 3 to 40 weeks gestational age.[19] At 4 weeks' gestation, mean doubling times of dimer hCG are 2.2 (SD ± 0.8) days, falling to 3.5 (SD ± 1.2) days at 9 weeks.[19] The peak median level is 108,800 mIU/ml at 10 weeks.[19] Between 12 and 16 weeks, median dimer hCG decreases rapidly, with a mean halving time of 2.5 (SD ± 1.1) days to 25 percent of first-trimester peak values. Levels continue to fall, from 16 to 22 weeks, at a slower mean halving rate of 4.1 (SD ± 1.8) days to become 10.7 percent of peak first-trimester median hCG.[19] During the third trimester, mean hCG rises gradually but significantly from 22 weeks until term.[19]

β-hCG subunit levels parallel dimer hCG (Fig. 1–10B). α-HCG, not detectable until about 6 weeks, rises in a sigmoid curve to reach peak levels in 36 weeks

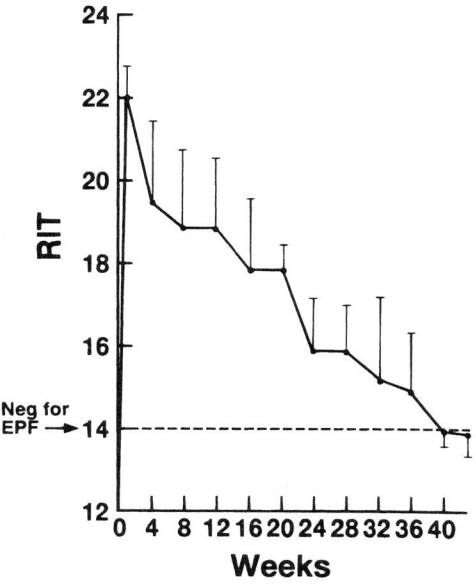

Figure 1–7. Early pregnancy factor (EPF) activity in serum tested before and at various times throughout pregnancy and after parturition. EPF activity is expressed as rosette inhibition titre (RIT; mean ±SEM). *Broken lines* indicate the RIT obtained with nonpregnant serum. (From Morton H, Rolfe BE, Cavanagh AC: Ovum factor and early pregnancy factor. Curr Top Dev Biol 23:73, 1987.)

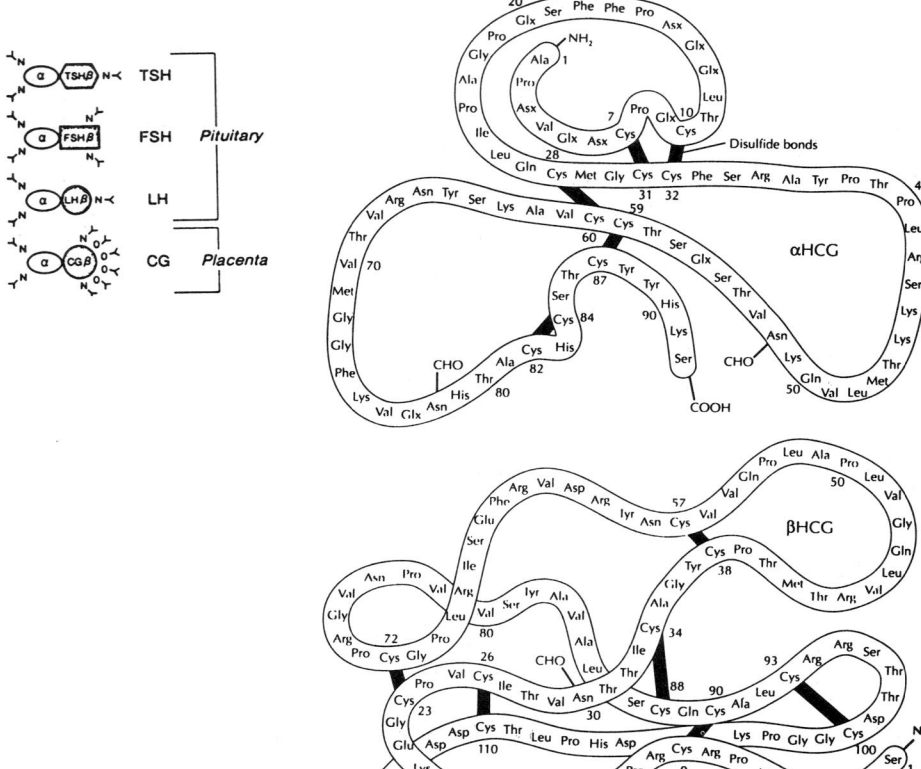

Figure 1–8. HCG and LH amino acid cores. They are structurally similar to one another except for a "tailpiece" at the terminus of the β side chain of hCG, which makes the latter structurally distinct. Disulfide bonds are marked with *dark lines.* Structural homology (*inset*) is shown for hCGs and three other pituitary glycoprotein hormones, LH, FSH, and TSH. The α-chain of hCG is biochemically and immunologically similar to the α-chain of the three pituitary glycoproteins. (Modified from Ren SG, Braunstein GD: Human chorionic gonadotropin. Semin Reprod Endocrinol 10:95, 1992; and Walker WH, Fitzpatrick SL, Barrera-Saldana HA, et al: The human placental lactogen genes: structure function, evolution and transcriptional regulation. Endocr Soc 4:316, 1991. © The Endocrine Society, with permission.)

tropboblasts, placental ACTH is produced by the syncytiotrophoblasts and secreted into the maternal circulation.[71-73]

Normal Variation and Function. Circulating maternal ACTH is increased above nonpregnancy levels, but remains within the upper normal range.[72,74] Placental ACTH stimulates an increase in circulating maternal free cortisol resistant to dexamethasone suppression.[71,74] Thus, the relative hypercortisolism of pregnancy occurs despite a high normal ACTH concentration. This regulation is made possible by two differences in endocrine relationships during pregnancy. First, maternal ACTH response to exogenous CRH is blunted.[74] Second, a paradoxical relationship exists between placental ACTH and CRH and their end-organ product, cortisol: glucocorticoids augment placental CRH and ACTH secretion.[74-76] Teleologically, this positive feedback mechanism allows an increase in glucocorticoid secretion in times of stress over and above the amount necessary if the mother was not pregnant.[76]

Human Somatomammotropin

Molecular Structure and Origin. Human chorionic somatomammotropin (hCS), or human placental lactogen (hPL), is a single-chain polypeptide with two intramolecular disulfide bridges and a molecular weight of 22.3 kDa. Of the 191 amino acids, 167 (85 percent) are identical to human pituitary growth hormone and human pituitary prolactin.[77,78] Accordingly, hCS shares biologic properties with both growth hormone and prolactin.[77,78] The hCS gene belongs to a superfamily of five closely related genes localized contiguously on chromosome 17.[79] HCS is produced in the syncytiotrophoblast.

Normal Variation. First detectable during the fifth week, hCS rises throughout pregnancy but maintains a con-

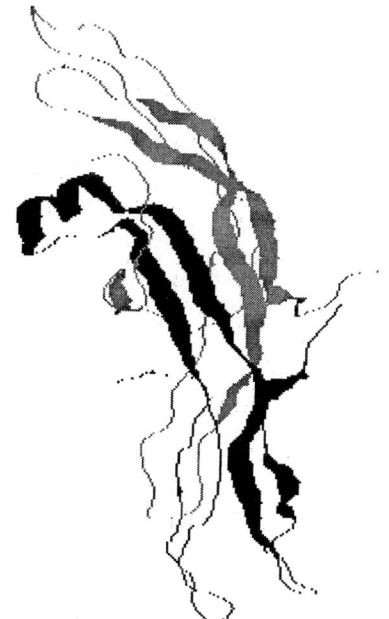

Figure 1–9. Tertiary structure of homodimer hCG by crystallography. This model represents two mature β subunits joined through the C-terminal peptide of the first β subunit. These β homodimer molecules can recombine with two free α subunits. The two β subunits are believed to fold upon each other as a globular structure. This model also illustrates the configurational impact of glycosylation. Desialization of intact pregnancy hCG reduces the molecule to its amino acid backbone and renders the hormone biologically inactive. β Subunits are represented by the dark shaded areas and α subunits by the lighter shaded areas. (From Lustbader JW, Pollak S, Lobel L, et al: Three-dimensional structures of gonadotropins. Mol Cell Endocrinol 125:21, 1996; and Lustbader JW, Lobel L, Wu H, et al: Structural and molecular studies of human chorionic gonadotropin and its receptor. Recent Prog Horm Res 53:395, 1998, with permission.)

stant hormone weight/placental weight relationship.[80] Concentrations reach their highest during the third trimester, from 3.3 μg/ml to 25 μg/ml at term[80] (Fig. 1–11). HCS levels rise and fall in response to fasting and glucose loading.[81]

Function. HCS antagonizes insulin action, inducing glucose intolerance, lipolysis, and proteolysis in the maternal system (see Chapter 32). The hormone is thought to promote transfer of glucose and amino acids to the fetus.[78] HCS is believed responsible for marked increases in maternal plasma IGF-1 concentrations as pregnancies approach term.[80–82] It enhances insulin secretion, impairs glucose tolerance, and promotes nitrogen retention in pregnant and nonpregnant women[79–83] (Fig. 1–12). Surprisingly, women without the hCS gene have no detectable hCS but experience normal pregnancy outcome.[84]

Human Chorionic Thyrotropin. HCT is structurally similar to pituitary TSH but does not have the common α subunit.[85] Placental content of hCT is very small.[20] HCG also has thyrotropic activity and probably has

more significant effects on maternal thyroid function than does hCT.[86]

HYPOTHALAMIC-LIKE HORMONES

Gonadotropin-Releasing Hormone

Molecular Structure and Origin. Placental GnRH is biologically and immunologically similar to the hypothalamic decapeptide GnRH.[16]

Origin. GnRH activity has been localized to the cytotrophoblastic cells along the outer surface layer of the syncytiotrophoblast.[16] HCG is localized to adjacent syncytiotrophoblast.

Normal Variation. GnRH histochemical activity peaks at 8 weeks and then decreases with advancing gestational age.[16–19] These changes parallel hCG concentration in both the placenta and maternal circulation.[19]

Function. Placental GnRH stimulates hCG release through a dose-dependent paracrine mechanism.[51] In first-trimester placental tissue culture, there is little hCG augmentation by GnRH because hCG production is already close to maximum.[51] In the second trimester, however, there is marked dose-dependent hCG augmentation of hCG release in vitro. This effect diminishes in the term placenta. In a superfusion system, 1-minute infusions of GnRH analog significantly increased pulse amplitude and frequency of hCG secretion.[51] GnRH administered intravenously during pregnancy does not increase serum hCG, presumably because placental GnRH receptors have low affinity and the GnRH is diluted in the maternal circulation. It is more likely that locally produced GnRH is the mechanism for stimulation of placental hCG.[51]

Corticotropin-Releasing Hormone

Molecular Structure. Placental CRH appears to be structurally similar to the 41-amino-acid hypothalamic CRH peptide,[87,88] and is therefore readily measured by radioimmunoassay in amniotic fluid, fetal plasma, and maternal plasma. Both hypothalamic and placental CRH are products of the same gene, which is located on the long arm of chromosome 8.[89]

Origin. Pro-CRH messenger RNA is present in the cytotrophoblast.[89] CRH activity is most intense in cytotrophoblasts during the first trimester and diminishes toward term.[15] Also, there is intense CRH immunoreactivity in the decidua.[15]

Normal Variation. CRH immunoreactivity has been measured in maternal plasma, fetal plasma, and amniotic fluid.[90,91] Maternal CRH increases sharply at 20 weeks' gestation, reaching highest concentrations at term[90] (Fig. 1–13). Although concentrations in umbilical plasma are lower than in maternal plasma, there is a highly significant correlation between maternal and umbilical plasma CRH.[90] In amniotic fluid, there is an

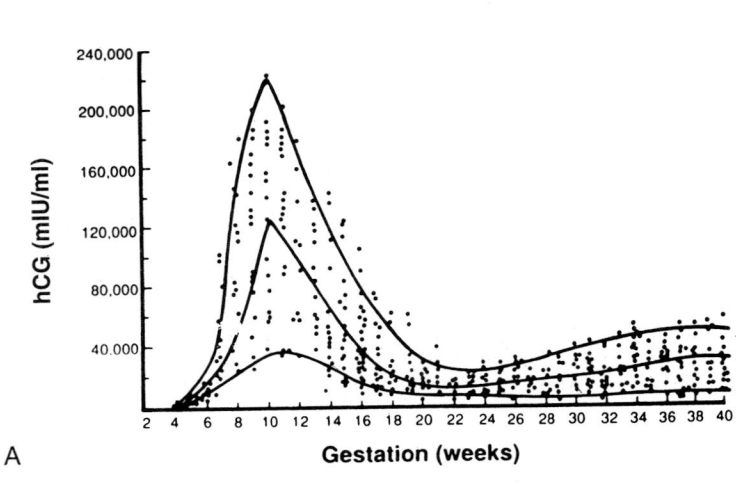

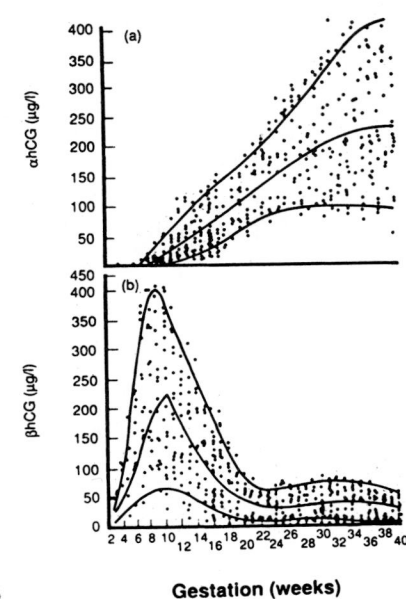

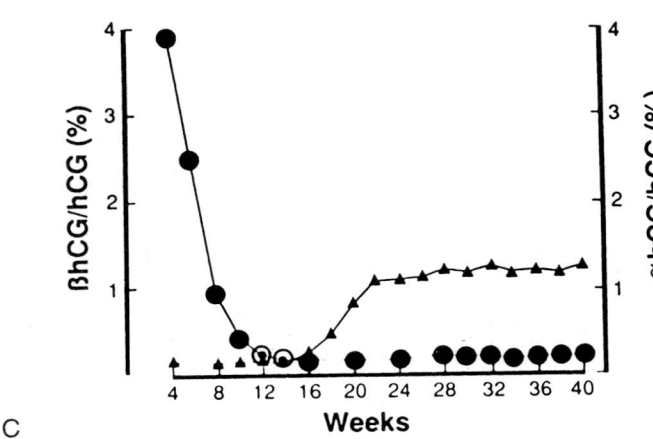

Figure 1–10. *A*, Dimeric hCG levels (mIU/ml) in 500 serum samples collected between 3 and 40 weeks' gestation (LMP) from 55 patients. The 5, 50, and 95 centiles are shown. *B*, Subunits of serum α-hCG (*a*) and β-hCG (*b*) measured directly without correcting for hCG cross-reaction; centiles 5, 50, and 95 are shown. *C*, The mean percentage α-hCG/dimer (▲) α-hCG/dimer (●) β-hCG/dimer ratios between 3 and 40 weeks' gestational age. (From Hay DL, Lopata A: Chorionic gonadotropin secretion by human embryos in vitro. J Clin Endocrinol Metab 67:1322, 1988, with permission.)

approximately threefold rise between the second and third trimesters.[90,91]

Function. Placental CRH stimulates placental ACTH release in vitro in a dose-dependent relationship.[52,76] Both CRH and ACTH are released into the fetal and maternal circulations, although their activity is moderated by a maternal CRH-binding protein.[92] Placental CRH participates in the surge of fetal glucocorticoids associated with late third-trimester fetal maturation.[52,90,92] Secretion of both CRH and ACTH increases when uterine blood flow is restricted. CRH is a potent uteroplacental vasodilator.[93,94] CRH is released into the fetal circulation in response to fetal stress and in conditions leading to growth restriction.[95–97] High circulating maternal CRH is believed responsible for the elevated plasma ACTH and cortisol in pregnant women, which renders them unresponsive to feedback suppression of plasma cortisol.[52,90–93] CRH stimulates prostaglandin synthesis in fetal membranes and placenta. Finally, CRH is fre-

quently elevated in preeclampsia, fetal asphyxia and premature labor, and various conditions causing growth restriction.[95–97]

Somatostatin. A substance similar to SRIF is identifiable in cytotrophoblasts and decidual stroma. Although it is logical to suggest that somatostatin is an hCS inhibiting factor, this cannot be confirmed in vitro.[99]

Thyrotropin-Releasing Hormone. TRH has been detected in the cytotrophoblast; however, the molecule is chromatographically different from the hypothalamic TRH tripeptide.[85] Because the principal placental thyroid-stimulator is believed to be hCG, a significant role for placental TRH is tenuous.[86]

GROWTH FACTORS

Inhibin and Activin

Molecular Structure. Inhibin and activin are heterodimeric glycoproteins each with α and β subunits.

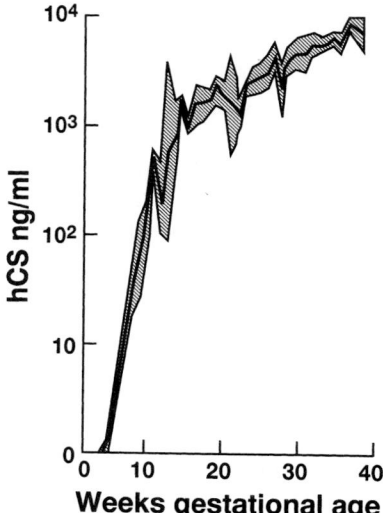

Figure 1–11. Weekly concentrations of hCS (ng/ml) in maternal plasma throughout pregnancy. Solid lines represents the geometric mean; shaded area represents predicted 95% confidence interval widths. (Modified from Braunstein GD, Rasor JL, Wade ME: Interrelationships of human chorionic gonadotropin, human placental lactogen, and pregnancy specific beta-1 glycoprotein throughout normal human gestation. Am J Obstet Gynecol 138:1205, 1980.)

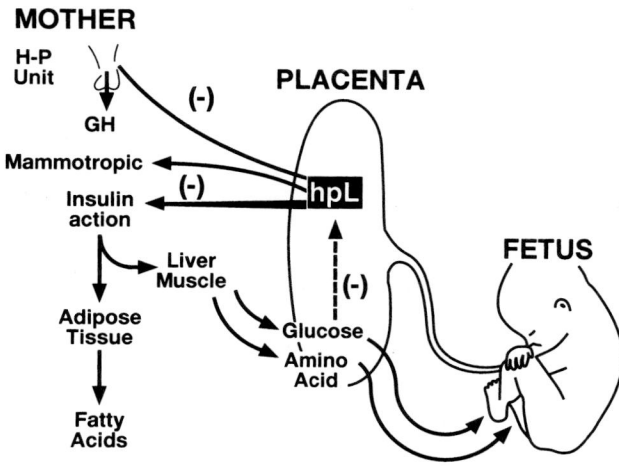

Figure 1–12. Physiologic role of hCS during pregnancy. The current model of the functional role of hCS in maternal metabolism is that hCS preferentially increases glucose availability for the fetus by its lipolytic and insulin antagonist activity. (Modified from Yen SCC: Endocrinology or pregnancy. *In* Creasy RK, Resnick R. [eds]: Maternal-Fetal Medicine: Principles and Practice. Philadelphia, WB Saunders Company, 1989, p 382.)

Origin. Inhibin and activin dimers have been localized to syncytiotrophoblast, with their subunits detected in both cytotrophoblasts and syncytiotrophoblasts.[100] Inhibin is secreted by the corpus luteum and has been detected in decidua.[101,102]

Normal Variation. Dimeric inhibin (α, β) in the maternal circulation begins to increase above nonpregnant levels by 12 days after conception, dramatically increasing at 5 gestational weeks to peak at 8 to 10 weeks. A subsequent decrease is observed at 13 weeks, stabilizes until 30 weeks, and then rises again with the approach of term[103] (Fig. 1–14). The early fluctuations in inhibin concentration probably reflect corpus luteum release, whereas the third-trimester increase probably reflects inhibin originating from the placenta and decidua. Inhibin disappears to nondetectable levels after delivery. Inhibin α dimer has a similar pattern throughout pregnancy.[103]

Function. Placental inhibin, functioning though a paracrine mechanism, is believed to inhibit the release of chorionic GnRH and hCG.[53,104] Activin stimulates release of GnRH and hCG. Decidual activin and inhibin probably have the same effects and appear to serve a role whereby maternal tissues modulate chorionic GnRH and hCG production. Potential immunosuppressive and mitogenic roles have been suggested.[104]

Insulin-like Growth Factor. The placenta is an important site of intrauterine IGF-1 and IGF-2 synthesis.[105] Syncytiotrophoblasts from second-trimester placentas transcribe IGF-1 mRNA; IGF-2 mRNA is found in placen-

tal fibroblasts. Human placental tissues are rich in IGF receptors.[106,107] IGF-1 stimulates prolactin synthesis in human decidual cells and may affect steroidogenesis.[78]

Transforming Growth Factor-β. TGF-β has been purified from placenta and is thought to be a paracrine regulator of mesenchyme–epithelium interactions.[55,108]

Epidermal Growth Factor. EGF is synthesized by the syncytiotrophoblast, and EGF receptors are observed

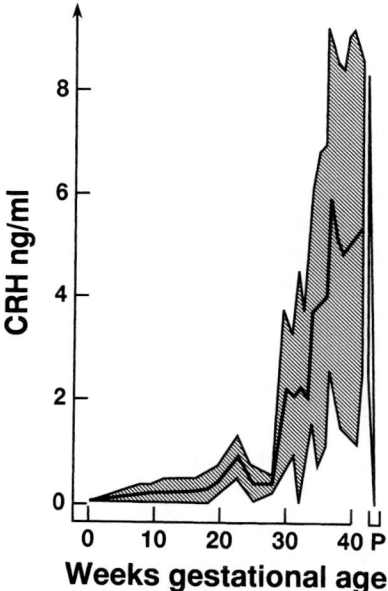

Figure 1–13. Maternal serum concentrations of immunoreactive CRH in 256 individual pregnant women in relation to gestational age and postpartum (mean ±SD). (Modified from Stalla GK, Bost H, Stalla J, et al: Human corticotropin releasing hormone during pregnancy. Gynecol Endocrinol 3:1, 1989, with permission.)

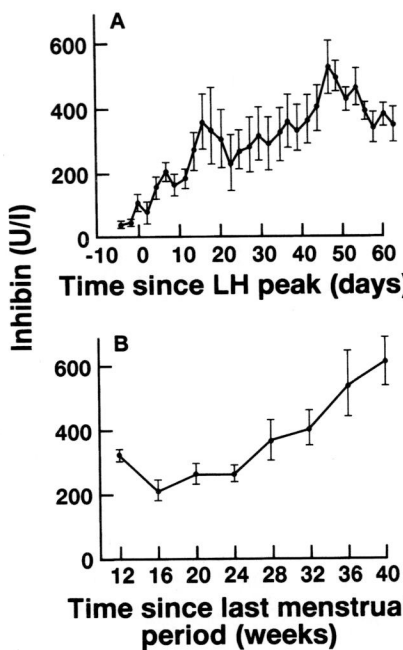

Figure 1–14. Geometric mean (67 percent confidence intervals) for plasma concentrations of inhibin. *A,* Data plotted from four subjects in early pregnancy from whom three weekly samples were obtained before and after conception. *B,* Data plotted from nine subjects in later pregnancy from whom samples were obtained at 4-week intervals starting at 12 weeks after the last menstrual period. (Modified from Tovanabutra S, Illingworth PJ, Ledger WL, et al: The relationship between peripheral immunoactive inhibin, human chorionic gonadotrophin, oestradiol and progesterone during human pregnancy. Clin Endocrinol 38:101, 1993.)

on these same cells. EGF has been shown to increase release of hCG and hCS.[55,109]

OTHER PREGNANCY-RELATED PEPTIDES

Besides the chorionic glycoproteins, which are analogous to pituitary glycoproteins present in the nonpregnant state, the placenta secretes a host of proteins with no known analog in the nonpregnant state. One group of these proteins was first identified by producing an antiserum to serum drawn in term pregnancy. Antiserum was then used to isolate and identify the pregnancy associated plasma proteins (PAPP) A through D. A second group was isolated by extraction of proteins from placental tissue that was later purified and characterized as pregnancy-specific β1-glycoprotein (Shwanger-schaftsspeziffische protein 1 [SP-1]).

Pregnancy Specific β1-Glycoprotein. This glycoprotein has a molecular weight of about 100 kDa. Secreted from trophoblastic cells, it is detected 18 to 23 days after ovulation.[110,111] Rising initially with an approximate 2- to 3-day doubling time, it reaches peak concentrations of 100 to 200 ng/ml at term. SP-1 is a potent immunosuppressor of lymphocyte proliferation and may help to prevent rejection of the conceptus.[112]

Pregnancy Associated Plasma Protein-A. PAPP-A, the largest of the pregnancy-related glycoproteins, has a molecular weight of 750 kDa. It originates principally from placental syncytiotrophoblasts.[113,114] It is first detected at a mean time of 33 days after ovulation. It then rises initially with a 3-day doubling time and continues to rise until term.[113] PAPP-A may serve an immunosuppressive role during pregnancy.[114]

Placental Protein-5. A glycoprotein with a molecular weight of 36 kDa, placental protein 5 (PP5) is believed to be produced in the syncytiotrophoblasts. It is detected about 42 days after ovulation, with a continuous rise until term.[115] Because PP5 has antithrombin and antiplasmic activities, it is believed to be a natural blood coagulation inhibitor active at the implantation site.[116]

Decidual Proteins

PROLACTIN

Molecular Structure. Decidual prolactin is a 197- to 199-amino-acid peptide with chemical and biologic properties identical to pituitary prolactin.[78]

Origin. Prolactin, produced by decidualized endometrium, is first detectable in the endometrium on cycle day 23, a time corresponding to implantation. Decidual prolactin secretion is thought to be induced by progesterone or a combination of estrogen and progesterone[117] with growth factors (e.g., IGF-1) and other polypeptide hormones (α-hCG) as co-regulators. Decidual prolactin is transported across intact amnion and chorion from adherent decidua and released into the amniotic fluid with little entering the fetal or maternal circulation.[118] Production, independent of dopaminergic control, is not affected by bromocriptine.[78] Circulating fetal prolactin is secreted by the fetal pituitary, while circulating maternal prolactin is secreted by the maternal pituitary under the influence of estrogens. Both are suppressed by maternal ingestion of bromocriptine.

Normal Variation. Decidual prolactin parallels the rapid rise in maternal serum prolactin until 10 weeks' gestation, rises rapidly until 20 weeks, and then falls as term approaches[119] (Fig. 1–15).

Function. Decidual prolactin regulates fluid and electrolyte flux through fetal membranes. Decidual prolactin reduces permeability of the amnion in the fetal to maternal direction.[78,117,118,120–124]

RELAXIN

Relaxin is a 6-kDa peptide hormone, structurally related to insulin, comprised of two short peptide chains that are linked by disulfide bridges.[125–127] It is believed that the corpus luteum is the major source of this hor-

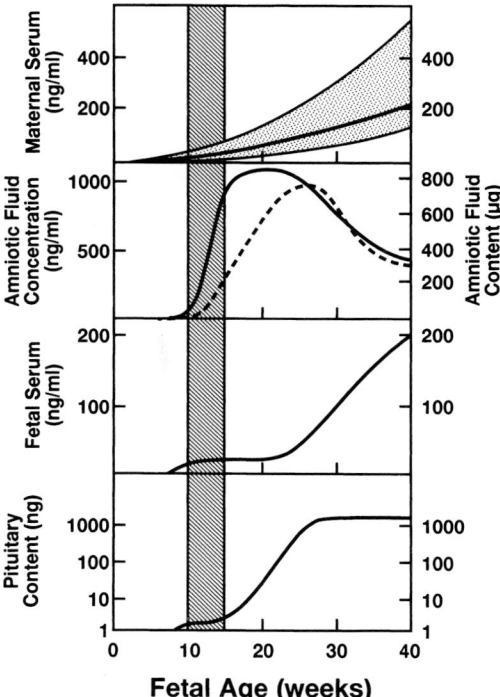

Figure 1–15. Amniotic fluid prolactin peaks in the second trimester and declines toward term. In contrast, maternal and fetal prolactin increase to maximum level during the third trimester. Solid line = amniotic fluid concentration; dotted line = amniotic fluid content. (From Clements JA, Reyes FI, Winter JS, et al: Studies on human sexual development, IV: fetal pituitary and serum, and amniotic fluid concentrations of prolactin. J Clin Endocrinol Metab 44:408, 1977, with permission.)

mone; however, relaxin has been identified in the placenta and decidua. Relaxin is undetectable in women without ovaries and appears nonessential in normal pregnancy outcome.[125–127]

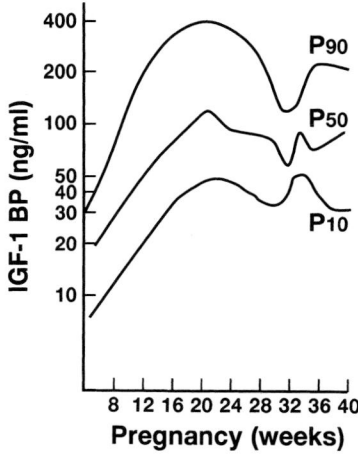

Figure 1–16. Maternal serum IGF-1BP levels throughout pregnancy as measured by radioimmunoassay. (From Rutanen E-M: Insulin-like growth factor binding protein-1. Semin Reprod Endocrinol 10:154, 1992, with permission.)

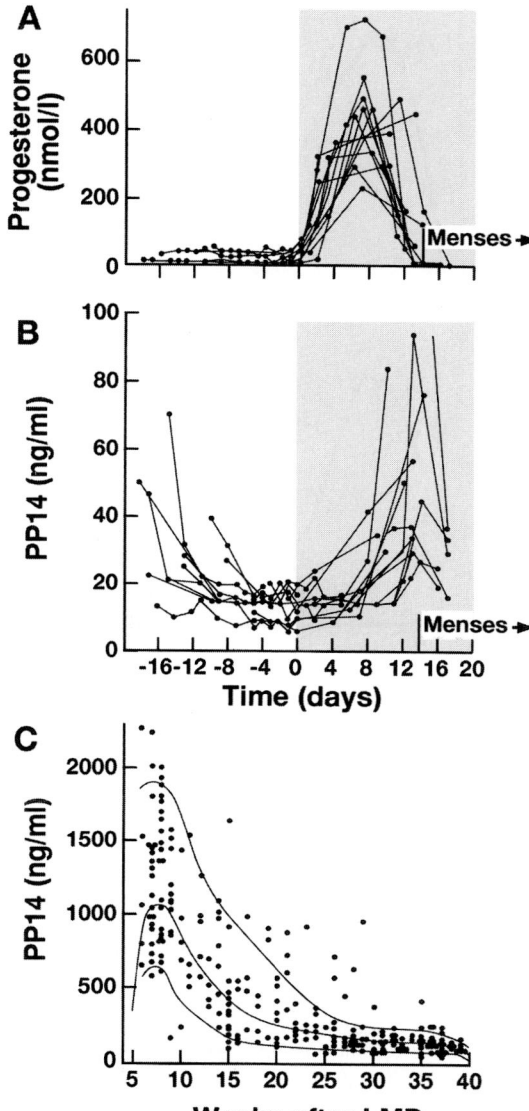

Figure 1–17. A, Serum progesterone and (B) PP14 concentrations in serum of normally ovulating women. PP14 rises approximately 8 days after the luteal phase rise of progesterone and remains elevated well into the next cycle. C, PP14 concentrations in maternal serum throughout pregnancy. (A and B from Seppala M, Riittinen L, Kamarainen M, et al: Placental protein 14/progesterone-associated endometrial protein revisited. Semin Reprod Endocrinol 10:164, 1992; C from Julkunen M, Rutanen EM, Koskimies A, et al: Distribution of placental protein 14 in tissues and body fluids during pregnancy. Br J Obstet Gynaecol 92:1145, 1985, with permission.)

IGF-1 BINDING PROTEIN (IGF-1BP OR PP12)

IGF-1 binding protein (IGF-1BP) contains 234 amino acids, with a molecular mass of approximately 25 kDa.[128] IGF-1BP is believed to originate from decidual stromal cells. In nonpregnant women, circulating IGF-1BP does not change with the cyclicity of the endometrium. However, during pregnancy, there is a severalfold increase in serum IGF-1BP levels that begins

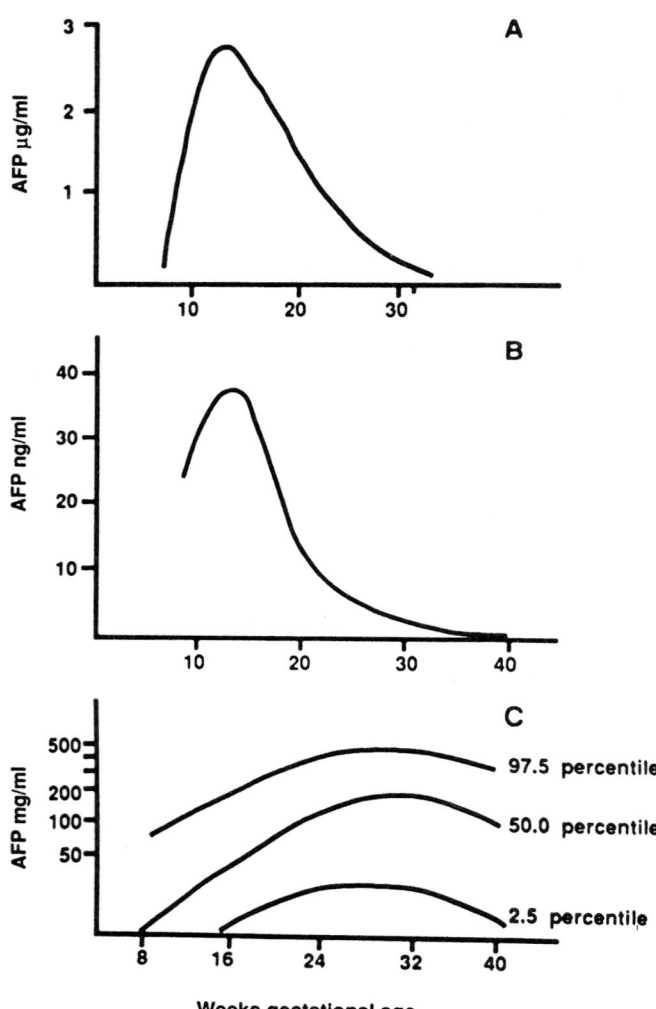

Figure 1–18. Normal median concentrations of AFP in fetal serum (*A*), amniotic fluid (*B*), and maternal serum (*C*), Maternal serum is shown with 2.5 and 97.5 percentile limits. (From Habib ZA: Maternal serum alpha-feto-protein: its value in antenatal diagnosis of genetic disease and in obstetrical-gynaecological care. Acta Obstet Gynecol Scand 61:1, 1977, with permission.)

during the first trimester, peaks during second trimester, falls, and then peaks a second time before term[129] (Fig. 1–16). IGF-1BP inhibits the binding of IGF-1 to receptors in the decidua.[129]

PLACENTAL PROTEIN

Placental protein (PP14) is a glycoprotein with 162 amino acids and a molecular weight of 28 kDa. It is synthesized in secretory and decidualized endometrium and is detectable on menstrual cycle day 24.[130] PP14 in serum rises sharply on days 22 to 24 of the cycle, reaches peak values at the onset of menstruation, and is maintained at high levels if pregnancy occurs.[131,132] In pregnant women, PP14 rises in parallel with hCG[130] (Fig. 1–17). PP14 levels are very low in patients with ectopic pregnancy, in which there is minimal decidual

reaction. PP14 is thought to be an immunosuppressant.[130]

Fetal Proteins

α-Fetoprotein (AFP) is a glycoprotein with a molecular weight of about 69 kDa.[133] AFP is believed to be synthesized sequentially in the yolk sac, gastrointestinal tact, and fetal liver.[128] It enters the fetal urine in abundance and is readily detected in the amniotic fluid. Concentrations of fetal plasma AFP, amniotic fluid AFP (AFAFP), and maternal serum AFP (MSAFP) are shown in Figure 1–18.[135] MSAFP peaks between 10 and 13 weeks' gestational age and then declines from 14 to 32 weeks. The rapid fall in fetal plasma AFP is believed due to increasing fetal blood volume and a decline in fetal production. AFP peaks at 12 and 14 weeks' gestation and then steadily declines to term.[135] The concentration gradient between fetal plasma AFP and MSAFP is about 150- to 200-fold. Detectable as early as 7 weeks' gestation, MSAFP reaches peak concentrations between 28 and 32 weeks.[135] The apparent paradoxical rise in MSAFP in association with decreasing AFAFP and fetal serum levels can be accounted for by increasing placental permeability to fetal plasma proteins that occurs with advancing gestation.[135]

Function. AFP regulates fetal intravascular volume as an osmoregulator[135] and may also be involved in immunoregulation.[135] AFAFP and MSAFP measurements are clinically important because they are elevated in association with neural tube defects.[137] MSAFP is decreased when the fetus has Down syndrome.[138]

PREGNANCY STEROIDS

The novel pregnancy peptides described above are in part responsible for the altered steroid milieu in pregnancy. In addition to stimulation of maternal hormones, the fetus and placenta produce and secrete steroids into the maternal circulation. The changes in maternal hormone concentrations are integrally related to metabolic and immunologic changes vital to intracorporeal gestation.

Ontogeny of Fetoplacental Steroid Production

Origins and amounts of fetoplacental steroid shift dramatically during gestation.

The Preimplantation Conceptus

Estradiol and progesterone secretion by the conceptus and its cumulus is detectable in vitro well before implantation.[139,140] There is little information on the regulation of conceptus steroid production. Mechanical removal of the corona cells is associated with cessation of secretion, whereas return of corona cells in co-culture restores steroid secretion.[139] Steroid production, therefore, is likely negligible by the time the conceptus reaches the endometrial cavity, since it has been mechanically denuded of cumulus during transport through the oviduct. Once implantation occurs and secretion of trophoblastic hCG and other pregnancy-related peptides is established, steroid production by the conceptus resumes.[139–141]

Progesterone production by the preimplantation conceptus is believed important in tubal and uterine transport, because receptor sites for progesterone are highest in concentration in the mucosal layer of the distal one third of the fallopian tube. The ova and sperm are most likely to meet at this location.[142]

The Decidua

Cortisol is secreted by decidual tissues.[143,144] In concert with hCG and progesterone secreted by the conceptus, decidual cortisol probably suppresses the maternal immune rejection response, helping to confer immunologic "privilege" to the implanted conceptus.[143,144]

The Corpus Luteum

Progesterone, 17α-hydroxyprogesterone, estradiol, and androstenedione are the principal steroid products of the corpus luteum. Progesterone is considered the steroid of greatest importance because progesterone alone given to a lutectomized woman in early pregnancy will maintain a pregnancy that would otherwise abort.[145] Likewise, exogenous progesterone given to an agonadal woman pregnant with donated embryos sustains viability through the early first trimester until the pregnancy can be maintained with its own placental progesterone production.[146] Although the human corpus luteum secretes up to 40 mg of progesterone a day during the midluteal phase of the ovarian cycle and into early pregnancy, surprisingly small amounts of progesterone are required to maintain donor embryo pregnancies when no corpus luteum is present.[147–149]

Low-density lipoprotein (LDL) cholesterol is the principal regulatory precursor of corpus luteum progesterone production.[150]

The Fetus and Placenta

The fetal adrenal cortex and placenta serve as incomplete but complementary steroidogenic organs, functioning in concert to become the principal sites of steroid production as gestation advances. After 7 weeks' gestational age, the placenta dominates steroid production. At this point, pregnancy continues even if the corpus luteum is excised, for in its stead is the beginning of the fetoplacental unit.[151] At this time of gestation, pituitary basophilic cells are producing significant amounts of fetal ACTH and stimulate the fetal adrenal cortex, whose cells have been amassed for 4 weeks, awaiting trophic stimulation to synthesize steroids.[152] This corresponds to the time in gestation when estriol is first detectable in the maternal circulation. The intricate interdependence of the fetal and adrenal cortex and the placenta allow these two relatively small organs to exchange, metabolize, and secrete more steroids than any other human endocrine tissue.

Because the fetal adrenal and placenta contain incomplete but complementary steroidogenic enzyme systems, they constantly exchange circulating steroid precursors, which produces the steroid profile that characterizes normal pregnancy. As one might expect, nature has also evolved an organ that exists only in pregnancy to handle this unique function—the fetal zone of the adrenal cortex (Fig. 1–19).[143,153] Between 32 and 36 weeks (Fig. 1–19B), a marked increase in fetal adrenal cortex growth velocity reflects the acceleration of fetal maturation processes just before parturition.[143,157] This fetal zone then rapidly involutes postpartum.[155,156]

The anatomic distribution of key steroidogenic enzymes involved in the production of circulating intrauterine steroids is diagrammed in Figure 1–20.[157,158] The fetal adrenal cortex is functionally deficient in 3β-hydroxysteroid dehydrogenase, the enzyme that converts pregnenolone and DHEA to progesterone and androstenedione, respectively.[159] Therefore, the fetus cannot make progesterone or androstenedione, the immediate precursor to the sex steroids. The placenta, however, has an abundance of 3β-hydroxysteroid dehydrogenase. Therefore, the fetal adrenal cortex extracts LDL from the fetal circulation and converts it to pregnenolone sulfate and DHEA-S.[157,160] Pregnenolone sulfate is delivered through the umbilical artery to the placenta. The placenta converts pregnenolone to progesterone and returns the latter to the fetus for synthesis into mineralocorticoids and glucocorticoids. Interestingly, the placenta contains a relative lack of 17α-hydroxylase.[158] Teleologically, this deficiency may exist to prevent placental metabolism of progesterone, which is the precursor of fetal adrenal cortex corticosteroids.[158] The placenta also has the enzymatic capability to extract LDL cholesterol and to convert it into progesterone without relying on the fetal adrenal cortex.

The other fetal steroid precursor, DHEA-S, is first delivered to the fetal liver, where it is converted into 16α-hydroxydehydroepiandrosterone sulfate (16α-OHDHEAS) before being converted in the placenta first to 16α-hydroxyandrostenedione and then further aro-

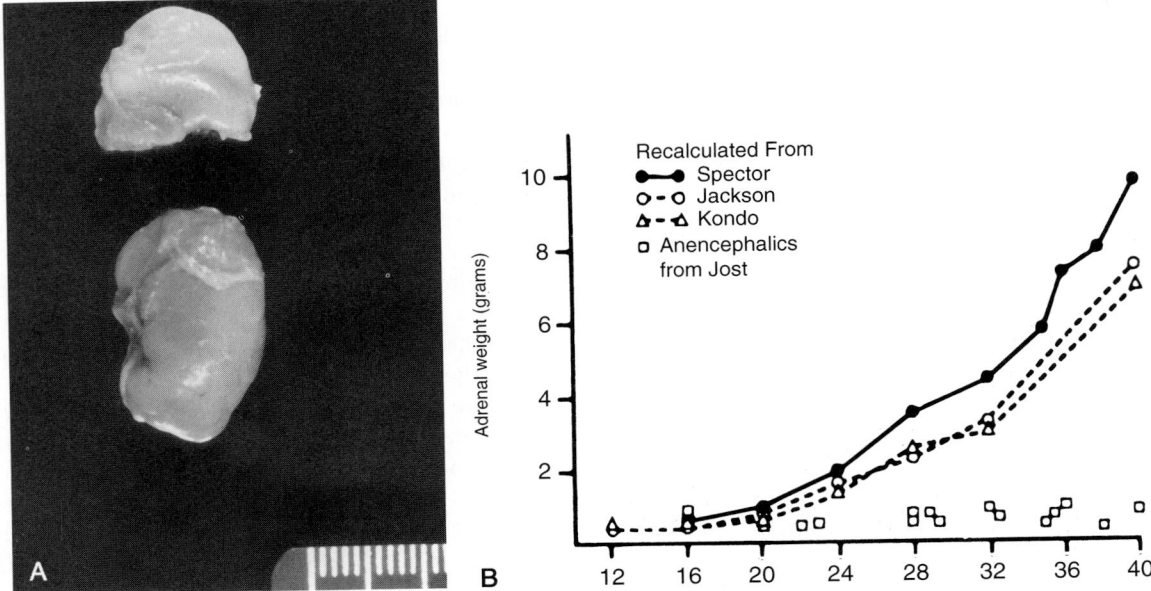

Figure 1–19. *A*, Fetal adrenal gland and kidney at 18 weeks. The adrenal cortex in fetal life is much larger relative to other organs in children and adults. (Courtesy of Dr. Steven Gabbe.) *B*, Growth of the fetal adrenal cortex. Total fetal adrenal mass is shown as a function of gestational age. Rapid increase in growth velocity occurs between 32 and 36 weeks' gestation. In anencephalic pregnancies, adrenal mass does not increase after the second trimester. (Data from Jost,[154] Kondo,[155] and Buster[157].)

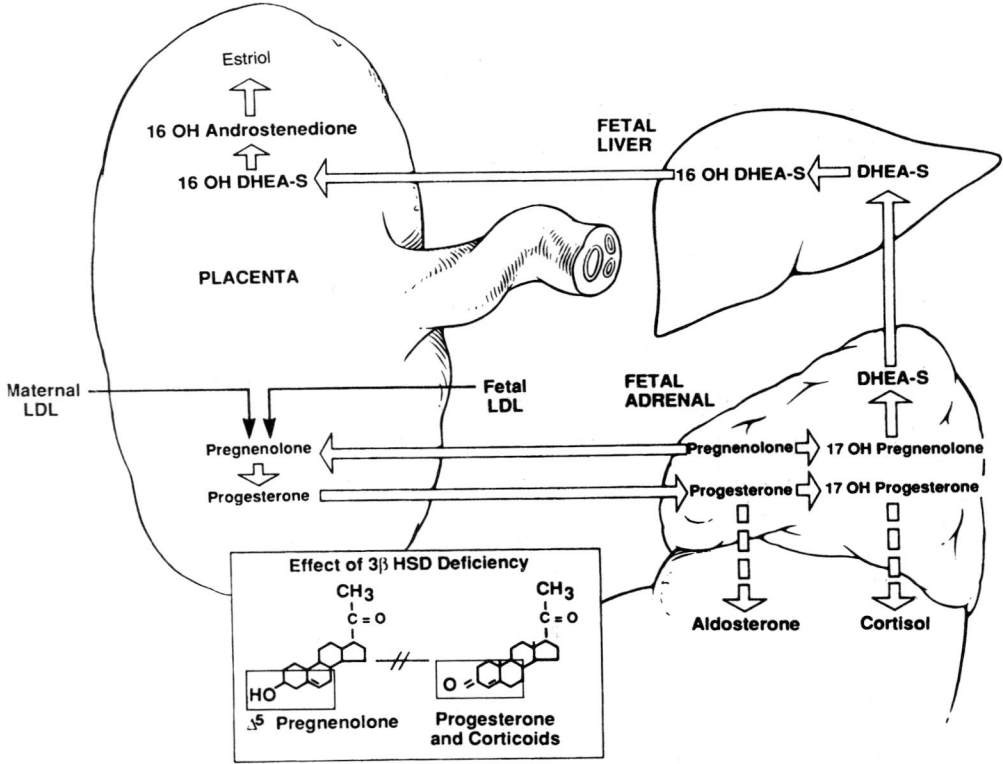

Figure 1–20. Exchange of circulating steroid intermediates between fetal zone and placenta. Steroidogenic enzyme deficiencies of the fetal zone are offset by enzyme activities of placenta enabling the two organs to work cooperatively to produce a massive and extensive profile of intrauterine steroids. The bulk of fetal zone steroids are secreted as sulfoconjugates.

matized into estriol.[158] The estrogens are subsequently secreted into the maternal and fetal circulations.[158]

Besides the obvious functional interdependence of these two organs, the placenta also acts as a structural stimulator of the fetal adrenal cortex. In the first 20 weeks of gestation, placental hCG and progesterone play important roles in fetal adrenal cortex maintenance and regulation.[161] HCG stimulates fetal adrenal cortex production of DHEA-S in vivo. Atrophy of the fetal zone after delivery may be in part due to removal of the trophic effect of hCG, although hCG appears to be less important after week 20 of gestation.[161,162] Indeed, the fetal adrenal cortex acquires increasing sensitivity to circulating ACTH, with advancing gestational age during the second half of gestation being primarily influenced by ACTH.[163,164] In addition, prolactin receptors have also been demonstrated in the adrenal cortex, and prolactin may therefore act in association with ACTH and hCG to regulate fetal adrenal cortex steroid production.[165-168]

Regulation of Fetoplacental Steroidogenesis

Steroidogenic regulation has been investigated extensively in vitro by study of fetal placental tissue explants. In vivo, regulation has been investigated in catheterized primate models, particularly the rhesus monkey and baboon. Factors emerging as major regulators of fetoplacental steroidogenesis include (1) LDL cholesterol, (2) pituitary regulatory hormones, (3) intraplacental regulators, and (4) intra-adrenal regulators.[167-169]

LDL CHOLESTEROL

LDL cholesterol, the principal lipoprotein utilized in fetal adrenal steroidogenesis, limits or augments steroid output by its availability. Between 50 and 70 percent of the cholesterol used for fetal adrenal steroidogenesis is extracted from circulating fetal LDL.[151,160,170] Fetal adrenal tissues contain high-affinity, low-capacity binding sites for LDL. In the presence of ACTH, adrenal-binding capacity for LDL is increased.[151,159,163] Cholesterol liberated from intra-adrenal hydrolysis of LDL is converted to steroids.

Simpson et al. proposed that fetal LDL cholesterol and the steroidogenic systems of the fetal adrenal and placenta may interact in a self-perpetuating positive feedback loop that becomes increasingly active with advancing gestation.[171] Most LDL cholesterol arises de novo from synthesis in the fetal liver[171] (Fig. 1–21). Fetal adrenal cortisol and placental estradiol (derived from fetal DHEA-S) augment de novo fetal liver biosynthesis of LDL.[96] All of these interacting elements increase with advancing fetal maturity in a chain-like sequence of self perpetuating loops that increase steroid production to meet the needs of a growing fetus.[171]

PITUITARY REGULATORY HORMONES

Fetal pituitary ACTH is detectable by 9 weeks' gestation.[162, 172–174] Plasma immunoreactive ACTH levels increase steadily until about 20 weeks. Levels remain relatively stable until approximately 34 weeks, when a significant decrement appears and persists until term.[163] Concentrations of ACTH over time therefore do not correlate with the increasing fetal adrenal mass or the increasing steroidogenic activities that characterize the third trimester.[163]

Fetal ACTH regulates steroidogenesis in both adrenal zones. ACTH receptor activity, present in both zones, is diminished somewhat in the fetal zone early in the sec-

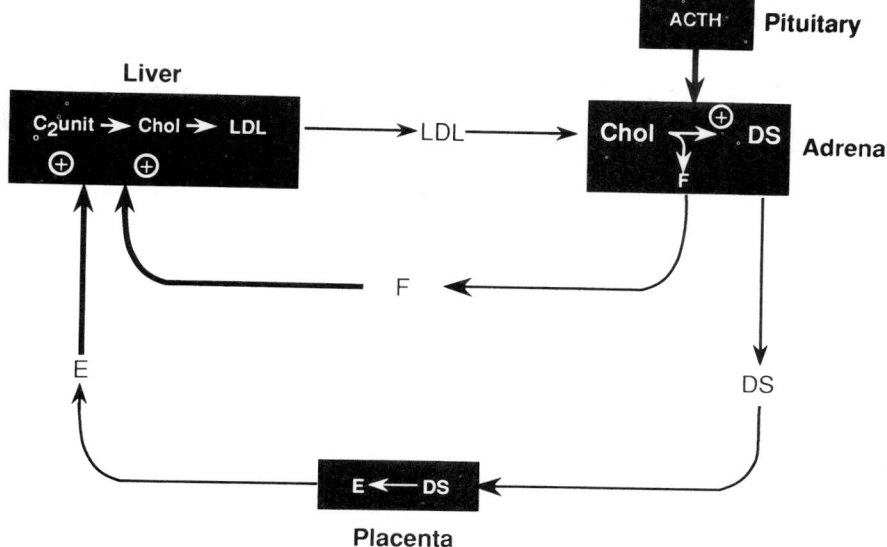

Figure 1–21. Proposed scheme for the regulation of steroidogenesis in the human fetal placental unit. Fetal adrenal cortisol (F) and estradiol (E) are produced in the placenta from dehydroepiandrosterone sulfate (DS) of fetal adrenal origin, which regulates de novo fetal hepatic synthesis of cholesterol (Chol). Cholesterol bound to LDL is then provided to the fetal adrenal for F and DS production, which is enhanced by ACTH of fetal pituitary origin. (From Simpson ER, Parker CR, Carr BR: Role of lipoproteins in the regulation of steroidogenesis by the human fetal adrenal. *In* Jaffe RB, Dell Acqua S [eds]: The Endocrine Physiology of Pregnancy and the Peripartal Period, Vol. 21. Serono Symposia Publications. New York, Raven Press, 1985, with permission.)

ond trimester when other trophic factors, such as hCG, are probably more important in the maintenance of this structure.[171] In vitro superfusion system studies of human fetal adrenal tissue show that ACTH stimulates the release of Δ5 pregnenolone sulfate and DHEA-S, whereas isolated definitive zones secrete only cortisol when stimulated by ACTH.[171] ACTH, in addition to its effect on LDL binding, acts on its own adrenal cell membrane receptor subunit and then adenyl cyclase to express its direct stimulatory effect on steroidogenic enzymes.[171]

ACTH 1-19 and ACTH 1-38 have been extracted from human fetal pituitaries and have been shown in vitro to stimulate the production of DHEA-S and cortisol.[162,173] Although fetal ACTH is clearly a major fetal adrenotropic principle, its activity is modulated by other tropic factors such as CRH and prolactin.

Fetal pituitary prolactin is detectable at 10 weeks.[174] Cord prolactin concentrations increase with advancing gestation in parallel with increased adrenal mass.[166] With prolactin receptors demonstrated in the adrenal cortex, prolactin may act as a co-regulator with ACTH, hCG, and growth factors in fetal adrenal steroid production.[165,175] In fetal baboon experiments, both in vivo and in vitro, prolactin augments ACTH-stimulated adrenal androgen production.[167,169]

INTRAPLACENTAL REGULATORS

As the secretor of *hCG, placental CRH, progesterone,* and *estradiol,* the placenta is an important fetal zone co-regulator.[153]

HCG receptor activity is present in the fetal zone, and hCG stimulates fetal adrenal production of DHEA-S both in vitro and in vivo.[67,164] HCG appears to be less important after the 20th week, when the fetal zone is primarily influenced by the ACTH. Fetal zone atrophy observed after delivery may be attributable to removal of placental hCG, but loss of other tropic factors is probably of similar importance.[162,171,175] Placental CRH, in a paracrine relationship with placental ACTH, probably participates with the fetal hypothalamus and pituitary in the surge of fetal glucocorticoids associated with the late third trimester.[91,176] This relationship is highlighted earlier in the chapter.

Placental progesterone inhibits the Δ5 to Δ4 steroid transformation in the fetal zone.[161,177] This effect is another explanation for the functional fetal adrenal 3βHSD deficiency.

Placental estradiol modifies metabolism and production of corticoids and progesterone. In chronically catheterized baboons, the placenta regulates maternal cortisol–cortisone interconversion, and fetal pituitary production of ACTH.[177,178] This effect occurs by modulation of maternal cortisol across the placenta into the fetus.

INTRA-ADRENAL REGULATORS

The fetal adrenal becomes more sensitive to circulating ACTH with advancing gestational age.[169] At least three factors are involved.

Fetal adrenal mass increases with advancing gestation[154,155] (Fig. 1–19B). At 8 weeks' gestation, a rudimentary but distinct adrenal cortex appears composed of two zones: the fetal zone, which comprises approximately 80% of fetal adrenal mass, and a surrounding definitive zone, a narrow capsular band of highly proliferative cells that corresponds to the adult zona glomerulosa.[178-182] Rapid growth that begins at approximately the 10th week of gestation consists almost entirely of enlargement of the fetal zone[178,179] (Fig. 1–22). By the 13th week of gestation, a third zone, the transitional zone, a layer residing between the above two zones, emerges and takes on the appearance of the zona fasciculata, the source of adult cortisol.[183] Between 32 and 36 weeks' gestation, the fetal zone increases its mass sharply (Fig. 1–19B).[178,179] This growth is thought to occur principally from hyperplasia in the definitive and transitional zones and from hypertrophy in the fetal zone (Fig. 1–22). The adrenal gland after birth shrinks abruptly by apoptosis occurring in the principally fetal zone.[178,179] During growth phases, an overall increase in cell numbers is thought to produce an increase in the number of ACTH receptors. The adrenal as a whole thus becomes more responsive to

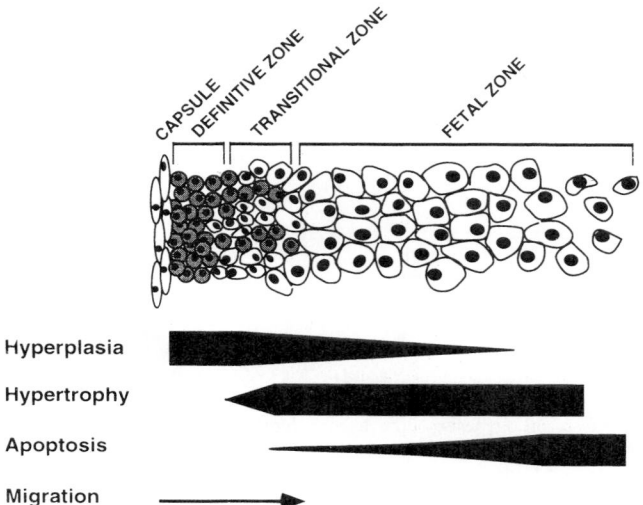

Figure 1–22. Zonation of the human fetal adrenal cortex at mid trimester. This schematic structure illustrates the three zones of the fetal cortex and their putative modes of growth in each zone. Hyperplasia is believed to be a predominant form of growth in the definitive zone; hypertrophy is believed to occur mainly in the fetal zone; apoptosis occurs mainly in the central areas of the fetal zone. Cells are believed to migrate from the periphery to the center of the gland. (From Mesiano S, Jaffe RB: Developmental and functional biology of the primate fetal adrenal cortex. Endocr Rev 18:378, 1997, with permission.)

circulating ACTH with resulting augmentation of steroid production. In late gestation, the definitive and transitional zones, with their 3βHSD steroidogenic activity, begin to produce Cortisol from cholesterol, as in the adult[183] (Fig. 1–23). After birth, these three zones survive: the definitive zone is transformed into the zona glomerulosa, the transitional zone evolves into the cortisol-secreting zona fasciculata, and the fetal zone envolves into the androgen-secreting zona reticularis[179] (Figs. 1–22 and 1–23).

Fetal adrenal blood flow, modulated by arterial oxygen tension, tropic hormones, and intra-adrenal vascular proliferation, exposes fetal adrenal receptors to increases in circulating tropic hormones. Beginning at 9 weeks' gestation, an extensive network of capillary sinuses forms between the cords of the fetal zone. The

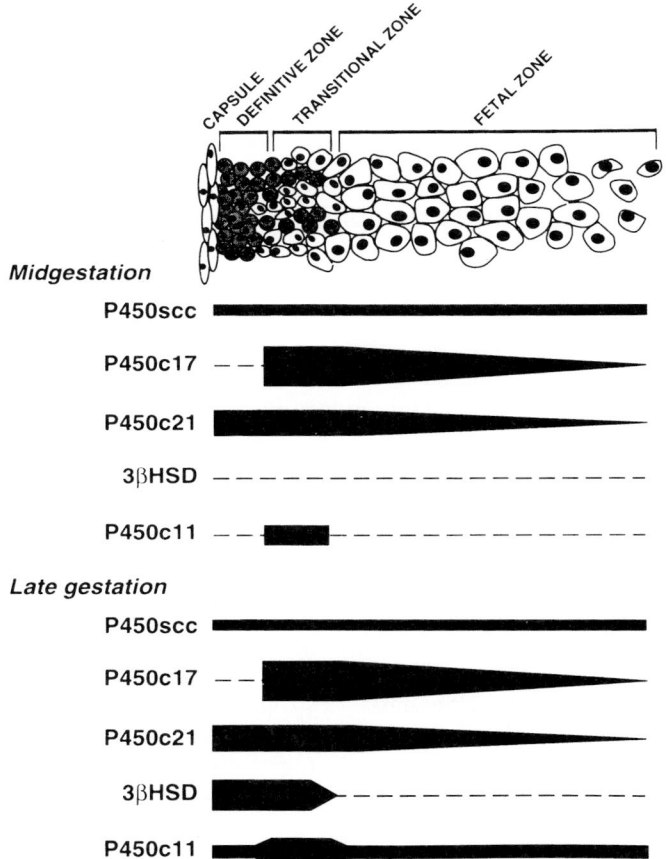

Figure 1–23. Expression of steroidogenic enzymes in the three zones of the fetal adrenal cortex. Relative amounts of steroidogenic enzyme activity are represented as line thickness and shown to change from mid gestation to late gestation for P450scc, P450c21, 3βHSD, and P450c11. *Dashed line* indicates lack of expression. Note the lack of P450c17 expression in the definitive zone at all stages of gestation and the ontogenic expression of 3βHSD only in the definitive and transitional zones in late pregnancy. (From Mesiano S, Jaffe RB: Developmental and functional biology of the primate fetal adrenal cortex. Endocr Rev 18:378, 1997, with permission.)

fetal cortex becomes one of the most highly vascularized fetal organs.[181]

Growth factors regulate the adrenal steroidogenic pathway by differential stimulation of zone growth. Basic fibroblastic growth factor (β-FGF) induces proliferation of cells in the definitive zone in preference to the fetal zone.[184,185] ACTH increases mRNA encoding for β-FGF by two- to three-fold.[186] Similarly, EGF, IGF-1 and IGF-2, activin/inhibin, and TGF-β induce total adrenal growth as well a preferential growth of specific zones.[187,192] These substances function as paracrine modulators to circulating fetal pituitary and placental ACTH.[178,179]

Physiology of Fetoplacental Steroids and Pregnancy

Fetoplacental estrogens, progestogens, and adrenocorticoids are secreted abundantly into *both* fetal and maternal circulations during pregnancy.

Estrogens

The origins and impact of estrogens in the maternal circulation vary with time in gestation and needs of the pregnancy.

VARIATION DURING PREGNANCY

Estradiol originates almost exclusively from the maternal ovaries for the first 5 to 6 weeks' gestation.[141] Later, the placenta secretes increasing quantities of estradiol, which it synthesizes from conversion of circulating maternal and fetal DHEA-S. After the first trimester, the placenta is the major source of circulating estradiol.[141] At term, approximately equal amounts of placental estradiol are converted from circulating maternal DHEA-S and fetal DHEA-S.[193,194] Estradiol concentrations are less than 0.1 ng/ml during the follicular phase and reach 0.4 ng/ml during the luteal phase of normal menstrual cycles.[195] Following conception, estradiol increases gradually to range from 6 to 30 ng/ml at term[196] (Fig. 1–24). In women with threatened first-trimester abortion, estradiol concentrations are abnormally low for gestational age. During the third trimester, low estradiol concentrations are associated with poor obstetric outcome.

For the first 4 to 6 weeks of pregnancy,[141] estrone originates primarily from maternal sources (ovaries, adrenals, peripheral conversion). After this time, the placenta secretes increasing quantifies of estrone from conversion of circulating maternal and fetal DHEA-S. For the remainder of pregnancy, the placenta remains the major source of circulating estrone.[141]

Estrone concentrations are less than 0.1 ng/ml during

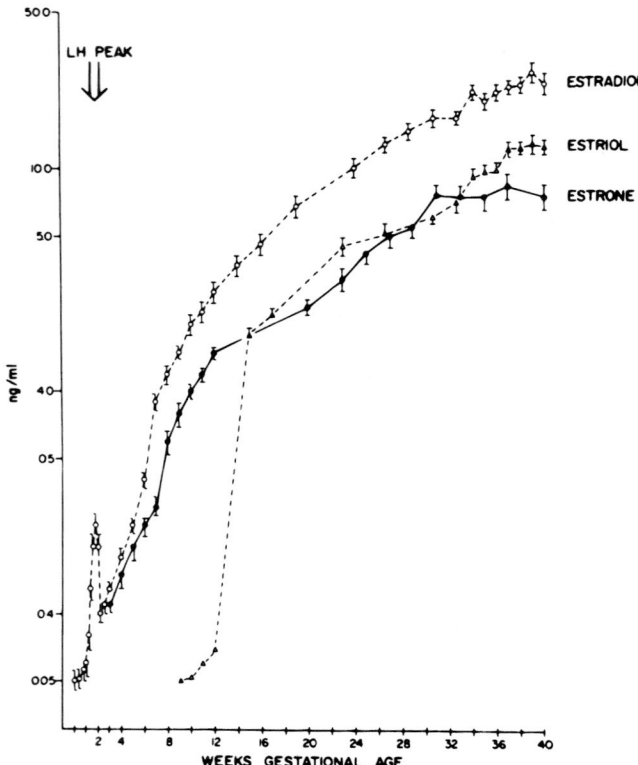

Figure 1–24. Mean concentrations (±SEM) of estrone, estradiol, and estriol from conception to term. Unconjugated estriol is first detectable at approximately 9 weeks' gestational age. Gestational ages are calculated from the last menstrual flow. (Composite adapted from Tulchinsky and Hobel,[141] Abraham et al.,[195] Lindbert et al.,[196] Buster et al.,[248,249] and Williams and Warwick.[250])

the follicular phase of a normal menstrual cycle.[197] Following conception, estrone concentrations remain within the luteal phase range through weeks 6 to 10. Subsequently, there is a gradual increase to a wide range of 2 to 30 ng/ml at term[141,196,197] (Fig. 1–24). Estrone concentrations probably reflect the same metabolic processes that are involved in the production of estradiol.

Estriol originates almost exclusively from the placenta and is produced principally from placental conversion of fetal 16α-DHEA-S.[158,198] Estriol is first detectable in maternal serum at 9 weeks.[141,193–199] This closely corresponds to the early steroidogenic evolution of the fetal adrenal cortex.[141] Its continued production is therefore dependent on the presence of a living fetus. The concentration of estriol is less than 0.01 ng/ml in nonpregnant women. First detectable at levels of approximately 0.05 ng/ml at 9 weeks,[141,197] estriol increases gradually to a range of approximately 10 to 30 ng/ml at term[157] (Fig. 1–24). Between 35 and 40 weeks' gestational age, estriol concentrations increase sharply in a pattern that reflects a final surge of intrauterine steroidogenesis just prior to term.

Maternal concentrations of estriol may reflect abnormalities in fetal and placental development including fetal compromise, fetal anomalies, and hydatidiform mole.[199] Fetal death at any time during the second or third trimester produces a striking drop in estriol concentrations within 1 to 2 hours.[199] Within 4 to 6 hours, concentrations are consistently less than 1 ng/ml in the second trimester and less than 2.5 ng/ml in the third trimester.[199] Fetal anomalies associated with adrenal atrophy, such as anencephaly and Down syndrome, are associated with low concentrations.[199] For this reason, evaluation of unexplained low estriol in the second and third trimesters should include ultrasonography and amniocentesis as appropriate. Hydatidiform moles are associated with low estriol.[199] Presumably this occurs because of the absence of a fetal adrenal and liver. The resultant deficiency of fetal 16α-hydroxylated sulfoconjugated precursors in molar pregnancy would account for the very low estriol values.[199]

Deteriorating fetoplacental health during the third trimester has long been associated with either falling or low estriol concentrations.[199–202] Chronically compromised infants have markedly elevated cord LDL concentrations, low DHEA-S values, and decreased movement, suggesting a depressed fetal central nervous system (CNS).[201,202]

HORMONAL FUNCTIONS DURING PREGNANCY

Estrogens affect uterine vasculature, placenta steroidogenesis, and parturition.

Uterine Vasculature. Estrogens augment uterine blood flow. In ovine models, direct estrogen injection into the uterine arteries through indwelling catheters produces striking increases in blood flow. Estradiol is the most potent estrogen in this role. Estrone and estriol, however, though less active, also produce the effect.[203] Because exposure of the uteroplacental bed to direct estriol secretion is massive, estriol may be the principal augmenter of uterine blood flow as described previously. This may be the dominant role of estriol in human pregnancy.[203]

Placental Steroidogenesis. Estrogen-regulated mechanisms may allow the fetus to govern production and secretion of progesterone during the third trimester. In the baboon, estrogen controls the biosynthesis of placental progesterone by regulating the availability of LDL cholesterol for conversion to pregnenolone and to its downstream steroid products.[204] Thus, in advanced pregnancy, the fetus may regulate placental progesterone production.

Parturition. Fetoplacental estrogens are closely linked to myometrial irritability, contractility, and labor. In primates, estrogens ripen the cervix, initiate uterine activity, and augment established labor.[205] Estrogens also increase the sensitivity of the myometrium to oxytocin by augmenting prostaglandin biosynthesis.[206,207] Because placental release of estrogens is linked to the fetal hypothalamus, pituitary, adrenals, and placenta, the fetal pituitary adrenal axis appears to fine tune parturition timing, in part through its effect on estrogen production.[205-208] Thus, in human pregnancy in which the fetus is anencephalic, labor is either too early or too late. Similarly, surgical anencephaly in the fetal macaque disrupts the normal timing of parturition.[209] Parturition in humans is a precise event with a well-defined frequency distribution surrounding a mean gestational age of 270 days. In macaques, labor most often begins after a preparturitional increase of fetal adrenal steroids (DHEA-S) that is maximal between 2300 and 0300 hours.[207] A diurnal rhythm in uterine activity is also evident in which the maximal hourly values of intrauterine pressure and contraction frequency surround midnight. In human studies, there is a similar entrainment of uterine activity with circulating maternal estrogens and progesterone as labor approaches.[209-211] There is firm evidence of increasing, rhythmic fetal adrenal and placental steroid output over the 5 weeks just before term that is important in preparing for the final cascade of oxytocin and prostaglandins that stimulate labor.[209-211]

The Progestogens

Progesterone and 17α-hydroxyprogesterone are the major progestogens in human pregnancy.

VARIATION DURING PREGNANCY

Progesterone. Progesterone originates almost entirely from the corpus luteum before 6 weeks' gestational age but shifts to the placenta after the seventh week. After 12 weeks, the placenta is the major source of progesterone.[141,197] The placenta produces progesterone from circulating maternal LDL cholesterol and is minimally dependant on fetal precursors.[141,150,158]

Progesterone concentrations are less than 1 ng/ml during the follicular phase of the normal menstrual cycle[195,197] (Fig. 1-25). In the luteal phase of conceptual cycles, progesterone concentrations rise from 1 to 2 ng/ml on the day of the LH peak to a plateau of 10 to 35 ng/ml over the subsequent 7 days. Progesterone concentrations remain within this luteal range through the 10th week (dated from last menstrual flow), and then show a sustained rise that continues until term. At term, progesterone concentrations range from 100 to 300 ng/ml.[141]

Low progesterone levels are well tolerated in patients without ovaries, carrying pregnancies with donor embryos.[147,149] In women with first-trimester threatened abortion, progesterone concentrations at the time of the initial evaluation are predictive of the ultimate outcome.[212] Abortion will occur in approximately 80 percent of those with progesterone concentrations under

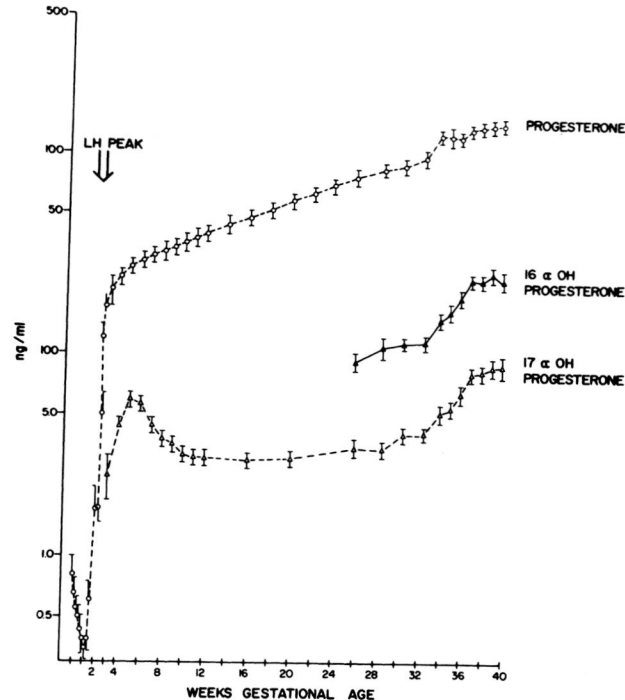

Figure 1-25. Mean concentrations (±SEM) of progesterone and 17α-hydroxyprogesterone from conception until term. Data are compiled from several reports. 17α-hydroxyprogesterone shows a marked rise in concentrations beginning at 32 weeks until term. Gestational ages are calculated from the last menstrual flow. (Composite adapted from Haluska and Novy,[208] Tulchinsky and Hobel,[141] Abraham et al.,[195] and Lindbert et al.[196])

10 ng/ml; viable pregnancies are virtually never observed at concentrations below 5.0 ng/ml.[213]

Conversely, in women with a hydatidiform mole, progesterone concentrations are significantly elevated above the normal range.[214] In women whose pregnancies are complicated by Rh isoimmunization, progesterone concentrations are elevated approximately twofold above values for normal pregnancies of comparable gestational ages.[197] This elevation may be related to a two- to threefold increase in placental mass associated with erythroblastosis.

Finally, progesterone concentrations are lower in women with an ectopic pregnancy. Single serum progesterone levels have been widely used in diagnostic algorithms with serum β-hCG and ultrasound in the diagnosis of ectopic pregnancy without laparoscopic surgery. Progesterone concentrations of less than 5 ng/ml are diagnostic of fetal death in the first trimester; thus, low progesterone levels prompt the performance of diagnostic curettage, which can help distinguish between ectopic pregnancy and intrauterine fetal demise. Direct visualization of the ectopic implantation is not required.[213]

17α-Hydroxyprogesterone. 17α-hydroxyprogesterone originates predominantly from the corpus luteum during the first trimester of pregnancy.[215] The ovaries continue to be a significant source of 17α-hydroxyprogesterone throughout pregnancy. During the third trimester, however, the placenta uses fetal Δ5-sulfoconjugated precursors to secrete increasing amounts of 17α-hydroxyprogesterone. The placenta is probably the major source of this hormone at term.[215]

17α-hydroxyprogesterone concentrations are less than 0.5 ng/ml during the follicular phase of normal menstrual cycles. In conceptual cycles, 17α-hydroxyprogesterone concentrations rise to about 1 ng/ml on the day of the LH peak, fall slightly for about 1 day, rise again over the subsequent 4 to 5 days to a level of 1 to 2 ng/ml, and then increase gradually to a mean of approximately 2 ng/ml (luteal phase levels) at the end of 12 weeks. This level remains relatively stable until a gestational age of about 32 weeks, when there begins an abrupt sustained rise to a mean of approximately 7 ng/ml at 37 weeks, a level that persists until term[215] (Fig. 1–25). The rise beginning at 32 weeks is strongly correlated with the activity of fetal maturational processes known to begin at this time.

During the first 7 weeks of gestation, through the time of the luteal-placental shift, 17α-hydroxyprogesterone concentrations reflect primarily the status of corpus luteum steroidogenesis.[215] In women undergoing spontaneous abortion, falling concentrations of 17α-hydroxyprogesterone parallel falling concentrations of progesterone.[215]

HORMONAL FUNCTIONS DURING PREGNANCY

Progestogens affect tubal motility, the endometrium, uterine vasculature, and parturition.

Tubal Motility. The preimplantation conceptus with its surrounding corona cells secretes progesterone long before implantation. Conceptus-secreted progesterone may itself affect tubal motility as the conceptus is carried to the uterus.[142] Progesterone, by action mediated through catecholamines and prostaglandins, is believed to relax uterotubal musculature. Estradiol, also secreted by these structures, may balance the progesterone, maintaining the desired level of tubal motility and tone.[142] Excess progesterone, as might occur from pharmacologically induced superovulation, may produce excessive relaxation of tubal musculature and could explain an apparent excess of ectopic pregnancies. Likewise, progesterone deficiency from blighted ova may cause accelerated oviduct transport with premature arrival of these ova to the uterus.

Endometrium. Progesterone inhibits T-lymphocyte–mediated tissue rejection and is believed to work in concert with hCG and decidual cortisol.[216,217] This inhibition of the rejection response may confer immunologic privilege to the implanted conceptus and developing placenta. It has been suggested that placental progesterone protects the pregnancy by inhibiting T-lymphocyte–mediated tissue rejection responses.[216,217] In rodents, progesterone extends the survival of transplanted human trophoblasts,[217] and high local intervillous concentrations of progesterone are of major importance in blocking the cellular immune rejection of the foreign protein originating from the pregnancy.[217]

Uterine Vasculature. Progesterone antagonizes estrogen-augmented uterine blood flow through depletion of cytoplasmic estrogen receptors.[218] Estrogen and progesterone appear to balance one another in the maintenance of blood flow at the implantation site.

Parturition Control. Progesterone and the estrogens are antagonistic in the parturition process. Progesterone produces uterine relaxation,[208] stabilizing lysosomal membranes and inhibiting prostaglandin synthesis and release. By contrast, estrogens labilize lysosomal membranes and augment the synthesis of prostaglandins and their release.[207]

Although gradual increase in cord DHEA-S and maternal estriol occurs toward term, there is no corresponding drop in either fetal or maternal progesterone concentrations.[219] That progesterone is important in the maintenance of uterine quiescence is not doubted, however, because in the first trimester removal of the corpus luteum leads rapidly to myometrial contractions.[145] Likewise, labor ensues following administration of antiprogesterone compounds in the third trimester.[220] The antiprogesterone agents occupy progesterone receptors and inhibit the action of progesterone, which is clearly essential for maintenance of uterine quiescence. Yet, progesterone administration to women, except in large doses, does not suppress human uterine contractions once begun.[220]

The ratios of estradiol and progesterone in various animals models are closely related to the stimulation of myometrial gap junction formation.[221]

Adrenocorticoids

VARIATION DURING PREGNANCY

Fetal plasma cortisol and amniotic fluid cortisol and cortisol sulfate concentrations increase considerably with advancing gestational age and approaching parturition.[222,223] With the exception of the amniotic membranes and decidua, virtually all fetal organs convert cortisol to cortisone.[143,144] The intracellular mechanisms of cortisol-to-cortisone interconversion and its regulatory effect on the biologic expression of cortisol are diagrammed in Figure 1–26. As parturition approaches, net conversion of cortisol to cortisone is decreased in many tissues such as fetal lung.[223] As cortisol-to-cortisone conversion decreases, there is increasing circulating cortisol available to maturing fetal tissues.

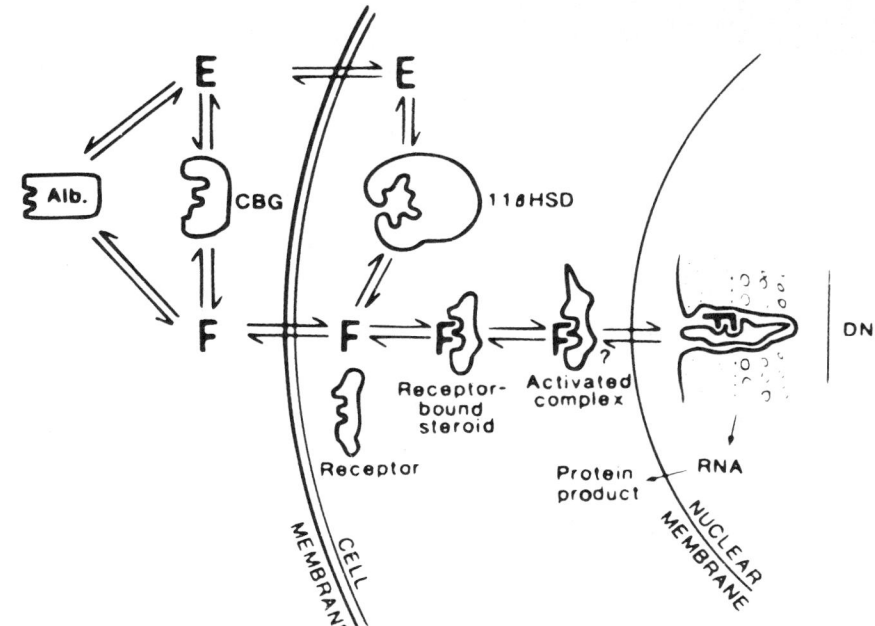

Figure 1–26. Mechanism of intrauterine cortisol (F) modulation. Target organ cells autoregulate F interaction with corticoid receptors by diverting F to E (cortisone) through 11 β-HSD interconversion. (From Murphy BEP: Cortisol economy in the human fetus. *In* James VHT, Serio M, Gusti G, et al [eds]: The Endocrine Function of the Human Adrenal Cortex. San Diego, Academic Press, 1978, p 509, with permission.)

The final increase in fetal cortisol in pregnancy may be limited to the increase in placental CRH (Fig. 1–13).

TARGET TISSUE INTERACTION DURING PREGNANCY

The profile of circulating adrenocorticoids in the fetoplacental circulation is determined extensively by steroid interconversions between cortisol and cortisone. The *placenta* contains abundant 11-dehydrogenase activity. Although much of circulating fetal cortisol derives from transplacental passage of maternal cortisol, approximately 80 percent of maternal cortisol is converted to cortisone on entering the fetal circulation.[222,223] Corticoid measurements in placental tissues indicate a cortisol/cortisone ratio of far less than 1.0, thus reconfirming active intraplacental conversion of cortisol to cortisone.[222,223]

Chorionic membranes contain an abundance of 11-ketoreductase activity and therefore convert cortisone to cortisol. First detectable at approximately 18 weeks' gestational age, this activity continues through term.[222,223] Activity is also found in the adherent decidua and in the juxtaposed myometrium. As a result of chorionic membrane and uterine peripheral interconversion, the concentration of cortisol in uterine tissues is nine times that detectable in nonpregnant myometrium.[222,223] It is plausible that the maintenance of high cortisol concentrations in myometrium is part of the same immunosuppressive process of pregnancy maintenance that involves hCG and progesterone.[222,223]

Fetal lung contains predominantly 11-dehydrogenase activity and therefore predominantly converts cortisol to cortisone. With advancing gestation, the fetal lung cortisol-to-cortisone interconversion diminishes.[222,223]

Lung tissue at birth shows no detectable cortisol-to-cortisone conversion. The net result of this transformation is increased pulmonary intracellular cortisol bioavailability, a process that may be related to maturation of the fetal lung, which is accelerating by 34 to 36 weeks' gestational age.[176]

HORMONAL FUNCTIONS DURING PREGNANCY

Adrenocorticoids impact with particular relevance on regulation of intrauterine maturation. In normally progressing human pregnancy, multiple enzyme systems accelerate, beginning at approximately 32 weeks' gestational age and finishing at approximately 37 weeks' gestational age.[176] Delivery at any time from 37 weeks to term generally produces a newborn free of the hazards of prematurity. Although a variety of interdependent hormonal events are involved, the weight of available evidence indicates that fetal cortisol is the major effector in the induction of these final and essential maturational systems involving fetal lung and liver, the nervous system, and the adrenal medulla.[176] Placental CRH, which increases over the last weeks of pregnancy, may be the final common endocrine modulator[224,225] (Fig. 1–13).

PREGNANCY DIAGNOSIS AND MONITORING

The novel hormones of pregnancy may be measured for diagnosis and clinical detection of abnormalities. A variety of assay techniques are available.

Human Chorionic Gonadotropin

There are four groups of hCG configurations that affect performance and interpretation of assays.

Dimeric hCG

Dimeric hCG and both subunits, α-hCG and β-hCG, rise sharply during the first trimester[19] (Fig. 1–10). The dimeric hCG is normally measured, either directly by sandwich-type assays or inferentially by detection of the β subunit for diagnosis and monitoring of early pregnancy. HCG is detectable in serum in approximately 5 percent of patients by 8 days after conception, and in virtually all patients by day 11.[12] Deviation from the normal doubling patterns suggests that the pregnancy is either an ectopic gestation or is undergoing spontaneous abortion. Thus, if hCG fails to rise 66 percent in 2 days, ancillary procedures are necessary to differentiate between the two conditions.[226]

Dimeric and free subunit hCG are produced in the pituitary and released in association with pituitary LH.[57,227] Levels are much higher in postmenopausal women (100 pg/ml vs. 10 pg/ml).[57] Nonpregnant levels of hCG are, however, well under the sensitivity (approximately 1 mIU/ml) detectable by the most sensitive clinical assays used in pregnancy monitoring.[228]

Free α- and β-hCG Subunits

Following in vitro fertilization and embryo transfer,[19] free β subunits of hCG may be detected as early as 7 days (1 day earlier than intact hCG). Free α subunits are first detectable at gestational week 6 and rise in sigmoid fashion to peak at 36 weeks' gestational age.[19] In general, α-hCG is rarely used in clinical interpretation, although the concentrations are elevated in persistent gestational trophoblastic neoplasia and are significantly lower in insulin-dependent diabetic women. Persistently elevated free β subunits in patients with trophoblastic disease may portend a poor prognosis.[229]

β-Subunit Core Fragment (β-Core)

β-Core is a major component of the immunoreactive hCG in urine, particularly during the second trimester.[47] β-Core circulates in small amounts because of its very short half-life. With a molecular weight of approximately 10.0 kDa, β-core consists of two polypeptide chains, composed of residues 6–40 disulfide bridges to residues 55–92 of the β subunit.[47] β-Core is detected in β-subunit assays. Despite the conformational differences of hCG measured through the β subunit, assays in either serum or urine of the same patient produce very similar results.[47]

Nicked hCG Subunits

Nicked hCG is an hCG subunit with deleted peptide linkages.[229] In the β subunit, these linkages are between residues 47–84 and between 44–45 or 46–57.[229] In the α subunits, they are between 70–71. As nicking increases, receptor binding decreases.[47] For this reason, nicked hCG is biologically less active. Disparities in levels of nicked versus non-nicked hCG account for major discrepancies in the hormone levels observed with different assay methods.[229–231] Test results between commercial assays are not necessarily interconvertible. For this reason, investigators in this field believe that hCG assay reports should include information about assay interaction with nicked hCG, free β subunit, and β-core fragment. In this way, the different standards, though not precisely interconvertible, can still be interpreted.[47]

hCG Standards

In comparing hCG measurements by different radioimmunoassays (RIAs), the standard must be specified. Two standards are commonly encountered. The Third International Standard (3rd IS), which is the same as First International Reference Preparation, is less contaminated with free α and β subunits of hCG than the Second International Standard (2nd IS). The discrepancy is irrelevant in hCG assays specified for the intact hCG molecule (whole molecule or sandwich assays) because neither detects free β subunits. However, the standards are important in interpreting results from RIAs that interact with the β subunit part of the molecule and are therefore unable to distinguish between free subunits and the intact molecule. Thus, the 3rd IS produces values approximately 1.5- to 2-fold greater for β-subunit radioimmunoassay than does the 2nd IS.[47] This difference, more or less uniform throughout pregnancy, is illustrated in Figure 1–27.

hCG Assays

The choice of hCG assay from the variety available depends on the demands required of the test.

Radioimmunoassays

RIAs are the traditional laboratory technique for measuring hCG. These assays bind at the β subunit and therefore measure combined concentrations of free β subunits plus dimeric hCG. HCG is labeled with a radioactive marker (e.g., ^{125}I) and is displaced from binding sites on an antibody directed against it by unlabeled hCG in the patient's serum. If no hCG is displaced, there is no detectable hCG in the patient's serum.[232–234]

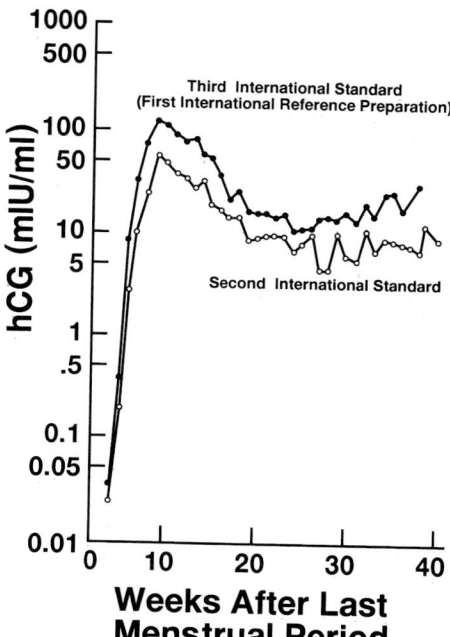

Figure 1-27. Serum concentrations of hCG measured using the 2nd IS as the reference preparation versus results obtained using the 3rd IS (1st IRP) as the standard in hCO radioimmunoassays. Note the 1.5- to 2-fold greater concentrations of hCG measured using the 3rd IS relative to those obtained with the 2nd IS. (From Ren SG, Braunstein GD: Human chorionic gonadotropin. Semin Reprod Endocrinol 10:95, 1992, with permission.)

If displacement does occur, the patient's serum will contain hCG in a quantitative relationship, resulting in displacement of labeled hCG from the antibody. Because RIAs are quantitative, they are useful in determining doubling times, as required for diagnosis of ectopic pregnancy, spontaneous abortion, or gestational trophoblastic neoplasia. Although precise, RIAs have limited sensitivity, require hours to perform, and involve use of radioisotopes.[232-234] RIAs have therefore been recently replaced in clinical laboratories by the technically simpler immunoradiometric assay (IRMA).

Immunoradiometric Assay

IRMA uses a sandwich principle to detect intact hCG (whole-molecule assay). IRMA hCG assays require only 30 minutes to complete and can detect very low concentrations of hCG.[231-235] IRMAs use a radioactive antibody labelled (^{125}I) to detect hCG in the serum. Briefly, anti-hCG antibodies are bound to a test tube. The patient's serum is added, and a second labeled antibody binds to the hCG–antibody complex already on the tube. The amount of labeled antibody bound to the tube is proportional to the amount of hCG in the patient's serum. The hCG molecule is thus "sandwiched" between two antibodies.[235] Commercial IRMA

assays can detect hCG levels as low as 0.05 mIU/ml. This "sandwich" principle is the technique used in the nonradioactive enzyme-linked immunosorbent assay (ELISA). Because IRMA requires ^{125}I-labeled hCG, a gamma counter is needed. For this reason, many commercial laboratories are switching to ELISA assays.

Enzyme Linked Immunosorbent Assay

ELISAs do not use radioisotopes.[236] The principle is the same as that of IRMA but instead of using a radiolabeled second antibody, the second antibody is labeled with a substance that can be detected by a color change after binding (alkaline phosphatase or horseradish peroxidase colorimetric reaction). Although not as precise as RIA, the assay is sensitive, quick, and ideal for the early diagnosis of pregnancy in urine where the level of hCG does not need to be known. Thus, with one commercial kit used for pregnancy diagnosis, a value exceeding greater than 30 mIU/ml in urine is reported as a positive test (Immulite). ELISA can also detect hCG in serum at concentrations as low as 1 to 2 mIU/ml, allowing for diagnosis of pregnancy as early as 5 days before first missed menses.[236] These assays are easily packaged for use in commercial laboratories or in a physician's office equipped with automated chemiluminescence equipment (e.g., Chiron Diagnostics ACS:180 total hGC). This equipment makes the assays quantitative so they can be used for both pregnancy diagnosis and monitoring.

Fluoroimmunoassay

This technique is another "sandwich" assay in which a second antibody is tagged with a fluorescent label. The fluorescence emitted, proportional to the amount of hCG in the test serum, allows for detection of concentrations as low as 1 mIU/ml.[237] The technique takes 2 to 3 hours, uses no radioactivity, and is highly precise. FIA is used to detect and follow hCG concentrations.

Clinical Application of hCG Measurements

Pregnancy Diagnosis

hCG is first detectable in maternal blood at approximately 8 to 11 days after conception using very sensitive research assays (sensitivity, 0.1 to 0.3 mIU/ml).[12,13,19] Most state-of-the-art rapid pregnancy tests are set to a sensitivity of 25 to 30 mIU/ml[238] (Fig. 1–28).

False-positive results occur in the range of 5 to 25 mIU/ml. False-positive results can occur in perimenopausal and postmenopausal women because of endogenous pituitary hCG secretion, which occurs in syn-

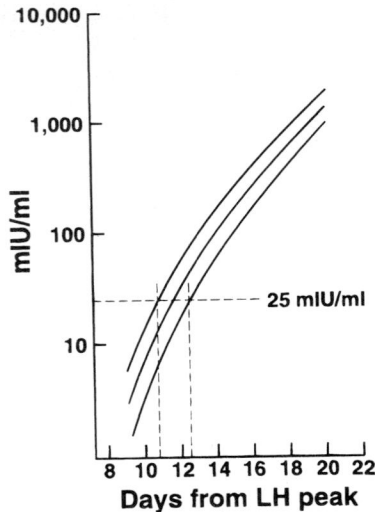

Figure 1–28. Levels of circulating hCG in early pregnancy showing that an assay with a sensitivity of 25 mIU/ml would become positive in some subjects 10 to 11 days after the LH peak and in most subjects 12 to 13 days after the LH peak. (From Chard T: Pregnancy tests: a review. Hum Reprod 7:701, 1992, with permisssion.)

chrony with LH. For practical purposes, a level of less than 5 mIU/ml can be confidently stated as negative. A level exceeding 25 mIU/ml can be confidently stated as positive.[238] When there is uncertainty, repeating the test in 2 days normally confirms a trend upwards, which documents the existence of a pregnancy.

Ectopic Pregnancy

With rare exceptions, patients with ectopic pregnancy have hCG titers exceeding 20 mIU/ml (3rd IS standard); 98 percent titers exceeding 40 mIU/ml. Serial hCGs, in combination with vaginal ultrasound and serum progesterone measurements, are used widely for nonsurgical diagnosis of ectopic pregnancy.[201]

Spontaneous Abortion

Serum hCG fails to double or falls in patients with spontaneous abortion. Serial hCG showing an abnormally slow rise or decrease may portend spontaneous abortion. Anembryonic gestation should be suspected when there is no fetal pole and the gestational sac exceeds 17 mm or β-hCG greater than or equal to 5,100 mIU/ml (3rd IS), and no fetal pole is seen.

Screening for Fetal Down Syndrome

HCG concentrations are elevated in women carrying a fetus affected with Down syndrome.[239] This finding has been used in various calculations using maternal age, AFP levels, and hCG concentrations, with or without unconjugated estriol to estimate the risk of carrying an affected fetus. Using serum analytes, one can identify approximately two thirds of affected fetuses with Down syndrome with a 6 percent false-positive (amniocentesis) rate.[239,240]

Gestational Trophoblastic Disease

Serial hCG measurements are used to monitor therapy for gestational trophoblastic disease. Disappearance of hCG is used to predict the course of the disease.[241]

Early Pregnancy Factor

Pregnancy diagnosis before implantation may be possible through measurement of EPF, which is detectable 26 to 24 hours after fertilization. EPF cannot be detected 24 hours after delivery or termination of either an ectopic or intrauterine pregnancy[1,2] (Fig. 1–7).

Detection of EPF currently depends on a cumbersome biologic assay, the rosette inhibition test.[1,2] Although recently EPF has been isolated, identified, and sequenced, the exact nature of the molecular species is uncertain and clinical assays are not yet available.[1,2]

Diagnosis of conception before implantation will open possibilities for contraception, preimplantation genetics through uterine lavage, and highly accurate dating of intrauterine pregnancies.

Progesterone

Single progesterone measurements in the first trimester are useful in screening for ectopic pregnancy and spontaneous abortion. A single progesterone measurement of less than or equal to 5 ng/ml rules out a viable intrauterine pregnancy[213,242,243] and allows the physician to perform a dilatation and curettage without fear of interfering with a viable pregnancy.[213] If villi are found, the patient is unlikely to have an ectopic pregnancy.[141] A value 25 ng/ml or more rules out 98 percent of ectopic pregnancies.[213] Values between 5 and 25 ng/ml are problematic and require further investigation with ultrasound.[243]

Combined Ultrasound and Hormone Measurements

Combined with hCG and progesterone, ultrasound is helpful in determining the viability and location of a pregnancy.[244,245] Transvaginal ultrasound allows detection of an intrauterine pregnancy as early as 4 weeks from the last menstrual period, when a gestational sac measures 4 to 5 mm[244] (Table 1–2). At 5 gestational

Table 1–2. GESTATIONAL AGE AT WHICH EMBRYOLOGIC STRUCTURES ARE DETECTABLE BY VAGINAL ULTRASOUND

Embryonic/Fetal Structure	Gestational Age of Detection
Gestational sac	4 weeks, 1–3 days
Yolk sac	5 weeks
Fetal cardiac activity	5 weeks, 6 days
Limb buds	8 weeks
Head	8 weeks
Ventricles	8 weeks, 2–4 days
Choroid plexus	9 weeks
Hand, fingers	12 weeks

Modified from Timor-Tritsch IE, Rottem S (eds): Transvaginal Sonography. New York, Elsevier Science, 1991.

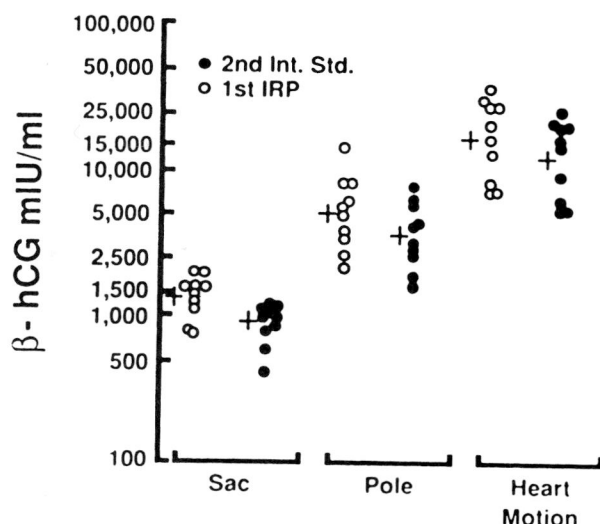

Figure 1–29. Range of β-hCG titers (IRP) and predicted developmental landmarks detected by vaginal ultrasound. (From Fossum GF, Davajan V, Kletzky OA: Early detection of pregnancy with transvaginal ultrasound. Fertil Steril 49:789, 1988. American Society for Reproductive Medicine, with permission.)

weeks, the yolk sac becomes visible; at the end of the fifth week, transvaginal ultrasound detects all intrauterine pregnancies with a 95 percent confidence limit.[244,245] Fetal cardiac activity is detected just before 6 gestational weeks. In a well-timed pregnancy, these ultrasonic milestones are useful in detecting deviations from the norm. Table 1–3 lists the appearance of key embryologic findings associated with rising hCG.[244,245] When combined with serum measurements of hCG, ultrasonographic findings are vital in the diagnosis of an ectopic gestation and impending abortion.[244,245]

Using transabdominal ultrasound, all patients with a healthy intrauterine pregnancy whose hCG measured 6,500 mIU/ml had a gestational sac visible by ultrasound.[244] Similarly, transvaginal ultrasound visualizes all intrauterine pregnancies when the hCG exceeds 2,400 mIU/ml[244,245] (Fig. 1–29). When hCG levels exceed these concentrations and no intrauterine pregnancy is detectable by ultrasound, either uterine curettage to exclude villi or laparoscopy to visualize an ectopic pregnancy is necessary.[245] Conversely, a heart beat detected at 8 gestational weeks assures a patient that her chance of continuing her pregnancy is over 95 per-

cent.[245] Algorithms have been devised utilizing rapid progesterone assay, serial β-hCG, and ultrasound to diagnose ectopic pregnancy nonsurgically.[246,247] This has been particularly important with the recent advancement of medical therapy for this condition, whereby laparoscopy is eschewed.

CONCLUSIONS

No biologic events can exceed the events considered in this chapter in the long-term importance to human development. Endocrine factors play important roles in the orchestration and outcome of these events. It is a privilege to detect, measure, observe, and occasionally assist nature in the nourishment and protection of the

Table 1–3. APPEARANCE OF KEY EMBRYOLOGIC STRUCTURES IN ASSOCIATION WITH RISING hCG TITERS*

Ultrasound Findings	Days from LMP	β-hCG (mIU/ml)	
		Third International Standard†	Second International Standard
Sac	34.8 ± 2.2	1,398 ± 155	914 ± 106
Fetal pole	40.3 ± 3.4‡	5,113 ± 298‡	3,783 ± 683
Fetal heart motion	46.9 ± 6.0	17,208 ± 3,772‡	13,178 ± 2,898‡

* Failure to identify these structures in the uterus as hCG rises above these levels suggests ectopic pregnancy.
† Third International Standard equal First International Reference Preparation.
‡ $p < 0.05$ when compared with sac.
From Fossum GT, Davajan V, Kletzky OA: Early detection of pregnancy with transvaginal ultrasound. Fertil Steril 49:789, 1988, with permission.

growing fetus in the otherwise invisible confines of the uterus.

Key Points

➤ Beginning with conception, a series of proteins specific for and secreted only during pregnancy evolve to facilitate invasion of half-foreign embryonic tissue into the uterine wall.

➤ Cytotrophoblasts, secreting hypothalamic peptides, function in juxtaposition to syncytiotrophoblast, secreting the corresponding pituitary-like peptides in an anatomic arrangement analogous to the hypothalamic-pituitary axis.

➤ Early pregnancy factor, an analogue of chaperonin 10, is the earliest known circulating marker of fertilization in pregnancy.

➤ Placental GnRH stimulates and is entrained to placental hCG production and release.

➤ Secretion of placental CRH and ACTH into the maternal circulation induces hypercortisolism mediated through the maternal hypothalamic-pituitary axis.

➤ hCG maintains the corpus luteum, stimulates adrenal and placental steroidogenesis, and modulates maternal immunologic response to the pregnancy.

➤ Human chorionic somatomammotropin antagonizes insulin action and induces maternal glucose intolerance, which promotes transfer of glucose and amino acids into the fetus.

➤ Decidual prolactin, a peptide similar to pituitary prolactin, regulates fluid and electrolyte flux through the fetal membranes; it is secreted independently of fetal or maternal dopaminergic control.

➤ Progesterone secreted by the preimplantation conceptus modulates tubal motility in early pregnancy; progesterone secreted by the placenta inhibits maternal–fetal tissue rejection, antagonizes the augmentation of uterine blood flow by estrogen, and induces uterine relaxation before parturition.

➤ When pregnancy tests are set to high sensitivity (<1 mIU/ml) of hCG, false-positives can occur because of endogenous pituitary hCG, which is released in synchrony with pituitary LH and is detected in the assay.

REFERENCES

1. Morton H: Early pregnancy factor: an extracellular chaperonin 10 homologue. Immunol Cell Biol 76:483, 1998.
2. Cavanagh AC: Identification of early pregnancy factor as chaperonin 10: implications for understanding its role. Rev Reprod 1:28, 1996.
3. Cavanagh AC, Morton H, Rolfe BE, et al: Ovum factor: a first signal of pregnancy? Am J Reprod Immunol 2:97, 1992.
4. Morton H, Rolfe BE, Cavanagh AC: Ovum factor and early pregnancy factor. Curr Top Dev Biol 23:73, 1987.
5. Croxatto HB, Oritz ME, Diaz S, et al: Studies on the duration of egg transport by the human oviduct, II: ovum location at various times following luteinizing hormone peak. Am J Obstet Gynecol 132:629, 1978.
6. Buster JE, Bustillo M, Rodi IA, et al: Biological and morphologic development of donated human ova recovered by nonsurgical uterine lavage. Am J Obstet Gynecol 153:211, 1985.
7. Bonduelle ML, Liebaers DR, Van Steiteghem A, et al: Chorionic gonadotrophin-beta mRNA, a trophoblasts maker, is expressed in human 8-cell embryos derived from tripronucleate zygotes. Hum Reprod 3:909, 1988.
8. Lopata A, Hay DL: The surplus human embryo: its potential for growth, blastulation, matching, and human chorionic gonadotropin production in culture. Fertil Steril 51:984, 1989.
9. Hay DL, Lopata A: Chorionic gonadotropin secretion by human embryos in vitro. J Clin Endocrinol Metab 67:1322, 1988.
10. Cross JC, Werb Z, Fisher SJ: Implantation and the placenta: key pieces of the development puzzle. Science 266:1508, 1994.
11. Navot D, Scott RT, Droesch K, et al: The window of embryo transfer and the efficiency of human conception in vitro. Fertil Steril 55:114, 1991.
12. Lenton EA, Neal LM, Sulaiman R: Plasma concentrations of human chorionic gonadotropin from the time of implantation until the second week of pregnancy. Fertil Steril 37:773, 1982.
13. Kosasa T, Levesque L, Goldstein DP, et al: Early detection of implantation using a radioimmunoassay specific for human chorionic gondotropin. J Clin Endocrinol Metab 36:622, 1973.
14. Chard T: Proteins of the human placenta: some general concepts. In Grudzinskas JC, Teisner BL, Sepala M (eds): Pregnancy Proteins: Biology, Chemistry and Clinical Application. San Diego, Academic Press, 1982, p 6.
15. Saijonmaa O, Laatikaninen T, Wahlstrom T: Corticotrophin-releasing factor in human placenta: localization, concentration and release in vitro. Placenta 9:373, 1988.
16. Khodr GS, Siler-Khodr TM: Placental luteinizing hormone-releasing factor and its synthesis. Science 207:315, 1980.
17. Shambaugh G III, Kubek M, Wilber JF: Thyrotrophin-releasing hormone activity in the human placenta. J Clin Endocrinol Metab 48:483, 1979.
18. Al-Timimi A, Fox H: Immunohistochemical localization of follicle-stimulating hormone, luteinizing hormone, growth hormone, adrenocoticotropic hormone and prolactin in the human placenta. Placenta 7:163, 1986.
19. Hay DL: Placental histology and the production of human choriogonadotropin and its subunits in pregnancy. Br J Obstet Gynaecol 95:1268, 1988.
20. Harada A, Hershman JM: Extraction of human chorionic thyrotropin (hCT) from term placentas: failure to recover thyrotropic activity. J Clin Endocrinol Metab 47:681, 1978.
21. Steuber DF: Peptide hormone precursors: biosynthesis, processing, and significance. In Parson JA (ed): Peptide Hormones. Baltimore, University Park Press, 1976, p 49.

22. Horshina M, Hussa R, Pattillo R, et al: The role of trophoblasts differentiation in the control of the hCG and hPL genes. Adv Exp Med Biol 176:299, 1984.
23. Hoshina M, Boime I, Mochizuki M: Cytological localization of hPL, hCG, and mRNA in chorionic tissues using in situ hybridization. Acta Obstet Gynecol Jpn 36:397, 1984.
24. Kurman RJ, Young RH, Norrie HJ, et al: Immunocytochemical localization of placental lactogen and chorionic gonadotropin in the normal placenta and trophoblastic tumors, with emphasis on intermediate trophoblasts and the placental site trophoblastic tumor. Int J Gynecol Pathol 3:101, 1984.
25. Kasai K, Shik SS, Yoshida Y: Production and localization of human prolactin in placenta and deciduas in early and at term normal pregnancy. Nippon Naika Gakkai Zasshi 56:1974, 1970.
26. Watkins WB, Yen SS: Somatostatin in cytotrophoblast of the immature human placenta: localization by immunoperoxidase cytochemistry. J Clin Endocrinol Metab 50:969, 1980.
27. Chard T, Grudzinskas JG: Pregnancy protein secretion. Semin Reprod Endocrinol 10:61, 1992.
28. Cavanagh AC, Morton H: The purification of early-pregnancy factor to homogeneity from human platelets and identification of chaperonin 10. Eur J Biochem 222:551, 1994.
29. Aranha C, Natraj U, Iyer KS, et al: Isolation and purification of an early pregnancy factor-like molecule from culture supernatants obtained from lymphocytes of pregnant women. J Assist Reprod Genet 15:117, 1998.
30. Aranha C, Bordekar A, Shahani S: Isolation and purification of an early pregnancy factor-like molecule from culture supernatants obtained from lymphocytes of pregnant women: II. Identification of the molecule as a Fc-receptor-like molecule: a preliminary report. J Assist Reprod Genet 15:619, 1998.
31. Zuo X, Su B, Wei D: Isolation and characterization of early pregnancy factor. Chin Med Sci J 9:34, 1994.
32. Bose R: An update on the identity of early pregnancy factor and its role in early pregnancy. J Assist Reprod Genet 14:497, 1997.
33. Di Trapani G, Orozeo C, Cock I, et al: A re-examination of the association of 'early pregnancy factor' activity with fractions of heterogeneous molecular weight distribution in pregnancy sera. Early Pregnancy 3:312, 1997.
34. Clarke FM: Identification of molecules and mechanisms involved in the 'early pregnancy factor' system. Reprod Fertil Dev 4:423, 1992.
35. Chard T, Grudzinskas JG: Early pregnancy factor. Biol Res Pregnancy 8:53, 1987.
36. Mesrogli M, Schneider J, Maas DHA: Early pregnancy factor as a marker for the earliest stages of pregnancy in infertile women. Hum Reprod 3:113, 1988.
37. Shahani SK, Moniz CL, Bordekar AD, et al: Early pregnancy factor as a marker for assessing embryonic viability in threatened and missed abortions. Gynecol Obstet Invest 37:73, 1994.
38. Straube W, Romer T, Zeemni L, et al: The early pregnancy factor (EPF) as an early marker of disorders in pregnancy. Zentralbl Gynakol 117:32, 1995.
39. Hubel V, Straube W, Loh M, et al: Human early pregnancy factor and early pregnancy associated protein before and after therapeutic abortion in comparison with beta-hCG, estradiol, progesterone and 17-hydroxyprogesterone. Exp Clin Endocrinol 94:171, 1989.
40. Shu-Xin H, Zhen-Qun Z: A study of early pregnancy factor activity in the sera of patients with unexplained spontaneous abortion. Am J Reprod Immunol 29:77, 1993.
41. Shahani SK, Moniz CL, Gokral JS, et al: Early pregnancy factor (EFE) as a marker for detecting subclinical embryonic loss in clomiphene citrate-treated women. Am J Reprod Immunol 33:350, 1995.
42. Fan XG, Zhang ZQ: A study of early pregnancy factor activity in preimplantetion. Am J Reprod Immunol 37:359, 1997.
43. Fan X, Yan L, Jia S, et al: A study of early pregnancy factor activity in the sera of women with trophoblastic tumor. Am J Reprod Immumol 41:204, 1999.
44. Morton H, Cavanagh AC, Athanasas-Platsis S, et al: Early pregnancy factor has immunosuppressive and growth factor properties. Reprod Fertil Dev 4:411, 1992.
45. Morton H, Rolfe BE, Cavanagh AC: Pregnancy proteins: basic concepts and clinical applications. Semin Reprod Endocrinol 10:72, 1992.
46. Summers KM, Murphy RM, Webb GC, et al: The human early pregnancy factor/chaperonin 10 gene family. Biochem Mol Med 58:52, 1996.
47. Ren SG, Braunstein GD: Human chorionic gonadotropin. Semin Reprod Endocrinol 10:95, 1992.
48. Lustbader JW, Pollak S, Lobel L, et al: Three-dimensional structures of gonadotropins. Mol Cell Endocrinol 125:21, 1996.
49. Elliott MM, Kardana A, Lustbader JW, et al: Carbohydrate and peptide structure of the alpha- and beta-subunit of human chorionic gonadotropin from normal and aberrant pregnancy and choriocarcinoma. Endocrine 7:15, 1997.
50. Lustbader JW, Lobel L, Wu H, et al: Structural and molecular studies of human chorionic gonadotropin and its receptor. Recent Prog Horm Res 53:395, 1998.
51. Barnea ER, Kaplan M: Spontaneous, gonadotropin-releasing hormone-induced, and progesterone-inhibited pulsatile secretion of human chorionic gonadotropin in the first trimester placenta in vitro. J Clin Endocrinol Metab 69:215, 1989.
52. Jones SA, Brooks AN, Challis JR: Steroids modulate corticotropin-releasing hormone production in human fetal membranes and placenta. J Clin Endocrinol Metab 68:825, 1989.
53. Mersol-Barg MS, Miller KF, Choi CM, et al: Inhibin suppresses human chorionic gonadotropin secretion in term, but not first trimester, placenta. J Clin Endocrinol Metab 71:1294, 1990.
54. Shi LT, Zhang ZW, Li WX: Regulation of human chorionic gonadotropin secretion and messenger ribonucleic acid levels by follistatin in the NUCC-3 choriocarcinoma cell line. Endocrinology 134:2431, 1994.
55. Prager D, Weber MM, Herman-Bonert V: Placental growth factors and releasing/inhibiting peptides. Semin Reprod Endocrinol 10:83, 1992.
56. Patton P, Hess DL, Cook DM, et al: Human chorionic gonadotropin production by the pituitary gland in a premenopausal woman. Am J Obstet Gynecol 178:1138, 1998.
57. Odell WD, Griffin J: Pulsatile secretion of human chorionic gonadotropin in normal adults. N Engl J Med 317:1688, 1987.
58. Daiter E, Braunstein GD, Snyder PJ, et al: Gonadotropin-releasing hormone-dependent chorionic gonadotropin secretion in a menopausal women. J Clin Endocrinol Metab 78:1293, 1994.
59. Willey KP: An elusive role for glycosylation in the structure and function of reproductive hormones. Hum Reprod Update 5:330, 1999.
60. Jameson JL, Hollenberg AN: Regulation of chorionic gonadotropin gene expression. Endocr Rev 14:203, 1993.
61. Petraglia F, de Micheroux AA, Florio P, et al: Steroid-protein interaction in human placenta. J Steroid Biochem Mol Biol 53:227, 1995.
62. Albanese C, Colin IM, Crowley WF, et al: The gonadotropin genes: evolution of distinct mechanisms for hormonal control. Recent Prog Horm Res 51:23, 1996.
63. Speroff L: Endocrinology of pregnancy. *In* Speroff L, Glass RH, Kase NG (eds): Clinical Gynecologic Endocrinology and

Infertility, 6th ed. Baltimore, Lippincott Williams & Wilkins, 1999, p 295.

64. Cole LA, Kardana A, Andrade-Gordon P, et al: The heterogeneity of human chorionic gonadotropin (hCG). III. The occurrence and biological and immunological activities of nicked hCG. Endocrinology 129:1559, 1991.

65. Knofler M: What factors regulate HCG production in Down's syndrome pregnancies? Regulation of HCG during normal gestation and in pregnancies affected by Down's syndrome. Mol Hum Reprod 5:895, 1999.

66. Hanson FW, Powell JE, Stevens VC: Effects of hCG and human pituitary LH on steroid secretion and functional life of the human corpus luteum. J Clin Endocrinol Metab 32:211, 1971.

67. Seron-Ferre M, Lawrence CC, Jaffee RB: Role of hCG in the regulation of the fetal adrenal gland. J Clin Endocrinol Metab 46:834, 1978.

68. Huhtaniemi IT, Korenbrot CC, Jaffee RB: HCG binding and stimulation of testosterone biosynthesis in the human fetal testis. J Clin Endocrinol Metab 44:963, 1977.

69. Adcock EW III, Teasdale F, August CS, et al: Human chorionic gonadotropin: its possible role in maternal lymphocyte suppression. Science 181:845, 1973.

70. Nishula BC, Ketelslegers JM: Thyroid stimulating activity and chorionic gonadotropin. J Clin Invest 54:494, 1974.

71. Rees LH, Burke CW, Chard T, et al: Possible placental origin of ACTH in normal human pregnancy. Nature 254:620, 1975.

72. Genazzani AR, Fraioli F, Hurlimann J, et al: Immune reactive ACTH and cortisol plasma levels during pregnancy. Detection and partial purification of corticotrophin-like placental hormone: the human chorionic corticotrophin (HCG). Clin Endocrinol 4:1, 1975.

73. Petraglia F, Sawchenko PE, Rivier J, et al: Evidence for local stimulation of ACTH secretion by corticotropin-releasing factor in human placenta. Nature 328:717, 1987.

74. Nolten WE, Reckert PA: Elevated free cortisol index in pregnancy: possible regulatory mechanism. Am J Obstet Gynecol 139:492, 1981.

75. Okamoto E, Takagi T, Azuma C, et al: Expression of the corticotropin-releasing hormone (CRH) gene in human placenta and amniotic membrane. Horm Metab Res 22:394, 1990.

76. Robinson BG, Emanuel RL, Frim DM, et al: Glucocorticoid stimulates expression of corticotropin-releasing hormone gene in human placenta. Proc Natl Acad Sci U S A 85:5244, 1988.

77. Niall HD, Hogan ML, Sauer R, et al: Sequences of pituitary and placental lactogenic and growth hormones: evolution from a primordial peptide by gene reduplication. Proc Natl Acad Sci U S A 68:866, 1971.

78. Handwerger S, Brar A: Placental lactogen, placental growth hormone, and decidual prolactin. Semin Reprod Endocrinol 10:106, 1992.

79. Walker WH, Fitzpatrick SL, Barrera-Saldana HA, et al: The human placental lactogen genes: structure function, evolution and transcriptional regulation. Endocr Soc 4:316, 1991.

80. Braunstein GD, Rasor JL, Wade ME: Interrelationships of human chorionic gonadotropin, human placental lactogen, and pregnancy specific beta-1 glycoprotein throughout normal human gestation. Am J Obstet Gynecol 138:1205, 1980.

81. Kim YJ, Felig P: Plasma human chorionic somatomammotropin levels during starvation in midpregnancy. J Clin Endocrinol Metab 32:864, 1971.

82. Furlanetto RW, Underwood LE, Van Wyk JJ, et al: Serum immunoreactive somatomedin-C is elevated late in pregnancy. J Clin Endocrinol Metab 47:695, 1978.

83. Yen SCC: Endocrinology or pregnancy. In Creasy RK, Res-

nick R (eds): Maternal-Fetal Medicine: Principles and Practice. Philadelphia, WB Saunders Company, 1989, p 382.

84. Simon P, Decoster G, Brocas H, et al: Absence of human chorionic somatomammotropin during pregnancy associated with two types of gene deletion. Hum Genet 74:235, 1986.

85. Youngblood WW, Humm J, Kizer S: Thyrotropin-releasing hormone-like bioactivity in placenta: evidence for the existence of substances other than Pyroglu-His-Pro-NH2 (TRH) capable of stimulating pituitary thyrotropin release. Endocrinology 106:541, 1980.

86. Taliadourous GS, Canfield RE, Nisula BC: Thyroid-stimulating activity of chorionic gonadotropin and luteinizing hormone. J Clin Endocrinol Metab 47:855, 1978.

87. Chrousos GP, Galabrese JR, Avgerinos P, et al: Corticotropin releasing factor: basic studies and clinical applications. Prog Neuropsychopharmacol Biol Psychiatry 9:349, 1985.

88. Stalla GK, Hartwimmer J, von-Werder K, et al: Ovine (o) and human (h) corticotropin releasing factor (CRF) in man: CRF-stimulation and CRF-immunoreactivity. Acta Endocrinol (Copenh) 106:289, 1984.

89. Shibahara S, Morimoto Y, Furutani Y, et al: Isolation and sequence analysis of the human corticotropin-releasing factor precursor gene. EMBO J 2:775, 1983.

90. Stalla GK, Bost H, Stalla J, et al: Human corticotropin releasing hormone during pregnancy. Gynecol Endocrinol 3:1, 1989.

91. Laatikainen TJ, Raisanen IJ, Salminen KR: Corticotropin-releasing hormone in amniotic fluid during gestation and labor and in relation to fetal lung maturation. Am J Obstet Gynecol 159:891, 1988.

92. Linton EA, Perkins AV, Woods RJ, et al: Corticotropin releasing hormone-binding protein (CRH-BP); plasma levels decrease during the third trimester of normal human pregnancy. J Clin Endocrinol Metab 76:260, 1993.

93. Sug-Tang A, Bocking AD, Brooks AN, et al: Effects of restricting uteroplacental blood flow on concentrations of corticotrophin-releasing hormone, adrenocorticotrophin, cortisol, and prostaglandin E2 in the sheep fetus during late pregnancy. Can J Physiol Pharmacol 70:1396, 1992.

94. Clifron VI, Read MA, Leitch IM, et al: Corticotrophin-releasing hormone-induced vasodilation in the human fetal placental circulation. J Clin Endocrinol Metal 79:666, 1994.

95. Perkins AV, Linton EA, Eben F, et al: Corticotrophin-releasing hormone and corticotrophin-releasing hormone binding protein in normal and pre-eclamptic human pregnancies. Br J Obstet Gynaecol 10:118, 1995.

96. Goland RS, Jozak S, Warren WB, et al: Elevated levels of umbilical cord plasma corticotropin-releasing hormone in growth-retarded fetuses. J Clin Endocrinol Metab 77:1174, 1993.

97. Ruth V, Hallman M, Laatikainen T: Corticotropin-releasing hormone and cortisol in cord plasma in relation to gestational age, labor, and fetal distress. Am J Perinatol 10:115, 1993.

98. Goland RS, Conwell IM, Warren WB, et al: Placental corticotropin-releasing hormone and pituitary-adrenal function during pregnancy. Neuroendocrinology 56:742, 1992.

99. Macaron C, Kyncl M, Rutsky L, et al: Failure of somatostatin to affect human chorionic somatomammotropin and human chorionic gonadotropin secretion in vitro. J Clin Endocrinol Metab 47:1141, 1978.

100. Petraglia F, Sawchenko P, Lim ATW, et al: Localization, secretion, and action of inhibin in human placenta. Science 237:187, 1987.

101. Abe Y, Hasegawa Y, Miyamoto K, et al: High concentration of plasma immunoreactive inhibin during normal pregnancy in women. J Clin Endocrinol Metab 71:133, 1990.

102. Tovanabutra S, Illingworth PJ, Ledger WL, et al: The relationship between peripheral immunoactive inhibin, human

chorionic gonadotrophin, oestradiol and progesterone during human pregnancy. Clin Endocrinol 38:101, 1993.

103. Muttukrishna S, George L, Fowlert PA, et al: Measurement of serum concentrations of inhibin-A (α-β_A dimer) during human pregnancy. Clin Endocrinol 42:391, 1995.

104. Khong TY, Healy DL, Findlay JK, et al: Inhibin and the human placenta: a critique. Reprod Fertil Dev 3:391, 1991.

105. Mills NC, D'Ercole AJ, Underwood LE, et al: Synthesis of somatomedin C/insulin-like growth factor I by human placenta. Mol Biol Rep 11:231, 1986.

106. Jonas HA, Harrison LC: The human placenta contains two distinct binding and immunoreactive species of insulin-like growth factor-I receptors. J Biol Chem 260:2288, 1985.

107. Grizzard JD, D'Ercole AJ, Wilkins JR, et al: Affinity-labeled somatomedin-C receptors and binding proteins from the human fetus. J Clin Endocrinol Metab 58:535, 1984.

108. Altman DJ, Schneider SL, Thompson DA, et al: A transforming growth factor beta 2 (TGF-beta 2) like immunosuppressive factor in amniotic fluid and localization of TGF-beta 2 mRNA in the pregnant uterus. J Exp Med 172:1391, 1990.

109. Brown MJ, Cook CL, Henry JL, et al: Levels of epidermal growth factor binding in third-trimester and term human placentas: elevated binding in term placentas of male fetuses. Am J Obstet Gynecol 156:716, 1987.

110. Lenton EA, Grudzinskas JG, Gordon YB, et al: Pregnancy specific β_1-glycoprotein and chorionic gonadotropin in early pregnancy. Acta Obstet Gynecol Scand 60:489, 1981.

111. Chou JY, Plouzek CA: Pregnancy-specific β_1-glycoprotein. Semin Reprod Endocrinol 10:116, 1992.

112. Tatarinov YS: Trophoblast-specific beta-glycoprotein as a marker for pregnancy and malignancies. Gynecol Obstet Invest 9:65, 1978.

113. Sinosich MJ, Teisner B, Folkersen J, et al: Radioimmunoassay for pregnancy associated plasma protein. Clin Chem 28:50, 1982.

114. Bischof P: Pregnancy-associated plasma protein-A. Semin Reprod Endocrinol 10:127, 1992.

115. Obiekwe B, Pendlebury DJ, Gordon YB, et al: The radioimmunoassay of placental protein 5 and circulating levels in maternal blood in the third trimester of normal pregnancy. Clin Chim Acta 95:509, 1979.

116. Salem HT, Seppala M, Chard T: The effect of thrombin on serum placental protein 5 (PP5): is PP5 the naturally occurring antithrombin III of the human placenta? Placenta 2:205, 1981.

117. Maslar IA, Ansbacher R: Effects of progesterone on decidual prolactin production by organ cultures of human endometrium. Endocrinology 188:2102, 1986.

118. Raabe MA, McCoshen JA: Epithelial regulation of prolactin effect on amnionic permeability. Am J Obstet Gynecol 154:130, 1986.

119. Clements JA, Reyes FI, Winter JS, et al: Studies on human sexual development, IV: fetal pituitary and serum, and amniotic fluid concentrations of prolactin. J Clin Endocrinol Metab 44:408, 1977.

120. Luciano AA, Varner MW: Decidual, amniotic fluid, maternal and fetal prolactin in normal and abnormal pregnancies. Obstet Gynecol 63:384, 1984.

121. Pullano JG, Cohen-Addad N, Apuzzio JJ, et al: Water and salt conservation in the human fetus and newborn, I: evidence for a role of fetal prolactin. J Clin Endocrinol Metab 69:1180, 1989.

122. Golander A, Kopel R, Lazebnik N, et al: Decreased prolactin secretion by decidual tissue of pre-eclampsia in vitro. Acta Endocrinol 108:111, 1985.

123. Healy DL, Herington AC, O'Herlihy C: Chronic polyhydramnios is a syndrome with a lactogen receptor defect in the chorion leave. Br J Obstet Gynaecol 92:461, 1985.

124. McCoshen JA, Barc J: Prolactin bioactivity following decidual synthesis and transport by amniochorion. Am J Obstet Gynecol 153:217, 1985.

125. Weiss G, O'Bryne EM, Hochman J, et al: Distribution of relaxin in women during pregnancy. Obstet Gynecol 52:569, 1978.

126. Fields PA, Larkin LH: Purification and immunohistochemical localization of relaxin in the human term placenta. J Clin Endocrinol Metab 52:79, 1981.

127. Goldsmith LT, Weiss G, Steinetz BG: Relaxin and its role in pregnancy. Endocrinol Metab Clin North Am 24:171, 1995.

128. Rutanen EM, Bohn H, Seppala M: Radioimmunossay of placental protein 12: levels in amniotic fluid, cord blood, and serum of healthy adults, pregnant women, and patients with trophoblastic disease. Am J Obstet Gynecol 144:460, 1982.

129. Rutanen E-M: Insulin-like growth factor binding protein-1. Semin Reprod Endocrinol 10:154, 1992.

130. Seppala M, Riittinen L, Kamarainen M, et al: Placental protein 14/progesterone-associated endometrial protein revisited. Semin Reprod Endocrinol 10:164, 1992.

131. Julkunen M, Rutanen EM, Koskimies A, et al: Distribution of placental protein 14 in tissues and body fluids during pregnancy. Br J Obstet Gynaecol 92:1145, 1985.

132. Seppala M, Julkunen M, Koistinen R, et al: Proteins in the human endometrium. *In* Naftolin F, DeCherney AH (eds): The Control of Follicle Development, Ovulation and Luteal Function: Lessons from In Vitro Fertilization. New York, Serono Symposia Publications, Raven Press 35:101, 1987.

133. Alpert E, Drysdale JW, Isselbacher KJ, et al: Human fetoprotein: isolation, characterization, and demonstration of microheterogeneity. J Biol Chem 247:3792, 1972.

134. Gitlin D, Perricelli A, Gitlin GM: Synthesis of fetoprotein by liver, yolk sac, and gastrointestinal tract of the human conceptus. Cancer Res 32:979, 1972.

135. Habib ZA: Maternal serum alpha-feto-protein: its value in antenatal diagnosis of genetic disease and in obstetrical-gynaecological care. Acta Obstet Gynecol Scand 61:1, 1977.

136. Murgita RA, Tomasi TB Jr: Suppression of the immune response by alpha-fetoprotein on the primary and secondary antibody response. J Exp Med 141:269, 1975.

137. Ferguson-Smith MA, May HM, Vince JD, et al: Avoidance of anencephalic and spina bifida births by maternal serum-alphafetoprotein screening. Lancet 1:330, 1978.

138. Wald N, Cuckle H: AFP and age screening for Down syndrome. Am J Med Genet 31:197, 1988.

139. Shutt DA, Lopata A: The secretion of hormones during the culture of human preimplantation embryos with corona cells. Fertil Steril 35:413, 1981.

140. Laufer N, DeCherney AH, Haseltine FP, et al: Steriod secretion by the human egg–corona cumulus complex in culture. J Clin Endocrinol Metab 58:1153, 1984.

141. Tulchinsky D, Hobel CJ: Plasma human chorionic gonadotropin estrone, estradiol, estriol, progesterone, and 17-hydroxyprogesterone in human pregnancy, III: early normal pregnancy. Am J Obstet Gynecol 117:884, 1973.

142. Punnonen R, Lukola A: Binding of estrogen and progestin in the human fallopian tube. Fertil Steril 36:610, 1981.

143. Murphy BEP: Cortisol economy in the human fetus. *In* James VHT, Serio M, Gusti G, et al (eds): The Endocrine Function of the Human Adrenal Cortex. San Diego, Academic Press, 1978, p 509.

144. Murphy BEP: Cortisol and cortisone in human fetal development. J Steroid Biochem 11:509, 1979.

145. Csapo AL, Pulkkinen MO, Wiest WG: Effects of luteectomy and progesterone replacement therapy in early pregnancy patients. Am J Obstet Gynecol 115:759, 1973.

146. Sauer MV, Paulson RJ, Lobo RA: A preliminary report on

oocytes donation extending reproductive potential to women over 40. N Engl J Med 323:1157, 1991.

147. Sultan KM, Davis OK, Liu HC, et al: Viable term pregnancy despite "subluteal" serum progesterone levels in the first trimester. Fertil Steril 60:363, 1993.

148. Schneider MA, Davies MC, Honour JW: The timing of placental competence in pregnancy after oocyte donation. Fertil Steril 59:1059, 1993.

149. Azuma K, Calderon I, Besanko M, et al: Is the luteoplacental shift a myth? Analysis of low progesterone levels in successful art pregnancies. J Clin Endocrinol Metab 77:195, 1993.

150. Carr BR, MacDonald PC, Simpson ER: The role of lipoproteins in the regulation of progesterone secretion by the human corpus luteum. Fertil Steril 38:303, 1982.

151. Carr BR, MacDonald PC, Simpson ER: The regulation of de novo synthesis of cholesterol in the human fetal adrenal gland by low density lipoprotein and adrenocorticotropin. Endocrinology 107:1000, 1980.

152. Baker BL, Jaffe RB: The genesis of cell types in the adenohypophysis of the human fetus as observed with immunocytochemistry. Am J Anat 143:137, 1975.

153. Johannison E: The fetal adrenal cortex in the human. Acta Endocrinol 58:130, 1968.

154. Jost A: The fetal adrenal cortex. In Greep RO, Astwood WB (eds): Handbook of Physiology. Washington, DC, Endocrinology American Physiology Society, 1975, p 426.

155. Kondo S: Developmental studies on the Japanese human adrenals, I: ponderal growth. Bull Exp Biol 9:51, 1959.

156. Soectir WS: Handbook of Biological Data. Philadelphia, WB Saunders Company, 1956.

157. Buster J: Fetal adrenal cortex. Clin Obstet Gynecol 23:803, 1980.

158. Dictalusy E: Steroid metabolism in the feto-placental unit. In Pecile A, Finzi C (eds): The Feto-Placental Unit. Amsterdam, Excerpta Medica, 1969.

159. Simpson ER, Carr BR, Parker CR, et al: The role of serum lipoproteins in steroidogenesis by the human fetal adrenal cortex. J Clin Endocrinol Metab 49:146, 1979.

160. Carr BR, Porter JC, MacDonald PC, et al: Metabolism of low density lipoprotein by human fetal-adrenal tissue. Endocrinology 107:1034, 1980.

161. Bloch E: Fetal adrenal cortex: function and steroidogenesis. Functions of the adrenal cortex. In McKerns KW (ed): Biochemical Endocrinology, Vol. 2. East Norwalk, CT, Appleton-Century-Crofts, 1968.

162. Seron-Ferre M, Lawrence CC, Siliteri PK, et al: Steroid production by definitive and fetal zones of the human fetal adrenal gland. J Clin Endocrinol Metab 39:269, 1974.

163. Winters AG, Oliver C, MacDonald JC, et al: Plasma ACTH levels in the human fetus and neonate as related to age and parturition. J Clin Endocrinol Metab 39:269, 1974.

164. Walsh SW, Normal RL, Novy MJ: In utero regulation of rhesus monkey fetal adrenals: effects of dexamethasone, adrenocorticotropin, thyrotropin-releasing hormone, prolactin, human chorionic gonadotropin and α-melanocyte stimulating hormone on fetal and maternal plasma steroids. Endocrinology 104:1805, 1979.

165. Katikineni M, Davies TF, Catt KJ: Regulation of adrenal and testicular prolactin receptors by adrenocorticotropin and luteinizing hormone. Endocrinology 108:2367, 1981.

166. Winters AJ, Colston C, MacDonald PC, et al: Fetal plasma prolactin levels. J Clin Endocrinol Metab 41:626, 1975.

167. Pepe GJ, Waddell BJ, Albrecht ED: The effects of adrenocorticotropin and prolactin on adrenal dehydroepiandrosterone secretion in the baboon fetus. Endocrinology 122:646, 1988.

168. Albrecht ED, Pepe GJ: Placental steroid hormone biosynthesis in primate pregnancy. Endocr Rev 11:124, 1990.

169. Pepe GJ, Albrecht ED: Regulation of the primate fetal adrenal cortex. Endocr Rev 11:151, 1990.

170. Parker RC, Carr BR, Winkel CA, et al: Hypercholesterolemia due to elevated low density lipoprotein-cholesterol in newborns with anencephaly and adrenal atrophy. J Clin Endocrinol Metab 57:37, 1983.

171. Simpson ER, Parker CR, Carr BR: Role of lipoproteins in the regulation of steroidogenesis by the human fetal adrenal. In Jaffe RB, Dell Acqua S (eds): The Endocrine Physiology of Pregnancy and the Peripartal Period, Vol. 21. Serono Symposia Publications. New York, Raven Press, 1985.

172. Begot M, Dubois MP, Dubois PM: Growth hormone and ACTH in the pituitary of normal and anencephalic human fetuses: immunocytochemical evidence for hypothalamic influences during development. Neuroendocrinology 24:208, 1977.

173. Baird AC, Kan DW, Solomon S: Role of pro-opiomelanocortin-derived peptides in the regulation of steroid production of human fetal adrenal cells in culture. Endocrinology 97:357, 1983.

174. Bugnon C, Lenys D, Bloch B, et al: Cyto-immunologic study of early cell differentiation phenomena in the human fetal anterior pituitary gland. C R Seances Soc Biol Fil 168:460, 1974.

175. Voutilaimem M, Miller WL: Coordinate tropic hormone regulation of mRNAs insulin-like growth factor II and the cholesterol side-chain-cleavage enzyme, P450scc, in human steroidogenic tissues. Proc Natl Acad Sci U S A 84:1590, 1987.

176. Liggins GC: Endocrinology of the foeto-maternal unit. In Sherman RP (ed): Human Reproductive Physiology. Oxford, Blackwell Scientific Publications, 1972.

177. Baggia S, Albrecht ED, Pep GJ: Regulation of 11 beta-hydroxysteroid dehydrogenase activity in the baboon placenta by estrogen. Endocrinology 126:2742, 1990.

178. Mesiano S, Jaffe RB: Developmental and functional biology of the primate fetal adrenal cortex. Endocr Rev 18:378, 1997.

179. Jaffe RB, Mesiano S, Smith R, et al: The regulation and role of fetal adrenal development in human pregnancy. Endocr Res 24:919, 1998.

180. Jaffe RB: Endocrinology of pregnancy. In Yem SCC, Jaffe RB (eds): Reproductive Endocrinology. Philadelphia, WB Saunders Company, 1999.

181. McClellan M, Brenner RM: Development of the fetal adrenals in nonhuman primates: Electron microscopy. In Novy MJ, Resko JA (eds): Fetal Endocrinology. New York, Academic Press, 1981, p 383.

182. McNutt NS, Jones AL: Observations of the ultrastructure of cytodifferentiation in the human fetal adrenal cortex. Lab Invest 11:513, 1970.

183. Mesiano S, Coulter CL, Jaffe RB: Localization of cytochrome P450 cholesterol side chain cleavage, cytochrome P450 17 β-hydroxylase/17,20-lyase, and 3 β-hydroxysteroid dehydrogenase-isomerase steroidogenic enzymes in the human and rhesus fetal adrenal gland: reappraisal of functional zonation. J Clin Endocrinol Metab 77:1184, 1992.

184. Crickard K, Ill CR, Jaffe RB: Control of proliferation of human fetal adrenal cells in vitro. J Clin Endocrinol Metab 53:790, 1981.

185. Hornsby PJ, Sturek M, Harris SE, et al: Serum and growth factor requirements for proliferation of human adrenocortical cells in culture: comparison with bovine adrenocortical cells. In Vitro 19:863, 1983.

186. Mesiano S, Mellon SH, Gospodarowicz D, et al: Basic fibroblast growth factor expression is regulated by ACTH in the human fetal adrenal: a model for adrenal growth regulation. Proc Natl Acad Sci U S A 88:5428, 1991.

187. Mesiano S, Jaffe RB: Interaction of insulin-like growth factor-II and estradiol directs steroidogenesis in the human fetal

adrenal toward dehydroepiandrosterone sulfate production. J Clin Endocrinol Metab 77:754, 1993.

188. Spencer SJ, Rabinovici J, Jaffe RB: Human recombinant activin-A inhibits proliferation of human fetal adrenal cells in vitro. J Clin Endocrinol Metab 71:1678, 1990.

189. Spencer SJ, Rabinovici J, Mesiano S, et al: Activin and inhibin in the human adrenal gland: regulation and differential effects in fetal and adult cells. J Clin Invest 90:142, 1992.

190. Roberts AB, Flanders KC, Kondalah P, et al: Transforming growth factor beta: biochemistry and roles in embryogenesis, tissue repair and remodeling and carcinogenesis. Recent Prog Horm Res 44:157, 1990.

191. Stankovic AK, Dion LD, Parker CR Jr: Effects of transforming growth factor-beta by human fetal adrenal steroid production. Mol Cell Endocrinol 99:145, 1994.

192. Stankovic AK, Parker CR Jr: Receptor binding of transforming growth factor-beta by human fetal adrenal cells. Mol Cell Endocrinol 109:159, 1995.

193. Siiteri PK, MacDonald PC: Placental estrogen biosynthesis during human pregnancy. J Clin Endocrinol Metab 26:751, 1966.

194. Tulchinsky D, Korenman SG: The plasma estradiol as an index of fetoplacental function. J Clin Invest 50:1490, 1971.

195. Abraham GE, Odell WD, Swerdloff RS, et al: Simultaneous radioimmunoassay of plasma FSH, LH, progesterone 17-hydroxyprogesterone, and estradiol-17β during the menstrual cycle. J Clin Endocrinol Metab 34:312, 1972.

196. Lindbert BS, Johansson EDB, Nilsson BA: Plasma levels of nonconjugated oestrone, oestradiol-17β and oestriol during uncomplicated pregnancy. Acta Obstet Gynecol Scand 32:21, 1974.

197. Tulchinsky D, Hobel CJ, Yeager E, et al: Plasma estrone estradiol, estriol, progesterone, and 17-hydroxyprogesterone in human pregnancy, I: normal pregnancy. Am J Obstet Gynecol 112:1095, 1972.

198. Klopper A, Masson G, Campbell D, et al: Estriol in plasma: a compartmental study. Am J Obstet Gynecol 117:21, 1973.

199. Tulchinsky D, Hobel CJ, Korenman SG: A radioligand assay for plasma unconjugated estriol in normal and abnormal pregnancies. Am J Obstet Gynecol 11:311, 1971.

200. Landon MB, Gabbe SG: Fetal surveillance in the pregnancy complicated by diabetes mellitus. Clin Obstet Gynecol 34:535, 1991.

201. Parker CR Jr, Simpson ER, Bilheimer DW, et al: Inverse relationship between LDL-cholesterol and dehydroisoandrosterone sulfate in human fetal plasma. Science 208:512, 1980.

202. Sadovsky E, Polshuk WZ: Fetal movements in utero. Obstet Gynecol 50:49, 1977.

203. Resnik R, Killam AP, Battaglia FC, et al: The stimulation of uterine blood flow by various estrogens. Endocrinology 94:1192, 1974.

204. Henson MC, Pepe GJ, Albrecht ED: Regulation of placental low-density lipoprotein uptake in baboons by estrogen: dose-dependent effects of the anti-estrogen ethamoxytriphetol (MER-25). Biol Reprod 45:43, 1991.

205. Novy MJ: Hormonal regulation of parturition in primates. In Sciara J (ed): Hormone Cell Interactions in Reproductive Tissues. New York, Masson Publishing, 1983.

206. Challis JR: Molecular aspects of preterm labor. Bull Mem Acad R Med Belg 153:263, 1998.

207. Olson DM, Zakar Tamas L: Intrauterine tissue prostaglandin synthesis: regulatory mechanisms. Semin Reprod Endocrinol 11:234, 1993.

208. Haluska GJ, Novy MJ: Hormonal modulation of uterine activity during primate parturition. Semin Reprod Endocrinol 11:272, 1993.

209. Ducsay CA, Seron-Ferre M, Germain AM, et al: Endocrine and uterine activity rhythms in the perinatal period. Semin Reprod Endocrinol 11:285, 1993.

210. Honnebier MB, Nathanielsz PW: Primate parturition and the role of the maternal circadian system. Eur J Obstet Gynecol Reprod Biol 55:193, 1994.

211. Patrick J, Challis J, Campbell K, et al: Circadian rhythms in maternal plasma cortisol and estriol concentrations at 30 to 31, 34 to 35, and 38 to 39 weeks' gestational age. Am J Obstet Gynecol 136:325, 1980.

212. Nygren KG, Johansson ED, Wide L: Evaluation of the prognosis of threatened abortion from the peripheral plasma levels of progesterone, estradiol, and human chorionic gonadotropin. Am J Obstet Gynecol 116:916, 1973.

213. Stovall TG, Ling FW, Carson SA, et al: Serum progesterone and uterine curettage in differential diagnosis of ectopic pregnancy. Fertil Steril 57:456, 1992.

214. Teoh ES, Das NP, Dawood MY, et al: Serum progesterone and serum chorionic gonadotropin in hydatidiform mole and choriocarcinoma. Acta Endocrinol 70:791, 1972.

215. Tulchinsky D, Simmer H: Sources of plasma 17β-hydroxyprogesterone in human pregnancy. J Clin Endocrinol Metab 35:799, 1972.

216. Siiteri PK, Febres F, Clemens LE, et al: Progesterone and maintenance of pregnancy: is progesterone nature's immunosuppressant? Ann N Y Acad Sci 286:3384, 1977.

217. Moriyama I, Sugawa T: Progesterone facilitates implantation of xenogenic cultured cells in hamster uterus. Nature 236:150, 1972.

218. Hsueh AJW, Peck EJ, Clark JH: Progesterone antagonism of the estrogen receptor and estrogen-induced uterine growth. Nature 254:337, 1977.

219. Parker CR, Leveno K, Carr BB, et al: Umbilical cord plasma levels of dehydroepiandrosterone sulfate during human gestation. J Clin Endocrinol Metab 54:1216, 1982.

220. Csapo AI: Antiprogesterones in fertility control. In Zatuchni GI, Sciarra JJ, Speidel JJ (eds): Pregnancy Termination: Procedures, Safety and New Developments. Hagerstown, Harper & Row, 1979, p 16.

221. Case ML, MacDonald PC: Human parturition: distinction between the initiation of parturition and the onset of labor. Semin Reprod Endocrinol 11:272, 1993.

222. Fencl MD, Stillman RJ, Cohen J, et al: Direct evidence of sudden rise in fetal corticoids later in human gestation. Nature 287:225, 1980.

223. Murphy BEP: Human fetal serum cortisol levels related to gestational age: evidence of a midgestational fall and a steep late gestational rise, independent of sex or mode of delivery. Am J Obstet Gynecol 144:276, 1982.

224. Majzoub JA, Karalis KP: Placental corticotropin-releasing hormone: function and regulation. Am J Obstet Gynecol 180:S242, 1999.

225. Fadalti M, Pezzani I, Cobellis L, et al: Placental corticotropin-releasing factor. An update. Ann N Y Acad Sci 900:89, 2000.

226. Kadar N, DeVore G, Romero R: Discriminatory hCG zone: its use in the sonographic evaluation for ectopic pregnancy. Obstet Gynecol 58:156, 1981.

227. Odell WD, Griffin J, Bashey HM, et al: Secretion of chorionic gonadotropin by cultured human pituitary cells. J Clin Endocrinol Metab 71:1318, 1990.

228. Griffin J, Odell WD: Ultrasensitive immunoradiometric assay for chorionic gonadotropin which does not cross-react with luteinizing hormone nor free beta chain of hCG and which detects hCG in blood of non-pregnant humans. J Immunol Methods 103:275, 1987.

229. Cole LA, Kardana A, Ying FC, et al: The biological and clinical significance of nicks in human chorionic gonadotropin and its free beta-subunit. Yale J Biol Med 64:627, 1991.

230. Cole LA, Seifer DB, Kardana A, et al: Selecting human chorionic gonadotropin immunoassays: consideration of cross-reacting molecules in first-trimester pregnancy serum and urine. Am J Obstet Gynecol 168:1580, 1993.

231. Kardana A, Cole LA: Polypeptide nicks cause erroneous results in assay of human chorionic gonadotropin free beta-subunit. Clin Chem 38:26, 1992.

232. Rasor JL, Braunstein GD: A rapid modification of the beta-hCG radioimmunoassay: use as an aid in the diagnosis of ectopic pregnancy. Obstet Gynecol 50:553, 1977.

233. Sturgeon CM, McAllister EJ: Analysis of hCG: clinical applications and assay requirements. Ann Clin Biochem 35:460, 1998.

234. Cole LA: Immunoassay of human chorionic gonadotropin, its free subunits, and metabolites. Clin Chem 43:2233, 1997.

235. Hales CN, Woodhead JS: Labelled antibodies and their use in the immunoradiomimetic assay. Methods Enzymol 70:334, 1980.

236. Joshi UM, Roy R, Sheth AR, et al: A simple and sensitive color test for the detection of human chorionic gonadotropin. Obstet Gynecol 57:252, 1981.

237. Stenman UH, Alfthan H, Myllynen L, et al: Ultrarapid and highly sensitive time-resolved fluoroimmunometric assay for chorionic gonadotropin. Lancet 2:647, 1983.

238. Chard T: Pregnancy tests: a review. Hum Reprod 7:701, 1992.

239. Phillips OP, Shulman ES, Andersen RN, et al: Maternal serum screening for fetal Down syndrome in women less than 35 years of age using alpha-fetoprotein, hCG, and unconjugated estriol: a prospective 2-year study. Obstet Gynecol 80:353, 1992.

240. Lambert-Messerlian GM, Canick JA: Endocrine analytes in multiple-marker screening. Clin Perinatol 25:963, 1998.

241. Yedema KA, Verheijen RH, Kenemans P, et al: Identification of patients with persistent trophoblastic disease by means of a normal human chorionic gonadotropin regression curve. Am J Obstet Gynecol 168:787, 1993.

242. Stovall TG, Ling FW, Andersen RN, et al: Improved sensitivity and specificity of a single mesurement of serum progesterone over serial quantitative beta-human chorionic gonadotrophin in screening for ectopic pregnancy. Hum Reprod 7:723, 1992.

243. Carson SA, Buster JE: Ectopic pregnancy. N Engl J Med 329:1174, 1993.

244. Timor-Tritsch IE, Rottem S (eds): Transvaginal Sonography. New York, Elsevier Science, 1991.

245. Fossum GT, Davajan V, Kletzky OA: Early detection of pregnancy with transvaginal ultrasound. Fertil Steril 49:789, 1988.

246. Mol BW, van Der Veen, Bossuyt PM: Implementation of probabilistic decision rules improves the predictive values of algorithms in the diagnostic management of ectopic pregnancy. Hum Reprod 14:2855, 1999.

247. Pisarska MD, Carson SA, Buster JE: Ectopic pregnancy. Lancet 351:1115, 1998.

248. Buster JE, Chang RJ, Preston DL, et al: Interrelationships of circulating maternal steroid concentrations in third trimester pregnancies. I. C21 steroids: progesterone, 16 alpha-hydroxyprogesterone, 17 alpha-hydroxyprogesterone, 20 alpha-dihydroprogesterone, delta 5-pregnenolone, delta 5-pregnenolone sulfate, and 17-hydroxy delta 5-pregnenolone. J Clin Endocrinol Metab 48:133, 1979.

249. Buster JE, Freeman AG, Tataryn IV, et al: Time trend analysis of unconjugated estriol concentrations in third-trimester pregnancy. Obstet Gynecol 56:743, 1980.

250. Williams L, Warwick L: Gray's Anatomy, 36th ed. Philadelphia, WB Saunders Company, 1980, p 125.

Placental and Fetal Physiology

MICHAEL G. ROSS, M. GORE ERVIN, AND
DONALD NOVAK

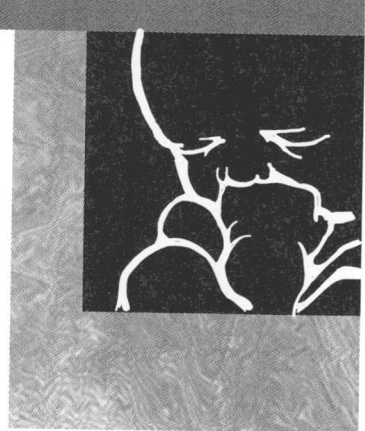

In obstetric practice, recognition of normal fetal growth, development, and behavior often suggests a nonintervention management plan. However, abnormalities may require clinical strategies for fetal assessment and/or intervention. The basic concepts of placental and fetal physiology provide the building blocks necessary for understanding pathophysiology, and thus mechanisms of disease. Throughout this chapter, we have reviewed the essential tenets of placental and fetal physiology, while relating this information to normal and abnormal clinical conditions.

Much of our knowledge of placental and fetal physiology derives from observations made in mammals other than humans. We have attempted to include only those observations reasonably applicable to the human placenta and fetus, and in most instances have not detailed the species from which the data were obtained. Should questions arise regarding the species studied, the reader is referred to the extensive bibliography.

PLACENTAL PHYSIOLOGY

The placenta provides the fetus with its essential nutrients, water and oxygen, and a route for clearance of fetal excretory products, and produces a vast array of protein and steroid hormones and factors essential to the maintenance of pregnancy.

Placental Metabolism and Growth

Anatomic and histologic aspects of placental growth are detailed in Chapter 1. This section focuses on the physiology of placental metabolism and growth, and its influence on the fetus.

The critical function of the placenta is illustrated by its high metabolic demands. For example, placental oxygen consumption equals that of the fetus, and exceeds the fetal rate when expressed on a weight basis (10 ml/min/kg).[1-3] Between 22 and 36 weeks of gestation, the number of trophoblast nuclei[4] increases four- to five-fold, placing increased metabolic demands on the placenta. Glucose is the principal substrate for oxidative metabolism by placental tissue.[2,5] Of the total glucose leaving the maternal compartment to nourish the uterus and its contents, placental consumption may represent up to 70 percent.[2,6,7] In addition, a significant fraction of placental glucose uptake derives from the fetal circulation,[8] and reflects placental oxidative metabolism. Although one third of placental glucose may be converted to the 3-carbon sugar lactate,[2,4,5,9] placental metabolism is not anaerobic. Instead, placental lactate is thought to be a fetal energetic substrate. The factors regulating short-term changes in placental oxygen and glucose consumption are at present incompletely understood.

The regulation of placental growth is also an area of incomplete understanding. Increases in trophoblast numbers exceed increases in fetal placental capillary endothelial cells[10] during the second half of gestation. Whether trophoblast cell proliferation is the primary event, or is dependent on endothelial cell growth is not known. Normal term placental weight averages 450 g, representing approximately one seventh, (one sixth with cord and membranes) of fetal weight. Large-appearing placentas, either ultrasonographically or at delivery, may prompt investigation into possible etiologies. Several clinical observations suggest a link between decreased tissue oxygen content and increased placental growth. Thus, increased placental size is associated with maternal anemia,[11-13] fetal anemia associated with erythrocyte isoimmunization, and hydrops fetalis secondary to fetal α-thalassemia with Bart's hemoglobin.

The association of a large placenta with maternal diabetes also has been recognized, possibly a result of insulin-stimulated mitogenic activity. An increased ratio of placental size to fetal weight is associated with increased morbidity, both in the neonatal period and subsequently.[14,15]

Receptors for growth-promoting peptide hormones (factors) characterized in placental tissue[16] include, among many, the insulin receptor,[17-22] receptors for insulin-like growth factors I and II (IGF-I, IGF-II), and epidermal growth factor (EGF).[23-27] IGF-I and IGF-II are polypeptides with a high degree of homology to human proinsulin.[28] Both IGF-I and IGF-II circulate bound to carrier proteins, and are 50 times more potent than insulin in stimulating cell growth.[28] EGF increases RNA and DNA synthesis and cell multiplication in a wide variety of cell types.[16] The observation that placental EGF binding is increased at term, relative to 8 to 18 weeks' gestation, led to a suggested role of EGF in placental growth regulation.[24] The integrated physiologic role of these and other potential placental growth factors[29-31] in regulating placental growth remains to be fully defined. However, the development of null-mutation mouse models for IGF-I, IGF-II, IGF-I receptor, and IGF-II receptor as well as for the EGF receptor has provided evidence in this regard.[32-37] Specifically, the EGF receptor appears important in placental development, as does IGF-II. Knockout of IGF-II results in diminished placental size, while deletion of the IGF-II receptor results in an increase in placental size. IGF-I does not appear to impact placental growth.

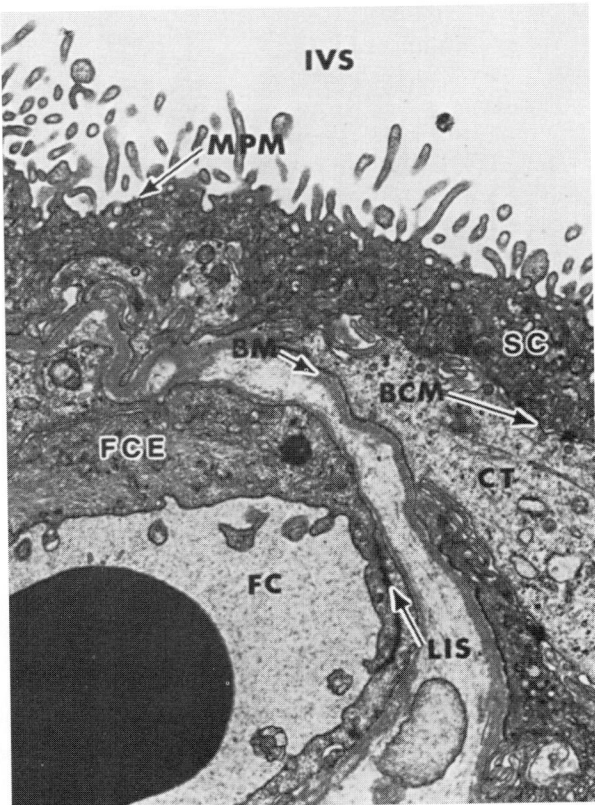

Figure 2–1. Electron micrograph of human placenta demonstrating the cellular and extracellular components with which solutes most interact in moving from the maternal intervillous space (IVS) to the lumen of the fetal capillary (FC). MPM, microvillous plasma membrane of the syncytiotrophoblast; SC, syncytiotrophoblast; BCM, basal cell membrane of the syncytiotrophoblast; BM, basement membrane; CT, cytotrophoblast cell; FCE, fetal capillary endothelial cell; LIS, lateral intercellular space of fetal endothelial cell. (Courtesy of Kent L. Thornburg, Ph.D., Department of Physiology, Oregon Health Sciences University, Portland, OR.)

Placental Transfer

General Considerations

In the hemochorial human placenta, maternal blood and solutes are separated from fetal blood by trophoblastic tissue and fetal endothelial cells. Thus, transit from the maternal intervillous space to the fetal capillary lumen takes place across a number of cellular structures (Fig. 2–1). The first step is transport across the microvillus plasma membrane of the syncytiotrophoblast. Since there are no lateral intercellular spaces in the syncytiotrophoblast, all solutes first interact with the placenta at this plasma membrane. The basal (fetal) syncytiotrophoblast membrane represents an additional step in the transport process. The discontinuous nature of the cytotrophoblast cell layer in later gestation suggests this layer should not limit maternal-to-fetal transfer. However, the presence of anionic sites on the glycoprotein backbone comprising the basal lamina[38] potentially may influence movement of large charged molecules. The fetal capillary endothelial cell imposes two additional plasma membrane surfaces.[39]

A number of specific mechanisms allow transit across the placental membranes, including passive diffusion, facilitated diffusion, active transport, and endocytosis/exocytosis. Solutes lacking specialized transport mechanisms cross by extracellular or transcellular diffusional transport pathways with permeability determined by size, lipid solubility, ionic charge, and maternal serum protein binding. Lipid-insoluble (hydrophilic) substances, which cross the trophoblast via extracellular pores, are restricted by molecular size in relation to the extracellular pore size. Up to a molecular weight of at least 5,000 daltons, placental permeability is proportional to the free diffusion of a molecule in water.[40] For example, urea (MW = 60) is at least 1,000 times more permeable than inulin (MW = 5,000).[40] Thus, transfer of small solutes will be governed primarily by the maternal–fetal concentration gradient. Because transfer is relatively slow, and the extracellular pore surface area is limited, transfer of these molecules is referred to as "diffusion-limited." Conversely, highly lipid-soluble (lipophilic) substances diffuse readily through the trophoblastic membrane. Thus, molecular weight is relatively less important in restricting diffusion. Ethanol, a molecule similar in size to urea, is 500 times more lipid soluble and 10 times more permeable.[41] Because the entire trophoblast surface is available for diffusion and the permeability is high, transfer rates for lipophilic substances to the fetus are limited primarily by placental intervillous and umbilical blood flows ("flow-limited"). Both facilitated diffusion and active transport utilize carrier-mediated transport systems, with the latter requiring energy, either directly or indirectly linked with ionic pump mechanisms. Carrier transport systems are specifically limited to unique classes of molecules (i.e., neutral amino acids). In addition, substances may traverse the placenta via endocytosis (invagination of the cell membrane to form an intracellular vesicle containing extracellular fluids) and exocytosis (release of the vesicle to the extracellular space).

Transfer of Individual Solutes

Respiratory Gases

The exchange or transfer of the primary respiratory gases, oxygen (O_2) and carbon dioxide (CO_2) is likely "flow limited." Thus, the driving force for placental gas exchange is the partial pressure gradient between the maternal and fetal circulations. Estimates of human placental diffusing capacities[42] would predict that placental efficiency as an organ of respiratory gas exchange will allow equilibrium of oxygen and carbon dioxide tensions at the maternal intervillous space and fetal capillary. However, this prediction varies from the observed 10 mm Hg difference in oxygen tension between the umbilical and uterine veins[43,44] and between the umbilical vein and intervillous space.[45] In addition, even though CO_2 is much more soluble than O_2 in water and tissues and will diffuse more readily than O_2, the P_{CO_2} difference from umbilical to uterine vein is small (3 mm Hg).[46] P_{O_2} differences could be explained by areas of uneven distribution of maternal to fetal blood flows or shunting, limiting fetal and maternal blood exchange. The most important contribution is likely the high metabolic rate of the placental tissues themselves. Thus, trophoblast cell O_2 consumption and CO_2 production lower umbilical vein O_2 tension and increase uterine vein CO_2 tension to a greater degree than could be explained by an inert barrier for respiratory gas transfer.

The arteriovenous difference in the uterine circulation (and venoarterial difference in the umbilical circulation) widens during periods of lowered blood flow. Proportionate O_2 uptake increases and O_2 consumption re-mains unchanged over a fairly wide range of blood flows.[47] Thus, both uterine and umbilical blood flows can fall significantly without decreasing fetal O_2 consumption.[48-50]

Carbon dioxide is carried in the fetal blood both as dissolved CO_2 and as bicarbonate. Due to its charged nature, fetal-to-maternal bicarbonate transfer is limited. However, CO_2 likely diffuses from fetus to mother in its molecular form, and $[HCO_3^-]$ does not contribute significantly to fetal carbon dioxide elimination.[51] Thus, diffusion is not limiting, and the important variables for fetal O_2 uptake and CO_2 excretion reside with uterine and umbilical blood flows, and carrying capacities of maternal and fetal bloods for O_2 and CO_2.

Glucose

Placental permeability for D-glucose is at least 50 times the value predicted on the basis of size and lipid solubility.[52] Thus, specialized transport mechanisms must be available on both the microvillous and basal membranes. Membrane proteins facilitating the translocation of molecules across cell membranes are termed "transporters." The human placental glucose transporter, originally identified as an approximately 55,000 MW component of the microvillous membranes[53-55] has subsequently been identified as GLUT1,[56,57] a sodium-independent transporter, as compared to the sodium-dependent transporters found in adult kidney[58] and intestine.[59,60] This transporter, in contrast to that found in human adipocytes (GLUT4)[61,63] is not insulin sensitive.[64-65] The placental D-glucose transporter is saturable at high substrate concentrations; 50 percent saturation is observed at sugar levels of approximately 5 mM (90 mg/dl).[54] Thus, glucose transfer from mother to fetus is not linear, and transfer rates decrease as maternal glucose concentration increases. This effect is reflected in fetal blood glucose levels following maternal glucose loading.[66] A second transporter, GLUT3, has also been noted in the fetal-facing placental endothelium. Its presence within the syncytiotrophoblast remains controversial.[67,68]

Amino Acids

Amino acid concentrations are higher in fetal umbilical cord blood than in maternal blood. Like monosaccharides, amino acids enter and exit the syncytiotrophoblast via transport-specific membrane proteins. These transport proteins allow amino acids to be transported against a concentration gradient into the placenta, and subsequently, in most cases, into the fetal circulation. Thus, amino acid transport is considered to be a "two-step" phenomenon.

Multiple systems mediate neutral, anionic, and cationic amino acid transport into the syncytiotrophoblast. These include both sodium-dependent and -independent transporters. Amino acid entry is, in many cases, coupled to sodium in co-transport systems located at the microvillous membrane facing the maternal intervillous space.[69,70] So long as an inwardly directed sodium gradient is maintained, trophoblast cell amino acid concentrations will exceed maternal blood levels. The sodium gradient is maintained by Na^+-K^+ATPase located on the basal or fetal side of the syncytiotrophoblast.[71] In addition, high trophoblast levels of amino acids transported by sodium-dependent transporters can "drive" uptake of other amino acids via transporters that function as "exchangers." Examples of these include System ASC, and System y^+L.[72-74] Still other transporters function in a sodium-independent fashion. Individual amino acids may be transported by single or multiple transport proteins. Transport systems that have been defined in human placenta are defined in Table 2-1.

Perhaps the most studied amino acid transporter within the placenta is the sodium-dependent System A, responsible for the transport of neutral amino acids with short polar or linear side chains. Trophoblast cells have two mechanisms of regulating amino acid uptake using the A system. The absence of amino acids increases cellular amino acid uptake,[75-77] partially because of an increase in carrier affinity.[75] Conversely, increases in trophoblast amino acid concentrations may suppress uptake (transinhibition). These mechanisms serve to maintain trophoblast cell amino acid levels constant during fluctuations in maternal plasma concentrations. Insulin has also been shown to up-regulate this transport activity,[20,78,79] as has IGF-I. System A is not the only sodium-dependent transporter identified on the microvillous membrane; others include that for β-amino acids such as taurine,[80] as well as perhaps glycine transport via System GLY.[81] Sodium-independent transporters mediating neutral amino acid transfer on the microvillous membrane include System L, which exhibits a high affinity for amino acids with bulky side chains such as leucine,[82] and perhaps Systems $b^{0,+}$ and y^+L, capable of transporting both neutral and cationic amino acids such as lysine and arginine.[83,84] Cationic amino acids are also transported by System y^+,[85,86]

while anionic amino acids (glutamate, aspartate) are transported by the sodium-dependent System X_{AG}^-. It is of interest that, as the proteins responsible for amino acid transport have been identified, it has become clear that more than one protein may mediate each previously defined transport activity within a single tissue. Examples include EAAT 1 to 5, associated with sodium-dependent anionic amino acid transfer (System X_{AG}^-), and CAT 1, 2, and 2a, associated with System y^+ activity.[85,87] The anionic amino acids glutamate and aspartate are poorly transported from mother to fetus.[88,89] Glutamate, however, is produced by the fetal liver from glutamine, and then taken up across the basolateral membrane of the placenta via System X_{AG}^-. Within the placenta, the majority of glutamate is metabolized and utilized as an energy source.[88] As a result, System X_{AG}^- activity is of particular importance on the basolateral membrane, as is System ASC activity, responsible for the uptake of serine, also produced by the fetal liver, into the placenta.[90] Abundant data now exist to suggest that placental amino acid transport is regulated in a variety of conditions resulting in altered fetal growth, including malnutrition, idiopathic small-for-dates pregnancies, and diabetes.[91-93] Mechanisms of regulation, however, remain to be completely elucidated.

Lipids

There is scant information regarding the transfer of maternal lipids across the placenta. Although maternal lipids cross the placenta, the relatively low transfer rates[94,95] suggest that the majority of fetal fatty acid accumulation in late pregnancy is not caused by placental transfer.[94] Due to their hydrophobic nature, free fatty acids are relatively insoluble in plasma and circulate bound to albumin. Fatty acid transfer involves dissociation from maternal protein, subsequent association with placental proteins (fatty acid–binding, translocase, and transport proteins) that have been identified in both microvillous and basolateral placental membranes, and then subsequent association with fetal plasma proteins.[96,97] These protein-binding steps are more important in determining mother-to-fetal fatty acid transfer

Table 2-1. PLACENTAL NEUTRAL AMINO ACID TRANSPORT SYSTEMS

Transport	A	L	ASC
Representative amino acids	Glycine, proline, alanine, serine, threonine, glutamine	Isoleucine, valine phenylalanine, alanine, serine, threonine, glutamine	Alanine, serine threonine, glutamine
Sodium dependency	+	—	+
Update increased by preincubation	+	—	+
Transinhibition	+	—	—

Data summarized from Enders et al.,[381] Smith et al.,[382] Smith and Depper,[383] and Steel et al.[384]

than interaction with the lipid layers of the placenta.[98,99] Placental fatty acid transfer increases logarithmically with decreasing chain length (C16 to C8) and then declines somewhat for C6 and C4. This latter effect is due to a decrease in lipid solubility of the shorter chain molecules.[99] Essential fatty acids are, in general, transferred more efficiently than are nonessential fatty acids.[100,101] In general, though, fatty acids transferred reflect those of the mother.[102] Placental uptake of cholesterol is discussed in the section Receptor-Mediated Endocytosis, below.

Water and Ions

Although water transfer across the placenta does not limit fetal water uptake during growth,[103] the factors regulating fetal water acquisition are poorly understood. Water transfer from mother to fetus is determined by a balance of osmotic, hydrostatic, and colloid osmotic forces at the placental interface. Calculation of osmotic pressure from individual solute concentrations is unreliable because osmotic pressure forces depend upon the membrane permeability to each solute. Thus, sodium and chloride, the principal plasma solutes, are relatively permeable across the placenta[104] and would not be expected to contribute important osmotic effects.[105] As a result, although human fetal plasma osmolality is equal to or greater than maternal plasma

osmolality,[106,107] these measured values do not reflect the actual osmotic force on either side of the membranes. Coupled with findings that hydrostatic pressure may be greater in the umbilical vein than in the intervillous space,[108,109] these data do not explain mechanisms for fetal water accumulation. Alternatively, colloid osmotic pressure differences[110] and active solute transport probably represent the main determinants of water fluxes. Water flux occurs through both transcellular and paracellular pathways. Water channels have been identified within the placenta, but their regulation and relative roles have not been discerned.[111,112]

In comparison with other epithelia, the specialized placental mechanisms for ion transport are incompletely understood.[113] Mechanisms for sodium transport in syncytiotrophoblast membranes are outlined in Figure 2–2. The maternal facing microvillous membrane contains, at a minimum, multiple amino acid co-transporters,[114] a sodium phosphate co-transporter in which two sodium ions are transported with each phosphate radical,[115] a sodium-hydrogen ion antiport that exchanges one proton for each sodium ion entering the cell,[116] as well as other nutrient transporters.[117,118] A membrane potential with the inside negative (−30 MV) would promote sodium entry from the intervillous space.[119] The fetal directed basal side of the cell contains the Na^+-K^+ATPase.[71] The microvillous or maternal facing trophoblast membrane has an anion exchanger

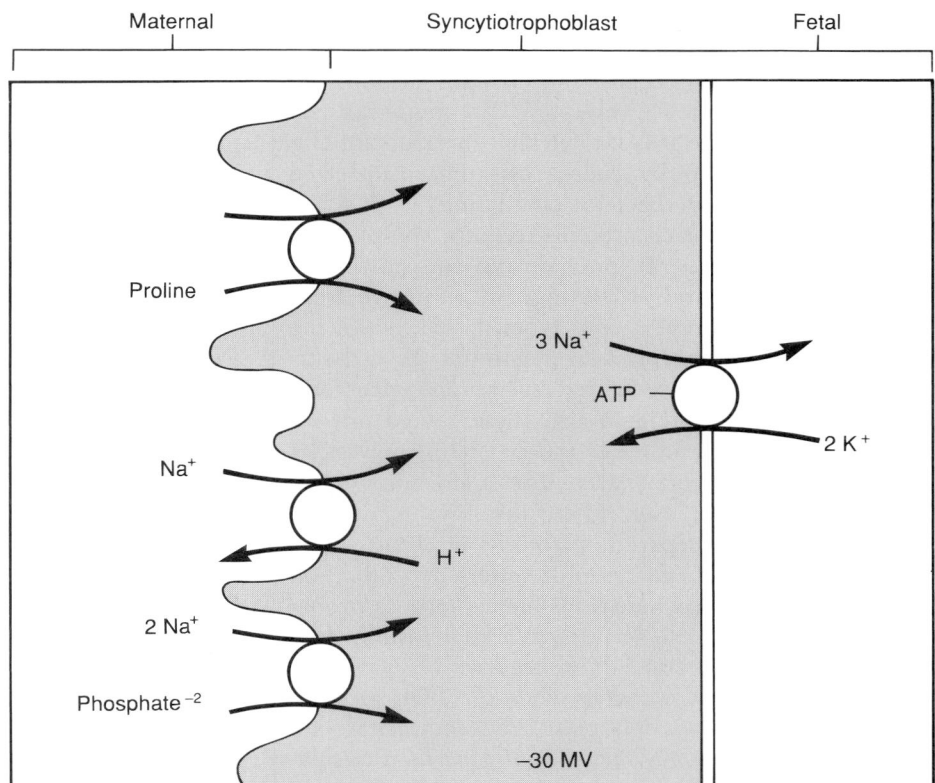

Figure 2–2. Pathways for sodium entry into syncytiotrophoblast and exit to the fetal circulation. (Data from Boyd et al.,[376] Whitsett and Wallick,[377] Lajeunesse and Brunette,[378] Balkovetz et al.,[379] and Bara et al.[380])

(AE1),[120] which mediates chloride transit across this membrane, in association with Cl⁻ conductance pathways (channels), present in both the microvillous and basolateral membranes.[121,122] Paracellular pathways also play an important role. The integration and regulation of these various mechanisms for sodium and chloride transport from mother to fetus are not completely understood.

Calcium

Ionized calcium levels are higher in fetal than in maternal blood.[106,123] Higher fetal calcium levels are caused by a syncytiotrophoblast basal membrane ATP-dependent Ca^{2+} transport system[124] exhibiting high affinity (nanomolar range) for calcium.[125] Calcium transport into the syncytiotrophoblast is mediated by a least one saturable transport process,[126,127] while transfer across the basal membrane is mediated by the ATPase denoted above, in addition to ATP-independent mechanisms.[128,129] Calcium transport across the placenta is increased by the calcium-dependent regulatory protein calmodulin[124]; transfer may be regulated by 1,25-dihydroxycholecalciferol, calcitonin, and parathyroid hormone.[113] A calcium-binding protein extracted from the placenta[130] differs from the human intestinal calcium-binding protein and may be an important regulator of maternal-to-fetal calcium transport.[131]

Receptor-Mediated Endocytosis/Exocytosis

The microvillous plasma membrane of the syncytiotrophoblast contains receptors specific for insulin,[17-21] low-density lipoprotein (LDL),[132-134] and transferrin.[135-137] In addition, it is known that immunoglobulin G (IgG) is taken up by endocytosis and transferred from the maternal to the fetal circulation.[138,139] While the precise steps for each protein–receptor complex are not yet defined, general mechanisms for postligand binding, cell entry, and processing can be drawn from available data in other cell types.[140-143] Following ligand binding, the receptors aggregate on the cell surface and collect in specialized membrane structures termed "coated pits" (Fig. 2–3). These coated pits invaginate, pinch-off, and enter the cell to form vesicles that fuse to form endosomes. The endosomes move deeper into the cytoplasm, where the lower endosome pH facilitates ligand separation from its receptor.

The fate of ligand and receptor differs depending on the specific substrate: whereas insulin receptor is probably recycled to the cell surface, maternal insulin does not reach the fetal circulation because of lysosomal degradation. Cholesterol enters with the LDL receptor and may be used for trophoblast pregnenolone/progesterone synthesis and/or is released into the fetal circulation.[144,145] IgG remains complexed to its receptor and is

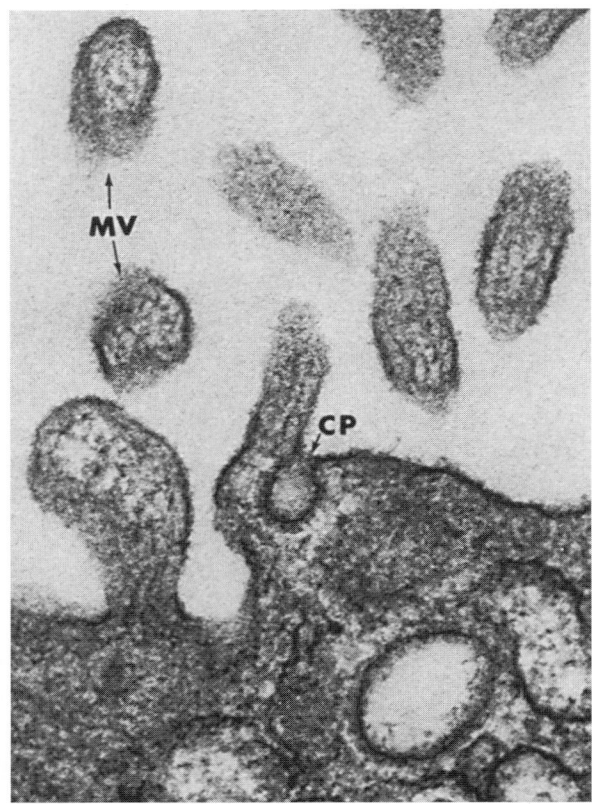

Figure 2–3. Electron micrograph of human placental microvillous plasma membrane demonstrating presence of a coated pit (CP). Note the presence of cytoskeletal components extending into the microvillous space (MV). (Courtesy of Kent L. Thornburg, Ph.D., Department of Physiology, Oregon Health Sciences University, Portland, OR.)

transferred to the fetus intact via exocytosis at the basal trophoblast membrane.[146] Ferrotransferrin carries two ferric ions per molecule and is unique in that it does not separate from the transferrin receptor. Rather, the iron dissociates and binds to ferritin, a cytoplasmic iron-storing protein.[135] Iron is then picked up at the basal side of the cell by fetal apotransferrin.

Placental Blood Flow

The transport characteristics of the placenta allow respiratory gases and many solutes to reach equal concentration between the maternal intervillous space blood (derived from uterine blood flow) and fetal capillary blood (derived from umbilical blood flow). Thus, the rate of blood flow in these two circulations is an important determinant of fetal oxygen and nutrient supply.

Uterine Blood Flow

Uterine blood flow during pregnancy supplies the myometrium, endometrium, and placenta, with the latter receiving nearly 90 percent of total uterine blood flow near term. Thus, interest has focused primarily on regulation of uteroplacental blood flow. Over the course of a normal singleton ovine gestation, uterine blood flow increases more than 50-fold above nonpregnant values.[142] This long-term increase in uterine blood flow is accompanied by a doubling of maternal cardiac output and a 40 percent increase in blood volume. Two primary factors contribute to this dramatic increase in uterine blood flow: placental growth and maternal arterial vasodilation. Along with fetal and placental growth, placental intervillous space volume almost triples between 22 and 36 weeks of gestation. Thus, the marked growth of the maternal placental vascular bed is consistent with the increase in placental diffusing capacity.[148,149] Second, the increase in blood flow is due in part to a direct estrogen-induced vasodilation of the uterine vasculature. This effect is mediated through the release of nitric oxide.[150] These combined effects provide uterine blood flow rates at term of at least 750 ml/min,[151,152] or 10 to 15 percent of maternal cardiac output.

The uterine artery behaves as a nearly maximally dilated system. Still, uterine blood flow is subject to short-term regulatory influences. Systemically administered vasodilator agents preferentially dilate systemic vessels, reducing uterine blood flow.[153] Thus, concerns regarding administration of antihypertensive agents or regional anesthesia with sympathetic blockade are well founded. Although pregnant women display a refractoriness to infused pressor agents,[154] pressor agent–induced increases in uterine vascular resistance may exceed increases in systemic vascular resistance, reducing uteroplacental blood flow. Thus, increased maternal plasma catecholamine levels during preeclampsia or pressor agents administered for treatment of maternal hypotension may have adverse effects on uterine blood flow. Although respiratory gases are important regulators of blood flow in a number of organs, there is no indication that either oxygen or carbon dioxide are responsible for short-term changes in uterine blood flow.[155] During uterine contractions, the relationship between uterine arterial and venous pressures and blood flow no longer holds. Since intrauterine pressures are directly transmitted to the intervillous space,[156] increases in intrauterine pressure are reflected by decreases in placental blood flow.

Umbilical Blood Flow

Fetal blood flow to the umbilical circulation represents approximately 40 percent of the combined output of both fetal ventricles.[157,158] Over the last third of gestation, increases in umbilical blood flow are proportional to fetal growth,[159] so that umbilical blood flow remains constant when normalized to fetal weight.[160] Human umbilical venous flow can be estimated through the use of triplex mode ultrasonography.[161] Although increases in villous capillary number represent the primary contributor to gestation-dependent increases in umbilical blood flow, the factors that regulate this change are not known. A number of important angiogenic peptides and factors have, however, been recently identified.[162,163] Short-term changes in umbilical blood flow are primarily regulated by perfusion pressure. The relationship between flow and perfusion pressure is linear in the umbilical circulation.[160,164] As a result, small (2 to 3 mm Hg) increases in umbilical vein pressure evoke proportional decreases in umbilical blood flow.[160,164] Since both the umbilical artery and vein are enclosed in the amniotic cavity, pressure changes caused by increases in uterine tone are transmitted equally to these vessels without changes in umbilical blood flow. Relative to the uteroplacental bed, the fetoplacental circulation is resistant to vasoconstrictive effects of infused pressor agents, and umbilical blood flow is preserved unless cardiac output decreases. Thus, despite catecholamine-induced changes in blood flow distribution and increases in blood pressure during acute hypoxia, umbilical blood flow is maintained over a relatively wide range of oxygen tensions.[165–168] Endogenous vasoactive autacoids have been identified; nitric oxide may also be important.[169,170]

Immunological Properties of the Placenta

The syncytiotrophoblast in contact with maternal blood in the intervillous space and the amniochorion in contact with maternal decidua represent the fetal tissues most prone to immunologic reactions from maternal factors. The rejection of tissue grafts is under genetic control, and the genes responsible for this phenomenon are termed "histocompatibility genes." Their products at the cell surface, major histocompatibility antigens, are integral to the host's recognition of self and nonself. Neither β_2-microglobulin (which is tightly associated with HLA antigens) nor the HLA antigens A, B, C, DR, or DC can be demonstrated on the surface of syncytiotrophoblast.[171,172] Invasive human cytotrophoblasts have been shown to express a trophoblast-specific, nonclassical class 1b antigen, HLA-G.[173] Postulated roles for HLA-G include protection of invasive cytotrophoblast from uterine natural killer cells, as well as containment of placental infection.[174] The chorionic sac in the first trimester exhibits HLA-A, -B, and -C antigens localized to nonvillous trophoblast of the cytotrophoblast cell columns and cytotrophoblastic shell.[175] In addition, histocompatibility antigens can be demonstrated on fetal stromal cells such as fibroblasts and fetal endothelial cells within the placental villi.[176] While the normal syncytiotrophoblast at the hemochorial interface within the interstitial space lacks major histocompatibility antigens, the observation that transformed trophoblast in vitro can manifest these antigens suggests the genetic information is present but suppressed in normal tissues in vivo.[176] Neither file A, B, or H blood group antigens[177] nor the H-Y antigens[171] are thought to be present on the syncytiotrophoblast surface. The presence of antigens in fetal stroma cells and endothelium of placental villi also may be important to maintenance of the fetus. For example,[178] this area may act as an immunologic sink to bind maternal antibodies so they do not reach the fetus.

The syncytiotrophoblast manifests unique antigens, termed trophoblast antigens and trophoblast-lymphocyte cross-reactive antigens.[176,178] Distinguishing the two groups is the latter's absorption by leukocytes. These trophoblast antigens are structural components of the plasma membrane and are distinct from soluble proteins produced by the placenta.[179] The trophoblast-lymphocyte cross-reactive antigens my be important for the induction of immunologic blocking factors in maternal serum during the second and third trimesters of normal pregnancy.[180] Antibodies against these antigens are thought to be important regulators of trophoblast growth.[181] The absence of trophoblast antigens, which the mother's immune system can recognize as non-self, may be related to a failure to produce these blocking factors, resulting in abortion.[176,181,184] Suppression of lymphocyte activation by local immunoregulatory responses in the decidua plays an important role in preventing rejection of the trophoblast. However, these same responses may also contribute to localized infections at this site in the absence of systemic effects.[185] In addition to the placenta, both the mother and the fetus make important contributions to the immunologic maintenance of pregnancy.[181,186,187]

Amniotic Fluid Volume

Mean amniotic fluid volume increases from 250 to 800 ml between 16 and 32 weeks' gestation. Despite considerable variability, the average volume remains stable up to 39 weeks and then declines to about 500 ml at 42 weeks.[188] The origin of amniotic fluid during the first trimester of pregnancy is uncertain. Possible sources include a transudate of maternal plasma through the chorioamnion or a transudate of fetal plasma through the highly permeable fetal skin, prior to keratinization.[189] The origin and dynamics of amniotic fluid are better understood beginning in the second trimester, when the fetus becomes the primary determinant. Amniotic fluid volume is maintained by a balance of fetal fluid production (lung liquid and urine) and fluid resorption (fetal swallowing and flow across the amniotic and/or chorionic membranes to the fetus or maternal uterus).

The fetal lung secretes fluid at a rate of 300 to 400 ml/day near term.[190] Chloride is actively transferred from alveolar capillaries to the lung lumen.[191] and water follows the chloride gradient. Thus, lung fluid represents a nearly protein-free transudate with an osmolarity similar to that of fetal plasma.[192] Fetal lung fluid does not appear to regulate fetal body fluid homeostasis, as fetal intravenous volume loading does not increase lung fluid secretion Rather, lung fluid likely serves to maintain lung expansion and facilitate pulmonary growth. Lung fluid must decrease at parturition to provide for the transition to respiratory ventilation. Notably, several hormones that increase in fetal plasma during labor (i.e, catecholamines, arginine vasopressin [AVP]) also decrease lung fluid production.[193–195] With the reduction of fluid secretion, the colloid osmotic gradient between fetal plasma and lung fluid results in lung fluid resorption across the pulmonary epithelium, and clearance via lymphatics. The absence of this process explains the increased incidence of transient tachypnea of the newborn, or "wet lung," in infants delivered by cesarean section in the absence of labor.

Fetal urine is the primary source of amniotic fluid, with outputs at term varying from 400 to 1,200 ml/day.[196,197] Between 20 and 40 weeks' gestation, fetal urine production increases about 10-fold,[197] in the presence of marked renal maturation. The urine is normally hypotonic[198] and the low osmolarity of fetal urine accounts for the hypotonicity of amniotic fluid in late gestation[198] relative to maternal and fetal plasma. Numerous fetal endocrine factors, including AVP, atrial natriuretic factor (ANF), angiotensin II (AII), aldosterone, and prostaglandins alter fetal renal blood flow, glomerular filtration rate, or urine flow rates.[199,200] In response to fetal stress, endocrine-mediated reductions in fetal urine flow may explain the association between fetal hypoxia and oligohydramnios. The regulation of fetal urine production is discussed further in the section Fetal Kidney, below.

Fetal swallowing is believed to be the major route of amniotic fluid resorption,[201–204] although swallowed fluid contains a mixture of amniotic and tracheal fluids.[205] Human fetal swallowing has been demonstrated by 18 weeks' gestation,[206] with daily swallowed volumes of 200 to 500 ml near term.[202,203] Similar to fetal urine flow, daily fetal swallowed volumes (per body weight) are markedly greater than adult values. With the development of fetal neurobehavioral states, fetal swallowing occurs primarily during active sleep states associated with respiratory and eye movements.[206,207] Moderate increases in fetal plasma osmolality increase the number of swallowing episodes and volume swallowed,[208,209] indicating the presence of an intact thirst mechanism in the near-term fetus.

Since amniotic fluid is hypotonic with respect to maternal plasma, there is a potential for bulk water removal at the amniotic-chorionic interface with maternal or fetal plasma. Although fluid resorption to the maternal plasma is likely minimal, intramembranous flow from amniotic fluid to fetal placental vessels may contribute importantly to amniotic fluid resorption.[210] Thus, intramembranous flow may balance fetal urine and lung liquid production with fetal swallowing to maintain normal amniotic fluid volumes.

FETAL PHYSIOLOGY

Growth and Metabolism

Substrates

Nutrients are utilized by the fetus for two primary purposes: oxidation for energy and tissue accretion. Under normal conditions, glucose is an important substrate for fetal oxidative metabolism. The glucose utilized by the fetus derives from the placenta rather than from endogenous glucose production.[211] However, based on umbilical vein–to–umbilical artery glucose and oxygen concentration differences,[212] glucose alone cannot account for fetal oxidative metabolism. In fact, glucose oxidation accounts for only two thirds of fetal carbon dioxide production.[213] Thus, fetal oxidative metabolism depends on substrates in addition to glucose. Because a large portion of the amino acids taken up by the umbilical circulation are used by the fetus for aerobic metabolism instead of protein synthesis, amino acids represent one of these substrates. Fetal uptake for a number of amino acids actually exceeds their accretion into fetal tissues.[214] In fetal sheep and likely the human fetus as well, lactate also is a substrate for fetal oxygen consumption.[213] Thus, the combined substrates glucose, amino acids, and lactate essentially provide the approximately 87 kcal/kg/day required by the growing fetus.

Metabolic requirements for new tissue accretion depend on the growth rate and the type of tissue acquired. Although the newborn infant has relatively increased body fat (16 percent),[215] fetal fat content is low at 26 weeks. Fat acquisition increases gradually up to 32 weeks, and rapidly thereafter ($\sim$ 82 g [dry weight] of fat per week). Since the necessary enzymes for carbohydrate to lipid conversion are present in the fetus,[216] fat acquisition reflects glucose utilization and not placental fatty acid uptake. In contrast, fetal acquisition of nonfat tissue is linear from 32 to 39 weeks, and may decrease to only 30 percent of the fat-acquisition rate in late gestation ($\sim$ 43 g [dry weight] per week).

Hormones

The role of select hormones in the regulation of placental growth was discussed previously in the section Placental Metabolism and Growth. Fetal hormones influence fetal growth through both metabolic and mitogenic effects. Although growth hormone and growth hormone receptors are present early in fetal life, and growth hormone is essential to postnatal growth,[217] growth hormone appears to have little role in regulating fetal growth. Instead, changes in IGF, IGF-binding proteins, or IGF receptors may explain the apparent reduced role of growth hormone on fetal growth.[218–222] Most if not all tissues of the body produce IGF-I and IGF-II,[223,224] and both IGF-I and IGF-II are present in human fetal tissue extracts after 12 weeks' gestation. Fetal plasma IGF-I and IGF-II levels begin to increase by 32 to 34 weeks' gestation.[225,226] The increase in IGF-I levels directly correlates with increase in fetal raze, and a reduction in IGF-I levels is associated with growth restriction. In contrast, there is no correlation between serum IGF-II levels and fetal growth. However, there is a correlation between small offspring and genetic manipulations resulting in only one allele and decreased IGF-II messenger RNA. Thus, tissue IGF-II concentrations and localized IGF-II release may be more important than circulating levels in supporting fetal growth.

A role for insulin in fetal growth is suggested from the increases in body weight, and heart and liver weights in infants of diabetic mothers.[227] Insulin levels within the high physiologic range increase fetal body weight,[228] and increases in endogenous fetal insulin significantly increase fetal glucose uptake.[229,230] In addition, fetal insulin secretion increases in response to elevations in blood glucose, although the normal rapid insulin response phase is absent.[230] Plasma insulin levels sufficient to increase fetal growth[228] also may exert mitogenic effects,[224] perhaps through insulin-induced IGF-II receptor binding.[231] Separate receptors for insulin and IGF-II are expressed in fetal liver cells by the end of the first trimester.[232] Hepatic insulin receptor numbers (per gram tissue) triple by 28 weeks, while IGF-II receptor numbers remain constant.[232] Thus, although children conceived of diabetic mothers are at increased risk of cardiac defects, the growth patterns of these infants[233,234] indicate insulin levels may be most important in late gestation. Though less common, equally dramatically low birth weights are associated with the absence of fetal insulin.[219] Experimentally induced hypoinsulinemia causes a 30 percent decrease in fetal glucose utilization and decreases fetal growth.[235,237]

As in the adult, β-adrenergic receptor activation increases fetal insulin secretion, while α-adrenergic activation inhibits insulin secretion.[238,239] Fetal glucagon secretion also is modulated by the β-adrenergic system.[238] However, the fetal glycemic response to glucagon is blunted, probably caused by a relative reduction in hepatic glucagon receptors.[240]

In addition to the insulin-like growth factors, a number of other factors including epidermal growth factor, transforming growth factor, fibroblast growth factor, and nerve growth factor are expressed during embryonic development and appear to exert specific effects during morphogenesis, For example, epidermal growth factor has specific effects on lung growth and growth and differentiation of the secondary palate,[241] and normal sympathetic adrenergic system development is dependent on nerve growth factor.[241] However, a specific role of these factors in regulating fetal growth remains to be defined. Similarly, the fetal thyroid also is not important for overall fetal growth, but is important for central nervous system development.[218,219]

Fetal Circulation

Anatomy

The first step in understanding fetal cardiovascular physiology is to recognize the peculiarities unique to fetal circulatory anatomy. Beginning with well-oxygenated blood from the placenta (Fig. 2–4), the umbilical vein gives off branches to the left lobe of the liver and then continues as the ductus venosus. A major branch to the right then joins the portal vein to supply the right lobe of the liver. Approximately half of the estimated umbilical blood flow (70 to 130 ml/min/kg feed weight[242] after 30 weeks' gestation) follows the ductus venosus.[243] Left hepatic vein blood combines with the well-oxygenated ductus venosus flow in the inferior vena cava to form a stream that is preferentially directed across the foramen ovale into the left atrium

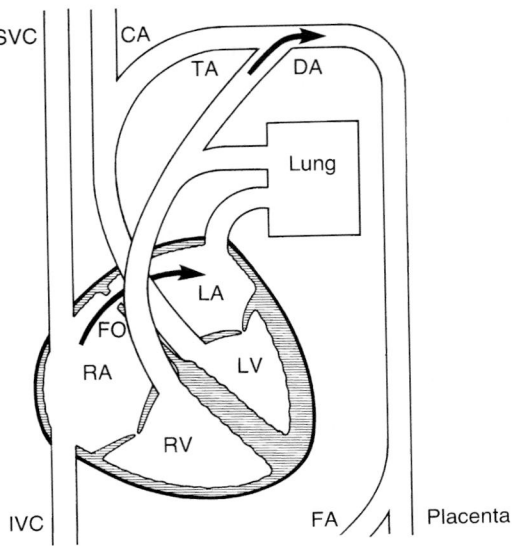

Figure 2–5. Anatomy of fetal heart and central shunts. SVC, superior vena cava; CA, carotid artery; TA, thoracic aorta; DA, ductus arteriosus; RA, right atrium; FO, foramen ovale; LA, left atrium; RV, right ventricle; LV, left ventricle; IVC, inferior vena cava; FA, femoral artery. (From Anderson DF, Bissonnette JM, Faber JJ, Thornburg KL: Central shunt flows and pressures in the mature fetal lamb. Am J Physiol 241:H60, 1981, with permission.)

(Figs. 2–4 and 2–5). As a result, blood with the highest oxygen content is delivered to the left ventricle, and ultimately supplies blood to the carotid circulation and upper body and brain. Flow across the foramen ovale is approximately one third of combined cardiac output.[244] Because blood from the ductus venosus to the right side of the liver combines with blood from the portal vein (only a small fraction of portal vein blood passes through the durum venosus), right hepatic vein blood is less oxygenated than its counterpart on the left.[243] Right hepatic vein blood joins with inferior vena caval flow (which further lowers the oxygen content) to form a stream that is preferentially directed through the tricuspid valve (Fig. 2–4) into the right ventricle (Fig. 2–5). Superior vena cava blood flow also is preferentially directed through the tricuspid valve to the right ventricle. Thus, right ventricular output, exceeding 50 percent of biventricular output,[244] is primarily directed through the ductus arteriosus to the descending aorta (Fig. 2–5). The high pulmonary vascular resistance and 2 to 3 mm Hg higher mean pulmonary artery pressure above aortic pressure directs flow to the ductus arteriosus, away from the pulmonary circulation,[244] which receives only 5 to 10 percent of the combined ventricular output.

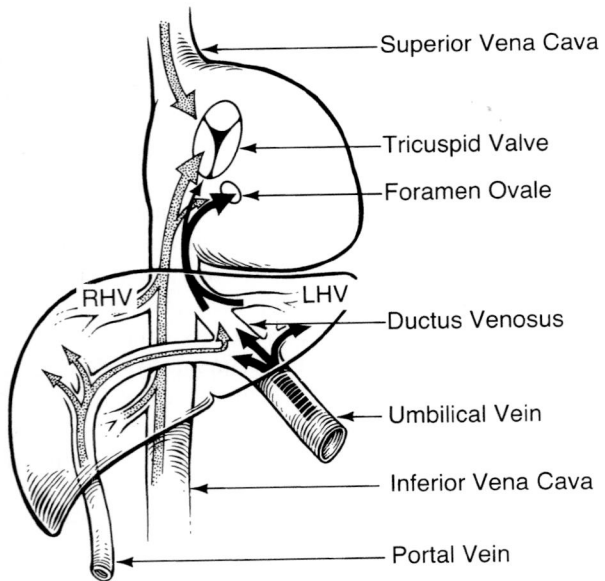

Figure 2–4. Anatomy of the umbilical and hepatic circulation. RHV, right hepatic vein; LHV, left hepatic vein. (From Rudolph AM: Hepatic and ductus venosus blood flows during fetal life. Hepatology 3: 254, 1983, with permission.)

Superior Vena Cava
Tricuspid Valve
Foramen Ovale
RHV **LHV**
Ductus Venosus
Umbilical Vein
Inferior Vena Cava
Portal Vein

Fetal Heart

Estimates of fetal left ventricular output average 20 ml/min/kg body weight.[245] If left ventricular output is 40 percent of the combined biventricular output,[244]

then total fetal cardiac output would be about 300 ml/min/kg. The distribution of the cardiac output to fetal organs is summarized in Table 2–2,[246,247] with fetal hepatic distribution reflecting only the portion supplied by the hepatic artery, In fact, hepatic blood flow derives principally from the umbilical vein and to a lesser extent the portal vein,[248] and represents about 25 percent of the total venous return to the heart.

Fetal ventricular output depends on contractility, pulmonary artery and aortic pressures, and the heart rate. The relationship between mean right atrial pressure (the index often used for ventricular volume at the end of diastole) and stroke volume is depicted in Figure 2–6. The steep ascending limb represents the length-active tension relationship for cardiac muscle in the right ventricle.[249] Under normal conditions, fetal right atrial pressure resides at the break point in this ascending limb; increases in pressure do not increase stroke volume. Thus, the contribution of Starling mechanisms to increasing right heart output in the fetus is limited. In contrast, decreases in venous return and right atrial pressure will decrease stroke volume. Because the right ventricle is sensitive to afterload, a linear inverse relationship exists between stroke volume and pulmonary artery pressure.[249] Thus, the fall in pulmonary artery pressure at birth contributes to the increase in right heart output. Compared to the left, the fetal right ventricle has a greater anteroposterior dimension, increasing both volume and circumferential radius of curvature. This anatomic difference increases the radius/wall thickness ratio for the right ventricle, producing increased wall stress in systole and a decrease in stroke volume when afterload increases.[250]

The relationship between atrial pressure and stroke volume in the left ventricle is similar to that shown in Figure 2–6 for the right ventricle. Although the break point occurs near the normal value for left atrial pressure, there is a small amount of preload reserve.[251] In

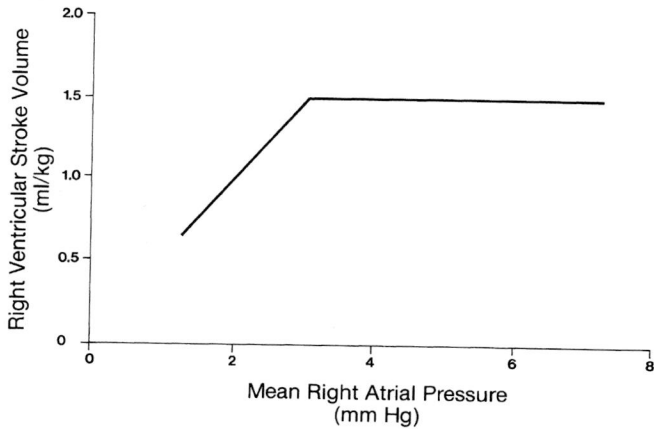

Figure 2–6. Stroke volume of the fetal right ventricle as a function of mean right atrial pressure. (From Thornburg KL, Morton MJ: Filling and arterial pressures as determinants of RV stroke volume in the sheep fetus. Am J Physiol 244:H656, 1983, with permission.)

distinction to the fetal right ventricle, the left side is not sensitive to aortic pressure increases. Thus, postnatal increases in systemic blood pressure do not increase stroke volume. Late-gestation fetal heart α-adrenergic receptor numbers are similar to the adult,[252] and increases in circulating catecholamine concentrations may increase stroke volume by 50 percent.[253] Blood flow to the myocardium reflects the greater stroke volume of the right side; right ventricular free wall and septal blood flows are higher than in the left ventricle.[254]

Glucose and lactate constitute the major substrates used for oxidative metabolism of the fetal heart. In contrast to the adult heart, free fatty acids are not metabolized in significant amounts by the myocardium in utero.[255] This may be a function of substrate availability, as palmitate can be oxidized by fetal heart muscle,[256] although to a lesser extent than in the neonate.

Fetal heart rate decreases during the last half of gestation, particularly between 20 and 30 weeks. If analysis is confined to episodes of low heart rate variability, mean heart rate decreases from 30 weeks to term. However, if all heart rate data are analyzed, mean heart rate is stable at 142 beats per minute over the last 10 weeks of gestation.[257] Variability in mean heart rate over 24 hours includes a nadir between 2 A.M. and 6 A.M. hours and a peak between 8 A.M. and 10 A.M. hours.[258] Most fetal heart rate accelerations occur simultaneous with limb movement, primarily reflecting central neuronal brain stem output. Also, movement-related decreases in venous return and a reflex tachycardia contribute.[259]

Because ventricular stroke volumes decrease with increasing heart rate, fetal cardiac output stays constant over a heart rate range of 120 to 180 beats per min.[260–262] The major effect of this inverse relationship between heart rate and stroke volume is an alteration in end-diastolic dimension. If end-diastolic dimension is

Table 2–2. DISTRIBUTION OF FETAL CARDIAC OUTPUT

Organ	Percentage of Biventricular Cardiac Output
Placenta	40
Brain	13
Heart	3.5
Lung	7
Liver	2.5 (hepatic artery)
Gastrointestinal tract	5
Adrenal glands	0.5
Kidney	2.5
Spleen	1
Body	25

Data from Rudolph and Heyman,[246] and Paton et al.[247]

kept constant, there is no fall in stroke volume and cardiac output goes up.[261,262]

Autonomic Regulation of Cardiovascular Function

Through reflex stimulation of peripheral baroreceptors, chemoreceptors, and central mechanisms, the sympathetic and parasympathetic systems have important roles in the regulation of fetal heart rate, cardiac contractility, and vascular tone. The fetal sympathetic system develops early, whereas the parasympathetic system develops somewhat later.[263-265] Nevertheless, in the third trimester, increasing parasympathetic tone accounts for the characteristic decrease in fetal heart rate with periods of reduced fetal heart rate reactivity. As evidence, fetal heart rate increases in the presence of parasympathetic blockade with atropine.[266] Opposing sympathetic and parasympathetic inputs to the fetal heart contribute to R-R interval variability from one heart cycle to the next, and to basal heart rate variability over periods of a few minutes. However, even when sympathetic and parasympathetic inputs are removed, a level of variability remains.[266]

Fetal sympathetic innervation is not essential for blood pressure maintenance when circulating catecholamines are present.[267] Nevertheless, fine control of blood pressure and fetal heart rate requires an intact sympathetic system.[268] In the absence of functional adrenergic innervation, hypoxia-induced increases in peripheral, renal, and splanchnic bed vascular resistances[269,270] and blood pressure are not seen.[271,272] However, hypoxia-related changes in pulmonary, myocardial, adrenal, and brain blood flows occur in the absence of sympathetic innervation, indicating that both local and endocrine effects contribute to regulation of blood flow in these organs.

Receptors in the carotid body and arch of the aorta respond to pressor or respiratory gas stimulation with afferent modulation of heart rate and vascular tone. Sensitivity of the fetal baroreflex response, in terms of the magnitude of decreases in heart rate per millimeter of mercury increase in blood pressure, is blunted relative to the adult.[273,274] However, fetal baroreflex sensitivity more than doubles in late gestation.[273] Although the set-point for fetal heart rate is not believed to depend on intact baroreceptors, fetal heart rate variability increases when functional arterial baroreceptors are absent.[275] The same observation has been made for fetal blood pressure. Thus, fetal arterial baroreceptors buffer variations in fetal blood pressure during body or breathing movements.[275,276] Changes in baroreceptor tone likely account for the increase in mean fetal blood pressure normally observed in late gestation.[276] In the absence of functional chemoreceptors, mean arterial pressure is maintained[275] while peripheral blood flow increases. Thus, peripheral arterial chemoreceptors may be important to maintenance of resting peripheral vascular tone. Peripheral arterial chemoreceptors also are important components in fetal reflex responses to hypoxia; the initial bradycardia is not seen without functional chemoreceptors.[277]

Hormonal Regulation of Cardiovascular Function

Adrenocorticotropic hormone (ACTH) and catecholamines are discussed in the section Fetal Adrenal and Thyroid, below.

ARGININE VASOPRESSIN. Significant quantities of AVP are present in the human fetal neurohypophysis by completion of the first trimester.[278] Ovine fetal plasma AVP levels increase appropriately in response to changes in fetal plasma osmolality induced directly in the fetus[279,280] or via changes in maternal osmolality.[281,282] Due to functional high and low-pressure baroreceptors and chemoreceptor afferents, decreases in fetal intravascular volume[283,284] or systemic blood pressure[285,286] also increase fetal AVP secretion. Thus, in the late-gestation fetus as in the adult, AVP secretion is regulated by both osmoreceptor and volume/baroreceptor pathways. Hypoxia-induced AVP secretion has been demonstrated beyond mid-pregnancy of ovine gestation,[287] and reductions in fetal PO_2 of 10 mm Hg (50 percent) evoke profound increases in fetal plasma AVP levels (200 to 400 pg/ml or more)[288,289] Thus, because fetal AVP responsiveness to hypoxia is augmented relative to the adult (as much as 40-fold), and fetal responsiveness appears to increase during the last half of gestation, hypoxemia is the most potent stimulus known for fetal AVP secretion.[288]

The cardiovascular response pattern to AVP infusion includes dose-dependent increases in fetal mean blood pressure and decreases in heart rate at plasma levels well below those required for similar effects in the adult.[289] Receptors distinct from those mediating AVP antidiuretic effects in the kidney account for AVP contributions to fetal circulatory, adjustments during hemorrhage,[290] hypotension,[291] and hypoxia.[292] Corticotropin-releasing factor (CRF) effects of AVP may contribute to hypoxia-induced increases in plasma ACTH and cortisol levels.[293-296] In addition to effects on fetal heart rate, cardiac output, and arterial blood pressure, AVP-induced changes in peripheral, placental, myocardial, and cerebral blood flows[297-300] directly parallel the cardiovascular changes associated with acute hypoxia. Because many of these responses are attenuated during AVP receptor blockade,[292] AVP effects on cardiac output distribution may serve to facilitate O_2 availability to the fetus during hypoxic challenges. However, other hypoxia-related responses, including decreases in renal and pulmonary blood flows, and increased adrenal blood flow are not seen in response to AVP infusions.[298]

RENIN–ANGIOTENSIN II. Fetal plasma renin levels are typically elevated during late gestation.[301] A variety of stimuli including changes in tubular sodium concentration,[302] reductions in blood volume,[303] vascular pressure or renal perfusion pressure,[304] and hypoxemia[305] all increase fetal plasma renin activity. The relationship between fetal renal perfusion pressure and log plasma renin activity is similar to that of adults.[306] Consistent with the effects of renal nerve activity on renin release in adults,[307] fetal renin gene expression is directly modulated by renal sympathetic nerve activity.[308]

Although fetal plasma AII levels increase in response to small changes in blood volume and hypoxemia,[309] fetal AII and aldosterone levels do not increase in proportion to changes in plasma renin activity.[301] This apparent uncoupling of the fetal renin-angiotensin-aldosterone system and the increase in newborn AII levels may relate to the significant contribution of the placenta to plasma AII clearance in the fetus relative to the adult.[310] Also, limited angiotensin converting enzyme (ACE) availability due to reduced pulmonary blood flow and direct inhibition of aldosterone secretion by the normally high circulating ANF levels may contribute. Thus, reductions in AII production and aldosterone responses to AII, augmented AII and aldosterone clearances, and the resulting reductions in AII and aldosterone levels and feedback inhibition of renin may account for the elevated renin and reduced AII and aldosterone levels typically observed during fetal life.

AII infusion increases fetal mean arterial blood pressure. In contrast to AVP-induced bradycardia, fetal AII infusion increases heat rate (after an initial reflex bradycardia) through both a direct effect on the heart,[311] and decreased baroreflex responsiveness. Both hormones increase fetal blood pressure similar to the levels seen with hypoxemia. However, AII does not reduce peripheral blood flow, perhaps because circulation to muscle, skin, and bone are always under maximum response to AII, thereby limiting increases in resting tone.[311] Angiotensin II infusions also decrease renal blood flow and increase umbilical vascular resistance, although absolute placental blood flow remains the same. While the adult kidney contains both AII receptor subtypes (AT_1 and AT_2), the AT_2 subtype is the only form present in the human fetal kidney.[312] Maturational differences in the AII receptor subtype expressed would be consistent with earlier studies demonstrating differing AII effects on fetal renal and peripheral vascular beds.[305] Thus, the receptors mediating AII responses in the renal and peripheral vascular beds differ during fetal life.

Fetal Hemoglobin

The fetus exists in a state of aerobic metabolism, with arterial blood PO_2 values in the 20 to 25 mm Hg range. However, there is no evidence of metabolic acidosis. Adequate fetal tissue oxygenation is achieved by several mechanisms. Of major importance are the higher fetal cardiac output and organ blood flows. A higher hemoglobin concentration (relative to the adult) and an increase in oxygen-carrying capacity of fetal hemoglobin also contribute. The resulting leftward shift in the fetal oxygen dissociation curve relative to the adult (Fig. 2–7) increases fetal blood oxygen saturation for any given oxygen tension. For example, at a partial pressure of 26.5 mm Hg, adult blood oxygen saturation is 50 percent, whereas fetal oxygen saturation is 70 percent. Thus, at a normal fetal PO_2 of 20 mm Hg, fetal whole blood oxygen saturation may be 50 percent.[313]

The basis for increased oxygen affinity of fetal whole blood resides in the interaction of fetal hemoglobin with intracellular organic phosphate 2,3-diphosphoglycerate (2,3-DPG). The fetal hemoglobin (HgbF) tetramere is comprised of two α-chains (identical to adult) and two γ-chains. The latter differ from the β-chain of adult hemoglobin (HgbA) in 39 of 146 amino acid residues. Among these differences is the substitution of serine in the γ-chain of HgbF for histidine at the β-143 position of HgbA, which is located at the entrance to the central cavity of the hemoglobin tetramere. Due to a positively charged imidazole group, histidine can bind with the negatively charged 2,3-DPG. Binding of 2,3-DPG to deoxyhemoglobin stabilizes the tetramere in the reduced form. Because serine is nonionized and does not interact with 2,3-DPG to the same extent as histi-

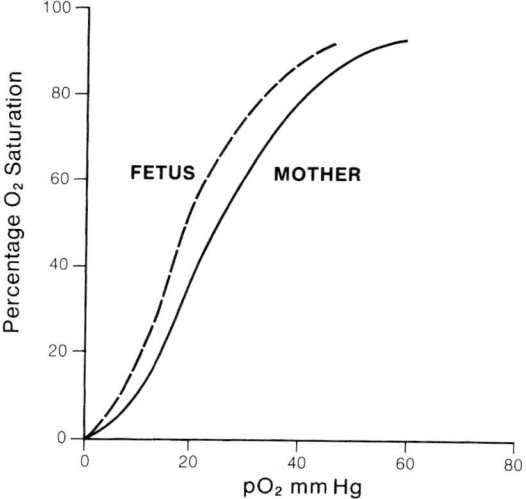

Figure 2–7. Oxyhemoglobin dissociation curves of maternal and fetal human blood at pH 7.4 and 37°C. (Adapted from Hellegers AE, Schruefer JJP: Normograms and empirical equations relating oxygen tension, percentage saturation, and pH in maternal and fetal blood. Am J Obstet Gynecol 81:377, 1961.)

dine,[314] the oxygen affinity of HgbF is increased and the dissociation curve is shifted to the left. If HgbA or HgbF is removed from the erythrocyte and stripped of organic phosphates, the oxygen affinity for both hemoglobins is similar. However, addition of equal amounts of 2,3-DPG to the hemoglobins decreases the oxygen affinity of HgbA (dissociation curve shifts to the right) to a greater extent than for HgbF. Thus, even though overall oxygen affinities are similar, differences in 2,3-DPG interaction result in a higher oxygen affinity for HgbF.

The proportion of HgbF to HgbA changes between 26 and 40 weeks of gestation, HgbF decreases linearly from 100 percent to about 70 percent, so that HgbA accounts for 30 percent of fetal hemoglobin at term.[315] This change in expression from γ- to β-globulin synthesis takes place in erythroid progenitor cells.[316] Although the basis for this switching is not yet known, our understanding of human globin gene regulation has provided important insights into several fetal hemoglobin disorders such as the thalassemias and sickle cell anemia. Duplication of the α-genes on chromosome 16 provides the normal fetus with four gene loci. The genes for the remaining globins are located on chromosome 11 and consist of $^G\gamma$, $^A\gamma$, δ, and β. The two γ-genes differ in the amino acid in position 36; glycine versus alanine. Hemoglobin A synthesis is dictated by the γ-and β-genes, HgbF by α and γ, and HgbA$_2$ by α and δ. Sequences in the δ region may be responsible for the relative expression of the γ-gene, such that fetal hemoglobin persists when these are absent.[317]

Fetal Kidney

Overall fetal water and electrolyte homeostasis is primarily mediated by fetal–maternal exchange across the placenta. However, urine production by the fetal kidney is essential to maintenance of amniotic fluid volume and composition. Although absolute glomerular filtration rate (GFR) increases during the third trimester, GFR per gram kidney weight does not change[318] because GFR and fetal kidney weight increase in parallel. The genesis of new glomeruli is complete by about 36 weeks.[319] Subsequent increases in GFR reflect increases in glomerular surface area for filtration, effective filtration pressure, and capillary filtration coefficient. Although glomerular filtration is related to hydrostatic pressure, and fetal blood pressure increases in the third trimester, both renal blood flow per gram of kidney weight and filtration fraction (GFR/renal plasma flow) remain constant.[318] Newborn increases in filtration fraction parallel increases in arterial pressure, suggesting the lower hydrostatic pressure within the glomerulus contributes to the relatively low filtration fraction and GFR of the intrauterine kidney.[318,320] A mild glomerulo-

tubular imbalance may describe the early gestation fetus. However, renal tubular sodium and chloride reabsorptions increase in late gestation, such that glomerulotubular balance is maintained in the third-trimester fetus.[320,321]

Although fetal GFR is low, the daily urine production rate is large (equaling 60 to 80 percent of the amniotic fluid volume). The large urine output results from the large portion of the filtered water (20 percent) that is excreted in the form of hypotonic urine. The positive free water clearance characterizing fetal renal function originally led to the hypothesis that the fetal kidney lacked AVP receptors. However, ovine fetal renal collecting duct responses to AVP can be demonstrated in the second trimester,[322] indicating diminished urine-concentrating ability is not caused by AVP receptor absence. Fetal renal V$_2$ receptors mediate AVP-induced tubular water reabsorption, and functional V$_2$ receptors are present in the fetal kidney by the beginning of the last third of gestation.[297,323] In addition, AVP-induced cyclic adenosine monophosphate (cAMP) production is not different from the adult,[324] and AVP-induced apical tubular water channels (aquaporin II) are expressed in the fetal kidney. In fact, the selective AVP V$_2$ receptor agonist [deamino^1,D-Arg^8]-vasopressin (dDAVP) appropriately increases fetal renal water reabsorption without affecting blood pressure or heart rate.[291] Thus, V$_2$ receptors mediate AVP effects on fetal urine production and amniotic fluid volume.[291,297] Instead, the reduced concentrating ability of the fetal kidney primarily reflects reductions in proximal tubular sodium reabsorption, short juxtamedullary nephron loops of Henle, and limited medullary interstitial urea concentrations.

Although fetal plasma renin activity levels are high, effective uncoupling of AII production from plasma renin activity and a high placental clearance rate for AII serve to minimize increases in fetal plasma AII levels. Limiting fluctuations in fetal plasma AII levels may be of advantage to the regulation of fetal renal function. For example, fetal AII infusion increases fetal mean arterial pressure, and renal and placental vascular resistances.[325] In contrast, fetal treatment with the ACE inhibitor captopril increases plasma renin activity and decreases arterial blood pressure, renal vascular resistance, and filtration fraction[326]; and urine flow effectively ceases.[327] Given the potential for AII to decrease placental blood flow,[299] uncoupling of renin-induced angiotensin I production, limited ACE activity, and augmented placental AII clearance may protect the fetal cardiovascular system from large increases in plasma AII levels. Collectively, plasma AII levels appear to be regulated within a very narrow range and this regulation may be important to overall fetal homeostasis.

Atrial natriuretic factor granules are present in the

fetal heart, and fetal plasma ANF levels are elevated relative to the adult.[328] Fetal plasma ANF levels increase in response to volume expansion,[329] and ANF infusion evokes limited increases in ovine fetal renal sodium excretion.[330,331] Fetal ANF infusion also decreases fetal plasma volume, with minimal effect on blood pressure.[328] These observations suggest ANF actions in the fetus are primarily directed at volume homeostasis, with minimal cardiovascular effects.

The ability of the fetal kidney to excrete titratable acid and ammonia is limited relative to the adult. In addition, the threshold for fetal renal bicarbonate excretion (defined as the excretion of a determined amount of bicarbonate per unit GFR) is much lower than in the adult. That is, fetal urine tends to be alkaline at relatively low plasma bicarbonate levels, despite the high fetal arterial P_{CO_2}.[332] Because fetal renal tubular mechanisms for glucose reabsorption are qualitatively similar to the adult, fetal renal glucose excretion is limited. In fact, the maximum ability of the fetal kidney to reabsorb glucose exceeds that of the adult when expressed as a function of GFR.[333]

Fetal Gastrointestinal System

Gastrointestinal Tract

Amniotic fluid contains measurable glucose, lactate, and amino acid concentrations, raising the possibility that fetal swallowing could serve as a source of nutrient uptake. Fetal swallowing contributes importantly to somatic growth and gastrointestinal development as a result of the large volume of ingested fluid. Ten to 15 percent of fetal nitrogen requirements may result from swallowing of amniotic fluid protein.[334] Amino acids and glucose are absorbed and utilized by the fetus if they are administered into the fetal gastrointestinal tract.[335,336] Furthermore, intragastric ovine fetal nutrient administration partially ameliorates fetal growth restriction induced by maternal malnutrition.[337] Further evidence for the role of swallowing in fetal growth results from studies demonstrating that impairment of fetal rabbit swallowing at 24 days gestation (term = 31 days) induces an 8 percent weight decrease (compared to controls) by 28 days.[338] The fetal gastrointestinal tract is directly impacted, as esophageal ligation of fetal rabbit pups results in marked reductions in gastric and intestinal tissue weight and gastric acidity.[1] Reductions in gastrointestinal and somatic growth were reversed by fetal intragastric infusion of amniotic fluid.[1] Similarly, esophageal ligation of 90-day ovine fetuses (term = 145 to 150 days) induces a 30 percent decrease of small intestine villus height[339] and a reduction in liver, pancreas, and intestinal weight.[340] Although ingestion of amniotic fluid nutrients may be necessary for opti-

mal fetal growth, trophic growth factors within the amniotic fluid also importantly contribute. Thus, the reduction in fetal rabbit weight induced by esophageal ligation is reversed by gastric infusion of epidermal growth factor.[166] Studies in human infants support the association of fetal swallowing and gastrointestinal growth as upper gastrointestinal tract obstructions are associated with a significantly greater rate of human fetal growth restriction as compared to fetuses with lower gastrointestinal obstructions.[341,342]

Blood flow to the fetal intestine does not increase during moderate levels of hypoxemia. The artery–mesenteric vein difference in oxygen content is also unchanged so that at a constant blood flow intestinal oxygen consumption can remain the same during moderate hypoxemia. However, with more pronounced hypoxemia, fetal intestinal oxygen consumption falls as blood flow decreases and the oxygen content difference across the intestine fails to widen. The result is a metabolic acidosis in the blood draining the mesenteric system.[343]

Liver

Near term, the placenta is the major route for bilirubin elimination. Less than 10 percent of an administered bilirubin load is excreted in the fetal biliary tree over a 10-hour period; about 20 percent remains in plasma.[334] Thus, the fetal metabolic pathways for bilirubin and bile salts remain underdeveloped at term. The cholate pool size (normalized to body surface area) is one third and the synthetic rate one half adult levels. In premature infants, cholate pool size and synthesis rates represent less than half and one third, respectively, of term infant values. In fact, premature infant intraluminal duodenal bile acid concentrations are near or below the level required to form lipid micelles.[344] The unique attributes of the fetal hepatic circulation were detailed during the earlier discussion of fetal circulatory anatomy. Notably, the fetal hepatic blood supply primarily derives from the umbilical vein. The left lobe receives its blood supply almost exclusively from the umbilical vein (there is a small contribution from the hepatic artery), while the right lobe receives blood from the portal vein as well. The fetal liver under normal conditions accounts for about 20 percent of total fetal oxygen consumption.[345] Because hepatic glucose uptake and release are balanced, net glucose removal by the liver under normal conditions is minimal.[345] During episodes of hypoxemia, α-adrenergic receptor–mediated increases in hepatic glucose release account for the hyperglycemia characteristic of short-term fetal hypoxemia.[239] Hypoxia severe enough to decrease fetal oxygen consumption selectively reduces right hepatic lobe oxygen uptake, which exceeds that of the fetus as a whole. In contrast, oxygen uptake by the left lobe of the liver is unchanged.[345]

Fetal Adrenal and Thyroid

Adrenal

The fetal pituitary secretes ACTH in response to "stress," including hypoxemia.[346] The associated increase in cortisol exerts feedback inhibition of the continued ACTH response.[347] In the fetus and adult, proopiomelanocortin posttranslational processing gives rise to ACTH, corticotropin-like intermediate lobe peptide (CLIP), and α-melanocyte–stimulating hormone (α-MSH). The precursor peptide preproenkephalin is a distinct gene product giving rise to the enkephalins. Fetal proopiomelanocortin processing differs from the adult. For example, although ACTH is present in appreciable amounts, the fetal pituitary contains large amounts of CLIP and α-MSH. The fetal ratio of CLIP plus α-MSH to ACTH decreases from the end of the first trimester to term.[348] Because pituitary corticotropin-releasing hormone (CRH) expression is relatively low until late gestation, AVP serves as the major CRF in early gestation. With increasing gestational age, fetal cortisol levels progressively increase secondary to hypothalamic-pituitary axis maturation. Cortisol is important to pituitary maturation because it shifts corticotrophs from the fetal to the adult type and to adrenal maturation through regulation of ACTH receptor numbers.[349]

On a body weight basis, the fetal adrenal gland is an order of magnitude larger than in the adult. This increase in size is due to the presence of an adrenal cortical definitive zone and a so-called fetal zone, which constitutes 85 percent of the adrenal at birth. Cortisol and mineralocorticoids are the major products of the fetal definitive zone, and fetal cortisol secretion is regulated by ACTH but not human chorionic gonadotrophin (hCG).[350,351] Low-density lipoprotein–bound cholesterol (see Receptor Mediated Endocytosis/Exocytosis, above) is the major source of steroid precursor in the fetal adrenal.[352,353] Because the enzyme 3β-hydroxysteroid dehydrogenase is lacking in the fetal adrenal, dehydroepiandrosterone sulfate (DHEAS) is the major product of the fetal zone. At mid-gestation, DHEAS secretion is determined by both ACTH and hCG.[350,351] Both fetal ACTH and cortisol levels are relatively low during most of gestation, and there is not a clear correlation between plasma ACTH levels and cortisol production. This apparent dissociation between fetal ACTH levels and cortisol secretion[354] may be explained by (1) differences in ACTH processing and the presence of the large-molecular-weight proopiomelanocortin processing products (CLIP and α-MSH) may suppress ACTH action on the adrenal until late gestation (when ACTH becomes the primary product), (2) fetal adrenal definitive zone ACTH responsiveness may increase, or (3) placental ACTH and/or posttranslational processing intermediates may affect the adrenal response to ACTH.

Resting fetal plasma norepinephrine levels exceed epinephrine levels approximately 10-fold.[355,356] The fetal plasma levels of both catecholamines increase in response to hypoxemia, with norepinephrine levels invariably in excess of the epinephrine levels.[356] Under basal conditions, norepinephrine is secreted at a higher rate than for epinephrine, and this relationship persists during a hypoxemic stimulus.[357] Plasma norepinephrine levels increase in response to acute hypoxemia, but decline to remain above basal levels with persistent (>5 minutes) hypoxemia. In contrast, adrenal epinephrine secretion begins gradually, but persists during 30 minutes of hypoxemia. These observations are consistent with independent sites of synthesis and regulation of the two catecholamines.[358] While the initial fetal blood pressure elevation during hypoxemia correlates with increases in norepinephrine, afterward, the correlation between plasma norepinephrine and hypertension is lost.[356]

Thyroid

The normal placenta is impermeable to thyroid-stimulating hormone (TSH), and triiodothyronine (T_3) transfer is minimal.[359] However, appreciable levels of maternal thyroxine (T_4) are seen in infants with congenital hypothyroidism.[360] By the 12th week of gestation, thyrotropin releasing hormone (TRH) is present in the fetal hypothalamus, and TRH secretion and/or pituitary sensitivity to TRH increases progressively during gestation. Extrahypothalamic sites including the pancreas also may contribute to the high TRH levels observed in the fetus.[359] Measurable TSH is present in the fetal pituitary and serum, and T_4 is measurable in fetal blood by week 12 of gestation. Thyroid function is low until about 20 weeks, when T_4 levels increase gradually to term. TSH levels increase markedly between 20 and 24 weeks, then slowly decrease until delivery. Fetal liver T_4 metabolism is immature, characterized by low T_3 levels until the 30th week. In contrast, reverse T_3 levels are high until 30 weeks, thereafter declining steadily until term.

Fetal Central Nervous System

Clinically relevant indicators of fetal central nervous system function are body movements and breathing movements. Fetal activity periods in late gestation are often termed active or reactive and quiet or nonreactive. The active cycle is characterized by clustering of gross fetal body movements, a high heart rate variability, heart rate accelerations (often followed by decelerations), and fetal breathing movements. The quiet cycle is noted by absence of fetal body movements and a low variability in the fetal heart period.[361,362] Fetal heart period variability in this context refers to deviations about the model heart rate period averaged over short (seconds) periods,[363] and is distinct from beat-to-beat variability. In the last 6 weeks of gestation, the fetus is in an active state 60 to 70 percent of total time. The average duration of quiet periods ranges from 15 to 23 minutes (see Table IV in Visser et al.[363] for a review).

The fetal electrocorticogram shows two predominant patterns. Low-voltage (high-frequency) electrocortical activity is associated with bursts of rapid eye movements and fetal breathing movements.[364] Similar to rapid eye movement sleep in the adult, inhibition of skeletal muscle movement is most pronounced in muscle groups having a high percentage of spindles. Thus, the diaphragm, which is relatively spindle free, is not affected. Fetal body movements during low-voltage electrocortical activity are reduced relative to the activity seen during high-voltage (low-frequency) electrocortical activity.[365] Polysynaptic reflexes elicited by stimulation of afferents from limb muscles are relatively suppressed when the fetus is in the low-voltage state.[366] Short-term hypoxia[365] or hypoxemia inhibit reflex limb movements, with the inhibitory neural activity arising in the midbrain area.[366] Fetal cardiovascular and behavioral responses to maternal cocaine use previously have been attributed to reductions in uteroplacental blood flow and resulting fetal hypoxia. However, recent fetal sheep studies indicate acute fetal cocaine exposure evokes catecholamine, cardiovascular, and neurobehavorial effects in the absence of fetal oxygenation changes.[367] It is not yet clear whether cocaine-induced reductions in fetal low-voltage electrocortical activity reflect changes in cerebral blood flow or a direct cocaine effect on norepinephrine stimulation of central regulatory centers. However, these observations are consistent with the significant neurologic consequences of cocaine use during pregnancy.

Fetal breathing patterns are rapid and irregular in nature, and are not associated with significant fluid movement into the lung.[364] The central medullary respiratory chemoreceptors are stimulated by carbon dioxide,[368] and fetal breathing is maintained only if central hydrogen ion concentrations remain in the physiologic range. That is, central (medullary cerebrospinal fluid) acidosis stimulates respiratory incidence and depth and alkalosis results in apnea.[369] Paradoxically, hypoxemia markedly decreases breathing activity, possibly due to inhibitory input from centers above the medulla.[370]

Glucose is the principal substrate for oxidative metabolism in the fetal brain under normal conditions.[371] During low-voltage electrocortical activity, cerebral blood flow and oxygen consumption are increased relative to high-voltage values,[372] with an efflux of lactate. During high voltage the fetal brain shows a net uptake of lactate.[373] The fetal cerebral circulation is sensitive to changes in arterial oxygen content. Despite marked hypoxia-induced increases in cerebral blood flow, cerebral oxygen consumption is maintained without widening of the arterial-venous oxygen content difference across the brain.[374] Increases in carbon dioxide also cause cerebral vasodilation. However, the response to hypercarbia is reduced relative to the adult.[375]

SUMMARY

The fetus and placenta depend upon unique physiologic systems to provide an environment supporting fetal growth and development, in preparation for transition to extrauterine life. Because specific functions of the various physiologic systems are often gestation specific, differences between the fetus and adult of one species are often larger than the differences between systems. Thus, the clinician or investigator concerned with fetal life or neonatal transition must fully appreciate these aspects of fetal physiology and their application to their area of study or treatment.

Key Points

➤ Pregnancy-associated cardiovascular changes include a doubling of maternal cardiac output and a 40 percent increase in blood volume.

➤ Uterine blood flow at term averages 750 ml/min, or 10 to 15 percent of maternal cardiac output.

➤ Normal term placental weight averages 450 g, representing approximately one seventh (one sixth with cord and membranes) of fetal weight.

➤ Mean amniotic fluid volume increases from 250 to 800 ml between 16 and 32 weeks, and decreases to 500 ml at term.

➤ Fetal urine production ranges from 400 to 1200 ml/day and is the primary source of amniotic fluid.

➤ The fetal umbilical circulation receives approximately 40 percent of fetal combined ventricular output (300 ml/mg/min).

➤ Umbilical blood flow is 70 to 130 ml/min after 30 weeks' gestation.

> ➤ Fetal cardiac output is constant over a heart rate range of 120 to 180 beats/min.

> ➤ The fetus exists in a state of aerobic metabolism, with arterial PO_2 values in the 20 to 25 mm Hg range.

> ➤ Approximately 20 percent of the fetal oxygen consumption of 8 ml/kg/min is required in the acquisition of new tissue.

REFERENCES

1. Chalier J-C, Schneider H, Dancis J: In vitro perfusion of human placenta. V. Oxygen consumption. Am J Obstet Gynecol 126:261, 1976.
2. Meschia G, Battaglia FC, Hay WW Jr, Sparks JW: Utilization of substrates by the ovine placenta in vivo. Fed Proc 39:245, 1980.
3. Hauguel S, Chalier J-C, Cedard L, Olive G: Metabolism of the human placenta perfused in vitro: glucose transfer and utilization, O2 consumption, lactate and ammomia production. Pediatr Res 17:729, 1983.
4. Teasdale F: Gestational changes in the functional structure of the human placenta in relation to fetal growth: a morphometric study. Am J Obstet Gynecol 137:560, 1980.
5. Holzman I, Phillips AF, Battaglia FC: Glucose metabolism, lactate and ammonia production by the human placenta in vitro. Pediatr Res 13:117, 1979.
6. Simmons MA, Battaglia FC, Meschia G: Placental transfer of glucose. J Dev Physiol 1:227, 1979.
7. Hay WW Jr, Myers SA, Sparks JW, et al: Glucose and lactate oxidation rates in the fetal lamb. Proc Soc Exp Biol Med 173:553, 1983.
8. Hay WW Jr, Sparks JW, Battaglia FC, Meschia G: Maternal-fetal glucose exchange: necessity of a three-pool model. Am J Physiol 246:E528, 1984.
9. Sparks JW, Hay WW Jr, Bonds D, et al: Simultaneous measurements of lactate turnover rate and umbilical lactate uptake in the fetal lamb. J Clin Invest 70:179, 1982.
10. Teasdale F: Gestational changes in the functional structure of the human placenta in relation to fetal growth: a morphometric study. Am J Obstet Gynecol 137:560, 1980.
11. Beischer NA, Holsman M, Kitchen WH: Relation of various forms of anemia to placental weight. Am J Obstet Gynecol 101:80, 1968.
12. Beischer NA, Sivasamboo R, Vohras S, et al: Placental hypertrophy in severe pregnancy anaemia. J Obstet Gynaecol Br Commonw 77:398, 1970.
13. Agboola A: Placental changes in patients with a low haematocrit. Br J Obstet Gynaecol 82:225, 1975.
14. Lao TT, Wong WM: The neonatal implications of a high placental ratio in small-for-gestational age infants. Placenta 20:723, 1999.
15. Barker DJ: The long-term outcome of retarded fetal growth. Clin Obstet Gynecol 40:853, 1997.
16. Gospodarowicz D: Growth factors and their action in vivo and in vitro. J Pathol 141:201, 1983.
17. Posner B: Insulin receptors in human and animal placental tissue. Diabetes 23:209, 1974.
18. Nelson DM, Smith RM, Jarett L: Nonuniform distribution and grouping of insulin receptors on the surface of human placental syncytial trophoblast. Diabetes 27:530, 1978.
19. Whitsett JA, Lenard JL: Characteristics of the microvillus brush border of human placenta: insulin receptor localization in brush border membranes. Endocrinology 103:1458, 1978.
20. Steel RB, Mosley JD, Smith CH: Insulin and placenta: degradation and stabilization, binding to microvillous membrane receptors, and amnio acid uptake. Am J Obstet Gynecol 135:522, 1979.
21. Deal CL, Guyda HJ: Insulin receptors of human term placental cells and choriocarcinoma (JEG-3) cells: characteristics and regulation. Endocrinology 112:1512, 1983.
22. Harrison LC, Itin A: Purification of the insulin receptor from human placenta by chromatography on immobilized wheat germ and receptor antibody. J Biol Chem 255:12066, 1980.
23. Richards RC, Beardmore JM, Brown PJ, et al: Epidermal growth factor receptors on isolated human placental syncytiotrophoblast plasma membrane. Placenta 4:133, 1983.
24. Lai WH, Guyda HJ: Characterization and regulation of epidermal growth factor receptors in human placental cell cultures. J Clin Endocrinol Metab 58:344, 1984.
25. Zhou J, Bondy CA: Insulin-like growth factor II and its binding proteins in placental development. Endocrinology 131:1230, 1992.
26. Holmes R, Porter H, Newcomb P, et al: An immunohistochemical study of type I insulin-like growth factor receptors in the placentae of pregnancies with appropriately grown or growth restricted fetuses. Placenta 20:325, 1999.
27. Fondacci C, Alsat E, Gabriel R, et al: Alterations of human placental epidermal growth factor receptor in intrauterine growth retardation. J Clin Invest 93:1149, 1994.
28. Zapf J, Rinderknecht E, Humbel RE, Froesch ER: Nonsuppressible insulin-like activity (NSILA) from human serum: recent accomplishments and their physiologic implications. Metab Clin Exp 27:1803, 1978.
29. Cooke NE, Ray J, Emery JG, Liebhaber SA: Two distinct species of human growth hormone-varient mRNA in the human placenta predict the expression of novel growth hormone proteins. J Biol Chem 263:9001, 1988.
30. Eriksson L, Frankenne F, Eden S, et al: Growth hormone secretion during termination of pregnancy. Further evidence of a placental variant. Acta Obstet Gynecol Scand 67:549, 1988.
31. Frankenne F, Closset J, Gomez F: The physiology of growth hormones (GHs) in pregnant women and partial characterization of the placental GH variant. J Clin Endocrinol Metab 66:1171, 1988.
32. Liu J-P, Baker J, Perkins AS, et al: Mice carrying null mutations of the genes encoding insulin-like growth factor I (Igf-l) and type I IGF receptor (Igflr). Cell 75:59, 1993.
33. Baker J, Liu J-P, Robertson EJ, Efstratiadis A: Role of insulin-like growth factors in embryonic and postnatal growth. Cell 75:73, 1993.
34. Lopez MF, Dikkes P, Zurakowski D, Villa-Komaroff L: Insulin-like growth factor II affects the appearance and glycogen content of glycogen cells in the murine placenta. Endocrinology 137:2100, 1996.
35. Wang ZQ, Fung MR, Barlow DP, Wagner EF: Regulation of embryonic growth and lysosomal targeting by the imprinted Igf2/Mpr gene. Nature 372:464, 1994.
36. Sibilia M, Wagner EF: Strain-dependent epithelial defects in mice lacking the EGF receptor. Science 269:234, 1995.
37. Threadgill DW, Dlugosz AA, Hansen LA, et al: Targeted disruption of mouse EGF reception: effect of genetic background on mutant phenotype. Science 269:230, 1995.
38. King BF: Distribution and characterization of the anionic sites

in trophoblast and capillary basal lamina of human placental villi. Anat Rec 212:63, 1985.

39. Leach L, Firth JA: Structure and permeability of human placental microvasculature. Microsc Res Tech 38:137, 1997.

40. Thornburg KL, Faber JJ: Transfer of hydrophilic molecules by placenta and yolk sac of the guinea pig. Am J Physiol 233: C111, 1977.

41. Bissonnette JM, Cronan JZ, Richards LL, Wickham WK: Placental transfer of water and nonelectrolytes during a single circulatory passage. Am J Physiol 236:C47, 1979.

42. Delivoria-Papadopoulos M, Coburn RF, Forster RE II: The placental diffusing capacity for carbon monixide in pregnant women at term. In Longo LD, Bartles H (eds): Respiratory Gas Exchange and Blood Flow in the Placenta. Bethesda MD, DHEW, 1972, p259.

43. Rooth G, Sjostedt S: The placental transfer of gases and fixed acids. Arch Dis Child 37:366, 1962.

44. Stenger V, Eitzman D, Anderson T, et al: Observations on the placental exchange of the respiratory gases in pregnant women in cesarean section. Am J Obstet Gynecol 88:45, 1964.

45. Sjostedt S, Rooth G, Caligara F: The oxygen tension of the blood in the umbilical cord and intervillous space. Arch Dis Child 35:529, 1960.

46. Wulf H: Der Gasaustausch in der reifen Plazenta des Menschen. Z Geburtsh Gynak 158:117, 1962.

47. Clapp JF III: The relationship between blood flow and oxygen uptake in the uterine and umbilical circulations. Am J Obstet Gynecol 132:410, 1978.

48. Wilkening RB, Meschia G: Fetal oxygen uptake, oxygenations, and acid-base balance as a function of uterine blood flow. Am J Physiol 244:H749, 1983.

49. Itskovitz J, LaGamma EF, Rudolph AM: Baroreflex control of the circulation in chronically instrumented fetal lambs. Circ Res 52:589, 1983.

50. Itskovitz J, LaGamma EF, Rudolph LAM: The effect of reducing umbilical blood flow on fetal oxygenation. Am J Obstet Gynecol 145:813, 1983.

51. Longo LD, Delivoria-Papadopoulos M, Foster RE II: Placental CO_2 transfer after fetal carbonic anhydrase inhibition. Am J Physiol 226:703, 1974.

52. Bissonnette JM: Studies in vivo of glucose transfer acorss the guinea-pig placenta. In Young M, Boyd RDH, Longo LD, Telegdy G (eds): Placental Transfer: Methods and Interpretations. Philadelphia, WB Saunders Company, 1981, p 155.

53. Johnson LW, Smith CH: Identification of the glucose transport protein of the microvillous membrane of human placenta by photoaffinity labeling. Biochem Biophys Res Common 109:408, 1982.

54. Ingermann RL, Bissonnette JM: Effect of temperature on kinetics of hexose uptake by human placental plasma membrane vesicles. Biochim Biophys Acta 734:329, 1983.

55. Ingermann RL, Bissonnette JM, Koch PL: D-Glucose-sensitive and-insensitive cytochalasin B binding proteins flora microvillous plasma membranes of human placenta: Identification of the D-glucose transporter. Biochim Biophys Acta 730:57, 1983.

56. Illsley NP, Sellers MC, Wright RL: Glycaemic regulation of glucose transporter expression and activity in the human placenta. Placenta 19:517, 1998.

57. Jansson T, Wennergreen M, Illsley P: Glucose transporter protein expression in human placenta throughout gestation and in intrauterine growth retardation. J Clin Endocrinol Metab 77:1554, 1993.

58. Turner RJ, Silverman M: Sugar uptake into brush border vesicles from normal human kidney. Proc Natl Acad Sci U S A 74:2825, 1977.

59. Wright EM, Loo DD, Panayotova-Heiermann M, et al: 'Active' sugar transport in eukaryotes. J Exp Biol 196:197, 1994.

60. Heilig CW, Brosius FC, Henry DN: Glucose transporters of the glomerulus and the implications for diabetic nephropathy. Kidney Int Suppl 60:S91, 1997.

61. Ciaraldi TP, Kolterman OE, Siegel JA, Olefsky JM: Insulin-stimulated glucose transport in human adipocytes. Am J Physiol 236:E621, 1979.

62. Charron MJ, Katz EB, Olson AL: GLUT4 gene regulation and manipulation. J Biol Chem 274:3253, 1999.

63. Livingstone C, Thomson FJ, Arbuckle MI, et al: Hormonal regulation of the insulin-responsive glucose transporter, GLUT4: some recent advances. Proc Nutr Soc 55:179, 1996.

64. Johnson LW, Smith CH: Monosaccharide transport across microvillous membrane of human placenta. Am J Physiol 236: E621, 1980.

65. Bissonnette JM, Ingermann RL, Thronburg KL: Placental sugar transport. In Yudilevich DL, Mann GE (eds): Carrier-Mediated Transport of Solutes from Blood to Tissue. London, Longman, 1985, p. 65.

66. Cordero L Jr, Yeh SY, Grunt JA, Anderson GG: Hypertonic glucose infusion during labor. Am J Obstet Gynecol 407:295, 1970.

67. Hahn T, Barth S, Graf R, et al: Placental glucose transporter expression is regulated by glucocorticoids. J Clin Endocrinol Metab 84:1445, 1999.

68. Hauguel-de Mouzon S, Challier JC, Kacemi A, et al: The GLUT3 glucose transporter isoform is differentially expressed within human placental cell types. J Clin Endocrinol Metab 82:2689, 1997.

69. Ruzycki SM, Kelly LK, Smith CH: Placental amino acid uptake. IV. Transport by microvillous membrane vesicles. Am J Physiol 234:C27, 1978.

70. Boyd CAR, Lund EK: L-Proline transport by brush border membrane vesicles prepared from human placenta. J Physiol 315:9, 1981.

71. Whitsett JA, Wallick ET: [3H] Oubain binding and Na+-K-ATpase activity in human placenta. Am J Physiol 238:E38, 1980.

72. Zerangue N, Kavanaugh MP: ASCT-1 is a neutral amino acid exchanger with chloride channel activity. J Biol Chem 271: 27991, 1996.

73. Chillaron J, Estevez R, Mora C, et al: Obligatory amino acid exchange via Systems $b^{o,+}$-like and y^+L-like. J Biol Chem 271: 17761, 1996.

74. Torres ZV, Leibach FH, Ganapathy V: Sodium-dependent homo- and hetero-exchange of neutral amino acids mediated by the amino acid transporter ATB degree. Biochem Biophys Res Commun 245:824, 1998.

75. Smith CH, Adcock EW, Teasdale F, et al: Placental amino acid uptake: tissue preparation, kinetics, and preincubation effect. Am J Physiol 224:558, 1973.

76. Smith CH, Depper R: Placental amino acid uptake. II. Tissue preincubation, fluid distribution and mechanisms of regulation. Pediatr Res 8:697, 1974.

77. Longo LD, Yuen P, Gusseck DJ: Anaerobic glycogen-dependent transport of amnio acids by the placenta. Nature 243: 531, 1973.

78. Karl PI, Alpy KL, Fisher SE: Amino acid transport by the cultured human placental trophoblast: effect of insulin on AIB transport. Am J Physiol 262:C834, 1993.

79. Karl PI: Insulin-like growth factor-1 stimulates amino acid uptake by the cultured human placental trophoblast. J Cell Physiol 165:83, 1995.

80. Karl PI, Fisher SE: Taurine transport by microvillous membrane vesicles and the perfused cotyledon of human placenta. Am J Physiol 258:C443, 1990.

81. Liu W, Leibach FH, Ganapathy V: Characterization of the glycine transport system GLYT 1 in human placental chorio-carcinoma cells (JAR). Biochim Biophys Acta 1194:176, 1994.

82. Johnson LW, Smith CH: Neutral amino acid transport systems of microvillous membrane of human placenta. Am J Physiol 254:C773, 1988.

83. Malandro MS, Beveridge MJ, Kilberg MS, Novak DA: Ontogeny of cationic amino acid transport systems in rat placenta. Am J Physiol 267:C804, 1994.

84. Novak DA, Beveridge MJ: Glutamine transport in human and rat placenta. Placenta 18:379, 1997.

85. Kamath SG, Furesz TC, Way BA, Smith CH: Identification of three cationic amino acid transporters in placental trophoblast: cloning, expression, and characterization of hCAT-1. J Membr Biol 171:55, 1999.

86. Furesz TC, Moe AJ, Smith CH: Lysine uptake by human placental microvillous membrane: comparison of system y+ with basal membrane. Am J Physiol 268:C755, 1995.

87. Matthews JC, Beveridge MJ, Malandro MS, et al: Activity and protein localization of multiple glutamate transporters in gestation-days-14 vs. -20 rat placenta. Am J Physiol 274:C603, 1998.

88. Moores RR, Vaughn PR, Battaglia FC, et al: Glutamate metabolism in fetus and placenta of late-gestation sheep. Am J Physiol 267:R89, 1994.

89. Vaughn PR, Lobo C, Battaglia FC, et al: Glutamine-glutamate exchage between placenta and fetal liver. Am J Physiol 268:705, 1995.

90. Cetin I, Fennessey PV, Quick AN Jr, et al: Glycine turnover and oxidation, and hepatic serine synthesis from glycine in fetal lambs. Am J Physiol 260:E371, 1991.

91. Glazier JD, Cetin I, Perugino G, et al: Association between the activity of the system A amino acid transporter in the microvillous plasma membrane of the human placenta and severity of fetal compromise in intrauterine growth restriction. Pediatr Res 42:514, 1997.

92. Harrington B, Glazier JD, D'Souza SW, Sibley CP: System A amino acid transporter activity in human placenta microvillous membrane vesicles in relation to various anthropometric measurements in appropiate (AGA) and small for gestational age (SGA) babies. Pediatr Res 45:810, 1999.

93. Kuruvilla AG, D'Souza SW, Glazier JD, et al: Altered activity of the System A amino acid transporter in microvillous membrane vesicles from placentas of macrosomic babies born to diabetic women. J Clin Invest 94:689, 1994.

94. Dancis J, Jansen V, Kayden HJ, et al: Transfer across perfused human placenta. II. Free fatty acids. Pediatr Res 7:192, 1972.

95. Booth C, Elphick MC, Hentrickse W, Hull D: Investigation of [14C] linoleic acid conversion into [14C] arachidonic acid and placental transfer of linoleic and palmitic acids across the perfused human placenta. J Dev Physiol 3:177, 1981.

96. Campbell FM, Dutta RA: Plasma membrane fatty acid-binding protein (FABPpm) is exclusively located in the maternal facing membranes of the human placenta. FEBS Lett 375:227, 1995.

97. Campbell FM, Bush PG, Veerkamp JH, Dutta RA: Detection and cellular localization of plasma membrane-associated and cytoplasmic fatty acid-binding proteins in human placenta. Placenta 19:409, 1998.

98. Dancis J, Jansen V, Kayden HJ, et al: Transfer across perfused human placenta 3. Effect of chain length on transfer of free fatty acids. Pediatr Res 8:796, 1974.

99. Dancis J, Jansen V, Levitz M: Transfer across perfused human placenta. IV. Effect of protein binding on free fatty acids. Pediatr Res 10:5, 1976.

100. Honda M, Lowy C, Thomas CR: The effects of maternal diabetes on placental transfer of essential and non-essential fatty acids in the rat. Diabetes Res 15:47, 1990.

101. Haggarty P, Page K, Abramovich DR, et al: Long-chain polyunsaturated fatty acid transport across the perfused human placenta. Placenta 18:635, 1997.

102. Stammers J, Stephenson T, Colley J, Hull D: Effect on placental transfer of exogenous lipid administered to the pregnant rabbit. Pediatr Res 38:1026, 1995.

103. Faber JJ, Thomburg KL: Fetal homeostatis in relation to placental water exchange. Ann Rech Vet 8:353, 1977.

104. Dancis J, Kammerman BS, Jansen V, et al: Transfer of urea, sodium, and chloride across the perfused human placenta. Am J Obstet Gynecol 141:677, 1981.

105. Faber JJ, Thornburg KL: Placental Physiology. New York, Raven Press, 1983, p 95

106. Faber JJ, Thornburg KL: The forces that drive inert solutes and water across the epitheliochorial placentae of the sheep and the goat and the haemochorial placentae of the rabbit and the guinea pig. In Young M, Boyd RDH, Longo LD, Teleydy G (eds): Placental Transfer: Methods and Interpretations. Philadelphia, WB Saunders Company, 1981, p 203.

107. Battaglia F: Fetal blood studies: XIII. The effect of the administration of fluids intravenously to mothers upon the concentrations of water and electrolytes in plasma of human fetuses. Pediatrics 25:2, 1960.

108. Reynolds SRM: Multiple simultaneous intervillous space pressures recorded in several regions of the hemochorial placenta in relation to functional anatomy of the fetal cotyledon. Am J Obstet Gynecol 102:1128, 1968.

109. Seeds AE: Water metabolism in the fetus. Am J Obstet Gynecol 92:727, 1965.

110. Anderson DF, Faber JJ: Water flux due to colloid osmotic pressures across the haemochorial placenta of the guinea pig. J Physiol 332:521, 1982.

111. Ma T, Yang B, Verkman AS: Cloning of a novel water and urea-permeable aquaporin from mouse expressed strongly in colon, placenta, liver, and heart. Biochem Biophys Res Commun 240:324, 1997.

112. Hasegawa H, Lian SC, Finkbeiner WE, Verkman AS: Extrarenal tissue distribution of CHIP28 water channels by in situ hybridization and antibody staining. Am J Physiol 266:C893, 1994.

113. Stulc J: Placental transfer of inorganic ions and water. Physiol Rev 77:805–836, 1997.

114. Moe AJ: Placental amino acid transport. Am J Physiol 268:C1321, 1995.

115. Lajeunesse D, Brunette MG: Sodium gradient-dependent phosphate transport in placental brush border membrane vesicles. Placenta 9:117, 1988.

116. Balkovetz DF, Leibach FH, Mahesh VB, et al: Na+-H+ exchanger of human placental brush-border membrane: identification and characterization. Am J Physiol 251:C852, 1986.

117. Wang H, Huang W, Fei YJ, et al: Human placental Na+-dependent multivitamin transporter. Cloning, functional expression, gene structure, and chromosomal localization. J Biol Chem 274:14875, 1999.

118. Prasad PD, Ramamoorthy S, Leibach FH, Ganapathy V: Characterization of a sodium-dependent vitamin transporter mediating the uptake of pantothenate, biotin and lipoate in human placental choriocarcinoma cells. Placenta 18:527, 1997.

119. Bara M, Challier JC, Guit-Bara A: Membrane potential and input resistance in syncytiotrophoblast of human term placenta in vitro. Placenta 9:139, 1988.

120. Powell TL, Lundquist C, Doughty IM, et al: Mechanisms of

chloride transport across the syncytiotrophoblast basal membrane in the human placenta. Placenta 19:315, 1998.

121. Doughty IM, Glazier JD, Greenwood SL, et al: Mechanisms of materno fetal chloride transfer across the human placenta perfused in vitro. Am J Physiol 271:R1701, 1996.

122. Doughty IM, Glazier JD, Powell TL, et al: Chloride transport across syncytiotrophoblast microvillous membrane of first trimester human placenta. Pediatr Res 44:226, 1998.

123. Care AD, Ross R, Pickard DW, et al: Calcium homeostasis in the fetal pig. J Dev Physiol 4:85, 1982.

124. Fisher GJ, Kelly LK, Smith CH: ATP-dependent calcium transport across basal plasma membranes of human placental trophoblast. Am J Physiol 252:C38, 1987.

125. Borke JL, Caride A, Verma AK, et al: Calcium pump epitopes in placental trophoblast basal plasma membrane. Am J Physiol 257:C341, 1989.

126. Brunette MG, Leclerc M: Ca2+ transport through the brush border membrane of human placenta syncytiotrophoblasts. Can J Physiol Pharmacol 70:835, 1992.

127. Kamath SG, Kelley LK, Friedman AF, Smith CH: Transport and binding in calcium uptake by microvillous membrane of human placenta. Am J Physiol 262:C789, 1992.

128. Kamath SG, Haider N, Smith CH: ATP independent calcium transport and binding by basal plasma membrane of human placenta. Placenta 15:147, 1994.

129. Kamath SG, Smith CH: Na+/Ca2+ exchange, Ca2+ binding, and electrogenic Ca2+ transport in plasma membranes of human placental syncytiotrophoblast. Pediatr Res 36:461, 1994.

130. Tuan RS: Identification and characterization of a calcium-binding protein from human placenta. Placenta 3:145, 1982.

131. Hershberger ME, Tuan RS: Placental 57-kDa Ca(2+)-binding protein: regulation of expression and function in trophoblast calcium transport. Dev Biol 199:80, 1998.

132. Wyne KL, Woollett LA: Transport of maternal LDL and HDL to the fetal membranes and placenta of the golden Syrian hamster is mediated by receptor-dependent and receptor-independent processes. J Lipid Res 39:518, 1998.

133. Grimes RW, Pepe GJ, Albrecht ED: Regulation of human placental trophoblast low-density lipoprotein uptake in vitro by estrogen. J Clin Endocrinol Metab 81:2675, 1996.

134. Wild AE: Trophoblast cell surface receptors. In Loke YW, Whyte A (eds): Biology of the Trophoblast. London, Elsevier Biomedical Press, 1983.

135. Douglas GC, King BF: Uptake and processing of 125I-labelled transferrin and 59Fe-labelled transferrin by isolated human trophoblast cells. Placenta 11:41, 1990.

136. van Dijk JP, Bierings MB, van der Zande FG: An investigation of placental transferrin processing: influence of N-ethylmaleimide. J Dev Physiol 14:49, 1990.

137. Loh TT, Higuchi DA, van Bockxmeer FM: Transferrin receptors on the human placental microvillus membrane. J Clin Invest 65:1182, 1980.

138. Ellinger I, Schwab M, Stefanescu A, et al: IgG transport across trophoblast-derived BeWo cells: a model system to study IgG transport in the placenta. Eur J Immunol 29:733, 1999.

139. Bright NA, Ockleford CD, Anwar M: Ontogeny and distribution of Fc gamma receptors in the human placenta. Transport or immune surveillance? J Anat 184:297, 1994.

140. Brown MA, Anderson RGW, Goldstein JL: Recycling receptors: the round trip itinerary of migrant membrane proteins. Cell 32:663, 1983.

141. Goldstein JL, Anderson RGW, Brown MS: Coated pits, coated vesicles and receptor-mediated endocytosis. Nature 279:679, 1979.

142. Pastan IH, Willingham MC: Journey to the center of the cell: role of the receptosome. Science 214:504, 1981.

143. Dautry-Varsat A, Cierchanover A, Lodish HF: pH and the recycling of transferin during receptor-mediated endocytosis. Proc Natl Acad Sci U S A 80:2258, 1983.

144. Woollet LA: Origin of cholesterol in the fetal golden Syrian hamster: contribution of de novo sterol synthesis and maternal-derived lipoprotein cholesterol. J Lipid Res 37:1246, 1996.

145. Lin DS, Pitkin RM, Connor WE: Placental transfer of cholesterol into the human fetus. Am J Obstet Gynecol 128:735, 1977.

146. Sooranna SR, Moss J, Contractor SF: Comparison of the intracellular pathways of immunoglobulin-G and low density lipoprotein in cultured human term trophoblast cells. Cell Tissue Res 274:619, 1993.

147. Rosenfeld CR: Circulatory changes in the reproductive tissues of ewes during pregnancy. Gynecol Invest 5:252, 1974.

148. Longo LD, Ching KS: Placental diffusing capacity for carbon monoxide and oxygen in unanesthetized sheep. J Appl Physiol 43:885, 1977.

149. Bissonnette JM, Wickham WK: Placental diffusing capacity for carbon monoxide in unanesthetized guinea pigs. Respir Physiol 31:161, 1977.

150. Rosenfeld CR, Cox BE, Roy T, Magness RR: Nitric oxide contributes to estrogen-induced vasodilation of the ovine uterine circulation. J Clin Invest 98:2158, 1996.

151. Assali NS, Douglas RA, Barid WW, et al: Measurement of uterine blood flow and uterine metabolism. Am J Obstet Gynecol 66:248, 1953.

152. Metcalfe J, Romney SL, Ramsey LH, et al: Estimation of uterine blood flow and uterine metabolism. J Clin Invest 34:1632, 1995.

153. Lumbers ER: Effects of drugs on uteroplacental blood flow and the health of the foetus. Clin Exp Pharmacol Physiol 24:864, 1997.

154. Rosenfeld CR, Naden RP: Responses of uterine and nonuterine tissues to angiotensin II in ovine pregnancy. Am J Physiol 257:H17, 1995.

155. Meschia G: Circulation to female reproductive organs. In Shepherd JT, Abboud FM (eds): Handbook of Physiology—The Cardiovascular System III. Peripheral Circulation and Organ Blood Flow. Bethesda, MD, American Physiological Society, 1983.

156. Hendricks CH, Quilligan EJ, Tyler CW, Tucker CJ: Pressure relationships between the intervillous space and the amniotic fluid in human term pregnancy. Am J Obstet Gynecol 77:1028, 1959.

157. Rudolph AM, Heymann MA: Circulatory changes during growth in the fetal lamb. Circ Res 26:289, 1970.

158. Wladimiroff JW, McGhie J: Ultrasonic assessment of cardiovascular geometry and function in the human fetus. Br J Obstet Gynecol 88:870, 1981.

159. Makowski EL, Meschia G, Droegemueller W, Battaglia FC: Measurement of umbilical arterial blood flow to the sheep placenta and fetus in utero. Circ Res 23:623, 1968.

160. Berman W Jr, Goodlin RC, Heymann MA, Rudolph AM: Relationships between pressure and flow in the umbilical and uterine circulations of the sheep. Circ Res 38:262, 1976.

161. Barbera A, Galan HL, Ferrazzi E, et al: Relationship of umbilical vein blood flow to growth parameters in the human fetus. Am J Obstet Gynecol 181:174, 1999.

162. Athanassiades A, Lala PK: Role of placenta growth factor (PIGF) in human extravillous trophoblast proliferation, migration and invasiveness. Placenta 19:465, 1998.

163. Cheung CY, Brace RA: Developmental expression of vascular

endothelial growth factor and its receptors in ovine placenta and fetal membranes. J Soc Gynecol Invest 6:179, 1999.

164. Thornburg KL, Bissonnette JM, Faber JJ: Absence of fetal placental waterfall phenomenon in chronically prepared fetal lambs. Am J Physiol 230:886, 1976.

165. Cohn HE, Piasecki GJ, Jackson BT: The effect of fetal heart rate on cardiovascular function during hypoxemia. Am J Obstet Gynecol 138:1190, 1980.

166. Cohn HE, Sacks EJ, Heymann MA, Rudolph AM: Cardiovascular responses to hypoxemia and acidemia in fetal lambs. Am J Obstet Gynecol 120:817, 1974.

167. Parer JT: Fetal oxygen uptake and umbilical circulation during maternal hypoxia in the chronically catheterized sheep. In Longo LD, Reneau DD (eds): Fetal and Newborn Cardiovascular Physiology, Vol 2. New York, Garland STPM Press, 1978, p 231.

168. Peeters LLH, Sheldon RE, Jones MD Jr, et al: Blood flow to fetal organs as a function of arterial oxygen content. Am J Obstet Gynecol 135:637, 1979.

169. Gude NM, King RG, Brennecke SP: Autacoid interactions in the regulation of blood flow in the human placenta. Clin Exp Pharmacol Physiol 25:706, 1998.

170. Boura AL, Walters WA, Read MA, Leitch IM: Autacoids and control of human placental blood flow. Clin Exp Pharmacol Physiol 21:737, 1994.

171. Galbraith RM, Kantor RRS, Ferra GB, et al: Differential anatomical expression of transplantation antigens within the normal human placental chorionic villus. Am J Reprod Immunol 1:331, 1981.

172. Ober C, van der Ven K: Immunogenetics of reproduction: an overview. Curr Top Microbiol Immunol 222:1, 1997.

173. Lebouteiller P: HLA-G: what's new? Am J Reprod Immunol 38:146, 1997.

174. Hammer A, Hutter H, Dohr G: HLA class I expression on the materno-fetal interface. Am J Reprod Immunol 38:150, 1997.

175. Sunderland CA, Redman CWG, Stirrat GM: HLA A,B,C antigens are expressed on nonvillous trophoblast of the early human placenta. J Immunol 127:2614, 1981.

176. Faulk WP, Hsi B-L: Immunology of human trophoblast membrane antigens. In Loke YW, Whyte A (eds): Biology of Trophoblast. New York, Elsevier, 1983, p 535.

177. Szulman AE: The ABH blood groups and development. Curr Top Dev Biol 14:127, 1980.

178. Faulk WP: Immunobiology of human extraembryonic membranes. In Wegman TG, Gill TJ (eds): Immunology of Reproduction. New York, Oxford University Press, 1983, p 253.

179. Klopper A: The new placental proteins. Placenta 1:77, 1980.

180. Rocklin RE, Kitzmiller JL, Farvoy MR: Maternal fetal relation. II. Further characterization of an immunologic blocking factor that develops during pregnancy. Clin Immunol Immunopathol 22:305, 1982.

181. Beer AE: Immunologic aspects of normal pregnancy and recurrent spontaneous abortion. Semin Reprod Endocinol 6:163, 1988.

182. Taylor C, Faulk WP: Prevention of recurrent abortions with leukocyte transfusions. Lancet 2:68, 1980.

183. Beer AE, Quebberman JF, Ayers JW, Haines RF: Major histocompatibility antigens maternal and paternal immune responses and chronic habitual abortion in humans. Am J Obstet Gynecol 141:987, 1981.

184. Komlos L, Zamir R, Joshua H, Halbrecht I: Common HLA antigens in couples with repeated abortions. Clin Immunol Immunopathol 7:330, 1977.

185. Redline RW, Lu CY: Role of local immunosuppression in murine fetoplacental listerosis. J Clin Invest 79:1234, 1987.

186. Jacoby DR, Olding LB, Oldstone MD: Immunologic regulation of fetal-maternal balance. Adv Immunol 35:157, 1984.

187. Torry DS, McIntyre JA, Faulk WP: Immunobiology of the trophoblast: mechanisms by which placental tissues evade maternal recognition and rejection. Curr Top Microbiol Immunol 222:127, 1997.

188. Brace RA, Wolf EJ: Normal amniotic fluid volume changes throughout pregnancy. Am J Obstet Gynecol 161:382, 1989.

189. Anderson DF, Faber JJ, Parks CM: Extraplacental transfer of waters in the sheep. J Physiol 406:75, 1988.

190. Mesher EJ, Platzker AC, Ballard PL, et al: Ontogeny of tracheal fluid, pulmonary surfactant, and plasma corticoids in the fetal lamb. J Appl Physiol 39:1017, 1975.

191. Olver RE, Schneeberger EE, Walters DV: Epithelial solute premeability, ion transport and tight junction morphology in the developing lung of the fetal lamb. J Physiol 315:395, 1981.

192. Adamson TM, Boyd RDH, Platt HS, Strang LB: Composition of alveolar liquid in the foetal lamb. J Physiol 204:159, 1969.

193. Walters DV, Olver RE: The role of catecholamines in lung fluid absorption at birth. Pediatr Res 12:239, 1978.

194. Perks AM, Cassin S: The effects of arginine vasopressin on lung fluid secretion in chronic fetal sheep. In Jones CT, Nathanielsz PW (eds): The Physiological Development of the Fetus and Newborn. London, Academic Press, 1985, p 252.

195. Castro R, Ervin MG, Ross MG, et al: Ovine fetal lung fluid response to atrial natriuretic factor. Am J Obstet Gynecol 161:1337, 1989.

196. Gresham EL, Rankin JHG, Makowski EL, et al: An evaluation of fetal renal function in a chronic sheep preparation. J Clin Invest 51:149, 1977.

197. Rabinowitz R, Peters MT, Vyas S, et al: Measurement of fetal urine production in normal pregnancy by real-time ultrasonography. Am J Obstet Gynecol 161:1264, 1939.

198. Canning JF, Boyd RDH: Mineral and water exchange between mother and fetus. In Beard RW, Nathanielsz PW (eds): Fetal Physiology and Medicine. New York, Marcel Dekker, 1984, p 481.

199. Robillard JE, Weitzman RE: Developmental aspects of the fetal renal response to exogenous arginine vasopressin. Am J Physiol 238:F407, 1980.

200. Lingwood B, Hardy KJ, Coghlan JP, Wintour EM: Effect of aldosterone on urine composition in the chronically cannulated ovine fetus. J Endocrinol 76:553, 1978.

201. Harding R, Bocking AD, Sigger JN, Wickham PJD: Composition and volume of fluid swallowed by sheep. Q J Exp Physiol 69:487, 1984.

202. Pritchard JA: Deglutition of normal and anencephalic fetuses. Obstet Gynecol 25:289, 1965.

203. Pritchard JA: Fetal swallowing and amniotic fluid volume. Obstet Gynecol 28:606, 1966.

204. Bradley RM, Mistretta CM: Swallowing in fetal sheep. Science 179:1016, 1973.

205. Harding R, Bocking AD, Sigger JN, Wickham PJD: Composition and volume of fluid swallowed by fetal sheep. Q J Exp Physiol 69:487, 1984.

206. Abramovich DR: Fetal factors influencing the volume and composition of liquor amnii. Br J Obstet Gynaecol 77:865, 1970.

207. Harding R, Sigger JN, Poore ER, Johnson P: Ingestion in fetal sheep and its relation to sleep states and breathing movements. Q J Exp Physiol 69:477, 1984.

208. Ross MG, Sherman DJ, Ervin MG, et al: Stimuli for fetal swallowing: systemic factors. Am J Obstet Gynecol 161:1559, 1989.

209. Abramovich DR, Page KR, Jandial L: Bulk flows through human fetal membranes. Gynecol Invest 7:157, 1976.

210. Gilbert WM, Brace RA: The missing link in amniotic fluid volume regulation: intramembranous flow. Obstet Gynecol 74:748, 1989.

211. Kalhan SC, D'Angelo LJ, Savin SM, Adam PAJ: Glucose production in pregnant women at term gestation: sources of glucose for human fetus. J Clin Invest 63:388, 1979.

212. Morris FH Jr, Makowski EL, Meschia G, Battaglia FC: The glucose/oxygen quotient of the term human fetus. Biol Neonate 25:44, 1975.

213. Hay WW Jr, Myers SA, Sparks JW, et al: Glucose and lactate oxidation rates in the fetal lamb. Proc Soc Exp Biol Med 173:553, 1983.

214. Lemons JA, Schreiner RL: Amino acid metabolism in the ovine fetus. Am J Physiol 244:E459, 1983.

215. Widdowson EH, Spray CM: Chemical development in utero. Arch Dis Child 26:205, 1951.

216. Warshaw JB: Fatty acid metabolism during development. Semin Perinataol 3:31, 1979.

217. Schoenle E, Zopf J, Humbel RE, Groesch ER: Insulin-like growth factor I stimulates growth in hypophysectomized rats. Nature 296:252, 1982.

218. Jost A: Fetal hormones and fetal growth. Contrib Gynecol Obstet 5:1, 1979.

219. Gluckman PD, Liggins GC: Regulation of fetal growth. *In* Beard RW, Nathanielsz PW (eds): Fetal Physiology and Medicine. New York, Marcel Dekker, 1984, p 511.

220. Gluckman PD: Functional maturation of the neuroendocrine system in the perinatal period: studies of the somatotrophic axis in the ovine fetus. J Dev Physiol 6:301, 1984.

221. Palmiter RD, Norstedt G, Gelinas RE, et al: Metallothionein–human GH fusion genes stimulate growth of mice. Science 222:809, 1983.

222. Browne CA, Thorburn CA: Endocrine control of fetal growth. Biol Neonate 55:331, 1989.

223. D'Ercole AJ, Stiles AD, Underwood LE: Tissue concentration of somatomedin C: further evidence for multiple sites of synthesis and paracrine or autocrine mechanism of action. Proc Natl Acad Sci U S A 81:935, 1984.

224. King GL, Kahn CR, Rechler MM, Nissley SP: Direct demonstration of separate receptors for growth and metabolic activities of insulin and multiplication stimulating activity (an insulin-like growth factor) using antibodies to the insulin receptor. J Clin Invest 66:130, 1980.

225. Bennett A, Wilson DM, Liu F, et al: Levels of insulin-like growth factors I and II in human cord blood. J Clin Endocrinol Metab 57:609, 1983.

226. Adams SO, Nissley SP, Handwerger S, Rechler MM: Developmental patterns of insulin-like growth factor I and II synthesis and regulation in rat fibroblasts. Nature 302:150, 1983.

227. Hill DE: Fetal effects of insulin. Obstet Gynecol Ann 11:133, 1982.

228. Susa JG, Gruppuso PA, Widness JA, et al: Chronic hyperinsulinemia in the fetal rhesus monkey: effects of physiologic hyperinsulinemia on fetal substrates, hormones, and hepatic enzymes. Am J Obstet Gynecol 150:415, 1984.

229. Philips AF, Dubin JW, Raye JR: Fetal metabolic responses to endogenous insulin release. Am J Obstet Gynecol 139:441, 1981.

230. Hay WW, Meznarich HK, Sparks JW, et al: Effect of insulin on glucose uptake in near-term fetal lambs. Proc Soc Exp Biol Med 78:557, 1985.

231. Oppenheimer CL, Pessin JE, Massague J, et al: Insulin action rapidly modulates the apparent affinity of the insulin-like growth factor II receptor. J Biol Chem 258:4824, 1983.

232. Sara VR, Hall K, Misaki M, et al: Ontogenesis of somatomedin and insulin receptors in the human fetus. J Clin Invest 71:1084, 1983.

233. Cardell BS: The infants of diabetic mothers; a morphological study. J Obstet Gynaecol Br Commonw 60:834, 1953.

234. Siddiqi TA, Miodovnik M, Mimouni F, et al: Biphasic intrauterine growth in insulin-dependent diabetic pregnancies. J Am Coll Nutr 8:225, 1989.

235. Fowden AL, Comline RS: The effects of pancreatectomy on the sheep fetus in utero. Q J Exp Physiol 69:319, 1984.

236. Fowden AL, Hay WW Jr: The effects of pancreatectomy on the rates of glucose utilization, oxidation and production in the sheep fetus. Q J Exp Physiol 73:973, 1988.

237. Fowden AL: The role of insulin in fetal growth. J Dev Physiol 12:173, 1989.

238. Sperling MA, Christensen RA, Ganguli S, Anand R: Adrenergic modulation of pancreatic hormone secretion in utero: studies in fetal sheep. Pediatr Res 14:203, 1980.

239. Jones CT, Ritchie JWK, Walker D: The effects of hypozia on glucose turnover in the fetal sheep. J Dev Physiol 5:223, 1983.

240. Devaskar SU, Ganuli S, Styer D, et al: Glucagon and glucose dynamics in sheep: evidence for glucagon resistance in the fetus. Am J Physiol 246:E256, 1984.

241. Gospodarowicz D: Epidermal and nerve growth factors in mammalian development. Annu Rev Physiol 43:251, 1981.

242. Jouppila P, Kirkinen P, Eik-Nes S, Koivula A: Fetal and intervillouos blood flow measurements in late pregnancy. *In* Kurjak A, Kratochwil A (eds): Recent Advances in Ultrasound Diagnosis. Amsterdam, Excerpta Medica, 1981, p 226.

243. Rudolph AM: Hepatic and ductus venosus blood flows during fetal life. Hepatology 3:254, 1983.

244. Anderson DF, Bissonnette JM, Faber JJ, Thornburg KL: Central shunt flows and pressures in the mature fetal lamb. Am J Physiol 241:H60, 1981.

245. Wladimiroff JW, McGhie J: Ultrasonic assessment of cardiovascular geometry and function in the human fetus. Br J Obstet Gynaecol 88:870, 1981.

246. Rudolph AM, Heymann MA: Circulatory changes during growth in the fetal lamb. Circ Res 26:289, 1970.

247. Paton JB, Fisher DE, Peterson EN: Cardiac output and organ blood flows in the baboon fetus. Biol Neonate 22:50, 1973.

248. Edelstone DI, Rudolph AM, Heymann MA: Liver and ductus venosus blood flows in fetal lambs in utero. Circ Res 42:426, 1978.

249. Thornburg KL, Morton MJ: Filling and arterial pressures as determinants of RV stroke volume in the sheep fetus. Am J Physiol 244:H656, 1983.

250. Pinson CW, Morton MJ, Thornburg KL: An anatomic basis for right ventricular dominance and arterial pressure sensitivity. J Dev Physiol 9:253, 1987.

251. Thornburg KL, Morton MG: Filling and arterial pressures as determinants of left ventricular stroke volume in fetal lambs. Am J Physiol 251:H961, 1986.

252. Cheng JB, Goldfien A, Cornett LE, Roberts JM: Identification of β-adrenergic receptors using [3H] dihydroalprenolol in fetal sheep heart: direct evidence of qualitative similarity to the receptors in adult sheep heart. Pediatr Res 15:1083, 1981.

253. Andersen PAW, Manning A, Glick KL, Crenshaw CC Jr: Biophysics of the developing heart. III. A comparison of the left ventricular dynamics of the fetal and neontal heart. Am J Obstet Gynecol 143:195, 1982.

254. Fisher DJ, Heymann MA, Rudolph AM: Regional myocardial blood flow and oxygen delivery in fetal, newborn and adult sheep. Am J Physiol 243:H729, 1982.

255. Fisher DJ, Heymann MA, Rudolph AM: Myocardial oxygen and carbohydrate consumption in fetal lambs in utero and in adult sheep. Am J Physiol 238:H399, 1980.

256. Werner JC, Sicard RE, Schuler HG: Palmitate oxidation by

isolated working fetal and newborn hearts. Am J Physiol 256: E315, 1989.

257. Visser GHA, Dawes GS, Redman CWG: Numerical analysis of the normal human antenatal fetal heart rate. Br J Obstet Gynaecol 88:792, 1981.

258. Patrick J, Campbell K, Carmichael L, Probert C: Influence of maternal heart rate and gross fetal body movements on the daily pattern of fetal heart rate near term. Am J Obstet Gynecol 144:533, 1992.

259. Bocking AD, Harding R, Wickham PJ: Relationship between accelerations and decelerations in heart rate and skeletal muscle activity in fetal sheep. J Dev Physiol 7:47, 1985.

260. Kenny J, Plappert T, Doubilet P, et al: Effects of heart rate on ventricular size, stroke volume, and output in the normal human fetus; a prospective Doppler echocardiographic study. Circulation 76:52, 1987.

261. Anderson PAW, Glick KL, Killam AP, Mainwaring RD: The effect of heart rate on in utero left ventricular output in the fetal sheep. J Physiol 372:557, 1986.

262. Anderson PAW, Killam AP, Mainwaring RD, Oakley AK: In utero right ventricular output in the fetal lamb: the effect of heart rate. J Physiol 387:297, 1987.

263. Nuwayhid B, Brinkman CR III, Su C, et al: Development of autonomic control of fetal circulation. Am J Physiol 228:337, 1975.

264. Assali NS, Brinkman CR III, Woods JR Jr, et al: Development of neurohumoral control of fetal, neonatal, and adult cardiovascular functions. Am J Obstet Gynecol, 129:748, 1977.

265. Walker AM, Cannata J, Dowling MH, et al: Sympathetic and parasympathetic control of heart rate in unanaesthetized fetal and newborn lambs. Biol Neonate 33:135, 1978.

266. Dalton KJ, Dawes GS, Patrick JE: The autonomic nervous system and fetal heart rate variability. Am J Obstet Gynecol 146:456, 1983.

267. Tabsh K, Nuwayhid B, Murad S, et al: Circulatory effects of chemical sympathectomy in fetal, neonatal and adult sheep. Am J Physiol 243:H113, 1982.

268. Jones CT, Roeback MM, Walker DW, et al: Cardiovascular, metabolic and endocrine effects of chemical sympathectomy and of adrenal demedullation in fetal sheep. J Dev Physiol 9: 347, 1987.

269. Cohn HE, Sacks EJ, Heymann MA, Rudolph AM: Cardiovascular responses in hypoxemia and acidemia in fetal lambs. Am J Obstet Gynecol 120:817, 1974.

270. Peeters LLH, Sheldon RE, Jones MD Jr, et al: Blood flow to fetal organs as a function of arterial oxygen content. Am J Obstet Gynecol 135:637, 1979.

271. Iwamoto HS, Rudolph AM, Miskin BL, Keil LC: Circulatory and humoral responses of sympathectomized fetal sheep to hypoxemia. Am J Physiol 245:H767, 1983.

272. Schuijers JA, Walkere DW, Browne CA, Thorburn GD: Effect of hypoxemia on plasma catecholamines in intact and immunosympathectomized fetal lambs. Am J Physiol 251:R893, 1986.

273. Shinebourne EA, Vapaavuori EK, Williams RL, et al: Development of baroreflex activity in unanesthetized fetal and neonatal lambs. Circ Res 31:710, 1972.

274. Dawes GS, Johnston BM, Walker DW: Relationship of arterial pressure and heart rate in fetal, newborn and adult sheep. J Physiol 309:405, 1980.

275. Itskovitz J, LaGamma EF, Rudolph AM: Baroreflex control of the circulation in chronically instrumented fetal lambs. Circ Res 52:589, 1983.

276. Yardley RW, Bowes G, Wilkinson M, et al: Increased arterial pressure variability after arterial baroreceptor denervation in fetal lambs. Circ Res 52:580, 1983.

277. Rudolph AM: The fetal circulation and its response to stress. J Dev Physiol 6:11, 1984.

278. Skowsky WR, Fisher DA: Fetal neurohypophysial arginine vasopressin and arginine vasotocin in man and sheep. Pediatr Res 11:627, 1977.

279. Weitzman RE, Fisher DA, Robillard JE, et al: AVP response to an osmotic stimulus in the fetal sheep. Pediatr Res 121:35, 1978.

280. Leake RD, Weitzman RE, Effros RM, et al: Maternal fetal osmolar homeostasis: fetal posterior pituitary autonomy. Pediatr Res 13:841, 1978.

281. Ervin MG, Ross MG, Youseff A, et al: Renal effects of ovine fetal arginine vasopressin secretion in response to maternal hyperosmolality. Am J Obstet Gynecol 155:1341, 1986.

282. Ross MG, Sherman DG, Ervin MG, et al: Maternal dehydration/rehydration: fetal plasma and urinary responses. Am J Physiol E674, 1988.

283. Robillard JE, Weitzman RE, Fisher DA, Smith FG: The dynamics of AVP release and blood volume regulation during fetal hemorrhage in the lamb fetus. Pediatr Res 13:606, 1979.

284. Rurak DW: Plasma vasopressin levels during hemorrhage in mature and immature fetal sheep. J Dev Physiol 1:91, 1979.

285. Rose JE, Meis PJ, Morris M: Ontogeny of endocrine (ACTH, vasopressin, cortisol) responses to hypotension in lamb fetuses. Am J Physiol 240:E656, 1981.

286. Ross MG, Ervin MG, Leake RD, et al: Isovolemic hypotension in the ovine fetus: plasma AVP response and urinary effects. Am J Physiol 250:E564, 1986.

287. Iwamoto HS, Kaufman TM, Rudolph AM: Response of young fetal sheep to acute hypoxemia. Soc Gynecol Invest 35: 62, 1988.

288. Stark R, Wardlow JL, Daniel SS, et al: Vasopressin secretion induced by hypoxia in sheep: developmental changes and relationship to β-endorphin release. Am J Obstet Gynecol 143: 204, 1982.

289. Rurak DW: Plasma vasopressin levels during hypoxemia and the cardiovascular effects of exogenous vasopressin in foetal and adult sheep. J Physiol 277:341, 1978.

290. Kelly RT, Rose JC, Meis PJ, et al: Vasopressin is important for restoring cardiovascular homeostasis in fetal lambs subjected to hemorrhage. Am J Obstet Gynecol 46:807, 1982.

291. Ervin MG, Terry KA, Calvario GC, Shaw S: Ovine fetal cardiovascular responses to acute hypotension during vasopressin VI receptor blockade [abstract]. Endoc Soc 789, 1993.

292. Perez R, Espinoza M, Riquelme R, et al: AVP mediates cardiovascular responses to hypoxemia in fetal sheep. Am J Physiol 256:R1011, 1989.

293. Norman LJ, Lye SJ, Wlodek MD, Challis JRG: Changes in pituitary responses to synthetic ovine corticotropin releasing factor in fetal sheep. Can J Pharmacol 63:1398, 1985.

294. Faucher DJ, Lowe TW, Magness RR, et al: Vasopressin and catecholamine secretion during metabolic acidemia in the ovine fetus. Pediatr Res 21:38, 1987.

295. Harper MA, Rose JC: Vasopressin-induced bradycardia in fetal and adult sheep is not dependent on an increase in blood pressure. Am J Obstet Gynecol 157:448, 1987.

296. Apostolakis EM, Longo LD, Yellon SM: Regulation of basal adrenocorticotropin and cortisol secretion by arginine vasopressin in the fetal sheep during late gestation. Endocrinology 129:295, 1991.

297. Ervin MG, Ross MG, Leake RD, Fisher DA: V1 and V2 receptor contributions to ovine fetal renal and cardiovascular responses to vasopressin. Am J Physiol 262:R636, 1992.

298. Iwamoto HS, Rudolph AM, Keil LC, Heymann MA: Hemodynamic responses of the sheep fetus to vassopressin infusion. Circ Res 44:430, 1979.

299. Irion GL, Mack CE, Clark KE: Fetal hemodynamic and feto-placental vascular response to exogenous arginine vasopressin. Am J Obstet Gynecol 162:1115, 1990.

300. Tomita H, Brace RA, Cheung CY, Longo LD: Vasopressin dose-response effects on fetal vascular presssures, heart rate and blood volume. Am J Physiol 249:H974, 1985.

301. Robillard JR, Nakamura KT: Neurohormonal regulation of renal function during development. Am J Physiol 254:F771, 1988.

302. Lumbers ER, Stevens AD: The effects of furosemide, saralasin and hypotension on fetal plasma renin activity and on fetal renal function. J Physiol 393:479, 1987.

303. Gomez RA, Robillard JE: Developmental aspects of the renal response to hemorrhage during converting-enzyme inhibition in fetal lambs. Circ Res 54:301, 1984.

304. Lumbers ER, Lewes J: The actions of vasoactive drugs on fetal and maternal plasma renin activity. Biol Neonate 35:23, 1979.

305. Nakamura KT, Ayres NA, Gomez A, Robillard JE: Renal response to hypoxemia during renin-angiotensin system inhibition in fetal lambs. Am J Physiol 249:R116, 1985.

306. Binder ND, Anderson DF: Plasma renin activity responses to graded decreases in renal perfusion pressure in fetal and newborn lambs. Am J Physiol 262:R524, 1992.

307. Kopp UC, Dibona GF: Interaction between neural and non-neural mechanisms controlling renin secretion rate. Am J Physiol 246:F620, 1984.

308. Page WV, Perlman VS, Smith FG, et al: Renal nerves modulate kidney renin gene expression during the transition from fetal to newborn life. Am J Physiol 262:R459, 1992.

309. Rudolph AM: Homeostasis of the fetal circulation and the part played by hormones. Ann Rech Vet 8:405, 1977.

310. Gresores A, Rosenfeld CR, Magness RR, Roy T: Metabolic clearance rate of angiotensin II in fetal and pregnant sheep. Pediatr Res 31:60A, 1992.

311. Iwamoto HS, Rudolph AM: Effects of angiotensin II on the blood flow and its distribution in fetal lambs. Circ Res 48:183, 1981.

312. Grone H-H, Simon M, Fuchs E: Autoradiographic characterization of angiotensin receptor subtypes in fetal and adult human kidney. Am J Physiol 262:F326, 1992.

313. Hellegers AE, Schruefer JJP: Normograms and empirical equations relating oxygen tension, percentage saturation, and pH in maternal and fetal blood. Am J Obstet Gynecol 81:377, 1961.

314. Bunn HF, Jandl JH: Control of hemoglobin function within the red cell. N Engl J Med 282:1414, 1970.

315. Bard H, Makowski EL, Meschia G, Battaglia FC: The relative rates of synthesis of hemoglobins A and F in immature red cells of newborn infants. Pediatrics 45:766, 1970.

316. Alter BP, Jackson BT, Lipton JM, et al: Control of the simian fetal hemoglobin switch at the progenitor cell level. J Clin Invest 67:458, 1981.

317. Bank A, Mears JG, Ramirez F: Disorders of human hemoglobin. Science 207:486, 1980.

318. Robillard JE, Weismann DN, Herin P: Ontogeny of single glomerular perfusion rate in fetal and newborn lambs. Pediatr Res 15:1248, 1981.

319. Potter EL: Developments of the human glomerulus. Arch Pathol 80:241, 1965.

320. Lumbers ER: A brief review of fetal renal function. J Dev Physiol 6:1, 1984.

321. Robillard JE, Sessions C, Kennedey RL, et al: Interrelationship between glomerular filtration rate and renal transport of sodium and chloride during fetal life. Am J Obstet Gynecol 128:727, 1977.

322. Abramow M, Dratwa M: Effect of vasopressin on the isolated human collecting duct. Nature 250:292, 1974.

323. Kullama LK, Ross MG, Lam R, et al: Ovine maternal and fetal and renal vasospressin receptor response to maternal dehydration. Am J Obstet Gynecol 167:1717, 1992.

324. Strandhoy JW, Giammattei CE, Rose JC: Stimulation of renal medullary cAMP production by vasopressin (AVP) in fetal sheep. FASEB J 6:A1745, 1992.

325. Iwamoto HS, Rudolph AM: Effects of angiotensin II on the blood flow and its distribution in fetal lambs. Circ Res 48:183, 1986

326. Robillard JE, Weismann RN, Gomez RA, et al: Renal and adrenal responses to converting enzyme inhibition in fetal and newborn life. Am J Physiol 262:R249, 1983.

327. Lumbers ER, Burrell JH, Menzies RI, Stevens AD: Effects of a converting enzyme inhibitor (captopril) and angiotensin II on fetal renal function. Br J Pharmacol 110:821, 1993.

328. Smith FG, Sata T, Vasille VA, Robillard JE: Atrial natriuretic factor during fetal and postnatal life: a review. J Dev Physiol 12:55, 1989.

329. Robillard JE, Weiner C: Atrial natriuretic factor in the human fetus: effect of volume expansion. J Pediatr 113:552, 1988.

330. Robillard JE, Nakamura KT, Varille VA, et al: Ontogeny of the renal response to ANF in sheep. Am J Physiol 254:F634, 1988.

331. Castro R, Ervin MG, Leake RD, et al: Fetal renal response to ANF decreases with maturation. Am J Physiol 260:R346, 1991.

332. Robillard JE, Sessions C, Burmeister L, Smith FG Jr: Influence of fetal extracellular volume contraction on renal reabsorption of bicarbonate in fetal lambs. Pediatr Res 11:649, 1977.

333. Robillard JE, Sessions C, Kennedy RL, Smith FG Jr: Maturation of the glucose transport process by the fetal kidney. Pediatr Res 12:680, 1978.

334. Pitkin R, Reynolds WA: Fetal ingestion and metabolism of amniotic fluid protein. Am J Obstet Gynecol 123:356, 1975.

335. Charlton VE, Reis BL: Effects of gastric nutritional supplementation on fetal umbilical uptake of nutrients. Am J Physiol 241:E178, 1981.

336. Charlton VE, Rudolph A: Digestion and absorption of carbohydrates by the fetal lamb in utero. Pediatr Res 13:1018, 1979.

337. Charlton V, Johengen M: Effects of intrauterine nutritional supplementation of fetal growth retardation. Biol Neonate 48:125, 1985.

338. Wesson D, Muraji T, Kent G, et al: The effect of intrauterine esophageal ligation on growth of fetal rabbits. J Pediatr Surg 19:398, 1984.

339. Trahair J, Harding R, Bocking A, et al: The role of ingestion in the development of the small intestine in fetal sheep. Q J Exp Physiol 71:99, 1986.

340. Avila C, Harding R, Robinson P: The effects of preventing ingestion on the development of the digestive system in the sheep fetus. Q J Exp Physiol 71:99, 1986.

341. Pierro A, Cozzi R, Colarossi G, et al: Does fetal gut obstruction cause hydramnios and growth retardation? J Pediatr Surg 22:454, 1987.

342. Cozzi F, Wilkinson A: Intrauterine growth rate in relation to anorectal and oesophageal anomalies. Arch Dis Child 44:59, 1969.

343. Edelstone DI, Holzman IR: Fetal intestinal oxygen consumption at various levels of oxygenation. Am J Physiol 242:H50, 1987.

344. Lester R, Jackson BT, Smallwood RA, et al: Fetal and neonatal hepatic function II. Birth Defects 12:307, 1976.

345. Bristow J, Rudolph AM, Itskovitz J, Barnes R: Hepatic oxygen and glucose metabolism in the fetal lamb. J Clin Invest 71:1047, 1983.

346. Jones CT, Ritchie JWK: The effects of adrenergic blockage on fetal response to hypoxia. J Dev Physiol 5:211, 1983.

347. Wood CE, Rudolph AM: Negative feedback regulation of adrenocorticotropin secretion by cortisol in ovine fetuses. Endocrinology 112:1930, 1983.

348. Silman RE, Chard T, Lowry PJ, et al: Human foetal pituitary peptide and parturition. Nature 260:716, 1976.

349. Challis JRG, Brooks AN: Maturation and activation of hypothalemic pituitary adrenal function in fetal sheep. Endocr Rev 10:182, 1989.

350. Challis JRG, Mitchell BF: Endocrinology of pregnancy and parturition. *In* Warshaw JB (ed): The Biological Basis of Reproductive and Developmental Medicine. New York, Elsevier, 1983, p 106.

351. Jaffe RB, Seron-Ferre M, Crickard K, et al: Regulation and function of the primate fetal adrenal gland and gonad. Recent Prog Horm Res 37P:41, 1981.

352. Carr BR, Parker CR Jr, Milewich L, et al: The role of law density, high density and very low density lipoproteins in steroidogenesis by the human fetal adrenal gland. Endocrinology 106:1854, 1980.

353. Simpson ER, Carr BR, Parker CR Jr, et al: The role of serum lipoproteins in steroidogenesis by the human fetal adrenal cortex. J Clin Endocrinol Metab 49:146, 1979.

354. Challis JRG, Mitchell BR, Lye SJ: Activation of fetal adrenal function. J Dev Physiol 6:93, 1984.

355. Nylund L, Langercrantz H, Lunell N-O: Catecholamines in fetal blood during birth in man. J Dev Physiol 1:427, 1979.

356. Cohen WR, Piasecki CJ, Jackson BT: Plasma catecholamines during hypoxemia in fetal lamb. Am J Physiol 243:R520, 1982.

357. Cohen WR, Piasecki GJ, Cohn HE, et al: Adrenal secretion of catecholamines during hypoxemia in fetal lambs. Endocrinology 114:383, l984.

358. Padbury J, Agata Y, Ludlow J, et al: Effect of fetal adrenalectomy on cathecholamine release and physiological adaptation at birth in sheep. J Clin Invest 80:1096, 1987.

359. Fisher DA: Maternal-fetal thyroid function in pregnancy. Clin Perinatol 10:615, 1983.

360. Vulsma T, Gons MH, de Vijlder JJ: Maternal-fetal transfer of thyroxine in congenital hypothyroidism due to a total organification defect of thyroid agenesis. N Engl J Med 321:13, 1989.

361. Timor-Tritsch IE, Dierker LJ, Hertz RH, et al: Studies of antepartum behavioral state in the human fetus at term. Am J Obstet Gynecol 132:524, 1978.

362. Martin CB Jr: Behavioral states in the human fetus. J Reprod Med 132:524, 1978.

363. Visser GHA, Goodman JDS, Levine DH, Dawes GS: Diurnal and other cyclic variations in human fetal heart rate near term. Am J Obstet Gynecol 142:535, 1982.

364. Dawes GS, Fox HE, Leduc BM, et al: Respiratory movements and rapid eye movement sleep in the foetal lamb. J Physiol 220:199, 1972.

365. Natale R, Clewlow F, Dawes GS: Measurement of fetal forelimb movements in the lamb in utero. Am J Obstet Gynecol 140:545, 1981.

366. Blanco CE, Dawes GS, Walker DW: Effect of hypoxia on polysynaptic hindlimb reflexes of unanesthetized foetal and newborn lambs. J Physiol 339:453, 1983.

367. Chan K, Dodd PA, Day L, et al: Fetal catecholamine, cardiovascular and neurobehavioral responses to cocaine. Am J Obstet Gynecol 167:1616, 1992.

368. Connors G, Hunse C, Carmichal L, et al: Control of fetal breathing in human fetus between 24 and 34 weeks gestation. Am J Obstet Gynecol 60:932, 1989.

369. Hohimer AR, Bissonnette JM, Richardson BS, Machida CM: Central chemical regulation of breathing movements in fetal lambs. Respir Physiol 52:99, 1983.

370. Dawes GS, Gardner WN, Johnson BM, Walker DW: Breathing activity in fetal lambs: the effect of brain stem section. J Physiol 335:535, 1983.

371. Jones MD Jr, Burd LI, Makowski EL, et al: Cerebral metabolism in sheep: a comparative study of the adult, the lamb, and the fetus. Am J Physiol 229:235, 1975.

372. Richardson BS, Patrick JE, Abduljabbar H: Cerebral oxidative metabolism in the fetal lamb: relationship to electrocortical state. Am J Obstet Gynecol 153:426, 1985.

373. Chao CR, Hohimer AR, Bissonnette JM: The effect of electrocortical state on cerebral carbohydrate metabolism in fetal sheep. Dev Brain Res 49:1, 1989.

374. Jones MD, Sheldon RE, Peeters LL, et al: Fetal cerebral oxygen consumption at different levels of oxygenation. J Appl Physiol 43:R1080, 1977.

375. Rosenberg AA, Jones MD Jr, Traystman RJ, et al: Response of cerebral blood flow to changes in PCO2 in fetal, newborn, and adult sheep. Am J Physiol 242:H862, 1982.

376. Boyd CAR, Lund EK: L-Proline transport by brush border membrane vesicles prepared from human placenta. J Physiol 315:9, 1981.

377. Whitsett JA, Wallick ET: [3H] Oubain binding and Na+-K-ATPase activity in human placenta. Am J Physiol 238:E38, 1980.

378. Lajeunesse D, Brunette MG: Sodium gradient-dependent phosphate transport in placental brush border membrane vesicles. Placenta 9:117, 1988.

379. Balkovetz DF, Leibach FH, Mahesh VB, et al: Na+-H+ exchanager of human placental brush-border membrane: identification and characterization. Am J Physiol 251:C852, 1986.

380. Bara M, Challier JC, Guit-Bara A: Membrane potential and input resistance in syncytiotrophoblast of human term placenta in vitro. Placenta 9:139, 1988.

381. Enders RH, Judd RM, Donohue TM, Smith CH: Placental amino acid uptake. III. Transport systems for neutral amino acids. Am J Physiol 230:706, 1976.

382. Smith CH, Adcock EW, Teasdale F, et al: Placental amino acid uptake: tissue preparation, kinetics, and preincubation effect. Am J Physiol 224:558, 1973.

383. Smith CH, Depper R: Placental amino acid uptake. II. Tissue preincubation, fluid distribution and mechanisms of regulation. Pediatr Res 8:697, 1974.

384. Steel RB, Smith CH, Kelly LK: Placental amino acid uptake. VI. Regulation by intracellular substrate. Am J Physiol 243:C46, 1982.

Maternal Physiology in Pregnancy

MICHAEL C. GORDON

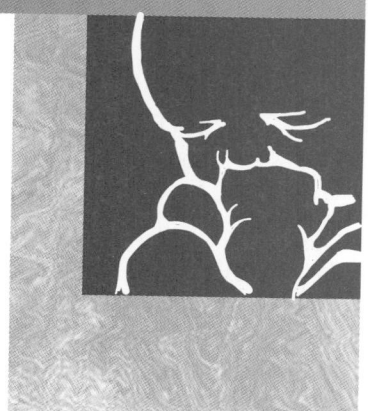

Major adaptations in maternal anatomy, physiology, and metabolism are required for a successful pregnancy. Hormonal changes, initiated before conception, significantly alter maternal physiology, and continue throughout the entire pregnancy. These alterations are needed to allow the development of a single diploid cell into an infant weighing 3.5 kg. These adaptations profoundly affect nearly every organ system and yet allow the woman to return to her prepregnancy state with minimal residual changes.[1] The obstetrician must fully understand these changes to determine what signs and symptoms are normal and which are potentially due to disease processes either unique to or exacerbated by pregnancy. This chapter will describe maternal adaptations in pregnancy and give examples of how these changes can affect the care of the pregnant woman.

BODY WATER METABOLISM

The increase in total body water of 6.5 to 8.5 L by the end of pregnancy represents one of the most significant adaptations of pregnancy. The water content of the fetus, placenta, and amniotic fluid at term accounts for about 3.5 L. Maternal blood volume is expanded by 1,500 to 1,600 ml, plasma volume by 1,200 to 1,300 ml, and red blood cells (RBCs) by 300 to 400 ml.[2] The remainder of the increase in water content is attributed to extravascular fluid, intracellular fluid in the uterus and breasts, and expanded adipose tissue. Thus, pregnancy is a condition of chronic volume overload in which hypervolemia is the result of active sodium and water retention due to changes in osmoregulation and the renin-angiotensin system. The increase in body water content is reflected in maternal weight gain and contributes to the hemodilution of pregnancy, physiologic

anemia of pregnancy, and elevation in maternal cardiac output.

Osmoregulation

The expansion in the plasma volume begins shortly after conception. It is associated with and partially mediated by a change in maternal osmoregulation and the control of the secretion of arginine vasopressin (AVP) by the posterior pituitary. Water metabolism is controlled by AVP (also known as antidiuretic hormone [ADH]) and thirst. Despite an overall increase in sodium retention of 900 mEq during pregnancy, the serum level of sodium decreases during a normal pregnancy by 3 to 4 mmol/L. In addition, the plasma osmolality decreases by 8 to 10 mOsm/kg by 10 weeks' gestation and remains at this lower level throughout pregnancy and until 1 to 2 weeks postpartum[3,4] (Fig. 3–1). The initial decline in serum sodium and osmolality begins at 5 weeks' gestation and is due to a resetting of the osmotic thresholds for both thirst and AVP secretion. The threshold for thirst changes early in pregnancy. Therefore, during gestational weeks 5 to 8, an increase in water intake occurs and results in increased urinary volume. This transient polyuria is the result of a lowered osmotic threshold for thirst prior to a change in the osmotic threshold for AVP release.[5]

Lowering the threshold to drink stimulates water intake and dilution of body fluids. Because AVP release is not suppressed at the usual body tonicity, the hormone continues to circulate and the ingested water is retained, increasing in total body water. After 8 weeks' gestation, when the threshold for AVP secretion has been reset and the new steady state for osmolality has been established, little change in water turnover occurs and pregnant women should not be polyuric or poly-

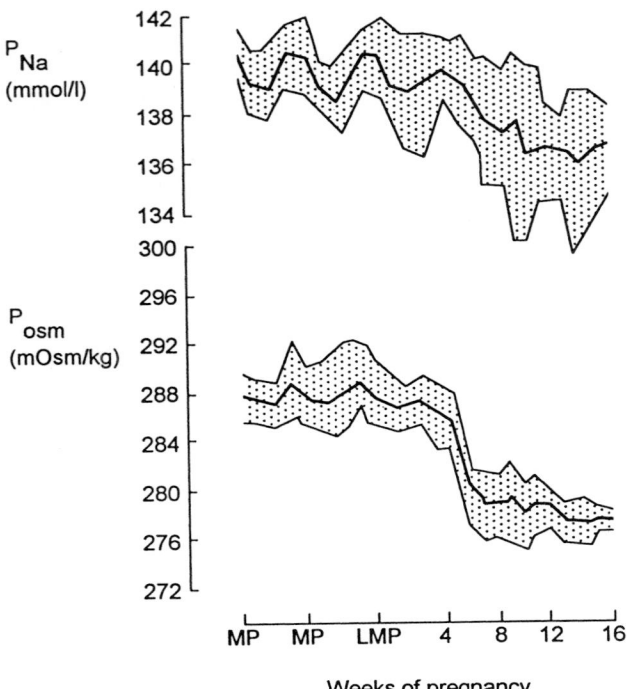

Figure 3–1. Plasma osmolality and plasma sodium during human gestation (n = 9: mean values ± SD). MP, menstrual period; LMP, last menstrual period. (From Davison JM, Vallotton MB, Lindheimer MD: Plasma osmolality and urinary concentration and dilution during and after pregnancy: evidence that the lateral recumbency inhibits maximal urinary concentration ability. Br J Obstet Gynaecol 88:472, 1981. Copyright Blackwell Science Ltd, with permission.)

dipsic. The pregnant woman perceives this decrease in plasma sodium and osmolality as normal and defends this lower steady state tonicity by concentrating and diluting normally around the new P_{osm}. Thus the gravid individual responds to fluid challenges or dehydration normally with changes in thirst and AVP secretion but at a new "osmostat."[6]

Plasma levels of AVP during pregnancy are similar to nonpregnant levels despite a three to fourfold increase in the metabolic clearance of AVP. The increased clearance is caused by the presence of a circulating vasopressinase synthesized by the placenta that rapidly inactivates AVP and oxytocin. This enzyme increases 1,000-fold from 4 weeks' gestation until term. Yet, plasma concentrations of AVP are unchanged due to its heightened production. The need for greater AVP production to maintain normal AVP levels and normal osmoregulation of pregnancy can unmask what are subclinical forms of diabetes insipidus and cause transient diabetes insipidus in pregnancy.[6] This is one example of how pregnancy may act as a stress test to uncover diseases that were previously latent or compensated when the woman is not pregnant. Gestational diabetes is another.

Salt Metabolism

Sodium metabolism is delicately balanced in pregnancy to permit a net accumulation of about 900 mEq of sodium. Sixty percent of the additional sodium enters the fetoplacental unit including the amniotic fluid and is lost at birth. Pregnancy increases the preference for salt and sodium intake, and this change accounts for some of the sodium accumulation. However, retention by the kidney is the main mechanism because of the enhanced tubular sodium reabsorption from early in pregnancy. During pregnancy, a 50 percent rise in the glomerular filtration rate leads to an increase in the filtered sodium load from 20,000 to about 30,000 mmol/day. Without an increase in tubular sodium reabsorption, greater sodium loss would occur. The adaptive rise in tubular reabsorption not only equals the increase in the filtered load but also is associated with an additional 2 to 6 mEq of sodium reabsorption. Renal sodium handling is another determinant of increased volume homeostasis and represents the largest renal adjustment that occurs during pregnancy.[7] The mechanisms responsible for the renal tubular adjustments are incompletely understood. Hormonal control of sodium balance is under the opposing actions of the renin-angiotensin-aldosterone system and atrial natriuretic peptide (ANP), and both are modified during pregnancy.

Renin-Angiotensin-Aldosterone System

In normal pregnancy, marked increases in all the components of this system occur. Plasma renin activity is 5 to 10 times the nonpregnant level. Likewise, renin substrate (angiotensinogen) and angiotensin levels are increased four to fivefold and lead to elevated levels of aldosterone.[8,9] In the third trimester, plasma aldosterone levels are twofold higher than in the nonpregnant state. This rise in aldosterone production is most likely the key factor in sodium reabsorption and prevention of sodium loss.[9] Despite the elevated aldosterone levels in late pregnancy, a normal homeostatic response occurs to changes in salt balance, fluid loss, and postural stimuli. In addition to aldosterone, other hormones might be responsible for increased tubular sodium retention, including deoxycorticosterone and estrogen.

Atrial Natriuretic Peptide

Secreted by atrial myocytes in response to atrial distention, ANP plays a major role in the regulation of extracellular fluid volume. It is a diuretic, a natriuretic, a vasorelaxant, and an antagonist to the renin-angiotensin system. Elevated levels of ANP are found in physiologic and pathologic conditions of volume overload. Whether ANP secretion is increased during gestation is controversial, as some authors have reported higher plasma levels during different stages of pregnancy, whereas others have reported no change.[10] In a meta-analysis by Castro et al., ANP levels were 40 percent higher during gestation and 150 percent higher during the first postpartum week. The authors speculated that the atrial stretch receptors sensed the expanded blood volume of pregnancy and thus increased production. The increase in postpartum ANP was felt to be consistent with the increased fluid volume postpartum and possibly contributed to postpartum diuresis.[11] By comparison, Sala et al. found that ANP levels were increased only in the first trimester and only in the supine position. These authors hypothesized that during pregnancy body posture can greatly affect ANP production. Normal ANP levels in later pregnancy may be caused by vena caval compression from the enlarged uterus with decreased atrial blood volume and a decreased stimulus for ANP secretion[10] (Fig. 3–2). Therefore, the discrepancies reported in these studies appear to be caused by the effects of body position on ANP secretion. ANP may also contribute to the systemic vasodilation of pregnancy by acting directly as a vasorelaxant or indirectly as an antagonist of the renin-angiotensin system.

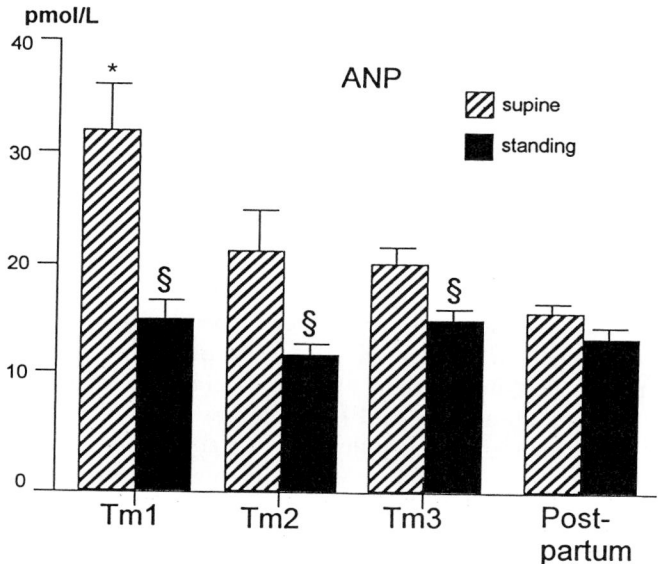

Figure 3–2. Bar graphs show plasma atrial natriuretic peptide (ANP) at each trimester (Tm) of pregnancy and postpartum in 15 healthy women in the supine and upright positions (mean ± SEM).* *p* <0.05 versus postpartum in the same position; § *p* <0.05 versus corresponding supine value. (From Sala C, Campise M, Ambroso G, et al: Atrial natriuretic peptide and hemodynamic changes during normal human pregnancy. Hypertension 25:631, 1995, with permission.)

CARDIOVASCULAR SYSTEM

Pregnancy causes profound physiologic changes in the cardiovascular system. In most women, these physiologic demands are well tolerated. However, in certain cardiac diseases, maternal morbidity and even mortality may occur.

Heart

Because of the displacement of the diaphragm and the effect of pregnancy on the shape of the rib cage, the heart is displaced to the left and upward. In addition, the heart is rotated on its long axis and as a result the apex is moved somewhat laterally. This results in an apparent increase in the size of the cardiac silhouette on radiographic studies even though no true change in the cardiothoracic ratio occurs. An apparent straightening of the left heart border occurs with increased prominence of the pulmonary conus. These radiographic changes make the diagnosis of cardiomegaly by simple radiography suspect.[12]

As a result of the expanded blood volume, there is an increase in left ventricular end-diastolic dimension as measured by M-mode echocardiography. This is observed in the first trimester, continues until term, and is accompanied by an increase in left ventricular wall mass consistent with mild myocardial hypertrophy. These structural changes in the heart are similar to those found in response to physical training and show that the structural heart changes during pregnancy are consistent with the effects of chronic strain on the heart.[13] The left and right atrial diameters also increase in dimension beginning early in gestation, with a plateau by 30 weeks. This increase is also a result of the rise in blood volume and suggests an increase in preload. Since there is no increase in the central venous pressure or the pulmonary capillary wedge pressure, there must be an increase in the capacitance of the systemic and pulmonary veins as reflected in a decrease in the systemic and pulmonary vascular resistances.

Cardiac Output

In a review of the literature on cardiac output in pregnancy, van Oppen et al. reviewed 33 cross-sectional and 19 longitudinal studies. They found greatly divergent results on when cardiac output peaked, the magnitude of the rise in cardiac output prior to labor, and the effect of the third trimester on cardiac output.[14] However, all of the studies agreed that cardiac output increased significantly during pregnancy by an average of 30 to 50 percent above nonpregnant values. In a longitudinal study by Robson et al. using Doppler echocardiography, cardiac output was found to increase by 50 percent at 34 weeks from a prepregnancy value of 4.88 L/min to 7.34 L/min[14,15] (Fig. 3–3). In twin gestations, cardiac output is raised an additional 15 percent above that of singleton pregnancies. In the review by van Oppen et al. cardiac output was found to increase by 5 weeks' gestation. By 12 weeks, the rise in output was 34 to 39 percent above nonpregnant levels, accounting for about 75 percent of the total increase in cardiac output during pregnancy. The numerous studies in the literature disagree on when cardiac output peaks, but the overall conclusion seems to be somewhere around 25 to 30 weeks of gestation, with a rise from the first to the second trimester. The data on whether the cardiac output continues to increase in the third trimester are very divergent, with equal numbers of good longitudinal studies showing a mild decrease, a slight increase, or no change.[14] The differences in these studies cannot be explained by differences in investigative techniques, position of the women during measurements, or study design. This apparent discrepancy appears to be explained by the small number of individuals in each study and the probability that the course of cardiac output during the third trimester is apparently determined by factors within individual women. If this is true, then within any given patient, cardiac output may rise, fall, or not changed during the third trimester[14,16] (Fig. 3–3).

Most of the increase in cardiac output is directed to the uterus and placenta, and the breasts. In the first trimester, as in the nonpregnant state, the uterus receives 2 to 3 percent of cardiac output and the breasts 1 percent. By term, the uterus receives 17 percent (450 to 650 ml/min) and the breasts 2 percent, mostly at the expense of a reduction of the fraction of the cardiac output going to the splanchnic bed and skeletal muscle. The absolute blood flow to the liver is not changed but the overall percentage of cardiac output is significantly decreased. The percentage of cardiac output going to the kidneys (20 percent), skin (10 percent), brain (10 percent), and coronary arteries (5 percent) remains at similar nonpregnant percentages, but because of the overall increase in cardiac output this results in an increase in absolute blood flow of approximately 50 percent.[17]

Cardiac output (CO) is the product of stroke volume (SV) and heart rate (HR) (CO = SV × HR), both of which increase during pregnancy and contribute to the overall rise in cardiac output. An initial rise in the heart rate occurs by 5 weeks' gestation and continues until it peaks at 32 weeks' gestation at 15 to 20 beats above the pregravid rate, an increase of 17 percent. The stroke volume begins to rise by 8 weeks' gestation and reaches its maximum at about 20 weeks, 20 to 30 percent above nonpregnant values. In the third trimester, it is the changes in the stroke volume that determine whether the cardiac output increases, decreases, or remains stable as described earlier[16,18] (Fig. 3–3).

Cardiac output in pregnancy depends on maternal position, being lowest in the sitting or supine position and highest in the right and left lateral and knee-chest positions. In a study in 10 normal gravid women in the third trimester, using pulmonary artery catheterization, the cardiac output was noted to be highest in the knee-chest position and lateral recombinant position at 6.6 to 6.9 L/min. The cardiac output decreased by 22 percent to 5.4 L/min in the standing position[19] (Fig. 3–4). In both the standing and the supine positions, a fall in stroke volume takes place as a result of decreased blood return to the heart, which results in the decrease in cardiac output.

In the supine position, the enlarged uterus compresses the inferior vena cava, reducing venous return to the heart and in turn the stroke volume and cardiac

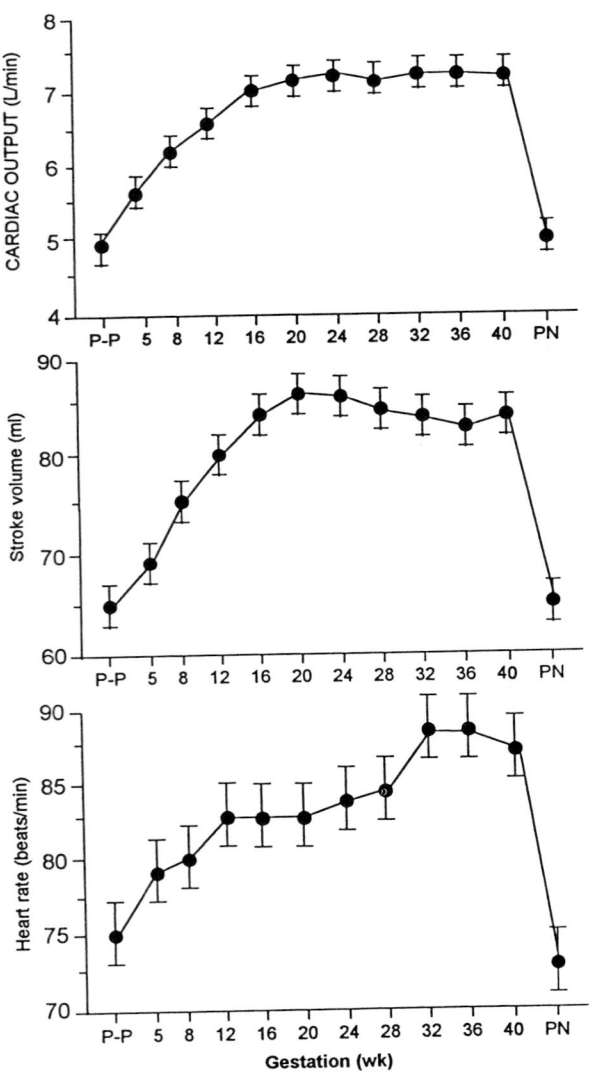

Figure 3–3. Increase in cardiac output from the nonpregnancy state throughout pregnancy. P-P, pre-pregnancy; PN, postnatal. (From Hunter S, Robson S: Adaptation of the maternal heart in pregnancy. Br Heart J 68:540, 1992, with permission.)

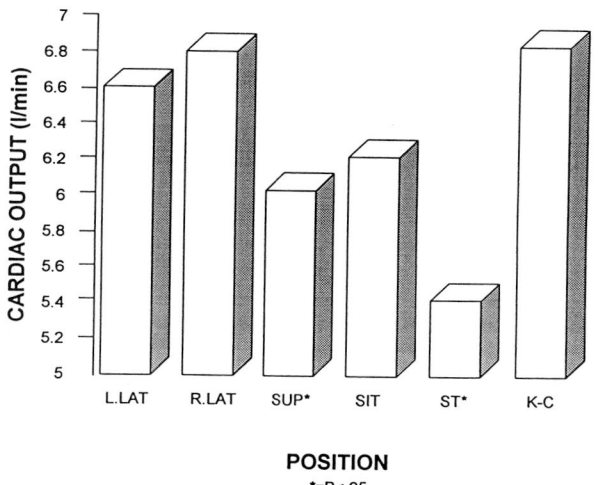

Figure 3–4. Effect of position change on cardiac output during pregnancy. L.LAT, left lateral; R.LAT, right lateral; SUP, supine; ST, standing; SIT, sitting; K-C, knee-chest. (From Clark S, Cotton D, Pivarnik J, et al: Position change and central hemodynamic profile during normal third-trimester pregnancy and postpartum. Am J Obstet Gynecol 164:883, 1991, with permission.)

output. In fact, in late pregnancy, the inferior vena cava is completely occluded in the supine position, with venous return from the lower extremities occurring through the dilated paravertebral collateral circulation.[20,21] The effect of the supine position on cardiac output is most marked in late pregnancy. The decrease in cardiac output in the supine position compared with the lateral recumbent position is 10 to 30 percent.[19,22] Prior to 24 weeks the effect of the supine position on cardiac output is not observed.

Despite the decrease in cardiac output in the supine position, the majority of women are not hypotensive or symptomatic because of the compensated rise in systemic vascular resistance (SVR). However, 5 to 10 percent of gravidas manifest supine hypotension with symptoms of dizziness, lightheadedness, nausea, and even syncope. Some investigators have proposed that the determination of whether women become symptomatic or not depends on the development of an adequate paravertebral collateral circulation. With inadequate collateral flow, a woman develops a vasovagal attack, with a decrease in heart rate and a fall in blood pressure (Fig. 3–5). Interestingly, with engagement of the fetal head, less of an effect on cardiac output is seen.[20] The ability to maintain a normal blood pressure in the supine position may be lost during epidural or spinal anesthesia because of an inability to increase the SVR.

Clinically, the effects of maternal position on cardiac output are important when maintenance of the cardiac output is vital, such as occurs with a nonreassuring fetal heart rate pattern or if the woman becomes hypotensive. Also, the finding of a decreased cardiac output in the standing position may give a physiologic basis for the observation of decreased birth weight and placental infarctions in working women who stand.[23]

Arterial Blood Pressure and Systemic Vascular Resistance

Blood pressure (BP) is the product of cardiac output and resistance (BP = CO × SVR). In spite of the large

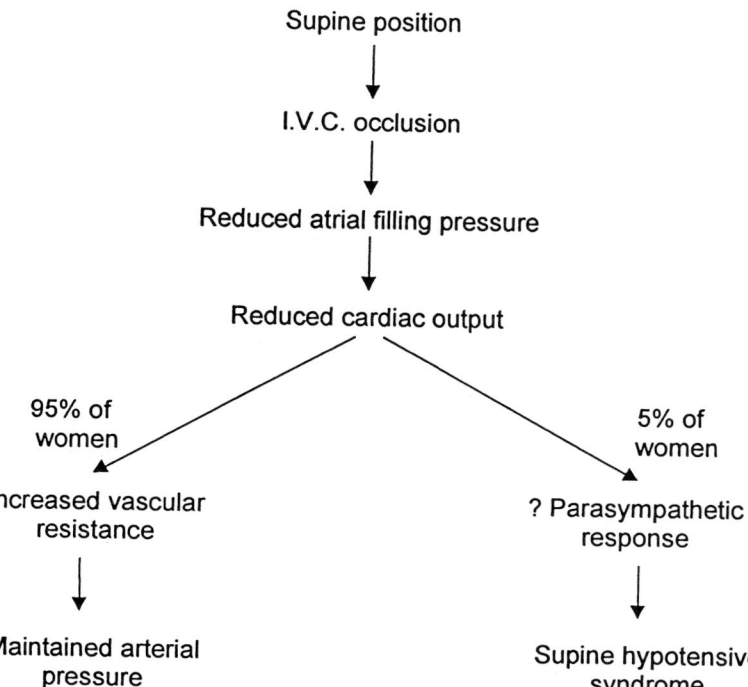

Figure 3–5. Summary of hemodynamic effects of supine position in late pregnancy. (From Kerr M: The mechanical effects of the gravid uterus in late pregnancy. J Obstet Gynaecol Br Commonw 72:513, 1965, with permission.)

increase in cardiac output, the maternal BP is decreased until later in pregnancy as a result of a decrease in SVR. The SVR decreases to a minimum at midpregnancy followed by a gradual rise until term, when it is still 21 percent lower than nonpregnant values[13,18,24] (Fig. 3–6). The most obvious cause for the decreased SVR is the smooth muscle–relaxing effects of the elevated progesterone level; however, the exact mechanism for the fall in SVR is poorly understood. The earlier notion of the uteroplacental circulation acting as an arteriovenous shunt seems unlikely. A more promising theory involves the presence of one or more circulating substances exerting a vasodilatory effect on the arterial and venous vasculature.[13] This may involve nitric oxide, prostaglandins, or ANP. In addition, despite the overall increase in the renin-angiotensin system in pregnancy, the normal pregnant woman is refractory to the hypertensive effects of angiotensin II. Gant et al. showed that nulliparous women who later become preeclamptic lose this refractoriness prior to developing clinical signs of preeclampsia.[25]

The decrease in maternal BP parallels that of SVR. A decrease occurs by at least 8 weeks' gestation or earlier. In the normal menstrual cycle, BP is decreased in the luteal phase and rises with menstruation.[26] The diastolic BP and the mean arterial pressure [MAP = (Systolic BP + Diastolic BP)/3] decrease more than the systolic BP, which changes minimally during pregnancy. The diastolic BP and the MAP nadir at midpregnancy (16 to 20 mm Hg) and return to prepregnancy levels by term. The overall decrease in diastolic BP and MAP is 5 to 10 mm Hg[27] (Fig. 3–7). In late pregnancy the BP in women without pregnancy-induced hypertension rarely exceeds the prepregnancy or postpartum BP.

The position of the women when the BP is taken and

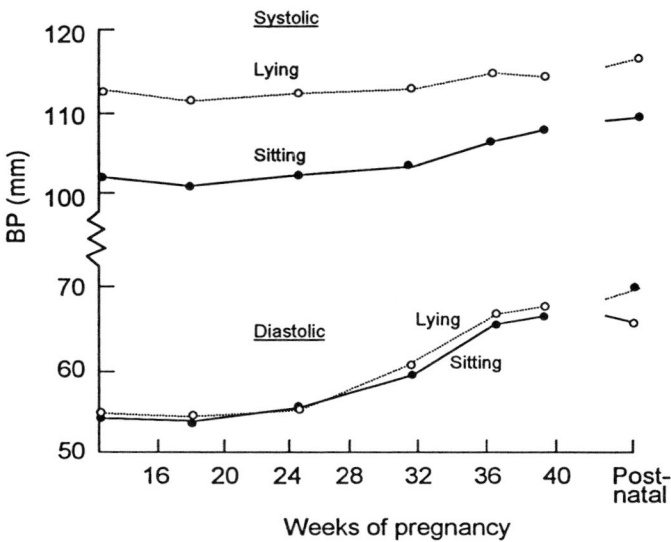

Figure 3–7. Blood pressure trends (sitting and lying) during pregnancy. Postnatal measures done six weeks postpartum. (From MacGillivray I, Rose G, Rowe B: Blood pressure survey in pregnancy. Clin Sci 37:395, 1969, with permission. © The Biochemical Society and the Medical Research Society.)

what Korotkoff sound is used to determine the diastolic BP is important. BP is lowest in the lateral recumbent position, and the BP of the superior arm in this position is 10 to 12 mm Hg lower than the inferior arm. In the clinic setting, BP should be measured in the sitting position and the Korotkoff 5 sound should be used. This is the diastolic BP when the sound disappears as opposed to the Korotkoff 4, when there is a muffling of the sound. In a study of 250 gravidas, the Korotkoff 4 sound could only be identified in 48 percent of patients, whereas the Korotkoff 5 sound could always be determined. The Korotkoff 4 should only be used when the Korotkoff 5 goes to zero.[28]

Venous Pressure

Venous pressure in the upper extremities remains unchanged in pregnancy but rises progressively in the lower extremities. Femoral venous pressure increases from values near 10 cm H_2O at 10 weeks' gestation to 25 cm H_2O near term.[29] From a clinical standpoint, it is this increase in pressure in addition to the obstruction of the inferior vena cava that leads to the development of edema, varicose veins, and an increased risk of deep venous thrombosis.

Central Hemodynamic Assessment and Left Ventricular Function

Clark et al. studied 10 carefully selected normal women at 36 to 38 weeks' gestation and again at 11 to 13 weeks postpartum with arterial lines and Swan-Ganz catheterization to characterize the central hemodynam-

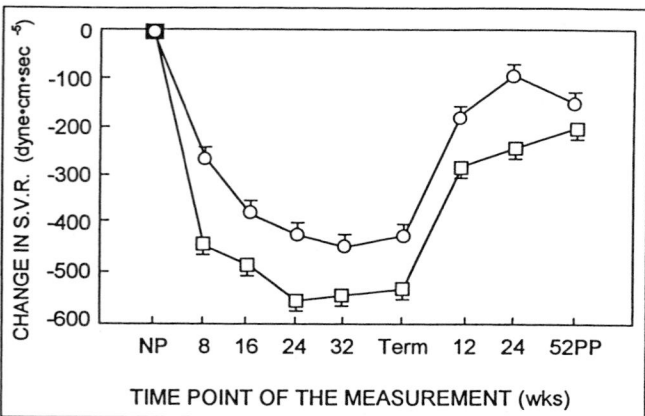

Figure 3–6. Change in systemic vascular resistance (S.V.R.) during normal pregnancy and the first year postpartum in nulliparous and parous women. *Open circles,* 15 nulliparous women; *open squares,* 15 parous women. Data are presented as mean ± SEM. 52PP, 52 weeks postpartum; NP, nonpregnant. (From Clapp J, Capeless E: Cardiovascular function before, during and after the first and subsequent pregnancies. Am J Cardiol 80:1469, 1997, with permission.)

ics of term pregnancy (Table 3–1). They found statistically significant increases in cardiac output and heart rate, accompanied by significant decreases in SVR, pulmonary vascular resistance (PVR), colloidal oncotic pressure (COP), and the COP − PCWP difference. No significant changes were found in MAP, pulmonary capillary wedge pressure (PCWP), central venous pressure (CVP), or left ventricular stroke work index.[24]

They postulated that the higher stroke volume of pregnancy was not associated with an increased end-diastolic pressure because of ventricular dilation. As a result of the marked fall in both SVR and PVR, the CVP and PCWP do not rise despite the increased blood volume of pregnancy. Their finding of a significantly decreased gradient between COP and PCWP (COP − PCWP) explains why pregnant women have a greater propensity for developing pulmonary edema with changes in capillary permeability or elevations in cardiac preload. When the PCWP is more than 4 mm Hg above the COP, the risk of pulmonary edema increases. The colloidal oncotic pressure can fall even further after delivery to 17 mm Hg and, if the pregnancy is complicated by preeclampsia, can reach levels as low as 14 mm Hg.[31] Therefore, unlike nonpregnant women who will rarely develop signs of pulmonary edema unless the PCWP is 24 mm Hg, pregnant women can experience pulmonary edema at a much lower PCWP, 18 to 20 mm Hg.

Evaluation of left ventricular function (contractility) is difficult in pregnancy because it is strongly influenced by changes in heart rate, preload, and afterload. Despite the increase in stroke volume and cardiac output, normal pregnancy is not associated with hyperdynamic left ventricular function during the third trimester as measured by ejection fraction or left ventricular stroke work index. However, some studies have shown that contractility might be slightly increased in the first two trimesters.[16]

Normal Changes That Mimic Heart Disease

The physiologic adaptations of pregnancy lead to a number of changes in maternal signs and symptoms that can mimic cardiac disease and make it difficult to determine if true cardiac disease is present.

- Dyspnea is common during pregnancy. Most pregnant women complain of dyspnea prior to 20 weeks, and 75 percent experience it by the third trimester. To differentiate the dyspnea of pregnancy from the much less common dyspnea of cardiac disease, certain distinguishing features should be considered. First, the dyspnea of pregnancy occurs early in pregnancy and does not worsen significantly as the pregnancy progresses, whereas the symptoms of heart disease usually worsen in the latter half of pregnancy. Second, physiologic dyspnea is usually mild and does not stop women from performing normal daily activities and does not occur at rest.[30]
- Other normal symptoms, that can mimic cardiac disease include decreased exercise tolerance, fatigue, occasional orthopnea, syncope, and chest discomfort. Symptoms that should not be attributed to pregnancy and need a more thorough investigation include hemoptysis, syncope or chest pain with exertion, and progressive orthopnea, or paroxysmal nocturnal dyspnea.
- Normal physical findings that could be mistaken as evidence of cardiac disease include peripheral edema, mild tachycardia, jugular venous distention after 20 weeks of gestation, and lateral displacement of the left ventricular apex.
- Pregnancy also alters normal heart sounds. At the end of the first trimester, both components of the first heart sound become louder, and there is exaggerated splitting. The second heart sound usually remains

Table 3–1. CENTRAL HEMODYNAMIC CHANGES*

	11–12 Weeks Postpartum	36–38 Weeks Gestation	Change from Nonpregnant State
Cardiac output (L/min)	4.3 ± 0.9	6.2 ± 1.0	+43%†
Heart rate (beats/min)	71 ± 10.0	83 ± 10.0	+17%†
Systemic vascular resistance (dyne·cm·sec⁻⁵)	1530 ± 520	1210 ± 266	−21%†
Pulmonary vascular resistance (dyne·cm·sec⁻⁵)	119 ± 47.0	78 ± 22	−34%†
Colloid oncotic pressure (mm Hg)	20.8 ± 1.0	18 ± 1.5	−14%†
Mean arterial pressure (mm Hg)	86.4 ± 7.5	90.3 ± 5.8	NS
Pulmonary capillary wedge pressure (mm Hg)	6.3 ± 2.1	7.5 ± 1.8	NS
Central venous pressure (mm Hg)	3.7 ± 2.6	3.6 ± 2.5	NS
Left ventricle stroke work index (g·m·m⁻²)	41 ± 8	48 ± 6	NS

*Data are presented as mean ± standard deviation. Although data are not presented, the pulmonary artery pressures were not significantly different.
†$p < 0.05$.
NS, not significant.
Adapted from Clark S, Cotton D, Lee W, et al: Central hemodynamic assessment of normal term pregnancy. Am J Obstet Gynecol 161:1439, 1989.

normal with only minimal changes. Up to 80 to 90 percent of gravid women demonstrate a third heart sound (S_3) after midpregnancy because of rapid diastolic filling. Rarely, a fourth heart sound may be ausculated, but typically phonocardiography is needed to detect this. Systolic ejection murmurs along the left sternal border develop in 96 percent of pregnancies and are thought to be caused by increased blood flow across the pulmonic and aortic valves. Most commonly these are midsystolic and less than grade 3. Diastolic murmurs have been found in up to 18 percent of pregnancies, but their presence is uncommon enough to warrant further evaluation. A continuous murmur in the second to fourth intercostal space may be heard in late pregnancy due to the so-called mammary soufflée caused by increased blood flow in the breast[32,33] (Fig. 3–8).

Effect of Labor and the Immediate Puerperium

In addition to the dramatic rise in cardiac output that occurs with normal pregnancy, even greater increases in cardiac output occur with labor and in the immediate puerperium. In a study by Robson et al. of 15 uncomplicated women without epidural anesthesia, using Doppler echocardiography, the cardiac output between contractions increased 12 percent during the first stage of labor[16,34] (Fig. 3–9). Early in the first stage of labor, the increase in cardiac output is caused primarily by an increased stroke volume, but later in labor heart rate also increases. MAP also rises in the first stage of labor, from 82 mm Hg to 91 mm Hg. Furthermore, with uterine contractions the cardiac output and MAP increase even further. By the end of the first stage of labor, the cardiac output during a contraction is 51 percent above baseline term pregnancy values (6.99 L/min to 10.57

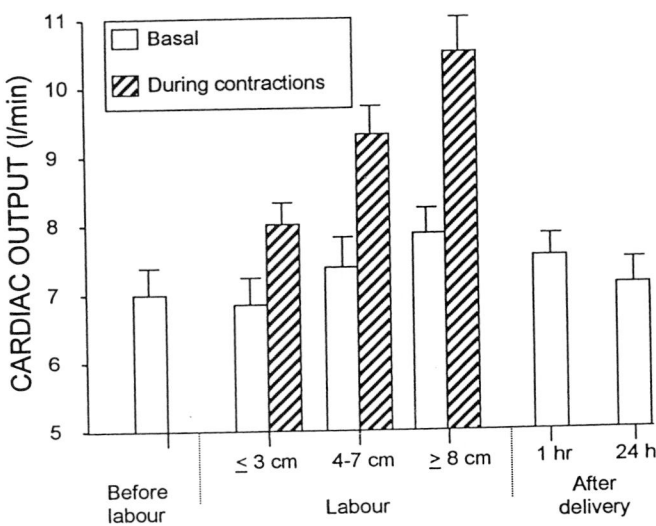

Figure 3–9. Changes in cardiac output and stroke volume during normal labor. (From Hunter S, Robson S: Adaptation of the maternal heart in pregnancy. Br Heart J 68:540, 1992, with permission.)

L/min) and the MAP is 102 mm Hg. The cardiac output with contractions increases as labor progresses from + 1.14 L/min at ≤ 3 cm to + 2.69 L/min at ≥ 8 cm. At the onset of a contraction, blood is expressed from the uterus, causing a 300 to 500 ml autotransfusion into the maternal circulation. This in turn increases the venous return and leads to a rise in stroke volume, BP, and cardiac output.[34,35]

Much of the increase in cardiac output and BP is due to pain and apprehension. With epidural anesthesia, the baseline increase in cardiac output is reduced, but the rise observed with contractions persists.[36] Maternal posture also influences hemodynamics during labor. Changing position from supine to lateral recumbent increases cardiac output. This change is greater than the increase seen prior to labor and suggests that during

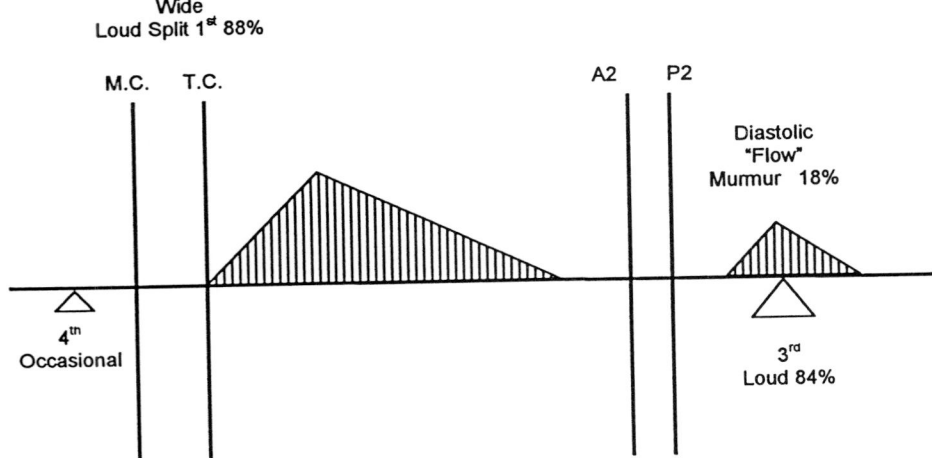

Figure 3–8. Summarization of the findings on auscultation of the heart in pregnancy. M.C., mitral closure; T.C., tricuspid closure; A_2 and P_2, aortic and pulmonary elements of the second sound. (From Cutforth R, MacDonald C: Heart sounds and murmurs in pregnancy. Am Heart J 71:741, 1966, with permission.)

labor cardiac output may be more dependent on preload. Therefore, it is important to avoid the supine position in laboring women.[37]

In the immediate postpartum period (10 to 30 minutes after delivery), cardiac output reaches its maximum, with a further rise of 10 to 20 percent. This increase is accompanied by a fall in the maternal heart rate that is thought to be caused by a greatly increased stroke volume. Traditionally, this rise was thought to be the result of the "squeezing" out of blood from the uterus as seen with contractions, but the validity of this concept is uncertain.[13] As with vaginal deliveries, in elective cesarean deliveries, the maximal increase in the cardiac output occurs at 10 to 30 minutes after delivery. The increase was 37 percent with epidural anesthesia, and 28 percent with general anesthesia. One hour following either vaginal delivery or cesarean delivery the cardiac output returns to prelabor baseline values.[38] Over the next 2 to 4 weeks, the cardiac hemodynamic parameters return to near prepregnant levels.[39]

RESPIRATORY SYSTEM

Upper Respiratory Tract

During pregnancy, the mucosa of the nasopharynx becomes hyperemic and edematous with hypersecretion of mucous due to increased estrogen. These changes often lead to marked nasal stuffiness; epistaxis is also common. Placement of nasogastric tubes may cause excessive bleeding if adequate lubrication is not used.[30] Polyposis of the nose and nasal sinuses develops in some individuals but regresses postpartum. Because of these changes, many gravid women complain of chronic cold symptoms. However, the temptation to use nasal decongestants should be avoided.[40]

Mechanical Changes

The configuration of the thoracic cage changes early in pregnancy, much earlier than can be accounted for by mechanical pressure from the enlarging uterus. Relaxation of the ligamentous attachments to the ribs may be responsible. The subcostal angle increases from 68 degrees to 103 degrees, the transverse diameter of the chest expands by 2 cm, and the chest circumference expands by 5 to 7 cm.[41] As gestation progresses, the level of the diaphragm rises 4 cm; however, diaphragmatic excursion is not impeded and actually increases 1 to 2 cm. Respiratory muscle function is not affected by pregnancy, and maximum inspiratory and expiratory pressures are unchanged.[42]

Lung Volume and Pulmonary Function

The described alterations in chest wall configuration and the diaphragm lead to changes in static lung volumes. In a review of studies with at least 15 subjects for whom nonpregnant controls were used, Crapo found the following changes in pregnancy[30]:

1. The elevation of the diaphragm decreases the volume of the lungs in the resting state, thereby reducing total lung capacity by 5 percent and the functional residual capacity (FRC) by 20 percent.
2. The FRC (the volume of air in the lungs at the end of quiet exhalation) can be subdivided into expiratory reserve volume and residual volume, and both decrease.
3. The inspiratory capacity, the maximum volume that can be inhaled from the FRC, increases 5 to 10 percent as a result of the reduction in the FRC.
4. The vital capacity does not change[30] (Fig. 3–10 and Table 3–2).

Spirometric measurements that assess flow are not altered in pregnancy. The forced expiratory volume in 1 second (FEV_1) and the ratio of FEV_1 to forced vital capacity are both unchanged in pregnancy, suggesting that airway function remains stable.[43] In addition, peak expiratory flow rates measured using a peak flowmeter seem to be unaltered in pregnancy at rates of 450 ± 16 L/min.[44] Therefore, during gestation both spirometry and peak flowmeters can be used in diagnosing and managing respiratory illnesses.

Because of the increased progesterone levels, pregnancy causes a state of chronic hyperventilation, as reflected by a 30 to 40 percent increase in both tidal volume and minute ventilation (Minute ventilation =

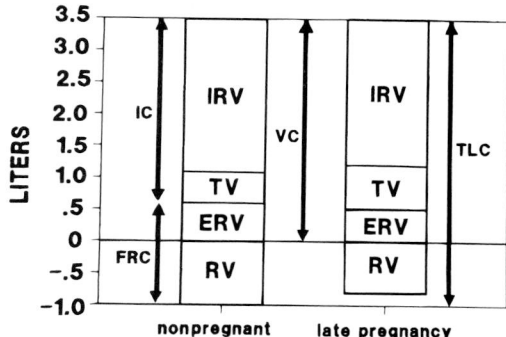

Figure 3–10. Lung volumes in nonpregnant and pregnant women. TLC, total lung capacity; VC, vital capacity; IC, inspiratory capacity; FRC, functional residual capacity; IRV, inspiratory reserve volume; TV, tidal volume; ERV, expiratory reserve volume; RV, residual volume. (From Cruickshank DP, Wigton TR, Hays PM: Maternal physiology in pregnancy. *In* Gabbe SG, Niebyl JR, Simpson JL [eds] Obstetrics: Normal and Problem Pregnancies, 3rd ed. New York, Churchill Livingstone, 1996, p 94, with permission.)

Table 3–2. LUNG VOLUMES AND CAPACITIES IN PREGNANCY

Measurement	Definition	Change in Pregnancy
Respiratory rate (RR)	Number of breaths per minute	Unchanged
Vital capacity (VC)	Maximum amount of air that can be forcibly expired after maximum inspiration (IC + ERV)	Unchanged
Inspiratory capacity (IC)	Maximum amount of air that can be inspired from resting expiratory level (TV + IRV)	Increased 5 to 10%
Tidal volume (TV)	Amount of air inspired and expired with normal breath	Increased 30 to 40%
Inspiratory reserve volume (IRV)	Maximum amount of air that can be inspired at end of normal inspiration	Unchanged
Functional residual capacity (FRC)	Amount of air in lungs at resting expiratory level (ERV + RV)	Decreased 20%
Expiratory reserve volume (ERV)	Maximum amount of air that can be expired from resting expiratory level	Decreased 15 to 20%
Residual volume (RV)	Amount of air in lungs after maximum expiration	Decreased 20 to 25%
Total lung capacity (TLC)	Total amount of air in lungs at maximal inspiration (VC + RV)	Decreased 5%

From Cruickshank DP, Wigton TR, Hays PM: Maternal physiology in pregnancy. *In* Gabbe SG, Niebyl JR, Simpson JL (eds): Obstetrics: Normal and Problem Pregnancies, 3rd ed. New York, Churchill Livingstone, 1996, p 95, with permission.

Tidal volume × Respiratory rate). The respiratory rate does not change. However, the increase in minute ventilation occurs by 8 to 11 weeks or earlier.

Gas Exchange

The rise in minute ventilation results in a 50 to 70 percent increase in alveolar ventilation with an increase in alveolar oxygen (PAO_2) and a decrease in alveolar carbon dioxide ($PACO_2$).[45] Hyperventilation results in a decreased $PaCO_2$ (arterial) from normal levels of 37 to 40 mm Hg to 27 to 32 mm Hg.[46] The drop in the $PaCO_2$ is important, as it increases the CO_2 gradient between the fetus and mother and facilitates transfer of CO_2 from the fetus to the mother. The low maternal $PaCO_2$ results in a chronic respiratory alkalosis. Partial renal compensation occurs through increased excretion of bicarbonate, which helps maintain the pH between 7.4 and 7.45 and lowers the serum bicarbonate levels to 18 to 21 mEq/L. Early in pregnancy, the arterial oxygen (PaO_2) increases (106 to 108 mm Hg) as the $PaCO_2$ decreases, but by the third trimester a slight decrease in the PaO_2 (101 to 104) occurs as a result of the enlarging uterus. The alveolar-to-arterial gradient $[P(A-a)O_2]$ increases slightly at the end of gestation from 14 mm Hg to 20 mm Hg. This decrease in the PaO_2 late in pregnancy is even more pronounced in the supine position, with a further drop of 5 to 10 mm Hg and an increase in the $P(A-a)O_2$ to 26 mm Hg.[30]

As the minute ventilation increases, a simultaneous but smaller increase in oxygen uptake and consumption occurs. Most investigators have found maternal oxygen consumption to be 20 to 40 percent above nonpregnant levels. This increase occurs as a result of the oxygen requirements of the fetus and placenta and the increased oxygen requirement of maternal organs. With exercise or during labor, an even greater rise in both minute ventilation and oxygen consumption takes place.[30] During a contraction, oxygen consumption can triple.[45] As a result of the increased oxygen consumption and because the functional reserve capacity is decreased, there is a lowering of the maternal oxygen reserve. Therefore, the pregnant patient is more susceptible to the effects of apnea. For example, during intubation, a more rapid onset of hypoxia, hypercapnia, and respiratory acidosis is seen.

Hankins et al. found that interpulmonary shunting was three times higher during gestation, increasing from 2 to 5 percent to 13 to 15 percent. These investigators attributed this observation to the anatomic changes of pregnancy that result in an overall decrease in lung volumes and greater ventilation-perfusion mismatches.[47] In a second study, Hankins et al. found no increase in oxygen delivery, oxygen extraction, or the arteriovenous oxygen content difference. Surprisingly, no increase in oxygen consumption was documented during pregnancy.[48]

HEMATOLOGIC CHANGES

Plasma Volume and Red Blood Cell Mass

Maternal blood volume begins to increase at about 6 weeks' gestation. Thereafter, it increases progressively until 30 to 34 weeks and then plateaus until delivery. The average expansion of blood volume is 40 to 50 percent, although increases of 20 to 100 percent may be found. Women with multiple pregnancies have a larger increase in blood volume than those with singletons.[49] Likewise, the blood volume expansion correlates with infant birth weight, but it is not clear whether this is a cause or an effect. The increase in blood volume results from a rise in both plasma volume and RBC mass. The plasma volume begins to increase by 6 weeks and expands at a steady pace until it plateaus at 30 weeks' gestation, 1,200 to 1,300 ml higher than prior to pregnancy (50 percent higher).

Erythrocyte mass also begins to increase at about 10 weeks' gestation, but initially at a rate slower than plasma volume. The erythrocyte mass grows progressively until term. The plateau seen in plasma volume after 30 to 34 weeks is not observed in RBC mass.[49] Without iron supplementation, RBC mass increases about 18 percent by term, from a mean nonpregnant level of 1,400 ml up to 1,650 ml. Women whose diet is supplemented with iron show a greater RBC mass increment, increasing about 400 to 450 ml or 30 percent.[49] Because plasma volume increases more than the RBC mass, maternal hematocrit falls. This so-called physiologic anemia of pregnancy reaches a nadir at 30 to 34 weeks. Since the RBC mass continues to increase after 30 weeks when the plasma volume expansion has plateaued, the hematocrit may rise somewhat after 30 weeks[50] (Fig. 3–11). The mean and fifth percentile hemoglobin concentrations for normal iron-supplemented pregnant women are listed in Table 3–3.[51] In pregnancy, erythropoietin levels increase two- to threefold, starting at 16 weeks. Moderate erythroid hyperplasia is found in the bone marrow, and the reticulocyte count is mildly elevated. These changes are thought to be due to the increased erythropoietin.[52]

The increased blood volume of pregnancy clearly protects the mother from the possibility of hemorrhage during pregnancy or at delivery. The larger blood vol-

Table 3–3. HEMOGLOBIN VALUES IN PREGNANCY

Weeks' Gestation	Mean Hemoglobin (g/dl)	Fifth Percentile Hemoglobin (g/dl)
12	12.2	11.0
16	11.8	10.6
20	11.6	10.5
24	11.6	10.5
28	11.8	10.7
32	12.1	11.0
36	12.5	11.4
40	12.9	11.9

From U.S. Department of Health and Human Services: MMWR Morb Mortal Wkly Rep 38:400, 1989.

ume also helps fill the expanded vascular system created by vasodilation and the large low-resistance vascular pool within the uteroplacental unit. This protects the mother and fetus from hypotension.[30]

Vaginal delivery of a singleton infant at term is associated with a mean blood loss of 500 ml; an uncomplicated cesarean birth, about 1,000 ml; and a cesarean hysterectomy, 1,500 ml.[49,53,54] In a normal delivery, almost all of the blood loss occurs in the first hour. Pritchard et al. found that over the next 72 hours only 80 ml of blood is lost. Gravid women respond to blood loss in a different fashion. In the nonpregnant state, with blood loss, the blood volume falls immediately and then expands via volume redistribution so that by 24 hours the blood volume approaches the prehemorrhage level. Therefore, isovolemia with anemia proportional to the blood loss occurs with an appropriate drop in hematocrit. In pregnancy, the blood volume drops after postpartum bleeding, but there is no reexpansion to the prelabor level, and there is less of a change in the hematocrit. After delivery with average blood loss, the hematocrit will drop moderately for 3 to 4 days followed by an increase. By days 5 to 7, the postpartum hematocrit will be similar to the prelabor hematocrit. If the postpartum hematocrit is lower than the prelabor hematocrit, then potentially the blood loss was larger than appreciated or the hypervolemia of pregnancy was less than normal as in preeclampsia.[49]

Iron Metabolism in Pregnancy

Iron is absorbed from the duodenum only in the ferrous (divalent) state, its form in iron supplements. Ferric (trivalent) iron from vegetable food sources must first be converted to the divalent state by the enzyme ferric reductase. If body iron stores are normal, only about 10 percent of ingested iron is absorbed, most of which remains in the mucosal cells or enterocytes until

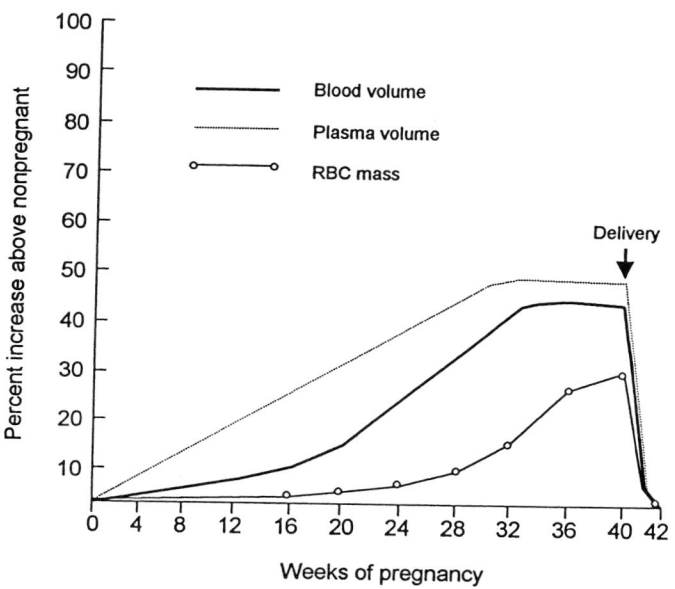

Figure 3–11. Blood volume changes during pregnancy. (From Scott D: Anemia during pregnancy. Obstet Gynecol Ann 1:219, 1972.)

sloughing leads to excretion in the feces.[55] Under conditions of increased iron needs, the fraction of iron absorbed increases. After absorption, iron is released from the enterocytes into the circulation, where it is carried bound to transferrin to the liver, spleen, muscle, and bone marrow. In those sites, iron is freed from transferrin and incorporated into hemoglobin (75 percent of iron), and myoglobin, or stored as ferritin and hemosiderin.[55] Menstruating women have about half the iron stores of men with total body iron of 2 to 2.5 g and iron stores of only 300 mg. Prior to pregnancy, 8 to 10 percent of women in Western nations have iron deficiency.[55]

The iron requirements of gestation are about 1,000 mg. This includes 500 mg used to increase the maternal RBC mass (1 ml of erythrocytes contains 1.1 mg iron), 300 mg transported to the fetus, and 200 mg to compensate for the normal daily iron losses by the mother (1 mg/day is lost from sloughing of enterocytes).[56] Thus, the normal expectant woman needs to absorb an average of 3.5 mg/day of iron. In actuality, the iron requirements are not constant but increase remarkably during the third trimester to 6 to 7 mg/day. The fetus receives its iron through active transport, primarily during the last trimester. Adequate iron transport to the fetus is maintained despite severe maternal iron deficiency. Thus, there is no correlation between maternal and fetal hemoglobin concentrations.

In the past, whether the nonanemic pregnant woman should receive routine iron supplementation was controversial. Most American obstetricians favored the practice, while those in Europe generally considered it unnecessary. With the availability of serum ferritin levels that closely mirror body iron stores, it has become apparent that the unsupplemented patient, although not anemic, is significantly iron deficient at term. Table 3–4, adapted from the work of Romslo et al. demonstrates that women who are not anemic at the beginning of gestation and who do not take iron supplementation have a significant drop in hemoglobin concentration, serum iron, serum ferritin, and transferrin saturation by term. The reason for these changes is the majority of women do not have sufficient iron stores to meet the demands of pregnancy. Such changes do not occur in women supplemented with iron (200 mg elemental iron given), although the total iron-binding capacity rises.[57-59]

It is important to remember that the purpose of iron supplementation during pregnancy is not to raise or even maintain the maternal hemoglobin level; instead, the goal is to maintain or restore normal maternal iron levels. Typically, this cannot be achieved by simply increasing the intake of iron-rich food such as meats, nongreen beans, iron-fortified cereals, egg yolk, dark green vegetables, and dried raisins. Therefore, iron supplementation is often needed during pregnancy, but

Table 3–4. EFFECT OF IRON SUPPLEMENTATION DURING PREGNANCY

	Iron-Treated	Placebo-Treated
Hemoglobin (g/dl)		
10 to 12 weeks	12.8	12.4
37 to 40 weeks	12.6	11.3*
Serum iron (μmol/L)		
10 to 12 weeks	19.2	20.4
37 to 40 weeks	21.9	9.5*
Serum ferritin (μg/L)		
10 to 12 weeks	28.0	27.0
37 to 40 weeks	24.0	6.0*
Serum iron-binding capacity (μm/dl)		
10 to 12 weeks	58.1	64.1
37 to 40 weeks	75.4*	92.3*

*Significant change between first trimester (10 to 12 weeks) and term (37 to 40 weeks).
Adapted from Romslo I, Haram K, Sagen N, et al: Iron requirement in normal pregnancy as assessed by serum ferritin, serum transferrin saturation and erythrocyte protoporphyrin determinations. Br J Obstet Gynaecol 90:101, 1983.

rarely needs to be started prior to 20 to 28 weeks. The recommended dose is 30 mg elemental iron per day, or one tablet of ferrous gluconate 325 mg. Taking iron prior to 20 weeks can worsen the nausea and vomiting of pregnancy. If a woman enters pregnancy with iron deficiency anemia, she will need to take additional iron above the 1,000 mg required for a normal pregnancy. Available iron supplements include ferrous sulfate 325 mg (65 mg elemental iron), ferrous gluconate 325 mg (35 mg elemental iron), and ferrous fumarate 325 mg (107 mg elemental iron). The usual dose to treat anemia is ferrous sulfate 325 mg twice daily, along with a stool softener such as docusate 100 mg twice daily.

Platelets

Prior to the introduction of automated analyzers, 11 studies of platelet counts during pregnancy reported conflicting results, with some showing a decrease, an increase, or no change with gestation. Unfortunately, even with the availability of automated cell counters, the data on the change in platelet count during pregnancy are still somewhat unclear.[60-62] Two studies have utilized true longitudinal methods with serial measurements in the same women. Pitkin et al. measured platelet counts in 23 women every 4 weeks and found that the counts dropped from $322 \pm 75 \times 10^3$/mm³ in the first trimester to $278 \pm 75 \times 10^3$/mm³ in the third trimester.[63] Similarly, O'Brien, in a study of 30 women, found a progressive decline in platelet counts.[64] Therefore, most recent studies show a decline in the platelet count during pregnancy possibly caused by increased destruction.[61] In addition to the mild decrease in the mean platelet count in pregnancy, Burrows and Kelton have demonstrated that in the third trimester approximately 8 percent of gravid women develop gestational thrombocytopenia, with platelet counts between 70,000 and 150,000/mm³. These women have no increased complications of pregnancy and their counts return to normal by 1 to 2 weeks postpartum. Gestational thrombocytopenia is thought to be due to accelerated platelet consumption similar to that seen in normal pregnancy, but more marked in this subset of women.[65,66]

Immune System and Leukocytes

The peripheral white blood cell (WBC) count rises progressively during pregnancy. During the first trimester, the mean WBC count is 8,000/mm³, with a normal range of 5,110 to 9,900/mm³. During the second trimester and third trimester, the mean is 8,500/mm³, with a range of 5,600 to 12,200/mm³.[63] In labor, the count may rise to 20,000 to 30,000/mm³, after which it gradually returns to the nonpregnant level by the end of the first week of the puerperium. The increase in the WBC count during pregnancy and delivery is largely because of increased numbers of circulating segmented neutrophils or granulocytes. The reason for the increased leukocytosis is unclear, but may be caused by the elevated estrogen and cortisol levels.

Successful pregnancy is dependent on maternal tolerance or immunononreactivity to paternal antigens. Maternal tolerance appears to be associated with the development of several specific mechanisms that protect the fetus from a maternal cytotoxic immune response.[67] Pregnancy is not a state of immunodeficiency but is a state of altered immune functions.[68] The major change observed is a modulation away from cell-mediated immune responses toward humoral or antibody-mediated immunity. T helper 1 cells and natural killer cells decline whereas T helper 2 cells increase. Clinically, the decrease in cellular immunity leads to the increased susceptibility to intracellular pathogens such as cytomegalovirus virus, varicella, and malaria. The decrease in cellular immunity may explain why women with rheumatoid arthritis frequently improve during gestation, since it is a cell-mediated immunopathologic disease.[67] Although pregnancy is characterized by enhanced antibody-mediated immunity, the levels of immunoglobulins A, G, and M all decrease in pregnancy.

Coagulation System

Pregnancy places women at increased risk for thromboembolic disease caused by increased venous stasis, vessel wall injury, and changes in the coagulation cascade that lead to hypercoagulability. In pregnancy, several procoagulant coagulation factors are increased, and changes occur to some of the natural inhibitors of coagulation. In addition, pregnancy causes a decrease in the fibrinolytic system with reduced levels of available circulating plasminogen activator.[1] These physiologic changes provide some defense against peripartum hemorrhage.

The majority of the procoagulant factors from the coagulation cascade are markedly increased, including factors I, VII, VIII, IX, and X. Factors II, V, and XII are unchanged or mildly increased and levels of factors XI and XIII decline[1,69,70] (Fig. 3–12). Plasma fibrinogen (factor I) levels begin to increase in the first trimester and peak in the third trimester at levels 50 percent higher than prior to pregnancy. The rise in fibrinogen is associated with an increase in the erythrocyte sedimentation rate.[71] The prothrombin time (PT), activated partial thromboplastin time (APTT), and thrombin time all fall slightly, but remain within the limits of normal nonpregnant values, whereas the bleeding time and whole blood clotting times are unchanged. Levels of coagulation factors normalize 2 weeks postpartum.

Increasingly in the medical literature, familial causes for thromboembolic diseases are being discovered that are related to isolated deficiencies of proteins involved in coagulation inhibition called thrombophilias. These disorders include abnormalities in the formation of natural inhibitors to coagulation such as antithrombin III, protein C, protein S, and activated protein C (APC) resistance. Resistance to APC is caused in the majority of individuals by a point mutation in the gene for procoagulant factor V, called the factor V Leiden mutation, that impairs inactivation of factor V by APC. This change prevents protein C from acting as an inhibitor to factor V.[72] Pregnancy has been shown to cause a progressive and significant decrease in the levels of total and free protein S from early in pregnancy but to have no effect on the levels of protein C and antithrombin III.[73,74] Pregnancy has also been shown to cause a decline in the APC sensitivity ratio (APC:SR), which is the ratio of the clotting time in the presence and the absence of APC. The APC:SR ratio is considered abnormal if less than 2.6. In a study of 239 women by Clark et al., the APC:SR ratio decreased from a mean of 3.12 in the first trimester to 2.63 by the third trimester. By the third trimester, 38 percent of women were found to have an acquired APC resistance, with APC:SR values below 2.6.[73] Whether the change in the protein S level and the APC:SR ratio are responsible for some of the hypercoagulability of pregnancy is unknown; however, if a work-up for familial thrombophilias is done during pregnancy, the clinician should use caution when attempting to interpret these levels if abnormal.

During pregnancy, some investigators have found evidence to support the theory that there is a state of low-

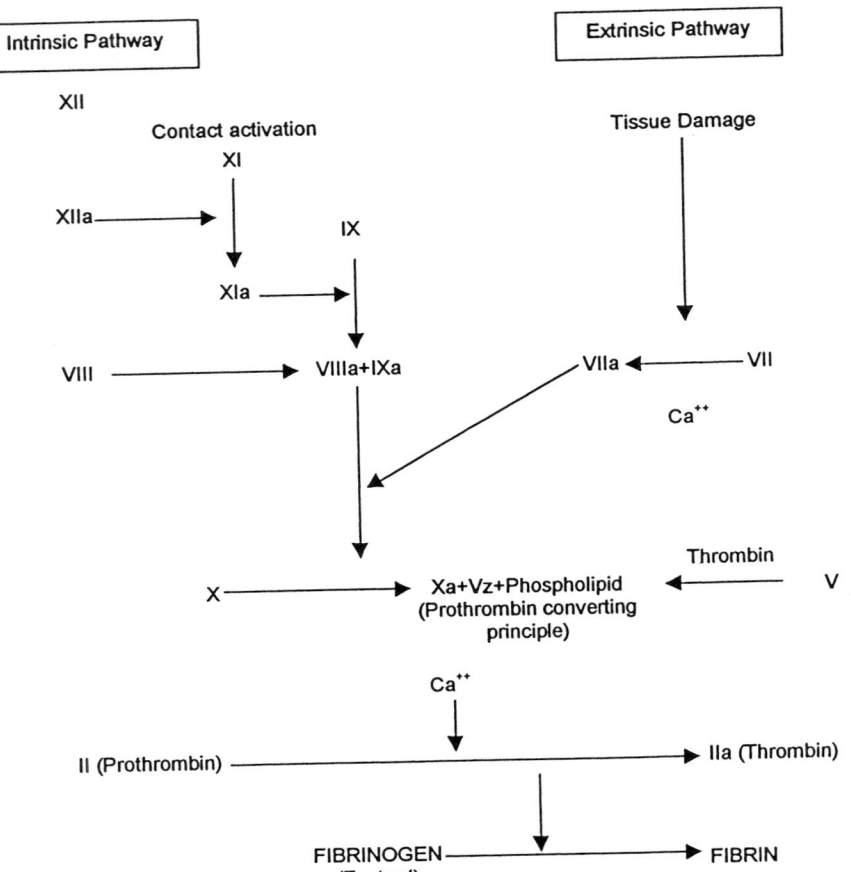

Figure 3–12. The normal components of the coagulation cascade. (From Johnson RL: Thromboembolic disease complicating pregnancy. *In* Foley MR, Strong TH [eds]: Obstetric Intensive Care: A Practical Manual. Philadelphia, WB Saunders Company, 1997, p 91, with permission.)

level intravascular coagulation. Investigators have found low concentrations of fibrin degradation products in maternal blood (markers of fibrinolysis), elevated levels of fibrinopeptide A (a marker for increased clotting), and increased levels of platelet factor 4 and β-thromboglobulin (markers of increased platelet activity).[75] The most likely cause for the low-level intravascular coagulation involves localized physiologic changes needed for maintenance of the uterine-placental interface.

URINARY SYSTEM

Anatomic Changes

The kidneys enlarge during pregnancy, with the length as measured by intravenous pyelography increasing about 1 cm. This growth in size and weight is due to increased renal vasculature, interstitial volume, and urinary dead space. The increase in urinary dead space is attributed to dilation of the renal pelvis, calyces, and ureters. Pelvicalyceal dilation by term averages 15 mm (range, 5 to 25 mm) on the right and 5 mm (range,

3 to 8 mm) on the left with the right greater than the left in most gravid women.[76]

The well-known dilation of the ureters and renal pelves begins by the second month of pregnancy and is maximal by the middle of the second trimester, when ureteric diameter may be as much as 2 cm. The right ureter is almost invariably dilated more than the left, and the dilation usually cannot be demonstrated below the pelvic brim. These findings have led some investigators to argue that the dilation is caused entirely by mechanical compression of the ureters by the enlarging uterus and ovarian venous plexus.[77] However, the early onset of ureteral dilation supports the hypothesis that smooth muscle relaxation caused by progesterone plays an additional role. Also supporting the role of progesterone is the finding of ureteral dilation in women with renal transplants and pelvic kidneys.[78] By 6 weeks postpartum, ureteral dilation resolves.[76] A clinical consequence of ureterocalyceal dilatation is an increased incidence of pyelonephritis among gravid women with asymptomatic bacteriuria. In addition, the ureterocalyceal dilatation makes interpretation of urinary radiographs more difficult when evaluating possible urinary tract obstruction or nephrolithiasis.

Anatomic changes are also observed in the bladder.

From midpregnancy on, an elevation in the bladder trigone occurs with increased vascular tortuousity throughout the bladder. This can cause an increased incidence of microhematuria during pregnancy. Due to the increasing size of the fetus and uterus, a decrease in bladder capacity develops, with an increased frequency of urinary incontinence.

Renal Hemodynamics

Renal plasma flow increases markedly from early in gestation. Dunlop showed convincingly that the effective renal plasma flow (ERPF) rises 75 percent over nonpregnant levels by 16 weeks' gestation[79] (Table 3–5). The increase is maintained until 34 weeks' gestation, when a decline in ERPF of about 25 percent occurs. The fall in ERPF has been demonstrated in subjects studied serially in both the sitting and the left lateral recumbent positions.[79,80] (Table 3–5).

Like ERPF, glomerular filtration rate (GFR) as measured by inulin clearance increases by 5 to 7 weeks. By the end of the first trimester, GFR is 50 percent higher than in the nonpregnant state, and this is maintained until the end of pregnancy. Three months postpartum, GFR values have declined to normal levels.[79,81] Because the ERPF increases more than the GFR early in pregnancy, the filtration fraction falls from nonpregnant levels until the late third trimester. At this time, because of the decline in ERPF, the filtration fraction returns to nonpregnant values of 20 to 21 percent.

Clinically, GFR is not determined by measuring the clearance of infused inulin (inulin is filtered by the glomerulus and is unaffected by the tubules), but rather by measuring endogenous creatinine clearance. This test gives a less precise measure of GFR, because creatinine is secreted by the tubules to a variable extent. Therefore, endogenous creatinine clearance is usually higher than the actual GFR. The creatinine clearance in pregnancy is greatly increased to values of 150 to 200 ml/min (normal nonpregnant, 120 ml/min). As with GFR, the increase in creatinine clearance occurs by 5 to 7 weeks' gestation, and in normal patients is maintained until the third trimester.

The clinical consequences of glomerular hyperfiltration are a reduction in maternal plasma levels of creatinine, blood urea nitrogen (BUN), and uric acid. Serum creatinine falls from a nonpregnant level of 0.8 mg/dl to 0.5 mg/dl by term. Likewise, BUN falls from nonpregnant levels of 13 mg/dl to 9 mg/dl by term.[7] Serum uric acid declines in early pregnancy because of the rise in GFR, reaching a nadir by 24 weeks with levels of 2.0 to 3.0 mg/dl.[82] After 24 weeks, the uric acid level begins to rise, and by the end of pregnancy, the levels in most women are essentially the same as before pregnancy. The rise in uric acid levels is caused by increased renal tubular absorption of urate. Patients with preeclampsia have elevated uric acid level concentrations; however, because uric acid levels normally rise during the third trimester, overreliance on this test should be avoided in the diagnosis and management of preeclampsia.[82]

During pregnancy nocturia is more common. In the standing position, sodium and water are retained and, therefore, during the daytime pregnant women tend to retain an increased amount of water.[83] At night, while in the lateral recumbent position, this added water is excreted, resulting in nocturia.

Renal Tubular Function/Excretion of Nutrients

Despite high levels of aldosterone, which would be expected to result in enhanced urinary excretion of potassium, pregnant women retain about 350 mmol of potassium. The majority of the excess potassium in stored in the fetus and placenta. The mean potassium concentrations in maternal blood are just slightly below nonpregnant levels. The kidney's ability to conserve potassium has been attributed to the increased progesterone levels of pregnancy.[84]

Glucose excretion increases in almost all pregnant women, and the presence of glycosuria during pregnancy is not necessarily abnormal. The urinary loss of glucose in the nonpregnant state is less than 100 mg/day, but 90 percent of pregnant women with

Table 3–5. SERIAL CHANGES IN RENAL HEMODYNAMICS

	Nonpregnant	Seated Position (n = 25)*			Left Lateral Recumbent Position (n = 17)†	
		16 wk	26 wk	36 wk	29 wk	37 wk
Effective renal plasma flow (ml/min)	480 ± 72	840 ± 145	891 ± 279	771 ± 175	748 ± 85	677 ± 82
Glomerular filtration rate (ml/min)	99 ± 18	149 ± 17	152 ± 18	150 ± 32	145 ± 19	138 ± 22
Filtration fraction	0.21	0.18	0.18	0.20	0.19	0.21

*Data from Dunlop W: Serial changes in renal haemodynamics during normal pregnancy. Br J Obstet Gynaecol 88:1, 1991.
†Data from Ezimokhai M, Davison J, Philips P, et al: Non-postural serial changes in renal function during the third trimester of normal human pregnancy. Br J Obstet Gynaecol 88:465, 1991.

normal blood glucose levels excrete 1 to 10 g of glucose per day.[85] The glycosuria is intermittent and not necessarily related to blood glucose levels or the stage of gestation. Glucose is freely filtered by the glomerulus, and with the 50 percent increase in GFR a greater load of glucose is presented to the proximal tubules. There may be a change in the reabsorptive capability of the proximal tubules themselves, but the old concept of pregnancy leading to an overwhelming of the maximum tubular reabsorptive capacity for glucose (Tm) is misleading and oversimplified.[85,86] The exact mechanisms underlying the altered handling of glucose by the proximal tubules remains obscure. Even though glycosuria is common during pregnancy, women with repetitive glycosuria should be screened for diabetes mellitus.

No increase in proteinuria occurs during a normal pregnancy in women without proteinuria prior to pregnancy. Higby et al. collected 24-hour urine samples on 270 gravid women over the course of pregnancy and determined the amount of proteinuria and albuminuria.[87] These investigators found that the amount of protein and albumin excreted in urine did not increase significantly by trimester (Table 3–6). They observed that in normal women without preeclampsia, underlying renal disease, or urinary tract infections the mean 24-hour urine protein across pregnancy is 116.9 mg with a 95 percent confidence limit of 259.4 mg. They also noted that patients do not normally have microalbuminuria, defined as urinary albumin excretion greater than 30 mg/dl.[87] In women with preexisting proteinuria, in the absence of preeclampsia, pregnancy causes increases in the amount of proteinuria in both the second and third trimesters and potentially in the first trimester. In a study by Gordon et al. of women with diabetic nephropathy, the amount of proteinuria increased from a mean of 1.74 ± 1.33 g/24 h in the first trimester to a mean of 4.82 ± 4.7 g/24 h in the third trimester.[88]

Other changes in tubular function during pregnancy include an increase in excretion of amino acids in the urine (aminoaciduria)[89] and an increase in calcium excretion (for more details, see Calcium Metabolism, below). Also, the kidney responds to the respiratory alkalosis of pregnancy by enhanced excretion of bicarbonate; however, renal handling of acid excretion is unchanged.[90]

ALIMENTARY TRACT

Appetite

Most women experience an increase in appetite throughout pregnancy. In the absence of nausea or "morning sickness," women eating according to appetite will increase food intake by about 200 kcal/day by the end of the first trimester.[91] The recommended dietary allowance (RDA) calls for an additional 300 kcal/day during pregnancy. Energy requirements vary depending on the population studied, and a greater increase may be necessary for pregnant teenagers and women with high levels of physical activity.[92]

Extensive folklore exists about dietary cravings and aversions during gestation. Many of these are undoubtedly due to an individual's perception of which foods aggravate or ameliorate such symptoms as nausea and heartburn. The sense of taste may be blunted in some pregnant women, leading to an increased desire for highly seasoned food. Pica, a bizarre craving for strange foods, is relatively common among pregnant women, and a history of pica should be sought in those with poor weight gain or refractory anemia. Examples of pica include the consumption of clay, starch, toothpaste, and ice.

Mouth

The pH and the production of saliva is probably unchanged during pregnancy.[93] Ptyalism, an unusual complication of pregnancy, most often occurs in women suffering from nausea and may be associated with the loss of 1 to 2 L of saliva per day. Most authorities believe ptyalism actually represents inability of the nauseated woman to swallow normal amounts of saliva rather than a true increase in the production of saliva. A decrease in the ingestion of starchy foods may help.

No evidence exists that pregnancy causes or acceler-

Table 3–6. COMPARISON OF 24-HOUR URINARY PROTEIN AND ALBUMIN EXCRETION FOR EACH TRIMESTER OF PREGNANCY*

	First Trimester (n = 19)	Second Trimester (n = 133)	Third Trimester (n = 118)	Significance
Protein (mg/24 h)	80.0 ± 60.6	116.7 ± 69.3	115.3 ± 69.2	$p = 0.13$
Albumin (mg/24 h)	9.9 ± 5.3	10.8 ± 6.9	12.8 ± 9.5	$p = 0.12$

*Values are expressed as mean $\pm$ SD.
From Higby K, Suiter C, Phelps J, et al: Normal values of urinary albumin and total protein excretion during pregnancy. Am J Obstet Gynecol 171:984, 1994, with permission.

ates the course of dental caries. However, the gums (gingiva) swell and may bleed after tooth brushing, giving rise to the so-called gingivitis of pregnancy.[94] At times a tumorous gingivitis may occur, presenting as a violaceous pedunculated lesion at the gum line that may bleed profusely. Called either epulis gravidarum or pyogenic granulomas, these lesions consist of granulation tissue and an inflammatory infiltrate. It is thought to be an abnormal tissue response to trauma and can occur elsewhere besides the mouth. These lesions usually remit 1 to 2 months after delivery. If the lesion persists or bleeds excessively during pregnancy, it should be excised.[95]

Stomach

The tone and motility of the stomach are decreased during pregnancy, probably because of the smooth muscle–relaxing effects of progesterone. Decreased levels of motilin, a gut hormone that stimulates smooth muscle, have also been noted.[96] Nevertheless, scientific evidence regarding delayed gastric emptying is inconclusive. Davison et al. showed that during pregnancy the mean total emptying time was significantly longer in pregnant women with heartburn versus a control group of nonpregnant women, but no clear evidence of a delay in emptying was found in gravid women without heartburn. More recently, Macfie and colleagues, using paracetamol absorption as an indirect measure of gastric emptying, failed to demonstrate a delay in gastric emptying when comparing 15 nonpregnant controls to 15 women in each trimester of pregnancy.[97] An increased delay was seen in laboring women, with the etiology ascribed to the pain and stress of labor.[98]

Pregnancy causes a decreased risk of peptic ulcer disease (PUD), but at the same time causes an increase in gastroesophageal reflux disease (GERD).[99] This apparent paradox can be partially explained by physiologic changes of the stomach and lower esophagus. The increase in GERD is attributed to esophageal dysmotility caused by gestational hormones and gastric compression from the enlarged uterus. In addition, the decrease in the tone of the gastroesophageal sphincter may also lead to increased reflux of stomach acids into the esophagus. Theories proposed to explain the decreased incidence of PUD include increased placental histaminase synthesis with lower maternal histamine levels; increased gastric mucin production leading to protection of the gastric mucosa; reduced gastric acid secretion; and enhanced immunological tolerance of *Helicobacter pylori*, the infectious agent that causes PUD.[99]

Intestines

Perturbations in the motility of the small intestines and colon are common in pregnancy, resulting in an increased incidence of constipation (11 to 38 percent) in some women and diarrhea in others. Up to 34 percent of pregnant women in one study noted an increased frequency of bowel movements, perhaps related to increased prostaglandin synthesis.[100,101] The motility of the small intestines is reduced in pregnancy, with increased orocecal transit times presumably caused by progesterone.[102,103] No studies on the colonic transit time have been performed in pregnancy, but limited information suggests reduced colonic motility.[101] Absorption of nutrients from the small bowel (with the exception of increased iron and calcium absorption) is unchanged, but the decreased transit times may allow for more efficient absorption. In the colon, Parry et al. demonstrated an increase in both water and sodium absorption.[104]

The enlarging uterus displaces the intestines and, most importantly, moves the position of the appendix. Thus, the presentation, physical signs, and type of surgical incision are affected in the management of appendicitis. Portal venous pressure is increased in gestation, leading to dilation wherever there are portosystemic venous anastomoses. This includes the gastroesophageal junction and the hemorrhoidal veins, which results in the common complaint of hemorrhoids.

Gallbladder

The function of the gallbladder is markedly altered during pregnancy because of the effects of progesterone. After the first trimester, the fasting and residual volumes are twice as great, and the rate at which the gallbladder empties is much slower.[105] In addition, the biliary cholesterol saturation is increased, and the chenodeoxycholic acid level is decreased.[106] This change in the composition of the bile fluid favors the formation of cholesterol crystals and, with incomplete emptying of the gallbladder, the crystals are retained and gallstone formation is more likely.

Liver

The size and histology of the liver are unchanged in pregnancy.[107] Many clinical and laboratory signs usually associated with liver disease are present in pregnancy, however. Spider angiomas and palmar erythema, caused by elevated estrogen levels, are normal and disappear soon after delivery. The serum albumin and total protein levels fall progressively during gestation. By term, albumin levels are 25 percent lower than nonpregnant levels. Despite an overall increase in total body protein, decreases in total protein and albumin concentrations occur as a result of hemodilution. In addition, serum alkaline phosphatase activity rises during the third trimester to levels two to four times that of nonpregnant women. Most of this increase is caused by placental production of the heat-stable isoenzyme.[1,108] During pregnancy, the serum concentrations of many proteins produced by the liver increase. These include elevations in fibrinogen, ceruloplasmin, and transferrin, and the binding proteins for corticosteroids, sex steroids, thyroid hormones, and vitamin D.[1]

With the exception of alkaline phosphatase, the other "liver function tests" are unaffected by pregnancy, including serum levels of bilirubin, aspartate aminotransferase (AST, formerly SGOT), alanine aminotransferase (ALT, formerly SGPT), γ-glutamyltransferase, 5'-nucleotidase, creatinine phosphokinase (CPK), and lactate dehydrogenase (LDH). In some studies the mean levels of ALT and AST are mildly elevated but still within normal nonpregnant values.[108,109] Levels of CPK and LDH can increase with labor.[1]

Finally, pregnancy may cause some changes in bile acid production and secretion. Pregnancy may be associated with mild subclinical cholestasis due to the high concentrations of estrogen. Reports on bile acid concentrations are conflicting, with some studies showing an increase and others no change. It does appear that the fasting levels are unchanged, and the measurement of a fasting level appears to be the best test for diagnosing cholestasis of pregnancy.[109]

Nausea and Vomiting of Pregnancy

Nausea and vomiting, or "morning sickness," complicate up to 70 percent of pregnancies. Typical onset is between 4 and 8 weeks' gestation, with improvement before 14 to 16 weeks.[110] Although the symptoms are often quite distressing, morning sickness seldom leads to significant weight loss, ketonemia, or electrolyte disturbances. The cause is not well understood, although relaxation of the smooth muscle of the stomach probably plays a role. Elevated levels of human chorionic gonadotropin (hCG) may be involved, although a good correlation between maternal hCG concentrations and the degree of nausea and vomiting does not exist.[111] Interestingly, women admitted to the hospital for nausea and vomiting more often have a female than a male fetus (56 vs. 44 percent).[112] Also of interest, pregnancies complicated by nausea and vomiting generally have a more favorable outcome than do those without such symptoms.[113] Treatment is largely supportive, consisting of reassurance, psychological support, avoidance of foods found to trigger nausea, and frequent small meals. Eating dry toast or crackers prior to getting out of bed may be beneficial. A recent review of alternative therapies to antiemetic drugs found that acupressure with wristbands and treatment with ginger root or vitamin B_6 may be helpful.[114]

Hyperemesis gravidarum, a more pernicious form of nausea and vomiting associated with weight loss, ketonemia, electrolyte imbalance, and dehydration, often persists throughout pregnancy. For these patients, the clinician must rule out other diseases such as pancreatitis, cholecystitis, hepatitis, and thyroid disease. Hospitalization with intravenous replacement of fluids and electrolytes is often needed. Options of antiemetics include the phenothiazines: promethazine (Phenergan), chlorpromazine (Thorazine), and prochlorperazine (Compazine) or metoclopramide (Reglan) or droperidol (Inapsine). On admission to the hospital, the patient should be kept totally NPO for 24 to 48 hours, given intravenous hydration, and tried on one of the above medications (intravenously or intramuscularly initially). Care must be given not to combine the phenothiazines with metoclopramide because of the additive risks of causing extrapyramidal reactions. Chlorpromazine given rectally (25 to 50 mg every 8 hours) may be highly effective in the more refractory cases. Recently, use of oral methylprednisolone, 16 mg three times daily for 3 days and then tapered over 2 weeks, has been shown to be more effective than promethazine.[115] Because of potential risks, use of parenteral calorie replacement should only be used after the patient has failed multiple antiemetic treatments and attempts at enteral tube feedings.

THE SKELETON

Calcium Metabolism

Pregnancy was initially thought to be a state of "physiologic hyperparethyroidism," with maternal skeletal calcium loss needed to supply the fetus with calcium. It was thought that this could result in long-term maternal calcium bone loss. This theory was shown to be incorrect and it is now evident that fetal calcium needs are met through a series of physiologic changes in calcium metabolism without long-term consequences to the maternal skeleton.[116] This allows the fetus to accumulate 21 g (range, 13 to 33 g) of calcium, 80 percent of this amount during the third trimester, when fetal skeletal mineralization is at its peak.[117,118] Calcium is actively transported across the placenta. In addition, calcium is excreted in greater amounts by the maternal kidneys so that by term the urinary loss of calcium is doubled.[119]

Maternal total calcium levels decline throughout pregnancy. However, the serum ionized calcium level is unchanged and constant during pregnancy. The fall in total calcium is caused by the reduced serum albumin concentration which results in a decrease in the albumin-bound fraction of calcium[116,120] (Fig. 3–13). Fifty percent of calcium is ionized, and it is this form that is physiologically important. It appears that the maternal serum calcium levels are maintained and the fetal cal-

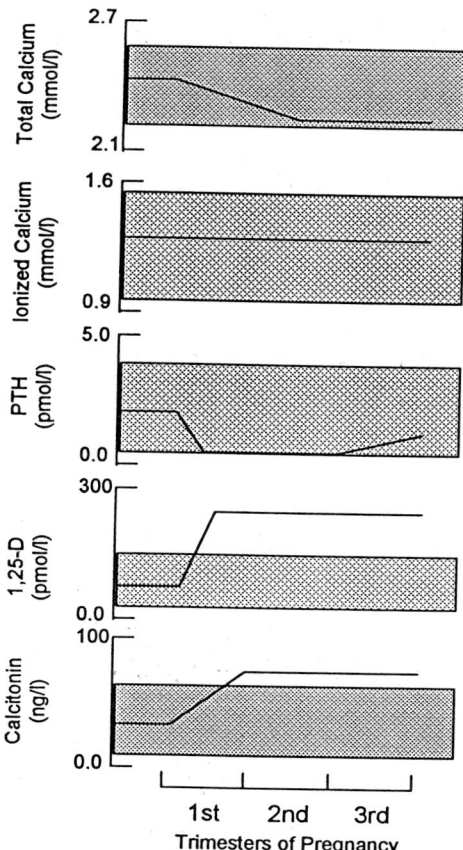

Figure 3–13. Schematic illustration of the longitudinal changes in calcium and calcitropic hormone levels that occur during human pregnancy. Normal adult ranges are indicated by the *shaded areas.* (From Kovacs C, Kronenberg H: Maternal-fetal calcium and bone metabolism during pregnancy, puerperium, and lactation. Endocr Rev 18:832, 1997.)

cium needs are met through increased intestinal calcium absorption. Calcium is absorbed through the small intestines and its absorption is doubled by 12 weeks' gestation.[116,121] The early increase in absorption may allow the maternal skeleton to store calcium in advance of the peak third-trimester fetal demands. Maternal serum phosphate levels are likewise unchanged.[116]

Older studies showed an increase in maternal parathyroid hormone (PTH) levels.[122] These studies used less sensitive PTH assays that measured multiple different fragments of PTH, most of which are biologically inactive. In five recent prospective studies, all utilizing the newer PTH assays, maternal levels of PTH were not elevated and actually remained in the low-normal range throughout gestation.[116] Therefore, pregnancy does not cause hyperparathyroidism (Fig. 3–13). Levels of 1,25-dihydroxyvitamin D increase during gestation, doubling in the first trimester as a result of increased production from the maternal kidneys and potentially the fetoplacental unit, which appears to be independent of PTH control.[119] The elevated levels of 1,25-dihydroxyvitamin

D are thought to be primarily responsible for the important increase in intestinal calcium absorption.[116] Calcitonin levels rise 20 percent during pregnancy and may help protect the maternal skeleton from bone loss.[116,123]

Skeletal and Postural Changes

Bone turnover appears to be low in the first half of gestation and then increase in the third trimester, corresponding to the peak rate of fetal calcium needs. This may represent turnover of previously stored skeletal calcium.[116] In the only study of bone biopsies performed in pregnant women, Shahtaheri et al. observed a change in the microarchitectural pattern of bone, but there was no change in overall bone mass by the end of pregnancy. This change in the microarchitectural pattern seems to result in a framework more resistant to the bending forces and biomechanical stresses needed to carry a growing fetus.[124]

Pregnancy results in a progressively increasing anterior convexity of the lumbar spine (lordosis). This compensatory mechanism keeps the woman's center of gravity over her legs, and prevents the enlarging uterus from shifting the center of gravity quite anteriorly. The unfortunate side effect of this necessary alteration is low back pain, a common complaint during gestation.

The ligaments of the pubic symphysis and sacroiliac joints loosen during pregnancy, probably from the effects of the hormone relaxin.[125] Marked widening of the pubic symphysis occurs by 28 to 32 weeks' gestation, with the width increasing from 3 to 4 mm in 7.7 to 7.9 mm.[126] This commonly results in pain near the symphysis that is referred down the inner thigh with standing and may result in a maternal sensation of snapping or movement of the bones with walking.

ENDOCRINE CHANGES

Thyroid

Despite alterations in thyroid morphology, histology, and laboratory indices, the pregnant woman remains euthyroid. These changes are primarily the result of increases in thyroxine-binding globulin (TBG) concentration and to the decrease in the size of the circulating pool of extrathyroidal iodide. Serum iodide levels fall because of increased renal loss of iodide. In addition, in the latter half of pregnancy, iodine is also transferred to the fetus, further decreasing maternal iodine levels. These alterations cause the thyroid to synthesize and secrete thyroid hormone actively.[127]

During pregnancy, the thyroid gland increases in size, but not as much as was commonly believed. If adequate iodine intake is maintained, the size of the thyroid gland remains unchanged or undergoes a small increase in size that can only be detected by ultrasound.[128,129] In pregnancy, the World Health Organization recommends that iodine intake be increased from 100 to 150 μg/day to 200 μg/day. In an iodine-deficient state, the thyroid gland is up to 25 percent larger, and goiters may be seen in 10 percent of women.[127] The development of a goiter during pregnancy is abnormal and should be evaluated.[130] Histologically, there is an increase in thyroid vascularity, with evidence of follicular hyperplasia.

Although there is increased uptake of iodine by the thyroid during gestation, the pregnant woman remains euthyroid by laboratory evaluation.[131] Total thyroxine (TT_4) and total triiodothyronine (TT_3) levels begin to increase in the first trimester and peak at midgestation as a result of increased TBG. The concentration of TT_4 increases from 5 to 12 μg/dl in nonpregnant women to 9 to 16 μg/dl during pregnancy. The increase in TBG is seen in the first trimester and plateaus at 12 to 14 weeks. Only a small amount of TT_4 and TT_3 is unbound, and it is these free (normally about 0.04 percent for T_4 and 0.5 percent for T_3) fractions that are the major determinant of whether an individual is euthyroid. The free T_4 levels rise slightly in the first trimester and then decrease so that by delivery the free T_4 levels are 10 to 15 percent lower than in nonpregnant women. However, these changes are small and in most pregnant women serum free T_4 concentrations remain within the normal nonpregnant range[127,132,133] (Fig. 3–14). Free T_3 levels follow a parallel pattern.

Thyroid-stimulating hormone (TSH) concentrations decrease transiently in the first trimester and then rise to prepregnant levels by the end of the first trimester. TSH levels then remain stable throughout the remainder of gestation.[127,132,133] The transient decrease in TSH coincides with the first-trimester increase in free T_4 levels, and both appear to be caused by the thyrotropic effects of hCG. Women with higher peak hCG levels have more TSH suppression. It clearly appears that hCG has some thyrotropic activity, but conflicting data on the exact role of hCG in maternal thyroid function remain.[127,132–134] While thyrotropin-releasing hormone (TRH) crosses the placenta, TSH does not.

The influence of maternal thyroid physiology on the fetus appears much more complex than previously thought. Whereas the maternal thyroid does not directly control fetal thyroid function, the systems interact by means of the placenta, which regulates the transfer of iodine and a small but important amount of thyroxine to the fetus. It was thought that little if any transplacental passage of T_4 and T_3 occurred.[135] It is now recognized that T_4 crosses the placenta and, in fact, in early pregnancy the fetus is critically dependent on the maternal T_4 supply for normal neurologic development.[136] Neonates with thyroid agenesis or a total defect in thyroid hormone synthesis were found to have umbilical cord thyroxine levels between 20 percent and 50 percent of those in normal infants.[137] These data demonstrate that the placenta is *not* impermeable to T_4. However, as a result of the deiodinase activity of the placenta, a large percentage of T_4 is broken down prior to transfer to the fetus. Evidence that the fetus is dependent on the maternal thyroid for normal development has recently been published. In women living in iodine-deficient areas, maternal hypothyroidism is associated with neonatal hypothyroidism and defects in long-term neurologic function and mental retardation or endemic cretinism. These abnormalities can be prevented if maternal iodine intake is initiated at the beginning of the second trimester.[138,139] Haddow et al. have found that maternal hypothyroidism during pregnancy results in slightly lower IQ scores in children at ages 7 to 9.[140]

Since iodine is actively transported across the placenta, the fetus is susceptible to iodine-induced goiters when the mother is given pharmacologic amounts of iodine. Similarly, radioactive iodine crosses the placenta, and, if given after 12 weeks' gestation, when the fetal thyroid is able to concentrate iodine, profound adverse effects on the fetus can occur.[132]

Adrenal Glands

Pregnancy is associated with marked changes in adrenocortical function, with increased serum levels of aldosterone, deoxycorticosterone (DOC), corticosteroid-binding globulin (CBG), cortisol, and free cortisol[141–143] (Table 3–7). Although the combined weight of the adrenal glands does not increase significantly in pregnancy, expansion of the zona fasciculata, which primarily produces glucocorticoids, is observed. The plasma concentration of CBG doubles by the end of the sixth

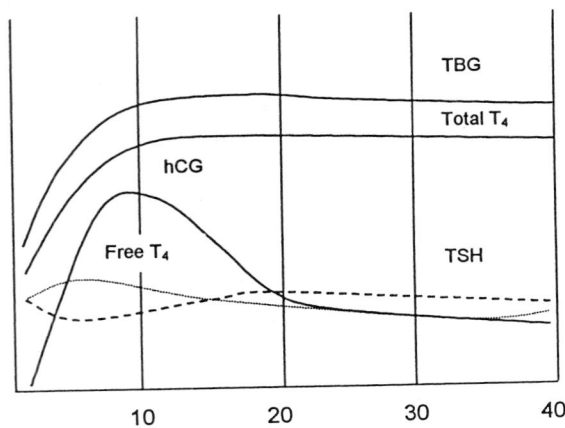

Figure 3–14. Relative changes in maternal thyroid function during pregnancy. (From Burrow G, Fisher D, Larsen P: Maternal and fetal thyroid function. N Engl J Med 331:1072, 1994, with permission.)

month of gestation when compared to nonpregnant values.[144] The increase in CBG results in elevated levels of total plasma cortisol concentrations. The levels of total cortisol rise after the first trimester, and by the end of pregnancy are nearly three times higher than nonpregnant values (12.5 ± 1.3 μg/dl vs. 30.1 ± 6.6 μg/dl).[141] During pregnancy, the diurinal variations in cortisol levels are maintained, with the highest values in the morning.

Only free cortisol, the fraction of cortisol not bound to CBG, is metabolically active, and direct measurements of free cortisol levels are difficult to perform. However, urinary free cortisol concentrations, the free cotisol index, and salivary cortisol concentrations, all of which reflect active free cortisol levels are all elevated after the first trimester.[141,143,145] In a study of 21 uncomplicated pregnancies, Goland et al. found that the urinary free cortisol concentration doubled from the first to the third trimester[143] (Table 3–7). Although the increase in total cortisol concentrations can be explained by the increase in CBG, this does not explain the higher free cortisol levels.

The elevation in free cortisol levels seems to be caused in part, by a marked increase in corticotropin-releasing hormone (CRH) during pregnancy. CRH levels are low in nonpregnant women and rise exponentially during the third trimester[143] (Table 3–7). CRH is produced by the placenta and fetal membranes and is secreted into the maternal circulation. It is thought to stimulate maternal pituitary production of ACTH. In support of this theory, Goland et al. have shown that despite the increased levels of total and free cortisol levels, maternal afternoon adrenocorticotropic hormone (ACTH) concentrations rise and mirror the third-trimester increase in CRH. These investigators observed a significant correlation between the rise in CRH levels and maternal ACTH and urinary free cortisol concentrations.[143,146] Other possible causes for the hypercortisolism of pregnancy include delayed plasma clearance

of cortisol as a result of changes in renal clearance and a resetting of the hypothalamic-pituitary sensitivity to cortisol feedback on ACTH production.[141]

DOC, like aldosterone, is a potent mineralocorticoid. Marked elevations in the maternal plasma concentrations of DOC are present by midgestation, reaching peak levels in the third trimester. In contrast to the nonpregnant state, plasma DOC levels in the third trimester do not respond to ACTH stimulation, dexamethasone suppression, or salt intake.[142] These findings suggest that an autonomous source of DOC, specifically the fetoplacental unit, may be responsible for the increased maternal concentrations of DOC.

Dehydroepiandrosterone sulfate (DHEAS) levels are decreased in gestation because of a marked rise in the metabolic clearance of this adrenal androgenic steroid. Most studies have found a modest decline in circulating levels of DHEA as well. Maternal plasma concentrations of testosterone and androstenedione are slightly higher, testosterone because of an elevation in sex hormone–binding protein and androstenedione because of a small increase in its synthesis.[147]

Pituitary Gland

The pituitary gland enlarges in pregnancy, principally because of proliferation of prolactin-producing cells in the anterior pituitary. Gonzalez et al. recently demonstrated that the mean pituitary volume increased by 136 percent at term.[148] The enlargement of the pituitary makes it more susceptible to alterations in blood supply and increases the risk of postpartum infarction (Sheehan's syndrome) should a large maternal blood loss occur.

The pituitary hormone levels are affected by pregnancy. Serum prolactin levels begin to rise a 5 to 8 weeks' gestation and by term are 10 times higher.[149] Despite the increase, prolactin levels remain suppressible by bromocriptine therapy.[150] The principal function

Table 3–7. SEQUENTIAL MEASUREMENTS OF PLASMA CRH, ACTH, CORTISOL, ALDOSTERONE, AND URINARY FREE CORTISOL DURING PREGNANCY

Weeks' Gestation	CRH (pg/ml)	ACTH (pg/ml)	Cortisol (μg/dl)	DHEAS (μg/dl)	Aldosterone (pg/ml)	Urinary Free Cortisol (μg/24 h)
11–15	115 ± 45	8.8 ± 2.8	10.5 ± 1.4	102 ± 14	412 ± 63.6	54.8 ± 7.3
21–25	145 ± 30	9.8 ± 1.5	20.0 ± 1.1*	85.1 ± 9.0	487 ± 42.8	84.4 ± 8.4
31–35	1,570 ± 349*	12.1 ± 2.0	22.0 ± 1.2*	62.6 ± 6.8*	766 ± 94	105 ± 8.8*
36–40	4,346 ± 754*	18.6 ± 2.6*	26.0 ± 1.1*	63.8 ± 7.1*	1,150 ± 170*	111 ± 8.7*

*$p < 0.05$ compared with mean hormone levels at weeks 11 to 15 of pregnancy.
CRH, corticotropin-releasing hormone; ACTH, adrenocorticotropic hormones; DHEAS, dehydroepiandrosterone sulfate.
From Goland R, Jozak S, Conwell I: Placental corticotropin-releasing hormone and the hypercortisolism of pregnancy. Am J Obstet Gynecol 171:1287, 1994, with permission.

of prolactin in pregnancy is to prepare the breast for lactation. Maternal follicle-stimulating hormone (FSH) and luteinizing hormone (LH) are decreased to undetectable levels as a result of feedback inhibition from the elevated levels of estrogen, progesterone, and inhibin.[150] Maternal growth hormone levels are also suppressed because of the action of placental growth hormone variant on the hypothalamus and pituitary.[150]

PANCREAS AND FUEL METABOLISM

Glucose

Pregnancy is associated with significant physiologic changes in carbohydrate metabolism. This allows for the continuous transport of nutrients from the gravid woman to the developing fetus and placenta. Pregnancy taxes maternal insulin and carbohydrate physiology, and in all pregnancies some deterioration in glucose tolerance occurs. In most women, only mild changes take place, whereas in others pregnancy is diabetogenic, with the impairment in glucose metabolism significant enough to result in gestational diabetes.[151] Overall, pregnancy results in fasting hypoglycemia, postprandial hyperglycemia, and hyperinsulinemia.[152] To accommodate the increased demand for insulin there is hypertrophy and hyperplasia of the β-cells (insulin-producing cells) within the islets of Langerhans in the maternal pancreas.[153]

Early in pregnancy, glucose homeostasis is affected by increased insulin release that appears to be caused by increased estrogen stimulation of the β-cells within the pancreas. During the first trimester, normal insulin sensitivity is maintained and this causes a 10 percent lowering of glucose levels because of the heightened peripheral muscle glucose utilization. Since insulin is lipogenic, the increased insulin levels favor enhanced lipogenesis, with storage of fat apparently in preparation for the rise in energy needs later in gestation.[154]

With the accelerated growth of the fetus, changes in maternal maintenance of the fasting state and insulin sensitivity take place. During normal pregnancy, maternal fasting is characterized by accelerated starvation. The fasting blood glucose level after a 12- to 14-hour fast is 10 mg/dl lower than that observed in the nonpregnant individual.[155,156] This exaggerated response to fasting is largely a result of the constant drain of maternal glucose by the fetoplacental unit. In the third trimester, glucose uptake by the fetus has been estimated to be approximately 6.0 mg/kg/min.[157] This results in a more rapid conversion from predominantly carbohydrate to predominantly fat utilization because of earlier depletion of liver glycogen stores. In addition, the fetus also withdraws amino acids from the maternal circulation and limits the availability of gluconeogenic amino acids such as alanine. Thus in pregnancy, during prolonged fasting increased utilization of fat stores occurs. Lipolysis generates glycerol, fatty acids, and ketones for gluconeogenesis and fuel metabolism.[155,156] This produces exaggerated starvation ketosis and preserves the utilization of glucose and amino acids for the maternal central nervous system and fetus. The increased utilization of fat stores is caused by decreased levels of insulin seen during prolonged fasting and the effects of human placental lactogen (hPL).[154] In summary, maternal hypoglycemia, hypoinsulinemia, hyperlipidemia, and hyperketonemia characterize the maternal response to starvation.

By contrast, hyperglycemia, hyperinsulinemia, hyperlipidemia, and reduced tissue sensitivity to insulin characterize the maternal response to feeding[152] (see Fig. 3–15). Insulin secretion rises progressively during gestation, with the maximal increase in the third trimester. The insulin response to an intravenous glucose tolerance test or an intravenous infusion of amino acids is also enhanced in pregnancy.[151] Insulin resistance is observed after the first trimester,[158,159] with a 50 to 80 percent decline in insulin sensitivity in the third trimester. Thus, despite this increase in postprandial hyperinsulinemia, the blood glucose response to the same carbohydrate load is greater in pregnancy.[151] In normal gestation, glucose homeostasis is maintained by the exaggerated response. If a woman has borderline pancreatic reserve prior to pregnancy and is unable to increase her insulin production, then gestational diabetes mellitus will be revealed during pregnancy.

The factors responsible for the diabetogenic effects of pregnancy include a variety of hormones secreted by the placenta, especially hPL. hPL is produced by syncytiotrophoblast cells and has strong lipolytic and anti-insulin actions. hPL secretion is proportional to total placental mass and parallels the development of insulin resistance. Other hormones potentially responsible for insulin resistance include cortisol, prolactin, estrogen, and progesterone. The diabetogenic effects of pregnancy are advantageous to the growing fetus, providing increased maternal levels of nutrients after a meal.[151,154]

The fetus is primarily dependent on maternal glucose for its fuel requirements. The concentration of glucose in the fetus is about 20 mg/dl less than maternal values.[160] Placental glucose transport occurs via carrier-mediated facilitated transporter that is energy-independent.[161] Normal maternal glucose levels are critically important in providing adequate glucose to the fetus. Maternal hyperglycemia can cause birth defects if present in the first trimester and fetal macrosomia if present in the latter half of pregnancy.[162]

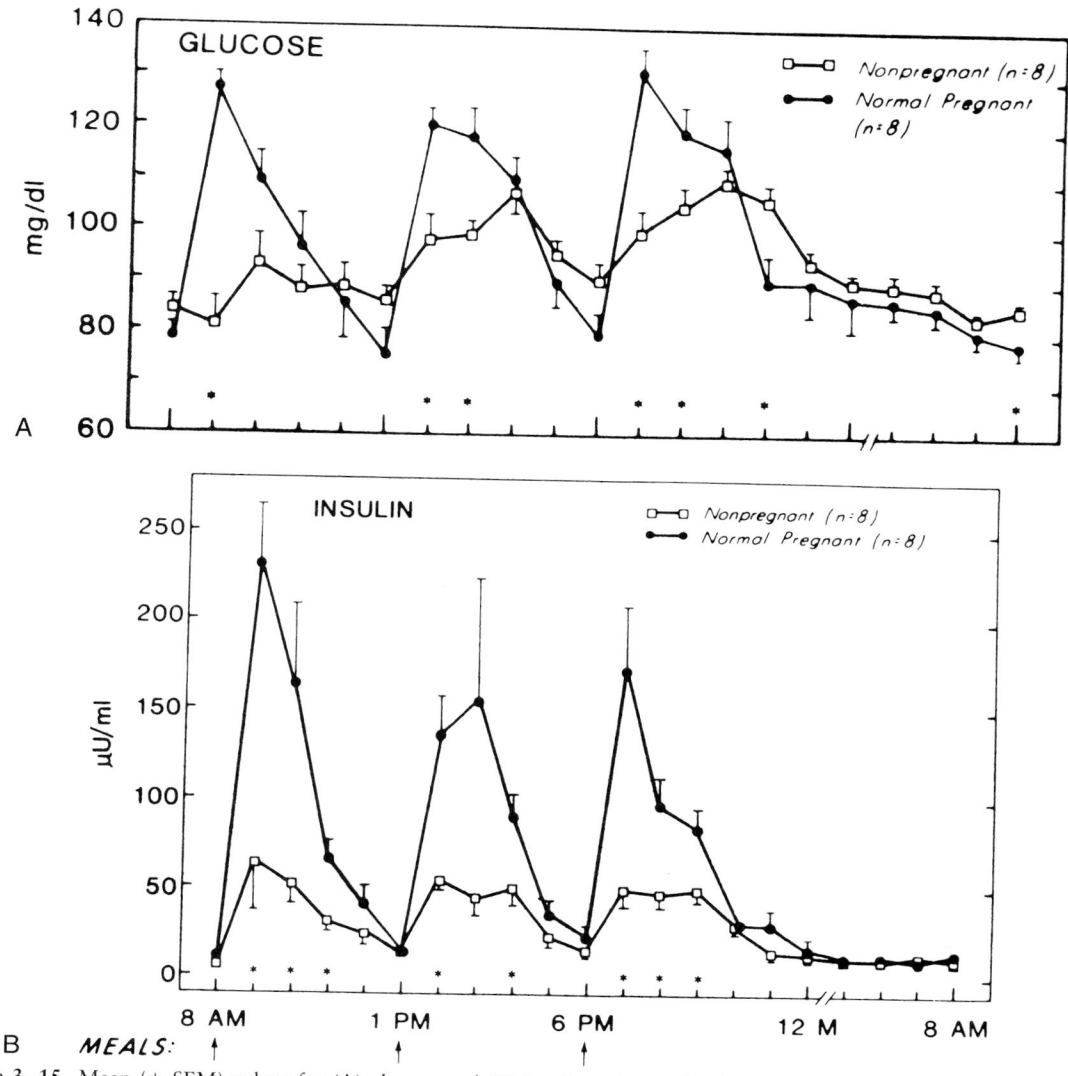

Figure 3–15. Mean (± SEM) values for (A) glucose and (B) insulin at intervals of 1 hour from 8:00 A.M. to midnight and 2 hours thereafter in eight nonpregnant and eight normal pregnant women in the third trimester. Mealtimes are indicated by arrows along the abscissa. Pregnant women demonstrate a greater amplitude in plasma glucose excursion after meals. The increased postprandial insulin secretion is apparent. (From Phelps R, Metzger B, Freinkel N: Carbohydrate metabolism in pregnancy. Am J Obstet Gynecol 140:730, 1981.)

Proteins

Amino acids are actively transported across the placenta, where they are used by the fetus for protein synthesis and as an energy source. In late pregnancy, the fetoplacental unit contains approximately 500 mg of protein. During pregnancy, fat stores are preferentially used as a substrate for fuel metabolism, and thus protein catabolism is decreased.

Fats/Lipids

Plasma lipids and lipoproteins increase in pregnancy. A gradual two- to threefold rise in triglyceride levels occurs by term and levels of 200 to 300 mg/dl are nor-

mal.[163] Total cholesterol and low-density lipoprotein (LDL) levels are also higher, so that by term a 50 to 60 percent increase from nonpregnant values takes place. High-density lipoprotein (HDL) levels initially rise in the first half of pregnancy and then fall in the second half. By term, HDL concentrations are 15 percent higher than nonpregnant levels. Both cholesterol and triglyceride concentrations return to normal by 6 weeks postpartum (Fig. 3–16) The mechanisms for the pregnancy-induced changes in lipids are not completely understood, but appear to be partly caused by the elevated levels of estrogen, progesterone, and hPL The rise in LDL appears to be necessary for placental steroidogenesis. Despite the increase in cholesterol and lipids during pregnancy, no increase in the long-term risk for atherosclerosis seems to occur.[163] However, pregnancy

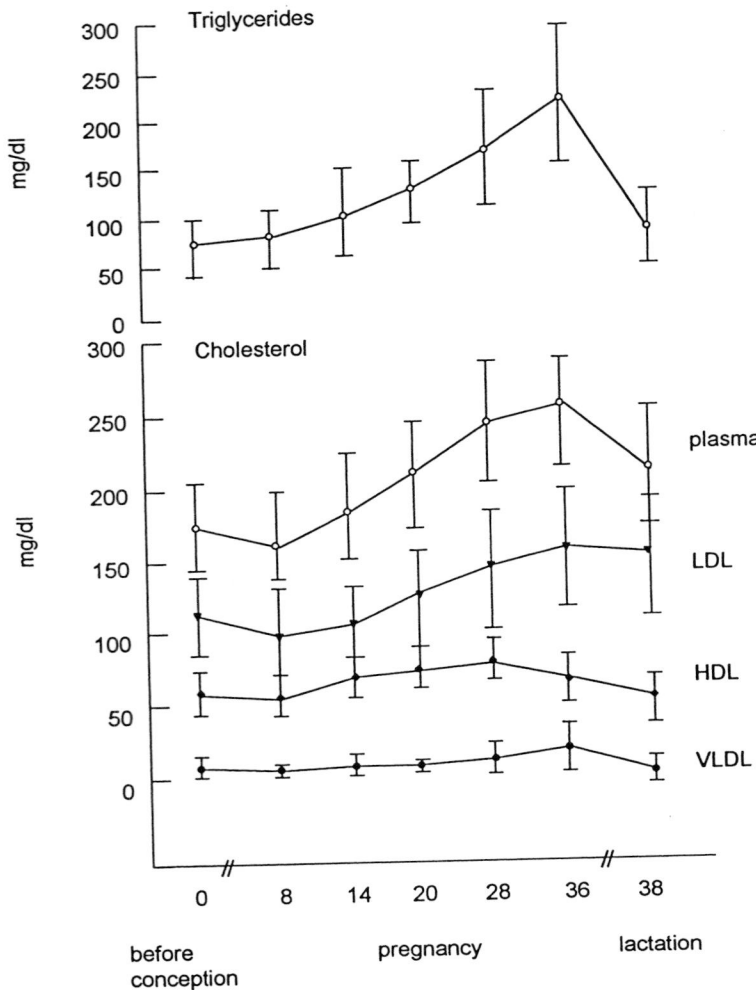

Figure 3-16. Triglycerides (*upper panel*) and cholesterol (*lower panel*) in plasma and in lipoprotein fractions before, during, and after pregnancy. (From Salameh W, Mastrogiannis D: Maternal hyperlipidemia in pregnancy. Clin Obstet Gynecol 37:66, 1994.)

can worsen the lipid profiles of women with preexisting hyperlipidemia.

THE BREASTS

The breasts begin to change early in pregnancy, with tenderness, tingling sensations, and a feeling of heaviness within 4 weeks of the last menstrual period. The breasts rapidly enlarge in the first 8 weeks as a result of vascular engorgement. Thereafter, breast size increases progressively throughout pregnancy because of both ductal growth stimulated by estrogen and alveolar hypertrophy stimulated by progesterone. Little if any of the increase in breast size is attributed to the deposition of fat. The degree of breast enlargement is quite variable.[164] The nipples enlarge and become more mobile during pregnancy. Likewise, the areolae enlarge and are more deeply pigmented.

The interaction of numerous hormones including estrogen, progesterone, prolactin, hPL, cortisol, and insulin are all necessary to prepare the breasts for milk production. The profound drop in estrogen and progesterone levels after delivery seems to be the initiating stimulus for lactation. In the latter half of gestation, colostrum, a thick yellow fluid, may leak or be expressed from the nipples. This normal finding is more common in parous women.

SKIN CHANGES

Pigmentation

Hyperpigmentation occurs in approximately 90 percent of pregnancies.[165] It may be generalized or localized only to areas of increased melanocyte density. Darkening of the areolae, umbilicus, vulva, and perianal skin may occur as early as the first trimester. The linea alba often becomes the hyperpigmented linea nigra. Pigmented nevi, freckles, and recent scars may also deepen in color. Hyperpigmentation on the face, known as melasma or chloasma, will often prompt complaints from pregnant women. Chloasma is usually manifested by well-defined hyperpigmented centrofacial patches and appears in various shades of brown. Chloasma occurs in at least 70 percent of women and affects all races equally.[166] The role of hormonal factors such as melanocyte-stimulating hormone is unclear.[95] Chloasma normally regresses or disappears; however, nearly 30 percent of women will have persistent hyperpigmentation at 10-year follow-up.[165] During pregnancy, some nevi may increase in size and new nevi may develop. A biopsy may be necessary if there is clinical suspicion for melanoma. In general, no evidence exists that pregnancy causes malignant transformation of nevi to melanoma.[167]

Hair Changes

Mild degrees of hirsutism are common during pregnancy. The face is frequently affected, although hair growth may be pronounced on the extremities as well. Abdominal hair growth is less common but may be exacerbated in women with a prominent male pattern escutcheon. Hirsutism is believed to be primarily an endocrinologic phenomenon and may result from placental androgen production as well as elevated levels of cortisol. Mild hirsutism rarely requires therapy. It normally regresses following delivery but does recur with subsequent pregnancies. Excessive hirsutism with virilization should warrant investigation for an androgen-secreting tumor. Occasionally, pelvic examination or ultrasound imaging will reveal large ovarian tumors in such women. These usually are luteomas of pregnancy, which represent exaggerated luteinization of normal ovaries rather than true neoplasms. Because luteomas regress after pregnancy, surgical intervention is not indicated.

The anagen (growing) phase of normal scalp hair lasts 2 to 6 years, after which hair enters the telogen (resting) phase. After about 3 months of telogen, the old hair strand is lost, and a new one grows to replace it. During normal pregnancy, the proportion of hair in the anagen phase is increased compared to that in telogen. Then after delivery, the number of hairs entering telogen increases remarkably. Therefore, it is normal to see a marked increase in scalp hair loss 2 to 4 months after delivery called telogen effluvium. Patients should be reassured of the normality of this phenomenon and told that their hair will regrow in 6 to 12 months.

Striae Distensae

Striae distensae begin to appear in the late second trimester in up to 90 percent of pregnant women.[95] Striae are thin atrophic pink or purple linear bands that are found on the abdomen, breasts, and thighs. Striae are believed to result from a combination of two factors. Stretching is necessary to produce striae; however, adrenocorticosteroids and estrogen also promote tearing in the collagen matrix of the dermis and weakening of elastic fibers.[165] While many creams and ointments have been employed to treat striae distensae, these therapies are not believed to be of any benefit. Striae are permanent, yet the purplish color most often fades with time and becomes white or silvery.

Vascular Changes

Vascular changes are evident within the skin of most pregnant women. High levels of estrogen are believed to be responsible for proliferation of blood vessels and congestion. Vasomotor instability may also produce pallor, flushing, and mottling of the skin in response to temperature changes. Increased capillary fragility is common in late pregnancy. Scattered petechiae are often seen on the lower extremities as a result of increased capillary hydrostatic pressure and capillary fragility. Spider angiomata may be observed in up to 70 percent of Caucasian women. These lesions consist of a central red arteriole with tortuous radiating branches resembling a spider. Also common to liver disease, spider angiomata are found on the face, trunk, and upper extremities in the areas drained by the superior vena cava. Most lesions fade during the first 3 postpartum months. Similar to spider angiomata, palmar erythema is more common in Caucasians than in black women, with nearly two thirds of pregnancies affected. It typically resolves following delivery.[168]

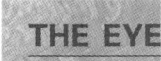

THE EYE

The two consistent and significant ocular changes during pregnancy are increased thickness of the cornea and decreased intraocular pressure. Edema causes a 3 percent increase in corneal thickness. It is apparent by 10 weeks' gestation and regresses by the sixth postpartum week. This change in corneal thickness may cause women to have problems with contact lenses and is the reason patients should be advised to wait several weeks postpartum for new eyeglass or contact prescriptions.[169] Intraocular pressure falls by about 10 percent during pregnancy, and individuals with preexisting glaucoma typically improve. Pregnancy either does not cause or minimally decreases visual fields Therefore, any complaints of visual field changes are atypical and need further evaluation.[169]

Key Points

➤ Plasma osmolality decreases during pregnancy as a result of reduction in the serum concentration of sodium and associated anions. The osmolality set point for AVP release and thirst is decreased in pregnancy.

➤ Cardiac output increases 30 to 50 percent during pregnancy. This is dependent on maternal position. Supine positioning and standing are both associated with a fall in cardiac output. The cardiac output is maximal during labor and the immediate postpartum period.

➤ As a result of the marked fall in systemic vascular resistance and pulmonary vascular resistance, pulmonary capillary wedge pressure does not rise, despite an increase in blood volume.

➤ Maternal blood pressure decreases early in pregnancy. The diastolic blood pressure and the mean arterial pressure nadir at midpregnancy (16 to 20 weeks) and return to prepregnancy levels by term.

➤ $PACO_2$ and $PaCO_2$ fall during pregnancy secondary to increased minute ventilation. This facilitates transfer of CO_2 from the fetus to the mother and results in a mild respiratory alkalosis.

➤ Maternal plasma volume increases 50 percent during pregnancy. As RBC volume increases approximately 18 to 30 percent, the hematocrit normally decreases during gestation, but not below 30 percent.

➤ Pregnancy is a hypercoagulable state, with increases in the levels of the majority of the procoagulant factors and a decrease in the fibrinolytic system and in some of the natural inhibitors of coagulation.

➤ BUN and creatinine normally decrease during pregnancy as a result of the increased glomerular filtration rate.

➤ Despite alterations in thyroid morphology, histology, and laboratory indices, the normal pregnant woman is euthyroid, with the levels of free T_4 and TSH within nonpregnant norms.

➤ Pregnancy is associated with a peripheral resistance to insulin, primarily mediated by human placental lactogen. Insulin resistance increases as pregnancy advances and results in hyperglycemia, hyperinsulinemia, and hyperlipidemia in response to feeding, especially in the third trimester.

REFERENCES

1. Lockitch G: Clinical biochemistry of pregnancy. Crit Rev Clin Lab Sci 34:67, 1997.
2. Theunissen I, Parer J: Fluid and electrolytes in pregnancy. Clin Obstet Gynecol 37:3, 1994.
3. Lindheimer M, Davison J: Osmoregulation, the secretion of arginine vasopressin and its metabolism during pregnancy. Eur J Endocrinol 132:133, 1995.
4. Davison JM, Vallotton MB, Lindheimer MD: Plasma osmolality and urinary concentration and dilution during and after pregnancy: evidence that the lateral recumbency inhibits maximal urinary concentration ability. Br J Obstet Gynaecol 88:472, 1981.
5. Lindheimer M, Barron W, Davison J: Osmoregulation of thirst and vasopressin release in pregnancy. Am J Physiol 257:F159, 1989.
6. Dürr J: Diabetes insipidus in pregnancy. Am J Kidney Dis 9:276, 1987.
7. Schobel H: Pregnancy-induced alterations in renal function. Kidney Blood Press Res 21:276, 1998.
8. Chesley LC: Renin, angiotensin, and aldosterone in pregnancy. In Chesley LC (ed): Hypertensive Disorders in Pregnancy. New York, Appleton-Century-Crofts, 1978, p. 236.
9. Miyamoto S, Shimokawa H, Sumioki H, et al: Circadian rhythm of plasma atrial natriuretic peptide, aldosterone, and blood pressure during the third trimester in normal and preeclamptic pregnancies. Am J Obstet Gynecol 158:393, 1998.
10. Sala C, Campise M, Ambroso G, et al: Atrial natriuretic peptide and hemodynamic changes during normal human pregnancy. Hypertension 25:631, 1995.
11. Castro L, Hobel C, Gornbein J: Plasma levels of atrial natriuretic peptide in normal and hypertensive pregnancies: a meta-analysis. Am J Obstet Gynecol 71:1642, 1994.
12. Bhagwat A, Engel P: Heart disease and pregnancy. Cardiol Clin 13:163, 1995.
13. Duvekot J, Peeters L: Maternal cardiovascular hemodynamic adaptation to pregnancy. Obstet Gynecol Surv 49:S1, 1994.
14. van Oppen A, Stigter R, Bruinse H: Cardiac output in normal pregnancy: a critical review. Obstet Gynecol 87:310, 1996.
15. Robson S, Hunter S, Boys R, et al: Serial study of factors influencing changes in cardiac output during human pregnancy. Am J Physiol 256:H1061, 1989.
16. Hunter S, Robson S: Adaptation of the maternal heart in pregnancy. Br Heart J 68:540, 1992.
17. McAnolty J, Metcalfe J, Ueland K: Heart disease and pregnancy. In Hurst JN (ed): The Heart, 6th ed. New York, McGraw-Hill, 1985, p. 1383.
18. Clapp J, Capeless E: Cardiovascular function before, during and after the first and subsequent pregnancies. Am J Cardiol 80:1469, 1997.
19. Clark S, Cotton D, Pivarnik J, et al: Position change and central hemodynamic profile during normal third-trimester pregnancy and postpartum. Am J Obstet Gynecol 164:883, 1991.
20. Kerr M: The mechanical effects of the gravid uterus in late pregnancy. J Obstet Gynaecol Br Commonw 72:513, 1965.
21. Kerr M, Scott D, Samuel E: Studies of the inferior vena cava in late pregnancy. Br Med J 1:532, 1964.
22. Elkayam U, Gleicher N: Cardiovascular physiology of pregnancy. In Elkayam U, Gleicher N (eds): Cardiac Problems in Pregnancy: Diagnosis and Management of Maternal and Fetal Disease. New York, Alan R Liss, 1982, p 5.
23. Naeye R, Peters E: Working during pregnancy effects on the fetus. Pediatrics 69:724, 1982.
24. Clark S, Cotton D, Lee W, et al: Central hemodynamic as-

sessment of normal term pregnancy. Am J Obstet Gynecol 161:1439, 1989.

25. Gant N, Daley G, Chand S, et al: A study of angiotensin II pressor response throughout primigravid pregnancy. J Clin Invest 52:2682, 1973.

26. Dunne F, Barry D, Ferris J, et al: Changes in blood pressure during the normal menstrual cycle. Clin Sci 81:515, 1996.

27. MacGillivray I, Rose G, Rowe B: Blood pressure survey in pregnancy. Clin Sci 37:395, 1969.

28. de Swiet M, Shennan A: Blood pressure measurement in pregnancy. Br J Obstet Gynaecol 103:862, 1996.

29. McLennan C: Antecubital and femoral venous pressure in normal and toxemia pregnancy. Am J Obstet Gynecol 45:568, 1943.

30. Crapo R: Normal cardiopulmonary physiology during pregnancy. Clin Obstet Gynecol 39:3, 1996.

31. Zinaman M, Rubin J, Lindheimer M: Serial plasma oncotic pressure levels and echoencephalography during and after delivery in severe pre-eclampsia. Lancet 1:1245, 1985.

32. Cutforth R, MacDonald C: Heart sounds and murmurs in pregnancy. Am Heart J 71:741, 1966.

33. O'Rourke R, Ewy G, Marcus F, et al: Cardiac auscultation in pregnancy. Med Ann D C 39:92, 1970.

34. Robson S, Dunlop W, Boys R, et al: Cardiac output during labour. BMJ 295:1169, 1987.

35. Kerr M: Cardiovascular dynamics in pregnancy and labour. Br Med Bull 24:19, 1968.

36. Ueland K, Hansen J: Maternal cardiovascular dynamics. III. Labor and delivery under local and caudal analgesia. Am J Obstet Gynecol 103:8, 1969.

37. Danilenko-Dixon D, Tefft L, Cohen R, et al: Positional effects on maternal cardiac output during labor with epidural analgesia. Am J Obstet Gynecol 175:867, 1996.

38. James C, Banner T, Caton D: Cardiac output in women undergoing cesarean section with epidural or general anesthesia. Am J Obstet Gynecol 160:1178, 1989.

39. Robson S, Boys R, Hunter S, et al: Maternal hemodynamics after normal delivery and delivery complicated by postpartum hemorrhage. Obstet Gynecol 74:234, 1989.

40. Schatz M, Zieger R: Diagnosis and management of rhinitis during pregnancy. Allergy Proc 9:545, 1988.

41. Thompson K, Cohen M: Studies on the circulation in pregnancy, II: vital capacity in normal pregnant women. Surg Gynecol Obstet 66:591, 1938.

42. Gilroy R, Mangura B, Lavietes M: Rib cage displacement and abdominal volume displacement during breathing in pregnancy. Am Rev Respir Dis 137:668, 1988.

43. Weinberger S, Weiss S, Cohen W, et al: Pregnancy and the lung. Am Rev Respir Dis 121:L559, 1980.

44. Brancazio L, Laifer S, Schwartz T: Peak expiratory flow rate in normal pregnancy. Obstet Gynecol 89:383, 1997.

45. Elkus K, Popovich J: Respiratory physiology in pregnancy. Clin Chest Med 13:555, 1992.

46. Lucius H, Gahlenbeck H, Kleine H, et al: Respiratory functions, buffer system, and electrolyte concentration of blood during human pregnancy. Respir Physiol 9:311, 1970.

47. Hankins G, Harvey C, Clark S, et al: The effects of maternal position and cardiac output on intrapulmonary shunt in normal third-trimester pregnancy. Obstet Gynecol 88:327, 1996.

48. Hankins G, Clark S, Uckan E, et al: Maternal oxygen transport variables during the third trimester of normal pregnancy. Am J Obstet Gynecol 180:406, 1999.

49. Pritchard J: Changes in blood volume during pregnancy and delivery. Anesthesiology 26:393, 1965.

50. Scott D: Anemia during pregnancy. Obstet Gynecol Ann 1:219, 1972.

51. U. S. Department of Health and Human Services: MMWR Morb Mortal Wkly Rep 38:400, 1989.

52. Ireland R, Abbas A, Thilaganathan B, et al: Fetal and maternal erythropoietin levels in normal pregnancy. Fetal Diagn Ther 7:21, 1992.

53. Pritchard J, Baldwin R, Dickey J, et al: Blood volume changes in pregnancy and the puerperium. II. Red blood cell loss and changes in apparent blood volume during and following vaginal delivery, cesarean section, and cesarean section plus total hysterectomy. Am J Obstet Gynecol 84:1271, 1962.

54. Ueland K: Maternal cardiovascular dynamics. VII. Intrapartum blood volume changes. Am J Obstet Gynecol 126:671, 1976.

55. Andrews N: Disorders of iron metabolism. N Engl J Med 341:1986, 1999.

56. McFee J: Iron metabolism and iron deficiency during pregnancy. Clin Obstet Gynecol 22:799, 1979.

57. Romslo I, Haram K, Sagen N, et al: Iron requirement in normal pregnancy as assessed by serum ferritin, serum transferrin saturation and erythrocyte protoporphyrin determinations. Br J Obstet Gynaecol 90:101, 1983.

58. Taylor D, Mallen C, McDougall N, et al: Effect of iron supplementation on serum ferritin levels during and after pregnancy. Br J Obstet Gynaecol 89:1011, 1982.

59. Van Eijk H, Kroos M, Hoogendoorn G, et al: Serum ferritin and iron stores during pregnancy. Clin Chim Acta 83:81, 1978.

60. Tygart S, McRoyan D, Spinnato J, et al: Longitudinal study of platelet indices during normal pregnancy. Am J Obstet Gynecol 154:883, 1986.

61. Fay R, Hughes A, Farron N: Platelets in pregnancy: hyperdestruction in pregnancy. Obstet Gynecol 61:238, 1983.

62. Sejeny S, Eastham R, Baker S: Platelet counts during normal pregnancy. J Clin Pathol 28:812, 1975.

63. Pitkin R, Witte D: Platelet and leukocyte counts in pregnancy. JAMA 242:2696, 1979.

64. O'Brien JR: Platelet count in normal pregnancy. J Clin Pathol 29:174, 1976.

65. Burrows R, Kelton J: Incidentally detected thrombocytopenia in healthy mothers and their infants. N Engl J Med 319:142, 1988.

66. American College of Obstetricians and Gynecologists: ACOG practice bulletin. Thrombocytopenia in pregnancy. Number 6, September 1999. Clinical management guidelines for obstetrician-gynecologists. Washington, DC, ACOG-1999.

67. Wilder R: Hormones, pregnancy, and autoimmune diseases. Ann N Y Acad Sci 840:45, 1998.

68. Stirrat G: Pregnancy and immunity: changes occur, but pregnancy does not result in immunodeficiency. BMJ 308:1385, 1994.

69. Hytten F, Lind T: Volume and composition of the blood. *In* Hytten FE, Lind T (eds): Diagnostic Indices in Pregnancy. Basel, Documenta Geigy, 1973, p 36.

70. Johnson RL: Thromboembolic disease complicating pregnancy. *In* Foley MR, Strong TH (eds): Obstetric Intensive Care: A Practical Manual. Philadelphia, WB Saunders Company, 1997, p 91.

71. Ozanne P, Linderkamp O, Miller F, et al: Erythrocyte aggregation during normal pregnancy. Am J Obstet Gynecol 147:576, 1983.

72. Bauer K: Hypercoagulability—a new cofactor in the protein C anticoagulant pathway. N Engl J Med 330:566, 1994.

73. Clark P, Brennand J, Conkie J, et al: Activated protein C sensitivity, protein C, protein S, and coagulation in normal pregnancy. Thromb Haemost 79:1166, 1998.

74. Faught W, Garner P, Jones G, et al: Changes in protein C and protein S levels in normal pregnancy. Am J Obstet Gynecol 172(1 Pt 1):147, 1995.

75. Gerbasi F, Bottoms S, Farag A, et al: Increased intravascular coagulation associated with pregnancy. Obstet Gynecol 75:385, 1990.

76. Fried A, Woodring J, Thompson D: Hydronephrosis of pregnancy: a prospective sequential study of the course of dilatation. J Ultrasound Med 2:255, 1983.

77. Hytten F, Lind T: Indices of renal function. *In* Hytten FE, Lind T (eds): Diagnostic Indices in Pregnancy. Basel, Documenta Geigy, 1973, p 18.

78. Davison J: The effect of pregnancy on kidney function in renal allograft recipients. Kidney Int 27:74, 1985.

79. Dunlop W: Serial changes in renal haemodynamics during normal pregnancy. Br J Obstet Gynaecol 88:1, 1981.

80. Ezimokhai M, Davison J, Philips P, et al: Non-postural serial changes in renal function during the third trimester of normal human pregnancy. Br J Obstet Gynaecol 88:465, 1981.

81. Davison J, Noble F: Glomerular filtration during and after pregnancy. J Obstet Gynaecol Br Commonw 81:588, 1974.

82. Lind T, Godfrey K, Otun H: Changes in serum uric acid concentrations during normal pregnancy. Br J Obstet Gynaecol 91:128, 1984.

83. Chesley L, Sloan D: The effect of posture on renal function in late pregnancy. Am J Obstet Gynecol 89:754, 1964.

84. Lindheimer M, Richardson D, Ehrlich E, et al: Potassium homeostasis in pregnancy. J Reprod Med 32:517, 1987.

85. Davison J, Hytten F: The effect of pregnancy on the renal handling of glucose. Br J Obstet Gynaecol 82:374, 1975.

86. Kurtzman N, Pillay V: Renal reabsorption of glucose in health and disease. Arch Intern Med 131:901, 1973.

87. Higby K, Suiter C, Phelps J, et al: Normal values of urinary albumin and total protein excretion during pregnancy. Am J Obstet Gynecol 171:984, 1994.

88. Gordon M, London M, Samuels P, et al: Perinatal outcome and long-term follow-up associated with modern management of diabetic nephropathy. Obstet Gynecol 87:401, 1996.

89. Hytten F, Cheyne G: The aminoaciduria of pregnancy. J Obstet Gynaecol Br Commonw 79:424, 1972.

90. Dafnis E, Sabatini S: The effect of pregnancy on renal function: physiology and pathophysiology. Am J Med Sci 303:184, 1992.

91. Hytten F, Lind T: Indices of alimentary function. *In* Hytten FE, Lind T (eds): Diagnostic Indices in Pregnancy. Basel, Documenta Geigy, 1973, p 13.

92. Catalano P, Hollenbeck C: Energy requirements in pregnancy: a review. Obstet Gynecol Surv 47:368, 1992.

93. Kallender D, Sonesson B: Studies on saliva in menstruating, pregnant and postmenopausal women. Acta Endocrinol (Copenh) 48:329, 1965.

94. Parmley T, O'Brien T: Skin changes during pregnancy. Clin Obstet Gynecol 33:713, 1990.

95. Winston G, Lewis C: Dermatosis of pregnancy, J Am Acad Dermatol 6:977, 1982.

96. Christofides N, Ghatei M, Bloom S, et al: Decreased plasma motilin concentrations in pregnancy. Br Med J 285:1453, 1982.

97. Macfie A, Magides A, Richmond M, et al: Gastric emptying in pregnancy. Br J Anaesth 67:54, 1991.

98. Davison J, Davison M, Hay D: Gastric emptying time in late pregnancy and labour. J Obstet Gynaecol Br Commonw 77:37, 1970.

99. Cappell M, Garcia A: Gastric and duodenal ulcers during pregnancy. Gastroenterol Clin North Am 27:169, 1998.

100. Levy N, Lemberg E, Sharf M: Bowel habits in pregnancy. Digestion 4:216, 1977.

101. Bonapace E, Fisher R: Constipation and diarrhea in pregnancy. Gastroenterol Clin North Am 27:197, 1998.

102. Parry E, Shields R, Turnbull A: Transit time in the small intestine in pregnancy. J Obstet Gynaecol Br Commonw 77:900, 1970.

103. Wald A, Van Thiel D, Hoechstetter L, et al: Effect of pregnancy on gastrointestinal transit. Dig Dis Sci 27:1015, 1982.

104. Parry E, Shields R, Turnbull A: The effect of pregnancy on the colonic absorption of sodium, potassium and water. J Obstet Gynaecol Br Commonw 77:616, 1970.

105. Braverman D, Johnson M, Kern F: Effects of pregnancy and contraceptive steroids on gallbladder function. N Engl J Med 302:362, 1980.

106. Kern F, Everson G, DeMark B, et al: Biliary lipids, bile acids, and gallbladder function in the human female: effects of pregnancy and the ovulatory cycle. J Clin Invest 68:1229, 1981.

107. Combes B, Abarns R: Disorders of the liver in pregnancy. *In* Assali (ed): Pathophysiology of Gestation. San Diego, Academic Press, 1971, p 297.

108. Carter J: Liver function in normal pregnancy. Aust N Z J Obstet Gynaecol 30:296, 1990.

109. Bacq Y, Zarka O, Brechot J-F, et al: Liver function tests in normal pregnancy: a prospective study of 103 pregnant women and 103 matched controls. Hepatology 23:1030, 1996.

110. Jamfelt-Samsioe A, Velinder F-M: Nausea and vomiting in pregnancy: a contribution to its epidemiology. Gynecol Obstet Invest 15:221, 1983.

111. Soulos M, Hughes C, Garcia J, et al: Nausea and vomiting of pregnancy: role of human chorionic gonadotropin and 17-hydroxyprogesterone. Obstet Gynecol 55:696, 1980.

112. Askling J, Erlandsson G, Kaijser M, et al: Sickness of pregnancy and sex of child. Lancet 354:2053, 1999.

113. Medalie J: Relationship between nausea and/or vomiting in early pregnancy and abortion. Lancet 2:117, 1957.

114. Murphy A: Alternative therapies for nausea and vomiting of pregnancy. Obstet Gynecol 91:149, 1998.

115. Safari H, Fassett M, Souter I, et al: The efficacy of methylprednisolone in the treatment of hyperemesis gravidarum: a randomized, double-blind, controlled study. Am J Obstet Gynecol 179:921, 1998.

116. Kovacs C, Kronenberg H: Maternal-fetal calcium and bone metabolism during pregnancy, puerperium, and lactation. Endocr Rev 18:832, 1997.

117. Givens M, Macy I: The chemical composition of the human fetus. J Biol Chem 102:7, 1933.

118. Trotter M, Hixon B: Sequential changes in weight, density, and percentage ash weight of human skeletons from an early fetal period through old age. Anat Rec 179:1, 1974.

119. Hojo M, August P: Calcium metabolism in normal and hypertensive pregnancy. Semin Nephrol 15:504, 1995.

120. Pitkin R, Gebhardt M: Serum calcium concentrations in human pregnancy. Am J Obstet Gynecol 127:775, 1977.

121. Cross N, Hillman L, Allen S, et al: Calcium homeostasis and bone metabolism during pregnancy, lactation, and postweaning: a longitudinal study. Am J Clin Nutr 61:514, 1995.

122. Pitkin R, Reynolds W, Williams G, et al: Calcium metabolism in normal pregnancy, a longitudinal study. Am J Obstet Gynecol 133:781, 1979.

123. Samaan N, Anderson G, Adam-Mayne M: Immunoreactive calcitonin in the mother, neonate, child, and adult. Am J Obstet Gynecol 121:622, 1975.

124. Shahtaheri S, Aaron J, Johnson D, et al: Changes in trabecular bone architecture in women during pregnancy. Br J Obstet Gynaecol 106:432, 1999.

125. Hall K: Relaxin. J Reprod Fertil 1:369, 1960.

126. Abramson D, Roberts S, Wilson P: Relaxation of the pelvic joints in pregnancy. Surg Gynecol Obstet 58:595, 1934.

127. Glinoer D: The regulation of thyroid function in pregnancy: pathways of endocrine adaptation from physiology to pathology. Endocr Rev 18:404, 1997.

128. Berghout A, Endert E, Ross A, et al: Thyroid function and thyroid size in normal pregnant women living in an iodine replete area. Clin Endocrinol 42:375, 1994.

129. Nelson M, Wickus G, Caplan R, et al: Thyroid gland size in pregnancy. An ultrasound and clinical study. J Reprod Med 32:888, 1987.

130. Mazzaferri E: Evaluation and management of common thyroid disorders in women. Am J Obstet Gynecol 176:507, 1997.

131. Pochin E: The iodine uptake of the human thyroid throughout the menstrual cycle and in pregnancy. Clin Sci 11:441, 1952.

132. Burrow G, Fisher D, Larsen P: Maternal and fetal thyroid function. N Engl J Med 331:1072,1994.

133. Ballabio M, Poshyachinda M, Ekins R: Pregnancy-induced changes in thyroid function: role of human chorionic gonadotropin as putative regulator of maternal thyroid. J Clin Endocrinol Metab 73:824, 1996.

134. Kennedy R, Darne J, Cohn M, et al: Human chorionic gonadotropin may not be responsible for thyroid-stimulating activity in normal pregnancy serum. J Clin Endocrinol Metab 74:260, 1992.

135. Fisher D, Lehman H, Lackey D: Placental transport of thyroxine. J Clin Endocrinol Metab 24:393, 1964.

136. Ekins R, Sinha A, Ballabio M, et al: Role of the maternal carrier proteins in the supply of thyroid hormones to the feto-placental unit: evidence of a feto-placental requirement for thyroxine. *In* Delange F, Fisher DA, Glinoer D (eds): Research in Congenital Hypothyroidism. New York, Plenum Press, 1989, p. 45.

137. Vulsma T, Gons M, de Vijlder J: Maternal-fetal transfer of thyroxine in congenital hypothyroidism due to a total organification defect or thyroid agenesis. N Engl J Med 321:13, 1989.

138. Xue-Yi C, Xin-min J, Zhi-hong D, et al: Timing of vulnerability of the brain to iodine deficiency in endemic cretinism. N Engl J Med 331:1739, 1994.

139. Utiger R: Maternal hypothyroidism and fetal development. N Engl J Med 341:601, 1999.

140. Haddow J, Palomaki G, Allan W, et al: Maternal thyroid deficiency during pregnancy and subsequent neuropsychological development of the child. N Engl J Med 341:549, 1999.

141. Nolten W, Lindheimer M, Rueckert P, et al: Diurnal patterns and regulation of cortisol secretion in pregnancy. J Clin Endocrinol Metab 51:466, 1980.

142. Nolten W, Lindheimer M, Oparil S, et al: Desoxycorticosterone in normal pregnancy. I. Sequential studies of the secretory patterns of desoxycorticosterone, aldosterone, and cortisol. Am J Obstet Gynecol 132:414, 1978.

143. Goland R, Jozak S, Conwell I: Placental corticotropin-releasing hormone and the hypercortisolism of pregnancy. Am J Obstet Gynecol 171:1287, 1994.

144. Doc R, Fernandez R, Seal U: Measurements of corticosteroid-binding globulin in man. J Clin Endocrinol Metab 24:1029, 1964.

145. Scott E, McGarrigle H, Lachelin G: The increase in plasma and saliva cortisol levels in pregnancy is not due to the increase in corticosteroid-binding globulin levels. J Clin Endocrinol Metab 71:639, 1990.

146. Goland R, Conwell I, Warren W, et al: Placental corticotropin-releasing hormone and pituitary-adrenal function during pregnancy. Neuroendocrinology 66:742, 1992.

147. Belisie S, Osaihanondh R, Tulchinsky D: The effect of constant infusion of unlabelled dehydroepiandrosterone sulfate on maternal plasma androgens and estrogens. J Clin Endocrinol Metab 45:544, 1977.

148. Gonzalez J, Elizondo G, Saldivar D, et al: Pituitary gland growth during normal pregnancy: an in vivo study using magnetic resonance imaging. Am J Med 85:217, 1988.

149. Tyson J, Hwang P, Guyda H, et al: Studies of prolactin secretion in human pregnancy. Am J Obstet Gynecol 113:14, 1972.

150. Prager D, Braunstein G: Pituitary disorders during pregnancy. Endocrinol Metab Clin North Am 24:1, 1995.

151. Kuhl C: Etiology and pathogenesis of gestational diabetes. Diabetes Care 21:19B, 1998.

152. Phelps R, Metzger B, Freinkel N: Carbohydrate metabolism in pregnancy. Am J Obstet Gynecol 140:730, 1981.

153. Van Assche F, Aerts L, De Prins F: A morphologic study of the endocrine pancreas in human pregnancy. Br J Obstet Gynaecol 85:818, 1978.

154. Boden G: Fuel metabolism in pregnancy and in gestational diabetes mellitus. Obstet Gynecol Clin North Am 23:1, 1996.

155. Felig P, Lynch V: Starvation in human pregnancy: hypoglycemia, hypoinsulinemia, and hyperketonemia. Science 170:990, 1970.

156. Tyson J, Austin K, Farinholt J, et al: Endocrine-metabolic response to acute starvation in human gestation. Am J Obstet Gynecol 125:1073, 1976.

157. Page E: Human fetal nutrition and growth. Am J Obstet Gynecol 104:378, 1969.

158. Catalano P, Tyzbir E, Roman N, et al: Longitudinal changes in insulin release and insulin resistance in non-obese pregnant women. Am J Obstet Gynecol 165:1667, 1991.

159. Fisher P, Sutherland H, Bewsher P: The insulin response to glucose infusion in normal human pregnancy. Diabetologia 19:15, 1980.

160. Economides D, Nicolaides K: Blood glucose and oxygen tension levels in small-for-gestation fetuses. Am J Obstet Gynecol 160:385, 1989.

161. Bell G, Burant C, Takeda J, et al: Structure and function of mammalian facilitative sugar transporters. J Biol Chem 268:19161, 1993.

162. Cordero L, Landon M: Infant of the diabetic mother. Clin Perinatol 20:635, 1993.

163. Salameh W, Mastrogiannis D: Maternal hyperlipidemia in pregnancy. Clin Obstet Gynecol 37:66, 1994.

164. Hytten F, Leitch I: Preparations for breastfeeding. *In* Hytten FE, Leitch I (eds): The Physiology of Human Pregnancy. Oxford, Blackwell Scientific Publications, 1971, p 234.

165. Wong R, Ellis C: Physiologic skin changes in pregnancy. J Am Acad Dermatol 10:929, 1984.

166. Sanchez N, Pathak M, Sato S, et al: Melasma: a clinical, light microscopic, ultrastructural, and immunofluorescence study. J Am Acad Dermatol 4:698, 1981.

167. Lemer A, Nordlund J, Kirkwod J: Effects of oral contraceptives and pregnancy on melanoma. N Engl J Med 301:47, 1979.

168. Mattison M: Transdermal drug absorption during pregnancy. Clin Obstet Gynecol 33:718, 1990.

169. Sunness J: The pregnant woman's eye. Surv Ophthalmol 32:219, 1988.

Physiology and Endocrinology of Term and Preterm Labor

JOHN R.G. CHALLIS AND STEPHEN J. LYE

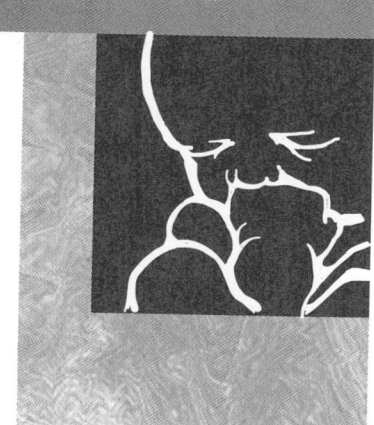

Preterm birth occurs in approximately 5 to 10 percent of all pregnancies in North America. This figure is even higher in certain population groups. Although some preterm births may be elective, approximately 30 percent occur in association with an underlying infectious process, and about 50 percent are so-called idiopathic preterm births, of unknown cause. In the developed world the incidence of preterm birth is, in fact, increasing. There are no effective diagnostic indicators of preterm birth, and there are no effective treatments for this condition. Thus, the direction of current research remains to understand this condition, to use that information to develop diagnostic and prognostic indicators, and to develop better methods of therapeutic management.

Currently, preterm birth is associated with 70 percent of neonatal deaths and up to 75 percent of neonatal morbidity. Infants born preterm have an increased incidence of cerebral palsy, neurologic handicap, and pulmonary disorders. The cost of caring for preterm babies in the United States has been estimated at around $8 billion annually.

Recent studies have shown that the incidence of spontaneous preterm labor in a very large population base relates to fetal size (R. Gagnon, unpublished information). Studies of over 30,000 deliveries in a tertiary care center in southwestern Ontario, Canada, showed that only 10.9 percent of spontaneous preterm labors were appropriate for gestational age. Remarkably, 24.6 percent of infants with spontaneous labor showed marked fetal growth restriction ($<$ 5th percentile), while 19.8 percent of spontaneous preterm deliveries were associated with "large-for-gestational-age" (LGA) ($>$ 95th percentile) weights at delivery. This study clearly indicates that preterm labor can arise through different causal mechanisms. The growth-restricted babies had reduced cord oxygen tensions, and were likely chronically hypoxemic, with precocious activation of the fetal stress responses in utero. The LGA babies had appropriate cord blood gases, and their premature delivery was likely associated with alternative mechanisms, including mechanical stretch of the uterus.

PHASES OF UTERINE ACTIVITY

For descriptive purposes it is helpful to think of different patterns of uterine contractility during pregnancy as being divisible into different phases. Thus, phase 0 of parturition corresponds to pregnancy, with relative *quiescence* of the myometrium maintained through the separate or combined activities of one or more inhibitors of uterine contractility. Phase 1 of parturition is associated with activation of uterine function, wherein mechanical stretch or uterotrophic priming leads to up-regulation of a cassette of contraction-associated protein (CAP) genes, essential for the development of myometrial contractility. CAP genes include Connexin-43 (Cx-43), the major constituent protein of GAP junctions, agonist receptors, and proteins encoding myometrial cell ion channels. In phase 2 of parturition, the activated uterus can then be *stimulated* through one or more uterotonins including prostaglandins, oxytocin, and potentially corticotropin-releasing hormone (CRH; see below). Phase 3 of parturition includes *expulsion* of the placenta and the involution process and has been attributed primarily to the effects of oxytocin. In this sequence, the "initiation" of parturition corresponds to the transition from phase 0 to phase 1 (uterine quiescence to uterine activation), although it is clear that the initiation process evolves gradually, rather than precipitously at a specific time in gestation. This sequence of events is also helpful in developing strategies for managing uterine activity during gestation. While current therapies have been directed at diminishing the stimulus to the uterus, it is evident that maintenance of quiescence or attenuation of the activation phase might be preferable treatment strategies. Of course, that strategy requires delineation of those pregnancies where fetal compromise is such that delivery preterm remains the preferred outcome.

Regulation of uterine quiescence during pregnancy has been discussed extensively in several review articles.[1,2] The major agents appear to include progesterone, relaxin, prostacyclin (PGI₂), parathyroid hormone–related peptide (PTH-rP), nitric oxide, and potentially CRH. These agents act in different ways, but in general increase the intracellular levels of cyclic nucleotides cyclic adenosine monophosphate (cAMP) or cyclic guanosine monophosphate (cGMP). In turn, these nucleotides inhibit release of calcium from intracellular stores, and/or reduce the activity of the enzyme myosin light chain kinase (MLCK) that is required for shortening of the myofilaments.

ACTIVATION OF MYOMETRIAL FUNCTION

It has been proposed[1] that activation of myometrial function can proceed through endocrine or mechanical pathways, driven through the fetal genotype. Studies involving embryo transfer clearly indicate that the fetal genotype controls the length of gestation. The classical view of parturition described in species such as the sheep through pioneering studies of Liggins and Thorburn (and others) reveals that fetal neuroendocrine signals originating in the hypothalamus initiate a cascade of events that activate the fetal hypothalamic-pituitary-adrenal (HPA) axis to increase fetal glucocorticoid production.[3] The fetal glucocorticoids then act on the placenta to effect changes in placental steroidogenesis and prostaglandin output. Maternal plasma concentrations of progesterone fall, estrogen increases, and this alteration in the estrogen/progesterone ratio is considered central to activation of the myometrium. In species such as the rat, expression of putative CAP genes is low during pregnancy and increases just before the onset of labor in association with an increase in the estrogen/progesterone ratio. Expression of CAP genes can be induced experimentally by uterine stretch, ovariectomy, or administration of the progesterone receptor antagonist RU-486.[1] In contrast, exogenous progesterone given to prevent the normal prepartum fall in the plasma progesterone concentration inhibited the increase in Cx-43, oxytocin receptor, and F-prostaglandin receptor (FP) mRNA in the myometrium, and blocked

the onset of labor. Recent studies suggest that the action of estrogen to increase Cx-43 mRNA in rat myometrium is effected indirectly through one or more transcription factors, including *c-fos*. Levels of *c-fos* in myometrium are highly correlated with *Cx-43* during labor, and manipulation of CAP gene expression is associated with coincident changes in *c-fos*. The promoters of both Cx-43 and oxytocin receptor contained putative Fos-binding sites and mutation at this site reduces basal promoter activity for Cx-43.[1]

It is likely that fetal growth contributes to uterine stretch and increases uterine wall tension. During gestation, uterine growth follows an initial phase of hyperplasia regulated by endocrine factors, a second phase in the 2nd and 3rd trimesters during which uterine growth is closely matched to fetal growth, and a final, third phase during which the rate of uterine growth declines relative to increasing fetal growth. Lye and colleagues[1] have speculated that with the fall in progesterone at term (in most species), uterine stretch no longer stimulates uterine growth and the increase in wall tension caused by continued fetal growth becomes translated into increased expression of CAP genes.

ACTIVATION: THE FETAL ENDOCRINE PATHWAY

The classic description of parturition in species such as sheep is that increased levels of fetal cortisol during late pregnancy up-regulate expression of the enzyme P450C17 hydroxylase in the placenta.[2,3] This allows metabolism of progesterone through to C19 steroids, which in turn can be converted to estrogen. Thus, progesterone output from the placenta falls and estrogen increases. The altered estrogen/progesterone ratio provokes increased prostaglandin synthesis and birth. Over the past few years it became evident that there were reasons to challenge this hypothesis. For example, fetal placental expression of prostaglandin H synthase type 2 (PGHS-2) mRNA increases progressively over the last 25 days of late gestation, coincident with the rise in fetal PGE₂ concentrations, and preceding changes in placental output of estrogen and progesterone.[4] Furthermore, using immunohistochemistry and Western blotting techniques, we showed that expression of P450C17 in placental trophoblast uninucleate cells followed rather than preceded expression of PGHS-2.[5] Finally, while estrogen administration increases expression of PGHS-2 in uterine tissues of nonpregnant sheep, intrafetal estrogen administration completely failed to increase levels of placental PGHS-2 in late-gestation sheep. In contrast, intrafetal cortisol administration at amounts that reproduced the circulating levels of cortisol in the fetal plasma near term provoked an increase in placental PGHS-2 mRNA and a subsequent increase in PGHS-2 protein.[6] In the placenta, immunoreactive PGHS-2 localizes exclusively to the trophoblast cells, and is absent from the maternal component. In the uterus, PGHS-2 localizes predominantly to the maternal endometrial epithelium.

To examine the relationship between cortisol, estrogen, and increased PGHS-2 expression more closely, we treated late pregnant sheep with either cortisol or cortisol and 4-hydroxyandrostenedione, an inhibitor of aromatase activity. After 72 to 80 hours' treatment of cortisol infusion alone, there were increased concentrations of PGE_2 in the fetal circulation, increased 13, 14-dihydro-15-keto-$PGF_{2\alpha}$ (PGFM, reflecting $PGF_{2\alpha}$ levels) in the maternal circulation, and increased PGHS-2

mRNA and protein in the placenta and maternal intercaruncular endometrium. However, in animals treated with cortisol and 4-hydroxyandrostenedione there was no increase in maternal PGFM concentrations and no increase in PGHS-2 mRNA or protein levels in the maternal tissues, although placental PGHS-2 expression increased in a manner similar to that in animals treated with cortisol alone. Thus, we have proposed a new model to explain the sequence of events occurring at the time of parturition in sheep[5,7,8] (Fig. 4–1). We describe this model in some detail, because its underlying characteristics coincide more closely with key steps in the control of human labor. We propose that increased fetal cortisol up-regulates PGHS-2 gene expression in fetal trophoblast cells. These cells express glucocorticoid receptors (GR) that are absent from the maternal

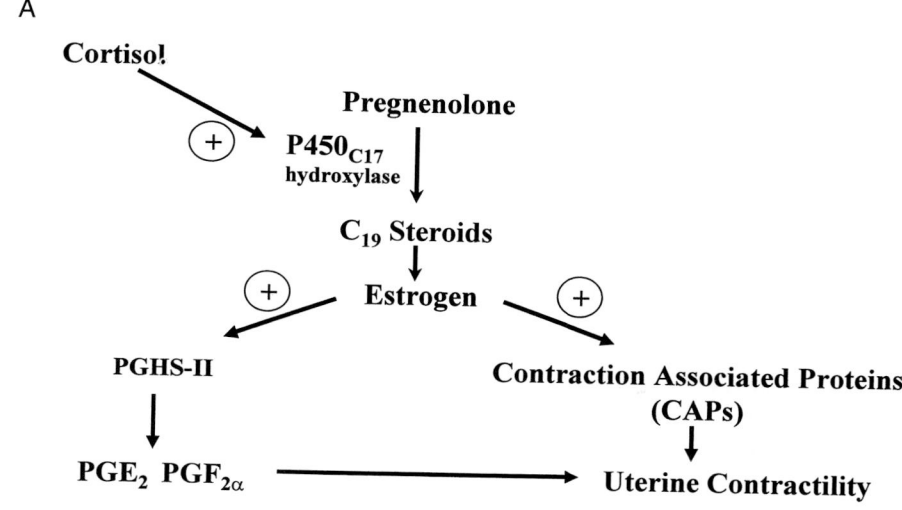

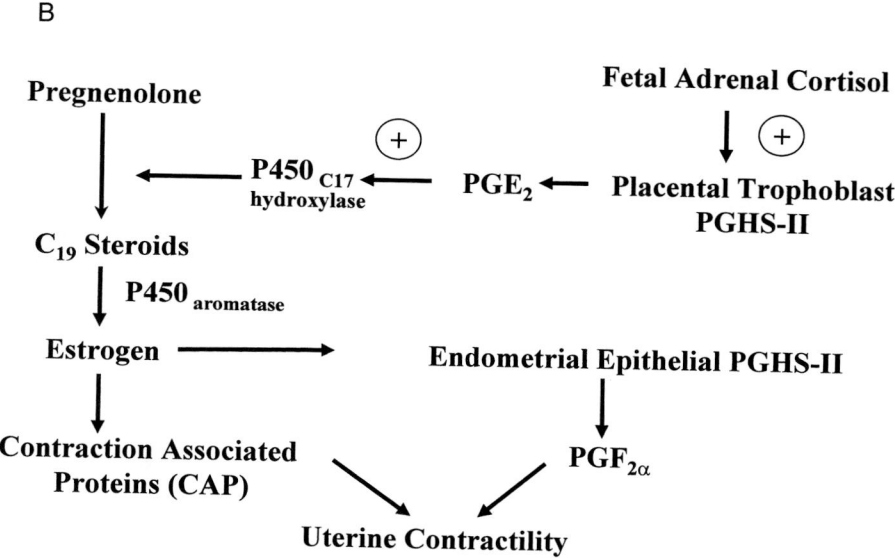

Figure 4–1. Current (*A*) and proposed (*B*) sequence of events occurring at the time of parturition in sheep.

component of the placenta. Increased placental expression of PGHS-2 results in a progressive increase in PGE_2 output from the placenta into the fetal compartment during late gestation. This accounts for the close temporal association between rising levels of cortisol and PGE_2 in the fetal circulation during late pregnancy. Furthermore, this relationship is suggestive of a positive feed-forward loop by which placental PGE_2 activates and stimulates activity of the fetal HPA axis, the end product of which, cortisol, promotes further placental PGE_2 production. We propose that in an autocrine or paracrine fashion, placental PGE_2 in turn up-regulates expression of P450C17. This enzyme co-localizes with PGHS-2 in fetal trophoblast cells. Up-regulation of this enzyme allows conversion of pregnenolone to C19 steroids and subsequently to estrogen. Thus, increased placental production of PGHS and P450C17 depends upon the elevation of fetal cortisol, but is independent of changes in estrogen. Support for a direct effect of PGE_2 on P450C17 expression is derived from studies in bovine adrenal tissue, and from measurements showing expression of EP (E-prostaglandin) receptor subtypes in ovine placental tissue.

Within the placenta, C19 steroids, formed locally from pregnenolone, are converted to estrogen. Estrogen up-regulates CAP gene expression in maternal uterine tissues. Estrogen is also critical for up-regulation of PGHS-2 in maternal endometrium, since increased endometrial PGHS-2 expression is blocked in animals treated with cortisol plus an aromatase inhibitor. Endometrial expression of PGHS-2 results in increased output into the maternal circulation of $PGF_{2\alpha}$ (reflected in concentrations of PGFM). The dependence of this response on estrogen is clear from experimental observations showing that the cortisol-induced increase in maternal PGFM concentrations does not occur after inhibition of placental aromatase activity.[8]

Thus, parturition in sheep (as in the human, see below) depends upon increased expression of PGHS-2 in intrauterine tissues. This finding immediately offers new therapeutic possibilities. We and others have shown that infusion of specific PGHS-2 inhibitors results in a rapid inhibition of uterine activity in sheep, either in the basal state, or after administration of RU-486 to induce uterine contractions.[9] The inhibition of uterine activity with PGHS-2 inhibitors such as meloxicam or nimesulide is associated with decreased output of PGE_2 into the fetal circulation and of PGFM into the maternal circulation. Importantly, while RU-486–induced preterm labor in sheep is associated with increased activity of the fetal HPA axis, attenuation of uterine contractility by administration of PGHS-2 inhibitor is associated with reduced concentrations of fetal plasma adrenocorticotropic hormone (ACTH) and cortisol. Thus, suppression of uterine activity is associated with a basal level of fetal HPA axis activity, compatible with pregnancy maintenance. The effect of meloxicam in inhibiting uterine activity is prolonged through at least 48 hours. This is clearly superior to the reappearance of uterine activity that occurs during β-sympathomimetic administration. Further studies are required to address the efficacy, safety, and reversibility of meloxicam action before this drug can be utilized in clinical therapeutic management.

FETAL HPA ACTIVATION IN PRIMATES

There is now an increasing body of evidence to suggest that the primate fetus exerts similar controls on gestation length through increased activity of the HPA axis.[10] The pattern of steroids produced by the primate fetal adrenal gland differs, however, from that in the sheep. In the latter species, there is no hypertrophied fetal zone, and cortisol is the major steroid produced. In the primate fetus, however, cortisol is produced from the transitional zone of the fetal adrenal cortex, whereas the predominant fetal zone, which lacks 3β-hydroxysteroid dehydrogenase, produces mainly $\Delta5$ steroids, especially dehydroepiandrosterone (DHEA). There is now convincing evidence for increased concentrations of fetal adrenal steroids in the circulation of primate fetuses in late gestation. In the fetal baboon there is increased expression of proopiomelanocortin (POMC) in the pars distalis of the fetal pituitary, and this appears to be driven by fetal hypothalamic CRH.[11] In the primate, especially the human, the placenta is an additional source of CRH, and expression of prepro-CRH mRNA increases exponentially in placental tissue during the latter part of gestation (see below). Recent studies have suggested that in addition to effects of placental CRH at the level of the fetal pituitary, this neuropeptide may also have a direct stimulatory effect on the fetal adrenal gland, promoting increased output of $\Delta5$-DHEA during the latter part of gestation. The regulation of placental CRH is discussed below.

Several studies have led investigators to argue strongly in favor of cortisol, presumably of fetal origin, having a major role to play in the mechanisms associated with human parturition. In particular, fetal glucocorticoids affect the expression and/or activity of enzymes of prostaglandin synthesis and metabolism, and promote, paradoxically, up-regulation of placental CRH gene expression.[6]

PROSTAGLANDINS AND HUMAN PARTURITION

There is now extensive evidence for a role of prostaglandins in the labor process of animals and humans.[10]

Mice lacking the ability to generate prostaglandins (PGHS-1 knockouts) have protracted labors. There is an increased capacity for prostaglandin synthesis by intrauterine tissues at the time of parturition, whether at term or preterm. Inhibitors of prostaglandin synthesis, such as indomethacin, block uterine contractility and prolong gestational length in subhuman primates and in women. Furthermore, the primate uterus is exquisitely sensitive to the stimulatory effect of exogenously applied prostaglandins.

The production of prostaglandins in human intrauterine tissues is compartmentalized discretely within the tissues of the pregnant uterus.[10] PGE_2 is formed predominantly in amnion, and its output increases at the time of labor. Chorion also produces predominantly PGE_2, although in chorion trophoblasts the metabolizing enzyme 15-hydroxyprostaglandin dehydrogenase (PGDH) metabolizes eicosanoids extensively, and may serve as a metabolic barrier to prevent passage of prostaglandins generated in amnion or chorion to the underlying decidua and myometrium. Decidua and myometrium both produce prostaglandins. Recent studies on changes in myometrial prostaglandin production in women at the time of labor have led to divergent findings, with some investigators reporting increased prostaglandin output, while others have reported no change or even decreased prostaglandin production.

Primary prostaglandins are formed from arachidonic acid through the activity of the PGHS enzyme complex. There are two forms of PGHS: PGHS-1 and PGHS-2. The former has been described as constitutive, the latter as an inducible gene product. Both forms may be up-regulated in response to certain stimuli, but it is apparent that major increases in PGHS-2 in amnion and chorion occur at the time of labor at term; PGHS-2 is also up-regulated in amnion collected from patients in preterm labor. Prostaglandin action is effected through specific receptors including the four main subtypes: EP1, EP2, EP3 and EP4 for PGE_2, and FP for $PGF_{2\alpha}$. EP1 and EP3 receptors mediate contractions of smooth muscle in a number of tissues through mechanisms that include increased calcium mobilization and inhibition of intracellular cAMP generation. EP3 receptors exist as a number of isoforms produced after alternative splicing of a single gene product. Activation of EP2 and EP4 receptors increases cAMP formation and relaxes smooth muscle. Theoretically, inhibition of uterine activity might be achieved through antagonism of EP1, EP3, or FP receptor action, or through agonist activation of the inhibitory EP2 and EP4 receptors. At present, however, there is little information concerning regulation and regional changes in any prostaglandin receptor subtype in human myometrial tissue at the time of parturition.[10]

Regulation of PGHS activity is a key step controlling conversion of arachidonic acid to biologically active prostaglandins. Experimental studies have shown that PGHS can be up-regulated in response to a variety of growth factors including epidermal growth factor (EGF), cytokines, interleukin-1 (IL-1), tumor necrosis factor (TNF), and interleukin-6 (IL-6). The action of cytokines appears to be mediated through an NF-κB consensus sequence in the promoter region of PGHS-2. This promoter also contains a cAMP response element, and early studies demonstrated convincingly that β-mimetics and cAMP analogs were capable of increasing PGE_2 output by human decidual cells and fetal membranes. Glucocorticoid also appeared to stimulate prostaglandin output and up-regulate levels of PGHS-2 mRNA in primary cultures of human amnion cells and in chorion trophoblast cells.[12] The mechanism of this action remains particularly controversial, since glucocorticoids appear to decrease PGHS expression in some other cell types. However, there is a consensus sequence corresponding to a glucocorticoid response element (GRE) at approximately +760 base pairs from the PGHS-2 transcription start site, and it has been speculated that, in trophoblasts, glucocorticoids may act either directly through this site, or through some other intermediate transcription factor.

Gibb and Lavoie were the first to show that human amnion cells, maintained in mixed monolayer culture, increased output of PGE_2 in a dose-dependent manner with increased exposure to dexamethasone.[13] This effect was observed once the cells had reached confluency; glucocorticoids inhibited PGE_2 output in freshly dispersed amnion cells. Several other investigators have subsequently confirmed this observation, although others have recently reported an inhibitory effect of glucocorticoids on amnion epithelial cells. Whittle and colleagues[12] developed techniques to separate human amnion and mesenchymal cells prior to in vitro culture. They found that the basal output of PGE_2 was considerably higher by mesenchymal fibroblast cells than by epithelial cells. Addition of arachidonic acid stimulated PGE_2 output by the epithelial cells, and glucocorticoids stimulated a further increase in PGE_2 accumulation into the incubation medium. This observation contrasts with the apparent stimulatory effect of glucocorticoids on fibroblast cells of mixed amnion cultures reported by Economopoulos et al.[14] This work has shown increased PGE_2 output and increased immunoreactive (ir)-PGHS-2 staining predominantly in cells derived from the amnion mesenchymal layer after exposure to corticosteroids. Clearly, this action of glucocorticoids is of great interest and the discrepancies in the literature as well as the mechanism of glucocorticoid action urgently need resolution.

Proinflammatory cytokines increase PGHS-2 gene expression, mRNA, protein, and PGE_2 output by cultured amnion and chorion cells. The opposing action of anti-inflammatory cytokines on prostaglandin output has recently been described. Pomini et al.[15] showed that interleukin-10 (IL-10) alone generated a modest stimulatory effect on PGHS-2 gene expression in villous and chorion trophoblast cells, but IL-10 completely attenuated stimulation of PGHS-2, mRNA, protein, and PGE_2 output produced by addition of interleukin-1β (IL-1β). Thus, in vivo it is apparent that the relative amounts of eicosanoids and cytokines produced from an interactive cytokine–eicosanoid cascade will be critical in regulating the final response of the tissue and level of prostaglandin produced.

The effect of cytokines on prostaglandin production is particularly important in circumstances of preterm labor associated with an underlying infections. Many investigators have suggested that approximately 30 percent of preterm labor is associated with an infection, although some have maintained that infection-driven prostaglandin release is a result rather than a cause of preterm birth.[16,17] Others have maintained that subclinical inflammatory responses with elevated cytokine production is a more common event, and may contribute to term labor as well as preterm labor. Infection-associated preterm labor is associated with increased concentrations of cytokines, including IL-1, IL-6, and TNF in the amniotic fluid. Administration of cytokines such as IL-1 or of bacterial endotoxin to pregnant mice provokes premature delivery, and this is associated with increased output of prostaglandin by intrauterine tissues. Cytokines increase phospholipase A_2 and PGHS-2 gene expression in a time- and dose-dependent fashion by amnion and choriodecidual tissue maintained in vitro. Thus, a currently accepted model is that, in the presence of an ascending bacterial infection, organisms pass between the fetal membranes and later reach the amniotic cavity.[16] Bacterial organisms may release phospholipases, which in turn stimulate prostaglandin production within the membranes. They may also release endotoxins such as lipopolysaccharide (LPS), which provoke prostaglandin or further cytokine release from macrophages. These cytokines would in turn stimulate PGHS-2 expression and prostaglandin output from amnion and/or decidual stroma cells. IL-1 stimulates output of other cytokines including IL-6 and IL-8 from decidua, thereby establishing a positive feed-forward cascade. IL-1 may also elicit release of other uterotonins including CRH and oxytocin from the decidua, membranes, and/or placenta.[18]

PROSTAGLANDIN METABOLISM

Recent studies have placed cortisol as a central mechanism of human parturition.[10] Glucocorticoids may stimulate prostaglandin synthesis. It is now apparent that glucocorticoids may also decrease prostaglandin metabolism (thereby allowing increased output of unmetabolized prostaglandin). Glucocorticoids in turn stimulate

CRH output from human intrauterine tissues, and CRH in turn increases PGHS-2 expression by fetal membranes in culture (see below).

A substantial body of evidence has revealed that the prostaglandin-metabolizing enzyme PGDH is extensively localized throughout the chorion trophoblast layer.[19] Of particular interest was the observation that immunostaining for PGDH was decreased in membranes collected from patients in idiopathic preterm labor, and in patients where preterm labor was associated with an underlying infective process and infiltration of leukocytes into the chorion trophoblast layer. In the latter circumstance, the number of trophoblast cells was diminished. In stage 3 chorioamnionitis, there was further loss of trophoblast cells and corresponding decrease in ir-PGDH. In situ hybridization studies showed that changes in PGDH protein reflected the pattern of change in PGDH mRNA in chorion trophoblast cells. In addition, the activity of PGDH in chorion was assessed by measurement of the conversion of $PGF_{2\alpha}$ to its metabolites 13,14-dihydro-$PGF_{2\alpha}$ and 13,14-dihydro-15-keto-$PGF_{2\alpha}$. PGDH activity in chorion was greatest in tissue collected from patients at term in the absence of labor.[20] There was a modest decrease in PGDH activity in chorion from patients at term in the presence of labor and a further decrease in mean PGDH activity in tissue collected from patients in preterm labor in the absence of an underlying infection. In this latter group, however, a subset of approximately 15 percent of patients had essentially undetectable PGDH activity, even though abundant chorion trophoblast cells were present. Thus, we surmised that deficient or diminished expression of PGDH in chorion trophoblasts might be causal to preterm labor in this subset of patients. PGDH activity was further reduced in preterm labor in association with infection; this was an expected observation, given the loss of trophoblast cells in membranes from such patients. Importantly, changes in PGDH in these chorion cell types were specific to chorion because there were no significant differences in PGDH activity in placental preparations from the same four groups of patients. Thus, we[19,20] proposed that during pregnancy, chorion PGDH effectively metabolizes prostaglandins generated within amnion and chorion, preventing their passage to decidua and myometrium. In this circumstance it is likely that prostaglandins responsible for stimulating myometrial contractility are generated within decidua or within the myometrium itself. In a subset of patients, PGDH activity in chorion trophoblasts is diminished in preterm labor in the absence of infection, allowing transmembrane passage of bioactive prostaglandins. In preterm labor with an underlying infective process, loss of trophoblasts is associated with loss of PGDH activity, and allows increased prostaglandin transfer through the membranous layer.

We used in vitro tissue culture techniques to examine regulation of PGDH expression and activity in trophoblast cells.[19,21] We found that cortisol inhibited PGDH activity and lowered PGDH mRNA levels in placenta and chorion trophoblast cells collected from patients at term spontaneous labor or at term elective cesarean delivery. Thus, glucocorticoids, which increase PGHS-2 expression in these cell types, decrease expression of the metabolizing enzyme PGDH. We reasoned that the availability of glucocorticoids within membranes could be altered through the activity of the steroid-metabolizing enzyme 11β-hydroxysteroid dehydrogenase-1 (11β-HSD-1). 11β-HSD exists in at least two isoforms; 11β-HSD-2, which acts predominantly as a dehydrogenase to inactivate cortisol by conversion to cortisone, and 11β-HSD-1, which acts predominantly as a reductase, converting cortisone to cortisol, and is present in kidney and placenta, where it may reduce transplacental transfer of cortisol from mother to fetus. In intrauterine tissues, 11β-HSD-1 predominates in amnion and in chorion trophoblast cells. We found that cortisone was equally effective as cortisol in decreasing PGDH activity in human chorion cells maintained in culture. However, the effect of cortisone, but not that of cortisol, was completely abolished in the presence of carbenoxolone, an inhibitor of the 11β-HSD-1 enzyme. Thus, while cortisone can influence PGDH expression in fetal membranes, it does so through conversion to cortisol.[22]

In our initial experiments, we were surprised that progesterone appeared to have no significant effects on PGDH activity. However, the fetal membranes and syncytiotrophoblasts of the placenta express 3β-HSD and synthesize abundant progesterone from available pregnenolone. Given that glucocorticoids might affect PGDH activity in an autocrine fashion, we considered the possibility that progesterone might act similarly. Placenta and chorion trophoblast cells were treated,

therefore, with trilostane, an inhibitor of 3β-HSD. In the presence of trilostane, PGDH activity was reduced in a dose-dependent fashion. When the highest concentration of trilostane was held constant, and progesterone was added back to the cells, PGDH activity could be restored again in a dose-dependent fashion. The effect of trilostane on PGDH activity was associated with a significant reduction in levels of PGDH mRNA in both chorion and placental trophoblast cells. The stimulatory effect of progesterone in the presence of trilostane was associated with a parallel increase in PGDH mRNA levels. Thus, we have concluded that progesterone may regulate PGDH activity in trophoblast cells but in a tonic matter; local generation of progesterone appears important for sustained PGDH activity.

Further support for these observations was derived from studies showing that PGDH activity and expression in chorion trophoblasts were increased by progesterone agonists, R5020 and medroxyprogesterone acetate (Fig. 4–2). Basal PGDH output was inhibited in the presence of progesterone receptor antagonists onapristone and RU-486. Synthetic glucocorticoids, betamethasone and dexamethasone, mimic the action of cortisol in inhibiting PGDH activity, and glucocorticoids were able to modulate the effects of progesterone on this enzyme. In related studies we showed that cytokines such as IL-1 and TNF decreased PGDH activity, whereas IL-10 stimulated PGDH activity. Others have reported that cAMP decreases PGDH. Thus, the actions of glucocorticoids, cAMP, and cytokines on PGDH (inhibition) are the same, and the opposite of the effects of these compounds on prostaglandin synthesis (PGHS-2 expression and stimulation) (Table 4–1).

To investigate further whether there might be regional changes in PGDH activity, chorion was obtained from the cervical, middle, and placental region of the uterus from patients at cesarean section in the absence

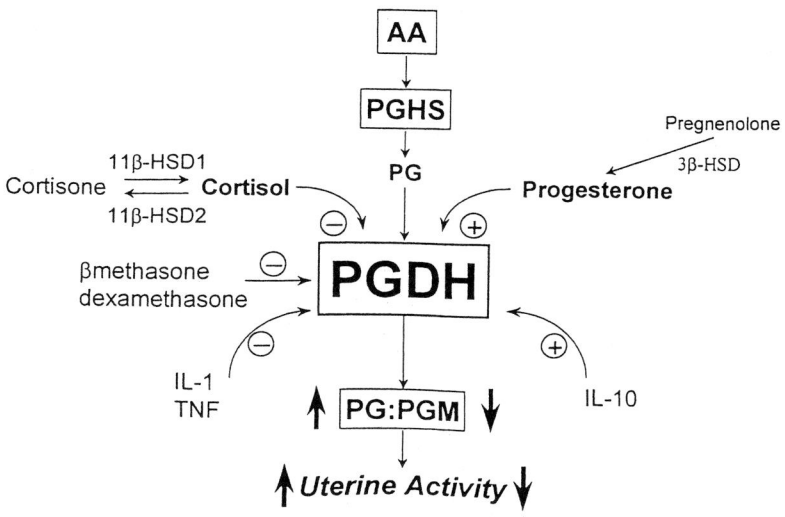

Figure 4–2. Regulation of 15-hydroxyprostaglandin dehydrogenase (PGDH) by glucocorticoids, cytokines, and progestins results from a balance between these different activities. We suggest that alterations in PGDH expression locally in chorion or villous trophoblasts alter the ratio of primary prostaglandin (PG) to prostaglandin metabolite (PGM), and the level of uterotonin available to alter myometrial contractility. AA, arachidonic acid; PGHS, prostaglandin H synthase; IL-1, interleukin-1; IL-10, interleukin-10; TNF, tumor necrosis factor; 11β-HSD, 11β-hydroxysteroid dehydrogenase type 1 or type 2; 3β-HSD 3β-hydroxysteroid dehydrogenase.

Table 4–1. OPPOSING EFFECTS OF AGONISTS/ANTAGONISTS ON PGHS AND PGDH IN HUMAN INTRAUTERINE TISSUES

PGHS	Agonist	PGDH
↑	Glucocorticoids	↓
↑	cAMP	↓
↑	Proinflammatory cytokines	↓
↓	Anti-inflammatory cytokines	↑
↔	Progesterone	↑

PGHS, prostaglandin H synthase; PGDH, 15-hydroxyprostaglandin dehydrogenase; cAMP, cyclic adenosine monophosphate.

or presence of labor. PGDH was highest in cervical chorion from patients not in labor. However, the activity of PGDH in cervical chorion from patients in labor was significantly lower than in the other two regions of the uterus. These were not significantly different between "labor" and "not in labor" patients. We speculated that the marked diminution in PGDH of the cervical chorion at the time of labor might reflect inhibition of PGDH expression by cytokines generated within the local environment of the vagina and cervix. The correlation between PGDH activity and 3β-HSD in midregion chorion suggested that alternative regulation (e.g., by progesterone) might be more important at this site. It was speculated that the reduction in PGDH activity of cervical chorion at the time of labor may have considerable physiologic importance. If prostaglandin synthesis is specifically up-regulated in this region, then those prostaglandins would not be metabolized by PGDH in chorion trophoblasts. There is only residual adherent decidual tissue in the cervical region, hence prostaglandins generated within amnion or chorion would find easy passage to the cervix, where they might participate in the process of effacement and dilatation. If this thesis is correct, it clearly offers opportunity for therapeutic regulation of PGDH activity in the cervical membranes, and potentially for chemical regulation of cervical function.

In addition to individual uterotonic actions, there is evidence to suggest that different myometrial stimulants might interact to regulate their own expression and action. For example, oxytocin has been shown to stimulate production of PGE_2 and $PGF_{2\alpha}$ from human and rat decidua, an effect blocked by oxytocin antagonists. Inhibitors of prostaglandin synthesis or antagonists of prostaglandin action have been reported to block oxytocin-stimulated contractions of uterine strips in rabbits. Oxytocin and CRH may also interact to increase myometrial contractions in human myometrium, although this action may also involve increased prostaglandin output.[1]

CRH AND HUMAN PARTURITION

Over the past decade there has been considerable interest in the role of placental CRH in the processes of parturition, and in the regulation of placental function.[18] Prepro-CRH mRNA increases in placental tissue exponentially during late gestation, and concentrations of CRH in maternal peripheral plasma rise with a similar time course. In maternal blood, CRH is associated with a high-affinity circulating CRH-binding protein (CRH-BP) produced in the liver, placenta, and also in other sites including brain. CRH-BP effectively blocks the action of placental CRH on the maternal pituitary and on maternal myometrium. However, near term and in association with preterm labor, CRH-BP concentrations decline, whereas CRH concentrations continue to increase. Thus, it has been surmised that there is a dramatic increase in free CRH concentrations in these different circumstances. Regulation of CRH output from placenta and fetal membranes has been examined mostly through the use of in vitro experiments. Placental CRH output and gene expression is inhibited by progesterone and nitric oxide; stimulated by oxytocin, cytokines, and catecholamines; and paradoxically markedly up-regulated by glucocorticoids. Thus, it has been suggested that increases in circulating cortisol concentration, within either the maternal compartment in response to stress or in the fetal compartment in response to HPA activation or stresses such as hypoxemia, would result, in the human, in a stimulus to increase placental CRH generation. Several groups have suggested that within placenta and fetal membranes CRH increases expression of PGHS-2 and thus output of biologically active prostaglandins. In vivo evidence in support of these observations has been obtained in two independent studies in which increased maternal plasma CRH concentrations were measured in patients who had presented in preterm labor and had received antenatal glucocorticoids for fetal lung maturation.[10] As discussed earlier, CRH and corticosteroids increased PGHS-2 expression by intrauterine tissues, and glucocorticoids decreased PGDH activity in human fetal membranes. These results suggest a close interrelationship between glucocorticoids, CRH, and prostaglandin production, and might provide an explanation of the transient increase in uterine activity seen in patients with multiple gestations treated prenatally with corticosteroids.[23]

Various studies have suggested that maternal plasma CRH concentrations are markedly elevated in patients at risk of preterm labor. Thus, McLean et al.[24] described elevations in circulating CRH concentrations in maternal blood as early as 14 to 15 weeks of gestation in patients destined to enter preterm labor. CRH concentrations in maternal blood were lower in those patients who subsequently delivered postterm. In our own studies, we found that CRH concentrations were not different, at 22 to 26 weeks of gestation, in the plasma of patients in preterm labor from those whose pregnancies would continue to term. However, maternal CRH concentrations were elevated significantly in the plasma of patients with the diagnosis of preterm labor at 28 to 32 weeks' gestation and 32 to 36 weeks' gestation.[25] This study suggested that maternal plasma CRH might be valuable as a means of discriminating those patients truly in preterm labor and requiring tocolytic management from those patients with a diagnosis of preterm labor but in whom uterine contractions would subsequently subside, and pregnancy continue through until close to term. Several clinical trials are currently underway to test this possibility and to compare the value of CRH measurements with those of other markers of preterm labor, including salivary estriol, cervical length, and oncofetal fibronectin.

The action of CRH on intrauterine tissues is mediated by specific CRH receptors. It is now apparent that there is an extensive network of high-affinity CRH receptors of different specificities within human myometrium, and there are several distinct receptor subtypes.[26] The predominant form in human myometrium is CRH-R1, which exists in at least two variant forms. The type II CRH receptors have tissue distribution distinct from the type I receptors, and exist in at least three splice-variant forms. These receptors couple with G-protein subtypes and activate adenylate cyclase. Human myometrial cells stimulated with CRH produced increased amounts of cAMP in culture. One would envisage that this activity should decrease calcium availability and decrease uterine contractility in vivo. However, as indicated above, cAMP may also stimulate PGHS-2 gene expression, and addition of CRH to human fetal membranes leads to increased output of PGE_2, and up-regulation of PGHS-2 mRNA. The CRH receptor appears to exist in different affinity forms during gestation; during pregnancy the receptors change to a high-affinity state and this is reversed at term. It appears that oxytocin may exert an inhibitory influence on myometrial adenylate cyclase activity and switch the CRH receptor to a low-affinity state and uncouple it from adenylate cyclase.[26] Thus, further studies on the effects of CRH on the human myometrium are clearly warranted.

Stevens and colleagues showed that the expression of CRH-R1 was increased in myometrium collected from patients at term, and preterm.[27] Of particular importance in that study, however, was the observation that expression of CRH-R1 in myometrium from pregnant women, and in tissue from a patient at term, was significantly higher in the lower uterine segment than in the fundal region. This observation would be compatible with CRH acting through CRH-R1 to stimulate adenylate cyclase and promote uterine relaxation in the lower uterine segment at term. CRH may then act in conjunction with other uterotonins to promote prostaglandin production, which would affect contractility in the fundal region of the uterus at this time. We have suggested that the failure to determine up-regulation of other CAP genes in the lower uterine segments of women at term is indicative of regional activation of the human uterus.[1] This suggestion may be of particular importance in relation to the continuing conundrum concerning changes in circulating progesterone concentrations before birth. In virtually all animal species, maternal plasma progesterone levels decline prior to parturition, an observation described by Csapo as withdrawal of the progesterone block that exists to reduce myometrial contractility during pregnancy (see Thorburn and Challis[2]). In primates, and particularly in the human, attempts to describe a similar decrease in maternal progesterone concentrations have been unsuccessful. Various investigators have proposed mechanisms for local withdrawal of progesterone that would obviate the need for a systemic change in hormone concentrations. We have suggested recently, however, the possibility that withdrawal of systemic progesterone in human gestation in fact should not occur in order to maintain the lower uterine segment in a nonquiescent state at the time of labor.[1] Withdrawal would then be confined to the upper segment, the region of greater activation and excitability. Verification of this proposition would give considerable importance in generating a unifying hypothesis for the control of labor between different animal species.

OXYTOCIN

Oxytocin is a nonapeptide, synthesized in the hypothalamus and released in a pulsatile fashion from the posterior pituitary into the systemic circulation. Pulses of oxytocin secretion increase in late pregnancy, but more important, the expression and numbers of oxytocin receptors in intrauterine tissues rises substantially; hence, increased end-organ response does not appear to require systemic oxytocin concentrations. It is clear that while oxytocin cannot be considered as an initiator of parturition, increased secretion through a neuroendocrine reflex occurs in stage 2 and 3 and contributes to expulsion of the placenta and uterine involution. Recent reports have suggested that mice bearing a null mutation in the oxytocin gene have a normal pregnancy and labor, raising some question as to the importance of this peptide in the labor process, certainly in small rodent species.

Oxytocin may also act as a local mediator of parturition. Oxytocin gene expression has been demonstrated in the pregnant rat uterus and fetal membranes and, at term, uterine oxytocin mRNA transcripts increase to values that were higher than those in the hypothalamus. Oxytocin is also synthesized in human fetal membranes, chorion, and decidua, and levels of oxytocin mRNA increase in these tissues at the time of parturition. In vitro studies with rat and human choriodecidual tissue have suggested that estrogen up-regulates oxytocin gene expression. More recently, studies from Hillhouse and colleagues have suggested that oxytocin may promote uterine activity by antagonizing the relaxant effect of CRH through receptors coupled to adenylate cyclase (see above).

GLUCOCORTICOIDS: GOOD NEWS AND BAD NEWS

The preceding argument has been that activation of HPA function with the resultant increase in glucocorticoids promotes parturition through increased prostaglandin synthesis, increased CRH expression, and decreased prostaglandin metabolism. Evidence is accumulating in support of this proposition. Glucocorticoids also participate in maturation of those organ systems, including the lung, that are required for postnatal survival. Glucocorticoids, however, may exert adverse effects on the developing fetal organism, and the elevations of fetal corticoids may occur with potential inhibition of fetal growth and altered programming of the fetal cardiovascular system, pancreas, and brain, particularly the hippocampus. It is imperative, therefore, that the fetus is protected from the excesses of maternal glucocorticoids through the activity of the 11β-HSD-2 enzyme in the placenta. Regulation of this enzyme is multifactorial. In vitro studies indicate that it is inhibited by progesterone, and inhibited by nitric oxide through a pathway that is partially dependent on the generation of cGMP. In contrast, 11β-HSD-2 in placental tissue is up-regulated by cAMP and by adenylate cyclase agonists. It is also up-regulated by transforming growth factor-β (TGF-β). Evidence has been presented in several species, including the rat and rhesus monkey, that the level of placental 11β-HSD-2 may be critical in determining the amount of glucocorticoid passing from the mother to the fetus. Maternal glucocorticoids affect the development of the fetal HPA axis. In addition, elevations of maternal glucocorticoid and/or decreased levels of placental 11β-HSD-2 result in growth restriction at birth and predispose to the development of hypertension in later life.[28]

In related experiments, we have examined regulation of 11β-HSD-1 in human fetal membranes. Previous studies have failed to demonstrate changes in 11β-HSD-1 mRNA levels or activity with cyclic nucleotides, nitric oxide, or steroids. However, Alfaidy and Challis (unpublished observations) have shown that $PGF_{2\alpha}$ up-regulates 11β-HSD-1 activity in a dose-dependent fashion in human chorion trophoblast cells maintained in culture. Moreover, this is a direct effect on 11β-HSD-1 activity, since it is observed within a very short time frame (minutes) and involves increased levels of intracellular calcium, apparently from intracellular stores rather than from an extracellular source. Thus, it appears that within the fetal membranes there exists a local feed-forward mechanism that results in elevated levels of glucocorticoid. Cortisol promotes prostaglandin synthesis and decreases prostaglandin metabolism, hence increasing output of prostaglandin from chorion trophoblast cells. If that prostaglandin, in turn, elevates 11β-HSD-1 expression, it would result in increased conversion of cortisone to cortisol, locally by these cells, and lessened opportunity for cortisol oxidation by this enzyme. It remains unclear whether this pathway is primarily concerned with the generation of prostaglandins required for myometrial activity, or whether it leads to the stimulated expression of various matrix metalloproteinases within the membranes, which in turn contribute to collagen breakdown and membrane rupture.

The effectiveness of the placental 11β-HSD barrier is reduced by the use of synthetic glucocorticoids, which are poor substrates for 11β-HSD. Studies in southwestern Australia have shown that pregnant sheep treated with clinically relevant amounts of betmethasone at 1-week intervals, on days 104, 111, and 118 of gestation (term, 145 days), produced lambs of reduced weight at day 125 and at term. At term, these lambs have decreased femur length, abdominal circumference, brain weight, liver weight, kidney weight, adrenal weight, but increased brain/liver weight ratio. At 6 and 12 months of life they have altered HPA responses to CRH stimulation tests. At 6 months and at 12 months of life the insulin response to a glycemic load is much greater than in controls, despite achieving similar circulating glucose concentrations, and is consistent with the acquisition of early insulin resistance.

These observations are not only of physiologic interest, they are of clinical importance.[29] Exogenous glucocorticoids are utilized, with very great benefit, in clinical practice to promote fetal pulmonary maturity. These observations, however, suggest the necessity of utilizing exogenous glucocorticoids with caution. They also indicate the necessity of distinguishing clearly those patients who truly are in preterm labor and warrant treatment with glucocorticoids as opposed to those patients with an initial diagnosis of preterm labor, but in whom pregnancy will continue to term, and weekly corticosteroid administration is unwarranted. An understanding of the processes of term and preterm labor should facilitate identification of appropriate markers (such as CRH). An understanding of the processes of labor should also facilitate development of new and more effective management protocols for suppressing uterine activity in those patients in true preterm labor where the health of the fetus is enhanced by continued intrauterine development.

Acknowledgments

Work in the authors' laboratory has been supported by the Canadian Institute of Health Research (CIHR Group in Fetal and Neonatal Health and Development, CIHR Group in Fetal Development and Health).

Key Points

➤ Preterm birth is a major problem in obstetrics for which there are currently no good diagnostic tests or effective management strategies.

➤ During pregnancy (phase 0 of parturition), relative uterine quiescence is maintained by a variety of endocrine and paracrine/autocrine factors.

➤ Labor is associated with myometrial activation (in response to uterine stretch and endocrine stimuli) and myometrial stimulation (in response to increased uterotonin production and/or action).

➤ Uterine activation involves increased hypothalamic-pituitary-adrenal (HPA) activity in the fetus at term. Increased fetal (and maternal) HPA function in response to stress may contribute to preterm labor.

➤ Prostaglandins have a key role in phase 2 of parturition as uterotonins. In women, prostaglandin production in the fetal membranes is increased, and prostaglandin metabolism in the chorion is decreased at term and preterm labor.

➤ Corticotropin-releasing hormone (CRH) is produced by human placenta and fetal membranes at term, and in response to elevated glucocorticoids. CRH may inhibit (via cAMP) or stimulate (through increased prostaglandin output) uterine activity.

➤ Factors leading to preterm birth may vary in different patients, and different factors may be of greater importance at different times in gestation.

➤ The human uterus at term may undergo regionalization into a lower segment that is relatively relaxed, and a contractile fundal region. Regional differences in the production/action of various agonists likely drive this process.

➤ Concern is expressed about the long-term effects on the fetus/newborn of repeated administration of maternal glucocorticoid during pregnancy; hence, the further need to differentiate patients in true preterm labor from those who are not and should not receive glucocorticoid treatment.

➤ Further basic research in animals and in humans should improve our understanding of birth, at term and preterm, leading to better diagnosis of this condition and its treatment.

REFERENCES

1. Lye SJ, Ou C-W, Teoh T-G, et al: The molecular basis of labour and tocolysis. Fetal Matern Med Rev 10:121, 1998.
2. Thorburn GD, Challis JRG: Endocrine control of parturition. Physiol Rev 59:863, 1979.
3. Liggins GC, Thorburn GD: Initiation of parturition. In Lamming G (ed): Marshall's Physiology of Reproduction, 4th ed, Vol 3, Pregnancy and Lactation Part 2. London, England, Chapman & Hall, 1994, p 863.
4. Gibb W, Matthews SG, Challis JRG: Localization of prostaglandin H synthase (PGHS) and PGHS mRNA in ovine placenta throughout gestation. Biol Reprod 54:654, 1996.
5. Gyomorey S, Lye SJ, Gibb W, Challis JRG: The fetal to maternal progression of PGHS-2 in ovine intrauterine tissues during the course of labor. Biol Reprod 62:797, 2000.
6. Challis JRG, Lye SJ, Gibb W: Prostaglandins and parturition. The uterus: endometrium and myometrium. Ann N Y Acad Sci 828:254, 1997.
7. Gyomorey S, Gupta S, Lye SJ, et al: Temporal expression of PGHS-2 and P450$_{C17}$ in ovine placentomes with the natural onset of labour. Placenta 21:478, 2000.
8. Whittle WL, Holloway AC, Lye SJ, et al: Prostaglandin production at the onset of ovine parturition in regulated by both estrogen-independent and estrogen-dependent pathways. Endocrinology 141:3783, 2000.
9. Lye SJ, Adamson SL, Booking AD, et al: The COX-2 inhibitor, meloxicam, effectively blocks preterm labour in sheep without adverse effects of fetal/maternal cardiovascular or GI function. Society for Gynecologic Investigation, 46th Annual Meeting, Atlanta, GA, Abstract #20, March 10–13, 1999.
10. Challis JRG: Characteristics of parturition. In Creasy RK, Resnick R (eds): Maternal-Fetal Medicine: Principles and Practice, 4th ed. Philadelphia, WB Saunders Company, 1998, p 434.
11. Pepe GJ, Albrecht ED: Actions of placental and fetal adrenal steroid hormones in primate pregnancy. Endocr Rev 16:608, 1995.

12. Whittle WL, Gibb W, Challis JRG: The characterization of human amnion epithelial and mesenchymal cell culture; the cellular expression, activity and glucocorticoid regulation of prostaglandin synthesis. Placenta 21:394, 2000.

13. Gibb W, Lavoie JC: Effects of glucocorticoids on prostaglandin formation by human amnion. Can J Physiol Pharmacol 68:671, 1990.

14. Economopoulos P, Sun M, Purgina B, Gibb W: Glucocorticoids stimulate prostaglandin H synthase type-2 (PGHS-2) in the fibroblast cells in human amnion cultures. Mol Cell Endocrinol 117:141, 1996.

15. Pomini F, Caruso A, Challis JRG: Interleukin-10 modifies the effect of interleukin 1-β and tumor necrosis factor α on the activity and expression of prostaglandin H synthase-2 and the NAD⁺-dependent 15-hydroxyprostaglandin dehydrogenase in cultured term human villous trophoblast and chorion trophoblast cells. J Clin Endocrinol Metab 84:4645, 1999.

16. Romero R, Avila C, Brekus CA, Morotti R: The role of systemic and intrauterine infection in preterm parturition. Ann N Y Acad Sci 622:355, 1991.

17. MacDonald PC, Casey ML: The accumulation of prostaglandins (PG) in amniotic fluid is an after-effect of labor and not indicative of a role for PGE$_2$ or PGF$_{2\alpha}$ in the initiation of human parturition. J Clin Endocrinol Metab 77:805, 1993.

18. Petraglia F, Florio P, Nappi C, Genazzani AR: Peptide signaling in human placenta and membranes: autocrine, paracrine and endocrine mechanisms. Endocr Rev 17:156, 1996.

19. Challis JRG, Patel FA, Pomini F: Prostaglandin dehydrogenase and the initiation of labor. J Perinat Med 27:26, 1999.

20. van Meir CA, Matthews SG, Keirse MJNC, et al: 15-Hydroxyprostaglandin dehydrogenase (PGDH): implications in preterm labor with and without ascending infection. J Clin Endocrinol Metab 82:969, 1997.

21. Patel FA, Clifton VL, Chwalisz K, Challis JRG: Steroidal regulation of prostaglandin dehydrogenase activity and expression in human term placenta and choriodecidua in relation to labor. J Clin Endocrinol Metab 84:291, 1999.

22. Patel FA, Sun K, Challis JRG: Local modulation by 11β-hydroxysteroid dehydrogenase of glucocorticoid effects on the activity of 15-hydroxyprostaglandin dehydrogenase in human chorion and placental trophoblast cells. J Clin Endocrinol Metab 84:395, 1999.

23. Elliott JP, Padan TG: The effect of corticosteroid administration on uterine activity and preterm labor in high-order multiple gestations. Obstet Gynecol 85:250, 1995.

24. McLean M, Bisits A, Davies J, et al: A placental clock controlling the length of human pregnancy. Nat Med 1:460, 1995.

25. Korebrits C, Ramirez MM, Watson L, et al: Maternal CRH as a predictor of impending preterm birth. J Clin Endocrinol Metab 83:1585, 1998.

26. Grammatopoulos DK, Hillhouse E: Hypothesis: role of corticotropin-releasing hormone in onset of labor. Lancet 354:1546, 1999.

27. Stevens YM, Challis JRG, Lye SJ: Corticotropin-releasing hormone receptor subtype 1 (CRH-R1) is significantly upregulated at the time of labor in the human myometrium. J Clin Endocrinol Metab 83:4107, 1998.

28. Sun K, Yang K, Challis JRG: Glucocorticoid actions and metabolism in pregnancy: implications for placental function and fetal cardiovascular activity. Placenta 19:353, 1998.

29. Norwitz ER, Robinson JN, Challis JRG: The control of labor. N Engl J Med 341:660, 1999.

Chapter 5

Physiology of Lactation and Breast-Feeding

EDWARD R. NEWTON

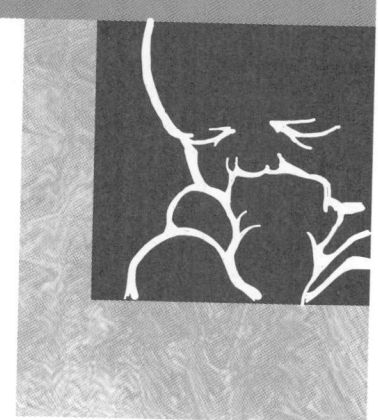

Breast-feeding and breast milk are the global standard for infant feeding in undeveloped and developed countries. This statement is supported by the World Health Organization, the U.S. Surgeon General, the American Academy of Pediatrics, the American College of Obstetrics and Gynecology, the American Academy of Family Practice, and the Academy of Breastfeeding Medicine. The American Academy of Pediatrics has recently published an endorsement for breast-feeding at least through the first year of life and as an exclusive method for the first 6 months.[1] Unfortunately, the majority of American infants are not given this opportunity. Figure 5-1 describes the incidence of breast-feeding in the United States. These data are the result of serial mail surveys sent to postpartum women. The response rate is consistently about 50 percent and minority women are underrepresented. The data for minority women are derived by major statistical manipulation. Despite the potential bias, no other national database exists. The latest survey (1995)[2] reports that 59.7 percent of women initiate breast-feeding in the hospital and only 21.6 percent of those are still breast-feeding at 6 months. Less than 10 percent of American infants meet the standard of breast-feeding 1 year or more.

Specific populations are at greater risk for the failure to initiate and continue breast-feeding. Lower socioeconomic classes, lack of education, and teenagers initiate breast-feeding at about one half to two thirds the rate of middle and upper class, mature high school graduates (Table 5-1). Fortunately, since 1989 more women at greatest risk for feeding their infants artificial breast milk are initiating breast-feeding in the hospital.[2] Perceived breast milk insufficiency, sore nipples and breasts, the lack of family and professional support, and the decision to return to work are the most often cited reasons for early weaning. Cultural attitudes underlie many of these risk factors for failure to breast-feed successfully.

Dysfunctional cultural and familial attitudes are outside the direct control of medicine, and may directly affect the care delivered by physicians. The normal function of the breasts, to produce breast milk, is muted by two cultural attitudes. One cultural attitude is the association of breasts with sexual attraction. The media is replete with examples that show beautiful, well-formed breasts as a sexual ideal. A corollary, of this attitude is that breast-feeding will cause the breasts to sag and lose their sex appeal. The other opposing cultural attitude is that breast-feeding restricts self-fulfillment; mothers who stay at home to breast-feed and care for their babies are considered poor examples of the modern, independent professional woman. These attitudes are exacerbated by a lack of knowledge about breast-feeding and lactation. The normal function of the breasts is excluded from the curriculum of primary and secondary schools on the basis of the connection between breasts and sex. After completion of their education, few women experience any examples of successful breast-feeding. Only 25 percent of grandmothers initiated breast-feeding, and few of the new mothers have breast-fed more than a few weeks. The lack of exposure to successful, experienced breast-feeding mothers seriously compromises the chances of success for the women who attempt to breast-feed.

Physicians are products of the same culture of the women they help. Unfortunately, many have the same cultural biases as their patients and the same lack of primary and secondary education regarding the normal physiology of breast-feeding. The curricula of medical school and residency training programs compound the lack of education. Most physicians reflecting on their own education on breast-feeding will identify neither a structured curriculum nor practical experiences with successfully breast-feeding mother–infant dyads. At most, he or she has experienced only one or two lectures regarding breast-feeding, often focused on breast anatomy or the endocrinology of lactation. In fact, the most commonly cited resource for physicians is another nonmedical individual or their breast-feeding spouse. On obstetric rotations, medical students and obstetrics residents rarely see normal breast-feeding dyads longer than 1 to 3 days postpartum. On pediatric rotations, learners often see the baby only in the nursery and rarely see the normal mother breast-feed as an inpatient or at newborn visits. While pediatric residents observe and support the mother who pumps or nurses her growing preterm infant, the exposure is not normal, and often is negative. As a result, there are serious gaps in physician knowledge as they attempt to serve the over 2 million newborns and mothers per year who attempt to breast-feed. A recent national survey of physician knowledge revealed that 20 to 40 percent of physicians (obstetricians, pediatricians, and family practitioners) did not know that breast-feeding is the "gold standard" for infant feeding, and similar percentages have serious and sometimes dangerous gaps in their knowledge in the management of breast-feeding problems.[3] A 1999 survey of fellows of the American Academy of Pediatricians revealed that only 65 percent recommended exclusive breast-feeding during the first month of life, and more than half agreed with or had a neutral opinion about the statement that breast-feeding and formula-feeding are equally acceptable methods for feeding infants.[4]

The purpose of this chapter is to begin the educational process through which obstetricians will adopt the lactating mother as their patient. In order to support the breast-feeding mother, the obstetrician must be

Table 5–1. DEMOGRAPHIC PREDICTORS OF BREAST-FEEDING: USA 1995

		In Hospital (%)	At 6 Months (%)
Race	White	64.3	24.1
	African-American	37.0	11.2
	Hispanic	61.0	19.6
Age	<20 years	42.8	9.1
	>35 years	70.0	33.8
Family income	<$10,000 per year	41.8	11.4
	≥$25,000 per year	71.0	28.5
Education	Grade school	43.8	17.1
	College	74.4	31.2
Employment	Full-time	60.7	14.3
	Not employed	58.0	25.0

Adapted from Ryan AS: The resurgence of breastfeeding in the United States. Pediatrics 99:E12, 1997. Copyright 1997 American Academy of Pediatrics, with permission.

convinced of the biologic superiority of breast-feeding and human breast milk over artificial breast milk (formula). This chapter discusses the limitations of the current research and reviews the morbidity and mortality associated with infant feeding using artificial breast milk. Subsequently, this chapter addresses breast anatomy and physiology of lactation in a framework pertinent to breast-feeding management. This chapter describes the vast differences between breast milk and artificial breast milk, a difference directly related to unique needs of the human infant. Specific issues related to the obstetrician (or other health care provider) will be addressed and include the role of the obstetrician in preconceptional counseling, prenatal care, delivery room management, and postpartum care for the breast-feeding mother.

LIMITATIONS OF BREAST-FEEDING RESEARCH

In the past there have been major flaws in the designs and conclusions of epidemiologic research regarding the benefits (or lack of benefits) of breast-feeding. In the last 10 years the quality has improved, but several cautions are warranted. A major confounder is the difference in the demographic characteristics between women who breast-feed and women who use artificial breast milk (Table 5–1). Many breast-feeding outcomes, such as infections and chronic diseases, are also more prevalent in the latter population. When comparing outcomes between breast-feeding and artificial breast milk feeding, the effect of demographic differences should be analyzed and controlled in the analysis. In addition,

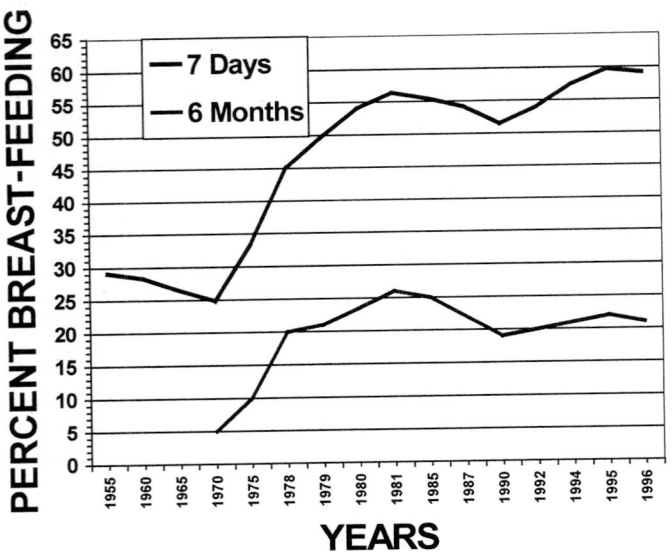

Figure 5–1. Incidence of breast-feeding.

cultural support and demographic differences of women who breast-feed their infants have changed. In the 1950s and 1960s cultural pressures pushed better educated, more wealthy middle class women away from breast-feeding; the incidence of initiation of breast-feeding reached its nadir in the early 1970s. This change is important when considering recall data used in studies evaluating differences in chronic diseases in the older adult, especially breast cancer.

Much of the older epidemiologic research has relied on self-report and recall data, usually long after the event has occurred. Memory is not perfect and biases are often introduced, such as combining events into convenient ages or socially acceptable times of weaning. One major area of recall bias is the definition of partial breast-feeding. An example of the confounding nature of this bias is a serial survey of nurses.[5] The study showed no significant benefit of breast-feeding in the reduction of premenopausal breast cancer, which was touted by the authors as evidence of no relationship between infant feeding and breast cancer. As this was a population of nurses, where a significant number were working at the time they were feeding their infant (this was not measured), the definition of breast-feeding may reflect intent more than actual degree of breast-feeding.

After statistical control for demographic variables, an unavoidable bias remains self-selection. Intrinsic personality characteristics may be determinants of feeding choice; a random allocation of feeding method is not possible. There is also evidence that women who breast-feed exhibit more nurturant behavior than women who feed their infants artificial breast milk.[6]

When analyzing any article involving breast-feeding, it is important to understand the author's definition of breast-feeding. Exclusive breast-feeding is considered when the infant does not receive any additional food or nutriment other than breast milk. Partial breast-feeding needs to be defined by the proportion of feeds that are breast milk or artificial breast milk. If an infant consumes 700 ml of artificial breast milk per day, then the proportion of breast milk consumed is small regardless of the frequency of breast-feeding episodes. Control for the "dose" effect is important in physiologic as well as epidemiologic studies. The content and character of breast milk are affected by the frequency of feeds, the duration of the feed, when in the feed the breast milk is collected, the method of breast milk collection, and the time of day of the collection.

One common design mistake is the failure to understand the effect of duration of breast-feeding. Breast-feeding has immediate and long-term benefits. The immediate benefits accrue only when a significant proportion of the infant's diet is breast milk. For example, the protection against gastroenteritis is afforded by the presence of antigen-specific immunoglobulin A (IgA) in breast milk. This protection is present only when the infant is breast-feeding. On the other hand, breast milk modulates the infant's immune system and improves response to infection well after breast-feeding has ceased. While it appears there is a dose-dependent relationship between the duration of exclusive breast-feeding and many long-term benefits, the effective dose (duration of exclusive breast-feeding) varies by benefit and is unknown. Most studies have arbitrarily determined the "effective" dose and challenge the benefits of breast-feeding based on that "effective" dose. For example,[7] Agre concluded that exclusive breast-feeding for 3 months had no bearing on the frequency of infection in the first year of life. However, his outcome variable, frequency of infection in first 12 months, did not stratify the outcome by when the infant was actually breast-feeding. An episode of gastroenteritis at 10 months was counted as a breast-feeding "failure" even though the infant breast-fed only 6 months.

In summary, good breast-feeding research must demonstrate appropriate definitions of breast-feeding, control for the "dose" effect, control for demographic differences between breast-feeding and non–breast-feeding populations, and appropriate linkage between behavior and outcomes.

BENEFITS OF BREAST-FEEDING

Epidemiologic research shows that human milk and breast-feeding of infants provide significant advantages to general health, growth, and development. In contrast, infant feeding with artificial breast milk is associated with higher incidences of acute and chronic diseases than in infants who are fed human milk through breast-feeding. The studies of predominantly, middle class populations in developed countries show that infant feeding with artificial breast milk is associated with higher incidences and greater severity of diarrhea,[8–12] lower respiratory infection,[13–15] otitis media,[9,16–18] bacteremia,[19,20] bacterial meningitis,[19,21] urinary tract infection,[22] and necrotizing enterocolitis[23,24] than similar populations who were breast-fed. Numerous studies show higher incidences of sudden infant death syndrome,[25–27] type I (insulin-dependent) diabetes,[28,29] adolescent obesity,[30] Crohn's disease,[31,32] ulcerative colitis,[32] lymphoma,[33] allergic diseases,[34–38] and other chronic digestive diseases among infants fed artificial breast milk.[36–38] In high-risk populations, preterm infants, and phenylketonurics, as well as healthy middle class populations of infants, breast-feeding has been associated with enhancement of cognitive development and intelligence quotients.[39–44]

Increase in acute medical diseases will manifest as increased costs of medical care for those families who choose to feed their infant artificial breast milk. Among Medicaid populations in Colorado,[45] California,[46] and health maintenance organizations in Arizona,[47] the medical cost of artificial breast milk feeding amounts to $300 to $500 dollars per year per infant. Among patients who belonged to a large health maintenance organization in Tucson, Arizona, the excess yearly medical costs of 1,000 never-breast-fed infants versus 1,000 infants who were exclusively breast-fed for at least 3 months was $331,041[48] (Table 5–2).

The nonmedical costs of artificial breast milk feeding are considerably higher than breast-feeding. The direct costs of artificial breast milk feeding includes the cost of the artificial formula (900 ml/day), bottles, and supplies. In eastern North Carolina (January 2000), the average retail cost of 900 ml of prepared formula was $4.45 daily ($1,622 yearly); of concentrate, $3.25 daily ($1,181 yearly); and of powdered formula, $2.74 daily ($1,001 yearly). A major indirect cost of artificial breast milk feeding is the environmental impact of large dairy herds to supply the milk substrate.

Breast-feeding provides the right amount of a superior product at precisely the right time and at the right temperature. The nonmedical costs of breast-feeding include the cost of increased calorie and protein needs ($1 to $2 daily), nursing bras and breast pads, and increased number of diapers in the first 2 to 3 months. If an electric breast pump is used when the woman returns to work, the cost of breast-feeding will increase $2 to $4 per day.

Breast-feeding accrues multiple benefits to the mother that are not shared by women who feed their infants artificial breast milk. Breast-feeding through increased release of oxytocin results in faster uterine involution and less postpartum blood loss[49]; the incidence of postpartum anemia may be reduced. Breast-feeding is associated with 1 to 3 kg (more in African-American women) less retained postpartum weight.[49,50] Decreased retained postpartum weight may reduce or delay the onset of chronic disease in older women, obesity,[49] type II (insulin-resistant) diabetes,[49] and hypertension.[49] Recent research demonstrates that exclusive breast-feeding delays ovulation with increased child spacing,[51] improved bone mineralization postpartum with reduction in hip fractures in the postmenopausal period,[52–54] a reduced risk of ovarian cancer[50] and premenopausal breast cancer.[50,54,55]

BREAST ANATOMY AND DEVELOPMENT

The size and shape of the breast vary greatly by stage of development, physiologic state, and phenotype. The breast is located in the superficial fascia between the second rib and sixth intercostal cartilage in the midclavicular line. There is usually a projection of the central disk into each axilla, the *tail of Spence*. The mature breast weighs about 200 g in the nonpregnant state; during pregnancy, 500 g; and during lactation, 600 to 800 g. As long as glandular tissue and the nipple are present, the size or shape of the breast has little to do with the functional success of the breast. The adequacy of glandular tissue for breast-feeding is ascertained by inquiring whether a woman's breasts have enlarged during pregnancy. If there is failure of the breast to enlarge as the result of pregnancy, especially if associated with minimal breast tissue on examination, the clinician should be wary of primary failure of lactation.

The nipple, or *papilla mammae*, is a conical elevation in the middle of the areola, or *areola mammae*. The areola is a circular pigmented area, which darkens during pregnancy. The contrast with the fairer skin of the body provides a visual cue for the newborn who is attempting to latch-on. The areola contains multiple small elevations, *Montgomery's tubercles*, which enlarge during pregnancy and lactation. Montgomery's tubercles contain multiple ductular openings of sebaceous and sweat glands. These glands secrete lubricating and anti-infective substances (IgA) that protect the nipples and areola during nursing. These substances are washed away when the breasts and nipples are washed with soap or alcohol-containing compounds, leaving the nipple prone to cracking and infection.

Unlike the dermis of the body of the breast, which includes fat, the areola and nipple contain smooth muscle and collagenous and elastic tissue. With light touch or anticipation, these muscles contract and the nipple erects to form a teat. The contraction pulls the lactifer-

Table 5–2. EXCESS MEDICAL COST (U.S. DOLLARS) AMONG 1,000 NEVER–BREAST-FED VERSUS 1,000 EXCLUSIVE (>3 MONTHS) BREAST-FED INFANTS

	Excess Services per year/1,000 Never–Breast-Fed	Total Excess Cost
Office visits	1,693	$111,315
Follow-up visits	340	$22,355
Medications*	609	$7,669
Chest radiography	51	$1,836
Days of hospitalization†	212	$187,866
Total excess cost per year		$331,031

*Lower respiratory infection, otitis media.
†Lower respiratory infection, gastroenteritis.
Adapted from Ball TM, Wright AL: Health care costs of formula-feeding in the first year of life. Pediatrics 103:870, 1999. Copyright 1999 American Academy of Pediatrics, with permission.

ous sinuses into the nipple–areola complex, which allows the infant to milk the breast milk from these reservoirs.

The tip of the nipple contains the openings (0.4 to 0.7 mm in diameter) of 15 to 20 milk ducts (2 to 4 mm in diameter). Each of the milk ducts empties one tubuloalveolar gland, which is embedded in the fat of the body of the breast. A sphincter mechanism at the opening of the duct limits the ejection of milk from the breast. The competency of this mechanism is variable. About 20 percent of women do not demonstrate milk ejection from the contralateral breast when milk ejection is stimulated. If milk leakage is demonstrated from the contralateral breast during nursing, there is supporting evidence of milk transfer to the infant.

Five to 10 mm from their exit, the milk ducts widen (5 to 8 mm) into the lactiferous sinuses (Fig. 5–2). When these sinuses are pulled into the teat during nursing, the infant's tongue, facial muscles, and mouth squeeze the milk from the sinuses into the infant's oropharynx.[56,57] The tubuloalveolar glands (15 to 20) form lobi, which are arranged in a radial fashion from the central nipple–areola complex. The lobi and lactiferous ducts extend into the tail of Spence. Ten to 40 lactiferous ducts connect to each lactiferous sinus, each forming a lobulus. Each lobulus arborizes into 10 to 100 alveoli for tubulosaccular secretory units. The alveoli are the critical units of the production and ejection of milk. A sac of alveolar cells is surrounded by a basket of myoepithelial cells. The alveolar cells are stimulated by prolactin to produce milk. The myoepithelial cells are stimulated by oxytocin to contract and eject the recently produced milk into the lactiferous ducts, lactiferous sinuses, and beyond.

The radial distribution of lactiferous ducts prompts important considerations relative to breast surgery on women who are breast-feeding or who will breast-feed. Surgical skin incisions parallel to the circumareolar line, especially at the circumareolar line, have better cosmetic healing and are often chosen by surgeons. However, if the incision is taken deep into the parenchyma, the lactiferous ducts may be compromised; a superficial, parallel skin incision and a radial deep incision are preferred. In women who intend to breast-feed, a circumareolar incision is to be avoided. The incision compromises breast-feeding in three ways: occlusion of lactiferous ducts, restriction of the formation of a teat during nursing, and injury to the lateral cutaneous branch of the fourth intercostal nerve.

Surgical disruption of the lateral cutaneous branch of the fourth intercostal nerve can have devastating effects on the success of breast-feeding.[58,59] This nerve is critical to the production and ejection of breast milk (see The Physiology of Lactation, below). Furthermore, the nerves provide organ-specific control of regional blood flow, and a tremendous increase in mammary blood flow occurs during a nursing episode.[60] Disruption of this autonomic control may severely compromise lactation performance. The rate of breast-feeding failure is two to three times higher when a circumareolar incision is performed.[58] The obstetrician needs to be alert to old surgical incisions when a pregnant patient expresses a desire to breast-feed or when a breast biopsy is anticipated in a reproductive-aged woman.

As a mammal, humans have the potential to develop mammary tissue, glandular or nipple tissue, anywhere along the milk line (*galactic band*). The milk line extends from the axilla and inner upper arm to its current position, down the abdomen along the midclavicular line to the upper lateral mons and upper inner thigh. When accessory glands occur, this is termed hypermastia. This may involve accessory glandular tissue, supernumerary nipples, or both. Two to 6 percent of women have hypermastia, and the response to pregnancy and lactation is variable. The most common site for accessory breast tissue is the axilla. These women may present at 2 to 5 days postpartum (galactogenesis) with painful enlargements in the axilla. Ice and symptomatic therapy for 24 to 48 hours is sufficient. Supernumerary nipples (*polythelia*) are associated with renal abnormalities (11 percent).

Full alveolar development and maturation of the breast must await the hormones of pregnancy (progesterone, prolactin, and human placental lactogen) for completion of the developmental process. By midpregnancy, the gland is competent to secrete milk (colostrum), although full function is not attained until the tissues are released from the inhibition of high levels of circulating progesterone. This is termed *lactogenesis stage 1*. Lactogenesis stage 2 occurs as the progesterone levels fall after delivery of the placenta, during the first 2 to 4 days after birth. Stage 2 includes dramatic increases in mammary blood flow and oxygen/glucose uptake by the breast. At 2 to 3 days postpartum, the secretion of milk is copious and "the milk comes in." This is the most common time for engorgement if the breasts are not drained by efficient, frequent nursing. Until lactogenesis stage 2 is developed, the breasts secrete colostrum. Colostrum is very different than mature milk in volume and constituents.[61,62] Colostrum has more protein, especially secretory immunoglobulins, lactose, and lower fat content than mature milk. Prolactin and glucocorticoids play important promoter roles in this stage of development.

After lactogenesis stage 2 (4 to 6 days postpartum) lactation enters an indefinite period of milk production formerly called galactopoiesis, now termed lactogenesis stage 3. The duration of this stage is dependent on the continued production of breast milk and the efficient transfer of the breast milk to the infant. Prolactin ap-

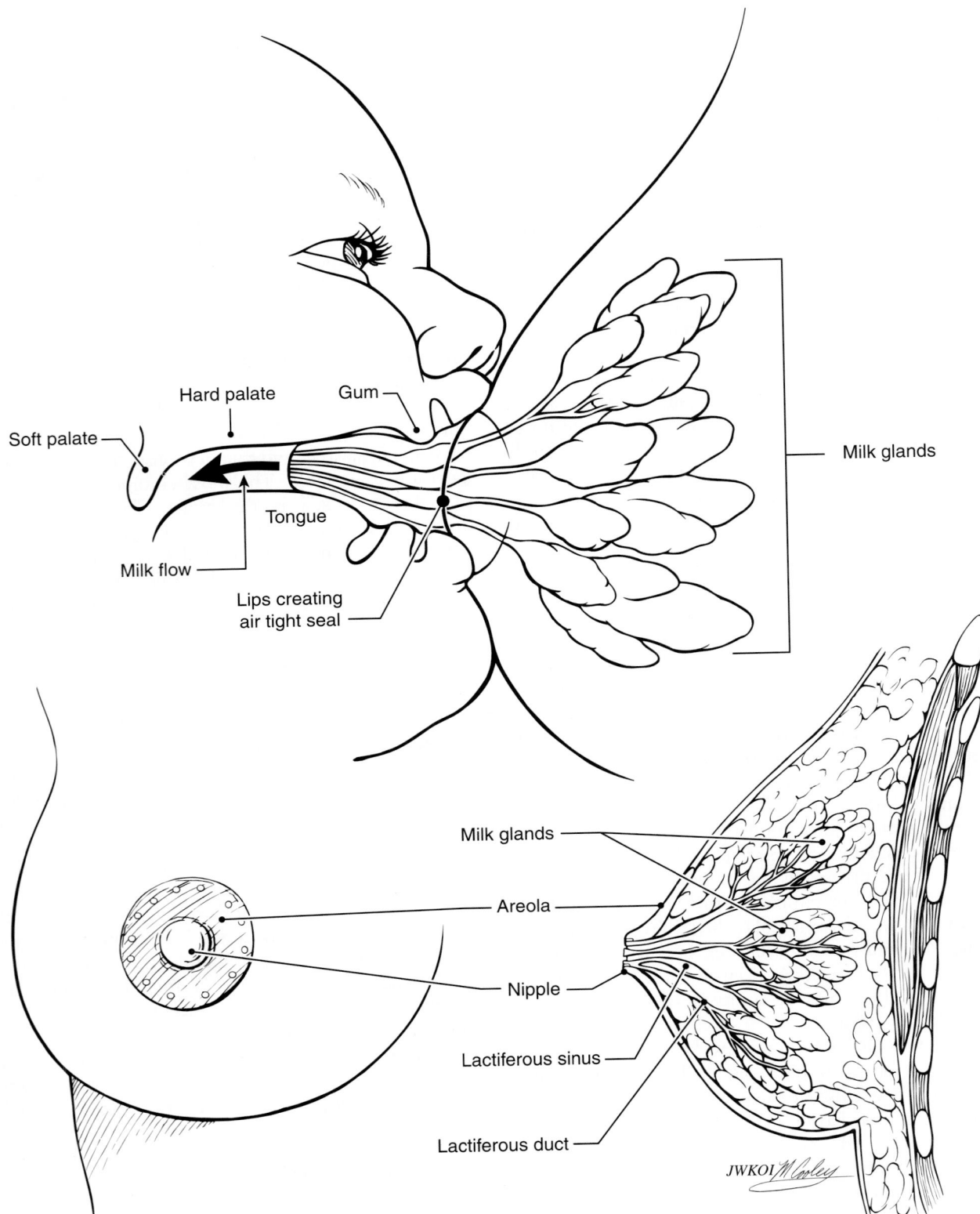

Soft palate

Hard palate

Gum

Milk glands

Tongue

Milk flow

Lips creating
air tight seal

Milk glands

Areola

Nipple

Lactiferous sinus

Lactiferous duct

JWKOI M Cooley

Figure 5–2. Anatomy of the breast.

pears to be the single most important galactopoietic hormone, since selective inhibition of prolactin secretion by bromocriptine disrupts lactogenesis. Oxytocin appears to be the major galactokinetic hormone. Stimulation of the nipple and areola or behavioral cues cause a reflex contraction of the myoepithelial cells that surround the alveoli and ejection of milk from the breast.

The final stage of development is involution and cessation of breast-feeding. As the frequency of breast-feeding is reduced to less than six episodes in 24 hours and milk volume is less than 400 ml/24 h, prolactin levels fall and a cyclic pattern ends in the total cessation of milk production. After 24 to 48 hours of no transfer of breast milk to the infant, intraductal pressure[63] and lactation inhibitory factor[64] appear to initiate apoptosis of the secretory epithelial cells and proteolytic degradation of the basement membrane. Lactation inhibitory factor is a protein secreted in the milk, whose increasing concentration in the absence of drainage appears to decrease milk production by the alveolar cells.[64-66] It counterbalances pressures to increase milk supply (increased frequency of nursing) and allows for the day-to-day adjustment in infant demands.

THE PHYSIOLOGY OF LACTATION

Prolactin is the major hormone promoting milk production. Prolactin induces the synthesis of mRNAs for the production of enzymes and milk proteins by binding to membrane receptors of the mammary epithelial cells. Thyroid hormones selectively enhance the secretion of lactalbumin. Cortisol, insulin, parathyroid hormone, and growth hormone are supportive metabolic hormones in the production of carbohydrates and lipids in the milk. Ovarian hormones are not required for the maintenance of established milk production and are suppressed by high levels of prolactin.

The alveolar cell is the principal site for the production of milk. Neville[67] describe five pathways for milk synthesis and secretion in the mammary alveolus, including four major transcellular and one paracellular pathway. They are (1) exocytosis (merocrine secretion) of milk protein and lactose in Golgi-derived secretory vesicles, (2) milk fat secretion via milk fat globules (apocrine secretion), (3) secretion of ions and water across the apical membrane, (4) pinocytosis-exocytosis of immunoglobulins, and (5) paracellular pathway for plasma components and leukocytes. During lactation as opposed to during pregnancy, very few of the constituents of breast milk are transferred directly from maternal blood. The junctions between cells, *tight junctions,* are closed. As weaning occurs, the tight junctions are released and sodium and other minerals easily cross to the milk, changing the taste of the milk.

The substrates for milk production are primarily absorbed from the maternal gut or produced in elemental form by the maternal liver. Glucose is the major substrate for milk production. Glucose serves as the main source of energy for other reactions and is a critical source of carbon. The synthesis of fat from carbohydrates plays a predominant role in fat production in human milk. Proteins are built from free amino acids derived from the plasma.

A sizable proportion of breast milk is produced during the nursing episode. In order to supply the substrates for milk production, there is increased blood flow to the mammary glands (20 to 40 percent), gastrointestinal tract, and liver. Cardiac output is increased by 10 to 20 percent during a nursing episode.[60] The vasodilation of the regional vascular beds is under the control of the autonomic nervous system. Oxytocin may play a critical role in directing the regional distribution of maternal cardiac output through an autonomic, parasympathetic action.

Given that milk is produced during the nursing episode, variation in content during a feed is expected. During a feeding episode the lipid content of milk rises by more than two to threefold (1 to 5 percent) with a corresponding 5 percent fall in lactose concentration.[68] The protein content remains relatively constant. At the extreme, there can be a 30 to 40 percent difference in the volume obtained from each breast.[69,70] Likewise, there are intra-individual variations in lipid and lactose concentrations.

The rising lipid content during a feed has practical implications in breast-feeding management. If a woman limits her feeds to less than 4 minutes, but nurses more frequently, the calorie density of the milk is lower and the infant's hunger may not be satiated. The infant wishes to feed sooner and the frequency of nursing accelerates. This stimulates more milk production and creates a scenario of a hungry infant despite apparent good volume and milk transfer.[71] Lengthening the nursing episode or using one breast for each nursing episode often solves the problem.

The volume and concentration of constituents also vary during the day.[69,70] Volume per feed increases by 10 to 15 percent in the late afternoon and evening. Nitrogen content peaks in the late afternoon and falls to a nadir at 5 A.M. Fat concentrations peak in the early morning and reach a nadir at 9 P.M. Lactose levels stay relatively stable throughout the day. The variation in milk volume and content in working women who nurse only when at home has not been studied. Presumably, the variation in volume and content is preserved if the woman pumps during the day.

Does diet affect the volume and constitution of breast milk? For the average American woman with the range of diets from teenagers to mature, health-conscious adults, the answer is "no." There is no convincing evidence that the macronutriments in breast milk, protein, fats, and carbohydrates, vary across the usual range of American diets. Volume may vary in the extremes. In developing countries where there is widespread starvation and daily calorie intake is less than 1,600 kcal during prepregnancy and pregnancy in underweight breast-feeding mothers, milk volume and calorie density are minimally decreased (5 to 10 percent), if at all.[72] In a controlled experiment,[73] well-nourished European women reduced their calorie intake by 33 percent for 1 week. Milk volume was not reduced when the diet was maintained at greater than 1,500 kcal/day. If the daily energy intake was less than 1,500 kcal/day, milk volume was reduced 15 percent. Moderate dieting and weight loss postpartum (4.5 lb/mo) are not associated with changes in milk volume,[50] nor does aerobic exercise have any adverse effect.[74]

In the first year of life, the infant undergoes tremendous growth; infants double their birth weight in 180 days. Infants fed artificial breast milk lose up to 5 percent of their birthweight during the first week of life, while breast-milk-fed infants lose about 7 percent of their birthweight. A maximum weight loss of 10 percent of birthweight is tolerated in the first week of life in breast-fed infants. If this threshold is exceeded, the breast-feeding dyad needs immediate intervention by a trained health care provider. While supplementation with donor breast milk or artificial breast milk may be a necessary part of the intervention, the key focus of intervention is establishing good breast milk transfer by ensuring adequate production, correct nursing behavior, and adequate frequency. Once stage 3 of lactogenesis occurs, "the milk has come in"; the term breast-fed infant will gain about 1 oz/day with adequate milk transfer. By 14 days, the breast-fed infant should have returned to birthweight.

Food intake and energy needs are not constant. The infant's need for energy and/or fluids varies by day or week with growth spurts, greater activity, fighting illness, or greater fluid losses as in hot weather. Mammals have developed an extremely efficient mechanism to adjust milk supply within 24 to 48 hours depending on demand via oxytocin and the let-down reflex, and prolactin production. The prolactin and oxytocin travel to their target cells, prolactin to the alveolar epithelium in the breast, oxytocin to the myoepithelial cells that shroud the alveolar epithelium. The pituitary's prolactin and luteinizing hormone (LH) response to nursing frequency is depicted in Figure 5–3. In lactating women, baseline prolactin levels are 200 ng/ml at delivery, 75 ng/ml between 10 and 90 days postpartum, 50 ng/ml between 90 and 180 days postpartum, and 35 ng/ml after 180 days postpartum. Maternal serum prolactin levels rise by 80 to 150 percent of baseline levels within seconds of nipple stimulation. As long as nursing frequency is maintained at greater than eight times for 10 to 20 minutes with each episode in 24 hours, the serum prolactin levels will suppress the LH surges and ovarian function.[75]

Serum oxytocin levels also rise with nipple stimulation. However, the oxytocin response is much more affected by operant conditioning, and its response may precede the rise in prolactin levels. The maternal cerebrum is influenced by exposure to nursing cues as well as the influences of nipple stimulation. The cerebrum either stimulates or inhibits the hypothalamus to increase or decrease the production of prolactin inhibitory factor (dopamine) and, subsequently, the release of oxytocin from the posterior pituitary. Cerebral influences have a lesser effect on the release of prolactin. Positive sights, sounds, or smells related to nursing often stimulate the production of oxytocin, which, in turn, causes the myoepithelial cells to contact and milk to leak from the breasts. This observation is a good clinical clue indicating an uninhibited *let-down reflex*.

In a classic series of experiments, Newton and Egli[76] demonstrated the power of noxious influences to inhibit the release of oxytocin and to reduce milk transfer to the infant. The baseline milk production per feed was measured in controlled situations, about 160 g per feed. During a consecutive feed, a noxious event (i.e., saline injection) was administered during the feed. The amount of milk produced was cut in half, 80 to 100 g. Subsequently, the milk production was measured in a trial where a noxious event was administered and intranasal oxytocin was given concomitantly. The milk production was restored to almost 90 percent of baseline production, 130 to 140 g. A wide variety of noxious events were able to elicit the same decrease in milk production. The noxious events included placing the mother's feet in ice water, applying electric shocks to her toes, having her trace shapes while looking only through a mirror, or requiring her to proofread a document in a timed fashion. These observations have important implications concerning the management of breast-feeding. Pain, anxiety, and insecurity may be hidden reasons for breast-feeding failure through the inhibitions of the let-down reflex. In contrast, the playing of a soothing motivational/educational audiotape to women who were pumping milk for their premature infants has improved milk yields.[77] These observations have been confirmed by measuring the inhibition of oxytocin release by psychological stress.[78] The positive and negative influences of the cerebrum are further highlighted by the observation[79] that 75 percent of women who had a positive attitude during pregnancy were likely to be successful at breast-feeding. In contrast, 75 percent of women who had a negative attitude

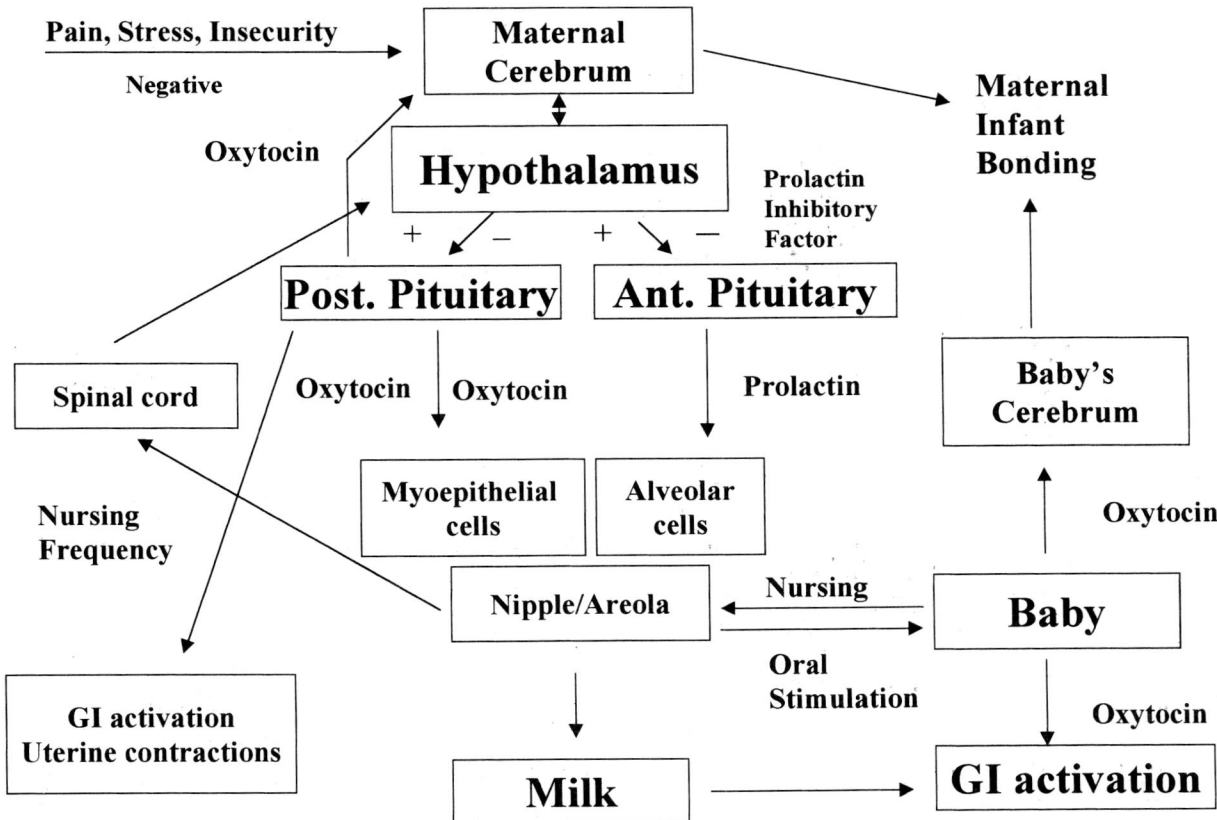

Figure 5–3. Ovarian function postpartum and during weaning. As nursing frequency falls, prolactin falls and ovarian function returns. (From Rolland R, DeJong FH, Schellekens LA, et al: The role of prolactin in the restoration of ovarian function during the early postpartum period in the human: a study during inhibition of lactation by bromergocryptine. Clin Endocrinol 4:23, 1975, with permission.)

during pregnancy had an unsuccessful breast-feeding experience.

Oxytocin has additional target cells in the mother. The effect of oxytocin on uterine activity is well known. Uterine involution is enhanced with breast-feeding. Animal and human research suggests that oxytocin is a neurohormone. Oxytocin is associated with an anti-fight/flight response in the autonomic nervous system, the mother tolerates stress better, and maternal–infant bonding is improved. In addition, gastrointestinal mobility and absorption are enhanced.[80,81]

In addition to the antistress effect, surges in oxytocin levels are associated with the release of gastrointestinal hormones and increased gastrointestinal motility.[80] In the mother, these actions enhance the absorption of substrates necessary for lactogenesis. In infants, there is a growing body of knowledge that indicates similar associations with oxytocin surges. Skin-to-skin contact and the oral stimulation of nursing stimulate a parasympathetic, anti-fight/flight response in the infant. Kangaroo care of premature newborns (skin-to-skin contact) is associated with a physiologically stable state,

improved stress responses, and improved weight gain.[80,81] Oxytocin appears to mediate this response.[82] Breast-feeding is associated with far more skin-to-skin contact and maternal behaviors than bottle-feeding.

While the central nervous system locus for imprinting is unknown, imprinting immediately after birth is an important predictor of breast-feeding success. The survival of lambs depends on nursing within an hour after birth. If the lamb has not nursed during the critical period, maternal–infant bonding becomes dysfunctional and the lamb suffers failure to thrive. In humans, the consequences are not nearly as drastic. Several trials with random assignment of subjects to early nursing (delivery room) or late nursing (2 hours after birth) demonstrated a 50 to 100 percent increase in the number of mothers who are breast-feeding at 2 to 4 months postpartum who nursed in the delivery room.[83] One of the keys to obstetric management is have the mother nurse her newborn in the delivery room.

Milk transfer to the infant is a key physiologic principle in lactation. The initial step of this process is good latch-on. With light tactile stimulation of the cheek and lateral angle of the mouth, the infant reflexively turns its head and opens its mouth, as in a yawn (Fig. 5–4). The nipple is tilted slightly downward using a "C-hold", or *palmar grasp*. In this hand position, the fingers support the breast from underneath and the thumb lightly grasps the upper surface 1 to 2 cm above the areola-breast line. The infant is brought firmly to the breast by the supporting arms while being careful to not push the back of the baby's head. The nipple and areola are drawn into the mouth as far as the areola-breast line (Figs. 5–5 and 5–6). The posterior areola may be less visible than the anterior areola, and the lower lip of the infant is often curled out. The infant's lower gum lightly fixes the teat over the lactiferous sinuses. A slight negative pressure exerted by the oropharynx and mouth holds the length of the teat and breast in place and reduces the "work" to refill the lactiferous sinuses after they are drained. The milk is extracted, not by negative pressure, but by a peristaltic action from the tip of the tongue to the base. There is no stroking, friction, or in-and-out motion of the teat; it is more of an undulating action. The buccal mucosa and tongue mold around the teat, leaving no space.

The peristaltic movement of the infant's tongue is most frequent in the first 3 minutes of a nursing epi-

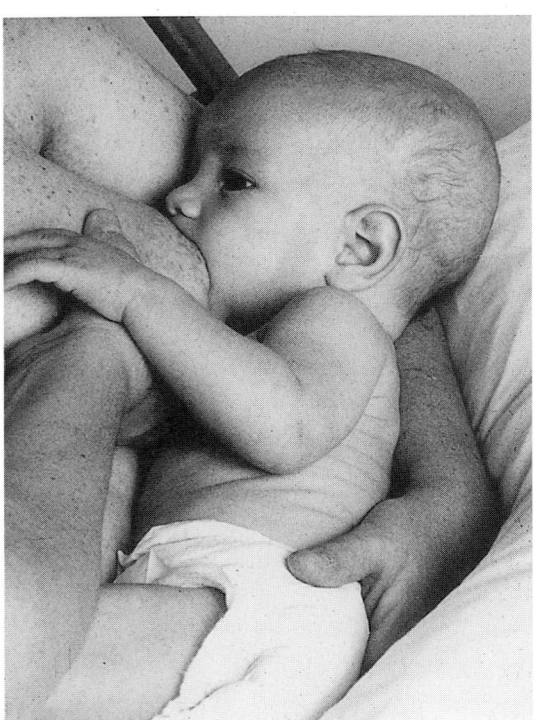

Figure 5–5. Appropriate latch-on.

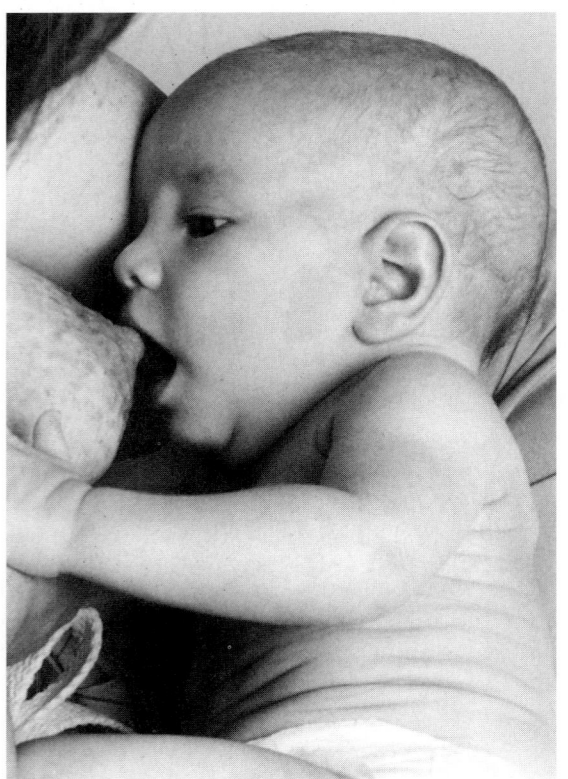

Figure 5–4. The latch-on reflex.

sode; the mean latency from latch-on to milk ejection is 2.2 minutes. After milk flow is established, the frequency of sucking falls to a much slower rate.[84] The change in cadence is recognizable as "suck-suck-swallow-breath." Audible swallowing of milk is a good sign of milk transfer. At the start of a feed the infant obtains 0.10 to 0.20 ml per suck. As the infant learns how to suck and as he matures he becomes more efficient at obtaining more milk in a shorter period of time. Eighty to 90 percent of the milk is obtained in the first 5 minutes the infant nurses on each breast, but the fat-rich and calorie-dense hind milk is obtained in the remainder of the time sucking at each breast, usually less than 20 minutes total.[85,86] A bottle-feeding infant sucks steadily in a linear fashion, receiving about 80 percent of the artificial breast milk in the first 10 minutes.

Sucking on a bottle is mechanically very different than nursing on the human teat (Fig. 5–7). The relatively inflexible artificial nipple resists the milking motion of the infant's tongue and mouth. The diameter of the artificial nipple expands during a suck, whereas the human teat collapses during the milk flow. The infant who is sucking on a bottle learns to generate strong negative pressures (> 100 mm Hg) in order to suck the milk out of the bottle. Since rapid flow from the bottle can gag the infant, he or she quickly learns to use the tongue to regulate the flow. When the infant who has learned to bottle-feed is put to the breast, the stopper

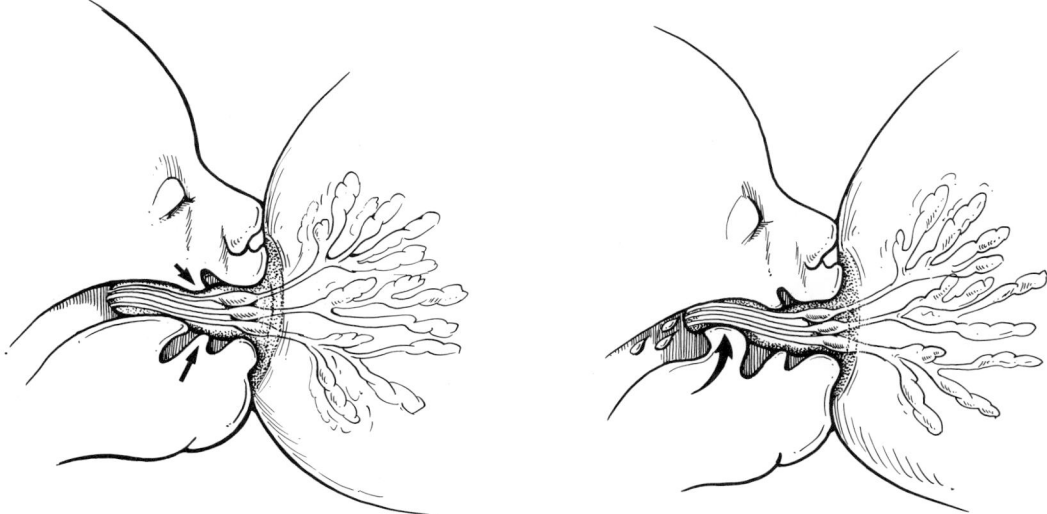

Figure 5–6. The mechanics of nursing.

function of the tongue may abrade the tip of the nipple and force the nipple out of the infant's mouth. The efficiency of milk transfer falls drastically and the hungry infant becomes frustrated and angry. A similar rejection may occur at 4 to 8 weeks when the exclusively breast-feeding infant is given a bottle in preparation for the mother's return to work.

Milk transfer is made more efficient by proper positioning of the infant to the breast. Proper positioning places the infant and mother chest-to-chest. The infant's ear, shoulder, and hip are in line. The three most common maternal positions are cross arm chest-to-chest, side-lying, or the football hold (Figs. 5–5, 5–8, 5–9). Each has their advantages. Rotating positions of nursing allows improved drainage of different lobules, an observation important in the management of a "plugged" duct. Maternal comfort and conven-

ience are the major reasons for changing nursing positions; the football hold position and the side-lying position are more comfortable if there is an abdominal incision

Baseline prolactin levels appear to be the major determinant of the hormonal state during lactation, a state of high-prolactin, low-estrogen, and low-progesterone levels. As the frequency of nursing decreases below eight in 24 hours, the baseline prolactin levels drop to below a level where ovulation is suppressed (35 to 50 ng/ml), LH levels rise, and menstrual cycling is initiated.[74,85,87] The intensity (adjusted odds ratio [OR]) of factors that initiate the onset of menses are the dura-

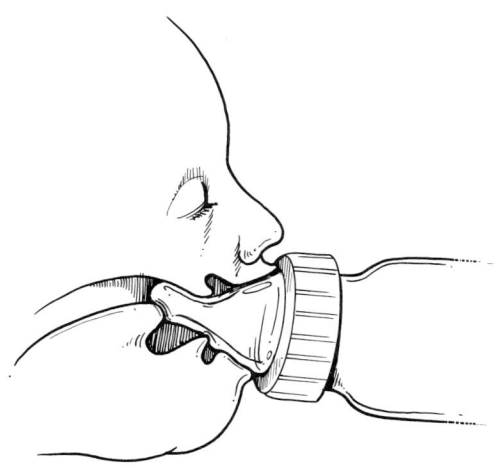

Figure 5–7. The mechanics of bottle-feeding.

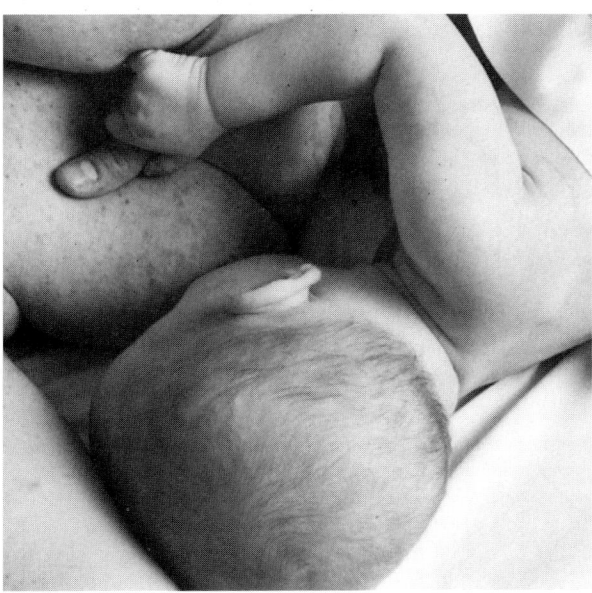

Figure 5–8. Side-lying nursing.

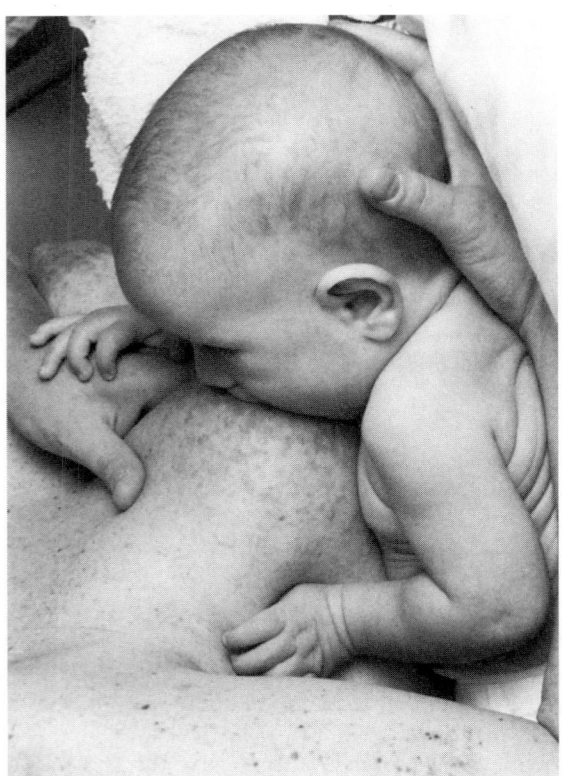

Figure 5–9. The football hold.

tion of sucking episodes less than 7 minutes (OR 2.4), night feeds less than four per 24 hours (OR 2.3), maternal age 15 to 24 years (OR 2.1), maternal age 25 to 34 years (OR 1.7), and day feeds less than seven per 24 hours (OR 1.6).[88] Serum prolactin levels in women who feed their infants artificial breast milk exclusively drop to prepregnant levels (8 to 14 ng/ml) within days. The total number of nursing episodes per day (more than eight per 24 hours) and night nursings are critical to the successful management of breast-feeding.

One of the major determinants of nursing frequency is the introduction of substitute nutriment sources for the infant, artificial breast milk or solids. Breast milk has the nutritional content to satisfy the growth needs of the infant for at least 6 months postpartum. In the first 6 months, feeding with artificial breast milk affects the physiology of successful lactation in three ways. Substitution with artificial breast milk reduces proportionally the nutriment requirements from breast milk, increases the gastric emptying time (slower digestion than breast milk) with a subsequent decrease in frequency of nursing episodes, and reduces the efficiency of nursing by the use of an opposing sucking technique on the artificial nipple. As depicted in Figure 5–3, prolactin falls and menses resumes.

Solid food (e.g., eggs, cereals, pureed food) have a

similar effect on the hormonal milieu of the lactating woman. One of the errors in Western child care is the early, forced introduction of solids. In most cases, the infant's gut is filled with slowly digesting food with less nutritional quality than either artificial breast milk or breast milk. The long-term result may be childhood and adolescent obesity. The most logical time to start solid food substitution is when the infant has reached the neurologic maturity to grasp and bring food to its mouth from his or her mother's plate. The required neurologic maturity to perform this behavior usually occurs at about 6 months. As the infant matures, his or her ability to feed improves and the proportion of the diet supplied by solid food gradually increases.

The failure to develop good milk transfer is the major cause of lactational failure and breast pain, especially in the neonatal period. Inhibition of the let-down reflex and failure to empty the breasts completely leads to ductal distention and parenchymal swelling (engorgement). Engorgement compromises the mechanics of nursing (Fig. 5–10) and alveolar distention reduces secretion of milk by the alveolar cells. Without adequate transfer of milk to the infant, lactation is doomed to fail. Distention of the alveoli by retained milk causes a rapid (6 to 12 hours) decrease in milk secretion and enzyme activity by the alveolar epithelium. The decreased production of milk is explained by pressure inhibition and by an inhibitor that is secreted in breast milk.[63–66] Distention of the alveoli inhibits secretion di-

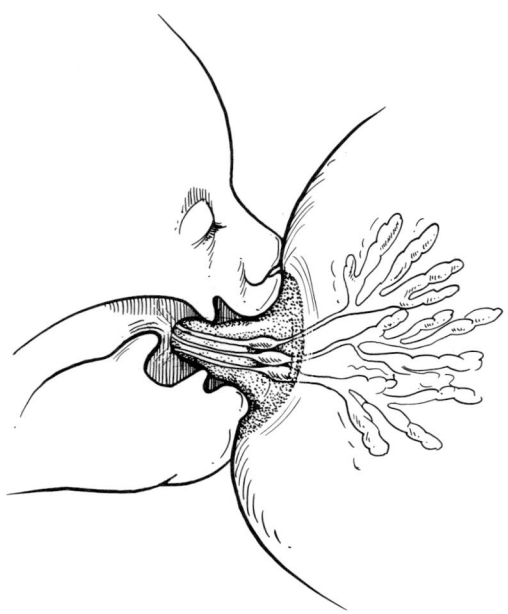

Figure 5–10. Breast-feeding and engorgement. The firm swollen breast parenchyma pushes the newborn's face away and she is unable to pull the teat into her mouth. Her tongue abrades the tip of the nipple.

rectly rather than indirectly by a decrease in nutriment or hormonal access.

BREAST MILK: THE GOLD STANDARD

One of the most common misperceptions by physicians and the lay public is that modern formulas for artificial breast milk are equivalent to breast milk. Human breast milk is uniquely suited to our biologic needs and remains the best source of nutrition for the human infant. It has a composition very different than that of bovine milk or soybean plants from which artificial breast milk is produced.

In contrast with most other animals, the human secretory immune system is not completely functional at birth. While the passive transplacental transfer of maternal IgG starts at 20 weeks, fetal levels do not approach maternal levels until term. By 3 months of age, the infant must rely on its own secretory response. The newborn's IgM and IgA responses are naive and incomplete. For example, in the presence of active antigen-positive cytomegalovirus infection at birth, 20 percent of infants will be IgM negative. A newborn's cellular response is likewise immature; functional impairment is evident for months after birth. Breast milk provides necessary support for the developing immune system.[89,90] The powerful anti-infective qualities of breast milk are measured by decreased infant mortality in developing countries, where exclusive breast-feeding is the norm. In first-world countries, the anti-infective benefits of exclusive breast-feeding are measured by decreased morbidity[35] and fewer hospitalizations.[48]

The composition of mature human milk is very different than artificial breast milk or "formula." Most artificial breast milk products use bovine milk as a substrate. Minerals, vitamins, protein, carbohydrates, and fats are added to pasteurized bovine milk for perceived nutritional needs as well as marketing needs in order to make a product that will successfully compete with human breast milk. Human breast milk appears "thinner" than bovine milk. Artificial breast milk manufacturers add constituents to make artificial breast milk appear rich and creamy. Fats such as palm or coconut oil are useful in producing a thick, creamy appearance.

Extensive research describes the unique composition of human milk. The infant formula industry has produced even greater volumes of data concerning their attempts to exactly reproduce human milk. The complete review of the composition of human milk requires the reading of textbooks and chapters specific to human milk, a challenge that is well beyond the scope of this chapter. In 1980, the U.S. Congress passed the Infant Formula Act (with revisions in 1985) as the result of severe health consequences when artificial breast milk failed to include key vitamins and minerals in new formula compositions.[91] This law now requires that all formulas for artificial breast milk contain minimum amounts of essential nutriments, vitamins, and minerals. Although life-threatening omissions are unlikely, current formulas for artificial breast milk have major differences in the total quantities and qualities of proteins, carbohydrates, and fats when compared to human milk.[92–96]

The nutritional differences between artificial breast milk and human milk are reflected in differences in the growth patterns of infants who are exclusively breast-fed for 4 to 6 months and infants who are fed artificial breast milk.[97] In general, breast-fed infants have faster linear and head growth, whereas artificial breast milk–fed infants tend to have greater weight gain and fat deposition. The greater deposition in fat may relate in part to the earlier introduction of solid foods in the infant fed artificial breast milk, a factor that has not been adequately controlled in current studies. Regardless of the cause, greater fat deposition in infants fed artificial breast milk has important adverse effects on the child and the future health of the society. Infant feeding using artificial breast milk is associated with a higher incidence of adolescent obesity,[30,36] which predicts significant increases in adult morbidity such as obesity, type II (insulin-resistant) diabetes, coronary heart disease, and hypertension.[98]

At birth, the fetus enters an unsterile world with an immature immune system. Full development of the immune system may take up to 6 years. Breast milk has a wide array of anti-infective properties that will support the developing immune system.[89,90] The major mechanisms for the protective properties of breast milk include active leukocytes, antibodies, antibacterial products, and competitive inhibition. Active leukocytes[99] are completely eliminated by pasteurization or freezing. Breast milk contains 4,000 cells/mm^3: 90 percent macrophages, 5 percent T-cell lymphocytes, 3 percent B-cell lymphocytes, and 2 percent plasma cells/neutrophils. The concentration of these cells is higher in the first week of breast-feeding. Later, the concentration decreases, but the change in the absolute number is not dramatic.

A critical event in host resistance is the recognition of pathogenic agents in the environment and the production of an antigen-specific response. Breast-feeding provides a unique system to help the infant fight infection with antigen-specific responses. The infant is at risk for infection by the same organism that is likely to infect the mother. Through breast milk, the neonate takes advantage of maternal recognition of these infectious agents. This important mechanism is depicted in Figure 5–11 and reviewed by Slade and Schwartz.[100] An antigen or infectious agent (virus, bacteria, fungus, and protozoa) stimulates the activity of leukocytes in the gastrointestinal or respiratory tract of the mother. Lymphocytes, which are encoded with the antigen signature, travel to the nearest lymph node and stimulate lymphoblasts to develop cytotoxic T cells, helper T cells, and plasma cells programmed to destroy the initiating antigen through phagocytosis or complement/immunoglobulins produced by the B cells. The response is amplified by the migration of committed helper lymphocytes to other sites of white blood cell production, the spleen and bone marrow, where they stimulate the production of antigen-specific committed white blood cells. Some of the committed, antigen-specific helper lymphocytes travel to the mucosa of the breast in the lactating mother. They may migrate into the breast milk (macrophages) or may produce immunoglobulin (lymphocytes or plasma cells). Both are uniquely programmed to fight the specific infectious agent challenging the mother.

Immunoglobulins are a unique component to breast milk and absent in artificial breast milk.[89,90] Immunoglobulins constitute a sizable portion of protein content of early milk (colostrum) for the first 2 to 4 days. In serum, the concentration of monomeric IgA is one fifth the concentration of IgG. In breast milk, the ratio is reversed. During the first day of lactation, the concentrations of immunoglobulins are IgA, 600 mg/dl; IgM, 125 mg/dl; and IgG, 80mg/dl. By day 4, the concentration, but not absolute amount, has fallen to a steady level; IgA, 80 mg/dl; IgM, 30 mg/dl; and IgG, 16 mg/dl. Other immunoglobulin classes are found in small amounts, but their function is not well understood. In contrast to monomeric serum IgA, the secretory immunoglobulin A (sIgA) in breast milk is dimeric or polymeric. Polymerization improves transport across the mucous membrane into the breast milk. The sIgA is produced locally by plasma cells. Plasma cells, which produce sIgA, constitute 50 to 80 percent of the leukocytes in the breast submucosa.

The immunoglobulins in breast milk appear to be fully functional. Secretory immunoglobulin A does not activate complement or promote opsonic complement subfragments. As a consequence, sIgA is not bactericidal. It appears that sIgA blocks the mucosal receptors (adhesins) on the infectious agent. The virulence of pathogens is related to their ability to use adhesins capable of interacting with complementary epithelial cell-surface receptors. When the antigen-specific sIgA attaches, the pathogen is effectively neutralized.

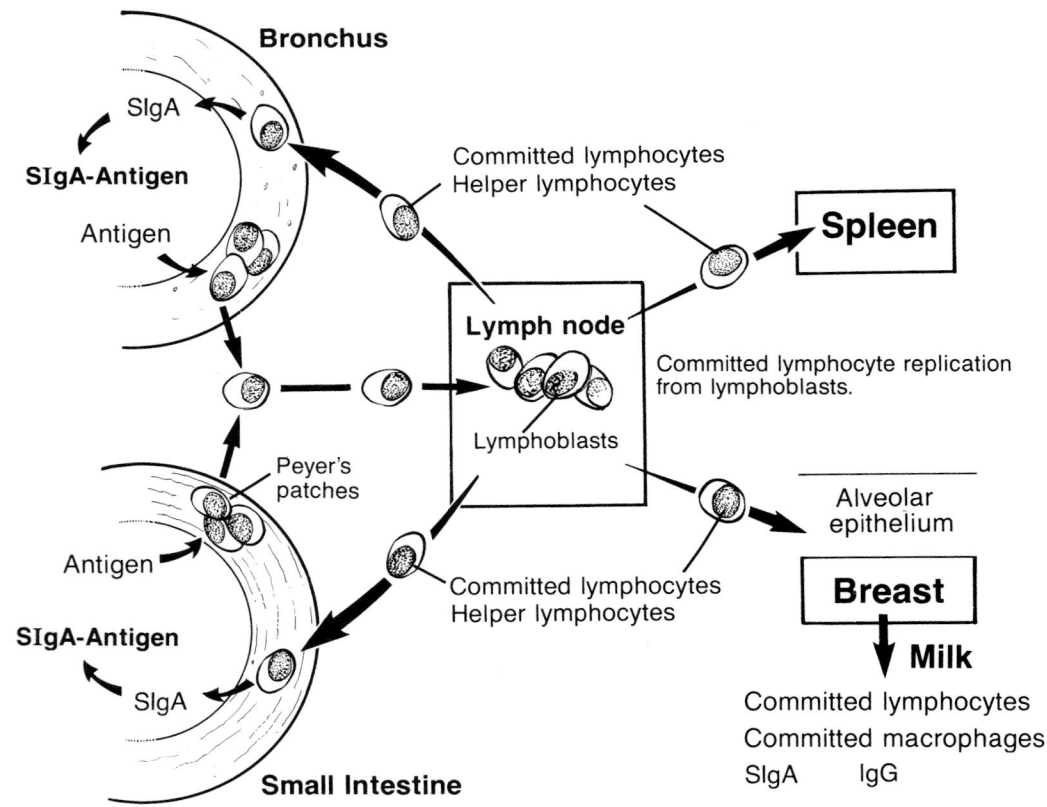

Figure 5–11. The immunology of the breast.

Certain vitamins and minerals are essential for the growth of pathogenic bacteria. A major mechanism by which breast milk protects the infant is the competition for "essential" nutriments for pathogenic bacteria. Iron and vitamin B_{12} are two essential nutriments for pathogenic bacteria that have been studied relative to breast milk. Breast milk contains lactoferrin, an iron-binding glycoprotein, in large quantities, 5.5 mg/ml in the colostrum to 1.5 mg/ml in mature milk, and is absent in artificial breast milk. The free iron form of lactoferrin competes with siderophilic bacteria for ferric iron,[101,102] and thus disrupts the proliferation of these organisms. The binding of iron to lactoferrin also enhances iron absorption; less iron is required in breast milk in order to satisfy the iron needs of the infant. The antibacterial role of lactoferrin is more complex than simple competition for ferric iron.[101] Lactoferrin causes a release of lipopolysaccharide molecules from the bacterial cell wall. This appears to sensitize the cell wall to attack by lysozyme. Lactoferrin and lysozyme work together to destroy the pathogenic organisms.

In summary, breast milk is uniquely composed to satisfy the biologic needs of the human infant. In particular, the uniquely human need for brain development and immune system support are provided by breast milk and not by artificial breast milk. Many of the documented benefits of breast-feeding are directly related to the unique composition of breast milk and the failure of artificial breast milk to replicate human milk.

THE ROLE OF THE OBSTETRICIAN

The obstetrician plays the primary role in the initiation of breast-feeding and is largely responsible for which women go home from their postpartum hospitalization breast-feeding. From then on, the obstetrician/gynecologist performs a critical supporting role to the pediatrician in the maintenance of breast-feeding. He or she provides the medical support for breast-specific problems or issues relative to maternal health, as pediatricians are uncomfortable with the examination of the adult breast and accepting the mother as their patient.

The obstetrician/gynecologist amplifies support for breast-feeding by community advocacy, office environment, and personal choices. The office environment needs to be "breast-feeding friendly." Visible, active support of breast-feeding includes the presence of breast-feeding mothers, patient educational programs on breast-feeding, a quiet area for nursing mothers, the absence of material supplied by formula companies, and visible support for office personnel who choose to breast-feed. The physician, especially the bright, young female obstetrician/gynecologist, is a powerful role model for patients. Women will ask the female gynecologist whether and how long she breast-fed her children. Her answers will have a powerful influence.

The support of the obstetrician continues at the first prenatal visit and continues through the mother's total breast-feeding experience. At the first prenatal visit, the method of infant feeding is identified, her choice to breast-feed is verbally reinforced, gaps in her knowledge are identified, and an educational plan is recommended. The educational plan may include reference reading, specific classes on breast-feeding, identification of a "breast-feeding–friendly pediatrician," and introduction to community resources, such as support groups (La Leche League International). At the initial physical examination the breasts are examined for anatomic abnormalities that might influence the success of breast-feeding, such as hypoplasia, nipple inversion and surgical scars.

At the 36-week visit, the obstetrician readdresses the mother's choice and knowledge regarding breast-feeding. Simple concepts of breast-feeding physiology are reinforced: early feeds, frequent feeds (>10 per day), reinforcing environment, and no supplementation unless directed by a pediatrician. The obstetrician reinforces the appropriate way to latch the baby to the breast and ensures that the increase in her breast size reflects the hormonal readiness for breast-feeding. The patient is warned of hospital policies and attitudes that interfere with breast-feeding success. The 36-week visit is a good time to address the appropriateness of medications and breast-feeding.

At delivery and during the postpartum hospitalization, the obstetrician is the champion for the application of breast-feeding physiology; early to the breast (<1 hour) after birth, frequent feeds (>10 per day), appropriate nursing behavior (latch-on), continuous mother–infant contact (rooming-in), and no infant supplementation unless directed by the infant's physician. As an advocate for breast-feeding the obstetrician must be willing to confront administrative and nursing protocols that are designed for control and efficiency rather than optimal care for the breast-feeding dyad.

National and international health organizations have long recognized the challenges and barriers that modern medical care and hospitals raise against successful breast-feeding. In 1989 the World Health Organization initiated the Baby Friendly Hospital initiative. The ten steps by which a hospital might be designated "baby friendly" are outlined in the highlighted box. The United States is the only developed country not to fully endorse the initiative, primarily as a result of the influence on congress by the powerful formula company lobby. As of the year 2000, less than 40 of the more than 1,500 hospitals worldwide who have been desig-

Ten Steps to Successful Breast-Feeding

1. Have a written policy to support breast-feeding.
2. Train all health care providers.
3. Inform all pregnant women about the benefits of management of breast-feeding.
4. Initiate breast-feeding within 1-hour after birth.
5. Show mothers how to breast-feed and maintain lactation even if they are separated from their infants.
6. Give newborn infants no food or drink other than breast milk, unless medically indicated.
7. Allow mothers and infants to remain together 24 hours a day (i.e., rooming in).
8. Encourage breast-feeding on demand.
9. Give no artificial teats or pacifiers.
10. Foster the establishment of breast-feeding support groups and refer mothers to them on discharge from the hospital or clinic.

Adapted from WHO/UNICEF: Protesting, Promoting, and Supporting Breastfeeding: The Special Role of Maternity Services, A Joint WHO/UNICEF Statement. Geneva, World Health Organization, 1989.

nated baby friendly are in the United States. The biggest challenge to hospitals in the United States in becoming baby friendly is the forebearance of artificial breast milk donations and direct in-hospital marketing by the artificial breast milk companies. The obstetrician has a role in supporting the baby-friendly initiative.

After postpartum discharge, the obstetrician is primarily focused on maternal concerns about breast-feeding: maternal diet, breast symptoms and signs, hormonal function postpartum, contraception, maternal medications, and as a breast-feeding advocate when the mother is referred to other specialists. A secondary but equally important focus is the growth and development of the infant. Traditionally, the obstetrician sees the mother at 4 to 6 weeks postpartum, but often the obstetrician and the mother communicate before that visit. By inquiring about the growth and feeding of her infant, the obstetrician provides an important reinforcement of the mother's decision to breast-feed and an important screen for the pediatrician regarding the growth and feeding of the infant. The obstetrician can identify critical or developing problems regarding infant growth and feeding for the pediatrician. The obstetrician must know the indicators of adequate infant growth and clinical indicators that milk is being pro-

duced and transferred. When the obstetrician remains a verbal participant in the mother's breast-feeding experience at the 4- to 6-week postpartum visit, the likelihood that the mother will continue to breast-feed at 16 weeks is almost doubled.[103]

SUCCESSFUL MANAGEMENT OF BREAST-FEEDING

The successful management of breast-feeding requires the active cooperation of the mother, her support group, the obstetric care provider, and infant care provider. In our current culture, a lactation consultant often becomes an active participant in the care of the breast-feeding dyad. There are numerous reliable reference texts for additional information. They include *Breast-feeding: a Guide For The Medical Profession*,[104] *The Breastfeeding Answer Book*,[105] *The Womanly Art of Breastfeeding*,[106] *Drugs In Pregnancy and Lactation*,[107] and *Medication and Mother's Milk*.[108]

ANATOMIC ABNORMALITIES OF THE BREAST

The relationship between breast anatomy and lactation should be addressed during the well-woman or family planning visits in women who anticipate future pregnancy. During pregnancy, infant feeding becomes a major focus, and the woman needs this issue addressed, as often there are hidden questions and concerns regarding her adequacy to breast-feed. The breast examination at the first prenatal visit is an excellent opportunity to address infant feeding concerns and myths relative to her breast anatomy. Self-doubt concerning the size or shape of the breasts should be addressed, and the patient should be reassured that less than 5 percent of lactational failures are caused by faulty anatomy.

Congenital abnormalities of the breasts (excluding inverted nipples) are rare, less than 1 in 1,000 women. The most significant defect is glandular hypoplasia. These women have no development or abnormal development of one or both breasts during sexual maturation. Women with no development of the breasts often have normally shaped and sized nipples and areolas, and they may have sought consultation from a plastic surgeon. One manifestation of abnormal development is referred to as the *tubular breast*. The nipple and areola, which are often normal in size, shape, and appearance, are attached to a tube of fibrous cords. Whatever the shape or size of the breasts in a nonpregnant woman, the final evaluation of adequate glandular tissue must await the expected growth during pregnancy. The size of the average breast will grow from 200 g to 600 g during pregnancy; most women will easily recognize this growth. A routine screening question at the 36-week prenatal visit should be, "Have your breasts grown during pregnancy?" If the response is negative in a woman with unusually small or abnormally shaped breasts, lactational failure is a possibility and prenatal consultation with a lactation expert is recommended. Unilateral abnormalities are usually not a problem except for increased asymmetry, as the normal breast can usually produce more than enough milk for the infant. The texture of the breast and tethering of the nipple are also assessed. An inelastic breast gives the impression that the skin is fixed to dense underlying tissue, whereas the elastic breast allows elevation of the skin and subcutaneous tissue from the parenchyma. Lack of elasticity may complicate nursing because of increased rigidity with engorgement. Massage of the periareolar tissue four times a day for 10 minutes is recommended. Engorgement should be assiduously avoided in the postpartum period by early, frequent nursing.

Congenital tethering of the nipple to underlying fascia is diagnosed by squeezing the outer edge of the areola (Fig. 5–12); normally, the nipple will protrude. Severe tethering is manifested by an inverted nipple. The most severe forms of tethering occur in less than 1 percent of women. While successful breast-feeding is possible in these severe cases, prenatal consultation and close follow-up are very important to identify and treat poor milk transfers. Flat or inverted nipples are much less likely to preclude successful breast-feeding. Three prenatal methods of treating tethered nipples have been described: nipple pulling, Hoffman's exercises, and nipple cups (shells). A recent controlled trial failed to demonstrate efficacy[109] of either shells or Hoffman's exercises and recommended that these should be abandoned.

In the early neonatal period, a breast pump may be of help in women with flat or inverted nipples. The breast is gently pumped at low settings until the teat is drawn out. The infant is immediately offered that breast. The same procedure is performed on the other side. Usually this is only required for a few days. If it is required for more than a few days, a relatively cheap alternative can be created from a 10- or 20-ml plastic syringe, the sizes depending on the size of the nipple.[110] The end of the syringe where the needle attaches is removed and the plunger is reversed. The nipple is placed in the smooth, plunger end of the syringe and gentle traction is applied until the nipple everts. While pumping and syringe suction are practical solutions, no controlled trials have supported their efficacy.

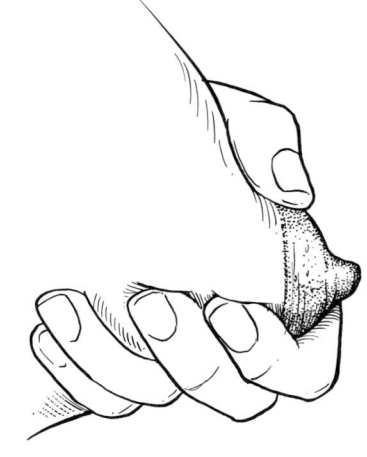

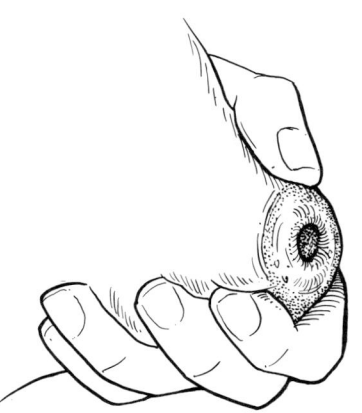

Figure 5–12. Assessment of nipple tethering.

Modern clothing (especially protective brassieres) prevents friction that toughens the skin and helps protect the nipple from cracking during early lactation. In the second half of pregnancy, nipple skin may be toughened by wearing a nursing brassiere with the flaps open. However, washing with harsh soaps; buffing the nipple with a towel; and using alcohol, benzoin, or other drying agents are not helpful and may increase the incidence of cracking. Normally, the breast is washed with clean water and should be left to air-dry. A cautiously used sunlamp or hair dryer may facilitate drying. Trials involving application of breast cream or expression of colostrum have not shown a reduction in nipple trauma or sensitivity, when compared to those with untreated nipples.

Previous breast surgery may have significant adverse effects on breast-feeding success. The major issues are loss of sensation in the nipple or areola by nerve injury or compromise of the lactiferous ducts. Women who have had breast surgery, breast biopsy, chest surgery, or augmentation, have a threefold higher incidence of unsuccessful breast-feeding.[58] Circumareolar skin incisions, which are used for cosmetic considerations in breast biopsies or breast augmentation, may compromise both the nerve and ducts. Breast augmentation has significant potential to disrupt breast-feeding.[111] In a carefully studied, prospective series, 27 of 42 (64 percent) of women who exclusively breast-fed after preconceptional breast augmentation had insufficient lactation, and the infant growth rate was less than 20 g/day. Circumareolar incision was the dominant predictor. One half of women with a submammary or axillary incision had insufficient lactation, whereas all 11 women after a circumareolar incision for breast augmentation had lactation failure. Compromise of the lactiferous ducts and loss of nipple sensation contribute to lactational insufficiency. Loss of nipple sensation occurs in one third to one half of patients after circumareolar incision. Circumareolar incisions between the 7 and 2 o'clock positions may reduce the loss of nipple sensation, but the effect of this maneuver on lactation insufficiency has not been studied. If the woman has had a silicone implant, she can be reassured that there is no evidence that breast-feeding places her infant at risk. The concentration of silicone in artificial formula or cow's milk is 5 to 10 times higher than in breast milk from women who have silicone implants.[112] Large epidemiologic studies of infants who have nursed from breasts with silicone implants have not shown excess adverse events.[113]

Reduction mammoplasty is always associated with lactation insufficiency if exclusive breast-feeding is relied upon for infant nutrition. If the reduction involves the removal of greater than 500 g per breast or the procedure uses the free nipple graph technique, the production of a nominal amount of breast milk is rare. If the nipple and areola are relocated on a pedicle of vascular tissue and ducts, partial breast-feeding is a small possibility. In any case of reconstructive surgery on the breast, augmentation or reduction, the breast-feeding dyad is considered at high risk for lactation failure. Prenatal referral to an expert on lactation is appropriate.

LABOR AND DELIVERY MANAGEMENT

Approximately 15 percent of women who state they wish to breast-feed at the onset of term labor are discharged either completely feeding their infant artificial breast milk or giving the majority of the infant's feeds as artificial breast milk. A combination of obstetric management, hospital policies, and pediatric management contribute to this attrition. Obstetric interventions are often critical for the health of the mother or infant, but they may affect the success of lactation. Few if any interventions directly inhibit the physiology of lactation. Most obstetric interventions reduce the success of lactation by indirect interference with physiology. Induction of labor is not associated with lactation failure, but a long, tiring induction and labor will reduce the likelihood that the mother will get appropriate amounts of infant contact in the delivery room and in the first 24 hours after birth. Cesarean delivery reduces the incidence of breast-feeding by 10 to 20 percent in the first week after birth. After most cesarean sections, the infant is not put to the breast immediately after birth nor will the mother breast-feed her infant more than eight times in the first 24 hours. Well-meaning nurses become concerned for the baby's nutrition and artificial breast milk is given to the infant until the mother "recovers." Labor analgesia (i.e., meperidine and promethazine) has long been associated with poor breast-feeding success. Intrapartum narcotics appear to adversely affect the infant's ability to nurse effectively.[82,114-116] Epidural anesthesia with local anesthetic agents seems to be better for breast-feeding than parenteral narcotics. Epidural anesthesia with local anesthetics does not appear to have a major effect. The effect of epidural or intrathecal narcotics on sucking behavior and/or lactation success has not been studied. The presence of a doula, or a labor companion other than family, appears to be an effective method to reduce the need for epidural anesthesia and operative deliveries.[117,118] An added benefit is earlier initiation and longer duration of breast-feeding.[118] Postsurgical pain control is best achieved with morphine rather than meperidine, which adversely affects neonatal behavior.[119] Obstetric and pediatric protocols can be very effective in separating mother and baby. Several prominent examples include magnesium sulfate therapy for preeclampsia, a positive maternal group B streptococcus culture, maternal fever work-up, and diabetes mellitus/hypoglycemia protocols. All of these medical interventions produce major barriers to delivery room nursing and an adequate frequency of nursing in the first 24 to 48 hours.

The peripartum period is critical for achieving successful lactation. The obstetrician must apply the five basic principles of lactation physiology: early imprinting, frequent nursing, good latch-on, a confident and comfortable mother, and no supplementation unless medically indicated. Nursing should be initiated within 30 minutes after birth, preferably in the delivery room.[83,114] Contraindications include (1) a heavily medicated mother; (2) an infant with a 5-minute Apgar test result less than 6; or (3) a premature infant at less than 36 weeks' gestation.

The instructor should pay special attention to the mother's position during the first feeding; she should be in a related, comfortable position. With skin-to-skin contact, the infant is presented to the breast with his ventral surface to the mother's ventral surface. A dry neonate, skin-to-skin contact, and supplemental radiant heating will prevent neonatal cold stress. Routine eye treatment should be delayed, as it may disrupt the important family bonding process.

In the recovery room and on the ward, the best place for the neonate is with the mother. This maximizes mother–infant bonding and allows "on-demand" feeding every 1 to 2 hours. Rooming-in allows the mother to participate in the care of her baby and gives her an opportunity to ask questions. The mother should be encouraged to sleep when the neonate sleeps. Since the hospital runs on an adult diurnal pattern, the patient should be discharged early in order to get her rest.

The frequency of early feeding is proportional to milk production and weight gain in neonates.[85,120–122] Therefore, supplementation with glucose or formula should be discouraged. Supplementation decreases milk production through a reduction in nursing frequency by satiation of the neonate and slower digestion of formula. Supplementation also undermines the mother's confidence about her lactational adequacy.[123–126] When obstetricians give information at the first prenatal visit about breast-feeding that was developed by makers of artificial breast milk, the duration of breast-feeding is significantly reduced when compared to packet information on breast-feeding developed by "breast-feeding–friendly" obstetricians and pediatricians. A randomized trial of giving or withholding free formula samples at the time of discharge demonstrated a significantly reduced incidence of breast-feeding at 1 month and an increased likelihood of solid food introduction by the mothers given the formula samples.[123] This was most significant in high-risk groups: those less educated, primiparas, and those reporting illness since leaving the hospital.

Other factors influencing the success of lactation are improper positioning and nursing technique, which can lead to increased nipple trauma and incomplete emptying. In the early postpartum period, nursing technique should be evaluated in three areas: presentation and latching-on, maternal–infant positioning, and breaking of the suction. The infant should not have to turn its head to nurse. A ventral surface–to–ventral surface presentation is necessary. When latching-on to the nipple, the neonate should take as much of the areola as possible into its mouth. This is facilitated by gently stimulating the baby's cheek to elicit a yawn-like opening of its mouth and rapid placement of the breast into it. A supporting hand on the breast helps; the C-hold involves four fingers cupping and supporting the weight of the breast, which is especially important in the weak or premature neonate whose lower jaw may be depressed by the weight of the breast. The thumb rests

above and 1 to 2 cm away from the areolar edge and points the nipple downward. Retraction by the thumb will pull the areola away from the mouth and cause an incorrect placement. Any position that is comfortable and convenient, while allowing the appropriate mouth-areola attachment, should be encouraged; the sitting position is the most common. In cesarean section patients in whom pressure on the abdomen is uncomfortable, a side-lying or football hold may be better. A rotation of positions is recommended to reduce focal pressure on the nipple and to ensure complete emptying. Removal of the nursing infant can be a problem; suction by the neonate can injure the nipple if it is not broken prior to disengagement. A finger inserted between the baby's lips and the breast will break the suction.

The single most difficult management issue is the control of routines and hospital attitudes detrimental to lactation. Winikoff et al.[127] studied in the early 1980s how feeding patterns were affected by routine procedures in a hospital. Policies that worked against the physiology of lactation included formula distribution and supplementation without a medical indication, constant questioning of the mother about breast-feeding, preprinted orders for lactation suppression medication, pediatric clearance prior to the first feeding, limited maternal access to the infant, and little educational material for new mothers or staff.

When providers are not well informed or are apathetic about lactation, success of lactation is unlikely. This theme underscores the role of the physician in educating patients, nursing staff, and support personnel about the physiology and benefits of lactation.

BREAST MASSES DURING LACTATION

Breast cancer is the most common cancer of the reproductive organs of the female. While the risk of breast cancer increases tremendously after the age of 40, 1 to 3 percent of all breast cancers occur during pregnancy and lactation. Breast cancer diagnosed during lactation may have its origin before or during pregnancy. As a result of this assumption and small numbers of pregnant or lactating women, most studies have lumped the populations together. Recently, researchers in Japan have analyzed breast cancer in age-matched control women (n = 192), women who were pregnant at diagnosis (n = 72), and women who were lactating at diagnosis (n = 120).[128] The prognosis for breast cancer that is diagnosed during pregnancy or lactation is poorer than for breast cancer diagnosed at other times. The 10-year survival for age-matched controls without lymph node metastasis was 93 percent; for women who were diagnosed during pregnancy or lactation the survival was 85 percent. When the lymph nodes are involved, the 10-year survival was 62 percent and 37 percent in controls and women who were diagnosed during pregnancy or lactation, respectively. The difference in survival is partially explained by a longer duration of symptoms prior to diagnosis (6.3 vs. 5.4 months), tumor size on palpation (4.6 vs. 3.0 cm), and tumor size on cut surface (4.3 vs. 2.6 cm), in lactating women versus control women, respectively. The delay in diagnosis and the greater size at diagnosis in lactating women is a failure of the obstetric care provider and/or the lactating woman to aggressively sample a breast mass.

The lactating woman is most likely to recognize a breast mass through her daily manipulations of her breasts. In her framework of reference, she usually considers this mass a "plugged duct." She should be encouraged to report a plugged duct that persists more than 2 weeks despite efforts to initiate drainage of that lobule. Her provider faces an expanded differential diagnosis. Fibromas and fibroadenomas are more common in young women. These solid tumors are rubbery, nodular, and mobile, and they may grow rapidly with the hormonal stimulation of pregnancy. The most common diagnosis is a dilated milk duct, a completely benign diagnosis.

A needle aspiration of the mass is the mainstay of diagnosis. Percutaneous fine-needle aspiration is performed in the same manner as in nonpregnant women. The use of local anesthetic is optional; infiltration of the area around a small lesion may increase the likelihood of a nondiagnostic aspiration. The area over the mass is swabbed with iodine or alcohol and, using sterile techniques, the lesion is fixed between the thumb and fingers of the nondominant hand. Using a 22-gauge needle attached to a 20-ml syringe, the center of the lesion is probed. Initial aspiration usually reveals the nature of the lesion. If milk or greenish fluid (fibrocystic disease) is found and the lesion disappears, no further diagnostic procedures need to be performed. If the tumor is solid or fails to disappear completely after aspiration, the needle is passed several times through the lesion under strong negative pressure. The aspirated tissue fluid is air-dried on a slide and sent for cytologic evaluation. The pathology requisition should note the age and lactating status. Fine-needle aspiration biopsy appears to have the same accuracy in pregnancy and lactation as in the nonpregnant, nonlactating woman. Gupta et al.[129] performed 214 fine-needle aspirations during pregnancy and lactation. Eight (13.7 percent) were cancer, and the sensitivity, specificity, and positive predictive value was 100, 81, and 61 percent, respectively.

Ultrasound is an expensive but accurate method of determining the cystic nature of a breast mass in lactating women. Mammography is more difficult to interpret during lactation. Young breasts are generally more dense, and the massive increase in functioning glands may obscure small cancers. However, the accuracy is still good if the films are interpreted by experienced radiologists. In general, mammography is a secondary diagnostic modality.

A core biopsy using ultrasound or radiographic guidance is a reasonable option to avoid a surgical procedure. If a surgical biopsy is required, the surgeon will usually need guidance regarding the management of lactation. Most breast biopsies can be performed under local anesthesia. If the mother nurses just before the procedure, she will empty the breast, which makes the surgery easier, and will allow 3 to 4 hours until the next feed. Local anesthetics are not absorbed orally and pose no risk to the infant. The mother should be allowed to nurse on schedule. Most anesthetics used for general anesthesia enter the breast milk in small amounts (1 to 3 percent) of the maternal dose, and minimal behavioral effects in infants have been observed. In most cases the mother can nurse within 4 hours of the anesthetic. The mother's breasts should be pumped 3 to 4 hours after the last feed regardless of the anesthetic status. She will begin to feel the discomfort of engorgement, and the fever of engorgement may confuse the postoperative picture as early as 8 or 10 hours. The failure to empty the breasts within 12 hours will begin to adversely affect milk supply.

Surgical biopsy usually has little effect on breast-feeding performance unless the procedure is done in the periareolar area or the nerves supplying the nipple are compromised. Circumareolar incisions are to be avoided if possible. Milk fistulas are an uncommon risk (5 percent) of central biopsy. The fistulas are usually self-limited and will spontaneously heal over several weeks. Prohibiting breast-feeding does not change the likelihood of ultimate healing.

MATERNAL NUTRITION

The efficiency of conversion of maternal foodstuff to milk is about 80 to 90 percent. If the average milk volume per day is 900 ml, and milk has an average energy content of 75 kcal/dl, the mother must consume an extra 794 kcal/day, unless stored energy is used. During pregnancy, most women store an extra 2 to 5 kg (19,000 to 48,000 kcal) in tissue, mainly as fat, in physiologic preparation for lactation. These calories and nutrients supplement the maternal diet during lactation. As a result, the required dietary increases are easily attainable in healthy mothers and infants.

In lactation, most vitamins and minerals should be increased 20 to 30 percent over nonpregnant requirements. Folic acid should be doubled. Calcium, phosphorus, and magnesium should be increased by 40 to 50 percent, especially in the teenager who is lactating. In practical terms, these needs can be supplied by the following additions to the diet: 2 cups of milk, 2 oz of meat or peanut butter, a slice of enriched or whole wheat bread, a citrus fruit, a salad, and an extra helping ($\frac{1}{2}$ to $\frac{3}{4}$ cup) of a dark green or yellow vegetable. The appropriate intake of vitamins can be ensured by continuing prenatal vitamins with 1 mg of folic acid through the lactation. The mother should drink at least 1 extra liter of fluid per day to make up for the fluid loss through milk.

Vegetarianism has become increasingly more common, and if this is the case, dietary deficiencies may include B vitamins (especially B_{12}), total protein, and the full complement of essential amino acids. The recommendation should be to take a good dietary history with the focus on protein, iron, calcium, and vitamins D and B; supplement with soy flour, molasses, or nuts; use complementary vegetable protein combinations; and avoid excess phytates and bran.

Many women are concerned about losing weight postpartum.[130,131] If 700 to 1,200 kcal are used daily to nourish an infant, a mother could lose weight by not increasing her caloric intake, but a thoughtful selection of food groups and the elimination of "empty calories" are necessary. A reduction of total calories (<25 kcal/kg) and total protein (<0.6 g/kg) may reduce the daily milk volume by 20 to 30 percent, but not the milk quality, unless the mother is more than 10 percent below her ideal body weight. Since dieting mobilizes fat stores that may contain environmental toxins, women with high exposure to such toxins should not lose weight during lactation.

BREAST AND NIPPLE PAIN

Breast or nipple pain is one of the most frequent complaints of lactating mothers. The frequency is related to failure in the initial management of lactation: late first feed, decreased frequency of feedings, poor nipple grasp, and/or poor positioning. The differential diagnosis of breast pain includes problems with latching-on, engorgement, nipple trauma, mastitis and, occasionally, the let-down reflex.

Symptoms assist with the differential diagnosis. One type of problem with latching-on is the anxious, vigorous infant who sucks strongly against empty ducts until the let-down occurs. The other is the nipple-confused infant who chews on the nipple and abrades the tip with his tongue. In these cases, the nipple and breast pain starts with latching-on and diminishes with let-down. Contact pain suggests nipple trauma and may persist as long as the nipple is manipulated. Engorgement causes a dull, generalized discomfort in the whole breast, worse just before a feed and relieved by it. Localized, unilateral, and continuous pain in the breast may be caused by mastitis. Occasionally, women describe the let-down reflex as painful; this occurs after the first minute of sucking and usually lasts only a minute or two as the ductal swelling is relieved by nursing.

A physical examination and observation of nursing technique can confirm the impression left by a good history. Through observation of a nursing episode, an infant's personality and nursing technique can be assessed. The whole of the nipple and much of the areola should be included in the infant's mouth. An examination of the nipple may reveal a fissure or blood blister. Bilateral breast firmness and tenderness may indicate engorgement. Engorgement may be peripheral, periareolar, or both. Mastitis is characterized by fever, malaise, localized erythema, heat, tenderness, and induration (see below).

Infection may be a co-factor associated with the pain of nipple injury. When the microbiology of the nipple/milk of 61 lactating women with nipple pain was compared to 64 lactating women without nipple pain and 31 nonlactating women, *Candida albicans* (19 percent) and *Staphylococcus aureus* (30 percent) were more common in women with pain and nipple fissures than in controls (3 to 5 percent).[132]

The management of breast pain consists of general as well as specific steps. Prevention is a key component. Appropriate nursing technique and positioning will prevent, or significantly decrease, the incidence of nipple trauma, engorgement, and mastitis. Rotation of nursing position will reduce the suction pressure on the same part of the nipple, as well as ensuring complete emptying of all lobes of the breast. Frequent nursing will reduce engorgement and milk stasis. The use of soaps, alcohol, and other drying agents on the nipples tends to increase nipple trauma and pain. The nipples should be air-dried for a few minutes after each feed, and clean water is sufficient to cleanse the breast, if necessary. Some experts recommend that fresh breast milk be applied to the nipples and allowed to dry after each feed.

Stimulating a let-down and manual expression of milk is useful in the management of many breast problems. The flow of milk can be improved by placing the mother in a quiet, relaxed environment.[77] The breast is massaged in a spiral fashion, staring at the top and moving toward the areola; the fingers are moved in a circular fashion from one spot to another, much like a breast examination. After the massage, the breast is stroked from the top of the breast to the nipple with a light stroke and shaken, while the woman leans forward. Once milk starts to flow, manual expression is begun.

Manual expression is performed by holding the thumb and first two fingers on either side of the areola, in a half circle, but the breast should not be cupped. The hand pushes the breast straight into the chest wall, as the thumb and fingers are rolled forward. Large, pendulous breasts may need lifting prior to this. The maneuver is repeated in all four quadrants of the areola to drain as many reservoirs as possible. The procedure is repeated rhythmically and gently, since squeezing, sliding, or pulling may injure the breast. The sequence of massage, stroke, shake, and express is useful in providing milk immediately for the vigorous infant, in allowing an improved latch-on by reducing periareolar engorgement, and in reducing high suction pressures on a traumatized nipple. The let-down produced by manual expression is never as complete as a normally elicited one. An effective let-down can by elicited by initiating nursing on the side without nipple trauma or mastitis. This will effectively reduce breast pain.

In the first 5 days after birth, about 35 percent of the nipples of breast-feeding mothers show damage, and 69 percent of mothers have nipple pain.[133,134] The management of painful, tender, or injured nipples includes prefeeding manual expression, correction of latching-on, rotation of positions, and initiation of nursing on the less painful side first, with the affected side exposed to air. Drying is facilitated by the application of dry heat (e.g., with hair dryer on low setting) for 20 minutes four times per day. Aspirin or codeine (15 to 30 mg) given $\frac{1}{2}$ hour before nursing may be helpful in severe cases. Engorgement can be avoided, but if it occurs, feeding frequency should be maintained or increased. A wide variety of preparations have been applied to traumatized nipples, including lanolin, A & D ointment, white petrolatum, antibiotics, vitamin E oil, and used tea bags, but few of these have been evaluated scientifically. Soap and alcohol have been shown to injure nipples.[133,134] Nipple shields should be used only as a last resort because of a 20 to 60 percent reduction in milk consumption. Thin latex shields may be better than the traditional red rubber ones, although milk flow is still reduced by 22 percent.[135]

Engorgement of the breast occurs when there is inadequate drainage of milk.[136] Swollen, firm, and tender breasts are caused by distention of the ducts and increased extravascular fluid. Aside from the discomfort, engorgement leads to dysfunctional nursing behavior and nipple trauma. The firm breast tissue pushes the infant's face away from the nipple. The widened base of the nipple disrupts the attachment, and the infant's thrusting tongue abrades the tip. This leads to further engorgement, decreased milk production and, in some cases, early termination of breast-feeding.

The best treatment is prevention, but when this has not occurred, management is centered on symptomatic support and relief of distention. Proper elevation of the breasts is important. The mother should wear a firm-fitting nursing brassiere, with neither thin straps nor plastic lining. A warm shower or bath, with prefeed manual expression, is effective. Frequent suckling (every 1 to 2 hours) is the most effective mechanism to relieve engorgement; postfeed electric pumping from each breast may be helpful. In selected cases, intranasal oxytocin may be given just prior to each feed if let-down seems to be inhibited.

GALACTOGOGUES: DRUGS TO IMPROVE MILK PRODUCTION

Obstetricians may interface with the breast-feeding dyad when there is a question of adequate milk production and transfer by the mother. The mother and/or the pediatrician will ask for a galactogogue to be prescribed by the obstetrician.

Numerous agents have been shown to increase prolactin production; and galactorrhea is a clinical issue for women on phenothiazines or metoclopramide. It is reasonable that these drugs might be used where milk supply seems insufficient.[137] The most understandable clinical scenarios include premature delivery requiring mechanical pumping, glandular hypoplasia, reduction mammoplasty, and relactation (nursing an adoptive child). The most common clinical presentation is perceived poor milk supply or inhibited milk let-down (oxytocin inhibition). Clinical trials with random assignment of subjects have demonstrated the effectiveness of metoclopramide,[138,139] sulpiride,[140,141] and nasal oxytocin[142] for increasing milk production.

Metoclopramide (Reglan) is used to promote gastrointestinal tone; however, a secondary effect is to increase prolactin levels. Most studies demonstrate a multiplefold increase in basal prolactin levels[143] and a 60 to 100 percent increase in milk volume.[137] The effects of metoclopromide are very dose dependent; the usual dose is 10 to 15 mg three times a day. The side effects, gastric cramping, diarrhea, and depression may limit its use. The incidence of depression increases with long-term use; treatment should be tapered over time and limited to less than 4 weeks. There appears to be little effect on the infant. In Kauppila's et al. study,[139] the dose that the infants received was much less than the amount used therapeutically to treat esophageal reflux, regardless of the time postpartum.

Sulpiride is a selective dopamine antagonist used in Europe as an antidepressant and antipsychotic. Smaller doses (50 mg twice daily) do not produce neuroleptic effects in the mother, but prolactin and milk production are increased significantly.[144] Clinical studies suggest an increase in milk production (20 to 50 percent) less than that seen with metoclopromide. In a placebo-controlled study with random assignment of 130 subjects, sulpiride 50 mg twice daily for the first 7 days postpartum increased the total milk yield from 916 ± 66 ml in the control group to 1211 ± 65 ml in the sulpiride-treated group.[141] The transfer of sulpiride to the breast milk was minimal and no adverse effects were seen in the infants. Sulpiride is not available in the United States.

Intranasal oxytocin substitutes for endogenous oxytocin to contract the myoepithelial cells and cause milk let-down. In theory, its use is to overcome an inhibited let-down reflex. Oxytocin is destroyed by gastrointestinal enzymes and is not given orally. Until recently, oxytocin intranasal spray was available commercially, but it has been taken off the market. A pharmacist can prepare an intranasal spray with a concentration of 2 IU per drop. The let-down dose is a spray (3 drops) to each nostril; the total let-down dose is approximately 12 IU. This is taken within 2 or 3 minutes of each nursing episode. The suggested duration of therapy is unclear. Underlying causes for an inhibited let-down reflex need to be identified and controlled.

There have been few clinical trials using oxytocin alone to improve milk production. In a double-blind group sequential trial, intranasal oxytocin alone was used to enhance milk production in women during the first 5 days after delivery of a premature infant. The cumulative volume of breast milk obtained between the second and fifth days was 3.5 times greater in primiparas given intranasal oxytocin than in primiparas given placebo.[142] Because of oxytocin's complementary mechanism to prolactin-stimulating medications, they are often used in combination.[145]

While metoclopramide, sulpiride, and oxytocin appear to be effective and relatively safe for the mother and infant, they are only secondary support interventions. The primary focus should be to enhance prolactin and oxytocin through the natural mechanisms, appropriate and frequent stimulation of the nipple and areola. Galactogogues should only be used for a short duration (2 to 4 weeks) and in conjunction with hands-on counseling by an individual with the time, energy, and knowledge to enhance the "natural" production of breast milk.

MASTITIS AND BREAST ABSCESS

Mastitis is an infectious process of the breast characterized by high fever (39° to 40°C), localized erythema, tenderness, induration, and palpable heat over the area. Often these signs are associated with nausea, vomiting, malaise, and other flu-like symptoms. Mastitis occurs most frequently in the first 2 to 4 weeks postpartum and at times of marked reduction in nursing frequency. Risk factors include maternal fatigue, poor nursing technique, nipple trauma, and epidemic *Staphylococcus aureus*. The most common organisms associated with mastitis are *S. aureus*, *S. epidermidis*, streptococci and, occasionally, gram-negative rods. The incidence of sporadic mastitis is 2 to 5 percent in lactating and less than 1 percent in nonlactating mothers.

Until recently, the management of mastitis has been directed by retrospective clinical reviews of experience. In most cases, this consisted of bed rest, continued lactation, and antibiotics, with an 80 to 90 percent cure rate, a 10 percent abscess rate, a 10 percent recurrence rate, and a 50 percent cessation of breast-feeding. Starting in 1982, Thomsen et al. published four important articles concerning pathophysiology, diagnosis, and treatment of mastitis.[146–149] He observed that the diagnosis and prognosis of inflammatory symptoms of the breast could be established by counts of leukocytes and bacteria in breast milk. This is obtained after careful washing of the mother's hands and breasts with a mild soap. The milk is manually expressed, and the first 3 ml discarded. When the leukocyte count was greater than 10^6 leukocytes/ml, and the bacterial count less than 10^3 bacteria/ml, the diagnosis was noninfectious inflammation of the breast. With no treatment, the inflammatory symptoms lasted 7 days; 50 percent developed mastitis, and only 21 percent returned to normal lactation. When the breast was emptied frequently by continued lactation, the symptoms lasted 3 days, and 96 percent returned to normal lactation.

If the breast milk showed greater than 10^6 leukocytes/ml and greater than 10^3 bacteria/ml, the diagnosis was mastitis. Delay in therapy resulted in abscess formation in 11 percent and only 15 percent returned to normal lactation. Frequent emptying of the infected breast by continued nursing eliminated abscess formation, but only 51 percent returned to normal lactation. Additional antibiotic therapy increased the return to normal lactation in 97 percent with resolution of symptoms in 2.1 days.

In summary, the management of mastitis includes the following: (1) breast support; (2) fluids; (3) assessment of nursing technique; (4) nursing initiated on the uninfected side first to establish let-down; (5) the infected side emptied by nursing with each feed (occasionally, a breast pump helps to ensure complete drainage); and (6) dicloxacillin, 250 mg every 6 hours for 7 days. Erythromycin may be used in patients allergic to penicillin. It is important to continue antibiotics for a full 7 days, since abscess formation is more likely with shorter courses. Hand washing before each feed and by nursing staff reduces nosocomial infection rates. Rooming-in does not reduce the acquisition of hospital strains of *S. aureus* or infection rates. During epidemics, early discharge may reduce infection rates.

Breast abscess will occur in about 10 percent of women who are treated for mastitis. The signs include a high fever (39° to 40°C), and a localized area of erythema, tenderness, and induration. In the center a fluctuant area may be difficult to palpate. The patient feels sick. Abscesses usually occur in the upper outer quadrants and *S. aureus* is usually cultured from the abscess cavity.

The management of breast abscess is similar to that for mastitis, except that (1) drainage of the abscess is indicated and (2) breast-feeding should be limited to the uninvolved side during the initial therapy. The infected breast should be mechanically pumped every 2 hours and with every let-down. The abscess can be drained by serial percutaneous needle aspiration under ultrasound guidance[150]; however, the most common method is surgical drainage. The skin incision should be made over the fluctuant area in a manner parallel to and as far as possible from the areolar edge. While the skin incision follows skin lines, the deeper extension should be made bluntly in a radial direction. Sharp dissection perpendicular to the lactational ducts increases blood loss, the risk of a fistula, and the risk of ductal occlusion. Once the abscess cavity is entered, all loculations are bluntly reduced and the cavity irrigated with saline. American surgeons pack the wound open for drainage and secondary closure. British surgeons advocate removal of the abscess wall and primary closure.[151] In either case, wide closure sutures should be avoided, as they may compromise the ducts. Patients have a protracted recovery of 18 to 32 days and recurrent abscess formation in 9 to 15 percent of cases. Breast-feeding from the involved side may be resumed, if skin erythema and underlying cellulitis have resolved, which may occur in 4 to 7 days.

Candida albicans infection is considered a common cause of breast pain. Candida infection of the breast is a commonly diagnosed by clinical presentation. Women describe severe pain when the infant nurses. She will describe the pain as "like a red hot poker being driven through my chest." Often she has received antibiotics recently, she is a diabetic, or the infant has evidence of oral thrush or diaper rash (*Candida albicans*). A potassium hydroxide (KOH) smear can confirm the diagnosis. A drop of midstream milk is combined with a drop of 10 percent KOH and examined under high-power light microscopy. A typical pattern of hyphae and spores will be visualized. The initial treatment is to massage nystatin cream or miconazole oral gel into both nipples after each feed and in the infant's mouth three times a day for 2 weeks. Recurrent or persistent candida mastitis can be treated by swabbing the infant's mouth with gentian violet liquid (0.5 percent) and immediately latching the baby to the breast, twice a day for 3 days. The major disadvantage of this therapy is the permanent staining associated with gentian violet. An alternative therapy in severe cases is oral fluconazole, 200-mg loading dose followed by 100 mg/day for 14 days.

DRUGS IN BREAST MILK

Most medications taken by the mother appear in the milk (see Chapter 9), but the calculated dose consumed by the nursing infant ranges from 0.001 to 5 percent of the standard therapeutic doses and are tolerated by infants without toxicity.[152,153] Two good references are *Drugs in Pregnancy and Lactation*[107] and *Medications in Mother's Milk*.[108] Very few drugs are absolutely contraindicated. These include anticancer agents, radioactive materials, lithium, chloramphenicol, phenylbutazone, atropine, and the ergot alkaloids.

The following guidelines are helpful:

1. Evaluate the therapeutic benefit of medication. Diuretics given for ankle swelling provide very different benefits from those for congestive heart failure. Are drugs really necessary, and are there safer alternatives?
2. Choose drugs most widely tested and with the lowest milk/plasma ratio.
3. Choose drugs with the lowest oral bioavailability.
4. Select the least toxic drug with the shortest half-life.
5. Avoid long-acting forms. Usually, these drugs are detoxified by the liver or bound to protein.
6. Schedule doses so that the least amount gets into the milk. The rate of maternal absorption and the peak maternal serum concentration are helpful in scheduling dosage. Usually, it is best for the mother to take the medication immediately after a feeding.
7. Monitor the infant during the course of therapy. Many pharmacologic agents for maternal use are also used for infants. This implies the availability of knowledge about therapeutic doses and the signs and symptoms of toxicity.

MATERNAL DISEASE

In the vast majority of cases of lactating mothers with intercurrent disease, there is no medical reason to stop breast-feeding. However, appropriate management requires individualizing the care of the nursing dyad in order to preserve the supply-and-demand relationship of lactation. For example, a hospitalized nursing mother should have her nursing baby with her in the hospital for on-demand feedings. This situation stretches the flexibility of hospital administrators and nursing services, but the problem can be overcome by education.

The first principle is to maintain lactation. An acute hospitalization for a surgical procedure is a common complication. If breast milk was the neonate's only source of nutrition, an acute reduction in nursing may lead to breast engorgement, confusing postoperative fever, and mastitis. The infant should be put to the breast just before premedication, and the breasts should be emptied in the recovery room. The most effective way is to have the mother nurse. Although some anesthetic may be present in the milk, most are compatible with lactation.[107,108,119,153] If there is legitimate concern or if the mother cannot communicate (on a ventilator), the breasts should be pumped mechanically and subsequently emptied every 2 to 3 hours by nursing or pumping.

The second principle is to adjust for the special nutritional requirements of nursing mothers. This principle is especially pertinent when intake is restricted postoperatively and when maternal diet must be manipulated, as in diabetes.[154] In the postoperative period, the surgeon must account for the calories and fluid required for lactation. Until oral intake is established, a lactating mother needs an additional 500 to 1,000 ml of fluid per day. Early return to a balanced diet is essential to offset the additional energy and protein requirements of lactation and wound healing.

The third principle is to ensure that the maternal disease will not harm the infant. This is most pertinent with infectious disease, but it is equally important in cases where a mother's judgment is in question, such as severe mental disease, substance abuse, or a history of physical abuse. The benefits of breast-feeding in the latter situations must be carefully evaluated, using the resources of the patient, her family and social services.

Infection is the most common area where breast-feeding is questioned. In general, the necessary exposure of the infant to the mother in day-to-day care is such that breast-feeding does not add to the risk. This recommendation assumes that appropriate therapy is being given to both mother and infant. Isolation of infected areas should still be practiced, such as a mask in the case of respiratory infection and lesion isolation in herpes. The three acute infections in which breast-feeding is contraindicated are herpes simplex lesions of the breast, untreated active (not just purified protein derivative [PPD]-positive) tuberculosis, and human immunodeficiency viral (HIV) disease.

The fourth principle is to evaluate adequately the need and type of medication used for therapy (see Chapter 9). The drug management of chronic hypertension illustrates this principle. First, the need for medication must be scrutinized. There is considerable controversy in the literature as to whether or not to treat patients with mild chronic hypertension (diastolic blood pressure 90 to 100 mm Hg). The desire of a mother with mild hypertension to breast-feed may change the risk/benefit ratio so that antihypertensive drug therapy should be delayed until after lactation. Second, the medication should be evaluated for its effect on milk production. In the first 3 to 4 months of therapy, diuretics reduce intravascular volume and, subsequently, milk volume. On the other hand, if a patient has been on low doses of thiazide diuretics for more than 6 months, the effect on milk volume is minimal as long as adequate oral intake is maintained. Third, the medication should be evaluated for its secretion in breast milk and its possible effects on the infant. Thiazide diuretics, ethacrynic acid, and furosemide also cross into breast milk in small amounts. These agents have the potential to displace bilirubin, and their use during lactation is of concern when the infant is less than 1 month old or is jaundiced. In general, most other antihypertensive drugs are compatible with breast-feeding. Although new drugs come onto the market frequently, it is wise to use drugs that have had a long history of clinical use.

MILK TRANSFER AND INFANT GROWTH

When is an exclusive diet of breast milk insufficient to supply the nutritional needs of the growing infant? Women who wean in the first 8 weeks most often say that insufficient milk is the reason for quitting, and well-meaning family members often ask, "When are you going to start feeding your child real food?"

Correct answers are not readily available.[97] Many nondietary factors affect the growth of infants, including high birth order, lower maternal age, low maternal weight, poor maternal nutrition during pregnancy, birth interval, birth weight less than 2.4 kg, multiple gestation, infection, death of either parent, and divorce or separation.

In addition, there are inconsistencies in the standard reference charts for growth or nutritional needs.[97] Most growth charts are based on formula-fed infants, who often receive solid food supplementation earlier and in greater proportion than comparable breast-fed infants. Reference charts with sufficiently large numbers of exclusively breast-fed infants from developed countries are lacking. As milk volume is a quantitative measure of nutrition, variations in volume and concentrations of constituents caused by individual variation and different methods of collection compound the interpretation.

Despite the latter concerns, it is apparent that a healthy and successfully breast-feeding mother can supply enough nutrition through breast milk alone for 6 months. The clinical markers for adequate breast milk transfer include an alert, healthy appearance, good muscle tone, good skin turgor, six wet diapers per day, eight or more nursing episodes per day, three or four loose stools per day, consistent evidence of a let-down with operant conditioning, and consistent weight gain.

The term "failure to thrive" has been used loosely to include all infants who show any degree of growth failure. For the breast-feeding mother, it may just be a matter of comparing the growth of her infant to growth charts compiled from formula-fed infants. The loosely applied term can seriously undermine the mother's confidence, and ill-advised supplementation further compromises milk volume and may mask other important underlying causes. The infant should be evaluated for failure to thrive or slowed growth if (1) it continues to lose weight after 7 days of life (after "the milk has come in" the infant should gain 1 oz/day); (2) does not regain birth weight by 2 weeks; or (3) gains weight at a rate below the 10th percentile beyond the first months of age. If the infant is premature, ill, or small for gestational age, weight, height, and skin-fold thickness can be used to define adequate growth. The cause of failure to thrive is often complex and is beyond the scope of this chapter.

JAUNDICE IN THE NEWBORN

Thirteen percent of breast-fed neonates will have jaundice defined by a peak serum bilirubin greater than 12 mg/dl in term infants.[155] Pediatric concerns include hemolysis, liver disease, or infection as underlying causes, and kernicterus as a consequence. Unconjugated serum bilirubin greater than 20 mg/dl is considered the critical level for the development of kernicterus in term infants. When the serum bilirubin is greater than 5 mg/dl in the first 24 hours, a serious disease process (hemolysis) may be present, and intervention is appropriate.

The focus on breast-feeding as related to neonatal jaundice results from the characterization of two syndromes, breast-feeding jaundice syndrome and breast milk jaundice syndrome.[155] In the early 1960s, 5 to 10 percent of lactating women were found to have a steroid metabolite of progesterone, 5β-pregnane-3(α), 20(β)-diol, in their icterogenic milk, but the compound was not found in the milk of women whose infants were normal (breast milk jaundice syndrome). This metabolite is associated with an inhibition of glucosyl transferase in the liver, differences in the metabolism of long-chain unsaturated fatty acids, and/or increased resorption of bile acids in jaundiced infants.

In breast milk jaundice syndrome, the neonates are healthy and active. The hyperbilirubinemia develops after the fourth day of life and may last several months, with a gradual fall in level. When breast-feeding is stopped for 24 to 48 hours, there is a 30 to 50 percent decline in bilirubin levels. With resumption of nursing, serum levels will rise slightly (1 to 2 mg/dl), plateau, and then start to fall slowly, regardless of feeding method. After excluding other causes of jaundice, and with careful monitoring of serum bilirubin, breast-feeding can continue.

Unfortunately, the focus on rare breast-milk jaundice cases, the concern about kernicterus, and the increased bilirubin in many breast-fed neonates between 2 and 7 days old led to routine supplementation of infants with water, glucose, and formula, even when bilirubin concentrations were in the moderate range of 8 to 12 mg/dl. These interventions have led to the breast-feeding jaundice syndrome, or starvation jaundice. The cause of the elevated bilirubin—reduced feeding frequency or low milk transfer—is often unrecognized. It has been clearly demonstrated that feeding frequency greater than eight feedings per 24 hours is associated with lower bilirubin levels.[121] Likewise, water supplementation studied in a controlled fashion does not decrease the peak serum bilirubin.[156] Management consists of prevention by improvement in the quality and frequency of nursing. Rooming-in and night feedings should be encouraged.

BACK-TO-WORK ISSUES

In 1984, approximately 26 percent of new mothers had full-time employment, and an additional 15 percent had part-time employment.[157] At 5 or 6 months postpartum, 12.3 percent of full-time employees were breast-feeding, as were 29 percent of part-time employees or unemployed mothers. Two thirds of the working mothers were supplementing their infants' diets with formula. In 1992, approximately 34 percent of new mothers had full-time employment, and an additional 15 percent had part-time employment. Full-time employees were breast-feeding at one half (13 percent) the rate of breast-feeding among part-time employees (26 percent) or the unemployed (27 percent).[104]

The separation between mother and infant adversely affects the psychology and physiology of lactation through a decrease in the frequency of nursing, breast engorgement, and unsatisfied needs of the baby. The anxiety and fatigue associated with the combination of employment and lactation inhibits the let-down reflex, weakens maternal host defenses, and disrupts family dynamics. The infant must adapt to another caregiver, a new sucking technique, and unfamiliar infectious agents found in day-care settings. Therefore, it is not surprising that formula feeding is viewed as an improvement in mothers' lives, but it does create feelings of inadequacy and guilt in some women.

Breast-feeding during employment is both possible and fulfilling.[157] Preparation, milk storage, and choice of child-care are the cornerstones to easy adaptation to employment. Preparation involves preemployment change in lifestyle to accommodate the increased stresses. Lactation should be well established with frequent nursing (10 to 14 times per day) and no supplementation prior to return to work. Return to full-time work prior to 4 months has a greater negative impact than return to work after 4 months.[157,158] Part-time work lessens the impact. About 2 weeks prior to work, the mother should change her nursing schedule at home. During the workday, she should express or pump her breasts two or three times, while increasing her nursing with short, frequent feeds before and after work times. The infant is fed bottles of stored breast milk by a different person in a different place to allow it to adapt more easily.

During the 2 weeks prior to employment, the day-care arrangements should be carefully selected and observed. In addition to references, several questions are pertinent to the selection of the day-care setting. Is the sitter a mother herself, and does the sitter have experience with nursing babies? Is the mother welcome to use the child-care site for a midday nursing? Does the day-care center provide in-arm feeding, or does it use high chairs and propped bottle-feedings. Is the time and activity of the center highly structured and rigid, or is it flexible to mother or infant needs and requests? Does the staff treat the parents and children with respect? Many of these questions can answered by an extended (1 to 2 hours) observation of the center and its children.

Fatigue is the number one enemy of the working mother. Emotional and physical support of the mother is critical. Some helpful suggestions include (1) bringing the infant's bed into the parent's room, or the construction of a temporary extension to the parents' bed; (2) use of labor saving devices, division of domestic chores, and the elimination of less important household chores to reduce the workload; and (3) taking naps and frequent rest periods to conserve energy.

Continued stimulation of the breast during working hours is important. Pumping not only improves milk supply but it also supplies human milk for the infant. Manual expression and/or mechanical pumping should be performed more frequently (two to three times) in the first 6 months postpartum. After 6 months, the frequency can be reduced and eliminated as the infant is supplemented by fluids or solids during the day.

The collection of breast milk has become simple with the wide variety of mechanical pumps available in the market. Mechanical pumps that employ a bulb syringe produce the least amount of milk and have the highest rate of bacterial contamination. Cyclic electric pumps produce the most milk with the least amount of nipple trauma. Water-driven pumps are both cheap and relatively effective. The most efficient pumps are not as effective as the efficiently nursing body in increasing milk volume and raising prolactin levels.[159]

The concern about bacterial growth in expressed and stored milk has been alleviated by recent studies showing that bacterial contamination does not increase significantly for up to 6 hours after expression, when the milk is stored at room temperature, nor were there differences in bacterial counts between specimens stored at room temperature and those stored under refrigeration for 10 hours.[160] Freshly refrigerated milk should be used within 2 days. Four to 6 oz of human milk can be frozen in partially filled resealable (Ziploc) plastic bags. When human milk is frozen, it should be cooled briefly prior to transfer to the freezer. The milk will keep for 2 to 4 weeks in the refrigerator freezer and up to 6 months in a freezer set at 0°F. The milk should be stored in layers and thawed quickly in warm tap water. Frozen milk should not be thawed in the microwave, as the heating is uneven and severe oral burns have been reported. After it is thawed it should be used within 6 to 8 hours.

WEANING

The American Academy of Pediatrics recommends exclusive breast-feeding for the first 6 months of life and continuation at least through the first 12 months of life. This recommendation in 1997 initiated a firestorm of controversy regarding "the excessive duration of breast-feeding." Breast-feeding is both a biologic process and a culturized activity. In the United States, breast-feeding has been culturized to no breast-feeding or breast-feeding for less than 6 months. From a broader biologic and historical perspective, the United States experience reflects cultural bias, not biologic reality. In a remarkable review, Dettwyler[161] makes a very cogent argument for the "natural" age of weaning in the human to be 3 to 4 years. She has several arguments. Traditional and prehistoric societies wean between the third and fourth year. Based on weaning when the infant weight is four times its birthweight, similar to other primates, weaning should occur between 2 and 3 years. If weaning corresponds to attainment of one third the adult weight, then weaning would occur between 3 and 4 years. If humans behaved like chimpanzees or gorillas and weaned at six times the gestational period, humans would wean at 4.5 years. The dental, neurologic, and immunologic systems are still developing until 6 years of age; breast-feeding and breast milk provide unique support for these systems up to 4 to 6 years. Developmentally, the infant is able to place solid food in its mouth at 6 months, but this intake, if left to the infant's own skills, would not reach a significant proportion of the nutritional requirements until 18 to 24 months. The ability to drink from a cup occurs close to the second year. As the infant supplements an increasing proportion of its nutritional needs with solid or liquid food, the mother will begin to ovulate. Subsequent pregnancy is increasingly more likely. Breast-feeding, through its suppression of gonadal function, mantains a birth interval of 3 to 4 years. Clearly, breast-feeding into the third or fourth year is a cultural exception in the United States, but prolonged breast-feeding does not constitute abnormal or deviant behavior as expressed by many "modern" Americans. As we learn more about the benefits of long-term lactation, our culture may return to more reasonable expectations for duration of breast-feeding.

Key Points

➤ The World Health Organization, the U.S. Surgeon General, the American Academy of Pediatrics, the American Academy of Family Practice, the American College of Obstetricians and Gynecologists, and the Academy of Breastfeeding Medicine endorse breast-feeding as the gold standard for infant feeding.

➤ Breast-feeding accrues many health benefits for the infant, including protection against infection, less allergy, better growth, better neurodevelopment, and lower rates of chronic disease such as insulin-dependent diabetes and childhood cancer.

➤ Breast-feeding accrues more health benefits for the mother, including faster postpartum involution, improved postpartum weight loss, less premenopausal breast cancer, better mother–infant bonding, and less economic burden.

➤ Artificial breast milk lacks key components including defenses against infection, hormones and enzymes to aid digestion, polyunsaturated fatty acids, which are necessary for optimal brain growth, and adequate composition for efficient digestion.

➤ Contact with the breast within one half hour after birth increases the duration of breast feeding. A frequency of nursing greater than eight per 24 hours, night nursing, and a duration of nursing longer than 15 minutes are needed to maintain adequate prolactin levels and milk supply.

➤ Prolactin is the major promoter of milk synthesis. Oxytocin is the major initiator of milk ejection. The release of prolactin and oxytocin results from the stimulation of the sensory nerves supplying the areola and nipple.

➤ Oxytocin released from the posterior pituitary can be operantly conditioned and is influenced negatively by pain, stress, or loss of self-esteem.

➤ The nursing actions on a human teat versus on an artificial teat are very different. Poor lactation is the major cause of nipple injury and poor milk transfer. Perceived or real lack of milk transfer is the major reason why lactation fails.

➤ Milk production is reduced by an autocrine pathway through a protein that inhibits milk production by the alveolar cells, and by distention and pressure against the alveolar cells.

REFERENCES

1. American Academy of Pediatrics, Work Group on Breastfeeding: Breastfeeding and the use of human milk. Pediatrics 100: 1035, 1997.
2. Ryan AS: The resurgence of breastfeeding in the United States. Pediatrics 99:E12, 1997.
3. Freed G, Clark S, Sorenson J, et al: National assessment of physicians' breast-feeding knowledge, attitudes, training and experience. JAMA 273:472, 1995.
4. Schanler RJ, O'Connor KG, Lawrence RA: Pediatricians' practices and attitudes regarding breastfeeding promotion. Pediatrics 103:E35, 1999.
5. Michels KB, Willett WC, Rosner BA, et al: Prospective assessment of breastfeeding and breast cancer incidence among 89 887 women. Lancet 347:431, 1996.
6. Crow RA, Fawcett JN, Wright P: Maternal behavior during breast- and bottle-feeding. J Behav Med 3:259, 1980.
7. Agre F: The relationship of mode of infant feeding and location of care to frequency of infection. Am J Dis Child 139: 809, 1985.
8. Howie PW, Forsyth JS, Ogston SA, et al: Protective effect of breast feeding against infection. BMJ 300:11, 1990.
9. Kovar MG, Serdual MK, Marks JS, et al: Review of the epidemiologic evidence for an association between infant feeding and infant health. Pediatrics 74:S615, 1984.
10. Popkin BM, Adair L, Akin JS, et al: Breastfeeding and diarrheal morbidity. Pediatrics 86:874, 1990.
11. Beaudry M, Dufour R, Marcoux S: Relation between infant

feeding and infections during the first six months of life. J Pediatr 126:191, 1995.

12. Golding J, Emmett PM, Rogers IS: Gastroenteritis, diarrhoea and breast feeding. Early Hum Dev 49:S83, 1997.

13. Frank AL, Taber LH, Glezen WP, et al: Breast-feeding and respiratory virus infection. Pediatrics 70:239, 1982.

14. Wright AI, Holberg CJ, Martinez FD, et al: Breast feeding and lower respiratory tract illness in the first year of life. BMJ 299:945, 1989.

15. Chen Y: Synergistic effect of passive smoking and artifical feeding on hospitalization for respiratory illness in early childhood. Chest 95:1004, 1989.

16. Duncan B, Ey J, Holberg CJ, et al: Exclusive breast-feeding for at least 4 months protects against otitis media. Pediatrics 91:867, 1993.

17. Owen MJ, Baldwin CD, Swank PR, et al: Relation of infant feeding practices, cigarette smoke exposure, and group child care to the onset and duration of otitis media with effusion in the first two years of life. J Pediatr 123:702, 1993.

18. Paradise JL, Rockette HE, Colborn DK, et al: Otitis media in 2253 Pittsburgh-area infants: prevalence and risk factors during the first two years of life. Pediatrics 99:318, 1997.

19. Cochi SL, Fleming DW, Hightower AW, et al: Primary invasive *Haemophilus influenzae* type b disease; a population-based assessment of risk factors. J Pediatr 108:887, 1986.

20. Takala AK, Eskola J, Palmgren J, et al: Risk factors of invasive *Haemophilus influenzae* type b disease among children in Finland. J Pediatr 115:694, 1989.

21. Istre GR, Conner JS, Broome CV, et al: Risk factors for primary invasive *Haemophilus influenzae* disease: increased risk from day care attendance and school-aged household members. J Pediatr 106:190, 1985.

22. Pisacane A, Graziano L, Mazzarella G, et al: Breast-feeding and urinary tract infection. J Pediatr 120:87, 1992.

23. Lucas A, Cole TJ: Breast milk and neonatal necrotizing enterocolitis. Lancet 336:1519, 1990.

24. Covert RF, Barman N, Domanico RS, et al: Prior enteral nutrition with human milk protects against intestinal perforation in infants who develop necrotizing enterocolitis. Pediatr Res 37:305A, 1995.

25. Ford RPK, Taylor BJ, Mitchell EA, et al: Breastfeeding and the risk of sudden infant death syndrome. Int J Epidemiol 22:885, 1993.

26. Mitchell EA, Taylor BJ, Ford RPK, et al: Four modifiable and other major risk factors for cot death: the New Zealand study. J Paediatr Child Health 28:S3, 1992.

27. Scragg LK, Mitchell EA, Tonkin SL, et al: Evaluation of the cot death prevention programme in South Auckland. N Z Med J 106:8, 1993.

28. Gerstein HC: Cow's milk exposure and type I diabetes mellitus: a critical overview of the clinical literature. Diabetes Care 17:13, 1994.

29. Gimeno SG, de Souza JM: IDDM and milk consumption. A case-control study in Sao Paulo, Brazil. Diabetes Care 20:1256, 1997.

30. Baker D, Taylor H, Henderson J, et al: Inequality in infant morbidity: causes and consequences in England in the 1990s. J Epidemiol Community Health 52:451, 1998.

31. Koletzko S, Sherman P, Corey M, et al: Role of infant feeding practices in development of Crohn's disease in childhood. BMJ 298:1617, 1994.

32. Rigas A, Rigas B, Glassman M, et al: Breast-feeding and maternal smoking in the etiology of Crohn's disease and ulcerative colitis in childhood. Ann Epidemiol 3:387, 1993.

33. Shu X-O, Clemens J, Zheng W: Infant breastfeeding and the risk of childhood lymphoma and leukemia. Int J Epidemiol 24:27, 1995.

34. Saarinen VM, Kajosaari M: Breast feeding as prophylaxis

35. Scariati PD, Grummer-Strawn LM, Fein SB: A longitudinal analysis of infant morbidity and the extent of breastfeeding in the United States. Pediatrics 99:5, 1997.

36. Wilson AC, Stewart-Forsyth J, Green SA, et al: Relation of infant diet to childhood health: seven year follow up of cohort of children in Dundee infant feeding study. BMJ 316:21, 1998.

37. Van den Bogaard C, van den Hoogen HJM, Huygen FJA, et al: Is the breast best for children with a family history of atopy? The relation between way of feeding and early childhood morbidity. Fam Med 25:471, 1993.

38. Wright AL, Holberg CJ, Taussig LM, et al: Relationship of infant feeding to recurrent wheezing at age 6 years. Arch Pediatr Adolesc Med 149:758, 1995.

39. Jamieson EC, Abbasi KA, Cockburn R, et al: Effect of diet on term infant cerebral cortex fatty acid composition. *In* Galli C, Simopoulis AP, Tremoli E (eds): Fatty Acids and Lipids: Biological Aspects. Basel, Karger 75:139, 1994.

40. Lucas A, Morley R, Cole TJ, et al: A randomized multicenter study of human milk versus formula and later development in preterm infant. Arch Dis Child 70:FI41, 1994.

41. Lucas A, Morley R, Cole TJ: Randomised trial of early diet in preterm babies and later intelligence quotient. BMJ 317:1481, 1998.

42. Taylor B, Wadsworth J: Breastfeeding and child development at five years. Dev Med Child Neurol 26:73, 1984.

43. Wigg NR, Tong S, McMichael AJ, et al: Does breastfeeding at six months predict cognitive development? Aust N Z J Public Health 22:232, 1998.

44. Riva E, Agostoni C, Biasucci G, et al: Early breastfeeding is linked to higher intelligence quotient scores in dietary treated phenylketonuric children. Acta Paediatr 85:56, 1996.

45. Montgomery D, Splett P: Economic benefit of breast-feeding infants enrolled in WIC. J Am Diet Assoc 97:379, 1997.

46. Tuttle CR, Dewey KG: Potential cost savings for Medi-Cal, AFDC, food stamps, and WIC programs associated with increasing breast-feeding among low-income among women in California. J Am Diet Assoc 96:885, 1996.

47. Chua S, Arulkumaran S, Lim I, et al: Influence of breastfeeding and nipple stimulation on postpartum uterine activity. Br J Obstet Gynaecol 101:804, 1994.

48. Ball TM, Wright AL: Health care costs of formula-feeding in the first year of life. Pediatrics 103:870, 1999.

49. Labbok MH: Health sequelae of breastfeeding for the mother. Clin Perinatol 26:491, 1999.

50. Dewey KG, Heinig MJ, Nommsen LA: Maternal weight-loss patterns during prolonged lactation. Am J Clin Nutr 58:162, 1993.

51. Short RV, Lewis PR, Renfree MB, et al: Contraceptive effects of extended lactational amenorrhoea; beyond the Bellagio consensus. Lancet 337:715, 1991.

52. Melton LJ, Bryant SC, Wahner HW, et al: Influence of breastfeeding and other reproductive factors on bone mass later in life. Osteoporos Int 3:76, 1993.

53. Cumming RG, Klineberg RJ: Breastfeeding and other reproductive factors and the risk of hip fractures in elderly woman. Int J Epidemiol 22:192, 1993.

54. Oski FA: What we eat may determine who we can be. Nutrition 13:220, 1997.

55. Newcomb PA, Storer BE, Longnecker MP, et al: Lactation and a reduced risk of premenopausal breast cancer. N Engl J Med 330:8187, 1994.

56. Smith WL, Erenberg A, Nowak A: Imaging evaluation of the human nipple during breastfeeding. Am J Dis Child 142:76, 1988.

57. Weber F, Woolridge MW, Baum JD: An ultrasonographic

study of the organization of sucking and swallowing by newborn infants. Dev Med Child Neural 28:19, 1986.

58. Neifert M, DeMarzo S, Seacat J, et al: The influence of breast surgery, breast appearance, and pregnancy-induced breast changes on lactation sufficiency as measured by infant weight gain. Birth 17:31, 1990.

59. Neifert MR: Clinical aspects of lactation: promoting breast-feeding success, Clin Perinatol 26:281, 1999.

60. Katz M, Creasy RK: Mammary blood flow regulation in the nursing rabbit. Am J Obstet Gynecol 150:497, 1984.

61. Saint L, Smith M, Hartmann PE: The yield and nutrient content of colostrum and milk of women from giving birth to 1 month post-partum. Br J Nutr 52:87, 1984.

62. Neville MC: Determinants of milk volume and composition. *In* Jensen RG (ed): Handbook for Milk Composition. San Diego, Academic Press, 1995.

63. Peaker M: The effect of raised intramammary pressure on mammary function in the goat in relation to the cessation of lactation. J Physiol (Lond) 310:415, 1980.

64. Wilde CJ, Addey CVP, Boddy LM, et al: Autocrine regulation of milk secretion by a protein in milk. Biochem J 305:51, 1995.

65. Lund LR, Romer J, Thomasset N, et al: Two distinct phases of apoptosis in mammary gland involution: proteinase-independent and -dependent pathways. Development 122:181, 1996.

66. Prentice A, Addey CP, Wilde CJ: Evidence for local feedback control of human milk secretion. Biochem Soc Trans 16:122, 1989.

67. Neville MC: Physiology of lactation. Clin Perinatol 26:251, 1999.

68. Hall B: Changing composition of human milk and early development of an appetite control. Lancet 1:779, 1975.

69. Neville MC, Keller R, Seacat J, et al: Studies in human lactation: milk volumes in lactating women during the onset of lactation and full lactation. Am J Clin Nutr 48:1375, 1988.

70. Neville MC, Keller RP, Seacat J, et al: Studies on human lactation. 1. Within-feed and between-breast variation in selected components of human milk. Am J Clin Nutr 40:635, 1984.

71. Woolridge MW, Fisher C: Colic, "overfeeding" symptoms of lactose malabsorption in the breast-fed baby a possible artifact of feed management. Lancet 2:382, 1988.

72. Rasmussen KM: Maternal nutritional status and lactational performance. Clin Nutr 7:147, 1988.

73. Strode MA, Dewey KG, Lonnerdal B: Effects of short-term caloric restriction on lactational performance of well-nourished women. Acta Paediatr Scand 75:222, 1986.

74. Dewey KG, Lovelady CA, Nommsen-Rivers LA, et al: A randomized study of the effects of aerobic exercise by lactating women on breast-milk volume and composition. N Engl J Med 330:449, 1994.

75. Rolland R, DeJong FH, Schellekens LA, et al: The role of prolactin in the restoration of ovarian function during the early postpartum period in the human: a study during inhibition of lactation by bromergocryptine. Clin Endocrinol 4:23, 1975.

76. Newton M, Egli GE: The effect of intranasal administration of oxytocin on the let-down of milk in lactating women. Am J Obstet Gynecol 76:103, 1958.

77. Feher SDK, Berger LR, Johnson JD, et al: Increasing breast milk production for premature infants with a relaxation/imagery audiotape. Pediatrics 83:57, 1989.

78. Ueda T, Yokoyama Y, Irahara M, et al: Influence of psychological stress on suckling-induced pulsatile oxytocin release. Obstet Gynecol 84:259, 1994.

79. Losch M, Dungy CI, Russell D, et al: Impact of attitudes on maternal decisions regarding infant feeding. J Pediatr 126:507, 1996.

80. Uvnas-Moberg K: Oxytocin linked antistress effects—the relaxation and growth response. Acta Physiol Scand Suppl 640:38, 1997.

81. Carter CS, Altemus M: Integrative functions of lactational hormones in social behavior and stress management. Ann N Y Acad Sci 807:164, 1997.

82. Kennel JH, Klaus MH: Bonding: recent observations that alter perinatal care. Pediatr Rev 19:4, 1998.

83. Lindenberg CS, Artola RC, Jimenez V: The effect of early postpartum mother-infant contact and breastfeeding promotion on the incidence and continuation of breastfeeding. Int J Nurs Stud 27:179, 1990.

84. Woolridge MW, How TV, Drewett RF, et al: The continuous measurement of milk intake at a feed in breast-babies. Early Hum Dev 6:365, 1982.

85. Howie PW, McNeilly AS, McArdle T, et al: The relationship between suckling-induced prolactin response and lactogenesis. J Clin Endocrinol Metab 50:670, 1980.

86. Lucas A, Lucas PI, Baum JD: Differences in the pattern of milk intake between breast and bottle fed infants. Early Hum Dev 5:195, 1981.

87. Anderson AN, Schioler V: Influence of breast-feeding pattern on the pituitary-ovarian axis of a woman in an industrialized country. Am J Obstet Gynecol 143:673, 1982.

88. Jones RE: A hazards model analysis of breastfeeding variables and maternal age on return to menses postpartum in rural Indonesian women. Hum Biol 60:853, 1988.

89. Goldman AS, Chheda S, Kenney SE, et al: Immunologic protection of the premature newborn by human milk. Semin Perinatol 19:495, 1994.

90. Garofalo RP, Goldman AS: Expression of functional immunomodulatory and anti-inflammatory factors in human milk. Clin Perinatol 26:361, 1999.

91. International code of marketing of breastmilk substitutes, Geneva, World Health Organization, 1981.

92. Tsang RC, Zlotkin SH, Nichols BL, Hansen JW (eds): Nutrition During Infancy: Principles and Practice, 2nd ed., Cincinnati, Digital Education Publisher, 1997.

93. National Academy of Sciences: Nutritional status and usual dietary intake of lactating women. *In* Nutrition Dining Lactation, Subcommittee on Nutrition During Lactation, Committee on Nutritional Status During Pregnancy and Lactation, Food and Nutrition Board, Institute of Medicine, National Academy of Sciences, National Academy Press, Washington, DC, 1991.

94. National Academy of Sciences: Meeting maternal nutrient needs during lactation. *In* Nutrition During Lactation Subcommittee on Nutrition During Lactation, Committee on Nutritional Status During Pregnancy and Lactation. Food and Nutrition Board, Institute of Medicine, National Academy of Sciences, National Academy Press, Washington, DC, 1991.

95. Kunz C, Rodriquez-Palmero M, Koletzko B, et al: Nutritional and biochemical properties of human milk, part I: general aspects, proteins, and carbohydrates. Clin Perinatol 26:307, 1999.

96. Rodriquez-Palmero M, Koletzko B, Kunz C, et al: Nutritional and biochemical properties of human milk, part II: lipids, micronutrients, and bioactive factors. Clin Perinatol 26:335, 1999.

97. Dewey KG, Peerson JM, Brown KH, et al: Growth of breast-fed infants deviates from current reference data: a pooled analysis of US, Canadian, and European data sets. Pediatrics 96:495, 1995.

98. Ravelli AC, van der Meulen JH, Osmond C, et al: Infant

feeding and adult glucose tolerance, lipid profile, blood pressure, and obesity. Arch Dis Child 82:248, 2000.

99. Xanthou M: Human milk cells. Acta Paediatr 86:1288, 1997.

100. Slade HB, Schwartz SA: Mucosal immunity: the immunology of breast milk. J Allergy Clin Immunol 80:346, 1987.

101. Ellison RT, Giehl TJ: Killing of gram-negative bacteria by lactoferrin and lysozyme. J Clin Invest 88:1080, 1991.

102. Iyer S, Lonnerdal B: Lactoferrin, lactoferrin receptors and iron metabolism. Eur J Clin Nutr 47:232, 1993.

103. Mansbach IK, Palti H, Pevsner B, et al: Advice from the obstetrician and other sources: do they affect women's breast feeding practices? A study among different Jewish groups in Jerusalem. Soc Sci Med 19:157, 1984.

104. Lawrence RA: Breastfeeding, A Guide for the Medical Profession, 4th edition. St. Louis, Mosby, 1994.

105. Mohrbacher N, Stock J: The Breastfeeding Answer Book, revised ed. Schaumburg, IL, La Leche League International, 1997.

106. The Womanly Art of Breastfeeding, 6th revised ed. Schaumburg, IL, La Leche League Internal, 1997.

107. Briggs GG, Freeman RK, Yaffe SJ: Drugs in Pregnancy and Lactation, 5th ed. Baltimore, Williams & Wilkins, 1998.

108. Hale TW: Medications and Mothers' Milk, 8th ed. Amarillo, TX, Pharmsoft Medical Publishers, 1999.

109. Alexander JM, Grant AM, Campbell MJ: Randomised controlled trial of breast shells and Hoffman's exercises for inverted and non-protractile nipples. BMJ 304:1030, 1990.

110. Kesaree N, Banapurmath CR, Banapurmath S, et al: Treatment of inverted nipples using a disposable syringe. J Hum Lact 9:27, 1993.

111. Hurst NM: Lactation after augmentation mammoplasty. Obstet Gynecol 87:30, 1996.

112. Semple JL, Lugowski SJ, Baines CJ, et al: Breast milk contamination and silicone implants: preliminary results using silicon as a proxy measurement for silicone. Plast Reconstr Surg 102:528, 1998.

113. Kjoller K, McLaughlin JK, Friis S, et al: Health outcomes in offspring of mothers with breast implants. Pediatrics 102:1112, 1998.

114. Righard L, Alade MO: Effect of delivery room routines on success of first breast-feed. Lancet 336:1105, 1990.

115. Righard L, Alade MO: Sucking technique and its effect on success of breastfeeding. Birth 19:185, 1992.

116. Hodgkinson R, Bhatt M, Wang CN: Double-blind comparison of the neurobehavior of neonates following the administration of different doses of meperidine to the mother. Can Anaesth Soc J 25:405, 1978.

117. Zhang J, Bernasko JW, Leybovich E, et al: Continuous labor support from labor attendant for primiparous women: a meta-analysis. Obstet Gynecol 88:739, 1996.

118. Hofmeyr CJ, Nikodem VC, Wolman WL, et al: Companionship to modify the clinical birth environment: effects on progress and perceptions of labour, and breastfeeding. Br J Obstet Gynaecol 98:756, 1991.

119. Wittels B, Scott DT, Sinatra RS: Exogenous opioids in human breast milk and acute neonatal neurobehavior: a preliminary study. Anesthesiology 73:864, 1990.

120. Christensson K, Nilsson BA, Stocks S, et al: Effect of nipple stimulation on uterine activity and on plasma levels of oxytocin in full term, healthy, pregnant women. Acta Obstet Gynecol Scand 68:205, 1989.

121. DeCarvalho M, Klaus MH, Merkatz RB: Frequency of breast-feeding and serum bilirubin concentration. Am J Dis Child 136:737, 1982.

122. Egli GE, Egli NS, Newton M: The influence of the number of breast-feedings on milk production. Pediatrics 27:314, 1961.

123. Bergeuim Y, Daugherty C, Kramer MS: Do infant formula samples shorten the duration of breastfeeding? Lancet 1:1148, 1983.

124. Wright A, Rice S, Wells S: Changing hospital practices to increase the duration of breastfeeding. Pediatrics 97:669, 1996.

125. Howard C, Howard F, Lawrence R, et al: Office prenatal formula advertising and its effect on breast-feeding patterns. Obstet Gynecol 95:296, 2000.

126. Howard FM, Howard CR, Weitzman ML: The physician a advertiser: the unintentional discouragement of breast-feeding. Obstet Gynecol 81:1048, 1993.

127. Winikoff B, Laukaran VH, Myers D: Dynamics of infant feeding: mothers, professional and institutional context in a large urban hospital. Pediatrics 77:357, 1986.

128. Ishida T, Yoke T, Kasumi F, et al: Clinicopathologic characteristics and prognosis of breast cancer patients associated with pregnancy and lactation: analysis of case-control study in Japan. Jpn J Cancer Res 83:1143, 1992.

129. Gupta RK, McHutchison AG, Dowle CS, et al: Fine-needle aspiration cytodiagnosis of breast masses in pregnant and lactating women and its impact on management. Diagn Cytopathol 9:156, 1993.

130. Brewer MM, Bates MR, Vannoy LP: Postpartum changes in maternal weight and body fat depots in lactating vs nonlactating women. Am J Clin Nutr 49:259, 1989.

131. Sadurskis A, Kabir N, Wager J, et al: Energy metabolism, body composition, and milk production in healthy Swedish women during lactation. Am J Clin Nutr 48:44, 1988.

132. Amir L, Garland SM, Dennerstein L, et al: *Candida albicans*: is it associated with nipple pain in lactating women? Gynecol Obstet Invest 41:30, 1996.

133. Brent N, Rudy SJ, Redd B, et al: Sore nipples in breast-feeding women. Arch Pediatr Adolesc Med 152:1077, 1998.

134. Cable B, Stewart M, Davis J: Nipple wound care: a new approach to an old problem. J Hum Lact 13:313, 1997.

135. Woolridge MW, Baum JD, Drewett RF: Effect of traditional and of a new nipple shield on sucking patterns and milk flow. Early Hum Dev 4:357, 1980.

136. Hill PD, Humenick SS: The occurrence of breast engorgement. J Hum Lact 10:79, 1994.

137. Emery MM: Galacatogogues: drugs to induce lactation. J Hum Lact 12:55, 1996.

138. de Gezelle H, Ooghe W, Thiery M, et al: Metoclopramide and breast milk. Eur J Obstet Gynecol Reprod Biol 15:31, 1983.

139. Kauppila A, Kivinen S, Ylikorkala O: A dose response relation between improved lactation and metoclopramide. Lancet 1:1175, 1981.

140. Aono T, Aki T, Koike K, et al: Effect of sulpiride on poor puerperal lactation. Am J Obstet Gynecol 143:927, 1982.

141. Aono T, Shioji T, Aki T, et al: Augmentation of puerperal lactation by oral administration of sulpiride. J Clin Endocrinol Metab 48:478, 1979.

142. Ruis H, Rolland R, Doesburg W, et al: Oxytocin enhances onset of lactation among mothers delivering prematurely. Br Med J 283:340, 1981.

143. Budd SC, Erdman SH, Long DM, et al: Improved lactation with metoclopramide. Clin Pediatr 32:53, 1993.

144. Wiesel FA, Alfredsson G, Ehrnebo M, et al: The pharmacokinetics of intravenous and oral sulpiride in healthy human subjects. Eur J Clin Pharmacol 17:385, 1980.

145. Aono T, Shioji T, Aki T, et al: Augmentation of puerperal lactation by oral administration of sulpiride. J Clin Endocrinol Metab 48:478, 1979.

146. Thomsen AC: Infectious mastitis and the occurrence of antibody-coated bacteria in milk. Am J Obstet Gynecol 144:350, 1982.

147. Thomsen AC, Hansen KPB, Moller BR: Leukocyte counts and microbiological cultivation in the diagnosis of puerperal mastitis. Am J Obstet Gynecol 146:938, 1983.

148. Thomsen AC, Espersen T, Maignard S: Course and treatment of milk stasis, non-infectious inflammation of the breast, and infectious mastitis in nursing women. Am J Obstet Gynecol 149:492, 1984.

149. Thomsen AC, Mogensen SC, Jepsen FL: Experimental mastitis in mice induced by coagulase-negative staphylococcus isolated from cases of mastitis in nursing women. Acta Obstet Gynecol Scand 64:163, 1985.

150. O'Hara RJ, Dexter SPL, Fox JN: Conservative management of infective mastitis and breast abscesses after ultrasonographic assessment. Br J Surg 83:1413, 1996.

151. Benson EA, Goodman MA: Incision with primary suture in the treatment of acute puerperal breast abscess. Br J Surg 57:55, 1970.

152. Rivera-Calimlim L: The significance of drugs in breast milk. Clin Perinatol 14:51, 1987.

153. Howard CR, Lawrence RA: Drugs and breastfeeding. Clin Perinatol 26:447, 1999.

154. Ferris AM, Dalindoquitz CK, Ingardia CM, et al: Lactation outcome in insulin-dependent diabetic women. Am Diabetic Assoc 88:314, 1988.

155. Gartner LM, Lee K: Jaundice in the breastfed infant. Clin Perinatol 26:431, 1999.

156. Scjitzam D, Jervada AR, Bramca PA: Effect of water supplementation on full-term newborns on arrival of milk in the nursing mother. Clin Pediatr 25:78, 1986.

157. Auerbach KG, Guss E: Maternal employment and breast-feeding. Am J Dis Child 138:958, 1984.

158. Fein SB, Roe B: The effect of work status on initiation and duration of breast-feeding. Am J Public Health 88:1042, 1998.

159. Zinaman MJ, Hughes V, Queenan JT, et al: Acute prolactin and oxytocin responses and milk yield to infant suckling and artificial methods of expression in lactating women. Pediatrics 89:437, 1992.

160. Hamosh M, Ellis LA, Pollock DR, et al: Breastfeeding and the working mother: effect of time and temperature of short-term storage on proteolysis, lipolysis, and bacterial growth in milk. Pediatrics 97:492, 1996.

161. Dettwyler KA: A time to wean: the hominid blueprint for the natural age of weaning in modern human populations. *In* Stuart-MacAdam P, Dettwyler KA (eds): Breastfeeding: Biocultural Perspectives. New York, Aldine de Gruyter, 1995.

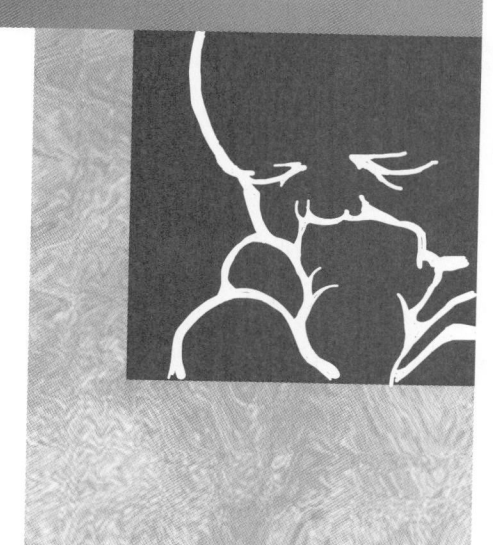

Prenatal Care

Chapter 6

Preconception and Prenatal Care: Part of the Continuum

TIMOTHY R. B. JOHNSON AND JENNIFER R. NIEBYL

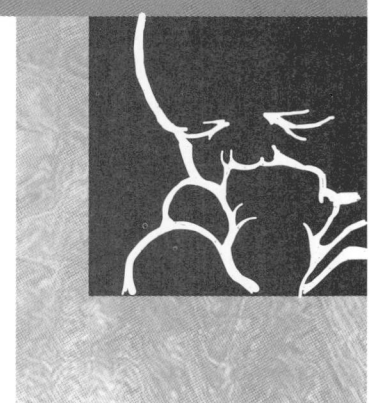

Primary care is defined as follows:

> Integrated, accessible health care services by clinicians who are accountable for addressing a large majority of personal health care needs, developing a sustained partnership with patients, and practicing in the context of family and community.[1]

It is obvious that pregnancy and child birth are major life events. Preconception and prenatal care are not only part of the pregnancy continuum that culminates in delivery, the postpartum period, and parenthood, but they should increasingly be considered in the context of women's health throughout the life span.

Prenatal care is an excellent example of preventive medicine and is very much a phenomenon of the 20th century. In 1929, the Ministry of Health of Great Britain issued a memorandum on the conduct of prenatal clinics. In 1942, vitamin tablets were provided for all women in the last 6 months of pregnancy. Maternal mortality declined from 319 per 100,000 live births in 1936 to 15 per 100,000 live births in 1985. The decline in maternal mortality was partly attributed to prenatal care and partly to medical advances in availability of blood transfusions, antibiotics, and management of fluid and electrolyte balance.

Recent guidelines addressing the content and efficacy of prenatal care have focused on the medical and the psychosocial and educational aspects of the prenatal care system. Prenatal care satisfies the definition of primary care from the Institute of Medicine.[1] In fact, prenatal care services can be used by obstetricians/gynecologists and other primary care providers as a general model for primary care.[2] Prenatal care satisfies other criteria for primary care in that it is comprehensive and continuous, and provides coordinated health care.[3] Preconception care—planning to ensure the healthiest possible pregnancy outcome—is consistent with this model. We will further argue that the preconception and prenatal care periods—just as labor, delivery, and the puerperium—must be seen as episodes in a woman's life and that they provide important opportunities to advance wellness and prevention. A medical model of care with separate encounters and ambulatory and inpatient visits does not represent any personal reality. It must be recognized that for pregnant women all these events are part of a life continuum with birth leading to the multiple challenges of parenting. They are opportunities to introduce and reinforce habits, knowledge, and life-long skills in self-care, health education, and wellness, to inculcate principles of routine screening, immunization, and regular assessment for psychological, behavioral, and medical risk factors.

The prenatal care record describes in a consistent fashion the comprehensive care that is provided and allows for documentation of coordinated services.

The goal of prenatal care is to help the mother maintain her well-being and achieve a healthy outcome for herself and her infant. Education about pregnancy, childbearing, and childrearing is an important part of prenatal care, as are detection and treatment of abnormalities. This process is best realized when begun even before pregnancy. Two documents[1,5] addressing the content and efficacy of prenatal care have suggested changes in the current prenatal care system, and current standards are continuously evolving.[6-13] Many services provided traditionally during the intrapartum hospital stay will be provided at prenatal and postpartum outpatient visits.[14] Too often, hospitalization for childbirth has been seen as an opportunity for education about self-care, child-care and parenting, and parenthood rather than as a time to ensure safe passage. Educational interventions have thus far been targeted for the intrapartum stay, when they can better and more cheaply be performed in the preconceptional, antenatal, or home care environment.[14,15]

MATERIAL MORTALITY

Maternal death is the demise of any woman from any pregnancy-related cause while pregnant or within 42 days of termination of pregnancy, irrespective of the duration and the site of pregnancy. A direct maternal death is an obstetric death resulting from obstetric complications of the pregnancy state, labor, or puerperium. An indirect maternal death is an obstetric death resulting from a disease previously existing or developing during the pregnancy, labor, or puerperium; death is not directly due to obstetric causes but may be aggravated by the physiologic effects of pregnancy. A nonmaternal death is an obstetric death resulting from accidental or incidental causes unrelated to the pregnancy or its management.

The maternal mortality rate is the number of maternal deaths (direct, indirect, or nonmaternal) per 100,000 women of reproductive age but, since this denominator is difficult to determine precisely, the National Center for Health Statistics,[16] the World Health Organization, and others utilize the maternal mortality ratio defined as the number of maternal deaths (indirect and direct) per 100,000 live births.

Direct obstetric deaths arise from six major areas: hypertensive diseases of pregnancy, hemorrhage, infections/sepsis, thromboembolism and, in developing countries, obstructed labor and complications from illegal abortion. There are other direct causes of death, such as ectopic pregnancy, complications of anesthesia, and amniotic fluid embolism. The main causes of indirect obstetric deaths are asthma, heart disease, type I diabetes, systemic lupus erythematosus, and other conditions that are aggravated by pregnancy to the point of death.[17]

Maternal mortality has been an underrecognized issue worldwide despite an estimated 600,000 maternal deaths per year from pregnancy-related causes.[18,19] Put in numerical perspective, this is equivalent to six jumbo jet crashes per day with the deaths of all 250 passengers on board, all of them women in the reproductive years of life. There is also a marked inequity in geographic distribution, since 95 percent of these deaths occur in developing countries (Fig. 6–1).

The Centers for Disease Control and Prevention (CDC) and the American College of Obstetricians and Gynecologists (ACOG) have introduced the concept that pregnancy-associated mortality is defined as "the death of a woman, from any cause, while she is pregnant or within one year of termination of pregnancy." Unfortunately, the United States is seeing an increase in nonmaternal deaths of pregnant women resulting from trauma and violence, many of these related to illegal drugs (Fig. 6–2).

In North Carolina from 1992 to 1994, 167 deaths to pregnant and postpartum women were identified through an enhanced surveillance system. When all deaths to pregnant women were categorized, direct and indirect obstetric deaths (classically defined maternal deaths) accounted for only 37 percent of deaths to pregnant and postpartum women. Injuries accounted for 38 percent of deaths to pregnant women, with homicide being the most common (36 percent), followed by motor vehicle accidents (32 percent), drug-related death (13 percent), other (11 percent), and suicide (8 percent).[20–23] Acceptance of pregnancy-associated mortality as the appropriate measure will

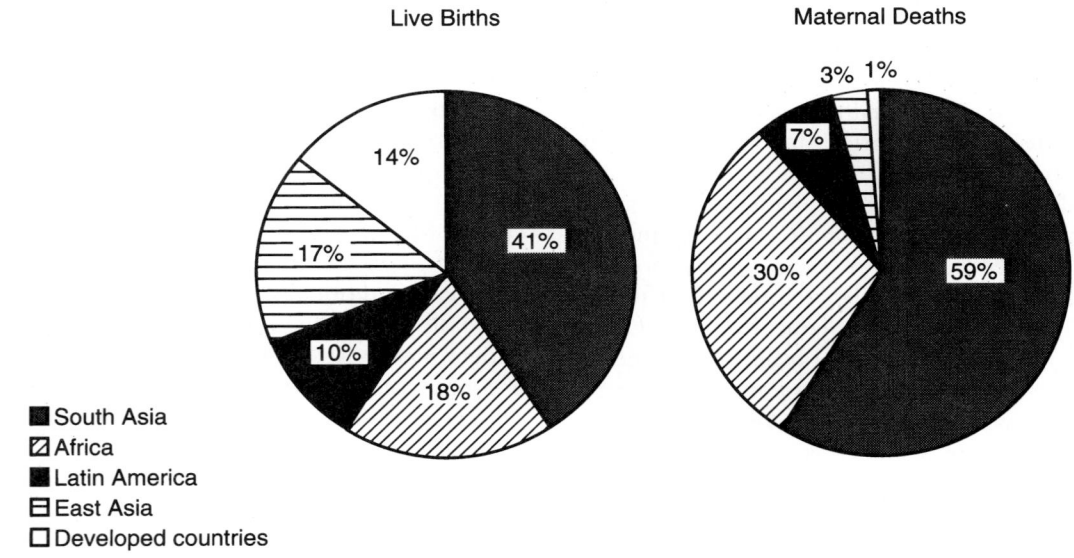

Figure 6–1. Worldwide distribution of live births and maternal deaths by region. (From WHO 861663.)

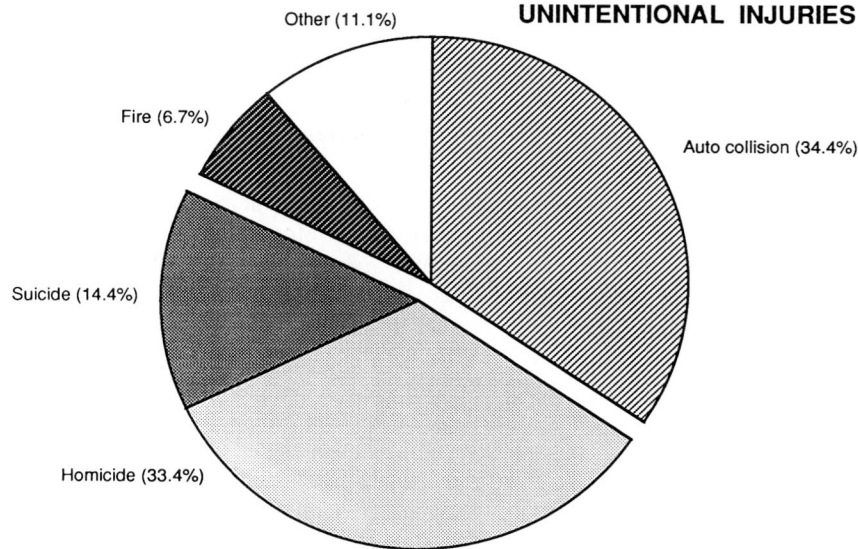

Figure 6–2. Distribution of deaths due to injury in the United States, 1980–1985 (N = 90). (From MMWR Morb Mortal Wkly Rep 37:[SS5]:26, 1988.)

lead to increased recognition of these important problems.

The prenatal care provider can play a role in preventing these common causes of death in women by advocating use of seat belts and screening for alcohol, drug use, depression, and violence.

Significant disparities exist between the maternal mortality ratios of white and black women. In the United States, maternal mortality occurs four times more often in black women than in white women. In a *Morbidity and Mortality Weekly Report* review of maternal deaths in 1990, the maternal mortality ratio for white women was 5.7; for black women it was 18.6, a 3.3-times greater mortality. On a state by-state basis, maternal mortality ratios for black women were higher in every state.[24,25]

NEONATAL MORTALITY AND MORBIDITY

Historically, in developed countries, when decreased maternal mortality was achieved, attention was then turned to fetal mortality and later to fetal morbidity. The stillbirth rate (fetal death rate) is the number of stillborn infants per 1,000 infants born. The neonatal mortality rate is the number of neonatal deaths (deaths in the first 28 days of life) per 1,000 live births. The perinatal mortality combines these two—the number of fetal deaths (stillbirths) plus neonatal deaths per 1,000 total births.

In 1990, the U.S. infant mortality rate was 9.2 per 1,000 live births, ranking the United States 19th inter-

nationally.[26] However, there are international differences in the way live births are classified, as some countries exclude infants weighing less than 1 kg and those with fatal anomalies.

PRENATAL CARE

During the past 20 years, new technology has been introduced to assess the fetus antepartum, including electronic fetal monitoring, sonography, and amniocentesis, with the fetus emerging as a patient in utero. Prevention of morbidity as well as mortality is now the goal. This has made the task of the prenatal clinic more complex, since mother and fetus now require an increasingly sophisticated level of care. At the same time, pregnancy is basically a physiologic process, and the normal pregnant patient may not benefit from application of advanced technology.

Prenatal care is provided at a variety of sites, ranging from the private office, to the public health and county hospital clinics, to the patient's home. Obstetricians must optimize their efforts by resourceful use of other professionals and support groups, including nutritionists, childbirth educators, public health nurses, nurse practitioners, family physicians, nurse midwives, and specialty medical consultants. Most pregnant women are healthy, with normal pregnancies, and can be followed by an obstetric team including nurses, nurse practitioners, and nurse-midwives, with an obstetrician available for consultation. These women can be followed by practitioners who have adequate time to spend on patient education and parenting preparation, while physicians can appropriately concentrate on complicated problems requiring their medical skills. This also provides for improved continuity of care, which is recognized as extremely important for patient satisfaction.[10]

There have been no prospective controlled trials demonstrating efficacy of prenatal care overall. However, many individual components have been shown to be effective (e.g., treatment with corticosteroids to prevent respiratory distress syndrome and screening for and treating asymptomatic bacteriuria for prevention of pyelonephritis).[27] In retrospective studies, however, patients with increased numbers of visits have improved maternal and fetal outcomes. This may be because of self-selection of patients for care who are motivated to take care of themselves in other ways, as women with no prenatal care often come from underprivileged socioeconomic groups.

Efficacy of prenatal care also depends on the quality of care provided by the caretaker. If a blood pressure is recorded as elevated and no therapeutic maneuvers are recommended, this will not change the outcome. Recommendations must be made and must be carried out by the patient, whose compliance is essential to alter outcome.

RISK ASSESSMENT

The concept of risk in obstetrics can be examined at many levels. All the problems that arise in pregnancy, whether common complaints or more hazardous diseases, convey some risk to the pregnancy, depending on how they are managed by the patient and her care provider. Risk assessment has received detailed attention in recent years. It has been shown that most women and infants suffering morbidity and mortality will come from a small segment of women with high-risk factors; by reassessing risk factors before pregnancy, during pregnancy, and again in labor, our ability to identify those at highest risk increases.[28] However, previous preterm birth is the most significant risk factor for prematurity; thus, risk scoring of primigravidas is of limited value.[29,30] Cervical length assessment, fetal fibronectin, and salivary estriol determination have been proposed to assess risk of prematurity (see Chapter 23), and prevention programs have been proposed.[31]

It is important to individualize patient care and to be thorough. The initial visit will include a detailed history and physical and laboratory examinations. The initial history requires that the patient be seen in an office setting. She should not be first seen undressed sitting on an examining table.

PRECONCEPTIONAL EDUCATION

We have reached a level in prenatal care where the optimal time to assess, manage, and treat many pregnancy conditions and complications is before pregnancy occurs.[32,33] The best time to see a woman for prenatal care is when she is considering pregnancy. At gynecologic visits, patients should be asked about their plans for pregnancy. At that time, much of the risk assessment described later in this chapter can be performed, as well as the basic physical and laboratory evaluations. If there are questions about the history, such as diethylstilbestrol (DES) exposure, family history of fetal anomaly, or previous cesarean delivery, further details can be obtained from family members or the appropriate medical facility. This is the time to draw a rubella titer and immunize the susceptible patient. Varicella titers or immunization is recommended in women with no history of chickenpox. Patients need to use contraception for 3 months thereafter (see Chapter 40). Toxoplasmosis screening may be indicated at this time. Patients who have negative screens are at risk for congenital toxoplasmosis and should be counseled to avoid risks such as contact with wild felines and ingestion of raw meat. Patients who screen positive can be reassured of lack of risk. Hepatitis B immunization can be given to appropriate patients and human immunodeficiency virus (HIV) testing offered.

Before pregnancy is the time to screen appropriate populations for genetic disease carrier states such as Tay-Sachs disease, Canavan's disease, cystic fibroisis, or hemoglobinopathies.[34] Resolution of these issues is much easier and less hurried without the time limits placed by an advancing pregnancy. Medical conditions such as anemia, urinary tract infection, or hypothyroidism can be fully evaluated and the woman medically treated before pregnancy. If the patient is obese, weight reduction should be attempted before pregnancy. Patients in whom risks are very serious should be so counseled, and every attempt should be made to let them make a fully informed decision about pregnancy. Often, significant risk factors can be treated or managed so as to reduce risk during pregnancy.

The value of prepregnancy counseling needs to be emphasized to all those who treat women at significant risk for pregnancy problems. Women who are followed by other physicians (family physicians, pediatricians, general internists) for such problems as diabetes, hypertension, or systemic lupus erythematosus should be seen, evaluated, and counseled before pregnancy.

There is evidence that for some conditions, such as diabetes mellitus and phenylketonuria, medical disease management before conception can positively influence pregnancy outcome. Medical management to normalize the biochemical environment should be discussed with the patient and appropriate management plans outlined before conception. This is also the time to review drug usage and other practices, such as alcohol ingestion and smoking (see Chapter 9). Advice can be given about avoiding medications in the first trimester, and general advice can be given concerning diet, exercise, and occupational exposures.

Periconceptional supplements with folic acid can reduce the incidence of neural tube defects (NTDs). In a randomized prospective trial of women with a previously affected child, 4 mg folic acid daily lowered the recurrence risk of neural tube defects by 72 percent.[35] In a prospective trial of women planning their first pregnancy, 0.8 mg of folic acid daily prevented first-occurrence neural tube defects and other defects.[36] The CDC recommends that all women of childbearing age who are capable of becoming pregnant should consume 0.4 mg of folic acid daily, which is most easily achieved by taking a supplement. For women with a previously affected child, the recommendation is that the patient take 4 mg daily from 4 weeks before conception through the first 3 months of pregnancy.

The importance of gestational age dating can be discussed with the patient. Great precision can be achieved with an accurate menstrual calendar predating pregnancy.

THE INITIAL PRECONCEPTIONAL OR PRENATAL VISIT

Social and Demographic Risks

Extremes of age are obstetric risk factors. The pregnant teenager has particular nutritional and emotional needs. She is at special risk for sexually transmitted diseases; it has been shown that she benefits particularly from education in areas of childbearing and contraception. The pregnant woman over age 35 is at increased risk for a chromosomally abnormal child,[37] and she must be so advised. Patients should be asked about family histories of Down syndrome, neural tube defects, hemophilia, hemoglobinopathies, and other birth defects, as well as mental retardation (see Chapter 8). Consultation for genetic counseling and genetic testing, if desired, may be appropriate. The age of the father may be important, as there may be genetic risks to the fetus when the father is older than 55 years.[38] Certain diseases may be race related. Black patients should be screened for sickle cell disease; those of Jewish and French Canadian heritage should be screened for Tay-Sachs disease, Canavan's disease, and cystic fibrosis; and those of Mediterranean descent should be screened for β-thalassemia.

Low socioeconomic status should be identified and attempts to improve nutritional and hygienic measures undertaken. Appropriate referral to federal programs, such as that for women, infants, and children (WIC), and to public health nurses can have real benefits. If a patient has a history of previous neonatal death or stillbirth, records should be carefully reviewed so that the correct diagnosis is made and recurrence risk appropriately assessed. A history of drug abuse or recent blood transfusion should be elicited. The history of the patient's mother's reproductive record may lead to discovery of DES exposure. The history of medical illnesses should be detailed and records obtained if possible. A new rapid procedure for diagnosing mental disorders in primary care may be useful in pregnancy.[39]

Occupational hazards should be identified. If a patient works in a laboratory with chemicals, for example, she should be advised to limit her exposure. Patients whose occupations require heavy physical exercise or excess stress should be informed that they may need to decrease such activity.

Tobacco, alcohol, and recreational drug use can all adversely affect pregnancy and are a critical part of the history. Specific questions concerning smoking, alcohol, and drugs (prescriptive, over-the-counter, and illicit) should be asked.[40] Regular screening for alcohol and substance use should be carried out using such tools as the T-ACE questionnaire (Table 6–1)[41] or other simple screening tools, and appropriate directed therapy should be made available to those women who screen positive. Women should be urged to stop smoking prior to pregnancy and to drink not at all or minimally once they are pregnant. Drug addiction confers a particularly

Table 6–1. ALCOHOL ABUSE SCREENING: THE T-ACE QUESTIONNAIRE*

T	How many drinks does it take to make you feel "high" (can you hold)? (*tolerance;* a positive response consists of two or more drinks)
A	Have people *annoyed* you by criticizing your drinking?
C	Have you ever felt you ought to *cut down* on your drinking?
E	Have you ever had a drink first thing in the morning to steady your nerves or to get rid of a hangover (*eye-opener*)?

Scoring: The tolerance question has substantially more weight (2 points) than the three other questions (1 point each).

*These questions were found to be significant identifiers of risk drinking in pregnancy (i.e., alcohol intake potentially sufficient to damage the embryo/fetus).

From Sokol RJ, Martier SS, Ager JW: The T-ACE questions: practical prenatal detection of risk-drinking. Am J Obstet Gynecol 160:863, 1989, with permission.

high risk, and addicted mothers require specialized care throughout pregnancy (see Chapter 9).

Violence against women is increasingly recognized as a problem that should be addressed, with reports suggesting that abuse occurs during 3 to 8 percent of pregnancies. Questions addressing personal safety and violence should be included during the prenatal period, and such tools as the Abuse Assessment Score (Fig. 6–3) are recommended.[41-43]

Medical Risk

Family history of diabetes, hypertension, tuberculosis, seizures, hematologic disorders, multiple pregnancies, congenital abnormalities, and reproductive wastage should be elicited. Often, a family history of mental retardation, birth defect, or genetic trait is difficult to elicit; these areas should be emphasized at the initial history. A better history may be obtained if patients are asked to fill out a preinterview questionnaire or history form. Any significant maternal cardiovascular, renal, or metabolic disease should be defined. Infectious diseases such as urinary tract disease, syphilis, tuberculosis, or herpes genitalis should be identified. Surgical history with special attention to any abdominal or pelvic operations should be noted. A history of previous cesarean birth should include indication, type of uterine incision, and any complications. A copy of the surgical report may be informative. Allergies, particularly

Abuse Assessment Screen (Circle YES or NO for each question)

1. Have you ever been emotionally or physically abused by your partner or someone important to you? . . . . YES NO

2. Within the last year, have you been hit, slapped, kicked, or otherwise physically hurt by someone? . . . . YES NO

   If YES, by whom (circle all that apply)

   Husband   Ex-husband   Boyfriend   Stranger   Other   Multiple

   Total No. of times _____

3. Since you've been pregnant, have you been hit, slapped, kicked, or otherwise physically hurt by someone? . . . . YES NO

   If YES, by whom (circle all that apply)

   Husband   Ex-husband   Boyfriend   Stranger   Other   Multiple

   Total No. of times _____

   Mark the area of injury on a body map

   Score each incident according to the following scale:

   1 = Threats of abuse, including use of a weapon
   2 = Slapping, pushing; no injuries and/or lasting pain
   3 = Punching, kicking, bruises, cuts, and/or continuing pain
   4 = Beaten up, severe contusions, burns, broken bones
   5 = Head, internal, and/or permanent injury
   6 = Use of weapon, wound from weapon

   (If any of the descriptions for the higher number apply, use the higher number)

4. Within the last year, has anyone forced you to have sexual activities? . . . YES NO

   If YES, by whom (circle all that apply)

   Husband   Ex-husband   Boyfriend   Stranger   Other   Multiple

   Total No. of times _____

5. Are you afraid of your partner or anyone you listed above? . . . . YES NO

Figure 6–3. Determination of frequency and severity of physical abuse during pregnancy. (From McFarlane J, Parker B, Soeken K, Bullock L: Assessing for abuse during pregnancy. JAMA 267:3176, 1992, with permission. Copyright 1992, American Medical Association.)

drug allergies, should be prominent on the problem list.

Obstetric Risk

Previous obstetric and reproductive history are essential to care in subsequent pregnancy. The gravidity and parity should be noted and the outcome for each prior pregnancy recorded in detail. Previous miscarriages not only confer risk and anxiety for another pregnancy loss but can increase the risk of genetic disease as well as preterm delivery.[44]

Previous preterm delivery is strongly associated with recurrence; it is important to delineate the events surrounding the preterm birth. Did the membranes rupture before labor? Were there painful uterine contractions? Was there bleeding? Were there fetal abnormalities? What was the neonatal outcome? All these questions are vital in determining the etiology and prognosis of the condition, although specific recommendations will vary and the efficacy of routine prevention programs is not clear.[31,45,46] DES exposure, incompetent cervix, and uterine anomalies are all conditions that may be known from a previous pregnancy. Previous fetal macrosomia makes glucose screening essential.

After all the specific questions, it is recommended to ask the patient a few simple questions: What important items haven't I asked? What else about you and your pregnancy do I need to know? What problems and questions do you have? Leaving time for open-ended questions is the best way to complete the initial visit.

Physical and Laboratory Evaluation

Physical examination should include a general physical examination as well as a pelvic examination. Baseline height and weight as well as prepregnancy weight are recorded. Special attention should be given to the initial vital signs, cardiac examination, and reflexes, since many healthy young women have not had a physical examination immediately before becoming pregnant. Any physical finding that might have an impact on pregnancy (e.g., DES changes in the cervix) or that might be affected by pregnancy (e.g., mitral valve prolapse) should be defined. Any factor that might become important later in pregnancy in assessing pathology or disease (e.g., reflexes) should be carefully noted. It is particularly important to perform and record a complete physical examination at this initial visit, since less emphasis will be placed on nonobstetric portions of the examination as pregnancy progresses in the absence of specific problems or complaints.

The pelvic examination should focus on the uterine size. Before 12 to 14 weeks, size can give a fairly accurate estimate of gestational age. Papanicolaou smear and culture for gonorrhea and chlamydia are done. Bacterial vaginosis should be recognized. The cervix should be carefully palpated, and any deviation from normal should be noted. Clinical pelvimetry should be performed and the clinical impression of adequacy noted. The pelvic examination is limited by examiner and patient variation as well as by obesity. If there is difficulty in examining the uterus, an ultrasound study is indicated.

Basic laboratory studies are routinely performed (Table 6–2). Some studies need not be repeated if recent normal values have been obtained, such as at an initial visit following a preconceptional visit or a recent gynecologic examination. Blood studies should include Rh type and screening for irregular antibodies, hemoglobin level, or hematocrit and serologic tests for syphilis and rubella. A urine sample should be obtained and tested for abnormal protein and glucose levels. Screening for asymptomatic bacteriuria has been traditionally done by urine culture, but screening may be simplified by testing for nitrites and leukocyte esterase.[47] Tuberculosis screening should also be performed in areas of disease prevalence.

The triple screen (α-fetoprotein, human chorionic gonadotropin [hCG], and estriol) or maternal serum α-fetoprotein screening is offered at 15 to 16 weeks' gestation to screen for neural tube defects (see Chapter 8).

The laboratory evaluations outlined above are the minimum standard tests. Specific conditions will require further evaluation. A history of thyroid disease will lead to thyroid function testing. Anticonvulsant therapy requires blood level studies to determine adequacy of medication. Identification of problems on screening (e.g., anemia, abnormal glucose screen) will mandate further testing. Screening for varicella has been suggested for women with no known history of chickenpox.

The ACOG has recommended routine screening of all pregnant women for hepatitis B.[34] At high risk are women of Asian descent, health care workers exposed to blood or blood products, women with previously undiagnosed jaundice or liver disease, parenteral drug abusers, prostitutes, women with tatoos, women with a history of blood transfusion, dialysis or renal transplant patients, women who work or reside in institutions for the retarded, and household contacts of persons infected with hepatitis B. HIV screening in high-risk populations should also be offered, since maternal therapy with azidothymidine (AZT) can reduce vertical transmission (see Chapter 40).[34]

Recommendations of the Public Health Service[4] for the content of prenatal care are summarized in Table 6–2.

Table 6-2. RECOMMENDATIONS FOR ALL WOMEN FOR PRENATAL CARE

	Preconception or First Visit	Weeks								
		6-8*	14-16	24-28	32	36	38	39	40	41
History										
Medical, including genetic	X									
Psychosocial	X									
Update medical and psychosocial		X	X	X	X	X	X	X	X	X
Physical examination										
General	X									
Blood pressure	X	X	X	X	X	X	X	X	X	X
Height	X									
Weight	X	X	X	X	X	X	X	X	X	X
Height and weight profile	X									
Pelvic examination and pelvimetry	X	X								
Breast examination	X	X								
Fundal height			X	X	X	X	X	X	X	X
Fetal position and heart rate			X	X	X	X	X	X	X	X
Cervical examination	X									
Laboratory tests										
Hemoglobin or hematocrit	X	X		X		X				
Rh factor, type blood	X									
Antibody screen	X			X						
Pap smear	X									
Diabetic screen				X						
MSAFP			X							
Urine										
Dipstick	X									
Protein	X									
Sugar	X									
Culture		X								
Infections										
Rubella titer	X									
Syphilis test	X									
Gonococcal culture	X	X				X				
Hepatitis B	X									
HIV (offered)	X	X								
Toxoplasmosis	X									
Illicit drug screen (offered)	X									
Genetic screen	X									

*If preconception care has preceded.
MSAFP, maternal serum α-fetoprotein; HIV, human immunodeficiency virus.

REPEAT PRENATAL VISITS

A plan of visits is outlined to the patient. This has been traditionally every 4 weeks for the first 28 weeks of pregnancy, every 2 to 3 weeks until 36 weeks, and weekly thereafter, if the pregnancy progresses normally. The Public Health Service[4] suggested that this number of visits can be decreased, especially in parous, healthy women, and another study suggests that this can be done safely.[9,46] If there are any complications, the intervals can be increased appropriately. For example, patients with hypertensive disease may require weekly visits. Fetal heart tones can be documented before the 12th week by Doppler devices and generally by the 20th week by Hillis-Delee stethoscope, and this information can be used for gestational dating purposes.

At regular visits, the patient is weighed, the blood pressure is recorded, and the presence of edema is evaluated. Fundal height is regularly measured with a tape measure, fetal heart tones are recorded, and fetal position is noted. The goal of subsequent pregnancy visits is to assess fetal growth and maternal well-being. In addition, at each prenatal visit, time should be allowed for the following questions: Do you have any problems? Do you have any questions? Family members should be encouraged to come to prenatal visits, ask questions, and participate to the degree that the patient wishes.

A pelvic examination is usually only performed on

the first visit. In patients at risk of prematurity or in those with a history of DES exposure, however, frequent cervical checks may reveal premature dilation or effacement.

Prenatal screening to include early ultrasound for genetic screening, triple test screening for NTDs and aneuploidy, as well as fetal anatomic survey at 18 to 20 weeks are also common practice.

Further laboratory evaluations are routinely performed at 28 weeks, when the hemoglobin or hematocrit and Rh type and the screen for antibodies, as well as the serologic test for syphilis and possibly HIV testing, can be repeated. If the patient is Rh negative and unsensitized, she should receive Rhesus immune globulin (RhIG) prophylaxis at this time. A glucose screening test for diabetes is also appropriately performed at this time (see Chapter 32),[48] and routine fetal movement counting can begin using a organized system.[49] At 36 weeks, a repeat hematocrit, especially in those women with anemia or at risk for peripartum hemorrhage (multipara, repeat cesarean), may be performed. Also, appropriate cultures for sexually transmitted disease (gonorrhea, chlamydia) should be obtained as indicated in the third trimester.

After 41 weeks from the last menstrual period, the patient should be entered into a screening program for fetal well-being, which may include electronic monitoring tests or ultrasound evaluation (see Chapter 27).

nancy in order to accept and explain the normal, but also to manage aggressively any abnormal changes.

Proteinuria reflects urinary tract disease, generally either infection or glomerular dysfunction, possibly the result of preeclampsia. Urinary tract infection should be looked for, and the degree of protein quantitated in a 24-hour urine collection.

Glycosuria, while common because of increased glucose filtered through the kidney in pregnancy, warrants evaluation for diabetes with a measurement of capillary glucose.

Fetal abnormalities are usually first detected by deviation from the clinical expectation. In some conditions, risk of fetal anomaly will be so high as to prompt some kind of baseline screening or testing (e.g., amniocentesis, sonography, fetal echocardiography). At other times, risk only becomes evident during the course of prenatal care. Growth restriction and macrosomia can often be suspected clinically, usually on the basis of an abnormality in fundal growth. For the patient who has a history of these conditions or other predisposing factors, such as hypertension, renal disease, or diabetes, particular vigilance is in order. Excess amniotic fluid is another condition that can be clinically detected, and an etiology for the hydramnios should be sought. In addition to maternal conditions, hydramnios may be caused by fetal disease that can also be defined using sonography and that may alter management of the pregnancy.

INTERCURRENT PROBLEMS

It is the practice in prenatal care to evaluate the pregnant patient for the development of certain complications. Inherent in these checks is surveillance for intervening problems, an important one being preeclampsia. If a patient shows a tendency to blood pressure elevation at 28 weeks, for example, she should be seen again in a week, not a month. Blood pressure will change physiologically in response to pregnancy, but development of hypertension must be recognized and evaluation and hospitalization appropriately instituted.

Weight gain in pregnancy has been shown to be an important correlate of fetal weight gain and is therefore closely monitored. Too little weight gain should lead to an evaluation of nutritional factors and an assessment of associated fetal growth. Excess weight gain is one of the first signs of fluid retention, but it may also reflect increased dietary intake or decreased activity. Dependent edema is physiologic in pregnancy, but generalized or facial edema can be a first sign of disease. It is critical here, as in all areas, for the practitioner to understand the normal changes associated with preg-

THE PRENATAL RECORD

Prenatal care should be documented by a prenatal record of good quality such as the antepartum record designed by the ACOG.[6] Many of the advances in risk assessment and in regionalization result directly from an improvement in this record. Technology allows sophisticated recording, display, and retrieval (often computer-based) of prenatal care records, but quality relies on accurate compiling and recording of the information. The record must be complete, yet simple; directive, but flexible; and transmittable, legible, and able to display necessary data rapidly. European nations often have one record for uniform care; many states and regions have adopted records to permit internal consistency.

The commonly used records accurately reflect the following:

1. Demographic data, obstetric history
2. Medical and family history, including genetic screening

3. Baseline physical examination, with emphasis on gynecologic examination
4. Menstrual history, especially last normal menstrual period
5. Record of individual visits
6. Routine laboratory data
7. Problem list
8. Space for special notations and plans

These records must be made available to consultants, and they should be available at the facility where delivery is planned. If transfer is expected, a copy of the prenatal record should accompany the patient.

PRENATAL EDUCATION

Patient education leads to better self-care. As maternal and neonatal outcomes improve, efforts become more sophisticated to improve understanding, involvement, and satisfaction with pregnancy and the perinatal period. In this area, more than any other, the options for paramedical support have expanded. Practitioners and patients have access to a vast array of support persons and groups to assist and advise in the pregnancy and subsequent parenthood. The wise practitioner stays abreast of these advances and integrates them into practice. Patients should be educate about care options and participate in decision-making.

Informed Consent and VBAC

During the educational components of prenatal care there is significant opportunity to accomplish most if not all the informed consent required for the delivery process. There are also advantages to securing documentation of appropriate informed consent for management of labor and associated obstetric procedures, possible interventions, and risks and benefits when they can be thoroughly reviewed and discussed rather than in the throes of labor It is our practice to obtain consent, whenever possible, in the third trimester for "delivery and related procedures including IV fluids, fetal monitoring, labor augmentation, operative vaginal delivery including forceps and vacuum and cesarean delivery," and this is documented on institutional consent forms and signed by the patient (Fig. 6–4). Consent for anesthesia can also be obtained prior to admission.

The special benefits and risks of vaginal birth after cesarean section are particularly important to discuss prior to labor, and it is common to document both the components of the informed consent process as well as the patient's choice with respect to route of delivery (Fig. 6–5).

Drugs and Teratogens

At the preconceptional or first prenatal visit, recommendations for nonpharmacologic remedies for common ailments can be given. This can often be integrated into a discussion of the common side effects of pregnancy. Because of widespread use of over-the-counter drugs, the patient should be warned to take only those drugs specifically approved or prescribed by her practitioner (see Chapter 9).

Radiologic Studies

Dental and radiologic diagnostic procedures should be performed during pregnancy when they are indicated. Dental restorative work especially should be performed to allow optimal maternal nutrition. Elective radiologic studies can safely be delayed until completion of the pregnancy.

Nutrition

One of the earliest purposes of prenatal care was to counsel and ensure that women received adequate nutrition for pregnancy. The health care provider may be influential in correcting inappropriate dietary habits.[50] Strict vegetarians may need supplemental vitamin B_{12}. Occasionally, consultation with a registered dietitian may be necessary when there is poor compliance or a special medical need such as diabetes mellitus.

The U.S. Department of Agriculture has published the new food guide pyramid.[51] Americans are encouraged to eat 6 to 11 servings per day of bread, cereal, rice, and pasta; three to five servings per day of vegetables; two to four servings per day of fruit; two to three servings per day of milk, yogurt, and cheese; and two to three servings per day of meat, poultry, fish, beans, eggs, and nuts. Fats, oils, and sweets should be used sparingly. Pregnant women need three servings per day of dairy products, a serving being a cup of milk or yogurt, $1\frac{1}{2}$ oz of natural cheese, or 2 oz processed cheese.

Dietary allowances for most substances increase during pregnancy. According to the 1989 recommended dietary allowances (RDAs), only the recommendations for iron, folic acid, and vitamin D double during gestation.[52] The RDA for calcium and phosphorus increase by one half; the RDA for pyridoxine and thiamine increase by about one third. The RDA for protein, zinc, and riboflavin increase by about one fourth. The RDA for all other nutrients except vitamin A increase by less than 20 percent (Tables 6–3 and 6–4) and vitamin A not at all, as that is felt to be stored adequately. All of these nutrients, with the exception of iron, are supplied by a well-balanced diet.

The National Academy of Sciences currently recom-

Pregnancy Information

Both the obstetric patient and her physicians and nurses want the same things for every pregnancy. They are: a comfortable pregnancy free of complications, an easy labor and delivery, and a healthy mother and baby when all is over. In our practice, to a greater or lesser extent, most patients achieve such outcomes. Complications can occur, however, and bad things at times do happen to good people.

The rationale for prenatal care is to prevent complications if possible, to identify complications if they occur, and to manage identified complications so as to minimize their adverse effects. Much of this is <u>our</u> job, but it is <u>your</u> job to keep your appointments, to avoid exposures to chemicals and drugs of abuse including cigarettes, and to use your seatbelts.

Mother Although pregnancy is a stress on you, most women tolerate pregnancy well. Depending on your situation, we may recommend a modification of your activities. Death of the mother during pregnancy is very unusual, but can occur either in mothers with serious underlying illnesses or from rare, but extremely serious obstetric problems. Other risks to the mother include organ injuries (for example, rectum or bladder), infections and hemorrhage. You may require blood transfusions if you have heavy bleeding. Blood is very safe, and the donors are tested for AIDS and hepatitis, but the risk of acquiring infections from blood transfusions is not zero. This is why we are conservative in our use of blood products.

Baby Babies are healthiest if they are full term and appropriately grown. This is why we will instruct you about warning signs of premature labor (cramping, intermittent back pain, vaginal spotting or change in discharge, and pressure in the pelvis), and why we measure the uterus (to get an idea of the size of the baby) at the time of your prenatal visits.

In the latter part of pregnancy, if you are worried about a decrease or lack of the baby's movements, call it to our attention promptly. Do not wait for your next appointment.

All parents fear malformations or birth defects. Although often these can be identified by testing, this is not always so. For example, just because an ultrasound examination does not indicate a particular problem, this does not mean with certainty that it is not there. One in 25 babies is born with a malformation. Many of these are minor or can be successfully corrected.

Cesarean Birth Fifteen to twenty percent of patients in our hospital are delivered by this operation. This is a very safe operation, but is a major operation nonetheless. Cesareans are done for complications in the mother or baby, and are only done with your permission. Risks include injury to normal structures, hemorrhage, infection and anesthetic complications. Most of these can be managed without lasting harm, but occasionally are associated with the need for additional surgery, including hysterectomy, or with continuing difficulties. Rarely, death or severe, permanent problems, including brain damage, may result.

VBAC Most women with previous cesarean births are candidates for attempted vaginal birth after cesarean, or VBAC. Most women successfully complete VBAC trials. If so, the discomforts and risks of cesarean birth are avoided. Approximately one-quarter to one-third of the time, the VBAC attempt will be unsuccessful, and repeat cesarean birth will be required. The most serious complication specifically attributable to VBAC is rupture of the uterus. This occurs less than 1% of the time, but is serious for both mother and baby and emergency surgery is required.

The purpose of the preceding paragraphs is not to frighten you, but to make certain you understand that complications can occur. We will be happy to answer your questions regarding this pregnancy information today or in the future.

I have read the above information and have had opportunity to have my questions answered. I realize that the practice of obstetrics is not an exact science and that no guarantees have been made.

PATIENT: _____

PHYSICIAN: _____

Figure 6–4. Example of prenatal education and consent form. (Courtesy of Dr. Frank Zlatnik.)

UNIVERSITY OF MICHIGAN HOSPITALS
Department of Obstetrics & Gynecology
Consent Form for
Trial of Labor/Repeat Cesarean Section

Date:_____

You have had a previous cesarean section. Although "once a cesarean always a cesarean section" used to be the rule, some women may choose to attempt a vaginal delivery, called a "trial of labor". The American College of Obstetricians and Gynecologists recommend that women with one previous cesarean delivery with a low transverse incision should be encouraged to attempt labor.

Your doctor or nurse-midwife will review the records of your cesarean section to determine whether or not you may safely attempt labor. A safe attempt to deliver vaginally is based on the type of uterine scar that you have. The previous incision in your uterus may have been transverse (back and forth) or vertical (up and down); this may be different from the incision in your skin.

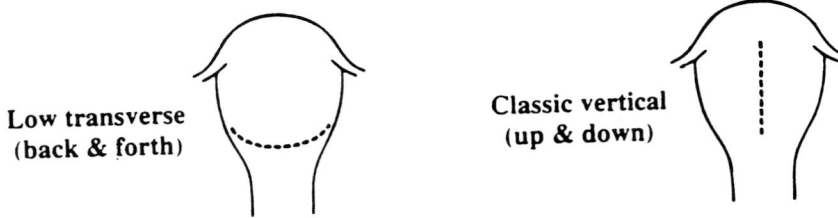

Low transverse   **Classic vertical**
(back & forth)   **(up & down)**

Some vertical incisions are known to be weaker and at greater risk of opening or rupturing during labor. Therefore, women with vertical uterine scars should not be allowed to labor. If you have had more than one cesarean section, it will be necessary to examine the operative note from each of your deliveries.

Large studies have found a success rate of vaginal deliveries in 70%-80% for women who have a trial of labor. The alternative to a trial of labor is to have a repeat cesarean section, without labor. Most obstetricians recommend a repeat cesarean section if the baby is expected to be very large, if the baby is in a breech or transverse position, or for twins.

There are benefits and risks of a trial of labor. The benefits of a vaginal delivery after cesarean section include a shorter hospital stay and recovery period for you. A vaginal delivery is considered safer than a cesarean section for the mother, with less blood loss and less risk of infection. The baby may benefit from vaginal birth by less remaining lung fluid after the first breath.

The risks of vaginal delivery after cesarean section should be understood as well. You may require a cesarean section during labor. If you do, you have a higher risk of infection. Cesarean section, however, does not guarantee a healthy/normal baby. Finally, there is a small (<1-2%) risk of the uterus opening in the area of the old incision. If this happens, it could cause distress, permanent injury or death to your baby, excessive bleeding, and rarely may require a hysterectomy (removal of the uterus).

If you qualify for a vaginal delivery after cesarean section, then you may choose to either plan a trial of labor or a repeat cesarean section. Your doctor or nurse-midwife will answer any questions that you may have.

_____ Please initial here that you have read and understand the risks and benefits of each procedure.

I have had the opportunity to have my questions answered and I elect:

☐   A trial of labor,

☐   A repeat cesarean section delivery.

_____ _____	_____ _____
signature date	witness signature date

PS2317 7/98 MEDICAL RECORDS	University of Michigan Medical Center	TRIAL OF LABOR/REPEAT CESAREAN

Figure 6–5. Consent form for trial of labor/repeat cesarean section.

Table 6-3. 1989 RECOMMENDED DIETARY ALLOWANCES

| | Nonpregnant Women | | | | Lactation (Months) | |
	15-18	19-24	25-50	Pregnancy	1-6	7-12
Calories (kcal)						
Protein (g)	44	46	50	60	65	62
Vitamin A (μg RE)	800	800	800	800	1,300	1,200
Vitamin D (μg)	10	5	5	10	10	10
Vitamin E (mg TE)	8	8	8	10	12	11
Vitamin C (mg)	60	60	60	70	95	90
Thiamin (mg)	1.1	1.1	1.1	1.5	1.6	1.6
Riboflavin (mg)	1.3	1.3	1.3	1.6	1.8	1.7
Niacin (mg NE)	15	15	15	17	20	20
Vitamin B_6 (mg)	1.5	1.6	1.6	12.2	2.1	2.1
Folate (μg)	180	180	180	400	280	260
Vitamin B_{12} (μg)	2.0	2.0	2.0	2.2	2.6	2.6
Calcium (mg)	1,200	1,200	800	1,200	1,200	1,200
Phosphorus (mg)	1,200	1,200	800	1,200	1,200	1,200
Magnesium (mg)	300	280	280	320	355	340
Iron (mg)	15	15	15	30	15	15
Zinc (mg)	12	12	12	15	19	16
Iodine (μg)	150	150	150	175	200	200
Selenium μg	50	55	55	65	75	75

Data from Spitzer RL, Williams JBW, Kroenke K, et al: Utility of a new procedure for diagnosing mental disorders in primary care. JAMA 272:1749, 1994.

mends that 30 mg of ferrous iron supplements be given to pregnant women daily, since the iron content of the habitual American diet and the iron stores of many women are not sufficient to provide the increased iron required during pregnancy. For those at high nutritional risk, such as some adolescents, those with multiple gestation, heavy cigarette smokers, and drug and alcohol abusers, a vitamin/mineral supplement should be given. Increased iron is needed both for the fetal needs and for the increased maternal blood volume. Thus, iron-containing foods should also be encouraged. Iron is found in liver, red meats, eggs, dried beans, leafy green vegetables, whole-grain enriched bread and cereal, and dried fruits. The 30-mg iron supplement is

Table 6-4. SUMMARY OF RECOMMENDED DIETARY ALLOWANCES FOR WOMEN AGED ≥ 25-50 YEARS, CHANGES FROM NONPREGNANT TO PREGNANT, AND FOOD SOURCES

Nutrient	Nonpregnant	Pregnant	Percent Increase	Dietary Sources
Energy (kcal)	2,200	2,500	+13.6	Proteins, carbohydrates, fats
Protein (g)	50	60	+20	Meats, fish, poultry, dairy
Calcium (mg)	800	1,200	+50	Dairy products
Phosphorus (mg)	800	1,200	+50	Meats
Magnesium (mg)	280	320	+14.3	Seafood, legumes, grains
Iron (mg)	15	30	+100	Meats, eggs, grains
Zinc (mg)	12	15	+25	Meats, seafood, eggs
Iodine (μg)	150	175	+16.7	Iodized salt, seafood
Vitamin A (μg RE)	800	800	0	Dark green, yellow, or orange fruits and vegetables, liver
Vitamin D (IU)	200	400	+100	Fortified dairy products
Thiamin (mg)	1.2	1.5	+36.3	Enriched grains, pork
Riboflavin (mg)	1.3	1.6	+23	Meats, liver, enriched grains
Pyridoxine (mg)	1.6	2.2	+37.5	Meats, liver, enriched grains
Niacin (mg NE)	15	17	+13.3	Meats, nuts, legumes
Vitamin B_{12} (μg)	2.0	2.2	+10	Meats
Folic acid (μg)	180	400	+122	Leafy vegetables, liver
Vitamin C (mg)	60	70	+16.7	Citrus fruits, tomatoes
Selenium (μg)	55	65	+18.2	

From National Academy of Sciences: Recommended Dietary Allowances, 10th ed. Washington, DC, National Academy Press, 1989.

contained in approximately 150 mg of ferrous sulfate, 300 mg of ferrous gluconate, or 100 mg of ferrous fumarate. Taking iron between meals on an empty stomach will facilitate its absorption.

Since women of higher socioeconomic status have better reproductive performance and fewer low-birth-weight babies than do women of lower socioeconomic status, and since they also consume more protein, it is probably prudent to continue to recommend a generous amount of dietary protein. However, it has not been documented that protein supplementation will improve pregnancy outcome.[53] Acute caloric restriction in a well-nourished population such as occurred during the Dutch famine of 1944 to 1945 caused the average birth weight to drop about 250 g, yet no adverse effect on long-term outcome was observed. These mothers ate a calorie-restricted, balanced diet in their second and third trimesters.

Weight Gain

The total weight gain recommended in pregnancy is 25 to 35 lb for normal women.[54] Underweight women may gain up to 40 lb, and overweight women should limit weight gain to 15 to 25 lb. About 2 to 3 lb are from increased fluid volume, 3 to 4 lb from increased blood volume, 1 to 2 lb from breast enlargement, 2 lb from enlargement of the uterus, and 2 lb from amniotic fluid. At term, the infant weighs approximately 6 to 8 lb and the placenta 1 to 2 lb. A 4- to 6-lb increase in maternal stores of fat and protein are important for lactation. Usually, 3 to 6 lb are gained in the first trimester and $\frac{1}{2}$ to 1 lb per week in the last two trimesters of pregnancy.

If the patient does not show a 10-lb weight gain by midpregnancy, her nutritional status should be reviewed. Inadequate weight gain is associated with an increased risk of a low-birth-weight infant (Fig. 6–6). Inadequate weight gain seems to have its greatest effect in woman who are of low or normal weight before pregnancy. Underweight mothers must gain more weight during pregnancy to produce infants of normal weight. Patients should be cautioned against weight loss during pregnancy. Total weight gain in the obese can be modified downward to 15 lb, but less weight gain is associated with lack of expansion of plasma volume and the risk of intrauterine growth retardation.

When excess weight gain is noted, an assessment for fluid retention is also performed. In the assessment of edema, some dependent edema in the legs is normal as pregnancy advances because of venous compression by the weight of the uterus. Elevation of the feet and bed rest on the left side will help correct this problem. Turning the patient from her back to her left side increases venous return from the legs as the pressure on

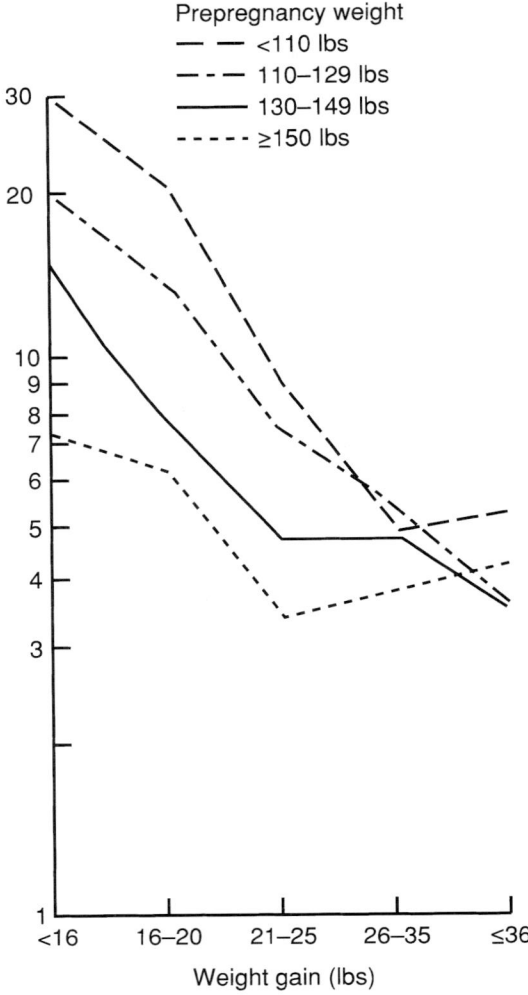

Figure 6–6. Percentage of live-born infants of low birth weight by maternal weight gain during pregnancy according to the mother's prepregnancy weight. Low birth weight is defined as birth weight of less than 2,500 g or 5 lb, 8 oz. (From the National Natality Survey—United States. DHHS Pub No. [PHS] 86-1922, 1980.)

the vena cava is relieved. This maneuver increases the effective circulating blood volume, cardiac output, and thus the blood flow to the kidney. A diuresis will follow as well as increased blood flow to the uterus.

Limitation of fluids will neither prevent nor correct fluid retention. Salt is not restricted, although patients with hypertension may be advised to decrease salt load.

Rest

During the first trimester, patients are often more tired and should be advised to go to bed earlier or to try to take a nap during the day, if possible. Fatigue often lessens in the second trimester but, in general, most patients need additional rest during pregnancy.

Activity and Employment

Most patients are able to maintain their normal activity levels in pregnancy. Mothers tolerate pregnancy with considerable physical activity, such as looking after small children, but heavy lifting and excessive physical activity should be avoided. Modification of activity level as the pregnancy progresses is seldom needed, except if the job involves physical danger. Recreational exercises should be encouraged, such as those available in prenatal exercise classes. The patient should be counseled to discontinue activity whenever she experiences discomfort.

Healthy pregnant women may work until their delivery, if the job presents hazards no greater than those encountered in daily life. Strenuous physical exercise, standing for prolonged periods, and work on industrial machines as well as other adverse environmental factors may be associated with increased risk of poor pregnancy outcome, and these should be modified as necessary.[55-57]

Travel

The patient should be advised against prolonged sitting during car or airplane travel because of the risk of venous stasis and possible thromboembolism. The usual recommendation is a maximum of 6 hours per day driving, with stopping at least every 2 hours for 10 minutes to allow the patient to walk around and increase venous return from the legs. Support stockings are also recommended.

The patient should be instructed to wear her seat belt during car travel, but under the abdomen as pregnancy advances. It may also be helpful to take pillows along in a car to increase comfort.

If the patient is traveling a significant distance, it might be helpful for her to carry a copy of her medical record with her in case an emergency arises in a strange environment. She could also check into the medical facilities in the area or perhaps obtain the name of an obstetrician in the event of a problem.

Immunizations

Because of a theoretical risk to the fetus, pregnant women or women likely to become pregnant should not be given live, attenuated-virus vaccines. Yellow fever and oral polio may be given to women exposed to these infections. Despite theoretical risks, no evidence of congenital rubella syndrome in infants born to mothers inadvertently given rubella vaccine has been reported. Measles, mumps, and rubella viruses are not transmitted by those immunized and can be given to children of pregnant women. There is no evidence of fetal risk from inactivated virus vaccines, bacterial vaccines, toxoids, or tetanus immunoglobulin, which should be administered if appropriate.

Nausea and Vomiting in Pregnancy

Nonpharmacologic measures are usually recommended initially to treat nausea and vomiting in early pregnancy. Patients should avoid eating greasy or spicy foods. In addition, frequent small feedings in order to keep some food in the stomach at all times is helpful. A protein snack at night is advised, and the patient is instructed to keep crackers at her bedside so that she can have these before arising in the morning. Drug therapy for nausea in pregnancy is covered in Chapter 9.

Heartburn

Heartburn is a common complaint in pregnancy because of relaxation of the esophageal sphincter. Overeating contributes to this problem, as do spicy foods. The patient should be advised to save part of her meal for later if she is experiencing postprandial heartburn and also not to eat immediately before lying down. Pillows at bedtime may help. If necessary, antacids may be prescribed. Liquid antacids coat the esophageal lining more effectively than do tablets.

Hemorrhoids

Hemorrhoids are varicose veins of the rectum. Since straining during bowel movements contributes to their aggravation, avoidance of constipation is preventive, and prolonged sitting should also be avoided. Hemorrhoids will often regress after delivery but usually will not disappear completely.

Constipation

Constipation is physiologic during pregnancy with decreased bowel transit time, and the stool may be hardened. Dietary modification with increased bulk such as with fresh fruit and vegetables and plenty of water can usually help this problem. Constipation is aggravated by the addition of iron supplementation; if dietary measures are inadequate, patients may require stool softeners. Additional dietary fibers such as Metamucil (psyllium hydrophilic muciloid) or surface-active agents such as Colace (docusate) are recommended. Laxatives are rarely necessary.

Urinary Frequency

Often during the first 3 months of pregnancy, the growing uterus places increased pressure on the bladder. Urinary frequency usually will improve as the uterus rises out of the pelvis by the second trimester. However, as the head engages near the time of delivery, urinary frequency may return as the head presses against the bladder. If the patient experiences pain with urination, it is appropriate to check for infection.

Round Ligament Pain

Frequently, patients will notice sharp groin pains caused by spasm of the round ligaments associated with movement. This is more frequently felt on the right side as a result of the usual dextrorotation of the uterus. The pain may be helped by application of local heat such as with hot soaks or a heating pad. Patients may awaken at night with this pain after having suddenly rolled over in their sleep without realizing it. During the daytime, however, modification of activity with gradual rising and sitting down, as well as avoidance of sudden movement, will decrease problems with this type of pain. Analgesics are rarely necessary.

Syncope

Compression of the veins in the legs from the advancing size of the uterus places patients at risk of venous pooling associated with prolonged standing. This may lead to syncope. Measures to avoid this possibility include wearing support stockings and exercising the calves to increase venous return. In later pregnancy, patients may have problems with supine hypotension, a distinct problem when undergoing a medical evaluation or an ultrasound examination. A left lateral tilt position with wedging below the right hip will help keep the weight of the pregnancy off the inferior vena cava.

Backache

Backache can be prevented to a large degree by avoidance of excessive weight gain. Exercises to strengthen back muscles can also be helpful. Posture is important, and sensible shoes, not high heels, should be worn.

Sexual Activity

No restriction need generally be placed on sexual intercourse. The patient is instructed that pregnancy may cause changes in comfort and sexual desire. Frequently, increased uterine activity is noted after sexual intercourse; it is unclear whether this is due to breast stimulation, female orgasm, or prostaglandins in male ejaculate. For women at risk for preterm labor or with a history of previous pregnancy loss and who note such increased activity, use of a condom or avoidance of sexual activity may be recommended.

Cirumcision

Newborn circumcision prevents phimosis and other penile problems. It results in a decreased incidence of urinary tract infections in the first year of life. The American Academy of Pediatrics does not recommend routine neonatal circumcision.[58] Education in good personal hygiene offers many of the advantages of circumcision without the risks.

Circumcision in the newborn is an elective procedure and should be performed only if the infant is stable and healthy. Local anesthesia is recommended, as it reduces the observed physiologic response to the newborn's pain.[59]

Breast-Feeding

During prenatal visits, the patient should be encouraged to breast-feed her infant (see Chapter 5). Human milk is the most appropriate nutrient for human infants and also provides significant immunologic protection against infection. Infants who are breast-fed have a lower incidence of infection and require fewer hospitalizations than do infants who are fed formula exclusively.

Other advantages of lactation include economy, convenience, more rapid involution of the uterus, and natural child spacing. The reasons a woman decides to bottle-feed should be explored, as they may be based on a misconception. Encouragement will sometimes convince a hesitant mother who may then be able to nurse successfully.

Working outside the home need not be a contraindication to breast-feeding. Many women who previously would not have considered nursing an option, such as those with careers, are now finding time to breast-feed their infants. Women should be aware that alternative ways of breast-feeding can be used to correspond with their work schedules. They can decrease the frequency of lactation to a few times a day in most cases and still continue to nurse. Other women may pump their breasts at work, leaving milk for the child's caretaker during the day and thus providing breast milk to the infant even more frequently. The milk may be collected in containers and, if refrigerated, is safe to use for 24 hours. For a longer duration, the milk should be frozen. Because freezing and thawing destroy the cellular content, fresh milk is preferred.

There is no need for specific nipple preparation during pregnancy. In one study, women prepared one nipple and not the other with a variety of techniques, including massage and breast creams, and found no difference in the two.[60] Soap and drying agents should not be used on the nipples, which should be washed only with water.

Preparation for Childbirth

The introduction of childbirth education and consumerism has had significant impact on the practice of obstetrics. The success of obstetric practice in preventing disasters has allowed interest to focus on the quality of the child and of the perinatal experience. Studies have shown that prepared childbirth can have a beneficial effect on performance in labor and delivery.[61,62] The prenatal period should be one in which the patient is exposed to information about pregnancy, normal labor and delivery, anesthesia and analgesia, obstetric complications, and obstetric operations (e.g., episiotomy, cesarean delivery, and forceps or vacuum delivery). The prenatal clinic is an appropriate place to obtain informed consent from the patient for her intrapartum care and management. Certainly, this affords a more dispassionate, quiet, and pain-free environment than the labor and delivery suite.

The education mentioned above is more than can be transmitted by the obstetrician at the initial or the shorter return visits, and patients expect more personal involvement than to be given a book or handout to read. The appropriate place for such education is a series of planned, structured prenatal education classes taught by informed, qualified individuals. These classes can be given in the physician's office, at the hospital, or in free-standing classes. National organizations such as the Childbirth Education Association and the American Society for Psychoprophylaxis in Obstetrics have recognized the need for such instruction and teach prepared childbirth. There are also advantages to office- and hospital-based programs, if the patient volume permits it, since specifics of management and alternatives offered by that practice or hospital can be discussed in these programs. On the other hand, free-standing classes offer the advantage of open-endedness and of presenting many options to the patient, who can then discuss them with her care provider. Many advances in family-centered practice (e.g., allowing fathers in the delivery room and operating room) have come from consumer requests and demands. A pregnant patient often makes a list of what she would like in the peripartum period, to discuss with her practitioner. Thus, the care provider can understand her needs and desires, better address these needs and desires if labor and delivery do not proceed normally or as planned, and, finally, explain why certain requests are not possible or reasonable.

Signs of Labor

It is important to instruct the patient about certain warning signs that should trigger a call to her care provider or a visit to the hospital. All women should be informed of what to do if contractions become regular, if rupture of membranes is suspected, or if vaginal bleeding occurs. Patients should be given a number to call where assistance is available 24 hours a day.

Prepared Parenthood and Support Groups

Routine classes on newborn child care and parenting should be part of the prenatal care program. Many parents are completely unprepared for the myriad of changes in their lives, and some idea of what to expect is beneficial. As pregnancy progresses, special needs can arise. Support groups for families with Down's syndrome infants, for mothers of twins or triplets, and for women who have had cesarean delivery have all shown that they can meet the special needs of these parents. Unsuccessful pregnancies lead to special problems and needs, for which social workers, clergy, and specialized support groups can be invaluable. Miscarriage, stillbirth, and infant death are particularly devastating events, best managed by a team approach, with special attention to the grieving process. Referral to such groups as Compassionate Friends of Miscarriage, Infant Death, and Stillbirth is recommended. Careful follow-up for depression should be part of the postpartum care for all and especially women.

ASSESSMENT OF GESTATIONAL AGE

During the course of the prenatal interview, assessment of gestational age begins with the question, "What was the first day of the last menstrual period?" From that point, the establishment of an estimated date of delivery and confirmation of that date by accumulation of supportive information remains one of the most important tasks of good prenatal care.

Human pregnancy has a duration of 280 days, measured from the first day of the last menstrual period (LMP) until delivery. The standard deviation is 14 days. It is important to remember that clinicians are measuring menstrual weeks (not conceptional weeks) with an assumption of ovulation and conception based on day 14 of a 28-day cycle. This gives pregnancy the 40-week gestational period in common clinical use. Much confusion exists among patients who try to measure pregnancy in terms of 9 months (40/4 = 10) or who try to measure in conceptional weeks. Another problem exists in women whose menstrual cycles do not follow a 28-day cycle and who therefore do not conceive on day 14 of the menstrual cycle.

It is often helpful to explain to patients and their families that their pregnancy will be described in terms of weeks, rather than months, and that the pregnancy can be broken into three trimesters lasting 1 to 14 weeks, 14 to 28 weeks, and 28 weeks to delivery. The commonly used term "4 months pregnant" has no meaning (one does not know whether this is 16 or 20 weeks) and has no place on a contemporary prenatal record. Every effort should be made to be consistent in usage to prevent confusion among patients and among clinicians who may assume care of the pregnancy.

Knowledge of gestational age is critical for obstetric decision-making. Generally, in a normal pregnancy, we can extrapolate from gestational age to estimate fetal weight. Throughout pregnancy, these are the two most important determinants of fetal viability and survival. Without accurate knowledge of gestational age, diagnosis of such conditions as postterm pregnancy and intrauterine growth retardation is often impossible. Multiple gestation is most often detected early when the size of the uterine fundus is greater than expected for gestation. Appropriate management of preterm labor or a medically complicated pregnancy depends on an accurate estimate of fetal age and size. Within regional perinatal systems, records of gestational age are important for flow of information, and rapid access to consistent, clear data is vital. In such situations, and during prolonged hospitalization, it is sometimes helpful to define gestational age further by using the notation of fractional weeks ($27\frac{4}{7}$ weeks). It must be remembered, however, that we are describing a biologic system and that such precision is being used more for ease of communication and organization than for any ability to date the pregnancy with such a degree of accuracy.

Clinical Dating

The most reliable clinical estimator of gestational age is an accurate LMP. Using Naegele's rule, the estimated date of confinement is calculated by subtracting 3 months and adding 1 week from the first day of the LMP. A careful history must be taken from the patient verifying that the date given is the first day of the period as well as whether the period was normal, heavy, or light. The date of the previous menstrual period will help ascertain the length of the cycle. History should also be taken about previous use of oral contraceptives, which might influence ovulation.

Other clinical tools can be used to confirm and support LMP data and, in cases in which the LMP is inaccurate or unknown, it has been shown that accumulated clinical information from early pregnancy can predict gestational age with an accuracy approaching that of menstrual dating.[63]

The size of the uterus on early pelvic examination, or by direct measurement of the abdomen from the pubic symphysis to the top of the uterine fundus (over the curve), provides useful information. Experienced practitioners can assess the early pregnancy with reproducibility before 12 to 14 weeks. Fundal height measurement in centimeters using the over-the-curve technique approximates the gestational age from 16 to 38 weeks within 3 cm (Fig. 6–7).

The uterus also tends to reach the umbilicus at about 20 weeks, and this too can be assessed when uterine fundal measurements are made.[48] The uterus may be elevated in early pregnancy in a patient with a previous cesarean delivery, making the fundal height appear abnormally high. Considerable variations in the level of the umbilicus and in the height of patients make this clinical marker variable. Quickening, the first perception of fetal movement by the mother, occurs at predictable times in gestation. In the first pregnancy, quickening is usually noted at about 19 weeks; in subsequent pregnancies, probably because of the experience of the observer, it tends to occur about 2 weeks earlier.[63] It is helpful to ask the woman to mark on a calendar the first time she feels the baby move and to report this date.

Audible fetal heart tones, in addition to being absolute evidence of pregnancy, are another marker of gestational age. Using an unamplified Hillis-DeLee fetoscope, they are generally audible at 19 to 20 weeks.[48] Observer experience, acuity, and the time spent listening can all affect this number, so this guideline may need to be adapted individually.

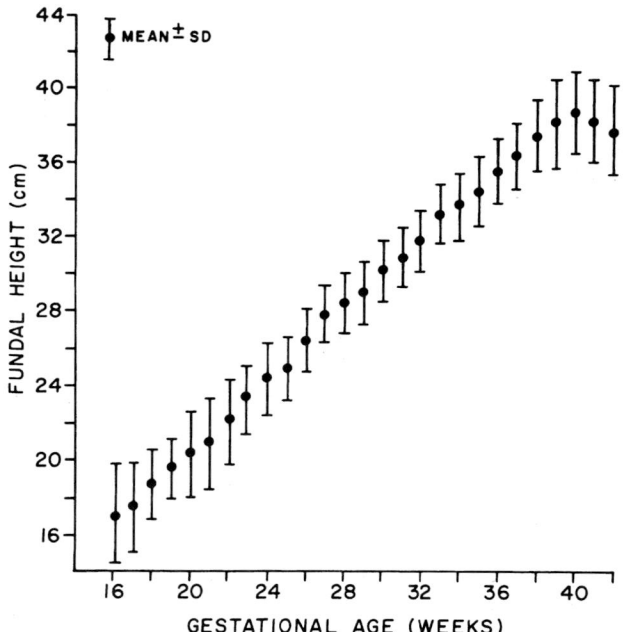

Figure 6–7. Fundal height versus gestational age. (From Knox AJ, Sadler L, Pattison WS, et al: An obstetric scoring system: its development and application in obstetric management. Obstet Gynecol 81: 195, 1993, with permission.)

Use of the electronic Doppler device is widespread and permits detection of the fetal heart by 11 to 12 weeks. Practitioners can set a standard individualized to their own equipment, which can be used as a gestational age marker. If fetal heart tones are not heard at the expected time, an sonogram is appropriate to look for date/examination discrepancy, polyhydramnios, fetal viability, and twins.

The conversion of a negative urinary pregnancy test to a positive one may be helpful in assessing gestational age, but the sensitivity of the test used must be known in order to interpret the data accurately (see Chapter 1). These tests may be negative if they are performed too early.

Comparison of the various clinical estimators shows a known LMP date to be the most precise predictor. The clinical estimators can be ranked according to decreasing order of accuracy as follows: (1) last menstrual period; (2) the uterus reaching umbilicus; and (3) fetal heart tone documentation, fundal height measurements, and quickening. Because of inherent biologic variability and differences in the examiner acuity, the estimated date of confinement can be predicted with 90 percent certainty only within ±3 weeks by even the best single estimator.[64]

Ultrasound

Ultrasound plays a major role in assessment of size and duration of pregnancy. The National Institutes of Health (NIH) consensus conference in 1984 concluded that in a low-risk pregnancy followed from the first trimester, routine ultrasound examination was not justified for determining gestational age. However, a long list of indications justify an ultrasound examination.[65]

A randomized trial has shown that the risk of being called overdue was reduced from 8 percent to 2 percent for patients who received early ultrasound.[66] Also, twins were detected more often and perinatal mortality was reduced in the ultrasound group. The Routine Antenatal Diagnostic Imaging with Ultrasound (RADIUS) study reported no improvement in perinatal outcome with use of routine ultrasound in normal, low-risk women.[67,68] However, 61 percent of women were excluded for many reasons such as an uncertain menstrual history, and only 35 percent of anomalies were detected in the ultrasound-screened group (only 17 percent before 24 weeks). The meta-analysis by Bucher and Schmidt[69] indicated that routine scanning can detect many more anomalies. The authors' practice is to perform ultrasound at 16 to 20 weeks for a baseline gestational age measurement and as a screening for fetal abnormality or multiple gestation. If ultrasound is not done routinely, the caregiver must be vigilant in detecting problems that are indications for a scan, and more frequent scans may be necessary.

Ultrasound is an accurate means of estimating gestational age in the first half of pregnancy.[70] The crown-rump length, biparietal diameter, and femur length in the first half of pregnancy correlate closely with age. As pregnancy progresses, fetal size varies considerably, and measurement of the fetus is a poor tool for estimation of gestational age, especially in the third trimester (see Chapter 10).

SUMMARY

Prenatal care is an effective, if incompletely understood and studied, intervention. It provides a model for primary care services for both obstetricians/gynecologists and other primary care providers. It satisfies the Institute of Medicine criteria for primary care, as it is comprehensive, and continuous, and provides coordinated services. Preconceptional care will introduce changes and improve it. Risk assessment, with subsequent elimination or management of risks, health education, advocacy, and disease prevention, as well as appropriate medical management of complications, remain the core of the process, changes in number of visits and improved understanding of the successful components of prenatal care will improve services and efficiency without altering the substance of what has been developed and achieved. Prenatal care should reinforce the importance of lifelong disease surveillance and prevention as well as active participation in personal wellness behavior for women.

Key Points

➤ Maternal mortality is the demise of any woman from any pregnancy-related cause while pregnant or within 42 days of termination of a pregnancy. The most frequent causes of maternal death are hemorrhage and embolism. The perinatal mortality combines the number of fetal deaths (stillbirths) plus neonatal deaths per 1,000 total births.

➤ Preconception evaluation should include rubella testing, hepatitis testing, and possibly toxoplasmosis and HIV testing, in addition to medical and family history. Further tests may be indicated depending on historical genetic risk factors identified.

➤ Preconception supplementation with folic acid can reduce the incidence of NTDs and other

➤ defects. All women of childbearing age should consume 0.4 mg of folic acid daily. Women who have had a child previously affected by an NTD should take 4 mg daily from 4 weeks before conception through the first 3 months of pregnancy.

➤ The triple screen (α-fetoprotein, hCG, and estriol) can detect women younger than 35 years of age at increased risk for chromosomal abnormalities.

➤ The number of prenatal visits can be decreased in healthy parous women with safety.

➤ The total weight gain recommended for healthy women is 25 to 35 lb. Underweight women may gain up to 40 lb, and overweight women should limit weight gain to 15 to 25 lb.

➤ Bed rest on the side increases venous return from the legs, as pressure on the vena cava is relieved. This maneuver increases the effective circulating blood volume, cardiac output and, thus, the blood flow to the kidney. A diuresis follows, as well as increased blood flow to the uterus.

➤ The pregnant woman should be advised against prolonged sitting during car or airplane travel because of the risk of venous stasis and possible thromboembolism.

➤ For infant nutrition, breast is best.

➤ Ultrasound evaluation between 16 and 20 weeks allows accurate assessment of gestational age and screening for fetal abnormality and multiple gestation.

REFERENCES

1. Donaldson M, Yordy K, Vanselow N (eds): Defining Primary Care: An Interim Report. Washington, DC, National Academy Press, 1994
2. American College of Obstetricians and Gynecologists: The Obstetrician-Gynecologist and Primary-Preventive Health Care. ACOG, 1993.
3. Starfield B: Primary care: Concept, Evaluation, and Policy. New York, Oxford University Press, 1992.
4. Public Health Service: Caring for Our Future: The Content of Prenatal Care—A Report of the Public Health Service Expert Panel on the Content of Prenatal Care. Washington, DC, PHS-DHRS, 1989.
5. Chalmers I, Enkin M, Keirse M: Effective Care in Pregnancy and Childbirth. Oxford, Oxford University Press, 1989.
6. Peoples-Sheps MD, Kalsbeck WD, Siegal WC: Prenatal records: a national survey of content. Am J Obstet Gynecol 164:514, 1991.
7. Rooney C: Antenatal care and maternal health: How effective is it? WHO/MSM/Divisional Family Health, Sept 1992, pp 1–74.
8. Huntington J, Connell FA: For every dollar spent—the cost-savings argument for prenatal care. N Engl J Med 331:1303, 1994.
9. McDuffie RS Jr, Bischoff KJ, Beck A, Orleans M: Does reducing the number of prenatal office visits for low-risk women result in increased use of other medical services? Obstet Gynecol 90:68, 1997.
10. Khan-Neelofur D, Gulmezoglu M, Villar J: Who should provide routine antenatal care for low-risk women, and how often? A systematic review of randomised controlled trials, WHO Antenatal Care Trial Research Group. Paediatr Perinat Epidemiol 12(Suppl 2):7, 1998.
11. Kogan MD, Martin JA, Alexander GR, et al: The changing pattern of prenatal care utilization in the United States, 1981–1995, using different prenatal care indices. JAMA 279:1623, 1998.
12. Misra DP, Guyer B: Benefits and limitations on prenatal care from counting visits to measuring content. JAMA 279:1661, 1998.
13. MacArthur C: What does prenatal care do for women's health? Lancet 353:343, 1999.
14. Johnson TRB, Zettelmaier MA, Warner PA, et al: A competency based approach to comprehensive pregnancy care. Women's Health Issues 10:240, 2000.
15. Johansen KS, Hod M: Quality development in perinatal care—the OBSQID project. Int J Gynecol Obstet 64:167, 1999.
16. Centers for Disease Control and Prevention: Maternal mortality—United States, 1982–1996. MMWR Morb Mortal Wkly Rep 47:705, 1998.
17. Berg CJ, Atrash HK, Koonin LM, Tucker M: Pregnancy related mortality in the United States, 1987–1990. Obstet Gynecol 88:161, 1996.
18. Rosenfield A: Maternal mortality in developing countries. An ongoing but neglected "epidemic." JAMA 262:376, 1989.
19. Revised 1990 Estimates of Maternal Mortality. A new approach by WHO and UNICEF, World Health Organization, April 1996.
20. Frautschi S, Cerulli A, Maine D: Suicide during pregnancy and its neglect as a component of maternal mortality. Int J Gynecol Obstet 47:275, 1994.
21. Center for Disease Control and Prevention: Enhanced maternal mortality surveillance—North Carolina, 1988 and 1989. MMWR Morb Mortal Wkly Rep 40:469, 1996
22. Harper M, Parsons L: Maternal death due to homicide and other injuries in North Carolina: 1992–1994. Obstet Gynecol 90:920, 1997.
23. Dannenberg AL, Carter DM, Lawson HW, et al: Homicide and other injuries as causes of maternal death in New York City, 1987 through 1991. Am J Obstet Gynecol 172:1557, 1995.
24. Centers for Disease Control and Prevention: Differences in maternal mortality among black and white women—United States, 1990. MMWR Morb Mortal Wkly Rep 44:6, 13, 1995.
25. Centers for Disease Control and Prevention: Differences in maternal mortality among black and white women—United States, 1987–1996. MMWR Morb Mortal Wkly Rep 48:492, 1999.
26. Sachs BP, Fretts RC, Gardner R, et al: The impact of extreme prematurity and congenital anomalies on the interpretation of international comparisons of infant mortality. Obstet Gynecol 85:941, 1995.

27. Enkin MW: Randomized controlled trials in the evaluation of antenatal care. Int J Technol Assess Health Care 8(Suppl 1):40, 1992.
28. Knox AJ, Sadler L, Pattison NS, et al: An obstetric scoring system: its development and application in obstetric management. Obstet Gynecol 81:195, 1993.
29. Mueller-Heubach E, Guzick DS: Evaluation of risk scoring in a preterm birth prevention study of indigent patients. Obstet Gynecol 160:829, 1989.
30. Kogan MD, Alexander GR, Kotelchuck M, Nagey DA: Relation of the content of prenatal care to the risk of low birth weight. JAMA 271:134, 1994.
31. Carey JC, Klebanoff MA, Hauth JC, et al: Metronidazole to prevent preterm delivery in pregnant women with asymptomatic bacterial vaginosis. N Engl J Med 342:534, 2000.
32. Moos MK, Cefalo RC: Preconceptional health promotion: a focus for obstetric care. Am J Perinatol 4:63, 1987.
33. Adams EM, Bruce C, Shulman MS, et al: The PRAMS Working Group: pregnancy planning and pre-conceptional counseling. Obstet Gynecol 82:955, 1993.
34. 2000 Compendium of Selected Publications, American College of Obstetricians and Gynecologists, 2000.
35. MRC Vitamin Study Research Group: Prevention of neural tube defects: results of the Medical Research Council Vitamin Study. Lancet 338:131, 1991.
36. Czeizel AE, Dudas I: Prevention of the first occurrence of neural-tube defects by periconceptional vitamin supplementation. N Engl J Med 327:1832, 1992.
37. Hook EB: Rates of chromosome abnormalities at different maternal ages. Obstet Gynecol 58:282, 1981.
38. Stene J, Fischer G, Steve E, et al: Paternal age effect in Down's syndrome. Am J Hum Genet 40:299, 1977.
39. Spitzer RL, Williams JBW, Kroenke K, et al: Utility of a new procedure for diagnosing mental disorders in primary care. JAMA 272:1749, 1994.
40. Moore RD, Bone LR, Geller G, et al: Prevalence detection and treatment of alcoholism in hospitalized patients. JAMA 261:403, 1989.
41. Sokol RJ, Martier SS, Ager JW: The T-ACE questions: practical prenatal detection of risk-drinking. Am J Obstet Gynecol 160:863, 1989.
42. McFarlane J, Parker B, Soeken K, Bullock L: Assessing for abuse during pregnancy. JAMA 267:3176, 1992.
43. Chang G, Wilkins-Haug L, Berman S, et al: Alcohol use and pregnancy: improving identification. Obstet Gynecol 91:892, 1998.
44. Creasy RC, Gummer BA, Liggins GC: System for predicting spontaneous preterm birth. Obstet Gynecol 55:692, 1980.
45. Main D, Richardson DK, Hadley CB, Gabbe S: Controlled trial of a preterm labor detection program: efficacy and costs. Obstet Gynecol 74:823, 1989.
46. McDuffie R, Bischoff K, Cross J, et al: An evaluation of risk-based prenatal care: a randomized controlled trial. Am J Obstet Gynecol 172:270, 1995.
47. Abbasi IA, Hess LW, Johnson TRB Jr, et al: Leukocyte esterase activity in the rapid detection of urinary tract and lower genital tract infection in pregnancy. Am J Perinatol 2:311, 1985.
48. Chang G, Wilkins-Haug L, Berman S, et al: Alcohol use and pregnancy: improving identification. Obstet Gynecol 91:892, 1998.
49. Grant A, Elbourne D, Valentin L, Alexander S: Routine fetal movement counting and risk of antepartum rate death in normally formed singletons. Lancet 2:345, 1989.
50. Kulier R, de Onis M, Gulmezoglu AM, Villar J: Nutritional interventions for the prevention of maternal morbidity. Int J Gynecol Obstet 63:231, 1998.
51. U.S. Department of Agriculture: The Food Guide Pyramid. Home and Garden Bulletin. Washington, DC, USDA, 1992.
52. National Academy of Sciences: Recommended Dietary Allowances, 10th ed. Washington, DC, National Academy Press, 1989.
53. Zlatnik FJ, Burmeister LF: Dietary protein in pregnancy: effect on anthropometric indices of the newborn infant. Am J Obstet Gynecol 146:199, 1983.
54. Food and Nutrition Board Institute of Medicine, National Academy of Sciences: Nutrition During Pregnancy. Washington, DC, National Academy Press, 1990, p 10.
55. Mamelle N, Laumon B, Lazar P: Prematurity and occupational activity during pregnancy. Am J Epidemiol 119:309, 1984.
56. Luke B, Mamelle N, Keith L, et al: The association between occupational factors and preterm birth: a U.S. nurses' study. Am J Obstet Gynecol 173:849, 1995.
57. Mozurkewich E, Luke B, Avni M, Wolf FM: Working conditions and adverse pregnancy outcome: a meta-analysis. Obstet Gynecol 95:623, 2000.
58. American Academy of Pediatrics: Circumcision Policy Statement (RE9850) 103:686, 1999.
59. Maxwell LG, Yaster M, Wetzel RC, et al: Penile nerve block for newborn circumcision. Obstet Gynecol 70:415, 1987.
60. Brown MS, Hurloch JT: Preparation of the breast for breast feeding. Nurs Res 24:449, 1975.
61. Scott JR, Rose NB: Effect of psychoprophylaxis (Lamaze preparation) on labor and delivery in primiparas. N Engl J Med 294:1205, 1976.
62. Villar J, Farnot U, Barros F, et al: A randomized trial of psychosocial support during high-risk pregnancies. The Latin American Network for Perinatal and Reproductive Biology Research. N Engl J Med 327:1266, 1992.
63. Andersen HF, Johnson TRB, Flora JD, et al: Gestational age assessment. II. Prediction from combined clinical observations. Am J Obstet Gynecol 140:770, 1981.
64. Kramer MS, McLean FH, Boyd ME, Usher RH: The validity of gestational age estimation by menstrual dating in term, preterm and postterm gestations. JAMA 260:3306, 1988.
65. U.S. Department of Health and Human Services: Ultrasound Imaging in Pregnancy. NIH Publication No. 84-667. Washington, DC, National Institutes of Health, 1984.
66. Eik-Nes SH, Okland O, Aure JC: Ultrasound screening in pregnancy: a randomized controlled trial. Lancet 1:1347, 1984.
67. Ewigman BG, Crane JP, Frigoletto FD, et al: Effect of prenatal ultrasound screening on perinatal outcome. N Engl J Med 329:821, 1993.
68. LeFevre ML, Bain RP, Ewigman BG, et al: A randomized trial of prenatal ultrasonographic screening: impact on maternal management and outcome. Am J Obstet Gynecol 169:483, 1993.
69. Bucher HC, Schmidt JG: Does routine ultrasound scanning improve outcome in pregnancy? Meta-analysis of various outcome measures. BMJ 307:13, 1993.
70. Reece EA, Gabrielli S, Degennaro N, Hobbins JC: Dating through pregnancy: a measure of growing up. Obstet Gynecol Surv 44:544, 1989.

Occupational and Environmental Perspectives of Birth Defects

JOE LEIGH SIMPSON AND JENNIFER R. NIEBYL

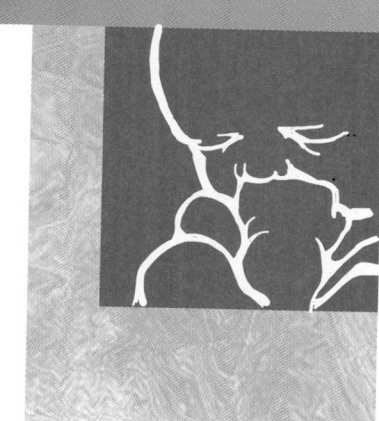

Pregnant women want to have a normal baby who develops into a healthy child and adult. Unfortunately, this wish is not always fulfilled. This chapter considers prenatal environmental influences acting maternally as potential causes of adverse development. The focus is on structural malformations (birth defects), but some attention is paid to aberrations in behavior and to other adverse reproductive outcomes. The importance of birth defects as a cause of infant mortality, the etiology of birth defects, and basic concepts of teratology, epidemiologic methods used to evaluate possible adverse effects of environmental exposures on reproductive outcomes, and data about some specific environmental and occupational exposures are reviewed.

BASIC PRINCIPLES OF TERATOLOGY

To understand the etiology of birth defects, it is important to consider what is known about the principles of abnormal development (teratogenesis). Although only a small percentage of birth defects currently can be linked to environmental agents, the search for other agents is important.

Teratology has been defined as the study of abnormal development; it is directed at understanding the causes and mechanisms of maldevelopment. A teratogen is a substance, organism, or physical agent capable of causing abnormal development. A teratogen can cause abnormalities of structure or function, growth **restriction,** or death of the organism.

Traditionally, the identification and definition of teratogenic agents was based on the production of struc-

tural defects. More recently, the concept has been expanded to include agents acting during embryonic or fetal development that lead to deviation from normal morphology or function. There is growing interest in exploring the role of prenatal factors in more subtle or difficult-to-ascertain effects, such as growth **restriction** and functional abnormalities. Wilson's six general principles of teratogenesis[1] provide a framework for understanding how structural or functional teratogens may act. These principles provide a conceptual framework to understand and investigate maldevelopment.

Genotype and Interaction with Environmental Factors

The first principle is that susceptibility to a teratogen depends on the *genotype of the conceptus* and on the manner in which the genotype interacts with environmental factors. This is perhaps most clearly shown by experiments in which different genetic strains of mice have varied greatly in their susceptibility to teratogens that lead to oral clefts.[2] Some of the variability in responses to human teratogens, such as to anticonvulsant drugs like valproic acid and hydantoin, probably relates to genotype of the embryo. The increasing complexity of these potential interactions is illustrated by a series of elegant studies by Musselman and colleagues.[3]

Timing of Exposure

The second principle is that susceptibility of the conceptus to teratogenic agents varies with the developmental stage at the time of exposure. This concept of *critical stages of development* is particularly applicable to alterations in structure. It is during the second to the eighth weeks of development after conception—the embryonic period—that most structural defects occur. For

This chapter substantially reflects the contribution in the previous edition by Lowell E. Sever and Mary Ellen Mortensen.

such defects, it is believed that there is a critical stage in the developmental process, after which abnormal embryogenesis cannot be initiated. For example, most investigators believe that the neural tube defects anencephaly and spina bifida result from the failure of the neural tube to close. Since this process occurs between 22 and 28 days postconception, any exogenous effect on development must be present at or before this time. Van Allen et al.[4] put forward convincing evidence that the neural tube has five distinct closure sites that may respond to different agents and that differ in their timing. Investigations of thalidomide teratogenicity have clearly shown that the effects of the drug differ as a function of the developmental stage at which the pregnant woman took it.[5]

Mechanisms of Teratogenesis

The third principle is that teratogenic agents act in specific ways (*mechanisms*) on developing cells and tissues in initiating abnormal embryogenesis (pathogenesis). Teratogenic mechanisms are considered separately below.

Manifestations

Irrespective of the specific deleterious agent, the final manifestations of abnormal development are death, malformation, growth restriction, and functional disorder. The manifestation is thought to depend largely on the stage of development at which exposure occurs; a teratogen may have one effect if exposure occurs during embryogenesis and another if the exposure is during the fetal period. Embryonic exposure is likely to lead to structural abnormalities or embryonic death; fetal exposure is likely to lead to functional deficits or growth restriction.

Agent

The fifth principle is that access of adverse environmental influences to developing tissues depends on the nature of the influence (*agent*). This principle relates to such pharmacologic factors as maternal metabolism and placental passage. While most clearly understood for chemical agents or drugs, the principle also applies to physical agents such as radiation or heat. For an adverse effect to occur, an agent must reach the conceptus, by being transmitted indirectly through maternal tissues or by directly traversing the maternal body.

Dose Effect

The final principle is that manifestations of abnormal development increase in degree from the no-effect level to the lethal level as *dosage* increases. What this means

is that the response (e.g., malformation, growth restriction) may be expected to vary according to the dose, duration, or amount of exposure. For most human teratogens, this dose-response is not clearly understood but, along with the principle of critical stages of development, these concepts are important in supporting causal inferences about human reproductive hazards. Data regarding in utero exposure to ionizing radiation clearly show the importance of dose on observed effects.[6] The potential complexity of relationships between dose and observed effects for teratogens has been discussed by Selevan and Lemasters.[7]

MECHANISMS OF TERATOGENESIS

In identifying human teratogens, it is important to consider the mechanisms of teratogenesis. A teratogenic insult can initiate changes in developing cells or tissues that can be categorized into nine mechanisms. An agent acts via a mechanism that alters normal cellular or biochemical processes; different alterations can produce similar defects through final common pathways. Among proposed mechanisms are gene mutation, chromosomal abnormalities (e.g., breaks and nondisjunction), mitotic interference, altered nucleic acid integrity or function, lack of normal precursors or substrates, altered energy sources, changes in membrane characteristics, osmolar imbalance, and enzyme inhibition. With these mechanisms in mind, it may be easier to understand why such diverse etiologies for spina bifida as maternal hyperthermia, valproic acid exposure, and folic acid deficiency have been suggested.

In identifying reproductive hazards, relationships among teratogenesis, mutagenesis, and carcinogenesis should be considered, since these processes may occur through similar mechanisms.[7] Hemminki and associates[8] illustrated how various manifestations, classified as teratogenic, mutagenic, or carcinogenic, could result from alterations of DNA.

ANIMAL MODELS FOR THE STUDY OF HUMAN TERATOGENS

Premarket testing of drugs and food additives involves animal testing to determine potential teratogenicity. Although important in recognizing potential reproductive toxicants and teratogens, such studies have a number of significant limitations. Extrapolation from animal data may not be relevant to human exposures to an agent because of interspecies differences in metabolism, end-organ response, transport across the placenta, and sensitivity of fetal structures, to name a few. For example, humans and rabbits are sensitive to the teratogenic effect of thalidomide, but rats are relatively insensitive.[9] There are also problems extrapolating from high doses to low doses, as most teratologic experiments involve exposure at high doses. Since human exposures typically involve lower doses, effects must then be extrapolated. The assumption is often made that teratogenic risk is identical at high- and low-dose exposures (e.g., linearity of dose-response). This may not be true, and it is not surprising that there is little or no evidence for human teratogenicity at low doses for many substances teratogenic in animals at high doses (e.g., arsenic and some solvents).[10]

Among regulatory agencies, there is increasing interest in the use of risk assessment methods for developmental toxicants. For example, the Environmental Protection Agency has published *Guidelines for the Health Assessment of Suspect Developmental Toxicants.*[11]

While teratologic testing of drugs and chemicals in animals serves an extremely important public health function, it does not necessarily prevent exposure of pregnant women to teratogens. Two drugs shown to be human teratogens (isotretinoin [Accutane] and valproic acid [Depakene]) were known to be teratogenic based on animal studies, but it was only through human exposure that their teratogenicity in humans was established. Tens of thousands of chemicals have never been tested for reproductive toxicity or teratogenicity.[7] The limitations of animal testing and the immense number of potentially hazardous substances underscore the need for human studies, the subject of the remainder of this chapter.

CONTRIBUTION OF EPIDEMIOLOGY

Environmental agents are of particular interest and concern because exposure of the conceptus to these factors is considered to be preventable by reducing or eliminating exposure of pregnant women. The combined forces of epidemiology and teratology are needed to study the effects of environmental exposures on reproductive outcomes.

Although most birth defects of public health significance probably involve the interaction of genetic and environmental factors (multifactorial etiology), the relative contributions and specific mechanisms of genetics and environmental agents remain unknown. By applying epidemiologic methods we attempt to determine the relative contributions of both factors to the etiology of these defects. Importantly, epidemiologic methods permit identification of specific agents associated with malformations or other adverse outcomes of pregnancy.[12]

Epidemiologic Concepts

A fundamental concept is that variation between populations exists in the frequency of disease occurrence. Epidemiology is based on comparisons, determining what is occurring at one place compared with another place, what is going on at one time compared with another time, and what is going on with one group of people compared with another group of people. Rates of occurrence are compared; how these rates are determined is of major importance in epidemiology.

Occurrence rates for birth defects are usually expressed in terms of either rates of incidence or prevalence at birth. An incidence rate, calculated using cases occurring during a specified period of time, consists of a numerator, the number of new cases of a defect; and a denominator, the population at risk of developing the defect. Incidence rates are expressed in terms of some base population, such as per 1,000 births, and give a measure of the risk of the defect occurring within the population. Many investigators believe it is inappropriate to refer to birth defect rates as incidence rates, since the true population at risk, that is, the number of embryos, is unknown. Thus, there is an increasing tendency to refer to the occurrence of birth defects as prevalence at birth.[13] Prevalence requires knowing the number of cases that exist at a point in time, in this case defined as birth. Thus, we determine prevalence at birth, since we can obtain information on the number of cases born in a population and the total number of births.

Examination of the occurrence rates for birth defects often shows geographic differences.[14] Such differences are found both between countries and between regions within countries. These differences are studied in an effort to identify possible etiologic factors. Detailed information on birth defect rates in the United States[15] and internationally[16,17] have been published.

Temporal variations in birth defect rates may occur within a population, and the interpretation of such variation may give insights into etiology. Two kinds of time-related changes are of particular interest: short-term increases that may be termed "epidemics" and long-term secular trends. Examples of the former are the epidemic of phocomelia in several European populations during the early 1960s[14] and a more recent epidemic of anencephalus in South Texas.[18] An example of the latter is the recent decline in neural tube defect (NTD) rates in several areas of the world.[19] The increase in phocomelia was found to be associated with the introduction of the drug thalidomide. The decline in NTD rates has not been explained and is an example of a trend whose contributing factors need to be identified through epidemiologic study.

EPIDEMIOLOGIC APPROACHES TO THE STUDY OF BIRTH DEFECTS

Epidemiology is the study of the distribution and determinants of disease. Understanding disease distribution often provides insights into disease determinants. Understanding uneven distribution can lead to the identification of factors involved in disease etiology.[20] While epidemiologic studies usually are unable to establish causal relationships, such as can be done through animal experiments, associations between exposures and an outcome from well-conducted studies can provide strong, compelling evidence that the outcome results from the exposure.

Three major issues are involved in epidemiologic studies of birth defects that evaluate potential associations between exposures and outcomes: (1) the definition and ascertainment of outcomes of interest; (2) the definition, identification, and quantification of exposures or of other risk factors; and (3) the use of epidemiologic and statistical techniques to determine the strength of that association.[20]

Epidemiologic studies of birth defects and other adverse reproductive outcomes often present special challenges in terms of case definition and ascertainment (identification) and determination of exposure. The definition of what constitutes a case can present major problems in studies of birth defects. The completeness of ascertainment may vary by source and by defect. For example, one can argue that recent increases observed in the rates of patent ductus arteriosus (PDA) are due to increases in the incidence of the defect, better diagnosis, or increased survival of low-birth-weight infants in whom PDA frequently occurs. Even for defects that are readily recognizable at birth, such as NTDs, differences in sources of case ascertainment can lead to apparent differences in rates of occurrence,[21] which may be unrelated to differences in incidence.

There are three general categories of epidemiologic studies: descriptive, analytical, and experimental. The following discussion briefly considers some of the major features of these study designs, relating them to studies of birth defects and other adverse reproductive outcomes.

Descriptive Epidemiology

Case Reports

Most known teratogens and reproductive toxicants have been identified through case reports of an unusual number of cases or a constellation of abnormalities. These have often come from astute clinicians, who observed something out of the ordinary.[22–24] Although the importance of astute observations of abnormal aggregations of cases or patterns of malformations must be recognized, we cannot rely on such methods for identifying health hazards. Furthermore, etiologic speculations based on case reports or case series usually do not lead to a causal agent and are often false-positive speculations. Whereas case reports may identify a new teratogen, they can never provide an estimate of the risk of disease after exposure.

Descriptive Studies

Descriptive epidemiologic studies can be used to provide information about the distribution and frequency of some outcome of interest, resulting in rates of occurrence that can be compared among populations, places, or times. Defining the population at risk is the first step in a descriptive study. The population at risk can be defined geographically, such as residents within a state, or medically, such as being a patient at a particular hospital. Definition of the population at risk includes the time period under consideration. The population at risk constitutes the *denominator* for calculating rates of the occurrence of outcomes of interest.

The second step in a descriptive study is to determine the *numerator* for calculating rates for comparison. This involves two important concepts: (1) case definition (what defines a case to be counted) and (2) case ascertainment (how are cases to be identified).

Descriptive studies determine rates so that they can be compared. Possible differences in case ascertainment methods must be kept in mind. Some of the important issues associated with the determination of rates and their comparison have been discussed extensively by Borman and Cryer.[25]

Surveillance Programs

In surveillance programs, an at-risk population is identified and then followed over time to detect outcomes of interest. As they occur, cases are included in the database. Surveillance programs provide rates that can be examined for changes over time. They develop baseline data and subsequently permit early recognition of potential problems, based on ongoing data collection and analysis.

Birth defect surveillance (monitoring) systems (BDMSs) are designed to identify cases occurring in a defined population, usually by reviewing vital records or hospital record abstracts or charts. The defined population often is a sociopolitical unit, such as a state, but some monitoring programs have been based on discharge data from particular groups of hospitals or births to women residing in a specified metropolitan area.

Two BDMSs are operated by the Division of Birth Defects and Developmental Disabilities, National Center for Environmental Health, Centers for Disease Control and Prevention (CDC), Atlanta, Georgia. These two systems—the Birth Defects Monitoring Program (BDMP) and the Metropolitan Atlanta Congenital Defects Program (MACDP)—perform important surveillance functions.[26] The two systems follow populations defined differently and differ in sources of case ascertainment. Descriptions and comparisons of both systems are available.[27]

In the last 20 years, there has been a dramatic increase in the number of state-based birth defect surveillance systems. As of 1995, approximately half the states have some type of birth defect surveillance system.[28] These programs conduct routine reviews of occurrence rates of specific malformations and attempt to identify increases in rates or clusters of cases. Several of the states conducted case-control studies using cases from their surveillance program, and others have linked outcome data with environmental databases in an attempt to identify environmental reproductive hazards.[29-32] The use of cases from surveillance programs for hypothesis testing studies leads to a consideration of analytical epidemiology.

Analytical Epidemiology

Analytical epidemiologic studies are designed to generate or test hypotheses about associations between exposures and outcomes. The detection and quantification of such associations are major epidemiologic concerns. Such associations can be examined at either the group or individual level.

Ecologic Studies

Ecologic studies are important for generating hypotheses about the causes of an outcome such as a birth defect. In such studies, occurrence rates for an outcome are compared between groups thought to differ in terms of some exposure. Studies of this type do not collect information about exposures of individuals and are often used in environmental epidemiology, where residence in a particular area is used as an indicator of exposure. Lack of specific individual exposure data can be a critical limitation of this study design.

Examples of ecologic studies relevant to reproductive outcome include studies of congenital malformations in communities with vinyl chloride production facilities[33,34] and in communities with solvent-contaminated drinking water.[35] Ecologic studies often lead to hypotheses that can be tested using other study designs. Studies that allow associations between exposure and outcome to be assessed in particular individuals play a much more important role in epidemiologic research.

Case-Control Studies

The case-control study design, where groups of individuals with some outcome or disease of interest (cases), such as a congenital malformation, are compared to controls with regard to a history of one or more exposures, is the one most widely used in reproductive outcomes research. The controls are individuals as similar as possible to the cases, except that they are without the outcome of interest.

After cases and controls have been identified, the hypothesis to be tested is whether these two groups differ in exposure as well as outcome. How accurately exposure and its timing are determined may vary greatly among studies, but in any study the same methods must be used to establish the exposure of both cases and controls.[20]

Case-control studies are frequently used in epidemiology for several reasons. In testing etiologic hypotheses, they are applicable to outcomes of infrequent occurrence, and they can be conducted relatively rapidly and inexpensively. A disadvantage is that they have a potential for several important types of bias, including bias in recalling exposure, in selecting appropriate controls, and in ascertaining cases.

These problems can be addressed in part by use of two control groups, one "normal" and the second "abnormal." Any of several abnormal controls seem equally useful, for example, infants with mendelian disorders as well as infants with no specific malformation.[36] In the former, mothers have incentive to recall but teratogenesis is not the etiology.

Most human studies of potential teratogens following descriptive studies have been case-control studies. After suspecting on the basis of case observations that thalidomide was teratogenic, Lenz[37] conducted a case-control study. Following ecologic studies of ambient exposure to vinyl chloride, the hypothesis of an association between vinyl chloride exposure and congenital malformations was tested using case-control studies.[34,38,39] The association between valproic acid use and spina bifida was verified by case-control studies.[40]

Cohort Studies

Cohort studies use the reverse approach from case-control studies; individuals who differ in exposure history are examined for differences in the occurrence of outcomes of interest. The groups are defined by the presence or absence of exposure to a given factor and then are followed over time and compared for rates of occurrence (i.e., incidence rates) of the outcome of interest.

Cohort studies have three advantages: (1) the cohort is classified by exposure before the outcome is determined, thereby eliminating the exposure recall bias; (2) incidence rates can be calculated among those exposed; and (3) multiple outcomes can be observed simultaneously.

Cohort studies, often called *prospective studies,* require that groups differing in exposure be followed through time, with outcomes observed. Therefore, these studies tend to be time consuming and expensive. In addition, since occurrence rates for many adverse reproductive outcomes, such as congenital malformations, are low, large samples must be followed for long periods of time. Two main types of cohort studies have been developed: (1) those that identify a cohort and follow it into the future (concurrent cohort study), and (2) those that identify a cohort at some time in the past and follow it to the present (nonconcurrent cohort study).

In both cases, the risks of adverse outcomes are then compared between groups. Cohort studies enable investigators to calculate incidence rates that provide a measure of the risk of an outcome after the exposure. Risk in the exposed group can be compared with the risk in an unexposed group. Most frequently, the ratio of the incidence rate among the exposed to the rate among the unexposed is determined. This ratio, referred to as *relative risk,* is a measure of how much the presence of exposure increases the risk of the outcome.

Only a few large-scale concurrent cohort studies of problems of pregnancy outcome have been conducted. Probably the best known is the Collaborative Perinatal Project, conducted by the National Institute of Neurological and Communicative Disorders and Stroke. In this study, conducted between 1959 and 1966, about 55,000 women and their subsequently born children were studied extensively: the children were examined through age 8 years.[41] This study has provided considerable information on the use of drugs in pregnancy and birth defects and on many other topics (see Chapter 9).

Numerous studies of reproductive outcome have been conducted by the noncurrent cohort approach. These studies, also known as *historical prospective studies,* begin by identifying groups who differ in terms of some past exposure and follow them to the present and determine outcomes; exposure groups are defined before outcomes are known. A major advantage is that although the time frame is prospective, investigators do not have to follow the cohort into the future, waiting for events to occur. A disadvantage is that these studies require the ability to determine exposure status retrospectively.

A series of noncurrent cohort studies tested associations between smelters and spontaneous abortions.[42] Nordstrom and co-workers[43] compared histories of spontaneous abortions between women who differed in terms of occupational exposure to smelting processes. Later, Beckman and Nordstrom[44] surveyed exposed and unexposed male workers about their wives' histories of spontaneous abortions. In both instances, the findings supported a hypothesis of an association between the smelter and spontaneous abortions.

Experimental Epidemiology

Clinical Trials

The most common experimental study design in epidemiology is the clinical trial, in which the efficiency of a prevention or treatment regimen is evaluated. Ideally, subjects are randomly assigned to different treatment groups. The individuals must be as similar as possible in terms of unknown factors that may affect the response before they are randomly assigned to the treatment groups and receive the different regimens.[45]

The role of vitamin supplements taken during the periconception period in preventing NTDs has been evaluated in experimental studies. Smithells and co-workers[46,47] suggested that recurrence risks for NTDs were reduced in women who took the supplements during the period. In the original study, subjects were not randomized into different treatment groups, and because of this the conclusions have been criticized. More recent clinical trials of both NTD recurrence[48] and occurrence[49] have shown a protective effect of periconceptional folic acid supplementation, findings that have led to key public health recommendations regarding the use of folic acid to reduce the risk of these often devastating defects.[50]

In summary, experimental studies in epidemiology are unique in that they involve intervention as well as observation. In this way, they compare with approaches used in animal studies of teratology and other life sciences and yield results that can be analyzed like other experimental findings. They are limited, however, in what can be ethically tested, namely, treatment or preventive measures, rather than etiologic hypotheses.

Exposure Assessment

As a prerequisite to evaluating the reproductive hazards associated with an occupational or environmental agent, one must be able to measure or estimate exposure to potential hazards. A number of investigators have recently addressed the problems associated with this exposure assessment.[20,51–54]

Considerations concerning occupational exposure can be categorized into three areas: defining and determining exposure, timing of exposure, and problems of mixed exposures.[20] In the first area, which can also be labeled exposure occurrence and measurement,[53] the problems relate to determining what a particular worker is exposed to and then determining the amount of exposure, if possible. Workers often may not be aware of the chemical substances to which they are exposed. If possible, determining exposure history should begin by questioning the worker and taking a job history. Ideally, this should be augmented by reviewing the occupational and job history records that the employer maintains. The job history may make it possible for the investigator to determine the substances to which the worker was exposed. If so, the exposure records the employer maintains may include data from environmental monitoring.

Timing of exposure is crucial in studies of reproductive outcome. The critical stages in human development for teratogenesis were discussed earlier in this chapter. Except for exposures associated with mutational events, damage to the reproductive or endocrine systems, or storage of a substance for long periods in body tissues such as bone (lead) or fat (PCBs), exposures must occur within a limited period to produce teratogenic effects. For example, an agent suspected of causing an NTD could not be implicated as the cause of an infant's neural tube's failing to close if the mother had been exposed to the agent after the tube should have closed.

Employees may be exposed to a variety of potentially hazardous substances, leading to difficulty in demonstrating that a specific substance is a reproductive hazard. Most occupational exposures are to more than one substance, and it may not be possible to determine the reproductive effects of one agent—often occupational groups rather than specific exposures are studied. Studies of birth defects and other adverse reproductive outcomes associated with occupational groups have been reviewed recently.[55–57]

It is particularly difficult to determine exposures in studies of the ambient environment. There is growing interest and research activities in the use of biologic markers of exposure in studies of adverse reproductive outcomes.[58–61]

An additional concern is confounding by nonoccupational exposure(s) and lifestyle factors, for example, alcohol and tobacco use. Family history also may affect risk of adverse outcomes.

EXPOSURES THAT MAY LEAD TO ADVERSE REPRODUCTIVE OUTCOMES

We shall now review what is known about the effects of prenatal exposure to certain occupational and environmental agents. Agents were selected on the basis of the availability of human data and on the authors'

impressions of public concern that the agents may cause adverse reproductive effects.

Known human teratogens number about 30.[62] To date, only two have caused human maldevelopment (cerebral palsy and mental retardation) as a result of environmental contamination: high-dose ionizing radiation and methylmercury. Agents suspected of being teratogens on the basis of animal studies and limited epidemiologic studies are more numerous. When these agents are found to be polluting the environment, there is justifiable concern about potential prenatal exposure and adverse reproductive effects (Table 7–1). The difficulty of demonstrating an association between an environmental hazard and any adverse reproductive outcome must be appreciated.[63]

Several recent publications have addressed epidemiologic aspects of studying health effects of environmental contamination, including reproductive effects.[63–65] In a concise review, Heath[66] summarized some of the problems in epidemiologic studies of environmental hazards. Using as examples the childhood leukemia cluster in Woburn, Massachusetts, and the population exposure to waste chemicals at Love Canal, Heath identified three problems relevant to our discussion: low-dose, nonquantifiable exposures; the long and variable latency between exposure and outcome (disease); and the nonspecific nature of the outcome or disease. As a corollary to the last problem, Heath[66] pointed out that multiple factors probably play a causative role in most outcomes of interest including birth defects, low birth weight, spontaneous abortion, and cancer.

Ionizing Radiation

Acute High Dose

During the 1920s and 1930s, ionizing radiation was used to treat women with pelvic disease; soon afterward, it was identified as the first known environmental human teratogen.[67] Systematic studies of atomic bomb survivors in Japan showed that in utero exposure to high-dose radiation increased the risk of microcephaly and mental and growth **restriction** in the offspring.[6,68–71]

Studies of the Japanese survivors clearly show that distance from the hypocenter—the area directly beneath the detonated bomb—and the gestational age at the time of exposure were directly related to microcephaly and mental and growth restriction in the infant. Nine and 20 years after exposure, the greatest number of children with microcephaly and mental retardation and growth restriction were in the group exposed at 15 weeks' gestation or earlier. These findings contrast with those of children exposed in utero during the third trimester and whose mothers were farthest from the hypocenter at the time of exposure. Of 55

Table 7–1. OCCUPATIONAL AND ENVIRONMENTAL AGENTS THAT MAY BE ASSOCIATED WITH HUMAN ADVERSE REPRODUCTIVE OUTCOMES

Agent	Outcome
Ionizing radiation	
Acute high-dose	Microcephaly, mental retardation, growth restriction
Chronic low-dose or before pregnancy	?Down syndrome
Methylmercury	Mental retardation, cerebral palsy, deafness, blindness, seizures (abnormal neuronal migration)
Mercury vapor	Cranial defects, spontaneous abortion, ?stillbirth
Lead	
High-dose	Infertility, spontaneous abortion, growth restriction, psychomotor retardation, seizures, stillbirth
Chronic low-dose	Lower IQ, cognitive impairment in speech and language, attention deficit
Polychlorinated biphenyls	
High-dose	Spontaneous abortion, low birth weight, neuroectodermal dysplasia (skin staining, natal teeth, dysplastic nails, developmental and psychologic deficits), abnormal bone calcification
Chronic low-dose	Lower birth weight, smaller head circumference, ?cognitive impairment
Polybrominated biphenyls	
Chronic low-dose	?Lower birth weight, ?smaller head circumference, ?cognitive impairment
Anesthetic gases	
Chronic low-dose	Spontaneous abortion
Birth defects	
Organic solvents	
Chronic high-dose	Developmental impairment, facial dysmorphism, growth restriction (similar to fetal alcohol embryopathy)
Chronic low-dose	Spontaneous abortion, CNS malformations, orofacial clefts

such children evaluated 20 years later, only 1 was found to be microcephalic, and all were of normal intelligence.[69] Although teratogenic effects have been found in several organ systems of animals exposed to acute, high-dose radiation, no structural malformations other than those mentioned above have been reported among humans exposed prenatally.

Using data from animals and from outcomes of reported human exposures at various times during pregnancy, DeKaban[72] constructed a timetable for extrapolating acute, high-dose radiation (>250 rad) to various reproductive outcomes in humans. Similarities between animal and known human effects support DeKaban's proposal.

Chronic Low Dose

Effects of chronic low-dose radiation on reproduction have not been identified in animals or humans. Increased risk of adverse outcomes was not detected among animals with continuous low-dose exposure (<5 rad) throughout pregnancy.[73]

The relationship between human structural malformations and background radiation has been examined in several epidemiologic studies in different geographic areas. Cosmic radiation was thought to be one factor that contributed to increased rates of anencephalus between 1950 and 1969 in several Canadian cities.[74] Using geologic estimates of natural radioactivity, some investigators have attributed increased malformation rates, including the rate for Down syndrome, to higher radioactivity levels.[75,76] Other studies of the association between estimated cosmic radiation exposure and congenital malformation rates have produced negative results.[77,78] Given that low-dose radiation could be one of a multitude of environmental factors that affect the risk of birth defects, perhaps it is not surprising that no consistent relationship is evident.

Mutagenesis

Children exposed in utero to radiation from the atomic bomb were studied over several years for evidence of genetic damage. No evidence for effects was found when six indicators were evaluated: congenital malformations, stillbirths and neonatal death rates, birth weight, sex ratio at birth, anthropomorphic measurements during the first year of life, and mortality in offspring (F1 generation).[67,79–81]

In contrast to the atomic bomb follow-up studies, other investigations have found that mutagenic effects may occur when women are exposed prenatally to diagnostic radiation. These effects include altered sex ratios among the offspring—slightly more females than expected[82]—and abnormal karyotypes in spontaneously aborted fetuses.[83]

Mutagenic effects in the offspring of irradiated women may be manifested years after the birth of the infant. Compared with nonirradiated controls, the estimated risk of leukemia was increased 50 percent for children exposed in utero to radiation during maternal pelvimetry examinations.[84–86] Although this increase seems considerable, it translates into an approximate risk of 1 in 2,000 for exposed versus 1 in 3,000 for unexposed children. As Brent[73] points out, if one were to recommend that pregnancies be terminated whenever exposure from diagnostic radiation occurred because of the increased probability of leukemia in the offspring, 1,999 exposed pregnancies would have to be terminated to prevent a single case of leukemia.

Questions have been raised about potential risks to children associated with parental (paternal) occupational exposure to low-dose radiation.[87] A case-control study by Gardner et al.[88,89] in the area around the Sellafield Nuclear Facility in the United Kingdom found a statistically significant association between paternal preconception radiation dose and childhood leukemia risk. A similar association had been observed between paternal preconception radiation and risk in workers at the Hanford Nuclear Facility in the United States.[90] The finding regarding childhood leukemia risk is a particularly contentious issue, contradicting studies of the children born to atomic bomb survivors who do not show genetic effects, such as increased risks of childhood cancers.[81] A study in the vicinity of nuclear facilities in Ontario also failed to demonstrate an association between childhood leukemia risk and paternal preconception dose (exposure).[91]

Video Display Terminals

Since the 1980s, there has been concern about video display terminals (VDTs) linked to adverse reproductive outcomes. Much of the early concern grew out of reports of spontaneous abortion clusters among groups of women who used VDTs at work, and some of the reported clusters also included birth defects.[92] While it was suggested that these "unexpected" clusters were actually expected based on the frequency of occurrence of spontaneous abortions (10 to 15 percent of recognized pregnancies) and the extremely large number of women working with VDTs,[93] several large epidemiologic studies were carried out to examine the association.[94,95] Numerous papers have been published on this topic, along with a number of reviews.[56,92,93] Our interpretation of these studies is that VDT use does not increase the risk of adverse reproductive outcomes.

Organic Mercury—Methylmercury

Exposure to organic mercury compounds, such as methyl- or ethylmercury, is not common. In the United States, methylmercury was widely used as a fungicide until the 1960s, when U.S. production was halted because of the compound's toxicity and bioaccumulation. Today in the United States, exposure mainly occurs through the consumption of contaminated fish. Fish may become contaminated when organomercurials are present in water or when bacteria in water convert inorganic mercury to organic mercury, part of a complex environmental mercury cycle.[96]

Methylmercury effects were discovered in 1959 after an epidemic of poisoning in Minamata, Japan, that resulted in fetal neurologic damage with psychomotor retardation, seizures, cerebral palsy, blindness, and deafness.[97] In 1972, similar fetal effects were observed in Iraq after an epidemic of methylmercury poisoning.[98] In both epidemics, breast-fed infants had additional exposure through maternal milk.[97]

Unintentional human exposures have permitted a more thorough study of the reproductive effects of methylmercury than of any other environmental pollutant.[99-101] The persistence of organic mercury in the body (biologic half-life about 70 days) and its accumulation in hair further make it possible to reconstruct prenatal exposure.[102] Methylmercury crosses the placenta easily and accumulates in embryonic and fetal tissues, particularly brain tissues, at concentrations exceeding those in the mother.[103,104] Methylmercury does not cause obvious structural malformations in humans; thus, the devastating effects are not apparent at birth and are manifested only as the child ages. The developing nervous system of the conceptus and infant is more sensitive to the toxic effects of organic mercury than that of the adult or older child,[97] and the infant of an asymptomatic mother can be affected severely.[98,101,105]

Little is known of the human effects of methylmercury at low levels of exposure. Minor neurologic differences, mainly brisker deep tendon reflexes, were found among native Quebec boys exposed in utero compared with boys who had no such exposure.[106] Low-level methylmercury exposure may be associated with an increased frequency of chromosomal abnormalities[107]; the significance of this finding for adverse health or reproductive effects is unknown.

Nonhuman primates chronically treated with low-dose methylmercury were more likely to experience reproductive failure (nonconception, spontaneous abortion) than nontreated controls.[108] Prenatal exposure of nonhuman primates resulted in offspring with impaired visual recognition that was consistent with a developmental teratogenic effect.[109-111]

While there appears to be no association between congenital malformations and human environmental exposure, methylmercury is embryolethal in laboratory animals and causes various structural malformations (exencephaly, limb abnormalities) when high doses are given during critical periods in development.[112] Mattison et al.[113] have reviewed experimental and human epidemiologic data regarding mercury and other metals, listing the site(s) of action or reproductive outcome studied. A recent review by Weiss[114] includes a quantitative risk assessment of the developmental neurotoxicology of methylmercury.

Elemental Mercury (Vapor)

Mercury is an unusual element. At room temperature it is liquid, with a high vapor pressure, and vapor concentrations can rise rapidly to toxic concentrations in closed or poorly ventilated areas. The vapor is odorless and colorless, making it virtually nondetectable without special equipment.

Women at risk for exposure work primarily in health-related occupations such as nursing, medicine, dentistry, and dental hygiene. Exposure may occur when dental amalgams are prepared and when thermometers or manometers are broken or mercury is spilled. In recent years, encapsulated amalgam preparations and electronic methods for measuring blood pressure and temperature have been developed. Consequently, mercury exposure in medicine and dentistry in the United States has probably decreased.

Given that large numbers of women of childbearing age may have been exposed occupationally to mercury vapor, there is a surprising dearth of animal and human epidemiologic studies of reproductive effects. In one study, mercury vapor exposure at 0.5 mg/m^3 throughout pregnancy resulted in cranial defects in 2 of 115 fetal rats.[115] Exposure during days 10 through 15 of gestation produced increased fetal resorption.[115] This vapor concentration is 10 times greater than the occupational limit of 0.05 mg/m^3 established by the Occupational Safety and Health Administration[116] and probably caused maternal toxicity that contributed to the observed fetal effects. To protect the developing conceptus, Koos and Longo[99] recommend that women of childbearing age should not be exposed to vapor concentrations exceeding 0.01 mg/m^3.

Animal studies demonstrate the ease with which elemental mercury crosses the placenta. Following mercury vapor exposure, fetal rat blood mercury concentrations were 65 times higher than the corresponding maternal values, and the highest mercury concentrations were found in the rat placenta.[117] Placental and fetal membranes from mercury-exposed dental workers contained two to three times more mercury than tissues taken from unexposed women.[118] The fetal and maternal blood mercury concentrations were similar in both groups, implying that the placenta and fetal tissues may act as a barrier at low levels of mercury vapor.[118]

Epidemiologic studies of reproductive effects have been conducted with dental assistants and female dentists. Radiation and anesthetic gases are potential confounding exposures overlooked in many studies. Other methodologic problems, such as nonverification of the outcome, absence of exposure data, and low survey response rates, often are not considered. The limited studies to date do not provide conclusive evidence that occupational exposure to mercury vapor is teratogenic or results in other adverse reproductive outcomes. The need for more animal and human studies of reproductive effects has been recognized.[119]

At least one case report has suggested a possible association between occupational exposure to mercury vapor and severe brain damage in a newborn.[120] A female dental surgeon, who worked in a surgery with mercury levels above the threshold limit value, gave birth to a small-for-dates baby with severe brain damage, not otherwise specified. The authors stress that a case report can only suggest an effect, but the finding is consistent with animal teratology.

Rowland[121] reviewed the reproductive effects of mercury vapor and presented data from studies of female dental assistants in California. Women who prepared 50 or more dental amalgams per week had a statistically insignificantly increased risk for spontaneous abortion. Women who prepared 30 or more amalgams a week in offices with poor mercury hygiene showed evidence of reduced fecundity. A detailed analysis of fecundity, assessed as time to pregnancy in this cohort of dental assistants, was published recently.[122] To our knowledge, there are no published data on congenital malformations among births to dental assistants in the United States.

Lead

Since the 19th century, exposure to high levels of lead has been known to cause embryotoxicity, growth restriction and mental retardation, increased perinatal mortality, and developmental disability.[123] These adverse reproductive effects were seen when women in occupational settings were exposed to concentrations of lead in air that far exceeded levels allowable today. As a matter of historic interest, unscrupulous vendors sold pills containing lead as an abortifacient at the turn of the century.[124]

Sources of nonoccupational lead exposure commonly encountered by U.S. women are unlikely to result in detectable effects. Regulatory and public health efforts are directed at reducing preconceptional and prenatal exposure in order to reduce maternal-to-fetal lead transmission.

Twenty-five years of public health efforts have produced a striking reduction in lead exposure in the United States. The average blood lead level has decreased to less than 20 percent of levels measured in the 1970s. However, elevated blood lead (>20 μg/dl) has a higher incidence among immigrants to Southern California. In Los Angeles, 25 of the 30 cases of elevated blood lead occurred in immigrants.[125]

High lead concentration in maternal blood is associated with an increased risk of delivery of a small-for-gestational-age infant.[126] The frequency of preterm birth was also almost three times higher among women who had umbilical cord levels greater than or equal to

5.1 μg/dl, compared with those who had levels below that cutoff. This was observed in nulliparous women, but not in multiparous women in Mexico City.[127] One study in Norway found an increased risk of low birth weight and also neural tube defects.[128]

Eating lead-glazed clay pots (pica) resulted in lead toxicity in pregnancy in a Mexican-American mother.[129] Asking pregnant women about risk factors for lead exposure can aid in assessing prenatal exposure risk. A questionnaire that combined housing conditions, smoking status, and high consumption of canned foods had a sensitivity of 89.2 percent and a negative predictive value of 96.4 percent.[130] Consumption of calcium and avoidance of the use of lead-glazed ceramics resulted in lowering of blood lead, especially in pregnant women of low socioeconomic status in Mexico City.[131]

Because the nervous system may be more susceptible to the toxic effects during the embryonic and fetal periods than at any other time of life[104] and because maternal and cord blood lead concentrations are directly correlated,[132] lead concentrations in blood should not exceed 25 μg/dl in women of reproductive age.[133]

Ideally, the maternal blood lead level should be less than 10 μg/dl to ensure that a child begins life with minimal lead exposure. A dose–response relationship is strongly supported by numerous epidemiologic studies of children showing a reduction in IQ with increasing blood lead concentrations above 10 μg/dl. Of note, these studies measured blood lead concentrations over time (often 2 years or more) and reported averaged values. Other neurologic impairments associated with increased blood lead concentrations include attention deficit disorder ("hyperactivity"), hearing deficits, learning disabilities, and shorter stature. Thus, for public health purposes, childhood lead poisoning has been defined as a blood lead level of 10 μg/dl or higher.[134]

In occupational settings, federal standards mandate that women should not work in areas where air lead concentrations can reach 50 μg/cm^3, since this may result in blood concentrations above 25 to 30 μg/dl.[135] Subtle but permanent neurologic impairment in children may occur at lower blood lead concentrations.[136,137] Although controversial, such studies raise the possibility that the occupational standard may inadequately protect the fetus. Protection of fetuses from lead exposure was an important concern raised in the Johnson Controls case in the U.S. Supreme Court.[138] The issues of the neurodevelopmental effects of prenatal lead exposure have been discussed by Bellinger and Needleman.[139]

Lead screening of pregnant women is highly controversial and not presently recommended. Lead is mobilized from the maternal skeleton during pregnancy and the postpartum period.[140] In the absence of excessive exposure, most of the lead in blood comes from bone stores, and no intervention is available to reduce the blood lead.[141] Chelation therapy is potentially hazardous, and some agents are teratogenic.[142] On the other hand, screening could identify women who may benefit from environmental or other interventions to reduce their lead exposure.

The Phenoxy Herbicide 2,4,5-Trichlorophenoxyacetic acid and Dioxins/Agent Orange

These compounds are considered together because 2,3,7,8-tetrachlorodibenzodioxin (TCDD or dioxin) and other chlorinated dibenzodioxins were produced as contaminants during production of the herbicide 2,4,5-trichlorophenoxyacetic acid (2,4,5-T).[143] This herbicide is no longer marketed in the United States, largely because of concerns about possible teratogenic and fetotoxic effects (seen after high doses are administered to animals during critical periods of organogenesis).[144]

Agent Orange, a defoliant used in Vietnam, was a mixture of herbicides, including 2,4,5-T. During the later years of the Vietnam War, public opinion against the ecologic effects of Agent Orange was fueled by reports of birth defects in South Vietnamese babies born to mothers who lived in areas where Agent Orange had been sprayed. The ensuing debate about the potential human teratogenicity of Agent Orange involved numerous federal agencies, and the use of 2,4,5-T containing any chlorodioxin contaminants was cancelled in 1970.[145]

Because 2,4,5-T contained small amounts of TCDD and since long-term human effects were unknown, the U.S. Public Health Service began an immense follow-up of Vietnam veterans. One portion of the study evaluated Vietnam veterans' risks of fathering infants with birth defects. The investigators concluded that "Vietnam veterans who had greater estimated opportunities for Agent Orange exposure did not seem to be at greater risk for fathering babies with all types of defects combined."[146] Vietnam service was associated with a few defects, however; Agent Orange exposure, other Vietnam-related experience, or some unidentified risk factor may have been responsible for the associations.[146] In a subsequent follow-up study, Vietnam and non-Vietnam veterans were interviewed regarding congenital malformations in their offspring. Although Vietnam veterans were more likely to report birth defects in their offspring, hospital records showed similar rates of birth defects for children born to both veteran groups.[147] In contrast, increased central nervous system (CNS), skeletal, and cardiovascular malformations and disease were reported among Australian Vietnam veterans.[148] This study was less rigorous than its American counterparts, since it was an unconventional case-control design and relatively few children had diagnoses confirmed by medical record review.

Concerns about the reproductive effects of dioxins continue to be expressed. The Environmental Protection Agency has included an extensive discussion of these issues in a recent reassessment of 2,3,7,8-TCDD.[149] Overall, the data appear inadequate to support allegations of adverse reproductive outcomes following human exposure to the dioxin-contaminated herbicide, although this is a topic of continuing discussion.[145] The 1996 Institute of Medicine report concluded that "limited/suggestive evidence exists of an association between dioxin exposure in veterans and offspring they sired with spina bifida."[150] The strength of even this tenuous statement seems arguable to us.

Polychlorinated Biphenyls

Polychlorinated biphenyls (PCBs) were widely used in industry because of their thermal stability and heat transfer properties.[151] PCBs are also extremely stable and resistant to metabolic or biologic degradation and have become ubiquitous in the environment because of past dumping or disposal in unregulated landfills and failure to recycle. PCBs are highly lipid soluble, accumulate in fat, and can be found at high concentrations in the breast milk of women despite low concentrations in their blood.[152] Details of PCB biochemistry and toxicology are available elsewhere.[153,154] Jacobson and Jacobson provide a thorough discussion of clinical effects of in utero PCB exposure.[155]

Two epidemics of cooking oil contamination provide evidence that high-dose PCBs are hazardous to human reproduction. In these epidemics, adults consumed cooking oil tainted with thermally degraded PCBs and developed a disease termed "Yusho" (in Japan) and "Yu-cheng" (in Taiwan). The disease was characterized by chloracne (an acneform rash), eyelid swelling and discharge, and skin hyperpigmentation.[156] Although PCBs alone are usually blamed for these and subsequent health problems, it is clear that heat-degradation products of PCBs (polychlorodibenzofurans [PCDEs] and polychlorinated quarterphenyls [PCQs]) contributed significantly to toxicity.[157,158] A follow up in 1999 compared 795 subjects exposed postnatal to 693 controls.[159] Lifetime prevalences in the former were increased for chloracne, abnormal nails, hyperkeratosis, skin allergy, goiter, headache, gum pigmentation, broken teeth, anemia in women, arthritis, and herniated intervertebral disks in men. For other medical conditions no differences were observed.

A teratogenic effect was observed as well, as reviewed by Jacobson and Jacobson.[155] High-dose transplacental exposure to the cooking oil resulted in congenital anomalies and low birth weight.[160] Skin and mucosal hyperpigmentation were the most often noted abnormalities.[160] Other anomalies included natal teeth, gingival hyperplasia, exophthalmos, skull calcifications, and delayed bone age.[160]

In 1985, Rogan and coworkers[161] examined 117 children with prenatal and/or breast milk exposure to the PCB/PCDF/PCQ-contaminated oil. Compared with unexposed children, those exposed demonstrated delayed developmental milestones, psychological deficits, and behavioral abnormalities. Physical abnormalities included shorter stature, lighter weight, and epidermal disorders such as acne, hyperpigmentation, deformed nails, gingival hypertrophy, and tooth chipping.[161] Developmentally, exposed children in Taiwan demonstrated cognitive impairment that persisted up to age 7 years.[162] "Catch-up" growth occurred in most of the surviving infants, with attainment of normal body weight by 2 years of age.[153,163] In aggregate, these findings suggest a neuroectodermal dysplasia due to combined effects of the PCBs and contaminants.[161]

In addition to the teratogenic effects, the contaminated oils led to excessive reproductive losses among exposed women. Increased risks for spontaneous abortion, stillbirth, and infant mortality were documented in follow-up study of a group of Taiwanese women.[163] A recent follow-up of 368 of the 596 living Yu-cheng women was performed, comparing reproductive outcome to that of 312 controls. The women exposed in 1979 reported more stillbirths (4.2 percent vs. 1.7 percent controls), more abnormal menstrual bleeding (16 percent vs. 8 percent), and more offspring dying during childbirth (10.2 percent vs. 6.1 percent).[164]

Effects of high-level cooking oil contamination should be distinguished from those of ambient or low-level exposure to PCBs. Low-level PCB maternal exposure can occur throughout life by consumption of fish from PCB-contaminated waters as well as other dietary sources. While transplacental transfer of PCBs occurs,[165] the largest dose is delivered to the nursing infant via breast milk.[152,166] Maternal exposure and PCB tranfer to nursing infants has resulted in justifiable concern about reproductive and developmental effects. Studies ongoing in the Great Lakes region are examining such effects.

In these studies, maternal PCB exposure via fish consumption, defined as 11.8 kg of Lake Michigan fish in the 6 years before delivery, was reported to be associated with a slight decrease in infant birth weight (160 to 190 g) and head circumference, relative to unexposed controls.[167] Neonatal assessment of the same infants provides some evidence that at low concentrations, PCBs may be behavioral teratogens.[168] Short-term memory impairment noted in infancy persisted at 4 years of age only in those children whose cord blood PCB concentrations were in the top 5 percent of values for the cohort.[166] A later study on the Lake Michigan–exposed cases also showed a small decrease in IQ in children exposed to in utero.[169] The difference was 6.2 points in the most highly exposed group, and only one child was mentally retarded. Others have criticized this conclusion on grounds of the small observed difference and the relatively small subset of the original exposed sample available for study (potential selection bias).[170,171]

A cohort of North Carolina children followed since birth appears to be representative of the general population, that is, without unusual PCB exposure. Periodic developmental evaluations, including standardized developmental tests, behavioral ratings, and school report card evaluations,[170,171] up to school age have not demonstrated a relationship between prenatal or postnatal (breast-feeding) PCB exposure.

A Dutch cohort of children exposed 42 months earlier in utero reported that scores on the Kaufman Assessment Battery for Children were lowered by 4 points.[172] The same cohort showed birth weight to be 165 g less.[173]

Overall, the developmental effect of low-level PCB exposure remains unclear. Any deleterious effect is not substantive and potentially explainable on the basis of confounding variables. Additional studies of congener-specific effects on a variety of reproductive and developmental endpoints are desirable, especially in determining propriety of breast-feeding.[174]

Polybrominated Biphenyls

Polybrominated biphenyl (PBB) compounds are structurally similar to PCBs and share characteristics of high lipid solubility and resistance to metabolic or biologic degradation. Fortunately, PBBs are not as widespread environmental contaminants as PCBs because their use has been more limited.

PBBs were used as fire-retardants in the United States until 1974. In 1973 and 1974, cattle feed distributed in Michigan inadvertently became contaminated with PBBs. Before the contamination was recognized, people in the state consumed PBB-tainted meat and poultry. Reviews of the incident and subsequent health studies are available.[175–178]

Fetal mortality in high- versus low-exposure regions of Michigan was not appreciably different after the PBB contamination.[179] The study of fetal mortality is not conclusive because of potential inaccuracies in exposure estimates, the inability to control for confounding variables, and the possibility that fetal mortality may not be the best indicator of PBB reproductive effects. In addition, this study was based on fetal deaths occurring at greater than 20 weeks gestation, and risks for early fetal losses could be different than those for later deaths.[180]

Transplacental and breast milk exposure of infants was documented in the Michigan incident.[181] An early follow-up study reported that children with higher PBB body burdens scored lower on standardized tests of perceptual motor, attentional, and verbal abilities.[182] Later testing of these children showed that their overall developmental scores were within the normal range.[183]

Nitrates and Nitrite

Nitrate contamination of drinking water supplies may result from agricultural (fertilizer) run-off, sewerage, or industrial waste. Nitrates and nitrite appear not to be teratogenic in animals.[184,185] Administration of sodium nitrite to pregnant mice stimulated fetal erythropoiesis but did not affect fetal mortality, resorptions, average weight, number of offspring, or incidence of skeletal malformations.[186]

Although some results are suggestive, human epidemiologic studies provide no conclusive evidence that pregnant women who consume low levels of nitrates from drinking water are at increased risk for having a malformed baby. In South Australia, an excess of birth defects prompted a case-control study examining the relationship between maternal drinking water source (groundwater vs. rainwater) and risk of malformations.[187] The risk of having a malformed infant was increased among women who drank groundwater. Risks for NTDs and oral clefts particularly were increased. Using estimated nitrate concentration, a dose–response relationship was found with a threefold increased risk at 5 to 15 mg/L nitrates and fourfold increased risk for greater than 15 mg/L nitrates. Study strengths include case ascertainment and monitoring of water nitrate concentrations during the study period; limitations include the assumption that water concentrations were constant during monitoring intervals and that subjects used the same source of drinking water throughout pregnancy. Most notable is the assumption that nitrates rather than some unmeasured drinking water contaminant was responsible. In fact, the seasonal variation in malformation risks suggests that dietary, nutritional, or other environmental factors may have contributed to the increased malformation rates.

A Canadian case-control study found that nitrate exposure from private wells was associated with an increased risk for delivering an infant with a CNS malformation. However, the opposite was found with drinking water obtained from other sources: increased nitrates were associated with a decrease in CNS malformations. To assess exposure, the investigators analyzed nitrates in water samples collected at addresses where study subjects lived at the time of delivery. Once again, the study is limited by the lack of information about other possible water contaminants. The contradictory risks associated with drinking water source, independent of nitrate concentration, also suggests that other factors contributed to the observed effects.[54]

The Iowa Health Department guidelines state that there is no toxicity under 10 parts per million of nitrates. The reason for toxicity is that infants under 6 months of age exposed to higher levels of nitrates are at risk of methemoglobinemia. Toxic effects of nitrates on pregnant women and fetuses have not been studied extensively, but no adverse effects have been found.

Organic Solvents

Large numbers of women are employed in industries that use organic solvents, and women also may be exposed through use of household products or drinking water contamination. Not surprisingly, concerns have arisen that such exposures may cause any of several adverse reproductive outcomes.

Acute human health effects of high-dose solvent exposure are well known. Central nervous system effects including cortical atrophy, cerebellar degeneration, and loss of intellectual functioning have been documented as a result of chronic, high-dose solvent abuse ("sniffing" or "huffing").[188] Solvent intoxication is an established occupational hazard in such diverse groups as painters and rubber, semiconductor, and dry-cleaning workers. Symptoms may follow inhalation, dermal, or ingestion exposure routes and may include headache, nausea, dizziness, and confusion progressing to CNS depression with loss of consciousness. Chronic exposure to low levels of solvents may lead to neuropsychiatric impairment and peripheral nerve damage.[189]

Analogous to the health effects described above, maternal solvent abuse by "sniffing" is reported to cause an embryopathy similar to the fetal alcohol syndrome (FAS), Hersch and associates[190] described three children with developmental and intellectual impairment, facial dysmorphism, and intrauterine growth restriction whose mothers abused spray paint throughout their pregnancies. Similar dysmorphic features and neurologic impairment have been described in other children born to mothers who chronically abused toluene or unnamed solvents during pregnancy.[191–193] A fetal solvent syndrome and toluene embryopathy have been described that may be similar in pathogenesis to FAS.[194,195]

At lower levels of maternal exposure there is no clear evidence of embryopathic, fetal, or neurobehavioral adverse effects. Epidemiologic studies have examined reproductive outcomes of occupationally as well as environmentally exposed women. Most occupational studies of this subject are case-control studies, with exposure status based on job descriptions and no actual exposure data available (e.g., air concentrations or duration of exposure). Multiple solvent exposures often are likely.[196]

Using occupational codes from birth certificates, Olsen[197] reported that mothers who were painters or worked in a laboratory were no more likely than unexposed mothers to have children with CNS, gastrointestinal, or congenital limb anomalies. Heidam[198] surveyed Danish women in selected occupations that could result in various chemical exposures. Compared with unexposed women, female painters had a slightly higher risk for spontaneous abortion. In a study of pregnancy outcomes among women employed at a semiconductor manufacturer, Pastides and associates[199] found an increased risk of spontaneous abortions for women working in the diffusion area. Materials used in the diffusion area include glycol ethers, toxic gases, and various solvents, providing potentially numerous and mixed exposures. Given the small number of pregnancies in exposed and unexposed groups, the authors consider their results as tentative, pointing out the need for larger prospective studies that include monitoring data to quantity exposure.[199]

Two subsequent studies have supported the earlier findings of associations between semiconductor manufacturing and spontaneous abortion risk. In a study of IBM employees, investigators from Johns Hopkins University reported an association between spontaneous abortion risk and working with ethylene glycol ethers in "clean rooms" (R.H. Gray, personal communication, 1993). Similarly, a study by investigators at the University of California, Davis, carried out for the Semiconductor Industry Association, found a significant increase in spontaneous abortion risk among fabrication workers. This increase was suggested to be associated with exposure to glycol ethers.[200]

Occupational exposure to organic solvents in the first trimester of pregnancy is also associated with an increased risk of major fetal malformation[201] (relative risk, 13.0; 95 percent confidence interval, 1.8 to 99.5). The risk is increased in women with symptoms associated with the exposure.[201]

On numerous occasions, drinking water contamination by organic solvents has resulted from storage tank leaks or hazardous waste leachate. Affected communities may identify a temporal or geographic clustering of adverse reproductive effects, believing that the contamination has caused the epidemic. To date, there is no published evidence to support such a cause-and-effect relationship, but at least one study demonstrated an increased risk of spontaneous abortions among women during the time that their drinking water supply was contaminated with trichloroethane and other organic solvents.[35] A hospital-based study also was undertaken in response to community concerns that there were increased numbers of children born with congenital cardiac anomalies to women living in the contaminated area. The increased prevalence of cardiac anomalies was confirmed but found to be temporally unrelated to the drinking water contamination, making a causal relationship unlikely.[202]

With all the limitations of a questionnaire study, one author found an association between spontaneous abortion and the number of hours worked per day in cosmetology, the number of chemical services performed, and work in salons where nail sculpturing was performed. There was no association among cosmetologists who performed few chemical services or who worked less than 35 hours per week.[203]

In conclusion, toluene and possibly other organic solvents are probably teratogenic at high exposure levels seen with solvent abuse. The risk for the "fetal solvent syndrome" is unknown, and no exposure threshold for effect can be identified at this time. Occupational exposure to organic solvents in the first trimester is also associated with an increased risk of major fetal malformations,[204] especially in women with symptoms.

In a similar vein, when a pregnant woman asks if it is safe for her to paint the baby's nursery, Scialli[204] wisely advises counseling to minimize exposure without giving the impression that paint is an established developmental toxicant. Similar advice can be offered to women who want to color their hair, (e.g., recommending a well-ventilated area).

Anesthetic Gases

Large numbers of women working in medical and dental professions may be exposed occupationally to anesthetic gases, raising serious concerns about the reproductive hazards of such exposures. There is evidence that chronic first-trimester exposure may increase the risk of spontaneous abortion.[205,206] Despite numerous studies, the question of whether or not a mother's exposure to anesthetic gas increases the risk of her bearing a congenitally malformed infant is still debated. One argument against a causal relationship is that no pattern of malformations has been found in studies reporting increased birth defect rates following maternal exposure during pregnancy.[207] On the other hand, animal studies have shown that anesthetic gases can be teratogenic at concentrations similar to those experienced by operating room personnel in the absence of gas scavenging systems.[208–210] Some investigators have found increased rates of birth defects in infants born to exposed women and have observed a dose-related effect.[205,206,211] In two studies, the rate of congenitally malformed infants was increased among female anesthetists who worked during the first 6 months of pregnancy compared with the rate among female anesthetists who did not work during pregnancy.[212,213] A criteria document prepared by the National Institute for

Occupational Safety and Health (NIOSH) reviews animal data and epidemiologic studies published before 1977.[206] More recent reviews are also available.[214,215]

In a retrospective study of reproductive outcomes and anesthetic gas exposure in Ontario hospital personnel, Guirguis et al.[216] observed significantly more congenital malformations among female workers with anesthesia exposure than among a comparison group without such exposure. Increases were also observed in wives of exposed males. These findings were based on self-reports, with an excess of minor malformations, and reporting bias is a potential problem. Statistically significantly increased risk of spontaneous abortion was also observed in the exposed cohort.

A recent study in France compared the rates of spontaneous abortions and birth defects in nurses who worked in operating rooms with those of nurses who worked in other departments of the same hospitals.[217] A total of 776 pregnancies was identified among 418 nurses. The rate of spontaneous abortions among nurses who worked in operating rooms during the pregnancy was significantly higher than among nurses working in other parts of the hospital. Self-reported first-trimester exposures to anesthetics, ionizing radiation, formol, and all three were also significantly associated with increased risks of spontaneous abortion. While an increased risk following exposure to antineoplastic agents was reported, it was not statistically significant. The only significantly increased risk of birth defects was observed with formol exposure. Adjusted odds ratios based on logistic regression showed a significantly increased risk of birth defects associated with the combination exposure of anesthetics, ionizing radiation, and formol. The methods suggest that there may be potential recall bias associated with exposures to specific agents that do not apply to the general work location, such as the operating room.

Using a case-control approach, Matte et al.[218] studied potential associations between parental employment in health care occupations and birth defects. Cases for the study came from the Metropolitan Atlanta Congenital Defects Program registry and controls were randomly selected from live births without malformations occurring in the five-county metropolitan Atlanta area. A statistically significant association was observed between maternal employment as a nurse and congenital defects as a group. The risks for several specific birth defects were also significantly elevated for nurses. Of particular relevance to our discussion here, potential maternal exposure to anesthetic gases was significantly associated with risk of spina bifida, based on three exposed cases.

Virtually all epidemiologic studies of exposure to waste anesthetic gas and reproductive outcomes have design problems that affect the interpretation of reported results. Crude estimates of anesthetic gas exposure have been used because no actual measurements of gas concentrations were available. The specific gases were usually not identified, and exposure to mixtures of anesthetic agents is likely.[206] Many studies have been conducted by survey, with no validation of the responses and, often, poor response rates. In such studies, selection bias cannot be evaluated because there is no information about nonresponders. Also, not validating the reproductive history can lead to misleading results for several reasons. Study subjects may forget or inaccurately recall events that took place years before. Women who think they are exposed to an adverse environmental agent may be more likely to recall having a spontaneous abortion or a child with a minor malformation than are unexposed women.[219] One last problem pertains to the inherent difficulty of studying spontaneous abortions. To avoid the criticism that reported spontaneous abortions were not validated, investigators in one study considered only patients whose spontaneous abortions required them to be hospitalized.[219] The problem with this approach is that women who have spontaneous abortions do not always require hospitalization, particularly if the abortion occurred during the first trimester or before pregnancy was diagnosed.

Specific data are accumulating regarding risks of occupational exposure to nitrous oxide. Rowland et al.[210] reported that exposure to 5 or more hours of unscavenged nitrous oxide per week among a cohort of female dental assistants was statistically significantly associated with reduced fertility. This was based on assessment of time to pregnancy and self-reported nitrous oxide exposure. In a subsequent report from the same cohort, Rowland et al.[219] observed an increased risk of spontaneous abortion among women in the cohort working with nitrous oxide 3 or more hours per week in offices not using scavenging equipment. This recent cohort study has not provided any information on malformation risks. The number of exposed births is too small ($n = 98$) to have sufficient statistical power to yield meaningful results for infrequent events.

Despite problems in study design, epidemiologic evidence supports the view that repeated maternal exposure to waste anesthetic gases during pregnancy should be minimized. Women who work in areas with a potential for repeated anesthetic gas exposure (no gas scavenger system in place) should be aware of the possibility of adverse reproductive effects and decide whether they want to continue to work in the same area during pregnancy or request to be transferred. In settings where anesthetic gases are administered, a gas scavenger system should be used, and particular attention must be given to maintaining that system. A properly functioning gas scavenging system should provide adequate protection from exposure.[206,222,223] Because

there is always uncertainty about completely avoiding exposure to anesthetic gases, however, a woman with a history of pregnancy loss or having a child with congenital malformations may want to transfer to another work area.[211]

Environmental Contamination and Hazardous Waste Sites

What is the possible role of environmental contamination in causing birth defects? While the topic is controversial and the data are equivocal, there is some evidence that suggests that further study is warranted. Much of the concern focused around specific hazardous waste sites such as Love Canal, New York, and Woburn, Massachusetts. Studies at Love Canal showed an effect on birth weight[224–226] but no increased risk of congenital malformations. A study at Woburn suggested increased risks of selected birth defects associated with consumption of water from specific wells that had been contaminated with volatile organic compounds.[227] The original Woburn study has been criticized on methodologic grounds,[228] and recently completed studies by the Massachusetts Department of Public Health failed to show elevated birth defect risks.[229]

Three recent studies examined residential proximity to hazardous waste sites, as surrogates for exposure, and the risk of birth defects. Since one of the studies received considerable press coverage, it is worthwhile to examine this issue briefly.

Shaw et al.[32] carried out a case-control study using cases from the California Birth Defects Monitoring Program and controls randomly selected using birth certificate files. Cases and controls came from a five-county area in metropolitan San Francisco. Exposure was defined on the basis of various types of hazardous waste facilities found in the census tract of the mother's residence at the time of the birth of the case or control. It appeared that risk for cardiac/circulatory malformations was increased for women living near the facilities. When risks were examined by contaminant chemical class, the odds ratios for heart/circulatory malformations were elevated for each class except hydrocarbon solvents, with the odds ratio for cyanides being the highest. Gastrointestinal malformations were associated with hydrocarbon solvents and metals.

In a widely cited study, Geschwind et al.[31] examined birth defect cases from the New York State Congenital Malformation Registry based on proximity to hazardous waste sites. Cases and controls came from 20 counties in upstate New York, and information on exposure to hazardous waste sites was based on geographic proximity to sites included in a large database. Statistically significant associations were observed between hazardous waste sites and all birth defects combined and several groups of birth defects (nervous system, musculoskeletal system, and skin). In addition, statistically significant associations were observed between specific types of contaminants and some types of birth defects: pesticides and musculoskeletal system; metals and nervous system; solvents and nervous system; and plastics and chromosomal anomalies. Notably, the observed increases in risk were for the most part small, control of confounding was minimal, there was considerable heterogeneity within the birth defect categories, and the methods used to assign exposure were subject to exposure misclassification.

The potential importance of some of these factors in influencing the results of the Geschwind et al. study is illustrated by a second study in upstate New York. As a follow up, Marshall et al.[230] studied musculoskeletal system and central nervous system malformations in 18 counties of upstate New York. Their cases included some of the cases studied by Geschwind et al.,[31] plus additional cases from 2 more recent years. Exposure assessment was based on residential proximity to hazardous waste sites using similar but more precise methods than those employed by Geschwind et al.[31] In contrast to the earlier study, Marshall et al.[230] failed to find significant associations between waste site proximity and either group of defects. They did, however, find a statistically significant association between central nervous system malformations and proximity to active industrial facilities. Marshall et al.[230] attribute the differences between their findings and those reported earlier to uncontrolled confounding, systematic misclassification, or chance. An important difference between the two studies is that the geographic data for the latter study were more refined, allowing for a more accurate determination of residential location.

Dolk et al.[231] generated more systematic data from seven research centers in five European countries. The seven centers maintained population-based registries of congenital anomalies as part of the EUROCAT Network. Among those within 7 km of a landfill site a total of 1,089 pregnancies with nonchromosomal anomalies occurred; 2,366 control births occurred without malformation. Next, the zone within 3 km was considered the exposed one, and in this zone there was a significantly increased risk for a congenital anomaly. The odds ratio (OR) for residence within 3 km of a landfill site was increased for neural-tube defects (OR, 1.86) cardiac septal defects (OR, 1.49), hypospadias (OR, 1.96), gastroschisis (OR, 3.19), and tracheoesophageal fistula (OR, 2.25); the former two were statistically significant. It was not possible to compare results among individual landfill sites, which obviously were heterogeneous as to composition.

THE OBSTETRICIAN'S ROLE IN EVALUATING REPRODUCTIVE RISKS IN AND BEYOND THE WORKPLACE

Clinical questions about environmental or occupational exposures causing adverse reproductive outcomes are extremely difficult to answer, and the answers are seldom as helpful as they need to be. The difficulty occurs because the exposure for the patient and fetus is seldom known or measurable. If the exposure is known, there is almost never a study of similar exposure, with a sufficient sample size, that enables a physician to give a reliable estimate of risk or lack thereof.

For all the environmental exposures discussed in this chapter, no threshold is known below which no adverse reproductive outcome can be expected. Except for ionizing radiation and mercury, maximum recommended exposure levels are difficult to quantify.

Human data usually consist of case reports, which seldom can establish a hazard and never can quantitate the magnitude of the risk. Epidemiologic studies, when available, often have limitations in design, execution, analysis, or interpretation. Thus, in most cases, the questions must be answered on the basis of reasoned judgments in the face of inadequate data.

The process by which a reasoned judgment can be made is summarized in Table 7–2 and the steps are described below. Paul and Himmelstein[51] provide a more detailed description of a similar evaluation process, and recent books[222,223] provide helpful guidance for clinicians.

Paul and Welch[234] have developed a number of recommendations related to improving education and resources about occupational reproductive hazards. They identify problems in clinical risk evaluation and management and develop proposed solutions, including improving information resources for clinicians and improving education for health care providers.

Assessment of potential adverse health effects or toxicity from a chemical exposure begins with correct identification of the agent(s) (Table 7–2). As workers increasingly demanded their right to know the identity and toxicity of chemicals, the U.S. Occupational Safety and Health Administration (OSHA) drafted a regulation and state and local governments have passed so-called worker right-to-know laws.[235] One intent of the regulation and laws is to provide workers and physicians with toxicity information about each chemical used in a given workplace. An information sheet, the Material Safety Data Sheet (MSDS), is developed by the chemical manufacturer or distributor and includes basic identifying and specific toxicity information. Other details of the OSHA regulation and right-to-know laws are reviewed elsewhere.[235,236]

Table 7–2. STEPS IN EVALUATING EXPOSURES THAT MAY RESULT IN BIRTH DEFECTS OR OTHER ADVERSE REPRODUCTIVE OUTCOMES

Step/Action	Information Resources
1. Identify the exposure(s)	Material Safety Data Sheet (MSDS)
	Industry (supervisors, industrial hygienists)
2. Characterize extent of exposure(s)	Description of job activities
	Monitoring data (e.g., air sampling, radiation badge)
	Assess exposure routes
	Biologic sampling (e.g., lead, mercury)
3. Hazard evaluation	Health professionals (occupational/industrial physicians, medical toxicologists, geneticists)
	Regional poison control centers
	Teratology information services (National Institute for Occupational Safety and Health [NIOSH] Criteria Documents, Technical Bulletins) State Health Departments
	On-line databases (National Library of Medicine, Environmental Teratology Information Center, Environmental Mutagen, Carcinogen and Teratogen Department, ReproTox)
	Textbooks, periodicals
4. Risk assessment/judgment	Steps 1–2
	Patient's family, medical, and reproductive history, other relevant exposures (e.g., alcohol, tobacco, drugs of abuse), background risk

Obstetricians should be aware that copies of MSDSs are available upon request from an employer to any woman who may be occupationally exposed to a hazardous chemical. Unfortunately, these MSDSs have been found to be of very limited usefulness for assessing reproductive hazards.[237] Supervisors, managers, and industrial hygienists may be able to provide additional identification, particularly when chemicals are mixed or modified through heating or industrial processes.

The next step is to characterize the extent to which the patient may be exposed. This can be relatively easy for substances such as lead and other heavy metals quantifiable in blood or urine. The radiation badge properly worn can provide exposure monitoring and should be checked frequently during pregnancy. OSHA has published occupational exposure standards for a large number of chemicals associated with adverse health effects.[116] These chemicals and agents must be monitored in the workplace, and such data may be helpful for exposure assessment.

Most often, however, no biologic or environmental data are available. Instead, the clinician must rely on a detailed description of the patient's job activities, precautions taken to avoid exposure (e.g., gloves, respirator, protective clothing, hand washing), and any clinical signs or symptoms suggesting excess exposure. All feasible routes of exposure should be considered, including ingestion (common if handwashing is not done before eating), inhalation (especially if hot vapors or odorless gases are produced), and dermal absorption (increased through irritated skin or prolonged contact with contaminated clothing). Similar considerations apply to nonoccupational exposures as well.

The third step is hazard evaluation. In this context, the physician must determine what is known of the reproductive effects of the chemicals or agents. Since no one can be all-knowing and no single information resource is sufficient for all patient questions, prudence dictates consulting a variety of sources. Physicians specializing in occupational or industrial medicine, medical toxicology, and genetics can be helpful. Such physicians may be affiliated with regional genetics centers or certified regional poison control centers. These centers may be able to recommend other helpful consultants as well. Numerous teratology information services (TISs) provide no-cost physician and patient telephone consultation. These services may vary considerably in how the consultation is provided, whether follow-up is done, nature of the staff qualifications, and the extent of medical supervision. In 1994, the Council of Regional Networks for Genetic Services and the Organization of Teratology Information Services developed a framework for the provision of teratology information services.[238] This framework is an important step toward the development of recommendations for strengthening existing programs and approaches to quality assurance.

Some TISs provide a written copy of the consultation to the referring obstetrician. One university-affiliated TIS maintains and updates a reproductive toxicology database (ReproTox) containing summaries of more than 3,000 chemicals and agents.[239] Obstetricians who choose to refer patients to any of these services should be familiar with the kinds of information and follow-up provided.

The National Library of Medicine in Bethesda, Maryland, maintains several files on the TOXNET database system, including reproductive and developmental toxicology information in bibliographic or text form. Examples include Developmental and Reproductive Toxicology (DART), GENE-TOX (genetic toxicology), and Environmental Mutagen Information Center (EMIC).

A variety of options are available for searching these databases, including personal computer software (Grateful Med, commercial services) and CD-ROM copies in medical libraries or leased from commercial versions. Information is available from a TOXNET representative, National Library of Medicine, Specialized Information Services, 8600 Rockville Pike, Bethesda, MD 20894, (301)496-6531.

Another federal resource is NIOSH, which publishes current recommendations for occupational exposure to a variety of agents or compounds. NIOSH also has a technical information service at its Cincinnati, Ohio, headquarters that may be able to provide in-house reports of investigations as well as NIOSH technical bulletins and criteria documents.

The American College of Obstetricians and Gynecologists publishes guidelines for several occupational exposures during pregnancy.[223] These guidelines include information about metals, solvents, and radiation—agents that also may be found as environmental contaminants.

Many state health or labor departments have a division responsible for occupational health issues. Staff may have expertise in industrial hygiene and safety, occupational medicine, and reproductive epidemiology and toxicology. Specific concerns about hazardous occupational exposures or adverse reproductive outcomes related to workplace exposures should be addressed to this division. In addition, state health departments may be helpful in evaluating associations between environmental exposures and adverse reproductive outcomes. Numerous off-the-shelf information resources include texts,[9,10,196,232,233,240,241] review articles,[51,73,141,244,246–248] and periodicals.

The final and most difficult step is formulating an assessment of risk. Chemical identity, extent of exposure, and the reproductive toxicity of the agent must be known. Unfortunately, all these necessary pieces of information are rarely available. If the exposure is known, available information rarely enables a physician to give a reliable estimate of risk. Thus, risk assessment is really a process of reasoned judgment as opposed to a quantitative estimate of risk. Formulating this judgment requires consideration of many factors, including the best estimate of the nature, extent, duration, and timing of exposure; the patient's medical, reproductive, and genetic history; lifestyle habits (especially tobacco, alcohol, and drugs-of-abuse); and, of course, reproductive toxicity information about the agent. Equally important, the patient should understand that with every pregnancy there is always a background risk for an adverse outcome. Birth defects and other adverse outcomes of pregnancy are relatively common events; approximately 12 to 15 percent of pregnancies result in a spontaneous abortion, and birth defects are observed in approximately 3 percent of all newborns. Frustrating though it is, the fact remains that it is usual *not* to know the cause for a given adverse outcome.

After completing this assessment process, the physician will be more familiar with and understand limitations of available information about a particular agent or chemical. The patient's exposure can be considered in the context of other relevant medical information, and this should be explained to the patient in nontechnical language. The physician may be able to recommend ways to decrease or minimize maternal exposure and determine if closer monitoring of the pregnancy is warranted.

CONCLUSION

Experimental studies in laboratory animals have identified a number of agents that are capable of causing abnormal development. While we know less about substances that are teratogenic in humans, a limited number of teratogenic drugs and chemicals have been identified. There is increasing evidence that some chemicals found in the occupational setting or in the ambient environment may be reproductive or developmental toxicants. While some of this evidence is for associations between exposures and congenital malformations, our interpretation is that there is more evidence for spontaneous abortions associated with occupational exposures than for congenital malformations. Since we believe that spontaneous abortion is one part of a spectrum of outcomes potentially associated with teratogenic exposures, agents that increase risks for spontaneous abortion are also likely to increase risks for congenital malformations.

It is important to refine exposure assessment and to improve outcome ascertainment to enhance epidemiologic studies that help determine the extent to which occupational and environmental exposures may contribute to birth defects and other adverse reproductive outcomes. This is particularly the case for studies of environmental contamination where residential location has commonly been used as a surrogate for exposure. Better exposure assessment and outcome ascertainment may also lead us to an improved understanding of how such teratogens produce their effects so we can design and test intervention/prevention strategies. In the meantime, prenatal counseling about most occupational and environmental exposures requires a large measure of reasoned judgment and interpretation of imperfect/imprecise animal and epidemiologic data.

Key Points

➤ Teratogens and high-dose occupational toxins have been shown to cause not only structural birth defects but also intrauterine death, growth restriction, and functional abnormalities.

➤ Understanding the principles of teratogenesis can help in identifying and understanding the causes of abnormal development.

➤ Exposure to high-dose ionizing radiation during gestation has been shown to cause microcephaly and mental retardation, but effects of low-dose exposures on the conceptus have not been identified.

➤ Prenatal exposure to metals, such as lead and mercury, has been shown to have adverse effects on the development and function of the central nervous system. Doses required for deleterious effects are high, usually above ambient exposures.

➤ The herbicides dioxin and Agent Orange are unlikely to increase the frequency of birth defects in offspring subsequently sired by Vietnam war veterans exposed during combat, despite the politically charged nature of allegations.

➤ High doses of polychlorinated biphenyls (PCBs), once ingested in Taiwan through contaminated cooking oil, cause a recognizable pattern of abnormalities: postnatal and prenatal low birth weight, skin hyperpigmentation, and skull calcifications.

➤ Effects of low-dose PCB contamination, through environmental contamination (e.g., eating Great Lakes fish contaminated with PCBs) is uncertain; however, even the largest effect reported alleges no more than a 6.2-point decrease in IQ.

➤ Organic solvent exposure in high doses (e.g., chronic "sniffing") causes teratogenic effects similar to the fetal alcohol syndrome; in lower level exposure (e.g., occupational), the risk is less, although some reports suggest an increased risk for spontaneous abortion.

➤ Concerns have been raised about the reproductive and developmental effects of pregnancies near toxic waste sites. Data are difficult to generate, but increased anomalies plausibly have been observed close to the site.

➤ Occupational exposures to anesthetic gases have been associated with increased risks for spontaneous abortions and birth defects in some studies.

REFERENCES

1. Wilson JG: Current status of teratology—general principles and mechanisms derived from animal studies. *In* Wilson JG, Fraser FC (eds): Handbook of Teratology. Vol 1. New York, Plenum, 1977, p 47.
2. Fraser FC: Relation of animal studies to the problem in man. *In* Wilson JG, Fraser FC (eds): Handbook of Teratology. Vol 1. New York, Plenum, 1977, p 75.
3. Musselman AC, Bennett GD, Greer KA, et al: Preliminary evidence of phenytoin-induced alterations in embryonic gene expression in a mouse model. Reprod Toxicol 8:383, 1994.
4. Van Allen MI, Kalousek DK, Chernoff GF, et al: Evidence for multi-site closure of the neural tube in humans. Am J Med Genet 47:723, 1993.
5. Lenz W, Knapp K: Foetal malformations due to thalidomide. Geriatr Med Monthly 7:253, 1962.
6. Sever LE: Neuroepidemiology of intrauterine radiation exposure. *In* Molgaard C (ed): Neuroepidemiology: Theory and Method. San Diego, Academic Press, 1993, p 241.
7. Selevan SG, Lemasters OK: The dose-response fallacy in human reproductive studies of toxic exposures. J Occup Med 29:451, 1987.
8. Hemminki K, Sorsa M, Vainio H: Genetic risks caused by occupational chemicals. Scand J Work Environ Health 5:307, 1979.
9. Shepard TH (ed): Catalog of Teratogenic Agents. 5th ed. Baltimore, The Johns Hopkins University Press, 1986, p 549.
10. Friedman JM, Prolifka JE: Teratogenic Effects of Drugs: A Resource for Clinicians (TERIS). Baltimore, The Johns Hopkins University Press, 1994.
11. Environmental Protection Agency: Guidelines for the health assessment of suspect developmental toxicants. Fed Reg 51:34028, 1986.
12. Sever LE: Epidemiologic approaches to reproductive hazards of the workplace. Birth Defects 18:33, 1982.
13. Sever LE: Incidence and prevalence as measures of the frequency of birth defects. Am J Epidemiol 118:608, 1983.
14. Leck I: Correlations of malformation frequency with environmental and genetic attributes in man. *In* Wilson JG, Fraser FC (eds): Handbook of Teratology. Vol 3. New York, Plenum, 1977, p 243.
15. Centers for Disease Control and Prevention: Congenital malformations surveillance. Teratology 48:545, 1993.
16. A Report from the International Clearinghouse for Birth Defects Monitoring Systems: Congenital Malformations Worldwide. Amsterdam, Elsevier, 1990.
17. EUROCAT Working Group: Surveillance of Congenital Anomalies 1980–1990. Brussels, Institute of Hygiene and Epidemiology, 1993.
18. Sever LE: The conundrum of birth defect clusters. Health Environ Digest 7:10, 1994.
19. Sever LE, Strassburg MA: Epidemiologic aspects of neural tube defects in the United States: changing concepts and their importance for screening and prenatal diagnostic programs. *In* Mizejewski GJ, Porter IH (eds): Alpha-Fetoprotein and

Congenital Disorders. San Diego, Academic Press, 1985, p 243.

20. Sever LE, Hessol NA: Overall design considerations in male and female occupational reproductive studies. Prog Clin Biol Res 160:15, 1984.

21. Sever LE, Sanders M, Monsen R: An epidemiologic study of neural tube defects in Los Angeles County. I. Prevalence at birth based on multiple sources of case ascertainment. Teratology 25:315, 1982.

22. Gregg NM: Congenital cataract following German measles in the mother. Trans Ophthalmol Soc Aust 3:35, 1941.

23. Lenz W: Discussion contribution by Dr. W. Lenz, Hamburg, on the lecture by Pfeiffer RA, Kosenow K: on the exogenous origin of malformations of the extremities. Tagung der Rheinisch-Westfalischen Kinderarztevereinigung in Dusseldorf, 1961.

24. McBride WG: Thalidomide and congenital abnormalities. Lancet 2:1358, 1961.

25. Borman B, Cryer C: Fallacies of international and national comparisons of disease occurrence in the epidemiology of neural tube defects. Teratology 42:405, 1990.

26. Edmonds LD, Layde PM, James LM, et al: Congenital malformation surveillance: two American systems. Int J Epidemiol 10:247, 1981.

27. Lynberg MC, Edmonds LD: Surveillance of birth defects. *In* Halperin W, Baker EL (eds): Public Health Surveillance. New York, Van Nostrand Reinhold, 1992, p 157.

28. Lynberg MC, Edmonds LD: State use of birth defects surveillance. *In* Wilcox LS, Marks JS (eds): From Data to Action: CDC's Public Health Surveillance for Women, Infants, and Children. Atlanta, Public Health Service, Centers for Disease Control and Prevention (no date).

29. Bove F, Fulcomer M, Klotz J, et al: Report on Phase IV-A: Public Drinking Water Contamination and Birthweight and Selected Birth Defects: A Cross-Sectional Study. New Jersey Department of Health, 1992.

30. Bove F, Fulcomer M, Klotz J, et al: Report on Phase IV-B: Public Drinking Water Contamination and Birthweight and Selected Birth Defects: A Case-Control Study. New Jersey Department of Health, 1992.

31. Geschwind SA, Stolwijk AJ, Bracken M, et al: Risk of congenital malformations associated with proximity to hazardous waste sites. Am J Epidemiol 135:1197, 1992.

32. Shaw G, Schulman J, Frisch J, et al: Congenital malformations and birthweight in areas with potential environmental contamination. Arch Environ Health 47:147, 1992.

33. Infante PF: Oncogenic and mutagenic risks in communities with polyvinyl chloride production facilities. Ann N Y Acad Sci 271:49, 1976.

34. Theriault G, Iturra H, Gingras S: Evaluation of the association between birth defects and ambient vinyl chloride. Teratology 27:359, 1983.

35. Deane M, Swan SH, Harris JA, et al: Adverse pregnancy outcomes in relation to water contamination, Santa Clara County, California 1980–1981. Am J Epidemiol 129:894, 1989.

36. Lieff S, Olshan AF, Werler M, et al: Selection bias and the use of controls with malformations in case-control studies of birth defects. Epidemiology 10:238, 1999.

37. Lenz W: Thalidomide and congenital abnormalities. Lancet 1:45, 1962.

38. Edmonds LD, Falk H, Nissim JE: Congenital malformations and vinyl chloride. Lancet 2:1098, 1975.

39. Edmonds LD, Anderson CE, Flynt JW Jr, James LM: Congenital central nervous system malformations and vinyl chloride

40. Lammer EJ, Sever LE, Oakley GP: Teratogen update: valproic acid. Teratology 35:465, 1987.

41. Sever LE, Olsen AR, Hinds NR, et al: NINCDS Collaborative Perinatal Project: A User's Guide to the Project and Data. Vol I. An Introduction to the History, Scope and Methodology of the Project. National Institute of Neurological and Communicative Disorders and Stroke, Contract NO1-NS-2-2311, 1983.

42. Nordstrom S, Beckman L, Nordenson I: Occupational and environmental risks in and around a smelter in Northern Sweden. III. Frequencies of spontaneous abortion. Hereditas 88:41, 1978.

43. Nordstrom S, Beckman I, Nordenson I: Occupational and environmental risks in and around a smelter in Northern Sweden. V. Spontaneous abortion among female employees and decreased birth weight in their offspring. Hereditas 90:291, 1979.

44. Beckman L, Nordstrom S: Occupational and environmental risks in and around a smelter in Northern Sweden. IX. Fetal mortality among wives of smelter workers. Hereditas 97:1, 1982.

45. Bracken MB: Design and conduct of randomized clinical trials in perinatal research. *In* Bracken MB (ed): Perinatal Epidemiology. New York, Oxford University Press, 1984, p 397.

46. Smithells RW, Sheppard S, Schorah CJ, et al: Apparent prevention of neural tube defects by periconceptional vitamin supplementation. Arch Dis Child 56:911, 1981.

47. Smithells RW, Sheppard S, Schorah CJ, et al: Possible prevention of neural-tube defects by periconceptional vitamin supplementation. Lancet 1:339, 1980.

48. MRC Vitamin Study Research Group: Prevention of neural tube defects: results of the Medical Research Council Vitamin Study. Lancet 338:131, 1991.

49. Czeizel AE, Dudas I: Prevention of the first occurrence of neural tube defects by periconceptional vitamin supplementation. N Engl J Med 327:1832, 1992.

50. Centers for Disease Control and Prevention: Recommendations for the use of folic acid to reduce the number of cases of spina bifida and other neural tube defects. Morbidity Mortality Weekly Reports (MMWR) 41(RR-14):1, 1992.

51. Paul M, Himmelstein J: Reproductive hazards in the workplace: what the practitioner needs to know about chemical exposures. Obstet Gynecol 71:921, 1988.

52. Lemasters GK, Selevan SG: Types of exposure models and advantages end disadvantages of sources of exposure data for use in occupational reproductive studies. Prog Clin Biol Res 160:67, 1984.

53. Gordon JE: Assessment of occupational and environmental exposures. *In* Bracken MB (ed): Perinatal Epidemiology. New York, Oxford University Press, 1984, p 450.

54. Sever LE: Epidemiologic aspects of environmental hazards to reproduction. *In* Talbott E, Craun G (eds): Introduction to Environmental Epidemiology. Boca Raton, FL, CRC Press, 1995, p 63.

55. Gold EB, Sever LE: Childhood cancers associated with parental occupational exposures. Occup Med 9:495, 1994.

56. Gold EB, Tomich E: Occupational hazards to fertility and pregnancy outcome. Occup Med 9:435, 1994.

57. Sever LE: Congenital malformations related to occupational reproductive hazards. Occup Med 9:471, 1994.

58. National Research Council Committee on Biological Markers: Biological Markers in Reproductive Toxicology. Washington, DC, National Academy Press, 1989.

59. Hulka BS, Wilcosky T: Biological markers in epidemiologic research. Arch Environ Health 43:83, 1988.

monomer exposure: a community study. Teratology 17:137, 1978.

60. Lemasters GK, Schulte PA: Biologic markers in the epidemiology of reproduction. *In* Schulte PA, Perara FP (eds): Molecular Epidemiology: Principles and Practices. San Diego, Academic Press, 1993, p 385.

61. Lynberg MC, Khoury MJ: Interaction between epidemiology and laboratory sciences in the study of birth defects: design of birth defects risk factor surveillance in metropolitan Atlanta. J Toxicol Environ Health 40:435, 1993.

62. Shepard T: Human teratogenicity. Adv Pediatr 33:225, 1986.

63. National Research Council: Environmental Epidemiology. Washington, DC, National Academy Press, 1991.

64. Lybarger JA, Spengler RF, DeRosa CT: Priority Health Conditions: An Integrated Strategy to Evaluate the Relationship between Illness and Exposure to Hazardous Substances. ATSDR, Atlanta, 1993.

65. Marsh GM, Caplan RJ: Evaluating health effects of exposure at hazardous waste sites: a review of state-of-the-art, with recommendations for future research. *In* Andelman JB, Underhill DW (eds): Health Effects from Hazardous Waste Sites. Chelsea, MI, Lewis Publishing, 1987, p 3.

66. Heath CW Jr: Epidemiology of dump exposures. *In* Finberg L (ed): Chemical and Radiation Hazards to Children. Report of the 84th Ross Conference on Pediatric Research. Columbus, OH, Ross Laboratories, 1982, p 10.

67. Miller RW: Measures of reproductive effects. *In* Finberg L (ed): Chemical and Radiation Hazards to Children. Report of the 84th Ross Conference on Pediatric Research. Columbus, OH, Ross Laboratories, 1982, p 88.

68. Miller RW: Effects of ionizing radiation from the atomic bomb on Japanese children. Pediatrics 41:257, 1968.

69. Kirsch-Volders M (ed): Mutagenicity, Carcinogenicity, and Teratogenicity of Industrial Pollutants. New York, Plenum, 1984.

70. Wood JW, Johnson KG, Omori Y, et al: Mental retardation in children exposed in utero to the atomic bombs in Hiroshima and Nagasaki. Am J Public Health 57:1381, 1967.

71. Miller RW: Delayed effects occurring within the first decade after exposure of young individuals to the Hiroshima atomic bomb. Pediatrics 18:1, 1956.

72. DeKaban AS: Abnormalities in children exposed to x-radiation during various stages of gestation: tentative timetable of radiation injury to the human fetus, part I. J Nucl Med 9:471, 1968.

73. Brent RL: The effects of embryonic and fetal exposure to x-ray, microwaves, and ultrasound. Clin Perinatol 13:615, 1986.

74. Archer VE: Anencephalus, drinking water, geomagnetism and cosmic radiation. Am J Epidemiol 109:88, 1979.

75. Gentry J, Parkhurst E, Bulin G: An epidemiologic study of congenital malformations in New York state. Am J Public Health 49:497, 1959.

76. Kochupiluai N, Verma IC, Grewal MS, Ramalingaswami V: Down's syndrome and related abnormalities in an area of high background radiation in coastal Kenya. Nature 262:60, 1976.

77. Brent RL: Radiations and other physical agents. *In* Wilson JG, Fraser FC (eds): Handbook of Teratology. Vol 1. New York, Plenum, 1977, p 208.

78. Segall A, MacMahon B, Hannigan M: Congenital malformations and background radiation in northern New England. J Chronic Dis 17:915, 1964.

79. Wood JW, Keehn RJ, Kawamoto S, Johnson KC: The growth and development of children exposed in utero to the atomic bombs in Hiroshima and Nagasaki. Am J Public Health 57:1374, 1967.

80. Neel JV, Kato H, Schull WJ: Mortality in the children of atomic bomb survivors and controls. Genetics 76:311, 1974.

81. Neel JV: Problem of "false positive" conclusions in genetic epidemiology: lessons from the leukemia cluster near the Sellafield nuclear installation. Genet Epidemiol 11:213, 1994.

82. Meyer MB, Diamond EL, Merz T: Sex ratio of children born to mothers who had been exposed to x-rays in utero. Johns Hopkins Med J 123:123, 1968.

83. Alberman E, Polani PE, Fraser-Roberts JA, et al: Parental x-irradiation and chromosome constitution in their spontaneously aborted foetuses. Ann Hum Genet Lond 36:185, 1972.

84. Stewart A, Kneale GW: Radiation dose effects in relation to obstetric x-rays and childhood cancers. Lancet 1:1185, 1970.

85. Stewart A, Webb D, Giles D, Hewitt D: Malignant disease in childhood and diagnostic irradiation in utero. Lancet 2:447, 1956.

86. Stewart A, Webb D, Hewitt D: A survey of childhood malignancies. BMJ 1:1495, 1958.

87. Sever LE: Parental radiation exposure and children's health: are there effects on the second generation? Occup Med 6:613, 1991.

88. Gardner MJ, Snee MP, Hall AJ, et al: Results of case-control study of leukaemia and lymphoma among young people near Sellafield nuclear plant in West Cumbria. BMJ 300:423, 1990.

89. Gardner MJ, Hall AJ, Snee MP, et al: Methods and basic data of case-control study of leukaemia and lymphoma among young people near Sellafield nuclear plant in West Cumbria. BMJ 300:429, 1990.

90. Sever LE, Gilbert ES, Hessol NA, McIntyre JM: A case-control study of congenital malformations and occupational exposure to low-level ionizing radiation. Am J Epidemiol 127:226, 1988.

91. McLaughlin JR, King WD, Anderson TW, et al: Paternal radiation exposure and leukaemia in offspring: the Ontario case-control study. BMJ 307:959, 1993.

92. Marcus M: Epidemiologic studies of VDT use and pregnancy outcome. Reprod Toxicol 4:51, 1990.

93. Blackwell R, Chang A: Video display terminals and pregnancy. A review. Br J Obstet Gynaecol 95:446, 1988.

94. Goldhaber MK, Polen MR, Hiatt RA: The risk of miscarriage and birth defects among women who use visual display terminals during pregnancy. Am J Ind Med 13:695, 1988.

95. Schnorr TM, Grajewski BA, Hornung RW, et al: Video display terminals and the risk of spontaneous abortion. N Engl J Med 324:727, 1991.

96. World Health Organization: Environmental Health Criteria 1: Mercury. Geneva, WHO, 1976, p 48.

97. Harada M: Minamata disease: a medical report. *In* Smith WE, Smith AM (eds): Minamata. New York, Holt, Rinehart, 1975, p 130.

98. Bakir F, Damluji SF, Amin-Zaki M, et al: Methylmercury poisoning in Iraq. Science 181:230, 1973.

99. Koos BJ, Longo LD: Mercury toxicity in the pregnant woman, fetus, and newborn infant. Am J Obstet Gynecol 126:390, 1976.

100. Choi BH: Effects of prenatal methylmercury poisoning upon growth and development of fetal central nervous system. *In* Clarkson TW, Nordberg GF, Sager PR (eds): Reproductive and Developmental Toxicology of Metals. New York, Plenum, 1983, p 473.

101. Marsh DO, Myers GT, Clarkson TW, et al: Fetal methylmercury poisoning: clinical and toxicologic data on 29 cases. Ann Neurol 7:348, 1980.

102. Clarkson TW: The pharmacology of mercury compounds. Annu Rev Pharmacol 12:375, 1972.

103. Tsuchiya H, Mitani K, Kodama K, Nakata T: Placental transfer of heavy metals in normal pregnant Japanese women. Arch Environ Health 39:11, 1984.

104. Sandstead HH, Doherty RA, Mahaffey KA: Effects and metabolism of toxic trace metals in the neonatal period. *In* Clarkson TW, Nordberg GF, Sager RP (eds): Reproductive and Developmental Toxicology of Metals. New York, Plenum, 1983, p 207.

105. Pierce PE, Thompson JF, Likosky WH, et al: Alkyl mercury poisoning in humans: report of an outbreak. JAMA 220: 1439, 1972.

106. McKeown-Eyssen G, Ruedy J, Neims A: Methylmercury exposure in northern Quebec. II. Neurologic findings in children. Am J Epidemiol 118:470, 1983.

107. Skerfving S, Hansson K, Mangs C, et al: Methylmercury-induced chromosome damage in man. Environ Res 7:83, 1974.

108. Burbacher TM, Monnett C, Grant KS, Mottet NK: Methylmercury exposure and reproductive dysfunction in the nonhuman primate. Toxicol Appl Pharmacol 75:18, 1984.

109. Gunderson VM, Grant KS, Burbacher TM, et al: The effect of low-level prenatal methylmercury exposure on visual recognition memory in infant crab-eating macaques. Child Dev 57: 1076, 1986.

110. Mottet NK, Shaw CM, Burbacher TM: Health risks from increases in methylmercury exposure. Environ Health Perspect 63:133, 1985.

111. Gunderson VM, Grant-Webster KS, Burbacher TM, Mottet NK: Visual recognition memory deficits in methylmercury-exposed *Macaca fascicularis* infants. Neurotoxicol Teratol 10: 373, 1988.

112. Gilani SH: Congenital abnormalities in methylmercury poisoning. Environ Res 9:128, 1975.

113. Mattison DR: Female reproductive system. *In* Clarkson TW, Nordberg GW, Sager PR (eds): Reproductive and Developmental Toxicology of Metals. New York, Plenum, 1983, p 43.

114. Weiss B: The developmental neurotoxicity of methyl mercury. *In* Needleman HL, Bellinger D (eds): Prenatal Exposure to Toxicants: Developmental Consequences. Baltimore, The Johns Hopkins University Press, 1994, p 112.

115. Steffek AJ, Clayton R, Siew C, et al: Effects of elemental mercury vapor exposure on pregnant Sprague-Dawley rats. Teratology 35:59A, 1987.

116. American Conference of Governmental Industrial Hygienists: Threshold Limit Values and Biological Exposure Indices for 1988–1989. Cincinnati, ACGIH, 1988.

117. Clarkson TW, Magos L, Greenwood MR: The transport of elemental mercury into fetal tissues. Biol Neonate 21:239, 1972.

118. Wannag A, Skjaerasen J: Mercury accumulation in placenta and foetal membranes. A study of dental workers and their babies. Environ Physiol Bioehem 5:348, 1975.

119. Agency for Toxic Substances and Disease Registry: Toxicological Profile for Mercury. Atlanta, U.S. Public Health Service, ATSDR, 1989, p 90.

120. Gelbier S, Ingram J: Possible foetotoxic effects of mercury vapour: a case report. Public Health 103:35, 1989.

121. Rowland AS: Reproductive effects of mercury vapor. Fundam Appl Toxicol 19:326, 1992.

122. Rowland AS, Baird DD, Weinberg CR, et al: The effect of occupational exposure to mercury vapour on the fertility of female dental assistants. Occup Environ Med 51:28, 1994.

123. Rom WN: Effects of lead on the female and reproduction: a review. Mt Sinai J Med 43:542, 1976.

124. Hall A: The increasing use of lead as an abortifacient. BMJ 1: 584, 1905.

125. Rothenberg SJ, Manalo M, Jiang J, et al: Maternal blood lead level during pregnancy in South Central Los Angeles. Arch Environ Health 54:151, 1999.

126. Pietrzyk JJ, Nowak A, Mitkowska Z, et al: Prenatal lead exposure and the pregnancy outcome. A case-control study in southern Poland. Przegl Lek 53:342, 1996.

127. Torres-Sanchez LE, Berkowitz G, Lopez-Carrillo L, et al: Intrauterine lead exposure and preterm birth. Environ Res 81: 297, 1999.

128. Irgens A, Kruger K, Skorve AH, et al: Reproductive outcome in offspring of parents occupationally exposed to lead in Norway. Am J Ind Med 34:431, 1998.

129. Fourtes LJ, Weismann D, Niebyl K: Pregnancy, pica, pottery, and Pb (lead). J Am Coll Toxicol 15:445, 1996.

130. Stefanak MA, Bourguet CC, Benzies-Styka T: Use of the Centers for Disease Control and Prevention childhood lead poisoning risk questionnaire to predict blood lead elevations in pregnant women. Obstet Gynecol 87:209, 1996.

131. Farias P, Borja-Aburto VH, Rios C, et al: Blood lead levels in pregnant women of high and low socioeconomic status in Mexico City. Environ Health Perspect 104:1070, 1996.

132. Creason JP, Svensgaard DJ, Baumgarner JE, et al: Maternal-fetal tissue levels of sixteen trace elements in eight communities. USEPA Report EPA No. 600:1-78-033, 1978.

133. Centers for Disease Control: Preventing lead poisoning in young children—United States. Morbidity Mortality Weekly Reports (MMWR) 34:66, 1985.

134. Centers for Disease Control: Preventing lead poisoning in young children. U.S. Department of Health and Human Services. Atlanta, Public Health Service, Centers for Disease Control, 1991, p 7.

135. Occupational Safety and Health Administration: Occupational exposure to lead. Final standard. Fed Reg 43:52952, 1978.

136. Needleman HL, Schell A, Bellinger D, et al: The long term effects of exposure to low doses of lead in childhood. An 11-year follow-up report. N Engl J Med 322:83, 1990.

137. Bellinger D, Leviton A, Waternaux C, et al: Longitudinal analyses of prenatal and postnatal lead exposure and early cognitive development. N Engl J Med 316:1037, 1987.

138. Clauss CA, Berzon M, Bertin J: Litigating reproductive and developmental health in the aftermath of UAW *versus* Johnson Controls. Environ Health Perspect Suppl 2:205, 1993.

139. Bellinger D, Needleman HL: The neurotoxicity of prenatal exposure to lead: kinetics, mechanisms, and expressions. *In* Needleman HL, Bellinger D (eds): Prenatal Exposure to Toxicants: Developmental Consequences. Baltimore, The Johns Hopkins University Press, 1994, p 89.

140. Gulson BL, Pounds JG, Mushak P, et al: Estimation of cumulative lead releases (lead flux) from maternal skeleton during pregnancy and lactation. J Lab Clin Med 134:631, 1999.

141. Gulson BL, Mahaffey KR, Mizon K, Murray C: Contribution of tissue lead to blood lead in adult female subjects. J Lab Clin Med 125:703, 1995.

142. Brownie CF, Brownie E, Noben D, et al: Teratogenic effect of calcium edetate (CaEDTA) in rats and the protective effect of zinc. Toxicol Appl Pharmacol 82:426, 1986.

143. Courtney KD, Gaylor DW, Hogan MD, et al: Teratogenic evaluation of 2,4,5-T. Science 168:864, 1970.

144. Kimbrough RD: Some fat-soluble stable industrial chemicals. *In* Finberg L (ed): Chemical and Radiation Hazards to Children. Report of the 84th Ross Conference on Pediatric Research. Columbus, OH, Ross Laboratories, 1982, p 23.

145. Institute of Medicine: Veterans and Agent Orange: Health Effects of Herbicides Used in Vietnam. Washington, DC, National Academy Press, 1993.

146. Erickson JD, Mulinare J, McClain PW, et al: Vietnam veterans risks for fathering babies with birth defects. JAMA 252: 903, 1984.

147. Centers for Disease Control: Centers for Disease Control Vietnam experience study: health status of Vietnam veterans.

III. Reproductive outcomes and child health. JAMA 259:2715, 1988.

148. Field B, Kerr C: Reproductive behavior and consistent patterns of abnormality in offspring of Vietnam veterans. J Med Genet 25:819, 1988.

149. U.S. EPA: Health Assessment Document for 2,3,7,8-Tetrachlorodibenzo-P-Dioxin (TCDD) and Related Compounds (Review Draft). Washington, DC, EPA, 1994.

150. Institute of Medicine, Division of Health Promotion and Disease Prevention, Committee to Review the Health Effects in Vietnam Veterans of Exposure to Herbicides: Veterans and Agent Orange: Update 1996. Washington, DC, National Academy Press, 1996.

151. Letz G: The toxicology of PCB's—an overview for clinicians. West J Med 138:534, 1983.

152. Schwartz PM, Jacobson SW, Fein G, et al: Lake Michigan fish consumption as a source of polychlorinated biphenyls in human cord serum, maternal serum, and milk. Am J Public Health 73:293, 1983.

153. Safe S: Polychlorinated biphenyls (PCBs) and polybrominated biphenyls (PBBs): biochemistry, toxicology, and mechanism of action. Crit Rev Toxicol 13:319, 1985.

154. Kimbrough RD: Human health effects of polychlorinated biphenyls (PCBs) and polybrominated biphenyls (PBBs). Annu Rev Pharmacol Toxicol 27:87, 1987.

155. Jacobson JL, Jacobson SW: The effects of perinatal exposure to polychlorinated biphenyls and related contaminants. In Needleman NL, Bellinger D (eds): Prenatal Exposure to Toxicants: Developmental Consequences. Baltimore, The Johns Hopkins University Press, 1994, p 130.

156. Kuratsune M, Yoshimura Y, Matsuzaka J, Yamagushi A: Epidmiologic study on yusho, a poisoning caused by ingestion of rice oil contaminated with a commercial brand of polychlorinated biphenyls. Environ Health Perspect 1:119, 1972.

157. World Health Organization: Assessment of Health Risks in Infants Associated with Exposure to PCBs and PCDFs in Breast Milk. Report on a WHO Working Group. Copenhagen, World Health Organization, 1988.

158. Buser HR: Polychlorinated dibenzofurans (PCDFs) found in yusho oil and used in Japanese PCB. Chemosphere 7:439, 1978.

159. Guo YL, Yu ML, Hsu CC, et al: Chloracne, goiter, arthritis, and anemia after polychlorinated biphenyl poisoning: 14-year follow-up of the Taiwan Yucheng cohort. Environ Health Perspect 107:715, 1999.

160. Yamashita F, Hayashi M: Fetal PCB syndrome: clinical features, intrauterine growth restriction and possible alteration in calcium metabolism. Environ Health Perspect 59:41, 1985.

161. Rogan WJ, Gladen BC, Hung KL, et al: Congenital poisoning by polychlorinated biphenyls and their contaminants in Taiwan. Science 241:334, 1988.

162. Chen Y-CJ, Guo Y-L, Hsu C-C, Rogan WJ: Cognitive development of Yu-Cheng ("oil disease") in children prenatally exposed to heat-degraded PCBs. JAMA 268:3213, 1992.

163. Yen YY, Lan SJ, Ko YC, Chen CJ: Follow-up study of reproductive hazards of multiparous women consuming PCBs-contaminated rice oil. Bull Environ Contam Toxicol 43:647, 1989.

164. Yu ML, Guo YL, Hsu CC, et al: Menstruation and reproduction in women with polychlorinated biphenyl (PCB) poisoning: long-term follow-up interviews of the women from the Taiwan Yucheng cohort. Int J Epidemiol 29:672, 2000.

165. Jacobson JL, Fein GG, Jacobson SW, et al: The transfer of polychlorinated biphenyls and polybrominated biphenyls across the human placenta and into maternal milk. Am J Public Health 74:378, 1984.

166. Jacobson JL, Jacobson SW, Humphrey HE: Effect of in utero exposure to polychlorinated biphenyls and related contaminants on cognitive functioning in young children. J Pediatr 116:38, 1990.

167. Fein GG, Jacobson JL, Jacobson SW, et al: Prenatal exposure to polychlorinated biphenyls: effects on birth size and gestational age. J Pediatr 105:315, 1984.

168. Jacobson JL, Jacobson SW, Fein GG, et al: Prenatal exposure to an environmental toxin: a test of the multiple effects model. Dev Psychol 20:523, 1984.

169. Jacobson JL, Jacobson SW: Intellectual impairment in children exposed to polychlorinated biphenyls in utero. N Engl J Med 335:783, 1996.

170. Middaugh JP, Egeland GM: Intellectual function of children exposed to polychlorinated biphenyls in utero. N Engl J Med 336:660, 1997.

171. Rogan WJ, Gladen BC: Neurotoxicity of PCBs and related compounds. Neurotoxicology 12:27, 1992.

172. Patandin S, Lanting CI, Mulder PG, et al: Effects of environmental exposure to polychlorinated biphenyls and dioxins on cognitive abilities in Dutch children at 42 months of age. J Pediatr 134:33, 1999.

173. Patandin S, Koopman-Esseboom C, de Ridder MA, et al: Effects of environmental exposure to polychlorinated biphenyls and dioxins on birth size and growth in Dutch children. Pediatr Res 44:538, 1998.

174. Frank JW, Newman J: Breast-feeding in a polluted world: uncertain risks, clear benefits. Can Med Assoc J 149:33, 1993.

175. Fries GF: The PBB episode in Michigan: an overall appraisal. Crit Rev Toxicol 16:105, 1985.

176. Anderson HA, Lilis R, Selikoff IJ, et al: Unanticipated prevalence of symptoms among dairy farmers in Michigan and Wisconsin. Environ Health Perspect 23:217, 1978.

177. Bekesi JG, Roboz JP, Fischbein A, Mason P: Immunotoxicology: environmental contamination by polybrominated biphenyls and immune dysfunction among residents of the state of Michigan. Cancer Detect Prevent Suppl 1:29, 1987.

178. Roboz J, Greaves J, Bekesi JG: Polybrominated biphenyls in model and environmentally contaminated human blood: protein binding and immunotoxicological studies. Environ Health Perspect 60:107, 1985.

179. Humble CG, Speizer FE: Polybrominated biphenyls and fetal mortality in Michigan. Am J Public Health 74:1130, 1984.

180. Sever LE: The state of the art and current issues regarding reproductive outcomes potentially associated with environmental exposures: reduced fertility, reproductive wastage, congenital malformations, and birth weight. U.S. EPA Workshop on Reproductive and Developmental Epidemiology: Issues and Recommendations. U.S. EPA 600/8-89-103, Cincinnati, 1989.

181. Eyster JT, Humphrey HEB, Kimbrough RD: Partitioning of polybrominated biphenyls (PBBs) in serum, adipose tissue, breast milk, placenta, cord blood, biliary fluid, and feces. Arch Environ Health 38:47, 1983.

182. Seagull EAW: Developmental abilities of children exposed to polybrominated biphenyls (PBB). Am J Public Health 73:281, 1983.

183. Schwartz EM, Rae WA: Effect of polybrominated biphenyls (PBB) on developmental abilities in young children. Am J Public Health 73:277, 1983.

184. Ema M, Kanoh S: Studies on the pharmacological bases of fetal toxicity of drugs. Fetal toxicity of potassium nitrate in two generations of rats. Folia Pharmacol Jpn 81:469, 1983.

185. Sleight SD, Sinha DP, Uzoukwu M: Effect of sodium nitrite on reproductive performance of pregnant sows. J Am Ved Med Assoc 61:819, 1972.

186. Globus M, Samuel D: Effect of maternally administered so-

dium nitrite on hepatic erythropoesis in fetal CD-1 mice. Teratology 18:367, 1978.

187. Dorsch MM, Scragg RKR, McMichael AJ, et al: Congenital malformations and maternal drinking water supply in rural South Australia: a case-control study. Am J Epidemiol 119: 473, 1984.

188. King MD: Neurological sequelae of toluene abuse. Hum Toxicol 1:281, 1982.

189. Andrews LS, Snyder R: Toxic effects of solvents and vapors. *In* Klaassen CD, Amdur MO, Doull J (eds): Casarett and Doull's Toxicology. The Basic Science of Poisons. 3rd ed. New York, Macmillan, 1986, p 636.

190. Hersh JH, Podruch PE, Rogers R, Weisskopf B: Toluene embryopathy. J Pediatr 106:922, 1985.

191. Hersh JH: Toluene embryopathy: two new cases. J Med Genet 26:333, 1989.

192. Toutant C, Lippmann S: Fetal solvents syndrome [Letter] Lancet 1:1356, 1979.

193. Goodwin TM: Toluene abuse and renal tubular acidosis in pregnancy. Obstet Gynecol 71:715, 1988.

194. Pradhan S, Ghosh TK, Pradhan SN: Teratological effects of industrial solvents. Drug Dev Res 13:205, 1988.

195. Pearson MA, Hoyme HE, Seaver LH, Rimsza ME: Toluene embryopathy: delineation of the phenotype and comparison with fetal alcohol syndrome. Pediatrics 93:211, 1994.

196. Barlow SM, Sullivan FM: Reproductive Hazards of Industrial Chemicals. San Diego, Academic Press, 1982.

197. Olsen J: Risk of exposure to teratogens amongst laboratory staff and painters. Dan Med Bull 30:24, 1983.

198. Heidam LZ: Spontaneous abortions among dental assistants, factory workers, painters, and gardening workers: a follow-up study. J Epidemiol Comm Health 38:149, 1984.

199. Pastides H, Calabrese EJ, Hosmer DW, Harris DR: Spontaneous abortion and general illness symptoms among semiconductor manufacturers. J Occup Med 30:543, 1988.

200. Schenker M, Beaumont J, Gold E, et al: Epidemiologic Study of Reproductive and Other Health Effects Among Workers Employed in the Manufacture of Semiconductors: Final Report to the Semiconductor Industry Association. Davis, CA, University of California, Davis, 1992.

201. Khattak S, K-Moghtader G, McMartin K, et al: Pregnancy outcome following gestational exposure to organic solvents. JAMA 281:1106, 1999.

202. Swan SH, Shaw G, Harris JA, Neutra RR: Congenital cardiac anomalies in relation to water contamination, Santa Clara County, California, 1981–1983. Am J Epidemiol 129:885, 1989.

203. John EM, Savitz DA, Shy CM: Spontaneous abortions among cosmetologists. Epidemiology 5:147, 1994.

204. Scialli AR: Who should paint the nursery? Reprod Toxicol 3: 159, 1989.

205. Spence AA, Cohen EN, Brown BW, et al: Occupational hazards for operating room-based physicians. Analysis of data from the United States and the United Kingdom. JAMA 238: 955, 1977.

206. National Institute for Occupational Safety and Health: Criteria for a Recommended Standard: Occupational Exposure to Waste Anesthetic Gases and Vapors. DHEW Publ. No. 77-140. Washington, DC, NIOSH, 1977.

207. Spence AA, Knill-Jones RP: Is there a health hazard in anaesthetic practice? Br J Anaesth 50:713, 1978.

208. Mazze RE, Wilson AI, Rice SA, Baden JM: Reproduction and fetal development in rats exposed to nitrous oxide. Teratology 30:259, 1984.

209. Corbett TH: Cancer and congenital anomalies associated with anesthetics. Ann N Y Acad Sci 271:58, 1976.

210. Edling C: Anesthetic gases as an occupational hazard—a review. Scand J Work Environ Health 6:85, 1980.

211. Vessey MP, Nunn JF: Occupational hazards of anesthesia. BMJ 281:696, 1980.

212. Corbett TH, Cornell RG, Endres JL, Lieding K: Birth defects among children of nurse-anesthetists. Anesthesiology 41:341, 1974.

213. Knill-Jones RP, Moir DD, Rodrigues LV, Spence AA: Anesthetic practice and pregnancy—controlled survey of woman anesthetists in the United Kingdom. Lancet 1:1326, 1972.

214. Friedman JM: Teratogen update: anesthetic agents. Teratology 37:69, 1988.

215. Infante PF, Tsongas TA: Anesthetic gases and pregnancy: a review of evidence for an occupational hazard. *In* Hemminki K, Sorsa M, Vainio H (eds): Occupational Hazards and Reproduction. Washington, DC, Hemisphere Publishing Corporation, 1985.

216. Guirguis SS, Pelmear PL, Roy ML, Wong L: Health effects associated with exposure to anaesthetic gases in Ontario hospital personnel. Br J Ind Med 47:490, 1990.

217. Saurel-Cubizolles MJ, Hays M, Estryn-Behar M: Work in operating rooms and pregnancy outcomes among nurses. Int Arch Occup Environ Health 66:235, 1994.

218. Matte TD, Mulinare J, Erickson JD: Case-control study of congenital defects and parental employment in health care. Am J Ind Med 24:11,1993.

219. Axelsson GA, Rylander R: Exposure to anaesthetic gases and spontaneous abortion: response bias in a postal questionnaire study. Int J Epidemiol 11:250, 1982.

220. Rowland AS, Baird DD, Weinberg CR, et al: Reduced fertility among women employed as dental assistants exposed to high levels of nitrous oxide. N Engl J Med 327:993, 1992.

221. Rowland AS, Baird DD, Shore DL, et al: Nitrous oxide and spontaneous abortion in female dental assistants. Am J Epidemiol 141:531, 1995.

222. Mattia MA: Anesthesia gases and methylmethacrylate. Am J Nurs 83:73, 1983.

223. American College of Obstetricians and Gynecologists: Guidelines on Pregnancy and Work. Chicago, The American College of Obstetricians and Gynecologists, 1977.

224. Curtiss JRB, Ginevan ME, Brown CD: Spatio/temporal analysis of human birth weight: an indicator of subtle environmental stress? *In* Health Impacts of Different Sources of Energy. Vienna, International Atomic Energy Agency, 1982, p 33.

225. Goldman LR, Paigen B, Magnant MM, Highland JH: Low birth weight, prematurity and birth defects in children living near the hazardous waste site, Love Canal. Haz Waste Haz Mat 2:209, 1985.

226. Vianna NJ, Polan AK: Incidence of low birth weight among Love Canal residents. Science 226:1217, 1984.

227. Lagakos SW, Wessen BJ, Zelen M: An analysis of contaminated well water and health effects in Woburn, Massachusetts. J Am Stat Assoc 81:583, 1986.

228. MacMahon B: Comment. J Am Stat Assoc 81:596, 1986.

229. Massachusetts Department of Public Health: Woburn Environment and Birth Study, 1994.

230. Marshall EG, Gensburg LJ, Geary NS, et al: Analytic study to evaluate associations between hazardous waste sites and birth defects. Final Report for ATSDR grant H75/ATH 290110012. Albany, NY, New York State Department of Health, 1995.

231. Dolk H, Vrijheid M, Armstrong B, et al: Risk of congenital anomalies near hazardous-waste landfill sites in Europe: the EUROHAZCON study. Lancet 352:423, 1998.

232. Paul M: Occupational and Environmental Reproductive Hazards: A Guide for Clinicians. Baltimore, Williams & Wilkins, 1993.

233. Scialli AR: A Clinical Guide to Reproductive and Developmental Toxicology. Boca Raton, FL, CRC Press, 1992.

234. Paul M, Welch L: Improving education and resources for health care providers. Environ Health Perspect Suppl 2:191, 1993.

235. Occupational Safety and Health Administration: Hazard Communication Guidelines for Compliance. Publication No. OSHA 3111, U.S. Department of Labor. Washington, DC, OSHA, 1988.

236. Himmelstein JS, Frumkin H: The right to know about toxic exposures. Implications for physicians. N Engl J Med 312:687, 1985.

237. Paul M, Kurtz S: Analysis of reproductive health hazard information on material safety data sheets for lead and the ethylene glycol ethers. Am J Ind Med 25:403, 1994.

238. Council of Regional Genetic Networks: Framework for provision of teratology information services. Reprod Toxicol 8:439, 1994.

239. ReproTox Database: The Reproductive Toxicology Center, 2425 L Street, NW, Washington, DC, 20037.

240. Richardson M: Reproductive Toxicology. New York, VCH Publishers, 1993.

241. Sullivan FM, Watkins WJ, van der Venne MTR: Reproductive Toxicity. Vol 1. Summary Reviews of the Scientific Evidence. Luxembourg, Office for Publications of the European Communities, 1993.

242. Koren G: Maternal-Fetal Toxicity, A Clinician's Guide. 2nd ed. New York, Marcel Dekker, 1994.

243. Schardein JL: Chemically Induced Birth Defects. 2nd ed. New York, Marcel Dekker, 1993.

244. Brent RL, Beckman DA: Environmental teratogens. Bull N Y Acad Med 66:123, 1990.

245. U.S. General Accounting Office: Reproductive and Developmental Toxicants: Regulatory Actions Provide Uncertain Protection. GAO/PEMD-92-3. Washington, DC, GAO, 1991.

246. Strobino B, Kline J, Stein ZA: Chemical and physical exposures of parents: effects on human reproduction and offspring. J Early Hum Dev 1:371, 1978.

247. Council on Scientific Affairs: Effects of toxic chemicals on the reproductive system. JAMA 253:3431, 1985.

248. Brent RL, Beckman DA: The contribution of environmental teratogens to embryonic and fetal loss. Clin Obstet Gynecol 37:646, 1994.

Chapter 8

Genetic Counseling and Prenatal Diagnosis

JOE LEIGH SIMPSON

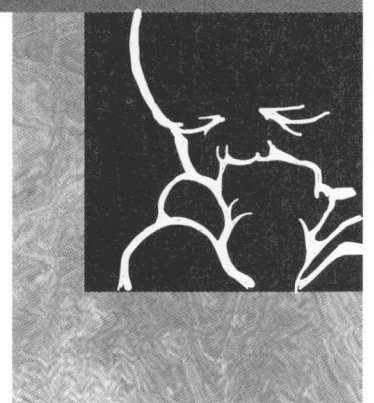

Approximately 3 percent of liveborn infants have a major congenital anomaly. About one half of these anomalies are detected at birth; the remainder become evident later in childhood or, less often, adulthood. Although nongenetic factors may cause malformations, genetic factors are usually responsible. In addition, more than 50 percent of first-trimester spontaneous abortions and at least 5 percent of stillborn infants show chromosomal abnormalities (see Chapter 22). Given such an important role for genetic factors, knowledge of medical genetics clearly becomes integral to the practice of modern obstetrics.

This chapter first considers the principles of genetic counseling and genetic screening. Thereafter, disorders amenable to genetic screening and prenatal diagnosis are discussed.

FREQUENCY OF GENETIC DISEASE

Phenotypic variation—normal or abnormal—may be considered in terms of several etiologic categories: (1) chromosomal abnormalities, numerical or structural; (2) single-gene or mendelian disorders; (3) polygenic and multifactorial disorders, polygenic implying an etiology resulting from cumulative effects of more than one gene and multifactorial implying interaction as well with environmental factors; and (4) teratogenic disorders, caused by exposure to exogenous factors (e.g., drugs) that deleteriously affect an embryo otherwise destined to develop normally. Principles of these mechanisms are reviewed elsewhere.[1]

Chromosomal Abnormalities

From surveys of more than 50,000 liveborn neonates, it has been established that the incidence of chromosomal aberrations is 1 in 160. Table 8–1 shows the incidences of individual abnormalities.[2]

Single-Gene Disorders

Approximately 1 percent of liveborns are phenotypically abnormal as a result of a single-gene mutation. Several thousand single-gene (mendelian) disorders have been recognized, and many more are suspected.[3] However, even the most common mendelian disorders (cystic fibrosis in whites, sickle cell anemia in blacks, β-thalassemia in Greeks and Italians, α-thalassemia in Southeast Asians, Tay-Sachs disease in Ashkenazi Jews) are individually rare. In aggregate, however, mendelian disorders account for 40 percent of the congenital defects seen in liveborn infants.

Polygenic/Multifactorial Disorders

Another 1 percent of neonates are abnormal but possess a normal chromosomal complement and have not undergone mutation at a *single* genetic locus. As will be discussed below, it can be deduced that several different genes are involved (polygenic/multifactorial inheritance).[1]

Disorders in this etiologic category include most common malformations limited to a single organ system. These include hydrocephaly, anencephaly, and spina bifida (neural tube defect [NTDs]); facial clefts (cleft lip and palate); cardiac defects; pyloric stenosis; omphalocele; hip dislocation; uterine fusion defects; and club foot (see the box, Polygenic/Multifactorial Traits). After the birth of one child with such anomalies, the

187

Table 8–1. CHROMOSOMAL ABNORMALITIES IN LIVEBORN INFANTS

Type of Abnormality	Incidence
Numerical aberrations	
Sex chromosomes	
47,XYY	1/1,000 MB
47,XXY	1/1,000 MB
Other (males)	1/1,350 MB
47,X	1/10,000 FB
47,XXX	1/1,000 FB
Other (females)	1/2,700 FB
Autosomes	
Trisomies	
13–15 (D group)	1/20,000 LB
16–18 (E group)	1/8,000 LB
21–22 (G group)	1/800 LB
Other	1/50,000 LB
Structural aberrations	
Balanced	
Robertsonian	
t(Dq;Dq)	1/1,500 LB
t(Dq;Gq)	1/5,000 LB
Reciprocal translocations and insertional inversions	1/7,000 LB
Unbalanced	
Robertsonian	1/14,000 LB
Reciprocal translocations and insertional inversions	1/8,000 LB
Inversions	1/50,000 LB
Deletions	1/10,000 LB
Supernumeraries	1/5,000 LB
Other	1/8,000 LB
Total	1/160 LB

LB, live births; MB, male births; FB, female births.
Pooled data tabulated by Hook and Hamerton.[2]

Polygenic/Multifactorial Traits*

Hydrocephaly (excepting some forms of aqueductal stenosis and Dandy-Walker syndrome)

Neural tube defects (anencephaly, spina bifida, encephalocele)

Cleft lip, with or without cleft palate

Cleft lip (alone)

Cardiac anomalies (most types)

Diaphragmatic hernia

Pyloric stenosis

Omphalocele

Renal agenesis (unilateral or bilateral)

Ureteral anomalies

Posterior urethral values

Hypospadias

Müllerian fusion defects

Müllerian aplasia

Limb reduction defects

Talipes equinovarus (clubfoot)

*Relatively common traits considered to be inherited in polygenic/multifactorial fashion. For each, normal parents have recurrence risks of 1 to 5 percent after one affected child. After two affected offspring, the risk is higher.

recurrence risk in subsequent progeny is usually 1 to 5 percent.[1] This frequency is less than would be expected if only a single gene were responsible but greater than that for the general population. The recurrence risks for malformations are also 1 to 5 percent for offspring of affected parents. That recurrence risks are similar for both siblings and offspring diminishes the likelihood that environmental causes are the exclusive etiologic factor because it is unlikely that households in different generations would be exposed to the same teratogen. Further excluding environmental factors as sole etiologic agents are observations that monozygotic twins are much more often concordant (similarly affected) than are dizygotic twins, despite both types of twins sharing a common intrauterine environment.

The above observations are best explained on the basis of polygenic/multifactorial inheritance. Although more than one gene is involved, only a few genes are necessary to produce the number of genotypes necessary to explain recurrence risks of 1 to 5 percent. That is, large numbers of genes and complex mechanisms need *not* be invoked. Polygenic/multifactorial etiology can thus plausibly be assumed responsible for most liveborns who have an anomaly of a single organ system and who have neither a chromosomal abnormality nor a mendelian mutation.

Teratogenic Disorders

Perhaps 20 proved teratogens are known, as reviewed in Chapter 9. Although many other agents are suspected teratogens, the quantitative contribution of known teratogens to the incidence of anomalies seems relatively small (with the possible exception of alcohol).

CLINICAL SPECTRUM OF CHROMOSOMAL ABNORMALITIES

A few generalizations concerning chromosomal disorders can be offered that may prove helpful to the obstetrician, who may encounter such abnormalities during prenatal studies or in the delivery room. In this section we briefly review the clinical and cytogenetic features characteristic of the common numerical chromosomal abnormalities. Standard genetic texts cover the broader spectrum of rare (mosaic) trisomies and autosomal duplications or deficiency syndromes.

Autosomal Trisomy

Trisomy 21

Trisomy 21 (Down syndrome, mongolism) is the most frequent autosomal chromosomal syndrome, occurring in 1 of every 800 liveborn infants (Table 8–1). The relationship to advanced maternal age is well known. Characteristic craniofacial features include brachycephaly, oblique palpebral fissures, epicanthal folds, broad nasal bridge, a protruding tongue, and small, low-set ears with an overlapping helix and a prominent antihelix (Fig. 8–1). The mean birth weight in Down syndrome, 2,900 g, is decreased but not so much as in some other autosomal syndromes. At birth, these infants are usually hypotonic. Other features include iridial Brushfield's spots, broad short fingers (brachymesophalangia), clinodactyly (incurving deflections resulting from an abnormality of the middle phalanx), a single flexion crease on the fifth digit, and an unusually wide space between the first two toes. A single palmar crease (simian line) is not pathognomonic, being present in only 30 percent of individuals with trisomy 21 and in 5 percent of normal individuals. Relatively common internal anomalies include cardiac lesions and duodenal atresia. Cardiac anomalies and increased susceptibility

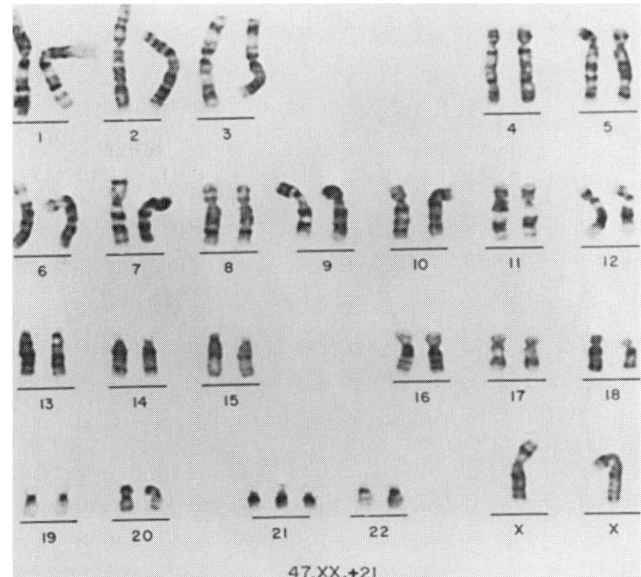

Figure 8–2. Karyotype of a trisomy 21 cell. Trypsin-Giemsa (GTG) banding. (From Simpson JL, Elias S: Genetics in Obstetrics and Gynecology, 3rd ed. Philadelphia, WB Saunders Company, [in press], with permission.)

to both respiratory infections and leukemia contribute to a reduced life expectancy. However, the mean survival is still into the fifth decade, and many affected individuals survive to older ages.

Patients with Down syndrome who survive beyond infancy invariably exhibit mental retardation. However, the degree of retardation is generally not as severe as that of many other chromosomal aberrations. Mean IQ ranges approximately from 25 to 70; 46/47,+21 mosaicism should be suspected if Down syndrome cases show IQs in the 70 to 80 range. Females are fertile. Although relatively few trisomic mothers have reproduced, about 30 percent of their offspring are also trisomic. Except possibly very exceptional cases, affected males are not fertile.

Several different cytogenetic mechanisms may be associated with Down syndrome, which is actually the result of triplication of a small portion of chromosome 21, namely, band q22. This triplication may be caused either by the presence of an entire additional chromosome 21 or by addition of only band q22. Of all cases of Down syndrome, 95 percent have primary trisomy (47 instead of the normal 46 chromosomes) (Fig. 8–2). These cases show the well-known relationship to maternal age effect. Autosomal trisomies usually originate in maternal meiosis, especially meiosis I.

Translocations show no definite relationship to parental age and may be either sporadic or familial. The translocation most commonly associated with Down syndrome involves chromosomes 14 and 21. With translocation Down syndrome [t(14q;21q)], one parent

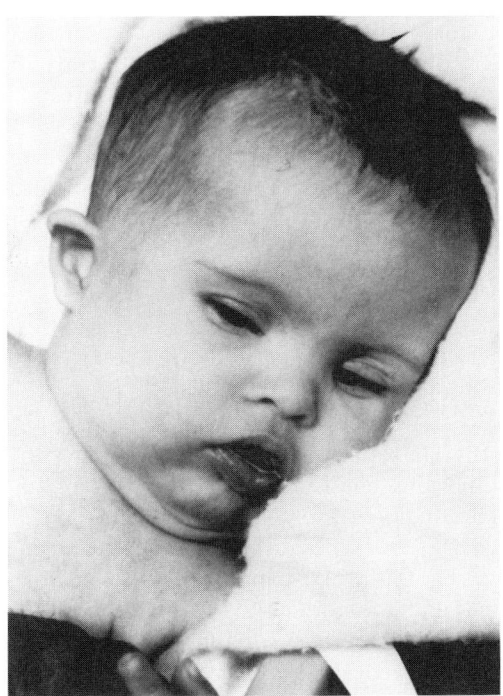

Figure 8–1. An infant with trisomy 21. (From Simpson JL, Elias S: Genetics in Obstetrics and Gynecology, 3rd ed. Philadelphia, WB Saunders Company, [in press], with permission.)

may have the same translocation chromosome, that is, 45,t(14q;21q). For parents with a translocation, the recurrence risk for a child with an unbalanced chromosome complement far exceeds the risk for recurrence of nondisjunction (1 percent). Empiric risks are approximately 10 percent for offspring of female translocation heterozygotes and 2 percent for offspring of male translocation heterozygotes.

Other structural rearrangements resulting in Down syndrome include t(21q;21q), t(21q;21q), and translocations involving chromosome 21 and chromosomes other than a member of group D (13 to 15) or G (21 to 22). In t(21q;21q) no normal gametes can be formed. Thus, only trisomic or monosomic zygotes are produced, the latter presumably appearing as preclinical embryonic losses. Parents having the other translocations have a low empiric risk of having offspring with Down syndrome.

Trisomy 13

Trisomy 13 occurs in about 1 per 20,000 live births. Intrauterine and postnatal growth retardation are pronounced, and developmental retardation is severe. Nearly 50 percent of affected children die in the first month, and relatively few survive past 3 years of age. Characteristic anomalies include holoprosencephaly, eye anomalies (microphthalmia, anophthalmia, or coloboma), cleft lip and palate, polydactyly, cardiac defects, and low birth weight. Other relatively common features include cutaneous scalp defects, hemangiomata on the face or neck, low-set ears with an abnormal helix, and rocker-bottom feet (convex soles and protruding heels).

Trisomy 13 is usually associated with nondisjunctional (primary) trisomy (47,+13). As in trisomy 21, a maternal age effect exists. Translocations are responsible for less than 20 percent of cases, invariably associated with two group D (13 to 15) chromosomes joining at their centromeric regions (robertsonian translocation). If neither parent has such a rearrangement, the risk for subsequent progeny is not increased. If either parent has a balanced 13q;14q translocation, the recurrence risk for an affected offspring is increased, but only to 1 to 2 percent. Homologous 13q;13q parental translocation carries the same dire prognosis as 21q;21q translocation.

Trisomy 18

Trisomy 18 occurs in 1 per 8,000 live births. Among liveborn infants, females are affected more often than males (3:1). Among stillborns and abortuses, however, the sex distribution is more equal.

Facial anomalies characteristic of trisomy 18 include microcephaly, prominent occiput, low-set and pointed "fawn-like" ears, and micrognathia. Skeletal anomalies include overlapping fingers (V over IV, II over III), short sternum, shield chest, narrow pelvis, limited thigh abduction or congenital hip dislocation, rocker-bottom feet with protrusion of the calcaneum, and a short dorsiflexed hallux ("hammer toe"). Cardiac and renal anomalies are common.

Mean birth weight (2,240 g) is below average. The mean survival time for these infants is only a few months. Those surviving show pronounced developmental and growth retardation. Fetal movement is feeble, and approximately 50 percent develop fetal distress during labor. Trisomy 18 is often detected among stillborn infants not clinically suspected of being trisomic.

Approximately 80 percent of trisomy 18 cases are caused by primary nondisjunction (47,XX,+18 or 47,XY,+18). In such cases, the recurrence risk is about 1 percent.

Other Autosomal Trisomies

Trisomies exist for all autosomes, but usually these terminate as abortuses. Trisomies for several chromosomes (8, 9, 14, 16, and 22) exist in nonmosaic forms. Mosaic trisomy exists for chromosome 16 and other chromosomes. All show mental retardation, various somatic anomalies, and intrauterine growth retardation. The extent of retardation and the spectrum of anomalies vary.

Autosomal Deletions or Duplications

Deletions or duplications of portions of autosomes also exist. All are characterized by mental retardation and somatic anomalies, but their specific features vary. One example will suffice for illustrative purposes.

In counseling, one should exclude parental chromosomal rearrangements like a balanced translocation or inversion (see Chapter 7). If the deletion is sporadic, the recurrence risk is no greater than that for any other couple of comparable parental ages.

Sex Chromosomal Abnormalities

Monosomy X (45,X)

45,X individuals account for approximately 40 percent of gonadal dysgenesis cases ascertained by gynecologists. The incidence of 45,X in liveborn females is about 1 in 10,000. Because monosomy X accounts for 10 percent of all first-trimester abortions, it can be calculated that more than 99 percent of 45,X conceptuses must end in early pregnancy loss.

Gonadal dysgenesis is usually associated with an abnormal sex chromosomal constitution. Associated complements include not only monosomy X but structural abnormalities of the X. Mosaicism is frequent, usually involving a coexisting 45,X cell line. Both the long arm and the short arm of the X chromosome contain determinants necessary for ovarian differentiation and for normal stature, as discussed in detail elsewhere.[4]

45,X individuals not only have streak gonads but invariably are short (<150 cm). Growth hormone treatment increases the final adult height 6 to 8 cm. Various somatic anomalies exist: renal and cardiac defects, skeletal abnormalities like cubitus valgus and clinodactyly, vertebral anomalies, pigmented nevi, nail hypoplasia, and a low posterior hairline. Performance IQ is lower than verbal IQ, but mentation should be considered normal. Adult-onset diseases include hypertension and diabetes mellitus.

Klinefelter Syndrome

Males with two or more X chromosomes have small testes, azoospermia, elevated follicle-stimulating hormone (FSH) and luteinizing hormone (LH) levels, and decreased testosterone. The most frequent chromosomal complement associated with this phenotype—Klinefelter syndrome—is 47,XXY; 48,XXXY and 49,XXXXY occur less often.

Mental retardation is uncommon in 47,XXY Klinefelter syndrome, although behavioral problems and dyslexia are not rare. Mental retardation is invariably associated with 48,XXXY and 49,XXXXY. Skeletal, trunk, and craniofacial anomalies occur infrequently in 47,XXY but are commonly observed in 48,XXXY and 49,XXXXY. Regardless of the specific chromosomal complement, patients with Klinefelter syndrome all have unquestioned male phenotypes. The penis may be hypoplastic, but hypospadias is uncommon. Sterility has traditionally been considered certain, but with intracytoplasmic sperm injection (ICSI) and other assisted reproductive technologies (ART) the prognosis is more hopeful.

Polysomy X in Females (47,XXX; 48,XXXX; 49,XXXXX)

About 1 in 800 liveborn females has a 47,XXX complement. 47,XXX individuals are more likely to show mental retardation than are individuals in the general population, and they show IQs 10 to 15 points lower than their sibs. However, the absolute risk for mental retardation does not exceed 5 to 10 percent, and even then IQ is usually 60 to 80. Most 47,XXX patients have a normal reproductive system. The theoretical risk of 47,XXX women delivering an infant with an abnormal chromosomal complement is 50 percent, given one half the maternal gametes carrying 24 chromosomes (24,XX). However, the empiric risk is much less. Somatic anomalies may or may not be more frequent in 47,XXX individuals than in 46,XX females. However, 48,XXXX and 49,XXXXX individuals are invariably retarded and more likely to have somatic malformations than 47,XXX individuals.

Polysomy Y in Males (47,XYY and 48,XXYY)

The presence of more than one Y chromosome is also a frequent chromosomal abnormality in liveborn males (1 in 1,000). Controversy notwithstanding, 47,XYY males seem more likely than 46,XY males to be tall and display sociopathic behavior. The precise prevalence of these features is unknown, but one estimate is that 1 percent of 47,XYY males will be incarcerated compared with 0.1 percent of 46,XY males. 47,XYY males usually have normal male external genitalia.

GENETIC HISTORY

All obstetrician-gynecologists must attempt to determine whether a couple, or anyone in their family, has a heritable disorder or is at increased risk for abnormal offspring. To address this question, some obstetricians find it helpful to elicit genetic information through the use of questionnaires or check lists that are often constructed in a manner that requires action only to positive responses. Figure 8–3 reproduces a form that has been modified from that recommended by the American College of Obstetricians and Gynecologists (ACOG).

One should inquire into the health status of first-degree relatives (siblings, parents, offspring), second-degree relatives (nephews, nieces, aunts, uncles, grandparents), and third-degree relatives (first cousins, especially maternal). Adverse reproductive outcomes such as repetitive spontaneous abortions, stillbirths, and anomalous liveborn infants should be pursued. Couples having such histories should undergo chromosomal studies in order to exclude balanced translocations. Genetic counseling may prove sufficiently complex to warrant referral to a clinical geneticist, or it may prove simple enough for the well-informed obstetrician to manage. If a birth defect exists in a second-degree relative (uncle, aunt, grandparent, nephew, niece) or third-degree relative (first cousin), the risk for that anomaly will usually not prove substantially increased over that in the general population. For example, identification of a second- or third-degree relative with an autosomal recessive trait places the couple at little increased risk for an affected offspring, an exception being if the patient and her husband are consanguineous. However, a maternal first cousin with an X-linked recessive disorder would

Prenatal Genetic Screen

Name _____ Patient# _____ Date _____

1. Will you be 35 years or older when the baby is due?   Yes ___ No ___
2. Have you, the baby's father, or anyone in either of your families ever had any of the following disorders?
   Down syndrome (mongolism)   Yes ___ No ___
   Other chromosomal abnormality   Yes ___ No ___
   Neural tube defect, i.e., spina bifida (meningomyelocele or open spine), anencephaly   Yes ___ No ___
   Hemophilia   Yes ___ No ___
   Muscular dystrophy   Yes ___ No ___
   Cystic fibrosis   Yes ___ No ___
   If yes, indicate the relationship of the affected person to you or to the baby's father:
   _____
3. Do you or the baby's father have a birth defect?   Yes ___ No ___
   If yes, who has the defect and what is it?_____
4. In any previous marriages, have you or the baby's father had a child born, dead or alive, with a birth defect not listed in question 2 above?   Yes ___ No ___
5. Do you or the baby's father have any close relatives with mental retardation?   Yes ___ No ___
   If yes, indicate the relationship of the affected person to you or to the baby's father:
   _____
   Indicate the cause, if known: _____
6. Do you, the baby's father, or a close relative in either of your families have a birth defect, any familial disorder, or a chromosomal abnormality not listed above?   Yes ___ No ___
   If yes, indicate the condition and the relationship of the affected person to you or to the baby's father:
   _____
7. In any previous marriage, have you or the baby's father had a stillborn child or three or more first-trimester spontaneous pregnancy losses?   Yes ___ No ___
   Have either of you had a chromosomal study?   Yes ___ No ___
8. If you or the baby's father is of Jewish ancestry, have either of you been screened for Tay-Sachs disease, Canavan disease, or cystic fibrosis?   Yes ___ No ___
   If yes, indicate who and the results: _____
9. If you or the baby's father is black, have either of you been screened for sickle cell trait?   Yes ___ No ___
   If yes, indicate who and the results: _____
10. If you or the baby's father is of Italian, Greek, or Mediterranean background, have either of you been tested for β–thalassemia?   Yes ___ No ___
    If yes, indicate who and the results: _____
11. If you or the baby's father is of Philippine or Southeast Asian ancestry, have either of you been tested for α–thalassemia?   Yes ___ No ___
    If yes, indicate who and the results: _____
12. Irrespective of ethnic group, have you or the baby's father been screened for cystic fibrosis?   Yes ___ No ___
13. Excluding iron and vitamins, have you taken any medications or recreational drugs since becoming pregnant or since your last menstrual period? (include nonprescription drugs)
    If yes, give name of medication and time taken during pregnancy: _____
    _____
14. Have you currently been taking folic acid supplements?   Yes ___ No ___

Figure 8–3. Questionnaire for identifying couples having increased risk for offspring with genetic disorders. (Modified from a form recommended by the American College of Obstetricians and Gynecologists: Antenatal Diagnosis of Genetic Disorders. Technical Bulletin No. 108. Washington, DC, ACOG, 1987.)

identify a couple at increased risk for a similar occurrence.

Parental ages should also be recorded. Advanced maternal age (Table 8–2) warrants discussion irrespective of a physician's personal convictions regarding pregnancy termination, as knowledge of an abnormality may affect obstetric management. Ethnic origin should be recorded. The above applies for both gamete donors as well as couples achieving pregnancy by natural means.

GENETIC COUNSELING

Although genetic counseling may require referral to a clinical geneticist, it is impractical for obstetricians to refer all patients with genetic inquiries. Indeed, obstetricians performing diagnostic procedures such as amniocentesis must counsel their patients before such a procedure. Salient principles of the genetic counseling process will therefore be described.

Table 8–2. MATERNAL AGE AND CHROMOSOMAL ABNORMALITIES (LIVE BIRTHS)*

Maternal Age	Risk for Down Syndrome	Risk for Any Chromosome Abnormalities[†]
20	1/1,667	1/526[†]
21	1/1,667	1/526[†]
22	1/1,429	1/500[†]
23	1/1,429	1/500[†]
24	1/1,250	1/476[†]
25	1/1,250	1/476[†]
26	1/1,176	1/476[†]
27	1/1,111	1/455[†]
28	1/1,053	1/435[†]
29	1/1,100	1/417[†]
30	1/952	1/384[†]
31	1/909	1/385[†]
32	1/769	1/322[†]
33	1/625	1/317[†]
34	1/500	1/260
35	1/385	1/204
36	1/294	1/164
37	1/227	1/130
38	1/175	1/103
39	1/137	1/82
40	1/106	1/65
41	1/82	1/51
42	1/64	1/40
43	1/50	1/32
44	1/38	1/25
45	1/30	1/20
46	1/23	1/15
48	1/18	1/12
48	1/14	1/10
49	1/11	1/7

*Because sample size for some intervals is relatively small, confidence limits are sometimes relatively large. Nonetheless, these figures are suitable for genetic counseling.
[†]47,XXX excluded for ages 20 to 32 (data not available).
Data from Hook[112] and Hook et al.[113]

Communication

A first principle of counseling is to communicate in terms that are readily comprehensible to patients. It is useful to preface remarks with a few sentences recounting the major causes of genetic abnormalities—cytogenetic, single-gene, polygenic/multifactorial (can be labeled "complex"), and environmental (teratogens). Writing unfamiliar words and using tables or diagrams to reinforce important concepts is helpful. Repetition is essential. Allow the couple not only to ask questions but to talk with one another to formulate their concerns.

Written information (letters or brochures) can serve as a couple's permanent record, allaying misunderstanding and assisting in dealing with relatives. Preprinted forms describing common problems (e.g., advanced maternal age) have the additional advantage of emphasizing that the couple's problem is not unique. More complicated scenarios require a letter.

Irrespective of how obvious a diagnosis may seem, confirmation is always obligatory. Accepting a patient's verbal recollection does not suffice, nor would accepting a diagnosis made by a physician not highly knowledgeable about the condition. The anomalous individual may need to be examined by the appropriate authority, and examining first-degree relatives may be required as well if the possibility of an autosomal dominant disorder (e.g., neurofibromatosis) exists. If a definitive diagnosis cannot be made, the physician should not hesitate to say so. Proper counseling requires proper diagnosis.

Nondirective Counseling

In genetic counseling, one should provide accurate genetic information yet ideally dictate no particular course of action. Of course, completely nondirective counseling is probably unrealistic. For example, a counselor's unwitting facial expressions may expose his or her unstated opinions. Merely offering antenatal diagnostic services implies approval. Despite the difficulties of remaining truly objective, one should attempt merely to provide information and then support the couple's decision.

Psychological Defenses

Psychological defenses permeate genetic counseling. If not appreciated, these defenses can impede the entire counseling process. Anxiety is low in couples counseled for advanced maternal age or for an abnormality in a distant relative. As long as the anxiety level remains low, comprehension of information is usually not impaired. However, couples who have experienced a stillborn infant, an anomalous child, or multiple repetitive abortions are more anxious. Their ability to retain information may be hindered.

Couples experiencing abnormal pregnancy outcomes manifest the same grief reactions that occur after the death of a loved one: denial, anger, guilt, bargaining, resolution. One should pay deference to this sequence by not attempting definitive counseling immediately after the birth of an abnormal neonate. Parents must be supported at that time, and the obstetrician should avoid discussing specific recurrence risks for fear of adding to the immediate burden. By 4 to 6 weeks the couple has begun to cope and is more receptive to counseling.

An additional psychological consideration is that of parental guilt. One naturally searches for exogenous factors that might have caused an abnormal outcome. In the process of such a search, guilt may arise. Conversely, a tendency to blame the spouse may be seen. Usually, guilt or blame is not justified, but occasionally the "blame" is realistic (e.g., in autosomal dominant traits). Fortunately, most couples can be assured that nothing could have prevented a given abnormal pregnancy.

Appreciating the psychological defenses described above helps one to understand the failure of ostensibly intelligent and well-counseled couples to comprehend genetic information.

GENETIC SCREENING

Genetic screening implies routine monitoring for the presence or absence of a given condition in apparently normal individuals. Screening is now offered routinely for (1) all individuals of certain ethnic groups to identify those individuals heterozygous for a given autosomal recessive disorder (Table 8–3), (2) all pregnant women to detect elevated maternal serum α-fetoprotein for diagnosis of fetal neural tube defects, (3) all pregnant women 35 years of age and above to undergo invasive tests and to detect Down syndrome, and (4) all pregnant women *under* age of 35 years to undergo maternal serum screening to detect Down syndrome.

Neonatal Screening

One could theoretically screen neonates for many other genetic disorders. On the other hand, screening is actually recommended for relatively few disorders because prerequisites essential for initiating screening programs are not usually met. A first prerequisite is that widespread testing is ordinarily performed only if an abnormal finding would alter clinical management. In the United States, neonates are mandated to be evaluated for phenylketonuria and hypothyroidism, both amenable to dietary or hormonal treatment. Many states screen for additional disorders, such as sickle cell anemia, 21-hydroxylase deficiency (congenital adrenal hyperplasia), and other metabolic disorders. A recent addition is deafness, which is often genetic in origin. Screening is not attempted for neonates with untreatable disorders. Thus, neonatal screening is not recom-

Table 8–3. GENETIC SCREENING IN VARIOUS ETHNIC GROUPS

Ethnic Group	Disorder	Screening Test	Definitive Test
Ashkenazi Jews	Tay-Sachs disease	Decreased serum hexosamidase-A, possibly molecular analysis	Chorionic villus sampling (CVS) or amniocentesis for enzymatic assay or molecular analysis to detect affected fetus
	Canavans disease	DNA analysis to detect most common alleles	CVS or amniocentesis for molecular analysis to detect affected fetus
African-Americans	Sickle cell anemia	Presence of sickle cell hemoglobin, confirmatory hemoglobin electrophoresis	CVS or amniocentesis for genotype determination (direct molecular analysis)
Mediterranean people	β-Thalassemia	Mean corpuscular volume (MCV) < 80%, followed by hemoglobin electrophoresis	CVS or amniocentesis for genotype determination (direct molecular analysis or linkage analysis)
Southeast Asians and Chinese (Vietnamese, Laotian, Cambodian, Filipino)	α-Thalassemia	MCV < 80%, followed by hemoglobin electrophoresis	CVS or amniocentesis for genotype determination; (direct molecular studies) (direct linkage analysis)
All ethnic groups	Cystic fibrosis	DNA analysis of specified panel of 25 CFTR mutations (those present in $\geq 0.1\%$ of the general U.S. population)	CVS or amniocentesis for genotype determination; definitive diagnosis on all fetuses is not possible, sensitivity varying by ethnic group
	In Caucasians and Ashkenazi Jews should be offered; in other ethnic groups (Asians, Hispanics, African-Americans should be made available)		

mended for chromosomal abnormalities, Tay-Sachs disease, and Duchenne muscular dystrophy.

Adult Screening

Adult population screening for Tay-Sachs disease, α- and β-thalassemia, and sickle cell anemia is reasonable in order to determine whether they are heterozygous for autosomal recessive disorders amenable to prenatal diagnosis. Table 8–3 lists disorders for which screening is currently recommended. The most well-known example in the United States is Tay-Sachs disease, an autosomal recessive disorder for which Ashkenazi Jews are at increased risk (heterozygote frequency, 1 in 27). In the United States, Jewish individuals may be uncertain whether they are of Ashkenazic or Sephardic descent (90 percent are Ashkenazi); thus, obstetricians should screen all Jewish couples, and possibly also couples in which only one partner is Jewish. The most recent conditions for which genetic screening can be considered standard are cystic fibrosis (see below) and Canavans disease. Ashkenazi Jews may also benefit from screening for Gaucher disease and Nieman-Pick disease (as well as Tay-Sachs, Canavans, and cystic fibrosis [CF]).[5] In aggregate, the likelihood of an Ashkenazi Jewish individual being heterozygous for one of these five autosomal recessive disorders is 1 in 7. Heterozygote detection for β-thalassemia in Italians and Greeks relies on measurement of mean corpuscular volume (MCV), as does screening for α-thalassemia in Southeast Asians and Filipinos. Greater than 80 percent excludes heterozygosity for α- or β-thalassemia. Values less than 80 percent are more likely to reflect iron deficiency anemia than heterozygosity, so additional confirmatory tests are indicated to exclude heterozygosity for the thalassemias. Genes for all the above disorders have been isolated and cloned. However, molecular heterogeneity is enormous for all except sickle cell anemia (see below for further discussion). Thus, screening preferentially still utilizes the methods listed in Table 8–3. Possible exceptions include sickle cell anemia and Tay-Sachs disease. In the latter, molecular testing is equal but not superior to enzyme testing in the Ashkenazi Jewish population.[6]

Population Screening for Cystic Fibrosis

Routine screening is now standard for cystic fibrosis, but not without difficulty. Recommendations have recently become available as a result of a joint effort of ACOG, the American College of Medical Genetics (ACMG), and the National Institutes of Health (NIH) Genome Center. The gene is large (27 exons) and its gene product is a chloride channel. About 75 percent of the cystic fibrosis mutations are caused by deletion of amino acid 508 (ΔF508), resulting in loss of a phenylalanine residue (Fig. 8–4). About 50 percent of couples at risk for cystic fibrosis offspring can be identified by screening solely for this mutation, offering unequivocal prenatal diagnosis. However, detecting the remaining couples at risk for cystic fibrosis is more difficult. Screening only for ΔF508 would uncover couples in which one parent has the ΔF508 mutation but the other does not. If one parent has ΔF508 but the other does not, the actual risk of that couple having an affected child is 1 in 400. Amniotic fluid analysis for the cystic fibrosis gene product (protein) is not yet available, meaning prenatal diagnosis is not possible except to exclude the fetus who inherited the ΔF508 from the known heterozygous parent.

The obvious solution is to detect other mutations within the cystic fibrosis locus. Unfortunately, except for one specific mutation (W1282X) in Ashkenazi Jews, all other mutations are individually rare. Figure 8–5 shows increasing detection rate in northern European Caucasian and Ashkenazi Jewish populations as increasing numbers of CF-causing alleles are sought. Sensitivity reaches an asymptote, not exceeding 90 to 97 percent in the two ethnic groups, respectively. Thus, not all at-risk pregnancies will be identified.

NORMAL

DNA	..GAA	AAT	ATC	ATC	TTT	GGT	GTT	TCC..
PROTEIN	Glu	Asn	Ile	Ile	Phe	Gly	Val	Ser
POSITION	504	505	506	507	508	509	510	511

CYSTIC FIBROSIS

DNA	..GAA	AAT	ATC	AT-	--T	GGT	GTT	TCC..
PROTEIN	Glu	Asn	Ile	Ile		Gly	Val	Ser

Figure 8–4. Schematic drawing illustrating ΔF508 mutation, which accounts for 75 percent of cystic fibrosis cases in couples of northern European ancestry.

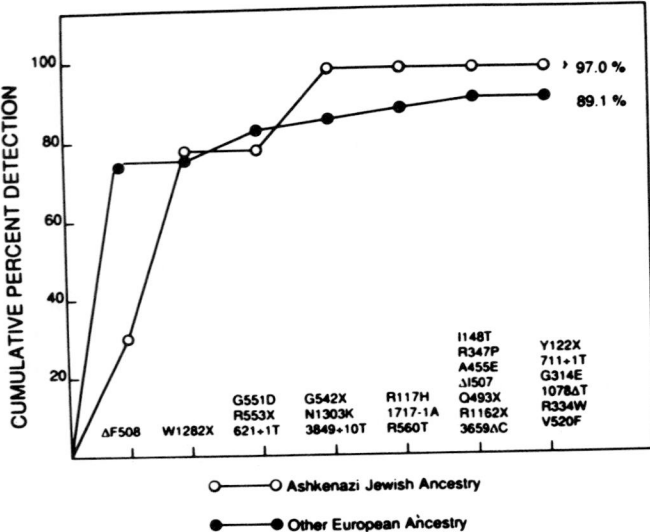

Figure 8–5. Increasing detection rate in northern European Caucasian and Ashkenazi Jewish populations as increasing numbers of CF-causing alleles are sought. Cystic Fibrosis Foundation.

Newly codified recommendations have been made by the ACOG, the American College of Medical Genetics, and NIH.[7] These guidelines are "to offer" CF heterozygote screening to non-Jewish Caucasians and Ashkenazi Jews, both of which show carrier frequencies of 1 in 25 to 30. In other ethnic group (Asian-Americans, Hispanics, African-Americans) the carrier frequency is lower; thus, it is recommended CF carrier screening be "made available" and that couples "be informed of their detectability through educational brochures." In Caucasians and Ashkenazi Jews, the overall heterozygote detection rates are 90 and 97 percent, respectively, whereas in the three other ethnic groups it approximates 70 percent even using a panel of ethnic-specific markers to maximize detection.[8–10] At present it is recommended that a panethnic mutation panel be used that includes all mutant CF alleles having a frequency of 0.1 percent in the general U.S. population. This encompasses 25 mutations at present (Table 8–4) and is subject to yearly review. Screening for other alleles is not discouraged (e.g., as part of ethnic-specific panels);

however, screening for more than the 25 alleles is optional.

Of specific note to obstetrician-gynecologists is allele R117H, even though this allele is more commonly associated with congenital bilateral absence of the vas deferens (CBAVD) than the classic cystic fibrosis phenotype characterized by pulmonary, hepatic, and pancreatic complications. CBAVD males usually have two dysfunctional CF alleles. One but not both could be ΔF508[9] (otherwise, the phenotype would not be CBAVD but classic CF). In CBAVD, the other allele is often R117H. If a male with CBAVD is ΔF508/R117H, the spouse could be heterozygous for ΔF508; thus, the likelihood is 25 percent that any given fetus will have a severe form of CF (ΔF508/ΔF508). The other major CF perturbation contributing to CBAVD involves a polymorphism (5T/7T/9T) in intron 8.[11] The 5T (thymine) and 7T variants may be observed in CBAVD in homozygous or compound heterozygous forms, or in complementation with ΔF508 or R117H. The 5T and to a lesser extent 7T polymorphisms are deleterious because they lead to splice-junction perturbation and, hence, a truncated dysfunctional CFTR gene product. If R117H is detected on the panel, testing for the 5T/7T/9T polymorphism is recommended. The reason is that 5T/R117H heterozygosity has been observed with classic CF.[12] If R117H is not detected, testing for the 5T/7T/9T polymorphism is not necessary.

If a couple has already had a child with cystic fibrosis, or recounts an affected close relative, screening as described above is not germane. Rather, case detection strategies become appropriate. The index case, or the couple if the proband is unavailable, should be screened not just for the panel in Table 8–4 but, if uninformative, for a larger panel totaling up to 70 CF mutations. If the mutation is still not evident, family studies to identify polymorphic loci informative for linkage analysis should be considered if prenatal genetic diagnosis are planned (see Disorders Detectable by Molecular Methods, below).

The complexity engendered in cystic fibrosis screening will be repeated for most mendelian disorders because molecular heterogeneity is the rule rather than the exception for single-gene disorders.

Table 8–4. RECOMMENDED PANEL OF MUTATIONS IN THE CYSTIC FIBROSIS TRANSMEMBRANE REGULATORY (CFTR) GENE THAT SHOULD BE SOUGHT IN CARRIER DETECTION PROGRAMS*

ΔF508	ΔI507	G542X	G551D	W1282X	N1303K
R553X	621 + 1G > T	R117H	1717 − 1G > A	A455E	R560T
R1162X	G85E	R334W	R347P	711 + 1G > T	1898 + 1G > A
2184delA	1078delT	3849 + 10kbC > T	2789 + 5G > A	3659delC	I148T
3120 + 1G > A					

* The panel is applicable in all ethnic groups. If R117H is detected, status of the 5T-7T-9T polymorphism should be determined.

Maternal Serum α-Fetoprotein Screening for Neural Tube Defects

Relatively few (5 percent) NTDs occur in families who have had previously affected offspring. Thus, a method other than a positive family history is needed to identify couples in the general population at risk for an NTD. Maternal serum α-fetoprotein (MSAFP) serves this purpose, identifying couples with a negative family history who nonetheless have sufficient risk to justify amniocentesis.

MSAFP is greater than 2.5 multiples of the median (MOM) in 80 to 90 percent of pregnancies in which the fetus has an NTD. Because considerable overlap exists between MSAFP in normal pregnancies and MSAFP in pregnancies characterized by a fetus with an NTD, systematic protocols for evaluating elevated MSAFP values are necessary. Elevated MSAFP occurs for reasons other than an NTD: (1) underestimation of gestational age, inasmuch as MSAFP increases as gestation progresses; (2) multiple gestation (60 percent of twins and almost all triplets having MSAFP values that would be elevated if judged on the basis of singleton values); (3) fetal demise, presumably caused by fetal blood extravasating into the maternal circulation; (4) Rh isoimmunization, cystic hygroma, and other conditions associated with fetal edema; and (5) anomalies other than NTD, usually characterized by edema or skin defects.

The initial MSAFP assay should be performed at 15 to 20 weeks' gestation. Corrections for maternal weight and some other factors are necessary, using various algorithms that provide a weight-adjusted MSAFP appropriate for gestational age. (Without weight adjustment, dilutional effects can result in heavier women having a spuriously low value when in fact MSAFP might actually be elevated for women of their weight.)

Maternal serum values above either 2.0 or 2.5 MOM are usually considered elevated. The precise value above which MSAFP is considered elevated is less important than setting a consistent policy per program. Values above 2.0 MOM are definitely considered elevated in insulin-dependent diabetic women, but in twin gestations MSAFP is judged abnormal only at 4.5 to 5.0 MOM or greater.

Approximately 5 percent of women will have an elevated MSAFP value. If gestational age assessment is determined accurately before MSAFP sampling, the number of women having an abnormal serum value will be lower (3 percent). A second MSAFP sample may or may not be necessary. There is virtue in reassaying MSAFP if the value lies between 2.50 and 2.99 MOM and if gestational age is 18 weeks or less. If not already performed, ultrasound is obviously required to exclude erroneous gestational age, multiple gestations,

or fetal demise. Amniocentesis for AFP and acetylcholinesterase (AChE) is necessary if no explanation for elevated MSAFP is evident on ultrasound. The presence of AChE indicates an open NTD or other anomalies.

MSAFP screening identifies 90 percent anencephaly and 80 to 85 percent of spina bifida, albeit at the cost of 1 to 2 percent of all pregnant women undergoing amniocentesis. Approximately 1 in 15 women having an unexplained elevated serum AFP will prove to have a fetus with an NTD. Not well appreciated is that sensitivity of detecting an NTD in twin gestations is less than in singleton gestations, being only about 30 percent for spina bifida given a threshold of 4.5 MOM. The poor sensitivity exists because twins are usually discordant for an NTD. Liberal use of comprehensive ultrasound is recommended in twin gestations.

Second-trimester MSAFP screening to detect neural tube defects is necessary even if first-trimester screening to detect aneuploidy (see below) is employed. First-trimester MSAFP is not a sensitive method of detecting NTDs. Some physicians prefer to utilize comprehensive ultrasound immediately after elevated MSAFP. Thus, amniocentesis might not be performed in the absence of ultrasound evidence of an NTD. Although a logical approach, the sensitivity of NTD detection cannot be assumed to be as high as with MSAFP followed by amniocentesis.

Maternal Serum Screening for Detecting Fetal Trisomy

Soon after maternal serum screening for the detection of NTDs was introduced, it became clear that a low MSAFP level was associated with trisomy 21.[13] The possibility arose that maternal serum screening could be offered to women under the age of 35 for detection of Down syndrome. Low serum values could confer a risk sufficiently high that women who are not otherwise candidates for invasive procedures like amniocentesis or chorionic villus sampling (CVS) might wish to undergo such. This proposition is attractive because only 25 percent of infants with Down syndrome are born to women aged 35 and above. Thus, decreasing the population incidence requires identifying younger women at sufficient risk to justify an invasive procedure. However, screening for Down syndrome is more complicated than screening for NTDs because the risk of Down syndrome is age specific. An MSAFP value of, say, 0.4 easily raises the age-associated risk of a 34-year-old high enough to justify amniocentesis; however, the same value would not necessarily increase the risk similarly for a 25-year-old woman. For this reason the preferable way to identify couples with sufficient risk to justify invasive procedures is to utilize likelihood ratios. For example, a maternal serum value for AFP of 0.4

MOM carries a likelihood ratio of 3.81 for having a child with Down syndrome. If the a priori (age-specific) risk is 1 in 581 (for a 25-year-old woman), the recalculated risk after taking into account MSAFP is 1 in 148.

In addition to the association between low MSAFP and Down syndrome, an association exists for other maternal serum analytes. The analyte having the greatest discriminatory value is human chorionic gonadotropin (hCG), which is elevated in Down syndrome pregnancies.[14] In the second trimester, either intact hCG or free β-hCG will suffice for assay. Irrespective, the combination of hCG, AFP, and maternal age, when analyzed with appropriate software to derive likelihood ratios, allows detection of some 60 percent of cases of Down syndrome at an amniocentesis rate of 5 percent.[15] Other analytes offer slight added value. Inhibin A (see below) and unconjugatad estriol (uE$_3$) are most widely added. Adding either of these analytes, the sensitivity of detecting trisomy 21 in the general population (all ages) increases to 65 to 70 percent.

Importantly, for accurate counseling, sensitivity of detecting Down syndrome is age dependent; thus, not all cohort studies will show identical results. Detection rates are 90 percent for women aged 35 and above, but much lower for those in their early third decade. Women should be given *precise* answers as to the sensitivity of detecting trisomy in their pregnancy; 65 percent detection is not the correct information to impart to a 25-year-old who inquires about her own detection rate. Confounding factors can affect serum screening. Corrections for maternal weight and ethnic group are routine, but adjustments for other confounding variables are not. Maternal weight affects AFP, uE$_3$, and hCG levels, all of which decrease with increasing weight. Insulin-dependent diabetes in mothers results in slightly decreased uE$_3$ and hCG levels. Maternal smoking increases MSAFP by 3 percent and decreases maternal serum uE$_3$ and hCG levels by 3 percent and 23 percent, respectively.[16] Maternal serum hCG has been found to be higher and MSAFP lower in pregnancies that were conceived in vitro when compared with pregnancies that were conceived spontaneously.[17] The effect of changes other than weight and ethnic group is not great, and may or may not be enough to warrant adjustment. Maternal serum screening to detect Down syndrome in twin gestations has become available. Down syndrome occurs more frequently (20 percent) in twin pregnancies than in singleton pregnancies, which is predictable given the known positive correlation between twinning and maternal age. Unfortunately, Down syndrome screening using multiple serum markers is not as sensitive in twin pregnancies as it is for singleton pregnancies. Using singleton cutoffs, 73 percent of monozygotic twin pregnancies but only 43 percent of dizygotic twin pregnancies with Down syndrome

should be detected, with a 5 percent false-positive rate.[18] The lower sensitivity in dizygotic twins reflects the blunting effect of the concomitant presence of one normal and one aneuploid fetus. Thus, patients should be informed that the detection rate is less than in singleton pregnancies. It may simply be preferable to perform invasive procedures, say in women 32 years or older.[19] Younger women may still wish to avail themselves of noninvasive screening despite its lower sensitivity.

Despite different policies in other venues (e.g., Europe), the ACOG continues to recommend that women aged 35 years or older be offered invasive procedures without prior serum screening. Women under 35 years of age should be counseled about serum screening. If older women insist on maternal serum screening in lieu of an invasive procedure, they must appreciate that detection is not 100 percent but only 90 percent at best.

Screening for Trisomy 18

Trisomy 18 can also be detected by triple-marker screening. This aneuploidy is associated with decreased hCG, AFP, and uE$_3$ levels, a pattern that differs from trisomy 21, in which hCG is elevated. One recommendation is to offer invasive prenatal diagnosis whenever serum screening shows each of these three markers to fall below certain thresholds (MSAFP $\leq$ 0.6 MOM; hCG $\leq$ 0.55 MOM; uE$_3$ $\leq$ 0.5 MOM).[20] Screening for trisomy 18 by simply using these thresholds would detect 60 to 80 percent of trisomy 18 fetuses, with a 0.4 percent amniocentesis rate.[21] Calculating individual risk estimation on the basis of three markers and maternal age, Palomaki and colleagues reported that 60 percent of trisomy 18 pregnancies can be detected, with an amniocentesis (false-positive) rate of about 0.2 percent.[20] One in nine pregnancies identified as being at increased risk for trisomy 18 by serum screening would be expected to be actually affected.

Other Markers

One attractive option for maternal screening is dimeric inhibin-A.[22] Alluded to already, inhibin-A is a dimeric glycoprotein with an α-subunit and a β^A-subunit linked by a disulfide bond. During pregnancy, inhibin-A is produced by the corpus luteum and the placenta. Serum inhibin-A levels from women carrying fetuses with Down syndrome are elevated, as are hCG levels.

Urinary (as opposed to serum) markers might also be useful in detecting fetal Down syndrome. Canick et al.[23] compared levels of a metabolite of hCG and urinary gonadotropin peptide (UGP) from 14 women carrying fetuses affected with Down syndrome with urinary samples from 91 control pregnancies and found the MOM to be 5.34. Cole et al.[24] believe hyperglycosolated hCG is useful.

First-Trimester Screening

Screening in the first trimester is highly desirable because patients at increased risk can be offered CVS, avoiding the increased late-pregnancy terminations if fetal abnormalities are detected. Associations exist between Down syndrome and low MSAFP, low pregnancy-associated placental protein A (PAPP-A), and elevated free β-hCG. Using PAPP-A and free β-hCG for first-trimester Down syndrome screening gives a 62 percent detection rate with a 5 percent false-positive rate.[25]

Another approach is to measure nuchal translucency thickening, a reproducible method of measurement pioneered by Nicolaides and Snijders in London.[26] This group has measured nuchal translucency in over 100,000 pregnancies in London and in surrounding district general hospitals. Risk of trisomy is derived by multiplying the background maternal age and gestational-related risk by a likelihood ratio, which reflects the deviation of nuchal translucency from the normal mean for gestation. In a study of 96,127 pregnant women of median age 31 years, a calculated risk of 1 in 300 or higher for Down syndrome was observed in 8.3 percent. The detection rate was 82.2 percent for trisomy 21 and 77.9 percent for other chromosomal abnormalities. A few of these may have aborted spontaneously had not intervention occurred, but sensitivity is still well over 70 percent.

First-trimester screening with maternal serum analytes (PAPP-A) and free β-hCG can be combined with fetal nuchal translucency screening to further refine risks for fetal trisomies.[27] In addition, sequential first-trimester (PAPP-A and β-hCG; nuchal translucency) and second-trimester (maternal serum so-called integrated test) screening is possible. This approach should theoretically detect nearly 90 percent, with a false-positive rate of 5 percent.[28] Alternatively, one can accept a detection rate of 80 percent for a lower (1 percent) rate of amniocentesis. The algorithm utilized by current proponents has the major disadvantage of requiring that first-trimester results be withheld until second-trimester results are obtained. In addition to failing to disclose information in a timely fashion, termination would be deferred until the second trimester, when risks are higher (see Chapter 42). The stated justification is that sensitivity is lowered if calculated with first-trimester serum screening or with first-trimester nuchal translucency alone;[23] however, the magnitude of the decreased detection rate has not been made available, making it difficult to comment objectively.

DIAGNOSTIC PROCEDURES FOR PRENATAL GENETIC DIAGNOSIS

Prenatal genetic diagnosis usually requires obtaining fetal tissue, necessitating an invasive procedure like amniocentesis or CVS. In this section we shall consider common techniques and their safety.

Traditional Amniocentesis

Technique

In amniocentesis, amniotic fluid is aspirated, often for the purpose of genetic diagnosis at 15 to 16 weeks' gestation (menstrual weeks). While the procedure has traditionally been performed at 15 to 16 weeks, it can be performed earlier (especially 12 to 14 weeks).[27] A 22-gauge spinal needle with stylet is usually used. Ultrasound examination is obligatory in order to determine gestational age, placental position, location of amniotic fluid, and number of fetuses. Ultrasound should be performed concurrently with amniocentesis. Rh-immune globulin should be administered to the Rh-negative, Du-negative, unsensitized patient.

Bloody amniotic fluid is aspirated occasionally; however, this blood is almost always maternal in origin and does not adversely affect amniotic cell growth. By contrast, brown, dark red, or wine-colored amniotic fluid is associated with an increased likelihood of poor pregnancy outcome. The dark color indicates that intra-amniotic bleeding has occurred earlier in pregnancy, with hemoglobin breakdown products persisting; pregnancy loss eventually occurs in about one third of such cases. If the abnormally colored fluid is characterized by elevated AFP, the outcome is almost always unfavorable (fetal demise or fetal abnormality). Greenish amniotic fluid is the result of meconium staining and is apparently not associated with poor pregnancy outcome.

In multiple gestations, amniocentesis can usually be performed on all fetuses. Following aspiration of amniotic fluid from the first sac, 2 to 3 ml of indigo carmine, diluted 1:10 in bacteriostatic water, is injected before the needle is withdrawn. A second amniocentesis is then performed at a site determined after visualizing the membranes separating the two sacs. It is important to note the locations of each sac in case selective termination is later required. Aspiration of clear fluid confirms that the second (new) sac was entered. Triplets and other multiple gestations can be managed similarly, sequentially injecting dye into successive sacs. Although cross-contamination of cells in multiple gestations appears to be rare, confusion may sometimes arise in interpreting amniotic fluid AChE or AFP results. Some obstetricians aspirate the second sac without dye injection or use a single-puncture technique; however, I still prefer dye injection for confirmation.

After amniocentesis, the patient may resume all normal activities. Common sense dictates that strenuous exercise such as jogging or "aerobic" exercise be deferred for a day or so. The patient should report persistent uterine cramping, vaginal bleeding, leakage of amniotic fluid, or fever; however, physician intervention is almost never required, unless overt abortion occurs.

If only one fetus in a multiple gestation is abnormal, parents should be prepared to choose between aborting all fetuses or continuing the pregnancy with one or more normal and one abnormal fetus. Selective termination in the second trimester is possible, but success of this procedure is greater in the first trimester.[30]

Safety of Traditional Amniocentesis

Any procedure that involves entering the pregnant uterus logically carries risk to the fetus. Amniocentesis is no exception. Amniocentesis carries potential danger to both mother and fetus. Maternal risks are quite low, with symptomatic amnionitis occurring only rarely (0.1 percent). Minor maternal complications such as transient vaginal spotting or minimal amniotic fluid leakage occur in 1 percent or fewer of cases, but almost always these are self-limited in nature. Other very rare complications include intra-abdominal viscus injury or hemorrhage.

The safety of traditional amniocentesis has been addressed by several large collaborative studies. In 1976, the U.S. National Institute of Child Health and Human Development (NICHD)[31] published the first major prospective study of genetic amniocentesis, encompassing 1,040 subjects and 992 matched controls. Of all women who underwent amniocentesis, 3.5 percent experienced fetal loss between the time of the procedure and delivery compared with 3.2 percent of controls; the small difference was not statistically significant and disappeared completely when corrected for maternal age. In Canada, a collaborative study did not include a concurrent control group,[32] assessing 1,223 amniocenteses performed during 1,020 pregnancies in 900 women. The pregnancy loss rate was 3.2 percent, similar to that reported in the U.S. collaborative study.

None of the collaborative studies cited above was conducted with high-quality ultrasonography as defined by today's standards, nor was concurrent ultrasonography ever universally applied. A 1986 Danish study was a true randomized, controlled study of 4,606 women aged 25 to 34 years who were without known risk factors for fetal genetic abnormalities;[33] a control group underwent no procedure. Women with three or more previous spontaneous abortions, diabetes mellitus, multiple gestation, or uterine anomalies or who used intra-

uterine contraceptive devices were excluded. Maternal age, social group, smoking history, number of previous induced and spontaneous abortions, stillbirths, livebirths, and low-birth-weight infants were comparable in the study and control groups, as was gestational age at time of entry into the study. Amniocentesis was performed under real-time ultrasound guidance with a 20-gauge needle by experienced operators. The spontaneous abortion rate after 16 weeks was 1.7 percent in the amniocentesis study group compared with 0.7 percent in controls ($p < 0.01$); a 2.6-fold relative risk of spontaneous abortion was observed if the placenta was traversed. The frequency of fetal postural deformations did not differ between the two groups. However, respiratory distress syndrome was diagnosed more often (relative risk [RR] = 2.1) in the amniocentesis group, and more of these infants were treated for pneumonia (RR = 2.5).

Studies conducted within the past decade have universally shown no statistical difference between outcomes following amniocentesis groups and controls. In British Columbia, children delivered of women who had second-trimester amniocentesis and were identified by a population-based database of congenital anomalies showed disabilities at the same rate as matched controls (i.e., offspring of women who had not undergone amniocentesis).[34] In Thailand, a randomized study found no statistically significant difference between women undergoing and not undergoing amniocentesis between 15 and 24 weeks; in 2,045 matched pairs the fetal loss rates were 3.18 percent and 2.79 percent, respectively.[35]

Unfortunately, a sample must be very large (perhaps 5,000 or 10,000 in each arm) in order to distinguish between the loss rate of 0.5 percent and the perhaps 0.2 percent loss rate that many have the clinical impression more closely approximates reality. In the absence of data substantiating the lower risk figure, it may be hazardous to state the lower risk without caveats.

In conclusion, it still seems wise to continue to counsel that the risk of pregnancy loss secondary to amniocentesis is low but in some hands is potentially up to 0.5 percent. At the author's medical center, serious maternal complications and fetal injuries are stated to be "remote" risks. Concurrent ultrasound is now essential.

Early Amniocentesis

Technique

Early amniocentesis is performed with basically the same technique as that used for traditional amniocentesis. A smaller amount of amniotic fluid is removed, usually 1 ml for each completed gestational week. Careful ultrasound needle guidance is essential, given the relatively small target area and the need to avoid the bladder and bowel. One problem is membrane "tenting," probably the most common reason for failing to obtain amniotic fluid in early amniocentesis. Membrane testing becomes increasingly problematic the earlier in gestation one attempts amniocentesis, reflecting incomplete fusion of the chorion and amnion.

Safety of Early Amniocentesis

The safety and efficacy of the procedure is still unknown. Early experiences suggested early amniocenteses could be a promising technique. In 1992, Hanson et al.[36] performed 936 amniocenteses at 12.8 weeks' gestation, reporting a loss rate of 0.7 percent (7 of 936) within 2 weeks of amniocentesis, an additional 2.2 percent before 28 weeks, and a final 0.5 percent stillbirths or neonatal deaths. Total losses (32 of 936 or 3.4 percent) were considered comparable to the 2.1 percent to 3.2 percent observed in ultrasonographically normal pregnancies not undergoing a procedure; however, maternal age and precise gestational age were not taken into account. Henry and Miller[37] also reported favorable early results in amniocentesis at 12, 13, and 14 weeks' gestation. Pregnancy losses prior to 28 weeks were 5 of 193 (2.6 percent), 5 of 426 (1.2 percent), and 18 of 1172 (1.5 percent), respectively.

More recently, it has become evident that amniocentesis prior to 13 weeks cannot be recommended. Although preliminary work had been encouraging,[38,39] the definitive study from the same investigators with the Canadian Early and Mid-Trimester Amniocentesis Trial (CEMAT) cohort proved different.[40] The salient comparison involved 1,916 women having an amniocentesis before 13 gestational weeks versus 1,775 having amniocentesis after 15 gestational weeks. Total fetal loss rates were 7.5 percent versus 5.9 percent ($p = 0.012$). Even more troubling, talipes equinovarus occurred in 1.3 percent in the early amniocentesis group, compared to the expected population incidence of 0.1 percent in the traditional amniocentesis group. Technical factors associated with these adverse results were difficult-to-perform procedures (e.g., multiple needle insertions) and post procedure amniotic fluid leakage.[41] The ACOG and others recommend that amniocentesis not be performed prior to 12 gestational weeks.[42]

Chorionic Villus Sampling

CVS allows prenatal diagnosis in the first trimester to permit pregnancy termination early in gestation and also protect patient privacy. Both chorionic villi analysis and amniotic fluid cell analysis offer the same information concerning chromosomal status, enzyme levels, and DNA patterns. The one major difference is that assays requiring amniotic fluid, specifically AFP, necessitate amniocentesis.

Technique

CVS can be performed by transcervical, transabdominal, or transvaginal approaches. *Transcervical* CVS is usually performed with a flexible polyethylene catheter that encircles a metal obturator extending just distal to the catheter tip. The outer diameter is usually about 1.5 mm. Introduced transcervically under simultaneous ultrasonographic visualization (Fig. 8–6), the catheter/obturator is directed toward the trophoblastic tissue surrounding the gestational sac. After withdrawal of the obturator, 10 to 25 mg of villi are aspirated by negative pressure into a 20- or 30-ml syringe containing tissue culture media. The optimal time for transcervical sampling is 10 to 12 completed gestational weeks.

In *transabdominal* chorionic villus sampling (Fig. 8–7), concurrent ultrasound is used to direct an 18- or 20-gauge spinal needle into the long axis of the placenta. After removal of the stylet, villi are aspirated into a 20-ml syringe containing tissue culture media. Unlike transcervical CVS, transabdominal CVS can be performed throughout pregnancy, therefore serving as an alternative to cordocentesis (percutaneous umbilical blood sampling [PUBS]) later in pregnancy. If oligohydramnios is present, transabdominal CVS is preferable to PUBS. The former is widely utilized in Europe in lieu of amnioinfusion techniques prior to PUBS.

A final technique is *transvaginal* CVS, using a spinal needle as in transabdominal CVS. This technique may

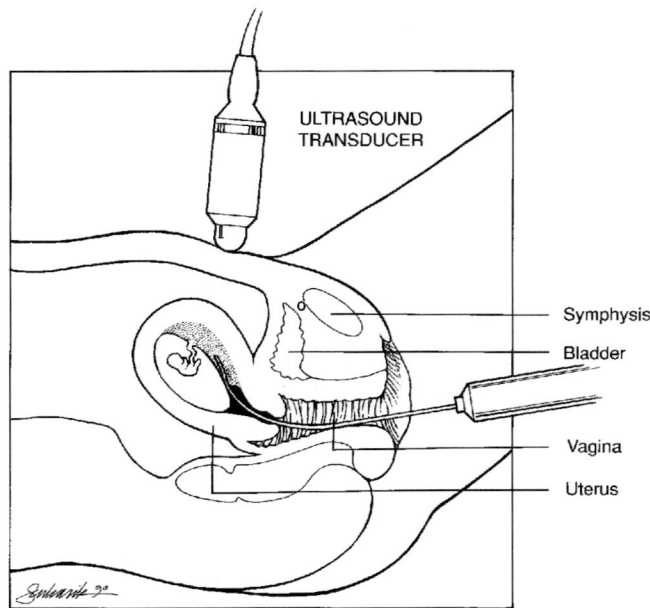

Figure 8–6. Transcervical chorionic villus sampling.

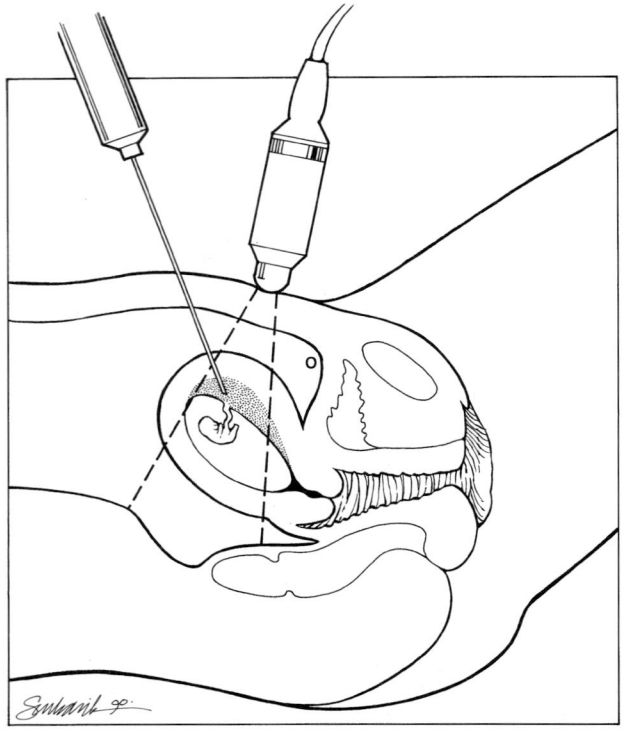

Figure 8–7. Transabdominal chorionic villus sampling.

be useful for a retroflexed uterus having a posterior placenta.

In the author's opinion, facility to perform both transcervical and transabdominal CVS is very helpful. In about one half to three fourths of cases either approach is possible, but in the remaining cases either transabdominal or transcervical CVS is greatly preferable to the other approach. For example, cervical myomas or angulated uteri may preclude transcervical passage of the catheter, whereas transabdominal CVS would permit sampling. The transabdominal approach is obviously preferable in the presence of genital herpes, cervicitis, or bicornuate uteri. A larger sample can more predictably be obtained with transcervical CVS. With either approach sampling women sensitized to Rh(D) should probably be deferred until later in gestation. Sensitization following CVS is probably no greater than that following amniocentesis.

Pregnancy Losses

The U.S. Cooperative Clinical Comparison of Chorionic Villus Sampling and Amniocentesis study[43] and the Canadian Collaborative CVS-Amniocentesis Trial Group study[44] have reported that pregnancy loss rates after CVS are no different from loss rates after amniocentesis. In the U.S. study,[43] 2,278 women self-selected transcervical CVS; 671 women similarly recruited in the first trimester selected amniocentesis. Randomization did not prove possible. The excess loss rate in the CVS group was 0.8 percent, not statistically significant. In a Canadian randomized study,[44] 1,391 subjects were assigned to transcervical CVS and 1,396 to amniocentesis. The excess loss rate in the former was also 0.8 percent and again not statistically different. Variables shown to influence fetal loss rates adversely in CVS include fundal location of the placenta, number of catheter passages, small sample size, and prior bleeding during the current pregnancy. Almost all except the last are surrogates for technical difficulty. The frequency of intrauterine growth retardation, placental abruption, and premature delivery are no higher in women undergoing CVS than expected in the general population.[45]

Transcervical CVS and transabdominal CVS appear to be equally safe procedures.[46] In another U.S. NICHD collaborative study, 1,194 patients were randomized to transcervical CVS and 1,929 patients to transabdominal CVS. The loss rates of cytogenetically normal pregnancies through 28 weeks were 2.5 percent and 2.3 percent, respectively.[47] Of considerable interest, the overall loss rate (i.e., background plus procedure-related) following CVS decreased by about 0.8 percent compared with rates observed during the earlier (1985 to 1987) transcervical versus amniocentesis self-selection study. This decrease in procedure-related loss rate probably reflects increasing operator experience as well as availability of both transcervical and transabdominal approaches. In a small randomized trial conducted in Italy, Brambati et al.[48] also found no difference between transabdominal and transcervical CVS.

The one major investigation substantively differing from all others is the United Kingdom Medical Research Council Study.[49] In this multicenter randomized study, comparison was made between second-trimester amniocentesis and first-trimester CVS performed in any fashion deemed suitable by the obstetrician. The outcome variable assessed was completed pregnancies. The 4.4 percent fewer completed pregnancies in the CVS cohort reflected both unintended and intended pregnancy terminations. The experience with CVS of the Medical Research Council Study operators was moreover considerably less than in the U.S. studies. For example, the only requirement for participation in the Medical Research Council study was 30 "practice" CVS procedures.

Finally, less formal data exist on the safety of CVS in multiple gestation, but in experienced hands this is quite feasible. In a major U.S. study involving four medical centers, the total loss rate of chromosomally normal fetuses (spontaneous abortions, stillborns, neonatal deaths) was 5.0 percent,[50] only slightly higher than the 4.0 percent absolute rate observed for singleton pregnancies.[43] If the placental mass appears fused, amniocentesis is probably a preferred choice. However,

CVS is appropriate in twin gestations when distinct placentas can be visualized by ultrasonography.

CVS is widely used prior to selective reduction in multiple gestation. It is desirable to test the inferior fetus (destined to remain to minimize risk of ascending infection) and at least two or three other fetuses to maximize normalcy in the requisite number.

Limb Reduction Defects

Controversy about the safety of CVS has more recently shifted focus from concerns about the risk of fetal loss to its being the possible cause for congenital abnormalities. In 1991, Firth and colleagues[51] reported that 5 of 289 (1.7 percent or 17 of 1,000) infants exposed to CVS between 56 and 66 days of gestation (i.e., 42 to 50 days after fertilization) had severe limb reduction deformities (LRDs). Four of the five infants had oromandibular–limb hypogenesis; the fifth had a terminal transverse limb reduction alone. There quickly followed a number of reports both supporting and refuting such an association.[52–55] In the United States, Burton et al.[56] reported a second cluster among 394 infants whose mothers had undergone CVS. Thirteen infants (3.3 percent) had major congenital abnormalities, including four with transverse LRD (10 of 1,000 or 1 percent). All four LRDs were transverse distal defects involving hypoplasia or absence of the fingers and toes. Three of these cases followed transcervical sampling, using a device that in the hands of the reporting physicians was associated with an 11 percent fetal loss rate.

Teratogenic mechanisms by which CVS might cause LRDs can be readily hypothesized. These include (1) decreased blood flow caused by fetomaternal hemorrhage or pressor substances released by disturbance of villi or the chorion; (2) embolization of chorionic villus material or maternal clots into the fetal circulation; and (3) amniotic puncture and limb entrapment in exocoelomic gel.

Given this concern, the potential association of LRD with CVS has been explored through various registries. In the Italian Multicenter Birth Defects Registry,[57] eight cases of oromandibular–limb hypogenesis complex were entered into the registry from January 1988 through December 1991. Of 166 cases of transverse limb defects alone, 4 were exposed to CVS compared with 36 cases among 8,445 controls. A 1994 update of this study, based on 11 CVS-exposed cases, continued to reveal an association with transverse limb defects.[58] The greatest risk was associated with procedures performed at less than 70 days' gestation (odds ratio [OR], 23.2; 95 percent confidence interval [CI], 1.31 to 41.0); a lower but still increased risk with procedures at 70 to 76 days (OR 17.1; 95 percent CI, 6.7 to 44.0); over 84 days there were no exposed cases, and the risk was interpreted as considerably lower. In contrast, analysis of other European registries in aggregate involving over 600,000 births showed that only 4 of 336 cases (1.2 percent) with limb reduction abnormalities had been exposed to CVS compared with 78 of 11,883 (0.66 percent) cases with other malformations (OR, 1.8; 95 percent CI, 0.7 to 5.0).[59] A publication from Taiwan reported a number of LRD cases associated with CVS, usually performed at less than 9 weeks.[60]

In an effort to quantify the risk for LDR associated with CVS, Olney et al.[61] conducted a case-control study in the United States. Case subjects consisted of 131 infants with nonsyndromic limb deficiency, identified in seven population-based birth defects surveillance programs. Controls consisted of 131 infants with other birth defects, matched to case subjects by the infant's year of birth, mother's age, race, and state of residence. The odds ratio for limb deficiency after CVS from 8 to 12 weeks' gestation was 1.7. This was not significantly increased because the 95 percent confidence limit crosses 1 (95 percent CI, 0.4 to 6.3); however, subsequent analysis by anatomic subtypes revealed a significant association for transverse digital deficiency (OR, 6.4; 95 percent CI, 1.1 to 38.6), an observation that was widely promulgated. There are three problems with this conclusion: (1) only seven exposed cases existed; (2) in several cases procedures were performed earlier than the 10 weeks that is the accepted lower limit for gestational age; and (3) if overall there is no association between CVS and *all* LRD, but there is between CVS and *transverse* LRD, the converse and illogical deduction is that CVS would be protective for longitudinal limb reduction defects. Irrespective, it was concluded that the absolute risk for such defects was approximately 1 in 3,000, a figure that can be considered the upper limit of risk. The World Health Organization (WHO) Committee on Chorionic Villus Sampling has for years analyzed data collected through an international voluntary registry.[62–65] In the 1998 report,[65] 77 LRD cases were detected among 138,996 infants born after CVS, reported from 63 registering centers. Types of limb reduction defects were compared to those in a population from British Columbia.[66] Defects following CVS involved the upper limb in 65 percent, lower limb in 13 percent, and both 23 percent; in the general population, frequencies were 68, 23, and 9 percent, respectively. Transverse limb defects occurred in 41 percent of infants in the cohort exposed to CVS, compared to 43 percent in the general population. Longitudinal limb deficiencies were found in 59 percent of cases, compared to 57 percent in the general population. Thus, pattern analysis of the types of limb defects and calculation of overall incidences failed to reveal a difference between the CVS and background populations. The 1999 WHO[64] report continued to confirm these results.

In 1995, the Committee on Genetics of the American College of Obstetricians and Gynecologists[67] reached these conclusions.

1. Transcervical CVS and transabdominal CVS performed at 10 to 12 weeks of gestation are relatively safe and accurate procedures that may be considered acceptable alternatives to second-trimester genetic amniocentesis.
2. CVS should not be performed before 10 weeks' gestation.
3. Chorionic villus sampling requires appropriate counseling before the procedure, an experienced operator, and a laboratory experienced in processing the specimen and interpreting the results. Counseling should contrast the risks and benefits of amniocentesis and CVS.
4. Although further studies were stated as needed to determine whether there is truly an increased risk of transverse digital deficiency following CVS performed at 10 to 12 weeks of gestation, it was considered prudent to counsel patients that such a complication is possible; the estimated risk may be on the order of 1 in 3,000 births.

At Baylor we still follow these 1995 ACOG guidelines, even while doubting that limb reduction defects are actually increased when CVS is performed by experienced hands at 10 gestational weeks and above. We counsel that fetal loss rates are the same as CVS and traditional amniocentesis, and state explicitly that the rate of limb reduction defects *could* be as high as 1 in 3,000 (3 per 10,000) over the background of 6 per 10,000.

Fetal Blood Sampling

Access to the fetal blood circulation was initially accomplished by fetoscopy, a method of directly visualizing the fetus, umbilical cord, and chorionic surface of the placenta using endoscopic instruments. Fetoscopy for this purpose has now been replaced by ultrasound-directed PUBS, also termed cordocentesis or funipuncture.

Fetal blood chromosome analysis is used most commonly in genetics to help clarify chromosome mosaicism detected in cultured amniotic fluid cells or chorionic villi. Fetal blood sampling is used in the prenatal evaluation of many fetal hematologic abnormalities. Fetal blood hematocrit level can be measured directly to assess hemolysis resulting from Rh or other blood antigen isoimmunization states. Fetal blood has been used for the diagnosis of blood factor abnormalities (gene products) like hemophilia A, hemophilia B, or von Willebrand's disease. Recovery of fetal blood permits assessment of viral, bacterial, or parasitic infections of the fetus. Serum studies of fetal blood permit quantification of antibody titers, and serum can be used to initiate viral, bacterial, or parasitic culture.

Cordocentesis (PUBS) is usually performed from perhaps 18 weeks onward, although successful procedures have been reported as early as 12 weeks.[68,69] Preliminary ultrasonographic examination of the fetus is performed to assess fetal viability, placental and umbilical cord location, fetal position, and presence or absence of fetal or placental anomalies. Maternal sedation is not usually required, but oral benzodiazepine given before the procedure may be of benefit to the anxious patient.

There are various potential sampling sites, but given its fixed position the placental cord root is the optimal site. Free loops of cord or the intrahepatic vein are alternatives.[70] The spinal needle is percutaneously inserted into the fetal blood vessel under direct ultrasound guidance, and a small amount of blood is aspirated.

Maternal complications are rare, but include amnionitis and transplacental hemorrhage.[71,72] Fetal risks are more substantive. Data from several large perinatal centers estimate the risk of in utero death or spontaneous abortion to be 3 percent or less following PUBS.[73-77] Other collaborative data from 14 North American centers sampling 1,600 patients at varying gestational ages for a variety of indications revealed an uncorrected fetal loss rate of 1.6 percent.[79] In selected fetal diagnosis and treatment units in the United States and Japan, the procedure-related fetal loss rate in 1,260 cases was 0.9 percent; excluding diagnoses other than chromosomal abnormalities and severe growth restriction, the procedure-related fetal loss rate was only 0.2 percent. Overall, loss rates for patients undergoing PUBS varies greatly by procedure indication, far more so than in amniocentesis or CVS. However, definitive statements will not be possible until studies directly comparing loss rates in control and treated groups are conducted, unlike CVS and amniocentesis.

INDICATIONS FOR PRENATAL GENETIC STUDIES

Cytogenetic Disorders

Every chromosomal disorder is potentially detectable in utero. It is not appropriate, however, to perform amniocentesis or CVS in every pregnancy because for many couples the risk of an invasive procedure outweighs diagnostic benefits. In addition to couples tested as a result of positive findings in population screening programs (see above), certain indications are considered standard.

Advanced Maternal Age

The most common indication for antenatal cytogenetic studies is advanced maternal age. The incidence of trisomy 21 is 1 per 800 liveborn births in the United States, but the frequency increases with age (see Table 8–2). Trisomy 13, trisomy 18, 47,XXX, and 47,XXY also increase with advanced age.

For approximately 20 years it has been standard medical practice in the United States to offer invasive chromosomal diagnosis to all women who at their expected delivery date will be 35 years or older. The choice of age 35 is largely arbitrary, however, having been chosen during an interval when risk figures were available only in 5-year intervals (i.e., 30 to 34 years, 35 to 39 years, 40 to 44 years). Flexibility is thus appropriate when answering inquiries from women younger than 35 years for, indeed, increasing numbers of women aged 33 or 34 years seek prenatal diagnosis.

The risk figures shown in Table 8–2 are applicable only for liveborns. The prevalence of abnormalities at the time when CVS or amniocentesis is performed is somewhat higher.[79,80] For example, the risk for a 35-year-old woman is 1 in 270 for Down syndrome at the time of amniocentesis (second trimester). (Most maternal serum screenings for Down syndrome detection report risks at the time of screening, i.e., second trimester.) That the frequency of chromosomal abnormalities is lower in liveborn infants than in first- or second-trimester fetuses is because to the disproportionate likelihood that fetuses lost spontaneously have chromosomal abnormalities. That is, some abnormal fetuses would have died in utero had iatrogenic intervention not occurred in the second trimester. In fact, 5 percent of stillborn infants show chromosomal abnormalities. (see Chapter 22)

Recall that maternal serum screening is recommended by the ACOG and other groups for women under age 35 years, the goal being identifying couples at sufficient risk for fetal trisomy to justify an invasive procedure. The logical corollary might be that a normal or slightly elevated MSAFP level decreases the risk of aneuploidy for older women to the extent that amniocentesis could be avoided. Most U.S. authorities do not agree because of the potential litigious hazard and because detection rates are not 100 percent but 90 percent. Still, noninvasive screening may be desired by some women, particularly if difficulty has occurred in becoming pregnant. This is most likely to be applicable for women ages 35 to 37; almost all women older than that will prove "screen positive" by maternal serum screening and still eventually require amniocentesis anyway.

Previous Child with Chromosomal Abnormality

After the occurrence of one child or abortus with autosomal trisomy, the likelihood that subsequent progeny will also have autosomal trisomy is increased, even if parental chromosomal complements are normal. Recurrence risks are perhaps 1 percent.[81] The risk is not so high as once believed, but antenatal chromosomal studies should be offered for couples having a prior trisomic pregnancy.

Recurrence risk data following the birth of a liveborn infant trisomic for a chromosome other than 21 are limited. Counseling that the risk is 1 percent for either the same or for a different chromosomal abnormality seems appropriate. Thus, antenatal studies will usually be necessary.

Parental Chromosomal Rearrangements

An uncommon but important indication for prenatal cytogenetic studies is the presence of a parental chromosomal abnormality. A balanced translocation is the usual indication, but inversions and other chromosomal abnormalities exist. As discussed above (Clinical Spectrum of Chromosomal Abnormalities), empirical data invariably reveal that theoretical risks for abnormal (unbalanced) offspring are greater than empirical risks. Empirical risks approximate 12 percent for offspring of either male or female heterozygotes having reciprocal translocations.[82] For robertsonian (centric fusion) translocations, risks vary according to the chromosomes involved. For t(14q;21q), risks are 10 percent for offspring of heterozygous mothers and 2 percent for offspring of heterozygous fathers (Fig. 8–8).[82] For other nonhomologous robertsonian translocations, empirical risks for liveborns are less than 1 percent. For homologous translocations (e.g., 21q;21q), all liveborn offspring should have trisomy 21. For other homologous robertsonian translocations (13q;13q or 22q;22q), almost all pregnancies result in abortions.

Diagnostic Dilemmas in Prenatal Cytogenetic Diagnosis (Amniotic Fluid Cells or Chorionic Villi)

The obstetrician-gynecologist should be aware of the common pitfalls associated with the analysis of chorionic villi or amniotic fluid cells. An obvious problem is that cells may not grow, or growth may be insufficient for proper analysis. Analysis of maternal rather than fetal cells is another theoretical problem, which fortunately has proved uncommon in experienced hands. In amniocentesis, maternal cell contamination can be minimized by discarding the first few drops of aspirated amniotic fluid. In CVS, examination under a dissecting microscope allows one to distinguish villi from decidua.

A more vexing concern is the possibility that chromosomal abnormalities detected in villi or amniotic fluid may fail to reflect fetal status. One reason is that chromosomal aberrations may arise in culture (in vitro). This possibility should be suspected whenever an abnormality is restricted to only one of the several culture flasks or clones from a single amniotic fluid or

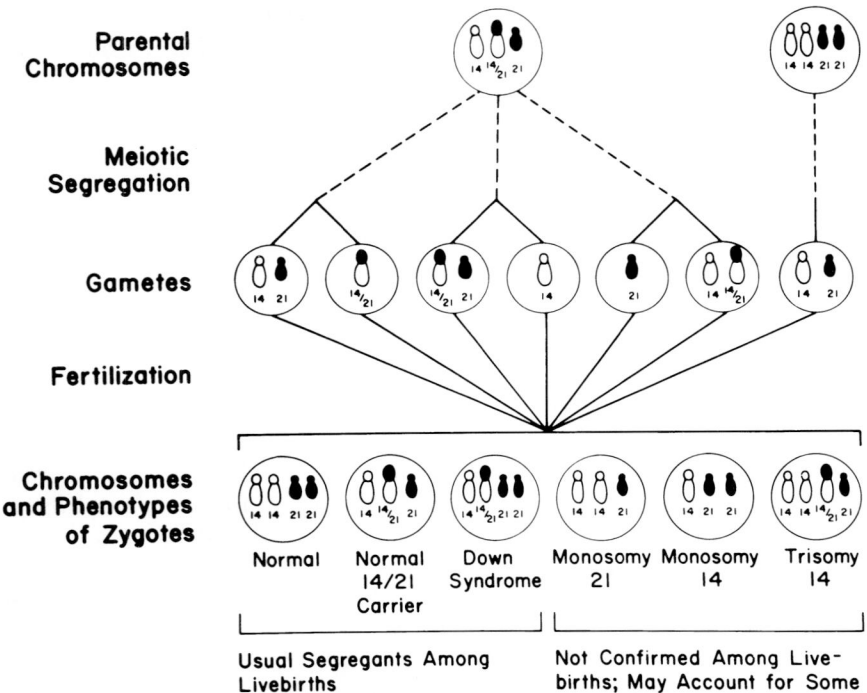

Figure 8–8. Diagram of possible gametes and progeny of a phenotypically normal individual heterozygous for a robertsonian translocation between chromosomes 14 and 21 (a form of D/G translocation). Three of the six possible gametes are incompatible with life. The likelihood that an individual with such a translocation would have a child with Down syndrome is theoretically 33 percent. However, the empirical risk is considerably less. (From Gerbie AT, Simpson JL: Antenatal diagnosis of genetic disorders. Postgrad Med 59:129, 1976, with permission.)

CVS specimen. In fact, cells containing at least one additional structurally normal chromosome are detected in 1 to 2 percent of amniotic fluid or chorionic villus specimens.[83] If these abnormal cells are restricted to a single culture or clone, the phenomenon is termed *pseudomosaicism;* no clinical significance is attached. Defined by the presence of the same abnormality in more than one clone or culture flask, true fetal mosaicism is rarer in amniotic fluid and villi but clinically significant. True mosaicism can be confirmed by studies of the abortus or liveborn in at least 70 to 80 percent of cases[84] and cannot be truly excluded in the remainder because the abnormality could exist in a tissue not readily analyzable.

Chorionic villi divide more rapidly than amniotic fluid cells. Metaphases from trophoblasts derived from villi can be accumulated within hours of sampling. Analysis of these cells can provide rapid answers. However, discrepancies may arise between short-term trophoblast cultures and long-term cultures initiated from the mesenchymal core of the villi.[85] Discrepancies may further exist between CVS preparations of either type (short-term or long-term) and the embryo. Fortunately, it is possible to recognize and manage these discrepancies, usually by confirmatory amniocentesis and assessment of the expected interval growth. In most discrepancies, the fetus proves normal at amniocentesis, having shown normal interim growth between 10 and 16 weeks.

The U.S. NICHD Collaborative Study involved 11,473 chorionic villus samples evaluated by direct methods, long-term culture, or both. There were no incorrect sex predictions.[85] No diagnostic errors occurred in 148 common autosomal trisomies (+13, +18, +21), 16 sex chromosomal aneuploidies, and 13 structural aberrations; a normal cytogenetic diagnosis with CVS was never followed by birth of a trisomic infant. Not confirmed were several rare trisomies (+16, +22, +7), findings consistent with those in other investigations.[86] Overall, the accuracy of CVS is comparable to that of amniocentesis, but additional tests may be necessary before definitive establishment of nonmosaic rare trisomies and, as in amniotic fluid analysis, polyploidies. Of interest is that the U.S. NICHD study observed increased late loss rates (8.6 percent) in pregnancies showing confirmed placental mosaicism compared with 3.4 percent in pregnancies without mosaicism.[87] However, no increased frequency of pregnancy complications was observed.

The clinical significance of the above is that the obstetrician must realize that the neonatal phenotype cannot always be predicted on the basis of the amniotic fluid cells or chorionic villi complement.

Structural Chromosomal Abnormalities

If a phenotypically normal parent carries the same balanced translocation as the fetus, reassurance is usually appropriate. On the other hand, if an ostensibly balanced inversion or translocation is detected in the fetus but in neither parent (de novo rearrangement), the likelihood is increased that the neonate will be phenotypically abnormal at birth. Presumably, the inversion or translocation is not actually balanced, appearances to the contrary. The risk for the fetus being abnormal has been calculated at 6 percent for de novo reciprocal inversion and 10 to 15 percent for de novo translocation.[89] These risks are not chromosome specific but represent pooled date involving many chromosomes. These risks apply only to structurally anatomic abnormalities evident at birth and do not take into account developmental delay (mental retardation) that would be evident only later in life.

Marker chromosomes, also called supernumerary chromosomes, are those that by definition cannot be fully characterized on the basis of standard cytogenetic analyses. These small chromosomes usually contain a centromere, and a high proportion derive from the short arms of the acrocentric chromosomes (13, 14, 15, 21, and 22). Marker chromosomes are observed in approximately 0.06 percent of the population.[90]

More specific information can be anticipated in the future because, with the advent of fluorescence in situ hybridization (FISH), the chromosomal origin of marker chromosomes can often be established. Analogous to translocations and inversions, the risk for phenotypic abnormality in a fetus with a marker chromosome depends on whether the marker is de novo or familial. Risk is higher when de novo markers are encountered. Studying 15 cases of marker chromosomes ascertained from 12,699 prenatal samples (11,055 amniotic fluids, 1,644 chorionic villus samples), Brondum-Nielsen and Mikkelson[91] used FISH techniques to characterize marker chromosomes. Five cases were familial, all were derived from acrocentric chromosomes (13, 14, 15, 21, and 22), and all resulted in phenotypically normal offspring. The other nine cases represented de novo abnormalities. In two cases, pregnancies resulted in phenotypically normal infants at birth; however, in one of the two, minimal psychomotor retardation at age 2 years was evident. The seven other pregnancies having de novo markers were terminated; three showed significant abnormalities at autopsy.

In reviewing 15,522 prenatal diagnostic procedures, Hume et al.[92] ascertained 19 marker chromosomes, 5 from CVS specimens and 14 from amniotic fluid samples. Monitoring these pregnancies with high-resolution ultrasonography revealed an association between a de novo marker chromosome and anomalies. When ultrasound examination was normal, the likelihood of a phenotypically normal offspring was high.

Fluorescence In Situ Hybridization (FISH) in Prenatal Diagnosis

FISH merges molecular genetics with cytogenetics. Using DNA sequences unique to the chromosome in question, chromosome-specific probes (e.g., chromosomes 13, 18, 21, the X, or the Y) can be created (see Fig. 8–3). The probe is then labeled with a fluorochrome and used to challenge unknown DNA. Disomic cells (metaphase or interphase) should show two separate signals; trisomic cells should show three signals. Because of geometric vicissitudes, not every trisomic cell will show three signals; however, the modal count readily indicates probes permitting simultaneous assessment of multiple chromosomes. The appeal of FISH is that its use in interphase cells permits rapid (same day) diagnosis of aneuploidy. This is particularly important when a rapid diagnosis is needed to aid in the management of a high-risk fetus (e.g., with ultrasound findings of multiple anomalies).

Mendelian Disorders

Increasing numbers of mendelian disorders are now detectable in utero. Initially, only metabolic disorders were detectable on the basis of enzyme analysis. Antenatal diagnoses of hemoglobinopathies and hemophilia were later accomplished with fetal blood, originally obtainable only by fetoscopic sampling. DNA analysis now permits many diagnoses using any available nucleated cell (chorionic villi, amniotic fluid cells). The nature of the mutant or absent gene product need not necessarily even be known. We can predict confidently that in the foreseeable future all common mendelian disorders will be detectable. The rapid progress and increasing complexity required to diagnose mendelian traits dictate close liaison between the obstetrician-gynecologist and geneticist. Tabulated lists of detectable disorders should be considered suspect for timeliness.

Inborn Errors of Metabolism

Antenatal diagnosis is possible for approximately 100 inborn errors of metabolism. Most are transmitted in autosomal recessive fashion, although a few display X-linked recessive or autosomal dominant inheritance. Couples at increased risk will usually be identified because they previously had an affected child. Most metabolic disorders are so rare that it is unreasonable to expect obstetricians who are not geneticists to be fully cognizant of diagnostic possibilities.

Detection of a metabolic error requires that the enzyme be expressed in amniotic fluid cells or chorionic villi. This requirement is fulfilled by most metabolic disorders, a prominent exception being phenylketonuria (PKU). Fortunately, PKU can be detected by the molecular techniques described below. All metabolic disorders detectable in amniotic fluid have proved detectable as well in chorionic villi. Although cultured cells are usually necessary for diagnosis, occasionally one can arrive at a diagnosis on the basis of a product in amniotic fluid. The most prominent example is a 17α-hydroxyprogesterone, an elevated value of which indicates adrenal 21-hydroxylase deficiency (congenital adrenal hyperplasia). This disorder can also be detected by analysis of linked human leukocyte antigen (HLA) markers in nuclei obtained by CVS or amniocentesis, and treated in utero by administration of dexamethasone to the mother.[93]

Disorders Detectable Solely by Tissue Sampling

If a gene causing a given disorder is not expressed in amniotic fluid or chorionic villi, enzymatic analysis of such tissues will provide no information concerning presence or absence of the disorder. However, the gene might still be expressed in other tissues—blood, skin, muscle, or liver. Initially, skin was obtained through fetoscopically directed biopsy, under direct vision; however, currently ultrasound-directed sampling permits use of smaller (14-gauge) instruments. Procedure-related losses following skin biopsy or other invasive procedures are presumed to be greater than that following CVS or amniocentesis; however, the severity of some disorders justifies tissue sampling if no other diagnostic method is available. Counseling a procedure-related loss of about 2 to 3 percent seems appropriate.[94]

Increasingly, molecular advances have made tissue sampling obsolete. Sampling fetal skin was once the only available method for diagnosing certain dermatologic abnormalities such as epidermolysis bullosa or congenital ichthyosis (harlequin ichthyosis).[94,95] Increasingly, molecular advances have allowed prenatal diagnosis simply by CVS or amniocentesis. Occasionally, histologic and electron microscopic analyses of fetal skin are necessary. Muscle biopsy may also be necessary to detect Duchenne, muscular dystrophy if DNA markers are not informative.

Disorders Detectable by Molecular Methods

The power of molecular prenatal diagnosis is that any available nuclear cell can be utilized for diagnosis. All cells contain the same DNA, and the gene need not be expressed, unlike the situation when a gene product (enzyme protein) must be analyzed. Thus, molecular techniques are now widely applicable. Duchenne, muscular dystrophy, CF, adult-onset polycystic kidney disease, Huntington's chorea, and most other undetectable disorders have become diagnosable.

To appreciate these advances, the obstetrician-gynecologist must be aware of the analytic techniques that made possible diagnosis by molecular methods. Principles and applications are now routinely applied and widely taught in medical school curricula. The reader can now find the topic covered in much greater detail elsewhere, ranging from single chapters in volumes intended for obstetrician-gynecologists with no prior knowledge in the field, to definitive volumes designed for the investigator. Here we shall almost perfunctorily define key principles whose understanding is crucial to the application of prenatal genetic diagnosis.

Pivotal was the discovery of *restriction endonucleases*. These bacterial enzymes recognize specific nucleotide sequences five to seven nucleotides in length and cut DNA only at those sites. Use of restriction enzymes permits DNA to be divided into fragments of reproducible lengths (Fig. 8–9).

Also pivotal to clinical diagnosis was development of the *polymerized chain reaction* (PCR) procedure. In PCR, a target sequence can be amplified severalfold (10^5 to 10^6) (Fig. 8–10). For most purposes, PCR amplification utilizes unique DNA primers that flank and are specific for the DNA region in question; thus, the sequence must be known. The region in question may consist of a portion of a gene containing a mutation, a polymorphic DNA sequence closely linked to a given locus, or a repetitive DNA sequence characteristic of a given chromosomal region. Irrespective, a heat-stable DNA polymerase extracted from *Thermas aquaticus* (*Taq* polymerase) is placed in a single tube with the DNA in question, excess deoxyribonucleoside triphosphates (adenine, thymine, guanine, cytosine), and the unique primers specific for the region being studied. DNA synthesis (amplification) is initiated (cycle 1 in Fig. 8–10). Raising the temperature denaturates the newly amplified double-stranded DNA back into single-stranded DNA. Upon cooling, another amplification cycle can occur (cycle 2 in Fig. 8–10), this time with twice as many strands. The DNA sequence between primers amplifies in geometric fashion with each replication. In 3 to 4 hours, 30 to 40 amplifications are achieved. PCR can be used not only to amplify DNA, but for diagnosis. If a DNA sequence is absent (e.g.,

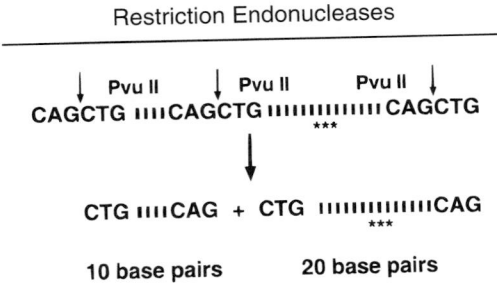

Restriction Endonucleases

Figure 8–9. Simplified diagram illustrating the manner in which a restriction endonuclease cuts DNA at a specific nucleotide sequence. Pvu II recognizes the sequence CAGCTG and only that sequence. DNA is separated into fragments of different lengths on the basis of distances between restriction enzyme recognition sites. The farther the distance between sites, the longer the length of intervening DNA (i.e., 20 vs. 30 base pairs). Shorter DNA fragments (e.g., 20 base pairs) show greater mobility and migrate farther in an agarose cell.

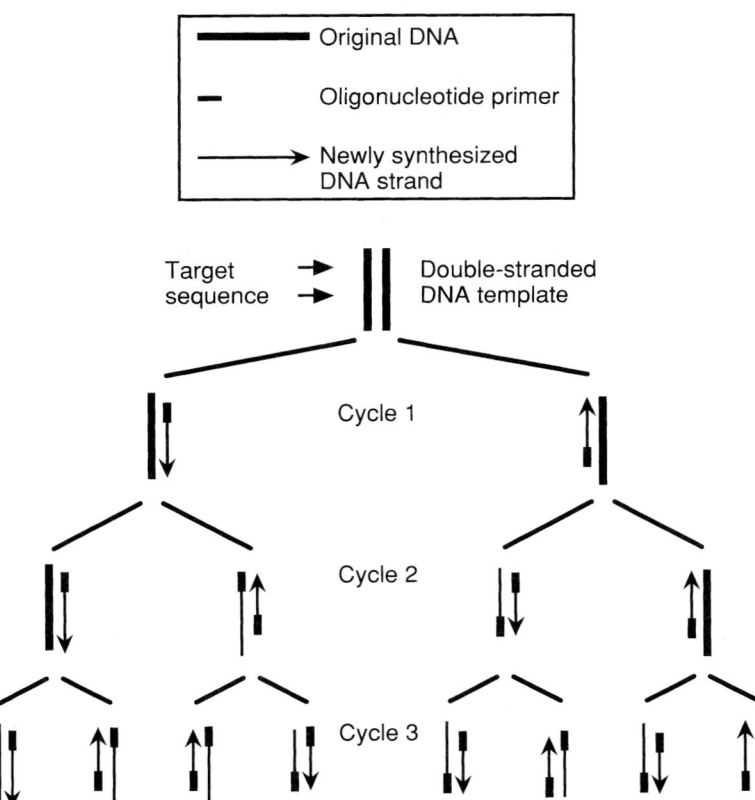

Figure 8–10. Polymerized chain reaction (PCR). Placing the DNA in question, unique primers, and *Taq* polymerase together results in amplification (cycle 1). When the temperature is raised, denaturation into single-stranded DNA occurs. Upon cooling, a second amplification cycle continued. Continued amplification increases the amount of DNA located between primers in logarithmic fashion.

α-thalassemia), no DNA is available with which the primers could anneal; thus, no hybridization (reaction) is observed. One can perform PCR concurrently for multiple sequences (multiplex PCR), an approach that permits assessment of presence or absence of deletions throughout a given region.

A modification of this approach involves use of synthetic oligonucleotides 15 to 18 in length, called *allele-specific oligonucleotides* (ASO). An ASO is designed to hybridize to an unknown sample if and only if the latter is characterized by all 15 to 18 nucleotides. ASOs that recognize normal DNA and any known mutant sequence can be designed and used for "dot-blot" DNA analysis or "slot-blot" analysis.

In addition to results of PCR per se (presence or absence of a sequence), several other diagnostic approaches are commonly applied. In Southern blotting (Fig. 8–11), agarose gel electrophoresis is used to separate DNA fragments by size, after exposure to restriction endonucleases. The DNA is then denatured and transferred from the agarose gel to a nitrocellulose filter, on which specific fragments can be located by hybridization. Labeled strands of known DNA sequences act as probes, hybridizing a specific complementary sequence from among the many DNA fragments on the filter. Fragments that contain the sequence that hybridizes with the probe can be detected as bands. Use of size standards facilitates determining whether a particular-sized fragment is or is not present. This technique is called *Southern blotting*.

Diagnosis When the Molecular Basis Is Known

Other molecular techniques taking advantage of hybridization as end points can also be used for diagnosis. Use of FISH to detect numerical chromosomal abnormalities (aneuploidy) in interphase cells has already been noted, and exactly the same principle can be applied to detect presence of a gene. For example, an SRY probe can detect presence of the testes determining region in newborns with genital ambiguity. Two FISH signals can detect gene duplications, such as exists in Charcot-Marie-Tooth disease.

It is convenient for heuristic purposes to divide mendelian disorders into those in which the molecular basis (i.e., precise nucleotide abnormality) is known and those in which the gene is localized to a given chromosomal region but in which the molecular basis is not known. Known causes of mendelian disorders include absence of the gene or point mutations. If a disorder is known to be characterized by absence of DNA, one can determine whether a probe does or does not hybridize with the relevant sequence of DNA from an individual of unknown genotype. Again, failure of am-

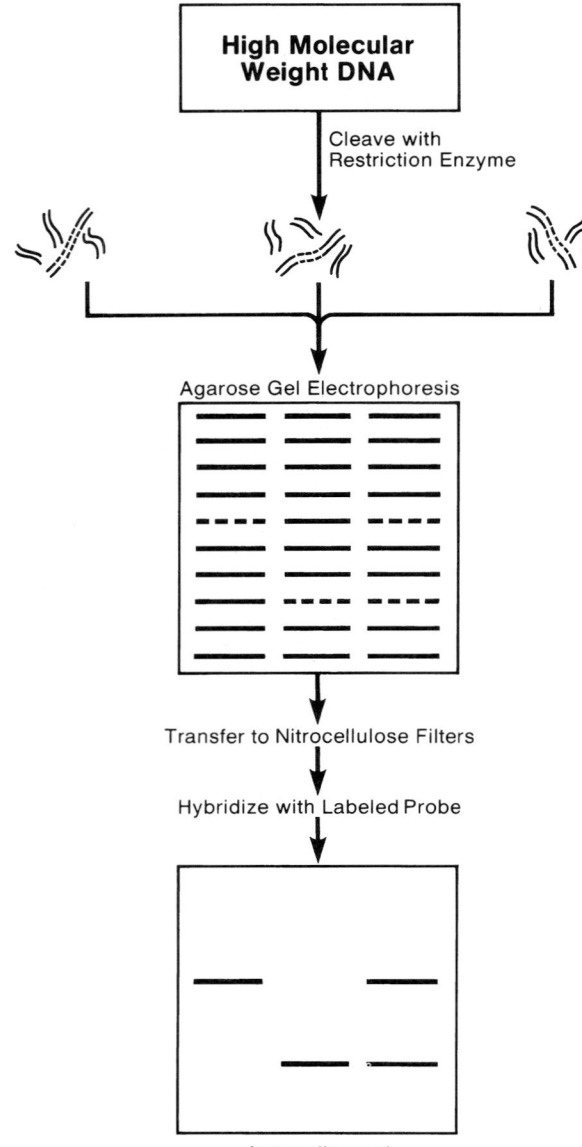

High Molecular Weight DNA

Cleave with Restriction Enzyme

Agarose Gel Electrophoresis

Transfer to Nitrocellulose Filters

Hybridize with Labeled Probe

Autoradiograph

Figure 8–11. Southern blotting cuts DNA at a specific sequence of nucleotides. After DNA is cleaved with restriction enzymes, the cleaved DNA is separated by size using agarose gel electrophoresis. The gel is then laid on a piece of nitrocellulose and buffer allowed to flow through the gel into the nitrocellulose. DNA fragments migrate out of the gel and bind to the filter. A replica of the gel's DNA fragment pattern is thus made on the filter. The filter can then be hybridized to a suitable radioactivity-labeled probe, with DNA fragments hybridizing to the probe identified after autoradiography.

plification (by PCR) or hybridizaton (by ASO) indicates that the individual lacks the DNA sequence in question; thus, the disorder is assumed present. This approach is currently used to diagnose all forms of α-thalassemia, many cases of Duchenne-Becker muscular dystrophy, some cases of β-thalassemia, and some forms of hemophilia.

A second general approach becomes applicable if the

molecular basis involves a point mutation whose nucleotide sequence is known. Sometimes, the mutation to be sought is obvious, and clinical diagnosis by molecular means is very straightforward. A clear example is sickle cell anemia, in which the triplet (codon) designating the sixth amino acid has undergone a mutation from adenine to guanine. As a result, codon 6 connotes valine rather than glutamic acid, leading to the abnormal protein (β^S). Several different molecular approaches can be exploited to make a diagnosis. For example, restriction enzymes recognize the normal but not the mutant DNA sequence at codons 5, 6, and 7. One could also construct ASOs designed to hybridize only if every single nucleotide is present. Use of a β^S oligonucleotide probe will confirm the specific mutant DNA sequence. Diagnosis with limited amounts of DNA can be achieved by the use of PCR amplification. A hybridized ASO usually appears as a "dot blot" (Fig. 8–12) or "slot blot."

As already discussed in the context of genetic screening, sickle cell anemia is very atypical for mendelian disorders in that its molecular basis is homogeneous. Far more commonly, many different molecular mutations are responsible (heterogeneity), as illustrated by cystic fibrosis. We have already considered this concept with respect to cystic fibrosis, but analogous findings exist for almost all mendelian traits. In the near future, sequencing the entire gene or selected exons is likely to become more widely available. This is more complex technically, but to most obstetricians the diagnostic approach will become more simple conceptually. However, at present, geneticists must often consider the diagnostic approach for prenatal diagnosis case by case. The approach discussed below may become applicable even if the location of the mutant gene responsible for a condition desired to be tested is known.

Diagnosis When the Molecular Basis Is Not Known

The molecular approaches described above are applicable only when the precise molecular basis of a disorder is known. Unfortunately, this requirement is fulfilled less often than one would desire. Certain genes are not yet cloned and isolated. Even if the chromosomal location is known, an interval passes before the sequence is determined. A second reason is the considerable heterogeneity noted previously to exist at the molecular level. Mutations at multiple nucleotide sites within the gene can all produce a dysfunctional product. Given that genes are often very large, diagnostic complexities may be daunting. Sequencing the entire gene for every diagnostic situation is not practical, and even then the mutation might not be detected if it were located in a promoter region or involved in translation.

The problem cited above can be addressed by linkage

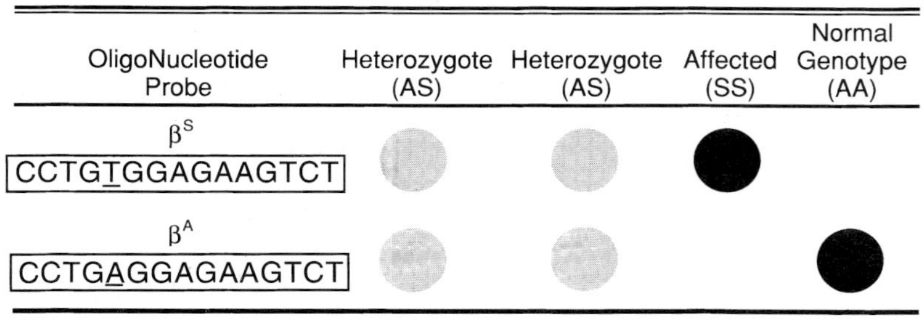

Figure 8–12. Dot blot analysis. Oligonucleotides are constructed for sequences complementary to normal DNA (β^A) and mutant DNA (β^S). DNA challenged by the oligonucleotide probe will be hybridized if and only if the DNA contains all nucleotides connoted by the probe. Thus, AS individuals will respond to both β^A and β^S probes, whereas AA or SS individuals will respond only to one of the two probes (β^A and β^S, respectively). Homozygous individuals respond with a stronger (darker) signal than heterozygous individuals.

OligoNucleotide Probe	Heterozygote (AS)	Heterozygote (AS)	Affected (SS)	Normal Genotype (AA)
β^S CCTG**T**GGAGAAGTCT			●	
β^A CCTG**A**GGAGAAGTCT				●

analysis, taking advantage of the ostensibly innocuous differences in DNA that exist among individuals in the general population. These differences are called *polymorphisms* and are analogous to such well-known polymorphisms as the ABO blood group locus. The initial molecular approach utilized restriction fragment length polymorphisms (RFLPs). The approach was initially possible because of the existence among normal individuals of clinically insignificant differences in DNA fragment lengths following exposure to a given restriction endonuclease, thus the term "restriction fragment length polymorphisms."

More recently, commonly used markers are dinucleotide or trinucleotide polymorphisms. Throughout the genome there exist polymorphisms in which the number of nucleotide repeats (e.g., the dinucleotides cytosine and adenine [CA]) vary among individuals at a given locus. For example, some individuals may show 6 CA repeats, others 8, others 10 at a given locus. The almost innumerable number of such polymorphisms underlies the scientific basis of DNA analysis being used for forensic pathology. In linkage analysis, a diagnosis is made not on the basis of analyzing the mutant gene per se but rather on the basis of the presence or absence of a nearby marker. In RFLPs, the marker is a DNA variant capable of being recognized following exposure to a given endonuclease.

To illustrate, let us assume that a given RFLP or nucleotide repeat is known to lie close to or preferably within the mutant gene of interest. One next needs to deduce the relationship of the mutant to the status of the marker. Starting with an individual of known genotype, usually an affected fetus or child, one determines on which parental chromosome a given DNA marker is located (*cis-trans* relationship). Is the marker located on the chromosome carrying the mutant gene, and is it located on the chromosome carrying the normal gene? Figure 8–13 illustrates a simple example using RFLPs. The principle would be exactly the same using dinucleotide or trinucleotide repeats as the DNA polymorphic marker.

Pitfalls exist in linkage analysis using RFLP or nucleotide repeats. First, the marker may or may not be informative in a given family. If all family members show identical DNA fragment patterns at a given locus,

that locus is obviously useless because affected and unaffected individuals cannot be distinguished from each other. If a given marker is uninformative, one searches for another marker that may prove informative. Fortunately, a potentially limitless number of markers exist. Second, the distance between the mutant gene and the marker is crucial because the likelihood of meiotic recombination is inversely related to this distance. Recall that during meiosis I recombination can occur between homologous chromosomes. Genes are linked to one another if, after meiosis I, they remain together more often than expected by chance. Recombination can occur even between closely linked loci; thus, prenatal diagnosis based on linkage analysis is never 100 percent accurate. Using polymorphic markers on both sides of the mutant can minimize but not exclude the possibility of a recombinational event.

Despite these caveats, linkage analysis permits prenatal diagnosis in many situations not otherwise possible. Linkage analysis is particularly applicable to the increasing numbers of single-gene (mendelian) disorders with considerable molecular heterogeneity. These include Huntington disease; hemophilia A and B; adult-onset polycystic kidney disease; and some forms of neurofibromatosis, Duchenne-Becker muscular dystrophy, and β-thalassemia.

Polygenic/Multifactorial Disorders

Amniotic Fluid α-Fetoprotein

Failure of the neural tube to close during embryogenesis leads to anencephaly, spina bifida (myelomeningocele or meningocele), encephalocele, and other less common midline defects (e.g., lipomeningocele). Anencephaly is almost never compatible with long-term survival. Spina bifida is compatible with long-term survival, although it is frequently associated with hemiparesis, urinary incontinence, and hydrocephalus.

Anencephaly and spina bifida represent different manifestations of the same pathogenic process and reflect the same genetic etiology. Couples who have had a child with an NTD have approximately a 1 percent risk for any subsequent offspring having spina bifida and a 1 percent risk for subsequent offspring having anen-

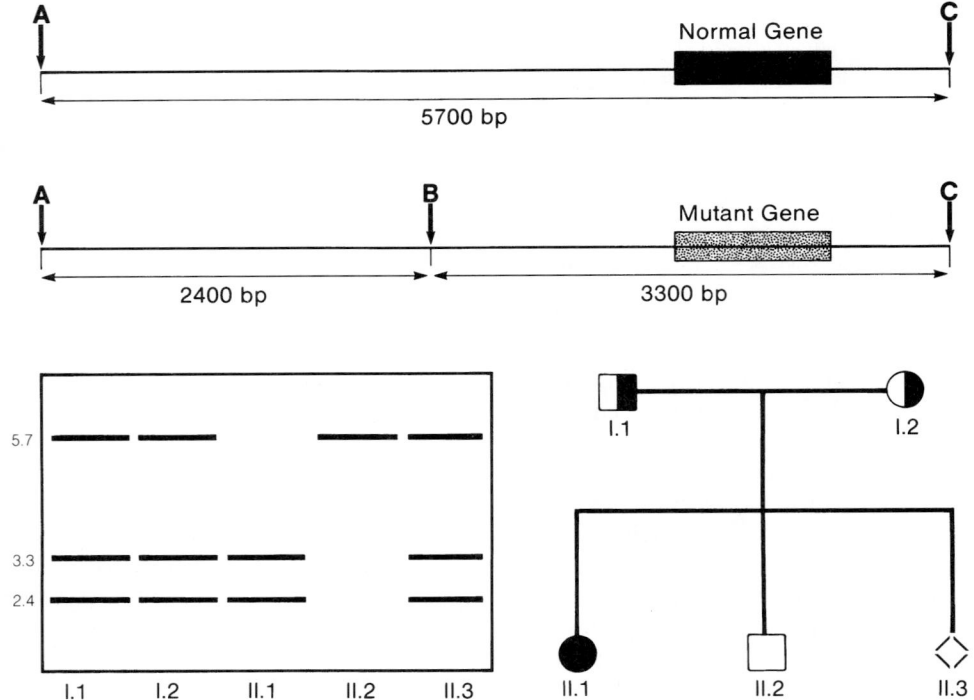

Figure 8–13. Restriction fragment length polymorphisms (RFLPs), which are invaluable for certain prenatal diagnoses. Suppose one mutant gene is linked to another gene (B) that governs whether or not a restriction site (B) is present. If the restriction site is present, DNA is cut by a certain restriction enzyme (*arrow*) to produce 3,300- and 2,400-bp-long fragments. If the segment conferring the restriction site is not present, the total fragment is 5,700 bp long. The different lengths can serve as markers to allow genotypes to be deduced. Suppose two obligate heterozygotes 1.1 and 1.2 have one affected child. Suppose further that a probe for the gene hybridizes to the region *A* to *C*. The probe can thus identify three fragments (2,400, 3,300, and 5,700 bp). If the affected child shows only the 2,400- and 3,300-bp fragments, it can be deduced that the mutant allele is in association (i.e., on the same chromosome) with the gene-conferring restriction site *B* and thus is producing both 2,400- and 3,300-bp fragments. The normal allele must be in association with the allele not conferring restriction *B* and thus is designated by the 5,700-bp fragment. Genotypes can thus be predicted from DNA analysis of chorionic villi and amniotic fluid cells. Fetus 11.3 can be assumed to be heterozygous because all three fragments (2,400, 3,300, and 5,700 bp) are present.

cephaly (2 percent for any NTD).[96] This holds true irrespective of the type of NTD present in the index case (proband). If a prospective parent has an NTD, the risk is also about 2 percent. Second-degree relatives (nieces, nephews, grandchildren) and third-degree relatives (first cousins) are less likely to be affected. A woman whose sister or brother had a child with an NTD carries a lower 0.5 to 1.0 percent risk for NTD offspring.[96] For reasons that are unclear, risks are slightly lower if the father's sibling had an NTD.

Antenatal diagnosis of an NTD is best accomplished by amniotic fluid α-fetoprotein (AF-AFP) assay. Through AF-AFP analysis, diagnosis of an NTD is possible in all anencephaly cases and in all spina bifida cases except the 5 to 10 percent in which skin covers the lesion. Closed lesions are somewhat more common in encephaloceles. Ultrasonography by experienced physicians should readily exclude anencephaly, and spina bifida theoretically can be detected by serial views of the vertebral column, shape of the cranium, ventricles, cerebellum, and cisternal magna. Unfortunately, few ultrasonographers know the sensitivity or specificity for detecting NTDs. Until such data are available, AF-AFP analysis should be considered the standard method for detecting an NTD despite frequent hopes and statements to the contrary.

AF-AFP may be spuriously elevated if the amniotic fluid is contaminated with fetal blood. This pitfall can be eliminated if AChE is assayed concurrently. AChE is present in the amniotic fluid of fetuses with open NTDs but is absent in normal amniotic fluid. If AChE is absent but fetal hemoglobin is present, the elevated AFP is probably because of fetal blood. Some confusion may arise if amniocentesis is performed earlier than 13 weeks.

Elevated AFP is also associated with certain other polygenic/multifactorial anomalies (e.g., omphalocele, gastroschisis, cystic hygroma). In these disorders, AChE may or may not be elevated. With certain mendelian traits (e.g., congenital nephrosis), AFP is elevated but

AChE is not. Ultrasonographic studies should therefore be undertaken to corroborate elevated AF-AFP and to determine the nature of any defect present. On the other hand, failure to detect an anomaly by ultrasound does not necessarily indicate that elevated AF-AFP was spurious. If AF-AFP is elevated and AChE is present, the fetus should be considered abnormal irrespective of ultrasound findings.

Folic acid deficiency is a major cause of NTD. This conclusion has been accepted for a decade, after a prospective, randomized study that found that folic acid supplementation decreased the recurrence rate of NTD, by 71 percent in women who had a previous child with an NTD.[97] The ACOG recommends 0.4 mg folate daily, beginning at least 1 month prior to conception.[97] In women who have had a child with a prior NTD, 4 mg daily is recommended.

Disorders Detectable Only by Ultrasound

Anomalies inherited in polygenic/multifactorial fashion usually carry recurrence risks of 1 to 5 percent for first-degree relatives (siblings, offspring, parent), a risk sufficiently high to justify prenatal diagnosis for many couples. The number of genes responsible for these defects is unknown, but presumably more than one; thus, diagnosis on the basis of enzyme assays or DNA cannot seriously be entertained at present. Except for the few conditions amenable to AF-AFP analysis, the principal method of assessment involves visualization of fetal anatomy by ultrasound.

The typical couple at risk already has had a child with the anomaly in question, thus incurring a 1 to 5 percent risk for another affected child. To alter clinical management, a diagnosis should be made by 20 to 24 weeks' gestation. This is sufficiently early to weigh the alternative options of termination, fetal surgery, or preterm delivery followed by neonatal surgery. PUBS and second-trimester transabdominal CVS can exclude chromosomal abnormalities if either of the latter options are contemplated. A careful search for other defects is also necessary. For some anomalies (e.g., hydrocephaly), an isolated anomaly is rare, but for others (e.g., posterior urethral values), only a single malformation may be present.

Antenatal ultrasonography for anomaly detection should be performed only by highly experienced physicians. Physicians scanning obstetric patients only for fetal viability, multiple gestations, and placental location should explicitly inform their patients that anomaly assessment is not being attempted. Casual reassurance of fetal normalcy should be eschewed. It should further be realized that almost no individual has sufficient experience to calculate his or her own specificities or sensitivities.

FUTURE DIRECTIONS: PREIMPLANTATION DIAGNOSIS

Despite the advantage CVS offers for first-trimester prenatal diagnosis, even earlier diagnosis may be desirable. One reason is that one can envision certain treatment regimens (metabolic, gene insertion). A second reason is that some couples at risk for affected offspring may undergo repeated prenatal diagnosis and termination. Other couples strongly wish to avoid clinical terminations.

These disadvantages can be addressed by preimplantation genetic diagnosis, utilizing access to gametes (oocytes) or embryos before 6 days, the time at which implantation occurs. Potential approaches include (1) polar body biopsy, (2) aspiration of one to two cells from the six- to eight-cell embryo at 2 to 3 days, and (3) trophectoderm biopsy of the 5- to 6-day blastocyst.

Obtaining Cells for Preimplantation Genetic Diagnosis

Preimplantation genetic diagnosis requires access to gametes (oocytes) or embryos by 6 days after conception or less, the time when implantation occurs. There are three potential approaches: (1) polar body biopsy, (2) blastomere biopsy or aspiration of one to two blastomeres from the six to eight-cell embryo (2 to 3 days), and (3) trophectoderm biopsy from the 5- to 6-day blastocyst. The first two are most widely applied.

Blastomere (Six to Eight Cells) Biopsy

Blastomere biopsy involves aspirating one to two of the six to eight cells contained within the zona pellucida. This can be accomplished by mechanical (razor), laser, or chemical (pronase, ethylenediaminetetraacetic acid [EDTA]) means, followed by aspiration with a second pipette. The sentinel work in this area was conducted by Handyside and colleagues over a decade ago.[98,99]

In the initial work of Handyside et al.,[98] a single cell was removed through a hole made in the zona pellucida by a drilling pipette (10 to 20 mm in diameter) containing acid Tyrode's solution. Removal of one or two cells did not affect glucose or pyruvate uptake or delay spontaneous hatching of blastocysts, the traditional indicator of normal embryonic development.[100]

Polar Body Biopsy

A second approach is to remove either the first or second polar biopsy, or both.[101] Literally, this is preconceptional rather than preimplantation diagnosis. If a woman and her mate were heterozygous for an autosomal recessive disorder, a polar body showing the mutant allele should be complemented by a primary oocyte having the normal allele. The normal oocyte could thus be allowed to fertilize in vitro and then transferred for potential implantation. Conversely, if the polar body were normal, fertilization would not be allowed to proceed because the oocyte would be deduced to contain the mutant allele. Similarly, a polar body containing only one chromosome 21 (as determined by FISH with a chromosome-specific probe) should be complemented by a primary oocyte also containing a single chromosome 21. If the first polar body failed to show a chromosome 21, however, the oocyte can be presumed to have two 21 chromosomes. This would lead to a trisomic zygote.

Polar body biopsy has the theoretical advantage of no reduction in cell number following biopsy. There should also be less likelihood of contamination with sperm. Disadvantages include inability to assess the paternal genotype, precluding application if a father has an autosomal dominant disorder. Lacking information about paternal transmission is also less efficient reproductively. Deducing a mutant autosomal recessive allele in the oocyte (by its absence in the polar body) precludes permitting an oocyte to be fertilized, whereas any resulting embryo would actually be affected only if the fertilizing sperm contained the same mutant allele.

A major potential disadvantage is recombination, that meiotic phenomenon occurring routinely between homologous chromosomes. If crossing over involves the region containing the gene in question, the single chromosome in the primary oocyte would contain DNA sequences encoding both alleles. That is, the two chromatids of the single chromosome would differ in genotype (heterozygosity). Genotype of the secondary oocyte could thus not be predicted without either biopsy of the second polar body or biopsy of the embryo per se (blastomere or blastocyst biopsy). Recombination can be addressed by performing biopsy on both the first and second polar bodies.[102] Actually, the "problem" of recombination then actually can be beneficial because presence of two alleles at the first polar body excludes allele dropout (failure of one allele to amplify) at that stage. Thus, one could be confident of the accuracy of a second polar body biopsy showing only one allele.

Technical Considerations in Diagnosing Chromosomal Abnormalities

Cytogenetic analysis in preimplantation genetic diagnosis would be useful for a variety of reasons. Sex determination (XX or XY) may be desirable for couples at risk for an X-linked recessive trait, in which an exact diagnosis is not possible. Detection of aneuploidy is also possible. Translocations and other chromosomal rearrangements are also detectable by FISH, using specifically selected break-point–specific or a combination of telomeric and centromeric FISH probes.[103] FISH accuracy in blastomeres seems at least as high as in amniotic fluid or chorionic villus cells.

Experience from individual preimplantation genetic diagnosis (PGD) centers is still limited, but anomaly rates and spontaneous abortion rates following PGD appear to be similar to those in conventional ART without embryo biopsy.[101] As of June 2000, there are approximately 2,500 PGD cycles worldwide, with a pregnancy rate of 20 to 25 percent.[104] The anomaly rates do not seem to be increased over that in the general population.[101,104,105]

Diagnostic accuracy is also achievable for mendelian traits, but single-cell diagnosis requires specialized technology (nested primer or fluorescent PCR; heteroduplex analysis). It cannot be assumed that a routine genetics or diagnostic laboratory can perform single-cell PCR just because they perform the techniques on samples containing many cells.

A major worry is the risk of contamination from ambient cells. Failed PCR also occurs, but this is less catastrophic than contamination, for only the latter would ordinarily lead to a false-negative diagnosis. If in an autosomal recessive disorder the embryo were a heterozygote, failure to amplify the normal allele would erroneously indicate the embryo to be affected; therefore, no transfer would occur. The clinical consequence would be limited to a missed opportunity to achieve a pregnancy. Conversely, failing to amplify the abnormal allele would result in transfer of an embryo assumed erroneously to be homozygously normal but actually heterozygous. In either cases, allele-specific PCR failure would not result in a clinically significant error (i.e., false-negative diagnosis). These problems are especially acute when attempting to diagnose compound heterozygosity.

A promising new use of PGD is to increase pregnancy in assisted reproductive technology by training on euploid embryos. This is most helpful in women 37 years or older or with prior history of ART failure.[106]

FUTURE DIRECTIONS: FETAL CELLS IN MATERNAL BLOOD

Fetal cells circulate in the maternal blood during pregnancy, and their analysis represents a new approach to noninvasive prenatal genetic diagnosis. Consensus has already developed that detection is possible for fetal aneuploidy and for selected mendelian disorders. The issue is sensitivity compared to other noninvasive approaches.

Using nested primer PCR for Y-specific DNA, signals

can be detected early in pregnancy in the peripheral blood of pregnant women carrying male fetuses. Y-specific signals were detected by 33 days' gestation by Thomas and colleagues.[107] By 6 weeks' gestation, all pregnancies having a male fetus show a Y-specific signals in maternal blood.

Diagnosis of chromosomal abnormalities requires fetal interphase cell analysis by FISH with chromosome-specific probes. Given the rarity of fetal cells in maternal blood ($1:10^7$), one must enrich for the rare fetal cells. This requires targeting a specific fetal cell type. Targets include fetal trophoblasts, lymphocytes, granulocytes, and nucleated red blood cells (NRBCs). The latter is generally considered to be the most attractive cell type because these cells (NRBCs) comprise about 10 percent of red cells in the 11-week fetus and 0.5 percent in the 19-week fetus. Nucleated red blood cells persist no longer than perhaps 5 days in the adult, and are rare in peripheral adult blood.

One concern is that fetal cells from a prior pregnancy could persist in the maternal circulation and, hence, lead to diagnostic error. This would especially be troublesome if aneuploid cells were to persist after a chromosomally abnormal liveborn offspring or a chromosomally abnormal spontaneous abortion. However, fetal cells usually disappear rapidly after delivery. Using the usual selection criteria, cells from prior pregnancies do not appear to be a major confounder.

Our group was the first to detect fetal aneuploidy by maternal blood analysis. Analyzing interphase cells by FISH with chromosome-specific probes we detected first trisomy 18[108] and then trisomy 21[109] in 1992. At present, the detection rate for aneuploidy using fetal cells recovered from maternal blood is estimated to be 40 to 59 percent, on the basis of an ongoing NICHD collaborative study.[110] Diagnosis is usually made on the basis of one to three trisomic (and, hence, fetal) cells recovered from a 20- to 30-ml specimen. Given that 1 ml of maternal blood is estimated to contain one fetal cell, many fetal cells must be lost. Improved sensitivity would be expected with increased fetal cell recovery and especially better cell separated selection criteria. Active collaborative work is in progress.

Detection of fetal mendelian disorders by analysis of fetal cells in maternal blood does not necessarily require enrichment and, thus, does not necessitate targeting for any specific fetal cell type. PCR-based technology alone may suffice, since the DNA may be derived from any type of fetal cell. Diagnosis can also be made from analysis of plasma, which contains fetal DNA.

In several situations, fetal cell analysis might be useful. First, determining fetal sex is useful in couples at risk for X-linked recessive traits. Second, certain point mutations (mendelian disorders) can be detected. One useful circumstance arises when the father is heterozy-gous (Aa) and the mother homozygously abnormal (aa) for an autosomal recessive trait. The normal allele may or may not be transmitted by the heterozygous father; but if it is, detection by PCR should be possible. If blood from the homozygous mother reveals the normal paternal allele (A), the fetus can be deduced to be heterozygous. Particularly applicable for obstetricians is diagnosis of fetal rhesus (D) through PCR of maternal blood. The molecular basis of Rh(D) negativity (dd) is usually a gene deletion, *d* representing lack of the DNA sequence that if present encodes *D*. This makes distinguishing Rh(D)-positive (DD or Dd) from Rh(D)-negative (dd) simple by molecular techniques. If the mother is Rh-negative and the father homozygous for Rh(D) (Rh-positive), all fetuses must be heterozygous (Dd); every pregnancy would then be at risk for RhD-isoimmunization. If the father is heterozygous, however, the likelihood is only 50 percent that the fetus would inherit his RhD gene and, hence, be affected; the other 50 percent of pregnancies would not be at risk for Rh-isoimmunization. If Rh(D) sequences are found in a pregnant Rh-negative woman (dd), their origin must be fetal; thus, the fetus is Dd.

The inconvenience of working with rare fetal cells could be overcome if these fetal cells could be cultured in vitro from a maternal blood sample. Given that maternal stem cells are also present in maternal blood, techniques designed to stimulate fetal cells differentially would be desirable. Several groups have reported the successful fetal cells in culture.[111]

Key Points

➤ The frequency of major birth defects is 2 to 3 percent. Major etiologic categories include chromosomal abnormalities (1 per 160 live births), single-gene or mendelian disorders, polygenic/multifactorial disorders, and teratogenic disorders. Of the chromosomal abnormalities, approximately half represent autosomal trisomy and half sex chromosomal abnormalities.

➤ Principles of genetic counseling include adequate communication, appreciation of psychological defenses, and philosophy of nondirective counseling.

➤ Genetic screening for heterozygote detection in the nonpregnant and, if not already evaluated, pregnant population is appropriate for only selected autosomal recessive disorders: Tay-Sachs disease in Jewish populations, α-thalassemia in Asians, β-thalassemia in Mediterranean peoples

(Greek and Italian), sickle cell in African-American blacks.

➤ The ACOG and major genetic organizations have recently recommended that screening for cystic fibrosis be offered to Caucasian and Ashkenazi Jewish individuals, and made available to other ethnic populations. Detection rates are 80 to 95 percent in the two former groups, and 70 percent in African-Americans, Hispanics, and Asians. Screening for a defined panel of alleles is considered the minimal standard.

➤ In all pregnancies, genetic screening should be performed for chromosomal abnormalities and NTDs. All women aged 35 years and above at delivery should be offered prenatal cytogenetic diagnosis. For younger women, maternal serum screening should be offered to detect autosomal trisomies. The profile of decreased MSAFP, elevated hCG, and decreased unconjugated serum estriol favors Down syndrome. Maternal serum analyte screening in combination with maternal age can detect 60 percent of Down syndrome cases, but the frequency varies according to maternal age (90 percent over age 35 but about 25 percent in the early third decade). Screening for NTDs involves elevated MSAFP followed by amniotic fluid analysis; approximately 80 to 90 percent of NTDs can be detected at a cost of 5 percent amniocentesis.

➤ All invasive procedures carry risks. Amniocentesis at 15 weeks and above carries a procedure-related risk of perhaps 0.2 to 0.5 percent loss. Amniocentesis before 14 to 15 weeks has been subjected to rigorous trials to determine safety, and use before 13 weeks is not recommended because of the unacceptable 1 to 2 percent risk of clubfoot. CVS is considered, in experienced hands, equal to amniocentesis in terms of loss rates and diagnostic accuracy. Transcervical and transabdominal CVS are equivalent in safety.

➤ Controversy exists concerning LRDs associated with CVS. If a risk exists, it appears to be greatest below 10 weeks' gestation, for which reason, in general, the procedure should generally be available at 10 weeks and beyond. A maximum limb reduction risk of 1 in 3,000 has been reported, and many believe that the risk is not greater than that of the general population.

➤ The complication rate associated with fetal blood sampling is uncertain, but appears to be 1 to 2 percent. The rate varies according to the diagnosis being assessed. No studies have directly compared loss rates in control and tested pregnancies.

➤ Many single-gene disorders are detectable. Some can be detected by enzymatic analysis, whereas others can be recognized best or only through molecular methodologies.

➤ Two principal types of molecular analysis are employed. Direct analysis is possible if the gene sequence is known. Linkage analysis is necessary if the gene has been localized but not yet sequenced. Linkage analysis takes advantage of markers lying close to the gene in question; accuracy is not 100 percent because recombination can occur between the marker and the mutant gene.

➤ Preimplantation genetic diagnosis has been performed in approximately 2,500 cycles, principally by removing a single cell (blastomere) from the eight-cell embryo. Diagnosis requires special molecular techniques for mendelian disorders or FISH for chromosomal abnormalities (trisomy). Accuracy is near 100 percent, and safety does not seem to be a major concern.

➤ Fetal cells have been recovered from maternal blood and fetal trisomies detected, with detection rates for autosomal trisomy of about 40 to 50 percent. Improving sensitivity compared with other noninvasive methods (e.g., maternal serum screening) is underway.

REFERENCES

1. Simpson JL, Elias S: Genetics in Obstetrics and Gynecology, 3rd ed. Philadelphia, WB Saunders Company, (in press).
2. Hook EB, Hamerton JL: The frequency of chromosome abnormalities detected in consecutive newborn studies—differences between studies—results by sex and by severity of phenotypic involvement. *In* Hook EB, Porter IH (eds): Population Cytogenetic Studies in Humans. San Diego, Academic Press, 1977, p 63.
3. McKusick VA: Mendelian Inheritance in Man, 12th ed. Baltimore, The Johns Hopkins University Press, 1998.
4. Simpson JL, Rajkovic A: Ovarian differentiation and gonadal failure. Am J Med Genet 89:186, 1999.
5. DeMarchi JM, Caskey CT, Richards CS: Population-specific screening by mutation analysis for diseases frequent in Ashkenazi Jews. Hum Mutat 8:116, 1996.
6. Kaback M, Lim-Steele J, Dabholkar D, et al: Tay-Sachs disease—carrier screening, prenatal diagnosis, and the molecular era. An international perspective, 1970 to 1993. The International TSD Data Collection Network. JAMA 270:2307, 1993.
7. American College of Medical Genetics/American College of Obstetrics and Gynecology/National Institute of Health

Steering Committee: Preconceptional and prenatal carrier screening for cystic fibrosis. 2001 (in press).

8. Cystic Fibrosis Foundation Annual Report, New York, 1996.
9. Abeliovich D, Lavon IP, Lerer I, et al: Screening for five mutations detects 97% of cystic fibrosis (CF) chromosomes and predicts a carrier frequency of 1:29 in the Jewish Ashkenazi population. Am J Hum Genet 51:951, 1992.
10. Macek M Jr, Mackova A, Hamosh A, et al: Identification of common cystic fibrosis mutations in African-Americans with cystic fibrosis increases the detection rate to 75%. Am J Hum Genet 60:1122, 1997.
11. Chillon M, Casals T, Mercier B, et al: Mutations in the cystic fibrosis gene in patients with congenital absence of the vas deferens. N Engl J Med 332:1475, 1995.
12. Kiesewetter S, Macek M Jr, Davis C, et al: A mutation in CFTR produces different phenotypes depending on chromosomal background. Nat Genet 5:274, 1993.
13. Merkatz IR, Nitowsky HM, Macri JN, et al: An association between low maternal serum alpha fetoprotein and fetal chromosome abnormalities. Am J Obstet Gynecol 148:886, 1984.
14. Bogart MH, Pandiani MR, Jones OW: Abnormal maternal serum chorionic gonadotropin levels in pregnancies with fetal chromosome abnormalities. Prenat Diagn 7:623, 1987.
15. Wald NJ, Cuckle HS, Densen JW, et al: Maternal serum screening for Down syndrome in early pregnancy. BMJ 297:883, 1988.
16. Palomaki GE, Knight GJ, Haddow JE, et al: Cigarette smoking and levels of maternal serum alpha-feto-protein unconjugated estriol, and hCG: impact on Down syndrome screening. Obstet Gynecol 81:675, 1993.
17. Barkai G, Goldman B, Ries L, et al: Down's syndrome screening marker levels following assisted reproduction. Prenat Diagn 16:111, 1996.
18. Neveux LM, Palomaki GE, Knight GJ, et al: Multiple marker screening for Down syndrome in twin pregnancies. Prenat Diagn 16:29, 1996.
19. Rodis JF, Egan JF, Craffey A, et al: Calculated risk of chromosomal abnormalities in twin gestations. Obstet Gynecol 76:1037, 1990.
20. Palomaki GE, Knight GJ, Haddow JE, et al: Prospective intervention trial of a screening protocol to identify fetal trisomy 18 using maternal serum alpha-fetoprotein, unconjugated oestriol, and human chorionic gonadotropin. Prenat Diagn 12:925, 1992.
21. Palomaki GE, Haddow JE, Knight GL, et al: Risk-based prenatal screening for trisomy 18 using alpha-feto-protein, unconjugated oestriol and human chorionic gonadotropin. Prenat Diagn 15:713, 1995.
22. Wenstrom KD, Owen J, Chu DC, et al: Alpha-fetoprotein, free beta-human chorionic gonadotropin, and dimeric inhibin A produce the best results in a three-analyte, multiple-marker screening test for fetal Down syndrome. Am J Obstet Gynecol 177:987, 1997.
23. Canick JA, Kellner LH, Saller DN, et al: Second-trimester levels of maternal urinary gonadotropin peptide in Down syndrome pregnancy. Prenat Diagn 15:739, 1995.
24. Cole LA, Shahabi S, Oz UA, et al: Urinary screening tests for fetal Down syndrome: II. Hyperglycosylated hCG. Prenat Diagn 19:35, 1999.
25. Wald NJ, Kennard A, Hackshaw AK: First trimester serum screening for Down's syndrome. Prenat Diagn 15:1227, 1995.
26. Snijders RJM, Noble P, Sebire A, et al: UK multicentre project on assessment of risk of trisomy 21 by maternal age and fetal nuchal-translucency thickness at 10–14 weeks of gestation. Lancet 352:343, 1998.
27. Nicolaides KH, Cicero S, Liao AW: One-stop clinic for as-

sessment of risk of chromosomal defects at 12 weeks of gestation. Prenat Neonat Med 5:145, 2000.
28. Wald NJ, Watt HC, Hackshaw AK: Integrated screening for Down's syndrome on the basis of tests performed during the first and second trimesters. N Engl J Med 341:461, 1999.
29. Elias S, Simpson JL, Bombard AT: Amniocentesis. In Milunsky A (ed): Genetic Disorders and the Fetus, 4th ed. Baltimore, The Johns Hopkins University Press, 1998, p 53.
30. Evans MI, Dommergues M, Timor-Tritsch I, et al: Transabdominal versus transcervical and transvaginal multifetal pregnancy reduction: international collaborative experience of more than one thousand cases. Am J Obstet Gynecol 170:902, 1994.
31. National Institute of Child Health Development National Registry for Amniocentesis Study Group: Midtrimester amniocentesis for prenatal diagnosis: safely and accuracy. JAMA 236:1471, 1976.
32. Simpson NE, Dellaire L, Miller JR, et al: Prenatal diagnosis of genetic disease in Canada: report of a collaborative study. Can Med Assoc J 15:739, 1976.
33. Tabor A, Philip J, Madsen MI, et al: Randomized controlled trial of genetic amniocentesis in 4,606 low-risk women. Lancet 1:1287, 1986.
34. Baird PA, Yee IML, Sadnovnick AD: Population-based study of long-term outcomes after amniocentesis. Lancet 334:1134, 1994.
35. Tongsong T, Wanapirak C, Sirivatanapa P, et al: Amniocentesis-related fetal loss: a cohort study. Obstet Gynecol 92:64, 1998.
36. Hanson FW, Tennant F, Hune S, Brookhyser K: Early amniocentesis: outcome, risks, and technical problems at ≤12.8 weeks. Am J Obstet Gynecol 166:1707, 1992.
37. Henry GP, Miller WA: Early amniocentesis. J Reprod Med 37:396, 1992.
38. Johnson JM, Wilson RD, Winsor EJT, et al: The early amniocentesis study: a randomized clinical trial of early amniocentesis vs midtrimester amniocentesis. Fetal Diagn Ther 11:85, 1996.
39. Wilson RD, Johnson J, Windrim E, et al: The early amniocentesis study: a randomized clinical trial of early amniocentesis vs mid-trimester amniocentesis. II. Evaluation of procedure details and neonatal congenital anomalies. Fetal Diagn Ther 12:97, 1997.
40. The Canadian Early and Mid-Trimester Amniocentesis Trial (CEMAT) Group: Randomized trial to assess safety and fetal outcome of early and mid-trimester amniocentesis. Lancet 351:242, 1998.
41. Johnson JM, Wilson RD, Singer J, et al: Technical factors in early amniocentesis predict adverse outcome. Results of the Canadian Early (EA) versus Mid-trimester (MA) Amniocentesis Trial. Prenat Diagn 19:732, 1999.
42. American College of Obstetricians and Gynecologists: Early amniocentesis. ACOG Newsletter, March 1997. Washington, DC, American College of Obstetricians and Gynecologists.
43. Rhoads GG, Jackson LG, Schlesselman SE, et al: The safety and efficacy of chorionic villus sampling for early prenatal diagnosis of cytogenetic abnormalities. N Engl J Med 320:609, 1989.
44. Canadian Collaborative CVS–Amniocentesis Clinical Trial Group: Multicentre randomized clinical trial of chorionic villus sampling. Lancet 337:1491, 1991.
45. Golbus MS, Simpson JL, Fowler SE, et al: Risk factors associated with transcervical CVS losses. Prenat Diagn 12:373, 1991.
46. Jackson L, Wapner RJ: Chorionic villus sampling. In Simpson JL, Elias S (eds): Essentials of Prenatal Diagnosis. New York, Churchill Livingstone, 1993, p 45.

47. Jackson LG, Zachary JM, Desnik RJ, et al: A randomized comparison of transcervical and transabdominal chorionic villus sampling. N Engl J Med 327:594, 1992.

48. Brambati B, Lanzani A, Tului L: Transabdominal and transcervical chorionic villus sampling: efficiency and risk evaluation of 2,411 cases. Am J Med Genet 35:160, 1990.

49. MRC Working Party on the Evaluation of Chorionic Villus Sampling: Medical Research Council European Trial of Chorion Villus Sampling. Lancet 337:1491, 1991.

50. Pergament E, Schulman JD, Copeland K, et al: The risk and efficacy of chorionic villus sampling in multiple gestations. Prenat Diagn 12:377, 1992.

51. Firth HV, Boyd PA, Chamberlin P, et al: Severe limb abnormalities after chorion villus sampling at 55–66 days' gestation. Lancet 337:762, 1991.

52. Mahoney MJ, and USNICHD Collaborators: Limb abnormalities and chorionic villus sampling. Lancet 337:1422, 1991.

53. Jackson LG, Wapner RJ, Brambai B: Limb abnormalities and chorionic villus sampling. Lancet 337:1423, 1991.

54. Mastroiacovo P, Cavalcanti DP: Limb reduction defects and chorion villus sampling. Lancet 337:1091, 1991.

55. Hsieh F-J, Chen D, Tseng L-H, et al: Limb-reduction defects and chorionic villus sampling. Lancet 337:1091, 1991.

56. Burton BK, Schulz CJ, Burd L: Limb anomalies associated with chorionic villus sampling. Obstet Gynecol 79:726, 1992.

57. Mastroiacovo P, Botto LD, Cavalcanti DP, et al: Limb anomalies following chorionic villus sampling: a registry based case-control study. Am J Med Genet 44:856, 1992.

58. Mastroiacovo P, Botto LD: Chorionic villus sampling and limb deficiencies. Review of case control and cohort studies. In Zakut H (ed): 7th International Conference on Early Prenatal Diagnosis of Genetic Disease. Jerusalem, Israel, 22–27 May 1994, p 71.

59. Dolk H, Beatrand F, Lechat MF: Chorionic villus sampling and limb abnormalities. Lancet 339:876, 1992.

60. Hsieh FJ, Shyu MK, Sheu BC, et al: Limb defects after chorionic villus sampling. Obstet Gynecol 85:84, 1995.

61. Olney RS, Khoury MJ, Alo CJ, et al: Increased risk for transverse digital deficiency after chorionic villus sampling (CVS): results of the US multistate case-control study, 1988–1992 [abstract]. Teratology 49:376, 1994.

62. Brambati B, Tului L: Prenatal genetic diagnosis through chorionic villus sampling. In Mulinsky A (ed): Genetic Disorders and The Fetus, 4th ed. Baltimore, The Johns Hopkins University Press, 1998, p 150.

63. Kuliev A, Jackson L, Froster U, et al: Chorionic villus sampling safety. Report of World Health Organization/EURO meeting in association with the Seventh International Conference on Early Prenatal Diagnosis of Genetic Diseases, Tel-Aviv, Israel, May 21, 1994. Am J Obstet Gynecol 174:807, 1996.

64. Kuliev A, Jackson L, Froster U, et al: Evaluation of chorionic villus sampling safety. Prenatal Diag 19:97, 1999.

65. Froster UG, Jackson L: Limb defects and chorionic villus sampling: results from an international registry, 1992–94. Lancet 347:489, 1996.

66. Froster-Ikenius UG, Baird PA: Limb reduction defects in over one million consecutive live births. Teratology 39:127, 1989.

67. American College of Obstetrics and Gynecology, Committee on Genetics. Chorionic Villus Sampling. Committee Opinion No. 169. Washington, DC, ACOG, 1995.

68. Orlandi F, Damiani G, Jakil C, et al: Clinical results and fetal biochemical data on 140 early second trimester diagnostic cordocentesis. Acta Eur Fertil 18:329, 1987.

69. Orlandi F, Damiani G, Jakil C, et al: The risks of early cordocentesis (12–21 weeks): analysis of 500 procedure. Prenat Diagn 10:425, 1990.

70. Nicolini U, Nicolaidis P, Fisk NM, et al: Fetal blood sampling from the intrahepatic vein: analysis of safety and clinical experience with 214 procedures. Obstet Gynecol 76:47, 1990.

71. Weiner CP, Grant SS, Huson J, et al: Effect of diagnostic and therapeutic cordocentesis upon maternal serum alpha fetoprotein concentration. Am J Obstet Gynecol 161:706, 1989.

72. Nicolini U, Kochenour NK, Greco P, et al: Consequences of fetomaternal haemorrhage after intrauterine transfusion. BMJ 297:1379, 1988.

73. Weiner CP: Cordocentesis for diagnostic indications: two years experience. Obstet Gynecol 70:664, 1987.

74. Rodeck CH, Nicolini U: Fetal blood sampling. Eur J Obstet Gynecol Reprod Biol 28:85, 1988.

75. Daffos F: Fetal blood sampling. Annu Rev Med 40:319, 1989.

76. Wilson RD, Farquharson DF, Wittmann BK, Shaw D: Cordocentesis: overall pregnancy loss rate as important as procedure loss rate. Fetal Diagn Ther 9:142, 1994.

77. Weiner CP, Okamura K: Diagnostic fetal blood sampling-technique related losses. Fetal Diagn Ther 11:169–75, 1996.

78. Nicolini U, Rodeck C: Fetal blood and tissue sampling. In Brock DJH, Rodeck CH, Ferguson-Smith MA (eds): Prenatal Diagnosis and Screening. Edinburgh, Churchill Livingstone, 1992, p 39.

79. Hook EB, Cross PK, Jackson L, et al: Maternal age specific rates of 47,+21 and other cytogenetic abnormalities diagnosed in the first trimester of pregnancy of chorionic villus biopsy specimens: comparison with rates expected from observations at amniocentesis. Am J Hum Genet 42:797, 1988.

80. Hook EB, Cross PK: Maternal age-specific rates of chromosome abnormalities at chorionic villus study: a revision [letter]. Am J Hum Genet 45:474, 1989.

81. Stene J, Stene E, Mikkelsen M: Risk for chromosome abnormality at amniocentesis following a child with a non-inherited chromosome aberration. Prenat Diagn 4:81, 1984.

82. Boué A, Gallano P: A collaborative study of the segregation of inherited chromosome structural rearrangements in 13356 prenatal diagnoses. Prenat Diagn 4:45, 1984.

83. Simpson JL, Martin AO, Verp MS, et al: Hypermodel cells in amniotic fluid cultures: frequency, interpretation, and clinical significance. Am J Obstet Gynecol 143:250, 1982.

84. Hsu LYF: Prenatal diagnosis of chromosomal abnormalities through amniocentesis. In Milunsky A (ed): Genetic Disorders and the Fetus, 4th ed. Baltimore, The Johns Hopkins University Press, 1998, p 179.

85. Ledbetter DH, Zachary JM, Simpson JL, et al: Cytogenetic results from the U.S. Collaborative Study on CVS: high diagnostic accuracy in over 11,000 cases. Prenat Diagn 12:317, 1992.

86. Association of Clinical Cytogeneticists Working Party on Chorionic Villi in Prenatal Diagnosis: Cytogenetic analysis of chorionic villi for prenatal diagnosis: an ACC collaborative study of U.K. data. Prenat Diagn 14:363, 1994.

87. Wapner R, Simpson JL, Golbus MS, et al: Confined chorionic mosaicism: association with fetal loss but not with adverse perinatal outcome. Prenat Diagn 12:357, 1992.

88. Warburton D: Outcome of cases of de novo structural rearrangements diagnosed at amniocentesis. Prenat Diagn 4:69, 1984.

89. Warburton D: De novo balanced chromosome rearrangements and extra marker chromosomes identified at prenatal diagnosis: clinical significance and distribution of break points. Am J Hum Genet 49:995, 1991.

90. Sachs ES, Van Hemel JO, Den Hollander JC, et al: Marker chromosomes in a series of 10,000 prenatal diagnoses: cytogenetic and follow-up studies. Prenat Diagn 7:81, 1987.

91. Brondum-Nielsen K, Mikkelson M: A 10-year survey, 1980–

1990, of prenatally diagnosed small supernumerary marker chromosomes. Outcome and follow-up of 14 cases diagnosed in a serious of 13699 prenatal samples. Prenat Diagn 15:615, 1995.

92. Hume RF Jr, Drugan A, Ebrahim SA, et al: Role of ultrasonography in pregnancies with marker chromosome aneuploidy. Fetal Diagn Ther 10:182, 1995.

93. Speiser PW, Laforgia N, Kato K, et al: First trimester prenatal treatment and molecular genetic diagnosis of congenital hyperplasia (21-hydroxylase deficiency). J Clin Endocrinol Metab 70:838, 1990.

94. Elias S, Easterly N: Prenatal diagnosis of hereditary skin disorders. Clin Obstet Gynecol 4:24:1069, 1981.

95. Bakhavev VA, Aivazyan AA, Karetnikova NA, et al: Fetal skin biopsy in prenatal diagnosis of some genodermatoses. Prenat Diagn 10:1, 1990.

96. Milunsky A: Maternal serum screening for neural tube and other defects. *In* Milunsky A (ed): Genetic Disorders and the Fetus, 4th ed. Baltimore, The Johns Hopkins University Press, 1998, p 635.

97. MRC Vitamin Study Research Group: Prevention of neural tube defects: results of the Medical Research Council Vitamin Study. Lancet 338:131, 1991.

98. Handyside AH, Pattinson JK, Penketh RJ, et al: Biopsy of human preimplantation embryos and sexing by DNA amplification. Lancet 1:347, 1989.

99. Handyside AH, Komtogianni EH, Hardy K, Winston RML: Pregnancies from biopsied human preimplantation embryos sexed by DNA amplification. Nature 344:768, 1990.

100. Hardy J, Martin JL, Leese HJ, et al: Human preimplantation development *in vitro* is not adversely affected by biopsy at 8-cell stages. Hum Reprod 5:708, 1990.

101. Verlinsky Y, Kuliev A: Preimplantation genetic diagnosis. Reprod Med Rev 7:1, 1999.

102. Verlinsky Y, Rechitsky S, Cieslak J, et al: Preimplantation diagnosis of single gene disorders by two-step oocyte genetic analysis using first and second polar body. Biochem Mol Med 62:182, 1997.

103. Munne S, Sandalinas M, Escudero T, et al: Outcome of preimplantation genetic diagnosis of translocations. Fertil Steril 73:1209, 2000.

104. Verlinsky Y: Present status of preimplantation diagnosis. Third International Symposium on Preimplantation Genetics. Mol Cell Endocrinol (in press).

105. ESHRE PGD Consortium Steering Committee: ESHRE Preimplantation Genetic Diagnosis (PGD) Consortium: preliminary assessment of data from January 1997 to September 1998. Hum Reprod 14:3138, 1999.

106. Simpson JL: Preimplantation diagnosis—an alternative to prenatal diagnosis. Third International Symposium on Preimplantation Genetics. Mol Cell Endocrinol (in press).

107. Thomas MR, Williamson R, Craft I: Y chromosome sequence DNA amplified from peripheral blood of women in early pregnancy. Lancet 343:413, 1994.

108. Price J, Elias S, Wachtel SS, et al: Prenatal diagnosis using fetal cells isolated from maternal blood by multiparameter flow cytometry. Am J Obstet Gynecol 165:1731, 1992.

109. Elias S, Price J, Docketer M, et al: First trimester prenatal diagnosis of trisomy 21 in fetal cells from maternal blood. Lancet 340:1033, 1992.

110. Bianchi DW, Simpson JL, Jackson LG, et al: Fetal cells in maternal blood: NIFTY clinical trial interim analysis. DM-STAT. NICHD fetal cell study (NIFTY) group. Prenat Diagn 19:994, 1999.

111. Valerio D, Aiello R, Altieri V, et al: Culture of fetal erythroid progenitor cells from maternal blood for non-invasive prenatal genetic diagnosis. Prenat Diagn 16:1073, 1996.

112. Hook EB: Rates of chromosomal activities of different maternal ages. Obstet Gynecol 58:282, 1981.

113. Hook EB, Cross PK, Schreinemachers DM, et al: Chromosomal abnormality rates at amniocentesis and liveborn infants. JAMA 249:2043, 1983.

Chapter 9

Drugs in Pregnancy and Lactation

JENNIFER R. NIEBYL

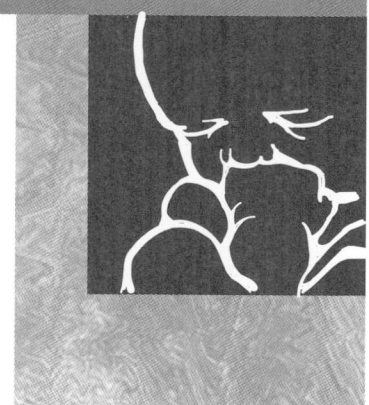

Caution with regard to drug ingestion during pregnancy is usually advised. Until recently, the fetus was thought to rest in a privileged site with little exposure to the environment experienced by the mother. The term *placental barrier* has been in widespread use but is truly a contradiction, as the placenta allows the transfer of many drugs and dietary substances.

Lipid-soluble compounds readily cross the placenta, and water-soluble substances pass less well the greater their molecular weight. The degree to which a drug is bound to plasma protein also influences the amount of drug that is free to cross the placenta. Virtually all drugs cross the placenta to some degree, with the exception of large organic ions such as heparin and insulin.

Developmental defects in humans may be from genetic, environmental, or unknown causes. Approximately 25 percent are known to be genetic in origin; drug exposure accounts for only 2 to 3 percent of birth defects. Approximately 65 percent of defects are of unknown etiology but may be from combinations of genetic and environmental factors (see Chapter 8).

The incidence of major malformations in the general population is usually quoted as 2 to 3 percent.[1] A major malformation is defined as one that is incompatible with survival, such as anencephaly, or one requiring major surgery for correction, such as cleft palate or congenital heart disease, or one producing major dysfunction (e.g., mental retardation). If minor malformations are also included, such as ear tags or extra digits, the rate may be as high as 7 to 10 percent. The risk of malformation after exposure to a drug must be compared with this background rate.

There is a marked species specificity in drug teratogenesis.[2] For example, thalidomide was not found to be teratogenic in rats and mice but is a potent human teratogen. On the contrary, in certain strains of mice,

corticosteroids produce a high percentage of offspring with cleft lip, although no studies have shown these drugs to be teratogenic in humans. The Food and Drug Administration (FDA) lists five categories of labeling for drug use in pregnancy:

A. Controlled studies in women fail to demonstrate a risk to the fetus in the first trimester, and the possibility of fetal harm appears remote.

B. Animal studies do not indicate a risk to the fetus; there are no controlled human studies, or animal studies do show an adverse effect on the fetus, but well-controlled studies in pregnant women have failed to demonstrate a risk to the fetus.

C. Studies have shown the drug to have animal teratogenic or embryocidal effects, but no controlled studies are available in women, or no studies are available in either animals or women.

D. Positive evidence of human fetal risk exists, but benefits in certain situations (e.g., life-threatening situations or serious diseases for which safer drugs cannot be used or are ineffective) may make use of the drug acceptable despite its risks.

X. Studies in animals or humans have demonstrated fetal abnormalities, or evidence demonstrates fetal risk based on human experience, or both, and the risk clearly outweighs any possible benefit.

The classic teratogenic period is from day 31 after the last menstrual period in a 28-day cycle to 71 days from the last period (Fig. 9–1). During this critical period, organs are forming, and teratogens may cause malformations that are usually overt at birth. The timing of exposure is important. Administration of drugs early in the period of organogenesis will affect the organs developing at that time, such as the heart or neural tube. Closer to the end of the classic teratogenic

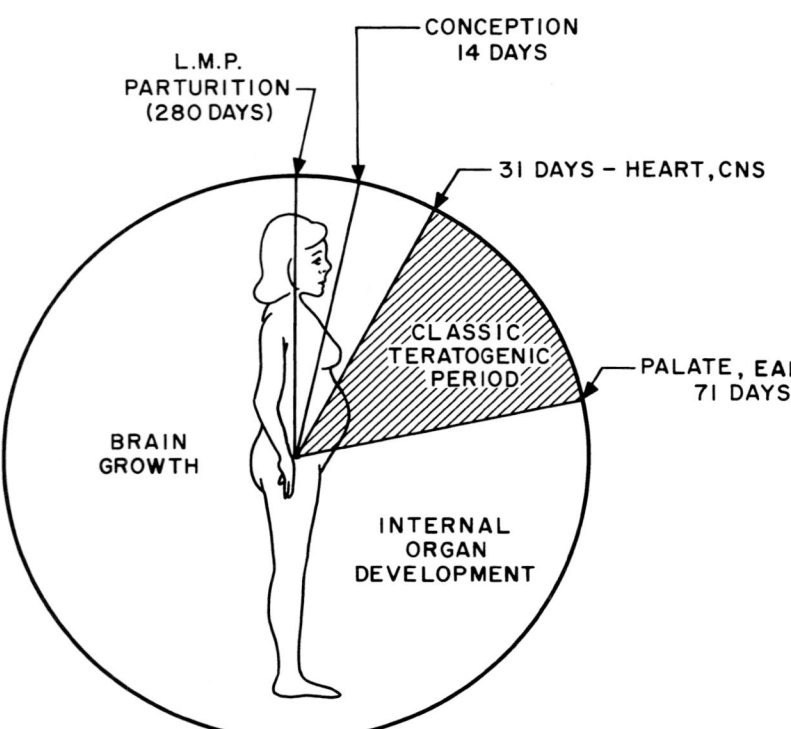

Figure 9–1. Gestational clock showing the classic teratogenic period. (From Blake DA, Niebyl JR: Requirements and limitations in reproductive and teratogenic risk assessment. *In* Niebyl JR (eds): Drug Use in Pregnancy, 2nd ed. Philadelphia, Lea & Febiger, 1988, p 1, with permission.)

period, the ear and palate are forming and may be affected by a teratogen.

Before day 31, exposure to a teratogen produces an all-or-none effect. With exposure around conception, the conceptus usually either does not survive or survives without anomalies. Because so few cells exist in the early stages, irreparable damage to some may be lethal to the entire organism. If the organism remains viable, however, organ-specific anomalies are not manifested, because either repair or replacement will occur to permit normal development. A similar insult at a later stage may produce organ-specific defects.

Patients should be educated about avenues other than the use of drugs to cope with tension, aches and pains,

Table 9–1. TERATOGEN INFORMATION SERVICES AND COMPUTER DATABASES

Organization of Teratogen Information Services:
http://orpheus.ucsd.edu/ctis, Telephone 801-328-2229.
Computer databases:
MICROMEDEX, Inc., 6200 South Syracuse Way, Suite 300, Englewood, CO 80111-4740.
Reproductive Toxicology Center, REPROTOX, Columbia Hospital for Women Medical Center, 2440 M Street NW, Suite 217, Washington, DC 20037-1404.
Teratogen Information Service, TERIS, University of Washington, Office of Technology Transfer, 4225 Roosevelt Way NE Suite 301, Seattle, WA 98105.

and viral illnesses during pregnancy. Drugs should be used only when necessary. The risk/benefit ratio should justify the use of a particular drug, and the minimum effective dose should be employed. As long-term effects of drug exposure in utero may not be revealed for many years, caution with regard to the use of any drug in pregnancy is warranted.

TERATOGEN INFORMATION SERVICES

An organization of teratology information services and several computer databases are available to physicians who counsel pregnant women (Table 9–1).

EMBRYOLOGY

During the first 3 days after ovulation, development takes place in the fallopian tube. At the time of fertilization, a pronuclear stage exists during which the nuclei from the egg and the sperm retain their integrity within the egg cytoplasm. After the pronuclei fuse, the fertilized egg begins a series of mitotic cell divisions (cleavage). The two-cell stage is reached about 30 hours after fertilization. With continued division, the cells develop into a solid ball of cells (morula), which reaches the endometrial cavity about 3 days after fertilization. Thereafter, a fluid-filled cavity forms within the cell mass, at which time the conceptus is called a *blastocyst*. The number of cells increases from approximately 12 to 32 by the end of the third day to 250 by the sixth day.

Until approximately 3 days after conception, any cell is thought to be totipotential, that is, capable of initiating development of any organ system. For example, separation of cells during this period can give rise to monozygotic twins, each normal. At the blastocyst stage, cells first begin to differentiate. The blastocyst is located in the uterus, where implantation occurs 6 to 9 days after conception.

One group of cells forms the inner cell mass that will ultimately develop into the fetus. Different tissues will arise from each of the three cell layers. The brain, nerves, and skin will develop from the ectoderm; the lining of the digestive tract, respiratory tract, and part of the bladder, as well as the liver and pancreas from the endoderm, and connective tissue, cartilage, muscle, blood vessels, the heart, kidneys, and gonads develop from the mesoderm. The group of cells forming the periphery of the blastocyst is termed the *trophoblast*. The placenta and the fetal membranes will develop from this outer cell layer.

The trophoblast continues to grow, and lacunae form within the previously solid syncytiotrophoblast. The lacunae are the precursors of the intervillous spaces of the placenta, and by 2 weeks after conception maternal blood is found within them. Meanwhile, the cytotrophoblast is forming cell masses that will become chorionic villi.

From the third to the eighth week after conception, the embryonic disk undergoes major developments that lay the foundation for all organ systems. By 4 weeks after conception, the fertilized ovum has progressed from one cell to millions of cells. The rudiments of all major systems have differentiated, and the blueprints are set for developmental refinements. The embryo has been transformed into a curved tube approximately 6 mm long and isolated from the extraembryonic membranes.

At 5 weeks after conception, the embryo first begins to assume features of human appearance. The face is recognizable, with the formation of discernible eyes, nose, and ears. Limbs emerge from protruding buds; digits, cartilage, and muscles develop. The cerebral hemispheres begin to fill the brain area, and the optic stalk becomes apparent. Nerve connections are established between the retina and the brain. The digestive tract rotates from its prior tubular structure, and the liver starts to produce blood cells and bile. Two tubes emerge from the pharynx to become bronchi, and the

lungs have lobes and bronchioles. The heart is beating at 5 weeks and is almost completely developed by 8 weeks after conception. The diaphragm begins to divide the heart and lungs from the abdominal cavity. The kidneys approach their final form at this time. The urogenital and rectal passages separate, and germ cells migrate toward the genital ridges for future transformation into ovaries or testes. Differentiation of internal ducts begins, with persistence of either müllerian or wolffian ducts. Virilization of external genitalia occurs in males. The embryo increases from approximately 6 to 33 mm in length and increases 50 times in weight.

Structurally, the fetus has become straighter, and the tubular neural canal along which the spinal cord develops becomes filled with nerve cells. Ears remain low on the sides of the head. Teeth are forming, and the two bony plates of the palate fuse in the midline. Disruptions during the latter part of the embryonic period lead to various forms of cleft lip and palate. By 10 weeks after the last menstrual period, all major organ systems have become established and integrated.

Development of other organs continues in the second and third trimesters of pregnancy. Therefore, we need to be concerned about drug use at this time in pregnancy, although the effects may not be recognized until later in life. Some of the uterine anomalies resulting from diethylstilbestrol (DES) occurred with exposure as late as 20 weeks but were not recognized until after puberty. The brain continues to develop throughout pregnancy and the neonatal period. Fetal alcohol syndrome may occur with chronic exposure to alcohol in the later stages of pregnancy.

EFFECTS OF SPECIFIC DRUGS

Estrogens and Progestins

Oral contraceptives and progestins given in the first trimester have been blamed in the past for a variety of birth defects, but recent studies have not confirmed any teratogenic risk for these drugs.

Data from the Collaborative Perinatal Project, a prospective study of 50,282 pregnancies between 1958 and 1965, initially supported the possibility of a risk of cardiac defects after first-trimester exposure to female hormones and oral contraceptives.[3] However, a reevaluation of these data has questioned this result.[4] Careful review of the records indicated that some patients had taken the medication too early or too late to affect the cardiovascular system. When infants with Down syndrome were excluded, no significant difference in the risk of cardiovascular anomalies remained. Another study of 2,754 infants born to mothers after bleeding in the first trimester suggested no increased risk associated with first-trimester exposure to progestogens.[5] A meta-analysis of first-trimester sex hormone exposure revealed no association between exposure and fetal genital malformations.[6] However, because of the medicolegal climate and the conflicting literature, it is wise to do a sensitive pregnancy test before refilling a prescription for pills or giving progestins to an amenorrheic patient.

Androgenic Steroids

Androgens may masculinize a developing female fetus. Progestational agents, most often the synthetic testosterone derivatives, may cause clitoromegaly and labial fusion if given before 13 weeks of pregnancy.[7] Danazol (Danocrine) has been reported to produce mild clitoral enlargement and labial fusion when given inadvertently for the first 10 to 12 weeks after conception (Fig. 9–2).[8] The abnormality was correctable by surgery.

Spermicides

A reported increased risk of abnormal offspring in mothers who had used spermicides for contraception

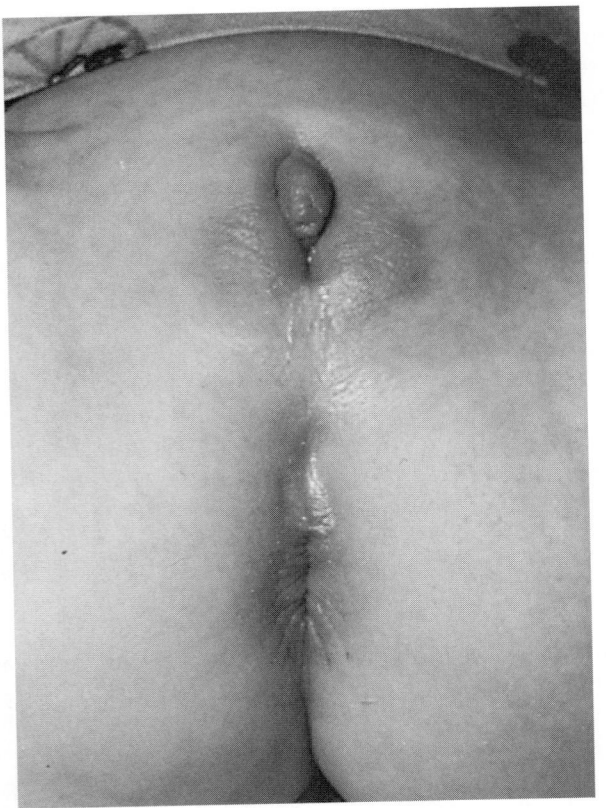

Figure 9–2. Perineum of a female fetus exposed to danazol in utero. (From Duck SC, Katayama KP: Danazol may cause female pseudohermaphroditism. Fertil Steril 35:230, 1981, with permission.)

has not been confirmed. In the Collaborative Perinatal Project data,[9] 462 women reported spermicide use in the first 4 lunar months, with 438 also describing use during the month preceding the last menstrual period. The exposed women had 23 infants with anomalies (5 percent) compared with 4.5 percent in the nonexposed controls, not a significant difference.

In the study of Mills et al.,[10] the malformation rate in women using spermicides after their last menstrual period was 4.8 in 1,000 compared with 6.4 in 1,000 in the controls, not significantly different. The risk of preterm delivery, a low-birth-weight infant, and spontaneous abortion was no higher in the spermicide-exposed group. The study of Linn et al.[11] of 12,440 women found no relationship between contraceptive method and the occurrence of malformations.

Anticonvulsants

Epileptic women taking anticonvulsants during pregnancy have approximately double the general population risk of malformations. Compared with the general risk of 2 to 3 percent, the risk of major malformations in epileptic women on anticonvulsants is about 5 percent, especially cleft lip with or without cleft palate and congenital heart disease. Valproic acid (Depakene) and carbamazepine (Tegretol) each carry approximately a 1 percent risk of neural tube defects and possibly other anomalies.[12,13] In addition, the offspring of epileptic women have a 2 to 3 percent incidence of epilepsy, five times that in the general population.

Whenever a drug is claimed to be a teratogen, one always can raise the issue of whether the drug actually is a teratogen or the disease for which the drug was prescribed in some way contributed to the defect. Even when they take no anticonvulsant drug, women with a convulsive disorder have an increased risk of delivering infants with malformations; this information supports a role for the epilepsy itself rather than the anticonvulsant drug as a contributor to the birth defect.[14] Of infants born to 305 epileptic women on medication in the Collaborative Perinatal Project, 10.5 percent had a birth defect. Of the offspring of women who had a convulsive disorder and who had taken no phenytoin at all, 11.3 percent had a malformation. In contrast, the total malformation rate was 6.4 percent for the control group of women who did not have a convulsive disorder and who therefore did not take any antiepileptic drugs. The issue remains unresolved, as patients who take more drugs during pregnancy usually have more severe convulsive disorders than do those who do not take any anticonvulsants. A combination of more than three drugs or a high daily dose increases the chance of malformations.[14]

Possible causes of anomalies in epileptic women on anticonvulsants include the disease itself, a genetic predisposition to both epilepsy and malformations, genetic differences in drug metabolism, the specific drugs themselves, and deficiency states induced by drugs such as decreased serum folate. Phenytoin (Dilantin) decreases folate absorption and lowers the serum folate, which has been implicated in birth defects.[15] Therefore, folic acid supplementation should be given to these mothers, but may require adjustment of the anticonvulsant dose. Although epileptic women were not included in the Medical Research Council study, most authorities would recommend 4 mg/day folic acid for high-risk women[16] (see Chapter 6). One study suggested that folic acid at doses of 2.5 to 5 mg daily could reduce birth defects in women on anticonvulsant drugs.[17]

Fewer than 10 percent of offspring show the fetal hydantoin syndrome,[18] which consists of microcephaly, growth deficiency, developmental delays, mental retardation, and dysmorphic craniofacial features (Fig. 9–3). In fact, the risk may be as low as 1 to 2 percent.[19] While several of these features are also found in other syndromes, such as fetal alcohol syndrome, more common in the fetal hydantoin syndrome are hypoplasia of the nails and distal phalanges (Fig. 9–4), and hypertelorism. Carbamazepine (Tegretol) is also associated with an increased risk of a dysmorphic syndrome.[20]

A genetic metabolic defect in arene oxide detoxification in the infant may increase the risk of a major birth defect.[21] Epoxide hydrolase deficiency may indicate susceptibility to fetal hydantoin syndrome.[22]

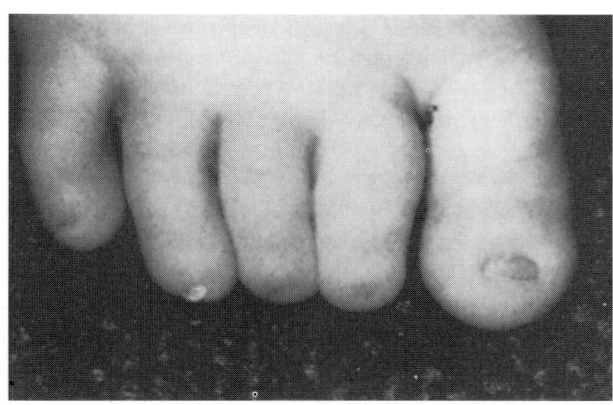

Figure 9–4. Hypoplasia of toenails and distal phalanges. (From Hanson JWM: Fetal hydantoin syndrome. Teratology 13:186, 1976, with permission.)

In a follow-up study of long-term effects of antenatal exposure to phenobarbital and carbamazepine, anomalies were not related to specific maternal medication exposure. There were no neurologic or behavioral differences between the two groups.[23] However, children exposed in utero to phenytoin scored 10 points lower on IQ tests than children exposed to carbamazepine or nonexposed controls.[24] Also, prenatal exposure to phenobarbitol decreased verbal IQ scores in adult men.[25]

Newer Antiepileptic Drugs

Lamotrigine (Lamictal) has been studied in a registry[26] established by the manufacturer, Glaxo Wellcome. Eight of 123 infants (6.5 percent; 95 percent confidence interval [CI] 3.1 to 12.8 percent) born to women treated with lamotrigine during the first trimester and followed prospectively to birth were found to have congenital anomalies.[26] All of the mothers of children with malformations had a seizure disorder and some took at least one other medication during the pregnancy.

Lamotrigine is an inhibitor of dihydrofolate reductase and decreases embryonic folate levels in experimental animals, so it is theoretically possible that this drug would be associated with an increased malformation risk like the other antiepileptic drugs.[27] The limited human data to date do not appear to indicate a major risk for congenital malformations or fetal loss following first-trimester exposure to lamotrigine.

There are no epidemiologic studies of congenital anomalies among children born to women treated with felbamate, gabapentin, oxcarbazepine, tiagabine, topiramate, or vigabatrin.[28]

Some women may have taken anticonvulsant drugs for a long period without reevaluation of the need for continuation of the drugs. For patients with idiopathic epilepsy who have been seizure free for 2 years and

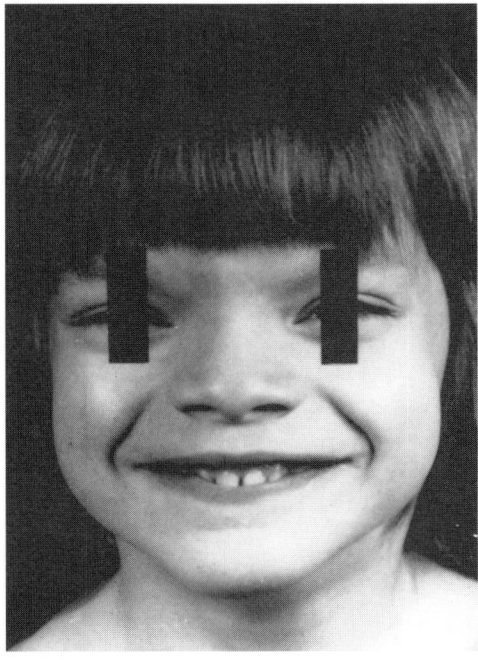

Figure 9–3. Facial features of the fetal hydantoin syndrome. Note broad, flat nasal ridge, epicanthic folds, mild hypertelorism, and wide mouth with prominent upper lip. (Courtesy of Dr. Thaddeus Kelly, Charlottesville, VA.)

who have a normal electroencephalogram (EEG), it may be safe to attempt a trial of withdrawal of the drug before pregnancy.[29]

Most authorities agree that the benefits of anticonvulsant therapy during pregnancy outweigh the risks of discontinuation of the drug if the patient is first seen during pregnancy. The blood level of drug should be monitored to ensure a therapeutic level but minimize the dosage. If the patient has not been taking her drug regularly, a low blood level may demonstrate her lack of compliance and she may not need the drug. Because the albumin concentration falls in pregnancy, the total amount of phenytoin measured is decreased, as it is highly protein bound. However, the level of free phenytoin, which is the pharmacologically active portion, is unchanged. Neonatologists need to be notified when a patient is on anticonvulsants, because this therapy can affect vitamin K–dependent clotting factors in the newborn. Vitamin K supplementation at 10 mg daily for these mothers has been recommended for the last month of pregnancy.[30]

Isotretinoin

Isotretinoin (Accutane) is a significant human teratogen. This drug is marketed for treatment of cystic acne and unfortunately has been taken inadvertently by women who were not planning pregnancy.[30] It is labeled as contraindicated in pregnancy (FDA category X) with appropriate warnings that a negative pregnancy test is required before therapy. Of 154 exposed human pregnancies to date, there have been 21 reported cases of birth defects, 12 spontaneous abortions, 95 elective abortions, and 26 normal infants in women who took isotretinoin during early pregnancy. The risk of structural anomalies in patients studied prospectively is now estimated to be about 25 percent. An additional 25 percent have mental retardation alone.[32] The malformed infants have a characteristic pattern of craniofacial, cardiac, thymic, and central nervous system anomalies. They include microtia/anotia (small/absent ears) (Fig. 9–5), micrognathia, cleft palate, heart defects, thymic defects, retinal or optic nerve anomalies, and central nervous system malformations including hydrocephalus.[31] Microtia is rare as an isolated anomaly yet appears commonly as part of the retinoic acid embryopathy. Cardiovascular defects include great vessel transposition and ventricular septal defects.

Unlike vitamin A, isotretinoin is not stored in tissue. Therefore, a pregnancy after discontinuation of isotretinoin is not at risk, as the drug is no longer detectable in serum 5 days after its ingestion. In 88 pregnancies prospectively ascertained after discontinuation of isotretinoin, no increased risk of anomalies was noted, in contrast to etretinate (see below).[33] Topical tretinoin (Retin-A) has not been associated with any teratogenic risk.[34]

Etretinate (Tegison)

This drug is marketed for use in psoriasis and may well have a teratogenic risk similar to that of isotretinoin. Case reports of malformation, especially central nervous system,[35] have appeared, but the absolute risk is

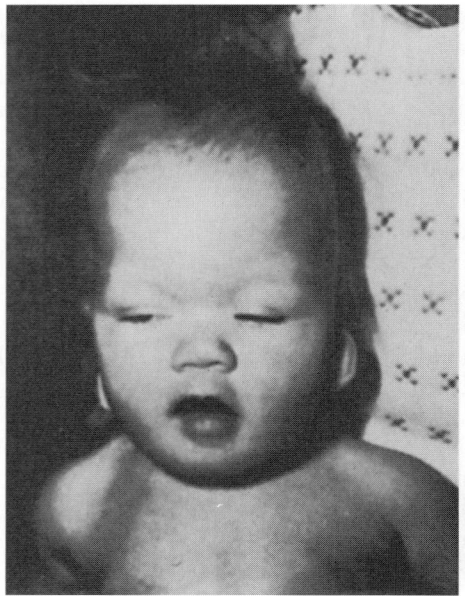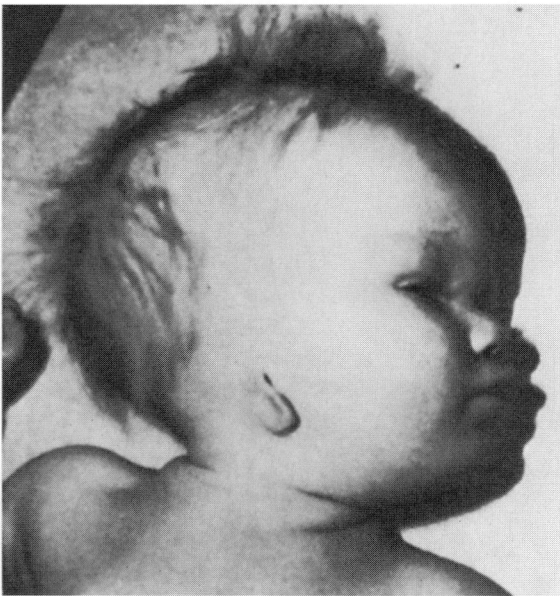

Figure 9–5. Infant exposed to Accutane in utero. Note high forehead, hypoplastic nasal bridge, and abnormal ears. (From Lot IT, Bocian M, Pribam HW, Leitner M: Fetal hydrocephalus and ear anomalies associated with use of isotretinoin. J Pediatr 105:598, 1984, with permission.)

unknown. The half-life of several months makes levels cumulative, and the drug carries a warning to avoid pregnancy within 6 months of use.

Vitamin A

There is no evidence that vitamin A itself in normal doses is teratogenic, nor is betacarotene. The levels in prenatal vitamins (5,000 IU/day orally) have not been associated with any documented risk. Eighteen cases of birth defects have been reported after exposure to levels of 25,000 IU of vitamin A or greater during pregnancy. Vitamin A in doses greater than 10,000 IU/day was shown to increase the risk of malformations in one study,[35] but not in another.[36]

Psychoactive Drugs

There is no clear risk documented for most psychoactive drugs with respect to overt birth defects. However, effects of chronic use of these agents on the developing brain in humans is difficult to study, and so a conservative attitude is appropriate. Lack of overt defects does not exclude the possibility of behavioral teratology.

Tranquilizers

Conflicting reports of the possible teratogenicity of the various tranquilizers, including meprobamate (Miltown) and chlordiazepoxide (Librium), have appeared, but in prospective studies no risk of anomalies has been confirmed.[37] In most clinical situations, the risk/benefit ratio does not justify the use of benzodiazepines in pregnancy.

A fetal benzodiazepine syndrome has been reported in 7 infants of 36 mothers who regularly took benzodiazepines during pregnancy.[38] However, the high rate of abnormality occurred with concomitant alcohol and substance abuse and may not be caused by the benzodiazepine exposure.[39] Perinatal use of diazepam (Valium) has been associated with hypotonia, hypothermia, and respiratory depression.

Lithium (Eskalith, Lithobid)

In the International Register of Lithium Babies,[40] 217 infants are listed as exposed at least during the first trimester of pregnancy, and 25 (11.5 percent) were malformed. Eighteen had cardiovascular anomalies, including six cases of the rare Ebstein's anomaly, which occurs in only 1 in 20,000 in the nonexposed population. Of 60 unaffected infants who were followed to age 5 years, no increased mental or physical abnormalities were noted compared with unexposed siblings.[41]

However, two other reports suggest that there was a bias of ascertainment in the registry and that the risk of anomalies is much lower than previously thought. A case-control study of 59 patients with Ebstein's anomaly showed no difference in the rate of lithium exposure in pregnancy from a control group of 168 children with neuroblastoma.[42] A prospective study of 148 women exposed to lithium in the first trimester showed no difference in the incidence of major anomalies compared with controls.[43] One fetus in the lithium-exposed group had Ebstein's anomaly, and one infant in the control group had a ventricular septal defect. The authors concluded that lithium is not a major human teratogen. Nevertheless, we do recommend that women exposed to lithium be offered ultrasound and fetal echocardiography.

Lithium is excreted more rapidly during pregnancy; thus, serum lithium levels should be monitored. Perinatal effects of lithium have been noted, including hypotonia, lethargy, and poor feeding in the infant. Also, complications similar to those seen in adults on lithium have been noted in newborns, including goiter and hypothyroidism.

Two cases of polyhydramnios associated with maternal lithium treatment have been reported.[44,45] Because nephrogenic diabetes insipidus has been reported in adults taking lithium, the presumed mechanism of this polyhydramnios is fetal diabetes insipidus. Polyhydramnios may be a sign of fetal lithium toxicity.

It is usually recommended that drug therapy be changed in pregnant women on lithium to avoid fetal drug exposure. Tapering over 10 days will delay the risk of relapse.[46] However, discontinuing lithium is associated with a 70 percent chance of relapse of the affective disorder in 1 year as opposed to 20 percent in those who remain on lithium. Discontinuation of lithium may pose an unacceptable risk of increased morbidity in women who have had multiple episodes of affective instability. These women should be offered appropriate prenatal diagnosis with ultrasound, including fetal echocardiography.

Antidepressants

Imipramine (Tofranil) was the original tricyclic antidepressant claimed to be associated with cardiovascular defects, but the number of patients studied remains small. Of 75 newborns exposed in the first trimester, 6 major defects were observed, 3 being cardiovascular.[47]

Amitriptyline (Elavil) has been more widely used. Although occasional reports have associated the use of this drug with birth defects, the majority of the evidence supports its safety. In the Michigan Medicaid study, 467 newborns had been exposed during the first trimester, with no increased risk of birth defects.[48]

Fluoxetine (Prozac) is being used with increasing frequency as an antidepressant. No increased risk of major malformations has been found after first-trimester exposure to fluoxetine in over 500 pregnancies.[49,50]

Nulman and colleagues[51] evaluated the neurobehavioral effects of long-term fluoxetine exposure during pregnancy and found no abnormalities among 228 children aged 16 to 86 months (average age, 3 years). Theoretically, some psychiatric or neurobehavioral abnormality might occur as a result of exposure, but it would be very difficult to ascertain because of all of the confounding variables. In mice, some behavioral effects have been observed.[52]

Chambers and associates[53] found more minor malformations and perinatal complications among infants exposed to fluoxetine throughout pregnancy, but this study is difficult to interpret because the authors did not control for depression. When a group whose mothers received tricyclic agents was used as a control for depression, infants exposed to fluoxetine in utero did not appear to have more minor malformations or perinatal complications.[49]

The newer selective serotonin reuptake inhibitors—fluvoxamine, paroxetine, and sertraline—were also studied during the first trimester in 267 women; there was no increased risk of birth defects.[54]

Anticoagulants

Warfarin (Coumadin) has been associated with chondrodysplasia punctata, which is similar to the genetic Conradi-Hünermann syndrome. This syndrome, occurring in about 5 percent of exposed pregnancies, includes nasal hypoplasia, bone stippling seen on radiologic examination, ophthalmologic abnormalities including bilateral optic atrophy, and mental retardation (Fig. 9–6). The ophthalmologic abnormalities and mental retardation may occur,[55] even with use only beyond the first trimester. Fetal and maternal hemorrhage have also been reported in pregnant women on warfarin, although the incidence can be lowered with careful control of the prothrombin time.

The alternative drug, heparin, does not cross the placenta, as it is a large molecule with a strong negative charge. Because heparin does not have an adverse effect on the fetus when given in pregnancy, it should be the drug of choice for patients requiring anticoagulation. In one study, heparin treatment was associated with more thromboembolic complications and more bleeding complications than warfarin therapy.[56] Therapy with 20,000 units/day for greater than 20 weeks has also been associated with bone demineralization.[57] Thirty-six percent of patients had more than a 10 percent decrease from baseline bone density to postpartum values.[58] The risk of spine fractures was 0.7 percent with low-dose heparin and 3 percent with a high-dose regimen.[59] Heparin can also cause thrombocytopenia.

Low-molecular-weight heparins may have substantial benefits over standard unfractionated heparin.[60] The molecules are still relatively large, and do not cross the placenta.[61] The half-life is longer, allowing for once-

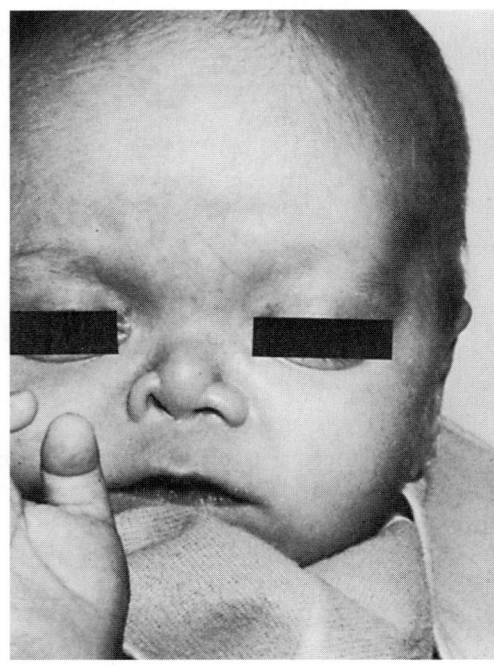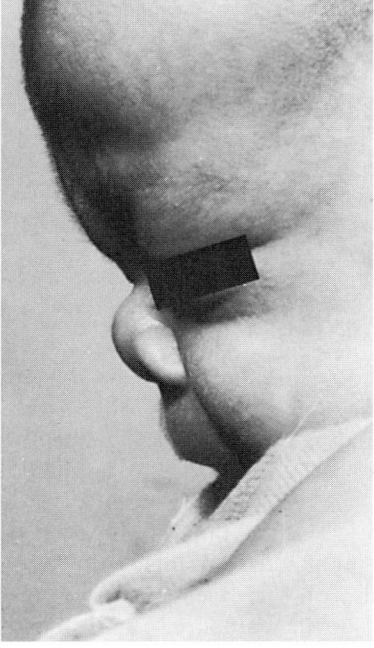

Figure 9–6. Warfarin embryopathy. Note small nose with hypoplastic bridge. (From Shaul W, Hall JG: Multiple congenital anomalies associated with oral anticoagulants. Am J Obstet Gynecol 127:191, 1977, with permission.)

daily administration. However, enoxaparin is cleared more rapidly during pregnancy, and so twice-daily dosing may be advised. They have a much more predictable dose–response relationship, obviating the need for monitoring. There is less risk of heparin-induced thrombocytopenia and clinical bleeding at delivery, but studies suggesting less risk of osteoporosis are preliminary. The cost is substantially higher than standard heparin.[62,63]

The risks of heparin during pregnancy may not be justified in patients with only a single episode of thrombosis in the past.[64,65] Certainly, conservative measures should be recommended, such as elastic stockings and avoidance of prolonged sitting or standing.

In patients with cardiac valve prostheses, full anticoagulation is necessary, as low-dose heparin resulted in three valve thromboses (two fatal) in 35 mothers so treated.[66]

Thyroid and Antithyroid Drugs

Propylthiouracil (PTU) and methimazole (Tapazole) both cross the placenta and may cause some degree of fetal goiter. In contrast, the thyroid hormones triiodothyronine (T_3) and thyroxine (T_4) cross the placenta poorly, so that fetal hypothyroidism produced by antithyroid drugs cannot be corrected satisfactorily by administration of thyroid hormone to the mother. Thus, the goal of such therapy during pregnancy is to keep the mother slightly hyperthyroid to minimize fetal drug exposure. Methimazole has been associated with scalp defects in infants;[67] as well as a higher incidence of maternal side effects. However, PTU and methimazole are equally effective and safe for therapy of hyperthyroidism.[68]

Radioactive iodine (^{131}I or ^{125}I) administered for thyroid ablation or for diagnostic studies is not concentrated by the fetal thyroid until after 12 weeks of pregnancy.[69] Thus, with inadvertent exposure, usually around the time of missed menses, there is no specific risk to the fetal thyroid from ^{131}I or ^{125}I administration.

The need for thyroxine increases in many women with primary hypothyroidism when they are pregnant, as reflected by an increase in serum thyroid-stimulating hormone (TSH) concentrations.[70] In one study, the mean thyroxine dose before pregnancy was 0.10 mg/day; it was increased to a mean dose of 0.15 mg/day during pregnancy.[70] As hypothyroidism in pregnancy may adversely affect the fetus,[71] it is prudent to monitor thyroid function throughout pregnancy and to adjust the thyroid dose to maintain a normal TSH level. Topical iodine preparations are readily absorbed through the vagina during pregnancy, and transient hypothyroidism has been demonstrated in the newborn after exposure during labor.[72]

Digoxin (Lanoxin)

In 52 exposures, no teratogenicity of digoxin was noted.[73] Blood levels should be monitored in pregnancy to ensure adequate therapeutic maternal levels.

Digoxin-like immunoreactive substances may be mistaken in assays for fetal concentrations of digoxin. In one study of fetuses with cardiac anomalies,[74] there was no difference in the immunoreactive digoxin levels whether or not the mother had received digoxin. In hydropic fetuses, digoxin may not easily cross the placenta.[75]

Antihypertensive Drugs

α-Methyldopa (Aldomet) has been widely used for the treatment of chronic hypertension in pregnancy. Although postural hypotension may occur, no unusual fetal effects have been noted. Hydralazine (Apresoline) has also had widespread use in pregnancy, and no teratogenic effect has been observed (see also Chapter 28).

Sympathetic Blocking Agents

Propranolol (Inderal) is a β-adrenergic blocking agent in widespread use for a variety of indications. Theoretically, propranolol might increase uterine contractility. However, this has not been reported, presumably because the drug is not specific for β_2-receptors in the uterine wall. No evidence of teratogenicity has been found. Bradycardia has been reported in the newborn as a direct effect of a dose of the drug given to the mother within 2 hours of delivery of the infant.[76]

Several studies of propranolol use in pregnancy show an increased risk of intrauterine growth restriction or at least a skewing of the birth weight distribution toward the lower range.[77] Ultrasound monitoring of patients on this drug is prudent. Studies from Scotland suggest improved outcome with the use of atenolol (Tenormin) to treat chronic hypertension during pregnancy.[78]

Angiotensin-Converting Enzyme Inhibitors

Angiotensin-converting enzyme inhibitors (e.g., enalapril [Vasotec], captopril [Capoten]) can cause fetal renal tubular dysplasia in the second and third trimesters, leading to oligohydramnios, fetal limb contractures, craniofacial deformities, and hypoplastic lung development.[79] Fetal skull ossification defects have also been described.[80] For these reasons, pregnant women on these medications should be switched to other agents.

Antineoplastic Drugs and Immunosuppressants

Methotrexate, a folic acid antagonist, appears to be a human teratogen, although experience with it is limited.

Infants of three women known to receive methotrexate in the first trimester of pregnancy had multiple congenital anomalies, including cranial defects and malformed extremities. Eight normal infants were delivered to seven women treated with methotrexate in combination with other agents after the first trimester. When low-dose oral methotrexate (7.5 mg/week) was used for rheumatoid disease in the first trimester, five full-term infants were normal, and three patients experienced spontaneous abortions.[81]

Azathioprine (Imuran) has been used by patients with renal transplants or systemic lupus erythematosus. The frequency of anomalies in 80 women treated in the first trimester was not increased.[82] Two infants had leukopenia, one was small for gestational age, and the others were normal.

No increased risk of anomalies in fetuses exposed to cyclosporine (Sandimmune) in utero has been reported.[83] An increased rate of prematurity and growth restriction has also been noted, but it is difficult to separate the contributions of the underlying disease and the drugs given to these transplant patients. The B-cell line may be depleted more than the T-cell line,[84] and one author recommends that infants exposed to immunosuppressive agents be followed for possible immunodeficiency.[84]

Eight malformed infants have resulted from first-trimester exposure to cyclophosphamide (Cytoxan), but these infants were also exposed to other drugs or radiation.[85] Low birth weight may be associated with use after the first trimester, but this may also reflect the underlying medical problem.

Chloroquine (Aralen) is safe in doses used for malarial prophylaxis, and there was no increased incidence of birth defects among 169 infants exposed to 300 mg once weekly.[86] However, after exposure to larger anti-inflammatory doses (250 to 500 mg/day), two cases of cochleovestibular paresis were reported.[87] No abnormalities were noted in an additional 14 infants.[88]

When cancer chemotherapy is used during embryogenesis there is an increased rate of spontaneous abortion and major birth defects. Later in pregnancy there is a greater risk of stillbirth and intrauterine growth restriction, and myelosuppression is often present in the infant.[89]

Antiasthmatics

Theophylline (Theo-Dur, Slo-Bid) and Aminophylline

Both theophylline and aminophylline are safe for the treatment of asthma in pregnancy. No evidence of teratogenic risk was found in 76 exposures in the Collaborative Perinatal Project.[73] Because of increased renal clearance in pregnancy, dosages may need to be increased.

Epinephrine (Adrenalin)

Minor malformations have been reported with sympathomimetic amines as a group in 3,082 exposures in the first trimester, usually in commercial preparations used to treat upper respiratory infections.[73]

Terbutaline (Brethine)

Terbutaline has been widely used in the treatment of preterm labor (see Chapter 23). It is more rapid in onset and has a longer duration of action than epinephrine and is preferred for asthma in the pregnant patient. No risk of birth defects has been reported. Long-term use has been associated with an increased risk of glucose intolerance.[90]

Cromolyn Sodium (Intal)

Cromolyn sodium may be administered in pregnancy, and the systemic absorption is minimal. Teratogenicity has not been reported in humans.

Isoproterenol (Isuprel) and Metaproterenol (Alupent)

When isoproterenol and metaproterenol are given as topical aerosols for the treatment of asthma, the total dose absorbed is usually not significant. With oral or intravenous doses, however, the cardiovascular effects of the agents may result in decreased uterine blood flow. For this reason, they should be used with caution. No teratogenicity has been reported.[73]

Corticosteroids

All steroids cross the placenta to some degree, but prednisone (Deltasone) and prednisolone are inactivated by the placenta. When prednisone or prednisolone are maternally administered, the concentration of active compound in the fetus is less than 10 percent of that in the mother. Therefore, these agents are the drugs of choice for treating medical diseases such as asthma. Inhaled corticosteroids are also effective therapy, and very little drug is absorbed. When steroid effects are desired in the fetus, for example, to accelerate lung maturity, betamethasone (Celestone) and dexamethasone (Decadron) are preferred, as these are minimally inactivated by the placenta. In several hundred infants exposed to corticosteroids in the first trimester, no increase in abnormalities was noted.[73,82]

Iodide

Iodide such as is found in a saturated solution of potassium iodide (SSKI) expectorant crosses the placenta and may produce a large fetal goiter, enough to produce respiratory obstruction in the newborn (Fig. 9–7).[69] Before a patient is advised to take a cough medicine, one should be sure to ascertain that it does not contain iodide.

Antiemetics

Remedies suggested to help nausea and vomiting in pregnancy without pharmacologic intervention include taking crackers at the bedside upon first awakening in the morning before getting out of bed, getting up very slowly, omitting the use of iron tablets, consuming frequent small meals, and eating protein snacks at night. Faced with a self-limited condition occurring at the time of organogenesis, the clinician is well advised to avoid the use of medications whenever possible and to encourage these supportive measures initially.

Vitamin B$_6$

Vitamin B$_6$ (pyridoxine) 25 mg three times a day has been reported in two randomized placebo controlled trials to be effective for treating the nausea and vomiting of pregnancy.[91,92] In several other controlled trials there was no evidence of teratogenicity.

Doxylamine

Doxylamine (Unisom) is an effective antihistamine for nausea in pregnancy and can be combined with vitamin B$_6$ to produce a therapy similar to the former preparation Bendectin. Vitamin B$_6$ (25 mg) and Unisom (25 mg) at bedtime, and one half of each in the morning and afternoon, is an effective combination.

Ginger

Ginger has been used with success for treating hyperemesis,[93] when defined as vomiting during pregnancy that was severe enough to require hospital admission. A significantly greater relief of symptoms was found after ginger treatment than with placebo. Patients took 250-mg capsules containing ginger as powdered root four times a day. Although there are no teratogenic effects known for other antiemetics, much less information is available.

Meclizine (Bonine)

In one randomized, placebo-controlled study, meclizine gave significantly better results than placebo.[94] Prospec-

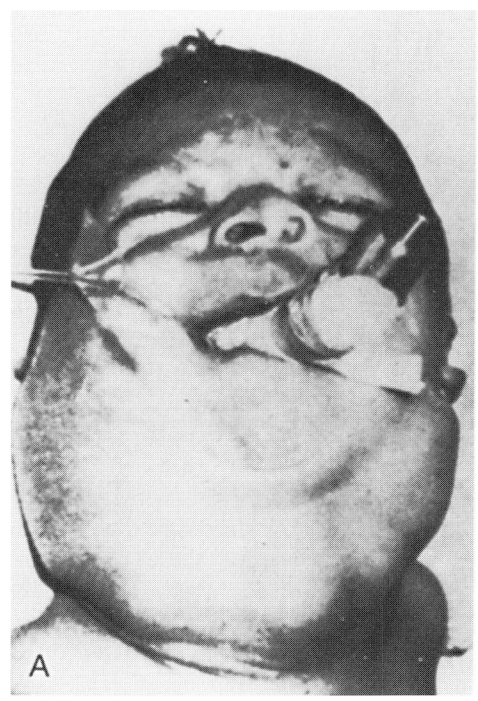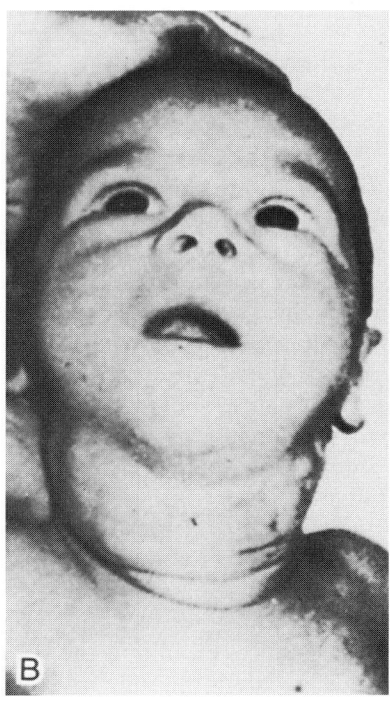

Figure 9–7. Iodide-induced neonatal goiter. *A,* Appearance on the first day of life. *B,* Appearance at 2 months of age. (From Senior B, Chernoff HL: Iodide goiter in the newborn. Pediatrics 47:510, 1971, with permission.)

tive clinical studies have provided no evidence that meclizine is teratogenic in humans. In 1,014 patients in the Collaborative Perinatal Project[73] and an additional 613 patients from the Kaiser Health Plan,[95] no teratogenic risk was found.

Dimenhydrinate (Dramamine)

No teratogenicity has been noted with dimenhydrinate, but a 29 percent failure rate and a significant incidence of side effects, especially drowsiness, has been reported.[96]

Diphenhydramine (Benadryl)

In 595 patients treated in the Collaborative Perinatal Project, no teratogenicity was noted with diphenhydramine.[73] Drowsiness can be a problem.

Trimethobenzamide (Tigan)

Trimethobenzamide, an antinauseant not classified as either an antihistamine or a phenothiazine, has been used for nausea and vomiting in pregnancy. The data collected from a small number of patients are conflicting. In 193 patients in the Kaiser Health Plan study[95] exposed to trimethobenzamide, there was a suggestion of increased congenital anomalies ($p < 0.05$); no concentration of specific anomalies was observed in these children, however, and some of the mothers took other drugs as well. In 340 patients in the Collaborative Perinatal Project,[73] no evidence for an association between this drug and malformations was found.

Phenothiazines

Because of the potential for severe side effects, the phenothiazines have not been used routinely in the treatment of mild or moderate nausea and vomiting, but have been reserved for the treatment of hyperemesis gravidarum. Chlorpromazine (Thorazine) has been shown to be effective in hyperemesis gravidarum, with the most important side effect being drowsiness.

Teratogenicity does not appear to be a problem with the phenothiazines when evaluated as a group. In the Kaiser Health Plan Study,[95] 976 patients were treated, and in the Collaborative Perinatal Project[73] 1,309 patients were treated; no evidence of association between these drugs and malformations was noted. Suspicion of an association between phenothiazines and cardiovascular malformations was observed, however, but this was considered of borderline significance and, in the context of multiple comparisons, of doubtful import. In one study,[97] chlorpromazine seemed to be associated with an increased risk of malformations in 141 exposed mothers. In 58 mothers treated with promethazine (Phenergan) and in 48 mothers given prochlorperazine (Compazine), no increased risk of malformations was found.

Ondansetron (Zofran)

Ondansetron is no more effective than promethazine (Phenergan), has not been evaluated for teratogenicity, and is considerably more costly.[98]

Methylprednisolone

Forty patients with hyperemesis admitted to the hospital were randomized to oral methylprednisolone or oral promethazine, and methylprednisolone was more effective.[99] Corticosteroids may act centrally in the brain stem to exert an antiemetic effect.

Acid-Suppressing Drugs

The use of cimetidine, omeprazole, and ranitidine has not been found to be associated with any teratogenic risk in 2,261 exposures.[100]

Antihistamines and Decongestants

No increased risk of anomalies has been associated with most of the commonly used antihistamines, such as chlorpheniramine (Chlor-Trimeton). However, in the Collaborative Perinatal Project,[73] the risk of malformations increased after exposure to brompheniramine (Dimetane) (10 of 65 infants), an effect that was not found for other antihistamines.

Terfenadine (Seldane) has been associated in one study with an increased risk of polydactyly.[101] Astemizole (Hismanal) did not increase the risk of birth defects in 114 infants exposed in the first trimester.[102]

An association between exposure to antihistamines during the last 2 weeks of pregnancy in general and retrolental fibroplasia in premature infants has been reported.[103]

In the Collaborative Perinatal Project,[73] an increased risk of birth defects was noted with phenylpropanolamine (Entex LA) exposure in the first trimester. In one retrospective study, an increased risk of gastroschisis was associated with first-trimester pseudoephedrine (Sudafed) use.[104] Although these findings have not been confirmed, use of these drugs for trivial indications should be discouraged, as long-term effects are unknown. If decongestion is necessary, topical nasal sprays will result in a lower dose to the fetus than systemic medication.

Patients should be educated that antihistamines and decongestants are only symptomatic therapy for the common cold and have no influence on the course of the disease. Other remedies should be recommended, such as use of a humidifier, rest, and fluids. If medications are necessary, combinations with two drugs should not be used if only one drug is necessary. If the situation is truly an allergy, an antihistamine alone will suffice.

Antibiotics and Anti-infective Agents

As pregnant patients are particularly susceptible to vaginal yeast infections, antibiotics should only be used when clearly indicated. Therapy with antifungal agents may be necessary during or after the course of therapy.

Penicillins

Penicillin, ampicillin, and amoxicillin (Amoxil) are safe in pregnancy. In the Collaborative Perinatal Project,[73] 3,546 mothers took penicillin derivatives in the first trimester of pregnancy, with no increased risk of anomalies. There is little experience in pregnancy with the newer penicillins such as piperacillin (Pipracil) and mezlocillin (Mezlin). These drugs, therefore, should be used in pregnancy only when another better-studied antibiotic is not effective.

Most penicillins are primarily excreted unchanged in the urine, with only small amounts being inactivated in the liver. Patients with impaired renal function require a reduction in dosage.

Serum levels of the penicillins are lower and their renal clearance is higher throughout pregnancy than in the nonpregnant state.[105] The increase in renal blood flow and glomerular filtration rate results in increased excretion of these drugs. The expansion of the maternal intravascular volume during the late stages of pregnancy is another factor that affects antibiotic therapy. If the same dose of penicillin or ampicillin is given to both nonpregnant and pregnant women, lower serum levels are attained during pregnancy as a result of the distribution of the drug in a larger intravascular volume.

Transplacental passage of penicillin is by simple diffusion. The free circulating portion of the antibiotic crosses the placenta, resulting in a lower maternal serum level of the unbound portion of the drug. Administration of penicillins with high protein binding (e.g., oxacillin, cloxacillin [Cloxapen], dicloxacillin [Pathocil], and nafcillin [Unipen]) to a pregnant woman leads to lower fetal tissue and amniotic fluid levels than the administration of poorly bound penicillins (e.g., penicillin G and ampicillin).

The antibiotic is ultimately excreted in the fetal urine and thus into the amniotic fluid. The delay in appearance of different types of penicillins in the amniotic fluid depends primarily on the rate of transplacental diffusion, the amount of protein binding in fetal serum, and the adequacy of fetal enzymatic and renal function. A time delay may occur before effective levels of the antibiotic appear in the amniotic fluid.

Cephalosporins

In a study of 5,000 Michigan Medicaid recipients, there was a suggestion of possible teratogenicity (25 percent increased birth defects) with cefaclor, cephalexin, and cephradine, but not other cephalosporins.[106] Because other antibiotics that have been used extensively (e.g., penicillin, ampicillin, amoxicillin, erythromycin) have not been associated with an increased risk of congenital defects, they should be first-line therapy when such treatment is needed in the first trimester.

Maternal serum levels of cephalosporins are lower than in nonpregnant patients receiving equivalent dosages due to a shorter half-life in pregnancy, an increased volume of distribution, and increased renal elimination. They readily cross the placenta to the fetal bloodstream and ultimately the amniotic fluid.

Sulfonamides

Among 1,455 human infants exposed to sulfonamides during the first trimester, no teratogenic effects were noted.[73] However, the administration of sulfonamides should be avoided in women deficient in glucose-6-phosphate dehydrogenase (G6PD), as a dose-related toxic reaction may occur, resulting in red cell hemolysis.

Sulfonamides cause no known damage to the fetus in utero, as the fetus can clear free bilirubin through the placenta. These drugs might theoretically have deleterious effects if present in the blood of the neonate after birth, however. Sulfonamides compete with bilirubin for binding sites on albumin, thus raising the levels of free bilirubin in the serum and increasing the risk of hyperbilirubinemia in the neonate. Although this toxicity occurs with direct administration to the neonate, kernicterus in the newborn following in utero exposure has not been reported.[107] The sulfonamides are easily absorbed orally, and readily cross the placenta, achieving fetal plasma levels 50 to 90 percent of those attained in the mother.[108]

Sulfasalazine (Azulfidine)

Sulfasalazine is used for treatment of ulcerative colitis and Crohn's disease because of its relatively poor oral absorption. However, it does cross the placenta, leading to fetal drug concentrations approximately the same as those of the mother, although both are low. Neither kernicterus nor severe neonatal jaundice have been reported following maternal use of sulfasalazine even when the drug was given up to the time of delivery.[109]

Sulfamethoxazole with Trimethoprim (Bactrim, Septra)

Trimethoprim is often given with sulfa to treat urinary tract infections. Two published trials including 131 women failed to show any increased risk of birth defects after first-trimester exposure to trimethoprim.[110,111] However, one unpublished study of 2,296 Michigan Medicaid recipients suggested an increased risk of cardiovascular defects after exposure in the first trimester.[112] In a retrospective study of trimethoprim with sulfamethoxazole, the odds ratio for birth defects was 2.3.[113]

Nitrofurantoin (Macrodantin)

Nitrofurantoin is used in the treatment of acute uncomplicated lower urinary tract infections as well as for long-term suppression in patients with chronic bacteriuria. Nitrofurantoin is capable of inducing hemolytic anemia in patients deficient in G6PD. However, hemolytic anemia in the newborn as a result of in utero exposure to nitrofurantoin has not been reported.

No reports have linked the use of nitrofurantoin with congenital defects. In the Collaborative Perinatal Project,[73] 590 infants were exposed, 83 in the first trimester, with no increased risk of adverse effects. More recent studies have confirmed these findings.[114,115]

Nitrofurantoin absorption from the gastrointestinal tract varies with the form administered. The macrocrystalline form is absorbed more slowly than the crystalline and is associated with less gastrointestinal intolerance. Because of rapid elimination, the serum half-life is 20 to 60 minutes. Therapeutic serum levels are not achieved, and therefore this drug is not indicated when there is a possibility of bacteremia. Approximately one third of an oral dose appears in the active form in the urine.

Tetracyclines

The tetracyclines readily cross the placenta and are firmly bound by chelation to calcium in developing bone and tooth structures. This produces brown discoloration of the deciduous teeth, hypoplasia of the enamel, and inhibition of bone growth.[116] The staining of the teeth takes place in the second or third trimesters of pregnancy, while bone incorporation can occur earlier. Depression of skeletal growth was particularly common among premature infants treated with tetracycline. First-trimester exposure to doxycycline is not known to carry any risk.[17] Alternate antibiotics are currently recommended during pregnancy.

Hepatotoxicity has been reported in pregnant women treated with tetracyclines in large doses, usually with intravenous administration for pyelonephritis. First-trimester exposure to tetracyclines has not been found to have any teratogenic risk in 341 women in the Collaborative Perinatal Project[73] or in 174 women in another study.[118]

Aminoglycosides

Streptomycin and kanamycin have been associated with congenital deafness in the offspring of mothers who took these drugs during pregnancy. Ototoxicity was reported with doses as low as 1 g of streptomycin biweekly for 8 weeks during the first trimester.[119] Of 391 mothers who had received 50 mg/kg of kanamycin for prolonged periods during pregnancy, nine children (2.3 percent) were found to have hearing loss.[120]

Nephrotoxicity may be greater when aminoglycosides are combined with cephalosporins. Neuromuscular blockade may be potentiated by the combined use of aminoglycosides and curariform drugs; therefore, the dosages should be reduced appropriately. Potentiation of magnesium sulfate–induced neuromuscular weakness has also been reported in a neonate exposed to magnesium sulfate and gentamicin (Garamycin).[121]

No known teratogenic effect other than ototoxicity has been associated with the use of aminoglycosides in the first trimester. In 135 infants exposed to streptomycin in the Collaborative Perinatal Project,[73] no teratogenic effects were observed. In a group of 1,619 newborns whose mothers were treated for tuberculosis with multiple drugs, including streptomycin, the incidence of congenital defects was the same as in a healthy control group.[122]

Aminoglycosides are poorly absorbed after oral administration and are rapidly excreted by the normal kidney. Because the rate of clearance is related to the glomerular filtration rate, dosage must be reduced in the face of abnormal renal function. The serum aminoglycoside levels are usually lower in pregnant than in nonpregnant patients receiving equivalent doses because of more rapid elimination.[123] Thus, it is important to monitor levels to prevent subtherapeutic dosing. Once-a-day dosing with gentamicin at 4 mg/kg, in treatment of puerperal infections, increases efficacy and decreases toxicity and cost.[124]

Antituberculosis Drugs

There is no evidence of any teratogenic effect of isoniazid (INH), para-aminosalicylic acid (PAS), rifampin (Rifadin), or ethambutol (Myambutol).

Erythromycin

No teratogenic risk of erythromycin has been reported. In 79 patients in the Collaborative Perinatal Project[73] and 260 in another study,[118] no increase in birth defects was noted.

Erythromycin is not consistently absorbed from the gastrointestinal tract of pregnant women, and the transplacental passage is unpredictable. Both maternal and fetal plasma levels achieved after the administration of the drug in pregnancy are low and vary considerably, with fetal plasma concentrations being 5 to 20 percent of those in maternal plasma.[125] Thus, some authors have recommended that penicillin be administered to every newborn whose mother received erythromycin for the treatment of syphilis.[126] Fetal tissue levels increase after multiple doses.[125] The usual oral dose is 250 to 500 mg every 6 hours, but the higher dose may not be well tolerated in pregnant women who are susceptible to nausea and gastrointestinal symptoms.

Clarithromycin

Of 122 first-trimester exposures, there was no significant risk of birth defects.[127]

Clindamycin (Cleocin)

Of 647 infants exposed to clindamycin in the first trimester, no increased risk of birth defects was noted.[128] Clindamycin is nearly completely absorbed after oral administration; a small percentage is absorbed after topical application. The drug crosses the placenta, achieving maximum cord serum levels of about 50 percent of the maternal serum.[125] Clindamycin is 90 percent bound to serum protein, and fetal tissue levels increase following multiple dosing.[125] Maternal serum levels after dosing at various stages of pregnancy are similar to those of nonpregnant patients.

Quinolones

The quinolones (e.g., ciprofloxacin [Cipro], norfloxacin [Noraxin]) have a high affinity for bone tissue and cartilage and may cause arthralgia in children. However, no malformations or musculoskeletal problems were noted in 38 infants exposed in utero in the first trimester.[129] Of 132 newborns exposed in the first trimester in the Michigan Medicaid data, no increased risk of birth defects was noted.[130] The manufacturer recommends against use in pregnancy and in children.

Metronidazole (Flagyl)

Studies have failed to show any increase in the incidence of congenital defects among the newborns of mothers treated with metronidazole during early or late gestation. In a study of 1,387 prescriptions filled, no risk of birth defects could be determined.[131] A recent meta-analysis confirmed no teratogenic risk.[132]

Controversy regarding the use of metronidazole during pregnancy was stirred when metronidazole was shown to be mutagenic in bacteria by the Ames test, which correlates with carcinogenicity in animals. However, the doses used were much higher than those used clinically, and carcinogenicity in humans has not been confirmed.[133] As some have recommended against its use in pregnancy, metronidazole should still be given only for clear-cut indications and its use deferred until after the first trimester if possible.

Acyclovir (Zovirax)

The Acyclovir Registry has recorded 581 first-trimester exposures during pregnancy, with no increased risk of abnormalities in the infants.[26] The Centers for Disease Control and Prevention recommends that pregnant women with disseminated infection (e.g., herpetic encephalitis or hepatitis or varicella pneumonia) be treated with acyclovir.[134]

Lindane (Kwell)

After application of lindane to the skin, about 10 percent of the dose used can be recovered in the urine. Toxicity in humans after use of topical 1 percent lindane has been observed almost exclusively after misuse and overexposure to the agent. Although no evidence of specific fetal damage is attributable to lindane, the agent is a potent neurotoxin, and its use during pregnancy should be limited. Pregnant women should be cautioned about shampooing their children's hair, as absorption could easily occur across the skin of the hands of the mother. An alternate drug for lice is usually recommended, such as pyrethrins with piperonyl butoxide (RID).

Antifungal Agents

Nystatin (Mycostatin) is poorly absorbed from intact skin and mucous membranes, and topical use has not been associated with teratogenesis.[118] The imidazoles are absorbed in only small amounts from the vagina. Clotrimazole (Lotrimin) or miconazole (Monistat) in pregnancy is not known to be associated with congenital malformations. However, in one study a statistically significantly increased risk of first-trimester abortion was noted after use of these drugs, but these findings were considered not to be definitive evidence of risk.[135] Of 7,266 newborns exposed in the first trimester in the Michigan Medicaid data, there was no increased risk of anomalies.[136]

An increased risk of limb deformities was reported in fetuses exposed to 400 to 800 mg/day of fluconazole in the first trimester.[137] In 460 who received a single 150-mg dose of fluconazole, no increased risk of defects was observed.[138,139]

Drugs for Induction of Ovulation

In more than 2,000 exposures, no evidence of teratogenic risk of clomiphene (Clomid) has been noted,[140] and the percentage of spontaneous abortions is close to the expected rate. Although infants are often exposed to bromocriptine (Parlodel) in early pregnancy, no teratogenic effects have been observed in more than 1,400 pregnancies.[141]

Mild Analgesics

Few pains during pregnancy justify the use of a mild analgesic. Pregnant patients should be encouraged to use nonpharmacologic remedies, such as local heat and rest.

Aspirin

There is no evidence of any teratogenic effect of aspirin taken in the first trimester.[73,142] Aspirin does have significant perinatal effects, however, as it inhibits prostaglandin synthesis. Uterine contractility is decreased, and patients taking aspirin in analgesic doses have delayed onset of labor, longer duration of labor, and an increased risk of a prolonged pregnancy.[143]

Aspirin also decreases platelet aggregation, which can increase the risk of bleeding before as well as at delivery. Platelet dysfunction has been described in newborns within 5 days of ingestion of aspirin by the mother.[144] Because aspirin causes permanent inhibition of prostaglandin synthetase in platelets, the only way for adequate clotting to occur is for more platelets to be produced.

Multiple organs may be affected by chronic aspirin use. Of note, prostaglandins mediate the neonatal closure of the ductus arteriosus. In one case report, maternal ingestion of aspirin close to the time of delivery was related to closure of the ductus arteriosus in utero.[145]

Low-dose aspirin (80 mg/day) may ultimately prove of benefit in prevention of fetal wastage associated with autoimmune diseases. Lubbe et al.[146] treated patients with lupus anticoagulant and fetal wastage with prednisone 40 to 60 mg/day and low-dose aspirin (75 mg/day) with improved fetal outcome (see Chapter 22). Cowchock et al.[147] have reported that in patients with antiphospholipid-associated fetal wastage, heparin is preferable to prednisone in combination with low-dose aspirin.

Although preliminary small studies suggested that low-dose aspirin might prevent preeclampsia, a large randomized trial has not shown any benefit.[148] Aspirin 60 mg/day did not prevent preeclampsia in women with twins, chronic hypertension, insulin-dependent diabetes, or a history of preeclampsia in a previous pregnancy.[149]

Acetaminophen (Tylenol, Datril)

Acetaminophen has also shown no evidence of teratogenicity.[150] With acetaminophen, inhibition of prostaglandin synthesis is reversible so that, once the drug has cleared, platelet aggregation returns to normal. The bleeding time is not prolonged with acetaminophen in contrast to aspirin,[151] and the drug is not toxic to the newborn. Thus, if a mild analgesic or antipyretic is indicated, acetaminophen is preferred over aspirin. Absorption and disposition of acetaminophen in normal doses is not altered by pregnancy.[152]

Other Nonsteroidal Anti-inflammatory Agents

No evidence of teratogenicity has been reported for other nonsteroidal anti-inflatmmatory drugs (e.g., ibuprofen[153] [Motrin, Advil], naproxen[154] [Naprosyn]), but limited information is available. Chronic use may lead to oligohydramnios, and constriction of the fetal ductus arteriosus or neonatal pulmonary hypertension as has been reported with indomethacin might occur.

Propoxyphene (Darvon)

Propoxyphene is an acceptable alternative mild analgesic with no known teratogenicity.[73] However, it should not be used for trivial indications, as it carries potential for narcotic addiction. Evidence of risk in late pregnancy comes from case reports of infants of mothers who were addicted to propoxyphene and had typical narcotic withdrawal in the neonatal period.[155]

Codeine

In the Collaborative Perinatal Project, no increased relative risk of malformations was observed in 563 codeine user.[73] Codeine can cause addiction and newborn withdrawal symptoms if used to excess perinatally.

Sumatriptan

Of 183 exposures in the first trimester,[26] seven infants (3.8 percent) had birth defects, not significantly different from the nonexposed population.

Smoking

Smoking has been associated with a fourfold increase in small size for gestational age as well as an increased prematurity rate.[156] The spontaneous abortion rate is up to twice that of nonsmokers. Abortions associated with maternal smoking tend to have a higher percentage of normal karyotypes and occur later than those with chromosomal aberrations[157] (see Chapter 22). The higher perinatal mortality rate associated with smoking is attributable to an increased risk of abruptio placentae, placenta previa, premature and prolonged rupture of membranes, and intrauterine growth restriction. The risks of complications and of the associated perinatal loss rise with the number of cigarettes smoked. Discontinuation of smoking during pregnancy can reduce the risk of both pregnancy complications and perinatal mortality, especially in women at high risk for other reasons.[158] Maternal passive smoking was also associated with a twofold risk of low birth weight at term in one study.[159]

There is also a positive association between smoking and sudden infant death syndrome (SIDS) and increased respiratory illnesses in children. In such reports, it is not possible to distinguish between apparent effects of maternal smoking during pregnancy and smoking after pregnancy, but both may play a role.

Smoking Cessation during Pregnancy

Tobacco smoke contains nicotine, carbon monoxide, and thousands of other compounds. Although nicotine is the mechanism of addiction to cigarettes, other chemicals may contribute to adverse pregnancy outcome. For example, carbon monoxide decreases oxygen delivery to the fetus, whereas nicotine decreases uterine blood flow.

Nicotine withdrawal may first be attempted with nicotine fading, switching to brands of cigarettes with progressively less nicotine over a 3-week period. Exercise may also improve quitting success rates.[160] Nicotine

medications are indicated for patients with nicotine dependence. This is defined as greater than one pack per day smoking, smoking within 30 minutes of getting up in the morning, or prior withdrawal symptoms.[161] Nicotine medications are available as patches, gum, or inhalers. Although one might question the propriety of prescribing nicotine during pregnancy, if the patient can stop smoking she eliminates many other toxins, including carbon monoxide, and nicotine blood levels are similar to that of smokers.[162] There are no studies of bupropion (Zyban) in human pregnancy for smoking cessation.

Alcohol

The fetal alcohol syndrome (FAS) has been reported in the offspring of alcoholic mothers and includes the features of gross physical retardation with onset prenatally and continuing after birth (Fig. 9–8).[163]

In 1980, the Fetal Alcohol Study Group of the Research Society on Alcoholism proposed strict criteria for the diagnosis of FAS.[164] At least one characteristic from each of the following three categories had to be present for a valid diagnosis of the syndrome:

1. Growth retardation before and/or after birth
2. Facial anomalies, including small palpebral fissures, indistinct or absent philtrum, epicanthic folds, flattened nasal bridge, short length of nose, thin upper lip, low-set, unparallel ears, and retarded midfacial development
3. Central nervous system dysfunction including microcephaly, varying degrees of mental retardation, or other evidence of abnormal neurobehavioral development, such as attention deficit disorder with hyperactivity.

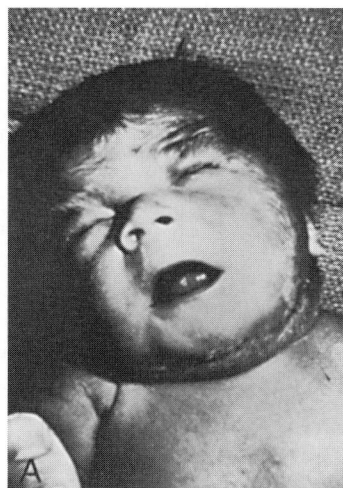 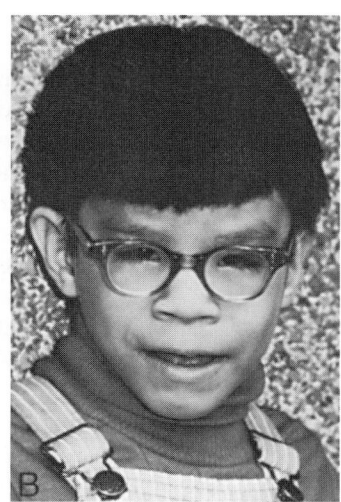 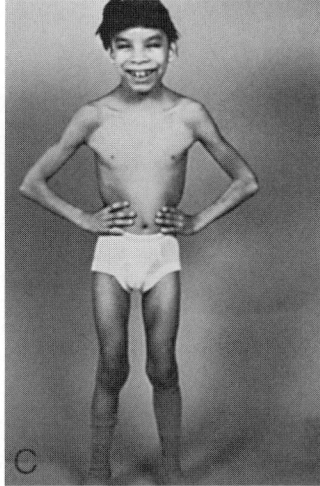

Figure 9–8. Fetal alcohol syndrome. Patient photographed at (*A*) birth, (*B*) 5 years, and (*C*) 8 years. Note short palpebral fissures, short nose, hypoplastic philtrum, thinned upper lip vermilion, and flattened midface. (From Streissguth AP: CIBA Foundation Monograph 105. London, Pitman, 1984, with permission.)

None of these features is individually pathognomonic for fetal alcohol exposure. Confirmatory evidence for this diagnosis is a history of heavy maternal drinking during pregnancy.

In the study of Jones et al.,[165] 23 chronically alcoholic women were matched with 46 controls and the pregnancy outcomes of the two groups compared. Among the alcoholic mothers, perinatal deaths were about eight times more frequent. Growth restriction, microcephaly, and IQ below 80 were considerably more frequent than among the controls. Overall outcome was abnormal in 43 percent of the offspring of the alcoholic mothers compared with 2 percent of the controls.

Ouellette et al.[166] addressed the risks of smaller amounts of alcohol. Nine percent of infants of abstinent or rare drinkers and 14 percent of infants of moderate drinkers were abnormal, not a significant difference. In heavy drinkers (average daily intake of 3 oz of 100-proof liquor or more), 32 percent of the infants had anomalies. Overall, including anomalies, growth restriction, and an abnormal neurologic examination, 71 percent of the children of heavy drinkers were affected, twice the frequency of abnormality found in the moderate and rarely drinking groups. In this study, an increased frequency of abnormality was not found until 45 ml of ethanol (equivalent to three drinks) daily were exceeded. The study of Mills and Graubard[167] also showed that total malformation rates were not significantly higher among offspring of women who had an average of less than one drink per day (77.3 in 1,000) or one to two drinks per day (83.2 in 1,000) than among nondrinkers (78.1 in 1,000). Genitourinary malformations increased with increasing alcohol consumption, however, so the possibility remains that for some malformations no safe drinking level exists.

Heavy drinking remains a major risk to the fetus, and reduction even in midpregnancy can benefit the infant. An occasional drink during pregnancy carries no known risk, but no level of drinking is known to be safe.

Sokol et al.[168] have addressed history taking for prenatal detection of risk drinking. Four questions help differentiate patients drinking sufficiently to potentially damage the fetus (Table 9–2). The patient is considered at risk if more than two drinks are required to make her feel "high." The probability of "risk drinking" increases to 63 percent for those responding positively to all four questions.

Marihuana

No teratogenic effect of marihuana has been documented. In a prospective study of 35 pregnancies,[169] infants born to marihuana users exhibited significantly more meconium staining (57 percent vs. 25 percent in

Table 9–2. THE T-ACE QUESTIONS FOUND TO IDENTIFY WOMEN DRINKING SUFFICIENTLY TO POTENTIALLY DAMAGE THE FETUS*

T	How many drinks does it take to make you feel high (can you hold) (*tolerance*)?
A	Have people *annoyed* you by criticizing your drinking?
C	Have you felt you ought to *cut down* on your drinking?
E	Have you ever had to drink first thing in the morning to steady your nerves or to get rid of a hangover (*eye-opener*)?

*Two points are scored as a positive answer to the tolerance question and one each for the other three. A score of 2 or more correctly identified 69 percent of risk drinkers.
From Sokol RJ, Martier SS, Ager JW: The T-ACE questions: practical prenatal detection of risk-drinking. Am J Obstet Gynecol 160:863, 1989, with permission.

nonusers). However, users tended to come from lower socioeconomic backgrounds. Most adverse outcomes of pregnancy were too infrequent to permit reliable comparisons between the groups. Marihuana users had an increased incidence of precipitate labor (<3 hours total), 29 percent compared with 3 percent in the control group.[169]

In another population in which the users and nonusers of marihuana were similar in general health, ethnic background, nutritional habits, and use of tobacco, these differences were not confirmed (19 patients in each group).[170] In this same small group of patients, average use of marihuana six or more times per week during pregnancy was associated with a reduction of 0.8 weeks in the length of gestation, although no reduction in birth weight was noted. One study suggested a mean 73-g decrease in birth weight associated with marihuana use, when urine assays were performed rather than relying on self-reporting.[171]

Cocaine

A serious difficulty in determining the effects of cocaine on the infant is the frequent presence of many confounding variables in the population using cocaine. These mothers often abuse other drugs, smoke, have poor nutrition, fail to seek prenatal care, and live under poor socioeconomic conditions. These factors are difficult to take into account in comparison groups. Another difficulty is the choice of outcome measures for infants exposed in utero. The neural systems likely to be affected by cocaine are involved in neurologic and behavioral functions that are not easily quantitated by standard infant development tests.

Cocaine-using women have a higher rate of spontaneous abortion than controls.[172] Three studies have suggested an increased risk of congenital anomalies after first-trimester cocaine use,[173–175] most frequently cardiac and central nervous system. In the study of Bingol et al.,[174] the malformation rate was 10 percent in cocaine users, 4.5 percent in polydrug users, and 2 percent in controls. MacGregor et al.[175] reported a 6 percent anomaly rate compared with 1 percent for controls.

Cocaine is a central nervous system stimulant and has local anesthetic and marked vasoconstrictive effects. Abruptio placentae has been reported to occur immediately after nasal or intravenous administration.[172] Several studies have also noted increased stillbirths, preterm labor, premature birth, and small-for-gestational-age infants with cocaine use.[171–173,176,177]

The impairment of intrauterine brain growth as manifested by microcephaly is the most common brain abnormality in infants exposed to cocaine in utero.[178] In one study, 16 percent of newborns had microcephaly compared with 6 percent of controls.[179] Somatic growth is also impaired, and so the growth restriction may be symmetric or characterized by a relatively low head circumference/abdominal circumference ratio.[180] Multiple other neurologic problems have been reported after cocaine exposure, as well as dysmorphic features and neurobehavioral abnormalities.[177]

Aside from causing congenital anomalies in the first trimester, cocaine has been reported to cause fetal disruption[181] presumably due to interruption of blood flow to various organs. Bowel infarction has been noted with unusual ileal atresia and bowel perforation. Limb infarction has resulted in missing fingers in a distribution different from the usual congenital limb anomalies. Central nervous system bleeding in utero may result in porencephalic cysts.

Narcotics

Menstrual abnormalities, especially amenorrhea, are common in heroin abusers, although they are not associated with the use of methadone. The goal of methadone maintenance is to bring the patient to a level of approximately 20 to 40 mg/day. The dose should be individualized at a level sufficient to minimize the use of supplemental illicit drugs, since they represent a greater risk to the fetus than do the higher doses of methadone required by some patients. Manipulation of the dose in women maintained on methadone should be avoided in the last trimester because of an association with increased fetal complications and in utero deaths attributed to fetal withdrawal in utero.[182] As management of narcotic addiction during pregnancy requires a host of social, nutritional, educational, and psychiatric interventions, these patients are best managed in specialized programs.

The infant of the narcotic addict is at increased risk of abortion, prematurity, and growth restriction. With-

drawal should be watched for carefully in the neonatal period.

Caffeine

There is no evidence of teratogenic effects of caffeine in humans. The Collaborative Perinatal Project[73] showed no increased incidence of congenital defects in 5,773 women taking caffeine in pregnancy, usually in a fixed-dose analgesic medication. There is still some conflicting evidence concerning the association between heavy ingestion of caffeine and increased pregnancy complications. Early studies suggested that the intake of greater than seven to eight cups of coffee per day (a cup of coffee contains about 100 mg of caffeine) was associated with low-birth-weight infants, spontaneous abortions, prematurity, and stillbirths.[183] However, these studies were not controlled for the concomitant use of tobacco and alcohol. In one report controlled for smoking, other habits, demographic characteristics, and medical history, no relationship was found between either low birth weight or short gestation and heavy coffee consumption.[184] Also, there was no excess of malformations among coffee drinkers. When pregnant women consumed over 300 mg of caffeine per day, one study suggested an increase in term low-birth-weight infants,[185] less than 2,500 g at greater than 36 weeks.

Concomitant consumption of caffeine with cigarette smoking may increase the risk of low birth weight.[186] Maternal coffee intake decreases iron absorption and may contribute to maternal anemia.[187]

Two other studies have shown conflicting results. One retrospective investigation reporting a higher risk of fetal loss was biased by ascertainment of the patients at the time of fetal loss, as these patients typically have less nausea and would be expected to drink more coffee.[188] A prospective cohort study found no evidence that moderate caffeine use increased the risk of spontaneous abortion or growth retardation.[189] Measurement of serum paraxanthine, a caffeine metabolite, revealed that only extremely high levels are associated with spontaneous abortions.[190]

Aspartame (NutraSweet)

The major metabolite of aspartame is phenylalanine,[191] which is concentrated in the fetus by active placental transport. Sustained high blood levels of phenylalanine in the fetus as seen in maternal phenylketonuria (PKU) are associated with mental retardation in the infant. Within the usual range of aspartame ingestion, peak phenylalanine levels do not exceed normal postprandial levels, and even with high doses phenylalanine concentrations are still very far below those associated with mental retardation. These responses have also been studied in women known to be carriers of PKU, and the levels are still normal. Thus, it seems unlikely that use of aspartame in pregnancy would cause any fetal toxicity.

Drugs in Breast Milk

Many drugs can be detected in breast milk at low levels that are not usually of clinical significance to the infant. The rate of transfer into milk depends on the lipid solubility, molecular weight, degree of protein binding, degree of ionization of the drug, and the presence or absence of active secretion. Nonionized molecules of low molecular weight such as ethanol cross easily.[192] If the mother has unusually high blood concentrations such as with increased dosage or decreased renal function, drugs may appear in higher concentrations in the milk.

The amount of drug in breast milk is a variable fraction of the maternal blood level, which itself is proportional to the maternal oral dose. Thus, the dose to the infant is usually subtherapeutic, approximately 1 to 2 percent of the maternal dose on the average. This amount is usually so trivial that no adverse effects are noted. In the case of toxic drugs, however, any exposure may be inappropriate. Allergy may also be possible. Long-term effects of even small doses of drugs may yet be discovered. Also, drugs are eliminated more slowly in the infant with immature enzyme systems. Short-term effects of most maternal medications on breast-fed infants are mild and pose little risk to the infants. As the benefits of breast-feeding are well known, the risk of drug exposure must be weighed against these benefits.

With respect to drug administration in the immediate few days postpartum before lactation is fully established, the infant receives only a small volume of colostrum, and thus little drug is excreted into the milk at this time. It is helpful to allay fears of patients undergoing cesarean deliveries that analgesics or other drugs administered at this time will have no known adverse effects on the infant. For drugs requiring daily dosing during lactation, knowledge of pharmacokinetics in breast milk may minimize the dose to the infant. For example, dosing after nursing will decrease the exposure, as the blood level will be lowest before the next dose.

The short-term effects, if any, of most maternal medications on breast-fed infants are mild and pose little risk to the infants.[193] Of 838 breast-feeding women, 11.2 percent reported minor infant adverse reactions in the infants, but these did not require medical attention. In 19 percent antibiotics caused diarrhea; in 11 percent narcotics caused drowsiness; in 9 percent antihistamines caused irritability; and in 10 percent sedatives, antidepressants, or antiepileptics caused drowsiness.[193]

The American Academy of Pediatrics has reviewed drugs in lactation[194] and categorized the drugs as listed below.

Drugs Commonly Listed as Contraindicated during Breast-Feeding

Cytotoxic Agents

Cyclosporine (Sandimmune), doxorubicin (Adriamycin), and cyclophosphamide (Cytoxan) might cause immune suppression in the infant, although data are limited with respect to these and other cytotoxic agents. In general, the potential risks of these drugs would outweigh the benefits of continuing nursing if these were required.

After oral administration to a lactating patient with choriocarcinoma, methotrexate was found in milk in low but detectable levels (0.26 μg/dl). Most individuals would elect to avoid any exposure of the infant to this drug. However, in environments in which bottle feeding is rarely practiced and presents practical and cultural difficulties, therapy with this drug would not in itself appear to constitute a contraindication to breast-feeding.[195] Busulphan (Myleran) has been reported to cause no adverse effect in nursing infants.[196]

Bromocriptine (Parlodel)

This agent is an ergot alkaloid derivative that has an inhibitory effect on lactation. However, in one report, a mother taking 5 mg/day for a pituitary tumor was able to nurse her infant.[197]

Ergotamine (Ergomar)

This medication has been reported to be associated with vomiting, diarrhea, and convulsions in the infant in doses used in migraine medications. However, short-term ergot therapy in the postpartum period for uterine atony is not a contraindication to lactation.

Lithium (Eskalith, Lithobid)

Lithium reaches one third to one half the therapeutic blood concentration in infants, who might develop lithium toxicity, with hypotonia and lethargy.[198]

Amphetamines

One report of 103 cases of exposure to amphetamines in breast milk noted no insomnia or stimulation in the infants.[199] However, amphetamines are concentrated in breast milk.

Radioactive Compounds That Require Temporary Cessation of Breast-Feeding

Radiopharmaceuticals require variable intervals of interruption of nursing to ensure that no radioactivity is detectable in the milk. Intervals generally quoted are, for ^{67}Ga, 2 weeks; ^{131}I, 5 days; radioactive sodium, 4 days; and ^{99}Tc, 24 hours. For reassurance, the milk may be counted for radioactivity before nursing is resumed.[200]

Drugs Whose Effects on Nursing Infants Are Unknown but May Be of Concern

Psychotropic drugs such as antianxiety, antidepressant, and antipsychotic agents are sometimes given to nursing mothers for long periods. Although there are no data about adverse effects in infants exposed to these drugs via breast milk, they could theoretically alter central nervous system function.[194] Fluoxetine (Prozac) is excreted in breast milk at low levels, so the infant receives approximately 6.7 percent of the maternal dose.[201] The level in the breast-fed newborn is certainly lower than the level during pregnancy.[202]

Sertraline causes a decline in 5-hydroxytryptamine levels in mothers, but not in their breast-fed infants.[203] This implies that the small amount of drug the infant ingests in breast milk is not enough to have a pharmacologic effect (Fig. 9–9).

Temporary cessation of breast-feeding after a single dose of metronidazole (Flagyl) may be considered. Its half-life is such that interruption of lactation for 12 to 24 hours after single-dose therapy usually results in negligible exposure to the infant. It is excreted into breast milk with a milk/plasma ratio of about 1:0. Therefore, even if a woman continued to nurse, the infant would get a trivial dose.

Drugs Usually Compatible with Breast-Feeding

Narcotics, Sedatives, and Anticonvulsants

In general, no evidence of adverse effect is noted with most of the sedatives, narcotic analgesics, and anticonvulsants. Patients may be reassured that, in normal doses, carbamazepine (Tegretol),[204] phenytoin (Dilantin), magnesium sulfate, codeine, morphine, and meperidine (Demerol) do not cause any obvious adverse effects in the infants,[205] since the dose detectable in the breast milk is approximately 1 to 2 percent of the mother's dose, which is sufficiently low to have no significant pharmacologic activity.

With diazepam (Valium), the milk/plasma ratio at peak dose is 0.68, with only small amounts detected in

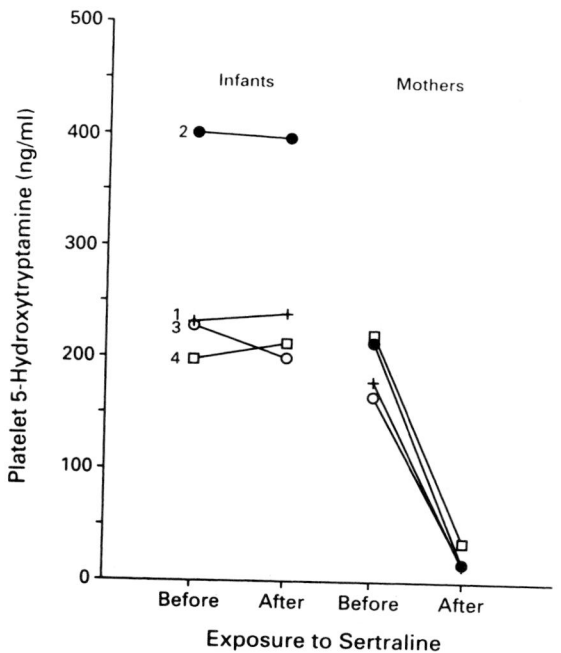

Figure 9–9. Effect of sertraline on platelet 5-hydroxytryptamine levels in four breast-fed infants and their mothers. (From Epperson CN, Anderson GM, McDougle CJ: Sertraline and breast-feeding. N Engl J Med 336:1189, 1997. Copyright 1997 Massachusetts Medical Society, with permission.)

the breast milk.[206] In two patients who took carbamazepine (Tegretol) while nursing, the concentration of the drug in breast milk at 4 and 5 weeks postpartum was similar, about 60 percent of the maternal serum level. Accumulation does not seem to occur, and no adverse effects were noted in either infant.[207]

In studies in which phenobarbital[208] and phenytoin (Dilantin) levels were measured, only small amounts of these drugs were detected in breast milk. Phenobarbital and diazepam (Valium) are slowly eliminated by the infant, however, and so accumulation may occur. Women consuming barbiturates or benzodiazepines should observe the infants for sedation.

In 10 preeclamptic patients receiving magnesium sulfate 1 g/h intravenously for 24 hours after delivery, magnesium levels in breast milk were 64 µg/ml compared with 48 µg/ml in controls.[209] Breast milk calcium levels were not affected by magnesium sulfate therapy.

Analgesics

Aspirin is transferred into breast milk in small amounts. Since acids exist primarily in the ionized form, salicylate transport from plasma into milk is not favored. The risk is related to high dosages (e.g., >16 300-mg tablets per day in the mother, when the infant may get sufficiently high serum levels to affect platelet aggregation or even cause metabolic acidosis).

No harmful effects of acetaminophen (Tylenol, Datril) have been noted. In one patient taking propoxyphene (Darvon) in a suicide attempt, the level in breast milk was half that of the serum. A breast-feeding infant could theoretically receive up to 1 mg of propoxyphene a day if the mother were to consume the maximum dose continually.[210] One infant was reported to have poor muscle tone when the mother was taking propoxyphene every 4 hours.

Antihistamines and Decongestants

Although studies are not extensive, no harmful effects have been noted from antihistamines or decongestants. Less than 1 percent of a pseudoephedrine dose or tripolidine dose ingested by the mother is excreted in the breast milk.[211]

Aminophylline

Maximum milk concentrations of aminophylline are achieved between 1 and 3 hours after an oral dose. The nursing infant has been calculated to receive less than 1 percent of the maternal dose with no noted adverse effects. To minimize neonatal drug exposure, however, a nursing mother should try to breast-feed her infant immediately before her doses of the drug.[212]

Antihypertensives

THIAZIDES. After a single 500-mg oral dose of chlorothiazide (Diuril), no drug was detected in breast milk at a sensitivity of 1 μg/ml.[213] In one mother taking 50 mg of hydrochlorothiazide (Hydrodiuril) daily, peak milk levels were about 25 percent of maternal blood levels. The drug was not detectable in the nursing infant's serum, and the infant's electrolytes were normal.[214] Thiazide diuretics may decrease milk production in the first month of lactation.[194]

β-BLOCKERS. Propranolol (Inderal) is excreted in breast milk, with milk concentrations after a single 40-mg dose less than 40 percent of peak plasma concentrations. In one patient on a continuous dosage of 40 mg four times daily,[215] plasma and breast milk concentrations peaked 3 hours after dosing and the peak breast milk concentration of 42 ng/ml was 64 percent of the corresponding plasma concentration. After a 30-day regimen of 240 mg/day of propranolol, the predose and 3-hour postdose propranolol concentrations in breast milk were 26 and 64 ng/ml, respectively. Thus, an infant consuming 500 ml/day of milk would ingest a maximum of 21 μg in 24 hours at a maternal dose of 160 mg/day and a maximum of 32 μg in 24 hours at a maternal dose of 240 mg/day. This amount represents

approximately 1 percent of a therapeutic dose, which is unlikely to cause any adverse effect.[216]

Atenolol (Tenormin) is concentrated in breast milk to about three times the plasma level.[217] One case has been reported in which a 5-day-old term infant had signs of β-adrenergic blockade with bradycardia (80 bpm) with the breast milk dose calculated to be 9 percent of the maternal dose.[218] Adverse effects in other infants have not been reported. As milk accumulation occurs with atenolol, infants must be monitored closely for bradycardia. Propranolol is a safer alternative.[219]

Clonidine (Catapres) concentrations in milk are almost twice maternal serum levels.[220] Neurologic and laboratory parameters in the infants of treated mothers are similar to those of controls.

ACE INHIBITORS. Captopril (Capoten) is excreted into breast milk in low levels, and no effects on nursing infants have been observed.[221]

CALCIUM CHANNEL BLOCKERS. Nifedipine is excreted into breast milk at a concentration of less than 5 percent of the maternal dose,[222] and verapamil at an even lower level. Neither have caused adverse effects in the infant.

Anticoagulants

Most mothers requiring anticoagulation may continue to nurse their infants with no problems. Heparin does not cross into milk and is not active orally.

At a maternal dose of warfarin (Coumadin) of 5 to 12 mg/day in seven patients with maternal plasma concentrations of 0.5 to 2.6 μg/ml, no warfarin was detected in infant breast milk or plasma at a sensitivity of 0.025 μg/ml. This low concentration is probably because warfarin is 98 percent protein bound. Thus, 1 L of milk would contain 20 μg of the drug at maximum, an insignificant amount to have an anticoagulant effect.[223] Another report confirms that warfarin appears only in insignificant quantities in breast milk.[224] The oral anticoagulant bishydroxycoumarin (dicumarol) has been given to 125 nursing mothers with no effect on the infants' prothrombin times and no hemorrhages.[225] Thus, with careful monitoring of maternal prothrombin time so that the dosage is minimized and of neonatal prothrombin times to ensure lack of drug accumulation, warfarin may be safely administered to nursing mothers.

This safety does not apply to all oral anticoagulant drugs, however. Phenindione,[226] a drug not used in the United States, has caused infant bleeding.

Corticosteroids

In one patient requiring corticosteroids, breast milk was obtained 2 hours after an oral dose of 10 mg of prednisone (Deltasone). The levels in the milk were 0.1 μg/dl of prednisolone and 2.67 μg/dl of prednisone. Thus, an infant taking 1 L of milk would obtain 28.3 μg of the two steroids, an mount not likely to have any deleterious effect.[227] In another study of seven patients,[228] 0.14 percent of a sample was secreted in the milk in the subsequent 60 hours, a negligible quantity. Thus, breast-feeding is allowed in mothers taking corticosteroids. Even at 80 mg/day, the nursing infant would ingest less than 0.1 percent of the dose, less than 10 percent of its endogenous cortisol.[229]

Digoxin (Lanoxin)

After a maternal dose of 0.25 mg, peak breast milk levels of 0.6 to 1 ng/ml occur, and the milk/plasma ratio at the 4-hour peak is 0.8 to 0.9. This represents a small amount due to significant maternal protein binding. In 24 hours, an infant would receive about 1 percent of the maternal dose.[230] No adverse effects in nursing infants have been reported.

Antibiotics

Penicillin derivatives are safe in nursing mothers. In the usual therapeutic doses of penicillin or ampicillin (Amoxil), the mother's milk/plasma ratios are only up to 0.2, and no adverse effects are noted in the infants. In susceptible individuals or with prolonged therapy, diarrhea and candidiasis are theoretical concerns.

Dicloxacillin (Pathocil) is 98 percent protein bound. If this drug is used to treat breast infections, very little will get into the breast milk, and nursing may be continued.

Cephalosporins appear only in trace amounts in milk. In one study after cefazolin 500 mg intramuscularly three times a day (Ancef, Kefzol), no drug was detected in breast milk.[231] After 2 g of cefazolin intravenously, 1.51 μg/ml was detected, for a milk/plasma ratio of 0.023 at the 3-hour peak level. Thus, the infant was exposed less than 1 percent of the maternal dose.

Tooth staining or delayed bone growth from tetracyclines have not been reported after the drug was taken by a breast-feeding mother. This finding is probably because of the high binding of the drug to calcium and protein, limiting its absorption from the milk. The amount in the milk is about half the level in the mother's plasma. Therefore, the amount of free tetracycline available is too small to be significant.

Sulfonamides only appear in small amounts in breast milk and are ordinarily not contraindicated during nursing. However, the drug is best avoided in premature infants or ill or stressed infants when hyper bilirubinemia may be a problem, as the drug may displace bilirubin from binding sites on albumin. In one study of sulfapyridine, the drug and its metabolites were detected in plasma and milk at levels of 4 to 7 μg/ml. Thus, the infant would receive less than 1 percent of the maternal dose. When a mother took sulfasalazine (Azulfidine) 500 mg every 6 hours, the drug was undetectable in all milk samples.

Gentamicin (Garamycin) is transferred into breast milk, and half of nursing newborn infants have the drug detectable in their serum. The low levels detected would not be expected to cause clinical effects.[232]

Nitrofurantoin (Macrodantin) is excreted into breast milk in very low concentrations. In one study the drug could not be detected in 20 samples from mothers receiving 100 mg four times a day.[233]

Erythromycin is excreted into breast milk in small amounts, with milk/plasma ratios of about 0.5. No reports of adverse effects on infants exposed to erythromycin in breast milk have been noted. Azithromycin (Zithromax) also appears in breast milk in low concentrations.[234] Clindamycin (Cleocin) is excreted into breast milk in low levels, and nursing is usually continued during administration of this drug.

There are no reported adverse effects on the infant of isoniazid (INH) administered to nursing mothers, and its use is considered compatible with breast-feeding.[194]

Acyclovir

Acyclovir is concentrated in breast milk with the average ratio of milk to serum 3.24.[235] The amount to which the infant would be exposed through breast milk will be less than 1 mg/day if the mother is taking 1,000 mg/day, which seems of low theoretical risk, provided the infant has normal renal function.

Antifungal Agents

No data are available with nystatin, miconazole, or clotrimazole in breast milk, but as only small amounts are absorbed vaginally, this would not be expected to be a problem.

Infant exposure to ketoconazole in human milk was 0.4 percent of the therapeutic dose, unlikely to cause adverse effects.[236]

Oral Contraceptives

Estrogen and progestin combination oral contraceptives cause a dose-related suppression of the quantity of milk produced. The use of oral contraceptives containing 50 μg and more of estrogen during lactation has been associated with shortened duration of lactation, decreased milk production, decreased infant weight gain, and decreased composition of nitrogen and protein content of the milk. However, the composition and volume of breast milk may vary considerably even in the absence of birth control pills. Lactation is inhibited to a lesser degree if the pill is started about 3 weeks postpartum and with lower doses of estrogen than 50 μg. Although the magnitude of the changes is low, the changes may be of nutritional importance, particularly in malnourished mothers. However, if the patient persists in taking birth control pills while nursing, there is no documented adverse effect of this practice.

An infant consuming 600 ml of breast milk daily from a mother using an oral contraceptive containing 50 μg of the ethinylestradiol receives a daily dose in the range of 10 ng of the estrogen.[237] The amount of natural estradiol received by infants who consume a similar volume of milk from mothers not using oral contraceptives is estimated at 3 to 6 ng during anovulatory cycles and 6 to 12 ng during ovulatory cycles. No consistent long-term adverse effects on children's growth and development have been described.

Evidence indicates that norgestrel (Ovrette) is metabolized rather than accumulated by the infants and, to date, no adverse effects have been identified as a result of progestational agents taken by the mother. Progestin-only contraceptives do not cause alteration of breast milk composition or volume,[238] making them ideal in the breast-feeding mother. When the infant is weaned, the mother should be switched to combined oral contraceptives for maximum contraceptive efficacy.

Alcohol

Alcohol levels in breast milk are similar to those in maternal blood. If a moderate social drinker had two cocktails and had a blood alcohol concentration of 50 mg/1 dl, the nursing infant would receive about 82 mg of alcohol, which would produce insignificant blood concentrations.[192] There is no evidence that occasional ingestion of alcohol by a mother is harmful to the infant. However, one study showed that ethanol ingested chronically through breast milk might have a detrimental effect on motor development, but not mental development, in the infant.[239] Also, alcohol in breast milk has an immediate effect on the odor of the milk, and this may decrease the amount of milk the infant consumes.[240]

Propylthiouracil

PTU is found in breast milk in small amounts.[241] If the mother takes 200 mg PTU three times a day, the child would receive 149 μg daily, or the equivalent of a 70-kg adult receiving 3 mg/day. Several infants have been studied up to 5 months of age with no changes in thyroid parameters, including TSH. Lactating mothers on PTU can continue nursing with close supervision of the infant.[241,242] PTU is preferred over methimazole (Tapazole) due to its high protein binding (80 percent) and lower breast milk concentrations.[243]

H₂-Receptor Blockers

In theory, H₂-receptor antagonists (e.g., ranitidine, cimetidine) might suppress gastric acidity and/or cause central nervous system stimulation in the infant, but these effects have not been confirmed in published studies. The American Academy of Pediatrics now considers H₂-receptor antagonists to be compatible with breast-feeding.[194] Famotidine, nizatidine, and roxatidine are less concentrated in breast milk and may be preferable in nursing mothers.[244]

Caffeine

Caffeine has been reported to have no adverse effects on the nursing infant, even after the mother consumes several cups of strong coffee.[243] In one study, the milk level contained 1 percent of the total dose 6 hours after coffee ingestion, which is not enough to affect the infant. In another report, no significant difference in 24-hour heart rate or sleep time was observed in nursing infants when their mothers drank coffee for 5 days or abstained for 5 days.[245]

Smoking

Nicotine and its metabolite cotinine enter breast milk. Infants of smoking mothers achieve significant serum concentrations of nicotine even if they are not exposed to passive smoking, and exposure to passive smoking further raises the levels of nicotine.[246] Women who smoke should be encouraged to stop smoking during lactation as well as during pregnancy.[247]

Conclusions

Many medical conditions during pregnancy and lactation are best treated initially with nonpharmacologic remedies. Before a drug is administered in pregnancy, the indications should be clear and the risk/benefit ratio should justify drug use. If possible, therapy should be postponed until after the first trimester. In addition, patients should be cautioned about the risks of social drug use such as smoking, alcohol, and cocaine during pregnancy. Most drug therapy does not require cessation of lactation, as the amount excreted into breast milk is sufficiently small to be pharmacologically insignificant.

Key Points

> ➤ Infants of epileptic women taking anticonvulsants have double the rate of malformations of

➤ unexposed infants; the risk of fetal hydantoin syndrome is less than 10 percent.

➤ The risk of malformations after in utero exposure to isotretinoin is 25 percent, and an additional 25 percent of infants have mental retardation.

➤ Heparin is the drug of choice for anticoagulation during pregnancy, although there is some risk of osteoporosis from its use.

➤ Angiotensin-converting enzyme inhibitors can cause fetal renal failure in the second and third trimesters, leading to oligohydramnios and hypoplastic lungs.

➤ Vitamin B_6 25 mg three times a day is a safe and effective therapy for first-trimester nausea and vomiting; doxylamine (Unisom) 12.5 mg three times a day is also effective in combination with B_6.

➤ Most antibiotics are generally safe in pregnancy. Cephalosporins and trimethoprim may carry an increased risk in the first trimester, and tetracyclines cause tooth discoloration in the second and third trimesters. Aminoglycosides can cause fetal ototoxicity.

➤ Aspirin in analgesic doses inhibits platelet function and prolongs bleeding time; thus, alternate analgesics are preferred in pregnancy.

➤ Fetal alcohol syndrome occurs in infants of mothers drinking heavily during pregnancy. A safe level of alcohol intake during pregnancy has not been determined.

➤ Cocaine has been associated with increased risk of spontaneous abortions, abruptio placentae, and congenital malformations, in particular, microcephaly.

➤ Most drugs are safe during lactation, as subtherapeutic amounts appear in breast milk, approximately 1 to 2 percent of the maternal dose.

REFERENCES

1. Wilson JG, Fraser FC (eds): Handbook of Teratology. New York, Plenum, 1979.
2. Blake DA, Niebyl JR: Requirements and limitations in reproductive and teratogenic risk assessment. *In* Niebyl JR (ed): Drug Use in Pregnancy, 2nd ed. Philadelphia, Lea & Febiger, 1988.
3. Heinonen OP, Slone D, Monson RR, et al: Cardiovascular birth defects and antenatal exposure to female sex hormones. N Engl J Med 296:67, 1977.
4. Wiseman RA, Dodds-Smith IC: Cardiovascular birth defects and antenatal exposure to female sex hormones: a reevaluation of some base data. Teratology 30:359, 1984.
5. Katz Z, Lancet M, Skornik J, et al: Teratogenicity of progestagens given during the first trimester of pregnancy. Obstet Gynecol 65:775, 1985.
6. Raman-Wilms L, Tseng AL, Wighardt S, et al: Fetal genital effects of firm-trimester sex hormone exposure: a meta-analysis. Obstet Gynecol 85:141, 1995.
7. Wilkins L: Masculinization of female fetus due to use of orally given progestins. JAMA 172:1028, 1960.
8. Duck SC, Katayama KP: Danazol may cause female pseudohermaphroditism. Fertil Steril 35:230, 1981.
9. Shapiro S, Slone D, Heinonen OP, et al: Birth defects and vaginal spermicides. JAMA 247:2381, 1982.
10. Mills JL, Reed GF, Nugent RP, et al: Are there adverse effects of periconceptional spermicide use? Fertil Steril 43:442, 1985.
11. Linn S, Schoenbaum SC, Monson RR, et al: Lack of association between contraceptive usage and congenital malformations in offspring. Am J Obstet Gynecol 147:923, 1983.
12. Robert E, Guibaud P: Maternal valproic acid and congenital neural tube defects. Lancet 2:937, 1982.
13. Rosa FW: Spina bifida in infants of women treated with carbamazepine during pregnancy. N Engl J Med 324:674, 1991.
14. Nakane Y, Okuma T, Takashashi R, et al: Multi-institutional study on the teratogenicity and fetal toxicity of antiepileptic drugs: a report of a collaborative study group in Japan. Epilepsia 21:663, 1980.
15. Dansky LV, Rosenblatt DS, Andermann E: Mechanisms of teratogenesis: folic acid and antiepileptic therapy. Neurology 42:32, 1992.
16. Centers for Disease Control: Recommendations for the use of folic acid to reduce the number of cases of spina bifida and other neural tube defects. MMWR Morb Mortal Wkly Rep 41:1, 1992.
17. Biale Y, Lewenthal H: Effect of folic acid supplementation on congenital malformations due to anticonvulsive drugs. Eur J Obstet Gynecol Reprod Biol 18:211, 1984.
18. Hanson JW, Smith DW: The fetal hydantoin syndrome. J Pediatr 87:285, 1975.
19. Gaily E, Granstrom M-L, Hiilesmaa V, et al: Minor anomalies in offspring of epileptic mothers. J Pediatr 112:520, 1988.
20. Jones KL, Lacro RV, Johnson KA, et al: Pattern of malformations in the children of women treated with carbamazepine during pregnancy. N Engl J Med 320:1661, 1989.
21. Strickler SM, Miller MA, Andermann E, et al: Genetic predisposition to phenytoin-induced birth defects. Lancet 2:746, 1985.
22. Buehler BA, Delimont D, VanWaes M, et al: Prenatal prediction of risk of the fetal hydantoin syndrome. N Engl J Med 322:1567, 1990.
23. Van der Pol MC, Hadders-Algra M, Huisjes JH, et al: Antiepileptic medication in pregnancy: late effects on the children's central nervous system development. Am J Obstet Gynecol 164:121, 1991.
24. Scolnik D, Nulman I, Rovet J, et al: Neurodevelopment of children exposed in utero to phenytoin and carbamazepine monotherapy. JAMA 271:767, 1994.
25. Reinisch JM, Sanders SA, Mortensen EL, et al: In utero exposure to phenobarbital and intelligence deficits in adult men. JAMA 274:1518, 1995.
26. Reiff-Eldridge R, Heffner CR, Ephross SA, et al: Monitoring pregnancy outcomes after prenatal drug exposure through

prospective pregnancy registries: a pharmaceutical company commitment. Am J Obstet Gynecol 182:159, 2000.

27. Briggs GG, Freeman RK, Yaffe SJ: Drugs in Pregnancy and Lactation, 5th ed. Baltimore, Williams & Wilkins, 1998, p 592.

28. Morrell MJ: The new antiepileptic drugs and women: efficacy, reproductive health, pregnancy, and fetal outcome. Epilepsia 37:S34, 1996.

29. Callaghan N, Garrett A, Goggin T: Withdrawal of anticonvulsant drugs in patients free of seizures for two years. N Engl J Med 318:942, 1988.

30. Deblay MF, Vert P, Andre M, et al: Transplacental vitamin K prevents haemorrhagic disease of infant of epileptic mother. Lancet 1:1247, 1982.

31. Lammer EJ, Chen DT, Hoar RM, et al: Retinoic acid embryopathy. N Engl J Med 313:837, 1985.

32. Adams J: High incidence of intellectual deficits in 5 year old children exposed to isotretinoin "in utero." Teratology 41: 614, 1990.

33. Dai WS, Hsu M-A, Itri L: Safety of pregnancy after discontinuation of isotretinoin. Arch Dermatol 125:362, 1989.

34. Jick SS, Terris BZ, Jick H: First trimester topical tretinoin and congenital disorders. Lancet 341:1181, 1993.

35. Rothman KJ, Moore LL, Singer MR, et al: Teratogenicity of high vitamin A intake. N Engl J Med 333:1369, 1995.

36. Mills JL, Simpson JL, Cunningham GC, et al: Vitamin A and birth defects. Am J Obstet Gynecol 177:31, 1997.

37. Czeizel A: Lack of evidence of teratogenicity of benzodiazepine drugs in Hungary. Reprod Toxicol 3:183, 1988.

38. Laegreid L, Olegard R, Wahlstrom J, et al: Abnormalities in children exposed to benzodiazepines in utero. Lancet 1:108, 1987.

39. Bergman V, Rosa F, Baum C, et al: Effects of exposure to benzodiazepine during fetal life. Lancet 340:694, 1992.

40. Linden S, Rich CL: The use of lithium during pregnancy and lactation. J Clin Psychiatry 44:358, 1983.

41. Weinstein MR, Goldfield MD: Cardiovascular malformations with lithium use during pregnancy. Am J Psychiatry 132:529, 1975.

42. Zalzstein E, Koren G, Einarson T, et al: A case-control study on the association between first trimest exposure to lithium and Ebstein's anomaly. Am J Cardiol 65:817, 1990.

43. Jacobson SJ, Jones K, Johnson K, et al: Prospective multicentre study of pregnancy outcome after lithium exposure during first trimester. Lancet 339:530, 1992.

44. Krause S, Ebbesen F, Lange AP: Polyhydramnios with maternal lithium treatment. Obstet Gynecol 75:504, 1990.

45. Ang MS, Thorp JA, Parisi VM: Maternal lithium therapy and polyhydramnios. Obstet Gynecol 76:517, 1990.

46. Cohen LS, Friedman MJ, Jefferson JW: A reevaluation of risk of in utero exposure to lithium. JAMA 271:146, 1994.

47. Briggs GC, Freeman RK, Jaffe SJ: Drugs in Pregnancy and Lactation, 5th ed. Baltimore, Williams & Wilkins, 1998, p 529.

48. Briggs GC, Freeman RK, Yaffe SJ: Drugs in Pregnancy and Lactation, 5th ed. Baltimore, Williams & Wilkins, 1998, p 46.

49. Pastuszak A, Schick-Boschetto B, Zuber C, et al: Pregnancy outcome following first-trimester exposure to fluoxetine (Prozac). JAMA 269:2446, 1993.

50. Goldstein DJ, Corbin LA, Sundell KL: Effects of first-trimester fluoxetine exposure on the newborn. Obstet Gynecol 89:713, 1997.

51. Nulman I, Rovert J, Stewart DE, et al: Neurodevelopment of children exposed in utero to antidepressant drugs. N Engl J Med 336:258, 1997.

52. Coleman FH, Christensen HD, Gonzalez CL, et al: Behavioral changes in developing mice after prenatal exposure to paroxetine (Paxil). Am J Obstet Gynecol 181:1166, 1999.

53. Chambers CD, Johnson KA, Dick LM, et al: Birth outcomes in pregnant women taking fluoxetine. N Engl J Med 335: 1010, 1996.

54. Kulin NA, Pastuszak A, Sage SR, et al: Pregnancy outcome following maternal use of the new selective serotonin reuptake inhibitors: a prospective controlled multicenter study. JAMA 279:609, 1998.

55. Hill RM, Stern L: Drugs in pregnancy: effects on the fetus and newborn. Drugs 17:182, 1979.

56. Sbarouni E, Oakley CM: Outcome of pregnancy in women with valve prostheses. Br Heart J 71:196, 1994.

57. deSwiet M, Ward PD, Fidler J, et al: Prolonged heparin therapy in pregnancy causes bone demineralization. Br J Obstet Gynaecol 90:1129, 1983.

58. Barbour LA, Kick SD, Steiner JF, et al: A prospective study of heparin-induced osteoporosis in pregnancy using bone densitometry. Am J Obstet Gynecol 170:862 1994.

50. Dahlman TC: Osteoporotic fractures and the recurrence of thromboembolism during pregnancy and the puerperium in 184 women undergoing thromboprophylaxis with heparin. Am J Obstet Gynecol 168:1265, 1993.

60. Nelson-Piercy C, Letsky EA, deSwiet M: Low-molecular-weight heparin for obstetric thromboprophylaxis: experience of sixty-nine pregnancies in sixty-one women at high risk. Am J Obstet Gynecol 176:1062, 1997.

61. Casele HL, Laifer SA, Woelkers DA, et al: Changes in the pharmacokinetics of the low-molecular-weight heparin enoxaparin sodium during pregnancy. Am J Obstet Gynecol 181: 1113, 1999.

62. Ginsberg JS, Hirsh J: Use of antithrombotic agents during pregnancy. Chest 114:524S, 1998.

63. Chan WS, Ray JG: Low molecular weight heparin use during pregnancy: issues of safety and practicality. Obstet Gynecol Survey 54:649, 1999.

64. Tengborn L, Bergqvist D, Matzsch T, et al: Recurrent thromboembolism in pregnancy and puerperium: is there a need for thromboprophylaxis? Am J Obstet Gynecol 160:90, 1989.

65. Lao TT, deSwiet M, Letsky E, et al: Prophylaxis of thromboembolism in pregnancy: an alternative. Br J Obstet Gynaecol 92:202, 1985.

66. Iturbe-Alessio I, del Carmen Fonseca M, Mutchinik O, et al: Risks of anticoagulant therapy in pregnant women with artificial heart valves. N Engl J Med 315:1390, 1986.

67. Mujtaba Q, Burrow GN: Treatment of hyperthyroidism in pregnancy with propylthiouracil and methimazole. Obstet Gynecol 46:282, 1975.

68. Wing DA, Millar LK, Koonings PP, et al: A comparison of propylthiouracil versus methimazole in the treatment of hyperthyroidism in pregnancy. Am J Obstet Gynecol 170:90, 1994.

69. Burrow GN: Thyroid diseases. In Burrow GN, Ferris TF (eds): Medical Complications During Pregnancy. Philadelphia, WB Saunders Company, 1988, p 229.

70. Mandel SJ, Larsen PR, Seely EW, et al: Increased need for thyroxine during pregnancy in women with primary hypothyroidism. N Engl J Med 323:91, 1990.

71. Haddow JE, Palomaki GE, Allan WC, et al: Maternal thyroid deficiency during pregnancy and subsequent neuropsychological development of the child. N Engl J Med 341:549, 1999.

72. l'Allemand D, Gruters A, Heidemann P, et al: Iodine-induced alterations of thyroid function in newborn infants after prenatal and perinatal exposure to povidone iodine. J Pediatr 102: 935, 1983.

73. Heinonen OP, Slone S, Shapiro S: Birth Defects and Drugs in Pregnancy. Littleton, MA, Publishing Sciences Group, 1977.

74. Weiner CP, Landas S, Persoon TJ: Digoxin-like immunoreactive substance in fetuses with and without cardiac pathology. Am J Obstet Gynecol 157:368, 1987.

75. Weiner CP, Thompson MIB: Direct treatment of fetal supraventricular tachycardia after failed transplacental therapy. Am J Obstet Gynecol 158:570, 1988.

76. Pruyn SC, Phelan JP, Buchanan GC: Long-term propranolol therapy in pregnancy: maternal and fetal outcome. Am J Obstet Gynecol 135:485, 1979.

77. Redmond GP: Propranolol and fetal growth retardation. Semin Perinatol 6:142, 1982.

78. Rubin PC, Clark DM, Sumner DJ: Placebo-controlled trial of atenolol in treatment of pregnancy-associated hypertension. Lancet 1:431, 1983.

79. Hanssens M, Keirse MJNC, Vankelecom F, et al: Fetal and neonatal effects of treatment with angiotensin-converting enzyme inhibitors in pregnancy. Obstet Gynecol 78:128, 1991.

80. Piper JM, Ray WA, Rosa FW: Pregnancy outcome following exposure to angiotensin-converting enzyme inhibitors. Obstet Gynecol 80:429, 1992.

81. Kozlowski RD, Steinbrunner JV, MacKenzie AH, et al: Outcome of first-trimester exposure to low-dose methotrexate in eight patients with rheumatic disease. Am J Med 88:589, 1990.

82. Haugen G, Fauchald P, Sodal G, et al: Pregnancy outcome in renal allograft recipients: influence of cyclosporin A. Eur J Obstet Gynecol Reprod Biol 39:25, 1991.

83. Armenti VT, Ahlswede BA, Ahlswede JR, et al: National transplantation pregnancy registry: analysis of outcome/risks of 394 pregnancies in kidney transplant recipients. Transplant Proc 26:2535, 1994.

84. Takahashi N, Nishida H, Hoshi J: Severe B cell depletion in newborns from renal transplant mothers taking immunosuppressive agents. Transplantation 57:1617, 1994.

85. Briggs GC, Freeman RK, Yaffe SJ: Drugs in Pregnancy and Lactation, 5th ed. Baltimore, Williams & Wilkins, 1998, p 272.

86. Wolfe MS, Cordero JF: Safety of chloroquine in chemosuppression of malaria during pregnancy. BMJ 290:1466, 1985.

87. Hart CW, Naunton RF: The ototoxicity of chloroquine phosphate. Arch Otolaryngol 80:407, 1964.

88. Levy M, Buskila D, Gladman DD, et al: Pregnancy outcome following first trimester exposure to chloroquine. Am J Perinatol 8:174, 1991.

89. Zemlickis D, Lishner M, Degendorfer P, et al: Fetal outcome after in utero exposure to cancer chemotherapy. Arch Intern Med 152:573, 1992.

90. Main EK, Main DM, Gabbe SG: Chronic oral terbutaline therapy is associated with maternal glucose intolerance. Obstet Gynecol 157:644, 1987.

91. Sahakian V, Rouse D, Sipes S, et al: Vitamin B$_6$ is effective therapy for nausea and vomiting of pregnancy: a randomized double-blind, placebo-controlled study. Obstet Gynecol 78:33, 1991.

92. Vutyavanich T, Wongtra-Rjan S, Ruangsri R: Pyridoxine for nausea and vomiting of pregnancy: a randomized double-blind placebo-controlled trial. Am J Obstet Gynecol 173:881, 1995.

93. Fischer-Rasmussen W, Kjaer SK, Dahl C, et al: Ginger treatment of hyperemesis gravidarum. Eur J Obstet Gynecol Reprod Biol 38:19, 1990.

94. Diggory PLC, Tomkinson JS: Nausea and vomiting in pregnancy: a trial of meclozine dihydrochloride with and without pyridoxine. Lancet 2:370, 1962.

95. Milkovich L, Van Den Berg BJ: An evaluation of the teratogenicity of certain antinauseant drugs. Am J Obstet Gynecol 125:244, 1976.

96. Cartwright EW: Dramamine in nausea and vomiting of pregnancy. West J Surg Obstet Gynecol 59:216, 1951.

97. Rumeau-Rouquette C, Goujard J, Huel G: Possible teratogenic effect of phenothiazines in human beings. Teratology 15:57, 1977.

98. Sullivan CA, Johnson CA, Roach H, et al: A pilot study of intravenous ondansetron for hyperemesis gravidarum. Am J Obstet Gynecol 174:2565, 1996.

99. Safari HR, Fassett MJ, Souter IC, et al: The efficacy of methylprednisolone in the treatment of hyperemesis gravidarum: a randomized, double-blind, controlled study. Am J Obstet Gynecol 179:921, 1998.

100. Ruigomez A, Garcia Rodriguez LA, Cattaruzzi C, et al: Use of cimetidine, omeprazole, and ranitidine in pregnant women and pregnancy outcomes. Am J Epidemiol 150:476, 1999.

101. Briggs GG, Freeman RK, Yaffe SJ: Drugs in Pregnancy and Lactation, 5th ed. Baltimore, Williams & Wilkins, 1998, p 1009.

102. Pastuszak A, Schick B, D'Alimonte D, et al: The safety of astemizole in pregnancy. J Allergy Clin Immunol 98:748, 1996.

103. Zierler S, Purohit D: Prenatal antihistamine exposure and retrolental fibroplasia. Am J Epidemiol 123:192, 1986.

104. Werler MM, Mitchell AA, Shapiro S: First trimester maternal medication use in relation to gastroschisis. Teratology 45:361, 1992.

105. Philipson A: Pharmacokinetics of antibiotics in pregnancy and labour. Clin Pharmacokinet 4:297, 1979.

106. Briggs GG, Freeman RK, Yaffe SJ: Drugs in Pregnancy and Lactation, 5th ed. Baltimore, Williams & Wilkins, 1988, p 152.

107. Briggs GG, Freeman RK, Yaffe SJ: Drugs in Pregnancy and Lactation, 5th ed. Baltimore, Williams & Wilkins, 1998, p 987.

108. Monif GFG: Infectious Diseases in Obstetrics and Gynecology. New York, Harper & Row, 1974.

109. Jarnerot G, Into-Malmberg MB, Esbjorner E: Placental transfer of sulfasalazine and sulfapyridine and some of its metabolites. Scand J Gastroenterol 16:693, 1981.

110. Ochoa AG: Trimethoprim and sulfamethoxazole in pregnancy. JAMA 217:1244, 1971.

111. Brumfitt W, Pursell R: Double-blind trial to compare ampicillin, cephalexin, co-trimoxazole, and trimethoprim in treatment of urinary infection. Br Med J 2:673, 1972.

112. Briggs GG, Freeman RK, Yaffe SJ: Drugs in Pregnancy and Lactation, 5th ed. Baltimore, Williams & Wilkins, 1998, p 1061.

113. Czeizel A: A case-control analysis of the teratogenic effects of co-trimoxazole. Reprod Toxicol 4:305, 1990.

114. Hailey FJ, Fort H, Williams JR, et al: Foetal safety of nitrofurantoin macrocrystals therapy during pregnancy: a retrospective analysis. J Int Med Res 11:364, 1983.

115. Lenke RR, VanDorsten JP, Schifrin BS: Pyelonephritis in pregnancy: a prospective randomized trial to prevent recurrent disease evaluating suppressive therapy with nitrofurantoin and close surveillance. Am J Obstet Gynecol 146:953, 1983.

116. Cohlan SQU, Bevelander G, Tiamsic T: Growth inhibition of prematures receiving tetracycline. Am J Dis Child 105:453, 1963.

117. Czeizel AE, Rockenbauer M: Teratogenic study of doxycyline. Obstet Gynecol 89:524, 1997.

118. Aselton P, Jick H, Mulnsky A, et al: First-trimester drug use and congenital disorders. Obstet Gynecol 65:451, 1985.

119. Robinson GC, Cambon KG: Hearing loss in infants of tuberculous mothers treated with streptomycin during pregnancy. N Engl J Med 271:949, 1964.

120. Nishimura H, Tanimura T: Clinical Aspects of the Teratogenicity of Drugs. Amsterdam, Excerpta Medica, 1976.

121. L'Hommedieu CS, Nicholas D, Armes DA, et al: Potentiation of magnesium sulfate-induced neuromuscular weakness by gentamicin, tobramycin, and amikacin. J Pediatr 102:629, 1983.

122. Marynowski A, Sianozecka E: Comparison of the incidence of congenital malformations in neonates from healthy mothers and from patients treated because of tuberculosis. Ginekol Pol 43:713, 1972.

123. Zaske DE, Cipolle RJ, Strate RG, et al: Rapid gentamicin elimination in obstetric patients. Obstet Gynecol 56:559, 1980.

124. Mitra AG, Whitten MK, Laurent SL, et al: A randomized, prospective study comparing once-daily gentamicin versus thrice-daily gentamicin in the treatment of puerperal infection. Am J Obstet Gynecol 177:786, 1997.

125. Philipson A, Sabath LD, Charles D: Transplacental passage of erythromycin and clindamycin. N Engl J Med 288:1219, 1973.

126. South MA, Short DH, Knox JM: Failure of erythromycin estolate therapy in in utero syphilis. JAMA 190:70, 1964.

127. Einarson A, Phillips E, Mawji F, et al: A prospective controlled multicentre study of clarithromycin in pregnancy. Am J Perinatol 15:523, 1998.

128. Briggs GC, Freeman RK, Jaffe SJ: Drugs in Pregnancy and Lactation. Baltimore, Williams & Wilkins, 1998, p 223.

129. Berkovitch M, Pastuszak A, Gazarian M, et al: Safety of the new quinolones in pregnancy. Obstet Gynecol 84:535, 1994.

130. Briggs GG, Freeman RK, Yaffe SJ: Drugs in Pregnancy and Lactation, 5th ed. Baltimore, Williams & Wilkins, 1998, p 212.

131. Piper JM, Mitchel EF, Ray WA: Prenatal use of metronidazole and birth defects: no association. Obstet Gynecol 82:348, 1993.

132. Burtin P, Taddio A, Ariburnu O, et al: Safety of metronidazole in pregnancy: a meta-analysis. Am J Obstet Gynecol 172:525, 1995.

133. Beard CM, Noller KL, O'Fallon WM, et al: Lack of evidence for cancer due to use of metronidazole. N Engl J Med 301:519, 1979.

134. Andrews EB, Yankaskas BC, Cordero JF, et al: Acyclovir in pregnancy registry: six years' experience. Obstet Gynecol 79:7, 1992.

135. Rosa FW, Baum C, Shaw M: Pregnancy outcomes after first trimester vaginitis drug therapy. Obstet Gynecol 69:751, 1987.

136. Briggs GG, Freeman RK, Yaffe SJ: Drugs in Pregnancy and Lactation, 5th ed. Baltimore, Williams & Wilkins, 1998, p 728.

137. Pursley TJ, Blomquist IK, Abraham J, et al: Fluconazole-induced congenital anomalies in three infants. Clin Infect Dis 22:336, 1996.

138. Jick SS: Pregnancy outcomes after maternal exposure to fluconazole. Pharmacotherapy 19:221, 1999.

139. Mastroiacovo P, Mazzone T, Botto LD, et al: Prospective assessment of pregnancy outcomes after first-trimester exposure to fluconazole. Am J Obstet Gynecol 175:1645, 1996.

140. Asch RH, Greenblatt RB: Update on the safety and efficacy of clomiphene citrate as a therapeutic agent. J Reprod Med 17:175, 1976.

141. Riuz-Velasco V, Tolis G: Pregnancy in hyperprolactinemic women. Fertil Steril 41:793, 1984.

142. Werler MM, Mitchell AA, Shapiro S: The relation of aspirin use during the first trimester of pregnancy to congenital cardiac defects. N Engl J Med 321:1639, 1989.

143. Collins E, Turner G: Salicylates and pregnancy. Lancet 2:1494, 1973.

144. Stuart JJ, Gross SJ, Elrad H, et al: Effects of acetylsalicyclic acid ingestion on maternal and neonatal hemostasis. N Engl J Med 307:909, 1982.

145. Areilla RA, Thilenius OB, Ranniger K: Congestive heart failure from suspected ductal closure in utero. J Pediatr 75:74, 1969.

146. Lubbe WF, Butler WS, Palmer SJ, et al: Lupus anticoagulant in pregnancy. Br J Obstet Gynaecol 91:357, 1984.

147. Cowchock FS, Reece EA, Balaban D, et al: Repeated fetal losses associated with antiphospholipid antibodies: a collaborative randomized trial comparing prednisone with low-dose heparin treatment. Am J Obstet Gynecol 166:1318, 1992.

148. Sibai BM: Prevention of preeclampsia: a big disappointment. Am J Obstet Gynecol 179:1275, 1998.

149. Caritis SN, Sibai BM, Hauth J, et al: Low-dose aspirin therapy for the prevention of preeclampsia in high-risk women. N Engl J Med 338:701, 1998.

150. Thulstrup AM, Sorensen HT, Nielsen GL, et al: Fetal growth and adverse birth outcomes in women receiving prescriptions for acetaminophen during pregnancy. Am J Perinatol 16:321, 1999.

151. Waltman T, Tricomi V, Tavakoli FM: Effect of aspirin on bleeding time during elective abortion. Obstet Gynecol 48:108, 1976.

152. Rayburn W, Shukla U, Stetson P, et al: Acetaminophen pharmacokinetics: comparison between pregnant and nonpregnant women. Obstet Gynecol 155:1353, 1986.

153. Briggs GG, Freeman RK, Yaffe SJ: Drugs in Pregnancy and Lactation, 5th ed. Baltimore, Williams & Wilkins, 1998, p 524.

154. Briggs GG, Freeman RK, Yaffe SJ: Drugs in Pregnancy and Lactation, 5th ed. Baltimore, Williams & Wilkins, 1998, p 1061.

155. Tyson HK: Neonatal withdrawal symptoms associated with maternal use of propoxyphene hydrochloride (Darvon). J Pediatr 85:684, 1974.

156. Shah NR, Bracken MB: A systematic review and meta-analysis of prospective studies on the association between interval cigarette smoking and preterm delivery. Am J Obstet Gynecol 182:465, 2000.

157. Alberman E, Creasy M, Elliott M, et al: Maternal factors associated with fetal chromosomal anomalies in spontaneous abortions. J Obstet Gynecol 83:621, 1976.

158. Dolan-Mullen P, Ramierez G, Groff JY: A meta-analysis of randomized trials of prenatal smoking cessation interventions. Am J Obstet Gynecol 171:1328, 1994.

159. Martin TR, Bracken MB: Association of low birth weight with passive smoke exposure in pregnancy. Am J Epidemiol 124:633, 1986.

160. Marcus BH, Albrecht AE, King TK, et al: The efficacy of exercise as an aid for smoking cessation in women. Arch Intern Med 159:1229, 1999.

161. Tonnesen P, Norregaard J, Simonsen K, et al: A double-blind trial of a 16-hour transdermal nicotine patch in smoking cessation. N Engl J Med 325:311, 1991.

162. Ogburn PL, Hurt RD, Croghan IT, et al: Nicotine patch use in pregnant smokers: nicotine and cotinine levels and fetal effects. Am J Obstet Gynecol 181:736, 1999.

163. Jones KL, Smith DW, Ulleland CN, et al: Patterns of malformation in offspring of chronic alcoholic mothers. Lancet 2:1267, 1973.

164. Rosett HL: A clinical perspective of the fetal alcohol syndrome. Alcohol Clin Exp Res 4:119, 1980.

165. Jones KL, Smith DW, Streissguth AP, et al: Outcome of offspring of chronic alcoholic women. Lancet 2:1076, 1974.

166. Ouellette EM, Rosett HL. Rosman NP, et al: Adverse effects on offspring of maternal alcohol abuse during pregnancy. N Engl J Med 297:528, 1977.

167. Mills JL, Graubard BI: Is moderate drinking during pregnancy associated with an increased risk of malformations? Pediatrics 80:309, 1987.

168. Sokol RJ, Martier SS, Ager JW: The T-ACE questions: practical prenatal detection of risk-drinking. Am J Obstet Gynecol 160:863, 1989.

169. Greenland S, Staisch KJ, Brown N, et al: The effects of marijuana use during pregnancy: part 1—a preliminary epidemiologic study. Am J Obstet Gynecol 143:408, 1982.

170. Fried PA, Buckingham M, Von Kulmiz P: Marijuana use during pregnancy and perinatal risk factors. Am J Obstet Gynecol 146:992, 1983.

171. Zuckerman B, Frank DA, Hingson R, et al: Effects of maternal marijuana and cocaine use on fetal growth. N Engl J Med 320:762, 1989.

172. Acker D, Sachs BP, Tracey KJ, et al: Abruptio placentae associated with cocaine use. Am J Obstet Gynecol 146:220, 1983.

173. Little BB, Snell LM, Klein VR, et al: Cocaine abuse during pregnancy: maternal and fetal implications. Obstet Gynecol 73:157, 1989.

174. Bingol N, Fuchs M, Diaz V, et al: Teratogenicity of cocaine in humans. J Pediatr 110:93, 1987.

175. MacGregor SN, Keith LG, Chasnoff IJ, et al: Cocaine use during pregnancy: adverse perinatal outcome. Am J Obstet Gynecol 157:686, 1987.

176. Keith LG, MacGregor S, Friedell S, et al: Substance abuse in pregnant women: recent experience at the perinatal center for chemical dependence of Northwestern Memorial Hospital. Obstet Gynecol 73:715, 1989.

177. Chasnoff IJ, Griffith DR, MacGregor S, et al: Temporal patterns of cocaine use in pregnancy. JAMA 261:1741, 1989.

178. Volpe JJ: Effect of cocaine use on the fetus. N Engl J Med 327:399, 1992.

179. Handler A, Kistin N, Davis F, et al: Cocaine use during pregnancy: perinatal outcomes. Am J Epidemiol 133:818, 1991.

180. Little BB, Snell LM: Brain growth among fetuses exposed to cocaine in utero: asymmetrical growth retardation. Obstet Gynecol 77:361, 1991.

181. Chasnoff IJ, Chisum GM, Kaplan WE: Maternal cocaine use and genitourinary tract malformations. Teratology 37:201, 1988.

182. Finnegan LP, Wapner RJ: Narcotic addiction in pregnancy. *In* Niebyl JR (ed): Drug Use in Pregnancy. Philadelphia, Lea & Febiger, 1988, p 203.

183. Van den Berg BJ: Epidemiologic observations of prematurity: effects of tobacco, coffee and alcohol. *In* Reed DM, Stanley FJ (eds): The Epidemiology of Prematurity. Baltimore, Urban & Schwarzenberg, 1977.

184. Linn S, Schoenbaum SC, Monson RR, et al: No association between coffee consumption and adverse outcomes of pregnancy. N Engl J Med 306:141, 1982.

185. Martin TR, Bracken MB: The association between low birth weight and caffeine consumption during pregnancy. Am J Epidemiol 126:813, 1987.

186. Beaulac-Baillargeon L, Desrosiers C: Caffeine-cigarette interaction on fetal growth. Am J Obstet Gynecol 157:1236, 1987.

187. Munoz LM, Lonnerdal B, Keen CL, et al: Coffee consumption as a factor in iron deficiency anemia among pregnant women and their infants in Costa Rica. Am J Clin Nutr 48:645, 1988.

188. Infante-Rivard C, Fernandez A, Gauthier R, et al: Fetal loss associated with caffeine intake before and during pregnancy. JAMA 270:2940, 1993.

189. Mills JL, Holmes LB, Aarons JH, et al: Moderate caffeine use and the risk of spontaneous abortion and intrauterine growth retardation. JAMA 269:593, 1993.

190. Klebanoff MA, Levine RJ, DerSimonian R, et al: Maternal serum paraxanthine, a caffeine metabolite, and the risk of spontaneous abortion. N Engl J Med 341:1639, 1999.

191. Sturtevant FM: Use of aspartame in pregnancy. Int J Fertil 30:85, 1985.

192. Wilson JT, Brown RD, Cherek DR, et al: Drug excretion in human breast milk: principles of pharmacokinetics and projected consequences. Clin Pharmacokinet 5:1, 1980.

193. Ito S, Blajchman A, Stephenson M, et al: Prospective follow-up of adverse reactions in breast-fed infants exposed to maternal medication. Am J Obstet Gynecol 168:1393, 1993.

194. American Academy of Pediatrics: Committee on Drugs. The transfer of drugs and other chemicals into human milk. Pediatrics 93:137, 1994.

195. Johns BG, Rutherford CD, Laighton RC, et al: Secretion of methotrexate into human milk. Am J Obstet Gynecol 112:978, 1972.

196. Bounaneaux Y, Duren J: Busulphan in nursing infants. Ann Soc Belg Med Trop 44:381, 1964.

197. Canales ES, Garcia IC, Ruiz JE, et al: Bromocriptine as prophylactic therapy in prolactinoma during pregnancy. Fertil Steril 36:524, 1981.

198. Linden S, Rich CL: The use of lithium during pregnancy and lactation. J Clin Psychiatry 44:358, 1983.

199. Ayd FJ Jr: Excretion of psychotrophic drugs in human breast milk. Int Drug Ther News Bull 8:33, 1973.

200. Berlin CM: The excretion of drugs in human milk. *In* Schwartz RH, Yaffe SJ (eds): Drug and Chemical Risks to the Fetus and Newborn. New York, Alan R Liss, 1980, p 125.

201. Nulman I, Koren G: The safety of fluoxetine during pregnancy and lactation. Teratology 53:304, 1996.

202. Burch KJ, Wells BG: Fluoxetine/norfluoxetine concentrations in human milk. Pediatrics 89:676, 1992.

203. Epperson CN, Anderson GM, McDougle CJ: Sertraline and breast-feeding. N Engl J Med 336:1189, 1997.

204. Niebyl JR, Blake DA, Freeman JM, et al: Carbamezapine levels in pregnancy and lactation. Obstet Gynecol 53:139, 1979.

205. Briggs GG, Freeman RK, Yaffe SJ: Drugs in Pregnancy and Lactation, 5th ed. Baltimore, Williams & Wilkins, 1998.

206. Cole AP, Hailey DM: Diazepam and active metabolite in breast milk and their transfer to the neonate. Arch Dis Child 50:741, 1975.

207. Pynnonen S, Sillanpaa M: Carbamazepine and mother's milk. Lancet 2:563, 1975.

208. Nau H, Rating D, Hauser I, et al: Placental transfer and pharmacokinetics of primidone and its metabolites phenobarbital, PEMA and hydroxyphenobarbital in neonates and infants of epileptic mothers. Eur J Clin Pharmacol 18:31, 1980.

209. Cruikshank DP, Varner MW, Pitkin RM: Breast milk magnesium and calcium concentrations following magnesium sulfate treatment. Am J Obstet Gynecol 143:685, 1982.

210. Ananth J: Side effects in the neonate from psychotrophic agents excreted through breastfeeding. Am J Psychiatry 135:801, 1978.

211. Findlay JWA, Butz RF, Sailstad JM, et al: Pseudoephedrine and triprolidine in plasma and breast milk of nursing mothers. Br J Clin Pharmacol 18:901, 1984.

212. Yurchak AM, Jusko NJ: Theophylline secretion into breast milk. Pediatrics 57:518, 1976.

213. Weithmann MW, Krees SV: Excretion of chlorothiazide in human breast milk. J Pediatr 81:781, 1972.

214. Miller ME, Cohn RD, Burghart PH: Hydrochlorothiazide disposition in a mother and her breast-fed infant. J Pediatr 101: 789, 1982.

215. Bauer JH, Pope B, Zajicek J, et al: Propranolol in human plasma and breast milk. Am J Cardiol 43:860, 1979.

216. Anderson PO, Salter FJ: Propranolol therapy during pregnancy and lactation. Am J Cardiol 37:325, 1976.

217. White WB, Andreoli JW, Wong SH, et al: Atenolol in human plasma and breast milk. Obstet Gynecol 63:42S, 1984.

218. Schmimmel MS, Eidelman AJ, Wilschanski MA, et al: Toxic effects of atenolol consumed during breast feeding. J Pediatr 114:476, 1989.

219. Briggs GG, Freeman RK, Yaffe SJ: Drugs in Pregnancy and Lactation, 5th ed. Baltimore, Williams & Wilkins, 1998, p 84.

220. Hartikainen-Sorri AL, Heikkinen JE, Koivisto M: Pharmacokinetics of clonidine during pregnancy and nursing. Obstet Gynecol 69:598, 1987.

221. Devlin RG, Fleiss PM: Selective resistance to the passage of captopril into human milk. Clin Pharmacol Ther 27:250, 1980.

222. Ehrenkranz RA, Ackerman BA, Hulse JD: Nifedipine transfer into human milk. J Pediatr 114:478, 1989.

223. Orme ME, Lewis PJ, deSwiet M, et al: May mothers given warfarin breastfeed their infants? Br Med J 1:1564, 1977.

224. deSwiet M, Lewis PJ: Excretion of anticoagulants in human milk. N Engl J Med 297:1471, 1977.

225. Brambel CE, Hunter RE: Effect of dicumarol on the nursing infant. Am J Obstet Gynecol 59:1153, 1950.

226. Eckstein HB, Jack B: Breastfeeding and anticoagulant therapy. Lancet 1:672, 1970.

227. Katz FH, Duncan BR: Entry of prednisone into human milk. N Engl J Med 293:1154, 1975.

228. MacKenzie SA, Seeley JA, Agnew JE: Secretion of prednisolone into breast milk. Arch Dis Child 50:894, 1975.

229. Ost L, Wettrell G, Bjorkhem I, et al: Prednisolone excretion in human milk. J Pediatr 106:1008, 1985.

230. Loughnan PM: Digoxin excretion in human breast milk. J Pediatr 92:1019, 1978.

231. Yoshioka H, Cho K, Takimoto M, et al: Transfer of cefazolin into human milk. J Pediatr 94:151, 1979.

232. Celiloglu M, Celiker S, Guven H, et al: Gentamicin excretion and uptake from breast milk by nursing infants. Obstet Gynecol 84:263, 1994.

233. Hosbach RE, Foster RB: Absence of nitrofurantoin from human milk. JAMA 202:1057, 1967.

234. Kelsey JJ, Moser LR, Jenning JC, et al: Presence of azithromycin breast milk concentrations: a case report. Am J Obstet Gynecol 170:1375, 1994.

235. Meyer LJ, de Miranda P, Sheth N, et al: Acyclovir in human breast milk. Am J Obstet Gynecol 158:586, 1988.

236. Moretti ME, Ito S, Koren G: Disposition of maternal ketoconazole in breast milk. Am J Obstet Gynecol 173:1625, 1995.

237. Nilsson S, Nygren KG, Johansson EDB: Transfer of estradiol to human milk. Am J Obstet Gynecol 132:653, 1978.

238. Grimes DA, Wallach M: Modern Contraception. Totowa, NJ, Emron, 1997, p 249.

239. Little RE, Anderson KW, Ervin CH, et al: Maternal alcohol use during breastfeeding and infant mental and motor development at one year. N Engl J Med 321:425, 1989.

240. Mennella JA, Beauchamp GK: The transfer of alcohol to human milk. Effects on flavor and the infant's behavior. N Engl J Med 325:981, 1991.

241. Kampmann JP, Hansen JM, Johansen K, et al: Propylthiouracil in human milk. Lancet 1:736, 1980.

242. Cooper DS: Antithyroid drugs: to breast-feed or not to breast-feed. Am J Obstet Gynecol 157:234, 1987.

243. Illingsworth RS: Abnormal substances excreted in human milk. Practitioner 171:533, 1953.

244. Anderson PO: Drug use during breast-feeding. Clin Pharm 10: 594, 1991.

245. Ryu JE: Effect of maternal caffeine consumption on heart rate and sleep time of breast-fed infants. Dev Pharmacol Ther 8: 355, 1985.

246. Luck W, Nau H: Nicotine and cotinine concentrations in serum and urine of infants exposed via passive smoking or milk from smoking mothers. J Pediatr 107:816, 1985.

247. Labrecque M, Marcoux S, Weber J-P, et al: Feeding and urine cotinine values in babies whose mothers smoke. Pediatrics 83: 93, 1989.

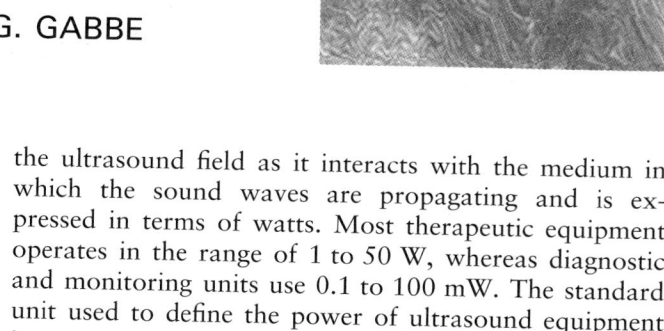

Chapter 10

Obstetric Ultrasound: Assessment of Fetal Growth and Anatomy

FRANK A. CHERVENAK AND STEVEN G. GABBE

Diagnostic ultrasound has emerged as an important tool for antepartum fetal surveillance. This technology has permitted the most accurate assessment of gestational age and has enabled the obstetrician to follow fetal growth serially and to detect fetal growth disorders. In addition, ultrasound has become an essential aid in the safe performance of a variety of diagnostic procedures, including amniocentesis, chorionic villus sampling, and cordocentesis. Finally, the use of real-time ultrasound has permitted the obstetrician to assess fetal well-being through the evaluation of fetal movements, breathing activity, tone, and the volume of amniotic fluid.

BIOPHYSICS OF ULTRASOUND

To use ultrasound most effectively, the obstetrician should understand the basic biophysics of the technique.[1] Sound is a waveform of energy that causes small particles in a medium to oscillate. The frequency of sound refers to the number of peaks or waves that traverse a given point per unit of time and is expressed in hertz. Sound with a frequency of one cycle or one peak per second would have a frequency of 1 Hz. Ultrasound applies to high-frequency sound waves exceeding 20,000 Hz. Diagnostic ultrasound instruments operate in a higher range of frequencies, varying from 2 to 10 million Hz, or 2 to 10 MHz.

Ultrasound energy is produced by a transducer containing crystal structures that convert electrical energy to ultrasound waves and the returning echoes to electrical energy. Therefore, each crystal in the transducer acts as both a transmitter and a receiver. The power of ultrasound refers to the amount of work being done by the ultrasound field as it interacts with the medium in which the sound waves are propagating and is expressed in terms of watts. Most therapeutic equipment operates in the range of 1 to 50 W, whereas diagnostic and monitoring units use 0.1 to 100 mW. The standard unit used to define the power of ultrasound equipment is watts per square centimeter, which describes the amount of energy delivered per given surface area.

Diagnostic ultrasound equipment generates a sound pulse every 1 msec, and the duration of the pulse is 1 μsec. The time the sound pulse is off is 1,000 times greater than the time it is on. Therefore, the duty factor of diagnostic ultrasound, defined as the ratio between the emission of a sound wave and the reception of the sound wave, is 1:1,000 or 0.001. During a 15-minute diagnostic evaluation, the fetus is exposed to only 1 second of ultrasound energy. The safety of diagnostic ultrasound is discussed later in more detail.

PRINCIPLES OF IMAGING

A two-dimensional picture is created when the returning ultrasound echoes are displayed on an oscilloscope screen.[1] The ultrasound signal returning to the transducer is converted to an electrical impulse, and the strength of that electrical impulse is directly proportional to the strength of the returning echo. The density of the medium into which the sound wave has been transmitted and through which it is reflected will determine the strength of the signal. The velocity of the reflected sound wave will be faster and its signal on the oscilloscope brighter after reflection off bone than off tissues that are less dense, such as muscle, fat, brain, or water. Air greatly decreases the transmission of sound waves. For this reason, a coupling medium or gel is applied between the surface of the transducer and the skin or vaginal mucosa.

Ultrasound can be used to produce diagnostic images in several ways. With M mode (motion mode), the reflected echo is displayed as a spot that generates a horizontal line on a moving display. In this way, one can examine the motion of structures against time. This technique has been widely applied in the assessment of cardiac anatomy, including the dimensions of the cardiac chambers, ventricular wall thickness, and valvular motion. B mode (brightness modulation) converts the strength of the returning echoes into signals of varying brightness that are proportional to the amplitude of the returning echoes. A storage oscilloscope is used to create a compounded image of the target and, in this way, produce a two-dimensional picture. Real-time array transducer systems create these images within a fraction of a second. When the image of the fetus is compounded at a rate faster than the flicker fusion rate of the eye, the fetus will appear to be moving in real time. In a linear array transducer, a series of crystals are aligned along the transducer. The standard transducer used in these systems is 3.5 MHz. The higher the frequency of the sound the better the reproduction and resolution, but the shallower the depth of penetration. Sector scanning uses a moving transducer head containing the crystals or a wheel containing multiple transducers that moves through a prescribed sector. Sector scanning facilitates the visualization of structures behind the symphysis pubis. The obstetrician will often use a curvilinear transducer, incorporating the advantages of both the linear array and the sector transducers. Recently, three-dimensional ultrasound has been used to better define surface rendering of normal fetal anatomy and fetal anomalies. Its role in clinical practice is uncertain at this time.[2,3]

Doppler ultrasound differs significantly from the imaging techniques that have been described. In this application of ultrasound, used in Doppler velocimetry (see Chapter 12) and antepartum and intrapartum fetal heart rate monitoring (see Chapters 12 and 14), the receiver detects shifts in the frequency of the returning sound waves rather than in the amplitude of these reflected echoes. Targets moving toward the receiving transducer produce an increase in the frequency of the echo, whereas objects moving away decrease the frequency. Doppler ultrasound uses a continuous beam of sound rather than intermittent transmission, which characterizes real-time ultrasound.

SAFETY OF ULTRASOUND

Concern has been expressed by basic scientists, physicians, and consumers about the safety of diagnostic ultrasound.[4–6] The dissipation of energy from ultrasound can produce heating of the exposed tissues.[7,8] Ultrasound may also create cavitation or the formation of bubbles and microstreaming, the flow of liquid around these oscillating bubbles. In experimental systems, exposure to high-intensity ultrasound has been associated with alterations in immune response, increases in sister chromatid exchange frequencies,[9] fetal malformations, and growth restriction. However, these effects have *not* been seen with diagnostic ultrasound.

The total ultrasound exposure for a fetus will depend on the number of ultrasound examinations performed, the type of equipment used, and the amount of energy received, which is dependent on the duration of the examination. It has been recommended that the length of each ultrasound study and the type of equipment used be recorded.[5]

The amount of ultrasound energy received by the fetus varies directly with the intensity of the ultrasound signal and is inversely related to the square of its distance from the emitting source. If one is using a 3.5-MHz transducer, which focuses at approximately 8 cm, exposed tissues will receive only 1/64th of the energy originally emitted from the transducer. Thus far, the safe level of ultrasound intensity has been defined as less than 100 mW/cm^2 for unfocused ultrasound and below 1 W/cm^2 for focused ultrasound. Most instruments in use today produce maximum power levels less than 50 mW/cm^2 in a standard scan mode.[10]

Studies of clinical outcomes of infants exposed to ultrasound have failed to demonstrate any significant effects. No effect on neurologic function, including speech, hearing, and vision, or on school performance, or on the incidence of childhood leukemia has been observed.[11–13] In 1993, the American Institute of Ultrasound in Medicine (AIUM) Bioeffects Committee concluded[10]:

Diagnostic ultrasound has been in use since the late 1950s. Given its known benefits and recognized efficacy for medical diagnosis, including use during human pregnancy, the American Institute of Ultrasound in Medicine (AIUM) herein addresses the clinical safety of such use:

No confirmed biological effects on patients or instrument operators caused by exposure at intensities typical of the present diagnostic ultrasound instruments have ever been reported. Although the possibility exists that such biological effects may be identified in the future, current data indicate that the benefits to patients of the prudent use of diagnostic ultrasound outweigh the risks, if any, that may be present.

In considering the safety of any diagnostic procedure, one must also consider the skill with which the examination is conducted and the way in which the results are interpreted and utilized. False-positive and false-negative diagnoses appear to be the greatest risk for the patient undergoing an obstetric ultrasound examination. What guidelines should be followed to ensure that an obstetrician is adequately trained in the application of ultrasound? The AIUM has published guidelines for training in diagnostic ultrasound.[14] These recommendations call for completion of an approved residency program, fellowship, or postgraduate training with a minimum of 3 months' supervised experience. The guidelines also specify involvement in the evaluation and interpretation of at least 500 diagnostic ultrasound examinations. Most recently, AIUM has broadened these guidelines to accredit ultrasound laboratories or practices including the experience of the sonographers, quality and maintenance of the equipment, record keeping, facilities, and quality assurance. Many managed care plans now require these or similar accreditation standards be met by their providers.

TRANSVAGINAL ULTRASOUND

Transvaginal ultrasound, with its ability to use higher frequency transducers, can result in better visualization of the early pregnancy.[15-17] The gestational sac, yolk sac, and embryo can be seen earlier and with more detail than transabdominal ultrasound. Extrauterine pathology, such as an ectopic pregnancy or an ovarian mass, can be better evaluated. This enhanced visualization with vaginal ultrasound is especially important in the obese patient and when there is a retroverted or myomatous uterus.

A gestational sac can be seen with transvaginal ultrasound as early as 4.5 menstrual weeks[18]. This sac is surrounded by an echogenic ring that represents trophoblastic tissue. The normal gestational sac is located in the upper uterine body and has a smooth contour and a round shape. Once seen, the gestational sac grows at a fairly constant rate of 1 mm in mean diameter per day.[19]

The yolk sac is visualized when the gestational sac is 10 mm or larger. Visualization of a yolk sac documents that an anechoic area in the uterus represents a true gestational sac and not the pseudogestational sac seen in ectopic pregnancy. Between the 7th and the 13th menstrual weeks, the yolk sac gradually increases in diameter from about 3 mm to 6 mm (Figs. 10-1 and 10-2).[20,21]

The amnion develops about the same time as the yolk sac but, because it is thinner, the amnion is more difficult to visualize. It surrounds the embryo and is opposite the yolk sac. The amnion grows rapidly during early pregnancy, and fusion with the chorion is usually complete by the 16th week. At that time, the extraembryonic coelom is obliterated.

Cardiac activity is usually the first manifestation of the embryo at about 6 menstrual weeks. Once the embryo is 5 mm, cardiac activity should be present; its absence is indicative of early demise.[22-24] If cardiac activity is absent and the embryo is less than 5 mm, the findings are not conclusive. At a gestational age of about 6.2 weeks, the normal heart rate is about 100 bpm, and at 6.3 to 7.0 weeks, about 120 bpm. A slow fetal heart rate is associated with a 35 to 50 percent rate of fetal loss. However, a slow fetal heart

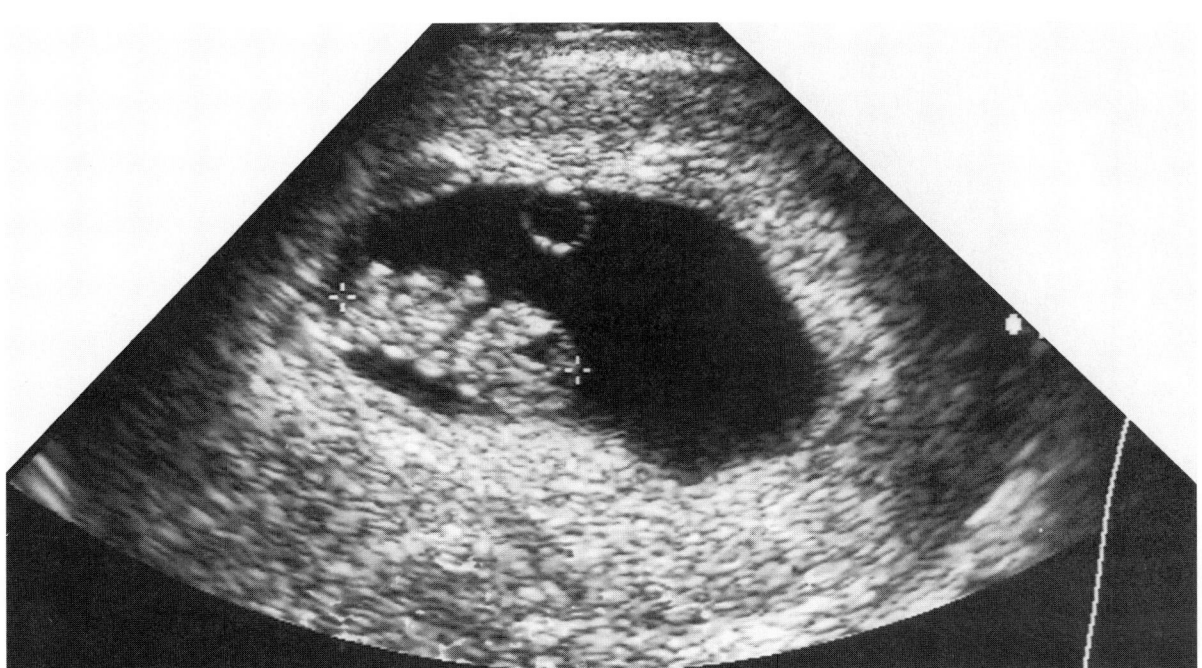

Figure 10-1. Sonogram demonstrating crown-rump length (between crosses) of 8-week fetus. Yolk sac is in the near field.

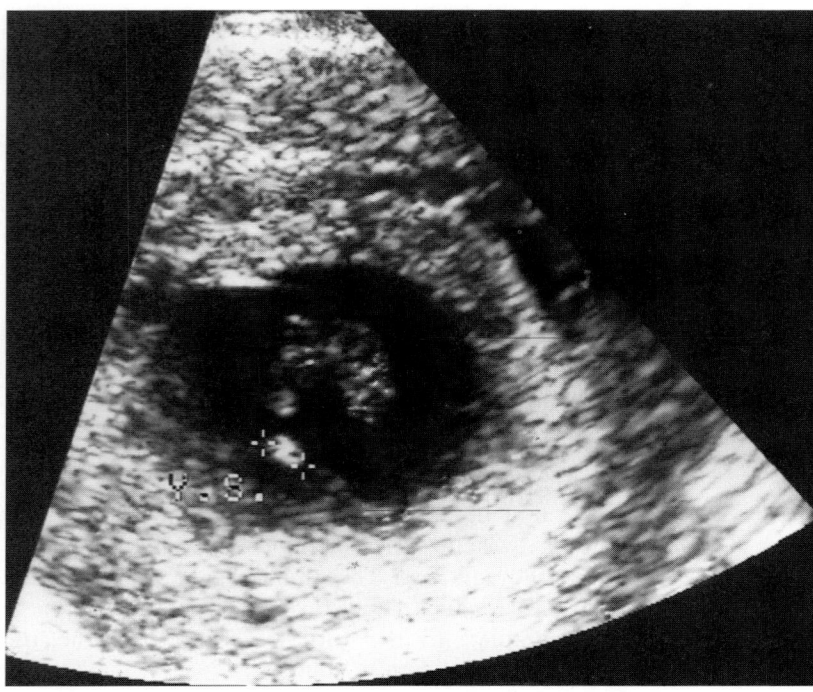

Figure 10–2. Sonogram demonstrating embryonic demise in 7-week embryo. No heart activity was present. Calcified yolk sac is outlined by crosses.

rate at or before 7 weeks in a pregnancy continuing beyond the first trimester is likely to be associated with a normal outcome.[25] Embryonic movements can be seen between 7 and 8 menstrual weeks.

Although the gestational sac can be used to date an early pregnancy, the most accurate sonographic measure is the crown–rump length.[23] During the first tri-

mester, this method is accurate to within 4 to 5 days. As this is the single best tool to assess gestational age at any time in pregnancy, it should be considered for patients at risk for growth restriction and other complications of pregnancy.

The embryonic pole, a flat, echogenic structure, can be visualized when it is 2 to 4 mm during the seventh

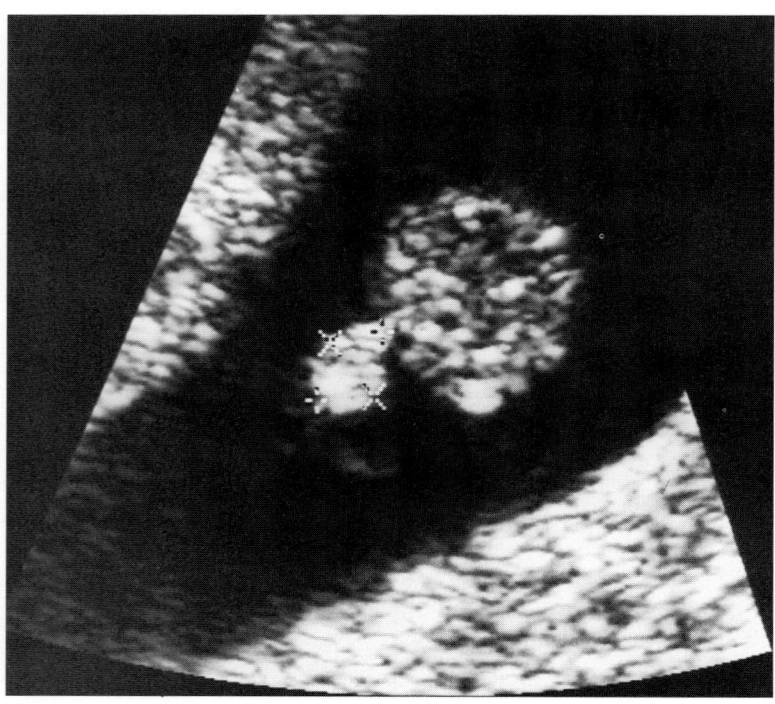

Figure 10–3. Crosses outline normal midgut herniation in 10-week fetus.

menstrual week. During the eighth week, a large head with a posterior cystic space, representing the rhomben-cephalon, can be visualized, together with the spinal column and the lower and upper extremities. By the 9th week, the falx cerebri and the choroid plexus can be seen, and, by the 11th week, the echogenic choroid plexus fills the prominent ventricles. The cerebellum may not be visualized until after 12 weeks.[15-17]

Between the 8th and 12th weeks, there is a normal midgut herniation (Fig. 10-3). This should not be confused with an omphalocele, which can be diagnosed with certainty after that time. The liver can be seen at 9 to 10 weeks; the stomach, at 10 to 12 weeks; the bladder, at 11 to 13 weeks; and the four chambers of the heart, at about 12 weeks.[15-17]

Many of the fetal anomalies identified during a trans-

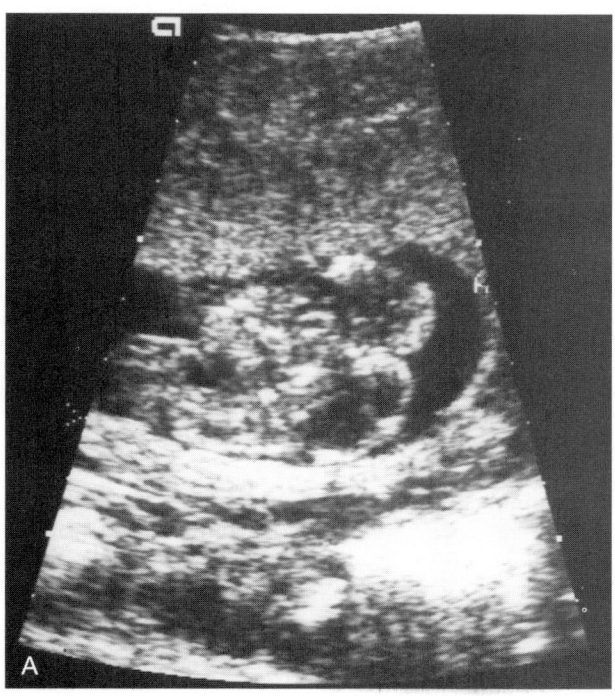

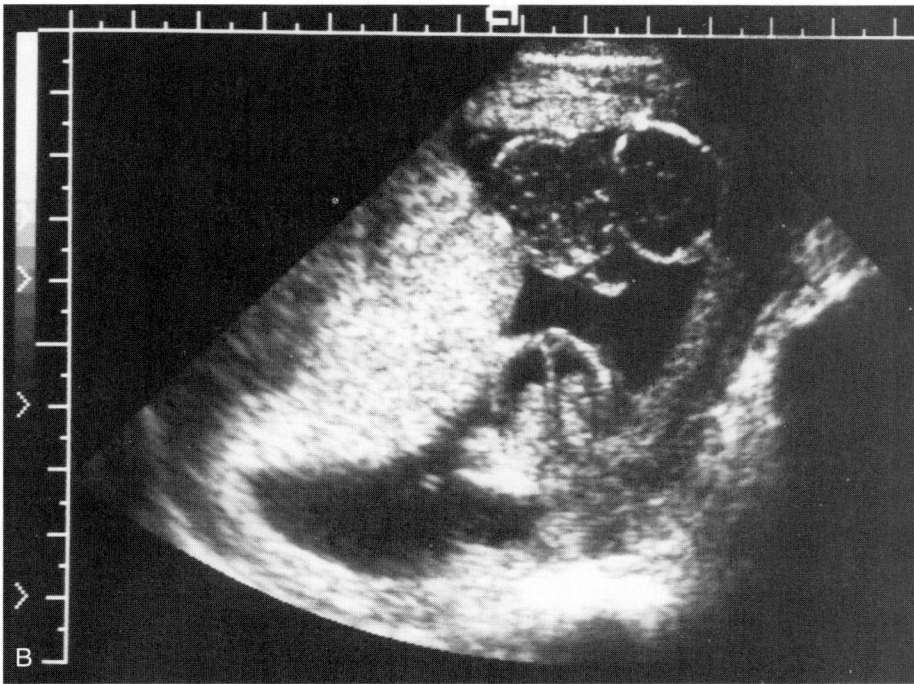

Figure 10-4. *A,* Sonogram at 11 weeks demonstrating conjoined twins. *B,* Sonogram showing conjoined twins in near field and normal triplet in far field.

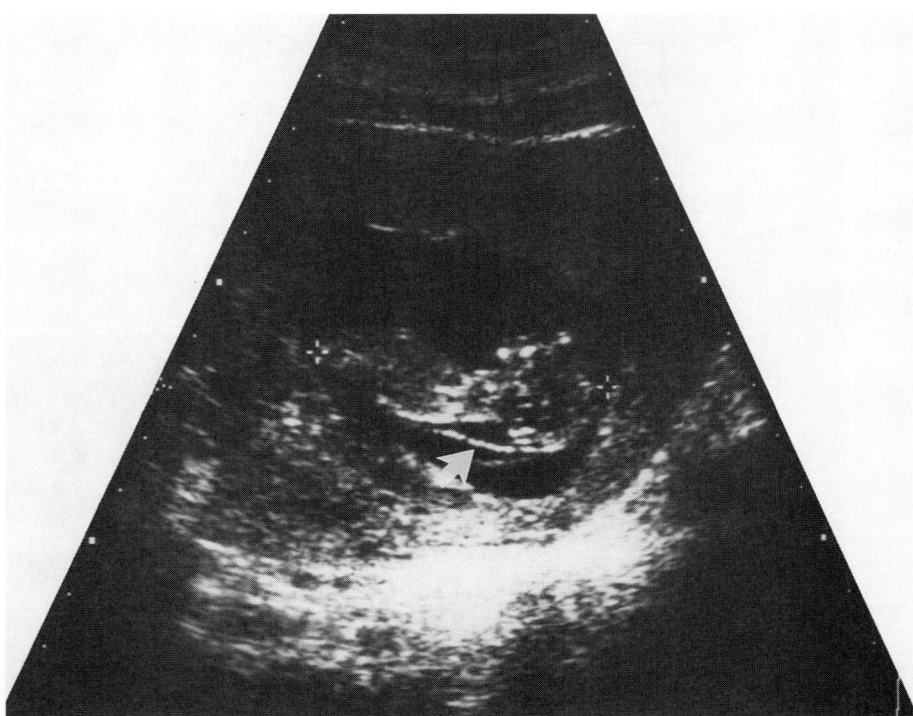

Figure 10–5. Sonogram demonstrating nuchal translucency (*arrow*) greater than 3 mm in 10-week embryo.

abdominal anatomic survey at 18 to 20 weeks can be diagnosed earlier with transvaginal ultrasound. The anomalies with the most serious disruptions of anatomy, such as anencephaly, holoprosencephaly, cystic hygroma, and conjoined twins, may be detected (Fig. 10–4).[15–17] However, at this time, first-trimester vaginal ultrasound is not as accurate in detecting anomalies. This is because some structures, such as the brain, are not as well developed and other structures, such as the heart, are too small to be adequately evaluated. Therefore, first-trimester ultrasound should not be used as a substitute for a second-trimester evaluation of anatomy.

An important aspect of first-trimester ultrasound is the evaluation of nuchal translucency (Fig. 10–5) to predict chromosomal aberrations. Nicolaides[26] and others have shown that nuchal translucency when combined with maternal age and/or serum analytes such as free β-human chorionic gonadotropin and pregnancy-associated plasma protein A have a combined sensitivity exceeding 90 percent in detecting chromosomal abnormalities including Down syndrome.[27–30] It is essential that the nuchal translucency be measured in a standardized manner.

Although the main value of vaginal ultrasound is in early pregnancy, it may be of clinical use later in gestation. Vaginal ultrasound permits direct visualization of the internal cervical os and therefore permits accurate assessment of the location of the placenta and its distance from the internal os. The diagnosis or exclusion of placenta previa is therefore facilitated.[31] In addition, because the cervix can be accurately visualized, vaginal ultrasound may identify early signs of preterm labor or incompetent cervix, such as funneling or shortening of the cervical length,[32,33] and thereby directly aid in patient care (see Chapter 23). Lastly, vaginal ultrasound can improve visualization of intracranial anatomy when the head is engaged and permits enhanced views of cranial structures in coronal and sagittal planes.

SECOND TRIMESTER

Assessment of Gestational Age

When performed during the first trimester, ultrasound permits an extremely accurate assessment of gestational age. The early studies of Robinson and Fleming[34] demonstrated that a fetal crown–rump length, a measurement from the top of the fetal head to its rump, could define gestational ages between 6 and 10 weeks with an error of ±3 to 5 days (Table 10–1).[35] In general, the gestational age of the pregnancy in weeks is equal to 6.5 plus the crown–rump length of the fetus in centimeters. When performing a crown–rump length measurement, care must be taken to avoid confusing the yolk sac with the fetal head. Beyond 12 weeks, the fetus begins to curve and the crown–rump length loses its accuracy.

Table 10–1. ULTRASONOGRAPHIC ASSESSMENT OF FETAL AGE

Measurement	Gestational Age (Menstrual Weeks)	Range (Days)
Crown–rump length	5–12	±3
Biparietal diameter	12–20	±8
	20–24	±12
	24–32	±15
	>32	±21
Femur length	12–20	±7
	20–36	±11
	>36	±16

From Gabbe SG, Iams JD: Intrauterine growth retardation. *In* Iams JD, Zuspan FP (eds): Manual of Obstetrics and Gynecology. St. Louis, CV Mosby, 1990, p 169.

The biparietal diameter (BPD) is the measurement most often used for establishing fetal gestational age. Campbell et al.[36] found the BPD to be the most accurate predictor of the estimated date of confinement (EDC) when performed between 12 and 18 weeks' gestation. The transaxial or transverse BPD is best obtained at the level of the thalami and cavum septum pellucidum (Fig. 10–6). The BPD measurement is made from the outer edge of the skull to the inner edge of the opposite side.

Assessment of gestational age in the second trimester is especially important because a routine obstetric ultrasound examination is commonly performed at this time. Gestational age assessment by ultrasound has recently been assessed in populations of patients with precisely dated pregnancies that resulted from in vitro fertilization (IVF).[37,38] Head circumference improved the accuracy of the dating equation (random error, 3.35 days). Most dating formulas had systematic errors of less than 1 week. The systematic error was −0.32 day when using the average singleton-based prediction for twins and −1.26 days for triplets.[37] The clinical practice in many units has been that, when gestational age by last menstrual period disagrees by more than 10 or 14 days from that derived from fetal biometry in the second trimester, the last menstrual period is superseded by fetal biometry. These data derived from an IVF population suggest that, in the face of a discrepancy of more than 7 days (2 SD), the sonographic biometric prediction should be given preference, provided there is no anomaly or severe growth delay. Other authorities would recommend that the biometric prediction should be given preference in every case.[38,39]

From 12 to 28 weeks' gestation, the relationship between BPD and gestational age is linear.[40] The error when measuring the BPD using a 3.5-MHz transducer is ±1 to 1.5 mm. This error will be least significant early in gestation when the fetal head is growing rapidly (Table 10–1). However, late in gestation, growth of the fetal head slows, and errors of several weeks may be made in estimating gestational age. In addition, later in gestation, the fetal head becomes more elongated in its anterior posterior plane. Such dolichocephaly may be assessed by measuring the cephalic index, the ratio of the BPD divided by the occipital frontal diameter. This ratio should normally be 0.75 to 0.85. If the ratio falls outside this range, the BPD should not be used to estimate gestational age. Femur length may be applied in such cases.

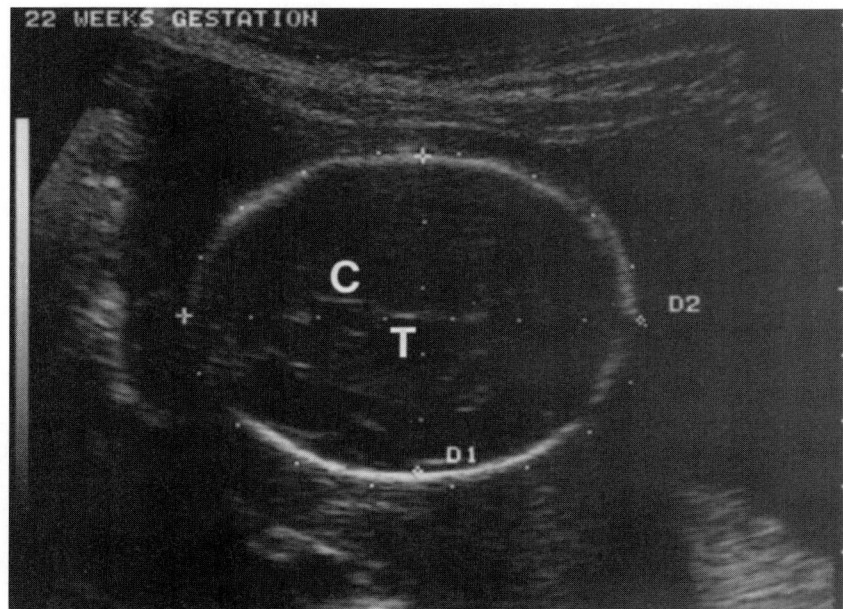

Figure 10–6. A determination of the BPD at the level of the thalami (T) and cavum septum pellucidum (C). The BPD measurement is made from the outer edge of the skull to the opposite inner edge (D1) and on a line perpendicular to the midline. The occipitofrontal diameter (D2) is also shown. The electronic calipers (*dots*) have been placed to obtain a measurement of the HC.

Assessment of Fetal Viability

Real-time ultrasound can be used to confirm the presence of fetal death in utero. The absence of fetal cardiac motion as well as the presence of fetal scalp edema and overlapping of the fetal cranial bones confirms fetal death.

THIRD TRIMESTER

Evaluation of Fetal Growth

When establishing gestational age and evaluating fetal growth, it is best to evaluate a variety of parameters, including the BPD, long bones, especially the femur and humerus, as well as the abdominal circumference (AC) (Fig. 10–7), outer and inner orbital diameters, and transcerebellar diameter. The uniformity of fetal growth that characterizes early gestation is lost after 20 weeks. Therefore, a single ultrasound study performed late in pregnancy cannot accurately establish gestational age (Table 10–1). The fetal AC or perimeter measured at the level of the umbilical vein has been used not only to assess gestational age, but to detect the presence of intrauterine growth restriction (IUGR) and macrosomia (Fig. 10–7). Composite tables estimating fetal weight have been constructed by several authors and are usually based on a combination of (1) head size, as measured by BPD or head circumference (HC); (2) femur

length (FL); and (3) AC.[41] Tables by Hadlock et al.[42] and Shepard et al.[43] are currently in most common use. Shepard et al. demonstrated that the BPD and fetal AC may be combined to calculate estimates of fetal weight that are likely to be within 10 percent of actual weight.

Abnormal Fetal Growth

Fetal growth restriction is discussed in Chapter 25.

Fetal Macrosomia (see Chapters 16 and 27)

Macrosomia has been defined by some investigators as a birth weight in excess of 4,000 to 4,500 g.[44] Other studies, using population-specific growth curves, categorize infants with a birth weight above the 90th percentile as large for gestational age (LGA). Excessive fetal growth resulting in macrosomia has long been recognized as an important cause of perinatal morbidity and mortality, especially in the pregnancy complicated by diabetes mellitus. At delivery, the macrosomic fetus is more likely to suffer shoulder dystocia, traumatic injury, and asphyxia.

Macrosomia in the infant of the diabetic mother (IDM) is characterized by selected organomegaly, with increases in both fat and muscle mass resulting in a disproportionate increase in the size of the abdomen and shoulders. However, brain growth is not altered, and, therefore, the HC is usually normal. Thus, the macrosomia of the IDM is asymmetric. The macrosomic infant of an obese woman without glucose intol-

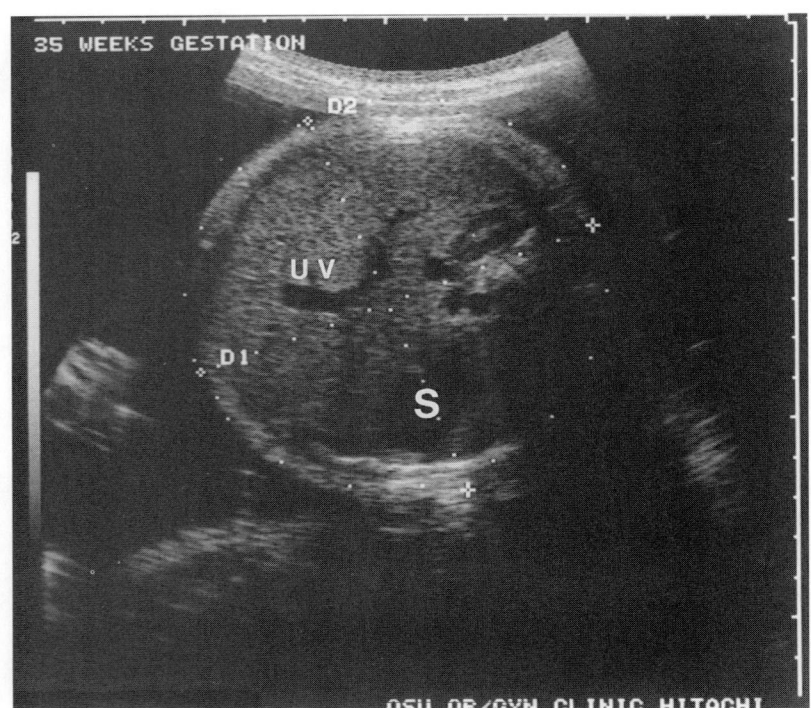

Figure 10–7. Transverse or axial view of the abdomen demonstrates the fetal stomach (S) and umbilical vein (UV). Note that the abdomen is round and the umbilical vein is well within the substance of the liver. This is the proper level for determination of the fetal AC; electronic calipers (*dots*) have been placed to make this measurement. The AC may also be calculated using measurements of the anteroposterior (D1) and transverse (D2) abdominal diameters using the following formula: AC = D1 + D2 × 1.57.

erance will demonstrate excessive growth of *both* the AC and HC, or symmetric macrosomia.

Antenatal sonographic detection of the LGA fetus could allow optimal selection of the route of delivery to reduce the likelihood of birth trauma. Unfortunately, our clinical ability to evaluate fetal size at term remains poor, with only 35 percent of large infants being identified by excessive symphysis–fundal height measurements.[45]

Sonographic estimation of fetal weight has been used to improve the detection of excessive growth. Using Shepard's formula, Ott and Doyle[46] determined fetal weight in 595 patients undergoing real-time ultrasound estimation within 72 hours of delivery. Overall, almost 75 percent of LGA infants were detected using an estimated fetal weight (EFW) above the 90th percentile as the cut-off for diagnosis. There were a significant number of false-positives, as the predictive value of a positive test was only 63.2 percent. An EFW below the 90th percentile predicted a normally grown fetus in 96 percent of cases, emphasizing the high negative predictive value of ultrasound.

Several studies have emphasized the limited predictive value of ultrasound to identify the macrosomic fetus and the unnecessary interventions that may be undertaken for suspected macrosomia.[47–51] Overall, both the sensitivity and positive predictive value in these reports range between 50 and 60 percent. It must be remembered that formulas for estimation of fetal weight are associated with a 95 percent confidence range of at least 10 to 15 percent.[42] Thus, the predicted weight using ultrasonography would have to exceed 4,700 g for all fetuses with weights in excess of 4,000 g to be accurately identified!

Measurement of the AC is probably the most reliable sonographic parameter for the detection of macrosomia. Using an AC above the 90th percentile obtained within 2 weeks of delivery, Tamura et al.[47] correctly identified 78 percent of LGA fetuses. When both the AC and EFW exceeded the 90th percentile, an LGA infant was correctly diagnosed in 88.8 percent of cases. Bochner et al.[52] used early third-trimester ultrasound measurements of the AC to determine the risk for both macrosomia and birth trauma at term. In a series of 201 women with gestational diabetes mellitus, 36 of 41 cases of macrosomia were identified by the presence of an AC above the 90th percentile at 30 to 33 weeks' gestation. The false-positive rate was high, with 28 normally grown fetuses having large AC measurements. Of note, the risk for shoulder dystocia was 9.3 percent in the suspected LGA group versus 0.8 percent in the group with a normal AC measurement at 30 to 33 weeks.

The HC/AC ratio has been used for the detection of asymmetric macrosomia. The HC/AC ratio should be reduced in cases of asymmetric macrosomia seen in diabetes mellitus, since abdominal size is disproportionately large compared with head growth (Fig. 10–8).[53] The HC/AC ratio does require an accurate knowledge of gestational age, since the ratio varies throughout pregnancy. Using a similar approach, Cohen has reported that when the difference between the abdominal diameter and BPD is 2.6 cm or more in IDMs weighing 3,800 to 4,200 g, the risk of significant shoulder dystocia is 30 percent.[54]

In summary, detection of the macrosomic infant using both clinical *and* ultrasonographic techniques remains challenging. In patients at risk for fetal macrosomia—women who have diabetes mellitus, are obese, or whose pregnancies go beyond 41 weeks—a "growth profile" including ultrasound measurements of estimated fetal weight and the HC/AC ratio may improve the identification of excessive fetal growth.[55] In patients at low risk for macrosomia, a fundal height measurement of 4 cm or more than expected for gestational age should signal the need for an ultrasound study.

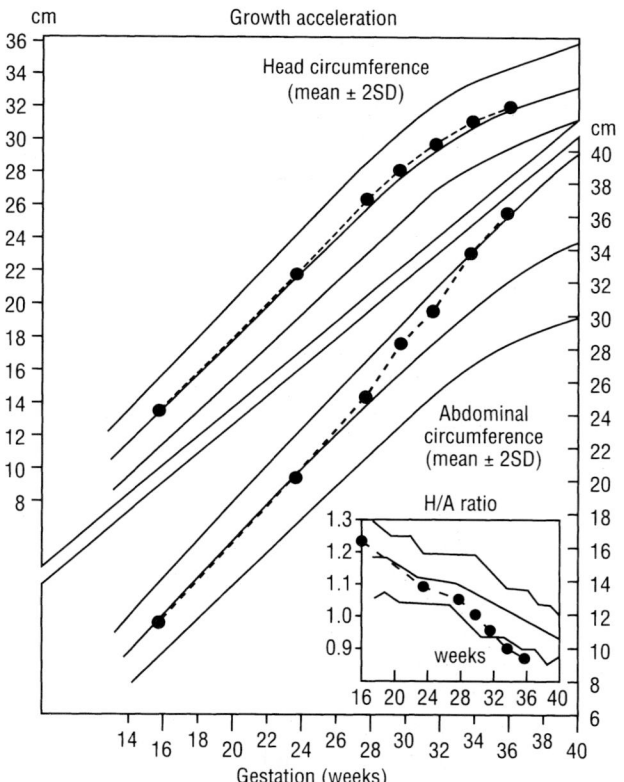

Figure 10–8. Growth chart in a case of asymmetric macrosomia. While HC growth is preserved, AC growth is accelerated in the third trimester. For this reason, the HC/AC or H/A ratio shown in the lower right corner of the graph is reduced. This growth pattern is characteristic of the accelerated growth of the fetus of the diabetic mother. (From Chudleigh P, Pearce JM [eds]: Obstetric Ultrasound. Edinburgh, Churchill Livingstone, 1986.)

Assessment of Amniotic Fluid Volume

Ultrasound has proved valuable in the evaluation of amniotic fluid volume. Early application of this technology included measurements of the largest vertical pocket of fluid. Oligohydramnios, a reduction in amniotic fluid volume, was diagnosed when the largest pocket of amniotic fluid measured in two perpendicular planes was less than 1 cm. Chamberlain et al.[56] reported this degree of oligohydramnios in 0.85 percent of more than 7,500 patients evaluated. When defined in this way, oligohydramnios was associated with a 40-fold increase in perinatal mortality (187.5 per 1,000); a 17-fold increase in lethal congenital anomalies such as renal agenesis, polycystic kidney disease, or complete obstruction of the genitourinary system (9.4 percent); and an eight-fold increase in growth restriction (39 percent). Hydramnios or excessive amniotic fluid was diagnosed when the largest pocket of amniotic fluid exceeded 8 cm in two perpendicular planes[57] (see Table 1–2).

Several investigators have questioned the diagnostic accuracy of the largest or maximum vertical pocket concept as an index of overall amniotic fluid volume and perinatal outcome. Bottoms et al.[58] reported that subjective assessment of amniotic fluid volume was as valuable as measurements of the maximum vertical pocket. They did note that suspected fetal growth restriction and suspected postterm gestation were negatively correlated with the maximum vertical pocket, whereas suspected fetal growth acceleration and increasing birth weight were positively correlated. Hoddick et al.[59] reported poor sensitivity when applying the 1-cm vertical pocket as an index of oligohydramnios for the detection of IUGR.

In an effort to find a more reproducible and quantitative technique to assess amniotic fluid volume, Phelan and colleagues[60,61] developed the amniotic fluid index (AFI). The AFI measurement is performed with the patient in the supine or semi-Fowler's positive position. The maternal abdomen is divided into quadrants (Figs. 10–9 and 10–10). The umbilicus is used as one reference point to divide the uterus into upper and lower halves, and the linea nigra is used as the midline to divide the uterus into right and left halves. The ultrasound transducer head is then placed on the maternal abdomen along the longitudinal axis. The transducer head is maintained perpendicular to the floor, and the vertical diameter of the largest amniotic fluid pocket in each quadrant is identified and measured. The total of each of these measurements is summed to obtain the AFI in centimeters. If a fetal extremity or portion of the umbilical cord is observed in the quadrant to be measured, the transducer head is moved slightly to exclude these structures. A linear array, sector, or curvilinear transducer may be used to determine the AFI.[52] Care

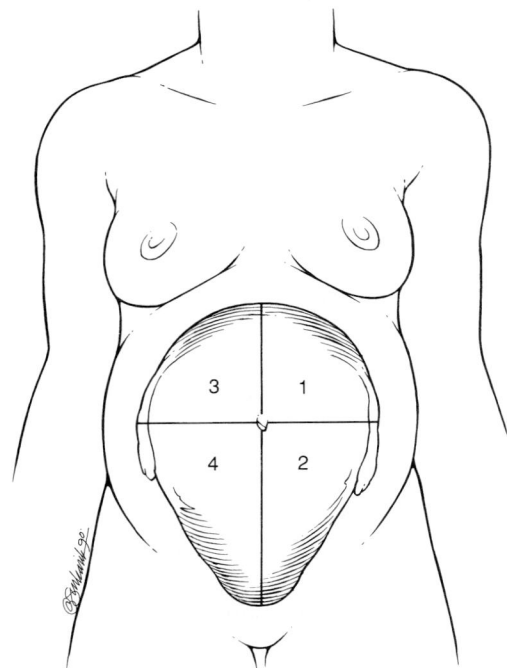

Figure 10–9. The AFI measurement utilizes ultrasound to assess the depth of fluid pockets in each quadrant of the uterus. Note that the umbilicus divides the uterus into upper and lower halves, and the linea nigra divides the uterus into right and left halves.

must be taken to avoid excessive pressure on the transducer, as this might decrease the AFI.[63] Moore and Cayle[64] have modified this approach by measuring only those amniotic fluid pockets completely clear of cord or extremities. The technique is extremely reproducible, with intraobserver and interobserver variations averaging 1.0 and 2.0 cm, respectively.[64–66] When the AFI is determined in a patient at 20 weeks' gestation or lower, the uterus is divided into halves using the linea nigra, and the largest pocket identified in each half is added to produce an AFI.

Using this technique, Phelan et al.[60] found that the mean AFI in over 350 pregnancies at 36 to 42 weeks was 12.9 ± 4.6 cm. Patients with an AFI less than 5.0 cm at term were considered to have oligohydramnios, and those with an AFI of 20 cm or greater were considered to have polyhydramnios. When the AFI fell below 5 cm, Rutherford et al.[65] noted that the frequency of nonreactive nonstress tests, fetal heart rate decelerations, meconium staining, cesarean sections for fetal distress, and low Apgar scores increased. Based on a maximum vertical pocket of 8 cm or more to define polyhydramnios, fetal structural anomalies have been observed in 36 to 63 percent of cases with polyhydramnios.[67,68]

Moore and his colleagues have demonstrated the validity of the AFI and established normative values for this measurement. In a pregnant sheep model, Moore and Brace[69] first found that the AFI demonstrated a

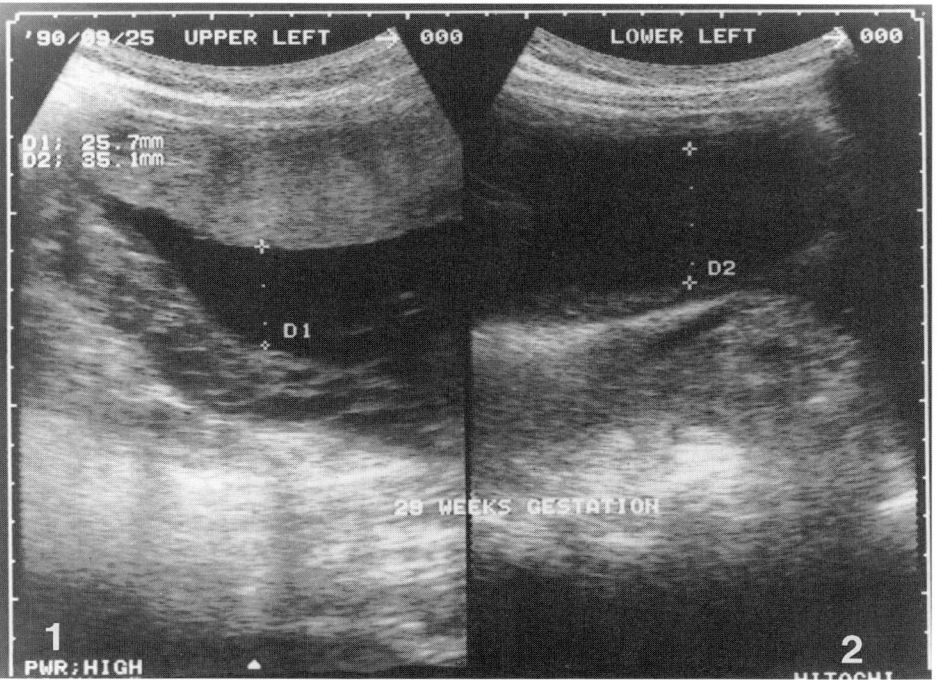

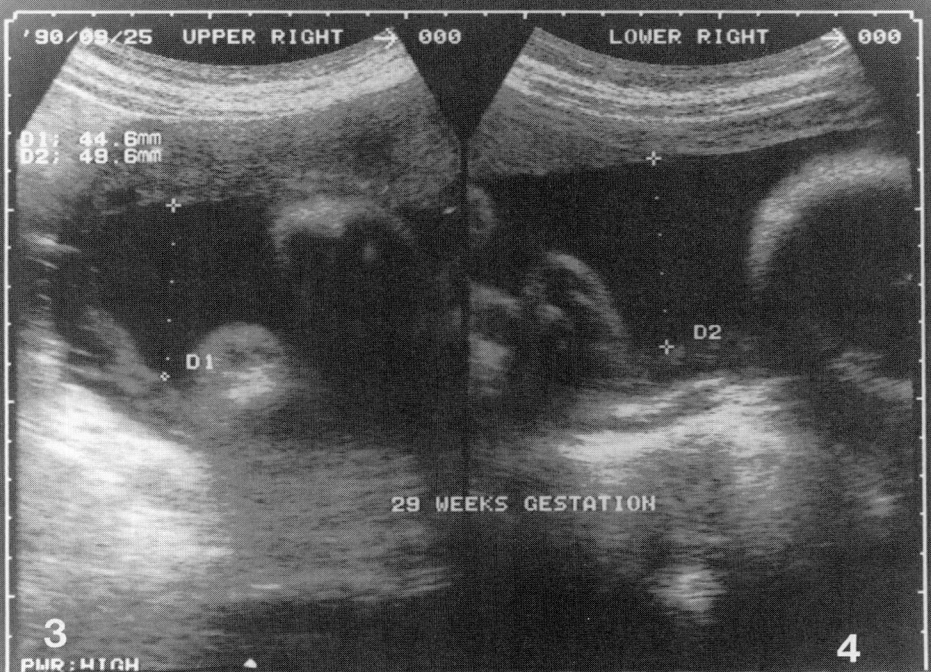

Figure 10–10. Ultrasound determination of the AFI at 29 weeks' gestation. The numbers in the corner of each ultrasound section correspond to those in Figure 10–9. The AFI was 15.6 cm, which is normal at this gestational age (see Table 10–2).

close linear relationship to the actual amount of amniotic fluid and was 88 percent accurate in quantitating amniotic fluid volume. Moore and Cayle[64] next studied 791 uncomplicated pregnancies prospectively to establish normal values for the AFI (Table 10–2). At term, the mean AFI was 11.5 cm, and the 5th and 95th percentiles were 6.8 and 19.6 cm, respectively. These values are similar to those reported by Phelan and co-workers. Moore[70] has also demonstrated the superiority of the AFI over the maximum vertical pocket in detecting abnormalities of amniotic fluid volume. In this study of 1,178 high-risk patients, oligohydramnios was defined as an AFI less than the 5th percentile for gestational age, whereas hydramnios was defined as an AFI greater than the 95th percentile for gestational age. The ability of a maximum vertical pocket of 3 cm or less to

Table 10-2. AMNIOTIC FLUID INDEX PERCENTILE VALUES (mm)

Week	Percentile					
	2.5th	5th	50th	95th	97.5th	n
16	73	79	121	185	201	32
17	77	83	127	194	211	26
18	80	87	133	202	220	17
19	83	90	137	207	225	14
20	86	93	141	212	230	25
21	88	95	143	214	233	14
22	89	97	145	216	235	14
23	90	98	146	218	237	14
24	90	98	147	219	238	23
25	89	97	147	221	240	12
26	89	97	147	223	242	11
27	85	95	146	226	245	17
28	86	94	146	228	249	25
29	84	92	145	231	254	12
30	82	90	145	234	258	17
31	79	88	144	238	263	26
32	77	86	144	242	269	25
33	74	83	143	245	274	30
34	72	81	142	248	278	31
35	70	79	140	249	279	27
36	68	77	138	249	279	39
37	66	75	135	244	275	36
38	65	73	132	239	269	27
39	64	72	127	226	255	12
40	63	71	123	214	240	64
41	63	70	116	194	216	162
42	63	69	110	175	192	30

From Moore TR, Cayle JE: The amniotic fluid index in normal human pregnancy. Am J Obstet Gynecol 162:1168, 1990, with permission.

identify cases with oligohydramnios by AFI was poor, with a sensitivity of only 42 percent and a positive predictive value of 51 percent. Moore[70] noted that 58 percent of cases with oligohydramnios by AFI had normal values when using the largest vertical pocket technique. The detection of polyhydramnios, defined as a maximum vertical pocket of 8.0 cm or greater, was also limited in cases identified to have excessive amniotic fluid by this method.

In summary, whereas there is reasonably good correlation between quantitation of amniotic fluid volume using subjective assessment of amniotic fluid volume, measurements of the maximum vertical pocket, and AFI, the AFI appears to have significant advantages. This index appears highly reproducible and may, therefore, be more uniformly used by a number of different examiners. Furthermore, the AFI may be applied with greater reliability at each gestational age using the normative values that have been developed by Moore and Cayle.[64] Finally, the AFI has greater sensitivity and predictive value in evaluating the pregnancy at risk for oligohydramnios and polyhydramnios.

SONOGRAPHIC EVALUATION OF FETAL AND PLACENTAL ANATOMY

Evaluation of fetal and placental anatomy is an integral part of ultrasound examinations during the second and third trimesters. A basic ultrasound examination that documents fetal life, fetal number, fetal presentation, gestational age and growth, amniotic fluid volume, and placental localization without an evaluation of fetal anatomy, therefore, should be considered incomplete. The following is meant to represent the examination of fetal anatomy that should be part of the basic study. A comprehensive sonographic examination of fetal anatomy is often more detailed when it is targeted to look for a certain anomaly.[72-74]

The fetal skull should be elliptical, with the cranium ossified and intact. The ventricular system should be evaluated by assessment of the width of the atrium (Fig. 10-11), and the cerebellum should be visualized (Fig. 10-12) and nuchal thickness measured. An attempt should be made to visualize the face, especially

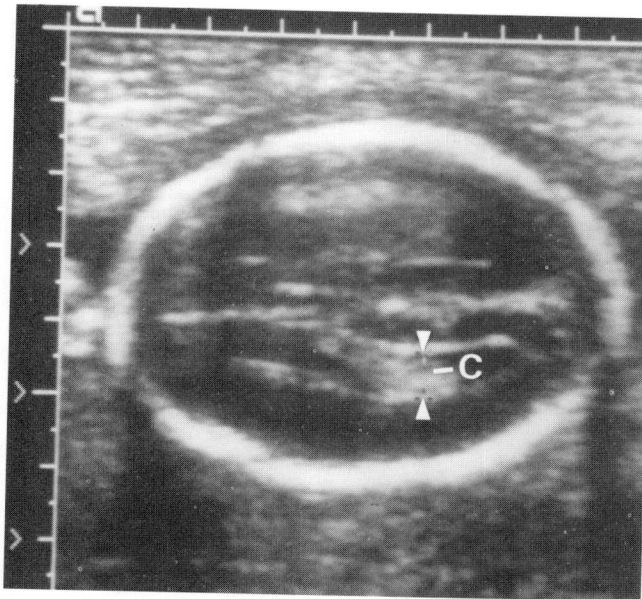

Figure 10–11. Transverse sonogram of fetal skull demonstrating normal ovoid contour. Arrows define width of the atrium of the lateral ventricle. C, choroid plexus.

senting venous blood flow. As gestation advances, the basal layer reveals more calcifications. A system of placental grading based on the characteristics of the chorionic plate, placental substance, and basal layer has been used in the past to predict fetal pulmonary maturity (see Chapter 12).

Placental thickness can be directly related to gestational age, with the thickness of the placenta in millimeters corresponding approximately to the weeks of gestation. For example, at 20 weeks' gestation, the placenta will be approximately 20 mm thick. Placentomegaly, a placenta of greater than normal thickness, has been associated with maternal diabetes mellitus, fetal hydrops, placental hemorrhage, intrauterine infection including syphilis, chromosomal abnormalities, and hydatidiform mole (Fig. 10–27), or a placental chorioangioma (Fig. 10–28).

Currently, placenta accreta can be suspected with ultrasound and may be of value in high-risk patients who have a placenta previa in conjunction with a prior cesarean delivery (see Fig. 17–8). However, a normal ultrasound examination does not exclude the possibility of an accreta, as sonographic diagnosis is imperfect.[78,79]

to rule out a facial cleft (Fig. 10–13). The spine is easier to evaluate in its entirety in the second trimester than in the third. A sagittal sonogram should be complemented by a series of transverse sonograms to identify normal anterior and normal posterior ossification elements (Figs. 10–14 and 10–15). A four-chambered view of the heart should be obtained.[75] Ventricles and atria of equal and appropriate sizes and an intact ventricular septum should be observed (Fig. 10–16). Evaluation of outflow tracts should be attempted (Fig. 10–17). The fetal bladder (Fig. 10–18), stomach (Fig. 10–19), and kidneys (Fig. 10–20) should be visualized. The abdominal wall should be intact (Fig. 10–21). The long bones of at least the lower extremities should be visualized (Figs. 10–22 and 10–23). Although fetal gender often may be identified in the second and third trimesters, this should not be considered an integral part of the examination (Figs. 10–24 and 10–25).

In addition to the assessment of placental location, ultrasound can provide an evaluation of placental anatomy[76,77] (Fig. 10–26; see also Fig. 1–5). Although difficult during the first trimester, the location of the placenta can be clearly established by the second trimester. Early in gestation, the placental substance is homogeneous but, as pregnancy advances, echospared areas corresponding to flow of blood from the maternal spiral arterioles and calcium deposition can be seen. The chorionic plate, the fetal surface of the placenta, is initially straight and well defined, but develops indentations as gestation progresses. The basal layer of the placenta is characterized by a hypoechoic area repre-

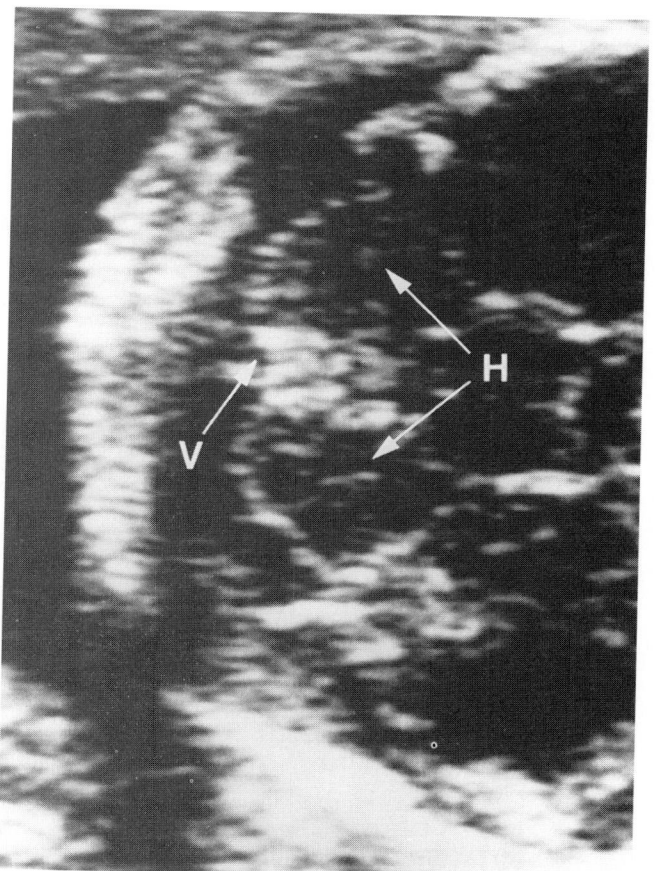

Figure 10–12. Sonogram demonstrating cerebellar hemispheres (H). V, cerebellar vermis.

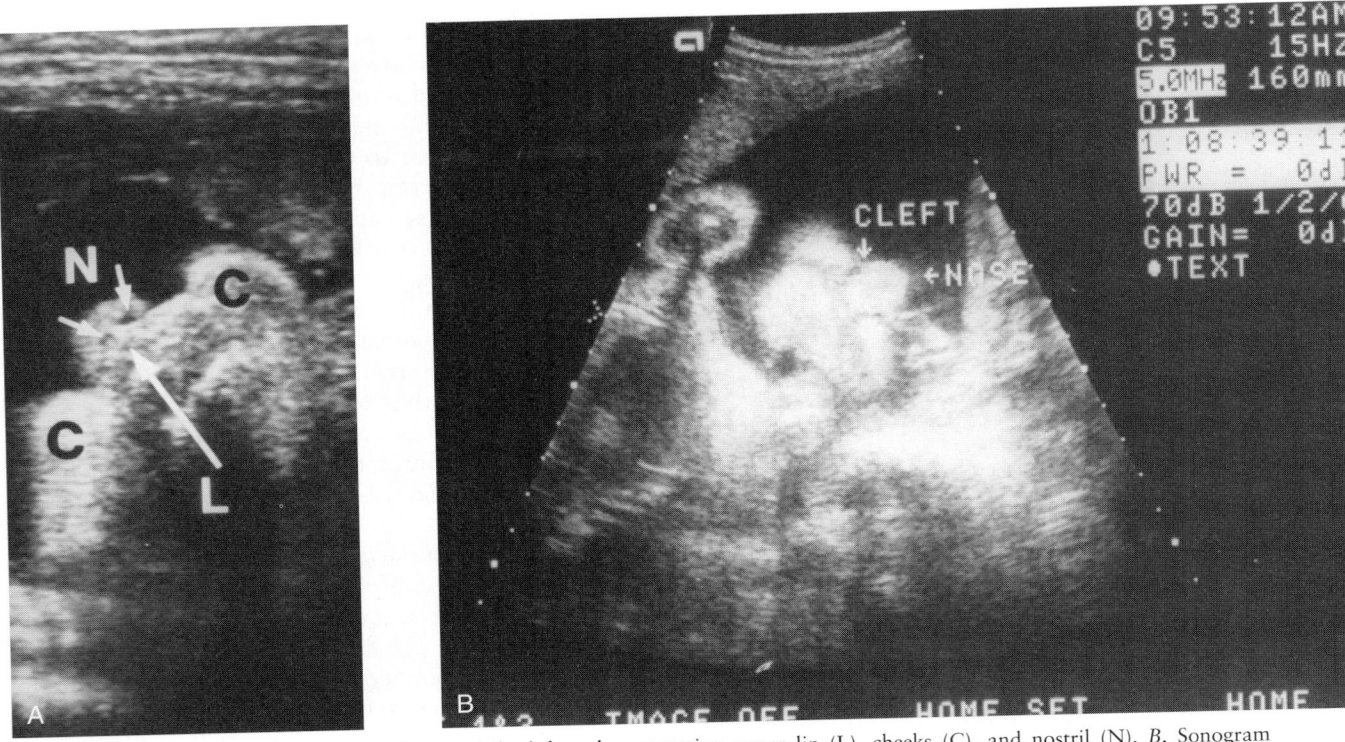

Figure 10–13. *A,* Sonogram of normal fetal face demonstrating upper lip (L), cheeks (C), and nostril (N). *B,* Sonogram demonstrating cleft lip (*arrow*).

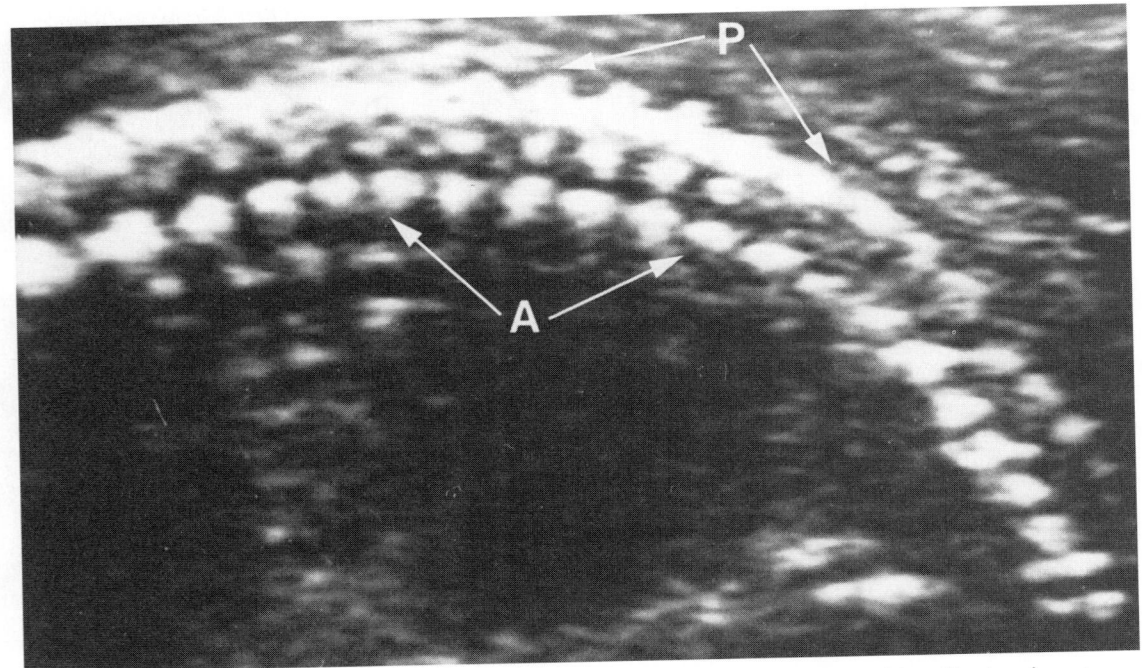

Figure 10–14. Longitudinal view of the spine demonstrating anterior (A) and posterior (P) ossification elements.

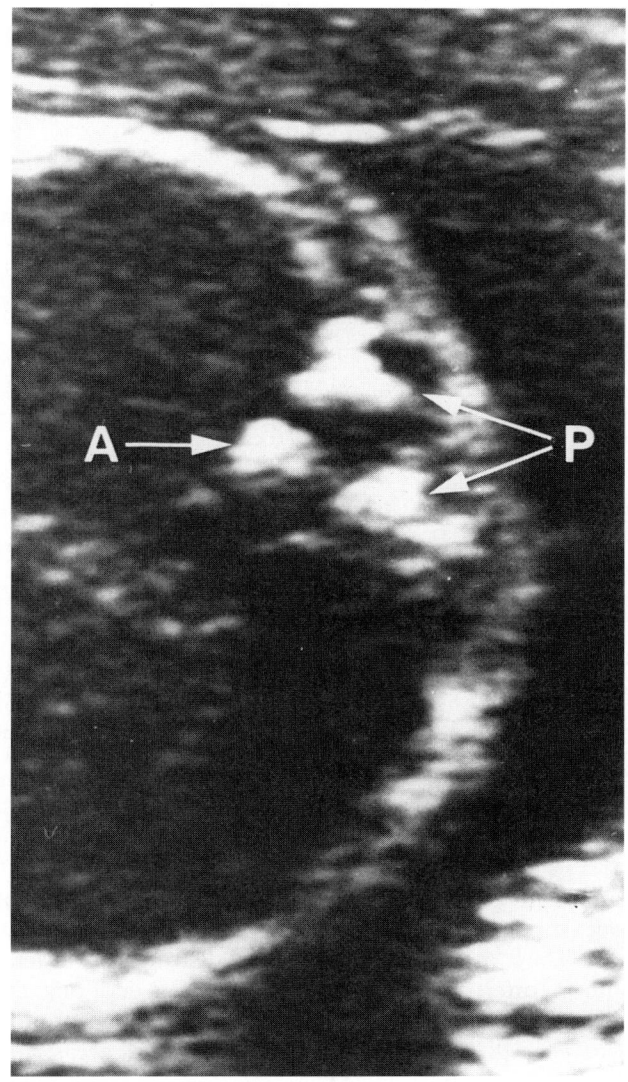

Figure 10-15. Transverse view of the spine demonstrating anterior (A) and posterior (P) ossification elements.

ULTRASOUND DIAGNOSIS OF FETAL ANOMALIES

Antenatal ultrasound scanning at about 18 to 20 weeks of gestation permits the detection of most major fetal structural anomalies.[80-82] It is important to appreciate, however, that even a thorough ultrasound evaluation during the second trimester will not detect all structural malformations. Anomalies such as hydrocephalus caused by aqueductal stenosis, duodenal atresia, microcephaly, achondroplasia, and polycystic kidneys may not manifest until the third trimester, when the degree of anatomic distortion is sufficient to be sonographically detectable.

What fetal malformations should be identified during a basic ultrasound examination? Nelson et al.[83] surveyed 27 radiologists and 15 obstetricians with expertise in this field who were told that the patient was referred for a dating scan between 20 and 24 weeks' gestation and had no complicating obstetric problems. The anomalies believed to be observable in the majority of cases included anencephaly, hydranencephaly, ventriculomegaly of greater than 15 mm, alobar holoprosencephaly, open spina bifida, a large amount of ascites, bilateral hydronephrosis greater than 20 mm, omphalocele, gastroschisis, and hydrothorax with a mediastinal shift. A useful classification of fetal anomalies is based on the nature of the dysmorphology that permits sonographic detection.

Absence of a Normally Present Structure

A dramatic example of the absence of a structure normally detected by ultrasound is anencephaly, the absence of calvaria and forebrain (Fig. 10-29). Ultrasound clearly reveals the absence of echogenic skull bones and the presence of a heterogeneous mass of cystic tissue, called the area cerebrovasculosa, which replaces well-defined cerebral structures. In 1972, anencephaly was the first fetal anomaly to be diagnosed with sufficient certainty to support a decision to terminate a pregnancy.[84]

Alobar holoprosencephaly is the absence of midline cerebral structures, resulting from incomplete cleavage

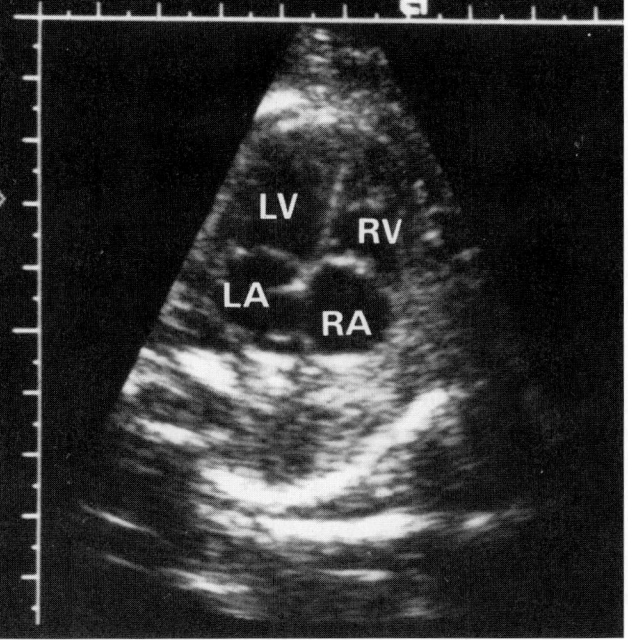

Figure 10-16. Four-chamber view of the heart. LA, left atrium; LV, left ventricle; RA, right atrium; RV, right ventricle.

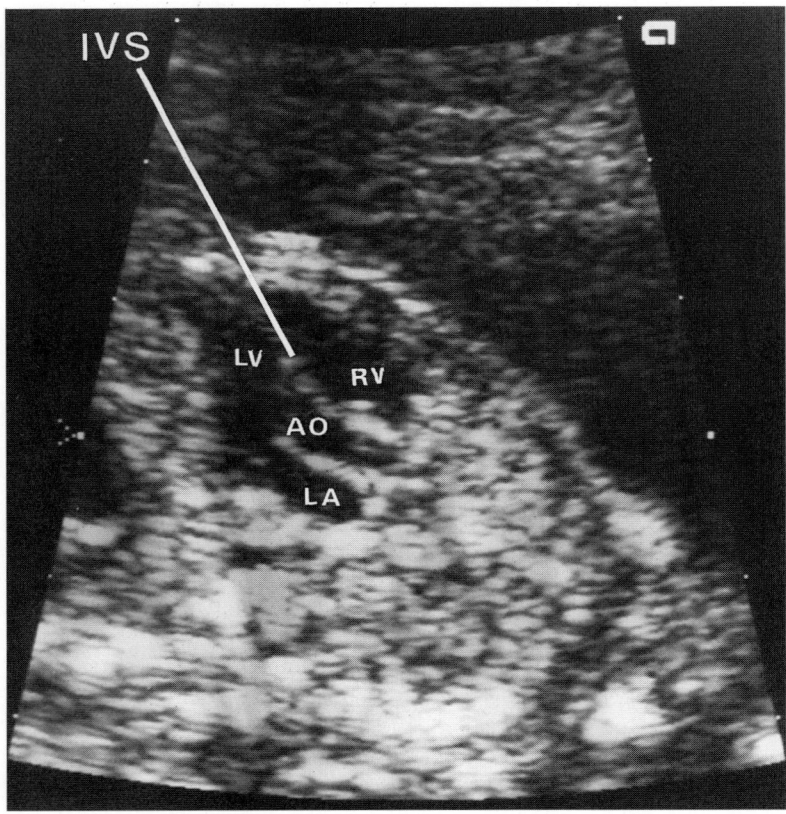

Figure 10–17. Sonogram demonstrating outflow tract (AO), left ventricle (LV), left atrium (LA), and right ventricle (RV). The anterior wall of the aortic outflow tract is contiguous with the interventricular septum (IVS).

of the primitive forebrain. The "midline echo" of the fetal head, normally generated by acoustic interfaces in the area of the interhemispheric fissure, is absent. However, absence of a midline echo is not specific to alobar holoprosencephaly; an additional sonographic sign should be sought to confirm a diagnosis, which may include hypotelorism, nasal anomalies, and facial clefts. The detection of the facial aberration helps to confirm the diagnosis of alobar holoprosencephaly (Fig. 10–30).[85]

The kidneys are normally visualized as bilateral, ovoid, paraspinal masses with echospared renal pelves. When not visualized, the diagnosis of renal agenesis should be suspected. Severe oligohydramnios and the inability to visualize the bladder support the diagnosis of renal agenesis. Although antenatal diagnosis of renal agenesis is possible, false-positive and false-negative diagnoses occur from inadequate visualization because of the presence of oligohydramnios and simulation of the sonographic appearance of kidneys by the ovoid-shaped adrenal glands.[86]

Presence of an Additional Structure

Masses that distort normal fetal anatomy can be readily identified with ultrasound. Teratomas are the most common neoplasms of fetuses. They are derived from pluripotent cells and are composed of a diversity of tissue foreign to the anatomic site from which they arise. They may be visualized as distortions of fetal contour, often in the sacrococcygeal area or along the fetal midline. The internal sonographic appearance, characterized by irregular cystic and solid areas and occasional calcifications, helps to identify the lesion (Fig. 10–31).[87]

Fetal cystic hygromas are fluid-filled masses of the fetal neck that arise from abnormal lymphatic development. They are generally anechoic, with scattered septations and the presence of a midline septum arising from the nuchal ligament. If the lymphatic disorder causing the hygromas is widespread, it may produce fetal hydrops and intrauterine death[88,89] (Fig. 10–32).

Fetal hydrops or fetal anasarca may be identified by the distortion of the normal fetal surface by skin edema. Ascites, pleural effusions, and pericardial effusions also may be identified. The etiologies of fetal hydrops are many and varied[90–92] (Fig. 10–33).

Herniation Through Structural Defects

A common theme in the development of the fetus is the formation of compartments containing vital structures by folding and midline fusion. Incomplete fusion in a

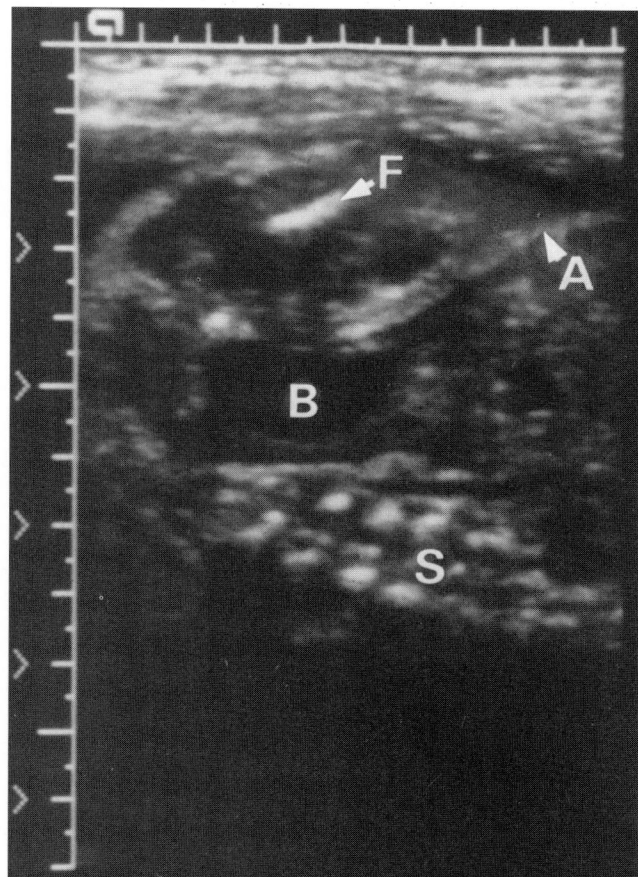

Figure 10–18. Sonogram demonstrating fetal bladder (B), spine (S), abdominal wall (A), and femur (F).

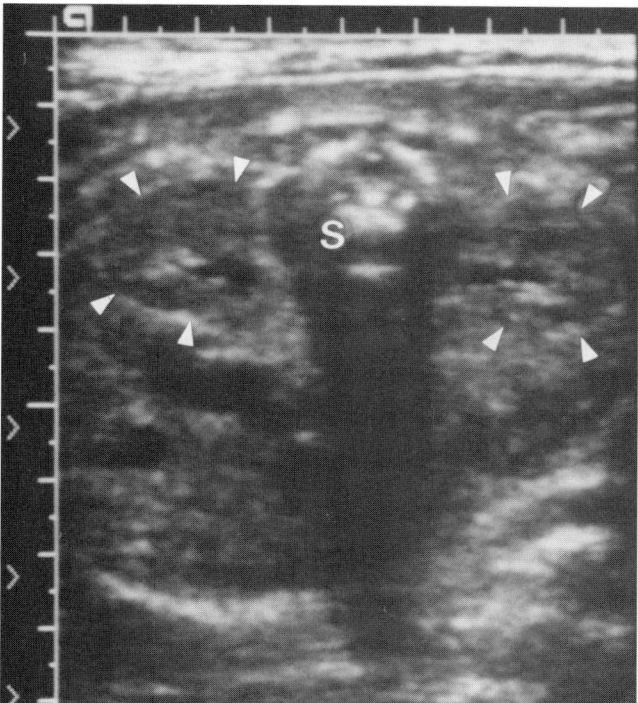

Figure 10–20. Sonogram demonstrating fetal kidneys outlined by *arrows*. S, fetal spine.

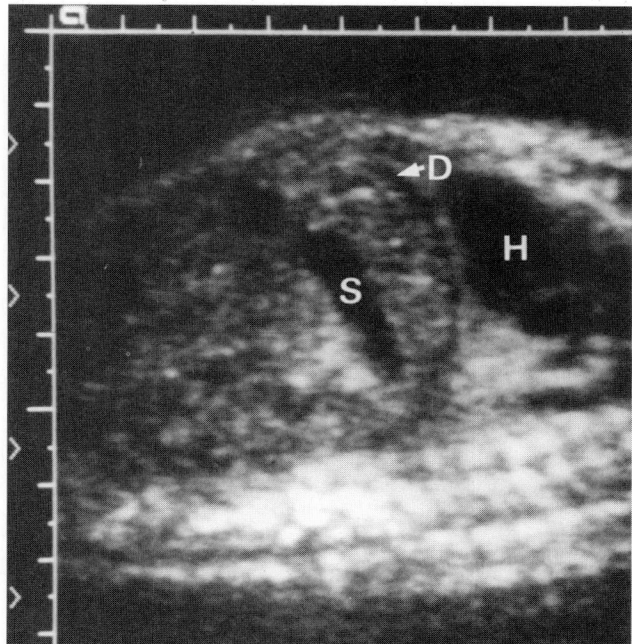

Figure 10–19. Sonogram demonstrating fetal stomach (S), diaphragm (D), and heart (H).

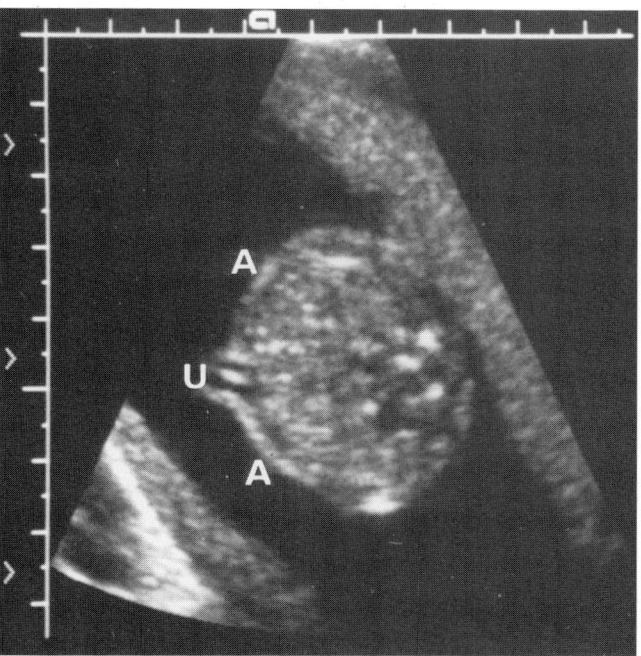

Figure 10–21. Sonogram demonstrating intact abdominal wall (A) and umbilical cord insertion (U).

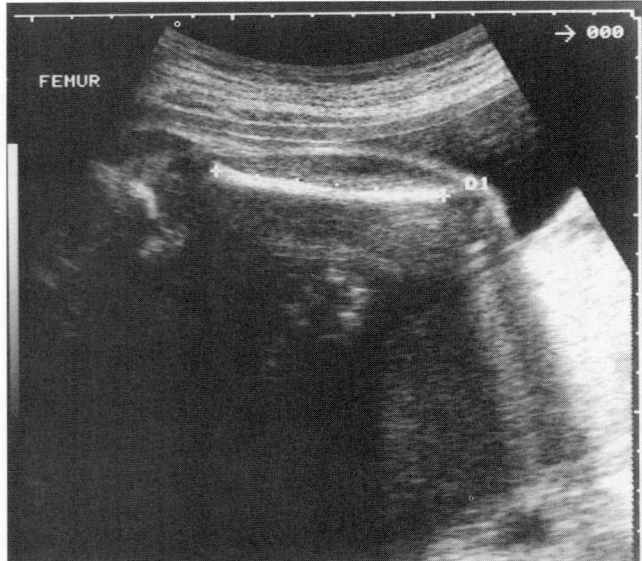

Figure 10–22. Sonogram demonstrating femur.

variety of locations can lead to defects and herniations of contained structures.[93]

The neural tube and overlying mesoderm begin their closure in the region of the fourth somite, with fusion extending both rostrally and caudally during the fourth week of fetal life.[93] Incomplete closure at the rostral end produces cephaloceles, with herniations of meninges and, frequently, of brain substance through a defect in the cranium (Fig. 10–34).[94] Failed fusion at the caudal end produces spina bifida with protruding meningoceles and meningomyeloceles (Fig. 10–35). Sonographic diagnosis of each of these anomalies depends on the

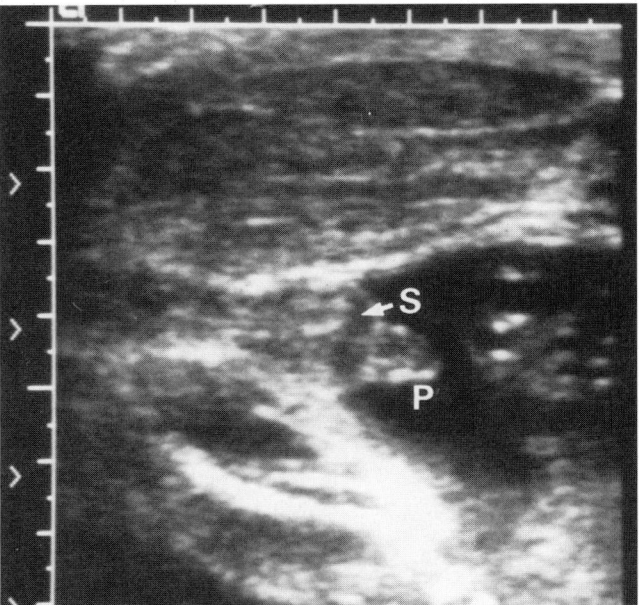

Figure 10–24. Sonogram demonstrating male genitalia. P, penis; S, scrotum.

demonstration of a defect in the normal structure of the cranium or spine and of a protruding sac, often containing tissue.[95,96]

The Arnold-Chiari malformation is an anomaly of the hindbrain that has two components. The first is a variable displacement of a tongue of spinal canal. The second is a similar caudal dislocation of the medulla

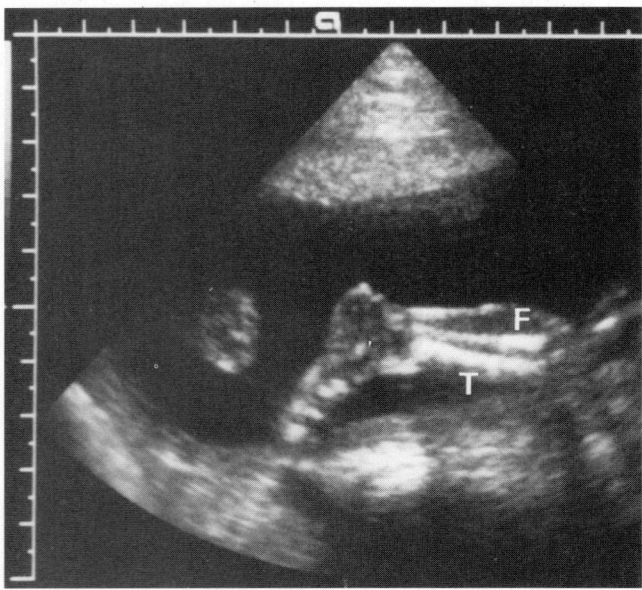

Figure 10–23. Sonogram demonstrating tibia (T) and fibula (F).

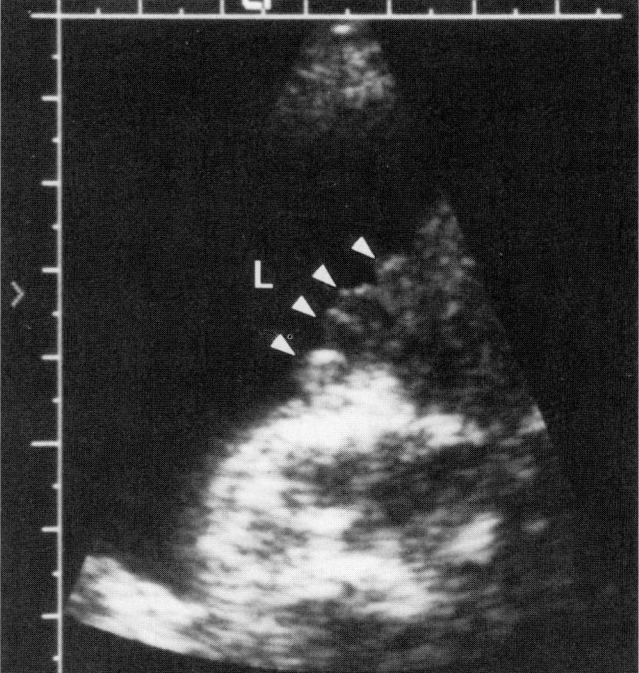

Figure 10–25. Sonogram demonstrating female genitalia. L, labia.

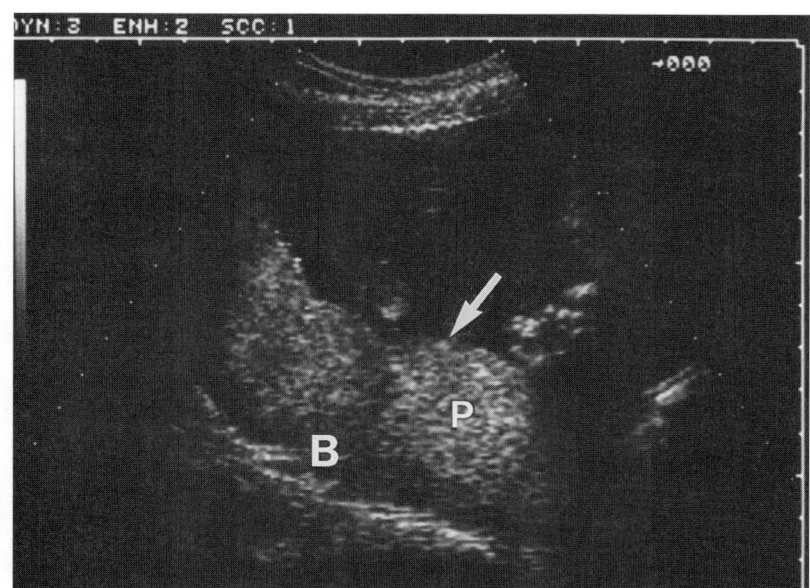

Figure 10–26. Ultrasound of a normal placenta at 24 weeks' gestation, demonstrating homogeneous placenta substance (P), smooth chorionic plate (*arrow*), and hypoechoic basal layer (B).

and fourth ventricle. Most, if not all, cases of spina bifida are complicated by the Arnold-Chiari malformation.[97] The Arnold-Chiari malformation can serve, therefore, as an important marker for spina bifida. Two characteristic sonographic signs (the "lemon" and the "banana") of the Arnold-Chiari malformation have been described.[98] A scalloping of the frontal bones can give a lemon-like configuration, in axial section, to the skull of an affected fetus during the second trimester. The caudal displacement of the cranial contents within

a pliable skull is thought to produce this scalloping effect. Similarly, as the cerebellar hemispheres are displaced into the cervical canal, they are flattened rostrocaudally, and the cisterna magna is obliterated, thus producing a flattened, centrally curved, banana-like sonographic appearance. In extreme instances, the cerebellar hemispheres may be absent from view during fetal head scanning. These characteristic cranial signs are valuable adjuncts to the sonographer in the search for spina bifida (Fig. 10–36).[98]

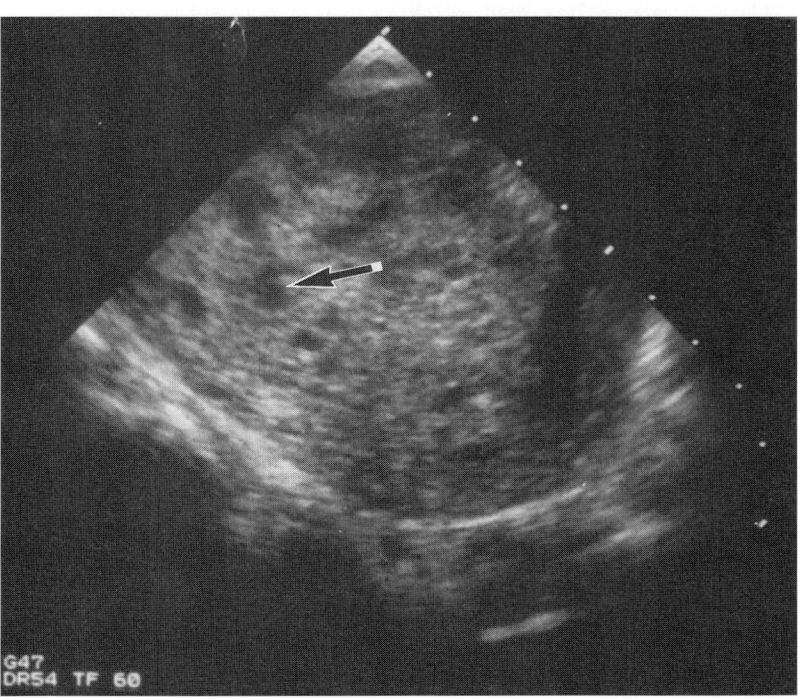

Figure 10–27. On ultrasound, a hydatidiform mole reveals hypoechoic structures (*arrow*) corresponding to enlarged, hydropic villi.

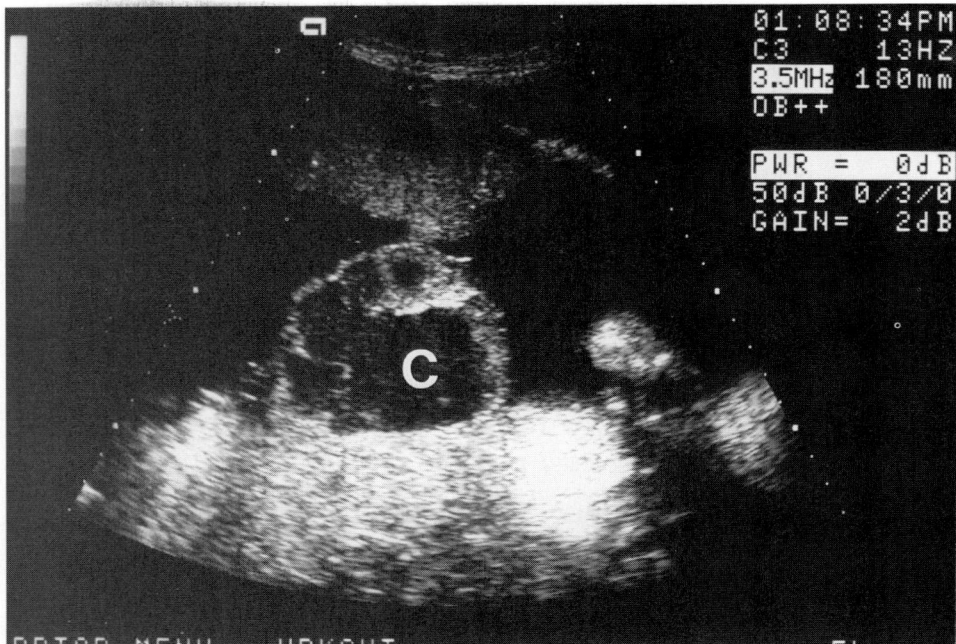

Figure 10–28. Ultrasound of a chorioangioma (C), a benign hemangioma of the fetal vasculature, demonstrates a large, hypoechoic mass. Large chorioangiomas, those greater than 5 cm in diameter, may be associated with hydramnios and preterm labor.

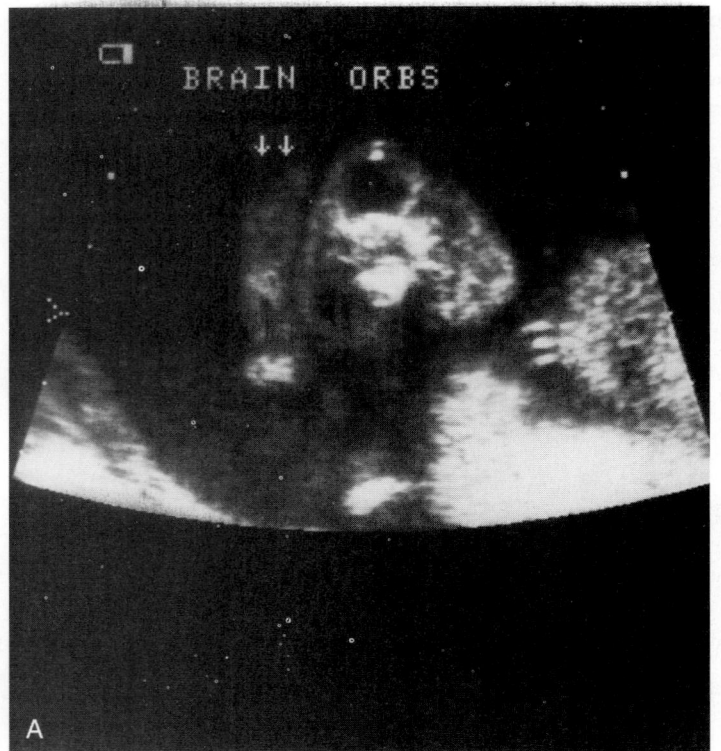

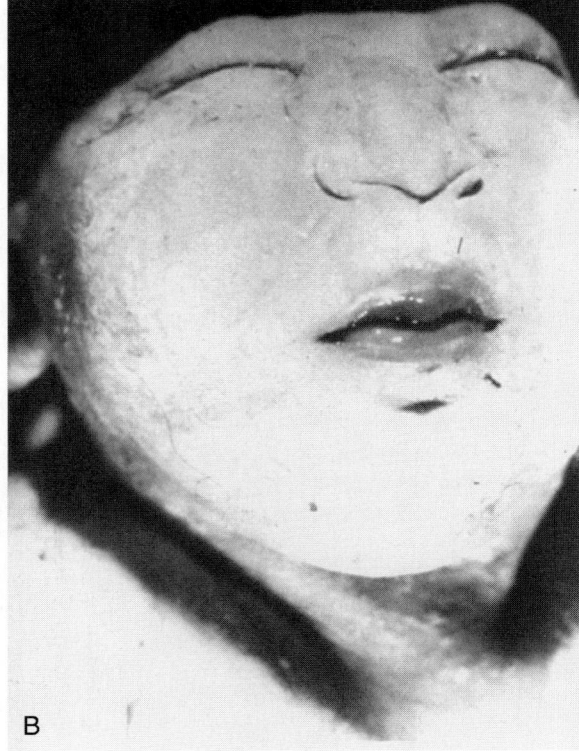

Figure 10–29. *A,* Coronal sonogram of fetal head demonstrating anencephaly. *B,* Postmortem photograph of infant with anencephaly demonstrating prominent area cerebrovasculosa.

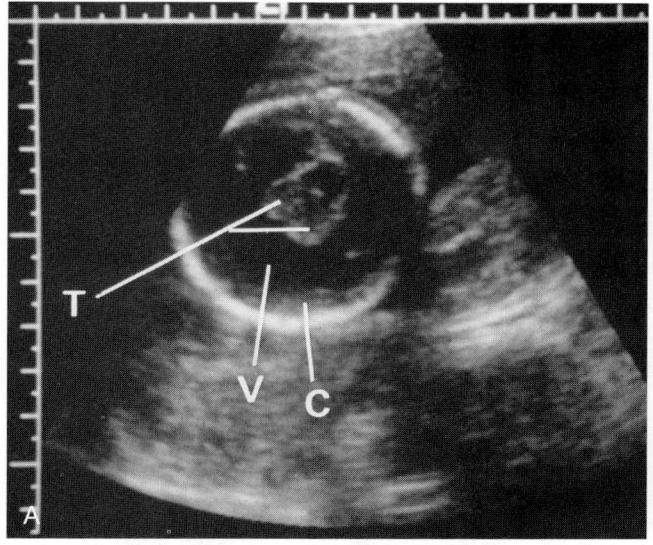
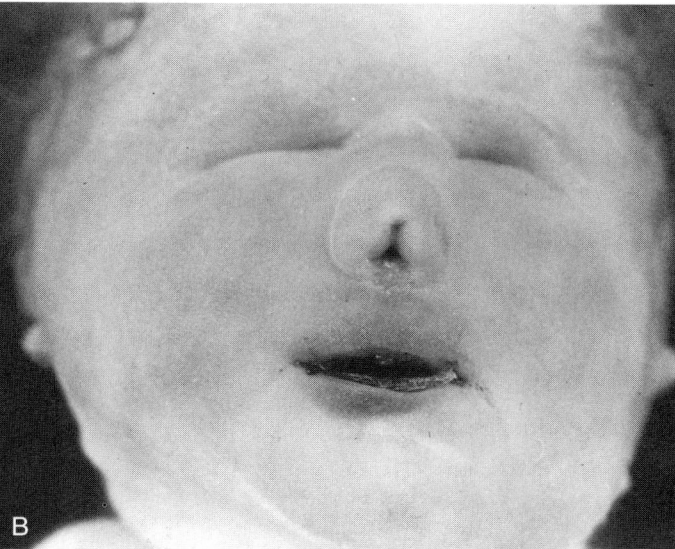

Figure 10–30. *A,* Cranial sonogram demonstrating alobar holoprosencephaly. V, common ventricle; T, prominent fused thalamus; C, compressed cerebral cortex. *B,* Cebocephaly with hypotelorism and normally placed nose with a single nostril. (From Chervenak FA, Isaacson G, Mahoney MJ, et al: The obstetric significance of holoprosencephaly. Obstet Gynecol 63: 115, 1984. American College of Obstetricians and Gynecologists, with permission.)

Omphaloceles result from failure of the intestines to retract from their temporary location in the umbilical cord and the subsequent herniation of other abdominal contents, including both hollow and solid structures contained within a peritoneal sac. Insertion of the um-bilical cord into the sac helps to differentiate an om-phalocele from gastroschisis, which has no covering membrane. Nonetheless, distinguishing these two enti-ties may be difficult[99] (Figs. 10–37 and 10–38).

The diaphragm forms from four separate structures

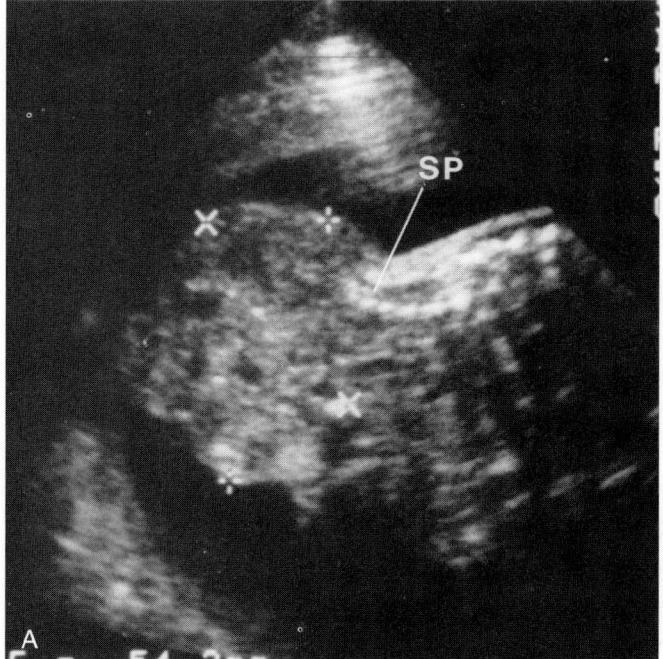
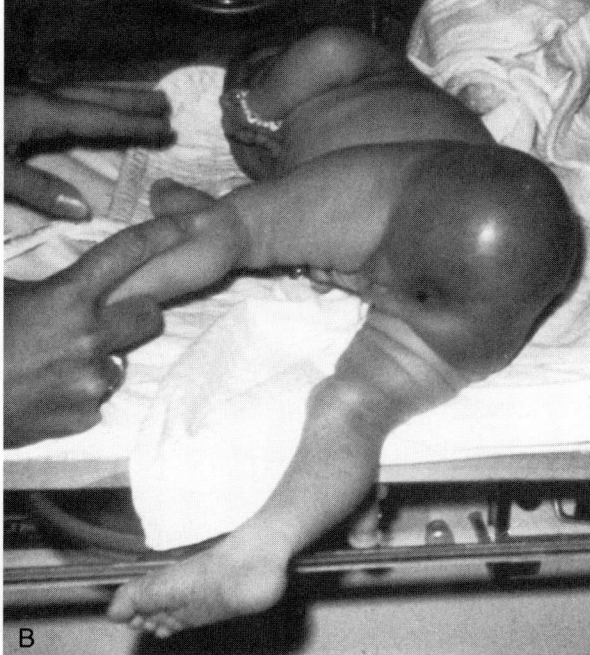

Figure 10–31. *A,* Sonogram of sacrococcygeal teratoma outlined by Xs protruding beneath fetal spine (SP). *B,* Neonate with sacrococcygeal teratoma. (From Chervenak FA, Isaacson G, Touloukian R, et al: The diagnosis and management of fetal teratomas. Obstet Gynecol 66:666, 1985. American College of Obstetricians and Gynecologists, with permission.)

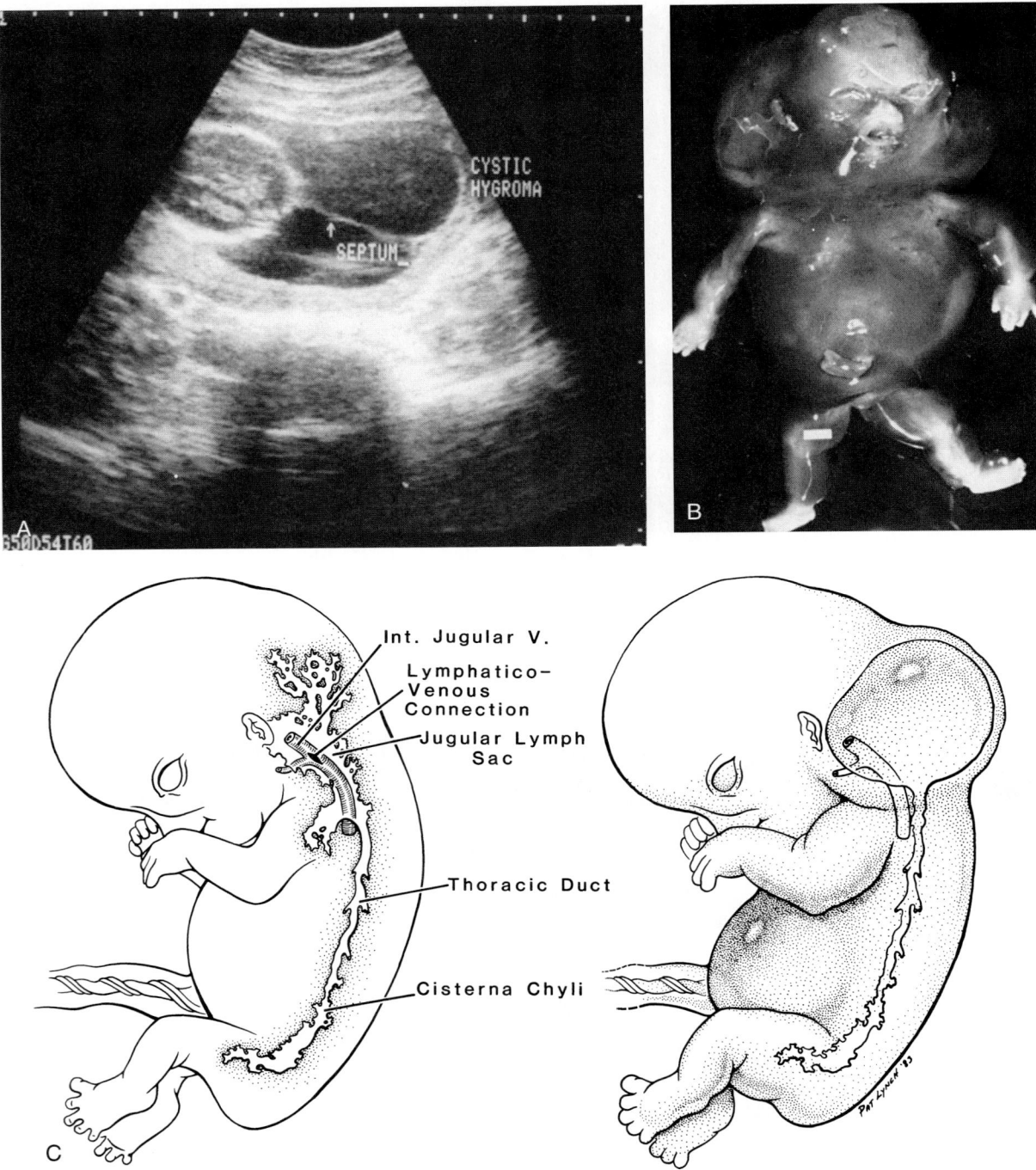

Figure 10–32. *A,* Sonogram demonstrating nuchal cystic hygroma divided by midline septum. *B,* Postmortem photograph demonstrating fetus with cystic hygroma protruding from posterolateral neck. (From Chervenak FA, Isaacson G, Lorber J: Anomalies of the Fetal Head, Neck and Spine: Ultrasound Diagnosis and Management. Philadelphia, WB Saunders Company, 1988, with permission.) *C,* Lymphatic system in normal fetus with patent connection between jugular lymph sac and internal jugular vein (*left*), and fetus with cystic hygroma and hydrops from failed lymphaticovenous connection (*right*). (From Chervenak FA, Isaacson G, Blakemore KJ, et al: Fetal cystic hygroma: cause and natural history. N Engl J Med 309: 822, 1984, with permission.)

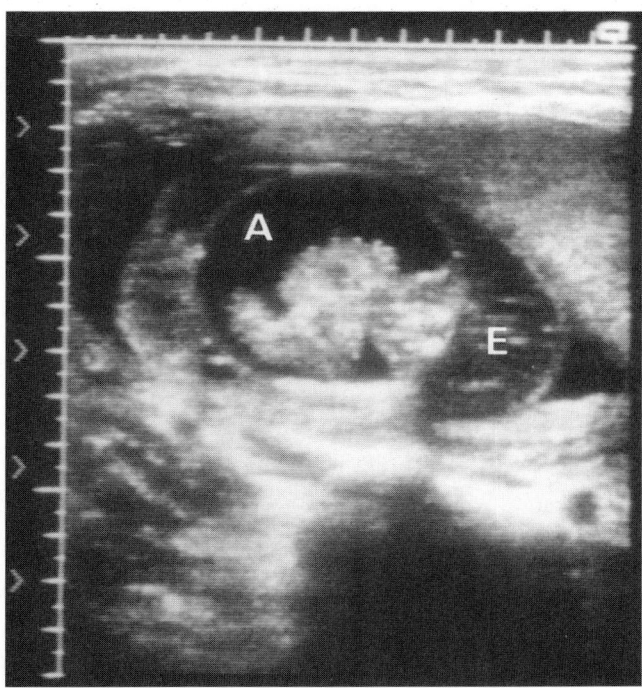

Figure 10–33. Transverse sonogram through fetal abdomen demonstrating fetal hydrops. E, edema of abdominal wall; A, ascites.

that fuse to separate the pleural and peritoneal cavities. When a diaphragmatic hernia is present, abdominal contents may be visualized within the chest on transverse sonographic scanning. A disruption in this development of the diaphragm may be seen in the sagittal plane.[100,101]

Dilatation Behind an Obstruction

In this class of anomalies, the structural defect itself is rarely seen. Rather, what is observed is the distention of structures behind a defect. Such dilatation is caused by obstruction to the normal flow of cerebrospinal fluid, urine, or swallowed amniotic fluid.

Hydrocephalus is characterized by a relative enlargement of the cerebroventricular system with an accompanying increase of pressure of the cerebrospinal fluid within the fetal head. Hydrocephalus is suggested by a lateral ventricular atrial width greater than 1 cm,[102–104] a dangling choroid plexus,[105] and an asymmetric appearance of the choroid plexus.[104,105] The location of the obstruction may be determined by observing which portions of the ventricular system are enlarged (Fig. 10–39). There is a frequent association of fetal hydrocephalus with other anomalies, especially spina bifida.[106]

Fetal small bowel obstruction may cause dilatation proximal to the area of obstruction. Duodenal atresia

has been observed to produce its characteristic "double-bubble" sign, consisting of enlarged duodenum and stomach with narrowing at the pylorus and duodenum and is commonly associated with Down syndrome[107,108] (Fig. 10–40). Obstruction in the lower gastrointestinal tract (e.g., imperforate anus) is generally not detected on antenatal ultrasound unless there is an associated lesion.

Obstructions to urinary flow with proximal dilatation can occur at the uteropelvic and uterovesicular junctions (Fig. 10–41). These are commonly unilateral defects, whereas obstruction at the urethra from posterior urethral valves characteristically produces bilateral dilatation of the ureters and renal pelves.[109–111] When a posterior urethral valve produces a complete obstruction, renal dysplasia and pulmonary hypoplasia may result (see Chapter 11).

Abnormal Fetal Biometry

Several fetal anomalies are best diagnosed not by observing alterations in shape or consistency, but by determining abnormalities in size. The science of fetal biometry has generated many nomograms defining normal values for parts of the fetal anatomy at various gestational ages.[109]

Fetal microcephaly is usually the result of an underdeveloped brain. Although commonly associated with cerebral structural malformations, microcephaly may be produced by a brain that is normal in configuration but merely small. The accurate diagnosis of microcephaly has proved challenging because compressive forces within the uterus may distort the shape of the fetal head. The best correlation between microcephaly diagnosed in utero and neonatal microcephaly is made when multiple parameters are measured and suggest a small head.[112,113]

A variety of skeletal dysplasias may affect the growth of long bones. Measurement may suggest a particular skeletal dysplasia, depending on which bones are foreshortened. The shape of these bones, their density, the presence of fractures, or the absence of specific bones may aid in differentiating the various bony abnormalities.[114]

When interorbital distances are inconsistent with gestational age, hypotelorism or hypertelorism may be suggested. Abnormal distance between the orbits may serve as a clue to several malformation syndromes (e.g., alobar holoprosencephaly[82] and median cleft face syndrome[115]) (Fig. 10–42).

The internal architecture of the kidneys may be difficult to assess in the presence of oligohydramnios. The diagnosis of polycystic kidneys thus is aided by renal measurement. In addition to being echogenic, polycystic kidneys usually are enlarged and display an abnormally

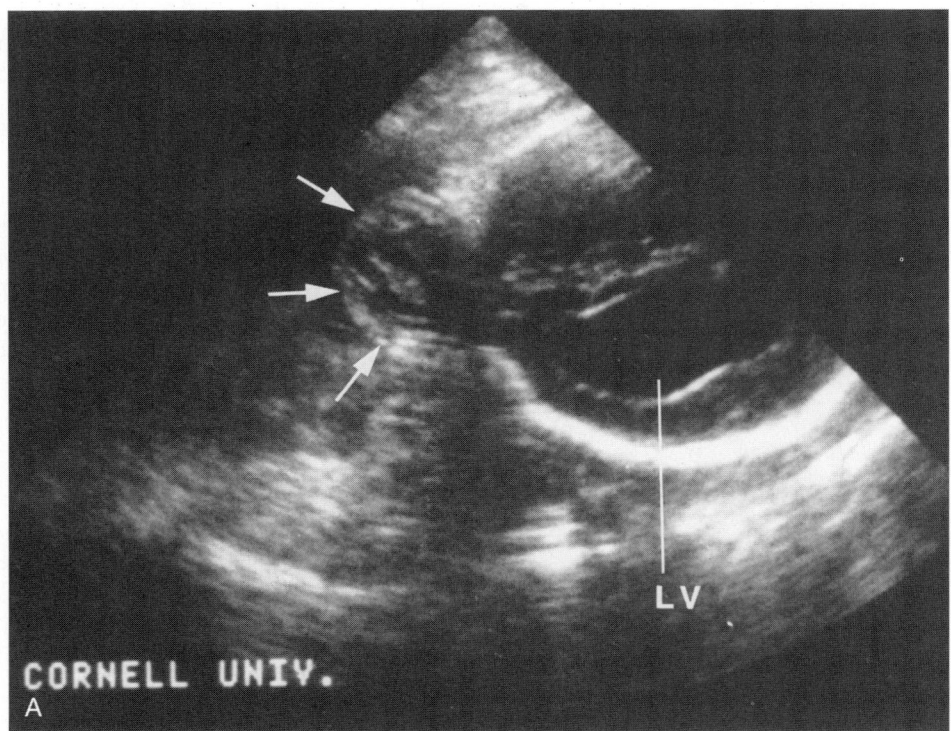

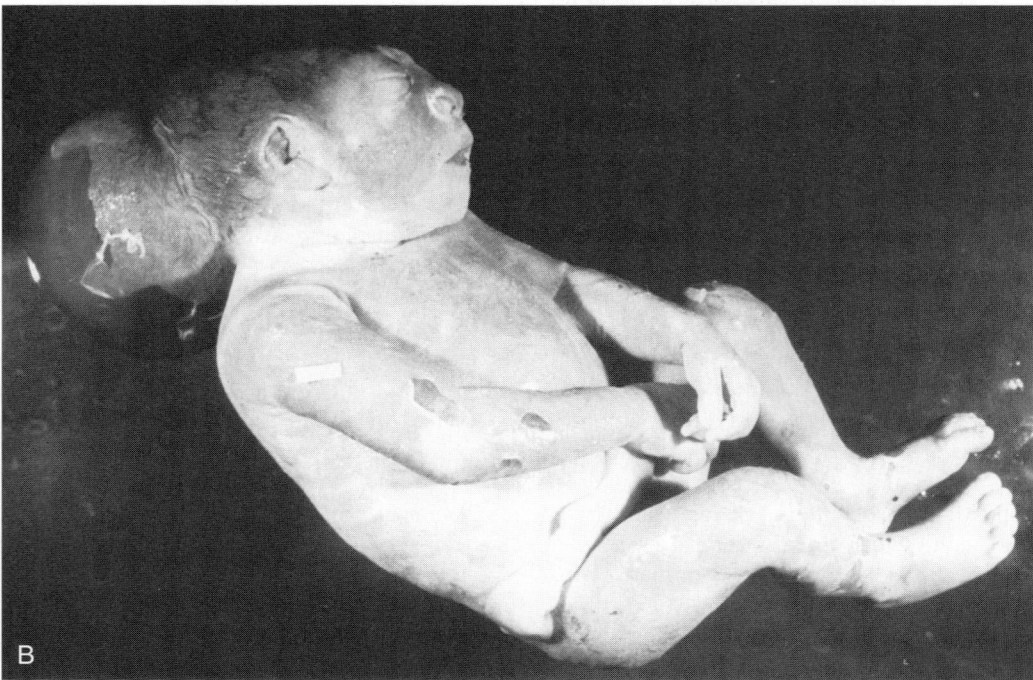

Figure 10–34. *A,* Occipital encephalocele (outlined by *arrows*). LV, dilated lateral ventricle. *B,* Large encephalocele with resultant microcephaly. (From Chervenak FA, Isaacson G, Mahoney MJ, et al: The diagnosis and management of fetal cephalocele. Obstet Gynecol 64:86, 1984. American College of Obstetricians and Gynecologists, with permission.)

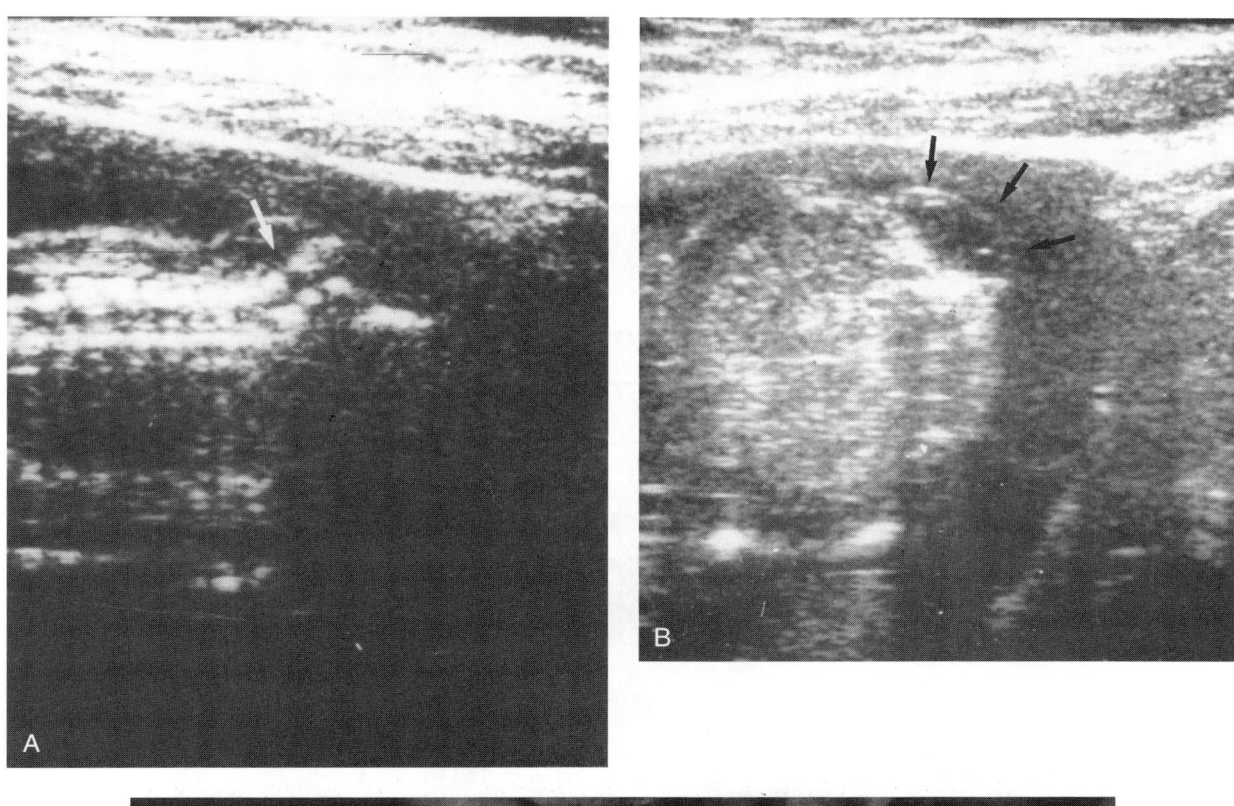

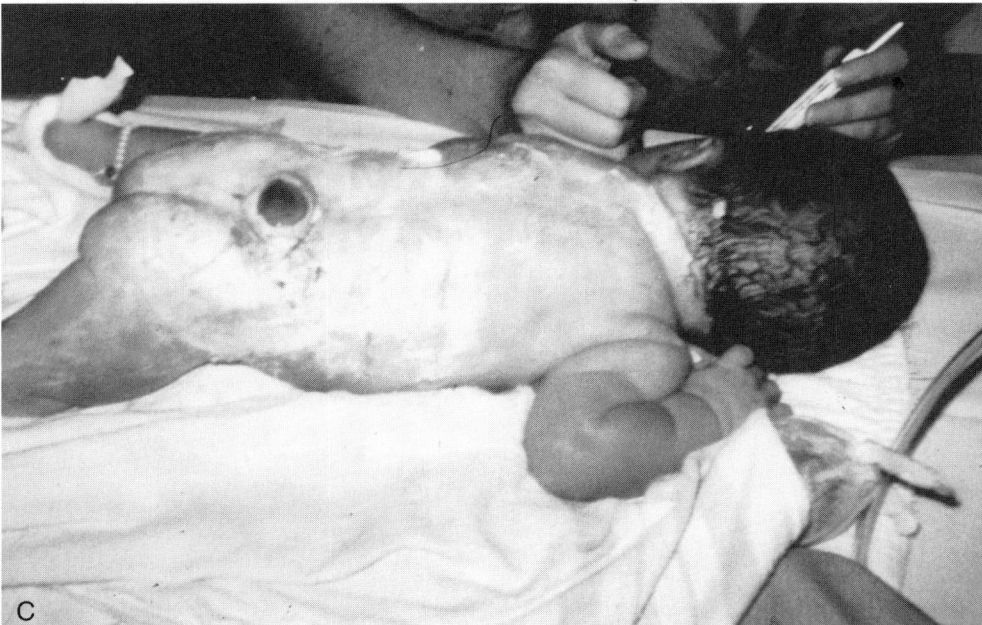

Figure 10–35. *A,* Longitudinal sonogram of fetal spine with *arrow* pointing to meningomyelocele. *B,* Transverse sonogram through fetal spine with *arrows* pointing to meningomyelocele. *C,* Intact lumbosacral meningomyelocele in neonate. (From Chervenak FA, Isaacson G, Lorber J: Anomalies of the Fetal Head, Neck and Spine: Ultrasound Diagnosis and Management. Philadelphia, WB Saunders Company, 1988, with permission.)

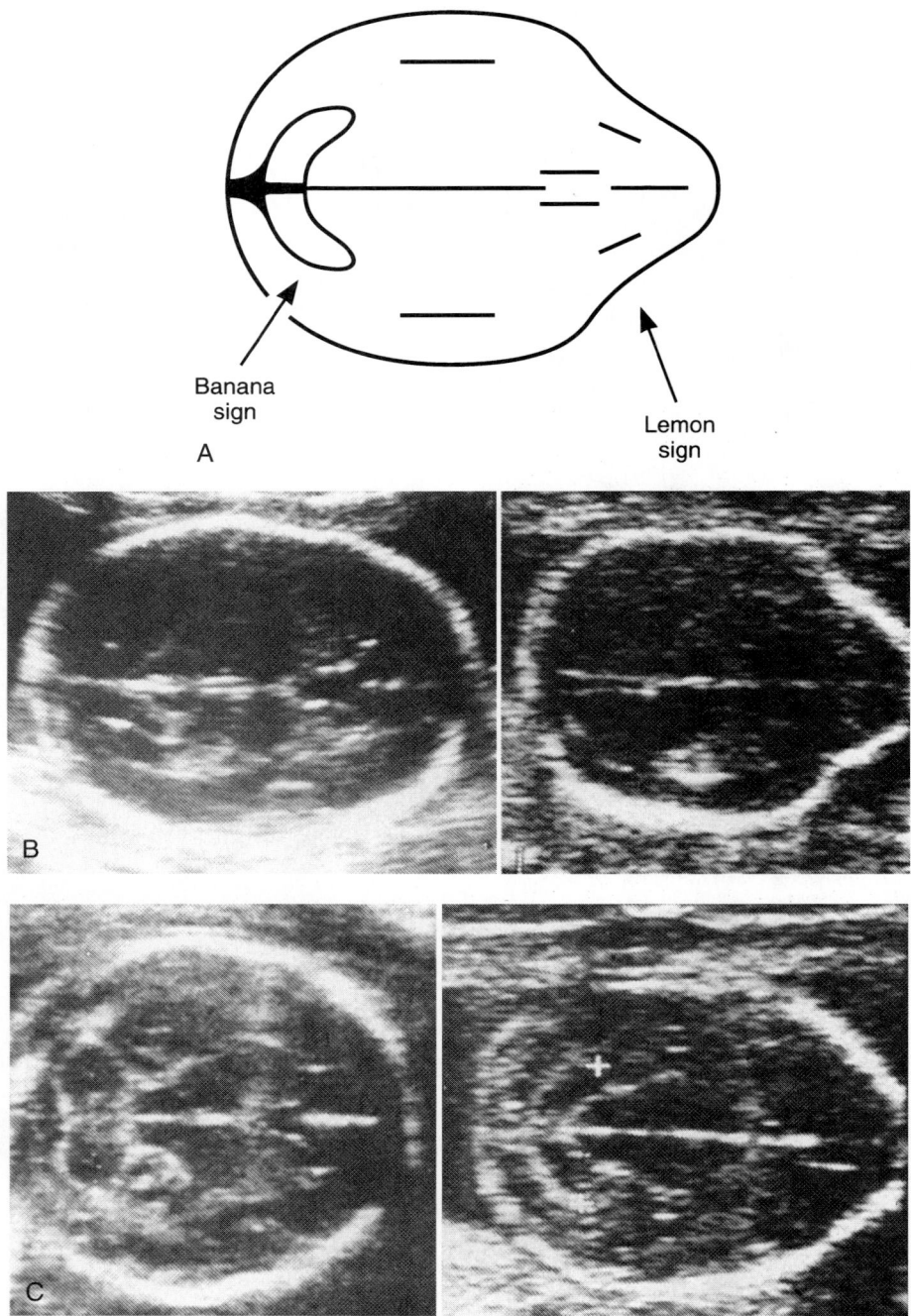

Figure 10–36. *A,* Diagrammatic representation of "banana" and "lemon" signs in fetus with spina bifida. *B,* Transverse section of normal fetal head in an 18-week fetus at level of cavum septi pellucidi (*left*). Transverse section of fetal head at level of cavum septi pellucidi in an 18-week fetus with open spina bifida showing "lemon" and "banana" sign (*right*). *C,* Suboccipital bregmatic view of fetal head in an 18-week fetus with normal cerebellum and cisterna magna (*left*). Suboccipital bregmatic view of fetal head in an 18-week fetus with open spina bifida, demonstrating "banana" sign (+). (From Nicolaides KM, Campbell S, Gabbe SG, Guidetti R: Ultrasound screening for spina bifida: cranial and cerebellar signs. Lancet 2:72, 1986. Copyright 1986 The Lancet Ltd, with permission.)

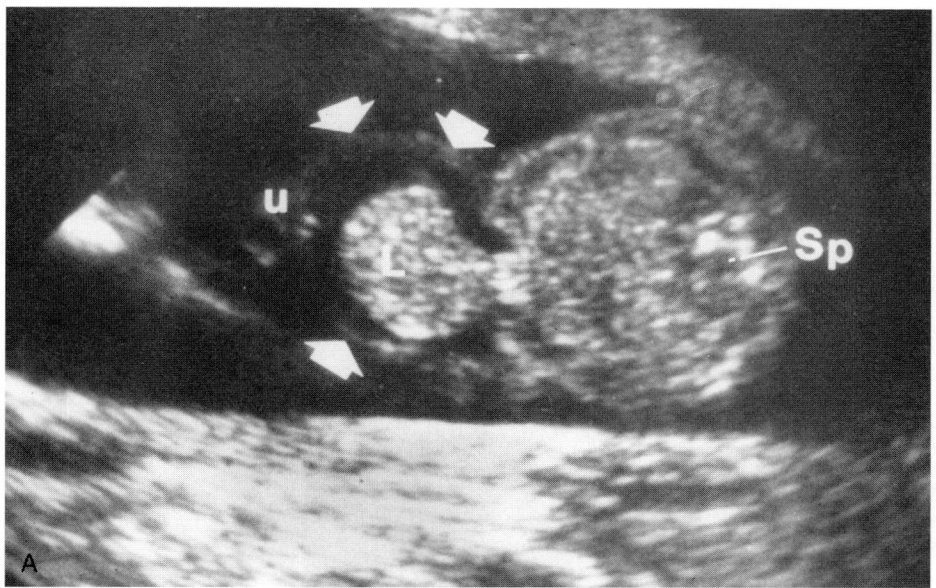

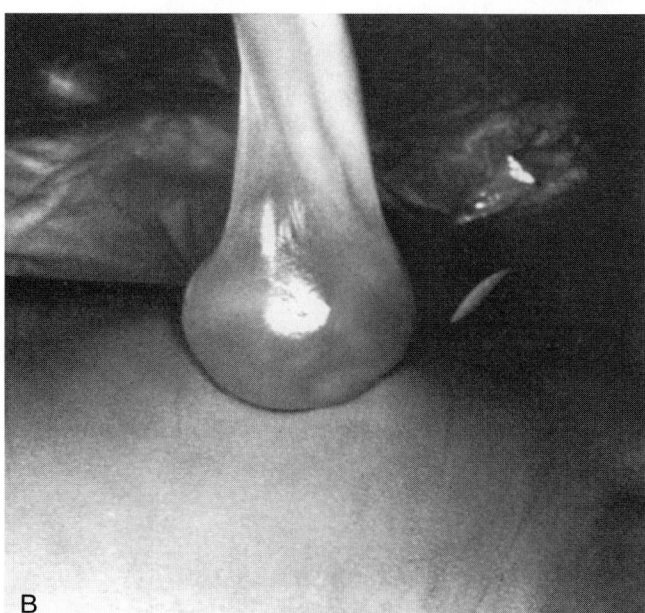

Figure 10–37. Omphalocele. *A*, The surrounding membrane (*arrowheads*), cord insertion into the apex of the omphalocele (u), liver (L) herniated into the omphalocele sac, and spine (Sp) can be seen. *B*, Gross picture of an omphalocele, although smaller than that illustrated in the accompanying ultrasound. Note that the abdominal contents are surrounded by a membrane and protrude into the base of the umbilical cord. (Courtesy of Dr. Harbhajan Chawla.)

increased kidney circumference/abdominal circumference ratio.[116,117]

Absent or Abnormal Fetal Motion

Abnormalities in fetal motion may suggest a malformation that cannot itself be seen. Although the fetus normally can assume contorted positions in utero, the persistence of such an unusual posture over time may suggest an orthopedic or neurologic anomaly such as clubfoot (Fig. 10–43)[118] or arthrogryposis.[119]

The fetal heart is the most conspicuously dynamic part of the fetus. Real-time ultrasound is invaluable in diagnosing most fetal cardiac anomalies (Fig. 10–44).

An attempt should be made to obtain a four-chamber view of the heart in any obstetric ultrasound examination in which fetal anatomy is surveyed.[75] Examination of the fetal outflow tracts increases the detection of heart anomalies. In cases of a suspected fetal arrhythmia, atrial and ventricular rates can be determined.[120,121]

Ultrasound Detection of Chromosomal Abnormalities in the Second Trimester

Ultrasound examination can suggest a chromosomal aberration. Sonographic markers for the most serious karyotype abnormalities are often present. Holoprosen-

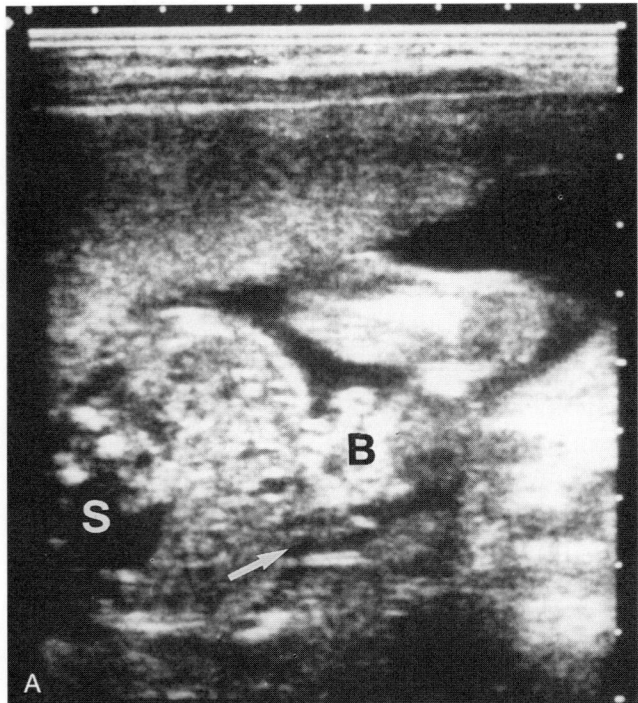

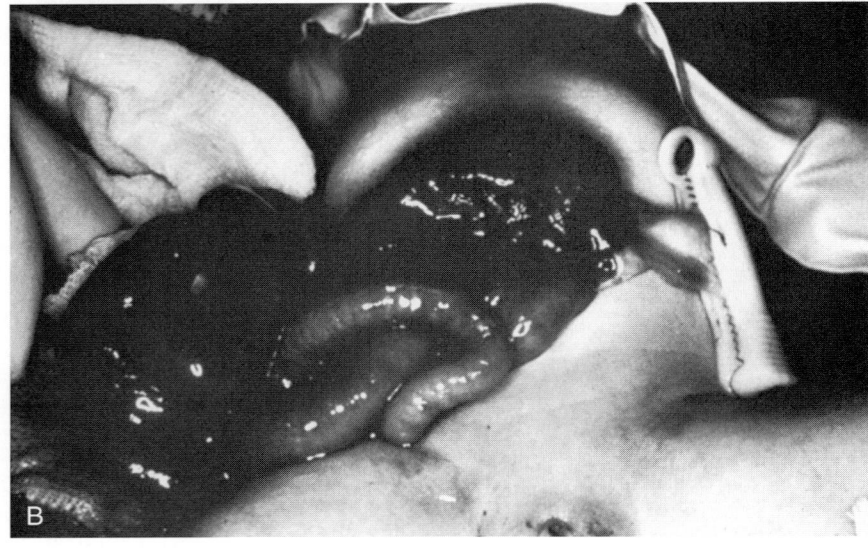

Figure 10–38. *A,* Loops of bowel (B) without a surrounding membrane are characteristic of gastroschisis. The *arrow* points to the insertion of the umbilical cord. Since the stomach (S) is on the left of the fetus, the site of the bowel herniation is to the right of the umbilical cord. *B,* Matted loops of bowel in a neonate with gastroschisis. Note the absence of a surrounding membrane. As in the ultrasound, the abdominal contents are seen to the right of the umbilical cord. (Courtesy of Dr. Harbhajan Chawla.)

cephaly, facial clefts, hypotelorism, omphalocele, polydactyly, and heart defects are associated with trisomy 13, whereas growth restriction, micrognathus, overlapping fingers, omphalocele, horseshoe kidney, and heart defects are associated with trisomy 18 (see Chapter 8). Early-onset severe growth restriction, large head, syndactyly, and heart defects suggest triploidy. Turner's syndrome (45,X) is classically associated with nuchal cystic hygroma, but this ultrasound finding can occur in a wide variety of genetic disorders.[122]

Major structural malformations, including hydrops, duodenal atresia, and heart defects, are associated with trisomy 21 but are detected sonographically in only about 30 percent of cases.[123,124] Nuchal skin thickness, defined as 6 mm or more, is a useful screening tool for trisomy 21 and other chromosomal malformations (Fig. 10–45).[121,125,126] Other sonographic signs used to screen for Down syndrome include short femur, short humerus, pyelectasis, mild cerebral ventriculomegaly, clinodactyly with hypoplastic middle phalanx of the fifth digit, widely spaced first and second toes, low-set ears, echogenic bowel, and a single palmar crease.[123,124,127] Scoring systems have been developed to include these sonographic markers, maternal age, and

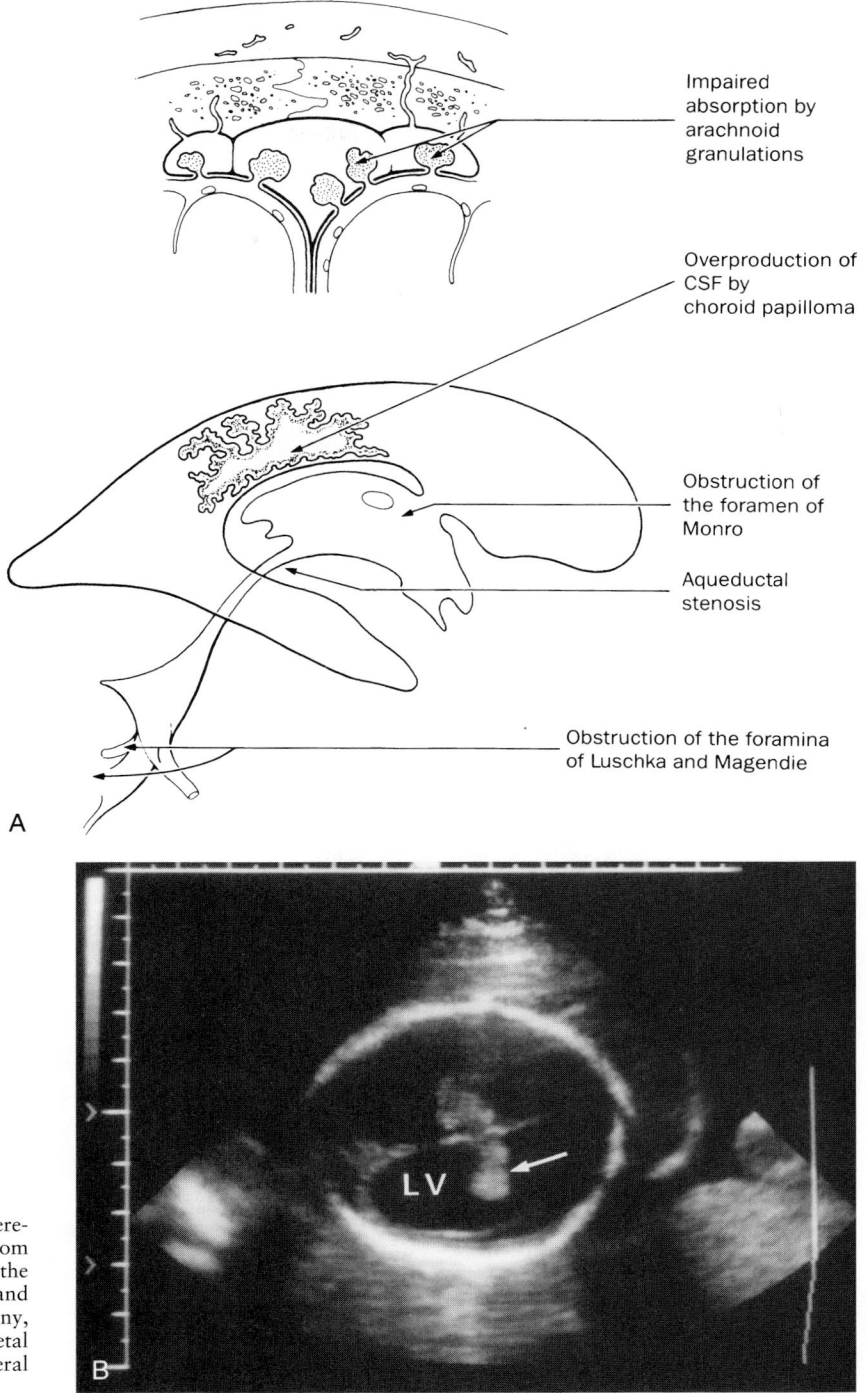

Figure 10–39. *A,* Common sites of obstruction of cerebrospinal fluid flow resulting in ventriculomegaly. (From Chervenak FA, Isaacson G, Lorber J: Anomalies of the Fetal Head, Neck and Spine: Ultrasound Diagnosis and Management. Philadelphia, WB Saunders Company, 1988, with permission.) *B,* Transverse sonogram of fetal head demonstrating hydrocephalus. LV, dilated lateral ventricle; *arrow* points to dangling choroid plexus.

serum markers to achieve a reported sensitivity of 90 percent.[128–131]

Choroid plexus cysts can occur in about 1 percent of fetuses and, although most are closely associated with trisomy 18, can be a marker for other chromosomal abnormalities[132,133] (Fig. 10–46). The need for a karyotype determination when the only structural abnormal-

ity seen is a choroid plexus cyst remains controversial.[134,135] Benaceraff et al.[133] have calculated that the performance of amniocentesis for choroid plexus cysts would result in more fetal loss than in detection of unsuspected chromosomal aberrations. In a study of over 30,000 patients, Boyd et al. found that the use of so-called soft markers for aneuploidy such as cho-

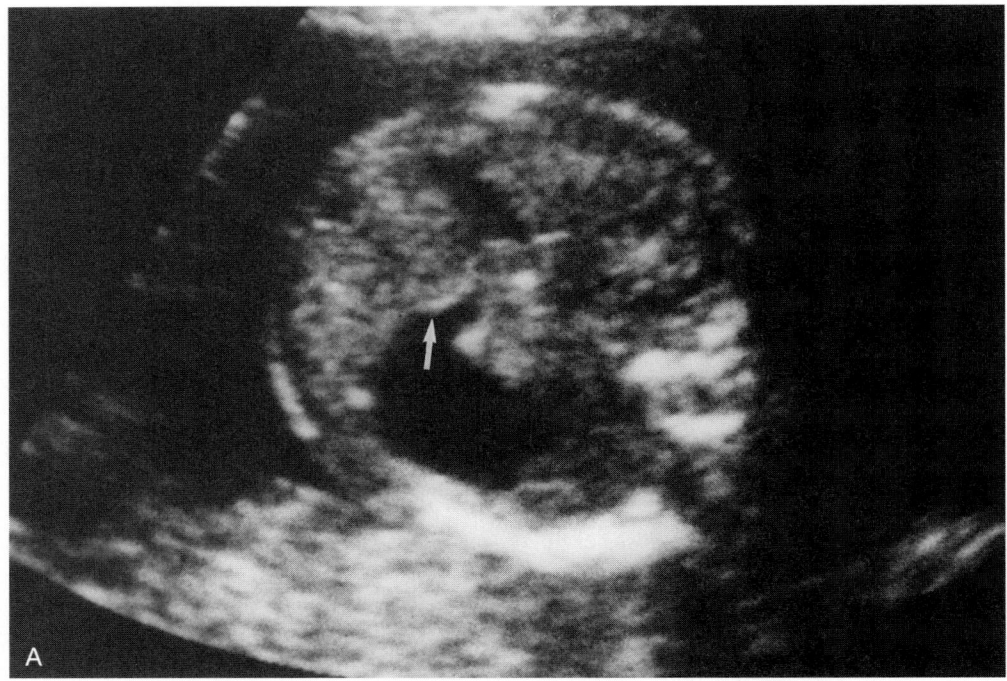

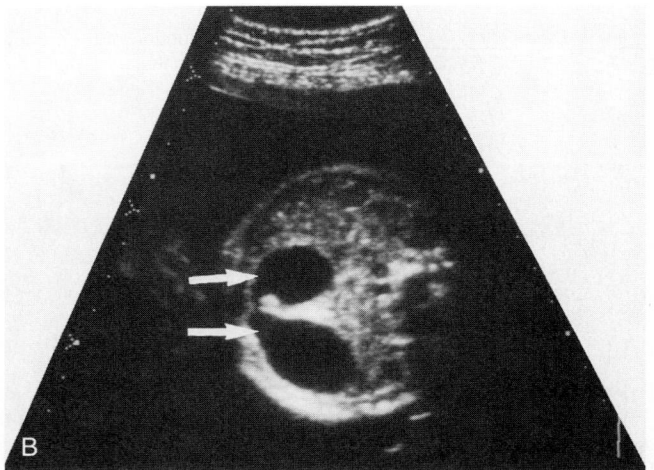
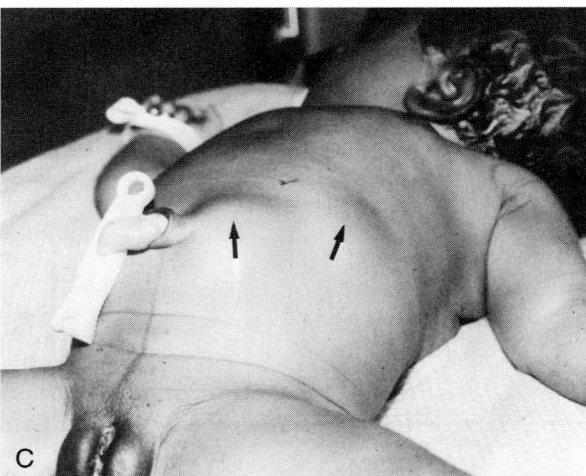

Figure 10–40. *A,* Sonogram demonstrating normal duodenum (*arrow*). *B,* Sonogram illustrating classic "double bubble" sign. The two echo-free areas (*arrows*) represent the stomach and proximal duodenum. *C,* Infant with "double bubble" sign (*arrows*) and duodenal atresia.

roid plexus cyst(s), echogenic bowel, and nuchal thickening led to a small increase in the detection rate for the abnormal fetus but increased the false-positive rate 12-fold![136]

In summary, if a major structural malformation is detected with ultrasound, karyotype determination should be considered by the pregnant woman. At the present time, nuchal thickness is a most clinically useful ultrasound marker for trisomy, with the relative value of other ultrasound markers under investigation.

MANAGEMENT OF A PREGNANCY COMPLICATED BY AN ULTRASONICALLY DIAGNOSED FETAL ANOMALY

If a fetal anomaly is diagnosed by obstetric ultrasound, the fetus should be carefully evaluated for other anomalies before management options can be considered.

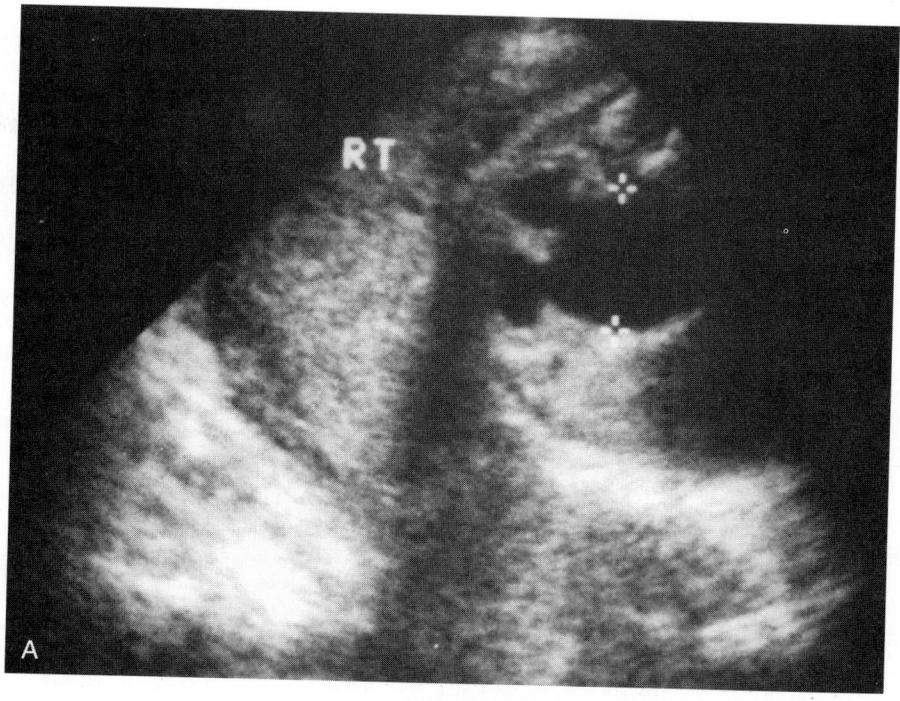

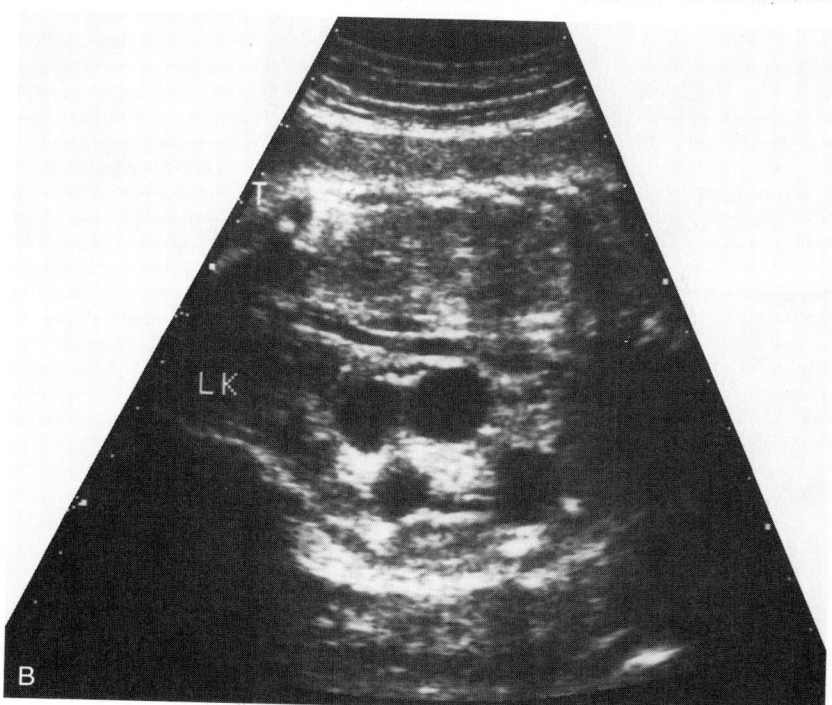

Figure 10–41. *A,* Sonogram demonstrating hydronephrosis with dilated renal pelvis and calyces. *B,* Sonogram demonstrating dysplastic left kidney with noncommunicating cysts (proximal) and normal right kidney (distal).

Echocardiography and karyotype determination should usually be part of this evaluation. Copel et al.[137] have shown that 23 percent of fetuses referred for echocardiography because of an extracardiac anomaly had congenital heart disease. Approximately one third of fetuses with structural anomalies have a chromosomal disorder.[138–141] This additional information is invaluable to define fetal prognosis. For example, the progno-

sis for isolated hydrocephalus is substantially better than that for hydrocephalus associated with alobar holoprosencephaly and trisomy 13.

After the fetal evaluation is completed, the certainties and uncertainties of fetal prognosis should be explained to the pregnant woman and her partner. The disclosure requirements of the informed consent process require the physician to present information about the range of

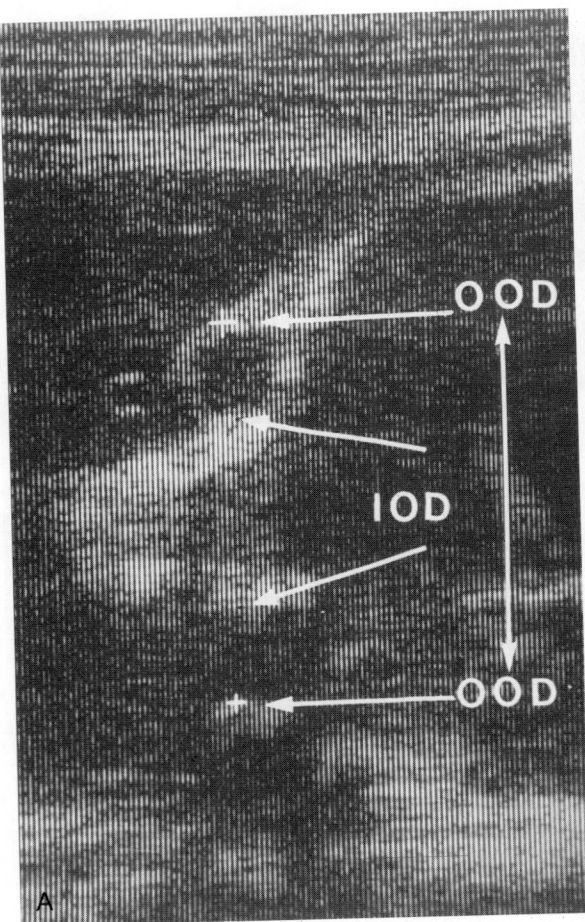

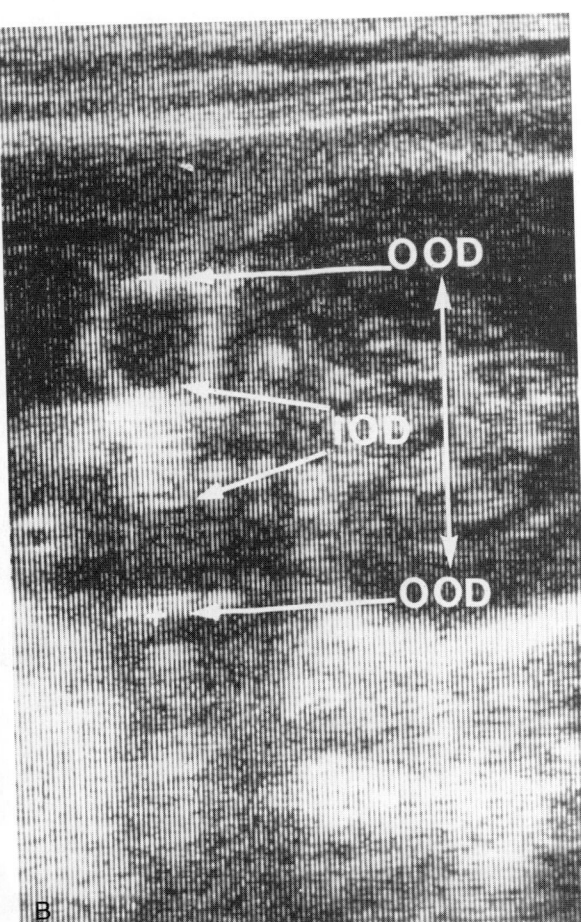

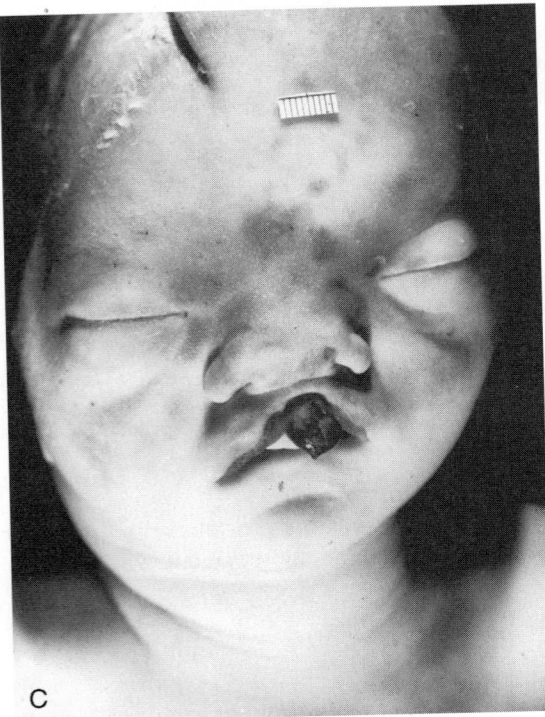

Figure 10–42. *A,* Transverse scan through orbits of fetus affected with median cleft face syndrome demonstrates hypertelorism. Inner orbital distance (IOD) and outer orbital distance (OOD) are increased for gestational age of 31 weeks. *B,* Transverse scan through orbits of normal fetus at 37 weeks of gestation demonstrates normal IOD and OOD. *C,* Infant with median cleft face syndrome at postmortem examination. Severe hydrocephalus, collapsed cranial bones, flattened nose, and cleft lip with protruding mass are demonstrated. (From Chervenak FA, Tortora M, Mayden K, et al: Antenatal diagnosis of median cleft face syndrome: sonographic demonstration of cleft lip and hypotelorism. Am J Obstet Gynecol 149:94, 1984, with permission.)

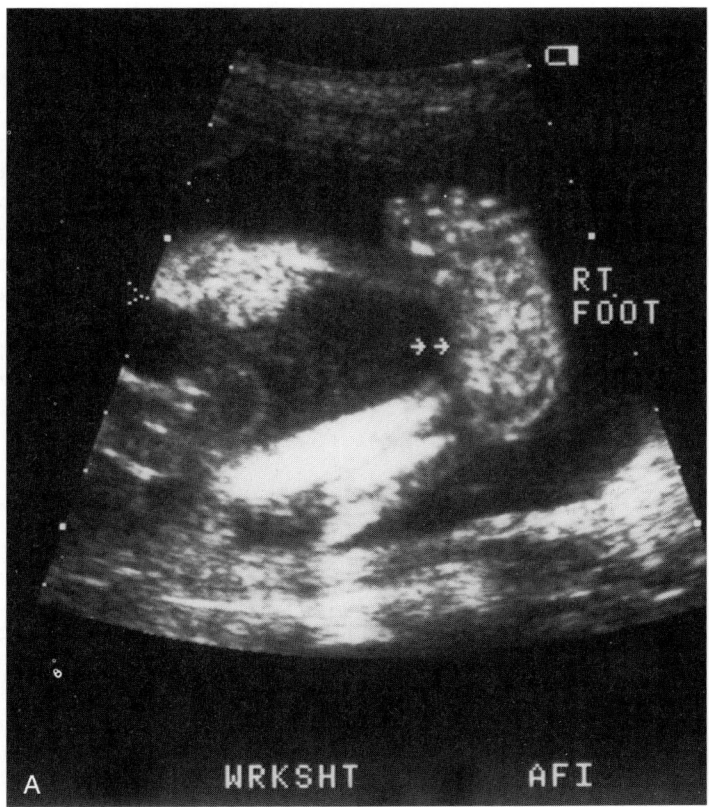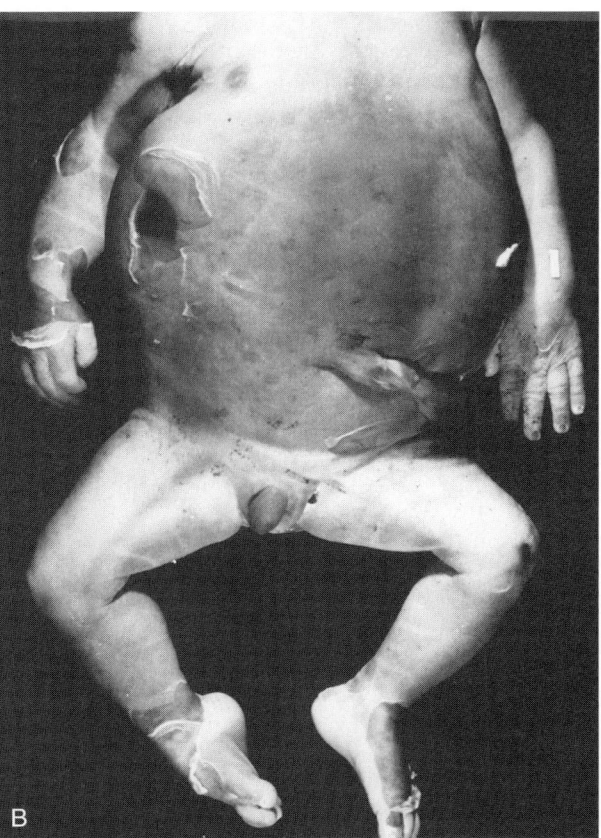

Figure 10–43. *A,* Sonogram demonstrating clubfoot (*arrows*). *B,* Postmortem photograph demonstrating clubfoot.

available management options: aggressive management, termination of pregnancy, nonaggressive management, and cephalocentesis.[142] These disclosure requirements obligate the physician to be objective when presenting this information. That is, the physician is not justified in withholding information about available management options to which he or she might object for reasons of personal conscience.[143]

Aggressive Management (see Chapter 11)

To optimize fetal outcome, there should be an interdisciplinary approach, including specialists in maternal–fetal medicine, neonatology, genetics, pediatric surgery, and pediatric cardiology.[144–146] Social work services may provide important support to the family before as well as after birth. Such a team approach is best equipped to address the important questions of where, when, and how the infant should be delivered, as well as the role of invasive fetal therapy.

Most infants with anomalies are best delivered in a referral center with a neonatal intensive care unit experienced in caring for such infants. In such a setting there is immediate access to diagnostic and therapeutic medical and surgical interventions.

Delivery at term is optimal for most fetal anomalies. For some malformations, however, such as hydrocephalus, delivery as soon as fetal lung maturation has occurred may be advisable in order to expedite corrective neonatal surgery.[147] Rarely, because of the risk of imminent fetal death, an anomaly such as progressive fetal hydrops may necessitate delivery prior to fetal lung maturity.[145]

Most fetuses with anomalies can be delivered vaginally. Cesarean delivery may be necessary to avoid dystocia if conditions such as a sacrococcygeal teratoma or conjoined twins are present. For other anomalies, such as spina bifida, cesarean delivery may be recommended in order to minimize trauma to fetal tissues and preserve neurologic function.[148]

Rarely, an invasive approach such as shunt placement may be considered to optimize outcome during the antenatal period. This strategy should only be considered when the natural history of the anomaly diagnosed is dismal and a relatively simple intrauterine correction is possible. The sonographic and karyotypic evaluations described above are especially important before an invasive approach can be considered. The disclosure requirements of the informed consent process necessitate that the experimental nature of invasive fetal therapy and the potential harms to the fetus and the mother be carefully explained. In addition, it is generally agreed that after 32 weeks of gestation such efforts offer no clear advantage over delivery and neonatal treatment. Given the risk of iatrogenic premature delivery as well as the experimental nature of these procedures, a normal coincident twin is considered to be a contraindication to this approach.[144,145,149]

The most common form of invasive fetal therapy has been intrauterine shunt placement. The purpose of such a shunt is to drain fluid under high pressure in a fetal organ to the lower pressure of the amniotic fluid. Such a shunt may have a role in the treatment of a complete bladder outlet obstruction that would be expected to result eventually in renal failure and pulmonary hypoplasia.[149-151] Analysis of fetal urine after bladder aspiration may help to define which fetuses are candidates for this vesiculoamniotic shunt.[151-153] Intrauterine aspiration or shunt placement may also be of value in cases of isolated pleural effusions[154-156] (Fig. 10–47). In fetal hydrocephalus, however, current experience does not demonstrate a clear benefit, and ventriculoamniotic shunt placement should be avoided unless performed under a research protocol.[149,157,158]

Harrison and colleagues have pioneered open fetal surgery to manage such conditions as congenital diaphragmatic hernia, sacrococcygeal teratoma with hydrops, cystic adenomatoid malformation of the lung, and spina bifida. In such cases, hysterotomy and exteriorization of the fetus is followed by repair of the abnormality, replacement of the fetus, and continuation of the pregnancy.[144,159] More recently, endoscopic procedures have been used to avoid hysterotomy.[142,159,160-166] At this time, it is not possible to make a final judgment concerning the place of this fascinating modality in fetal therapy. More clinical experience is needed to better define the benefits to the fetus and the risks to the mother.

Termination of Pregnancy

Prior to fetal viability, abortion of any pregnancy is a woman's right as established by *Roe v. Wade.*[167] The option of abortion prior to fetal viability is, therefore, available to a pregnant woman when *any* fetal anomaly is diagnosed by ultrasound. Ethically, this option is supported by an approach that holds that all of obstetric ethics is essentially a function of the pregnant woman's autonomy[168,169] as well as an approach that holds that autonomous-based obligations to the pregnant woman should be balanced against beneficence-based obligations to her and the fetus she is carrying (see Chapter 41).[143]

After fetal viability, there is limited legal access in the United States to termination of pregnancy because of a fetal anomaly. Ethically, the option of terminating third-trimester pregnancies complicated by fetal anomalies has been defended when there is (1) certainty of diagnosis and (2) either (a) certainty of death as an outcome of the anomaly diagnosed or (b) short-term survival but certainty of the absence of cognitive developmental capacity as a result of the anomaly diagnosed. Anencephaly is a clear example of a sonographically diagnosed anomaly that meets these criteria.[170] Trisomy 21 is a clear example of an anomaly that does *not* meet these criteria.[171,172]

Nonaggressive Management

The above-mentioned criteria for termination of pregnancy for fetal anomalies during the third trimester are quite restrictive. In addition, even if ethical criteria for third-trimester termination of pregnancy were met, it may not be possible to perform termination in some situations because of legal concerns. Nonaggressive management is the noninclusion of obstetric interventions to benefit the fetus, such as fetal surveillance, tocolysis, cesarean delivery, or delivery in a referral center.[173] Ethically, the option of nonaggressive management for third-trimester pregnancies complicated by fetal anomalies has been defended when there is (1) a very high probability of a correct diagnosis and (2) either (a) a very high probability of death as an outcome of the anomaly diagnosed or (b) a very high probability of severe irreversible deficit of cognitive developmental capacity as a result of the anomaly diagnosed.

Cephalocentesis

When a pregnancy is complicated by fetal hydrocephalus with macrocephaly, there may be a role for cephalocentesis, which is the transabdominal or transvaginal aspiration of cerebrospinal fluid to avoid cesarean delivery. Ethical justification for this procedure can be based on an analysis of beneficence-based and autonomy-based obligations to the pregnant woman and the fetus she is carrying. Such an analysis needs to respect the heterogeneity of fetal hydrocephalus: isolated fetal hydrocephalus, hydrocephalus with severe associated anomalies (such as alobar holoprosencephaly), and hydrocephalus with other associated anomalies (such as an arachnoid cyst)[174,175] (Fig. 10–48).

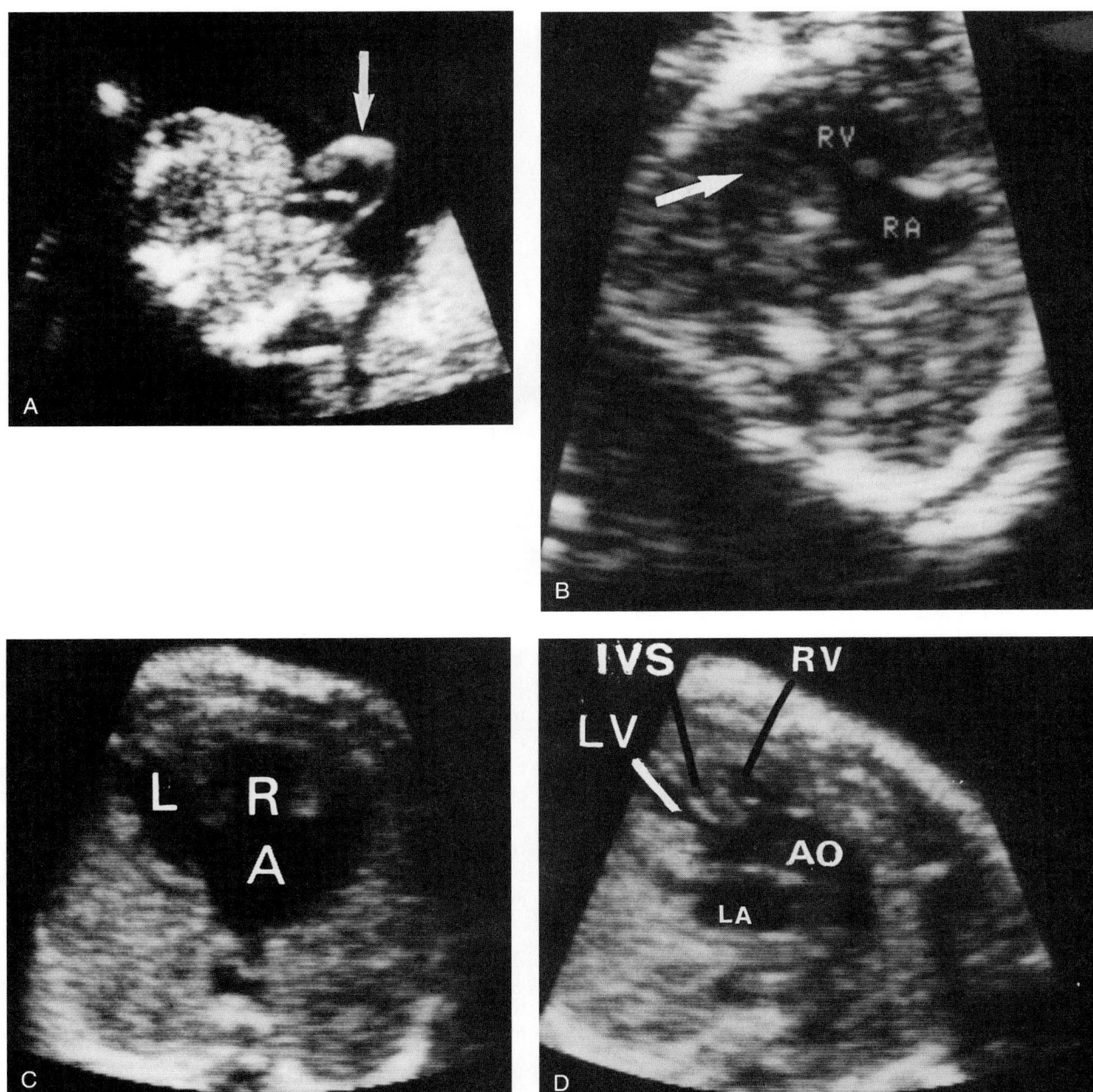

Figure 10-44. *A,* Sonogram demonstrating ectopic cordis with *arrow* pointing to heart outside the chest. *B,* Sonogram demonstrating hypoplastic left heart. RV, right ventricle; RA, right atrium. *Arrow* points to region of hypoplastic left ventricle. *C,* Sonogram demonstrating arteriovenous canal in fetus with Down syndrome. L, left ventricle; R, right ventricle; A, common atrium. *D,* Sonogram of fetus with tetralogy of Fallot demonstrating enlarged aortic outflow tract (AO). Its anterior wall overrides the interventricular septum (IVS). RV, right ventricle; LV, left ventricle; LA, left atrium.

WHO SHOULD HAVE AN OBSTETRIC ULTRASOUND EXAMINATION?

Routine performance of obstetric ultrasound examinations, the performance of an ultrasound study on every obstetric patient at approximately 18 weeks' gestation, remains controversial. A routine obstetric ultrasound examination describes what the American College of Obstetricians and Gynecologists (ACOG) has called a *basic* ultrasound examination, which would include the following information: fetal number, fetal presentation, documentation of fetal life, placental location, assessment of amniotic fluid volume, assessment of gestational age, survey of fetal anatomy for gross malfor-

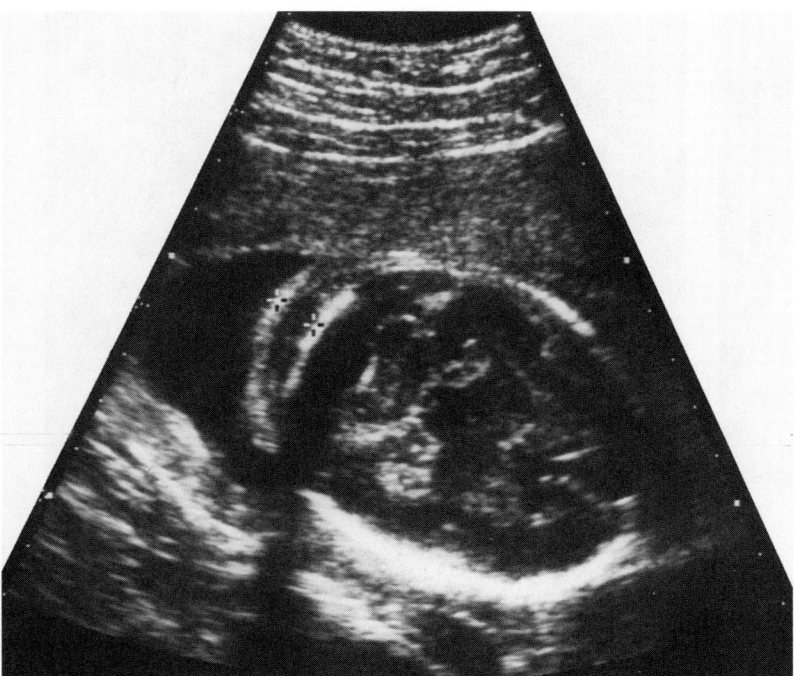

Figure 10–45. Sonogram demonstrating nuchal skin thickness greater than 6 mm.

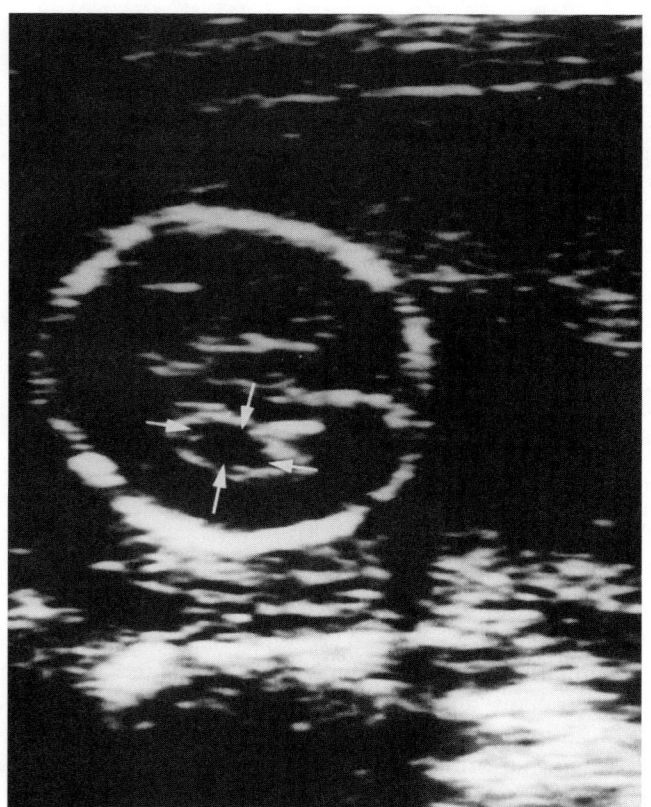

Figure 10–46. Sonogram demonstrating choroid plexus cyst outlined by *arrows*.

mations, and an evaluation for maternal pelvic masses.[171,176] When the findings of a basic ultrasound examination suggest a fetal abnormality or in patients at greater risk of a fetal abnormality, a comprehensive ultrasound examination may be indicated. As noted by the ACOG, the comprehensive ultrasound study should be conducted by an individual experienced in these evaluations.

At the present time, routine obstetric ultrasound is practiced in many European countries. The Royal College of Obstetricians and Gynaecologists has concluded that a routine obstetric ultrasound examination is justifiable.[4] Routine obstetric ultrasound has become widely used in the United States. This practice offers at least six advantages: accurate dating of all pregnancies; accurate evaluation of maternal serum levels of α-fetoprotein, human chorionic gonadotropin, and unconjugated estriol (triple screening); early detection of multiple pregnancies; placental localization to rule out placenta previa; detection of structural abnormalities of the fetus; and psychological benefit to the parents.[177,178]

The ideal timing for a routine ultrasound study would appear to be approximately 18 weeks' gestation. At this gestational age, the pregnancy can be accurately dated and fetal anatomy well visualized. Should a fetal abnormality be identified, sufficient time is available to perform a comprehensive ultrasound, obtain a fetal karyotype if necessary, and counsel the patient and her partner.

A large number of clinical studies support the value

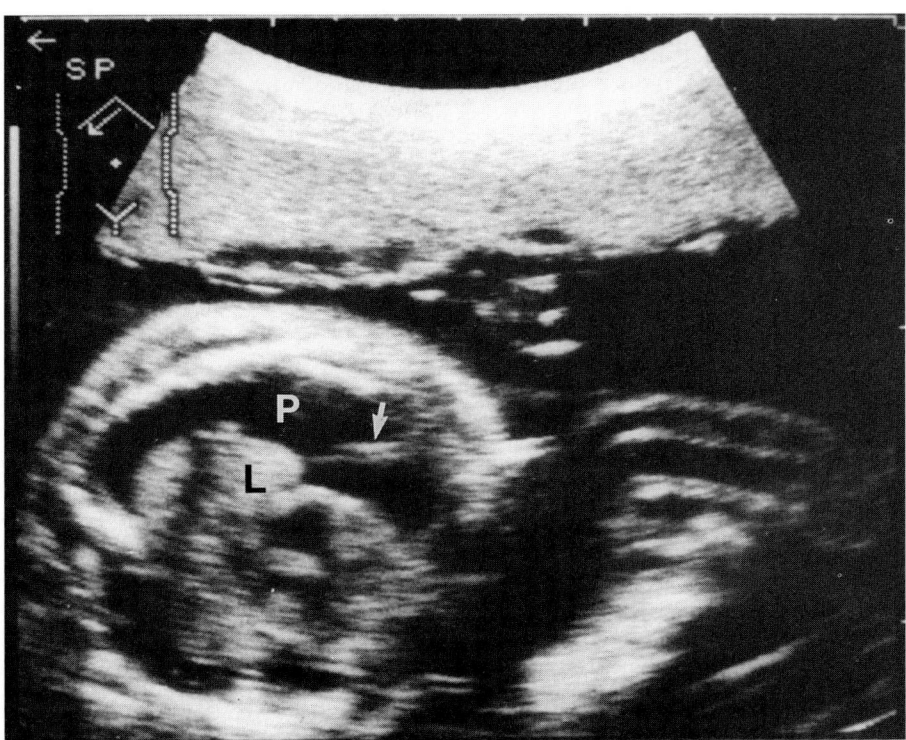

Figure 10–47. A shunt (*arrow*) has been placed to drain a pleural effusion (P) in a fetus at 24 weeks' gestation. Note the compressed lung (L).

of routine obstetric ultrasound.[179] In an investigation of 11,045 women for whom an ultrasound at 16 to 18 weeks was used as the standard for dating a pregnancy, Kramer et al.[180] found that obstetric dating based on the patient's last menstrual period was most likely to be in error in identifying a preterm or postterm pregnancy. Kramer et al.[180] concluded that the mistakes made in dating using menstrual gestational age "support the argument for routine gestational dating with an early ultrasound examination," particularly when one considers

the clinical consequences of poor dating. Reviewing their experience with maternal serum markers to screen for Down syndrome in over 25,000 women, Haddow et al.[181] noted that "Universal dating by ultrasonography before screening would greatly lessen the number of women who are wrongly told that their pregnancies are high risk, and it would allow subsequent diagnostic steps to be taken more expeditiously."

Routine ultrasound performed at 18 weeks' gestation will detect nearly all multiple pregnancies.[182–184] Clini-

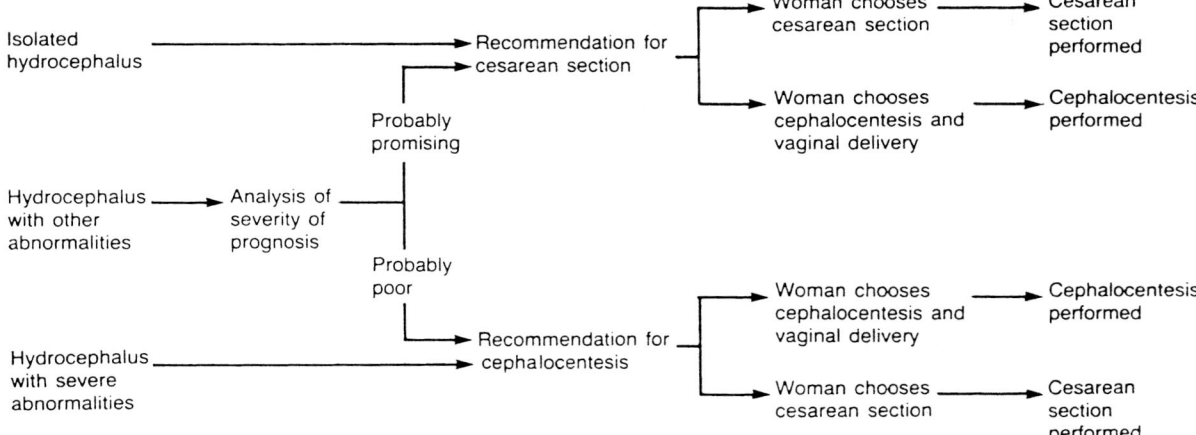

Figure 10–48. Resolution strategies for conflicts in the intrapartum management of hydrocephalus with macrocephaly. (From Chervenak FA, McCullough LB: Ethical challenges in perinatal medicine: the intrapartum management of pregnancy complicated by fetal hydrocephalus with macrocephaly. Semin Perinatol 11:232, 1987, with permission.)

cal experience gained in Sweden as well as in the United States indicates that earlier identification of a twin gestation can reduce perinatal mortality and morbidity, perhaps by allowing more close observation and intervention.

An ultrasound performed at 18 weeks' gestation will reveal that approximately 10 percent of placentas overlie the cervical os, allowing the obstetrician to exclude placenta previa in the remaining 90 percent of cases. Of patients with a low-lying placenta at 18 weeks, only those women in whom the placenta completely covers the os are at risk for a placenta previa in the third trimester. The risk of placenta previa in this group is 41 percent, and a repeat ultrasound evaluation should be performed in these cases.[176-185]

One of the most important benefits of routine ultrasound appears to be the identification of major congenital malformations. Major anomalies occur in 2 to 3 percent of all births, and data from the Centers for Disease Control and Prevention demonstrate that birth defects are a leading cause of infant mortality, accounting for 22 percent of all infant deaths in 1995 (see Chapter 12). Cardiac abnormalities result in one third of infant deaths caused by birth defects, with respiratory, central nervous system, and chromosomal abnormalities each responsible for approximately 15 percent of these losses. Systematic examination of fetal structure as part of the basic ultrasound study outlined by the ACOG can identify a significant proportion of these abnormalities. In six European studies, including 52,295 patients scanned between 1980 and 1991, routine ultrasound had a sensitivity of 52.9 percent and a positive predictive value of 95.9 percent in identifying major structural anomalies.[186] The specificity and negative predictive value were 99.9 and 99.2 percent, respectively. Recent data from 61 European obstetric units participating in the Eurofetus study demonstrate a sensitivity of 61.4 percent for the detection of 3,685 malformed fetuses.[187] Similar sensitivities and predictive values have been reported by experienced groups in this country.[188,189]

Several investigations have confirmed the psychological benefit of routine ultrasound, revealing that women who have undergone a scan are more likely to follow the recommendations of their health care providers to stop smoking cigarettes and drinking alcohol.[190,191]

Until recently, the proposed benefits of routine ultrasound had not been evaluated in large, prospective, randomized studies. Six small studies did reveal that routine ultrasound was associated with fewer inductions for suspected prolonged pregnancy, less morbidity in postdate infants, greater birth weight in twins, and fewer cases of unexpected bleeding from placenta previa.[192-197]

To determine the value of an ultrasound scan at the first prenatal visit, Crowther and her colleagues in Aus-

tralia performed a prospective randomized clinical trial of 648 women presenting at 10 to 11 weeks' gestation.[198] Women who had no previous ultrasound and no indication for a scan were randomized to have an ultrasound performed at that time or to a control group. The main outcome measures included the number of women who needed adjustment in their dates by 10 days or more when an ultrasound was later performed to assess fetal anatomy at 18 to 20 weeks, as well as the number of women who were scheduled for their fetal anatomy scan or who had maternal serum screening tests at inappropriate gestational ages. Women in both study groups also completed a questionnaire at the first prenatal visit to assess their feelings about the pregnancy.

For those women randomized to receive an ultrasound at the first prenatal visit, 24 percent required a correction in gestational dating by 10 days or more. Among women who said they were certain of the date of their last menstrual period, 18 percent needed adjustment of their dates. As expected, significantly fewer women who had an ultrasound at their first visit needed an adjustment of their due date when an ultrasound was performed at 18 to 20 weeks (9 percent vs. 18 percent). In the control group, 25 percent of women did have a scan before 18 to 20 weeks, most often for vaginal bleeding or uncertain gestational age. No significant differences were observed in the number of control group women who were scheduled inappropriately for their 18- to 20-week scan or the number of repeat maternal serum screening tests required because of incorrect dating, the number of nonviable pregnancies detected, the number of twins diagnosed at an earlier gestational age, or the number of major anomalies detected. Women who had an ultrasound at the first visit were less worried about their pregnancy. These investigators concluded that a routine ultrasound assessment for dating at the first antenatal visit allowed a more accurate estimation of gestational age and decreased the need to adjust dating later in pregnancy.

Saari-Kemppainen et al.[199] reported the results of a prospective, randomized investigation of routine ultrasonography performed in the early second trimester including 9,000 Finnish women. The study compared routine ultrasound screening between 16 and 20 weeks, with selective screening performed for usual practice standards. Routine ultrasonography was associated with fewer outpatient clinic visits and antenatal hospitalizations, improved early detection of twins, and identification of patients at risk for placenta previa. There were no differences in the number of labor inductions or mean birth weights in the two groups. Perinatal mortality was significantly lower in the screened than in the control group (4.6 per 1,000 vs. 9.0 per 1,000). This reduction by almost one half was due primarily to early detection of major malformations that led to induced abortion. Additional benefits were correction of the expected date of delivery by 10 or more days in over 11 percent of the screened group and a decrease in the rate of prolonged pregnancy. The authors concluded that their findings justified routine ultrasound screening of all pregnancies at 16 to 20 weeks for the detection of major congenital abnormalities under circumstances in which induced abortion was acceptable.

The Routine Antenatal Diagnostic Imaging with Ultrasound Study (RADIUS) is the largest prospective randomized investigation evaluating the efficacy of routine ultrasound screening.[200–202] To determine if routine ultrasound could improve the detection of congenital malformations, pregnancies with multiple gestations, abnormal fetal growth, placental abnormalities, and errors in the estimation of gestational age and reduce the frequency of adverse perinatal outcomes, Ewigman and his colleagues[200] studied 15,151 low-risk patients recruited from 92 obstetric and 17 family medicine practices in six states. Ultrasound screening was performed twice in 7,812 study subjects, first at 15 to 22 weeks and again at 31 to 35 weeks, whereas the 7,718 women in the control group had an ultrasound only if medically indicated. The adverse outcomes evaluated included fetal or neonatal deaths, severe morbidity such as the need for mechanical ventilation for more than 48 hours, a stay of more than 30 days in the special care nursery, and moderate morbidity including a brachial plexus injury.

Women in the experimental group had an average of 2.2 ultrasound studies. Forty-five percent of control subjects also had an ultrasound, for an average of 0.6 studies per control patient. No statistically significant difference was noted in the rate of adverse perinatal outcomes in this investigation: 5.0 percent in the experimental group and 4.9 percent for the control subjects.[200] No difference was observed in the rate of preterm births or in birth weight distribution. Of 187 major anomalies in the infants of ultrasound-screened patients, 65 (34.8 percent) were detected. Of these, 31 (16.6 percent) were identified before 24 weeks' gestation. In the control group, only 18 of 163 major malformations (11 percent) were recognized, 8 (4.9 percent) before 24 weeks' gestation.[202] When outcomes were examined in subgroups of patients with postdate pregnancies, multiple gestations, or infants with a birth weight below the 10th percentile, no differences were observed. In an analysis of data on maternal management and outcome, LeFevre et al.[201] noted no significant differences in the rates of induced abortion, amniocentesis, tests of fetal well-being, external version, induction, cesarean delivery, and the distribution of total hospital days. However, the use of tocolytics and the rate of postdate pregnancy were both slightly lower in the screened group. These investigators concluded that screening ultrasonography did not improve perinatal outcome compared with ultrasonography performed only for medical indications.

Although the RADIUS trial is an important study, a number of significant concerns have been raised in applying the results to general obstetric practice.[186,203] The adverse perinatal outcomes studied were caused primarily by prematurity or birth trauma. Clearly, prematurity cannot be reduced by routine ultrasound, nor will a second ultrasound examination performed as early as 31 to 35 weeks help to identify the macrosomic fetus at risk for birth trauma. As noted by Berkowitz[203] in an accompanying editorial, the study population was at extremely low risk for perinatal problems. Women who were eligible for the study had to be at least 18 years of age and speak English. Only 13 percent of them smoked, and more than 40 percent of them had graduated from college.[200] When O'Day et al.[204] applied these criteria to 1,000 Medicaid patients at the University of Texas, Houston, only 78 women met the eligibility criteria for the RADIUS trial! Accurate dating of all pregnancies has been cited as an advantage of routine ultrasound. Yet, in the RADIUS trial, women had to know their last menstrual period within 1 week. Not surprisingly, gestational age was reassigned in only 11 percent of the study subjects.[187] Even in those women assigned to the routine ultrasound group, the detection of major anomalies was poor, only 34.8 percent, and of the 65 malformations identified, only 31 were recognized before 24 weeks.

Why do these results differ from the large clinical experiences of many centers? The answer may be that there is nothing "routine" about a routine ultrasound examination. A basic ultrasound study must be carefully performed by an experienced sonographer. Of note, the rate of detection of fetal malformations at tertiary centers in the RADIUS trial was 35 percent (19 of 54), but only 13 percent (8 of 64) in nontertiary centers. Few women in the RADIUS trial who had a fetal malformation identified elected to terminate their pregnancies.[200] This choice may be based on cultural differences compared with the study in Helsinki,[199] on the severity of the anomalies recognized, or, perhaps, on lack of confidence in the diagnosis.[186] Unfortunately, the RADIUS trial did not evaluate the psychological benefits of routine ultrasound screening, which have been recognized in other prospective studies. Clinicians caring for patients in the routine ultrasound arm of the RADIUS trial, although having the results of the ultrasound studies available, did not follow established protocols in their management of pregnancies complicated by growth restriction, prolonged pregnancy, or multiple gestations.[201] Furthermore, the number of cases in each of these high-risk groups was limited. These shortcomings make it difficult to evaluate whether routine ultrasound is useful in the care of such patients. Finally, it is important to point out that ultrasound screening did not *increase* the risk of adverse perinatal outcomes.

In their discussion of the results of the RADIUS trial, the authors note that the cost of screening more than 4 million pregnant women annually in the United States at $200 per ultrasound scan would be more than $1 billion. This figure could be reduced to $500 million, since only 40 percent of all pregnancies screened were eligible for the study. However, several other factors should be considered in calculating this cost. Barrett and Brinson[205] found that a routine ultrasound performed at the first prenatal visit was the most cost-effective of all prenatal laboratory assessments performed. DeVore[206] has examined the cost of detecting a malformed fetus in the RADIUS trial compared with the California MSAFP screening program. For tertiary centers in the RADIUS trial with a detection rate for fetal anomalies of 6.8 per 1,000, the cost was $29,533 compared with a detection rate of 1.7 per 1,000 and a cost of $115,575 for nontertiary centers. The detection rate in the California MSAFP program is 1.3 per 1,000, yielding a cost of $40,338 for each identified malformed fetus. One must compare this expense with those of caring for a severely malformed infant. Vintzileos and his colleagues recently performed a cost–benefit analysis of routine second-trimester sonograms in 1 million American women.[207] When performed in tertiary care centers, routine studies resulted in a net savings of $1.35 to $1.70 for every dollar spent, with an annual net benefit of $97 to $189 million. In contrast, the reduced sensitivity observed in the nontertiary sites in the RADIUS trial would lead to expected net losses of $69 to $161 million.

In its 1993 Technical Bulletin, the ACOG[176] offered the following recommendations concerning routine ultrasound:

> Routine ultrasonography in early pregnancy can help to reduce the incidence of labor induction for suspected postdatism, and decrease the frequency of undiagnosed major fetal anomalies and undiagnosed twins. However, significant effects on infant outcome are not confirmed by randomized, controlled trials. Although obstetric ultrasound studies are performed routinely in many European countries, in the United States the routine use of ultrasonography cannot be supported from a cost-benefit standpoint.

More recently, in the summary of its Practice Pattern on routine ultrasound in low-risk pregnancy, the ACOG concluded[208]:

- The specificity of a fetal anatomic survey in detecting fetal anomalies can be anticipated to exceed 99 percent.
- The sensitivity of a fetal anatomic survey in detecting fetal anomalies cannot be estimated with precision; rather, it should be acknowledged that sensitivity may vary in different clinical settings and with different levels of skill of professionals performing the examination.
- It is uncertain whether an improvement in the survival of fetuses with life-threatening anomalies can be expected from routine ultrasound in low-risk pregnancy.
- In a population of women with low-risk pregnancy, neither a reduction in perinatal morbidity and mortality nor a lower rate of unnecessary interventions can be expected from routine diagnostic ultrasound. Thus ultrasound should be performed for specific indications in low-risk pregnancy.

While the debate concerning routine obstetric ultrasound continues, a reasonable strategy for this dilemma is the concept that prenatal informed consent for sonogram be considered.[209] Shortly after the pregnancy is diagnosed, the woman should be provided with information about the actual and theoretical benefits and harms of a routine ultrasound examination. Because the sonographic detection of fetal anomalies has been recognized as a benefit of routine ultrasound, withholding this information from the pregnant patient would not appear to be justified. Thus, a routine obstetric ultrasound examination is *offered*, but not necessarily recommended.

CONCLUSION

In summary, studies of routine ultrasound have failed to demonstrate any associated adverse effects on the mother or fetus. Routine ultrasound has a high positive predictive value for conditions known to be associated with poor perinatal outcome such as twins, placenta previa, and congenital malformations. To date, several large, prospective, randomized studies have evaluated the benefits of routine ultrasound in obstetric practice.[199–202] One, performed in Finland,[199] demonstrated a reduction in perinatal mortality, resulting from the identification of major fetal anomalies. The RADIUS trial,[201,202] performed in the United States, failed to show an improvement in perinatal outcome. Nevertheless, a large clinical experience from centers both in the United States and in Europe has repeatedly found that routine ultrasound screening at 18 weeks can improve gestational dating in approximately 10 to 25 percent of patients, detect nearly all multiple gestations, exclude placenta previa in most patients and recognize those at greatest risk for this condition, detect one third to one half of major fetal malformations, and reduce parental anxiety and increase compliance with the recommendations of health care providers. The cost of routine ultrasound screening must be compared with the costs created by false-positive diagnoses, which may lead to unnecessary patient anxiety and further intervention,[210] and to the cost savings resulting from reduction in the rate of inductions for suspected prolonged pregnancy, a decrease in the rate of preterm delivery for twins, and the identification of a fetus with an anomaly likely to survive but with a poor quality of life. Finally, like any analytic technique, the value of ultrasound screening is dependent on the skill with which the study is performed and the manner in which the results are interpreted and used in clinical care.[178]

Key Points

➤ Ultrasound energy is produced by a transducer containing crystal structures that convert electrical energy to ultrasound waves and the returning echoes to electrical energy.

➤ No deleterious effects on the pregnant woman or fetus caused by exposure to ultrasound at the intensities used for imaging have ever been reported.

➤ Although the gestational sac can be used to date an early pregnancy, measurement of the crown–rump length is the single best method to assess gestational age at any time in pregnancy.

➤ From 12 to 28 weeks' gestation, the relationship between the biparietal diameter and gestational age is linear.

➤ Formulas for estimation of fetal weight are associated with a 95 percent confidence range of at least 10 to 15 percent.

➤ Measurement of the fetal abdominal circumference is probably the most reliable sonographic parameter for the detection of macrosomia.

➤ At term, an AFI less than 5.0 cm indicates oligohydramnios and greater than 20 cm polyhydramnios.

➤ The thickness of the placenta in millimeters corresponds to the number of weeks gestation.

➤ The "lemon" and "banana" signs are important cranial markers for spina bifida.

➤ Major structural malformations, including hydrops, duodenal atresia, and cardiac anomalies, are observed in 30 percent of cases of Down syndrome (trisomy 21).

REFERENCES

1. Manning F: General Principals and Applications of Ultrasonography. *In* Creasy RK, Resnik R (eds): Maternal-Fetal Medicine: Principles and Practice. Philadelphia, WB Saunders Company, 1999, p 169.
2. Johnson DD, Pretorius DH, Riccabona M, et al: Three-dimensional ultrasound of the fetal spine. Obstet Gynecol 89: 434, 1997.
3. Mueller GM, Weiner CP, Yankowitz J: Three-dimensional ultrasound in the evaluation of fetal head and spine anomalies. Obstet Gynecol 88:372, 1996.
4. Report of the Royal College of Obstetricians and Gynaecologists Working Party on Routine Ultrasound Examination in Pregnancy, December 1984.
5. U.S. Department of Health and Human Services: Diagnostic Ultrasound in Pregnancy. NIH Publ. No. 84-667. Washington, DC, National Institutes of Health, 1984.
6. Fowlkes JB, Holland CK: Mechanical bioeffects from diagnostic ultrasound: AIUM Consensus statements. J Ultrasound 19: 68–154, 2000.
7. Maulik D: Biologic effects of ultrasound. Clin Obstet Gynecol 32:645, 1989.
8. Miller MW, Brayman AA, Abramowicz JS: Obstetric ultrasonography: a biophysical consideration of patient safety—the "rules" have changed. Am J Obstet Gynecol 179:241, 1998.
9. Porfirio B, Dallapiccola B, Cittanti C, et al: Sister chromatid exchanges in cultured amniocytes exposed to diagnostic ultrasound in vitro. Acta Radiol 35:58, 1994.
10. American Institute of Ultrasound in Medicine: Bioeffects & Safety of Diagnostic Ultrasound, 1993.
11. Salvesen KA, Vatten LJ, Jacobsen G, et al: Routine ultrasonography in utero and subsequent vision and hearing at primary school age. Ultrasound Obstet Gynecol 2:243, 1992.
12. Salvesen KA, Vatten LJ, Bakketeig LS, Eik-Nes SH: Routine ultrasonography in utero and speech development. Ultrasound Obstet Gynecol 4:101, 1994.
13. Naumberg E, Bellocco R, Cnattingius S, et al: Prenatal ultrasound examinations and risk of childhood leukaemia: case-control study. BMJ 320:282, 2000.
14. Nelson LH III, Kurtz AB, Hissong SL, Lawrence H: Training guidelines for physicians who interpret diagnostic ultrasound examinations. AIUM Reporter, May 1993.
15. Timor-Tritsch IE, Rottem S (eds): Transvaginal Sonography. 2nd ed. New York, Elsevier Science, 1991.
16. Fleischer AC, Kepple DM: Transvaginal Sonography. A Clinical Atlas. Philadelphia, JB Lippincott, 1992.
17. Timor-Tritsch IE, Rottem S: Normal and abnormal fetal anatomy in the first fifteen weeks. *In* Timor-Tritsch IE, Rottem S (eds): Diagnostic Ultrasound Applied to Obstetrics and Gynecology. 3rd ed. Philadelphia, JB Lippincott, 1994, p 353.
18. Fossum GT, Davajan V, Kletzky OA: Early detection of pregnancy with transvaginal ultrasound. Fertil Steril 49:788, 1988.
19. Nyberg DA, Mack LA, Laing FC, Palten RM: Distinguishing normal from abnormal gestational sac growth in early pregnancy. J Ultrasound Med 6:23, 1987.
20. Reece EA, Scioscia A, Pinta E, et al: Prognostic significance of the human yolk sac assessed by ultrasonography. Am J Obstet Gynecol 159:1191, 1988.
21. Lindsay DJ, Lyons EA, Levi CS, et al: Yolk sac diameter and shape at endovaginal US: predictors of pregnancy outcome. Radiology 183:115, 1992.
22. Levi CS, Lyons EA, Zheng XH: Endovaginal ultrasound:

demonstration of cardiac activity in embryos of less than 5 mm in crown-rump length. Radiology 176:71, 1990.

23. Brown DL, Emerson DS, Felker RE: Diagnosis of early embryonic demise by endovaginal sonography. J Ultrasound Med 9:631, 1990.

24. Simpson JL, Mills JL, Holmes LB, et al: Low fetal loss rates after ultrasound-proved viability in early pregnancy. JAMA 258:2555, 1987.

25. Doubilet PM, Benson CB, Crow JS: Long-term prognosis of pregnancies complicated by slow embryonic heart rates in the early first trimester. J Ultrasound Med 18:537, 1999.

26. Nicolaides KM: Fetal nuchal translucency: ultrasound screening for fetal trisomy in the first trimester of pregnancy. Br J Obstet Gynaecol 101:782, 1994.

27. Spencer K, Souter V, Tull N, et al: A screening program for trisomy 21 at 10–14 weeks using fetal nuchal translucency, maternal serum free beta-human chorionic gonadotropin and pregnancy-associated plasma protein-A. Ultrasound Obstet Gynecol 13:231, 1999.

28. Taiplae P, Hiilesmaa V, Salonen R, Ylostalo P: Increased nuchal translucency as a marker for fetal chromosomal defects. N Engl J Med 337:1654, 1997.

29. Zosmer N, Souter VL, Chan CS, et al: Early diagnosis of major cardiac defects in chromosomally normal fetuses with increased nuchal translucency. Br J Obstet Gynaecol 106:829, 1999.

30. Spencer K, Spencer CE, Power M, et al: One stop clinic for assessment of risk for fetal anomalies: a report of the first year of prospective screening for chromosomal anomalies in the first trimester. Br J Obstet Gynaecol 107:1271, 2000.

31. Farine D, Fox HE, Timor-Tritsch IE: Vaginal approach to the ultrasound diagnosis of placenta previa. In Chervenak FA, Isaacson G, Campbell S (eds): Ultrasound in Obstetrics and Gynecology. Boston, Little, Brown, 1993, p 1503.

32. Iams JD, Goldenberg RL, Meis PJ, et al: The length of the cervix and the risk of spontaneous premature delivery. N Engl J Med 334:567, 1996.

33. Heath VC, Southall TR, Souka AP, et al: Cervical length at 23 weeks of gestation: prediction of spontaneous preterm delivery. Ultrasound Obstet Gynaecol 12:312, 1998.

34. Robinson HP, Fleming JEE: A critical evaluation of sonar crown-rump length measurement. Br J Obstet Gynaecol 82:702, 1975.

35. Gabbe SG, Iams JD: Intrauterine growth retardation. In Iams JD, Zuspan FP (eds): Manual of Obstetrics and Gynecology. St. Louis, CV Mosby, 1990, p 169.

36. Campbell S, Warsof S, Little D, et al: Routine ultrasound screening for the prediction of gestational age. Obstet Gynecol 65:613, 1985.

37. Chervenak FA, Skupski DW, Romero R, et al: How accurate is fetal biometry in the assessment of fetal age. Am J Obstet Gynecol 178:678, 1998.

38. Mul T, Mongelli M, Gardosi J: A comparative analysis of second-trimester ultrasound dating formulas in pregnancies conceived with artificial reproduction techniques. Ultrasound Obstet Gynecol 8:397, 1996.

39. Geirsson RT, Have G: Comparison of actual and ultrasound estimated second trimester gestational length in in vitro fertilized pregnancies. Aota Obstet Gynecol Scand 72:344, 1993.

40. Kurtz A, Wapner R, Kurtz R, et al: Analysis of biparietal diameter as an accurate indicator of gestational age. J Clin Ultrasound 8:319, 1980.

41. Chien PFW, Owen R, Khan KS: Validity of ultrasound estimation of fetal weight. 95:856, 2000.

42. Hadlock EP, Harrist RB, Carpenter RJ, et al: Sonographic estimation of fetal weight. Radiology 150:535, 1984.

43. Shepard M, Richard V, Berkowitz R, et al: An evaluation of two equations for predicting fetal weight by ultrasound. Am J Obstet Gynecol 142:47, 1982.

44. Macrosomia: American College of Obstetricians and Gynecologists, Technical Bulletin, Number 159, 1991.

45. Persson B, Stangenberg M, Lunnell NO, et al: Prediction of size of infants at birth by measurement of symphysis fundus height. Br J Obstet Gynaecol 93:206, 1986.

46. Ott WJ, Doyle S: Ultrasonic diagnosis of altered fetal growth by use of a normal ultrasound fetal weight curve. Obstet Gynecol 63:201, 1984.

47. Tamura RK, Sabbagha RE, Depp R, et al: Diabetic macrosomia: accuracy of third trimester ultrasound. Obstet Gynecol 67:828, 1986.

48. Chervenak JL, Divon MY, Hirsch J, et al: Macrosomia in the postdate pregnancy: is routine ultrasonographic screening indicated? Am J Obstet Gynecol 161:753, 1989.

49. Pollack RN, Hauer-Pollack G, Divon MY: Macrosomia in postdates pregnancies: the accuracy of routine ultrasonographic screening. Am J Obstet Gynecol 167:7, 1992.

50. Delpapa EH, Mueller-Heubach E: Pregnancy outcome following ultrasound diagnosis of macrosomia. Obstet Gynecol 78:340, 1991.

51. Sandmire HF: Whither ultrasonic prediction of fetal macrosomia? Obstet Gynecol 82:860, 1993.

52. Bochner CJ, Medearis AL, Williams J, et al: Early third-trimester ultrasound screening in gestational diabetes to determine the risk of macrosomia and labor dystocia at term. Am J Obstet Gynecol 157:703, 1987.

53. Chudleigh P, Pearce JM (eds): Obstetric Ultrasound. Edinburgh, Churchill Livingstone, 1986.

54. Cohen B, Penning S, Major C, et al: Sonographic prediction of shoulder dystocia in infants of diabetic mothers. Obstet Gynecol 88:10, 1996.

55. Deter RL, Hadlock FP: Use of ultrasound in the detection of macrosomia: a review. J Clin Ultrasound 13:519, 1985.

56. Chamberlain P, Manning F, Morrison I, et al: Ultrasound evaluation of amniotic fluid volume. I. The relationship of marginal and decreased amniotic fluid volumes to perinatal outcome. Am J Obstet Gynecol 150:245, 1984.

57. Chamberlain P, Manning F, Morrison I, et al: Ultrasound evaluation of amniotic fluid volume. II. The relationship of increased amniotic fluid volume to perinatal outcome. Am J Obstet Gynecol 150:250, 1984.

58. Bottoms SF, Welch RA, Zador IE, et al: Limitations of using maximum vertical pocket and other sonographic evaluations of amniotic fluid volume to predict fetal growth: technical or physiologic? Am J Obstet Gynecol 155:154, 1986.

59. Hoddick WK, Callen PW, Filly RA, et al: Ultrasonographic determination of qualitative amniotic fluid volume in intrauterine growth retardation: reassessment of the 1 cm rule. Am J Obstet Gynecol 149:758, 1984.

60. Phelan JP, Smith CV, Broussard P, Small M: Amniotic fluid volume assessment using the four-quadrant technique in the pregnancy between 36 and 42 weeks' gestation. J Reprod Med 32:540, 1987.

61. Phelan FP, Ahn MO, Smith CV, et al: Amniotic fluid index measurements during pregnancy. J Reprod Med 32:601, 1987.

62. Del Valle GO, Bateman L, Gaudier FL, Sanchez-Ramos L: Comparison of three types of ultrasound transducers in evaluating the amniotic fluid index. J Reprod Med 39:869, 1994.

63. Flack NJ, Dore C, Southwell D, et al: The influence of operator transducer pressure on ultrasonographic measurements of amniotic fluid volume. Am J Obstet Gynecol 171:218, 1994.

64. Moore TR, Cayle JE: The amniotic fluid index in normal human pregnancy. Am J Obstet Gynecol 162:1168, 1990.

65. Rutherford SE, Smith CV, Phelan JP, et al: Four-quadrant

assessment of amniotic fluid volume. J Reprod Med 32:587, 1987.

66. Bruner JP, Reed GW, Sarno AP, et al: Intraobserver and interobserver variability of the amniotic fluid index. Am J Obstet Gynecol 168:1309, 1993.

67. Carlson DE, Platt LD, Medearis AL, et al: Quantifiable polyhydramnios: diagnosis and management. Obstet Gynecol 75:989, 1990.

68. Damato N, Filly RA, Goldstein RB, et al: Frequency of fetal anomalies in sonographically detected polyhydramnios. J Ultrasound Med 12:11, 1993.

69. Moore TR, Brace RA: Amniotic fluid index (AFI) in the term ovine pregnancy: a predictable relationship between AFI and amniotic fluid volume. *In* Proceedings of the 35th Annual Meeting of the Society for Gynecologic Investigation, Baltimore, Maryland, March 1988.

70. Moore TR: Superiority of the four-quadrant sum over the single-deepest-pocket technique in ultrasonographic identification of abnormal amniotic fluid volumes. Am J Obstet Gynecol 163:762, 1990.

71. Chervenak FA, Isaacson G, Lorber J: Anomalies of the Fetal Head, Neck and Spine: Ultrasound Diagnosis and Management. Philadelphia, WB Saunders Company, 1988.

72. Ultrasound in Pregnancy. ACOG Technical Bulletin 116. Washington, DC, American College of Obstetricians and Gynecologists, 1988.

73. Filly RA: Level 1, level 2, level 3 obstetric sonography: I'll see your level and raise you one. Radiology 172:312, 1989.

74. Campbell S: The obstetric ultrasound examination. *In* Chervenak FA, Isaacson G, Campbell S (eds): Ultrasound in Obstetrics and Gynecology. Boston, Little, Brown, 1993, p 187.

75. AIUM Technical Bulletin. Performance of the Basic Fetal Cardiac Ultrasound Examination. J Ultrasound Med 17:601, 1998.

76. Jauniaux E, Campbell S: Ultrasonographic assessment of placental abnormalities. Am J Obstet Gynecol 163:1650, 1990.

77. Jauniaux E, Ramsay B, Campbell S: Ultrasonographic investigation of placental morphologic characteristics and size during the second trimester of pregnancy. Am J Obstet Gynecol 170:130, 1994.

78. Finberg HJ, Williams JW: Placenta accreta: prospective sonographic diagnosis in patients with placenta previa and prior cesarean section. J Ultrasound Med 11:333, 1992.

79. Levine D, Hilka CA, Ludmir J, et al: Placenta accreta: evaluation with color Doppler US, Doppler US and MR imaging. Radiology 205:773, 1997.

80. Sabbagha R (ed): Diagnostic Ultrasound Applied to Obstetrics and Gynecology. Philadelphia, JB Lippincott, 1994.

81. Chervenak FA, Isaacson G, Campbell S (eds): Ultrasound in Obstetrics and Gynecology. Boston, Little, Brown, 1993.

82. Manning FA: The anomalous fetus. *In* In Fetal Medicine. Principles and Practice. Norwalk, CT, Appleton & Lange, 1995, p 451.

83. Nelson NL, Filly RA, Goldstein RB, Callen PW: The AIUM/ACR antepartum obstetrical sonographic guidelines: expectations for detection of anomalies. J Ultrasound Med 4:189, 1993.

84. Campbell S, Johnstone FD, Hold EM, et al: Anencephaly: early ultrasonic diagnosis and active management. Lancet 2:1226, 1972.

85. Chervenak FA, Isaacson G, Mahoney MJ, et al: The obstetric significance of holoprosencephaly. Obstet Gynecol 63:115, 1984.

86. Romero R, Cullen M, Grannum P, et al: Antenatal diagnosis of renal anomalies with ultrasound. III. Bilateral renal agenesis. Am J Obstet Gynecol 151:38, 1985.

87. Chervenak FA, Isaacson G, Touloukian R, et al: The diagno-

sis and management of fetal teratomas. Obstet Gynecol 66:666, 1985.

88. Chervenak FA, Isaacson G, Blakemore KJ, et al: Fetal cystic hygroma: cause and natural history. N Engl J Med 309:822, 1984.

89. Johnson MP, Johnson A, Holzgreve W, et al: First trimester cystic hygromas: cause and outcome. Am J Obstet Gynecol 168:156, 1993.

90. Holzgreve W, Curry CJR, Golbus MS: Investigation of nonimmune hydrops fetalis. Am J Obstet Gynecol 150:805, 1984.

91. Machin GA: Hydrops revisited: literature review of 1414 cases published in the 1980s. Am J Med Genet 34:366, 1989.

92. Santolaya J, Alley D, Jaffe R, Warsof SL: Antenatal classification of hydrops fetalis. Obstet Gynecol 79:256, 1992.

93. Arey LB: Developmental Anatomy. Philadelphia, WB Saunders Company, 1974, pp 245, 465.

94. Chervenak FA, Isaacson G, Mahoney MJ, et al: The diagnosis and management of fetal cephalocele. Obstet Gynecol 64:86, 1984.

95. Hobbins JC, Venus I, Tortora M, et al: Stage II ultrasound examination for the diagnosis of fetal abnormalities with an elevated amniotic fluid alpha-fetoprotein concentration. Am J Obstet Gynecol 142:1026, 1982.

96. Platt LD, Feuchtbaum L, Filly R, et al: The California maternal serum alpha-fetoprotein screening program: the role of ultrasonography in the detection of spina bifida. Obstet Gynecol 166:1328, 1992.

97. McIntosh R: The incidence of congenital malformations: a study of 5964 pregnancies. Pediatrics 14:505, 1954.

98. Nicolaides KM, Campbell S, Gabbe SG, Guidetti R: Ultrasound screening for spina bifida: cranial and cerebellar signs. Lancet 2:72, 1986.

99. Nakayama DK, Harrison RM, Gross BH, et al: Management of the fetus with an abdominal wall defect. J Pediatr Surg 19:408, 1984.

100. Marwood RP, Dawson MR, Gross BH, et al: Antenatal diagnosis of diaphragmatic hernias. Br J Obstet Gynaecol 88:71, 1981.

101. Sharlane GK, Lockhart SM, Heward AJ, Allan P: Prognosis in fetal diaphragmatic hernia. Am J Obstet Gynecol 166:9, 1992.

102. Cardoza JD, Goldstein RB, Filly RA: Exclusion of fetal ventriculomegaly with a single measurement: the width of the lateral ventricular atrium. Radiology 169:711, 1988.

103. Cardoza JD, Filly RA, Podarsky AE: The dangling choroid plexus: a sonographic observation of value in excluding ventriculomegaly. Am J Radiol 151:767, 1988.

104. Benaceraff BR, Birnholz JC: The diagnosis of fetal hydrocephalus prior to 22 weeks. J Clin Ultrasound 15:531, 1987.

105. Benaceraff BR: Fetal hydrocephalus: diagnosis and significance. Radiology 169:858, 1988.

106. Chervenak FA, Duncan C, Ment LR, et al: The outcome of fetal ventriculomegaly. Lancet 2:179, 1984.

107. Lees RF, Alford BA, Brenbridge NAG, et al: Sonographic appearance of duodenal atresia in utero. AJR Am J Roentgenol 131:701, 1978.

108. Romero R, Jeanty P, Pilu G, et al: The prenatal diagnosis of duodenal atresia. Does it make any difference? Obstet Gynecol 71:739, 1988.

109. Hobbins JC, Romero R, Grannum P, et al: Antenatal diagnosis of renal anomalies with ultrasound. I. Obstructive uropathy. Am J Obstet Gynecol 148:868, 1984.

110. Corteville JE, Gray DL, Crane JP: Congenital hydronephrosis: correlation of fetal ultrasonographic findings with infant outcome. Am J Obstet Gynecol 165:384, 1991.

111. Mandell J, Blyth B, Peters CA, et al: Structural genitourinary defects detected in utero. Radiology 178:193, 1991.

112. Chervenak FA, Jeanty P, Cantraine F, et al: The diagnosis of fetal microcephaly. Am J Obstet Gynecol 149:512, 1984.

113. Chervenak FA, Rosenberg J, Brightman RC, et al: A prospective study of the accuracy of ultrasound in predicting fetal microcephaly. Obstet Gynecol 69:908, 1987.

114. Romero R, Pilu G, Jeanty P, et al: Prenatal Diagnosis of Congenital Anomalies. Norwalk, CT, Appleton & Lange, 1988, p 311.

115. Chervenak FA, Tortora M, Mayden K, et al: Antenatal diagnosis of median cleft face syndrome: sonographic demonstration of cleft lip and hypotelorism. Am J Obstet Gynecol 149: 94, 1984.

116. Grannum P, Bracken M, Silverman R, et al: Assessment of fetal kidney size in normal gestation by comparison of ratio of kidney circumference to abdominal circumference. Am J Obstet Gynecol 136:249, 1980.

117. Romero R, Cullen JM, Jeanty P, et al: The diagnosis of congenital renal anomalies with ultrasound. II. Infantile polycystic kidney disease. Am J Obstet Gynecol 150:259, 1984.

118. Chervenak FA, Tortora MN, Hobbins JC: Antenatal sonographic diagnosis of clubfoot. J Ultrasound Med 4:49, 1985.

119. Goldberg JD, Chervenak FA, Lipman RA, et al: Antenatal sonographic diagnosis of arthrogryposis multiplex congenita. Prenat Diagn 6:45, 1986.

120. Copel JA, Pilu G, Green J, et al: Fetal echocardiographic screening for congenital heart disease: the importance of the four-chamber view. Am J Obstet Gynecol 157:648, 1987.

121. Kleinman CS, Copel JA: Fetal cardiac dysrhythmias: diagnosis and therapy. In Chervenak FA, Isaacson G, Campbell S (eds): Ultrasound in Obstetrics and Gynecology. Boston, Little, Brown, 1993, p 195.

122. Hill LM: Chromosomal abnormalities. In McGahan JP, Porto M (eds): Diagnostic Ultrasound. Philadelphia, JB Lippincott, 1994, p 449.

123. Benacerraf BR, Gelman R, Frigoletto FD: Sonographic identification of second-trimester fetuses with Down syndrome. N Engl J Med 317:1371, 1987.

124. Nyberg DA, Resta RG, Luthy DA, et al: Prenatal sonographic findings of Down syndrome: review of 94 cases. Obstet Gynecol 76:370, 1990.

125. Crane JP, Gray DL: Sonographically measured nuchal skinfold as a screening tool for Down syndrome: results of a prospective clinical trial. Obstet Gynecol 77:533, 1991.

126. Benacerraf BR, Neuberg D, Bromley B, Frigoletto FD: Sonographic scoring index for prenatal detection of chromosomal abnormalities. J Ultrasound Med 11:449, 1992.

127. Hill LM, Gurzevich D, Belfar ML, et al: The current role of sonography in the detection of Down syndrome. Obstet Gynecol 74:620, 1989.

128. Benacerraf BR, Neuberg D, Bromley B, Frigoletto DF Jr: Sonographic scoring index for prenatal detection of chromosomal abnormalities. J Ultrasound Med 11:449, 1992.

129. Bromley B, Lieberman E, Benacerraf BR: The incorporation of maternal age into the sonographic scoring index for the detection at 14–20 weeks of fetuses with Down syndrome. Ultrasound Obstet Gynecol 10:321, 1997.

130. Vintzileos AM, Campbell WA, Rodis JF, et al: The use of second-trimester genetic sonogram in guiding clinical management of patients at increased risk for fetal trisomy 21. Obstet Gynecol 87:948, 1996.

131. Bahado-Singh R, Oz U, Kovanci E, et al: A high-sensitivity alternative to "routine" genetic amniocentesis: multiple urinary analytes, nuchal thickness and age. Am J Obstet Gynecol 180:169, 1999.

132. Platt LD, Carlson DE, Medearis AL, et al: Fetal choroid plexus cysts in the second trimester of pregnancy. A cause for concern. Am J Obstet Gynecol 64:1652, 1991.

133. Benacerraf BR, Hanlon B, Frigoletto F: Are choroid plexus cysts an indication for second-trimester amniocentesis? Am J Obstet Gynecol 162:1001, 1990.

134. Chitty LS, Chudleigh P, Wright E, et al: The significance of choroids plexus cysts in an unselected population: results of a multicenter study. Ultrasound Obstet Gynecol 12:391, 1998.

135. Gupta JK, Cave M, Lilford RJ, et al: Clinical significance of fetal choroid plexus cysts. Lancet 346:724, 1995.

136. Boyd PA, Chamberlain P, Hicks NR: 6-year experience of prenatal diagnosis in an unselected population in Oxford, UK. Lancet 352:1577, 1998.

137. Copet JA, Pilu G, Kleinmann CS: Congenital heart disease and extracardiac anomalies: associations and indications for fetal echocardiography. Am J Obstet Gynecol 154:1121, 1986.

138. Palmer CG, Miles JH, Howard-Peebles PN, et al: Fetal karyotype following ascertainment of fetal anomalies by ultrasound. Prenat Diagn 7:551, 1987.

139. Platt LD, DeVore GR, Lopez E, et al: Role of amniocentesis in ultrasound-detected fetal malformations. Obstet Gynecol 68:153, 1986.

140. Williamson RA, Weiner CP, Patil S, et al: Abnormal pregnancy sonogram: selective indication for fetal karyotype. Obstet Gynecol 69:15, 1987.

141. Nicolaides K, Shawwa L, Brizot M, Snijders R: Ultrasonographically detectable markers of fetal chromosomal defects. Ultrasound Obstet Gynecol 3:56, 1993.

142. Chervenak FA, McCullough LB: An ethically justified, clinically comprehensive management strategy for third-trimester pregnancies complicated by fetal anomalies. Obstet Gynecol 75:311, 1990.

143. Chervenak FA, McCullough LB: Does obstetric ethics have any role in the obstetrician's response to the abortion controversy? Am J Obstet Gynecol 163:1425, 1990.

144. Harrison M, Golbus M, Filly R: The Unborn Patient. New York, Grune & Stratton, 1984.

145. Seeds JW, Azizkhan RG: Congenital Malformations. Antenatal Diagnosis, Perinatal Management, and Counseling. Rockville, MD, Aspen Publishers, 1990.

146. Romero R, Oyarzun E, Sirtori M, Hobbins JC: Detection and management of anatomic congenital anomalies. Obstet Gynecol Clin North Am 15:215, 1988.

147. Chervenak FA, Berkowitz RL, Tortora M, et al: The management of fetal hydrocephalus. Am J Obstet Gynecol 151:933, 1985.

148. Luthy DA, Wardinsky T, Shurtleff DB, et al: Cesarean section before the onset of labor and subsequent motor function in infants with open spina bifida. N Engl J Med 162:662, 1991.

149. Manning FA, Harrison MR, Rodeck C, et al: Catheter shunts for fetal hydronephrosis and hydrocephalus: special report. N Engl J Med 315:336, 1986.

150. Manning FA: The anomalous fetus. In Manning FA (ed): Fetal Medicine. Principles and Practice. Norwalk, CT, Appleton & Lange, 1995, p 451.

151. Albar H, Manning FA, Harman CR: Treatment of urinary tract and CNS obstruction. In Harman CR (ed): Invasive Fetal Testing and Treatment. Cambridge, Blackwell Scientific, 1995, p 259.

152. Anderson RL, Golbus MS: Bladder aspiration. In Chervenak FA, Isaacson G, Campbell S (eds): Textbook of Ultrasound in Obstetrics and Gynecology. Boston, Little, Brown, 1993.

153. Freedman AL, Johnson MP, Smith CA, et al: Long-term outcome in children after antenatal intervention for obstructive uropathies. Lancet 354:374, 1999.

154. Rodeck CH, Fisk NM, Fraser DI, Nicolini U: Long-term in

utero drainage of fetal hydrothorax. N Engl J Med 319:1135, 1988.

155. Nicolaides KH, Azar G: Thoracoamniotic shunting. *In* Chervenak FA, Isaacson G, Campbell S (eds): Textbook of Ultrasound in Obstetrics and Gynecology. Boston, Little, Brown, 1993, p 1289.

156. Vaughn JI, Fisk NM, Rodeck CM: Fetal pleural effusions. *In* Harman CR (ed): Fetal Testing and Treatment. Cambridge, Blackwell Scientific, 1995, p 219.

157. Clewell WH, Johnson ML, Meier PR, et al: A surgical approach to the treatment of fetal hydrocephalus. N Engl J Med 306:1320, 1982.

158. Clewell W: Current status of ventriculo-amniotic shunt placement. *In* Kurjak A, Comstock C, Chervenak FA (ed): Ultrasound and the Fetal Brain. Carnforth, Parthenon, 1996.

159. Harrison MR, Adzick NS, Longaker MT, et al: Successful repair in utero of a fetal diaphragmatic hernia after removal of herniated viscera from the left thorax. N Engl J Med 322:1582, 1990.

160. Hedrick MH, Estes JM, Sullivan KM, et al: Plug the lung until it grows (PLUG): a new method to treat congenital diaphragmatic hernia in utero. J Pediatr Surg 29:612, 1994.

161. Adzick NS, Harrison MR, Crombleholme TM, et al: Fetal lung lesions: management and outcome. Am J Obstet Gynecol 179:884, 1998.

162. Nilner R, Adzick NS: Perinatal management of fetal malformations amenable to surgical correction. Curr Opin Obstet Gynecol 11:177, 1999.

163. Bruner JP, Richard WO, Tulipan NB, Arney TL: Endoscopic coverage of fetal myelomeningocele in utero. Am J Obstet Gynecol 180:153, 1999.

164. Deprest JA, Gratacos E: Obstetrical endoscopy. Curr Opin Obstet Gynecol 11:195, 1999.

165. Johnson MP, Bukowski TP, Reitlerman C, et al: In utero surgical treatment of fetal obstructive uropathy: a new compression approach to identify appropriate candidates for vesicoamniotic shunt therapy. Am J Obstet Gynecol 170:1770, 1994.

166. Quintero RA, Hume R, Smith C, et al: Percutaneous fetal cystoscopy and endoscopic fulguration of posterior urethral valves. Am J Obstet Gynecol 172:206, 1995.

167. *Roe v. Wade,* 410 US 113, 1973.

168. Elias S, Annas GJ: Reproductive Genetics and the Law. Chicago, Year Book Medical Publishers, 1987.

169. Annas GJ: Protecting the liberty of pregnant patients. N Engl J Med 316:1213, 1987.

170. Chervenak FA, Farley MA, Walters L, et al: When is termination of pregnancy during the third trimester morally justifiable? N Engl J Med 310:501, 1984.

171. Chervenak FA, McCullough LB, Campbell S: Is third trimester abortion justified? Br J Obstet Gynaecol 102:434, 1995.

172. Chervenak FA, McCullough LB: Third trimester abortion: is compassion enough? Br J Obstet Gynaecol 106:293, 1999.

173. Chervenak FA, McCullough LB: Nonaggressive obstetric management. An option for some fetal anomalies during the third trimester. JAMA 261:3439, 1989.

174. Chervenak FA, McCullough LB: Ethical challenges in perinatal medicine: the intrapartum management of pregnancy complicated by fetal hydrocephalus with macrocephaly. Semin Perinatol 11:232, 1987.

175. Chervenak FA, McCullough LB: Fetal destructive procedures in operative obstetrics. *In* O'Grady JP, Gimovsky ML, McIlhargie LJ (eds): Operative Obstetrics. Baltimore, Williams & Wilkins, 1995, p 354.

176. Ultrasonography in Pregnancy. ACOG Technical Bulletin, No.

177. Washington, DC, American College of Obstetricians and Gynecologists, 1993.

177. Warsof SL, Pearce JM, Campbell S: The present place of routine ultrasound screening. Clin Obstet Gynaecol 10:445, 1985.

178. Gabbe SG: Routine versus indicated scans. *In* Sabbagha RE (ed): Diagnostic Ultrasound Applied to Obstetrics and Gynecology. 3rd ed. Philadelphia, JB Lippincott, 1994, p 67.

179. Levi S, Chervenak FA: Ultrasound screening for fetal anomalies: is it worth it? Ann N Y Acad Sci 847, 1998.

180. Kramer MS, McLean FH, Boyd ME, Usher RH: The validity of gestational age estimation by menstrual dating in term, preterm, and postterm gestations. JAMA 260:3306, 1988.

181. Haddow JE, Palomaki GE, Knight GJ, et al: Prenatal screening for Down's syndrome with use of maternal serum markers. N Engl J Med 327:588, 1992.

182. Grennert L, Persson P-H, Gennser G: Benefits of ultrasonic screening of a pregnant population. Acta Obstet Gynecol Scand 78(Suppl):5, 1978.

183. Persson P-H, Kullander S: Long-term experience of general ultrasound screening in pregnancy. Am J Obstet Gynecol 146:942, 1983.

184. Hughey MJ, Olive DL: Routine ultrasound scanning for detection and management of twin pregnancy. J Reprod Med 30:427, 1985.

185. Sanderson DA, Milton PJD: The effectiveness of ultrasound screening at 18–20 weeks gestational age for prediction of placenta praevia. J Obstet Gynecol 11:320, 1991.

186. Romero R: Routine obstetric ultrasound. Utrasound Obstet Gynecol 3:303, 1993.

187. Grandjean H, Larroque D, Levi S: The performance of routine ultrasonographic screening of pregnancies in the Eurofetus Study. Am J Obstet Gynecol 181:446, 1999.

188. Skupski DW, Newman S, Edersheim T, et al: The impact of routine obstetric ultrasonographic screening in a low-risk population. Am J Obstet Gynecol 175:1142, 1996.

189. Magriples U, Copel J: Accurate detection of anomalies by routine ultrasonography in an indigent clinic population. Am J Obstet Gynecol 179:978, 1998.

190. Reading AE, Campbell S, Cox DN, Sledmere CM: Health beliefs and health care behaviour in pregnancy. Psychol Med 12:379, 1982.

191. Waldenstrom U, Nilsson S, Fall O, et al: Effects of routine one-stage ultrasound screening in pregnancy: a randomised controlled trial. Lancet 2:585, 1988.

192. Bennett MJ, Little G, Dewhurst SJ, Chamberlain G: Predictive value of ultrasound measurement in early pregnancy: a randomized controlled trial. Br J Obstet Gynaecol 89:338, 1982.

193. Eik-Nes SH, Okland O, Aure JC, Ulstein M: Ultrasound screening in pregnancy: a randomised controlled trial. Lancet 1:1347, 1984.

194. Bakketeig LS, Jacobsen G, Brodtkorb CJ, et al: Randomised controlled trial of ultrasonographic screening in pregnancy. Lancet 2:207, 1984.

195. Neilson JP, Munjanja SP, Whitfield CR: Screening for small for dates fetuses: a controlled trial. BMJ 289:1179, 1984.

196. Belfrage P, Fernstrom I, Hallenberg G: Routine or selective ultrasound examinations in early pregnancy. Obstet Gynecol 69:747, 1987.

197. Ewigman B, LeFevre M, Hesser J: A randomized trial of routine prenatal ultrasound. Obstet Gynecol 76:189, 1990.

198. Crowther CA, Kornman L, O'Callaghan S, et al: Is an ultrasound assessment of gestational age at the first antenatal visit of value? A randomized clinical trial. Br J Obstet Gynaecol 106:1273, 1999.

199. Saari-Kemppainen A, Karjalainen O, Ylostalo P, et al: Ultrasound screening and perinatal mortality: controlled trial of

systematic one-stage screening in pregnancy. Lancet 336:387, 1990.

200. Ewigman BG, Crane JP, Frigoletto FD, et al: Effect of prenatal ultrasound screening on perinatal outcome. N Engl J Med 329:821, 1993.

201. LeFevre ML, Bain RP, Ewigman BG, et al: A randomized trial of prenatal ultrasonographic screening: impact on maternal management and outcome. Am J Obstet Gynecol 169:483, 1993.

202. Crane JP, LeFevre ML, Winborn RC, et al: A randomized trial of prenatal ultrasonographic screening: impact on the detection, management, and outcome of anomalous fetuses. Am J Obstet Gynecol 171:392, 1994.

203. Berkowitz RL: Should every pregnant woman undergo ultrasonography? N Engl J Med 329:874, 1993.

204. O'Day M, Ivey T, Bianchi A, Wilkins I: Application of RADIUS study criteria to a low-income obstetric population [SPO abstract 305]. Am J Obstet Gynecol 172:345, 1995.

205. Barrett JM, Brinson J: Evaluation of obstetric ultrasonography at the first prenatal visit. Am J Obstet Gynecol 165:1002, 1991.

206. DeVore GR: The routine antenatal diagnostic imaging with ultrasound study: another perspective. Obstet Gynecol 84:622, 1994.

207. Vintzileos AM, Ananth CV, Smulian JC, et al: Routine second-trimester ultrasonography in the United States: a cost-benefit analysis. Am J Obstet Gynecol 182:655, 2000.

208. ACOG Practice Patterns: Routine ultrasound in low-risk pregnancy. Washington, DC, American College of Obstetricians and Gynecologists, 1997, p 1.

209. Chervenak FA, McCullough LB, Chervenak JL: Prenatal informed consent for sonogram: an indication for obstetric ultrasonography. Am J Obstet Gynecol 161:857, 1989.

210. Filly RA: Obstetrical sonography: The best way to terrify a pregnant woman. J Ultrasound Med 19:1, 2000.

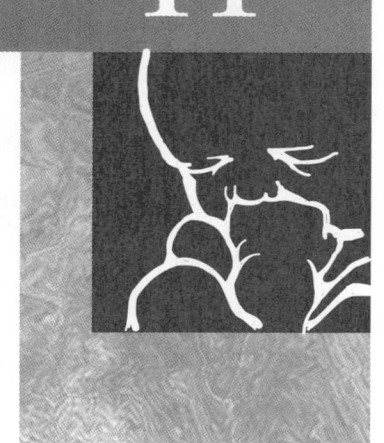

Chapter 11

Fetal Therapeutic Intervention

MARK I. EVANS, MICHAEL R. HARRISON,
ALAN W. FLAKE, AND MARK P. JOHNSON

For close to 30 years, obstetricians have developed a number of approaches to diagnose both structural and functional fetal anomalies.[1] When such abnormalities are severe or lethal, pregnancy termination may provide a reasonable management option for couples. In less severe cases, obstetric care can be tailored to optimize outcomes and prevent secondary complications. In certain situations, prenatal correction of the underlying problem has become possible. Structural malformations can sometimes be approached surgically, while metabolic disorders may benefit from pharmacologic or genetic therapy. Over the past decade, fetal therapy has evolved into four major areas: open surgical approaches, "closed" endoscopic surgical approaches, pharmacologic therapy, and stem cell/gene therapy. Advances in the field have been characterized by alternating exuberance at dramatic successes, but also periods of intense frustration at technical challenges needing to be overcome to bring new approaches on line.

Perhaps the single most misunderstood issue about fetal therapy is why before and not after birth. There is not one single answer, but rather a series of disorder-specific considerations. If something can be treated well and safely postnatally, then there is no justification for prenatal intervention. However, for the conditions discussed below, profound and irreparable damage occurs before birth, making fetal intervention the best, or sometimes only, way to ameliorate the damage. Some of those procedures have been quite rare. Others are more common, but the expectation is that with improvements and increasing utilization of prenatal diagnosis, more women will chose to avail themselves of opportunities to treat fetuses with discernable problems.

SURGICAL THERAPY

In Utero "Closed" Fetal Surgery

The most efficacious percutaneous in utero fetal surgery has been for the evaluation and treatment of obstructive uropathy. Lower urinary tract obstruction (LUTO) is a heterogeneous entity that affects 1 in 5,000 to 1 in 8,000 newborn males. Posterior urethral valves (PUV) or urethral atresias are the most common causes for LUTO, although other etiologies such as stenosis of the urethral meatus, anterior urethral valves, ectopic insertion of a ureter, and tumors of the bladder have been observed. LUTO can result in massive distention of the bladder with compensatory hypertrophy and hyperplasia of the smooth muscle within the bladder wall, leading to a loss of compliance and elasticity, and poor postnatal function generally requiring surgical reconstruction.[2] Elevated intravesicular pressures prevent urine inflow from the ureters; distortion of the uretero-vesical angles contributes to eventual reflux hydronephrosis. Progressive pyelectasis and calycectasis compress the delicate renal parenchyma within the encasing serosal capsule, leading to functional abnormalities within the medullary and eventually the cortical regions (Fig. 11–1). Focal compressive hypoxia likely contributes to the progressive fibrosis and perturbations in tubular function resulting in the urinary hypertonicity that is observed. Obstructive processes can lead to type IV cystic dysplasia and renal insufficiency.

The effects are not limited to the genitourinary (GU) tract. Progressive oligo-/anhydramnios leads to compressive deformations as seen in Potter sequence, in-

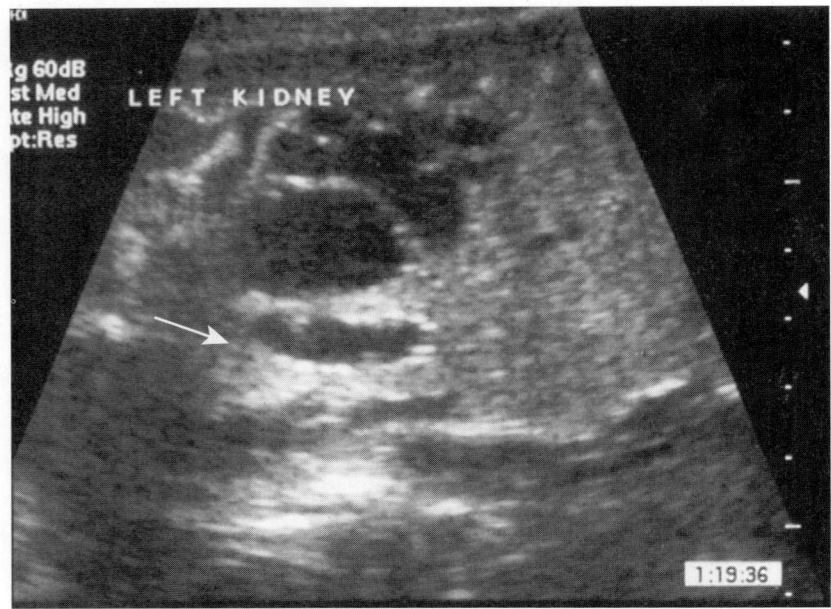

Figure 11–1. Oligohydramnios and dilated ureters (*arrow*) in a fetus at 23 weeks with poor electrolytes.

cluding extremity contractures and facial dysmorphology. Absence of normal amniotic fluid volume also interferes with pulmonary growth and development. Constant compressive pressure on the fetal thorax leads to restriction of expansion of the chest through normal physiologic "breathing movements." Babies born with LUTO generally die due to pulmonary complications and not renal failure.

The prenatal sonographic diagnosis of LUTO includes a dilated and thickened wall bladder, hydronephrosis, and oligohydramnios (Fig. 11–2). Urethral strictures or atresia, urethral agenesis, megalourethra, ureteral reflux, and cloacal anomalies may be present and have a very similar appearance on ultrasound. The typical "keyhole sign" of proximal urethral dilation is secondary to urethral obstruction present in PUV or atresia. However, the precise diagnosis can only be made after birth.[3]

The prenatal evaluation and management of fetuses with the sonographic findings of LUTO is complex. Ruling out other congenital anomalies such as cardiac and neural tube defects is necessary before intervention can be considered. Karyotyping is essential to confirm a normal male chromosomal status, as cases of LUTO

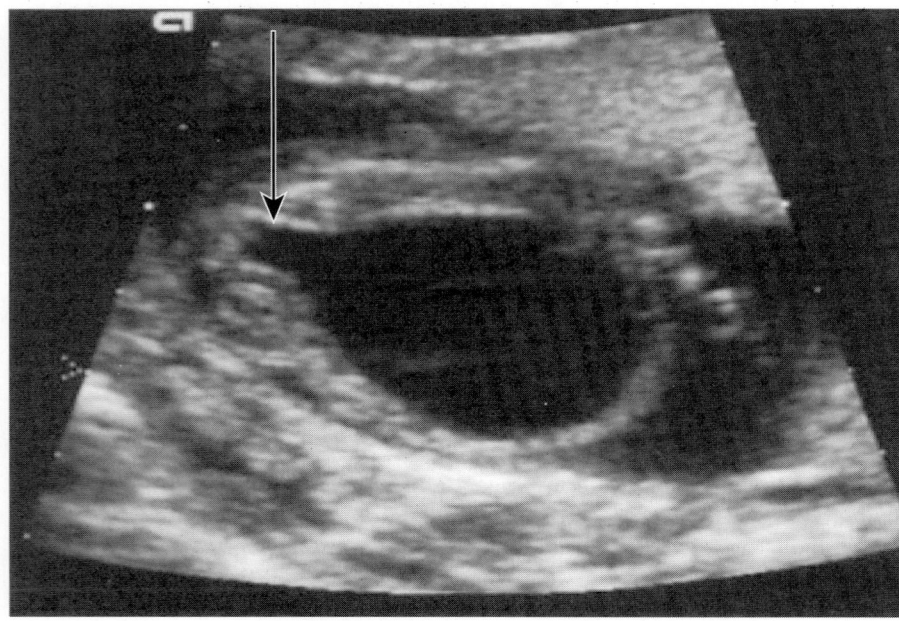

Figure 11–2. Ultrasound image of an obstructed fetal bladder at 15 weeks' gestation with classic keyhole sign (*arrow*).

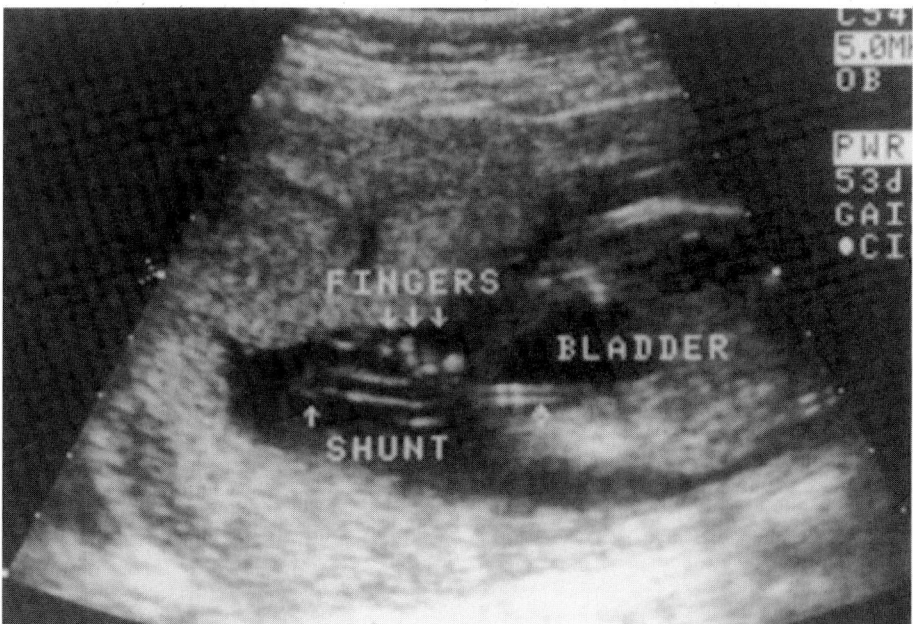

Figure 11–3. Vesicoamniotic shunt with the proximal portion lying within the fetal bladder (*right arrows*) while the distal portion lies within the amniotic fluid space (*left arrow*), allowing diversionary draining of urine into the appropriate space.

have an increased incidence of aneuploidy. Female fetuses almost always represent more complex syndromes of cloacal malformations, which do not benefit from in utero shunt therapy. Because of the presence of oligo-/anhydramnios, we commonly obtain karyotypes by transabdominal chorionic villus sampling. This approach yields reliable results within 5 days, during which the remainder of the prenatal evaluation is underway.

Perhaps the most important, complicated, and poorly understood aspect of the prenatal work-up is the evaluation of underlying renal status in the fetus. We use a multicomponent approach to the analysis of fetal urine that evaluates proximal tubular and possible glomerular status using sodium, chloride, osmolality, calcium, β_2-microglobulin, albumin, and total protein concentrations.[4] We have demonstrated that predictive reliability can be significantly improved by sequential samplings at 48- to 72-hour intervals.[5] Using such an approach, one can directly correlate the degree of impaired renal function and damage with the extent of urinary hypertonicity and proteinuria. As such, the ability to counsel patients about the renal status of their fetus and the long-term prognosis has been dramatically improved.

The function of the vesicoamniotic catheter is to bypass the urethral obstruction, diverting urine into the amniotic space to allow appropriate drainage of the upper urinary tract and prevention of pulmonary hypoplasia and physical deformations (Fig. 11–3). In fetuses with isolated LUTO, a normal male karyotype, and progressively improving urinary profile that meet threshold parameters (Table 11–1), we have been very

successful in salvaging fetuses using percutaneous vesicoamniotic shunt therapy.

Subsequent experience in humans has been widely variable and appears to be related to the extent of prenatal evaluation prior to shunt placement, as well as the etiology of obstruction. Freedman et al. found that prune belly infants without complete urethral obstructions have very good renal outcomes following vesicoamniotic shunt therapy.[6] They also observed significant improvement in survival and renal function in infants with PUVs treated by shunting; however, many of these children have mild to moderate renal insufficiency at birth, and several progressed to renal failure, dialysis, and transplantation. The worst outcomes are observed in infants with urethral atresia. In the Wayne State University series, there have been two survivors following early shunt intervention, both with stable mild to moderate renal insufficiency. These findings support animal studies that indicate that early-onset,

Table 11–1. UPPER THRESHOLD VALUES FOR SELECTING FETUSES THAT MIGHT BENEFIT FROM PRENATAL INTERVENTION

Sodium	<100 mg/dl
Chloride	<90 mg/dl
Osmolality	<190 mOsm/L
Calcium	<8 mg/dl
β_2-Microglobulin	<6 mg/L
Total protein	<20 mg/dl

complete obstructions resulted in more severe renal damage than later onset or partial obstructions, and emphasizes the necessity for early diagnosis, evaluation, and intervention in such cases.

Although vesicoamniotic shunting has certainly improved survival and renal function in cases of early obstructive uropathy, complications of this procedure remain unacceptably high. We have found that in 48 percent of our cases the shunts have become physically displaced into the amniotic or intraperitoneal space, or have become obstructed with loss of drainage function, necessitating replacement. Concerns also remain about the physiologic consequences of chronic shunt drainage on the normal development process of the lower urinary tract, given the presence of this foreign body and absence of normal filling and emptying cycles in the bladder.

Because of these concerns we have looked for alternate ways to approach LUTO. Using thin, fiberoptic endoscopes we have recently been able to perform in utero fetal cystoscopy and antegrade urethroscopy using simple needle systems and techniques similar to vesicocentesis.

Early therapeutic removal of a LUTO due to posterior urethral valves should improve physiologic development of the urinary tract. Reestablished patency of the penile urethra should improve the urethral hypoplasia distal to the site of obstruction, which is encountered postnatally at the time of retrograde resection. Normal filling and emptying of the fetal bladder should help in normal bladder development and may eliminate the need for reconstructive procedures postnatally. Also, this may reduce the need for temporary vesicostomy placement postnatally, which carries a high incidence of infectious febrile morbidity and accumulative renal damage. On balance, intervention for LUTO has saved fetuses who would otherwise have surely died. Many have normal to moderately impaired renal function. A carefully balanced approach in counseling is required for patients to determine what is right for them.

Other Shunt Approaches

Originally, shunting was attempted in cases of obstructive hydrocephalus. Attempts in the late 1970s and early 1980s at ventriculoamniotic shunting were nearly uniformly dismal. However, in retrospect, most operated patients were, in fact, poor candidates for intervention. Many had multisystem syndromic disorders, including aneuploidy, and hopeless congenital anomalies such as holoprosencephaly.

Ventriculoamniotic shunts were abandoned in the early 1980s. With better understanding of the poor natural history of the anomaly,[7] and more accurate diagnostic techniques, there may now be limited applications for prenatal neurologic shunting in cases of early-onset, isolated, progressive obstructive hydrocephaly.

The other use of percutaneously placed shunts has been for thoracic abnormalities. The macrocystic form of congenital cystic adenomatous malformation can present with a large, dominant macrocyst that causes mediastinal shift with its potential hemodynamic changes, as well as pulmonary compression and risk of lung hypoplasia (Fig. 11–4). Such dominant cysts can be approached using pleuroamniotic shunts to chronically drain these structures, reducing their volume, and diminishing their space-occupying effects.

Isolated pleural effusions can also accumulate, causing mediastinal hemodynamic changes and onset of generalized hydrops as well as pulmonary compression, which interferes with normal lung development, increasing the risk of hypoplasia (Fig. 11–5). Small, unilateral effusions generally do not warrant intervention, but must be followed closely, as they have the potential for rapid progression and initiation of generalized hydrops.[8]

Prenatal evaluation prior to intervention is critical for appropriate case selection, as isolated effusions may be the first sign of a cardiac malformation, aneuploidy, anemia, or an infectious process. Thoracoamniotic shunting is effective in carefully evaluated cases when the risk of pulmonary hypoplasia from large effusions early in gestation is present, or early signs of progressive hydrops (unilateral or bilateral effusions, skin or scalp edema, ascites, pericardial effusion) appear. Fetal anemia is not an indication for thoracoamniotic effusion shunting, as hydropic changes will usually resolve with timely fetal transfusion therapy. Also, if one waits

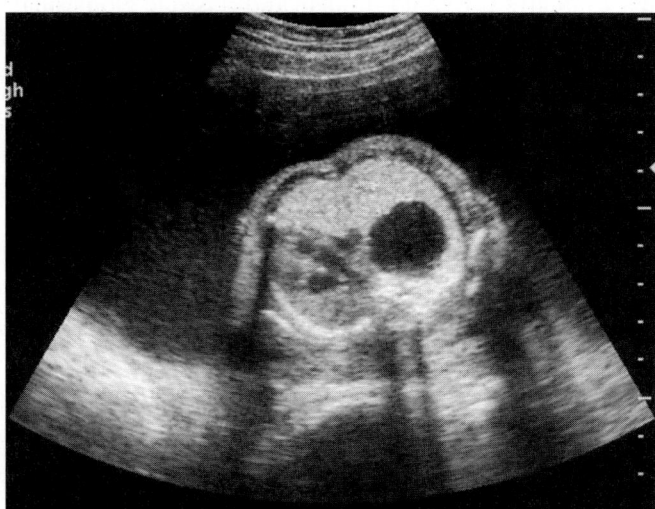

Figure 11–4. Microcystic congenital cystic adenomatous malformation (microcystic) with beginnings of hydrops (rim underskin).

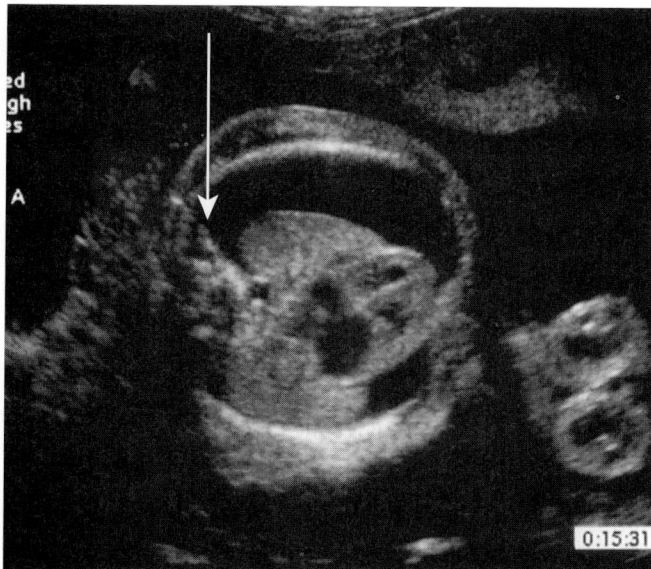

Figure 11–5. Sonographic image of a pleural effusion with needle (*arrow*) entering from top left.

to intervene until the fetus develops significant ascites, the prognosis becomes much poorer despite successful shunt intervention.[9] Nevertheless, several cases with suddenly progressive pleural effusions and onset of generalized hydrops (skin and/or scalp edema, pericardial effusion, and moderate ascites) have been treated with complete resolution of all hydropic complications and normal postnatal outcomes.

Positioning of the thoracoamniotic shunt is critical for success, and great care must be taken to avoid mediastinal structures. Shunts have the potential for displacement and obstruction, so continued ultrasound surveillance throughout the remainder of the pregnancy is necessary.[8] In most cases, postnatal management involves simple removal of the shunt in the nursery, as most of these cases represent transient chylothorax that require no additional therapy.

OPEN SURGICAL APPROACHES

Open fetal surgery has been performed for a limited number of indications for over 15 years, primarily at the University of California, San Francisco, with later expansion to a few other sites. Its application has been limited by the appropriate concern for maternal risk, rigorous selection criteria, and somewhat frustrating results. During this time, there has been continuing innovation and development of instruments and techniques,

motivated by the clinical necessity to improve the feasibility and safety of open fetal surgery for both the fetus and the mother.

The Fetal Operation—General Considerations

Opening the Gravid Uterus

Open fetal surgery is performed through a maternal hysterotomy, preferentially performed in the lower uterine segment. The uterine incision must provide optimal exposure of a specific fetal part or region, avoid the placenta, and provide hemostasis with absolute control of the fetal membranes. The consequences of a poorly placed or technically inadequate hysterotomy include technical failure of the fetal procedure, intra- or postoperative fetal demise, postoperative amniotic fluid leak, chorioamnionitis, and associated preterm labor.

For all fetal surgical procedures, exposure of the uterus is facilitated by a large, true transverse, lower abdominal incision with division of the rectus muscle. Exposure is enhanced by placement of a large, circular, fixed retraction system and exteriorization of the uterus. Pre- and intraoperative sonographic assessment is essential for planning the hysterotomy to identify the position and size of the placenta, as well as other potentially disastrous anatomic abnormalities such as a velamentous insertion of the umbilical cord. Complete uterine relaxation facilitates fetal version when necessary and is essential for hysterotomy and the entire period of the fetal operation. Various regimens have proven effective, including a combination of preoperative indomethacin, with intraoperative isoflurane and nitroglycerin, supplemented with intravenous terbutaline or magnesium sulfate as required.

After adequate uterine relaxation is confirmed by palpation, the planned hysterotomy is initiated by placement of full-thickness, monofilament, absorbable traction sutures on large needles, under ultrasound guidance at the anticipated midpoint of the planned hysterotomy. The traction sutures are then used to elevate the uterine wall, which is grasped and compressed to assist in hemostasis. A large metal trocar is inserted under ultrasound guidance through this area into the amniotic space. The myometrium and membranes are then incised over the trocar for a distance of 2 to 4 cm. The full thickness of the uterus and membranes is grasped on each side with broad Allis clamps. This results in a circumferentially controlled, full-thickness puncture site in the uterine wall. A commercially available uterine stapler is then passed through the opening and fired once in each direction. The absorbable staples hemostatically compress and divide the layers of the uterus, including the membranes, with each application.[10,11]

Fetal Monitoring and Homeostasis

Reliable intraoperative monitoring of the fetus and uterus has been very difficult to achieve. The confined space and small amount of exposed fetal tissue in combination with the poor tissue integrity of the fetus early in gestation make sutured electrodes unsatisfactory. Originally, pulse oximetry was utilized, but the inherent problems and limitations of this technology are amplified in the fetus. Radiotelemetry systems have been developed in cooperation with the National Aeronautics and Space Administration, which allow fetal heart rate, temperature, intra-amniotic pressure, and other parameters such as blood pH and tissue oxygenation to be monitored.[12] A small radiotelemeter sutured to the fetal skin sends a continuous signal to an outside antenna. This can be left in place postoperatively for monitoring and is more sensitive for detection of uterine contractions than standard tocodynamometry. At this time, however, the use of intraoperative ultrasound remains the most reliable method of assessing fetal status, providing information on fetal heart rate, volume status, and contractility.

Fetal homeostasis is maintained by protection of uteroplacental blood flow through continued uterine relaxation and careful monitoring, and control of maternal volume status and blood pressure. Care is taken to avoid umbilical cord compression, which may occur at the margins of the hysterotomy or if inadequate amniotic fluid surrounds the fetus. Intra-amniotic volume is maintained by exteriorization of only the necessary part of the fetus, and by continuous high-volume perfusion of the amniotic space with warm lactated Ringer's solution. Without such high-volume flow, loss of uterine volume could initiate uterine contractions.

Congenital Diaphragmatic Hernia

The repair of congenital diaphragmatic hernia (CDH) in the fetus has undergone continuous evolution since it was first attempted in 1986.[13,14] Definitive repair of CDH by reduction of viscera from the chest, diaphragmatic patch placement, and abdominal silo construction to reduce intra-abdominal pressure had unacceptable mortality, particularly when the liver was herniated into the chest. The definitive repair was therefore abandoned as an option for CDH, and in utero tracheal occlusion was utilized. Tracheal occlusion induces lung growth through accumulation of pulmonary secretions, which reduces the herniated viscera from the chest and alleviates lung hypoplasia. The tracheal occlusion procedure is relatively simple, consisting of exposure of the fetal neck in hyperextension, dissection of the trachea circumferentially (Fig. 11–6) taking care to avoid the recurrent laryngeal nerves, and placement of occlusive hemoclips. The fetus is then gently placed back into the uterus, and the uterine incision close, paying careful attention to hemostasis.

Experience with tracheal occlusion likewise proved to have a significant learning curve. Multiple attempts were made to find an appropriate polymer to use as a tracheal plug inserted through the fetal mouth. Experience quickly showed that unless there was 100 percent occlusion, the pulmonary secretions would seep out, thereby defeating the purpose of the plug. Eventually, it was decided that procedures would best be done using an external tracheal clip to make sure the occlusion was complete, and for the past several years, all cases have been done using this method.

A principal divergence in methodology has come be-

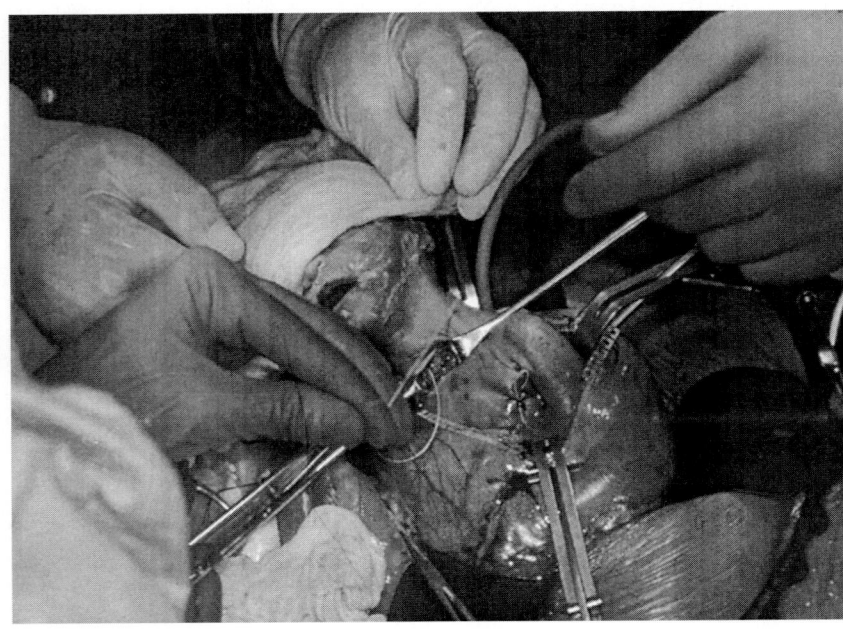

Figure 11–6. Surgical isolation of the fetal trachea prior to placement of hemoclips in a tracheal occlusion procedure for congenital diaphragmatic hernia.

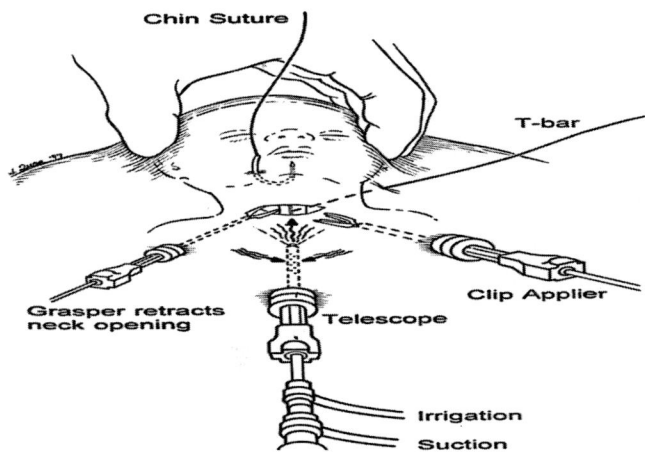

Figure 11–7. Schematic of FETENDO endoscopic approach to tracheal ligation clip for diaphragmatic hernia.

tween two camps. One favors the open surgical approach to this problem, while the other favors a more technically difficult endoscopic surgical approach to minimize the complications of open fetal surgery (Fig. 11–7). Published data on the two methods so far have been somewhat comparable, although it will take several more years of experience to have a definitive answer as to the best approach.

Congenital Cystic Adenomatoid Malformation

Congenital cystic adenomatoid malformation (CCAM) is a space-occupying congenital cystic lesion of the lung that may grow and induce hydrops by causing mediastinal shift and compromising venous return to the heart. Fetuses with CCAM who develop hydrops have a mortality approaching 100 percent. Fetal resection of CCAM reverses hydrops and has improved survival dramatically.[15] The fetal operation is performed by exposure of the arm and chest wall on the side of the lesion through the maternal hysterotomy. A large thoracotomy is performed through midthorax of the fetus and the lobe containing the CCAM is exteriorized. The attachments of the lobe to adjacent lung tissue are bluntly divided and the lobar hilum is divided by application of a stapler or a bulk ligature. The thoracotomy is quickly closed. Although a major operative procedure, operative time is short compared to repair of CDH, and blood loss and fetal stress relatively minimal.

Sacrococcygeal Teratoma

Fetal sacrococcygeal teratoma (SCT) arises from the presacral space and may grow to massive proportions. In some fetuses, high-output cardiac failure results from tumor vascular steal. Fetal SCT and high-output failure

with associated placentomegaly or hydrops uniformly result in fetal demise. Ligation of vessels to the SCT may reduce the vascular steal and high-output failure. The fetal operation is performed by exteriorization of the fetal buttocks with the attached tumor.[16] Every attempt is made to keep the head, torso, and lower extremities of the fetus in the uterus. Since the tumor can sometimes be larger than the fetus, significant loss of uterine volume occurs, and the uterus may contract. After exteriorization of the fetus, the anus is identified, and the fetal skin incised posterior to the anorectal sphincter complex to avoid injury to the continence mechanism. A tourniquet is then applied to the base of the tumor and gradually compressed. The vascular pedicle is ligated with suture ligatures or stapled depending on the width of the pedicle. The entire fetal procedure can be performed in less than 15 minutes with minimal blood loss. Because of the increase in afterload following ligation of the low-resistance tumor circuit, fetal hemodynamic status must be monitored by ultrasound closely during and in the immediate period following the ligation.

The EXIT Procedure

The EXIT procedure is a modified fetal delivery and may be used for the delivery of fetuses after surgical procedures such as tracheal ligation, or for fetuses with difficult airway problems such as massive cervical teratomas or cystic hygromas. The most important component of the EXIT procedure is maintenance of uteroplacental perfusion until the fetal airway is secured and ventilation is established. In direct contrast to cesarean section, where uterine contraction for hemostasis is encouraged, uterine relaxation is maintained by active tocolysis. With this approach, clips can be removed, bronchoscopy performed, and stable airway access established in otherwise difficult circumstances. Once the fetus is ready for transport to the nursery or operating suite, the cord is clamped and cut and the cesarean delivery completed.

Meningomyelocele

It has long been appreciated that babies with meningomyeloceles have impaired motor function and loss of bowel and bladder control. A significant percentage develop obstructive hydrocephalus, which requires ventriculoperitoneal shunting which, in and of itself, is fraught with complications. Experience from the 1970s and 1980s has shown that babies with meningomyeloceles delivered atraumatically by cesarean section maintain a better level of motor function for the given level of anatomic defect than those babies delivered through the vaginal canal.[17] Such data suggest that compression of the cord in the delivery process can have permanent

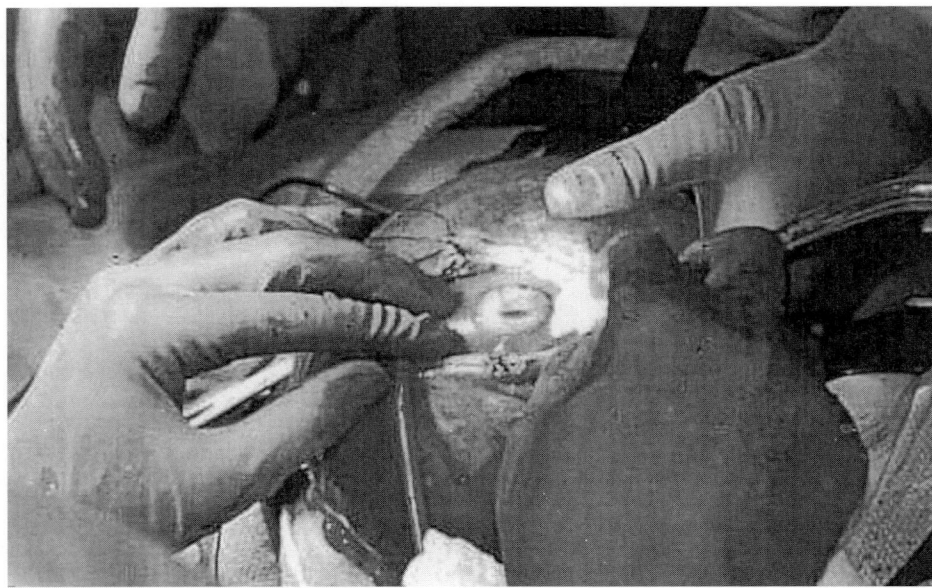

Figure 11–8. Open repair of fetal meningomyelocele. Uterus is opened over open meningomyelocele. (Courtesy of Dr. N. Scott Adzick.)

long-term sequelae on motor function. It therefore follows that trauma to the spinal cord in utero, either from the uterine wall, or perhaps even the amniotic fluid could be detrimental to the function of the spinal cord. It was generally believed that an abnormally developed spinal cord prevented the normal proper development of the bony spinal column, leading to a meningomyelocele. It is now understood that the primary defect is likely to be the bony spinal column, which exposes a perfectly normal spinal cord, that is then damaged by the trauma of amniotic fluid and the uterine environment. Thus, the rationale was formed for attempts to patch over, or at least to protect the spinal cord in utero to minimize these sequelae.[18]

Two groups at Vanderbilt and the Children's Hospital of Philadelphia have done considerable work in this area. The two groups have attempted to repair meningomyeloceles in utero (Figs. 11–8 and 11–9), both as an open surgical procedure and endoscopically.[19,21] The principal benefit of the surgery is secondary (i.e., significant reduction in the number of babies requiring ventriculoperitoneal shunting for obstructive hydrocephalus has been observed). It is currently too early in the experience to understand whether or not there will be significant improvements in long-term lower motor function. A randomized controlled trial would be the optimal way to answer important questions about the efficacy of this therapy.

Closing the Uterus

The obvious difference between fetal surgery and a cesarean delivery is that the fetus must be returned to the uterus, and remain in utero for several weeks. The primary criteria of an adequate closure are strength, healing, and avoidance of amniotic fluid loss. The described approach has been applied in many cases and has resulted in strong closures that heal well with minimal risk of anmiotic fluid leak. The closure is initiated by placement of large, interrupted, full-thickness monofilament retention sutures the length of the wound. This allows elevation of the wound edges during closure to minimize hemorrhage. The staple lines are then cut

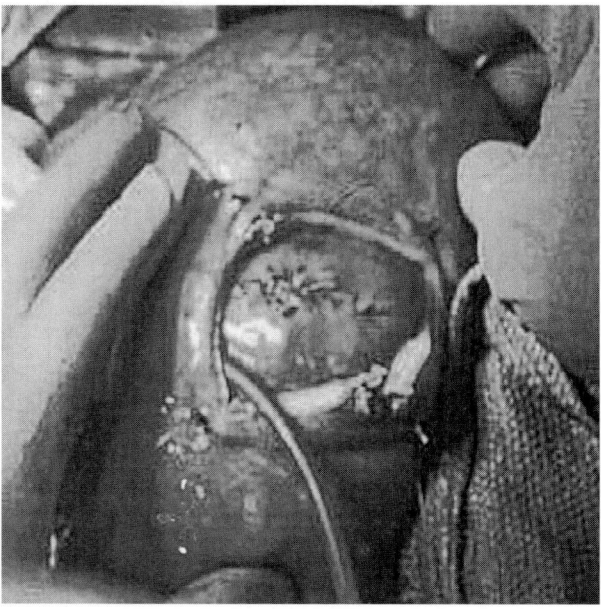

Figure 11–9. Same patient as Figure 11–8 after meningomyelocele repair. (Courtesy of Dr. N. Scott Adzick.)

away to freshen the edges and allow apposition of muscle tissue. A fine running monofilament is used to approximate the membranes. A small catheter is left in the amniotic space to reconstitute amniotic fluid and instill antibiotics prior to the completion of the closure. A second running layer of larger monofilament absorbable suture is placed through the myometrium to achieve broad musclular approximation. Finally, the retention sutures are tied to relieve tension on the wound and provide strength. Fibrin glue has been used as an additional sealant but has not been proven to be necessary. Prior to tying the last stitch, the amniotic fluid volume is reconstituted with warm lactated Ringer's solution under ultrasound guidance. Antibiotics are then instilled, and the catheter is removed.

MEDICAL THERAPY

Congenital Adrenal Hyperplasia

Congenital adrenal hyperplasia (CAH) was the first example of an inborn error of metabolism treated in utero with the primary goal of preventing malformations. Prenatal diagnosis became possible in the early 1980s by using the accumulation of 17-hydroxyprogesterone in the amniotic fluid as a marker. Later, the diagnosis became possible by linkage analysis, as the CAH gene was known to lie within the human leukocyte antigen (HLA) region of chromosome 6. More recently, the gene has been located, and the diagnosis has been made directly using molecular probes.

The 21-hydroxylase enzyme defect most commonly present in CAH impairs the metabolism of cholesterol to cortisol, generating excessive 17-hydroxyprogesterone. Alternate metabolism of this precursor shifts to androstenedione and other androgens (Fig. 11–10). Consequently, genetic females are exposed to high levels of androgens and can become masculinized. The resulting abnormal differentiation can vary from mild clitoral hypertrophy to formation of a phallus with labial fusion, giving rise to an apparent scrotum and misclassification of the newborn's sex.

The clinical spectrum of disease associated with CAH ranges from a severe salt-wasting variety to milder forms with simple precocious virilization in males or genital ambiguity in females. Since virilization of the female fetus was thought to occur during weeks 10 to 16 of gestation, prenatal in utero therapy aimed at preventing these changes must be started prior to determination of gender or disease status.[21,24] Prenatal treatment for this problem has been aimed at pharmacologically suppressing the fetal adrenal by giving the mother dexamethasone, which readily crosses the placenta.

In the first attempt to prevent this birth defect, Evans and colleagues[24] administered dexamethasone, a fluorinated steroid, to an at-risk mother, beginning in the 10th week of gestation. Maternal estriol and cortisol values indicated rapid and sustained fetal and maternal adrenal gland suppression. Forrest and David,[22,24] using the same protocol of 0.25 mg of dexamethasone four times a day, but beginning at 9 weeks, reported the successful prevention of masculinization of the external genitalia in several pregnancies at risk for the severe form of 21-hydroxylase deficiency.

Utilization of chorionic villus sampling and molecular markers for the diagnosis of CAH can now assign disease status and gender sooner than amniocentesis, allowing maternal steroid therapy to be discontinued in males or unaffected females, all of whom have to be started on therapy before the diagnosis can be performed. Because masculinization has now been reported in a few cases following the start of therapy at 9 weeks, it is important to begin steroid suppression at 7 weeks, and continue treatment until delivery, or confirmation of an unaffected fetus.

The fundamental principles addressed in attempts to prevent masculinization of the female fetus with CAH are logically extended to other fetal therapies. The concepts of a thorough informed consent for innovative treatments as well as detailed documentation of obstetric management and outcomes have generally been followed by investigators in this field.

Methylmalonic Acidemia

Methylmalonic acidemia is related to a functional vitamin B_{12} deficiency. Coenzymatically active vitamin B_{12} is required for the conversion of methylmalonyl-coenzyme A to succinylcoenzyme A. Genetically determined etiologies for methylmalonic acidemia include defects in methylmalonyl-coenzyme A mutase or in the metabolism of vitamin B_{12} to the conenzymatically active form, adenosylcobalamin by the converting enzyme. Some patients respond to high-dose vitamin B_{12} therapy, which can enhance the amount of the active holoenzyme (mutase apoenzyme plus adenosylcobalamin). There are at least five complementation groups in this enzymatic classification.

Ampola and colleagues[25] were the first to attempt prenatal diagnosis and treatment of a vitamin B_{12}–responsive variant of methylmalonic acidemia. Cyanocobalamin (10 mg/day) was administered orally to the mother in divided doses. The maternal serum B_{12} level rose sixfold above normal, and the maternal urinary excretion of methylmalonic acid progressively decreased to slightly above normal by delivery. Amniotic fluid methylmalonic acid levels were three to four times the normal mean, despite prenatal treatment. Postnatally,

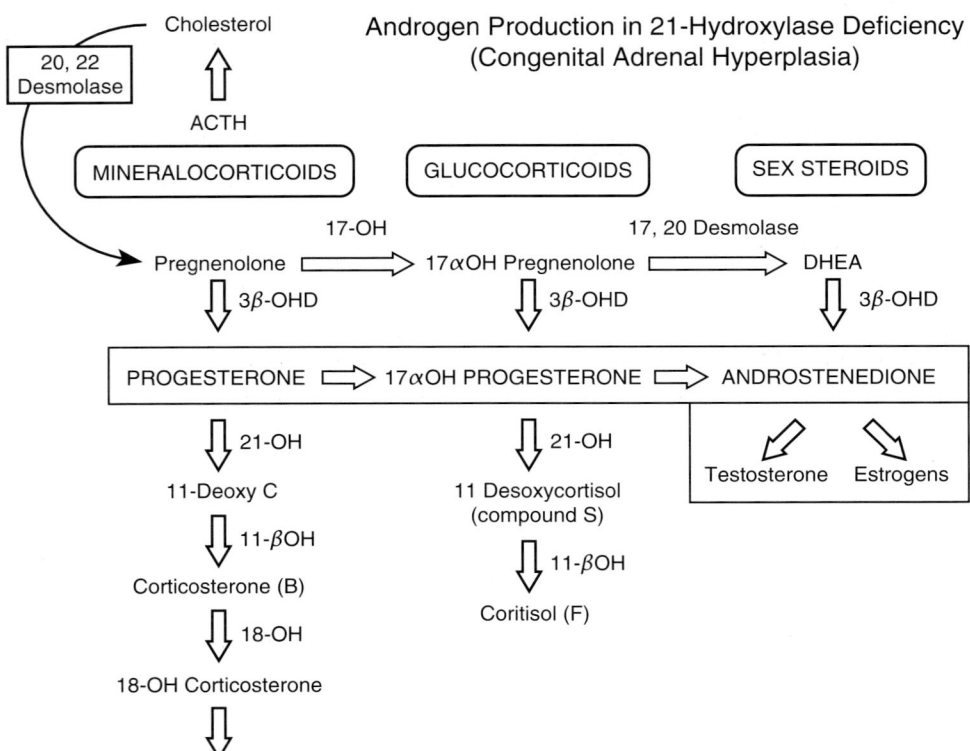

Androgen Production in 21-Hydroxylase Deficiency (Congenital Adrenal Hyperplasia)

Figure 11–10. Pathway of metabolism of cholesterol to cortisol. Blockage of 21-hydroxylase leads to excess 17-hydroxyprogesterone.

the diagnosis of methylmalonic acidemia was confirmed. The newborn suffered no acute neonatal complications, and had an extremely high serum level of vitamin B_{12}. In this case, the prenatal therapy certainly improved the fetal biochemical status and secondarily the maternal status as well. Whether this represented a direct clinical benefit to this fetus cannot be sufficiently ascertained.

Evans and colleagues followed a dose-response vitamin B_{12} regimen in the treatment of methylmalonic acidemia and showed a need for an increasingly higher dose as the pregnancy progressed.[26] In order to maintain plasma and urinary methylmalonic acid within the normal range, vitamin B_{12} doses needed to be increased sevenfold from the early second through the third trimester.

The report of Ampola and colleagues[25] was the first example of the treatment of a vitamin-responsive inborn error of metabolism in utero. Further studies are needed to establish the risk/benefit ratio of this therapeutic approach.

Multiple Carboxylase Deficiency

Biotin-responsive multiple carboxylase deficiency is an inborn error of metabolism in which the mitochondrial biotin-dependent enzymes, pyruvate carboxylase, pro-

pionyl-coenzyme A carboxylase, and β-methylcrotonyl coenzyme A carboxylase have decreased activity. Affected patients present as newborns or in early childhood with dermatitis, severe metabolic acidosis, and a characteristic pattern of organic acid excretion in their urine.[27] Metabolism in patients and in cells cultured in vitro can be restored toward normal levels by biotin supplementation. Such therapy has been utilized for fetuses affected with this severe disorder of metabolism. Roth and colleagues[28] empirically treated a fetus prenatally in a family in which two siblings had died of multiple carboxylase deficiency. No untoward maternal effects were noted, and the maternal urinary biotin excretion increased 100-fold. Dizygotic twins were subsequently delivered at term. Cord blood and urinary organic acid profiles were normal in both newborns. Cord blood biotin concentrations, however, were four- and sevenfold greater than normal. Metabolically, the immediate neonatal courses were unremarkable for both infants. Cultured fibroblasts from twin B had virtually complete deficiency of all three carboxylase activities, whereas those obtained from twin A were normal.

Biotin administration effectively prevents neonatal complications in certain patients with biotin-responsive multiple carboxylase deficiency. No fetal or maternal toxicity has been observed. Further experience with vitamin-responsive disorders will be useful in the determination of the optimal mode and dose interval for fetal therapy.

Smith-Lemli-Opitz Syndrome

Smith-Lemli-Opitz syndrome (SLOS) was first reported in 1964.[29] In 1993, an inborn error of cholesterol biosynthesis in a patient with SLOS was confirmed to be a deficiency of the hepatic enzyme 7-dehydrocholesterol (7-DHC) reductase.[30-32]

Characteristic features of SLOS include facial phenotype; growth and mental retardation; and anomalies of the heart, kidneys, central nervous system, and limbs. Cleft palate, postaxial polydactyly, 2–3 syndactyly of the toes, and cataracts are often seen in affected patients. The 2–3 syndactyly of the toes is very specific for this disorder and is seen in over 90 percent of affected patients. The facial phenotype is absolutely characteristic of the syndrome. Affected patients typically present with a narrow forehead, ptosis, anteverted nares, low-set ears, and micrognathia.

Patients with SLOS are deficient in cholesterol, and therefore also most likely have low levels of the steroid hormones necessary for masculinization of the male genitalia. The ambiguous genitalia seen in SLOS are the result of undermasculinization of male genitalia.

The biochemical defect in SLOS is due to deficiency of the enzyme 7-dehydrocholesterol reductase, which is responsible for the conversion of 7-DHC to cholesterol in the last step of cholesterol biosynthesis. Deficiency of this enzyme results in the characteristic biochemical pattern of low cholesterol and elevated 7-DHC and 8-dehydrocholesterol (8-DHC), its isomer. The values seen in affected patients are extremely variable. The diagnosis is made primarily by elevated levels of 7-DHC and not by a deficiency of cholesterol. The level of 7-DHC in affected patients is 100 to 1,000 times normal. Infants with more severe clinical manifestations have cholesterol levels that are quite low (usually < 10 to 15 mg/dl), while those with mild manifestations may present with levels of 40 to 70 mg/dl.

Prenatal diagnosis is possible by either amniocentesis at or after 13 weeks' gestation or chorionic villus sampling (CVS) at 10 to 12 weeks.

Fetal treatment has focused on providing cholesterol to the mother or to the fetus.[32-35] The former is not possible because cholesterol does not easily cross the placenta in the third trimester. Cholesterol is available only in a crystalline form that cannot be given intravenously or intramuscularly. It cannot be placed in the amniotic fluid because it would precipitate. However, cholesterol can be administered to the fetus in the form of low-density lipoprotein (LDL) cholesterol in fresh frozen plasma. Investigators at Tufts have attempted treatment in two patients late in pregnancy.[34] The re-

sults are inconclusive. In general, if fetal therapy is to be successful, the earlier the diagnosis, the better.

Neural Tube Defects

Animal studies suggest that neural tube defects (NTDs) can arise from a variety of vitamin or mineral deficiencies. There are historical data in humans suggesting increased NTD frequencies in subjects with poor dietary histories or with intestinal bypasses. Biochemical evidence of suboptimal nutrition is present in some women bearing infants with NTDs. In 1980, Smithells et al. suggested that vitamin supplementation containing 0.36 mg folate can reduce the frequency of NTD recurrence by sevenfold in women with one or more prior affected children.[36,37] For almost a decade, there was a great deal of controversy regarding the benefit of folate supplementation for the prevention of NTDs.[38-40] Finally, in 1991, a randomized double-blinded trial designed by the MRC Vitamin Study Research Group demonstrated that preconceptional folate reduced the risk of recurrence in high-risk patients.[41] Subsequently, it was shown that preparations containing folate and other vitamins also reduced the occurrence of first-time NTDs.[42] In response to these findings, the Centers for Disease Control (CDC) issued guidelines calling for consumption of 4.0 mg/day folic acid by women with a prior child affected with an NTD, for at least 1 month prior to conception through the first 3 months of pregnancy. In addition, 0.4 mg/day folic acid is recommended preconceptionally for *all women* of reproductive age. (Over half of all pregnancies in the United States are not planned.) The data on NTD recurrence prevention are now very well established, and routine for women with prior affected offspring. The majority of experts believe that the primary incidence of NTDs could be cut by perhaps half by folic acid supplementation. As of January 1998, the U.S. Food and Drug Administration has mandated that breads and grains be supplemented with folic acid. It is one of the largest public health experiments ever performed. It is hoped that a 30 to 50 percent reduction of NTDs will be seen.

Future Developments

Vitamin therapy has been utilized in the two vitamin-responsive genetic errors of metabolism discussed above. A significant number of other vitamin-responsive defects are known. The in utero treatment approach would seem to be a possibility for these conditions, especially those with neonatal manifestations. We speculate that in addition to these disorders there may be genetic defects for which prenatal vitamin E administration may be justifiable. Postnatally, vitamin E administration prevents abnormalities of leukocyte function and improves shortened red blood cell (RBC) survival in glutathione synthetase deficiency. Because lowered intracellular glutathione levels in this mutant state seem to predispose to oxidant-mediated cellular damage, it might be desirable to consider prenatal antioxidant therapy with vitamin E. Most patients with glutathione synthetase deficiency have neurologic impairment, which can be progressive.

In betalipoproteinemia, which is associated with very low serum vitamin E levels, progressive and fatal neurologic impairment develops. It is now known that high-dose vitamin E supplementation can slow or prevent these neurologic changes. Prenatal treatment might therefore be justifiable in these disorders on an experimental basis. However, at present it is not known when this damage begins and therefore when in utero treatment should optimally be initiated.

Genetic Therapies

Genetic approaches to fetal therapy using preimplantation injection of deoxyribonucleic acid (DNA) into the male pronucleus of an in vitro fertilized embryo have been successful in ewes but are not likely to be used in the near future in humans. This subject has been reviewed extensively elsewhere and will not be reported here.[11,43,44]

PRENATAL HEMATOPOIETIC STEM CELL TRANSPLANTATION

Hematopoietic stem cell therapy has recently been shown to be successful in the prenatal treatment of X-linked severe combined immunodeficiency disorder (SCID).[45] Hematopoietic stem cell (HSC) therapy for the treatment of congenital disease has tremendous theoretical appeal. The replacement of defective cells with normal cells during specific periods of organ development and cellular ontogeny may have significant advantages over postnatal transplantation.

The engraftment and clonal proliferation of a relatively small number of normal HSCs can sustain normal hematopoiesis for a lifetime. This observation provides the compelling rationale for bone marrow transplantation (BMT) and is now supported by thousands of long-term survivors of BMT who otherwise would have succumbed to lethal hematologic disease. Realization of the full potential of BMT, however, continues to be limited by a critical shortage of immunologically compatible donor cells, the inability to control the recipient or donor immune response, and the requirement for recipient myeloablation to achieve engraftment. The price of HLA mismatch remains high: the greater the mismatch, the higher the incidence of graft failure, graft-versus-host disease (GVHD), and delayed immunologic reconstitution. Current methods of myeloablation have high morbidity and mortality. In combination, these problems remain prohibitive for most patients who might theoretically benefit from BMT. A potentially attractive alternative that could address many of the limitations of BMT is in utero transplantation of HSC. This approach may be applicable to any congenital hematopoietic disease that can be diagnosed prenatally and can be cured or improved by engraftment of normal HSCs.

Rationale for In Utero Transplantation

The rationale for in utero transplantation is to take advantage of the window of opportunity created by normal ontogeny of hematopoietic cell lines. There is a period, prior to population of the bone marrow and prior to thymic processing of self-antigen, when the fetus theoretically should be receptive to engraftment of foreign HSC without rejection and without the need for myeloablation. In the human fetus, the ideal window would appear to be prior to 14 weeks' gestation, before release of differentiated T lymphocytes into the circulation and while the bone marrow is just beginning to develop sites for hematopoiesis. The window certainly may extend beyond that in immunodeficiency states, particularly when T-cell development is abnormal. During this time, presentation of foreign antigen by thymic dendritic cells theoretically should result in clonal deletion of reactive T cells during the negative selection phase of thymic processing. Recent advances in prenatal diagnosis have made possible the diagnosis of a large number of congenital diseases during the first trimester. Technical advances in fetal intervention make transplantation feasible by 12 to 14 weeks' gestation. The ontologic window of opportunity falls well within these diagnostic and technical constraints, making application of this approach a realistic possibility.

Because of the unique fetal environment, prenatal HSC transplantation could theoretically avoid many of the current limitations of postnatal BMT. There would be no requirement for HLA matching, resulting in expansion of the donor pool. Transplanted cells would not be rejected, and space would be available in the bone marrow, eliminating the need for toxic immunosuppressive and myeloablative drugs. The mother's uterus may ultimately prove to be the ultimate sterile isolation chamber, eliminating the high risk and costly 2 to 4 months of isolation required after postnatal BMT and prior to immunologic reconstitution. Finally, prenatal transplantation would preempt the clinical manifestations of the disease, avoiding the recurrent infections, multiple transfusions, growth delay, and other complications that cause immeasurable suffering for the patient and often compromise postnatal treatment.

Source of Donor Cells

The source of donor cells may prove to be critical for the success of engraftment. The most obvious advantage of the use of fetal HSCs is the minimal number of mature T cells in fetal liver-derived populations prior to 14 weeks' gestation. This alleviates any concern about GVHD and avoids the necessity of T-cell depletion processes, which can negatively impact potential engraftment.

Although there may be important homing, proliferative, and developmental advantages to the use of fetal cells, there are practical and ethical advantages to the use of cord blood or postnatal HSC sources. Legitimate ethical concerns regarding the use of fetal tissue for transplantation must be addressed by the medical and lay community. Fetal tissue obtained by the usual methods at the time of elective abortion has a high degree of microbial contamination.[46] Transplantation of transmissible viral, fungal, or bacterial disease could have disastrous consequences for the recipient fetus or mother. Although the fetal liver is a rich source of HSC, small size limits total cell yield, and current technology does not yet allow undifferentiated expansion of donor cells. In contrast, use of adult-derived cells would allow a renewable, relatively infection-free, ethically acceptable source of donor cells. Tolerance induction by in utero transplantation of highly purified adult bone marrow HSC from a living related donor, followed by a single or multiple postnatal "booster" injections offers an intriguing approach in situations where postnatal BMT is necessary but an HLA-matched donor is not available.

Diseases Amenable to Prenatal Treatment

Generally speaking, any disease that can be diagnosed early in gestation, that is improved by BMT, and for which postnatal treatment is not entirely satisfactory is a target disease. Some diseases, however, are far more likely to benefit from prenatal transplantation than others. The list can be divided into three general categories: hemoglobinopathies, immunodeficiency disorders, and inborn errors of metabolism. Each of the diseases has unique considerations for treatment, and in fact each disease may respond differently. Issues such as availability of engraftment sites within the bone marrow at the time of transplantation, and capacity of a needed enzyme to cross the blood-brain barrier at a particular gestational age must be considered. Of particular relevance to the prenatal approach, in which experimental levels of engraftment have been relatively low, is the observation that in many of the target diseases, engrafted normal cells would be predicted to have a significant survival advantage over diseased cells. This would have the clinical effect of amplification of the level of engraftment in the peripheral circulation. In addition, even with minimal levels of engraftment, specific tolerance for donor antigen should be induced, allowing additional cells from the same donor to be given to the tolerant recipient after birth.

Hemoglobinopathies

The sickle cell anemia and thalassemia syndromes make up the largest patient groups potentially treatable by prenatal stem cell transplantation. Both groups can be diagnosed within the first trimester. Both have been cured by postnatal BMT, but BMT is not recommended routinely because of its prohibitive morbidity and mortality and the relative success of modern postnatal medical management. In both diseases, the success of BMT is indirectly related to the morbidity of the disease, that is, the younger the patient, the fewer transfusions received, and the less organ compromise from iron overload, the better the results. With both diseases the primary questions relevant to prenatal transplantation are: (1) what levels of normal peripheral cell expression are necessary to alleviate clinical disease, and (2) can adequate levels of donor cell engraftment be achieved by in utero HSC transplantation? At present, only indirect evidence exists to answer these questions.

In sickle cell disease (SCD), the pathophysiology is directly related to the concentration of hemoglobin S (HbS) within red blood cells, which results in marked rheologic abnormality, including hyperviscosity, cellular adherence, and sickling, with a result of vaso-occlusion and tissue ischemia. In examining the in vitro relationships between hematocrit (Hct) and viscosity using mixtures of sickle and normal RBCs, Schmalzer et al. observed that the primary determinant of viscosity is the sickle Hct (fraction of RBCs that contain HbS).[47] Adverse effects of Hct on viscosity were seen at a sickle Hct level in the low 20s. Oxygen delivery, as gauged by the maximal point on the Hct versus viscosity curve, was markedly improved by exchanging normal for sickle RBCs (even when the total Hct was held constant). The clinical correlate of this in vitro information presently is chronic exchange transfusion therapy with its inherent discomfort and potential complications. However, prenatal transplantation of normal HSCs may offer a solution to this problem. Normal cells may have a developmental advantage over HbS cells such that overall production of Hb-normal RBCs may exceed that of HbS cells. This could potentially decrease the overall HbS fraction, reducing the risk of hyperviscosity and vaso-occlusive/ischemic complications.

Clinical manifestations of thalassemia are secondary

to hypoxia related to severe anemia and ineffective erythropoiesis. It is now standard therapy to transfuse patients with thalassemia major chronically from an early age. This process suppresses endogenous erythropoiesis and maintains oxygen delivery. When instituted at an early age, it effectively prevents the bone marrow expansion and secondary bony changes, as well as the hemodynamic and cardiac manifestations of the disease. The necessary normal Hb level required is controversial, but good results have been achieved with maintenance of a Hb of 9 g/dl.

Although these levels of normal Hb are higher than have been achieved experimentally (30 percent donor Hb is maximal), there would be a significant survival advantage of normal cells in both diseases. In SCD, erythrocytes have a circulating half-life of 10 to 20 days (normal half-life, 120 days) prior to destruction. In thalassemia, most cells (80 percent) never leave the bone marrow and also have shortened survival in the periphery. Therefore, engraftment of even a relatively small number of normal HSCs could result in significantly increased levels of peripheral donor cell expression.

Immunodeficiency Diseases

These represent an extremely heterogeneous group of diseases, which differ in their likelihood of cure by their capacity to develop hematopoietic chimerism. Once again, the most likely to benefit from even low levels of donor cell engraftment are those diseases in which a survival advantage exists for normal cells. The best example of this situation is SCID. Several different molecular causes of SCID have been identified, with approximately two thirds of cases being of X-linked recessive inheritance (X-SCID). The genetic basis of X-SCID has been defined recently[48] as a mutation of the gene encoding the common -γ chain (-γc), which is a common component of several members of the cytokine receptor superfamily, including those for interleukin-2 (IL-2), IL-4, IL-7, IL-9, IL-15, and possibly IL-13. Children affected with X-SCID have simultaneous disruption of multiple cytokine systems, resulting in a block in thymic T-cell development and diminished T-cell response. Although present in normal or even increased numbers, B cells are dysfunctional, secondary to either the lack of helper T-cell function or an intrinsic defect in B-cell maturation. Another form of SCID is secondary to adenosine deaminase (ADA) deficiency. Clinical experience with HLA-matched sibling bone marrow, fetal liver, or thymus transplantation generally has been successful without myeloablative therapy, suggesting that the lymphoid progeny of relatively few engrafted normal HSC have a selective growth advantage in vivo over genetically defective cells.[49] The competitive advantage of normal cell populations in X-SCID is best supported by the discovery of skewed X-inactivation in female carriers.[50] Only T cells containing the normal X chromosome were found to be present in the circulation of recipients. Evidence that ADA production confers a survival advantage derives from the early experience with gene therapy for ADA deficiency SCID. ADA-gene-corrected autologous T cells have persisted for prolonged periods despite discontinuation of the T-cell infusions. Transfer of ADA-gene-corrected cells versus uncorrected cells from the same SCID patient into an immunodeficient BNX mouse results in survival of the corrected cells and death of the uncorrected cells, confirming a survival advantage for ADA-producing cells even when there is normal ADA production in the surrounding environment. Unfortunately, other diseases such as chronic granulomatous disease would not be expected to provide a competitive advantage for donor cells. Nevertheless, in all these conditions even a partial engraftment and expression of normal cell phenotype might at least partially ameliorate the clinical manifestations of the disease and should result in donor-specific tolerance for later transplantation. If higher levels of engraftment are needed, further HSC transplants from the same donor could be performed after birth without fear of rejection.

Flake et al. successfully treated a fetus with X-linked SCID in a family where a previously afflicted child died at 7 months of age. Diagnosis by CVS in the second pregnancy showed another affected male. For this couple, abortion was not an option. After lengthy informed consent, paternal bone marrow was harvested, T cells depleted, and enriched stem cell populations injected intraperitoneally into the fetus beginning at about 16 weeks' gestation. Subsequent injections were performed at 17 and 18 weeks. The baby presently shows a split chimerism with all of his T cells being his father's, whereas the majority of B cells are his. He has achieved normal milestones and immune progress through 2 years of age.[45] Other cases have been recently tried using less T-cell–depleted populations resulting in higher T-cell concentrations. This approach has resulted in fetal demise.[51]

Inborn Errors of Metabolism

An even more heterogeneous group of diseases, inborn errors of metabolism, can be caused by a deficiency of a specific lysosomal hydrolase, which results in the accumulation of substrates such as mucopolysaccharide, glycogen, or sphingolipid. Depending on the specific enzyme abnormality and the compounds that accumulate, certain patterns of tissue damage and organ failure occur. These include central nervous system (CNS) deterioration, growth failure, dysostosis multiplex and joint abnormalities, hepatosplenomegaly, myocardial or cardiac disease, upper airway obstruction, pulmonary infiltration, corneal clouding, and hearing loss. The potential efficacy of prenatal HSC transplantation for the treatment of these diseases must be considered on an individual disease basis. The purpose of BMT in these diseases is to provide HSC-derived mononuclear cells that can repopulate various organs in the body, including the liver (Kupffer cells), skin (Langerhans' cells), lung (alveolar macrophages), spleen (macrophages), lymph nodes, tonsils, and the brain (microglia). Patients with disorders that have been corrected by postnatal BMT, such as Gaucher's disease or Maroteaux-Lamy syndrome (minimal CNS involvement), are certainly reasonable candidates for prenatal treatment. In many cases, postnatal BMT has corrected the peripheral manifestations of the disease and has arrested the neurologic deterioration. However, postnatal BMT has not reversed neurologic injury that is present in such disorders as metachromatic leukodystrophy and Hurler's disease. In these cases, the neurologic injury may begin well before birth. Postnatal maturation of the blood-brain barrier restricts access to the CNS of transplanted cells or the deficient enzyme. These considerations suggest that prenatal treatment may be beneficial and offer the possibility for a cure. The primary unanswered question is whether donor HSC-derived microglial elements would populate the CNS, providing the necessary metabolic correction inside the blood-brain barrier. To date, the only definitively successful transplants have been for SCID. All others have either failed to take or were afflicted with GVHD. More work needs to be done to determine the optimal dosing, timing, and specific protocols for these different conditions.

CONCLUSION

There are an increasing number of congenital and genetic abnormalities for which in utero treatment is possible. Advances in therapies have progressed at different paces for different disorders, but there is great hope and enthusiasm that progress will continue to expand the number of disorders for which therapy can be effective.

Key Points

➤ Fetal therapy is possible for some anomalies, but only after proper diagnosis.

➤ Fetal therapy can ameliorate the effect of some anomalies, for which waiting until birth can be too late.

➤ Surgical techniques have been greatly refined over the years with a gradual shift to the endoscopic approach.

➤ Indications for intervention in diaphragmatic hernia now focus on liver position, with only the worst cases (liver up) being candidates for fetal surgical intervention.

➤ Surgery for congenital cystadenomatoid malformation and sacrococcygeal teratomas has reduced mortality in these conditions.

➤ Surgery for meningomyelocele is showing promise, but will require many cases for proper evaluation.

➤ Prenatal medical therapy with dexamethasone can prevent external genital masculinization in 21-hydroxylase deficiency congenital adrenal hyperplasia.

➤ Folic acid supplementation of diet can reduce both the recurrence risk and the primary incidence of neural tube defects, but must begin preconceptionally.

➤ Stem cell transplantation can achieve engraftment and correction of immunodeficiencies, such as SCID.

➤ Stem cells have not yet been effective in nonimmunodeficiency disorders.

REFERENCES

1. Evans MI (ed): Reproductive Risks and Prenatal Diagnosis. Norwalk, CT, Appleton & Lange, 1992.
2. Johnson MP, Flake AW, Quintero RA, Evans MI: Shunt Procedures. In Evans MI, Johnson MP, Moghissi KS (eds): Invasive Outpatient Procedures in Reproductive Medicine. New York, Raven Press, 1997.
3. Evans MI, Sacks AL, Johnson MP, et al: Sequential invasive assessment of fetal renal function, and the in utero treatment of fetal obstructive uropathies. Obstet Gynecol 77:545, 1991.
4. Johnson MP, Bukowski TP, Reitlerman C, et al: In utero surgical treatment of fetal obstructive uropathy: a new comprehensive approach to identify appropriate candidates for vesicoamniotic shunt therapy. Am J Obstet Gynecol 170:1770, 1994.
5. Johnson MP, Corsi P, Bradfield WB, et al: Sequential fetal urine analysis provides greater precision in the evaluation of fetal obstructive uropathy. Am J Obstet Gynecol 173:59, 1995.
6. Freedman AL, Bukowski TP, Smith CA, et al: Fetal therapy for obstructive uropathy: specific outcomes diagnosis. J Urol 156:720, 1996.
7. Drugan A, Krause B, Canady A, et al: The natural history of prenatally diagnosed ventriculomegaly. JAMA 261:1785, 1989.
8. Ahmad FK, Sherman SJ, Hagglund KH, et al: Isolated unilateral pleural effusion: the role of sonographic surveillance and in utero therapy. Fetal Diagn Ther 11:383, 1996.

9. Nicolaides KH, Azar GB: Thoracoamniotic shunting. Fetal Diagn Ther 5:153, 1990.

10. Adzick N, Harrison M, Flake A, et al: Automatic uterine stapling devices in fetal surgery: experience in a primate model. Surg Forum 36:479, 1985.

11. Jennings RW, Adzick NS, Longaker MT, et al: New techniques in fetal surgery. J Pediatr Surg 27:1329, 1992.

12. Jennings RW, Adzick NS, Longaker MT, et al: Radiotelemetric fetal monitoring during and after open fetal operation. Surg Gynecol Obstet 176:59, 1993.

13. Harrison MR, Longaker MT, Adzick NS, et al: Successful repair in utero of a fetal diaphragmatic hernia after removal of herniated viscera from the left thorax. N Engl J Med 322:1582, 1990.

14. Harrison MR, Adzick NS, Flake AW, et al: Correction of congenital diaphragmatic hernia in utero: VI. Hard-learned lessons. J Pediatr Surg 28:1141, 1993.

15. Adzick NS, Harrison MR, Flake AW, et al: Fetal surgery for cystic adenomatoid malformation of the lung. J Pediatr Surg 28:806, 1993.

16. Flake AW: Fetal sacrococcygeal teratoma. Eur J Med 2:113, 1993.

17. Lemire RJ: Neural tube defects. JAMA 259:558, 1988.

18. Meuli M, Meuli-Simmen C, Hutchins GM, et al: In utero surgery rescues neurological function at birth in sheep with spina bifida. Nat Med 1:342, 1995.

19. Bruner JP, Tulipan N, Paschall RL, et al: Fetal surgery for myelomeningocele and the incidence of shunt-dependent hydrocephalus. JAMA 282:1819, 1999.

20. Sutton LN, Adzick NS, Bilaniuk LT, et al: Improvement in hindbrain herniation demonstrated by serial fetal magnetic resonance imaging following fetal surgery for myelomeningocele. JAMA 282:1826, 1999.

21. Evans MI, Chrousos GP, Mann DL, et al: Pharmacologic suppression of the fetal adrenal gland in utero: attempted prevention of abnormal, external genital masculinization in suspected congenital adrenal hyperplasia. JAMA 253:1015, 1985.

22. David M, Forrest M: Prenatal treatment of congenital adrenal hyperplasia resulting from 21-hydroxylase deficiency. J Pediatr 105:799, 1984.

23. Pang S, Pollack MS, Marshall RN, Immken LD: Prenatal treatment of congenital adrenal hyperplasia due to 21-hydroxylase deficiency. N Engl J Med 322:111, 1990.

24. Forrest MG, David M: Prevention of sexual ambiguity in children with 21-hydroxylase deficiency by treatment in utero. Pediatrics 47:351, 1992.

25. Ampola MG, Mahoney MJ, Nakamura E: Prenatal therapy of a patient with vitamin B responsive methylmalonic acidemia. N Engl J Med 293:313, 1975.

26. Evans MI, Duquette DA, Rinaldo P, et al: Modulation of B12 dosage and response in fetal treatment of methylmalonic aciduria (MMA); titration of treatment dose to serum and urine MMA. Fetal Diagn Ther 12:21, 1997.

27. Scriver C, Beaudet A, Valle D (eds): The Metabolic Basis of Inherited Disease. 7th ed. New York, McGraw-Hill, 1994.

28. Roth KS, Yang W, Allen L: Prenatal administration of biotin: biotin responsive multiple carboxylase deficiency. Pediatr Res 16:126, 1982.

29. Smith DW, Lemli L, Opitz JM: A newly recognized syndrome of multiple congenital anomalies. J Pediatr 64:210, 1964.

30. Irons M, Elias ER, Salen G, et al: Defective cholesterol biosynthesis in Smith-Lemli-Opitz syndrome. Lancet 341:1414, 1993.

31. Tint GS, Irons M, Elias E, et al: Defective cholesterol biosynthesis associated with the Smith-Lemli-Opitz syndrome. N Engl J Med 330:107, 1994.

32. Shefer S, Salen G, Batta AK, et al: Markedly inhibited 7-dehydrocholesterol-reductase activity in liver microsomes from Smith-Lemli-Opitz homozygotes. J Clin Invest 96:1779, 1995.

33. Irons M, Elias E, Tint GS, et al: Abnormal cholesterol metabolism in the Smith-Lemli-Opitz syndrome: report of clinical and biochemical findings in 4 patients and treatment in 1 patient. Am J Med Genet 50:347, 1994.

34. Irons M, Elias ER, Abuelo D, et al: Treatment of Smith-Lemli-Opitz syndrome: results of a multicenter trial. Am J Med Genet 68:311, 1997.

35. Elias ER, Irons MB, Hurley AD, et al: Clinical effects of cholesterol supplementation in six patients with the Smith-Lemli-Opitz syndrome (SLOS). Am J Med Genet 68:305, 1997.

36. Smithells RW, Sheppard S, Schorah CJ, et al: Possible prevention of neural tube defects by preconceptual vitamin supplementation. Lancet 1:399, 1980.

37. Smithells RW, Nevin NC, Seller MJ, et al: Further experience of vitamin supplementation for prevention of neural tube defect recurrences. Lancet 1:1027, 1983.

38. Mills JL, Rhoads GG, Simpson JL, et al: The absence of a relation between the periconceptional use of vitamins and neural-tube defects. N Engl J Med 321:430, 1989.

39. Mulinare J, Cordero JF, Erickson JD, Berry RJ: Periconceptional use of multivitamins and the occurrence of neural tube defects. JAMA 260:3141, 1988.

40. Schulman JD: Treatment of the embryo and the fetus in the first trimester: current status and future prospects. Am J Med Genet 35:197, 1990.

41. MRC Vitamin Study Research Group: Prevention of neural tube defects: results of the MRC vitamin study. Lancet 338:132, 1991.

42. Czeizel AE, Dudas I: Prevention of the first occurrence of neural-tube defects by preconceptional vitamin supplementation. N Engl J Med 327:1832, 1992.

43. Yaron Y, Kramer R, Johnson MP, Evans MI: Gene therapy: is the future here yet? Obstet Gynecol Clin North Am 24:179, 1997.

44. Evans MI, Johnson MP: Multifetal pregnancy reduction. In Reece EA, Hobbins J (eds): Medicine of the Fetus and Mother. 2nd ed. Philadelphia, Lippincott-Raven, 1999, p 1433.

45. Flake AW, Puck JM, Almieda-Porada G, et al: Successful in utero correction of X-linked recessive severe combined immuno-deficiency (X-SCID): fetal intraperitoneal transplantation of CD34 enriched paternal bone marrow cells (EPPBMC). N Engl J Med 335:1806, 1996.

46. Jennings RW, Adzick NS, Harrison MR: Fetal surgery. In Evans MI (ed): Reproductive Risks and Prenatal Diagnosis. Norwalk, CT, Appleton & Lange, 1992, p 311.

47. Schmalzer EA, Lee JO, Brown AK, et al: Viscosity of mixtures of sickle and normal red cells at varying hematocrit levels. Implications for transfusion. Transfusion 27:228, 1987.

48. Noguchi M, Yi H, Rosenblatt HM, et al: Interleukin-2 receptor gamma chain mutation results in X-linked severe combined immunodeficiency in humans. Cell 73:147, 1993.

49. Buckley RH, Schiff SE, Schiff RI, et al: Haploidentical bone marrow stem cell transplantation in human severe combined immunodeficiency [Review]. Semin Hematol 30:92, 1993.

50. Puck JM, Stewart CC, Nissbaum RL: Maximum-likelihood analysis of human T-cell X chromosome inactivation patterns: normal women versus carriers of X-linked severe combined immunodeficiency. Am J Hum Genet 50:742, 1992.

51. Blakemore K, Bambach B, Moser H, et al: Engraftment following in utero bone marrow transplantation for globoid cell leukodystrophy. Am J Obstet Gynecol 174:312, 1996.

Antepartum Fetal Evaluation

MAURICE L. DRUZIN, STEVEN G. GABBE, AND KATHRYN L. REED

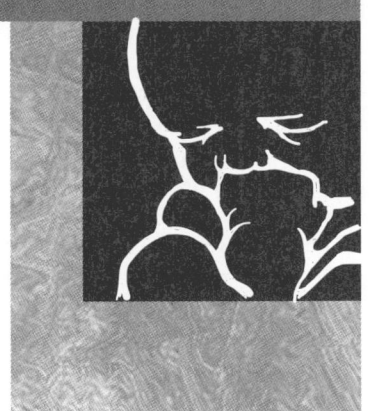

Not too long ago, the first aim of obstetric care was to prevent maternal death due to tuberculosis, syphilis, difficult deliveries, and haemorrhage. When this battle was won, at least in developed countries, and when perinatal mortality had dropped spectacularly, more time and interest could be focused on the fetus.[1]

Antepartum fetal deaths now account for 48 percent of all perinatal mortality in the United States.[2] The obstetrician must be concerned not only with prevention of this mortality, but with the detection of fetal compromise and the timely delivery of such infants in an effort to maximize their future potential.[3] This chapter reviews the definition and causes of perinatal mortality, the techniques available for assessing fetal condition, how one may evaluate their diagnostic accuracy, and the clinical application of these techniques to obstetric practice.

THE ETIOLOGY OF PERINATAL MORTALITY

The perinatal mortality rate (PMR) has been defined by the National Center for Health Statistics (NCHS) as the number of late fetal deaths (fetal deaths of 28 weeks' gestation or more) plus early neonatal deaths (deaths of infants 0 to 6 days of age) per 1,000 live births plus fetal deaths.[4] A live birth is the complete expulsion or extraction of a product of conception from its mother, irrespective of the duration of the pregnancy, that, after separation, breathes or shows any evidence of life, such as beating of the heart, pulsation of the umbilical cord,

or definite movement of voluntary muscles, whether or not the umbilical cord has been cut or the placenta is attached; each product of such a birth is considered liveborn. According to the NCHS, the neonatal mortality rate is defined as the number of neonatal deaths (deaths of infants 0 to 27 days of age) per 1,000 live births; the postneonatal mortality rate, the number of postneonatal deaths (the number of infants 28 to 365 days of age) per 1,000 live births; and the infant mortality rate, the number of infant deaths (deaths of infants under 1 year of age) per 1,000 live births. The definition of PMR provided by the World Health Organization (WHO) is somewhat different, including the number of fetuses and live births weighing at least 500 g or, when birth weight is unavailable, the corresponding gestational age (22 weeks) or body length (25 cm crown–heel) dying before day 7 of life per 1,000 such fetuses and infants. The American College of Obstetricians and Gynecologists (ACOG) has recommended that only deaths of fetuses and infants weighing 500 g or more at delivery be used to compare data among states in the United States.[5] For international comparisons, only deaths of fetuses and infants weighing 1,000 g or more at delivery should be included.[5]

Since 1965, the PMR in the United States has fallen steadily. Using the NCHS definition, the PMR reported in 1997 was 7.3 per 1,000.[2] The neonatal mortality rate was 3.8 per 1,000, with fetal deaths at 3.5 per 1,000. The PMR for blacks, 13.2 per 1,000, was more than twice that of whites, 6.3 per 1,000. The significantly greater PMR in blacks results from higher rates of *both* neonatal and fetal deaths.

Although the majority of fetal deaths occur before 32 weeks' gestation, in planning a strategy for antepartum fetal monitoring, one must examine the risk of fetal death in the population of women who are still pregnant at that point in pregnancy.[6,7] When this approach is taken, one finds that fetuses at 40 to 41 weeks are at a threefold greater risk and those at 42 or more weeks are at a 12-fold greater risk for intrauterine death than fetuses at 28 to 31 weeks.

The overall pattern of perinatal deaths in the United States has changed considerably during the past 30 years. Data collected between 1959 and 1966 by the Collaborative Perinatal Project revealed that 30 percent of perinatal deaths could be attributed to complications of the cord and placenta.[8] Other major causes of perinatal loss were maternal and fetal infections (17 percent), prematurity (10 percent), congenital anomalies (8 percent), and erythroblastosis fetalis (4 percent). In this series, 21 percent of the deaths were of unknown causes. In 1982, the major cause of early neonatal death was attributed to conditions originating in the perinatal period, such as infections, intraventricular hemorrhage, hydrops, meconium aspiration, and maternal complications such as diabetes mellitus and hypertension.[3] Congenital anomalies were the second leading cause of early neonatal death, accounting for 23 percent of such losses, whereas intrauterine hypoxia and birth asphyxia were responsible for 5 percent.

The infant mortality rate has fallen progressively from 47.0 per 1,000 in 1940 to 26.0 per 1,000 in 1960, 12.6 per 1,000 in 1980, 9.2 per 1,000 in 1990, and 7.2 per 1,000 in 1997.[9] Although the infant mortality rate includes all deaths of infants under 1 year of age, 50 percent of all infant deaths occur in the first week of life, and 50 percent of these losses result during the first day of life.[5] Clearly, perinatal events play an important role in infant mortality. In 1994, the leading cause of infant mortality reported by the NCHS was "perinatal conditions not separately listed," including maternal complications such as hypertension and substance abuse, multiple pregnancy, placenta previa and abruption, breech delivery, prolonged pregnancy and macrosomia, congenital pneumonia and viral infections, meconium aspiration, and Rh isoimmunization. This diverse category accounted for 25.4 percent of infant mortality, whereas congenital anomalies and sudden infant death syndrome were responsible for 20.3 and 14.8 percent, respectively. Short gestation and low birth weight contributed 12.3 percent and respiratory distress syndrome 6.7 percent. Only 2.1 percent of infant mortality was attributed to intrauterine hypoxia–birth asphyxia. Birth defects have been the single most important contributor to infant mortality for the past 20 years. In 1995, malformations were responsible for 22 percent of all infant deaths, with one third caused by cardiac abnormalities and respiratory, central nervous system, and chromosomal defects each contributing approximately 15 percent.[11]

Fetal deaths may be divided into those that occur during the antepartum period and those that occur during labor, intrapartum stillbirths. From 70 to almost 90 percent of fetal deaths occurred before the onset of labor.[12] Manning et al.[13] point out that antepartum deaths may be divided into four broad categories: (1) chronic asphyxia of diverse origin; (2) congenital malformations; (3) superimposed complications of pregnancy, such as Rh isoimmunization, placental abruption, and fetal infection; and (4) deaths of unexplained cause. If it is to succeed, a program of antenatal surveillance must identify malformed fetuses (see Chapter 10) and recognize those at risk for asphyxia.

Recent data describing the specific etiologies of fetal deaths in the United States are not available. Fretts and colleagues[14,15] have analyzed the causes of deaths in fetuses weighing more than 500 g in 94,346 births at the Royal Victoria Hospital in Montreal from 1961 to 1993. The population studied was predominantly white and included patients from all socioeconomic groups. Approximately 95 percent made four or more prenatal visits. The autopsy rate in this series was greater than 95 percent. Overall, the fetal death rate declined by 70 percent, from 11.5 per 1,000 in the 1960s to 3.2 per 1,000 during 1990 to 1993.[15] The decline in the fetal death rate may be attributed to the prevention of Rh sensitization, antepartum fetal surveillance, improved detection of intrauterine growth restriction (IUGR) and fetal anomalies with ultrasound, and improved care of maternal diabetes mellitus and preeclampsia. Fetal deaths attributable to intrapartum asphyxia and Rh isoimmunization fell dramatically, from 13.1 to 1.2 per 1,000 for intrapartum asphyxia and 4.3 to 0.7 per 1,000 for Rh disease.[14] Deaths caused by lethal anomalies declined by 50 percent, 10.8 to 5.4 per 1,000, because early terminations of pregnancy were performed for anencephaly. Whereas fetal mortality resulting from IUGR fell 60 percent, 17.9 to 7.0 per 1,000 births, the growth-restricted fetus still had a more than 10-fold greater risk for fetal death than an appropriately grown fetus (see Chapter 25).

Fretts et al. noted that most of these deaths occurred between 28 and 36 weeks' gestation and that the diagnosis of IUGR was rarely identified before death. In addition to IUGR, leading causes of fetal death after 28 weeks' gestation included abruption and unexplained antepartum losses. Despite a marked fall in unexplained fetal deaths, 38.1 to 13.6 per 1,000, these losses were still responsible for more than 25 percent of all stillbirths. Fetal–maternal hemorrhage may occur in 10 to 15 percent of cases of unexplained fetal deaths. Fetal deaths caused by infection, most often associated with premature rupture of the membranes before 28 weeks' gestation, did not decline over the 30 years of the study. Fretts et al.[11] also noted that, after controlling for risk factors such as multiple gestation, hypertension, diabetes mellitus, placenta previa and abruption, previous abortion, and prior fetal death, women 35 years of age or older had a nearly twofold greater risk for fetal death than women under 30. Data from Denmark have confirmed the J-shaped curve relationship between maternal age and fetal deaths with the highest rates in teenagers and women over age 35.[16,17]

Schauer et al.[18] summarized data from seven studies evaluating the causes of fetal death after 20 weeks. The largest group was unexplained, mostly asphyxial intrauterine deaths, 9 to 50 percent; major anomalies, 7 to 21 percent; antepartum hemorrhage with or without verified abruption (as in the Fretts et al. data the single largest known cause of fetal death), 12 to 17 percent; IUGR, 7 to 15 percent; hypertension, 1.9 to 15.7 percent; isoimmunization, 2.3 to 7.7 percent; diabetes mellitus, less than 1 to 4.8 percent; and infection, 2.1 to 6.1 percent. In a prospective study of 107 late fetal deaths, all of which had a full autopsy, Schauer et al.[18] observed a similar distribution of causes: asphyxia, 66 percent; multiple anomalies, 6 percent; chromosomal disorders, 6 percent; infection, 3 percent, and unknown, 19 percent. The chromosomal abnormalities included trisomy 21, trisomy 18, and 45,XO.

In summary, based on available data, approximately 30 percent of antepartum fetal deaths may be attributed to asphyxia (IUGR, prolonged gestation), 30 percent to maternal complications (placental abruption, hypertension, preeclampsia, and diabetes mellitus), 15 percent to congenital malformations and chromosomal abnormalities, and 5 percent to infection. At least 20 percent of stillbirths will have no obvious etiology.

Can these antepartum fetal deaths be prevented? Grant and Elbourne[7] have noted that "antepartum late fetal death is the component of perinatal mortality that has shown greatest resistance to change over recent years. In part, this reflects its relative unpredictability; in part, it reflects the relatively long period of time over which it can occur." Obstetric and pediatric assessors reviewed the circumstances surrounding each case of perinatal death in the Mersey region of England to identify any avoidable factors contributing to the death.[19] There were 309 perinatal deaths in this population, consisting of 157 stillbirths and 152 deaths in the first week of life. Of the 309 perinatal deaths, 182 (58.9 percent) were considered to have had avoidable factors. Most avoidable factors were found to be obstetric rather than pediatric or maternal and social. A high proportion (73.8 percent) of normal-birth-weight infants with no fetal abnormalities and no maternal complications had avoidable factors. The failure to re-

spond appropriately to abnormalities during pregnancy and labor, including results from the monitoring of fetal growth or intrapartum fetal well-being, significant maternal weight loss, or reported reductions in fetal movement, constituted the largest groups of avoidable factors. Kirkup and Welch[20] confirmed these results in an analysis of avoidable factors contributing to fetal death in nonmalformed infants weighing 2,500 g or more. Patients at highest risk for fetal death included women of a parity of 3 or more and those who had no prenatal care before 20 weeks. The Mersey Region Working Party on Perinatal Mortality concluded that, in light of increasing public awareness about obstetric management and, in some instances, an antipathy toward modern procedures, the failure to act on abnormalities discovered during monitoring would assume greater importance.[19] These workers found that in no case was the induction of labor as a result of such monitoring considered an avoidable factor.

A large clinical experience has demonstrated that antepartum fetal assessment can have a significant impact on the frequency and causes of antenatal fetal deaths. Schneider and colleagues[21] reviewed a decade of experience with antepartum fetal heart rate monitoring from 1974 through 1983. The contraction stress test was used primarily during the first 2 years of the study, followed by the nonstress test. Overall, the perinatal mortality rate was found to be 22.4 per 1,000 in the nontested population and 11.8 per 1,000 in the tested high-risk population, a highly significant difference. The stillbirth rate in the nontested population, 11.1 per 1,000, was twice that of patients who were followed with antepartum surveillance. When corrected for congenital anomalies, the stillbirth rate in the tested high-risk population was only 2.2 per 1,000. Of 18 stillbirths within 7 days of testing, the majority were because of congenital anomalies and placental abruption.

In a carefully performed study, Stubblefield and Berek[22] reviewed the causes of perinatal death in term and postterm births at the Boston Hospital for Women. The most frequent cause of death of a term or postterm infant was extrinsic perinatal hypoxia, and the second most common cause was a lethal malformation. Overall, extrinsic perinatal hypoxia accounted for 56.1 percent of the deaths of term infants and 71.4 percent of the deaths of postterm infants. Major malformations were implicated in 26.3 percent of the deaths of term infants. Twenty-nine of the 32 antenatal deaths occurred between 37 and 42 weeks' gestation. The authors concluded that two thirds of the antenatal deaths were associated with chronic processes such as placental infarction that might have been detected had routine antepartum fetal surveillance been used. In obstetric populations in which high-risk patients are monitored, the majority of stillbirths now occur in what had previously been considered normal pregnancies.

APPLICATION OF ANTEPARTUM FETAL TESTING

Before using antepartum fetal testing, the obstetrician must ask several important questions[23]:

1. Does the test provide information not already known by the patient's clinical status?
2. Can the information be helpful in managing the patient?
3. Should an abnormality be detected, is there a treatment available for the problem?
4. Could an abnormal test result lead to increased risk for the mother or fetus?
5. Will the test ultimately decrease perinatal morbidity and mortality?

Unfortunately, few of the tests commonly employed today in clinical practice have been subjected to prospective and randomized evaluations that can answer these questions.[24-27] In most cases, when the test has been applied and good perinatal outcomes were observed, the test has gained further acceptance and has been used more widely. In such cases, one cannot be sure whether it is actually the information provided by the test that has led to the improved outcomes or whether it is the total program of care that has made the difference. When prospective randomized investigations are conducted, large numbers of patients must be studied, since many adverse outcomes such as intrauterine death are uncommon even in high-risk populations.[25] Although several controlled trials have failed to

---

Aspects of Fetal Condition That Might Be Predicted by Antepartum Testing

Perinatal death

Intrauterine growth restriction (IUGR)

Nonreassuring fetal status, intrapartum

Neonatal asphyxia

Postnatal motor and intellectual impairment

Premature delivery

Congenital abnormalities

Need for specific therapy

Adapted from Chard T, Klopper A: Introduction. *In* Placental Function Tests. New York, Springer-Verlag, 1982, p 1.

Obstetric Management That Might Be Influenced by Antepartum Testing

Preterm delivery

Route of delivery

Bed rest

Observation

Drug therapy

Operative intervention in labor

Neonatal intensive care

Termination of pregnancy for a congenital anomaly

Adapted from Chard T, Klopper A: Introduction. *In* Placental Function Tests. New York, Springer-Verlag, 1982, p 1.

---

demonstrate improved outcomes with nonstress testing, the study populations ranged from only 300 to 530 subjects.[28-31]

The information one might predict from an antepartum fetal test is listed in the box "Aspects of Fetal Condition that Might Be Predicted by Antepartum Testing." Although one would want to detect IUGR or discover the presence of a significant congenital malformation, the most valuable information provided by antepartum fetal assessment may be that the fetus is well and requires no intervention. In this way, the pregnancy may be safely prolonged and the fetus allowed to gain further maturity.[27] The second box lists those aspects of obstetric management that might be influenced by antepartum testing. Certainly, one would not want to begin a program of testing unless one were prepared to use the information.

Using the information has invariably meant prompt intervention by delivery that may not be indicated and could lead to potentially avoidable complications of prematurity. A more current approach is to use the term *intervention* to describe other types of procedures short of premature delivery. This strategy would include using combinations of antepartum tests in an organized sequence to evaluate the fetus further; administration of antenatal steroids; bed rest; prolonged oxygen therapy; and correction of maternal metabolic, cardiopulmonary, or other medical disorders. *Intervention* may also refer to fetal therapy such as intrauterine transfusion for anemia, removal of fluid from body cavities, diagnostic procedures, and direct administration of medication to the fetus.

Testing can be initiated at early gestational ages, 25 to 26 weeks, to identify the fetus at risk. Maternal and fetal interventions can then be considered. Obviously, prolongation of intrauterine life is the primary goal,

Indications for Antepartum Fetal Monitoring

1. Patients at high risk of uteroplacental insufficiency

   Prolonged pregnancy
   Diabetes mellitus
   Hypertension
   Previous stillbirth
   Suspected IUGR
   Advanced maternal age
   Multiple gestation with discordant growth
   Antiphospholipid syndrome

2. When other tests suggest fetal compromise

   Suspected IUGR
   Decreased fetal movement
   Oligohydramnios

3. Routine antepartum surveillance

and better understanding of the pathophysiology of the premature fetus and the use of combinations of tests will allow this to be accomplished. In the event of impending in utero death or severe compromise, premature delivery, although the last resort, is a reasonable option, given the remarkable survival statistics being reported in modern neonatal intensive care units (see Chapters 20 and 23). The use of postnatal surfactant and improved mechanical ventilators are only some of the advances leading to survival and intact neurologic survival statistics that would have been incomprehensible a decade ago.[32–34]

In selecting the population of patients for antepartum fetal evaluation, one would certainly include those pregnancies known to be at high risk of uteroplacental insufficiency (see the box "Indications for Antepartum Fetal Monitoring").[27]

The question of routine antepartum fetal surveillance must be carefully examined. Antepartum fetal testing can more accurately predict fetal outcome than antenatal risk assessment using an established scoring system.[35] Patients judged to be at high risk based on known medical factors but whose fetuses demonstrated normal antepartum fetal evaluation had a lower PMR than did patients considered at low risk, whose fetuses had abnormal antepartum testing results. Routine antepartum fetal evaluation would be necessary to detect most infants dying in utero as the result of hypoxia and asphyxia.[22] It would seem reasonable, therefore, to consider extending some form of antepartum fetal surveillance to all obstetric patients. As described below, as-

sessment of fetal activity by the mother may be an ideal technique for this purpose.

STATISTICAL ASSESSMENT OF ANTEPARTUM TESTING

To determine the clinical application of antepartum diagnostic testing, the predictive value of the tests must be considered.[36,37] This information can most easily be presented in a 2 × 2 matrix. Table 12–1 presents this matrix using the contraction stress test (CST) and intrauterine fetal death as examples. The sensitivity of the test is the probability that the test will be positive or abnormal when the disease is present. The specificity of the test is the probability that the test result will be negative when the disease is not present. Note that the sensitivity and specificity refer not to the actual numbers of patients with a positive or abnormal result, but to the proportion or probability of these test results. The predictive value of an abnormal test would be that fraction of patients with an abnormal test result who have the abnormal condition, and the predictive value of a normal test would be the fraction of patients with a normal test result who are normal (Table 12–1).

Antepartum fetal tests may be used to screen a large obstetric population to detect fetal disease. In this setting, a test of high sensitivity is preferable, since one would not want to miss patients whose fetuses might be compromised. One would be willing to overdiagnose the problem, that is, accept some false-positive diagnoses. In further evaluating the patient whose fetus may be at risk and when attempting to confirm the presence of disease, one would want a test of high specificity. One would not want to intervene unnecessarily and deliver a fetus that was doing well. In this setting, multiple tests may be helpful. When multiple test results are normal, they tend to exclude disease. When all

Table 12–1. TWO-BY-TWO MATRIX OF POSSIBLE RESULTS FOR THE CST

Test Result	Perinatal Outcome	
	Normal (Normal Newborn)	Abnormal (Intrauterine Fetal Death)
Normal (negative CST)	A True-negative	B False-negative
Abnormal (positive CST)	C False-positive	D True-positive

Sensitivity = D/(D + B).
Specificity = A/(A + C).
Predictive value of a positive test = D/(C + D).
Predictive value of a negative test = A/(A + B).

Table 12–2. FIFTY PERCENT PREVALENCE

| | Perinatal Outcome | |
Test Result	Normal	Abnormal
Normal	490	125
	True-negative	False-negative
Abnormal	10	375
	False-positive	True-positive

Sensitivity = 75%.
Specificity = 98%.
Predictive value of a positive test = 97.4% (375 of 385).
Predictive value of a negative test = 79.6% (490 of 615).

Table 12–3. TWO PERCENT PREVALENCE

| | Perinatal Outcome | |
Test Result	Normal	Abnormal
Normal	960	5
	True-negative	False-negative
Abnormal	20	15
	False-positive	True-positive

Sensitivity = 75%.
Specificity = 98%.
Predictive value of a positive test = 42.8% (15 of 35).
Predictive value of a negative test = 99.4% (960 of 965).

are abnormal, however, they tend to support the diagnosis of fetal disease.

The prevalence of the abnormal condition has great impact on the predictive value of anterpartum fetal tests. Table 12–2 presents data for a population of 1,000 patients in whom the prevalence of the disease is 50 percent. The sensitivity of the test being evaluated is 75 percent, and its specificity is 98 percent. These figures are similar to those observed for several antepartum tests now in use. In this setting, an abnormal test result is likely to be associated with a true fetal abnormality. The predictive value of a positive test is 97.4 percent. However, when the prevalence of the disease falls to 2 percent, as it may be for intrauterine fetal deaths, even tests with a high sensitivity and specificity are associated with many false predictions (Table 12–3). In this circumstance, an abnormal test is more likely to indicate a false-positive diagnosis ($n = 20$) than it is a true-positive diagnosis ($n = 15$).

In interpreting the results of studies of antepartum testing, the obstetrician must consider the application of that test to his or her own population. If the study has been done in a population of patients at great risk,

it is more likely that an abnormal test will be associated with an abnormal fetus. If the obstetrician is practicing in a community with patients who are, in general, at low risk, however, an abnormal test result would more likely be associated with a false-positive diagnosis.

For most antepartum diagnostic tests, a cut-off point used to define an abnormal result must be arbitrarily established.[38] The cut-off point is selected to maximize the separation between the normal and diseased populations (Fig. 12–1). Changing the cut-off will have a great impact on the predictive value of the test. For example, suppose that 10 accelerations in 10 minutes were required for a fetus to have a reactive nonstress test (threshold A). The fetus who fulfilled this rigid definition would almost certainly be in good condition. However, many fetuses who failed to achieve 10 accelerations in 10 minutes would also be in good condition, but would be judged to be abnormal by this cut-off. In this instance, the test would have many abnormal results. It would be highly sensitive and capture all of the abnormal fetuses, but it would have a low specificity. If the number of accelerations required

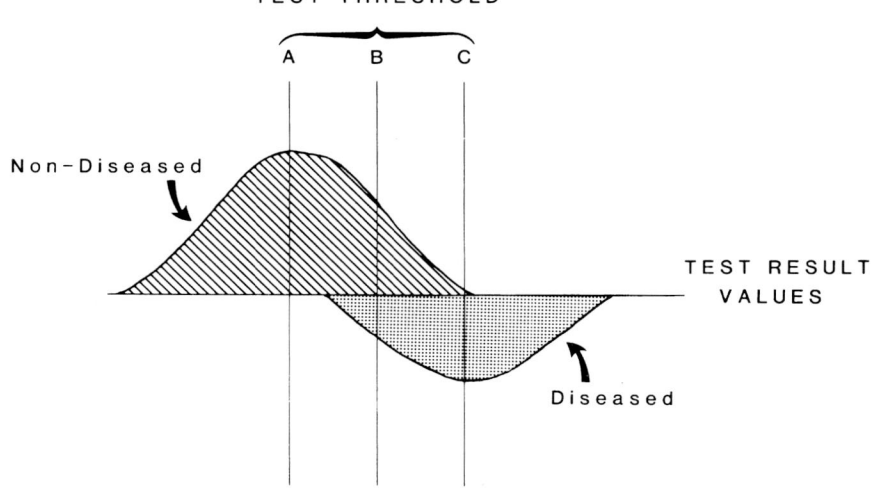

Figure 12–1. Hypothetical distribution of test results in a normal and diseased population, demonstrating the differences in test sensitivity and specificity with a change in test threshold. Making it more difficult for the fetus to pass the test by raising the test threshold (A) will increase the sensitivity, but decrease the specificity, of the test. On the other hand, making the test easier to pass by decreasing the test threshold (C) will increase the specificity of the test, but decrease the sensitivity. (Adapted from Carpenter M, Coustan D: Criteria for screening tests for gestational diabetes. Am J Obstet Gynecol 144:768, 1982.)

to pass a nonstress test were lowered to 1 in 10 minutes, it would decrease the sensitivity of the test (threshold C). That is, one might miss a truly sick fetus. At the same time, however, one would improve the specificity of the test or its ability to predict that percentage of the patients who are normal. Using the criterion of two accelerations of the fetal heart rate in 20 minutes for a reactive nonstress test (threshold B), one hopes to have a test with both high sensitivity and high specificity.

BIOPHYSICAL TECHNIQUES OF FETAL EVALUATION

Fetal State

When interpreting tests that monitor fetal biophysical characteristics, one must appreciate that, during the third trimester, the normal fetus may exhibit marked changes in its neurologic state.[39,40] Four fetal states have been identified. The near-term fetus spends approximately 25 percent of its time in a quiet sleep state (state 1F) and 60 to 70 percent in an active sleep state (state 2F). Active sleep is associated with rapid eye movement (REM). In fetal lambs, electrocortical activity during REM sleep is characterized by low-voltage, high-frequency waves. The fetus exhibits regular breathing movements and intermittent abrupt movements of its head, limbs, and trunk. The fetal heart rate in active sleep (state 2F) exhibits increased variability and frequent accelerations with movement. During quiet, or non-REM, sleep, the fetal heart rate slows and heart rate variability is reduced. The fetus may make infrequent breathing movements and startled movements. Electrocortical activity recordings at this time reveal high-voltage, low-frequency waves. Near term, periods of quiet sleep may last 20 minutes, and those of active sleep approximately 40 minutes.[40] The mechanisms that control these periods of rest and activity in the fetus are not well established. External factors such as the mother's activity, her ingestion of drugs, and her nutrition may all play a role.

When evaluating fetal condition using the nonstress test or the biophysical profile, one must ask whether a fetus that is not making breathing movements or shows no accelerations of its baseline heart rate is in a quiet sleep state or is neurologically compromised. In such circumstances, prolonging the period of evaluation will usually allow a change in fetal state, and more normal parameters of fetal well-being will appear.

Maternal Assessment of Fetal Activity

Maternal assessment of fetal activity is a simple yet valuable method for monitoring fetal condition. Most patients can understand and follow protocols for counting fetal activity, and this method is obviously inexpensive. Therefore, maternal assessment of fetal activity may be ideal for routine antepartum fetal surveillance.

Studies performed using real-time ultrasonography have demonstrated that during the third trimester the human fetus spends 10 percent of its time making gross fetal body movements and that 30 such movements are made each hour.[41] Periods of active fetal body movement last approximately 40 minutes, whereas quiet periods last about 20 minutes. Patrick et al.[41] noted that the longest period without fetal movements in a normal fetus was approximately 75 minutes. The mother is able to appreciate about 70 to 80 percent of gross fetal movements. The fetus does make fine body movements such as limb flexion and extension, hand grasping, and sucking, which probably reflect more coordinated central nervous system (CNS) function. However, the mother is generally unable to perceive these fine movements. Fetal movement appears to peak between 9:00 P.M. and 1:00 A.M., a time when maternal glucose levels are falling.[34] In a study in which maternal glucose levels were carefully controlled with an artificial pancreas, Holden et al.[42] found that hypoglycemia was associated with increased fetal movement. Fetal activity does not increase after meals or after maternal glucose administration.[43,44]

Maternal evaluation of fetal activity may reduce fetal deaths caused by asphyxia. Using a sheep model, Natale et al.[45] demonstrated that fetal activity is extremely sensitive to a decrease in fetal oxygenation. A small fall in fetal PO_2 was associated with a cessation of limb movements in the fetal lamb.

Several methods have been used to monitor fetal activity in clinical practice. In general, the presence of fetal movements is a reassuring sign of fetal health. However, the absence of fetal activity requires further assessment before one can conclude that fetal compromise exists. Sadovsky et al.[46] recommended that mothers count fetal activity for 30 to 60 minutes each day, two or three times daily. If the mother has fewer than three movements in 1 hour, or if she appreciates no movements for 12 hours, the movement alarm signal, further evaluation of fetal condition must be made. Rayburn et al.[47] suggested that patients count fetal activity at least 60 minutes each day. Fewer than three movements an hour for 2 consecutive days may be a sign of fetal compromise. Pearson and Weaver[48] advocated the use of the Cardiff Count-to-Ten chart. They found that only 2.5 percent of 1,654 daily movement counts recorded by 61 women who subsequently delivered healthy infants fell below 10 movements per 12 hours. Therefore, they accepted 10 movements as the minimum amount of fetal activity the patient should perceive in a 12-hour period. The patient is asked to start counting the movements in the morning and to record the time of day at which the 10th movement has been perceived. Should the patient not have 10 movements during 12 hours, or should it take longer each day to reach 10 movements, the patient is told to contact her obstetrician. Sadovsky et al.[49] found that, of those techniques currently used in clinical management, the movement alarm signal and the technique of Pearson and Weaver are the most valuable.

Whatever technique is used must be carefully explained to the patient. Although most women are reassured by keeping a fetal activity chart and maternal–fetal attachment may be enhanced, some patients do become more anxious.[50,51] Women who were concerned about monitoring fetal movement complained that they were not given adequate information about variations in fetal activity patterns and maternal perception of movement.

Although there will be a wide but normal range in fetal activity, with fetal movement counting, each mother and her fetus serve as their own control.[7] Fetal and placental factors that influence maternal assessment of fetal activity include placental location, the length of fetal movements, the amniotic fluid volume, and fetal anomalies.[52] If the placenta is anterior, maternal perception of fetal movements may be decreased. Movements lasting 20 to 60 seconds are most likely to be felt by the mother.[53] Hydramnios will reduce the mother's appreciation of fetal activity. Hydramnios may be associated with a fetal anomaly and should be further evaluated using ultrasonography. Rayburn and Barr[54] reported that 26 percent of fetuses with major malformations show decreased fetal activity compared with only 4 percent of normal fetuses. Anomalies of the CNS are most commonly associated with decreased activity.

Approximately 80 percent of all mothers will be able to comply with a program of counting fetal activity.[7,55] Maternal factors that influence the evaluation of fetal movement include maternal activity, obesity, and medications. Mothers appear to appreciate fetal movements best when resting in the left lateral recumbent position. Patients should therefore be told to lie down when counting fetal movement, an additional benefit of this approach to fetal evaluation. Obesity decreases maternal appreciation of fetal activity. Maternal medications such as narcotics or barbiturates may depress fetal movement.

Several large clinical studies have demonstrated the efficacy of maternal assessment of fetal activity in preventing unexplained fetal deaths. In a prospective randomized study, Neldam[55,56] asked one group of 1,562 pregnant patients at 32 weeks' gestation to count fetal activity three times each week for 2 hours after their main meals. Fewer than three fetal movements each hour was regarded as a sign of potential fetal compromise and was further evaluated with an ultrasound examination and a nonstress test. In the monitored group

of patients, only one stillbirth occurred. Ten stillbirths were noted in a control population of 1,549 women. Overall, 4 percent of patients in the monitored group reported their baby was not moving adequately, a low figure, but one similar to that observed in other studies. Of these 60 patients, almost 25 percent were found to have a fetus in distress based on further antepartum testing. Neldam[56] attributed the prevention of 14 fetal deaths to the use of maternal assessment of fetal activity.

Rayburn[57] found that in the 5 percent of his patients who reported decreased fetal activity the incidence of stillbirths was 60 times higher, the risk of fetal distress in labor 2 to 3 times higher, the incidence of low Apgar scores at delivery 10 times greater, and the incidence of severe growth restriction 10 times higher. Rayburn also observed that the normal fetus does *not* decrease activity in the week before delivery.

Using the Cardiff Count-to-Ten chart, Liston et al.[58] noted that 11 of 150 high-risk patients (7.3 percent) reported fewer than 10 movements in a 12-hour period. Two of these patients suffered perinatal deaths, and 33 percent experienced fetal distress in labor. Overall, 60 percent of patients who reported decreased fetal activity did exhibit evidence of fetal compromise. The number of false alarms was quite manageable.

Two prospective studies have yielded conflicting results regarding the efficacy of fetal movement counting as a technique for preventing fetal deaths. Grant and co-workers[59] recruited 68,000 European women who were randomly allocated within 33 pairs of clusters to either routine fetal movement counting using the Cardiff Count-to-Ten method or to standard care. Women counted for an average of almost 3 hours per day, and about 7 percent of the charts showed at least one alarm. Of concern, the rate of compliance for reporting decreased fetal movement was only 46 percent. Furthermore, compliance for charting movements and reporting alarms was lower among women who had a late fetal death. The antepartum death rates for nonmalformed singleton fetuses were equal in both experimental groups. However, in none of the 17 cases in which reduced movements were recognized and the fetus was still alive when the patient arrived at the hospital was an emergency delivery attempted. Why? Grant et al.[59] believe that intervention was not undertaken because of false reassurance from follow-up testing, especially heart rate monitoring, and because of errors in clinical judgment. One might conclude that this large prospective study failed to demonstrate a reduction in the antepartum fetal death rate as a result of fetal movement counting. However, what it seems to prove most clearly is that patient compliance is an essential part of this program as is appropriate evaluation of the patient who presents with decreased fetal activity.

In contrast, an investigation by Moore and Piacquadio[60]

demonstrated an impressive reduction in fetal deaths resulting from a formal program of fetal movement counting. Patients used the Count-to-Ten approach but were told to monitor fetal activity in the evening, a time of increased fetal movement. Most women observed 10 movements in an average of 21 minutes, and compliance was greater than 90 percent. Patients who did not perceive 10 movements in 2 hours, a level of fetal activity slightly more than 5 SD below the mean, were told to report immediately for further evaluation. During a 7-month control period, a fetal mortality rate of 8.7 per 1,000 was observed in 2,519 patients, and 11 of 247 women who came to the hospital with a complaint of decreased fetal movement had already suffered an intrauterine death. During the study period, the fetal death rate fell to 2.1 per 1,000, and only 1 of 290 patients with decreased fetal movement presented after fetal death had occurred. The number of antepartum tests required to assess patients with decreased fetal activity rose 13 percent during the study period. This investigation has been expanded to include almost 6,000 patients, and a fetal death rate of 3.6 per 1,000, less than half that found in the control period, has been achieved.[61]

In conclusion, there appears to be a clearly established relationship between decreased fetal activity and fetal death. Therefore, it would seem prudent to request that *all* pregnant patients, regardless of their risk status, monitor fetal activity starting at 28 weeks' gestation (Fig. 12–2). The Count-to-Ten approach developed by Moore and Piacquadio[61] seems ideal.

Contraction Stress Test

The CST, also known as the oxytocin challenge test (OCT), was the first biophysical technique widely applied for antepartum fetal surveillance. It was well known that uterine contractions produced a reduction in blood flow to the intervillous space. Analyses of intrapartum fetal heart rate monitoring had demonstrated that a fetus with inadequate placental respiratory reserve would demonstrate late decelerations in response to hypoxia (see Chapter 14). The CST extended these observations to the antepartum period.

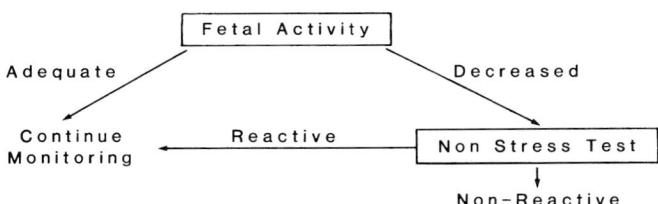

Figure 12–2. Maternal assessment of fetal activity is a valuable screening test for fetal condition. Should the mother report decreased fetal activity, a NST is performed. In this situation most NSTs will be reactive.

The response of the fetus at risk for uteroplacental insufficiency to uterine contractions formed the basis for this test.

Performing the CST

The CST may be conducted in the labor and delivery suite or in an adjacent area, although the likelihood of fetal distress requiring immediate delivery in response to uterine contractions or hyperstimulation is extremely small. The CST should be performed by staff familiar with the principles and technique of such testing. In many institutions, an antenatal diagnostic unit has been developed for this purpose. The patient is placed in the semi-Fowler's position at a 30- to 45-degree angle with a slight left tilt to avoid the supine hypotensive syndrome. The fetal heart rate is recorded using a Doppler ultrasound transducer, and uterine contractions are monitored with the tocodynamometer. Maternal blood pressure is determined every 5 to 10 minutes to detect maternal hypotension.[62] Baseline fetal heart rate and uterine tone are first recorded for a period of approximately 10 to 20 minutes. In some cases, adequate uterine activity will occur spontaneously, and additional uterine stimulation will not be necessary. An adequate CST requires uterine contractions of moderate intensity lasting approximately 40 to 60 seconds with a frequency of three in 10 minutes. These criteria were selected to approximate the stress experienced by the fetus during the first stage of labor. If uterine activity is absent or inadequate, nipple stimulation is used to initiate contractions or intravenous oxytocin is begun. Oxytocin is administered by an infusion pump at 0.5 mU/min. The infusion rate is doubled every 20 minutes until adequate uterine contractions have been achieved.[27] One does not usually need to exceed 10 mU/min to produce adequate uterine activity. After the CST has been completed, the patient should be observed until uterine activity has returned to its baseline level. With nipple stimulation, the test may take approximately 30 minutes. If oxytocin is needed, 90 minutes may be required to perform the CST.

Contraindications to the test include those patients at high risk for premature labor, such as patients with premature rupture of the membranes, multiple gestation, and cervical incompetence, although the CST has not been associated with an increased incidence of premature labor.[63] The CST should also be avoided in conditions in which uterine contractions may be dangerous, such as placenta previa and a previous classical cesarean section or uterine surgery.

Interpreting the CST

Most clinicians utilize the definitions proposed by Freeman to interpret the CST[63,64] (Table 12–4). In an at-

Table 12–4. INTERPRETATION OF THE CONTRACTION STRESS TEST

Interpretation	Description	Incidence (%)
Negative	No late decelerations appearing anywhere on the tracing with adequate uterine contractions (three in 10 minutes)	80
Positive	Late decelerations that are consistent and persistent, present with the majority (>50 percent) of contractions without excessive uterine activity; if persistent late decelerations seen before the frequency of contractions is adequate, test interpreted as positive	3–5
Suspicious	Inconsistent late decelerations	5
Hyperstimulation	Uterine contractions closer than every 2 minutes or lasting >90 seconds, or five uterine contractions in 10 minutes; if no late decelerations seen, test interpreted as negative	5
Unsatisfactory	Quality of the tracing inadequate for interpretation or adequate uterine activity cannot be achieved	5

tempt to decrease the frequency of suspicious tests that would require further evaluation, Martin and Schifrin[65] developed the "10-minute window" concept. A positive test would be any 10-minute segment of the tracing that includes three contractions, all showing late decelerations. A negative test is one in which no positive window is seen and there is at least one negative window, three uterine contractions in 10 minutes with no late decelerations (Figs. 12–3 and 12–4). The CST would be read as negative and not suspicious if an occasional late deceleration were seen, but a negative window was also present. They used the term *equivocal* rather than *suspicious* for a CST with an occasional late deceleration but no negative window. Equivocal implies that one is unable to make a determination of fetal condition based on the available information. A CST with both a positive and negative window would be interpreted as positive.

Variable decelerations that occur during the CST may indicate cord compression often associated with oligohydramnios. In such cases, ultrasonography should be performed to assess amniotic fluid volume. However, even if the amniotic fluid volume is demonstrated to be adequate, cord compression patterns need careful follow-up, because cord accidents with subsequent fetal death may occur in the presence of normal amounts of amniotic fluid on sonography. What appears to be a normal volume of amniotic fluid may contain meconium, which has a specific gravity different from clear amniotic fluid and therefore does not allow the cord to float freely. In cases of early placental insufficiency, the amount of Wharton's jelly in the umbilical cord may be diminished prior to the clinical appearance of oligohydramnios. The loss of the protective Wharton's jelly may make the umbilical vessels vulnerable to compression and lead to diminished blood flow.

A negative CST has been consistently associated with good fetal outcome. A negative result therefore permits the obstetrician to prolong a high-risk pregnancy safely. Nageotte et al.[66] reported only one preventable fetal death in 1,337 high-risk patients within 7 days after a negative CST. In a series of 679 pregnancies complicated by a prolonged gestation, Freeman et al.[67] observed no perinatal deaths when the CST was used as the primary method of surveillance. Of 337 women with a previous intrauterine fetal death, none had a stillbirth during a pregnancy in which they were followed with CSTs.[68] Druzin et al.[69] reported no antepartum deaths in a series of 819 patients tested at 280

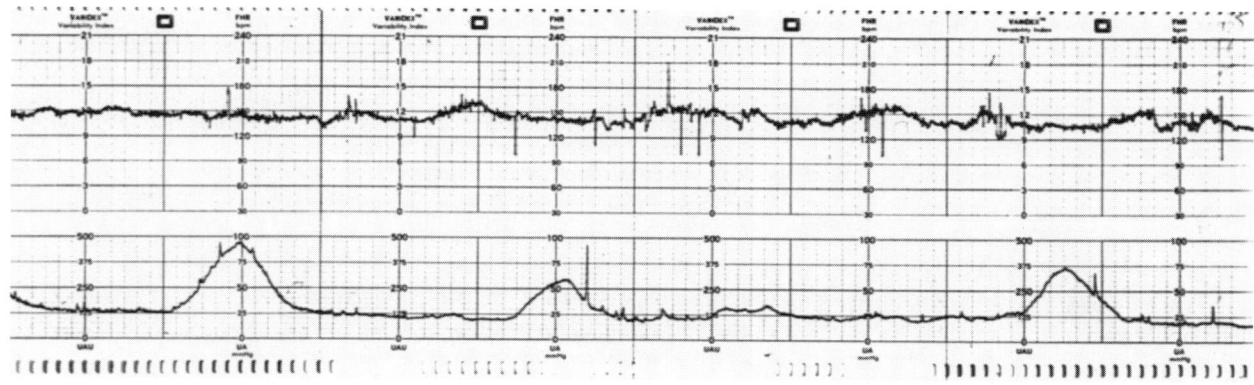

Figure 12–3. A reactive and negative CST. With this result, the CST would ordinarily be repeated in 1 week.

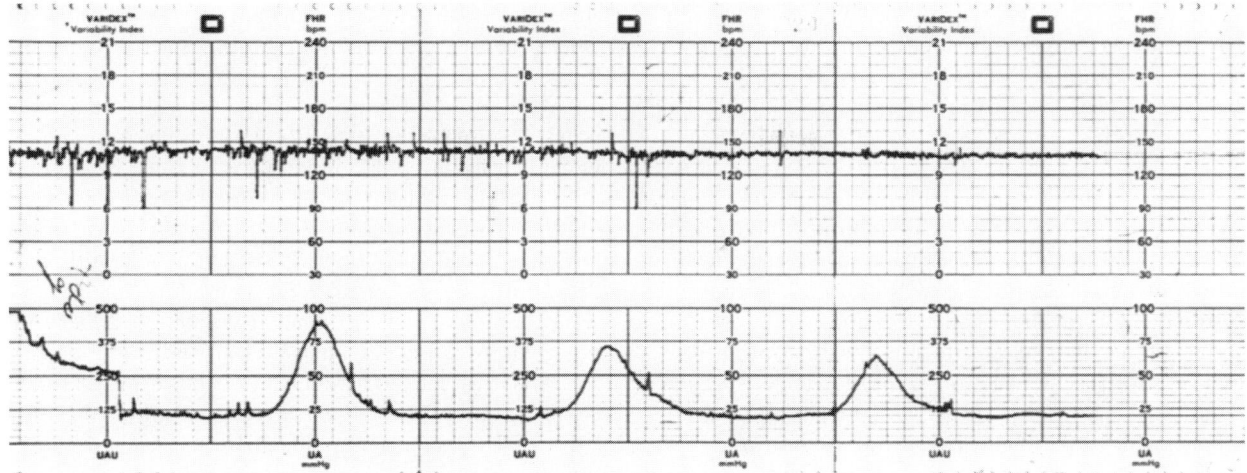

Figure 12–4. A nonreactive and negative CST. After this result, the test would ordinarily be repeated in 24 hours.

days or more gestation, using both the nonstress test (NST) and nipple stimulation CST. There were no differences in perinatal outcome in the group with a reactive NST, irrespective of the CST result. Similarly, Gabbe et al.[70] and Lagrew et al.[71] have reported only one fetal death within 1 week of a negative CST in 811 pregnancies complicated by type 1 diabetes mellitus. Other studies have shown the incidence of perinatal death within 1 week of a negative CST to be less than 1 per 1,000.[72-74] Many of these deaths, however, can be attributed to cord accidents, malformations, placental abruption, and acute deterioration of glucose control in patients with diabetes. Thus, the CST, like most methods of antepartum fetal surveillance, cannot predict acute fetal compromise. If the CST is negative, a

repeat study is usually scheduled in 1 week. Although testing patients with a weekly CST is practical, it is also arbitrary. Changes in the patient's clinical condition may warrant more frequent studies.

A positive CST has been associated with an increased incidence of intrauterine death, late decelerations in labor, low 5-minute Apgar scores, IUGR, and meconium-stained amniotic fluid (Fig. 12–5).[74] In a prospective and blinded study, Ray et al.[75] observed 3 fetal deaths in 15 patients with positive CSTs. The incidence of low Apgar scores in this group was 53 percent. Overall, the likelihood of perinatal death after a positive CST has ranged from 7 to 15 percent. On the other hand, there has been a significant incidence of false-positive CSTs that, depending on the endpoint used, will average ap-

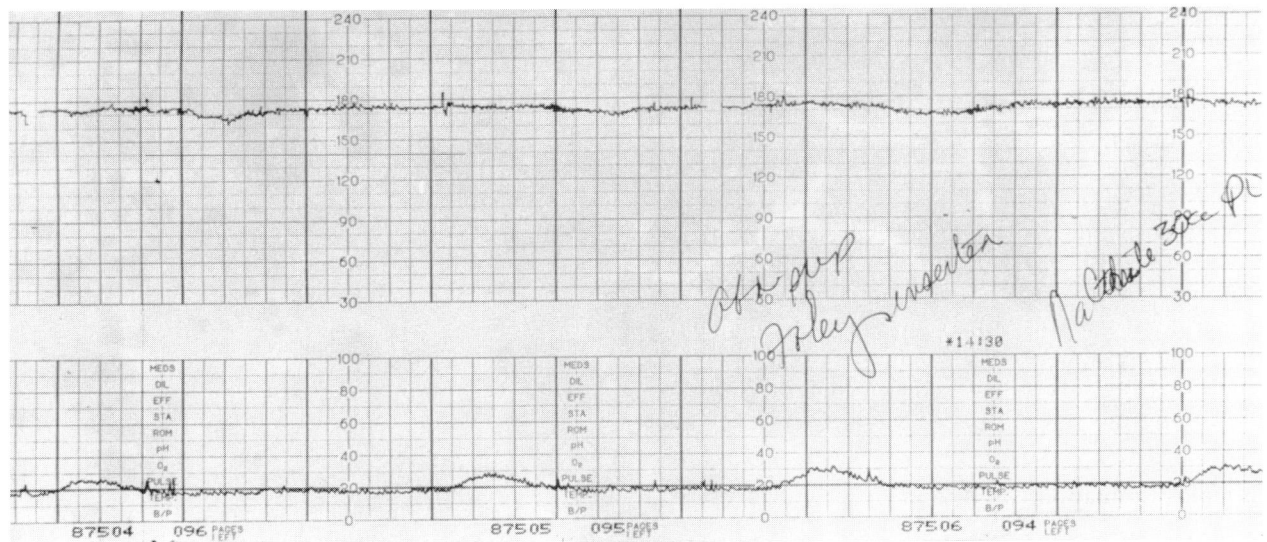

Figure 12–5. A nonreactive and positive CST with fetal tachycardia. At 34 weeks, a poorly compliant patient with type 1 diabetes mellitus, reported decreased fetal activity. The NST revealed a fetal tachycardia of 170 bpm and was nonreactive. The CST was positive, and a BPP score was 2. The patient's cervix was unfavorable for induction. The patient underwent a low transverse cesarean delivery of a 2,200-g male infant with Apgar scores of 1 and 3. The umbilical arterial pH was 7.21.

proximately 30 percent.[76] The positive CST is more likely to be associated with fetal compromise if the baseline heart rate lacks accelerations or "reactivity" and the latency period between the onset of the uterine contractions and the onset of the late deceleration is less than 45 seconds.[77,78]

There is no doubt that the high incidence of false-positive CSTs is one of the greatest limitations of this test, as such results could lead to unnecessary premature intervention. False-positive CSTs may be attributable to misinterpretation of the tracing; supine hypotension, which decreases uterine perfusion; uterine hyperstimulation, which is not appreciated using the tocodynamometer; or an improvement in fetal condition after the CST has been performed. The high false-positive rate also indicates that a patient with a positive CST need not necessarily require an elective cesarean delivery. If a trial of labor is to be undertaken after a positive CST, the cervix should be favorable for induction so that direct fetal heart rate monitoring and careful assessment of uterine contractility with an intrauterine pressure catheter can be performed. False-positive results are not increased when the CST is used early in the third trimester.[76] A negative or positive CST obtained between 28 and 33 weeks' gestation appears to have the same diagnostic significance as it would later in gestation. Merrill et al.[79] reported prolongation of pregnancy for up to 13 days in the presence of a nonreactive nonstress test and a positive CST test if the biophysical profile (BPP) score was 6 or greater. This approach should only be used in the premature fetus and when careful follow-up with daily assessment, using the nonstress test, CST, and BPP can be reliably performed.

A suspicious or equivocal CST should be repeated in 24 hours. Most of these tests will become negative. Bruce et al.[80] did observe that 5 of 67 patients (7.5 percent) with an initially suspicious CST exhibited positive tests on further evaluation. In 36 patients, the CST became negative, whereas in 26 patients it remained suspicious. Like the suspicious CST, a test that is unsatisfactory or shows hyperstimulation should be repeated in 24 hours.

In follow-up studies of children who demonstrated a positive CST, few have exhibited abnormalities in neurologic and psychological development.[81–83] An important determinant in the long-term outcome for these children would be the early recognition of nonreassuring fetal heart rate patterns and the prevention of intrapartum compromise.

The Nipple Stimulation CST

Many centers utilize nipple stimulation to produce the uterine contractions needed for the CST. With nipple stimulation, the CST can generally be completed in less time, and an intravenous infusion is not required. Therefore, this approach would appear to be an ideal first step in performing a CST.

Several methods have been used to induce adequate uterine activity.[27,84,85] The patient may first apply a warm moist towel to each breast for 5 minutes. If uterine activity is not adequate, the patient is asked to massage one nipple for 10 minutes. Using this protocol, Oki et al.[84] achieved adequate uterine contractions in 30 minutes or less in 87.5 percent of 657 patients tested. The incidence of negative tests (72 percent) and positive tests (2 percent) was not different from that seen with the oxytocin-induced CST. Huddleston et al.[86] reported great success using intermittent nipple stimulation. The patient gently strokes the nipple of one breast with the palmar surface of her fingers through her clothes for 2 minutes and then stops for 5 minutes. This cycle is repeated only as necessary to achieve adequate uterine activity. In a series of 193 patients and 345 CSTs, 97 percent of the tests required only three cycles of stimulation. The average time for a CST performed in this way was 45 minutes, and 67.5 percent of the patients completed their tests in 40 minutes or less. The nipple stimulation CST was negative in 80.3 percent of patients and positive in 2.6 percent of patients. All the patients in the Huddleston et al.[86] series were able to achieve adequate uterine contractions with nipple stimulation, and none required an oxytocin infusion. Intermittent rather than continuous nipple stimulation is important in avoiding hyperstimulation. Defined as contractions lasting more than 90 seconds or five or more contractions in 10 minutes, hyperstimulation has been reported in approximately 2 percent of tests when intermittent nipple stimulation is employed.[87,88]

The Nonstress Test

In 1969, Hammacher[89] noted that "the fetus can be regarded as safe, especially if reflex movements are accompanied by an obvious increase in the amplitude of oscillations in the basal fetal heart rate." This observation that accelerations of the fetal heart rate in response to fetal activity, uterine contractions, or stimulation reflect fetal well-being has formed the basis for the NST, the most widely applied technique for antepartum fetal evaluation.

In late gestation, the healthy fetus exhibits an average of 34 accelerations above the baseline fetal heart rate each hour.[90] These accelerations, which average 20 to 25 bpm in amplitude and approximately 40 seconds in duration, require intact neurologic coupling between the fetal CNS and the fetal heart.[90] Fetal hypoxia will disrupt this pathway. At term, fetal accelerations are associated with fetal movement more than 85 percent of the time, and more than 90 percent of gross movements are accompanied by accelerations. Fetal heart rate accelerations may be absent during periods of quiet fetal sleep. Studies by Patrick et al.[90] demonstrated that the longest time between successive accelerations in the healthy term fetus is approximately 40 minutes. However, the fetus may fail to exhibit heart rate accelerations for up to 80 minutes and still be normal.

Although an absence of fetal heart rate accelerations is most often attributable to a quiet fetal sleep state, CNS depressants such as narcotics and phenobarbital, as well as the β-blocker propranolol, can reduce heart rate reactivity.[91,92] Chronic smoking is known to decrease fetal oxygenation through an increase in fetal carboxyhemoglobin and a decrease in uterine blood flow. Fetal heart rate accelerations are also decreased in smokers.[93]

The NST is usually performed in an outpatient setting. In most cases, only 10 to 15 minutes are required to complete the test. It has virtually no contraindications, and few equivocal test results are observed. The patient may be seated in a reclining chair, with care being taken to ensure that she is tilted to the left to avoid the supine hypotensive syndrome.[27,94] The patient's blood pressure should be recorded before the test is begun and then repeated at 5- to 10-minute intervals. Fetal heart rate is monitored using the Doppler ultrasound transducer, and the tocodynamometer is applied to detect uterine contractions or fetal movement. Fetal activity may be recorded by the patient using an event marker or noted by the staff performing the test. The most widely applied definition of a reactive test requires that at least two accelerations of the fetal heart rate of 15 bpm amplitude and 15 seconds' duration be ob-

served in 20 minutes of monitoring (Fig. 12–6).[94] Since almost all accelerations are accompanied by fetal movement, fetal movement need not be recorded with the accelerations for the test to be considered reactive. However, fetal movements do provide another index of fetal well-being.

If the criteria for reactivity are not met, the test is considered nonreactive (Fig. 12–7). The most common cause for a nonreactive test will be a period of fetal inactivity or quiet sleep. Therefore, the test may be extended for an additional 20 minutes with the expectation that fetal state will change and reactivity will appear. Keegan et al.[95] noted that approximately 80 percent of tests that were nonreactive in the morning became reactive when repeated later the same day. In an effort to change fetal state, some clinicians have manually stimulated the fetus or attempted to increase fetal glucose levels by giving the mother orange juice. There is no evidence that such efforts will increase fetal activity.[96,97] If the test has been extended for 40 minutes, and reactivity has not been seen, a BPP or CST should be performed. Of those fetuses that exhibit a nonreactive NST, approximately 25 percent will have a positive CST on further evaluation.[94,98,99] Reactivity that occurs during preparations for the CST has proved to be a reliable index of fetal well-being.

Overall, on initial testing, 85 percent of NSTs will be reactive and 15 percent will be nonreactive (Fig. 12–8).[94] Fewer than 1 percent of NSTs will prove unsatisfactory because of inadequately recorded fetal heart rate data. On rare occasions, a sinusoidal heart rate pattern may be observed as described in Chapter 14. This undulating heart rate pattern with virtually absent variability has been associated with fetal anemia, fetal

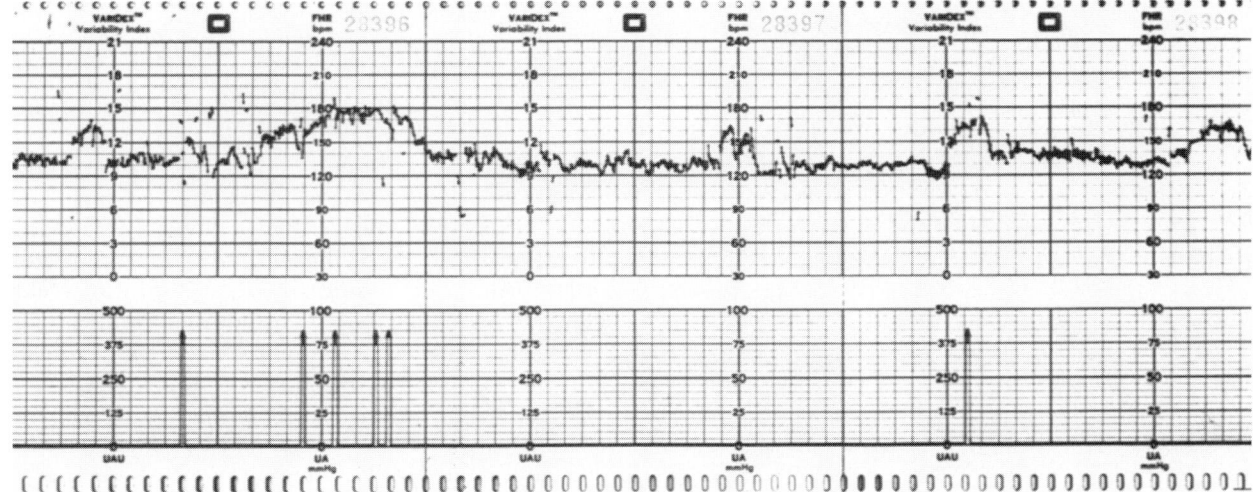

Figure 12–6. A reactive NST. Accelerations of the fetal heart that are greater than 15 bpm and last longer than 15 seconds can be identified. When the patient appreciates a fetal movement, she presses an event marker on the monitor, creating the arrows on the lower portion of the tracing.

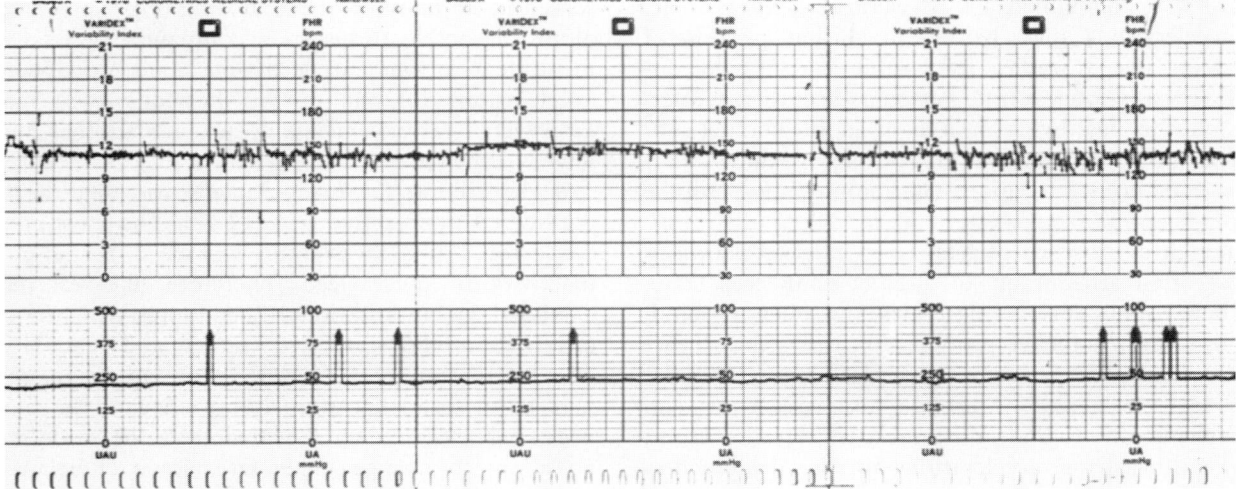

Figure 12-7. A nonreactive NST. No accelerations of the fetal heart rate are observed. The patient has perceived fetal activity as indicated by the arrows in the lower portion of the tracing.

asphyxia, congenital malformations, and medications such as narcotics. In one of the earliest reports on the use of the NST, Rochard et al.[100] described a sinusoidal pattern in 20 of 50 pregnancies complicated by Rh isoimmunization. One half of these pregnancies ended in a perinatal death, and 40 percent of the surviving infants required prolonged hospitalization. Only 10 percent of the babies with a sinusoidal pattern had an uncomplicated course.

The NST is most predictive when normal or reactive. Overall, a reactive NST has been associated with a perinatal mortality of approximately 5 per 1,000.[94,101] At least one half of the deaths of babies dying within 1 week of a reactive test may be attributed to placental abruption or cord accidents. The perinatal mortality rate associated with a nonreactive NST, 30 to 40 per

1,000, is significantly higher, for this group includes those fetuses who are truly asphyxiated. On the other hand, when considering perinatal asphyxia and death as endpoints, a nonreactive NST has a considerable false-positive rate. Most fetuses exhibiting a nonreactive NST will not be compromised but will simply fail to exhibit heart rate reactivity during the 40-minute period of testing. Malformed fetuses also exhibit a significantly higher incidence of nonreactive NSTs.[102] Overall, the false-positive rate associated with the nonreactive NST is approximately 75 to 90 percent.[94]

The likelihood of a nonreactive test is substantially increased early in the third trimester.[103] Between 24 and 28 weeks' gestation, approximately 50 percent of NSTs are nonreactive.[104] Fifteen percent of NSTs remain nonreactive between 28 and 32 weeks.[105,106] After 32 weeks, the incidences of reactive and nonreactive tests are comparable to those seen at term. In summary, when accelerations of the baseline heart rate are seen during monitoring in the late second and early third trimesters, the NST has been associated with fetal well-being.

Before 27 weeks' gestation, the normal fetal heart rate response to fetal movement may in fact be a bradycardia.[107] However, in some settings such as IUGR associated with antiphospholipid syndrome, bradycardia at a gestational age of 26 to 28 weeks may be a predictor of fetal compromise and impending fetal death. Druzin et al.[108] reported three cases in which antenatal steroid administration and elective premature delivery led to good perinatal outcome. In these challenging cases, the entire clinical situation needs to be evaluated, and a full discussion with the patient, including neonatal consultation, should be initiated prior to intervention and delivery of the very preterm fetus exhibiting fetal heart rate decelerations.

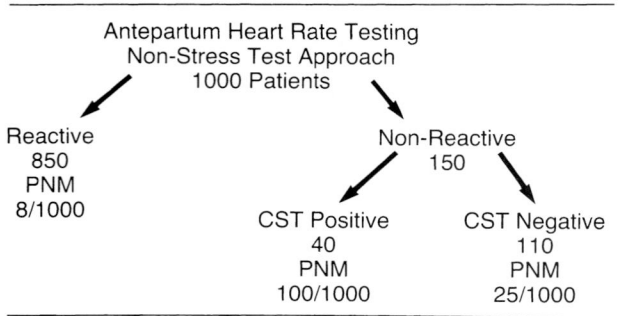

Figure 12-8. Results of nonstress testing in 1,000 high-risk patients. In general, 85 percent of the NSTs will be reactive and 15 percent nonreactive. Of those patients with a nonreactive NST, approximately 25 percent will have a positive CST on further evaluation. The highest perinatal mortality (PNM) will be observed in patients with a nonreactive NST and positive CST. Patients with a nonreactive NST and negative CST will have a perinatal mortality rate higher than that found in patients whose NST is initially reactive. (PNM rates based on data from Evertson et al.[99])

When nonreactive, the NST is extended in an attempt to separate the fetus in a period of prolonged quiet sleep from those who are hypoxemic or asphyxiated.[109-111] In three studies, approximately 3 percent of fetuses tested remained nonreactive after 80 to 90 minutes of evaluation. Brown and Patrick[109] noted that all NSTs that were to become reactive did so by 80 minutes or remained nonreactive for up to 120 minutes. Two stillbirths and one neonatal death occurred in seven cases with prolonged absence of reactivity. The mean arterial cord pH at delivery in this group was 6.95! In 27 pregnancies in which the fetus failed to exhibit accelerations during 80 minutes of monitoring, Leveno et al.[110] reported 11 perinatal deaths. In this study, IUGR was documented in 74 percent of cases, oligohydramnios in 81 percent, fetal acidosis in 41 percent, meconium staining of the amniotic fluid in 30 percent, and placental infarction in 93 percent. Therefore, if the NST is extended and a persistent absence of reactivity is observed, the fetus is likely to be severely compromised.

Vibroacoustic stimulation (VAS) may be utilized to change fetal state from quiet to active sleep and shorten the length of the NST (Fig. 12–9). Most studies have employed an electronic artificial larynx that generates sound pressure levels measured at 1 m in air of 82 dB with a frequency of 80 Hz and a harmonic of 20 to 9,000 Hz.[112] Whether it is the acoustic or vibratory component of this stimulus that alters fetal state is unclear. Gagnon et al.[113] reported that a low-frequency vibratory stimulus applied at term changed fetal state within 3 minutes and was associated with an immediate and sustained increase in long-term fetal heart rate variability, heart rate accelerations, and gross fetal body movements. VAS may produce a significant increase in the mean duration of heart rate accelerations, the mean amplitude of accelerations, and the total time spent in accelerations.[114] Using VAS, the incidence of nonreactive NSTs was reduced from 12.6 to 6.1 percent in a retrospective study and from 14 to 9 percent in a prospective investigation.[115,116] A reactive NST after VAS stimulation appears to be as reliable an index of fetal well-being as spontaneous reactivity. However, those fetuses that remain nonreactive even after VAS may be at increased risk for poor perinatal outcome.[117] Intrapartum fetal distress, growth restriction, and low Apgar scores were increased in fetuses that were nonreactive after acoustic stimulation.[118] Auditory brain stem response appears to be functional in the fetus at 26 to 28 weeks' gestation.[117] VAS significantly increases the incidence of reactive NSTs after 26 weeks' gestation.[119]

In most centers that use VAS, the baseline fetal heart rate is first observed for 5 minutes.[112] If the pattern is nonreactive, a stimulus of 3 seconds or less is applied near the fetal head. If the NST remains nonreactive, the stimulus is repeated at 1-minute intervals up to three times. If there continues to be no response to VAS, further evaluation should be carried out with a BPP or CST. In summary, VAS may be helpful in shortening the time required to perform an NST and may be especially useful in centers where large numbers of NSTs are done.

Could the sound generated by an electronic artificial larynx damage the fetal ear? Using intrauterine microphones, Smith and colleagues[120] documented baseline intrauterine sound levels of up to 88 dB during labor. Transabdominal stimulation with an electronic artificial larynx increased these levels minimally, up to 91 to

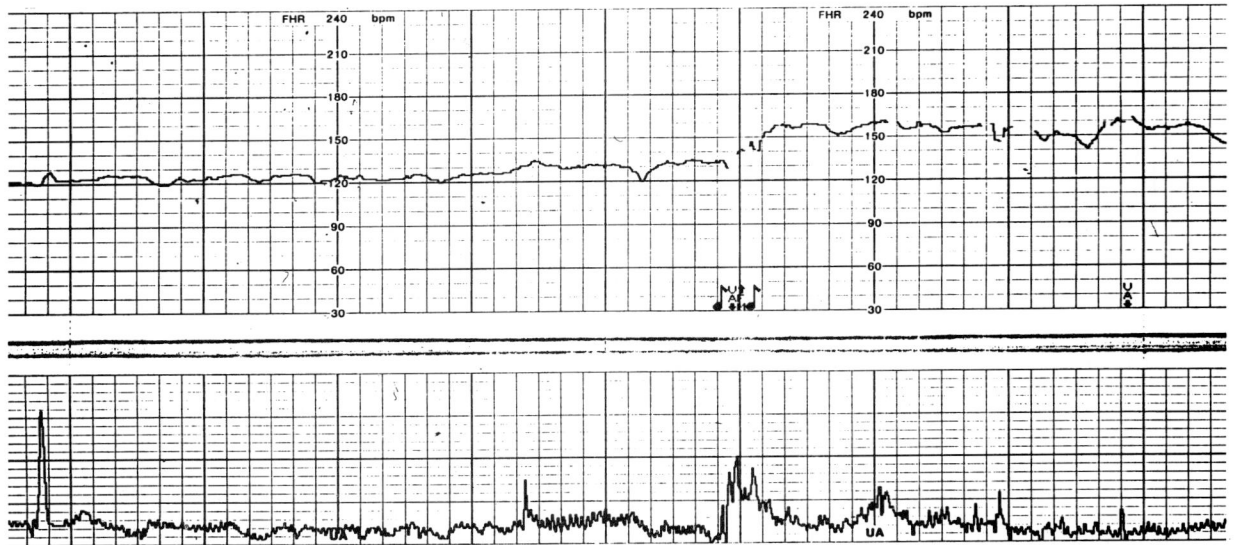

Figure 12–9. Reactive NST after VAS. The stimulus was applied in panel 54042 at the point marked by the musical notes. A sustained fetal heart rate acceleration was produced.

111 dB. Sound vibrations and intensity are attenuated by amniotic fluid.[121] Therefore, a 90-dB sound pressure produced by VAS in air results in exposure of the fetal ear to the equivalent of 40 dB, the level of normal conversation at about 3 feet. Arulkumaran et al.[121] concluded that intrauterine sound levels from VAS were not hazardous to the fetal ear. Two studies have confirmed the safety of VAS use during pregnancy with no long-term evidence of hearing loss in children followed in the neonatal period and up to 4 years of age.[122,123]

Significant fetal heart rate bradycardias have been observed in 1 to 2 percent of all NSTs.[124–129] Druzin et al.[124] defined such bradycardias as a fetal heart rate of 90 bpm or a fall in the fetal heart rate of 40 bpm below the baseline for 1 minute or longer (Fig. 12–10). This definition has been most widely applied. In a review of 121 cases, bradycardia was associated with increased perinatal morbidity and mortality, particularly antepartum fetal death, cord compression, IUGR, and fetal malformations.[130] Although about one half of the NSTs associated with bradycardia were reactive, the incidence of a nonreassuring fetal heart rate pattern in labor leading to emergency delivery in this group was identical to that of patients exhibiting nonreactive NSTs. Clinical management decisions should be based on the finding of bradycardia, *not* on the presence or absence of reactivity. Bradycardia has a higher positive predictive value for fetal compromise (fetal death or fetal intolerance of labor) than does the nonreactive NST. In this setting, antepartum fetal death is most likely because of a cord accident.[124,128,129]

If a bradycardia is observed, an ultrasound examination should be performed to assess amniotic fluid volume and to detect the presence of anomalies such as renal agenesis. Expectant management in the setting of a bradycardia has been associated with a perinatal mortality rate of 25 percent. Several reports have therefore recommended that delivery be undertaken if the fetus is mature. When the fetus is premature, one might elect to administer corticosteroids to accelerate fetal lung maturation before delivery. Continuous fetal heart rate monitoring is necessary if expectant management is followed.

In most cases, mild variable decelerations are not associated with poor perinatal outcome. Meis et al.[131] reported that variable decelerations of 20 bpm or more below the baseline heart rate but lasting less than 10 seconds were noted in 50.7 percent of patients having an NST. Whereas these decelerations were more often associated with a nuchal cord, they were not predictive of IUGR or a nonreassuring fetal heart rate pattern, or more severe variable decelerations during labor. Phelan[112] has added, however, that when mild variable decelerations are observed, even if the NST is reactive, an ultrasound examination should be done to rule out oligohydramnios. A low amniotic fluid index and mild variable decelerations increase the likelihood of a cord accident.

In selected high-risk pregnancies, the false-negative rate associated with a weekly NST may be unacceptably high.[132,133] Boehm et al.[134] reported a reduction in the fetal death rate in their high-risk population from 6.1 to 1.9 per 1,000 when the frequency of the NST was increased from once to twice weekly. Barrett et al.[132] have emphasized that in pregnancies complicated by IUGR and diabetes mellitus, twice-weekly testing should be utilized. In reviewing the literature, they noted that the fetal death rate within 1 week after a

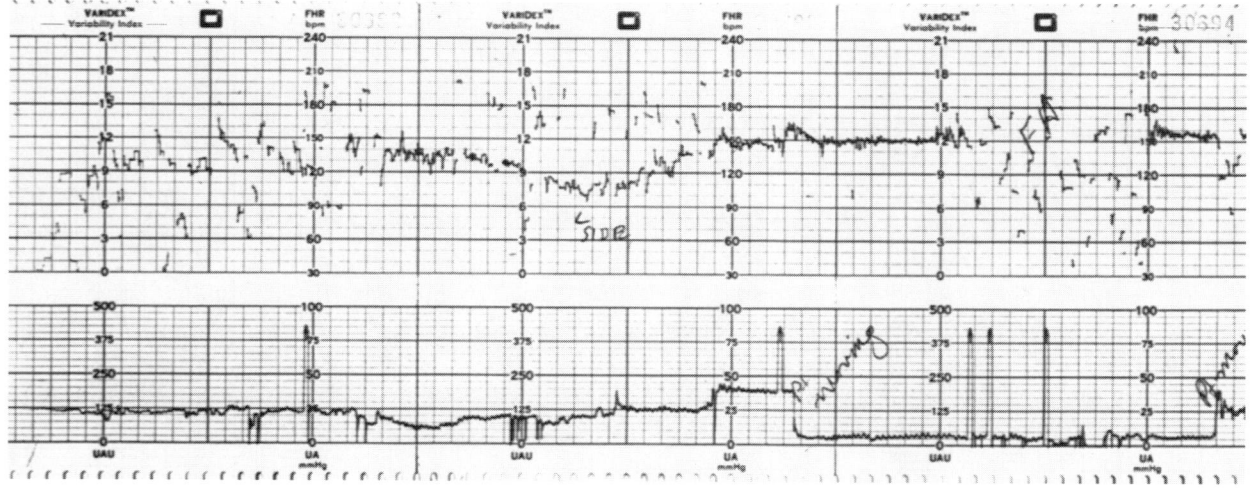

Figure 12–10. A NST in this primigravid patient of 43 weeks' gestation reveals a spontaneous bradycardia (panel 30692). The fetal heart rate has fallen from a baseline of 150 to 100 bpm. Upon induction of labor, the patient required cesarean delivery for fetal distress associated with severe variable decelerations. The amniotic fluid was decreased in amount and was meconium stained.

nonreactive NST was significantly increased in both diabetes mellitus (14 per 1,000) and IUGR (20 per 1,000). Miyazaki and Miyazaki,[135] reported an 8 percent false-negative rate in 125 prolonged gestations evaluated with the NST. In the prolonged pregnancy and IUGR, oligohydramnios may occur, leading to cord compression and fetal demise. The assessment of amniotic fluid volume has clearly proved important in such cases. Barss and co-workers[136] reviewed the incidence of stillbirths within 1 week of a reactive test in patients with a prolonged gestation. For the general high-risk population, a false-negative rate of 2.7 per 1,000 was reported. Although the incidence in pregnancies complicated by a prolonged gestation was not higher (2.8 per 1,000), Barss et al.[136] noted that even this low rate can be considered excessively high in view of the fact that these fetuses are otherwise normal and mature. In summary, it appears that the frequency of the NST should be increased to *twice* weekly in pregnancies complicated by diabetes mellitus, prolonged gestation, and IUGR.[134]

Which antepartum heart rate test is best? The NST has proved to be an ideal screening test and remains the primary method for antepartum fetal evaluation at most centers. It can be quickly performed in an outpatient setting and is easily interpreted. In contrast, the CST is usually performed near the labor and delivery suite, may require an intravenous infusion of oxytocin, and may be more difficult to interpret. In initial studies, a reactive NST appeared to be as predictive of good outcome as a negative CST. Nevertheless, as more data have been gathered, it appears that the ability of the CST to stress the fetus and evaluate its response to intermittent interruptions in intervillous blood flow provides an earlier warning of fetal compromise. Murata et al.[137] found that, in the dying fetal rhesus monkey, the fetal pH at which late decelerations appear is significantly higher (7.32) than the pH at which fetal heart rate accelerations disappear (7.22). In a large collaborative project in which 1,542 patients were evaluated primarily with the NST and 4,626 with the CST, Freeman et al.[138] observed that the corrected perinatal mortality associated with a reactive NST, 3.2 per 1,000, was significantly higher than that observed with a negative CST, 1.4 per 1,000. Whereas both fetal death rates are extremely low for a high-risk population, that associated with the CST is clearly better.

The healthy fetus should exhibit a reactive baseline heart rate with no late decelerations when a CST is performed. However, as the fetus deteriorates, one will first observe late decelerations, and, finally, the most ominous fetal heart rate pattern, the nonreactive NST and positive CST[72,78,139] (Fig. 12–5). When a nonreactive NST is followed by a positive CST, the incidence of perinatal mortality has been approximately 10 percent, a nonreassuring fetal heart rate pattern has occurred in most laboring patients, and IUGR has been reported in 25 percent of cases. The unusual combination of a reactive NST and a positive CST has been associated with a higher incidence of IUGR and late decelerations in labor than that seen with a negative CST.[140] The likelihood of fetal death is increased in patients demonstrating a nonreactive NST followed by a negative CST.[73,141,142] Consequently, repeating the NST in 24 hours appears the prudent course in such cases (Fig. 12–11).

Finally, arguments about the "best test" are counterproductive. Each test has its strengths and weaknesses, and a thorough understanding of the nature of the antepartum test, taking into consideration its advantages and disadvantages, is essential. The type of test and its application should be "condition" or diagnosis specific in which a similar basic screening approach is used, adding different types of evaluation and increased

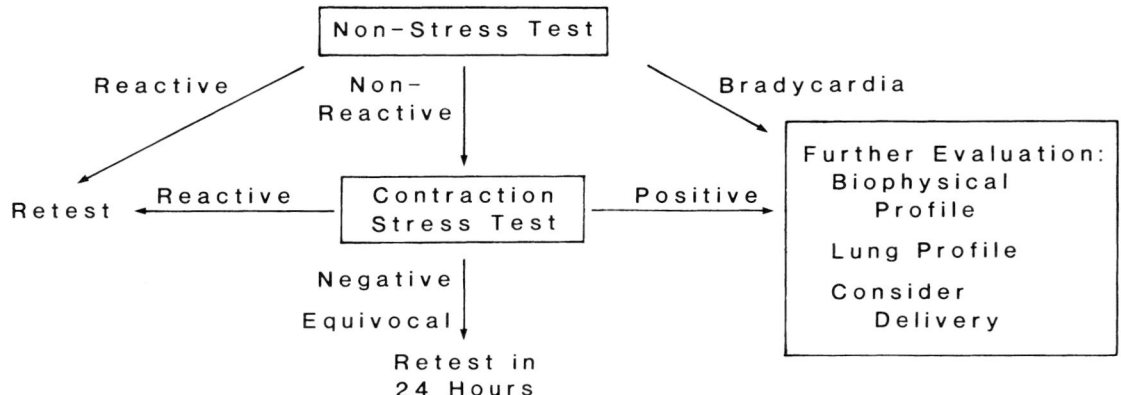

Figure 12–11. A branched testing scheme using the NST, CST, and BPP. Delivery is considered when the NST is nonreactive and the CST is positive. Delivery is also considered when a bradycardia is observed during the NST. The fetal BPP may be used to decrease the incidence of unnecessary premature intervention.

frequency of testing as appropriate for the clinical situation.

Fetal Biophysical Profile

The use of real-time ultrasonography to assess antepartum fetal condition has enabled the obstetrician to perform an in utero physical examination and evaluate dynamic functions reflecting the integrity of the fetal CNS.[143] As emphasized by Manning et al.,[144] "fetal biophysical scoring rests on the principle that the more complete the examination of the fetus, its activities, and its environment, the more accurate may be the differentiation of fetal health from disease states."

Fetal breathing movements were the first biophysical parameter to be assessed using real-time ultrasonography. It is thought that the fetus exercises its breathing muscles in utero in preparation for postdelivery respiratory function. With real-time ultrasonography, fetal breathing movement (FBM) is evidenced by downward movement of the diaphragm and abdominal contents and by an inward collapsing of the chest. Fetal breathing movements become regular at 20 to 21 weeks and are controlled by centers on the ventral surface of the fourth ventricle of the fetus.[145] They are observed approximately 30 percent of the time, are seen more often during REM sleep, and, when present, demonstrate intact neurologic control. Although the absence of FBMs may reflect fetal asphyxia, this finding may also indicate that the fetus is in a period of quiet sleep.[39,40]

Several factors other than fetal state and hypoxia can influence the presence of FBM. As maternal glucose levels rise, FBM becomes more frequent, and, during periods of maternal hypoglycemia, FBM decreases. Maternal smoking will also reduce FBM, probably as a result of fetal hypoxemia.[146] Narcotics that depress the fetal CNS will also decrease FBM.

Platt and colleagues[147] were among the first to examine the ability of FBM to predict perinatal outcome. Using real-time ultrasonography, they judged FBM to be present if at least one episode of FBM of at least 60 seconds' duration was observed within any 30-minute period of observation. Of 136 fetuses studied, 116 (85 percent) exhibited FBM. The incidence of fetal distress was significantly higher in fetuses without FBM, 60 percent (12 of 20), as was the incidence of low Apgar scores at 5 minutes, 50 percent (10 of 20). The comparable figures for fetuses demonstrating FBM were 3 percent (4 of 116) for a nonreassuring fetal heart rate pattern and 4 percent (5 of 116) for low Apgar scores.

Further research demonstrated that the evaluation of FBM could be used to distinguish the truly positive CST from a false-positive CST. Those fetuses that displayed FBM but had a positive CST were unlikely to exhibit fetal distress in labor. However, when a fetus failed to show FBM and demonstrated late decelerations during the CST, the likelihood of fetal compromise was great. A pattern emerged from these studies that as long as one antepartum biophysical test was normal, the likelihood that the fetus would have a normal outcome was high.[148,149] As the number of abnormal tests increased, however, the likelihood that fetal asphyxia was present increased as well.

Using these principles, Manning et al.[150] developed the concept of the fetal BPP score. These workers elected to combine the NST with four parameters that could be assessed using real-time ultrasonography: FBM, fetal movement, fetal tone, and amniotic fluid volume. FBM, fetal movement, and fetal tone are mediated by complex neurologic pathways and should reflect the function of the fetal CNS at the time of the examination. On the other hand, amniotic fluid volume should provide information about the presence of chronic fetal asphyxia. Finally, the ultrasound examination performed for the BPP has the added advantage of detecting previously unrecognized major fetal anomalies.

Vintzileos et al.[145] stressed that those fetal biophysical activities that are present earliest in fetal development are the last to disappear with fetal hypoxia. The fetal tone center in the cortex begins to function at 7.5 to 8.5 weeks. Fetal tone would therefore be the last fetal parameter to be lost with worsening fetal condition. The fetal movement center in the cortex-nuclei is functional at 9 weeks and would be more sensitive than fetal tone. As noted above, FBM becomes regular at 20 to 21 weeks. Finally, fetal heart rate control, residing within the posterior hypothalamus and medulla, becomes functional at the end of the second trimester and early in the third trimester. An alteration in fetal heart rate would theoretically be the earliest sign of fetal compromise.

A BPP score was developed that is similar to the Apgar score used to assess the condition of the newborn.[150] The presence of a normal parameter, such as a reactive NST, was awarded 2 points, whereas the absence of that parameter was scored as 0. The highest score a fetus can receive is 10, and the lowest score is 0. The BPP may be used as early as 26 to 28 weeks' gestation. The time required for the fetus to achieve a satisfactory BPP score is closely related to fetal state, with an average of only 5 minutes if the fetus is in a 2F state but over 25 minutes if it is in a 1F state.[151] Twice-weekly testing is recommended in pregnancies complicated by IUGR, diabetes mellitus, prolonged gestation, and hypertension with proteinuria. The criteria proposed by Manning et al.,[150] and the clinical actions recommended in response to these scores, are presented in Tables 12–5 and 12–6. Regardless of a low score on the BPP, Manning et al. have emphasized that vagi-

Table 12–5. TECHNIQUE OF BIOPHYSICAL PROFILE SCORING

Biophysical Variable	Normal (Score = 2)	Abnormal (Score = 0)
Fetal breathing movements	At least one episode of >30 seconds' duration in 30 minutes' observation	Absent or no episode of ≥30 seconds' duration in 30 minutes
Gross body movement	At least three discrete body/limb movements in 30 minutes (episodes of active continuous movement considered a single movement)	Up to two episodes of body/limb movements in 30 minutes
Fetal tone	At least one episode of active extension with return to flexion of fetal limb(s) or trunk; opening and closing of hand considered normal tone	Either slow extension with return to partial flexion or movement of limb in full extension or absent fetal movement
Reactive fetal heart rate	At least two episodes of acceleration of ≥15 bpm and 15 seconds' duration associated with fetal movement in 30 minutes	Fewer than two accelerations or acceleration <15 bpm in 30 minutes
Qualitative amniotic fluid volume	At least one pocket of amniotic fluid measuring 2 cm in two perpendicular planes	Either no amniotic fluid pockets or a pocket <2 cm in two perpendicular planes

Adapted from Manning FA: Biophysical profile scoring. *In* Nijhuis J (ed): Fetal Behaviour. New York, Oxford University Press, 1992, p 241.

nal delivery is attempted if other obstetric factors are favorable.

In a prospective blinded study of 216 high-risk patients, Manning and colleagues[150] found no perinatal deaths when all five variables described above were normal, but a perinatal mortality rate of 60 percent in fetuses with a score of zero. Fetal deaths were increased 14-fold with the absence of fetal movement, and the perinatal mortality rate was increased 18-fold if FBM was absent. Any single test was associated with a significant false-positive rate ranging from 50 to 79 percent. However, combining abnormal variables significantly decreased the false-positive rate to as low as 20 percent. The false-negative rate, that is, the incidence of babies who were compromised but who had normal testing, was quite low, ranging from a perinatal mortality rate of 6.9 per 1,000 for infants with normal amniotic fluid volume to 12.8 per 1,000 for fetuses demonstrating a reactive NST. These investigators found that,

in most cases, the ultrasound-derived BPP parameters and NST could be completed within a relatively short time, each requiring approximately 10 minutes.

Manning et al.[152] have presented their experience with 26,780 high-risk pregnancies followed with the BPP. In Manning et al.'s protocol, a routine NST is not performed if all of the ultrasound parameters are found to be normal for a score of 8.[153] An NST is performed when one ultrasound finding is abnormal. The corrected PMR in this series was 1.9 per 1,000, with less than 1 fetal death per 1,000 patients within 1 week of a normal profile. Of all patients tested, almost 97 percent had a score of 8, which means that only 3 percent required further evaluation for scores of 6 or less. In a study of 525 patients with scores of 6 or less, poor perinatal outcome was most often associated with either a nonreactive NST and absent fetal tone or a nonreactive NST and absent FBM.[154] A significant inverse linear relationship was observed between the last BPP

Table 12–6. MANAGEMENT BASED ON BIOPHYSICAL PROFILE

Score	Interpretation	Management
10	Normal infant; low risk of chronic asphyxia	Repeat testing at weekly intervals; repeat twice weekly in diabetic patients and patients at ≥41 weeks' gestation
8	Normal infant; low risk of chronic asphyxia	Repeat testing at weekly intervals; repeat testing twice weekly in diabetics and patients at ≥41 weeks' gestation; oligohydramnios is an indication for delivery
6	Suspect chronic asphyxia	If ≥36 weeks' gestation and conditions are favorable, deliver; if at >36 weeks and L/S <2.0, repeat test in 4–6 hours; deliver if oligohydramnios is present
4	Suspect chronic asphyxia	If ≥36 weeks' gestation, deliver; if <32 weeks' gestation, repeat score
0–2	Strongly suspect chronic asphyxia	Extend testing time to 120 minutes; if persistent score ≤4, deliver, regardless of gestational age

Adapted from Manning FA, Harman CR, Morrison I, et al: Fetal assessment based on fetal biophysical profile scoring. Am J Obstet Gynecol 162:703, 1990; and Manning FA: Biophysical profile scoring. *In* Nijhuis J (ed): Fetal Behaviour. New York, Oxford University Press, 1992, p 241.

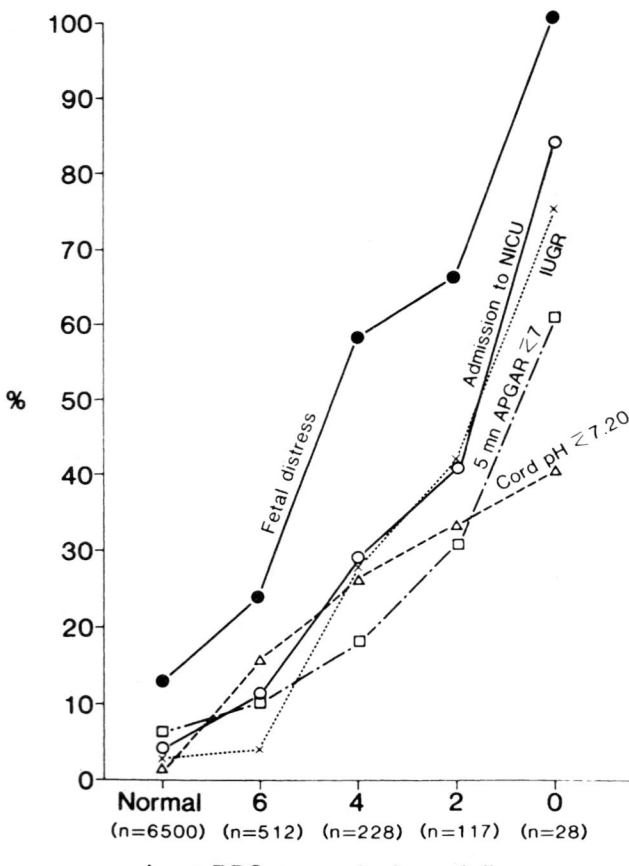

Figure 12–12. The relationship between five indices of perinatal morbidity and last biophysical profile score before delivery. A significant inverse linear correlation is observed for each variable. (From Manning FA, Harman CR, Morrison I, et al: Fetal assessment based on fetal biophysical profile scoring. Am J Obstet Gynecol 162:703, 1990, with permission.)

Recent studies have demonstrated that antenatal corticosteroid administration may have an effect on the BPP, decreasing the profile score. Because corticosteroids are used in cases of anticipated premature delivery (24 to 34 weeks), any false-positives on biophysical testing may lead to inappropriate intervention and delivery. Kelly et al. reported that BPP scores were decreased in more than one third of the fetuses tested at 28 to 34 weeks' gestation. This effect was seen within 48 hours of corticosteroid administration. Neonatal outcome was not affected. Repeat BPPs within 24 to 48 hours were normal in cases in which the BPP score had decreased by 4 points. The most commonly affected variables were FBM and the NST.[157] Similarly Deren et al.[158] and Rotmensch et al.[159] reported transient suppression of FBM, fetal body movements, and heart rate reactivity following corticosteroid administration at less than 34 weeks' gestation. These changes were transient and returned to normal by 48 to 96 hours after corticosteroid treatment. This effect must be considered at institutions where daily BPPs are used to evaluate the

score and both perinatal morbidity and mortality (Figs. 12–12 and 12–13).[152] The false-positive rate, depending on the endpoint used, ranges from 75 percent for a score of 6 to less than 20 percent for a score of 0. Manning[155] has summarized the data reported in eight investigations using the BPP for fetal evaluation. Overall, 23,780 patients and 54,337 tests were reviewed. The corrected perinatal mortality rate, excluding lethal anomalies, was 0.77 per 1,000.

The BPP correlates well with fetal acid–base status. Vintzileos et al.[156] studied 124 patients undergoing cesarean birth *before* the onset of labor. Deliveries were undertaken for severe preeclampsia, elective repeat cesarean section, growth restriction, breech presentation, placenta previa, and fetal macrosomia. Acidosis was defined as an umbilical cord arterial pH less than 7.20. The earliest manifestations of fetal acidosis were a nonreactive NST and loss of FBM. With scores of 8 or more, the mean arterial pH was 7.28, and only 2 of 102 fetuses were acidotic. Nine fetuses with scores of 4 or less had a mean pH of 6.99, and all were acidotic.

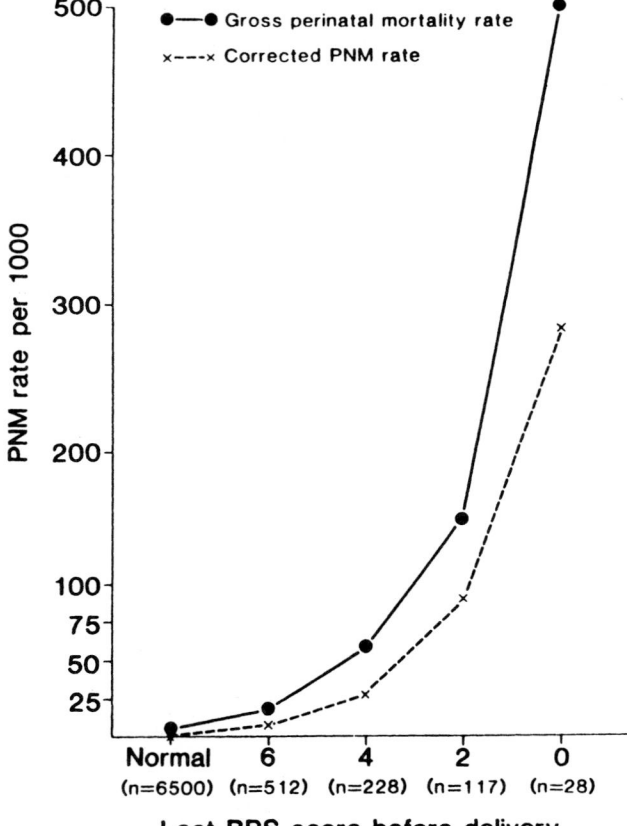

Figure 12–13. The relationship between perinatal mortality, both total and corrected for major anomalies, and the last BPP score before delivery. A highly significant inverse and exponential relationship is observed. (From Manning FA, Harman CR, Morrison I, et al: Fetal assessment based on fetal biophysical profile scoring. Am J Obstet Gynecol 162:703, 1990, with permission.)

fetus in cases of preterm labor or preterm premature rupture of the membranes.

There has been some controversy concerning the utility of the BPP in predicting chorioamnionitis in pregnancies complicated by preterm labor or preterm premature rupture of the membranes. Sherer et al.[160] reported that the absence of FBM is associated with histologic evidence of fetal inflammation and intrauterine infection in patients with preterm labor and intact membranes before 32 weeks' gestation. However, they recommend that this finding not be used to guide clinical management because of the low positive predictive value of absent FBM. Lewis et al.[161] performed a randomized trial of daily NSTs versus BPP in the management of preterm premature rupture of the membranes. They concluded that neither daily NSTs nor BPPs had high sensitivity in predicting infectious complications in these patients. Daily BPPs increased cost without apparent benefit.

Manning et al. have described the correlation between biophysical scoring and the incidence of cerebral palsy in Manitoba. In patients referred for a BPP, there was an inverse, exponential, and highly significant relationship between last BPP score and the incidence of cerebral palsy. Scores of 6 or less had a sensitivity of 49 percent. The more abnormal the last BPP, the greater the risk of cerebral palsy. Gestational age, birth weight, or assumed timing of the injury were not related to the incidence of cerebral palsy. The incidence of cerebral palsy ranged from 0.7 per 1,000 live births, for a normal BPP score; to 13.1 per 1,000 live births, for a score of 6; and 333 per 1,000 live births, for a score of 0.[162]

Is an NST needed if all ultrasound parameters of the BPP are normal? Prospective and blinded studies by Platt et al.[163] and Manning et al.[164] using both the BPP and NST have demonstrated that each of these tests is a valuable predictor of normal outcome. In the experience of Manning et al., an NST was needed in less than 5 percent of tests. As emphasized by Eden et al.,[165] however, the NST will allow the detection of fetal heart rate decelerations. In the presence of reduced amniotic fluid, these decelerations may be associated with a cord accident. Eden et al. reported that when spontaneous fetal heart rate decelerations lasting at least 30 seconds with a decrease of at least 15 bpm are seen in the presence of normal amniotic fluid, there is an increased likelihood of late decelerations in labor and cesarean delivery for fetal distress.

Several drawbacks of the BPP should be considered. Unlike the NST and CST, an ultrasound machine is required, and, unless the BPP is videotaped, it cannot be reviewed. If the fetus is in a quiet sleep state, the BPP can require a long period of observation. The present scoring system does not consider the impact of hydramnios. In a pregnancy complicated by diabetes mellitus, the presence of excessive amniotic fluid is of great concern.

The false-positive (false-abnormal) rate of a particular test has always been of concern because of the possibility of unnecessary intervention (usually delivery) and subsequent iatrogenic complications. The BPP was developed in part to address the issue of the high false-abnormal rate of the CST and the NST. There has been little attention paid to the possible false-positive rate of the abnormal or equivocal BPP. This is particularly relevant because the BPP is most commonly used as the final backup test in the NST and CST sequence of testing and is critically important when dealing with the premature fetus. As noted above, the false-positive rate of a score of 0 is less than 20 percent, but for a score of 6 is up to 75 percent. Inglis et al.[166] used VAS to define fetal condition with BPP scores of 6 or less in 81 patients at 28 to 42 weeks. Obstetric and neonatal outcomes of 41 patients whose score improved to normal after VAS were compared with those of 238 patients who had normal scores without VAS. The obstetric and neonatal outcomes were not significantly different between the two groups. VAS improved the BPP in about 80 percent of cases. Use of VAS for an equivocal BPP did not increase the false-negative rate and may reduce the likelihood of unnecessary obstetric intervention.[166]

DOPPLER ULTRASOUND

With the introduction of Doppler ultrasound, noninvasive assessment of the fetal, maternal, and placental circulations became possible. Evaluation of blood flow in the fetus and placenta had previously entailed such invasive procedures as injection of radioactive microspheres or direct application of transducers, with the potential of jeopardy to the fetus and mother. Investigators could now examine the association of changes in umbilical blood flow with fetal morbidity in the ongoing human pregnancy.

The Doppler principle is based on changes in the frequency of sound (or light) produced by a changing relationship between two objects. The frequency of sound produced by an object moving away from an observer is perceived as lower than the same frequency of sound produced by an object moving toward the observer.[167] A common example of this is the sound of a train horn as it moves toward, then past and away from the listener. Ultrasound waves beamed with a particular frequency will return to a receiver at a lower frequency when the target is moving away from the transducer, and at a higher frequency when the target is moving towards the transducer. The speed and direc-

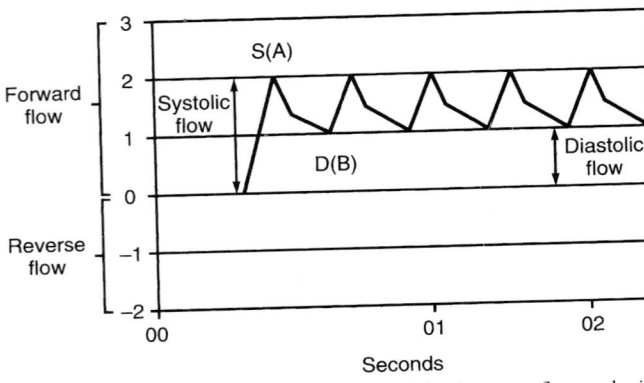

Figure 12–14. Diagram of a normal umbilical artery flow velocity waveform. Note the forward flow during both systole and diastole, the latter indicating low resistance in the placental bed. (Adapted from Warsof SL, Levy DL: Doppler blood flow and fetal growth retardation. *In* Gross TL, Sokol RJ (ed): Intrauterine Growth Retardation, A Practical Approach. Chicago, Year Book, 1989, p 158.)

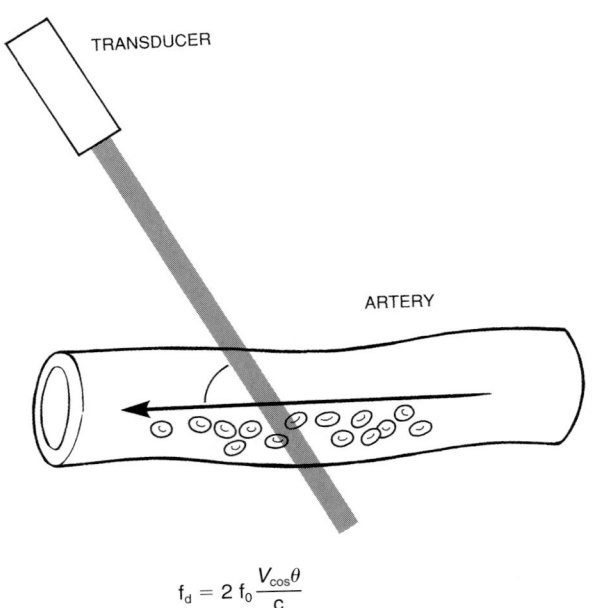

$$f_d = 2\, f_0 \frac{V\cos\theta}{c}$$

Figure 12–16. Application of the Doppler principle to determine blood flow velocity. The frequency (f_0) of the ultrasound beam directed at a moving column of red blood cells with velocity V will be increased to f_d in proportion to V and the cosine of the angle of intersection of the vessel by the beam (θ).

tion of moving red blood cells have been investigated using this information, and converting it into waveforms interpretable by the human eye and ear. By convention, information received from objects moving away from the transducer is recorded below a zero line, and information received from objects moving toward the transducer is recorded above a zero line (Figs. 12–14 and 12–15). The frequency of the reflected sound is proportional to the velocity of the moving red blood cells. Information about blood flow velocity provides an indirect assessment of changes in blood flow. Calculation of flow velocity is derived from the equation

$$f_d = 2\, f_0 \frac{V_{\cos}\theta}{c},$$

where f_d is the change in ultrasound frequency or Doppler shift, f_0 is the transmitted frequency of the

ultrasound beam, V is the velocity of the red blood cells, θ is the angle between the beam and the direction of movement of the reflector or red blood cells, and c is the velocity of sound in the medium (Fig. 12–16). The speed of sound in tissues is 1,540 m/sec. The number 2 in the equation accounts for the time spent from the transmission of the sound signal at its origin to its return. Volume flow may be calculated by multiplying the mean velocity by the cross-sectional area of the vessel. Velocities are measured in meters per second.

The combination of real-time ultrasound imaging

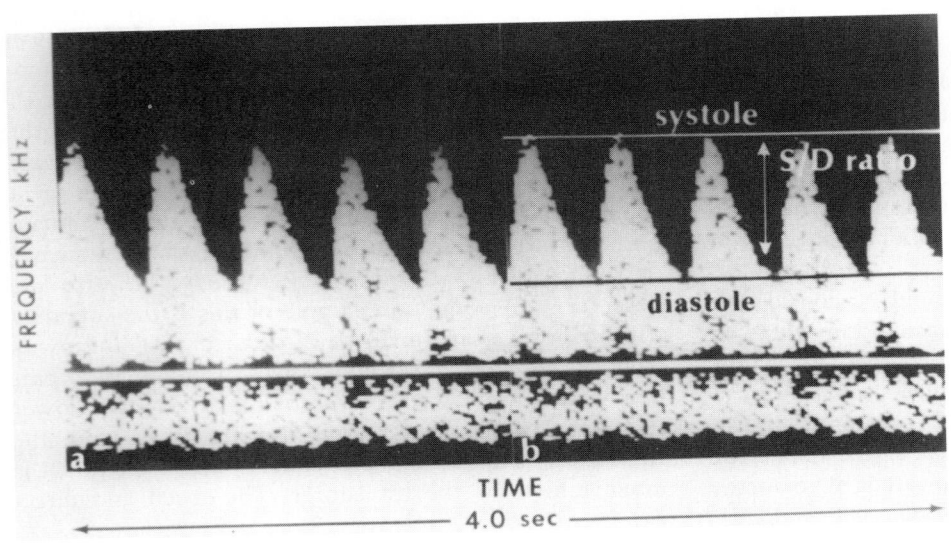

Figure 12–15. Doppler flow velocity waveforms of the normal umbilical artery. Note that umbilical arterial flow velocities are recorded above the baseline, whereas nonpulsatile umbilical vein flow in the opposite direction is found below the baseline (a). Measurement of the S/D ratio is also illustrated (b). (From Bruner JP, Gabbe SG, Levy DW, et al: Doppler ultrasonography of the umbilical cord in normal pregnancy. J South Med Assoc 86:52, 1993, with permission.)

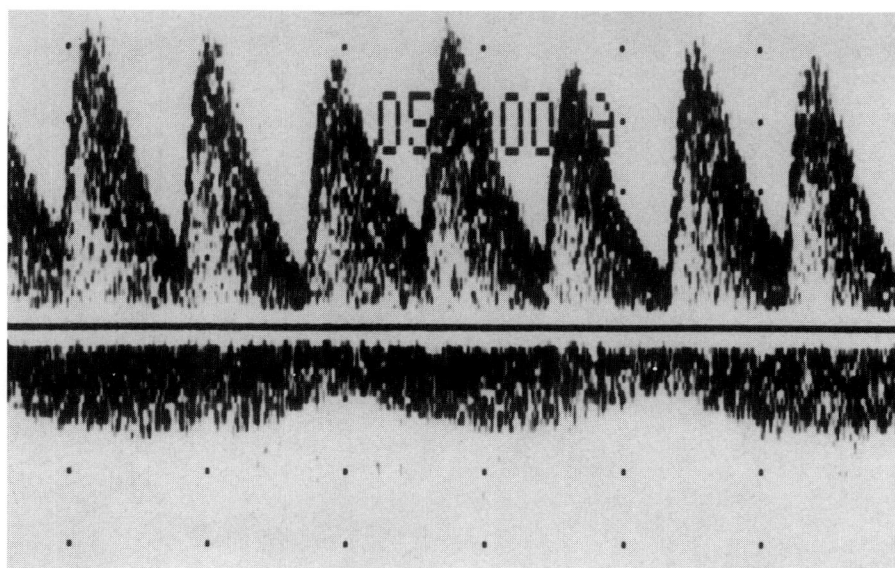

Figure 12–17. Umbilical arterial and venous Doppler flow velocity waveforms during an episode of fetal breathing. Venous velocities vary with every two to three arterial waveforms.

with pulsed wave Doppler allows the identification of a specific area or vessel for sampling. A vessel can be identified, and the ultrasound beam placed across that vessel using range gating. Ideally, the angle between the beam and the insonated vessel should less than 30 degrees. As the angle increases, large errors may be made in estimating flow velocity. Determinations of the volume of blood flow require accurate measurements of the diameter of the vessel studied in order to calculate its cross-sectional area. A small error in the measurement of the diameter can produce substantial errors in the determination of the volume of blood flow, since the radius is squared to calculate the area of the blood vessel. If blood flow is expressed in milliliters per kilogram per minute, fetal weight must be accurately estimated. Usually, a minimum of three to five waveforms is used to obtain measurements. In umbilical vessels, multiple sites are sampled.

Given the difficulty of estimating the angle between the Doppler ultrasound beam and the direction of blood flow in a particular vessel, a variety of angle-independent indices have been developed to characterize flow velocity waveforms produced. Indices rely on systolic, diastolic, and mean velocities. Systolic velocities are peak velocities that result from cardiac contraction. Diastolic velocities result from an interaction between peak flows, vessel compliance, heart rate, and the vascular impedance of the sites perfused. These indices do not measure the volume of blood flow. A commonly used index is the systolic (S)/diastolic (D) velocity ratio, the S/D ratio (Figs. 12–14 and 12–15). The pulsatility index is calculated as the systolic minus diastolic values divided by the mean of the velocity waveform (S–D/mean). An additional ratio, the resistance index, or Pourcelot ratio, is expressed as S–D/S. The latter two ratios are useful when the diastolic flow is absent or

reversed. Higher indices occur with relatively lower diastolic velocities that are thought to be the result of increased resistance or vascular impedance.[170]

Variations in umbilical artery blood flow occur during episodes of fetal breathing (Fig. 12–17).[171] Changes in abdominal and thoracic pressure that occur with fetal breathing produce changes in preload, stroke volume, and afterload. Variations in fetal heart rate may shorten or lengthen diastole, with changes in stroke volume and less or more time for diastolic run-off, resulting in subsequent changes in both systolic and diastolic velocities. Sites closer to the fetal abdomen have relatively higher diastolic velocities, and sites closer to the placenta have relatively lower diastolic velocities.[172] For these reasons, it is recommended that umbilical velocity studies be performed in midportions of the umbilical cord while fetuses are relatively quiet.

Values of normal umbilical artery flow velocity waveforms during pregnancy have been reported by many investigators (Fig. 12–18).[173,174] Prior to 15 weeks' gestation, diastolic flow is not consistently identified in the umbilical artery.[175] As the normal pregnancy progresses, there is proportionately more blood flow during diastole, and indices decrease. The normal decrease in umbilical artery velocity indices is consistent with a decrease in placental resistance with advancing gestational age.[176]

The main application of umbilical artery Doppler flow velocity measurements has been in the pregnancy at risk for or demonstrating IUGR (see Chapter 25).[177] Intrauterine growth restriction is seen more often in fetuses with umbilical artery velocity indices that are elevated for their gestational age.[178] In some cases, end-diastolic flow is absent or reversed (Figs. 12–19 and 12–20).

The association of umbilical artery flow velocity

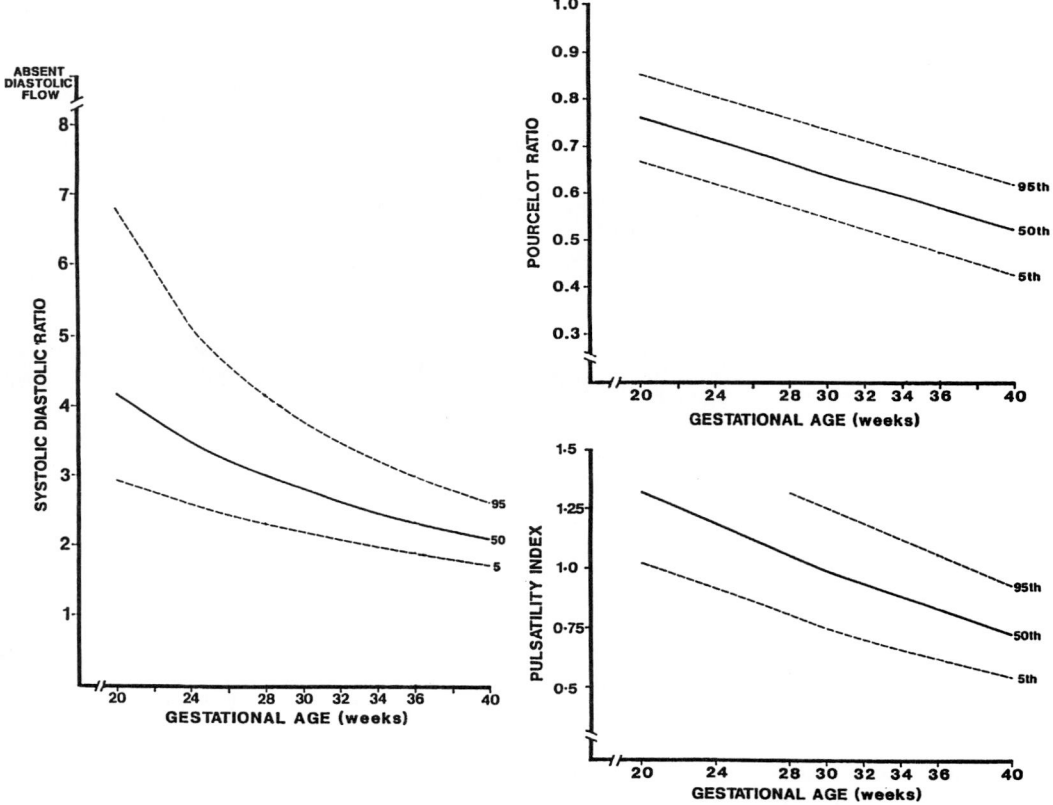

Figure 12–18. Normal ranges for the various indices used to quantify the flow velocity waveform patterns of the umbilical artery during pregnancy. (Derived from Thompson et al.[173])

waveform indices with alterations in placental blood flow was examined by Trudinger et al. in a sheep model.[179] The umbilical placental circulation was embolized with microspheres each day for 9 days in late gestation. The umbilical artery S/D ratio increased at 4 days, as did vascular resistance in the placental bed. The volume of umbilical blood flow did not fall significantly until the end of the study period. Using a similar

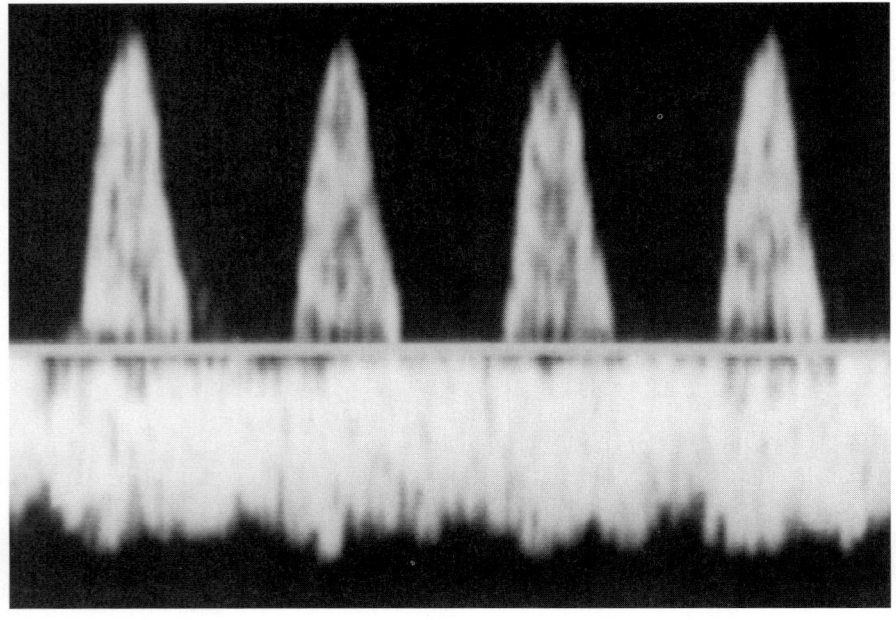

Figure 12–19. Umbilical arterial waveforms with absent end-diastolic velocities. In this case, venous velocities also demonstrate variation with the arterial waveforms.

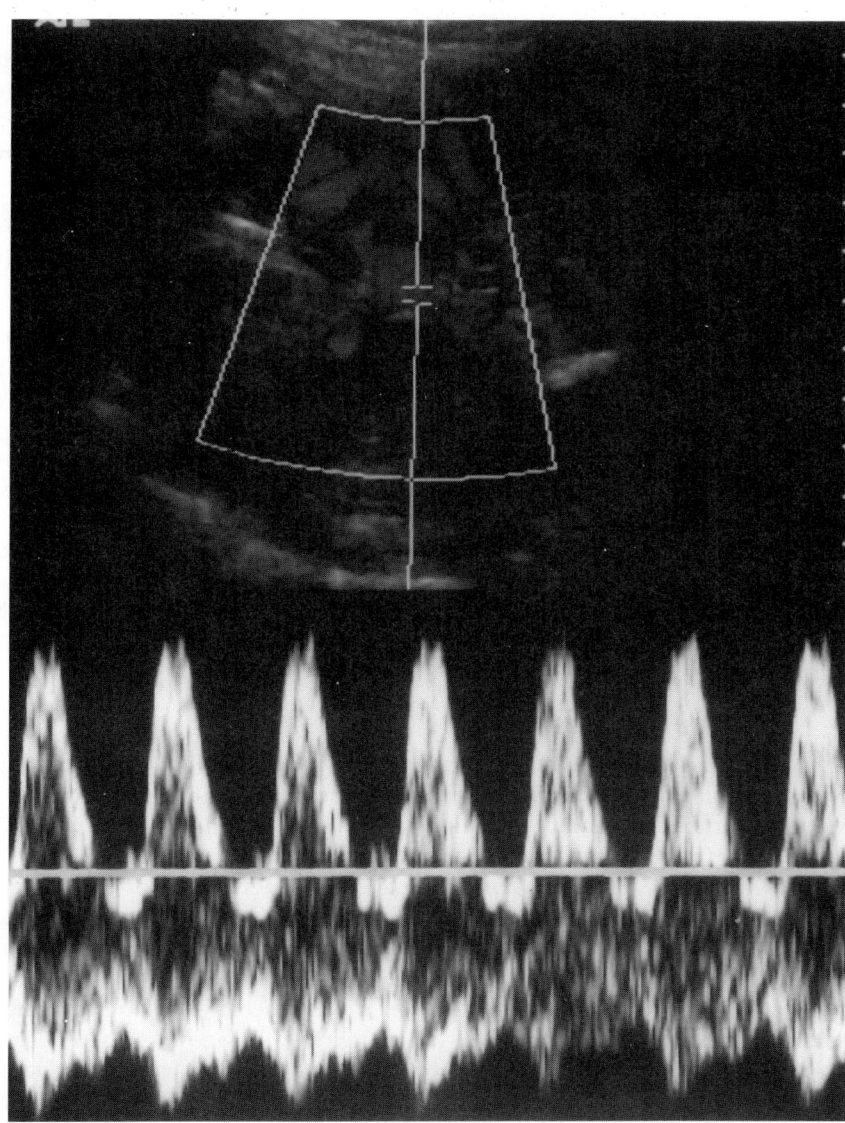

Figure 12–20. Umbilical arterial waveforms with reverse flow at end-diastole. Umbilical venous velocities have marked pulsations.

experimental model, Morrow and Ritchie,[180] reported a progressive increase in the S/D ratio leading to absent and then reversed diastolic flow. Hypoxia did not alter the S/D ratio, an observation also reported by Copel et al.[181] using a sheep model in which umbilical blood flow and S/D ratio were measured shortly after placental embolization. Copel et al. reported normal umbilical artery S/D ratios in the presence of fetal acidosis. Therefore, the umbilical artery S/D ratio more likely reflects placental vascular resistance than acute fetal hypoxemia.

The most extreme abnormalities in umbilical artery waveforms are those in which the velocities are absent or reversed.[183] Absence of end-diastolic velocities is associated with an increase in perinatal morbidity and mortality. Reverse flow is even more predictive of poor perinatal outcome than absent diastolic flow. In addi-

tion to an association with intrauterine growth restriction, markedly abnormal Doppler studies have been reported in fetuses with congenital malformations, including chromosomal abnormalities. Farine et al. summarized information from 31 studies with a total of 904 fetuses demonstrating absent or reversed end-diastolic velocities.[183] They found a perinatal mortality of 36 percent. Eighty percent of the fetuses were below the 10th percentile in weight for gestational age. Abnormal karyotypes were found in 6 percent, and malformations in 11 percent. The average duration from diagnosis to delivery ranged from 0 to 49 days, averaging 6 to 8 days. Absence or reversal of end-diastolic flow velocities in the umbilical artery, although not an indication for immediate delivery, is considered an indication for immediate and intensive ongoing fetal surveillance. Delivery is usually based on the results of fetal heart rate monitoring or the BPP, with consideration of maternal condition and gestational age.

Most Doppler ultrasound studies of the fetus have focused on the umbilical arterial circulation. Examination of the fetal venous circulation has allowed some refinement in our understanding of the normal fetal circulation as well as fetal well-being. Most commonly, the fetal umbilical venous blood flow is monophasic (Fig. 12–15). Fetuses with abnormal arterial velocities, or with abnormal cardiac function, may develop "pulsations" in the venous velocity waveform (Fig. 12–19).[184] These pulsations occur during late diastole, and can be distinguished from breathing changes produced during fetal breathing episodes by their regularity, persistence, and association with the fetal heart rate. Umbilical venous pulsations can be produced in fetal lambs by volume-loading the venous circulation, and are associated with increases in central venous pressure.[185] Serial studies of human fetuses with absent end-diastolic velocities in the umbilical artery showed that the development of umbilical venous pulsations was associated with a shorter time between diagnosis and delivery with the deliveries performed for abnormal fetal heart rate patterns.[186] Fetuses with abnormally high umbilical artery velocity indices have a higher perinatal morbidity and mortality if abnormal venous velocities also develop.[187] Umbilical venous pulsations have been demonstrated in fetuses with late decelerations, during the deceleration itself.[188] These findings suggest that fetuses with abnormal umbilical arterial velocities may develop higher central venous pressures and umbilical venous pulsations as their condition deteriorates. Furthermore, fetuses with abnormal cardiac function or cardiac failure may demonstrate umbilical venous velocity pulsations even when umbilical arterial velocities are normal. Prospective clinical studies utilizing umbilical venous velocities will be needed before the value of this parameter can be determined.

The effectiveness of umbilical artery Doppler studies as an antepartum fetal surveillance technique has been summarized in an editorial by Divon and Ferber, in which the results of several meta-analyses were reviewed.[182] A meta-analysis by Giles and Bisit of six published, peer-reviewed, randomized controlled, clinical trials showed a reduction in perinatal mortality in the 2,102 fetuses studied with Doppler compared with the 2,133 fetuses not evaluated with this technique.[189] An analysis of 12 published and unpublished randomized controlled clinical trials in 7,474 high-risk patients revealed fewer antenatal admissions, inductions of labor, cesarean deliveries for fetal distress, and perinatal mortality in high-risk pregnancies monitored with Doppler velocimetry.[190] A recent report by Neilson and Alfirevic confirmed these findings.[191] Divon and Ferber conclude that Doppler ultrasound is useful in high-risk pregnancies and will decrease perinatal mortality without increasing maternal or neonatal morbidity. Studies of low-risk pregnancies have not shown a benefit from the use of Doppler ultrasound.[192]

THE ASSESSMENT OF FETAL PULMONARY MATURATION

This section reviews those techniques that enable the obstetrician to predict accurately the risks of respiratory distress syndrome (RDS) for the infant requiring premature delivery and to avoid the unnecessary tragedy of iatrogenic prematurity.

RDS is caused by a deficiency of pulmonary surfactant, an antiatelectasis factor that is able to maintain a low stable surface tension at the air–water interface within alveoli. Surfactant decreases the pressure needed to distend the lung and prevents alveolar collapse (see Chapter 20). The type II alveolar cell is the major site of surfactant synthesis. Surfactant is packaged in lamellar bodies, discharged into the alveoli, and carried into the amniotic cavity with pulmonary fluid.

Phospholipids account for more than 80 percent of the surface active material within the lung, and more than 50 percent of this phospholipid is dipalmitoyl lecithin. The latter is a derivative of glycerol phosphate and contains two fatty acids as well as the nitrogenous base choline. Other phospholipids contained in the surfactant complex include phosphatidylglycerol (PG), phosphatidylinositol (PI), phosphatidylserine (PS), phosphatidylethanolamine (PE), sphingomyelin, and lysolecithin. PG is the second most abundant lipid in surfactant and significantly improves its properties.

An accurate assessment of gestational age and fetal maturity is essential before an elective induction of labor or cesarean delivery or before the delivery of a patient whose fetus may not have matured normally such as a growth-restricted fetus or the fetus of a poorly controlled diabetic mother. Many of the techniques used in clinical practice in the past not only failed to predict gestational age, but provided little information about fetal pulmonary maturation.[193]

Prior to the now-common practice of using ultrasound to establish gestational age and amniotic fluid studies to assess fetal pulmonary maturation, iatrogenic prematurity was an important clinical problem. In 1975, Goldenberg and Nelson[194] concluded that untimely or unwarranted intervention was responsible for 15 percent of their cases of RDS. In a similar study, Hack et al.[195] observed that 12 percent of all infants with RDS in their neonatal intensive care unit were born after elective deliveries. None of these infants had had documentation of pulmonary maturation before delivery.

Several changes in clinical practice appear to have decreased the incidence of RDS caused by iatrogenic prematurity. More patients who have had a previous low transverse cesarean delivery are attempting a vaginal birth. In such cases, since the onset of spontaneous labor is awaited, documentation of fetal pulmonary maturation prior to elective intervention is not required. Most importantly, ultrasound documentation of gestational age in the first trimester or early in the second trimester has proven extremely reliable in timing elective inductions or cesarean deliveries (see Chapter 10).

Assessment of Fetal Pulmonary Maturity

Available methods for evaluating fetal pulmonary maturity can be divided into three categories: (1) quantitation of pulmonary surfactant, such as the lecithin/sphingomyelin (L/S) ratio; (2) measurement of surfactant function including the shake test; and (3) evaluation of amniotic fluid turbidity.[196,197]

With the exception of amniotic fluid specimens obtained from the vaginal pool, the evaluation of fetal pulmonary maturation requires that a sample of amniotic fluid be obtained by amniocentesis. In the past, third-trimester amniocentesis was associated with significant fetal and maternal risks. Fetal complications have included fetal bleeding from laceration of the placenta or umbilical cord, fetomaternal bleeding, premature labor and premature rupture of the membranes, placental abruption, and fetal injury. Maternal complications, though rare, have included hemorrhage, in some cases from perforation of the uterine vessels, abdominal wall hematomas, Rh sensitization, and infection.

Ultrasound guidance for third-trimester amniocentesis has significantly decreased the risks of the procedure. In a review of seven studies that included 4,115 third-trimester amniocenteses, the frequency of complications was 3 percent for rupture of the membranes within 24 hours, 7 percent for a bloody tap, 4.4 percent for failed amniocentesis, 3.3 percent for labor within 24 hours, 1 percent for fetal trauma, and 0.05 percent for fetal death.[198]

A bloody tap warrants careful observation.[199] At term, the fetal blood volume is relatively small, and fetal bleeding may have disastrous consequences. When a bloody tap occurs, the patient should be evaluated with continuous electronic fetal heart rate monitoring until an Apt test or Kleihauer-Betke test confirms that the blood is of maternal origin and the fetus has demonstrated no evidence of compromise. Should a nonreassuring fetal heart rate pattern be observed, cesarean delivery is performed. When fetal blood is recovered, the fetus is delivered if its pulmonary status is mature even if it has not exhibited fetal distress. For those fetuses with pulmonary immaturity, treatment with corticosteroids and delivery thereafter is recommended.[219]

Quantitation of Pulmonary Surfactant

Lecithin/Sphingomyelin Ratio

The L/S ratio was the first reliable assay for the assessment of fetal pulmonary maturity.[200,201] The amniotic fluid concentration of lecithin increases markedly at approximately 35 weeks' gestation, whereas sphingomyelin levels remain stable or decrease. Rather than determine the concentration of lecithin that could be altered by variations in amniotic fluid volume, Gluck and coworkers used sphingomyelin as an internal standard and compared the amount of lecithin to that of sphingomyelin. Amniotic fluid sphingomyelin exceeds lecithin until 31 to 32 weeks, when the L/S ratio reaches 1. Lecithin then rises rapidly, and an L/S ratio of 2.0 is observed at approximately 35 weeks. Wide variation in the L/S ratio at each gestational age has been noted. Nevertheless, a ratio of 2.0 or greater has repeatedly been associated with pulmonary maturity. In more than 2,100 cases, a mature L/S ratio predicted the absence of RDS in 98 percent of neonates.[202] With a ratio of 1.5 to 1.9, approximately 50 percent of infants will develop RDS. Below 1.5, the risk of subsequent RDS increases to 73 percent. Thus, the L/S ratio, like most indices of fetal pulmonary maturation, rarely errs when predicting fetal pulmonary maturity, but is frequently incorrect when predicting subsequent RDS.[203] Many neonates with an immature L/S ratio will not develop RDS.

Several important variables must be considered in interpreting the predictive accuracy of the L/S ratio. A prolonged interval between the determination of an immature L/S ratio and delivery will necessarily increase the number of falsely immature results. It is probably best to discard amniotic fluid samples heavily contaminated by blood or meconium, because the effects of these compounds on the determination of the L/S ratio are quite unpredictable.[204,205] Blood has been reported to both increase and decrease the ratio, and meconium can produce falsely mature results. The presence of PG in a bloody or meconium-stained amniotic fluid sample remains a reliable indicator of pulmonary maturity.[206] PG is not normally found in blood, and meconium generally does not interfere with the identification of PG.[207,208] Finally, it is essential that the obstetrician know the analytic technique used and the predictive value of a mature L/S ratio in his or her laboratory.

Many perinatal processes alter the final interpretation of the L/S ratio. Surfactant deficiency, immaturity, and intrapartum complications are the prime factors in determining the pathogenesis of RDS.[209] Birth asphyxia may lead to RDS in many infants despite an L/S ratio greater than 2.0. In earlier studies, infants with severe Rh disease and infants of diabetic mothers were reported to have developed RDS despite mature L/S ratios. More recent data indicate that the L/S ratio is reliable in both high-risk conditions.[210,211] Kjos and colleagues[211] found no cases of RDS caused by surfactant deficiency in a study of women with pregestational and gestational diabetes.

PG, which does not appear until 35 weeks' gestation and increases rapidly between 37 to 40 weeks, is a marker of completed pulmonary maturation.[212] Most infants who lack PG but who have a mature L/S ratio fail to develop RDS. However, PG may provide further insurance against the onset of RDS despite intrapartum complications.

Slide Agglutination Test for PG

A rapid immunologic semiquantitative agglutination test (Amniostat-FLM) can be used to determine the presence of PG.[213] This assay can detect PG at a concentration greater than 0.5 μg/ml of amniotic fluid. The test takes 20 to 30 minutes to perform and requires only 1.5 ml of amniotic fluid. Besides being highly sensitive, several studies have found a positive Amniostat-FLM to correlate well with the presence of PG by thin-layer chromatography and the absence of subsequent RDS. In a study evaluating samples from the vaginal pool and those obtained by amniocentesis, the overall concordance for the Amniostat-FLM and thin-layer chromatography results was 89 percent.[213] No cases of RDS were observed when the Amniostat-FLM assay demonstrated PG. This technique can be applied to samples contaminated by blood and meconium.

Fluorescence Polarization

TDx Test (Surfactant Albumin Ratio)

The TDx analyzer, an automated fluorescence polarimeter, has been utilized to assess surfactant content in amniotic fluid.[215-217] The test requires 1 ml of amniotic fluid and can be run in less than 1 hour. The surfactant albumin ratio (SAR) is determined with amniotic fluid albumin used as an internal reference. A value of 70 was considered mature with the original assay, whereas with the newer FLM-II test, 55 is the mature cut-off.[196] A mature value reliably predicts the absence of RDS requiring intubation in infants of diabetic mothers.[218] The TDx test correlates well with the L/S ratio and has few falsely mature results, making it an excellent screening test.[219] The TDx assay proved to be reliable in predicting fetal lung maturity in vaginal pool specimens in patients with preterm premature rupture of the membranes at 30 to 36 weeks.[220] Approximately 50 percent of infants with an immature TDx result will develop RDS.

Measurement of Surfactant Function

Foam Stability Index

The test is based on the manual foam stability index (FSI), and is a variation of the shake test.[221] The kit currently available contains test wells with a predispensed volume of ethanol. The addition of 0.5-ml amniotic fluid to each test well in the kit produces final ethanol volumes of 44 to 50 percent. A control well contains sufficient surfactant in 50 percent ethanol to produce an example of the stable foam endpoint. The amniotic fluid/ethanol mixture is first shaken, and the FSI value is read as the highest value well in which a ring of stable foam persists.[222]

This test appears to be a reliable predictor of fetal lung maturity.[223] Subsequent RDS is very unlikely with an FSI value of 47 or higher. The methodology is simple, and the test can be performed at any time of day by persons who have had only minimal instruction. The assay appears to be extremely sensitive, with a high proportion of immature results being associated with RDS, as well as moderately specific, with a high proportion of mature results predicting the absence of RDS. Contamination of the amniotic fluid specimen by blood or meconium invalidates the FSI results. The FSI can function well as a screening test.

Evaluation of Amniotic Fluid Turbidity

Visual Inspection

During the first and second trimesters, amniotic fluid is yellow and clear. It becomes colorless in the third trimester. By 33 to 34 weeks' gestation, cloudiness and flocculation are noted, and, as term approaches, vernix appears. Amniotic fluid with obvious vernix or fluid so turbid it does not permit the reading of newsprint through it will usually have a mature L/S ratio.[224]

Lamellar Body Counts

Lamellar bodies are the storage form of surfactant released by fetal type II pneumocytes into the amniotic fluid. Because they have the same size as platelets, the amniotic fluid concentration of lamellar bodies may be determined using a commercial cell counter.[225-228] The test requires less than 1 ml of amniotic fluid and takes only 15 minutes to perform. A lamellar body count greater than 30,000 to 55,000/μl is highly predictive of pulmonary maturity, whereas a count below 10,000/μl suggests a significant risk for RDS. Lewis et al. have recently reported that a lamellar body count of less than 8,000 predicted an immature L/S and PG assay in all cases, whereas a value over 32,000 predicted a mature L/S or PG assay in 99 percent of cases.[229] The cutoff used to predict fetal pulmonary status will depend on the type of cell counter used and the speed of centrifugation of the amniotic fluid specimen. Neither meconium nor lysed blood has a significant effect on the lamellar body count.

Determination of Fetal Pulmonary Maturation in Clinical Practice

A large number of techniques are now available to assess fetal pulmonary maturation.[196] Several rapid screening tests, including the TDx test, Amniostat-FLM, and lamellar body count appear to be highly reliable when mature. In an uncomplicated pregnancy, when a screening test such as the TDx demonstrates fetal pulmonary maturation, one can safely proceed with delivery.[217,229] This sequential approach is also extremely cost effective.[196,197,230,231] However, when the screening test is immature, the L/S ratio should be used. Similarly, in complicated pregnancies such as those with diabetes mellitus, IUGR, and Rh isoimmunization, the L/S ratio should be determined to assess fetal pulmonary maturation.

A PRACTICAL APPROACH TO TESTING

How can one most efficiently use all the techniques available for antepartum fetal surveillance? Obstetricians should take a "diagnosis-specific" approach to testing. That is, they must consider the pathophysiology of the disease process that will be evaluated and then select the best method or methods of testing for that problem. For example, in the pregnancy complicated by significant Rh isoimmunization, one might want to use serial evaluations of fetal hemoglobin. In a pregnancy complicated by diabetes mellitus, careful monitoring of maternal glucose levels should accompany antepartum heart rate testing. In contrast, in a pregnancy complicated by suspected growth restriction, one would want to make serial evaluations of amniotic fluid volume with ultrasound to detect oligohydramnios.

In a prolonged pregnancy, one would use a parallel testing scheme. In this situation, the obstetrician is not concerned with fetal maturity, but rather with fetal well-being. Several tests are performed at the same time, such as antepartum fetal heart rate testing and the BPP. It is acceptable in this high-risk situation to intervene when a single test is abnormal. One is willing to accept a false-positive test result to avoid the intrauterine death of a mature and otherwise healthy fetus. In a

study of prolonged gestations in Canada between 1980 and 1995, Sue-A-Quan et al. reported a decline in the stillbirth rate for deliveries at 41 or more weeks' gestation that they attribute to an increased rate of labor induction.[232] Patients may have been induced electively or selectively for abnormal tests of fetal well-being.

In most other high-risk pregnancies, such as those complicated by diabetes mellitus or hypertension, it is preferable to allow the fetus to remain in utero as long as possible. In these situations, a branched testing scheme is used. To decrease the likelihood of unnecessary premature intervention, the obstetrician uses a series of tests and, under most circumstances, would only deliver a premature infant when all parameters suggest fetal compromise. In this situation, one must consider the likelihood of neonatal RDS as predicted by the evaluation of amniotic fluid indices and review these risks with colleagues in neonatology.

Maternal assessment of fetal activity would appear to be an ideal first-line screening test for both high-risk and low-risk patients. The use of this approach may decrease the number of unexpected intrauterine deaths in so-called normal pregnancies. Although a negative CST has been associated with fewer intrauterine deaths than a reactive NST, the NST appears to have significant advantages in screening high-risk patients. It can be easily and rapidly performed in an outpatient setting. Most clinicians use the BPP or CST to assess fetal condition in patients exhibiting a persistently nonreactive NST. This sequential approach may be particularly valuable in avoiding unnecessary premature intervention.

Figure 12–21 presents a practical testing scheme that has been utilized successfully by several centers.[112,143,233,234] The NST, an indicator of present fetal condition, may be combined with the amniotic fluid index (AFI) (see Chapter 10), a marker of long-term status, in a modified BPP. In this setting, an AFI greater than 5 cm is usually considered normal, although different criteria have been applied.[235] VAS may be used to shorten the time required to achieve a reactive NST. While most patients are evaluated weekly, patients with diabetes mellitus, IUGR, or a prolonged gestation are tested twice weekly. If the NST is nonreactive despite VAS or extended monitoring, or if the AFI is abnormal, either a full BPP or CST is performed. Using this approach, Clark et al.[233] found no unexpected antepartum fetal deaths in a series of 2,628 high-risk pregnancies. VAS shortened the mean testing time to 10 minutes. Only 2 percent of all NSTs were nonreactive. However, 17 percent of these were followed by a positive CST or BPP score of 4 or less. Clark et al. have extended their experience with this technique to include an additional 3,005 tests. One fetus died 2 days after a reactive NST because of a cord accident. Therefore, only one fetal death has been observed in almost 9,000 tests after a

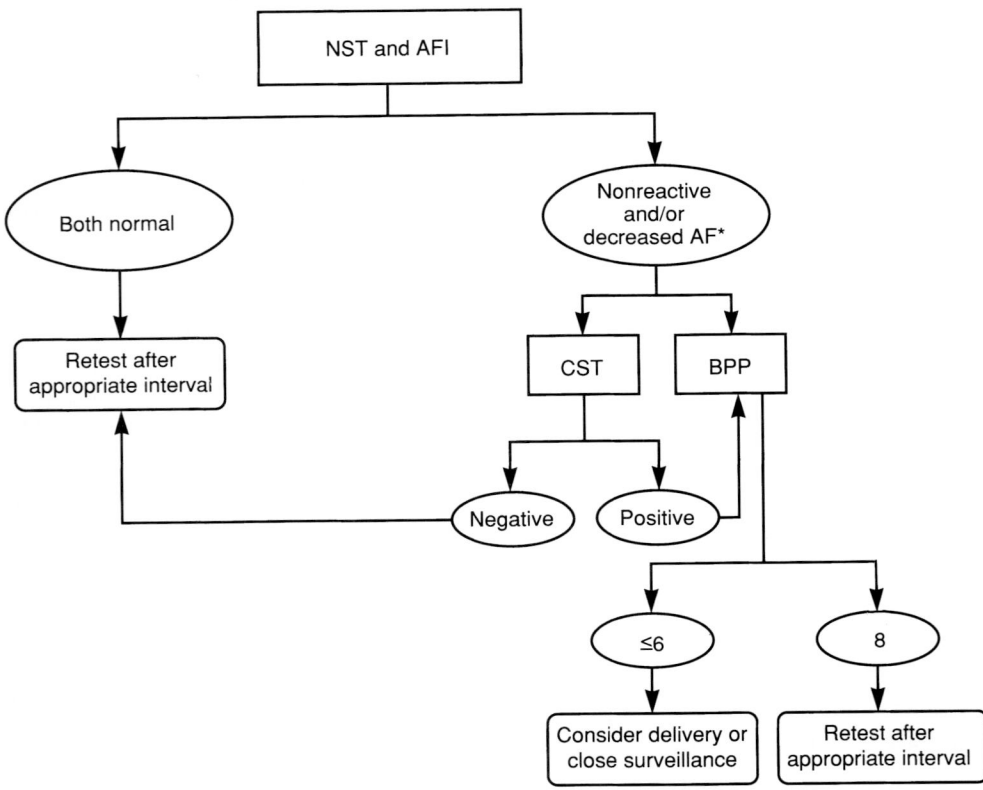

Figure 12–21. Flow chart for antepartum fetal surveillance in which the NST and AFI are used as the primary methods for fetal evaluation. A nonreactive NST and/or decreased AF are further evaluated using either the CST or the BPP. Further details regarding the use of the BPP are provided in Table 12–7. *If the fetus is mature and amniotic fluid volume is reduced, delivery should be considered before further testing is undertaken. (Adapted from Finberg HJ, Kurtz AB, Johnson RL, et al: The biophysical profile: a literature review and reassessment of its usefulness in the evaluation of fetal well-being. J Ultrasound Med 9:583, 1990.)

reactive NST and normal AFI! In a series of 6,543 fetuses, Vintzileos et al.[236] reported no fetal deaths attributable to hypoxia within 1 week of a reactive NST and an ultrasound study demonstrating normal amniotic fluid. Nageotte et al.[237] demonstrated that the modified BPP was as good a predictor of adverse fetal outcome as a negative CST. Furthermore, the CST as a backup test was associated with a higher rate of intervention for an abnormal test than the use of a complete BPP as a backup test. Miller et al. described 56,617 antepartum tests in 15,482 women identified as high risk.[238] Six indications (postdates pregnancy, diabetes mellitus, decreased fetal movement, suspected IUGR, hypertension, and a history of previous stillbirth) accounted for over 90 percent of patients tested. The modified BPP including the NST and AFI was used primarily with the full BPP as a backup test. Sixty percent of those delivered for an abnormal test had no evidence of fetal compromise. However, false-positive tests led to preterm deliveries in only 1.5 percent of those tested before 37 weeks. The false-negative rate was similar to that of the CST and complete BPP, 0.8 per 1,000 women tested. Overall, the modified BPP had a false-positive rate comparable to the NST but higher than the CST and full BPP. The low false-negative rate and ease of performance of the modified BPP make it an excellent approach for the evaluation of large numbers of high-risk patients.

STRATEGIES TO REDUCE ANTEPARTUM FETAL DEATHS

What strategies can be utilized to reduce antepartum fetal deaths?[239] (See the box "Strategies to Reduce An-

> ### Strategies to Reduce Antepartum Fetal Deaths
>
> Determination of the cause of fetal death
>
> Antepartum fetal evaluation in all pregnancies with routine fetal movement counting
>
> Surveillance for fetal malformations in all pregnancies with a triple screen and routine ultrasound at 18–20 weeks
>
> Surveillance for detection of IUGR with fundal height measurements and ultrasound at 30–32 weeks in high-risk patients and patients with lagging growth
>
> Programs to identify and treat cocaine abuse in pregnancy
>
> From Gabbe SG: Prevention of antepartum fetal deaths. OB/GYN Clinical Alert, April 1998, p 94, with permission.

tepartum Fetal Deaths.") First, it is important to determine the cause of a fetal death so that the patient and her partner can be counseled, the risk of recurrence described, and a plan of care for subsequent pregnancies developed. The obstetrician should write a detailed note describing the stillborn fetus, amniotic fluid, umbilical cord, placenta, and membranes. If the infant is malformed, growth restricted, or hydropic, chromosomal studies should be obtained. An autopsy should be requested.[239,240] Incerpi et al. observed that an autopsy and evaluation of the placenta were the most valuable tests in determining the cause of fetal death.[241] Tests for syphilis, antiphospholipid antibodies, and lupus anticoagulant should be done. If the patient has not been screened for diabetes mellitus during gestation, a fasting glucose should be ordered. Because significant fetal–maternal hemorrhage has been observed in approximately 5 percent of all fetal deaths, a Kleihauer-Betke test should be obtained.

To prevent antepartum deaths, routine fetal movement counting should be considered in all pregnancies, starting at 28 weeks' gestation. The modified Count-to-Ten method developed by Moore and Piacquadio is a simple and valuable technique.[60] To reduce fetal deaths resulting from fetal malformations, a triple analyte screen should be offered and routine ultrasound performed at 18 to 20 weeks (see Chapters 8 and 10). To detect IUGR, careful serial measurements of fundal height should be performed with an ultrasound examination at 30 to 32 weeks in high-risk patients including those with vascular disease and in patients with lagging uterine growth (see Chapter 25). Finally, to reduce fetal deaths caused by placental abruption, patients who are known to be abusing cocaine should be counseled and enrolled in treatment programs.

Key Points

➤ The prevalence of an abnormal condition (i.e., fetal death) has great impact on the predictive value of antepartum fetal tests.

➤ The near-term fetus spends approximately 25 percent of its time in a quiet sleep state (state 1F) and 60 to 70 percent in an active sleep state (state 2F).

➤ Approximately 5 percent of women monitoring fetal movement will report decreased fetal activity.

➤ The incidence of perinatal death within 1 week of a negative CST is less than 1 in 1,000.

➤ The observation that accelerations of the fetal heart rate in response to fetal activity, uterine contractions, or stimulation reflect fetal well-being is the basis for the NST.

➤ The frequency of the NST should be increased to twice weekly in pregnancies complicated by diabetes mellitus, prolonged gestation, and IUGR.

➤ Use of VAS for an equivocal BPP does not increase the false-negative rate and may reduce the likelihood of unnecessary obstetric intervention.

➤ Reversed end-diastolic flow in the umbilical artery flow velocity waveform has been associated with an increased perinatal mortality rate.

➤ Most amniotic fluid indices of fetal pulmonary maturation rarely err when predicting maturity, but are frequently incorrect when predicting subsequent RDS.

➤ The NST, an indicator of present fetal condition, and the amniotic fluid index, a marker of long-term fetal status, have been combined in the modified BPP.

REFERENCES

1. Eskes TKAB: Introduction. *In* Nijhuis J (ed): Fetal Behaviour. New York, Oxford University Press, 1992, p xv.
2. Centers for Disease Control and Prevention, NCHS, National Vital Statistics System: Vital statistics of the United States, vol. II, mortality, Part A; Infant mortality rates, fetal mortality rates, and perinatal mortality rates, according to race: United States, selected years 1950–1998. Public Health Service, Washington, DC, U.S. Govt. Printing Office.
3. Chard T, Klopper A: Introduction. *In* Placental Function Tests. New York, Springer-Verlag, 1982, p 1.
4. Friede A, Rochat R: Maternal mortality and perinatal mortality: definitions, data, and epidemiology. *In* Sachs B (ed): Obstetric Epidemiology. Littleton, MA, PSG Publishing Company, 1985, p 35.
5. American College of Obstetricians and Gynecologists: Perinatal and infant mortality statistics. Committee Opinion 167, December 1995.
6. Cotzias CS, Paterson-Browm S, Fisk NM: Prospective risk of unexplained stillbirth in singleton pregnancies at term: population based analysis. BMJ 319:287, 1999.
7. Grant A, Elbourne D: Fetal movement counting to assess fetal well-being. *In* Chalmers I, Enkin M, Keirse MJNC (eds): Effective Care in Pregnancy and Childbirth. Oxford, Oxford University Press, 1989, p 440.
8. Naeye RL: Causes of perinatal mortality in the United States Collaborative Perinatal Project. JAMA 238:228, 1977.
9. Guyer B, Strobino DM, Ventura SJ, Singh GK: Annual summary of vital statistics 1994. Pediatrics 96:1029, 1995.
10. March of Dimes Perinatal Profiles: Health Indicators, 1990–

1997. New York, The March of Dimes Perinatal Data Center and Planning and Community Services Divison, 2000.

11. Morbidity and Mortality Weekly Report: Trends in infant mortality attributable to birth defects-United States, 1980–1995. Boston, Massachusetts Medical Society, 2000.

12. Lammer EJ, Brown LE, Anderka MT, Guyer B: Classification and analysis of fetal deaths in Massachusetts. JAMA 261: 1757, 1989.

13. Manning FA, Lange IR, Morrison I, Harman CR: Determination of fetal health: methods for antepartum and intrapartum fetal assessment. *In* Leventhal J (ed): Current Problems in Obstetrics and Gynecology. Chicago, Year Book Medical Publishers, 1983.

14. Fretts RC, Boyd ME, Usher RH, Usher H: The changing pattern of fetal death, 1961–1988. Obstet Gynecol 79:35, 1992.

15. Fretts RC, Schmittdiel J, McLean FH, et al: Increased maternal age and the risk of fetal death. N Engl J Med 333:953, 1995.

16. Andersen AMN, Wohlfahrt J, Christens P, et al: Maternal age and fetal loss: population based register linkage study. BMJ 320:1708, 2000.

17. Stein Z, Susser M: The risks of having children in later life. BMJ 320:1681, 2000.

18. Schauer GM, Kalousek DK, Magee JF: Genetic causes of stillbirth. Semin Perinatol 16:341, 1992.

19. Mersey Region Working Party on Perinatal Mortality. Perinatal health. Lancet 1:491, 1982.

20. Kirkup B, Welch G: "Normal but dead": perinatal mortality in the non-malformed babies of birthweight 2–5 kg and over in the Northern Region in 1983. Br J Obstet Gynaecol 97: 381, 1990.

21. Schneider EP, Hutson JM, Petrie RH: An assessment of the first decade's experience with antepartum fetal heart rate testing. Am J Perinatol 5:134, 1988.

22. Stubblefield P, Berek J: Perinatal mortality in term and postterm births. Obstet Gynecol 56:676, 1980.

23. Duenhoelter J, Whalley P, MacDonald P: An analysis of the utility of plasma immunoreactive estrogen measurements in determining delivery time of gravidas with a fetus considered at high risk. Am J Obstet Gynecol 125:889, 1976.

24. Mohide P, Keirse MJNC: Biophysical assessment of fetal wellbeing. *In* Chalmers I, Enkin M, Keirse MJNC (eds): Effective Care in Pregnancy and Childbirth. Oxford, Oxford University Press, 1989, p 477.

25. Thornton JG, Lilford RJ: Do we need randomised trials of antenatal tests of fetal wellbeing? Br J Obstet Gynaecol 100: 197, 1993.

26. Divon MY, Ferber A: Evidence-based antepartum fetal testing. *In* Prenatal and Neonatal Medicine. New York, The Parthenon Publishing Group, 2000.

27. American College of Obstetricians and Gynecologists: Antepartum fetal surveillance. Practice Bulletin 9, October 1999.

28. Flynn AM, Kelly J, Mansfield H, et al: A randomized controlled trial of non-stress antepartum cardiotocography. Br J Obstet Gynaecol 89:427, 1982.

29. Brown VA, Sawers RS, Parsons RJ, et al: The value of antenatal cardiotocography in the management of high-risk pregnancy: a randomized controlled trial. Br J Obstet Gynaecol 89:716, 1982.

30. Lumley J, Lester A, Anderson I, et al: A randomized trial of weekly cardiotocography in high-risk obstetric patients. Br J Obstet Gynaecol 90:1018, 1983.

31. Kidd LC, Patel NB, Smith R: Non-stress antenatal cardiotocography: a prospective randomized clinical trial. Br J Obstet Gynaecol 92:1156, 1985.

32. Ferrera TB, Hoekstra RF, Couser RJ, et al: Survival and follow-up of infants born at 23–26 weeks gestational age: effects of surfactant therapy. J Pediatr 124:119, 1994.

33. Allen M, Donohue P, Dushman A: The limit of viability: neonatal outcome of infants born at 22–25 weeks gestation. N Engl J Med 329:1597, 1993.

34. Schwartz RM, Luby AM, Scanlon JW, Kellog RJ: Effect of surfactant on morbidity, mortality and resource use in newborn infants weighing 500–1500 grams. N Engl J Med 330: 1476, 1994.

35. Schifrin B, Foye G, Amato J, et al: Routine fetal heart rate monitoring in the antepartum period. Obstet Gynecol 54:21, 1979.

36. Stempel L: Eenie, meenie, minie, mo . . . what do the data really show? Obstet Gynecol 144:745, 1982.

37. Peipert JF, Sweeney PJ: Diagnostic testing in obstetrics and gynecology: a clinician's guide. Obstet Gynecol 82:619, 1993.

38. Carpenter M, Coustan D: Criteria for screening tests for gestational diabetes. Am J Obstet Gynecol 144:768, 1982.

39. Manning FA: Assessment of fetal condition and risk: analysis of single and combined biophysical variable monitoring. Semin Perinatol 9:168, 1985.

40. Van Woerden EE, VanGeijn HP: Heart-rate patterns and fetal movements. *In* Nijhuis J (ed): Fetal Behaviour. New York, Oxford University Press, 1992, p 41.

41. Patrick J, Campbell K, Carmichael L, et al: Patterns of gross fetal body movements over 24-hour observation intervals during the last 10 weeks of pregnancy. Am J Obstet Gynecol 142:363, 1982.

42. Holden K, Jovanovic L, Druzin M, Peterson C: Increased fetal activity with low maternal blood glucose levels in pregnancies complicated by diabetes. Am J Perinatol 1:161, 1984.

43. Phelan JP, Kester R, Labudovich ML: Nonstress test and maternal glucose determinations. Obstet Gynecol 67:4, 1982.

44. Druzin ML, Foodim J: Effect of maternal glucose ingestion compared with maternal water ingestion on the nonstress test. Obstet Gynecol 67:4, 1982.

45. Natale R, Clewlow F, Dawes G: Measurement of fetal forelimb movements in the lamb in utero. Am J Obstet Gynecol 140:545, 1981.

46. Sadovsky E, Yaffe H, Polishuk W: Fetal movement monitoring in normal and pathologic pregnancy. Int J Gynaecol Obstet 12:75, 1974.

47. Rayburn W, Zuspan F, Motley M, Donaldson M: An alternative to antepartum fetal heart rate testing. Am J Obstet Gynecol 138:223, 1980.

48. Pearson J, Weaver J: Fetal activity and fetal well being: an evaluation. BMJ 1:1305, 1976.

49. Sadovsky E, Ohel G, Havazeleth H, et al: The definition and the significance of decreased fetal movements. Acta Obstet Gynecol Scand 62:409, 1983.

50. Draper J, Field S, Thomas H: Women's views on keeping fetal movement charts. Br J Obstet Gynaecol 93:334, 1986.

51. Mikhail MS, Freda MC, Merkatz RB, et al: The effect of fetal movement counting on maternal attachment to fetus. Am J Obstet Gynecol 165:988, 1991.

52. Sorokin Y, Kierker L: Fetal movement. Clin Obstet Gynecol 25:719, 1982.

53. Johnson TRB, Jordan ET, Paine LL: Doppler recordings of fetal movement: II. Comparison with maternal perception. Obstet Gynecol 76:42, 1990.

54. Rayburn W, Barr M: Activity patterns in malformed fetuses. Am J Obstet Gynecol 142:1045, 1982.

55. Neldam S: Fetal movements as an indicator of fetal well being. Lancet 1:1222, 1980.

56. Neldam S: Fetal movements as an indicator of fetal well being. Dan Med Bull 30:274, 1983.

57. Rayburn W: Antepartum fetal assessment. Clin Perinatol 9: 231, 1982.

58. Liston R, Cohen A, Mennuti M, Gabbe S: Antepartum fetal evaluation by maternal perception of fetal movement. Obstet Gynecol 60:424, 1982.

59. Grant A, Valentin L, Elbourne D, Alexander S: Routine formal fetal movement counting and risk of antepartum late death in normally formed singletons. Lancet 2:345, 1989.

60. Moore TR, Piacquadio K: A prospective evaluation of fetal movement screening to reduce the incidence of antepartum fetal death. Am J Obstet Gynecol 160:1075, 1989.

61. Moore TR, Piacquadio K: Study results vary in count-to-10 method of fetal movement screening. Am J Obstet Gynecol 163:264, 1990.

62. Collea J, Holls W: The contraction stress test. Clin Obstet Gynecol 25:707, 1982.

63. Braly P, Freeman R, Garite T, et al: Incidence of premature delivery following the oxytocin challenge test. Am J Obstet Gynecol 141:5, 1981.

64. Freeman R: The use of the oxytocin challenge test for antepartum clinical evaluation of uteroplacental respiratory function. Am J Obstet Gynecol 121:481, 1975.

65. Martin C, Schifrin B: Prenatal fetal monitoring. *In* Aladjem S, Brown A (eds): Perinatal Intensive Care. St. Louis, CV Mosby, 1977, p 155.

66. Nageotte MP, Towers CV, Asrat T, et al: The value of a negative antepartum test: contraction stress test and modified biophysical profile. Obstet Gynecol 84:231, 1994.

67. Freeman R, Garite T, Modanlou H, et al: Postdate pregnancy: utilization of contraction stress testing for primary fetal surveillance. Am J Obstet Gynecol 140:128, 1981.

68. Freeman RK, Dorchester W, Anderson G, Garite TJ: The significance of a previous stillbirth. Am J Obstet Gynecol 151: 7, 1985.

69. Druzin ML, Karver ML, Wagner W, et al: Prospective evaluation of the contraction stress test and non stress tests in the management of posterm pregnancy. Surg Gynecol Obstet 174:507, 1992.

70. Gabbe SG, Mestman JH, Freeman RK, et al: Management and outcome of diabetes mellitus, classes B-R. Am J Obstet Gynecol 129:723, 1977.

71. Lagrew DC, Pircon RA, Towers CV, et al: Antepartum fetal surveillance in patients with diabetes: when to start? Am J Obstet Gynecol 168:1820, 1993.

72. Evertson L, Gauthier R, Collea J: Fetal demise following negative contraction stress tests. Obstet Gynecol 51:671, 1978.

73. Grundy H, Freeman RK, Lederman S, Dorchester W: Non-reactive contraction stress test: clinical significance. Obstet Gynecol 64:337, 1984.

74. Freeman R, Anderson G, Dorchester W: A prospective multi-institutional study of antepartum fetal heart rate monitoring. I. Risk of perinatal mortality and morbidity according to antepartum fetal heart rate test results. Am J Obstet Gynecol 143:771, 1982.

75. Ray M, Freeman R, Pine S, et al: Clinical experience with the oxytocin challenge test. Am J Obstet Gynecol 114:1, 1972.

76. Gabbe S, Freeman R, Goebelsmann U: Evaluation of the contraction stress test before 33 weeks' gestation. Obstet Gynecol 52:649, 1978.

77. Bissonnette J, Johnson K, Toomey C: The role of a trial of labor with a positive contraction stress test. Am J Obstet Gynecol 135:292, 1979.

78. Braly P, Freeman R: The significance of fetal heart rate reactivity with a positive oxytocin challenge test. Obstet Gynecol 50:689, 1977.

79. Merrill PM, Porto M, Lovett SM, et al: Evaluation of the non-reactive positive contraction stress test prior to 32 weeks: the role of the biophysical profile. Am J Perinatol 12:229, 1995.

80. Bruce S, Petrie R, Yeh S-Y: The suspicious contraction stress test. Obstet Gynecol 51:415, 1978.

81. Scanlon J, Suzuki K, Shea E, Tronick E: A prospective study of the oxytocin challenge test and newborn neurobehavioral outcome. Obstet Gynecol 54:6, 1979.

82. Crane J, Anderson B, Marshall R, Harvey P: Subsequent physical and mental development in infants with positive contraction stress tests. J Reprod Med 26:113, 1981.

83. Beischer N, Drew J, Ashton P, et al: Quality of survival of infants with critical fetal reserve detected by antenatal cardiotocography. Am J Obstet Gynecol 146:662, 1983.

84. Oki EY, Keegan KA, Freeman RD, Dorchester W: The breast-stimulated contraction stress test. J Reprod Med 32:919, 1987.

85. Keegan KA, Helm DA, Porto M, et al: A prospective evaluation of nipple stimulation techniques for contraction stress testing. Am J Obstet Gynecol 157:121, 1987.

86. Huddleston J, Sutliff G, Robinson D: Contraction stress test by intermittent nipple stimulation. Obstet Gynecol 63:669, 1984.

87. Curtis P, Evens S, Resnick J, et al: Patterns of uterine contractions and prolonged uterine activity using three methods of breast stimulation for contraction stress tests. Obstet Gynecol 73:631, 1989.

88. Devoe LD, Morrison J, Martin J, et al: A prospective comparative study of the extended nonstress test and the nipple stimulation contraction stress test. Am J Obstet Gynecol 157: 531, 1987.

89. Hammacher K: The clinical significance of cardiotocography. *In* Huntingford P, Huter K, Saling E (eds): Perinatal Medicine. 1st European Congress, Berlin. San Diego, Academic, 1969, p 80.

90. Patrick J, Carmichael L, Chess L, Staples C: Accelerations of the human fetal heart rate at 38 to 40 weeks' gestational age. Am J Obstet Gynecol 148:35, 1984.

91. Margulis E, Binder D, Cohen A: The effect of propranolol on the nonstress test. Am J Obstet Gynecol 148:340, 1984.

92. Keegan K, Paul R, Broussard P, et al: Antepartum fetal heart rate testing. III. The effect of phenobarbital on the nonstress test. Am J Obstet Gynecol 133:579, 1979.

93. Phelan J: Diminished fetal reactivity with smoking. Am J Obstet Gynecol 136:230, 1980.

94. Lavery J: Nonstress fetal heart rate testing. Clin Obstet Gynecol 25:689, 1982.

95. Keegan K, Paul R, Broussard P, et al: Antepartum fetal heart rate testing. V. The nonstress test: an outpatient approach. Am J Obstet Gynecol 136:81, 1980.

96. Druzin M, Gratacos J, Paul R, et al: Antepartum fetal heart rate testing. XII. The effect of manual manipulation of the fetus on the nonstress test. Am J Obstet Gynecol 151:61, 1985.

97. Eglinton G, Paul R, Broussard P, et al: Antepartum fetal heart rate testing. XI. Stimulation with orange juice. Am J Obstet Gynecol 150:97, 1984.

98. Keegan K, Paul R: Antepartum fetal heart rate testing. IV. The nonstress test as a primary approach. Am J Obstet Gynecol 136:75, 1980.

99. Evertson L, Gauthier R, Schifrin B, et al: Antepartum fetal heart rate testing. I. Evolution of the nonstress test. Am J Obstet Gynecol 133:29, 1979.

100. Rochard F, Schifrin B, Goupil F, et al: Nonstressed fetal heart rate monitoring in the antepartum period. Am J Obstet Gynecol 126:699, 1976.

101. Phelan J: The nonstress test: a review of 3,000 tests. Am J Obstet Gynecol 139:7, 1981.

102. Phillips W, Towell M: Abnormal fetal heart rate associated with congenital abnormalities. Br J Obstet Gynaecol 87:270, 1980.

103. Natale R, Nasello C, Turliuk R: The relationship between movements and accelerations in fetal heart rate at twenty-four to thirty-two weeks' gestation. Am J Obstet Gynecol 148:591, 1984.

104. Bishop E: Fetal acceleration test. Am J Obstet Gynecol 141: 905, 1981.

105. Lavin J, Miodovnik M, Barden T: Relationship of nonstress test reactivity and gestational age. Obstet Gynecol 63:338, 1984.

106. Druzin ML, Fox A, Kogut E, et al: The relationship of the nonstress test to gestational age. Am J Obstet Gynecol 153: 386, 1985.

107. Aladjem S, Vuolo K, Pazos R, et al: Antepartum fetal testing: evaluation and redefinition of criteria for clinical interpretation. Semin Perinatol 5:145, 1981.

108. Druzin ML, Lockshin M, Edersheim T, et al: Second trimester fetal monitoring and preterm delivery in pregnancies with systematic lupus erythematosus and/or circulating anticoagulant. Am J Obstet Gynecol 157:1503, 1987.

109. Brown R, Patrick J: The nonstress test: how long is enough? Am J Obstet Gynecol 141:646, 1981.

110. Leveno K, Williams M, DePalma R, et al: Perinatal outcome in the absence of antepartum fetal heart rate acceleration. Obstet Gynecol 61:347, 1983.

111. DeVoe L, McKenzie J, Searle N, et al: Clinical sequelae of the extended nonstress test. Am J Obstet Gynecol 151:1074, 1985.

112. Phelan JP: Antepartum fetal assessment: new techniques. Semin Perinatol 12:57, 1988.

113. Gagnon R, Foreman J, Hunse C, et al: Effects of low-frequency vibration on human germ fetuses. Am J Obstet Gynecol 161:1479, 1989.

114. Gagnon R, Hunse C, Foreman J: Human fetal behavioral states after vibratory stimulation. Am J Obstet Gynecol 161: 1470, 1989.

115. Smith CV, Phelan JP, Paul RH, et al: Fetal acoustic stimulation testing: a retrospective experience with the fetal acoustic stimulation test. Am J Obstet Gynecol 153:567, 1985.

116. Smith CV, Phelan JP, Platt LD, et al: Fetal acoustic stimulation testing. II. A randomized clinical comparison with the nonstress test. Am J Obstet Gynecol 155:131, 1986.

117. Kuhlman KA, Depp R: Acoustic stimulation testing. Obstet Gynecol Clin North Am 15:303, 1988.

118. Trudinger BJ, Boylan P: Antepartum fetal heart rate monitoring: value of sound stimulation. Obstet Gynecol 55:265, 1980.

119. Druzin ML, Edersheim TG, Hutson JM, et al: The effect of vibroacoustic stimulation on the nonstress test at gestational ages of thirty-two weeks or less. Am J Obstet Gynecol 1661: 1476, 1989.

120. Smith CV, Satt B, Phelan JP, et al: Intrauterine sound levels: intrapartum assessment with an intrauterine microphone. Am J Perinatol 7:312, 1990.

121. Arulkumaran S, Talbert D, Hsu TS, et al: In-utero sound levels when vibroacoustic stimulation is applied to the maternal abdomen: an assessment of the possibility of cochlea damage in the fetus. Br J Obstet Gynaecol 99:43, 1992.

122. Arulkumaran S, Mircog B, Skurr BA, et al: No evidence of hearing loss due to fetal acoustic stimulation test. Obstet Gynecol 78:2, 1991.

123. Ohel G, Horowitz E, Linder N, et al: Neonatal auditory acuity following in utero vibratory acoustic stimulation. Am J Obstet Gynecol 157:440, 1987.

124. Druzin M, Gratacos J, Keegan K, et al: Antepartum fetal heart rate testing. VII. The significance of fetal bradycardia. Am J Obstet Gynecol 139:194, 1981.

125. Druzin ML: Antepartum Fetal Assessment. Cambridge, MA, Blackwell Scientific Publications, 1992, p 13.

126. Phelan J, Lewis P: Fetal heart rate decelerations during a nonstress test. Obstet Gynecol 57:288, 1981.

127. Pazos R, Vuolo K, Aladjem S, et al: Association of spontaneous fetal heart rate decelerations during antepartum nonstress testing and intrauterine growth retardation. Am J Obstet Gynecol 144:574, 1982.

128. Dashow E, Read J: Significant fetal bradycardia during antepartum heart rate testing. Am J Obstet Gynecol 148:187, 1984.

129. Bourgeois F, Thiagarajah S, Harbert G: The significance of fetal heart rate decelerations during nonstress testing. Am J Obstet Gynecol 150:215, 1984.

130. Druzin ML: Fetal bradycardia during antepartum testing, further observations. J Reprod Med 34:47, 1989.

131. Meis P, Ureda J, Swain M, et al: Variable decelerations during non-stress tests are not a sign of fetal compromise? Am J Obstet Gynecol 154:586, 1994.

132. Barrett J, Salyer S, Boehm F: The nonstress test: an evaluation of 1,000 patients. Am J Obstet Gynecol 141:153, 1981.

133. Miller JM Jr, Horger EO III: Antepartum heart rate testing in diabetic pregnancy. J Reprod Med 30:515, 1985.

134. Boehm FH, Salyer S, Shah DM, et al: Improved outcome of twice weekly nonstress testing. Obstet Gynecol 67:566, 1986.

135. Miyazaki F, Miyazaki B: False reactive nonstress tests in postterm pregnancies. Am J Obstet Gynecol 140:269, 1981.

136. Barss V, Frigoletto F, Diamond F: Stillbirth after nonstress testing. Obstet Gynecol 65:541, 1985.

137. Murata Y, Martin C, Ikenoue T, et al: Fetal heart rate accelerations and late decelerations during the course of intrauterine death in chronically catheterized rhesus monkeys. Am J Obstet Gynecol 144:218, 1982.

138. Freeman R, Anderson G, Dorchester W: A prospective multi-institutional study of antepartum fetal heart rate monitoring. II. Contraction stress test versus nonstress test for primary surveillance. Am J Obstet Gynecol 143:778, 1982.

139. Slomka C, Phelan J: Pregnancy outcome in the patient with a nonreactive nonstress test and a positive contraction stress test. Am J Obstet Gynecol 139:11, 1981.

140. Devoe L: Clinical features of the reactive positive contraction stress test. Obstet Gynecol 63:523, 1984.

141. Druzin M, Gratacos J, Paul R: Antepartum fetal heart rate testing. VI. Predictive reliability of "normal" tests in the prevention of antepartum death. Am J Obstet Gynecol 137:746, 1980.

142. Kadar N: Perinatal mortality related to nonstress and contraction stress tests. Am J Obstet Gynecol 142:931, 1982.

143. Finberg HJ, Kurtz AB, Johnson RL, et al: The biophysical profile: a literature review and reassessment of its usefulness in the evaluation of fetal well-being. J Ultrasound Med 9:583, 1990.

144. Manning FA, Morrison I, Lange IR, et al: Fetal assessment based on fetal biophysical profile scoring: experience in 12,620 referred high-risk pregnancies. Am J Obstet Gynecol 151:343, 1985.

145. Vintzileos A, Campbell W, Ingardia C, Nochimson D: The fetal biophysical profile and its predictive value. Obstet Gynecol 62:271, 1983.

146. Gennser G, Marsal K, Brantmark B: Maternal smoking and fetal breathing movements. Am J Obstet Gynecol 123:861, 1975.

147. Platt L, Manning F, Lemay M, Sipos L: Human fetal breathing: relationship to fetal condition. Am J Obstet Gynecol 132:514, 1978.

148. Manning F, Platt L, Sipos L, Keegan K: Fetal breathing movements and the nonstress test in high-risk pregnancies. Am J Obstet Gynecol 135:511, 1979.

149. Schifrin B, Guntes V, Gergely R, et al: The role of real-time scanning in antenatal fetal surveillance. Am J Obstet Gynecol 140:525, 1981.

150. Manning F, Platt L, Sipos L: Antepartum fetal evaluation: development of a fetal biophysical profile. Am J Obstet Gynecol 136:787, 1980.

151. Pillai M, James D: The importance of behavioral state in biophysical assessment of the term human fetus. Br J Obstet Gynaecol 97:1130, 1990.

152. Manning FA, Harman CR, Morrison I, et al: Fetal assessment based on fetal biophysical profile scoring. Am J Obstet Gynecol 162:703, 1990.

153. Manning FA, Morrison I, Lange IR, et al: Fetal biophysical profile scoring: selective use of the nonstress test. Am J Obstet Gynecol 156:709, 1987.

154. Manning FA, Morrison I, Harman CR, et al: The abnormal fetal biophysical profile score. V. Predictive accuracy according to score composition. Am J Obstet Gynecol 162:918, 1990.

155. Manning FA: Biophysical profile scoring. *In* Nijhuis J (ed): Fetal Behaviour. New York, Oxford University Press, 1992, p 241.

156. Vintzileos AM, Gaffney SE, Salinger LM, et al: The relationship between fetal biophysical profile and cord pH in patients undergoing cesarean section before the onset of labor. Obstet Gynecol 70:196, 1987.

157. Kelly MK, Schneider EP, Petrikovsky BM, Lesser ML: Effect of antenatal steroid administration on the fetal biophysical profile. J Clin Ultrasound 28:224, 2000.

158. Deren O, Karaer C, Önderoglu L, et al: The effect of steroids on the biophysical profile of the healthy preterm fetus and its relationship with time. Am J Obstet Gynecol 185:S108, 2000.

159. Rotmensch S, Liberati M, Celentano C, et al: The effect of betamethasone on fetal biophysical activities and Doppler velocimetry of umbilical and middle cerebral arteries. Acta Obstet Gynecol Scand 78:768, 1999.

160. Sherer DM, Spong CY, Salafia CM: Fetal breathing movements within 24 hours of delivery in prematurity are related to histologic and clinical evidence of amnionitis. Am J Perinatol 14:337, 1997.

161. Lewis DF, Adair CD, Weeks JW, et al: A randomized clinical trial of daily nonstress testing versus biophysical profile in the management of preterm premature rupture of the membranes. Am J Obstet Gynecol 181:1495, 1999.

162. Manning FA: Fetal biophysical profile. Obstet Gynecol Clin North Am 26:557, 1999.

163. Platt L, Eglinton G, Sipos L, et al: Further experience with the fetal biophysical profile. Obstet Gynecol 61:480, 1983.

164. Manning F, Lange I, Morrison I, et al: Fetal biophysical profile score and the nonstress test: a comparative trial. Obstet Gynecol 64:326, 1984.

165. Eden RD, Seifert LS, Kodack LD, et al: A modified biophysical profile for antenatal fetal surveillance. Obstet Gynecol 71:365, 1988.

166. Inglis SR, Druzin ML, Wagner WE, Kogut E: The use of vibroacoustic stimulation during the abnormal or equivocal biophysical profile. Obstet Gynecol 82:371, 1993.

167. Hatle L, Angelsen B: Doppler Ultrasound in Cardiology. Philadelphia, Lea & Febiger, 1985, p 1.

168. Warsof SL, Levy DL: Doppler blood flow and fetal growth retardation. *In* Gross TL, Sokol RJ (ed): Intrauterine Growth Retardation, A Practical Approach. Chicago, Year Book, 1989, p 158.

169. Bruner JP, Gabbe SG, Levy DW, et al: Doppler ultrasonography of the umbilical cord in normal pregnancy. J South Med Assoc 86:52, 1993.

170. Morrow RJ, Hill AA, Adamson SL: Experimental models used to investigate the diagnostic potential of Doppler ultrasound in the umbilical circulation. *In* Copel JA, Reed KL (eds): Doppler Ultrasound in Obstetrics and Gynecology. New York, Raven Press, 1995, p 5.

171. Indik JH, Reed KL: Variation and correlation in human fetal umbilical velocities with fetal breathing: evidence of the cardiac-placental connection. Am J Obstet Gynecol 163:1792, 1990.

172. Sonesson SE, Fouron JC, Drblik SP, et al: Reference values for Doppler velocimetric indices from the fetal and placental ends of the umbilical artery during normal pregnancy. J Clin Ultrasound 21:317, 1993.

173. Thompson RS, Trudinger BJ, Cook CM, et al: Umbilical artery velocity waveforms: normal reference values for A/B ratio and Pourcelot ratio. Br J Obstet Gynaecol 95:589, 1988.

174. Hendricks SK, Sorensen TK, Wang KY, et al: Doppler umbilical artery waveform indices—normal values from fourteen to forty-two weeks. Am J Obstet Gynecol 161:761, 1989.

175. Rizzo G, Arduini D, Romanini C: First trimester fetal and uterine Doppler. *In* Copel JA, Reed KL (eds): Doppler Ultrasound in Obstetrics and Gynecology. New York, Raven Press, 1995, p 105.

176. Itskovitz J: Maternal-fetal hemodynamics. *In* Maulik D, McNellis D (eds): Reproductive and Perinatal Medicine (VIII) Doppler Ultrasound Measurement of Maternal-Fetal Hemodynamics. Ithaca, NY, Perinatology Press, 1987, p 13.

177. McCowan LME, Harding JE, Stewart AW: Umbilical artery Doppler studies in small for gestational age babies reflect disease severity. Br J Obstet Gynaecol 107:916, 2000.

178. Pollock RN, Divon MY: Intrauterine growth retardation: diagnosis. *In* Copel JA, Reed KL (eds): Doppler Ultrasound in Obstetrics and Gynecology. New York, Raven Press, 1995, p 171.

179. Trudinger BJ, Stevens D, Connelly A, et al: Umbilical artery flow velocity waveforms and placental resistance: the effects of embolization of the umbilical circulation. Am J Obstet Gynecol 157:1443, 1987.

180. Morrow R, Ritchie K: Doppler ultrasound fetal velocimetry and its role in obstetrics. Clin Perinatol 16:771, 1989.

181. Copel JA, Schlafer D, Wentworth R, et al: Does the umbilical artery systolic/diastolic ratio reflect flow or acidosis? Am J Obstet Gynecol 163:751, 1990.

182. Divon MY, Ferber A: Evidence-based antepartum fetal testing. Perinatal Neonatal Med 5:3, 2000.

183. Farine D, Kelly EN, Ryan G, et al: Absent and reversed umbilical artery end-diastolic velocity. *In* Copel JA, Reed KL (eds): Doppler Ultrasound in Obstetrics and Gynecology. New York, Raven Press, 1995, p 187.

184. Indik JH, Chen V, Reed KL: Association of umbilical venous with inferior vena cava blood flow velocities. Obstet Gynecol 77:551, 1991.

185. Reed KL, Chaffin D, Anderson CF: Umbilical venous Doppler velocity pulsations and inferior vena cava pressure elevations in fetal lambs. Obstet Gynecol 87:617, 1996.

186. Arduini D, Rizzo G, Romanini C: The development of abnormal heart rate patterns after absent end-diastolic velocity in umbilical artery: analysis of risk factors. Am J Obstet Gynecol 168:50, 1993.

187. Hecher K, Campbell S, Doyle P, et al: Assessment of fetal compromise by Doppler investigation of the fetal circulation. Circulation 91:129, 1995.

188. Damron DP, Chaffin DG, Anderson CF, Reed KL: Umbilical artery velocity ratios and venous pulsations in fetuses with late decelerations. Obstet Gynecol 84:1038, 1994.

189. Giles WB, Bisits A: Clinical use of Doppler in pregnancy: information from six randomized trials. Fetal Diagn Ther 8: 247, 1993.

190. Alfirevic Z, Neilson JP: Doppler ultrasonography in high-risk pregnancies: systematic review with meta-analysis. Am J Obstet Gynecol 172:1379, 1995.

191. Neilson JP, Alfirevic Z: Doppler ultrasound in high-risk pregnancies (Cochrane Review). In The Cochrane Library, Issue 4. Oxford, Update Software, 1999.

192. Goffinet F, Paris-Llado J, Nisand I, Breart G: Umbilical artery Doppler velocimetry in unselected and low risk pregnancies: a review of randomized controlled trials. Br J Obstet Gynaecol 104:425, 1997.

193. Strassner H, Nochimson D: Determination of fetal maturity. Clin Perinatol 9:297, 1982.

194. Goldenberg R, Nelson K: Iatrogenic respiratory distress syndrome. Am J Obstet Gynecol 123:617, 1975.

195. Hack M, Fanaroff A, Klaus M, et al: Neonatal respiratory distress following elective delivery: a preventable disease? Am J Obstet Gynecol 126:43, 1976.

196. Assessment of Fetal Lung Maturity, ACOG Educational Bulletin, Number 230, 1996.

197. Dunn LR: The clinical use of fetal lung maturity testing. Resident Reporter 3:32, 1998.

198. Newton ER, Cetrulo CL, Kosa DJ: Biparietal diameter as a predictor of fetal lung maturity. J Reprod Med 28:480, 1983.

199. Golde S, Platt L: The use of ultrasound in the diagnosis of fetal lung maturity. Clin Obstet Gynecol 27:391, 1984.

200. Gluck L, Kulovich M, Borer R, et al: The interpretation and significance of the lecithin/sphingomyelin ratio in amniotic fluid. Am J Obstet Gynecol 120:142, 1974.

201. Kulovich M, Hallman M, Gluck L: The lung profile. Am J Obstet Gynecol 135:57, 1979.

202. Harvey D, Parkinson C, Campbell S: Risk of respiratory distress syndrome. Lancet 1:42, 1975.

203. Creasy G, Simon N: Sensitivity and specificity of the L/S ratio in relation to gestational age. Am J Perinatol 1:302, 1984.

204. Buhi W, Spellacy W: Effects of blood or meconium on the determination of the amniotic fluid lecithin/sphingomyelin ratio. Am J Obstet Gynecol 121:321, 1975.

205. Tabsh K, Brinkman C, Bashore R: Effect of meconium contamination on amniotic fluid lecithin:sphingomyelin ratio. Obstet Gynecol 58:605, 1981.

206. Stedman C, Crawford S, Staten E, et al: Management of preterm premature rupture of membranes: assessing amniotic fluid in the vagina for phosphatidylglycerol. Am J Obstet Gynecol 140:34, 1981.

207. Strassner H, Golde S, Mosley G, et al: Effect of blood in amniotic fluid on the detection of phosphatidylglycerol. Am J Obstet Gynecol 138:697, 1980.

208. Hill L, Ellefson R: Variable interference of meconium in the determination of phosphatidylglycerol. Am J Obstet Gynecol 147:339, 1983.

209. Thibeault D, Hobel C: The interrelationship of the foam stability test, immaturity, and intrapartum complications in the respiratory distress syndrome. Am J Obstet Gynecol 118:56, 1974.

210. Horenstein J, Golde SH, Platt LD: Lung profiles in the isoimmunized pregnancy. Am J Obstet Gynecol 153:443, 1985.

211. Kjos SL, Walther FJ, Montoro M, et al: Prevalence and etiology of respiratory distress in infants of diabetic mothers: predictive value of fetal lung maturation tests. Am J Obstet Gynecol 163:898, 1990.

212. Kulovich M, Gluck L: The lung profile. II. Complicated pregnancy. Am J Obstet Gynecol 135:64, 1979.

213. Towers CV, Garite TJ: Evaluation of the new Amniostat-FLM test for the detection of phosphatidylglycerol in contaminated fluids. Am J Obstet Gynecol 160:298, 1989.

214. Steinfeld JD, Samuels P, Bulley MA, et al: The utility of the TDx test in the assessment of fetal lung maturity. Obstet Gynecol 79:460, 1992.

215. Bayer-Zwirello LA, Jertson J, Rosenbaum J, et al: Amniotic fluid surfactant-albumin ratio as a screening test for fetal lung maturity: two years of clinical experience. J Perinatol XIII: 354, 1993.

216. Apple FS, Bilodeau L, Preese LM, Benson P: Clinical implementation of a rapid, automated assay for assessing fetal lung maturity. J Reprod Med 39:883, 1994.

217. Bonebrake RG, Towers CV, Rumney PJ, Peimbold P: Is fluorescence polarization reliable and cost efficient in a fetal lung maturity cascade? Am J Obstet Gynecol 177:835, 1997.

218. Livingston EG, Herbert WNP, Hage ML, et al: Use of the TDx-FLM assay in evaluating fetal lung maturity in an insulin-dependent diabetic population. Obstet Gynecol 86:826, 1995.

219. Liu KZ, Shaw RA, Dembinski TC, et al: Comparison of infrared spectroscopic and fluorescence depolarization assays for fetal lung maturity. Am J Obstet Gynecol 183:181, 2000.

220. Edwards RK, Duff P, Ross KC: Amniotic fluid indices of fetal pulmonary maturity with preterm premature rupture of membranes. Obstet Gynecol 96:102, 2000.

221. Sher G, Statland B, Freer D, Hisley J: Performance of the amniotic fluid foam stability-50 percent test. A bedside procedure for the prenatal detection of hyaline membrane disease. Am J Obstet Gynecol 134:705, 1979.

222. Sher G, Statland B: Assessment of fetal pulmonary maturity by the Lumadex Foam Stability Index Test. Obstet Gynecol 61:444, 1983.

223. Lockitch G, Wittmann BK, Snow BE, et al: Prediction of fetal lung maturity by use of the Lumadex-FSI test. Clin Chem 32: 361, 1986.

224. Strong TH Jr, Hayes AS, Sawyer AT, et al: Amniotic fluid turbidity: a useful adjunct for assessing fetal pulmonary maturity status. Int J Gynecol Obstet 38:97, 1992.

225. Ashwood ER, Palmer SE, Taylor JS, Pingree SS: Lamellar body counts for rapid fetal lung maturity testing. Obstet Gynecol 81:619, 1993.

226. Fakhoury G, Daikoku NH, Benser J, Dubin NH: Lamellar body concentrations and the prediction of fetal pulmonary maturity. Am J Obstet Gynecol 170:72, 1994.

227. Greenspoon JS, Rosen DJD, Roll K, Dubin SB: Evaluation of lamellar body number density as the initial assessment in a fetal lung maturity test cascade. J Reprod Med 40:260, 1995.

228. Dalence CR, Bowie LJ, Dohnal JC, et al: Amniotic fluid lamellar body count: a rapid and reliable fetal lung maturity test. Obstet Gynecol 86:235, 1995.

229. Lewis PS, Lauria MR, Dzieczkowski J, et al: Amniotic fluid lamellar body count: cost-effective screening for fetal lung maturity. Obstet Gynecol 93:387, 1999.

230. Garite TJ, Freeman RK, Nageotte MP: Fetal maturity cascade: a rapid and cost-effective method for fetal lung maturity testing. Obstet Gynecol 67:619, 1986.

231. Herbert WNP, Chapman JF: Clinical and economic considerations associated with testing for fetal lung maturity. Am J Obstet Gynecol 155:820, 1986.

232. Sue-A-Quan AK, Hannah ME, Cohen MM, et al: Effect of labour induction on rates of stillbirth and cesarean section in post-term pregnancies. Can Med Assoc J 160:1145, 1999.

233. Clark SL, Sabey P, Jolley K: Nonstress testing with acoustic stimulation and amniotic fluid volume assessment: 5973 tests without unexpected fetal death. Am J Obstet Gynecol 160: 694, 1989.

234. Mills MS, James KD, Slade S: Two-tier approach to biophysical assessment of the fetus. Am J Obstet Gynecol 163:12, 1990.

235. Magann EF, Isler CM, Chauhan SP, Martin JN: Amniotic fluid volume estimation and the biophysical profile: a confusion of criteria. Obstet Gynecol 96:640, 2000.

236. Vintzileos AM, Campbell WA, Nochimson DJ, et al: The use and misuse of the fetal biophysical profile. Am J Obstet Gynecol 156:527, 1987.

237. Nageotte MP, Towers CV, Asrat T, Freeman RK: Perinatal outcome with the modified biophysical profile. Am J Obstet Gynecol 170:1672, 1994.

238. Miller DA, Rabello YA, Paul RH: The modified biophysical profile: antepartum testing in the 1990s. Am J Obstet Gynecol 174:812, 1996.

239. Bove KE: Autopsy Committee of the College of American Pathologists: Practice Guidelines for Autopsy Pathology. Arch Pathol Lab Med 121:368, 1997.

240. Doyle LW: Effects of perinatal necropsy on counselling. Lancet 355:2093, 2000.

241. Incerpi MH, Miller DA, Samadi R, et al: Stillbirth evaluation: what tests are needed? Am J Obstet Gynecol 178:1121, 1998.

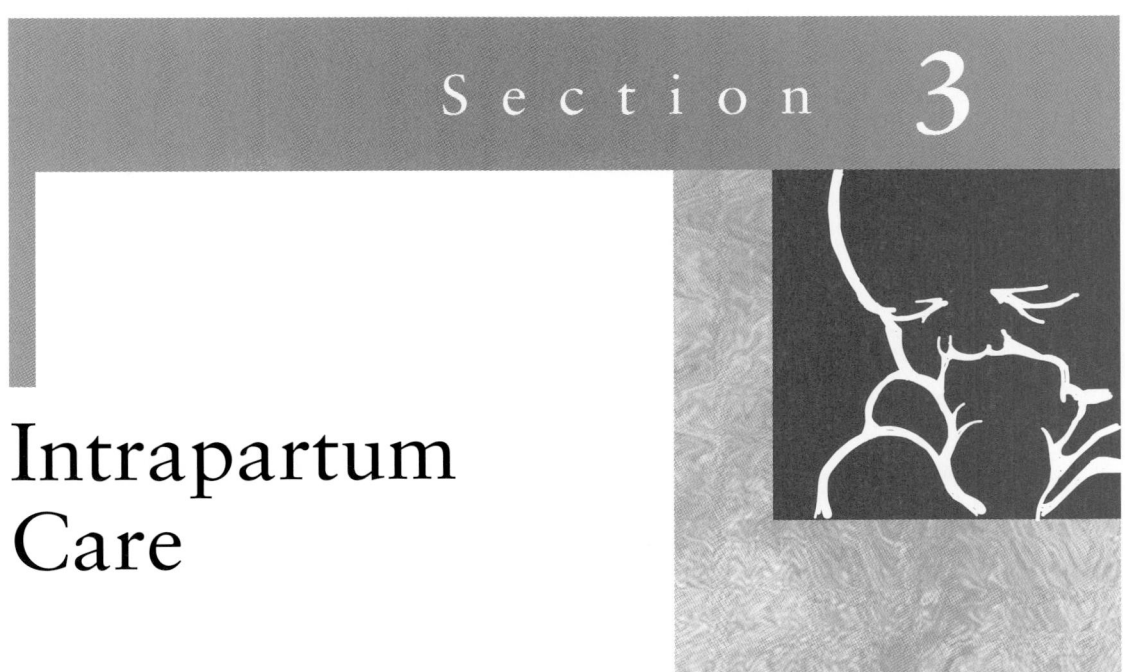

Intrapartum Care

Labor and Delivery

ERROL R. NORWITZ, JULIAN N. ROBINSON, AND
JOHN T. REPKE

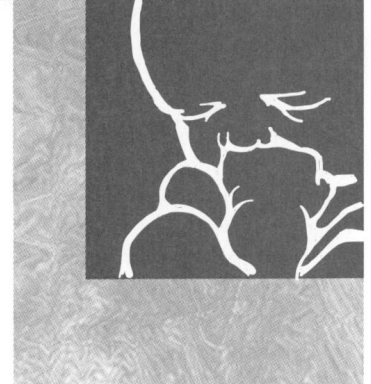

DEFINITIONS

Labor is the physiologic process by which a fetus is expelled from the uterus to the outside world. Labor is defined as an increase in myometrial activity or, more precisely, a switch in the myometrial contractility pattern from "contractures" (long-lasting, low-frequency activity) to "contractions" (frequent, high-intensity, high-frequency activity),[1] resulting in effacement and dilatation of the uterine cervix. In normal labor, there appears to be a time-dependent relationship between the biochemical connective tissue changes in the cervix, which usually precede uterine contractions and cervical dilatation. All of these events usually occur before rupture of the membranes. Spontaneous rupture of the fetal membranes prior to the onset of uterine activity is seen in only 8 percent of term pregnancies.[2]

The mean duration of human singleton pregnancy is 280 days (40 weeks) from the first day of the last menstrual period. "Term" is defined as the period from 36 completed (37.0) to 42.0 weeks of gestation. "Preterm" (premature) labor refers to the onset of labor prior to 36 completed weeks' gestation (see Chapter 23). "Postterm" (prolonged) pregnancy refers to pregnancies continuing beyond 42.0 weeks' gestation (see Chapter 27).

Diagnosis

Labor is a clinical diagnosis. The classic diagnosis of labor includes regular painful uterine contractions, progressive cervical effacement and dilatation, and a show (bloody discharge). Cervical dilatation in the absence of

The reader is referred to the Appendix for illustrations of anatomy relevant to this discussion.

uterine contractions is seen most commonly in the second trimester and is suggestive of cervical incompetence (see Chapter 23). Similarly, the presence of uterine contractions in the absence of cervical change does not meet criteria for the diagnosis of labor.

PHYSIOLOGY OF NORMAL LABOR AT TERM

Historical Perspective

Considerable evidence suggests that, in most viviparous animals, the fetus is in control of the timing of labor.[3–5] During the Hippocratic period, it was believed that the fetus presented head first so that it could kick its legs up against the fundus of the uterus, thereby propelling itself through the birth canal. While we have moved away from this simple mechanical view of labor, the factors responsible for the initiation and maintenance of labor at term are not well defined.

The last few decades have seen a marked change in the nature of the hypotheses to explain the onset of labor. Initial investigations centered on changes in the profile of circulating hormone levels in the maternal and fetal circulations (i.e., endocrine events). More recent studies have focused on the dynamic biochemical dialogue that exists between the fetus and the mother (i.e., paracrine and autocrine events) in an attempt to understand in detail the molecular mechanisms that regulate such interactions.

Phases of Parturition

Labor at term may be regarded physiologically as a release from the inhibitory effects of pregnancy on the

353

myometrium rather than as an active process mediated by uterine stimulants. Strips of quiescent myometrium obtained from a uterus at term and placed in an isotonic water bath, for example, will contract vigorously and spontaneously without added stimuli.[6,7] In vivo, however, it is likely that both inhibitory and stimulatory mechanisms are important.

It is useful to consider the regulation of uterine activity during pregnancy as being divided into four distinct physiologic phases (Fig. 13–1).[8,9] During pregnancy, the uterus is maintained in a state of functional quiescence (phase 0) through the action of various putative inhibitors including, but not limited to, progesterone, prostacyclin (prostaglandin I_2 [PGI_2]), relaxin, parathyroid hormone–related peptide, nitric oxide, calcitonin gene–related peptide, adrenomedullin, and vasoactive intestinal peptide. Before term, the uterus undergoes activation (phase 1) and stimulation (phase 2). Activation occurs in response to uterotopins, including estrogen, and is characterized by increased expression of a series of contraction-associated proteins (including myometrial receptors for prostaglandins and oxytocin), activation of certain ion channels, and an increase in connexin-43 (a key component of gap junctions). An increase in gap junctions between adjacent myometrial cells leads to electrical synchrony within the myometrium and allows for effective coordination of contractions. Following activation, the "primed" uterus can be stimulated to contract by the action of uterotopins such as the stimulatory prostaglandins (PGE_2 and $PGF_{2\alpha}$) and oxytocin. Involution of the uterus after delivery occurs during phase 3 and is mediated primarily by oxytocin.

The Endocrine Control of Labor

Horse–donkey crossbreeding experiments performed in the 1950s resulted in a gestational length intermediate between that of horses (340 days) and that of donkeys (365 days), suggesting a role for the fetal genotype in the initiation of labor.[5,10] The hypothesis that the fetus is in control of the timing of labor has been elegantly demonstrated in domestic ruminants, such as sheep and cows, and involves activation at term of the fetal hypothalamic-pituitary-adrenal axis.[1,11–14] However, this mechanism does not apply to humans. The slow progress in our understanding of the biochemical mechanisms involved in the process of labor in humans in large part reflects the difficulty in extrapolating from the endocrine-control mechanisms in various animals to the paracrine/autocrine mechanisms of parturition in humans, processes that preclude direct investigation.

Regardless of whether the trigger for labor begins within the fetus or outside the fetus, the final common pathway for labor ends in the maternal tissues of the uterus and is characterized by the development of regular phasic uterine contractions. As in other smooth muscles, myometrial contractions are mediated through the adenosine triphosphate (ATP)-dependent binding of myosin to actin. In contrast to vascular smooth muscle, however, myometrial cells have a sparse innervation,

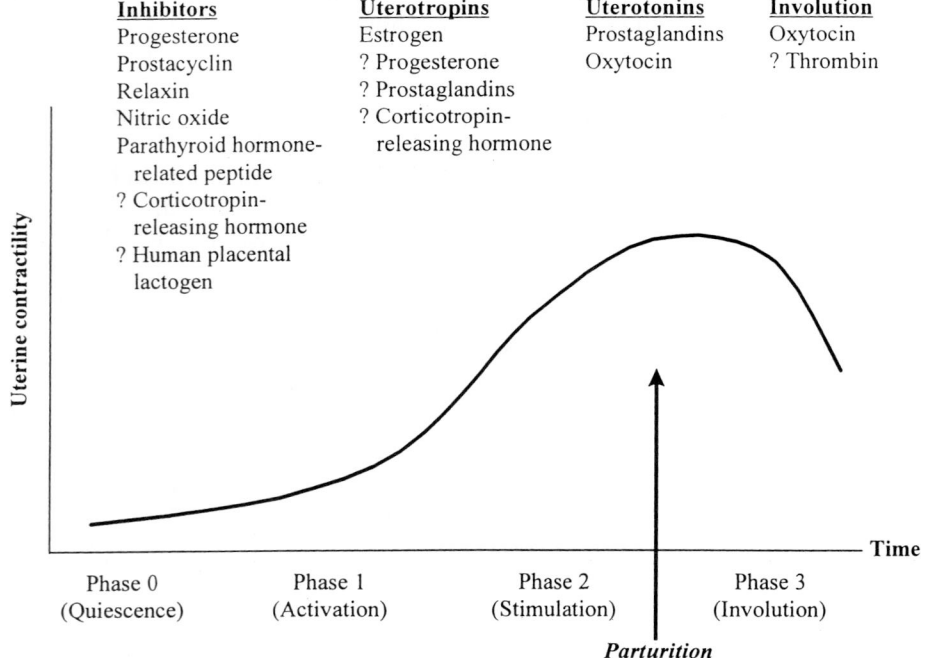

Figure 13–1. Regulation of uterine activity during pregnancy and labor. (Adapted from Challis JRG, Gibb W: Control of parturition. Prenat Neonat Med 1:283, 1996.)

which is further reduced during pregnancy.[15] The regulation of the contractile mechanism of the uterus is therefore largely humoral and/or dependent on intrinsic factors within myometrial cells.

It is likely that there is a "parturition cascade" at term that removes the mechanisms maintaining uterine quiescence and recruits factors promoting uterine activity (Fig. 13–2).[16] Given its teleologic importance, such a cascade would likely have multiple redundant loops to ensure a fail-safe system of securing pregnancy success and ultimately the preservation of the species. In such a model, each element is connected to the next in a sequential fashion, and many of the elements demonstrate positive feed-forward characteristics typical of a cascade mechanism. The sequential recruitment of signals that serve to augment the labor process suggest that it may not be possible to single out any one signaling mechanism as being responsible for the initiation of labor. It may therefore be prudent to describe such mechanisms as being responsible for *promoting*, rather than *initiating*, the process of labor.[17] A comprehensive analysis of each of the individual paracrine/autocrine pathways implicated in the process of labor have been reviewed in detail elsewhere.[8-10,16-19] In brief, human labor at term is a multifactorial physiologic event involving an integrated set of changes within the maternal tissues of the uterus (myometrium, decidua, and uterine cervix) that occur gradually over a period of days to weeks. Such changes include, but are not limited to, an increase in prostaglandin synthesis and release within the uterus, an increase in myometrial gap junction formation, and up-regulation of myometrial oxytocin receptors (uterine activation). Once the myometrium and cervix are prepared, endocrine and/or paracrine/autocrine factors from the fetoplacental unit bring about a switch in the pattern of myometrial activity from irregular contractures to regular contractions (uterine stimulation). The fetus may coordinate this switch in myometrial activity through its influence on placental steroid hormone production, through mechanical distention of the uterus, and through secretion of neurohypophyseal hormones and other stimulators of prostaglandin synthesis. The final common pathway towards labor appears to be activation of the fetal hypothalamic-pituitary-adrenal axis, and is probably common to all species. In the human, the fetal adrenal provides abundant C19 estrogen precursor (dehydroepiandrostenedione) directly from its intermediate (fetal) zone. This is because the human placenta is an incomplete steroidogenic organ and estrogen synthesis by the human placenta has an obligate need for C19 steroid precursor[20] (Fig. 13–2). In the rhesus monkey, infusion of C19 precursor (androstenedione) leads to preterm delivery.[21,22] This effect is blocked by concurrent infusion of an aromatase inhibitor,[23] demonstrating that conversion to estrogen is important. However, systemic infusion of estrogen failed to induce delivery, suggesting that the action of estrogen is likely paracrine/autocine.[21,22]

MECHANICS OF LABOR

Mechanics of Normal Labor at Term

Labor and delivery are not passive processes in which uterine contractions push a rigid object through a fixed aperture. The ability of the fetus to successfully negotiate the pelvis during labor and delivery is dependent on the complex interaction of three variables: the powers, the passenger, and the passage.

The Powers

The powers refer to the forces generated by the uterine musculature. Uterine activity is characterized by the frequency, amplitude (intensity), and duration of contractions. Assessment of uterine activity may include simple observation, manual palpation, external objective assessment techniques (such as external tocodynamometry), and direct measurement of intrauterine pressure (using either internal manometry or pressure transducers). External tocodynamometry measures the change in shape of the abdominal wall as a function of uterine contractions and, as such, is qualitative rather than quantitative. Although it permits graphic display of uterine activity and allows for accurate correlation of fetal heart rate patterns with uterine activity, external tocodynamometry does not allow measurement of contraction intensity or basal intrauterine tone. The most precise method for determination of uterine activity is the direct measurement of intrauterine pressure. Such techniques, however, require insertion of a fluid-filled catheter and/or pressure transducer directly into the uterine cavity usually through the cervix after rupture of the fetal membranes. A risk of uterine injury (perforation) exists during placement of the catheter and such catheters may be associated with an increased incidence of intrauterine infection.

Despite technological improvements, the definition of "adequate" uterine activity during labor remains unclear. Classically, three to five contractions in 10 minutes has been used to define adequate labor, and is seen in around 95 percent of women in spontaneous labor at term. In the active management of labor protocols, seven contractions in 15 minutes is regarded as adequate.[24,25] The more recent introduction of intrauterine pressure transducers has enabled objective measurement

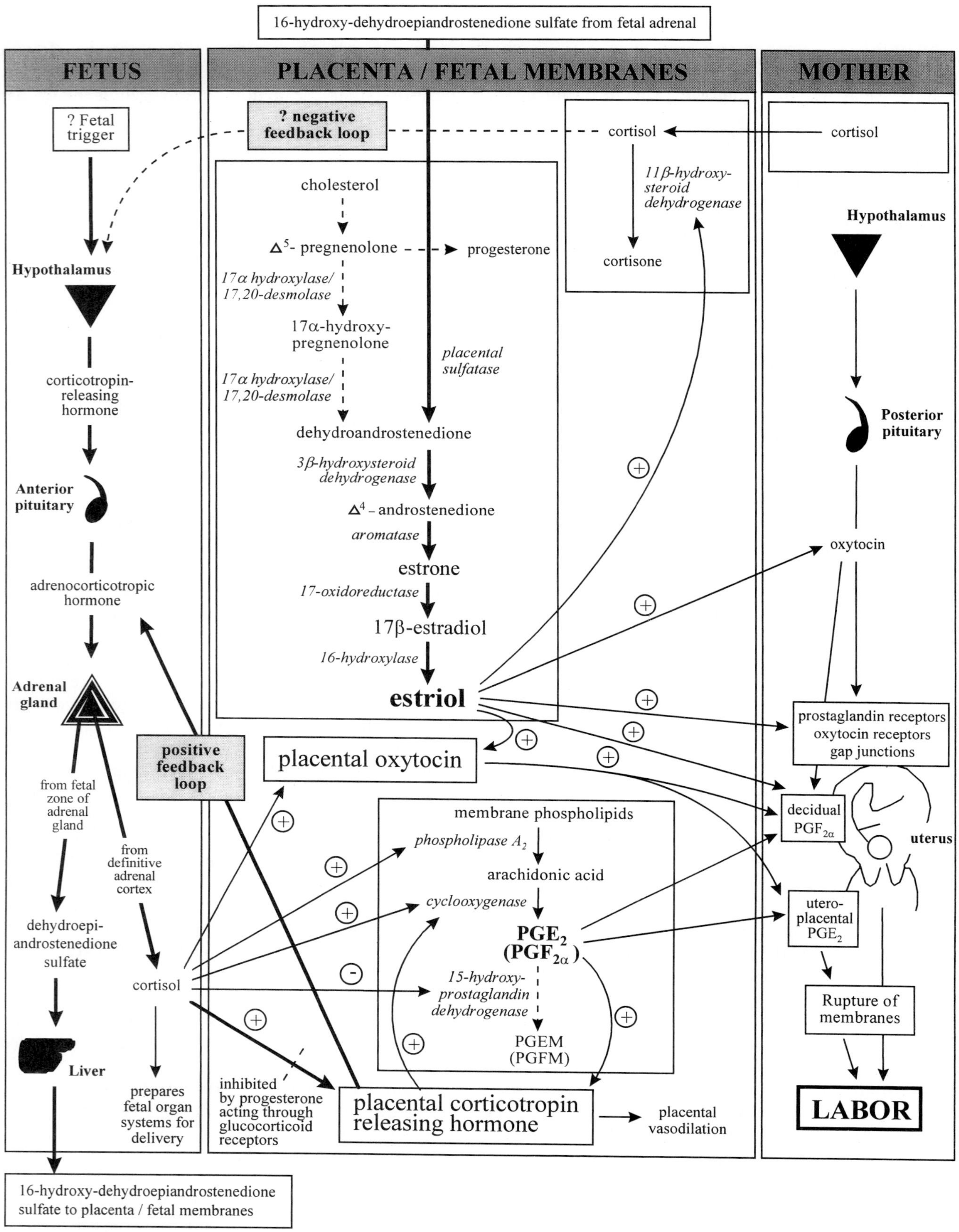

Figure 13–2. Proposed "parturition cascade" for labor induction at term. The spontaneous induction of labor at term in the human is regulated by a series of paracrine/autocrine hormones acting in an integrated parturition cascade responsible for promoting uterine contractions. PGE_2, prostaglandin E_2; PGEM, 13, 14-dihydro-15-keto-PGE_2; $PGF_{2\alpha}$, prostaglandin $F_{2\alpha}$; PGFM, 13,14-dihydro-15keto-$PGF_{2\alpha}$. (Modified from Norwitz ER, Robinson JN, Repke JT: The initiation of parturition: a comparative analysis across the species. Curr Prob Obstet Gynecol Fertil 22:41, 1999.)

of uterine activity.[26] Various units have been devised to objectively measure uterine activity, the most common of which is *Montevideo units* (the average strength of contractions in millimeters of mercury multiplied by the number of contractions per 10 minutes), which is a measure of average frequency and amplitude above basal tone. Two hundred to 250 Montevideo units defines adequate labor.[26,27] It is generally believed that the more optimal the powers, the more likely a successful outcome. However, there are no data to support this statement. The ultimate measure of uterine activity is a clinical one. If uterine contractions are "adequate" to effect vaginal delivery, one of two things will happen. Either the cervix will efface and dilate and the fetal head will descend, or there will be worsening caput succedaneum (scalp edema) and/or moulding of the fetal head (overlapping of the skull bones) without cervical effacement and dilatation. The latter situation suggests the presence of cephalopelvic disproportion (CPD), which can be either absolute (in which a given fetus is simply too large to negotiate a given pelvis) or relative (in which delivery of a given fetus through a given pelvis would be possible under optimal conditions but is precluded by malposition or abnormal attitude of the fetal head).

The Passenger

The passenger is the fetus. There are several fetal variables that influence the course of labor and delivery. These are summarized below.

1. Absolute fetal *size* can be estimated both clinically by abdominal palpation or with ultrasound, but both are subject to a large degree of error. Fetal macrosomia (defined by the American College of Obstetricians and Gynecologists (ACOG) as an absolute fetal size $\geq$ 4,500 g[28]) may be associated with failure to progress in labor.

2. *Lie* refers to the longitudinal axis of the fetus relative to the longitudinal axis of the uterus. Fetal lie can be either longitudinal, transverse, or oblique (Fig. 13–3). In a singleton pregnancy, only fetuses in a longitudinal lie can be safely delivered vaginally.

3. *Presentation* refers to the fetal part that directly overlies the pelvic inlet. In a fetus presenting in the longitudinal lie, the presentation can be either cephalic (vertex), breech, or (rarely) shoulder. Compound presentation refers to the presence of more than one fetal part overlying the pelvic inlet. Funic presentation refers to presentation of the umbilical cord, and is rare at term. In a cephalic fetus, the presentation is classified according to the leading bony landmark of the skull, which can be either the occiput, the mentum (chin), or the brow (Fig. 13–4). *Malpresentation* refers to any presentation that is

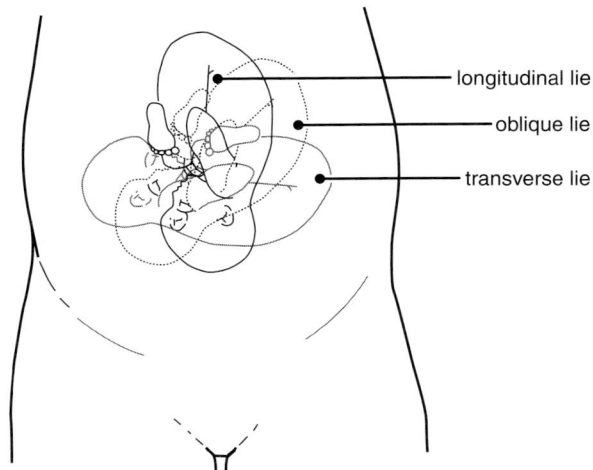

Figure 13–3. Examples of different fetal lie.

not cephalic with the occiput leading, and is seen in around 5 percent of all term labors (see Chapter 16).

4. *Attitude* refers to the position of the head with regard to the fetal spine (i.e., the degree of flexion and/or extension of the fetal head). Flexion of the head is important to facilitate *engagement* of the head in the maternal pelvis. When the fetal chin is optimally flexed onto the chest, the suboccipitobregmatic diameter (9.5 cm) presents at the pelvic inlet (Fig. 13–5). This is the smallest possible presenting diameter in the cephalic presentation. As the head deflexes (extends), the diameter presenting to the pelvic inlet progressively increases even before the malpresentations of brow and face are encountered (Fig. 13–5), and may contribute to failure to progress in labor. The architecture of the pelvic floor along with increased uterine activity may correct deflexion in the early stages of labor.

5. *Position* of the fetus refers to the relationship of a nominated site of the presenting part to a denominating location on the internal pelvis, and can be assessed most accurately on transvaginal examination. In a cephalic presentation, the nominated site is the occiput (e.g., right occiput anterior [ROA]). In the breech presentation, the nominated site is the sacrum (e.g., right sacrum anterior [RSA]). The various positions of a cephalic presentation are illustrated in Figure 13–6. *Malposition* refers to any position in labor which is not ROA, OA, or LOA.

6. *Station* is a measure of descent of the presenting part of the fetus through the birth canal (Fig. 13–7). The old classification was an arbitrary subjective assignment of seven stations (−3 to +3), whereas the new classification (−5 to +5) is an attempt to quantitate in centimeters the distance of the leading bony edge from the ischial spines. In both classifications,

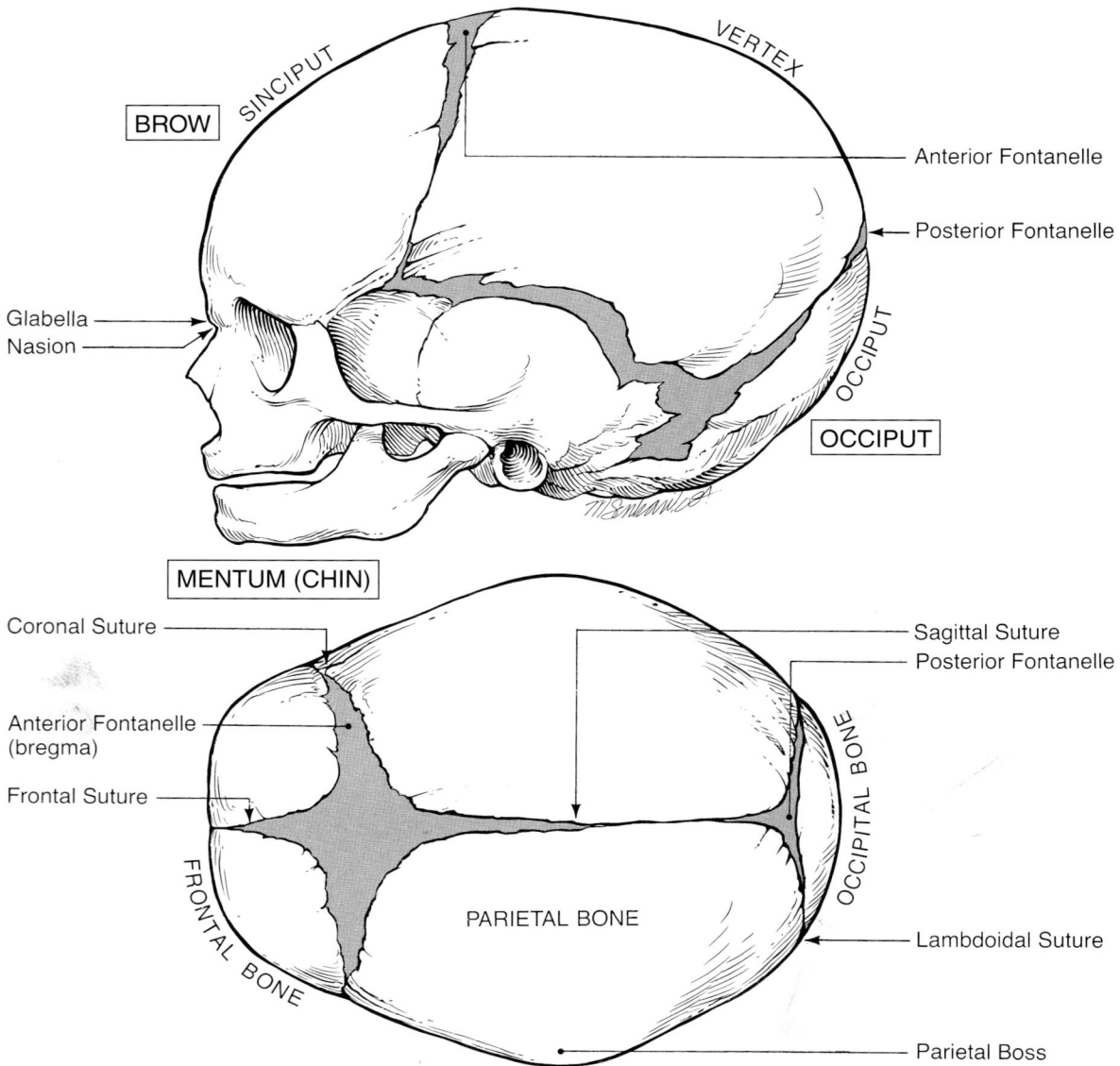

Figure 13–4. Landmarks on the fetal skull for determination of fetal position. (Modified from O'Brien WF, Cefalo RC: Labor and delivery. *In* Gabbe SG, Niebyl JP, Simpson JL [eds]: Obstetrics: Normal and Problem Pregnancies, 3rd ed. New York, Churchill Livingstone, 1996, p 393.)

the midpoint (0 station) is defined as the plane of the maternal ischial spines.

7. *Multifetal pregnancies* (twins, triplets, and/or higher order multifetal pregnancies) increase the probability of abnormal lie and malpresentation in labor.

Abnormality in any of the above fetal variables may influence the decision of whether or not to proceed with vaginal delivery, and may affect the course of labor. Failure to progress in labor should prompt a careful reevaluation of the above fetal parameters to exclude absolute or relative CPD.

The Passage

The passage consists of the bony pelvis (composed of the sacrum, ilium, ischium, and pubis) and the resistance provided by the soft tissues. The bony pelvis is divided into the false (greater) and true (lesser) pelvis by the pelvic brim, which is demarcated by the sacral promontory, the anterior ala of the sacrum, the arcuate line of the ilium, the pectineal line of the pubis, and the pubic crest culminating in the symphysis (Fig. 13–8). Measurements of the various parameters of the bony female pelvis have been made with great precision, directly in cadavers and using radiographic imaging in living women. Such measurements have divided the true

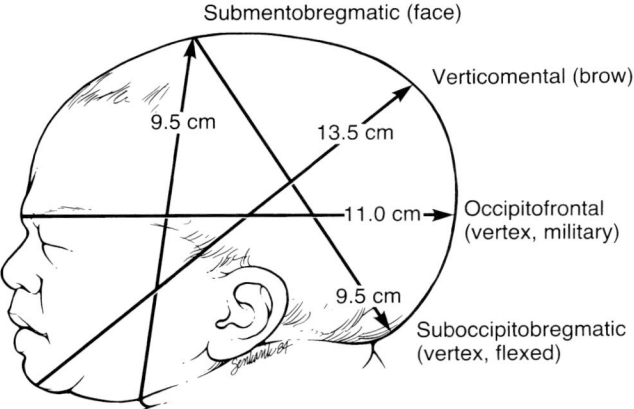

Figure 13–5. Presenting diameters of the average term fetal skull. (From O'Brien WF, Cefalo RC: Labor and delivery. *In* Gabbe SG, Niebyl JR, Simpson JL [eds]: Obstetrics: Normal and Problem Pregnancies, 3rd ed. New York, Churchill Livingstone, 1996, p 377, with permission.)

pelvis into a series of planes that must be negotiated by the fetus during passage through the birth canal, which can be broadly classified into the pelvic inlet, midcavity and outlet. X-ray pelvimetry[29] has defined average and critical limit values for the various parameters of the bony pelvis (Table 13–1). Critical limit values are measurements that are associated a high probability of CPD.[30] X-ray pelvimetry is now rarely used, having been replaced in large part by a clinical trial of the pelvis (a "trial of labor"). Computed tomography (CT) has the potential for highly reproducible measurements of the bony pelvis.[31] However, concerns over cost and exposure of the fetus to even small mounts of ionizing radiation have limited its use. Clinical pelvimetry is currently the only method of assessing the shape and dimensions of the bony pelvis in labor. A useful protocol for clinical pelvimetry is detailed in Figure 13–9, and involves assessment of three parameters of the pelvic inlet, midcavity, and outlet. The inlet of the true pelvis is largest in its transverse diameter (usually ≥ 12.0 cm). The *diagonal conjugate* (the distance from the sacral promontory to the inferior margin of the symphysis pubis as assessed on bimanual examination)

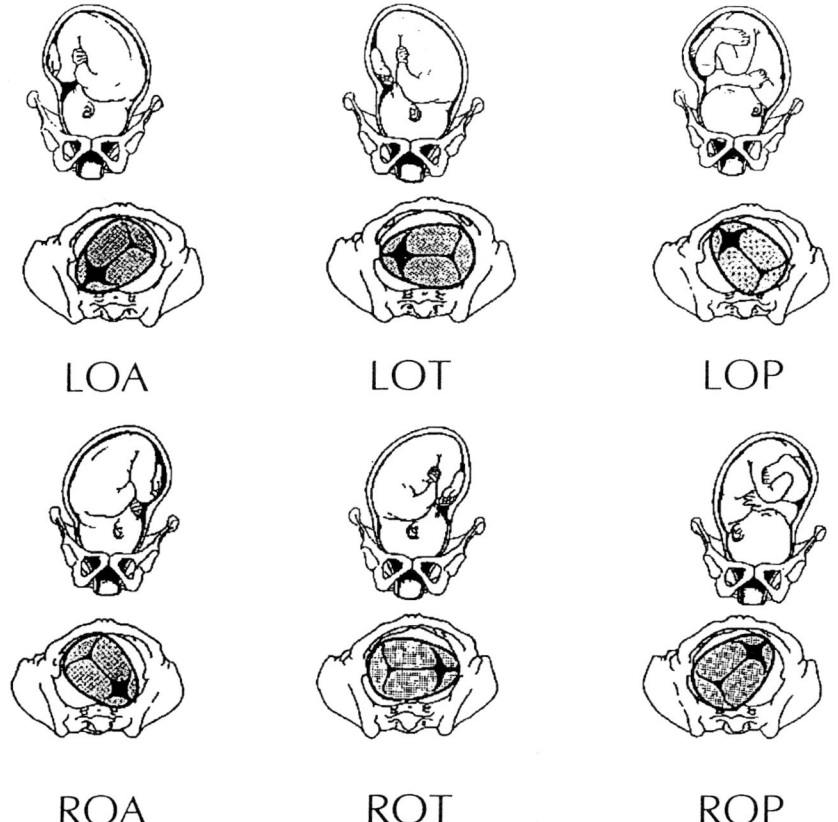

Figure 13–6. Fetal presentations and positions in labor. LOA, left occiput anterior; LOT, left occiput transverse; LOP, left occiput posterior; OA, occiput anterior; OP, occiput posterior; ROA, right occiput anterior; ROT, right occiput transverse; ROP, right occiput posterior. (Adapted from Norwitz ER, Robinson J, Repke JT: The initiation and management of labor. *In* Seifer DB, Samuels P, Kniss DA [eds]: The Physiologic Basis of Gynecology and Obstetrics. Baltimore, Lippincott Williams & Wilkins, 2000 [in press].)

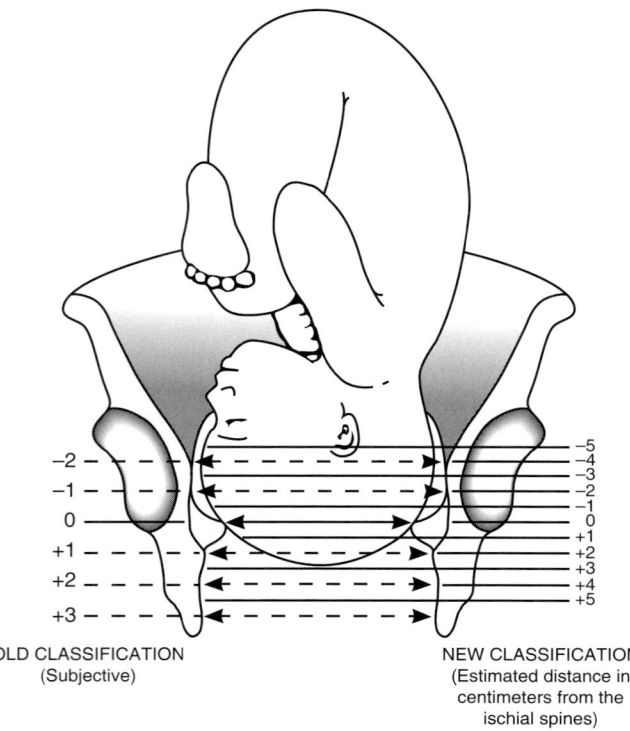

OLD CLASSIFICATION
(Subjective)

NEW CLASSIFICATION
(Estimated distance in
centimeters from the
ischial spines)

Figure 13-7. The relationship of the leading edge of the presenting part of the fetus to the plane of the maternal ischial spines determines the station. Station +1/+3 (old classification) or +2/+5 (new classification) is illustrated.

Table 13-1. AVERAGE AND CRITICAL LIMIT VALUES FOR PELVIC MEASUREMENTS BY X-RAY PELVIMETRY

Diameter	Average Value	Critical Limit*
Pelvic inlet		
Anteroposterior (cm)	12.5	10.0
Transverse (cm)	13.0	12.0
Sum (cm)	25.5	22.0
Area (cm²)	145.0	123.0
Pelvic midcavity		
Anteroposterior (cm)	11.5	10.0
Transverse (cm)	10.5	9.5
Sum (cm)	22.0	19.5
Area (cm²)	125.0	106.0

*The critical limit values cited imply a high likelihood of cephalopelvic disproportion.
Adapted from O'Brien WF, Cefalo RC: Labor and delivery. *In* Gabbe SG, Niebyl JR, Simpson JL (eds): Obstetrics: Normal and Problem Pregnancies, 3rd ed. New York, Churchill Livingstone, 1996, p 377.

is a clinical representation of the anteroposterior diameter of the pelvic inlet. The *true conjugate* (or *obstetric conjugate*) of the pelvic inlet is the distance from the sacral promontory to the superior aspect of the symphysis pubis. This measurement cannot be made clinically, but can be estimated by subtracting 1.5 to 2.0 cm from the obstetric conjugate. This is the smallest diameter of the inlet, and usually measures around 10 to 11 cm. The limiting factor in the midcavity is the interspinous diameter (the measurement between the is-

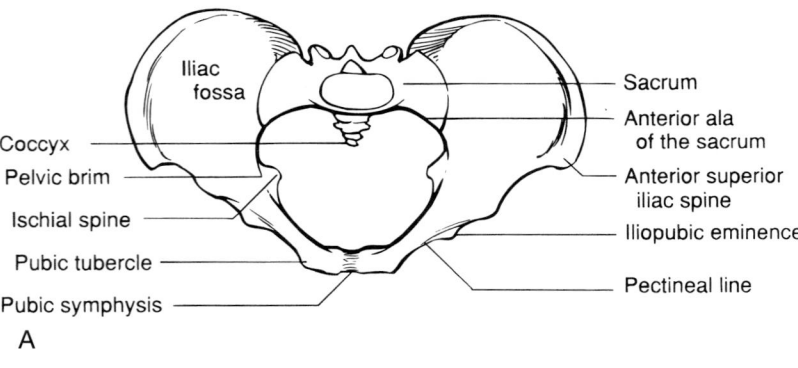

A

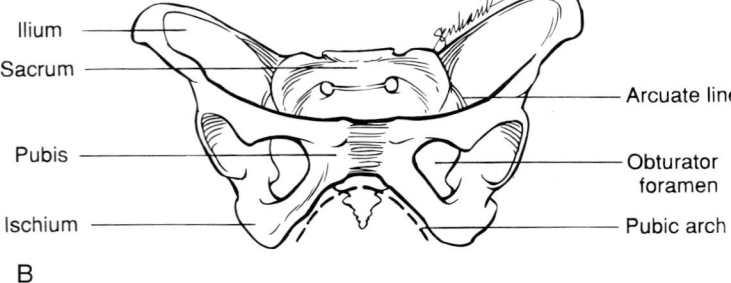

B

Figure 13-8. Superior (*A*) and anterior (*B*) view of the female pelvis. (From Repke JT: Intrapartum Obstetrics. New York, Churchill Livingstone, 1996, p 68, with permission.)

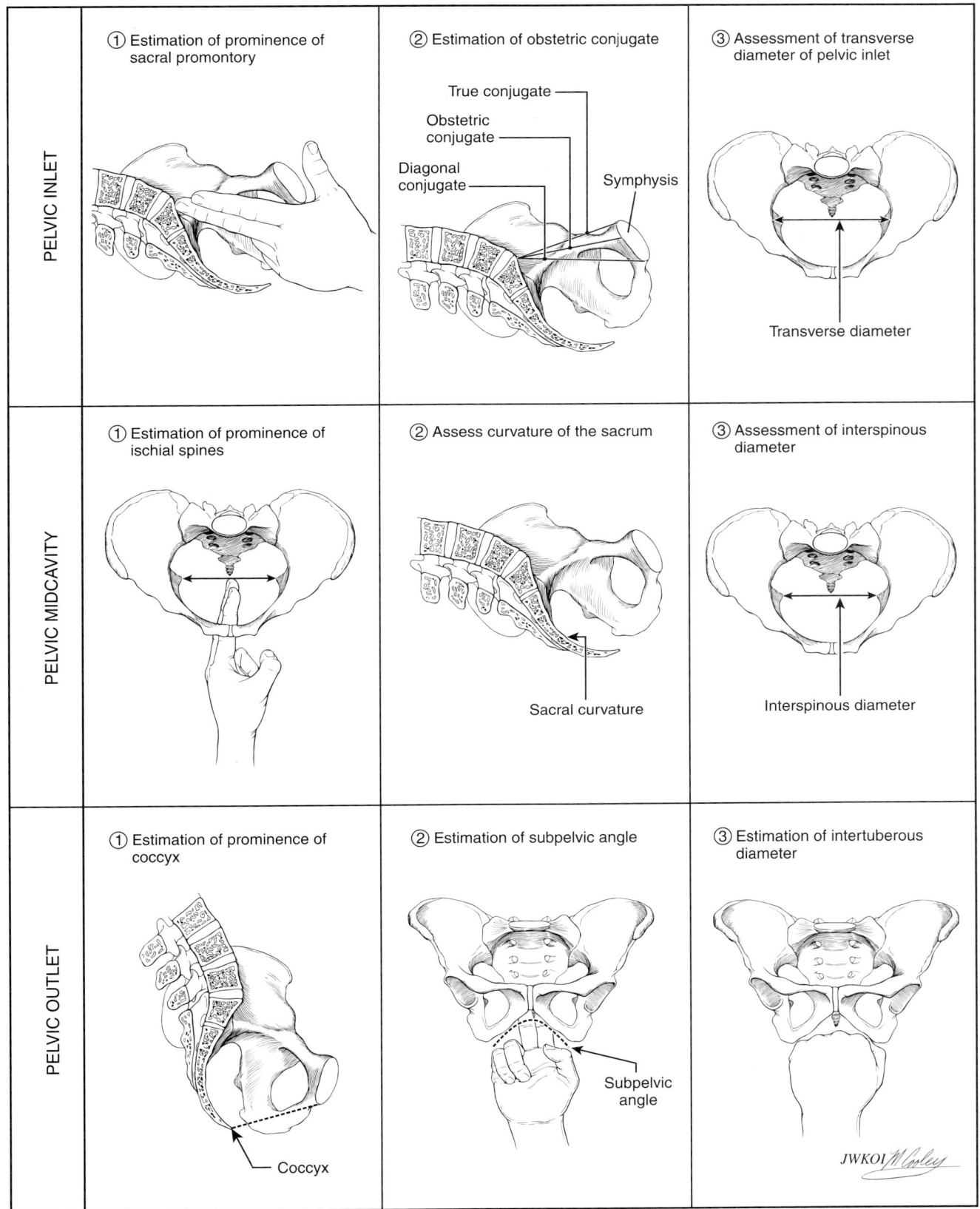

Figure 13–9. A protocol for clinical pelvimetry.

chial spines), which is usually the smallest diameter of the pelvis, but should be greater than 10 cm. The pelvic outlet is rarely of clinical significance. The anteroposterior diameter from the coccyx to the symphysis pubis is usually around 13 cm, and the transverse diameter between the ischial tuberosities around 8 cm.

The shape of the female bony pelvis can be classified into one or more of four broad categories: gynecoid, anthropoid, android, and platypelloid (Fig. 13–10). This classification, based on the radiographic studies of Caldwell and Moloy,[32] separates those with favorable characteristics (gynecoid, anthropoid) from those that are less favorable for vaginal delivery (android, platypelloid). In reality, however, many women fall into intermediate classes and the distinctions become arbitrary. The gynecoid pelvis is the classic female shape with an oval-shaped inlet, diverging midpelvic sidewalls, and far-spaced ischial spines. The anthropoid pelvis has an exaggerated oval shape to the inlet with the largest diameter being anteroposterior, and with limited anterior capacity to the pelvis. Such pelves are more often associated with delivery in the occiput posterior position. The android pelvis is male in pattern, with a heart-shaped inlet, prominent sacral promontory and ischial spines, shallow sacral hollow, and converging midpelvic sidewalls. Women with such pelves are at increased risk of CPD. The platypelloid pelvis is a broad, flat pelvis with an exaggerated oval-shaped inlet, but with the largest diameter being the transverse diameter. Although the assessment of fetal size along with pelvic shape and capacity is useful to predict women at risk of CPD in labor, it is an inexact science. An adequate trial of labor is the only way to determine whether a given fetus will be able to safely negotiate a given pelvis.

Pelvic soft tissues may provide resistance in both the first and second stages of labor. In the first stage, resistance is offered primarily by the cervix; whereas in the second stage, it is by the muscles of the pelvic floor. It has been proposed that rapid labors result from low pelvic resistance rather than from high myometrial activity.[33] Indeed, intrauterine pressures are lower when cervical ripening is used prior to augmentation of labor with oxytocin as compared with augmentation alone.[34] However, this hypothesis has not received wide acceptance. In the second stage of labor, the resistance of the pelvic musculature is believed to play an important role

		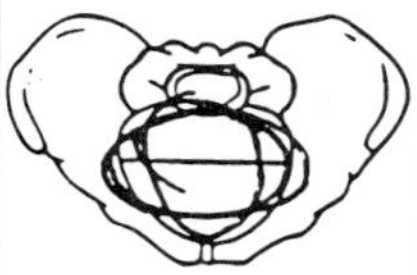 Gynecoid	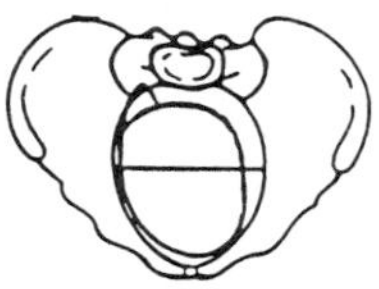 Anthropoid	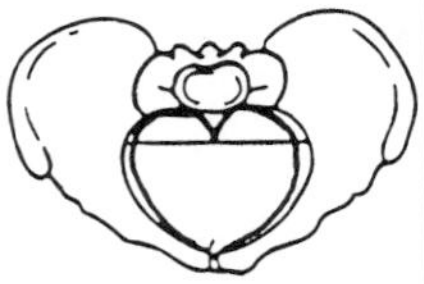 Android	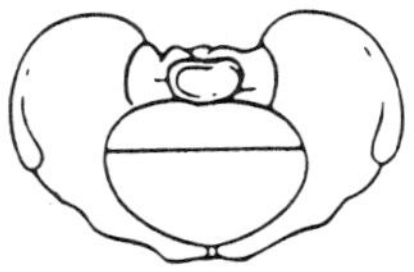 Platypelloid
Pelvic inlet 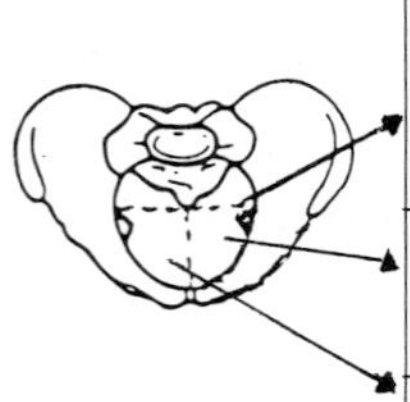	Widest transverse diameter of inlet	12 cm	< 12 cm	12 cm	12 cm
	Anteroposterior diameter of inlet	11 cm	> 12 cm	11 cm	10 cm
	Forepelvis	Wide	Divergent	Narrow	Straight
Pelvic midcavity 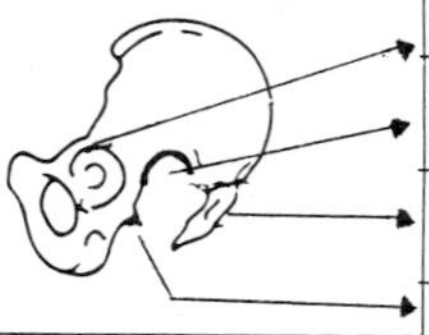	Side walls	Straight	Narrow	Convergent	Wide
	Sacrosciatic notch	Medium	Backward	Narrow	Forward
	Inclination of sacrum	Medium	Wide	Forward (lower third)	Narrow
	Ischial spines	Not prominent	Not prominent	Not prominent	Not prominent
Pelvic outlet 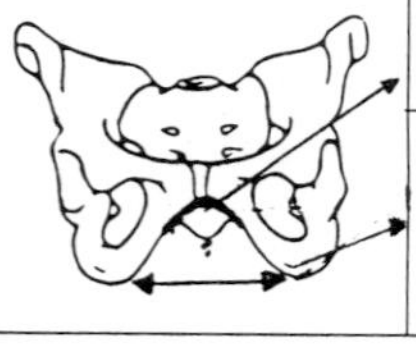	Subpubic arch	Wide	Medium	Narrow	Wide
	Transverse diameter of outlet	10 cm	10 cm	< 10 cm	10 cm

Figure 13–10. Characteristics of the four types of female bony pelvis. (Modified from Callahan TL, Caughey AB, Heffner LJ [eds]: Blueprints in Obstetrics & Gynecology. Malden, MA, Blackwell Science, 1998, p 45.)

in the rotation and movement of the presenting part through the pelvis.

Stages of Labor

Although labor is a continuous process, for reasons of study and to assist in clinical management it has traditionally been divided into three stages, with the first stage further subdivided into three phases.

First Stage

The first stage of labor refers to the interval between the onset of labor and full cervical dilatation. It has been subdivided by Friedman[35,36] in his classic studies on the course of labor in primigravida into three phases according to the rate of cervical dilatation (Fig. 13–11). The *latent phase* is defined as the period between the onset of labor and a point at which a change in the slope of the rate of cervical dilatation is noted.[35,36] It is characterized by slow cervical dilatation and is of variable duration. The *active phase* is associated with a greater rate of cervical dilatation and usually begins at around 2 to 3 cm dilatation.[35–37] The active phase is further subdivided into an acceleration phase, a phase of maximum slope, and a deceleration phase. A *descent phase* was described in the original manuscript that usually coincides with the second stage of labor. Not all investigators accept the existence of a separate descent phase. Subsequent studies have shown that the characteristics of the labor curve do not differ

between various ethnic groups,[38] although there are significant differences between the labor curve of primigravid and multiparous women. Friedman[35,36] has described averages and a statistical maximum (2 SD greater than the mean) for each phase (Table 13–2). As evidenced in Table 13–2, the minimum rate of cervical dilatation of 1.2 cm/h for a nulliparous patient represents 2 SD from the mean, and not the average rate of dilatation. From the normal profile produced by Friedman, it is possible to identify abnormal labor patterns and thereby pregnancies at risk for adverse events in labor. For any individual patient, the clinician responsible for managing the labor should have a sense at any point in time of where on the normal labor curve the patient is. This task can be facilitated by the use of the partogram,[39] a graphical representation of the labor curve against which a patient's progress in labor is plotted. In this way, abnormal labor patterns can easily be identified and appropriate measures taken.

Second Stage

The second stage of labor is the interval between full cervical dilatation (10 cm) and delivery of the infant. It is characterized by descent of the presenting part through the maternal pelvis culminating in expulsion of the fetus. The mother can assume a more active role in the second stage, using maternal effort to aid descent of the fetus. In modern obstetric practice, the nulliparous patient is recommended to push for a maximum of 2 hours without regional anesthesia (or 3 hours with re-

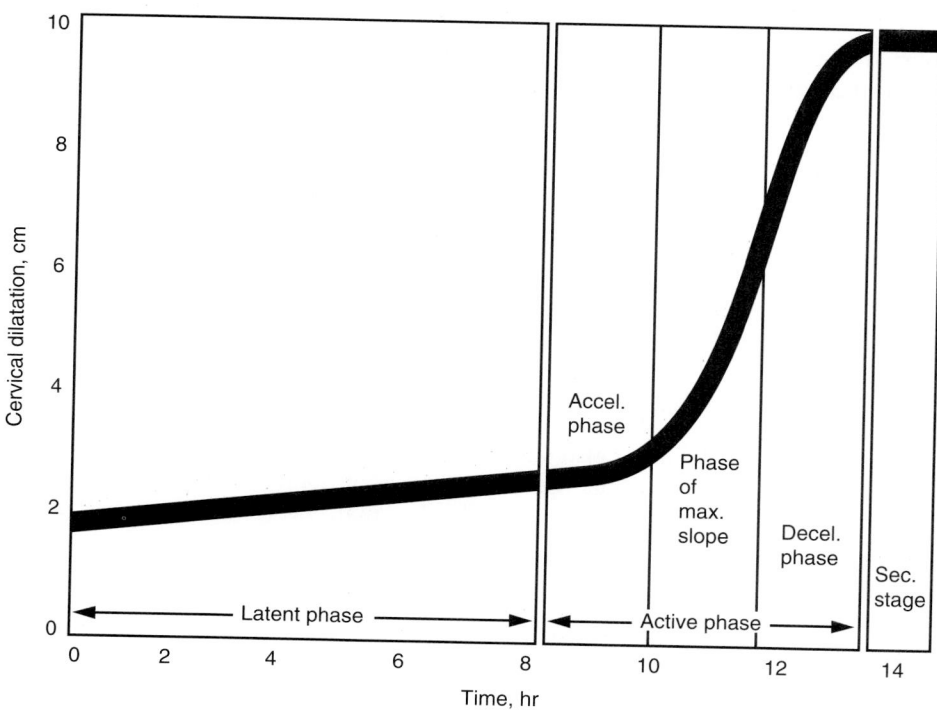

Figure 13–11. Characteristics of the average cervical dilatation curve for nulliparous labor. (Adapted from Friedman EA: Labor: Clinical Evaluation and Management, 2nd ed. Norwalk, CT, Appleton-Century-Crofts, 1978.)

Table 13–2. PROGRESSION OF SPONTANEOUS LABOR AT TERM

Parameter	Mean	5th Percentile
Nulliparas		
Total duration of labor	10.1 h	25.8 h
Stage of labor		
Duration of the first stage	9.7 h	24.7 h
Duration of the second stage	33.0 min	117.5 min
Duration of latent phase	6.4 h	20.6 h
Rate of cervical dilatation during active phase	3.0 cm/h	1.2 cm/h
Duration of the third stage	5.0 min	30.0 min
Multiparas		
Total duration of labor	6.2 h	19.5 h
Stage of labor		
Duration of the first stage	8.0 h	18.8 h
Duration of the second stage	8.5 min	46.5 min
Duration of latent phase	4.8 h	13.6 h
Rate of cervical dilatation during active phase	5.7 cm/h	1.5 cm/h
Duration of the third stage	5.0 min	30.0 min

Data from Friedman EA: Labor: Clinical Evaluation and Management, 2nd ed. Norwalk, CT, Appleton-Century-Crofts, 1978.

gional anesthesia). The multiparous patient is recommended to push for a maximum of 1 hour without regional anesthesia (or 2 hours with regional anesthesia).[40] In practice, full cervical dilatation is not a prerequisite for descent of the presenting part and descent can commence during the first stage. However, no active intervention (either maternal expulsive efforts or obstetric intervention) should be attempted until full cervical dilatation has been achieved.

Third Stage

The third stage of labor refers to delivery of the placenta and fetal membranes. The third stage usually lasts less than 10 minutes, but up to 30 minutes may be allowed before active intervention is considered, as long as blood loss is not excessive.

Cardinal Movements in Labor

The mechanisms of labor, also known as the cardinal movements, refer to the changes in position of fetal head during its passage through the birth canal. Because of the asymmetry of the shape of both the fetal head and the maternal bony pelvis, such rotations are required for the fetus to successfully negotiate the birth canal. Although labor and birth is a continuous process, seven discrete cardinal movements of the fetus are described: engagement, descent, flexion, internal rota-

tion, extension, external rotation or restitution, and expulsion (Fig. 13–12).

Engagement

Engagement refers to passage of the widest diameter of the presenting part to a level below the plane of the pelvic inlet (Fig. 13–13). In the cephalic presentation with a well-flexed head, the largest transverse diameter of the fetal head is the biparietal diameter (9.5 cm). In the breech, the widest diameter is the bitrochanteric diameter. Clinically, engagement can be confirmed by palpation of the presenting part both abdominally and vaginally. With a cephalic presentation, engagement is achieved when only two fifths of the fetal head are palpable abdominally or when the presenting part is at 0 station (at the level of the maternal ischial spines) on bimanual examination. This is because the average distance between the plane of the pelvic inlet and the ischial spines is approximately 5 cm, while the distance between the biparietal plane and the occiput averages 3 to 4 cm. Engagement is considered an important clinical parameter as it demonstrates that, at least at the level of the pelvic inlet, the maternal bony pelvis is sufficiently large to allow descent of the fetal head. In nulliparas, engagement of the fetal head usually occurs by 36 weeks' gestation and the inability of the head to engage by this time may be an early sign of CPD. In multiparas, however, engagement can occur later in gestation or even during labor.

Descent

Descent refers to the downward passage of the presenting part through the pelvis. Descent of the fetus, however, is not continuous, with the greatest rate of descent occurring during the deceleration phase of the first stage of labor and during the second stage of labor.

Flexion

Flexion of the fetal head occurs passively as the head descends due to the shape of the bony pelvis and the resistance offered by the soft tissues of the pelvic floor. Although flexion of the fetal head onto the chest is present to some degree in most fetuses before labor, complete flexion usually only occurs during the course of labor. The result of complete flexion is to present the smallest diameter of the fetal head (the suboccipitobregmatic diameter) for optimal passage through the pelvis.

Internal Rotation

Internal rotation refers to rotation of the presenting part from its original position (usually transverse with

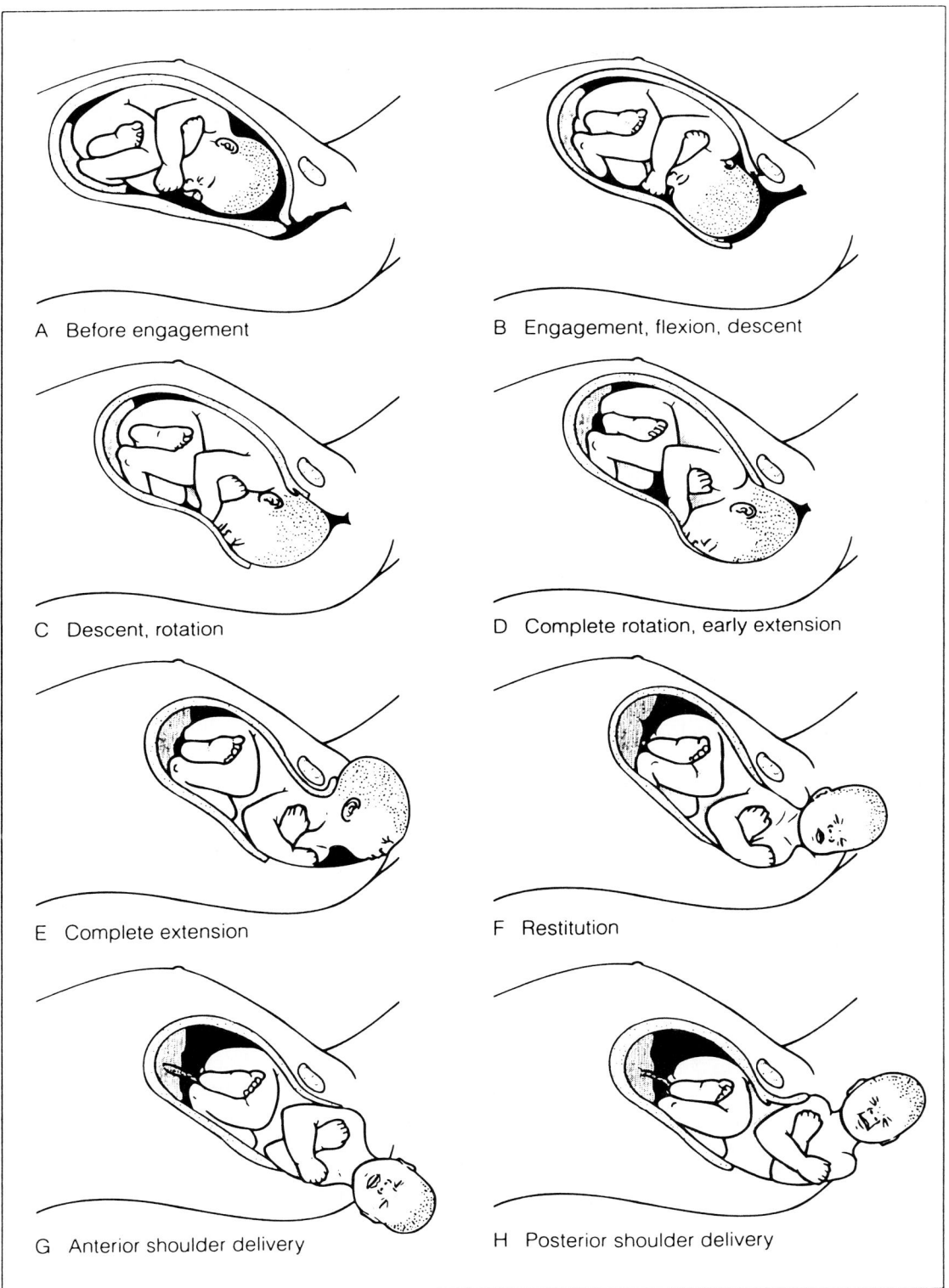

Figure 13–12. Cardinal movements of labor.

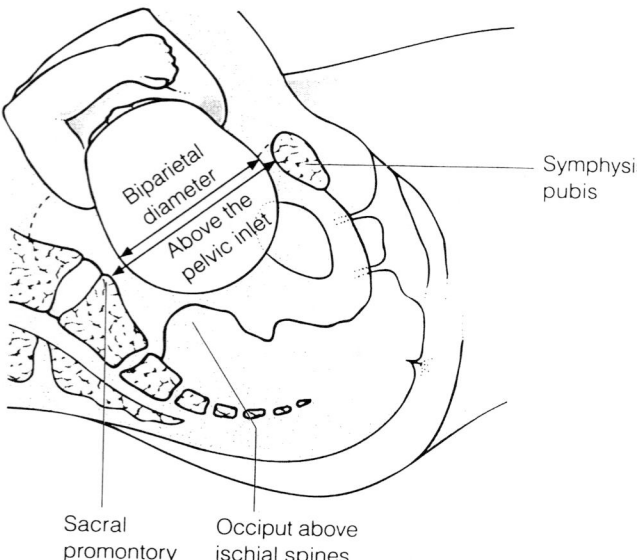

Figure 13–13. Engagement of the fetal head.

regard to the birth canal) to the anteroposterior position as it passes through the pelvis. As with flexion, internal rotation is a passive movement resulting from the shape of the pelvis and the pelvic floor musculature. The pelvic floor musculature, including the coccygeus and ileococcygeus muscles, form a V-shaped hammock that diverges anteriorly. As the head descends, the occiput of the fetus rotates towards the symphysis pubis (or, less commonly, towards the hollow of the sacrum), thereby allowing the widest portion of the fetus to negotiate the pelvis at its widest dimension. Due to the angle of inclination between the maternal lumbar spine and pelvic inlet, the fetal head engages in an asynclitic fashion (i.e., with one parietal eminence lower than the other). With uterine contractions, the leading parietal eminence descends and is first to engage the pelvic floor. As the uterus relaxes, the pelvic floor musculature causes the fetal head to rotate until it is no longer asynclitic.

Extension

Extension occurs once the fetus has descended to the level of the introitus. This descent brings the base of the occiput into contact with the inferior margin at the symphysis pubis. At this point, the birth canal curves upwards. The fetal head is delivered by extension and rotates around the symphysis pubis. The forces responsible for this motion are the downward force exerted on the fetus by the uterine contractions along with the upward forces exerted by the muscles of the pelvic floor.

External Rotation

External rotation, also known as restitution, refers to the return of the fetal head to the correct anatomic position in relation to the fetal torso. This can occur to either side depending on the orientation of the fetus. This is again a passive movement resulting from a release of the forces exerted on the fetal head by the maternal bony pelvis and its musculature and mediated by the basal tone of the fetal musculature.

Expulsion

Expulsion refers to delivery of the rest of the fetus. After delivery of the head and external rotation, further descent brings the anterior shoulder to the level of the symphysis pubis. The anterior shoulder is delivered in much the same manner as the head, with rotation of the shoulder under the symphysis pubis. After the shoulder, the rest of the body is usually delivered without difficulty.

MANAGEMENT OF NORMAL LABOR AND DELIVERY

Initial Assessment in Labor

Initial assessment in labor should include a review of the patient's prenatal information, a focused history (including the time of onset of contractions, status of fetal membranes, presence or absence of vaginal bleeding, perception of fetal movement), physical examination, and necessary laboratory testing as indicated. Physical examination should include documentation of the patient's vital signs; notation of fetal position and presentation; an assessment of fetal well-being; and an estimation of the frequency, duration, and quality of uterine contractions. The size, presentation, and lie of the fetus can be assessed by abdominal palpation. A systematic method of examination of the gravid abdomen was first described by Leopold and Sporlin in 1894.[41] Although abdominal examination has several limitations (small fetus, maternal obesity, multifetal pregnancies, polyhydramnios), it is safe, well tolerated, and may add valuable information in the management of labor. Palpation is divided into four separate Leopold's maneuvers (Fig. 13–14). Each maneuver is designed to identify specific fetal landmarks or to reveal a specific relationship between the fetus and the mother. These are summarized below.

Leopold's maneuver #1. The gravid uterus is slightly dextrorotated (deviated to the right) because of the

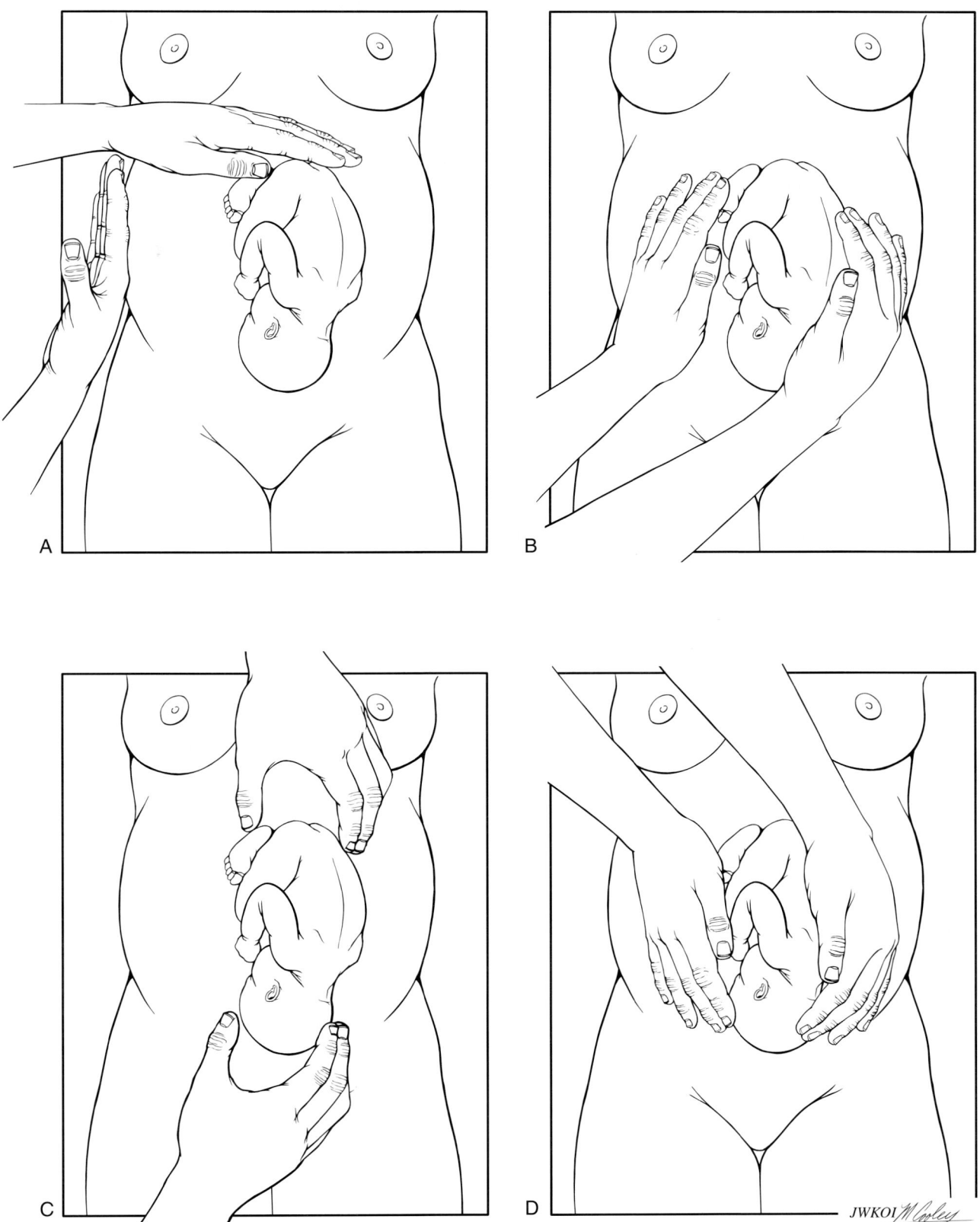

Figure 13–14. Leopold's maneuvers for palpation of the gravid abdomen.

position of the sigmoid colon. With the patient lying supine and her knees comfortably flexed, the examiner corrects for dextrorotation of the uterus with the back of one hand and delineates the fundus of the uterus with the other. The "fundal height" refers to a midline measurement from the symphysis pubis to the top of the uterine fundus. This is a useful measurement to estimate gestation age, although it has some limitations (multifetal pregnancies, poly- or oligohydramnios, uterine fibroids).

Leopold's maneuver #2. The examiner runs their hands down the maternal abdomen on either side of the fetus to determine the fetal lie, and uses their fingers to locate the fetal spine and small parts (extremities). Fetal parts can usually be identified by palpation at 25 to 26 weeks' gestation. If fetal movements are noted, these should be documented.

Leopold's maneuver #3. Also known as Pawlik's grip, this maneuver involves the examiner firmly grasping the upper and lower poles of the fetus by placing their fingers laterally above the symphysis pubis and at the fundus. In this way, the characteristics of the two fetal poles can be determined and compared, and the presentation documented. The fetal breech is often larger, softer, less well defined, and less ballottable than the cranium. This maneuver also allows an estimation of amniotic fluid volume and fetal size. If the estimated fetal weight is less than expected for gestational age, if the head is disproportionately firm in a small fetus, and/or if the fetal parts can be very easily felt (a clinical proxy for low amniotic fluid volume), a diagnosis of intrauterine growth restriction should be entertained.

Leopold's maneuver #4. In this maneuver, the examiner faces the patient's feet and moves their hands in bilaterally from the anterior superior iliac crests to determine whether or not the presenting part of the fetus is engaged in the maternal pelvis. In a cephalic presentation, the head is regarded as unengaged (greater than three fifths above the pelvic brim) if the examiner's hands are seen to converge below the fetal head. If the examiner's hands are noted to diverge as they trace the fetal head into the pelvis, the vertex is regarded as engaged (greater than three fifths below the pelvic brim). This procedure also allows the practitioner to assess the attitude (degree of flexion/extension) of the fetal head.

In most pregnant women, abdominal palpation will be sufficient to determine the lie, presentation, and engagement of the fetus. However, abdominal palpation cannot accurately assess fetal position or station. If there are no contraindications to pelvic examination, the degree of cervical dilatation, effacement, status of the fetal membranes, and the position and station of the presenting part should be noted. If the practitioner is still uncertain about fetal presentation or if the clinical examination suggests an abnormality (such as a multifetal pregnancy, low amniotic fluid volume, or intrauterine growth restriction), an ultrasound examination is indicated. At term, estimation of fetal weight by the physician, and even the mother, is at least as good as sonographic estimations, with an error of 15 to 20 percent.[42]

Intrapartum Management

Approximately 25 to 30 percent of pregnancies will be identified either antenatally or during the course of labor as being at high risk for adverse perinatal outcome because of the presence of underlying maternal or fetal conditions. Such pregnancies account for 75 to 80 percent of all perinatal morbidity and mortality.[43] However, the remaining 20 to 25 percent of perinatal morbidity and mortality arise from pregnancies with no underlying risk factors for adverse outcome. As such, all pregnant women require adequate surveillance throughout labor and delivery.

After the patient has been admitted in labor, she and her family should be introduced to the members of the health care team responsible for her care. The patient and her family should be consulted and involved in such decisions as the use of oxytocin to augment labor, the choice of agent for intrapartum pain management, and the need for assisted vaginal delivery. Emotional support of the patient during the birthing process has been shown repeatedly to lower intrapartum analgesia requirements, to decrease intrapartum complications, and to minimize postpartum emotional difficulties,[44,45] and is strongly encouraged.

Assessment of the quality of the uterine contractions as well as cervical examinations at appropriate intervals should be performed in order to follow the progress of labor. Vaginal examinations should be kept to a minimum to avoid promoting intra-amniotic infection. Cleansing of the perineum with an antiseptic and the use of a sterile lubricant may decrease potential contamination. Although walking during the first stage of labor is often recommended and may reduce patients' discomfort, it does not alter the duration of labor, the need for labor augmentation with oxytocin, the use of analgesia, or the rate of assisted vaginal delivery and cesarean section.[46] During the first stage of labor, the fetal heart rate should be recorded at least every 30 minutes and should be auscultated during and immediately after a contraction.

During the second stage of labor, the fetal heart should be auscultated at least every 15 minutes, and after each uterine contraction. Either manual auscultation or continuous electronic fetal monitoring is acceptable.[47] Maternal oral intake is usually limited during this period because of the risk of aspiration pneumonitis, a major cause of anesthetic-associated morbidity and mortality. Some authors have suggested that, since the pneumonitis results from the acidity of the aspirated gastric contents, a clear antacid (such as 0.3 M sodium citrate) be administered to all women in labor. However, neither of these protocols are universally recommended.

Clinical Assistance at Delivery

Preparation for delivery should take into account the patient's parity, the progression of labor, presentation of the fetus, and complications of the labor. If it is anticipated that fetal manipulation may be necessary (such as women at risk for shoulder dystocia, breech presentation, or twin pregnancies), it may be appropriate to transfer the patient to a large and better equipped delivery room. It may also be appropriate to remove the foot of the bed and to encourage delivery in the lithotomy position. If no complications are anticipated, delivery can be accomplished with the mother in almost any position. Common positions include the lateral (Sims) position or the partial sitting position.

The goals of clinical assistance at spontaneous delivery are the reduction of maternal trauma, prevention of fetal injury, and initial support of the newborn if required. When the fetal head crowns and delivery is imminent, pressure from the accoucheur's hand is used to hold the head flexed and to control delivery, thereby preventing precipitous expulsion, which has been associated with perineal tears as well as intracranial trauma. If there is a delay in delivery of the fetal head, a modified Ritgen's maneuver may be attempted. Using a sterile towel, the fetal chin is palpated through the perineum or rectum, and upward pressure is applied to facilitate extension of the fetal head. Once the fetal head is delivered, external rotation (restitution) is allowed to occur. If the cord is around the neck, it should be looped over the head or, if not reducible, doubly clamped and transected. Mucus can then be gently suctioned from the fetal mouth, oropharynx, and nares using a bulb syringe. In the presence of meconium, aspiration with a DeLee suction catheter may reduce the risk of meconium aspiration syndrome. However, care should be taken not to suction too vigorously, as posterior pharyngeal stimulation can cause a vagal response and fetal bradycardia. Once the fetal airway has been cleared, a hand is placed on each parietal eminence and the anterior shoulder is delivered with the next contraction by downward traction towards the mother's sacrum in concert with maternal expulsive efforts. In this way, the anterior shoulder is

encouraged to slip under the symphysis pubis. The posterior shoulder is then delivered by upward traction. These movements should be performed with as little downward or upward force as possible to avoid perineal injury and/or traction injuries to the brachial plexus. The infant should be cradled as delivery is completed, either spontaneously or with a gentle maternal push. After delivery, there is a net transfer of blood from the placenta to the fetus. Spasm of the umbilical artery occurs within approximately 1 minute of birth. However, the remaining communication between the neonate and placenta, the umbilical vein, permits passage of blood for up to 3 minutes after birth. Delay in clamping of the cord will allow an increase in the volume of transfusion. In most instances, however, the volume of transfusion is not clinically significant. As such, the timing of cord clamping is dictated by convenience and is usually performed immediately after delivery. The infant should be held securely and wiped dry with a sterile towel, while any mucus remaining in the airway is suctioned.

Delivery of the Placenta and Fetal Membranes

The third stage of labor can be managed either passively or actively. Passive management is characterized by patiently waiting for the three classic signs of placental separation: (1) lengthening of the umbilical cord, (2) a gush of blood from the vagina signifying separation of the placenta from the uterine wall, and (3) a change in the shape of the uterine fundus from discoid to globular with elevation of the fundal height.

In active management, uterotonic agents such as oxytocin can be administered at delivery of the anterior shoulder or after the fetus is out (either intramuscularly, intravenously, or infused into the umbilical vein) to hasten delivery of the placenta and reduce blood loss. Active management of the third stage of labor has been shown to reduce total blood loss and the incidence of postpartum hemorrhage,[48] but can complicate management in cases involving an undiagnosed second twin or placenta accreta. In addition, two techniques of controlled cord traction are described to facilitate separation and delivery of the placenta: the *Brandt-Andrews maneuver* (in which an abdominal hand secures the uterine fundus to prevent uterine inversion while the other hand exerts sustained downward traction on the umbilical cord [Fig. 13–15]) or the *Créde maneuver* (in which the cord is fixed with the lower hand while the uterine fundus is secured and sustained upward traction is applied using the abdominal hand). Care should be taken to avoid avulsion of the cord.

After delivery, the placenta, umbilical cord, and fetal membranes should be examined. Placental weight (excluding membranes and cord) varies with fetal weight,

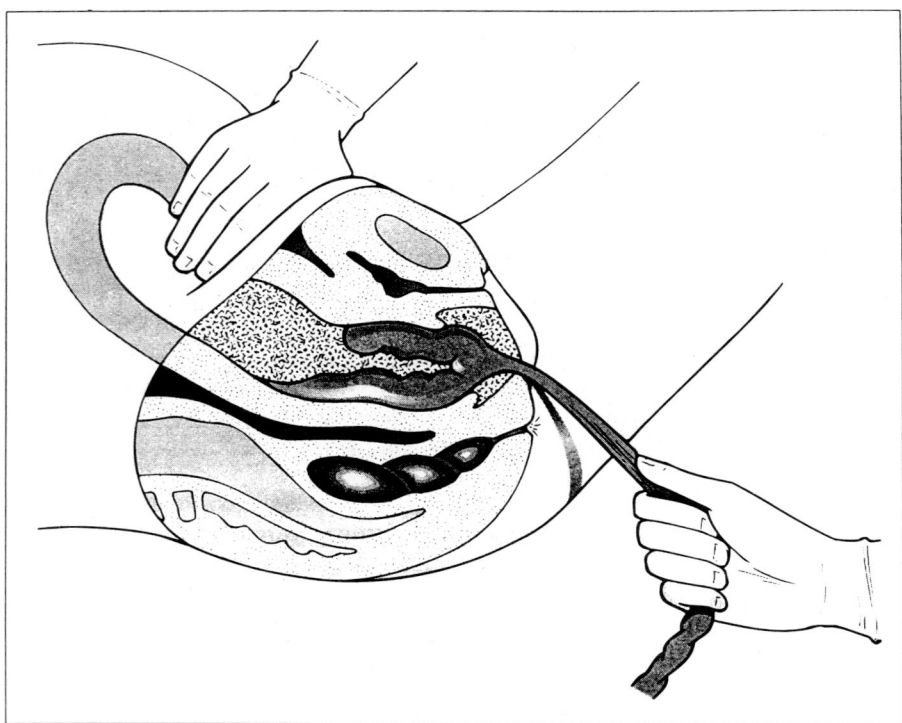

Figure 13–15. Delivery of the placenta and fetal membranes using controlled traction on the cord and suprapubic pressure with the abdominal hand to prevent uterine inversion.

with a ratio of approximately 1:6. Abnormally large placentae are associated with such conditions as fetal hydrops fetalis and congenital syphilis. Inspection and palpation of the placenta should include the fetal and maternal surfaces and may reveal areas of fibrosis, infarction, or calcification. Although each of these conditions may be seen in the normal term placenta, excessive loss of surface area can result in impairment of exchange between mother and fetus. Abnormalities of lobulation (a missing placental cotyledon or a membrane defect suggesting a missing succenturiate lobe) may suggest retention of a portion of placenta, which can lead to postpartum hemorrhage or infection. The classic hallmark of placental abruption is a depressed area on the maternal side of the placenta with an attached blood clot. The absence of such a finding, however, does not exclude the diagnosis. The site of insertion of the umbilical cord into the placenta should be noted. Abnormal insertions include marginal insertion (in which the cord inserts into the edge of the placenta) and membranous insertion (in which the vessels of the umbilical cord course through the membranes prior to attachment to the placental disk). The cord itself should be inspected for length, the correct number of umbilical vessels (normally two arteries and one vein), true knots, hematomas, and strictures. The average cord length is 50 to 60 cm. Extremes of length have been associated with a number of clinical entities, including oligohydramnios and cord compression. A single umbilical artery is associated with other structural anomalies in 20

percent of cases.[49] The fetal membranes should also be examined for meconium staining and for opacification of the membranes, which may suggest chorioamnionitis. A membrane defect might provide the only clue to a retained accessory lobe.

Following delivery of the placenta, the cervix, vagina, and perineum should be carefully examined for evidence of birth injury. If a laceration is seen, its length and position should be noted and repair initiated. Adequate analgesia (either regional or local) is essential for repair (see Chapter 17). Special attention should be paid to repair of the perineal body, the external anal sphincter, and the rectal mucosa. Failure to recognize and repair rectal injury can lead to serious long-term morbidity, most notably fecal incontinence.

The need for manual and/or surgical exploration of the uterus after delivery is controversial. Adequate analgesia is essential for any such procedure. Although it has been proposed by some investigators that manual exploration be performed after all deliveries,[50] it is usually reserved for women in whom there is suspicion of retained products of conception, where there is excessive vaginal bleeding, and in cases of premature delivery or vaginal birth after cesarean (VBAC).[51] If a transmural defect in a prior cesarean scar is palpated following delivery, it should be repaired only if there is excessive bleeding. In the absence of bleeding, the patient can be managed expectantly, although a subsequent vaginal birth after cesarean should probably be discouraged.

ABNORMAL PATTERNS OF LABOR

Abnormalities of the First Stage

Abnormalities of the first stage of labor imply a deviation from the normal pattern of cervical dilatation described by Friedman[35,36,52] (Fig. 13–11). The abnormality may be either protraction or arrest, and may occur during the latent or active phases of the first stage.

Disorders of the Latent Phase

Latent phase arrest implies simply that labor has not truly begun. *Prolonged latent phase* refers to a latent phase of 20 hours or longer in the nulliparous patient or 14 hours or longer in the multiparous patient.[53] Although the duration of the latent phase of labor is highly variable and prolongation of the latent phase does not correlate with adverse perinatal outcome, this situation can be taxing to both the mother and the practitioner. The management of the prolonged latent phase should be individualized. Unless there is a maternal or fetal indication for expediting delivery, expectant management is usually recommended. On occasion, administration of an analgesic agent such as 15 to 20 mg of morphine may allow the patient to rest for a few hours or days (so-called therapeutic rest). If the decision is made to proceed with augmentation of labor, oxytocin infusion is the technique of choice. Amni-

otomy in such patients should be deferred because of the association between prolonged rupture of the membranes (defined as >18 hours) and intra-amniotic infection. Prolonged latent phase is not itself an indication for cesarean delivery.

Disorders of the Active Phase

Disorders of the active phase of the first stage of labor are classified into three broad categories according to the pattern of their departure from the norm. All such diagnoses are retrospective. Once identified, the underlying etiology should be sought.

A diagnosis of *primary dysfunctional labor* implies that the gravida has entered the active phase of labor but that the rate of active phase cervical dilatation is less than the fifth percentile, defined as less than 1.2 cm/h in nulliparas and less than 1.5 cm/h in multiparas[35,36,52] (Table 13–2 and Fig. 13–16). Although such pregnancies are at risk for secondary arrest and poor perinatal outcome, primary dysfunctional labor is not itself an indication for cesarean delivery. In the nulliparous patient, inadequate uterine activity is the most common cause of primary dysfunctional labor. Once diagnosed, augmentation with amniotomy and/or oxytocin infusion should be attempted. Reports from the National Maternity Hospital in Dublin[54] suggest that this approach is effective, but not all in-

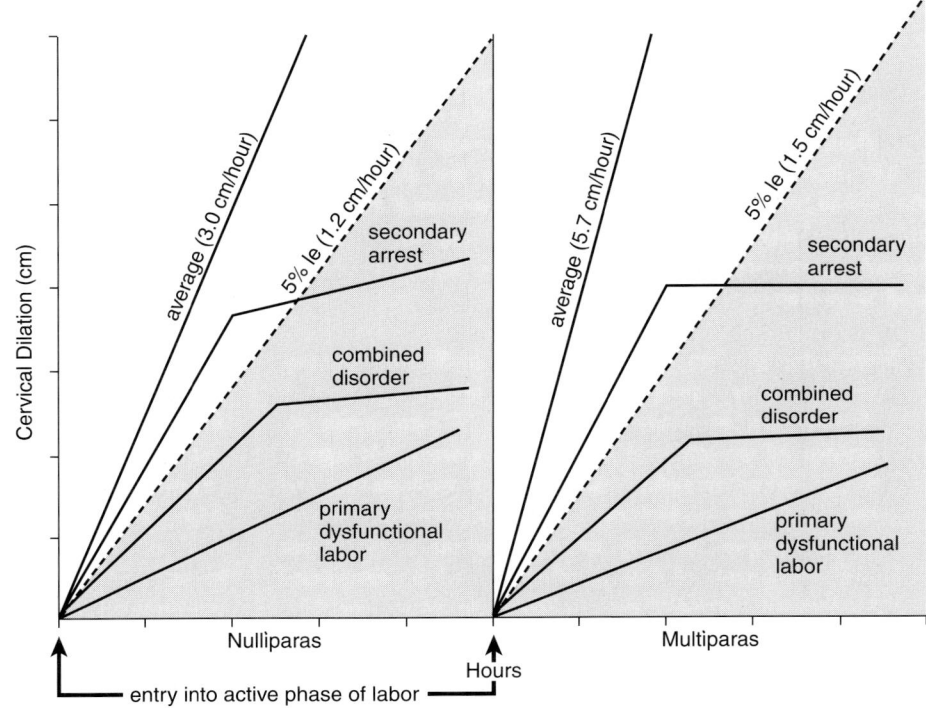

Figure 13–16. Disorders of the first stage of labor. Combined disorder implies an arrest in a gravida previously exhibiting primary dysfunctional labor.

vestigators have been able to confirm these results.[55] In the multiparous patient, CPD due to malposition is the most common cause.

Secondary arrest is defined as cessation of previously normal active phase cervical dilatation for a period of 2 hours or more.[56] The duration of arrest of normal cervical dilatation is somewhat arbitrary, and arrest of only 1 hour has been associated with an increase in second-stage abnormalities and fetal morbidity. A hypothetical "action line" has been proposed by Studd[39] that attempts to define labor dystocia in primigravid patients. In this model, a delay in cervical dilatation of greater than or equal to 2 hours over that expected in the presence of adequate uterine contractions suggests labor dystocia and requires further evaluation. Intrapartum management should include confirmation of adequate uterine contractions and exclusion of CPD. Vaginal examination should be performed to verify cervical dilatation as well as fetal presentation, position, and station. Clinical pelvimetry should be performed with notation of pelvic type and overall pelvic capacity. If uterine activity is suboptimal, amniotomy and/or oxytocin infusion should be initiated. The majority of gravidas with secondary arrest (70 to 80 percent) will respond to such maneuvers and resume progression of cervical dilatation, although such pregnancies remain at increased risk of second-stage abnormalities and operative deliveries. Continued arrest over 2 to 4 hours with adequate uterine contractions is an indication for cesarean delivery.

A *combined disorder* of active phase dilatation is defined as arrest of dilatation occurring when the patient has previously exhibited primary dysfunctional labor. This pattern is associated with a less favorable outcome with regard to vaginal delivery than in gravidas with secondary arrest alone.[56]

An alternative classification system for disorders of the active phase of labor has been proposed based on the electromechanical state of the uterus.[25,57] Two broad categories are described on the basis of clinical and monometric criteria:

Hypotonic dysfunction reflects an inefficient generation and/or propagation of action potentials though the myometrium or lack of contractile response of myometrial cells to the contractile signal. It can occur in either nulliparas or multiparas, and may indicate underlying CPD, malposition, or maternal fatigue. In this setting, uterine contractions are infrequent, of low amplitude, and accompanied by low or normal basal intrauterine pressures. Maternal discomfort is minimal.

Hypertonic dysfunction is primarily a condition of primiparas and usually occurs in early labor. It is characterized by the presence of regular uterine contractions that fail to effect cervical effacement and dilatation. Frequent contractions of low amplitude are often associated with an elevated basal intrauterine pressure. As such, maternal discomfort is significant and backache frequent.

Abnormalities of the Second Stage

The second stage of labor is the interval between full cervical dilatation and delivery of the infant. Abnormalities of the second stage can be classified into two broad categories:

Protraction of Descent

Protraction of descent is defined as descent of the presenting part during the second stage of labor occurring at less than 1 cm/h in nulliparas and less than 2 cm/h in multiparas.[58] This diagnosis relies on the subjective assessment of station at vaginal examination, which is subject to wide interobserver error. Despite these limitations, it is clear that labors complicated by protraction of descent leading to prolonged second stage are associated with increased perinatal mortality and morbidity. Review of electronic fetal heart rate tracings obtained during prolonged second stage labors have documented a high incidence of variable decelerations and prolonged decelerations[59] (see Chapter 14). The gradual fall in fetal scalp capillary pH that occurs throughout labor is accelerated during the second phase.[60] Deliveries complicated by prolonged second stage therefore place the fetus at increased risk of acidosis. For these reasons, the ACOG has recommended that intervention be considered once the second stage of labor is prolonged, defined as greater than or equal to 2 hours in nulliparas without regional analgesia ($\geq$3 hours with regional analgesia) and greater than or equal to 1 hour in multiparas without regional analgesia ($\geq$2 hours with regional analgesia).[40] In practice, however, a short period of expectant management is reasonable provided that electronic fetal monitoring is reassuring, descent is progressive, and vaginal delivery is imminent.[61-64]

Arrest of Descent

Arrest (failure) of descent is more accurately diagnosed (especially when examinations are limited to a single examiner) than protraction of descent. As in arrest of dilatation, arrest of descent requires prompt reevaluation of uterine contractions, maternal and fetal well-being, and cephalopelvic relationships (including clinical pelvimetry, fetal station, position, and the presence of caput succedaneum and/or moulding of the skull bones). Obvious problems such as inadequate uterine contractions, overdistended bladder, ineffectual maternal expulsive efforts, dense conduction anesthesia, or strong perineal resistance (soft-tissue dystocia) should be managed appropriately and are associated with a high expectation of success. In the absence of such factors, however, good clinical judgment is the cornerstone of management. The decision to continue oxytocin infusion or to proceed with operative intervention (assisted vaginal delivery or cesarean) should be individualized. If the practitioner is uncertain how to proceed, consultation may prove useful.

Abnormalities of the Third Stage

Separation of the placenta is a consequence of continued uterine contractions following expulsion of the fetus. These contractions reduce the area of the uterine placental bed with subsequent disruption of the placental attachment along a plane in the spongiosa layer of the decidua vera. Continued powerful and prolonged contractions serve to expel the placenta and control blood loss through compression of the spiral arterioles. Since placental separation relies exclusively on uterine contractions, interference with this process by either fundal pressure or excessive traction on the umbilical cord can increase the incidence of complications such as hemorrhage, cord avulsion, or uterine inversion (see Chapter 17).

The interval between delivery of the infant and delivery of the placenta and fetal membranes usually lasts less than 10 minutes and is complete within 15 minutes in 95 percent of all deliveries. After 30 minutes, intervention is indicated to expedite delivery of the placenta. Controlled trials have demonstrated that dilute intravenous oxytocin is superior to intravenous or intramuscular ergometrine in this regard.[65] If bleeding is excessive or if there is no response to uterotonic agents, manual removal of the placenta may be required. Prophylactic antibiotics should be administered to such patients to prevent postpartum endomyometritis.

INDUCTION OF LABOR

Induction of Labor

Induction of labor refers to the initiation of uterine contractions before the spontaneous onset of labor by medical and/or surgical means for the purpose of delivery. The patient and her family should be actively involved in the decision to proceed with induction, and should be informed of the risks, benefits, and potential complications of the various options available, including the possibility of cesarean delivery. Induction of labor may be either indicated or elective.

Indicated Induction of Labor

In general, induction of labor is indicated when the benefits of delivery to the mother and/or fetus outweigh the potential risks of continuing the pregnancy. The appropriate timing for induction is the point at which the benefits to the mother and/or the fetus are greater if the pregnancy is interrupted than if the pregnancy is continued, and is gestational-age dependent. If obstetric criteria confirm that the pregnancy is at term or if fetal pulmonary maturity has been documented (Table 13–3), the decision to induce labor is not difficult. The decision to induce labor prior to term, on the other hand, is far more difficult. In such cases, there should be clear benefit to the fetus of premature delivery, which outweighs the potential problems associated with iatrogenic prematurity.

Table 13–3. CRITERIA FOR CONFIRMATION OF GESTATIONAL AGE AND/OR FETAL PULMONARY MATURITY IN PREPARATION FOR INDUCTION OF LABOR

Parameters

Clinical criteria
1. ≥39 weeks' gestation have elapsed since the first day of the last menstrual period in a woman with a regular menstrual cycle and no immediate antecedent use of oral contraceptives.
2. Fetal heart tones have been documented for ≥20 weeks' gestation by nonelectronic fetoscope or for ≥30 weeks by Doppler ultrasound.

Laboratory determinations
1. ≥36 weeks' gestation have elapsed since a positive serum human chorionic gonadotropin pregnancy test.
2. Ultrasound estimation of gestational age is considered accurate if it is based on crown-rump measurements obtained at 6 to 11 weeks' gestation or it is based on biparietal diameter measurements obtained before 20 weeks' gestation.

Fetal pulmonary maturity
According to the Guidelines for Perinatal care,* term gestation can be confirmed if two or more of the above obstetric clinical or laboratory criteria are present. If term gestation cannot be confirmed, amniotic fluid analysis can be used to provide evidence of fetal lung maturity. A number of tests are available:
1. Lecithin/sphingomyelin (L/S) ratio >2.1 is regarded as evidence of pulmonary maturity.
2. Phosphatidylglycerol if present, fetal pulmonary maturity can be assumed.
3. TDx-FLM assay ≥70 mg surfactant per 1 g albumin is regarded as evidence of pulmonary maturity, <50 is regarded as evidence of pulmonary immaturity, and 50 to 69 is a borderline result and a secondary test is indicated (usually L/S ratio).
4. Saturated phosphatidylcholine (SPC) ≥500 ng/ml is regarded as evidence of fetal lung maturity (≥1,000 ng/ml in pregestational diabetic patients).

*Data from the American Academy of Pediatrics and The American College of Obstetricians and Gynecologists publication: Guidelines for Perinatal Care, 4th ed., 1997.

Table 13-4. INDICATIONS FOR INDUCTION OF LABOR

Absolute Indications	Relative Indications
Maternal indications	
Preeclampsia/eclampsia	Chronic hypertension
Pregnancy-induced hypertension	Gestational diabetes
Maternal medical problems	Logistic factors
Diabetes mellitus	Risk of rapid labor
Chronic renal disease	Distance from the hospital
Chronic pulmonary disease	Psychosocial indications
Fetal indications	
Chorioamnionitis	Premature rupture of
	membranes
Abnormal (nonreassuring)	Fetal macrosomia
antepartum fetal testing	
Intrauterine growth restriction	Fetal demise
Postdates pregnancy	Previous stillbirth
(>42 weeks)	
Isoimmunization	Fetus with a major
	congenital anomaly
Uteroplacental indications	
Placental abruption	Unexplained
	oligohydramnios

Adapted from Norwitz ER, Robinson JN, Repke JT: The initiation and maintenance of normal labor. *In* Seifer DB, Samuels P, Kniss DA (eds): The Physiologic Basis of Gynecology and Obstetrics. Baltimore, Lippincott Williams & Wilkins, 2000 (in press).

Table 13-5. CONTRAINDICATIONS FOR INDUCTION OF LABOR

Absolute Contraindications	Relative Contraindications
Maternal contraindications	
Active genital herpes	Cervical carcinoma
Serious chronic medical conditions	Grandmultiparity
Absolute cephalopelvic	Uterine overdistention
disproportion (such as women	(secondary to
with pelvic deformities)	polyhydramnios or
	multiple gestation)
Fetal contraindications	
Malpresentation (transverse or	Malpresentation (breech)
oblique lie)	
Extreme fetal compromise	Fetal macrosomia
Uteroplacental contraindications	
Cord prolapse	Low-lying placenta
Placenta previa	Unexplained vaginal
Vasa previa	bleeding
Prior high vertical hysterotomy	Cord presentation
("classical" cesarean section)	Myomectomy involving
	the uterine cavity

Adapted from Norwitz ER, Robinson JN, Repke JT: The initiation and maintenance of normal labor. *In* Seifer DB, Samuels P, Kniss DA (eds): The Physiologic Basis of Gynecology and Obstetrics. Baltimore, Lippincott Williams & Wilkins, 2000 (in press).

With recent technologic advances, the therapeutic armamentarium available to the obstetrician has increased, as has the temptation to intervene. A firm indication for delivery is a prerequisite for induction. In the absence of a clear indication, intervention may not be in the best interest of the mother or the fetus. Indications and contraindications for induction of labor at term are detailed in Tables 13-4 and 13-5, respectively. Indications for delivery may be absolute or relative. If relative, a staged approach may be taken, and an attempted induction may be deferred or stopped if not successful. Having made the decision to induce labor, a number of factors should be documented to determine a patient's suitability for induction (Table 13-6).

Elective Induction of Labor

Elective induction of labor is defined as termination of pregnancy without an acceptable medical indication. In general, elective induction of labor should not be attempted simply for the convenience of the patient and practitioner, although such a strategy may be appropriate in select patients (such as patients who live a great distance from the hospital or who have a history of rapid labors). The major potential complication of elective induction is iatrogenic prematurity, which can be minimized by using strict criteria for gestational age (Table 13-3). Although it has traditionally been taught that elective induction of labor at term is associated with an increased incidence of cesarean delivery resulting from failed induction,[66,67] more recent studies[68-70] have demonstrated that routine induction of labor at 41 weeks' gestation is not associated with an increased risk of cesarean section overall or in any subgroup of women, regardless of parity, state of the cervix, or method of induction. Prerequisites for elective induction of labor are similar to those for indicated induction.

Cervical Ripening

The success of a labor induction is determined, in large part, by the initial state of the cervix. When induction

Table 13-6. PATIENT ASSESSMENT PRIOR TO INDUCTION OF LABOR

Maternal Parameters	Fetal Parameters
Confirm indication for induction	Confirm gestational age
Review for contraindications to labor and/or vaginal delivery	Estimate fetal weight (clinically or by ultrasound)
Assess shape and adequacy of bony pelvis (clinical pelvimetry)	Determine fetal position
	Confirm fetal well-being
Assess cervical exam (Bishop score)	Assess need for documentation of fetal lung maturity
Review risks and benefits of induction of labor with the patient and her family	

Table 13–7. ASSESSMENT OF ANTEPARTUM CERVICAL STATUS BY MODIFIED BISHOP SCORE

Parameter	Score 0	1	2	3
Dilatation (cm)	Closed	1–2	3–4	5 or more
Effacement (%)	0–30	40–50	60–70	80 or more
Station	−3	−2	−1 or 0	+1 or +2
Consistency	Firm	Medium	Soft	
Cervical position	Posterior	Midposition	Anterior	

Adapted from Bishop EH: Pelvic scoring for elective induction. Obstet Gynecol 24:266, 1964; American College of Obstetricians and Gynecologists, with permission.

of labor is attempted against an unfavorable cervix, the likelihood of a successful outcome is reduced.[71–74] In 1964, Bishop[75] developed a scoring system to evaluate multiparous patients for elective induction of labor at term. The scoring system is based on the properties of the cervix that can be assessed clinically; namely, dilatation, effacement, station, consistency, and position (Table 13–7). Although the original goal of this scoring system was to prevent iatrogenic prematurity in the preultrasound era, it has subsequently been used to predict the success of induction of labor at term.[72,76] When the cervical score exceeded 8, the incidence of vaginal delivery subsequent to induction was similar to that for spontaneous labor. Based on such studies, the ACOG has recommended that a Bishop score of greater than or equal to 6 be deemed favorable and likely to result in a successful induction of labor.[77] It would seem logical, therefore, that enhancement of cervical maturation would be an appropriate first step toward induction of labor when the cervix is unfavorable. Indeed, preinduction cervical maturation is associated with fewer failed inductions, fewer serial inductions, lower fetal and ma-

ternal morbidity, a shorter hospital stay, lower medical cost, and (possibly) a lower rate of cesarean delivery.[73,74,78,79]

Cervical maturation (or cervical "ripening") describes a complex series of hormonally mediated biochemical events that alter both cervical collagen and ground substance, resulting in a softer and more pliable cervix prior to induction of labor.[80] A number of agents are available to facilitate cervical maturation (Table 13–8).

Methods of Cervical Maturation and Labor Induction

The choice of which method to use to promote cervical maturation and to induce labor should be individualized. A single technique is rarely effective on its own, and a combination of maneuvers may be required. The options available for induction of labor are reviewed in Table 13–9.

Nonpharmacologic Methods

Nonpharmacologic methods for cervical maturation and/or labor induction include surgical techniques (stripping of the membranes, amniotomy) and mechanical dilatation.

STRIPPING OF THE MEMBRANES. Stripping or sweeping of the fetal membranes refers to digital separation of

Table 13–8. METHODS OF CERVICAL RIPENING

Pharmacologic Methods	Nonpharmacologic Methods
Hormonal techniques	Membrane stripping
Prostaglandins	
Prostaglandin E₂ (dinoprostone [Prepidil])	Mechanical dilators
Prostaglandin E₁ (misoprostol [cytotec])	Hygroscopic dilators (laminaria, lamicel, Dilapan)
Oxytocin	Balloon catheter (alone, with traction, with infusion)
Estrogen	
Steroid receptor antagonists (?)	
RU-486 (Mifepristone)	Amniotomy
ZK98299 (Onapristone)	
Relaxin (?)	
Dehydroepiandrostenedione sulfate (?)	

Table 13–9. METHODS OF INDUCTION OF LABOR

Medical (Hormonal) Techniques	Surgical Techniques
Hormonal techniques	Amniotomy
Oxytocin	
Prostaglandins	
Prostaglandin E₂ₐ (dinoprost)	
Prostaglandin E₂ (dinoprostone [Prepidil])	
Prostaglandin E₁ (misoprostol [cytotec])	
RU-486 (Mifepristone) (?)	

the chorioamniotic membrane from the wall of the cervix and lower uterine segment, and was first reported for induction of labor at term in 1810.[81] In order for stripping of the membranes to be successful, the vertex should be well applied to the cervix and the cervix must be dilated sufficiently to admit the practitioner's finger. Stripping of the membranes is believed to work by release of endogenous prostaglandins from the membranes and adjacent decidua.[82] Indeed, levels of 13,14-dihydro-15-keto-prostaglandin $F_{2\alpha}$, the primary metabolite of decidual $PGF_{2\alpha}$, increase markedly in the maternal circulation within a short time after stripping of the membranes and/or amniotomy.[83] Prostaglandins may be involved in stimulating myometrial contractions and in the onset of labor. In addition, manual exploration of the cervix may trigger an autonomic neural reflex, the Ferguson reflex, which promotes the release of oxytocin from the maternal posterior pituitary,[84] although the existence of such a reflex remains controversial. Several trials have demonstrated a benefit of this procedure,[85–87] whereas others have not been able to reproduce these favorable results.[88] A recent meta-analysis suggests that sweeping of the membranes is able to reduce the interval to spontaneous onset of labor, but there is no evidence of a reduction in operative vaginal delivery, cesarean section rates, or maternal or neonatal morbidity.[89] Since the effects of membrane stripping are not predictable and the efficacy of this method has not been proven, it should not be relied on as the sole method of labor induction.

AMNIOTOMY. The technique of amniotomy, artificial rupture of the membranes, involves perforation of the chorioamniotic membranes using either a toothed clamp (Allis) or a plastic hook (Amniohook, Hollister, Chicago, IL). Before amniotomy is performed, the vertex should be seen to be engaged in the pelvis and well applied to the cervix to prevent prolapse of the umbilical cord. The membranes should be swept away from the cervix and the instrument of choice gently applied to the membranes and turned so as to hook or scratch the membranes. The opening in the membranes should be widened by blunt dissection using the examining finger to retract the membranes over the vertex without dislodging the vertex. The amount and character of released amniotic fluid should be noted. Since a degree of cervical dilatation is necessary to perform the procedure, amniotomy can only be carried out once the cervix is favorable.

Amniotomy was introduced into clinical practice by Kreis in 1929.[90] Despite its wide acceptance, there is a paucity of scientific literature on the efficacy of amniotomy in inducing labor. In patients with a favorable cervical examination (a high Bishop score) at term, amniotomy alone has been reported to be effective in inducing labor in 88 percent of cases[91] and to shorten the interval to delivery by around 0.8 to 2.3 hours.[92,93] There are a small number of controlled trials in the literature comparing amniotomy alone to combined amniotomy and oxytocin.[92–96] All of these trials report a shorter induction to delivery time with combined amniotomy and oxytocin, with no apparent difference in safety profile. Whether this reduction in time to delivery translates into an improvement in clinical outcome is not clear.[96] The timing of oxytocin augmentation, however, remains controversial and should be individualized.

Amniotomy is associated with benefits and risks. Advantages of amniotomy include (1) a high success rate for induction of labor; (2) observation of the amniotic fluid for blood or meconium; and (3) ready access to the intrauterine cavity and to the fetus for placement of an intrauterine pressure catheter, a fetal scalp electrode, or for fetal scalp blood sampling. Although early amniotomy has been shown to reduce the incidence of labor dystocia and the length of labor, it does not appear to lower the rate of cesarean delivery.[92,93,97] Complications of amniotomy include (1) umbilical cord prolapse, (2) fetal injury, (3) prolonged rupture of the membranes and resultant increased risk of intra-amniotic infection, (4) adverse change in fetal position as amniotomy is associated with a greater frequency of malposition and asynclitism,[93] and (5) rupture of vasa previa and subsequent fetal hemorrhage. With due caution, many of the risks can be avoided. The fetal heart rate should be monitored electronically or by auscultation during and immediately after amniotomy. A transient fetal tachycardia is common after amniotomy, but decelerations or bradycardia are rare in the absence of overt or occult cord prolapse. Contraindications to early amniotomy include maternal infection with human immunodeficiency virus, an active perineal herpes simplex viral infection, and possibly viral hepatitis.

MECHANICAL DILATORS. Mechanical dilators all rely on release of endogenous prostaglandins from the membranes and maternal decidua to promote cervical maturation and/or labor induction. When compared with no preinduction cervical ripening, an intracervical balloon catheter has been shown to significantly shorten the induction to delivery interval and to increase the rate of vaginal delivery.[98] A more recent randomized comparison between intracervical PGE_2 gel and intracervical Foley catheter for cervical ripening at term showed them to be equally effective, with no difference in side-effect profile, intrapartum complications, or mode of delivery.[99] Hygroscopic dilators—including laminaria (desiccated seaweed), Dilapan (polyacrilonitrile), and lamicel (magnesium sulfate in polyvinyl alcohol)—rely on absorption of water to swell and forcibly dilate the cervix, and have been found to be at least as effective in promoting cervical maturation as PGE_2 gel.[100–102] A significant disadvantage of mechanical dilators, however, is patient discomfort both at the time of insertion and with progressive cervical dilatation. With equally efficacious pharmacologic agents available, there is no obvious advantage to the routine use of mechanical dilators. However, in specific clinical circumstances where prostaglandins should be avoided (such as glaucoma or pulmonary disease) or where other products are unavailable because of supply or cost, mechanical dilators can be used both safely and effectively.

Pharmacologic Methods

Pharmacologic methods available for cervical maturation and/or induction of labor are summarized in Tables 13–8 and 13–9, respectively.

PROSTAGLANDINS. The use of prostaglandins to induce cervical ripening at term was introduced in the 1970s in an attempt to mimic events that occur during spontaneous labor.[103–105] Prostaglandins are a family of 20-carbon bioactive lipids. Human uterine tissues are selectively enriched with arachidonic acid, an essential fatty acid and the obligate precursor of prostaglandins of the 2 series.[106] An increase in the biosynthesis of prostaglandins of the E and F series in the uterus is a consistent element in the transition into labor, both at term and preterm.[106–108] Prostaglandins are predominantly paracrine/autocrine hormones, meaning that they act locally at their site of production on contiguous cells. Their half-life in the peripheral circulation is approximately 1 to 2 minutes. The production of prostaglandins is discreetly compartmentalized within the uterus. The maternal decidua is the main source of $PGF_{2\alpha}$ in the uterus; the fetal membranes, especially the amnion, produce primarily PGE_2; and the myometrium produces predominantly prostacyclin (PGI_2).[106] In vitro, both $PGF_{2\alpha}$ and PGE_2 cause myometrial contractions. In vivo, however, decidual $PGF_{2\alpha}$ acts primarily to promote myometrial contractility, whereas PGE_2 appears to be important for cervical maturation. Indeed, exogenous PGE_2 preparations have been shown to be more potent at promoting cervical maturation than $PGF_{2\alpha}$.[104,109] Unlike oxytocin, the response of the uterus to prostaglandins does not change significantly throughout gestation. This has led to the widespread use of prostaglandins to effect midtrimester pregnancy termination or induction of labor following intrauterine death remote from term.

Initial clinical trials using transvaginal PGE_2 gel preparations (240 to 2,000 mg) to promote cervical maturation 1 day prior to induction of labor suggested that the rate of failed induction, defined as the inability to establish labor, was only 0.8 to 6.3 percent.[105,110–113] In a recent meta-analysis of all randomized, placebo-controlled trials on the effect of prostaglandins on preinduction cervical ripening and on subsequent induction success, Keirse[114] demonstrated that PGE_2 administered by any route improved the rate of spontaneous vaginal delivery and decreased the rate of both cesarean and operative vaginal delivery. Gastrointestinal side effects from PGE_2 are reported with all routes of administration, but appeared to be minimized with vaginal administration. Local application of PGE_2 gel has now become the gold standard for cervical ripening in clinical practice. The most commonly used transvaginal PGE_2 preparation is 0.5 mg dinoprostone gel (Prepidil), which received Food and Drug Administration (FDA) approval for this indication in the United States in 1992. Placement of PGE_2 within the cervical canal will have a more marked effect on cervical maturation than placement in the posterior fornix of the vagina, but with no significant difference in labor delivery outcomes.[115,116] In 1995, a sustained release preparation of 10 mg PGE_2 (Cervidil) was approved by the FDA. The advantage of this preparation is that, unlike the gel, it can be easily removed if clinical complications such as tachysystole or uterine hypertonus ensue.[117]

More recent attention has been focused on the use of the PGE_1 analogues such as misoprostol (Cytotec) for cervical ripening. Although such preparations are FDA approved only for the treatment of peptic ulcer disease and have not received approval for use during pregnancy, they have been used for induction of labor. They can be administered either transvaginally (50 μg every 3 hours to a maximum of six doses,[118] or 25 μg every 3 hours to a maximum of eight doses[119]) or orally (50 μg every 4 hours[120]). To date, there has been no evidence of teratogenic or carcinogenic effects in animal studies.[121] Results of clinical trials suggest that misoprostol is as effective as PGE_2 for cervical ripening and labor induction,[118–120] and at least two groups have found it to be more effective.[122,123] The cost of misoprostol is a fraction that of any of the PGE_2 preparations. The optimal dosage regimen for PGE_1 preparations has yet to be determined. However, the less-frequent, higher dosage schedules appear to be associated with shorter intervals to delivery, less requirement for oxytocin infusion, and fewer failed inductions.[124] On a cautionary note, the authors would like to emphasize that this drug is not approved by the FDA for use in pregnancy, and that a higher prevalence of tachysystole, meconium passage, and possibly uterine rupture has been reported with its use.[118] Misoprostol is not recommended for patients with a previous cesarean birth due to the possibility of uterine rupture.

Oxytocin

Oxytocin is a potent endogenous uterotonic agent that is capable of stimulating uterine contractions at intravenous infusion rates of 1 to 2 mIU/min at term.[125] Maternally derived oxytocin is a peptide hormone synthesized in the hypothalamus and released from the posterior pituitary in a pulsatile fashion. Its biologic half-life is approximately 3 to 4 minutes, but appears to be shorter when higher doses are infused. Oxytocin is inactivated largely in the liver and kidney. During pregnancy, oxytocin is degraded primarily by placental oxytocinase. Concentrations of oxytocin in the maternal circulation do not change significantly during pregnancy or prior to the onset of labor, but do rise late in the second stage of labor.[125,126] Studies on fetal pituitary oxytocin production, the umbilical arteriovenous difference in plasma oxytocin, amniotic fluid oxytocin levels, and fetal urinary oxytocin output demonstrate conclusively that the fetus secretes oxytocin that reaches the maternal side of the placenta.[125,127] Furthermore, the calculated rate of oxytocin secretion from the fetus increases from a baseline of 1 mIU/min prior to labor to around 3 mIU/min after spontaneous labor, a level similar to that normally administered to women to induce labor at term (2 to 8 mIU/min). Specific receptors for oxytocin are present in the myometrium, and there appear to be regional differences in oxytocin receptor distribution, with large numbers of receptors in the fundal area and few receptors in the lower uterine segment and cervix.[128]

Myometrial oxytocin receptor concentrations increase on average 100- to 200-fold during pregnancy, reaching a maximum during early labor.[125,126,129,130] This rise in receptor concentration is paralleled by an increase in uterine sensitivity to circulating levels of oxytocin. Specific high-affinity oxytocin receptors have also been isolated from human amnion and decidua parietalis, but not decidua vera.[125,128] Neither amnion nor decidual cells are contractile, and the action of oxytocin on these tissues remains uncertain. It has been suggested that oxytocin plays a dual role in parturition. It may act directly through both oxytocin receptor–mediated and nonreceptor, voltage-mediated calcium channels to affect intracellular biochemical pathways and promote uterine contractions. It may also act indirectly through stimulation of amniotic and decidual prostaglandin production.[128,131,132] Indeed, induction of labor at term is successful only when the oxytocin infusion is associated with an increase in $PGF_{2\alpha}$ production, in spite of seemingly adequate uterine contractions in both induction failures and successes.[128]

Oxytocin in the form of crude pituitary extracts has been used in clinical obstetrics since the early 1900s. Intravenous oxytocin for induction of labor was initiated by Theobald et al.[133] in 1948. Oxytocin was subsequently successfully purified in 1951, and synthetic preparations became available 2 years later. Only intravenous preparations are approved by the FDA for induction and augmentation of labor. Continuous low-dose (1 to 4 mIU/min) oxytocin infusion has been shown to be effective in promoting cervical maturation,[134] and appears to be as effective as PGE_2 gel preparations in this regard.[135] High-dose oxytocin significantly shortens labor without any adverse fetal effect[136] (see Active Management of Labor, below). With continuous intravenous oxytocin infusion, plasma oxytocin concentrations increase during the first 20 to 30 minutes. After 30 minutes, the concentration of oxytocin reaches a steady state in maternal plasma and does not change significantly. Because of its short half-life, plasma levels of oxytocin fall rapidly after the intravenous infusion is discontinued.[137]

Overall, PGE_2 gel is probably a better agent for preinduction cervical ripening than oxytocin, being equally if not more effective, easier to administer, and possibly safer for the fetus.[138] The incidence of neonatal hyperbilirubinemia, for example, is higher with oxytocin than with prostaglandins.[139] However, the use of continuous low-dose oxytocin is still considered safe, and is a reasonable treatment alternative in most circumstances.

Progesterone Receptor Antagonists

RU-486 (Mifepristone) is a competitive steroid receptor antagonist that affects the action of both progesterone and glucocorticoids. ZK98299 (Onapristone) is a more selective progesterone receptor antagonist. Pretreatment with RU-486 (200 mg vaginally daily for 2 days) prior to planned induction of labor has been shown to produce cervical maturation, to cause uterine contractions and cervical dilatation,[140–143] to diminish oxytocin requirements in labor,[144] and to lower the cesarean section rate.[142] More recently, a placebo-controlled study using RU-486 for labor induction after cesarean delivery demonstrated that it is an effective agent at term and, furthermore, can diminish oxytocin requirements in labor.[145] There were no differences in terms of mode of delivery or neonatal outcome. Further clinical studies are awaited.

MANAGEMENT OF ABNORMAL LABOR AND DELIVERY

Augmentation of Labor at Term

Abnormalities of the first stage of labor may be either protraction or arrest disorders, and many occur during the latent or active phases of the first stage (Fig. 13–16). When such an abnormality is noted and uterine activity is suboptimal, administration of an oxytocic agent is recommended. Care should be taken to exclude other possible contributing factors such as malpresentation, especially in multiparous patients.

Intravenous oxytocin infusion is the agent of choice. Variability in patient sensitivity and response to intravenous oxytocin is the rule rather than the exception. As such, the recommended rate of oxytocin administration is that which produces contractions every 2 to 3 minutes, lasting 60 to 90 seconds with a peak intrauterine pressure of 50 to 60 mm Hg and a resting uterine tone of 10 to 15 mm Hg if intrauterine pressure monitoring is used. Dosage may vary from 0.5 to 30 to 40 mIU/min of oxytocin. Control of the intravenous dose is best achieved by using a constant-infusion pump. A number of different low-dose oxytocin protocols have been investigated.[138,146,147] Augmentation is usually started at 0.5 mIU/min, and the rate is doubled every 15 to 20 minutes until adequate uterine contractions are observed. Approximately 30 to 40 minutes are needed for the full effect of an increase in dosage to be reflected in the contraction pattern. A slow rate of increase in oxytocin administration is as effective for inducing labor as a fast rate of increase, while at the same time minimizing oxytocin requirements.[146] Similar results are seen with pulsatile oxytocin administration.[147] Recent studies have demonstrated that, when used in patients demonstrating a protraction disorder, oxytocin infusion rates greater than 6 mIU/min are rarely required.[148] It is unusual for a patient to require more than 30 to 40 mIU/min of oxytocin to achieve adequate uterine contractions, and some authorities recommend a maximal rate of 20 mIU/min.[149,150] As labor progresses, the frequency and intensity of contractions may increase, and the oxytocin infusion may need to be reduced.

The decision to initiate oxytocin infusion in the setting of a protraction disorder with adequate contractions is controversial. Nevertheless, it is clear that the use of oxytocin infusion is associated with a high rate of success. Overall, around 80 percent of patients with documented disorders of labor will respond to oxytocin infusion with subsequent progression of labor and vaginal delivery.[56,151]

The advantages of intravenous oxytocin lie in its cost, its familiarity for the clinician, and its short half-life, which allows for titration of infusion rate against uterine contractions. Monitoring of uterine contractions and fetal heart rate is recommended throughout the induction and is best accomplished with continuous electronic monitoring. A number of complications of intravenously administered oxytocin are described.

Uterine Hyperstimulation

The most frequently encountered problem is *uterine hyperstimulation,* which refers to excessive frequency of contractions (polysystole) or increased uterine tone (hypertonia). Uterine hyperstimulation may produce a nonreassuring fetal heart rate tracing, placental abruption, or uterine rupture. The use of electronic fetal monitoring has increased the early detection of these potentially damaging maternal or fetal complications. The detection of fetal heart rate abnormalities secondary to uterine hyperstimulation should prompt discontinuation of the oxytocin infusion, positioning of the patient on her left side, and oxygen administration.

Water Intoxication

Oxytocin is structurally and functionally related to vasopressin (antidiuretic hormone). Although rarely seen in low-dose infusion protocols, high-dose oxytocin infusions (30 to 40 mIU/min) have been associated with excessive fluid retention caused by binding of oxytocin to vasopressin and oxytocin receptors in the kidney leading to *water intoxication,* characterized by hyponatremia, confusion, convulsions, coma, congestive heart failure, and death. A slight elevation in blood pressure may also be noted. Fluid overload and hyponatremia can be prevented by strict recordings of fluid intake and output, use of balanced salt solutions, and by avoiding prolonged administration of high-dose oxytocin infusion.

Hypotension

Bolus injections of oxytocin may cause *hypotension.* When administered intravenously as dilute solutions at recommended rates, few cardiovascular side effects are noted.

Uterine Rupture

Uterine rupture has been associated with excessive oxytocin administration, although how much oxytocin constitutes "excessive" is not clear. Other risk factors for uterine rupture include prior uterine surgery, fetal malpresentation, grandmultiparity, and a markedly overdistended uterus. After uterine rupture, contractions may cease even if the oxytocin infusion is continued.

Prostaglandins have been compared with oxytocin infusion for augmentation of labor at term. These studies have generally failed to demonstrate a superiority of prostaglandins over oxytocin in terms of efficacy.[136,138,152] Since prostaglandins have more side effects and are more difficult to titrate, it is unlikely that prostaglandins will replace oxytocin for augmentation of labor.

Episiotomy

Episiotomy is an incision into the perineal body made during the second stage of labor to facilitate delivery. It is still performed in over 50 percent of vaginal deliveries in the United States.[153–156] Although there is general agreement that episiotomy is indicated (1) in cases of arrested or protracted descent, (2) in association with an instrumental delivery, or (3) to expedite delivery in the setting of fetal heart rate abnormalities, the use of prophylactic episiotomy is widely debated. Cited advantages of prophylactic episiotomy include substitution of a straight surgical incision for a ragged spontaneous laceration, reduction in the duration of the second stage, and reduction of trauma to the pelvic floor musculature that would reduce the likelihood of subsequent pelvic relaxation. However, the data to support these contentions are limited.[157]

Episiotomy can be classified into two broad categories: median and mediolateral. *Median (midline) episiotomy* refers to a vertical midline incision from the posterior forchette towards the rectum, and is preferred in the United States. The incision should be performed when the fetal head has distended the vulva to 2 to 3 cm, and once adequate analgesia, either local or regional, has been achieved. A straight Mayo scissors is generally used to perform the episiotomy, although a scalpel may be used. Care should be taken to displace the perineum from the fetal head. The size of the incision will depend on the length of the perineum but is generally around one half of the length of the perineum, and should be extended vertically up the vaginal mucosa for a distance of 2 to 3 cm. Every effort should be made to avoid injury to the anal sphincter. Complications of median episiotomy include increased blood loss, especially if the incision is made too early, fetal injury, and localized pain. Furthermore, in contrast to the stated goal of reducing perineal trauma, recent studies have demonstrated conclusively that median episiotomies are associated with an increased incidence of third- and fourth-degree lacerations (see Chapter 17).[153,156] Such injuries are associated with a high incidence of long-term incontinence and pelvic prolapse. *Mediolateral episiotomy* is performed by incision at a 45 degree angle from the inferior portion of the hymeneal ring. The length of the incision is less critical than with median episiotomy, but longer incisions require more lengthy repair. The side to which the episiotomy is performed is usually dictated by the dominant hand of the practitioner. Such incisions are favored in Europe, and do not appear to increase the incidence of third- and fourth-degree lacerations. Indeed, a number of studies suggest that such procedures are less likely to be associated with damage to the anal sphincter and the rectal mucosa. Since such incisions appear to protect against severe perineal trauma, they are the procedure of choice for women with inflammatory bowel disease because of the critical need to prevent rectal injury. Chronic complications such as unsatisfactory cosmetic results and inclusions within the scar may be more common with mediolateral episiotomies, and blood loss is greater. Although it is often said that mediolateral episiotomy causes more pain in the postpartum period than medial episiotomy and that they are associated with prolonged dyspareunia, the literature does not support this statement.[158] Bilateral mediolateral episiotomies are rarely, if ever, indicated. *Anterior episiotomy* is rarely performed, and is reserved for women with prior female genital mutilation or female circumcision.

Primary approximation of the episiotomy affords the best opportunity for functional repair, especially if there is evidence of rectal sphincter injury. The external anal sphincter should be repaired by direct apposition or overlapping the cut ends and securing them using interrupted sutures (see Chapter 17).

In view of the lack of objective evidence of benefit of prophylactic episiotomy and the data suggesting that median episiotomy is associated with an increased incidence of severe perineal trauma, prophylactic median episiotomy should be discouraged.

Assisted Vaginal Delivery

Assisted vaginal delivery refers to any operative procedure designed to effect vaginal delivery, and includes forceps delivery and vacuum extraction. Randomized studies comparing forceps with vacuum have not shown a significant difference in success rate.[159-161] The choice of which method to use is dependent largely on clinician preference and experience. Manual rotation is described, but results vary considerably.

Forceps-Assisted Vaginal Delivery

Forceps were invented by the Chamberlain family in the 17th century in Europe. Obstetric forceps vary greatly in design, but all consist of two separate blades that are inserted into the vagina sequentially. Each half consists of the blade proper, which has a cephalic curvature designed to be applied to the fetal head, a shank, and a handle. The halves are joined by a lock usually located at the junction of the shanks and the handle. The angle of the blade to the shank defines the pelvic curvature, designed to compensate for the curvature of the birth canal. Several different types of forceps have since been developed (Fig. 13–17). These can be classified into three broad categories according to their intended use.

"Classical" forceps have a cephalic curvature, a pelvic curve yielding a concave longitudinal axis, and an "English" lock in which the articulation is fixed. Examples include (1) Simpson forceps, which have fenestrated blades and separated (nonoverlapping) shanks; (2) Tucker-McLane forceps, which have solid (nonfenestrated) blades and overlapping shanks; and (3) Elliot forceps, which have fenestrated blades, overlapping shanks, and a greater cephalic curvature. Forceps in

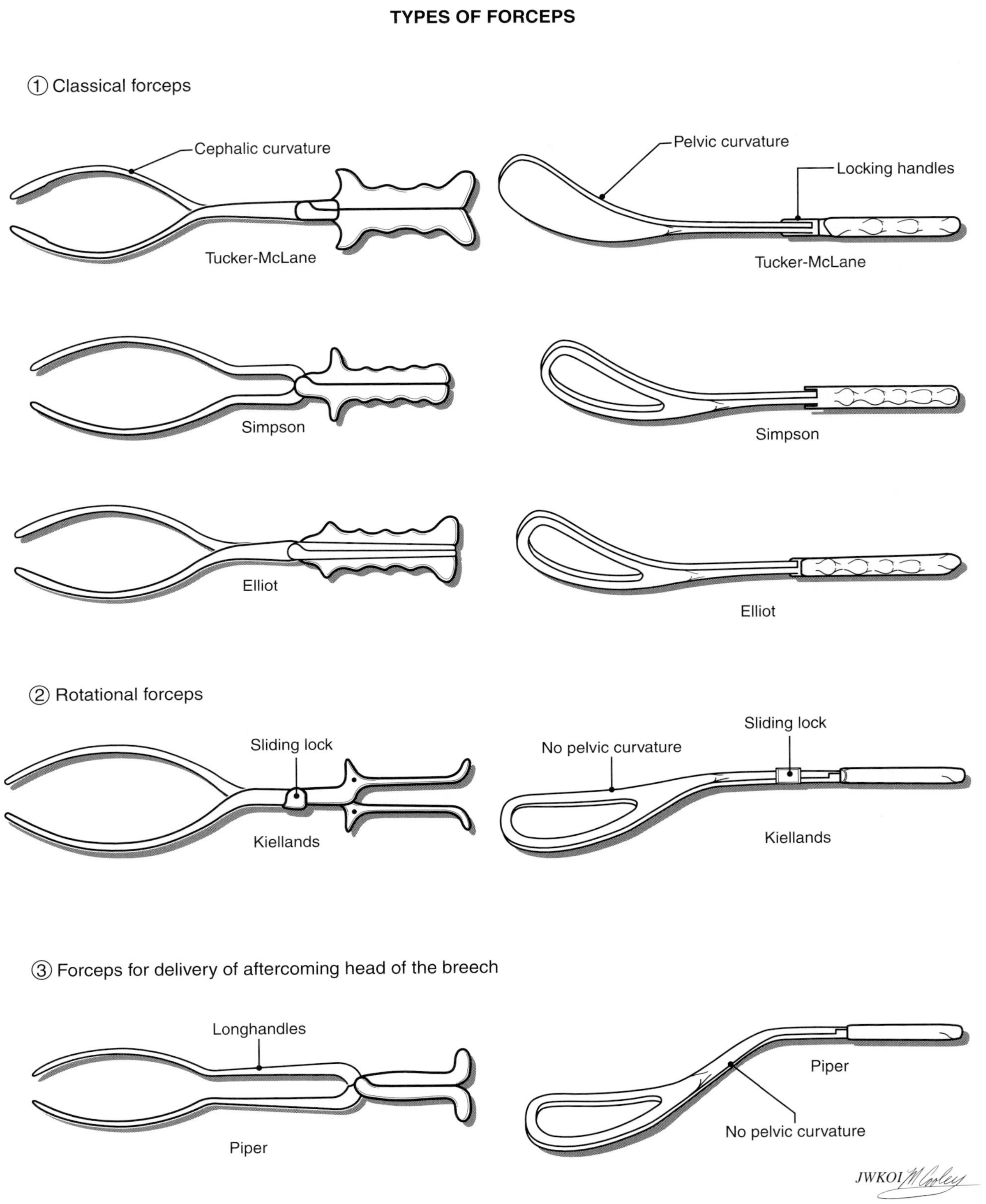

TYPES OF FORCEPS

① Classical forceps

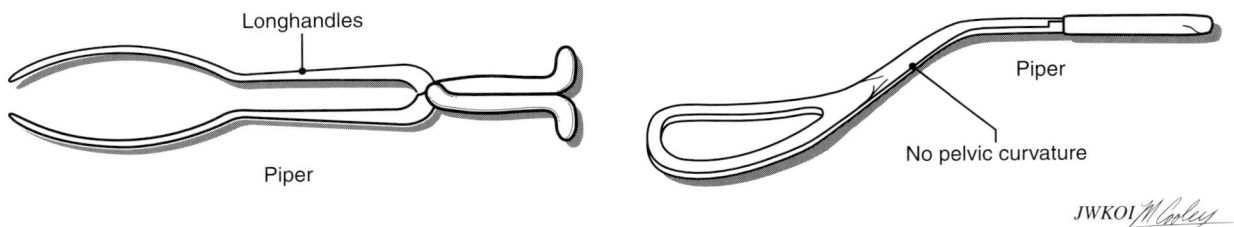

Cephalic curvature

Tucker-McLane

Pelvic curvature

Locking handles

Tucker-McLane

Simpson

Simpson

Elliot

Elliot

② Rotational forceps

Sliding lock

Kiellands

No pelvic curvature

Sliding lock

Kiellands

③ Forceps for delivery of aftercoming head of the breech

Longhandles

Piper

Piper

No pelvic curvature

JWKOI MCooley

Figure 13–17. Classification of forceps.

this category are primarily intended for use when the fetal head does not require rotation prior to delivery, but they may be used for rotation as in the Scanzoni-Smellie maneuver.

Rotational forceps have a cephalic curvature to grasp the fetal head, but no pelvic curvature and a "sliding" lock, which permits movement between the forceps halves along the longitudinal axis of the shanks to correct for asynclitism of the fetal head. Examples include Kielland and Barton forceps. Kielland forceps also have blades that lie below rather than above the plane of the shanks. This modification, along with the lack of pelvic curvature, facilitates rotation of the forceps around a point rather than around a circle as is required with the classical instruments. Once the fetal head has been rotated into the anteroposterior position, it is recommended that the rotational forceps be replaced by classical forceps, as the pelvic curvature of the classical forceps will minimize perineal trauma. Barton forceps were designed for use in a platypelloid pelvis, since they allow traction of the fetal head in a transverse position until the introitus has been reached, but are rarely, if ever, used in modern obstetric practice.

Forceps designed to assist vaginal breech deliveries such as Piper forceps lack a pelvic curve and have blades below the plane of the shanks. These modifications are designed to facilitate application to the aftercoming head of the breech. In addition, the shanks are elongated, which allows the practitioner to rest the body of the breech on the shanks while effecting delivery of the aftercoming head.

Forceps deliveries are classified according to the station of the fetal head at the time of application. In 1988, the Committee on Obstetrics: Maternal and Fetal Medicine of the ACOG[162] proposed a new classification of obstetric forceps deliveries (Table 13–10) that correlates better with short-term maternal and neonatal morbidity than did the older classifications.[40,163] The old category of "high-forceps," in which forceps were placed with the fetal head floating and ballottable above the brim of the true pelvis, has been abandoned because of excessive fetal risk.

Table 13–10. CLASSIFICATION OF OPERATIVE VAGINAL DELIVERIES

Type of Procedure	Criteria
Outlet forceps	Scalp is visible at the introitus without separating the labia
	Fetal skull has reached the level of the pelvic floor
	Sagittal suture is in the direct anteroposterior diameter or in the right or left occiput anterior or posterior position
	Fetal head is at or on the perineum
	Rotation is ≤45 degrees
Low forceps	Leading point of the fetal skull (station) is +2 or more but has not as yet reached the pelvic floor
	1. Rotation is ≤45 degrees
	2. Rotation is >45 degrees
Midforceps	The head is engaged in the pelvis but the presenting part is above +2 station
High forceps	(Not included in this classification)

Adapted from American College of Obstetricians and Gynecologists: Operative vaginal delivery, ACOG Technical Bulletin No. 196. Washington, DC, American College of Obstetricians and Gynecologists, 1994.

Few areas in obstetrics have been surrounded with as much controversy as the use of obstetric forceps. The ACOG has concluded that the use of elective outlet forceps to shorten the second stage of labor does not adversely affect either the mother or the fetus.[40,164] The use of low or midforceps deliveries, however, should be limited to women with an absolute indication for assisted vaginal delivery (Table 13–11). Midforceps deliveries should be performed only by competent operators and after careful consideration of alternative approaches (such as oxytocin administration, cesarean delivery, or simply expectant management) and of the potential fetal risks. Cases in which instrumental rotation is considered may prove amenable to digital or manual rotation.

Once the decision has been made to proceed with forceps delivery, several criteria (summarized in Table

Table 13–11. INDICATIONS FOR OPERATIVE VAGINAL DELIVERY

Maternal Indications	Fetal Indications	Other Indications
Maternal exhaustion	Nonreassuring fetal testing	Prolonged second stage of labor
Inadequate maternal expulsive efforts (such as women with spinal cord injuries or neuromuscular diseases)		Nulliparas: ≥2 h without regional analgesia, ≥3 h with regional analgesia
Need to avoid maternal expulsive efforts (such as women with certain cardiac or cerebrovascular diseases)		Multiparas: ≥1 h without regional analgesia, ≥2 h with regional analgesia
? Lack of maternal expulsive effort		? Elective shortening of the second stage of labor using outlet forceps

Data from American College of Obstetricians and Gynecologists: Operative vaginal delivery, ACOG Technical Bulletin No. 196. Washington, DC, American College of Obstetricians and Gynecologists, 1994.

Table 13–12. PREREQUISITES FOR OPERATIVE VAGINAL DELIVERY: A NUMBER OF CRITERIA NEED TO BE FULFILLED PRIOR TO ATTEMPTING OPERATIVE VAGINAL DELIVERY

Maternal Criteria	Fetal Criteria	Uteroplacental Criteria	Other Criteria
Adequate analgesia	Vertex presentation	Cervix fully dilated	Experienced operator who is fully
Lithotomy position	The fetal head must be engaged in the	Membranes ruptured	acquainted with the use of the
Bladder empty	pelvis	No placenta previa	instrument
Clinical pelvimetry must be	The position of the fetal head must		The capability to perform an
adequate in dimension	be known with certainty		emergency cesarean delivery if
and size to facilitate an	The station of the fetal head must be		required
atraumatic delivery	≥+2		
Verbal or written consent	The attitude of the fetal head and the		
	presence of caput succedaneum		
	and/or moulding should be noted		

13–12) must be met before application of the forceps. The patient should be placed in the modified lithotomy position and cleansed and draped in the usual fashion. The bladder should be emptied by catheterization. Adequate analgesia is mandatory for both maternal indications and fetal safety. Estimated fetal weight should be compatible with a high probability of successful vaginal delivery. A thorough examination of the fetal presenting part and characteristics of the maternal pelvis should follow. Exact knowledge of fetal position, station, and degree of asynclitism is essential to proper application. A "phantom application" should be performed by the operator by positioning the forceps in front of the perineum in the correct position of the final application. The phantom application aids in the evaluation of proper placement. There are three broad categories of forceps deliveries, and the technique used to place the forceps and to effect delivery is different for each.

Nonrotational forceps delivery is delivery that is effected without rotation or with rotation of less than 45 degrees (Fig. 13–18). Following separation of the blades of the classical forceps, two fingers of the operator's right hand should be placed transvaginally along the fetal head to protect the vaginal tissues. The left forceps blade is then passed over the palmar aspect of the fingers in the following manner: the handle is held loosely by the left hand of the operator so that the initial position of the blade is essentially vertical over the maternal pubis; the handle is then allowed to drop, almost under its own weight, in a wide arc as the blade is guided along the parietal eminence of the fetal head by the operator's right (intravaginal) hand. The right blade is then applied in a similar manner. The handles are then locked comfortably together. All classical forceps are designed such that the lock will articulate only if the left forceps blade is placed prior to the right-handled blade. Before

traction is initiated, it is mandatory that the application be checked for correct positioning. This will ensure that the compressive and traction forces to the fetal skull will occur in the biparietal or bimalar position thereby minimizing cranial or neurologic damage. Proper application is determined by assessing the position of the forceps in relation to three landmarks on the fetal skull, the posterior fontanelle, the sagittal suture, and the parietal bones. An illustration of proper application is shown in Fig. 13–19. If rotation is required, it should be performed at this time. The fetal head should be flexed by lowering the handles of the forceps, and the handles rotated in an arc until the sagittal suture rests in the direct anteroposterior position. After rotation, the position of the forceps should be rechecked before traction. After application of the forceps, delivery is accomplished according to the principle of axis traction. The pelvis is curved in a J shape, and it is in this direction that the series of force vectors should be applied. When the fetal head lies at the midpelvis, the initial traction is directly posteriorly at a 45-degree angle. Once the head has reached the pelvic floor, the traction is directed horizontally and, finally, upward (anteriorly) to facilitate expulsion of the fetal head by extension. Such force vectors can be achieved either manually using the Saxtorph-Pajot maneuver, in which one hand pulls downwards on the handles while the other hand directs the traction upward or downward at the level of the shanks, or by axis-traction attachments.

Scanzoni-Smellie maneuver refers to complete instrumental rotation of the fetal head from an occiput posterior to anterior position. This was described first by Smellie in 1752 and subsequently modified by Scanzoni in 1853.[165] Classical forceps are placed over the occiput posterior as detailed above. The forceps are then locked and the handles elevated to flex the fetal head. Rotation from the

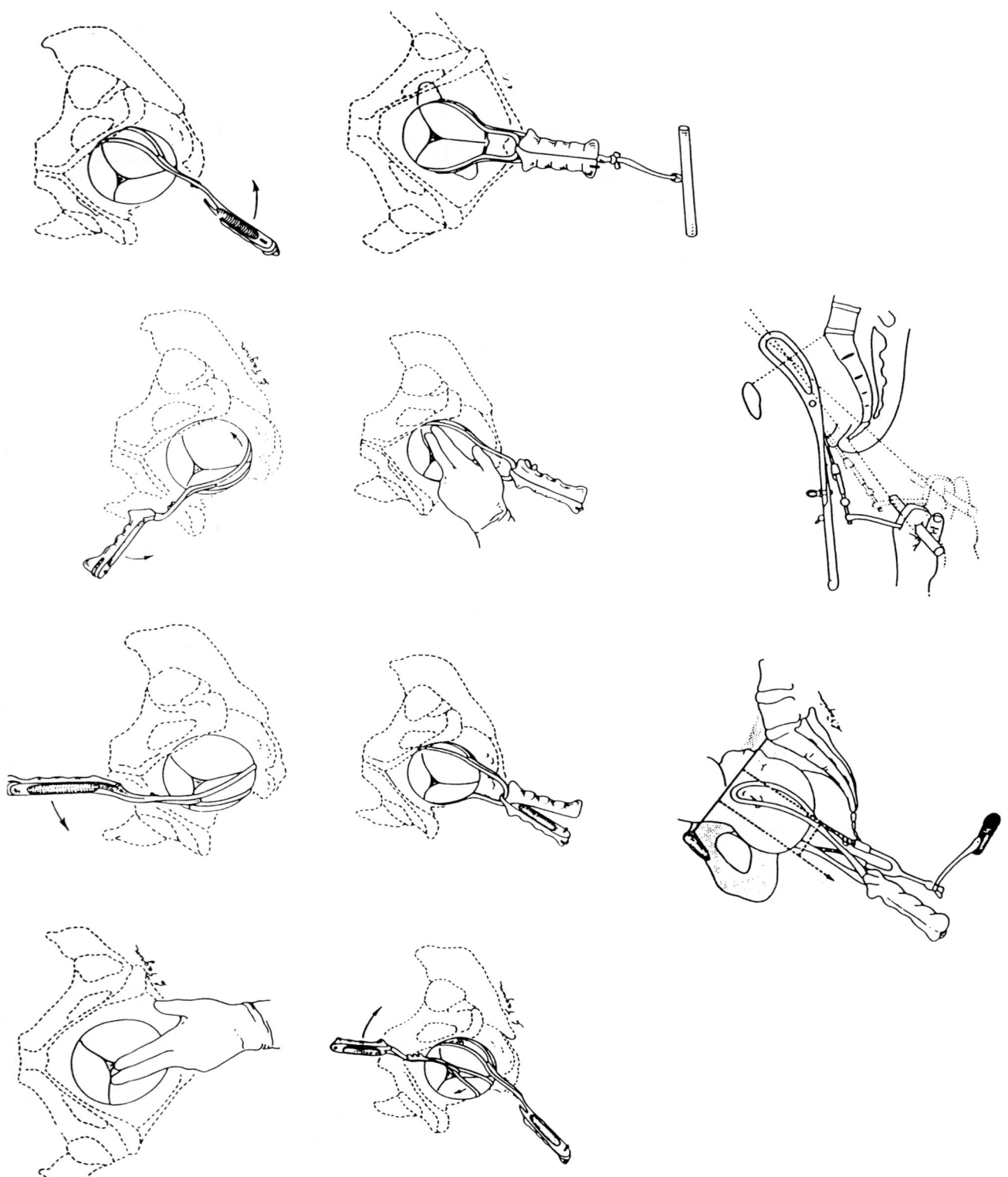

Figure 13–18. Stepwise approach to application of obstetric forceps.

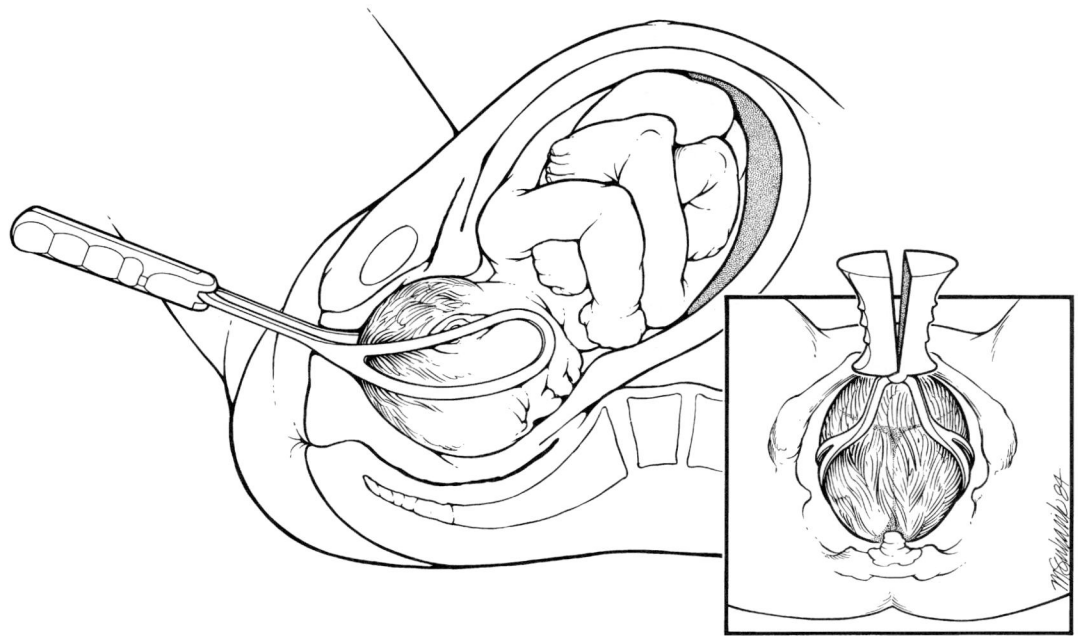

Figure 13–19. Proper application of obstetric forceps. (From O'Brien WF, Cefalo RC: Labor and delivery. *In* Gabbe SG, Niebyl JR, Simpson JL [eds]: Obstetrics: Normal and Problem Pregnancies, 3rd ed. New York, Churchill Livingstone, 1996 p 377, with permission.)

occiput posterior to anterior position is facilitated by dislodging the fetal head very slightly upwards. *The head should not be disengaged from the pelvis.* Rotation should be carried out in a wide arc toward the fetal back (commonly in the direction of the shortest distance to the symphysis pubis) to avoid cervical spine injury. Once the occiput anterior position is reached, the blades will be upside down with the pelvic curve facing the sacrum. To facilitate traction and prevent maternal perineal trauma, it is then necessary to replace the blades in the correct position before traction is applied. In the original description, both blades were removed and replaced. On occasion, however, the head would rotate back toward the original position before reapplication could be attempted. For this reason, the anterior blade is initially removed and repositioned while the posterior blade is temporarily retained to "splint" the head in the anterior position. Thereafter, the posterior blade is removed and repositioned. After the head has been rotated to the occiput anterior position, the reapplication is checked and, if found to be satisfactory, traction is begun. An alternative to the Scanzoni-Smellie maneuver, which is currently the preference of most clinicians, is to deliver the fetus in the direct occiput posterior position.

Rotational forceps deliveries should be reserved for practitioners with the requisite experience. Indications for rotational forceps are limited. The classic indication is arrest of descent in the occiput transverse position (so-called deep transverse arrest), which is often accompanied by asynclitism of the fetal head. In this setting, rotational forceps (such as Kielland forceps) are able to correct the asynclitism (because of their sliding lock) and rotate the fetal head to the anteroposterior position. The same criteria should be fulfilled as for classic forceps (Table 13–12). A "phantom application" of the forceps should be performed with the knobs on the posterior surfaces of the handles facing the occiput. The anterior blade is applied first in one of three ways: (1) the *wandering technique,* in which the blade is held vertically with the handle pointing upwards (the blade is then inserted posteriorly and wandered 180 degrees across the fetal face to its anterior position); (2) the *direct technique,* in which the blade is held vertically with the handle pointing downwards towards the floor, and inserted directly over the parietal eminence of the fetal head with the handle coming to rest in the horizontal position; and (3) the *classical technique* used by Kielland in his original description in 1916,[166] in which the blade is held vertically with the handle pointing towards the ceiling. The blade is then slipped under the symphysis pubis until it comes to rest with the handle in the horizontal position and the cephalic curvature of the blade facing upwards. The blade is then rotated 180 degrees until the cephalic curve of the forceps articulates with the head of the fetus. This application is of historical interest only, and should not be used because of the high incidence of maternal injury. After the anterior blade is in place, the posterior blade is held vertically with the handle pointing toward the ceiling and inserted in the standard fashion. Keeping the handles depressed down against the perineum, the handle tips are brought into alignment correcting the asynclitism and the head is rotated to the anteroposterior position, either OA or OP. The position is then rechecked, and traction is applied with contractions. Some practitioners recommend replacing the rotational forceps with classic forceps after the rotation is complete to facilitate traction and delivery of the head.

Vaginal breech delivery is reviewed in detail in Chapter 16. Delivery of the aftercoming head of the breech can be facilitated by the application of forceps. The Piper forceps were designed specifically to assist the obstetrician in delivering the aftercoming head of the breech. These forceps are placed directly on either side of the fetal head after the body has been delivered, and the body is draped over the elongated shanks. A controlled delivery of the head is then effected by raising the handles of the forceps to facilitate flexion of the fetal head. This instrument is particularly useful if the obstetrician is not assisted. If an assistant is available to lift the legs of the breech, it may be easier to use classic forceps to flex the aftercoming head of the breech.

Following delivery, the fetus and the maternal perineum should be carefully examined. Common fetal findings include facial bruising and, on occasion, facial laceration. Facial nerve palsy, skull fractures, cervical spine injuries, and intracranial hemorrhage are extremely rare, and almost never seen with low or outlet forceps.[164] Maternal perineal injury including sulcus tears and third- and fourth-degree lacerations are increased with forceps deliveries, especially if a forceps rotation is performed.

Vacuum-Assisted Vaginal Delivery

Vacuum extraction was first described by James Yonge in 1705,[167] well before the invention of the forceps. First popularized by Malmström[168] during the mid-1950s, the use of vacuum extraction-assisted delivery has become widespread in Europe. The first classical Malmström vacuum extractor or "ventouse" used a metal disk-shaped cup (the "M" cup) through which a vacuum of up to 0.8 kg/cc^2 is applied to the fetal scalp. The suction induces an artificial caput succedaneum or chignon within the cup to which a traction force is applied in concert with uterine contractions. Current instruments are disposable and made of plastic, poly-

ethylene, or silicone. There are two general types: those with a firm, mushroom-shaped cup similar to the M cup, the rigid cup available in three sizes (40, 50, and 60 mm); or with a pliable, funnel-shaped cup, the soft cup. Manual or electronically operated vacuum sources are available.

A number of technical considerations should be borne in mind when performing a vacuum extraction-assisted delivery. The suction cup should be placed on the fetal scalp symmetrically astride the sagittal suture with the posterior margin of the cup around 1 to 3 cm anterior to the posterior fontanelle, the so-called median flexing point. It should not be placed over the fontanelle. This placement will promote flexion of the fetal head with traction. After application, a low suction (100 mm Hg) is applied to establish a vacuum of around 0.2 kg/cc^2 as the cup is held in place. After ensuring that no maternal soft tissue is trapped between the cup and the fetal head, suction is increased slowly by 0.2 kg/cc^2 every 2 minutes to a final vacuum of 0.7 to 0.8 kg/cc^2 (500 to 600 mm Hg). These slow increments in vacuum are necessary for the proper development of the chignon. Once a proper vacuum has been reached, sustained downward traction is applied along the pelvic curve using a two-handed technique in concert with uterine contractions and maternal expulsive efforts. Suction is released between contractions. Ideally, an episiotomy should be avoided, as pressure of the perineum on the vacuum cup will help to keep it applied to the fetal head and assist in flexion and rotation. It is suggested that the procedure be abandoned if the cup detaches three times, if no descent of the head is achieved, or if delivery is not effected within 30 minutes.

Indications for vacuum extraction-assisted delivery are similar to those for forceps delivery. One potential advantage of vacuum extraction is that delivery can be accomplished with minimal maternal analgesia. Relative contraindications include extreme prematurity (<34 weeks' gestation), suspected fetal coagulation disorder, and suspected fetal macrosomia. Although the overall rate of complications is similar between forceps and vacuum deliveries, the complication profile is different. Failed delivery is commonly encountered using the vacuum extractor, and may be more common with the soft cup (10 to 54 percent) as compared with the M cup (4 to 30 percent).[169,170] Maternal perineal injuries are less common than with forceps deliveries. However, there is an increased incidence of fetal cephalohematoma or bleeding into the scalp which, if large, may be associated with neonatal jaundice, scalp lacerations (especially so-called cookie-cutter injuries which result from attempts by the operator to manually rotate the head with the vacuum), and scalp bruising.[160,169,170] Whether the incidence of fetal intracerebral hemorrhage is increased with vacuum extraction is not clear. In response to reports of 12 fetal deaths and 9 serious injuries over a 4-year period, the FDA issued a Public Health Advisory on May 21, 1998,[171] delineating the fetal risks associated with vacuum extraction and urging physicians to use caution when employing these devices. A follow-up statement by the ACOG[172] argued that "while no medical procedure is risk-free, vacuum extraction has an extraordinary low risk for adverse outcomes" (i.e., 5 adverse events per 228,354 vacuum deliveries per year, or 1 in 45,455 vacuum extractions per year), and strongly recommended the continued use of vacuum-assisted devices in appropriate clinical settings. A recent study by Towner et al. found that the rate of intracranial hemorrhage was higher in infants delivered by vacuum extraction, forceps, or cesarean section during labor than in infants delivered by cesarean section before labor, suggesting that abnormal behavior rather than the mode of delivery was the most important risk factor.[173]

Congenital Neurological Birth Injuries

Facial nerve paralysis results from pressure on the facial nerve (cranial nerve VII) as it exits the skull through the stylomastoid foramen. It is the most common neurologic birth injury, with an incidence of 0.1 to 7.5 per 1,000 live births.[174,175] These injuries are usually associated with operative vaginal (forceps) delivery, although up to a third of cases follow spontaneous vaginal delivery. Facial paralysis may be immediately apparent or may develop within hours of birth. Resolution is usually complete within a few days.

Injuries to the neck and spine are rare, but may result from excessive traction and/or rotation of the spinal cord at delivery. There may be a fracture or dislocation of the vertebral column with resultant neurologic injury (usually at C1–C3), and such injuries may prove fatal. Risk factors for cervical spinal cord injuries include vaginal breech delivery and forceps-assisted vaginal delivery involving a rotation of greater than 90 degrees.[181] The true incidence of spinal injuries is not known.

INTRAPARTUM COMPLICATIONS

Cord Prolapse

Cord prolapse refers to passage of the umbilical cord into the vagina ahead of the presenting part following rupture of the fetal membranes. It is a true obstetric emergency, with a reported perinatal mortality rate of 50 percent.[176] Fetal perfusion is rapidly diminished either by mechanical distortion in the vagina and/or by vasospasm triggered by the precipitous drop in temper-

ature outside the uterus. Cord prolapse is a rare event in term cephalic pregnancies (0.4 percent), but is more common with malpresentations (0.5 percent of frank breech, 4 to 6 percent of complete breech, and 15 to 18 percent of footling breech presentations, and probably greater than 20 percent in pregnancies complicated by transverse lie).[176,178] Other risk factors include a small fetus and prematurity.[177,179] Diagnosis is made by palpation of the cord on vaginal examination with or without fetal bradycardia. Management involves manual replacement of the cord, pushing the presenting part up away from the cord, and immediate delivery, usually by emergent cesarean section. Prevention of iatrogenic cord prolapse can be achieved by performing amniotomy with fundal pressure and only when the vertex is well applied to the cervix.[179]

CONTROVERSIAL ISSUES IN LABOR MANAGEMENT

Active Management of Labor

The increasing incidence of cesarean deliveries in the United States since the 1970s has prompted a systematic examination of labor management. There are two established methods of managing labor at term, traditional management and active management. The major difference between these two approaches is in the definition of failure to progress and in the oxytocin protocol chosen for labor augmentation.

Traditional Management

Traditional management uses a lower dose oxytocin regimen as compared with active management protocols, with longer intervals between dose increments. Low-dose oxytocin infusion, starting at an infusion rate of 1 mIU/min and increasing by 1 to 2 mIU/min at intervals of not less than 30 minutes, significantly shortens the interval from initiation of oxytocin augmentation to full dilation as compared with physician-directed regimens.[77,148] There has been considerable debate as to whether a low-dose or high-dose oxytocin protocol is more effective for augmentation of labor at term, but there are few publications that directly compare these two protocols. High-dose oxytocin (starting at an infusion rate of 4 mIU/min and increasing by 4 mIU/min every 15 minutes "until adequate uterine contractility were obtained") may shorten the length of labor in both nulliparous and multiparous patients as compared with low-dose protocols.[136,182] It remains unclear, however, whether high-dose oxytocin actually improves obstetric outcome or whether it merely produces the same outcome in a shorter period of time.

Active Management of Labor

Active management of labor refers to a philosophy of labor management based on the premise that optimizing uterine contractions will improve the progress of labor and subsequent outcome.[24,54] An extension of this philosophy is the belief that fetal and maternal injuries are less with propulsion than with traction. It applies specifically to nulliparous patients in spontaneous labor with a cephalic presentation, and is not applicable to the multiparous patient, to patients undergoing induction of labor, or the management of patients attempting vaginal delivery after cesarean.

Active management describes a pragmatic protocol of clinical management that focuses on the first stage of labor. It is based on the premise that, by foreshortening the first stage of labor, the outcome of the second stage can be improved.[24,54] The popularized view of the active management of labor is that of a high-dose oxytocin regimen. However, there are many other important components to this approach of management. The basic principles of active management include the following:

Strict criteria for admission to labor and delivery. In active management of labor protocols, labor is defined strictly as the presence of regular, painful contractions in conjunction with at least one further finding (complete cervical effacement, bloody show, or rupture of the fetal membranes).

Early amniotomy.

Hourly cervical examinations.

Early diagnosis of inefficient uterine activity. If the patient does not achieve and maintain a cervical dilatation rate of greater than or equal to 1.0 cm/h, a diagnosis of inefficient uterine activity is made and augmentation with intravenous oxytocin infusion is initiated immediately.

High-dose oxytocin infusion. In patients requiring oxytocin augmentation, a high-dose oxytocin infusion protocol is used. Oxytocin infusion is initiated at a rate of 6 mIU/min and increased by the same amount every 15 minutes until a uterine contraction frequency of seven contractions per 15 minutes is achieved or until the maximum oxytocin infusion rate of 36 mIU/min is reached.

Active intervention. Using this protocol, the expected duration of the first stage of labor is less than 12 hours and less than 2 hours for the second stage. If these expectations are not met, active intervention, operative vaginal or cesarean delivery, is recommended.

Patient education. The logistic component of the active management protocol aimed at allaying patient fear and anxiety is often overlooked. Emphasis has been placed on antenatal education with a view to realistic expectations for the patient, close supervision by a senior obstetrician, and one-on-one nursing care. An emphasis on peer review of all cesarean sections was highlighted in the original protocol.

Since its introduction in 1968, adherence to these principles at the National Maternity Hospital in Dublin, Ireland, through 1980 has been associated with a sustained primary cesarean section rate in nulliparous women of around 5 percent to 6 percent.[183] It should not be forgotten that the initial objective of the active management protocol was to shorten the length of nulliparous labor, not to lower the cesarean section rate. Since the rate of cesarean deliveries is dependent on a number of demographic factors, including maternal age and race, extrapolation from one population to another is difficult. Despite these limitations, trials of active management have been carried out in several institutions around the world, some of whom have reported a decrease in cesarean deliveries as compared with historic controls.[184–185] However, there have been only two randomized trials comparing the active management of labor with preexisting management strategies.[187,188] In 1992, Lopez-Zeno et al.[187] reported a controlled trial carried out in the United States in which 705 nulliparous, term, singleton pregnancies were randomized to either active management or to a more traditional management protocol. The active management protocol was similar to that carried out in previous trials, with strict criteria for the diagnosis of labor, amniotomy within an hour of labor onset, augmentation when cervical dilatation was not maintained at greater than or equal to 1.0 cm/h, and a high-dose oxytocin augmentation regimen (initial infusion rate of 6 mIU/min that was increased by the same amount every 15 minutes with a maximum oxytocin infusion rate of 36 mIU/min). Less emphasis was placed on antenatal education and individualized obstetric nursing care than in the original Dublin studies. Results of this trial suggested that the active management group had a 26 percent reduction in the rate of cesarean deliveries when compared with controls (10.5 percent vs. 14.1 percent, respectively; odds, ratio 0.57; 95% confidence interval, 0.36, 0.95). The length of labor was decreased by an average of 1.66 hours in the active management group. There was also decrease in maternal infectious morbidity, but no other differences in maternal or neonatal morbidity or morality. The second randomized trial, that of Frigoletto et al.[188] in 1995, adhered more strictly to the logistic concerns of the active management protocol, with greater patient participation, antenatal classes, improved patient education, and individualized nursing. The oxytocin augmentation protocol was slightly different from the study by Lopez-Zeno et al., with a starting rate of 4 mIU/min and a 4 mIU/min incremental rate every 15 minutes to a maximum of 40 mIU/min; 1,934 nulliparous, low-risk women were randomly assigned to either active management or usual care prior to 30 weeks' gestation. Outcome data included cesarean delivery rates and various measures of maternal and neonatal morbidity and mortality. Results showed that the cesarean delivery rates were similar between the two groups (19.4 percent vs. 19.5 percent, respectively). Again, the length of labor and infectious morbidity were decreased with active management. The evidence regarding the rate of cesarean delivery rates and active management of labor is therefore contradictory. Multivariate analysis by the Oxford Collaborative Group[189] aimed at dissecting apart the individual components of the active management of labor strategy showed that oxytocin augmentation, either on its own or in combination with amniotomy, did not reduce the rate of cesarean delivery. The authors did find, interestingly, that psychological support during labor was associated with a decrease in operative delivery, but only when the patient's partner was not present. In support of the argument that active management does not decrease the rate of cesarean deliveries, attention has been drawn to centers with similar cesarean section rates to that reported in the original active management studies using a minimal intervention management style.[190,191]

Regardless of the effect on cesarean section rates, the active management strategy is associated with a shortening in the duration of labor. Whether this is a result of the presence of a supportive "doula-like" figure, to the lower incidence of epidural anesthesia, to the more aggressive oxytocin augmentation protocol, to the delayed diagnosis of labor, or to a combination of these factors, is not clear. It has also been suggested that the aggressive introduction of high-dose oxytocin may overcome early, subclinical labor dystocia before uterine infection and fatigue make it less responsive to augmentation.[192]

The Effect of Epidural Analgesia on the Progress of Labor

The question of whether or not epidural analgesia prolongs the length of labor and increases the incidence of operative delivery is controversial (see Chapter 15). The mode of pain relief during labor should be individualized and is a decision that is best left in the hands of the patient and her care provider.

Premature Rupture of the Membranes at Term

Premature rupture of the membranes is defined as rupture of the fetal membranes prior to the onset of labor, and occurs in 8 percent of term pregnancies.[2] The man-

agement of this condition is controversial. Immediate delivery is indicated if there is evidence of chorioamnionitis, vaginal bleeding, and/or fetal compromise. It may also be prudent to expedite delivery in women colonized with group B streptococci, because of the increased risk of neonatal sepsis.[193] Premature rupture of the membranes is not a contraindication to cervical ripening using transvaginal prostaglandin preparations.[194,195]

Initial studies suggested that expectant management of women with premature rupture of the membranes at term in the absence of obstetric complications was associated with a lower rate of cesarean delivery as compared with active management.[196,197] Subsequent larger and better designed studies[198,199] as well as a recent meta-analysis[200] have refuted these observations. These investigations conclude that immediate induction of labor with intravenous oxytocin, induction of labor with vaginal PGE_2 gel, and expectant management are all reasonable options for women and their babies if membranes rupture before the start of labor at term, since they result in similar rates of neonatal infection and cesarean delivery.[199,200] However, an increase in maternal chorioamnionitis and endometritis with expectant management was a consistent finding in all of the trials. In one large randomized trial, women themselves viewed induction of labor more positively than expectant management.[199]

Key Points

➤ Labor is a clinical diagnosis.

➤ The classical diagnosis of labor includes regular painful uterine contractions, progressive cervical effacement and dilatation, and a show (bloody discharge).

➤ It is likely that the fetus is in control of the timing of labor, although the precise mechanism by which this occurs is not clear.

➤ The ability of the fetus to successfully negotiate the pelvis during labor and delivery is dependent on the complex interaction of three variables: the powers, the passenger, and the passage.

➤ The two major potential complications of elective induction of labor are iatrogenic prematurity and increased cesarean delivery resulting from failed induction. Recent studies have demonstrated that routine induction of labor at 41 weeks' gestation is not associated with an increased risk of cesarean section regardless of parity, state of the cervix, or method of induction.

➤ When induction of labor is attempted against an unfavorable cervix, the likelihood of a successful outcome is reduced. The choice of which method to use to promote cervical maturation and to induce labor should be individualized. A single technique is rarely effective on its own, and a combination of maneuvers may be required.

➤ In view of the lack of objective evidence of benefit of prophylactic episiotomy and the data suggesting that median episiotomy is associated with an increased incidence of severe perineal trauma, prophylactic median episiotomy should be discouraged.

➤ Abnormal labor itself, not the mode of delivery, may be the most important risk factor for intracranial hemorrhage in the neonate.

➤ Active management of labor refers to a philosophy of labor management based on the premise that optimizing uterine contractions will improve the progress of labor and subsequent outcome.

➤ Induction of labor with intravenous oxytocin, induction of labor with vaginal PGE$_2$ gel, and expectant management are all reasonable options for women and their babies if membranes rupture before the start of labor at term, since they result in similar rates of neonatal infection and cesarean delivery.

REFERENCES

1. Nathanielsz PW, Giussani DA, Wu WX: Stimulation of the switch in myometrial activity from contractures to contractions in the pregnant sheep and nonhuman primate. Equine Vet J 24(Suppl):83, 1997.
2. Duff P, Huff RW, Gibbs RS: Management of premature rupture of membranes and unfavorable cervix in term pregnancy. Obstet Gynecol 63:697, 1984.
3. Thorburn GD, Challis JRG, Robinson JS: The endocrinology of parturition. In Wynn RM (ed): Cellular Biology of the Uterus. New York, Plenum Press, 1977, p 653.
4. Casey LM, MacDonald PC: The initiation of labour in women: regulation of phospholipid and arachidonic acid metabolism and of prostaglandin production. In Creasy RK, Warshaw JB (eds): Seminars in Perinatology, Vol 10. Orlando, FL, Grune & Stratton, 1986, p 270.
5. Liggins GC: The onset of labour: An overview. In McNellis D, Challis JRG, MacDonald PC, et al (eds): The Onset of Labour: Cellular and Integrative Mechanisms. A National Institute of Child Health and Human Development Research Planning Workshop (November 29–December 1, 1987). Ithaca, NY, Perinatology Press, 1988, p 1.
6. López Bernal A, Rivera J, Europe-Finner GN, et al: Parturition: activation of stimulatory pathways or loss of uterine quiescence? Adv Exp Med Biol 395:435, 1995.
7. Garrioch DB: The effect of indomethacin on spontaneous activity in the isolated human myometrium and on the response to oxytocin and prostaglandin. Br J Obstet Gynaecol 85:47, 1978.
8. MacDonald PC: Parturition: biomolecular and physiologic process. In Cunningham FG, MacDonald PC, Gant NF, et al (eds): Williams Obstetrics, 19th ed. Norwalk, CT, Appleton & Lange, 1993, p 298.
9. Challis JRG, Gibb W: Control of parturition. Prenat Neonat Med 1:283, 1996.
10. Liggins GC: Initiation of labor. Biol Neonate 55:366, 1989.
11. Liggins BJ, Fairclough RJ, Grieves SA, et al: The mechanism of initiation of parturition in the ewe. Rec Prog Horm Res 29:111, 1973.
12. Flint APF, Anderson ABM, Steele PA, et al: The mechanism by which fetal cortisol controls the onset of parturition in the sheep. Biochem Soc Trans 3:1189, 1975.
13. Matthews SG, Challis JRG: Regulation of the hypothalamo-pituitary-adreno-cortical axis in fetal sheep. Trends Endocrinol Metab 4:239, 1996.
14. Norwitz ER, Robinson JN, Repke JT: The initiation of parturition: a comparative analysis across the species. Curr Probl Obstet Gynecol Fertil 22:41, 1999.
15. Pauerstein CJ, Zauder HL: Autonomic innervation, sex steroids and uterine contractility. Obstet Gynecol Surv. (Suppl) 25:617, 1970.
16. Norwitz ER, Robinson JN, Challis JRG: The control of labor. N Engl J Med 341:660, 1999.
17. Myers DA, Nathanielsz PW: Biologic basis of term and preterm labor. Clin Perinatol 20:9, 1993.
18. Honnebier MB, Nathanielsz PW: Primate parturition and the role of the maternal circadian system. Eur J Obstet Gynecol Reprod Biol 55:193, 1994.
19. Nathanielsz PW: Comparative studies on the initiation of labor. Eur J Obstet Gynecol Reprod Biol 78:127, 1998.
20. Challis JRG: Characteristics of parturition. In Creasy RK, Resnick R (eds): Maternal-Fetal Medicine: Principles and Practice, 3rd ed. Philadelphia, WB Saunders Company, 1994, p 482.
21. Mecenas CA, Giussani DA, Owiny JR, et al: Production of premature delivery in pregnant rhesus monkeys by androstenedione infusion. Nat Med 2:443, 1996.
22. Figueroa JP, Honnebier MBOM, Binienda Z, et al: Effect of 48 hour intravenous Δ^4 androstenedione infusion on pregnant rhesus monkeys in the last third of gestation: changes in maternal plasma estradiol concentrations and myometrial contractility. Am J Obstet Gynecol 161:481, 1989.
23. Nathanielsz PW, Jenkins SL, Tame JD, et al: Local paracrine effects of estradiol are central to parturition in the rhesus monkey. Nat Med 4:456, 1998.
24. O'Driscoll K, Meagher D: Induction. In O'Driscoll K, Meagher D (eds): Active Management of Labour, 2nd ed. Eastbourne, United Kingdom, Balliere Tindall, 1986, p 96.
25. Caldeyro-Barcia R, Posiero JJ: Physiology of uterine contractions. Clin Obstet Gynecol 3:386, 1960.
26. Caldeyro-Barcia R, Sica-Blanco Y, Poseiro JJ, et al: A quantitative study of the action of synthetic oxytocin on the pregnant human uterus. J Pharmacol Exp Ther 121:18, 1957.
27. Miller FC: Uterine activity, labor management, and perinatal outcome. Semin Perinatol 2:181, 1978.
28. American College of Obstetricians and Gynecologists: Fetal

macrosomia, ACOG Practice Bulletin No. 22. Washington, DC, American College of Obstetricians and Gynecologists, 2000.

29. O'Brien WF, Cefalo RC: Evaluation of x-ray pelvimetry and abnormal labor. Clin Obstet Gynecol 25:157, 1982.

30. Joyce DN, Giva-Osagie F, Stevenson GW: Role of pelvimetry in active management of labor. Br Med J 4:505, 1975.

31. Morris CW, Heggie JC, Acton CM: Computed tomography pelvimetry: accuracy and radiation dose compared with conventional pelvimetry. Australas Radiol 37:186, 1993.

32. Caldwell WE, Moloy HC: Anatomical variations in the female pelvis and their effect in labor with a suggested classification. Am J Obstet Gynecol 26:479, 1933.

33. Crawford JW: Computor monitoring of fetal heart rate and uterine pressure. Am J Obstet Gynecol 21:342, 1975.

34. Lamont RF, Neave S, Baker AC, et al: Intrauterine pressures in labours induced by amniotomy and oxytocin or vaginal prostaglandin gel compared with normal labour. Br J Obstet Gynaecol 98:441, 1991.

35. Friedman EA: The graphic analysis of labor. Am J Obstet Gynecol 68:1568, 1954.

36. Friedman EA: Primigravid labor: a graphicostatiscal analysis. Obstet Gynecol 6:567, 1955.

37. Peisner DB, Rosen MG: Transition from latent to active labor. Obstet Gynecol 68:448, 1986.

38. Duignan NM, Studd JWW, Hughes AO: Characteristics of normal labour in different racial groups. Br J Obstet Gynaecol 82:593, 1975.

39. Studd J: Partograms and nomograms of cervical dilatation in the management of primigravid labour. Br Med J 4:451, 1973.

40. American College of Obstetricians and Gynecologists: Operative vaginal delivery, ACOG Technical Bulletin No. 196. Washington, DC, American College of Obstetricians and Gynecologists, 1994.

41. Sporlin L: Conduct of normal births through external examination alone. Arch Gynaekol 45:337, 1894.

42. Chauhan SP, Lutton PM, Bailey KJ, et al: Intrapartum clinical, sonographic, and parous patients' estimates of newborn birth weight. Obstet Gynecol 79:956, 1992.

43. Friedman EA: Labor: Clinical Evaluation and Management. New York, Appleton-Century-Crofts, 1967, p 34.

44. Kennell J, Klaus M, McGrath S, et al: Continuous emotional support during labor in a US hospital. A randomized controlled trial. JAMA 265:2197, 1991.

45. Wolman WL, Chalmers B, Hofmeyr GJ, et al: Postpartum depression and companionship in the clinical birth environment: a randomized, controlled study. Am J Obstet Gynecol 168:1388, 1993.

46. Bloom SL, McIntire DD, Kelly MA, et al: Lack of effect of walking on labor and delivery. N Engl J Med 339:76, 1998.

47. Thacker SB, Stroup DF, Peterson HB: Efficacy and safety of electronic fetal monitoring: an update. Obstet Gynecol 86:613, 1995.

48. Rogers J, Wood J, McCandlish R, et al: Active versus expectant management of third stage of labour: the Hinchingbrooke randomised controlled trial. Lancet 351:693, 1998.

49. Romero R, Pilu G, Jeanty P, et al: Prenatal Diagnosis of Congenital Anomalies. Norwalk, CT, Appleton & Lange, 1988.

50. Thierstein ST, Jahn HC, Lange K: Routine third-stage exploration of the uterus. Obstet Gynecol 10:269, 1957.

51. Blanchette H: Elective manual exploration of the uterus after delivery: a study and review. J Reprod Med 19:13, 1977.

52. Friedman EA: The functional divisions of labor. Am J Obstet Gynecol 109:274, 1971.

53. Friedman EA, Sachtelben MR: Dysfunctional labor. I. Pro-

54. longed latent phase in the nullipara. Obstet Gynecol 17:135, 1961.

54. O'Driscoll K, Meagher P: Active Management of Labor. Philadelphia, WB Saunders Company, 1980.

55. Friedman EA, Sachtelben MR: Dysfunctional labor. II. Protracted active phase dilatation in the nullipara. Obstet Gynecol 17:566, 1961.

56. Friedman EA, Sachtelben MR: Dysfunctional labor. III. Secondary arrest of dilatation in the nullipara. Obstet Gynecol 19:576, 1962.

57. Jocoate TN, Baker K, Martin RB: Inefficient uterine activity. Surg Gynecol Obstet 95:257, 1952.

58. Friedman EA, Sachtelben MR: Station of the fetal presenting part. V. Protracted descent patterns. Obstet Gynecol 36:558, 1970.

59. Gaziano EP, Freeman DW, Bendel RP: FHR variability and other heart rate observations during second stage labor. Obstet Gynecol 56:42, 1980.

60. Jacobson L, Rooth G: Interpretative aspects on the acid-base composition and its variation in fetal scalp blood and maternal blood during labour. J Obstet Gynaecol Br Commonw 78:971, 1971.

61. Cohen W: Influence of the duration of the second stage of labor on perinatal outcome and puerperal morbidity. Obstet Gynecol 49:266, 1977.

62. Menticoglou SM, Manning F, Harman C, et al: Perinatal outcome in relation to second stage-stage duration. Am J Obstet Gynecol 173:906, 1995.

63. Albers LL, Schiff M, Gorwoda JG: The length of active labor in normal pregnancies. Obstet Gynecol 87:355, 1996.

64. Rouse DJ, Owen J, Hauth JC: Active-phase labor arrest: oxytocin augmentation for at least 4 hours. Obstet Gynecol 93:323, 1999.

65. Sorbe B: Active pharmacologic management of the third stage of labor. Obstet Gynecol 52:694, 1978.

66. Smith LP, Nagourney BA, McLean FH, et al: Hazards and benefits of elective induction of labor. Am J Obstet Gynecol 148:579, 1984.

67. Macer JA, Macer CL, Chan LS: Elective induction versus spontaneous labor: a retrospective study of complications and outcomes. Am J Obstet Gynecol 166:1690, 1992.

68. Hannah ME, Hannah WJ, Hellman J, et al: Induction of labor as compared with serial antenatal monitoring in postterm pregnancy. N Engl J Med 326:1587, 1992.

69. McNellis D, Medearis AL, Fowler S, et al, for The National Institute of Child Health and Human Development Network of Maternal-Fetal Medicine Units: A clinical trial of induction of labor versus expectant management in postterm pregnancy. Am J Obstet Gynecol 170:716, 1994.

70. Yeast JD, Jones A, Poskin M: Induction of labor and the relationship to cesarean delivery: a review of 7001 consecutive inductions. Am J Obstet Gynecol 180:628, 1999.

71. Cocks DP: Significance of initial condition of cervix uteri to subsequent course of labour. Br Med J 1:327, 1955.

72. Friedman EA, Niswander KR, Bayonet-Rivera NP, et al: Relation of prelabor evaluation in inducibility and the course of labor. Obstet Gynecol 28:495, 1966.

73. Brindley BA, Sokol RJ: Induction and augmentation of labor: basis and methods for current practice. Obstet Gynecol Surv 43:730, 1988.

74. Xenakis EMJ, Piper JM, Conway DL, et al: Induction of labor in the nineties: conquering the unfavorable cervix. Obstet Gynecol 90:235, 1997.

75. Bishop EH: Pelvic scoring for elective induction. Obstet Gynecol 24:266, 1964.

76. Hughey MJ, McElin TW, Bird CC: An evaluation of preinduction scoring systems. Obstet Gynecol 48:635, 1976.

77. American College of Obstetricians and Gynecologists: Induction of labor, ACOG Technical Bulletin No. 217. Washington, DC, American College of Obstetricians and Gynecologists, 1995.

78. Poma PA: Cervical ripening: a review and recommendations for clinical practice. J Reprod Med 44:657, 1999.

79. Kierse MJNC, Chalmers I: Methods for inducing labour. *In* Chalmers I, Enkin M, Kierse MJNC (eds): Effective Care in Pregnancy and Childbirth. Oxford, Oxford University Press, 1989, p 1057.

80. Leppert PC: Anatomy and physiology of cervical ripening. Clin Obstet Gynecol 38:267, 1995.

81. Kerr JMM, Johnstone RW, Phillips MH: Historical Review of British Obstetrics and Gynaecology, 1800–1950. London, E&S Livingston, 1954, p 34.

82. McColgin PG, Bennet WA, Roach H, et al: Parturitional factors associated with membrane stripping. Am J Obstet Gynecol 169:71, 1993.

83. Mitchell MD, Flint APF, Bibby J, et al: Rapid increase in plasma prostaglandins after vaginal examination and amniotomy. Br Med J 2:1183, 1977.

84. Ferguson JKW: A study of the motility of the intact uterus at term. Surg Gynecol Obstet 73:359, 1941.

85. Swann RO: Induction of labor by stripping membranes. Obstet Gynecol 11:74, 1958.

86. Wiriyasirivaj B, Vutyavanich T, Ruangsri RA: A randomized controlled trial of membrane stripping at term to promote labor. Obstet Gynecol 87:767, 1996.

87. Berghella V, Rogers RA, Lescale K: Stripping of membranes as a safe method to reduce prolonged pregnancies. Obstet Gynecol 87:927, 1996.

88. Crane J, Bennett K, Yound D, et al: The effectiveness of sweeping membranes at term: a randomized trial. Obstet Gynecol 89:586, 1997.

89. Boulvain M, Irion O, Marcoux S, et al: Sweeping of the membranes to prevent post-term pregnancy and to induce labour: a systematic review. Br J Obstet Gynaecol 106:481, 1999.

90. Kreis J: L'accouchement médical. Rev Fr Gynecol Obstet 24:604, 1979.

91. Booth JH, Kurdizak VB: Elective induction of labor: a controlled study. Can Med Assoc 103:245, 1970.

92. Fraser WD, Marcoux S, Moutquin J-M, et al: Effect of early amniotomy on the risk of dystocia in nulliparous women. N Engl J Med 328:1145, 1993.

93. Brisson-Carroll G, Fraser W, Bréart G, et al: The effect of routine early amniotomy on spontaneous labor: a meta-analysis. Obstet Gynecol 87:891, 1996.

94. Patterson WM: Amniotomy, with or without simultaneous oxytocin infusion. J Obstet Gynaecol Br Commonw 78:310, 1971.

95. Saleh YZ: Surgical induction of labor with and without oxytocin infusion. Aust N Z J Obstet Gynaecol 15:80, 1975.

96. Moldin PG, Sundell G: Induction of labour: a randomised clinical trial of amniotomy versus amniotomy with oxytocin infusion. Br J Obstet Gynaecol 103:306, 1996.

97. Baumgarten K: Advantages and disadvantages of low amniotomy. J Perinatal Med 4:3, 1976.

98. Embery MP, Mollison BC: The unfavourable cervix and the induction of labor using a cervical balloon. J Obstet Gynaecol Br Commonw 74:44, 1967.

99. Onge RD, Connors GT: Preinduction cervical ripening: a comparison of intracervical prostaglandin E2 gel versus the Foley catheter. Am J Obstet Gynecol 172:687, 1995.

100. Sanchez-Ramos L, Kaunitz AM, Connor PM: Hygroscopic cervical dilators and prostaglandin E2, gel for preinduction cervical ripening. J Reprod Med 37:355, 1992.

101. Rouben D, Arias F: A randomized trial of extra-amniotic saline infusion plus intracervical Foley catheter balloon versus prostaglandin E2 vaginal gel for ripening of the cervix and inducing of labor in patients with unfavorable cervices. Obstet Gynecol 82:290, 1993.

102. Sullivan CA, Benton LW, Roach H, et al: Combining medical and mechanical methods of cervical ripening: does it increase the likelihood of successful induction of labor? J Reprod Med 41:823, 1993.

103. Calder AA, Embery MP, Tait T: Ripening of the cervix with extra-amniotic prostaglandin E2 in viscous gel before induction of labor. Br J Obstet Gynaecol 84:264, 1977.

104. MacKenzie IZ, Embery MP: A comparison of PGE2 and PGF2α vaginal gel for ripening the cervix before induction of labor. Br J Obstet Gynaecol 85:657, 1979.

105. Shepherd JH, Pearce JMF, Sims C: Induction of labor using prostaglandin E2 pessaries. Br Med J 2:108, 1979.

106. Keirse MJNC: Endogenous prostaglandins in human parturition. *In* Keirse MJNC, Anderson ABM, Bennebroek-Gravenhorst J (eds): Human Parturition. Leiden, Leiden University Press, 1979, p 101.

107. Keirse MJNC, Turnbull AC: Prostaglandins in amniotic fluid during late pregnancy and labour. J Obstet Gynaecol Br Commonw 80:970, 1973.

108. Romero R, Munoz H, Gomez R, et al: Increase in prostaglandin bioavailability precedes the onset of human parturition. Prostaglandins Leukot Essent Fatty Acids 54:187, 1996.

109. Neilson DR, Prins RP, Bolton RN, et al: A comparison of prostaglandin E2 gel and prostaglandin F2α gel for pre-induction cervical ripening. Am J Obstet Gynecol 146:526, 1983.

110. Calder AA, Embery MP, Hillier K: Extra-amniotic prostaglandin E2 for induction of labor at term. Br J Obstet Gynaecol 81:39, 1974.

111. O'Herlihy C, MacDonald HN: Influence of pre-induction prostaglandin E2 gel on cervical ripening and labour induction. Obstet Gynecol 54:708, 1979.

112. Shepherd JH, Knuppel RA: The role of prostaglandins in ripening the cervix and inducing labor. Clin Perinatol 8:49, 1986.

113. Ulmsten U, Wingerup L, Belfrage P, et al: Intracervical application of prostaglandin gel for induction of term labor. Obstet Gynecol 59:336, 1982.

114. Keirse MJNC: Prostaglandins in preinduction cervical ripening: meta-analysis of world wide clinical experience. J Reprod Med 38:89, 1993.

115. Ekman G, Forman A, Marsal K, et al: Intravaginal versus intracervical application of prostaglandin E2 in viscous gel for cervical priming and induction of labor at term in patients with an unfavourable cervical state. Am J Obstet Gynecol 147:657, 1983.

116. Keirse JNC, de Koning Gans HJ: Randomized comparison of the effects of endocervical and vaginal prostaglandin E2 gel in women with various degrees of cervical ripeness. Am J Obstet Gynecol 173:1859, 1995.

117. Rayburn WF, Wapner RJ, Barss VA, et al: An intravaginal controlled release prostaglandin E2 pessary for cervical ripening and initiation of labor at term. Obstet Gynecol 79:374, 1992.

118. Wing DA, Jones MM, Rahall A, et al: A comparison of prostaglandin E2 gel for preinduction cervical ripening and labor induction. Am J Obstet Gynecol 172:1804, 1995.

119. Wing DA, Rahall A, Jones MM, et al: Misoprostol: an effective agent for cervical ripening and labor induction. Am J Obstet Gynecol 172:1811, 1995.

120. Windrim R, Bennett K, Mundle W, et al: Oral administration of misoprostol for labor induction: a randomized controlled trial. Obstet Gynecol 89:392, 1997.

121. Garris RE, Kirkwood CF: Misoprostol: A prostaglandin E₁ analogue. Clin Pharm 8:627, 1999.

122. Varaklis K, Gumina R, Stubblefield PG: Randomized controlled trial of vaginal misoprostol and intracervical prostaglandin E₂ gel for induction of labor at term. Obstet Gynecol 86:541, 1995.

123. Chuck FJ, Huffaker BJ: Labor induction with intravaginal misoprostol versus intracervical prostaglandin E₂ gel: randomized comparison. Am J Obstet Gynecol 173:1137, 1995.

124. Wing DA, Paul RH: A comparison of differing dosing regimens of vaginally administered misoprostol for preinduction cervical ripening and labor induction. Am J Obstet Gynecol 175:158, 1996.

125. Zeeman GG, Khan-Dawood FS, Dawood MY: Oxytocin and its receptor in pregnancy and parturition: current concepts and clinical implications. Obstet Gynecol 89:873, 1997.

126. Fuchs A-R, Fuchs F: Endocrinology of human parturition: a review. Br J Obstet Gynaecol 91:948, 1984.

127. Dawood MY, Wang CF, Gupta R, et al: Fetal contribution to oxytocin in human labor. Obstet Gynecol 52:205, 1978.

128. Fuchs A-R: The role of oxytocin in parturition. *In* Huszar G (ed): The Physiology and Biochemistry of the Uterus in Pregnancy and Labour. Boca Raton, FL, CRC Press, 1986, p 163.

129. Fuchs AR, Fuchs F, Husslein P, et al: Oxytocin receptors and human parturition: a dual role for oxytocin in the initiation of labor. Science 215:1396, 1982.

130. Fuchs AR, Fuchs F, Husslein P, et al: Oxytocin receptors in the human uterus during pregnancy and parturition. Am J Obstet Gynecol 150:734, 1984.

131. Husslein P, Fuchs A-R, Fuchs F: Oxytocin and the initiation of human parturition. I. Prostaglandin release during induction of labor with oxytocin. Am J Obstet Gynecol 141:688, 1981.

132. Fuchs A-R, Husslein P, Fuchs F: Oxytocin and the initiation of human parturition. II. Stimulation of prostaglandin production in human decidua by oxytocin. Am J Obstet Gynecol 141:694, 1981.

133. Theobald GW, Graham A, Campbell J, et al: The use of posterior pituitary extract in physiological mounts in obstetrics. Br Med 2:123, 1948.

134. Valentine BV: Intravenous oxytocin and oral prostaglandin E₂ for ripening the unfavourable cervix. Br J Obstet Gynaecol 84:846, 1977.

135. Magann EF, Perry KG, Dockery JR, et al: Cervical ripening before medical induction of labor: a comparison of prostaglandin E₂ gel, estradiol and oxytocin. Am J Obstet Gynecol 172:1702, 1995.

136. Merrill DC, Zlatnick FJ: Double-masked comparison of oxytocin dosage in induction and augmentation of labor. Obstet Gynecol 94:455, 1999.

137. Perry RL, Saatin AJ, Barth WH, et al: The pharmacokinetics of oxytocin as they apply to labor induction. Am J Obstet Gynecol 174:1590, 1996.

138. Pollnow DM, Broekhuizen FF: Randomized, double-blind trial of prostaglandin E2 intravaginal gel versus low-dose oxytocin for cervical ripening before induction of labor. Am J Obstet Gynecol 174:1910, 1996.

139. Chew WC: Neonatal hyperbilirubinaemia: a comparison between prostaglandin E₂ and oxytocin inductions. Br Med J 2:679, 1977.

140. Johnson N, Bryce FC: Could antiprogesterones be used as alternative cervical ripening agents? Am J Obstet Gynecol 162:688, 1990.

141. Swahn ML, Brydgeman M: The effect of the antiprogestin mifepristone on uterine contractility and sensitivity to prostaglandin and oxytocin. Br J Obstet Gynaecol 95:126, 1988.

142. Sanchez-Ramos L, Kaunitz AM, Wears RL, et al: Misoprostol for cervical ripening and labor induction: a meta-analysis. Obstet Gynecol 89:633, 1997.

143. Cabrol D, Dubois C, Cronje H, et al: Induction at labor with mifepristone (RU486) in intrauterine fetal death. Am J Obstet Gynecol 163:540, 1990.

144. Frydman R, Lelaidier C, Baton-Saint-Mleux C, et al: Labor induction in women at term with mifepristone (RU486): a double-blind, randomized, placebo-controlled study. Obstet Gynecol 80:972, 1992.

145. Lelaidier C, Baton C, Benifla JL, et al: Mifepristone for labor induction after caesarean section. Br J Obstet Gynaecol 101:501, 1994.

146. Blakemore KI, Qin N, Petrie RH, et al: A prospective comparison of hourly and quarter hourly oxytocin increase intervals for the induction of labor at term. Obstet Gynecol 75:757, 1990.

147. Willcourt RJ, Pager D, Wendel J, et al: Induction of labor with pulsatile oxytocin by a computercontrolled pump. Am J Obstet Gynecol 170:603, 1994.

148. Seitchik J, Castillo M: Oxytocin augmentation of dysfunctional labor. I. Clinical data. Am J Obstet Gynecol 144:899, 1982.

149. Tumbull AC, Anderson ABM: Induction of labour. III. Results with amniotomy and oxytocin "titration." J Obstet Gynaecol Br Commonw 75:32, 1968.

150. Toaff ME, Herzoni J, Toaff R: Induction of labour by pharmacological and physiological doses of intravenous oxytocin. Br J Obstet Gynaecol 85:101, 1978.

151. Seitchik J, Amico J, Robinson AG, et al: Oxytocin augmentation of dysfunctional labor. Am J Obstet Gynecol 150:225, 1984.

152. Simons CL: Prostaglandins and labor: problems and benefits. Contemp Obstet Gynecol 12:91, 1978.

153. Helwig JT, Thorp JM Jr, Bowes WA Jr: Does midline episiotomy increase the risk of third- and fourth-degree lacerations in operative vaginal deliveries? Obstet Gynecol 82:276, 1993.

154. Homsi R, Daikoku NH, Littlejohn J, et al: Episiotomy: risks of dehiscence and rectovaginal fistula. Obstet Gynecol Surv 49:803, 1994.

155. Klein MC, Janssen PA, MacWilliams L, et al: Determinants of vaginal-perineal integrity and pelvic floor functioning in childbirth. Am J Obstet Gynecol 176:403, 1997.

156. Robinson JN, Norwitz ER, Cohen AP, et al: Epidural analgesia and the occurrence of third and fourth degree obstetric laceration in nulliparas. Obstet Gynecol 94:259, 1999.

157. Goodlin RC: On protection of the maternal perineum during birth. Obstet Gynecol 62:393, 1983.

158. Coates PM, Chan KK, Wilkins M, et al: A comparison between midline and mediolateral episiotomies. Br J Obstet Gynaecol 87:408, 1980.

159. Williams MC, Knuppel RA, O'Brien WF, et al: A randomized comparison of assisted vaginal delivery by obstetric forceps and polyethylene vacuum cup. Obstet Gynecol 78:789, 1991.

160. Johanson RB, Rice C, Doyle M, et al: A randomised prospective study comparing the new vacuum extractor policy with forceps delivery. Br J Obstet Gynaecol 100:524, 1993.

161. Bofill JA, Rust OA, Schorr SJ, et al: A randomized prospective trial of the obstetric forceps versus the M-cup vacuum extractor. Am J Obstet Gynecol 175:1325, 1996.

162. Committee on Obstetrics: Maternal and Fetal Medicine: Obstetric forceps, ACOG Committee Opinion No. 59. Washington, DC, American College of Obstetricians and Gynecologists, 1988.

163. Hagadom-Freathy AS, Yeomans ER, Hankins GDV: Validation of the 1988 ACOG forceps classification system. Obstet Gynecol 77:356, 1991.

164. Carmona F, Martinez-Roman S, Manau D, et al: Immediate

maternal and neonatal effects of low-forceps delivery according to the new criteria of the American College of Obstetricians and Gynecologists compared with spontaneous vaginal delivery in term pregnancies. Am J Obstet Gynecol 173:55, 1995.

165. Scanzoni FW: Lehrbuch der Geburtshülfe, 3rd ed. Vienna, Seidel, 1853, p 838.

166. Kjelland C: On the application of forceps to the unrotated head, with description of a new model of forceps. Monatsschr Geburt Gynkol 43:48, 1916.

167. Sjostedt JE: The vacuum extractor and forceps in obstetrics: a clinical study. Acta Obstet Gynecol Stand 46:1, 1967.

168. Malmström T: Vacuum extractor: an obstetrical instrument. Acta Obstet Gynecol Scand 33(Suppl):3, 1954.

169. Kuit JA, Eppinga HG, Wallenberg HCS, et al: A randomized comparison of vacuum extraction delivery with a rigid and a pliable cup. Obstet Gynecol 82:280, 1993.

170. Bofill JA, Rust OA, Schorr SJ, et al: A randomized trial of two vacuum extraction techniques. Obstet Gynecol 89:758, 1997.

171. FDA Public Health Advisory: Need for CAUTION when using vacuum assisted delivery devices. Food and Drug Administration of the United States, May 21, 1998.

172. Committee on Obstetric Practice: Delivery by vacuum extraction, ACOG Committee Opinion No. 208. Washington, DC, American College of Obstetricians and Gynecologists, 1998.

173. Towner D, Castro MA, Eby-Wilkiens E, et al: Effects of mode of delivery in nulliparous women on neonatal intracranial injury. N Engl J Med 341:1709, 1999.

174. Levine MG, Holroyde LT, Woods JR, et al: Birth trauma: incidence and predisposing factors. Obstet Gynecol 63:792, 1984.

175. Curran JS: Birth-associated injury. Clin Perinatol 8:111, 1981.

176. Rhodes P: Prolapse of the umbilical cord. Proc R Soc Med 49:937, 1956.

177. Pathak UN: Presentation and prolapse of the umbilical cord. Am J Obstet Gynecol 101:401, 1968.

178. Savage EW, Schuyler GK, Wynn RM: Prolapse of the umbilical cord. Obstet Gynecol 36:502, 1970.

179. Roberts WE, Martin RW, Roach HH, et al: Are obstetric interventions such as cervical ripening, induction of labor, amnioinfusion, or amniotomy associated with umbilical cord prolapse? Obstet Gynecol 176:1181, 1997.

180. Benedetti TJ, Gabbe SG: Shoulder dystocia: a complication of fetal macrosomia and prolonged second stage of labor with midpelvic delivery. Obstet Gynecol 52:526, 1978.

181. Menticoglou SM, Perlman M, Manning FA: High cervical spinal cord injury in neonates with forceps: report of 15 cases. Obstet Gynecol 86:589, 1995.

182. Xenakis EMJ, Langer O, Conway D, et al: Low-dose versus high-dose oxytocin augmentation of labor: a randomized trial. Am J Obstet Gynecol 173:1874, 1995.

183. O'Driscoll K, Foley M, MacDonald D: Active management of labour as an alternative to cesarean section for dystocia. Obstet Gynecol 33:485, 1984.

184. Turner MJ, Brassil M, Gordon H: Active management of labor associated with a decrease in the cesarean section rate in nulliparas. Obstet Gynecol 71:150, 1988.

185. Akoury HA, Brodie G, Caddick R, et al: Active management of labor and operative delivery in nulliparous women. Am J Obstet Gynecol 158:255, 1988.

186. Boylan P, Frankowski R, Roundtree R, et al: Effect of active management of labor on the incidence of cesarean section for dystocia in nulliparas. Am J Perinatol 8:373, 1991.

187. Lopez-Zeno JA, Peaceman AM, Adashek JA, et al: A controlled trial of a program for the active management of labor. N Engl J Med 326:450, 1992.

188. Frigoletto FD, Lieberman E, Lang JM, et al: A clinical trial of active management of labor. N Engl J Med 333:745, 1995.

189. Thornton JG, Lilford RJ: Active management of labour: current knowledge and research issues. BMJ 309:366, 1994.

190. Rochenschaub A: Technology-free obstetrics at the Semmelweiss clinic. Lancet 335:977, 1990.

191. van Alten D, Eskes M, Treffers PE: Midwifery in the Netherlands. The Wormerveer study: selection, mode of delivery, perinatal mortality and infant morbidity. Br J Obstet Gynaecol 96:656, 1989.

192. Satin AJ, Mayberry MC, Leveno KJ, et al: Chorioamnionitis: a harbinger of dystocia. Obstet Gynecol 79:913, 1992.

193. Seaward PGR, Hannah ME, Myhr TL, et al: International multicenter term PROM study: evaluation of predictors of neonatal infection in infants born to patients with premature rupture of membranes at term. Am J Obstet Gynecol 179:635, 1998.

194. Chua S, Arulkumaran S, Yap C, et al: Premature rupture of membranes in nulliparas at term with unfavorable cervices: a double-blind randomized trial of prostaglandin and placebo. Obstet Gynecol 86:550, 1995.

195. Wing DA, Paul RH: Induction of labor with misoprostol for premature rupture of membranes beyond thirty-six weeks' gestation. Am J Obstet Gynecol 179:94, 1998.

196. Duff P, Huff RW, Gibbs RS: Management of premature rupture of membranes and unfavorable cervix in term pregnancy. Obstet Gynecol 63:697, 1984.

197. Grant JM, Serle E, Mahmood T, et al: Management of prelabour rupture of the membranes in term primigravidae: report of a randomised prospective trial. Br J Obstet Gynaecol 99:557, 1992.

198. Natale R, Milne JK, Campbell MK, et al: Management of premature rupture of membranes at term: randomized trial. Am J Obstet Gynecol 171:936, 1994.

199. Hannah ME, Ohlsson A, Farine D, et al: Induction of labor compared with expectant management for prelabor rupture of the membranes at term. N Engl J Med 334:1005, 1996.

200. Mozurkewich EL, Wolf FM: Premature rupture of membranes at term: a meta-analysis of three management schemes. Obstet Gynecol 89:1035, 1997.

Chapter 14

Intrapartum Fetal Evaluation

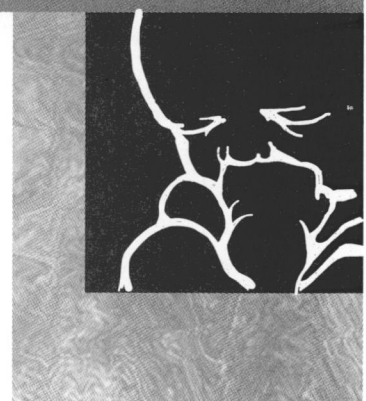

THOMAS J. GARITE

The question being asked by the clinician evaluating the fetus in labor is quite simple: What is the status of fetal oxygenation? If hypoxia is severe enough and lasts long enough, fetal tissue and organ damage will result, which may result in long-term injuries and/or death. Hypoxia severe enough to cause tissue damage virtually always occurs only in the face of a significant metabolic acidosis, and the term "asphyxia" is used in this situation (Fig. 14–1). To clarify the terminology used in these situations, a Glossary is provided.

Although there are other less frequent causes of fetal injury and/or death in labor (e.g., infection, hemorrhage), hypoxia is by far the most common etiology and the one for which medical and surgical interventions have the potential for preventing injury and death. Prior to intensive intrapartum fetal heart rate (FHR) monitoring, relatively uniform intrapartum fetal death rates of 3 to 4 per 1,000 were reported.[1] Thus, on an obstetric service of 200 to 300 monthly deliveries, 1 intrapartum death would occur each month; but now such events are extremely rare in monitored fetuses. Fetal hypoxia that is severe and associated with metabolic acidosis, but not sufficient to result in death, may alternatively cause asphyxial injury to the fetus and newborn. The fetal central nervous system (CNS) is the organ system most vulnerable to long-term injury. However, the fetus destined to have permanent neurologic damage will virtually always have multiorgan dysfunction in the newborn period. Usually, complications such as seizures, respiratory distress, pulmonary hypertension with persistent fetal circulation, renal failure, bowel dysfunction, and pulmonary hemorrhage are seen in the baby who will ultimately have permanent neurologic injury.[2] Babies who recover from these complications and survive may be normal or may develop cerebral palsy. Cerebral palsy is defined as a movement disorder, usually spastic in nature, that is present at birth, nonprogressive and often, but not always, associ-

ated with varying degrees of mental retardation.[3] Seizures are often seen in children with cerebral palsy. However, mental retardation or seizures, in the absence of spasticity, are rarely the result of peripartum asphyxia. It is still unclear whether other neurologic dysfunction in children, such as learning and behavioral disorders, can be the result of perinatal asphyxia. Cerebral palsy will develop in 0.5 percent of all births and is prevalent in about 0.1 percent of all school-age children.[3,4] Prematurity remains the leading cause of cerebral palsy. It is estimated that peripartum events contribute to no more than 25 percent of the overall rate of this disease.[5]

Thus, the goal of intrapartum monitoring is to detect hypoxia in labor and allow the clinician to implement nonoperative interventions such as positioning and oxygen (O_2) administration to correct or ameliorate the oxygen deficiency. If this is unsuccessful, the monitor should help the clinician to determine the severity and duration of the hypoxia and whether there is a metabolic acidosis. And finally, if there is sufficient hypoxia and metabolic acidosis present, the monitor should give adequate warning and time to permit the clinician to deliver the baby expeditiously, whether by operative vaginal means or cesarean section, to prevent damage or death from occurring. Unfortunately, the fetus is quite inaccessible, and until recently we have had crude and limited tools available to determine all of the above information necessary to make correct and timely decisions to accomplish these goals.

HISTORY OF FETAL MONITORING

Because of the inaccessible location of the fetus, evaluating fetal well-being, or more specifically, fetal oxygen

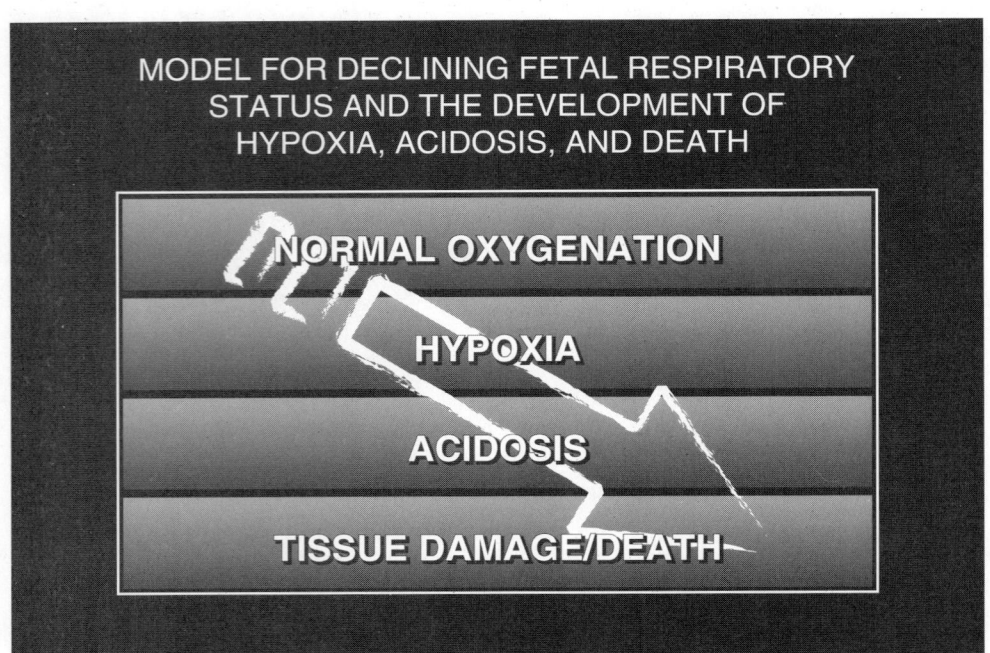

Figure 14–1. The purpose of FHR monitoring is to detect fetal hypoxia and metabolic acidosis. Many fetuses develop hypoxia intermittently but never progress to metabolic acidosis. The ideal is to avoid intervention for hypoxia, but to intervene in the presence of early metabolic acidosis before it can result in tissue damage or fetal death.

status, has been an ongoing and difficult challenge. In the 1600s, Kilian first proposed that the fetal heart rate might be used to diagnose fetal distress and to indicate when the clinician should intervene on behalf of the fetus. The sound of the fetal heart had first been detected by Marsac of France in the 1600s and described in a poem by his colleague, Phillipe LeGaust. This observation went unnoticed until 1818, when Mayor, and subsequently Kergaradec, described the fetal heart sounds by placing an ear on the maternal abdomen. Kergaradec suggested that auscultation of the fetal heart could be used to determine fetal viability and fetal lie. In 1893, VonWinckel described the criteria for fetal distress that were to remain essentially unchanged until the arrival of electronic FHR monitoring. These included tachycardia (FHR >160 bpm), bradycardia (FHR <100 bpm), irregular heart rate, passage of meconium, and gross alteration of fetal movement.[1]

These criteria went unquestioned until 1968, when Benson et al. published the results of the Collaborative Project.[6] These authors reviewed the benefits of auscultation in over 24,000 deliveries and concluded "there was no reliable indicator of fetal distress in terms of fetal heart rate save in extreme degree." Thus, it became apparent that other, more sophisticated means of intrapartum fetal evaluation were required. In 1906, Cremer described the use of the fetal electrocardiogram (ECG) using abdominal and intravaginal electrical leads.[7] Several investigators made attempts using ECG waveforms to detect fetal hypoxia, but ultimately concluded that there was no consistent fetal electrocardiographic changes with fetal distress.[8] The subsequent history of electronic FHR monitoring (EFM) is a story of technological development and empiric observations of

alterations in FHR associated with various causes of fetal hypoxia and acidosis.

In 1958, Edward Hon (the "father of EFM" in the United States) reported on the instantaneous recording of the fetal ECG from the maternal abdomen.[9] He and his colleagues painstakingly measured R-R intervals from a continuous ECG tracing and mathematically converted these to rate, in beats per minute (bpm), and then hand-recorded each interval on graph paper. From these efforts Hon, Caldeyro-Barcia in Uruguay, and Hammacher in Germany began to describe various FHR patterns associated with fetal distress.[10–12] Despite attempts by these and subsequent leaders in the field, universal standards for monitoring and terminology were never really established. For example, Europeans tend to refer to electronic fetal heart rate monitoring (EFM in the United States) as "cardiotocography" (CTG) and run their tracings at a paper speed of 1 cm/min as compared to 3 cm/min in this country. The first commercially available electronic fetal monitor was produced in the late 1960s, and by the mid-1970s, EFM was in use in most labor and delivery units in the United States. Today, the vast majority of all women giving birth in the United States have electronic FHR monitoring during labor.

INSTRUMENTATION FOR EFM

Many technological advances have been made since the first monitors were produced. External FHR monitoring using electrocardiography did not work in labor, and

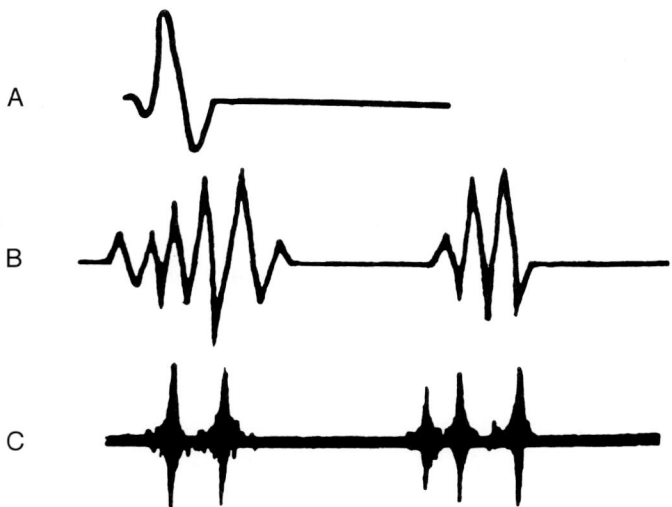

Figure 14–2. These complexes represent the types of signals that the FHR may be required to count. *A,* ECG; *B,* Doppler; *C,* phonocardiogram. Note the complexity of the Doppler signal. To consistently count the same place in the signal complex and avoid artifactually increasing variability, complex signal processing formulas are required.

phonocardiography was subject to fetal and maternal movement and other external noise. Doppler became the dominant modality for external monitoring. Initially, this modality was difficult to use because the complex Doppler signal made it difficult to determine which point within that signal the computer should use

to measure the interval from beat to beat to convert to rate (Fig. 14–2). Logic, or computer processing formulas, were used to get apparently good continuous signals, but this process introduced artifact, and the apparent variability and other aspects of the FHR were often inaccurate. Ultimately, better Doppler devices coupled with autocorrelation formulas for processing the signal have resulted in excellent external FHR signals that can be relied upon clinically. External monitoring is necessary at all times when the membranes are intact and cannot or should not be ruptured (Fig. 14–3). In addition, certain clinical situations make it unwise to puncture the skin with a fetal electrode for fear of vertical transmission of infection to the fetus. Such conditions include maternal infection with human immunodeficiency virus (HIV), hepatitis C, and herpes simplex.

It is often necessary to apply an internal electrode to obtain a high-quality, accurate, continuous FHR tracing. This is especially true in patients who are obese, those with a premature fetus, or when the mother or fetus is moving too much to obtain an adequate signal. The original internal electrode was made from a modified skin clip that required a special instrument to place on the fetal scalp. In the mid-1970s, an easier to insert and less traumatic spiral electrode was introduced (Fig. 14–4). This is applied to the fetal scalp manually without additional instruments and without the requirement for a speculum to visualize the scalp. The electrical

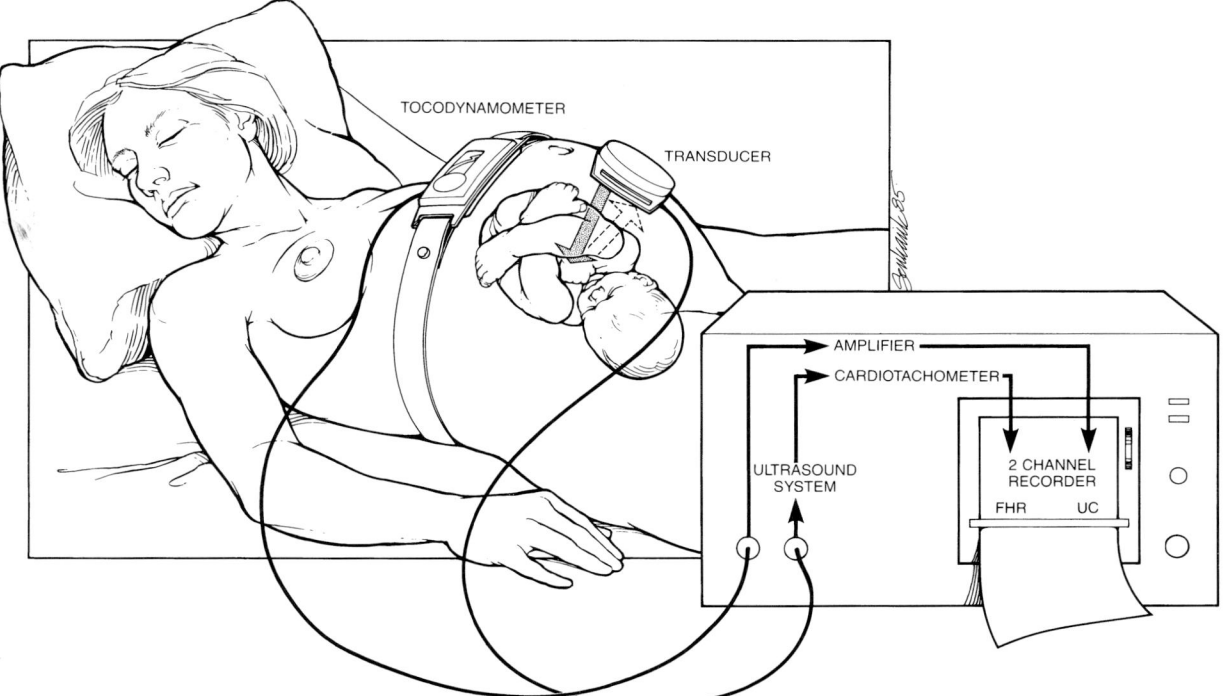

Figure 14–3. Instrumentation for external monitoring. Contractions are detected by the pressure-sensitive tocodynamometer, amplified, and then recorded. Fetal heart rate is monitored using the Doppler ultrasound transducer, which both emits and receives the reflected ultrasound signal that is then counted and recorded.

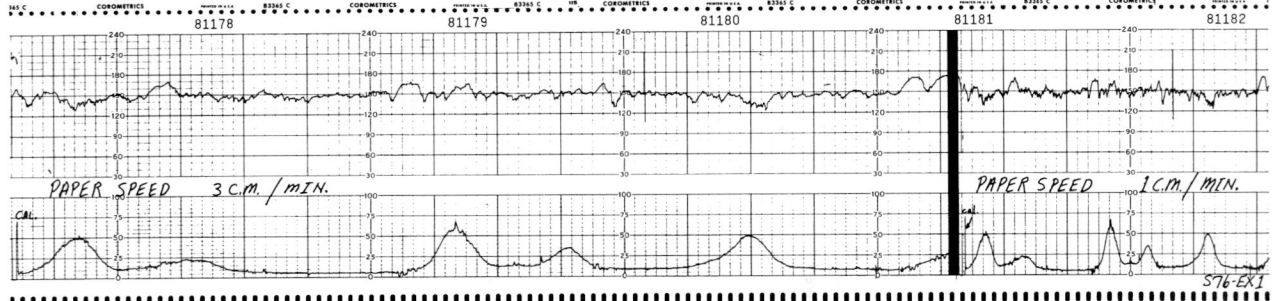

Figure 14–4. Internal fetal heart rate data gathered at the standard recording speed of 3 cm/min for the first portion. The same data are being recorded at a speed of 1 cm/min in the last segment. Normal long-term and short-term variabilities are present. Note that the uterine activity channel has been calibrated so that the intrauterine pressure readings can be measured correctly.

circuit for this electrode includes the spiral electrode for one pole and a small metal bar at the base of the plastic which, bathed in vaginal secretions, completes the circuit through the mother's body. The spiral electrode has remained in use without substantial change since its introduction. The FHR tracing results from the signal processor, which counts every R-R interval of the ECG from the scalp electrode, converts this interval to rate, and displays every interval (in rate as beats per minute) on the top channel of the two-channel fetal monitor recording paper. The signal is amplified by an automatic gain amplifier, which increases the amplitude (gain) until an adequate signal is available to count

(Fig. 14–5). It must be remembered that when the fetus is dead, the amplifier may increase the gain of the small maternal ECG transmitted through the dead fetus, and this may be easily misinterpreted as a fetal bradycardia (Fig. 14–6).

It is clear that the term "electronic fetal monitoring," unlike the European version "cardiotocography," undervalues the lower channel of the fetal monitor tracing, which provides information about the uterine contractions in labor. Contractions can also be monitored externally or internally. The external monitoring device, or tocodynamometer, is basically a ring-style pressure transducer attached to the maternal abdomen via a belt

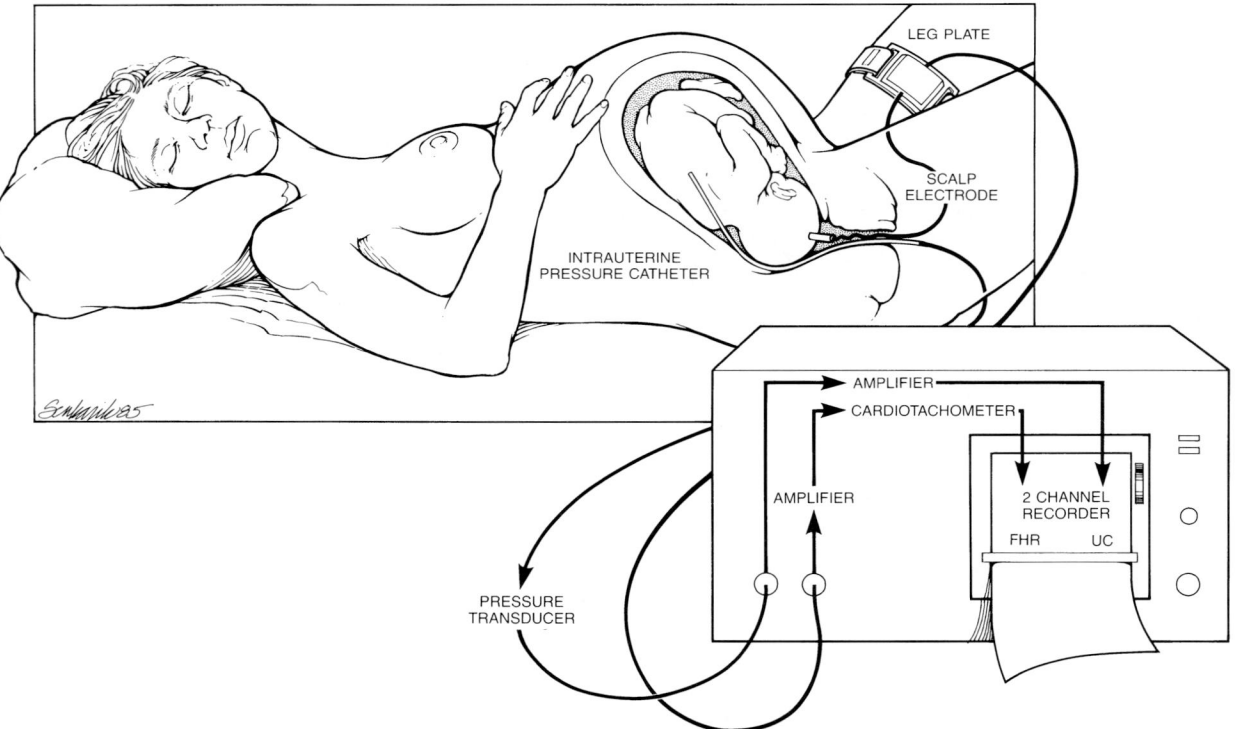

Figure 14–5. Techniques used for direct monitoring of fetal heart rate and uterine contractions. Uterine contractions are assessed with an intrauterine pressure catheter connected to a pressure transducer. This signal is then amplified and recorded. The fetal electrocardiogram is obtained by direct application of the scalp electrode, which is then attached to a leg plate on the mother's thigh. The signal is transmitted to the monitor, where it is amplified, counted by the cardiotachometer, and then recorded.

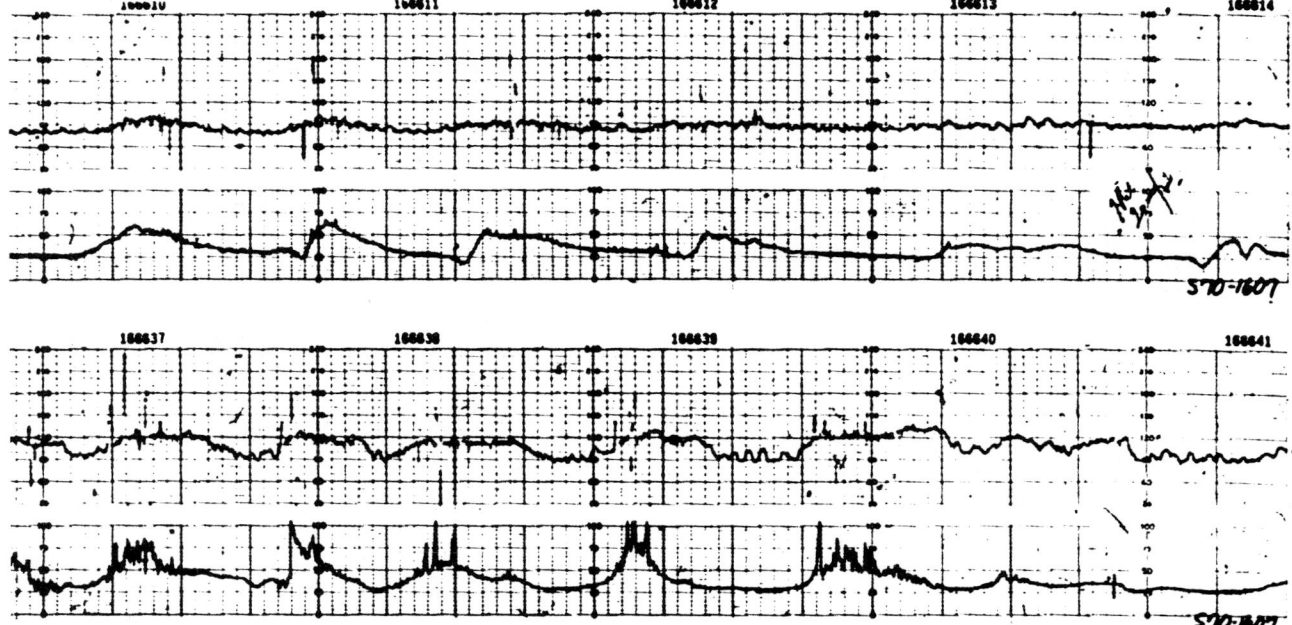

Figure 14–6. This is a tracing from an internal electrode demonstrating an apparent bradycardia with a rate of about 90 bpm. In actuality, this tracing is from a dead fetus, and the automatic gain amplifier increases the amplitude of the maternal ECG signal, allowing the monitor to count and display maternal heart rate.

that maintains tight continuous contact. When the uterus contracts, the change in shape and rigidity depresses the plunger of the sensor, which changes the voltage of the electrical current. The change in voltage is proportional to the strength of the uterine contractions. The tocodynamometer depicts the frequency of the contractions accurately, but the strength of the contractions only relatively, since it cannot measure actual intrauterine pressure. In addition, the apparent duration of the contraction varies with the sensitivity of the monitor, which is negatively affected by variables such as maternal obesity and premature gestational age (Fig. 14–7). The advantage of the external monitor is that it can be used when membranes are intact and it is noninvasive. Its disadvantages, in addition to its inherently limited accuracy, is that it is more uncomfortable for the mother and limits her mobility. Contractions can be more accurately monitored via an intrauterine pressure catheter. The catheters require that the membranes be ruptured and are inserted transcervically beyond and above the fetal presenting part to rest within the uterine cavity. The original pressure catheters were open water-filled systems attached to a pressure transducer adjacent to the fetal monitor. These systems, while accurate, required frequent adjustments and flushing. Newer catheters have closed systems with the strain gauges in the tips or with sensors that relay the signal to a strain gauge at the base of the catheter. While more expensive, they are easier to use and require less nursing attention. Once the catheter is electronically "zeroed" (calibrated), the contractions are accurately recorded in

terms of frequency, duration, and intensity on the lower channel of the two-channel recording paper or television monitor. This channel is conveniently calibrated at 0 to 100 mm Hg on its vertical scale, from which contraction amplitude can be read. These catheters also are often made with a second port through which saline can be infused for amnioinfusion (see below).

The goal of monitoring is to maintain adequate, high-quality, continuous FHR and contraction tracings while maintaining maximum maternal comfort and

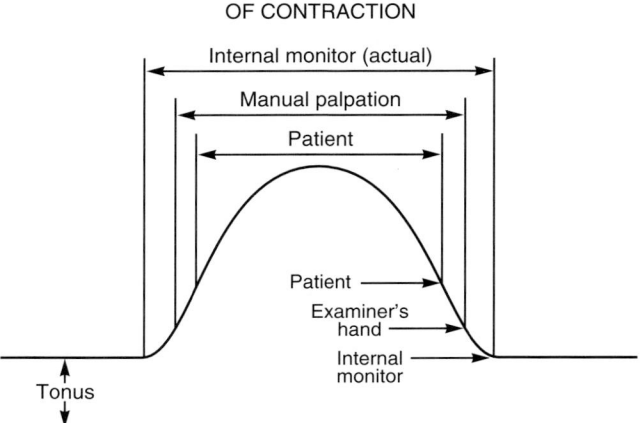

APPARENT DURATION
OF CONTRACTION

Figure 14–7. The sensitivity of the device used to monitor a uterine contraction can affect not only the apparent strength of the contraction but also the apparent duration of the contraction.

avoiding the risk of trauma and/or infection to the fetus and mother. External devices minimize risk but often give less accurate information and are more uncomfortable for the mother. In general, when the FHR is reassuring and there is an adequate tracing and when the progress of labor is adequate, the external devices are fine. When better quality FHR monitoring is required or it becomes important to accurately assess uterine contraction duration and intensity, then internal device(s) may be necessary.

THE PHYSIOLOGIC BASIS OF FHR MONITORING

The basis of FHR monitoring is, in a real sense, fetal brain monitoring. The fetal brain is constantly responding to stimuli, both peripheral and central, with signals to the fetal heart that alter the heart rate on a moment-to-moment basis. Such stimuli to which the brain responds include chemoreceptors, baroreceptors, and direct effects of metabolic changes within the brain itself. The benefit for the brain to modulate the FHR is derived from its goal of maintaining optimal perfusion to the brain without compromising blood flow to other organs any more than is necessary. It should be intuitively obvious, therefore, that the use of FHR to monitor fetal oxygenation is inherently crude and nonspecific, as many stimuli other than oxygen will either cause the brain to alter the fetal heart rate or may have a direct effect on the fetal heart itself. This really explains the most important basic premise of EFM: when the FHR is normal in appearance, one can be assured with high reliability that the fetus is well oxygenated, but when the FHR is not entirely normal, it may be the result of hypoxia or of other variables that may also affect fetal heart rate. In the past when the FHR became abnormal and the clinician decided intervention was necessary because of concern over fetal hypoxia, the term "fetal distress" was used. More often than not, however, such intervention results in the delivery of a well-oxygenated, nonacidotic, vigorous newborn. Thus, more recently, on the basis of recommendations of the American College of Obstetricians and Gynecologists (ACOG), the terminology was changed to reflect the inherent inaccuracy of the abnormal FHR. The term "fetal distress" has been abandoned in favor of the more intellectually honest term, "nonreassuring fetal status" (NRFS).[13]

Fetal oxygenation is determined by many factors. The placenta functions as the fetal lung. Oxygen transfer across the placenta, as in the lung or any membrane, is proportional to the difference between partial pressures of oxygen between the mother and the fetus,

the blood flow to the placenta, a coefficient of diffusion for the gas, and the surface area of the placenta. Transfer is inversely proportional to the thickness of the membrane (placenta). Thus, under normal circumstances during labor, the only variable that alters fetal oxygenation is the temporary interruption in blood flow to the placenta that occurs as a result of the compression of the spiral arteries by the wall of the uterus at the peak of the contraction. The duration that the spiral arteries will be compressed will thus depend on the duration and strength of the contraction (Fig. 14–8). Under normal circumstances, the fetus tolerates these periods of stasis well without a significant change in its oxygen content. Contractions that are unusually long or unusually strong may, however, result in transient periods of fetal hypoxemia.

Other variables that have the potential for altering fetal oxygenation most commonly include those that affect uterine perfusion. A laboring woman in the supine position can develop supine hypotension as a result of vena caval compression from the uterus. Maternal hypotension with redistribution of blood flow away from the placenta occurs not infrequently with regional anesthesia. Maternal hemorrhage, such as in placenta previa or abruptio placentae, may have similar effects. There are several forms of microvascular disease that can impair fetal oxygenation from poor perfusion within the uteroplacental vascular bed. Examples include hypertension, preeclampsia/eclampsia, collagen vascular disease, diabetic vasculopathy, and postmaturity. Abruptio placentae may compromise fetal oxygenation in several ways. These include maternal hypotension, as previously mentioned; a decrease in the surface area of the placenta; and uterine hyperactivity.

While the placenta functions as the fetal lung, the umbilical cord functions as its trachea, leading oxygen to the baby and carbon dioxide (CO_2) away. Alteration in umbilical cord blood flow is a very common occurrence during labor, either from direct compression or from stretch. Direct compression may occur when the cord becomes impinged between any part of the fetal body and the uterine wall, either with contractions or with fetal movement. This is especially more common when there is oligohydramnios, as there is less amniotic fluid to provide a cushion for the cord.[14] Alternatively, cord stretch may occur as the fetus descends into the pelvis. Typically, this is seen just prior to complete dilation, when descent of the vertex normally occurs. There are three potent stimuli that produce spasm of the umbilical vessels and are intended to allow cessation of fetal umbilical cord blood flow following birth. These include a lower ambient temperature, a higher oxygen tension as the baby begins breathing, and the stretch of the umbilical cord as the baby falls from the birth canal.[15] Thus, it should not be surprising that transient cessation of cord blood flow will occur with

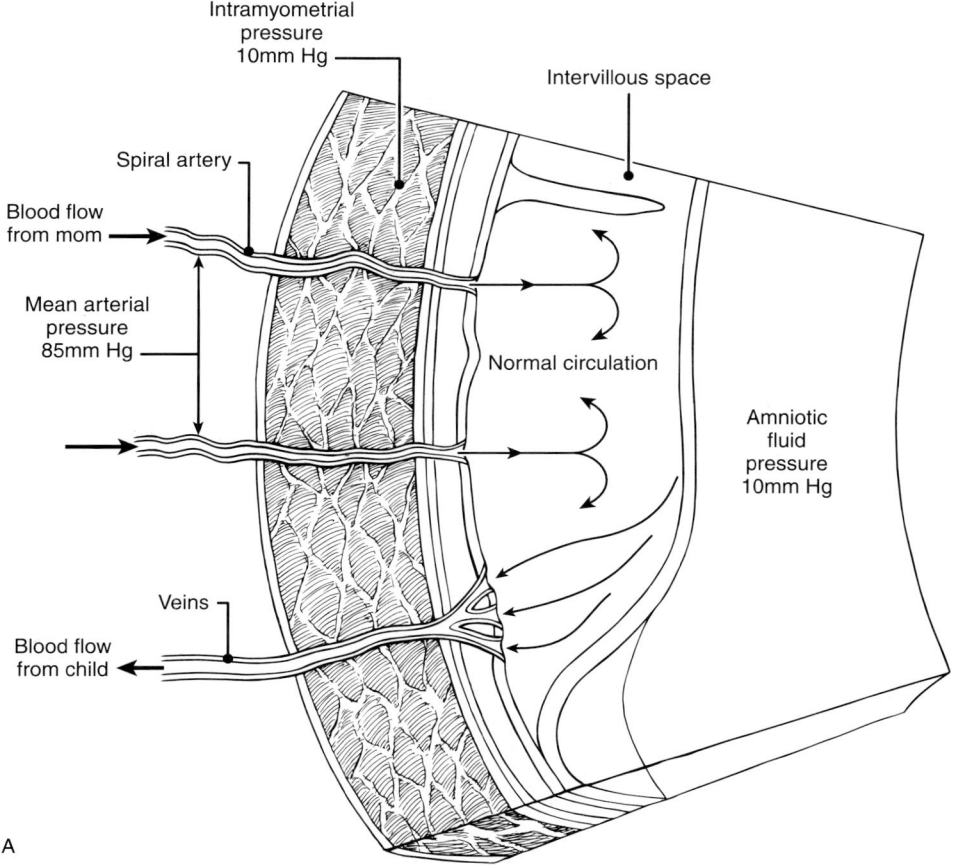

Intramyometrial
pressure
10mm Hg

Intervillous space

Spiral artery

Blood flow
from mom

Mean arterial
pressure
85mm Hg

Normal circulation

Amniotic
fluid
pressure
10mm Hg

Veins

Blood flow
from child

A

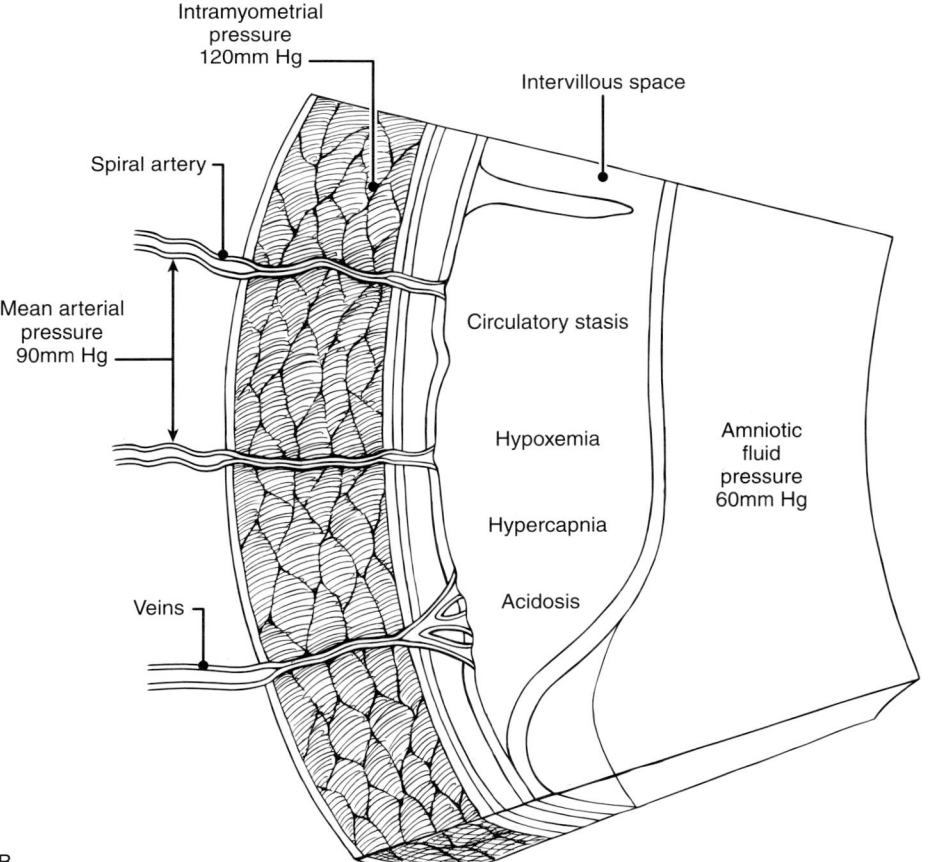

Intramyometrial
pressure
120mm Hg

Intervillous space

Spiral artery

Mean arterial
pressure
90mm Hg

Circulatory stasis

Hypoxemia

Amniotic
fluid
pressure
60mm Hg

Hypercapnia

Veins

Acidosis

Figures 14–8. In the resting state between contractions *A*, the intraluminal pressure within the spiral arteries exceeds the intramyometrial pressure. Thus uteroplacental blood flow is sustained. However, at the peak of a uterine contraction *B*, the myometrial pressure can exceed the arterial pressure and uterine blood flow will be transiently interrupted, temporarily halting oxygen delivery to the placenta.

B

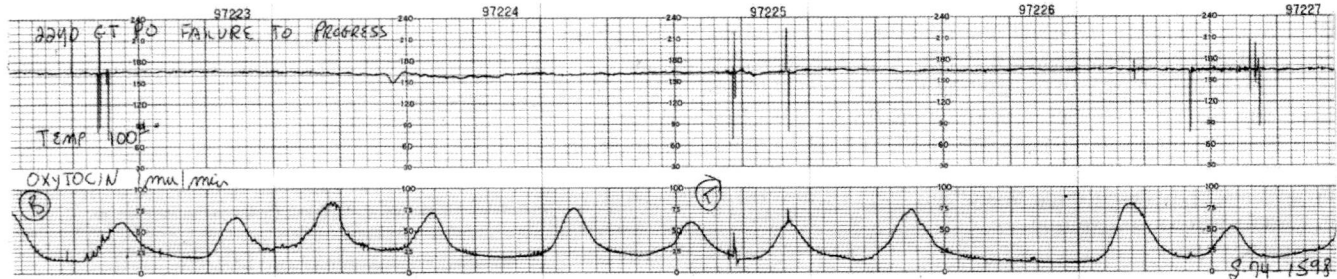

Figure 14–9. A tachycardia with a fetal heart rate of 170 bpm seen in association with a maternal fever of 100.4°F.

stretching of the cord during descent if the cord is looped around the baby's neck and descent of the vertex occurs.

It becomes important, therefore, to understand the physiologic mechanisms that control the fetal heart rate. This is so not only because the FHR may be used to determine the severity of the hypoxia and whether a metabolic acidosis is ensuing, but also because the FHR pattern can elucidate the mechanism of the reduction in fetal oxygenation. Thus, by knowing the cause of any hypoxia, the treatment, when possible, can be more specifically directed at the cause. Finally, an understanding of the mechanism and progression of the FHR pattern can often also provide an opportunity to predict how fetal oxygenation will progress over time.

The FHR has many characteristics that we are able to use to accomplish this interpretation. These include the *baseline rate;* the *variability* of the FHR from beat to beat; transient alterations below the baseline, termed *decelerations;* and transient alterations above the baseline, termed *accelerations.* Rate and variability are generally included as *characteristics of the baseline* FHR, and decelerations and accelerations as *periodic changes.* *

Tachycardia

The baseline FHR is typically between 120 and 160 bpm. In very early gestation (15 to 20 weeks), the FHR is significantly higher than in the term fetus. The decline in fetal heart rate represents a maturation of fetal vagal tone with progressing gestation.[18] If atropine or other vagolytic drugs are administered, the FHR will regress to the higher baseline of 160 bpm. Thus, the baseline heart rate is largely a function of vagal activity. Many factors have the potential to alter the fetal baseline. Rates above 160 bpm are called *tachycardia.* Tachycardia may have great clinical significance. The

two most common causes of tachycardia are maternal fever and drugs that directly raise the fetal heart rate. Maternal fever raises the core temperature of the fetus, which is always about 1°F higher than the maternal temperature. With maternal fever, virtually all fetuses have tachycardia (Fig. 14–9). The FHR rises approximately 10 bpm for each 1°F increase in maternal temperature. Since at term with chorioamnionitis only 1 to 2 percent of fetuses are septic, the tachycardia is unlikely to indicate fetal sepsis, but rather is probably caused by an increase in fetal metabolic rate associated with the elevated temperature. Drugs that elevate the fetal heart rate fall into one of two categories: vagolytic and β-sympathomimetic. Commonly used drugs that are vagolytic include scopalomine, atropine and phenothiazines, and hydroxyzine. These drugs, however, rarely raise the FHR above 160 bpm. β-Sympathomimetics include terbutaline and ritodrine, used for preterm labor, and terbutaline and epinephrine, used for bronchospasm. Other less common causes of fetal tachycardia include fetal hyperthyroidism, fetal anemia, fetal heart failure, and fetal tachyarrhythmias. As fetal hypoxia becomes progressively worse and persists over time, fetal tachycardia often develops. However, when contractions are present, tachycardia is not the first physiologic response to hypoxia and, in the absence of decelerations, in the laboring patient, is rarely if ever caused by hypoxia.[19]

Bradycardia

An FHR less than 120 bpm is termed a *bradycardia.* One must distinguish between a baseline FHR less than 120 bpm and a deceleration from a previous normal baseline. Not only is a deceleration that is prolonged difficult to distinguish from a baseline change, but there is also some disagreement over terminology. This is an important issue, since a baseline bradycardia is usually innocuous (Fig. 14–10), whereas a prolonged deceleration to less than 120 bpm lasting more than 60 to 90 seconds may often indicate significant fetal hypoxia (Fig. 14–11). True fetal bradycardias are due to several possible causes. In the range of 90 to 120 bpm, a

---

*The terminology used in this chapter is fairly standard and is consistent with the most recent ACOG Technical Bulletin (Number 207–July, 1995)[16]; however, a recent publication from the National Institute of Child Health and Human Development Research Planning Workshop has some notable differences, and these are discussed.[17]

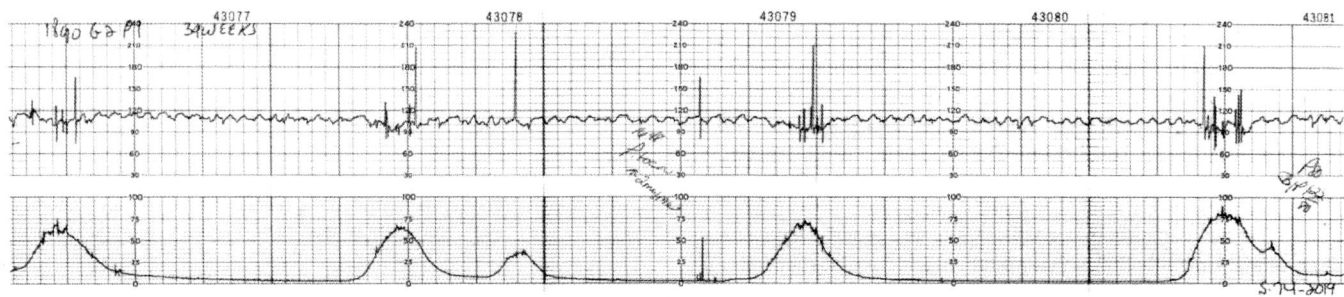

Figure 14–10. A bradycradia with a fetal heart rate of 110 bpm. This patient is in premature labor at 34 weeks' gestation and is being treated with magnesium sulfate. The fetal bradycardia is probably because of maternal hypothermia, which can be seen with vasodilation caused by the magnesium sulfate.

bradycardia may often be a normal variant, and these fetuses are usually bradycardic after birth, but are otherwise well oxygenated and normal. As with tachycardia and fever, maternal hypothermia may cause fetal bradycardia. This is commonly seen with patients on magnesium sulfate ($MgSO_4$) who are vasodilated and has also been described with maternal hypoglycemia and hypothermia.[20,21] A number of drugs may also result in fetal bradycardia. A fetal baseline heart rate in the range of 80 bpm or less, especially with reduced variability, may be caused by a complete heart block. Complete heart block may be caused by antibodies associated with maternal lupus erythematosus, may be seen with congenital cardiac anomalies, or is idiopathic.[22] Whereas a heart block is not associated with hypoxia, it makes the FHR essentially useless in monitoring fetal oxygenation, as the fetal brain is no longer communicating with the ventricle of the heart that is being monitored. Finally, when a patient is admitted with a baseline bradycardia, one should also consider the possibility of maternal heart rate being recorded with a dead fetus (whether internal or external monitor) (Fig. 14–6). Real-time ultrasound is used to verify that the bradycardia is fetal in origin.

Variability

The fetal cardiotachometer is unique among adult monitors in that it records the interval-to-interval difference in rate for every heart beat. Thus, differences in heart rate from beat to beat are recorded as "variability" reflected visually as a line that fluctuates above and below the baseline. This variability is a reflection of neuromodulation of the FHR by an intact and active CNS and also reflects normal cardiac responsiveness. Generally, the variability of the FHR is described as having two components: *short-term* and *long-term variability*. Short-term variability is the beat-to-beat irregularity in the FHR and is caused by the difference in rates between successive beats of the FHR. It is caused by the push–pull effect of sympathetic and parasympathetic nerve input, but the vagus nerve has the dominant role in affecting variability. Long-term variability is the waviness of the FHR tracing, and is generally seen in three to five cycles per minute. Previous texts spent considerable effort in distinguishing between the significance of short- and long-term variability, but in general they are reduced or increased together, and there is no clear evidence that distinguishing between the two is helpful clinically. The National Institute of Child Health and Human Development (NICHD) Research Planning Workshop also concluded that no distinction should be made between short- and long-term variability.[17]

This characteristic of the fetal baseline can be one of the most useful single parameters in determining the severity of fetal hypoxia if understood correctly. The simplest way to describe the causes of alterations, espe-

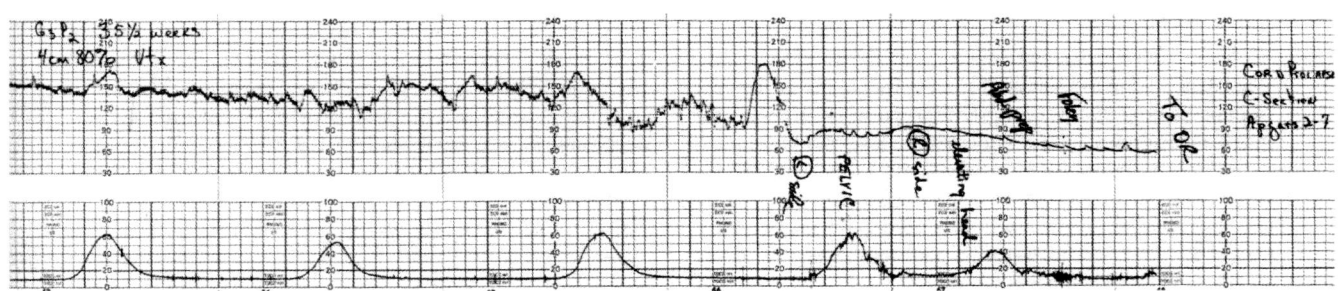

Figure 14–11. The prolonged deceleration to 60 bpm in this case due to umbilical cord prolapse should be distinguished from a fetal "bradycardia", which is defined as the baseline heart rate.

cially reductions, in FHR variability is to say that this parameter reflects the activity of the fetal brain. When the fetus is alert and active, the FHR variability is normal or increased. When the fetus is obtunded, due to whatever cause, the variability is reduced. Since severe hypoxia, especially when it reaches the level of metabolic acidosis, will always depress the CNS, normal variability reliably indicates the absence of severe hypoxia and acidosis (Fig. 14–12A). Unfortunately, the converse is not true, as there are many things that cause the CNS to be depressed (see box, Potential Causes of Decreased Variability of the FHR); thus, reduced variability is a very nonspecific finding and must

be interpreted in the context of other indicators of hypoxia, and other causes of reduced variability must be considered (Fig. 14–12B). In general, anything that is associated with depressed or reduced brain function will diminish variability. These include fetal sleep cycles; drugs, especially CNS depressants; fetal anomalies, especially of the CNS; and previous insults that have damaged the fetal brain. FHR variability is also affected by gestational age, and very immature fetuses of less than 26 weeks' gestation often have reduced variability from an immature CNS, although this varies from fetus to fetus. In addition, as heart rate increases with fetal tachycardia, variability is often reduced from the

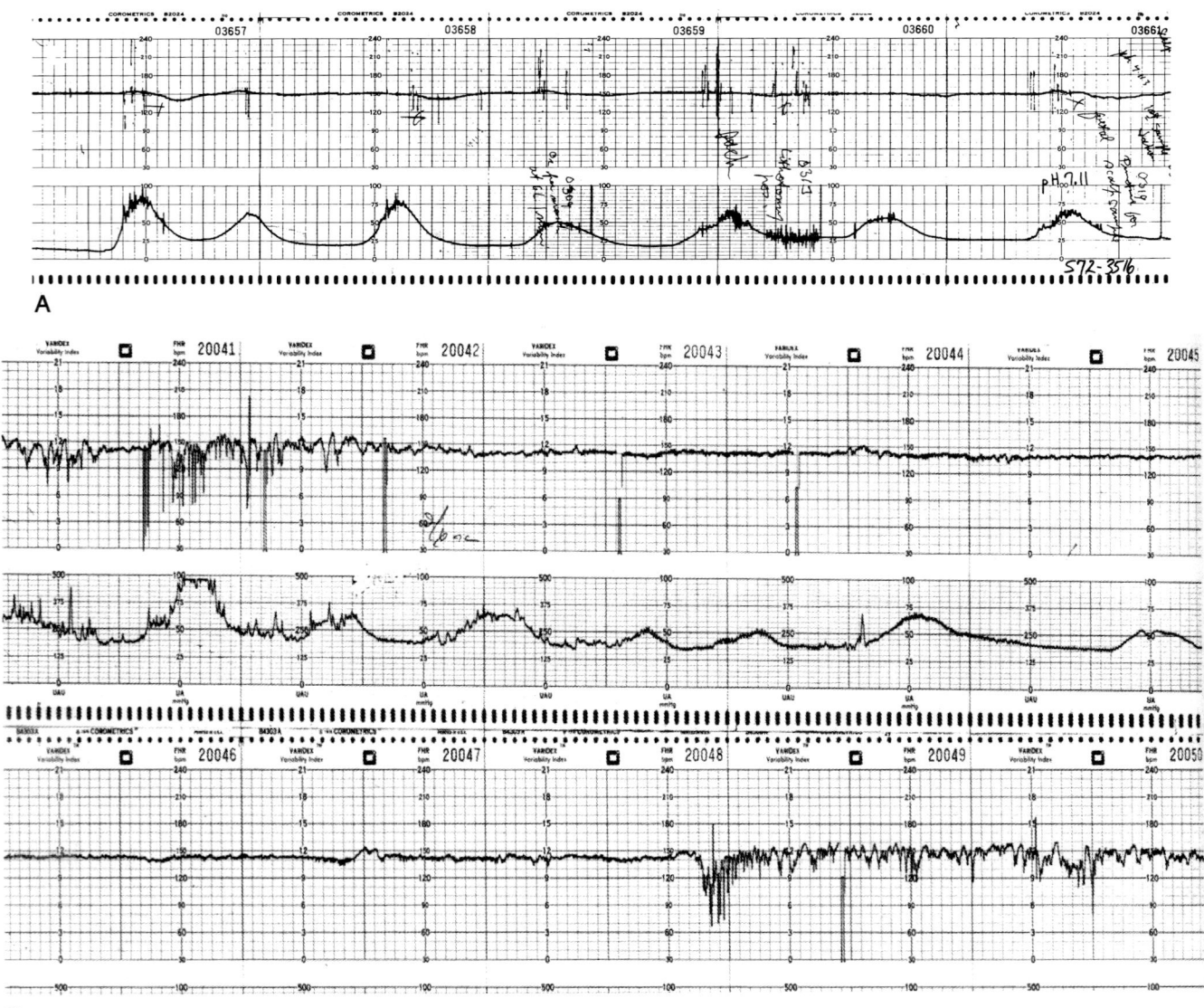

Figure 14–12. *A,* The markedly decreased variability seen in this case is in association with persistent late decelerations. A scalp pH of 7.11 confirms that the loss of variability is because of CNS depression caused by acidosis. *B,* The abrupt decrease in variability seen here, in contrast to *A,* is not seen in association with any decelerations that might suggest hypoxia. Thus, the decreased variability must be because of another reason, and in this case, given the equally abrupt return to normal variability in *B,* is probably caused by a fetal sleep cycle.

Potential Causes of Decreased Variability of the FHR

Depression due to hypoxia and acidosis
Fetal anomalies, especially of the CNS
Fetal sepsis
Tumors of the CNS
Fetal heart block
Tachycardia
Extreme prematurity
Previous neurologic insult
Fetal sleep cycles
Drugs/medications
    Narcotics
    Barbiturates
    Tranquilizers
    Phenothiazines
    Parasympatholytics
    General anesthetics

rate alone, as sympathetic dominance overrides the natural influence of the vagus. Increased FHR variability, original referred to as a "saltatory" FHR pattern, in nonlaboring animals has been shown to be associated with very early or minimal hypoxia.[23] This is a rare pattern and difficult to interpret. In labor, late, variable, or prolonged decelerations will virtually always be present with early hypoxia, and increased variability is not consistent with an acidotic fetus; so this finding can be interpreted in context with the entire FHR pattern.

Another problem with variability besides its nonspecificity is that the interpretation of variability is quite subjective. Variability is usually described quantitatively, as normal, increased, reduced, or absent. The NICHD Research Planning Workshop suggested that FHR variability be defined as follows:

Absent: amplitude undetectable
Minimal: amplitude > undetectable and ≤ 5 bpm
Moderate: amplitude 6 to 25 bpm

Marked: > 25 bpm.[17]

Experts given tracings to interpret often disagree on the quantification of variability even using just these four categories. Trying to categorize variability any further is fraught with even more potential for disagreement and does not appear to have predictive value.

PERIODIC CHANGES

Variability, tachycardia, and bradycardia are characteristic alterations of the baseline heart rate. Periodic changes of the FHR include decelerations and accelerations. These are transient changes in the fetal heart rate of relatively brief duration with return to the original baseline FHR. In labor, these usually occur in response to uterine contractions, but may also occur with fetal movement.

Decelerations

There are four principal types of decelerations: *early, late, variable,* and *prolonged.* These are named for their timing, relationship to contractions, duration, and shape, but are important distinctions more because they describe the cause of the decelerations.

Early Decelerations

Early decelerations are shallow, symmetric, uniform decelerations with onset and return that are gradual, resulting in a U-shaped deceleration (Fig. 14–13). They begin early in the contraction, have their nadir coincident with the peak of the contraction, and return to the baseline by the time the contraction is over. Early decelerations are not associated with accelerations that precede or follow the deceleration. These decelerations rarely descend more than 30 to 40 bpm below the baseline rate. They are thought to be caused by compression of the fetal head by the uterine cervix as it over-

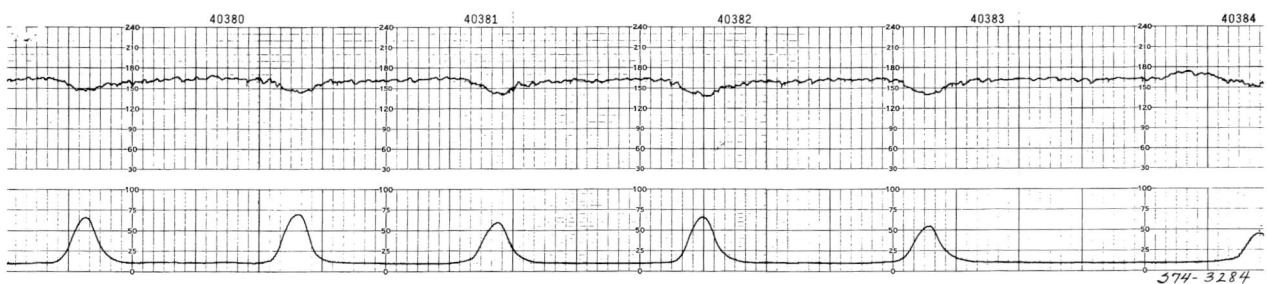

Figure 14–13. Early decelerations.

rides the anterior fontanel of the cranium.[24] This results in altered cerebral blood flow, precipitating a vagal reflex with the resultant slowing of the FHR. More nonspecific head compression can result in decelerations that are indistinguishable from variable decelerations. Because of the similar cause, these latter decelerations have often been called early decelerations, but are by definition not so. Because the cervix creates the pressure, these decelerations are usually seen between 4 and 6 cm of dilation (E.H. Hon, personal communication). They do not indicate fetal hypoxia and are only significant in that they may be easily confused with late decelerations because of their similar shape and depth. They are the most infrequent of decelerations, occurring in about 5 to 10 percent of all fetuses in labor.

Late Decelerations

Late decelerations are similar in appearance to early decelerations. They too are of gradual onset and return, U-shaped, and generally descend below the baseline no more than 30 to 40 bpm, although there are exceptions. However, in contrast to early decelerations, late decelerations are delayed in timing relative to the contraction. They begin usually about 30 seconds after the onset of the contraction or even at or after its peak. Their nadir is after the peak of the contraction. FHR variability may be unchanged or even increased during the decelerations. These decelerations are not associated with accelerations immediately preceding or following their onset and return (Fig. 14–14).

The physiology of late decelerations is quite complex, but an understanding of the physiology pays dividends in terms of interpreting and managing these important FHR changes. Late decelerations are generally said to be caused by "uteroplacental insufficiency." This implies that uteroplacental perfusion is temporarily interrupted during the peak of strong contractions. The fetus that normally will not become hypoxic with this temporary halt in blood flow may do so if there is insufficient perfusion and/or oxygen exchange at other times. Whereas this may be a correct idealized description, in reality any compromise of delivery, exchange, or uptake in fetal oxygen, other than by umbilical cord compression, can result in a late deceleration if the insult is sufficient. Physiologically, oxygen sensors within the fetal brain detect a relative drop in fetal oxygen tension in association with the uterine contraction. This change initially results in an increase in sympathetic neuronal response, causing an elevation in fetal blood pressure which, when detected by baroreceptors, produces a protective slowing in the FHR in response to the increase in peripheral vascular resistance. This has been referred to as the "reflex" type of late deceleration. This complex double reflex is probably the reason the deceleration is delayed.[25] During this type of reflex, the depth of the deceleration is proportional to the severity of the hypoxia and the deceleration moves closer to the contraction as the hypoxia becomes more severe. However, there is also a second type of late deceleration, caused by "myocardial depression." As the hypoxia continues and becomes more severe, late decelerations are no longer vagally mediated and are seen even with interruption of the vagus nerve; thus, they are directly myocardial in origin. These decelerations are *not* proportional in their depth to the severity of the hypoxia, and actually may become more shallow as the hypoxia becomes quite severe. Because of this latter type of deceleration, it is generally agreed that the depth of the late deceleration cannot be used to judge the severity of the hypoxia. Because of the mechanisms causing these changes, *late decelerations always indicate fetal hypoxia.* Only the severity of the hypoxia and the overall duration of the late decelerations will determine whether a metabolic acidosis will occur, and this is highly unpredictable. One reason this may be so is found in recent data suggesting that the oxygen threshold that triggers the brain to slow the fetal heart in this characteristic way may be more related to the relative

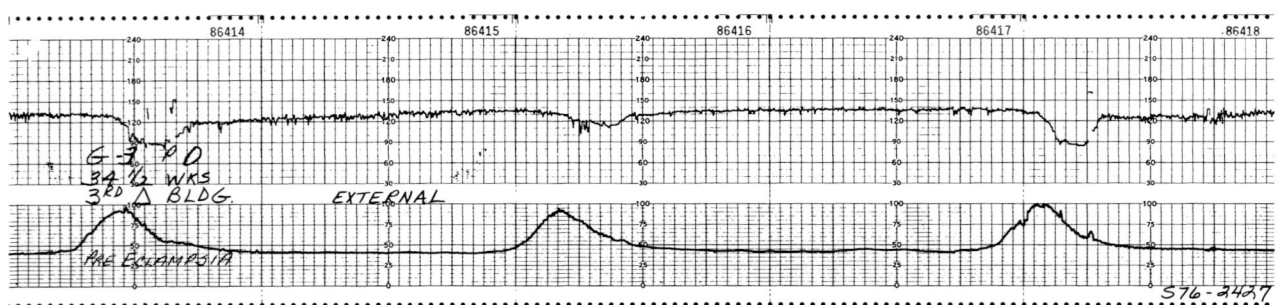

Figure 14–14. A case complicated by third-trimester bleeding in which the external heart rate and uterine activity data are collected. Note the presence of persistent late decelerations with only three contractions in 20 minutes as well as the apparent loss of variability of the fetal heart rate. The rise in baseline tone of the uterine activity channel cannot be evaluated with the external system.

drop from baseline oxygenation rather than an absolute number.[26] Thus, the fetus accustomed to higher than average oxygen saturation may have a drop in oxygen at or only slightly below the normal range; a level deep enough to signal a late deceleration, but not low enough to require anaerobic metabolism. Another important point in understanding the results of hypoxia associated with late decelerations is that the placenta's capacity for exchanging oxygen is substantially less than its capacity for exchanging carbon dioxide. In situations where there are persistent late decelerations and the fetus becomes sufficiently hypoxic to develop a metabolic acidosis, there may be no retention of carbon dioxide. This is quite analogous to the adult with lung but no airway disease where hypoxia is often seen without difficulty in eliminating CO_2. Thus, the metabolic acidosis is usually not mixed with a respiratory acidosis. The only common exception to this is with abruptio placentae, where CO_2 retention is seen with late decelerations.[27]

Causes of late decelerations include any factor that can alter delivery, exchange, or uptake of oxygen at the fetal–maternal interface within the placenta. Most commonly, late decelerations are observed in patients without inherent pathology. Excessive uterine contractions, usually seen with oxytocin, are the single most common cause of late decelerations. In these situations, the duration of interruption of uterine blood flow is prolonged and the hypoxia is more than the normal fetus can endure, and late decelerations are expressed. Conduction anesthesia (spinal or epidural) can cause either systemic or local hypoperfusion/hypotension, and thus the level of contractions required to interrupt uterine blood flow is lower, and again the duration of interruption of uterine blood flow is prolonged (Fig. 14–15). The most common pathologic conditions of the placenta associated with late decelerations are those characterized by either microvascular disease in the pla-

centa or local vasospasm compromising blood flow and thus exchange. Common causes include postmaturity, maternal hypertension (chronic hypertension or preeclampsia), collagen vascular diseases, and diabetes mellitus in its more advanced stages. Besides altering perfusion, abruptio placentae is an example of altered placental exchange caused by a combination of reduced placental surface area and increased contractions that typically result in late decelerations when the separation is sufficient to cause fetal hypoxia. Severe maternal anemia or maternal hypoxemia may compromise oxygen delivery and result in late decelerations. Conversely, chronic fetal anemia may diminish fetal oxygen uptake and be associated with late decelerations.

Variable Decelerations

The most common type of decelerations seen in the laboring patient are variable decelerations. Variable decelerations are, in general, synonymous with umbilical cord compression, and anything that results in the interruption of blood flow within the umbilical cord will result in a variable deceleration. The variable deceleration is the most difficult pattern to describe verbally, but the easiest to recognize visually. First and foremost, the term "variable" is by far the best single word to describe this type of deceleration. They are variable in all ways: size, shape, depth, duration, and timing relative to the contraction. The onset is usually abrupt and sharp. The return is similarly abrupt in most situations. The depth and duration are proportional to the severity and duration of interruption of cord blood flow. Variable decelerations are usually seen with accelerations immediately preceding the onset of the deceleration and immediately following the return to baseline. The NICHD Research Planning Workshop proposed that the duration of a variable deceleration should be limited to 2 minutes, and that beyond 2 minutes, it should

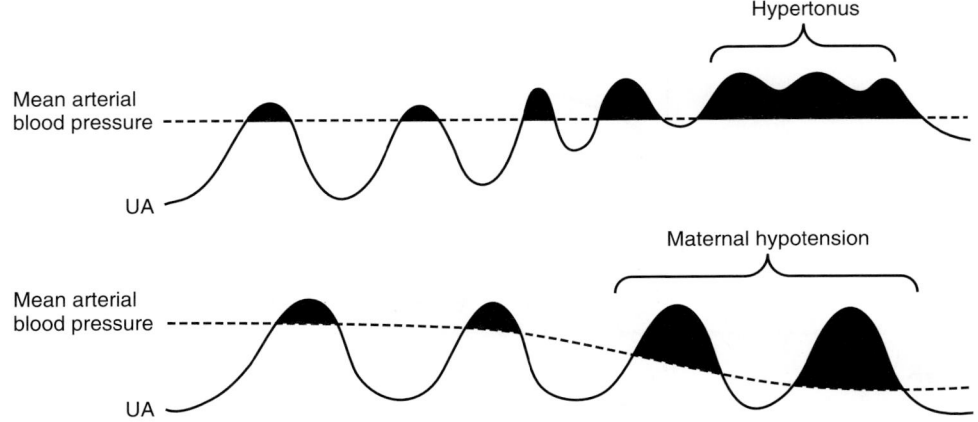

EFFECTS OF HYPERTONUS AND MATERNAL HYPOTENSION

Hypertonus

Mean arterial blood pressure

UA

Maternal hypotension

Mean arterial blood pressure

UA

Figure 14–15. The two most common causes of late decelerations in labor are excessive uterine contractions (usually caused by oxytocin) and maternal hypotension. Both result in decrease in uteroplacental perfusion, hypertonus by interrupting the transmyometrial perfusion for a prolonged period, and hypotension by dropping the perfusion pressure, thus increasing the amount of time perfusion is interrupted even with a normal contraction. UA, uterine artery.

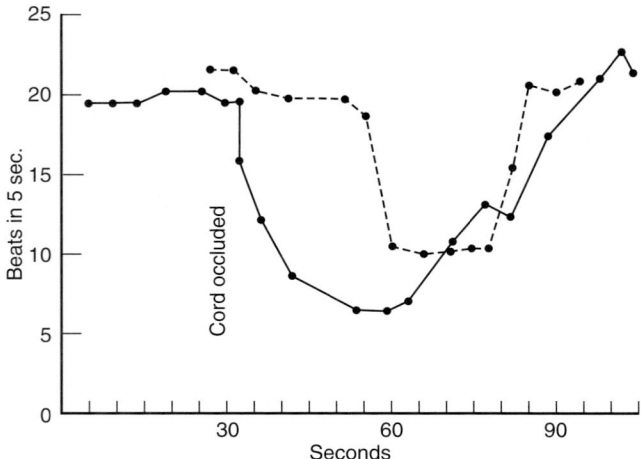

Figure 14–16. This is the original description of a variable deceleration in a fetal goat by Barcroft. The *solid line A* represents the fetal heart rate with temporary umbilical cord occlusion and the *dotted line B* is the fetal heart rate with temporary cord occlusion after the vagal nerve has been severed.

be called a prolonged deceleration.[17] However, most definitions in the past have not put a limit on duration but rely more on the appearance of the deceleration. More than 50 years ago, Barcroft first described the variable deceleration when he ligated the umbilical cord of a fetal goat (Fig. 14–16).[28] In 1975, Lee externalized the human umbilical cord at cesarean section prior to delivery and demonstrated that the reflex involved in the complex pattern of the variable deceleration is one that is caused primarily by changes in systemic blood pressure in the fetus and is mediated through baroreceptors (Fig. 14–17).[29] When the umbilical cord is gradually compressed, the thinner walled umbilical vein collapses first and blood flow returning to the fetus is interrupted. This results in decreased cardiac return, fetal hypotension, and a baroreceptor reflex that leads the brain to accelerate the heart rate in order to maintain cardiac output. This increase in heart rate is the acceleration that precedes the variable deceleration. With continuing compression, the umbilical artery is compressed, and the fetus detects an increase in systemic vascular resistance as the previously low-resistance placental bed, to which 50 percent of fetal cardiac output normally flows, is occluded. The baroreceptors detect the increase in resistance and the heart slows as a protective mechanism. As the cord vessels gradually open, the arteries open first and the heart rate returns to baseline; but if the flow in the vein is still blocked, an acceleration of the same mechanism of the one that preceded the deceleration occurs. While this model is idealized, one might surmise that the orderly occlusion of vein, vein and artery, vein does not always occur. This is probably the reason that with variable decelerations any combination of deceleration with acceleration preceding, preceding and following, following only, neither, or even acceleration alone may be seen with cord compression as in Figure 14–18.

In reality, although we refer to umbilical cord compression as the single mechanism for interruption of cord blood flow, there are probably several different mechanisms that may have the same end result. Compression may be the mechanism that occurs when the cord is impinged between a fetal body part and the uterine wall during contractions or with fetal movement. As previously mentioned, cord stretch may be the

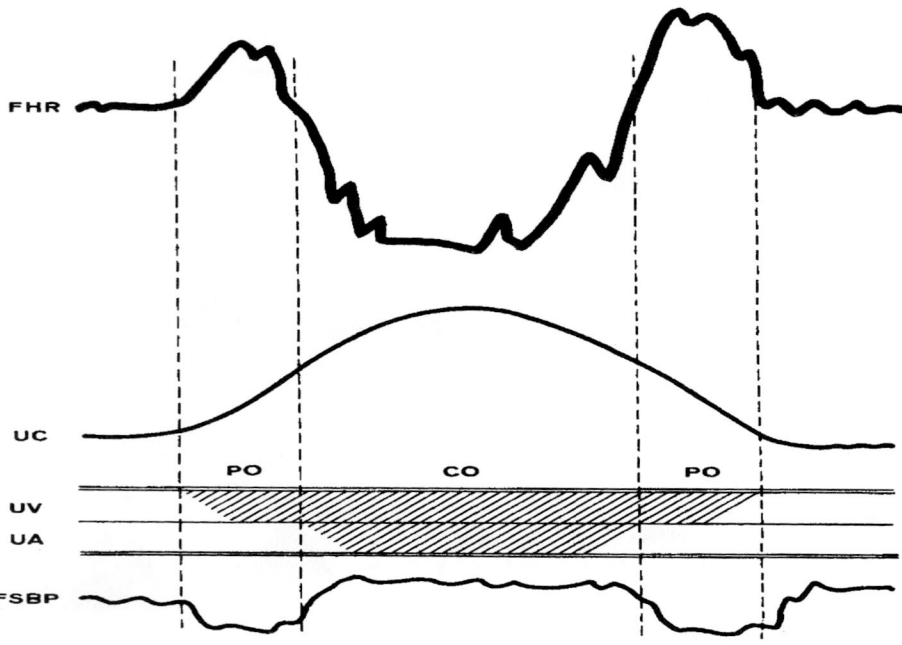

Figure 14–17. This figure represents FHR and fetal systemic blood pressure (FSBP) occurring during compression of the umbilical vein (UV) and umbilical artery (UA). UC is the uterine contraction. Note the acceleration of the FHR as the FSBP is decreased, marking a baroreceptor response to decreased cardiac return, and the deceleration of the FHR when the FSBP is increased, the baroreceptor response to increased peripheral resistance.

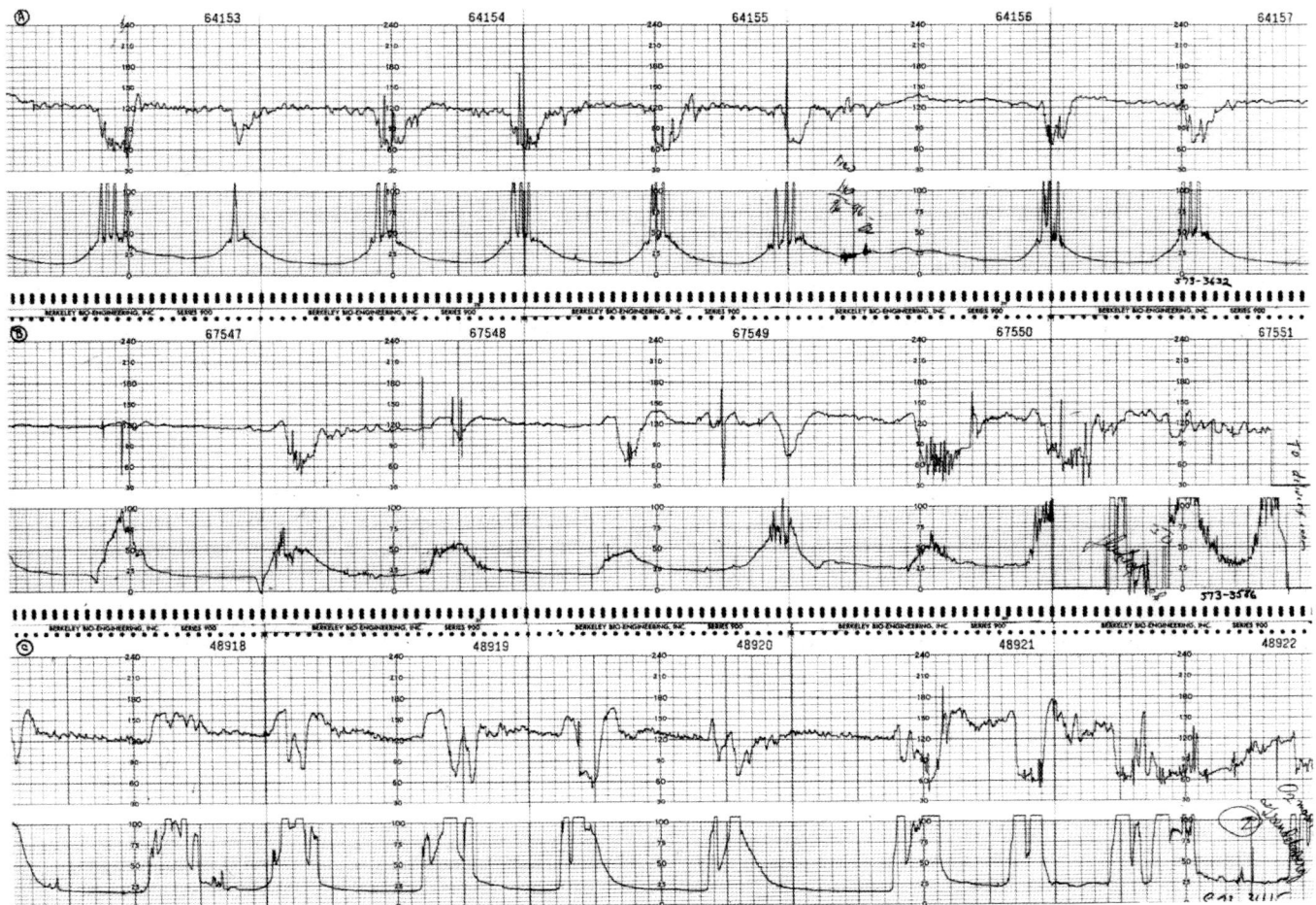

Figure 14–18. These are typical variable decelerations. Note that such decelerations are often recognized by the accelerations that precede and follow the decelerations.

reason the flow is compromised with nuchal cords and seen as the baby descends through the pelvis. If cold saline is infused too rapidly with amnioinfusion, the FHR may slow, presumably caused by cord spasm, the natural fetal reflex to cold stimulus. Whatever the mechanism, it is most important to realize that variable decelerations are initially caused by a reflex in response to changes in pressure and not hypoxia. Thus, variable decelerations (even deep and prolonged) can be seen in fetuses with no change in oxygen saturation (Fig. 14–19).

Variable decelerations are seen in the vast majority of all labors, and most often these decelerations occur without fetal hypoxemia. It is apparent that additional criteria are needed to separate those benign variable decelerations not likely to be associated with hypoxia from those that are. Kubli et al. described a category of mild, moderate, and severe variable decelerations based on depth and duration (see box, Classifications of the Severity of Variable Decelerations).[30] While there is indeed a correlation between the severity of these decelerations and the likelihood of hypoxia, one can see from

Figure 14–19 that it is difficult to pick a specific depth and duration that always predicts oxygen compromise. Therefore, in addition, characteristics of the fetal baseline are also used, including the development of tachy-

---

Classifications of the Severity of Variable Decelerations

Mild
  Deceleration of a duration of <30 seconds, regardless of depth
  Decelerations not below 80 bpm, regardless of duration
Moderate
  Deceleration with a level < 80 bpm
Severe
  Deceleration to a level < 70 bpm for > 60 seconds

Data from Kubli et al.[30]

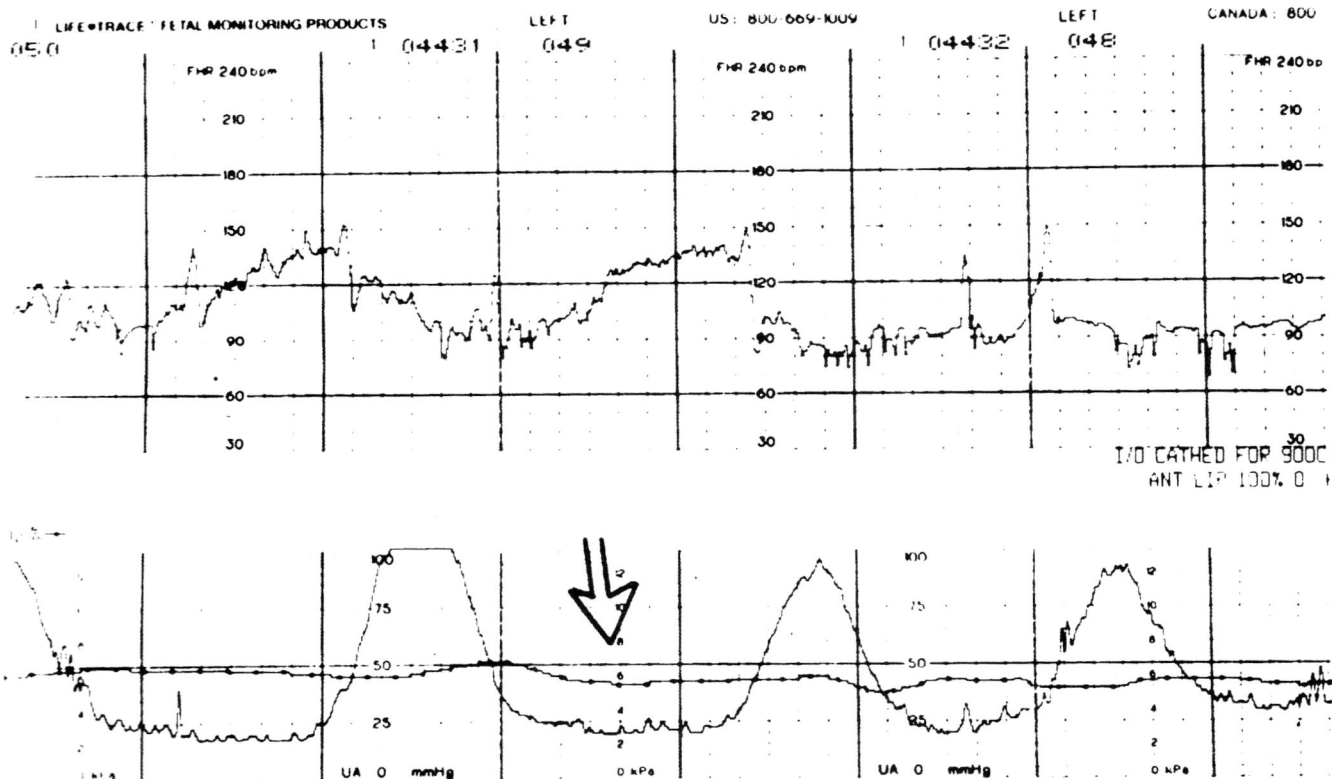

Figure 14–19. Superimposed on the contraction monitor tracing is a continuous tracing using a newly approved fetal pulse oximeter. The tracing shows an fetal oxygen saturation value ranging from 50 to 40 percent (normal = 35 to 60 percent). Note the consistently normal saturation values despite the prolonged FHR decelerations to 80 bpm.

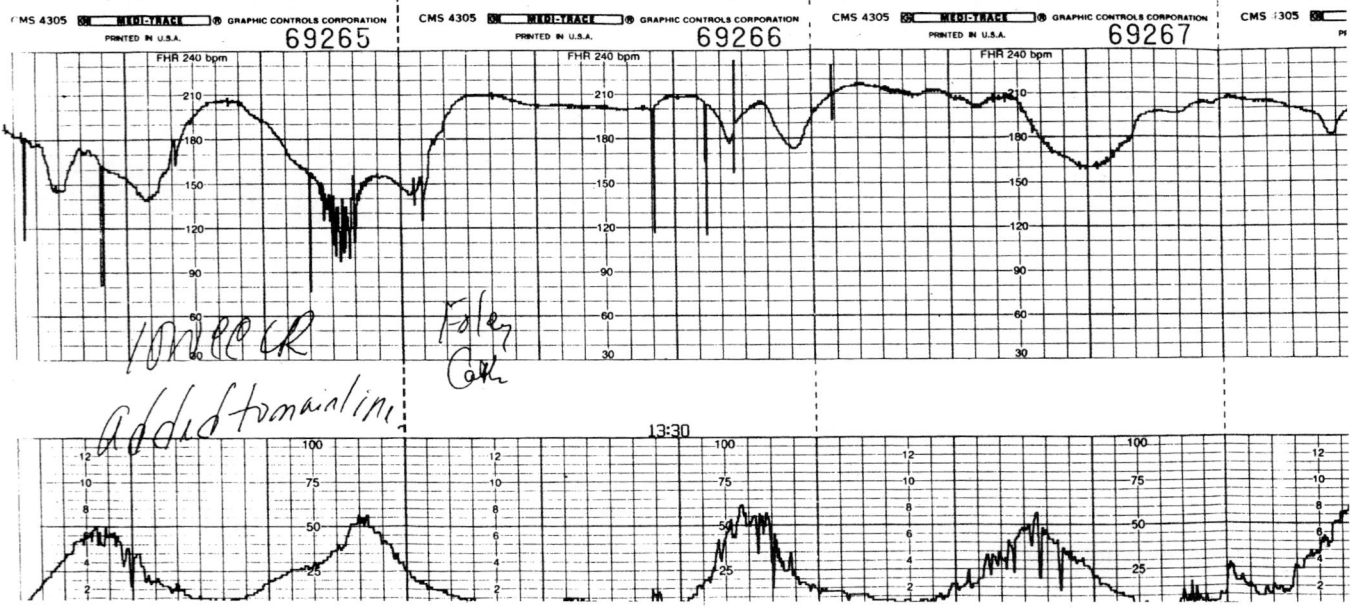

Figure 14–20. The association of loss of variability and tachycardia in association with these variable decelerations make this a nonreassuring FHR pattern.

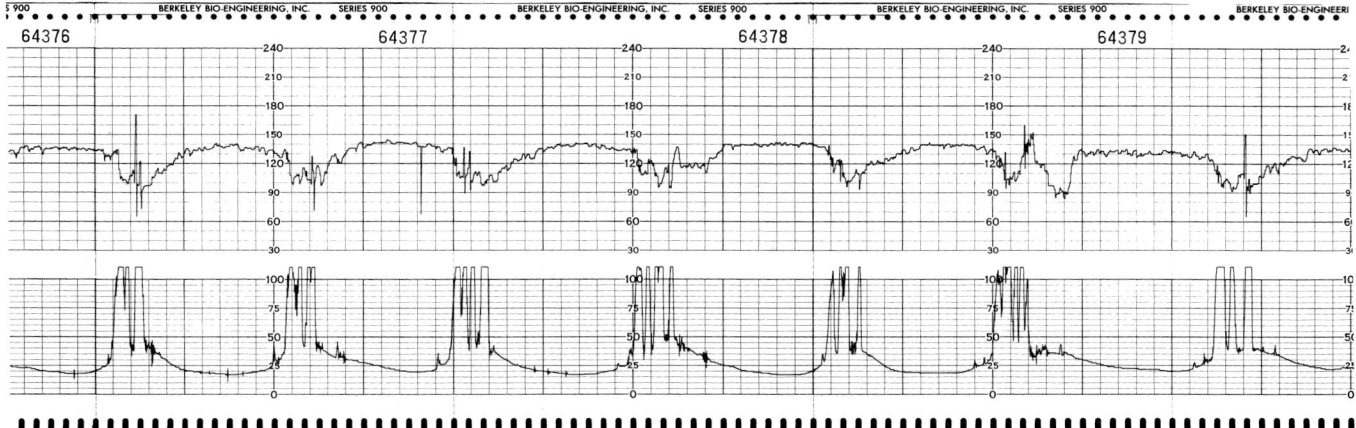

Figure 14–21. These variable decelerations, although mild in depth and duration, are associated with a slow, rather than abrupt, return to baseline. This may be a sign of developing hypoxia as a result of repetitive umbilical cord compression with inadequate opportunity to reoxygenate between events. Generally, this finding makes the variable decelerations non-reassuring.

cardia and loss of variability (Fig. 14–20). When cord compression occurs with each contraction and is sustained for a prolonged period of time, there will be a change from the usual abrupt return to baseline to a slow or delayed return to baseline (Fig. 14–21). This is also often called a late component, although a combined pattern of late and variable decelerations (Fig. 14–22) should be distinguished from progressive, severe variable decelerations that result in slow return to baseline, as the etiologies and thus the potential treatments will differ. This particular discriminator of vari-

able decelerations can be one of the most confusing aspects in all of fetal monitoring. Since a slow return to baseline can represent fetal hypoxia from either progressive cord compression or from a coincident late deceleration, the question is, Does this finding always represent hypoxia? Many times this sign appears without significant cord compression preceding its onset; therefore, it is unlikely that a substantial oxygen deficit has developed. Thus, many times these are benign findings and may represent more slow release of the cord or some other unexplained phenomenon. Finally, in ex-

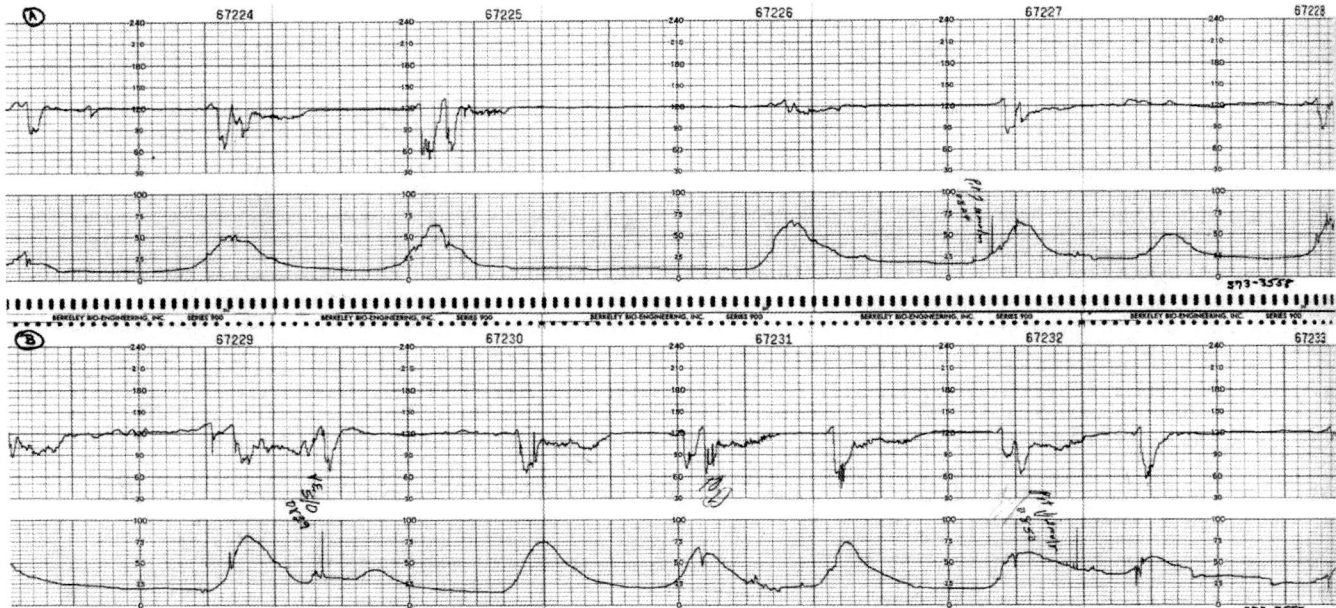

Figure 14–22. Here are repetitive variable decelerations with a slow return to baseline. However, the minimal depth and duration of the variable decelerations and the fact that one can see an independent late deceleration with the third contraction would suggest that this pattern is actually a combined one of mild variable and persistent late decelerations.

treme situations where there is profound fetal hypoxia and acidosis, the variable decelerations will appear smoother and rounded or "blunted" rather than having the usual abrupt changes seen with the more common benign decelerations. Such cases are virtually always seen in association with absent FHR variability and they can also be followed by a blunted acceleration following the return to baseline described by Goodlin and Lowe as "overshoot" (Fig. 14–23).[31] This is a rare situation, and is only seen when all criteria are met including absent variability, blunted variable decelerations, no acceleration preceding the variable deceleration, and no other spontaneous accelerations of the FHR.

There are four categories of causes of cord compression patterns that are useful to consider from a management standpoint. Variable decelerations appearing early in labor are often caused by oligohydramnios. Other variable decelerations often first appear when the patient reaches 8 to 9 cm of dilation, the time in labor when the curve for descent of the presenting part becomes steep. This is probably most often because of nuchal cords, wherein the cord becomes stretched with descent of the fetal head, and as previously described, cord stretch is a profound stimulus for vasospasm in the cord vessels.[15] Unusual types of abnormal umbilical cords, such as short cords, true knots, velamentous cord insertion, cord looped around the extremities, and occult cord prolapse, will produce variable decelerations. And finally, the rarest form of cord compression, and one that usually requires rapid delivery by cesarean section, is true umbilical cord prolapse.

Since the umbilical cord is most analogous to the adult trachea, interruption in cord flow results in both retention of CO_2 and cessation of O_2 delivery. When this becomes progressive, the intermittent compression often first leads to a progressive increase in fetal CO_2, which results in a respiratory acidosis. If the cord com-

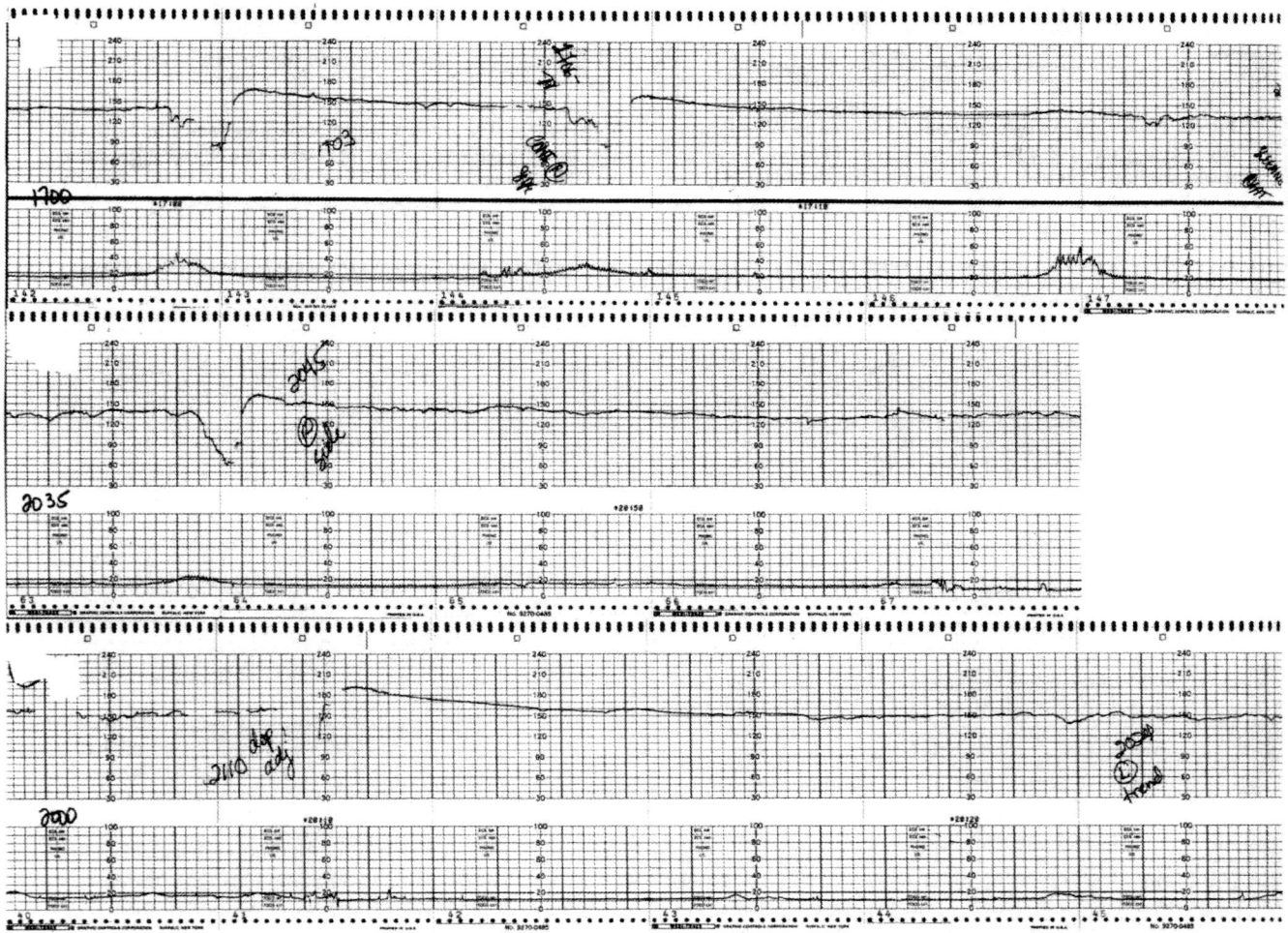

Figure 14–23. The accelerations following these variable decelerations, without any acceleration preceding, in association with absent variability fulfill the criteria to describe the accelerations as "overshoot." Such a finding can be an ominous finding and is often associated with marked metabolic acidosis.

pression continues and also is sufficiently severe to cause insufficient delivery of oxygen, then a metabolic acidosis can also develop. Thus, in a fetal acidosis resulting from cord compression, the acidosis can be respiratory or combined respiratory and metabolic, but should not be metabolic alone.

Prolonged Decelerations

Prolonged decelerations are isolated decelerations lasting 90 to 120 seconds or more. The NICHD Research Planning Workshop proposed that prolonged decelerations be defined as those lasting 2 to 10 minutes and that beyond 10 minutes this is a baseline change.[17] While this proposal is meant to create uniform definitions, it belies the pathophysiology of the deceleration, as the sudden drop in FHR is the result of some adverse afferent stimulus and if sustained will result in a prolonged decrease in FHR. Thus, this is not really a baseline change, as the FHR will return to or near its original baseline when the stimulus is removed. Unlike the other three decelerations, where the type of deceleration defines the pathophysiologic mechanism, prolonged decelerations may be caused by virtually any of the mechanisms previously described, but usually are of a more profound and sustained nature. Prolonged umbilical cord compression, profound placental insufficiency, or possibly even sustained head compression may lead to prolonged decelerations.

The presence of and severity of hypoxia are thought to correlate with the following variables with a prolonged deceleration: the depth and duration of the deceleration, how abruptly it returns to baseline, how much variability is lost during the deceleration, and whether there is a rebound tachycardia and loss of variability following the deceleration (Fig. 14–24). Examples of the more profound stimuli that may result in this type of deceleration include prolapsed umbilical cord or other forms of prolonged cord compression, prolonged uterine hyperstimulation, hypotension following conduction anesthesia, severe degrees of abruptio placentae, paracervical anesthesia, an eclamptic seizure, and rapid descent through the birth canal. Occasionally, less severe stimuli such as examination of the fetal head, Valsalva's maneuvers, or application of a scalp electrode may cause milder forms of prolonged decelerations.

Accelerations

Accelerations are periodic changes of the FHR above the baseline (Fig. 14–25). They are not classified by type. Except for those accelerations previously described that are associated with variable decelerations, virtually all accelerations are a physiologic response to fetal movement.[32] Accelerations are usually short in duration, lasting no more than 30 to 90 seconds, but in an unusually active fetus they can be sustained as long

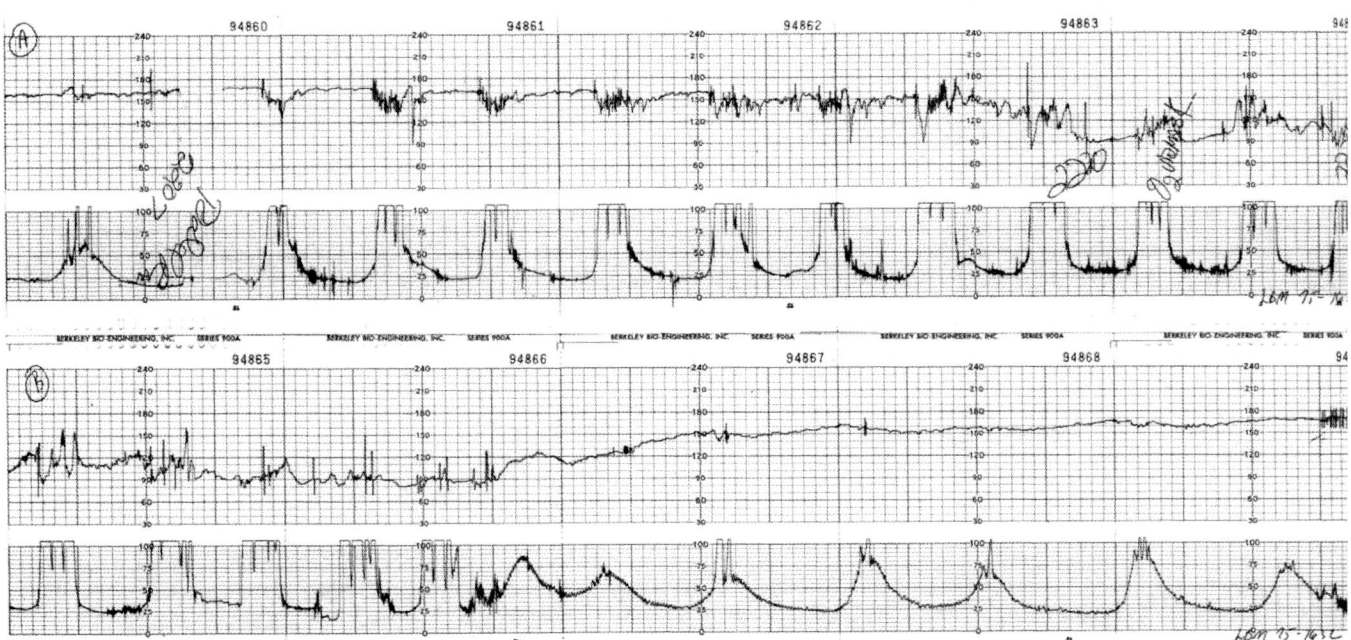

Figure 14–24. Often following a prolonged deceleration, as with the one shown in this figure, there is a temporary period of tachycardia and loss of variability. Such a response would suggest that this was a significant hypoxic event. The etiology of this deceleration is not clear but may have been because of excessive uterine contractions compounded by maternal pushing.

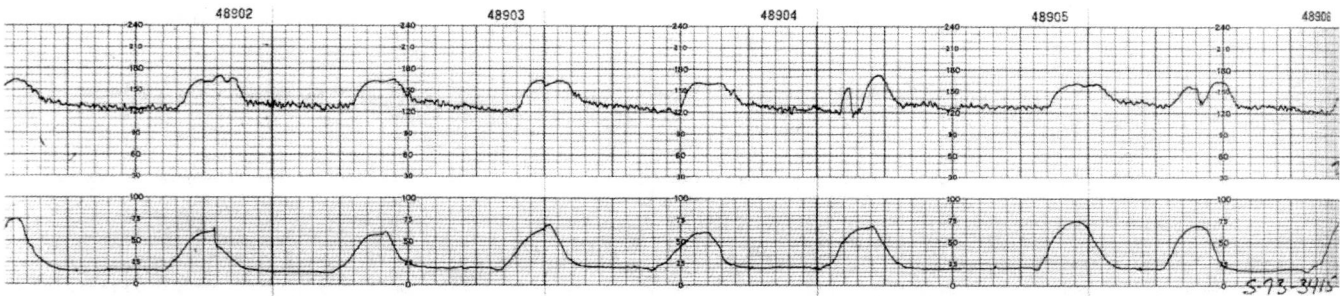

Figure 14–25. These are accelerations of the fetal heart. They are usually seen with fetal movement, and are often coincident with uterine contractions as well, as in this patient.

as 30 minutes or more. Again, the NICHD Research Planning Workshop disagrees somewhat on this definition, in that they propose that accelerations of more than 10 minutes be defined as a change in baseline.[17] However, sustained accelerations (Fig. 14–26) are associated with an actively moving fetus, and when the fetus becomes quiet, the FHR will return to baseline. It is important that this acceleration not be confused with a baseline change, because sustained accelerations, which are consistent with a well-oxygenated, vigorous fetus, can be confused visually with fetal tachycardia, and the return of the FHR to the original baseline can be confused with decelerations.

The presence of accelerations has virtually the same meaning as normal FHR variability, but the absence of accelerations means only that the baby is not moving.

Since accelerations can be quantified in beats per minute above the baseline and duration, their presence is less subjective than quantifying FHR variability. The 15 bpm above the baseline lasting for more than 15 seconds definition of an acceleration, first described with the nonstress test, is the definition usually used for defining accelerations in labor. Earlier in gestation, accelerations are less frequent and of lower amplitude. Fetuses of less than 32 weeks have been defined as having accelerations if they exceed 10 bpm for more than 10 seconds.[17] Clark et al. made the observation that in fetuses having otherwise nonreassuring FHR patterns, the presence of accelerations, using this definition, virtually always ruled out a pH less than 7.20 on scalp sampling.[33] Subsequently, these authors and others have confirmed that the presence of spontaneous accelera-

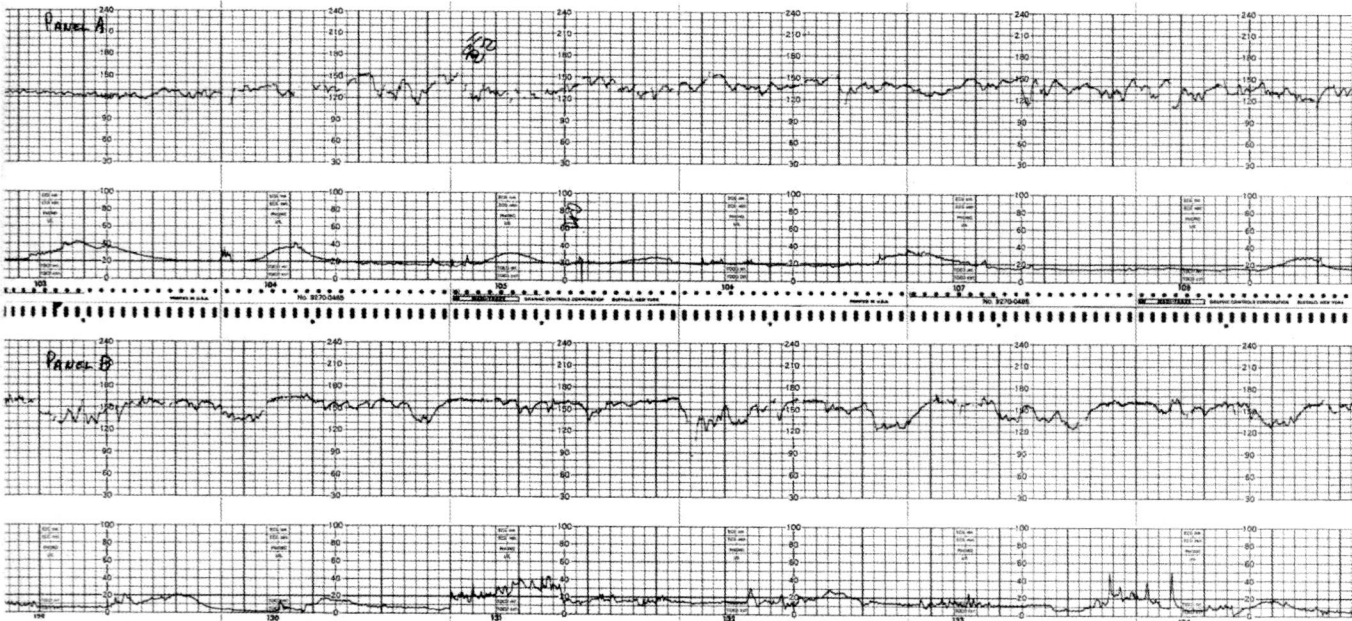

Figure 14–26. This figure shows prolonged and repetitive accelerations, especially on the lower panel. Accelerations that are sustained or confluent can be easily confused with a tachycardia and the return to baseline can be confused with decelerations.

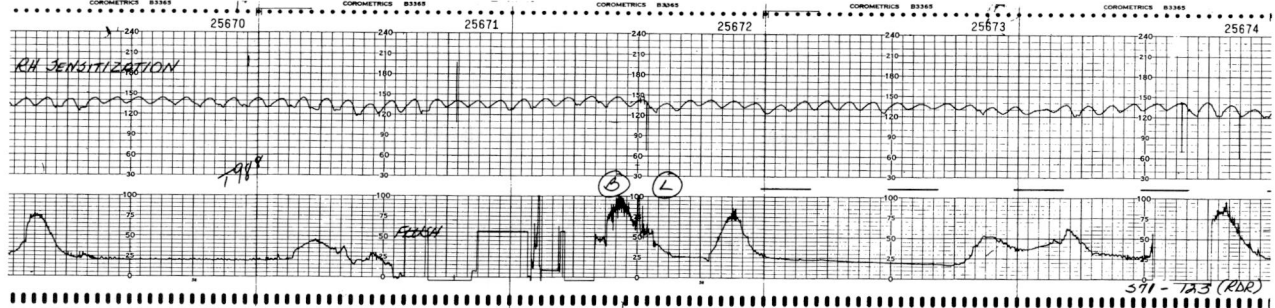

Figure 14–27. The sinusoidal heart rate pattern with its even undulations is demonstrated. Internal monitoring shows the absence of beat-to-beat variability characteristic of true sinusoidal patterns.

tions or accelerations induced by stimulation of the fetal scalp or acoustic stimulation with a vibroacoustic stimulator has the same reliability.[34,35] If there is no acceleration in the face of an otherwise nonreassuring FHR, most studies have shown that about 50 percent of these fetuses have an acidotic pH value on scalp sampling. However, the absence of accelerations in a fetus without a nonreassuring deceleration pattern rarely indicates fetal acidosis.

Sinusoidal Patterns

This pattern was originally described by Kubli et al. in 1972[36] and Shenker in 1973[37] and is rare, but significant. This pattern is strongly associated with fetal hypoxia, most often seen in the presence of severe fetal anemia. Using strict criteria for this pattern, defined by Modanlou et al., there will be a high correlation with significant fetal acidosis and/or severe anemia.[38] These criteria for identifying a sinusoidal FHR include (1) a stable baseline FHR of 120 to 160 bpm with regular sine wave–like oscillations, (2) an amplitude of 5 to 15 bpm, (3) a frequency of 2 to 5 cycles/min, (4) fixed or absent short-term variability, (5) oscillation of the sine wave above and below the baseline, and (6) ab-

sence of accelerations (Fig. 14–27). The pathophysiology of the sinusoidal pattern has been elucidated by Murata et al., who correlated the pattern with levels of fetal arginine vasopressin and subsequently reproduced the pattern with vagotomy and injection of arginine vasopressin.[39] Arginine vasopressin is elevated with hemorrhage or acidosis, and it appears that in such situations with a severely compromised fetus and little vagal activity, the hormone directly affects the fetal heart and this FHR pattern results. The sinusoidal pattern has also been described after injection of certain narcotics such as butorphanol (Stadol)[40] or meperidine (Demerol).[41]

Unfortunately, there are relatively commonly seen FHR patterns that mimic sinusoidal patterns (pseudosinusoidal) that are associated with well-oxygenated and nonanemic fetuses.[38] These can easily be confused with sinusoidal FHR patterns (Fig. 14–28); therefore, it is quite important to strictly apply all of the above six criteria before calling a pattern sinusoidal.

Evolution of FHR Patterns

One of the sources of greatest confusion regarding FHR pattern interpretation and management is that the pat-

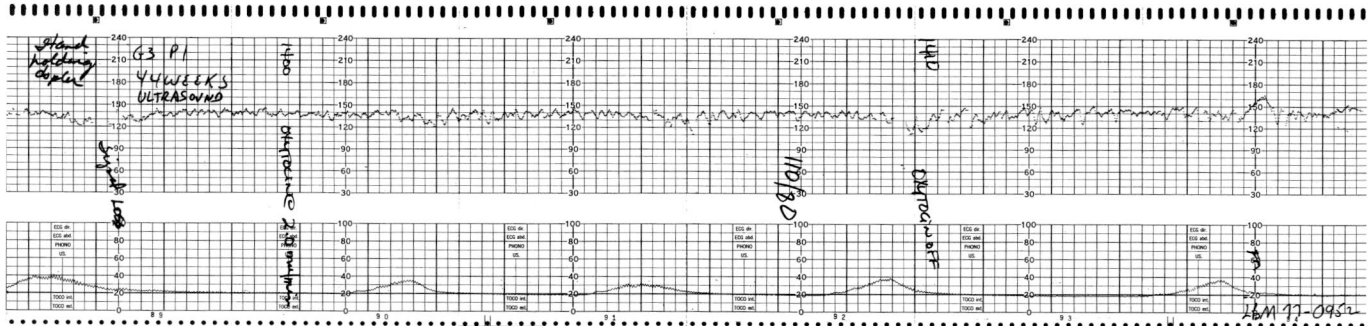

Figure 14–28. More common than sinusoidal tracings are those that are actually normal but can easily be confused with a sinusoidal pattern. There are often small accelerations or above-average variability that mimics the sine wave–like pattern. It is important to use the strict criteria defined in the text before interpreting a pattern as sinusoidal.

terns have very poor specificity in terms of predicting fetal hypoxia and acidosis, newborn depression, or need for resuscitation. When patterns are normal or "reassuring," there is almost always normal oxygenation and the baby is born vigorous, with normal pH and Apgar scores. However, when the pattern is nonreassuring, the baby is more often normal than depressed or acidotic.

In addition to the inherent problem we have in trying to use EFM, a nonspecific modality, to determine fetal oxygenation, there is another reason why many studies have demonstrated such poor correlation with adverse perinatal outcome. Investigators have tried to correlate specific FHR findings in isolation without taking into account the expected evolution of the FHR patterns.[19,30] For example, if one attempts to correlate FHR variability with acidosis or depression, normal variability will correlate well with a normal pH and normal Apgar scores, but reduced or absent variability will correlate poorly with acidosis or depression. This is partly because of the multiple causes of reduced variability. However, in the fetus with persistent late decelerations who then loses FHR variability, the correlation with acidosis and depression should improve substantially because there was evidence that *hypoxia led to the acidosis*. This is a critical

concept in understanding FHR monitoring. Murata and co-workers demonstrated in the fetal monkey, whose oxygenation was progressively reduced, that late decelerations consistently *preceded* the loss of variability and accelerations.[42] Decelerations are the indicators of hypoxia. If hypoxia is the cause of the reduced variability, then those decelerations indicative of hypoxia should *precede* the development of tachycardia, loss of variability, and/or disappearance of accelerations (Fig. 14–29). Furthermore, the duration and appearance of the decelerations should be of sufficient magnitude to suggest that CNS depression could have resulted.

Therefore, the fetus who develops one of the latter variables (e.g., loss of accelerations) in the absence of decelerations is not likely to have hypoxia, and another cause should be considered (e.g., drugs, sleep cycle). It must be remembered that when the fetus demonstrates one of these baseline changes or absence of accelerations on admission, it is not possible to know whether evidence of hypoxia preceded these changes. In addition, this approach does not apply antepartum, when the nonstress test is used. Contractions are not present, and there will not be an opportunity to assess for the presence or absence of decelerations in response to contractions.

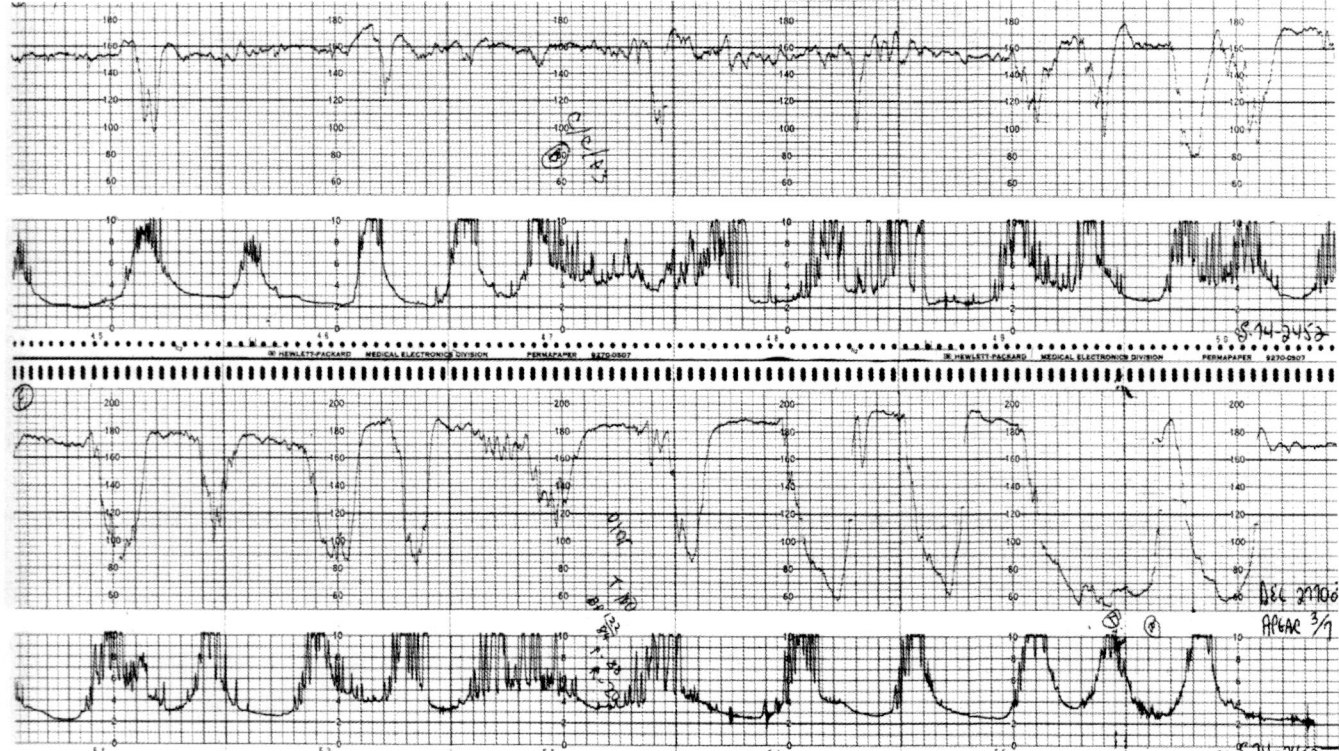

Figure 14–29. Loss of variability and tachycardia should only be interpreted as indicative of hypoxia and developing acidosis when they are associated with decelerations that suggest progressive hypoxia as with these variable decelerations, which are becoming deeper and more prolonged.

MANAGEMENT OF NONREASSURING FETAL HEART RATE PATTERNS

Traditionally, an FHR pattern that suggested fetal hypoxia would be called fetal distress if it was sufficiently concerning to warrant immediate operative intervention. But, as previously mentioned, in most cases, when a cesarean or forceps delivery was done for "fetal distress," the fetus was delivered without evidence of significant hypoxia or acidosis. This has led to the recommendation from the ACOG to use the term "nonreassuring fetal status" to indicate a more accurate description of the indication for such intervention.[13] This is also descriptive of the approach to the management of the fetus with concerning FHR patterns. That is, when the FHR pattern is suggestive of hypoxia, and therefore nonreassuring, other means of reassurance should be used when possible.

Interventions for Nonreassuring Fetal Status

The ideal intervention for fetal hypoxia is a cause-specific, noninvasive one that permanently reverses the problem. While not always possible, this should certainly be the goal. Obviously, the first step in achieving this goal is to recognize the cause of the abnormal FHR pattern. A thorough knowledge of the pathophysiology of FHR changes coupled with a careful clinical patient evaluation and a knowledge of common causes of specific FHR changes will maximize the opportunity for this goal to succeed. In addition to cause-specific types of interventions, virtually all cases of hypoxia should theoretically also benefit by more generic interventions that have the potential to maximize oxygen delivery and placental exchange.

Nonsurgical Interventions

OXYGEN ADMINISTRATION. One of the most obvious ways to maximize oxygen delivery to the fetus is to give additional oxygen to the mother. Whereas diffusion across the membrane is driven by PO_2 as opposed to oxygen content, and whereas maternal PO_2 can be raised substantially with mask O_2, it is not well demonstrated that fetal PO_2 is raised substantially by routine maternal oxygen administration. Recent evidence, while still preliminary, from fetuses being monitored with pulse oximetry, does not substantiate a significant rise in fetal arterial oxygen saturation (SaO_2) using regular face mask.[43] A tight-fitting rebreathing mask does appear to raise fetal SaO_2, at least somewhat.[43] Whereas this is the state of current knowledge, routine O_2 administration via face mask has become such standard practice with nonreassuring FHR patterns that it is difficult to recommend otherwise until further studies are available to substantiate these preliminary data.

LATERAL POSITIONING. Ideally, all patients should labor in the lateral recumbent position, at least from the standpoint of maximizing uterine perfusion. The reasons for this are, at least theoretically, twofold: (1) in being inactive and recumbent, the body is required to deliver the least amount of blood flow to other muscles; and (2) in the lateral position, there is no compression by the uterus on the vena cava or aorta, thus maximizing cardiac return and cardiac output.

HYDRATION. Most patients in labor are either restricted or prohibited from taking oral fluids for fear of requiring an urgent operative delivery in the presence of a full stomach. If not fluid restricted, individuals involved in sustained exercise, and possibly by inference in active labor, do not voluntarily ingest adequate amounts of fluid because of a phenomenon called "autodehydration,"[44] In addition, recent evidence would suggest that the usual amount of intravenous fluid of 125 ml/h is a gross underestimate of the replacement required in labor.[45] Thus, by increasing fluid administration, there is the potential to maximize intravascular volume and thus uterine perfusion.

OXYTOCIN. In a patient with a nonreassuring pattern, the more time there is between contractions, the more time to maximally perfuse the placenta and deliver oxygen. In patients receiving oxytocin, there is potential to improve oxygenation by decreasing or discontinuing oxytocin. Often, however, this becomes a difficult situation, as many patients will stop progressing in labor in terms of continued dilation and/or descent if the oxytocin is discontinued. It is often necessary to restart the oxytocin, and this may be appropriate especially if there are accelerations or other means to document the absence of acidosis (e.g., oxygen saturation). Written documentation explaining the necessity and appropriateness of continuing oxytocin in this situation is especially important. The situation with patients who develop persistently nonreassuring patterns, especially with loss of accelerations or absence of other reassurance, and who require discontinuation of oxytocin, but then fail to progress because adequate contractions cannot be sustained, is often referred to as "fetal intolerance to labor."

TOCOLYTICS. There are numerous references in the obstetric literature to the use of tocolytics to maximize oxygen delivery, by essentially the same mechanism described in the above paragraph on discontinuing oxytocin.[46–49] Tocolytics are appropriate in at least two situations: (1) When patients are having spontaneous excessive contractions leading to nonreassuring FHR

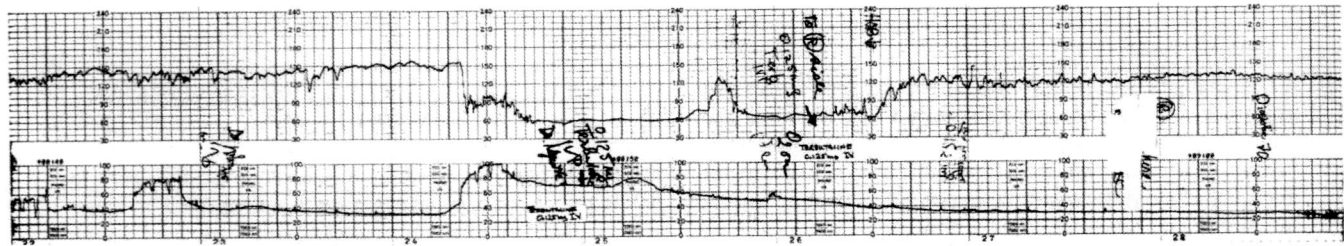

Figure 14–30. This prolonged deceleration in a patient with a spontaneous prolonged contraction is treated with subcutaneous terbutaline with apparent resolution of both the contraction and the deceleration.

patterns, especially prolonged decelerations (Fig. 14–30) (different tocolytics have been described, but the most commonly used one, and perhaps the one that provides the most rapid response, is subcutaneous terbutaline, 0.25 mg); and (2) intrauterine resuscitation after the decision is made to perform an operative delivery while waiting for preparations to be made. Subcutaneous terbutaline has been demonstrated to improve Apgar scores and cord pH values without apparent complications such as postpartum hemorrhage.[50]

AMNIOINFUSION. In situations where variable decelerations appear to be caused by oligohydramnios, reestablishing intrauterine fluid volume via a process called "amnioinfusion" has been demonstrated in numerous randomized studies to ameliorate the variable decelerations, improve Apgar scores and cord pH values, and even reduce the need for cesarean section for NRFS.[51–53] Reference to this idea can be found as far back as 1925,[54] but was rediscovered and proposed by Miyazaki and Taylor in 1983.[55] Intrauterine pressure catheters are now made with a port that allows the simultaneous administration of saline to accomplish this goal. Thus, in the patient with variable decelerations that suggest progression to more nonreasurring types, and where the cause is likely to be caused by oligohydramnios, the implementation of amnioinfusion is warranted. What has not yet been established is whether in some situations amnioinfusion should be started prophylactically when there is an unusually high risk for the development of variable decelerations from oligohydramnios, such as preterm premature rupture of membranes (PROM).

Theoretically, using amnioinfusion before the onset of the decelerations in certain fetuses, such as very premature ones or those with intrauterine growth restriction who will progress to acidosis and depression much more rapidly with cord compression, will prevent the rapid evolution of hypoxia and acidosis. No studies are available as of yet to compare therapeutic as opposed to prophylactic amnioinfusion. Amnioinfusion also has been proposed, in several prospective randomized trials, to be used to avoid the fetal/neonatal pulmonary prob-

lems in the presence of meconium.[56] The evidence for efficacy in this setting is good. However, clear evidence that this modality avoids the meconium aspiration syndrome is lacking, since this complication is relatively infrequent. Some of these problems will be avoided with good oropharyngeal suctioning on the perineum and neonatal suctioning below the vocal cords when necessary. The theory behind this use of amnioinfusion is that (1) it dilutes the meconium by increasing fluid volume, and (2) by avoiding fetal gasping, which can occur with significant hypoxic episodes (i.e., sustained cord compression), the likelihood of meconium aspiration prior to delivery is reduced. Surveys of university hospitals suggest that amnioinfusion is used for both variable decelerations and meconium in the vast majority.[57]

MECONIUM. The presence of meconium is an extremely confusing issue when evaluating the fetus in labor. The quandary arises from the fact that while a hypoxic insult eliciting a significant vagal response from the fetus often results in the passage of meconium from the fetal gut, passage of meconium can also occur in the absence of any significant or sustained hypoxia. Meconium is not only a potential sign of fetal hypoxia but is also a potential toxin if the fetus aspirates this particulate matter with a gasping breath in utero or when it takes its first breaths following birth. The thickness of the meconium is also a reflection of the amount of amniotic fluid, and thick meconium virtually always reflects some degree of oligohydramnios. Thus, there may be a vicious cycle in such a situation. Oligohydramnios often leads to cord compression; the vagal response to cord compression may also lead to further passage of meconium, but also when it is sustained or prolonged may lead to fetal gasping, increasing the likelihood that meconium aspiration can occur before birth. Furthermore, since oligohydramnios may be an indicator of failing placental function, meconium may also indicate that the fetus is at risk for placental insufficiency. In general, meconium should alert the clinician to the potential for oligohydramnios, umbilical cord compression, placental insufficiency, and meconium aspiration. Fortunately, a reassuring FHR tracing is generally reliable, and patients with meconium can be managed expectantly. But in the presence of meconium, especially thick meconium, the risk factors associated with meconium should be entered in the equation when managing relatively nonreassuring patterns, as should all clinical variables.

Alternatives for Evaluating the Fetus with a Nonreassuring FHR Pattern

In the fetus with a persistently nonreassuring FHR pattern, where nonsurgical efforts at reversing or improving the pattern fail, the next step is to attempt to find out whether the hypoxia has progressed to metabolic acidosis.

FETAL SCALP pH. Determination of fetal scalp pH is historically the oldest and most well-tested method for determining if the fetus is acidotic. Technically, a plastic cone is inserted transvaginally against the fetal vertex. The cervix needs to be at least 4 to 5 cm dilated and the vertex at a −1 station or below to accomplish this. Mineral oil or another lubricant is applied to the scalp so blood will bead, and then using a lancet, the scalp is pricked and blood is then collected in a long capillary tube (Fig. 14–31). The tube will hold about 100 μl of blood, and about 30 μl is needed to perform a pH test alone and 70 μl to determine PCO_2 as well. To determine if an acidosis is metabolic or respiratory, the PCO_2 is needed. This is an important distinction, as the question being asked is whether there has been sufficient hypoxia to lead to metabolic acidosis. Respiratory acidosis is far less concerning, but without determining PCO_2, this cannot be sorted out. Unfortunately, it is difficult to obtain enough blood for both pH and PCO_2 in most instances. PCO_2 determination is especially important when doing scalp pH for variable decelerations, as most acidosis is respiratory in this situa-

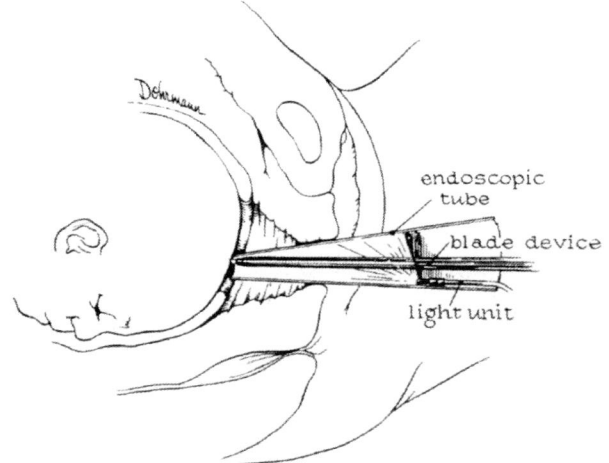

Figure 14–31. Technique of fetal scalp blood sampling.

tion. A scalp pH less than 7.20 is consistent with fetal acidosis and a pH of 7.20 to 7.25 is borderline and should be repeated immediately. A reassuring value over 7.25 must be repeated every 20 to 30 minutes as long as the pattern persists and the fetus is not acidotic. In practice, because this technique is cumbersome, fraught with technical inaccuracy, uncomfortable for the patient, and with the requirement to perform repeated samples, it is used very infrequently.[58] Even in large teaching services accustomed to using this technique, its abandonment, coupled with an appreciation for the utility of accelerations for predicting presence or absence of acidosis, does not appreciatably increase the need for operative intervention.[59]

ACCELERATIONS. In the fetus with a nonreassuring pattern, spontaneous accelerations have the same significance as those elicited by scalp or acoustic stimulation. Thus, any acceleration—spontaneous or induced—indicates the absence of acidosis. It should be emphasized that the absence of accelerations as well as the absence of decelerations or other patterns suggesting hypoxia should not elicit concern. The fetus is often not moving in labor; and from a pathophysiologic perspective, without evidence of hypoxia, the fetus cannot develop a metabolic acidosis. Thus, the application of the interpretation of accelerations should generally be restricted to the fetus with an otherwise nonreassuring FHR pattern, where the question is being asked: Hypoxia is present. Is the fetus now developing a metabolic acidosis?

FETAL PULSE OXIMETRY. One of the most exciting recent developments in obstetrics is the introduction of fetal pulse oximetry. Since FHR monitoring is specifically intended to monitor fetal oxygenation and since this modality is so nonspecific, it stands to reason that what we should be using ideally is a device that directly monitors fetal oxygenation and/or pH. Since the mid 1980s, the use of pulse oximetry has revolutionized monitoring of "air-breathing" adults, children, and neonates. Virtually all patients in the operating room and in intensive care units are monitored with this device, and direct benefit has been demonstrated in reducing hypoxia-related anesthetic deaths.[60] The application of this modality to the fetus has been hindered by several problems. The fetus is inaccessible. The vertex in labor poses problems for light transmission with pulse oximetry including hair, vernix, and meconium. Developing caput creates stasis, and the low pulse pressure of the fetus creates technical difficulty. Fetal hemoglobin will alter absorption curves of the normally used red and infrared wavelengths. It was not until a special sensor was developed that is placed transcervically to lie against the fetal cheek that many of these problems were overcome (Fig. 14–32). This device accurately de-

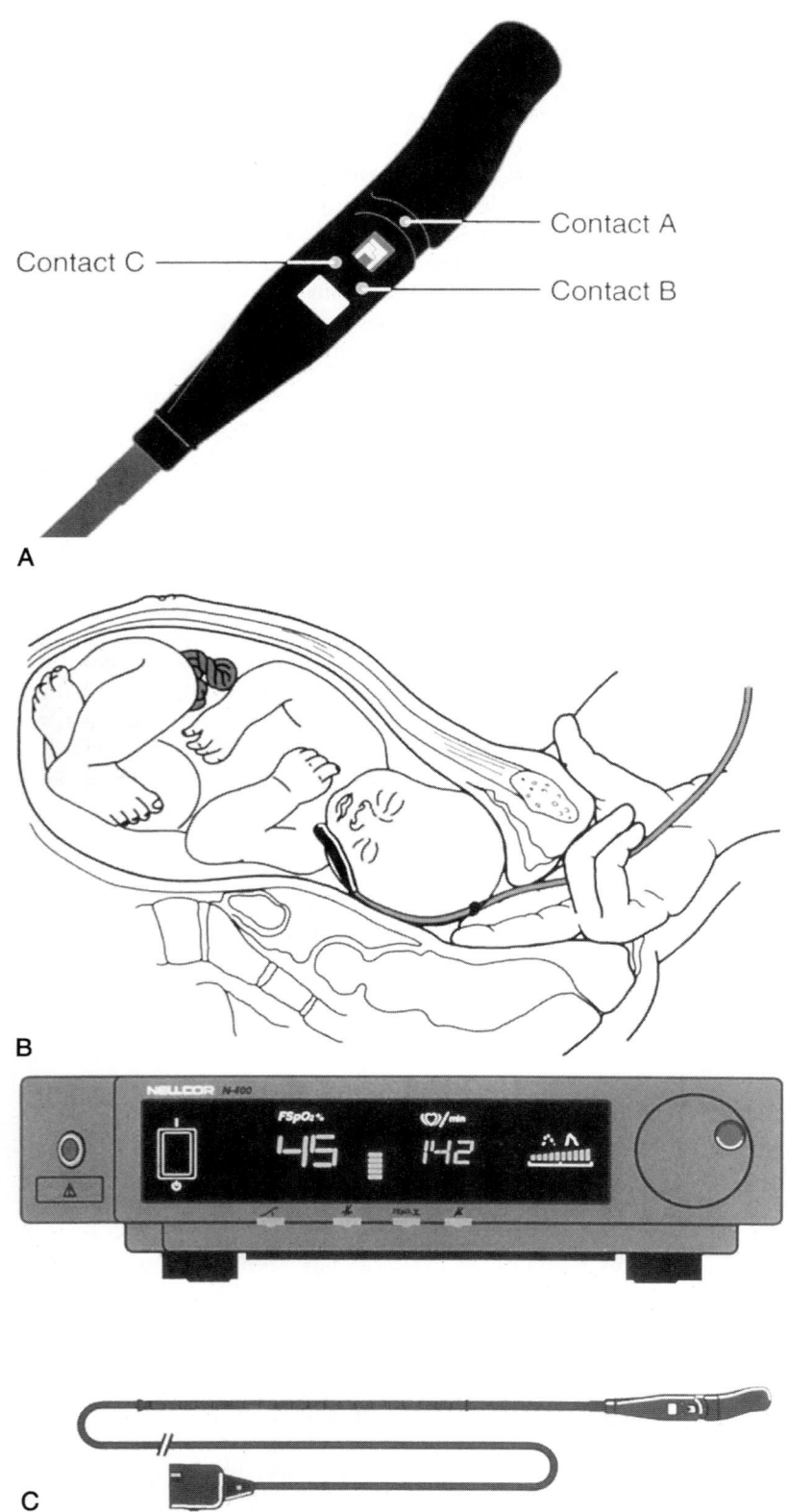

A

B

C

Figure 14–32. Technology for fetal pulse oximetry. *A,* This is the face of the sensor used to determine fetal oxygen saturation. On its surface are three gold-plated electrodes (contacts A, B, and C), which determine adequate electrical contact, and a photoemittor and photodector. *B,* This figure shows the technique for insertion of the sensor. The device is inserted transcervically, as with an intrauterine pressure catheter, to lie against the fetal face, where it is held in place simply by the pressure of the uterine cervix or pelvic sidewall. *C,* The sensor is connected to this monitor, which processes the signal and displays (left to right) fetal oxygen saturation, pulse amplitude, fetal heart rate, and adequacy of electrical contact. This device can be connected to a conventional fetal monitor that displays the oxygen saturation continuously on the contraction channel (see Fig. 14–19).

termines fetal oxygen saturation and continually records the value on the lower (contraction) channel of the electronic FHR monitor.

The second hurdle to overcome was to determine if there was a reliable "critical threshold" that could be determined. The concept of the critical threshold is that a fetal metabolic acidosis will not develop until the fetal oxygen saturation falls below a certain value. In multiple animal and human studies there is essentially uniform agreement that this critical threshold is a saturation of 30 percent.[61-63] Normal fetuses in labor have a range of oxygen saturation of about 40 to 70 percent.[64] In animals, a fetal metabolic acidosis will not develop until levels below 30 percent are reached.[61] In humans, this value has been compared to scalp pH in fetuses with nonreassuring FHR patterns, and there is an extremely high correlation between the cutoff value of 30 percent and the scalp pH value of 7.20.[62] Furthermore, Dildy and colleagues demonstrated that in over 1,100 umbilical cord pH samples, there were no cases of significant metabolic acidosis with a fetal oxygen saturation above 30 percent.[63] In addition, the saturation must remain below 30 percent for a substantial period of time (about 10 minutes or more) before a metabolic acidosis develops in most situations in labor.

Fetal pulse oximetry was approved by the Food and Drug Administration (FDA) for use in fetuses with nonreassuring FHR patterns in May 2000. The approval was made on the basis of the previously mentioned data and the results of a large multicenter trial of over 1,000 patients comparing FHR monitoring alone versus FHR monitoring backed up by pulse oximetry in fetuses already having nonreassuring FHR patterns.[65] Whereas the trial did not demonstrate an overall reduction in cesarean section, there was a reduction in cesarean section for NRFS and an improved specificity and sensitivity of operative intervention for the fetus with depression, acidosis, and in need of resuscitation. Most importantly, in following the fetus with a nonreassuring FHR tracing but a reassuring oxygen saturation value (>30 percent), there was no increase in babies with adverse outcomes.

Therefore, fetal pulse oximetry may prove to be an excellent alternative to fetal scalp pH monitoring in patients with nonreassuring FHR patterns and may allow continued monitoring and avoid intervention of fetuses with apparently nonreassuring FHR patterns but with normal oxygenation. Since at this time there is such limited clinical experience in this country and few confirmatory studies of its value in practice are available, it is difficult to determine how it will impact practice; however, its potential is quite promising. It is unlikely that this modality will replace EFM for many years to come for several reasons. It cannot be used until the membranes are ruptured, and the cervix is at least 2 to 3 cm dilated. FHR monitoring is highly reli-

able when reassuring, and in the current format the monitor is needed to correlate and prognosticate changes in fetal oxygen saturation. Fetal pulse oximetry in its current form only gives an adequate signal about 70 percent of the time, although this will improve as the technology continues to be perfected.[65] Finally, the FHR pattern gives some clues as to the mechanism of hypoxia, allowing specific therapy to be provided, and the pulse oximeter only quantifies the degree of hypoxia. These modalities are complementary, and the potential for improving intrapartum assessment of the hypoxic fetus is vast.

Operative Intervention for Nonreassuring Fetal Status

When the fetus is determined to have a persistently nonreassuring FHR pattern and backup methods (scalp pH, accelerations, pulse oximetry) cannot provide reassurance that the fetus is not acidotic, operative intervention is indicated to expeditiously deliver the baby to avoid further deterioration. Several questions arise when the decision has been made for intervention for NRFS. What is the best choice, operative vaginal delivery or cesarean section? How much time do we have to perform the delivery? What anesthetic should be used? What is the prognosis of the baby? And, finally, are there situations where the baby is already damaged or otherwise not likely to benefit from this intervention?

Choosing operative vaginal delivery or cesarean section is not difficult if the patient is in early labor. For the patient near or at complete dilation, this becomes a question of judgment. Which route is more likely to create the more rapid delivery while at the same time result in the least complications for mother and baby? When the clinician is unsure whether an attempt at operative vaginal delivery will succeed, the question is even more difficult. This decision will depend not only on the variables that predict success for an operative vaginal delivery (e.g., station, clinical pelvimetry, size of the baby, skill of the clinician) but also on the severity of the FHR pattern and whether there is time to find out whether an operative delivery will succeed. The time for intervention also is a question of judgment. Except for the situation of a prolonged deceleration to less than 70 bpm with loss of variability that will not recover and requires the most rapid intervention safely possible, most other situations require judgment and integration of the entire clinical picture of mother and baby.

The question of how much time is available to perform an operative intervention in the face of a nonreassuring FHR pattern is a complex one, muddied not only by the unpredictability of the nonreassuring pattern, but also by the medicolegal pressures that have arisen as a result of EFM. The ACOG recommends that "all hospitals have the capability of performing a cesarean delivery within 30 minutes of the decision to operate,"[66] but that "not all indications for a cesarean delivery will require a 30-minute response time." The examples given that mandate an expeditious delivery include hemorrhage from placenta previa, abruptio placentae, prolapse of the umbilical cord, and ruptured uterus. In some situations (e.g., sustained prolonged deceleration to <70 bpm with loss of variability), 30 minutes may be too long to avoid damage; in others, this may be too restrictive and may result in suboptimal anesthetic choices and compromised preoperative preparation. Thus, a judgment made on the basis of the severity of the FHR pattern and the overall clinical status of mother and baby must be integrated into this difficult decision.

MANAGEMENT OF NONREASSURING FHR PATTERNS— A PROPOSED PROTOCOL

The following algorithm for management of nonreassuring patterns is proposed.

1. When the pattern suggests the beginning development of hypoxia or is already nonreassuring:
   a. Identify when possible the cause of the problem (e.g., hypotension from an epidural).
   b. Correct the cause (e.g., fluids and ephedrine to correct the hypotension).
   c. Give measures to maximize placental oxygen delivery and exchange: oxygen by face mask, lateral positioning, hydration, consider decreasing or discontinuing oxytocin.
2. If the pattern becomes or remains nonreassuring and the above measures have been completed:
   a. Attempt to provide other measures of reassurance to rule out metabolic acidosis.
      • Accelerations—spontaneous or elicited
      • Scalp pH
      • Fetal pulse oximetry
   b. If reassurance using one of the above methods can be provided, and the pattern persists, continuous or intermittent (every 30 minutes) evidence of absence of acidosis must be ascertained.
   c. If reassurance of the absence of acidosis cannot be provided, deliver expeditiously by the safest and most reasonable means (operative vaginal or cesarean section).

Patterns that qualify as nonreassuring and cannot be corrected and therefore warrant evidence of the absence of metabolic acidosis include:

1. Persistent late decelerations (>50 percent of contractions).
2. Nonreassuring variable decelerations.
   a. Progressively severe.
   b. With developing tachycardia and loss of variability.
   c. With developing slow return to baseline.
3. Sinusoidal tracing.
4. Recurrent prolonged decelerations.
5. The confusing pattern.
   a. The patient presents with a pattern of absent variability but without explanatory decelerations.
   b. An unusual pattern that does not fit into one of the categories defined above but does not have elements of a reassuring pattern.

Several of the above presentations and others warrant additional discussion. Prolonged decelerations that will not return to baseline are a potentially ominous situation. Causes of these patterns include virtually any substantial insult that can cause severe hypoxia, especially when the FHR goes below 80 bpm. Examples include abruptio placentae, ruptured uterus, cord prolapse or sustained cord compression, profound hypotension, maternal seizure or respiratory arrest, and rapid descent and impending delivery of the fetus. Generally, the following approach to these sustained prolonged decelerations should be taken. First, be patient. Often these are noticed on the central monitor and caregivers unnecessarily run to the room and frighten the patient and family. Since the vast majority of these decelerations will spontaneously resolve in 1 to 3 minutes, such action is usually unwarranted. If the deceleration does not resolve, the patient should be examined to rule out cord prolapse or sudden descent. If these are not present, determine if there is an apparent cause that can be specifically corrected. If the cause cannot be found, the general explanation by process of elimination is sustained cord compression, and repositioning the patient, oxygen administration, and discontinuing oxytocin is all that can be provided. Should none of these work, operative delivery will be required unless spontaneous delivery is imminent. How long one should wait for the corrective measures and/or spontaneous recovery to occur is somewhat variable. This will be determined by the depth of the deceleration, the loss of variability during the deceleration, whether evidence of hypoxia preceded the deceleration, and whether the heart rate is intermittently returning toward baseline or is just staying down. Evidence to recommend a precise amount of time wherein intervention must occur is difficult to integrate, as the vast majority of time we are dealing with relative hypoxia rather than complete anoxia. Complete anoxia in real life probably occurs only with severe degrees of uterine rupture and complete abruption. Even with cord prolapse, the vast majority of time there is some cord blood flow. Windle performed the classic experiment using complete anoxia in fetal monkeys.[67] Monkeys allowed to breathe in 6 minutes or less showed no clinical or pathologic ill effects. Asphyxiation for 7 to 12 minutes resulted in transient motor and behavioral changes, with some scarring in certain specific brain areas in some animals. Those anoxic for 12 to 17 minutes, if death did not occur, had the most severe neurologic and clinical effects. Therefore, in the worst case of all, if delivery occurs in less than 12 minutes from the onset of the deceleration, damage will be unlikely, unless there was some hypoxia prior to the deceleration.

The most difficult pattern to manage is in the fetus with recurrent prolonged decelerations that do recover (Fig. 14–33). Generally, these can be managed using the same algorithm for nonreassuring patterns as described above. However, even if one can provide reassurance that acidosis does not exist following any of the decelerations, there is a concern that this pattern portends a deceleration that will recur and will not recover, and one will be placed in the situation described in the previous paragraph. Therefore, there will be occasions when the recurrent prolonged decelerations are concerning enough that operative intervention is warranted even if there is no concern about acidosis

at the present moment. One must integrate the frequency, severity, and duration of the deceleration; the fetal response in terms of tachycardia and loss of variability; and how much time is expected before spontaneous delivery will occur to make this difficult decision. Therefore, for example, in the nulliparous patient at 4 cm, having decelerations lasting 4 minutes to 70 bpm every 10 minutes, operative delivery may be warranted. Whereas in the multipara at 8 cm making normal progress with similar or less frequent decelerations, it may be justified to manage these expectantly, but with all preparations made for immediate delivery should one of the decelerations not recover.

Auscultation as an Alternative

Almost all randomized controlled trials have demonstrated that intermittent auscultation is as effective as EFM in detecting fetal hypoxia in labor. There are some limitations to this statement, however. Virtually all of these trials compared EFM to intermittent auscultation with one-on-one nursing, where the auscultation was performed every 15 minutes in the first stage and every 5 minutes in the second stage, and the auscultation was performed for a period of 60 seconds through and following an entire uterine contraction. This is a situation that is difficult to duplicate in everyday practice because of lower nurse/patient ratios and because

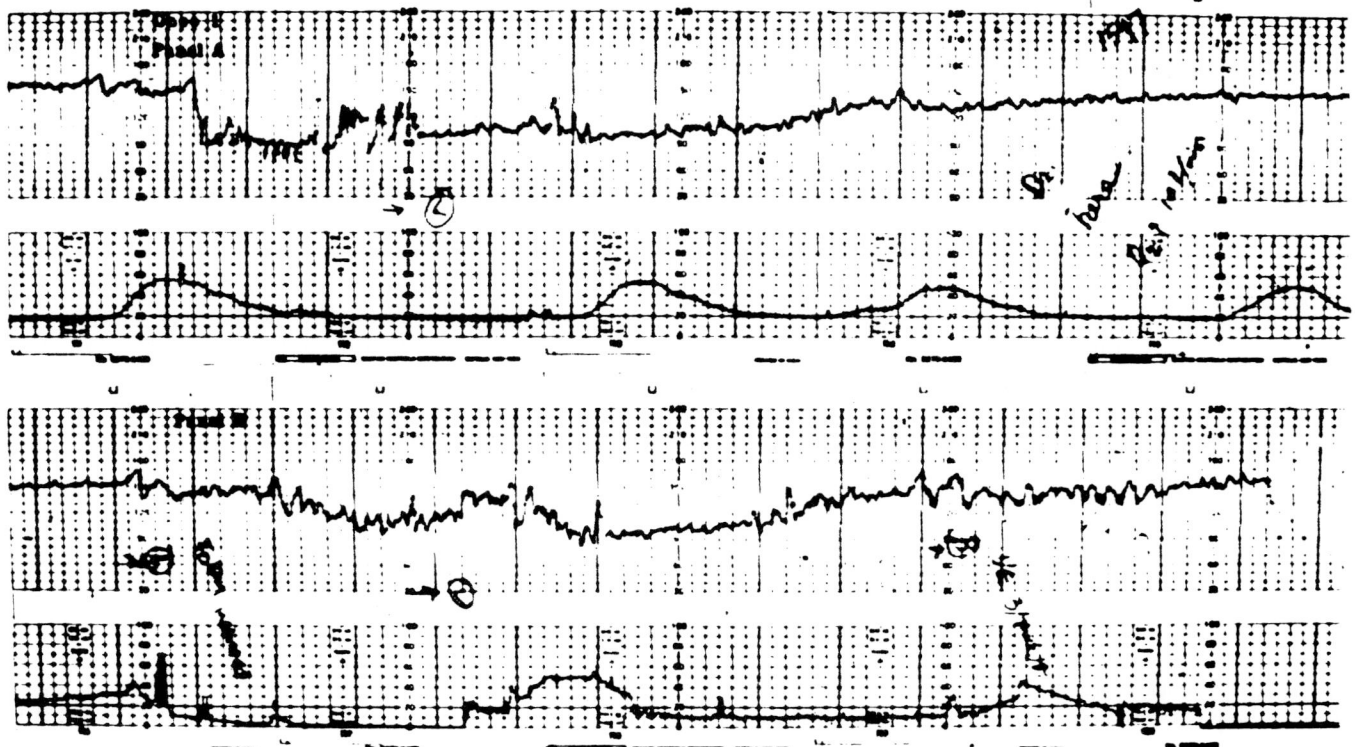

Figure 14–33. Recurrent unexplained prolonged decelerations.

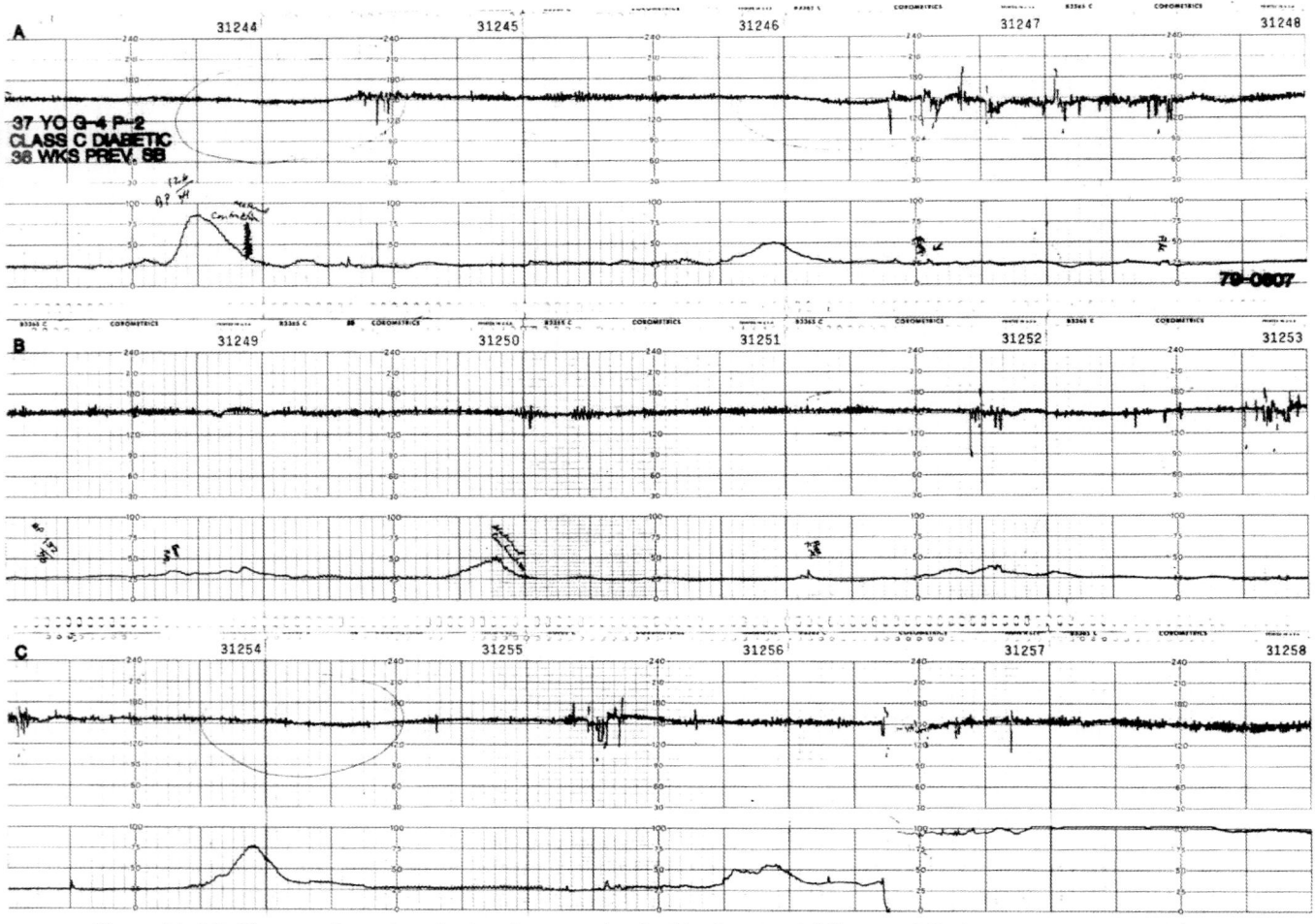

Figure 14–34. These persistent late decelerations associated with absent variability are difficult to recognize even with an internal electrode. This is a nonreassuring FHR pattern, which is often ominous. It is unlikely that such decelerations, associated with a normal baseline rate, would be recognized with intermittent auscultation.

emergencies with other patients often take a nurse away from the bedside for long periods of time. Second, in most of the studies, fetuses who entered labor may have been monitored electronically prior to randomization, and often very-high-risk patients were excluded from study. Ingemarsson et al. have shown that 50 percent of patients who will develop nonreassuring FHR patterns in labor will have a nonreassuring FHR pattern on admission.[68] And finally, in virtually all of the studies comparing EFM with auscultation, when the auscultated FHR was abnormal, the patient was then monitored electronically. Furthermore, there are nonreassuring FHR tracings that are quite indicative of hypoxia and acidosis that are not likely to be detected with auscultation (Fig. 14–34).

Therefore, it is reasonable to conclude that auscultation is an acceptable option for monitoring the fetus in labor when certain conditions are in place. The fetus should have a reassuring FHR on admission monitored electronically. The patient should have one-on-one nursing. The standards for frequency from the ACOG for auscultation are at least every 30 minutes in the first stage and every 15 minutes in the second stage for the low-risk patient and every 15 minutes in the first stage and every 5 minutes in the second stage for the high-risk patient.[16] Fetuses with abnormal FHR patterns on auscultation should have electronic monitoring to define the pattern and monitor for progression to worsening or nonreassuring patterns.

ASSESSMENT OF FETAL CONDITION AT BIRTH

The Apgar score was originally introduced as a tool to be used in guiding the need for neonatal resuscitation. Subsequently, this means of fetal assessment became used routinely for all births. However, the Apgar score has been expected to predict far more than was originally intended. Such expectations have included evaluating acid–base status at birth (i.e., the presence or absence of perinatal asphxia) and even predicting long-term prognosis. Unfortunately, the Apgar is a nonspecific measure of these parameters, as many other causes of fetal depression may mimic that seen with asphyxia, such as drugs, anomalies, prematurity, suctioning for meconium, and so forth. In situations where FHR patterns have been concerning and other back-up methods for evaluating fetal oxygenation or fetal acid–base status have been utilized, or in cases where the baby is unexpectedly depressed, it is important to specifically evaluate these parameters at birth, using umbilical cord blood gases. To accomplish this, a doubly clamped 10- to 30-cm section of umbilical cord is taken after the orginal cord clamping and separation of the baby from the cord. Using heparinized syringes, samples of umbilical artery and vein are separately obtained. These samples are evaluated for respiratory gases. Normal ranges for umbilical cord gases are shown in Table 14–1. Cord blood PO_2 or O_2 saturation is not useful, as many normal newborns are initially hypoxemic until normal extrauterine respiration is established. While cord pH, especially arterial, is the essential value, PCO_2 is also very important, as if the pH is low, the PCO_2 is used to determine whether the acidosis is respiratory or metabolic. Respiratory acidosis is not predictive of newborn or long-term injury and should correlate with little or no need for resuscitation. In addition, the cord gases should be used to correlate interpretation of the FHR patterns, as previously described in the sections on their pathophysiology and to determine the appropriateness of operative intervention or lack of it. These gases can help the pediatrician in determining the etiology of immediate complications and the need for more intense observation of the baby. In addition, these values are often useful if the baby develops any long-term neurologic injury in determining whether any such injury may have been related to peripartum asphyxia. Studies have shown that if such asphyxia is present, in order for it to result in long-term injury it must have been severe (metabolic acidosis with a pH <7.0 to 7.05) and be associated with multiple organ dysfunction in the newborn period.[2]

RISKS AND BENEFITS OF EFM

Electronic FHR monitoring was introduced with the hope that this modality would reduce or eliminate the devastating consequences of asphyxia. Enthusiasm for this new technology established the role of continuous FHR monitoring in labor before studies demonstrated its accuracy. Initial retrospective studies evaluated more that 135,000 patients and showed more than a threefold improvement in the intrapartum fetal death rate for patients monitored electronically.[1] However, the majority of subsequent prospective, randomized, controlled trials have failed to demonstrate an improvement in the intrapartum fetal death rate using EFM.[70–76] In these studies, however, electronic FHR monitoring was compared with frequent intermittent auscultation with one-on-one nursing, a standard that is difficult to maintain. Many patients with abnormal FHR patterns on admission were not randomized and, virtually always, patients with an abnormal FHR on auscultation were ultimately monitored electronically. A more recent randomized controlled trial of EFM versus intermittent auscultation did demonstrate a significant improvement in perinatal mortality in the electronically monitored group.[77] The past three decades have not shown a change in the 2 per 1,000 incidence of cerebral palsy, suggesting that the widespread use of EFM has not affected this problem. However, these data are somewhat difficult to analyze because of other changes occurring simultaneously. There has been a dramatic improvement in the survival of very-low-birthweight premature babies during this time period, and prematurity accounts for the majority of cerebral palsy. Second, term babies with asphyxia have had an increase in survival during this time period, thus allowing for a potential increase in surviving children with brain damage. Any of these factors may obscure an effect that FHR monitoring may have had in reducing the incidence of cerebral palsy. EFM has other potential benefits. These include an ability to understand the mechanism of developing hypoxia and treat it more specifically. It provides the ability to accurately monitor uterine contractions so we can better understand progress or lack of progress in labor as well as monitor the effects of oxy-

Table 14–1. NORMAL BLOOD GAS VALUES OF UMBILICAL ARTERY AND VEIN

	Mean Value	Normal Range*
Artery		
pH	7.27	7.15 to 7.38
PCO_2	50	35 to 70
Bicarbonate	23	17 to 28
Base excess	−3.6	−2.0 to −9.0
Vein		
pH	7.34	7.20 to 7.41
PCO_2	40	33 to 50
Bicarbonate	21	15 to 26
Base excess	−2.6	−1.0 to −8.0

*Values are ± 2 SD and represent a composite of multiple studies.
Data derived from Thorp and Rushing.[69]

tocin-stimulated contractions on fetal oxygenation. The monitor is ultimately, like all other monitors in intensive care situations, a labor-saving device allowing nurses to perform other tasks simultaneously.

EFM has several disadvantages, however. During the period in which FHR monitoring has risen in popularity, there was a parallel increase in the cesarean section rate. Certainly, this was not all caused by EFM, as there were many other changes in obstetric practice during this time period. In virtually all of the randomized controlled trials, EFM resulted in an increase in the cesarean section rate over intermittent auscultation without a concomitant improvement in outcome.[70-74] There is also, however, a desire to deliver babies before significant hypoxia has any potential to damage the baby, and the nonspecific changes in FHR only fuel this concern, setting up the current environment of excessive intervention. In reality, metabolic acidosis occurs in only about 2 percent of all labors, and even allowing for a reasonable amount of latitude in early intervention, cesarean section rates should not exceed 4 to 5 percent for this indication. Unfortunately, rates of 10 percent for NRFS are common. Thus, the need for better, more specific modalities to allow us to evaluate hypoxia and acidosis in the fetus with a nonreassuring FHR pattern are needed. Fetal pulse oximetry appears to have great potential, but its effect on cesarean section rates in real practice remains to be seen.

The second major problem associated with EFM is the fear of a lawsuit should the child be compromised in any way. The monitor has created an expectation of perfect outcome. The interpretation of abnormal FHR tracings is highly subjective and variable, and "experts" often give diametrically opposite interpretations of the same tracing. The modality itself is nonspecific, and babies with anomalies or preexisting brain damage will often have abnormal FHR tracings easily confused with ongoing hypoxia. Finally, a jury cannot help but be sympathetic to a family and baby with disfiguring and debilitating cerebral palsy, and large financial awards seem to be the only way at present to compensate these unfortunate victims. However, these outcomes are not consistent with what we know about asphyxia. More than 75 percent of brain-damaged children have causes that are *not* related to perinatal asphyxia. Many cases of asphyxia occur *prior to* labor or early in labor before the patient arrives in the hospital. Very few of these cases are truly preventable. Again, a modality such as fetal pulse oximetry would seem to have the potential to clarify whether an abnormal FHR pattern is truly hypoxic in origin and eliminate any subjectivity in interpretation. One can only hope that once these pressures are removed from the labor and delivery suite, the opportunity to do what is best for the fetus and mother will be enhanced and this will be the only motivating force.

SUMMARY

Electronic FHR monitoring has become the standard means for evaluating fetal oxygenation in labor. Because of fetal inaccessibility and the lack of alternatives to more specifically evaluate fetal oxygenation, this modality has been the only alternative. FHR monitoring is reliable when it tells us the fetus is well oxygenated, but more often unreliable when it suggests the fetus is "in distress." The recent change in terminology describing the abnormal FHR pattern as "nonreassuring" is a more accurate and honest depiction of the limitations of EFM in this situation. Despite or even because of these limitations, it is imperative that the clinician understand as much as possible about the underlying physiologic explanations of normal and abnormal FHR patterns, as this allows the only reasonable opportunity to appropriately evaluate and manage these changes. The goal of FHR monitoring should be to carefully and thoroughly monitor all patients in active labor; avoid unnecessary operative and nonoperative intervention for benign and innocuous FHR patterns; correct nonreassuring FHR patterns with noninvasive, etiology specific therapies when possible; or if not possible use appropriate means such as scalp pH, accelerations, or fetal pulse oximetry to rule out acidosis; and finally, if acidosis cannot be ruled out, operatively intervene in an expeditious manner appropriate for the entire clinical situation.

Key Points

➤ The goals of intrapartum fetal evaluation by electronic fetal heart rate monitoring and available back-up methods are to detect fetal hypoxia, reverse the hypoxia with nonsurgical means, or if unsuccessful, determine if the hypoxia has progressed to metabolic acidosis, and if so deliver the baby expeditiously to avoid the hypoxia and acidosis from resulting in any damage to the baby.

➤ EFM is an inherently suboptimal method of determining fetal hypoxia and acidosis, because many factors besides these variables may alter the FHR and mimic changes caused by hypoxia and acidosis. When the FHR is normal, its reliability in predicting the absence of fetal compromise is high, but when the FHR is abnormal, its reliability in predicting the presence of asphyxia is poor.

➤ The term "fetal distress" should be abandoned in favor of "nonreassuring fetal status," because when the fetal monitor suggests there may be a problem, in most circumstances we can only say that we are no longer reassured with a high degree of certainty that the fetus is well oxygenated.

➤ Late decelerations are always indicative of relative fetal hypoxia, and are caused by inadequate oxygen delivery, exchange, or uptake that is aggravated by the additional hypoperfusion of the placenta caused by contractions. Variable decelerations are caused by a decrease in umbilical cord flow resulting from cord compression or cord stretch. Prolonged decelerations may be caused by any mechanism that decreases fetal oxygenation.

➤ In labor, loss of variability, loss of accelerations, and tachycardia should only be interpreted as indicative of fetal compromise in the presence of nonreassuring decelerations (late, nonreassuring variable or prolonged decelerations), as signs of hypoxia should always precede signs of neurologic depression secondary to hypoxia.

➤ In the presence of oligohydramnios and variable decelerations, or with meconium, intrapartum amnioinfusion has been shown to decrease rates of cesarean delivery for NRFS and to decrease neonatal respiratory complications caused by meconium aspiration.

➤ In the presence of an otherwise nonreassuring FHR pattern, the presence of accelerations of the FHR, either spontaneous or elicited by scalp stimulation or vibroacoustic stimulation, indicate the absence of fetal acidosis. Their absence is associated with a 50 percent chance of fetal acidosis, but only in the setting of a nonreassuring FHR.

➤ Umbilical cord blood gases should be obtained and documented in situations where there is a nonreassuring or confusing FHR pattern during labor, where there is neonatal depression following birth, with premature babies, and when suctioning for meconium is performed. These values will help clarify the reasons for abnormal FHR patterns or for neonatal depression.

➤ Fetal pulse oximetry was approved in May 2000 by the FDA for use in term (≥36 weeks) patients with nonreassuring FHR patterns. This technology may improve our ability to more accurately interpret nonreassuring FHR patterns and may have the potential to decrease cesarean sections for NRFS.

➤ Although there is correlation between a nonreassuring FHR pattern and neonatal depression, the FHR is a poor predictor of long-term neurologic sequelae. Furthermore, fetuses with previous neurologic insults may have significantly abnormal FHR patterns even when they are well oxygenated in labor.

GLOSSARY

Acidemia – increased hydrogen ion concentration in blood.

Acidosis – increased hydrogen ion concentration in tissue.

Asphyxia – hypoxia with metabolic acidosis.

Base deficit – buffer base content below normal (this is calculated from a normogram using pH and P_{CO_2}).

Base excess – buffer base content above normal.

Hypoxemia – decreased oxygen concentration in blood.

Hypoxia – decreased oxygen concentration in tissue.

pH – the negative log of hydrogen ion concentration ($7.0 = 1 \times 10^{-7}$).

REFERENCES

1. Freeman RK, Garite TJ, Nageotte MP: Clinical management of fetal distress. *In* Fetal Heart Rate Monitoring, 2nd ed. Baltimore, Williams & Wilkins, 1991.
2. American College of Obstetricians and Gynecologists: Fetal and Neonatal Neurologic Injury. Technical Bulletin No. 163, January 1992.
3. Eastman NJ, Kohl SG, Maisel JE, et al: The obstetrical background of 753 cases of cerebral palsy. Obstet Gynecol Surv 17: 459, 1962.
4. Nelson KB, Ellenberg JH: Epidemiology of cerebral palsy. *In* Schoenberg BS (ed): Advances in Neurology, Vol. 19. New York, Raven Press, 1979.
5. Wegman M: Annual summary of vital statistics. Pediatrics 70: 835, 1982.
6. Benson RC, Shubeck F, Deutschberger J, et al: Fetal heart rate as a predictor of fetal distress: a report from the Collaborative Project. Obstet Gynecol 32:529, 1968.
7. Cremer M: Munch. Med Wochensem 58:811, 1906.
8. Hon EH, Hess OW: The clinical value of fetal electrocardiography. Am J Obstet Gynecol 79:1012, 1960.
9. Hon EH: The electronic evaluation of the fetal heart rate. Am J Obstet Gynecol 75:1215, 1958.
10. Hon EH: Observations on "pathologic" fetal bradycardia. Am J Obstet Gynecol 77:1084, 1959.

11. Caldeyro-Barcia R, Mendez-Bauer C, Poseiro JJ, et al: Control of human fetal heart rate during labor. *In* Cassels D (ed): The Heart and Circulation in the Newborn Infant. New York, Grune & Stratton, 1966.

12. Hammächer K: *In* Kaser O, Friedberg V, Oberk K (eds): Gynakologie v Gerburtshilfe BD II. Stutgart, Georg Thieme Verlag, 1967.

13. American College of Obstetricians and Gynecologists: Fetal Distress and Birth Asphyxia. Washington, DC, American College of Obstetricians and Gynecologists, ACOG Committee Opinion 137.

14. Vintzileos M, Campbell WA, Nochimson DJ, Weinbaum PJ: Degree of oligohydramnios and pregnancy outcome in patients with PROM. Obstet Gynecol 66:162, 1985.

15. Roach MR: The umbilical vessels. *In* Goodwin JM, Godden DO, Chance GW (eds): Perinatal Medicine. Baltimore, Williams & Wilkins, 1976, p 136.

16. American College of Obstetricians and Gynecologists: Fetal Heart Rate Patterns: Monitoring, Interpretation and Management. Technical Bulletin No. 207, July 1995.

17. Electronic Fetal Heart Rate Monitoring: Research Guidelines For Interpretation, National Institute of Child Health and Human Development Research Planning Workshop. Am J Obstet Gynecol 177:1385, 1997.

18. Schifferli P, Caldeyro-Barcia R: Effects of atropine and beta adrenergic drugs on the heart rate of the human fetus. *In* Boreus L (ed): Fetal Pharmacology. New York, Raven Press, 1973, p 259.

19. Bisonette JM: Relationship between continuous fetal heart rate patterns and Apgar score in the newborn. Br J Obstet Gynaecol 82:24, 1975.

20. Langer O, Cohen WR: Persistent fetal bradycardia during maternal hypoglycemia. Am J Obstet Gynecol 149:688, 1984.

21. Parsons MT, Owens CA, Spellacy WN: Thermic effects of tocolytic agents: decreased temperature with magnesium sulfate. Obstet Gynecol 69:88, 1987.

22. Gembruch U, Hansmann M, Redel DA, et al: Fetal complete heart block: antenatal diagnosis, significance and management. Eur J Obstet Gynecol Reprod Biol 31:9, 1989.

23. Druzen M, Ikenoue T, Murata Y, et al: A possible mechanism for the increase in FHR variability following hypoxemia. Presented at the 26th Annual Meeting of the Society for Gynecological Investigation, San Diego, California, March 23, 1979.

24. Paul WM, Quilligan EJ, MacLachlan T: Cardiovascular phenomenon associated with fetal head compression. Am J Obstet Gynecol 90:824, 1964.

25. Martin CB Jr, de Haan J, van der Wildt B, et al: Mechanisms of late deceleration in the fetal heart rate. A study with autonomic blocking agents in fetal lambs. Eur J Obstet Gynecol Reprod Biol 9:361, 1979.

26. Garite TJ: The relationship between late decelerations and fetal oxygen saturation. (Work in progress.)

27. Francis J, Garite T: The association between abruptio placentae and abnormal FHR patterns. (Submitted for publication.)

28. Barcroft J: Researches on Prenatal Life. Oxford, Blackwell Scientific Publications, 1946.

29. Lee ST, Hon EH: Fetal hemodynamic response to umbilical cord compression. Obstet Gynecol 22:554, 1963.

30. Kubli FW, Hon EH, Khazin AE, et al: Observations on heart rate and pH in the human fetus during labor. Am J Obstet Gynecol 104:1190, 1969.

31. Goodlin RC, Lowe EW: A functional umbilical cord occlusion heart rate pattern. The significance of overshoot. Obstet Gynecol 42:22, 1974.

32. Navot D, Yaffe H, Sadovsky E: The ratio of fetal heart rate accelerations to fetal movements according to gestational age. Am J Obstet Gynecol 149:92, 1984.

33. Clark S, Gimovsky M, Miller FC: Fetal heart rate response to scalp blood sampling. Am J Obstet Gynecol 144:706, 1982.

34. Clark S, Gimovsky M, Miller F: The scalp stimulation test: a clinical alternative to fetal scalp blood sampling. Am J Obstet Gynecol 148:274, 1984.

35. Smith C, Hguyen H, Phelan J, Paul R: Intrapartum assessment of fetal well-being: A comparison of fetal acoustic stimulation with acid base determinations. Am J Obstet Gynecol 155:776, 1986.

36. Kubli F, Ruttgers, H, Haller U, et al: Die antepartale fetale Herzfrequenz. II. Verhalten von Grundfrequenz, Fluktuation und Dezeratione bei antepartalem Fruchttod, Z. Gerburtshilfe Perinatol 176:309, 1972.

37. Shenker L: Clinical experience with fetal heart rate monitoring of 1000 patients in labor. Am J Obstet Gynecol 115:1111, 1973.

38. Modanlou H, Freeman RK: Sinusoidal fetal heart rate pattern: its definition and clinical significance. Am J Obstet Gynecol 142:1033, 1982.

39. Murata Y, Miyake Y, Yamamoto T, et al: Experimentally produced sinusoidal fetal heart rate pattern in the chronically instrumented fetal lamb. Am J Obstet Gynecol 153:693, 1985.

40. Angel J, Knuppel R, Lake M: Sinusoidal fetal heart rate patterns associated with intravenous butorphanol administration. Am J Obstet Gynecol 149:465, 1984.

41. Epstein H, Waxman A, Gleicher N, et al: Meperidine induced sinusoidal fetal heart rate pattern and reversal with naloxone. Obstet Gynecol 59:225, 1982.

42. Murata Y, Martin CB, Ikenoue T, et al: Fetal heart rate accelerations and late decelerations during the course of intrauterine death in chronically catheterized rhesus monkeys. Am J Obstet Gynecol 144:218, 1982.

43. Dildy G, Clark S, Loucks C: Intrapartum fetal pulse oximetry: the effects of maternal hyperoxia on fetal oxygen saturation mark. Am J Obstet Gynecol 171:1120, 1994.

44. Noakes TD: Fluid replacement during exercise. Exerc Sport Sci Rev 21:297, 1993.

45. Garite TJ, Weeks J, Peters-Phair K, et al: A randomized controlled trial of the effect of increased intravenous hydration on the course of labor in nulliparas. Am J Obstet Gynecol (in press).

46. Lipshitz J: Use of B2 sympathomimetic drug as a temporizing measure in the treatment of acute fetal distress. Am J Obstet Gynecol 129:31, 1977.

47. Tejani N, Verma UL, Chatterjee S, et al: Terbutaline in the management of acute intrapartum fetal acidosis. J Reprod Med 28:857, 1983.

48. Arias F: Intrauterine resuscitation with terbutaline: a method for the management of acute intrapartum fetal distress. Am J Obstet Gynecol 131:39, 1977.

49. Patriarcho MS, Viechnicki BN, Hutchinson TA: A study on intrauterine fetal resuscitation with terbutaline. Am J Obstet Gynecol 157:383, 1987.

50. Burke MS, Porreco RP, Day D, et al: Intrauterine resuscitation with tocolysis: an alternate month clinical trail. J Perinatol 10:296, 1989.

51. Miyazaki F, Nevarez F: Saline amnioinfusion for relief of repetitive variable decelerations: a prospective randomized study. Am J Obstet Gynecol 153:301, 1985.

52. Nageotte MP, Freeman RK, Garite TJ, et al: Prophylactic intrapartum amnioinfusion in patients with preterm premature rupture of membranes. Am J Obstet Gynecol 153:557, 1985.

53. Owen J, Henson BV, Hauth JC: A prospective randomized study of saline solution amnioinfusion. Am J Obstet Gynecol 162:1146, 1990.

54. Delee JB, Pollack C: Intrauterine injection of saline to replace the amniotic fluid. Obstet Gynecol 1925.

55. Miyazaki F, Taylor N: Saline amnioinfusion for relief of variable or prolonged decelerations. Am J Obstet Gynecol 14:670, 1983.

56. Pierce J, Gaudier FL, Sanchez-Ramos L: Intrapartum amnioinfusion for meconium-stained fluid: meta-analysis of prospective clinical trials. Obstet Gynecol 95:1051, 2000.

57. Wenstrom K, Andrews WW, Maher JE: Amnioinfusion survey: prevalence, protocols and complications. Obstet Gynecol 86:572, 1995.

58. Clark SL, Paul RH: Intrapartum fetal surveillance: the role of fetal scalp blood sampling. Am J Obstet Gynecol 153:717, 1985.

59. Goodwin TM, Milner-Masterson C, Paul R: Elimination of fetal scalp blood sampling on a large clinical service. Obstet Gynecol 83:971, 1994.

60. Johnson N: Development and potential of pulse oximetry. Contemp Rev Obstet Gynecol 3:193, 1991.

61. Nijiland R, Jongsma HW, Nijhuis JG, et al: Arterial oxygen saturation in relation to metabolic acidosis in fetal lambs. Am J Obstet Gynecol 172:810, 1995.

62. Kuhnert M, Seelbach-Gobel B, Butterwegge M: Predictive agreement between the fetal arterial oxygen saturation and fetal scalp pH: results of the German multicenter study. Am J Obstet Gynecol 178:330, 1998.

63. Dildy G, Thorp JA, Yeast JD, et al: The relationship between oxygen saturation and pH in umbilical blood: implications for intrapartum fetal oxygen saturation monitoring. Am J Obstet Gynecol 175:682, 1996.

64. Dildy GA, van den Berg PP, Katz M, et al: Intrapartum fetal pulse oximetry: fetal oxygen saturation trends during labor and relation to delivery outcome. Am J Obstet Gynecol 171:679, 1994.

65. Garite TJ, Dildy GA, McNamara H, et al: A multicenter controlled trial of fetal pulse oximetry in the intrapartum management of non-reassuring fetal heart rate patterns. Am J Obstet Gynecol 183:1049, 2000.

66. Guidelines for Perinatal Care: American Academy of Pediatrics and American College of Obstetricians and Gynecologists, 4th ed. Washington, DC, ACOG, 1997, p 112.

67. Windle WF: Neuropathology of certain forms of mental retardation. Science 140:1186, 1963.

68. Ingemarsson I, Arulkumaran S, Ingemarsson E, et al: Admission test: a screening test for fetal distress in labor. Obstet Gynecol 68:800, 1986.

69. Thorp JA, Rushing RS: Umbilical cord blood gas analysis. Obstet Gynecol Clin North Am 26:695, 1999.

70. Haverkamp AD, Thompson HE, McFee JG, et al: The evaluation of continuous fetal heart rate monitoring in high risk pregnancy. Am J Obstet Gynecol 125:310, 1976.

71. Haverkamp AD, Orleans M, Langendoerfer S, et al: A controlled trial of the differential effects of intrapartum fetal monitoring. Am J Obstet Gynecol 134:399, 1979.

72. Renou P, Chang A, Anderson I, et al: Controlled trial of fetal intensive care. Am J Obstet Gynecol 126:470, 1976.

73. Kelso IM, Parsons RJ, Lawrence GF, et al: An assessment of continuous fetal heart rate monitoring in labor: a randomized trial. Am J Obstet Gynecol 131:526, 1978.

74. Wood C, Renou P, Oates J, et al: A controlled trial of fetal heart rate monitoring in a low-risk population. Am J Obstet Gynecol 141:527, 1981.

75. McDonald D, Grant A, Sheridan-Pereira M, et al: The Dublin randomized control trial of intrapartum fetal heart rate monitoring. Am J Obstet Gynecol 152:524, 1985.

76. Leveno KJ, Cunningham FG, Nelson S, et al: A prospective comparison of selective and universal electronic fetal monitoring in 34,995 pregnancies. N Engl J Med 315:615, 1986.

77. Vintzileos AM, Antsaklis A, Varvarigos I, et al: A randomized trial of intrapartum electronic fetal heart rate monitoring versus intermittent auscultation. Obstet Gynecol 81:899, 1993.

Obstetric Anesthesia

JOY L. HAWKINS, DAVID H. CHESTNUT, AND CHARLES P. GIBBS

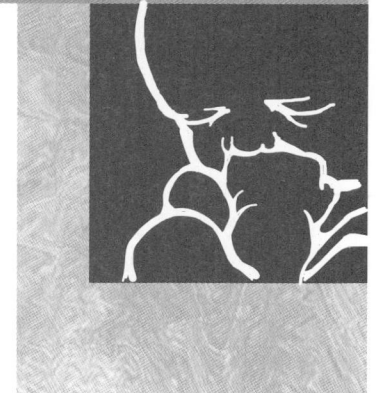

The word "anesthesia" encompasses all techniques used by anesthesiologists: general anesthesia, regional anesthesia, local anesthesia, and analgesia. Traditionally, general anesthesia includes four stages during which not only sensation but also consciousness and motor and reflex activities are gradually lost. During stage I, termed analgesia, memory and sensitivity to pain fade, yet consciousness and protective reflexes such as swallowing and laryngeal closure persist. Inhalation analgesia may be used for vaginal delivery, commonly in combination with local infiltration or pudendal block. Alone, this degree of anesthesia is not sufficient for even minor surgical incisions, including episiotomy. Stage II, the excitement stage, borders consciousness and unconsciousness. The patient may be agitated and uncooperative. Protective laryngeal reflexes may be either hyperactive or obtunded. Anesthesiologists avoid the second stage by keeping the patient in stage I or by rapidly inducing stage III with the aid of fast-acting barbiturates and muscle relaxants. The patient must also pass through this stage on awakening. Induction of and emergence from general anesthesia are usually the most dangerous times for the patient, because marked cardiovascular, respiratory, and laryngeal reflex changes occur.

Stage III, which is used for most surgical procedures, has four planes. As anesthesia deepens, it progressively depresses the central nervous, cardiovascular, and respiratory systems. Laryngeal reflexes nearly disappear; thus, vomiting or regurgitation render the patient particularly susceptible to aspiration unless her airway is protected by an endotracheal tube. Stage IV terminates in death.

Anesthesiologists can produce all stages of general

anesthesia. With the proper dose, concentration, and combination of agents, a specific anesthetic technique is matched to the requirements of a given procedure. The requirements for general anesthesia for cesarean delivery differ considerably from those for craniotomy, cholecystectomy, or exploratory laparotomy for a ruptured ectopic pregnancy, yet all these patients will be rendered unconscious, immobile, and pain free.

Balanced general anesthesia is the type of general anesthesia used for obstetrics; it usually refers to various combinations of barbiturates, inhalation agents, opioids, and muscle relaxants as opposed to high concentrations of potent inhalation agents alone. General anesthesia is used in obstetrics mainly for cesarean section and rarely is required for vaginal delivery.

Regional analgesia/anesthesia uses local anesthetics to provide sensory as well as various degrees of motor blockade over a specific region of the body. In obstetrics, regional techniques include major blocks, such as spinal and lumbar or caudal epidural, as well as minor blocks, such as paracervical, pudendal, and local infiltration (Fig. 15–1). In some cases, the anesthesiologist may combine a local anesthetic and opioid for epidural or spinal administration.

PAIN PATHWAYS

Pain during the first stage of labor results primarily from cervical dilation and secondarily from uterine contractions themselves. Painful sensations travel from the uterus via visceral afferent (sympathetic) nerves that enter the spinal cord through the posterior segments of thoracic spinal nerves 10, 11, and 12 (Fig. 15–1). Pain during the second stage of labor results primarily from

---

The reader is referred to the Appendix for illustrations of anatomy relevant to this discussion.

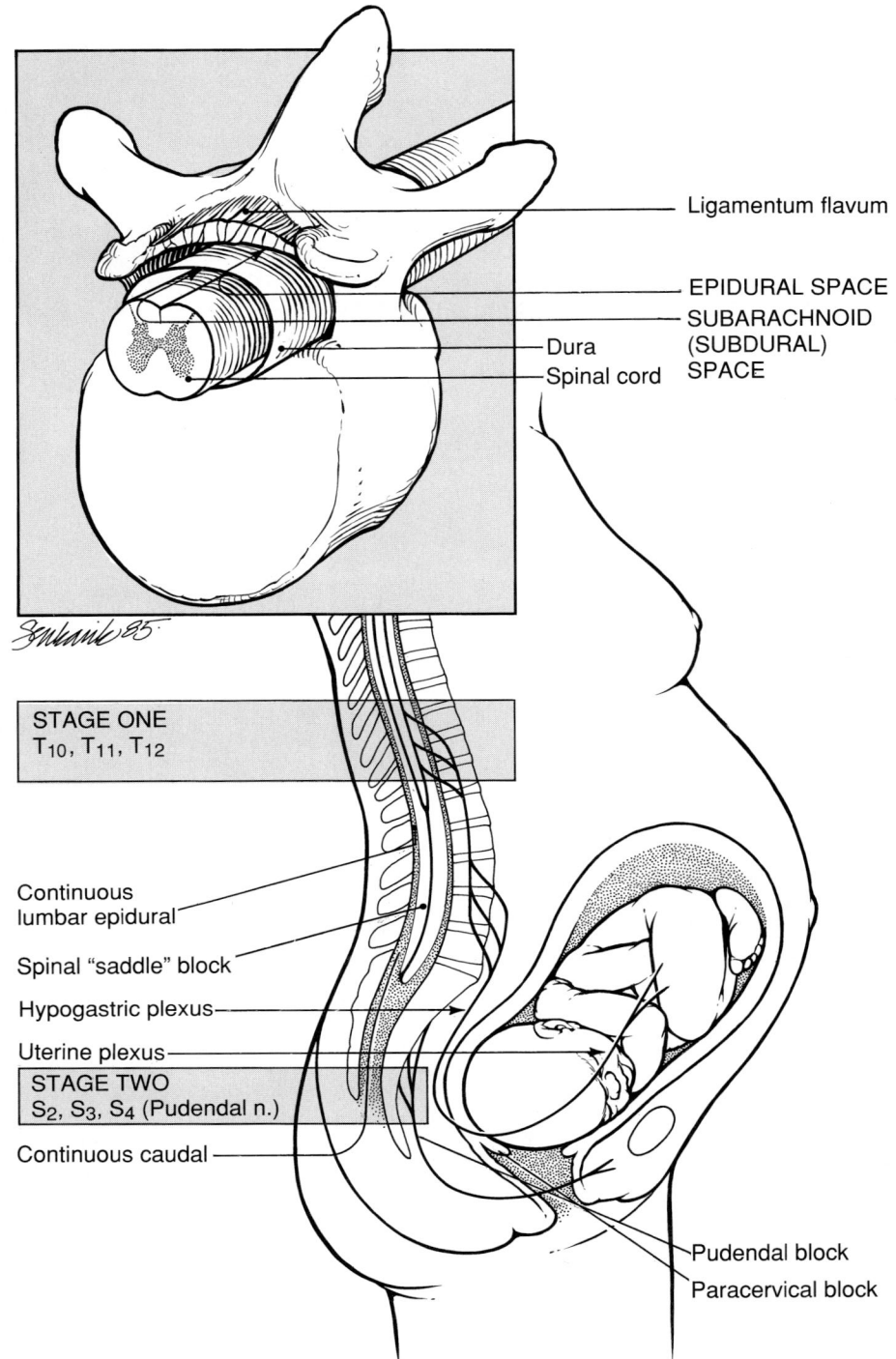

Ligamentum flavum

EPIDURAL SPACE

SUBARACHNOID
(SUBDURAL)
SPACE

Dura

Spinal cord

STAGE ONE
T₁₀, T₁₁, T₁₂

Continuous
lumbar epidural

Spinal "saddle" block

Hypogastric plexus

Uterine plexus

STAGE TWO
S₂, S₃, S₄ (Pudendal n.)

Continuous caudal

Pudendal block

Paracervical block

Figure 15–1. Pain pathways of labor and delivery and nerves blocked by various anesthetic techniques.

distention of the pelvic floor, vagina, and perineum by the presenting part of the fetus. (Some physicians contend that uterine contractions themselves may also contribute to pain during the second stage.) The sensory fibers of sacral nerves 2, 3, and 4 (i.e., the pudendal nerve) transmit painful impulses from the perineum to the spinal cord (Fig. 15–1).

PERSONNEL

An anesthesiologist is a physician who has completed 4 years of postgraduate residency training in anesthesia. A nurse anesthetist is a registered nurse (with variable background and training) who has completed a 2- to 3-year training program sponsored by the American Association of Nurse Anesthetists. Most states require that nurse anesthetists be supervised or directed by a physician. Ideally, an anesthesiologist assumes this role, which results in an efficient anesthesiologist/anesthetist team. Either an anesthesiologist working independently or an anesthesiologist/anesthetist team provides anesthesia for 96 percent of obstetric procedures in larger hospitals in the United States.[1] Nurse anesthetists, independent of anesthesiologists, provide anesthesia for 4 percent of operations in larger hospitals, but 59 percent of obstetric procedures in hospitals with fewer than 500 births per year.[1] Almost all hospitals with more than 300 beds will have an anesthesiologist on the medical staff, while only 16 percent of hospitals with fewer than 50 beds will have an anesthesiologist available.[2] In this situation, the operating surgeon or obstetrician must assume the role of supervisor. When anesthetic-related untoward events occur, the nonanesthesiologist supervising a nurse anesthetist often will be ultimately responsible for the treatment and outcome of those events. The American Society of Anesthesiologists and the American College of Obstetricians and Gynecologists (ACOG) issued the Joint Statement on the Optimal Goals for Anesthesia Care in Obstetrics.[3] That statement recommends that there be a qualified anesthesiologist responsible for all anesthetics in every hospital providing obstetric care. The statement notes: "There are obstetric units where obstetricians or obstetrician-supervised nurse anesthetists administer anesthetics. The administration of general or regional anesthesia requires both medical judgment and technical skills. Thus, a physician with privileges in anesthesiology should be readily available."[3]

PAIN AND STRESS

When considering obstetric anesthesia, reasonable questions include the following: How painful is labor? How stressful is labor? What are the effects of pain and stress? What role does anesthesia play? Melzack and colleagues[4] provided perhaps the most sophisticated, enlightened, and in-depth study of labor pain. Using the McGill Pain Questionnaire, which measures intensity and quality of pain, these investigators quantified and described the reaction of 87 nulliparous and 54 parous patients to labor pain. When pain rating index scores were assigned to each parturient's description of labor pain and compared with those of other patients suffering different kinds of pain, 59 percent of nulliparous and 43 percent of parous patients described their labor pain in terms more severe than did those suffering back

and cancer pain. More than 50 percent of the obstetric patients described their pain as sharp, cramping, and intense; more than 33 percent as aching, throbbing, stabbing, shooting, heavy, and exhaustive; and 25 percent of nulliparous patients and 9 percent of parous patients as horrible or excruciating. In contrast, only 24 percent of parous patients and 9 percent of nulliparous patients described the pain as relatively minor. Although those with childbirth training reported less pain than those without such training, the differences were small. Eighty-one percent of trained patients requested epidural anesthesia compared with 82 percent of those without training. The most substantial predictors of pain intensity proved to be socioeconomic status and prior menstrual difficulties.

How does the body respond to the pain and stress of labor? Does the response affect mother, fetus, or both? Most investigators have described and quantified the body's response to stress in terms of the release of certain hormones, namely, adrenocorticotropic hormone (ACTH), cortisol, catecholamines, and β-endorphins (Fig. 15–2).

What kind of response does labor invoke? The following have been reported: prolonged increases of plasma cortisol levels in early labor,[5] increases of both ACTH and cortisol during labor and immediately postpartum,[6] and increases in epinephrine, norepinephrine, and β-endorphins throughout labor.[7,8] These are the same responses described during other types of pain,[9] surgical stress,[10] and even hypoxia.[11] Thus, many of the hormones associated with stress are elevated during labor.

What are the effects of these hormones on pregnancy? Elevated epinephrine levels are found in patients with anxiety and prolonged labor, which is not surprising, considering the well-known uterine relaxant effects of β-adrenergic agents.[12] Animal studies indicate that both epinephrine and norepinephrine can decrease uterine blood flow and cause fetal asphyxia.[13–15] Furthermore, these alterations may occur without clinical signs, because uteroplacental blood flow can change in the absence of heart rate and blood pressure change.[14] Maternal psychological stress can detrimentally affect the fetal cardiovascular system and acid–base status as demonstrated in baboons and monkeys.[16–18] In pregnant sheep, catecholamines increase and uterine blood flow decreases after both painful and nonpainful stimuli (Fig. 15–3). In humans, sudden noise and flashing lights predictably increase maternal heart rate. Not so predictably, fetal heart rate responds similarly within 45 seconds.[19] Fear produces similar effects.[19]

If one accepts that anxiety, pain, and labor are forms of stress and that stress may be harmful, can anesthesia, by alleviating pain, minimize the effects of that stress? Postpartum women suffer objective deficits in cognitive and memory function.[20] Intrapartum analgesia

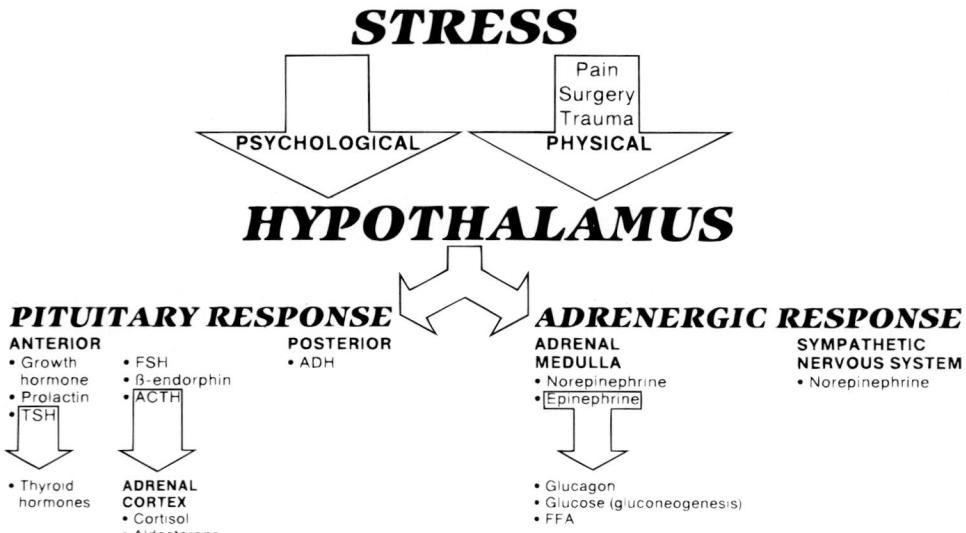

Figure 15–2. The stress response.

does not exacerbate, but rather *lessens* the defect compared to unmedicated parturients. Presumably, cognitive function is adversely affected by the stress of labor, which is mitigated by judicious use of analgesics. Epidural anesthesia prevents increases in both cortisol and 11-hydroxycorticosteroid levels during labor,[21,22] but systemically administered opioids do not.[23] Epidural anesthesia also attenuates elevations of epinephrine, norepinephrine,[7] and endorphin levels.[24] Presumably, regional anesthesia blocks afferent stimuli to the hypo-thalamus and thus inhibits the body's response to stress[25] (Fig. 15–4).

What of the fetus? There is convincing evidence that anesthesia, sedation, or both effectively decrease asphyxia-inducing effects of psychologically induced stress in monkey and baboon fetuses.[18,26] Furthermore, acid–base status of human infants whose mothers receive epidural anesthesia during the first stage of labor is altered less than infants of mothers who do not receive regional anesthesia. During the second stage of labor, the salutary effects of anesthesia may be limited to the mother.[27]

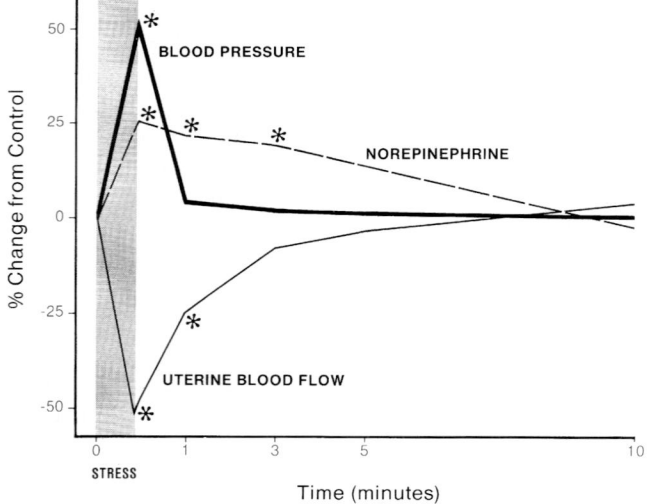

✳ Significantly different
from control, P<0.05

Figure 15–3. Effects of electrically induced stress (30 to 60 seconds) on maternal mean arterial blood pressure, plasma norepinephrine levels, and uterine blood flow. (Modified from Shnider SM, Wright RG, Levinson G, et al: Uterine blood flow and plasma norepinephrine changes during maternal stress in the pregnant ewe. Anesthesiology 50:526, 1979.)

ANESTHESIA FOR LABOR

Psychoprophylaxis

Psychoprophylaxis is a nonpharmacologic method of minimizing the perception of painful uterine contractions. Relaxation, concentration on breathing, gentle massage (effleurage), and partner participation contribute to its effectiveness. One of the method's most valuable contributions is that it is often taught in prepared childbirth classes where patients learn about the physiology of pregnancy and the normal processes of labor and delivery. In many instances, partner and wife may visit the hospital and the labor and delivery suites before labor, to mitigate the fear of the unknown.

Although psychoprophylactic techniques may discourage the use of drugs, not all patients are alike and not all will be satisfied with psychoprophylaxis.[28] The greatest disadvantage is the potential for believing the use of drug-induced pain relief is a sign of failure and

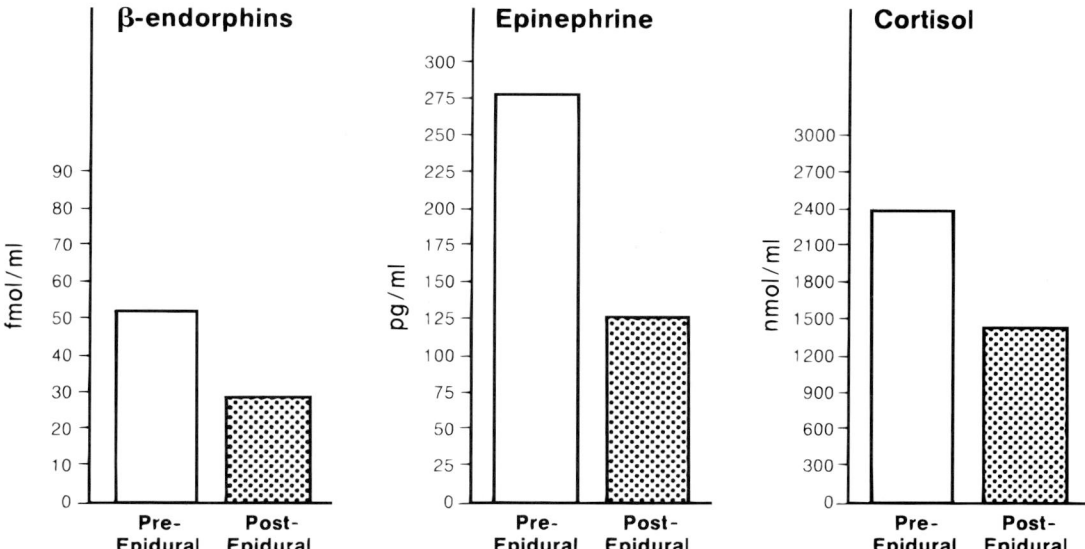

Figure 15–4. Effects of epidural analgesia on the response to stress.

will harm the child. Those who believe that accepting analgesia is a sign of failure do not understand that some labors are longer and/or more painful than others and that some patients have lower pain thresholds than others. Furthermore, there are times when anesthesia will be *required* for vaginal or cesarean delivery. In these instances, both mother and fetus should benefit from all that modern medicine can provide. Anyone who doubts that modern anesthetic techniques can be applied to the pregnant patient without harm to her or to her unborn child need only be aware that approximately 25 percent of all births in the United States today are cesarean births. All of these patients receive anesthesia, yet few believe that such anesthesia results in harm to the fetus, and no one would suggest that these patients avoid anesthesia.

Systemic Opioid Analgesia

Opioids (also known as narcotics) are drugs possessing morphine-like pharmacologic actions.[29] Morphine and codeine are natural alkaloids derived from opium. Opioids such as hydromorphone and heroin are semi-synthetic compounds made by a simple alteration of the morphine molecule. Meperidine, alphaprodine, and fentanyl are synthetic compounds resembling morphine.[29] All opioids provide pain relief and a sense of euphoria, hence their use in obstetrics. However, opioids also produce respiratory depression, the degree of which is usually comparable for equipotent analgesic doses. Also, all opioids freely cross the placenta to the newborn.[30,31] Therefore, the risk associated with opioids for obstetrics is obvious—all can produce respiratory depression in both mother and newborn.[32,33] Nevertheless, when used properly, they can be safe and effective.

In the past, because large doses of the long-acting opioids (e.g., morphine) were given intramuscularly throughout labor, depressant effects on the infant were observed.[34] Currently, morphine is rarely used for pain relief during labor. Instead, smaller doses of other opioids are used and are administered via the more predictable intravenous route. Therefore, recent reports detail little neonatal depression.[35,36] In addition, anesthesiologists recently have begun to give opioids (with or without local anesthetics) via the epidural or subarachnoid (i.e., spinal) space. Opioids may then bind to opioid receptors in the spinal cord and thereby produce segmental analgesia.

The immediate treatment for respiratory depression caused by opioids is ventilation. Infants depressed by opioids may be sleepy and may not breathe adequately. Initially, they typically are not hypoxic, hypercarbic, or acidotic; however, if they are not ventilated, then hypoxia, hypercarbia, and acidosis will result. Hypoxia and acidosis (not opioids per se) may cause neonatal injury. If properly cared for, infants with opioid-induced depression will suffer no ill effects. Proper care includes ventilation, oxygenation, gentle stimulation, and the judicious use of the opioid antagonist naloxone. Positive-pressure ventilation is the single most effective measure and can be provided via face mask or intubation. Without ventilation, other measures are fruitless.

Naloxone, 0.1 mg/kg, should be given intravenously if possible, but it can be given intramuscularly or subcutaneously. This dose (i.e., 0.1 mg/kg) is higher than that previously recommended and should ensure an increased likelihood of effectiveness.[37] It may be repeated in 3 to 5 minutes if there is no immediate response. If there is no response after two or three doses, the depression is most likely *not* due to opioid effect.[38] Nursery personnel should be advised when naloxone has been given because it has a short duration of action, and therefore repeat administration may be necessary in the nursery. Naloxone should not be used prophylactically. Specifically, it should not be given to the mother just before delivery. Pain relief afforded the mother by the opioid will be antagonized. Furthermore, because of the unpredictability of placental transfer, it is difficult to estimate how much naloxone would get to the infant. Indeed, naloxone may not be necessary at all. It should not be given routinely to all opioid-exposed newborns.[48] Finally, naloxone should not be given to infants of opioid-dependent mothers, because this may precipitate withdrawal in the physically dependent newborn infant.[48] Naloxone is a useful drug that should be available whenever opioids are used. However, it is an adjunct to ventilation, not a substitute for it.

Opioids also may produce neurobehavioral changes in the newborn, and these changes may persist for as long as 2 to 4 days.[39,40] Although some have indicated that the effects may persist and be influential in later life, such has not been proved true.[41] In fact, the significance of neurobehavioral changes in general is open to question.

An important and significant disadvantage of opioid analgesia is the prolonged effect of these agents on gastric emptying. When parenteral or epidural opioids are used, gastric emptying is prolonged, and if general anesthesia becomes necessary, the risk of aspiration is increased.[42-44]

Morphine

Morphine is now primarily used to provide sedation and rest during the early prodromal stages of labor. With intramuscular administration, the onset of analgesia occurs in 10 to 20 minutes and lasts for approximately 2.5 to 4 hours.[29] With intravenous administration, the onset of analgesia is less than 3 to 5 minutes and lasts approximately 1.5 to 2 hours. Occasionally, bradycardia will follow an injection of morphine. Also, histamine release may occur and result in orthostatic hypotension. One of the more frequent and bothersome side effects of morphine is nausea and vomiting. Urinary retention is also common. As with most opioids, a small amount of morphine is eliminated in the urine unchanged. The remainder is gradually detoxified by the liver.

Meperidine (Demerol)

Meperidine 100 mg is roughly equianalgesic to 10 mg morphine, but is reported to have a less depressive effect on respiration.[33] Usually, 25 mg is administered intravenously, or 50 to 75 mg is given intramuscularly.

Shnider and Moya[32] showed that both timing and dosage influence neonatal depression. When administered within 1 hour of delivery, little neonatal depression as reflected by Apgar scores or time to sustained respiration occurs. With a 50-mg intramuscular dose, the greatest depression occurs during the second hour; when 75 to 100 mg is administered, this effect extends through the second and third hours. Notably, when secobarbital, 100 mg, is added, depression extends even further to the fourth hour after administration.[32] The peculiar metabolism of meperidine may partially explain the lack of depression in the first hour. Normeperidine is an active metabolite of meperidine. Normeperidine concentrations increase slowly, and therefore it exerts its effect on the newborn during the second hour after administration.[30,45] Furthermore, Kuhnert and colleagues[46,47] observed that multiple doses of meperidine result in greater accumulation of both meperidine and normeperidine in fetal tissues.

The analgesic action of meperidine begins in approximately 10 to 20 minutes and persists for 2 to 3 hours after intramuscular administration. Lazebnik and colleagues[48] noted that plasma concentrations of meperidine are higher after deltoid injection than after gluteus muscle injection. They suggested that the deltoid muscle might be the preferred intramuscular site during labor. Intravenously, the onset of analgesia begins almost immediately and lasts approximately 1.5 to 2 hours. Side effects are similar to those of morphine except that tachycardia occasionally results rather than bradycardia. As with morphine, nausea and vomiting are frequent, and there is considerable delay in gastric emptying. Slightly less urinary retention occurs with meperidine than with morphine.[29]

Fentanyl

Fentanyl is a short-acting synthetic opioid with rapid pharmacokinetics and no active metabolites. In a randomized comparison with meperidine, fentanyl 50 to 100 μg every hour provided equivalent analgesia, with fewer neonatal effects and less maternal sedation and nausea.[36] The main drawback of fentanyl is its short duration of action requiring frequent redosing or the use of a patient-controlled intravenous infusion pump.[49,50]

Butorphanol (Stadol)

Butorphanol is a synthetic agonist-antagonist opioid analgesic drug. One to 2 mg is administered intravenously and compares favorably with 40 to 80 mg of meperidine.[35,51] Nausea and vomiting appear to occur less with butorphanol than with other opioids.[35] The major advantage is a ceiling effect for respiratory depression; that is, respiratory depression from multiple doses appears to plateau.[52,53] The major side effects are somnolence, dizziness, dysphoria, and opioid withdrawal syndrome in an opioid-dependent patient.

Nalbuphine (Nubain)

Nalbuphine is another synthetic agonist-antagonist opioid. Its analgesic potency is similar to that of morphine when compared on a milligram-per-milligram basis. As with butorphanol, a reported advantage of nalbuphine is its ceiling effect for respiratory depression.[54] It may cause less maternal nausea and vomiting than meperidine, but it tends to produce more maternal sedation and dizziness, as well as the risk of opioid withdrawal in susceptible patients.[55]

Patient-Controlled Opioid Analgesia

In some centers, opioids are administered by patient-controlled intravenous infusion. The infusion pump is programmed to give a predetermined dose of drug upon patient demand. The physician may program the pump to include a lock-out interval (i.e., there is a minimum interval between doses of drug). Thus, the physician may limit the total dose administered per hour. Advantages of this method include the sense of autonomy, which patients appreciate, as well as the fact that one avoids lengthy delays between doses. In general, this practice results in a decreased total dose of opioid during labor.[56,57]

Sedatives

Sedatives do not possess analgesic qualities and are most often used early in labor to relieve anxiety or to augment the analgesic qualities and reduce the nausea associated with opioids. All sedatives and hypnotics cross the placenta freely. Perhaps the most important property of these drugs is that, except for the benzodiazepines, they have no known antagonists. Those most frequently used are barbiturates, phenothiazines, and benzodiazepines.

Barbiturates

Because barbiturates and other sedatives are not analgesic, patients may be less able to cope with pain than if they had received no pharmacologic assistance at all; that is, normal coping mechanisms may be blunted.[58,59] Although barbiturates can depress both cardiovascular and respiratory functions in mother and newborn, low doses have little effect. The combination of barbiturate (100 mg secobarbital) with opioid (50 to 100 mg meperidine) increases the degree of neonatal depression.[32] In addition, effects that do occur may persist for a prolonged time. For example, attention span can be depressed for as long as 2 to 4 days.[60] Thus, these drugs should rarely be used during labor.

Phenothiazines

Promethazine is perhaps the most widely used phenothiazine. However, propiomazine, promazine, and hydroxyzine are also commonly administered. When given in small doses in combination with an opioid, these drugs do not seem to produce additional neonatal depression.[61,62] However, like the barbiturates, these agents rapidly cross the placenta and, in large doses, can depress the fetus for a significant period. Also like the barbiturates, they have no known antagonist.

Benzodiazepines

Diazepam was the first widely used benzodiazepine. A major disadvantage of diazepam is that it disrupts thermoregulation in newborns, which renders them less able to maintain body temperature.[63] The drug may persist in the fetal circulation for as long as 1 week.[64] As with many drugs, beat-to-beat variability of the fetal heart rate is reduced markedly even with a single intravenous dose (i.e., 5 to 10 mg). However, these doses have little effect on acid–base or clinical status of the newborn.[65] Sodium benzoate, a buffer in the injectable form of diazepam, competes with bilirubin binding to albumin. Thus, unbound bilirubin is increased and could be a threat to infants susceptible to kernicterus.[66] Unlike diazepam, midazolam is water soluble, and it is shorter acting than diazepam.[67] There are conflicting data regarding its effects on the fetus/neonate.[68,69]

A disadvantage of all the benzodiazepines is their tendency to cause maternal amnesia, a significant disadvantage if the drug is given near the time of delivery.[70] Flumazenil, a specific benzodiazepine antagonist, can reliably reverse benzodiazepine-induced sedation and ventilatory depression.[71]

PLACENTAL TRANSFER

Essentially, all analgesic and anesthetic agents except muscle relaxants cross the placenta,[72–75] although muscle relaxants cross in only small amounts. That muscle relaxants do not readily cross the placenta is one of the major factors that enables anesthesiologists to utilize general anesthesia for cesarean delivery without causing fetal paralysis.

Placental transfer of any agent begins with uptake of the agent into the bloodstream of the mother and thus distribution to all internal organs, one of which is the uterus. The distribution of uterine blood flow deter-

---

**Factors Influencing Placental Transfer
from Mother to Fetus**

Drug
  Molecular weight
  Lipid solubility
  Ionization, pH of blood
  Spatial configuration
Maternal
  Uptake into bloodstream
  Distribution via circulation
  Uterine blood flow
    Amount
    Distribution (myometrium vs. placenta)
Placental
  Circulation: intermittent spurting arterioles
  Lipid membrane: Fick's law of simple diffusion
Fetal
  Circulation: ductus venosus, foramen ovale,
    ductus arteriosus

---

mines the final common pathway to the uterus and placenta. Eighty percent of uterine blood flow goes to the placenta, while 20 percent is directed to the myometrium and thus never comes into contact with either placenta or fetus.[76] The intermittent spurting character of the maternal spiral arterioles also prevents a portion of the drug from reaching the placental circulation and fetus. Because not all these spiral arterioles are functioning at the same time, some of the anesthetic bypasses the area of exchange and remains in the maternal circulation.

Once in the fetal circulation, a part of the drug will travel directly to the liver, where some will be metabolized, eventually reaching the inferior vena cava. The other part will be shunted directly across the ductus venosus into the inferior vena cava. That portion of drug reaching the inferior vena cava will proceed to the right atrium, where some will enter the right ventricle, and hence the pulmonary artery. All but 10 percent will be shunted directly across the ductus arteriosus to the lower part of the systemic circulation, bypassing the cerebral circulation. The remainder of the drug that reaches the right atrium will be shunted across the foramen ovale into the left atrium, left ventricle, and out the aorta into the upper part of the fetal circulation, which includes the fetal brain, where the greatest effect occurs. Given the complexity of the fetal circulation, it is easy to see how the mother can be affected by a certain concentration of drug without the fetus being affected.

Because the placenta has the properties of a lipid membrane, most drugs and all anesthetic agents cross by a mechanism called simple diffusion. The physico-chemical factors governing transfer across a lipid membrane by simple diffusion is described by Fick's law[72]:

$$Q/T = [K\ A(C_m - C_f)]/X$$

where Q/T is the rate of diffusion, K is the diffusion constant of the drug, A is the available area, C_m is the maternal blood concentration, C_f is the fetal blood concentration, and X is the thickness of the membrane. Thus the amount of drug that crosses the placenta increases as concentrations in the maternal circulation and total area of the membrane increase and decreases as the thickness of the membrane increases. The effective surface area of the human placenta is approximately 11 m^2, and its thickness is approximately 3.5 μm. The diffusion constant, K, accounts for the properties of the drug itself, including molecular weight, spatial configuration, degree of ionization, lipid solubility, and protein binding. For example, bupivacaine is highly protein bound, a characteristic that some believe explains why fetal blood concentrations are so much lower than with other local anesthetics. On the other hand, bupivacaine is also highly lipid soluble. The more lipid soluble a drug is, the more freely it passes through a lipid membrane. Furthermore, once in the fetal system, lipid solubility enables the drug to be taken up by fetal tissues rapidly, which again contributes to the lower blood concentration of the agent.

The degree of ionization of a drug is also important. Most drugs exist in both an ionized and nonionized state. It is the nonionized state that freely crosses lipid membranes. Drugs such as muscle relaxants are highly ionized; thus little crosses to the fetus. The degree of ionization is influenced by the pH of the medium. For

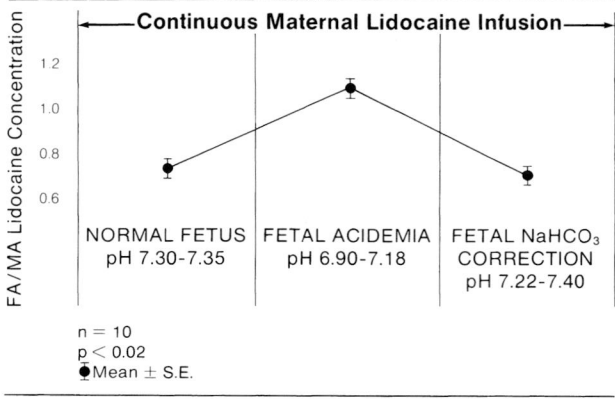

Figure 15–5. Fetal–maternal arterial (FA/MA) lidocaine ratios were significantly higher ($p < 0.02$) during fetal acidemia than during control or when pH was corrected with bicarbonate ($N = 10$; mean ± SE). (From Biehl D, Shnider SM, Levinson G, Callender K: Placental transfer of lidocaine: effects of fetal acidosis. Anesthesiology 48: 409, 1978, with permission.)

example, local anesthetics are more ionized at a lower pH. Such factors become clinically relevant in obstetrics, because occasionally the pH of the mother's blood will be 7.4, while that of the fetus will be 7.0 or less. In this instance, the nonionized portion of the drug in the maternal circulation crosses to the fetus, becomes ionized, and thus remains in the fetus (Fig. 15–5).[77]

Lumbar Epidural Analgesia/Anesthesia

Epidural blockade is a major regional anesthetic technique in which local anesthetic is injected into the epidural space. Epidural blockade may be used to provide *analgesia* during labor, or surgical *anesthesia* for vaginal or cesarean delivery. A large-bore needle (16-, 17-, or 18-gauge) is used to locate the epidural space. Next, a catheter is inserted through the needle, and the needle is removed over the catheter. Local anesthetic is injected through the catheter, which remains taped in place to the mother's back to enable subsequent injections throughout labor (Figs. 15–1 and 15–6). Thus, it is often called continuous epidural analgesia. A test dose of local anesthetic is given first to be certain the catheter has not been unintentionally placed in the subarachnoid (spinal) space or in a blood vessel. Single dose techniques are occasionally used for vaginal or cesarean delivery when the duration of pain is expected to be brief. For the single-dose technique, the catheter is omitted.

Two forms of epidural analgesia are used for labor: lumbar and caudal. The catheter is placed via a lumbar interspace in the former and via the sacral hiatus in the latter (Fig. 15–1). More local anesthetic is necessary for the caudal technique, because the local anesthetic must fill the entire sacral canal before filling the epidural space up to T10; 15 to 20 ml of local anesthetic is required. In contrast, for the lumbar technique, 8 to 10 ml (and often less) suffices, because the local anesthetic is injected much closer to its site of action.

For the caudal approach, because the local anesthetic is injected at the sacral area, sacral nerves 2, 3, and 4 are always affected. Because these nerves innervate the pelvic floor, the muscles of the pelvic floor will become insensitive and relaxed throughout labor. Moreover, the patient's legs will be affected and occasionally will be rendered immobile, depending on the strength of the local anesthetic. Pressure exerted on the pelvic floor by the descending vertex plays a major role in ensuring proper rotation of the fetal head to the occiput anterior position, and resistance may not be adequate to rotate the head when muscles of the pelvic floor are relaxed. Thus, an increase in occiput transverse or occiput posterior positions may result with the caudal technique. Also, because the patient's perception of pressure on the perineum by the presenting part is a stimulus for her to increase voluntary effort, blocking or minimizing

this perception may prolong the second stage. Because of the large volume of local anesthetic used, adverse effects on muscle tone in the legs and pelvic floor, and the highly variable anatomy of the sacral hiatus in adults, the caudal approach has fallen out of favor for labor analgesia. A rare but serious complication of caudal anesthesia is accidental injection of local anesthetic into the fetal head leading to newborn apnea, bradycardia, and convulsions.[78]

Most anesthesiologists now prefer the lumbar approach and use a technique described as segmental epidural analgesia (Fig. 15–7). Because nerves that carry painful impulses during the first stage of labor are small sympathetic nerves and because they are easily blocked, only the smallest amount and the weakest effective concentration of local anesthetic is injected via the L2-3, L3-4, or L4-5 interspace. Thus, both sensation and motor function of the perineum and lower extremities remain mostly intact. The patient can move about and perceive the impact of the presenting part on the perineum. If perineal anesthesia is needed for delivery, a larger concentration and dose of local anesthetic can be administered at that time through the catheter (Fig. 15–7). Alternatively, for perineal anesthesia, the obstetrician can perform a pudendal block or local infiltration of the perineum.

The segmental epidural technique, when performed properly, is effective and safe for both mother and fetus. In most instances, total or near total pain relief is accomplished without resorting to depressant and sometimes disorienting drugs. The mother remains awake, alert, and aware of her surroundings. She can communicate with her husband, her physician, and the nursing personnel. She will remember and appreciate her entire labor and delivery. Finally, because anesthesia can be extended to the perineum at the time of delivery, the obstetrician can accomplish whatever kind of delivery is necessary, spontaneous or instrumental, with or without an episiotomy.

A new technique of labor analgesia involves passing a small-gauge pencil-point spinal needle through the epidural needle prior to catheter placement. This combined spinal-epidural or coaxial technique provides rapid onset of analgesia using a very small dose of opioid or a local anesthetic and opioid combination.[79,80] Because the dose of drug used in the subarachnoid space is much smaller than that used for epidural analgesia, the risks of local anesthetic toxicity or high spinal block are avoided. Side effects are usually mild, and include pruritus and nausea. The risk of postdural puncture headache is no different than using epidural analgesia alone.[81] Some practitioners have used this technique to allow parturients to ambulate during labor since there is little or no interference with motor function.[79]

Even though the advantages would seem to make

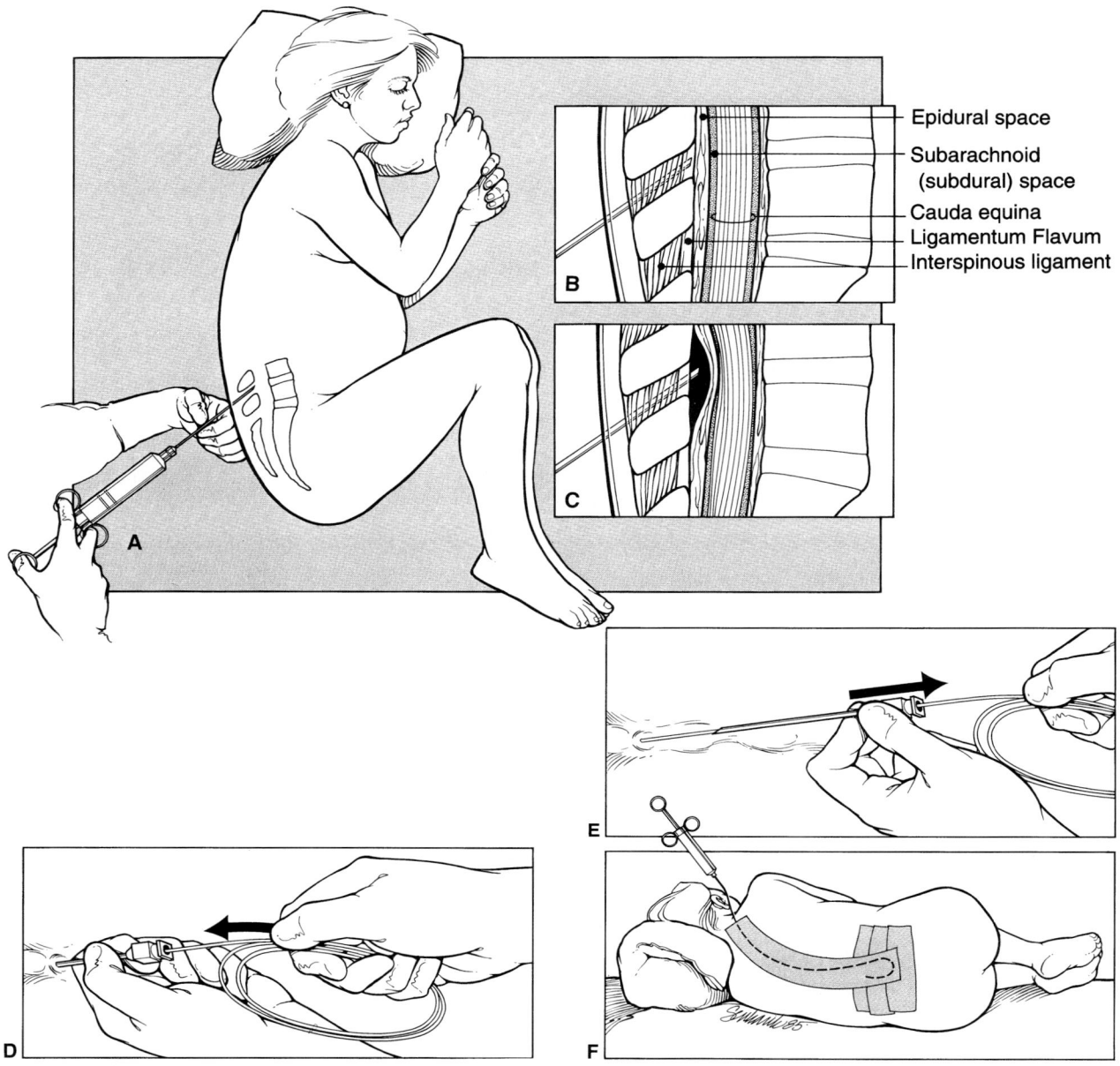

Epidural space
Subarachnoid (subdural) space
Cauda equina
Ligamentum Flavum
Interspinous ligament

Figure 15–6. Technique of lumbar epidural puncture by the midline approach. *A,* This side view shows left hand held against patient's back, with thumb and index finger grasping hub. Attempts to inject solution while point of needle is in the interspinous ligament meet resistance. *B,* Point of needle is in the ligamentum flavum, which offers marked resistance and makes it almost impossible to inject solution. *C,* Entrance of the needle's point into epidural space is discerned by sudden lack of resistance to injection of saline. Force of injected solution pushes dura-arachnoid away from point of needle. *D,* Catheter is introduced through needle. Note that hub of needle is pulled caudad toward the patient, increasing the angle between the shaft of the needle and the epidural space. Also note technique of holding the tubing: it is wound around the right hand. *E.* Needle is withdrawn over tubing and held steady with the right hand. *F,* Catheter is immobilized with adhesive tape. Note the large loop made by the catheter to decrease risk of kinking at the point where the tube exits from the skin. (From Bonica JJ: Obstetric Analgesia and Anesthesia. Amsterdam, World Federation of Societies of Anesthesiologists, 1980, with permission.)

epidural or combined spinal-epidural analgesia the ideal analgesic technique, and many believe it to be so, there are disadvantages. These include hypotension, local anesthetic toxicity, allergic reaction, high or total spinal anesthesia, neurologic injury, and spinal headache. Recent reports have not found an adverse effect on progress of labor when lower concentrations of anesthetic are used for regional analgesia.[82]

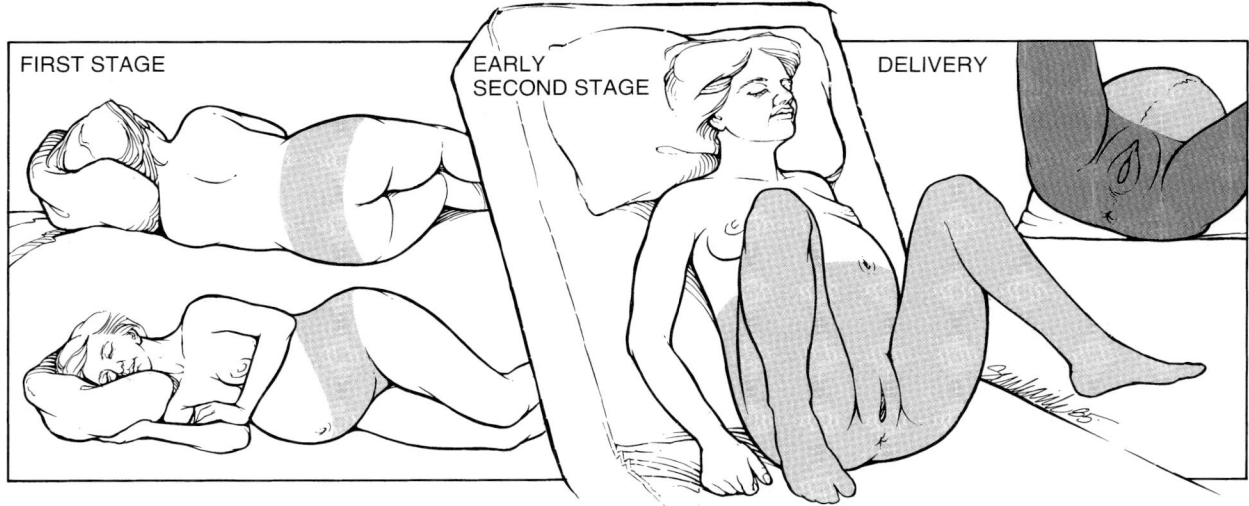

Figure 15–7. Segmented epidural analgesia for labor and delivery. A single catheter is introduced into the epidural space and advanced so that its tip is at L2. Initially, small volumes of low concentrations of local anesthetic are used to produce segmental analgesia. For the second stage, the analgesia is extended to the sacral segments by injecting a larger amount of the same concentration of local anesthetic, with the patient in the semirecumbent position. After internal rotation, a higher concentration of local anesthetic is injected to produce motor block of the sacral segments and thus achieve perineal relaxation and anesthesia. The wedge under the right buttock causes the uterus to displace to the left. (From Bonica JJ: Obstetric Analgesia and Anesthesia. Amsterdam, World Federation of Societies of Anesthesiologists, 1980, with permission.)

Hypotension

Hypotension is defined variably, but most often it as a systolic blood pressure less than 100 mm Hg or a 20 percent decrease from control measurements. It occurs after approximately 10 percent of epidural blocks given during labor, but the incidence has been reported to be as low as 1.4 percent in some large series.[83–85] Hypotension occurs primarily as a result of sympathetic blockade. Local anesthetics block not only pain fibers but sympathetic fibers as well, which normally maintain blood vessel tone. When these fibers are blocked, vasodilation results and blood pools in the lower extremities, decreasing the return of blood to the right side of the heart. Cardiac output then decreases, and hypotension results. Hypotension threatens the fetus by decreasing uterine blood flow and threatens the mother by decreasing cerebral blood flow. When hypotension is recognized promptly and treated effectively, few, if any, untoward effects accrue to either mother or fetus (Table 15–1).[86–88] However, in the acutely or chronically compromised fetus, hypotension could further worsen fetal status if not treated immediately.

Treatment of hypotension begins with prophylaxis, which demands an intravenous catheter and an infusion of isotonic crystalloid solution. The infusion fills the expanded vascular space caused by vasodilation. Glucose is easily transported across the placenta; therefore, dextrose-containing solutions are avoided for this purpose because they can lead to neonatal hypoglycemia.[89] Left uterine displacement must be maintained during the block because compression of the inferior vena cava and aorta may decrease cardiac output and/or uteroplacental perfusion. Proper treatment depends on immediate diagnosis. Therefore, the individual administering the anesthesia must be present and attentive. Once diagnosed, hypotension is corrected by increasing the rate of intravenous fluid infusion and exaggerating left uterine displacement. If these simple measures do not suffice, a vasopressor is indicated. The vasopressor of

Table 15–1. EPIDURAL ANALGESIA: HYPOTENSION VERSUS NO HYPOTENSION*

	Hypotension† ($N = 5$)	No Hypotension ($N = 20$)
Umbilical artery		
pH	17.269	7.311
BE (mEq/L)	1.4	1.3
PO$_2$ (mm Hg)	23.6	23.2
SaO$_2$ (%)	48.2	50.2
Umbilical vein		
pH	17.344	7.366
BE (mEq/L)	1.8	1.5
PO$_2$ (mm Hg)	41.0	33.7
SvO$_2$ (%)	84.6	72.0

*Values are means; they indicate that properly treated hypotension need not result in a compromised fetus.
†Hypotension was severe enough to be treated with the vasopressor ephedrine.
BE, base excess.
Modified from James FM III, Crawford JS, Hopkinson R, et al: A comparison of general anesthesia and lumbar epidural analgesia for elective cesarean section. Anesth Analg 56:228, 1977.

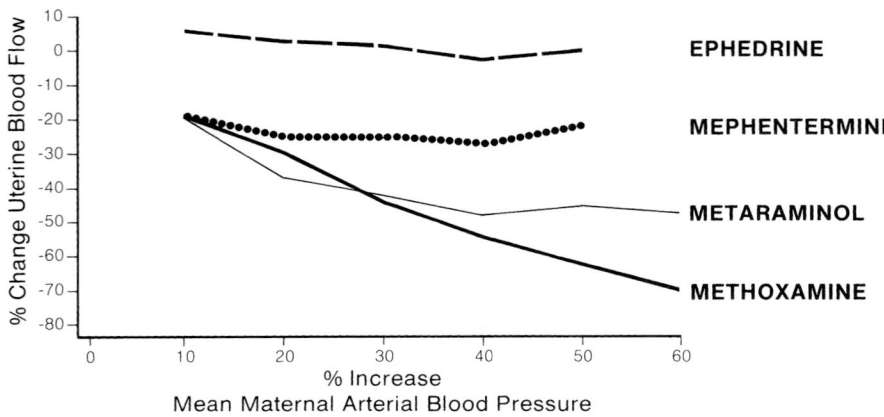

Figure 15–8. Changes in uterine blood flow at equal elevations of mean arterial blood pressure after vasopressor administration (pregnant ewes). (From Ralston DH, Shnider SM, deLorimier AA: Effects of equipotent ephedrine, metaraminol, mephentermine, and methoxamine on uterine blood flow in the pregnant ewe. Anesthesiology 40:354, 1974, with permission.)

choice is ephedrine, given in 5- to 10-mg doses. Ephedrine is a mixed α- and β- agonist, and it is less likely to compromise uteroplacental perfusion than the pure α-agonists.[90] α-Adrenergic agents such as methoxamine or phenylephrine are avoided in most cases (Fig. 15–8), although they may be useful when a parturient is excessively tachycardic in association with hypotension, or if tachycardia associated with ephedrine may be detrimental. Clinical studies have suggested that phenylephrine in small doses may be given safely to treat hypotension during regional anesthesia for cesarean delivery.[91]

Local Anesthetic Toxicity

The incidence of systemic local anesthetic toxicity (high blood concentrations of local anesthetic) after lumbar epidural analgesia is 0.01 percent.[92] However, convulsions due to local anesthetic toxicity were the most common damaging events in obstetric patients in the ASA Closed Claims Project database. In 83 percent of these cases, neurologic injury or death to the mother, newborn, or both occurred.[93] Maternal mortality data also show that local anesthetic toxicity is the most common cause of death resulting from regional anesthesia during cesarean delivery.[94] Most often, toxicity occurs when the local anesthetic is injected into a vessel rather than into the epidural space or when too much

is administered even though injected properly. Occasionally, the dosage can be miscalculated: 1 ml of 1 percent lidocaine contains 10 mg of lidocaine, not 1 mg. All local anesthetics have maximal recommended doses, and these should not be exceeded. For example, the maximum recommended dose of lidocaine is 4 mg/kg when used without epinephrine and 7 mg/kg when used with epinephrine. Epinephrine delays and decreases the uptake of local anesthetic into the bloodstream. Package inserts for all local anesthetics contain appropriate dosing information (Table 15–2).

Local anesthetic reactions have two components, central nervous system (CNS) and cardiovascular. Usually, the CNS component precedes the cardiovascular component. Prodromal symptoms of the CNS reaction include excitation, bizarre behavior, ringing in the ears, and disorientation. These symptoms may culminate in convulsions, which are usually brief. After the convulsions, depression follows and manifests predominantly by the postictal state. The cardiovascular component of the local anesthetic reaction usually begins with hypertension and tachycardia but is soon followed by hypotension, arrhythmias, and in some instances cardiac arrest. Thus, the cardiovascular component also has excitant and depressant characteristics. Usually, the CNS and cardiovascular components are widely separated, because it takes a significantly higher blood concentra-

Table 15–2. MAXIMAL RECOMMENDED DOSES OF COMMON LOCAL ANESTHETICS

| | With Epinephrine* | | Without Epinephrine | | |
Local Anesthetic	mg/kg	Dose (mg/70 kg)	mg/kg	Total (mg/70 kg)
Bupivacaine	2.5	175	3.0	225
Chloroprocaine	11.0	800	14.0	1,000
Etidocaine	4.0	300	5.5	400
Lidocaine	4.0	300	7.0	500
Mepivacaine	5.0	400	—	—
Tetracaine	1.5	100	—	—

*All epinephrine concentrations 1:200,000.

tion of local anesthetic to cause the cardiovascular symptoms than it does the CNS symptoms. Thus, one frequently sees the CNS component without the more serious cardiovascular component. Bupivacaine may represent an exception to this principle.[95,96] There are reports of several patients who experienced serious arrhythmias and marked cardiovascular depression after administration of 0.75 percent bupivacaine. Most anesthesiologists now believe there is little difference in the doses required to cause the two types of reactions to bupivacaine. Moreover, resuscitation of these patients was difficult or impossible, probably because of the drug's prolonged blocking effect on sodium channels.[97] Indeed there now is laboratory evidence that bupivacaine is more cardiotoxic than equianalgesic doses of other amide local anesthetics. Several manufacturers of bupivacaine have recommended that the 0.75 percent concentration not be used in obstetric patients or for paracervical block.[98] Of course, it is possible to give the same total dose of bupivacaine by giving a larger volume of 0.5 percent bupivacaine. However, use of a more dilute concentration of drug does not guarantee safety. Thus, it is important that the physician give bupivacaine, or any other local anesthetic, by slow, incremental injection.[99]

The bupivacaine controversy has resulted in greater emphasis on the administration of a safe and effective test dose to exclude unintentional intravenous or subarachnoid injection of local anesthetic before injection of a therapeutic dose of local anesthetic. Many anesthesiologists give a test dose that includes 15 μg of epinephrine.[100,101] An increase in heart rate of at least 25 to 30 bpm would signal intravascular injection. Others have questioned whether an epinephrine-containing test dose is the best choice in obstetric patients.[102]

Treatment of a local anesthetic reaction depends on recognizing the signs and symptoms as they occur. Again, to recognize this complication, the anesthesia-care provider must be present. If possible, once prodromal symptoms arise, the injection of local anesthetic should be stopped. However, if convulsions have already occurred, treatment is aimed at maintaining proper oxygenation and preventing the patient from harming herself. Convulsions use considerable amounts of oxygen, which results in hypoxia and acidosis (Table 15–3).[103] Adequate oxygenation is essential for both mother and fetus, because a hypoxic mother results in a hypoxic and acidotic fetus. Should the convulsions continue for more than a brief period, small intravenous doses of thiopental (25 to 50 mg) or midazolam (1 to 2 mg) are useful. In obstetrics, because of the adverse effects of benzodiazepines on the neonate, thiopental would be the agent of choice. Occasionally, succinylcholine is used for paralysis to prevent the muscular activity associated with the convulsions and to facilitate ventilation and perhaps intubation. Before using thiopental, diazepam, or succinylcholine, consideration must be given to the depressant effects that these agents will add to the depressant phase of the local anesthetic reaction. Therefore, appropriate equipment and personnel must be available to maintain oxygenation, a patent airway, and cardiovascular support. Re-

Table 15–3. BLOOD GAS DETERMINATIONS DURING AND AFTER LOCAL ANESTHETIC-INDUCED CONVULSIONS

Convulsion	Time	Oxygen	pH	P_{CO_2} (mm Hg)	P_{O_2} (mm Hg)	HCO_3 (mEq/L)	Base Excess (mEq/L)
Patient 1							
1st	19:50:00	10*	—	—	—	—	—
2nd	9:50:30		7.27	48	48	21.5	4
3rd	9:51:00		—	—	—	—	—
4th	9:53:00		7.09	59	33	17.1	−10
Cessation	9:54:00		—	—	—	—	—
	9:55:30	6†	7.01	71	210	17.2	−11
	10:22:00	Room air	7.25	48	99	20.5	−5
			7.56	25	106	22.5	0
Patient 2							
1st	19:47:00		—	—	—	—	—
2nd	9:47:30		6.99	76	87	17.4	−10.2
3rd	9:48:00		—	—	—	—	—
Cessation	9:50:00		—	—	—	—	—
	10:02:00	10*	7.16	54	140	18.5	−6.9

*Bag and mask with oral Guedel airway and artificial respiration.
†Nasal prongs.
Modified from Moore DC, Crawford RD, Scurlock JE: Severe hypoxia and acidosis following local anesthetic-induced convulsions. Anesthesiology 53:259, 1980.

suscitation of the pregnant patient is essentially the same as that of the nonpregnant patient except that left uterine displacement must be maintained. Usually, this means that the uterus will have to be elevated off the inferior vena cava manually for resuscitation with the patient supine. Delivery of the infant may facilitate maternal resuscitation. The American Heart Association has stated: "Several authors now recommend that the decision to perform a perimortem cesarean section should be made rapidly, with delivery effected within 4 to 5 minutes of the arrest."[104]

Allergy to Local Anesthetics

There are two classes of local anesthetics: amides and esters. A true allergic reaction to an amide-type local anesthetic (e.g., lidocaine, bupivacaine, ropivacaine) is extremely rare. Allergic reactions to the esters (2-chloroprocaine, procaine, tetracaine) are also uncommon but do occur more often. When a patient reports that is "allergic" to local anesthetics, she is frequently referring to a normal reaction to the epinephrine that is occasionally added to local anesthetics, particularly by dentists. Epinephrine can cause increased heart rate, pounding in the ears, and nausea, symptoms that may be interpreted as an allergy. It is therefore important to document any history of allergy. Was there a rash? Hives? Difficulty breathing? If so, which local anesthetic was used? If a specific local anesthetic can be identified, choosing one from the other class should be safe, or meperidine can be used as an alternative to local anesthetics in the subarachnoid space.[105]

High Spinal or "Total Spinal" Anesthesia

This complication occurs when the level of anesthesia rises dangerously high, resulting in paralysis of the respiratory muscles, including the diaphragm. The incidence of total spinal anesthesia after epidural anesthesia is less than 0.03 percent and after spinal anesthesia is 0.2 percent.[92,106] Total spinal anesthesia can result from a miscalculated dose of drug, unintentional subarachnoid injection during an epidural block, or improper positioning of a patient after spinal block with hyperbaric local anesthetic solutions. Motor nerves to the diaphragm, the major respiratory muscle, emanate from C3 to C5; therefore, the anesthetic must be at this level before phrenic nerve paralysis results. Moreover, the phrenic nerve is a large motor nerve, which requires considerable local anesthetic for complete block. Because the accessory muscles of respiration are paralyzed earlier, their paralysis may result in apprehension and anxiety. The patient usually can breathe adequately as long as the diaphragm is not paralyzed. However, treatment must be individualized, and dyspnea, real or imagined, should always be considered an effect of pa-

ralysis until proved otherwise. In addition to respiratory symptoms, cardiovascular components, including hypotension and even cardiovascular collapse, may occur.

Treatment of total spinal anesthesia includes rapidly assessing the true level of anesthesia. Therefore, individuals performing major regional anesthesia should be thoroughly familiar with dermatome charts (Fig. 15–9) and should also be able to recognize what a certain sensory level of anesthesia means with regard to innervation of other organs or systems. For example, a T4 sensory level may represent total sympathetic nervous system blockade. Numbness and weakness of the fingers and hands indicates that the level of anesthesia has reached the cervical level (C6 to C8), which is dangerously close to the innervation of the diaphragm. If the diaphragm is not paralyzed, the patient is breathing adequately, and cardiovascular stability is maintained, administration of oxygen and reassurance may suffice. If the patient remains anxious or if the level of anesthesia seems to be involving the diaphragm, then assisted ventilation is indicated. Occasionally, this can be accomplished with a bag and face mask without rendering the patient unconscious. Most often, however, endotracheal intubation will be necessary. If so, induction of general anesthesia will facilitate the process. Cardiovascular support is provided as necessary. If the person administering regional anesthesia is well acquainted with the signs and symptoms of high spinal anesthesia and its treatment, serious sequelae should be extremely rare. The onset can be easily recognized, and the treatment is relatively simple. However, the same admonition applies as with hypotension and local anesthetic toxicity: early symptoms cannot be diagnosed if the person administering the block is not present and attentive.

Paralysis and Nerve Injury

Paralysis after either epidural or spinal anesthesia is extremely rare; even minor injuries such as foot-drop and segmental loss of sensation are uncommon. Nerve injury occurs in 0.06 percent of spinal anesthetics and 0.02 percent of epidural anesthetics.[92] With commercially prepared drugs, ampules, and disposable needles, infection and caustic injury rarely occur. Several years ago there were several cases of neurologic deficit after use of 2-chloroprocaine, primarily after unintentional subarachnoid (i.e., spinal) injection of large volumes of the drug.[107–109] These cases prompted performance of several laboratory studies to evaluate any potential neurotoxicity of 2-chloroprocaine. The earlier formulation of 2-chloroprocaine contained the antioxidant 0.2 percent sodium bisulfite. Currently the consensus is that 2-chloroprocaine itself is not neurotoxic, but that the low pH of the local anesthetic solution and the inclusion of

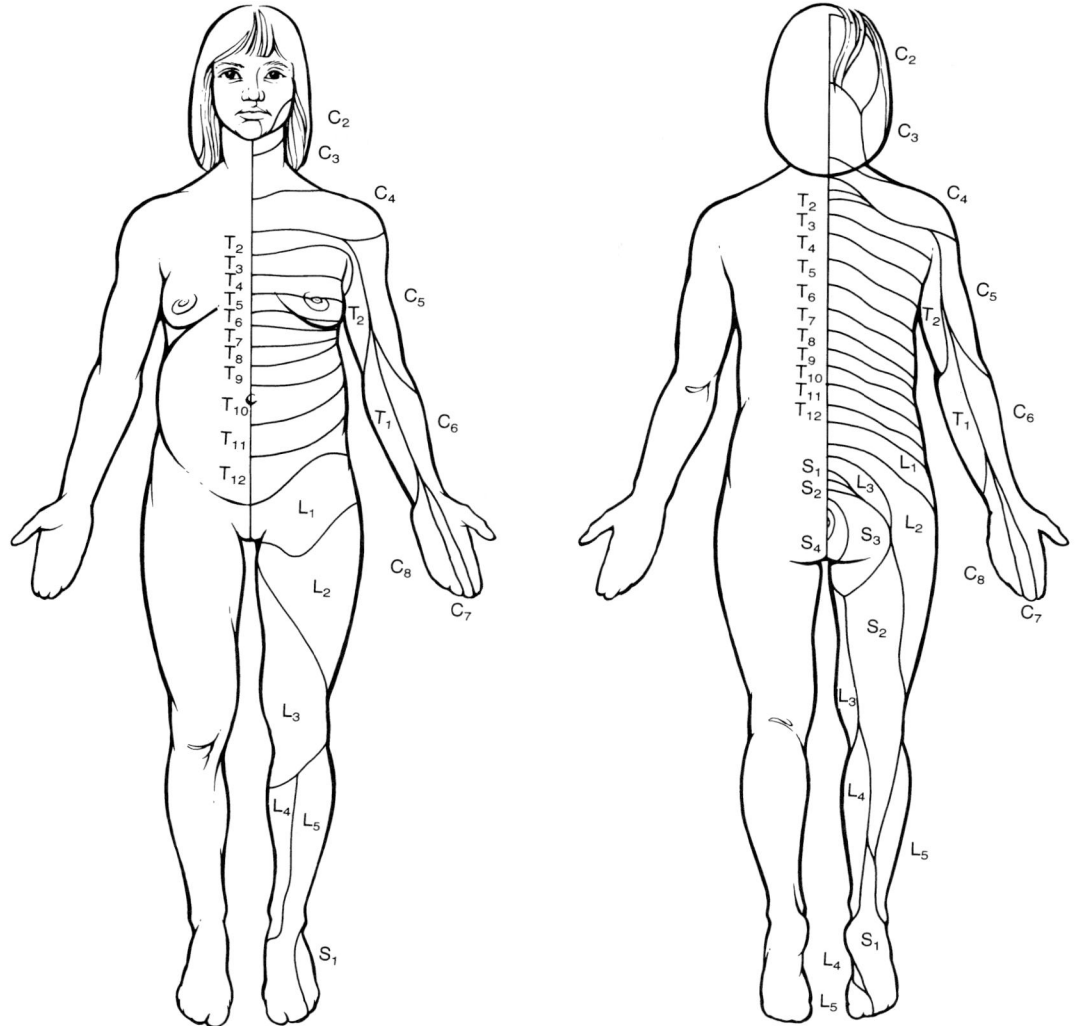

Figure 15–9. Dermatome chart. (Adapted from Haymaker L, Woodhall B: Peripheral Nerve Injuries. Philadelphia, WB Saunders Company, 1945.)

the sodium bisulfite together may produce neurologic dysfunction.[110] Following reformulation using ethylene diamine tetraaotic acid (EDTA) as a preservative, there were reports of transient back pain after epidural use of the new formulation of 2-chloroprocaine in nonpregnant patients.[111,112] This appeared to be due to the calcium chelating effects of EDTA in the paraspinous muscles causing tetany and painful muscle spasms. The current formulation does not contain preservatives.

When nerve damage follows regional analgesia during obstetric or surgical procedures, the anesthetic technique must be suspected. Nerve damage can result from other causes, however. For example, incorrectly positioned stirrups may cause nerve injury after both gynecologic and obstetric procedures.[113–115] Also, nerve damage can be secondary to a difficult forceps application. During abdominal procedures, overzealous or prolonged application of pressure with retractors on sensi-

tive nerve tissues may result in injury. Fortunately, most neurologic deficits after labor and delivery are minor and transient.[116] Nonetheless, one should consider consultation with a neurologist or neurosurgeon. Although patients are often concerned about the development of back pain following epidural anesthesia, the incidence of back pain in postpartum women is the same with or without the use of regional anesthesia. The incidence of back pain after childbirth is 44 percent at 1 to 2 months postpartum[117] and 49 percent at 12 to 18 months postpartum,[118] again unrelated to the use of epidural anesthesia.

One of the more dramatic and correctable forms of nerve damage follows compression of the spinal cord by a hematoma that has formed during the administration of spinal or epidural anesthesia, presumably from accidental puncture of an epidural vessel. If the condition is diagnosed early, usually with the aid of a neurologist or neurosurgeon, the hematoma can be removed by laminectomy and the problem resolved without permanent damage. Fortunately, this is a rare complication. Nonetheless, spinal and epidural blocks are contraindicated if coagulation is abnormal.[119,120] Any prolonged motor or sensory deficit after regional anesthesia should be investigated immediately and thoroughly.

Spinal Headache

Spinal headache may follow uncomplicated spinal anesthesia. This complication can also occur when, during the process of administering an epidural block, the dura is punctured and spinal fluid leaks out (i.e., "wet tap"). The incidence of this complication varies between 1 and 3 percent, and its occurrence depends an the experience of the person performing the epidural block.[121] Once a wet tap occurs, a spinal headache results in as many as 70 percent of patients. The incidence is much less following spinal anesthesia, because smaller needles are used. Characteristically the headache is more severe in the upright position and is relieved by the prone position. The headache is thought to be caused by loss of cerebrospinal fluid, which allows the brain to settle and thus meninges and vessels to stretch. Hydration, abdominal binders, and the prone position have all been advocated as prophylactic measures. However, most anesthesiologists now agree that these actions are of little value.[122] In some hands, epidural saline injected through the catheter has proven to be an effective prophylactic measure.[123]

Treatment of the headache, once it has occurred, may be initiated with oral analgesics, caffeine,[124] and continued hydration. If these simple measures do not prove immediately effective, an epidural blood patch is placed. Approximately 15 ml of the patient's own blood is placed aseptically into the epidural space; the blood coagulates over the hole in the dura and prevents further leakage.[125] Patients can be released within 1 to 2 hours.[126] Patients should be instructed to avoid coughing or straining at stool for the first several days after performance of the blood patch. The epidural blood patch has been found to be remarkably effective and nearly complication free.[127-129] There remains controversy regarding whether one should perform a prophylactic blood patch before the onset of spinal headache.[130-132]

Because epidural anesthesia is associated with these side effects and complications, those who administer it must be thoroughly familiar not only with the technical aspects of its administration but also with the signs and symptoms of complications and their treatment. Specifically, the American Society of Anesthesiologists and ACOG have stated: "Persons administering or supervising obstetric anesthesia should be qualified to manage the infrequent but occasionally life-threatening complications of major regional anesthesia such as respiratory and cardiovascular failure, convulsions due to toxic levels of local anesthetic, or vomiting and aspiration. Mastering and retaining the skills and knowledge necessary to manage these complications require adequate training and frequent application."[3]

Effects on Labor and Method of Delivery

One of the more controversial aspects of regional anesthesia for obstetrics is the question of whether these techniques influence the length and pattern of labor, the incidence of malposition, the use of forceps, and the rate of cesarean delivery. The perspectives of the anesthesiologist and the obstetrician differ when trying to answer these questions. The anesthesiologist is concerned primarily with relieving pain and sees regional anesthesia as the ideal method because it depresses neither mother nor fetus, provides exceptional pain relief, and even optimal operating conditions for the obstetrician. The obstetrician, although concerned with pain relief, is also concerned with the progress of labor and the method of delivery. Reports on the effects of epidural analgesia on labor are numerous and conflicting.

STUDY DESIGN. Most published studies on the effect of epidural analgesia on the progress of labor are retrospective and, if prospective, are nonrandomized. Studies that compare patients who received epidural analgesia versus those who did not are typically biased in favor of the nonepidural group of patients. Specifically, patients who have rapid, uncomplicated labor are less likely to ask for, and even if they ask for it are less likely actually to receive, epidural analgesia. In other words, the epidural group will include more patients with dysfunctional, difficult, and complicated labors. In fact, it is possible that the very reason why some, but not all, parturients request and receive epidural analgesia may relate to a greater likelihood of abnormal labor. For example, prolonged latent phase is associated with an increased need for cesarean delivery,[133] and rupture of membranes prior to the onset of labor increases the likelihood of operative delivery.[134] In both of these situations, labor may be prolonged, oxytocin use is more common, and epidural analgesia may be requested more often. Furthermore, severe pain during early labor also predicts an increased risk for abnormal labor and operative delivery.[135] It is also problematic when one attempts to evaluate the influence of epidural analgesia on labor by using historical controls. For example, if one compares the incidence of midforceps delivery after the introduction of epidural analgesia in a hospital (e.g., in 1989) versus the incidence of midforceps delivery before the use of epidural analgesia in that hospital (e.g., in 1979), one might note no change in the incidence of midforceps delivery and therefore conclude that the introduction of epidural analgesia did not affect the incidence of midforceps delivery. However, other changes in obstetric practice may have occurred during that 10-year interval. For example, some obstetricians are less willing to perform difficult midforceps delivery today than they were a decade ago. Therefore, it would be inappropriate to conclude that epidural analgesia did not influence the incidence of midforceps delivery in that hospital.

VARIATION IN EPIDURAL TECHNIQUE. A second difficulty with interpretation of existing studies is that epidural analgesia is not a generic procedure. The influence of epidural analgesia on the progress of labor may vary according to the technique used, as well as the choice and dose of the local anesthetic administered. The use of combined spinal-epidural (CSE) analgesia—with or without ambulation—has increased. Furthermore, anesthesiologists today use more dilute solutions of local anesthetic for epidural analgesia than were used a decade ago. Anesthesiologists now give greater attention to titrating the dose of the local anesthetic to the specific needs of the patient. For example, Naulty and colleagues[136] made an abrupt change in their epidural analgesia technique in June 1987. Specifically, they had been providing epidural analgesia during labor with either 1.5 percent lidocaine or 0.25 to 0.5 percent bupivacaine, but they changed their technique to include 0.125 to 0.25 percent bupivacaine with fentanyl. They then compared the results during the 9 months before the change versus those during the 9 months after the change. They noted a significant decrease in the percentage of patients admitted for labor who eventually underwent cesarean delivery. During the 9 months before the change, 20 percent of patients in labor were delivered by cesarean section, whereas after the change 15 percent required this procedure. Furthermore, there was a significant decrease in the percentage of patients who received epidural analgesia and who subsequently underwent cesarean delivery. Finally, the incidence of forceps deliveries decreased from 17 percent before the change to 6 percent after the change.

More recently, Olofsson et al.[137] randomized 1,000 women of mixed parity (who requested epidural analgesia during labor) to receive either 0.25 percent bupivacaine with 1:200,000 epinephrine or 0.125 percent bupivacaine with sufentanil. The incidence of cesarean delivery was 15 percent in the high-dose bupivacaine group and 10 percent in the low-dose bupivacaine group ($p < 0.05$).

Another potential source of variation in management and outcome is the timing of administration of epidural analgesia. Although controversial, many physicians believe that institution of analgesia during the latent phase of the first stage of labor is more likely to delay the progress of labor. Friedman[138] stated:

> Spinal anesthesia given prior to the onset of the phase of dilatation in the first stage of labor will impede progress of

the latent phase, and forestall the normal progressive changes of late labor. It would seem that spinal block given after the latent phase has ended, in a patient whose labor is otherwise normal, and to a level which does not exceed that necessary for uterine pain relief (tenth thoracic) should not influence labor. The general impression of caudal or epidural anesthesia as it affects labor is that of negligible influence unless misused.

The Committee on Obstetrics: Maternal and Fetal Medicine of the American College of Obstetricians and Gynecologists issued a statement about dystocia. Regarding the latent phase of labor, they stated: "The latent phase may be prolonged by excessive medication and inappropriate timing of conduction anesthesia." Regarding the active phase, they stated: "The normal active phase tends to be resistant to the inhibitory effects of the usual amounts of analgesia. At times, further sedation or epidural anesthesia, hydration, or ambulation may be advantageous." Furthermore, the Committee stated: "A hypertonic pattern may be observed in the active phase. Prolongation of a hypertonic pattern may result in maternal exhaustion, marked pain, and decreased uteroplacental blood flow. The combination of sedation, epidural anesthesia and oxytocin infusion may prove effective."[139]

The problem with delaying institution of epidural analgesia until the onset of the active phase of labor is that it is often difficult to make that diagnosis prospectively. Furthermore, it is also inappropriate to delay institution of epidural analgesia until the patient has reached an arbitrary cervical dilation.[140] For example, approximately 50 percent of patients will enter the active phase of labor by 4 cm cervical dilation, but a minority will not enter active labor until more than 5 cm cervical dilation.[140] If one delays institution of epidural analgesia until the patient reaches an arbitrary dilation (e.g., 5 cm cervical dilation), one will subject some patients to unnecessary periods of severe pain. Early institution of epidural analgesia may slow labor in some patients, but this can usually be corrected with the use of oxytocin.

MANAGEMENT OF THE SECOND STAGE. A third problem with interpretation of studies of epidural anesthesia and progress of labor relates to the indication for performance of instrumental delivery. In general, an obstetrician is more likely to perform elective forceps delivery in a comfortable patient with effective epidural anesthesia than in an uncomfortable patient with no anesthesia. Furthermore, heretofore some obstetricians have arbitrarily terminated the second stage at 2 hours in nulliparous patients and at 1 hour in parous patients. There is evidence that effective epidural analgesia may slightly prolong the second stage of labor.[141,142] However, a delay in the second stage is not necessarily harmful to infant or to mother, provided there is reassuring electronic fetal heart rate monitoring and adequate maternal hydration and analgesia.[141,143–145] Indeed, the ACOG has defined a prolonged second stage as more than 3 hours in nulliparous patients *with* regional anesthesia as compared with more than 2 hours in nulliparous patients without regional anesthesia.[146]

PROSPECTIVE STUDIES OF EPIDURAL ANESTHESIA AND PROGRESS OF LABOR. It is difficult to perform prospective, randomized studies of the effect of epidural analgesia on the progress of labor. The fact that epidural analgesia provides analgesia superior to other techniques causes physicians to be reluctant to randomize patients to a nonepidural group. Robinson and colleagues[147] randomized 386 parturients to receive either epidural anesthesia or systemic analgesia (i.e., meperidine with inhalation analgesia) during labor. They noted that "epidural block was more effective than systemic analgesia in the relief of pain and discomfort in all stages of labor." They also noted that there was a significant increase in the incidence of instrumental delivery in the epidural group. Unfortunately, the randomization occurred before final consent was obtained. Patients were free to withdraw from the study after they learned their group assignment, and many did. Only 93 of the original patients completed the study. One can suspect that more patients with a long, difficult labor dropped out of the systemic analgesia group. This suspicion is confirmed when one notes that there was a threefold increase in the incidence of induction of labor in the epidural group. Furthermore, patients in the epidural group received 0.5 percent bupivacaine, a concentration higher than that used by most anesthesiologists today. Finally, the authors did not report the incidence of cesarean delivery in either group.

Philipsen and Jensen[148] reported the second published study in which patients were randomized to receive either epidural analgesia or systemic opioid during the first stage of labor. Patients in the epidural group received 0.375 percent bupivacaine, although the authors noted that they attempted to produce a segmental block from T10 to L1. They also stated: "In an attempt to retain the bearing-down reflex and to allow the mother to take active part in the second stage of labor, the analgesic effect was allowed to wear off at the beginning of the second stage and a top-up dose was not given if the cervix was dilated beyond 8 cm." There was no significant difference between groups in the method of delivery.

There are several studies in which nulliparous patients already receiving epidural analgesia were randomized with respect to management of epidural analgesia during the second stage.[141,149–151] Phillips and Thomas[149] reported no increase in duration of the second stage, and a nonsignificant decrease in the incidence of instrumental delivery, in 28 nulliparous women who received additional epidural bupivacaine (i.e., 0.25 percent) at complete cervical dilatation compared with 28 women who received no additional bupivacaine. However, this study was randomized but nonblinded, and it is unclear as to how the two groups actually differed, as there was no significant difference between groups in total dose of bupivacaine or in mean number of doses of bupivacaine (i.e., four doses per patient in each group).

Chestnut and colleagues[150] performed a study in which nulliparous patients already receiving a continuous epidural infusion of 0.75 percent lidocaine were randomized to receive either additional 0.75 percent lidocaine or saline placebo after 8 cm cervical dilation. The epidural infusion of lidocaine or saline placebo was continued in all patients until delivery. Maintenance of the epidural infusion of 0.75 percent lidocaine until delivery did not prolong the second stage or increase the frequency of instrumental delivery, but it also did not reliably provide second-stage analgesia or perineal anesthesia. Specifically, women who continued to receive epidural lidocaine until delivery did not clearly perceive that they had better analgesia than did women who received saline placebo.

Subsequently, Chestnut and colleagues[141] performed a study in which nulliparous women already receiving a continuous epidural infusion of 0.125 percent bupivacaine were randomized to receive either additional 0.125 percent bupivacaine or saline placebo beyond 8 cm cervical dilation. Patients continued to receive the epidural infusion of bupivacaine or saline placebo until delivery. Maintenance of the epidural infusion of bupivacaine until delivery resulted in second-stage analgesia that was clearly superior to that provided by replacement of the bupivacaine with placebo. Infusion of bupivacaine until delivery prolonged the second stage of labor approximately 30 minutes, and it also increased the incidence of instrumental delivery. However, maintenance of epidural bupivacaine analgesia did not result in an increased incidence of abnormal position of the vertex, and it did not result in an increased incidence of cesarean delivery. Furthermore, there were nonsignificant tendencies toward better neonatal condition in the bupivacaine group as evaluated by umbilical cord blood acid–base status and Apgar scores.

CESAREAN DELIVERY RATE. Does the use of epidural analgesia for labor influence the cesarean delivery rate? Gribble and Meier found no difference in the cesarean delivery rate before and after the availability of "on-demand" epidural analgesia for labor.[152] The patients were managed by the same group of obstetricians using the same management techniques in both time intervals. Before the introduction of an epidural analgesia service, the cesarean delivery rate was 9.0 percent. After the use of epidural analgesia had risen from 0 percent to 48 percent, the cesarean delivery rate was 8.6 percent. A number of other authors have also shown that cesarean section rates can actually decrease while the use of epidural analgesia rises. Larson et al.[153] found the cesarean delivery rate actually fell from 28 percent to 23 percent ($p = 0.0007$) after a 24-hour in-house obstetric anesthesiology service was established. The use of epidural analgesia rose from 0 percent to 32 percent during the same time period.[153] Yancey et al.[154] compared operative vaginal and abdominal delivery rates in a large population (9,637 patients) before and after on-demand labor epidural analgesia became available. Despite an increase from less than 1 percent to 59 percent in labor epidural analgesia use, the rate of neither cesarean delivery nor operative vaginal delivery increased. In a study of 6,928 patients, Fogel et al.[155] found that expanded epidural analgesia use (from 1 percent to 29 percent) did not change the overall dystocia cesarean delivery rate, although dystocia was more common among women who chose epidural analgesia.

Iglesias et al.[156] and Socol et al.[157] assessed the impact of changes in obstetric management on the incidence of cesarean delivery. Both groups found that they could decrease the cesarean delivery rate at the same time that the use of epidural analgesia was increasing in their hospitals. The decline in cesarean delivery rates in these studies is achieved primarily by increasing the use of vaginal birth after cesarean (VBAC), active management of labor, and use of oxytocin. The availability of epidural analgesia may be an important factor in patient acceptance of VBAC and in the obstetrician's willingness to aggressively manage labor and use oxytocin. This active management of labor is exemplified by the National Maternity Hospital in Dublin. At that institution, the epidural rate rose from 10 percent in 1987 to 45 percent in 1992, whereas the cesarean section rate remained unchanged at 4 to 5 percent.[158] The practitioners in Dublin note that "epidural analgesia may be of major benefit in labor and need not reduce the chance of spontaneous vaginal delivery if the passive phase of second stage of labor is lengthened."

Other work has also shown that obstetric management influences outcome independent of the type of labor analgesia utilized. In a retrospective review of epidural analgesia *managed by obstetricians*, women having epidural analgesia for labor actually had a *decreased* risk of cesarean delivery.[159] Neuhoff and colleagues retrospectively investigated cesarean deliveries for failed progress in labor at their hospital. The cesarean birth rate on the resident clinic service was 5 percent versus 17 percent on the private service, while the use of epidural analgesia was comparable on both services (42 percent in each group).[160] Cesarean births were increased on the private service when epidural analgesia was used, but cesarean delivery rates remained stable on the clinic service whether or not epidural analgesia was used. Segal et al.[161] analyzed data

from 110 obstetricians at their institution over 5 years. They found no relationship between the frequency of epidural analgesia and rate of cesarean delivery for dystocia across practitioners. They concluded that obstetric practitioners and, to a limited extent, the characteristics of their patient populations are major determinants of these rates.

A series of articles by Thorp and colleagues on the relationship between epidural analgesia and cesarean section caused great concern among obstetricians, anesthesiologists, and parturients.[162–164] The first publication, a retrospective review of 711 consecutive nulliparous women in spontaneous labor at term,[162] reported that women who received epidural analgesia had a longer duration of labor, were more likely to receive oxytocin, and had a 10.3 percent cesarean delivery rate for dystocia versus 3.8 percent in the nonepidural group. A subsequent retrospective study of 500 consecutive patients again showed an increased cesarean delivery rate in the epidural versus nonepidural group (11.4 vs. 2.4 percent) and noted that nulliparous women who had epidural analgesia administered before 5 cm of cervical dilation seemed to have the greatest effect on the incidence of cesarean delivery.[163] The authors concluded that "epidural analgesia in first labors may have contributed significantly to the cesarean epidemic." Thorp and colleagues[164] subsequently published a prospective study in which nulliparous women were randomized to receive intravenous meperidine or epidural bupivacaine. Twelve of 48 (25 percent) women in the epidural group—versus 1 of 45 (2.2 percent) women in the meperidine group—underwent cesarean delivery. Eleven of the 12 cesarean deliveries in the epidural group occurred in women who had received epidural analgesia before 5 cm dilation. Neonatal outcome was similar in both groups, and pain relief was rated superior in the epidural group by nurses and patients.

Three prospective, randomized trials were performed at Parkland Hospital in Dallas. Ramin[165] randomized 1,330 women of mixed parity to receive either epidural bupivacaine-fentanyl or intravenous meperidine analgesia during labor. Approximately one third of the women in each group did not receive the allocated treatment. When the authors evaluated outcome according to intention-to-treat analysis, they noted that 60 (9 percent) of the 664 women in the epidural group, versus 35 (5 percent) of the 666 women in the meperidine group, underwent *operative* delivery for dystocia. However, operative delivery was defined as either cesarean or low-forceps delivery. Within the intention-to-treat analysis, the authors did not report the number of cesarean deliveries in the two groups. Thus, it is unclear that there was an increased incidence of cesarean delivery in the women randomized to an offer of epidural analgesia.

Sharma et al.[166] reported this group's second randomized trial of epidural versus intravenous meperidine analgesia during labor. The authors randomized 715 women of mixed parity in spontaneous labor at term to receive either epidural analgesia or patient-controlled intravenous analgesia (PCIA) with meperidine. Enrollment and randomization occurred when the patients were admitted to the nurse-midwifery service at Parkland Hospital. Subsequently, an anesthesiologist offered epidural analgesia to the patients randomized to the epidural group, but not to the patients randomized to the PCIA group. Among the 358 patients who were randomized to an offer of epidural analgesia, only 243 actually received epidural analgesia. Of the remaining 115 patients, 78 labored rapidly and never requested or received epidural analgesia, and the remaining 37 refused epidural analgesia. Among the 357 patients who were randomized to an offer of PCIA, only 259 patients completed the study as allocated. Of the remaining 98 patients, 73 labored rapidly and did not receive any analgesia, 20 refused PCIA, and 5 who received meperidine PCIA "crossed over" to epidural analgesia because of unsatisfactory pain relief.

Using an intention-to-treat analysis, the authors observed no difference between the two groups in the incidence of cesarean delivery (i.e., 4 percent in the epidural group and 5 percent in the PCIA group). The authors also observed no difference between the two groups in the incidence of cesarean section when they evaluated outcome for protocol-compliant patients (i.e., 5 percent in the epidural analgesia group and 6 percent in the PCIA group). Women in the epidural group had lower pain scores during both the first and the second stages of labor, and women in the PCIA group were more sedated. There was no difference between the two groups in neonatal outcome, except that more babies in the PCIA group received naloxone for treatment of respiratory depression at birth.[166]

Gambling et al.[167] reported this group's third randomized trial, in which patients received either CSE or intravenous meperidine analgesia during labor. Profound fetal bradycardia, which prompted emergency cesarean section within 1 hour of intrathecal administration of sufentanil, occurred in 8 of 400 parturients who received CSE analgesia, versus none of 352 women who received intravenous meperidine ($P < 0.01$). However, CSE analgesia did *not* increase the overall incidence of cesarean section or the incidence of cesarean delivery for dystocia. Similarly, Bofill et al.[168] and Clark et al.[169] observed no increase in the overall incidence of cesarean delivery in nulliparous women randomized to receive epidural bupivacaine analgesia, when compared with similar women randomized to receive intravenous opioid analgesia.

A 1994 meta-analysis suggested a strong association between epidural analgesia and an increased risk of cesarean section.[170] However, a 1998 meta-analysis of randomized controlled trials did *not* support the hypothesis that epidural analgesia causes an increase in the cesarean delivery rate.[171] A 1999 meta-analysis sponsored by the National Institute of Child Health and Human Development (NICHD) found that epidural analgesia with low-dose bupivacaine may increase the risk of oxytocin augmentation but not that of cesarean delivery.[172]

Chestnut et al.[173,174] performed two studies to assess the effect of the *timing* of epidural analgesia on the incidence of cesarean delivery. The first study included nulliparous women *already* receiving oxytocin for induction or augmentation of labor.[173] Patients were randomized to receive intravenous nalbuphine or epidural bupivacaine when they had achieved a cervical dilation of at least 3 but less than 5 cm. Patients in the nalbuphine group could receive epidural analgesia once they achieved a cervical dilation of 5 cm or more, or 1 hour after a second dose of nalbuphine (as a rescue alternative). Attempts were made to minimize motor block in the epidural group. Early administration of epidural analgesia did not prolong the first stage of labor or increase the incidence of malposition of the vertex, instrumental vaginal delivery, or cesarean delivery. The overall incidence of cesarean delivery was 18 percent in the early epidural group and 19 percent in the late epidural group. Umbilical cord blood pH measurements were slightly lower in the late epidural group.

Chestnut et al.[174] used a similar study design to determine whether early use of epidural analgesia affected obstetric outcome in nulliparous women in *spontaneous* labor.[175] Early use of epidural analgesia did not increase the use of oxytocin augmentation, prolong the first stage of labor, or increase the incidence of malposition or instrumental delivery. There was no increase in cesarean delivery rate in the early epidural group (10 percent) versus the late epidural group (8 percent). Umbilical cord blood pH measurements were slightly lower in the late epidural group. The higher overall cesarean delivery rate in the first of these two studies (i.e., in women requiring induction or augmentation of labor) supports the conclusion that these parturients are at higher risk for cesarean delivery and should be considered separately in outcome studies.[133,134]

What might cause the difference in outcome[175] between the prospective studies of Thorp et al.[164] and Chestnut et al.?[173,174] In the work of Chestnut et al., all patients ultimately received epidural analgesia, whereas in the study by Thorp et al., only one patient in the meperidine group ultimately received epidural analgesia. In the prospective study by Thorp et al.[164] the authors assumed responsibility for the obstetric management decisions and obviously were not blinded to the anesthetic group. Their study patients were limited to an indigent population, while those of Chestnut et al.[173,174] were evenly divided between indigent and private patients.

Chestnut et al. adjusted the epidural infusion to minimize the degree of motor block, but Thorp's group did not indicate the degree of maternal motor block or whether epidural analgesia was managed in such a way as to minimize excessive motor block.

RECOMMENDATIONS. What can be concluded from these studies of epidural analgesia and the progress of labor? *First,* it is probably preferable to avoid institution of epidural analgesia during early, latent-phase labor in most patients. In general, epidural analgesia should not be instituted until the obstetrician is satisfied that the labor is established, that is, until the patient is having regular contractions and the cervix is dilating progressively. However, it is difficult to assign a specific cervical dilation as indicating the time to administer epidural analgesia; for some patients it will be 3 to 4 cm and for others, 4 to 6 cm. Psychoprophylactic techniques are probably most effective during the latent phase of labor and will allow many patients to forego supplemental analgesia during that period. However, physicians should recognize that some patients experience severe pain during latent-phase labor. This is especially true if the patient is receiving intravenous oxytocin. It is best to individualize decisions regarding timing of epidural analgesia. Thus, in some patients, early institution of epidural analgesia may be appropriate. In these situations, it may be possible to utilize intrathecal or epidural opioids and allow the patient to ambulate until labor has become more active. The American Society of Anesthesiologists and the ACOG have written a joint statement on pain relief in labor that notes in part, "There is no other circumstance where it is considered acceptable for a person to experience severe pain, amenable to safe intervention, while under a physician's care."[176]

Second, it is preferable to use dilute solutions of local anesthetic rather than more concentrated solutions. For example, 0.125 percent or 0.25 percent bupivacaine will provide satisfactory analgesia in almost all parturients, and it is rarely necessary to give a more concentrated solution of bupivacaine for analgesia during labor. If a patient develops motor block, the local anesthetic solution can be made more dilute and supplemented with an opioid as needed.

Third, the obstetrician should recognize that a brief period of decreased uterine activity often follows the institution of epidural analgesia. In some patients, there is a brief period of decreased uterine activity followed by reestablishment of the contraction pattern and resumption of normal labor (Fig. 15–10).[177] This may actually be caused by the intravenous hydration given prior to epidural analgesia.[178,179] In one study, a 1,000-ml fluid load decreased uterine activity for a short period of time, whereas an epidural block without a fluid load was associated with increased uterine

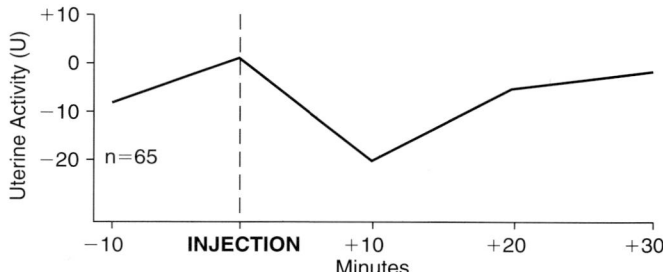

Figure 15–10. Effect of epidural injections of lidocaine with epinephrine on uterine activity levels in 65 cases. (From Lowenshon RI, Paul RH, Fales S, et al: Intrapartum epidural anesthesia: an evaluation of effects on uterine activity. Obstet Gynecol 44:388, 1974, with permission.)

activity.[178] In some patients, epidural analgesia may accelerate labor, perhaps by decreasing maternal concentrations of catecholamines. At least one study has documented a favorable influence of epidural analgesia in patients with discoordinate uterine contractions and prolonged labor.[180] However, in other patients, analgesia may seem to slow or to stop labor for more than a brief period. In such patients, the obstetrician should be willing to augment labor by giving oxytocin intravenously.

Fourth, there remains disagreement regarding whether it is advisable to add epinephrine to the therapeutic dose of local anesthetic. Some anesthesiologists add epinephrine to local anesthetic solutions to produce vasoconstriction in the area where the local anesthetic is injected. In this way, the blood absorbs smaller amounts of anesthetic over a longer time period. Thus, there is a decreased concentration of local anesthetic in the maternal blood, and less local anesthetic crosses the placenta to the fetus (Fig. 15–11). Also, the addition of epinephrine may result in a more solid block, especially if one is administering lidocaine. On the other hand, some studies have demonstrated that the addition of epinephrine to local anesthetic solution is more likely to decrease uterine activity than administration of local anesthetic without epinephrine (Fig. 15–12). Another study reported a similar effect of epinephrine on uterine activity but no significant effect of epinephrine on the duration of labor.[181] Other investigations have also suggested that the addition of epinephrine to local anesthetic does not prolong the duration of labor.[182–185] This is especially likely to be true if a very dilute concentration of epinephrine is administered.[182–185]

Fifth, should epidural analgesia be continued or discontinued during the second stage of labor? We believe that it is inappropriate to withhold analgesia routinely during the second stage. Johnson et al.[186] concluded: "Voluntary effort is decreased in some patients in the second stage of labor with spinal and peridural analgesia. Since this is not a consistent finding, and some patients actually exhibited increased capability for bear-

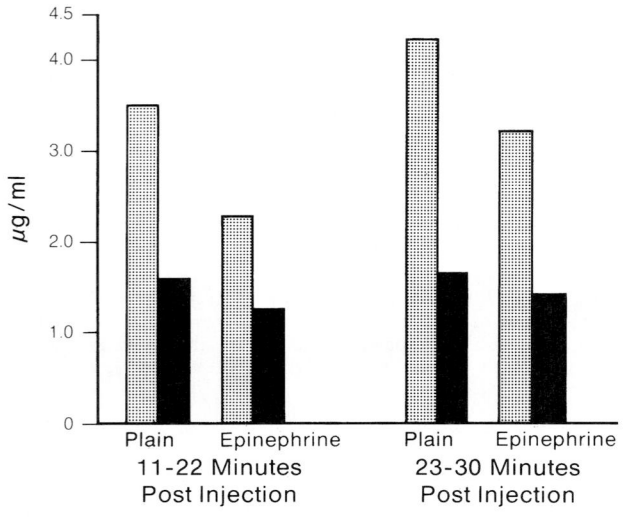

Figure 15–11. Histogram of mean maternal and cord plasma concentrations of lidocaine, 20 ml 2 percent solution with or without the addition of 1:250,000 epinephrine, in patients who were delivered 11 to 22 minutes or 23 to 30 minutes after administration of lidocaine by the lumbar epidural route. (From Thomas J, Climmie CR, Long G, Nighjoy LE: The influence of adrenaline on the maternal plasma levels and placental transfer of lignocaine following lumbar epidural administration. Br J Anaesth 41:1031, 1969, with permission.)

ing down after the anesthesia, it must be an individual reaction without the actual loss of ability." We should like to emphasize that epidural analgesia during labor is not a generic procedure. For example, in one study[150] maintenance of the infusion of local anesthetic until delivery did not prolong the second stage or increase the incidence of instrumental delivery, but it also did not reliably provide second-stage analgesia. In a similar study[141] performed at the same institution, infusion of a different local anesthetic until delivery provided excellent second-stage analgesia, but it prolonged the second stage and increased the incidence of instrumental delivery. In the first study,[150] the block during the second stage was clearly inadequate in most patients, while in the second study[141] the block was probably excessive in some patients. Clearly, a dense epidural block may decrease the ability of some patients to push effectively. On the other hand, other patients will push more effectively in the presence of analgesia. In clinical practice, it seems best to individualize patient management. If the block is too dense and the patient cannot push effectively, then there should be diminution of the level and/or intensity of analgesia. In other patients, the block should be maintained or strengthened. The optimal approach is to provide a reasonable level of analgesia consistent with the parturient's ability to push effectively. Of course, it is also important that patients be actively coached in pushing.

Sixth, one should avoid arbitrary termination of the second stage. As noted earlier, the ACOG has redefined the "normal" limits of the duration of the second stage in patients with and without regional anesthesia.[146] Indeed, in some patients with effective epidural analgesia, it may be appropriate to allow a second stage of more than 3 hours, provided that there is continued progress in descent of the vertex.

Seventh, it is important to recognize that risk to mother and infant of instrumental delivery performed under the ideal conditions provided by spinal or epidural anesthesia may differ from the risk of instrumental delivery performed without adequate anesthesia. Indeed, regional anesthesia may well allow for more complete cooperation by the patient, a more accurate application of the forceps, and a more gentle birth.

Finally, the weight of current evidence suggests that maternal–fetal factors and obstetric management are the most important determinants of the cesarean delivery rate.[159–161,187–189] Epidural analgesia during labor is not a generic procedure, and conclusions regarding the effect of one technique on the progress of labor may not be applicable to other techniques. We do *not* recommend withholding analgesia until the patient has achieved an arbitrary cervical dilation during the first stage of labor, and it is equally inappropriate to discontinue analgesia altogether during the second stage.

There remain several unresolved questions with regard to optimal management of epidural anesthesia during labor. *First,* does continuous infusion of local anesthetic affect labor differently than intermittent epidural bolus injection? Purported advantages of continuous epidural infusion during labor include (1) a more stable level of analgesia, (2) reduced risk of hypotension, (3) reduced risk of systemic toxicity, (4) reduced risk of total spinal block, and (5) convenience for the

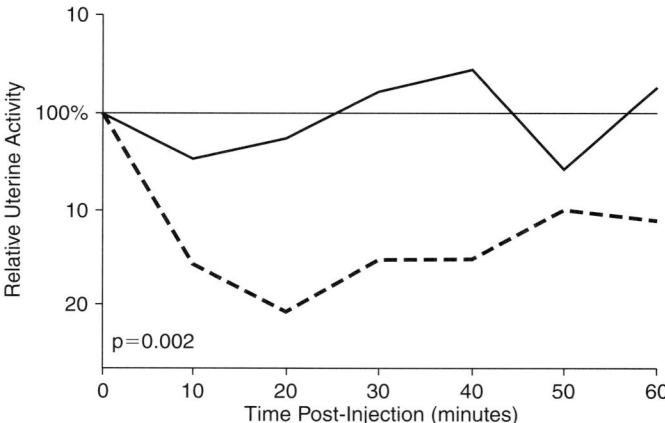

Figure 15–12. Mean values of uterine activity after epidural administration of lidocaine (*solid line*) or lidocaine with epinephrine (*dotted line*). (From Matadial L, Cibils LA: The effect of epidural anesthesia on uterine activity and blood pressure. Am J Obstet Gynecol 125: 846, 1976, with permission.)

anesthesiologist.[190] An infusion pump delivers a dilute solution of local anesthetic by continuous positive pressure. A potential disadvantage of continuous epidural infusion is that it tends to discourage individualization of the dose of local anesthetic in an individual patient. Thus, there is a tendency to give more local anesthetic than one would give if one were using the intermittent epidural bolus injection technique. For example, there have been at least five controlled comparisons of the continuous epidural infusion of bupivacaine versus intermittent epidural bolus injection of bupivacaine.[191–195] In each study, patients in the continuous infusion group received more bupivacaine than did patients in the intermittent bolus group. It is unclear whether the increased dose of bupivacaine is clinically significant and represents a disadvantage. Furthermore, it is unclear whether the continuous epidural infusion technique has more or less effect on the progress of labor and method of delivery than does the intermittent epidural bolus injection technique. Altogether, the weight of evidence suggests that the continuous epidural infusion technique is advantageous, provided the anesthesiologist uses a dilute solution of local anesthetic.

Second, is it advantageous to add opioid to the solution of local anesthetic and thereby reduce the total dose of local anesthetic and the extent of maternal motor block? Chestnut and colleagues[196] observed that the continuous epidural infusion of 0.0625 percent bupivacaine–0.0002 percent fentanyl produced first-stage analgesia similar to that provided by the infusion of 0.125 percent bupivacaine alone. Women who received bupivacaine and fentanyl experienced less intense motor block, but they did *not* have a shorter second stage or a lower incidence of instrumental delivery than did women who received bupivacaine alone. A legitimate criticism of that study is that the epidural infusion was discontinued at full cervical dilation in both groups. Had the infusion been continued until delivery, it is possible that there would have been a difference between groups in the method of delivery.

Vertommen et al.[197] performed a multicenter randomized study of epidural bolus administration of 0.125 percent bupivacaine with 1:800,000 epinephrine, with and without sufentanil, in 695 parturients of mixed parity. There was no difference between the two groups in the duration of the second stage of labor (33 ± 24 minutes in the sufentanil group vs. 27 ± 21 minutes in the control group). Women in the sufentanil group had a decreased incidence of instrumental vaginal delivery (24 percent vs. 36 percent, $p < 0.01$). The authors attributed this reduction to the decreased total dose of bupivacaine (34 ± 17 vs. 42 ± 19 mg) and the decreased intensity of motor block in the sufentanil group. The authors did not specifically assess and report the quality of analgesia during the second stage of labor. In an accompanying editorial, it was noted that

"no published study has shown that one can consistently provide effective analgesia *throughout the second stage of labor* without increasing the risk of instrumental delivery."[198]

Third, should there be more frequent use of oxytocin during the second stage of labor? Goodfellow and colleagues[199] noted a significant increase in maternal blood concentrations of oxytocin between the onset of full cervical dilation and crowning of the fetal head in patients without epidural anesthesia, but they did not observe a similar increase in patients with epidural anesthesia. Similarly, Bates and colleagues[200] observed significantly less uterine activity during the second stage in patients with epidural anesthesia compared with patients without epidural anesthesia. Both groups of investigators recommended increased utilization of oxytocin during the second stage in order to increase the chance of spontaneous vaginal delivery.

Fourth, is there a role for delayed pushing during the second stage? Maresh and colleagues[143] reported a study of 76 nulliparous women with epidural anesthesia who were randomly assigned to early pushing or late pushing in the second stage. There was a significant increase in the duration of the second stage but a nonsignificant decrease in the frequency of instrumental delivery in the late-pushing group. The increased second-stage duration was not associated with an increase in fetal heart rate abnormalities or a decrease in Apgar scores or umbilical cord blood pH. It is possible that patients become exhausted when asked to push too early during the second stage. Indeed, it may be preferable to allow the force of uterine contractions to deliver the vertex to a station at which maternal pushing might be effective.

Paracervical Block

Paracervical block analgesia, a simple, effective procedure when performed properly, is used most commonly by obstetricians. Usually, 5 to 6 ml of a dilute solution of local anesthetic without epinephrine (e.g., 1 percent lidocaine or 1 or 2 percent 2-chloroprocaine) is injected into the mucosa of the cervix at either the 4- and 8- or 3- and 9-o'clock positions; an Iowa trumpet prevents deep penetration of the needle (Fig. 15–13). The duration of analgesia depends on the local anesthetic used. Several manufacturers have stated that bupivacaine, the longest acting local anesthetic, is contraindicated for obstetric paracervical block. In the past, paracervical block enjoyed considerable favor, particularly when anesthesiologists were not available to provide major regional analgesia techniques. Disadvantages of the technique are that the block can only be applied during the first stage of labor and that it must be reapplied frequently during the course of a long labor. Furthermore, it has the widely recognized major disadvantage of fetal

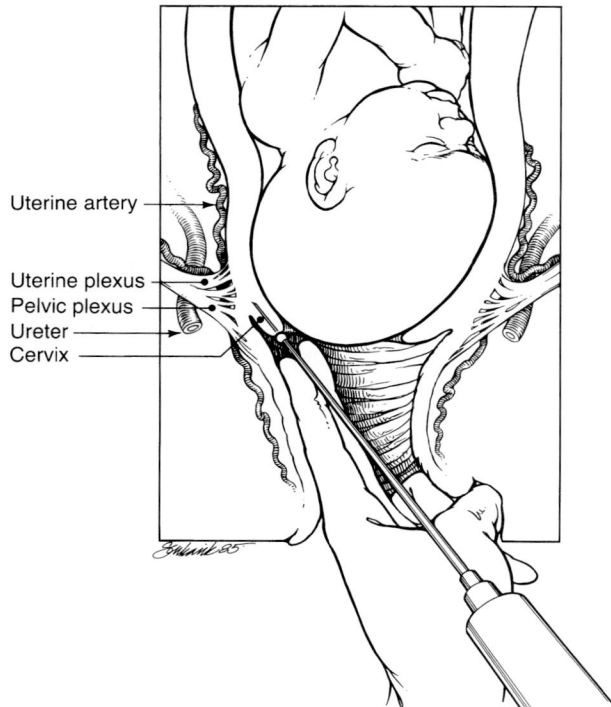

Figure 15–13. Technique of paracervical block. Schematic coronal section (enlarged) of lower portion of cervix and upper portion of vagina shows relation of needle to paracervical region. (Modified from Bonica JJ: Principles and Practice of Obstetric Analgesia and Anesthesia. Philadelphia, FA Davis, 1967, p 234.)

high blood concentration is feasible, because the local anesthetic is injected close to the uterine artery. The anesthetic would traverse the wall of the uterine artery, pass directly to the fetus, and thus result in a high blood concentration and subsequent bradycardia.[201] Clinical support for this theory is that infants who suffer bradycardia frequently have higher anesthetic blood concentrations than do their mothers.[201] Alternatively, the bradycardia may result from uterine artery vasoconstriction secondary to a direct effect of the local anesthetic on the uterine artery.[204,205] This effect has been demonstrated in vitro on human uterine arteries[204] (Fig. 15–14) and is supported by uterine blood flow studies in animals.[205] The fetal electrocardiogram (ECG) pattern during one of these episodes suggests hypoxia, a finding that supports the uterine artery vasoconstriction theory.[206] Furthermore, the high concentrations of local anesthetic required to produce vasoconstriction during the administration of a paracervical block can be achieved close to the uterine artery (Fig. 15–13). It is unlikely that such levels are obtained with other forms of regional anesthesia. The third theory is based on the possibility that local anesthetic injected directly into the uterine musculature increases uterine tone.

Some have suggested that manipulation of the fetal head, the uterus, or the uterine vasculature during institution of the block might produce reflex bradycardia. It is possible that no one theory is adequate to explain all cases of postparacervical block bradycardia. Regardless of etiology, the severity and duration of the bradycardia correlate with the incidence of fetal acidosis and subsequent neonatal depression. Freeman and colleagues[206] reported a significant fall in pH and a rise in base deficit only in those fetuses with bradycardia persisting more than 10 minutes. In summary, paracervical block should be used cautiously at all times and should not be used at all in mothers with fetuses in either acute or chronic distress.

bradycardia, which occurs in 2 to 70 percent of applications. It occurs within 2 to 10 minutes and lasts from 3 to 30 minutes. Although usually benign, it can be associated with fetal acidosis and occasionally with fetal death.[201–203]

There is no consensus regarding the mechanism of postparacervical block bradycardia. The theories include (1) high blood concentrations of local anesthetic in the fetus, (2) uterine artery vasoconstriction, and (3) postparacervical block increase in uterine activity. A

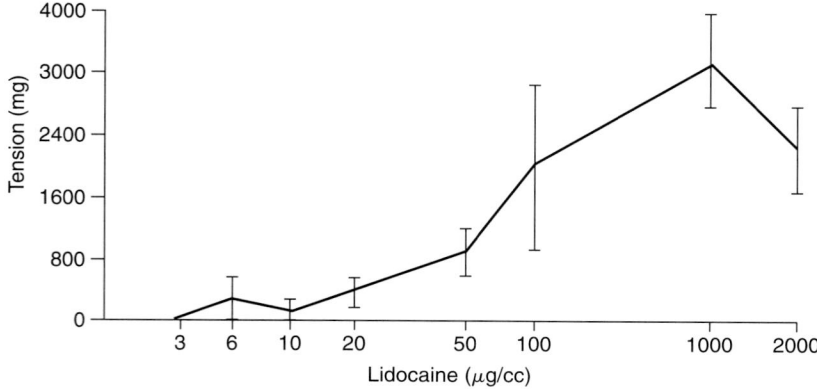

mean ±SEM, n=9

Figure 15–14. Dose–response curve of the pregnant human uterine artery to lidocaine hydrochloride (mean ± SEM; $N = 9$). (From Gibbs CP, Noel SC: Response of arterial segments from gravid human uterus to multiple concentrations of lignocaine. Br J Anaesth 45:409, 1977, with permission.)

Table 15-4. ANESTHETIC PROCEDURES USED FOR LABOR IN 1997 ACCORDING TO SIZE OF DELIVERY SERVICE

Delivery Service (births/year)	No Anesthesia (%)	Narcotics Barbiturates Tranquilizers (%)	Paracervical Block (%)	Spinal or Epidural Block (%)
<500	17	50	6	42
500-1,499	11	53	3	55
>1,500	11	39	2	66

From Hawkins JL, Beaty BR, Gibbs CP, et al: Update on U.S. obstetric anesthesia practices [abstract]. Anesthesiology 91:A1060, 1999.

Sterile Water Injection

A novel way to provide relief of severe lower back pain during the first stage of labor involves subcutaneous or intracutaneous injection of sterile water at four points on the lower back.[207] In a randomized controlled trial, the median reductions in the visual analogue scores were 4 to 5 compared to 1 in the placebo group.

Table 15-4 presents the frequency with which the various forms of analgesia are used during labor. The data are from a survey of 750 hospitals in the United States.[208]

ANESTHESIA FOR VAGINAL DELIVERY

Pain relief for vaginal delivery can be achieved in a number of ways. Some patients will require no anesthesia. For those who do, the goal is to match the patient's wishes with the requirements of the delivery without subjecting either mother or fetus to unnecessary risk.

Local Anesthesia

In the form of perineal infiltration, local anesthesia is widely used and very safe. Spontaneous vaginal deliveries, episiotomies, and perhaps use of outlet forceps can be accomplished with this simple technique. Local anesthetic toxicity may occur if large amounts of local anesthetic are used or in the unlikely event that an intravascular injection occurs. Usually, 5 to 15 ml of 1 percent lidocaine suffices. Philipson and colleagues[209] demonstrated the rapid and significant transfer of lidocaine to the fetus after perineal infiltration. In 5 of 15 infants, the concentration of lidocaine at delivery was greater in the umbilical vein than in the mother (Table 15-5).[209]

Pudendal Nerve Block

Pudendal nerve block is a minor regional block that also is widely used, reasonably effective, and very safe. The obstetrician, using an Iowa trumpet and a 20-gauge needle, injects 5 to 10 ml of local anesthetic just below the ischial spine. Because the hemorrhoidal nerve may be aberrant in 50 percent of patients,[210] some physicians prefer to inject a portion of the local anesthetic somewhat posterior to the spine (Fig. 15-15). For those inexperienced at identifying the ischial spine, the bony prominence at the inner canthus of one's eye provides a reasonable facsimile of a small and somewhat sharp ischial spine. Although a transperineal approach to the ischial spine is possible, most prefer the transvaginal approach. One percent lidocaine or 2 percent 2-chloroprocaine is used.

The technique is satisfactory for all spontaneous vaginal deliveries and episiotomies and for some outlet or low-forceps deliveries, but may not be sufficient for deliveries requiring additional manipulation. For example, a breech delivery or a delivery necessitating more

Table 15-5. LIDOCAINE CONCENTRATIONS AT DELIVERY IN MATERNAL PLASMA AND UMBILICAL CORD VEIN AFTER PERINEAL INFILTRATION

Sample (N = 15)	Concentration (ng/ml)	
	Mean ± SD	Range
Maternal plasma		
Peak concentration	648 ± 666	60-2,400
At delivery	548 ± 468	33-1,474
Umbilical cord vein	420 ± 406	45-1,380
Fetal/maternal ratio*	1.32 ± 1.46	0.05-4.66

*Ratio of level in cord vein to level in maternal vein at delivery (mean of individual ratios, not ratio of means).
From Philipson EH, Kuhnert BR, Syracuse CD: Maternal, fetal, and neonatal lidocaine levels following local perineal infiltration. Am J Obstet Gynecol 149: 403, 1984, with permission.

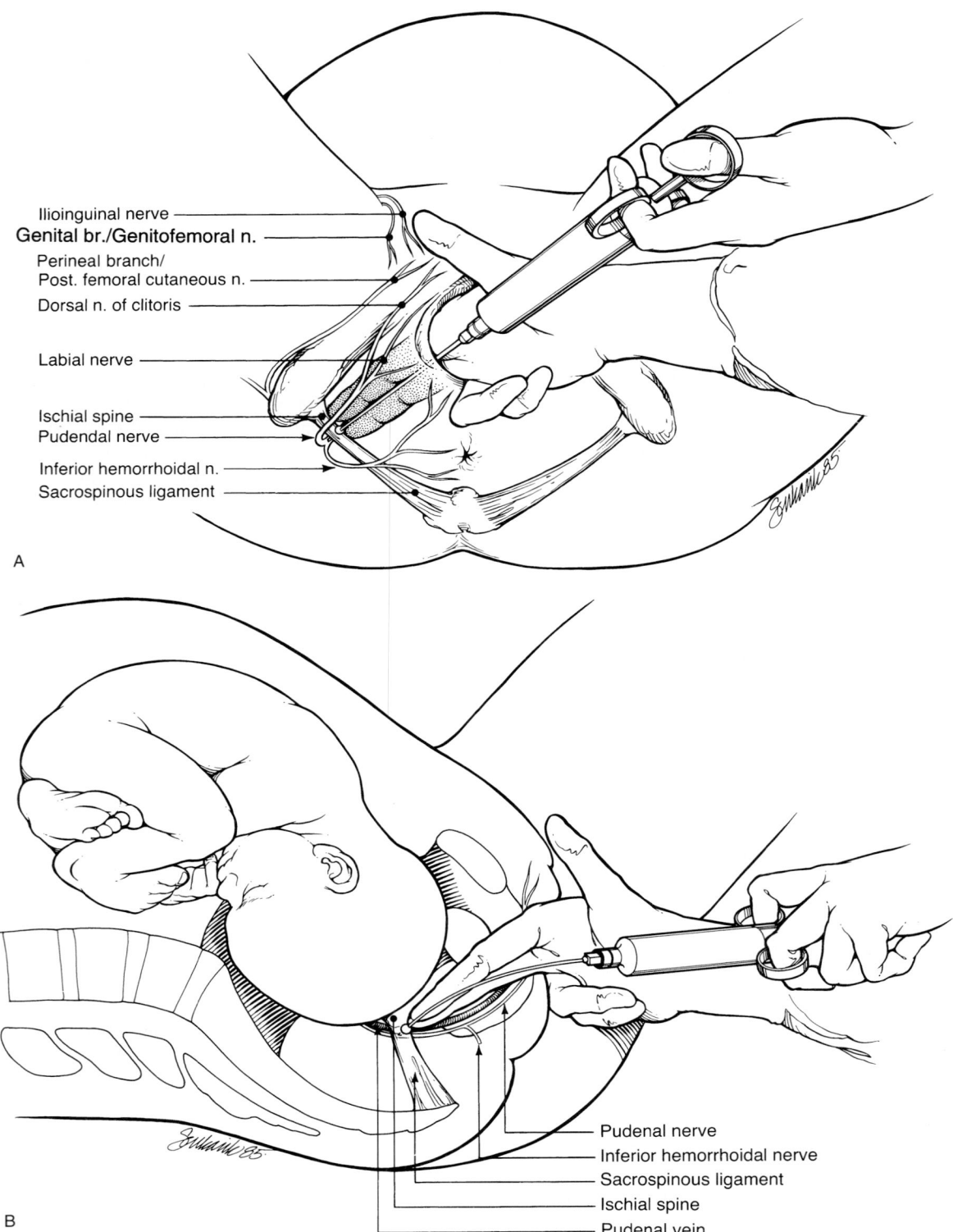

Ilioinguinal nerve

Genital br./Genitofemoral n.

Perineal branch/
Post. femoral cutaneous n.

Dorsal n. of clitoris

Labial nerve

Ischial spine
Pudendal nerve

Inferior hemorrhoidal n.

Sacrospinous ligament

A

Pudenal nerve
Inferior hemorrhoidal nerve
Sacrospinous ligament
Ischial spine
Pudenal vein

B

Figure 15–15. *A* and *B*, Anatomy of the pudendal nerve and techniques of pudendal block.

than outlet forceps may require more pain relief, relaxation, and cooperation than pudendal block can ensure. Likewise, a pudendal block may not provide enough anesthesia for the successful and controlled release of shoulder dystocia. In these instances, as in any others that require significant manipulation, more extensive anesthesia will be required. Ideally, such requirements should be anticipated before the event.

More than with perineal infiltration, the potential for local anesthetic toxicity exists with pudendal block because of the proximity of large vessels close to the site of injection (Fig. 15–15). Therefore, aspiration before injection is particularly important. Furthermore, the potential for large amounts of local anesthetic to be used increases when perineal and labial infiltration are required in addition to the pudendal block. In these instances, it is important to monitor closely the amount of local anesthetic given.

Inhalation or Intravenous Analgesia

An anesthesiologist or nurse anesthetist administers inhalation or intravenous analgesia (stage I anesthesia), which provides varying degrees of pain relief and amnesia but maintains protective laryngeal and cough reflexes. Most often the obstetrician will add local infiltration or a pudendal block. The anesthesiologist will frequently question the patient to determine the level of anesthesia and to ensure that deeper planes of anesthesia are avoided. Such precautions are important because, if the patient becomes unconscious and passes beyond stage I, all of the hazards associated with general anesthesia are possible, including inadequate airway, hypoxia, and aspiration. Because continual assessment of the patient's state of consciousness is required and is sometimes difficult, only anesthesiologists or nurse anesthetists should administer inhalation analgesia. Furthermore, this technique requires the use of the increasingly complicated anesthesia machine, misuse of which can prove disastrous. Most frequently, the anesthesiologist uses 40 or at most 50 percent nitrous oxide or, for intravenous analgesia, ketamine, 0.25 mg/kg. This latter agent may be particularly effective for the patient who cannot or will not tolerate an anesthetic face mask. Less commonly, the anesthesiologist may administer a subanesthetic concentration of a potent halogenated agent (e.g., sevoflurane) for a brief period.

Inhalation or intravenous analgesia alone will not be sufficient for performing episiotomies or repairing perineal lacerations. Therefore, these techniques usually require supplemental pudendal block or perineal infiltration. The combined effects of both techniques are additive and satisfactory for spontaneous vaginal deliveries, most outlet forceps deliveries, and even some manipulative deliveries. Inhalation or intravenous analgesia

renders some patients amnesic of the event, a characteristic that is often undesirable.

Spinal (Subarachnoid) Block

A saddle block is a spinal block in which the level of anesthesia is limited to little more than the perineum, that is, the saddle area. Spinal anesthesia is reasonably easy to perform and usually provides total pain relief in the blocked area. Therefore, spontaneous deliveries, forceps deliveries, and episiotomies can be accomplished without pain for the mother. Likewise, complicated deliveries that require extensive manipulation can be effected in a controlled and pain-free manner. Although the ability to push may be compromised somewhat, the advantage of having a cooperative patient who is receptive to suggestion and able to cooperate because she is pain-free may outweigh the disadvantage of moderately diminished strength.

Usually spinal anesthesia is achieved by injecting 25 to 50 mg hyperbaric lidocaine or 5 to 7.5 mg hyperbaric bupivacaine into the subarachnoid space through a 24 to 27-gauge spinal needle. It is preferable to use a pencil-point needle of the smallest possible gauge, because these needles reduce the risk of spinal headache. Fentanyl 10 to 25 μg may also be added to the spinal anesthetic. Because the solution is hyperbaric relative to cerebrospinal fluid, the most important determinant of anesthesia level is gravity. The level is most easily controlled by varying the position of the patient. For example, the sitting position causes the level to fall toward the sacral nerve roots for a perineal block. Other factors may also contribute to the level of anesthesia: amount of drug, volume injected, speed of injection, and height of the patient. Less controllable factors include the Valsalva maneuver, coughing, and straining, any of which will cause the level to rise. One should avoid injecting the local anesthetic during a contraction, because a higher than expected level of anesthesia may occur. Finally, left uterine displacement is maintained by a wedge or by some other effective device placed under the right hip after the local anesthetic has been injected.

Because spinal anesthesia is sometimes administered by persons other than anesthesiologists and is technically easy to perform, the single most important fact to understand is that it is a major regional block; it is not a procedure to be taken lightly. All hazards associated with major blocks are possible, including hypotension and "total spinal." Although these complications can occur, they should not result in disaster if diagnosed early and treated appropriately. The person who administers spinal anesthesia must never leave the patient unattended without ensuring that another competent individual will assume responsibility for monitoring the blood pressure and level of anesthesia. Usually, the level of the spinal block will be complete and fixed within 5 to 10 minutes. However, sometimes the level continues to creep upward for 20 minutes or longer.

Single-Dose Caudal and Lumbar Epidural Anesthesia

Single-dose epidural anesthesia techniques are used much less frequently than in the past. The relative difficulty and the large amounts of local anesthetic required are significant disadvantages for the caudal technique. Usually, when these techniques are used they are instituted during labor as continuous techniques and maintained or intensified for the delivery.

General Anesthesia

General anesthesia is rarely indicated for vaginal delivery. Whether given for a brief or a prolonged period of time, general anesthesia engenders considerable risk and should therefore not be used without strong indication. An unanticipated breech presentation, shoulder dystocia, or internal version and extraction of a second twin represent rare indications for general anesthesia. Also, general anesthesia may rarely be indicated for a difficult forceps delivery in a patient in whom major regional anesthesia is contraindicated. When general anesthesia is indicated, the technique specific for cesarean delivery is used, including administration by experienced and competent personnel, rapid sequence induction, and endotracheal intubation. For breech delivery or delivery of a second twin, one may administer a high concentration of a volatile halogenated agent (e.g., isoflurane, desflurane, or sevoflurane) to effect uterine and perhaps cervical relaxation. Equipotent doses of any of these three agents will provide equivalent uterine relaxation.[211] Table 15–6 lists the frequencies with which the various forms of anesthesia are used for vaginal delivery.

Table 15–6. ANESTHETIC PROCEDURES USED FOR CESAREAN DELIVERY IN 1997 ACCORDING TO SIZE OF DELIVERY SERVICE

Delivery Service (births/year)	Lumbar Epidural Block (%)	Spinal Block (%)	General Anesthesia (%)
<500	29	63	8
500–1,499	33	55	11
>1,500	43	49	8

From Hawkins JL, Beaty BR, Gibbs CP, et al: Update on U.S. obstetric anesthesia practices [abstract]. Anesthesiology 91:A1060, 1999.

ANESTHESIA FOR CESAREAN DELIVERY

The patient can be either asleep or awake during cesarean delivery. For those who wish to be awake, either spinal anesthesia or lumbar epidural anesthesia is used most commonly. In the United States, general anesthesia is used for 8 to 11 percent of cesarean births (depending on size of hospital), and spinal and epidural anesthetics are used for approximately 90 percent (Table 15–7).[208] Local anesthesia for cesarean delivery is possible but is only rarely used.[212]

Either general or regional anesthesia should be safe for the infant; studies have reported Apgar scores and blood gas measurements as essentially the same for infants of mothers choosing either technique (Table 15–8).[213–215,211] In recent years, some authors have suggested that Apgar scores and acid–base analysis evaluated brain stem activity, but not the higher centers. Therefore, neurobehavioral testing for the newborn was developed.[216] The testing involves eliciting and observing the quality of the infant's responses to certain stimuli in the early postpartum hours. A trained person can accomplish the testing in approximately 15 minutes. Results indicate that infants of mothers who receive regional anesthesia achieve somewhat higher scores than those whose mothers receive general anesthesia, and infants do somewhat better when ketamine is the induction agent for general anesthesia than when thiopental is used.[217] Regarding the choice of local anesthetic for regional anesthesia, infants were originally thought to do better after 2-chloroprocaine and bupivacaine than after lidocaine and mepivacaine.[216,218] Recently, however, lidocaine has been "exonerated" and is associated with neurobehavioral scores equal to those observed when mothers have received 2-chloroprocaine or bupivacaine.[83] When the Food and Drug Administration (FDA) appointed a committee to study neurobehavioral changes in newborns after anesthesia, the committee concluded that, although anesthetic agents can alter neurobehavioral performance, there was no evidence that they affect later development.[41] Therefore, neurobehavioral considerations do not weigh heavily in the choice of anesthesia or anesthetic agent; the choice can be based on the preferences of the mother, the obstetrician, and the anesthesiologist as well as on the demands of the particular clinical situation.

General Anesthesia

Although outcomes for the neonate are similar after regional or general anesthesia, failure to intubate and aspiration continue to be major causes of maternal mortality.[219–223] Because these two disadvantages of

Table 15-7. ELECTIVE CESAREAN SECTION—BLOOD GAS AND APGAR SCORES

	General Anesthesia* (N = 20)	Epidural Anesthesia* (N = 15)	Spinal Anesthesia† (N = 15)
Umbilical vein			
pH	7.38	7.359	7.34
PO_2 (mm Hg)	35	36	37
PCO_2 (mm Hg)	38	42	48
Apgar <6			
1	1	0	0
5	0	0	0
Umbilical artery			
pH	7.32	7.28	7.28
PO_2 (mm Hg)	22	18	18
PCO_2 (mm Hg)	47	55	63
BE (mEq/L)	−1.80	−1.60	−1.40

*Data from James FM III, Crawford JS, Hopkinson R, et al: A comparison of general anesthesia and lumbar epidural analgesia for elective cesarean section. Anesth Analg 56:228, 1977.
†Data from Datta S, Brown WU: Acid-base status in diabetic mothers and their infants following general or spinal anesthesia for cesarean section. Anesthesiology 47:272, 1977.
BE, base excess.

general anesthesia are a considerable and significant threat to the mother, many anesthesiologists now prefer regional anesthesia over general anesthesia. Data from both the ASA Closed Claims study[93] and the Centers for Disease Control and Prevention[223] indicate maternal mortality rates are higher during general anesthesia than during regional anesthesia, perhaps as much as 17 times higher. To understand how these complications arise, the obstetrician should be aware of the sequence of events during general anesthesia. Furthermore, there may be times when the obstetrician must participate in difficult decisions concerning anesthetic management. Those decisions may affect the lives and well-being of both mother and infant.

Premedication

Premedication using sedative or opioid agents is usually omitted because these agents cross the placenta and can depress the fetus. Sedation should be unnecessary if the procedure is explained well.

Antacids

Use of a clear antacid is considered routine for all parturients prior to surgery. Additional aspiration prophylaxis using an H_2-receptor blocking agent and/or metoclopramide may be given to parturients with risk factors such as morbid obesity, diabetes mellitus, a difficult airway, or those who have previously received narcotics. As soon as it is known that the patient requires cesarean delivery, be it with regional or general anesthesia, 30 ml of a clear, nonparticulate antacid, such as 0.3 M sodium citrate,[224] Bicitra,[225] or Alka Seltzer, 2 tablets in 30 ml water,[226] is administered to decrease gastric acidity and ameliorate the consequences of aspiration, should it occur. The chalky white partic-

Table 15-8. ARTERIAL BLOOD GAS TENSIONS AND pH OF DOGS 30 MINUTES AFTER ASPIRATION OF 2 CC/KG OF VARIOUS MATERIALS

Aspirate		Response		
Composition	pH	PO_2 (mm Hg)	PCO_2 (mm Hg)	pH
Saline	5.9	61	34	7.37
HCl	1.8	41	45	7.29
Food particles	5.9	34	51	7.19
Food particles	1.8	23	56	7.13

From Gibbs CP, Modell JH: Management of aspiration pneumonitis. *In* Miller RD (ed): Anesthesia, 3rd ed. New York, Churchill Livingstone, 1990, p 1293, with permission.

Advantages and Disadvantages of General Anesthesia for Cesarean Delivery

Advantages
  Patient does not have to be awake during a
    major operation.
  General anesthesia provides total pain relief.
  Operating conditions are optimal.
Disadvantages
  Patient will not be awake during childbirth,
    although there is a small risk of undesirable
    awareness.
  There is a slight risk of fetal depression.
  Intubation causes hypertension and tachycardia,
    which may be particularly dangerous in
    severely preeclamptic patients.
  Intubation can be difficult or impossible.
  Aspiration of stomach contents is possible.

ulate antacids are avoided because they can produce lung damage (Fig. 15–16).[227]

Left Uterine Displacement

As during labor, the uterus may compress the inferior vena cava and the aorta during cesarean delivery; aortocaval compression is detrimental to both mother and fetus. The duration of anesthesia has little effect on neonatal acid–base status when left uterine displacement is practiced; however, when patients remain supine, Apgar scores decrease as time of anesthesia increases.[228]

Regarding this latter point (i.e., anesthesia time or induction-to-delivery time), more recent data indicate that the induction-to-delivery time is not the crucial time. Rather, it is the uterine incision-to-delivery interval that is predictive of neonatal status.[229] A uterine-incision interval of less than 90 seconds is optimal, whereas an incision-to-delivery interval of 90 to 180 seconds is less satisfactory; after 180 seconds, the inci-

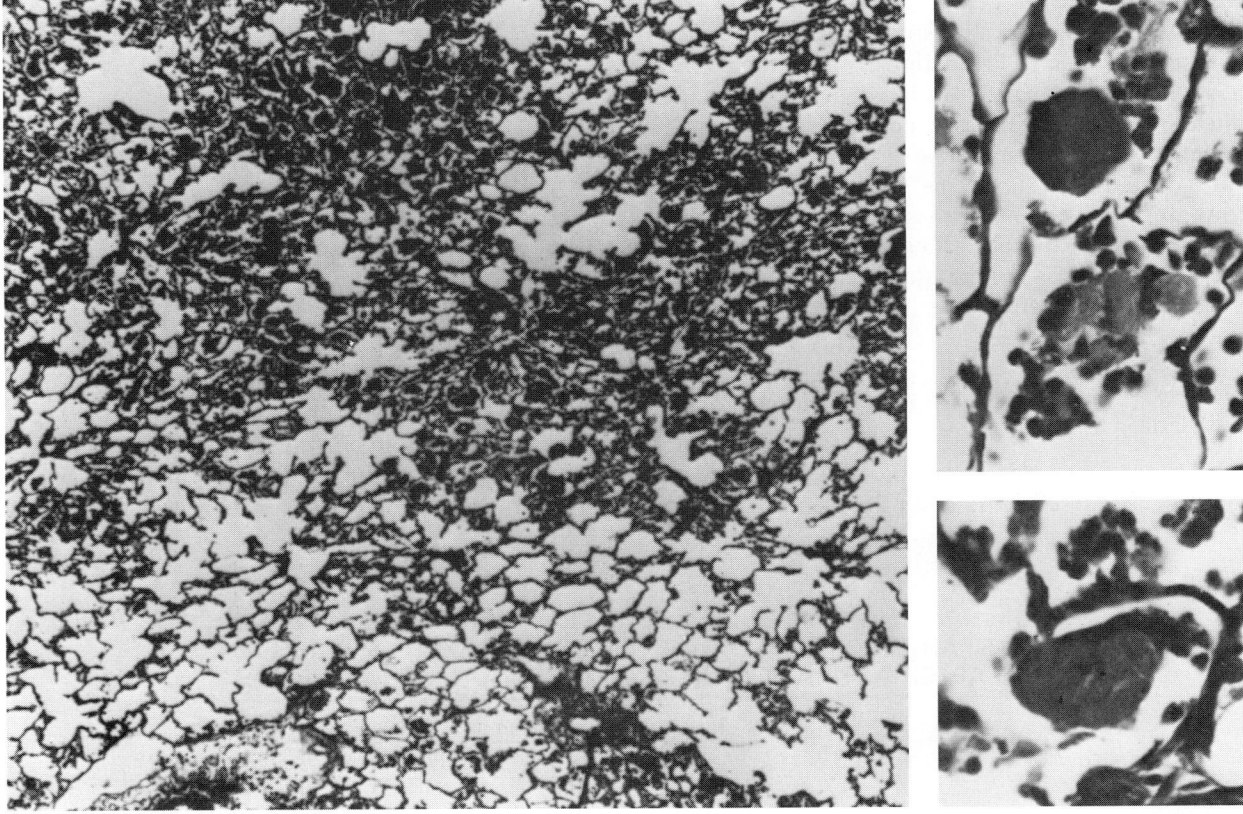

Figure 15–16. Lung after aspiration of particulate antacid. Note marked extensive inflammatory reaction. The alveoli are filled with polymorphonuclear leukocytes and macrophages in approximately equal numbers. Insets at right show large and small intra-alveolar particles surrounded by inflammatory cells (48 hours). Later, the reaction changed to an intra-alveolar cellular collection of clusters of large macrophages with abundant granular cytoplasm, in some of which were small amphophilic particles similar to those seen in the insets. No fibrosis or other inflammatory reaction was seen (28 days). (From Gibbs CP, Schwartz DJ, Wynne JW, et al: Antacid pulmonary aspiration in the dog. Anesthesiology 51:380, 1979, with permission.)

dence of newborn depression is significantly increased. Therefore, it seems that uterine manipulation and difficulty of the delivery are significant factors for the fetus during cesarean section.

Preoxygenation

Before patients become unconscious and paralyzed, it is best to wash all nitrogen from the lungs and replace it with oxygen. This is especially important in pregnant patients, because functional residual capacity is decreased and pregnant patients become hypoxemic more quickly than nonpregnant patients during periods of apnea.[230] Therefore, before starting induction, 100 percent oxygen is administered via face mask for 2 to 3 minutes. In situations of dire emergency, four vital capacity breaths of 100 percent oxygen via a tight circle system will provide similar benefit.[231] Thus, should untoward events occur, the patient can tolerate them for a longer period without becoming hypoxic.

Induction

The anesthesiologist rapidly administers thiopental (a short-acting barbiturate) or ketamine to render the patient unconscious. An appropriate dose of either agent has little effect on the fetus.[215,232–234]

Muscle Relaxant

Immediately after administration of thiopental or ketamine, the anesthesiologist gives a muscle relaxant to facilitate intubation. Succinylcholine, a rapid-onset, short-acting muscle relaxant, remains the agent of choice in most patients.

Cricoid Pressure

In rapid-sequence induction, as the thiopental or ketamine begins to take effect and the patient approaches unconsciousness, an assistant applies pressure to the cricoid cartilage, which is just below the thyroid cartilage, and does not release the pressure until an endotracheal tube is placed, its position verified, and the cuff on the tube inflated.[235,236] Pressure on the cricoid closes off the esophagus and is extremely important in preventing aspiration should regurgitation or vomiting occur. It is a simple, safe, effective maneuver that should not be omitted.

Intubation

Usually, intubation proceeds smoothly. However, in approximately 5 percent of patients, it will be difficult or delayed. In some (~0.3 percent of obstetric patients), it will be impossible. The incidence of failed intubation in obstetric patients is about seven times more common than in patients in the general operating room (i.e., 1:280 in obstetric patients vs. 1:2,230 in surgical patients).[237] When the delay is prolonged or the intubation impossible, the situation becomes a crisis in which the critical factor is to deliver oxygen to the now unconscious and paralyzed patient. Also, because it is during this induction sequence (i.e., before the airway is secured with an endotracheal tube) that the patient is most at risk from aspiration, any delay increases the risk.[93,220] It is therefore particularly important during a difficult intubation that the person applying cricoid pressure not release that pressure until told to do so by the anesthesiologist.

The patient at risk for a difficult or impossible intubation can often be identified prior to surgery. Examination of the airway is a critical part of the preanesthetic evaluation. The most important factors to assess are (1) the ability to visualize oropharyngeal structures (Mallampati classification[238]); (2) range of motion of the neck; (3) a receding mandible, which indicates the depth of the submandibular space; and (4) whether protruding maxillary incisors are present.[239] When airway abnormalities are recognized by the obstetrician, patients should be referred for an early preoperative evaluation by the anesthesiologist.

Proper Tube Placement

Before the operation begins, the anesthesiologist must ensure that the endotracheal tube is properly positioned within the trachea. End-tidal carbon dioxide analysis is the preferred method to confirm that the tube is within the trachea.[240] Of course, the anesthesiologist will also confirm that breath sounds are bilateral and equal. If the endotracheal tube is not in the trachea (and therefore is likely in the esophagus), the tube must be removed immediately and the entire situation reassessed. In some instances, the attempt will be repeated. Otherwise, the anesthesiologist will allow the patient to awaken (wherein lies the virtue of the short-acting drugs thiopental and succinylcholine), and another course of action will be chosen. Until the patient completely awakens, ventilation with bag and face mask and continuous application of cricoid pressure may be necessary. Once the patient is awake and breathing spontaneously, the anesthesiologist must choose between awake intubation or regional anesthesia. In most cases, if the endotracheal tube is incorrectly placed, the operation should not proceed until the airway is secure, because the patient cannot be allowed to awaken after the abdomen is opened. If the operation proceeds and ventilation cannot be accomplished, hypoxia, hypercarbia, and cardiac arrest can result; the fetus also will suffer.

When cesarean delivery is not urgent, the decision to

delay the operation and allow the mother to awaken is easy. However, if the operation is being done because of rapidly worsening fetal condition or maternal hemorrhage, allowing the mother to awaken may further jeopardize the fetus or mother. It is helpful if one continues fetal heart rate monitoring before and even during induction of anesthesia. In most situations, one can leave the fetal scalp electrode in place until delivery. At that time the circulating nurse can reach under the drapes and disconnect the scalp lead. Fetal heart rate monitoring may guide anesthetic and obstetric management in situations of failed intubation. Rarely, in situations of dire fetal compromise, the anesthesiologist and obstetrician may jointly decide to proceed with cesarean delivery while the anesthesiologist provides oxygenation, ventilation, and anesthesia by face mask ventilation with an additional person maintaining continuous cricoid pressure. In these emergency situations, it may be necessary to have additional trained personnel to provide assistance. After delivery, the obstetrician should obtain temporary hemostasis and then halt surgery while the anesthesiologist secures the airway by fiberoptic or blind nasal intubation.

The obstetrician and anesthesiologist should address these issues before they become emergent. Such instances should be the subject of combined obstetric/anesthesia conferences during which the concerns of all can be presented and discussed. An algorithm for management of failed intubation in the obstetric patient is shown in Figure 15–17. Equipment to manage the difficult airway must be immediately available in the labor and delivery suite.[241] The anesthesiologist performing a rapid-sequence induction is in a position comparable to the obstetrician confronted with the vaginal delivery of a breech presentation: the anesthesiologist has an un-

conscious and paralyzed mother whose airway is not yet established, and the obstetrician must deliver the largest part of the baby last. In both instances, one acts before the outcome is certain. In both instances, considerable clinical skill and judgment must be exercised.

Nitrous Oxide and Oxygen

Once the endotracheal tube is in place, a 50:50 mixture of nitrous oxide and oxygen is added to provide analgesia. Such a mixture is safe for both mother and fetus.[242]

Volatile Halogenated Agent

Usually, in addition to the nitrous oxide, an analgesic quantity (low concentration) of a volatile halogenated agent (e.g., isoflurane, sevoflurane, or desflurane) will be added to provide amnesia and additional analgesia. These agents, in low concentrations, are not harmful to mother or fetus. Also, uterine relaxation does not occur, and bleeding is not excessive.[211,215,243,244] If one does not add a potent inhalation agent, there will be an unacceptably high incidence of maternal awareness and recall. Even with the use of one of these agents, maternal awareness and recall occasionally occur. Therefore, it is important that all operating room personnel use discretion in conversation and conduct themselves as if the patient were awake.

Postdelivery

Usually the concentration of nitrous oxide can be increased after delivery. In addition, the volatile haloge-

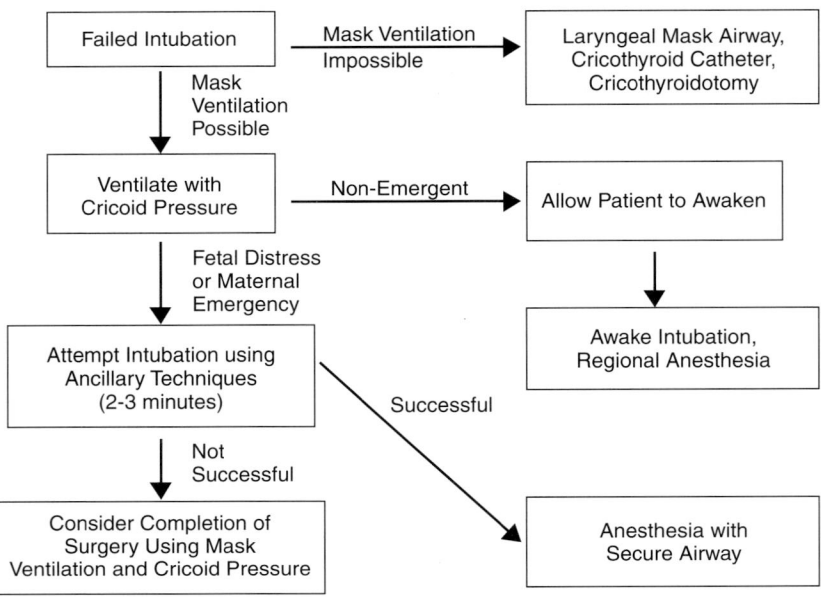

Figure 15–17. An algorithm for the management of failed intubation in the obstetric patient.

nated agent is continued, and an opioid is added to supplement the nitrous oxide and oxygen.

Oxytocin Administration

Ten to 30 U/L are infused intravenously. Bolus injections are avoided, because they can cause hypotension and tachycardia.[245]

Extubation

Because the patient can aspirate while awakening as well as during induction, extubation is not done until the patient is awake and can respond appropriately to commands. Coughing and bucking do not necessarily indicate that the patient is awake, merely that she is in the second stage—the excitement stage—of anesthesia. It is during this period of anesthesia that laryngospasm is most likely to occur should any foreign body, including the endotracheal tube or bits of stomach contents, stimulate the larynx. The patient must therefore be awake and conscious, not merely active, before extubation.

Recovery

The most important requirement of the recovery room is the presence of personnel trained appropriately and assigned no other duties than those required for the recovery process. The recovery room must contain adequate facilities such as suction, oxygen, and monitoring, and should provide care comparable to that provided patients who have received general or regional anesthesia for other surgical procedures.[3,246–250]

Aspiration

Aspiration is a serious and often fatal complication of general anesthesia and therefore deserves specific attention. In most instances it can be prevented. When it cannot, the consequences depend in part on the volume and nature of the aspirate. The conventional wisdom is that patients are at risk when their stomach contents are greater than 25 ml and when the pH of those contents is less than 2.5.[251] There are several reasons why the pregnant patient is particularly at risk. The enlarged uterus increases intra-abdominal pressure and thus intragastric pressure.[252] The gastroesophageal sphincter is distorted by the enlarged uterus, making it less competent, possibly explaining the high incidence of heartburn that occurs during pregnancy.[253,254] Concentrations of progesterone are increased during pregnancy. Progesterone is a smooth muscle relaxant, and thereby it delays gastric emptying and relaxes the gastroesophageal sphincter. Gastrin, the hormone that increases both acidity and volume of gastric contents, is increased during pregnancy,[255] and motilin, a hormone that speeds

gastric emptying, is decreased during pregnancy.[256] Labor itself delays gastric emptying,[257] primarily when patients have received opioids.[258] Many patients undergo cesarean section after a prolonged labor, during which they may have received several doses of opioids.[42]

Not all cases of aspiration are the same. The severities of lung damage, morbidity, and mortality vary and depend on the type of material aspirated. A less acidic liquid (pH >2.5) significantly decreases PaO_2 physiologically but has little histologic effect. Liquids with a pH of less than 2.5 decrease PaO_2 further and cause a burn in the lungs that results in hemorrhage, exudate, and edema histologically. The type of aspiration that produces the most severe physiologic and histologic alterations is partially digested food. PaO_2 decreases more than with any other type of aspiration, and lung damage is considerably more destructive[259] (see Table 15–9).

The variability of the effects is important to the obstetrician and the anesthesiologist. Because the necessity of a cesarean delivery cannot always be predicted, oral intake of anything but small sips of clear liquids or ice chips should be prohibited during labor.[241] Eating food during labor is unnecessary and dangerous and should not be encouraged or allowed.[241] Acidic liquid can be neutralized safely and effectively with clear antacids or an H_2-receptor antagonist.[224–226,260,261] Partially digested food, however, causes significant hypoxia and lung damage even at a pH level as high as 5.9.[259] Therefore, the most important and critical preventive measure by the obstetrician is the advice not to eat before coming to the hospital, which should be accompanied by a thorough explanation of the necessity for such advice.

Regional Anesthesia

Ongoing hemorrhage is a firm contraindication to regional anesthesia. The blood volume of a hemorrhaging patient is too low for the vascular tree. One compensatory mechanism is vasoconstriction, which reduces the size of the vasculature, making it more commensurate with the blood volume. Major regional anesthesia produces sympathetic blockade, which not only hampers the compensatory mechanism but also dilates the vasculature and makes the discrepancy between volume and vasculature even greater.

Other contraindications to regional anesthesia include infection at the site of needle insertion, coagulopathy, patient refusal, and perhaps some varieties of heart disease. For example, most obstetricians and anesthesiologists have considered epidural anesthesia to be the anesthetic technique of choice for patients with mitral valvular disease, but have considered regional anesthesia to be contraindicated in other patients with aortic stenosis, pulmonary hypertension, and/or a right-to-left shunt. The latter group of patients cannot tolerate a decrease in systemic vascular resistance and/or a de-

Advantages and Disadvantages of Regional Anesthesia

Advantages
  The patient is awake and can participate in the birth of her child.
  There is little risk of drug depression or aspiration and no intubation difficulties.
  Newborns generally have good neurobehavioral scores.
  The mother can be given 100 percent oxygen.
  The father is more likely to be allowed in the operating room.
Disadvantages
  Patients may prefer not to be awake during major surgery.
  An inadequate block may result.
  Hypotension, perhaps the most common complication of regional anesthesia, occurs during 25 to 75 percent of spinal or epidural procedures.*
  Total spinal anesthesia may occur.
  Local anesthetic toxicity may occur.
  Although extremely rare, permanent neurologic sequelae may occur.
  There are several contraindications.

*See Reisner and Lin,[215] James et al.,[262] Caritis et al.,[263] Corke et al.,[264] and Rout et al.[265]

crease in venous return of blood to the right side of the heart.[266] Recently, there have been several reports of successful administration of epidural anesthesia to patients with aortic stenosis[267] and Eisenmenger syndrome.[268] However, it must be remembered that these reports represent small numbers of cases. Because regional anesthesia results in widespread sympathetic blockade, the pathophysiology of these forms of heart disease would most often dictate that regional anesthesia not be provided. If one chooses to give regional anesthesia to such patients, it is clear that single-dose spinal or epidural anesthesia is inappropriate. Rather, there should be slow, careful induction of epidural anesthesia performed by an anesthesiologist with experience in the use of epidural anesthesia in high-risk obstetric patients. Intrathecal or epidural *opioid* analgesia does not decrease systemic vascular resistance and cause hypotension and has emerged as an attractive choice of analgesia during labor.[269–271] Because neuraxial opioids provide inadequate somatic anesthesia, they are not appropriate for cesarean delivery unless combined with a local anesthetic.

The use of regional anesthesia in patients with fetal compromise depends on the severity of fetal condition and the presence or absence of preexisting epidural anesthesia. If the situation is severe and acute, most often one should not take the additional time necessary to perform a regional technique de novo. Also, if hypotension occurs, the risk to the already compromised fetus is increased. Lesser degrees of fetal compromise may well be compatible with regional anesthesia.[272,273] For example, if an epidural catheter has been placed earlier, a partial level of anesthesia already exists, and there is hemodynamic stability, extension of epidural anesthesia may be appropriate for cesarean delivery. The anesthesiologist may give additional local anesthetic while the urethral catheter is inserted and the abdomen is prepared and draped. Often, there will be satisfactory anesthesia when the surgeon is ready to make the skin incision. If not, the ongoing fetal heart rate pattern will dictate whether a delay is acceptable. When partial but inadequate epidural anesthesia results, one may consider supplemental local infiltration of local anesthetic. Because the anesthesiologist may have already given a large dose of local anesthetic, the obstetrician should consult with the anesthesiologist to determine the proper choice and concentration of local anesthetic in order to avoid local anesthetic toxicity. For example, if the anesthesiologist has given lidocaine epidurally, and the patient has an area of inadequate anesthesia, the obstetrician might infiltrate the skin with 1 percent 2-chloroprocaine.

An improved fetal heart rate tracing may allow one to wait for satisfactory extension of epidural anesthesia, or it may allow the anesthesiologist to perform epidural or spinal anesthesia de novo. This must be done with caution, as there may be an increased risk of high spinal anesthesia when it is placed after an unsuccessful epidural anesthetic.[106] Again, this illustrates the usefulness of continuing fetal heart rate monitoring before and during induction of anesthesia. In the absence of satisfactory epidural anesthesia and in the presence of ongoing acute fetal deterioration, rapid sequence induction of general anesthesia is usually indicated for cesarean section. However, one should not indiscriminately perform rapid sequence induction of general anesthesia. A history and/or suspicion of difficult intubation should prompt performance of either awake intubation or regional anesthesia, despite the presence of fetal compromise. One should not endanger the mother, however. As noted in the ACOG Committee Opinion on Anesthesia for Emergency Deliveries, "the risk of general anesthesia must be weighed against the benefit for those patients who have a greater potential for complications. . . . Cesarean deliveries that are performed for a nonreassuring fetal heart rate pattern do not necessarily preclude the use of regional anesthesia."[274]

Finally, in healthy patients, the choice between epidural and spinal anesthesia will primarily rest with the anesthesiologist. With the recent availability of small-gauge spinal needles with pencil-point tip design, the risk of headache is no different after spinal or epidural anesthesia.[85,275] Most consider spinal block to be easier and quicker to perform, and most believe that the resulting anesthesia will be more solid and complete.[276] On the other hand, hypotension is more rapid in onset. Perhaps the most significant advantage of spinal anesthesia is that it requires considerably less local anesthetic, and therefore the potential for local anesthetic toxicity is less. Either technique is satisfactory, however, and should provide safe, effective anesthesia for mother, newborn, and obstetrician.

If spinal or epidural anesthesia is used for cesarean delivery, excellent postoperative analgesia can be obtained by addition of narcotics to the local anesthetic solution.[277] In general, the more lipid-soluble narcotics such as fentanyl or sufentanil provide fast onset of analgesia with minimal side effects but have a short duration of 2 to 4 hours. They are often used in combination with a local anesthetic in a continuous or patient-controlled epidural infusion to improve the quality of the block. In contrast, morphine is quite hydrophilic, which gives it a prolonged duration of up to 24 hours, and it can be given as a single dose at the time of cesarean delivery. Unfortunately, its water solubility gives it a long onset time and higher incidence of side effects. The most common side effects of spinal and epidural narcotics are itching and nausea. Respiratory depression is a rare but serious complication.[277,278]

Several studies have shown that spinal or epidural opioids provide superior pain relief when compared with parenteral (intramuscular or intravenous PCA) narcotics with a trend toward earlier hospital discharge and lower cost.[279,280]

Local Anesthesia

The obstetrician can use local anesthesia to perform a cesarean delivery but must be thoroughly familiar with the recommended maximal dosages of the anesthetic used because large amounts may be necessary (Table 15–2). The obstetrician should give a dilute solution of local anesthetic (e.g., 0.5 percent lidocaine or 1.0 percent 2-chloroprocaine) to allow for administration of a sufficiently large volume. It may be necessary to dilute a stock solution of 1 percent lidocaine or 2 percent 2-chloroprocaine to provide the recommended dilute solution. The patient must be familiar with the procedure and willing to cooperate. When the technique is used successfully, the operation must be done skillfully and with minimal tissue trauma. Such requirements are often difficult to meet during an emergency cesarean section, particularly one for severe fetal distress or massive hemorrhage. When a major operation proceeds with local anesthesia, the initial stages of the operation may be accomplished easily, but later the need may arise to

progress more rapidly or to use maneuvers that require more tugging and pulling than anticipated. For example, the fetal head may be impacted in the pelvis, or a uterine vein may be lacerated. In these situations, the obstetrician must proceed with extreme haste, and a patient under local anesthesia may not be able to tolerate the manipulation. With an anesthesiologist in attendance, general anesthesia can be instituted immediately and the situation resolved. Therefore, the obstetrician must seriously consider all consequences before beginning an emergency cesarean delivery without an anesthesiologist in attendance.

Occasionally local anesthesia is elected in the patient for whom a regional block is technically impossible or contraindicated (e.g., after back injury or surgery) so that the patient can be awake for the delivery of the infant. In these cases, after delivery of the infant general anesthesia is usually initiated, if necessary, for completion of the operation.

Key Points

➤ Analgesia during labor can reduce or prevent adverse hormonal and metabolic stress responses to the pain of labor.

➤ Use of parenteral opioids for labor analgesia can produce respiratory depression in the mother and newborn and delayed gastric emptying in the mother. However, when used appropriately, opioids are safe and effective.

➤ Placental transfer of a drug between mother and fetus is governed by the characteristics of the drug (including its size, lipid solubility, and ionization), maternal blood levels and uterine blood flow, placental circulation, and the fetal circulation.

➤ Regional analgesia is the most effective form of intrapartum pain relief currently available, and has the flexibility to provide additional anesthesia for spontaneous or instrumental delivery, cesarean delivery, and postoperative pain control.

➤ Spinal opioids provide excellent analgesia during much of the first stage of labor, while decreasing or avoiding the risks of local anesthetic toxicity, high spinal anesthesia, and motor block. Patients can often ambulate, although most will need additional analgesia later in labor and during the second stage.

➤ Side effects and complications of regional anesthesia include hypotension, local anesthetic toxicity, total spinal anesthesia, neurologic injury, and spinal headache. Personnel providing anesthesia must be available and competent to treat these problems.

➤ Epidural analgesia during labor is *associated* with an increased risk of prolonged labor and operative delivery, but whether there is a *cause-and-effect* relationship is controversial. Epidural analgesia is not a generic procedure, and use of a dilute solution of local anesthetic is less likely to result in prolonged labor and malposition of the fetal vertex.

➤ General anesthesia is utilized for 8 to 11 percent of cesarean deliveries. Although safe for the newborn, general anesthesia can be associated with failed intubation and aspiration, the leading causes of anesthesia-related maternal mortality.

➤ Aspiration of gastric contents causes the worst physiologic consequences when there are food particles present and/or pH is less than 2.5; therefore, patients should be encouraged not to eat during labor.

➤ Regional anesthesia may be an appropriate choice for cesarean section for nonreassuring fetal condition, especially if there is a suspicion of a difficult maternal airway.

REFERENCES

1. Hawkins JL, Gibbs CP, Orleans M, et al: Obstetric anesthesia work force survey, 1981 versus 1992. Anesthesiology 87:135, 1997.
2. Orkin FK: The geographic distribution of anesthesiologists during rapid growth in their supply [abstract]. Anesthesiology 81:A1295, 1994.
3. Joint Statement on the Optimal Goals for Anesthesia Care in Obstetrics: American Society of Anesthesiologists/American College of Obstetricians and Gynecologists, Park Ridge, IL, 2000.
4. Melzack R, Taenzer P, Feldman P, Kinch RA: Labour is still painful after prepared childbirth training. Can Assoc Med J 125:357, 1981.
5. Burns JK: Relation between blood levels of cortisol and duration of human labour. J Physiol (Lond) 254:12P, 1976.
6. Tuimala RJ, Kauppila JI, Haapalahti J: Response of pituitary-adrenal axis on partial stress. Obstet Gynecol 46:275, 1975.
7. Falconer AD, Powles AB: Plasma noradrenaline levels during labour: influence of elective lumbar epidural blockade. Anaesthesia 37:416, 1982.
8. Goland RS, Wardlaw SI, Stark RI, Frantz AG: Human plasma beta-endorphin during pregnancy, labor, and delivery. J Clin Endocrinol Metab 52:74, 1981.
9. Rossier J, French ED, Rivier C, et al: Foot-shock induced β-endorphin levels in blood but not brain. Nature 270:618, 1977.
10. Dubois M, Pickar D, Cohen MR, et al: Surgical stress in humans is accompanied by an increase in plasma beta-endorphin immunoreactivity. Life Sci 29:1249, 1981.
11. Wardlaw SL, Stark RI, Bazi L, Frantz AG: Plasma beta-endorphin and beta-lipotropin in human fetus at delivery: correlation with arterial pH and PO₂. J Clin Endocrinol Metab 49: 888, 1979.
12. Lederman RP, Lederman E, Work BA Jr, et al: The relationship of maternal anxiety, plasma catecholamines, and plasma cortisol to progress in labor. Am J Obstet Gynecol 132:495, 1978.
13. Adamsons K, Mueller-Heubach E, Myers RE: Production of fetal asphyxia in the rhesus monkey by administration of catecholamines to the mother. Am J Obstet Gynecol 109:248, 1971.
14. Rosenfeld CR, Barton MD, Meschia G: Effects of epinephrine on distribution of blood flow in the pregnant ewe. Am J Obstet Gynecol 124:156, 1976.
15. Roman-Ponce H, Thatcher WW, Caton D, et al: Effects of thermal stress and epinephrine on uterine blood flow in ewes. J Anim Sci 46:167, 1978.
16. Myers RE: Maternal psychological stress and fetal asphyxia: a study in the monkey. Am J Obstet Gynecol 122:47, 1975.
17. Morishima HO, Yeh M-N, James LS: Reduced uterine blood flow and fetal hypoxemia with acute maternal stress: experimental observation in the pregnant baboon. Am J Obstet Gynecol 134:270, 1979.
18. Morishima HO, Pedersen H, Finster M: The influence of maternal psychological stress on the fetus. Am J Obstet Gynecol 131:286, 1978.
19. Copher DE, Huber CP: Heart rate response of the human fetus to induced maternal hypoxia. Am J Obstet Gynecol 98: 320, 1967.
20. Eidelman AI, Hoffmann NW, Kaitz M: Cognitive deficits in women after childbirth. Obstet Gynecol 81:764, 1993.
21. Maltau JM, Eielsen OV, Stokke KT: Effect on the stress during labor on the concentration of cortisol and estriol in maternal plasma. Am J Obstet Gynecol 134:681, 1979.
22. Buchan PC, Milne MK, Browning MCK: The effect of continuous epidural blockade on plasma 11-hydroxy-corticosteroid concentrations in labour. J Obstet Gynaecol Br Commonw 80:974, 1973.
23. Thornton CA, Carrie LES, Sayers I, et al: A comparison of the effect of extradural and parenteral analgesia on maternal plasma cortisol concentrations during labour and the puerperium. Br J Obstet Gynaecol 83:631, 1976.
24. Abboud TK, Sarkis F, Hung TT, et al: Effects of epidural anesthesia during labor on maternal plasma beta-endorphin levels. Anesthesiology 59:1, 1983.
25. Abboud TK, Artal R, Henriksen EH, et al: Effects of spinal anesthesia on maternal circulating catecholamines. Am J Obstet Gynecol 142:252, 1982.
26. Myers R, Myers SE: Use of sedative, analgesic, and anesthetic drugs during labor and delivery: bane or boon? Am J Obstet Gynecol 133:83, 1979.
27. Pearson JF, Davies P: The effect of continuous lumbar epidural analgesia upon fetal acid-base status during the first stage of labour. J Obstet Gynaecol Br Commonw 81:971, 1974.
28. Talbot M: Pay on delivery. The New York Times Magazine, 10/31/99.
29. Jaffe JH, Martin WR: Opioid analgesics and antagonists. *In*

Goodman LS, Gilman A (eds): The Pharmacological Basis of Therapeutics, 7th ed. New York, Macmillan, 1985, p 491.

30. Kuhnert BR, Kuhnert PM, Tu AL, Lin DCK: Meperidine and normeperidine levels following meperidine administration during labor. II. Fetus and neonate. Am J Obstet Gynecol 133: 909, 1979.

31. Pittman KA, Smyth RD, Losada M, et al: Human perinatal distribution of butorphanol. Am J Obstet Gynecol 138:797, 1980.

32. Shnider S, Moya F: Effects of meperidine on the newborn infant. Am J Obstet Gynecol 89:1009, 1964.

33. Way WL, Costley EC, Way EL: Respiratory sensitivity of the newborn infant to meperidine and morphine. Clin Pharmacol Ther 6:454, 1965.

34. Walker PA: Drugs used in labour: an obstetrician's view. Br J Anaesth 45(suppl):787, 1973.

35. Quilligan EJ, Keegan KA, Donahue MJ: Double-blind comparison of intravenously injected butorphanol and meperidine in parturients. Int J Gynaecol Obstet 18:363, 1980.

36. Rayburn WF, Smith CV, Parriott JE, Woods RE: Randomized comparison of meperidine and fentanyl during labor. Obstet Gynecol 74:604, 1989.

37. Emergency Cardiac Care Committee and Subcommittees, American Heart Association: Neonatal resuscitation. JAMA 268:2276, 1992.

38. Committee on Obstetrics: Maternal and Fetal Medicine: Naloxone Use in Newborns. American College of Obstetricians and Gynecologists, Washington, DC, 1989.

39. Brackbill Y, Kane J, Manniello RL, Abramson D: Obstetric premedication and infant outcome. Am J Obstet Gynecol 118: 377, 1974.

40. Corke BC: Neurobehavioural responses of the newborn: the effect of different forms of maternal analgesia. Anaesthesia 32:539, 1977.

41. Kolata GB: Scientists attack report that obstetrical medications endanger children. Science 204:391, 1979.

42. Nimmo WA, Wilson J, Prescott LF: Narcotic analgesics and delayed gastric emptying during labour. Lancet 1:890, 1975.

43. Wright PMC, Allen RW, Moore J, et al: Gastric emptying during lumbar extradural analgesia in labour: effect of fentanyl supplementation. Br J Anaesth 68:248, 1992.

44. O'Sullivan GM, Sutton AJ, Thompson SA, et al: Noninvasive measurement of gastric emptying in obstetric patients. Anesth Analg 66:505, 1987.

45. Kuhnert BR, Kuhnert PM, Tu AL, et al: Meperidine and normeperidine levels following meperidine administration during labor. I. Mother. Am J Obstet Gynecol 133:904, 1979.

46. Kuhnert BR, Philipson EH, Kuhnert PM, Syracuse CD: Disposition of meperidine and normeperidine following multiple doses during labor. I. Mother. Am J Obstet Gynecol 151: 406, 1985.

47. Kuhnert BR, Kuhnert PM, Philipson EH, Syracuse CD: Disposition of meperidine and normeperidine following multiple doses during labor. II Fetus and neonate. Am J Obstet Gynecol 151:410, 1985.

48. Lazebnik N, Kuhnert BR, Carr PC, et al: Intravenous, deltoid, or gluteus administration of meperidine during labor? Am J Obstet Gynecol 160:1184, 1989.

49. Kleinman SJ, Wiesel S, Tessler MJ: Patient-controlled analgesia (PCA) using fentanyl in a parturient with a platelet function abnormality. Can J Anaesth 38:489, 1991.

50. Rosaeg OP, Kitts JB, Koren G, et al: Maternal and fetal effects of intravenous patient-controlled fentanyl analgesia during labour in a thrombocytopenic parturient. Can J Anaesth 39:277, 1992.

51. Maduska AL, Hajghassemali M: A double-blind comparison of butorphanol and meperidine in labour: maternal pain relief and effect on the newborn. Can Anaesth Soc J 25:398, 1978.

52. Nagashima H, Karamanian A, Malovany R, et al: Respiratory and circulatory effects of intravenous butorphanol and morphine. Clin Pharmacol Ther 19:738, 1976.

53. Kallos T, Caruso FS: Respiratory effects of butorphanol and pethidine. Anaesthesia 34:633, 1979.

54. Romagnoli A, Keats AS: Ceiling effect for respiratory depression by nalbuphine. Clin Pharmacol Ther 27:478, 1980.

55. Wilson CM, McClean E, Moore J, Dundee JW: A double-blind comparison of intramuscular pethidine and nalbuphine in labour. Anaesthesia 41:1207, 1986.

56. Podlas J, Breland BD: Patient-controlled analgesia with nalbuphine during labor. Obstet Gynecol 70:202, 1987.

57. Rayburn W, Leuschen MP, Earl R, et al: Intravenous meperidine during labor: a randomized comparison between nursing- and patient-controlled administration. Obstet Gynecol 174: 702, 1989.

58. Clutton-Brach JC: Some pain threshold studies with particular reference to thiopentone. Anaesthesia 15:71, 1960.

59. Dundee JW: Alterations in response to somatic pain associated with anaesthesia. II. The effect of thiopentone and pentobarbitone. Br J Anaesth 32:407, 1960.

60. Irving FC: Advantages and disadvantages of the barbiturates in obstetrics. R I Med J 28:493, 1945.

61. Powe CE, Kiem IM, Fromhagen C, Cavanagh D: Propiomazine hydrochloride in obstetrical analgesia: a controlled study of 520 patients. JAMA 181:290, 1962.

62. Zsigmond EK, Patterson RL: Double-blind evaluation of hydroxyzine hydrochloride in obstetric anesthesia. Anesth Analg 46:275, 1967.

63. Owen JR, Irani SF, Blair AW: Effect of diazepam administered to mothers during labour on temperature regulation of neonate. Arch Dis Child 47:107, 1972.

64. Cree JE, Meyer J, Hailey DM: Diazepam in labour: its metabolism and effect on the clinical condition and thermogenesis of the newborn. Br Med J 4:251, 1973.

65. Yeh SY, Paul RH, Cordero L, Hon EH: A study of diazepam during labor. Obstet Gynecol 43:363, 1974.

66. Schiff D, Chan G, Stern L: Fixed drug combinations and the displacement of bilirubin from albumin. Pediatrics 48:139, 1971.

67. Wilson CM, Dundee JW, Moore J, et al: A comparison of the early pharmacokinetics of midazolam in pregnant and nonpregnant women. Anaesthesia 42:1057, 1987.

68. Ravlo O, Carl P, Crawford ME, et al: A randomized comparison between midazolam and thiopental for elective cesarean section anesthesia. II. Neonates. Anesth Analg 68:234, 1989.

69. Bland BAR, Lawes EG, Duncan PW, et al: Comparison of midazolam and thiopental for rapid sequence anesthetic induction for elective cesarean section. Anesth Analg 66:1165, 1987.

70. Camann W, Cohen MB, Ostheimer GW: Is midazolam desirable for sedation in parturients? Anesthesiology 65:441, 1986.

71. Gross JB, Weller RS, Conard P: Flumazenil antagonism of midazolam-induced ventilatory depression. Anesthesiology 75: 179, 1991.

72. Moya F, Thorndike V: Passage of drugs across the placenta. Am J Obstet Gynecol 84:1778, 1962.

73. Dilts PV: Placental transfer. Clin Obstet Gynecol 24:555, 1981.

74. Finster M, Ralston DH, Pederson H: Perinatal pharmacology. *In* Shnider SM, Levinson G (eds): Anesthesia for Obstetrics, 3rd ed. Baltimore, Williams & Wilkins, 1993, p 71.

75. Alper MH: What drugs cross the placenta and what happens to them in the fetus? *In* Henry SG (ed): Refresher Courses in

Anesthesiology, Vol 4. Park Ridge, IL, American Society of Anesthesiologists, 1976, p 1.

76. Makowski EL, Meschia G, Droegemueller W, Battaglia FC: Distribution of uterine blood flow in the pregnant sheep. Am J Obstet Gynecol 101:409, 1968.

77. Biehl D, Shnider SM, Levinson G, Callender K: Placental transfer of lidocaine: effects of fetal acidosis. Anesthesiology 48:409, 1978.

78. Sinclair JC, Fox HA, Lentz JF, et al: Intoxication of the fetus by a local anesthetic. N Engl J Med 273:1173, 1965.

79. Eisenach JC: Combined spinal-epidural analgesia in obstetrics. Anesthesiology 91:299, 1999.

80. Honet JE, Arkoosh VA, Norris MC, et al: Comparison among intrathecal fentanyl, meperidine, and sufentanil for labor analgesia. Anesth Analg 75:734, 1992.

81. Norris MC, Grieco WM, Borkowski M, et al: Complications of labor analgesia: epidural versus combined spinal epidural techniques. Anesth Analg 79:529, 1994.

82. Beilin Y, Leibowitz AB, Bernstein HH, et al: Controversies of labor epidural analgesia. Anesth Analg 89:969, 1999.

83. Abboud TK, Khoo SS, Miller F, et al: Maternal, fetal, and neonatal responses after epidural anesthesia with bupivacaine, 2-chloroprocaine, or lidocaine. Anesth Analg 61:638, 1982.

84. Matadial L, Cibils LA: The effect of epidural anesthesia on uterine activity and blood pressure. Am J Obstet Gynecol 125:846, 1976.

85. Norris MC, Grieco WM, Borkowski M: Complications of labor analgesia: epidural versus combined spinal epidural techniques. Anesth Analg 79:529, 1994.

86. Datta S, Kitzmiller JL, Naulty JS, et al: Acid-base status of diabetic mothers and their infants following spinal anesthesia for cesarean section. Anesth Analg 61:662, 1982.

87. James FM, Greiss FC Jr, Kemp RA: An evaluation of vasopressor therapy for maternal hypotension during spinal anesthesia. Anesthesiology 33:25, 1970.

88. Brizgys RV, Dailey PA, Shnider SM, et al: The incidence and neonatal effects of maternal hypotension during epidural anesthesia for cesarean section. Anesthesiology 67:782, 1987.

89. Kenepp NB, Sheley WC, Kumar S, et al: Effects on newborn of hydration with glucose in patients undergoing caesarean section with regional anesthesia. Lancet 1:645, 1980.

90. Ralston DH, Shnider SM, deLorimier AA: Effects of equipotent ephedrine, metaraminol, mephentermine, and methoxamine on uterine blood flow in the pregnant ewe. Anesthesiology 40:354, 1974.

91. Moran DH, Perillo M, LaPorta RF, et al: Phenylephrine in the prevention of hypotension following spinal anesthesia for cesarean delivery. J Clin Anesth 3:301, 1991.

92. Auroy Y, Narchi P, Messiah A, et al: Serious complications related to regional anesthesia. Anesthesiology 87:479, 1997.

93. Chadwick HS, Posner K, Caplan RA, et al: A comparison of obstetric and nonobstetric anesthesia malpractice claims. Anesthesiology 74:242, 1991.

94. Hawkins JL, Koonin LM, Palmer SK, et al: Anesthesia-related deaths during obstetric delivery in the United States, 1979–1990. Anesthesiology 86:277, 1997.

95. Albright GA: Cardiac arrest following regional anesthesia with etidocaine or bupivacaine. Anesthesiology 51:285, 1979.

96. deJong RH, Gamble CA, Bonin JD: Bupivacaine-induced cardiac arrhythmias and plasma cation concentrations in normokalemic cats. Regional Anesth 8:104, 1983.

97. Clarkson CW, Hondeghem LM: Mechanism for bupivacaine depression of cardiac conduction: fast block of sodium channels during the action potential with slow recovery from block during diastole. Anesthesiology 62:396, 1985.

98. Abbott Laboratories: Letter to doctors: urgent new recom-

99. Writer WDR, Davies JM, Strunin L: Trial by media: the bupivacaine story. Can Anaesth Soc J 31:1, 1984.

100. Moore DC, Batra MS: The components of an effective test dose prior to epidural block. Anesthesiology 55:693, 1981.

101. Abraham RA, Harris AP, Maxwell LG, Kaplow S: The efficacy of 1.5 percent lidocaine with 7.5 percent dextrose and epinephrine as an epidural test dose for obstetrics. Anesthesiology 64:116, 1986.

102. Leighton BL, Norris MC, Sosis M, et al: Limitations of epinephrine as a marker of intravascular injection in laboring women. Anesthesiology 66:688, 1987.

103. Moore DC, Crawford RD, Scurlock JE: Severe hypoxia and acidosis following local anesthetic-induced convulsions. Anesthesiology 53:259, 1980.

104. Emergency Cardiac Care Committee and Subcommittees, American Heart Association: Guidelines for cardiopulmonary resuscitation and emergency cardiac care: recommendations of the 1992 national conference. JAMA 268:2249, 1992.

105. Camann W, Bader A: Spinal anesthesia with meperidine as the sole agent. Int J Obstet Anesth 1:156, 1992.

106. Furst SR, Reisner LS: Risk of high spinal anesthesia following failed epidural block for cesarean delivery. J Clin Anesth 7: 71, 1995.

107. Ravindran RS, Bond VK, Tasch MD, et al: Prolonged neural blockade following regional analgesia with 2-chloroprocaine. Anesth Analg 59:447, 1980.

108. Reisner LS, Hochman BN, Plumer MH: Persistent neurologic deficit and adhesive arachnoiditis following intrathecal 2-chloroprocaine injection. Anesth Analg 59:452, 1980.

109. Moore DC, Spierdijk J, Van Kleef JD, et al: Chloroprocaine neurotoxicity: four additional cases. Anesth Analg 61:155, 1982.

110. Gissen AJ, Datta S, Lambert D: The chloroprocaine controversy, II. Is chloroprocaine neurotoxic? Reg Anesth 9:135, 1984.

111. Fibuch EE, Opper SE: Back pain following epidurally administered Nesacaine-MPF. Anesth Analg 69:113, 1989.

112. Levy L, Randel GI, Pandit SK: Does chloroprocaine (Nesacaine MPF) for epidural anesthesia increase the incidence of backache? Anesthesiology 71:476, 1989.

113. Cole JT: Maternal obstetric paralysis. Am J Obstet Gynecol 52:374, 1946.

114. Martin JT: Lithotomy positions. In Martin JT, Warner MA (eds): Positioning in Anesthesia and Surgery. Philadelphia, WB Saunders Company, 1997, p 47.

115. Deppe G, Hercule J, Gleicher N: Sciatic nerve injury complicating surgical removal of retroperitoneal tumor. Acta Obstet Gynaecol Scand 63:369, 1984.

116. Ong BY, Cohen MM, Esmail A, et al: Paresthesias and motor dysfunction after labor and delivery. Anesth Analg 66:18, 1987.

117. Breen TW, Ransil BJ, Groves PA, et al: Factors associated with back pain after childbirth. Anesthesiology 81:29, 1994.

118. Groves PA, Breen TW, Ransil BJ, et al: Natural history of postpartum back pain and its relationship with epidural anesthesia [abstract]. Anesthesiology 81:A1167, 1994.

119. Heit JA, Horlocker TT (eds): Neuraxial anesthesia and anticoagulation: consensus statements. Richmond, VA, American Society of Regional Anesthesia, 1998.

120. Horlocker TT: Regional anesthesia and analgesia in the patient receiving thromboprophylaxis [editorial]. Reg Anesth 21: 503, 1996.

121. Stride PC, Cooper GM: Dural taps revisited. Anaesthesia 48: 247, 1993.

122. Carbaat PAT, van Crevel H: Lumbar puncture headache: con-

trolled study on the preventive effect of 24 hours' bed rest. Lancet 2:1133, 1981.

123. Craft JB, Epstein BS, Coakley CS: Prophylaxis of dural-puncture headache with epidural saline. Anesth Analg 52:228, 1973.

124. Camann WR, Murray RS, Mushlin PS, et al: Effects of oral caffeine on postdural puncture headache. Anesth Analg 70:181, 1990.

125. Szeinfeld M, Ihmeldan IH, Moser MM, et al: Epidural blood patch: evaluation of the volume and spread of blood injected into the epidural space. Anesthesiology 64:820, 1986.

126. Ravindran RS: Epidural autologous blood patch on an outpatient basis. Anesth Analg 63:962, 1984.

127. DiGiovanni AJ, Galbert MW, Wahle WM: Epidural injection of autologous blood for postlumbar-puncture headache. II. Additional clinical experiences and laboratory investigation. Anesth Analg 51:226, 1972.

128. Abouleish E, de la Vega S, Blendinger I, Tio TO: Long-term follow-up of epidural blood patch. Anesth Analg 54:459, 1975.

129. Abouleish E, Wadhwa RK, de la Vega S, et al: Regional analgesia following epidural blood patch. Anesth Analg 54:634, 1975.

130. Quaynor H, Corbey M: Extradural blood patch—why delay? Br J Anaesth 57:538, 1985.

131. Cheek TG, Banner R, Sauter J, Gutsche BB: Prophylactic extradural blood patch is effective. Br J Anaesth 61:340, 1988.

132. Berger CW, Crosby ET, Grodecki W: North American survey of the management of dural puncture occurring during labour epidural analgesia. Can J Anaesth 45:110, 1998.

133. Chelmow D, Kilpatrick SJ, Laros RK: Maternal and neonatal outcomes after prolonged latent phase. Obstet Gynecol 81:486, 1993.

134. Kong AS, Bates SJ, Rizk B: Rupture of membranes before the onset of spontaneous labour increases the likelihood of instrumental delivery. Br J Anaesth 68:252, 1992.

135. Wuitchik M, Bakal D, Lipshitz J: The clinical significance of pain and cognitive activity in latent labor. Obstet Gynecol 73:35, 1989.

136. Naulty JS, Smith R, Ross R: The effect of changes in labor analgesic practice on labor outcome [abstract]. Anesthesiology 69:A660, 1988.

137. Olofsson C, Ekblom A, Ekman-Ordeberg G, Irestedt L: Obstetric outcome following epidural analgesia with bupivacaine-adrenaline 0.25% or bupivacaine 0.125% with sufentanil—a prospective randomized controlled study in 1000 parturients. Acta Anesthesiol Scand 42:284, 1998.

138. Friedman EA: Effects of drugs on uterine contractility. Anesthesiology 26:409, 1965.

139. Committee on Obstetrics: Maternal and Fetal Medicine: Dystocia: Etiology, Diagnosis, and Management Guidelines. Washington, DC, American College of Obstetricians and Gynecologists, 1983.

140. Peisner DB, Rosen MG: Transition from latent to active labor. Obstet Gynecol 68:448, 1986.

141. Chestnut DH, Vandewalker GE, Owen CL, et al: The influence of continuous epidural bupivacaine analgesia on the second stage of labor and method of delivery in nulliparous women. Anesthesiology 66:774, 1987.

142. Kilpatrick SJ, Laros RK: Characteristics of normal labor. Obstet Gynecol 74:85, 1989.

143. Maresh M, Choong KH, Beard RW: Delayed pushing with lumbar epidural analgesia in labour. Br J Obstet Gynaecol 90:623, 1983.

144. Cohen WR: Influence of the duration of second stage labor

145. Pearson JF: The effect of continuous lumbar epidural analgesia on maternal acid-base balance and arterial lactate concentration during the second state of labour. J Obstet Gynaecol Br Commonw 80:225, 1973.

146. ACOG Technical Bulletin, #196: Operative Vaginal Delivery. Washington, DC, American College of Obstetricians and Gynecologists, 1994.

147. Robinson JO, Rosen M, Evans JM, et al: Maternal opinion about analgesia for labor. Anaesthesia 35:1173, 1980.

148. Philipsen T, Jensen NH: Epidural block or parenteral pethidine as analgesic in labour: a randomized study concerning progress in labour and instrumental deliveries. Eur J Obstet Gynecol Reprod Biol 30:27, 1989.

149. Phillips KC, Thomas TA: Second stage of labour with or without extradural analgesia. Anaesthesia 38:972, 1983.

150. Chestnut DH, Bates JN, Choi WW: Continuous infusion epidural analgesia with lidocaine: efficacy and influence during the second stage of labor. Obstet Gynecol 69:323, 1987.

151. Johnsrud ML, Dale PO, Loveland B: Benefits of continuous infusion epidural analgesia throughout vaginal delivery. Acta Obstet Gynecol Scand 67:355, 1988.

152. Gribble RK, Meier PR: Effect of epidural analgesia on the primary cesarean rate. Obstet Gynecol 78:231, 1991.

153. Larson DD: The effect of initiating an obstetric anesthesiology service on rate of cesarean section and rate of forceps delivery [abstract]. Society of Obstetric Anesthesia and Perinatology 13:1992.

154. Yancey MK, Pierce B, Schweitzer D, et al: Observations on labor epidural analgesia and operative delivery rates. Am J Obstet Gynecol 180:353, 1999.

155. Fogel ST, Shyken JM, Leighton BL, et al: Epidural labor analgesia and the incidence of cesarean delivery for dystocia. Anesth Analg 87:119, 1998.

156. Iglesias S, Burn R, Saunders LD: Reducing the cesarean section rate in a rural community hospital. Can Med Assoc J 145:1459, 1991.

157. Socol ML, Garcia PM, Peaceman AM: Reducing cesarean births at a primarily private university hospital. Am J Obstet Gynecol 168:1748, 1993.

158. Robson M, Boylan P, McFarland P, et al: Epidural analgesia need not influence the spontaneous vaginal delivery rate [abstract]. Am J Obstet Gynecol 168:364, 1993.

159. Farabow WS, Roberson VO, Maxey J, et al: A twenty-year retrospective analysis of the efficacy of epidural analgesia-anesthesia when administered and/or managed by obstetricians. Am J Obstet Gynecol 169:270, 1993.

160. Neuhoff D, Burke S, Porreco RP: Cesarean birth for failed progress in labor. Obstet Gynecol 73:915, 1989.

161. Segal S, Blatman R, Doble M, et al: The influence of the obstetrician in the relationship between epidural analgesia and cesarean section for dystocia. Anesthesiology 91:90, 1999.

162. Thorp JA, Parisi VM, Boylan PC, et al: The effect of continuous epidural analgesia on cesarean section for dystocia in nulliparous women. Am J Obstet Gynecol 161:670, 1989.

163. Thorp JA, Eckert LO, Ang MS, et al: Epidural analgesia and cesarean section for dystocia: risk factors in nulliparas. Am J Perinatol 8:402, 1991.

164. Thorp JA, Hu DH, Albin RM, et al: The effect of intrapartum epidural analgesia on nulliparous labor: a randomized, controlled, prospective trial. Am J Obstet Gynecol 169:851, 1993.

165. Ramin SM, Gambling DR, Lucas MJ, et al: Randomized trial of epidural versus intravenous analgesia during labor. Obstet Gynecol 86:783, 1995.

166. Sharma SK, Sidawi JE, Ramin SM, et al: Cesarean delivery: a

randomized trial of epidural versus patient-controlled meperidine analgesia during labor. Anesthesiology 87:487, 1997.

167. Gambling DR, Sharma SK, Ramin SM, et al: A randomized study of combined spinal-epidural analgesia versus intravenous meperidine during labor: impact on cesarean delivery rate. Anesthesiology 89:1336, 1998.

168. Bofill JA, Vincent RD, Ross EL, et al: Nulliparous active labor, epidural analgesia, and cesarean delivery for dystocia. Am J Obstet Gynecol 177:1465, 1997.

169. Clark A, Carr D, Loyd G, et al: The influence of epidural analgesia on cesarean delivery rates: a randomized, prospective trial. Am J Obstet Gynecol 179:1527, 1998.

170. Morton SC, Williams MS, Keeler EB, et al: Effect of epidural analgesia for labor on the cesarean delivery rate. Obstet Gynecol 83:1045, 1994.

171. Halpern SH, Leighton BL, Ohlsson A, et al: Effect of epidural vs parenteral opioid analgesia on the progress of labor: a meta-analysis. JAMA 280:2105, 1998.

172. Zhang J, Klebanoff MA, DerSimonian R: Epidural analgesia in association with duration of labor and mode of delivery: a quantitative review. Am J Obstet Gynecol 180:970, 1999.

173. Chestnut DH, Vincent RD, McGrath JM: Does early administration of epidural analgesia affect obstetric outcome in nulliparous women who are receiving intravenous oxytocin? Anesthesiology 80:1193, 1994.

174. Chestnut DH, McGrath JM, Vincent RD: Does early administration of epidural analgesia affect obstetric outcome in nulliparous women who are in spontaneous labor? Anesthesiology 80:1201, 1994.

175. Dewan DM, Cohen SE: Epidural analgesia and the incidence of cesarean section. Time for a closer look. Anesthesiology 80:1189, 1994.

176. American Society of Anesthesiologists and American College of Obstetricians and Gynecologists: Pain relief during labor, 1999.

177. Lowenshon RI, Paul RH, Fales S, et al: Intrapartum epidural anesthesia: an evaluation of effects on uterine activity. Obstet Gynecol 44:388, 1974.

178. Cheek TG, Samuels P, Tobin M, et al: Rapid intravenous saline infusion decreases uterine activity in labor. Br J Anaesth 77:632, 1996.

179. Zamora JE, Rosaeg OP, Lindsay MP, et al: Haemodynamic consequences and uterine contractions following 0.5 or 1.0 litre crystalloid infusion before obstetric epidural analgesia. Can J Anaesth 43:347, 1996.

180. Maltau JM, Andersen HT: Epidural anaesthesia as an alternative to caesarean section in the treatment of prolonged, exhaustive labour. Acta Anaesthesiol Scand 19:349, 1975.

181. Craft JB, Epstein BS, Coakley CS: Effect of lidocaine with epinephrine versus lidocaine (plain) on induced labor. Anesth Analg 51:243, 1972.

182. Abboud TK, David S, Nagappala S, et al: Maternal, fetal, and neonatal effects of lidocaine with and without epinephrine anesthesia in obstetrics. Anesth Analg 63:973, 1984.

183. Abboud TK, Sheik-ol-Eslam A, Yanagi T, et al: Safety and efficacy of epinephrine added to bupivacaine for lumbar epidural analgesia in obstetrics. Anesth Analg 64:585, 1985.

184. Abboud TK, DerSarkissian L, Terrasi J, et al: Comparative maternal, fetal, and neonatal effects of chloroprocaine with and without epinephrine for epidural anesthesia in obstetrics. Anesth Analg 66:71, 1987.

185. Eisenach JC, Grice SC, Dewan DM: Epinephrine enhances analgesia produced by epidural bupivacaine during labor. Anesth Analg 66:447, 1987.

186. Johnson WL, Winter WW, Eng M, et al: Effect of pudendal, spinal, and peridural block anesthesia on the second stage of labor. Am J Obstet Gynecol 113:166, 1972.

187. Chestnut DH: Does epidural analgesia during labor affect the incidence of cesarean delivery? Reg Anesth 22:495, 1997.

188. Chestnut DH: Epidural analgesia and the incidence of cesarean section: time for another close look [editorial]. Anesthesiology 87:472, 1997.

189. Chestnut DH: Epidural and spinal analgesia/anesthesia: effect on the progress of labor and method of delivery. In Obstetric Anesthesia: Principles and Practice, 2nd ed. St. Louis, Mosby, 1999, p 408.

190. Morrison DH, Smedstad KG: Continuous infusion epidurals for obstetric analgesia. Can Anaesth Soc J 32:101, 1985.

191. Nadeau S, Elliott RD: Continuous bupivacaine infusion during labour: effects on analgesia and delivery [abstract]. Can Anaesth Soc J 32:S70, 1985.

192. Bogod DG, Rosen M, Rees GAD: Extradural infusion of 0.125 percent bupivacaine at 10 ml h^{-1} to women during labour. Br J Anaesth 59:325, 1987.

193. Gaylard DG, Wilson IH, Balmer HGR: An epidural infusion technique for labor. Anaesthesia 42:1098, 1987.

194. Hicks JA, Jenkins JG, Newton MC, et al: Continuous epidural infusion of 0.075 percent bupivacaine for pain relief in labour: a comparison with intermittent top-ups of 0.5 percent bupivacaine. Anaesthesia 43:289, 1988.

195. Smedstad KG, Morrison DH: A comparative study of continuous and intermittent epidural analgesia for labour and delivery. Can J Anaesth 35:234, 1988.

196. Chestnut DH, Owen CL, Bates JN, et al: Continuous infusion epidural analgesia during labor: a randomized, double-blind comparison of 0.0625 percent bupivacaine/0.0002 percent fentanyl versus 0.125 percent bupivacaine. Anesthesiology 68:754, 1988.

197. Vertommen JD, Vandermeulen E, Van Aken H, et al: The effects of addition of sufentanil to 0.125% bupivacaine on the quality of analgesia during labor and on the incidence of instrumental deliveries. Anesthesiology 74:809, 1991.

198. Chestnut DH: Epidural anesthesia and instrumental vaginal delivery [editorial]. Anesthesiology 74:805, 1991.

199. Goodfellow CF, Hull MGR, Swaab DF, et al: Oxytocin deficiency at delivery with epidural analgesia. Br J Obstet Gynaecol 90:214, 1983.

200. Bates RG, Helm CW, Duncan A, Edmonds DK: Uterine activity in the second stage of labour and the effect of epidural analgesia. Br J Obstet Gynaecol 92:1246, 1985.

201. Shnider SM, Asling JH, Holl JW, Margolis AJ: Paracervical block anesthesia in obstetrics. I. Fetal complications and neonatal morbidity. Am J Obstet Gynecol 107:619, 1970.

202. Tafeen CH, Freedman HL, Harris H: Combination continuous paracervical and continued pudendal nerve block anesthesia in labor. Am J Obstet Gynecol 100:55, 1968.

203. Teramo K, Widholm O: Studies of the effects of anesthetics on fetus. I. The effect of paracervical block with mepivacaine upon fetal-base values. Acta Obstet Gynaecol Scand 46(Suppl 2):1, 1967.

204. Gibbs CP, Noel SC: Response of arterial segments from gravid human uterus to multiple concentrations of lignocaine. Br J Anaesth 45:409, 1977.

205. Greiss FC Jr, Still JG, Anderson SG: Effects of local anesthetic agents on the uterine vasculatures and myometrium. Am J Obstet Gynecol 124:889, 1976.

206. Freeman RK, Gutierrez NA, Ray ML, et al: Fetal cardiac response to paracervical block anesthesia. Part I. Am J Obstet Gynecol 113:583, 1972.

207. Martensson L, Wallin G: Labour pain treated with cutaneous injections of sterile water: a randomised controlled trial. Br J Obstet Gynaecol 106:633, 1999.

208. Hawkins JL, Beaty BR, Gibbs CP, et al: Update on U.S.

obstetric anesthesia practices, [abstract]. Anesthesiology 91: A1060, 1999.

209. Philipson EH, Kuhnert BR, Syracuse CD: Maternal, fetal, and neonatal lidocaine levels following local perineal infiltration. Am J Obstet Gynecol 149:403, 1984.

210. Klink EW: Perineal nerve block: an anatomic and clinical study in the female. Obstet Gynecol 1:137, 1953.

211. Gambling DR, Sharma SK, White PF, et al: Use of sevoflurane during elective cesarean birth: a comparison with isoflurane and spinal anesthesia. Anesth Analg 81:90, 1995.

212. Ranney B, Stanage WF: Advantages of local anesthesia for cesarean section. Obstet Gynecol 45:163, 1975.

213. James FM III, Crawford JS, Hopkinson R, et al: A comparison of general anesthesia and lumbar epidural analgesia for elective cesarean section. Anesth Analg 56:228, 1977.

214. Datta S, Alper MH: Anesthesia for cesarean section. Anesthesiology 53:142, 1980.

215. Reisner LS, Lin D: Anesthesia for cesarean section. In Chestnut DH (ed): Obstetric Anesthesia: Principles and Practice, 2nd ed. St. Louis, Mosby, 1999, p 465.

216. Scanlon JW, Brown WU Jr, Weiss JB, Alper MH: Neurobehavioral responses of newborn infants after maternal epidural anesthesia. Anesthesiology 40:121, 1974.

217. Hodgkinson R, Bhatt M, Kim SS, et al: Neonatal neurobehavioral tests following cesarean section under general and spinal anesthesia. Am J Obstet Gynecol 132:670, 1978.

218. McGuinness GA, Merkow AJ, Kennedy RL, Erenberg A: Epidural anesthesia with bupivacaine for cesarean section: neonatal blood levels and neurobehavioral responses. Anesthesiology 49:270, 1978.

219. Marx GF, Finster M: Difficulty in endotracheal intubation associated with obstetric anesthesia. Anesthesiology 51:364, 1979.

220. Gibbs CP, Rolbin SH, Norman P: Cause and prevention of maternal aspiration. Anesthesiology 61:111, 1984.

221. Lewis G, Drife J, Botting B, et al: Report on Confidential Enquiries Into Maternal Deaths in the United Kingdom 1994–1996. Her Majesty's Stationery Office, London, 1998, p 91.

222. Morgan M: Anaesthetic contribution to maternal mortality. Br J Anaesth 59:842, 1987.

223. Hawkins JL, Koonin LM, Palmer SK, et al: Anesthesia-related maternal deaths during obstetric delivery in the United States, 1979–1990. Anesthesiology 86:277, 1997.

224. Gibbs CP, Spohr L, Schmidt D: The effectiveness of sodium citrate as an antacid. Anesthesiology 57:44, 1982.

225. Gibbs CP, Banner TC: Effectiveness of Bicitra as a preoperative antacid. Anesthesiology 61:97, 1984.

226. Chen CT, Toung TJ, Cameron JL: Alka-Seltzer® for prophylactic use in prevention of acid aspiration pneumonia. Anesthesiology 57:A103, 1982.

227. Gibbs CP, Schwartz DJ, Wynne JW, et al: Antacid pulmonary aspiration in the dog. Anesthesiology 51:380, 1979.

228. Crawford JA, Burton M, Davies P: Time and lateral tilt at caesarean section. Br J Anaesth 44:477, 1972.

229. Datta S, Ostheimer GW, Weiss JB, et al: Neonatal effect of prolonged anesthetic induction for cesarean section. Obstet Gynecol 58:331, 1981.

230. Archer GW, Marx GF: Arterial oxygen tension during apnoea in parturient women. Br J Anaesth 46:358, 1974.

231. Norris MC, Dewan DM: Preoxygenation for cesarean section: a comparison of two techniques. Anesthesiology 62:827, 1985.

232. Kosaka Y, Takahashi T, Mark LC: Intravenous thiobarbiturate anesthesia for cesarean section. Anesthesiology 31:489, 1969.

233. Peltz B, Sinclair DM: Induction agents for cesarean section: a comparison of thiopental and ketamine. Anaesthesia 28:37, 1973.

234. Holdcroft A, Morgan M: Intravenous induction agents for caesarean section [editorial]. Anaesthesia 44:719, 1989.

235. Sellick BA: Cricoid pressure to control regurgitation of stomach contents during induction of anesthesia. Lancet 2:404, 1961.

236. Sellick BA: Rupture of the oesophagus following cricoid pressure? Anaesthesia 37:213, 1982.

237. Samsoon GLT, Young JRB: Difficult tracheal intubation: a retrospective study. Anaesthesia 42:487, 1987.

238. Mallampati SR, Gatt SP, Gugino LD, et al: A clinical sign to predict difficult tracheal intubation: a prospective study. Can Anaesth Soc J 32:429, 1985.

239. Rocke DA, Murray WB, Rout CC, et al: Relative risk analysis of factors associated with difficult intubation in obstetric anesthesia. Anesthesiology 77:67, 1992.

240. American Society of Anesthesiologists: Standards for Basic Anesthetic Monitoring. Park Ridge, IL, American Society of Anesthesiologists, 1998.

241. American Society of Anesthesiologists Task Force on Obstetrical Anesthesia: Practice guidelines for obstetrical anesthesia. Anesthesiology 90:600, 1999.

242. Marx GF, Joshi CW, Orkin LR: Placental transmission of nitrous oxide. Anesthesiology 32:429, 1970.

243. Kan K, Shigihara A, Tase C, et al: Comparison of sevoflurane and other volatile anesthetics for cesarean section. J Anesth 9: 363, 1995.

244. Warren TM, Datta S, Ostheimer GW, et al: Comparison of the maternal and neonatal effects of halothane, enflurane, and isoflurane for cesarean delivery. Anesth Analg 62:516, 1983.

245. Andersen TW, DePadua CB, Stenger V, Prystowsky H: Cardiovascular effects of rapid intravenous injection of synthetic oxytocin during elective cesarean section. Clin Pharmacol Ther 6:345, 1965.

246. Orkin LR, Shapiro G: Admission assessment and general monitoring. Int Anesthesiol Clin 21:3, 1983.

247. Aldrete JA, Kroulik D: A postanesthetic recovery score. Anesth Analg 49:924, 1970.

248. Fisher TL: Responsibility for care in recovery rooms. Can Med Assoc J 102:78, 1970.

249. Clark RB, Miller FC: Recovery room and postoperative complications of cesarean section. Anesth Clin North Am 8:173, 1990.

250. Cohen SE, Hamilton CL, Riley ET, et al: Obstetric postanesthesia care unit stays. Anesthesiology 89:1559, 1998.

251. Roberts RB, Shirley MA: Reducing the risk of acid aspiration during cesarean section. Anesth Analg 53:859, 1974.

252. Spence AA, Moir DD, Finlay WEI: Observations on intragastric pressure. Anaesthesia 22:249, 1967.

253. Greenan J: The cardio-oesophageal junction. Br J Anaesth 33: 432, 1961.

254. Williams MH: Variable significance of heartburn. Am J Obstet Gynecol 42:814, 1941.

255. Attia RR, Ebeid AM, Fisher JE, Goudsouzian NG: Maternal fetal and placental gastrin concentrations. Anaesthesia 37:18, 1982.

256. Christofides ND, Ghatei MA, Bloom SR, et al: Decreased plasma motilin concentrations in pregnancy. Br Med J 285: 1453, 1982.

257. Davison JS, Davison MC, Hay DM: Gastric emptying time in late pregnancy and labour. J Obstet Gynaecol Br Commonw 77:37, 1970.

258. O'Sullivan GM, Bullingham RE: Noninvasive assessment by radiotelemetry of antacid effect during labor. Anesth Analg 64:95, 1985.

259. Schwartz DJ, Wynne JW, Gibbs CP, et al: The pulmonary

consequences of aspiration of gastric contents at pH values greater than 2.5. Am Rev Respir Dis 121:119, 1980.

260. Eyler SW, Cullen BF, Murphy ME, Welch WD: Antacid aspiration in rabbits: a comparison of Mylanta and Bicitra. Anesth Analg 61:288, 1982.

261. Hodgkinson R, Glassenberg R, Joyce TH, et al: Comparison of cimetidine (Tagamet®) with antacid for safety and effectiveness in reducing gastric acidity before elective cesarean section. Anesthesiology 59:86, 1983.

262. James FM III, Dewan DM, Floyd HM, et al: Chloroprocaine vs. bupivacaine for lumbar epidural analgesia for elective cesarean section. Anesthesiology 52:488, 1980.

263. Caritis SN, Abouleish E, Edelstone DI, Mueller-Heubach E: Fetal acid-base state following spinal or epidural anesthesia for cesarean section. Obstet Gynecol 56:610, 1980.

264. Corke BC, Datta S, Ostheimer GW, et al: Spinal anaesthesia for caesarean section: the influence of hypotension on neonatal outcome. Anaesthesia 37:658, 1982.

265. Rout CC, Rocke DA, Levin J, et al: A reevaluation of the role of crystalloid preload in the prevention of hypotension associated with spinal anesthesia for elective cesarean section. Anesthesiology 79:262, 1993.

266. Mangano DT: Anesthesia for the pregnant cardiac patient. *In* Shnider SM, Levinson G (eds): Anesthesia for Obstetrics, 3rd ed. Baltimore, Williams & Wilkins, 1993, p 435.

267. Easterling TR, Chadwick HS, Otto CM, Benedetti TJ: Aortic stenosis in pregnancy. Obstet Gynecol 72:113, 1988.

268. Spinnato JA, Kraynack BJ, Cooper MW: Eisenmenger's syndrome in pregnancy: epidural anesthesia for elective cesarean section. N Engl J Med 304:1215, 1981.

269. Ahmad S, Hawes D, Dooley S, et al: Intrathecal morphine in a parturient with a single ventricle. Anesthesiology 54:515, 1981.

270. Abboud TK, Raya J, Noveihed R, Daniel J: Intrathecal morphine for relief of labor pain in a parturient with severe pulmonary hypertension. Anesthesiology 59:477, 1983.

271. Pollack KL, Chest DH, Wenstrom KD: Anesthetic management of a parturient with Eisenmenger's syndrome. Anesth Analg 70:212, 1990.

272. Marx GF, Luykx WM, Cohen S: Fetal-neonatal status following caesarean section for fetal distress. Br J Anaesth 56:1009, 1984.

273. Chestnut DH: Anesthesia for fetal distress. *In* Chestnut DH (ed): Obstetric Anesthesia: Principles and Practice, 2nd ed. St. Louis, Mosby, 1999, p 493.

274. Committee on Obstetrics: Maternal and fetal medicine: anesthesia for emergency deliveries. Washington, DC, American College of Obstetricians and Gynecologists, 1992.

275. Hurley RJ, Lambert D, Hertwig L, et al: Post dural puncture headache in the obstetric patient: spinal vs epidural anesthesia [abstract]. Anesthesiology 77:A1018, 1992.

276. Riley ET, Cohen SE, Macario A, et al: Spinal versus epidural anesthesia for cesarean section: a comparison of time efficiency, costs, charges, and complications. Anesth Analg 80: 709, 1995.

277. Abouleish E, Rawal N, Rashad MN: The addition of 0.2 mg subarachnoid morphine to hyperbaric bupivacaine for cesarean delivery: a prospective study of 856 cases. Reg Anesth 16: 137, 1991.

278. Ferouz, F, Norris MC, Leighton BL: Risk of respiratory arrest after intrathecal sufentanil. Anesth Analg 85:1088, 1997.

279. Cohen SE, Subak LL, Brose WG, et al: Analgesia after cesarean delivery: patient evaluations and costs of five opioid techniques. Reg Anesth 16:141, 1991.

280. Baysinger CL, Harkins TL, Horger EO, et al: Intrathecal morphine sulfate versus intravenous patient controlled analgesia following cesarean section: a comparison of hospital costs and duration of stay [abstract]. Anesth Analg 78:S22, 1994.

Malpresentations

SUSAN M. LANNI AND JOHN W. SEEDS

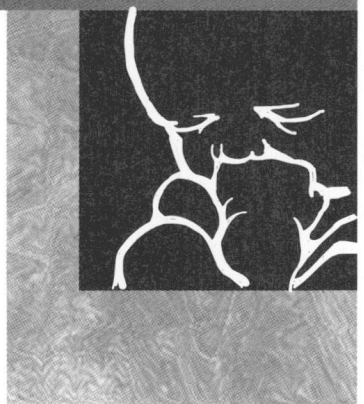

Near term or during labor, the fetus normally assumes a vertical orientation or lie and a cephalic presentation with the fetal vertex flexed on the neck (Fig. 16–1). In about 5 percent of cases, however, deviation occurs from this normal lie, presentation, and flexion attitude, and such deviation constitutes a fetal malpresentation. The word "malpresentation" suggests the possibility of adverse consequences and is typically associated with increased risk to both the mother and the fetus. Malpresentation once led to a variety of maneuvers intended to facilitate vaginal delivery, and early in the 20th century such interventions included destructive operations leading, predictably, to fetal death. Later, manual or instrumental attempts to convert the malpresenting fetus to a more favorable orientation were devised. Internal podalic version followed by a complete breech extraction was once advocated as a solution to many malpresentation situations. However, internal podalic version along with most manipulative efforts to achieve vaginal delivery were associated with a high fetal or maternal morbidity or mortality rate and have been largely abandoned. In contemporary practice, cesarean delivery has become the recommended alternative to manipulative vaginal techniques when normal progress toward vaginal delivery is not observed.

This chapter examines malpresentations, possible etiologies, and the mechanics of labor and vaginal delivery unique to each situation.

CLINICAL CIRCUMSTANCES ASSOCIATED WITH MALPRESENTATION

Generally, factors associated with malpresentation include (1) diminished vertical polarity of the uterine cav-

ity, (2) increased or decreased fetal mobility, or (3) obstructed pelvic inlet. The association of great parity with malpresentation is presumably related to laxity of maternal abdominal muscular support and therefore loss of the normal vertical orientation of the uterine cavity. Placentation either high in the fundus or low in the pelvis (Fig. 16–2) is another factor that diminishes the likelihood of a fetus comfortably assuming a longitudinal axis. Uterine myomata, intrauterine synechiae, and müllerian duct abnormalities such as septate uterus or uterus didelphys are likewise associated with a higher than expected rate of malpresentation. Because both prematurity and hydramnios permit increased fetal mobility, there is an increased probability of a noncephalic presentation if labor or rupture of membranes occurs. In contrast, conditions such as autosomal trisomies, myotonic dystrophy, joint contractures from various etiologies, arthrogryposis or oligohydramnios, and fetal neurologic dysfunction that result in decreased fetal muscle tone, strength, or activity are also associated with an increased incidence of fetal malpresentation. Furthermore, preterm birth involves a fetus that is small relative to the maternal pelvis and results in increased fetal mobility. In these cases, pelvic engagement and descent with labor or rupture of membranes can occur despite malpresentation. Finally, the cephalopelvic disproportion associated with severe fetal hydrocephalus or with a frankly contracted pelvis is frequently implicated as an etiology of malpresentation because normal engagement of the fetal head is prevented.

ABNORMAL AXIAL LIE

The fetal "lie" indicates the orientation of the fetal spine relative to the spine of the mother. The normal

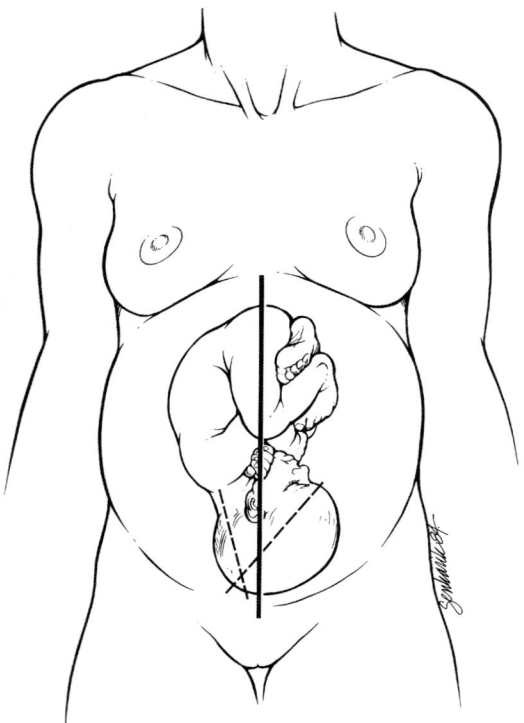

Figure 16–1. Frontal view of a fetus in a longitudinal lie with fetal vertex flexed on the neck.

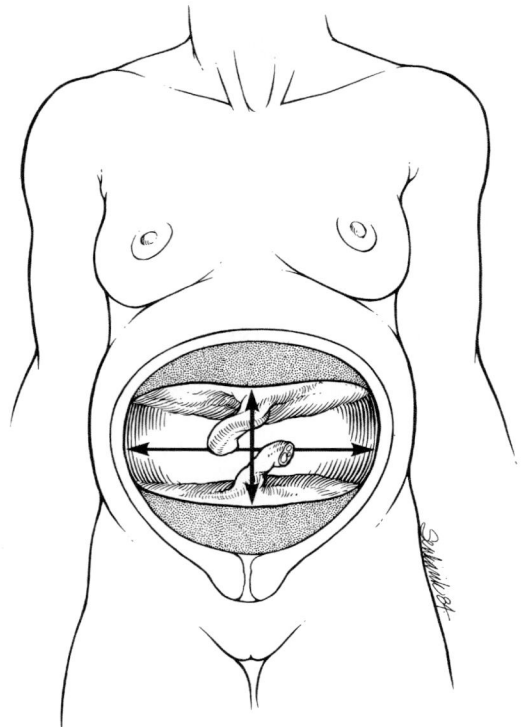

Figure 16–2. Either the high fundal or low implantation of the placenta illustrated here would normally be in the vertical orientation of the intrauterine cavity and increase the probability of a malpresentation.

fetal lie is longitudinal and by itself does not indicate whether the presentation is cephalic or breech. If the fetal spine or long axis crosses that of the mother, the fetus may be said to occupy a transverse or oblique lie (Fig. 16–3), resulting in a shoulder or arm presentation (Fig. 16–4). The lie may be termed unstable if the fetal membranes are intact and there is great fetal mobility resulting in frequent changes of lie or presentation.[1]

Abnormal fetal lie is diagnosed in approximately 1 in 300 cases, or 0.33 percent.[2–8] Prematurity is often a factor, with abnormal lie reported to occur in about 2 percent of pregnancies at 32 weeks, or six times the rate found at term.[9] Persistence of a transverse, oblique, or unstable lie beyond 37 weeks requires a systematic clinical assessment and plan for management, because rupture of membranes without a fetal part filling the inlet of the pelvis imposes a high risk of cord prolapse, fetal compromise, and maternal morbidity if neglected.

Great parity, prematurity, contraction or deformity of the maternal pelvis, and abnormal placentation are the most commonly reported clinical factors associated with abnormal lie,[2,5,9] although Cockburn and Drake[3] found many cases that manifested none of these. In fact, any condition that alters the normal vertical polarity of the intrauterine cavity will predispose to abnormal lie.

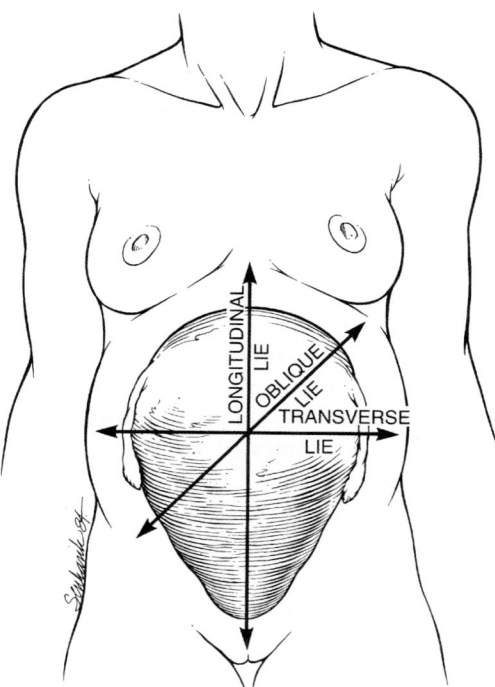

Figure 16–3. A fetus may occupy a longitudinal, oblique, or transverse axis, as illustrated by these vectors. The lie does not indicate whether the vertex or the breech is closest to the cervix.

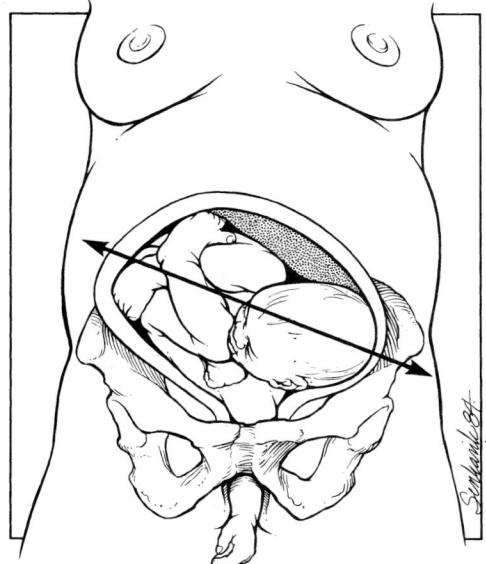

Figure 16–4. This fetus lies in an oblique axis with an arm prolapsing.

Diagnosis may be by palpation or vaginal examination. Routine use of Leopold's maneuvers may assist detection, but Thorp et al.[10] found the sensitivity of Leopold's maneuvers for the detection of malpresentation to be only 28 percent and the positive predictive value only 24 percent compared with immediate ultrasound verification. Others have observed prenatal detection in as few as 41 percent of cases before labor.[3] A fetal loss rate of 9.2 percent[3] with early diagnosis compares with a mortality of 27.5 percent when the diag-

---

Etiologic Factors in Malpresentation

Maternal
  Great parity
  Pelvic tumors
  Pelvic contracture
  Uterine malformation
Fetal
  Prematurity
  Multiple gestation
  Hydramnios
  Macrosomia
  Hydrocephaly
  Trisomies
  Anencephaly
  Myotonic dystrophy
  Placenta previa

---

nosis was delayed, indicating that early diagnosis improves fetal outcome.

Reported perinatal mortality for unstable or transverse lie (corrected for lethal malformations and extreme prematurity) varies from 3.9 percent[11] to 24 percent,[1] with maternal mortality as high as 10 percent. Maternal deaths are usually related to infection after premature rupture of membranes, hemorrhage secondary to abnormal placentation, complications of operative intervention for cephalopelvic disproportion, or traumatic delivery.[7,9] Fetal loss of phenotypically and chromosomally normal neonates from a pregnancy of gestational age such that viability is expected is primarily associated with neglect, prolapsed cord, or traumatic delivery.[9] Cord prolapse occurs 20 times as often with abnormal axial lie as it does with a cephalic presentation.

MANAGEMENT

The normally grown infant at term cannot undergo a safe vaginal delivery from an axial malpresentation.[4,7] Furthermore, a careful search for a potentially dangerous or compromising etiology of the malpresentation is indicated. A transverse/oblique or unstable lie late in the third trimester necessitates ultrasound examination to exclude a major fetal malformation and abnormal placentation. Elective hospitalization may permit observation and early recognition of cord prolapse.[6,11] Phelan et al.[12] reported 29 patients with transverse lie diagnosed at or beyond 37 weeks' gestation and managed expectantly. Eighty-three percent (24 of 29) spontaneously converted to breech (9 of 24) or vertex (15 of 24) before labor; however, the overall cesarean delivery rate was 45 percent, and there were two cases of cord prolapse, one uterine rupture, and one neonatal death. Such outcomes suggest that active intervention at or beyond 37 weeks or after confirmation of fetal lung maturity may be of benefit. External cephalic version with subsequent induction of labor, if successful, might diminish the risk of adverse outcome.

In cases of an abnormal lie, the risk of fetal death varies with the type of obstetric intervention. Fetal mortality of 0 to 10 percent has been reported for cesarean birth compared with 25 to 90 percent when internal podalic version and breech extraction are performed.[3,4,7–9,13] A mortality rate of only 6 percent was reported for successful external version and vertex vaginal delivery.[8,9] External cephalic version followed by induction of labor after 37 weeks in the case of abnormal lie is a reasonable alternative to both expectant management and elective cesarean delivery. Although disputed by some,[3,14] external cephalic version has been found to be safe, with close monitoring, and effective in the majority of cases.[15] Using such a protocol, Edwards and Nicholson[6] reported 86 of 96 cases delivered vaginally, with fetal compromise detected in only four and no fetal losses.

If external version is unsuccessful or unavailable, if spontaneous rupture of membranes occurs, or if active labor has begun with an abnormal lie, cesarean delivery is the treatment of choice for the potentially viable infant.[1,3,14] There is no place for internal podalic version and breech extraction in the management of transverse or oblique lie or unstable presentation in singleton pregnancies because of the unacceptably high rate of fetal and maternal complications.[2]

A persistent abnormal axial lie, particularly if accompanied by ruptured membranes, also alters the choice of uterine incision at cesarean delivery. Although a low transverse cervical incision has many surgical advantages, up to 25 percent of transverse incisions require vertical extension for delivery of an infant from an abnormal lie to allow access to and atraumatic delivery of the vertex entrapped in the muscular fundus.[3,14] Furthermore, the lower uterine segment is often poorly developed. It makes no sense to perform a cesarean section to minimize birth trauma, then choose a transverse uterine incision if that incision makes fetal extraction more difficult. Therefore, when managing a transverse or oblique lie with ruptured membranes or a poorly developed lower segment, a vertical incision is more prudent. Intraoperative cephalic version may allow the use of a low transverse incision, as reported by Pelosi et al.,[14] but ruptured membranes with oligohydramnios makes this difficult.

DEFLECTION ATTITUDES

"Attitude" refers to the position of the fetal head with relation to the neck. The normal attitude of the fetal vertex during labor is one of full flexion on the neck, with the fetal chin against the upper chest. Deflexed attitudes include various degrees of deflection or even extension of the fetal head on the neck (Fig. 16–5). Spontaneous conversion to a more normal flexed attitude or further extension of an intermediate deflection to a fully extended position will commonly occur as labor progresses due to resistance exerted by the pelvic bony and soft tissues. Although safe vaginal delivery is possible in most cases, experience indicates that cesarean delivery is the only appropriate alternative when arrest of progress is observed.

Face Presentation

A face presentation is characterized by a longitudinal lie and full extension of the fetal head on the neck,

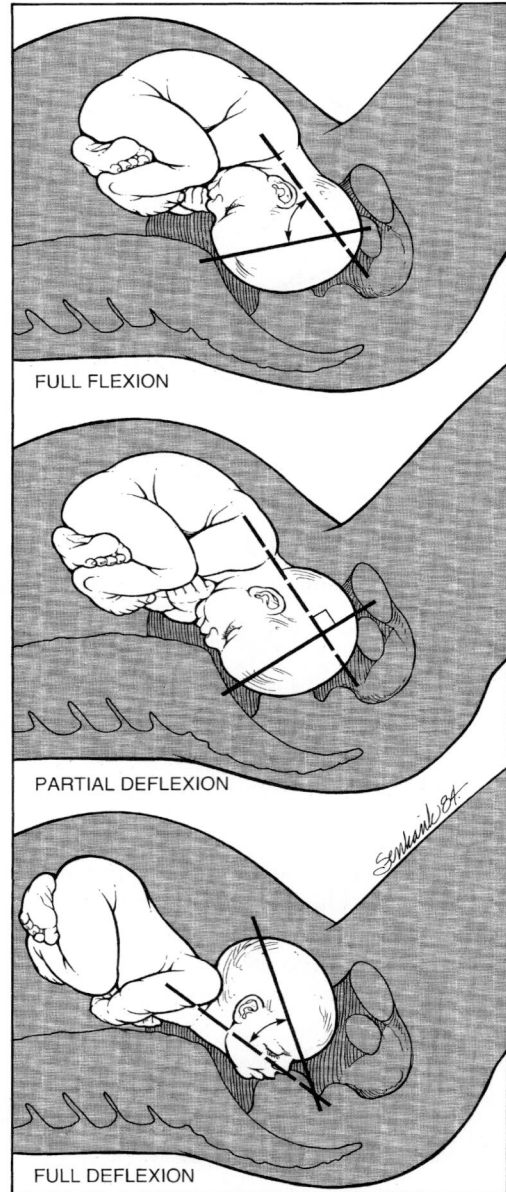

Figure 16–5. The normal "attitude" (*top view*) shows the fetal vertex flexed on the neck. Partial deflexion (*middle view*) shows the fetal vertex intermediate between flexion and extension. Full deflexion (*lower view*) shows the fetal vertex completely extended, with the face presenting.

with the occiput against the upper back (Fig. 16–6). The fetal chin is chosen as the point of designation at vaginal examination. For example, a fetus presenting by the face whose chin is in the right posterior quadrant of the maternal pelvis would be called a *right mentum posterior* (RMP) (Fig. 16–7). The reported incidence of face presentation ranges from 0.14 to 0.54 percent,[8,16–21] averaging about 0.2 percent, or 1 in 500 live births overall. Reported perinatal mortality, corrected for nonviable malformations and extreme prematurity,

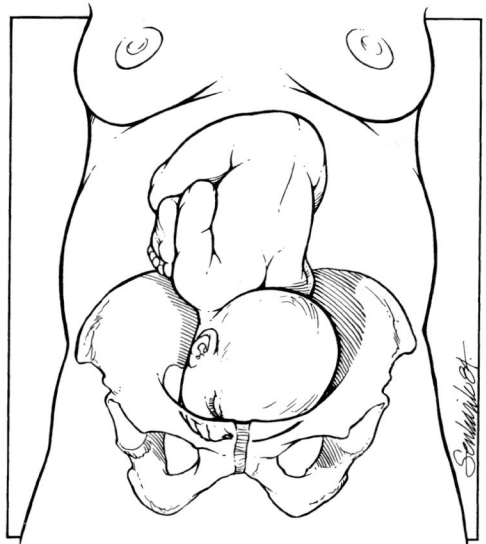

Figure 16–6. This fetus with the vertex completely extended on the neck enters the maternal pelvis in a face presentation. The cephalic prominence would be palpable on the same side of the maternal abdomen as the fetal spine.

varies from 0.6 percent[22] to 5 percent,[23] averaging about 2 to 3 percent.

All clinical factors known to increase the general rate of malpresentation (see box, Etiologic Factors in Malpresentation, above) have been implicated in face presentation, but Browne and Carney[24] emphasized that as many as 60 percent of infants with a face presentation were malformed. Anencephaly, for instance, is found in about one third of cases of face presentation.[5,25,26] Fetal goiter resulting from iodine deficiency or in cases of maternal Graves' disease with thyroid-stimulating immunoglobulin, as well as tumors of the soft tissues of the neck may also cause deflexion of the head. Frequently observed maternal factors include a contracted pelvis or cephalopelvic disproportion in 10 to 40 percent of cases.[17,20,23] In a review of face presentation,

Duff[18] found that one of these etiologic factors was found in up to 90 percent of cases.

Early recognition is important, and diagnosis can be suspected anytime abdominal palpation finds the fetal cephalic prominence on the same side of the maternal abdomen as the fetal back (Fig. 16–8); however, face presentation is more often discovered by vaginal examination and confirmed by radiography or ultrasound. In practice, fewer than 1 in 20 infants with face presentation is diagnosed abdominally.[22] In fact, only half of these infants are found to have a face presentation by any means prior to the second stage of labor,[5,20,22,26,27] and half of the remaining cases are undiagnosed until delivery.[20,23] Perinatal mortality may be higher, however, with late diagnosis.[17]

Mechanism of Labor

Knowledge of the early mechanism of labor for face presentation is incomplete. Many infants with a face presentation probably begin labor in the less extended brow position. With descent into the pelvis, the forces of labor press the fetus against maternal tissues; either flexion or full extension of the head on the spine then occurs. The labor of a face presentation must include engagement, descent, internal rotation generally to a mentum anterior position, and delivery by flexion as the chin passes under the symphysis (Fig. 16–9). However, flexion of the occiput may not always occur. Borrell and Fernstrom[28] have proposed that delivery in the fully extended attitude may be common.

The prognosis for labor with a face presentation depends on the orientation of the fetal chin. At diagnosis, 60 to 80 percent of infants with a face presentation are mentum anterior,[5,20,22,29] 10 to 12 percent are mentum transverse,[5,22,29] and 20 to 25 percent are mentum posterior.[5,20,22,29] Almost all average-sized infants presenting mentum anterior with adequate pelvic dimensions will achieve spontaneous or easily assisted vaginal delivery.[5,22,30,31] Furthermore, most mentum transverse in-

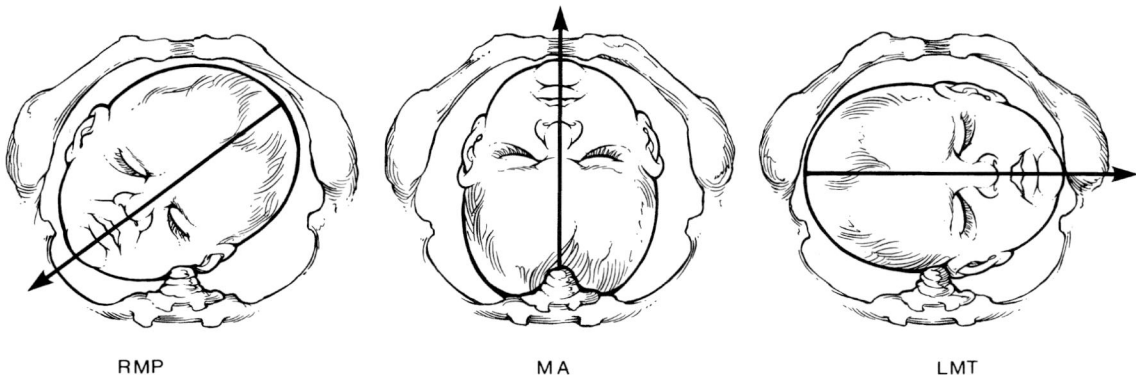

RMP   MA   LMT

Figure 16–7. The point of designation from digital examination in the case of a face presentation is the fetal chin relative to the maternal pelvis. *Left,* Right mentum posterior (RMP). *Middle,* Mentum anterior (MA). *Right,* Left mentum transverse (LMT).

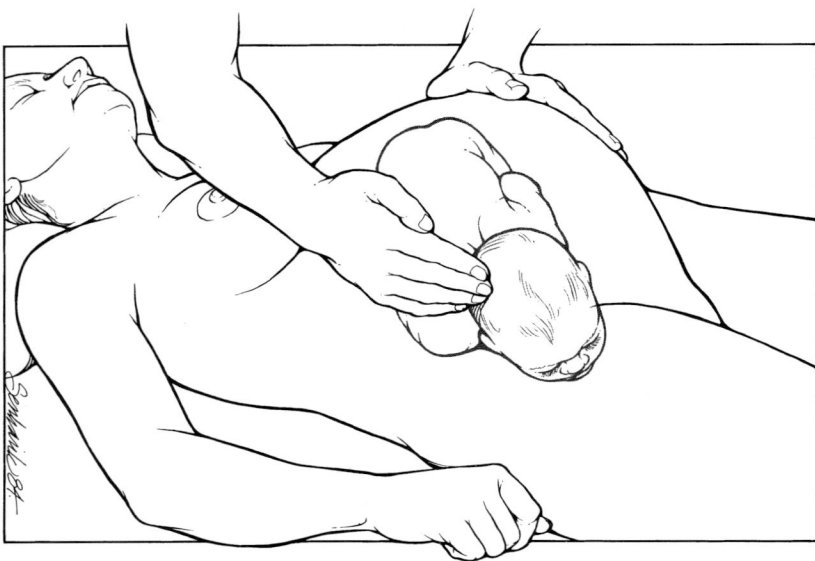

Figure 16–8. Palpation of the maternal abdomen in the case of a face presentation should find the fetal cephalic prominence on the side away from the fetal small parts instead of on the same side as in the case of a normally flexed fetal head.

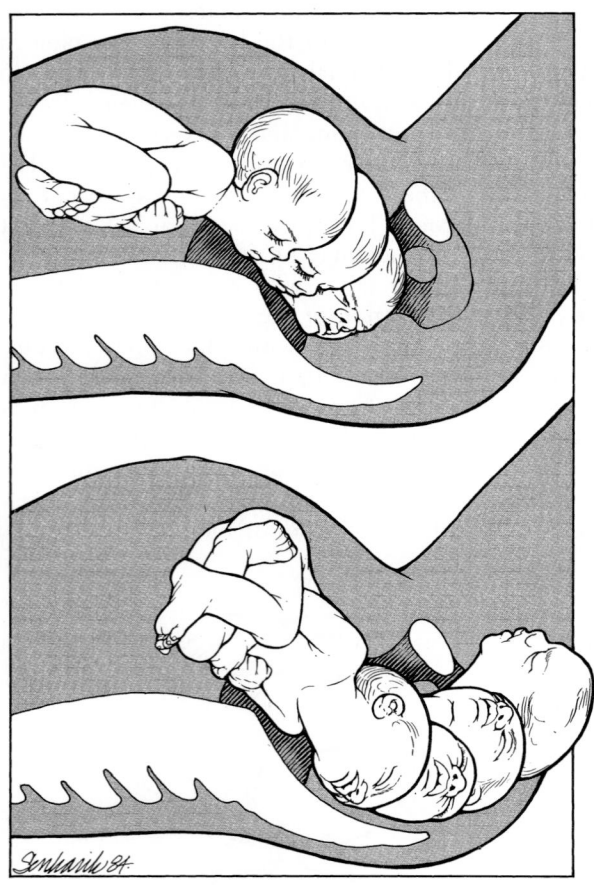

Figure 16–9. Engagement, descent, and internal rotation remain cardinal elements of vaginal delivery in the case of a face presentation, but successful vaginal delivery of a term size fetus presenting a face generally requires delivery by flexion under the symphysis from a mentum anterior position as illustrated here.

fants will rotate to the mentum anterior position and deliver vaginally, and even 25 to 33 percent of mentum posterior infants will rotate and deliver vaginally in the mentum anterior position.[5,16,20] In a review of 51 cases of persistent face presentation, Schwartz et al.[29] found that the mean birth weight of those infants in mentum posterior who did rotate and deliver vaginally was 3,425 g, compared with 3,792 g for those infants who did not rotate and deliver vaginally. Persistence of mentum posterior with an infant of normal size, however, makes safe vaginal delivery less likely. Overall, 70 to 80 percent[5,20,22,23] of infants with face presentation can be delivered vaginally, either spontaneously or by low forceps, while 12 to 30 percent require cesarean delivery. Manual attempts to convert the face to a flexed attitude or to rotate a posterior position to a more favorable mentum anterior are rarely successful and increase both maternal and fetal risks.[16,22,26,32] Internal podalic version and breech extraction as a remedy for face presentation is contraindicated. Campbell[22] reported fetal losses of up to 60 percent with this maneuver. Maternal deaths from uterine rupture and trauma after version with extraction have also bean documented. Spontaneous delivery or cesarean delivery are therefore the preferred routes for maternal safety as well.[16,22,26]

Prolonged labor is a common feature of face presentation[5,8] and has been associated with an increased number of intrapartum deaths.[17] Therefore, prompt attention to an arrested labor pattern is recommended. The choice between augmentation of a dysfunctional labor or primary cesarean delivery rests on an assess-

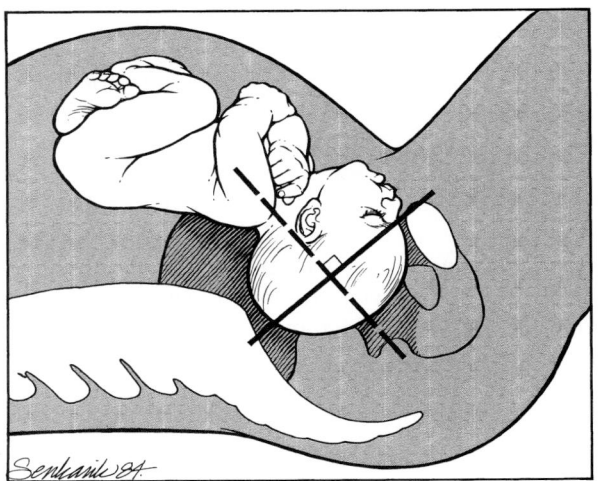

Figure 16–10. This fetus is a brow presentation in a frontum anterior position. The head is in an intermediate deflexion attitude.

No absolute contraindication to oxytocin augmentation of hypotonic labor in the case of a face presentation exists, but an arrest of progress despite adequate labor or nonreassuring fetal heart rate pattern should call for cesarean delivery.[8] Although cesarean delivery has been reported in up to 60 percent of cases of face presentation,[18,27] safe vaginal delivery may be accomplished in many, and a trial of labor with careful monitoring of fetal condition and progress is not contraindicated unless macrosomia or a small pelvis is identified. If cesarean delivery is warranted, care should be taken to flex the head gently both to accomplish elevation of the head through the hysterotomy incision as well as to avoid potential nerve damage to the neonate. However, forced flexion may also result in damage, especially with fetal goiter, or neck tumors.

Laryngeal and tracheal edema resulting from pressures of the birth process might require immediate nasotracheal intubation.[33] Nuchal tumors or simple goiter, fetal anomalies that might have caused the malpresentation, require expert neonatal management.

ment of uterine activity, pelvic adequacy, and fetal condition. In the case of an average or small fetus, adequate pelvis, and hypotonic labor, oxytocin may be considered. However, worsening of fetal condition during labor is common. Salzmann et al.[26] observed a 10-fold increase in fetal compromise with face presentation. Several other observers have also found that abnormal fetal heart rate patterns occur more often with face presentation.[16,18] Continuous intrapartum electronic fetal heart rate monitoring of a fetus with face presentation is considered mandatory, but extreme care must be exercised in the placement of an electrode, as ocular and cosmetic damage might result from this device. If external Doppler heart rate monitoring is inadequate and an internal electrode is considered necessary, placement of the electrode on the fetal chin is often recommended.

BROW PRESENTATION

An infant in a brow presentation occupies a longitudinal axis, with a partially deflexed cephalic attitude, midway between full flexion and full extension (Fig. 16–10).[24] The frontal bones are the point of designation. If the anterior fontanel is on the mother's left side, with the sagittal suture in the transverse pelvic axis, the fetus would be in a left frontum transverse (LFT) position (Fig. 16–11). The reported incidence of brow presentation varies widely, from 1 in 670[34] to 1 in 3,433,[35] averaging about 1 in 1,500 deliveries. Brow

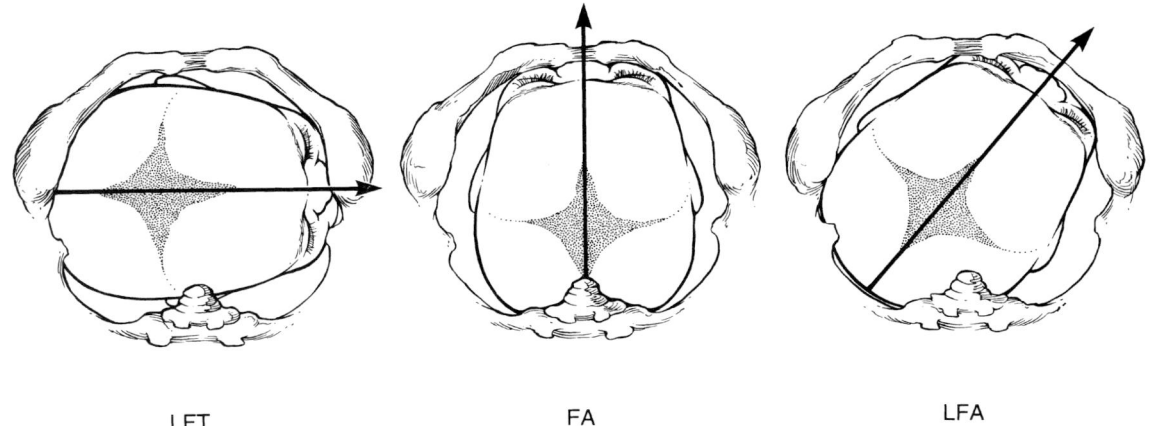

LFT   FA   LFA

Figure 16–11. In brow presentation, the anterior fontanel (frontum) relative to the maternal pelvis is the point of designation. *Left,* Fetus in left frontum transverse (LFT). *Middle,* Frontum anterior (FA). *Right,* Left frontum anterior (LFA).

presentation will be detected more often in early labor before flexion occurs to a normal attitude. Less frequently, further extension results in a face presentation.

Perinatal mortality corrected for lethal anomalies and very low birth weight varies from 1 to 8 percent.[36] In an examination of 88,988 deliveries, Ingolfsson[37] found that corrected perinatal mortality rates for fetuses presenting by the brow depended on the mode of delivery. The highest loss rate, 16 percent, was associated with manipulative vaginal birth.[37]

In general, factors that delay engagement are associated with persistent brow presentation. Cephalopelvic disproportion, prematurity, and great parity are often found and have been implicated in more than 60 percent of cases of persistent brow presentation.[5,35,38,39]

Detection of a brow presentation by abdominal palpation is unusual in practice. More often, a brow is detected on vaginal examination. As in the case of a face presentation, late diagnosis is more likely. Fewer than 50 percent of brow presentations are detected before the second stage of labor, with most of the remainder undiagnosed until delivery.[34,37–39] Frontum anterior is reportedly the most common position at diagnosis, occurring about twice as often as either transverse or posterior positions. Although the initial position at diagnosis may be of limited prognostic value, Skalley and Kramer[39] reported the cesarean delivery rate to be higher with frontum transverse or frontum posterior than with frontum anterior.

A persistent brow presentation requires engagement and descent of the largest (mento-occipital) diameter or profile of the fetal head.[40] This process is possible only with a large pelvis or a small infant or both. However, brow presentations convert spontaneously by flexion or further extension to either a vertex or a face presentation and are then managed accordingly.[34,35] The earlier the diagnosis is made, the more likely conversion will occur spontaneously. Fewer than half of infants with persistent brow presentations undergo spontaneous vaginal delivery, but in most cases a trial of labor is not contraindicated.[5,36]

Prolonged labors have been observed in 33 to 50 percent of brow presentations,[5,20,35,38,39] and secondary arrest is not uncommon.[34] Forced conversion of the brow to a more favorable position with forceps is contraindicated,[34,35,38] as are attempts at manual conversion. One unexpected cause of persistent brow presentation may be an open fetal mouth pressed against the vaginal wall, splinting the head and preventing either flexion or extension[28,35] (Fig. 16–12).

In most brow presentations, as with face presentations, minimal manipulation yields the best results[35,41] if the fetal heart rate pattern remains reassuring. Ingolfsson[37] concluded, however, that expectancy is justified only with a large pelvis, a small fetus, and adequate progress. If a brow presentation persists with a large baby, successful vaginal delivery is unlikely, and cesarean delivery may be most prudent.[20]

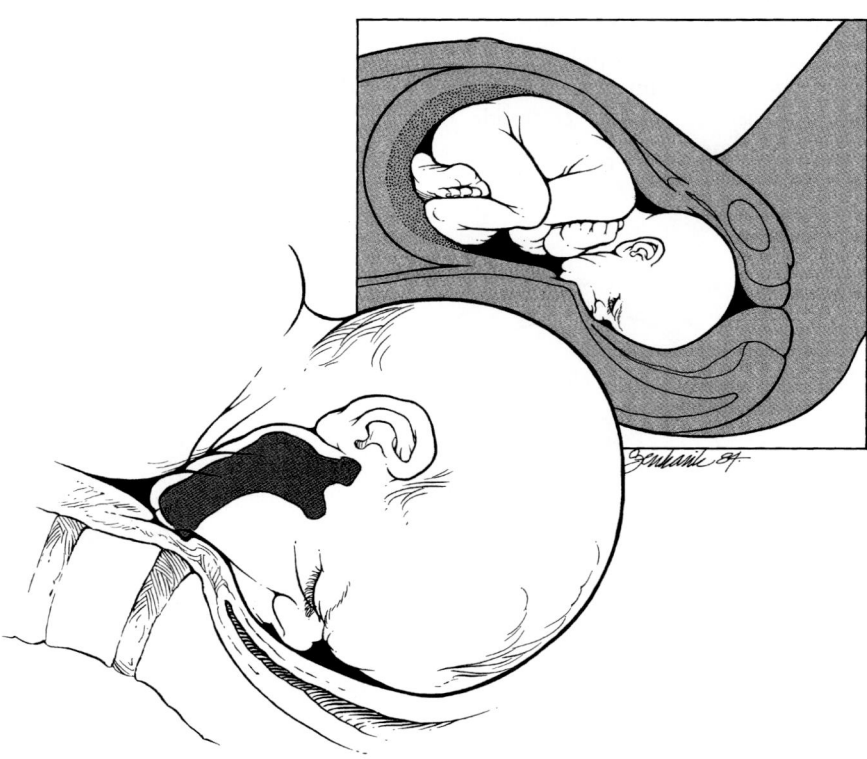

Figure 16–12. The open fetal mouth against the vaginal sidewall may brace the head in the intermediate deflexion attitude as shown here.

Although radiographic or computed tomographic pelvimetry might be helpful, Cruikshank and White[5] reported that while 91 percent of those cases with adequate pelvic dimensions converted to a vertex or a face and delivered vaginally, only 20 percent of those with some form of pelvic contracture did also. Therefore, regardless of pelvic dimensions, consideration of a trial of labor with careful monitoring of maternal and fetal condition may be appropriate. As in the case of a face presentation, oxytocin may be used cautiously to correct hypotonia, but prompt resumption of progress toward delivery should follow.

COMPOUND PRESENTATION

Whenever an extremity is found prolapsed beside the major presenting fetal part, the situation is referred to as a compound presentation[42] (Fig. 16–13). The reported incidence ranges from 1 in 377 to 1 in 1,213 deliveries.[5,42–45] The combination of an upper extremity and the vertex is the most common.

This diagnosis should be suspected with any arrest of labor in the active phase or failure to engage during active labor.[44] Diagnosis is made by vaginal examination that discovers an irregular mobile tissue mass adjacent to the larger presenting part. Recognition late in labor is common, and as many as 50 percent of persisting compound presentations are not detected until the second stage.[42] Delay in diagnosis may not be detrimental because it is likely that only the persistent cases require significant intervention.

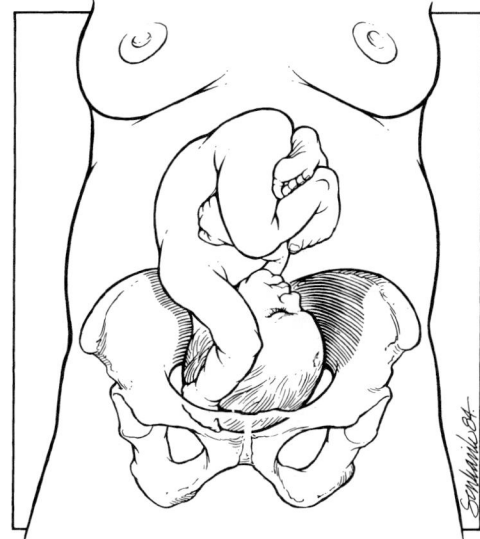

Figure 16–13. The compound presentation of an upper extremity and the vertex illustrated here most often spontaneously resolves with further labor and descent.

Although maternal age, race, parity, and pelvic size have all been associated with compound presentation,[43,44] prematurity is the most consistent clinical finding.[5,42] It is primarily the very small fetus that is at great risk of persistent compound presentation. In late pregnancy, external cephalic version of a fetus in breech position may increase the risk of a compound presentation.[46]

Perinatal mortality with a compound presentation is typically elevated, with an overall rate of 93 per 1,000 reported by Cruikshank and White.[5] Higher losses of 17 and 19 percent have been reported when the foot prolapses.[43] As with other malpresentations, fetal risk can be directly related to the method of management. A fetal mortality rate of 4.8 percent has been noted if no intervention is required compared with 14.4 percent with intervention other than cesarean delivery. A 30 percent fetal mortality rate has been observed with internal podalic version and breech extraction.[43] There is probably some selection bias in these figures, because it is likely that more difficult cases were chosen for manipulative intervention. When intervention is necessary, cesarean delivery appears to be the only safe choice.

Fetal risk in compound presentation is specifically associated with birth trauma and cord prolapse. Cord prolapse occurs in 11 to 20 percent of cases.[5,43,44] and is the most frequent single complication of this malpresentation. Prolapse probably occurs because the prolapsed extremity splints the presenting part, resulting in an irregular fetal aggregate that incompletely fills the pelvic inlet. In addition to the hypoxic risk of cord prolapse, common fetal morbidity includes neurologic and musculoskeletal damage to the involved extremity. Maternal risks include soft tissue damage and obstetric laceration.

Despite these dangers, labor is not necessarily contraindicated with a compound presentation; however, the prolapsed extremity should not be manipulated.[42–44,47] The accompanying extremity may retract as the major presenting part descends. Cruikshank and White[5] found that 75 percent of vertex/upper extremity combinations deliver spontaneously. Occult or undetected cord prolapse is possible, and therefore continuous electronic fetal heart rate monitoring is recommended.

The primary indications for surgical intervention are cord prolapse, nonreassuring fetal heart rate patterns, and failure to progress.[5] Cesarean delivery is the only appropriate clinical intervention,[42] since both version extraction and attempts to reposition the prolapsed extremity are associated with high fetal and maternal morbidity and mortality and are to be avoided.[43,44] Breen and Wiesmeien[42] found that 2 percent of patterns with compound presentation required abdominal delivery, whereas Weissberg and O'Leary[44] reported cesarean delivery to be necessary in 25 percent of cases. Protraction of the second stage of labor has been noted

Table 16-1. BREECH CATEGORIES

Type	Overall Percent of Breeches	Risk (%)	
		Prolapse	Premature
Frank breech	48–73[31,46,48,54,70]	0.5[68]	38[48]
Complete	4.6–11.5[31,48,54,70]	4–6[68]	12[48]
Footling	12–38[31,48,54]	15–18[68]	50[48]

to occur more frequently with persistent compound presentation, and dysfunctional labor patterns are said to be common.[42] Again, as in other malpresentations, spontaneous resolution occurs more often and surgical intervention is less frequently necessary in those cases diagnosed early in labor. Persistent compound presentation is more likely with a small infant, as is the prognosis for successful vaginal delivery. Persistent compound presentation with a term-sized infant has a poor prognosis for safe vaginal delivery, and cesarean delivery is usually necessary.

BREECH PRESENTATION

The infant presenting as a breech occupies a longitudinal axis with the cephalic pole in the uterine fundus. This presentation occurs in 3 to 4 percent of labors overall, although it is found in 7 percent of pregnancies at 32 weeks and in 25 percent of pregnancies of less than 28 weeks' duration.[48] The three types of breech are noted in Table 16–1. The infant in the frank breech position is flexed at the hips with extended knees. The complete breech is flexed at both joints, and the footling breech has one or both hips partially or fully extended (Fig. 16–14).

The diagnosis of breech presentation may be made by abdominal palpation or vaginal examination and confirmed by ultrasound. Prematurity, fetal malformation, müllerian anomalies, and polar placentation are commonly observed causative factors. High rates of breech presentation are noted in certain fetal genetic disorders, including trisomies 13, 18, and 21; Potter's syndrome; and myotonic dystrophy.[49] Thus, conditions that alter fetal muscular tone and mobility also increase the frequency of breech presentation.

Mechanism and Conduct of Labor and Vaginal Delivery

The two most important elements for the safe conduct of vaginal breech delivery are continuous electronic fetal heart rate monitoring and noninterference until spontaneous delivery of the breech to the umbilicus has occurred. Early in labor, the capability for immediate cesarean delivery should be established. Anesthesia should be available, the operating room readied, and appropriate informed consent obtained. Two obstetricians should be in attendance as well as a pediatric team. Appropriate training and experience with vaginal breech delivery are fundamental to success. The instrument table should be prepared in the customary manner, with the addition of Piper forceps and extra towels. There is no contraindication to epidural analgesia once labor is well established; many view epidural anesthesia as an asset in the control of the second stage.

The infant presenting in the frank breech position usually enters the pelvic inlet in one of the diagonal

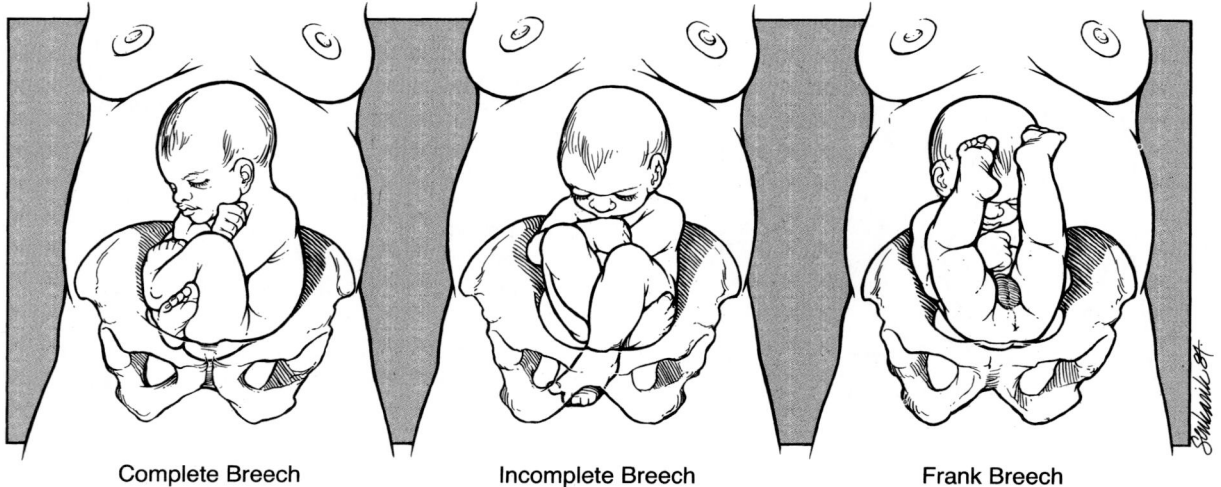

Complete Breech   Incomplete Breech   Frank Breech

Figure 16–14. The complete breech is flexed at the hips and flexed at the knees. The incomplete breech shows incomplete deflexion of one or both knees or hips. The frank breech is flexed at the hips and extended at the knees.

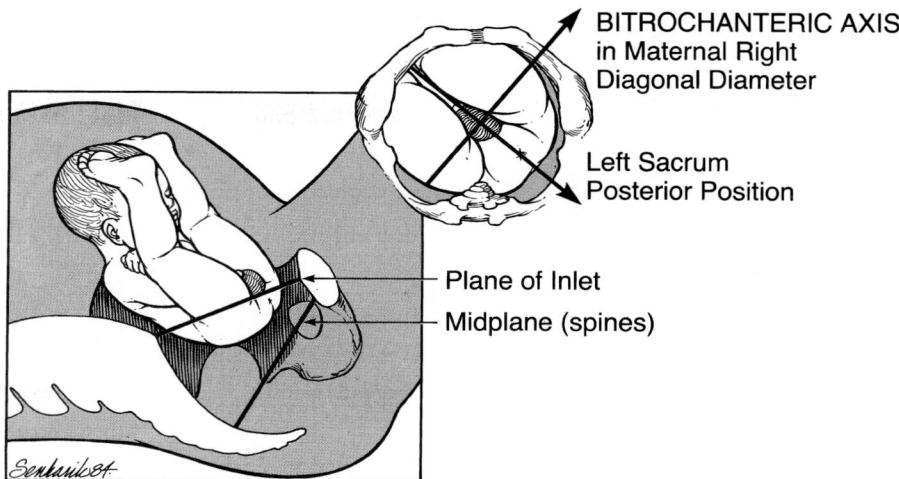

BITROCHANTERIC AXIS
in Maternal Right
Diagonal Diameter

Left Sacrum
Posterior Position

— Plane of Inlet
— Midplane (spines)

Figure 16–15. The breech typically enters the inlet with the bitrochanteric diameter aligned with one of the diagonal diameters, with the sacrum as the point of designation in the other diagonal diameter. This is a case of left sacrum posterior (LSP).

pelvic diameters (Fig. 16–15). Engagement has occurred when the bitrochanteric diameter of the fetus has passed the plane of the pelvic inlet, although by vaginal examination the presenting part may only be palpated at −2 to −4 station (out of 5) relative to the ischial spines. As the breech descends and encounters the levator ani muscular sling, internal rotation usually occurs to bring the bitrochanteric diameter into the anteroposterior (AP) axis of the pelvis. The point of designation in a breech labor is the fetal sacrum and, therefore, when the bitrochanteric diameter is in the AP axis of the pelvis, the fetal sacrum will lie in the transverse pelvic diameter (Fig. 16–16).

If normal descent occurs, the breech will present at the outlet and begin to emerge, first as a sacrum transverse, then rotate to a sacrum anterior. Crowning occurs when the bitrochanteric diameter passes under the pubic symphysis. An episiotomy in the midline to but not through the anal sphincter may facilitate delivery but should be delayed until crowning begins. Some ar-

gue that a mediolateral episiotomy offers more room and less risk of extension through the anal sphincter, but considerable skill and experience are required to repair a mediolateral episiotomy properly, and this incision is associated with greater blood loss and pain. Premature episiotomy will contribute to unnecessary blood loss and to the level of anxiety and perhaps a tendency to rush the delivery. As the infant emerges, rotation begins, usually toward a sacrum anterior position. This direction of rotation may reflect the greater capacity of the hollow of the posterior pelvis to accept the fetal chest and small parts. It is important to emphasize that operator intervention is not yet needed or helpful other than possibly to perform the episiotomy and encourage maternal expulsive efforts.

Premature or aggressive assistance may adversely affect the breech birth in at least two ways. First, cervical dilatation must be maximized and complete dilatation sustained for sufficient duration to retard retraction of the cervix and entrapment of the aftercoming fetal

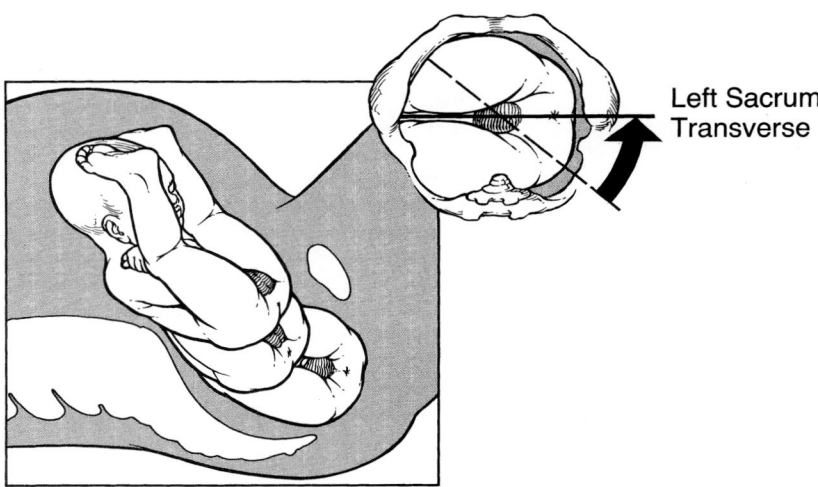

Left Sacrum
Transverse

Figure 16–16. With labor and descent, the bitrochanteric diameter generally rotates toward the anteroposterior axis and the sacrum toward the transverse.

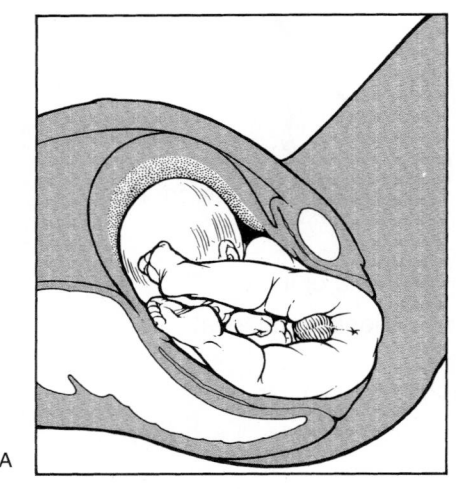
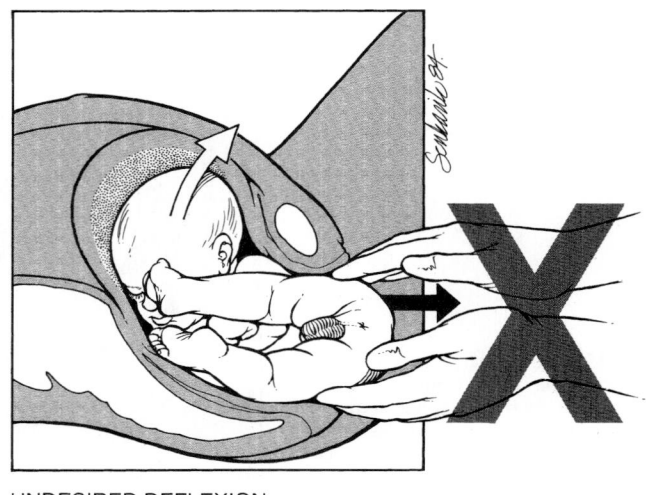

SPONTANEOUS EXPULSION   UNDESIRED DEFLEXION

Figure 16–17. The fetus emerges spontaneously (*A*), while uterine contractions maintain cephalic flexion. Premature aggressive traction (*B*) encourages deflexion of the fetal vertex and increases the risk of head entrapment or nuchal arm entrapment.

head. Rushing the delivery of the trunk may significantly diminish the effectiveness of this process. Second, the safe descent and delivery of the breech infant must be the result of expulsive forces from above to maintain flexion of the fetal vertex. Any traction from below in an effort to speed delivery would encourage deflexion of the vertex and result in the presentation of the larger occipitofrontal fetal cranial profile to the pelvic inlet (Fig. 16–17). Such an event could be catastrophic. Rushed delivery also increases the risk of a nuchal arm, with one or both arms trapped behind the head above the pelvic inlet. Entrapment of a nuchal arm makes safe

vaginal delivery much more difficult, as it dramatically increases the size of the aggregate object that must pass through the birth canal. Safe breech delivery of an average-sized infant, therefore, depends predominantly on maternal expulsive forces, and patience, not traction from below.

As the frank breech emerges farther, the fetal thighs are typically pressed firmly against the fetal abdomen, often splinting and protecting the umbilicus and cord. After the umbilicus appears over the maternal perineum, the operator may align his or her fingers medial to one thigh, then the other, pressing laterally as the

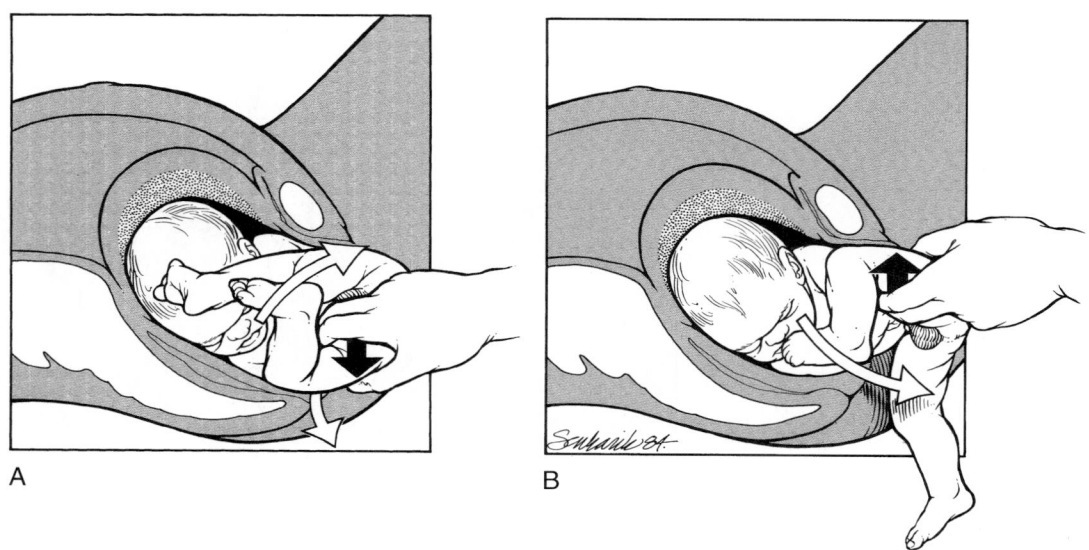

Figure 16–18. After spontaneous expulsion to the umbilicus, external rotation of each thigh (*A*) combined with opposite rotation of the fetal pelvis results in flexion of the knee and delivery of each leg (*B*).

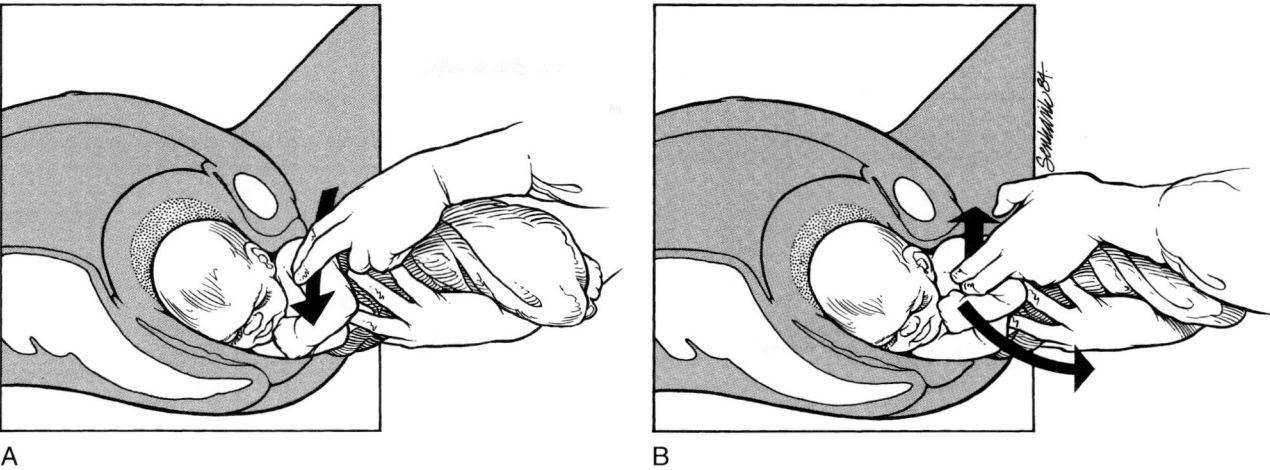

Figure 16–19. When the scapulae appear under the symphisis, the operator reaches over the left shoulder, sweeps the arm across the chest (*A*), and delivers the arm (*B*).

fetal pelvis is rotated away from that side (Fig. 16–18). This results in external rotation of the thigh at the hip, flexion of the knee, and delivery of one and then the other leg. The dual movement of counterclockwise rotation of the fetal pelvis as the operator externally rotates the right thigh and clockwise rotation of the fetal pelvis as the operator externally rotates the fetal left thigh is most effective in facilitating delivery. The fetal trunk is then wrapped with a towel to provide secure support of the body while further descent results from expulsive forces from the mother. The operator primarily facilitates the delivery of the fetus by guiding the body through the introitus. The operator is not applying outward traction on the fetus that might result in deflexion of the fetal head or nuchal arm.

When the scapulae appear at the outlet, the operator may slip a hand over the fetal shoulder from the back (Fig. 16–19), follow the humerus and, with a lateral

movement, sweep first one and then the other arm across the chest and out over the perineum. Gentle rotation of the fetal trunk counterclockwise assists delivery of the right arm, and clockwise rotation assists delivery of the left arm (turning the body "into" the arm). This accomplishes delivery of the arms by drawing them across the fetal chest in a fashion similar to that used for delivery of the legs (Fig. 16–20). Once both arms have been delivered, if the vertex has remained flexed on the neck, the chin and face will appear at the outlet, and the airway may be cleared and suctioned (Fig. 16–21).

With further maternal expulsive forces alone, spontaneous controlled delivery of the fetal head will often occur. If not, delivery may be accomplished with a

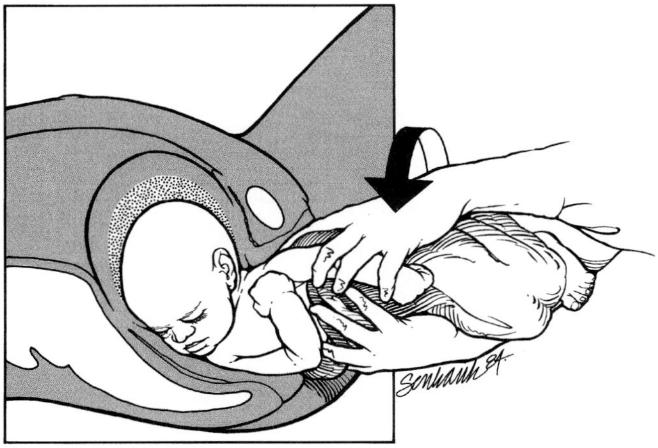

Figure 16–20. Gentle rotation of the shoulder girdle facilitates delivery of the right arm.

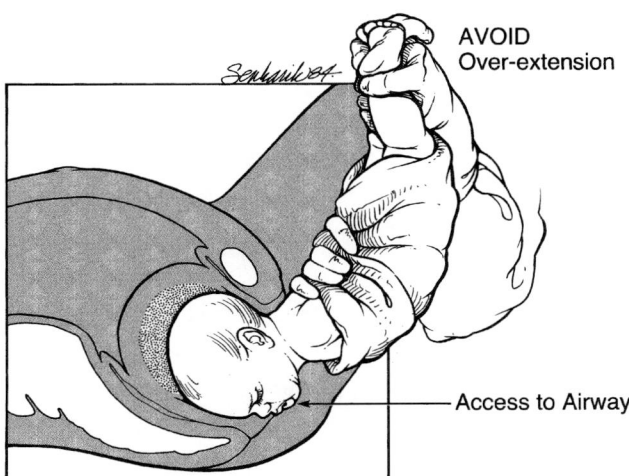

Figure 16–21. Following delivery of the arms, the fetus is wrapped in a towel for control and slightly elevated. The fetal face and airway may be visible over the perineum. Excessive elevation of the trunk is avoided.

simple manual effort to maximize flexion of the vertex using pressure on the fetal maxilla (not mandible; the Mauriceau-Smellie-Veit maneuver) along with suprapubic pressure (Credé's maneuver) and gentle downward traction (Fig. 16–22). Although maxillary pressure will maximize cephalic flexion, the main force effecting delivery remains the mother.

Alternatively, the operator may apply Piper forceps to the aftercoming head to facilitate delivery. The application requires very slight elevation of the fetal trunk by the assistant, while the operator kneels and applies the Piper forceps directly to the fetal head in the pelvis. The position of the operator for applying the forceps is depicted in Figure 16–23, which also demonstrates how *excessive* elevation by the assistant may potentially cause harm to the neonate. Hyperextension of the fetal neck from excessive elevation of the fetal trunk, shown in Figure 16–23, should be avoided.

Piper forceps are characterized by absence of pelvic curvature. This modification allows *direct* application to the fetal head and avoids conflict with the fetal body that would occur with the application of standard instruments from below. The forceps are inserted into the vagina from beneath the fetus. The blade to be placed on the maternal right is held by the handle in the operator's right hand and the blade inserted with the operator's left hand in the vagina along the right maternal sidewall and placed against the left fetal parietal bone. The handle of the left blade is then held in the operator's left hand and inserted by right hand along the left maternal sidewall and placed against the right fetal parietal bone. Forceps application controls the fetal head and prevents extension of the head on the neck. Gentle downward traction on the forceps with the fetal trunk supported on the forceps shanks results in controlled delivery of the vertex (Fig. 16–24). Routine use of Piper forceps to the aftercoming head may

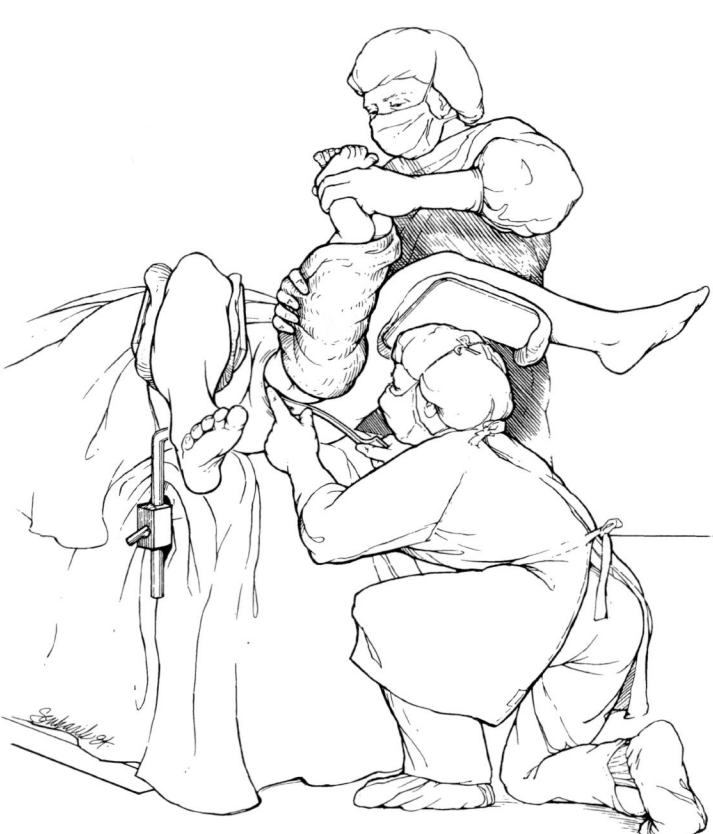

Figure 16–23. Demonstration of INCORRECT assistance during the application of Piper forceps; the assistant hyperextends the fetal neck. Positioning as such increases the risk for neurologic injury.

be advisable both to ensure control of the delivery and to maintain optimal operator proficiency in anticipation of deliveries that may require their use.

Arrest of spontaneous progress in labor with adequate uterine contractions necessitates consideration of cesarean delivery. Any evidence of fetal compromise or sustained cord compression on the basis of continuous

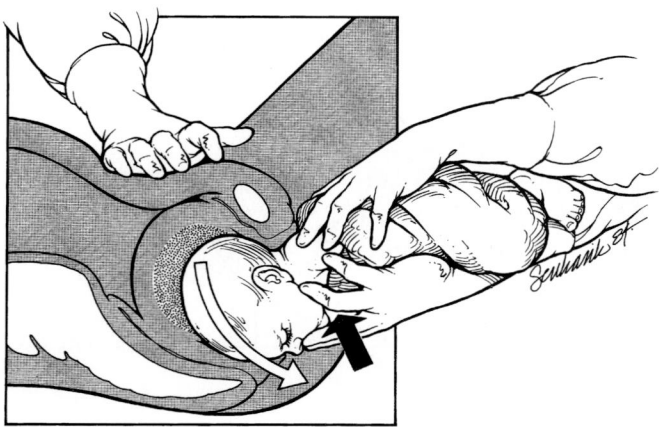

Figure 16–22. Cephalic flexion is maintained by pressure (*heavy arrow*) on the fetal maxilla (not mandible!). Often, delivery of the head is easily accomplished with continued expulsive forces from above and gentle downward traction.

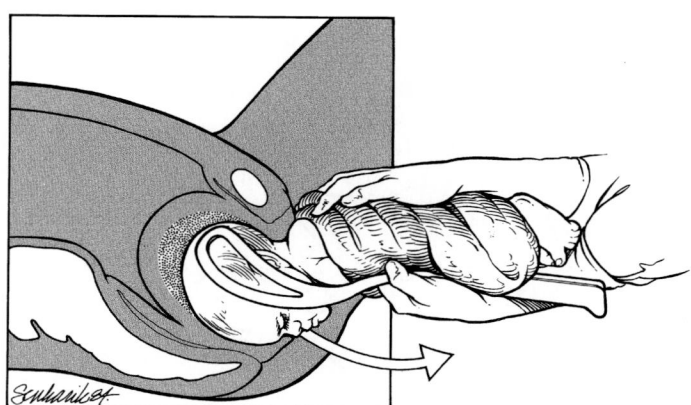

Figure 16–24. The fetus may be laid on the forceps and delivered with gentle downward traction as illustrated here.

electronic fetal monitoring also requires consideration of cesarean delivery. Vaginal interventions directed at facilitating delivery of the breech that is complicated by an arrest of spontaneous progress are discouraged, because fetal and maternal morbidity and mortality are both greatly increased. However, if labor is deemed to be hypotonic by internally monitored uterine pressures, oxytocin is not contraindicated.[50-52]

Mechanisms of descent and delivery of the footling and the complete breech are not unlike those of the frank breech described above, except one or both legs might already be extended and thus not require attention. The risk of cord prolapse or entanglement is greater and, hence, the possibility of emergency cesarean delivery increased. Furthermore, footling and complete breeches are not as effective a cervical dilator as either the vertex or the larger aggregate profile of the thighs and buttocks of the frank breech. Thus, the risk of entrapment of the aftercoming head is perhaps increased, and as a result primary cesarean delivery is often advocated for nonfrank breech presentations. However, the randomized trial of Gimovsky et al. found the vaginal delivery of the nonfrank breech to be reasonably safe as well.[53]

Management of the Term Breech

The reported perinatal mortality associated with breech presentation has varied from 9 to 25 percent,[54,55] three to five times that of the nonbreech infant at term.[56-58] The excess deaths associated with breech presentation are largely due to lethal anomalies and complications of prematurity, both of which are found more frequently among breech infants. Excluding anomalies and extreme prematurity, the corrected perinatal mortality reported by some investigators approaches zero regardless of the method of delivery, whereas others find that even with exclusion of these factors the term breech infant has been found to be at higher risk for birth trauma and asphyxia.[59-61] In order to assess the safety of breech delivery, an appropriately controlled randomized trial with sufficient number of study patients must be conducted. To date, only two randomized trials have been reported.[50,53] The remainder of reports surrounding the issue of safety of breech delivery is confined to cohort and observational types of studies, usually retrospective, and subject to significant risk of bias. Therefore, conclusions regarding safety of breech from a fetal standpoint will vary, but those reported are summarized in Table 16–2. Overall, consideration of a potential breech vaginal delivery often involves bias, and yet must be mutually agreed upon by the patient and the physician. A cooperative, compliant patient makes the most appropriate candidate for breech vaginal delivery.

At least a portion of the striking increase in the rate of cesarean deliveries over the past two decades is a

Table 16–2. INCIDENCE OF COMPLICATIONS SEEN WITH BREECH PRESENTATION

Complication	Incidence
Intrapartum fetal death	Increased 16–fold[65,67]
Intrapartum asphyxia	Increased 3.8–fold[65,67]
Cord prolapse	Increased 5– to 20–fold[48,55,68]
Birth trauma	Increased 13–fold[48]
Arrest of aftercoming head	8.8%[48]
Spinal cord injuries with extended head	21%[30,98]
Major anomalies	6–18%[55,65,67]
Prematurity	16–33%[31,54,60,63,69,82,83]
Hyperextension of head	5%[97]

response to the risk of morbidity and mortality associated with the breech presentation.[62-65] In 1980, Collea[48] observed that 29 percent of primary cesarean operations performed at his institution during a 12-month period were performed at least in part because of breech presentation. The National Institutes of Health Consensus Report in 1981 found that 12 percent of cesarean deliveries in 1978 were performed for breech presentation and that this indication contributed 10 to 15 percent to the overall rise in the rate of cesarean births. The overall rate of cesarean birth for breech in some institutions is as high as 94 percent, while in the United States generally the cesarean delivery rate for breech presentation increased from 11.6 percent to 79.1 percent between 1970 and 1985.[65,66] However, even though greater risks appear to face the breech infant,[67] the method of delivery alone has not been conclusively shown to contribute to those risks.[68,69] There remain many who believe that complete abandonment of vaginal delivery for the breech is not yet justified.[70,71]

In some series, improved perinatal survival has been reported for breeches born by cesarean delivery,[55,60,67,72,73] and there is some evidence, though inconsistent, that the method of delivery may also impact on the quality of survival. In 1979, Westgren et al.[74] found functional neurologic defects by 2 years of age in 24 percent of breech infants born vaginally, but only in 2.5 percent of those breech infants of similar weights and gestational ages born by cesarean delivery. However, in comparing 175 breech infants having a 94 percent cesarean delivery rate with 595 historical controls having a 22 percent rate of abdominal delivery, Green et al.[65] found no significant differences in outcome. Faber-Nijholt et al.[75] reviewed neurologic outcomes in 348 infants born in breech position. Examinations were performed on 239 children from 3 to 10 years of age. No statistically significant differences were noted between neonates delivered by vaginal breech versus matched vertex controls, thus concluding breech outcomes relate to degree of prematurity, impact of pregnancy complications, and presence of malformations as well as birth trauma or asphyxia. The benefit of elective cesarean delivery in the case of breech presentation therefore remains uncertain.

In the term breech, observational studies report increased neonatal morbidities including neonatal intensive care unit (NICU) admission, hyperbilirubinemia, bone fracture, intracranial hemorrhage, neonatal depression,[77] convulsions, and death.[78] However, Roman et al. found that emergent cesarean section was also associated with poor neonatal outcomes. On the other hand, in a review of outcomes of 705 singleton, nonmalformed breech presentations, Irion et al. reported similar neonatal outcomes, and concluded that as a result of the increased maternal morbidity associated with cesarean birth there was no firm evidence to recommend elective cesarean delivery for the term breech neonate.[79] This opinion was supported by Brown et al. in their prospective case series, noting corrected perinatal mortality rate did not differ for neonates weighing greater than or equal to 1,500 g.[52]

Special Clinical Circumstances and Risks—Preterm Breech, Hyperextended Head, Footling Breech

The various categories of breech presentation clearly demonstrate dissimilar risks, and management plans might vary among these situations.[80,81] The premature breech, the breech with a hyperextended head, and the footling breech are categories that have high rates of fetal morbidity or mortality. Complications associated with incomplete dilatation and cephalic entrapment may be more frequent. For these three breech situations, in general, cesarean delivery appears to optimize fetal outcome and is therefore recommended.

Low birth weight (<2,500 g) is a confounding factor in about one third of all breech presentations.[54,60,63,69,82,83] Whereas the benefit of cesarean delivery for the 1,500 to 2,500 g breech infant remains controversial,[11,35,52,55,82,84–89] some studies showed improved survival with abdominal delivery in the 1,000 to 1,500-g weight group.[60,86] A recent multicenter study of long-term outcomes of vaginally delivered 26 to 31-week pregnancies found no differences in rates of death or developmental disability within 2 years of follow-up.[90] Traumatic morbidity is reportedly decreased in both weight groups by the use of cesarean delivery, including a lower rate of both intra- and periventricular hemorrhage.[89] Although some advocate a trial of labor in the frank breech infant weighing over 1,500 g, others recommend labor only when the infant exceeds 2,000 g.[35,63,69,91] There are proportionately fewer frank breech presentations in the low-birth-weight group.[31,60] In fact, most infants weighing less than 1,500 g and

presenting as a breech are footling.[91] Although most deaths in the very-low-birth-weight breech group are due to prematurity or lethal anomalies,[82,85,91,92] cesarean delivery has been shown by some to decrease corrected perinatal mortality in this weight group compared with that in similar-sized vertex presentations.[60,93] Other authors suggest that improved survival in these studies relates to improved neonatal care of the premature infant when compared with the outcomes of historical controls.[94] When vaginal delivery of the preterm breech is chosen or is unavoidable, however, conduction anesthesia and the use of forceps for the delivery of the aftercoming head appear to decrease fetal morbidity and mortality.[82,95,96]

Premature rupture of the fetal membranes (PROM) is associated with prematurity and chorioamnionitis, both of which have been found to be independent risk factors for the development of cerebral palsy (CP). PROM is associated with a high rate of malpresentations because of the prematurity and decreased amniotic fluid. Knowing the association of chorioamnionitis with periventricular leukomalacia (PVL), a lesion found to precede development of CP in the premature neonate, Baud et al. correlated the mode of delivery with PVL, and subsequent CP in breech preterm deliveries. The authors found that in the presence of chorioamnionitis, delivery by elective cesarean section was associated with a dramatic decrease in the incidence of PVL.[76]

Hyperextension of the fetal head has been consistently associated with a high (21 percent) risk of spinal cord injury if the breech is delivered vaginally.[30,97,98] In such cases, it is important to differentiate simple deflexion of the head from clear hyperextension, given that Ballas et al.[99] have shown that simple deflexion carries no excess risk. The issue of simple deflexion of the fetal vertex as opposed to hyperextension is similar to the relationships between the occipitofrontal cranial plane and the axis of the fetal cervical spine illustrated in Figure 16–5. Often, as labor progresses, spontaneous flexion will occur in response to fundal forces.

Finally, the footling breech carries a prohibitively high (16 to 19 percent) risk of cord prolapse during labor. In many cases, cord prolapse is manifest only late in labor, after commitment to vaginal delivery has been made.[60,85] Cord prolapse necessitates prompt cesarean delivery. Furthermore, the footling breech is a poor cervical dilator, and cephalic entrapment becomes more likely.

Near-Term Frank or Complete Breech

Controversy continues surrounding the method of delivery for the frank or complete breech, as the cesarean delivery rate for breech presentation generally increases to over 90 percent without a continued or proportionate drop in perinatal mortality.[62–64] Maternal mortality is clearly higher with cesarean delivery, ranging from 0.2 to 0.43 percent.[68,80] Maternal morbidity is also higher with abdominal delivery. Some institutions report a 50 percent incidence of postoperative maternal morbidity[68,77] compared with as little as 5 percent with vaginal delivery.[68] In an attempt to balance both maternal and fetal risks, plans have been proposed to select appropriate candidates for a trial of labor.

Cheng and Hannah[100] examined some of the English language literature regarding breech term deliveries between 1966 and 1992. They reviewed 82 reports, rejecting 58 because of study design inconsistencies or flaws. The remaining 24 presented outcomes according to intended mode of delivery (vaginal or abdominal). Among the studies reviewed, perinatal mortality was higher for the planned vaginal delivery groups, with an odds ratio (OR) of 3.86 (95 percent confidence interval [CI] = 2.22 to 6.69). Neonatal short-term morbidity caused by trauma was higher in the planned vaginal delivery group, with an odds ratio of 3.96 (95 percent CI = 2.76 to 5.67). Likewise, long-term infant morbidity was more frequent in the planned vaginal delivery group (OR = 2.88, with a 95 percent CI = 1.04 to 7.97), but this finding barely achieved significance and resulted from only four foreign studies. Unfortunately, most of the 24 reports constituting this review were retrospective, and many presented data gathered without the use of continuous fetal monitoring. One of the most influential reports with a relatively high rate of adverse outcome with vaginal delivery was from West Africa, where continuous fetal monitoring was not used. The significance of statistical summaries that encompass data from such widely disparate practice patterns is unclear. The authors acknowledged that differences in outcomes might be caused by factors other than the planned method of delivery because of selection bias in most of the studies.[100]

In 1965, Zatuchni and Andros[83] retrospectively analyzed 182 breech births. Of those reviewed, 25 infants had poor outcomes. These investigators concluded that scoring six clinical variables at the time of admission (Table 16–3) identified those patients destined to manifest serious problems in labor and allowed prompt and appropriate intervention. The parturient herself could increase the score by presenting later in labor; other factors that affect the score are less modifiable. At least three subsequent prospective studies applied the Zatuchni-Andros system and found it to be both sensitive and accurate in selecting candidates for successful vaginal delivery.[101–103] A Zatuchni-Andros score of less than 4 in these studies accurately predicted poor outcomes in patients with infants presenting as a breech. Furthermore, in applying the scoring system, only 21 to 27 percent of patients failed to qualify for a trial of labor.[101,102] Previous breech delivery, one of the items scored in the Zatuchni-Andros system, has a significant odds ratio for recurrence of breech (4.32, 95 percent CI = 4.08 to 4.59) after one breech delivery, and up to 28.1 (95 percent CI = 12.2 to 64.8) after three. This study did not, however, control for recurrent causes of breech presentation such as uterine malformations and abnormal placentation.[104]

Because most reports of breech delivery are of level II to III evidence, their validity and, most importantly, universal applicability are called into question. Many data were gathered prior to electronic fetal heart rate monitoring becoming commonplace. Only one randomized trial (level I evidence) has examined term frank breech and method of delivery.[68] Singleton term frank breech infants with an estimated fetal weight between 2.5 and 3.8 kg of mothers with radiographically adequate pelvimetry were prospectively randomized into two groups. One hundred fifteen patients were randomized to a vaginal delivery compared with 93 randomized to elective cesarean delivery. One hundred twelve of the 115 women had time for x-ray pelvimetry; three delivered vaginally before pelvimetry was possible. Fifty-two of 112 women in the planned vaginal delivery group were not allowed to labor because of inadequate pelvimetry, leaving 60 for a planned vaginal delivery. Intrapartum monitoring was used in all patients. Eighty-three percent of patients allowed to labor delivered vaginally without a perinatal loss.[50] There were no maternal deaths, but 36 percent of patients experienced some postpartum morbidity.[68] The authors found no significant difference in perinatal outcome and concluded that a trial of labor is a safe option with the frank breech of average size, flexed head, adequate pelvis, reassuring heart rate monitoring, and normal progress in labor. The small numbers of patients studied, however, make their acceptance of the null hypothesis inconclusive.

In a similar study, O'Leary[105] allowed frank breeches estimated to be between 2.5 and 3.5 kg in women with a large pelvis to labor vaginally. He used radiographic pelvimetry, ultrasound, and the Zatuchni-Andros score and was attentive to the labor curve in selecting candidates for cesarean delivery. Results were similar to

Table 16–3. ZATUCHNI-ANDROS SYSTEM

Factor	0	1	2
Parity	Nullipara	Multipara	Multipara
Gestational age	39	38	37
Estimated fetal weight	8 lb	7–8 lb	7 lb
Previous breech	No	One	Two
Dilatation	2	3	4 or more
Station	−3 or >	−2	−1 or less

From Zatuchni GI, Andros GJ: Prognostic index for vaginal delivery in breech presentation at term. Am J Obstet Gynecol 93:237, 1965, with permission.

those of Collea et al.[50] Neither group of investigators found that oxytocin induction of labor was contraindicated if all other criteria were satisfied[50,105]; however, both groups concluded that augmentation of secondary arrest was not appropriate. Neither nulliparity nor multiparity was found to be an accurate prognostic indicator.[31,106] In a similar study, Gimovsky et al.[53] randomized 105 nonfrank term breech infants to cesarean section or trial of labor and found that 44 percent of those undergoing trial of labor achieved safe vaginal delivery with no differences in neonatal outcomes. Most cesarean deliveries were performed for arrested progress.

Flanagan et al.[51] reported a nonrandomized, retrospective study in which 244 women with breech infants at term (the majority were frank, with some complete, and footling breeches) underwent a trial of labor. Of these, 72 percent delivered vaginally. Of those cesarean deliveries ultimately required, 44 were for abnormal labor (64 percent of those delivered by cesarean), 14 for fetal distress (20 percent), and 11 for cord prolapse (16 percent). The authors noted no increased trauma related to vaginal delivery. However, one child had a facial nerve paralysis with facial asymmetry. The authors surmised this injury may be a result of in utero compressive damage, not from trauma at the time of the vaginal delivery. The authors estimated that with the application of external version to a known breech population and a trial of labor for selected frank breech infants, the cesarean section rate for these pregnancies could be cut in half.[51]

In conclusion, there appears to be a place for a trial of labor and attempted vaginal delivery of the uncomplicated term or near term frank breech of average size through a normal pelvis if there is normal progress in labor and fetal heart rate monitoring remains reassuring. The apparent safety of a trial of labor in selected cases, however, is not without dispute.[100,107]

Radiographic pelvimetry has been included in the management of the breech presentation with little objective validation. Regardless, it is expected to predict successful vaginal delivery when adequate pelvic dimensions are present. There are at least four techniques for pelvimetry that are presently in common usage worldwide, including conventional plain film radiography using up to three films, computed tomography (CT) with up to three views (lateral, AP, and axial slice), magnetic resonance imaging (MRI), and digital fluorography, not presently used in the United States. MRI is the only technique not associated with radiation exposure, and CT pelvimetry using a single lateral view results in the lowest exposure dose.[108] Air gap technique with conventional radiography will lower the radiation dosage. Current trends show a move towards the lower dose CT techniques of up to three images.[109]

The clinician must possess the necessary training and

experience to offer a patient with a persistent breech presentation a trial of labor. Furthermore, the relationship between the patient and the clinician should be well established and the discussions of risks and benefits must be objective and nondirective with accurate documentation of the discussion. If any of these factors are lacking, cesarean delivery becomes the safer choice. However, even if a clinician has made the choice that he or she will never prospectively offer a patient with breech presentation a trial of labor, the burden of responsibility to know and understand the mechanism and management of a breech delivery is not relieved. No one active in obstetrics will avoid the occasional emergency breech delivery. Regular review of principles, and practice with simulations using a mannekin and model pelvis with an experienced colleague, can increase the skills and improve the performance of anyone facing such an emergency.

Factors that impact on the decision to deliver a breech vaginally or by cesarean section are listed in the box, Management of the Breech. The obvious implication of the dramatically decreased experience in training programs with vaginal breech delivery is that inexperience itself will constitute an indication for cesarean delivery. Certainly, in no case should a woman with an infant presenting as a breech be allowed to labor unless (1) anesthesia coverage is immediately available, (2) cesarean delivery can be undertaken promptly, (3) contin-

---

Management of the Breech

Trial of labor may be considered if
Estimated fetal weight (EFW) = 2,000 to 3,800 g
Frank breech
Adequate pelvis
Flexed fetal head
Fetal monitoring
Zatuchni-Andros score ≥4
Rapid cesarean possible
Good progress maintained in labor
Experience and training available
Informed consent possible
Cesarean delivery may be prudent if
EFW <1,500 or >4,000 g
Footling presentation
Small pelvis
Hyperextended fetal head
Zatuchni-Andros score <4
Absence of expertise
Nonreassuring fetal heart rate pattern
Arrest of progress

uous fetal heart rate monitoring is used, and (4) the delivery is attended by a pediatrician and two obstetricians of whom at least one is experienced with vaginal breech birth.

Breech Second Twin

Approximately one third of all twin gestations present as vertex/breech (i.e., first twin is a vertex, and the second is a breech).[110] The management alternatives in the case of the vertex/breech twin pregnancy in labor include cesarean delivery, vaginal delivery of the first twin and attempted external cephalic version of the second twin, or internal podalic version and extraction of the second twin. Gocke et al.[111] examined the outcomes of management of 136 pairs of vertex/nonvertex twins weighing over 1,500 g and concluded that breech extraction of the second twin appeared to be a safe alternative to cesarean delivery.[111] Blickstein et al.[110] compared the obstetric outcomes of 39 cases of vertex/breech twins to the outcomes of 48 vertex/vertex twins. Although the breech second twin had a higher incidence of low birth weight and a longer hospital stay, the authors found no basis for elective cesarean delivery in this clinical circumstance. Laros and Dattel[112] studied 206 twin pairs and likewise found no clear advantage to arbitrary cesarean delivery because of a specific presentation. Fishman et al.[113] examined outcomes in 390 vaginally delivered second twins, 207 delivered as a vertex and 183 delivered breech. Ninety-five percent of the breech deliveries were total breech extractions. No significant differences were found between the vertex and breech infants even when stratified by birth weight. Any clinician uncomfortable with the prospective delivery of a singleton breech, however, would be unwise to consider a breech extraction of a second twin.

Vaginal delivery followed by external version is a viable alternative, using ultrasound in the delivery room to directly visualize the fetus. Often there is a transient decrease in uterine activity after the delivery of the first infant, which can be used to advantage in the performance of a cephalic version. Tchabo and Tomai[114] described an experience with 30 malpositioned second twins (12 transverse and 18 breech). Version after birth of the first twin was successful in 11 of the 12 transverse infants and in 16 of the 18 breech infants. These cases were all over 35 weeks' gestation, with intact membranes of the second twin after delivery of the first, no evidence of anomalies, and normal amniotic fluid volume.

Internal podalic version/extraction of the second twin can be facilitated by ultrasonic guidance. The goal is to insert a hand into the uterus, identify and grasp both fetal feet with membranes intact, and apply traction to bring the feet into the pelvis and out the introitus with maternal expulsive efforts remaining the major force in effecting descent of the fetus. Membranes are left intact until both feet are at the introitus.[115] Once membranes are ruptured, the delivery is subsequently managed as a footling breech delivery. If the operator has difficulty identifying the fetal feet, intrapartum ultrasound may be of assistance.

During breech extraction, and perhaps more often with a breech extraction of a smaller twin, the fetal head can become caught in the cervix. In such a case, with the operator's entire hand into the uterus the fetal head is cradled; as the hand is withdrawn, the head is protected.[116] This splinting technique has also been used for the safe extraction of the breech head at the time of cesarean delivery.

No randomized prospective trials involving preterm twins with vertex/nonvertex presentation have been performed. A small, prospective trial in the near-term gestation (>35 weeks) by Rabinovici et al.[115] found no difference in neonatal morbidity between vaginal delivery and cesarean birth. They did find increased maternal morbidity with cesarean delivery.

External Cephalic Version

External cephalic version is a third alternative to vaginal delivery or cesarean delivery for the breech infant.[15,54,56,117–120] Many have found that external cephalic version significantly reduces the incidence of breech presentation in labor and is associated with few complications such as cord compression or placental abruption.[15,120] Reported success with external version varies from 60 to 75 percent, with a similar percentage of these remaining vertex at the time of labor.[15,121–124] Ylikorkala and Hartikainen-Sorri[120] found that while many infants in breech presentation before 34 weeks will convert spontaneously to a cephalic presentation, few will do so afterward. Repetitive external version applied weekly after 34 weeks was successful in converting over two thirds of cases and reducing their breech presentation rate by 50 percent.[120] In a randomized trial of external cephalic version in low-risk pregnancies between 37 and 39 weeks, Van Dorsten and colleagues[117] were successful in 68 percent of 25 cases in the version group, whereas only 4 of the 23 controls converted to a vertex spontaneously before labor. All those in whom external version was successful presented in labor as a vertex.[117] Van Veelan et al.[126] reported a prospective, controlled study of external cephalic version performed weekly between 33 weeks and term, and 48 percent of the study group were vertex in labor compared with only 26 percent of controls. Hanss[127] reported experience with 112 patients seen for external version, with a success rate of 49 percent, and a cesarean delivery rate of 17 percent among those with successful version compared with 78 percent among those patients with an unsuccessful version attempt.

Zhang et al.[15] reviewed English language reports between 1980 and 1991 that reported the outcomes of pregnancies after external cephalic version and concluded that it was a safe and effective intervention. The overall success rate among investigators in the United States was 65 percent, with an average cesarean delivery rate of 37 percent among those undergoing an attempted version compared with 83 percent among controls. Successful version was reported more often in parous than nulliparous women and more often between 37 and 39 weeks than after 40 weeks.[15]

Gentle constant pressure applied in a relaxed patient with frequent fetal heart rate assessments are elements of the method stressed by all investigators.[54,56,117] Methodology varies, although the "forward roll" is more widely supported than the "back flip" (Fig. 16–25).[117] The mechanical goal is to squeeze the fetal vertex gently out of the fundal area to the transverse and finally into the lower segment of the uterus.

Tocolysis, epidural anesthesia, and ultrasound during the procedure may also be helpful. A number of tocolytics have been reported; however, the most experience has been reported using intravenous ritodrine. Because of maternal side effects, however, this agent has fallen out of favor in this country. Other agents used are hexaprenaline, salbutamol, nitroglycerin,[128] and terbutaline. A randomized trial of 103 nulliparous patients found success rates with subcutaneous terbutaline were 52 percent compared to 27 percent in the control group. No adverse maternal effects resulting from the drug were found.[129] Robertson et al.,[122] in a randomized trial including 58 patients at 37 to 41 weeks' gestation with breech presentation, found no benefit from β-mimetic tocolysis. The success rate was 66.7 percent with tocolysis and 67.8 percent without tocolysis.[122] Factors associated with failure of version included obesity, deep pelvic engagement of the breech, oligohydramnios, and posterior positioning of the fetal back.[123] The use of epidural anesthesia for external cephalic version has also been controversial. Many believe that operators might apply excessive pressure to the maternal abdomen when epidural anesthesia is employed, which will make fetal compromise more likely, caused by either fetal heart rate decelerations or placental abruption. However, a randomized trial of 69 women using epidural anesthesia demonstrated a better than twofold increase in success of the procedure when epidural was employed.[130] Fetomaternal transfusion has been reported to occur in up to 6 percent of patients undergoing external version,[131] and thus Rh-negative unsensitized women should receive Rh-immune globulin. Quantitation of fetomaternal hemorrhage with the Kleihauer-Betke test will determine the number of ampules of Rh immune globulin to be administered.

In the case of the gravida with a previous cesarean delivery, external cephalic version has also been controversial. Studies of limited sample size have concluded that external cephalic version is safe for mother and fetus and results in increased vaginal delivery rates. Flamm et al. quoted a success rate of 82 percent in patients with a previous cesarean delivery.[132] In 1994, Schachter et al. used intravenous ritodrine tocolysis in a study of 11 patients with history of previous low cervical transverse cesarean section. No uterine dehiscences were found either clinically or at the time of cesarean delivery. Of the five patients that needed cesarean delivery, three had fetuses with newborn weights of greater than 4 kg; all patients in the vaginal delivery group had newborns weighing 3.5 kg.[133]

Of interest is the recent randomized trial of moxibustion of accupoint BL 67 (Zhiyin; beside the outer corner of the 5th toenail) to resolve breech presentation. Moxibustion is a traditional Chinese method that uses the application of heat generated by the combustion of

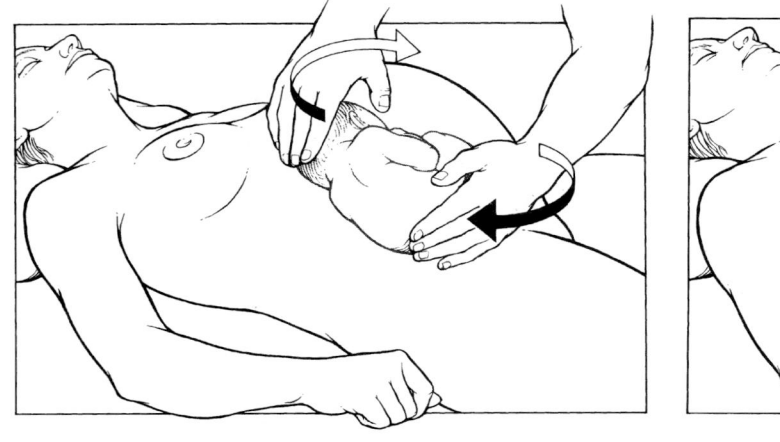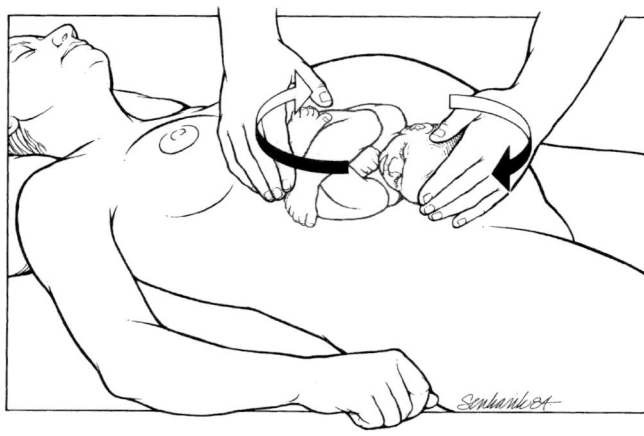

A   B

Figure 16–25. External cephalic version is accomplished by gently "squeezing" the fetus out of one area of the uterus and into another. Here, the "forward roll," often the most popular, is illustrated.

herbs to provide stimulation to the accupoints for a period of 1 to 2 weeks. The particular herb used is *Artemisia vulgaris* (mugwort), which is purported to work by stimulating fetal movements, which were found to be significantly increased in the intervention group. One of 130 patients in the treatment group required cephalic version, whereas 24 of 130 in the controls group required this procedure. Seventy-five percent of the treatment group, and 62 percent of the control group were cephalic at birth.[134] Such an approach is of uncertain value.

SHOULDER DYSTOCIA

Shoulder dystocia is diagnosed when, after delivery of the fetal head, further expulsion of the infant is prevented by impaction of the fetal shoulders within the maternal pelvis. Specific efforts are necessary to facilitate delivery (Fig. 16–26).

Although a difficult shoulder dystocia occurs infrequently, one does not soon forget the experience. Often, but not always, at the end of a difficult labor, the fetal head may be delivered spontaneously or by forceps, but the neck then retracts. The fetal head appears to be drawn back with the chin close to the maternal perineum or thigh, creating difficulty suctioning the infant's mouth. As maternal expulsive efforts are encouraged, the fetal head becomes plethoric, and the danger to the infant is apparent if delivery cannot be promptly accomplished.

Shoulder dystocia has been reported in 0.15 to 1.7 percent of all vaginal deliveries.[135,136] All investigators have documented increased perinatal morbidity and mortality with shoulder dystocia.[135,136] Mortality varies from 21 to 290 in 1,000 when shoulder girdle impaction occurs, and neonatal morbidity has been reported to be immediately obvious in 20 percent of infants.[135] In reviewing 131 macrosomic infants, Boyd et al.[137] found that only half of all cases of brachial palsy occurring in macrosomic infants also carried a diagnosis of shoulder dystocia. Obviously, brachial palsy was noted in half of these cases without a clinical diagnosis of shoulder dystocia. Severe asphyxia was observed in 143 of 1,000 births with shoulder dystocia compared with 14 of 1,000 overall.[137] Fetal morbidity is not always immediately apparent. McCall[138] found 28 percent of infants born with shoulder dystocia to demonstrate some neuropsychiatric dysfunction at 5- to 10-year follow-up. Fewer than one half of these children had immediate morbidity. The neonatal morbidity of greatest concern is brachial plexus injury, resulting from trauma to cervical nerve root V and VI. Fortunately, most cases are transient, with full recovery observed in 90 to 95 percent of infants.[139]

Although shoulder dystocia has traditionally been strongly associated with macrosomia, up to one half of cases of shoulder dystocia occur in neonates under 4,000 g.[140,141] However, Acker et al.[141] found that the relative probability of shoulder dystocia in the 7 percent of infants over 4,000 g was 11 times greater than the average, and in the 2 percent of infants over 4,500 g it was 22 times greater. With macrosomia or continued fetal growth beyond term, the trunk and particularly the chest grow larger relative to the head. Chest circumference exceeds the head circumference in 80 percent of cases.[140] Arms also contribute to the greater dimensions of the upper body. Macrosomia shows the strongest correlation with shoulder dystocia of any clinical factor and occurs more often with gestational diabetes and twice as often in postdate pregnancies. Other clinical factors associated with shoulder dystocia appear to be related to macrosomia as well and include maternal obesity,[137,142] previous birth of an infant weighing over 4,000 g,[137,140,142,143] diabetes mellitus,[142,143] prolonged second stage of labor,[141–143] prolonged deceleration phase (8 to 10 cm),[127] instrumental midpelvic delivery,[144] and previous shoulder dystocia,[143] which has been found to have a recurrence risk of almost 14 percent. Increased maternal age and excess maternal weight gain have been found by some but not all investigators[137,142–144] to increase the risk of macrosomia and shoulder dystocia.[143] Father's birthweight, and adult size during young adulthood have also been found to correlate with fetal weight in addition to the traditional determinants.[146]

Macrosomia has been variously defined as a birth weight over either 4,000 g or 4,500 g.[135,137,147,149] Male predominance is routinely observed, and the condition is associated with the clinical features described above.

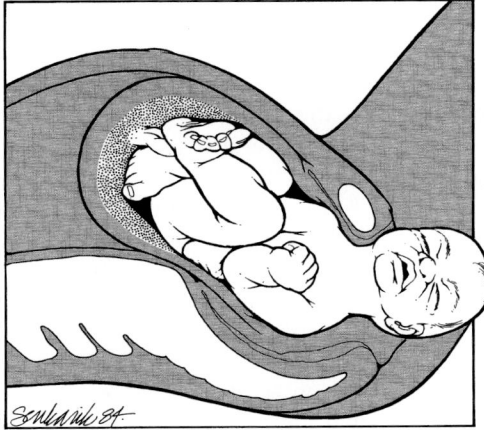

Figure 16–26. When delivery of the fetal head is not followed by delivery of the shoulders, the anterior shoulder has often become caught behind the symphysis as illustrated here. The head may retract toward the perineum. Desperate traction on the fetal head is not likely to facilitate delivery and may lead to trauma.

The two most common complications observed with macrosomia are postpartum hemorrhage and shoulder dystocia.[142] Golditch and Kirkman[148] observed shoulder dystocia in 3 percent of deliveries of infants weighing between 4,100 and 4,500 g and in 8.2 percent of those over 4,500 g. Benedetti and Gabbe[135] reported that fetal injury occurred in 47 percent of infants weighing over 4,000 g who were delivered from the midpelvis and had shoulder dystocia.

Clinical efforts to detect macrosomia prenatally could be helpful in anticipating problems with delivery of the shoulders. Such efforts, however, have been disappointing. Numerous sonographic markers have been assessed to determine their usefulness in predicting macrosomia. These include the estimation of fetal weight using a variety of fetal dimensions and the comparison of chest to head circumference. Most recently, the fetal abdominal diameter biparietal diameter difference (AD−BPD) was evaluated retrospectively both in diabetic and in nondiabetic women.[150] A difference of greater than or equal to 2.6 cm was found to predict shoulder dystocia with sensitivity and specificity of 100 and 46 percent, respectively, with positive and negative predictive values of 30 and 100 percent, respectively. Furthermore, a fetal abdominal circumference of 35 cm or greater has been found to identify more then 90 percent of macrosomic infants.[151] Both of these studies are retrospective and limited by difficulty measuring the fetal abdominal outline at advanced gestational age caused by acoustic shadowing. Parks and Ziel[142] found that of 110 macrosomic infants the diagnosis was made prenatally in only 20 percent. The clinical estimate of birth weight was more than 3 lb in error in 6 percent of cases. Numerous efforts in the literature repeatedly demonstrate the shortcomings of both clinical and ultrasonographic estimations of fetal weight, and have concluded that the best estimation is a combination of the two.

There is a growing trend to consider cesarean delivery of any infant with an estimated weight over 4,500 g or of any infant of a diabetic mother with an estimated weight over 4,000 g[141,144] to avoid birth trauma, particularly brachial plexus injury. Any consideration of elective abdominal delivery on the basis of estimated fetal weight alone, however, must consider the technical error of the method. If 90 percent confidence is desired that the actual fetal weight is at least 4,000 g, the sonographic estimate by most current methods must exceed 4,600 g. This is a result of the expected methodologic error of ±10 percent (±1 SD). Furthermore, the fetal vertex is often too deeply engaged in the pelvis to allow accurate measurement of head circumference. Estimated fetal weight should be only one of several factors considered in the management of the laboring patient. In the obsese diabetic patient with an estimated fetal weight over 4,500 g and showing poor progress in labor, cesarean delivery may be the most prudent course.

However, in most other cases, the risks of cesarean to the mother, the accuracy of prediction of macrosomia, and the alternative of a carefully monitored trial of labor should be discussed. Gross et al.[152] carefully reviewed the clinical characteristics of 394 mothers delivering infants over 4,000 g and concluded that, although birth weight, prolonged deceleration phase, and length of second stage were all individually predictive, no prospective model adequately discriminated the infant destined to sustain trauma from shoulder dystocia from the infant not so destined.[152] Taking this one step further, identifying macrosomic fetuses for the ultimate prevention of neurologic injury has been the subject of reports that report a significant increase in annual cost for routine cesarean deliveries for macrosomia in the nondiabetic population, but improved ratios of cost per brachial plexus injury prevented per year in the diabetic population. Ultrasound detection and elective cesarean delivery of the macrosomic infant of the nondiabetic has been predicted to result in $4.9 million of expenditure to prevent one permanent neurologic injury, whereas one maternal death would result from cesarean delivery for every 3.2 neonatal nerve injuries prevented.[153] Elective cesarean delivery for fetuses of diabetic mothers (both gestational and pregestational) has also been controversial. Langer et al. found that 76 percent of shoulder dystocias could be prevented if a policy of elective cesarean delivery was instituted at an estimated weight of 4,250 g,[154] while Acker found that using a fetal weight threshold of 4,000 g, 55 percent could be prevented in the diabetic poplation.[141] While many clinicians will perform an elective cesarean delivery in a patient with diabetes mellitus and an estimated fetl weight of 4,000 to 4,500 g,[154] Keller expressed concern about the inaccuracy of ultrasound estimation of fetal weight in the gestational diabetic population, with 50 percent of shoulder dystocias occurring in fetuses who weighed less than 4,000 g.[156]

The occurrence of brachial plexus injury in the absence of shoulder dystocia has been described and attributed to in utero forces, such as the posterior shoulder impacting on the sacral promontory (although anterior injuries have been described as well),[157] malpresentations,[158] and dysfunctional labor, mostly precipitate labor.[141,159] Interestingly, in neonates with brachial plexus injury without shoulder dystocia, there was a trend toward lower birth weight, more clavicular fractures, injuries to the brachial plexus of the posterior arm, and longer persistence of the condition than their counterparts in the shoulder dystocia-present group.[157]

The most effective preventive measure is to be familiar with the normal mechanism of labor and to be constantly prepared to deal with shoulder dystocia. Normally, after the delivery of the head, external rotation (restitution) occurs, returning the head to its natural perpendicular relationship to the shoulder girdle.

The fetal sagittal suture is usually oblique to the AP diameter of the outlet, and the shoulders occupy the opposite oblique diameter of the inlet (Fig. 16–27). As the shoulders descend in response to maternal pushing, the anterior shoulder emerges from its oblique axis under one of the pubic rami. If, however, the anterior shoulder descends in the AP diameter of the outlet and the fetus is relatively large for the outlet, impaction behind the symphysis can occur, and further descent is blocked.[136] Shoulder dystocia also occurs with an extremely rapid delivery of the head, as can occur with vacuum extraction or forceps or precipitous labor.

Successful treatment follows anticipation and preparation. Anticipation involves the prenatal suspicion of macrosomia by clinical and/or sonographic means. One must be aware of the clinical features that have been cited and consider a pregnancy at high risk for macrosomia and therefore for shoulder dystocia.

Such deliveries are best managed in a delivery room. Deliveries in bed increase the difficulty of reducing a shoulder dystocia because the bedding precludes fullest use of the posterior pelvis and outlet. Strong consideration for cesarean delivery is recommended when a prolonged second stage occurs in association with macrosomia.

Once a vaginal delivery has begun, the obstetrician must resist the temptation to rotate the head forcibly to a transverse axis. Maternal expulsive efforts should be used rather than traction. Gentle manual pressure on the fetal head inferiorly and posteriorly will push the posterior shoulder into the hollow of the sacrum, increasing the room for the anterior shoulder to pass under the pubis (Fig. 16–28). This pressure is not outward traction and must be symmetric. If the head is pressed asymmetrically, as if to "pry" the anterior shoulder out, brachial plexus injury is more likely.

If delivery is not accomplished, a deliberate, planned

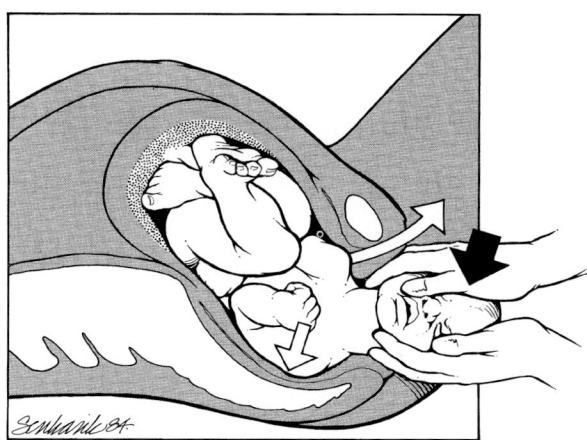

Figure 16–28. Gentle, symmetric pressure on the head will move the posterior shoulder into the hollow of the sacrum and encourage delivery of the anterior shoulder. Care should be taken not to "pry" the anterior shoulder out asymmetrically, as this might lead to trauma to the anterior brachial plexus.

sequence of efforts should then be initiated. One must not pull desperately on the fetal head. Fundal expulsive efforts, including maternal pushing and any fundal pressure, should be temporarily stopped. Aggressive fundal pressure prior to disimpaction or rotation of the shoulders will not facilitate delivery and may work against rotation and disimpaction.

The McRoberts maneuver[160] is a simple, logical, and usually successful measure to promote delivery of the shoulders. The McRoberts maneuver involves hyperflexion of maternal legs on the maternal abdomen that results in flattening of the lumbar spine and ventral rotation of the maternal pelvis and symphysis (Fig. 16–29). This maneuver may increase the useful size of the posterior outlet, resulting in easier disimpaction of the anterior shoulder. Gonik et al.[161] showed that the McRoberts maneuver significantly reduces shoulder extraction forces, brachial plexus stretching, and likelihood of clavicular fracture. In a retrospective review of shoulder dystocia, Gherman et al. found that the McRoberts maneuver was the only step required in 42 percent of 236 cases.[162] When shoulder dystocia occurs because of failure of the bisacromal diameter to engage, the Walcher position, which entails dropping the maternal legs down toward the floor with concurrent suprapubic pressure in a dorsal-caudal direction, has been advocated. Only then, while constant suprapubic pressure is being maintained, should the parturient be placed in the McRoberts position; this may allow for the disimpaction of the fetal shoulder from the symphysis by increasing the AP diameter of the inlet prior to increasing the outlet.[163] Additionally, the "all fours," or Gaskin maneuver, which differs from the knee-chest position, may relieve the dystocia.[164] Use of this maneuver is reasonable only in the setting of a mobile parturi-

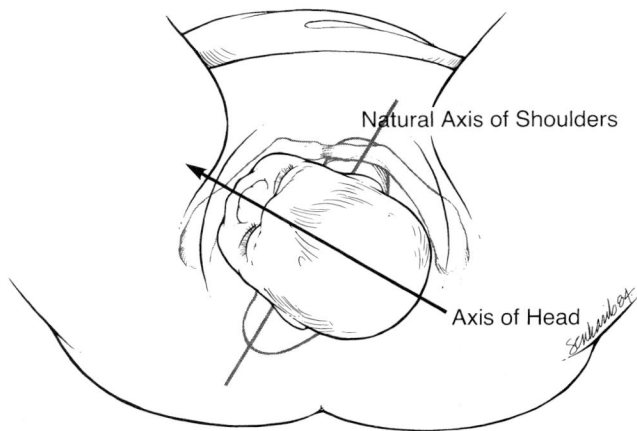

Figure 16–27. After delivery of the head, "restitution" results in the long axis of the head reassuming its normal orientation to the shoulders as seen here.

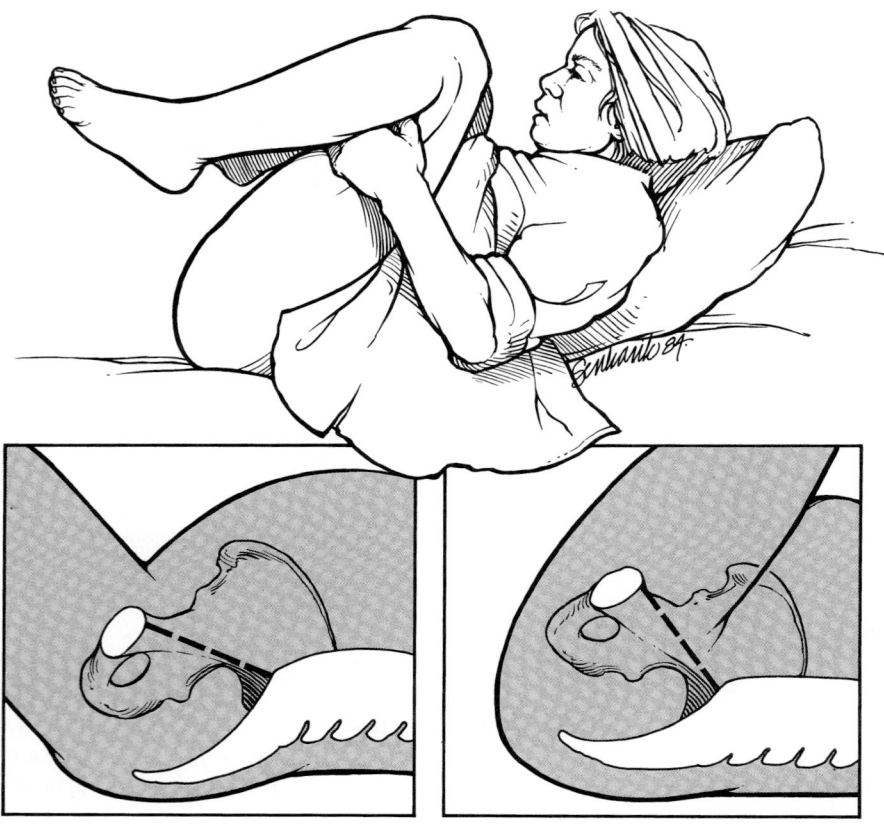

Figure 16–29. The least invasive maneuver to disimpact the shoulders is the McRoberts maneuver. Sharp ventral flexion of the maternal hips results in ventral rotation of the maternal pelvis and an increase in the useful size of the outlet.

ent with no significant motor blockade from regional anesthetic, and a stable and wide surface on which to assume this position in order to avoid the potential for injury during transition to this position.

If the shoulders remain undelivered, often only moderate suprapubic pressure is required to disimpact the anterior shoulder and allow delivery (Fig. 16–30). If this is not effective, the operator's hand may be passed

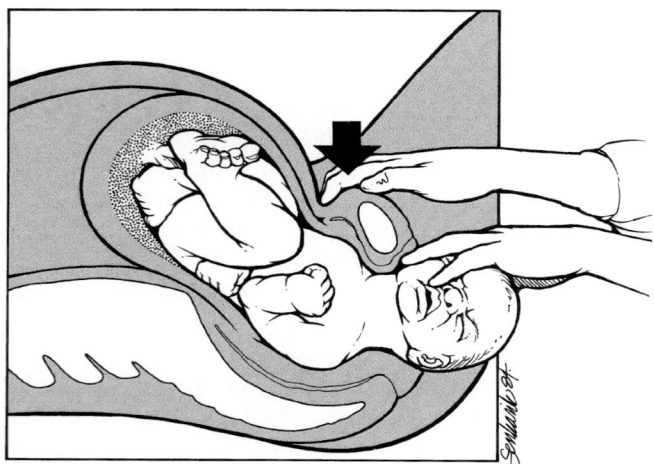

Figure 16–30. Moderate suprapubic pressure will often disimpact the anterior shoulder.

behind the occiput into the vagina, and the anterior shoulder may be pushed forward to the oblique, after which, with maternal efforts and gentle posterior pressure, delivery should occur (Fig. 16–31).[131] Alternatively, the posterior shoulder may be rotated forward, through a 180-degree arc, and passed under the pubic ramus as in turning a screw (Wood's screw maneuver). As the posterior shoulder rotates anteriorly, delivery will often occur.[165]

Many authorities have advocated delivery of the posterior arm and shoulder should the above methods fail. The operator's hand is passed into the vagina, following the posterior arm of the fetus to the elbow. The arm is flexed and swept out over the chest and the perineum (Fig. 16–32). In some cases, delivery will now occur without further manipulation. In others, rotation of the trunk, bringing the freed posterior arm anteriorly, is required.[131,140] These maneuvers are highly likely to fracture the clavicle (up to 25 percent), humerus (up to 15 percent), or both or result in transient or permanent nerve injury (up to approximately 9 percent).[165] Overall, similar rates of bone fracture were noted when any type of manipulation was performed to accomplish delivery of an impacted fetal shoulder.[166] Deliberate fracture of the clavicle is possible and will facilitate delivery by diminishing the rigidity and size of the shoulder girdle. It is best if the pressure is exerted in a direction away from the lung to avoid puncture. Sharp instrumental transection of the clavicle is not recommended, since lung puncture is common with such a method, and infection of the bone through the open wound is a serious possible complication.

Two techniques rarely used in the United States for the management of shoulder dystocia include vaginal replacement of the fetal head with cesarean delivery (Zavanelli maneuver) and subcutaneous symphysiotomy. Sandberg reviewed the Zavanelli maneuver for both the vertex- and breech-presenting undeliverable fetuses. Cephalic replacement was successful in 84 of 92 vertex-presenting fetuses, and in 11 of 11 breech-presenting, podalic replacement was successful. Maternal risks included soft tissue trauma and sepsis, but the fetal risks were described as "minimal," with no fetal injuries attributed to the maneuver; this may be misleading because of the presence of a multitude of etiologies for permanent injury or death, likely from attempts at disimpaction, prolonged delivery time, and hypoxia.[167] O'Leary and Cuva[168] described 35 cases, 31 of which were considered successful and 1 of which needed a hysterotomy incision to allow manual disimpaction of the fetal shoulders and facilitate vaginal delivery when the fetal head could not be replaced into the vagina from below.

Subcutaneous symphysiotomy has been practiced in remote areas of the world for many years as an expedient alternative to cesarean delivery with very good results.[169] In a case series of three symphysiotomies, the procedure was associated with death of all three neonates because of hypoxic complications but as a last resort. The procedure was concluded to be safe and

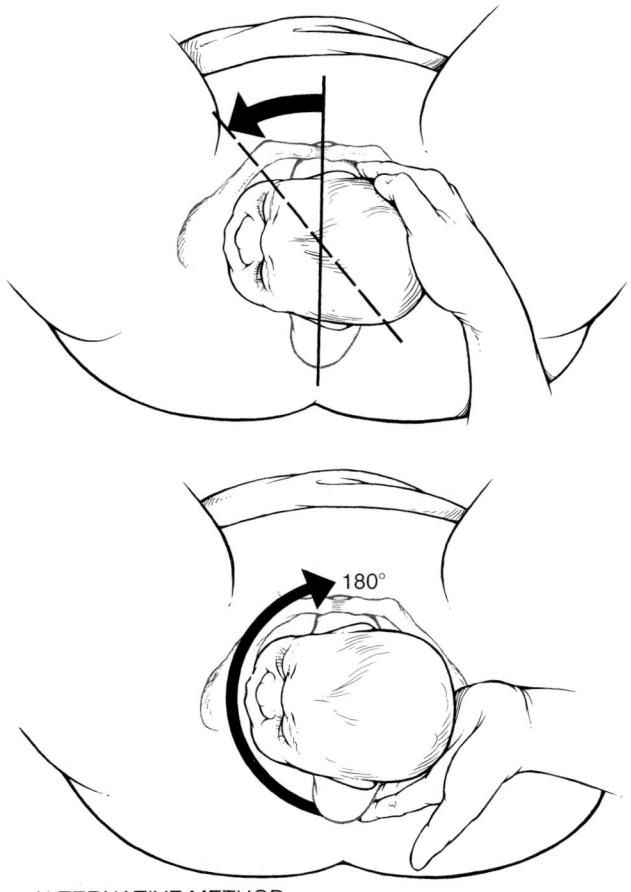

ALTERNATIVE METHOD

Figure 16–31. Rotation of the anterior shoulder forward through a small arc or the posterior shoulder forward through a larger one will often lead to descent and delivery of the shoulders. Forward rotation is preferred, as it tends to compress and diminish the size of the shoulder girdle, while backward rotation would open the shoulder girdle and increase the size.

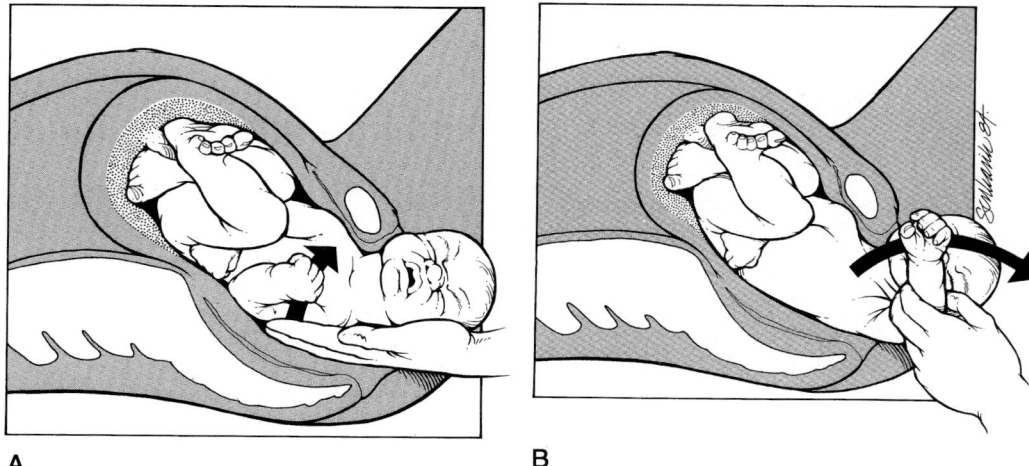

A   B

Figure 16–32. The operator here inserts a hand and sweeps the posterior arm across the chest and over the perineum. Care should be taken to distribute the pressure evenly across the humerus to avoid unnecessary fracture.

effective as long as attention is paid to the three main points in the procedure: lateral support of the legs, partial sharp dissection of the symphysis, and displacement of the urethra to the side with an indwelling urinary catheter.[170] However, neither cephalic replacement nor symphysiotomy has been widely or often used in obstetric practice in the United States. Attempted implementation of either method by the inexperienced practitioner before the trial of more conventional remedies may increase risk to the child, the mother, and the clinician.

In summary, shoulder dystocia is not precisely predictable, but may be anticipated in the case of a variety of predisposing clinical conditions. Shoulder dystocia will, in most cases, respond to any or all of several prudent interventions. The specific method used to disimpact the shoulder is probably not as critical as the practice of a careful, methodical approach to the problem and the avoidance of desperate, potentially traumatic or asymmetric traction. The maneuvers used should be carefully described in the delivery note. There may not be any complication of labor and delivery where forethought is more important to a successful outcome than shoulder dystocia.

Key Points

➤ The "fetal lie" indicates the orientation of the fetal spine relative to that of the mother. Normal fetal lie is longitudinal and by itself does not connote whether the presentation is cephalic or breech.

➤ Cord prolapse occurs 20 times as often with an abnormal axial lie as it does with a cephalic presentation.

➤ Fetal malformations are observed in more than half of infants with a face presentation.

➤ Fetal malpresentation requires timely diagnostic exclusion of major fetal or uterine malformations and/or abnormal placentation.

➤ With few exceptions, a closely monitored labor and vaginal delivery is a safe possibility with most malpresentations. However, cesarean delivery is the only acceptable alternative if normal progress toward spontaneous vaginal delivery is not observed.

➤ External cephalic version of the infant in breech presentation near term is a safe and often successful management option. Use of tocolytics and/or epidural anesthesia may improve success.

➤ Appropriate training and experience is a prerequisite to the safe vaginal delivery of selected infants in breech presentation.

➤ Shoulder dystocia cannot be precisely predicted or prevented but is often associated with macrosomia, maternal obesity, gestational diabetes, and a postdate pregnancy.

➤ The clinician must be prepared to deal with shoulder dystocia at every vaginal delivery with a deliberate, controlled sequence of interventions.

REFERENCES

1. Yates MJ: Transverse foetal lie in labour. J Obstet Gynaecol Br Commonw 71:237, 1964.
2. MacGregor WG: Aetiology and treatment of the oblique, transverse and unstable lie of the foetus with particular reference to antenatal care. J Obstet Gynaecol Br Commonw 71:237, 1964.
3. Cockburn KG, Drake RF: Trasnverse and oblique lie of the foetus. Aust N Z J Obstet Gynaecol 8:211, 1968.
4. Sandhu SK: Transverse lie. J Indian Med Assoc 68:205, 1977.
5. Cruikshank DP, White CA: Obstetric malpresentations— twenty years' experience. Am J Obstet Gynecol 116:1097, 1973.
6. Edwards RI, Nicholson HO: The management of the unstable lie in late pregnancy. J Obstet Gynaecol Br Commonw 76:713, 1969.
7. Flowers CE: Shoulder presentation. Am J Obstet Gynecol 96:145, 1966.
8. Johnson CE: Abnormal fetal presentations. Lancet 84:317, 1964.
9. Johnson CE: Transverse presentation of the fetus. JAMA 187:642, 1964.
10. Thorp JM, Jenkins TJ, Watson W: Utility of Leopold maneuvers in screening for malpresentation. Obstet Gynecol 78:394, 1991.
11. Hourihane MJ: Etiology and management of oblique lie. Obstet Gynecol 32:512, 1968.
12. Phelan JP, Boucher M, Mueller E, et al: The nonlaboring transverse lie. J Reprod Med 31:184, 1986.
13. Cackins LA, Pearce EWJ: Transverse presentation. Obstet Gynecol 9:123, 1957.
14. Pelosi MA, Apuzzio J, Fricchione D, et al: The intraabdominal version technique for delivery of transverse lie by low segment cesarean section. Am J Obstet Gynecol 136:1009, 1979.
15. Zhang J, Bowes WA, Fortney JA: Efficacy of external cephalic version: a review. Obstet Gynecol 82:306, 1993.
16. Benedetti TJ, Lowensohn RI, Trluscott AM: Face presentation at term. Obstet Gynecol 55:199, 1980.
17. Copeland GN, Nicks FI, Christakos AC: Face and brow presentations. N C Med J 29:507, 1968.
18. Duff P: Diagnosis and management of face presentation. Obstet Gynecol 57:105, 1981.
19. Groenig DC: Face presentation. Obstet Gynecol 2:495, 1953.
20. Magid R, Gillespie CF: Face and brow presentation. Obstet Gynecol 9:450, 1957.

21. Prevedourakis CN: Face presentation. Am J Obstet Gynecol 94:1092, 1966.
22. Campbell JM: Face presentation. Aust N Z J Obstet Gynaecol 5:231, 1965.
23. Dede JA, Friedman EA: Face presentation. Am J Obstet Gynecol 87:515, 1963.
24. Browne ADH, Carney D: Management of malpresentations in obstetrics. Br Med J 5393:1295, 1964.
25. Gomez HE, Dennen EH: Face presentation. Obstet Gynecol 8:103, 1956.
26. Salzmann B, Soled M, Gilmour T: Face presentation. Obstet Gynecol 16:106, 1960.
27. Cucco UP: Face presentation. Am J Obstet Gynecol 94:1085, 1966.
28. Borrell U, Fernstrom A: Face I: the mechanism of labor. Radiol Clin North Am 5:73, 1966.
29. Schwartz A, Dgani R, Lancet M, et al: Face presentation. Aust N Z J Obstet Gynaecol 26:172, 1986.
30. Abroms IF, Bresnan MJ, Zuckerman JE, et al: Cervical cord injuries secondary to hyperextension of the head in breech presentations. Obstet Gynecol 41:369, 1973.
31. Adams CM: Review of breech presentation. S D J Med 32:15, 1979.
32. Gold S: The conduct and management of face presentations. J Int Coll Surg 43:253, 1965.
33. Lansford A, Arias D, Smith BE: Respiratory obstruction associated with face presentation. Am J Dis Child 116:318, 1968.
34. Meltzer RM, Sachtleban MR, Friedman EA: Brow presentation. Am J Obstet Gynecol 100:255, 1968.
35. Kovacs SG: Brow presentation. Med J Aust 2:820, 1970.
36. Levy DL: Persistent brow presentation—a new approach to management. South Med J 69:191, 1976.
37. Ingolfsson A: Brow presentations. Acta Obstet Gynecol Scand 48:486, 1969.
38. Bednoff SL, Thomas BE: Brow presentation. N Y J Med 67:803, 1967.
39. Skalley TW, Kramer TF: Brow presentation. Obstet Gynecol 15:616, 1960.
40. Moore EJT, Dennen EH: Management of persistent brow presentation. Obstet Gynecol 6:186, 1955.
41. Jennings PN: Brow presentation with vaginal delivery. Aust N Z J Obstet Gynaecol 8:219, 1968.
42. Breen JL, Wiesmeien E: Compound presentation—a survey of 131 patients. Obstet Gynecol 32:419, 1968.
43. Goplerud J, Eastman NJ: Compound presentation. Obstet Gynecol 1:59, 1953.
44. Weissberg SM, O'Leary JA: Compound presentation of the fetus. Obstet Gynecol 41:60, 1973.
45. Dignam WJ: Difficulties in delivery, including shoulder dystocia and malpresentations of the fetus. Clin Obstet Gynecol 19:577, 1976.
46. Ang LT: Compound presentation following external version. Aust N Z J Obstet Gynaecol 19:213, 1978.
47. Douglas HGK, Savage PE: An unusual case of compound presentation. J Obstet Gynaecol Br Commonw 77:1036, 1970.
48. Collea JV: Current management of breech presentation. Clin Obstet Gynecol 23:525, 1980.
49. Braun FHT, Jones KL, Smith DW: Breech presentation as an indicator of fetal abnormality. J Pediatr 86:419, 1975.
50. Collea JV, Chein C, Quilligan EJ: The randomized management of term frank breech presentation—a study of 208 cases. Am J Obstet Gynecol 137:235, 1980.
51. Flanagan TA, Mulchahey KM, Korenbrot CC, et al: Management of term breech presentation. Am J Obstet Gynecol 156:1492, 1987.
52. Brown L, Karrison T, Cibils L: Mode of delivery and perinatal results in breech presentation. Am J Obstet Gynecol 171:28, 1994.
53. Gimovsky ML, Wallace RL, Schifrin BS, et al: Randomized management of the non-frank breech presentation at term—a preliminary report. Am J Obstet Gynecol 146:34, 1983.
54. Fall O, Nilsson BA: External cephalic version in breech presentation under tocolysis. Obstet Gynecol 53:712, 1979.
55. Kubli F: Risk of vaginal breech delivery. Contrib Gynecol Obstet 3:80, 1977.
56. Hibbard LT, Schumann WR: Prophylactic external cephalic version in an obstetric practice. Am J Obstet Gynecol 116:511, 1973.
57. Kauppila O, Gronroos M, Aro P, et al: Management of low birth weight breech delivery—should cesarean section be routine? Obstet Gynecol 57:289, 1981.
58. Rovinsky JJ, Miller JA, Kaplan S: Management of breech presentation at term. Am J Obstet Gynecol 115:497, 1973.
59. de la Fuente P, Escalante JM, Hernandez-Garcia JM: Perinatal mortality in breech presentations. Contrib Gynecol Obstet 3:108, 1977.
60. Goldenberg RL, Nelson KG: The premature breech. Am J Obstet Gynecol 127:240, 1977.
61. NIH consensus development statement on cesarean childbirth. Obstet Gynecol 57:537, 1981.
62. Mansani FE, Cerutti M: The risk in breech delivery. Contrib Gynecol Obstet 3:86, 1977.
63. Seitchik J: Discussion of "breech delivery—evaluation of the method of delivery on perinatal results and maternal morbidity" by Bowes et al. Am J Obstet Gynecol 135:970, 1979.
64. Wolter DF: Patterns of management with breech presentation. Am J Obstet Gynecol 125:733, 1976.
65. Green JE, McLean F, Smitt LP, et al: Has an increased cesarean section rate for term breech delivery reduced the incidence of birth asphyxia, trauma, and death? Am J Obstet Gynecol 142:643, 1982.
66. Croughan-Minihane MS, Petitt DB, Gordis L, Golditch I: Morbidity among breech infants according to method of delivery. Obstet Gynecol 75:821, 1990.
67. Brenner WE, Bruce RD, Hendricks CH: The characteristics and perils of breech presentation. Am J Obstet Gynecol 118:700, 1974.
68. Collea JV, Rabin SC, Weghorst GR, et al: The randomized management of term frank breech presentation—vaginal delivery versus cesarean section. Am J Obstet Gynecol 131:186, 1978.
69. De Crespigny LJC, Pepperell RJ: Perinatal mortality and morbidity in breech presentation. Obstet Gynecol 53:141, 1979.
70. Graves WK: Breech delivery in twenty years of practice. Am J Obstet Gynecol 137:229, 1980.
71. Niswander KR: Discussion of "the randomized management of term frank breech presentation—vaginal delivery versus cesarean section" by Collea et al. Am J Obstet Gynecol 131:193, 1978.
72. Lyons ER, Papsin FR: Cesarean section in the management of breech presentation. Am J Obstet Gynecol 130:558, 1978.
73. Spanio P, Elia F, DeBonis F, et al: Fetal-neonatal mortality and morbidity in cesarean deliveries. Contrib Gynecol Obstet 3:130, 1977.
74. Westgren M, Ingemarsson I, Svenningsen NW: Long-term follow up of preterm infants in breech presentation delivered by cesarean section. Dan Med Bull 26:141, 1979.
75. Faber-Nijholt R, Huisjes JH, Touwen CL, et al: Neurological follow up of 281 children born in breech presentation—a controlled study. BMJ 286:9, 1983.
76. Baud O, Ville Y, Zupan V, et al: Are neonatal brain lesions due to infection related to mode of delivery? Br J Obstet Gynaecol 105:121, 1998.

77. Diro M, Puangsricharem A, Royer L, et al: Singleton term breech deliveries in nulliparous and multiparous women: a 5 year experience at the University of Miami/Jackson Memorial Hospital. Am J Obstet Gynecol 181:247, 1999.

78. Roman J, Bakos O, Cnattingius S: Pregnancy outcomes by mode of delivery among term breech births: Swedish experience 1987–1993. Obstet Gynecol 92:945, 1998.

79. Irion O, Almagbaly PH, Morabia A: Planned vaginal delivery versus elective cesarean section: a study of 705 singleton term breech presentations. Br J Obstet Gynaecol 105:710, 1998.

80. Bowes WA, Taylor ES, O'Brien M, et al: Breech delivery—evaluation of the method of delivery on perinatal results and maternal morbidity. Am J Obstet Gynecol 135:965, 1979.

81. Lewis BV, Sene Viratne HR: Vaginal breech delivery or cesarean section. Am J Obstet Gynecol 134:615, 1979.

82. Cruikshank DP, Pitkin RM: Delivery of the premature breech. Obstet Gynecol 50:367, 1977.

83. Zatuchni GI, Andros GJ: Prognostic index for vaginal delivery in breech presentation at term. Am J Obstet Gynecol 93:237, 1965.

84. Cruikshank DP: Premature breech [letter to the editor]. Am J Obstet Gynecol 130:500, 1978.

85. Woods JR: Effects of low birth weight breech delivery on neonatal mortality. Obstet Gynecol 53:735, 1979.

86. Ulstein M: Breech delivery. Ann Chir Gynaecol Fenn 69:70, 1980.

87. Weissman A, Blazer S, Zimmer EZ, et al: Low birthweight breech infant: short term and long term outcome by method of delivery. Am J Perinatol 5:289, 1988.

88. Anderson G, Strong C: The premature breech: caesarean section or trial of labour? J Med Ethics 14:18, 1988.

89. Tejani N, Verma U, Shiffman R, et al: Effect of route of delivery on periventricular/intraventricular hemorrhage in the low birthweight fetus with a breech presentation. J Reprod Med 32:911, 1987.

90. Wolf H, Schaap HP, Brunise HW, et al: Vaginal delivery compared with cesarean section in early preterm breech delivery: a comparison of long term outcome. Br J Obstet Gynaecol 106:486, 1999.

91. Karp LE, Doney JR, McCarthy T, et al: The premature breech—trial of labor or cesarean section? Obstet Gynecol 53:88, 1979.

92. Mann LI, Gallant JM: Modern management of the breech delivery. Am J Obstet Gynecol 134:611, 1979.

93. Duenhoelter JH, Wells CE, Reisch JS, et al: A paired controlled study of vaginal and abdominal delivery of the low birth weight breech fetus. Obstet Gynecol 54:310, 1979.

94. Cox C, Kendall AC, Hommers M: Changed prognosis of breech-presenting low birthweight infants. Br J Obstet Gynaecol 89:881, 1982.

95. Milner RDG: Neonatal mortality of breech deliveries with and without forceps to the aftercoming head. Br J Obstet Gynaecol 82:783, 1975.

96. Milner RDG: Neonatal mortality of breech deliveries with and without forceps to the aftercoming head. Contrib Gynecol Obstet 3:113, 1977.

97. Caterini H, Langer A, Sama JC, et al: Fetal risk in hyperextension of the fetal head in breech presentation. Am J Obstet Gynecol 123:632, 1975.

98. Daw E: Hyperextension of the head in breech presentation. Am J Obstet Gynecol 119:564, 1974.

99. Ballas S, Toaff R, Jaffa AJ: Deflexion of the fetal head in breech presentation. Obstet Gynecol 52:653, 1978.

100. Cheng M, Hannah M: Breech delivery at term: a critical review of the literature. Obstet Gynecol 82:605, 1993.

101. Bird CC, McElin TW: A six year prospective study of term breech deliveries utilizing the Zatuchni-Andros prognostic scoring index. Am J Obstet Gynecol 121:551, 1975.

102. Mark C, Roberts PHR: Breech scoring index. Am J Obstet Gynecol 101:572, 1968.

103. Zatuchni GI, Andros GJ: Prognostic index for vaginal delivery in breech presentation at term. Am J Obstet Gynecol 98:854, 1967.

104. Albrechtsten S, Rasmussen S, Dalaker K, Irgens L: Reproductive career after breech presentation: subsequent pregnancy rates, interpregnancy interval and recurrence. Obstet Gynecol 92:345, 1998.

105. O'Leary JA: Vaginal delivery of the term frank breech. Obstet Gynecol 53:341, 1979.

106. Selvaggi L, Chieppa M, Loizzi P, et al: Intrapartum mortality among breech deliveries. Contrib Gynecol Obstet 3:99, 1977.

107. Bingham P, Lilford RJ: Management of the selected term breech presentation: assessment of the risks of selected vaginal delivery versus cesarean section for all cases. Obstet Gynecol 69:965, 1987.

108. Badr I, Thomas SM, Cotterill AD, et al: X-ray pelvimetry—which is the best technique? Clin Radiol 52:136, 1997.

109. Thomas SM, Bees NR, Adam EJ: Trends in the use of pelvimetry techniques. Clin Radiol 53:293, 1998.

110. Blickstein I, Schwartz-Shoham Z, Lancet M: Vaginal delivery of the second twin in breech presentation. Obstet Gynecol 69:774, 1987.

111. Gocke SE, Nageotte MP, Garite T, et al: Management of the nonvertex second twin: primary cesarean section, external version, or primary breech extraction. Am J Obstet Gynecol 161:111, 1989.

112. Laros RK, Dattel BJ: Management of twin pregnancy: the vaginal route is still safe. Am J Obstet Gynecol 158:1330, 1988.

113. Fishman A, Grubb DK, Kovacs BW: Vaginal delivery of the nonvertex second twin. Am J Obstet Gynecol 168:861, 1993.

114. Tchabo JG, Tomai T: Selected intrapartum external cephalic version of the second twin. Obstet Gynecol 79:421, 1992.

115. Rabinovici J, Reichman B, Serr DM, et al: Internal podalic version with unruptured membranes for the second twin in transverse lie. Obstet Gynecol 71:428, 1988.

116. Druzin ML: Atraumatic delivery in cases of malpresentation of the very low birthweight fetus at cesarean section: the splint technique. Am J Obstet Gynecol 154:941, 1986.

117. Van Dorsten JP, Schifrin BS, Wallace RL: Randomized control trial of external cephalic version with tocolysis in late pregnancy. Am J Obstet Gynecol 141:417, 1981.

118. Hanley BJ: Editorial—fallacy of external version. Obstet Gynecol 4:124, 1954.

119. Thornhill PE: Changes in fetal polarity near term spontaneous and external version. Am J Obstet Gynecol 93:306, 1965.

120. Ylikorkala O, Hartikainen-Sorri A: Value of external version in fetal malpresentation in combination with use of ultrasound. Acta Obstet Gynecol Scand 56:63, 1977.

121. Stine LE, Phalen JP, Wallace R, et al: Update on external cephalic version performed at term. Obstet Gynecol 65:642, 1985.

122. Robertson AW, Kopelman JN, Read JA, et al: External cephalic version at term: is a tocolytic necessary? Obstet Gynecol 70:896, 1987.

123. Fortunato SJ, Mercer LJ, Guzick DS: External cephalic version with tocolysis: factors associated with success. Obstet Gynecol 72:59, 1988.

124. Marchick R: Antepartum external cephalic version with tocolysis: a study of term singleton breech presentations. Am J Obstet Gynecol 158:1339, 1988.

125. Scaling ST: External cephalic version without tocolysis. Am J Obstet Gynecol 158:1424, 1988.

126. van Veelen AJ, van Cappellen AW, Flu PK, et al: Effect of external cephalic version in late pregnancy on presentation at delivery: a randomized control trial. Br J Obstet Gynaecol 96: 916, 1989.

127. Hanss JW: The efficacy of external cephalic version and its impact on the breech experience. Am J Obstet Gynecol 162: 1459, 1990.

128. Belfort MA: Intravenous nitroglycerine as a tocolytic for intrapartum exterenal cephalic version. S Afr Med J 83:656, 1993.

129. Fernandez CO, Bloom SL, Smulian JC, et al: A randomized placebo controlled evaluation of terbutaline for external cephalic version. Obstet Gynecol 90:775, 1997.

130. Schorr SJ, Speights SE, Ross EL, et al: A randomized trial of epidural anesthesia to improve external cephalic version success. Am J Obstet Gynecol 177:1133, 1997.

131. Marcus RG, Crewe-Brown H, Krawitz S, et al: Fetomaternal haemorrhage following successful and unsuccessful attempts at external cephalic version. Br J Obstet Gynaecol 82:578, 1975.

132. Flamm BL, Fried MW, Lonky NM, Giles SW: External cephalic version after previous cesarean section. Am J Obstet Gynecol 165:370, 1991.

133. Schachter M, Kogan S, Blickstein I: External cephalic version after previous cesarean section—a clinical dilemma. Int J Gynecol Obstet 45:17, 1994.

134. Cardini F, Weixin H: Moxibustion for the correction of breech presentation: a randomized controlled trial. JAMA 280:1580, 1998.

135. Benedetti TJ, Gabbe SG: Shoulder dystocia—a complication of fetal macrosomia and prolonged second stage of labor with midpelvic delivery. Obstet Gynecol 52:526, 1978.

136. Swartz DP: Shoulder girdle dystocia in vertex delivery—clinical study and review. Obstet Gynecol 15:194, 1960.

137. Boyd ME, Usher RH, McLean FH: Fetal macrosomia—prediction, risks, and proposed management. Obstet Gynecol 61: 715, 1983.

138. McCall JO: Shoulder dystocia—a study of after effects. Am J Obstet Gynecol 83:1486, 1962.

139. Sandmire HF, DeMott RK: The Green Bay cesarean section study IV. The physician factor as a determinant of cesarean birth rates for the large fetus. Am J Obstet Gynecol 174: 1557, 1996.

140. Seigworth GR: Shoulder dystocia—review of 5 years' experience. Obstet Gynecol 28:764, 1966.

141. Acker DB, Sachs BP, Friedman EA: Risk factors for Erb-Duchenne palsy. Obstet Gynecol 66:764, 1985.

142. Parks DG, Ziel HK: Macrosomia—a proposed indication for primary cesarean section. Obstet Gynecol 52:407, 1978.

143. Lewis DF, Edwards MS, Asrat T, et al: Can shoulder dystocia be predicted? J Reprod Med 43:654, 1998.

144. Acker DB, Gregory KD, Sachs BP, et al: Risk factors for Erb-Duchenne palsy. Obstet Gynecol 71:389, 1988.

145. Lewis DF, Raymond RC, Perkins MB, et al: Recurrence rate of shoulder dystocia. Am J Obstet 172:1369, 1995.

146. Klebanoff MA, Mednick BR, Schulsinger C, et al: Father's effect on infant birthweight. Am J Obstet Gynecol 178:1022, 1998.

147. Modanlou HD, Dorchester WL, Thorosian A, et al: Macrosomia-maternal, fetal, and neonatal implications. Obstet Gynecol 55:420, 1980.

148. Golditch IM, Kirkman K: The large fetus—management and outcome. Obstet Gynecol 52:26, 1978.

149. Modanlou HD, Komatsu G, Dorchester W, et al: Large for gestational age neonates: anthropometric reasons for shoulder dystocia. Obstet Gynecol 60:417, 1982.

150. Cohen B, Penning S, Major C, et al: Songraphic prediction of shoulder dystocia in infants of diabetic mothers. Obstet Gynecol 88:10, 1996.

151. Jazayeri A, Heffron JA, Phillips R, Spellacy WN: Macrosomia prediction using ultrasound fetal abdominal circumference of 35 centimeters or more. Obstet Gynecol 93:523, 1999.

152. Gross TL, Sokol RJ, Williams T, et al: Shoulder dystocia: a fetal-physician risk. Am J Obstet Gynecol 156:1408, 1987.

153. Rouse DJ, Owen J, Goldenberg RL, Cliver SP: The effectiveness and costs of elective cesarean delivery for fetal macrosomia diagnosed by ultrasound. JAMA 276:1480, 1996.

154. Langer O, Berkus MD, Huff RW, Samueloff A: Shoulder dystocia: should the fetus weighing >4000g be delivered by cesarean section? Am J Obstet Gynecol 165:831, 1991.

155. ACOG Practice Patterns, Shoulder Dystocia, No. 7, October 1997.

156. Keller JD, Lopez-Zano JA, Dooley SL, Socol ML: Shoulder dystocia and birth trauma in gestational diabetes: a five year experience. Am J Obstet Gynecol 165:928, 1991.

157. Gherman RB, Ouzounian JG, Miller DA, et al: Spontaneous vaginal delivery: a risk for Erb's palsy? Am J Obstet Gynecol 178:423, 1998.

158. Gilbert WM, Nesbitt TS, Danielsen B: Associated factors in 1611 cases of brachial plexus injury. Obstet Gynecol 93:536, 1999.

159. Sandmire HF, DeMott RK: Erb's palsy: concepts and causation. Obstet Gynecol 95:940, 2000.

160. Gonik B, Stringer CA, Held B: An alternate maneuver for management of shoulder dystocia. Am J Obstet Gynecol 145: 882, 1983.

161. Gonik B, Allen R, Sorab J: Objective evaluation of the shoulder dystocia phenomenon: effect of maternal pelvic orientation on force reduction. Obstet Gynecol 74:44, 1989.

162. Gherman RB, Goodwin TM, Souter I, et al: The McRobert's maneuver for the alleviation of shoulder dystocia: how successful is it? Am J Obstet Gynecol 176:656, 1997.

163. Pecorari D: A guest editorial from abroad: meditations on a nightmare of modern midwifery: shoulder dystocia. Obstet Gynecol Surv 54:353, 1999.

164. Brunner JP, Drummond SB, Meenan AL, Gaskin IM: All fours maneuver for reducing shoulder dystocia during labor. J Reprod Med 43:439, 1998.

165. Gross SJ, Shime J, Farine D: Shoulder dystocia: predictors and outcome. Am J Obstet Gynecol 156:334, 1987.

166. Gherman RB, Ouzounian JG, Goodwin TM: Obstetric maneuvers for shoulder dystocia and associated fetal morbidity. Am J Obstet Gynecol 178:1126, 1998.

167. Sandberg EC: The Zavanelli maneuver: 12 years of recorded experience. Obstet Gynecol 93:312, 1999.

168. O'Leary JA, Cuva A: Abdominal rescue after failed cephalic replacement. Obstet Gynecol 80:514, 1992.

169. Hartfield VJ: Symphysiotomy for shoulder dystocia [letter]. Am J Obstet Gynecol 155:228, 1986.

170. Goodwin TM, Banks E, Millar LK, Phelan JP: Catastrophic shoulder dystocia and emergency symphysiotomy. Am J Obstet Gynecol 177:463, 1997.

Chapter 17

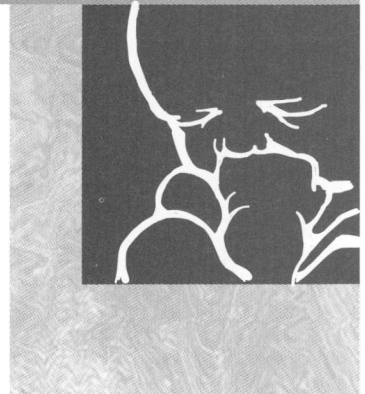

Obstetric Hemorrhage

THOMAS J. BENEDETTI

It is critical that the obstetrician be able to estimate rapidly the blood volume deficit in the pregnant patient. Although some have proposed that the pregnant woman fails to show the usual signs and symptoms of blood loss, there is little scientific evidence to support this hypothesis. This confusion may have arisen from an incomplete understanding of the physiologic responses to volume loss and lack of appreciation of normal volume expansion of pregnancy. The normal pregnant patient frequently loses 500 ml of blood at the time of vaginal delivery and 1,000 ml at the time of cesarean delivery. Appreciably more blood can be lost without clinical evidence of a volume deficit as a result of the 40 percent expansion in blood volume that occurs by the 30th week of pregnancy.

To understand why the pregnant patient does not exhibit early signs of volume loss, it is important to understand the normal physiologic responses to hemorrhage (Fig. 17–1). When 1,000 ml is rapidly removed from the circulatory blood volume, vasoconstriction occurs in both the arterial and venous compartments in order to preserve essential body organ flow. As illustrated in Figure 17–1, when intravascular volume is lost, blood pressure is initially maintained by increases in systemic vascular resistance. As volume loss exceeds 20 percent, the fall in cardiac output accelerates and blood pressure can no longer be maintained by increases in resistance. Blood pressure and cardiac output fall in parallel after this point. In addition, if the volume loss has occurred more than 4 hours earlier, significant fluid shifts from the interstitial space into the intravascular space will partially correct the volume deficit. This movement of fluid, termed *transcapillary refill,* can replace as much as 30 percent of lost volume. In more chronic bleeding states, the final blood volume deficit may amount to as little as 70 percent of the actual blood lost.

CLASSIFICATION OF HEMORRHAGE

A standard classification for volume loss secondary to hemorrhage is illustrated in Table 17–1. Hemorrhage can be classified as one of four groups, depending on the volume lost. The determination of the class of hemorrhage reflects the volume deficit, which may not be the same as the volume loss. The average 60-kg pregnant woman has a blood volume of 6,000 ml at 30 weeks, and an unreplaced volume loss of less than 900 ml falls into class 1. Such patients rarely exhibit signs or symptoms of volume deficit.

A blood loss of 1,200 to 1,500 ml is characterized as a class 2 hemorrhage. These individuals will begin to show expected physical signs, the first being a rise in pulse rate and/or a rise in respiratory rate. Tachypnea is a nonspecific response to volume loss and, although a relatively early sign of mild volume deficit, is frequently overlooked. A doubling of the respiratory rate may be observed in this circumstance. If the patient appears to be breathing rapidly, the minute ventilation is usually twice its normal value. This finding should not be interpreted as an encouraging sign, but rather one of impending problems.

Patients with class 2 hemorrhage will frequently have orthostatic blood pressure changes and may have decreased perfusion of the extremities. However, this amount of blood loss will not usually result in the classic cold, clammy extremities. Rather, a more subtle test is needed to document this phenomenon. One can simply squeeze the hypothenar area of the hand for 1 to 2 seconds and then release the pressure. A patient with normal volume status will have an initial blanching of the skin, followed within 1 to 2 seconds by a return to the normal pink coloration. A patient who

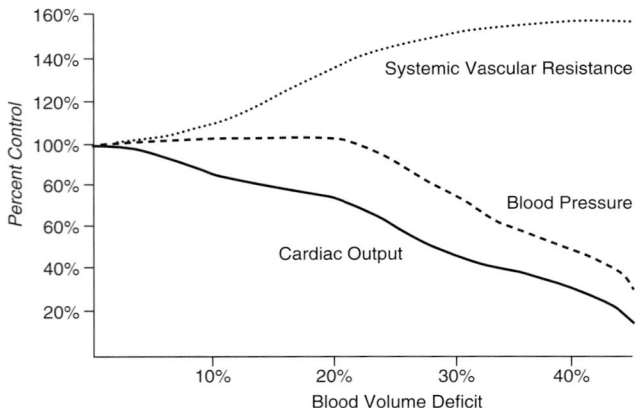

Figure 17–1. Relationships among systemic vascular pressure, cardiac output, and blood pressure in the face of progressive blood volume deficit.

has a volume deficit of 15 to 25 percent will have delayed refilling of the blanched area of the hand.

Narrowing of the pulse pressure is another sign of class 2 hemorrhage. A thorough understanding of blood pressure readings is necessary in order to interpret subtle volume changes in the pregnant patient. The blood pressure can be viewed as having three components: diastolic pressure, pulse pressure, and systolic pressure. The diastolic pressure reflects the amount of systemic vasoconstriction present, the pulse pressure indicates stroke volume, and the systolic pressure denotes the interrelationship between the level of vasoconstriction and the stroke volume. While pulse pattern is a good clinical approach to the assessment of stroke volume in a given patient, it is not a reliable method of monitoring stroke volume in larger groups of patients because of individual variations in the many factors that may alter stroke volume (age, aortic stiffness). However, monitoring this parameter in a given patient will provide earlier signs of hypovolemia and reduced blood flow than either systolic or diastolic pressure used individually.

When a patient loses blood, compensatory mecha-

Table 17–1. CLASSIFICATION OF HEMORRHAGE IN THE PREGNANT PATIENT*

Hemorrhage Class	Acute Blood Loss†	Percentage Lost
1	900	15
2	1,200–1,500	20–25
3	1,800–2,100	30–35
4	2,400	40

* Total blood volume = 6,000 ml.

† In the usual clinical setting, very few episodes of volume loss occur without some infusion of intravenous fluids, usually crystalloid-containing solutions such as lactated Ringer's solution, or normal saline. Therefore, the amount of blood loss preceding physical signs and symptoms will usually exceed the values listed.

Adapted from Baker R: Hemorrhage in obstetrics. Obstet Gynecol Annu 6:295, 1997.

nisms are activated that help ensure perfusion to vital body organs (brain, heart). The initial response, vasoconstriction, diverts blood away from nonvital body organs (skin, muscle, kidney). Blood loss results in sympathoadrenal stimulation, which causes a rise in diastolic pressure. Since the systolic pressure is usually maintained with small volume deficits (15 to 25 percent), the first blood pressure response seen with volume loss is narrowing of the pulse pressure (120/70 to 120/90 mm Hg). That is, pulse pressure changes from 50 mm Hg to 30 mm Hg. When pulse pressure drops to 30 mm Hg or less, the patient should be carefully evaluated for other signs of volume loss.

Class 3 hemorrhage is defined as blood loss sufficient to cause overt hypotension. In the pregnant patient, this usually requires a blood loss of 1,800 to 2,100 ml. These patients exhibit marked tachycardia (120 to 160 beats/min) and may have cold, clammy skin and tachypnea (respiratory rate of 30 to 50 breaths/min).

In class 4 patients, the volume deficit exceeds 40 percent. These patients are in profound shock and frequently have no discernible blood pressure. They may have absent pulses in their extremities and are oliguric or anuric. If volume therapy is not quickly begun, circulatory collapse and cardiac arrest will soon result.

The hematocrit is another clinical method frequently used to estimate blood loss. After acute blood loss, the hematocrit will not change significantly for at least 4 hours, and complete compensation requires 48 hours. Infusion of intravenous fluids can alter this relationship, resulting in earlier lowering of measured hematocrit. When significant hemorrhage is thought to have occurred, a hematocrit should always be obtained. If this result shows a significant fall from a previous baseline value, a large amount of blood has been lost. Measures should immediately be taken to evaluate the source of the loss and whether the hemorrhage is ongoing but unrecognized.

Cesarean delivery is a frequent cause of excessive blood loss. It must be remembered that narcotics, which are frequently used for pain relief in the immediate postoperative period, can significantly reduce the ability of the sympathetic nervous system to effect vasoconstriction of the arterial and venous compartments. If these medications are given to a hypovolemic patient, serious hypotension can result. Signs and symptoms of hypovolemia should always be sought before the postoperative patient is given narcotic analgesics on the first postpartum day.

URINE OUTPUT—"THE WINDOW OF BODY PERFUSION"

In hypovolemic patients, urine output must be carefully monitored. In many cases, the urine output will fall before other signs of impaired perfusion are manifest. In contrast, adequate urine volume in patients who have not received diuretics strongly suggests perfusion to vital body organs is adequate.

There is reasonable correlation between renal blood flow and urine output. If the urine output is low, renal blood flow is often low as well. When there is a rapid decrease in renal blood flow, there is usually a reduction in urine output. In such cases, renal blood flow tends to shift from the outer renal cortex to the juxtamedullary portion of the renal cortex. Glomerular filtration rate is further reduced, but absorption of water and sodium is increased because there are fewer glomeruli and longer loops of Henle in this region. Urine will become more concentrated and will have a lower concentration of sodium and a higher osmolarity. With a gradual fall in renal blood flow, the urine sodium and osmolarity will often be affected before any significant fall in urine output. A urine sodium concentration of less than 10 to 20 mEq/L or a urine/serum osmolar ratio of greater than 2 usually indicates reduced renal perfusion.

BLOOD LOSS IN SEVERE PREECLAMPSIA

Major blood loss in a patient with severe preeclampsia may present a confusing picture. One must be aware of the altered hemodynamic status of these patients to appreciate the extent of the volume loss and to ensure appropriate fluid replacement. In severe preeclampsia, the blood volume has frequently failed to expand and is similar to that in a nonpregnant woman. These patients will not have the protective effect of the usual volume expansion of pregnancy and will show signs of blood loss earlier. In these cases, however, blood pressure can be a misleading indicator of volume. A blood pressure appropriate for a previously normotensive patient could indicate serious volume depletion in the preeclamptic woman. It is especially important to record serial pressures. If the blood pressure shows a significant drop during the immediate postoperative or postpartum period, a volume deficit should be suspected because hypertension usually persists for days to weeks in patients with severe preeclampsia.

When significant hemorrhage occurs in the woman with hypertension, it may be important to supplement the crystalloid fluid resuscitation with colloidal fluids pending the availability of the best colloid, whole blood. Albumin (5 percent) may be given in the ratio of 500 ml of albumin for every 4 L of crystalloid. This form of therapy will help compensate for the low albumin and total protein concentrations present in the patient with severe preeclampsia. It is not uncommon for these women to have total protein levels less than 5.0 g/dl with an albumin concentration below 2.5 g/dl. If crystalloid fluids are given alone, massive fluid accumulation in the already overexpanded extravascular space can occur and may result in cerebral as well as pulmonary edema.[1]

TREATMENT

Patients showing signs of class 2 or greater volume loss should receive crystalloid intravenous fluids pending the arrival of blood and blood products. The infusion rate should be rapid, between 1,000 and 2,000 ml in 30 to 45 minutes, or faster if the patient is obviously hypotensive. This infusion may serve as a therapeutic trial to help determine the amount of blood loss. If the physical signs and symptoms return to normal and remain stable after this challenge, no further therapy may be needed. If blood loss has been severe and the patient continues to bleed, however, this favorable response may be only transient. In this situation, typed and cross-matched blood should be given. The initial administration of a balanced salt solution will reduce the amount of whole blood needed to restore an adequate blood volume.[2]

Blood and Blood Products

Whole Blood

The use of whole blood has been discouraged and in many instances discontinued by blood banking centers around the United States. In obstetrics, the main indication for whole blood rather than component therapy is massive blood loss requiring more than a 4,000-ml replacement (Table 17–2). New strategies and algorithms must now be developed to respond to clinical situations that, in the past, were treated with whole blood.

For many years, the anticoagulant cpda-1 has been used to preserve whole blood. This compound contains c, a calcium chelating agent; p, phosphate, to maintain adenosine triphosphate (ATP) levels; d, dextrose, food for red blood cells (RBCs) and for preservation of 2,3-diphosphoglyceric acid (2,3-DPG) levels; and a, adenine, to preserve ATP levels. Maintenance of ATP is essential to preserve the RBC sodium pump and cell shape, both of which affect cell survival. A by-product of the normal glycolytic pathway in the RBC, 2,3-DPG, causes a shift to the right of the oxyhemoglobin dissociation curve. This shift permits more oxygen to be dissociated from the hemoglobin molecule and released into the tissues. Despite these alterations, the useful life of a unit of whole blood is 35 days. Recently, a new system for red cell preservation has been developed. The red cell preservative Optisol is a crystalloid solu-

Table 17–2. BLOOD REPLACEMENT

Product	Cost/Unit	Contents	Volume (ml)	Effect
Whole blood (WB)	$97	Red blood cells (2,3—DPG) White blood cells (not functional after 24 hours) Coagulation factors (50%—V, VIII after 7 days) Plasma proteins	500	Increase volume (ml/ml) Increase hematocrit 3%/unit
Packed red cells	$97	Red blood cells—same as whole blood White blood cells—less than whole blood Plasma proteins—few	240	Same red blood cells as whole blood Less risk febrile, or WBC transfusion reaction Increase hematocrit 3%/unit
Platelets	$47	55×10^6 platelets/unit, few white blood cells	50	Increase platelet count 5,000–10,000 μl/unit Give 6 packs minimum
Fresh frozen plasma	$50	Clotting factors V and VIII, fibrinogen	250	Only source of factors V, XI, XII Increase fibrinogen 10 mg/dl/unit
Cryoprecipitate	$30	Factor VIII 25% Fibrinogen von Willebrand factor	40	Increase fibrinogen 10 mg/dl/unit
Albumin 5%	$54	Albumin	500	
Albumin 25%	$54	Albumin	50	

tion containing sodium, dextrose, adenine, and mannitol. The clinical advantages of this system are improved flow characteristics of the red cells, extension of the shelf life of red cells from 35 days to 42 days, and the ability to extract larger volumes of fresh frozen plasma (FFP) from each unit of whole blood. The expansion of the shelf life is a particular advantage and should make the autologous blood donation available to more patients. The main disadvantage of this system is that its adoption by the blood bank eliminates the availability of whole blood for transfusion. The other consideration is for neonates in whom large volumes of adenine and mannitol may be toxic.

Massive Blood Transfusion

Massive transfusion is an ill-defined term but can generally be thought of as the need to replace a patient's entire blood volume in 24 hours or less.[3] In a pregnant patient, this is usually 10 or more units of blood. Massive transfusion is a medical emergency that often requires the ultimate in surgical and medical skills. Administrative skills are also essential because usually a number of physicians from various medical specialties are involved in the care of such a patient. Events may be occurring rapidly and clinical circumstances changing from minute to minute. Clear lines of communication between the various health care providers must be maintained. During an acute hemorrhage requiring prolonged surgical management, such as a placenta accreta with bladder involvement or severe placental abruption,

it is optimal to have one member of the obstetric team whose job is to coordinate blood replacement and to monitor laboratory results, which are the basis for choosing which components to replace. Communication between the surgeon and the anesthesiologist regarding volume and coagulation status is essential and may be compromised if all physicians are heavily involved in their own work.

The essentials of management of the patient requiring massive transfusion are maintenance of circulation, blood volume, oxygen-carrying capacity, hemostasis, colloid osmotic pressure, and biochemical balance. At the University of Washington, we have addressed the problem of massive obstetric bleeding by the institution of an Emergency Bleeding Protocol. This is a series of prearranged actions that are put in place once a member of the health care team initiates the protocol. The attending anesthesiologist or obstetrician is usually this individual. Once activated, the protocol stipulates a designated on-call individual at the central blood center to be emergently notified. Two units of O-negative packed cells are immediately sent to the delivery suite from the hospital emergency supply and an order is sent to the blood center for immediate release of 4 units of uncross-matched packed red cells, 6 units of platelets, and 10 bags of cryoprecipitate. An emergency set of blood studies is done that includes coagulation studies, an arterial blood gas, and an additional tube for cross-match. An algorithm is used to guide transfusion of blood products once laboratory studies are available. (If platelets are <100,000, 6 units of platelets are transfused; if fibrinogen is <125 mg/dl, 10 bags of cryoprecipitate are transfused; if international normalized ratio [INR] is >1.5 or massive bleeding is encountered, then 4 units of AB plasma are thawed and transfused.) Specified individuals are designated to keep track of orders and results. A flow sheet is used to keep track of products used, medications given, laboratory results, and intravenous fluids.

In the last 2 years, our ability to standardize the response to these uncommon but life-threatening situations has been well received by all the providers involved in these situations. A predictable series of responses to this acute emergency has served to reduce the level of provider stress and anxiety that accompanies emergency bleeding.

Metabolic derangements are frequently mentioned when massive transfusion is discussed. However, traditional formulas for using alkylating agents or calcium supplements are probably unnecessary. Hypocalcemia is a theoretical problem, but clinical syndromes from this problem are infrequently described and the possible complications of prophylactic calcium infusion may be more harmful than hypocalcemia. Hypocalcemia can be clinically important when it is combined with hyperkalemia and hypothermia, a triad that can lead to cardiac arrhythmias. Hypothermia can be a problem if the recently refrigerated blood is administered at a rate of 1 unit every 5 to 10 minutes. If this rate of administration is required, attempts should be made to warm the blood above 4°C before transfusion. Close attention should be paid to the electrocardiogram. If arrhythmias are noted, supplemental calcium should be considered.

Acid–base problems may arise in the event of massive transfusion. However, citrate toxicity is rarely a problem because the healthy liver can metabolize the citrate in a unit of blood in 5 minutes. Unless transfusion rates exceed 1 unit per 5 minutes or the liver is previously diseased, citrate toxicity should not be a problem. Although stored blood has an acid pH, acidosis is uncommon because the metabolism of citrate produces alkalosis. Prolonged acidosis is more often the result of hypoperfusion and shock rather than blood replacement. Blood gas measurement should guide the therapy with bicarbonate in this instance.

Packed Red Blood Cells

Packed red blood cells (PRBCs) are the most effective and efficient way to provide increased oxygen-carrying capacity to the anemic patient. Unless a patient has suffered massive blood loss, PRBCs and crystalloid will satisfy most clinical needs. Oxygen-carrying capacity may become impaired in the euvolemic patient when the hemoglobin level drops below 7 g/dl. If adequate volume replacement has not been accomplished, patients may exhibit orthostatic blood pressure changes or other signs of impaired oxygen-carrying capacity at hemoglobin levels above 7 g/dl. Because a unit of PRBCs has small amounts of white blood cells (WBCs) and isohemagglutinins (anti-A and anti-B), its use reduces the incidence of nonhemolytic transfusion reactions compared with that of 1 unit of whole blood. However, care should be taken to administer PRBCs with normal saline rather than lactated Ringer's or dextrose solutions. These solutions can cause the blood to clot or the red cells to lyse.

Platelets

Platelets are necessary for the initial phase of hemostasis. They must be maintained at room temperature and agitated during storage. Platelet concentrates usually contain less than 100 ml of plasma and small numbers of RBCs and WBCs.

Platelet concentrates now exist in two forms: random donor concentrates and apheresis platelets. Pooled random donor platelets have been harvested by centrifuging units of whole blood. Although the usual dose is 4 to 6 units of pooled platelets, up to 8 units can be pooled into a single bag for transfusion. All units are the same ABO type and will expire 4 hours after pooling. Apharesis platelets are collected from a single donor and contain more plasma (200 to 400 ml) than the random pooled platelet concentrates. They can be collected as a random unit or for a specific recipient. As with the pooled donor concentrates, they expire 4 hours after release from the blood center.

A unit of platelets derived from a single unit of whole blood has a shelf life of 72 hours. Transfusion of a single unit of platelets can be expected to raise the platelet count between 5,000 and 10,000/μl in a patient without antiplatelet antibodies and a normal sized spleen. The survival of transfused platelets can be as long at 3 to 5 days but will be shorter if disseminated intravascular coagulation (DIC) is present. A single unit of platelets should never be given: the smallest single dose of clinical value is 4 to 6 units. Platelets should be administered rapidly, over 10 minutes, with repeat laboratory evaluation performed 2 hours after infusion. For the obstetric patient, it is important that the platelets be ABO and Rh specific. Sensitization can be prevented by concomitant administration of Rh-immune globulin. One 300-μg dose will prevent sensitization for 30 platelet packs. It must also be remembered that six packs of platelets have a volume effect if multiple doses are used. Each unit of random donor platelets carries the transfusion risk of a single unit of blood.

Platelet administration is frequently considered for patients with DIC, massive hemorrhage, severe preeclampsia, and idiopathic thrombocytopenic purpura (ITP). In each of these conditions, the absolute levels at which a platelet transfusion is indicated may vary depending on the time course of the thrombocytopenia (more chronic forms will result in less hemostatic defects than acute loss), the need to perform a surgical procedure, the etiology of the inciting event producing thrombocytopenia, and the level of blood pressure elevation and the bleeding time. In general, platelet counts below 50,000/μl will require transfusion prior to or during surgery. However, when the need for a cesarean delivery arises in patients with platelet counts ranging from 20,000 to 50,000 platelets, transfusion may be avoided or the amount reduced if the transfusion is delayed until the need becomes apparent. This is usually evident from bleeding from skin edges, as hemostasis in the uterus is primarily a function of uterine muscle contraction, not platelet function.

Cryoprecipitate

Prepared by warming fresh frozen plasma and collecting the precipitate, cryoprecipitate contains significant amounts of factor VIII, factor XIII, fibrinogen, and von Willebrands' factor. ABO compatibility is necessary only in infants because of their small size. In pregnant patients, whenever possible, Rh-compatible cryoprecipitate should be used. If this is not possible, RhoGAM should be administered within 72 hours of transfusion. One 20-ml unit of cryoprecipitate will contain 200 mg of fibrinogen. When attempting to calculate the expected rise in serum fibrinogen, one must take into account the anticipated recovery with transfusion and the plasma volume of the patient (approximately 4 L in a 70-kg pregnant patient). This should result in only a 5 mg/dl rise in fibrinogen per bag of cryoprecipitate transfused because only 75 percent of the fibrinogen remains in the intravascular space after transfusion. In the past, estimates were twice this level, and many patients were undertransfused with cryoprecipitate. This preparation should be used when significant hypofibrinogenemia must be treated. Multiple bags need to be pooled and suspended in normal saline.

Fresh Frozen Plasma

Fresh frozen plasma is the plasma harvested from a unit of whole blood. It is frozen within 8 hours of collection. FFP contains all coagulation factors in normal concentrations. It contains no platelets, leukocytes, or red blood cells. Transfusion of FFP need not be Rh compatible but should be ABO compatible. FFP has not been shown to transmit cyotomegalovirus (CMV). Fresh frozen plasma should be administered when both volume replacement and coagulation factors are needed. The main clinical indication for this therapy is the massively hemorrhaging patient. If bleeding continues after the transfusion of 4 to 5 units of blood, a

coagulation screen should be checked to see whether the replacement of clotting factors and platelets is indicated. If the prothrombin time (PT) or partial thromboplastin time (PTT) are at least 50 percent prolonged or the international normalized ratio (INR) is greater than 1.5, there is usually a 70 percent reduction in factor levels present. A 10 percent increase in factor levels will usually be required for significant change in coagulation status. The required dose of FFP in this instance will be 4 250-ml units.

A second type of FFP has recently been introduced to the market. Manufactured by the Vitex Corporation, solvent/detergent-treated plasma is produced by pooling approximately 2,500 units of donor plasma. It is then batch treated with a solvent and a detergent, which together are very effective in destroying the lipid envelope viruses. These viruses include human immunodeficiency (HIV)-1, HIV-2, hepatitis B, hepatitis C, and human T-lymphotrophic virus (HTLV) types I and II. Coagulation factors are equivalent to FFP. The obvious advantage of this approach is the elimination of the risk of viral transmission of the previously mentioned viruses. Disadvantages are the exposure of many donors because of the pooled nature of the preparation. Disease transmission of nonlipid envelope viruses hepatitis A and parvovirus has been reported. The second disadvantage is cost, which is approximately three times that of FFP ($125 vs. $44). Physicians should check with their respective blood centers regarding the availability and policies regarding the use of this product.

Autologous Transfusion

Primarily as the result of fear of acquiring the acquired immunodeficiency syndrome (AIDS) virus from blood transfusion, interest in autologous blood transfusion for pregnant patients was heightened in past years. Autologous transfusion can be accomplished in two ways. In the most common approach, blood is collected and stored during the weeks before delivery. In the past this presented some logistic problems for the pregnant patient, since 3 weeks was the longest time that blood can be stored. Currently, blood storage has been extended to 35 days and, with the advent of a new solution for blood storage, another week can be added to the shelf life of donated blood (see prior section). Although predelivery autologous blood donation is generally safe for both mother and fetus, the low incidence of blood transfusion in patients at the time of childbirth and the safety of allogeneic transfusion has limited enthusiasm on the part of health care professionals. Studies have questioned the cost effectiveness of autologous transfusion in general.[4] Since the incidence of transfusion in pregnant patients is significantly lower than the incidence of transfusion in operative patients, predelivery autologous blood donation in pregnant patients is probably not cost effective.

The chance of acquiring HIV from a unit of donated and screened blood is now approximately 1 in 700,000. Furthermore, when blood transfusion is clinically indicated, there is usually the need for more blood than the patient is able to donate unless the blood is frozen, which dramatically increases the cost of the procedure. Antepartum patients inquiring about this practice should be carefully counseled that the chance of needing a blood transfusion is about 1 in 80 overall. It exceeds 1 percent when emergency cesarean delivery becomes necessary or if placenta previa exists.[5-7] These data, coupled with the low risk of acquiring HIV from a donated unit of blood, makes the a priori risk of a low-risk patient needing a blood transfusion and subsequently acquiring HIV less than 1 in 20 million.

A second type of autologous donation, intraoperative blood salvage, can occur at the time of excessive blood loss. Intraoperative autotransfusion has been reported in obstetric patients at the time of ruptured ectopic pregnancy and after delayed cesarean hysterectomy. This technique has some limitations in the obstetric setting. Heavy bacterial contamination is a contraindication, and the use during cesarean delivery had been questioned because of the possibility of amniotic fluid, fetal debris, and bacterial contamination. Recently, a clinical report of 139 patients who were transfused with autologous blood has been published.[8] In all cases, Cell Saver technology (Haemonetics, Braintree, MA) was used either at cesarean section or during severe obstetric hemorrhage. Blood salvage was begun after delivery of the infant and after amniotic fluid was removed from the operative field. Median volumes infused were 500 ml, but a few patients had volumes refused over 4,000 ml and in one case over 11,000 ml were refused. There were no differences in infections, respiratory, or coagulation abnormalities when the autologous transfused patients were compared to patients with similar conditions transfused with donor blood products. This technique may be useful in patients in whom anticipated blood loss is high. It may be acceptable to Jehovah's Witness patients and has the potential to add a significant margin of safety for these patients.

Transfusion Risks

PRBCs, fresh frozen plasma, cryoprecipitate, and platelets have the same risk of transmitting infectious diseases as a unit of whole blood. See the box "Risks of Blood Transfusion" for common risks of blood transfusion when blood is procured from volunteer donors. Significant progress has been made in historical and laboratory screening for common infectious diseases.

Risks of Blood Transfusion: Transfusion Risks Table[9-11]

A. Viral infection	
HIV-1, HIV-2	1/700,000
Hepatitis B	1/140,000
Hepatitis C*	1/90,000
HTLV I and II	1/641,000
B. Bacterial contamination	
Red cells	1/500,000
Platelets	1/12,000
C. Reactions	
Acute hemolytic reaction	1/600,000
Delayed hemolytic reaction	1/1,000
Acute lung injury	1/5,000

*In 1999, trials were begun to screen blood with a PCR test for HCV RNA. It is anticipated that there will be a significant reduction in the transmission of hepatitis C but reliable data are not currently available.

The risks of serious complications from blood transfusion have fallen to very low rates. Blood obtained from paid sources can be expected to have higher rates of many of the complications listed in the box.

Transfusion Reactions

Transfusion of an incompatible blood component results in a hemolytic transfusion reaction. They are usually due to clerical errors or to misidentification of the patient or unit of blood. Naturally occurring antibodies in the ABO system are the usual causes. Hemolytic transfusion reactions may result in DIC or acute renal failure. The clinical signs of acute hemolytic transfusion reaction may include some or all of the following: severe anxiety, flushing, chest or back pain, fever, hypotension, tachycardia, or dyspnea. In an anesthetized patient, hemoglobinuria may be the first noticeable sign. A rapid diagnostic test is the discovery of reddish plasma after centrifugation of a red-top tube of blood. Upon recognition, the transfusion should be stopped, and the blood returned to the blood center along with a tube of the patient's blood. Treatment with fluids, diuretics, and transfusion support for bleeding are the cornerstone of therapy. A delayed hemolytic transfusion reaction can occur in patients who have been previously sensitized to an antigen through transfusion or pregnancy. This can result in a symptomatic or asymptomatic hemolysis within a week after a transfusion. Although more common than acute hemolytic reactions, the consequences are generally less severe.

Fever after or during transfusion is usually, but not

always, related to sensitization of antigens on cell components, usually leukocytes. However, fever can also be the first sign of sepsis related to bacterial contamination of red cells or platelets. Some authorities recommend empiric antibiotic therapy in patients who develop fever within 6 hours of transfusion of RBCs or platelets.[11]

Transfusion-related acute lung injury is an acute respiratory distress syndrome occurring within 4 hours of transfusion. It is characterized by dyspnea and hypoxemia secondary to noncardiogenic pulmonary edema and is estimated to occur with a frequency of greater than 1 in 5,000 transfusions. The mechanisms of injury to the pulmonary capillaries are varied and involve lipid products from donor red cell membranes and neutrophil reactions. The estimate of mortality secondary to this entity is felt to be underreported, but greater than 90 percent of patients can be expected to recover.

ANTEPARTUM HEMORRHAGE

Abruptio Placenta

The premature separation of the normally implanted placenta from the uterus is called *abruptio placenta* or *placental abruption*. Diagnosis of placental abruption is certain when inspection of the placenta shows an adherent retroplacental clot with depression or disruption of the underlying placental tissue; however, this frequently is not found if the abruption is of recent onset. Clinical findings indicating placental abruption include the triad of external or occult uterine bleeding, uterine hypertonus and/or hyperactivity, and fetal distress and/or fetal death. Placental abruption can be broadly classified into three grades that correlate with clinical and laboratory findings.

Grade 1: Slight vaginal bleeding and some uterine irritability are usually present. Maternal blood pressure is unaffected, and the maternal fibrinogen level is normal. The fetal heart rate pattern is normal.
Grade 2: External uterine bleeding is mild to moderate. The uterus is irritable, and tetanic or very frequent contractions may be present. Maternal blood pressure is maintained, but the pulse rate may be elevated and postural blood volume deficits may be present. The fibrinogen level may be decreased. The fetal heart rate often shows signs of fetal compromise.
Grade 3: Bleeding is moderate to severe but may be concealed. The uterus is tetanic and painful. Maternal hypotension is frequently present and fetal death has occurred. Fibrinogen levels are often reduced to less than 150 mg/dl; other coagulation abnormalities (thrombocytopenia, factor depletion) are present.

Incidence

The reported incidence of placental abruption varies from 1 in 86 to 1 in 206 births.[12–14] This variability reflects differing criteria for diagnosis as well as the increased recognition in recent years of milder forms of the disorder. Grade 1 placental abruption is found in about 40 percent, grade 2 in about 45 percent, and grade 3 in 15 percent of clinically recognized cases of placental abruption.[12,15] Eighty percent of all cases will occur before the onset of labor.[13]

Etiology

The primary etiology of placental abruption is unknown, but several reports have identified statistically significant correlations with common obstetric complications. Studies have suggested an increased incidence of abruption in patients with advanced parity or age, maternal smoking, poor nutrition, cocaine use, and chorioamnionitis.[15–19] However, some of these data may have been subject to selection bias, as only populations of low socioeconomic status were evaluated. The U.S. Perinatal Collaborative project performed during the years 1959 and 1966 and a recent population-based study in Washington state failed to show a relationship between placental abruption and either maternal age or parity.[14,20] However, a population-based study over 15 years in Norway was able to demonstrate a strong relationship between maternal age and placental abruption for all levels of parity.[21]

Maternal hypertension (>140/90 mm Hg) seems to be the most consistently identified factor predisposing to placental abruption.[22] This relationship is true for all grades of placental abruption but is most strongly associated with grade 3 abruption, in which 40 to 50 percent of cases are found to have hypertensive disease of pregnancy.[20,22] Intrapartum hypertension significantly increases the risk of abruption, but one study failed to show a relationship between the antenatal detection of hypertension and placental abruption.

Blunt external maternal trauma is an increasingly important cause of placental abruption. Two conditions account for the majority of blunt abdominal trauma leading to placental abruption: motor vehicle collision and maternal battering. Historically, 1 to 2 percent of grade 3 abruptions have been attributed to maternal trauma.[22,23] However, recent epidemiologic studies show an alarmingly high incidence of maternal battering in some populations.[24] These data make it incumbent on the obstetrician to consider placental abruption when a history of trauma is elicited and vice versa. The

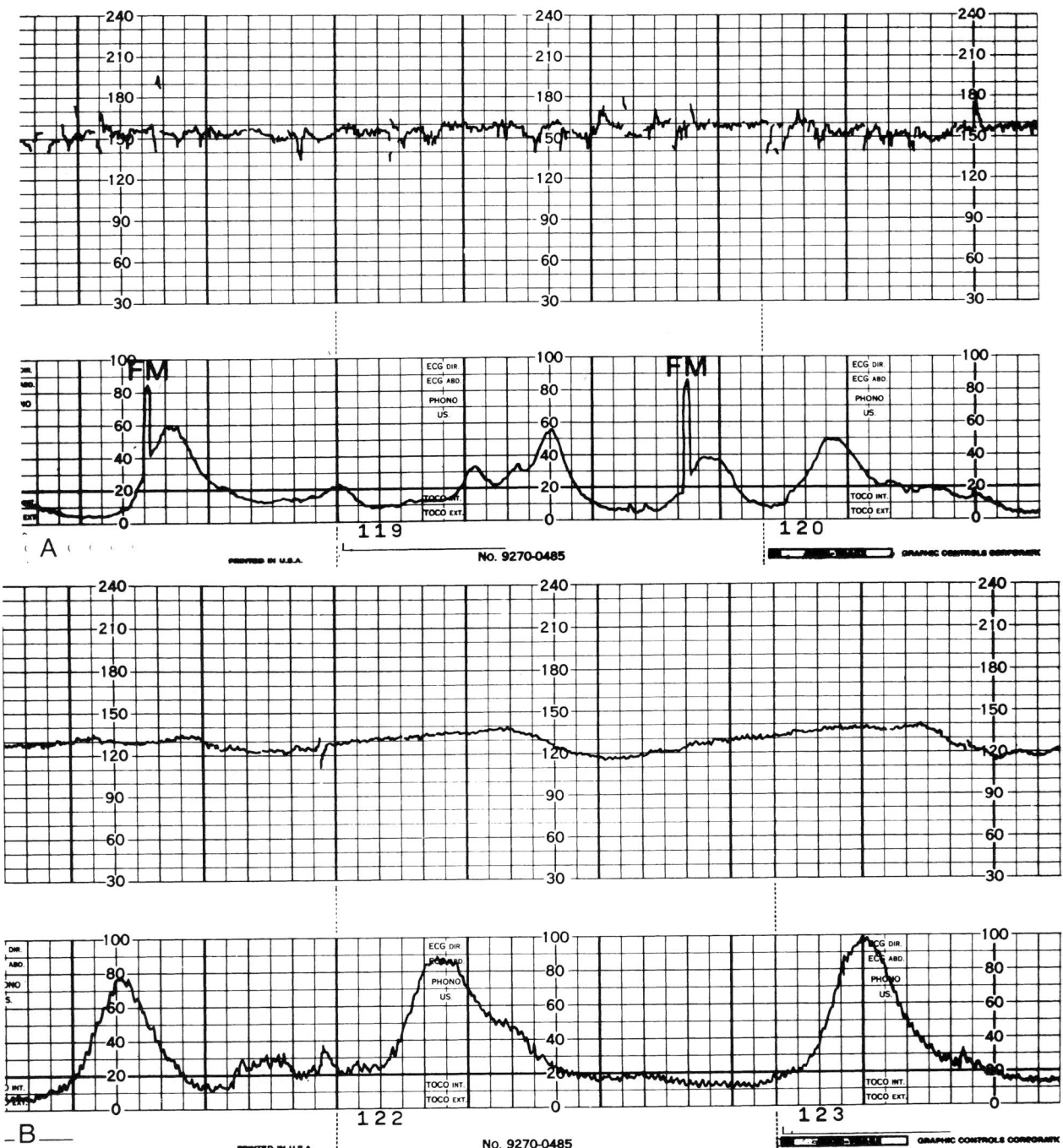

Figure 17–2. *A,* A fetal heart rate tracing at 37 weeks' gestation in a patient involved in an automobile accident in which the maternal abdomen struck the steering wheel. Fetal movements were present, and no periodic changes were observed. Uterine contractions were occurring every 2 to 3 minutes. *B,* Eight hours later, repetitive late decelerations are now present. An asphyxiated fetus was delivered, and evidence of grade 3 placental abruption was found at the time of delivery.

physical evidence of trauma may be minimal and yet still be associated with placental abruption that can progress from grade 1 to 3 within 24 hours. Figure 17–2 illustrates fetal heart rate tracings 8 hours apart in a patient involved in an automobile accident.

Rapid decompression of the overdistended uterus is an uncommon cause of placental abruption. This may occur in patients with multiple gestations and those with polyhydramnios. There is an increased risk of placental abruption associated with multiple gestation.[21] However, the timing of placental abruption in multiple gestations is difficult to ascertain. When rapid decompression of the uterus is apparent, abruption is usually observed after the delivery of the first fetus. Delivery of the second twin follows soon after, before a retroplacental clot has time to form. Rapid decompression of the uterus should be avoided in a patient with polyhydramnios. Amniotic fluid should be slowly released by amniocentesis before the induction of labor or once spontaneous labor has been established.

In the past, folic acid deficiency, a short umbilical cord, and the supine hypotensive syndrome had been suggested as etiologies for placental abruption. Further evidence has shown, however, that these factors are unlikely causes of placental abruption.

Recent evidence has implicated the presence of acquired or inherited thrombophilias as a significant factor in the etiology of placental abruption.[25] In that study of Jewish women, mutations of one or more of three thrombolphilic mutations (factor V Leiden mutation) were present in 60 percent of women who had suffered placental abruption. The presence of factor V Leiden mutation in the control population was much higher (17 percent) than in the comparable white United States population (5 percent). Furthermore, ethnic minority populations have even lower risk of this mutation.[26] Further study of this finding is necessary before definitive clinical recommendations can be made regarding screening and treatment.

The pathologic changes in the placental bed in patients with placental abruption show a high incidence of vascular abnormalities. Failure of transformation of uteroplacental arteries is the most common finding (60 percent). Anomalies in the vessels deep in the myometrium, including vessel occlusion with surrounding myometrial hemorrhage, were observed in 33 percent.[27] At the placental level, hemorrhage into the decidua basalis causes it to split, leaving a layer adherent to the myometrium. This decidual hematoma may then progress to cause further separation and compression of the adjacent placenta.

There is a significant recurrence rate for placental abruption. This figure has been reported to vary from 5 percent to 17 percent.[13,17,22] If a patient has suffered an abruption in two pregnancies, the chance for recurrence is 25 percent. In the largest series of placental abruption severe enough to result in fetal demise, the recurrence rate of severe placental abruption again resulting in fetal demise was 11 percent. Unfortunately, no published data are available to document a prospective plan of management that will reduce this unacceptably high risk. The following case illustrates one plan for such a patient.

Illustrative Case

A 32-year-old G5P4 presented at 6 weeks' gestation with the following history: She had suffered grade 3 placental abruption in her third pregnancy at 35 weeks'

gestation and had undergone cesarean delivery for severe maternal coagulopathy with a dead fetus. She required 8 units of blood and blood products because of a significant intraoperative hemorrhage and contracted hepatitis C. In her next pregnancy she had an uncomplicated antenatal course and was last seen for a clinic visit at 33 weeks. She was a one-pack-a-day smoker, but all efforts to eliminate smoking from her life had been unsuccessful. At 35 weeks' gestation she presented with syncope followed by severe abdominal pain with a dead fetus. This was the same clinical presentation and gestation as the previous pregnancy. She underwent induction of labor and had a successful vaginal delivery but required 12 units of blood and blood products. In the fifth pregnancy the following management plan was developed: enrollment in a smoking cessation program; clinic visits every 2 weeks; antenatal testing beginning at 28 weeks; amniocentesis at 34 weeks' gestation, and delivery by repeat cesarean section with tubal ligation if pulmonary maturity was documented, and, if pulmonary maturity was not present, maternal administration of glucocorticoids with continuous fetal monitoring for 48 hours, followed by cesarean delivery. The patient was unable to comply with the smoking cessation program but maintained her clinic visits. At 34 weeks, amniocentesis demonstrated pulmonary maturity, and cesarean section and tubal ligation were accomplished without complication. Her 2,500-g male infant had an uncomplicated neonatal course. While this case resulted in a favorable outcome for both mother and fetus, it has been shown that grade 3 placental abruption and fetal death can follow normal antepartum testing by as few as 4 hours.[28]

Diagnosis and Management

Vaginal bleeding in the third trimester of pregnancy is the hallmark of placental abruption and should always prompt an investigation to determine its etiology. After appropriate physical and laboratory examination of the mother and fetus, ultrasound evaluation of the uterus, placenta, and fetus has become the standard of care (Fig. 17–3). The other common and potentially life-threatening cause of third-trimester bleeding, placenta previa, should be recognized in nearly all cases in which it is present. If ultrasound examination fails to show a placenta previa and if other local causes of vaginal bleeding (including cervical or vaginal trauma, labor, or malignancy) have been ruled out, placental abruption becomes the most likely diagnosis.

In the initial studies evaluating ultrasound, less than 2 percent of cases were definitively identifiable with ultrasound. Recent advances in ultrasound imaging and interpretation have improved this rate so that more than 50 percent of patients with confirmed placental abruption will demonstrate ultrasound evidence of hemorrhage. However, even complete placental abrup-

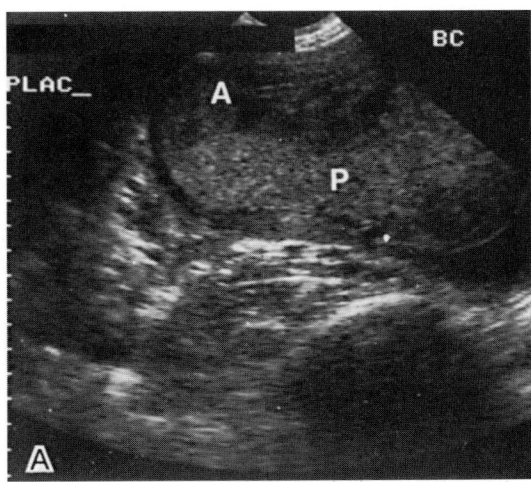 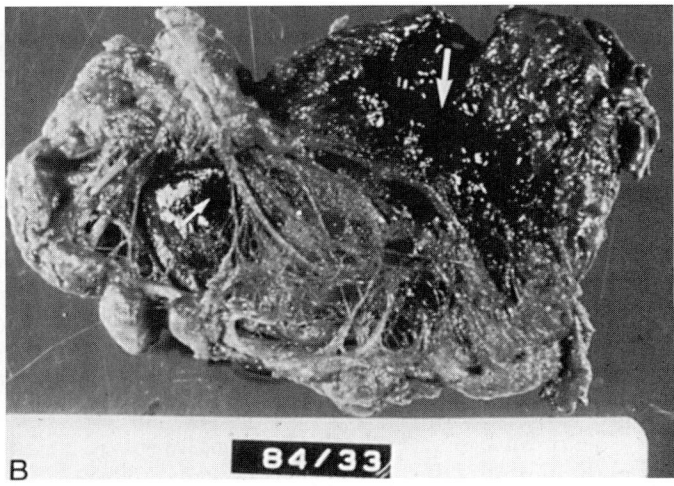

Figure 17–3. *A,* Ultrasound study at 18 weeks' gestation demonstrating a hypoechoic area (A) representing retroplacental bleeding and an enlarged placenta (P). This patient had chronic hypertension. She presented with intermittent dark red vaginal bleeding and abdominal pain, a picture consistent with a chronic abruption. *B,* At delivery, the placenta revealed a large clot (*small arrow*) and fresh hemorrhage (*large arrow*). The fibrous bands bridging the clot are also consistent with chronic abruption.

tion may be missed by ultrasound examination during the acute phase of placental abruption.

Ultrasound can identify three predominant locations for placental abruption. These are subchorionic (between the placenta and the membranes), retroplacental (between the placenta and the myometrium), and preplacental (between the placenta and the amniotic fluid). Hematomas identified by ultrasound during the early phases of vaginal bleeding and pain are most likely to be hyperechoic or isoechoic compared with the placenta. As the hematoma resolves, it will become hypoechoic within a week and sonolucent within 2 weeks.[29] Because of the changing character of the hematoma, misinterpretation of a hematoma as uterine myoma, succenturiate placental lobe, chorioangioma, or molar pregnancy has been reported.

The location and extent of the placental abruption identified on ultrasound has definite clinical significance. Retroplacental hematomas carry a worse prognosis for fetal survival than subchorionic hemorrhages. The size of the hemorrhage is also predictive of fetal survival. Large retroplacental hemorrhages (>60 ml) are associated with a 50 percent or greater fetal mortality, whereas similar sized subchorionic hemorrhages are associated with a 10 percent mortality.[30]

Nearly half of all placental abruptions will result in delivery at less than 37 weeks' gestation.[21] Gestational age at the time of presentation is an important prognostic factor. In patients presenting at less than 20 weeks, 82 percent can be expected to have a term delivery despite evidence of placental abruption. If the presentation occurs after 20 weeks' gestation, only 27 percent will deliver at term.

Nearly 80 percent of patients who eventually prove to have a placental abruption will present with vaginal bleeding. The remaining 20 percent of patients fail to exhibit external signs of bleeding. These patients have a concealed abruption and are commonly given the diagnosis of premature labor. Such cases must be watched very carefully. On some occasions, the abruption may progress despite successful tocolysis, and fetal death may result. Other classic signs of placental abruption include increased uterine tenderness and tone. These findings are uncommon (17 percent) unless the abruption is grade 2 or 3.[13]

Once the diagnosis of placental abruption has been made, precautions should be taken to deal with the possible life-threatening consequences for both mother and fetus. At least 4 units of blood should be available for maternal transfusions. A large-bore (16-gauge) intravenous line must be secured and the infusion of a crystalloid solution begun. Blood should be drawn for hemoglobin and hematocrit determinations and coagulation studies (fibrinogen, platelet count, fibrin degradation products, PT, PTT). A red-topped tube should also be obtained and used to perform a clot test. This test, a "poor man's" fibrinogen assay, will often give critical information before the laboratory can document a coagulation defect. If a clot does not form within 6 minutes or forms and lyses within 30 minutes, a coagulation defect is probably present and the fibrinogen level is less than 150 mg/dl. Continuous fetal monitoring should be used to record fetal heart rate and document uterine activity.

In the patient with a term fetus in whom the diagnosis of grade 1 abruption is made, close observation for signs of fetal or maternal compromise is essential. If the fetus is known to be mature, controlled delivery should be accomplished by induction of labor while the mother and fetus are in stable condition.

The occurrence of a grade 1 placental abruption with a preterm fetus presents greater challenge. Often, a vicious circle is established in which a small placental abruption stimulates uterine irritability, further separating the placenta until fetal compromise becomes evident. In patients remote from term, and with both mother and fetus clinically stable, inhibition of uterine contractions with tocolytic agents has been described. However, there are no randomized studies demonstrating improved fetal or maternal outcome using tocolysis in this condition. In three separate reports totaling 92 patients, no adverse maternal complications were reported and significant prolongation of gestation (>1 week) was accomplished in over 50 percent of patients.[31-32] No adverse fetal complications were reported, with mortality being attributable only to extreme prematurity. In the largest and most recent uncontrolled study, Towers et al. used tocolysis in over 70 percent of 131 patients presenting, with placental abruption. In patients stable enough to receive tocolysis, approximately one third of patients delivered within the first 48 hours, one third delivered within 7 days, and one third delivered greater than 1 week from initial presentation. Fetal death was related to prematurity and there were no cases of intrauterine fetal demise of a fetus alive on hospital admission. Tocolysis in this setting does not appear to be hazardous to the fetus, but its benefit may be limited to 48 hours, as is the case with tocolysis in preterm labor not associated with placental abruption. The maternal safety of tocolysis cannot be ascertained from the current studies, but physicians should keep in mind that placental abruption accounts for 6 percent of all maternal morality. Unproven therapies in the face of high-risk maternal conditions should be approached with caution and should be administered after careful consideration and counseling of risks and benefits to the mother and fetus. Any attempt to arrest preterm labor in known or suspected abruption should be weighed against the likelihood for survival, morbidity if the infant were delivered, and the severity of the abruption.

When tocolysis is used, magnesium sulfate has less adverse cardiovascular side effects than β-sympathomimetics. A comparison of other tocolytic agents or a comparison with observation alone has never been evaluated by a clinical trial. In many cases of placental abruption, delivery will be the treatment of choice. During labor, careful attention must be paid to several maternal and fetal parameters. Because 60 percent of fetuses may exhibit signs of intrapartum fetal distress, continuous fetal heart rate monitoring is essential. In a similar manner, continuous monitoring of maternal volume status is important. An indwelling Foley catheter will permit accurate assessment of maternal urine output. Serial maternal hematocrit determinations should be made regularly at intervals of 2 to 3 hours. The goal

of therapy should be to maintain a maternal urine output of 1 ml/min and a hematocrit of at least 30 percent. An updated flow sheet at the bedside permits the clinician to follow maternal vital signs, urine output, laboratory values, and critical clotting parameters.

Placental abruption frequently stimulates the clotting cascade, resulting in DIC. Intravascular fibrinogen is converted to fibrin by activation of the extrinsic clotting cascade. In the usual clinical setting, platelets and clotting factors V and VIII are also depleted. Serial measurements of plasma fibrinogen provide valuable information regarding the coagulation status of the patient and will help estimate the volume of blood loss that has occurred.

The normal maternal fibrinogen concentration in the third trimester is 450 mg/dl. In grade 1 abruptions, there is often no alteration in this value and no evidence of DIC. However, when the fibrinogen value drops below 300 mg/dl, significant coagulation abnormalities are usually present. Most women with significant falls in fibrinogen will require blood transfusion to maintain a normal circulating volume. If the presenting fibrinogen level is less than 150 mg/dl, most patients will have already lost 2,000 ml of blood. The signs and symptoms of such blood loss may not be obvious because, as noted earlier, the normal hypervolemia of pregnancy protects the mother from a volume loss that a nonpregnant individual could not tolerate. In the case of grade 3 placental abruption, the mean blood loss is 2,500 ml or more.[34] In patients with grade 2 and grade 3 abruption, rapid crystalloid infusion of at least 1,000 ml pending the availability of whole blood should be done. Two to 3 ml of crystalloid should be given for each 1 ml of blood lost to maintain euvolemia.

If urine output fails to reach 30 ml/h despite adequate volume replacement, consideration should be given to inserting a central venous pressure (CVP) catheter to determine the adequacy of intravascular volume. This catheter may be inserted through a site in the arm rather than the neck or subclavian area because of the severe coagulopathy that is often present. The absolute level of CVP is less important than the response of the CVP to volume infusion, as long as the CVP is less than 7 cm H_2O in response to the preceding 250-ml aliquot. If this response has been achieved but the urine output is still inadequate, consideration should be given to replacing the CVP catheter with a pulmonary artery catheter. This circumstance is uncommon unless there is intrinsic heart disease or severe preeclampsia or the patient has already suffered critical renal ischemia and is in acute renal failure.

Considerable controversy remains regarding the appropriate method of delivery in patients with placental abruption. Concern exists for the fetal outcome in such cases. A number of patients present with a live fetus, only to have that fetus die undelivered while awaiting vaginal delivery.[12,15] Retrospective reviews show a trend for increased fetal survival in patients who have undergone cesarean delivery once the maternal condition has been stabilized. However, none of these reports surveyed a period in which intrapartum fetal monitoring was routine. Currently, the use of continuous electronic fetal monitoring in this situation is associated with excellent fetal survival, and cesarean delivery can be reserved for cases with fetal distress or other traditional obstetric indications.[13] The cesarean section rate associated with placental abruption is 50 to 75 percent, depending on the clinical aggressiveness of the physicians managing the patient.[35]

The management of mothers with severe coagulopathy and/or fetal demise requires a thorough knowledge of the natural history of severe placental abruption. This information is best found in the classic paper of Pritchard and Brekken. Several important clinical observations first noted in 1967 are still important today. They observed that only 38 percent of patients with placental abruption severe enough to result in fetal demise will show DIC. They documented that patients destined to have severe placental abruption will show evidence of hypofibrinogenemia within 8 hours of initial symptoms. They did not observe any recovery from low fibrinogen levels in patients with severe hypofibrinogenemia without blood product transfusion. They also documented the time course for recovery from hypofibrinogenemia to be 10 mg/dl/h after delivery of the fetus and placenta.

Restoration of a normal blood volume and coagulation status is the sine qua non of treatment in these patients. It is important to remember that rather than exhibit shock out of proportion to the total blood loss, patients with severe placental abruption often appear resistant to the development of hypotension. They may have a blood pressure that appears quite normal. However, this is a false interpretation because 50 percent of patients will exhibit hypertension once adequate volume replacement has been accomplished. Adequate volume status in this situation is best achieved by ensuring a urine output of at least 30 ml/h.

After euvolemia has been achieved and appropriate coagulation factors administered, attention can be given to effecting delivery. Some clinicians believe that if placental abruption has progressed to fetal death and severe coagulopathy, cesarean delivery will result in the quickest resolution of maternal problems. However, operating in the presence of a coagulopathy can result in prolonged operative times secondary to surgically uncontrollable bleeding. Pritchard and Brekken observed that bleeding from all cut surfaces at the time of cesarean delivery occurred with fibrinogen levels of less than 150 mg/dl. Hemorrhage after vaginal delivery was not correlated with fibrinogen levels unless there were extensive vaginal lacerations or uterine atony. In their study, Pritchard and Brekken did not administer coagulation products unless they were performing laporotomy or there were extensive vaginal lacerations. In current obstetric practice, administration of coagulation factor replacement along with PRBCs is the treatment of choice in patients with DIC. Even in the face of a severe coagulopathy, induction to delivery times exceeding 18 hours may result in equal or better maternal outcome as long as maternal volume status and coagulation status can be maintained.[14]

As soon as adequate volume status is accomplished and blood products are available, induction of labor should be initiated. This can usually be accomplished with oxytocin. Many patients are already experiencing some uterine activity, oftentimes hypertonic in nature. Pritchard and Brekken noted that frequently there is generalized increased uterine tone without rhythmic uterine contractions being clinically detectable. It is important to judge the progress of labor in this instance by serial cervical exams with particular attention being given to cervical effacement. In patients with severe placental abruption, rapid cervical dilatation usually occurs only after complete effacement. Care must be taken not to prematurely abandon a vaginal trial because of the lack of early cervical dilatation.

Contrary to popular belief, the uterus does not need to be evacuated before coagulation status can be restored. Administering blood and blood products and delaying attempts at vaginal delivery for a few hours until hematologic parameters have improved is associated with good maternal outcome. There are now two reported cases of severe placental abruption with maternal coagulopathy in the second trimester in which blood and blood product administration completely reversed the syndrome, and live fetuses were subsequently delivered.[36,37]

When cesarean delivery is necessary, extravasation of blood into the uterine muscle to produce red to purple discoloration of the serosal surface will be found in 8 percent of patients. This finding, known as a Couvelaire uterus, has been feared to result in a high incidence of uterine hemorrhage secondary to atony. However, atony is the exception rather than the rule, and most patients with a Couvelaire uterus demonstrate an appropriate response to the infusion of oxytocin. Hysterectomy should be reserved for cases of atony and hemorrhage unresponsive to conventional uterotonics.

Neonatal Outcome

Increased perinatal mortality has been uniformly associated with placental abruption, with some groups reporting as high as 25 to 30 percent combined fetal and neonatal deaths.[38,39] Recent studies have shown a greater risk for adverse long-term neurobehavioral outcome in infants delivered after placental abruption.[40] In a case-control study of low-birth-weight infants, 40 infants born after placental abruption were compared with 80 infants matched for gestational age at delivery. There was a significant association between abruption and abnormal neonatal outcome (death or cerebral palsy). The chance of a completely normal neonatal outcome tended to decrease in relationship to the severity of the abruption, but small numbers of patients in each group limited the statistical significance of this finding. The most significant obstetric finding in this group was the high incidence of abnormal fetal heart rate tracings (45 percent) and emergency cesarean delivery (53 percent) compared with the control group (10 percent and 10 percent, respectively).

Placenta Previa

Placenta previa is defined as the implantation of the placenta over the cervical os. There are three recognized variations of placenta previa: total, partial, and marginal (Fig. 17–4). In total placenta previa, the cervical os is completely covered by the placenta. This type presents the most serious maternal risk, as it is associated with greater blood loss than either marginal or partial placenta previa. The frequency of total placenta previa has been reported to be as low as 20 percent[41] and as high as 43 percent.[42] Partial placenta previa is defined as the partial occlusion of the cervical os by the placenta and occurs in 31 percent of diagnosed cases. A marginal placenta previa is characterized by the encroachment of the placenta to the margin of the cervical os. It does not cover the os. The differentiation of the latter two degrees of placenta previa is dependent on the dilatation of the cervix and the method of diagnosis (ultrasound or direct examination).

A leading cause of third-trimester hemorrhage, placenta previa presents classically as painless bleeding. Bleeding is thought to occur in association with the development of the lower uterine segment in the third trimester. Placental attachment is disrupted as this area gradually thins in preparation for the onset of labor. When this occurs, bleeding occurs at the implantation site, as the uterus is unable to contract adequately and stop the flow of blood from the open vessels.

The incidence of placenta previa is stated to be 1 in 200 live births.[42,43] Significant epidemiologic risk factors are maternal age above 35 years (rate ratio, 4.7) and black or other minority races (rate ratio, 1.3). Whether the increased risk for older mothers is related to parity or to an independent risk factor is still uncertain. The most important obstetric risk factor in the development of placenta previa is previous cesarean delivery. The risk for placenta previa occurring in the pregnancy following a cesarean delivery has been reported to be between 1 and 4 percent.[41,44–47] There is a linear increase in placenta previa risk with the number of prior cesarean deliveries. In patients with four or more cesarean deliveries, the risk of placenta previa approaches 10 percent.[44]

The timing of the diagnosis of placenta previa has undergone significant change in the last decade. Whereas third-trimester bleeding was a common presentation for placenta previa, most cases of placenta previa are now detected antenatelly prior to the onset of significant bleeding. The common practice of second-trimester ultrasound for detection of fetal anomalies has led to this change. However, because most cases of placenta previa diagnosed in the second trimester will resolve, management of placenta previa diagnosed in the second trimester will differ from the same diagnosis in the third trimester. At 17 weeks' gestation, evidence of placental tissue covering the cervical os will be found in 5 to 15 percent of all patients.[42] More than 90

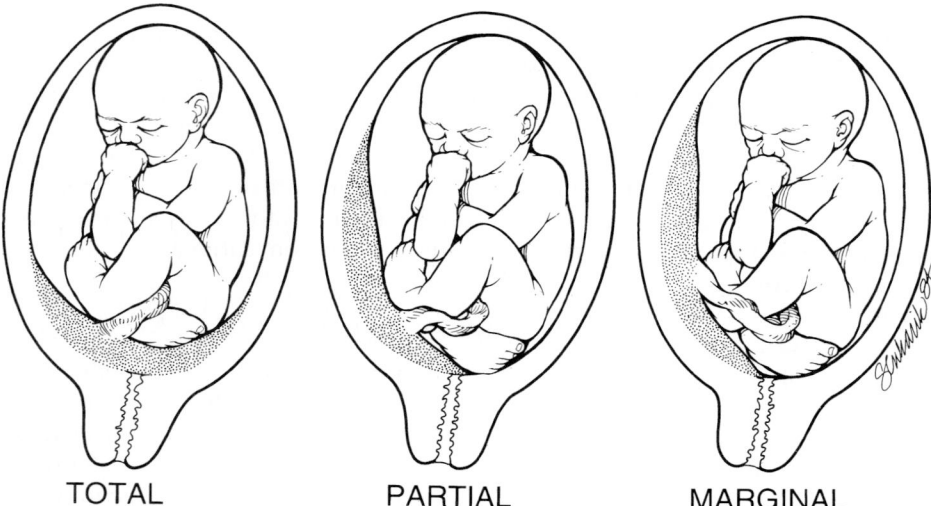

TOTAL   PARTIAL   MARGINAL

Figure 17–4. Three variations of placenta previa.

percent of these patients will have a normal ultrasound by 37 weeks' gestation.[48] This phenomenon has been termed *placental migration*. It is unlikely that the placenta actually separates and reattaches throughout the second and third trimesters. The changes in architecture secondary to differential growth of the lower uterine segment during the second and third trimesters probably account for this observation. Location of the placenta with reference to the cervix will influence the likelihood of resolution of placenta previa with advancing gestation. Total placenta previa diagnosed in the second trimester will persist into the third trimester in 26 percent of cases, while marginal or partial placenta previa will persist in only 2.5 percent of cases.[49]

In patients diagnosed prior to 24 weeks' gestation, a repeat ultrasound should be scheduled between 24 and 28 weeks' gestation to confirm the resolution of the radiographic diagnosis of placenta previa. However, if patients have vaginal bleeding during this time period, they should be managed as presumed cases of placenta previa. Placenta previa should be suspected in all patients presenting with bleeding after 24 weeks' gestation.

Changes in the antenatal course of placenta previa were documented by Wing et al. in their prospective randomized study.[50] Of 139 patients admitted with placenta previa diagnosed after 24 weeks, 23 percent experienced no bleeding episodes by 36 weeks. An additional 12 percent had an initial bleeding episode after 35 weeks and were delivered shortly after delivery. Therefore, at least one third of patients with placenta previa persisting after 24 weeks will suffer no significant bleeding episodes before 35 weeks. A small percentage of patients (5 percent) will present with bleeding so severe as to necessitate immediate delivery.

Patients with third-trimester bleeding should be treated in a manner similar to that outlined in the section on abruptio placenta (e.g., maternal stabilization, fetal monitoring). However, blood studies do not need to be as extensive as those ordered for patients with placental abruption. DIC is rare in cases of placenta previa and tests for maternal coagulation abnormalities do not need to be routinely performed. Once fetal and maternal status have been stabilized, ultrasound evaluation should be performed to establish or reconfirm the diagnosis. (Fig. 17–5).

Once the diagnosis of placenta previa is made, management decisions depend on the gestational age, amount of bleeding, fetal condition, and presentation. In the patient who is unequivocally at 37 weeks' gestation with evidence of uterine activity or with persistent bleeding, delivery is the treatment of choice. In previous years, a double setup examination was the initial step in this process. With the early diagnosis of placenta previa and rapid and reliable ultrasound availability and interpretation, this technique is now unnecessary in the majority of cases.

In uncommon patients, vaginal delivery may still be considered. Patients with marginal or partial placenta previa who present in labor with minimal bleeding are ideal candidates. It can also be considered for patients with previable gestations or intrauterine fetal demise. Appropriately conducted labor in these selected instances can be safe for both mother and fetus.[51]

When double setup examination is elected, it should be done in an operating room with full preparation made to perform emergency cesarean delivery should excessive vaginal bleeding follow the examination. In performing a double setup examination, the patient should be prepared and draped for cesarean delivery.

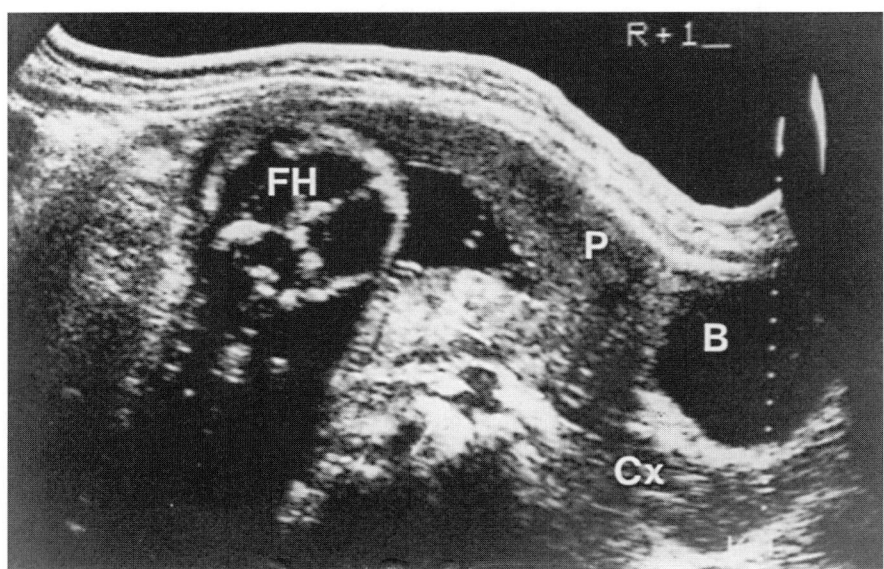

Figure 17–5. This ultrasound examination at 34 weeks' gestation in a patient with painless vaginal bleeding revealed placenta previa (P) covering the cervical os (Cx). The maternal bladder (B) and fetal head (FH) are also shown.

The anesthesiologist should be present and the operating room team ready. The patient should first undergo a careful speculum examination, which may reveal placental tissue in the cervical os. If the diagnosis of placenta previa cannot be made with a speculum examination, the obstetrician should next examine the vaginal fornices. Fullness in the fornices suggests the presence of the placenta extending down toward the cervix. Finally, examining fingers should be carefully introduced into the cervical os to detect the placenta.

For the patient who is remote from term (24 to 36 weeks' gestation), expectant management is the treatment of choice. The essence of this approach is maintenance of the fetus in a healthy intrauterine environment without jeopardizing maternal condition. Maternal blood loss should be replaced in order to maintain the maternal hematocrit between 30 and 35 percent. This RBC volume will provide a margin of safety in the event of a large hemorrhage. Even an initial blood loss in excess of 500 ml can be expectantly managed with adequate volume replacement.

Although obstetricians are most concerned about maternal hemorrhage, they must remember that fetal blood can also be lost during the process of placental separation. Rh-immune globulin should be given to all at-risk patients with third-trimester bleeding who are Rh-negative and unsensitized. A Kleihauer-Betke preparation of maternal blood should also be performed in all Rh-negative women. This test will detect the occasional patient with a fetomaternal hemorrhage of greater than 30 ml. Thirty-five percent of infants whose mothers require antepartum transfusion will themselves be anemic and require transfusion when delivered.[42]

Twenty percent of patients with placenta previa will show evidence of uterine contractions. Because a vaginal examination to document cervical dilatation is absolutely contraindicated, it is difficult to make a firm diagnosis of preterm labor. Although no controlled studies are available to show the efficacy of tocolytic therapy in such cases, some studies document that it can be safely attempted.[42,52] The choice of agents in this situation is controversial. If β-mimetics are used in the presence of maternal hypovolemia, serious maternal hypotension can result (Fig. 17–6). In addition, the use of β-mimetics will produce maternal tachycardia, making the evaluation of maternal volume status more difficult. Nonetheless some authors have reported the use of these agents for tocolysis in patients with placenta previa without excessive complications.[53–55]

Because of the reduced risk of cardiovascular complications, magnesium sulfate has become the agent of choice for the treatment of patients in preterm labor with placenta previa at many institutions. Infusion of a 6-g loading dose followed by 3 g/h or more are often necessary to control uterine irritability because of the increased maternal glomerular filtration rate. Once the patient has been stabilized on magnesium sulfate, the use of oral tocolytics has been advocated by some, although no conclusive studies demonstrate improved outcome with oral tocolytic therapy for any indication. Patients may occasionally require more than 1 week of continuous intravenous tocolytic therapy. Such treatment is considered justified since, before 33 weeks' gestation, each day that the fetus remains in utero reduces its stay in the neonatal intensive care nursery by 2 days.[56] The use of antenatal corticosteroids to accelerate fetal pulmonary maturity is effective in reducing the incidence of neonatal respiratory distress syndrome, in-

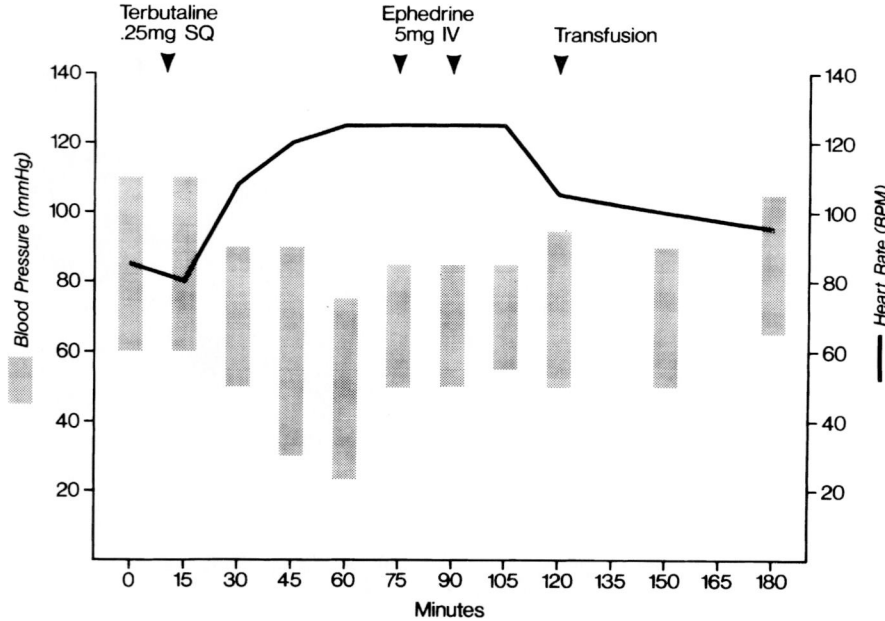

Figure 17–6. Blood pressure and heart rate response to terbutaline administration in a bleeding patient with placenta previa. Hypotension, which developed acutely, was somewhat resistant to ephedrine and crystalloid administration.

tracranial hemorrhage, and neonatal death.[57,58] Given a high incidence of respiratory distress syndrome in the infants of mothers requiring delivery after failed expectant management (24 to 41 percent),[42,59] antenatal steroids should be given in patients presenting between 25 and 33 weeks. Data on safety of repeated weekly doses of steroids are concerning enough that this practice is currently not recommended outside of investigational protocols.

If the mother responds to conservative management, she should be treated with bed rest, preferably in the hospital setting. Blood should always be available for maternal transfusion in the event of sudden hemorrhage. The length of maternal hospitalization in this instance is presently undergoing reevaluation. An initial study suggested that continued hospitalization until delivery was more cost effective than rest at home when total expenses for both mother and baby are calculated.[59] An additional reason for continued hospitalization was the observation that one half of all patients requiring early delivery because of failed expectant management do so because of excessive bleeding with or without uterine contractions.

Two recent studies have challenged this management plan.[60,61] In those retrospective studies, no significant advantage for either cost or morbidity was found with conservative hospital management until delivery.[50] Wing et al. showed that between 40 and 50 percent of patients presenting with bleeding placenta previa will be candidates for conservative management. Conservative management consisted of hydration, indicated blood transfusion, and magnesium sulfate tocolysis when uterine activity was apparent when the amniotic membranes were intact and the fetus exhibited a reactive nonstress test. After a 72 hour period of observed stability, patients with adequate resources (24-hour phone contact and 24-hour ability to rapidly return to the hospital) are candidates for home treatment. Treatment at home should include bed rest with bathroom privileges. In 15 percent of cases, the placenta previa will resolve radiographically in an average of 4 weeks. Treated conservatively, nearly 30 percent of patients with persistent placenta previa will progress to term without further bleeding. Approximately 70 percent of patients so treated can be expected to have at least one further episode of bleeding. However, only 10 percent will have a third episode. In patients with more than two episodes of significant bleeding, hospital treatment until delivery appears to be the safest strategy.

Approximately 25 to 30 percent of patients can be expected to complete 36 weeks' gestation without labor or repetitive bleeding forcing earlier delivery. In these patients, amniocentesis should be performed and, if the analysis of amniotic fluid documents pulmonary maturity, a cesarean delivery planned.

When encountering a patient with placenta previa, the possibility of a placenta accreta or one of its variations, placenta percreta or placenta increta, should be considered (Fig. 17–7).[62] In this condition, the placenta forms an abnormally firm attachment to the uterine wall. There is absence of the decidua basalis and incomplete development of the fibrinoid layer. The placenta can be attached directly to the myometrium (accreta), invade the myometrium (increta), or penetrate the myometrium (percreta). Antenatal diagnosis with ultrasound has been demonstrated by some authors.[63,64] However, in the largest reported series a false-positive diagnosis was reported in 20 percent of patients. Ultrasound findings most predictive of placenta accreta are thinning and distortion of the uterine serosa–bladder interface. Color Doppler imaging can also aid the detection of bladder invasion as illustrated in Figure 17–8.

Prior cesarean delivery and other uterine surgery are the factors most often associated with placenta accreta. In patients without prior uterine surgery who have placenta previa, the incidence of placenta accreta will be 4 percent. In patients with previous cesarean delivery who have placenta previa, the incidence of placenta accreta is approximately 10 to 35 percent.[44,47] In patients with multiple cesarean deliveries and placenta previa the risk of accreta is 60 to 65 percent. At least two thirds of the patients with placenta previa/placenta accreta will require cesarean hysterectomy.[42,65,66] However, in cases where uterine preservation is highly desired and no bladder invasion has occurred, bleeding after placental removal has been successfully controlled with a variety of surgical techniques. Packing of the lower uterine segment with subsequent removal of the pack through the vagina within 24 hours[66] has been successful. Interrupted circular suture of the lower uterine segment on the serosal surface of the uterus has

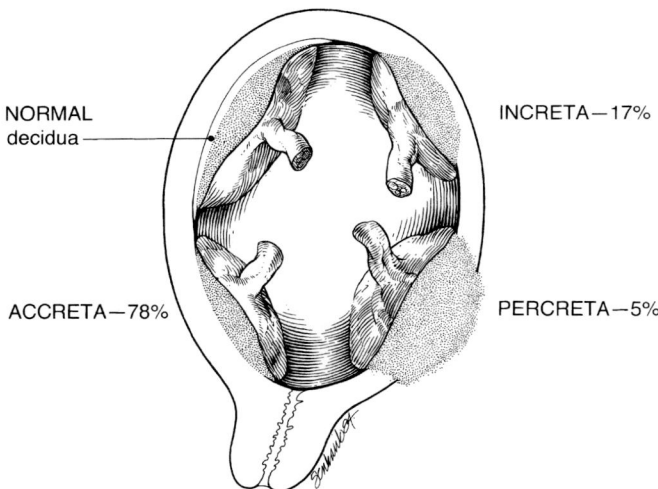

Figure 17–7. Uteroplacental relationships found in abnormal placentation.

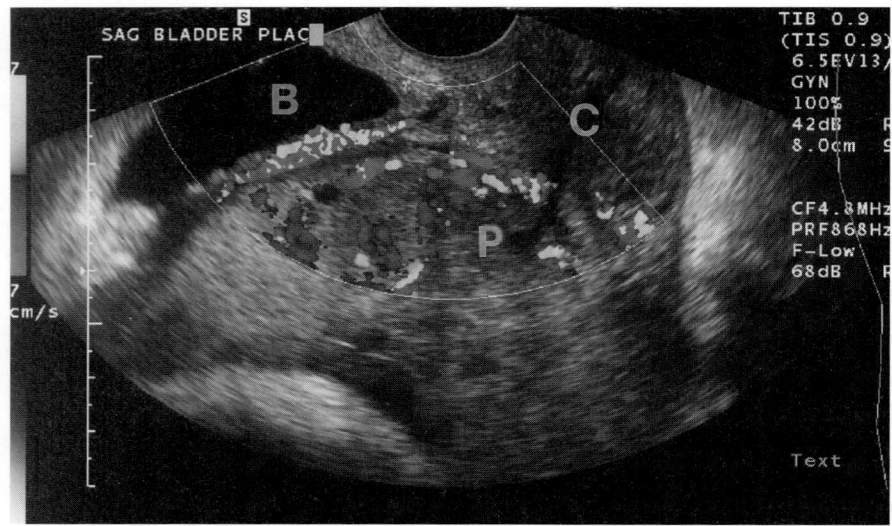

Figure 17–8. Color Doppler image of a placenta previa and placenta accreta with bladder invasion confirmed during operative delivery. Note the loss of the normal hyperechoic border between the placenta and the bladder. B, bladder; P, placenta; C, cervix.

also been reported to be successful.[67] Predelivery placement of catheters for angiographic embolization of pelvic vessels is another technique recently described.[68,69]

Complete placenta accreta suspected or confirmed before attempted placental removal may permit other treatment options. Bleeding may be minimal unless the placenta has partially separated. If no cleavage plane is identified and a placenta accreta is suspected, one should first make preparations for the possibility of major postpartum blood loss. At least 4 units of blood should be on hand and an anesthesiologist present in the delivery room. If vaginal delivery has occurred, the patient should be in a suite in which a laparotomy can be performed, and surgical instruments for hysterectomy should be sterilized and ready. Whenever possible, the obstetrician should discuss the likely diagnosis with the patient and review possible treatment options.

If uterine preservation is not important, or if maternal blood loss is excessive, hysterectomy offers the best chance for survival and will minimize morbidity.[70] If uterine preservation is important, four treatment options are available:

1. *Placental removal and oversewing the uterine defects.* After removing as much of the placenta as possible, the bleeding defects are oversewed and the patient treated with oxytocics and antibiotics (this option is probably most useful when there is significant bleeding from a partially separated placenta with only a focal accreta).
2. *Localized resection and uterine repair.*
3. *Curettage of the uterine cavity, and leaving the placenta in situ.* For the patient who wishes to maximize her chances for uterine preservation and who is not actively bleeding, the placenta may be left in situ. The umbilical cord should be ligated and cut as close to its base as possible. The patient should then

be treated with antibiotics. This approach has been successful when bleeding has not necessitated more aggressive surgical procedures.[71] Some authors have advocated treatment with methotrexate in this instance, but there is presently no consensus on whether this therapy is any more effective than observation.

4. In rare cases, placenta accreta invades the maternal bladder. In this instance, it is probably best to treat in a manner similar to abdominal pregnancy and avoid placental removal. However, this may not obviate the need for eventual hysterectomy and partial cystectomy.[72,73]

Third-Trimester Fetal Bleeding

A rare but important cause of third-trimester bleeding is that associated with rupture of a fetal vessel. Vasa previa is a condition in which the fetal vessels traverse the membranes in the lower uterine segment and cover the cervical os and occurs in approximately 1 in 1,000 to 1 in 5,000 pregnancies. With a velamentous insertion of the umbilical cord, its vessels often run between the chorion and amnion without the protection of Wharton's jelly. In other instances, a succenturiate placenta will have vascular communications between placental cotyledons. The classic presentation is spontaneous rupture of membranes, laceration of a fetal vessel, and rapid fetal death.

Ultrasound imaging now makes it possible to diagnose this condition in some instances, prior to the onset of fetal bleeding. The diagnosis of a succenturiate placental cotyledon or the discovery of an anomaly of the umbilical cord insertion should prompt the use of color Doppler examination of the membranes over the cervix. Both transabdominal and transcervical imaging have been used for this purpose. When umbilical arterial waveforms are documented at the same rate as the fetal heart rate, diagnosis is confirmed. When this occurs, careful observation and timing of elective cesarean section upon documentation of fetal pulmonary maturity should be considered.

When the fetal vessel ruptures, often acute vaginal bleeding is associated with an abrupt change in the fetal heart rate. The fetal heart rate pattern often shows an initial fetal tachycardia followed by bradycardia with intermittent accelerations. Short-term variability is frequently maintained.

One must have a high index of suspicion to make the correct diagnosis. In most instances, one must make the diagnosis rapidly and institute definitive therapy and delivery to optimize fetal outcome. The fetal mortality in this condition has been reported to be greater than 50 percent.[74,75] Figure 17-9 illustrates the fetal heart rate tracing of a successfully treated case of spontaneous rupture of a velamentous insertion of the fetal vessel.

On occasion when the fetal heart rate is not abnormal and the source of the bleeding is in question, an examination of the blood passed vaginally can be performed. Adult oxyhemoglobin is less resistant to alkali than fetal oxyhemoglobin. There are three tests for fetal hemoglobin using alkaline denaturation: Apt, Ogita, and Loendersloot.[76] All take from 5 to 10 minutes to perform. They all have good sensitivity for detection of pure fetal blood. However, when the blood is mixed with amniotic fluid, the Apt and the Loendersloot tests were not able to identify fetal blood at concentrations less than 60 percent. The Ogita test was able to detect fetal blood at levels of only 20 percent and requires less sample than the other tests.

To perform the Ogita test, one drop of sample is added to five drops of alkali (0.1 mole potassium hydroxide) and shaken for 2 minutes. Ten drops of precipitation solution (400 ml of 50 percent saturated ammonium sulfate and 1 ml of 10-mole hydrochloric acid) are added. The mixture is dropped on a filter paper with a capillary tube to make a 20-mm ring. Fetal hemoglobin will form a colored ring at the periphery of the deposited sample within 30 seconds.

In most cases, there is rarely time to perform this test. In the acute situation, the diagnosis is based on clinical findings unless there has been prior ultrasound suspicion of vasa previa.

POSTPARTUM HEMORRHAGE

Acute blood loss is the most common cause of hypotension in obstetrics. Hemorrhage usually occurs immediately preceding or after delivery of the placenta. Excessive blood loss most commonly results when the uterus fails to contract after the delivery of its contents. Effective hemostasis after separation of the placenta is dependent on contraction of the myometrium to compress severed vessels. Failure of the uterus to contract can usually be attributed to myometrial dysfunction and retained placental fragments. Factors predisposing to myometrial dysfunction include overdistention of the uterus as in multiple pregnancy, fetal macrosomia, hydramnios, oxytocin-stimulated labor, uterine relaxants, and amnionitis. At term, approximately 600 ml/min of blood flows through the placental site. However, blood loss from severe uterine atony can easily exceed this rate because blood is lost from the entire intrauterine surface when the uterus fails to contract.

Prevention

Reduction of excessive blood loss after vaginal birth or cesarean delivery can be aided by recognizing high-risk factors for postpartum hemorrhage (Table 17-3) and by applying proven methods to limit bleeding. Some techniques with demonstrated effectiveness have still not found their way into general use by many obstetric practitioners, including active management of the third stage of labor and spontaneous delivery of the placenta at time of cesarean delivery. Dilute solutions of oxytocin in addition to gentle cord traction reduces cesarean delivery associated blood loss by 31 percent compared with manual removal of the placenta.[77] Similarly, umbilical cord clamping within 30 seconds of delivery and gentle cord traction followed by administration of intramuscular or dilute solutions of intravenous oxytocin before delivery of the placenta reduce postpartum blood loss and postpartum transfusion requirements.[78] Administration of oxytocin before delivery of the placenta is associated with a reduction in the length of the third stage of labor (mean 5 minutes) and a low incidence of manual removal of the placenta (2 percent) compared with physiologic management of the third stage of labor (15 minutes and 2.5 percent, respectively).[78] When the placenta is retained for 30 minutes

Table 17-3. RISK FACTORS FOR OBSTETRIC HEMORRHAGE OF > 1,000 ml

Factor	Risk Increase
Placental abruption	12.6
Placenta previa	13.1
Multiple pregnancy	4.5
Obesity	1.6
Retained placenta	5.2
Induced labor	2.2
Episiotomy	2.1
Birth weight > 4 kg	1.9

From Stones RW, Paterson CM, Saunders NJ: Risk factors for major obstetric hemorrhage. Eur J Obstet Gynecol Reprod Biol 48:15, 1993, with permission.

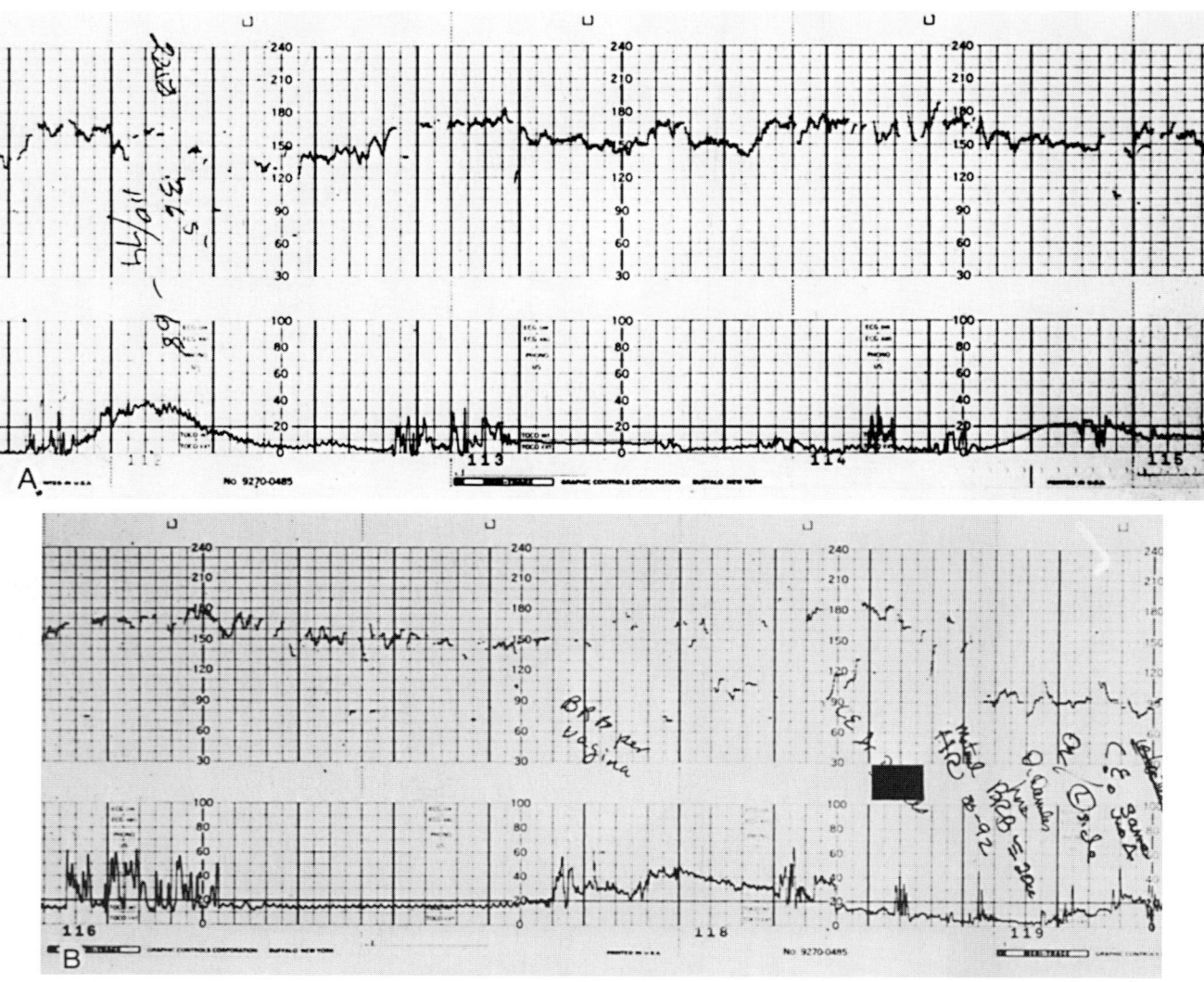

Figure 17–9. Fetal heart rate tracing after rupture of a velamentous insertion of the cord. *A,* Normal fetal heart rate tracing in early labor at term showing accelerations but no other changes. *B,* Just before panel 118, bright red vaginal bleeding is noted. Shortly thereafter, the fetal heart rate is noted to be 80 to 90 beats/min.

Illustration continued on opposite page

or longer, randomized studies have shown that injection of the umbilical cord with either saline or oxytocin has no significant benefit in effecting spontaneous delivery of the placenta. In the absence of significant maternal hemorrhage, an additional 30 minutes of expectant management can be allowed because half of the retained placentas will deliver spontaneously during this time, avoiding the need for manual removal, anesthesia, and excessive blood loss.

Spontaneous delivery of the placenta after administration of oxytocin is also associated with reduced blood loss during cesarean section. Randomized trials have shown that both the risk of endometritis and the mean blood loss are significantly lower when the placenta is delivered spontaneously. Blood loss was reduced by 30 percent and postpartum endometritis re-

duced sevenfold when compared to manual removal of the placenta.[79]

Upon encountering postpartum hemorrhage, manual digital exploration of the uterus should be quickly accomplished to rule out the possibility of retained placental fragments (Fig. 17–10). If retained tissue is not detected, manual massage of the uterus should be started (Fig. 17–11). Simultaneously, pharmacologic methods should be employed to control uterine bleeding. Initial therapy includes the administration of a dilute solution of oxytocin, usually 10 to 20 units of oxytocin in 1,000 ml of physiologic saline solution. The solution can be administered in rates as high as 500 ml in 10 minutes without cardiovascular complications. However, an intravenous bolus injection of as little as 5 units of oxytocin may be associated with maternal hy-

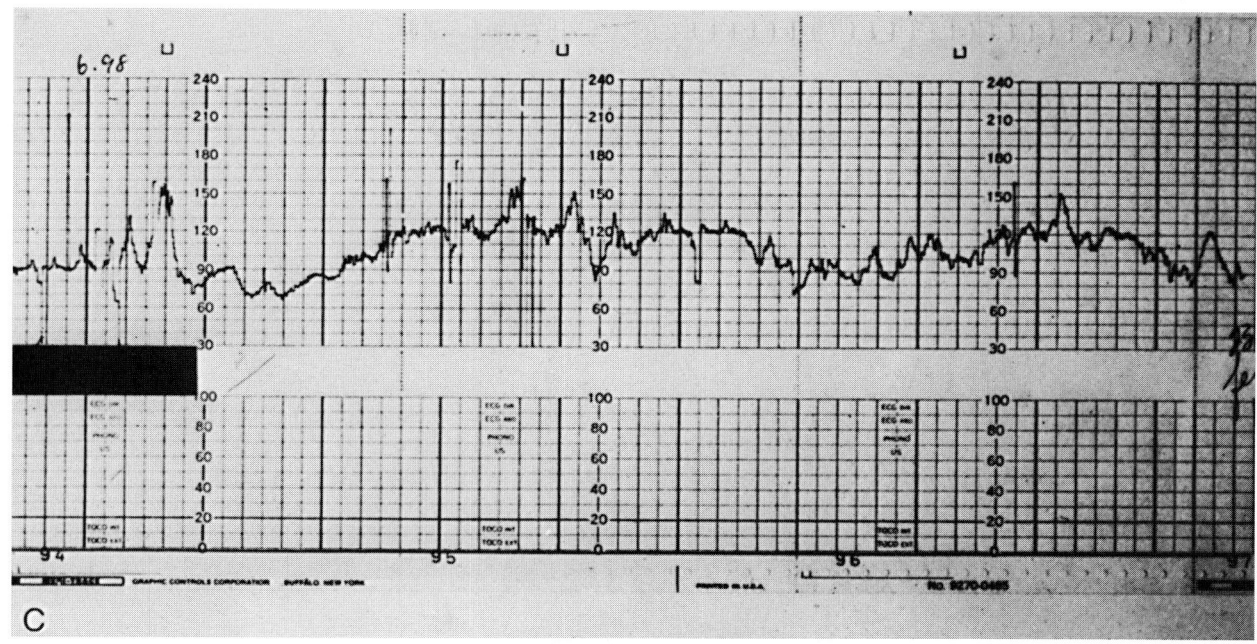

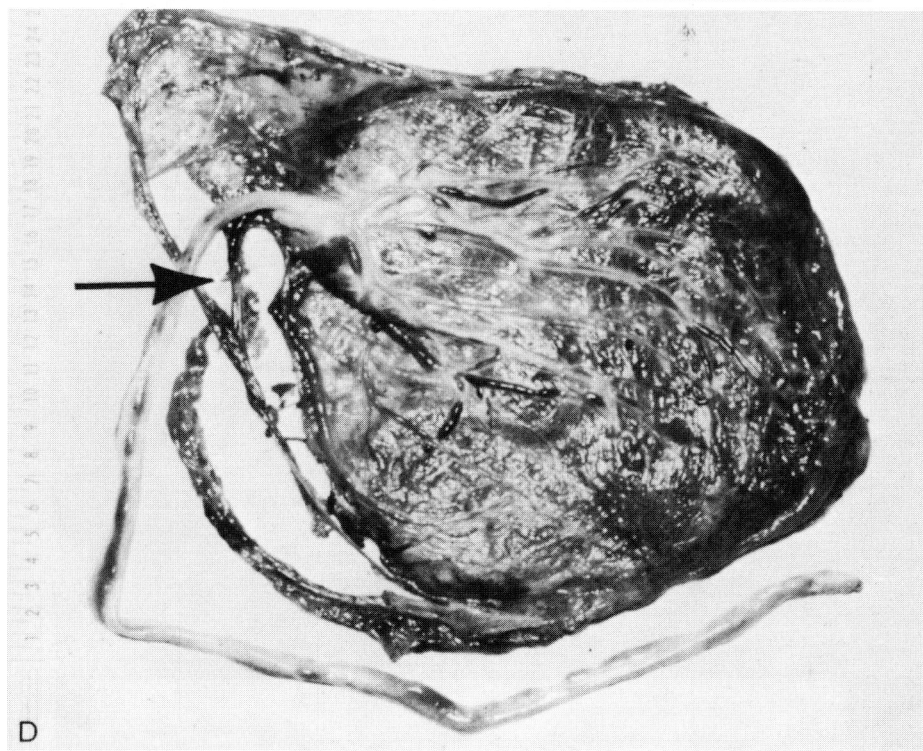

Figure 17–9. *(Continued) C,* In the delivery room, the fetal heart rate tracing shows the characteristic bradycardia-tachycardia heart rate response as the fetus attempts to compensate for acute blood loss. An emergency cesarean delivery was performed, and the infant was anemic. After rapid volume infusion and resuscitation, the infant survived and is developing normally. *D,* Examination of the placenta showed a velamentous insertion of the umbilical cord and a lacerated fetal vessel as a result of spontaneous rupture of the membranes. In this case, the unprotected fetal vessels passed over the cervical os, a vasa previa.

potension, further stressing an already compromised maternal cardiovascular system.

When oxytocin fails to produce adequate uterine contraction, most clinicians now administer synthetic 15-methyl-$F_{2\alpha}$-prostaglandin (Prostin, Upjohn). Although ergovine (0.2 mg intramuscularly) has been a standard second-line drug for many years, the efficacy and safety of prostaglandin medications in this instance have obviated the need to use ergonovine in most instances. Initial studies with prostaglandin medications for postpartum hemorrhage were performed with the naturally occurring $F_{2\alpha}$-prostaglandin compound, which required direct intrauterine injection. The total dose used was 1 to 2 mg diluted in 10 to 20 ml of saline.[80] Subsequently, clinical trials of the synthetic 15-methyl-$F_{2\alpha}$-prostaglandin produced promising results.[82] This

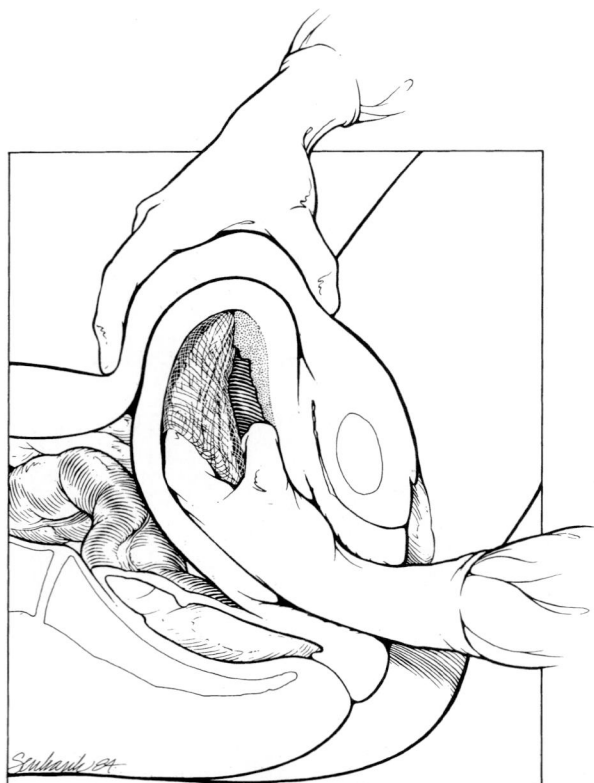

Figure 17–10. Digital exploration of the uterus and removal of retained membranes. A sponge has been wrapped around the examiner's fingers.

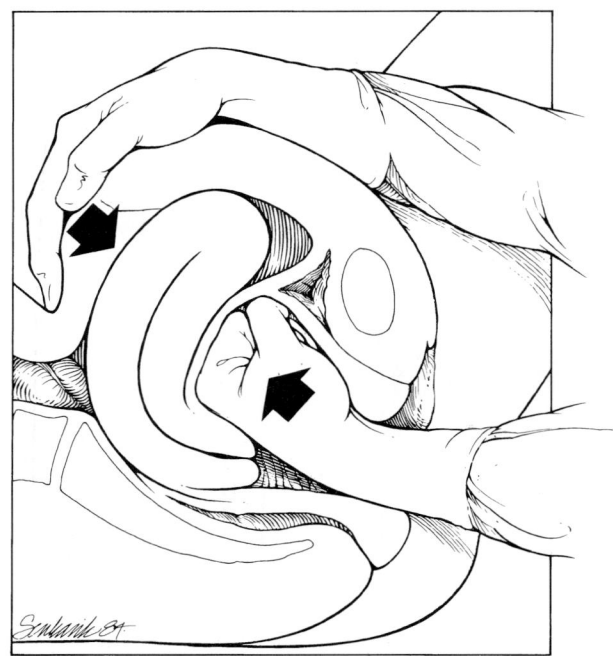

Figure 17–11. Manual compression and massage of the uterus to control bleeding from uterine atony.

compound should be given in 0.25-mg doses in the deltoid muscle every 1 to 2 hours. As many as five doses may be administered without adverse effect. Experience at the University of Washington would support these observations, as the routine availability of this agent in the delivery unit has arrested a number of otherwise uncontrollable hemorrhages.

A recent uncontrolled report of a newer agent, misoprostol, for the control of refractory hemorrhage may represent a promising new medical option. O'Brien et al. used 1,000 μg of misoprostol per rectum in patients with refractory uterine bleeding prior to the administration of 15-methyl-F$_{2\alpha}$-prostaglandin.[81] Control of uterine bleeding was reported in all cases and no further uterotonic medications were necessary. Further studies are necessary to determine the exact place and safety of misoprostol during postpartum hemorrhage from uterine atony.

When pharmacologic methods fail to control hemorrhage from atony, surgical measures should be undertaken to arrest the bleeding before it becomes life threatening. However, before a laparotomy, a careful inspection of the vagina and cervix should be made to confirm that the uterus is the source of the bleeding.

If the uterus is found to be contracted appropriately

and no placental fragments are retained within the uterus, a laceration of maternal soft tissues is the likely cause of continued vaginal bleeding. Careful inspection of the cervix and vagina will often indicate the source of the bleeding. Figures 17–12 through 17–15 illustrate second-, third-, and fourth-degree lacerations of the perineum and techniques for their repair. Adequate exposure for the repair of such lacerations is critical and, if needed, assistance should be summoned to aid in retraction.

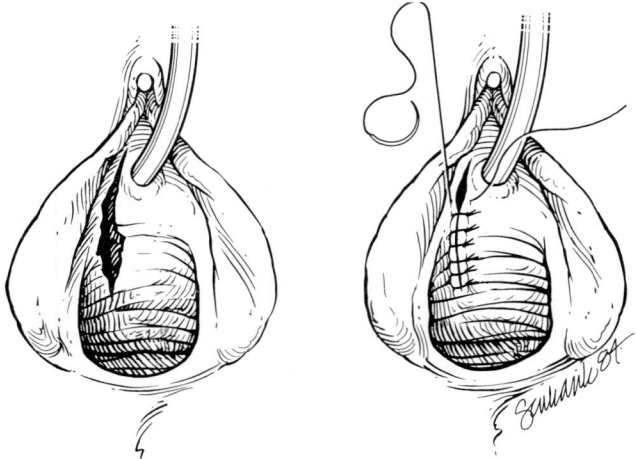

Figure 17–12. Repair of an anterior periurethral laceration. Either running or interrupted sutures can be used. An indwelling catheter is placed before the repair is made.

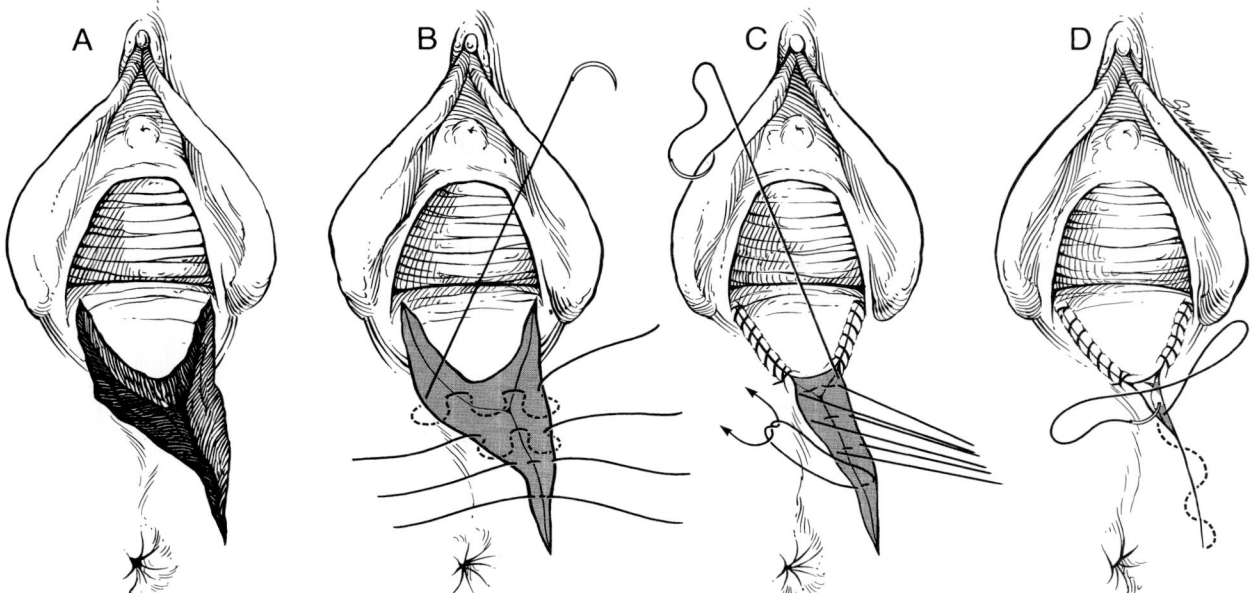

Figure 17–13. Repair of a second-degree laceration. A first-degree laceration involves the fourchet, the perineal skin, and the vaginal mucous membrane. A second-degree laceration also includes the muscles of the perineal body. The rectal sphincter remains intact.

In cervical laceration, it is important to secure the base of the laceration, which is often a major source of bleeding. However, this area is frequently the most difficult to suture. Valuable time can be lost trying to expose the angle of such a laceration. A helpful technique to use in these cases, especially when help is limited or slow in responding, is to start to suture the laceration at its proximal end, using the suture for trac-

tion to expose the more distal portion of the cervix until the apex is in view (Fig. 17–16). This technique has the added advantage of arresting significant bleeding from the edges of laceration.

When uterine bleeding is not responsive to pharmacologic methods and no vaginal or cervical lacerations are present, surgical exploration may be necessary. Laceration of uterine vessels during the birth process will

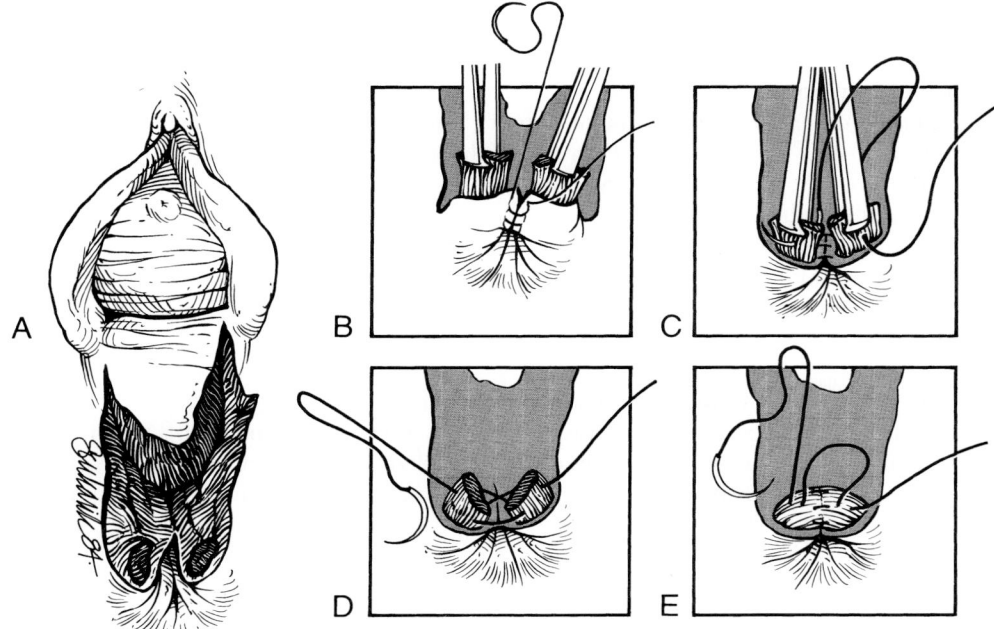

Figure 17–14. Repair of the sphincter after a third-degree laceration. A third-degree laceration extends not only through the skin, mucous membrane, and perineal body, but includes the anal sphincter. Interrupted figure-of-eight sutures should be placed in the capsule of the sphincter muscle.

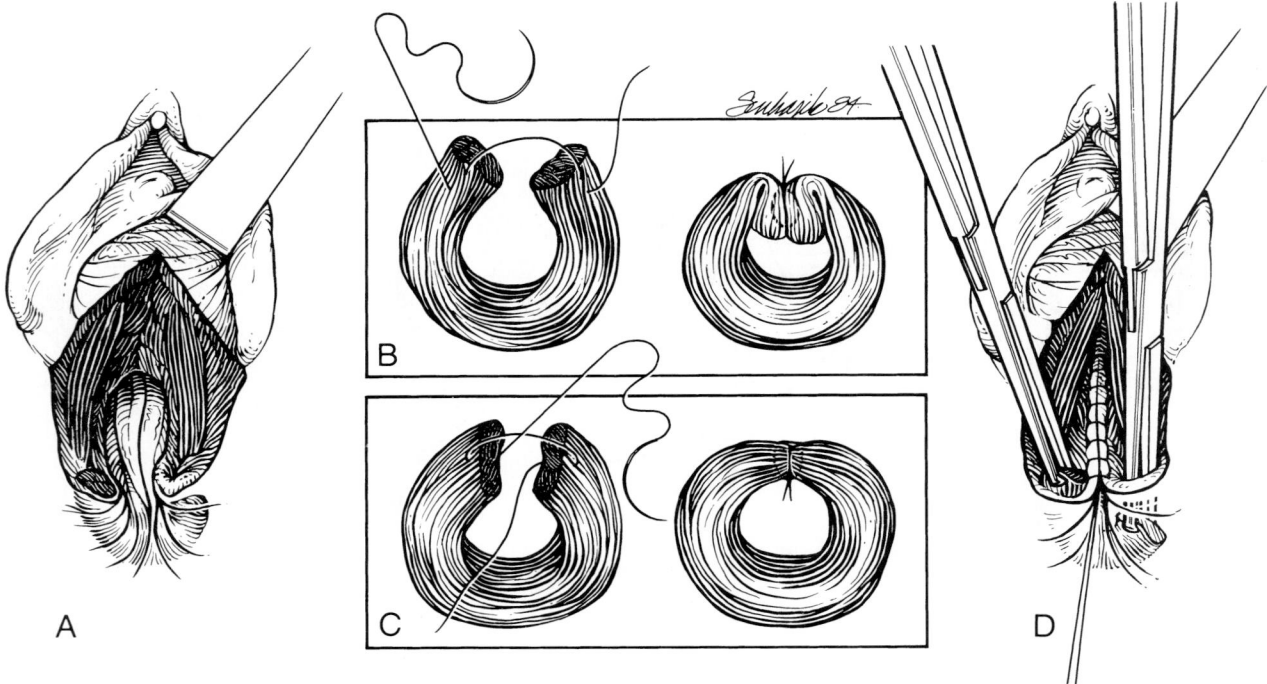

Figure 17–15. Repair of a fourth-degree laceration. This laceration extends through the rectal mucosa. *A,* The extent of this laceration is shown, with a segment of the rectum exposed. *B,* Approximation of the rectal submucosa. This is the most commonly recommended method for repair. *C,* Alternative method of approximating the rectal mucosa in which the knots are actually buried inside the rectal lumen. *D,* After closure of the rectal submucosa, an additional layer of running sutures may be placed. The rectal sphincter is then repaired.

occasionally be found. On occasion, bleeding will be similar to that from uterine atony, but the uterus will appear contracted. On other occasions, substantial episodic hemorrhage followed by periods of relatively little blood flow will occur. Hayashi et al. have recently documented 3- to 8 cm-longitudinal lacerations of the inner myometrium as a cause of bleeding refractory to the usual techniques.[83] Hysterectomy specimens have demonstrated longitudinal laceration of the lower uterine segment myometrium to depths of 3 to 10 mm. They have termed this condition inner myometrial laceration. It appears to be an incomplete type of uterine rupture. It is often difficult to diagnose this condition before the hysterectomy is performed. When the uterine arteries and the cardinal ligaments are clamped and cut in this condition, the uterine cavity will often be entered because of the attenuated nature of the myometrium in these areas.

If hemorrhage is secondary to atony, vascular ligation will often be necessary to control bleeding. Hypogastric artery ligation, a technique recommended for many decades to control postpartum hemorrhage, has fallen out of favor because of the prolonged operating time, technical difficulties associated with its performance, and an inconsistent clinical response. Instead, a stepwise progression of uterine vessel ligation should be

rapidly accomplished. Ligation of the ascending branch of the uterine arteries should be attempted as a first step if hemorrhage is unresponsive to oxytocin or prostaglandin[84,85] (Fig. 17–17*A* and *B*). The uterine artery should be located at the border between the upper and lower uterine segment and suture ligated with 0 or No. 1 chromic suture. The suture should be placed 2 cm medial to the uterine artery and the needle driven from the anterior surface of the uterus posteriorly and tied. Because the suture is placed high in the lower uterine segment, the ureter is not in jeopardy and the bladder usually does not need to be mobilized. In approximately 10 to 15 percent of cases of atony, unilateral ligation of the uterine artery is sufficient to control hemorrhage. Bilateral ligation will control an additional 75 percent.[85]

If bleeding continues, attention should next be paid to interrupting the blood flow to the uterus from the infundibulopelvic ligament (Fig. 17–17*C*). There are a number of techniques to accomplish this. The easiest involves ligation of the anastomosis of the ovarian and uterine artery, high on the fundus, just below the utero-varian ligament. A large suture on an atraumatic needle can be passed from the uterus, around the vessel, and tied. If bilateral uterovarian vessel ligation does not stop the bleeding, temporary occlusion of the infundi-

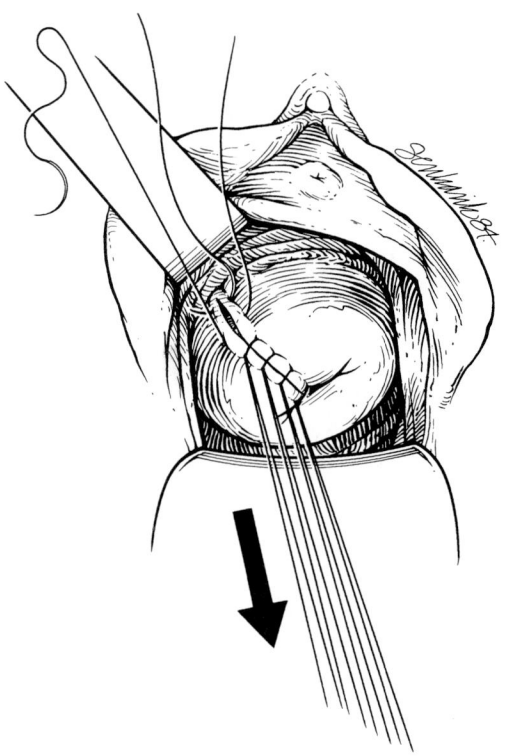

Figure 17–16. Repair of a cervical laceration, which begins at the proximal part of the laceration, using traction on the previous sutures to aid in exposing the distal portion of the defect.

bulopelvic ligament vessels may be attempted. This can be accomplished with digital pressure or with rubber-sleeved clamps. It may be an especially useful technique if the patient is of low parity and future childbearing is of great importance. If this appears to control hemorrhage, ligation of the infundibulopelvic ligament can be performed by passing an absorbable suture from anterior to posterior through the avascular area inferior to and including the ovarian vessels. Although the ovarian blood supply may be decreased, successful pregnancy has been reported after all major pelvic vessels were ligated to arrest postpartum hemorrhage.[72,73]

There are two recently described surgical techniques for the control of hemorrhage secondary to uterine atony: hemostatic suturing and the B-Lynch surgical technique.[87,88] Both of these techniques use surgical tamponade of the uterus to control bleeding. Neither has been subjected to randomized trials, but reports of cessation of hemorrhage secondary to atony is reported to be successful in clinical circumstances in which usual medical and surgical treatments have failed to control hemorrhage. These techniques may be considered prior to hysterectomy in women of low parity in whom preservation of childbearing is desired.

A prerequisite to successful use of the B-Lynch or brace suture technique is the control of uterine bleeding with manual compression of the uterus. Assessment of bleeding should be done by direct visualization through the vagina by placing the patient in a supine frogleg position during the operation. It is important to confirm cessation of bleeding with manual compression both before performing the B-Lynch procedure and after the procedure has been performed. Technical details of the procedure can be found in the original article.

Another hemostatic suturing technique recently described involves placing multiple 2- to 3-cm^2 sutures in the myometrium using a through-and-through suture of No. 1 chromic. With this procedure, segments of the anterior and posterior uterine wall are sewn together and tied tightly, compressing the intervening myometrium. This technique can be used in the upper portion of the uterus to control bleeding from atony or in the lower uterine segment to control bleeding from low-lying placental implantation.

Selective Arterial Embolization

Arterial embolization is currently an increasingly common therapeutic option for various types of obstetric hemorrhage. The radiographic approach to obstetric hemorrhage has a number of advantages over the surgical approach: anesthetic and surgical risks are reduced, specific vessels can be identified and selectively occluded, and hysterectomy can be avoided. In addition to embolization, transient transcatheter uterine artery balloon occlusion can aid in the management of surgical cases where extreme hemorrhage has been a common occurrence. The obstetric conditions in which arterial embolization have been successfully employed include postpartum bleeding from atony, bleeding from pelvic vessel laceration, postcesarean hemorrhage, and bleeding associated with extrauterine pregnancy. In the absence of coagulopathy, the success rate of arterial embolization has been reported to be greater than 90 percent.

Procedure-specific complications occur in less than 10 percent of cases. Postprocedure fever and pelvic infection are most commonly reported. Much less common, but potentially more serious, is reflux of embolic material to nontargeted pelvic structures. Currently, there are no procedure-related deaths described in obstetric patients.

In order to maximize the full potential of this technique, a close working relationship between the obstetric team and the interventional radiologists must exist. Preoperative identification of patients at high risk for life-threatening hemorrhage is the responsibility of the obstetrician. Such conditions will include, but not be limited to, placenta accreta, cervical pregnancy, and abdominal pregnancy. Prophylactic catheterization of the anterior division of the internal iliac arteries can be

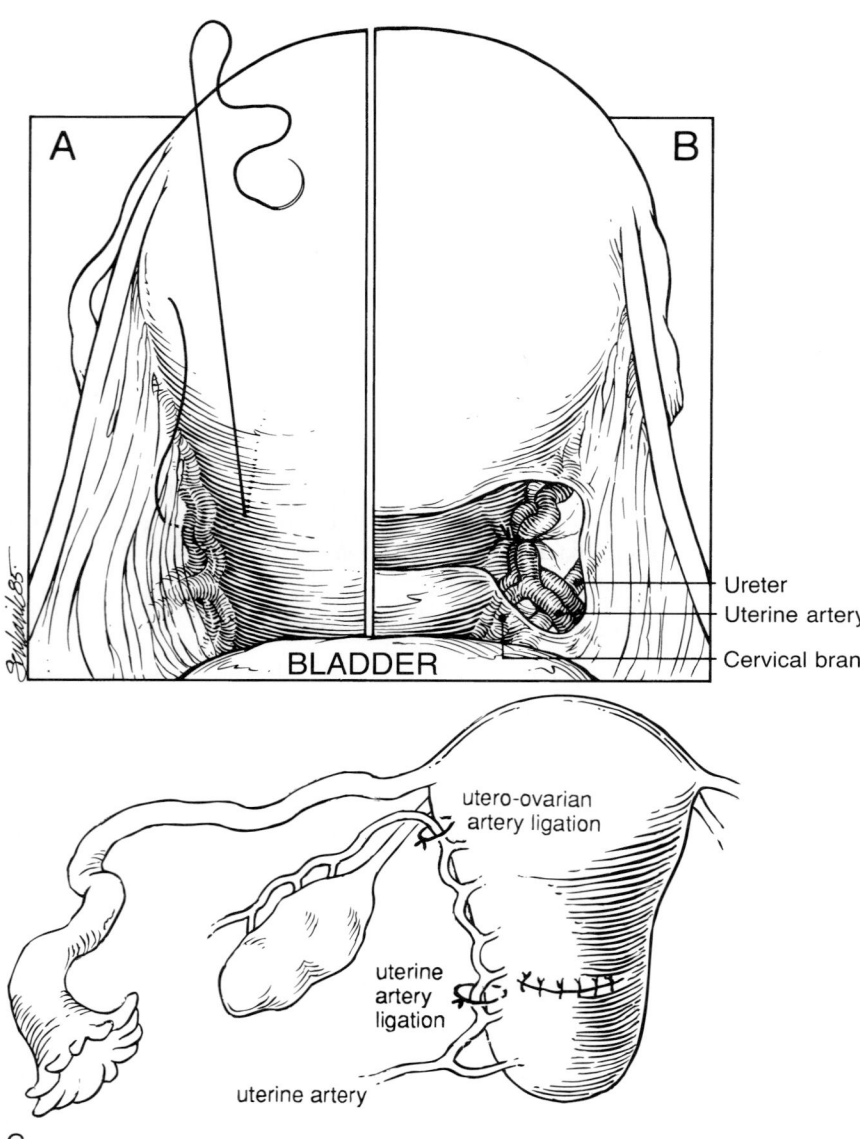

Ureter
Uterine artery
Cervical branch

BLADDER

utero-ovarian
artery ligation

uterine
artery
ligation

uterine artery

C

Figure 17–17. Ligation of the uterine artery. *A* and *B*, This anterior view of the uterus demonstrates the placement of a suture around the ascending branch of the uterine artery and vein as described by O'Leary and O'Leary. Note that 2 to 3 cm of myometrium medial to the vessels has been included in the ligature. The vessels are not divided. *C*, View of sutured uterus: ligated uterine artery, and ligated utero-ovarian artery.

done in less than 10 minutes with fluoroscopy. However, radiation exposures of 2 rad/min should be expected. Whether this potential fetal risk is justified by the opportunity to avoid life-threatening hemorrhage is a decision that must be made in consultation with the patient.[90–94]

Pelvic Hematoma

Blood loss leading to cardiovascular instability is not always visible. In some instances, traumatic laceration of blood vessels may lead to the formation of a pelvic hematoma. Pelvic hematomas may be divided into three main types: vulvar, vaginal, or retroperitoneal.

Vulvar Hematoma

This type of hematoma results from laceration of vessels in the superficial fascia of either the anterior or posterior pelvic triangle. The usual physical signs are subacute volume loss and vulvar pain. The blood loss in this case is limited by Colle's fascia and the urogenital diaphragm. In the posterior area, the limitations are the anal fascia. Because of these fascial boundaries, the mass will extend to the skin and a visible hematoma will result (Figs. 17–18 and 17–19).

Treatment in these cases requires the volume support outlined previously. Surgical management calls for wide linear incision of the mass through the skin and evacuation of blood and clots. As this condition is often the result of bleeding from small vessels, the lacerated ves-

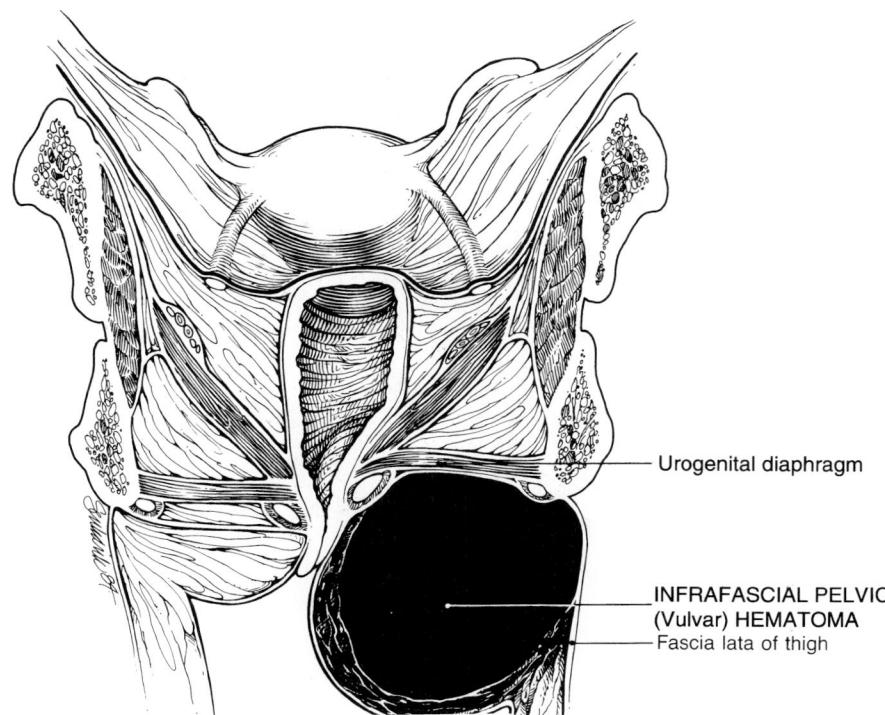

Urogenital diaphragm

INFRAFASCIAL PELVIC
(Vulvar) HEMATOMA
Fascia lata of thigh

Figure 17–18. Vulvar hematoma, showing anatomic landmarks.

sel will not usually be identified. Once the clot has been evacuated, the dead space can be closed with sutures. The area should then be compressed by a large sterile dressing and pressure applied. Efforts to pack the cavity are usually futile and only serve to create further bleeding. An indwelling catheter should be placed in the bladder at the start of the surgical evacuation and left in place for 24 to 36 hours. Compression can be removed after 12 hours.

Vaginal Hematoma

Vaginal hematomas may result from trauma to maternal soft tissues during delivery. These hematomas are frequently associated with a forceps delivery but may occur spontaneously. They are less common than vulvar hematomas. In this instance, blood accumulates in the plane above the level of the pelvic diaphragm (Fig. 17–20). It is unusual for large amounts of blood to collect in this space. The most frequent complaint in such cases is severe rectal pressure. Examination will reveal a large mass protruding into the vagina.

Vaginal hematomas should be treated by incision of the vagina and evacuation. Figure 17–21 shows an ultrasound of a vaginal hematoma recognized 3 weeks postpartum. Even with delayed recognition of a vaginal hematoma, evacuation should be undertaken. The accumulated blood will take many weeks to reabsorb and the patient's discomfort will usually be intolerable for such a long period of time. As with vulvar hematomas, it is uncommon to find a single bleeding vessel as the source of bleeding. The incision need not be closed, as the edges of the vagina will fall back together after the clot has been removed. A vaginal pack should be inserted to tamponade the raw edges. The pack is then removed in 12 to 18 hours.

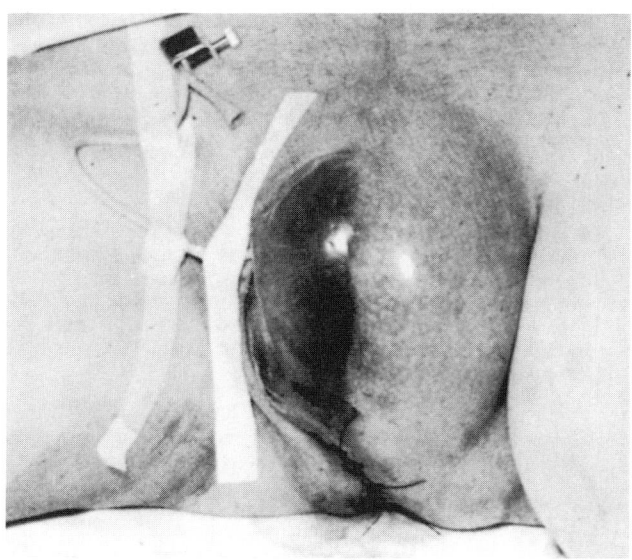

Figure 17–19. Photograph of vulvar hematoma before evacuation.

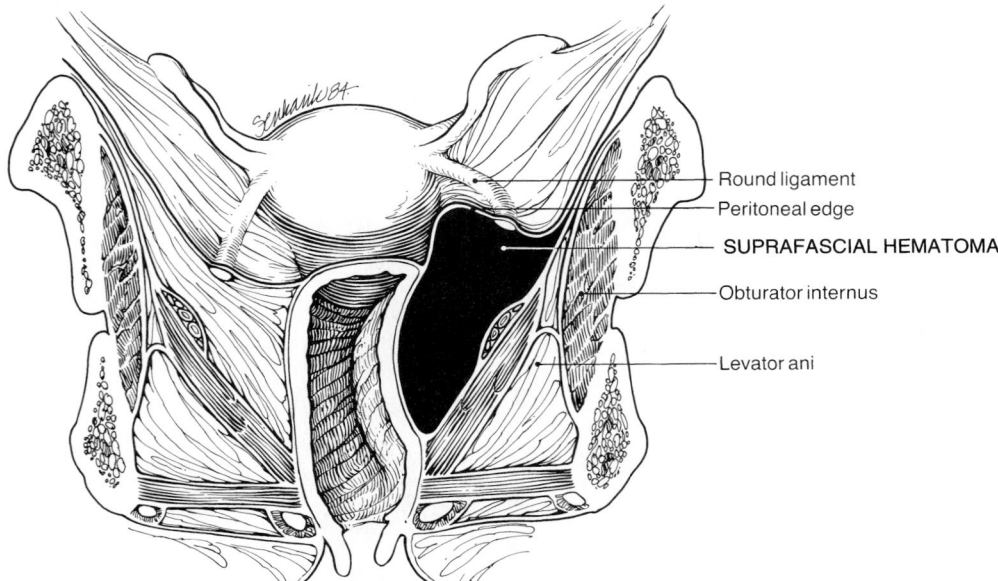

Figure 17–20. Vaginal hematoma showing anatomic landmarks.

Round ligament
Peritoneal edge
SUPRAFASCIAL HEMATOMA
Obturator internus
Levator ani

Retroperitoneal Hematoma

Retroperitoneal hematomas are the least common of the pelvic hematomas but are the most dangerous to the mother. Symptoms from a retroperitoneal hematoma may not be impressive until the sudden onset of hypotension or shock. A retroperitoneal hematoma occurs after laceration of one of the vessels originating from the hypogastric artery (Fig. 17–22). Such lacerations may result from inadequate hemostasis of the uterine arteries at the time of cesarean delivery or after rupture of a low transverse cesarean delivery scar dur-

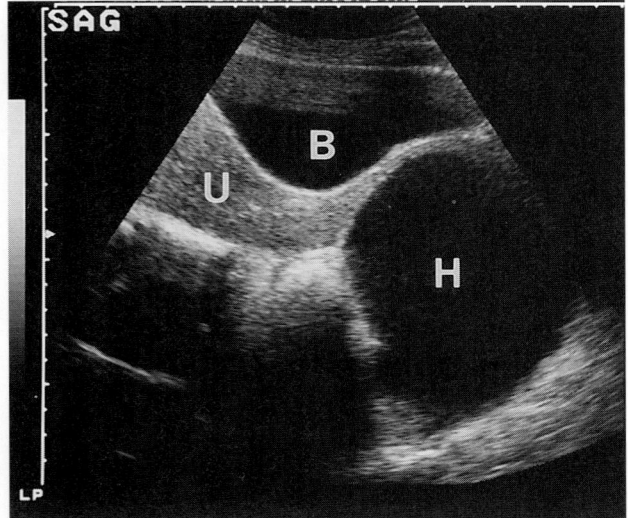

Figure 17–21. Abdominal ultrasound image of larger vaginal hematoma, approximately 3 weeks postpartum. B, bladder; U, uterus; H, hematoma.

ing a trial of labor. In these patients, blood may dissect up to the renal vasculature.

Treatment of this life-threatening condition involves surgical exploration and ligation of the hypogastric vessels on both the lacerated side and on the contralateral side if unilateral ligation does not arrest the bleeding. On occasion, it may be possible to open the hematomas and identify the bleeding vessel.

Umbrella Pack

The use of an umbrella pack to control bleeding after hysterectomy is a valuable technique in desperate situations (Fig. 17–23). This technique may be needed after cesarean hysterectomy complicated by persistent bleeding from the vaginal cuff. Such hemorrhage may be encountered after massive blood loss secondary to the washout of platelets or as a result of DIC. In either instance, it may be impossible to control the generalized oozing from the vaginal cuff except with pressure. The umbrella pack will often permit one to tamponade the bleeding surfaces until coagulation factors and platelets can be given and, in addition, enables the surgeon to close the abdomen without the fear of continued blood loss.

The pack itself should be a bag or sack of nonadhesive material. A small plastic bag serves the purpose very well. The bag can be inserted through the vagina or at laparotomy. When abdominal placement is possible, the bag should be filled with 2-in gauze packing through the vagina to ensure an orderly packing that will facilitate removal at a future time. The bag should be filled with enough gauze to occlude the open vaginal

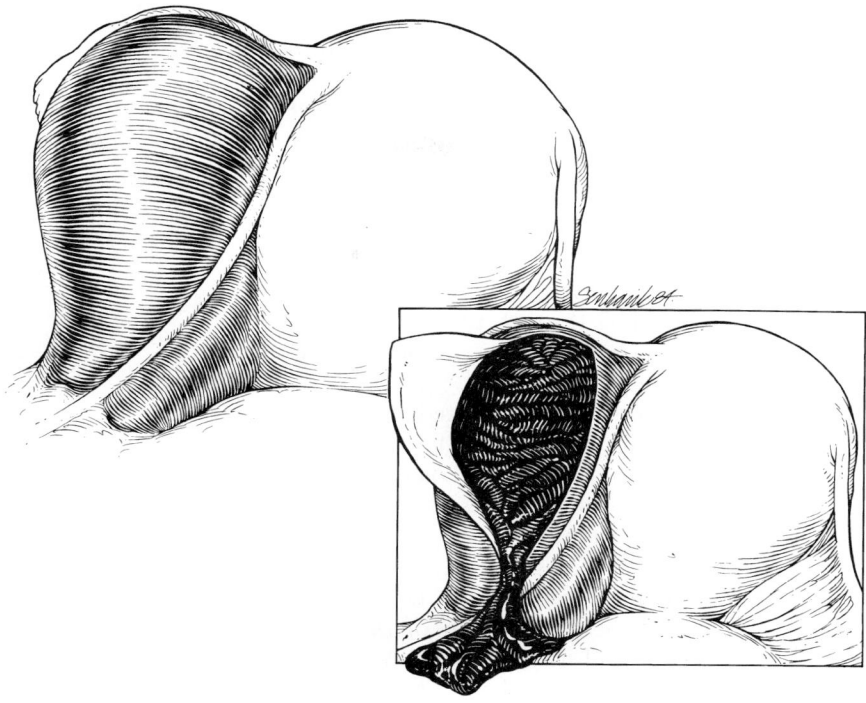

Figure 17–22. Retroperitoneal hematoma as a result of laceration of one of the branches of the hypogastric artery. Evacuation of the hematoma is illustrated in the accompanying panel.

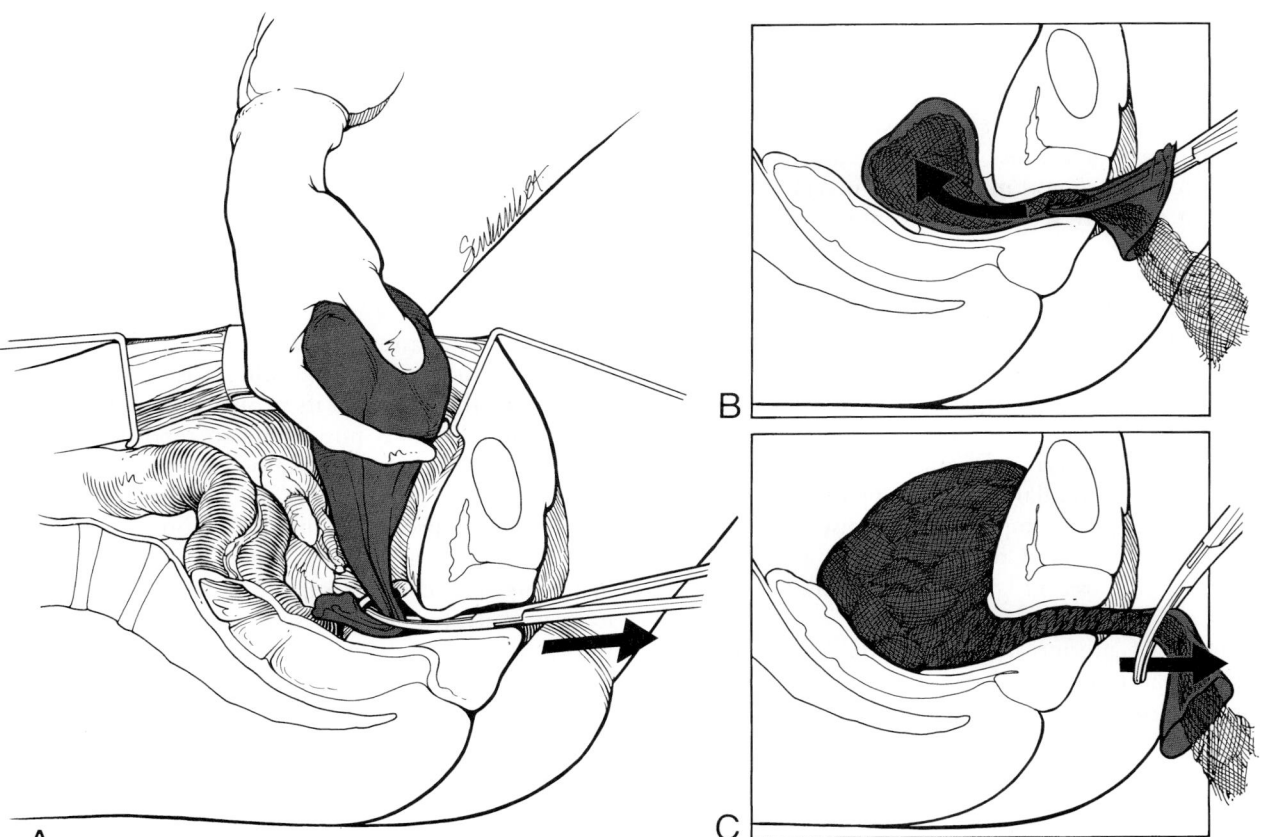

Figure 17–23. Abdominal placement of an umbrella pack to control hemorrhage from the vaginal cuff. *A*, Vaginal route for insertion of gauge packing. The pack is pulled downward over the vaginal cuff (*B*) and is secured (*C*).

cuff completely and present enough resistance to prevent expulsion when a weight is attached to the end of the pack.

Once the pack is in true pelvis and the gauze has been inserted, a 1,000-ml intravenous bag should be tied to the umbrella pack and traction applied. Traction should be maintained for 24 hours. After 24 hours, the traction may be relieved, but the bag should be left in place for an additional 12 hours. After 36 hours, the gauze packing should be removed by pulling on the tail that has been left protruding through the vagina. After the gauze has been evacuated, the bag should be removed.

Two major complications of this procedure include infection and urinary obstruction. The latter can be obviated by the use of an indwelling Foley catheter. The danger of infection is an ever-present one but is usually of secondary importance in the acute events surrounding such massive bleeding. Prophylactic antibiotics should be used in these cases. Since the publication of this technique in the first edition of this textbook, three cases of successful use of the umbrella pack in obstetric patients have been published.[95,96]

Inversion of the Uterus

Occasionally, the third stage of labor is complicated by partial delivery of the placenta followed by rapid onset of shock in the mother. These events characterize uterine inversion. Hypotension usually results before significant blood loss has occurred. The inexperienced obstetrician may mistake an inversion of the uterus for a partially separated placenta or aborted myoma.

Uterine inversion is an uncommon but life-threatening event. Since 1970, the reported incidence has been 1 in 2,000 deliveries.[97] Inversion of the uterus is termed incomplete if the corpus does not pass through the cervix, complete if the corpus passes through the cervix, and prolapsed if the corpus extends through the vaginal introitus. Uterine inversion usually occurs in association with a fundally inserted placenta. Although previous studies have implicated the use of excessive cord traction and the Crede maneuver as causes of uterine inversion, recent studies have failed to document this association.[97]

Treatment of uterine inversion should include fluid therapy for the mother and restoration of the uterus to its normal position. This latter is best accomplished using the technique illustrated in Figure 17–24 and should be attempted immediately upon recognition of the inversion. Separation of the placenta before replacement of the uterus will only increase maternal blood loss.[98] If possible, the uterus should be replaced without removing the placenta. Initial efforts to replace the uterus should be made without the use of uterine-relax-

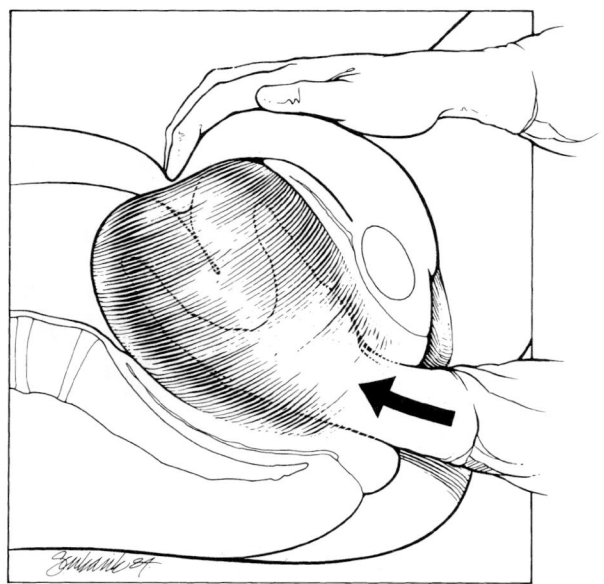

Figure 17–24. Manual replacement of an inverted uterus.

ing agents. If initial efforts fail, the use of either β-mimetic agents or magnesium sulfate should be tried. The choice of these agents depends on the maternal vital signs. In the case of severe maternal hypotension, magnesium sulfate is probably the best choice. These agents have been reported to be safe and associated with an 85 to 90 percent success rate in patients failing initial replacement without pharmacologic therapy. In 10 to 15 percent of remaining cases, general anesthesia should be employed.[99] Subacute inversion of the uterus occurs when the corpus has protruded through the cervix, and the cervix and lower uterine segment have subsequently contracted, thereby trapping the corpus. In this instance, general anesthesia is necessary for restoration of the uterus to its proper anatomic position.

Occasionally, it is impossible to reposition the subacutely inverted uterus vaginally and laparotomy is necessary. Figure 17–25 shows the surgical technique used to correct this problem. Initially, a combination of vaginal pressure and traction from above on the round ligaments should be attempted. However, this maneuver may not always be successful, and one may have to resort to a vertical incision on the posterior aspect of the lower uterine segment in order to replace the uterus.

Once the uterine inversion has been corrected, the anesthetic agents used for uterine relaxation should be discontinued and oxytocic agents given to produce uterine contraction. If oxytocin fails to contract the uterus, prostaglandin $F_2\alpha$ should be used. The same dosage and intervals used to arrest postpartum hemorrhage with uterine atony are appropriate in this circumstance.

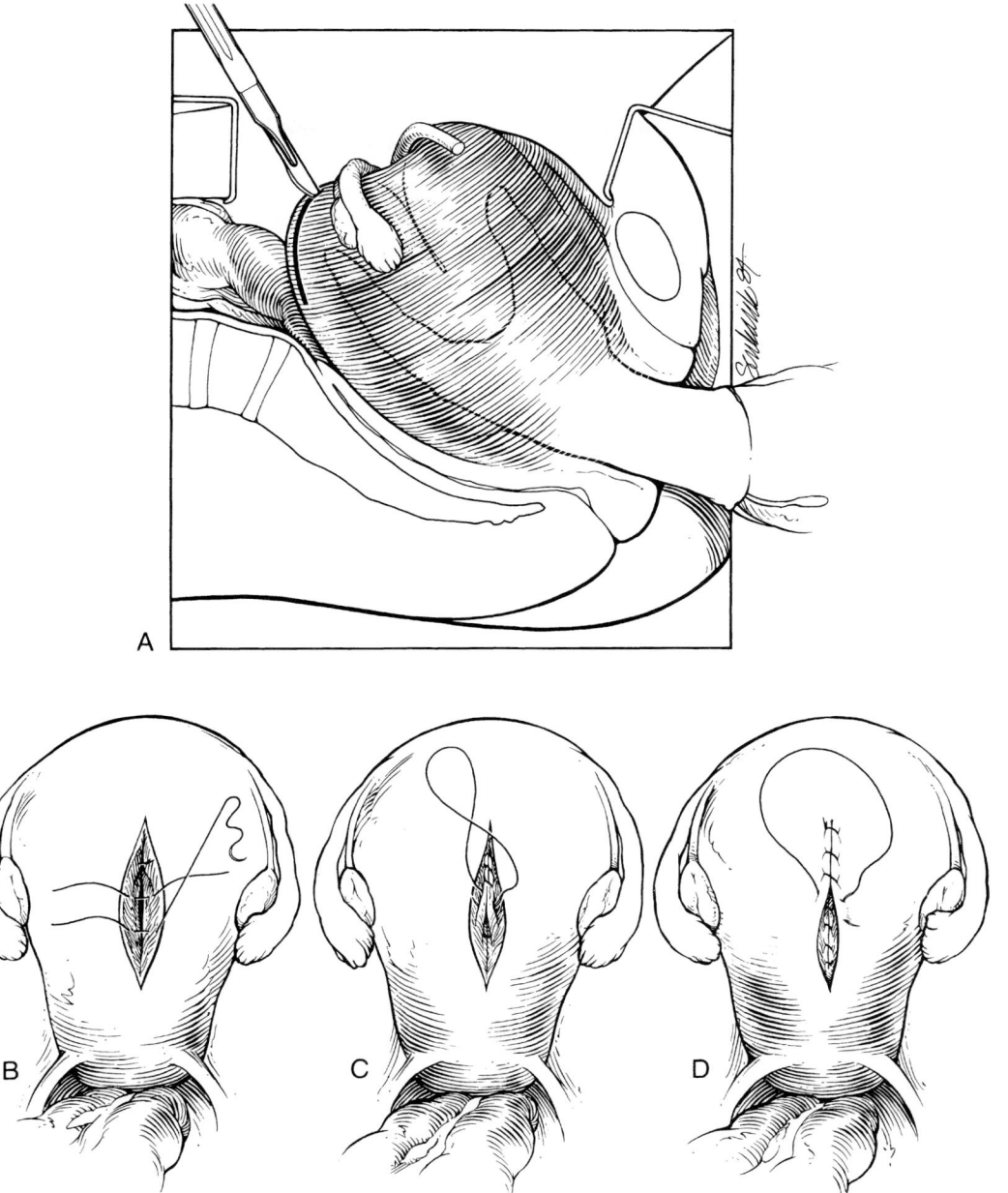

Figure 17–25. Surgical restoration of an inverted uterus. Note the incision on the posterior aspect of the uterus and subsequent repair.

Coagulation Disorders

Continued bleeding in the third stage of labor that is unresponsive to usual treatment should cause the clinician to consider uncommon but serious maternal coagulation disorders.

Von Willebrand's Disease

Von Willebrand's disease (VWD) is a hemorrhagic disorder that affects both men and women. This coagulopathy is inherited in an autosomal dominant pattern and is characterized by the following laboratory abnormalities: prolonged bleeding time, decreased factor VIII activity, decreased factor VIII–related antigen, and decreased von Willebrand factor. The latter is a plasma factor that is essential for proper platelet function and aggregation.

VWD is quite variable in its clinical course, severity, and laboratory abnormalities, even in the same patient. It is therefore possible for a patient with this disorder to go undetected throughout pregnancy until bleeding problems develop postpartum. The usual increase in factor VIII coagulant activity associated with pregnancy may also mask VWD. Only those patients with very low levels (<5 percent) before gestation fail to exhibit this rise.

When VWD is diagnosed before parturition, factor VIII activity should be monitored serially and transfusion with cryoprecipitate given to keep the factor VIII activity near term at 40 percent. If factor VIII levels are inadequate, the patient should be given one bag of cryoprecipitate per 10 kg body weight 24 hours before the planned induction of labor or cesarean delivery. This infusion will immediately restore the factor VIII activity level, but it will take 24 hours for the associated platelet defect to be corrected. If one suspects this disorder in a patient with unexplained postpartum hemorrhage, coagulation studies should be ordered and a hematologist consulted. However, since time is often limited, it would be prudent to notify the blood bank that cryoprecipitate may be needed emergently. In this situation, at least 6 units of cryoprecipitate are required, to be given every 12 hours for the next 3 to 5 days.[100]

Amniotic Fluid Embolism/Anaphylactoid Syndrome of Pregnancy

Amniotic fluid embolism (AFE) is a rare but frequently fatal obstetric emergency clinically recognized in approximately 1 in 8,000 to 1 in 80,000 births. The mortality rate for mothers suffering from AFE is 50 to 60 percent,[101–103] but an additional 30 percent (75 percent of survivors) can be expected to have long-term neurologic deficits.[104] The definitive diagnosis of AFE has traditionally been thought to require demonstration of fetal squames and lanugo in the pulmonary vascular space. However, in the most comprehensive study of this syndrome to date, only 73 percent of patients dying from this syndrome had this finding.[103] Based on mounting clinical and experimental evidence, Clark et al.[104] have suggested renaming this clinical syndrome the *anaphylactoid syndrome of pregnancy* to emphasize that the clinical findings are secondary to biochemical mediators rather than pulmonary embolic phenomenon.

The classic clinical presentation of the syndrome has been described by five signs that often occur in the following sequence: (1) respiratory distress, (2) cyanosis, (3) cardiovascular collapse, (4) hemorrhage, and (5) coma. In the previously mentioned paper, Clark et al.[104] described a more heterogenous clinical presentation.

The most important new findings are the certainty of fetal distress accompanying this syndrome and the high incidence of maternal coagulopathy. In many cases, fetal distress is the initial presenting symptom, rapidly followed by maternal distress (see Table 17–4).

The cardiorespiratory effects of acute intravascular

Table 17–4. INCIDENCE: SIGNS AND SYMPTOMS OCCURRING IN >50% OF PATIENTS WITH AFE

Sign or Symptom	No. of Patients	Percentage
Hypotension	43	100
Fetal distress	30	100
Pulmonary edema/ARDS	28	93
Cardiac arrest	40	87
Cyanosis	38	83
Coagulopathy	38	83
Dyspnea	22	49
Seizure	22	48

From Clark S, Morgan M: Amniotic fluid embolism. Anesthesia 34:20, 1979, with permission.

injection of amniotic fluid have been studied in pregnant ewes.[105] The initial response to the intravascular injection of amniotic fluid was hypotension. A 40 percent decrease in mean arterial pressure was followed by a 100 percent increase in mean pulmonary artery pressure. Little change occurred in the left atrial pressure or the pulmonary artery wedge pressure. A 40 percent fall in cardiac output was associated with the rapid rise in pulmonary artery pressure. These changes resulted in a two- to threefold increase in pulmonary vascular resistance and a two- to threefold decrease in systemic vascular resistance. In contrast to these findings in sheep, intravascular injection of amniotic fluid in rhesus monkeys failed to produce cardiovascular changes similar to the syndrome observed in humans.[103]

Classic teachings have emphasized the role of uterine hyperstimulation as a predisposing factor in this syndrome. More recent data[103] have shown this to be an erroneous conclusion. Uterine hyperstimulation was found in less than 10 percent of patients prior to the occurrence of AFE. Uterine tetany did occur in 50 percent of patients concomitant with respiratory distress. This most likely represents the uterine response to maternal hypoxemia rather than the event precipitating the AFE. Equally incorrect is the hypothesis that oxytocin administration is a risk factor for the development of the syndrome. There is no higher frequency of oxytocin use in patients suffering AFE than in laboring patients without this complication.

Only scanty information is available on which to base the treatment of the initial syndrome. Early airway control usually necessitating endotracheal intubation has been stressed in the few patients surviving the full-blown syndrome.[106,107] Once maximal ventilation and oxygenation have been achieved, attention should be paid to restoration of cardiovascular equilibrium. Central monitoring of fluid therapy with a pulmonary artery catheter is very helpful if the patient can be stabilized long enough to allow time for its placement. Pulmonary arterial blood may be aspirated and stained for the presence of fetal squames, lanugo hair, and mucin. However, these are found in only 50 percent of patients with the syndrome, and there are known false-positives. The treatment of shock in the early phase of the syndrome unaccompanied by massive blood loss has not been well studied. Recent data would suggest that the hypotension results from myocardial failure and that efforts should be used to provide myocardial support.[104] These would include inotropic agents such as dopamine, as well as volume therapy.[108] Other investigators have observed reduced systemic vascular resistance and have used vasopressor therapy such as ephedrine or levarterenol with success.[107] If the patient survives the initial cardiorespiratory collapse, there is a high likelihood that coagulopathy will develop if it has not been previously clinically apparent. DIC results in the depletion of fibrinogen, platelets, and coagulation factors, especially factors V, VIII, and XIII. The fibrinolytic system is activated as well.[109] Most patients will have profound hypofibrinogenemia, with values less than 200 mg/dl being the rule. PT and PTT will also be abnormal in nearly all patients. Platelet counts are more variable, with 60 percent having values less than 100,000/μl. Supportive coagulation and volume therapy (blood, fresh frozen plasma, or cryoprecipitate) should be administered as soon as they are available.

The neonatal outcome in patients suffering this catastrophe is better than the maternal outcome. If the fetus is alive at the time of the event, nearly 80 percent will survive the delivery. Unfortunately, 50 percent of the survivors will incur neurologic damage.[103] The two main factors influencing neonatal outcome are the presence or absence of maternal cardiac arrest and the time from arrest to delivery in the latter group. In general, fetal outcome is improved when maternal cardiac arrest does not occur. The shortest arrest to delivery time is associated with the best neonatal outcomes in the presence of maternal cardiac arrest.

Disseminated Intravascular Coagulation

DIC results from the loss of local control of the body's clotting mechanisms. Normally, there are four essential elements in the maintenance of local control of the hemostatic system: vascular integrity, platelet function, the coagulation system, and clot lysis.[110] The body must maintain vascular integrity for the survival of the organism. To minimize blood loss, any break in this system initiates the entire hemostatic cascade.

Platelets play an essential role in initiating and localizing clot formation. Platelets circulate until they encounter a break in vascular integrity. They then adhere to the damaged endothelium and release adenosine diphosphate (ADP), recruiting additional platelets to form an adhesive mass of platelets. Once the platelet plug extends past the site of damaged endothelium, platelets interact with the normal vessel wall and produce prostacyclin. This substance inhibits further platelet aggregation and localizes the platelet plug to the site of injury.

Platelets also localize the formation of fibrin by the coagulation cascade. Coagulation factors circulate in an inactive form. Aggregated platelets and injured tissue provide a phospholipid surface on which the coagulation factors can act. Once the factors are activated, fibrin is produced. The action of the coagulation cascade is limited to a localized area by a decrease in the mount of activated factors. These factors are reduced by (1) the reticuloendothelial system, (2) dilution by rapid blood flow, and (3) neutralization by a circulating protein (antithrombin 3).[110]

Once a clot has formed, the reestablishment of normal circulation depends on the orderly removal of the clot. Clot lysis is usually a localized process that must proceed in a timely fashion, since rapid lysis would lead to rebleeding. Clot lysis is limited in two ways. Since the coagulation cascade and lytic processes both depend on factor XII, they are triggered simultaneously. Second, activated plasminogen or plasmin is inactivated by antiplasmin, which circulates in concentrations 10 times that of plasminogen. The orderly progression of clot lysis is facilitated by the incorporation of plasminogen directly into the clot, protecting it from rapid neutralization by antiplasmin. Activation of plasminogen within the clot can then proceed at a local level.

During DIC, the body is forming and lysing fibrin clots throughout the circulation rather than in the localized physiologic process. Therefore, the loss of localization of the clotting process is the main defect in DIC. The lyric process may be activated as well but occurs only in response to the activation of the clotting system.

In obstetrics, DIC causing hemorrhage may involve any of the four mechanisms involved in the localization process. However, it is uncommon for DIC to be initiated by a failure of vascular integrity. Similarly, a platelet abnormality leading to diffuse platelet aggregation is an unlikely cause of hemorrhage in obstetrics. However, activation of the coagulation cascade by the presence of large amounts of tissue phospholipid is a common stimulus for DIC in obstetrics. Such conditions include abruptio placenta, retained dead fetus, and amniotic fluid embolism. These tissue phospholipids contribute to the utilization of large amounts of clotting factors and lead to a consumption coagulopathy. Once this widespread coagulation has taken place, the lytic process is called into action. The degradation of large amounts of fibrin produces fibrin split products, or fibrin degradation products (FDPs). These factors have their own physiologic activity and, when present in large amounts, contribute to bleeding by inhibiting fibrin cross-linking and producing platelet dysfunction.

The platelet count and fibrinogen level are the most

clinically useful tests in evaluating the patient with DIC. They may be repeated on an hourly to every 2-hour basis to provide an accurate reflection of the activity of the coagulation process. PT and PTT are usually abnormal during DIC but are less helpful in evaluating the ongoing severity of the disorder. Because platelets and fibrinogen have a half-life of 4 to 5 days, they are not immediately replaced by the body's own mechanisms and will give an accurate reflection of ongoing consumption as well as the effectiveness of factor replacement.

The sine qua non of successful management of DIC is treatment of the initiating event. Once the cause has been located and treated, the process should resolve. However, depleted factors must be restored to permit orderly repair of injured tissues. Successful therapy involves the replacement of essential factors faster than the body is consuming them. These factors are platelets, coagulation factors derived from fresh frozen plasma or cryoprecipitate, and fibrinogen supplied by cryoprecipitate of fresh frozen plasma. Monitoring replacement therapy should be initiated 20 minutes after the intravenous administration of these products. The obstetrician should attempt to achieve a platelet count of more than 100,000/μl and a fibrinogen level of greater than 100 mg/dl. In obstetric conditions complicated by hemorrhage, heparin has no use and will only cause the bleeding to worsen.

Key Points

➤ The rapid assessment of volume loss is dependent on basic vital signs and physical findings.

➤ Blood product use should be based on objectively determined needs rather than predetermined formulas.

➤ An action plan should be developed for situations in which massive blood transfusion is anticipated or arises unexpectedly.

➤ In patients with abruptio placentae, cesarean delivery usually should be performed for obstetric or fetal indications, not maternal coagulopathy.

➤ Expectant management of patients with abruptio placentae or placenta previa can be safely accomplished in many patients.

➤ In patients with postpartum hemorrhage secondary to uterine atony, dilute solutions of oxytocin (intravenous) and 15-methyl-F$_{2\alpha}$-prostaglandin (intramuscular) should be the first two drugs administered.

➤ The maternal risks from heterologous blood transfusion have decreased significantly in the last 5 years.

➤ The clinical presentation of amniotic fluid embolism is more heterogenous than previously described.

➤ When uterine inversion is encountered, the uterus should be replaced and reinverted before placental removal is attempted.

➤ Oxytocin should be given before placental expulsion and separation to minimize postpartum blood loss.

REFERENCES

1. Benedetti T, Quilligan E: Cerebral edema in severe pregnancy induced hypertension. Am J Obstet Gynecol 137:860, 1979.
2. Shires G: Management of hypovolemic shock. Bull N Y Acad Med 55:139, 1979.
3. Hewitt PE, Machin SJ: Massive blood transfusion. BMJ 300:107, 1990.
4. Etchason J, Petz L, Keeler E, et al: The cost effectiveness of preoperative autologous blood donations. N Engl J Med 332:719, 1995.
5. Grimes DA: A simplified device for intraoperative autotransfusion. Obstet Gynecol 72:947, 1988.
6. Chestnut DH, Dewan DM, Redick LF, et al: Anesthetic management for obstetric hysterectomy: a multi-institutional study. Anesthesiology 70:607, 1989.
7. Celayeta MA: Comment: Tocolysis in placenta previa. Drug Intell Clin Pharmacol 22:828, 1988.
8. Rebarber A, Lonser R, Jackson S, et al: The safety of intraoperative autologous blood collection and autotransfusion during cesarean section. Am J Obstet Gynecol 179:715, 1998.
9. Schreiber GB, Busch MP, Kleinman SH, et al: The risk of transmission related viral infections. N Engl J Med 337:1685, 1996.
10. Dodd RY: The risk of transfusion transmitted infection. N Engl J Med 327:419, 1992.
11. Goodnough LT, Ali S, Despotis M, et al: Transfusion medicine: blood transfusion. N Engl J Med 340:438, 1999.
12. Knab D: Abruptio placentae. Obstet Gynecol 52:625, 1978.
13. Pritchard J: Obstetric hemorrhage. In Pritchard J, MacDonald P (eds): Williams Obstetrics. New York, Appleton-Century-Crofts, 1980, p 485.
14. Krohn M, Voight L, McKnight B, et al: Correlates of placental abruption in birth certificate data. Br J Obstet Gynaecol 94:333, 1987.
15. Hurd W, Miodovnik M, Hertzberg V, Lavin J: Selective management of abruptio placentae: a prospective study. Obstet Gynecol 61:467, 1983.
16. Paterson M: The aetiology and outcome of abruptio placentae. Acta Obstet Gynecol Scand 58:31, 1979.
17. Hibbard B, Jeffcoate T: Abruptio placentae. Obstet Gynecol 27:155, 1966.
18. Townsend RR, Laing FC, Jeffrey RB: Placental abruption associated with cocaine abuse. AJR Am J Roentgenol 150:1339, 1988.
19. Darby MJ, Caritis SN, Shen-Schwarz S: Placental abruption

in the preterm gestation: an association with chorioamnionitis. Obstet Gynecol 74:88, 1989.

20. Naeye R, Harkness W, Utts J: Abruptio placentae and perinatal death: a prospective study. Am J Obstet Gynecol 128:740, 1977.

21. Rasmussen S, Irgens L, Bergsojo P, Dalaker K: The occurrence of placental abruption in Norway 1967–1991. Acta Obstet Gynecol Scand 75:222, 1996.

22. Pritchard J: The genesis of severe placental abruption. Am J Obstet Gynecol 208:22, 1970.

23. Douglas R, Stromme W: Operative Obstetrics. New York, Appleton-Century-Crofts, 1976.

24. Helton AS, McFarlane J, Anderson ET: Battered and pregnant: a prevalence study. Am J Public Health 77:1337, 1987.

25. Kupferminc MJ, Eldor A, Steinmen N, et al: Increased frequency of genetic thrombophilia in women with complications of pregnancy. N Engl J Med 340:9, 1999.

26. Redker PM, Miletich JP, Hennekens CH, Buring JE: Ethnic distribution of factor V Leiden in 4047 men and women: imlications of venous thromboembolism screening. JAMA 227:1305, 1997.

27. Dommisse J, Tiltman A: Placental bed biopsies in placental abruption. Br J Obstet Gynaecol 99:651, 1992.

28. Seski JC, Compton AA: Abruptio placenta following a negative oxytocin challenge test. Am J Obstet Gynecol 125:276, 1976.

29. Nyberg DA, Cyr DR, Mack LA, et al: Sonographic spectrum of placental abruption. AJR Am J Roentgenol 148:161, 1987.

30. Nyberg DA, Mack LA, Benedetti TJ, et al: Placental abruption and placental homorrhage: correlation of sonographic findings with fetal outcome. Radiology 358:357, 1987.

31. Bond A, Edersheim T, Curry L, et al: Expectant management of abruptio placentae before 35 weeks gestation. Am J Perinatol 6:121, 1989.

32. Combs C, Nyberg D, Mack L, et al: Expectant management after sonographic diagnosis of placental abruption. Am J Perinatol 9:170, 1992.

33. Saller DJ: Tocolysis in the management of third trimester bleeding. J Perinatol 10:125, 1990.

34. Pritchard J, Brekken A: Clinical and laboratory studies on severe abruptio placentae. Am J Obstet Gynecol 97:681, 1967.

35. Rasmussen T, Karegard M, Gennser G: Incidence and recurrence rate of abruptio plancentae in Sweden. Obstet Gynecol 67:523, 1986.

36. Olah D, Gee H, Deedham P: The management of severe disseminated intravascular coagulopathy complicating placental abruption in the second trimester. Br J Obstet Gynaecol 95:419, 1988.

37. Montaeiro AA, Onocencio AC, Jorge CS: Placental abruption with disseminated intravascular coagulopathy in the second trimester of pregnancy with fetal survival. Br J Obstet Gynaecol 94:811, 1987.

38. Lowe TW, Cunningham FG: Placental abruption. Clin Obstet Gynecol 33:406, 1990.

39. Saftlas A, Olson D, Atrash H, et al: National trends in the incidence of abruptio placenta. Obstet Gynecol 78:1081, 1991.

40. Spinillo A, Fazzi E, Stronati E, et al: Severity of abruptio placenta and neurodevelopmental outcome in low birth weight infants. Early Hum Dev 35:44, 1993.

41. Brenner W, Edelman D, Hendricks C: Characteristics of patients with placenta previa and results of "expectant management." Am J Obstet Gynecol 132:180, 1978.

42. Cotton D, Ead J, Paul R, Quilligan E: The conservative aggressive management of placenta previa. Am J Obstet Gynecol 17:687, 1980.

43. Iyasu S, Saftlas A, Rowley D, et al: The epidemiology of placenta previa in the United States, 1979. Am J Obstet Gynecol 168:1424, 1987.

44. Clark S, Koonings P, Phelan J: Placenta previa/accreta and prior cesarean section. Obstet Gynecol 66:89, 1985.

45. Nielsen TF, Hagberg H, Ljungblad U: Placenta previa and antepartum hemorrhage after previous cesarean section. Gynecol Obstet Invest 27:88, 1989.

46. Singh P, Rodrigues C, Gupta PA: Placenta previa and previous cesarean section. Acta Obstet Gynecol Scand 60:367, 1981.

47. Chattopadhyay S, Kharif H, Sherbeeni J: Placenta previa and accreta after previous cesarean section. Eur J Obstet Gynecol Reprod Biol 52:151, 1993.

48. Rizos N, Doran T, Miskin M, et al: Natural history of placenta previa ascertained by diagnostic ultrasound. Am J Obstet Gynecol 133:287, 1979.

49. Zelop C, Bromley B, Frigoletto FJ, Benacerraf B: Second trimester sonographically diagnosed placenta previa: prediction of persistent previa at birth. Int J Gynaecol Obstet 44:207, 1994.

50. Wing DA, Paul RH, Miller LK: Management of the symptomatic placenta previa: a randomized, controlled trial of inpatient versus outpatient expectant management. Am J Obstet Gynecol 175:806, 1996.

51. Chervenak F, Lee Y, Hendler M, et al: Role of attempted vaginal delivery in the management of placenta previa. Obstet Gynecol 64:798, 1984.

52. Watson P, Cefalo R: Magnesium sulfate tocolysis in selected patients with symptomatic placenta previa. Am J Perinatol 7:251, 1990.

53. Sampson M, Lastres O, Tomasi A, et al: Tocolysis with terbutaline sulfate in patients with placenta previa complicated by premature labor. J Reprod Med 29:248, 1984.

54. McShane P, Heyl P, Epstein M: Maternal and perinatal morbidity resulting from placenta previa. Obstet Gynecol 65:176, 1985.

55. Tomich P: Prolonged use of tocolytic agent in expectant management of placenta previa. J Reprod Med 30:745, 1985.

56. Perkins R: Discussion of paper. Am J Obstet Gynecol 149:323, 1984.

57. Liggins G, Howie R: A controlled trial of antepartum glucocorticoid treatment of RDS. Pediatrics 50:515, 1972.

58. Ballard R, Ballard P, Goanberg P, Sinderman S: Prenatal administration of betamethasone for prevention of respiratory distress syndrome. J Pediatr 94:97, 1979.

59. d'Angelo L, Irwin L: Conservative management of placenta previa: a cost benefit analysis. Am J Obstet Gynecol 149:320, 1984.

60. Droste S, Keil K: Expectant management of placenta previa: cost benefit analysis of outpatient treatment. Am J Obstet Gynecol 170:1254, 1994.

61. Mouer J: Placenta previa: antepartum conservative management inpatient vs. outpatient. Am J Obstet Gynecol 170:1685, 1994.

62. Breen J, Neubecker R, Gregori C, Franklin J: Placenta accreta, increta and percreta. Obstet Gynecol 49:51, 1977.

63. Hoffman-Tretin J, Koenigsberg M, Rabin A, Anyaebunam A: Placenta accreta. Additional sonographic observations. J Ultrasound Med 11:326, 1992.

64. Finberg H, Williams J: Placenta accreta: prospective sonographic diagnosis in patients with placenta previa and prior cesarean section. J Ultrasound Med 11:333, 1992.

65. Read J, Cotton D, Miller F: Placenta accreta: changing clinical aspects and outcome. Obstet Gynecol 56:31, 1980.

66. Druzin ML: Packing of lower uterine segment for control of postcesarean bleeding in instances of placenta previa. Surg Gynecol Obstet 169:543, 1980.

67. Cho J, Kim S, Cha K, et al: Interrupted circular suture: bleed-

ing control during cesarean delivery in placenta previa accreta. Obstet Gynecol 78:876, 1991.

68. Alvarez M, Lockwood C, Ghidini A, et al: Prophylactic and emergent arterial catheterization for selective embolization in obstetric hemorrhage. Am J Perinatol 9:441, 1992.

69. Mitty H, Sterling K, Alvarez M, Gendler R: Obstetric hemorrhage: prophylactic and emergency arterial catheterization and embolotherapy. Radiology 188:183, 1993.

70. Fox H: Placenta accreta. Obstet Gynecol Surv 27:475, 1972.

71. Gemmell A: Unusual case of adherent placenta treated in unorthodox manner. J Obstet Gynecol 49:43, 1947.

72. Jaffe R, DuBeshter B, Sherer D, et al: Failure of methotrexate treatment for term placenta percreta. Am J Obstet Gynecol 171:558, 1994.

73. Bakrai L: Placenta percreta with bladder invasion: report of three cases. Am J Perinatol 10:468, 1993.

74. Torrey E: Vasa previa. Am J Obstet Gynecol 63:146, 1952.

75. Sirivongs B: Vasa previa report of 3 cases. J Med Assoc Thai 57:261, 1974.

76. Odunsi K, Bullough C, Neenzel J, Polanska A: Evaluation of chemical tests for fetal bleeding from vasa previa. Int J Gynecol Obstet 55:207, 1996.

77. McCurdy C, Magann E, McCurdy C, Saltazman A: The effect of placental management at cesarean delivery on operative blood loss. Am J Obstet Gynecol 167:1363, 1992.

78. Prendiville W, Harding J, Elburne D, Stirrat G: The Briston third stage trial: active vs. physiological management of the third stage of labor. J Obstet Gynecol 95:3, 1988.

79. McCurdy CM, Magann EF, McCurdy CJ, Saltzman AK: The effect of placental management at cesarean delivery on operative blood loss. Am J Obstet Gynecol 167:1363, 1993.

80. Takagi S, Yuoshida T, Togo Y, et al: The effects of intramyometrial injection of prostaglandin $F_{2\alpha}$ on severe postpartum hemorrhage. Prostaglandins 12:565, 1980.

81. O'Brien P, El-Rafaey H, Gordon A, et al: Rectally administered misoprostol for the treatment of postpartum hemorrhage unresponsive to oxytocin and ergometrine: a descriptive study. Obstet Gynecol 92:212, 1998.

82. Hayashi R, Castillo M, Noah M: Management of severe postpartum hemorrhage due to uterine atony usng an analog of prostaglandin $F_{2\alpha}$. Obstet Gynecol 58:426, 1981.

83. Hayashi M, Mori Y, Nogami K, et al: A hypothesis to explain the occurrence of inner myometrial laceration causing massive postpartum hemorrhage. Acta Obstet Gynecol Scand 79:99, 2000.

84. O'Leary J, O'Leary J: Uterine artery ligation in control of intractable postpartum hemorrhage. Am J Obstet Gynecol 94:920, 1966.

85. Adrabbo F, Salah J: Stepwise uterine devascularization: a novel technique for management of uncontrollable postpartum hemorrhage with preservation of the uterus. Am J Obstet Gynecol 171:694, 1984.

86. Mengert W, Burchell R, Blumstein R, Daskal J: Pregnancy after bilateral ligation of internal iliac and ovarian arteries. Obstet Gynecol 34:664, 1969.

87. Cho JH, Jun HS, No Lee C: Hemostatic suturing technique for uterine bleeding during cesarean delivery. Obstet Gynecol 96:129, 2000.

88. B-Lynch C, Coker A, Lawal AH, et al: The B-Lynch surgical technique for the control of massive postpartum hemorrhage: an alternative to hysterectomy? Five cases reported. Br J Obstet Gynaecol 104:372, 1997.

89. Ferguson JE, Bourgeois J, Underwood PB: B-Lynch suture for postpartum hemorrhage. Obstet Gynecol 95:1020, 2000.

90. Brown BJ, Heaston DK, Poulson AM, et al: Uncontrollable postpartum bleeding: a new approach to hemostasis through angiographic arterial embolization. Obstet Gynecol 54:361, 1979.

91. Jander HP, Russinovich NAE: Transcatheter Gelfoam embolization in abdominal, retroperitoneal and pelvic hemorrhage. Radiology 16:337, 1980.

92. Chin HG, Scott DR, Resnik R, et al: Angiographic embolization of intractable puerperal hematomas. Am J Obstet Gynecol 160:434, 1989.

93. Hansch E, Chitkara U, McAlpine J, et al: Pelvic arterial embolization for control of obstetric hemorrhage: a five year experience. Am J Obstet Gynecol 180:1454, 1999.

94. Pelage JP, Le Dref O, Jacob D, et al: Selective arterial embolization of the uterine arteries in the management of intractable postpartum hemorrhage. Acta Obstet Gynecol Scand 78:698, 1999.

95. Cassels JJ, Greenberg H, Otterson W: Pelvic tamponade in puerperal hemorrhage. J Reprod Med 30:689, 1985.

96. Robie G, Morgan M, Payne G, Wasemiller-Smith L: Logothetopulos pack for the management of uncontrollable postpartum hemorrhage. Am J Perinatol 7:327, 1990.

97. Watson P, Desch N, Bowes W: Management of acute and subacute puerperal inversion of the uterus. Obstet Gynecol 55:12, 1980.

98. Kitchin JD III, Thiagarajah S, May HV Jr, Thornton WN Jr: Puerperal inversion of the uterus. Am J Obstet Gynecol 123:51, 1975.

99. Brar H, Greenspoon J, Platt L, Paul RH: Acute puerperal uterine inversion: new approaches to management. J Reprod Med 34:173, 1989.

100. Walker E, Dormandy K: The management of pregnancy in von Willebrand's disease. J Obstet Gynaecol Br Commonw 74:459, 1968.

101. Courtney L: Amniotic fluid embolism. Obstet Gynecol Surv 29:169, 1974.

102. Stolte L, van Kessel H, Seelen H, et al: Failure to produce the syndrome of amniotic fluid embolism by infusion of amniotic fluid and meconium into monkeys. Am J Obstet Gynecol 83:694, 1967.

103. Clark S, Hankins G, Dudley D, et al: Amniotic fluid embolism: analysis of the national registry. Am J Obstet Gynecol 172:1158, 1995.

104. Clark S, Montz F, Phelan J: Hemodynamic alterations associated with amniotic fluid embolism: a reappraisal. Am J Obstet Gynecol 151:617, 1985.

105. Reis R, Pierce W, Behrendt D: Hemodynamic effects of amniotic fluid embolism. Surg Gynecol Obstet 129:45, 1969.

106. Clark S, Morgan M: Amiotic fluid embolism. Anesthesia 34:20, 1979.

107. Resnik R, Swartz W, Plummer M, et al: Amniotic fluid embolism with survival. Obstet Gynecol 47:295, 1976.

108. Schaef R, Campo T, Civetta J: Hemodynamic alterations and rapid diagnosis in a case of amniotic fluid. Anesthesiology 45:155, 1977.

109. Ratnoff O, Vosburgh G: Observations on the dotting defect in amniotic fluid embolism. N Engl J Med 247:970, 1952.

110. Fishbach D, Fogdall R: Coagulation: The Essentials. Baltimore, Williams & Wilkins, 1981.

Cesarean Delivery

RICHARD DEPP

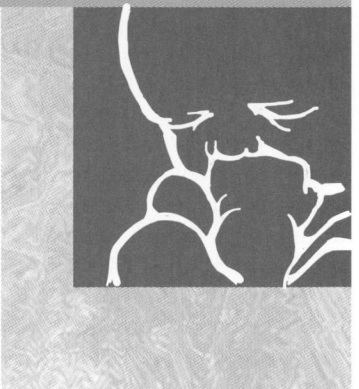

The terms *cesarean section, cesarean delivery,* and *cesarean birth* may be used to describe the delivery of a fetus through a surgical incision of the anterior uterine wall. This definition does not include nonsurgical expulsion of the embryo/fetus from the uterine cavity or tubes following uterine rupture or ectopic pregnancy. *Cesarean section* is a tautology; both words connote incision. Therefore, *cesarean birth* and *cesarean delivery* are preferable terms.

Cesarean birth has become the most common hospital-based operative procedure in the United States, accounting for more than 22 percent of all live births in 1999.[1-3] The increase has been attributed to the liberalization of indications for "fetal distress," cephalopelvic disproportion/failure to progress, breech presentations, as well as elective repeat cesarean delivery.[4] In many medical centers, the present overall rate would be significantly higher were it not for a recent change in attitude facilitating acceptance of vaginal birth after cesarean birth.[5]

The cesarean delivery–associated maternal mortality rate is approximately 20 per 100,000 births in the United States.[6] Taken as an isolated endpoint, it is an infrequent complication. Cesarean delivery has many possible immediate untoward consequences: an increased risk for postpartum infectious morbidity despite antibiotic prophylaxis, an increased risk of significant blood loss and need for transfusion with potential problems associated with blood and blood product replacement, and an increased risk of anesthetic complications. There are no reliable data regarding the cumulative long-term maternal morbidity associated with cesarean birth.

Despite a dramatic impact on society, little attention has been focused on the cumulative consequences of this major surgical procedure with its implications not only for the current pregnancy but also for future re-production. The increase in cesarean birth rates noted in the 1980s has had a dramatic impact on the reproductive future of women. As the percentage of laboring patients presenting with a prior cesarean birth has increased, there has been an associated increase in more difficult repeat cesarean deliveries and complications, including a higher incidence of placenta previa, placenta accreta, symptomatic uterine rupture, hemorrhage, requirement for transfusion, and need for unplanned hysterectomy.

This chapter presents indications for cesarean delivery and peripartum hysterectomy, surgical techniques and procedural complications, and issues surrounding candidacy for and management of a trial of labor (TOL) after a prior cesarean birth (VBAC).

HISTORY OF CESAREAN DELIVERY

Terms

The origin of the term *cesarean section* is likely the product of two separate reports in 1581 and 1598, the former making reference to *Cesarean* and the second to *Sections*. The origin of the term *cesarean* is somewhat uncertain. The hypothesis that Julius Caesar was the product of a cesarean birth is unlikely to be true in view of the probability of fatality associated with the procedure in ancient times and the observation that his mother, Aurelia, corresponded with him during his campaigns in Europe many years later. The term may have as its origin in the Latin verb *cadere,* to cut; the children of such births were referred to as *caesones.* It is also possible that the term stems from the Roman law known as Lex Regis, which mandated postmortem operative delivery so that the mother and child could be buried separately; the specific law is referred to historically as Lex Cesare.[7]

In 1876, Eduardo Porro, an Italian professor, recommended hysterectomy combined with cesarean birth to control uterine hemorrhage and prevent systemic infection.[8-10] The Porro procedure combined subtotal cesarean hysterectomy (see the section Peripartum Hysterectomy, below) with marsupialization of the cervical stump.[9] Fortunately, the need for such an extreme procedure was soon minimized by the proposal to close the uterine incision with sutures. The introduction of suture material, which enabled the surgeon to control bleeding, was of monumental importance in the evolution of the procedure. In 1882, Max Sänger from Leipzig published a monograph based largely on experience from surgeons in the United States who had used internal sutures, explaining the principles and technique of cesarean delivery, including aseptic preparation, with special emphasis on a two-step uterine closure using silver wire and silk and careful attention to hemostasis.[11,12] The use of silver wire stitches were developed by 19th century gynecologist J. Marion Sims, who invented his sutures to repair vaginal tears (fistulas) that had resulted from traumatic childbirth. Sänger thought that this approach would obviate the growing tendency for cesarean hysterectomy caused by fear of hemorrhage and infection. It is interesting to note that Sänger attributed much of the early development of suture material to American frontier surgeons, including Frank Polin of Springfield, Kentucky, who in 1852 had reported the use of silver wire sutures in surviving patients who had undergone cesarean delivery.[13]

The low transverse incision was trialed between 1880 and 1925 and was noted to reduce the risk of infection, as well as uterine rupture, in subsequent pregnancies.[8]

Death from peritonitis remained a major threat. Approximately 30 years later, extraperitoneal cesarean delivery was first described by Frank[14] (1907) and subsequently modified by Latzko[15] (1909) as a technique to reduce the risk of peritonitis in high-risk patients. Subsequently, Krönig[16] (1912) realized that extraperitoneal cesarean birth not only minimized the effects of peritonitis but also allowed access to the lower uterine segment through a vertical midline incision, which could then be covered with peritoneum, an approach that led to the modern-day low vertical procedure. Later, Beck[17] (1919) and DeLee and Cornell[18] (1922) modified the Krönig approach and popularized it in the United States. Finally, Kerr[19] (1926) developed the low transverse incision, which is most commonly employed throughout the world today. The need for an extraperitoneal procedure was essentially eliminated by the development of modern antibiotics.

As the risk-versus-benefit considerations changed, obstetricians became more confident in the use of cesarean section and began to argue against delaying surgery. Surgeons such as Robert Harris of the United States, Thomas Radford of England, and Franz von Winckel of Germany recommended cesarean delivery as an early solution to labor disorders to improve outcome. In turn, maternal and perinatal mortality rates were reduced as cesarean birth became viewed as one of several approaches to improve perinatal outcome.[8]

CESAREAN BIRTH RATES

The Changing Rate of Cesarean Birth

The early onset of a change in the overall cesarean delivery rate is dramatically demonstrated by data from the Chicago Lying-In Hospital, which had a fivefold increase in the cesarean rate from 0.6 percent in 1910 to 3 percent in 1928.[20] In the ensuing years, the reported rate of cesarean delivery in the United States increased in dramatic fashion, from 4.5 percent in 1965 to 16.5 percent in 1980, finally peaking at 24.7 percent in 1988.[21] Cesarean delivery rates have also increased worldwide during the past 20 years.[22,23] In a recent survey of obstetricians in London, 31 percent of female obstetricians and 8 percent of their male counterparts said they would prefer to deliver by cesarean section. The leading reason for this choice was fear of perineal injury with vaginal birth, followed by fear of damage to the baby, and the desire for an electively scheduled procedure.[24] However, the increase in international rates does not approach the high rates seen in the United States.

NICHD Task Force on Cesarean Childbirth

Cesarean births increase health care costs, pose considerable additional risk for maternal mortality and morbidity and, with few exceptions, provide only marginal proven fetal benefits. In 1979, the National Institute of Child Health and Human Development (NICHD) established a task force on cesarean childbirth and in 1980 sponsored a consensus development conference to consider the issue of cesarean delivery in the United States.[25] The task force recommended that efforts be made to diminish the impact of elective repeat cesarean delivery and the diagnosis of "dystocia" because these indications were the two major causes of the increase in cesarean birth rates that were likely to be susceptible to reduction.

Although an immediate slowing of the rate of increase of cesarean births was not readily apparent, the widespread dissemination of the consensus document did provide the medical community with reassurance that an attempt to reduce the escalating cesarean rate was a reasonable goal. The cesarean rate ultimately peaked at 24.7 percent in 1988.[1,26] Both the total cesarean rate and the primary rate have decreased since then to approximately 22.8 and 14.5 percent, respectively, in 1993.[2] Unfortunately, cesarean rates in some institutions continue to exceed 30 percent.

Is There an "Ideal" Cesarean Rate?

It is probably not possible to define an "ideal" cesarean rate. The desired rate will vary from institution to institution on the basis of multiple factors. Quilligan[27] has suggested that it may be better to define a range of values for each indication: failure to progress/cephalopelvic disproportion (2 to 4 percent); repeat cesarean delivery (2 to 6 percent); breech and abnormal lie (1.3 to 3.5 percent); nonreassuring fetal heart rate (FHR) (1.5 to 3 percent); and third-trimester bleeding (1 percent). Tertiary centers with associated higher rates of preterm birth and placenta previa can be expected to have higher cesarean rates. Recently, the U.S. Department of Health and Human Services, as part of its Healthy People 2000 program, identified a number of health-related objectives, including (1) reduction of the primary cesarean delivery rate to 12 percent and (2) increase of the number of VBACs to greater than or equal to 35 per 100 women who have had a prior cesarean section.[2,29]

In 1997, the American College of Obstetricians and Gynecologists (ACOG) appointed a task force on cesarean delivery rates to determine the factors that contribute to the cesarean delivery rates in the United States.[28] The task force noted that the highest variation in primary cesarean delivery rates occurred among nulliparous women with a singleton fetus in a cephalic presentation without other complications. The task force also observed that patients with a prior cesarean varied in the frequency with which they were offered a trial of labor and how often the trial of labor was successful. Using data from the National Center for Health Statistics, the task force established two benchmark rates based on the 25th to 75th percentiles of state rankings for these two patient groups. The task force advised that the targets for these two categories be set at the 25th percentile for primary cesarean delivery rates and the 75th percentile for VBAC rates. For nulliparous women at 37 weeks with a singleton fetus and a cephalic presentation, the national 1996 cesarean delivery rate was 17.9 percent. The group recommended a benchmark rate of 15.5 percent, at the 25th percentile. For multiparous women with one prior low transverse cesarean delivery at 37 weeks' gestation or greater with a singleton fetus and a cephalic presentation, the national 1996 VBAC rate was 30.3 percent. The task force recommended a benchmark rate of 37 percent, at the 75th percentile. The task force emphasized that in examining the cesarean rate of obstetricians or the institutions in which they practice it is essential that the rate be adjusted for the risk factors in the patient population. The task force proposed that using case-mix adjusted cesarean delivery rates and these benchmarks would be helpful in evaluating practice patterns and developing strategies to lower the rate of cesarean sections.[28]

Causes of Increased Cesarean Birth Rate

At least 90 percent of the increase between 1980 and 1985 was attributable to three factors: repeat cesarean deliveries (48 percent), dystocia (29 percent), and "fetal distress" (16 percent). There are many complex and interrelated reasons (Table 18–1) for the increase in the cesarean birth rate.[22]

Medical Advances

Early liberalization of the indications for cesarean delivery rose out of the increased availability of effective antibiotics, safer blood banking, and a greater tendency for obstetrics to be practiced in facilities delivering large numbers of patients. Even socioeconomic factors have played a role.

Table 18–1. CAUSES OF INCREASED CESAREAN RATE

Medical advances diminishing maternal risks
Labor- and delivery-related factors
   Repeat cesarean birth*
   Continuous electronic fetal monitoring*
   Dystocia diagnosis liberalized*
   Epidural analgesia/anesthesia
   Macrosomia (>4,000 vs. >4,500 g)
   Decreased use of forceps/vacuum[30]
Maternal factors
   More older childbearing women/delay in childbirth[21]
   More nulliparous women with attendant risk
   Increasing maternal risk
Fetal factors
   Fetus as a patient
   Breech presentation[21]
   VLBW fetus
   Active genital herpes
   Postterm pregnancy
   Multiple gestation (especially with nonvertex)
   Failed induction for fetal indication
Physician factors
   Fear of malpractice litigation
   Physician compensation (possible)
   Physician convenience (possible)

*Data from Taffel et al.,[21] Notzon et al.,[22] and Placek et al.[30]

Delay in Childbirth

The widespread availability of contraceptive and sterilization techniques has resulted in women giving birth at an older age.[21]

More Older and Often Nulliparous Patients

Older and often nulliparous patients constitute an increasing proportion of laboring women. In the United States between 1980 and 1985, the number of births in patients at least 30 years of age increased from 20 to 25 percent of all deliveries.[21] It is well known that the cesarean delivery rate increases with advancing age (Table 18–2) as a result of increased likelihood of dystocia and medical complications such as preeclampsia and gestational diabetes.

Dystocia Diagnosis Liberalized

The diagnostic criteria for dystocia accepted by some have been liberalized, and forceps deliveries have fallen into relative disfavor in some medical centers. For the interval 1972 to 1980, Placek et al.[30] reported a decline in forceps deliveries from 37 to 18 percent, which parallels the increase in the cesarean delivery rate from 7 to 17 percent.[30]

Fetus as a Patient

Historically, cesarean delivery had been performed primarily to reduce the likelihood of maternal morbidity and mortality. In the mid-1970s, the eventual health status of the fetus-neonate began to play a larger role in the decision process. Widespread use of techniques such as continuous electronic fetal monitoring, ultrasound evaluation of the fetus, and fetal karyotype determinations by amniocentesis or chorionic villus sampling resulted in a change in emphasis to "quality of survival" for newborns, not simply survival. The fetus became viewed more as a person and eventually a patient (see Chapter 11).

Table 18–2. TOTAL CESAREAN BIRTH RATES (%) BY AGE OF MOTHER

Age (years)	1980*	1989*	1991†
<20	14.5	18.1	18.2
20–24	15.8	21.1	21.0
25–29	16.7	24.8	24.3
30–34	18.0	26.6	26.7
≥35	20.6	30.3	28.4
Total	16.5	23.8	23.5

*Data from Taffel et al.[26]
†Data from National Center for Health Statistics.[291]

Nonreassuring FHR Indications

Despite dramatic advances in perinatal medicine, the widespread use of electronic fetal monitoring, and a significant increase in the cesarean birth rate in the last two decades, there has been no reported reduction in the rate of cerebral palsy. There is consensus that continuous electronic fetal monitoring (EFM) does not reduce the risk of newborn morbidity related to metabolic acidosis or cerebral palsy more than intermittent auscultation.[31–34] Since cesarean delivery for this indication commonly follows the observation of subtle EFM changes in FHR variability or late decelerations, both of which are not detectable by auscultation, the association of subtle findings with later developmental problems may indicate a preexisting fetal abnormality, not likely to benefit from a cesarean delivery. The previously "normal" fetus, except in extreme conditions (i.e., severe prolonged decelerations arising from cord prolapse or placental abruption), is likely to have sufficient physiologic adaptability to adjust to the stress responsible for the relatively subtle fetal heart rate patterns that are not detectable by intermittent auscultation (see Chapter 14). Support for this notion is provided by the obvious contrast between the relatively high frequency of significant FHR alterations but infrequent occurrence of cerebral palsy. The fetus with prior developmental abnormality is more likely to demonstrate nonreassuring FHR patterns during labor than is its neurologically normal peer.

Breech as an Indication

Vaginal breech deliveries have been abandoned by many clinicians in favor of cesarean delivery (see Chapter 16). Most breech presentations are now delivered by cesarean birth, with rates in some medical centers as high as 79 and 92 percent.[21,35] Hannah and her colleagues recently published a large prospective randomized trial comparing planned cesarean delivery with planned vaginal birth for term frank or complete breech presentations. Perinatal mortality, neonatal mortality, and serious neonatal morbidity were all significantly lower in the planned cesarean group.[36] This study certainly supports current patterns of practice. It should be remembered that extraction of a breech at cesarean delivery requires skills very similar to those used in a vaginal birth, including avoidance of hyperextension of the fetal head.

Fear of Litigation

Unfortunately, obstetric practice in the United States is adversely influenced by the high rate of malpractice litigation. Medicolegal pressures have forced a liberalization of indications. Concern regarding potential malpractice action for failure to intervene at an alleged "standard" time increased dramatically in the 1980s, particularly among physicians in traditional private practice. Statistics to support this concept indicate that private nulliparous patients are more likely than clinic patients to undergo cesarean delivery if dystocia or malpresentation or so-called fetal distress is diagnosed.[37]

The practice of obstetrics has become more defensive. Many American obstetricians have concluded that one of the best ways to reduce malpractice vulnerability is to "liberalize" indications for cesarean delivery. Obstetricians harbor a fear that they may be criticized in hindsight for failure to perform an earlier cesarean delivery that "may have" resulted in a better outcome. The result is a more defensive approach to practice, including a lower threshold for resorting to cesarean delivery.[38] Unfortunately, there are few data to support a benefit to this strategy.

The magnitude of "fear of litigation" as a contributing factor to the current cesarean rates can be inferred from a survey of British and American obstetricians, designed to determine the perceived reason for the rise in cesarean rates. Litigation was the leading reason given by 84 percent of American obstetricians but only 42 percent of British obstetricians.[39] Some physicians have used cesarean delivery as an answer to all potential problems; an extreme was reached in 1985, when the following was asked: "If an informed patient opts for prophylactic cesarean section at term, can it be denied?"[40,41] Tort reform is the only likely solution to this particular problem.

Prior Cesarean Birth

As the indications were expanded, it is not surprising that "prior cesarean delivery" became an ever-increasing indication for cesarean birth. Approximately 25 percent of all cesarean deliveries were for the indication of prior cesarean birth in 1970.[1,2] The percentage of all cesarean procedures attributable to this indication peaked at 37.2 percent in 1997.

Determinants of Rate Variation

Physician Factors

The etiology of differences in cesarean birth rates reported by different centers is as yet unresolved. For instance, Blumenthal et al.[42] noted a significant difference between the incidence of dystocia in public versus private patients and concluded that the difference was probably the result of differences in indications used by physicians in the two groups. Although it has been suggested that physician convenience or economic gain may be operative in the decision to perform a cesarean

delivery in private patients, Phillips et al.[43] were unable to demonstrate the predictable distribution of non-scheduled cesarean births that would support this hypothesis. Furthermore, this author's experience with a large number of private physicians in many centers suggests that this is not a major contributor. Rather, it is the fear of not performing a cesarean that is often the main culprit. Furthermore, the difference in compensation for cesarean and vaginal deliveries is small, and, in most cases well deserved, often following long or difficult labors.

Regional Differences

There are surprisingly dramatic regional differences in total cesarean rates in all hospitals as well as in teaching hospitals.[1,2,43,44] In 1993, the cesarean rate in the South was 25.9 percent, significantly higher than rates in the West (19.3 percent), Midwest (20.8 percent), and Northeast (23.4 percent).[1,2] Regional variations also exist among teaching hospitals.

Teaching Versus Nonteaching Hospitals

Women delivering in a teaching hospital are less likely to have a cesarean delivery than are those delivering in hospitals without resident programs. In 1990, the estimated rate in all hospitals with resident programs was 20.3 percent compared with an overall national rate of 23.5 percent; the estimated rate for nonteaching hospitals was 24.7 percent (odds ratio [OR], 0.77; 95 percent confidence interval [CI], 0.77–0.78; $p = 0.0001$). Of all cesarean deliveries conducted in teaching hospitals, 64.8 percent were primary and 35.2 percent were repeat.[44] The hypothesized basis for the lower rate in teaching hospitals includes routine consultation prior to performing nonelective cesareans, routine review conferences, and around-the-clock availability of physicians to manage labor, minimizing any tendency for physician time pressures to influence the decision process.

Obstacles to Rate Reduction

There is an ongoing need to continue to reduce the current cesarean birth rates. Despite an awareness that there is a potential problem, we may have entered a cycle that will make major rate reduction difficult. Respected clinicians vary greatly in their acceptance of procedures such as midforceps or vaginal delivery of the breech, whether it be a singleton or one of a multiple gestation. Many physicians recently trained in obstetrics have had insufficient exposure to operative vaginal procedures to develop a "comfort" level and consequently often opt for a procedure with which they are familiar, cesarean delivery. In 1999, residents completing their training in obstetrics and gynecology in the

United States performed, on average, 169 cesarean deliveries, 31 forceps deliveries, and 27 vacuum deliveries.[46] Furthermore, increasing concern has been raised about the safety of VBAC, leading to provider and patient preference for a repeat cesarean delivery.

BENEFITS AND RISKS OF CESAREAN BIRTH

Maternal Mortality

Maternal mortality as a result of cesarean delivery fortunately is an infrequent occurrence, but the overall rate is estimated to be severalfold higher than that following vaginal delivery. Approximately 300 maternal deaths occur annually in the United States in just over 4 million deliveries of all types per year, an overall rate less than 10 per 100,000 live births. Not surprisingly, the reported incidence of maternal mortality following cesarean delivery can vary greatly from series to series, particularly in single-institution reports. Maternal mortality following cesarean birth has been assessed in two publications[6,47] with a sufficient number of cesarean deliveries (400,000 and 121,000) to provide meaningful estimates. On the basis of these two reports, mortality can be estimated to range from 6.1 to 22 per 100,000 live births. Approximately one third to one half of maternal deaths of these patients can be attributed directly to the cesarean procedure itself.

Perinatal Morbidity and Mortality

The hypothesis that cesarean birth offers a major opportunity to improve perinatal outcome has, with few exceptions, not been proven. It is more likely that the improvement in perinatal mortality is the product of widespread changes in perinatal care. There are no well-documented prospective trials demonstrating benefit to the fetus or to the mother that would justify the extent of the increase in the primary cesarean delivery rate over the past two decades.

There has been a heated international debate regarding the role of cesarean birth in reducing perinatal mortality. O'Driscoll and Foley[48] do not attribute improvements in perinatal outcome to liberalization of cesarean indications. Cesarean delivery rates have remained stable at the National Maternity Hospital in Dublin, Ireland, at less than 5 percent between 1965 to 1980, whereas rates in the United States have increased from slightly less than 5 percent in 1965 to more than 15 percent in 1980. Because the perinatal mortality rate at the National Maternity Hospital has progressively fallen from 42.1 to 16.8 per 1,000 births despite a low cesarean delivery rate, one is forced to consider that,

although liberalization of cesarean delivery indicators may contribute to better perinatal outcome, it is likely to be less important than the overall improvement in obstetric and neonatal care.

Leveno et al.[50] subsequently countered that the data of O'Driscoll and Foley[48] are limited by their emphasis on mortality rather than morbidity. They suggested that their more liberal use of cesarean delivery (18 percent in 1983) was "associated with" decreased intrapartum deaths and neonatal seizures when compared with the National Maternity Hospital in Dublin.[48,49]

O'Driscoll and Foley, in their response to the critique by Leveno et al., indicated that in order to compare uncommon events, a larger number of births would be required. They compared data from more than 24,000 births with a 5.1 percent cesarean rate at the National Maternity Hospital with those from more than 22,000 deliveries with a 17.8 percent cesarean rate at Parkland Hospital. Despite the dramatic difference in cesarean rates, they could detect no difference in perinatal mortality.[51] During the study years (1982 to 1984), the incidence of neonatal seizures was similar in the two institutions. Caution was also raised regarding the precision of the diagnosis and etiology of seizures between the two institutions.

It is most likely that the decline in perinatal mortality is attributable to major advances in prenatal care (ultrasound, antepartum testing, amniotic fluid surfactant determinations, and so forth), as well as dramatic improvements in neonatal intensive care including the availability of surfactant implemented in the same time frame. Porreco[52] provided data to suggest little, if any, impact arising from cesarean birth. They divided unselected patients into two groups, one with management minimizing the use of cesarean delivery and the other with routine management. The cesarean rate in the first group (5.7 percent) was considerably less than that of the routine group (17.6 percent). Despite the dramatic difference in cesarean rates, the perinatal mortality and morbidity rates were not significantly different between the two groups.[52]

Cesarean Delivery as a Strategy To Reduce Cerebral Palsy

Scheller and Nelson[53] from the NICHD, in a review of the literature of the past 25 years, concluded that there is no evidence to support the hypothesis that the increased cesarean delivery rate has had a favorable impact on the rate of neurologic disorders or on cerebral palsy. When comparing the occurrence rates of cerebral palsy in nations with a broad range of cesarean rates (7 to 22 percent), the reported cerebral palsy rates in all countries were within a very narrow range of 1.1 to 1.3 per 1,000 in neonatal survivors with birth weights more than 2,500 g.[53] Furthermore, there is no evidence that continuous electronic fetal monitoring provides an advantage over periodic auscultation or reduces the rate of cerebral palsy.[31-33,54]

INDICATIONS FOR CESAREAN DELIVERY

Overview of Indications

In general, cesarean delivery is used when labor is contraindicated or vaginal delivery is unlikely to be accomplished safely or within a time frame necessary to prevent the development of fetal and/or maternal morbidity in excess of that expected following vaginal delivery.

Indications for cesarean delivery can be categorized (Table 18–3) in several ways. Some indications strictly benefit the fetus, whereas others are largely done for maternal benefit to avoid maternal hemorrhage, reduce the potential spread of malignancy, avoid the repeated need for additional procedures such as abdominal cer-clage in future pregnancies, and prevent uterine rupture. Some indications will benefit *both* mother and fetus. Some indications are well accepted even though selectively applied on a subjective basis. Placenta previa and conjoined twins are universally accepted as indications for cesarean birth. On the other hand, several indications such as a breech presentation or a VLBW fetus are controversial.

Fetal Indications

Fetal indications for cesarean birth are in large part designed to minimize neonatal morbidity and possibly long-term consequences of profound intrapartum metabolic or mixed metabolic acidemia and/or delivery-related trauma (including significant fetal thrombocytopenia) or transmission of infection.[55] Accepted indications, often used selectively, include the following: "significant" nonremediable and nonreassuring FHR patterns, especially when associated with progressive loss of variability; various categories of breech presentation at risk for head entrapment and/or cord prolapse; the VLBW fetus; and active genital herpes. The

Table 18–3. COMMONLY REPORTED INDICATIONS FOR CESAREAN DELIVERY

Indications	Selective	Subjective	Controversial*	Universally Accepted†
Fetal				
Nonreassuring FHR‡	√	√		√
Breech, frank	√		√	
Breech, nonfrank	√		√	
Breech, preterm	√		√	
Very low birth weight (<1,500 g)	√		√	
Herpes simplex virus	√			
Immune thrombocytopenic purpura	√			
Congenital anomalies, major	√		√	
Maternal–fetal				
Cephalopelvic disproportion (relative)	√	√		√
Cephalopelvic disproportion (absolute)		√		√
Failure to progress	√	√		√
Placental abruption	√	√		√
Placenta previa				√
Maternal				
Obstructive benign and malignant tumors	√	√		√
Large vulvar condyloma	√	√		
Cervical cerclage (abdominal)	√			
Prior vaginal colporrhaphy	√			
Conjoined twins				√

*Controversy regarding need for universal application.
†Universally accepted if selective/subjective criteria present.
‡Of a critical degree commonly associated with change in FHR variability.

decision to use cesarean delivery may be selective, based on the results of ultrasound or cordocentesis studies (i.e., major fetal congenital anomalies such as hydrocephalus, gastroschisis, or omphalocele). In such cases, a planned, controlled delivery with predictable access to pediatric surgical support may be desirable. However, at this time, there is no proven benefit in performing a cesarean delivery for gastroschisis or omphalocele.[56]

"Significant" Nonreassuring FHR Observations

Approximately 1 to 3 percent of all laboring patients undergo cesarean delivery for a nonremediable and nonreassuring FHR pattern (see Chapter 14). Some clinicians unfortunately continue to designate this indication as "fetal distress," a term not recommended by the ACOG.[56] The cesarean delivery rate and the precise criteria for "fetal distress" vary considerably from hospital to hospital and among individual practitioners. In large part, that variation reflects the subjective nature of the interpretation of continuous FHR. In 1978, Haddad and Lundy[57] estimated that approximately 50 percent of cesarean births performed for such nonreassuring FHR patterns in their hospital were not justified on independent peer review.

Infection as a Risk

The impact of vaginal delivery as a risk factor for transmission of infections such as human immunodeficiency virus (HIV) and herpes simplex virus (HSV) is organism/problem specific (see Chapter 40).

Maternal–Fetal Indications

Placental abnormalities such as placenta previa or placental abruption in which hemorrhage poses a significant risk to both mother and fetus (see Chapter 17), as well as labor "dystocia," are indications for which cesarean delivery offers a potential benefit to both mother and fetus. When extreme, each can pose one or more maternal risks, including hemorrhage, uterine rupture and infection, and fetal metabolic acidosis.

Dystocia is a term used to describe indications for cesarean birth arising from one or more of the "three Ps": relatively large fetus (passenger), relatively small "passage" (pelvis), or relatively insufficient or inefficient uterine contractions (power). Some add a fourth "P," the fearful physician. Included in dystocia are failure to progress (FTP), relative cephalopelvic disproportion (CPD), and absolute CPD on the rare occasion when the latter can be diagnosed (see Chapter 13). Some include failed inductions under this designation. CPD is almost always a relative term; the CPD diagnosis is made only after application of a number of diagnostic

and therapeutic measures including oxytocin. In most instances it involves a normal-sized fetus.[58]

Maternal Indications

There are only a few indications for cesarean delivery that are solely maternal. They include mechanical obstructions of the vagina from large vulvovaginal condylomata, advanced lower genital tract malignancy, and placement of a permanent abdominal cerclage with a desire for future pregnancies.

HOSPITAL REQUIREMENTS FOR CESAREAN DELIVERY

The requirements for hospitals offering cesarean delivery appear in several publications.[59–60]

Facility and Personnel Requirements

Any hospital that provides labor and delivery services should be equipped to perform an "emergency" cesarean delivery. In the past, it was recommended that a hospital offering obstetric services should provide the professional and institutional resources to respond to "acute obstetric emergencies" (i.e., a cesarean delivery) within 30 minutes, when indicated (see below), from the time a decision is made until the procedure is begun.[60] The nursing, anesthesia, neonatal resuscitation, and obstetric personnel required must be either in the hospital or readily available. In its 1999 Practice Bulletin, the ACOG has recommended that, if a VBAC-TOL is considered, a physician capable of monitoring the labor and performing an emergency cesarean delivery should be "immediately" available.[3] Will adverse outcomes be prevented if patients are delivered "immediately"? Data from a prospective study by Porter suggests that factors other than time to delivery are important in determining neonatal outcome associated with uterine rupture.[62] Porter described 26 cases of uterine rupture in VBAC-TOL patients laboring in large metropolitan hospitals, all with 24-hour in-house anesthesia. Six infants (23 percent) suffered either neonatal death or significant neurologic sequelae. The mean time from decision to delivery was 19 minutes for cases with a poor neonatal outcome and 41 minutes for those with a good result. Patients who demonstrated a bradycardia were delivered in less than 20 minutes, and one third still had a poor outcome.

At this time, there is no consensus standard that defines an acceptable time interval for performance of a cesarean delivery. In the presence of certain subjective, judgment-dependent, "clinically significant" nonreassuring FHR patterns that fulfill criteria and pose significant risk of profound fetal metabolic acidemia requiring rapid intervention, prolapse of the cord, symptomatic uterine rupture, and certain cases of obvious and symptomatic placental abruption and persistent hemorrhage secondary to placenta previa, an immediate response is warranted. Under most circumstances (i.e., protraction and arrest disorders of labor) cesarean delivery is not necessary within a 30-minute time frame. Indeed, in certain large units, triage may be necessary to determine priority of access to the operating room, anesthesiologists, and other resources.

Porreco and Meier[63] evaluated the likelihood of need for an urgent cesarean birth that would activate the 30-minute recommendation in patients with and without a prior cesarean birth. The need for a delivery within 30 minutes was similar in patients with no prior cesarean delivery (1.9 percent [two cases]) and in those with a previous low transverse incision (1.4 percent). The two patients with a prior low transverse incision who required an urgent cesarean birth were found to have an intact scar at the time of surgery. The Canadian Consensus Conference on Cesarean Childbirth (four prospective studies) made similar observations, noting the probability of urgent cesarean delivery to be only 2.7 percent among 11,819 births.[64] Symptomatic uterine dehiscence occurred in only 0.22 percent of births.

SURGICAL PRINCIPLES AND OPERATIVE PROCEDURE

Skin Preparation

An abdominal incision interrupts the body's first line of defense against infection. The primary objective of skin preparation for cesarean delivery is to reduce the risk of wound infection by decreasing the bacterial flora of the patient's abdominal wall along the anticipated incision site. It is impossible to sterilize skin. The preparation of the patient's intended incision site in the operating room ordinarily includes mechanical removal of obvious foreign material, application of soap or detergent scrub to remove surface dirt and oil, plus application of a topical antimicrobial agent to reduce the bacteria to a minimal level at the site and adjacent skinfolds and/or umbilicus.[65] In surgical patients, the duration and choice of the scrub have not been demonstrated to reduce the rate of wound infection significantly in either clean or clean-contaminated (cesarean delivery) wounds.[66–68] There is great variation in the duration of the clinical skin scrub among both physicians and hospitals. Some apply a surgical scrub for up to 5 minutes, whereas others simply scrub the intended site for approximately 30 seconds and apply a bacteri-

cidal solution. Overall, the rate of wound infection is approximately 6 to 8 percent whether the skin preparation is sprayed or mechanically scrubbed. It is likely that simple application by painting or spraying is as effective, if not more effective, than the traditional approach of long-term mechanical scrubbing.[69,70] There are also data that suggest that a rapid alcohol preparation followed by application of iodine-impregnated sterile drapes may safely reduce skin preparation time to 1 to 2 minutes.[71]

Bacteria such as *Staphylococcus aureus,* which may be normal inhabitants of the hair follicle, may be reduced in the preparation process, but are not totally eliminated.[72] Fortunately, "transient" flora are easier to remove from the skin than are the "resident" flora that are attached to the skin by adhesion or adsorption and require friction for removal. Under ordinary circumstances, the number of flora in any one area is relatively stable. The relative risk of infection with skin incisions varies, to some extent, according to the site of the incision; the availability of moisture, which promotes bacterial colonization; and the presence of lipid secretion by sebaceous glands. The indigenous "resident" flora of the skin are mainly diphtheroids and gram-positive rods, including aerobic *Corynebacterium* and anaerobic *Propionibacterium*. Gram-negative organisms can proliferate in moist areas such as under a panniculus or air-tight dressing.[73] The aerobic corynebacteria diphtheroids are the most common organisms in areas of moist skin. These diphtheroids seldom cause clinical infection and are actually important in the ecology of skin by suppressing *Staphylococcus epidermidis* and *S. aureus.*

In contrast to the normal resident skin flora whose numbers are normally stable, "transient" flora are deposited on the skin and in the incision/wound from the environment and, as a consequence, vary greatly in type and number. Other factors that determine whether a wound infection will occur include host resistance, virulence of the organisms deposited on the skin/incisional wound, presence and amount of tissue destruction, size and reactivity of the suture material, vascularity of the incision site, and length of the procedure. In the case of cesarean delivery, leakage of cervical and vaginal secretions into the pelvis and transmittal to the skin incision site are also contributing factors.

Preparation of the vagina prior to cesarean delivery is seldom an issue with the possible exception of cases in which a cesarean hysterectomy is planned. Preparation of the vagina is intended to reduce postoperative infection. However, if the clinician decides to use prophylactic antibiotics, it is doubtful that there is any additional benefit to be gained from preoperative preparation of the vagina with an antiseptic preparation. Should a cesarean hysterectomy be planned, simple irrigation of the vagina with a saline solution will dilute the concentration of bacteria in the vagina and may provide additional benefit.

Hair Removal

In general, the only reason to remove hair from the intended operative site is to eliminate hair that will mechanically interfere with the surgeon's approximation of the wound edges and with adhesion and removal of postoperative dressings.[74] Hair is sterile.[75] Removal of hair with a razor may increase wound infection rates by creating breaks in the skin for bacterial entry. Should shaving be required, it is best done in the operating room. Alexander et al.[76] have shown that clipping the hair the morning of surgery results in a significantly lower infection rate than does clipping the hair the evening prior to surgery or shaving at any time.

Suture Selection

Sutures may be synthetic or nonsynthetic in origin. The latter are derived from gut, cotton, or silk. Sutures can be further divided into absorbable and nonabsorbable types (Table 18–4). The *United States Pharmacopeia* categorizes suture materials as nonabsorbable if tensile strength is maintained for more than 60 days. In turn, synthetic suture types are braided or monofilament. The braided absorbable sutures are either coated (Vicryl or Dexon Plus) or noncoated (Dexon S).

Synthetic sutures offer the benefits of decreased tissue reactivity, prolonged and predictable strength, and low coefficients of friction. Monofilament synthetic sutures elicit somewhat less tissue reaction than their braided counterparts: both are less reactive than their nonsynthetic absorbable and nonabsorbable counterparts. The larger the gauge of the suture, the greater the likelihood of adhesion formation.[77] Knot security is maintained for several weeks longer with synthetic absorbable sutures than with chromic cat gut.

The ideal suture ties easily and offers knot security, minimal tissue inflammatory reaction, and tensile strength compatible with the inherent healing properties of the tissue to be reapproximated. It is also desirable that the suture be flexible, pliable, and easy to handle, resistant to infection, and reabsorbed at a predictable rate. The selection of the suture material to be used should also be based on how rapidly the particular tissue heals. For instance, chromic cat gut, a suture material that maintains tensile strength for a relatively short time, is often appropriate for visceral organs like the bladder, peritoneum, and vagina, surfaces that generally heal quickly, particularly in pregnancy.[78] In contrast, skin and fascia heal more slowly; thus, the suture selected should provide more long-term tensile strength. For example, fascia regains only 25 percent of its original strength after 20 days of healing, and the fascial layer is subject to dehiscence if not closed properly. Nonabsorbable synthetic sutures such as polypropylene (Prolene) and polybutester (Novafil) are strong and dependable and are frequently used to repair fascia and for mass closure. Monofilament nylons, braided absorbable (Vicryl) Maxon, and polydioxanone (PDS) are also useful.[79]

Each suture type has definite advantages and disadvantages. When using the synthetic sutures, it is recommended that the clinician add two more knots with longer tails to ensure knot security because these sutures may slip when knots are not properly tied. Manufacturers have introduced coated synthetic sutures (Dexon Plus, coated Vicryl) that have less memory and lie more easily. Should the clinician desire to maintain tensile strength in fascial and subcuticular tissue over longer intervals (e.g., patients who have diabetes mellitus, are infected, or on corticosteroid therapy), the newer synthetic monofilament absorbable sutures such as polyglyconate (Maxon) and PDS may be preferable because they support the tissues in the wound adequately for more than 6 weeks.

Nonabsorbable monofilament sutures such as Prolene and Novafil may be the suture of choice for closing the patient at risk of infection because they do not allow bacteria to invade and colonize the interstices of the braided polyfilament sutures. This feature is particularly

---

Table 18–4. CATEGORIES OF SUTURE MATERIAL POTENTIALLY AVAILABLE FOR CESAREAN DELIVERY AND/OR PERIPARTUM HYSTERECTOMY

	Absorbable	Nonabsorbable
Nonsynthetic	Plain gut	Silk
	Chromic gut	Cotton
Synthetic	Polyglycolic acid (Dexon)	Polypropylene monofilament (Surgilene, Prolene)
	Polyglactin (Vicryl) 910	Braided (Dacron, Mersilene)
	Polydioxanone (PDS)	Gore-Tex (Polytetrafluoroethylene)
	Polyglyconate (Maxon)	Nylon (Ethibond)
	Monocryl	

important for infected abdominal wall fascia, where tensile strength is crucial and chronic inflammation least desirable.

ABDOMINAL INCISIONS

Selection of Incision Type

The surgeon may choose either a vertical or a transverse skin incision (Fig. 18–1) when performing a cesarean delivery. The ultimate choice hinges on factors such as the urgency of the procedure, the presence of prior abdominal scars, and associated nonobstetric pathology, if any. To some degree the decision will be based on the surgeon's past experience and on consumer pressures favoring a low transverse incision.[80,81] The midline vertical, transverse Maylard, and transverse Pfannenstiel incisions are the three most commonly used types. Transverse Cherney and paramedian vertical incisions are seldom used.

There has been a significant increase recently in the use of transverse incisions as opposed to the traditional low vertical incision. The obstetrician, comfortable with several types of incision, is able to make a selective decision for each patient. The choice should be based on the relative simplicity and speed of the various incisions, the desired exposure, the estimated fetal weight, the anticipated cosmetic results, and the risk factors for infection or dehiscence. In general, vertical incisions al-

low more rapid access to the lower uterine segment, have less blood loss, provide greater feasibility for incisional extension around the umbilicus, and allow easier examination of the upper abdomen. In pregnancy, speed of entry through a midline vertical incision is facilitated by the common occurrence of diastasis of the rectus muscles.

Transverse incisions are somewhat more time consuming; the difference in time of entry between the two incision types is approximately 30 to 60 seconds in the hands of an experienced clinician. Transverse incisions are preferred cosmetically, are generally less painful, have been associated with a lower risk of subsequent herniation, and yet provide equal, if not better, visualization of the pelvis. Some argue that there is a lower incidence of postoperative pulmonary complications when a transverse incision is used, particularly in patients with preexisting pulmonary problems such as obstructive lung disease.[82] Whether a transverse incision is less subject to dehiscence and herniation remains controversial.[83,84]

A number of surgical principles are relevant regardless of the incision selected. The surgeon and surgical assistant should apply traction at right angles to the intended incision site in a symmetric manner so that the incision is developed in a uniform vertical plane through its length and depth. The "Allis" test may be used to determine if the abdominal incision will be large enough; if a 15-cm-long Allis clamp fits easily between retractors placed at the ends of the incision, little difficulty will be encountered in delivering the fetus.[85] There is no reason to disturb the fat from the adjacent fascia unless there is difficulty in exposing the fascial edges. Such efforts will simply increase the risk of postoperative seromas and develop unnecessary dead space.

The Pfannenstiel and Maylard incisions are the most commonly used transverse incisions for cesarean delivery. The Maylard incision is quicker, provides better lateral pelvic and midabdominal visualization, requires less dissection and retraction of the anterior abdominal wall during the procedure, and makes a repeat procedure somewhat easier than the Pfannenstiel.

The Maylard incision (Fig. 18–1) differs from the Pfannenstiel incision in that it involves transverse incision of the anterior rectus sheath and the rectus muscles bilaterally.[86] In the nonobese patient, the skin incision is ordinarily at least 3 to 4 cm above the symphysis. Should there be a large panniculus, the incision may be made considerably higher to avoid placement of the incision on the undersurface of the panniculus. The superficial inferior epigastric vessels, generally located in the lateral one third of the incision, may be individually ligated if necessary. Incision of the rectus muscles is accomplished by placing two fingers or clamps beneath each rectus muscle and lifting the mus-

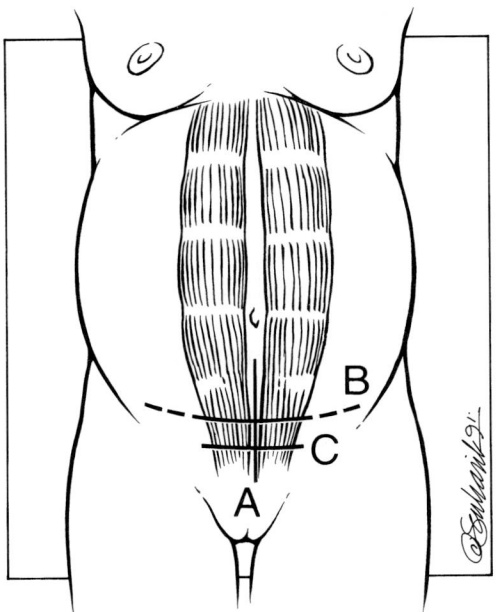

Figure 18–1. The obstetrician most commonly uses one of three abdominal incisions: (A) midline, (B) Maylard, and (C) Pfannenstiel. *Hatched lines* indicate possible extension. (Modified from Baker C, Shingleton HM: Incisions. Clin Obstet Gynecol 31:701, 1988.)

cles in such a way as to allow surgical incision with either a knife or cutting cautery between the fingers or clamps. In most cesarean procedures, pelvic exposure is sufficient if only the medial two thirds of the rectus muscles are incised. This avoids the necessity to ligate the deep inferior epigastric vessels, as may be necessary in more extensive gynecologic cases. Nonetheless, the surgeon should palpate for these vessels. Should extension of the incision be necessary, these vessels should be isolated and ligated to avoid hematoma formation. Those favoring a Cherney modification believe it is preferable to partial transsection of the rectus muscles, a technique required with the Maylard incision.[87] After separation of the rectus muscles from the pubic symphysis, the transversalis fascia and peritoneum are then incised transversely, as opposed to the Pfannenstiel incision in which they are incised vertically.

The Pfannenstiel incision (Fig. 18–1) is a curvilinear incision that is best suited for the nonobese patient. The incision is generally made approximately 3 cm above the symphysis pubis within the pubic hair line at its midpoint. The determination of its lateral extension should, to some extent, be a function of the estimated fetal size. Symmetry of the incision can be facilitated by traction of the skin in a cephalad direction during incision that, when released, will result in a curvilinear incision. The incision is generally extended to the lateral border of the rectus muscles at a point 2 to 3 cm inferior and medial to the anterior superior iliac crests. The inferior and superior margin of the fascial incision is elevated to facilitate blunt dissection of the fascial sheath from the underlying rectus muscles. Individual perforating blood vessels between muscle and fascia will require ligation or coagulation to achieve adequate hemostasis. Sharp separation of the muscles from the median raphe, which is facilitated by upward traction on the anterior rectus sheath, is extended superiorly to the level of the umbilicus. Once the rectus muscles are adequately exposed, they are retracted laterally to reveal the underlying transversalis fascia and peritoneum, which is entered via a midline vertical incision in a manner similar to that of a low vertical abdominal incision.

Abdominal Entry

Surgeons vary in their choice of technique for incising the fascia. Some prefer initial entry by scalpel with subsequent extension with scissors. Others use the scalpel for the entirety of the incision because it is theoretically less traumatic. Once the surgeon becomes familiar with this technique, it allows somewhat faster entry than does scissors. Nonetheless, either technique is appropriate. The site of initial peritoneal entry chosen should be approximately halfway between the umbilicus and symphysis so as to avoid bladder injury, particularly in patients undergoing a repeat cesarean procedure; the peritoneum should be "tented" between two hemostats or pickups and palpated to ascertain that there is no adherent bowel omentum, or even bladder. The peritoneal cavity may be entered using a scalpel or scissors. Should the planned peritoneal incision be in a vertical direction, the peritoneal incision is first extended superiorly for greater exposure and then inferiorly to a point just above the superior pole of the bladder.

SPECIAL CONSIDERATIONS

Skin Incision in the Obese Patient

The obese patient is at significant additional risk for wound complications. Reported wound complication rates are 4 and 29 percent in nonobese and obese patients, respectively.[88] Should the patient be massively obese, it may be better to use an incision that does not involve the underside of the panniculus, an area that is more heavily colonized with bacteria and is difficult to prepare surgically, to keep dry, and to inspect in the postoperative period. The objective is to enter the abdomen directly over the lower uterine segment. The surgeon may choose either a vertical midline incision, which is developed periumbilically both above and below the umbilicus or, alternatively, a transverse incision closer to the umbilicus. The actual selection of the site of incision, whether it be vertical or transverse, can be made by retracting the panniculus in a caudad direction so as to place the incision directly overlying the uterine segment.

In closing the fascia of an obese patient, placement of the sutures in the fascia should be at least 1.5 to 2 cm lateral to the cut margin of the fascia, with successive bites approximately 1.5 cm apart along the longitudinal axis of the incision. Should there be major risk factors other than obesity, the clinician may consider use of (1) Smead-Jones monofilament polypropylene internal retention sutures or (2) interrupted or figure-of-eight sutures using either polyglycolic acid or other delayed absorption sutures like monofilament polyglyconate or polydioxanone.

It is also acceptable to use a running continuous large-gauge monofilament polypropylene suture on a large needle in closing the fascial incision. This technique offers the theoretical advantages of distributing tension equally over the continuity of the incision line and increasing the speed of wound closure, thus minimizing the risk of foreign material within the wound. Sutures should not be locked, a technique that reduces vascularization and potentially slows wound healing. Shepherd et al.[89] encountered no wound dehiscences using a mass closure technique in over 200 high-risk gynecology patients. Some advocate placement of a clip on the short end of the suture to avoid knot disruption. Subcutaneous sutures may be used and the skin closed with suture staples, left in place for 7 to 10 days. Subcutaneous closure will reduce the risk of wound disruption in women with 2 cm or more of subcutaneous fat.[90]

Placenta Previa and Accreta

Although the incidence of placenta accreta has been reported to be approximately 1 in 2,500 deliveries, the incidence increases to approximately 4 percent in patients with a placenta previa.[91] This association is particularly marked in the patient with a previous cesarean birth. Under such circumstances, the incidence of placenta accreta may approach 25 percent.[92] For this reason the physician contemplating a cesarean delivery for placenta previa, particularly a repeat procedure, should consider the possibility of hysterectomy.

Selection of Lower Uterine Incision

The most commonly used uterine incisions (Table 18–5 and Fig. 18–2) are the low transverse incision originally advocated by Kerr[19] and the low vertical incision originally proposed by Krönig.[16] A low transverse (Kerr) incision is used in more than 90 percent of all cesarean births. The low transverse incision has the following advantages over a vertical incision: less risk of entry into the upper uterine segment, greater ease of entry, less bladder dissection, less operative blood loss, less repair, easier reperitonealization, and less likelihood of adhesion formation to bowel or omentum. Importantly, in subsequent pregnancies the obstetrician can feel more comfortable offering a VBAC trial because there is less likelihood of uterine rupture.[93]

Table 18–5. SURGICAL CONSIDERATIONS IN SELECTION OF UTERINE INCISION FOR CESAREAN DELIVERY

Low Segment Incisions	Transverse	Vertical
Technical ease of		
Extension of incision	–	+
Bladder dissection	+	–
Uterine closure	+	–
Reperitonealization	+	–
Anticipate hysterectomy	–	+
Benefits vs. risks		
Uterine rupture (subsequent)	+	–
Lateral extension into uterine vessels	–	+
Extension inferiorly	+	–
Intraoperative bleeding	+	–
Subsequent adhesions	+	–

+, Advantage to uterine incision type; –, disadvantage.

A vertical incision (classic or low vertical) may be advantageous if the patient has not been in labor and the lower uterus is narrow and poorly developed or if the fetus is not in a cephalic presentation, particularly a back-down transverse lie or preterm breech. Should a transverse incision be performed under such circumstances, there is a greater likelihood of lateral extension of the incision into the vessels of the broad ligament. However, individualization is reasonable. For instance, the author generally prefers a vertical incision for a transverse lie. However, a low transverse incision is certainly feasible if the lower uterine segment is well developed, as may be the case when the patient presents in active labor with advanced cervical dilatation. Other possible indications for a vertical incision include leiomyomata obstructing exposure to the lower segment and structural uterine anomalies.

The classic uterine incision involves the upper active uterine segment. Its primary advantage is the rapidity of entry into the uterus. Furthermore, some physicians believe that the incision is useful in the presence of an anterior placenta previa, reducing the potential for maternal and fetal hemorrhage.[94] Despite these advantages, this incision is used in no more than 10 percent of cases. A classic incision may be used when it is not possible to expose the lower uterine segment or when a hysterectomy is planned. More commonly encountered complications associated with classic incisions include subsequent adhesion formation and greater risk of uterine rupture with later pregnancies.[95] Patients who have had a prior classic incision should consider an appropriately timed elective repeat cesarean birth because of the risk of uterine rupture even before labor has started.

The theoretical advantages of the low vertical (Krönig) incision over the classic incision are similar to those of the low transverse incision. However, unlike the classic incision, there may occasionally be a caudad (inferior) extension of the incision into the cervix and vagina or even into the bladder. Although the low vertical (Krönig) incision is theoretically limited to the lower uterine segment, it often involves the upper segment.

PERFORMING THE CESAREAN DELIVERY

Development of Bladder Flap

After placement of a bladder catheter and entry into the peritoneal cavity, the obstetrician should palpate the uterus to determine the degree and direction of uterine rotation. In most instances, the uterus is dextrorotated such that the left round ligament may be visualized more anteriorly and closer to the midline than is

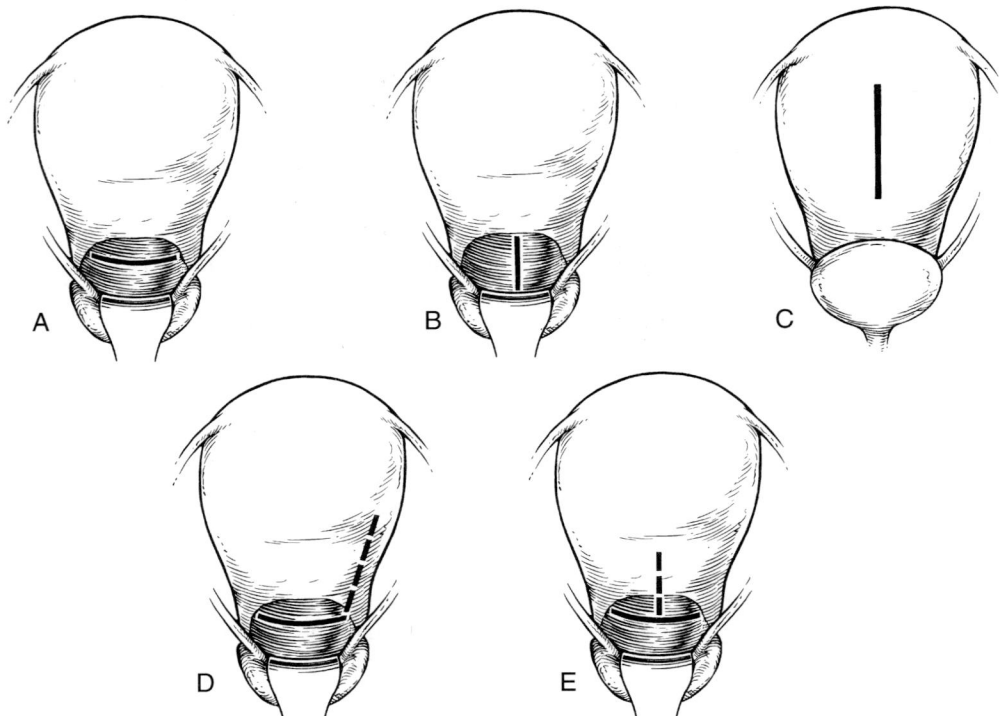

Figure 18–2. Uterine incisions for cesarean delivery. *A,* Low transverse incision. The bladder is retracted downward, and the incision is made in the lower uterine segment, curving gently upward. If the lower segment is poorly developed, the incision can also curve sharply upward at each end to avoid extending into the ascending branches of the uterine arteries. *B,* Low vertical incision. The incision is made vertically in the lower uterine segment after reflecting the bladder, avoiding extension into the bladder below. If more room is needed, the incision can be extended upward into the upper uterine segment. *C,* Classic incision. The incision is entirely within the upper uterine segment and can be at the level shown or in the fundus. *D,* J incision. If more room is needed when an initial transverse incision has been made, either end of the incision can be extended upward into the upper uterine segment and parallel to the ascending branch of the uterine artery. *E,* T incision. More room can be obtained in a transverse incision by an upward midline extension into the upper uterine segment.

the right. Some obstetricians insert moistened laparotomy pads into each lateral peritoneal gutter prior to making the uterine incision to absorb amniotic fluid and blood escaping from the incision, particularly when there is a strong suspicion of amnionitis. The uterovesical peritoneum (serosa) is grasped in the midline and undermined with Metzenbaum scissors inserted between the peritoneum and underlying myometrium to develop bluntly a retroperitoneal space bilaterally to the lateral margins of the lower uterine segment. The peritoneal reflection is then incised bilaterally in an upward direction and the vesicouterine fold is grasped with forceps and the bladder lifted anteriorly, allowing blunt separation of the bladder from the underlying lower uterine segment. Should adherent adhesions be noted in a repeat procedure, sharp dissection may be necessary to free-up the posterior aspect of the bladder. Once the dissection is complete in the midline, the fingers may be carefully swept laterally in each direction to free the bladder more completely. After the bladder flap is adequately developed, a universal retractor or bladder blade is used to retract the bladder anteriorly and infe-

riorly to facilitate exposure of the intended incision site. Use of a Richardson retractor to retract the superior margin of a transverse abdominal incision may help to facilitate exposure.

Low Transverse Cesarean Incision

The lower uterine segment incision (Fig. 18–2A) is begun 1 to 2 cm above the site of the original upper margin of the bladder. A small midline incision is first made with a scalpel through the lower uterine segment to the fetal membranes. Continuous suction should be available to facilitate visualization of the operative field and to evacuate amniotic fluid should the incision perforate through the fetal membranes. Care should be taken to avoid laceration of the fetus, which is an occasional complication, especially when the lower uterine segment is thin or when expeditious delivery of the fetus is required.

After suctioning, the incision may be extended laterally and slightly upward (cephalad) to the lateral margin of the lower uterine segment so as to maximize incisional length and avoid extension into the uterine vessels. Extension of the incision may be accomplished by either of two methods: (1) sharp dissection, taking care to avoid fetal fingers and toes; or (2) blunt dissection by spreading the incision with each index finger. Blunt splitting of the uterine incision, particularly if the lower uterine segment is thin, will result in more rapid entry; however, there is potential for unpredictable extension with this method, particularly if the lower segment is not fully effaced. The choice is largely a function of training and theoretical concerns regarding unintended extension. The relative merits of the two approaches were recently addressed in a prospective randomized study that could detect no difference in the incidence of unintended extension, estimated blood loss, or length of surgery between the two approaches. Rather, the frequency of unintended extensions correlated with the stage of labor (1.4, 15.5, and 35.0 percent for no labor, first stage of labor, and second stage, respectively).[96]

Low Vertical Incision

Should the fetus present as a breech or transverse lie, particularly back-down, there is often advantage to a low vertical (Figs. 18–2*B* and 18–3) uterine incision, particularly if the lower uterine segment is not well developed. The bladder is displaced downward to expose the lower uterine segment more inferiorly so that the low vertical incision will be less likely to extend into the upper segment. Once the anticipated site is exposed, an incision is made at the inferior margin of the lower segment and extended cephalad with either

bandage scissors or knife. Should it be necessary to extend the incision into the upper active uterine segment, it should be noted in the operative report.

Although vertical cesarean incisions are traditionally categorized into low vertical and classic types, the performance of a true low vertical incision that does not enter the upper contractile portion of the uterus is actually uncommon. The clinical implication is that the low vertical incision poses considerably less risk in a subsequent VBAC trial than would be the case with a classic incision; nonetheless, the risk of rupture is probably somewhat greater than that of a low transverse incision.

Classic Cesarean Incision

The initial incision (Fig. 18–2*C*) is made with a scalpel 1 to 2 cm above the bladder reflection. Once the fetus or membranes are visualized, the incision is extended cephalad with bandage scissors, the size of the incision varying with the estimated size of the fetus. The patient should also be advised of this occurrence and its importance to future pregnancies should a VBAC trial be considered.

Management of the Anterior Placenta

Should the placenta be located in the anterior lower uterine segment, entry can be accomplished by one of three methods. First, the clinician can simply dissect through the placenta; this carries the risk of short-term fetal hemorrhage. Second, the placenta can be separated from the lower uterine segment, facilitating lateral ex-

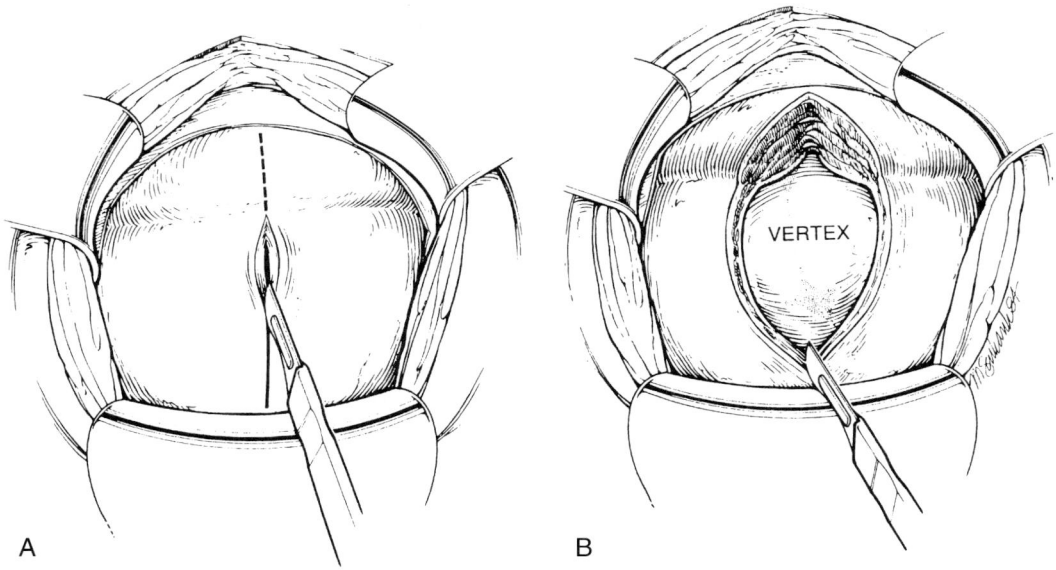

A   B

Figure 18–3. Low vertical incision. *A,* Ideally, a vertical incision is contained entirely in the lower uterine segment. *B,* Extension into the upper uterine segment, either inadvertently or by choice, is common.

posure of the fetus. Finally, a classic uterine incision can be used.

Delivery of the Fetus

Upon completion of the incision, the retractors are removed and a hand is inserted into the uterine cavity to elevate and flex the fetal head through the uterine incision. Initial efforts to deliver the presenting part through the uterine incision will indicate the adequacy of the uterine incision. Should the head be deeply wedged within the pelvis, it can be dislodged by an assistant applying upward pressure vaginally. Once the occiput presents into the incision, moderate fundal pressure may facilitate expulsion. On occasion the head may be delivered with shorthandled Simpson forceps or vacuum. Once delivery of the fetal head is completed, the nose and oropharynx are suctioned with a bulb syringe. If meconium is present, suction can be accomplished with continuous wall suction. When suctioning is complete, expulsion of the remainder of the newborn is facilitated by moderate uterine fundal pressure. The cord is then doubly clamped and cut, and the infant is transferred to the resuscitation team.

Umbilical cord blood gas data may be collected routinely or selectively in high-risk circumstances, such as fetal growth restriction, preterm birth, breech presentations, amnionitis, the presence of thick meconium, cesarean delivery for nonreassuring FHR findings, or unanticipated low Apgar scores. To facilitate collection of an adequate arterial sample, the umbilical cord is first clamped close to the placenta so as to maintain filling of the umbilical arteries and vein and then clamped close to the newborn. It is then doubly clamped in each location so as to isolate a 10- to 15-cm segment of cord for umbilical arterial and venous blood sampling.

Operative Techniques for the Preterm Fetus

The uterine incision to be used for the delivery of the preterm fetus is best selected after entry into the maternal abdomen. At least 50 percent of cases will require a low vertical or classic incision for indications such as malpresentation or a poorly developed lower uterine segment. Among 174 VLBW cesarean births at Los Angeles County Women's Hospital, a low transverse incision was performed in 31 percent of cases, a low vertical incision in 47 percent, and a classic uterine incision in 22 percent.[97] Using ultrasound, Morrison[98] prospectively evaluated the width of the lower uterine segment in the absence of labor and found its transverse dimension to be 0.5, 1.0, and 4.0 cm at 20, 28, and 34 weeks, respectively. Thus, without significant labor, the lower uterine segment will probably not be sufficiently developed to provide an adequate transverse dimension for removal of the fetus. The complications of performing a low transverse incision in the absence of adequate development of the lower uterine segment include difficult removal of the fetus, lateral extension of the incision into the broad ligament and uterine vessels, and downward extension of the incision into the cervix and the vagina. Boyle and Gabbe observed that 1.3 percent of low transverse cesarean incisions required a T or J extension (Fig. 18–2D and E) for malpresentation, usually of a preterm fetus, for a poorly developed lower uterine segment, or when the fetal head was deeply arrested in the midpelvis. Estimated blood loss was significantly greater in these cases.[99] It is noteworthy that intraoperative complications including injury to the bladder, broad ligament laceration, and uterine artery laceration are more common in preterm than in term cesarean births. The complication rate is independent of incision type.[100]

Cesarean Delivery of the Breech Presentation

Should an elective cesarean section be planned for a breech presentation, it is desirable, prior to performing the procedure, to confirm that the breech has not converted spontaneously to a vertex or to a more unfavorable transverse lie. The lie of the fetus can be verified by palpation prior to making the uterine incision. In the case of a transverse lie, the vertex or the buttocks of the breech can often be guided into a position underlying the planned site of the uterine incision. Should the lower uterine segment be well developed, a transverse or vertical uterine incision can be used. However, a vertical incision is often preferable should the cervix be long and closed, the lower uterine segment poorly developed, or the breech converted to a back-down transverse lie.

The head of a preterm breech infant may be trapped if the incision is not large enough.[97] Although cesarean delivery is often elected in an attempt to minimize fetal trauma, the actual delivery mechanism via the cesarean incision is essentially identical to that of the vaginal route. Should the fetus present as a nonfrank breech or back-up transverse lie, the first step is to identify and grasp a foot and extract the leg through the incision until the second foot can be identified. The surgeon should conduct the delivery process in such a way as to minimize hyperextension of the fetal neck and compression of fetal organs. The mechanism for delivery of the breech is discussed elsewhere (see Chapter 16). However, should there be evidence of head entrapment, the first action should be to extend the abdominal incision and to enlarge the uterine incision. Occasionally, it may be necessary to incise perpendicular to a transverse incision (inverted T-shaped incision) or to extend the transverse incision upward parallel to the uterine artery (J incision) (Fig. 18–2D and E). Both the inverted T and J incisions are more subject to uterine rupture with subsequent pregnancies.

Manual Versus "Spontaneous" Placental Expulsion

Following delivery of the fetus, 20 to 40 units of oxytocin can be administered in an isotonic crystaloid solution. Subsequent removal of the placenta is commonly done manually. McCurdy et al.[101] compared the manual option to spontaneous delivery of the placenta in a prospective randomized trial. The manual group demonstrated a significantly higher measured blood loss (967 vs. 666 ml) and a surprisingly higher incidence of endometritis (23 vs. 3 percent). Additional data suggesting a benefit for awaiting "spontaneous expulsion" are provided in a 1964 report from Queenan and Nakamoto[102] that demonstrated a reduction in Rh sensitization in the "spontaneous" group. Following its removal, the placenta should be inspected for possible missing cotyledons.

Repair of the Uterine Incision

Closure of the uterine incision may be aided by manual delivery of the uterine fundus through the abdominal incision.[103] Delivery of the uterine fundus through the abdominal incision facilitates uterine massage and observation of uterine tone, as well as routine examination of the adnexa and tubal ligation. The fundus may be covered with a moistened laparotomy pad and the uterine incision inspected for obvious bleeding points, which are controlled with either Ring forceps or Allis clamps until suture closure can be accomplished. The uterine cavity may then be inspected and wiped clean with a dry laparotomy sponge to remove fetal membranes and placental fragments.

The primary disadvantages of uterine exteriorization are possible peritoneal discomfort and nausea and/or vomiting in patients under inadequate regional anesthesia. Some have hypothesized that exteriorization may temporarily kink and occlude the uterine blood supply, resulting in a delayed onset of bleeding at the incision site. If possible, such a complication must be quite unusual. A prospective randomized study by Magann et al.[104] addressed the cumulative impact of delivery of the placenta and uterine exteriorization and confirmed that blood loss associated with "spontaneous" placental separation was significantly less than that associated with manual removal. When blood loss (uterus exteriorized vs. in situ) was compared, no difference was detectable between the spontaneous separation/expulsion and manual removal groups.

Midline placement of a ring forceps or Allis clamp may be used to elevate the lower portion of the low transverse uterine incision, facilitating visualization of the field and approximation of the incision. Although Allis clamps can be routinely placed at the angles of the incision to control bleeding and to identify the end of the incision, routine placement of more than the one midline clamp in the absence of bleeding simply clutters the field. The perimeter of the uterine incision is then inspected to locate bleeding vessels and to localize the true margins of the uterine incision. Control of uterine bleeding is facilitated by oxytocin administration and uterine massage. Oxytocin administration is particularly important following classic cesarean birth. If bleeding is encountered along the margins of the incision, a ring forceps or Allis clamp should be placed at the site of bleeding. If the incisional margin is not carefully identified, on occasion the posterior wall of the lower uterine segment may balloon anteriorly and be confused with the lower margin of the transverse incision, potentially resulting in complete closure of the uterine cavity (i.e., superior edge of the inferior incision margin sutured to the posterior uterine wall).

Reapproximation of the lower uterine incision may be performed in either one or two layers (Fig. 18–4) using 0 or double 0 chromic suture or similar absorbable synthetic suture such as Vicryl, the second layer inverting the first. The initial suture should be placed lateral to the angle of a transverse incision or inferior to the lower margin of a vertical incision. Subsequent stitches may be run in a continuous or continuous-locking manner to the opposite end of the incision. The sutures may be placed through the entire myometrium. Some have stressed the importance of avoiding incorporation of decidua in the suture for concern of later development of endometriosis in the scar; however, this is a remote possibility.[105] Although many routinely use a continuous-locking suture, there is questionable advantage to routine suture locking along the entire margin, except at sites of obvious oozing. Locking sutures potentially increase the likelihood of tissue ischemia and potentially may limit wound healing. It has been traditional to place a second continuous layer (Lembert or Cushing) of chromic or similar suture to invert the first layer, with either vertically or horizontally stitches, the latter requiring more frequent placement of the needle upon the needle holder. If the low transverse uterine segment is well effaced and hemostasis adequate, it is reasonable to reapproximate the uterine margins with a single suture layer. Hauth et al.[106] have, on the basis of a prospective ($n = 906$) randomized trial comparing traditional two-layer with single-layer closure, reported that the single-layer closure significantly decreased oper-

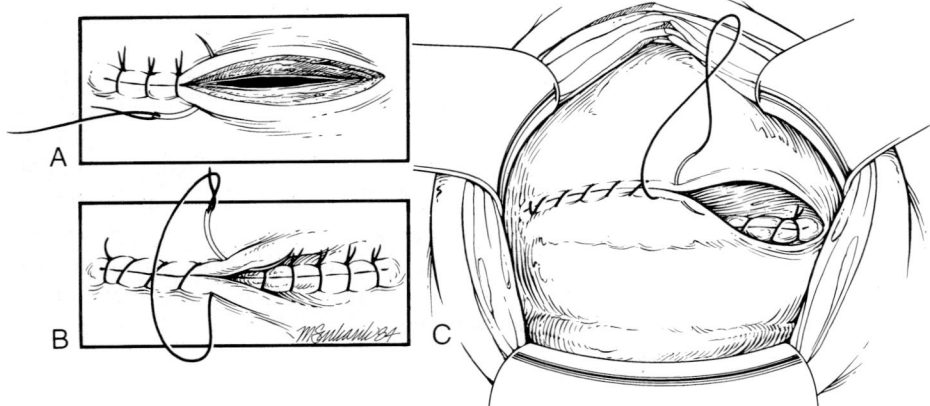

Figure 18–4. Closure of low transverse incision. *A,* The first layer can be either interrupted or continuous. A continuous locking suture is less desirable, despite its reputed hemostatic abilities, because it may interfere with incision vasculature and, hence, with healing and scar formation. *B,* A second inverted layer created by using a continuous Lembert's or Cushing's stitch is customary but is really needed only when apposition is unsatisfactory after application of the first layer. Inclusion of too much tissue produces a bulky mass that may delay involution and interfere with healing. *C,* The bladder peritoneum is reattached to the uterine peritoneum with fine suture.

ating time (39.2 vs. 44.8 minutes), had no increase in postoperative complications and, surprisingly, required fewer additional hemostatic sutures (beyond that expected in one or two layers) per patient. Uterine scar dehiscence or rupture does not appear to be increased with a single layer of closure. Tucker et al.[107] compared the outcomes of 149 women with a single-layer closure with 143 women with two-layer closure and found no complete uterine ruptures in any of the 292 trials of labor. Partial scar separation was detected in approximately 2 percent of patients in each group.

Closure of a classic cesarean incision (Fig. 18–5) involving the more thickened upper segment most often will require a two-layer closure. Should the uterine wall be unusually thick, it may be necessary to use a third layer. Repair of the incision can be done in several ways. A common method is to use continuous 0 or 1 chromic cat gut suture in layers, the first layer approximating the inner one half of the uterine wall thickness in a continuous or continuous-locking manner. A sec-

ond and occasionally a third layer is then used to approximate the uterine musculature. It may be desirable to bury the knot (at the superior end of the incision) of the outer suture line. The operative record should state the type of uterine incision, and the patient should be informed about the incision and its impact on care in subsequent pregnancies, including the advisability against a future attempt at a VBAC.[95]

Reapproximation of the Visceral (Bladder Flap) and Parietal Peritoneum

Most obstetricians no longer close the visceral (bladder flap) and parietal peritoneum, a principle long accepted in the surgical literature. Unrepaired mesothelial surfaces spontaneously reapproximate within 48 hours and demonstrate healing with no scar formation at 5 days. Clinically, this approach is associated with a reduced need for postoperative analgesia and quicker return of

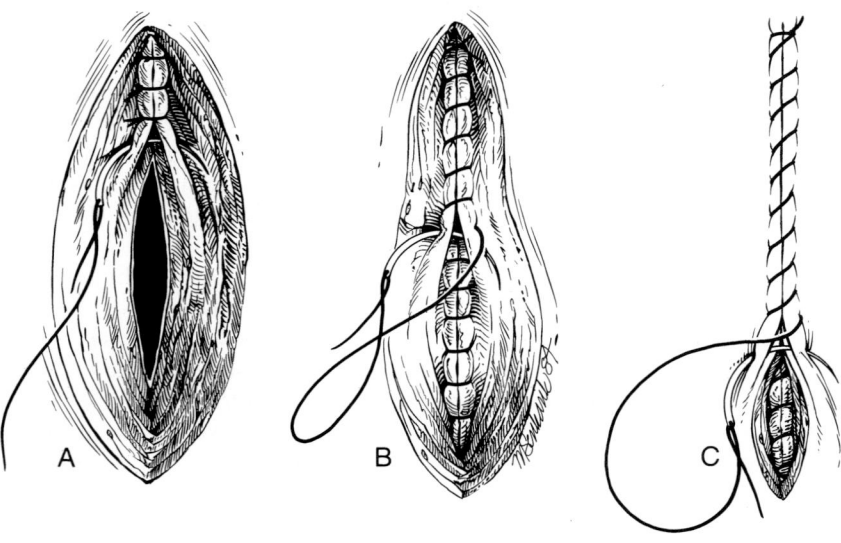

Figure 18–5. Repair of a classic incision. Three-layer closure of a classic incision, including inversion of the serosal layer to discourage adhesion formation. The knot at the superior end of the incision of the second layer can be buried by medial to lateral placement of the suture from within the depth of the incision and subsequent lateral to medial reentry on the opposing side with resultant knot placement within the incision.

bowel function.[108,109] Furthermore, this approach does not promote adhesion formation.[110–113]

Abdominal Closure

Once the uterine incisional reapproximation is completed, the incision should once again be inspected for bleeding points, which can be individually ligated, coagulated, or controlled with figure-of-eight sutures. Before closing the abdomen, the uterus, fallopian tubes, and ovaries should be examined for unsuspected pathology. Some routinely examine the appendix. When surgical sterilization or ovarian cystectomy is required, it is accomplished before replacing the uterus into the abdominal cavity. If used, laparotomy pads are removed and the abdominal contents, lateral gutters, and cul-de-sac are inspected and, where indicated, suctioned. The pelvis and lower abdomen may be irrigated, especially if there is coexistent chorioamnionitis or if there has been heavy spillage of meconium outside the operative field. The operating team should confirm that the needle and sponge counts are correct.

There is no need to reapproximate the parietal peritoneum or rectus muscles. The rectus fascia may be closed with either interrupted or continuous (nonlocking) sutures. Suture choice is important in fascial healing. If the suture is absorbed too rapidly, tensile strength may be reduced, thus increasing the likelihood of wound breakdown. Chromic suture should be avoided when possible. Selection of a suture for its duration of strength is particularly important for patients at risk for wound dehiscence. Unlike their chromic counterparts, synthetic braided sutures maintain tensile strength throughout fascial healing. They are predictably broken down by hydrolysis. In contrast, gut suture has less tensile strength and is degraded less predictably. Local infection may also result in more rapid loss of strength. If the surgeon is dealing with a patient at risk for wound breakdown from chronic corticosteroid therapy, for example, delayed absorbable material such as PDS or polyglyconate (Maxon) or permanent material such as nylon or polypropylene (Prolene) may have merit.

Once an appropriate suture is chosen, care should be taken in selecting the site of suture placement for fascial closure. In most instances of wound dehiscence, the suture remains intact but has cut through the tissue in which it has been placed. One study indicates that this problem is responsible for up to 88 percent of disrupted wounds.[114]

Large bites using larger gauge suture material are less likely to transect tissue than are small bites with narrow-gauge suture material. Suture entry and exit sites should be well beyond the 1-cm inner zone of collagenolysis at the margin of the wound. Should sutures be

placed within this inner zone, there is greater tendency for them to pull through, leading to dehiscence and possible evisceration. Sutures should be placed at approximately 1-cm intervals approximately 1.5 cm from the incision line.

It is acceptable to use a running suture in closing the fascia in patients with a clean incision. Fagniez et al.[115] were not able to demonstrate a difference in dehiscence rates in a randomized prospective trial of 3,135 patients using a running versus interrupted polyglycolic acid suture in midline incisions. Approximation of fascia should allow maintenance of adequate blood flow; unnecessarily tight sutures will cause hypoxia and potentially interfere with predictable wound healing.[116,117] Should a patient be at high risk for wound dehiscence, it is preferable that the fascia not be closed with continuous suturing, particularly on a vertical incision. If the patient is at high risk for abdominal distention and wound breakdown, a mass or Smead-Jones (Fig. 18–6) closure is preferable. This closure is mechanically more sound and allows for a 30 percent increase in abdominal girth.

It is generally not necessary to reapproximate the subcutaneous tissue unless the patient is markedly obese, in which case subcutaneous closure may reduce wound disruption. No difference in the rate of dehiscence was noted between obese patients who underwent peritoneal closure and those who did not in one large randomized trial.[116] Skin may be closed with staples or a subcuticular stitch. Steristrip adhesive tape (3M Surgical Products, St. Paul, MN) can be used to

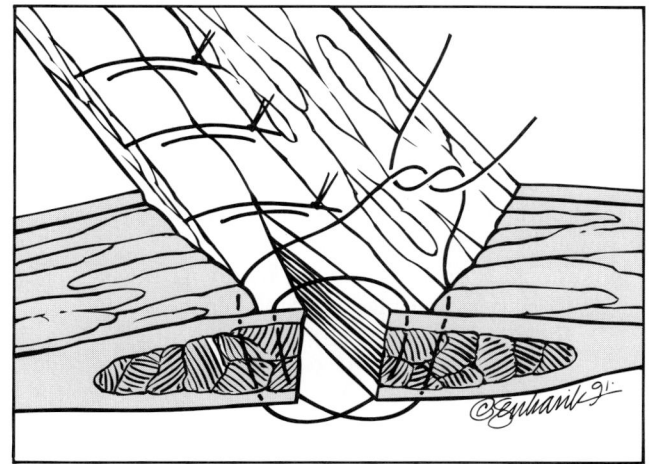

Figure 18–6. Modification of far-near, near-far Smead-Jones suture. Suture passes deeply through lateral side of anterior rectus fascia and adjacent fat, crosses the midline of the incision to pick up the medial edge of the rectus fascia, then catches the near side of the opposite rectus sheath, and, finally, returns to the far margin of the opposite rectus sheath and subcutaneous fat. (Modified from American College of Obstetricians and Gynecologists: Prolog. *In* Gynecologic Oncology and Surgery. Washington, DC, ACOG, 1991, p 187.)

reduce tension on subcuticular sutures. If staples are used, they may be replaced with Steristrips 3 or 4 days after surgery to decrease scarring.

INTRAOPERATIVE COMPLICATIONS

The patient undergoing cesarean delivery is at risk for many of the same intra- and postoperative complications as is the patient having a vaginal delivery. Management problems more commonly associated with cesarean delivery, as well as conditions such as uterine atony and placenta accreta, which are also discussed in Chapter 17, are briefly reviewed in this section.

Although injury to bladder, bowel, or ureters is uncommon, many competent obstetricians, despite careful surgical technique, will encounter complications. When they occur, the primary responsibility is to identify the injury and its extent, to repair the injury, and to obtain consultation should injuries be extensive or unusually complex.

Uterine Lacerations

Lacerations of the lower uterine incision are more common when a low transverse incision is used in the presence of a macrosomic fetus or a noncephalic presentation. Fortunately, these lacerations are usually easily sutured as long as they only extend laterally to the margin of the myometrium or inferiorly into the vagina. Care must be taken to avoid ligation of the ureters. In most circumstances, the lateral apex of the extension can be identified and the suture placed just lateral to that point. Should there be extension into the broad ligament in proximity to the ureters, on occasion it may be necessary to open the broad ligament and identify the ureters before suture placement. Rarely, there may be an advantage to retrograde placement of an 8-Fr ureteral catheter into the ureters. This can be accomplished transurethrally or by performing a vertical incision in the dome of the bladder to visualize the ureteral orifices. The bladder can then be repaired with an initial continuous 2-0 chromic suture followed by a second imbricating layer of 2-0 suture.

Bladder Injuries

Injury to the bladder is an infrequent but recognized complication of cesarean delivery. More widespread use of the transverse abdominal incision has increased the likelihood of bladder dome injury upon entering the abdomen. Although the risk of bladder injury can be minimized by preoperative catheterization of the bladder and careful entry into the peritoneal cavity, it is not always possible to avoid injury during a repeat procedure. When the bladder is more adherent than usual, sharp dissection of the "webbing" between the bladder base and the lower uterine segment and vagina, as opposed to blunt dissection with a sponge stick or gauze-covered finger, will reduce, but not eliminate, the incidence of unplanned cystotomy.

Bladder injury may also occur at the time of uterine rupture, particularly in patients with a prior cesarean delivery. Although rates as high as 10 to 14 percent have been reported, the incidence has decreased somewhat in women attempting VBAC.[118–120] Should hysterectomy be required, cystotomy as a complication of cesarean hysterectomy has been noted to occur in as many as 4 to 5 percent of procedures.[121,122] In most cases, the injury occurs at the bladder base. To some extent, if hysterectomy is anticipated, mobilizing the bladder from the lower uterine segment and upper vagina prior to making the uterine incision will diminish this risk.

Should a bladder laceration be encountered, the bladder may be repaired with a two-layer closure with 2-0 or 3-0 chromic. Surgeons may differ significantly in their surgical approach to repair. Controversies focus on the use of continuous versus interrupted sutures, on whether it is important to avoid including the mucosa in the suture line, and on the duration of catheter drainage. The issues are probably of little significance when the cystotomy is in the dome of the bladder. However, a cystotomy in the bladder base is more likely to present problems, because the bladder base is thinner and receives less blood flow. There is also a possibility of laceration into the trigone and injury to the ureteral orifices. Should the trigone be lacerated, there may be an advantage to inserting a ureteral catheter under direct visualization. After the bladder has been repaired, a catheter can be left in place for 7 to 10 days.[120,123]

Ureteral Injury

Although one does not frequently think of ureteral injury during cesarean delivery, this complication has been reported in up to 1 in 1,000 procedures.[120] Ureteral injury is also increased with cesarean hysterectomy, with rates of 0.2 to 0.5 percent being documented.[121,122] In most instances, injury occurs during efforts to control bleeding arising from lateral extension of the uterine incision. Opening the anterior leaf of the broad ligament while controlling blood loss with direct pressure will often facilitate more accurate suture placement, which will diminish the potential for ureteral injury. Unfortunately, the injury often goes unrecognized intraoperatively.

Gastrointestinal Tract Injury

Injuries to the bowel are also rare, but nonetheless are reported to occur in approximately 1 in 1,300 cesarean sections.[100] Prior abdominal surgery and pelvic/abdominal infection leading to adhesion formation are common risk factors. Sharp scalpel incision limited to a site of transparent peritoneum will reduce inadvertent bowel or bladder injury.

Should adhesions require lysis to gain access to the lower uterine segment, they should be sharply dissected with scissors tips pointed away from the bowel. Small defects in bowel serosa can be closed simply with interrupted silk sutures on an atraumatic needle. If these defects are very small, no closure may be necessary. Full-thickness lacerations should be repaired in a double-layer closure, using a transverse closure of a longitudinal laceration, to minimize the possibility of narrowing the bowel lumen. The mucosa can be closed with running or interrupted 3-0 absorbable sutures such as chromic or polyglactin. The muscular and serosal layers are then closed with a similar-sized interrupted silk suture.

In the event that there are multiple full-thickness small bowel injuries or the colon or sigmoid is entered, consultation with a gynecologic oncologist or general surgeon is appropriate. The small bowel may require resection and reanastomosis. Primary closure of a small laceration (<1 cm) of the colon is indicated using a double-layer closure as described above. More extensive injury associated with fecal contamination should be treated with copious lavage and may require a temporary colostomy. In either case, gram-negative aerobic and anaerobic antibiotic coverage should be provided. This is commonly provided by combination therapy with an aminoglycoside and either clindamycin or metronidazole (i.e., clindamycin/gentamicin) and/or cephalosporin with metronidazole. Some have recommended broad-spectrum monotherapy, which has the advantages of lower toxicity, lower drug costs, and lower cost of administration, including eliminating the need for monitoring of aminoglycoside blood levels. Ampicillin/sulbactam (3.0 g intravenously every 6 hours) is a reasonable first-line choice, with combination therapy reserved for patients with documented penicillin allergy.[124]

Uterine Atony

Initial efforts to control uterine atony include uterine massage and medical therapy with (1) intravenous oxytocin, 20 to 40 units/L; (2) methergotamine, 0.2 mg, or ergonovine administered intramuscularly; or (3) 15 methylprostaglandin $F_{2\alpha}$ (Hemabate), which can be administered either intramuscularly or directly into the myometrium. Should the initial dose of prostaglandin be insufficient, successive dosages of 250 μg, up to a total dose of 1.0 to 1.5 mg, can be used. Should medical treatment fail, the surgeon must decide between ligation of the uterine arteries (see Fig. 17–17), hypogastric artery ligation, and hysterectomy. Uterine or hypogastric artery ligation may be the desirable approach should the patient be stable cardiovascularly and desirous of future pregnancy. Hypogastric artery ligation can be accomplished by ligation of the ascending branch, which can usually be found at the inferior and lateral extreme of the low transverse incision ascending retroperitoneally within the broad ligament (Fig. 18–7). Unfortunately, even hypogastric artery ligation is actually successful in less than one half of the cases.[125] Should uterine or hypogastric artery ligation also fail to control the hemorrhage, it may be necessary to proceed to hysterectomy.

Placenta Accreta

Placenta accreta is now the most common indication for postcesarean hysterectomy. Approximately 25 percent of patients having a cesarean delivery for placenta previa in the presence of a prior uterine incision subsequently require cesarean hysterectomy for placenta accreta. The risk of placenta accreta appears to increase with the number of prior incisions. This obstetric complication may be rising because of the growing number of previous cesarean sections.[128,129]

If the accreta is focal and the patient desires future pregnancies, it may be possible to excise the site of trophoblastic invasion, oversewing bleeding areas with several figure-of-eight sutures. If that is not possible, hysterectomy should be initiated. A complete hysterectomy will usually be required because a placenta accreta commonly involves the lower uterine segment and, in such cases, a supracervical hysterectomy will not be effective in controlling the bleeding.

Drainage of the Abdominal Incision

The purpose of a drain is to remove the bacterial growth media that can act as a site of infection and reduce potential spaces within the wound. There are few indications for prophylactic drainage, because cesarean delivery is a relatively "short" procedure and operative time and tissue devitalization are ordinarily not an issue. Prophylactic drainage is most commonly used in situations in which there is an expectation of fluid accumulation in association with likely contamination of the wound, particularly in obese patients.[130] Therapeutic drainage is seldom, if ever, indicated with cesarean delivery or cesarean hysterectomy unless there

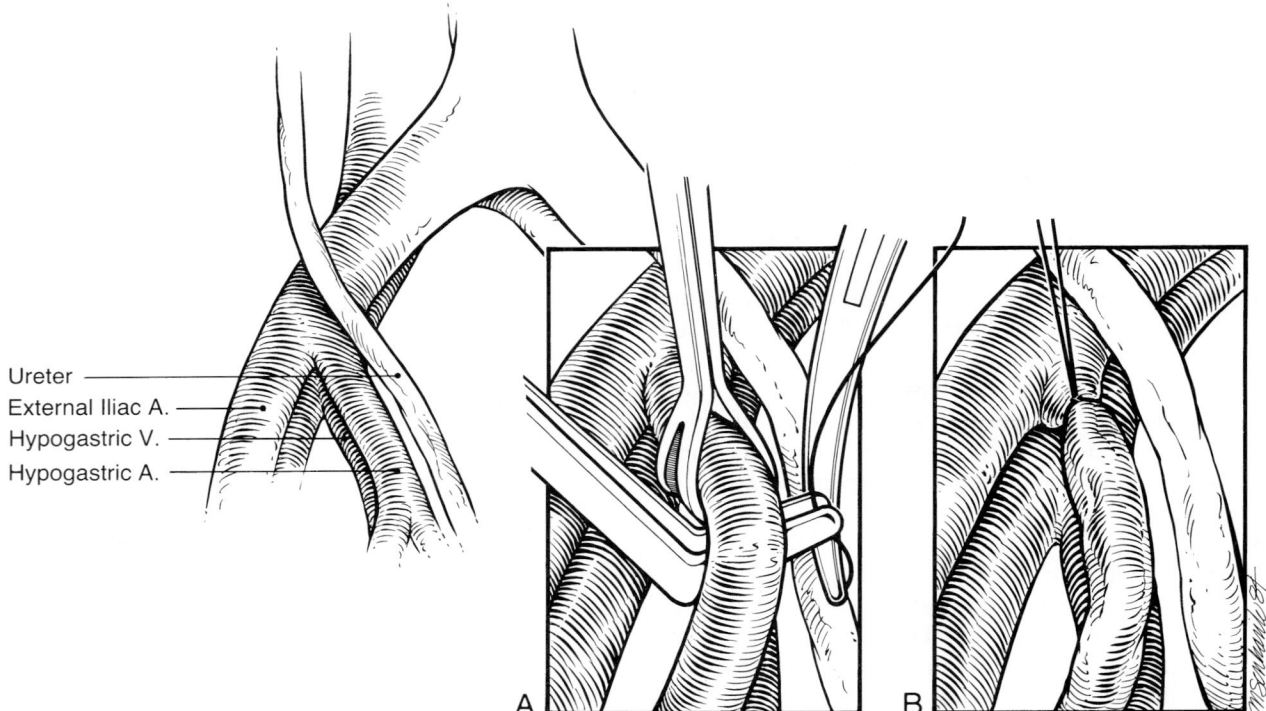

Ureter
External Iliac A.
Hypogastric V.
Hypogastric A.

A   B

Figure 18–7. Hypogastric artery ligation. Approach to the hypogastric artery via the peritoneum, parallel and just lateral to the ovarian vessels, exposing the interior surface of the posterior layer of the broad ligament. The ureter will be found attached to the medial leaf of the broad ligament. The bifurcation of the common iliac artery into its external and internal (hypogastric) branches is exposed by blunt dissection of the loose overlying areolar tissues. Identification of these structures is essential. *A* and *B*, To avoid traumatizing the underlying hypogastric vein, the hypogastric artery is elevated by means of a Babcock clamp before passing an angled clamp to catch a free tie. (Adapted from Breen J, Cregori CA, Kindzierski JA: Hemorrhage in Gynecologic Surgery. Hagerstown, MD, Harper & Row, 1981, p 438.)

is a coincidental abscess. Should an abscess be encountered, a continuous suction drain should be inserted via a separate stab wound at a site away from the incision.[131] In some instances in which there is a suspicion of heavy contamination, particularly in morbidly obese patients, it may be better to plan secondary wound closure as opposed to drainage.

POSTMORTEM CESAREAN DELIVERY

If clinically possible, a postmortem cesarean delivery should be started within 4 to 5 minutes after initiation of cardiopulmonary resuscitation for cardiac arrest. Delivery will increase the effectiveness of cardiopulmonary resuscitation by diminishing uterine compression of the inferior vena cava in the supine position.

If a postmortem cesarean delivery is contemplated, successful perinatal outcome will depend on knowledge of preexisting fetal status and realization that maternal demise can be reliably anticipated in the near future. There are a number of determinants that favorably affect outcome: (1) a gestational age compatible with fe-

tal survival, (2) delivery within 10 minutes of cessation of maternal circulation, (3) prompt availability of appropriately trained staff and equipment, and (4) access to personnel capable of neonatal resuscitation.

Unfortunately, in many instances it is not possible to provide one or more of the above, and for this reason outcome is most often poor. Katz et al.[132] described 269 cases of postmortem cesarean births between 1879 and 1986 in the English literature. Only 188 newborns survived. In recent history, normal survival following postmortem cesarean birth has been primarily limited to instances in which the baby was delivered within 5 minutes after maternal death. The likelihood of a normal outcome decreases to approximately 10 to 15 percent in the 6- to 15-minute interval and to less than 15 percent at 16 or more minutes after death. The current consensus is that postmortem cesarean delivery may be performed at any time that a viable fetus or the potential for one exists, even without the consent of a family member.

There are limited data with which to assess the ability of modern life-support equipment to maintain the mother for an extended period. A 1988 case report described a mother supported for 10 weeks to gain time for fetal maturation.[133]

PREOPERATIVE AND INTRAOPERATIVE FLUID GUIDELINES

Extracellular (interstitial and intravascular) water constitutes approximately one third of total body water and 20 percent of total body weight. Ordinary daily physiologic fluid needs are approximately 2,000 to 2,500 ml.[134] In the pregnant patient, daily physiologic fluid losses are estimated to be 1,000 ml in excess of urinary output and include urinary output (800 to 1,500 ml), insensible loss (800 ml) from both skin and lungs, and stool loss (200 ml). Insensible loss in the laboring patient can be considerably greater.

Because insensible fluid loss increases significantly in the laboring patient, the woman about to undergo a cesarean delivery for CPD may be quite dehydrated. She may have had insufficient fluid intake since the onset of labor and have increased fluid loss because of the physical exertion and rapid breathing movements associated with labor. The bleeding patient or the patient about to receive epidural anesthesia is particularly sensitive to the effects of dehydration.

There will be little problem with dehydration if intravenous fluid intake has been maintained at 100 to 125 ml/h during labor. Should this not be the case, fluid losses can be estimated based on the average hourly need (100 to 125 ml) times the cumulative number of hours since the time of last fluid intake. Adjustments, which may vary from center to center, should be made for ice chips and other fluid intake. An additional intravenous fluid load is required prior to the administration of epidural anesthesia.

Intravenous Fluids Commonly Used

1. Sodium chloride (0.9 percent isotonic saline) is an isotonic solution commonly used to expand plasma volume as well as to correct mild degrees of hyponatremia.
2. Lactated Ringer's solution is also an isotonic solution containing multiple electrolytes in a concentration similar to that found in human plasma. This solution is also used to expand plasma volume and may be preferable to isotonic saline during the first 24 postoperative hours.
3. Sodium chloride 0.45 percent is a hypotonic (half-normal) solution that is useful in the provision of postoperative fluid needs after the first 24 hours when volume expansion is no longer needed.

Fluid and Electrolyte Replacement

Should the patient be only mildly hypovolemic in the first 24 hours, normal isotonic saline or Ringer's lactate solution in 5 percent dextrose is preferable to more hypotonic solutions because there is greater retention of fluids in the intravascular space providing volume expansion. In contrast, infusion of a 5 percent dextrose in water solution ($D_5 W$) will result in distribution of fluid evenly throughout all water spaces, two thirds being in the intracellular space. Should hypovolemia be more significant, particularly in association with low intravascular colloid osmotic pressure, administration of an albumin-containing solution may minimize the effects of loss of fluids into the interstitial space. Under such circumstances, it may on occasion be advisable to use a central venous pressure line or a Swan-Ganz catheter.

Special Considerations for Preoperative Fluids

Some patients such as those with vomiting, diarrhea, or fever may require additional fluids. The presence of a fever may increase the need for intravenous fluid replacement, generally on the order of 15 percent above basal levels for every degree centigrade above normal body temperature.[130]

Intraoperative Fluids

Fluid needs during surgery are generally determined by the anesthesiologist or nurse anesthetist and are largely directed to the replacement of estimated blood loss, insensible losses, and urinary output. In general, isotonic solutions are used to maintain adequate circulating blood volume. Actual blood or plasma replacement is rarely needed during cesarean delivery.

Intraoperative fluid requirements, apart from blood replacement, range from 500 to 1,000 ml/h, up to a maximum of 3 L in a 4-hour interval under ordinary surgical conditions. Such replacement is associated with a low incidence of renal failure and pulmonary edema in instances in which there has been obstetric hemorrhage.[135,136]

POSTOPERATIVE COMPLICATIONS

Maternal Morbidity and Mortality

The previously noted increase in risk for maternal morbidity and mortality is in part a result of the complications leading to the cesarean delivery as well as the risk associated with any surgical procedure. Nonetheless, even when morbidity and mortality arising from the indication leading to cesarean delivery have been excluded, maternal morbidity and mortality remain severalfold higher for cesarean delivery than for vaginal delivery.[6,47,136]

In a review of approximately 400,000 cesarean births performed between 1965 and 1978, maternal death occurred in 1 in 1,635 (mortality rate was 6.1 per 100,000) procedures; approximately one half of the deaths were attributable to the procedure.[6,47] In another series, Sachs et al.[47] reviewed 121,000 cesarean births performed in Massachusetts from 1976 to 1984; 7 (5.8 per 100,000) of 27 total deaths (22 per 100,000) arose as a result of the procedure itself. Lower rates have been described, the most remarkable being a study from the Boston Hospital for Women reporting no maternal mortality in 10,231 cesarean deliveries.[137]

Major sources of morbidity and associated mortality relate to complications of maternal sepsis, anesthesia, and thromboembolic disease and its complications. Each has been discussed in Chapters 15 and 40. Much has been done in recent years to reduce the impact of anesthesia-related mortality largely through increased availability of qualified anesthesia personnel and the implementation of rigid protocols, including routine use of antacids prior to cesarean delivery, as well as routine protocols for intubation. Other common causes of morbidity arising from cesarean delivery include hemorrhage and injury to the urinary tract.[138,139] It is important to remember that data describing morbidity for a primary cesarean delivery do not include the consideration of long-term consequences such as the possible need for repeat cesarean births, the increased likelihood of placenta accreta, and the need for unplanned hysterectomy.

Endomyometritis

Postpartum infection is the most frequent complication arising from cesarean delivery, and indeed primary cesarean delivery is the greatest risk factor, with rates up to 20-fold that associated with vaginal delivery. Should prophylactic antibiotics not be used, the incidence of postcesarean endomyometritis varies from as low as 5 to 10 percent to as high as 70 to 85 percent, with a mean of 35 to 40 percent in most series.[140–142] The rate is largely dependent on socioeconomic status and on whether the cesarean delivery is a primary procedure. The lowest incidence occurs in middle- and upper-income women undergoing a scheduled cesarean delivery; the highest in the young indigent patient undergoing primary cesarean delivery after an extended labor and prolonged membrane rupture. Age and socioeconomic status may influence the incidence of infection because they reflect general health and host immunocompetence. The other major risk factors include length of labor, duration of membrane rupture, and number of vaginal examinations and presence of prior chorioamnionitis. These factors exert their effects by influencing the size of the bacterial inoculum. Other weaker risk factors include length of surgery, preoperative hematocrit, intraoperative blood loss, duration of internal fetal monitoring, experience of the surgeon, and type of anesthesia.

Prior to the advent of modern broad-spectrum antibiotics with activity against both anaerobic and aerobic gram-negative bacilli, the incidence of severe complications arising from endomyometritis was as high as 4 to 5 percent.[143,144] When blood cultures were obtained, the frequency of associated bacteremia was approximately 10 percent.[140] Prophylactic antibiotics at the time of cesarean delivery reduce the postoperative infection rate to approximately 5 percent.[143] With the advent of modern antibiotics, the incidence of life-threatening complications, including pelvic abscess, septic shock, and septic pelvic thrombophlebitis, is now less than 2 percent.

The microbiology, clinical diagnosis, laboratory aids, treatment, and approaches to reduce the rate of endometritis are detailed in Chapter 40.

Wound Complications

Risk Factors for Poor Wound Healing and Wound Infection

Identifiable medical risk factors that increase the likelihood of poor wound healing include diabetes mellitus and malnutrition. Surgical risk factors to be considered are the duration of surgery, the use of drains, the suture material chosen, and the closure technique employed. Postoperative factors include asthma, pulmonary complications and associated coughing, and vomiting.[145–146] In rare cases, other risk factors such as ascites, long-term corticosteroid therapy, anemia, and even prior irradiation may exist.

Wound infection rates following cesarean delivery vary, according to the patient population evaluated, from 2.5 to as high as 16.1 percent.[145] Determinants include local wound conditions and patient host resistance. Infection rates will vary according to whether the cesarean delivery is performed as an elective repeat (clean procedure) procedure with intact membranes or follows labor, particularly with ruptured membranes (clean contaminated procedure). Risk factors for wound infection interact in a complex manner, making it difficult to determine the independent contribution of any one factor. Clean procedures are generally associated with a wound infection rate of approximately 2 percent, whereas the corresponding rate for a clean contaminated case is on the order of 5 to 10 percent. Should chorioamnionitis (contaminated procedure) be present, the wound infection rate will approximate 20 percent.

Many studies demonstrate a substantial increase in wound infections with increasing duration of membrane rupture, long labors, and more frequent vaginal examinations.[147-150] Amnionitis and possibly meconium passage are additional risk factors. Up to 75 percent of amniotic fluid cultures done at the time of primary cesarean delivery are positive, with an average of 3.5 organisms, 44 percent being highly virulent bacteria.[151] Flora isolated from amniotic fluid and wound infections exist in a synergistic system of aerobes and anaerobes similar to the situation with endometritis. *S. aureus*, *Escherichia coli*, *Proteus mirabilis*, *Bacteroides* species, and group B streptococci are common isolates; clostridial species are infrequent.[152] Even in the absence of ruptured membranes, patients in preterm labor with unrecognized chorioamnionitis may have pathogens consistent with bowel flora.[153]

Methods To Reduce Wound Infection

Some determinants of wound infection (diabetes mellitus, amnionitis, obesity, and alcoholism) are to a large degree beyond the control of the obstetrician. However, the obstetrician who knows the potential risk factors does have the option to use a number of measures selectively in an attempt to reduce the risk of wound infection and wound breakdown. These measures include (1) hair removal at the incision site (as opposed to shaving pubic and abdominal hair) if the abdomen is prepared the night prior to surgery; (2) preoperative skin preparation, including careful cleansing of the umbilicus and abdomen prior to surgery; (3) sterile technique; (4) wound hemostasis; (5) selective use of prophylactic antibiotics; (6) avoidance of reactive (plain gut) or unnecessary suture material, particularly in the patient at risk for a wound infection or breakdown; (7) closed-system drainage if the patient is obese or the wound is "wet" in the absence of an obvious bleeder as opposed to open Penrose drains; (8) skin closure with suture rather than a skin stapler; and (9) delayed wound closure if the wound is grossly contaminated by bowel contents.

Although it is difficult to determine the magnitude of preventable wound infections, Emmons et al.[154] suggest that the approximately 25 percent of wound infections that are associated with *S. aureus* represent a potentially preventable condition that presumably arises from exogenous sources. Sixty consecutive wound infections (5.4 percent) were studied among 1,104 women undergoing cesarean delivery. Wound infections caused by cervical-vaginal flora were associated with prolonged labor, particularly with greater duration of continuous electronic FHR monitoring; with more frequent vaginal examinations; and with organisms isolated from the endometrium at cesarean section. In contrast, women with wound infections caused by *S. aureus* had neither prolonged labor nor *S. aureus* isolated at cesarean delivery.[154]

When closing the wound, a balance must be maintained between adequate hemostasis and significant tissue devitalization. Excessive use of electrocautery may result in unnecessary tissue damage and reduced host resistance. Seroma or hematoma formation reduces tissue oxygenation and phagocyte penetration. Tissues should be carefully reapproximated without major tension. Unnecessarily tight placement of sutures may interfere with adequate tissue oxygenation, which is essential to bacterial phagocytosis.[155]

Morbid obesity is a risk factor for wound infection, regardless of the degree of contamination and length of procedure.[156] Adipose tissue is relatively fragile and tends to heal poorly. As a result, careful handling of the subcutaneous tissue is important. However, there is uncertainty as to the best surgical approach. Gallup[84] recommends a midline incision, a superficial closed suction drain, a nonabsorbable monofilament fascial closure with a Smead-Jones technique, and avoidance of subcutaneous suture. Others favor a transverse incision[157] and the use of subcutaneous sutures.[90]

Diagnosis and Management of Wound Infection

The diagnosis of a wound infection is generally the result of daily inspection of the wound. Suspicion may be heightened should the patient, previously treated for endometritis, be unresponsive to antibiotic therapy. If fever develops, careful inspection of the wound will often lead to early diagnosis and treatment. Diagnosis of a wound infection is relatively obvious in the febrile patient if the wound is unusually tender, inflamed, and indurated or if drainage of purulent material is observed on palpation. The bacteriology and laboratory approach to diagnosis are discussed in Chapter 40.

Should an infection be found, the involved wound must be opened to allow drainage and debrided to clean the wound margins. A culture for anaerobic and aerobic organisms may be obtained and systemic antibiotics used to cover the anticipated organisms within the wound. Culturing tissue debris from the wound improves the likelihood of anaerobic organisms. Once the wound is opened, drained, irrigated, and possibly debrided to remove adherent purulent material, the wound can be packed with wet-to-dry dressing three times daily until there is a healthy margin of red granulation tissue. When the infection is controlled, the patient and surgeon must then decide between the inconvenience for the patient associated with healing by secondary intention versus the risk of recurrent infection should primary closure be elected.[158]

Fascial Dehiscence

Dehiscence of a wound through the fascia is infrequent, occurring in approximately 5 percent of wound infec-

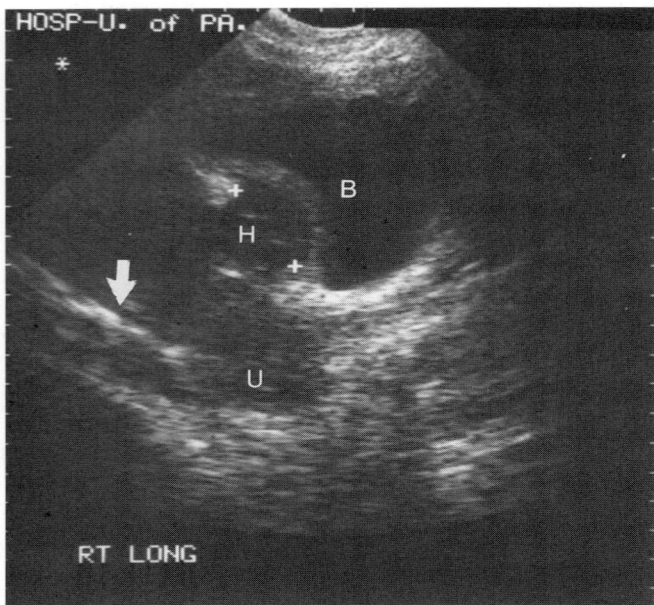

Figure 18–8. Ultrasound of infected bladder flap hematoma marked by cursors (+). The patient presented approximately 1 week after cesarean delivery with fever. She responded to antibiotics. Note that the full bladder (B) enhances visualization of the hematoma (H). The *arrow* designates the endometrial cavity of the uterus (U).

tions.[150] Dehiscence is suggested by the presence of a large amount of discharge from the wound. If loops of small bowel protrude through the incision, the small bowel should be immediately covered with wet sterile dressings. The wound should be opened and inspected and emergency closure performed in the operating room under sterile conditions. If a dehiscence is confirmed, the wound should be cleansed, debrided, and

closed with either Smead-Jones or retention sutures (Fig. 18–6).

Radiologic Imaging as Potential Diagnostic Aid

Resistance to antibiotic therapy, as evidenced by a persistent spiking febrile response, may be an indication for sonography or other imaging techniques (Figs. 18–8 to 18–10) to rule out retained uterine products, seromas, hematomas, or abscesses in the abdominal wall, pelvis, or occasionally the uterine incision. Whereas sonography offers immediate evaluation of the pelvis in the patient resistant to therapy, computed tomographic (CT) scanning may be preferable in some cases because it allows complete assessment of the entire peritoneal cavity and may identify fresh hemorrhage within a fluid collection as well as ovarian vein thrombosis. Sonography with a 5- or 7-MHz short-focus transducer also allows detailed examination of the abdominal wall for seromas, hematomas, and abscesses.

By the first postpartum day, the uterus will be at or below the level of the umbilicus. On ultrasound, the uterine wall thickness will vary from 3 to 6.5 cm, being slightly thicker in multiparous patients than in primiparas.[22] The uterine wall ordinarily appears homogenous with an occasional subtle irregularity.[159] The endometrial cavity often presents as a stripe whose anteroposterior diameter varies from 0.5 to 1.3 cm.[160] The uterine incision may present a variable sonographic appearance following cesarean section.[161] Strong echoes may arise from the suture material. It is not unusual to see small seromas and hematomas of the uterine incision under the bladder flap. Should a significant fluid collection be observed around the uterine incision in a

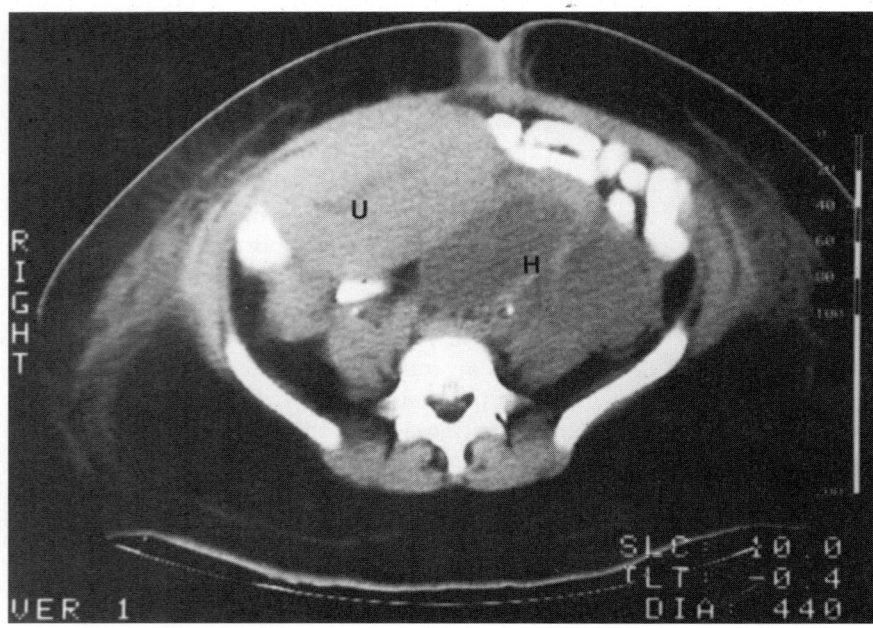

Figure 18–9. CT scan of pelvis 6 days after a cesarean section showing left-sided broad ligament hematoma (H). The uterus (U) is displaced to the right. The patient responded to antibiotics. (Courtesy of Dr. Michael Blumenfeld, Department of Obstetrics and Gynecology, Ohio State University, Columbus, OH.)

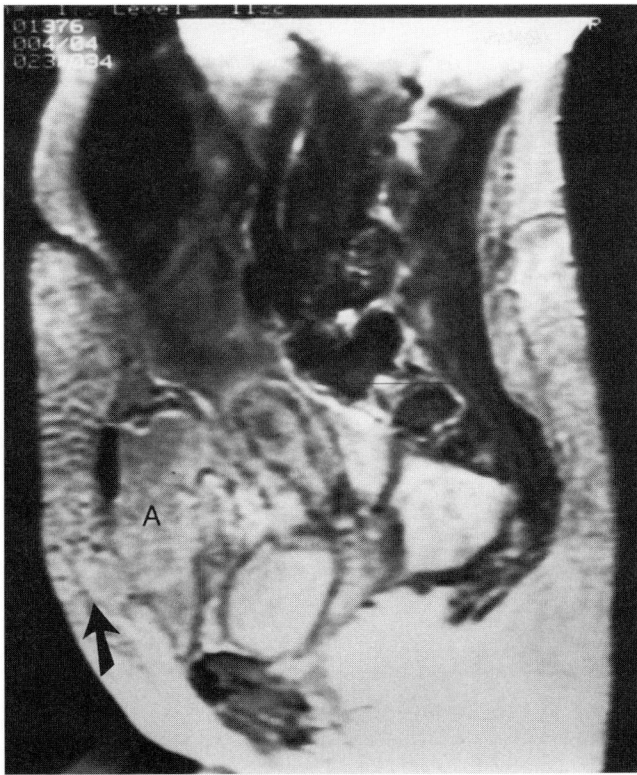

Figure 18–10. Magnetic resonance imaging (MRI) scan of abdominal wall abscess. This patient presented 1 week after a cesarean delivery with fever and an abdominal mass. The differential diagnosis included an intraperitoneal infection with extension or a wound abscess. This MRI shows a wound abscess (A) above fascia that extended to the abdominal wall (*arrow*). The abscess responded to drainage and antibiotics.

febrile patient, an abscess should be considered (Fig. 18–8).

When a postpartum abdominal ultrasound examination is performed, the patient should have a full bladder. This will facilitate displacement of the normal anteflexed puerperal uterus posteriorly, positioning the endometrial cavity at right angles to the sound waves and improving visualization.[162] In addition, bladder filling will frequently push any gas-filled loops of bowel out of the pelvis, thus facilitating visualization of the cul-de-sac, adnexa, and uterus. Transvaginal scanning may be helpful if the abdomen is distended, the incision site interferes with adequate abdominal imaging, or the patient is unable to tolerate the pressure of abdominal scanning.

Sonographic findings suggesting endometritis may include a dilated fluid- or gas-filled uterine cavity and fluid in the cul-de-sac. Sonographic evidence of an empty uterus will eliminate the possibility of retained products. However, an abnormal scan may represent either the normal retention of blood or retained products of conception.[163] Abscesses may present with characteristic fluid and gas collections, shaggy walls, and internal echoes in association with cul-de-sac fluid accumulations indicating peritonitis. If gas is detected on sonogram, gas-forming organisms such as *E. coli* or *Clostridium perfringens* may be present. CT scanning may be used to diagnose ovarian vein thrombophlebitis (see Fig. 40–4).[164]

Urinary Complications

Urinary tract infections rank second to endomyometritis as a cause of postcesarean febrile morbidity. The reported incidence varies from as low as 2 percent to as high as 16 percent.[165,166] In one study, approximately 7 percent of postoperative clean-catch urine specimens had at least 10^5 bacteria per milliliter in culture. One percent of patients had both bacteriuria and endomyometritis.[167] Urethral catheterization contributes to 80 percent of nosocomial urinary tract infections in hospitalized patients, particularly when indwelling catheters are used. The incidence is increased with longer duration of catheter use, in diabetic patients, and in patients who are critically ill.[164] Attention to detail in terms of proper preparation and insertion of the catheter and the use of a closed drainage system have decreased this risk.

Gastrointestinal Complications

Most patients undergoing cesarean delivery have little if any gastrointestinal problems postoperatively. However, anesthesia and narcotics employed to treat postoperative pain may contribute to bowel dysfunction. As a result, an occasional patient may have postoperative nausea or mild transient abdominal distention in the first 24 hours.

Ileus should be suspected if prolonged nausea or vomiting together with signs such as abdominal distention, absence of bowel sounds, and failure to pass flatus are persistent. Distended loops of bowel with or without air–fluid levels on radiography will provide confirmatory evidence. In most instances, simply withholding oral intake, providing adequate fluid replacement, and being observant are sufficient. If the ileus is persistent, nasogastric suction may be required.

Actual mechanical bowel obstruction may initially present as an ileus, but is commonly associated with peristaltic rushes and high-pitched bowel sounds in conjunction with symptoms of nausea, vomiting, and abdominal distention. Once again, some patients will respond to conservative management, including restriction of oral intake and placement of a nasogastric tube or possibly even a long tube. The key to success is maintenance not only of fluids and electrolytes but also of hematocrit and serum protein. Should conservative therapy fail, surgical consultation and possible exploration may be required.

Thromboembolic Disorders

The risk of thrombosis increases during pregnancy because of both higher levels of coagulation factors and diminished fibrinolysis. These changes peak near term and immediately after delivery. Deep venous thrombophlebitis (DVT) of the lower extremities occurs in approximately 0.24 percent of all deliveries.[168,169] The risk of DVT after cesarean delivery is approximately three to five times greater than after vaginal delivery.[170] Compounding risk factors include obesity, inability to ambulate, advanced maternal age, and higher parity. Should the DVT go untreated, approximately 15 to 25 percent of patients will develop pulmonary emboli, and 15 percent will sustain a fatal pulmonary embolus (PE). However, if recognized early and treated appropriately, the risks of PE and death are reduced to 4.5 and 0.7 percent, respectively.[169,171]

Classic symptoms for DVT include unilateral leg pain, tenderness, and swelling. A 2-cm difference in leg circumference between the affected and normal limb is generally required for diagnosis. Other clinical signs include edema, a palpable cord, and a change in limb color. A positive Homan's sign (calf pain on passive dorsiflexion of the foot) or a positive Lowenberg test (pain distal to the site of rapid inflation of a blood pressure cuff to 100 mm Hg) suggests DVT.

Unfortunately, the first sign of DVT may be the occurrence of a PE, which can present with symptoms of tachypnea (90 percent), dyspnea (80 percent), pleuritic chest pain with or without splinting (>70 percent), apprehension (~60 percent), tachycardia (40 percent), and cough (>50 percent).[172,173] Other findings include atelectatic rales, a friction rub, accentuated second heart sound, and a gallop. Patient evaluation is complicated in the postcesarean delivery patient, since splinting from incisional pain and tachypnea are not unusual findings. Doppler studies have a sensitivity of 90 percent for popliteal, femoral, or iliac thromboses, but only 50 percent for calf involvement because of abundant collateral vessels. Impedance plethysmography (IPG) is sensitive in approximately 95 percent of proximal thromboses, but is not as effective as Doppler for pelvic vessel thrombosis and will generally identify most cases, especially above the calves. Should Doppler and IPG be inconclusive, ascending venography, the most accurate of the three tests, should be performed. IPG can be used as a first-line test postpartum in the nonlactating mother. Should PE be suspected, a baseline arterial blood gas, chest radiograph, and electrocardiogram, as well as prothrombin time and partial thromboplastin time, should be obtained. Oxygen therapy should also be administered. Once the diagnosis has been established, heparin therapy should be started. The diagnosis and treatment of a PE are discussed in Chapter 30.

Septic Pelvic Thrombophlebitis

Approximately 0.5 to 2 percent of patients with endomyometritis or wound infection will develop septic pelvic thrombophlebitis, a more common complication of cesarean birth than of vaginal delivery. In large part, this is a result of the higher rate of endomyometritis in patients undergoing cesarean delivery.[174] Largely a diagnosis of exclusion, septic pelvic thrombophlebitis occurs most commonly on the right side and may be suspected should there be fever and unilateral pain. Although tenderness about the incision site may make detection difficult, occasionally one will be able to palpate a tender, rope-like abdominal mass extending laterally and cephalad from the uterus. Sonographic examination of the lower abdomen and pelvis or CT scan may be of assistance in the diagnosis (see Fig. 40–4).

POSTOPERATIVE MANAGEMENT

Postoperative Analgesia

Analgesia should be provided in a dose and at a frequency that will neither obtund nor cause respiratory depression and yet allow the patient (1) to avoid the consequences of extremes in analgesic blood levels resulting in unnecessary pain and (2) to cooperate with normal postoperative management. The patient receiving inadequate analgesia may, in an effort to protect her wound, maintain a shallow breathing pattern without deep breaths and, hence, develop atelectasis.[175]

Commonly used analgesics include meperidine (50 to 75 mg) or morphine (10 mg, depending on maternal size), administered intravenously or intramuscularly every 3 to 4 hours. Intrathecal or epidural narcotic administration used with agents such as morphine can also be used for postoperative anesthesia, which may last as long as 30 hours following delivery, providing an advantage to a patient who has undergone a regional block (see Chapter 15).[176]

Ambulation

Early ambulation is important in reinstitution of inflation of the most dependent alveoli and the prevention of pulmonary complications, particularly in the patient who has had general anesthesia. Early ambulation also promotes the return of normal urinary and bowel activity. Under most circumstances, the uncomplicated patient can be allowed to sit up within 8 to 12 hours following the procedure, even after epidural anesthesia. The patient generally can ambulate within the first day after surgery, and by the second day can shower without fear of injury to the incision.

Oral Intake

Active bowel sounds are commonly not observed until the second postoperative day. Nonetheless, in most instances the patient will easily tolerate oral fluids the day after surgery. Only rarely, when the patient has been septic or there has been extensive intra-abdominal manipulation, will there be a need to withhold oral fluids, even though the patient may have diminished bowel sounds and not pass gas. Most clinicians feel comfortable in providing clear liquids and ice chips with only a small amount of liquid as soon as nausea subsides to relieve complaints of a dry mouth. The progression of the diet also varies according to clinician. Some advance the patient rapidly to a regular diet, whereas others institute a progression to a full liquid diet by 48 hours, awaiting the return of normal bowel sounds and passage of flatus to indicate return of colonic function. Few wait beyond the third postoperative day to institute a regular diet.

Bladder Management

The urinary catheter is ordinarily removed within 12 to 24 hours following surgery unless there have been intraoperative complications.

Postoperative Wound Care

The incision is generally covered for the first day with a light dressing, until the wound is sealed. The dressing is removed after the first postoperative day.

Laboratory Studies

Blood loss arising from an uncomplicated cesarean delivery is approximately 1,000 ml.[177] As a consequence of blood loss as well as intra- and postoperative hydration, the postoperative hematocrit may be expected to drop by approximately 2 to 3 percentage points during the initial 2 days following surgery, independent of hydration status.

Postoperative Fluids

The normal postpartum period is generally characterized by mobilization of the physiologic accumulation of fluid during pregnancy. As a consequence, large volumes of intravenous fluids are seldom required after cesarean delivery. In the low-risk patient, fluid replacement needs during a 24-hour interval are generally only 1,000 ml above urinary output. Three liters of a salt-containing solution will thus generally suffice during the first 24 hours unless urinary output falls below 30 ml/h. Under certain circumstances there may be increased requirements for fluids: following prolonged labor, febrile illness, vomiting and diarrhea, or even prior use of diuretics or salt restriction. More complex patients may have additional needs. Potassium is ordinarily not required during the first 24 hours by uncomplicated patients because of intracellular potassium release from cell destruction. After the first 24 hours, intravenous fluid replacement with 5 percent dextrose in 0.45 percent sodium chloride is commonly used, unless volume expansion is an issue. If it is anticipated that the patient will require prolonged intravenous fluids, potassium may be administered as 60 to 80 mEq/day. Should the patient be oliguric, potassium is generally not given until the patient has a normal urinary output.

Average Length of Stay

Depending on postoperative morbidity/complications and availability of care at home, hospital discharge may occur as early as the second to as late as the fifth postoperative day. The average length of stay is approximately 3 days. The length of hospitalization associated with cesarean birth, like those associated with vaginal delivery, has declined dramatically.[1,2,26]

Discharge Management

Reduction in the length of stay, from over 6 to 7 days to fewer than 4, has had a dramatic impact on many patient-related programs. Table 18–6 provides an example of a typical management guideline that may be used by third-party payors as they extend their efforts to "manage care."[178] Elective cesarean patients are no longer admitted the night before the intended procedure. It is noteworthy that their goal for length of stay for a cesarean birth is 2 days. One would hope that the managed care payers will divert some of the savings from profit to patient support and medical supervision of the mother and newborn at home.

The mother's activities at home for the first week should be limited to personal care and to care of the newborn. By the third to fourth week, the patient can generally resume most activities at home.

REDUCING THE CURRENT CESAREAN BIRTH RATE

Possible Strategies To Reduce the Rate

National Strategies

A number of national strategies have been proposed to reduce the current cesarean birth rate: (1) equalize the reimbursement for vaginal and cesarean deliveries; (2) publish physician-specific cesarean rates; (3) publish

Table 18–6. TYPICAL MANAGED CARE GOALS FOR CESAREAN DELIVERY (S-350)

Protocol:	(CPT-4:58611, 59510, 59514, 59515, 59525) (ICD-9:74.0, 74.1, 74.4, 74.9) (ICD-9:054.11, 641, 642.5, 642.6, 652.2-652.6, 652.9, 653, 654, 654.2, 654.7, 654.8, 658.2, 658.3, 660, 662.2, 663)
Day 1:	Preadmission patient education and home care assessment. Operating room for cesarean delivery, parenteral fluids and medications, possible PCA or epidural analgesics
Day 2:	Clear liquids to advanced diet as tolerated. Discontinue passive cutaneous analgesics (PCA) or epidural analgesics. Discontinue IV and Foley if not done previously. Parenteral or oral medications. Ambulatory. Flatus present. Possible discharge
Day 3:	Afebrile, ambulatory, oral medications, regular diet. Discharge
Note:	Although most patients recover and may require no more than 36 hours as inpatients postoperatively, the variability in the hour of surgical delivery makes it uncertain how many patients may be able to go home on the first postpartum day. Some who deliver early in the day of delivery may do so

Data from Doyle and Schibanoff.[178]

hospital-specific cesarean rates; and (4) address physician malpractice concerns through legislation. The ACOG has indicated, with regard to the first strategy, that there is little or no evidence that the decision to perform a cesarean delivery or to offer a trial of labor is in any way motivated by a differential in payment. They recommend that financial incentives should not be used by payors to influence physician or patient decisions relative to the mode of delivery; rather, the decision should be based on standard obstetric indications and maternal fetal safety.[179]

Hospital Administrative Strategies

Bottoms et al.[180] concluded that cesarean delivery for dystocia and repeat cesarean deliveries should be points of primary review. If primary indications can be more tightly controlled, the number of candidates for repeat cesarean section will be reduced accordingly. Each hospital review committee should examine its institutional and individual physician cesarean rates. It is important that the review target each indication, since variation in total rate among physicians may not be associated with the same indication. Peer review conference screening should support the concept that, with the exception of a failed induction, cesarean delivery conducted on patients while still in the latent phase of labor should be an infrequent indication for cesarean birth. The validity of such a program is evident in a trial conducted in one hospital that evaluated the effects of selected clinical criteria and review mechanisms. Second opinions were required; VBAC-TOL was the preferred clinical approach; and peer review was implemented. After implementation of the program, the cesarean rate decreased from 17.5 percent in 1985 to 11.5 percent in 1987, a time when cesarean rates were rising.[181]

Clinical Strategies

Table 18–7 summarizes potential clinical strategies to reduce the current cesarean rate. The strategy most likely to have a significant impact is one that strongly encourages VBAC-TOL.

Indications Susceptible to Reduction

In 1993, 921,000 (22.8 percent) of approximately 4 million births were by cesarean delivery.[1,2] Of all cesarean deliveries, approximately 336,000 (36 percent) were associated with a prior cesarean birth and 585,000 (64 percent) were primary cesarean births.[1,2] The primary cesarean delivery rate of 16.3 percent is the lowest since 1985 but is still approximately four times the rate in 1985 of 4.2 percent.[1,2]

Reduction in the overall rate will occur only if a strategy is developed for each indication category. For example, O'Driscoll et al.[182] attributed much of their

Table 18–7. POTENTIAL APPROACHES TO REDUCE CESAREAN BIRTHS

Vaginal birth after cesarean trial of labor (VBAC-TOL)
Dystocia/CPD/FTP
Disciplined approach to labor management
Active management of labor
Breech presentation/transverse lie
External version
Selective vaginal delivery of breech
Fetal hypoxia/acidosis
Develop more predictive markers for acidosis
Fetal capillary blood gases for reassurance
Fetal stimulation for reassurance

Data from Taffel et al.[26]

success in maintaining a low cesarean rate to a lower rate of dystocia secondary to aggressive utilization of oxytocin, greater use of VBAC-TOL, and liberal criteria for vaginal breech deliveries. Brief mention will be made regarding the above clinical problems associated with cesarean birth with increased emphasis on VBAC-TOL as a strategy to reduce current cesarean rates.

Dystocia (Failure to Progress)/Cephalopelvic Disproportion

There is likely to be significant room for improvement in the current cesarean delivery rate for the clinical entity referred to as "dystocia," the most common indication for primary cesarean birth in the United States. The term includes a broad range of problems, including relative CPD and FTP encountered in the latent and active phases of labor (see Chapter 13). In 1993, of all women who had a cesarean section, 17.4 percent had an abnormal labor and 17 percent had CPD.[1,2] There is also some basis for a special designation for "failed induction," since a diagnosis of CPD/FTP is more common following labor induction.[183,184]

Determination of the cause of failure to achieve more vaginal deliveries is complex; as a result, any single strategy to reduce the impact of dystocia for cesarean delivery is unlikely to meet with major success.[21,26] Although failure to make sufficient progress in the active phase of the first stage (cervical dilatation) or the second stage (descent) has been attributed to deficiencies in uterine "power"/activity, "excess size" of the "passenger," or "relative-small size" of the "pelvic-passage," FTP may also potentially be the result of different "physician" approaches to the management of the latent and active phases of labor (see Safety of Active Labor Management as a Strategy, below).

Prior Cesarean Birth

A reduction in the cesarean birth rate can be achieved only by using VBAC-TOL as an approach to address and lower the self-perpetuating contribution of the indication of previous cesarean birth.[185] Few changes within the specialty of obstetrics and gynecology offer greater potential impact to more women than that of VBAC-TOL, since elective repeat cesarean delivery is estimated to be largely responsible for the increase in cesarean deliveries. The cesarean birth rate rose 44 percent between 1978 and 1984, and 47 percent of the rise was attributable to the performance of elective repeat cesarean deliveries.[1,2,4] The total cesarean rate in the United States peaked in 1988 at 24.7 percent; of these, 36.3 percent (351,000) were repeat cesarean deliveries. In the 1989 to 1991 interval, the cesarean rate appeared to reduce or plateau. Changing VBAC-TOL

rates appear to be largely responsible, increasing 47 percent from 1988 (12.6 percent) to 1989 (18.5 percent). The VBAC rate peaked in 1996 at 28.3 percent.

Breech Presentation

There is some potential for improvement in the current rate of cesarean deliveries. The management of both term and preterm breech presentations remains controversial. Nonetheless, the combination of fear of litigation and ever-decreasing opportunities to train residents in the proper approach to the management and technique for vaginal delivery has resulted in a continuing drift in practice toward cesarean births. In the United States, residents completing their training in obstetrics and gynecology perform, on average, eight breech deliveries including the delivery of the second twin.[46] The cesarean rate for breech presentations in this country increased from 67.2 percent in 1980 to 80.4 percent in 1985.[23] Given the recent report from Hannah and the Term Breech Trial Collaborative Group,[36] this rate is likely to be maintained or to increase.

Nonreassuring FHR and the Medicolegal Environment

Under better circumstances, physicians could reduce the impact of FHR-based indication for cesarean delivery. Some of the blame for the current increase in cesarean delivery is attributed to continuous electronic fetal monitoring and inappropriate overinterpretation of FHR data. However, it is likely that the root cause is physician fear of malpractice litigation. Most FHR alterations, including some rather dramatic (in a visual sense) variable decelerations, are likely to reflect only a temporary decrease in fetal oxygenation, as opposed to so-called fetal distress, a diagnosis lacking a consensus for diagnostic criteria. It is well known that such a diagnosis is associated with a high false-positive rate. There is fairly widespread fear of the medicolegal consequences of not performing a cesarean delivery in the presence of a nonreassuring FHR strip, despite the presence of indicators that ordinarily should provide reassurance. In a less litigious environment, the physician in doubt could gain reassurance that labor can be allowed to continue by a favorable response to fetal scalp or fetal acoustic stimulation or alternatively from a reassuring fetal capillary pH value. The goal is avoidance of rather severe fetal metabolic (cord arterial pH <7.00) or mixed acidosis as a means to reduce newborn morbidity and mortality.[186,187] Temporary fetal hypoxemia, without associated metabolic or mixed metabolic acidosis, poses little risk for significant newborn morbidity. Defensive medicine will continue to impact upon this indication. Although cesarean delivery for this indication is not a major contributor to the overall cesarean delivery rate, it is nonetheless likely that the impact of this indication can be reduced if tort reform can be enacted.

Active Management of Labor as a Reduction Strategy

Although the original intent of the active approach to the management of labor was to decrease the incidence of prolonged labor, in some centers its application has been associated with a significant reduction in the cesarean rate for dystocia.[182,188-191] Unfortunately, this has not been observed in all studies.[192] The active management of labor relies on utilization of strict criteria for the diagnosis of the active phase of labor and on a protocol using relatively high doses of oxytocin should there be diminished cervical dilatation in the first stage or inadequate descent in the second stage of labor. The benefits of the program are likely to accrue from avoidance of the clinical trap of overly aggressive management of the latent phase of labor as well as early intervention with oxytocin in patients with either protraction or arrest disorders. Patient education and one-on-one supervision by a personal nurse is also important (see Chapter 13).[182,188]

VAGINAL BIRTH AFTER CESAREAN BIRTH

Despite early reports in the 1960s that VBAC-TOL was both feasible and safe, the American obstetrician was initially reluctant to accept a significant modification in obstetric practice.[193] As late as 1987, more than 90 percent of women with a prior cesarean delivery had a repeat procedure.[4]

Benefits and Risks of VBAC-TOL

VBAC-TOL is successful in 60 to 80 percent of acceptable candidates.[194-197] If applied to all patients presenting with a prior cesarean procedure (8.2 to 8.5 percent), there is a potential to increase the rate of overall vaginal delivery by approximately 5 percent. Furthermore, there is evidence from a large multicenter trial that VBAC-TOL reduces the incidence of postpartum infection, the need for postpartum transfusion, and maternal length of stay; as a result, there is significant cost savings.[197,198] Adding further impetus is the observation that the associated perinatal mortality rate (7 per 1,000 live births) of the VBAC-TOL study group is not higher than that of the overall rate (10.1 per 1,000 live births).[197]

The potential financial savings arising from a successful national VBAC program was estimated at approximately $500 million in 1985, assuming a repeat cesarean birth rate of only 6 percent and 3.4 million births.[199] Data compiled for 1996 by the Health Insurance Association of America on 40,967 vaginal deliveries and 10,305 cesarean sections across the country reveal average charges of $11,450 for a cesarean delivery and $7,090 for a normal vaginal delivery, including both the hospital and physician components.[198]

Evolution of VBAC-TOL Acceptance

Cesarean rates appeared to have plateaued by 1991. One of the most important contributing factors has been a rejection of the historical dictum "once a cesarean section, always a cesarean section," which had been in practice since the early 1900s. It is logical that such an approach would eventually disappear. First, the clinical environment has changed dramatically since this policy was advocated. At that time only 2 percent of births resulted in a cesarean delivery; most often the procedure was performed following a diagnosis of cephalopelvic disproportion; and the procedure commonly used was a classic uterine incision. The advent of the low cervical segment incision together with better control of postcesarean infections has decreased the risk of uterine incision dehiscence during subsequent pregnancies. Second, there was a need to control rapidly rising national health care costs. Third, elective repeat cesarean delivery was the indication most responsible for the recent increase in cesarean births.

Although obstetricians in western European countries have encouraged VBAC-TOL, the concept did not begin to gain momentum in the United States until after 1981, when the NICHD Conference on Child Birth concluded that vaginal delivery after cesarean birth is an appropriate option.[25]

Initial reports indicated that successful VBAC could be achieved in 50 to 80 percent of patients with a prior low transverse uterine incision and in as many as 70 percent of women for whom the indication for the prior cesarean delivery was "failure to progress in labor."[5,204-206] Although uterine rupture was an infrequent possibility, it was noted to be rarely "catastrophic." Maternal and perinatal mortality rates for VBAC-TOL were no higher than those for elective repeat cesarean births.[5,200-206] Acceptance has become more widespread as numerous positive reports, documenting the efficacy and safety of VBAC under a wide variety of clinical settings, have been published.[5,195,207-212] Later reports documented no increase in maternal or fetal risk for candidates who had more than one prior cesarean.[209,210,213]

In 1988, the ACOG published *Guidelines for Vaginal Delivery After a Previous Cesarean Birth*, recommending VBAC-TOL as an option that should be selected based on available evidence available at that time.[61] They further recommended that "each hospital develop its own protocol for management of VBAC-TOL patients; and a woman with one prior cesarean delivery with a low transverse incision should be counseled and encouraged to attempt labor in the absence of a contraindication, such as a prior classical uterine incision." At the time there were insufficient data to provide a complete cost–benefit analysis for patients presenting with a prior low vertical incision, more than one fetus, a breech presentation, or estimated fetal weight greater than 4,000 g. The 1988 Committee Opinion indicated that the use of oxytocin to augment labor does not confer greater risk in a VBAC-TOL in a patient with a prior low transverse incision than would be the case in a general obstetric population; however, it did acknowledge that some physicians would not choose to use oxytocin in VBAC-TOL.[61] Epidural anesthesia was considered appropriate. Suggested 1988 guidelines include the following:

1. Repeat cesarean birth should be by specific indication.
2. Women with two or more prior cesarean deliveries should not be discouraged from attempting a VBAC-TOL.
3. Normal patient activity should be encouraged during the latent phase of labor. There is no need for restriction prior to the onset of the active phase of labor.
4. Professional and institutional resources should be available to respond to "intrapartum obstetric emergencies" such as performing a cesarean delivery within 30 minutes from the time the decision is made until the "surgical procedure is begun."
5. A physician capable of evaluating labor and performing a cesarean delivery should be "readily available."

As noted earlier, ACOG has recently modified its recommendations. VBAC after one prior low transverse cesarean delivery is encouraged, and after two it may be allowed recognizing the increased risk of uterine rupture.[213] The ACOG advises that the use of prostaglandin gel or oxytocin require close monitoring. Patients with a true low vertical incision are candidates for VBAC. The major change has been the recommendation that the obstetrician be "immediately available" to provide emergency care.[3]

VBAC Trends

VBAC-TOL Rates

Acceptance of the VBAC-TOL concept has not been uniform. Approximately 40 to 50 percent of eligible

Table 18–8. TRIAL OF LABOR IN WOMEN WITH PRIOR CESAREAN BIRTHS (C/S): TRENDS IN EMPLOYMENT AND SUCCESS

	1983 (%)	1992 (%)
Percent total deliveries	8.1	14.1
With 1 prior C/S	6.1	11.3
With 2 prior C/S	1.6	2.2
With at least 3 prior C/S	0.4	0.6
Trial of labor used	68	79
With 1 prior C/S	81	85
With 2 prior C/S	31	65
With ≥3 prior C/S	12	33
Trial of labor success	82	87
All prior C/S → vaginal delivery	56	69
Repeat C/S as percent of total deliveries	3.5	4.4

Data from Miller et al.[211]

women who are offered a VBAC-TOL choose the alternative, to have a repeat cesarean delivery.[214–217] A meta-analysis of 29 studies involving 8,770 VBAC-TOLs reflects wide variation in approach as evidenced by "remarkable variation in the percentage of patients accepted for trial of labor, ranging from 16–81%." Of interest, regression analysis indicated that the acceptance and success rates were not significantly associated.[218] Table 18–8 summarizes the dramatic change in acceptance of the validity of the VBAC-TOL concept at a large university hospital in the 10-year interval from 1983 to 1992. Although the percentage of all patients with a prior cesarean delivery increased, the effect was neutralized by an increase in use of TOL (68 to 79 percent). The increase was especially evident in patients with two or more prior cesareans.[211]

Evaluating the VBAC-TOL Data

U.S. Preventive Task Force Scoring System

Typically, under such an approach a Medline database search is conducted for reports of studies published in a predetermined time interval in one or more languages. The selected studies are evaluated, and the quality of the evidence obtained is then assessed on the basis of a scoring system (Table 18–9) scale. The evidence was graded (Table 18–9) according to the three categories of (A) "good" evidence, (B) fair evidence, and (C) insufficient evidence; but the recommendation can be made on other grounds.

Meta-Analysis as a Tool To Evaluate Infrequent Endpoints

Meta-analysis is a statistical tool that provides access to pooled data from multiple similar selected nonrandom-

Table 18–9. U.S. PREVENTIVE SERVICES TASK FORCE SCORING SYSTEM FOR EVIDENCE QUALITY

Score	Required Evidence
I	At least one properly designed randomly controlled trial
II-1	Well-designed controlled trial without randomization
II-2	Well-designed cohort or case-control analytic studies, preferably from more than one medical center or research group
II-3	Multiple time series with or without the intervention. Dramatic results in uncontrolled experiments
III	Opinion of respected authorities, based on clinical experience, descriptive studies, or reports of expert committees

Adapted from Rosen MG, Dickinson JC, Westhoff CL: Vaginal birth after cesarean: a meta-analysis of morbidity and mortality. Obstet Gynecol 77:465, 1991.

ized studies deemed appropriate by the reporting investigators. This approach provides the most readily available means with which to accumulate sufficient data to evaluate the impact of selected uncommon risk factors or endpoints. Odds ratios for each of the outcomes of interest can be calculated for each individual study, as well as for the pooled data. In the case of VBAC-TOL data, an odds ratio that is far from 1.0 (i.e., 0.5 or 2.5) indicates a strong relationship between the TOL group and the outcome analyzed. In contrast, an odds ratio that is close to 1 indicates a weak relationship. Similarly a narrow confidence interval indicates that the summary odds ratio is a precise estimate of the effect, whereas a wide confidence interval or one that includes the null hypothesis value (1.0) indicates that the observed odds ratio is not a precise effect estimator, which is most often observed when the outcome is a rare event. When outcome measures are rare, the odds ratio for any one particular outcome may appear to reveal a substantial difference between the various birth routes (TOL vs. VBAC vs. elective repeat cesarean delivery); however, when such outcomes are rare, the risk difference between the birth routes will be small. The primary limitation of meta-analysis is that both physician and patient choice are involved in each study and likely to be inconsistent from study to study.

Relevant VBAC-TOL Comparison Groups

To best determine the most appropriate prospective clinical management for patients presenting with a prior cesarean birth, the elective repeat cesarean group is the appropriate reference group with which to evaluate the safety of VBAC-TOL. Prospectively, the outcome of the elective group should be compared with the outcome of all patients undergoing TOL. In hindsight, after completion of the TOL, the TOL group may be subdivided into (1) successful TOL (VBAC) and (2) failed TOL.

Preexisting Conditions as Predictors of VBAC-TOL Success

One of the first questions to be raised by a patient when considering a VBAC-TOL is, what is the likelihood for a successful vaginal birth according to the indication for the prior cesarean birth? The overall VBAC success rate for all candidates is 60 to 80 percent (Evid. Qual. II-2 and II-3).[195–198] Obstetric history regarding preexisting conditions is helpful in the prediction of VBAC success. Women who have previously given birth vaginally or women whose prior cesarean delivery was for nonrecurring conditions are more likely to succeed (Evid. Qual. II-3).[196,218–220] Despite providing some assistance, there is no system to predict the specific patient who will achieve a VBAC success; even x-ray pelvimetry cannot predict success (Evid. Qual. II-1 and II-3).[221,222] Furthermore, success rates vary because of nonclinical variables and patient self-selection, which influences (Evid. Qual. Level II-2 and II-3) VBAC-TOL attempt rates.[215,223,224]

Recurring Versus Nonrecurring Indications

The likely success of a VBAC trial will depend to some degree on whether the indication for the prior cesarean is a recurring or nonrecurring one. Patients with a nonrecurring indication (breech presentation, so-called fetal distress–nonreassuring FHR pattern, and conditions such as placenta previa, abruption, or maternal hemorrhage) are more likely (82 to 86 percent) to achieve success than is the patient who has undergone a prior cesarean for a potentially recurring condition (70 percent) such as dystocia (failure to progress and/or CPD), approximating the success rate for the so-called low-risk nulliparous patient.[208,218,225]

Rosen used meta-analysis of 29 individual studies reported between 1982 and 1989 (Table 18–10) to evaluate the association between preexisting conditions and achievement of vaginal delivery (successful VBAC) for the entire subset; the effect of not attempting a VBAC-TOL is included.[218] VBAC-TOL success rates are similar (63 to 85 percent) among the subsets. However, when each subset is considered as a whole, a trial was offered apparently less often or when offered was refused more frequently when the prior indication was dystocia (OR, 0.5) and when oxytocin was used (OR, 0.3). The odds ratios of achieving vaginal delivery (when one condition is compared with all other preexisting conditions) are listed in Table 18–10 in decreasing order.

Table 18-10. META-ANALYSIS OF 29 STUDIES (RANGE, 6-24 FOR EACH INDICATOR) INVOLVING 8,770 VBAC-TOL

Preexisting Indicator in Prior Pregnancy	No. of Studies	Average Success Rate (%)	Odds Ratio*	95% CI	Studies Analyzed (Cases)
Previous breech	17	85	2.1	1.8-2.3	17 (1,720)
Prior vaginal delivery	12	84	2.1	1.7-2.5	12 (834)
Prior cesarean	6	75	0.7	0.5-0.9	6 (1,015)
Dystocia†	24	67	0.5	0.5-0.6	24 (3,582)
Oxytocin used‡	10	63	0.3	0.3-0.4	10 (2,289)

*Cephalopelvic disproportion, failure to progress.
†Odds ratio for a successful trial of labor after cesarean with various preexisting indications.
‡Used in current pregnancy.
Data from Rosen and Dickinson.[218]

Prior Breech

Sixteen of 17 studies selected for meta-analysis indicate that the highest success rate (OR, 2.1; 95 percent CI, 1.8 to 2.3) with the current trial of labor is achieved when the prior indication for cesarean is breech presentation, indicating that the chance of achieving vaginal delivery was more than twice as great for a woman who had had a prior cesarean for a breech than if she had had a cesarean for all other reasons.[218] Only one study found no association.[201]

Prior Vaginal Delivery

Although all patients have a relatively high rate of successful VBAC attempt, the success rate is increased to over 80 percent for women who have had a prior vaginal birth.[125,226,227] An early report was unable to demonstrate a significant impact of prior vaginal birth on an already high overall success rate (>80 percent).[208] It may be that the impact of a prior vaginal birth exerts its effect only in patient populations in which VBAC trial management was less aggressive. Eleven of 12 available studies selected for meta-analysis indicate that a prior vaginal delivery improves the likelihood (OR, 2.1; 95 percent CI, 1.7 to 2.5) of a successful trial of labor.[218] Only one selected study indicated that a prior vaginal delivery did not improve the likelihood.[228] Two studies have examined the issue in greater detail, controlling for the order of these deliveries, and determined that vaginal delivery following the prior cesarean is a stronger predictor of success than vaginal delivery before the prior cesarean.[118,208]

More Than One Prior Cesarean (Multiple Prior Cesarean Births)

In 1999, the ACOG Practice Bulletin for vaginal delivery after a previous cesarean birth specified that "Women with two previous low-transverse cesarean deliveries and no contraindications who wish to attempt VBAC may be allowed a trial of labor. They should be advised that the risk of uterine rupture increases as the number of cesarean deliveries increases."[3] The safety of VBAC-TOL in women having had two or more cesareans is now well established; they can be managed in a manner similar to that for patients with only one prior incision, with few complications.[5,193,201,208-211,213,214,220,229] Meta-analysis of six studies, providing data (Table 18-10) on 1,015 women who had more than one prior cesarean before a trial of labor, indicates that such patients have historically been 30 percent less likely (OR, 0.7; 95 percent CI, 0.5 to 0.9) to be successful than all other trials of labor.[218] A report by Miller et al.[211] (Table 18-11) emphasizes the importance of inclusion of patients with two or three prior cesareans if reduction of the total cesarean rate is to be considered a serious goal. They constitute approximately 1.8 and 0.5 percent of the entire obstetric patient population, respectively, and are highly likely (75 and 79 percent, respectively) to achieve vaginal delivery. Although uterine rupture is more likely in this group (OR, 3.06), there is no appreciable increase in perinatal mortality.[211]

Currently available data on the outcome of TOL with three or more prior cesareans are limited; however, VBAC success rate was 79 percent in one study.[211] As noted by the ACOG, women with more than two prior procedures should be informed that they may possibly be at greater risk for uterine rupture if they choose TOL. However, they should not be discouraged from attempting a VBAC-TOL. As many as 33 percent of such patients will accept the VBAC-TOL option, and approximately 80 percent of those who do so will be successful.[211]

Prior Dystocia (CPD/FTP)

Absolute cephalopelvic disproportion is virtually never present. Inherent clinical biases would suggest that patients with a previous cesarean delivery for dystocia

Table 18–11. USE AND SUCCESS RATES OF A VBAC-TOL ACCORDING TO THE NUMBER OF PRIOR CESAREAN BIRTHS

| | No. of Prior Cesareans | | | |
	One	Two	Three	Total
No. of prior cesareans	13,594	2,936	792	17,332
Percent toal population	8.2	1.8	0.5	10.5
Trial of labor (TOL) (%)	80	54	30	73
Success (VBAC) (%)	83	75*	79*	82
Percent potential reduction in total cesarean rate	5.5	0.8	0.1	6.4

*Success rate with ≥2 prior cesareans was 75.3%, significantly lower than with 1 prior cesarean (OR, 0.612; 95% CI, 0.54–0.69; $p < 0.001$).
Data from Miller et al.[211]

(FTP or CPD and failed induction) would not only be less likely to achieve a VBAC-TOL, but also would not attempt a trial as often. Meta-analysis of 24 studies involving 3,582 trials in women with a prior cesarean for dystocia (Table 18–10) indicates that if such women attempt a trial, they achieve a 67 percent VBAC-TOL success rate. However, when the entire group with prior dystocia is considered, they have the lowest success rate for vaginal delivery (OR, 0.5 to 50 percent of the rate of success [11 to 16 fewer vaginal deliveries per 100 cases]) achieved by all other women presenting with a history of prior cesarean for other indications (95 percent CI, 0.5 to 0.6).[218] A more recent multicenter study (Evid. Qual. II-2) indicates that the patients with prior dystocia (CPD, FTP) who attempted a trial were successful in approximately two of three trials.[197] One study in which 58 patients received oxytocin therapy prior to cesarean delivery for "failure to progress" in the first term pregnancy labors is particularly instructive.[26] Despite the seeming importance of a well-managed initial pregnancy labor trial, 40 (69 percent) of the 58 women achieved vaginal delivery in their subsequent VBAC trial.

Impact of Dystocia-Related Factors

The likelihood of VBAC success is increased in the absence of a prior dystocia diagnosis. Similarly, success is increased by the presence of factors predicting the absence of dystocia, such as absolute fetal weight less than 4,000 g, smaller relative fetal weight than the index pregnancy, and response to oxytocin stimulation within 2 hours.[227] Should oxytocin be required, the absence of a prior CPD diagnosis increases the likelihood of VBAC success.[226] Furthermore, if the issue is indirectly assessed by evaluating other factors possibly related to dystocia, such as the length of the labor prior to the primary cesarean, the fetal birth weight, and the extent of dilatation at the time of the prior cesarean, there is no improvement in predictability, as described below.[230]

Length of Labor Preceding Prior Cesarean

Two studies reported a tendency for a shorter labor immediately prior to the primary cesarean in women who are successful in a subsequent VBAC-TOL.[230,231]

Fetal Birth Weight

One might hypothesize a linkage between fetal birth rate and VBAC success. Jarrell et al.[228] reported a lower trial success rate in women with prior CPD delivering a newborn weighing more than 3,900 g. In contrast, Phelan et al.[204] in a report involving 140 trials of labor with "macrosomic" (> 4,000 g) infants, reported that 67 percent of the women delivered vaginally. A statistically significant association between a higher average birth weight and a higher failure rate could not be identified in a subsequent meta-analysis of 10 selected studies providing sufficient data to determine average birth weights (average birth weight ranged from 3,123 to 3,642 g) of VBAC-TOL candidates.[218]

Cervical Dilatation upon Admission for Current Pregnancy

Cervical dilatation greater than 4 cm upon admission has been reported to increase the likelihood of a successful trial of labor significantly in one study but not in the other.[230,231]

Extent of Cervical Dilatation During Prior Primary Cesarean

Should the history indicate that the prior cesarean was for "failure to progress" following a failed induction or in a patient who did not enter the active phase of labor, one might anticipate the success rate to be similar to that of the general VBAC-TOL population. In contrast, should the history indicate that the patient entered the second stage and despite adequate contractile activity and pushing was unable to deliver, one could reasonably hypothesize such a patient to be less likely to achieve success. Despite the possible rationality of the thought process, the data are not supportive. Two studies found no association between the extent of dilatation at the time of the primary cesarean and subsequent success in the present trial of labor.[230,232] Most recently, Jongen et al. reported that 80 percent of 103 women who underwent VBAC-TOL after a prior cesarean delivery for failure of descent in the second stage had a successful trial.[234]

Considerations in Management of VBAC-TOL

Management of the patient undergoing a VBAC-TOL is similar to that of patients attempting to achieve a vaginal delivery.[3,233] As a consequence, it is appropriate to use oxytocin and epidural anesthesia as one would in other labors. Potential problems such as suspected fetal macrosomia will be encountered and management will be no different from that in normal labor. The major difference will arise from some heightening of concern for uterine dehiscence and/or rupture. Even that concern need not be extreme; the risk is low and, should dehiscence or rupture occur, in most cases the outcome is favorable for both the mother and fetus.

Prior Uterine Incision

Prior Lower Uterine Segment Incision

The presence of a preexisting incision confined to the lower uterine segment engenders minimal risk of uterine rupture, and the risk does not appear to be modified by the route of delivery.[211,212] Only in hindsight (i.e., should there have been a failed TOL) does the 95 percent confidence interval (1.4 to 5.4) exceed and not overlap the reference value of 1.0, indicating increased risk.

Prior Low Vertical Incision

A prior low vertical uterine incision, limited to the lower, more passive, noncontractile portion of the uterine segment, is not a contraindication for a VBAC-TOL.[60,212] Candidacy for a TOL in a patient with a prior low vertical scar is somewhat controversial. Low vertical incisions are not necessary as often, and most investigators have excluded women with low vertical scars from their reported series of patients. As a consequence, the available data are limited, and the data reported are possibly biased, since they are not the product of prospective studies. Some clinicians believe that it is not possible to confine a vertical incision to the lower uterine segment. Some consider any uterine incision that extends into the upper, more contractile

portion of the myometrium to be a contraindication to subsequent labor.[235] The theoretical concern does not appear to be warranted. Rosen et al.,[212] in a meta-analysis of 170 VBAC patients with a prior low vertical incision, reported that the combined risk of dehiscence and rupture (two cases) was not different from that of VBAC patients with a prior low transverse incision.

Prior Classic Incision

It is likely that we will continue on occasion to be confronted with patients who have had a prior classic incision. A TOL should be strongly discouraged in such cases.[60] Fortunately, classic cesarean incisions are uncommon, and as a result the need to conduct a repeat cesarean in this population subset will make only a small contribution to the overall repeat cesarean rate. Patients with prior classic incision have an associated 12 percent (SE 6 percent) risk (3 cases in 26 women who underwent unplanned TOL) of symptomatic uterine rupture during labor.[212,236] Since approximately one third of ruptures occur prior to labor, it is currently recommended that women who have a prior classic cesarean delivery be delivered by repeat cesarean procedure upon achieving fetal pulmonary maturity prior to the onset of labor. Such patients should be warned of the hazards of an unintended labor and the signs of possible uterine rupture.[237]

Known Versus Unknown Incision Type

In an era when prior medical records are not always readily available, it is reassuring that the overall risk of dehiscence or rupture is low even among women undergoing a TOL with an unknown prior cesarean incision type. In large part this is a function of observation that 90 to 95 percent of women with unknown scars will have had a low transverse incision.[202] Some believe that if the extent of an incision is unknown or poorly documented, a TOL is probably not a reasonable approach.[235] However, this is not very practical and is probably unnecessary. Meta-analysis reveals no statistically significant difference in rates ($p = 0.95$) between those with versus those without known incision types.[212]

Oxytocin Usage in VBAC Trial

Use of oxytocin is contraindicated only if the patient has a prior classic incision; the indications for use of oxytocin are the same as those for patients without a history of one or more prior cesarean births.[212,238] Oxytocin use should be in general accordance with the guidelines described in Chapter 13 and ACOG Technical Bulletin No. 218.[239] Its use during a VBAC-TOL for augmentation does not increase risk and is not associated with an increase in perinatal mortality.[60,240] Some discussion of theoretical questions relating to benefits and risks justifying this conclusion is worthwhile.

Does the Use of Oxytocin Provide Clinical Benefit?

If oxytocin is not used selectively, a significant number of VBAC-TOLs will end up as repeat cesarean procedures. However, when VBAC-TOL patients receiving oxytocin are compared with those not receiving oxytocin, failure is significantly higher in the oxytocin group. Unfortunately, it is not possible to predict prospectively which patient will derive benefit. If there is an early response to oxytocin, one can expect a greater probability of success. In contrast, if a patient fails to progress within approximately 2 hours, cesarean delivery becomes considerably more likely.[227]

Benefit accrues from its use when employed for either induction or augmentation; vaginal delivery can be accomplished in 60 and 68 percent, respectively.[241] Meta-analysis of 10 selected studies indicates that the success rate among TOL patients requiring oxytocin is approximately one third the rate of success in patients not receiving oxytocin (OR, 0.3; 95 percent CI, 0.3 to 0.4).[218] Only 1 of the 10 studies suggested a higher, but not significantly higher, success rate following the administration of oxytocin.[201] Although the data are not available, selection bias may explain the discrepancy; oxytocin augmentation is seldom used unless there is recognition of delayed progress in either cervical dilatation in the first stage or descent in the second stage, and induction may be indicated in patients with an unfavorable cervix.

Are There Contraindications to Oxytocin Usage?

With the exception of a prior classic uterine incision, currently there are no absolute contraindications to the use of oxytocin in an appropriate VBAC-TOL candidate. Each case must be considered on the basis of the clinical presentation and a judgment made regarding the relative benefits and risks of its use under the circumstances of the case.

Spontaneous Versus Induced Uterine Contractions as Risk Factors

Uterine contraction patterns, whether spontaneous or oxytocin induced, may demonstrate hypercontractility (tachysystole or tetany); on occasion there may be associated FHR decelerations. Hypercontractility, if persistent, may potentially increase fetal risk, a risk that is independent of the presence of a prior uterine scar.

Does Oxytocin "Significantly" Increase the Risk of Uterine Rupture and Perinatal Mortality in a VBAC-TOL?

Initial concern that oxytocin usage would significantly increase the risk of uterine rupture/dehiscence has not been confirmed. First, the risk is quite low. Its use is not associated with an increase in perinatal mortality.[58] However, a case-control study found that "excessive (overuse of)" oxytocin infusion rates increased the risk for rupture or dehiscence.[242] Although it is known that use of oxytocin is "associated" with an increase in risk of uterine rupture, this risk must be interpreted in an overall clinical context that may include other factors also associated with rupture. Use and duration of administration do not significantly increase the risk above that expected in the absence of oxytocin.[5,92,199,212,241] Meta-analysis of selected studies indicates that the use of oxytocin during a VBAC-TOL does not appear to influence the risk of a dehiscence or rupture ($p = 0.7$), nor does it increase perinatal mortality rates.[212] In a recent large series, Miller et al.[211] report that oxytocin was used in only 68 percent of 118 cases of uterine rupture (74 percent of 69 ruptures in women with one prior cesarean and 67 percent of 39 ruptures in women with two prior cesarean deliveries). The risk of rupture may be increased in patients who receive oxytocin in the latent phase of labor or have dysfunctional labor.[242]

Prostaglandin Gel and Misoprostol Usage

Although the use of prostaglandin E_2 gel for cervical ripening is extensive and is likely to have been employed in many prior VBAC candidates, reported data are limited. Three authors have reported experience with prostaglandin E_2 gel for cervical ripening.[243–245] At this point, its use appears justified. In contrast, misoprostol has been associated with an increased risk of uterine rupture and should not be used in VBAC-TOL patients.[246]

Possible Fetal Macrosomia

Prospective management of potential fetal macrosomia presents a significant clinical dilemma in any labor. Estimated fetal weight (EFW) of more than 4,000 g is not a contraindication to a TOL.[60,212] Although clinicians might strategically reduce exposure to litigation by routine repeat cesarean delivery when the EFW is greater than 4,000 g, the strategy is flawed. It incorrectly assumes that fetal weight can be predicted reliably and ignores data that indicate that vaginal delivery can be accomplished safely in a large proportion of patients.[204] The decision to perform a cesarean in all patients with an EFW of more than 4,000 g would result in many cesarean deliveries for actual weight less than 4,000 g and with little or no improvement in outcome. The 1999 ACOG Practice Bulletin states that whether a trial of labor should be encouraged in the patient with an estimated fetal weight of more than 4,000 g "is controversial" as it is for patients with multiple previous cesarean deliveries, an unknown uterine scar, breech presentation, twin gestation, and a postterm pregnancy as well.[3]

The only way to address the question conclusively is to review retrospectively the outcomes of VBAC-TOLs in which the birth weight is known to be in excess of 4,000 g. Flamm and Goings[247] reviewed the outcomes of 1,776 patients who attempted a TOL in eight California hospitals; 301 newborns weighed at least 4,000 g. Fifty-eight percent of newborns weighing 4,000 to 4,500 g and 43 percent of those with birth weights of at least 4,500 g delivered vaginally. Of interest, when the outcomes of the 301 "macrosomic" TOLs were compared with the outcomes of the 1,475 TOLs with birth weights less than 4,000 g, there was no significant difference in maternal or perinatal morbidity or mortality. This clinical issue should be explored further.

Fetal Monitoring

In most cases, a significant alteration in FHR pattern is the presenting sign (Fig. 18–11); on occasion, an alteration (increased frequency and/or intensity) in uterine contraction pattern (if monitored externally) or a loss of intrauterine pressure (if monitored with an internal pressure catheter) is the presenting sign.[199] The clinical detection and management of a possible uterine rupture will involve interpretation and reaction to a nonreassuring FHR observation (i.e., a sudden prolonged deceleration, late decelerations, or repetitive "significant" variable deceleration of a degree requiring intervention under the circumstances of the case). Although repetitive "significant" variable decelerations or a prolonged deceleration occur all too frequently in non–VBAC-TOL, detection of these findings during a VBAC-TOL strategically may justify a heightened response. It would appear prudent to proceed more rapidly to cesarean delivery under such circumstances than would be the case in the absence of a prior uterine incision. Undoubtedly, such a recommendation will result in some cesarean deliveries in which there is no rupture. However, the occurrence of a significantly nonreassuring FHR observation in a VBAC candidate is so infrequent as to have little impact on the overall cesarean rate of only one institution.

Intrauterine Pressure Catheters

One of the primary justifications for early recommendations by some that intrauterine pressure catheters be used was the potential to detect intrauterine pressure changes (abrupt change in intrauterine activity or pressure) associated with uterine rupture. Unfortunately, use of intrauterine pressure catheters does not reliably assist in the diagnosis of rupture.[248,249]

Epidural Anesthesia

On the basis of available information, there appears to be little reason to withhold epidural anesthesia in a VBAC-TOL.[5,195,206–208,220] The experience to date suggests that the use of epidural anesthesia does not delay the diagnosis of uterine rupture and does not decrease the likelihood of a successful VBAC-TOL.[60,206] Although there was natural concern that the use of epidural anesthesia in the first and second stages of labor may obscure symptomatology (pain, tenderness) of an otherwise painful uterine rupture and delay its diagnosis, the safety of epidural anesthesia in patients with a prior low transverse cesarean incision is now well established. Regional anesthesia does not appear to obscure the symptoms associated with uterine rupture.[199,250–252] Furthermore, only a minority of patients experience pain and bleeding.[195,206] Even in the unanesthetized patient, uterine or scar tenderness, a sign of uterine rupture, occurs in only 25 percent of cases.[253]

Routine Uterine Exploration

The relative merits of routine uterine exploration of the lower uterine segment following a successful VBAC is a subject of some controversy, an area where reasonable people may disagree reasonably. Advocates of routine exploration argue that failure to identify a defect does not allow for rational consideration of risk and benefits should a subsequent VBAC trial be considered. It is their belief that should routine exploration detect a "significant defect" that is connected with the peritoneal cavity, laparotomy should be performed either to repair the defect or to perform a hysterectomy. The logic supporting an approach not involving routine exploration is based on two observations. It is not clear how such information would modify future pregnancy management. If active bleeding is suspected, a laparotomy must be performed regardless of pelvic findings. Most agree it is not necessary to repair a small defect dehiscence unless there is significant bleeding or the patient develops significant symptomatology, because these asymptomatic scar dehiscences will heal well.[3] If a small defect is detected and there are no supporting signs or symptoms, the patient can be followed expectantly with careful observation of vital signs and serial hematocrit determinations.[61,214] Second, should routine exploration occur in a patient with a "uterine window" (the lower uterine segment is intact, but very thin), there is the possibility that the exploration could disrupt an intact but thin lower segment. Although disrup-

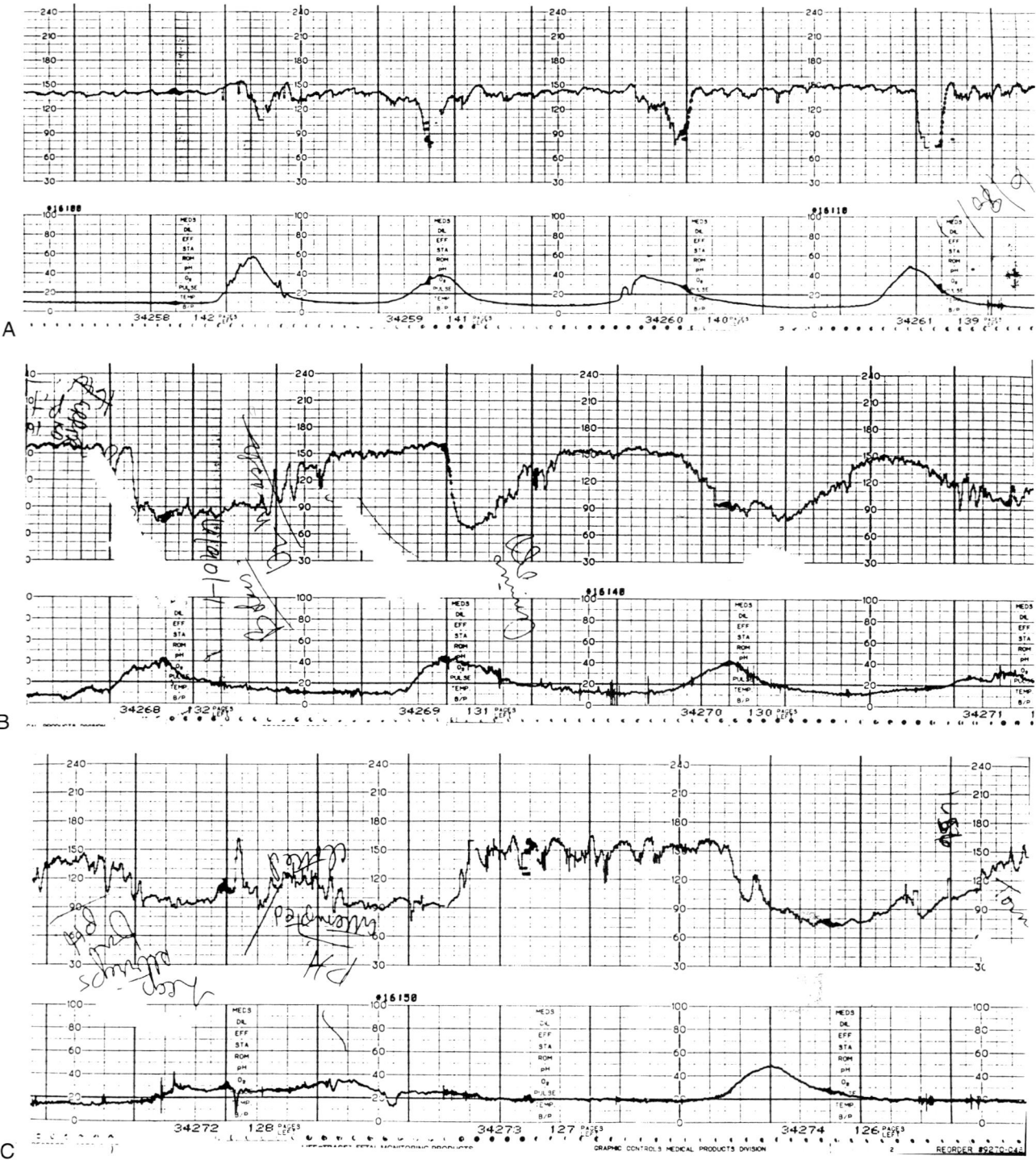

Figure 18–11. *A,* The patient is a 37-year-old gravida 7 para 3 AB3 woman at 41 weeks' gestation who presented for induction of labor. She had had two prior vaginal deliveries but her last baby was born at 33 weeks by low transverse cesarean section for nonimmune hydrops caused by a cardiac malformation. The patient's induction was begun with prostaglandin gel. Her cervix changed from fingertip dilated, 50 percent effaced, to 1 cm dilated, 70 percent effaced with a cephalic presentation at −2 station. Oxytocin was then begun at 1 milliunit/min. The patient progressed well, and epidural anesthesia was administered at 4 to 5 cm dilatation, 90 percent effaced, and 0 station. The patient was at 6 cm dilatation with a tracing demonstrating normal heart rate variability and variable decelerations. *B,* 30 minutes after the above tracing was recorded, the fetal heart rate pattern changed to severe variable decelerations. *C,* The tracing then demonstrated prolonged decelerations at 90 bpm. The patient was taken to the operating room for an emergency cesarean delivery. Uterine rupture had occurred along the site of the previous uterine incision. A female fetus weighing 3,200 g with Apgar scores of 7 and 8 was delivered. The umbilical arterial pH was 7.17 and the venous pH 7.22. The uterine incision had not extended and was easily closed. The baby did well.

Table 18–12. CANDIDACY FOR VBAC-TOL: CLINICAL CONDITIONS FOR WHICH THERE ARE INSUFFICIENT DATA TO MAKE A CONCLUSIVE RECOMMENDATION

Condition	Evidence Quality
Prior vertical cesarean (low segment)	II-3
Multiple gestation	II-3
Breech	II-3
EFW >4,000 g (nondiabetic)	II-2
External version	II-2
Prior myomectomy	No data

Adapted from American College of Obstetricians and Gynecologists: Vaginal Delivery After Previous Cesarean Birth. Practice Patterns, No 1. Washington, DC, ACOG, 1995.

tion of such a window would be unlikely to result in a significant problem, should abdominal exploration not be performed, one can easily predict an unnecessary sense of anxiety and anticipation by the patient in the ensuing hours until the clinician is confident that the patient will not develop signs or symptoms that would require abdominal exploration.

The ACOG VBAC Practice Pattern

In 1995, the ACOG published its first of a series entitled *Practice Patterns* on management of VBAC-TOL candidates.[214] It was revised in 1999.[3] The Practice Patterns are intended to serve as an acceptable clinical guideline to assist practitioners and patients in making decisions regarding appropriate care. They do not offer an exclusive course of management, but provide a detailed analysis, including meta-analysis, of factors that should help to determine a reasonable course of action to be chosen after taking into consideration available resources, patient risk factors, and desires of the pa-

tient. The relative merits of available data were evaluated using the U.S. Preventative Task Force Scoring System (Table 18–12) and the evidence (based on the highest level of data available) was graded (Tables 18–13 and 18–14) according to the following categories: (A) "good" evidence; (B) fair evidence; and (C) insufficient evidence, but the recommendation can be made on other grounds.

Candidacy for VBAC-TOL

Most patients with a prior cesarean birth are candidates (Table 18–12, Evid. Level A).[61,194,195,197] The only established contraindication is a prior classic incision (Evid. Level A).[214,241] Patients with more than one prior cesarean may be selectively offered a VBAC-TOL (Evid. Level B).[194,220,254–256] Clinical conditions for which there are insufficient data to make a conclusive recommendation are noted in Table 18–12. Limited data (Evid. Level B) support a VBAC-TOL for patients with a prior low vertical incision.

Uterine Dehiscence and Uterine Rupture

Unfortunately, many studies do not define or differentiate between uterine rupture and dehiscence, and as a result most available data do not reliably specify the risks of rupture vs. dehiscence. Dehiscence has a distinctly different clinical connotation from "uterine rupture," which historically has been associated with prolonged oxytocin use in multiparous patients or following obstetric manipulations such as internal version or extraction.[257,258] Despite this limitation, the combined threat of uterine dehiscence and rupture during a TOL is not sufficiently high (when compared with the elective repeat cesarean group) to deny women the well-accepted advantages of vaginal delivery.

Table 18–13. THE ACOG VBAC PRACTICE PATTERN SUMMARY

Clinical Issue	Conclusion from Trial	Evidence Level: Quality
Success rate	60–80%	A:II-2
Benefits of VBAC-TOL	Outweigh risks	A:II-2
Candidates		
Prior LT C/S	Encourage trial	A:II-2
≥2 LT C/S	Do not discourage	B:II-2
Contraindications	Prior classic incision	C:III
Clinical problems		
Suspect macrosomia (in nondiabetic)	Not disqualified from VBAC trial	B:II-2
Multiple gestation	Insufficient data	C:II-2; II-3
Breech presentation	Insufficient data	C:II-2; II-3
Nonsubspecialty hospital	Appropriate site	A:II-3

LT C/S, low transverse uterine incision with no contraindications.
Data from ACOG.[214]

Table 18–14. THE ACOG VBAC PRACTICE PATTERN: POSSIBLE COMPONENTS OF MANAGEMENT PLAN

	Indication	Evidence Level: Quality
Latent/early active phase		
Activity: no restriction	Routine	—
Oxytocin induction	As needed	B:II-3
Prostaglandins	As needed (insufficient data)	C:II-2
Active phase of labor		
FHR every 15 minutes	Routine	NA:III
Epidural anesthesia	As needed (not contraindicated)	A:II-2
Oxytocin augmentation	As needed	B:II-3
Second stage of labor		
FHR every 5 minutes	Routine	NA:III
Epidural anesthesia	As needed	A:II-2
Third stage of labor		
Manual exploration for rupture/dehiscence	Not addressed	NA

NA, not available.
Data from ACOG.[3,214]

Definitions (Dehiscence Versus Rupture)

Uterine incisional dehiscence is commonly used to describe the occult or asymptomatic scar separation or thinning that is occasionally observed at surgery in patients with a prior low transverse incision. A useful operational definition of *dehiscence* is a uterine scar separation that does not penetrate the uterine serosa, does not produce hemorrhage, and does not cause major clinical problems.[5] Dehiscence is most often detected among women who have experienced a failed TOL. Some patients may develop dehiscence during labor that on occasion may lead to the need for repeat cesarean. The first indication may be observation of a scar defect, a separation, or only a near-transparent uterine "window" at the time of a cesarean procedure. Incomplete ascertainment of uterine dehiscence is likely in women having a successful VBAC-TOL.

Uterine rupture, on the other hand, is symptomatic and may have presenting signs that require acute intervention. Since dehiscence is uncommon (≤ 2 percent) and rupture is relatively rare (< 1 percent), most reported studies provide limited statistical power to detect small changes in the risk of dehiscence or rupture among relevant prior cesarean birth comparison groups.[218] It is, however, unlikely that there is a major increased risk, since dehiscence or rupture is infrequent in all groups.

Combined Risk for Uterine Dehiscence and Rupture

Patients with a prior cesarean delivery who attempt a VBAC-TOL are at no higher risk, antepartum or early intrapartum, for uterine scar disruption (dehiscence and rupture) than are those having an elective repeat cesarean delivery.[5,212,248,259,260] A recent meta-analysis that assessed the relative impact of VBAC-TOL on the combined risk of true rupture and asymptomatic dehiscence detected no difference ($p = 0.5$) in the combined risk between patients undergoing a VBAC-TOL (1.8 percent of 2,771) and those undergoing an elective repeat cesarean procedure (1.9 percent of 3,611).[212] However, in hindsight the risk of dehiscence or rupture in the subset that had a failed TOL was 2.8 times that following an elective repeat cesarean ($p < 0.01$). The use of oxytocin did not ($p > 0.1$) influence the risk.

Risk for Dehiscence

Asymptomatic dehiscence is found incidentally in up to 2 percent of prior cesarean patients.[218] The rate is similar in patients with a prior low transverse and low vertical incision.[210] In a series of more than 2,600 patients, dehiscence was noted in only 1.5 percent of 1,465 patients having a successful VBAC-TOL versus 5.1 percent of 331 patients undergoing cesarean delivery for a failed VBAC-TOL. The difference may be partially a function of incomplete ascertainment in the VBAC success group. Nonetheless, these rates were not significantly different from the dehiscence rates in control patients who did not plan a TOL.[5] A study (Table 18–15) involving more than 17,000 patients presenting with a prior cesarean, 12,000 of whom underwent a TOL, may give a more accurate assessment of the true prevalence of dehiscence; the status of the scar was routinely assessed visually or manually, and scar defects were categorized as either dehiscence or rupture. Among 17,332 women, there were 193 (1.1 percent) uterine dehiscences and 117 (0.7 percent) ruptures, for a combined risk in all women of 1.8 percent. The trial-

Table 18-15. UTERINE RUPTURE VERSUS DEHISCENCE AMONG 17,332 WOMEN WITH ONE OR MORE PRIOR CESAREAN BIRTHS

| | Trial of Labor | | | | Total | |
| | No | | Yes | | | |
	No.	Percent	No.	Percent	No.	Percent
Total prior cesarean cases	4,615		12,707		17,322	
Uterine dehiscence	NA		NA		193	1.1
Uterine rupture	22	0.5*	95	0.7†	117	0.7
Combined risk	NA	NA	NA	NA	310	1.8

NA, not available.
*Thirteen non-TOL cases diagnosed at emergency cesarean for FHR indications immediately after admission; nine discovered at nonemergent cesarean.
†One prior cesarean = 0.5%; two prior cesareans = 1.3%; three prior cesareans = 1.1%.
Data from Leung et al.[242]

related risk of uterine rupture was 0.5 percent with one prior cesarean, 1.3 percent with two prior cesareans, and 1.1 percent with three or more prior cesareans.[211]

Risk for Uterine Rupture

Two series, one involving more than 11,000 and one more than 17,000 women with prior cesarean births, provide data specific for risk of rupture.[195,197,211] In one series, the overall risk (Table 18-15) of rupture (117 cases) was 0.7 percent (0.5 percent for those not undergoing a trial and 0.7 percent for those attempting a trial) in all women presenting with a prior cesarean.[211] In the two other reports summarizing experience from Kaiser-Permanente Hospitals in California, the overall incidence of rupture during the past decade was 0.5 percent ([10 of 5,733] in the interval between 1984 and 1988 and 0.8 percent [39 of 5,022] during the 1990 to 1992 interval).[195,197]

Prospective Risk Scoring for Uterine Dehiscence or Rupture

Unfortunately, there are insufficient data for factors other than prior uterine incision type to provide a basis for prospectively identifying the specific patient who is likely to develop uterine rupture. Despite this limitation in prospective clinical care, VBAC-TOL continues to be viewed in a positive manner, largely because of the likelihood of VBAC success, the associated reduction in cesarean deliveries, and reduction in morbidity arising from cesarean delivery.

Certain risk factors, including exposure to "excessive amounts" (dose not defined) of oxytocin, dysfunctional labor, and a history of two or more prior cesarean procedures (Evid. Qual. II-2), have been "associated" with uterine rupture.[242] It is noteworthy that in one case-control study of 70 patients with prior cesarean

delivery, the term *excessive amounts* of oxytocin was, in the authors' judgment, injudicious initiation (overutilization) of oxytocin during the latent phase of labor without delay following failure of uterine contractions to respond to hydration; the majority of such patients received oxytocin before they had confirmed dysfunctional labor (at 1 to 4 cm dilatation).[242] The frequency and relative impact of a number of possible clinical risk factors, using elective repeat cesarean delivery as a reference, is summarized from a meta-analysis of more than 6,000 VBAC-TOLs in Table 18-16.

Maternal Morbidity and Mortality

Maternal Mortality

Because maternal mortality is a rare complication, estimation of relative risk between prior cesarean comparison groups is difficult. In one review of American studies involving 5,400 patients published prior to 1980, there were no maternal deaths arising from uterine rupture, even those involving classic uterine scars.[261] A 1985 summary report of 6,258 women undergoing a TOL over a span of more than 30 years (1950 to 1984) indicated that 5,356 (86 percent) were successful with no maternal mortality, comparing favorably with an expected mortality rate of approximately 1 death per 1,000 cesarean deliveries.[199] Even the increased use of oxytocin during VBAC has not increased the risk of morbidity or mortality.[5,212,226] Other more recent studies support the prior observations of no significant increase in maternal mortality or morbidity.[195,212,255,262] A meta-analysis (Table 18-17), summarizing maternal morbidity (dehiscence, rupture, fever) and mortality data from 11,417 VBAC-TOLs and 6,147 elective repeat cesareans reported in 31 VBAC studies between 1982 and 1989, confirms low maternal mortality and morbidity rates for both the elective repeat cesarean and TOL groups.[212] There were only two deaths among

Table 18–16. RISK FOR UTERINE DEHISCENCE (D) OR RUPTURE (R)*

Potential Risk Factors	R or D Cases	Odds Ratio	Freq./1,000 Births	95% CI	Studies: (Trials) Comments:
Elective cesarean	69	1.0‡	19	—	11: (n = 3,611)
All trials	50	0.8	18	0.6–1.2	11: (n = 2,771)
VBAC-TOL success†	19	0.7	12	0.4–1.2	11: (n = 1,613); p = 0.3
VBAC-TOL failure	19	2.8	33	1.4–5.4	11: (n = 584) p <.01
Oxytocin use	23	1.2	23	0.7–2.1	5: (n = 995); p = 0.7
Oxytocin not used	32	—	15	—	5: (n = 2,130)
Indications, recurrent	3	0.4	7	0.1–1.1	4: (n = 443)
Indications, nonrecurrent	16	—	26	—	4: (n = 607)
Uterine scar known	25	0.8	11	0.4–1.8	7: (n = 2,315)
Uterine scar unknown	26	—	22	—	7: (n = 1,181)
Low vertical scar	2	—	20	—	5: (n = 170)
Classic cesarean scar	3	—	120	—	2: (n = 26)

*Meta-analysis of 11 VBAC studies with more than 6,000 VBAC-TOL (1982–1989).
†Relative risk versus elective repeat cesarean delivery.
‡Standard error is 6%, or 60 per 1,000 births.
Data from Rosen et al.[212]

all TOLs and elective repeat cesarean deliveries. As one would expect, the observed maternal deaths derived from 10 studies were associated with postoperative surgical complications such as pulmonary embolus or following an obstetric complication such as placenta accreta. McMahon recently compared maternal morbidity in women undergoing VBAC-TOL with a group having an elective cesarean delivery. The higher rate of morbidity in the VBAC group was attributable to those patients who had had unsuccessful TOL.[263]

Maternal Febrile Morbidity

Mothers with successful TOLs (Table 18–17) have the lowest febrile morbidity, whereas those with a failed TOL (labor plus cesarean) have the highest (p < 0.001).[212] Because such a large percentage of women undergoing a trial of labor following a prior cesarean have a subsequent vaginal delivery, most women undergoing a VBAC-TOL will have less febrile morbidity and are thus likely to require a shorter hospital stay and fewer days lost from employment and family care responsibilities.

The perinatal risk for patients considering VBAC is no higher than that for patients delivering by elective repeat cesarean birth.[195,197,208,212,254,262] The overall uncorrected perinatal death rate arising from more than 5,500 women presenting with a prior cesarean birth (Table 18–18) was 1.4 percent (14 per 1,000) in a meta-analysis of 10 studies.[212] The uncorrected total

Table 18–17. MATERNAL MORBIDITY AND MORTALITY: META-ANALYSIS OF 31 VBAC STUDIES INVOLVING 11,417 VBAC-TOL AND 6,147 ELECTIVE REPEAT (ER) CESAREAN DELIVERIES (1982–1989)

	ER Cesarean	All TOL	Failed TOL	Successful TOL	Studies: (Trials)
Prior cesarean cases	3,831	4,617	1,206	3,411	31: (11,417)
Febrile morbidity/1,000*	173	96	271	34	17: (N/A)
Odds ratio	1.0	0.5	2.0	0.2	
95% CI	—	0.5–0.6	1.7–2.5	0.2–0.2	
Dehiscence/rupture (%)†		2.0			11: (>6,000)
No./1,000 births	19	18	33	12	
Odds ratio	1.0	0.8	2.8	0.7	
95% CI	—	0.6–1.2	1.4–5.4	0.4–1.2	
p Value	—	0.5	<0.01	0.3	
Maternal mortality/10,000	2.4‡	2.8§			10: (7,830)

*Febrile morbidity: amniotic infection, urinary tract infection, endometritis, wound infection/1,000 births.
†Combined risk (i.e., data not subdivided).
‡One death from placenta accreta after ER cesarean.
§One death from pulmonary embolus after failed TOL.
Data from Rosen et al.[212]

Table 18–18. COMPOSITE PERINATAL MORBIDITY (5-MINUTE APGAR SCORE ≤6) AND MORTALITY RATES*

	Elective Repeat Cesarean (n = 2,929)	All TOL (n = 2,549)	Failed TOL (n = NA)	Successful TOL (n = NA)
Perinatal deaths				
No./1,000 births	4	3	—	—
Odds ratio	1.0[†]	0.8[‡]	—	—
95% CI	—	0.3–2.1	—	—
5-minute Apgar score ≤6				
No./1,000 births	16	24	38	17
Odds ratio	1.0[†]	2.1[§]	2.6[§]	1.8[§]
95% CI	—	1.2–3.6	1.2–5.6	0.8–4.6
p Value			0.03	0.2

*Ten studies involving more than 5,000 births for perinatal endpoint.
[†]Reference group.
[‡]Excludes antenatal death <750 g, congenital anomalies.
[§]Includes <750 g, congenital anomalies.
Data from Rosen et al.[212]

perinatal death rate for the subset of women undergoing a TOL was 2.1 times that of women who underwent an elective repeat cesarean (p < 0.001); however, when unrelated causes, such as antepartum fetal death (prior to labor), very low birth weight (< 750 g) and congenital anomalies incompatible with life, were excluded, this difference in perinatal mortality disappeared. The corrected perinatal mortality rate was 3 per 1,000 following a TOL and 4 per 1,000 following elective repeat cesarean (OR, 0.8; p = 0.9). When the perinatal outcome of "true" uterine ruptures was compared (only antepartum deaths excluded) with the outcome with no ruptures, there were 3 (13.6 percent) deaths after 22 ruptures and 28 (0.5 percent) after no rupture in 5,463 trials. Oxytocin use during a TOL did not influence perinatal mortality rate (OR, 1.5; 95 percent CI, 0.5 to 4.4).

Perinatal Morbidity and Mortality Arising from Dehiscence or Rupture

Intrapartum fetal deaths arising in the subset of patients who experience dehiscence of a low transverse uterine incision are uncommon. Although uterine rupture does occur infrequently, it is rarely catastrophic because of the availability of modern fetal monitoring, anesthesia, and obstetric support services. Data associated with rupture of a classic fundal incision are less reassuring. No maternal deaths were reported in an early review of published American VBAC studies involving 5,400 patients prior to 1980; fetal deaths were observed in 17 (56.7 percent) cases in which there was dehiscence or rupture of a fundal incision.[261] In contrast, lower uterine segment dehiscence occurred in 25

instances (0.46 percent), with no maternal deaths and only 3 (12 percent) fetal losses; the overall fetal mortality risk was 0.37 percent. Most fetal deaths arising from uterine dehiscence occurred either prior to admission or prior to the advent of widespread employment of continuous electronic FHR monitoring. More recent data suggest that maternal and perinatal outcomes are generally good following uterine rupture. However, uterine rupture under certain circumstances can have serious sequelae. Two reports have summarized the outcomes of 20 uterine ruptures. There were no maternal deaths in either reports, but only 14 of 20 (70 percent) had good perinatal outcomes. There were four perinatal deaths and four cases with newborn neurologic sequelae. Unfortunately, three of the four perinatal deaths involved women who were laboring at home without fetal monitoring.[248,260] Table 18–19 summarizes the risks of uterine rupture and related perinatal deaths from a series of more than 17,000 women according to the number of prior cesarean births.

Newborn Depression as Morbidity Endpoint

The uncorrected odds radio for a 5-minute Apgar score of 6 or less following a VBAC-TOL was 2.1 (p < 0.001) versus the elective repeat group (Table 18–18). However, the absolute risk for the same score is low in both groups (2 percent in VBAC-TOL vs. 1.6 percent in the elective repeat group). These outcome data are flawed, since they include newborns weighing less than 750 g and those with serious congenital anomalies.[212] Should there be a failed TOL, the risk for a low Apgar score is 2.6 times that following an elective repeat cesarean section (p = 0.03). However, should the TOL

Table 18–19. VBAC-TOL: RISK OF A UTERINE RUPTURE AND RELATED PERINATAL DEATHS PER 1,000 TRIALS ACCORDING TO NUMBER OF PRIOR CESAREAN BIRTHS

	No. of Prior Cesarean Births							
	One		Two		Three		Total	
	No.	Percent	No.	Percent	No.	Percent	No.	Percent
Uterine rupture*	63	0.6	29	1.8†	3	1.2†	95	0.7
Related perinatal death (per 1,000 trials)	2	0.2	1	0.6	0	—	3	0.2

*In women undergoing a trial of labor.
†Incidence of uterine rupture with two or more prior cesarean births was 1.7%, significantly greater than with one prior cesarean (OR, 3.06; 95% CI, 1.95–4.79; $p < 0.001$).
Data from Miller et al.[211]

succeed, there is no greater risk than after a repeat cesarean delivery ($p = 0.2$). Use of oxytocin does not increase the risk (OR, 1.6; 95 percent CI, 0.8 to 3.2; $p = 0.2$).

Documenting the Medical Record

Unknown Uterine Incision

Although it is highly likely that a prior uterine incision of unknown type involved the lower uterine segment, the best strategy is to make a reasonable effort to document the nature of the prior incision.[60] The medical records office of the prior hospital in many cases can provide the necessary information. In those instances when the clinician is unable to determine the nature of the prior incision, the inability per se should not serve as a contraindication to a TOL.

The Operative Report

A description of the extent of a vertical uterine incision (low vertical vs. classic) in the cesarean operative report can be important in deliberations regarding the decision to pursue a VBAC-TOL in future pregnancies.

Timing of Elective Repeat Cesarean Delivery

Should the patient refuse a VBAC-TOL or have a recurring indication for cesarean delivery, the clinician has four possible options to determine when elective cesarean delivery should occur. According to the ACOG, fetal maturity may be assumed and amniocentesis need not be performed if the criteria of one of the four options in Table 18–20 are met.[237,264] The criteria do not preclude use of menstrual dating, particularly if one of the four confirm menstrual dates in a patient with normal menstrual cycles and no immediately re-

cent use of oral contraceptives. Ultrasound is considered confirmatory if there is agreement between menstrual-gestational age and crown–rump age at 6 to 11 weeks or by the average gestational age determined by multiple measurements at 12 to 20 weeks within 1 week and within 10 days, respectively.

Table 18–20. FETAL MATURITY ASSESSMENT PRIOR TO ELECTIVE REPEAT CESAREAN DELIVERY

Option 1 (FHR)	One or more of the following is present for the stated duration: For 20 weeks: FHR by nonelectronic fetoscope For 30 weeks: FHR by Doppler
Option 2 (hCG)	For 36 weeks: positive serum or urine pregnancy test
Option 3* (Ultrasound)	At 6–12 weeks' gestation: Ultrasound crown–rump length supports gestational age of ≥39 weeks
Option 4* (Ultrasound)	At 12–20 weeks, multiple ultrasound measures confirm gestational age of ≥39 weeks as determined by clinical history and physical examination
Option 5	Await spontaneous onset of labor
Option 6	Fetal pulmonary maturity documented by amniotic fluid surfactant assessment

*Does not preclude use of menstrual age with agreement within 7 days (option 3) or 10 days (option 4).
Data from ACOG.[264]
Adapted from American College of Obstetricians and Gynecologists, Committee Opinion: Fetal Maturity Assessment Prior to Elective Repeat Cesarean Delivery. No. 98. September 1991.

Desire for Permanent Sterilization as an Indication for Repeat Cesarean

Approximately 42 percent of patients refuse the VBAC option.[217] The decision to attempt a VBAC-TOL is often clouded by other clinical factors such as the need for a postpartum tubal ligation. Some would argue that a patient's desire for a permanent sterilization is not an appropriate indication for a repeat cesarean procedure. In most cases, such a view is appropriate; the morbidity of vaginal delivery and subsequent postpartum tubal ligation is less than that of a repeat cesarean. In one study, 13 percent of successful VBAC patients had a postpartum tubal ligation with only minor prolongation of their hospital stay.[265]

Many patients, however, will find such an argument unattractive, particularly if the prior cesarean for dystocia was performed after a long labor including extended pushing. Unfortunately, ligation may not be feasible immediately postpartum following a successful VBAC. Other reasons for refusal are fear of "another long labor" resulting in a cesarean; concern about the likely need for one anesthesia for the cesarean/vaginal delivery and another for the tubal ligation; a preference not to reinitiate contraception; and concern that they cannot easily take time away from family or professional activities, even for an outpatient tubal ligation. More predictable access to tubal ligation immediately following a successful VBAC could potentially blunt the influence of many of the above. This access will vary according to hospital resources, particularly at night and on weekends.

Indication for Repeat Cesarean Delivery

Nearly two thirds of all repeat cesarean procedures are performed without a trial of labor. The most common indications are listed in Table 18–21.[211]

Table 18–21. MOST COMMON INDICATIONS FOR REPEAT CESAREAN DELIVERY WITHOUT LABOR IN 17,322 WOMEN WITH PRIOR CESAREANS

Indication	Occurrence (%)
Elective repeat	47*
Malpresentation	20
FHR indication	14
Macrosomia	5
Placenta previa	3
Multiple gestation	2

*21% in women with 1 prior cesarean delivery; 56% in women with two prior cesarean deliveries; 68% in women with ≥3 prior cesarean deliveries.
Data from Miller et al.[211]

INFORMED CONSENT

Informed Consent Is a Process

Informed consent should be considered a process that includes sharing of information and discussion of the choices reflected in the informed consent document.[266] Ordinarily, effective informed consent requires active participation by both the physician and the patient. It is the physician's responsibility to make sure that the patient is well informed; has under ordinary circumstances reasonable time to contemplate the information provided; and is encouraged to ask questions when necessary. It is the patient's responsibility to provide accurate and complete information and, if matters are unclear, to pose questions.[267]

The patient and her partner should participate in the decision-making process leading to cesarean delivery. There is considerable variation in both the style and substance of obtaining informed consent for cesarean birth. Although there is certainly merit to nondirected counseling, it should be somewhat obvious that it is difficult to transmit a minimum of 8 years of training and a number of years of clinical experience into a 5- to 10-minute discussion for informed consent, particularly when stress and emotions are high. The provision of informed consent involves walking a fine line; it is part of the so-called art of medicine. Much of the information provided will depend on whether the procedure is scheduled or unplanned. A key feature in the process is physician–patient rapport and associated patient trust of the managing physician. Current practice patterns often dictate that the patient receive care from several members of a large group practice, in which case rapport is not always optimal. Some patients want a detailed explanation, whereas others desire whatever the doctor advises. Sadly, much of what is discussed is often not understood or is forgotten when stress is high. Provision of too much information may overwhelm the patient. On the other hand, provision of inadequate or unbalanced information may result in a decision that the patient later regrets.

Content Disclosure Guidelines

There may be variation from state to state regarding the degree of disclosure required for a valid surgical consent (i.e., what is adequate information?). Most states use the "professional" or "reasonable physician standard," whereas others use the "materiality" or "patient viewpoint standard."

"Professional" Approach

The "professional" approach to consent is determined by what is customary practice in the medical community. Less information is provided, that is, extremely remote risk even with serious consequences may not necessarily be disclosed. In the case of an anticipated cesarean delivery when time is not an issue, the patient would be informed about the commonly encountered risks of any operative procedure, namely, infection and hemorrhage, as well as major complications associated with anesthesia. Injury to nearby organs, including bladder and ureters, at the time of cesarean delivery is a rare complication that is not ordinarily discussed. Should vaginal delivery be an acceptable alternative, the patient may benefit from knowledge regarding the relative risks and benefits of that approach.

Should primary cesarean delivery be considered for conditions such as a frank breech presentation, much of the focus of the discussion commonly may relate to the potential and theoretical fetal advantages, if any, of cesarean birth. Some mention of the severalfold increase in maternal morbidity and mortality associated with a cesarean delivery and its complications is also appropriate.

The patient should *not* be asked, "Do you want to do everything possible for your baby?" There are as yet few data to suggest that a cesarean birth, except in the presence of selective indications, has a beneficial effect with regard to survival and long-term outcome. Should cesarean delivery be considered for a very low birthweight fetus, it may be advantageous to review the anticipated weight and gestational age-specific rate of intact survival by either route. If the procedure would not follow labor, discussion of the potentially higher risk of respiratory distress with an elective cesarean birth may be appropriate.

Contingencies can also be important. Should the physician anticipate a repeat cesarean procedure in a patient with a current diagnosis of anterior placenta previa, informed consent may include some discussion regarding the potential need for hysterectomy for placenta accreta, as well as the potential need for transfusion and its associated risks (see Chapter 17). When an elective cesarean delivery likely to require blood replacement is anticipated, the option of autologous transfusion is a possible topic for discussion.[268]

Patient Viewpoint Approach

There may be an evolution to a new conceptual framework, the "materiality" or "patient viewpoint standard." Under the "materiality" or "patient viewpoint standard," even if the risk of a procedure is extremely remote, but has serious consequences, the risk would be disclosed, i.e., the amount of information provided should be based on what a "reasonable person in the patient's position" would "want to know in similar circumstances." This approach would then be based on what a patient would "need to know" to make a decision rather than on professional perception of what a patient "should know." The problem with such an approach is that the "needs" and "the reasonable patient" have not been objectively defined; clearly, there are many patients who, in foresight, are happy to rely on the physician's advice, but, in hindsight, would want to know virtually everything. Clearly, there are degrees of ability of the physician to communicate and of the patient to comprehend and remember. Such an approach would require physicians to discard their experience regarding what patients are capable of comprehending under similar circumstances or even what the experienced physician, who has an ongoing relation with the patient, believes the patient or most patients would like to know or understand.

Possible Components of Consent

Under either approach, the physician should not guarantee or even suggest a guarantee of outcome. To obtain fully informed consent, the physician should explain the following:

1. The diagnosis and nature of the condition calling for the intervention
2. The nature and the purpose of the treatment/procedure recommended
3. The material risks and potential complications associated with the recommended treatment/procedure
4. Feasible alternative treatments/procedures, including the option of taking no action
5. Description of material risks and potential complications associated with the alternatives
6. A relative probability of success for the treatment/procedure in understandable terms

Patient Refusal of Treatment/Procedure

On occasion, a patient may refuse a cesarean delivery that is perceived by the physician to be necessary to save either her life or that of the fetus; in most cases there are either religious or ethical considerations. Although there is no "correct" way to manage such a circumstance, the record should reflect the fact that the patient was informed of the benefits anticipated and that the patient refused the procedure. The ACOG Committee on Ethics has released a Committee Opinion that addresses such a situation: "Every reasonable effort should be made to protect the fetus, but the pregnant woman's autonomy should be respected. . . . The role of the obstetrician should be one of an informed educator and counselor, weighing the risks and benefits to both patients, as well as realizing that tests, judgments, and decisions are fallible. Consultation with others, including an institutional ethics committee, should be sought when appropriate, to aid the patient and obstetrician in making decisions. The use of the courts to resolve these conflicts is warranted only in extraordinary circumstances."[269]

Is Informed Consent a Prerequisite for VBAC-TOL?

The need for specific consent from a patient attempting VBAC seems somewhat superfluous if one acknowledges that the inherent risks of a VBAC are less than or equal to those of an attempted vaginal delivery in other patients. Because likelihood of a successful VBAC is only minimally dependent on the indication for the prior cesarean delivery, the physician should present the chances of success in a positive manner. An increasing number of clinicians now obtain written consent. However, an equally reasonable approach would be to indicate in the patient's prenatal record that the patient has been informed that labor following a prior cesarean delivery is an acceptable alternative to routine repeat cesarean delivery with only minor attendant risks that are not significantly greater than those of a repeat cesarean procedure.[3]

Patient Refusal of VBAC-TOL

Despite increasingly widespread acknowledgement that VBAC-TOL is safe and has a high success rate, only 40 to 50 percent of eligible candidates are reported to request an elective repeat procedure.[215,216] A desire to avoid labor-related pain and the convenience of a scheduled elective repeat cesarean are the most common reasons.[270] A woman should not be coerced to undergo a VBAC-TOL. Certain social, geographic, and past obstetric complications may justify the patient's electing to have a repeat cesarean birth. ACOG has recently stated that "the ultimate decision to attempt this procedure (VBAC) or undergo a repeat cesarean delivery should be made by the patient and her physician. . . . Global mandates for a trial of labor after a previous cesarean delivery are inappropriate because individual risk factors are not considered. . . ."[3]

PERIPARTUM HYSTERECTOMY

Peripartum or obstetric hysterectomy is the surgical removal of the uterus at the time of a planned or unplanned cesarean delivery or in the immediate postpartum period. Peripartum hysterectomies can be classified as total, subtotal or, occasionally, as radical (with or without node dissection and/or adnexectomy) or alternatively as "unplanned" (emergency), "planned" (scheduled), or "elective" (sterilization being the only indication). Such distinctions are critical when comparing the relative benefits and operative risks of hysterectomy with alternative management options.

Historically, the first cesarean hysterectomy was performed by H.R. Storer, in Boston, in a patient who expired on the third postpartum day.[271] Eduardo Porro (1876) performed the first procedure on a surviving patient.[9] In that case, subtotal hysterectomy (amputation of the uterine fundus following hysterotomy with subsequent marsupilization of the stump to the anterior abdominal wall) was performed to increase the likelihood of survival.[272] Twenty-five percent of cesarean deliveries were performed as Porro cesarean hysterectomies as late as 1922.[273]

Incidence

Two reports from the same institution over a 10-year span summarize a possible trend of increasing incidence of hysterectomy following cesarean delivery. The rate following cesarean delivery increased from 7.0 (1989) to 8.3 (1993) per 1,000 and continues to be dramatically higher than the rate following vaginal delivery (0.2 per 1,000 births in 1984 and 0.09 per 1,000 in 1993).[125,274] The increased rate following cesarean births may reflect the change in prevalence of prior cesarean deliveries. In the early series, only 44 percent of patients requiring hysterectomy had a prior cesarean delivery, whereas 67 percent had a prior cesarean in the more recent cases from 1985 to 1990.

Unplanned Emergency Indications

Most peripartum hysterectomies are unplanned (Table 18–22) and follow cesarean delivery.[125] Most are performed after more conservative efforts to control bleeding have been unsuccessful. Although hysterectomy may be the ultimate remedy for control of obstetric hemorrhage, conservative measures remain the primary approach; hysterectomy is reserved for circumstances in which these efforts either fail or are not applicable as would often be the case with abnormal placentation.[274]

Risk Factors for Emergency Hysterectomy

Sixty percent of emergency hysterectomies performed at Harvard were done in women with a history of a prior cesarean delivery.[275] Prior cesarean delivery heightens the risk for subsequent placenta previa, placenta accreta, and symptomatic uterine rupture, each of which increases the likelihood for an emergency hysterectomy.[272,275] The adverse impact of placenta previa as a

Table 18-22. INDICATIONS FOR UNPLANNED PERIPARTUM HYSTERECTOMY

Indication	Clark et al.[128] (1978-82)		Stanco et al.[274] (1985-90)		Zelop et al.[275] (1983-91)	
	No.	Percent	No.	Percent	No.	Percent
Placenta accreta	21	30	55	45	75	64*
Placenta percreta	—		6	5	—	
Uterine atony	30	43	25	20	25	21
Bleeding	—		19	16	—	
Uterine rupture	9	13	14	11	10	9
Fibroids with bleeding	3	4	3	2	2	2
Uterine infection	—		1	1	3	3
Scar extension/other	7	10	—		2	2
Total	70	100	123	100†	117	101

*"Abnormal placentation."
†82 (67%) had at least one prior cesarean.

risk factor for unplanned hysterectomy in patients with a prior cesarean is established.[91,276]

The importance of both previa and prior cesarean delivery as risk factors is supported by several studies from the same institution. In the first of three reports from southern California, a strong association (25 to 30 percent) between placenta accreta and a preexisting cervical uterine scar was reported.[89] The linkage was even greater in the subset who required hysterectomy. In the second of the series, 52 percent of hysterectomies performed for placenta accreta were associated with a previous cesarean scar.[125] In the third report, 69 percent of 58 patients with placenta previa had one or more prior cesarean births. In that series, peripartum hysterectomy followed cesarean delivery in 94 percent of cases; 67 percent had a prior cesarean delivery, 47 percent had a placenta previa, and 50 percent had an accreta or percreta.[274] In another series from Massachusetts, the risk of peripartum hysterectomy in association with placenta previa increased from 7 per 1,000 deliveries in nulliparous women to 1 in 4 deliveries in women with a history of 4 or more prior births ($p < 0.001$).[275]

Placenta Accreta/Percreta

Placenta accreta/percreta with or without previa is now the most common indication for peripartum hysterectomy.[242,274,275]

In the past, the most common indication for peripartum hysterectomy had been uterine atony. The introduction of prostaglandin $F_{2\alpha}$ as a therapeutic intervention has reduced the relative impact of uterine atony as an indication for hysterectomy. Furthermore, hysterectomy is seldom performed solely for a Couvelaire uterus in the absence of other more pressing complications or for asymptomatic cesarean scar dehiscence. The shift to abnormal placentation as the most com-

mon indication for hysterectomy also reflects the dramatic increase in cesarean deliveries, including repeat cesarean procedures.[85] The shift in relative importance is illustrated (Table 18-22) by two reports from southern California.[128,274] In the first report, uterine atony was the most common indication; however, in the more recent series from the same institution, Stanco et al.[274] found that abnormal implantation of the placenta had assumed greater relative importance as the most common indication. In a recent series from Harvard, 64 percent of 117 cases were performed for this indication, whereas only 21 percent were done for uterine atony.[275]

Uterine Dehiscence and Rupture

Uterine rupture requiring hysterectomy is reported to occur in 0.2 percent (1 in 555) to 0.8 percent (1 in 122) of VBAC-TOL.[242,274]

In one series, 14 (11 percent) of 123 peripartum hysterectomies (Table 18-22) were performed for uterine rupture in patients undergoing a VBAC-TOL, the institutional incidence in such patients being 0.18 percent.[274] These data complement a report from the same institution in which uterine rupture occurred in 0.8 percent of 7,598 patients with a prior cesarean delivery undergoing a TOL.[207]

In early years, hysterectomy for asymptomatic uterine dehiscence was accepted practice. However, this is no longer the case. Should symptomatic rupture occur, hysterectomy is not always necessary, particularly if the patient has a desire for future fertility and the rupture site is in a favorable location where repair is feasible. The clinician may simply repair the defect or, should dehiscence be discovered at routine exploration following vaginal delivery, it may be followed by expectant observation as detailed above.

Extension of Uterine Incision

Extension of a uterine incision into the uterine vessels is an uncommon indication for hysterectomy. However, such extensions can pose a therapeutic dilemma. Should hemorrhage be significant, consideration should be given to the alternative of hypogastric or uterine artery ligation (as opposed to hysterectomy), depending on the patient's parity and desire for future pregnancy. Ligation of the anterior division of one or both hypogastric or internal iliac arteries may decrease the arterial pulse pressure up to 85 percent distal to the point of the ligation, thus allowing clot formation.[277] Alternatively, it is possible to ligate the uterine arteries.[278] In some cases it may be advisable to attempt to identify the ureter, which may be in close proximity, by either palpation or direct visualization before ligating the uterine vessels.[118]

Elective Procedures

Permanent sterilization combined with elimination of potential long-term risks for later uterine pathology were acceptable indications for cesarean hysterectomy in the 1950s and 1960s. Elective procedures were commonly performed for sterilization.[120,121] Justification for hysterectomy was based on an observed need for hysterectomy in 20 percent of patients within a mean interval of 6.3 years from the most recent cesarean delivery.[279] Several reports supported the safety of the planned/elective hysterectomy subset based on a low morbidity rate (Table 18–23).[280,281] Despite the relative safety of this subset, the incidence of elective cesarean hysterectomy has fallen dramatically in recent years. As other contraceptive options became available, authors such as Brenner et al.[282] suggested that if hysterectomy is performed primarily for sterilization, the morbidity of a scheduled procedure will outweigh its benefits.

Nonemergency Cesarean Hysterectomy

Some have included "elective" procedures in this category; however, it is not appropriate to consider planned procedures as "elective"—a term that would imply that there is no indication. In most cases, a planned hysterectomy is performed when a woman requiring cesarean delivery also has a gynecologic problem that is appropriately managed by hysterectomy. Large or symptomatic uterine leiomyomas and cervical intraepithelial neoplasia are the most common indications as well as benign gynecologic conditions, occasional pelvic malignancy, and prior uterine scars.[283] Several investigators have reported their experience with a scheduled procedure for women referred for cervical cancer and early cervical neoplasia complicating pregnancy.[284,285] Because invasive disease can be excluded by colposcopy during pregnancy, some prefer vaginal delivery after carcinoma in situ of the cervix is confirmed as the most serious lesion. However, in some cases the patient may desire a single procedure or be noncompliant, in which case cesarean hysterectomy is a reasonable option. An occasional cesarean hysterectomy may be performed for microinvasive disease. Rarely, invasive cancer of the cervix may be treated with a primary cesarean delivery followed by radical hysterectomy with pelvic lymphadenectomy.[286,287]

Total Versus Subtotal Hysterectomy

The relative merits of subtotal versus total peripartum hysterectomy will vary according to whether the procedure is a planned or unplanned one. Should the proce-

Table 18–23. PLANNED HYSTERECTOMY MORBIDITY

	Ward and Smith[280] (1953–64)		McNulty[283] (1972–82)		Yancey et al.[290] (1979–90)	
	No.	Percent	No.	Percent	No.	Percent
No. of cases	254		80		43	
Operative time	90–120*		—		123 ± 36†	
Patients transfused	195	77‡	15	19	17	40§
Pelvic hematoma	6	2	4	5	2	5
Febrile morbidity	—		5	6	—	
Pelvic cellulitis	9	4			4	9
Pyelitis	2	1	—		—	
Cystotomy	8	3	4	5	1	2
Ureteral injury	0		0		0	

*Minutes skin to skin.
†Mean ± standard deviation.
‡126 of 195 received 1 unit; indication = Hct < 35%.
§7 of 17 received 1 unit transfusions.

dure be planned, total hysterectomy is most commonly performed; contrarily, if the procedure is unplanned, a larger fraction will be subtotal. Some have viewed subtotal hysterectomy as a faster procedure, one to be used particularly when the patient is unstable, based on the belief that subtotal hysterectomy has less blood loss and requires less operative time. A recent publication does not support this hypothesis; the authors were unable to detect a significant difference between total and subtotal procedures with respect to blood loss, operating time, or length of hospital stay.[128] Clark et al.[128] did suggest that this observation was attributable to a selection bias, reflecting the indication and its management prior to the decision to proceed to hysterectomy. This possible bias is most evident should the indication be uterine atony or placenta accreta.

Uterine Atony

In one series, a subtotal procedure was performed in 77 percent of 30 cases associated with uterine atony.[128] Uterine atony requiring hysterectomy is commonly associated with amnionitis, oxytocin augmentation, preoperative magnesium sulfate infusion, increased fetal weight, and cesarean delivery for an arrest of labor; however, 23 percent of patients undergoing a hysterectomy for atony have no identifiable risk factors. Not surprisingly, both blood loss and operating time may be increased in patients undergoing hysterectomy for uterine atony.[121] The surgeon, when faced with uterine atony, commonly follows a predetermined series of pharmacologic interventions (oxytocin, methergine, and prostaglandin $F_{2\alpha}$ [Hemabate, Upjohn Co., Kalamazoo, MI]), as well as other maneuvers including curettage and hypogastric artery ligation in an effort to control bleeding and maintain fertility. Such procedures may be effective in controlling hemorrhage; however, if control is not achieved, blood loss experienced prior to the time the procedure is initiated would tend to be greater and the time spent on conservative measures is reflected in a longer operative time, both commonly attributed to the unplanned hysterectomy.

Placenta Accreta/Percreta

In contrast to atony as an indicator, only 23 percent of 21 hysterectomies performed for placenta accreta were of the subtotal variety.[128] Since placenta accreta is less often amenable to conservative management, the transition to a decision for hysterectomy may be somewhat more rapid. Only rarely can accreta be managed by curetting or oversewing the placental bed (see Chapter 17). Implantation site involvement is usually too extensive to respond to treatment other than hysterectomy, particularly when it is associated with placenta previa. Subtotal hysterectomy is also less likely to be effective should placentation be in the lower uterine segment, presumably because blood flow via the cervical branch of the uterine artery remains uncontrolled.

Maternal Morbidity and Mortality

It is important to distinguish those procedures performed primarily for gynecologic indications plus or minus sterilization from those performed for obstetric problems requiring emergency intervention, most commonly hemorrhage. Maternal morbidity (Table 18–23) and mortality (Table 18–24) associated with peripartum hysterectomy is not simply the product of the procedure itself. Maternal mortality and morbidity will in large part depend on whether (1) the procedure is a planned/scheduled or an unplanned/emergency procedure, (2) the patient was previously in labor and had significant risk factors for infection, or (3) the patient had coincidental pregnancy-related complications. Unplanned hysterectomies have a greater risk for maternal mortality than planned procedures, since they are commonly performed in response to life-threatening hemorrhage with independent morbidity and mortality consequences. Nonetheless, the risk is very low for both types, and as a result, single-institution reports seldom report mortality. Only one death (Table 18–23) was noted in three studies (series of 123 and 70 emergency cases from California[128,274] and 117 emergency procedures from Massachusetts[275]). The combined mortality rate for the three series is 3.2 per 100,000 (1 in 310).

Unfortunately, population-based mortality data specific for indication/procedure type are not available. However, Wingo et al.[288] assessed data collected by the Commission on Professional and Hospital Activities (1979 and 1980) to determine risk factors for 477 deaths among more than 317,000 women having abdominal hysterectomies. Not surprisingly, mortality rates for hysterectomy, when standardized for age and race, were higher when the procedure was associated with pregnancy or cancer than if not associated with these conditions. Although only 8 percent of all hysterectomies performed are associated with pregnancy or cancer, they account for approximately 61 percent of all deaths. The authors estimated the minimum and maximum standardized mortality rates for pregnancy-related abdominal hysterectomy to be 22.8 and 32.0 per 10,000 procedures, respectively.[288] Although not strictly applicable, the minimum and maximum rate estimates should provide some insight into rates to be associated with planned and unplanned procedures, respectively.

Operative Technique

Should the procedure be an emergency one in which there has been preexisting and ongoing rapid blood

Table 18–24. UNPLANNED HYSTERECTOMY MORBIDITY AND MORTALITY

	Clark et al.[128] (1978–82)		Stanco et al.[274] (1985–90)		Zelop et al.[275] (1983–91)	
	No.	Percent	No.	Percent	No.	Percent
Procedures	70		123		117	
Subtotal	38	54	65	53	25	21
Operative time (Mean)	3.1 h		NA		3.0	
Blood loss (Mean)	3,575 ml		3,000 ml		3,000 ml*	
Hemorrhagic					102	87
Transfused patients	67	96	102	83	102	87
Reexplored	—				3	1
Infect Morbidity					58	50
Febrile	35	50	NA		39	33
UTI			NA		7	6
Wound	8	12	11	9	4	6
Urologic injury	3	4	4	3	10	9
Cystotomy		0	12†		9	8
Ureteral	3	4	—		3	3
Maternal death	1§	1	0		0	

*Median value 50% ≥3,000 ml and 50% <3,000 ml.
†Intentional cystotomies for ureteral stent passage.
§Cardiac arrest secondary to amniotic fluid embolus.
Data from Clark et al.,[128] Stanco et al.,[274] and Zelop et al.[275]

loss, it may be necessary to compress the aorta manually until the operative field can be suctioned sufficiently to allow identification and clamping of bleeding points. In some cases, bilateral internal iliac, anterior hypogastric, or uterine artery ligation may be required to reduce arterial bleeding from the uterine, vesicle, and pudendal arteries. The operative technique for peripartum hysterectomy uses the general principles applicable to abdominal hysterectomy in the nongravid state. In initiating the surgical procedure, the surgeon should direct attention to (1) early adequate displacement of the bladder from the lower uterine segment and cervix, (2) use of overlapping sutures for successive vascular pedicles, (3) selective as opposed to mass placement of clamps and sutures to control bleeders, (4) periodic inspection of the bladder for an inadvertent cystotomy, (5) possible localization of the ureter should a lateral extension/laceration of the incision be the indication for the procedure, and (6) avoidance of excessive removal of vaginal length, particularly when the cervix is completely effaced.

There is considerable variation in operative technique. Variation involves the use of two versus three clamps for pedicles above the cardinal ligament, use of single versus double ligation of vascular pedicles, the relative desirability for skeletonization of vessels in the broad ligament, and the relative need for an additional step to separate and individually ligate the uterosacral ligaments.

Although the uterine vessels are considerably larger in the pregnant than in the nonpregnant state, tissue planes are more easily developed. Blood loss from a peripartum procedure is greater than (500 to 1,000 ml) that associated with hysterectomy in the nongravid patient, particularly if it is an unplanned one. The altered hemodynamics of normal pregnancy as well as associated obstetric problems are largely responsible. The uterus is enlarged and highly vascular. The associated collateral circulation results in prominence of vessels that would be of little concern in the nonpregnant state. It is for this reason that some surgeons use a three-clamp rather than a two-clamp technique for pedicle development above the cardinal ligaments. In the case of the three-clamp technique the incision is made between a single medial clamp (to reduce the likelihood of retrograde blood loss from the medial pedicle) and two lateral clamps (to prevent clamp slippage from the lateral pedicle).

Planned Hysterectomy Considerations

Should the hysterectomy be a planned one, the cesarean procedure is performed in the usual manner except that the initial peritoneal/vesicle uterine fold incision may be extended more laterally to the round ligaments. There is also advantage to early mobilization and separation of the bladder from the underlying lower segment in the midline with gentle blunt dissection to a point approximately 1 to 2 cm below the cervical vaginal junction and to some extent laterally. On occasion, the bladder may be adherent, requiring sharp dissection with down-turned scissors. This will result in displacement of the bladder and ureters caudad or inferiorly. There is also some advantage in use of a low vertical incision, particularly if the lower segment is not completely developed, to reduce the possibility of extension into the broad ligament and provide a site for placement of the surgeon's finger in the apex of the incision to facilitate later traction and manipulation of the uterus.

Procedure

Upon completion of the cesarean delivery, the placenta may be delivered and the lower uterine incision quickly reapproximated, or alternatively the surgeon may simply proceed rapidly to gain control of the vascular supply of the uterus while the placenta spontaneously separates. Polyglycolic acid or chromic catgut suture (0 or 1 gauge) may be used throughout the procedure.

Placement of an O'Conner-O'Sullivan retractor or perhaps a large Balfour retractor in the abdominal wall may be helpful, particularly should the patient be obese or exposure difficult. The uterine fundus is then delivered through the incision, and constant traction is maintained on the uterus to maximize pedicle exposure, facilitate development of tissue planes, and stretch the uterine veins, thereby narrowing their lumen and reducing venous blood loss. If a vertical uterine incision has been made, it is often convenient for the assistant to hook an index finger in the upper extreme of the uterine incision to manipulate the fundus and to expose the operative site. If the placenta is still in place, it can be removed. If bleeding of the uterine incision is excessive, further bleeding can be controlled by a variety of techniques, including use of oxytocin, ligation of individual bleeders, or even closure of the uterine incision. In many instances, however, it is possible to complete the isolation of the uterine pedicles in a time period that approximates that required to close the uterine incision.

If the bladder has not been previously mobilized, this can be done with blunt and sharp dissection. Once the bladder separation is completed, the round ligaments (Fig. 18–12) are then clamped with Heaney or Kocher clamps, cut, and ligated with transfixing sutures. If not done earlier, the previously made vesicouterine peritoneum incision is extended laterally and cephalad across the anterior leaf of the broad ligament through the point of the previously incised round ligaments.

The ovaries should be inspected; it is seldom necessary to remove them. If the ovaries are normal, placement of the utero-ovarian clamps and a free tie at the intended site is facilitated by perforation of the avascular portion of the posterior leaf of the broad ligament adjacent to the uterus just inferior to the fallopian tube, utero-ovarian ligaments, and ovarian vessels with a curved Kelly clamp. The intent is to provide enough room to insert two or three clamps, either atraumatic (e.g., Masterston) or crushing (e.g., Heaney), across the utero-ovarian ligament and fallopian tube between the previously placed utero-ovarian free tie and the uterus. The utero-ovarian ligament and tube may then be ligated with clamps or free tie. An attempt should be made to avoid placement of the clamps or ligature across ovarian tissue, which may result in immediate or delayed bleeding. If the intent is to place three Kocher/Ochsner or Heaney/Masterson clamps on the utero-ovarian ligament and fallopian tube, sequential placement of clamps should move in the direction of the dorsum of the surgeon's dominant hand so as to avoid placement of the surgeon's hand between clamps. If the three-clamp technique is used, the pedicle is incised between the single medial clamp and the two lateral clamps.

If a lateral free tie is used, the utero-ovarian/adnexal pedicle is then doubly clamped medial to the free tie. The pedicle is incised between the clamps and the lateral pedicle and ligated with a transfixing suture (Fig. 18–12B). Some surgeons also ligate the opposing medial pedicle so as to remove the most medial clamp from the operative field, while avoiding back-bleeding.

Some surgeons then incise the avascular portion of the broad ligaments and skeletonize the large uterine veins. This is more difficult in a cesarean hysterectomy than in a simple abdominal hysterectomy. The ascending uterine vessels adjacent to the uterus near their origin are then identified near the junction of the cervix and uterus and doubly or triply clamped with Heaney or Masterson clamps, incised, and ligated, either singularly or doubly. The surgeon should attempt to place the clamp tip snuggly against the uterine margin at a right angle to the ascending uterine vessels to reduce the likelihood of back-bleeding. Placement of the clamp tip on this vascular pedicle against the lower segment is easy should the cervix be long and uneffaced. However, if the lower segment is well developed, soft, and without distinct margins, palpation of the lateral margin of the lower uterine segment (between thumb and forefinger straddling the intended broad ligament pedicle) may be required to facilitate closer approximation of the clamp tip to the uterine margin. Prior to placement of the clamps on the uterine vessel, it is often useful to confirm that the bladder is displaced inferiorly and, should ureteral location be an issue, the ureter can occasionally be palpated between the forefinger and thumb.

The incision of the uterine vessel pedicle should occur in such a manner as to leave a small portion of tissue medial to the clamp to diminish the likelihood of clamp or later suture slippage. Before incising the uterine pedicle there may be advantage to placement of a medial Heaney or Ochsner/Kocher clamp on the uterine vessels above the intended site of incision of the vascular pedicle. Others prefer isolation of the uterine vessels

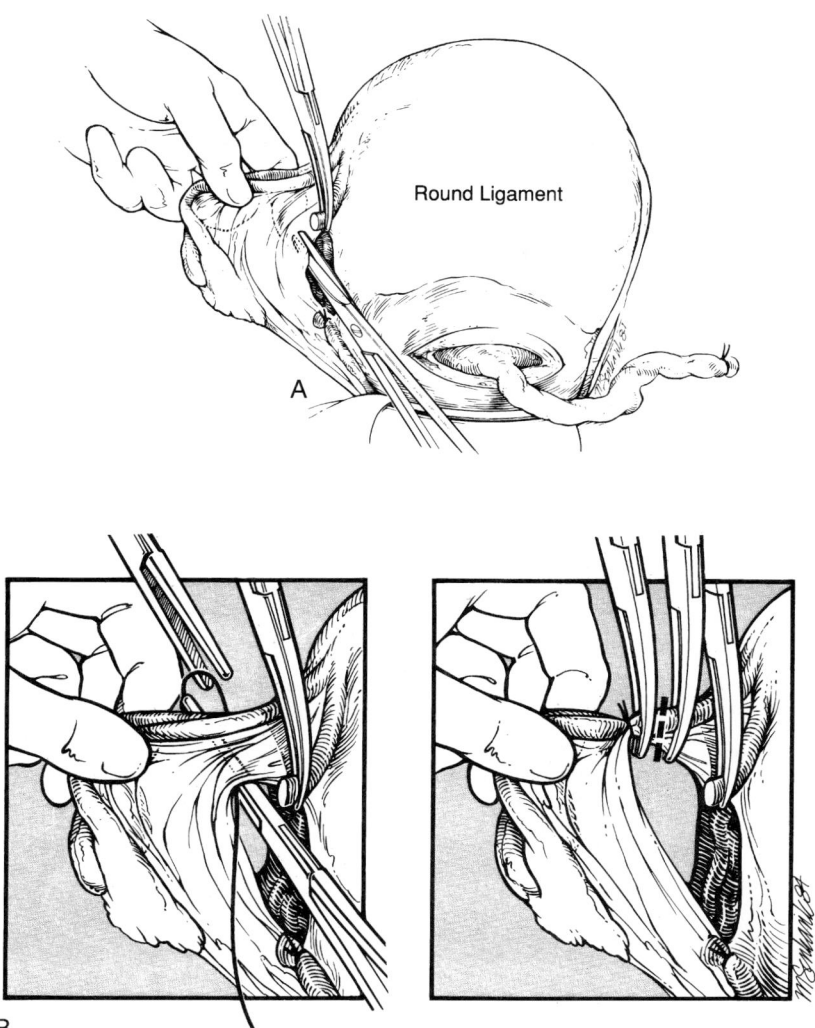

Figure 18–12. Cesarean hysterectomy. *A,* After extending the bladder flap, each round ligament is cut and ligated. The posterior leaf of the broad ligament can be opened for a short distance, taking care to incise only the surface layer. The avascular space beneath the utero-ovarian ligament may be opened by blunt finger dissection to isolate the adnexal pedicle. *B,* (left) A free tie is passed through the avascular space and firmly tied. The advantage of this tie is to secure the vessels within the pedicle before it is cut. (right) The adnexal pedicle is doubly clamped and cut. In addition, a transfixing suture will then be placed around the pedicle.

bilaterally prior to incising either pedicle as a technique to avoid back-bleeding. A variation of the two-clamp technique is presented in Figure 18–13.

Subtotal Hysterectomy

Supracervical/subtotal hysterectomy may be a consideration at this point either as a transitional step to remove the fundus and provide better visualization of the lower pelvis or as a permanent strategy (i.e., should the patient be unstable or dissection unusually difficult). The obstetrician should usually plan to perform a total hysterectomy. However, should the patient be unstable or the procedure unusually difficult, a subtotal hysterectomy may occasionally be desirable because it is sim-

pler, particularly should the pathology be confined to the upper uterine segment and the surgeon judge that prolongation of the procedure associated with removal of the cervix will adversely affect the patient.

Once the ascending uterine artery and vein are doubly clamped and the pedicles cut and ligated as in a total hysterectomy, the cervix is amputated at the level of the pedicles. In amputating the cervix it may be useful to cone the amputation downward toward the canal (Fig. 18–14A). The resultant cervical stump can be closed with several interrupted figure-of-eight sutures. Some surgeons doubly suture ligate the ascending uterine vessels by the angles of the cervix (Fig. 18–14B) to minimize the risk of angle bleeding. Additional bleeding points are ligated and reperitonealization per-

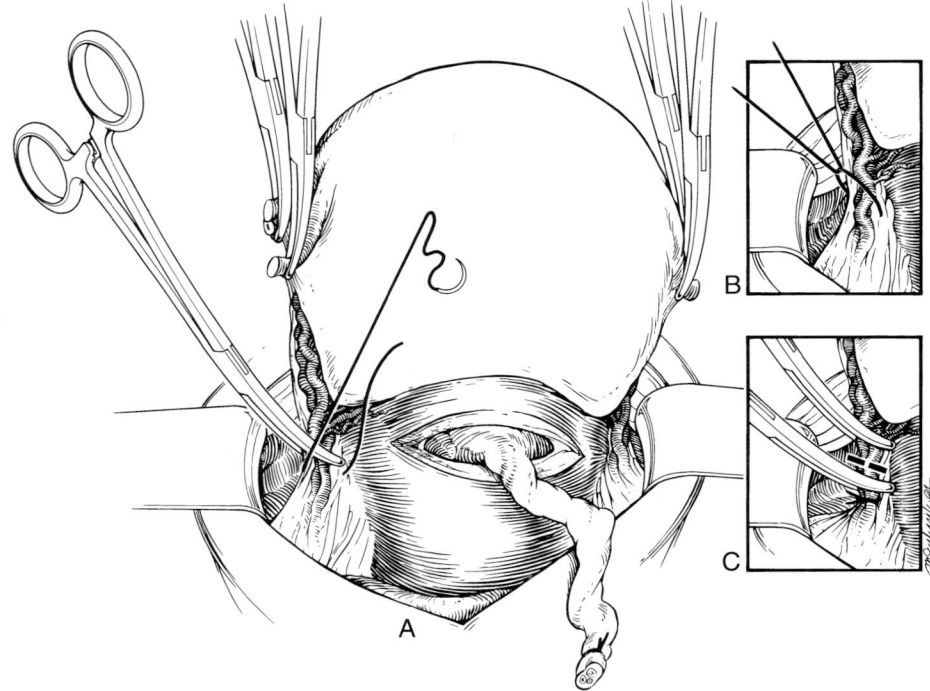

Figure 18–13. *A,* The ascending branches of the uterine artery are clamped, cut, and a suture is placed just below the tip of the clamp and immediately next to the uterine wall. *B,* After removing the clamp, the suture is tied, thus securing the vessels before they are cut. *C,* The pedicle is regrasped just above the tie and then doubly ligated.

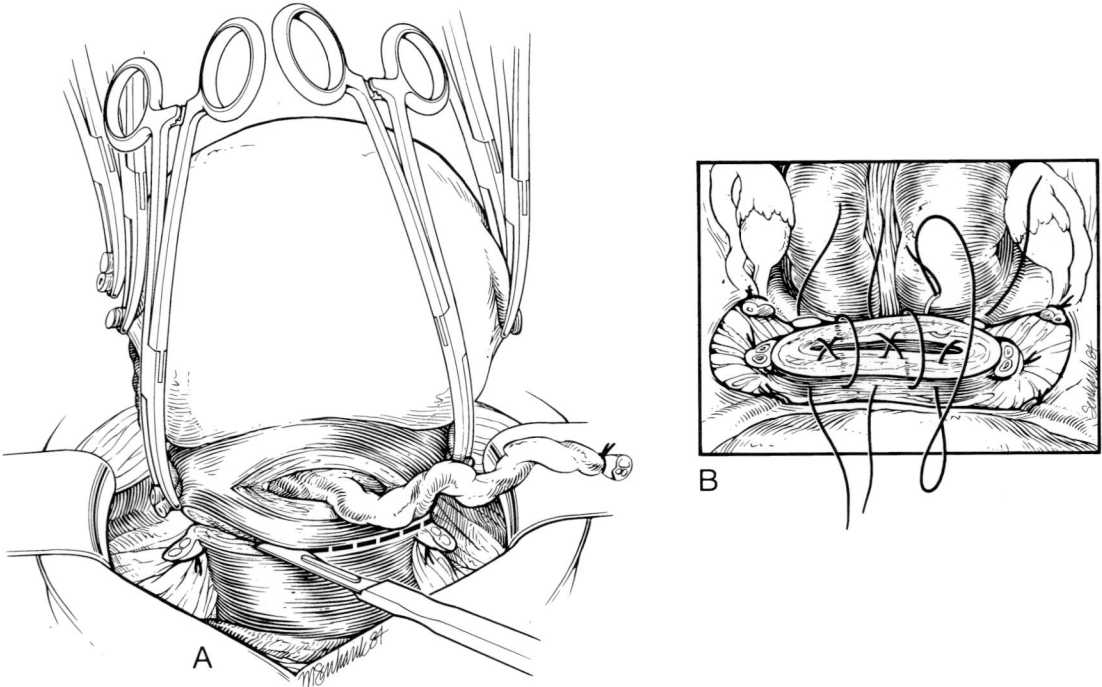

Figure 18–14. Subtotal hysterectomy. *A,* The cervix is incised just below the level of the ligated pedicles of the uterine arteries, amputating the uterine corpus from its cervical stump. *B,* The cervical stump may be closed with several interrupted figure-of-eight sutures; reperitonealization is then accomplished as in a total hysterectomy.

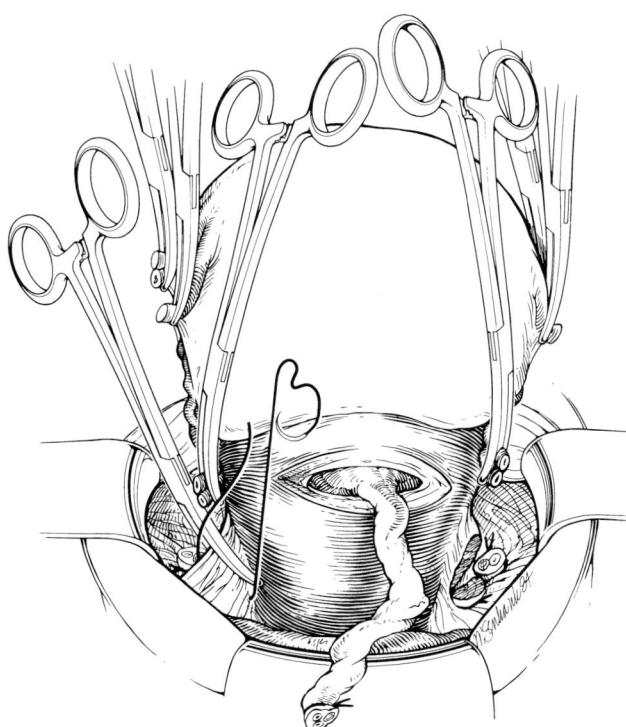

Figure 18–15. The cardinal ligaments are clamped at their point of insertion, cut, and singly ligated. Because these structures are hypertrophied, several bites may be necessary. Some physicians clamp, cut, and ligate the uterosacral ligaments separately.

formed in a fashion similar to that required for total hysterectomy.

Total Hysterectomy

Should the patient be stable after removal of the fundus, two or more Ochsner/Kocher clamps may be placed on the remaining cervical stump to control bleeding and provide traction for later manipulation while completing the hysterectomy. After the ascending uterine vessels have been ligated, the cervix is separated from the supporting cardinal and uterosacral ligaments and vagina. Pedicles containing descending branches of the uterine vessels and the cardinal and uterosacral ligaments are clamped (doubly or singularly) with either Heaney-type curved clamps or Ochsner/Kocher-type straight clamps, attempting to place the clamps as close to the cervix as possible. Approximately 1.0 to 1.5 cm of cardinal pedicle tissue should be encompassed within the instrument with each "bite." Placement of the Heaney or Kocher straight clamps should be done in such a manner that the progressively closing jaws of the clamp slide off the firm body of the cervix to decrease the likelihood of inclusion of the adjacent ureters. Should the lower segment be well developed and thinned out, delineation of the margin can be accomplished by palpating the tissues between forefinger and thumb. The

resultant wedge-shaped pedicle is then incised and sutured. Inclusion of a portion of the adjacent more superior uterine pedicle in the tie may reduce bleeding between the two pedicles.

Should the lower uterine segment be well developed, it is often necessary to develop more than one pedicle for each cardinal ligament. Successive clamps are placed medial to the preceding clamp, with care to avoid the possibility of unsecured tissue between successive bites. After reconfirming that the bladder reflection is retracted away from the site of intended clamp placement, successive more inferior pedicles are clamped, incised, and suture ligated until the surgeon is confident that the supporting cardinal and uterosacral ligaments have been separated and the level of the lateral vaginal fornix is reached (Fig. 18–15). Although some surgeons attempt to identify and ligate the uterosacral ligaments individually, the uterosacral ligaments are generally not as distinct at this time as would be the case in the nonpregnant state. In most cases they are included in the cardinal ligament pedicles.

The vagina may be entered anteriorly (or posteriorly) in the midline with the scalpel or alternatively following placement of a curved Heaney clamp just below the inferior margin of the cervix at the lateral angle. Separation of the cervix from its vaginal attachments can be quite difficult should the lower uterine segment be thinned out and long as a result of effacement. One should avoid both incomplete removal of the cervix and excessive removal of the upper vagina. In some instances it is possible to palpate and milk superiorly the lower margin of the cervix by palpating the approximate site with thumb and forefinger placed anteriorly and posteriorly about the cervicovaginal junction. Should identification of the cervicovaginal junction not be possible by external palpation, there are several alternatives. The surgeon may insert an index finger through a vertical incision in the anterior lower uterine segment/cervical canal into the upper vagina to locate the cervical vaginal margin (Fig. 18–16). Should the index-finger method to locate the lower margin of the cervix be used, the circulating nurse may reglove the surgeon. After the vagina is entered, the vagina and cervix are circumferentially separated under direct visualization with large curved Mayo scissors, attempting to maintain the full length of the vagina. Once the cervix is freed from the vagina, the specimen is then inspected to ensure that the cervix has been completely excised. The two angles of the resultant vaginal cuff are identified and clamped with Kocher/Heaney clamps (Fig. 18–17). The vaginal angle containing the vaginal artery can then be secured by a variety of techniques.

The apex of the vaginal cuff is then supported by approximating the vaginal angles to the cardinal ligament pedicle and the uterosacral ligament if previously incised separately. Some incorporate the vaginal angle

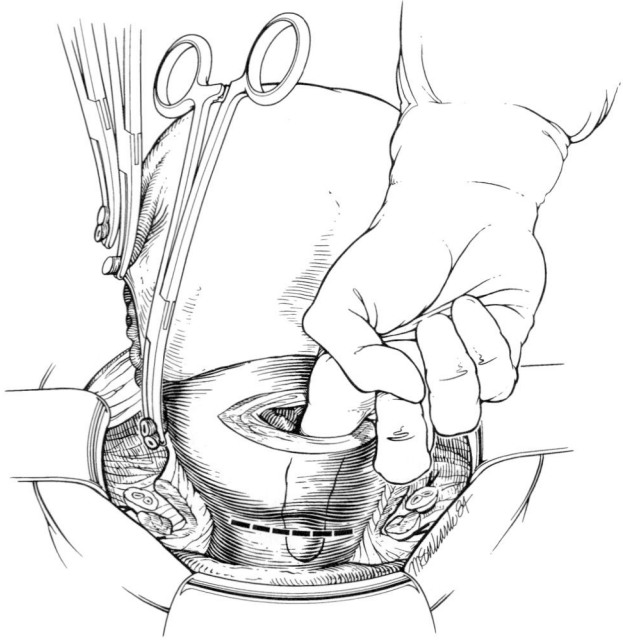

Figure 18–16. Because the cervix is elongated, it may be useful to insert an index finger through the cervical canal to demarcate the vaginal incision and to ensure complete removal of the cervix and avoid unnecessary removal of vaginal length.

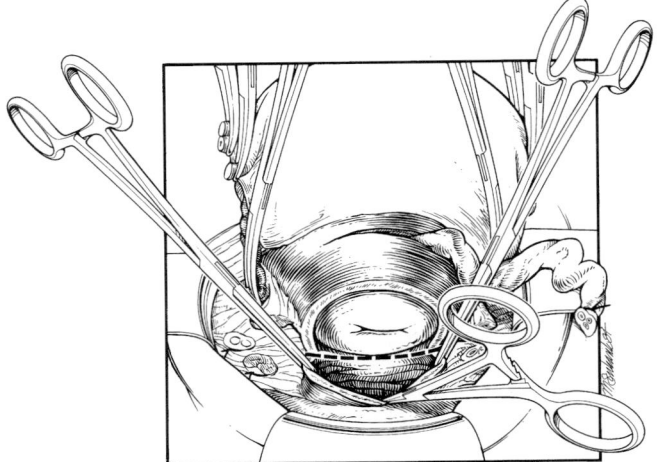

Figure 18–17. The vagina is circumferentially incised at its cervical attachment and grasped with four clamps.

to the cardinal and uterosacral ligaments via a lock loop suture (Fig. 18–18). The vaginal cuff may be left open or closed. The decision to leave the vaginal cuff open in most instances will depend on the presence of adequate hemostasis and absence of obvious infection. The open cuff will allow excess blood or serous material to drain from the lower pelvis. The vaginal cuff may be closed in either one or two layers, particularly if the pelvis is dry and there are no major additional risks for cuff infection, using either interrupted figure-of-eight sutures or a continuous closure (Fig. 18–19).

Alternatively, the cuff can be left open by running a locking circumferential suture about the cuff margins to minimize vaginal cuff bleeding and facilitate drainage; some prefer figure-of-eight sutures.

The cul-de-sac and peritoneal gutters are suctioned of blood and accumulated debris and all previous pedicles examined for bleeding points. Bleeding sites should be individually controlled by picking up as little tissue as possible to avoid ligation or kinking of the ureters. Once the surgeon is assured that hemostasis is adequate and that there have been no lacerations of the bladder, the pelvis may be irrigated.

Should the surgeon decide to reperitonealize the pelvic floor (Fig. 18–20), this can be accomplished in several ways using a continuous suture. The end result is inversion of the pedicle of the ligated fallopian tube and ovarian ligament and round ligament retroperito-

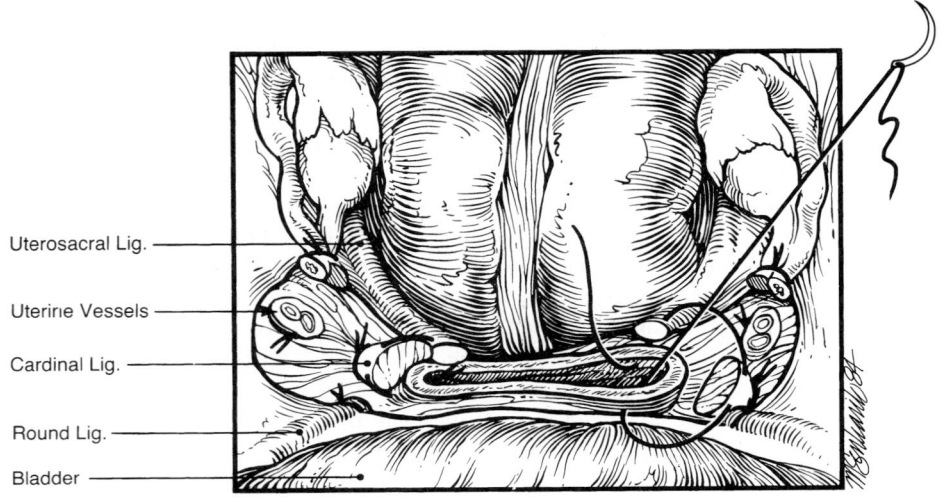

Uterosacral Lig.

Uterine Vessels

Cardinal Lig.

Round Lig.

Bladder

Figure 18–18. The angles of the vaginal cuff are closed with sutures to include the cardinal and uterosacral ligaments, thus providing fascial support to the vaginal vault. A simple loop suture is commonly used at this location to reduce the likelihood of breakage during the stage of postoperative edema.

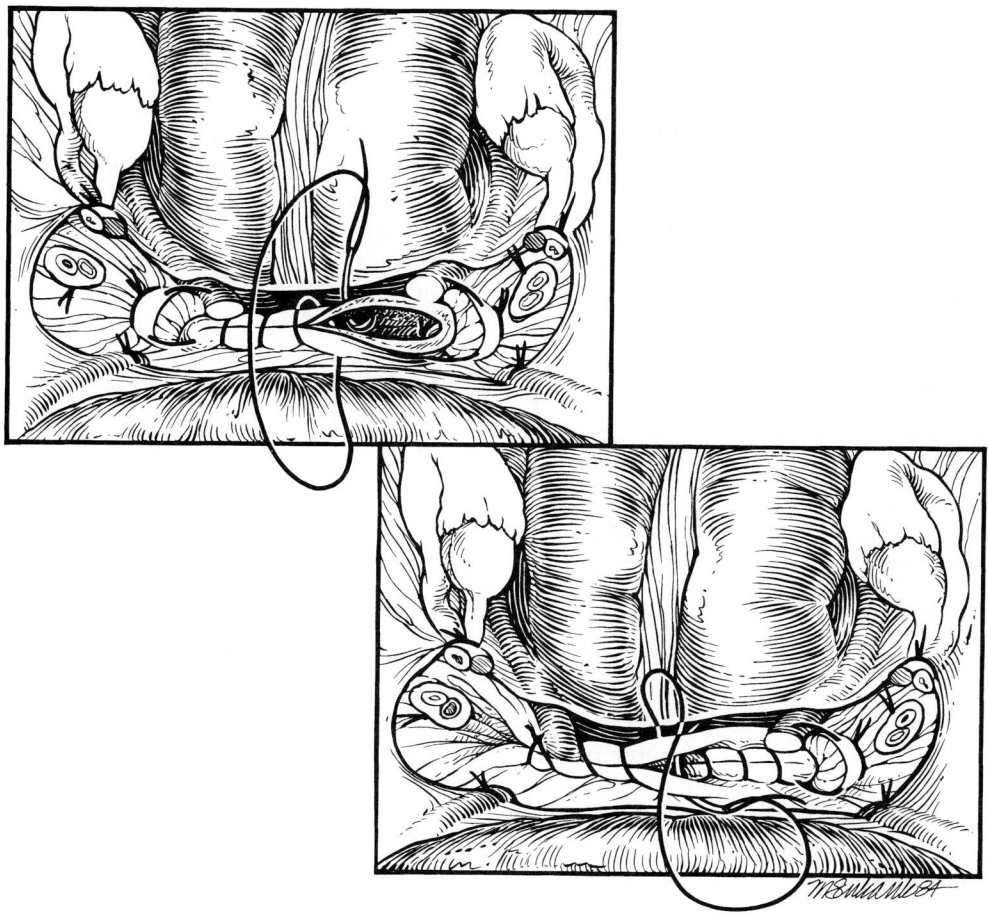

Figure 18–19. There are a number of methods of closing the vaginal cuff. Illustrated is a two-layer closure. The first layer closes the vagina, and the second layer closes the endopelvic fascia. Many operators prefer to leave the cuff "open" by using one continuous suture that circles the cuff, approximating the cut edge to its surrounding fascia.

neally, avoiding fixation of the ovary to the cuff in the cul-de-sac. A continuous suture reapproximates the medial and lateral leaves of the broad ligament, burying the round ligament stump and approximating the anterior vesicouterine peritoneum over the vaginal vault to the cul-de-sac peritoneum on the posterior margin of the vagina. The procedure is then conducted in reverse order on the opposing side. Some accomplish the dual goals of reperitonealization and support of the apex of the vaginal vault by successive placement of the suture on the anterior vaginal wall to the cardinal ligament to the round ligament pedicle and back to the uterosacral ligaments/posterior vaginal wall, which is then drawn down to the cuff. Many surgeons have discontinued the process of reperitonealizing the pelvic floor and simply allow the sigmoid and bladder to fall into place over the vaginal cuff, an approach that may also minimize the admittedly small chance of suturing the ureter during reperitonealization. The surgeon may avoid attachment of the ovarian pedicles to the angle of the vagina

by suturing the ovarian pedicle to the ipsilateral round ligament.

Intraoperative Complications

Intraoperative complications associated with peripartum hysterectomy, although similar to those following nonobstetric total abdominal hysterectomy, occur with greater frequency, especially in unplanned procedures. Total hysterectomy may add 30 to 60 minutes to the operating and anesthesia times (Tables 18–23 and 18–24), depending on (1) the surgeon's experience, (2) whether the procedure is emergent or elective, (3) the degree of development of the lower uterine segment, (4) coincidental pelvic pathology such as leiomyomata or obesity, and (5) the presence of ureteral or bladder laceration.

Increased blood loss and occasional injury to either bladder or ureters are the two most commonly encountered intraoperative complications.[289] There is an asso-

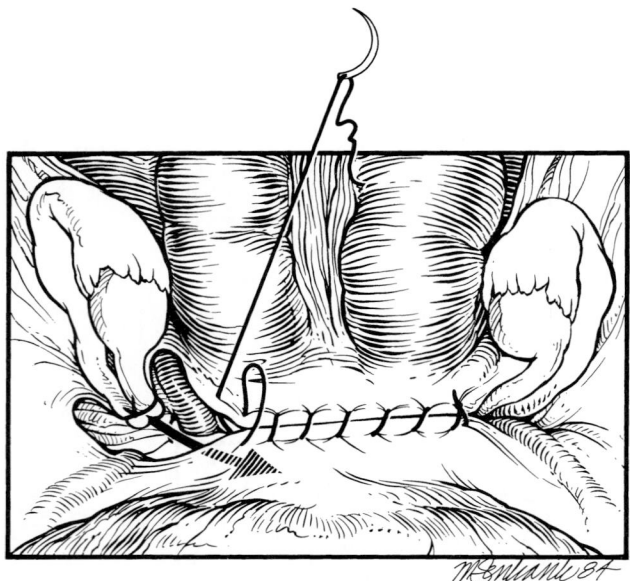

Figure 18–20. The bladder flap is closed with a continuous suture that inverts the pedicles of the round ligaments and adnexae. Note that these structures have not been attached to the vaginal cuff.

ciated additional blood loss of 500 to 1,000 ml, depending on preexisting blood loss and whether the procedure is planned or unplanned. In emergency procedures, a major portion of the blood loss can be attributed to the indication for the procedure. This is particularly true for uterine atony that has been unresponsive to more conservative obstetric interventions, including prostaglandin $F_{2\alpha}$. Intraoperative blood loss may be secondary to slippage of a clamp off a pedicle or bleeding between pedicles and may be a function of the type of clamp and/or suture placement. It may involve the utero-ovarian or the uterine pedicles, or there may be bleeding at the angle of the vagina and cardinal ligament. On occasion, the adnexal bleeding is the result of suture placement through an ovarian vessel. This can often be avoided by the placement of a free-tie suture at the site of the most lateral of two or three clamps and subsequent placement of a transfixing suture at the site of the more medial (middle) clamp of the lateral pedicle. On occasion it may be necessary to perform a salpingo-oophorectomy to control hematoma formation. In a recent series from Harvard, 17 percent of 117 women who underwent emergency hysterectomy required removal of their adnexa.[275]

Injuries to the bladder and ureter are most common during unplanned/emergency procedures. Most bladder injuries are easily recognized and repaired, since they most often occur when dissecting the bladder from the lower uterine segment, particularly in patients with multiple prior cesarean births. The bladder is infrequently included in the lateral margin of the vaginal cuff at the time of the separation of the cardinal liga-

ments. Rarely, spontaneous laceration of the bladder may occur coincident with uterine rupture.

Cystotomy as a complication of cesarean hysterectomy occurred in approximately 4 to 5 percent of procedures in early series.[120,121] Bladder injury can be minimized at two points—first, by separation and downward displacement of the bladder from the anterior vaginal wall prior to the cesarean delivery while the anterior vaginal wall is still taut; and second, by rolling the Oschner/Kocher clamps off the cervix when developing the cardinal pedicles.

The incidence of ureteral injury during cesarean delivery is reported to be approximately 1 in 1,000 cesarean deliveries.[119] The risk of ureteral injury is increased even further with cesarean hysterectomy, with rates of 0.2 to 0.5 percent being observed in early series including planned procedures.[120,121] In more recent series typically involving emergency unplanned hysterectomies (Table 18–23), most urinary tract injuries involve the bladder, although on occasion the ureter may be incised or incorporated within a pedicle. Stanco et al.,[274] in a 5-year review of 123 (1.3 per 1,000 births) emergency peripartum hysterectomies, found a 3.2 percent incidence of urinary tract injury; in addition, they performed 12 (10 percent) intentional cystotomies to facilitate passage of a ureteral stent. Zelop et al.,[275] in an 8-year review of 117 (1.55 per 1,000 births) emergency peripartum hysterectomies, found that 10 (8.5 percent) patients sustained urologic injuries. Of these, there were nine (7.7 percent) cystotomies and three (2.5 percent) ureteral injuries that required stenting.

Injury to the ureter is more common in cases where there is a necessity to control a broad ligament bleeding or hematoma formation or to dissect a pelvic tumor. In the case of pelvic tumors, careful dissection of the mass, palpation of the lateral cervical margins, and careful placement of the clamps as close to the cervical margin as possible with successive bites more medial to the preceding pedicle will make inclusion of the ureter highly unlikely. Should the surgeon be concerned about the possibility of a ureteral injury, intentional cystotomy in the bladder dome and placement of retrograde ureteral catheters may be used to assess the patency and integrity of the ureter.

Postoperative Complications

As is the case in any hysterectomy, infection and bleeding are the most common major postoperative complications. The incidence of infectious complications is closely linked to the presence of preexisting risk factors for infection and whether the procedure is planned or unplanned. The incidence of urinary tract infection in the absence of preexisting amnionitis is strongly linked to the duration of indwelling catheter placement. Scheduled procedures performed before labor have an associated incidence of febrile morbidity less than 10 percent; most cases involve the urinary tract, with an occasional wound or vaginal cuff infection. In contrast, febrile morbidity rates approach 30 percent for unplanned procedures.[274,275,290] Postoperative infectious morbidity may be reduced by prophylactic antibiotics to women who have been either in labor or at risk for infection and early removal of indwelling catheters. Prophylactic antibiotics are generally administered intraoperatively, immediately following delivery of the fetus.

The pelvic tissues, if there has been hemorrhage or infection, are frequently quite friable and may tear easily. There may be later ligature slippage as tissue edema resolves. Vaginal bleeding is commonly associated with a bleeder at the lateral angle/junction of the vagina and cardinal ligament; it also may involve the uterine vessels. In some instances, bleeding will involve the formation of a broad ligament hematoma arising from the uterine or ovarian vessels. Should the hematoma be small, stable, and asymptomatic, such patients may require no further treatment. The surgeon may evaluate the patient serially using sonography; on occasion, it may be necessary to use CT scan or magnetic resonance imaging.

Reexploration for bleeding following a peripartum hysterectomy has been reported to be necessary in as many as 2.6 to 4 percent of cases.[274,275] Reexploration may be indicated should the hematoma progressively enlarge. Alternatively, it may be necessary if the patient remains unstable or demonstrates a progressive unanticipated fall in serial hematocrit determinations, after taking into account preoperative and intraoperative blood loss and replacement. Evacuation of the pelvic hematoma and identification and ligation of bleeders are the surgical goals; in some cases it may not be possible to isolate a definite bleeder. On occasion, it may be necessary to place cervical drains postoperatively.

ELECTIVE MYOMECTOMY AND APPENDECTOMY

The propriety of performing an elective myomectomy or appendectomy during a cesarean delivery is a matter of dispute. The majority opinion is that, with the possible exception of a subserosal myoma on a thin pedicle, myomectomy is contraindicated because achieving hemostasis may be difficult. Others assert that hemostasis will be excellent because of the action of the contracting uterus. A better argument for abstention is the knowledge that most myomas will involute to an insignificant size during the puerperium. Although the risk

of elective appendectomy is quite low, there are no statistics to prove that the benefits to be gained are greater than the possible surgical complications.

COINCIDENTAL OVARIAN NEOPLASMS AT CESAREAN DELIVERY

Should an ovarian neoplasm be discovered at the time of cesarean delivery, the surgeon should first rule out the possibility of a theca-lutein cyst or the rare luteoma of pregnancy. Other ovarian neoplasms should be excised, sparing the ovary whenever possible.

Key Points

➤ Even when morbidity and mortality arising from the indications leading to cesarean delivery are excluded, maternal morbidity and mortality remain many times higher for cesarean delivery than for vaginal delivery.

➤ As the percentage of laboring patients presenting with prior cesarean births has increased, there have been associated increases in more difficult repeat cesarean deliveries and complications, including a higher incidence of placenta previa, placenta accreta, symptomatic uterine rupture, hemorrhage, requirement for transfusion, and need for unplanned hysterectomy.

➤ The reported incidence of maternal mortality following cesarean delivery is estimated to range from 6.1 to 22 per 100,000 live births. Approximately one third to one half of maternal deaths can be attributed directly to the cesarean procedure itself.

➤ There are no well-documented prospective trials demonstrating benefit to the fetus or to the mother that would justify the extent of the increase in the primary cesarean delivery rate over the past two decades. Although perinatal mortality rates have decreased as cesarean birth rates have increased, the improvement is largely attributable to major advances in prenatal and intrapartum care, as well as dramatic improvements in neonatal intensive care implemented in the same time frame.

➤ If the patient is massively obese, it may be better to use an incision directly over the lower uterine segment that does not involve the underside of the panniculus, an area that is more heavily colonized with bacteria and that is difficult to prepare surgically, to keep dry, and to inspect in the postoperative period.

➤ The physician contemplating a cesarean delivery for placenta previa, particularly a repeat procedure, should consider the possibility of hysterectomy. The reported incidence of placenta accreta (1 in 2,500 deliveries) increases to approximately 4 percent in patients with a placenta previa and may approach 25 percent in patients with a prior cesarean birth.

➤ Although cesarean delivery is often elected to minimize trauma to the preterm breech fetus, the actual delivery mechanism via the cesarean incision is essentially identical to that of the vaginal route. Should head entrapment be encountered, the first action should be to extend the abdominal incision and to enlarge the uterine incision.

➤ Elective repeat cesarean delivery is estimated to be responsible for a significant proportion of the increase in the cesarean birth rate during the past two decades. VBAC-TOL lowers the self-perpetuating contribution of the indication of previous cesarean birth.

➤ Most patients with a prior cesarean birth are candidates for VBAC. The only established contraindication is a prior classical incision. VBAC reduces the incidence of postpartum infection, the need for postpartum transfusion, maternal length of stay and, as a result, offers the potential to generate significant cost savings.

➤ VBAC trial candidates are no more likely to require a cesarean delivery than a population of women with no prior cesarean deliveries. VBAC trial of labor is successful in 60 to 80 percent of acceptable candidates.

REFERENCES

1. Curtin SC, Park MM: Trends in the attendant, place, and timing of births, and in the use of obstetric interventions: United States, 1989–1997. National Vital Health Statistics Reports. Vol 47, No 27. Hyattsville, MD, National Center for Health Statistics, 1999.
2. National Center for Health Statistics: Rates of cesarean delivery—United States, 1993. MMWR Morb Mortal Wkly Rep 44:303, 1995.
3. American College of Obstetricians and Gynecologists: ACOG Practice Bulletin: Vaginal Birth after Previous Cesarean Delivery. No 5. Washington, DC, ACOG, 1999.
4. Shiono PA, McNellis D, Rhoads GS: Reasons for the rising cesarean delivery rates 1978–1984. Obstet Gynecol 69:696, 1987.
5. Phelan JP, Clark SL, Diaz F, et al: Vaginal birth after cesarean. Am J Obstet Gynecol 157:1510, 1987.
6. Petitti DB: Maternal mortality and morbidity in cesarean section. Clin Obstet Gynecol 28:763, 1985.
7. Horley JMG: Cesarean section. Clin Obstet Gynecol 7:529, 1980.
8. Sewell JE: Cesarean Section—A Brief History. Washington, DC, American College of Obstetricians and Gynecologists, 1993.
9. Porro E: Della Amputazione Utero-ovarica. Milan, 1876.
10. Harris RP: The results of the first fifty cases of cesarean ovarohysterectomy 1869–1880. Am J Med Sci 80:129, 1880.
11. Sänger M: Speaking before the German Gynecology Association 1885. Am J Obstet Dis Women Child 19:883, 1886.
12. Sänger M: My work in reference to the cesarean operation. Am J Obstet Dis Women Child 20:593, 1887.
13. Eastman NJ: The role of Frontier America in the development of cesarean section. Am J Obstet Gynecol 24:919, 1932.
14. Frank F: Suprasymphysial delivery and its relation to other operations in the presence of contracted pelvis. Arch Gynaekol 81:46, 1907.
15. Latzko W: Ueber den extraperitonealen Kaiserschnitt. Zentralbl Gynaekol 33:275, 1909.
16. Krönig B: Transperitonealer Cervikaler Kaiser-Schnitt. *In* Doderlein A, Kronig B (eds): Operative Gynakologie. Stuttgart, F Enke, 1912, p 879.
17. Beck AC: Observations on a series of cesarean sections done at the Long Island College Hospital during the past six years. Am J Obstet Gynecol 79:197, 1919.
18. DeLee JB, Cornell EL: Low cervical cesarean section laparotracheotomy. JAMA 79:109, 1922.
19. Kerr JMM: The technique of cesarean section with special reference to the lower uterine segment incision. Am J Obstet Gynecol 12:729, 1926.
20. DeLee JB: Principles and Practice of Obstetrics. 6th ed. Philadelphia, WB Saunders Company, 1933.
21. Taffel SM, Placek PJ, Liss T: Trends in the United States cesarean section rate for the 1980–1985 rise. Am J Public Health 77:955, 1987.
22. Notzon FC, Placek PJ, Taffel SM: Comparisons of national cesarean-section rates. N Engl J Med 316:386, 1987.
23. Notzon FC: International differences in the use of obstetric interventions. JAMA 264:3286, 1990.
24. Al-Mufti R, McCarthy A, Fisk NM: Obstetricians personal choice and mode of delivery. Lancet 347:544, 1996.
25. Cesarean Childbirth: Report of a Consensus Development Conference Sponsored by the National Institute of Child Health and Human Development. DHHS Publ No 82-2067. Washington, DC, U.S. Government Printing Office, October 1981.
26. Taffel SM, Placek PJ, Moien M, Kosary CL: 1989 US cesarean section rate steadies-VBAC rises to nearly one in five. Birth 18:73, 1991.
27. Quilligan EJ: Making inroads against the C-section rate. Contemp Obstet Gynecol Jan:221, 1983.
28. American College of Obstetricians and Gynecologists: ACOG Executive Summary: Evaluation of Cesarean Delivery. Washington, DC, ACOG, 2000.
29. U.S. Department of Health and Human Services: Healthy Children 2000, DHHS Publ No HRSA-M-CH 91-2. Washington, DC, U.S. Government Printing Office, 2000.
30. Placek PJ, Taffel SM, Keppel KG: Maternal and infant char-

acteristics associated with cesarean section delivery. Department of Health and Human Services. Publ No PHS 84-1232. Hyattsville, MD, National Center for Health Statistics, December 1983.

31. Freeman JM, Nelson KB: Intrapartum asphyxia and cerebral palsy. Pediatrics 82:240, 1988.

32. Freeman R: Intrapartum fetal monitoring—a disappointing story. N Engl J Med 322:624, 1990.

33. Shy KK, Luthy DA, Bennett FC, et al: Effects of electronic fetal heart rate monitoring, as compared with periodic auscultation, on the neurologic development of premature infants. N Engl J Med 322:588, 1990.

34. American College of Obstetricians and Gynecologists, Committee on Obstetrics: Fetal and neonatal neurologic injury. Technical Bulletin No 163. Washington, DC, ACOG, 1992.

35. Green JE, McLean F, Smith LP, et al: Has an increased cesarean section rate for term breech delivery reduced the incidence of birth asphyxia, trauma and death? Am J Obstet Gynecol 142:643, 1982.

36. Hannah ME, Hannah WJ, Hewson SA, et al, and the Term Breech Trial Collaborative Group: Planned cesarean section versus planned vaginal birth for breech presentation at term: a randomised multicentre trial. Lancet 356:1375, 2000.

37. Haynes de Regt RH, Minkoff HL, Feldman J, Schwarz RH: Relation of private or clinic care to the cesarean birth rate. N Engl J Med 315:619, 1986.

38. NIH consensus development statement on cesarean childbirth. The Cesarean Birth Task Force. Obstet Gynecol 57:537, 1981.

39. Savage W, Francome C: British CS rates: have we reached a plateau? Br J Obstet Gynaecol 100:493, 1993.

40. Feldman GB, Freiman JA: Prophylactic cesarean section at term? N Engl J Med 312:1264, 1985.

41. Sachs BP, Kobelin C, Castro MA, Frigoletto F: The risks of lowering the cesarean delivery rate. N Engl J Med 340:54, 1999.

42. Blumenthal NJ, Harris RS, O'Connor MC, et al: Changing caesarean section rates experience at a Sydney obstetric teaching hospital. Aust N Z J Obstet Gynaecol 24:246, 1984.

43. Phillips RN, Thornton J, Gleicher N: Physician bias in cesarean sections. JAMA 248:1082, 1982.

44. Sanchez-Ramos L, Moorhead RI, Kaunitz AM: Cesarean section rates in teaching hospitals: a national survey. Birth 21:194, 1994.

45. Oleske DM, Glandon GL, Giacomelli GJ, Hohmann SF: The cesarean birth rate: influence of hospital teaching status. Health Serv Res 26:325, 1991.

46. Residency Review Committee for Obstetrics/Gynecology: Resident Obstetric Experience-Program Mean Comparison. Chicago, IL, Accreditation Council for Graduate Medical Education, 1999.

47. Sachs BP, Yeh J, Acker D, et al: Cesarean section-related maternal mortality in Massachusetts, 1954–1985. Obstet Gynecol 71:385, 1988.

48. O'Driscoll K, Foley M: Correlation of decrease in perinatal mortality and increase in cesarean section rate. Obstet Gynecol 61:1, 1983.

49. Leveno KJ, Cunningham FG, Pritchard JA: Cesarean section: an answer to the House of Horne. Am J Obstet Gynecol 153:838, 1985.

50. Leveno KJ, Cunningham FG, Prithchard JA: Cesarean section: the House of Horne revisited. Am J Obstet Gynecol 160:78, 1989.

51. O'Driscoll K, Foley M, MacDonald D, Stronge J: Cesarean section and perinatal outcome: response from the House of Horne. Am J Obstet Gynecol 158:449, 1988.

52. Porreco RP: High cesarean section rate: a new perspective. Obstet Gynecol 65:307, 1985.

53. Scheller J, Nelson K: Does cesarean delivery prevent cerebral palsy or other neurologic problems of childhood? Obstet Gynecol 83:624, 1994.

54. Nelson KB, Dambrosia JM, Ting TY, Grether JK: Uncertain value of electronic fetal monitoring in predicting cerebral palsy. N Engl J Med 334:613, 1996.

55. American College of Obstetricians and Gynecologists: Fetal Distress and Birth Asphyxia. Committee Opinion No 137. Washington, DC, ACOG, 1994.

56. How HY, Harris BJ, Pietrantoni M, et al: Is vaginal delivery preferable to elective cesarean delivery in fetuses with a known ventral wall defect? Am J Obstet Gynecol 182:1527, 2000.

57. Haddad H, Lundy LE: Changing indications for cesarean section: a 38 year experience at a community hospital. Obstet Gynecol 51:133, 1978.

58. NIH Consensus Development Task Force: Statement on Cesarean Childbirth. Am J Obstet Gynecol 139:902, 1981.

59. American Academy of Pediatrics, American College of Obstetricians and Gynecologists: Guidelines for Perinatal Care. 4th ed. Washington, DC, ACOG, 1997, p 112.

60. American College of Obstetricians and Gynecologists: Guidelines for Vaginal Delivery After a Previous Cesarean Birth. Committee Opinion No 64. Washington, DC, ACOG, 1988.

61. American College of Obstetricians and Gynecologists: Vaginal Delivery After a Previous Cesarean Birth. Committee Opinion No 143 [replaces No. 64, October 1988]. Washington, DC, ACOG, 1994.

62. Porter TF, Clark SL, Esplin MS, et al: Timing of delivery and neonatal outcome in patients with clinically overt uterine rupture during VBAC. Am J Obstet Gynecol 178:S31, 1998.

63. Porreco RP, Meier RP: Repeat cesarean—most unnecessary. Contemp Obstet Gynecol 21:55, 1984.

64. Hannah W: Final statement of the panel from the National Consensus Conference on Aspects of Cesarean Birth. Hamilton, Ontario, Canada, 1986.

65. Goodenough RD, Molnar JA, Burke JF: Surgical infections. In Hardy JD (ed): Hardy's Textbook of Surgery. Philadelphia, JB Lippincott, 1983, p 123.

66. Cruse PJE, Foord R: The epidemiology of wound infection. Surg Clin North Am 60:27, 1980.

67. Dineen P: An evaluation of the duration of the surgical scrub. Surg Gynecol Obstet 129:118, 1969.

68. Mead PB, Pories SE, Hall P, et al: Decreasing the incidence of surgical wound infections. Arch Surg 121:458, 1986.

69. Ritter MS, French MLV, Eitzen HE, Gioe TJ: The antimicrobial effectiveness of operative-site preparative agents. J Bone Joint Surg 62:826, 1980.

70. Brown TR, Ehrlich CE, Stehman FB, et al: A clinical evaluation of chlorhexidine gluconate spray as compared with iodophor scrub for preoperative skin preparation. Surg Gynecol Obstet 158:363, 1984.

71. Alexander JW, Aerni S, Plettner JP: Development of a safe and effective one-minute preoperative skin preparation. Arch Surg 120:1357, 1985.

72. Masterson BJ: Skin preparation. Clin Obstet Gynecol 31:736, 1988.

73. Larson E: Handwashing and skin physiologic and bacteriologic aspects. Infect Control 6:14, 1985.

74. Garner JS: CDC guidelines for the prevention and control of nosocomial infections: guideline for prevention of surgical wound infections, 1985. Am J Infect Control 14:71, 1986.

75. Price PB: The bacteriology of normal skin; a new quantitative test applied to a study of the bacterial flora and the disinfec-

tant action of mechanical cleansing. J Infect Dis 63:301, 1938.

76. Alexander JW, Fischer JE, Boyajian M, et al: The influence of hair-removal methods on wound infections. Arch Surg 118:347, 1983.

77. Holtz C: Adhesion induction by suture of varying tissue reactivity and caliber. Int J Fertil 27:134, 1982.

78. Kenady DE: Management of abdominal wounds. Surg Clin North Am 64:803, 1984.

79. Bucknall TE: Abdominal wound closure: choice of suture. J R Soc Med 74:580, 1981.

80. Ellis H, Coleridge-Smith PD, Joyce AD: Abdominal incisions—vertical or transverse? Postgrad Med J 60:407, 1984.

81. Greenall MJ, Evans M, Pollack AV: Mid-line or transverse laparotomy? A random controlled clinical trial. Br J Surg 67:188, 1980.

82. Becquemin J-P, Piquet J, Becquemin M-H, et al: Pulmonary function after transverse or midline incision in patients with obstructive pulmonary disease. Int Care Med 11:247, 1985.

83. Mowat J, Bonnar J: Abdominal wound dehiscence after cesarean section. BMJ 2:256, 1971.

84. Gallup DG: Modification of celiotomy techniques to decrease morbidity in the obese gynecologic patient. Am J Obstet Gynecol 150:171, 1984.

85. Finan MA, Mastrogiannis DS, Spellacy WN: The "Allis" test for easy cesarean delivery. Am J Obstet Gynecol 164:772, 1991.

86. Maylard AE: Direction of abdominal incisions. BMJ 2:895, 1907.

87. Cherney LS: A modified transverse incision for low abdominal operations. Surg Gynecol Obstet 72:92, 1941.

88. Pitkin RM: Abdominal hysterectomy in obese women. Surg Gynecol Obstet 142:532, 1976.

89. Shepherd JH, Cavanagh D, Riggs D, et al: Abdominal wound closures using a nonabsorbable single layer technique. Obstet Gynecol 61:248, 1983.

90. Naumann RW, Hauth JC, Owen J, et al: Subcutaneous tissue approximation in relation to wound disruption after cesarean delivery in obese women. Obstet Gynecol 85:412, 1995.

91. Read JA, Cotton DB, Miller FC: Placenta accreta: changing clinical aspects and outcome. Obstet Gynecol 56:31, 1980.

92. Clark SL, Koonings PP, Phelan JP: Placenta previa-accreta and previous cesarean section. Obstet Gynecol 66:89, 1985.

93. Tahilramaney MP, Boucher M, Eglinton GS, et al: Previous cesarean section and trial of labor. Factors related to uterine dehiscence. J Reprod Med 29:17, 1984.

94. Pritchard JA, McDonald PC, Gant NF (eds): Williams Obstetrics. 17th ed. Norwalk, CT, Appleton-Century-Crofts, 1985.

95. Pedowitz P, Schwartz RM: The true incidence of silent rupture of cesarean section scars: a prospective analysis of 403 cases. Am J Obstet Gynecol 74:1701, 1957.

96. Rodriguez AI, Porter KB, O'Brien WF: Blunt versus sharp expansion of the uterine incision in low-segment transverse cesarean section. Am J Obstet Gynecol 171:1022, 1994.

97. Jovanovic R: Incision of the pregnant uterus and delivery of low birthweight infants. Am J Obstet Gynecol 152:971, 1985.

98. Morrison J: The development of the lower uterine segment. Aust N Z J Med 12:182, 1972.

99. Boyle JG, Gabbe SG: T and J vertical extensions in low transverse cesarean births. Obstet Gynecol 87:238, 1996.

100. Nielson TF, Hokegard KH: Cesarean section and intraoperative surgical complications. Acta Obstet Gynaecol Scand 63:103, 1984.

101. McCurdy CM Jr, Magann EF, McCurdy CJ, Saltzman AK: The effect of placental management at cesarean delivery on operative blood loss. Am J Obstet Gynecol 167:1363, 1992.

102. Queenan JT, Nakamoto M: Postpartum immunization: the hypothetical hazard of manual removal of the placenta. Obstet Gynecol 23:392, 1964.

103. Hershey DW, Quilligan EJ: Extraabdominal uterine exteriorization at cesarean section. Obstet Gynecol 52:189, 1978.

104. Magann EF, Dodson MK, Allbert JR, et al: Blood loss at time of cesarean section by method of placental removal and exteriorization versus in situ repair of the uterine incision. Surg Gynecol Obstet 177:389, 1993.

105. Chatterjee SK: Scar endometriosis: a clinicopathologic study of 17 cases. Obstet Gynecol 56:81, 1980.

106. Hauth JC, Owen J, Davis RO: Transverse uterine incision closure: one versus two layers. Am J Obstet Gynecol 167:1108, 1992.

107. Tucker JM, Hauth JC, Hodgkins P, et al: Trial of labor after a one- or two-layer closure of a low transverse uterine incision. Obstet Gynecol 168:545, 1993.

108. Hull DB, Varner MW: A randomized study of closure of the peritoneum at cesarean delivery. Obstet Gynecol 77:818, 1991.

109. Pietrantoni M, Parsons MT, O'Brien WF, et al: Peritoneal closure or non-closure at cesarean. Obstet Gynecol 77:293, 1991.

110. Ellis H: The aetiology of post operative abdominal adhesions, an experimental study. Br J Surg 50:10, 1962.

111. Ellis H, Heddle R: Does the peritoneum need to be closed at laparotomy? Br J Surg 64:733, 1977.

112. Elkins TE, Stovall TG, Warren J: Histological evaluation of peritoneal injury and repair: implications for adhesion formation. Obstet Gynecol 70:225, 1987.

113. Tulandi T, Hum HS, Gelfand MM: Closure of laparotomy incisions with or without peritoneal suturing and second-look laparoscopy. Am J Obstet Gynecol 158:536, 1988.

114. Sanz LE: Choosing the right wound closure technique. Contemp Obstet Gynecol 21:142, 1983.

115. Fagniez PL, Hay JM, Lacaine F, et al: Abdominal midline incision closure. Arch Surg 120:1351, 1985.

116. Sanders RJ, Diclementi D, Ireland K: Principles of abdominal wound closure. II. Prevention of wound dehiscence. Arch Surg 112:1184, 1977.

117. Stone IK, von Fraunhofer JA, Masterson BJ: The biomechanical effects of tight suture closure upon fascia. Surg Gynecol Obstet 163:448, 1986.

118. Raghaviah NV, Devi AI: Bladder injury associated with rupture of the uterus. Obstet Gynecol 46:573, 1975.

119. Eglinton GS, Phelan JP, Yeh S-Y, et al: Outcome of a trial of labor after prior cesarean delivery. J Reprod Med 29:3, 1984.

120. Eisenkop SM, Richman R, Platt LD, et al: Urinary tract injury during cesarean section. Obstet Gynecol 60:591, 1982.

121. Mickal A, Begneaud WP, Hawes TP Jr: Pitfalls and complications of cesarean section hysterectomy. Clin Obstet Gynecol 12:660, 1969.

122. Barclay DL: Cesarean hysterectomy. A thirty year experience. Obstet Gynecol 35:120, 1970.

123. Everett HS, Mattingly RF: Urinary tract injuries resulting from pelvic surgery. Am J Obstet Gynecol 71:502, 1956.

124. Levin S: Selected overview of nongynecologic surgical intraabdominal infections: prophylaxis and therapy. Am J Med Suppl 79:146, 1985.

125. Clark SL, Phelan JP, Yeh SY, et al: Hypogastric artery ligation for the control of obstetric hemorrhage. Obstet Gynecol 66:353, 1985.

126. Zaki AMS, Bahar AM, Ali ME, et al: Risk factors and morbidity in patients with placenta previa accreta compared to placenta previa nonaccreta. Acta Obstet Gynecol Scand 77:391, 1998.

127. Bakshi S, Meyer BA: Indications for and outcomes of emergency peripartum hysterectomy: a five-year review. J Reprod Med 44:733, 2000.

128. Clark SL, Yeh S-Y, Phelan JP, et al: Emergency hysterectomy for obstetric hemorrhage. Obstet Gynecol 64:376, 1984.

129. Hayashi RH, Castillo MS, Noah ML: Management of severe postpartum hemorrhage due to uterine atony using an analogue of prostaglandin F_2. Obstet Gynecol 58:426, 1981.

130. Shaffer D, Benotti PN, Bothe A Jr, et al: Subcutaneous drainage in gastric bypass surgery. Infect Surg 5:716, 1986.

131. Cruse PJE, Foord R: A five-year prospective study of 23,649 surgical wounds. Arch Surg 107:206, 1973.

132. Katz VL, Dotters DJ, Droegemueller W: Perimortem cesarean delivery. Obstet Gynecol 68:571, 1986.

133. Field DR, Gates EA, Creasy R, et al: Maternal brain death during pregnancy: medical and ethical issues. JAMA 260:816, 1988.

134. Metheny NM: Fluid Balance. Philadelphia, JB Lippincott, 1984.

135. Shires GT, Canizaro PC: Fluid and electrolyte management of the surgical patient. *In* Schwartz S (ed): Principles of Surgery. New York, McGraw-Hill, 1984, p 45.

136. Rubin GL, Peterson HB, Rochat RW, et al: Maternal death after cesarean section in Georgia. Am J Obstet Gynecol 139: 681, 1981.

137. Frigoletto FD Jr, Phillipe M, Davies IJ, Ryan KJ: Avoiding iatrogenic prematurity with elective repeat cesarean section without the use of routine amniocentesis. Am J Obstet Gynecol 137:521, 1980.

138. Baskett TF, McMillen RM: Cesarean section: trends and morbidity. Can Med Assoc J 125:723, 1981.

139. Danforth DN: Cesarean section. JAMA 253:811, 1985.

140. Duff P: Pathophysiology and management of postcesarean endomyometritis. Obstet Gynecol 67:269, 1986.

141. Vorherr H: Puerperal genitourinary infection. *In* Sciarra J (ed): Gynecology and Obstetrics. Vol 2. Philadelphia, Harper & Row, 1982, p 1.

142. Brumfield CG, Hauth JC, Andrews WW: Puerperal infection after cesarean delivery: evaluation of a standardized protocol. Am J Obstet Gynecol 182:1147, 2000.

143. Schwartz WH, Grolle K: The use of prophylactic antibiotics in cesarean section. A review of the literature. J Reprod Med 26:595, 1981.

144. Cartwright PS, Pittaway DE, Jones HE, et al: The use of prophylactic antibiotics in obstetrics and gynecology: a review. Obstet Gynecol Surv 39:537, 1984.

145. Mead PB: Managing infected abdominal wounds. Contemp Obstet Gynecol 14:69, 1979.

146. Wallace D, Hernandez W, Schlaerth JB, et al: Prevention of abdominal wound disruption utilizing the Smead-Jones closure technique. Obstet Gynecol 56:26, 1980.

147. Green SL, Sarubbi FA: Risk factors associated with postcesarean section febrile morbidity. Obstet Gynecol 49:686, 1977.

148. Hawrylyshyn PA, Bernstein P, Papsin FR: Risk factors associated with infection following cesarean section. Am J Obstet Gynecol 139:294, 1981.

149. Nielson TF, Hokegard KH: Postoperative cesarean section morbidity: a prospective study. Am J Obstet Gynecol 146: 911, 1983.

150. Gibbs RS, Blanco JD, St Clair PJ: A case-control study of wound abscess after cesarean delivery. Obstet Gynecol 62: 498, 1983.

151. Gall SA Jr, Gall SA: Diagnosis and management of postcesarean wound infections. *In* Phelan JP, Clark SL (eds): Cesarean Delivery. New York, Elsevier Publishers, 1985, p 388.

152. Sweet RL, Yonekura ML, Hill G, et al: Appropriate use of antibiotics in serious obstetric and gynecologic infections. Am J Obstet Gynecol 136:719, 1983.

153. Gall SA: Infections in the female genital tract. Compr Ther 9: 34, 1983.

154. Emmons SL, Krohn M, Jackson M, Eschenbach DA: Development of wound infections among women undergoing cesarean section. Obstet Gynecol 72:559, 1988.

155. Kuhn HH, Ullman U, Kuhn FW: New aspects on the pathophysiology of wound infection and wound healing—the problem of lowered oxygen pressure in the tissue. Infection 13:52, 1985.

156. Polk HC: Operating room acquired infection: a review of pathogenesis. Am Surg 45:349, 1979.

157. Krebs HB, Helmkamp BF: Transverse periumbilical incision in the massively obese patient. Obstet Gynecol 63:241, 1984.

158. Dodson MK, Magann EF, Meeks GR: A randomized comparison of secondary closure and secondary intention in patients with superficial wound dehiscence. Obstet Gynecol 80:321, 1992.

159. Gross BH, Callen PW: Ultrasound of the uterus. *In* Callen PW (ed): Ultrasonography in Obstetrics and Gynecology. Philadelphia, WB Saunders Company, 1982, p 227.

160. Lee CY, Madrazo BL, Drukker GH: Ultrasonic evaluation of the postpartum uterus in the management of postpartum bleeding. Obstet Gynecol 58:227, 1981.

161. Burger NF, Dararas B, Boes EGM: An echographic evaluation during the early puerperium of the uterine wound after cesarean section. J Clin Ultrasound 10:271, 1982.

162. Lavery J, Gadwood KA: Postpartum sonography. *In* Sanders RC, Jones E (eds): Ultrasonography in Obstetrics and Gynecology. 4th ed. Norwalk, CT, Appleton-Century-Crofts Medical, 1991, p 509.

163. Malvern J, Campbell S, May P: Ultrasonic scanning of the puerperal uterus following secondary postpartum haemorrhage. Br J Obstet Gynaecol 80:320, 1973.

164. Shaffer PB, Johnson JC, Bryan D, et al: Diagnosis of ovarian vein thrombophlebitis by computed tomography. J Comput Assist Tomogr 5:436, 1981.

165. Farrell SJ, Andersen HF, Work BA Jr: Cesarean section: indications and postoperative morbidity. Obstet Gynecol 56:696, 1980.

166. Schwartz MA, Wang CC, Eckert LO, Critchlow CW: Risk factors for urinary tract infection in the postpartum period. Am J Obstet Gynecol 181:547, 1999.

167. Rehu M, Nilsson CG: Risk factors for febrile morbidity associated with cesarean section. Obstet Gynecol 56:269, 1980.

168. Bonnar J: Venous thromboembolism and pregnancy. Clin Obstet Gynecol 8:455, 1981.

169. Villasanta U: Thromboembolic disease in pregnancy. Am J Obstet Gynecol 93:142, 1965.

170. Stead RB: Regulation of hemostasis. *In* Goldhaber AZ (ed): Pulmonary Embolism and Deep Venous Thrombosis. Philadelphia, WB Saunders Company, 1985, p. 27.

171. Hirsh J, Cade JF, Gallus AS: Anticoagulants in pregnancy: a review of indications and complications. Am Heart J 83:301, 1972.

172. Laros RK, Alger LS: Thromboembolism and pregnancy. Clin Obstet Gynecol 22:871, 1979.

173. Rosenow ED III, Osmundson PJ, Brown ML: Pulmonary embolism. Mayo Clin Proc 56:161, 1981.

174. Duff P, Gibbs RS: Pelvic vein thrombophlebitis: diagnostic dilemma and therapeutic challenge. Obstet Gynecol Surv 38: 365, 1983.

175. Bartlette RH, Brennan ML, Gazzaniga AB, et al: Studies on the pathogenesis and prevention of postoperative pulmonary complications. Surg Gynecol Obstet 137:925, 1973.

176. Rosen MA, Hughes SC, Shnider SM: Epidural morphine for the relief of postoperative pain after cesarean delivery. Anesth Analg 62:666, 1983.

177. Metcalfe J, Ueland K: Maternal cardiovascular adjustments to pregnancy. Prog Cardiovasc Dis 16:363, 1974.

178. Doyle RL, Schibanoff JM (eds): Healthcare Management Guidelines. Vol 1. Inpatient and Surgical Care. Albany, NY, Milliman & Robertson, 1995.

179. American College of Obstetricians and Gynecologists: Financial Influences on Mode of Delivery. Committee Opinion No 149, Washington, DC, ACOG, 1994.

180. Bottoms SF, Rosen MG, Sokol RJ: The increase in the cesarean birth. N Engl J Med 302:559, 1980.

181. Myers SA, Gleicher N: A successful program to lower cesarean-section rates. N Engl J Med 319:1511, 1988.

182. O'Driscoll K, Foley M, MacDonald D: Active management of labor as an alternative to cesarean for dystocia. Obstet Gynecol 63:485, 1984.

183. Bergsjo P, Bakketeig LS, Eikhom SN: Case-control analysis of post-term induction of labour. Acta Obstet Gynaecol Scand 61:317, 1982.

184. Gibb DMF, Cardozo LD, Studd JWW, Cooper DJ: Prolonged pregnancy: is induction of labour indicated? A prospective study. Br J Obstet Gynaecol 89:292, 1982.

185. Hage ML, Helms MJ, Hammond WE, Hammond CB: Changing rates of cesarean delivery: the Duke experience, 1978–1986. Obstet Gynecol 72:98, 1988.

186. Low JA, Panagiotopoulos C, Derrick EJ: Newborn complications after intrapartum asphyxia with metabolic acidosis in the term fetus. Am J Obstet Gynecol 170:1081, 1994.

187. Low JA, Panagiotopoulos C, Derrick EJ: Newborn complications after intrapartum asphyxia with metabolic acidosis in the preterm fetus. Am J Obstet Gynecol 172:805, 1995.

188. Boylan PC, Frankowski R, Rountree R, et al: Effective active management of labor on the incidence of cesarean section for dystocia in nulliparous. Am J Perinatol 8:373, 1991.

189. Socol ML, Garcia PM, Peaceman AM, Dooley SL: Reducing cesarean births at a primarily private university hospital. Am J Obstet Gynecol 168:1748, 1993.

190. Satin AJ, Leveno KJ, Sherman ML, et al: High-versus low-dose oxytocin for labor stimulation. Obstet Gynecol 80:111, 1992.

191. Lopez-Zeno JA, Peaceman AM, Adashek JA, et al: A controlled trial of a program for the active management of labor. N Engl J Med 326:450, 1992.

192. Frigoletto FD, Lieberman E, Lang JM, et al: A clinical trial of active management of labor. N Engl J Med 333:745, 1995.

193. Riva H, Teich J: Vaginal delivery after cesarean section. Am J Obstet Gynecol 81:501, 1961.

194. Cowan RK, Kinch RAH, Ellis B, Anderson R: Trial of labor following cesarean delivery. Obstet Gynecol 83:933, 1994.

195. Flamm BL, Newman LA, Thomas SJ, et al: Vaginal birth after cesarean delivery: results of a 5-year multicenter collaborative study. Obstet Gynecol 76:750, 1990.

196. Nguyen TV, Dinh TV, Suresh MS, et al: Vaginal birth after cesarean section at the University of Texas. J Reprod Med 37:880, 1992.

197. Flamm B, Goings J, Yunbao L, Wolde-Tsadik G: Elective repeat cesarean delivery versus trial of labor: a prospective multicenter study. Obstet Gynecol 83:927, 1994.

198. Costs of uncomplicated cesarean and vaginal deliveries, Met Life Claims Data, 1996, Health Insurance Association of America, Source Book of Health Insurance Data, 1999–2000.

199. Flamm BL: Vaginal birth after cesarean section: controversies old and new. Clin Obstet Gynecol 28:735, 1985.

200. Lavin JP, Stephens RJ, Miodovnik M, et al: Vaginal delivery in patients with a prior cesarean section. Obstet Gynecol 59:135, 1982.

201. Martin JN Jr, Harris BA Jr, Huddleston JF, et al: Vaginal delivery following previous cesarean birth. Am J Obstet Gynecol 146:255, 1983.

202. Beall M, Eglinton GS, Clark SL, et al: Vaginal delivery after cesarean section in women with unknown types of uterine scar. J Reprod Med 29:31, 1984.

203. Boucher M, Tahilramaney MP, Eglinton GS, et al: Maternal morbidity as related to trial of labor after previous cesarean delivery: a quantitative analysis. J Reprod Med 29:12, 1984.

204. Phelan JP, Eglinton GS, Horenstein JM, et al: Previous cesarean birth: trial of labor in women with macrosomic infants. J Reprod Med 29:36, 1984.

205. Stovall TG, Shaver DC, Solomon SK, Anderson GD: Trial of labor in previous cesarean section patients, excluding classical cesarean sections. Obstet Gynecol 70:713, 1987.

206. Flamm BL, Lim OW, Jones C, et al: Vaginal birth after cesarean section: results of a multicenter study. Am J Obstet Gynecol 158:1079, 1988.

207. Farmer RM, Kirschbaum T, Potter D, et al: Uterine rupture during a trial of labor after previous cesarean section. Am J Obstet Gynecol 165:996, 1991.

208. Paul RH, Phelan JP, Yeh S: Trial of labor in the patient with a prior cesarean birth. Am J Obstet Gynecol 151:297, 1985.

209. Farmakides G, Duvivier R, Schulman H, et al: Vaginal birth after two or more previous cesarean sections. Am J Obstet Gynecol 154:565, 1987.

210. Pruett K, Kirshon B, Cotton D: Unknown uterine scar in trial of labor. Am J Obstet Gynecol 159:807, 1988.

211. Miller DA, Diaz FG, Paul RH: Vaginal birth after cesarean: a 10-year experience. Obstet Gynecol 84:255, 1994.

212. Rosen MG, Dickinson JC, Westhoff CL: Vaginal birth after cesarean: a meta-analysis of morbidity and mortality. Obstet Gynecol 77:465, 1991.

213. Porreco RP, Meier PR: Trial of labor in patients with multiple previous cesarean sections. J Reprod Med 28:770, 1983.

214. American College of Obstetricians and Gynecologists: Vaginal Delivery After Previous Cesarean Birth. Practice Patterns, No 1. Washington, DC, ACOG, 1995.

215. Hueston WJ, Rudy M: Factors predicting elective repeat cesarean delivery. Obstet Gynecol 83:741, 1994.

216. Joseph GF Jr, Stedman CM, Robichaux AG: Vaginal birth after cesarean section: the impact of patient resistance to a trial of labor. Am J Obstet Gynecol 164:1441, 1991.

217. American College of Obstetricians and Gynecologists: Vaginal Birth After Cesarean section: Report of 1990 Survey of ACOG's membership. Washington, DC, ACOG, 1990.

218. Rosen MG, Dickinson JC: Vaginal birth after cesarean: a meta-analysis of indicators for success. Obstet Gynecol 76:865, 1990.

219. Shiono PH, Fielden JR, McNellis D, et al: Recent trends in cesarean birth and trial of labor rates in the United States. JAMA 257:494, 1987.

220. Phelan JP, Ahn MO, Diaz F, et al: Twice a cesarean always a cesarean? Obstet Gynecol 73:161, 1989.

221. Thubisi M, Ebrahim A, Moodley J, Shweni PM: Vaginal delivery after previous caesarean section: is x-ray pelvimetry necessary? Br J Obstet Gynaecol 100:421, 1993.

222. Krishnamurthy S, Fairlie F, Cameron AD, et al: The role of postnatal x-ray pelvimetry after caesarean section in the management of subsequent delivery. Br J Obstet Gynaecol 98:716, 1991.

223. Goldman G, Pineault R, Pitvin L, et al: Factors influencing the practice of vaginal birth after cesarean section. Am J Public Health 83:1104, 1993.

224. Stafford RS: The impact of nonclinical factors on repeat cesarean section. JAMA 265:59, 1991.

225. Eglinton GS: Effect of previous indications for cesarean on subsequent outcome. *In* Phelan JP, Clark SL (eds): Cesarean Delivery. New York, Elsevier, 1988.

226. Horenstein JP, Phelan JP: Previous cesarean section: the risks and benefits of oxytocin usage in a trial of labor. Am J Obstet Gynecol 151:564, 1985.

227. Silver RK, Gibbs RS: Prediction of vaginal delivery in patients with a previous cesarean section who require oxytocin. Am J Obstet Gynecol 156:57, 1987.

228. Jarrell MA, Ashmead GG, Mann LI: Vaginal delivery after cesarean section: a five year study. Obstet Gynecol 65:628, 1985.

229. Saldana LR, Schulman H, Reuss L: Management of pregnancy after cesarean section. Am J Obstet Gynecol 135:555, 1979.

230. Seitchik J, Rao VRR: Cesarean delivery in nulliparous women for failed oxytocin-augmented labor: route of delivery in subsequent pregnancy. Am J Obstet Gynecol 143:393, 1982.

231. Whiteside DC, Mahan CS, Cook JC: Factors associated with successful vaginal delivery after cesarean delivery after cesarean section. J Reprod Med 28:785, 1983.

232. Ollendorff DA, Goldberg JM, Minoque JP, Socol ML: Vaginal birth after cesarean section for arrest of labor: is success determined by maximum cervical dilatation during the prior labor? Am J Obstet Gynecol 159:636, 1988.

233. American College of Obstetricians and Gynecologists: Practice perspective: Guidelines for vaginal delivery after previous cesarean birth. Newsletter, February. Washington, DC, ACOG, 1985.

234. Jongen VHWM, Halfwerk MGC, Brouwer WK: Vaginal delivery after previous ceasarean section for failure of second stage of labour. Br J Obstet Gynecol 105:1079, 1998.

235. Hankins GDV, Clark SL, Cunningham FG, Gitstrap LC III (eds): Operative Obstetrics. Norwalk, CT, Appleton & Lange, 1995.

236. Halperin ME, Moore DC, Hannah WJ: Classical vs. low-segment transverse incision for preterm cesarean section: maternal complications and outcome of subsequent pregnancies. Br J Obstet Gynaecol 95:990, 1988.

237. American College of Obstetricians and Gynecologists, Committee on Obstetrics: Maternal and Fetal Medicine: Assessment of Fetal Maturity Prior to Repeat Cesarean Delivery or Elective Induction of Labor. No 77. Washington, DC, ACOG, 1990.

238. Flamm BL, Goings JR, Fuelberth NJ, et al: Oxytocin during labor after previous cesarean section: results of a multicenter study. Obstet Gynecol 70:709, 1987.

239. American College of Obstetricians and Gynecologists: ACOG Technical Bulletin: Dystocia and the Augmentation of Labor. No 218. Washington, DC, ACOG, 1995.

240. Arulkumaran S, Chua S, Ratnam SS: Symptoms and signs with scar rupture—value of uterine activity measurements. Aust N Z J Obstet Gynaecol 32:208, 1992.

241. Horenstein J, Phelan JP: Vaginal birth after cesarean: the role of oxytocin. *In* Phelan JP, Clark SL (eds): Cesarean Delivery. New York, Elsevier, 1988.

242. Leung AS, Farmer RM, Leung EK, et al: Risk factors associated with uterine rupture during trial of labor after cesarean delivery: a case controlled study. Am J Obstet Gynecol 168:1358, 1993.

243. Mackenzie IZ, Bradley S, Embrey MP: Vaginal prostaglandins and labor induction for patients previously delivered by cesarean section. Br J Obstet Gynaecol 91:7, 1984.

244. Norman M, Ekman G: Preinductive cervical ripening with prostaglandin E_2 in women with one previous cesarean section. Acta Obstet Gynecol Scand 71:351, 1992.

245. Blanco JD, Collins M, Willis D, Prien S: Prostaglandin E_2 gel induction of patients with a prior low transverse cesarean section. Am J Perinatol 9:80, 1992.

246. Wing DA, Lovett K, Paul RH: Disruption of prior uterine incision following misoprostol for labor induction in women with previous cesarean delivery. Obstet Gynecol 91:828, 1998.

247. Flamm BL, Goings JR: Vaginal birth after cesarean section: is suspected fetal macrosomia a contraindication? Obstet Gynecol 74:694, 1989.

248. Jones R, Nagashima A, Hartnett-Goodman M, Goodlin R: Rupture of low transverse cesarean scars during trial of labor. Obstet Gynecol 77:815, 1991.

249. Rodriguez M, Masaki D, Phelan J, Diaz F: Uterine rupture: are intrauterine pressure catheters useful in the diagnosis? Am J Obstet Gynecol 161:666, 1989.

250. Crawford JS: The epidural sieve and MBC, minimal blocking concentration: a hypothesis. Anaesthesia 31:1278, 1976.

251. Carlson C, Lybell-Lindahl G, Ingemarsson I: Extradural block in patients who have previously undergone cesarean section. Br J Anaesth 52:827, 1980.

252. Uppington J: Epidural analgesia and previous caesarean section. Anaesthesia 38:336, 1983.

253. Golan A, Sandbank O, Rubin A: Rupture of the pregnant uterus. Obstet Gynecol 56:349, 1980.

254. Hansell RS, McMurray KB, Huey GR: Vaginal birth after two or more cesarean sections: a five-year experience. Birth 17:146, 1990.

255. Chattopadhyay SK, Sherbeeni MM, Anokute CC: Planned vaginal delivery after two previous caesarean sections. Br J Obstet Gynaecol 101:498, 1994.

256. Ganovsky-Grisaru S, Shaya M, Diamant YZ: The management of labor in women with more than one uterine scar: is a repeat cesarean section really the only "safe" option? J Perinat Med 22:13, 1994.

257. Plauché WC, Von Almen W, Mueller R: Catastrophic uterine rupture. Obstet Gynecol 64:792, 1984.

258. Eden RD, Parker RT, Gall SA: Rupture of the pregnant uterus: a 53 year review. Obstet Gynecol 68:671, 1986.

259. Pitkin RM: Once a cesarean? Obstet Gynecol 77:939, 1991.

260. Scott J: Mandatory trial of labor after cesarean delivery: an alternative viewpoint. Obstet Gynecol 77:811, 1991.

261. Brundenell M, Chakravarti S: Uterine rupture in labour. BMJ 2:122, 1975.

262. Eriksen NL, Buttino L Jr: Vaginal birth after cesarean: a comparison of maternal and neonatal morbidity to elective repeat cesarean section. Am J Perinatol 6:375, 1989.

263. McMahon MJ, Luter ER, Bowes WA Jr, Olshan AF: Comparison of a trial of labor with an elective second cesarean section. N Engl J Med 335:689, 1996.

264. American College of Obstetricians and Gynecologists: Assessment of Fetal Lung Maturity. Educational Bulletin No 230. Washington, DC, ACOG, 1996.

265. Meier P, Porreco R: Trial of labor following cesarean section: a two year experience. Am J Obstet Gynecol 144:671, 1982.

266. American College of Obstetricians and Gynecologists: Ethical Dimensions of Informed Consent. Committee Opinion No 108. Washington, DC, ACOG, 1992.

267. Department of Professional Liability, The American College of Obstetricians and Gynecologists: Informed Consent: The Assistant. 1234/89/1 35 40. Washington, DC, ACOG, 1987.

268. American College of Obstetricians and Gynecologists: ACOG Technical Bulletin. Blood component therapy. No 199 Washington, DC, ACOG, 1994.

269. American College of Obstetricians and Gynecologists: ACOG Committee Opinion: Patient Choice and the Maternal-Fetal Relationship. No 214. Washington, DC, ACOG, 1999.

270. Abitol MM, Castillo I, Taylor UB, et al: Vaginal birth after cesarean section: the patient's point of view. Am Fam Physician 47:129, 1993.

271. Bixby GH: Extirpation of the puerperal uterus by abdominal section. J Gynaecol Soc (Boston) 1:223, 1986.

272. Speert H: Eduardo Poor and cesarean hysterectomy. Surg Gynecol Obstet 106:245, 1958.

273. Harris JW: A study of the results obtained in sixty-four cesarean sections terminated by supravaginal hysterectomy. Bull Johns Hopkins Hosp 33:318, 1922.

274. Stanco LM, Schrimmer DB, Paul RH, Mishell DR Jr: Emergency peripartum hysterectomy and associated risk factors. Am J Obstet Gynecol 168:879, 1993.

275. Zelop CM, Harlow BL, Frigoletto FD Jr, et al: Emergency peripartum hysterectomy. Am J Obstet Gynecol 168:1443, 1993.

276. Fox H: Placenta accreta, 1945–1969. Obstet Gynecol Surv 17:475, 1972.

277. Burchell DR: Physiology of internal iliac artery ligation. J Obstet Gynaecol Br Commonw 75:642, 1968.

278. Clark SL, Phelan JP: Surgical control of obstetric hemorrhage. Contemp Obstet Gynecol 24:70, 1984.

279. Weed JC: The fate of post cesarean uterus. Obstet Gynecol 14:780, 1959.

280. Ward SV, Smith H: Cesarean total hysterectomy: combined section and sterilization. Obstet Gynecol 26:858, 1965.

281. Schneider GT, Tyrone CH: Cesarean total hysterectomy: experience of 160 cases. South Med J 59:927, 1968.

282. Brenner P, Sall S, Sonnenblick D: Evaluation of cesarean section hysterectomy as a sterilization procedure. Am J Obstet Gynecol 108:335, 1970.

283. McNulty JV: Elective cesarean hysterectomy—revisited. Am J Obstet Gynecol 149:29, 1984.

284. Park RC, Duff WP: Role of cesarean hysterectomy in modern obstetric practice. Clin Obstet Gynecol 23:601, 1980.

285. Hoffman NS, Roberts WS, Fiorica JV, et al: Elective cesarean hysterectomy for treatment of cervical neoplasia: an update. J Reprod Med 38:186, 1993.

286. Sall S, Rini S, Pineda A: Surgical management of invasive carcinoma of the cervix in pregnancy. Obstet Gynecol 118:1, 1974.

287. Thompson JD, Caputo TA, Franklin EW III, et al: The surgical management of invasive cancer of the cervix in pregnancy. Am J Obstet Gynecol 121:853, 1975.

288. Wingo PA, Huezo CM, Rubin GL, et al: The mortality risk associated with hysterectomy. Am J Obstet Gynecol 152:803, 1985.

289. Plauché WC, Gruich FG, Bourgeois MO: Hysterectomy at the time of cesarean section: analysis of 108 cases. Obstet Gynecol 58:459, 1981.

290. Yancey MK, Harlass FE, Benson W, Brady K: The perioperative morbidity of scheduled cesarean hysterectomy. Obstet Gynecol 81:206, 1993.

291. National Center for Health Statistics: Rates of cesarean delivery—United States, 1991. MMWR Morb Mortal Wkly Rep 42:285, 1993.

Surgical Procedures in Pregnancy

JACK LUDMIR AND PHILLIP G. STUBBLEFIELD

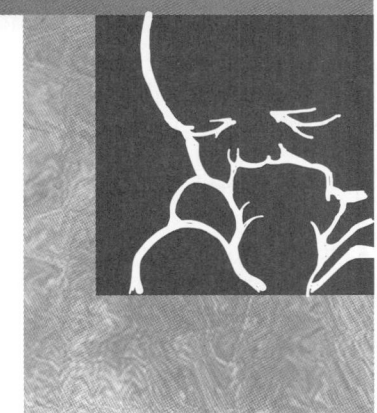

Approximately 0.2 to 2.2 percent of pregnant women require surgery in pregnancy.[1-3] Changes in the maternal cardiovascular system and increased uterine perfusion and size during gestation require special adaptation of anesthesia and surgical technique to the pregnant patient (see the box "Maternal Physiologic Changes Relevant to Surgery").[4-10] During advanced pregnancy, abdominal pain and symptoms of gastrointestinal disease are difficult to assess secondary to a large uterus. Advances in diagnostic modalities, including computed tomographic (CT) imaging, magnetic resonance imaging (MRI), high-resolution ultrasound, and Doppler studies have improved our ability to make the diagnosis of surgical conditions during gestation.[11-14] Furthermore, new surgical therapeutic modalities, including laparoscopy, well established in the gynecologic and surgical arena, are now being evaluated in the management of the pregnant patient with a surgical condition.[15-22] The patient and physician facing the possibility of surgery during pregnancy are concerned about the possible ill effects of anesthesia and surgery on the developing fetus versus the consequences of delaying such surgery. In the largest study to date of surgical procedures in pregnancy, Mazze and Kallen in Sweden[23] studied the effects of 5,405 nonobstetric procedures performed in 720,000 pregnant Swedish women during the 1970s and 1980s. These authors found that surgery was performed in the first trimester in 41 percent, compared with 35 percent in the middle, and 24 percent in the third trimester. Abdominal surgery constituted one fourth of all operations, and almost 20 percent were gynecologic and urologic procedures. Although laparoscopy was the most commonly performed first-trimester operation to rule out ectopic gestation, appendectomy was the most common procedure in the second trimester. One half of the surgeries were performed using general anesthesia, and in 90 percent of the cases, nitrous oxide was given. To determine the effects of the surgery and anesthesia on the 5,405 pregnancies, the authors compared the outcomes to the total database of 720,000 pregnancies for the study period. The rate of congenital malformation and stillbirth were not significantly increased. However, the rate of low-birth-weight infants, as well as neonatal deaths during the first 7 days of life in patients undergoing surgery, was significantly increased. These authors concluded that surgery, in particular nonobstetric, during pregnancy could increase the rate of poor obstetric outcomes. This increase in perinatal morbidity was thought to be secondary to the surgical disease process affecting the pregnancy rather than to the adverse effects of anesthesia or surgery. In approaching the pregnant patient requiring surgery, reassurance can be given regarding the rate of birth defects and stillbirths, but prematurity and growth restriction may be significantly increased, secondary to the ill-effects of the underlying condition requiring surgery.

This chapter will describe the most common obstetric and nonobstetric surgical procedures performed during gestation.

CERVICAL CERCLAGE

Few subjects in obstetrics are as controversial as the ubiquitous term cervical incompetence. The term was initially used by Lash and Lash[24] while describing repetitive abortion presenting with painless extrusion of the products of conception. The work by Iams et al.[25] and others[26-29] using sonography to evaluate the cervix in pregnancy, have challenged the historical notion that the cervix is either competent or incompetent, to one of

Maternal Physiologic Changes Relevant to Surgery

Cardiovascular changes
  Increased cardiac output
  Increased blood volume
  Decreased systematic vascular resistance
  Decreased venous return from the lower
    extremities
Respiratory changes
  Increased minute ventilation
  Decreased functional residual capacity
Gastrointestinal changes
  Decreased gastric motility
  Delayed gastric emptying
Coagulation changes
  Increased clotting factors II, V, VII, VIII, IX, X,
    and XII
  Increased fibrinogen
  Increased risk for thromboembolic disease
Renal changes
  Increased renal plasma flow and glomerular
    filtration rate
  Ureteral dilatation
  Increased bladder capacity

variable cervical competence. Cervical function in gestation is described by a bell-shaped curve that correlates to length.[25] Cervical function could change secondary to interaction with different variables, such as physical activity, infection, uterine distention, and uterine contractility.[30] This new concept of a continuum in cervical competence could be helpful to explain why a cervix that appears and feels long and closed could result in an early pregnancy loss, whereas a cervix that feels short and soft could carry a pregnancy to term. The traditional criteria used for performing a cervical cerclage are a classic history of painless dilatation with delivery of a premature infant, history of rapid labors, history of recurrent premature rupture of membranes (particularly in patients with prior history of cervical surgeries or trauma), or a history of diethylstilbestrol (DES)-exposure. These criteria are currently being challenged as the only criteria (see the box "Diagnostic Criteria for Cervical Incompetence").[31-37] The use of vaginal sonography in gestation to evaluate the cervix longitudinally may be a more objective way of screening patients at risk for cervical incompetence and of helping the clinician to decide which women would benefit from a cerclage. Sonographic parameters such as cervical shortening and/or funneling (Figs. 19–1 and 19–2)[38-43] may be particularly helpful in the patient in whom a classic history of painless dilatation cannot be

elucidated and the benefit of placing a prophylactic cerclage remains unclear. We have used this technology to follow patients with historical risk factors such as prior surgical conization, uterine anomalies, and DES exposure in utero.[42] Recent studies by Guzman et al.[43] suggest that following patients at risk for cervical incompetence with vaginal ultrasound, and placing a cerclage only in those patients demonstrating sonographic changes, results in the same obstetric outcomes as in a group of women who have a prophylactic cerclage placed between 12 and 16 weeks. Contrary to this study, Berghella et al.[44] in an observational study of 168 singleton pregnancies at risk for preterm labor did not show benefit in placing cerclage in patients with sonographic changes compared with those without intervention. The ideal cervical length at which to place a cerclage has not been determined. Studies have recommended cerclage for cervical lengths varying from as low as 1.5 to 2.5 cm in length.[43-45] Currently, randomized studies to determine the value of therapeutic cerclage based on sonographic cervical changes are being performed both in patients at risk for cervical incompetence and in low-risk patients in whom a short cervix is found during routine ultrasound obstetric evaluation.[46,47] It remains to be seen if cerclage, pessary, or bed rest are justifiable therapeutic interventions in patients demonstrating sonographic cervical change.

Cerclage Technique

Prophylactic Cerclage

In 1950, Lash and Lash described repair of the cervix in the nonpregnant state involving partial excision of the cervix to remove the area of presumed weakness.[24] Unfortunately, this technique had a high incidence of subsequent infertility. In 1955, Shirodkar reported successful management of cervical incompetence with the

Diagnostic Criteria for Cervical Incompetence

Historical factors
  History of painless cervical dilatation with
    preterm delivery
  History of forceful cervical dilatation and
    evacuation
  History of obstetric trauma: cervical lacerations,
    prolonged second stage followed by cesarean
  Prior cervical surgery: cone, loop
  DES exposure in utero
Cervical sonography
  Short cervical length
  Cervical funneling

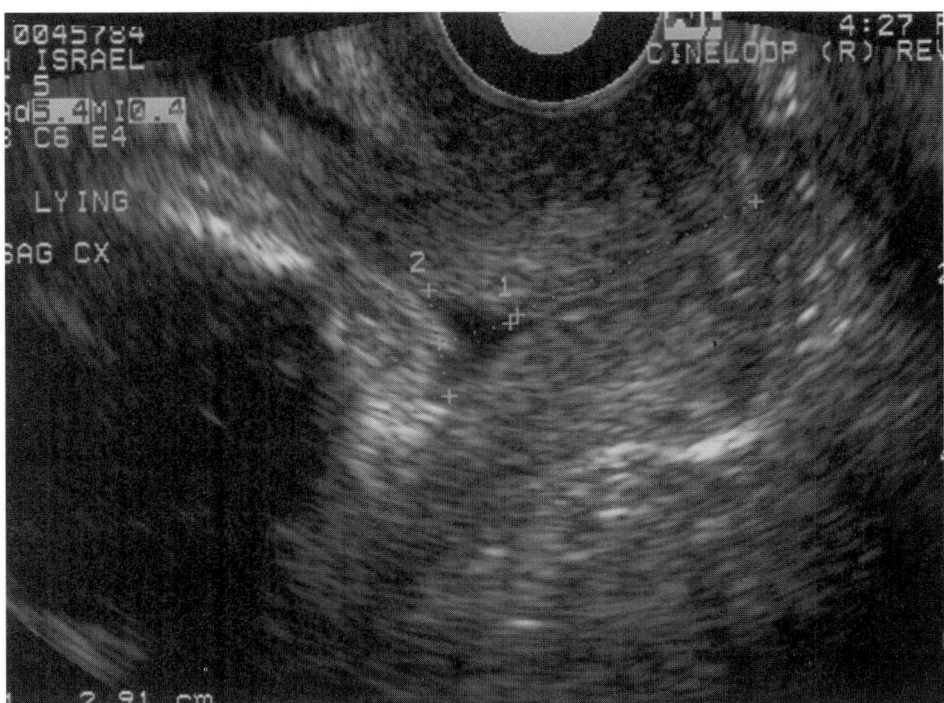

Figure 19–1. Transvaginal sonogram of the cervix at 22 weeks' gestation. Patient is at risk for cervical incompetence. Note minimal evidence of cervical funneling.

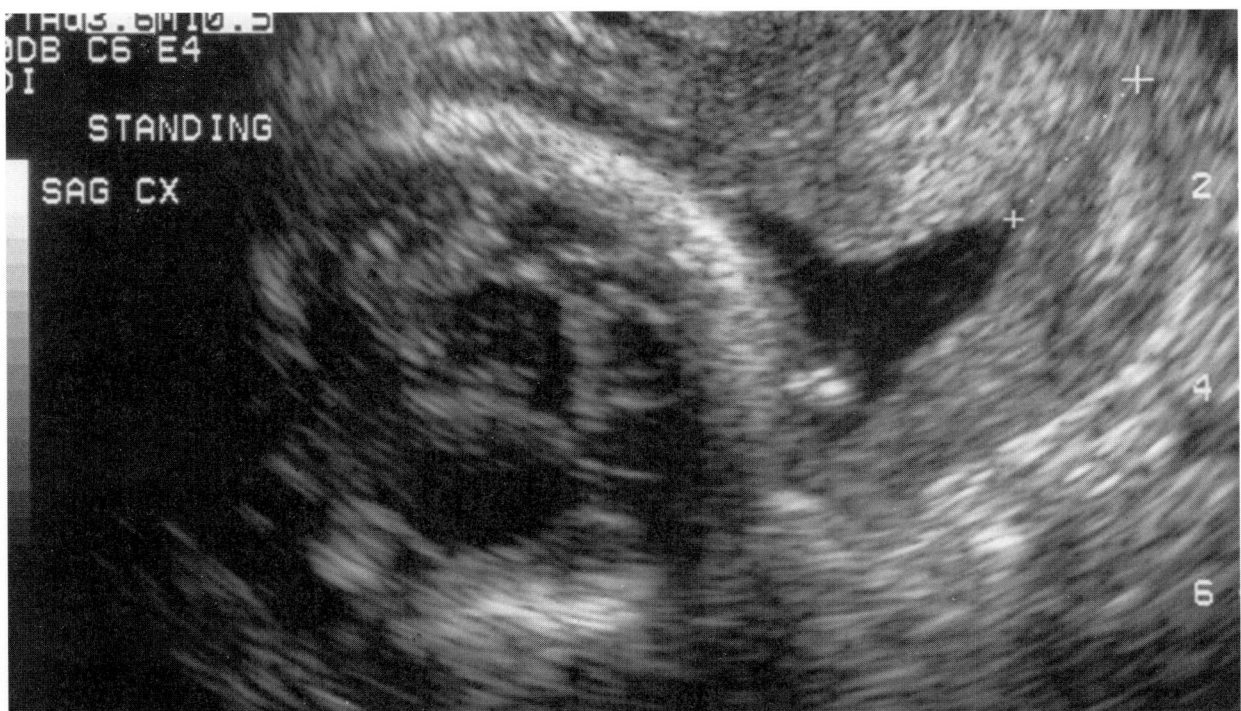

Figure 19–2. Transvaginal sonogram of the same patient as Figure 19–1 after standing up for 15 minutes. Note cervical funneling and decreased cervical length.

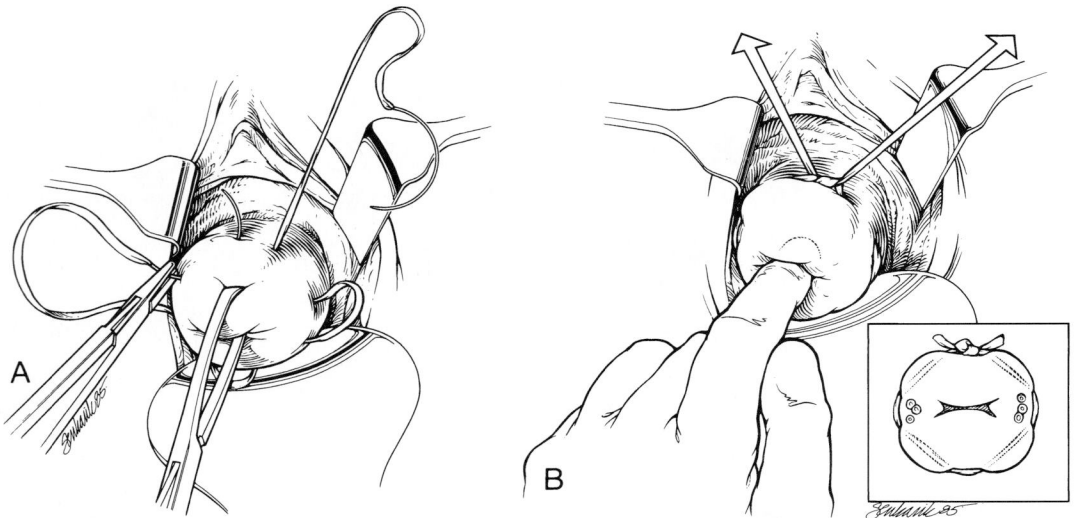

Figure 19–3. Placement of sutures for McDonald cervical cerclage. *A,* We use a double-headed Mersilene band with four "bites" in the cervix, avoiding the vessels. *B,* The suture is placed high upon the cervix close to the cervical-vaginal junction, approximately the level of the internal os.

use of a submucosal band.[48] Initially, he used catgut as suture material, and later he used Mersilene placed at the level of the internal cervical os. The procedure required anterior displacement of the bladder in an attempt to place the suture as high as possible at the level of cervical internal os. This type of procedure resulted in a greater number of patients being delivered via cesarean section because of the difficulty in removing the suture buried under the cervical surface and may require leaving the suture in place postpartum. Several years later, McDonald described a suture technique in the form of a purse string, not requiring cervical dissection, easily placed during pregnancy.[49] This technique involves taking four or five bites as high as possible in the cervix, trying to avoid injury to the bladder or the rectum, with placement of a knot anteriorly to facilitate removal (Fig. 19–3). Several types of suture material have been used.[50] We have been successful in using a Mersilene tape. However, the use of thinner suture material, such as Prolene or other synthetic nonabsorbable sutures like Ethibond is advocated by others, with the argument that the width of the Mersilene tape places the patient at greater risk for infection.[50,51] Currently, there is no evidence that placing two sutures results in better outcomes than placing one.[52–54] Preoperative patient preparations, including the use of prophylactic antibiotics or tocolytics, have not been proven to be of benefit. We perform a culture for group B streptococcus and give preoperative penicillin to the patient with a positive culture. Prophylactic cerclage placement is performed after the first trimester, to avoid the risk of spontaneous loss most likely attributable to chromosomal abnormalities.[52,53] The choice of anesthesia for cerclage varies.[55] Chen et al.[56] did not show difference

in outcome between general versus regional anesthesia. In our experience, a short-acting regional anesthetic is sufficient. We advise patients to remain on bed rest for the first 48 hours after cerclage and to avoid intercourse until follow-up postoperative visit. Decisions regarding physical activity and intercourse are individualized and based on the status of the cervix as determined by outpatient digital evaluation or sonographic findings (Fig. 19–4)[39,40,57–59] The suture is usually removed at 37 weeks electively.[52,53]

In patients with a hypoplastic cervix, such as those exposed to DES in utero, history of large cervical conization, or prior history of failed vaginal cerclage, an abdominal cerclage has been recommended.[60] This procedure is usually done at 11 weeks and requires a laparotomy. A bladder flap is created and a Mersilene tape is placed at the level of the junction between the lower uterine segment and the cervix. Novy et al. have reported extensive experience with this procedure, with low morbidity and favorable outcome.[61] Greater morbidity including injury to the uterine vessels requires expertise with this procedure. Delivery by cesarean section is necessary. We have described the placement of a transvaginal cerclage when there is a hypoplastic cervix, or the cervix is flush against the vaginal wall.[62] Under ultrasound guidance, the supravaginal portion of the cervix is dissected away from the bladder and a suture is placed either in a purse-string fashion, or in cross fashion from 12 to 6 o'clock and 3 to 9 o'clock (Fig. 19–5). We have performed this procedure in 18 patients, avoiding an abdominal procedure with successful pregnancy outcome. Fifty percent of patients delivered by cesarean section and the rest delivered vaginally after the suture was cut through a small posterior colpot-

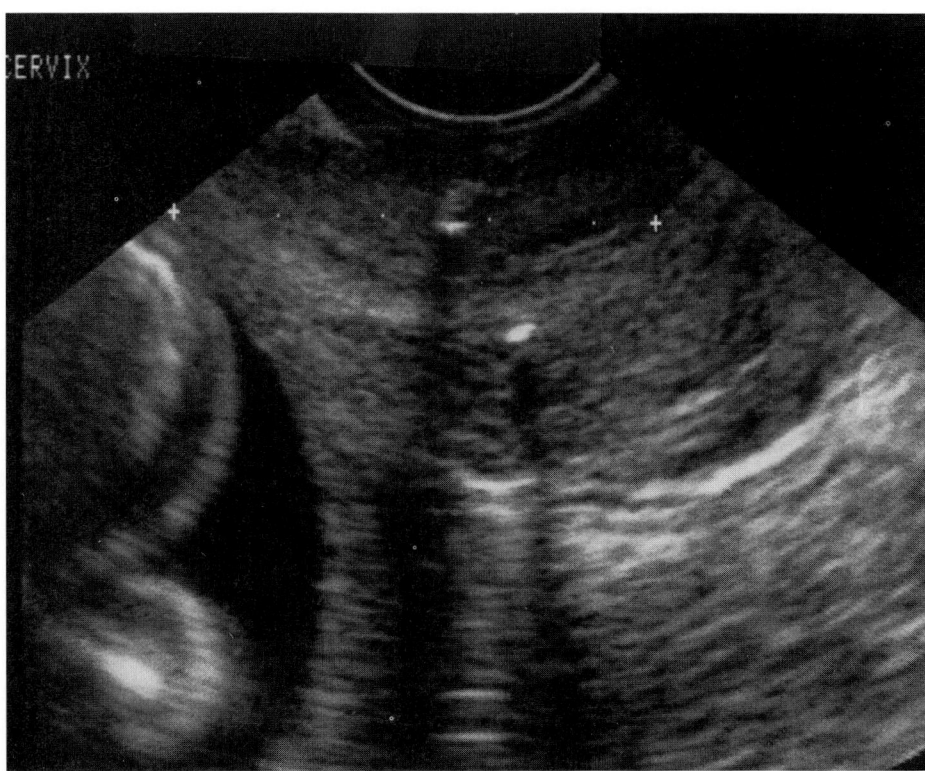

Figure 19–4. Transvaginal sonogram picture of the cervix after cerclage placement. Internal os closed and no funneling. Echogenic spots in the cervix correspond to cerclage.

omy incision. Recently, a laparoscopic abdominal approach to the cervix has been described using the same principles as an abdominal cerclage.[63] A need for randomized trials evaluating this new technique compared with a vaginal approach is necessary to determine the best approach to patients with a history of failed cerclage.

Therapeutic and Emergent Cerclage

Patients demonstrating cervical change either by digital evaluation or transvaginal sonography may benefit from a therapeutic cerclage.[32,34,35,37,39,43] The gestational age limit for cerclage placement is ill defined. Although some clinicians will offer this therapeutic modality up to 28 weeks,[64] we do not advocate the use of therapeutic cerclage beyond 24 weeks' gestation, because of fetal viability concerns and potentially causing a preterm delivery while placing the cerclage. Some of these patients have been managed successfully with strict bed rest.[44] If the decision is made to place a cerclage, we treat preoperatively with antibiotics and nonsteroidal anti-inflammatory agents, such as indomethacin. The patient is placed on strict bed rest for the first 72 hours and is advised to refrain from intercourse and strenuous physical activity for the remainder of the pregnancy. We follow these patients with frequent sonographic assessment of the cervix and recommend strict bed rest if the membranes are prolapsing to the level of

the suture.[58] Prophylactic tocolytics are not used after the procedure.

In situations in which the cervix has dilated enough to allow visualization of the membranes or the membranes have prolapsed into the vagina, placing an emergent cerclage constitutes a heroic maneuver.[64–68] These patients are at high risk of having a subclinical infection and subsequent poor outcome.[65,69] To rule out infection, some clinicians advocate amniocentesis prior to cerclage placement.[70] Several techniques have been described to reduce the prolapsing membranes, including the following: placing the patient in Trendelenburg position; the use of a pediatric Foley catheter to tease the membranes into the endocervical canal, and instilling 1 L of saline into the bladder with upper displacement of the lower uterine segment.[67,68,70,71] Although the efficacy of antibiotics or tocolytics has not been properly studied, some case series advocate their use. Although clinicians have been reluctant to offer cerclage in patients with protruding membranes, some reports have suggested salvage rate in excess of 70 percent despite advanced cervical dilatation.[72–74]

Risks of Cerclage

Cervical lacerations at time of delivery are one of the most common complications from a cerclage, occurring in 1 to 13 percent of patients.[52] Three percent of patients require cesarean birth because of the inability of

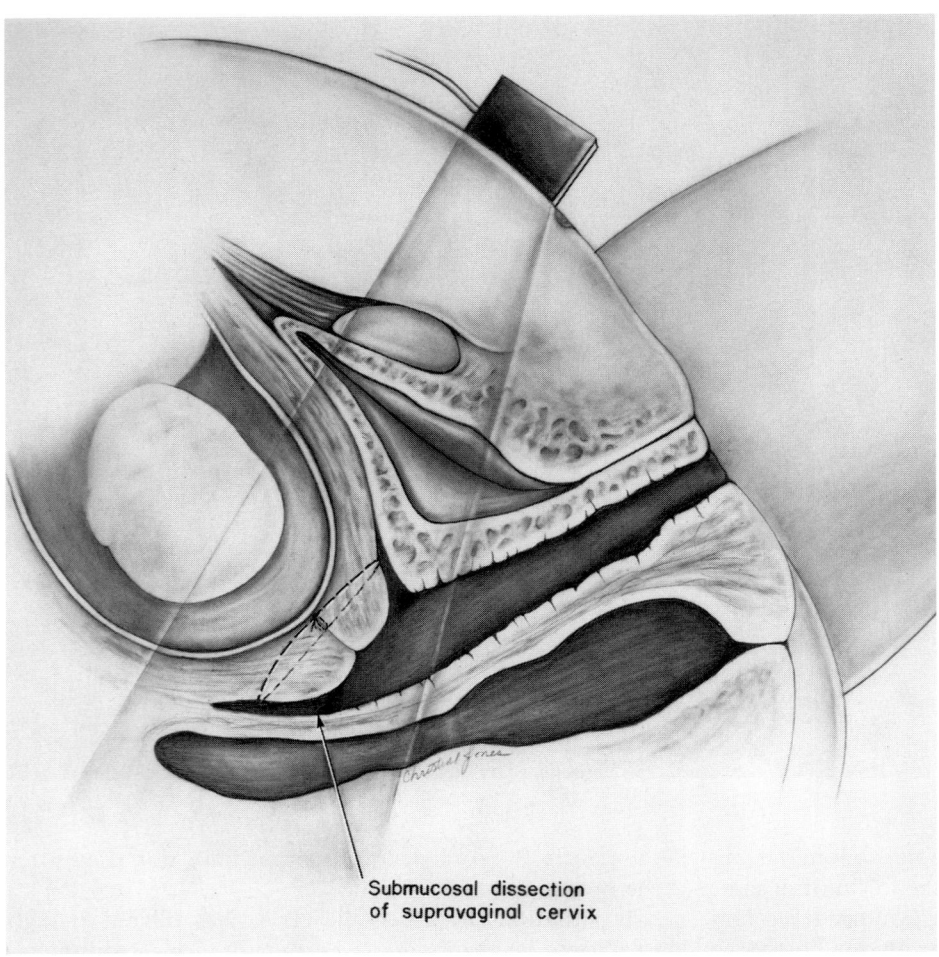

Submucosal dissection
of supravaginal cervix

Figure 19–5. Transvaginal cerclage under ultrasound guidance. (Modified from Ludmir J, Jackson GM, Samuels P: Transvaginal cerclage under ultrasound guidance in cases of severe cervical hypoplasia. Obstet Gynecol 78: 1067, 1991.)

the cervix to dilate secondary to cervical scarring and dystocia.[52] Although the risk of infection is minimal with a prophylactic cerclage, the risk increases significantly in cases of advanced dilatation with exposure of membranes to the birth canal.[69] Cervical cerclage displacement occurs in a small number of patients. We have not performed revision of the cerclage during the index pregnancy, although small series have reported successful surgical treatment of failed cerclage.[54] When the clinician is faced with premature rupture of membranes distant from term in a patient with cerclage, the decision to remove or leave the suture is controversial. Our own data suggests that with suture retention, there is an increased period of latency, at the expense of increased risk for neonatal sepsis and mortality.[75] These data have been recently challenged by reports suggesting increased latency period without increase in neonatal morbidity.[76,77] Decisions to remove the suture at time of ruptured membranes should be individualized until more information becomes available. Finally, even though cerclage placement is considered a benign procedure, a maternal death secondary to sepsis in a patient with retained cerclage has been reported.[78] The

liberal use of this surgical procedure should be carefully balanced against potential harm, in particular for patients in whom the indications for cerclage are not clear.

Efficacy of Cervical Cerclage

Most reports demonstrating improvement in pregnancy outcome with cerclage placement have done so by using each patient as her own historical control. Four prospective, randomized, controlled trials of cerclage, including one for multiple gestations, failed to demonstrate significant improvement in pregnancy outcome in patients receiving prophylactic cerclage.[79–82] Unfortunately, these trials did not involve patients with classic indications for cerclage, but used as criteria for randomization increased risk for preterm birth, or cases in which obstetricians were unsure as to whether a cerclage should be placed. The introduction of sonography in assessing the cervix during gestation will provide additional diagnostic criteria to help the clinician decide if therapeutic intervention with cerclage is indicated.[43–45] Initial information from ongoing randomized trials in patients at high risk for cervical incompetence do not demonstrate differences in preterm delivery between prophylactic cerclage versus sonographically indicated therapeutic cerclage.[43] Based on this new information, it seems prudent to incorporate cervical sonography in the management of patients at risk for cervical incompetence. Further recommendations regarding patient selection and treatment require continuing research in this evolving area.

MYOMECTOMY

Uterine myomas (fibroids) are the most common pelvic masses found in gestation. Myomas can increase in size during gestation, and place the patient at risk for preterm birth, abruption, dystocia, and bleeding.[83] When myomas outgrow their blood supply, they can develop cystic areas of red degeneration resulting in severe pain requiring nonsteroidal agents or narcotic medication.[83] Follow-up of myoma size by ultrasound has been studied extensively.[84] Lev-Toaff and colleagues[85] found that small fibroids increased in size during the second trimester, but during the third trimester, most fibroids decrease in size, regardless of their initial size. Most of the complications in pregnant patients with myomas are secondary to myoma location in the uterus.[86-88] The removal of a fibroid in pregnancy is contraindicated unless there is the presence of a pedunculated myoma twisting its stalk and giving the patient severe discomfort. Laparoscopic removal of this type of fibroid could be considered, but lack of experience with this situation precludes its routine use. The finding of myomas at time of cesarean section constitutes a challenge to the obstetrician.[88,89] If the myomas are encountered on the uterine incision line, careful myomectomy may be performed,[89] but may cause profuse bleeding and even may require hysterectomy to control hemorrhage. To avoid massive hemorrhage, routine myomectomy at time of cesarean section should be avoided; most myomas will involute in size in the nonpregnant state.

OOPHORECTOMY

The frequent use of ultrasound in early gestation has resulted in a significant number of asymptomatic adnexal masses diagnosed early in pregnancy. This knowledge creates a dilemma for the clinician: the appropriate management of an asymptomatic adnexal mass on the pregnant patient.[90] Ovarian masses in pregnancy could undergo torsion, rupture, and cause obstruction of labor (Fig. 19–6).[91] They also carry a small risk of malignancy.[92] If the clinical presentation is consistent with torsion, rupture, or hemorrhage, immediate surgical intervention is indicated. Hess and associates[91] found that if surgery for an adnexal mass was delayed until onset of severe symptoms, pregnancy outcome was worse compared with those patients that had elective surgery. If an adnexal mass is identified coincidentally at the time of cesarean section, Koonings and colleagues[93] advocate its removal including those smaller than 5 cm. In their study, only 2 of 41 masses smaller than 5 cm were functional cysts. Some authors have advocated aspiration and cytologic evaluation of cysts in selected cases. Rodin et al.[94] caution against this approach, in particular if the cyst is greater than 5 cm,

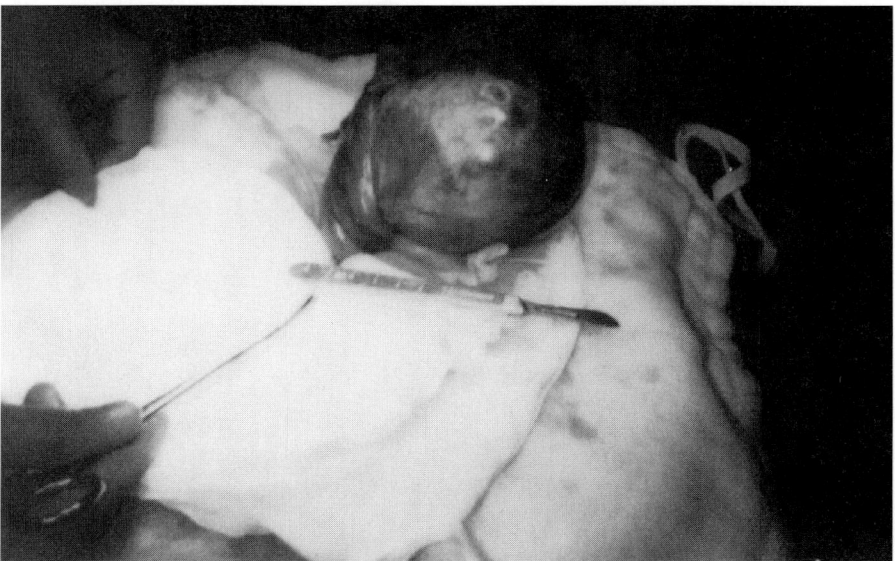

Figure 19–6. Laparotomy for 12-cm ovarian serous cystadenoma at 16 weeks' gestation.

Table 19–1. RISK OF OVARIAN MALIGNANCY BASED ON SONOGRAPHIC FINDINGS

Low risk of malignancy	Simple smooth wall cyst
	Size <5 cm
Increased risk of malignancy	Solid mass
	Nodules
	Thick septations
	Size >5 cm

because malignancy could be missed even with simple smooth-walled cysts. The patient with a simple sonographic cyst, smaller than 5 cm, has a very small risk for malignant change.[95] This patient can be followed during gestation without surgical intervention.[96,97] For those patients demonstrating masses greater that 5 cm, and with presence of solid elements, surgical intervention should be considered during the early second trimester, to minimize fetal risk. Surgery in the second trimester is felt to be the safest time to perform an oophorectomy or ovarian cystectomy via laparotomy. However, the risk of surgical intervention may favor a conservative approach on the basis of sonographic findings (Table 19–1). Laparoscopy offers a newer approach to the pregnant patient with an adnexal mass. A recent report by Soriano et al.[17] described 88 pregnant women who underwent 93 operations for suspected adnexal pathology. Laparoscopy was performed during the first trimester in 39 patients. The remaining 54 patients underwent laparotomy, 25 during the first trimester and 29 during the second trimester. The authors concluded that laparoscopic surgery during pregnancy appears to be safe in the management of adnexal masses, but cautioned against its liberal use until prospective controlled studies to determine the safety of this procedure in pregnancy are performed. We recently performed operative laparoscopy in a patient at 20 weeks' gestation presenting with symptoms of adnexal torsion (Fig. 19–7). On the basis of recent studies that seem to indicate that adnexal torsion can be safely managed by untwisting the ovarian pedicle,[98] we untwisted the adnexal mass laparoscopically and the patient continued with an uneventful pregnancy to term. With increased knowledge of the role of laparoscopy in pregnancy, the management of the adnexal mass in pregnancy may change in the future, favoring a laparoscopic approach instead of the traditional open laparotomy.

TUBAL STERILIZATION

Surgical approach to tubal sterilization is influenced by whether the procedure is being performed on a postpartum or on an interval basis. Advantages to the postpartum approach include the use of one anesthesia for labor, delivery, and sterilization, and only one hospital-

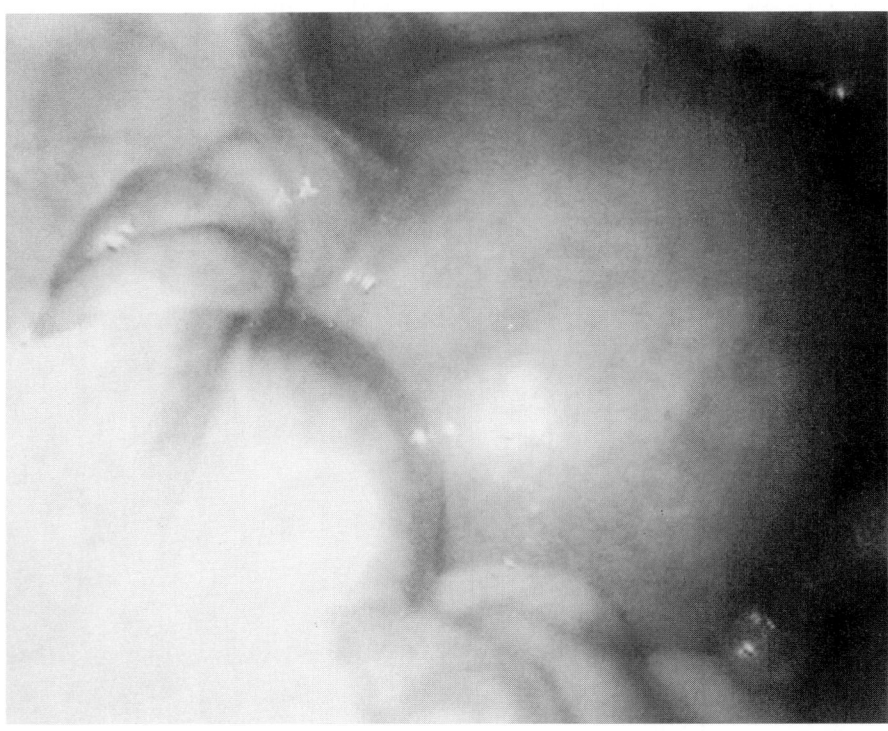

Figure 19–7. Laparoscopic appearance of adnexal torsion at 20 weeks' gestation.

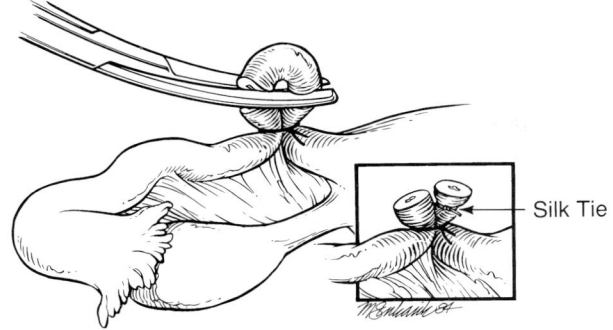

Figure 19–8. Pomeroy sterilization. A knuckle of tube is ligated with absorbable suture, and a small segment is being excised. Note that the ligation is performed at a site that will favor reanastomosis, should that become desirable. Some surgeons place an extra tie of nonabsorbable suture around the proximal stump as added protection against recanalization.

Silk Tie

ization.[99] Tubal ligations after vaginal delivery are performed through a minilaparotomy incision at the level of the uterine fundus, usually subumbilically. The same surgical techniques are applied if tubal ligation is performed at time of cesarean section. Interval sterilizations are performed by laparoscopy or minilaparotomy.

The choice of surgical approach influences the choice of methods of tubal occlusion. For example, most procedures performed via minilaparotomy use some type of partial salpingectomy technique as the method of tubal occlusion. Most laparoscopic sterilizations use either coagulation, application of silicone rubber bands, or application of clips as the method of tubal occlusion.[100] The long-term failure rate is approximately 1 percent overall.

Modified Pomeroy

The method of tubal occlusion used by Pomeroy was described in 1930,[101] and is the most popular means of postpartum tubal ligation because of its simplicity. The Pomeroy technique as originally described included grasping the fallopian tube at its midportion, creating a small knuckle, and then ligating the loop of tube with a double strand of No. 1 chromic catgut suture. It is critical that the fallopian tube be conclusively identified. Visualizing the fimbriated portion of the tube and identifying the round ligament as a separate structure can accomplish this. Absorbable sutures are used so that the tubal ends will separate quickly after surgery, leaving a gap between the proximal and distal ends. The most popular modification of the Pomeroy technique involves the use of No. 1 catgut suture instead of chromic catgut suture. Other modifications include placing nonabsorbable suture in the proximal ends of each resected tube. In performing the procedure, care should be taken to make the loop of fallopian tube sufficient in size to ensure that complete transection of the tubal

lumen will occur. After the loop of fallopian tube is ligated, the mesosalpinx of the ligated loop should be perforated using scissors, and the knuckle of the tube is transected (Fig. 19–8). It is important not to resect the fallopian tube so close to the suture that the remaining portion of the fallopian tube slips out of the ligature and causes delayed bleeding.

The Irving Procedure

Irving first reported his sterilization technique in 1924, with a modification in 1950.[102] In the modified procedure, a window is created in the mesosalpinx and the fallopian tube is doubly ligated with No. 1 chromic catgut. The fallopian tube is then transected approximately 4 cm from the uterotubal portion; the two free ends of the ligation stitch on the proximal tubal segment are held long. The proximal portion of the fallopian tube is dissected free from the mesosalpinx and then buried into the incision into the myometrium of the posterior uterine wall, near the uterotubal junction. This is accomplished by first creating a tunnel approximately 2 cm in length with a mosquito clamp in the uterine wall. The two free ends of the ligation stitch on the proximal tubal segment are then brought deep into the myometrial tunnel, and brought out through the uterine serosa. Traction is then placed on the sutures to

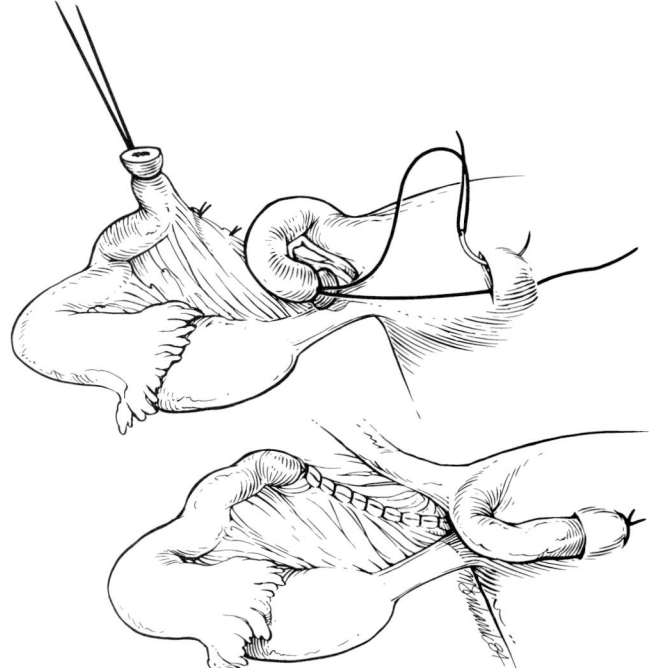

Figure 19–9. Irving sterilization. The tube is transected 3 to 4 cm from its insertion, and a short tunnel is created by means of a sharp-nosed hemostat in either the anterior or posterior uterine wall. The cut end of the tube can then be buried in the tunnel and, if necessary, further secured by an interrupted suture at the opening of the tunnel. The distal cut end is buried between the leaves of the broad ligament.

draw the proximal tubal stump into the myometrial tunnel; tying the free sutures fixes the tube in that location. No treatment of the distal tubal stump is necessary, but some choose to bury the segment in the mesosalpinx (Fig. 19–9). Although this technique is slightly more complicated than the others, it has the lowest failure rate.[103]

The Uchida Procedure

In this sterilization procedure,[104] the fallopian tube muscular portion is separated from its serosal cover and grasped approximately 6 to 7 cm from the uterotubal junction, saline solution is injected subserosally, and the serosa is then incised. The muscular portion of the fallopian tube is grasped with a clamp and divided. The serosa over the proximal tubal segment is bluntly dissected toward the uterus, exposing approximately 5 cm

of the proximal tubal segment. The tube is then ligated with chromic suture near the uterotubal junction, and approximately 5 cm of the tube is resected. The shortened proximal tubal stump is allowed to retract into the mesosalpinx. The serosa around the opening in the mesosalpinx is sutured in a purse-string with a fine absorbable stitch; when the suture is tied the mesosalpinx is gathered around the distal tubal segment (Fig. 19–10). Some surgeons choose to excise only 1 cm of fallopian tube rather than the recommended 5 cm in case the patient wishes tubal reanastomosis in the future.

Kroener Fimbriectomy

This technique consists of excising the distal tube and fimbriae and ligating the cut ends of the tube with silk sutures. In one series, the failure rate was 3 percent.

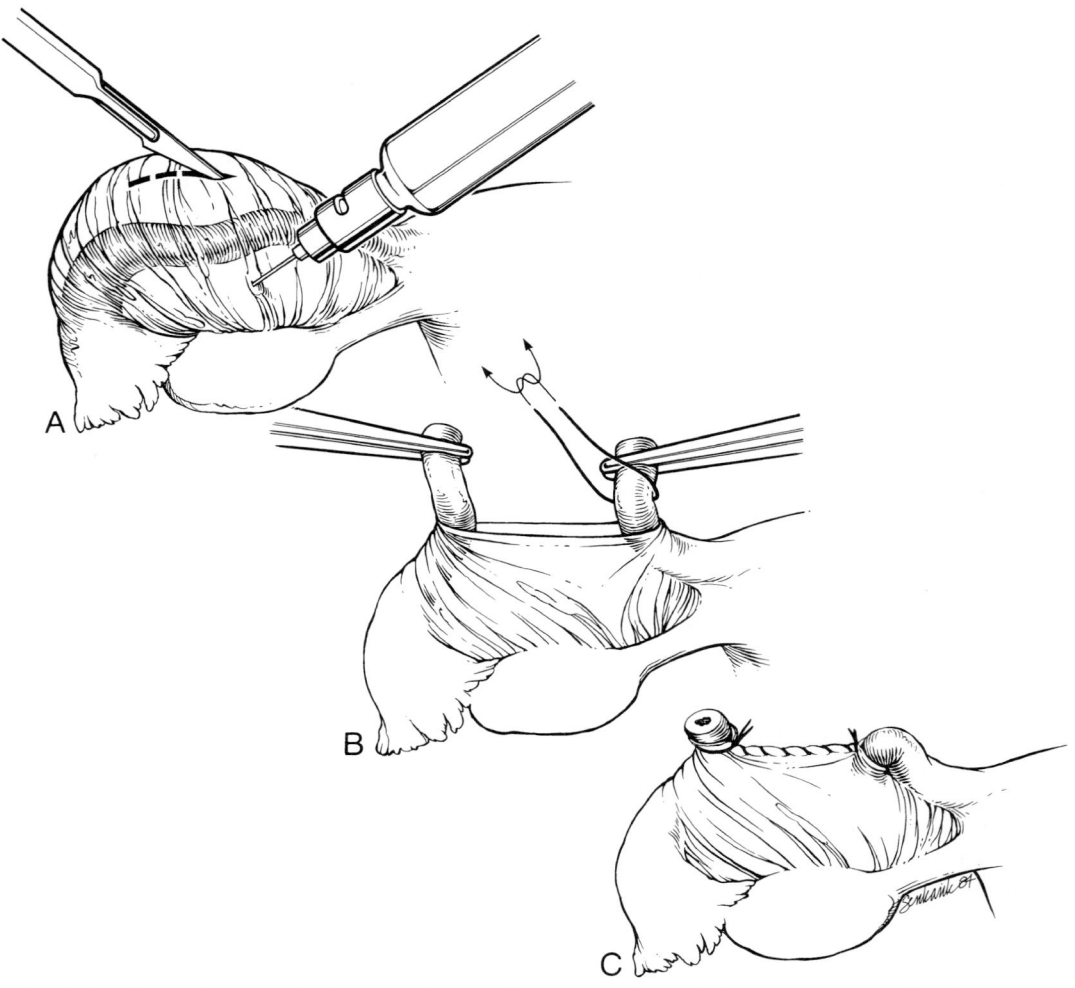

Figure 19–10. Uchida sterilization. The leaves of the broad ligament and peritubal peritoneum are infiltrated with saline so that the tube can be easily isolated from these structures, divided, and ligated. The broad ligament is then closed, burying the proximal stump between the leaves and including the distal stump in the line of closure.

SPECIFIC SURGICAL PROBLEMS IN PREGNANCY

Appendicitis

Appendicitis is one of the most common surgical complications of pregnancy, with an incidence of 1 to 2 per 1,000 gestations.[105] This incidence is roughly similar to that in the nonpregnant population. There is no evidence that pregnancy appears to increase the risk for appendicitis.[106] Baer in 1932[107] described the change in appendiceal location as pregnancy progresses with upper displacement of the appendix with advancing gestation (Fig. 19–11). The change in appendiceal location with advancing gestation would change the location of perceived pain toward the patient's right upper quadrant or right flank. Mourad et al.,[108] in a retrospective review of 66,993 deliveries, found 68 pregnancies complicated by appendicitis, and challenged this concept. Pain in the right lower quadrant of the abdomen was

the most common symptom of appendicitis regardless of gestational age. The diagnosis of appendicitis in pregnancy is difficult secondary to a clinical picture mimicking common symptoms in gestation including nausea, vomiting, and abdominal discomfort.[109]

Early in the course of appendicitis, temperature and pulse rate may be normal; later, a low-grade temperature elevation or even a normal temperature may be present. Only 20 percent of patients exhibit rectal or vaginal tenderness. The normal leukocytosis of pregnancy (14,000/mm³) might mask appendicitis. Radiographic studies are rarely helpful, but most recently ultrasound and CT scan of the abdomen have been advocated as another objective way of making the diagnosis.[14,110] Even though the diagnosis is only found in 50 percent of patients undergoing surgery, it is better to operate unnecessarily rather than postpone surgery until generalized peritonitis has developed. Surgery can minimize maternal–fetal morbidity by preventing progression to appendiceal rupture and peritonitis.[105,106,109] Fetal mortality is low when acute appendicitis is diagnosed and treated, but could rise significantly in the presence of peritonitis. Maternal death may occur in the presence of peritonitis and overwhelming intra-abdominal sepsis. Mazze and Kallen, using the Swedish registry of surgery during pregnancy, performed a review of 778 cases of appendectomy during gestation.[105] The diagnosis was confirmed in 64 percent of cases. These findings showed an increase in the risk for delivery the week after appendectomy when the operation was performed after 23 weeks' gestation. Cesarean section is rarely indicated at the time of appendectomy. A recent abdominal incision presents no problem during labor and vaginal delivery. Recently, several small case series of laparoscopic appendectomies in pregnancy have been reported demonstrating success during all trimesters, without complications (Fig. 19–12).[15,18,19,111] Some investigators note that laparoscopy expands the ability to explore the abdomen with less uterine manipulation. Further studies evaluating laparoscopic appendectomy in pregnancy are necessary prior to determining the safety of this procedure.

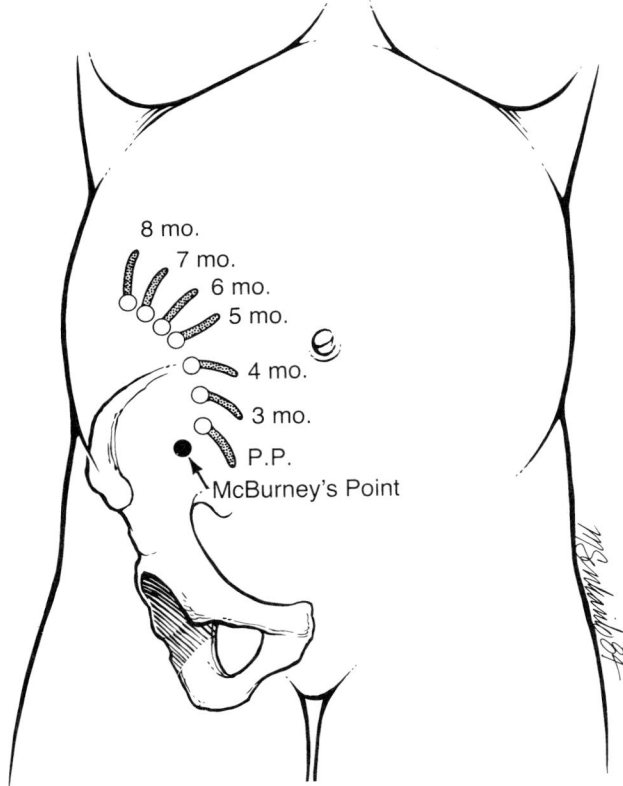

8 mo.
7 mo.
6 mo.
5 mo.
4 mo.
3 mo.
P.P.
McBurney's Point

Figure 19–11. Locations of the appendix in pregnancy. As modified from Bauer et al., the approximate location of the appendix during succeeding months of pregnancy is diagrammed. In planning an operation, it is better to make the abdominal incision over the point of maximum tenderness unless there is a great disparity between that point and the theoretical location of the appendix. (Modified from Baer JL, Reis RA, Arens RA: Appendicitis in pregnancy with changes in position and axis of the normal appendix in pregnancy. JAMA 98: 1359, 1932.)

Acute Cholecystitis

After appendicitis, biliary tract disease is the second most common general surgical condition encountered in pregnant women. Its incidence varies from 1 in 2,000 to 1 in 4,000 pregnancies.[112] Pregnancy increases the risk of gallstones, probably secondary to high progesterone levels that inhibit smooth muscle contractility. This results in greater gallbladder volume with retention of cholesterol crystals prerequisite for gallstone formation.[113]

Cholecystitis during pregnancy usually develops when

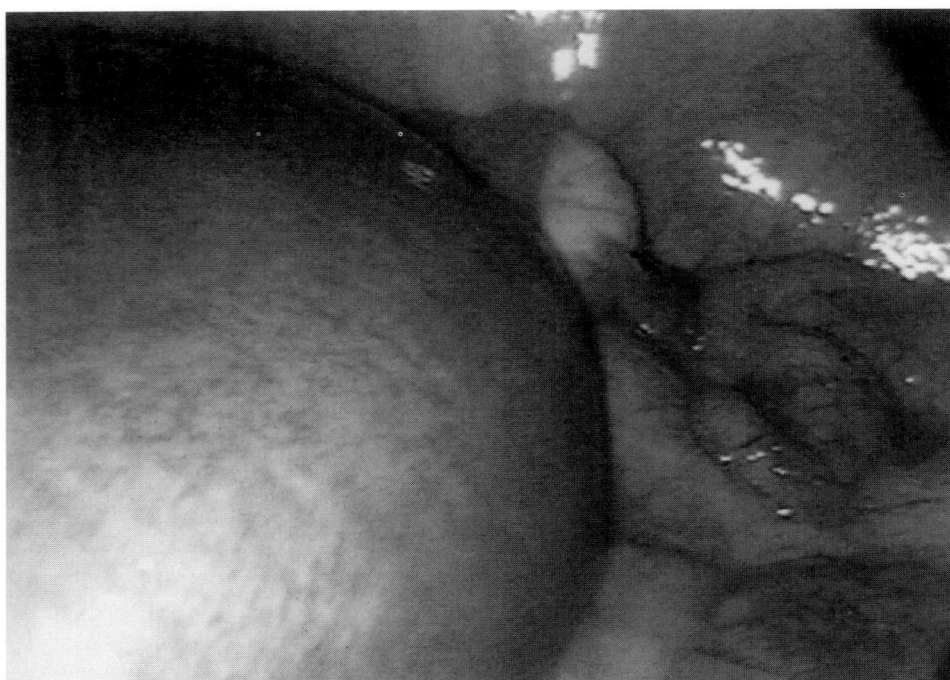

Figure 19–12. Laparoscopic appearance of appendix at 18 weeks' gestation.

there is obstruction of the cystic duct. This clinical entity ranges from intermediate attacks of biliary colic to persistent pain radiating into the subcapsular area in cases where the common duct is obstructed by a stone. There is usually right subcostal tenderness along with a low-grade fever. Ultrasound is helpful in detecting the presence of stones as small as 2 mm, and confirms the diagnosis of gallstones in about 90 percent of patients.[11] The differential diagnoses for cholecystitis include conditions unique to pregnancy such as acute fatty liver of pregnancy and severe preeclampsia. Initial attacks of cholecystitis should be treated conservatively, with intravenous fluids, nasogastric suction, antibiotics, and antispasmodics. Without prompt resolution of symptoms, surgery should be considered. Eighty percent of patients with an initial attack will get relief with conservative medical treatment. In the presence of common duct obstruction or pancreatitis, cholecystectomy is necessary and should not be delayed.[114]

Laparoscopic cholecystectomies have revolutionized the management of the pregnant patient with cholecystitis.[16,115,116] Small case series demonstrate the same good outcomes compared with open laparotomies. Our own experience demonstrates that delaying surgery for cholecystitis results in increased perinatal morbidity, with lower morbidity found in those patients managed surgically, particularly in cases of bile duct obstruction.[117] Larger studies are needed to recommend the laparoscopic approach to cholecystectomy in pregnancy, once the diagnosis of cholecystitis is made.[115,118]

Intestinal Obstruction

The incidence of bowel obstruction in pregnancy is similar to that of the general population, approximately 1 in 3,000 deliveries.[119] Intestinal obstruction usually involves the small bowel, and is commonly caused by an adhesive band or hernia (Table 19–2).[120] Prior abdominal and pelvic surgery are the most frequent causes for intestinal obstruction. Ludmir et al.[121] reported a case of spontaneous bowel obstruction in a patient carrying triplets, without risk factors for bowel obstruction. Intestinal obstruction is a grave complication of pregnancy and results from pressure of the growing uterus on intestinal adhesions. Patients with bowel obstruction

Table 19–2. CAUSES OF INTESTINAL OBSTRUCTION IN PREGNANCY

Cause	%
Adhesions	60
Volvulus	25
Ileus	8
Intussusception	5
Hernia, appendicitis	6

From Perdue PW, Johnston HW Jr, Stafford PW: Intestinal obstruction complicating pregnancy. Am J Surg 164:384, 1992, with permission.

present with colicky midabdominal pain associated with hyperactive peristalsis. Nausea and vomiting is found in 80 percent of cases as reported by Perdue et al.[122] As time passes, the intestinal peristalsis decreases and the abdomen finally becomes silent. Bowel distention may be marked, and difficult to access in pregnancy. Limited radiography are clearly indicated. In cases of small bowel obstruction, radiologic findings include dilatation of small bowel loops with air–fluid levels. Initial treatment of intestinal distention includes decompression with nasogastric tube or long tube, adequate fluid resuscitation, and correction of electrolyte imbalance. Perdue and colleagues reported a maternal mortality rate of 6 percent primarily caused by sepsis and shock, with a 26 percent incidence of fetal demise. If after 6 to 8 hours of treatment there is no satisfactory patient response, laparotomy should be performed before bowel necrosis and perforation occur. The uterus rarely interferes with the surgery, and if preterm labor follows the procedure, tocolytics can be used.

Ogilvie's syndrome, or pseudo-obstruction of the colon, is caused by an adynamic colonic ileus; about 10 percent of cases follow delivery. The syndrome is characterized by massive abdominal distention with cecal dilation. Laparotomy may be indicated,[117] and colonoscopy for decompression has been described in a postpartum patient.[123]

Trauma

Trauma from accidental injuries complicates 6 to 7 percent of all pregnancies.[124] The majority of these patients suffer only minor injuries and would not require hospital admission in the absence of pregnancy.[125] Unfortunately, trauma is the leading nonobstetric cause of maternal mortality, accounting for 20 percent of maternal deaths.[126] Fort and Harlen report that the risk of fetal demise from major blunt trauma increases from 8.7 percent in the first trimester, to 40 to 50 percent during the second and third trimesters.[127] Poole and associates,[128] in a recent study of trauma in pregnancy, determined that 31.5 percent of patients were victims of domestic violence, in most cases from the husband or boyfriend. The authors concluded that interpersonal violence during pregnancy is an increasingly common cause of maternal injury.

Automobile restraint systems with a shoulder harness prevent forward flexion of the maternal torso, and when used correctly reduce fetal death rates by preventing ejection of the mother from the vehicle. A waist-type seat belt can produce distortion of the uterus produced by the sudden compression of the belt resulting in placental abruption (Fig. 19–13).[129,130] Blunt trauma may result in rupture of the membranes and preterm labor. Placental abruption is the most common cause of fetal demise when the maternal injuries are not lethal.[131] The placenta separation may manifest at the time of injury or later, with the great majority of them in the first 24 hours. For this reason, even moderate blunt trauma should be an indication for fetal heart rate monitoring and close observation.[132–134]

Uterine rupture resulting from trauma is an infrequent event reported in about 0.6 percent of trauma cases in pregnancy.[124] In early pregnancy, the uterus is resistant to injury, but after the first trimester the uterus becomes an abdominal organ and is susceptible to injury. Prompt diagnosis of rupture is imperative to reduce the risk of maternal and fetal mortality. It is important to emphasize that normal vital signs in the mother do not preclude the possibility of uterine rupture, and fetal heart rate abnormalities could be the first sign of a rupture.

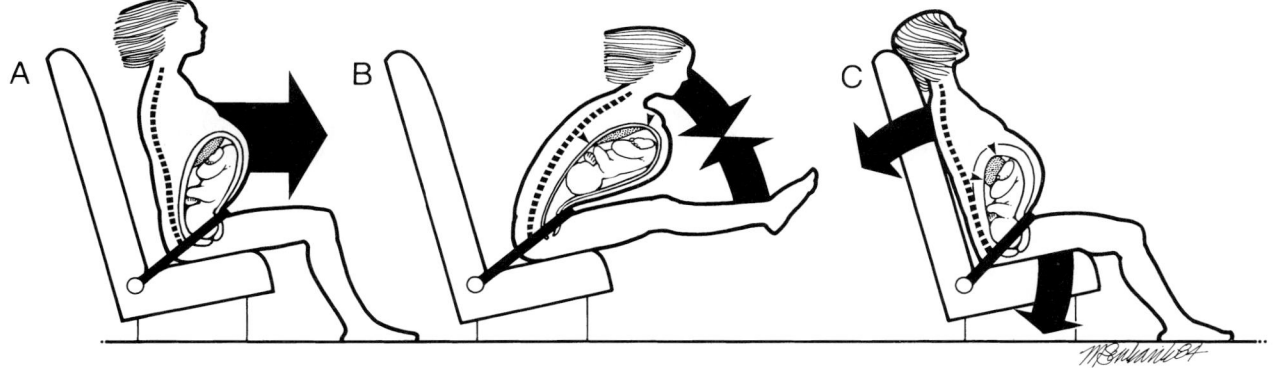

Figure 19–13. Seat belt injury. The mechanisms by which placental separation might be produced by a waist-type seat belt are illustrated. *A*, The force of a collision propels the body forward. *B*, Acute flexion of the trunk results in elongation of the uterus, including elongation of the site of placental attachment. *C*, As the trunk recoils, the placental site is shortened and the posterior wall of the uterus collides with the vertebral column. (Redrawn from Lees DH, Singer A: Gynecologic Survey. Vol 6. London, Wolfe Medical, 1983, with permission.)

Penetrating injuries to the maternal upper abdomen may cause damage to intra-abdominal organs. Franger et al. recommended conservative management of the these injuries if (1) the mother is hemodynamically stable, (2) the entrance wound is below the uterine fundus, (3) there is no evidence of blood in the gastrointestinal and urinary tracts, and (4) the bullet can be demonstrated within the uterus.[135]

Management of the pregnant trauma patient requires a team effort and complete understanding of the physiologic changes unique to gestation. Initially, the "ABCs" (airway, breathing, and circulation) should be assessed. If possible, the injured pregnant woman who is more than 20 weeks' gestation should be kept in the lateral decubitus position. Once the maternal vital signs have been stabilized, appropriate diagnostic studies to rule out internal injury, including CT scan and MRI are performed, if necessary. Fetal assessment with continuous electronic monitoring is advocated, as well as uterine contraction monitoring.[133,134] Possible placental abruption is predicted by using continuous electronic monitoring and findings of frequent uterine contractions.[124]

The American College of Obstetricians and Gynecologists (ACOG) recommends that any pregnant woman sustaining trauma beyond 22 to 24 weeks' gestation should undergo fetal monitoring for a minimum of 24 hours. In the presence of ruptured membranes, bleeding, fetal arrhythmia, fetal heart rate deceleration, or more than four contractions per hour, the patient should be admitted with continuous fetal monitoring for at least 24 hours.[136] Ultrasound is useful to determine gestational age, to determine fetal well-being if monitoring is equivocal, and to confirm fetal death.

A recent study attempted to elucidate risk factors that would predict adverse outcome in pregnant trauma patients, and would require monitoring greater than 4 to 6 hours. Curet and colleagues[137] studied 271 pregnant patients admitted after blunt trauma. The following risk factors were predictive of fetal death: ejections, motorcycle and pedestrian collisions, maternal death, maternal tachycardia, abnormal fetal heart rate, and lack of restraints. Risk factors significantly predictive for contractions or preterm labor included assaults and pedestrian collisions.

Several studies have established that fetal maternal hemorrhage is increased in women who have suffered trauma in pregnancy.[124] The use of the Kleihauer-Betke test is advocated in particular in RhD-negative women, so adequate anti-D immune globulin can be administered. The role of a routine Kleihauer-Betke test after trauma in predicting adverse outcome is not clear. A recent study by Pak et al. found negative results in all 85 pregnant patients with blunt abdominal trauma that had a Kleihauer-Betke test.[134]

Burns

Thermal burns occur with the same frequency as in the nonpregnant state. Most authors feel that pregnancy does not alter the chances for survival.[138,139] Amy et al.[138] reported that mothers with second- and third-degree burns involving less than 20 percent body surface area, as well as their fetuses, survived the burn period. Of the mothers with 20 to 50 percent body surface area burns, all survived but the fetal survival rate was only 70 percent because of frequent preterm delivery. Burns greater than 50 percent body surface area were associated with high mortality rate, with subsequent high fetal death rate. Complications such as inhalation injury with hypoxemia, sepsis, and hypovolemic shock require aggressive management of maternal airway and fluid status with concurrent assessment of fetal condition. These patients are at high risk for preterm delivery, and the severely burned patient may not tolerate the use of tocolytic agents.[140]

LAPAROSCOPY IN PREGNANCY

Laparoscopic surgery has revolutionized the management of many surgical disorders.[15-22] However, during the 1980s and early 1990s, pregnancy remained a relative contraindication to laparoscopy, with most surgeons performing open laparotomy. As more case reports and small series of laparoscopic surgery in pregnancy appeared in the literature, the initial reluctance by surgeons for this approach changed to one of cautious optimism.[15,116,141] Laparoscopy offers several advantages over traditional laparotomy,[15,18,20] including better visualization, especially with small incisions. Total operative time for laparoscopic procedures is less, and postoperative pain is reduced (see the box "Advantages of Laparoscopic Surgery"). Unfortunately, access

---

Advantages of Laparoscopic Surgery

Better visualization
Small incision
Less pain
Less operative time
Postoperative convalescence reduced
Less use of postoperative analgesics
Earlier ambulation
Decreased risk of thromboembolic disease
Shorter hospital stay

Relative Contraindications to Laparoscopy in Pregnancy

Access issues
  Late second or third trimester
  Multiple gestations
  Advanced disease process (e.g., walled-off abscess)
  Retrocecal location of appendix
Medical complications
  Intra-abdominal sepsis
  Bleeding disorders
  Ileus

Laparoscopy During Pregnancy Guidelines (SAGES)

Pneumatic compression devices
Lead shield with selective fluoroscopy
Dependent position
Obstetric consultation
Intraoperative fetal monitoring
Minimal pneumoperitoneum (8–12 mm Hg)
Serial arterial blood gas analysis
Second-trimester deferment
Open technique

Modified from Guidelines for laparoscopic surgery during Pregnancy. Surg Endosc 4:100, 1998.

issues in late and second or third trimester in pregnancy are still considered a relative contraindication to this approach (see the box "Relative Contraindications to Laparoscopy in Pregnancy"). Limited published physiologic data exist concerning maternal–fetal interactions during laparoscopic surgery.[142,143] The normally decreased maternal $PaCO_2$ during pregnancy may be important in ensuring adequate transplacental CO_2 diffusion from the fetus to the mother. CO_2 pneumoperitoneum may cause maternal and fetal hypercarbia because of decreased maternal ventilation and increased transplacental CO_2 absorption by the mother. Hunter and associates, studying pregnant ewes,[143] demonstrated that carbon dioxide pneumoperitoneum induced maternal hypercarbia, which led to fetal hypercarbia, acidosis, and tachycardia when pneumoperitoneum pressure exceeded 15 mm Hg. These effects were minimized by using a low pneumoperitoneum pressure or by using nitrous oxide as the distending gaseous agent. The significance of these findings for humans is debatable, but on the basis of these findings, in 1998, the Society of American Gastrointestinal Endoscopic Surgeons (SAGES) published a list of guidelines for laparoscopic surgery during pregnancy (see the box "Laparoscopy During Pregnancy Guidelines [SAGES]").[144] Affleck et al.[19] have recently modified these criteria, recommend-

ing a maternal end-tidal CO_2 within physiologic range (30 to 40 mm Hg) instead of performing serial arterial blood gases, and raising the pneumoperitoneum pressure from a minimal of 8 to 12 mm Hg to a pressure of 10 to 15 mm Hg. These authors also recommend the use of tocolytic agents only for uterine irritability and not prophylactically.[19]

Laparoscopic appendectomy during pregnancy continues to be controversial. Case reports and small series have reported success during all trimesters, when compared with an open approach.[18,141,145] In the largest series to date of laparoscopic appendectomies in pregnancy, Affleck et al. reported 19 patients.[19] Six underwent surgery in the first trimester, nine in the second, and four in the third. Three patients delivered preterm, one prior to 35 weeks. There were no uterine injuries, spontaneous abortions, or fetal losses (Table 19–3).

Several small series of laparoscopic cholecystectomies in pregnancy suggest that the procedure may be performed safely, without major complications.[18,19,146,147] In an attempt to analyze a large number of patients undergoing cholecystectomy in pregnancy, Barone et al.[115] obtained data from the Connecticut Laparoscopic

Table 19–3. LAPAROSCOPIC APPENDECTOMY VARIABLES

	Term, n = 16	Preterm, n = 3	p Value
Patient age	26.3 ± 5.3	27 ± 2.6	NS (0.9)
Gestational age at surgery	16.4 ± 7.7	21.7 ± 10.9	NS (0.4)
Length OR (min)	51 ± 12.9	58 ± 25.5	NS (0.4)
Pathology, number positive	10/16	1/3	NS (0.5)
Fetal losses	0	0	NS

Modified from Affleck DG, Handrahan DL, Egger MJ, et al: The laparoscopic management of appendicitis and cholelithiasis during pregnancy. Am J Surg 178:523, 1999.

Table 19–4. CHOLECYSTECTOMY DURING PREGNANCY

	Laparoscopic, n = 20	Open, n = 26	p Value
Maternal age	25.4 ± 9.9	24.8 ± 4.7	NS (0.78)
Gestational age at surgery	18.4 ± 6.7	23.7 ± 6.5	0.01
Duration of procedure (min)	82.8 ± 37.9	118.5 ± 145.4	NS (0.20)
Gestational age at delivery (weeks)	39.3 ± 1.4	38.3 ± 3.8	NS (0.27)

Modified from Barone JE, Bears S, Chen S, et al: Outcome study of cholecystectomy during pregnancy. Am J Surg 177:232, 1999.

Cholecystectomy Registry and data from the Connecticut Hospital Association for the years 1992 through 1996. Complete data were available for 46 patients, 20 laparoscopic and 26 open cases (Table 19–4). The groups were comparable, except for the timing of cholecystectomy, which was performed earlier for the laparoscopic group, 18.4 ± 6.7 weeks, compared with 24.0 ± 4.7 weeks for the open cases. The authors concluded that laparoscopic cholecystectomy does not lead to increased numbers of fetal complications; furthermore, preterm labor was more common in the open cholecystectomy group (eight vs. one, p = 0.057) compared with the laparoscopy group. Unfortunately, this large study found a maternal fatality 2 weeks after laparoscopic cholecystectomy at 20 weeks. The death was secondary to intra-abdominal hemorrhage, but the source of bleeding could not be identified. Complications from laparoscopic surgery are well recognized and should always be considered (Table 19–5). On the basis of this experience, it seems prudent that when a laparoscopic approach to appendectomy or cholecystectomy is considered during pregnancy, specific guidelines for monitoring maternal and fetal condition should be established in individual institutions.[19,115] Large studies with long-term follow-up of infants exposed to laparoscopy in utero are needed before establishing the true safety of this surgical procedure.

Table 19–5. LAPAROSCOPIC COMPLICATIONS

Anesthesia Related	Procedure Related
Failed endotracheal intubation	Abdominal wall hematoma
Gastric aspiration	Bladder or bowel perforation
Cardiac arrhythmias	Vascular injury
(SVT, PVC)	Peritonitis/sepsis
Cardiac arrest	Ureteral injuries
	Urinary retention
	Vesicocutaneous fistula
	Pneumothorax
	Hypercarbia
	Hypotension
	Hemorrhage

FERTILITY CONTROL AND HEALTH

Pregnancy can result in illness and death. The U.S. maternal mortality rate is about 9 per 100,000 live births. Risk of death from legal abortion in the United States is less than 1 death per 100,000 induced abortions.[148] Pregnancy risk for women with preexisting illnesses can be much greater. Women in their 40s are seven times more likely to die in pregnancy than are women in their early 20s, the safest time to have a baby.[149] Fertility control, or lack of it, also impacts on child health. When pregnancies are too close together, the risk of prematurity and perinatal mortality increase.[150] Higher order births to young mothers are at very great risk. Second births to mothers under 20 are more likely to be premature and to die than are first-born children, and the risk is still higher for a third-born infant to a woman under 20.[151,152]

Legal Abortion and Voluntary Control of Fertility

Modern methods of contraception can be highly effective but fail more often than we usually appreciate. Only about half of U.S. pregnancies are intended.[153] Young people are much more likely to experience contraceptive failure[154] because they are more fertile, and because they are more likely to have unexpected intercourse. Contraception is preventive medicine, and as such requires advance motivation. Abortion, on the other hand, is sought after the fact, when pregnancy has occurred. For all of these reasons, induced abortion is essential for a high level of voluntary control of fertility.

History of Abortion

Some means for attempting abortion can be found in all cultural groups and are evident in the artifacts of ancient civilizations.[155,156] Folk methods in use today include ingested wild plants, insertion of sticks through the cervix into the uterus, and forceful massage of the uterus.[157] Abortion was common in the 19th century United States. The complications of these procedures, and the competition from lay abortionists, so concerned the "regular" physicians that medical societies carried out intensive campaigns that resulted in the passage of laws making abortion illegal in most states by the end of the century.[158] These laws remained on the books until 1973, when the Supreme Court legalized abortion throughout the land.[158]

Duty of Health Professionals

As health professionals, we have a duty "to put health first, to do so by respecting the best available scientific evidence, and to be frank when we put aside such evidence for other considerations, be they moral, or religious, or economic, or simply expedient."[159] We are not required to perform abortions if this is against our ethical principles, but we have a duty to our patients to help them assess pregnancy risks and make appropriate referrals.

LEGAL ABORTION IN THE UNITED STATES

Overview

Approximately 1,200,000 abortions are reported to the Centers for Disease Control each year in the United States, a number that has been declining since 1990. In 1996, the national abortion ratio was 314 abortions for every 1,000 live births, and the national abortion rate was 20 per 1,000 women aged 15 to 44.[148] The majority of women who obtain abortions are unmarried (78.7 percent in 1996), and the ratio of abortions to live births is eight times higher for unmarried women than for married women. Utilization of abortion varies markedly with age. Twenty percent of women obtaining abortions were 19 or younger and 52 percent were 24 or younger in 1996. In 1996, the abortion ratio for women under 15 was 723 per 1,000 live births, almost as many abortions as births (Fig. 19–14). Abortion ratios for black women are almost three times those for whites, although 59 percent of abortions nationally are performed for white women.[148]

Risk of death from legal abortion in the United States is 0.7 per 100,000 induced abortions. The risk of death from legal abortion prior to 16 weeks is 5- to 10-fold less than that from continuing the pregnancy. As shown in Table 19–6, the risk of death increases with gestational age.[160] For individual women with high-risk conditions, for example, cyanotic heart disease, even late abortion is undoubtedly a safer alternative. Because of the availability of low-cost, out-of-hospital first-trimester abortion, 88 percent of legal abortions are performed in the first trimester, when abortion is the safest.[148] Type of procedure also determines risk. First-trimester abortions are virtually all performed by vacuum curettage; however, early medical abortion induced with methotrexate/misoprostol is practiced in some centers, and may increase when mifepristone, the antiprogesterone, becomes available in the United States. Currently, 93 percent of abortions after 12 weeks are performed by variations of "dilatation and evacuation" (D&E), the surgical evacuation of the uterus through the vagina.[148] Risk of death from abortion by the various techniques at different gestational ages is given in Table 19–7. The data clearly show the greater safety of D&E over other procedures, especially in the early midtrimester. Anesthesia is another determinant of risk. General anesthesia increases the risk for perforation of the uterus, visceral injury, hemorrhage,

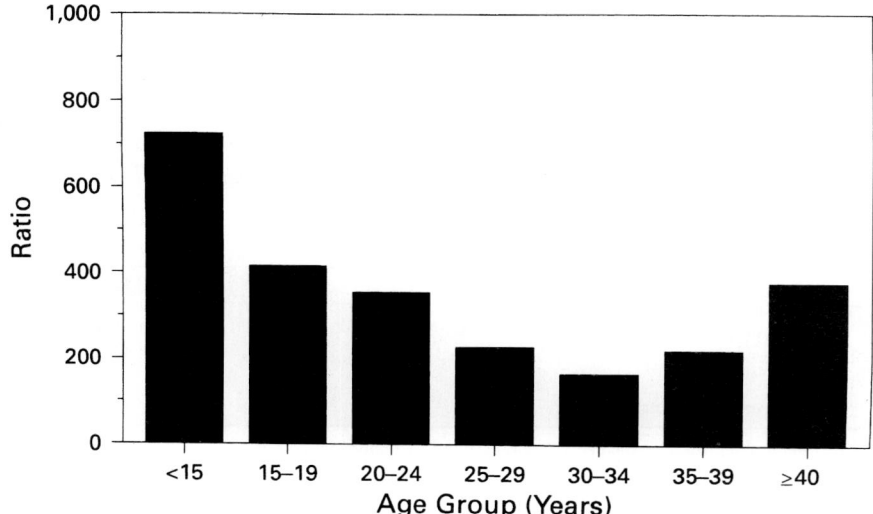

Figure 19–14. Abortion ratio (per 1,000 live births by age group—United States 1996). (From Koonin LM, Strauss LT, Chrisman CE, et al: Abortion surveillance. United States, 1996. MMWR Morb Mortal Wkly Rep 48:1, 1999.)

Table 19–6. DEATH TO CASE RATES FOR LEGAL ABORTION MORTALITY BY WEEKS OF GESTATION, UNITED STATES, 1972–1987

Weeks of Gestation	Deaths	Abortions	Rate*	Relative Risk
≤8 weeks	33	8,673,759	0.4	Referent
9–10	39	4,847,321	0.8	2.1
11–12	33	2,360,768	1.4	3.7
13–15	28	962,185	2.9	7.7
16–20	74	794,093	9.3	24.5
≥21	21	175,395	12.0	31.5

* Legal abortion deaths per 100,000 procedures; excludes deaths from ectopic pregnancies or pregnancy with gestation length unknown.
From Lawson HW, Frye A, Atrash HK, et al: Abortion mortality, United States, 1972–1987. Am J Obstet Gynecol 171:1365, 1994, with permission.

hysterectomy, and death.[161–163] Paracervical block augmented with conscious sedation is preferred.

Benefits of Legal Abortion

In the 1940s, more than 1,000 women died each year from abortion complications.[164] In 1996, the last year for which complete data are available, there were 17 deaths from spontaneous abortion, 10 deaths from abortion legally induced, and no deaths from illegal abortion (abortion induced by a nonprofessional) in the entire United States.[148] The American Medical Association attributes the decline in deaths to the introduction of antibiotics; the widespread use of effective contraception beginning in the 1960s, which reduced the number of unwanted pregnancies; and more recently, the shift from illegal to legal abortion.[165]

Indications for Abortion

Since 1973, the only legal condition necessary for abortion in the first trimester is that the woman consult with her physician. The critical question has become: when should abortion of a **desired** pregnancy be recommended on medical grounds? In some situations, for example, congenital heart disease with pulmonary hypertension, the risk of death in late pregnancy is so great that any prudent physician would recommend abortion. Similarly, if major fetal malformation leaves no hope for meaningful life, most would recommend abortion. However, in the majority of cases of maternal illness or fetal malformation, the patient and her family can determine how much risk they are willing to take and make their own informed choice with medical advice. Tables 19–8 and 19–9 list some fetal and maternal indications for abortion of a desired pregnancy.[166] This list is meant only as a guide, and is by no means all inclusive.

First-Trimester Abortion

Dilatation and curettage is an ancient procedure.[155] Vacuum curettage was described for the first time by two Chinese physicians in 1954.[167] The vacuum technique was introduced in England in the 1960s and then brought to the United States by Burdick. After 1973, it quickly became the procedure of choice. Subsequent comparative trials have demonstrated that vacuum curettage is quicker, less traumatic, and safer than sharp curettage.[168]

Table 19–7. DEATH TO CASE RATES* FOR LEGAL ABORTIONS BY TYPE OF PROCEDURE AND WEEKS OF GESTATION, UNITED STATES, 1974–1987

Procedure	Weeks of Gestation					
	≤8	9–10	11–12	13–15	16–20	≥21
Vacuum curettage†	0.3	0.7	1.1	NA	NA	NA
D & E	NA	NA	NA	2.0	6.5	11.9
Instillation‡	—	—	—	3.8	7.9	10.3
Hysterectomy/hysterotomy	18.3	30.0	41.2	28.1	103.4	274.3

* Legal induced abortion deaths per 100,000 legal induced abortions.
† Includes all suction and sharp curettage procedures.
‡ Includes all instillation methods (saline, prostaglandin, other).
From Lawson HW, Frye A, Atrash HK, et al: Abortion mortality, United States, 1972–1987. Am J Obstet Gynecol 171:1365, 1994, with permission.

Table 19–8. FETAL INDICATIONS FOR TERMINATION OF A DESIRED PREGNANCY

Category	Examples
Known major fetal malformation	Anencephaly, myelomeningocele, severe hydrocephaly, porencephaly, severe cardiac disease, bilateral cystic kidney disease
Chromosomal abnormality	Down syndrome
Inherited metabolic defect	
Autosomal recessive	Tay-Sachs disease
X-linked recessive	Classic hemophilia
	Duchenne's muscular dystrophy
Fetal exposure to known teratogen	
Infectious illness	Maternal infection with rubella, cytomegalovirus, toxoplasmosis
Drugs	Folate antagonists, warfarin, thalidomide, ethanol in high doses
Irradiation	X-ray exposure of 15 rads or more
Preterm premature rupture of the membranes prior to 24 weeks	
Fetal death in utero	

Modified from Stubblefield PG: Induced abortion: indications, counseling, and services. *In* Sciarra JJ, Zatuchni GI, Daly MJ (eds): Gynecology and Obstetrics. Vol 6. Philadelphia, Harper & Row, 1982, p 2.

Manual Vacuum Procedures

In 1972, Karman and Potts described a small-bore, flexible vacuum cannula used with a 50-ml syringe to evacuate the uterus through 7 menstrual weeks with only minimal cervical dilatation.[169] The procedure is readily accomplished in the physician's office. The only instruments required in addition to speculum and tenaculum are the Karman cannula and modified 50-ml syringe (Fig. 19–15).

Technique for Manual Vacuum Procedures (see Fig. 19–16)

After examination to determine uterine position and to be sure that pregnancy is 7 weeks or less, the cervix is exposed with a speculum, infiltrated with local anesthetic, and grasped with a tenaculum placed vertically at 12 o'clock. Four- and 5-mm-diameter cannulas are passed through the cervical canal as dilators, and then a 6-mm cannula is inserted and attached to the evacuated 50-ml syringe to establish suction. The 4- and 5-mm cannulas are not large enough to dependably evacuate the uterus in pregnancy, but are useful as atraumatic dilators and for endometrial biopsies in the nonpregnant state. The 6-mm cannula is rotated and pushed in and out with gentle strokes, taking care to rotate the cannula only on the outstroke so as to avoid twisting off the flexible tip by rotating it when it is pressed against the uterine fundus. When no more tissue comes through, the cannula is withdrawn, its tip cleared in a sterile fashion, and it is reinserted and vacuum reestablished for a final, check curettage to

Table 19–9. MATERNAL INDICATIONS FOR TERMINATION OF A DESIRED PREGNANCY

Category	Examples
Cardiovascular disease	Pulmonary hypertension, Eisenmenger's syndrome, history of myocardial infarction, history of pregnancy cardiomyopathy, severe hypertensive disease
Genetic disease	Marfan's syndrome
Hematologic disease	Thrombotic thrombocytopenic purpura
Infection	Human immunodeficiency virus
Metabolic disease	Proliferative diabetic retinopathy
Neoplastic disease	Invasive carcinoma of the cervix, any neoplasm in which maternal survival depends on prompt treatment with chemotherapy with teratogenic agents or in which the fetus will receive a dangerous dose of radiation
Neurologic disease	Untreated cerebrovascular malformation or berry aneurysm
Renal disease	Deterioration of renal function in early pregnancy
Pregnancy-specific disorder in present pregnancy	Intrauterine infection, severe preeclampsia or eclampsia

Modified from Stubblefield PG: Induced abortion: indications, counseling, and services. *In* Sciarra JJ, Zatuchni GI, Daly MJ (eds): Gynecology and Obstetrics. Vol 6. Philadelphia, Harper & Row, 1982, p 2.

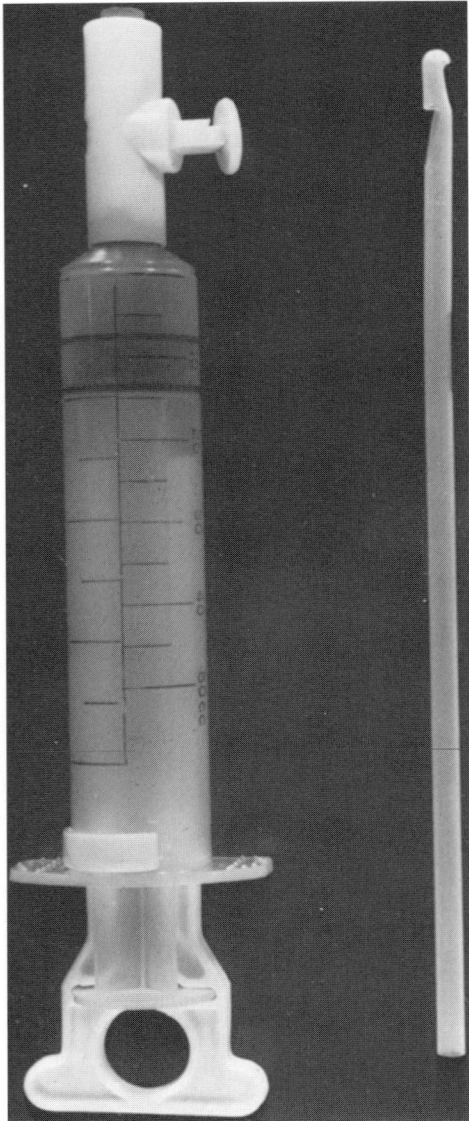

Figure 19–15. Instruments for early abortion: 6-mm Karman cannula and modified 50-ml plastic syringe. (Photo courtesy of International Projects Assistance, Chapel Hill, NC.)

prove the uterus empty. The operator must then carefully examine the aspirated tissue to identify the gestational sac, to prevent failed abortion, to diagnose molar pregnancy, and to detect ectopic pregnancy.[170] The fresh exam is best accomplished by floating the aspirated tissue in a clear plastic dish over a light source. Figure 19–17 demonstrates the appearance of an early pregnancy.

This same procedure allows treatment of incomplete spontaneous abortion in an office or emergency department without need for an operating room and general anesthesia. A double-valve version of the instrument accommodates vacuum cannulas as large as 10 mm and makes possible manual vacuum evacuation of the uterus through 12 weeks of pregnancy.

Edwards and Carson have modified the manual vacuum technique and applied it to pregnancies as early as 3 weeks from last menstrual period.[171] The cervix is dilated to 7 mm with Pratt dilators and then a 7-mm rigid curved vacurette is used with a hand-held 60-ml syringe as vacuum source (Mylex, Chicago). An intracervical block of 20 ml 0.5 percent lidocaine with 2 units of vasopressin and conscious sedation with midazolam and nalbuphine intravenously are used for analgesia. A series of 1,530 patients were treated prior to 6 weeks from last menstrual period after preoperative ultrasound and with careful examination of the aborted tissue and follow-up with serial β-human chorionic gonadotropin (β-hCG) titers to ensure diagnosis of ectopic pregnancy. No serious complications occurred and nine unsuspected ectopic pregnancies were diagnosed and treated.

Technique for Standard Vacuum Curettage

Standard vacuum curettage applies essentially the same technique as manual vacuum, but uses larger cannulas, from 7 to 12 mm, with an electric vacuum pump. After establishing a paracervical block as above, the operator dilates the cervical canal, using serial insertion of tapered rods that increase progressively in size. We favor the Denniston dilators pictured in Figure 19–18 for their blunt tips, gentle taper, and semirigid "fee." Dilatation is continued to a diameter 1 mm less than the estimated length of gestation in menstrual weeks and then a vacuum cannula of that same outside diameter is inserted. After aspiration is complete, we gently insert a sharp curette and use it as a finger to gently explore the cavity and prove it empty. Finally, the suction cannula is reintroduced for a final few seconds to remove any additional tissue remaining. Finally, the operator must perform a careful fresh examination of the aspirated tissue. An instrument kit sufficient for all first-trimester procedures is pictured in Figure 19–19.

Pain Control for First-Trimester Abortion

Most first-trimester abortions are performed out of hospital, without a major anesthetic. This practice has contributed to the remarkable safety record of U.S. abortion services. Local anesthetic is injected around or into the cervix to produce paracervical block. There is residual pain in spite of this. Pain is increased for women who exhibit preprocedure anxiety, for the youngest women, and for procedures done prior to 8 weeks or at the end of the first trimester.[172] Premedication with naproxen[173] or ibuprofen[174] is helpful. Lidocaine, chloroprocaine, and bupivacaine are equally effective for paracervical anesthesia. Lidocaine is most widely used and

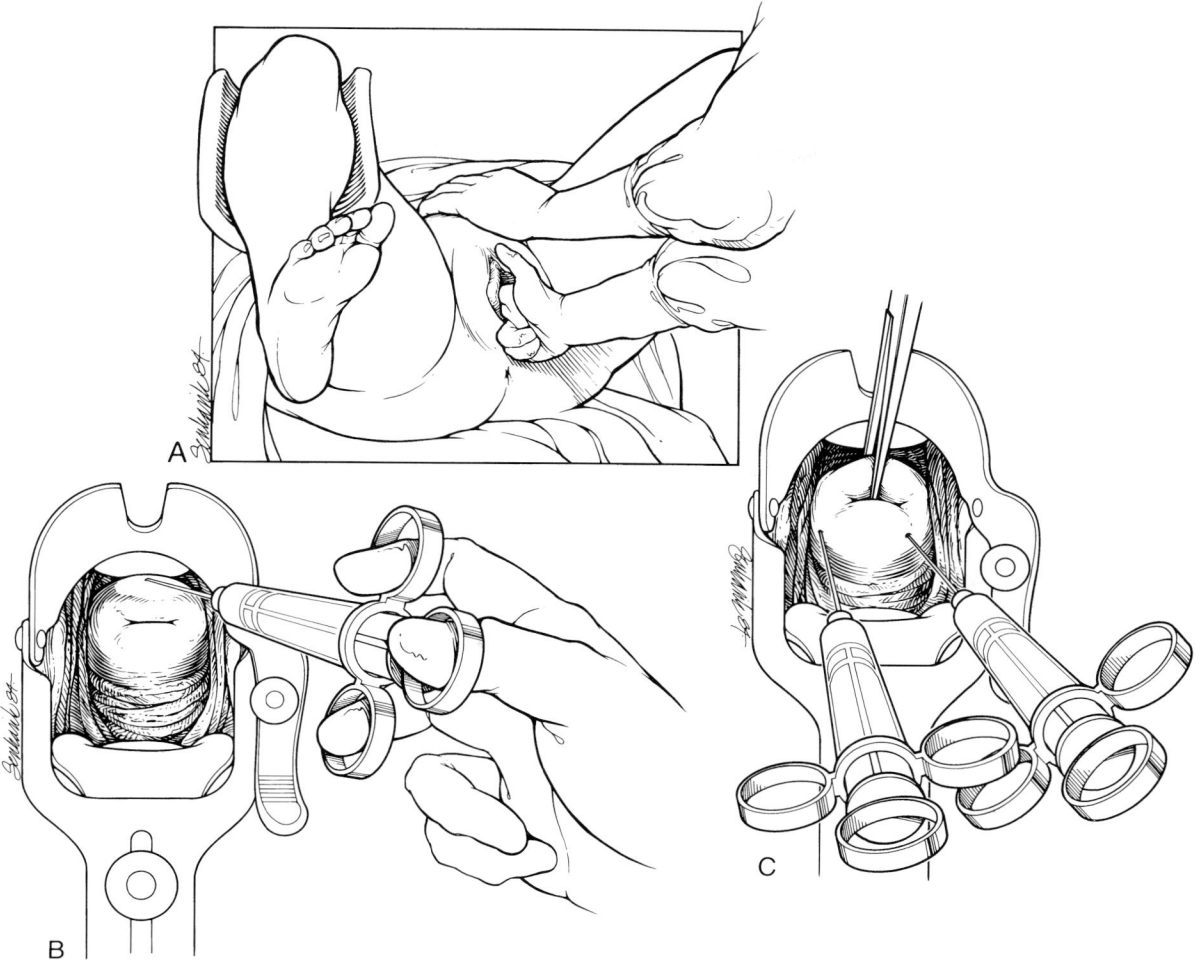

Figure 19–16. Early vacuum curettage abortion. *A,* Examining the patient. *B,* Administering paracervical block and superficial injection into the cervix at 12 o'clock to anesthetize tenaculum site. *C,* Completing paracervical block and injecting local anesthetic superficially, just under the vaginal mucosa, at the lateral margins of the cervix, 4 and 8 o'clock.

Illustration continued on following page

is least expensive. Buffering the lidocaine solution by adding 2 ml of 8.4 percent sodium bicarbonate to 18 ml of 1 percent lidocaine reduces the pain of injection.[174] Where the local anesthetic is injected is more important than what is injected. Glick described a combination superficial and deep injection technique at multiple sites around the cervix.[175] Wiebe demonstrated the superior pain relief of injections deep into the cervical stroma as compared with superficial submucosal injection.[176] We use a modification of Glick's technique. The cervix is infiltrated superficially at 12 o'clock with 2 to 3 ml of the anesthetic solution. The needle is then advanced through the anesthetized area for 3 cm to reach the junction of cervix and lower uterine segment, where an additional 3 ml are injected. The tenaculum is placed in the anesthetized area and used to steady the cervix for placement of an additional anesthetic at 4 and 8 o'clock, again injecting first superficially, and then advancing the needle 3 cm into the cervical stroma

for the deep injection[177] (Fig. 19–20). Aspiration is performed prior to each injection to prevent intravascular injection. To avoid systemic toxicity, the initial dose of lidocaine should not exceed 200 mg for the average weight patient (20 ml of 1 percent solution). Vasopressin, 2 units, is added to each 10 ml of lidocaine to reduce blood loss during the procedure.

Conscious Sedation

Conscious sedation is the use of drugs to reduce pain while maintaining consciousness, protective airway reflexes, and the ability to respond to commands. We use midazolam 2 mg intravenously, then 0.050 mg of fentanyl, a short-acting narcotic, given intravenously and repeated in a few minutes as needed. Respiratory depression occurs with both drugs at higher doses,[178] and we routinely use a pulse oximeter for monitoring. If oxygen saturation falls, it is usually only necessary to

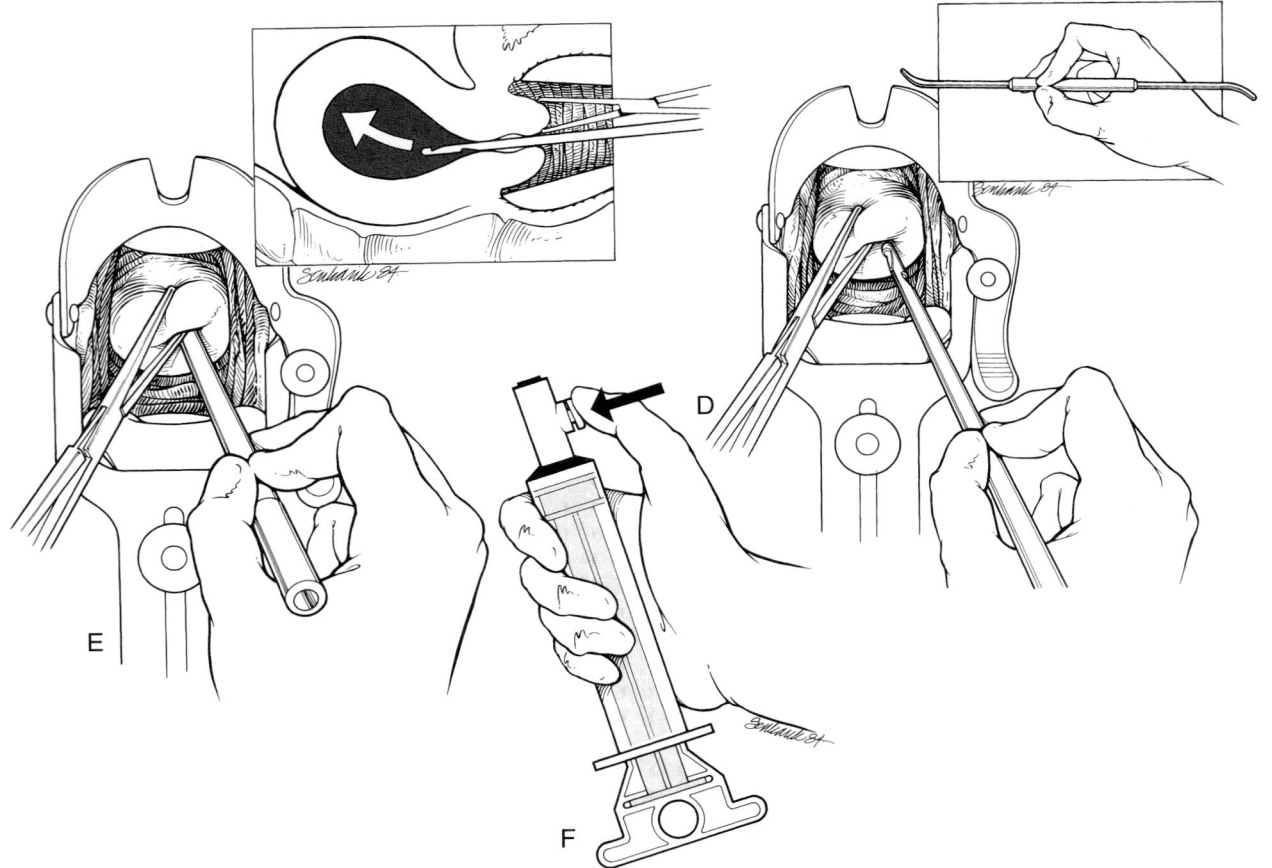

Figure 19–16. *Continued. D,* Dilatation, using a 4-mm Karman cannula. This will be followed by the 5-mm Karman and then the 6-mm cannula. Alternatively, the Denniston dilators 4, 5, and 6 can be used (*inset*). *E,* Insertion of the 6-mm Karman cannula, as far as the top of the cavity (inset). *F,* Preparing the syringe by closing the pinch valve.

Illustration continued on opposite page

tell the patient to take a deep breath. Occasionally, supplemental oxygen is briefly required. Patients who receive intravenous sedation must be under constant observation until fully recovered.

Cervical Dilatation

Forcible dilatation with tapered rods is the standard. We place a single tooth tenaculum vertically with one branch inside the cervical canal to provide traction near the internal os, the region of greatest resistance. Traction straightens the angle between cervix and uterus, helping to avoid perforation (Fig. 19–21). Then dilators are inserted slowly and carefully. The dilator tip must negotiate a curve where cervix and uterus join, and to guide the dilator properly with an anteflexed uterus, the operator's hand must follow a downward curve (Fig. 19–22). The direction is reversed if the uterus is retroverted. If the cervical os is very small, use the small, semirigid plastic os finder instrument (Cheshire Medical Specialties, Inc., Branford, CT) or misoprostol treatment as described below.

Osmotic Dilators

Osmotic dilators reduce the risk of perforation, although they do not completely prevent it. A fivefold reduction in cervical lacerations[179] and in uterine perforations was seen when laminaria were used instead of forcible dilatation in a large national study.[180] Use of laminaria has not been associated with increased risk for infection.[181]

Laminaria is a genus of seaweed. The stems are inserted into the cervical canal as small dry sticks. They take up water and swell, exerting gentle pressure (Fig. 19–23). Over several hours, this produces softening of the cervix and considerable dilatation. If the laminaria are left in place overnight, additional forcible dilatation will not be needed. Medical laminaria are either of two species: *L. japonicum* and *L. digitatum*. *L. japonicum* tents are preferred, as they retain their integrity when wet. The main drawbacks of laminaria are the need for insertion by a skilled practitioner and the requirement of several hours for dilatation to be accomplished. Hypan,[182] a plastic dilator, achieved greater cervical dilatation than laminaria among primigravid women.

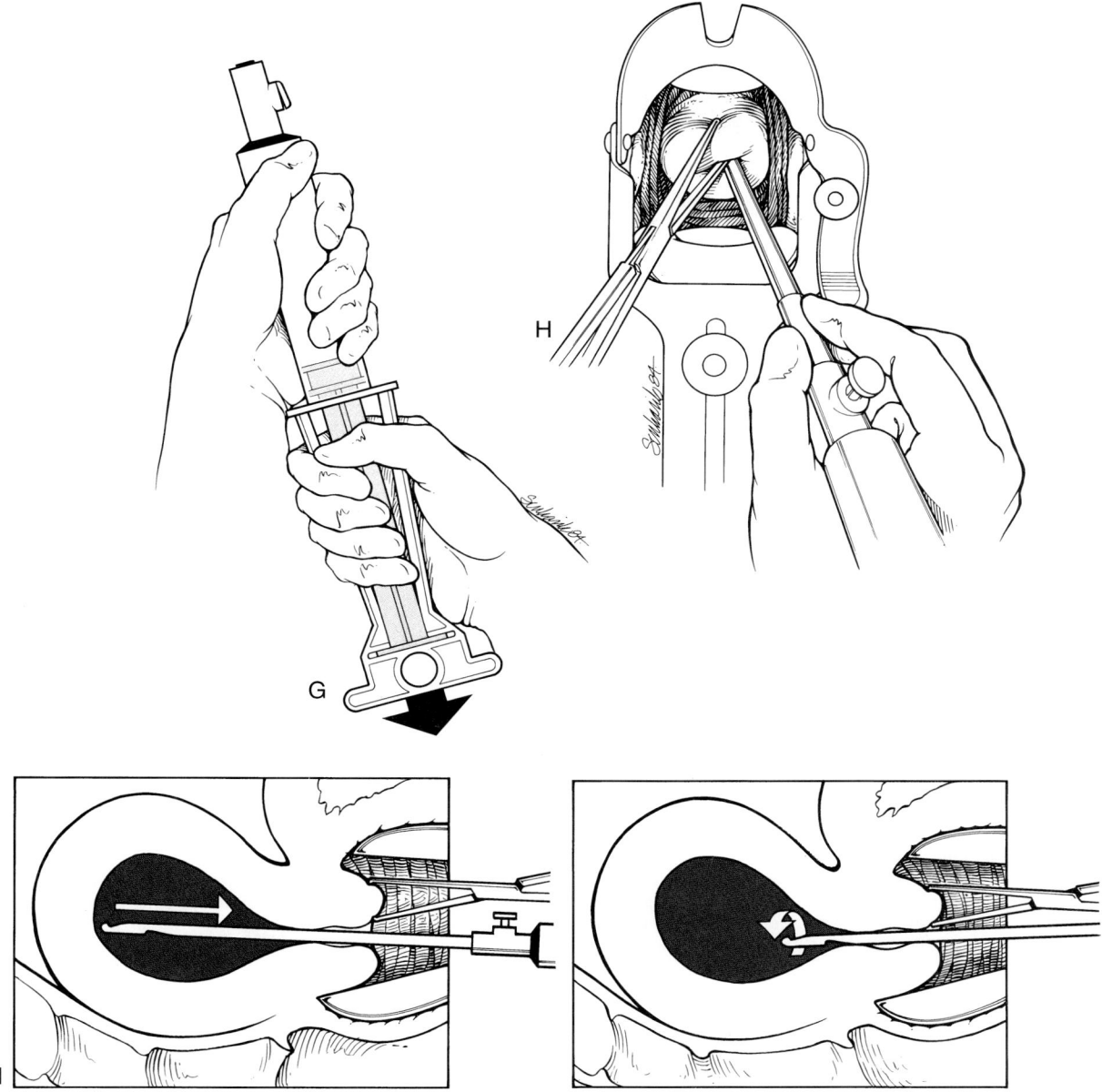

Figure 19–16. *Continued. G,* Evacuating the syringe, with side arms on the plunger assembly locking it in the withdrawn position, maintaining vacuum. *H,* Uterine evacuation through the Karman cannula into the syringe. *I,* The cannula is rotated and is slid in and out of the cavity in a pistonlike fashion. Care must be taken to rotate only on the out stroke, when the cannula tip is withdrawn away from the top of the uterus. Rotation when the cannula is pressed against the top of the fundus may cause the tip of the cannula to break off inside the uterine cavity.

Illustration continued on following page

Prostaglandin for Dilatation

Until recently, vomiting, diarrhea, and pain limited the usefulness of prostaglandins for preoperative cervical dilation.[185] Misoprostol, the 15-methyl analogue of prostaglandin E_1(PGE_1), produces effective dilatation with few side effects and low cost. Vaginal misoprostol, 400 μg given 3 hours prior to surgery, produces adequate dilation for first-trimester procedures, with few side effects.[183] Misoprostol (Cytotec) is sold in the United States for the indication of prevention of ulcers of the stomach and duodenum. It is stable at room temperature, unlike the other prostaglandins which must be refrigerated.

Rh Prophylaxis

Risk of Rh sensitization is said to be 2 percent after spontaneous abortion and 4 to 5 percent after induced abortion.[184] All Rh-negative women are given 50 μg of

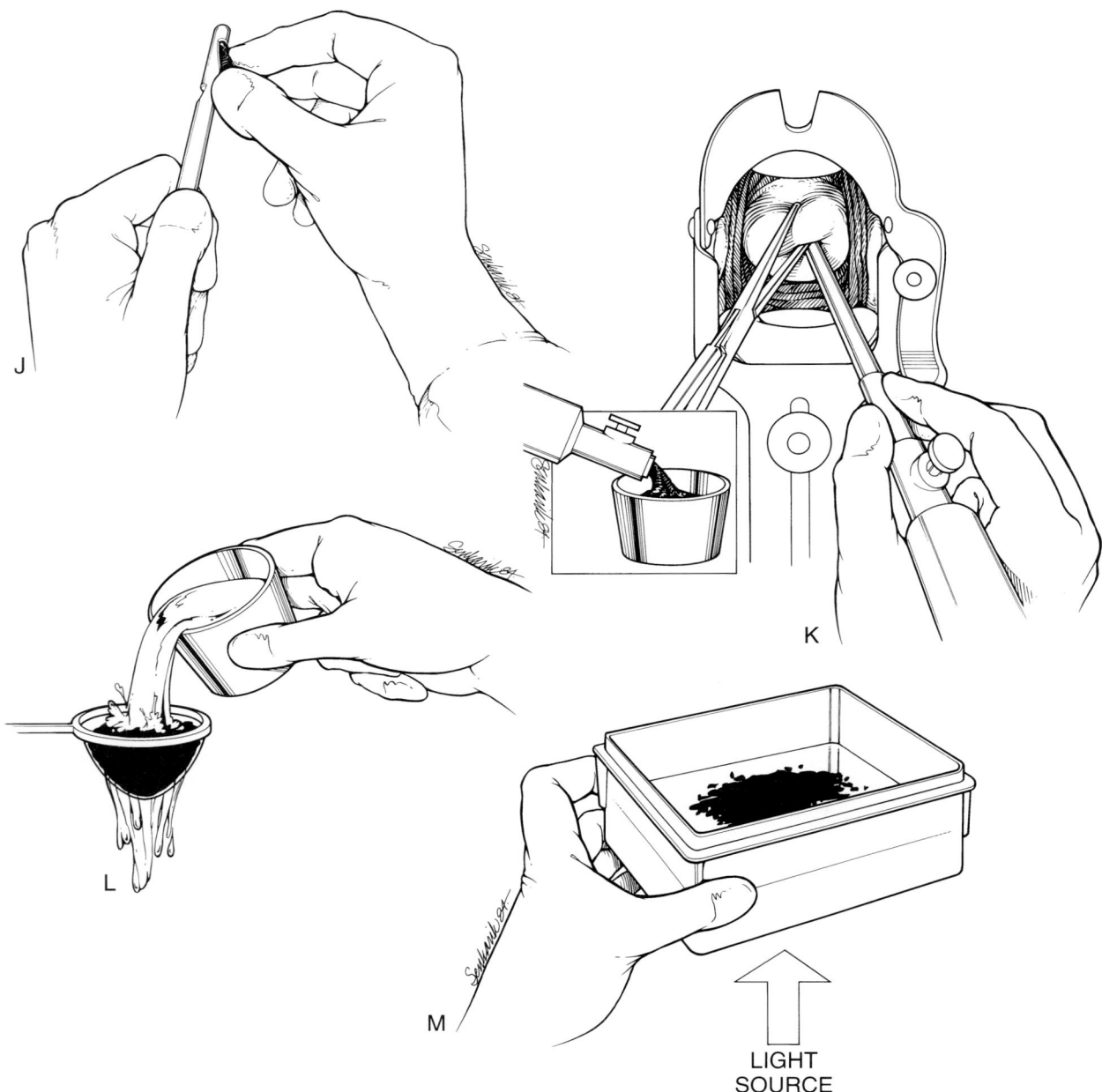

Figure 19–16. *Continued. J,* When no further tissue comes through the cannula, it is withdrawn; using a sterile glove, the tip is cleared. *K,* Repeat aspiration. After clearing the tip, the cannula is reinserted, the syringe emptied (*inset*) and reevacuated, and vacuum established for a final check to ensure that the uterus is empty. Omission of this step results in incomplete abortion. *L,* Preparing the tissue for examination. The tissue is emptied into a tea strainer and washed with saline. *M,* Fresh examination. The tissue is floated in saline in a clear plastic dish over a light source. The gestational sac must be identified.

Rh immune globulin within 72 hours of induced or spontaneous first-trimester abortion. Whether this is necessary for the earliest procedures has not been determined. Patients in the midtrimester, 13 weeks or more, are routinely given a full dose, 300 μg. If administration of Rh immune globulin is accidentally omitted, it should still be given, even as late as 2 weeks after the procedure, because partial protection will still be provided.

Medical Means for First-Trimester Abortion

Historically, women have eaten a variety of plant substances in attempts to produce abortion.[155] The prostaglandins were the first modern means for pharmacologic induction of abortion.[185] Misoprostol, the analog of PGE_1, has many fewer side effects than other prostaglandins, and as described below, is an effective abortifacient when combined with mifepristone or methotrexate.

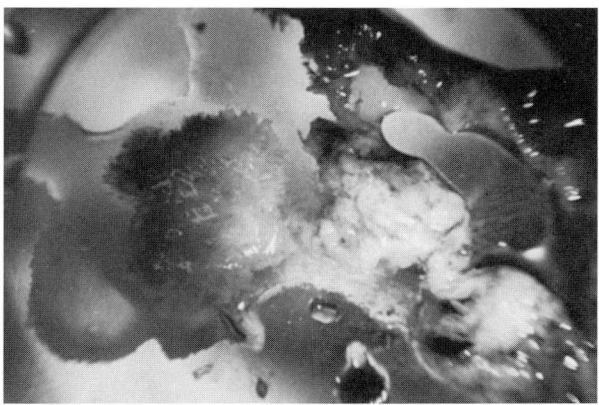

Figure 19–17. Tissue specimen in a 6-week pregnancy, as seen without magnification. The conceptus is on the left, and to the right is the decidual lining of the uterus. (From Stubblefield PG: Induced abortion: indications, counseling, and services. *In* Sciarra JJ, Zatuchni GI, Daly MJ [eds]: Gynecology and Obstetrics. Vol 6. Philadelphia, Harper & Row, 1982, p 2.)

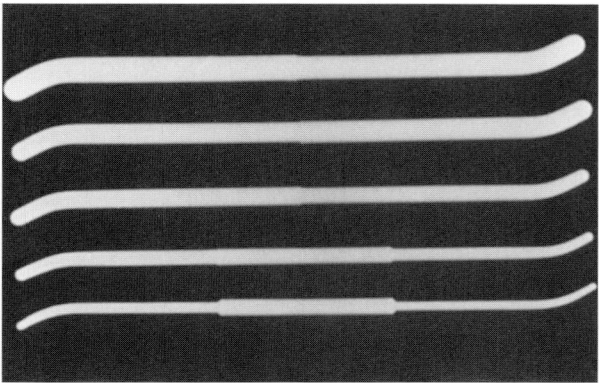

Figure 19–18. Denniston dilators. (Photo courtesy of International Projects Assistance, Chapel Hill, NC.)

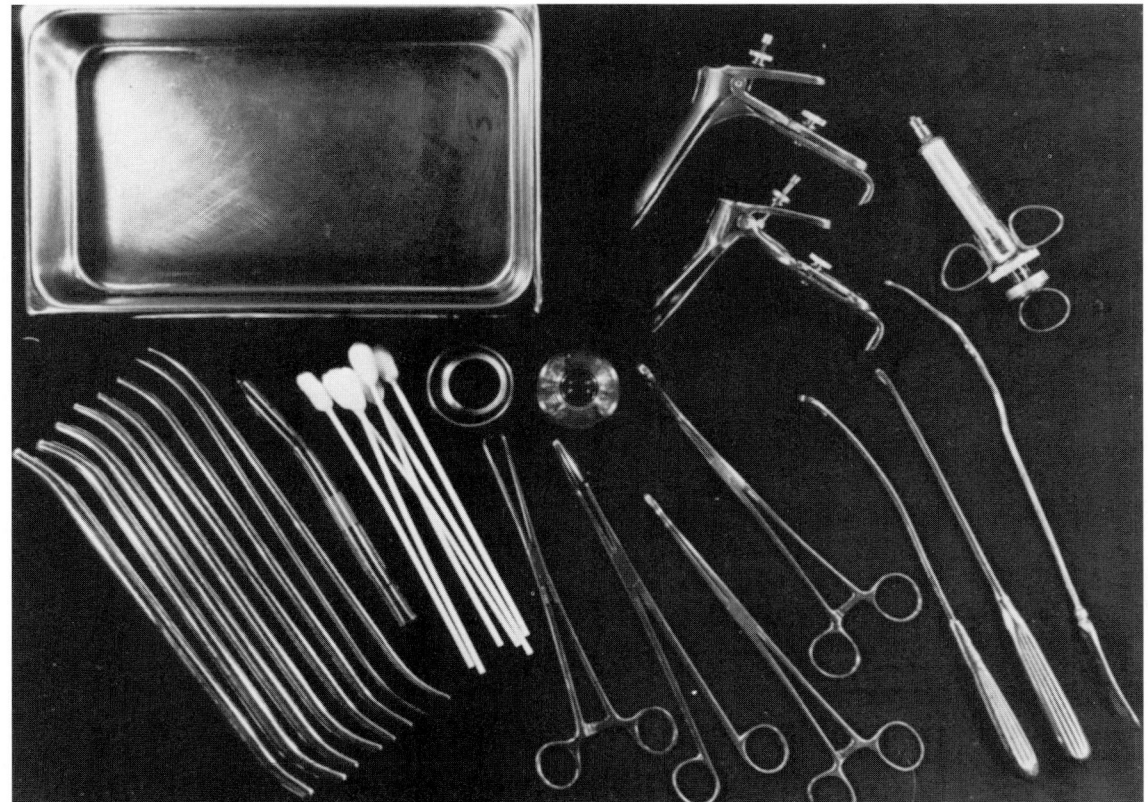

Figure 19–19. Instrument kit for vacuum curettage abortion. Clockwise (left to right): sterile tray, Graves speculum, Moore speculum, control syringe, uterine sound, No. 1 curette, No. 3 curette, curved Foerrester forcep, straight Forrester forcep, Moore avum forcep, single-toothed tenaculum, medicine glasses, cotton swabs, plastic vacurette, Pratt cervical dilators. (From Stubblefield PG: Induced abortion: indications, counseling, and services. *In* Sciarra JJ, Zatuchni GI, Daly MJ [eds]: Gynecology and Obstetrics. Vol 6. Philadelphia, Harper & Row, 1982, p 2.)

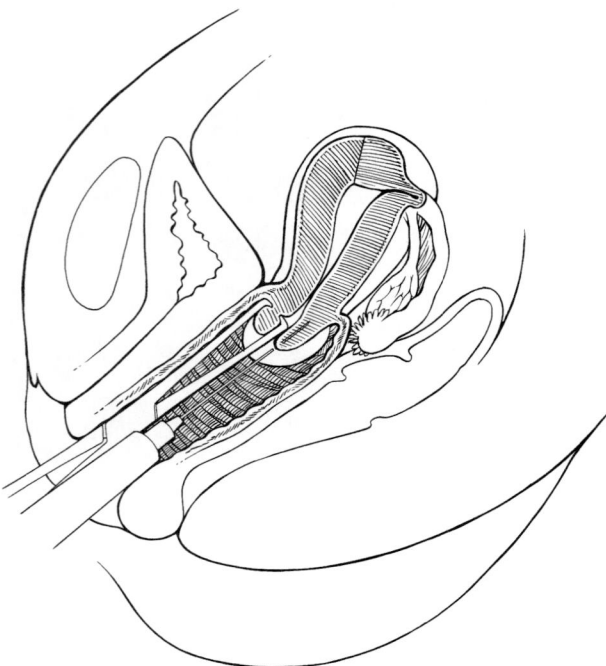

Figure 19–20. Deep technique for paracervical block. Infiltration of the lower uterine segment at the 4 o'clock position.

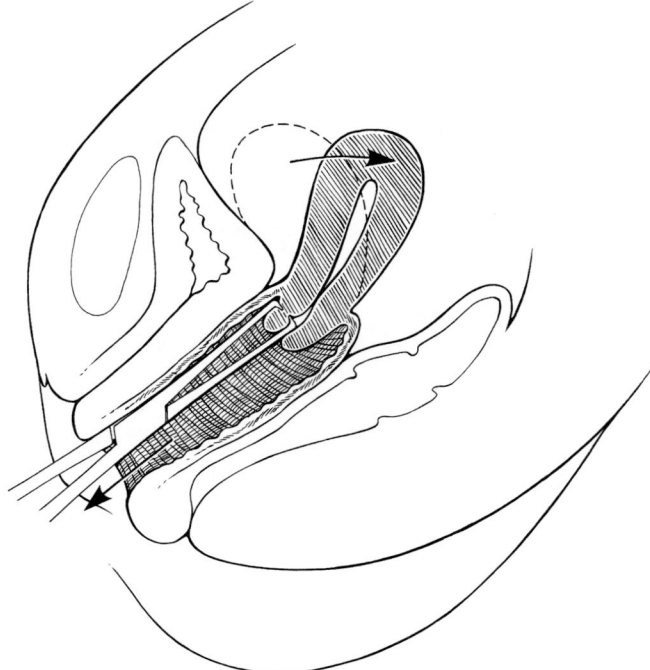

Figure 19–21. Effect of proper tenaculum placement in straightening the angle between the cervix and uterus by traction.

Mifepristone (RU-486)

Mifepristone, an analog of the progestin norethindrone, has strong affinity for the progesterone receptor, but acts as an antagonist, blocking the effect of natural progesterone.[186] Addition of a low dose of prostaglandin improves efficacy.[187] The standard protocol is as follows: women with amenorrhea of less than 50 days and pregnancy confirmed by serum β-hCG or ultrasonography receive an oral dose of 600 mg of mifepristone on day 1. On day 3, the patient returns for the prostaglandin: sulprostone (a PGE_2 analog), gemeprost (a PGE_1 analog), or misoprostol. Rh-negative patients receive Rh immune globulin. Patients remain in the clinic for 4 hours, during which expulsion of the pregnancy often occurs. They return 8 to 15 days later for measurement of β-hCG or ultrasonography.[188–190] If treatment fails or if the patient bleeds excessively, vacuum curettage is performed. In a series of almost 17,000 cases, 600 mg of mifepristone orally followed in 36 to 48 hours by either sulprostone or gemeprost produced complete abortion in 95 percent of cases.[188,189] About 2 percent abort incompletely and will require curettage; 1 percent require urgent curettage for bleeding, and about 1 percent do not respond at all and will require vacuum curettage. Three myocardial infarctions and one death have occurred with mifepristone/prostaglandin of a total of 60,000 women treated.[190] The myocardial infarctions were attributed to coronary artery spasm from sulprostone in women over age 35

who were smokers. Age greater than 35 and smoking or history of cardiovascular disease are now considered contraindications to mifepristone/sulprostone for abortion. No myocardial infarctions have occurred with the PGE_1 analogues gemeprost and misoprostol. The mife-

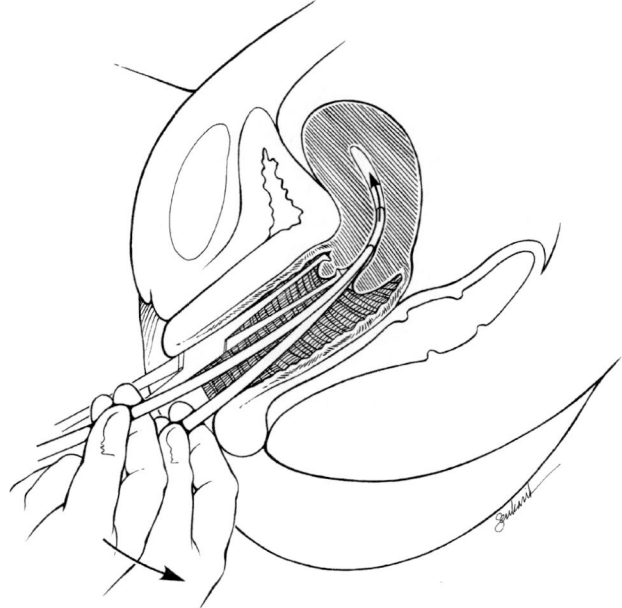

Figure 19–22. Inserting the dilator along the proper curved path to avoid perforation.

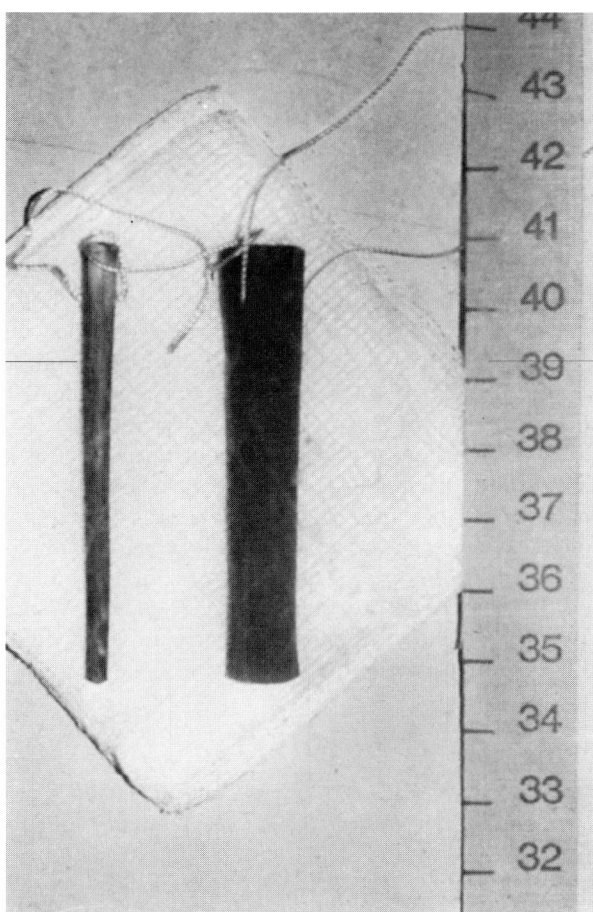

Figure 19–23. Tents of *Laminaria japonicum.* Dry tent (*left*) as it would be just before insertion. Wet tent (*right*) as it would be after several hours exposed to water. (Photo courtesy of Mildred Hanson, MD, Mount Sinai Hospital, Minneapolis, MN.)

pristone/misoprostol combination is highly effective.[191,192] Mifepristone has been used by more than 3 million women in Europe and China. For additional details of management, see Creinin and Aubeny's summary.[193] Mifepristone can also be used to trigger cervical softening and dilatation before surgical abortion.[194]

Methotrexate and Misoprostol

The antifolate methotrexate provides another medical approach to pregnancy termination. Widely used to treat ectopic pregnancies without surgery,[195] it can also be used with intrauterine gestations. Creinin and Darney proved that methotrexate, 50 mg/m^2 intramuscularly followed by vaginal misoprostol 800 μg, effectively terminated early intrauterine pregnancies.[196] In a subsequent study, 300 women received methotrexate at or before 56 days of gestation, followed 7 days later with vaginal misoprostol.[197] Misoprostol was repeated at 24 hours if the patient had not aborted. Fifty-three percent aborted after the first dose of misoprostol, an

additional 15 percent after the second dose, and a total of 92 percent aborted by 35 days. The methotrexate/misoprostol regimen takes longer than mifepristone/misoprostol, but the regimen is inexpensive and already available in the United States.

Selective Termination of Anomalous Twins and Reduction of Multifetal Pregnancies

Multifetal pregnancies are likely to lead to extreme prematurity with resultant perinatal loss or serious neonatal handicap. Reduction of multifetal pregnancies in the first trimester and selective termination of second-trimester anomalous twins have become standard practices in many centers.[198–202] The most effective technique is transabdominal intracardiac instillation of potassium chloride (see Chapter 24). A 22-gauge spinal needle is advanced through the maternal abdominal and uterine walls toward the fetal cardiac echo under guidance with high-resolution ultrasound. In the first trimester, 0.2 to 0.4 ml of a 2-mmol solution of potassium chloride (KCl) is injected at a time until cardiac asystole is seen. The amount required is 0.2 to 1.8 ml.[199] Observation is continued for 2 minutes, and the needle is then redirected into another gestational sac. In the second trimester, 0.5 ml is injected at a time, and 0.5 to 3 ml will be needed. Cardiac activity resumed 30 minutes later in 2 of 42 first-trimester cases and one of four second-trimester cases in Wapner's series and were successfully reinjected the same day.[199] Evans and colleagues described 463 pregnancies with multifetal gestation treated at nine centers in four countries.[200] There were no failed procedures. The rate of pregnancy loss was 3.9 percent at 2 weeks or less after procedure, and 4.6 percent at 4 weeks or less. A total of 16.2 percent were lost before 24 weeks of gestation. Eighty-three percent of the pregnancies delivered at 33 weeks or later, and there was no evident damage to any surviving fetus. Gestational age at delivery was principally determined by the number of fetuses remaining. Multifetal pregnancies are usually reduced to two gestations, since the morbidity of diamniotic twins is acceptable. Selective reduction improves outcome for triplet pregnancies as well. In a comparative study, Lipitz and colleagues found that reduction of triplets to twins decreased rates of prematurity, low birth weight, very low birth weight, neonatal morbidity, neonatal mortality, and pregnancy complications.[201]

Selective termination is also performed for one anomalous fetus of a multifetal gestation. The procedure was first reported in 1978.[202] Evans' group described 183 completed cases of selective termination for fetal anomalies.[203] One hundred sixty-nine were twins, 11 were triplets, and 3 were quadruplets. Termination of the affected fetus was successful in all cases. Injection of KCl was a safer means for termination than air embolization, producing an 8.3 percent rate of loss as compared with a 41.7 percent rate of loss. Twelve percent of the pregnancies subsequently miscarried before 24 weeks, and 83 percent of viable pregnancies delivered after 33 weeks. The most recent report from this group describes a total of 402 patients treated with intracardiac or intrafunic KCl. Three hundred forty-five were twin gestations, 39 were triplets, and 18 were quadruplets or greater. All were believed to be dyzogotic. There were no procedural failures. Rates of pregnancy loss after procedure by gestational age at the time of procedure were 5.4 percent at 9 to 12 weeks, 8.7 percent at 13 to 18 weeks, 6.8 percent from 19 to 24 weeks, and 9.1 percent for procedures performed at 25 weeks or more. No maternal coagulopathy occurred and no ischemic damage or coagulopathies were seen in the surviving neonates. In one case at the beginning of the series, the wrong fetus was terminated in a trisomy 21 pregnancy. When there is no distinct morphologic abnormality detectable by ultrasound at the time of procedure, a direct determination of karyotype is advised.[204]

Selective reduction should not be tried with monoamniotic twins, or for twin–twin transfusion syndrome, as embolization or exsanguination through the shared circulation to the remaining twin is likely. Maternal serum α-fetoprotein remains elevated into the second trimester after first-trimester procedures.[53]

First-Trimester Abortion Complications and their Prevention

For a more detailed description of the management of postabortal complications, the reader is referred to Pearlman and Tintinalli's text.[205]

Complications of Local Anesthesia

Intravascular injection or an overdose of the medication can produce a severe systemic response: convulsions, cardiorespiratory arrest, and death.[205] Management requires endotracheal intubation and support of respiration plus anticonvulsive therapy. Care must be taken to aspirate before injecting each dose of the local anesthetic to guard against intravascular injection. Epinephrine-containing solutions should not be used for paracervical block. Fatal anaphylaxis from allergy to the metabisulfite preservative in epinephrine solutions can occur in asthmatic patients.[206]

Cervical Shock

Vasovagal syncope produced by stimulation of the cervical canal can be seen even after paracervical block.

Although brief tonic-clonic activity is observed, this is distinguished from a true seizure by the presence of a very slow pulse, the patient's rapid recovery, and the absence of any postictal state. Routine use of low-dose vasopressin mixed with the paracervical anesthetic prevents "cervical shock."

Cervical Lacerations

Minor lacerations are common during forcible dilatation when the cervical tenaculum pulls off, but more serious injury can also be inflicted with actual full-thickness tearing of the cervical wall. A superficial laceration that is bleeding minimally may not need to be sutured if bleeding stops with pressure. If bleeding persists in spite of pressure or the tear is full thickness, then it should be sutured. A long laceration extending through the internal os may well be a partial or complete perforation, and if lateral, may involve the descending branch of the uterine artery. Cervical lacerations are prevented by use of gently tapered dilators and by use of osmotic dilators.

Perforation

Perforation may cause injury to major blood vessels, bowel, or bladder and endanger the patient's life. In a study of U.S. national data from 67,175 abortions, the rate of perforation was 0.9 per 1,000.[207] Laminaria use reduced the risk of perforation to less than one in five, and performance by a resident as opposed to an attending physician was associated with a fivefold increase in risk.[60] Each 2-week increase in gestational age was associated with a 1.4-fold increase in risk of perforation. A much lower rate of perforation (1 in 10,625) in a series of 170,000 abortions was accomplished without laminaria, by a small group of very experienced clinicians with predominantly first-trimester procedures.[208]

Management of Perforation

Suspected perforation can often be confirmed by inserting a sterile blunt instrument through the cervix into the suspect area with ultrasound guidance. The best management of perforation is immediate laparoscopy to determine the extent of the injury and complete the abortion under laparoscopic guidance.[209] Perforations of the cervix, either at the junction of the cervix and lower uterine segment, or lower down the canal, produce two different clinical syndromes, depending on the precise anatomic location of the perforation (Fig. 19–24).[210] Perforations at the junction of the cervix and lower uterine segment can lacerate the ascending branch of the uterine artery within the broad ligament, giving rise to severe pain, a broad ligament hematoma, and intra-abdominal bleeding. These perforations are

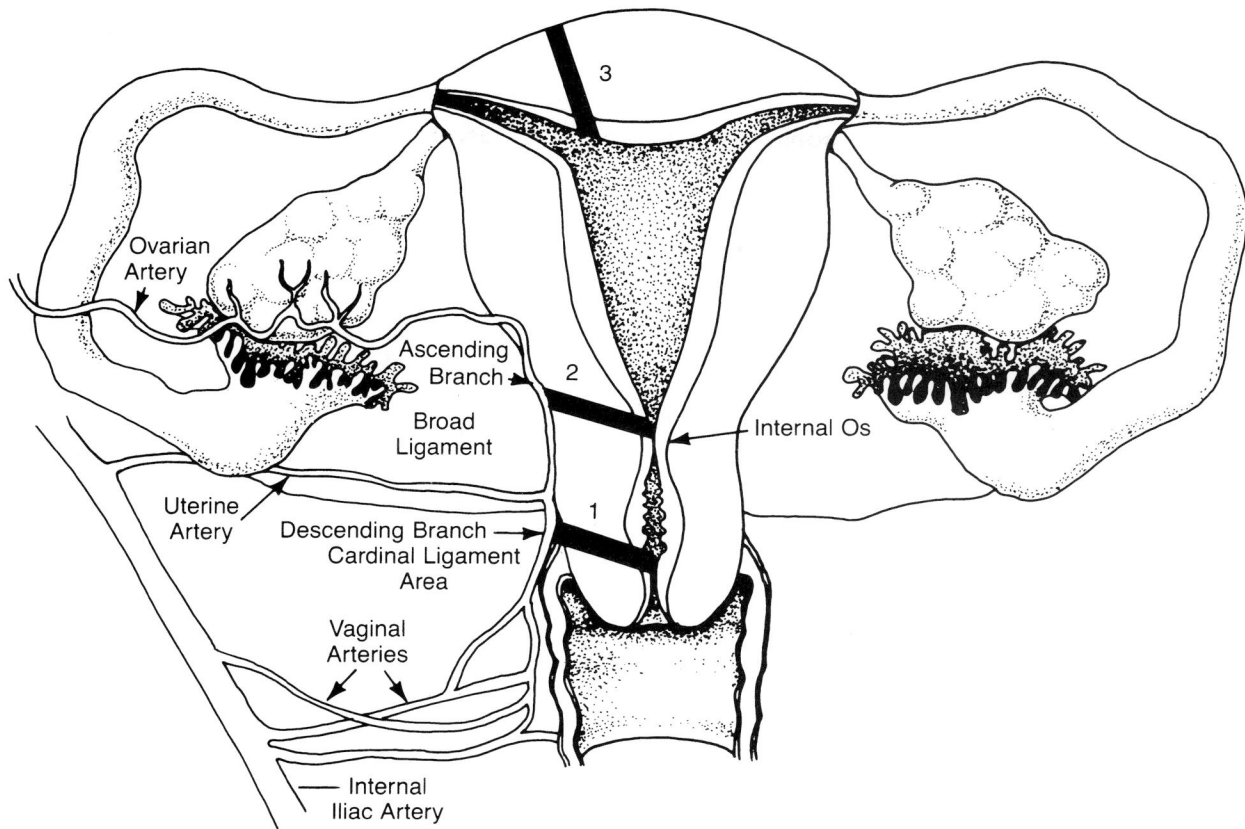

Figure 19–24. Possible sites of uterine perforation at abortion. 1, Low cervical perforation with laceration of descending branches of uterine artery; 2, perforation at junction of cervix and lower uterine segment with laceration of ascending branch of uterine artery; 3, fundal perforation. (Redrawn from Berek JS, Stubblefield PG: Anatomical and clinical correlations of uterine perforations. Am J Obstet Gynecol 135:181, 1979.)

usually recognized at the time. They are managed by laparoscopy to confirm the injury, and then by laparotomy to ligate the severed vessels and repair the uterine injury. Hysterectomy should not be required for injury in this location. Low cervical perforations, on the other hand, may injure the descending branch of the uterine artery within the dense collagenous substance of the cardinal ligaments. In this case, there is no intra-abdominal bleeding; the bleeding is only outwards, through the cervical canal, and may subside temporarily as the artery goes into spasm. Deaths have occurred when a low cervical perforation was not appreciated and the patient bled again later. If low cervical perforation is suspected, bleeding can be controlled by inflating the balloon of a Foley catheter in the cervical canal while the patient is transferred for x-ray anteriography with selective embolization of the injured vessel. Otherwise, hysterectomy may be needed.

Bowel Injury

If perforation is not recognized, the bowel may be grasped with the vacuum cannula or forceps and lacer-ated or stripped off its mesentery. A suspected bowel injury must be completely visualized. An experienced operator may accomplish this at laparoscopy, but laparotomy is indicated if the site of injury cannot be completely visualized. Small areas of injury can be managed by oversewing the lesion, irrigating thoroughly, and leaving a large intra-abdominal drain. Full-thickness injury or stripping of the mesentery will require segmental resection and anastomosis. High-dose antibiotics are given prophylactically. Larger injuries to the colon will require diverting colostomy after anastomosis.

Bladder Injury

The evaluation of a major perforation includes catheterization of the bladder to look for gross hematuria, a sign of bladder laceration. The injury is confirmed at laparoscopy, but laparotomy is required for management. Injuries to the dome are closed in two layers with catheter drainage for 7 days. Injuries to the trigone must not be repaired directly, but require an ample cystotomy incision in the dome for good visualization of the injury, catheterization of the ureters, and then closure in two layers. The best possible operative consultation with an experienced surgical specialist is advised for management of these more extensive injuries. Inadequate initial management of major injury adds markedly to the patient's problems and may jeopardize survival.

Hemorrhage

Excessive bleeding during vacuum curettage may indicate uterine atony, uterine trauma, cervical pregnancy, or a pregnancy of more advanced gestational age than anticipated. Bleeding from atony is common with general anesthesia using halothane or enfluorane. Management requires a rapid reassessment of gestational age by examination of the fetal parts already extracted, and gentle exploration of the uterine cavity with curette or forceps to confirm that there is no perforation. Intravenous oxytocin is administered and the abortion completed. The uterus is then massaged between two hands to ensure contraction. Intracervical administration of 10 units of vasopressin diluted to 10 ml helps to reduce bleeding and produce a strong uterine contraction. Misoprostol, 800 μg given rectally, is an important adjunct. When these measures fail, adequate fluid resuscitation is begun and the patient is transferred immediately to the hospital. Insertion of a Foley urinary catheter into the uterine cavity and inflating the 30-ml balloon may be an effective temporizing measure. Persistent postabortal bleeding suggests retained tissue or clot (hematometra), cervical or uterine laceration or perforation, uterine atony, or (rarely in the first trimester) disseminated intravascular coagulopathy (DIC). If bleeding persists, tests are drawn to rule out DIC and the patient is prepared for laparoscopy. Cervical pregnancy and low cervical perforation described above are best managed with arteriography and selective embolization of the bleeding vessels.[211]

Postabortal Syndrome (Hematometra)

This syndrome is a type of uterine atony.[212] In the classic presentation, the patient begins to complain of increasing lower abdominal pain a half hour or so after abortion and may develop tachycardia and diaphoresis. On exam, the uterus is large, globular, and tense, and could be mistaken for a broad ligament hematoma except that the mass is midline and arises from the cervix. The treatment is immediate reevacuation. The uterus will then contract to its normal postabortal size. Sands, Burnhill, and colleagues reported that pretreatment with ergot, 0.1 mg intramuscularly, reduces the incidence of this phenomenon.[212]

Failed Abortion, Continued Pregnancy, and Ectopic Pregnancy

Failure to interrupt the pregnancy is more often a problem with very early abortions. Pregnancy may continue in spite of the aspiration of histologically proven chorionic villi. The problem is prevented by insistence on identification of the gestational sac in the fresh exam of the aborted tissue.[213] When no chorionic villi are found in the fresh exam, ectopic pregnancy is a risk. Death from ectopic pregnancy is five times more likely when it is associated with attempted abortion than when it is not, presumably because the history of apparent induced abortion delays diagnosis.[214] Various plans of management to reduce risk from ectopic pregnancy have been proposed.[171] Evaluation with quantitative β-hCG levels and vaginal probe ultrasound are essentials. Women with unruptured ectopics 3.5 cm or less in diameter can be treated with methotrexate, 50 mg/m² intramuscularly.[195] Patients with larger ectopics or peritoneal signs indicating rupture are offered immediate laparoscopy.

Postabortal Triad

The most common postabortal problem is the triad of pain, bleeding, and low-grade fever. Although these symptoms may be managed successfully by oral antibiotics and ergot preparations, the great majority of cases will exhibit some retained gestational tissue or clot in the uterine cavity. The best management is repeat uterine evacuation, performed under local anesthesia in the ambulatory setting. Results obtained in 54 consecutive reaspirations performed for these symptoms are displayed in Table 19–10.

Incomplete Abortion

Retained tissue will produce increased postabortal bleeding and places the patient at risk for infection.

Table 19–10. FINDINGS AT REPEAT UTERINE EVACUATION IN 53 CONSECUTIVE CASES OF PATIENTS PRESENTING WITH PAIN, BLEEDING, AND LOW-GRADE FEVER AFTER FIRST-TRIMESTER ABORTION

Findings	No.
Retained tissue	24
Scant fragments of gestational tissue or decidua	4
Clot and gestational tissue mixture	10
Blood clot only (hematometra)	9
Continued pregnancy (intact gestational sac)	6
Total	53

From Stubblefield PG: Current technology for abortion. Curr Probl Obstet Gynecol 2:1, 1978, with permission.

Management is by repeat curettage. If the uterus is larger than 12 weeks, it is wise to obtain a preoperative ultrasound to determine the amount of tissue remaining. Where fever is present, a cervical Gram's stain and appropriate cultures are taken; then, high-dose intravenous antibiotic therapy is initiated and the curettage is performed shortly thereafter. There should be no delay in evacuating the uterus. Women have gone into septic shock in spite of antibiotic therapy while awaiting curettage.[215]

Endometritis, myometritis, and pelvic peritonitis can be seen without any retained tissue. This is probably most likely in patients with preexisting cervical colonization with gonorrhea, chlamydia, or mycoplasma. A small, firm uterus on pelvic exam suggests that the uterus is empty and the curettage will not be needed. Where there is a question as to retained tissue, ultrasound is useful in making the decision whether to perform curettage or to treat with antibiotics alone.

Management of Septic Abortion

Delay in initiating adequate therapy may result in preventable death. We review management in the box, "Management of Septic Abortion."[215] Clostridial sepsis, not uncommon as a complication of illegal abortion, is occasionally seen as a complication of legal abortion. This should be suspected from the presence of large gram-positive rods on Gram's stain of the cervical secretions or curetted tissue, when tachycardia seems out of proportion to the fever, and especially when hematuria and shock develop rapidly. These patients can rapidly develop a severe adult respiratory distress syndrome. Initial treatment requires high-dose penicillin, vacuum aspiration of the uterus, and fluid management. A superficial clostridial infection will respond to these measures, but if hemolysis is present, indicating systemic release of clostridial toxins, prompt hysterectomy will be probably necessary if the patient is to survive.[215–217] Hyperbaric oxygenation may play a role in addition to effective surgical and medical management of clostridial sepsis.[218]

Choice of Antibiotics for Postabortal Infection

A number of different species of bacteria, chlamydia, and mycoplasma have been implicated in postabortal sepsis. No one agent or even pair of agents is effective against all possible organisms. When the patient is seriously ill, we have used three drugs: ampicillin (2 to 3 g intravenously every 6 hours), clindamycin (900 mg intravenously every 8 hours), and gentamicin (loading dose of 2 mg/kg of body weight, followed by 1.5 mg/kg every 8 hours, depending on the blood level and renal status).[215] Once-a-day dosing is recommended currently for gentamicin, as it increases efficacy and decreases toxicity and cost.

Prophylactic Antibiotics

The use of perioperative doxycycline with induced abortion is advisable.[219–223] The major determinant of postabortal infection is previous chlamydia colonization of the cervix. Both chlamydia-positive and chlamydia-

Management of Septic Abortion

1. Be suspicious when a woman of childbearing age presents with unexplained fever, vaginal bleeding, and a history of amenorrhea
2. Make the diagnosis with a sensitive pregnancy test and pelvic examination
3. Eradicate the infection
   Obtain cultures by endometrial biopsy or uterine evacuation
   Start high-dose, broad-spectrum antibiotics
4. Empty the uterus
   First trimester: vacuum curettage under local anesthesia with conscious sedation
   Midtrimester: D&E, with ultrasound guidance or prostaglandin induction (carboprost 250 μg IM q2h or misoprostol 200 μg vaginally q12h) or high dose oxytocin regimen
5. Laparotomy if no response to uterine evacuation and adequate medical therapy, or perforation with suspected bowel injury, pelvic abscess, or clostridial myometritis. Hysterectomy, bilateral salpingoophorectomy for severe myometritis. Copious irrigation of abdominal cavity, drainage, closure with Smead-Jones or similar stay sutures, delayed primary closure
6. Supportive care
   Severe sepsis and septic shock require intensive care unit management
   Provide cardiovascular support to restore close to normal blood pressure. Monitor with arterial line, balloon-flotation right heart catheter. Fluid resuscitation plus dopamine and dobutamine as needed if pulmonary wedge pressure becomes elevated before target mean arterial pressure is reached.
   Manage adult respiratory distress syndrome. Monitor tissue oxygenation and begin ventilation if oxygen saturation falls below 90 percent or if pulmonary compliance begins to decrease

After Stubblefield PG, Grimes DA: Septic abortion. N Engl J Med 331:310, 1994.

Table 19–11. RATES OF POSTABORTAL PELVIC INFECTION (PID) IN A PLACEBO-CONTROLLED TRIAL OF PROPHYLACTIC DOXYCYCLINE

	Doxycycline		Placebo	
	No.	%	No.	%
In women with negative *Chlamydia* screening				
PID Yes	2	0.4	15	3.0
PID No	500	99.6	482	97.3
$p = 0.001$				
In women with positive *Chlamydia* screening				
PID Yes	1	3.0	11	26.2
PID No	32	97.0	31	73.8

Data from Levellois and Rioux.[223]

negative patients have almost 10-fold reduction in risk of postabortal pelvic inflammation if they receive perioperative oral doxycycline (Table 19–11).[223]

Second-Trimester Abortion

D&E is the most commonly used method through 20 menstrual weeks in the United States, with labor induction methods favored only for those procedures performed after 20 weeks.[148] The abandonment of older labor induction methods in favor of D&E was strongly stimulated by Centers for Disease Control publications documenting the greater safety of early midtrimester D&E over other methods of the time.[223]

Dilatation and Evacuation in the Midtrimester

The variety of techniques that have been used for D&E are summarized elsewhere.[224–226] These differ primarily in the preparatory steps that precede the evacuation, whether one stage, with forcible dilation and followed by forceps evacuation of the fetus; two stage, with initial dilation of the cervix using laminaria tents, followed by instrumental evacuation; or multistage, with several sets of laminaria over 40 to 48 hours.

Choice of technique becomes more important as gestational age advances. Preoperative ultrasound is routine prior to midtrimester abortion. Pregnancies at 13 to 14 menstrual weeks are readily evacuated using the 12-mm vacuum cannula.[227] Dilatation of this amount is usually readily accomplished with Pratt's or Deniston's dilators. We advise the routine use of laminaria tents after 13 weeks. The actual evacuation of the uterine content is usually accomplished with long, heavy forceps, whereas the vacuum curette is used as an adjunct, to rupture the fetal membranes and drain amniotic fluid, and then to ensure evacuation is complete at the end of the procedure. The 16-mm vacuum system

(Rocket of London, Branford, CT) allows standard vacuum curettage to be performed through 16 menstrual weeks.

Anesthesia for D&E

With good psychological support from trained counselors, midtrimester D&E can be performed under paracervical block with conscious sedation. The necessary psychological support may be difficult to provide in the operating rooms of a busy general hospital, oriented toward major anesthetics. In a multicenter study, general anesthesia increased the risk for cervical laceration and hemorrhage with D&E.[228] On the other hand, large series have been reported with very low rates of uterine injury with general anesthesia.[229,230] When general anesthesia is used, it is all the more critical to have adequate preparation of the cervix with osmotic dilators. When general anesthesia is used, full compliance with current standards for monitoring tissue oxygen levels, end-expiratory CO_2, and frequent vital signs is mandatory.[231] When these procedures will take place out of hospital, more stringent patient selection is required. Combinations of short-acting intravenous barbiturates and inhaled nitrous oxide/oxygen mixtures or intravenous propofol combined with small doses of short-acting intravenous narcotic agents with inhaled air/oxygen mixtures are preferred regimens. Potent inhalant agents are avoided altogether, or used in very low concentrations to avoid uterine relaxation. Close observation during recovery is essential. Use of intravenous sedation or general anesthesia requires personnel trained in cardiorespiratory support.

An Approach to D&E

Most patients perceive the procedure as relatively minor, especially as compared with the alternatives of labor or major surgery.[229] When all goes well, as it usually does, the procedure takes only 10 to 20 minutes, the patient recovers for an hour or two, and goes home. Yet, the potential for sudden, life-threatening complications is always there: perforation and intestinal or bladder injury, amniotic fluid embolism, and DIC. The D&E procedure must be approached with caution and gentleness in the handling of instruments, and the patient must know that serious injury is possible, although not likely.

We describe our own technique in hopes this will help others to prevent complications. For a more detailed description, the reader is referred to Hern's excellent monograph,[226] and to Haskell, Easterling, and Lichtenberg.[232] After adequate counseling, complete menstrual and medical history, and physical examination with attention to uterine size and ultrasound dating history, osmotic dilators are inserted into the cervical canal and held in place with two 4 × 4-inch gauze sponges tucked into the fornices. At menstrual ages 13 to 15 weeks, two laminaria tents will suffice; at 16 to 20 weeks we insert four or more tents, and use 8 to 10 tents after 20 weeks. Paracervical anesthesia is produced with 10 ml of 1 percent lidocaine for the insertion. The patient is kept lying down for a few minutes after insertion to avoid syncope and then goes home. For gestations of 13 to 20 menstrual weeks, the abortion procedure will be performed the following day. At menstrual ages 20 weeks and beyond, the laminaria may be left in place for 48 hours. The additional dilatation greatly facilitates the procedure (P. D. Darney, MD, personal communication). A narcotic analgesic is prescribed, as approximately half of patients will experience significant cramping during laminaria dilatation. Doxycycline is given routinely, 100 mg after the insertion, an additional 100 mg with food before sleep and then 100 mg twice a day after the procedure for 2 days. Occasionally, the fetal membranes rupture a few hours after laminaria insertion. The laminaria are left in place and the abortion performed as scheduled the following day. Ultrasound guidance during the surgery is helpful for the more advanced cases and has been found to reduce the risk of perforation for new operators.[233]

Uterine evacuation is performed as follows. An intravenous line is established and the anesthetic of choice is begun. The patient is placed in lithotomy position, avoiding the Trendelenburg or head-down position, which might increase negative pressure in the uterine veins and increase risk for embolic phenomena. The previously placed vaginal sponges and laminaria are removed. Occasionally, especially in the young, primigravid patient at 13 to 15 weeks, the cervix is quite resistant to dilatation and the laminaria tents may be entrapped. This is more often a problem when a single large laminaria or Dilapan has been used, and is obviated by using two or more tents. If the laminaria cannot be removed with gentle traction, it is best to stop and wait 6 hours for additional cervical softening to occur. Next, the vagina and cervix are cleansed with povidone-iodide and paracervical block established with 20 ml of lidocaine 1 percent with 10 units of vasopressin injected deeply into the cervix at the 12-, 4-, and 8-o'clock positions.[234] If general anesthesia is used, the Xylocaine is omitted, and the vasopressin is diluted in 10 ml of saline and injected into the cervix as above. Two single-toothed tenaculi are placed vertically, each with one branch inside the cervical canal. Intravenous infusion of oxytocin, 40 units/1,000 ml, is begun at 150 to 200 ml/h. A large dilator is gently inserted to confirm dilatation. The vacuum cannula is then inserted and vacuum established briefly to rupture membranes

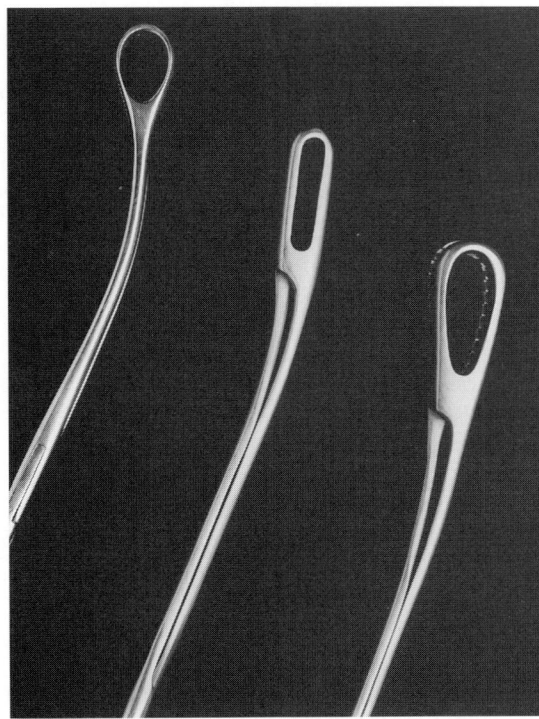

Figure 19–25. Instruments for D&E. Kelly placental forceps, Sopher forceps, and Bierer forceps (left to right).

and drain amniotic fluid. The cannula is then removed and replaced with an ovum forceps of appropriate size: Forester forceps for 13 to 15-week procedures; and Bierer, Sopher, or Kelly placental forceps for more advanced procedures (Fig. 19–25). The forceps are manipulated within the lower uterine segment to remove the pregnancy tissue. The vacuum cannula is reinserted as needed to pull tissue downward, where it can be grasped with the forceps. When the procedure feels complete, a large sharp curette is inserted and used to explore the cavity. If any additional tissue is encountered, the forceps or cannula is reinserted to remove it. After the procedure, the operator carefully examines the fetal parts to be sure all have been evacuated. On occasion, the fetal calvarium is retained in the uterus. If gentle attempts at extraction fail, operative ultrasound is used. If ultrasound is not available, it is best to stop, administer an oxytocin infusion for 2 hours, and then try again. By then, the remaining fetal parts will have been pushed down to the internal os, where they can be easily extracted.

Attempting evacuation of a pregnancy of gestational age beyond the operator's skill and experience poses serious risk. The chance that this will occur is reduced by routine use of preoperative ultrasound. However, if the procedure has begun, the operator can tell gestational age by the size of the fetal parts (Table 19–12). Where multiple laminaria tents have been used and the

Table 19–12. RECOMMENDED VALUES FOR FETAL MEASUREMENTS, BY MENSTRUAL AGE

Weeks	Foot Length (mm)	Fetal Weight (g)	Placental Weight (g)	Sonographic BPD (mm)
10	6			
11	7			
12	8	14	26	18
13	10	18	38	23
14	14	36	63	25
15	18	66	87	30
16	21	97	105	34
17	23	122	117	35
18	25	150	130	38
19	30	234	160	43
20	33	294	178	46
21	35	338	191	47
22	39	434	215	50

From Hern WM: Abortion Practice. Philadelphia, JB Lippincott, 1984, with permission.

cervix is widely dilated, a surgeon familiar with D&E can satisfactorily extract a pregnancy up to 20 or 21 weeks. Beyond this, we feel the procedure should be abandoned unless the surgeon routinely performs these more advanced procedures. The patient can be treated instead with high-dose intravenous oxytocin or systemic prostaglandins (see below). Perforation with midtrimester D&E is more likely to result in major visceral injury than is perforation in first-trimester procedures and will usually require a laparotomy.

Facilitating D&E

Modifications of technique are often used to facilitate D&E in the late midtrimester. Wright inserts multiple laminaria tents into the cervix, and injects 1.5 mg digoxin into the fetal heart to produce fetal death. The D&E is carried out under brief general anesthesia the following day. Oxytocin is administered as 50 to 100 units/1,000 ml during the procedure. In his series of 2,400 cases at 19 to 23 weeks, there were no perforations.[230] Hern described a personal series of gestations with anomalies at 15 to 34 weeks managed as outpatients with a similar technique.[235] After multistage laminaria treatment and ultrasound-guided intrafetal injection of 1.5 to 2.0 mg digoxin, membranes are ruptured on day 3, intravenous oxytocin (167 mU/min) is started, and assisted delivery is performed after a few hours.

Intact D&E

This variation of D&E is typically used at 20 to 24 weeks. Paracervical block is placed, the cervix is dilated to 9 to 11 mm with Pratt dilators and then several laminaria or Dilapan dilators are inserted. The next day, the original osmotic dilators are removed, and 15 to 25 Dilapan dilators are inserted into the cervical canal. On the third day, uterine evacuation is performed. Ultrasound is used to determine fetal position and presentation. In the variation described by Haskell, the membranes are ruptured and a large grasping forceps such as a Hern or Bierer forceps are inserted through the dilated cervix and a fetal foot is grasped and pulled downward, converting the presentation to breech.[232] The surgeon manually delivers the second lower extremity into the vagina, then the torso, and then the upper extremities, rotating the fetus so the dorsum remains up. The calvarium remains at the internal cervical os. Next, traction is applied to the shoulders of the fetus with the surgeon's fingers while elevating the cervical lip with one finger, and a scissors is advanced into the base of the fetal skull. A suction catheter is introduced and the central nervous system aspirated. With the calvarium thus decompressed, the fetus is delivered intact. McMahon described a similar procedure, with dilatation followed by laminaria placement twice a day for 2 days or more, followed by rupture of the membranes, administration of 250 mg of carboprost, and then 20 minutes later, fetal evacuation, as described above if the fetus is breech or transverse. If the fetus is in vertex presentation, the calvarium is allowed to descend into the cervical canal by uterine contractions and then decompressed by insertion of a trocar and aspiration of the cerebrospinal fluid and central nervous system followed by forceps extraction of the collapsed calvarium and intact fetus.[236]

Labor Induction Methods

Hypertonic Saline

Amnioinfusion of hypertonic saline is historically important as one of the oldest of the labor induction methods for abortion. There are serious hazards unique to hypertonic saline: cardiovascular collapse, pulmonary and cerebral edema, and renal failure occur if the solution is injected intravenously, and all patients are at risk for DIC. Hypertonic saline produces mean times from instillation to abortion of 33 to 35 hours.[237,238] Augmentation with high doses of intravenous oxytocin reduces instillation to abortion time, and results in fewer failed abortions, fewer retained placentas, less blood loss, and less risk of infection. Unfortunately, the addition of oxytocin increases the rate of occurrence of DIC and adds risk for water intoxication, uterine rupture, and annular detachment of the cervix.[237] When saline is used as a primary method, 200 ml of a 20 percent solution is administered. In current practice, much lower doses are used to augment prostaglandin abortion, and the amnioinfusion is performed under ultrasound guidance.

Hypertonic Urea

Hypertonic urea is attractive as an alternative to saline because of its greater safety, but the interval from injection to abortion is prolonged. In a series of papers, a group from Johns Hopkins explored this method, augmenting it at first with intravenous oxytocin, and subsequently with low doses of prostaglandin $F_{2\alpha}$. The combination of 5 mg of $PGF_{2\alpha}$ and 80 g of urea instilled into the amniotic sac produces abortion in a mean time of 17.5 hours, with 80 percent of the patients aborting within 24 hours.[239] Fetal survival appears to be very rare with abortion by this method. In a comparative study, urea-prostaglandin produced shorter times from instillation to abortion and fewer serious complications than hypertonic saline.[240]

Prostaglandins

Prostaglandins, oxygenated metabolites of C_{20} carboxylic acid, are found naturally in most biologic tissues, where they act as modulators of cell function. They act via specific receptors of the G-protein family, which are coupled to a variety of intracellular signaling mechanisms that may stimulate or inhibit adenyl cyclase or phosphatidylinositol.[241] Prostaglandins of the E and F series can cause uterine contraction at any stage of gestation. Pioneering work by Karim demonstrated that intravenous infusion of prostaglandins produced abortion,[185] but this route proved impractical because of associated vomiting and diarrhea. Side effects were much reduced when $PGF_{2\alpha}$ was given by the intra-amniotic route, and a clinically useful means for midtrimester abortion developed.

Intra-amniotic Prostaglandins

Though initially hailed as a better alternative than intra-amniotic saline, acceptance of intra-amniotic $PGF_{2\alpha}$ was limited because of problems with incomplete abortion, the need for a second injection in many cases, the risk for cervical rupture in the primigravida, and the lack of a direct toxic effect on the fetus. Results with intra-amniotic $PGF_{2\alpha}$ are much improved if overnight treatment with laminaria is used prior to infusion: mean times to abortion are reduced from 29 hours to 14 hours, many fewer require a second dose, and cervical rupture becomes rare.[242] $PGF_{2\alpha}$ was withdrawn by the manufacturer after intense picketing by "antichoice" extremists, but can be replaced with the analogue 15(s)-15-methyl prostaglandin $F_{2\alpha}$ (carboprost tromethamine [Hemabate]). An extensive experience

with midtrimester abortion induced by intra-amniotic carboprost has been reported by Osathanondh from Brigham and Womens' Hospital in Boston.[243] Patients are pretreated overnight with multiple intracervical laminaria tents. The following morning, the tents are removed and an intra-amniotic injection of 2 mg of carboprost combined with 64 mg of 23.4 percent sodium chloride is given. Four hours later, the membranes are artificially ruptured and, unless the cervix is found to be well effaced and dilated, a prostaglandin E_2 suppository is placed into the cervical canal on the end of an osmotic dilator. Subsequently, vaginal suppositories of the PGE_2 are given at 3-hour intervals. All patients have a brief exploration of the uterine cavity and curettage under low-dose intravenous sedation after expulsion of the placenta. If the patient has not aborted by 14 hours, a D&E procedure is performed. The Boston group reports a mean time from instillation to abortion of 8 hours and no cervical lacerations or uterine rupture in over 4,000 consecutive cases treated with this protocol. Ferguson and colleagues report a similar procedure, with laminaria placed in the cervical canal and then immediate administration of 80 g of urea and 2.0 mg of carboprost by the intra-amniotic route.[244] The mean time to abortion was 13 hours for a group of 62 patients. One patient sustained a transverse cervical laceration.

Systemic Prostaglandins

Dinoprostone (prostaglandin E_2) by vaginal suppository and intramuscular carboprost are approved by the U.S. Food and Drug Administration for induction of abortion. Both are easy to administer, and are highly effective. With vaginal dinoprostone, 20 mg every 3 hours, the mean time to abortion is 13.4 hours, with 90 percent of patients aborting by 24 hours.[245] When carboprost is given as 250 μg intramuscularly every 2 hours, the mean times to abortion are 15 to 17 hours, with about 80 percent aborting by 24 hours.[246] Gastrointestinal side effects are common, with 39 percent of dinoprostone-treated patients experiencing vomiting and 25 percent experiencing diarrhea in one large trial.[245] These side effects are more common with carboprost: 83 percent had vomiting and 71 percent had diarrhea in the trial cited above.[246] Fever is more common with dinoprostone than with carboprost. About one third of patients treated with dinoprostone 20 mg every 3 hours will have a temperature elevation of 1°C or more. In abortions induced by prostaglandins of the F series, pretreatment with overnight placement of osmotic dilators shortens the length of prostaglandin treatment, reduces the dose of the drug required, and hence reduces the prostaglandin-related side effects.[247] Whether there is benefit from laminaria for abortion induced by E prostaglandins appears not to have been demonstrated, although laminaria is commonly used prior to dino-prostone treatment.

Misoprostol for Midtrimester Abortion

A randomized comparison of vaginal dinoprost supposi-tories (20 mg every 3 hours) and vaginally adminis-tered misoprostol (200 μg every 12 hours) in patients 12 to 22 weeks pregnant showed equal efficacy. The patients receiving misoprostol had fewer side effects of fever, uterine pain, vomiting, and diarrhea. The miso-prostol cost much less and was easier to administer.[248] Fifty-seven percent of patients treated with misoprostol aborted after a single 200-μg vaginal dose. Both patient groups included women with fetal death and intact ges-tations. The mean time intervals from start of treatment to fetal expulsion for fetal death and intact pregnancies were 9.1 and 13.2 hours, respectively, for those receiv-ing dinoprost, and 10.4 and 15.4 hours, respectively, for those receiving misoprostol. More than half of pa-tients in both groups needed manual or instrumental extraction for retained placentae, as is usual with pros-taglandin abortions. In a subsequent study, these au-thors found laminaria inserted at the same time as the misoprostol did not shorten the treatment-to-abortion interval.[249] Whether overnight pretreatment with lami-naria would improve efficacy of the misoprostol method seems not to have been investigated.

High-Dose Oxytocin

Winkler and colleagues compared dinoprost supposito-ries to a high-dose oxytocin protocol at 17 to 24 weeks and found equal efficacy with fewer side effects from the oxytocin.[250] Patients initially received an infusion of 50 units oxytocin in 500 ml of 5 percent dextrose and normal saline over 3 hours, 1 hour of no oxytocin, followed by a 100-units/500 ml solution over 3 hours, another hour of rest, then a 150-units/500 ml solution over 3 hours, etc., alternating 3 hours of oxytocin with 1 hour of rest, increasing the oxytocin by 50 units in each successive time period until a final concentration of 300 units/500 ml was reached. Fifty-nine percent of the oxytocin patients had either fetal death or ruptured membranes, which could be expected to make the uterus more responsive to induction.

Complications of Labor Induction Abortions and Their Management

The labor induction methods share common hazards: failure of the primary procedure to produce abortion within a reasonable time, incomplete abortion, retained placenta, hemorrhage, infection, and embolic phenom-ena. Failed abortion can lead to serious infection and continued blood loss. Intramuscular injections of carbo-prost or vaginal suppositories of PGE$_2$ are important second-line therapies when the primary method has not produced abortion within a reasonable time period. If dinoprost vaginal suppositories have been used initially and the patient does not abort by 14 to 16 hours, it is reasonable to change to intramuscular carboprost. Also, blood or amniotic fluid may dilute vaginally adminis-tered prostaglandin and limit efficacy; hence, early change to intramuscular carboprost is advised. For-merly, hysterotomy was used to manage these cases, but experienced physicians can safely use D&E tech-niques, sparing the patient major surgery.[251] Failed sa-line or prostaglandin abortions are technically easier to manage by D&E than is a primary procedure at the same gestational age, because the cervix is usually widely dilated, the uterus is well contracted, and the fetus and placenta are compacted into the lower uterine segment. All labor induction methods can lead to fetal expulsion through a rent in the cervix above the exter-nal os, a cervicovaginal fistula, or even annular detach-ment of the lower cervix. Use of laminaria tents helps protect the cervix. The protection is greatest with 12 or more hours of exposure to laminaria prior to uterine stimulation. Uterine rupture may occur when saline, urea, or prostaglandins are augmented with high-dose oxytocin infusion.[252] Easy availability of a treatment room outfitted with a uterine aspirator to allow for early instrumental removal of retained placenta using conscious sedation improves care and avoids the need for an operating room and a major anesthetic. Prosta-glandin abortions are frequently incomplete and hence associated with late bleeding. If the placenta has not delivered within 1 hour after fetal expulsion, further waiting is not advised. Either routine exploration of the uterus with ring forceps and vacuum curettage after all abortions, or routine ultrasound to confirm the uterus is empty, appear to reduce rates of postabortal hemor-rhage and infection to low levels. Oxytocin should be used with caution in prostaglandin-treated patients in order to avoid uterine rupture.

DIC is rare after first-trimester vacuum curettage, where the incidence is 8 per 100,000 procedures.[253] The incidence is higher after midtrimester D&E, 191 per 100,000, and highest for saline instillation proce-dures, 658 per 100,000. DIC must be considered when-ever postabortal hemorrhage is seen and, if present, must be managed aggressively with infusions of fresh frozen plasma and packed red cells. Heparin therapy is not helpful in these cases.

With increasing use of D&E for the early midtrimes-ter, labor induction methods primarily are reserved for late procedures, when concerns about fetal viability and transient fetal survival are the greatest. In our experi-ence with prostaglandins, 7 to 10 percent of fetuses exhibit some transient survival. For this reason, and to improve efficacy, reduced doses of intra-amniotic hypertonic saline or urea may be used to augment prostaglandin abortion. If the fetus is near viability, intracardiac injection of digoxin or KCl should be performed under ultrasound guidance, prior to the prostaglandin.[235]

Choice of Midtrimester Procedure

Many different procedures are available in the United States for midtrimester abortion. Resident physicians on our service have been able to terminate 16- to 20-week pregnancies consistently and safely by D&E under the following conditions: overnight placement of multiple laminaria tents, use of the 16-mm vacuum cannula system, good nursing support, and direct hands-on supervision by a small group of experienced faculty.[254] Robbins and Surrago[255] have found D&E to be safer and more effective than a prostaglandin method. Therefore, we see little indication for any procedure other than D&E prior to 17 menstrual weeks.

When the entire midtrimester is considered, D&E appears safer than the alternatives but, as noted by Kafrissen et al.[256] in their comparison of D&E to urea-$PGF_{2\alpha}$, the advantage of D&E is for procedures performed at 13 to 16 weeks. Thereafter, the risks for major complications and death are comparable. Urea, prostaglandins, and saline infusion all involve overnight hospitalization, which greatly increases expense. As documented by Kaltreider et al.,[229] the psychological impact on the patient is much greater with labor induction abortion than with D&E. Several skilled surgeons offer D&E techniques to 24 weeks and beyond. Indeed, the lowest reported rate of complications for any late abortion technique is that of Hern[235]: serial multiple laminaria over several days to achieve wide cervical dilatation, amniotomy, intravenous oxytocin, and then D&E. For the operator faced with the need to perform an occasional abortion in the midtrimester, we would suggest ultrasound-guided intracardiac injection of 1.5 mg of digoxin and then vaginal misoprostol, 200 μg every 12 hours.

Induced Abortion and Subsequent Reproduction

Hogue et al.[257] reviewed current literature on this topic and concluded that legal abortion as currently practiced in the United States has no measurable adverse effect on later reproduction. A single induced abortion appears safe as far as later reproduction is concerned. Studies of reproductive outcome are difficult because of the need to control for multiple confounding factors that are frequently present among women who report multiple abortions. Our group found that women with two or more induced abortions appeared at greater risk for later first- or second-trimester spontaneous loss, even after appropriate control for other factors.[258] In a separate study, we found that women who reported two or more induced abortions prior to their present pregnancy appeared initially to have more pregnancy complications. However, statistical control by multiple logistic regression analysis found multiple abortions to be associated only with first-trimester bleeding, abnormal presentations, and premature rupture of the membranes prior to labor, but not with low birth weight, prematurity, or increased perinatal loss.[259] A large Hawaiian study found even two or more induced abortions to have no detectable adverse effect.[260] Concerns about infertility as a result of induced abortion seem largely unfounded, except for the rare severe complication managed by hysterectomy. A prospective follow-up study found no reduction in subsequent pregnancy rates when an abortion group was compared with two control groups.[261] The lack of adverse effects on later pregnancy probably reflects the safety of current abortion technology in the United States: most abortions are performed by vacuum curettage under local anesthesia in the first trimester. The safety of midtrimester methods for subsequent pregnancy remains to be demonstrated and unquestionably varies with the method. Forcible dilation of the cervix to large diameters for D&E in the late midtrimester may well increase the risk of midtrimester loss or prematurity later.[262] We have shown that by 2 weeks after laminaria dilation, the cervical canal has recovered to an internal diameter smaller than that found prior to abortion.[263] We feel strongly that laminaria tents, their synthetic alternative, or low-dose prostaglandins should be used to prepare the cervix prior to late abortion and that forcible dilation to large diameters should be avoided.

Pregnancy Termination After Fetal Death In Utero

Whereas fetal death in utero can be managed exactly as induced abortion in the first and second trimesters, there are some differences. After fetal death, laminaria treatment may result in onset of labor. This is not a problem if the patient knows this may happen and has been instructed to return to the hospital. DIC is more common after D&E or induction of labor after a fetal death than with a living fetus. The amniotic sac may be more permeable after fetal death, and intra-amniotic injection becomes technically more difficult. Systemic reactions from hypertonic saline or intra-amniotic prostaglandin are more common in these cases. Indeed, it was this experience that spurred the development of vaginal PGE_2 suppositories to treat fetal death. In cases of fetal death, the response to prostaglandins is faster than with intact gestations, and treatment-to-expulsion times are shorter. Special caution is required for managing fetal death after 28 weeks with prostaglandins. A full dose of 20 mg of PGE_2 has produced fatal uterine rupture. Our protocol, used successfully for many years, is to cut the suppository into fourths and treat the patient with one fourth of the suppository (approximately 5 mg of PGE_2) at 2-hour intervals. The same protocol allows safe, effective treatment for women with severe asthma.

The Limit to Midtrimester Abortion

Women must have access to legal abortion. Efforts to ban abortion by making it illegal do not reduce the number of abortions performed but rather results in expensive and dangerous procedures with many complications and high rates of maternal mortality.[264] However, our society will not countenance infanticide. Inevitably, there must be a gestational age limit for abortion. The U.S. Supreme Court used viability as the limit for abortion based on the decision of the women and allowed states to limit abortion thereafter.[265] With the use of surfactant treatment and current U.S. neonatal intensive care practice, 23-week infants that survive to reach the nursery have at most a 35 percent probability of survival to leave the hospital, and 24-week infants have approximately a 60 percent probability of survival, but infants born prior to 23 weeks almost never survive.[266] In our opinion, 23 weeks should be considered the threshold of viability. We would avoid performing abortion after 22 weeks unless the mother's life were endangered or unless the fetus had major malformations so severe as to preclude prolonged survival. Current ultrasound techniques combine measurements of several fetal dimensions to give more reliable estimates of gestational age than previous techniques that relied on the biparietal diameter alone.[267] When abortion is performed just prior to viability, a method that ensures fetal demise should be selected to avoid the anguished decisions occasioned by the live birth of a fetus of borderline viability. When termination of pregnancy will be undertaken at or after 23 weeks because of serious risk to maternal health, the fetus must be considered as well. Each case must be managed individually, based on the mother's status, and intervention delayed until survival of the fetus is probable, if maternal condition permits.

The ethics of abortion after viability have been explored by Chervanek and colleagues.[268] They conclude that abortion should be considered ethical in cases of fetal conditions with no prospect for prolonged survival after birth and when there is a completely accurate means for diagnosing the conditions. Fetal anencephaly was cited as such a condition.

Key Points

➤ Surgery in pregnancy requires knowledge and understanding of the physiologic alterations in gestation.

➤ Symptoms of gastrointestinal disease during gestation can mimic pregnancy-related symptomatology. Careful evaluation of the patient with abdominal pain in pregnancy is mandatory.

➤ Delay in surgical intervention for patients with intra-abdominal surgical pathology results in increased maternal and fetal morbidity and mortality.

➤ Elective surgery early during the second trimester is associated with the most favorable outcome for both mother and fetus.

➤ Decisions regarding cervical cerclage placement require careful evaluation of the patient's history and cervical status.

➤ Evaluation of the cervix by ultrasound is helpful in the management of patients at risk for cervical incompetence.

➤ Surgery for asymptomatic adnexal masses in pregnancy should include sonographic evaluation of the mass.

➤ High index of suspicion for appendicitis is required for the pregnant patient presenting with right lower quadrant abdominal pain.

➤ Recent series of laparoscopic appendectomies and cholecystectomies during gestation demonstrate similar outcomes to an open approach.

➤ The performance of laparoscopic surgery in gestation should be subject to specific guidelines to ensure maternal and fetal well-being. Further studies are necessary before making absolute recommendations regarding the safety of this technique.

➤ The risk of death from legal abortion in the United States performed prior to 16 weeks is 5- to 10-fold less than that of continuing the pregnancy.

➤ Mifepristone (RU-486) and low-dose prostaglandin provide a medical means for terminating early pregnancy, producing complete abortion in 95 percent of cases.

➤ Selective termination of multifetal pregnancies is practical and improves perinatal outcome.

➤ In the United States, midtrimester abortion is most often accomplished with D&E as opposed to labor induction abortion. Safety with D&E requires close attention to procedural details.

➤ Induced abortion as currently practiced in the Unites States does not increase risk of loss in later pregnancies.

REFERENCES

1. Allen JR, Helling TS, Langenfeld M: Intraabdominal surgery during pregnancy. Am J Surg 158:567, 1989.
2. Brodsky JB, Cohen EN, Brown BW Jr, et al: Surgery during pregnancy and fetal outcome. Clin Obstet Gynecol 138:1165, 1980.
3. Brodsky JB: Anesthesia and surgery during early pregnancy and fetal outcome. Clin Obstet Gynecol 26:449, 1983.
4. Monga M, Creasy RK: Cardiovascular and renal adaptation to pregnancy. In Creasy RK, Resnick R (eds): Maternal-Fetal Medicine: Principles and Practice. 3rd ed. Philadelphia, WB Saunders Company, 1994, p 758.
5. Pritchard JA: Changes in blood volume during pregnancy and delivery. Anesthesiology 26:393, 1965.
6. Prowse CM, Gaensler EA: Respiratory and acid-base changes during pregnancy. Anesthesiology 26:381, 1965.
7. Weinberger SE, Weiss ST, Cohen WR, et al: Pregnancy and the lung. Am Rev Respir Dis 121:559, 1980.
8. Davison JS, Davison MC, Hay DM: Gastric emptying time in late pregnancy and labour. Br J Obstet Gynaecol 77:37, 1970.
9. Bellina JH, Dougherty CM, Mickal A: Pyeloureteral dilation and pregnancy. Am J Obstet Gynecol 108:356, 1970.
10. Todd ME, Thompson JH Jr, Bowie EJW, et al: Changes in blood coagulation during pregnancy. Mayo Clin Proc 40:370, 1965.
11. Chesson RR, Gallup DG, Gibbs RL, et al: Ultrasonographic diagnosis of asymptomatic cholelithiasis in pregnancy. J Reprod Med 30:921, 1985.
12. McCarthy SM, Stark DD, Filly RA, et al: Obstetrical magnetic resonance imaging: maternal anatomy. Radiology 154:421, 1985.
13. McRobbins D, Foster MA: Pulsed magnetic field exposure during pregnancy and implications for NMR foetal imaging: a study with mice. Magn Reson Imaging 3:231, 1985.
14. Puylaert JBCM, Rutgers PH, Lalisang RI, et al: A prospective study of ultrasound in the diagnosis of appendicitis. N Engl J Med 317:666, 1987.
15. Gurbuz AT, Peetz ME: The acute abdomen in the pregnant patient. Surg Endosc 11:98, 1997.
16. Morrell DG, Mullins JR, Harrison PB: Laparoscopic cholecystectomy during pregnancy in symptomatic patients. Surgery 112:856, 1992.
17. Soriano D, Yefet Y, Seidman DS, et al: Laparoscopy versus laparotomy in the management of adnexal masses during pregnancy. Fertil Steril 71:955, 1999.
18. Curet MJ, Allen D, Josloff RK, et al: Laparoscopy during pregnancy. Arch Surg 131:546, 1996.
19. Affleck DG, Handrahan DL, Egger MJ, et al: The laparoscopic management of appendicitis and cholelithiasis during pregnancy. Am J Surg 178:523, 1999.
20. Soper NJ, Brunt LM, Kerbl K: Laparoscopic general surgery. N Engl J Med 330:455, 1994.
21. Chung RS, Broughan RA: The phenomenal growth of laparoscopy cholecystectomy: a review. Cleve Clin J Med 59:186, 1992.
22. Nezhat FR, Tazuke S, Nezhat CH, et al: Laparoscopy during pregnancy: a literature review. J Soc Laparosc Surg 1:17, 1997.
23. Mazze RI, Kallen B: Reproductive outcome after anesthesia and operation during pregnancy: a registry study of 5404 cases. Obstet Gynecol 161:1178, 1989.
24. Lash AF, Lash SR: Habitual abortion: the incompetent internal os of the cervix. Am J Obstet Gynecol 59:68, 1950.
25. Iams JD, Goldenberg RL, Meis PJ, et al: The length of the cervix and the risk of spontaneous premature delivery. N Engl J Med 334:567, 1996.
26. Andersen HF, Nugent CE, Wanty SD, et al: Prediction of risk for preterm delivery by ultrasonographic measurement of cervical length. Am J Obstet Gynecol 163:859, 1990.
27. Gomez R, Galasso M, Romero R, et al: Ultrasonographic examination of the uterine cervix is better than cervical digital examination as a predictor of the likelihood of premature delivery in patients with preterm labor and intact membranes. Am J Obstet Gynecol 171:956, 1994.
28. Iams JD, Parakos J, Landon MG, et al: Cervical sonography in preterm labor. Obstet Gynecol 84:40, 1994.
29. Andersen HF: Transvaginal and transabdominal ultrasonography of the uterine cervix during pregnancy. J Clin Ultrasound 19:77, 1991.
30. Iams JD, Johnson F, Sonek J, et al: Cervical competence as a continuum: a study of sonographic cervical length and obstetrical performance. Am J Obstet Gynecol 172:1097, 1995.
31. Cousins L: Cervical incompetence, 1980: a time for reappraisal. Clin Obstet Gynecol 23:467, 1980.
32. Harger JH: Cervical cerclage: patient selection, morbidity, and success rates. Clin Perinatol 10:321, 1983.
33. Rechberger T, Uldbjerg N, Oxlund H: Connective tissue changes in the cervix during normal pregnancy and pregnancy complicated by cervical incompetence. Obstet Gynecol 71:563, 1988.
34. Zlatnik FJ, Burmeister LF: Interval evaluation of the cervix for predicting pregnancy outcome and diagnosing cervical incompetence. J Reprod Med 38:365, 1993.
35. Ludmir J, Landon MB, Gabbe SG, et al: Management of the diethylstilbestrol-exposed pregnant patient: a prospective study. Am J Obstet Gynecol 157:665, 1987.
36. Crombleholme W, Minkoff H, Delke I, et al: Cervical cerclage: an aggressive approach to threatened or recurrent pregnancy wastage. Am J Obstet Gynecol 146:168, 1983.
37. Cardosi RJ, Chez RA: Comparison of elective and empiric cerclage and the role of emergency cerclage. J Matern Fetal Med 7:230, 1998.
38. Michaels WH, Montgomery C, Karo J, et al: Ultrasound differentiation of the competent from the incompetent cervix: prevention of preterm delivery. Am J Obstet Gynecol 154:537, 1986.
39. Michaels WH, Montgomery C, Karo J, et al: Ultrasound differentiation of the competent from the incompetent cervix: prevention of preterm delivery. Am J Obstet Gynecol 154:537, 1986.
40. Andersen HF, Karimi A, Sakala EP, et al: Prediction of cervical cerclage outcome by endovaginal ultrasonography. Am J Obstet Gynecol 171:1102, 1994.
41. Guzman ER, Rosenberg JC, Houlihan C, et al: A new method using ultrasound and transfundal pressure to evaluate the asymptomatic incompetent cervix. Obstet Gynecol 83:248, 1994.

42. Wong G, Levine D, Ludmir J: Maternal postural challenge as a functional test for cervical incompetence. J Ultrasound Med 16:169, 1997.

43. Guzman ER, Forster JK, Vintzileos AM, et al: Pregnancy outcomes in women treated with elective versus ultrasound-indicated cervical cerclage. Ultrasound Obstet Gynecol 12:323, 1998.

44. Berghella V, Daly SF, Toloso JE, et al: Prediction of preterm delivery with transvaginal ultrasonography of the cervix in patients with high-risk pregnancies: does cerclage prevent prematurity? Am J Obstet Gynecol 181:809, 1999.

45. Heath VCF, Souka AP, Erasmus I, et al: Cervical length at 23 weeks of gestation: the value of Shirodkar suture of the short cervix. Ultrasound Obstet Gynecol 12:318, 1998.

46. Rust O, Atlas R, Jones K, et al: A randomized trial of cerclage vs no cerclage in patients with sonographic detected 2nd trimester premature dilation of the internal os [abstract]. Presented at the 20th Annual Meeting of the Society for Maternal-Fetal Medicine, Miami Beach, FL, 2000.

47. Althuisius SM, Dekker GA, van Geijin HP, et al: Cervical incompetence prevention randomized cerclage trial, preliminary results [abstract]. Presented at the 20th Annual Meeting of Society for Maternal-Fetal Medicine, Miami Beach, FL, 2000.

48. Shirodkar VN: A new method of operative treatment for habitual abortion in the second trimester of pregnancy. Antiseptic 52:299, 1955.

49. McDonald IA: Suture of the cervix for inevitable miscarriage. J Obstet Gynecol Br Commonw 64:346, 1957.

50. Abdelhak YE, Sheen JJ, Kuczynski E, et al: Comparison of delayed absorbable suture v nonabsorbable suture for treatment of incompetent cervix. J Perinatol Med 27:250, 1999.

51. Aarnoudse JG, Huisjes HJ: Complications of cerclage. Acta Obstet Gynecol Scand 58:225, 1979.

52. Harger JH: Comparison of success and morbidity in cervical cerclage procedures. Obstet Gynecol 53:543, 1980.

53. McDonald IA: Incompetence of the cervix. Aust N Z J Obstet Gynaecol 18:34, 1978.

54. Schulman H, Farmakides G: Surgical approach to failed cervical cerclage: a report of three cases. J Reprod Med 30:626, 1985.

55. Steinberg ES, Santos AC: Surgical anesthesia during pregnancy. Int Anesthesiol Clin 28:58, 1990.

56. Chen L, Ludmir J, Miller FL, et al: Is regional better than general anesthesia for cervical cerclage? Nine years experience. Anesth Analg 70:S1, 1990.

57. Andersen HG: Transvaginal and transabdominal ultrasonography of the uterine cervix during pregnancy. J Clin Ultrasound 19:77, 1991.

58. Althuisius SM, Dekker GA, van Geijin HP, et al: The effect of therapeutic McDonald cerclage on cervical length as assessed by transvaginal ultrasonography. Am J Obstet Gynecol 180:366, 1999.

59. Funai EF, Paidas MJ, Rebarber A, et al: Change in cervical length after prophylactic cerclage. Obstet Gynecol 94:117, 1999.

60. Novy MJ: Transabdominal cervicoisthmic cerclage for the management of repetitive abortion and premature delivery. Am J Obstet Gynecol 143:44, 1982.

61. Novy MJ: Transabdominal cervicoisthmic cerclage: a reappraisal 25 years after its introduction. Am J Obstet Gynecol 164:163, 1991.

62. Ludmir J, Jackson GM, Samuels P: Transvaginal cerclage under ultrasound guidance in cases of severe cervical hypoplasia. Obstet Gynecol 78:1067, 1991.

63. Scarantino SE, Reilly JG, Moretti ML, et al: Laparoscopic removal of a transabdominal cervical cerclage. Am J Obstet Gynecol 182:1086, 2000.

64. Benifla JL, Goffinet F, Darai E, et al: Emergency cervical cerclage after 20 weeks gestation: a retrospective study of 6 years' practice in 34 cases. Fetal Diagn Ther 12:27408, 1997.

65. Minakami H, Matsubara S, Izumi A, et al: Emergency cervical cerclage: relation between its success, perioperative serum level of C-reactive protein and WBC count, and degree of cervical dilatation. Gynecol Obstet Invest 47:157, 1999.

66. Aarts JM, Brons JT, Bruinse HW, et al: Emergency cerclage: a review. Obstet Gynecol Surv 50:459, 1995.

67. Caruso A, Trivellini C, DeCarolis S, et al: Emergency cerclage in the presence of protruding membranes: is pregnancy outcome predictable? Acta Obstet Gynaecol Scand 79:265, 2000.

68. Barth WH Jr, Yeomans ER, Hankins GDV, et al: Emergent cerclage. Surg Gynecol Scand 58:225, 1979.

69. Charles D, Edwards WR: Infectious complications of cerclage. Am J Obstet Gynecol 141:1065, 1981.

70. Mays JK, Figueroa R, Shah J, et al: Amniocentesis for selection before rescue cerclage. Obstet Gynecol 95:652, 2000.

71. Scheerer LJ, Lam F, Barotolucci L, et al: A new technique for reduction of prolapsed fetal membranes for emergency cervical cerclage. Obstet Gynecol 74:408, 1989.

72. Kurup M, Goldkrand JW: Cervical incompetence: elective, emergent, or urgent. Am J Obstet Gynecol 181:240, 1999.

73. Wu MY, Yang YS, Huang SC, et al: Emergent and elective cervical cerclage for cervical incompetence. Int J Gynaecol Obstet 54:23, 1996.

74. Lipitz S, Libshitz A, Oelsner G, et al: Outcome of second-trimester, emergency cervical cerclage in patients with no history of cervical incompetence. Am J Perinatol 13:419, 1996.

75. Ludmir J, Bader T, Chen L, et al: Poor perinatal outcome associated with retained cerclage in patients with premature rupture of membranes. Obstet Gynecol 84:823, 1994.

76. Norwitz ER, Lieberman ES, Heffner LJ: Cervical cerclage and preterm premature rupture of the membranes: should the stitch be removed? [abstract]. Presented at the 20th Annual Meeting of Society for Maternal-Fetal Medicine, Miami Beach, FL, 2000.

77. Berghella V, McIntyre C, Pollock M, et al: Timing of cerclage removal after PPROM-maternal and neonatal outcomes [abstract]. Presented at the 20th Annual Meeting of the Society for Maternal-Fetal Medicine, Miami Beach, FL, 2000.

78. Dunn LE, Robinson JC, Steer CM: Maternal death following suture of incompetent cervix during pregnancy. Am J Obstet Gynecol 78:335, 1959.

79. Dor J, Shalev J, Mashiach S, et al: Elective cervical suture of twin pregnancies diagnosed ultrasonically in the first trimester following induced ovulation. Gynecol Obstet Invest 13:55, 1982.

80. Lazar P, Gueguen S, Dreyfus J, et al: Multicentred controlled trial of cervical cerclage in women at moderate risk of preterm delivery. Br J Obstet Gynaecol 91:731, 1984.

81. Rush RW, Issacs S, McPherson K, et al: A randomized controlled trial of cervical cerclage in women at high risk of spontaneous preterm delivery. Br J Obstet Gynaecol 91:724, 1984.

82. MRC/RCOG Working Party on Cervical Cerclage: Final report of the Medical Research Council/Royal College of Obstetricians and Gynaecologists multicentre randomized trial of cervical cerclage. Br J Obstet Gynaecol 100:516, 1993.

83. Ahavoni A, Reiter A, Golan D, et al: Patterns of growth of uterine leiomyomas during pregnancy. A prospective longitudinal study. Br J Obstet Gynaecol 95:510, 1988.

84. Bezjian AA: Pelvic masses in pregnancy. Clin Obstet Gynecol 27:402, 1984.

85. Lev-Toaff AS, Coleman BG, Arger PH, et al: Leiomyomas in pregnancy: sonographic study. Radiology 164:375, 1987.

86. Roberts WE, Fulp KS, Morrison JC, et al: The impact of leiomyomas on pregnancy. Aust N Z J Obstet Gynaecol 39: 43, 1999.

87. Szamatowicz J, Laudanski T, Bulkszas B, et al: Fibromyomas and uterine contractions. Acta Obstet Gynecol Scand 76:973, 1997.

88. Coronado GD, Marshall LM, Schwartz SM: Complications in pregnancy, labor, and delivery with uterine leiomyomas: a population-based study. Obstet Gynecol 95:764, 2000.

89. Omar SZ, Sivanesaratnam V, Damodaran P: Larger lower segment myoma—myomectomy at lower segment cesarean section—a report of two cases. Singapore Med J 40:109, 1999.

90. Marino T, Craigo S: Managing adnexal masses in pregnancy. Contemp Obstet Gynecol 45:130, 2000.

91. Hess LW, Peaceman A, O'Brien WF, et al: Adnexal masses occurring with intrauterine pregnancy. Am J Obstet Gynecol 158:1029, 1988.

92. Beischer NA, Buttery BW, Fortune DW: Growth and malignancy of ovarian tumors in pregnancy. Aust N Z J Obstet Gynaecol 11:208, 1971.

93. Koonings PP, Laurence P, Wallace R, et al: Incidental adnexal neoplasm at cesarean section. Obstet Gynccol 72:767, 1988.

94. Rodin A, Coltart TM, Chapman MG: Needle aspiration of simple ovarian cysts in pregnancy. Br J Obstet Gynaecol 96: 994, 1989.

95. Moyle JW, Rochester D, Sider L, et al: Sonography of ovarian tumors: predictability of tumor type. AJR Am J Roentgenol 141:985, 1983.

96. Thornton JG, Wells M: Ovarian cysts in pregnancy: does ultrasound make traditional management inappropriate? Obstet Gynecol 69:717, 1987.

97. Hogston P, Lilford RJ: Ultrasound study of ovarian cysts in pregnancy: prevalence and significance. Br J Obstet Gynaecol 93:625, 1986.

98. Shalev E, Peley D: Laparoscopic treatment of adnexal torsion. Surg Gynecol Scand 65:583, 1993.

99. Viscomi CM, Rathmell JP: Labor epidural catheter reactivation or spinal anesthesia for delayed postpartum tubal ligation: a cost comparison. J Clin Anesth 7:380, 1995.

100. Peterson HB, Xia Z, Hughes JM, et al: The risk of pregnancy after tubal sterilization: findings from the U.S. Collaborative Review of Sterilization. Am J Obstet Gynecol 174:1161, 1996.

101. Bishop E, Nelms WF: A simple method of tubal sterilization. N Y State J Med 30:214, 1930.

102. Irving FC: Tubal sterilization. Am J Obstet Gynecol 60:1101, 1950.

103. Lopez-Zeno JA, Muallem NS, Anderson JB: The Irving sterilization technique: a report of a failure. Int J Fertil 35:23, 1990.

104. Uchida H: Uchida tubal sterilization. Am J Obstet Gynecol 121:153, 1975.

105. Mazze RI, Kallen B: Appendectomy during pregnancy: a Swedish registry study of 778 cases. Obstet Gynecol 77:835, 1991.

106. Weingold AB: Appendicitis in pregnancy. Clin Obstet Gynecol 26:801, 1983.

107. Baer JL, Reis RA, Arens RA: Appendicitis in pregnancy with changes in position and axis of the normal appendix in pregnancy. JAMA 98:1359, 1932.

108. Mourad J, Elliott JO, Erickson L, et al: Appendicitis in pregnancy: new information that contradicts long-held clinical beliefs. Am J Obstet Gynecol 182:1027, 2000.

109. Gomez A, Wood M: Acute appendicitis in pregnancy. Am J Surg 137:180, 1979.

110. Barloon TJ, Brown BP, Abu-Yousef MM, et al: Sonography of acute appendicitis in pregnancy. Abdom Imaging 20:149, 1995.

111. Anderson B, Neilsen TF: Appendicitis in pregnancy: diagnosis, management and complications. Acta Obstet Gynaecol Scand 78:758, 1999.

112. Landers D, Carmona R, Crombleholme W, Lin T: Acute cholecystitis in pregnancy. Obstet Gynecol 69:131, 1987.

113. Mazze RI, Kallen B: Reproductive outcome after anesthesia and operation during pregnancy: a registry study of 5405 cases. Obstet Gynecol 161:1178, 1989.

114. Dixon NF, Faddis DM, Silberman H: Aggressive management of cholecystitis during pregnancy. Am J Surg 154:294, 1987.

115. Barone JE, Bears S, Chen S, et al: Outcome study of cholecystectomy during pregnancy. Am J Surg 177:232, 1999.

116. Lanzafame RJ: Laparoscopic cholecystectomy during pregnancy. Surgery 118:627, 1995.

117. Goldthorp WO: Intestinal obstruction during pregnancy and the puerperium. Br J Clin Pract 20:367, 1966.

118. Rusher AH, Fields B, Henson K: Laparoscopic cholecystectomy in pregnancy. Contraindicated or indicated? A Ark Med Soc 89:383, 1993.

119. Davis MR, Bohon CJ: Intestinal obstruction in pregnancy. Clin Obstet Gynecol 26:832, 1983.

120. Hill LM, Symmonds RE: Small bowel obstruction in pregnancy: a review and report of four cases. Obstet Gynecol 49: 170, 1977.

121. Ludmir J, Samuels P, Armson BA, et al: Spontaneous small bowel obstruction associated with a spontaneous triplet gestation: a case report. J Reprod Med 34:985, 1989.

122. Perdue PW, Johnston HW Jr, Stafford PW: Intestinal obstruction complicating pregnancy. Am J Surg 164:384, 1992.

123. Spira IA, Wolff WI: Colonic pseudo-obstruction following termination of pregnancy and uterine operation. Am J Obstet Gynecol 126:7, 1976.

124. Pearlman MD, Tintinalli JE, Lorenz RP: Blunt trauma during pregnancy. N Engl J Med 323:1609, 1990.

125. Esposito TJ, Gens DR, Gerber-Smith L, et al: Evaluation of blunt abdominal trauma occurring during pregnancy. J Trauma 29:1628, 1989.

126. Connolly AM, Katz VL, Bash KL, et al: Trauma and pregnancy. Am J Perinatol 14:331, 1997.

127. Fort AT, Harlin RS: Pregnancy outcome after noncatastrophic maternal trauma during pregnancy. Obstet Gynecol 35:912, 1970.

128. Poole GV, Martin JN Jr, Perry KG Jr, et al: Trauma in pregnancy: the role of interpersonal violence. Am J Obstet Gynecol 174:1873, 1996.

129. Lees DH, Singer A: Gynecologic Survey. Vol 6. London, Wolfe Medical, 1983.

130. Crosby WM, Costiloe JP: Safety of lap-belt restraint for pregnant victims of automobile collisions. N Engl J Med 284:632, 1971.

131. Dahmus MA, Sibai MB: Blunt abdominal trauma: are there any predictive factors for abruptio placentae or maternal-fetal distress? Am J Obstet Gynecol 169:1054, 1993.

132. Pearlman MD, Tintinalli JE: Evaluation and treatment of the gravida and fetus following trauma during pregnancy. Obstet Gynecol Clin North Am 18:371, 1991.

133. Williams JK, McClain L, Rosemary AS, et al: Evaluation of blunt abdominal trauma in the third trimester of pregnancy: maternal and fetal considerations. Obstet Gynecol 75:33, 1990.

134. Pak LL, Reece EA, Chan L: Is adverse pregnancy outcome predictable after blunt abdominal trauma? Am J Obstet Gynecol 179:1140, 1998.

135. Franger AL, Buchsbaum HJ, Peaceman AM: Abdominal gunshot wounds in pregnancy. Am J Obstet Gynecol 160:1124, 1989.

136. ACOG Educational Bulletin Number 251: Obstetric aspects of trauma management. Compendium of Selected Publications. Washington, DC, ACOG, 2000.

137. Curet MJ, Schermer CR, Demarest GB, et al: Predictors of outcome in trauma during pregnancy: identification of patients who can be monitored for less than 6 hours. J Trauma 49:18, 2000.

138. Amy BW, McManus WF, Goodwin CW, et al: Thermal injury in the pregnancy patient. Surg Gynecol Obstet 161:209, 1985.

139. Benmeir P, Sagi A, Gerber CB, et al: Burns during pregnancy: our experience. Burns Incl Term Inj 14:233, 1988.

140. Matthews RN: Obstetric implications of burns in pregnancy. Br J Obstet Gynaecol 89:603, 1982.

141. Amos D, Schorr SJ, Norman PF, et al: Laparoscopic surgery during pregnancy. Am J Surg 171:435, 1996.

142. Reedy MB, Galan HL, Bean-Lijewski JD, et al: Maternal and fetal effect of laparoscopic insufflation in the gravid baboon. J Am Assoc Gynecol Laparosc 2:399, 1995.

143. Hunter JG, Swanstrom L, Thomburg K: Carbon dioxide pneumoperitoneum induces fetal acidosis in a pregnant ewe model. Surg Endosc 9:272, 1995.

144. Guidelines for laparoscopic surgery during pregnancy. Surg Endosc 12:189, 1998.

145. Schreiber JH: Laparoscopic appendectomy in pregnancy. Surg Endosc 4:100, 1990.

146. Steinbrook RA, Brooks DC, Datta S: Laparoscopic cholecystectomy during pregnancy. Surg Endosc 10:511, 1996.

147. Grahan G, Baxi L, Tharakan T: Laparoscopic cholecystectomy during pregnancy: a case series and review of the literature. Obstet Gynecol Survey 53:566, 1998.

148. Koonin LM, Strauss LT, Chrisman CE, et al: Abortion surveillance. United States, 1996. MMWR Morb Mortal Wkly Rep 48:1, 1999.

149. Tietze C: New estimates of mortality associated with fertility control. Fam Plann Perspect 9:74, 1977.

150. Eisner V, Brazie JV, Pratt MW, Hexter AC: The risk of low birth weight. Am J Public Health 69:887, 1979.

151. Puffer RR, Serrano CV: Birth weight, maternal age and birth order: three important determinants in infant mortality. Pan Am Health Organization, Scientific Publ. No. 294, 1975.

152. Bakketieg LS, Hoffman HJ: Epidemiology of preterm birth: results from a longitudinal study of births in Norway. In Elder MG, Hendricks CH (eds): Preterm Labour, London, Butterworths, 1981, p 17.

153. Henshaw SK: Unintended pregnancy in the United States. Fam Plann Perspect 30:24, 1998.

154. Forrest JD, Henshaw SK: What US women think and do about contraception. Fam Plann Perspect 15:157, 1983.

155. Potts M, Diggory P, Peel J: Abortion. Cambridge, Cambridge University Press, 1977.

156. Deveraux G: A Study of Abortion in Primitive Societies. New York, International Universities Press, 1976.

157. Narkavonnakit T, Bennett T: Health consequences of induced abortion in rural Northeast Thailand. Stud Fam Plann 12:58, 1981.

158. Mohr JC: Abortion in America: The Origins and Evolution of National Policy. New York, Oxford University Press, 1978.

159. Susser M: Induced abortion and health as a value. Am J Public Health 82:1323, 1992.

160. Lawson HW, Frye A, Atrash HK, et al: Abortion mortality, United States, 1972–1987. Am J Obstet Gynecol 171:1365, 1994.

161. Peterson HB, Grimes DA, Cates W Jr, et al: Comparative risk of death from induced abortion at 12 weeks or less gestation performed with local versus general anesthesia. Am J Obstet Gynecol 141:763, 1981.

162. Atrash HK, Cheek TG, Hogue CJ: Legal abortion mortality and general anesthesia. Am J Obstet Gynecol 158:420, 1988.

163. Osborn JF, Arisi E, Spinelli A, et al: General anesthesia, a risk factor for complications following induced abortion. Eur J Epidemiol 6:419, 1989.

164. Cates W Jr, Rochat RW: Illegal abortions in the United States: 1972–1974. Fam Plann Perspect 8:86, 1976.

165. Council on Scientific Affairs, American Medical Association: Induced termination of pregnancy before and after Roe v Wade: trends in the mortality and morbidity of women. JAMA 268:3231, 1992.

166. Stubblefield PG: Induced abortion: indications, counseling, and services. In Sciarra JJ, Zatuchni GI, Daly MJ (eds): Gynecology and Obstetrics. Vol 6. Philadelphia, Harper & Row, 1982, p 2.

167. Wu YT: Suction in artificial abortion: 300 cases. Chin J Obstet Gynecol 6:447, 1958.

168. Andolsek L (ed): The Ljubljana Abortion Study, 1971–1973. Bethesda, MD, National Institutes of Health, Center for Population Research, 1974.

169. Karman H, Potts M: Very early abortion using syringe as vacuum source. Lancet 1:7759, 1972.

170. Burnhill MS, Armstead JW: Reducing the morbidity of vacuum aspiration abortion. Int J Gynecol Obstet 16:204, 1978.

171. Edwards J, Carson SA: New technologies permit safe abortion at less than six weeks gestation and provide timely diagnosis of ectopic gestation. Am J Obstet Gynecol 1076:1101, 1987.

172. Smith GM, Stubblefield PG, Chirchirillo L, et al: Pain of first trimester abortion: its quantification and relations with other variables. Am J Obstet Gynecol 133:489, 1979.

173. Suprato K, Reed S: Naproxen sodium for pain relief in first trimester abortion. Am J Obstet Gynecol 150:1000, 1984.

174. Wiebe ER, Rawling M: Pain control in abortion: a comparison of various local anesthetics, preoperative analgesics and techniques. Presented at National Abortion Federation Risk Management Seminar: Pain Management: Reducing patient discomfort and provider anxiety. September 18, 1994, Philadelphia, PA.

175. Glick E: Paracervical and lower uterine field block anesthesia for therapeutic abortion and office D&C. Presented at the 11th Annual Convention of the National Abortion Federation. Salt Lake City, UT, May 18, 1987.

176. Wiebe ER: Comparison of the efficacy of different local anesthetics and techniques of local anesthesia in therapeutic abortion. Am J Obstet Gynecol 167:131, 1992.

177. Stubblefield PG: Control of pain for women undergoing abortion. Int J Gynecol Obstet 3 (Suppl):131, 1989.

178. Bell GP, Morden A, Coady T, et al: A comparison of diazepam and midazolam as endoscopy premedication: assessing changes in ventilation and oxygen saturation. Br J Clin Pharmacol 26:595, 1988.

179. Schulz, KF, Grimes DA, Cates W Jr: Measures to prevent cervical injury during suction curettage abortion. Lancet 1:1182, 1983.

180. Grimes DA, Schulz KF, Cates W Jr: Prevention of uterine perforation during curettage abortion. JAMA 25:2108, 1984.

181. Gold J, Schulz KR, Cates W Jr, Tyler CW: The safety of *Laminaria* and rigid dilators for cervical dilatation prior to suction curettage for first trimester abortion: a comparative analysis. In Naftolin F, Stubblefield PG (eds): Dilatation of the Uterine Cervix: Connective Tissue Biology and Clinical Management. New York, Raven Press, 1980, p 363.

182. Darney PD, Dorward K: Cervical dilatation before first-trimester election abortion: a controlled comparison of meteneprost, *Laminaria* and hypan. Obstet Gynecol 70:397, 1987.

183. Ngai SW, Chan YM, Tang OS: The use of misoprostol for preoperative cervical dilatation prior to vacuum curettage abortion: a randomized trial. Hum Reprod 14:21, 1999.

184. Bowman JM: Controversies in Rh prophylaxis. Am J Obstet Gynecol 151:289, 1985.

185. Karim SMM: The use of prostaglandins in abortion. *In* Lewit S (ed): Abortion Techniques and Services. Amsterdam, Excerpta Medica, 1972, p 68.

186. Couzinet B, LeStrat N, Ulman A, et al: Termination of early pregnancy by the progesterone antagonist RU 486 (mifepristone). N Engl J Med 315:1565, 1986.

187. Bygdeman M, Swahm ML: Progesterone receptor blockage: effect on uterine contractility and early pregnancy. Contraception 32:45, 1985.

188. Silvestre L, Dubois C, Renault M, et al: Voluntary interruption of pregnancy with mifepristone (RU486) and a prostaglandin analogue. N Engl J Med 322:645, 1990.

189. Ulmann A, Silvestre L, Chemama L, et al: Medical termination of early pregnancy with mifepristone (RU486) followed by a prostaglandin analogue: study in 16,639 women. Acta Obstet Scand 71:278, 1992.

190. Noticeboard: A death associated with mifepristone/sulprostone. Lancet 337:969, 1991.

191. Peyron R, Aubeny E, Targosz V, et al: Early termination of pregnancy with mifeprisone (RU486) and the orally active prostaglandin misoprostol. N Engl J Med 328:1509, 1993.

192. El-Rafaey H, Rajasekar D, Abdala M, et al: Induction of abortion with mifepristone (RU486) and misoprostol. N Engl J Med 332:983, 1995.

193. Creinin M, Aubeny MD: Medical abortion in early pregnancy. *In* Paul M, Lichtenberg ES, Borgatta L, et al (eds): A Clinician's Guide to Medical and Surgical Abortion. New York, Churchill Livingstone, 1999, p 91.

194. Lefebvre Y, Proulx L, Elie R, et al: The effects of RU38486 on cervical ripening. Am J Obstet Gynecol 162:61, 1990.

195. Stovall TG, Ling FW: Single dose methotrexate: an expanded clinical trial. Am J Obstet Gynecol 168:1759, 1993.

196. Creinin MD, Darney PD: Methotrexate and misoprostol for early abortion. Contraception 48:339, 1993.

197. Creinin MD, Vittinghoff E, Keder L, et al: Methotrexate and misoprostol for early abortion: a multicenter trial. I. Safety and efficacy. Contraception 53:321, 1996.

198. Berkowitz RL, Lynch L, Chitkara U, et al: Selection reduction of multifetal pregnancies in the first trimester. N Engl J Med 318:1043, 1988.

199. Wapner RJ, Davis GH, Johnson A, et al: Selective reproduction of multifetal pregnancies. Lancet 335:90, 1990.

200. Evans MI, Dommergues M, Wapner RJ, et al: Efficacy of transabdominal multifetal pregnancy reduction: collaborative experience among the world's largest centers. Obstet Gynecol 82:61, 1993.

201. Lipitz S, Reichman B, Uval J, et al: A prospective comparison of the outcome of triplet pregnancies managed expectantly or by multifetal reduction to twins. Am J Obstet Gynecol 170:874, 1994.

202. Aberg A, Metelman R, Canz M, et al: Cardiac puncture of fetus with Hurler's disease avoiding abortion of unaffected co-twin. Lancet 2:990, 1978.

203. Evans MI, Goldberg JD, Dommergues M, et al: Efficacy of second trimester selective termination for fetal anomalies: international collaborative experience among the world's largest centers. Am J Obstet Gynecol 171:90, 1994.

204. Evans MI, Goldberg JD, Horenstein J, et al: Selective termination for structural, chromosomal and mendelian anomalies: international experience. Am J Obstet Gynecol 181:893, 1999.

205. Stubblefield PG: Complications of induced abortion. *In* Pearlman MD, Tintinalli JE (eds): Emergency Care of the Woman. New York, McGraw-Hill, 1998, p 37.

206. US Food and Drug Administration: Warning for prescription drugs containing sulfite. Drug Bull 17:2, 1987.

207. Grimes DA, Schulz KF, Cates WJ: Prevention of uterine perforation during curettage abortion. JAMA 251:2108, 1984.

208. Hakim-Elahi E, Tovell HMM, Burnhill MS: Complications of first trimester abortion: a report of 170,000 cases. Obstet Gynecol 76:129, 1990.

209. Lauersen NJ, Birnbaum S: Laparoscopy as a diagnostic and therapeutic technique in uterine perforations during first-trimester abortions. Am J Obstet Gynecol 117:522, 1973.

210. Berek JS, Stubblefield, PG: Anatomical and clinical correlations of uterine perforations. Am J Obstet Gynecol 135:181, 1979.

211. Vedantham S, Goodwin SC, McLucas B, et al: Uterine artery embolization: an underused method of controlling pelvic hemorrhage. Am J Obstet Gynecol 176:938, 1997.

212. Sands RX, Burnhill MS, Hakim Elahi E: Post-abortal uterine atony. Obstet Gynecol 43:595, 1974.

213. Fielding WL, Lee WY, Borten N, Friedman EA: Continued pregnancy after failed first trimester abortion. Obstet Gynecol 63:421, 1984.

214. Rubin GL, Peterson EB, Dorfman SF, et al: Ectopic pregnancy in the United States, 1970 through 1978. JAMA 249:1725, 1983.

215. Stubblefield PG, Grimes DA: Septic abortion. N Engl J Med 331:310, 1994.

216. Hoyme UB, Eschenback DA: Postoperative infection. *In* Iffy L, Charles D (eds): Operative Perinatology. New York, Macmillan, 1984, p 821.

217. Faro S, Pearlman M: Infections and Abortion. New York, Elsevier, 1992.

218. Grimm PS, Gottlieb LJ, Bodie A, et al: Hyperbaric oxygen therapy. JAMA 263:2216, 1990.

219. Hodgson JE, Major B, Portman K, et al: Prophylactic use of tetracycline for first trimester abortions. Obstet Gynecol 45:574, 1975.

220. Grimes DA, Schulz KF, Cates W: Prophylactic antibiotics for curettage abortion. Am J Obstet Gynecol 150:689, 1984.

221. Park TK, Flock M, Schulz KF, et al: Preventing febrile complications of suction curettage abortion. Am J Obstet Gynecol 152:252, 1985.

222. Sonne-Holme S, Heisterberg L, Hebjorn S, et al: Prophylactic antibiotics in first trimester abortion: a clinical controlled trial. Am J Obstet Gynecol 139:693, 1981.

223. Levallois P, Rioux JE: Prophylactic antibiotics for suction curettage abortion: results of a clinical controlled trial. Am J Obstet Gynecol 158:100, 1988.

224. Grimes DA, Schulz KF, Cates W Jr, Tyler CW: Mid-trimester abortion by dilatation and evacuation: a safe and practical alternative. N Engl J Med 296:1141, 1977.

225. Stubblefield PG: Midtrimester abortion by curettage procedures: an overview. *In* Hodgson JE (ed): Abortion and Sterilization: Medical and Social Aspects. San Diego, CA, Academic Press, 1981, p 277.

226. Hern WM: Abortion Practice. Philadelphia, JB Lippincott, 1984.

227. Stubblefield PG, Albrecht BH, Koos B, et al: A randomized study of 12 mm vs. 15.9 mm vacuum cannulas in midtrimester abortion Laminaria and vacuum curettage. Fertil Steril 29:512, 1978.

228. MacKay HT, Schulz KR, Grimes DA: The safety of local

versus general anesthesia for second trimester dilatation and evacuation abortion. Obstet Gynecol 66:661, 1985.

229. Kaltreider NB, Goldsmith S, Margolis AJ: The impact of midtrimester abortion techniques on patients and staff. Am J Obstet Gynecol 135:235, 1979.

230. Wright PC: Late midtrimester abortion by dilatation and evacuation using dilapan and digoxin. Presented at the 13th Annual Meeting of the National Abortion Federation, San Francisco, CA, April 4, 1989.

231. Eichorn JH, Cooper JB, Cullen DJ, et al: Standards for patient monitoring during anesthesia at Harvard Medical School. JAMA 256:1017, 1986.

232. Haskell WM, Esterling TR, Lichtenberg ES: Surgical abortion after the first trimester. In Paul M, Lichtenberg ES, Borgatta L, et al (eds): A Clinician's Guide to Medical and Surgical Abortion. New York, Churchill Livingstone, 1999, p 123.

233. Darney PD, Sweet RL: Routine intraoperative ultrasonography for second trimester abortion reduces incidence of uterine perforation. J Ultrasound Med 8:71, 1989.

234. Schulz KF, Grimes DA, Christensen DD: Vasopressin reduces blood loss from second trimester dilatation and evacuation abortion. Lancet 2:353, 1985.

235. Hern WM, Ferguson KA, Hart V, et al: Outpatient abortion for fetal anomaly and fetal death from 15–34 menstrual weeks' gestation: techniques and clinical management. Obstet Gynecol 81:301, 1993.

236. McMahon JT: Intact D & E. The first decade. Presented at the National Abortion Federation Annual Meeting. New Orleans, LA, April 2, 1995.

237. Kerenyi TD, Mandelman N, Sherman DH: Five thousand consecutive saline abortions. Am J Obstet Gynecol 116:593, 1973.

238. Berger GS, Edelman DA: Oxytocin administration, instillation to abortion time, and morbidity associated with saline instillation. Am J Obstet Gynecol 121:941, 1975.

239. Burkeman RT, King TM, Atienza MF: Hyperosmolar urea. In Berger GS, Brenner WE, Keith LG (eds): Second Trimester Abortion: Perspectives After a Decade of Experience. Boston, John Wright, PSG, Inc, 1981.

240. Binkin NJ, Schulz KF, Grimes DA, Cates W Jr: Urea-prostaglandin versus hypertonic saline for instillation abortion. Am J Obstet Gynecol 146:947, 1983.

241. Negishi M, Sugimoto YI, Ichikawa A: Prostanoid receptors and their biological actions. Prog Lipid Res 32:417, 1993.

242. Stubblefield PG: Current technology for abortion. Curr Probl Obstet Gynecol 2:1, 1978.

243. Osathanondh R: Conception control. In Ryan KJ, Barbieri R, Berkowitz RS (eds): Kistner's Gynecology. 5th ed. Chicago, Year Book Medical Publishers, 1989, p 480.

244. Ferguson JE, Burkett BU, Pinkerton JV, et al: Intraamniotic 15(s)-15-methyl prostaglandin $F_{2\alpha}$ and terminatio of middle and late second trimester pregnancy for genetic indications: a contemporary approach. Am J Obstet Gynecol 169:332, 1993.

245. Surrago EJ, Robins J: Midtrimester pregnancy termination by intravaginal administration of prostaglandin E_2. Contraception 26:285, 1976.

246. Robins J, Mann LI: Second generation prostaglandins: midtrimester pregnancy termination by intramuscular injection of a 15-methyl analog of prostaglandins $F_{2\alpha}$ for midtrimester pregnancy termination. Prostaglandins 10:413, 1975.

247. Stubblefield PG, Naftolin F, Lee EY, et al: Combination therapy for midtrimester abortion: Laminaria and analogues of prostaglandin. Contraception 13:723, 1976.

248. Jain JK, Mishell DR: A comparison of intravaginal misoprostol with prostaglandin E_2 for termination of second trimester pregnancy. N Engl J Med 331:290, 1994.

249. Jain JK, Mishell DR Jr: A comparison of misoprostol with and without laminaria tents for induction of second trimester abortion. Am J Obstet Gynecol 175:173, 1996.

250. Winkler CL, Gray SE, Hauth JC, et al: Mid-second-trimester labor induction: concentrated oxytocin compared with prostaglandin E_2 suppositories. Obstet Gynecol 77:297, 1991.

251. Burkeman RT, Atienza M, King TM, Burnett LS: The management of midtrimester abortion failures by vaginal evacuation. Obstet Gynecol 49:233, 1977.

252. Propping D, Stubblefield PG, Golub J: Uterine rupture following midtrimester abortion by Laminaria, prostaglandin $F_{2\alpha}$ and oxytocin: report of two cases. Am J Obstet Gynecol 128:689, 1977.

253. Kafrissen ME, Barke MW, Workman P, et al: Coagulopathy and induced abortion methods: rates and relative risks. Am J Obstet Gynecol 147:344, 1983.

254. Altman A, Stubblefield PG, Parker K, et al: Midtrimester abortion by Laminaria and evacuation (L&E) on a teaching service: a review of 789 cases. Adv Plann Parent 16:1, 1981.

255. Robbins J, Surrago EJ: Early midtrimester pregnancy termination: a comparison of dilatation and evacuation and intravaginal prostaglandins $F_{2\alpha}$. J Reprod Med 27:415, 1982.

256. Kafrissen ME, Schulz KR, Grimes DA, et al: A comparison of intraamniotic instillation of hyperosmolar urea and prostaglandin $F_{2\alpha}$ vs dilatation and evacuation for midtrimester abortion. JAMA 251:916, 1984.

257. Hogue CJR, Cates W Jr, Tietze C: The effects of induced abortion on subsequent reproduction. Epidemiol Rev 4:66, 1982.

258. Levin AA, Schoenbaum SC, Monson RR, et al: The association of induced abortion with subsequent pregnancy loss. JAMA 243:2395, 1980.

259. Linn S, Schoenbaum SC, Monson RR, et al: The relationship between induced abortion and outcome of subsequent pregnancies. Am J Obstet Gynecol 146:136, 1983.

260. Chung CS, Steinhoff PG, Smith RG, et al: The effects of induced abortion on subsequent reproductive function and pregnancy. Papers of the East-West Population Institute, No. 86, June 1983, East-West Institute, Honolulu, HI.

261. Stubblefield PG, Monson RR, Schoenbaum SC, et al: Fertility after induced abortion: a prospective follow-up study. Obstet Gynecol 63:186, 1984.

262. Hogue CJR, Peterson WF: Late effects of late D&E. Presented at the National Abortion Federation Postgraduate Symposium on D&C. San Francisco, CA, September 20, 1981.

263. Stubblefield PG, Altman AM, Goldstein SP: Randomized trial of one versus two days of Laminaria treatment prior to late midtrimester abortion by uterine evacuation: a pilot study. Am J Obstet Gynecol 143:481, 1982.

264. The Alan Guttmacher Institute: Clandestine abortion: a Latin American Reality. New York, The Alan Guttmacher Institutes, 1994.

265. Roe v. Wade. 410 U.S. 113, 1973.

266. Hack M, Franoff AA: Outcomes of children with extremely low birthweight and gestational age in the 1990s. Early Hum Dev 53:193, 1999.

267. Hohler CW: Ultrasound estimation of gestational age. Clin Obstet Gynecol 27:314, 1984.

268. Chervenak FA, Farley MA, Walters L, et al: When is termination of pregnancy during the third trimester morally justifiable? N Engl J Med 310:501, 1984.

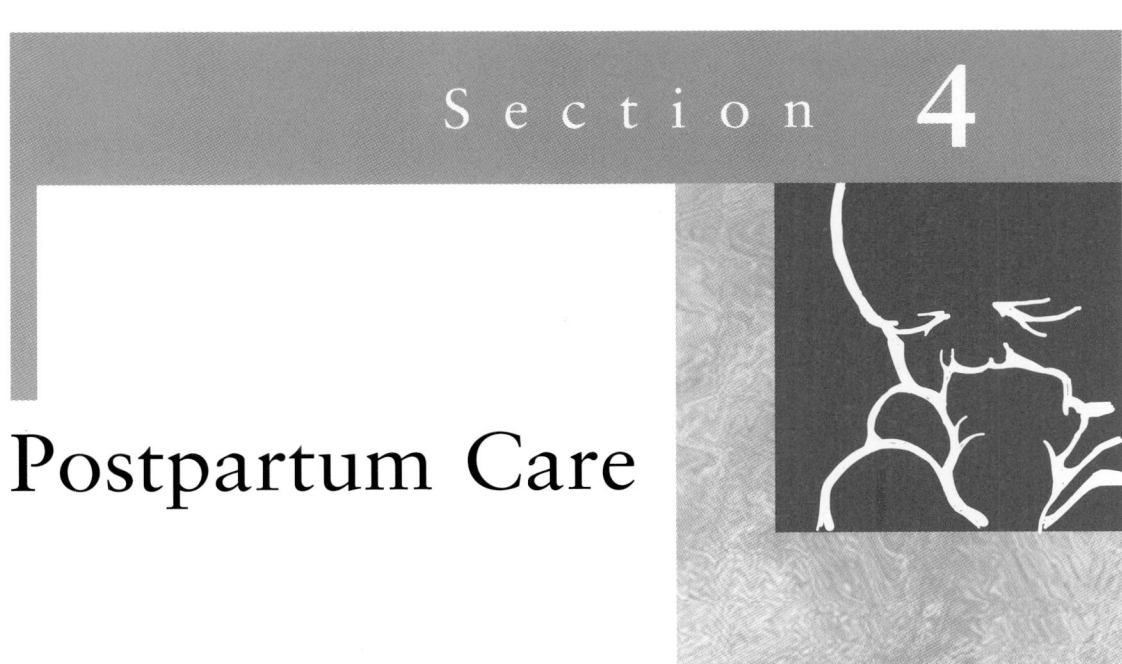

Section 4

Postpartum Care

Chapter 20

The Neonate

ADAM A. ROSENBERG

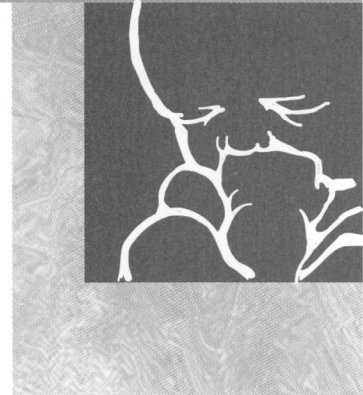

The first 4 weeks of an infant's life, the neonatal period, are marked by the highest mortality rate in all of childhood. The greatest risk occurs during the first several days after birth. Critical to survival during this period is the infant's ability to adapt successfully to extrauterine life. During the early hours after birth, the newborn must assume responsibility for thermoregulation, metabolic homeostasis, and respiratory gas exchange, as well as undergo the conversion from fetal to postnatal circulatory pathways. This chapter reviews the physiology of a successful transition as well as the implications of circumstances that disrupt this process. Implicit in these considerations is the understanding that the newborn reflects the sum total of its genetic and environmental past as well as any minor or major insults to which it was subjected during gestation and parturition. The period of neonatal adaptation is then most meaningfully viewed as continuous with fetal life.

CARDIOPULMONARY TRANSITION

Pulmonary Development

Lung development and maturation require a carefully regulated interaction of anatomic, physiologic, and biochemical processes. The outcome of these events provides an organ with adequate surface area, sufficient vascularization, and the metabolic capability to sustain oxygenation and ventilation during the neonatal period. Five stages of morphologic lung development have been identified in the human fetus[1]:

1. Embryonic period—conception to 7 weeks
2. Pseudoglandular period—8th to 16th weeks
3. Canalicular period—17th to 27th weeks
4. Saccular period—28th to 35th weeks
5. Alveolar period—at or after 36 weeks

The lung arises as a ventral diverticulum from the foregut during the fourth week of gestation. During the ensuing weeks, branching of the diverticulum occurs, leading to a tree of narrow tubes with thick epithelial walls composed of columnar-type cells. By 16 weeks, the conducting portion of the tracheobronchial tree up to and including terminal bronchioles has been established. The vasculature derived from the pulmonary circulation develops concurrently with the conducting airways, and by 16 weeks preacinar blood vessels are formed. The canalicular stage is characterized by differentiation of the airways, with widening of the airways and thinning of epithelium. In addition, primitive respiratory bronchioles begin to form, marking the start of the gas-exchanging portion of the lung. Vascular proliferation continues, along with a relative decrease in mesenchyme, bringing the vessels closer to the airway epithelium. The saccular stage is marked by the development of the gas-exchanging portion of the tracheobronchial tree (acinus) composed of respiratory bronchioles, alveolar ducts, terminal saccules, and finally alveoli. During this stage, the pulmonary vessels continue to proliferate with the airways and surround the developing air sacs. The final phase of prenatal lung development (alveolar) is marked by the formation of thin secondary alveolar septae and the remodeling of the capillary bed. Several million alveoli will form before birth, which emphasizes the importance of this last few weeks of pregnancy to pulmonary adaptation. Postnatal lung growth is characterized by generation of alveoli. At birth, there are approximately 50 million airspaces and by 8 years of age, 300 million.[2]

In early gestation, respiratory epithelial cells are simple and columnar in type. A slow transition from co-

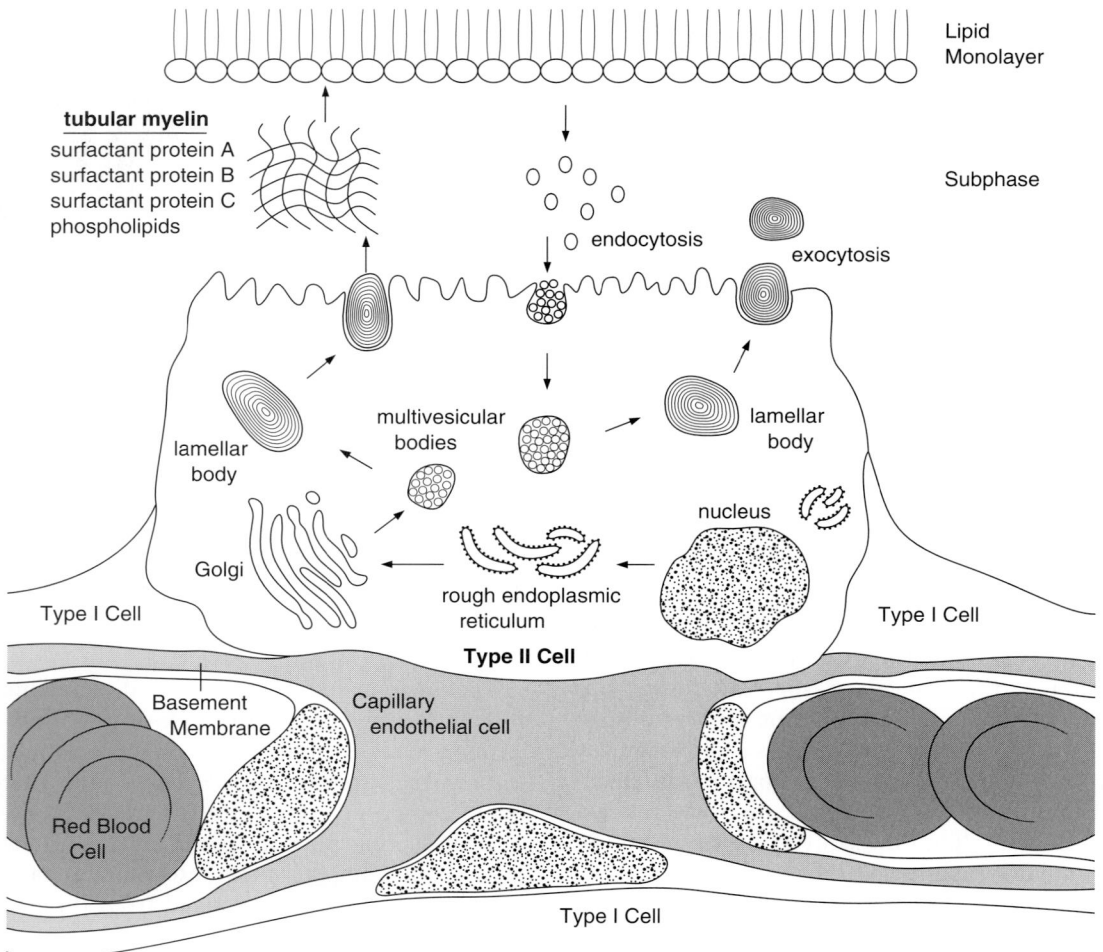

Figure 20–1. Metabolism of surfactant. Surfactant phospholipids are synthesized in the endoplasmic reticulum, transported through Golgi apparatus to multivesicular bodies, and finally packaged in lamellar bodies. After lamellar body exocytosis, phospholipids are organized into tubular myelin before aligning in a monolayer at the air–fluid interface in the alveolus. Surfactant phospholipids and proteins are taken up by type II cells and either catabolized or reutilized. Surfactant proteins are synthesized in polyribosomes, modified in endoplasmic reticulum, Golgi apparatus, and multivesicular bodies. (Adapted from Whitsett JA, Pryhuber GS, Rice WR, et al: Acute respiratory disorders. *In* Avery GB, Fletcher MA, MacDonald MG (eds): Neonatology: Pathophysiology and Management of the Newborn, 5th ed. Philadelphia, Lippincott Williams & Wilkins, 1999, p 485, with permission.)

lumnar epithelium to the lining of a fully developed alveolus starts during the fifth month.[3] By the time of birth, the epithelial lining of the gas-exchanging surface is thin and continuous with two alveolar cell types (types I and II). Type I cells contain few subcellular organelles, while type II cells contain abundant mitochondria, endoplasmic reticulum, Golgi apparatus, and osmiophilic lamellar bodies known to contain surfactant. A scheme for the synthesis of surfactant is presented in Figure 20–1. The kinetics of movement of surfactant from synthesis to lamellar body storage and secretion is slow. Surfactant is secreted as lamellar bodies that unravel into tubular myelin. Tubular myelin is a loose lattice of phospholipids and surfactant-specific proteins. The surface active component of surfactant then adsorbs at the alveolar interface between air and

water in a monolayer.[4] With repetitive expansion and compression of the surface monolayer, material is extruded that is either cleared by alveolar macrophages via endocytic pathways or taken up by the type II cell for recycling back into lamellar bodies.[5]

Because of the development of high surface forces along the respiratory epithelium when breathing begins, the availability of surfactants in terminal airspaces is critical to postnatal lung function. Just as surface tension acts to reduce the size of a bubble in water, so too it acts to reduce lung inflation, promoting atelectasis. This is described by the LaPlace relationship, which states that the pressure, P, within a sphere is directly proportional to surface tension, T and inversely proportional to the radius of curvature, r (Fig. 20–2). Surfactant has the physical property of variable surface ten-

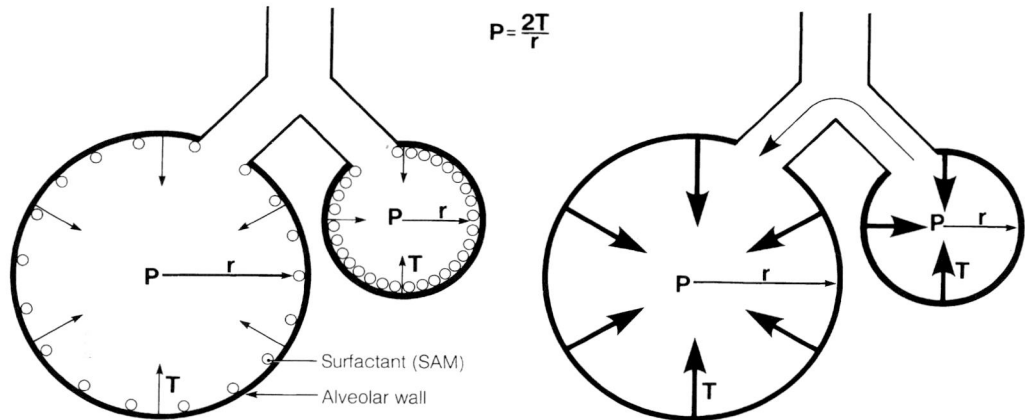

$$P = \frac{2T}{r}$$

Surfactant (SAM)

Alveolar wall

Figure 20–2. LaPlace's law. The pressure, P, within a sphere is directly proportional to surface tension, T, and inversely proportional to the radius of curvature, r. In the normal lung, as alveolar size decreases, surface tension is reduced because of the presence of surfactant. This serves to decrease the collapsing pressure that needs to be opposed and maintains equal pressures in the small and large interconnected alveoli. (Adapted from Netter FH: The Ciba Collection of Medical Illustrations. The Respiratory System, Vol 7. Summit, NJ, Ciba-Geigy, 1979.)

sion dependent on the degree of surface area compression. In other words, as the radius of the alveolus decreases, surfactant serves to reduce surface tension, preventing collapse of the alveolus. If this property is extrapolated to the lung, smaller alveoli will remain stable because of lower surface tension than other larger alveoli. This feature is emphasized in Figure 20–3, which compares pressure–volume curves from surfactant-deficient and surfactant-treated preterm rabbits. Surfactant deficiency is characterized by high opening pressure, low maximal lung volume, and lack of deflation stability at low pressures.[6]

Saturated phosphatidylcholine (the surface tension–reducing component of surfactant) is found in lung tissue of the human fetus earlier in gestation than in other species (Fig. 20–4).[7] Tissue stores of surfactant are considerable at term. Surfactant is released from storage

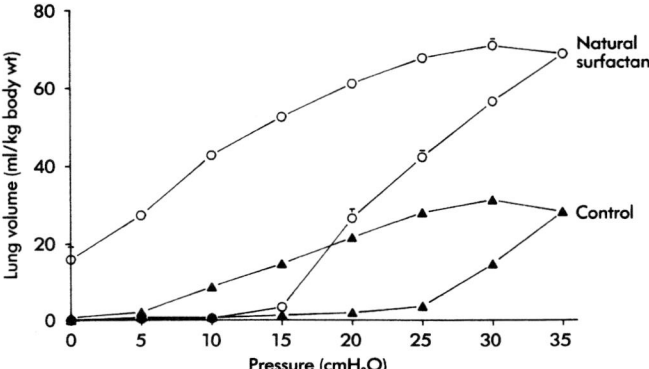

Figure 20–3. Pressure–volume relationships for the inflation and deflation of surfactant-deficient and surfactant-treated preterm rabbit lungs. (Adapted from Jobe AH: Lung development. *In* Fanaroff AA, Martin RI [eds]: Neonatal-Perinatal Medicine: Diseases of the Fetus and Infant, 6th ed. St. Louis, CV Mosby, 1997, p 991.)

pools into fetal lung fluid at a basal rate during late gestation. Secretion is stimulated by labor and the initiation of air breathing.[8]

Natural surfactant contains 80 percent phospholipids, 10 percent neutral lipids, and 10 percent protein (Fig. 20–5).[6,9] Approximately half of the protein is specific for surfactant. The principal classes of phospholipids are saturated phosphatidylcholine compounds, 45 percent (more than 80 percent of which are dipalmitoylphosphatidylcholine [DPPC]); 25 percent unsaturated phosphatidylcholine compounds; and 10 percent phosphatidylglycerol, phosphatidylinositol, and phosphatidylethanolamine. Four unique surfactant-associated proteins have been identified.[10] All are synthesized and secreted by type II alveolar cells. DPPC is the molecule critical to the surface tension–lowering property of surfactant at the air–liquid interface in the alveolus. Surfactant protein (SP)-A functions cooperatively with the other surfactant proteins and lipids to improve surface properties and regulate secretory and reuptake pathways.[10,11] SP-B and SP-C are lipophilic proteins that facilitate the adsorption and spreading of lipid to form the surfactant monolayer.[10,11] SP-D is the least well-described surfactant-associated protein, but appears to function in pulmonary host defense mechanisms.[12]

Several hormones and growth factors contribute to the regulation of pulmonary phospholipid metabolism and lung maturation: glucocorticoids, thyroid hormone, thyrotropin-releasing hormone, prolactin, cyclic adenosine monophosphate (cAMP), epidermal growth factor, and others. Glucocorticoids are the most important of the stimulating factors. They augment the synthesis of all surfactant components and accelerate morphologic development.[9,13]

Pregnant women with anticipated preterm delivery have received corticosteroid treatment since 1972.[14]

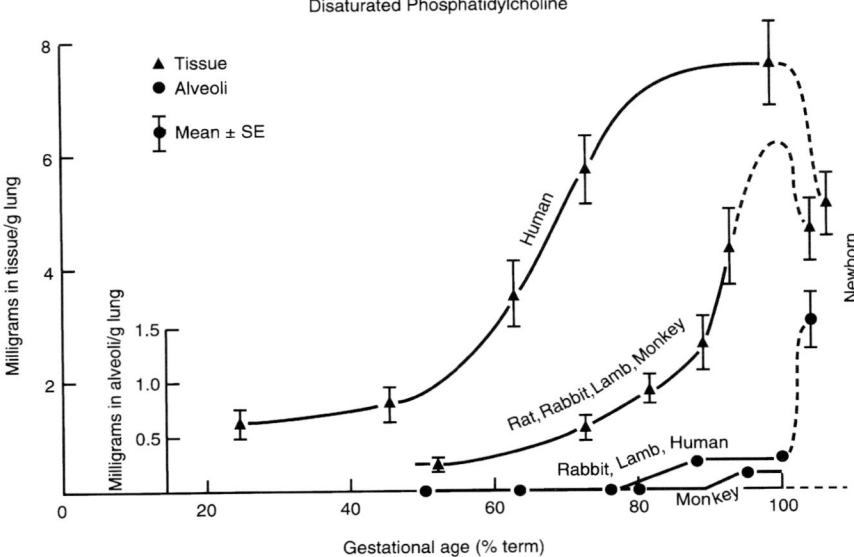

Disaturated Phosphatidylcholine

Figure 20–4. Accumulation of saturated phosphatidylcholine during gestation. Gestational age is plotted as percentage of term. (Adapted from Clements JA, Tooley WH: Kinetics of surface-active material in the fetal lung. *In* Hodson WA [ed]: Development of the Lung. New York, Marcel Dekker, 1977.)

Numerous controlled trials have since been done and have been cumulatively evaluated using meta-analysis.[15] Meta-analysis uses quantitative methods to summarize results from a systematic review of randomized controlled trials. Based on such analysis, a significant reduction of about 50 percent in the incidence of respiratory distress syndrome (RDS) is seen in infants born to mothers who received antenatal corticosteroids. In secondary analysis, a 70 percent reduction in RDS was seen among babies born between 24 hours and 7 days after corticosteroid administration. In addition, evidence suggests a reduction in mortality and RDS even with treatment started less than 24 hours before delivery. Although most babies in the trials were between 30 and 34 weeks' gestation, clear reduction in RDS was evident when the population of babies less than 31

weeks was examined. Gender and race do not influence the protective effect of corticosteroids. In the population of patients with preterm premature rupture of the membranes, antenatal corticosteroids also reduce the frequency of RDS.

Corticosteroids also accelerate maturation of other organs in the developing fetus, including cardiovascular, gastrointestinal, and central nervous system. Corticosteroid therapy reduces the chances of both periventricular–intraventricular hemorrhage and necrotizing enterocolitis.[15,16] The significant reductions in serious neonatal morbidity are also reflected in a reduction in the risk of early neonatal mortality. The short-term beneficial effects of antenatal corticosteroids are enhanced by reassuring reports about long-term outcome. The children of mothers treated with antenatal cortico-

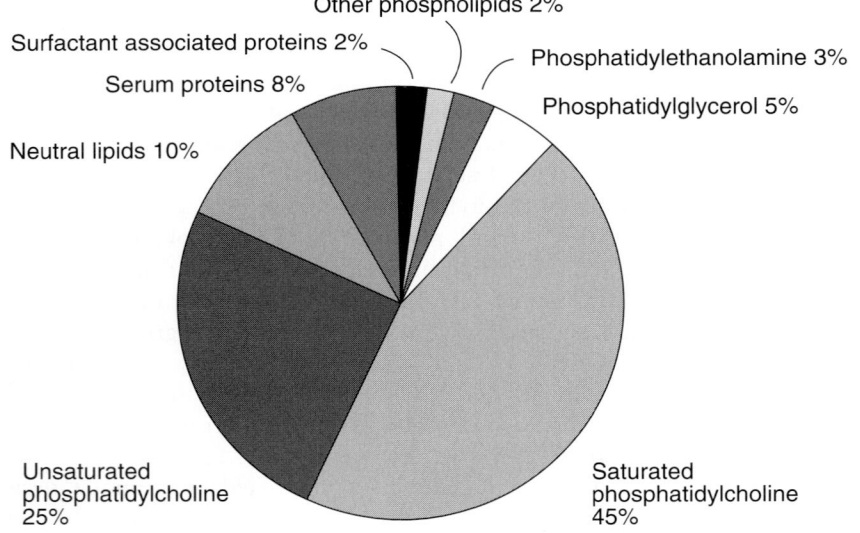

Figure 20–5. Composition of pulmonary surfactant. (Adapted from Ballard PL: Hormonal regulation of pulmonary surfactant. Endocr Rev 10:165, 1989.)

steroids show no lag in intellectual or motor development, no increase in learning disabilities or behavioral disturbances, and no effect on growth compared with untreated infants.[17,18]

Since the advent of antenatal steroids for the prevention of RDS, other maternal and neonatal therapies have been introduced that decrease mortality and morbidity. Surfactant replacement therapy to treat specifically the surfactant deficiency that is the cause of RDS has been shown to decrease mortality and the severity of RDS.[19–22] The effects of antenatal corticosteroids and postnatal surfactant appear to be additive in terms of decreasing the severity of and mortality caused by RDS.[23] Finally, in recent years thyroid-releasing hormone (TRH) has been introduced as an agent to accelerate lung maturation. TRH efficiently crosses the placenta and elicits a striking fetal TSH response.[24] Animal studies have demonstrated improvement in fetal pulmonary maturation after maternal administration of TRH.[25] In addition, thyroid hormone has an additive effect with glucocorticoid on choline incorporation into phosphatidylcholine[26] and is synergistic with cortisol and prolactin in increasing lung compliance and surfactant production.[27] However, the only large double-blind, placebo-controlled trial performed during the era of routine surfactant replacement in newborns showed that TRH and glucocorticoid is no more beneficial than glucocorticoid alone in altering the frequency of RDS—death at 28 days and chronic lung disease.[28] In addition, initial follow-up data from a previous Australian trial suggest that antenatal TRH may be associated with delays in early developmental milestones.[29] Currently, routine use of TRH in women at risk for preterm delivery cannot be recommended.

The First Breaths

A critical step in the transition from intrauterine to extrauterine life is the conversion of the lung from a dormant fluid-filled organ to one capable of gas exchange. This requires aeration of the lungs, establishment of an adequate pulmonary circulation, ventilation of the aerated parenchyma, and diffusion of oxygen and carbon dioxide through the alveolar-capillary membranes. This process has its roots in utero as fetal breathing.

Fetal Breathing

Fetal breathing has been demonstrated in a large number of mammalian species.[30] Fetal breathing has been most extensively studied in fetal sheep and to a lesser degree in humans. Fetal breathing in third-trimester fetal sheep occurs primarily during periods of low-voltage electrocortical activity (rapid-eye-movement [REM] sleep).[31,32] The predominant respiratory pattern is one of rapid, irregular movements varying in amplitude at a rate of 60 to 120 per minute. Isolated deep inspiratory efforts can occur at one to three times per minute unassociated with any particular stage of sleep. During high-voltage electrocortical activity (quiet sleep), only occasional breaths occur after tonic muscular discharges associated with body movements. During non-REM sleep, the breathing movements are inhibited by a mechanism situated in the midbrain and pons.[33,34] Developmental studies on the ontogeny of fetal breathing have been conducted primarily in the fetal lamb and to a lesser extent the human fetus. The onset of breathing in the fetal sheep has been noted as early as 40 days of gestation. By days 90 through 115, breathing is almost continuous, with rare apneic pauses of less than 2 minutes' duration. From day 115 to term, breathing is episodic as described above. Human fetal breathing is quite similar to that observed in fetal sheep.[35] Respiratory activity is initially detectable at 11 weeks. The most prevalent pattern is rapid, small-amplitude movements (60 to 90 per minute) present 60 to 80 percent of the time. Less commonly, irregular low-amplitude movements interspersed with slower larger amplitude movements are seen.

Initially, fetal breathing was thought to depend on behavioral influences. However, subsequent work has shown responses to chemical stimuli and other agents. Acute hypercapnea stimulates breathing in both human and sheep fetuses.[36,37] Hypoxia abolishes fetal breathing,[37] while an increase in oxygen tension to levels above 200 mm Hg induces continuous fetal breathing.[38] Hyperglycemia after bolus injections of glucose to the mother or after ingestion of a meal increases fetal breathing in humans.[39,40] Of the pulmonary reflexes, the inflation reflex (decreasing frequency of breathing) is active in fetal life.[41] Peripheral and central chemoreflexes as well as vagal afferent reflexes can be demonstrated in the fetus, but their role in spontaneous fetal breathing appears minimal.[42]

Breathing is intermittent in the fetus and becomes continuous after birth. The mechanism responsible for this transition is unknown. In the fetal lamb, the REM sleep dependence of breathing can be overcome in a number of ways. The most profound continuous intrauterine breathing is caused by prolonged infusion of large doses of prostaglandin synthesis inhibitors,[43] suggesting that prostaglandins may be involved in the transition to continuous postnatal respiration. Other factors surrounding birth, including blood gas changes and various sensory stimuli, are also postulated to be involved.[42,44] Another factor possibly involved is the "release" from a placental inhibitory factor that is removed after cord occlusion.[45]

The role of fetal breathing in the continuum from fetal to neonatal life is still not completely understood. Fetal respiratory activity is probably essential to the development of chest wall muscles (including diaphragm) and serves as a regulator of lung fluid volume and thus lung growth.[42]

Mechanics of the First Breath

With its first breaths, the neonate must overcome several forces resisting lung expansion: (1) viscosity of fetal lung fluid, (2) resistance provided by lung tissue itself, and (3) the forces of surface tension at the air–liquid interface.[46] Viscosity of fetal lung fluid is a major factor as the neonate attempts to displace fluid present in the large airways. As the passage of air moves toward small airways and alveoli, surface tension becomes more important. Resistance to expansion by the lung tissue itself is less significant. The process begins as the infant passes through the birth canal. The intrathoracic pressure caused by vaginal squeeze is up to 200 cm H_2O.[47,48] With delivery of the head, approximately 5 to 28 ml of tracheal fluid is expressed. Subsequent delivery of the thorax causes an elastic recoil of the chest. With this recoil, a small passive inspiration (no more than 2 ml) occurs.[47] This is accompanied by glossopharyngeal forcing of some air into the proximal airways (frog breathing)[49] and the introduction of some blood into pulmonary capillaries.[50,51] This pulmonary vascular pressure may have a role in producing initial continuous surfaces throughout the small airways of the lung into which surfactant can deploy.[51]

The initial breath is characteristically a short inspiration followed by a more prolonged expiration (Fig. 20–6).[47,52,53] The initial breath begins with no air volume and no transpulmonary pressure gradient. Considerable negative intrathoracic pressure during inspiration is provided by diaphragmatic contraction and chest wall expansion. An opening pressure of about 25 cm H_2O usually is necessary to overcome surface tension in the smaller airways and alveoli before air begins to enter. The volume of this first breath varies between 30 and 67 ml and correlates with intrathoracic pressure. The expiratory phase is quite prolonged, as the infant's expiration is opposed by intermittent closure at the pharyngolaryngeal level[49] with the generation of large positive intrathoracic pressure. This pressure serves to aid both in maintenance of a functional residual capacity (FRC) and with fluid removal from the air sacs. The residual volume after this first breath ranges between 4 and 30 ml, averaging 16 to 20 ml. There are really no major systematic differences among the first three breaths, demonstrating similar pressure patterns of decreasing magnitude. The FRC rapidly increases with the first several breaths and then more gradually. By 30 minutes of age, most infants attain a normal FRC with uniform lung expansion.[54] The presence of functional surfactant is instrumental in the accumulation of an FRC.[7,8]

In utero, alveoli are open and stable at nearly neonatal lung volume because they are filled with fetal lung liquid, probably produced by ultrafiltration of pulmonary capillary blood as well as by secretion by alveolar cells.[55] Transepithelial chloride secretion appears to be a major factor responsible for the production of luminal liquid in the fetal lung.[56,57] Normal expansion and aeration of the neonatal lung is dependent on removal of fetal lung liquid. This process begins before a normal term birth because of decreased fluid secretion and increased absorption.[58] Factors involved in this process postnatally are (1) the thoracic squeeze during delivery, (2) a marked increase in pulmonary lymph flow, and (3) removal via the pulmonary circulation.[58,59] The role of the thoracic squeeze in fluid removal is thought to be minimal during a normal birth.[58] With the onset of breathing, residual liquid from the lung lumen moves into the interstitium. Puddling of fluid in connective tissue spaces away from sites of gas exchange allows time for the pulmonary microcirculation and lymphatics to remove the fluid.[60,61] In normal circumstances, the process is complete within 6 hours of birth. Cesarean-delivered infants without benefit of labor and premature infants have delayed lung fluid clearance. In both groups, the prenatal decrease in lung water does not occur.[58,62] In addition, in the premature, fluid clearance is diminished by increased alveolar surface tension, increased left atrial pressure, and hypoproteinemia.[58,63] Overall, lymphatic pathways remove about 10 percent of lung liquid, with most fluid taken up by the pulmonary circulation.[61] The stimulus for absorption of lung liquid with birth appears to be active sodium transport across the pul-

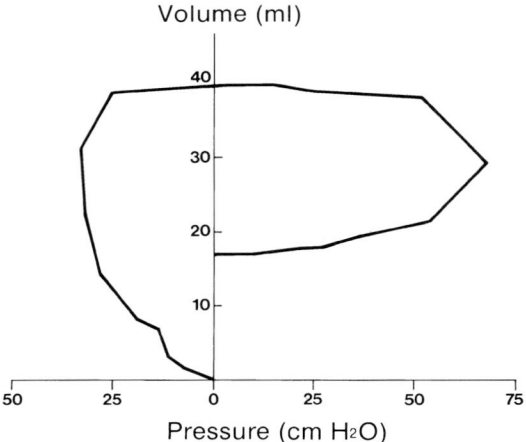

Figure 20–6. Pressure–volume loop of the first breath. Air enters the lung as soon as intrathoracic pressure falls and expiratory pressure greatly exceeds inspiratory pressure. (Modified from Milner AD, Vyas H: Lung expansion at birth. J Pediatr 101:879, 1982.)

monary epithelium driving fluid into the pulmonary interstitium.[58,64]

Circulatory Transition

The circulation in the fetus (Fig. 20–7) has been studied in a variety of species using several techniques (see Chapter 2). These studies have been the subject of a number of excellent reviews.[65–68]

Umbilical venous blood, returning from the placenta, has a PO_2 of about 30 to 35 mm Hg. Because of the left shift of the oxyhemoglobin disassociation curve caused by fetal hemoglobin, this corresponds to a saturation of 80 to 90 percent. About 50 percent of this blood passes through the liver (mainly to the middle and left lobes). This blood will ultimately enter the inferior vena cava (IVC) through the hepatic veins. The remainder bypasses the hepatic circulation via the duc-

tus venosus, which empties directly into the IVC. Because of streaming in the IVC, the more oxygenated blood from the ductus venosus and left hepatic vein, as it enters the heart, is deflected by the crista dividens through the foramen ovale to the left atrium. The remainder of left atrial blood is the small amount of venous return from the pulmonary circulation. The remainder of return from the IVC, less oxygenated blood from the lower body, renal, mesenteric, and right hepatic veins, streams across the tricuspid valve to the right ventricle. Almost all the return from the superior vena cava (SVC) and the coronary sinus passes through the tricuspid valve to the right ventricle, with only 2 to 3 percent crossing the foramen ovale. In the near-term fetus, the combined ventricular output is about 450 ml/kg/min. Two thirds of the cardiac output is from the right ventricle, and one third is from the left ventricle. The blood in the left ventricle has a PO_2 of

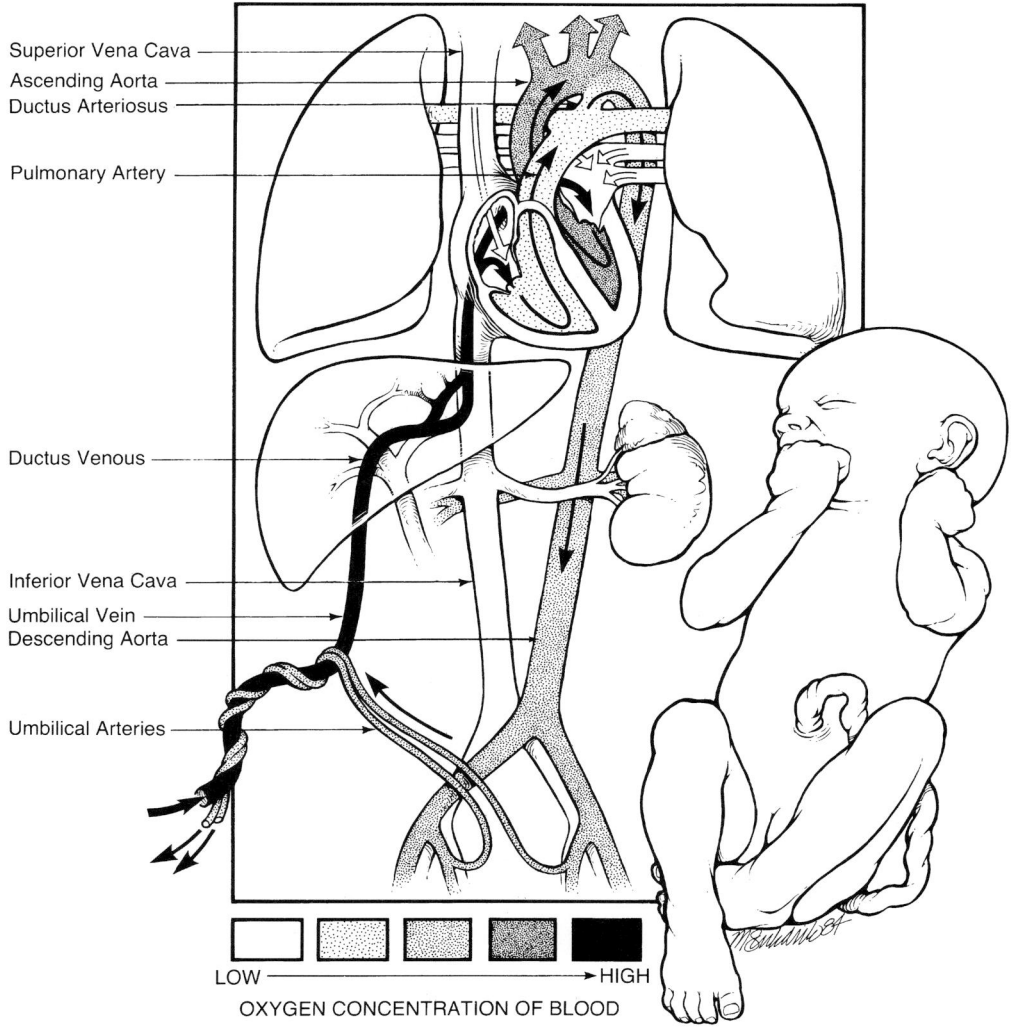

Figure 20–7. The fetal circulation.

25 to 28 mm Hg (saturation of 60 percent) and is distributed to the coronary circulation, brain, head, and upper extremities, with the remainder (10 percent of combined output) passing into the descending aorta. The major portion of the right ventricular output (60 percent of combined output) is carried by the ductus arteriosus to the descending aorta, with only 7 percent of combined output going to the lungs. Thus, 70 percent of combined output passes through the descending aorta, with a PO_2 of 20 to 23 mm Hg (saturation of 55 percent) to supply the abdominal viscera and lower extremities. Forty-five percent of combined output will go through the umbilical arteries to the placenta. This arrangement provides blood of a higher PO_2 to the critical coronary and cerebral circulations and serves to divert venous blood to where oxygenation occurs.

The diversion of right ventricular output away from the lungs through the ductus arteriosus is caused by the very high pulmonary vascular resistance (PVR) in the fetus. This high pulmonary pressure results from chronic exposure to a low PO_2 causing vasoconstriction and an increase in the medial muscle layer in pulmonary arteries.[66,69] In addition, compression of capillaries by fetal lung liquid may contribute to pulmonary vascular resistance.[70] With advancing gestational age, an increase in the number of small pulmonary vessels occurs that increases the cross-sectional area of the pulmonary vasculature. This contributes to the gradual decline in PVR that begins during later gestation (Fig. 20–8). With delivery, a variety of factors interact to

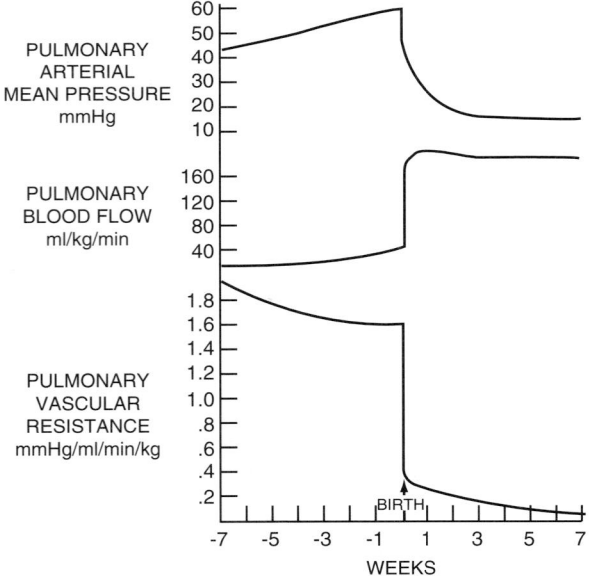

Figure 20–8. Representative changes in pulmonary hemodynamics during transition from the late-term fetal circulation to the neonatal circulation. (Adapted from Rudolph AM: Fetal circulation and cardiovascular adjustments after birth. *In* Rudolph AM, Hoffman JIE, Rudolph CD [eds]: Rudolph's Pediatrics, 20th ed. Stamford, CT, Appleton & Lange, 1996, p 1409.)

Table 20–1. PRESSURES IN THE PERINATAL CIRCULATION

	Fetal (mm Hg)	Neonatal (mm Hg)
Right atrium	4	5
Right ventricle	65/10	40/5
Pulmonary artery	65/40	40/25
Left atrium	3	7
Left ventricle	60/7	70/10
Aorta	60/40	70/45

Modified from Nelson NM: Respiration and circulation after birth. *In* Smith CA, Nelson NM (eds): The Physiology of the Newborn Infant, 4th ed. Springfield, IL, Charles C Thomas, 1976, p 117.

decrease PVR acutely. Mechanical expansion of the lungs with a hypoxic gas mixture causes a decrease in PVR and a fourfold increase in pulmonary blood flow.[71] When oxygen was used to ventilate in this study, a further increase in pulmonary blood flow was seen, caused by an increase in oxygen tension of the blood. Finally, various hormones and vascular mediators may be involved in the decrease in PVR after birth. Increased production of endothelium-derived relaxing factor or nitric oxide appears to play an important role in this regard.[72,73]

With the increase in pulmonary flow, left atrial return increases with a rise in left atrial pressure (Table 20–1). In addition, with the removal of the placenta, inferior vena cava return to the right atrium is diminished. The foramen ovale is a flap valve, and, when left atrial pressure increases over that on the right side, the opening is functionally closed. It is still possible to demonstrate patency with insignificant right-to-left shunts in the first 12 hours of life in a human neonate, but in a 7- to 12-day newborn such a shunt is rarely seen, although anatomic closure is not complete for a longer time.

With occlusion of the umbilical cord, the large runoff of blood to the placenta is interrupted, causing an increase in systemic pressure. This, coupled with the decrease in right-sided pressures, serves to reverse the shunt through the ductus arteriosus to a predominantly left-to-right shunt. By 15 hours of age, shunting in either direction is physiologically insignificant.[74] Although functionally closed by 4 days of age,[75] the ductus is not irreversibly and anatomically occluded for 1 month. The role of an increased oxygen environment in ductal closure is well established.[76] Prostaglandin metabolism has also been shown to play an important role in ductal patency in utero and in closure after birth.[77] Ductal closure appears to occur in two phases: constriction and destruction. Initially, the muscular wall constricts followed by permanent closure achieved by endothelial destruction, subintimal proliferation, and connective tissue formation.[78] The ductus venosus is functionally occluded shortly after the umbilical circulation is interrupted.[65]

Shortly after birth in the neonatal lamb, resting cardiac output is about 350 ml/kg/min.[66] This represents an increase in left ventricular output from about 150 (fetal) to 350 (postnatal) ml/kg/min, while right ventricular output increases from 300 (fetal) to 350 (postnatal) ml/kg/min. The most dramatic increase in individual organ blood flow is that to the lungs (30 to 350 ml/kg/min). Myocardial, renal, and gastrointestinal blood flows also increase, while adrenal, cerebral, and carcass flows decrease.[79]

ABNORMALITIES OF CARDIOPULMONARY TRANSITION

Birth Asphyxia

Even normal infants may experience some asphyxia during the birth process. A variety of circumstances can exaggerate the degree of asphyxia, resulting in a depressed infant, including (1) acute interruption of umbilical blood flow, as occurs during cord compression; (2) premature placental separation; (3) maternal hypotension or hypoxia; (4) any of the above superimposed on chronic uteroplacental insufficiency; and (5) failure to execute a proper resuscitation.[80] Other contributing factors include anesthetics and analgesics used in the mother, mode and difficulty of delivery, maternal health, and prematurity.

Fortunately, some characteristics of the newborn provide protection from these insults. The fetus and neonate are more resistant to asphyxia than are adults.[81] In response to asphyxia, the mature fetus redistributes blood flow to the critical cardiac, cerebral, and adrenal circulations.[82] Unlike adults, who develop tachycardia in response to hypoxia, the fetus responds initially with a reflex bradycardia.[83] As the fetus becomes more hypoxic, it becomes dependent on anaerobic glycolysis to meet energy requirements. During asphyxia, glucose can be released from glycogen stores into the circulation to increase substrate availability.[84,85] In addition, in response to hypoxia, there is a reduction in body movements, a cessation of fetal breathing, and diminished energy utilization by the brain.[86,87] Cumulatively, these features may serve to protect vital organ function.

The neonatal response to asphyxia follows a predictable pattern demonstrable in a number of species. Dawes[88] investigated the responses of the newborn rhesus monkey (Fig. 20–9). After delivery, the umbilical cord was tied and the monkey's head was placed in a plastic bag. Within about 30 seconds, a short series of respiratory efforts began. These were interrupted by a convulsion or a series of clonic movements accompa-

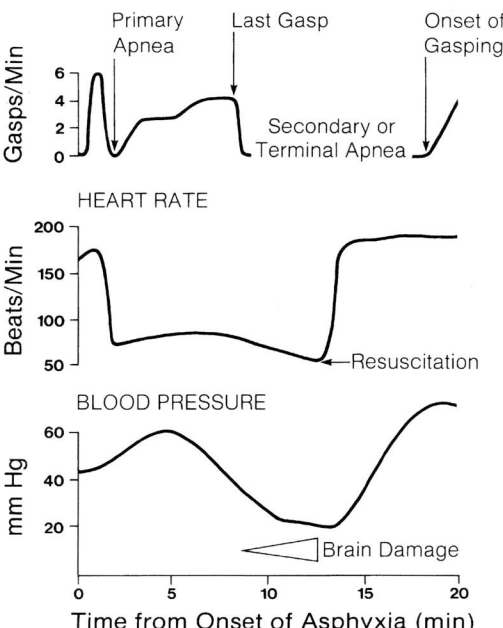

Figure 20–9. Schematic depiction of changes in rhesus monkeys during asphyxia and on resuscitation by positive-pressure ventilation. (Adapted from Dawes GS: Foetal and Neonatal Physiology. Chicago, Year Book, 1968.)

nied by an abrupt fall in heart rate. The animal then lay inert with no muscle tone. Skin color became progressively cyanotic and then blotchy because of vasoconstriction in an effort to maintain systemic blood pressure. This initial period of apnea lasted about 30 to 60 seconds. The monkey then began to gasp at a rate of three to six per minute. The gasping lasted for about 8 minutes, becoming weaker terminally. The time from onset of asphyxia to last gasp could be related to postnatal age and maturity at birth; the more immature the animal, the longer the time. Secondary or terminal apnea followed and, if resuscitation was not quickly initiated, death ensued. As the animal progressed through the phase of gasping and then on to terminal apnea, heart rate and blood pressure continued to fall, indicating hypoxic depression of myocardial function. As the heart failed, blood flow to critical organs decreased, resulting in organ injury.

The response to resuscitation has also been described in great detail and is qualitatively similar in all species, including humans.[89,90] During the first period of apnea, almost any physical or chemical stimulus will cause the animal to breathe. If gasping has already ceased, the first sign of recovery with initiation of positive-pressure ventilation is an increase in heart rate. The blood pressure then rises, rapidly if the last gasp has only just passed, but more slowly if the duration of asphyxia has been longer. The skin then becomes pink, and gasping ensues. Rhythmic spontaneous respiratory efforts become established after a further interval. For each 1 minute past the last gasp, 2 minutes of positive-pressure breathing is required before gasping begins and 4 minutes to reach rhythmic breathing. Not until some time later do the spinal and corneal reflexes return. Muscle tone gradually improves over the course of several hours.

Delivery Room Management of the Newborn

A number of situations during pregnancy, labor, and delivery place the infant at increased risk for asphyxia: (1) maternal diseases, such as diabetes and hypertension, third-trimester bleeding, and prolonged rupture of membranes; (2) fetal conditions, such as prematurity, multiple births, growth retardation, fetal anomalies, and rhesus isoimmunization; and (3) conditions related to labor and delivery, including fetal distress, meconium staining, breech presentation, and administration of anesthetics and analgesics.

When an asphyxiated infant is expected, a resuscitation team should be in the delivery room. The team should have at least two persons, one to manage the airway and one to monitor heart rate and provide whatever assistance is needed. The necessary equipment for an adequate resuscitation is listed in Table 20–2. The equipment should be checked regularly and should be in a continuous state of readiness.

Steps in the resuscitation process[91,92] are as follows (Fig. 20–10):

1. Dry the infant well and place under the radiant heat source on the back or side with the neck slightly extended.
2. Gently suction the oropharynx and nose.
3. Assess the infant's condition (Table 20–3). The best criteria to assess are the infant's respiratory effort (apneic, gasping, regular) and heart rate (more or less than 100). A depressed heart rate indicative of hypoxic myocardial depression is the single most reliable indicator of the need for resuscitation.[90,93]
4. Generally, infants who are breathing with heart rates over 100 bpm will require no further intervention. If the infant is breathing with an adequate heart rate, but is cyanotic, provide supplemental oxygen. Infants with heart rates less than 100 bpm with apnea or irregular respiratory efforts should be vigorously stimulated by rubbing the baby's back with a towel while blowing oxygen over the face.
5. If the baby fails to respond rapidly to tactile stimulation, proceed to bag and face mask ventilation, using a soft mask that seals well around the mouth and nose. Choice of ventilation bags in-

cludes a flow-inflating bag (500 to 750 ml) with a pressure gauge and flow control valve or a self-inflating bag (240 to 750 ml) with an oxygen reservoir and pressure release valve (Fig. 20–11). For the initial inflations, pressures of 30 to 40 cm H_2O may be necessary to overcome surface active forces in the lungs. Adequacy of ventilation is assessed by observing expansion of the infant's chest with bagging and a gradual improvement in color, perfusion, and heart rate. After the first few breaths, attempts should be made to lower the peak pressure to 15 to 20 cm H_2O. Rate of bagging should not exceed 40 to 60 bpm.
6. Most neonates can be effectively resuscitated with a bag and face mask. If the infant does not initially respond to bag and mask ventilation, try to reposition the head (slight extension), reapply the mask to achieve a good seal, consider suctioning the mouth and oropharynx, and try ventilating with the mouth open. It may be necessary to increase the pressure used. However, if there is not favorable response in 30 to 40 seconds, one must proceed to intubation:

Table 20–2. EQUIPMENT FOR NEONATAL RESUSCITATION

Clinical Needs	Equipment
Thermoregulation	Radiant heat source with platform, mattress covered with warm sterile blankets, servo control heating, temperature probe
Airway management	*Suction:* bulb suction, meconium aspirator, wall vacuum suction with sterile catheters
	Ventilation: manual infant resuscitation bag connected to pressure manometer capable of delivering 100% oxygen, appropriate masks for term and preterm infants, oral airways, stethoscope, gloves
	Intubation: neonatal laryngoscope with #0 and #1 blades; extra bulbs and batteries; endotracheal tubes 2.5, 3.0, and 3.5 mm OD with stylet; scissors, adhesive tape
Gastric decompression	Nasogastric tube, 8.0 Fr
Administration of drugs/volume	Sterile umbilical catheterization tray, umbilical catheters (3.5 and 5.0 Fr), volume expanders (lactated Ringer's, normal saline), drug box with appropriate neonatal vials and dilutions (see Table 20–5), sterile syringes, and needles
Transport	Warmed transport isolette with oxygen source

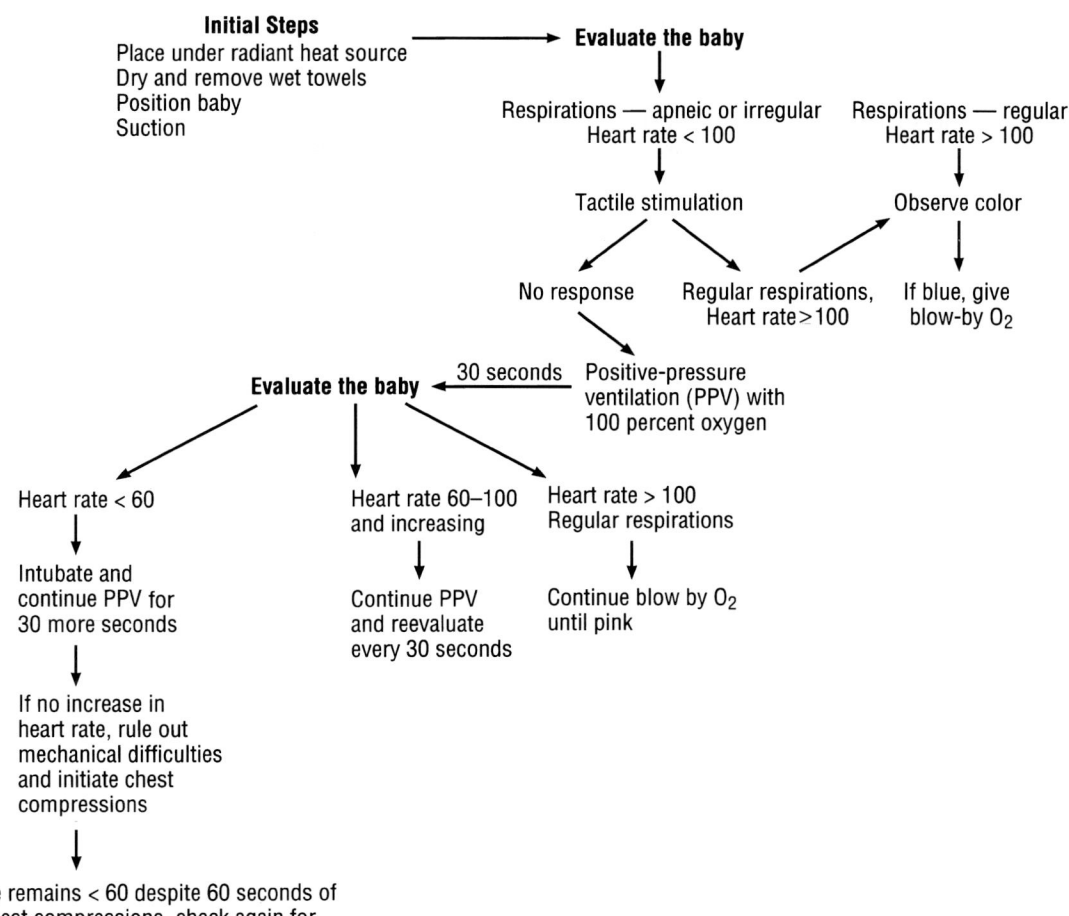

Initial Steps
Place under radiant heat source
Dry and remove wet towels
Position baby
Suction

Evaluate the baby

Respirations — apneic or irregular
Heart rate < 100

Respirations — regular
Heart rate > 100

Tactile stimulation

Observe color

No response

Regular respirations,
Heart rate > 100

If blue, give
blow-by O₂

30 seconds

Positive-pressure
ventilation (PPV) with
100 percent oxygen

Evaluate the baby

Heart rate < 60

Heart rate 60–100
and increasing

Heart rate > 100
Regular respirations

Intubate and
continue PPV for
30 more seconds

Continue PPV
and reevaluate
every 30 seconds

Continue blow by O₂
until pink

If no increase in
heart rate, rule out
mechanical difficulties
and initiate chest
compressions

If heart rate remains < 60 despite 60 seconds of
PPV ± chest compressions, check again for
mechanical difficulties and initiate medications

Figure 20–10. Delivery room management of the newborn. PPV, positive-pressure ventilation.

Table 20–3. THE APGAR SCORING SYSTEM

Sign	0	1	2
Heart rate	Absent	<100 bpm	>100 bpm
Respiratory effort	Apneic	Weak, irregular, gasping	Regular
Reflex irritability*	No response	Some response	Facial grimace, sneeze, cough
Muscle tone	Flaccid	Some flexion	Good flexion of arms and legs
Color	Blue, pale	Body pink, hands and feet blue	Pink

* Elicited by suctioning the oropharynx and nose.
Modified from Apgar V: A proposal for a new method of evaluation of the newborn infant. Anesth Analg 32:260, 1953.

a. The head should be stable, with the nose in the sniffing position (pointing straight upward).
b. Insert the laryngoscope blade, and sweep the tongue to the left.
c. Advance the blade to the base of the tongue, and identify the epiglottis.
d. Pick up the proper size endotracheal tube (2.5 mm OD for infants <1,000 g, 3.0 mm for infants 1,000 to 2,000 g, and 3.5 mm for larger infants) with the right hand.
e. Slide the laryngoscope anterior to the epiglottis, and gently lift along the angle of the handle of the laryngoscope (Fig. 20–12).
f. Identify the vocal cords.
g. Insert the tube in the right side of the mouth, and visualize the tube passing through the vocal cords. The tube should be located 7 cm at the lip for a 1,000-g infant, 8 cm for a 2,000-g infant, and 9 cm for a 3,000-g infant.
h. Ventilate as described above.
i. Failure to respond to intubation and ventilation

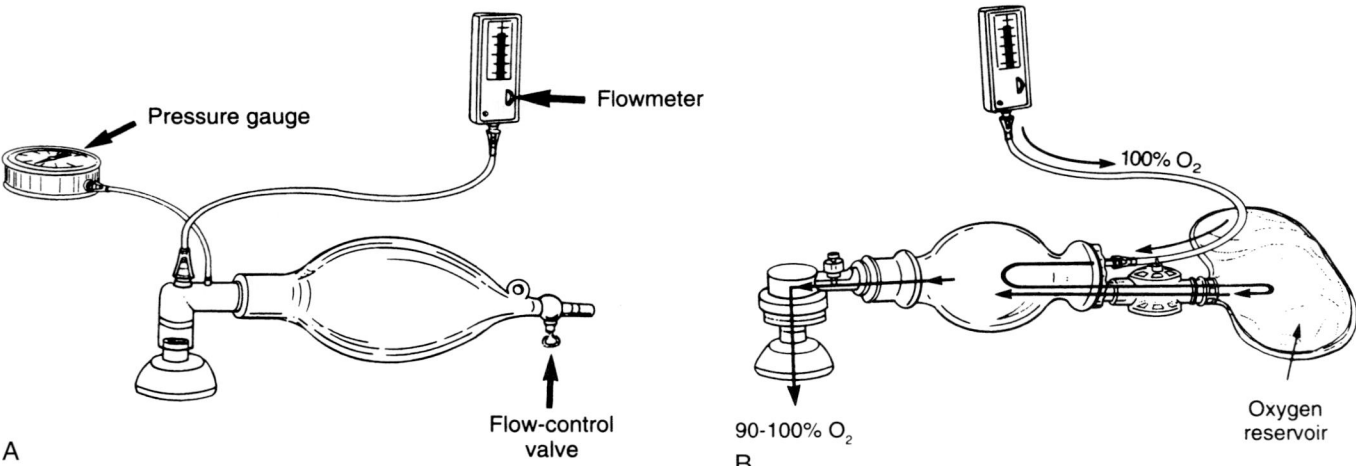

A

B

Figure 20–11. Bags used for neonatal resuscitation. Panel *A*, A flow-inflating bag with a pressure gauge and flow control valve. *B*, A self-inflating bag with an oxygen reservoir to maintain 90 to 100 percent oxygen. (From the American Heart Association and American Academy of Pediatrics: Textbook of Neonatal Resuscitation. Washington, DC, American Heart Association, 1994, with permission.)

can result from (i) mechanical difficulties (Table 20–4), (ii) profound asphyxia with myocardial depression, and (iii) inadequate circulating blood volume.

j. The mechanical causes listed in Table 20–4 should be quickly ruled out. Check to be sure the endotracheal tube passes through the vocal cords. Occlusion of the tube should be suspected when there is resistance to bagging and no chest wall movement. If the endotracheal tube is in place and not occluded, and the equipment is functioning, a trial of bagging with higher pressures is indicated. The other causes listed in Table 20–4 are rare compared with equipment failure or tube problems. A pneumothorax is characterized by asymmetric breath sounds not corrected by repositioning the tube above the carina. Pleural effusions usually occur with fetal hydrops, while a diaphragmatic hernia should be ruled out in the setting of asymmetric breath sounds and a scaphoid abdomen. Pulmonary hypoplasia should be considered if the pregnancy has been complicated by oligohydramnios. It is very unusual for a neonatal resuscitation to require either cardiac massage or drugs. Almost all newborns respond to ventilation with 100 percent oxygen.

7. If mechanical causes are ruled out, external cardiac massage should be performed for persistent heart rate at less than 60 bpm. Compression of ⅓ the anterior-posterior diameter of the chest should be performed, interposed with ventilation at a 3:1 ratio (90 compressions, 30 breaths per minute).

8. If drugs are needed for a persistent heart rate less than 60 bpm after ventilation and chest compressions (Table 20–5), the drug of choice is 0.1 to 0.3 ml/kg of 1:10,000 epinephrine through the endotracheal tube or preferably an umbilical

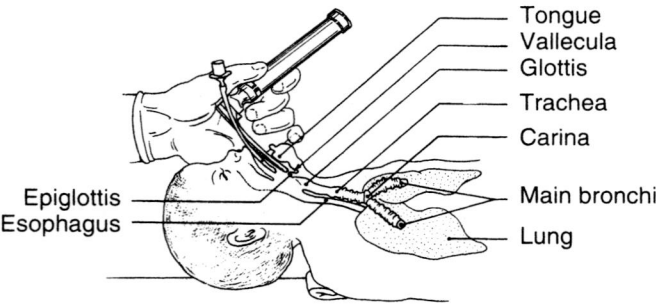

Figure 20–12. Anatomy of laryngoscopy for endotracheal intubation. (From the American Heart Association and American Academy of Pediatrics: Textbook of Neonatal Resuscitation. Washington, DC, American Heart Association, 1994, with permission.)

Table 20–4. MECHANICAL CAUSES OF FAILED RESUSCITATION

Category	Examples
Equipment failure	Malfunctioning bag, oxygen not connected or running
Endotracheal tube malposition	Esophagus, right mainstem bronchus
Occluded endotracheal tube	
Insufficient inflation pressure to expand lungs	
Space-occupying lesions in the thorax	Pneumothorax, pleural effusions, diaphragmatic hernia
Pulmonary hypoplasia	Extreme prematurity, oligohydramnios

Table 20–5. NEONATAL DRUG DOSES

Drug	Dose	Route	How Supplied
Epinephrine	0.1–0.3 ml/kg	IV or ET	1 : 10,000 dilution
Sodium bicarbonate*	1–2 mEq/kg	IV	0.5 mEq/ml (4.2% solution)
Volume†	10 ml/kg	IV	Whole blood, lactated Ringer's, normal saline
Naloxone (Narcan)‡	0.1 mg/kg	IV, ET, IM, or SC	1 mg/ml

* For correction of metabolic acidosis only after adequate ventilation has been achieved; give slowly over several minutes.
† Infuse slowly over several minutes.
‡ After proceeding with proper airway management and other resuscitative techniques.
IV, intravenous; ET, endotracheal; IM, intramuscular; SC, subcutaneous.
Modified from American Heart Association and American Academy of Pediatrics: Neonatal Resuscitation Textbook. American Academy of Pediatrics and American Heart Association, 2000.

venous line. Sodium bicarbonate 1 to 2 mEq/kg of the neonatal dilution (0.5 mEq/ml) can be used in prolonged resuscitation efforts in which response to other measures is poor or with a documented metabolic acidosis. If volume loss is suspected (e.g., documented blood loss with clinical evidence of hypovolemia), 10 ml/kg of a volume expander (normal saline) should be administered through an umbilical venous line. The appropriateness of continued resuscitative efforts should always be re-evaluated in an infant who fails to respond to all of the above efforts. Today, resuscitative efforts are made even in "apparent stillbirths," that is, infants whose 1-minute Apgar scores are 0 to 1. However, efforts should not be sustained in the face of little or no improvement over a reasonable period of time (i.e., 10 to 15 minutes).[94]

A few special circumstances merit discussion at this point. Infants in whom respiratory depression secondary to narcotic administration is suspected may be given naloxone (Narcan). However, this should not be done until the airway has been managed and the infant resuscitated in the usual fashion. In addition, naloxone should not be given to the infant of an addicted mother, as it will precipitate withdrawl. A second special group are preterm infants. Minimizing heat loss improves survival, so prewarmed towels should be available, and the environmental temperature of the delivery suite should be raised. In the extremely-low-birth-weight infant (<1,000 g), proceed quickly to intubation. Volume expanders and sodium bicarbonate should be infused slowly to avoid rapid swings in blood pressure.

Finally, there is the issue of meconium-stained amniotic fluid. Meconium aspiration syndrome (MAS) is a form of aspiration pneumonia that occurs most often in term or postterm infants who have passed meconium in utero (10 to 15 percent of all deliveries[95]). Overall, 4 to 6 percent of children born through meconium-stained fluid will be diagnosed with meconium aspiration syn-

drome, and an additional 4 to 9 percent will be diagnosed with other respiratory disorders.[95] Delivery room management of meconium in the amniotic fluid has been based on the notion that aspiration takes place with the initiation of extrauterine respiration and that the pathologic condition is related to the aspirated contents. This resulted in the practice of oropharyngeal suction on the perineum after delivery of the head followed by airway visualization and suction by the resuscitator after delivery.[96] Both of these assumptions are now being questioned. Meconium is found below the vocal cords in 35 percent of births from meconium-stained fluid.[97] In utero aspiration has been induced in animal models[97,98] and confirmed in autopsies of human stillbirths.[97,99] In addition, the combined suction approach to prevention of MAS has not been uniformly successful in decreasing the incidence of MAS.[97,100,101] Further concern has been raised by the experience that routine suctioning of the neonatal airway has been associated itself with respiratory morbidity.[102,103] Of note as well is the finding that infants with meconium-stained fluid in whom only pharyngeal suctioning is performed suffer no increase in the incidence of MAS.[102,103] Recently, a large multicenter, prospective, randomized controlled trial assessing selective intubation of apparently vigorous meconium-stained infants was completed.[95,104] Compared with expectant management, intubation and tracheal suction did not result in a decreased incidence of MAS or other respiratory disorders.

In terms of the role of meconium in the genesis of MAS, 35 percent of infants born with meconium in the amniotic fluid will have meconium in the lungs. Up to 55 percent will have abnormal chest radiographs, yet respiratory distress develops in only 5 to 10 percent of these infants.[97] Severe MAS is associated with persistent pulmonary hypertension of the newborn and is likely the result of a long-standing intrauterine process with meconium only a marker of intrauterine hypoxia.[105,106]

Current clinical and experimental data support that MAS is the result of intrauterine asphyxia. The best method of prevention is to identify the fetus at risk (postterm, oligohydramnios). Intrapartum management should emphasize treatments that enhance uteroplacental perfusion. Aminoinfusion in cases with oligohydramnios may reduce cord compression, gasping, and intrapartum aspiration.[107] The management of the infant's airway remains controversial, although postnatal prevention of MAS will often not be possible. A reasonable approach is as follows:

1. The obstetrician carefully suctions the oro- and nasopharynx after delivery of the head with a suction apparatus, hooked to wall suction.
2. The delivery is then completed and the baby given to the resuscitator.
3. If the baby is active and breathing and requires no resuscitation, the airway need not be inspected, thus avoiding the risk of inducing vagal bradycardia.
4. Any infant in need of resuscitation should have the airway inspected and suctioned before instituting positive-pressure ventilation.
5. Suction the stomach when airway management is complete and vital signs are stable.

Sequelae of Birth Asphyxia

The incidence of birth asphyxia varies between 1 and 5 percent, depending on criteria utilized in making the diagnosis.[108,109] As would be expected, the incidence increases in infants of lower gestational age. In a study involving more than 38,000 deliveries, MacDonald et al.[108] reported an incidence of 0.4 percent in infants more than 38 weeks and 62.3 percent in those less than 27 weeks. The acute sequelae that need to be managed in the neonatal period are listed in Table 20–6. It is evident that widespread organ injury occurs.[110] Management focuses on supportive care and treatment of

Table 20–6. THE ACUTE SEQUELAE OF ASPHYXIA

System	Manifestations
Central nervous system	Cerebral edema, seizures, and hemorrhage
Cardiac	Papillary muscle necrosis–transient tricuspid insufficiency, cardiogenic shock
Pulmonary	Aspiration syndromes (meconium, clear fluid), acquired surfactant deficiency, persistent pulmonary hypertension, pulmonary hemorrhage
Renal	Acute tubular necrosis
Adrenal	Hemorrhage with adrenal insufficiency
Hepatic	Enzyme elevations, liver failure
Gastrointestinal	Necrotizing enterocolitis
Metabolic	Hypoglycemia, hypocalcemia
Hematologic	Coagulation disturbances, thrombocytopenia

specific abnormalities. This includes careful fluid management, blood pressure support, intravenous glucose, and treatment of seizures. Phenobarbital (40 mg/kg) 1 to 6 hours after the event given as neuroprotective therapy is associated with an improved neurologic outcome.[111] The roles of hypothermia (in particular selective head cooling), oxygen free radical scavengers, excitatory amino acid antagonists, and calcium channel blockers in minimizing cerebral injury after asphyxia are still investigational.[112–114] If the infant survives, the major long-term concern is permanent central nervous system (CNS) damage. The challenge is identifying criteria that can provide information about the risk of future problems for a given infant. A variety of markers have been examined to identify birth asphyxia and risk for adverse neurologic outcome.[97,115–121] Meconium in the amniotic fluid considered in isolation does not increase the risk of unfavorable outcome.[97] Marked fetal bradycardia is associated with some increase in risk, but use of electronic fetal monitoring and cesarean delivery have not altered the incidence of cerebral palsy over the last several decades.[115–118] Low Apgar scores at 1 and 5 minutes are not very predictive of outcome, but infants with low scores that persist at 15 and 20 minutes after birth have a 50 percent chance of manifesting cerebral palsy if they survive.[119] Cord pH is predictive of adverse outcome only after the pH is less than 7.00.[120] The best predictor of outcome is the severity of the neonatal neurologic syndrome.[121] Infants with mild encephalopathy all survive and are normal on follow-up examination. Moderate encephalopathy carries a 5 percent mortality risk and a 15 percent chance of late disability, while the severe syndrome carries a 100 percent risk of death or disability. Diagnostic aids including electroencephalograms, evoked potentials, computed tomography (CT) and magnetic resonance imaging (MRI) scans, and Doppler flow studies can also aid in predicting outcome.[122] It is also important to keep in mind that the circulatory response to hypoxia is to redistribute blood flow to provide adequate oxygen delivery to critical organs (e.g., brain, heart) at the expense of other organs. Thus, it is hard to imagine an insult severe enough to damage the brain without evidence of other organ dysfunction. In particular, renal dysfunction correlates with neurologic outcome.[123]

The long-term neurologic sequelae of intrapartum asphyxia are cerebral palsy with or without associated cognitive deficits and epilepsy.[115,124,125] Although cerebral palsy can be related to intrapartum events, the large majority of cases are of unknown cause.[125,126] Furthermore, cognitive deficits and epilepsy, unless associated with cerebral palsy, cannot be related to asphyxia or to other intrapartum events.[124,125] To attribute cerebral palsy to peripartum asphyxia, there must be an absence of other demonstrable causes, substantial or prolonged intrapartum asphyxia (fetal heart rate abnormalities, fetal acidosis), and clinical evidence during the first days of life of neurologic dysfunction in the infant.[121,124]

BIRTH INJURIES

Birth injuries are defined as those sustained during labor and delivery. Although significant birth injury accounts for fewer than 2 percent of neonatal deaths and stillborns, the frequency is 6 to 8 injuries per 1,000 live births (excluding cephalohematomas).[127] Factors predisposing to birth injury include macrosomia, cephalopelvic disproportion, shoulder dystocia, prolonged or difficult labor, precipitous delivery, abnormal presentations (including breech), and use of forceps (especially midforceps). Injuries range from minor (requiring no therapy) to life threatening (Table 20–7).

Soft tissue injuries are most common. Most are related to dystocia and to the use of forceps. Accidental lacerations of the scalp, buttocks, and thighs may be inflicted with the scalpel during cesarean delivery. Cumulatively, these injuries are of a minor nature and respond well to therapy. Hyperbilirubinemia, particularly in the premature, is the major neonatal complication related to soft tissue damage.

A cephalhematoma occurs in 0.2 to 2.5 percent of live births.[128] Caused by rupture of blood vessels that traverse from the skull to the periosteum, the bleeding is subperiosteal and therefore limited by suture lines, with the most common site of bleeding being over the parietal bones. Associations include prolonged or difficult labor and mechanical trauma from forceps. Linear skull fractures beneath the hematoma have been reported in 5.4 percent of cases,[128] but are of no major consequence except in the unlikely event that a leptomeningeal cyst develops. Most cephalhematomas are reabsorbed in 2 weeks to 3 months. Subgaleal bleeds, which are not limited by suture lines, can occur in association with vacuum extraction and difficult forceps deliveries, and can result in life-threatening anemia, hypotension, or consumptive coagulopathy. Depressed skull fractures are also seen in neonates, but most do not require surgical elevations.

Intracranial hemorrhages related to trauma include subdural and subarachnoid bleeds.[129] With improvements in obstetric care, subdural hemorrhages fortunately are now rare. Three major varieties of subdural bleeds have been described: (1) tentorial laceration with rupture of the straight sinus, vein of Galen, or lateral sinus; (2) falx laceration, with rupture of the inferior sagittal sinus; and (3) rupture of the superficial cerebral veins. The clinical symptomatology is related to the location of bleeding. With tentorial laceration, bleeding is infratentorial, causing brain stem signs and a rapid progression to death. Falx tears will cause bilateral cerebral signs until blood extends infratentorially to the brain stem. Subdural hemorrhage over the cerebral convexities can cause several clinical states, ranging from an asymptomatic newborn to one with seizures and focal neurologic findings. Infants with lacerations of the tentorium and falx have a poor outlook. In contrast, the prognosis for rupture of the superficial cerebral veins is much better, with more than one half the survivors being normal. Primary subarachnoid hemorrhage is the most common variety of neonatal intracranial hemorrhage.[129] Clinically, these infants are often asymptomatic, although they may present with a characteristic seizure pattern. The seizures begin on day 2 of life, and the infants are "well" between convulsions. In general, the prognosis for subarachnoid bleeds is good.

Trauma to peripheral nerves produces another major group of birth injuries. Brachial plexus injuries are caused by stretching of the cervical roots during delivery, usually when shoulder dystocia is present. Upper arm palsy (Erb-Duchenne), the most common brachial plexus injury, is caused by injury to the fifth and sixth cervical nerves; lower arm paralysis (Klumpke) results from damage to the eighth cervical and first thoracic nerves. Damage to all four nerve roots produces paralysis of the entire arm. Outcome for these injuries is variable, with some infants left with significant residual.[130,131] Horner's syndrome may accompany Klumpke's palsy, and approximately 5 percent of patients with Erb's palsy have an associated phrenic nerve

Table 20–7. BIRTH INJURIES

Classification	Example
Soft tissue injuries*	Lacerations, abrasions, bruising, fat necrosis
Skull injuries	Cephalhematoma,* fractures
Intracranial hemorrhage	Subdural, subarachnoid
Nerve injuries	Facial n.,* brachial plexus,* phrenic n., recurrent laryngeal n. (vocal cord paralysis), Horners' syndrome
Fractures	Clavicle,* facial bones, humerus, femur
Dislocations	
Eye injuries	Subconjunctiva* and retinal hemorrhages
Torticollis†	
Spinal cord injuries	
Visceral rupture	Liver, spleen
Scalp laceration*	Fetal scalp electrode, pH
Scalp abscess*	Fetal scalp electrode, pH

* More common occurrences.
† Secondary to hemorrhage into the sternocleidomastoid muscle.

paresis.[127] Facial palsy is another fairly common injury caused either by pressure from the sacral promontory as the infant passes through the birth canal or by forceps. Most of these palsies resolve, although in some infants paralysis is persistent.

The majority of bone fractures resulting from birth trauma involve the clavicle and result from shoulder dystocia or breech extractions that require vigorous manipulations. Clinically, many of these fractures are asymptomatic, and symptoms when present are mild. Prognosis for clavicular as well as limb fractures is uniformly good. The most commonly fractured long bone is the humerus.

Spinal cord injuries are a relatively infrequent but often severe form of birth injury. Accurate incidence is difficult to assess, because symptomatology mimics other neonatal diseases and autopsies often do not include a careful examination of the spine. Depressed tone and hyporeflexia are clues to this diagnosis. Excessive longitudinal traction and head rotation during forceps delivery predispose to spinal injury, and hyperextension of the head in a footling breech is particularly dangerous. Outcomes include death or stillbirth caused by high cervical or brain stem lesions, long-term survival of infants with paralysis from birth, and minimal neurologic symptoms or spasticity.[132]

NEONATAL THERMAL REGULATION

Physiology

The human newborn is a homeotherm possessing the ability to maintain a stable core body temperature over a range of environmental temperatures.[133] The range of environmental temperatures over which the neonate can operate is narrower than that of an adult as a result of the infant's inability to dissipate heat effectively in warm environments and, more critically, to maintain temperature in response to cold.

Heat Production

The heat production within the body is a by-product of metabolic processes and must equal heat losses through the skin and lungs. In the adult, heat production in response to cold can come from voluntary muscle activity, involuntary muscle activity (shivering), and nonshivering chemical thermogenesis. While some increases in activity and shivering have been observed, nonshivering thermogenesis is the most important means of increased heat production in the cold-stressed newborn.[134,135] Nonshivering thermogenesis can be defined as an increase in total heat production without detectable (visible or electrical) muscle activity. From both animal[136] and human[137] observations, it has been inferred that the site of this increased heat production is brown fat. More abundant in newborns than adults, brown fat accounts for 2 to 6 percent of total body weight.[133] This fat is located between the scapulae; around the muscles and blood vessels of the neck, axillae, and mediastinum; between the esophagus and trachea; and around the kidneys and adrenal glands. Brown fat differs both morphologically and metabolically from white fat. Brown fat cells contain more mitochondria and fat vacuoles and have a richer blood and sympathetic nerve supply. Brown fat metabolism is stimulated by norepinephrine released through sympathetic innervation causing triglyceride hydrolysis.[136,138] The initiation of nonshivering thermogenesis at birth depends on cooling, separation from the placenta, and a euthyroid state. Sympathetic nervous system stimulation by cold increases local catecholamine turnover within brown fat, resulting in a marked increase in oxygen consumption.[139]

Heat Loss

Heat loss to the environment is dependent on both an internal temperature gradient (from within the body to the surface) and an external gradient (from the surface to the environment). The infant can change the internal gradient by altering vasomotor tone and, to a lesser extent, by postural changes that decrease the amount of exposed surface area. The external gradient is dependent on purely physical variables. Heat transfer from the surface to the environment involves four routes: radiation, convection, conduction, and evaporation. Radiant heat loss, heat transfer from a warmer to a cooler object that is not in contact, depends on the temperature gradient between the objects. Heat loss by convection to the surrounding gaseous environment depends on air speed and temperature. Conduction or heat loss to a contacting cooler object is minimal in most circumstances. Heat loss by evaporation is cooling secondary to water loss at the rate of 0.6 cal/g water evaporated and is affected by relative humidity, air speed, exposed surface area, and skin permeability. In infants in excessively warm environments, under overhead radiant heat sources, or in very immature infants with thin, permeable skin, evaporative losses increase considerably.

Compared with an adult, the newborn is compromised in the ability to conserve as well as dissipate heat. Conservation of heat is impaired because of a large surface area/body weight ratio and less tissue insulation because of less subcutaneous fat.[140] With a cold stress, heat is conserved chiefly by vasoconstriction in both mature and immature neonates. When the environment is too warm, heat loss is augmented by vaso-

Table 20–8. NEONATAL RESPONSE TO THERMAL STRESS

Stressor	Response	Term	Preterm
Cold	Vasoconstriction	+ +	+ +
	↓ Exposed surface area (posture change)	±	±
	↑ Oxygen consumption	+ +	+
	↑ Motor activity; shivering	+	–
Heat	Vasodilation	+ +	+ +
	Sweating	+	–

+ +, Maximum response; +, intermediate; ±, may have a role; –, no response.

dilation of skin vessels and an increase in evaporative heat loss by sweating. Sweating is present in term infants when rectal temperatures rise above 37.2°C.[141] With sweating, evaporative heat losses can increase two- to fourfold in term babies, but this is not enough to prevent a rise in core temperature. Table 20–8 summarizes the neonate's efforts to maintain a stable core temperature in the face of cold or heat stress.

Neutral Thermal Environment

Although most available information confirms that the human neonate is a homeotherm, the range of temperatures over which core body temperature remains stable is narrower than in an adult and decreases with decreasing gestational age. It is therefore advantageous to maintain an infant in a neutral thermal environment (Fig. 20–13). A neutral thermal environment makes minimal demands on the neonate's energy reserves, core body temperature being regulated by changes in skin blood flow and posture. Body temperature remains normal, while oxygen consumption and heat production are minimal and match heat loss.[142] With a drop in environmental temperature out of the thermoneutral range, the infant will increase oxygen consumption and thus heat production to keep up with heat losses and maintain a stable core temperature. Core temperature will be maintained until heat loss exceeds the infant's ability to increase heat production further. When the infant is placed in an environment warmer than neutral thermal zone, hyperthermia rapidly occurs because of the neonate's inability to dissipate heat and an increase in oxygen consumption that ensues as the infant's body temperature rises. The neutral thermal environment for a given infant depends on size, gestational age, and

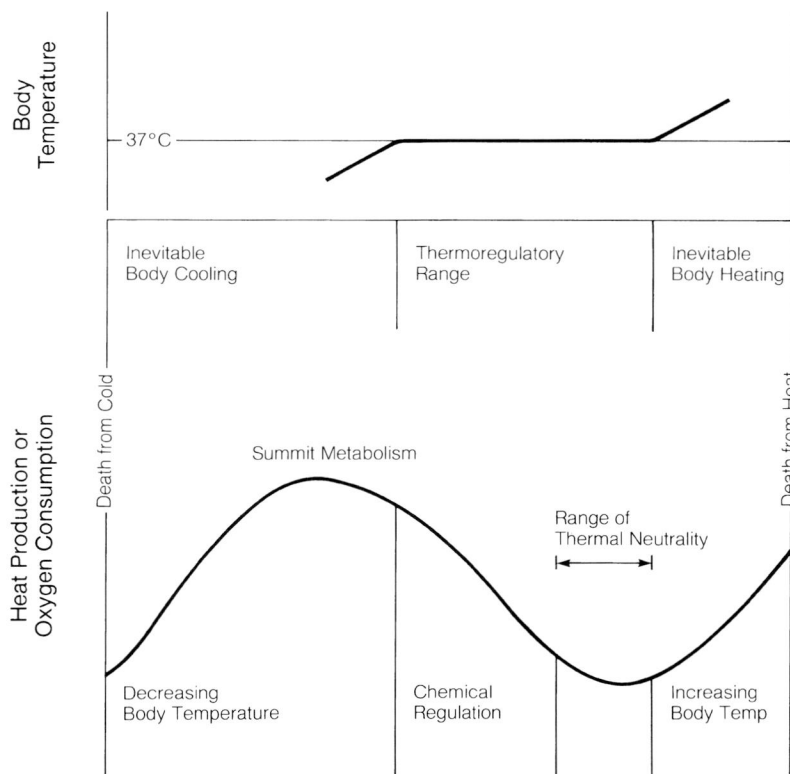

Figure 20–13. Effect of environmental temperature on oxygen consumption and body temperature. (Adapted from Klaus MH, Martin RJ, Fanaroff AA: The physical environment. *In* Klaus MH, Fanaroff AA [eds]: Care of the High-Risk Neonate, 4th ed. Philadelphia, WB Saunders Company, 1993, p 114.)

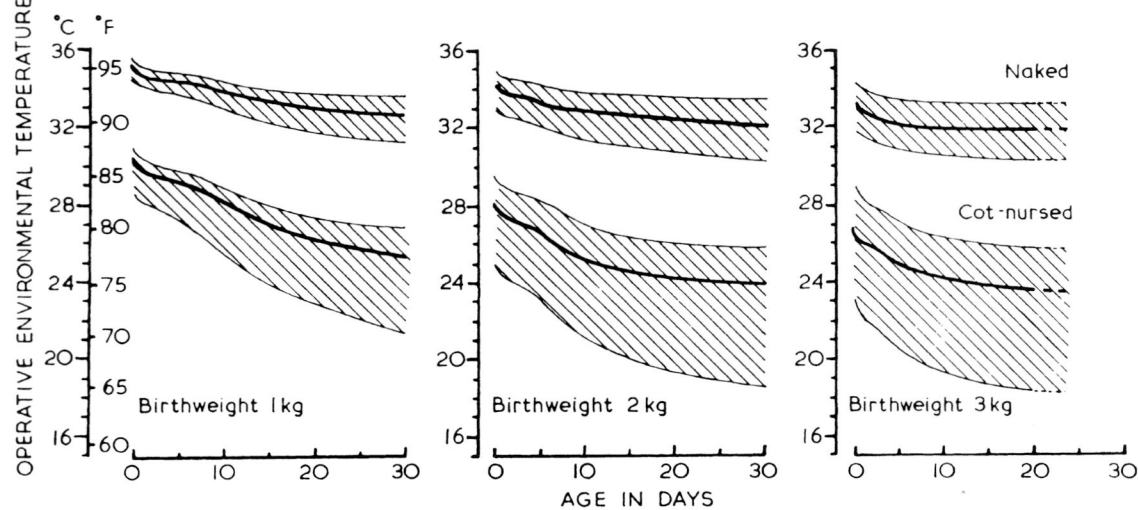

Figure 20–14. Range of environmental temperatures to maintain naked or cot-nursed 1-kg, 2-kg, and 3-kg infants in a neutral thermal environment. (From Hey EN, Katz G: The optimum thermal environment for naked babies. Arch Dis Child 45:328, 1970.)

postnatal age.[143] The optimal thermal environment for naked babies and cot-nursed (dressed and bundled) babies has been defined (Fig. 20–14).[142,144] It is important to note that the environmental temperatures shown in Figure 20–14 are operative temperatures for an infant in an incubator. The operative temperature can differ from the measured environmental temperature because of changes in relative humidity and temperature of the incubator walls. Incubator wall temperature will vary as a function of room temperature. In general, maintaining the abdominal skin temperature at 36.5°C minimizes oxygen consumption.[145]

CLINICAL APPLICATIONS

Delivery Room

In utero, fetal thermoregulation is the responsibility of the placenta and is dependent on maternal core temperature, with fetal temperature 0.5°C higher than maternal temperature.[146] At birth, the infant's core temperature drops rapidly from 37.8°C because of evaporation from its wet body and radiant and convective losses to the cold air and walls of the room. Heat loss can occur at a rate of 0.2 cal/kg/min in the term infant and at a greater rate in premature and sick or unstable infants.[146,147] Even with an increase in oxygen consumption to the maximum capability of the newborn (15 ml/kg/min), the infant can produce only 0.075 cal/kg/min and will rapidly lose heat. Measures taken to reduce heat loss after birth depend on the clinical situation. For the well term infant, drying the skin and wrapping the baby with warm blankets is

sufficient. When it is necessary to leave an infant exposed for close observation or resuscitation, the infant should be dried and placed under a radiant heat source. Room temperature can be elevated as an added precaution for the low-birth-weight infant.

Nursery

Babies are cared for in the newborn nursery wrapped in blankets in bassinets (cot nursed), in isolettes, or under a radiant heat source. Healthy full-term infants (weighing >2.5 kg) need only be clothed and placed in a bassinet under a blanket. A nursery temperature of 25°C should be adequate (Fig. 20–14). Infants weighing 2 to 2.5 kg who are either slightly premature or growth retarded should be allowed 12 to 24 hours to stabilize in an isolette and then advanced to a bassinet. Lower birth weight babies (<2 kg) will require care in either isolettes or under radiant heat sources. Adequate thermal protection of the low-birth-weight infant is essential. Several groups have demonstrated decreased mortality in low-birth-weight infants kept in warmer environments.[148–150] This is especially important for the very-low-birth-weight infant (<1.5 kg), who often does not behave like a mature homeotherm. These neonates can react to a small change in environmental temperature with a change in body temperature rather than a change in oxygen consumption. In addition, warmer environments have also been shown to hasten growth of the premature.[151]

The isolette, which heats by convection, is the most commonly used heating device for the low-birth-weight nude infant. The major source of heat loss while in a neutral thermal environment is radiant to the walls of the isolette. The magnitude of this loss is predictable if room temperature is known. These losses can be minimized using double-walled isolettes in which the inner wall temperature is very close to the air temperature within the isolette. An isolette permits adequate observation of the infant and is suitable for caring for the most sick low-birth-weight or full-sized infants. Once clinical status has been stabilized the child can be dressed, which will afford increased thermal stability.

Radiant warmers can also be used to ensure thermal stability of both low-birth-weight and full-sized infants. Radiant warmers are used most effectively for short-term warming during initial resuscitation and stabilization as well as for performing procedures. They provide easy access to the infant while ensuring thermal stability. The main heat losses are convection, which can be quite significant because of variable air speed in a room, and evaporation. Evaporative heat loss resulting in significant fluid losses is a major concern for the very-low-birth-weight premature cared for under a radiant warmer. Placing a plastic shield over the infant or covering the skin with a semipermeable membrane can minimize these fluid losses.[152,153]

The most economical means of thermal support for the low-birth-weight infant is skin-to-skin contact with a parent. This "kangaroo" care has been shown to reduce serious illness and enhance lactation while providing adequate thermal support.[154-157]

Hypothermia and Neonatal Cold Injury

Hypothermia is seen in low-birth-weight infants, particularly following delivery room resuscitation. Hypothermia may also be a sign of infection or intracranial pathology. Neonatal cold injury is a consequence of excessive cold exposure most commonly seen in both term and preterm infants born unexpectedly outside the hospital. Clinical features include poor feeding, lethargy, coolness of skin, bright red color, edema, and occasionally sclerema (hardening of the skin associated with reddening and edema), slow and shallow respiratory effort, and bradycardia.[158] Metabolic derangements include metabolic acidosis, hypoglycemia, hyperkalemia, and elevated blood urea nitrogen. The infant should be warmed slowly in an isolette set at an operative temperature of 2°C higher than the infant's core body temperature.

NEONATAL NUTRITION AND GASTROENTEROLOGY

At birth, the newborn infant must assume various functions performed during fetal life by the placenta. Cardiopulmonary transition and thermoregulation have already been discussed. The final critical task for the newborn is the assimilation of calories, water, and electrolytes.

Nutritional Requirements

The required caloric, water, and electrolyte intake of the newborn depends on body stores and normal rate of energy expenditure. Body composition varies considerably with gestational age (Fig. 20–15).[159,160] The average 1-kg neonate consists of 85 percent water, 10 percent protein, and 3 percent fat as compared with 74 percent water, 12 percent protein, and 11 percent fat at term. Carbohydrate stores in the term infant are eight times higher. Rates of energy expenditure differ as well. Although basal metabolic rate is lower in premature than in term infants, the premature infant frequently has increased metabolic demand secondary to cold stress and work of breathing. The small-for-gestational-age (SGA) infant provides another special consideration, possessing a higher basal metabolic rate per kilogram than a normally grown infant.[161]

Water and Electrolyte

Maintenance water requirements are dependent on metabolic rate (evaporative losses to dissipate the heat of oxidation) and the necessary water to excrete the renal solute load. Other pertinent factors, especially for the premature infant, include environmental variation in insensible water losses and diminished ability to concentrate urine.[162,163] An individual infant's water requirement can be determined by measuring urine and stool losses and estimating insensible losses through skin and mucosa. It is normal during the first 3 to 4 postnatal days for an infant to experience a weight loss

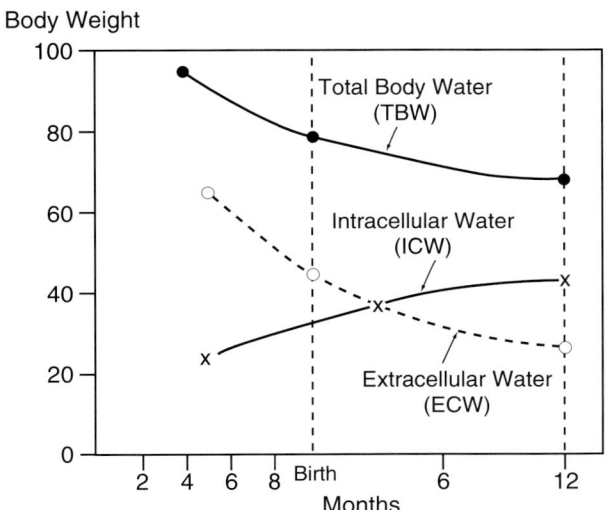

Figure 20–15. Changes in body water during gestation and infancy. (Adapted from Friis-Hansen B: Water distribution in the foetus and newborn infant. Acta Paediatr Scand Suppl 305:7, 1983.)

of up to 10 percent as the physiologic contraction of extracellular body fluid takes place. Maintenance electrolyte requirements are 2 to 3 mEq/kg/day for sodium, chloride, and bicarbonate and 1 to 2 mEq/kg/day for potassium. During periods of rapid growth, requirements will be higher.

Calories

Caloric needs are primarily dependent on oxygen consumption. The character of the feeding also affects caloric needs by altering specific dynamic action and fecal losses. The average caloric requirement for a normal full-term infant is estimated to be about 100 to 110 kcal/kg/day. The needs of the low-birth-weight infant are more variable, but usually 105 to 130 kcal/kg/day is adequate.[164] Standard infant formulas and breast milk provide approximately 20 kcal/oz. Therefore, volumes of 150 to 180 ml/kg/day will provide the necessary caloric intake of 100 to 120 kcal/kg/day for the average term or preterm infant beyond 32 to 34 weeks' gestation. However, infants less than 1,500 g should be fed with either formulas designed specifically for the premature (20 to 24 kcal/oz) or fortified breast milk.

Protein

Both the quantity and quality of protein intake are important for adequate growth, particularly for the premature infant.[165] Suggested intakes range from 2.25 to 4.0 g/kg/day (3.5 g/kg/day for the premature).[164] The "gold standard" for amino acid content is that which provides a plasma amniogram as close as possible to that seen with human milk.[166]

Fat and Carbohydrate

Fat intake plays several important roles in infant nutrition. It is a major energy source, a component of cellular membranes, a carrier of fat-soluble vitamins, and a source of essential fatty acids.[164] Long-chain polyunsaturated fatty acids such as arachidonic acid and docosahexaenoic acid play an important role in infant retinal and brain development. Because mammalian cells lack the enzymes to insert a double bond at the ω-6 or ω-3 position, a dietary source of these fatty acids is required. The precursors are linoleic and linolenic acids, but the newborn is not able to effectively lengthen the fatty acid chain and produce these long-chain molecules. Breast milk contains the ω-6 and ω-3 long-chain fats, and ongoing work is assessing the need for supplementation in formulas.[167] Fat is also not completely absorbed; more so in the premature than in the term infant.[164,168] For that reason, preterm formulas provide a portion of the fat energy as medium-chain triglycerides. Fat represents 40 to 50 percent of the caloric intake in the newborn, with 3 percent of total calories in the form of linoleic acid.[164]

Intestinal disaccharidases develop early in fetal life, with lactase reaching mature levels at term.[169] Both term and preterm infants can digest lactose, the major sugar in human milk and standard infant formulas, although there is some evidence that digestion may not be fully efficient the first several days of life.[164] Carbohydrate represents 40 to 50 percent of total calories in most formulas as well as human milk. These levels are more than adequate to maintain normal blood glucose levels and prevent ketosis.

Vitamins and Minerals

Published requirements are available for all major minerals and vitamins for term and preterm infants.[164,170,171] Information on trace minerals[164,170,171] is available as well.

Infant Feeding

For the well term or slightly preterm infant, institution of oral feeds within the first 2 to 4 hours of life is reasonable practice. For infants who are SGA or large for gestational age (LGA), feeds within the first hour or two of life may be indicated to avoid hypoglycemia. Premature infants (<34 weeks' gestation) who are unable to nipple feed present a more complex set of circumstances. In addition to an inability to suck and swallow efficiently, such infants face a number of problems: (1) relatively high caloric demand; (2) small stomach capacity; (3) incompetent esophageal-cardiac sphincter, leading to gastroesophageal reflux; (4) poor gag reflex, creating a tendency for aspiration; (5) decreased digestive capability (especially for fat); and (6) slow gastric emptying and intestinal motility. These infants can initially be supported adequately with parenteral nutrition followed by institution of nasogastric tube feedings when their cardiopulmonary status is stable.

Although a wide range of infant formulas satisfy the nutritional needs of most neonates, breast milk remains the standard on which formulas are based. The distribution of calories in human milk is 7 percent protein, 55 percent fat, and 38 percent carbohydrate. The whey/casein ratio is 60:40, allowing ease of protein digestion, while fat digestion is augmented by the presence of a breast milk lipase. In addition to easy digestibility, the amino acid make-up is well suited for the newborn. Despite the low levels of several vitamins and minerals, bioavailability is high. Besides the nutritional features, breast milk's immunochemical and cellular components provide protection against infection.[164,172]

The major area of controversy regarding breast milk has been its use for the small premature infant. The growth demands of the low-birth-weight infant exceed the contents of human milk for protein, calcium, phosphorus, sodium, zinc, copper, and possibly other nutrients.[173] These shortcomings can be addressed through the addition of human milk fortifiers to mother's preterm breast milk.[173] Advantages of breast milk for the premature include its anti-infective properties, possible protection against necrotizing enterocolitis, and its role in enhancing neurodevelopmental outcome.[174–177]

Under certain circumstances, breast-feeding might be deleterious. For example, phenylketonuria (PKU), a condition requiring special nutritional products, precludes breast-feeding. The presence of environmental pollutants has been documented in breast milk, but to date no serious side effects have been reported. Most drugs do not contraindicate breast-feeding, but there are a few exceptions (see Chapter 9). Transmission of some viral infections via breast milk is a concern as well. Mothers who are hepatitis B surface antigen (HB$_s$Ag) or human immunodeficiency virus (HIV) positive should not breast-feed. Finally, there is the insufficient milk syndrome and breast-feeding failure. Monographs that deal with this as well as other minor breast-feeding problems are available for mother and physician.[178] The obstetrician and pediatrician should serve as a source of knowledge and, most importantly, support. Table 20–9 illustrates what a mother can expect as she breast-feeds her infant.

Neonatal Hypoglycemia

Glucose is a major fetal fuel transported by facilitated diffusion across the placenta. After birth, before an appropriate supply of exogenous calories is provided, the newborn must maintain blood glucose through endogenous sources. This homeostasis depends on an adequate supply of gluconeogenic substrates (amino acids, lactate, glycerol), functionally intact hepatic glycogenolytic and gluconeogenic enzyme systems, and a normal endocrine counterregulatory hormone system (glucagon, catacholamines, growth hormone, cortisol) integrating and modulating these processes. Hepatic glycogen stores are almost entirely depleted within the first several hours before birth. Fat and protein stores are then used for energy, while glucose levels are maintained by hepatic gluconeogenesis.

In utero, fetal blood glucose concentration is 15 mg/dl lower than maternal levels. In the healthy unstressed neonate, glucose falls over the first 1 to 2 hours after birth, stabilizes at a minimum of about 40 mg/dl, and then rises to 50 to 80 mg/dl by 3 hours of life.[179] Hypoglycemia can be defined as blood glucose levels less than 40 mg/dl.[180] Infants at risk for hypoglycemia and in whom glucose should be monitored include preterm infants, SGA infants, hyperinsulinemic (LGA) infants, and infants with perinatal as-

phyxia. As in term babies, blood sugar drops after birth in preterm babies, but the latter are less able to mount a counterregulatory response.[181] In addition, the presence of respiratory distress, hypothermia, and other factors can increase glucose demand, exacerbating hypoglycemia. SGA infants are at risk for hypoglycemia resulting from decreased glycogen stores as well as impaired gluconeogenesis and ketogenesis.[182] Onset of hypoglycemia in SGA and preterm infants usually occurs at 2 to 6 hours of life. Hyperinsulinemia occurs in the infant of a diabetic mother as well as other rare conditions, including Beckwith-Weidemann syndrome and islet cell dysregulation syndrome (nesidioblastosis).[179] Onset of hypoglycemia in these infants can be in the first 30 to 60 minutes after birth. In the case of perinatal asphyxia, hypoglycemia is the result of excessive glucose demand.[180]

Symptoms of hypoglycemia include jitteriness, seizures, cyanosis, respiratory distress, apathy, hypotonia, and eye rolling.[179] However, many infants, particularly prematures, are asymptomatic. Because of the risk of subsequent brain injury,[183,184] hypoglycemia, when present, should be aggressively treated. However, the single best treatment is prevention by identifying infants at risk, including prematures, SGA, LGA, and any stressed infant. These newborns should have blood glucose screened with a bedside glucose meter. All values less than or equal to 40 mg/dl should be confirmed with a laboratory or rapid glucose analyzer measurement of whole blood glucose.[185] Treatment is provided by early institution of feeds or an intravenous glucose bolus (2 ml/kg of D$_{10}$W solution) followed by a glucose infusion at a rate of 6 mg/kg/min.

Congenital Gastrointestinal Surgical Conditions

Several congenital surgical conditions of the gastrointestinal tract interfere with a normal transition. Many of these conditions can be diagnosed with antenatal ultrasound, allowing transfer of the mother to a perinatal center for delivery.

Gastrointestial Tract Obstruction

Tracheoesophageal fistula and esophageal atresia are characterized by a blind esophageal pouch and a fistulous connection between either the proximal or distal esophagus and the airway.[186] Eighty-five percent of infants with these conditions have the fistula between the distal esophagus and the airway. Polyhydramnios is common because of the high level of gastrointestinal obstruction. Infants present in the first hours of life with copious secretions, choking, cyanosis, and respiratory distress. Diagnosis can be confirmed with chest radiography after careful placement of a nasogastric

Table 20–9. GUIDELINES FOR SUCCESSFUL BREAST FEEDING

	First 8 Hours	8–24 Hours	Day 2	Day 3	Day 4	Day 5	Day 6 Onward
Milk Supply	You may be able to express a few drops of milk.		Milk should come in between the 2nd & 4th day.			Milk should be in. Breasts may be firm and/or leak milk.	Breasts should feel softer after nursing.
Baby's Activity	Baby is usually wide awake in the first hour of life. Put baby to breast within $\frac{1}{2}$ to 1 hour of birth.	Wake up your baby. Babies may not wake up on their own to feed.	Baby should be more cooperative and less sleepy.	Look for early feeding cues such as rooting, lip smacking, and hands to face.		You should be able to hear your baby swallow your milk.	Baby should appear satisfied after feedings.
Feeding Routine	Baby may go into a deep sleep 2–4 hours after birth.		Use chart on back side of page to write down time and length of each feeding.			May go one longer interval (up to 5 hours) between feeds in a 24-hour period.	
		Feed your baby every 1 to 4 hours, as often as wanted, a minimum of 8–12 times each day.					
Breast-Feeding	Baby will wake up and be alert and responsive for several more hours after initial deep sleep.	As long as Mom is comfortable, nurse at both breasts as long as baby is actively sucking.	Try to nurse both sides each feeding, aiming for 10 minutes each side. Expect some nipple tenderness.	Consider hand expressing or pumping a few drops of milk to soften the nipple if the breast is too firm for the baby to latch on.	Nurse a minimum of 10–20 minutes each side every feeding for the first few weeks of life.	Once your milk supply is well established, allow your baby to finish the first breast before offering the second.	Mom's nipple tenderness is improving or is gone.
Baby's Urine Output		Baby must have a minimum of 1 wet diaper in first 24 hours.	Baby must have at least one wet diaper every 8–12 hours.	You should see an increase in wet diapers to 4–6 times in 24 hours.	Baby's urine should be light yellow or clear.	Baby should have 6–8 wet diapers each day.	
Baby's Stools		Baby should have a black-green stool (meconium stool).	Baby may have a second very dark (meconium) stool.	Baby's stools should be changing color from black-green to yellow.		Baby should have 3–4 yellow, soft stools a day.	The number of stools may decrease gradually after 4–6 weeks of life.

Courtesy of Beth Gabrielski, RN: The Children's Hospital, Denver, 1994, with permission.

tube to the point where resistance is met. The tube will be seen in the blind pouch. If a tracheoesophageal fistula is present to the distal esophagus, gas will be present in the abdomen.

Infants with high intestinal obstruction present early in life with either bilious or nonbilious vomiting.[187] A history of polyhydramnios is common and the amniotic fluid, if bile stained, can easily be confused with thin meconium staining. In duodenal atresia, vomitus may or may not contain bile, whereas malrotation with midgut volvulus and high jejunal atresia are characterized by bilious vomiting. Malrotation and midgut volvulus involve torsion of the intestine around the superior mesenteric artery, causing occlusion of the vascular supply to most of the small intestine. If not treated promptly, the infant can lose most of the small bowel because of ischemic injury. Therefore, bilious vomiting in the neonate demands immediate attention and evaluation. Diagnosis of high intestinal obstruction can be confirmed with radiographs. Duodenal atresia is characterized by a "double-bubble sign" (stomach and dilated duodenum). Diagnosis of midgut volvulus can be confirmed with an upper gastrointestinal tract series, looking for contrast not to pass the ligament of Treitz. Approximately 30 percent of cases of duodenal atresia are associated with Down syndrome.[187]

Low intestinal obstruction presents with increasing intolerance of feeds (spitting progressing to vomiting), abdominal distention, and decreased or absent stool.[187] Differential diagnosis of lower intestinal obstruction includes imperforate anus, Hirschsprung's disease, meconium plug syndrome, small left colon, colonic and ileal atresia, and meconium ileus. Plain x-ray film of the abdomen will show gaseous distention, with air through a considerable portion of the bowel and air–fluid levels. Diagnosis of meconium ileus, meconium plug, and small left colon syndrome can be made by appearance on contrast enema. Rectal biopsy searching for absence of ganglion cells will confirm the diagnosis of Hirschsprung's disease. Infants with meconium ileus and meconium plug should be screened for cystic fibrosis.

Abdominal Wall Defects

Omphaloceles[188] are formed by incomplete closure of the anterior abdominal wall after return of the midgut to the abdominal cavity. The size of the defect is variable, but usually the omphalocele sac contains some intestine, stomach, liver, and spleen. The abdominal cavity is small and underdeveloped. The umbilical cord can be seen to insert onto the center of the omphalocele sac. There is a high incidence of associated anomalies, including cardiac, other gastrointestinal anomalies, and chromosomal syndromes (trisomy 13). Delivery room treatment involves covering the defect with sterile warm saline to prevent fluid loss and nasogastric tube decompression.[189]

Gastroschisis[188] a defect in the anterior abdominal wall lateral to the umbilicus with no covering sac, with the herniated viscera usually limited to intestine. Furthermore, the intestine has been exposed to amniotic fluid and has a thickened, beefy red appearance. The herniation is thought to occur as a rupture through an ischemic portion of the abdominal wall. Other than intestinal atresia, associated anomalies are uncommon. Delivery room management is as described for omphalocele.

Diaphragmatic Hernia

In diaphragmatic hernia,[190] herniation of abdominal organs into the hemithorax (usually left) occurs because of a posterolateral defect in the diaphragm. Infants usually present in the delivery room with respiratory distress, cyanosis, decreased breath sounds on the side of the hernia, and shift of the mediastinum to the side opposite the hernia. The rapidity and severity of presentation with respiratory distress is dependent on the degree of associated pulmonary hypoplasia. The ipsilateral and to some extent contralateral lung are compressed in utero because of the hernia. Delivery room treatment is to intubate, to ventilate, and to decompress the gastrointestinal tract with a nasogastric tube. A chest radiograph will confirm the diagnosis. See Chapter 11 for a discussion of fetal surgical approaches to diaphragmatic hernia aimed at minimizing lung hypoplasia.[191,192]

Necrotizing Enterocolitis

Necrotizing enterocolitis (NEC) is the most common acquired gastrointestinal emergency in the neonatal intensive care unit. This disorder predominantly affects premature infants, with higher incidences present with decreasing gestational age, although it is seen in term infants with polycythemia, congenital heart disease, and birth asphyxia.[193,194] The pathogenesis is multifactorial with intestinal ischemia, infection, provision of enteral feedings, and gut maturity playing roles to varying degrees in individual patients.[193,195] Tocolysis with indomethacin presumably related to changes in intestinal circulation has been associated with an increased incidence of NEC and isolated intestinal perforation, while antenatal betamethasone may decrease the incidence.[15,196,197]

Clinically, there is a varied spectrum of disease, from a mild gastrointestinal disturbance to a rapid fulminant course characterized by intestinal gangrene, perforation, sepsis, and shock. The hallmark symptoms are abdominal distention, ileus, delayed gastric emptying, and bloody stools. The radiographic findings are bowel wall edema, pneumatosis intestinalis, biliary free air, and free peritoneal air. Associated symptoms include apnea, bradycardia, hypotension, and temperature instability.

NEONATAL JAUNDICE

The most common "problem" encountered in a term nursery population is jaundice. Neonatal hyperbilirubinemia occurs when the normal pathways of bilirubin metabolism and excretion are altered. Figure 20–16 demonstrates the metabolism of bilirubin.[198] The normal destruction of circulating red cells accounts for about 75 percent of the newborn's daily bilirubin production. The remaining sources include ineffective erythropoiesis and tissue heme proteins. Heme is converted to bilirubin in the reticuloendothelial system. Unconjugated bilirubin is lipid soluble and transported in the plasma reversibly bound to albumin. Bilirubin enters the liver cells by dissociation from albumin in the hepatic sinusoids. Once in the hepatocyte, bilirubin is conjugated with glucuronic acid in a reaction catalyzed by uridine diphosphoglucuronosyl transferase (UDPGT). The water-soluble conjugated bilirubin is sufficiently polar to be excreted into bile or filtered through the kidney. After conjugation, bilirubin is excreted rapidly into the bile canaliculi and into the small intestine. The enzyme β-glucuronidase is present in small bowel and hydrolyzes some of the conjugated bilirubin. This unconjugated bilirubin can be reabsorbed into the circulation, adding to the total unconjugated bilirubin load (enterohepatic circulation). Major predisposing factors of neonatal jaundice are (1) increased bilirubin load because of increased red cell vol-

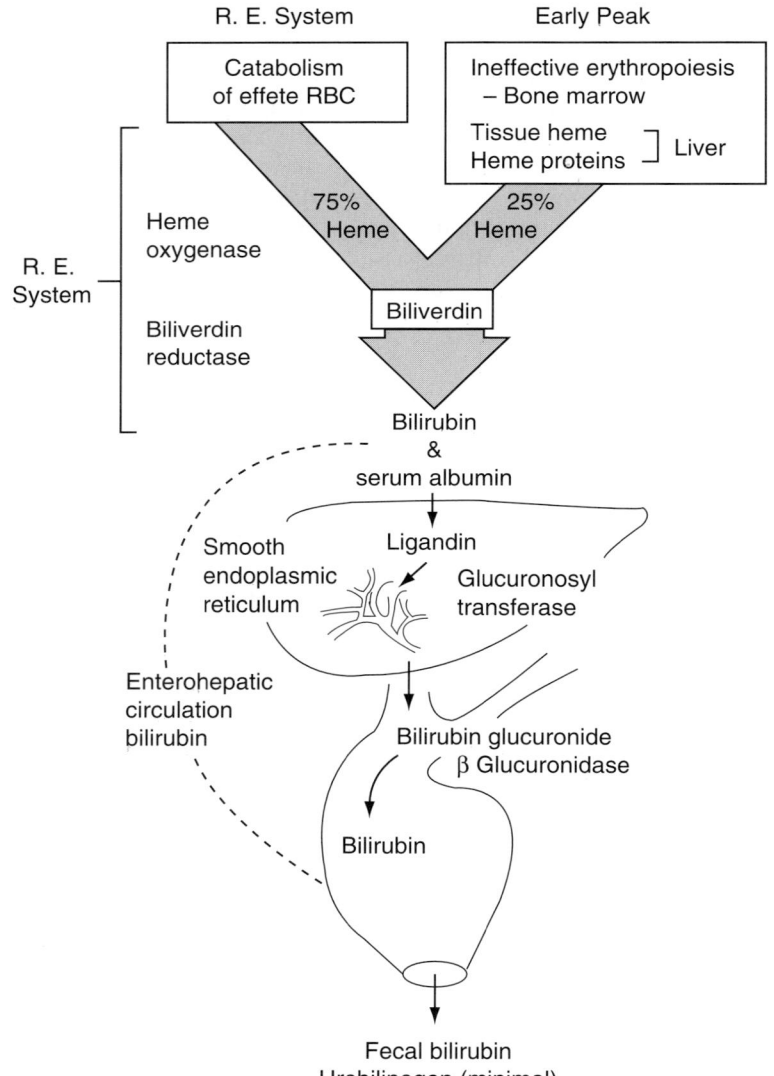

Figure 20–16. Neonatal bile pigment metabolism. (Adapted from Maisels MJ: Jaundice. *In* Avery GB, Fletcher MA, MacDonald MG [eds]: Neonatology: Pathophysiology and Management of the Newborn. 5th ed. Philadelphia, Lippincott Williams & Wilkins, 1999, p 765, with permission.)

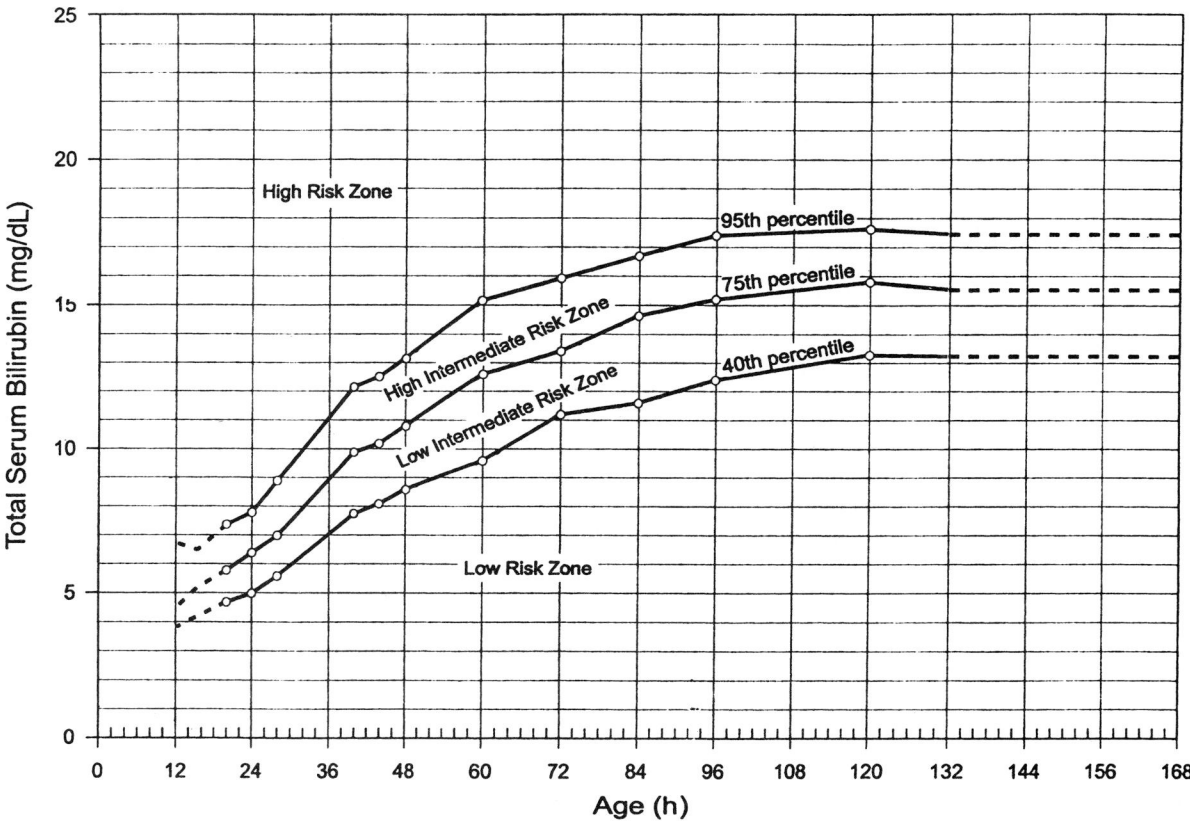

Figure 20–17. Risk of developing significant hyperbilirubinemia in term and near-term infants based on hour-specific bilirubin determinations. (From Bhutani VK, Johnson L, Sivieri EM: Predictive ability of a predischarge hour-specific serum bilirubin for subsequent significant hyperbilirubinemia in healthy term and near-term newborns. Pediatrics 103:6, 1999. Copyright 1999 American Academy of Pediatrics, with permission.)

ume with decreased cell survival, increased ineffective erythropoiesis, and the enterohepatic circulation; and (2) decreased hepatic uptake, conjugation, and excretion of bilirubin. These factors result in the presence of clinically apparent jaundice in approximately two thirds of newborns during the first week of life.[198] This transient jaundice has been called physiologic jaundice. Infants whose bilirubin levels are above the 95th percentile for age in hours require close follow-up (Fig. 20–17).[199]

Pathologic jaundice during the early neonatal period is indirect hyperbilirubinemia usually caused by overproduction of bilirubin. The leading cause in this group of patients is hemolytic disease, of which fetomaternal blood group incompatibilities (Rh and ABO) are the most common (see Chapter 26). Other causes of hemolysis include genetic disorders much as hereditary spherocytosis and nonspherocytic hemolytic anemias, such as glucose-6-phosphate dehydrogenase (G6PD) deficiency. Other etiologies of bilirubin overproduction include extravasated blood (bruising, hemorrhage), polycythemia, and exaggerated enterohepatic circulation of bilirubin because of mechanical gastrointestinal obstruction or reduced peristalsis from inadequate oral intake. Disease

states involving decreased bilirubin clearance must be considered in the patients in whom no cause of overproduction can be identified. Causes of indirect hyperbilirubinemia in this category include familial deficiency of UDPGT (Crigler-Najjar syndrome), Gilbert syndrome, breast milk jaundice, and hypothyroidism. Mixed or direct hyperbilirubinemia are rare during the first week of life.

A strong association exists between breast-feeding and neonatal hyperbilirubinemia. The syndrome of breast milk jaundice is characterized by full-term infants who have jaundice that persists into the second and third weeks of life with maximal bilirubin levels of 10 to 30 mg/dl. If breast-feeding is continued, the levels persist for 4 to 10 days and then decline to normal by 3 to 12 weeks. Interruption of breast-feeding is associated with a prompt decline in 48 hours.[200] In addition to this syndrome, breast-fed infants as a whole have higher bilirubin levels over the first 3 to 5 days of life than their formula-fed counterparts (Fig. 20–18).[201] Rather than interrupting breast-feeding, this early jaundice is responsive to increased frequency of breast-feeding. Suggested mechanisms for breast-feeding–associated jaundice include decreased early caloric intake,

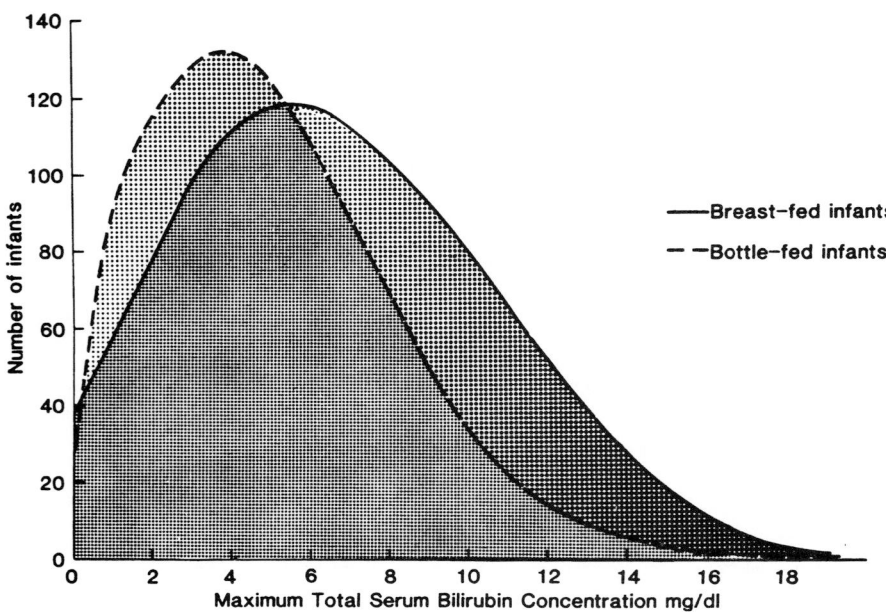

Figure 20–18. Distribution of maximum serum bilirubin concentrations in white infants who weigh more than 2,500 g. (Adapted from Maisels MJ, Gifford KL: Normal serum bilirubin levels in the newborn and the effect of breast-feeding. Pediatrics 78:837, 1986.)

inhibitors of bilirubin conjugation in breast milk, and increased intestinal reabsorption of bilirubin.[201,202] In some patients, there is considerable overlap in these described syndromes.

The overriding concern with neonatal hyperbilirubinemia is the development of bilirubin toxicity causing the pathologic entity of kernicterus, the staining of certain areas of the brain (basal ganglia, hippocampus, geniculate bodies, various brain stem nuclei, and cerebellum) by bilirubin. Neuronal necrosis is the dominant histopathologic feature at 7 to 10 days of life. The clinical syndrome in term infants is marked by refusal to feed, high-pitched cry, hypertonicity, and opisthotonos. Survivors usually suffer sequelae, including athetoid cerebral palsy, high-frequency hearing loss, paralysis of upward gaze, and dental dysplasia.[203] The risk of kernicterus in a given infant is not well defined. The only group that one can speak of with any certainty is those infants with Rh isoimmunization in whom a level of 20 mg/dl has been associated with an increased risk of kernicterus.[204] This observation has been extended to the management of other neonates with hemolytic disease, although no definitive data exist regarding these infants. The risk is probably small for term infants without hemolytic disease even at levels higher than 20 mg/dl.[205–207] Recent descriptions of kernicterus in breast-fed infants with dehydration and hyperbilirubinemia in whom an adequate supply of breast milk has not been established mandates close follow-up of all breast-feeding mothers.[208,209] The true risk for nonhemolytic hyperbilirubinemia to produce brain damage in the preterm in the current era of liberal use of phototherapy that prevents marked elevation of severe bilirubin in these infants is unknown. However, most cur-

rently available data would suggest this risk is low.[198,210]

NEONATAL HEMATOLOGY

Anemia

Early hematopoietic cells originate in the yolk sac. By 8 weeks' gestation, erythropoiesis is taking place in the liver, which remains the primary site of erythroid production through the early fetal period. By 6 months of gestation, the bone marrow becomes the principal site of red cell development.[211] Normal hemoglobin levels at term range from 13.7 to 20.1 g/dl.[212] In the very preterm infant, values as low as 12 g/dl are acceptable.[213] Anemia at birth or appearing in the first few weeks of life is the result of blood loss, hemolysis, or underproduction of erythrocytes.[214] Blood loss resulting in anemia can occur prenatally, at the time of delivery, or postnatally. In utero blood loss can be the result of fetomaternal bleeding, twin-to-twin transfusion, or blood loss resulting from trauma (maternal trauma, amniocentesis, external cephalic version). The diagnosis of fetomaternal hemorrhage large enough to cause anemia can be made using the Kleihauer-Betke technique of acid elution to identify fetal cells in the maternal circulation. Blood loss at delivery can be caused by umbilical cord rupture, incision of the placenta during cesarean delivery, placenta previa, or abruptio placentae. Internal hemorrhage can occur in the newborn, often related to a difficult delivery. Sites include intracranial, cephalhematomas, subgaleal space, retroperitoneal, liver capsule, and ruptured spleen. When blood loss has been chronic (e.g., fetomaternal), infants will be pale at birth but well compensated and without signs of volume loss. The initial hematocrit will be low. Acute bleeding will present with signs of hypovolemia (tachycardia, poor perfusion, hypotension). The initial hematocrit can be normal or decreased, but after several hours of equilibration it will be decreased. Anemia caused by hemolysis from blood group incompatibilities is common in the newborn period. Less common causes of hemolysis include erythrocyte membrane abnormalities, enzyme deficiencies, and disorders of hemoglobin synthesis. Impaired erythrocyte production is an unusual cause of neonatal anemia.

Polycythemia

Elevated hematocrits occur in 1.5 to 4 percent of live births.[215] Although 50 percent of polycythemic infants are appropriate for gestational age (AGA), the proportion of polycythemic infants is greater in the SGA and LGA populations.[215] Causes of polycythemia include twin-to-twin transfusion, maternal-to-fetal transfusion, intrapartum transfusion from the placenta associated with fetal distress, chronic intrauterine hypoxia (SGA infants, LGA infants of diabetic mothers), delayed cord clamping, and chromosomal abnormalities.[216] The consequence of polycythemia is hyperviscosity, resulting in impaired perfusion of capillary beds. Therefore, clinical symptoms can be related to any organ system (see Box). As viscosity measurements are not routinely performed at most institutions, hyperviscosity is inferred from hematocrit because the major factor influencing viscosity in the newborn is red cell mass. Cord blood

Table 20–10. DIFFERENTIAL DIAGNOSIS OF NEONATAL THROMBOCYTOPENIA

Diagnosis	Comments
Immune	Passively acquired antibody (e.g., idiopathic thrombocytopenic purpura, systemic lupus erythematosus, drug induced)
	Alloimmune sensitization to HPA-1a antigen
Infections	Bacterial; congenital viral infections (e.g., cytomegalovirus, rubella)
Syndromes	Absent radii; Fanconi's anemia
Giant hemangioma	
Thrombosis	
High-risk infant with respiratory distress syndrome, pulmonary hypertension, and so forth	Disseminated intravascular coagulation
	Isolated thrombocytopenia

hematocrit greater than or equal to 57 percent[217] and capillary hematocrit of at least 70 percent are indicative of polycythemia. Confirmation of the diagnosis is a peripheral venous hematocrit of at least 64 percent.[217] Reduction of venous hematocrit to less than 60 percent may improve acute symptoms, but it has not been shown to improve long-term neurologic outcome.[218-220]

Thrombocytopenia

Neonatal thrombocytopenia can be isolated or occur associated with deficiency of clotting factors. A differential diagnosis is presented in Table 20–10. The immune thrombocytopenias have important implications for perinatal care. In idiopathic thrombocytopenic purpura (ITP), maternal antiplatelet antibodies that cross the placenta lead to destruction of fetal platelets. Correlation between the degree of thrombocytopenia in mother and fetus is not good[221,222]; thus, the severity of thrombocytopenia in an individual fetus cannot be predicted with certainty. The incidence of severe neonatal thrombocytopenia varies from 5 to 20 percent of cases.[223,224] However, even in the presence of severe neonatal thrombocytopenia, there is a very low rate of significant bleeding complications in these infants including intracranial bleeds, irrespective of route of delivery.[223-225] In alloimmune thrombocytopenia, maternal antibody to paternal platelet antigen on fetal platelets crosses the placenta and causes destruction of fetal platelets. In the largest series of cases of suspected alloimmune thrombocytopenia, the majority were caused by HPA-1a alloantibodies.[226] As the maternal platelet count is normal, the diagnosis is suspected on the basis of a history of a previously affected pregnancy. Intracranial hemorrhage is more common with

Organ-Related Symptoms of Hyperviscosity

Central nervous system	Irritability, jitteriness, seizures, lethargy
Cardiopulmonary	Respiratory distress caused by congestive heart failure or persistent pulmonary hypertension
Gastrointestinal	Vomiting, heme-positive stools, abdominal distention, necrotizing enterocolitis
Renal	Decreased urine output, renal vein thrombosis
Metabolic	Hypoglycemia
Hematologic	Hyperbilirubinemia, thrombocytopenia

this condition than in maternal ITP (10 to 20 percent) and can occur in the antenatal or intrapartum periods.[227,228] Recurrence risk is 75 percent. Percutaneous umbilical blood sampling (PUBS) at 18 to 20 weeks can be done to measure platelet count. If severe thrombocytopenia is present, intravenous immunoglobulin can be given weekly to the mother.[227,228] Other treatment options include serial in utero platelet transfusions and combination therapy with intravenous immune globulin (IVIG) and steroids.[227] Route of delivery is determined by fetal platelet count on a PUBS sample. Cesarean delivery is done for counts less than 50,000/μl.

Vitamin K Deficiency

Vitamin K_1 oxide (1 mg) should be given intramuscularly to all newborns to prevent hemorrhagic disease caused by a deficiency in vitamin K–dependent clotting factors.[229] Babies born to mothers who are on anticonvulsant medication are particularly at risk of having vitamin K deficiency. Oral vitamin K has been shown to be effective in raising vitamin K levels, but is not as effective in preventing late hemorrhagic disease of the newborn (presenting at 4 to 6 weeks of age). Late hemorrhagic disease of the newborn most commonly occurs in breast-fed infants whose courses have been complicated by diarrhea.

PERINATAL INFECTION

See Chapter 40.

RESPIRATORY DISTRESS

The establishment of respiratory function at birth is dependent on expansion and maintenance of air sacs, clearance of lung fluid, and provision of adequate pulmonary perfusion. In many premature and other high-risk infants, developmental deficiencies or unfavorable perinatal events hamper a smooth respiratory transition. Furthermore, a neonate has a limited number of ways to respond symptomatically to a variety of pathophysiologic insults. The presentation of respiratory distress is among the most common symptom complexes seen in the newborn and may be secondary to both noncardiopulmonary and cardiopulmonary etiologies (Table 20–11). The symptom complex includes an elevation of the respiratory rate to greater than 60 bpm with or without cyanosis, nasal flaring, intercostal and sternal retractions, and expiratory grunting. The retrac-

tions are the result of the neonate's efforts to expand a lung with poor compliance utilizing a very compliant chest wall. The expiratory grunt is caused by closure of the glottis during expiration in an effort to increase expiratory pressure to help maintain functional residual capacity. The evaluation of such an infant requires utilization of history, physical examination, and laboratory data to arrive at a diagnosis. It is important to consider causes other than those related to the heart and lungs, because one's natural tendency is to focus immediately on the more common cardiopulmonary etiologies.

Cardiovascular Causes

Cardiovascular causes of respiratory distress in the neonatal period can be divided into two major groups— those with structural heart disease and those with persistent right-to-left shunting through fetal pathways and a structurally normal heart. The two presentations of serious structural heart disease in the first week of life are cyanosis and congestive heart failure. Examples of cyanotic heart disease include transposition of the great vessels, tricuspid atresia, certain types of truncus arteriosus, total anomalous pulmonary venous return, and right-sided outflow obstruction including tetralogy of Fallot and pulmonary stenosis or atresia. Although cyanosis is the central feature in these disorders, tachypnea will develop in many infants because of increased pulmonary blood flow or secondary to metabolic acidosis from hypoxia. Infants with congestive heart failure generally have some form of left-sided outflow obstruction. Left-to-right shunt lesions such as ventricular septal defect do not present with increased pulmonary blood flow and congestive heart failure until pulmonary vascular resistance is low enough to permit a significant shunt (usually 3 to 4 weeks of age at sea level). Infants with left-sided outflow obstruction generally do well the first day or so until the source of systemic flow, the ductus arteriosus, closes. With ductal narrowing, dyspnea, tachypnea, and tachycardia develop, followed by rapid progression to congestive heart failure and metabolic acidosis. On examination, these infants all have pulse abnormalities. With hypoplastic left heart syndrome and critical aortic stenosis, pulses are profoundly diminished in all extremities, while infants with coarctation of the aorta and interrupted aortic arch will have differential pulses when the arms and legs are compared.

The syndrome of persistent pulmonary hypertension of the newborn (PPHN) occurs when the normal postnatal decrease in pulmonary vascular resistance does not occur, maintaining right-to-left shunting across the patent ductus arteriosus and foramen ovale. Most infants with PPHN are full term or postmature and have experienced perinatal asphyxia. Other clinical associations include hypothermia, MAS, hyaline membrane

Table 20–11. RESPIRATORY DISTRESS IN THE NEWBORN

Noncardiopulmonary	Cardiovascular	Pulmonary
Hypo- or hyperthermia	Left-sided outflow obstruction	Upper airway obstruction
Hypoglycemia	Hypoplastic left heart	Choanal atresia
Metabolic acidosis	Aortic stenosis	Vocal cord paralysis
Drug intoxications; withdrawal	Coarctation of the aorta	Meconium aspiration
Polycythemia	Cyanotic lesions	Clear fluid aspiration
Central nervous system insult	Transposition of the great vessels	Transient tachypnea
Asphyxia	Total anomalous pulmonary venous return	Pneumonia
Hemorrhage	Tricuspid atresia	Pulmonary hypoplasia
Neuromuscular disease	Right-sided outflow obstruction	Primary
Werdnig-Hoffman disease		Secondary
Myopathies		Hyaline membrane disease
Phrenic nerve injury		Pneumothorax
Skeletal abnormalities		Pleural effusions
Asphyxiating thoracic dystrophy		Mass lesions
		Lobar emphysema
		Cystic adenomatoid malformation

disease, polycythemia, neonatal sepsis, chronic intrauterine hypoxia, pulmonary hypoplasia, and premature closure of the ductus arteriosus in utero.[230–232]

On the basis of developmental considerations, these infants can be separated into three groups[231]: (1) acute vasoconstriction caused by perinatal hypoxia, (2) prenatal increase in pulmonary vascular smooth muscle development, and (3) decreased cross-sectional area of the pulmonary vascular bed caused by inadequate vessel number. In the first group, an acute perinatal event leads to hypoxia and failure of pulmonary vascular resistance to drop. In the second, abnormal muscularization of the pulmonary resistance vessels results in PPHN after birth. The third circumstance includes infants with pulmonary hypoplasia (e.g., diaphragmatic hernia). Clinically, the syndrome is characterized by cyanosis, often unresponsive to increases in FIO_2, respiratory distress, an onset at less than 24 hours, evidence of right ventricular overload, systemic hypotension, acidosis, and no evidence of structural heart disease.

Infants with PPHN make up the majority of patients who are treated in some centers with extracorporeal membrane oxygenation (ECMO).[233] When conventional medical therapy (ventilator, systemic pressors, respiratory alkalosis) fails, infants are placed on bypass, with blood exiting the baby from the right atrium and returning to the aortic arch after passing through a membrane oxygenator. Over several days, pulmonary hypertension resolves, and the infants are weaned from ECMO back to conventional ventilator therapy. In recent years, new modes of treatment have been introduced that are decreasing the need for ECMO.[234] Specifically, use of high-frequency ventilators and inhaled nitric oxide have shown great promise.[235–237] Nitric oxide is identical or similar to endogenously produced endothelium-derived relaxing factor and is used as a

selective pulmonary vasodilator in infants with PPHN.[236]

Pulmonary Causes

Of the causes of respiratory distress related to the airways and pulmonary parenchyma listed in Table 20–11, the differential diagnosis in a term infant includes transient tachypnea, aspiration syndromes, congenital pneumonia, and spontaneous pneumothorax. The syndrome of transient tachypnea (wet lung or type II RDS) presents as respiratory distress in nonasphyxiated term infants or slightly preterm infants. The clinical features include various combinations of cyanosis, grunting, nasal flaring, retracting, and tachypnea during the first hours after birth. The chest radiograph is the key to the diagnosis, with prominent perihilar streaking and fluid in the interlobar fissures. The symptoms generally subside in 12 to 24 hours, although they can persist longer. The preferred explanation for the clinical features is delayed reabsorption of fetal lung fluid.[238] Transient tachypnea is seen more commonly in infants delivered by elective cesarean section or in the slightly preterm infant (see Mechanics of the First Breath, above).

At delivery, the neonate may aspirate clear amniotic fluid or fluid mixed with blood. Whether infants can aspirate a sufficient volume of clear fluid to cause symptoms is controversial. However, there are a group of infants whose clinical course is more prolonged (4 to 7 days) and severe than that of infants with transient tachypnea. These infants have a radiologic picture similar to transient tachypnea often associated with more marked hyperexpansion. Occasionally, the infiltrates are quite impressive, with evidence of far more fluid than is seen with transient tachypnea.

MAS occurs in full-term or postmature infants. The perinatal course is often marked by fetal distress and low Apgar scores. These infants exhibit tachypnea, retractions, cyanosis, overdistended and barrel-shaped chest, and coarse breath sounds. Chest radiography reveals coarse, irregular pulmonary densities with areas of diminished aeration or consolidation. There is a high incidence of air leaks, and many of the infants exhibit persistent pulmonary hypertension.[97,105]

The lungs represent the most common primary site of infection in the neonate. Both bacterial and viral infections can be acquired before, during, or after birth. The most common route of infection, particularly for bacteria, is ascending from the genital tract before or during labor. Thus, prolonged rupture of the membranes in excess of 12 to 18 hours is a major predisposing factor.[239,240] Major pathogens include group B β-hemolytic *Streptococcus,* gram-negative enterics, and *Listeria monocytogenes.*[241,242] Infants with congenital pneumonia present with symptomatology from very early in life, including tachypnea, retractions, grunting, nasal flaring, and cyanosis. The chest radiograph pattern is often indistinguishable from other causes of respiratory distress, particularly hyaline membrane disease (HMD).[243]

Spontaneous pneumothorax occurs in 1 percent of all deliveries, but a much lower percent result in symptoms.[244] The risk is increased by manipulations such as positive-pressure ventilation. Respiratory distress is usually present from shortly after birth, and breath sounds may be diminished on the affected side. The majority of these resolve spontaneously without specific therapy.

Despite improved understanding and recent advances, HMD remains the most common etiology for respiratory distress in the neonatal period. HMD affects approximately 20,000 infants per year in the United States, developing in 50 percent of infants at 26 to 28 weeks of gestation and in 30 percent of those at 30 to 31 weeks. It was the initial reports of Avery and Mead[245] demonstrating a high surface tension in extracts of lungs from infants dying of RDS that led to the present understanding of the role of surfactant in the pathogenesis of HMD. The deficiency of surfactant in the premature infant increases alveolar surface tension and, according to LaPlace's law (Fig. 20–2) increases the pressure necessary to maintain patent alveoli. The end result is poor lung compliance, progressive atelectasis, loss of FRC, alterations in ventilation–perfusion mismatch, and uneven distribution of ventilation.[244] HMD is further complicated by the weak respiratory muscles and compliant chest wall of the premature. Hypoxemia and respiratory and metabolic acidemia contribute to increased pulmonary vascular resistance, right-to-left ductal shunting, and worsening ventilation–perfusion mismatch that exacerbate hypoxemia. Hypoxemia and hypoperfusion result in alveolar

epithelial damage, with increased capillary permeability and leakage of plasma into alveolar spaces. Leakage of protein into airspaces serves to inhibit surfactant function, exacerbating the disease process.[246] The materials in plasma and cellular debris combine to form the characteristic hyaline membrane seen pathologically. The recovery phase is characterized by regeneration of alveolar cells, including type II cells, with an increase in surfactant activity.

Clinically, neonates with HMD demonstrate tachypnea, nasal flaring, subcostal and intercostal retractions, cyanosis, and expiratory grunting. As the infant begins to tire with progressive disease, apneic episodes occur. If some intervention is not undertaken at this point, death ensues. The radiologic appearance of the lungs is what would be expected in an extensive atelectatic process. The infiltrate is diffuse, with a ground-glass appearance. Major airways are air filled and contrast with the atelectatic alveoli, creating the appearance of air bronchograms, while the diaphragms are elevated because of profound hypoexpansion. Acute complications of HMD include infection, air leaks, and persistent patency of the ductus arteriosus.

Of more concern than acute complications are the long-term sequelae suffered by infants with HMD. The major long-term consequences are chronic lung disease requiring prolonged ventilator and oxygen therapy and significant neurologic impairment. In 1967, Northway et al.[247] first described the syndrome of bronchopulmonary dysplasia in infants surviving severe HMD requiring mechanical ventilation. Today, many infants who develop chronic lung disease are extremely-low-birthweight infants who require prolonged ventilation for apnea and poor respiratory effort. The incidence is now estimated at about 20 percent in preterm infants weighing less than 1,000 g requiring mechanical ventilation.[248] The severity is variable, ranging from very mild pulmonary dysfunction to severe disease with prolonged mechanical ventilation, frequent readmissions for respiratory exacerbations after nursery discharge, and a higher incidence of neurodevelopmental sequelae compared with very-low-birth-weight controls.[249] Although pulmonary function improves over time and most children do quite well, long-term pulmonary sequelae are evident.[250,251] Factors involved in the etiology of chronic lung disease are gestational age, elevated inspired oxygen concentration, positive-pressure ventilation, severity of underlying disease, inflammation, and infection.[252]

One of the exciting areas in neonatology is the development of surfactant replacement therapy for the management of hyaline membrane disease. Modified natural surfactant, which is extracted by alveolar lavage or from lung tissue (usually bovine) and then modified by selective addition and/or removal of components, and true artificial surfactant, which is a mixture of synthetic

Table 20–12. CUMULATIVE RESULTS OF PLACEBO-CONTROLLED SURFACTANT TRIALS*

	Modified Natural[†] (%)		Synthetic[‡] (%)	
	Surfactant	Control	Surfactant	Control
Mortality	15	24	11	18
Patent ductus arteriosus	46	43	44	48
Severe ICH	19	19	7	8
Chronic lung disease	37	37	11	11

* Higher incidences of intracranial hemorrhage (ICH) and chronic lung disease in modified natural surfactant studies reflects the lower gestational age on average in both groups in these studies compared to the artificial surfactant studies.
[†] Studies with Survanta, Curosurf, and Infasurf; 2,000 patients.
[‡] Studies with Exosurf; 4,400 patients.

compounds that may or may not be components of natural surfactant, have been extensively studied.[19–22,253] In most studies, these agents (administered intratracheally) have shown efficacy in decreasing the severity of acute HMD and the frequency of air leak complications. Efficacy has been demonstrated when used in the delivery room to "prevent" or when used as a rescue treatment for established HMD. Although surfactant replacement therapy has decreased mortality and acute pulmonary morbidity, this therapy has not affected the frequency of other complications of prematurity (Table 20–12). Of note is that, despite resulting in lower ventilator settings and FiO_2 concentration over the first several days of life, the incidence of chronic lung disease has not been changed. However, the severity of long-term pulmonary complications is less. Long-term neurodevelopment follow-ups show rates of handicap similar to placebo-treated infants.[254]

NEONATAL NEUROLOGY

Intraventricular Hemorrhage

Although related most closely to degree of prematurity, periventricular hemorrhage (PVH) and intraventricular hemorrhage (IVH) should also be considered within the context of sequelae of asphyxia. The incidence of this complication is 20 to 30 percent in infants weighing less than 1,500 g or at 31 weeks' gestation. The highest incidence is seen in babies of the lowest gestational age ($\leq$26 weeks).[255,256]

Bleeding originates in the subependymal germinal matrix located ventrolateral to the lateral ventricles in the caudothalamic groove. The germinal matrix is made up of a rete or meshwork of thin-walled vessels in the process of remodeling into a capillary network and a mass of undifferentiated cells that are destined to become cortical neurons, astrocytes, and oligodendroglia.

Rupture of a germinal matrix hemorrhage into the ventricular system leads to intraventricular hemorrhage. A proposed pathogenesis derived from a review of available information is presented in Figure 20–19. The critical predisposing event is likely an ischemia-reperfusion injury to the capillaries in the germinal matrix. Physiologic data from beagle puppies have shown that the germinal matrix is a low blood flow region prone to ischemia.[257] Furthermore, IVH is most reliably produced in these puppies by a sequence of hemorrhagic hypotension followed by hypertension.[258] The amount of bleeding is then influenced by a variety of factors that affect the pressure gradient across the injured capillary wall. This pathogenic scheme also applies to intraparenchymal bleeding (venous infarction in a region rendered ischemic) and periventricular leukomalacia (PVL; ischemia in a watershed region of arterial supply).[259] Periventricular hemorrhagic infarction is most often an asymmetric lesion, with the more affected areas occurring on the same side as the larger amount of intraventricular blood, PVL can develop independent of IVH and is usually bilateral and symmetric. PVL has a peak incidence in babies born between 28 and 32 weeks' gestation and is associated with maternal chorioamnionitis.[260,261] Up to 50 percent of bleeds occur at less than 24 hours of age, and virtually all occur by day 4 of life.[262] Bleeds are graded according to severity as indicated in Table 20–13.[263] Diagnosis is confirmed with real-time ultrasound.

The neurodevelopmental outcome of infants with IVH is determined by the severity of the original bleed, development of posthemorrhagic hydrocephalus, and the degree of associated parenchymal injury. Infants with grade I or II IVH have neurodevelopmental outcomes similar to preterm infants without IVH, although recent reports of outcome in school-aged children do show that survivors of mild IVH display a variety of subtle neurologic and cognitive abnormalities, including motor incoordination, hyperactivity, attention and learning deficits, and visual motor difficulties.[264,265] On

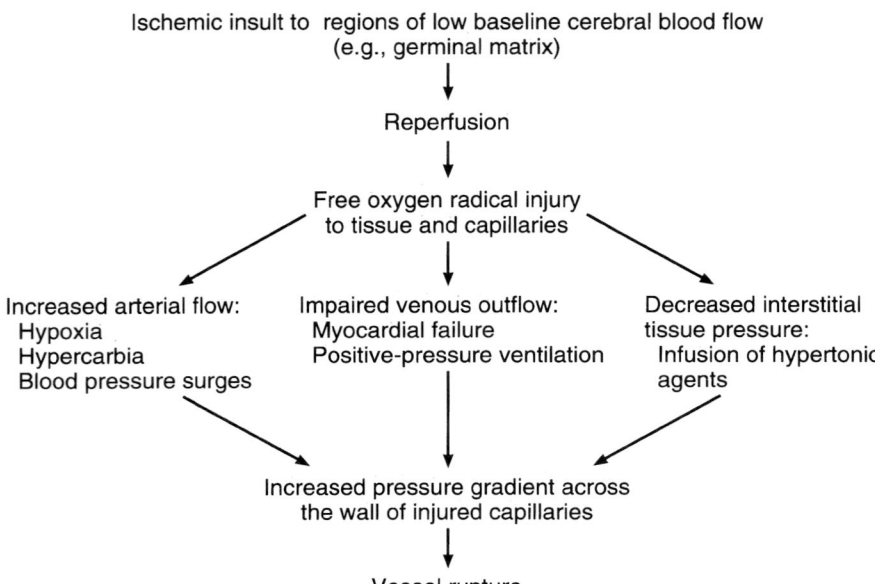

Ischemic insult to regions of low baseline cerebral blood flow (e.g., germinal matrix)

↓

Reperfusion

↓

Free oxygen radical injury to tissue and capillaries

Increased arterial flow:
 Hypoxia
 Hypercarbia
 Blood pressure surges

Impaired venous outflow:
 Myocardial failure
 Positive-pressure ventilation

Decreased interstitial tissue pressure:
 Infusion of hypertonic agents

↓

Increased pressure gradient across the wall of injured capillaries

↓

Vessel rupture

Figure 20–19. Pathogenesis of periventricular/intraventricular hemorrhage in the preterm infant.

the other hand, infants with progressive ventricular dilatation (grade III) or periventricular hemorrhagic infarction (grade IV) are at high risk for major neurodevelopmental handicap as well as less severe neurologic and cognitive disabilities.[266,267] In addition, the presence of severe PVL carries an ominous prognosis.[268,269]

Although incidence and severity of intracranial hemorrhage have progressively decreased as a result of advances in both obstetric and neonatal care, the therapeutic focus continues to be on strategies to prevent this complication of prematurity (see Box). Both antenatal and postnatal approaches have been developed. Postnatal pharmacologic strategies have for the most part not had a major effect in decreasing the incidence and severity of IVH. The prostaglandin synthesis inhibitor indomethacin has been most widely studied and has shown some promise when used in the first several hours after birth.[270] Since IVH and PVL are likely peri-

natal events, antenatal prevention holds the most promise. Both vitamin K and phenobarbital have been administered in this way.[271] Antenatal phenobarbital has resulted in a decrease in both frequency and severity of IVH. The proposed mechanism of action is thought to be scavenging of oxygen free radicals, although pheno-

Table 20–13. CLASSIFICATION OF INTRAVENTRICULAR HEMORRHAGE

Grade	Definition
I	Subependymal hemorrhage
II	Intraventricular hemorrhage without ventricular dilatation
III	Intraventricular hemorrhage with ventricular dilatation
IV	Intraventricular hemorrhage with associated parenchymal hemorrhage

From Papile L-A, Burstein J, Burstein R, Koffler H: Incidence and evolution of subependymal and intraventricular hemorrhage: a study of infants with birth weights less than 1500 gm. J Pediatr 92:529, 1978, with permission.

Interventions for the Prevention of Periventricular/Intraventricular Hemorrhage

Antenatal interventions
Pharmacologic
 Phenobarbital
 Vitamin K
 Corticosteroids
Obstetric
 Prevention of prematurity
 Optimal management of preterm labor and delivery
Postnatal interventions
Pharmacologic
 Indomethacin
Optimal NICU care
 Aggressive resuscitation
 Careful ventilation to avoid airleaks
 Blood pressure management avoiding hypotension and sudden changes
 Correction of coagulation abnormalities

NICU, neonatal intensive care unit.

Table 20–14. DIFFERENTIAL DIAGNOSIS OF NEONATAL SEIZURES

Diagnosis	Comments
Hypoxic-ischemic encephalopathy	Most common etiology (60%, onset first 24 hours)
Intracranial hemorrhage	≤15% of cases; PVH/IVH, subdural or subarachnoid bleeds, stroke
Infection	12% of cases
Hypoglycemia	SGA, IDM
Hypocalcemia, hypomagnesemia	Low-birth-weight infant, IDM
Hyponatremia	Rare, seen with syndrome of inappropriate secretion of antidiuretic hormone (SIADH)
Disorders of amino and organic acid metabolism, hyperammonemia	Associated acidosis, altered level of consciousness
Pyridoxine dependency	Seizures refractory to routine therapy; cessation of seizures after administration of pyridoxine
Developmental defects	Other anomalies, chromosomal syndromes
Drug withdrawal	
Benign familial neonatal seizures	
No cause found	10% of cases

PVH/IVH, periventricular/intraventricular hemorrhage; SGA, small for gestational age; IDM, infant of diabetic mother.

barbital does decrease both brain blood flow and cerebral metabolic rate. However, two large randomized prospective studies failed to confirm the positive effects of phenobarbital shown in smaller studies.[272,273] One reason for the discrepancy may be the widespread use of antenatal corticosteroids in the more recent studies. Antenatal corticosteroids, although not used specifically to decrease the incidence of IVH and PVL, do appear to decrease the frequency of these complications and likely represent the most important antenatal strategy to prevent intracranial hemorrhage.[15,16] Phenobarbital may still have a role in the mother who has not been "prepared" and is delivering at under 28 weeks' gestation. The route of delivery may also play a role, with infants delivered by cesarean section showing a decreased rate of intracranial bleeds, but this issue is controversial.[274]

Seizures

Newborns rarely have well-organized tonic-clonic seizures because of incomplete cortical organization and a preponderance of inhibitory synapses. Newborn seizures can be classified into four subtypes.[275] The first is the subtle seizure characterized by ocular phenomena, oral-buccal-lingual movements, peculiar limb movements (e.g., bicycling movements), autonomic alterations, and apnea. Clonic seizures are characterized by rhythmic (one to three jerks per second) movements that can be focal or multifocal. The third seizure type is focal or generalized tonic seizures marked by extensor posturing. The fourth seizure type is myoclonic activity that is distinguished from clonic seizures by the more rapid speed of the myoclonic jerk and the predilection for flexor muscle groups. The differential diagnosis of neonatal seizures is presented in Table 20–14. The most frequent cause of neonatal seizures is hypoxic ischemic encephalopathy, with the second leading cause being intracranial hemorrhage. The prognosis for neonatal seizures depends on the cause. Difficult-to-control seizure activity caused by hypoxic ischemic encephalopathy and hypoglycemic seizures in particular have a high incidence of long-term sequelae.

CLASSIFICATION OF NEWBORNS BY GROWTH AND GESTATIONAL AGE

In assessing the risk for mortality or morbidity in a given neonate, evaluation of birth weight and gestational age together provide the clearest picture. This requires an accurate assessment of the infant's gestational age. When large populations are considered, maternal dates remain the single best determinant of gestational age. Early obstetric ultrasound is also a very useful adjunct in determining pregnancy dating. However, in the individual neonate, especially when dates are uncertain, a reliable postnatal assessment of gestational age is necessary. A scoring system appraising gestational age on the basis of physical and neurologic criteria was developed by Dubowitz et al.[276] and later simplified and updated by Ballard et al.[277,278] (Fig. 20–20). The Ballard exam is less accurate before 28 weeks' gestation,[279] but additional features can be examined to aid in the determination of an accurate gestational age. The anterior vascular capsule of the lens reveals complete coverage of the lens by vessels at 27 to 28 weeks. Foot length (from the heel to the tip of the largest toe) is 4.5 cm at 25 weeks and increases by 0.25 cm/wk. Infants can then be classified, using growth parameters and gestational age, by means of intrauterine growth curves such as those developed by Lubchenco et al.[280] (Fig. 20–21). Infants born between 38 and 42 weeks are classified as term; less than 38 weeks, preterm; and greater than 42 weeks, postterm. In each grouping, infants are then identified according to growth as AGA if birth weight falls between the 10th to 90th percentile, SGA if birth weight is below the 10th percentile, and LGA if birth weight is above the 90th percentile. On

Neuromuscular Maturity

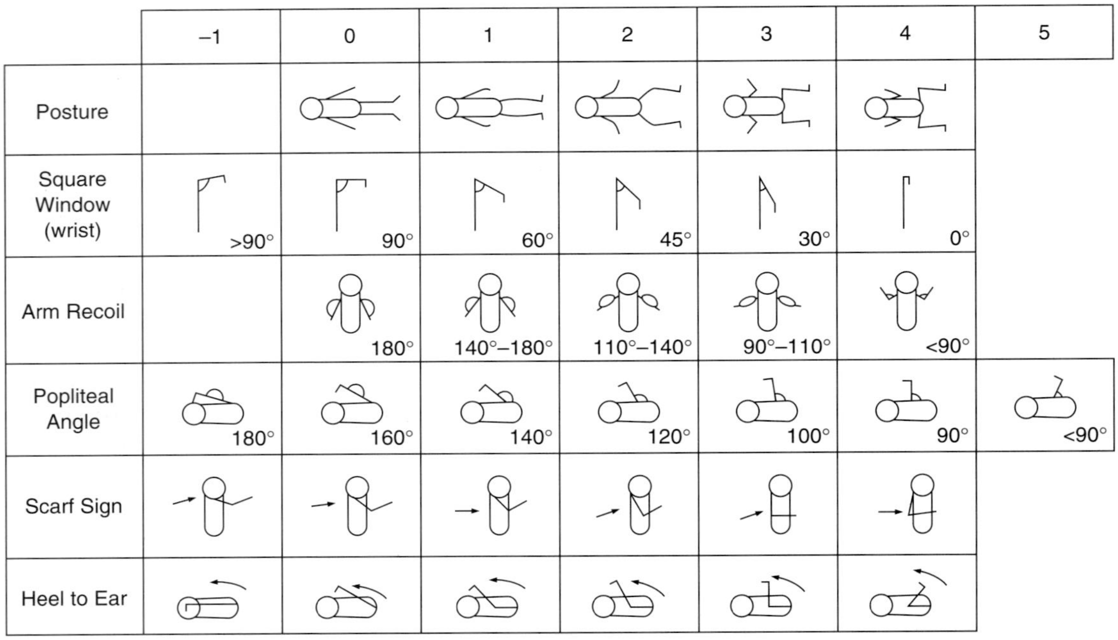

	−1	0	1	2	3	4	5
Posture							
Square Window (wrist)	>90°	90°	60°	45°	30°	0°	
Arm Recoil		180°	140°–180°	110°–140°	90°–110°	<90°	
Popliteal Angle	180°	160°	140°	120°	100°	90°	<90°
Scarf Sign							
Heel to Ear							

Physical Maturity

Skin	sticky friable transparent	gelatinous red, translucent	smooth pink, visible veins	superficial peeling &/or rash, few veins	cracking pale areas rare veins	parchment deep cracking no vessels	leathery cracked wrinkled
Lanugo	none	sparse	abundant	thinning	bald areas	mostly bald	
Plantar Surface	heel-toe 40–50 mm: −1 < 40 mm: −2	> 50 mm no crease	faint red marks	anterior transverse crease only	creases ant. 2/3	creases over entire sole	
Breast	imperceptible	barely perceptible	flat areola no bud	stippled areola 1–2 mm bud	raised areola 3–4 mm bud	full areola 5–10 mm bud	
Eye/Ear	lids fused loosely: −1 tightly: −2	lids open pinna flat stays folded	sl. curved pinna; soft; slow recoil	well-curved pinna; soft but ready recoil	formed & firm instant recoil	thick cartilage ear stiff	
Genitals male	scrotum flat, smooth	scrotum empty faint rugae	testes in upper canal rare rugae	testes descending few rugae	testes down good rugae	testes pendulous deep rugae	
Genitals female	clitoris prominent labia flat	prominent clitoris small labia minora	prominent clitoris enlarging minora	majora & minora equally prominent	majora large minora small	majora cover clitoris & minora	

Maturity Rating

score	weeks
−10	20
-5	22
0	24
5	26
10	28
15	30
20	32
25	34
30	36
35	38
40	40
45	42
50	44

Figure 20–20. Assessment of gestational age. (From Ballard JL, Khoury JC, Wedig K, et al: New Ballard Score, expanded to include extremely premature infants. J Pediatr 119:417, 1991, with permission.)

the basis of a given infant's classification, the risk of mortality[281,282] (Fig. 20–22) can be assessed. Not only does mortality risk vary, but specific clinical problems can also be anticipated by an infant's birth weight/ gestational age distribution.

There are numerous causes of growth restriction (see Chapter 25). Those operative early in pregnancy such as chromosomal aberrations, congenital viral infections, and some drug exposures induce symmetric restriction of weight, length, and head circumference. In most

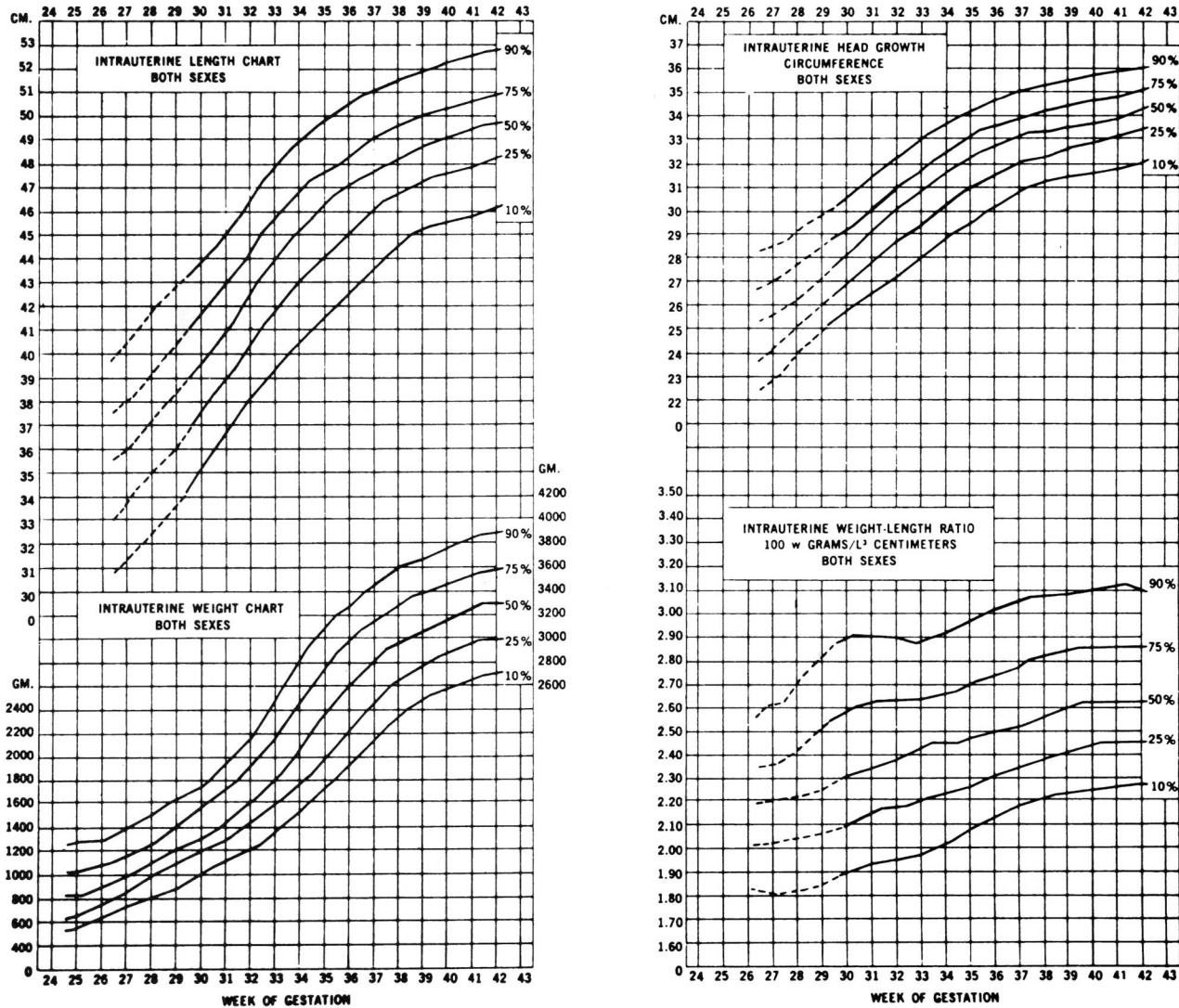

Figure 20–21. Intrauterine growth curves for weight, length, and head circumference for singleton births in Colorado. (From Lubchenco LO, Hansman C, Boyd E: Intrauterine growth in length and head circumference as estimated from live births at gestational ages from 26 to 42 weeks. Pediatrics 37:403, 1966, with permission.)

cases, the phenomenon occurs later in gestation and leads to more selective restriction of birth weight alone. Such factors include hypertension or other maternal vascular disease and multiple gestation.[283] Neonatal problems besides chromosomal abnormalities and congenital viral infections common in SGA infants include birth asphyxia, hypoglycemia, polycythemia, and hypothermia. In addition, congenital malformations are seen more frequently among undergrown infants.[284]

The most common identifiable conditions leading to excessive infant birth weight are maternal diabetes and maternal obesity. Other conditions associated with macrosomia are erythroblastosis fetalis, other causes of fetal hydrops, and Beckwith-Weidemann syndrome. LGA infants are at risk for hypoglycemia, polycythe-

mia, congenital anomalies, cardiomyopathy, hyperbilirubinemia, and birth trauma.

NURSERY CARE

Nurseries are classified on the basis of level of care provided. Level I nurseries care for infants presumed healthy, with an emphasis on screening and surveillance. Level II nurseries can care for infants more than 30 weeks' gestation, who weigh at least 1,200 g, and who require special attention short of the need for circulatory or ventilator support and major surgical proce-

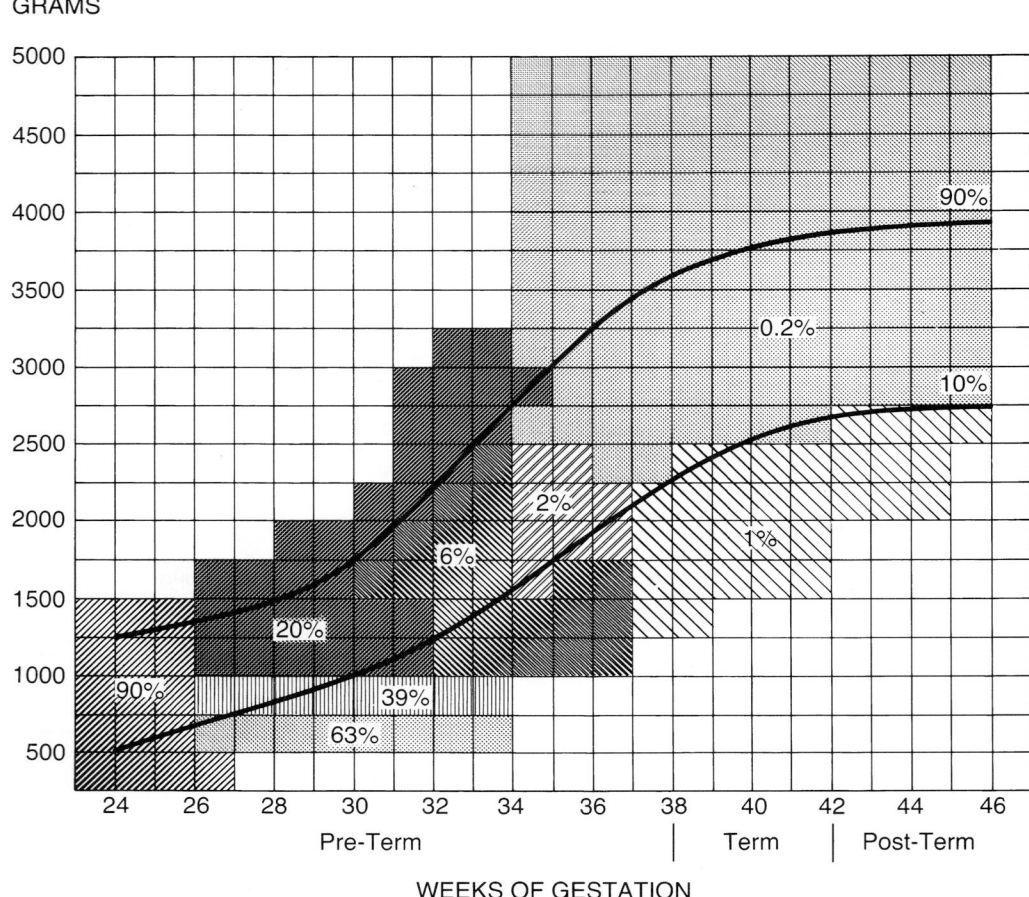

GRAMS

WEEKS OF GESTATION

Pre-Term | Term | Post-Term

Figure 20–22. Neonatal mortality risk by birth weight and gestational age based on 14,413 live births at the University of Colorado Health Sciences Center, 1974–1980. (From Koops BL, Morgan LJ, Battaglia FC: Neonatal mortality risk in relation to birth weight and gestational age: update. J Pediatr 101:969, 1982, with permission.)

dures. Level III nurseries care for all newborn infants who are critically ill regardless of the level of support required. A perinatal center encompasses both high-risk obstetric services and level III nursery services.

Care of the normal newborn involves observation of transition from intra- to extrauterine life, establishing breast- or bottle-feeds, noting normal patterns of stooling and urination, and surveillance for neonatal problems. Signs suggestive of illness include temperature instability, change in activity, refusal to feed, pallor, cyanosis, jaundice, tachypnea and respiratory distress, delayed (beyond 24 hours) passage of first stool or void, and bilious vomiting. In addition, the following laboratory screens should be performed: (1) blood type and direct and indirect Coombs' test on infants born to mothers with type O or Rh-negative blood; (2) glucose screen in infants at risk for hypoglycemia; (3) hematocrit in infants with signs and symptoms of anemia or polycythemia; (4) serologic test for syphilis; and (5) mandated screening for inborn errors of metabolism, such as PKU, maple syrup urine disease, homocystinuria, galactosemia, sickle cell disease, hypothyroidism,

cystic fibrosis, and congenital adrenal hyperplasia. All newborns should also have an initial hearing screen performed prior to discharge.[285] Finally, babies routinely receive 1 mg intramuscular of vitamin K to prevent vitamin K–deficient hemorrhagic disease of the newborn and either 1 percent silver nitrate or erythromycin ointment to prevent gonococcal ophthalmia neonatorum. Hepatitis B vaccine and hepatitis B immunoglobulin are administered to infants born to HB$_s$Ag-positive mothers.

Infants should be positioned supine or lying on the right side with the dependent arm forward for sleep to minimize the risk of sudden infant death syndrome.[286]

It is now common on most services for mothers and babies to be discharged within 24 to 36 hours of delivery. Criteria for early discharge at the University of Colorado are presented in the Box.[287] These criteria have been adapted from those of the American Academy of Pediatrics.[288] Discharge at 24 to 36 hours appears safe and appropriate for most infants without contraindications, provided a follow-up at 48 to 72 hours after discharge is ensured.[287]

Infant Criteria for Early Discharge

1. Delivery is vertex, single, sterile, and vaginal.
2. Apgar scores at 1 and 5 minutes are ≤7.
3. The infant is term (38 to 42 weeks) and weighs 2,700 to 4,000 g.
4. Minimum length of stay is 20 hours. A transition to normal thermoregulation in an open crib, completion of two successful feedings, evidence of stool and void, completion of neonatal screening for metabolic disease, and blood type and Coombs' test (Rh-negative and O mothers) prior to discharge.
5. Vital signs within normal ranges at discharge; axillary temperature, 36.1° to 37.2°C; heart rate, 110 to 150 bpm; respiratory rate, 40 to 60 breaths/min.
6. The infant has a normal neonatal hospital course and presents no signs or symptoms that require continuous observation:

    Blood glucose maintained, >45 mg/dl ABO-incompatible infants usually held 48 hours and released only if not requiring therapy for jaundice. These infants may leave at 24 hours with good follow-up examination if no jaundice is present. Jaundice at <24 hours for any reason mandates a longer stay.
7. Infants born to group B *Streptococcus*-positive mothers with inadequate antenatal chemoprophylaxis or born to mothers with >12 hours ruptured membranes are observed for 48 hours.
8. Physical examination is completed by physician or trained physician's assistant.
9. Minimum 2 hours of observation after circumcision with no bleeding.
10. Mother demonstrates understanding and ability to provide adequate care for her newborn; infant care education is provided on a one-to-one or classroom basis by the nursing staff before discharge.
11. Signed documentation by the mother that states her obligation to participate in follow-up care within 48 hours of discharge.

Circumcision is an elective procedure to be performed only in healthy, stable infants. The procedure probably has medical benefits, including prevention of phimosis, paraphimosis, and balanoposthitis as well as a decreased incidence of cancer of the penis, cervical cancer (in partners of circumcised men), sexually transmitted diseases (including HIV), and urinary tract infection in male infants.[289] Most parents, however, make the decision regarding circumcision for nonmedical reasons. The risks of the procedure include local infection, bleeding, removal of too much skin, and urethral injury. The combined incidence of these complications is less than 1 percent. Local anesthesia (dorsal penile nerve block or circumferential ring block) with 1 percent lidocaine without epinephrine or topical application of an anesthetic cream are safe and effective and should always be used.[289] Techniques that allow visualization of the glans throughout the procedure (Plastibell and Gomco clamp) are preferred to a "blind" technique (Mogen clamp) because of occasional amputation of the glans with the latter. Circumcision is contraindicated in infants with genital abnormalities. Appropriate lab evaluation should be performed prior to the procedure in infants with a family history of bleeding disorders.

Care of the Parents

Klaus and Kennell[290] outline these steps in maternal–infant attachment: (1) planning the pregnancy; (2) confirming the pregnancy; (3) accepting the pregnancy; (4) noting fetal movement; (5) accepting the fetus as an individual; (6) going through labor; (7) giving birth; (8) hearing and seeing the baby; (9) touching, smelling, and holding the baby; (10) caretaking; and (11) accepting the infant as a separate individual. Numerous influences can affect this process. A mother's and father's actions and responses are derived from their own genetic endowment, their own interfamily relationships, cultural practices, past experiences with this or previous pregnancies, and, most importantly, how they were raised by their parents.[290] Also critical is the in-hospital experience surrounding the birth—how doctors and nurses act, separation from the baby, and hospital practices.

The 60- to 90-minute period after delivery is a very important time. The infant is alert, active, and able to follow with his or her eyes,[291] allowing meaningful interaction to transpire between infant and parents. The infant's array of sensory and motor abilities evokes responses from the mother and initiates communication that may be helpful for attachment and induction of reciprocal actions. Whether a critical time period for these initial interactions exists is not clear, but improved mothering behavior does seem to occur with increased contact over the first 3 postpartum days.[292] The practical implications of this information are that labor and delivery should pose as little anxiety as possible for the mother, and parents and baby should have time together immediately after delivery if the baby's medical condition permits. Eye prophylaxis for gonococcal ophthalmitis should ideally be withheld until after the initial bonding has taken place. It can be performed safely within 1 hour of birth.

Mothers with high-risk pregnancies are at increased risk for subsequent parenting problems. It is important for both obstetrician and pediatrician alike to be involved prenatally, allowing time to prepare the family for anticipated aspects of the baby's care as well as providing reassurance that the odds are heavily in favor of a live baby who will ultimately be healthy. If before birth one can anticipate a need for neonatal intensive care (known congenital anomaly, refractory premature labor), maternal transport to a center with a unit that can care for the baby should be planned. In this way, a mother can be with her baby during its most critical care. Before delivery it is also very helpful to allow the parents to tour the unit their baby will occupy. This practice greatly reduces anxiety after the baby is born.

The single basic principle in dealing with parents of a sick infant is to provide essential information clearly and accurately to both parents, preferably when they are together. With improved survival rates, especially in prematures, most babies, despite early problems, will do well. It is therefore reasonable in most circumstances to be positive about the outcome. There is also no reason to emphasize problems that might occur in the future or to deal with individual worries of the physician. Questions, if asked, need to be answered honestly, but the list of parents' worries does not need to be voluntarily increased.

Before the parents' initial visit to the unit, a physician or nurse should describe what the baby and the equipment look like. When they arrive in the nursery, this can again be reviewed in detail. If a baby must be moved to another hospital, the mother should be given time to see and to touch her infant prior to transfer. The father should be encouraged to meet the baby at the receiving hospital so he can become comfortable with the intensive care unit. He can serve as a link between baby and mother with information and photographs.

As a baby's course proceeds, the nursery staff can help the parents to become comfortable with their infant. This can include participation in caretaking as well as skin-to-skin contact with the infant (Kangaroo care).[293] Individualized developmentally based care has also shown some benefit for high-risk infants.[294] It is also important for the staff to discuss among themselves any problems that parents may be having as well as to keep a record of visits and phone calls. This approach will allow early intervention to deal with potential problems.

The birth of an infant with a congenital malformation provides another situation in which staff support is essential. Parents' reactions to the birth of a malformed infant follow a predictable course. For most, there is

initial shock and denial, a period of sadness and anger, gradual adaptation, and finally an increased satisfaction with and the ability to care for the baby. The parents must be allowed to pass through these stages and, in effect, to mourn the loss of the anticipated normal child.[295]

The death of an infant or a stillborn is a highly stressful family event. This fact has been emphasized by Cullberg,[296] who found that psychiatric disorders developed in 19 of 56 mothers studied 1 to 2 years after the deaths of their neonates. One of the major predispositions was a breakdown of communication between parents. The health care staff need to encourage the parents to talk with each other, discuss their feelings, and display emotion. The staff should talk with the parents at the time of death and then several months later to review the findings of the autopsy, answer questions, and see how the family is doing.

OUTCOME OF NEONATAL INTENSIVE CARE

More sophisticated neonatal care has resulted in improved survival of very-low-birth-weight ($\geq$1,500 g) infants, in particular those less than 1,000 g (Fig. 20–23). Current survival rates are 90 percent or greater for infants greater than 1,000 g and 28 weeks' gestation, 80 percent at 800 to 1,000 g and 26 to 27 weeks' gestation, and nearly 70 percent for infants 700 to 800 g and 25 week's gestation, with a considerable drop in survival below 700 g and 25 weeks.[297] It is important to note that survival in terms of best obstetric estimate is greater at very low gestational ages than survival in terms of postnatal assessment of gestational age. The numbers in terms of best obstetric estimate should be referred to for antenatal counseling. This improved survival comes with a price, as a variety of morbidities are seen in these infants. However, concern that improved survival would be associated with an increased rate of neurologic sequelae has been largely unfounded. Major neurologic morbidities seen in very-low-birth-weight infants include cerebral palsy (spastic diplegia, quadriplegia, hemiplegia, or paresis), cognitive delay, and hydrocephalus. Lesser disabilities include learning and behavior difficulties that can cause problems when school age is attained. The rate of significant neurologic disability is fairly constant at 10 to 25 percent of all very-low-birth-weight (<1,500 g) survivors. The number trends toward the higher side in infants of extremely low birth weight (<1,000 g).[298–300] In addition to a slight increase in severe disability, extremely-low-birth-weight infants have an increased rate of lesser

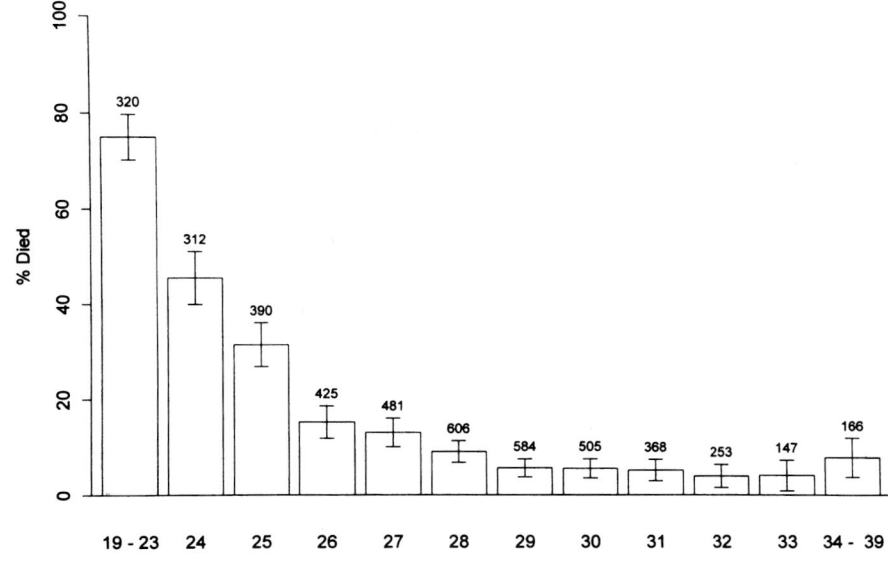

Figure 20–23. Survival by gestational age according to best obstetric measures among infants born in National Institute of Child Health and Human Development Neonatal Research Network centers between January 1993 and December 1994. Data are expressed as percentage who died with 95 percent confidence intervals. (From Stevenson DK, Wright LL, Lemons JA, et al: Very low birth weight outcomes of the National Institute of Child Health and Human Development Neonatal Research Network, January 1993 through December 1994. Am J Obstet Gynecol 179:1632, 1998, with permission.)

disabilities, including subnormal mental performance and the need for special education in school (Fig. 20–24).[301,302] Risk factors for neurologic morbidity include seizures, major intracranial hemorrhage or periventricular leukomalacia, severe intrauterine growth retardation, need for mechanical ventilation, poor early head growth, and low socioeconomic class.[302–308]

There are other morbidities that need to be considered as well. As the number of survivors weighing less than 1,000 g has increased, a reemergence of retinopathy of prematurity has been seen. This disorder, caused by retinal vascular proliferation leading to hemorrhage, scarring, retinal detachment, and blindness, originally was thought to be caused solely by inappro-

priate exposure to high concentrations of oxygen. It is now thought that the origin is multifactorial, with extreme prematurity a critical factor.[309] Incidence of acute proliferative retinopathy by birth weight is less than 10 percent in infants weighing more than 1,250 g, 15 percent in those 1,000 to 1,250 g, 40 percent in those 750 to 1,000 g, and 50 percent in those less than 750 g.[310] Severe retinopathy is evident in 5 percent of the infants 1,000 to 1,250 g, in 15 percent of infants 750 to 1,000 g, and 25 percent of infants less than 750 g. Of the infants with severe retinopathy, 10 percent (4 percent of the total population) will go on to have severe visual problems. The other major neurosensory morbidity is hearing loss, which occurs in 2 percent of neonatal

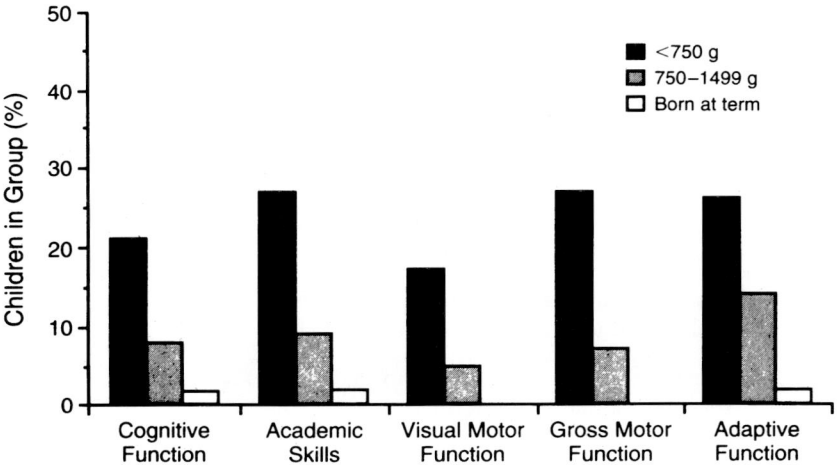

Figure 20–24. Percentage of children at different birth weights with subnormal functioning. (From Hack M, Taylor G, Klein N, et al: School-age outcomes in children with birth weights under 750 g. N Engl J Med 331:753, 1994, with permission.)

intensive care unit survivors.[311] Other sequelae of neonatal intensive care include chronic lung disease, growth failure, short gut, and need for postdischarge rehospitalization.

Key Points

➤ Surfactant maintains lung expansion on expiration by lowering surface tension at the air–liquid interface in the alveolus.

➤ Respiratory distress syndrome in premature infants is in part caused by a deficiency of surfactant and can be treated with surfactant replacement therapy.

➤ Antenatal corticosteroids accelerate fetal lung maturation and decrease neonatal mortality and respiratory distress syndrome in preterm infants. In addition, corticosteroids are associated with a decrease in intracranial hemorrhage and necrotizing enterocolitis.

➤ Transition from intra- to extrauterine life requires removal of fluid from the lungs, switching from a fetal to neonatal circulation, and establishment of a normal neonatal lung volume.

➤ The most important step in neonatal resuscitation is to achieve adequate expansion of the lungs.

➤ Meconium aspiration syndrome likely is the result of intrauterine asphyxia with mortality related to associated persistent pulmonary hypertension.

➤ The best predictor of neurologic sequelae of birth asphyxia is the presence of hypoxic ischemic encephalopathy in the neonatal period. The neurologic sequelae of birth asphyxia is cerebral palsy. Moreover, the large majority of cerebral palsy is of unknown origin.

➤ The major neurologic complications seen in premature infants are periventricular/intraventricular hemorrhage and periventricular leukomalacia.

➤ Hypoglycemia is a predictable and preventable complication in the newborn.

➤ Survival, in particular for infants less than 1,000 g, has increased with improved methods of neonatal intensive care, including provision of exogenous surfactant.

REFERENCES

1. Hodson WA: Normal and abnormal structural development of the lung. In Polin RA, Fox WW (eds): Fetal and Neonatal Physiology, 2nd ed. Philadelphia, WB Saunders Company, 1998, p 1033.
2. Thurlbeck WM: Postnatal growth and development of the lung. Am Rev Respir Dis 111:803, 1975.
3. Campiche MA, Gautier A, Hernandez EI, Reymond A: An electron microscope study of the fetal development of human lung. Pediatrics 32:976, 1963.
4. Wright JR, Clements JA: Metabolism and turnover of lung surfactant. Am Rev Respir Dis 136:426, 1987.
5. Rider ED, Ikegami M, Jobe AH: Localization of alveolar surfactant clearance in rabbit lung cells. Am J Physiol 283:L201, 1992.
6. Jobe AH: Lung development. In Fanaroff AA, Martin RI (eds): Neonatal-Perinatal Medicine: Diseases of the Fetus and Infant, 6th ed. St. Louis, CV Mosby, 1997, p 991.
7. Clements JA, Tooley WH: Kinetics of surface-active material in the fetal lung. In Hodson WA (ed): Development of the Lung. New York, Marcel Dekker, 1977.
8. Jobe AH: The role of surfactant in neonatal adaptation. Semin Perinatol 12:113, 1988.
9. Ballard PL: Hormonal regulation of pulmonary surfactant. Endocr Rev 10:165, 1989.
10. Creuwels LAJM, van Golde LMJ, Haagsman HP: The pulmonary surfactant system: biochemical and clinical aspects. Lung 175:1, 1997.
11. Possmayer F: The role of surfactant-associated proteins. Am Rev Respir Dis 142:749, 1990.
12. Kuan S, Rust K, Crouch E: Interaction of surfactant protein D with bacterial lipopolysaccharides. J Clin Invest 90:97, 1992.
13. Ballard PL, Ballard RA: Scientific basis and therapeutic regimens for use of antenatal glucocorticoids. Am J Obstet Gynecol 173:254, 1995.
14. Liggins GC, Howie RN: A controlled trial of antepartum glucocorticoid treatment for prevention of the respiratory distress syndrome in premature infants. Pediatrics 50:515, 1972.
15. Crowley PA: Antenatal corticosteroid therapy: a meta-analysis of the randomized trials, 1972–1994. Am J Obstet Gynecol 173:322, 1995.
16. Leviton A, Kuban KC, Pagano M, et al: Antenatal corticosteroids appear to reduce the risk of postnatal germinal matrix hemorrhage in intubated low birth weight newborns. Pediatrics 91:1083, 1993.
17. Schmand B, Neuvel J, Smolders-de-Haas H, et al: Psychological development of children who were treated antenatally with corticosteroids to prevent respiratory distress syndrome. Pediatrics 86:58, 1990.
18. Smolders-de-Haas H, Neuvel J, Schmand B, et al: Physical development and medical history of children who were treated antenatally with corticosteroids to prevent respiratory distress syndrome: a 10- to 12-year follow-up. Pediatrics 86:65, 1990.
19. Halliday HL: Overview of clinical trials comparing natural and synthetic surfactants. Biol Neonate 67(Suppl 1):32, 1995.
20. Jobe AH: Pulmonary surfactant therapy. N Engl J Med 328:861, 1993.
21. Pramanik AK, Holtzman RB, Merritt TA: Surfactant replacement therapy for pulmonary diseases. Pediatr Clin North Am 40:913, 1993.
22. Merritt TA, Soll RF, Hallman M: Overview of exogenous

surfactant replacement therapy. J Intensive Care Med 8:205, 1993.

23. Jobe AH, Mitchell BR, Gunkel JH: Beneficial effects of the combined use of prenatal corticosteroids and postnatal surfactant on preterm infants. Am J Obstet Gynecol 168:508, 1993.

24. Thorpe-Beeston JG, Nicolaides KH, Snijders RJM, et al: Fetal thyroid stimulating hormone response to maternal administration of thyrotropin-releasing hormone. Am J Obstet Gynecol 164:1244, 1991.

25. Rooney SA, Marino PA, Gobran LJ, et al: Thyrotropin-releasing hormone increases the amount of surfactant in lung lavage from fetal rabbits. Pediatr Res 13:623, 1979.

26. Gross I, Dynia DW, Wilson CW, et al: Glucocorticoid-thyroid hormone interaction in the fetal rat lung. Pediatr Res 18:191, 1984.

27. Schellenberg J, Liggins GC, Manzai M, et al: Synergistic hormonal effects on lung maturation in fetal sheep. J Appl Physiol 65:94, 1988.

28. Ballard RA, Ballard PL, Cnaan A, et al: Antenatal thyrotropin-releasing hormone to prevent lung disease in preterm infants. N Engl J Med 338:493, 1998.

29. Crowther CA, Hiller JE, Studs DS, et al: Australian collaborative trial of antenatal thyrotropin-releasing hormone: adverse effects at 12-month follow-up. Pediatrics 99:311, 1997.

30. Jansen AH, Chernick V: Development of respiratory control. Physiol Rev 63:437, 1983.

31. Dawes GS, Fox HE, Leduc BM, et al: Respiratory movements and rapid eye movement sleep in the foetal lamb. J Physiol (Lond) 220:119, 1972.

32. Rigatto H, Moore M, Cates D, et al: Fetal breathing and behavior measured through a double-wall Plexiglas window in sheep. J Appl Physiol 61:160, 1986.

33. Dawes GS, Gardner WN, Johnston BM, Walker DW: Breathing in fetal lambs: the effect of brainstem section. J Physiol (Lond) 335:535, 1983.

34. Hanson MA, Moore PJ, Nijhuis JG, Parkes MJ: Effects of pilocarpine on breathing movements in normal, chemodenervated and brainstem-transected fetal sheep. J Physiol (Lond) 400:415, 1988.

35. Kaplan M: Fetal breathing movements, an update for the pediatrician. Am J Dis Child 137:177, 1983.

36. Connors G, Hunse C, Carmichael L, et al: The role of carbon dioxide in the generation of human fetal breathing movements. Am J Obstet Gynecol 158:322, 1988.

37. Boddy K, Dawes GS, Fisher R, et al: Foetal respiratory movements, electrocortical and cardiovascular responses to hypoxaemia and hypercapnia in sheep. J Physiol (Lond) 243:599, 1974.

38. Baier RJ, Hasan SU, Cates DB, et al: Effects of various concentrations of O_2 and umbilical cord occlusion on fetal breathing and behavior. J Appl Physiol 68:1597, 1990.

39. Goodman JDS: The effect of intravenous glucose on human fetal breathing measured by Doppler ultrasound. Br J Obstet Gynaecol 87:1080, 1980.

40. Patrick J, Campbell K, Carmichael L, et al: Patterns of human fetal breathing during the last 10 weeks of pregnancy. Obstet Gynecol 56:24, 1980.

41. Maloney JE, Adamson TM, Brodecky V, et al: Modification of respiratory center output in the unanesthetized fetal sheep "in utero." J Appl Physiol 39:552, 1975.

42. Jansen AH, Chernick V: Fetal breathing and development of control of breathing. J Appl Physiol 70:1431, 1991.

43. Kitterman JA, Liggins GC, Clements JA, Tooley WH: Stimulation of breathing movements in fetal sheep by inhibitors of prostaglandin synthesis. J Dev Physiol 1:453, 1979.

44. James LS, Weisbrot IM, Prince CE, et al: The acid-base status of human infants in relation to birth asphyxia and the onset of respiration. J Pediatr 52:379, 1958.

45. Alvaro RE, de Almeida V, Al-Alaiyan S, et al: A placental factor inhibits breathing induced by umbilical occlusion in fetal sheep. J Dev Physiol 19:23, 1993.

46. Agostoni E, Taglietti A, Agostoni AF, Setnikar I: Mechanical aspects of the first breath. J Appl Physiol 13:344, 1958.

47. Milner AD, Vyas H: Lung expansion at birth. J Pediatr 101:879, 1982.

48. Karlberg P, Adams FH, Geubelle F, Wallgren G: Alteration of the infant's thorax during vaginal delivery. Acta Obstet Gynaecol Scand 41:223, 1962.

49. Bosma J, Lind J: Upper respiratory mechanisms of newborn infants. Acta Paediatr Scand (Suppl 135):132, 1962.

50. Jäykkä S: Capillary erection and lung expansion. Acta Paediatr Scand 46(suppl 112):9, 1957.

51. Talbert DG: Role of pulmonary vascular pressure in the first breath: engineering reassessment of Jaykka's experimental findings. Acta Paediatr Scand 81:737, 1992.

52. Karlberg P, Cherry RB, Escardó FE, Koch G: Respiratory studies in newborn infants. II. Pulmonary ventilation and mechanics of breathing in the first minutes of life, including the onset of respiration. Acta Paediatr Scand 51:121, 1962.

53. Karlberg P: The adaptive changes in the immediate postnatal period, with particular reference to respiration. J Pediatr 56:585, 1960.

54. Klaus M, Tooley WH, Weaver KH, Clements JA: Lung volume in the newborn infant. Pediatrics 30:111, 1962.

55. Oliver RE, Strang LB: Ion fluxes across the pulmonary epithelium and the secretion of lung liquid in the foetal lamb. J Physiol (Lond) 241:327, 1974.

56. Carlton DP, Cummings JJ, Chapman DL, et al: Ion transport regulation of lung liquid secretion in foetal lambs. J Dev Physiol 17:99, 1992.

57. Carlton DP, Cummings JJ, Poulain FR, et al: Increased pulmonary vascular filtration pressure does not alter lung liquid secretion in fetal sheep. J Appl Physiol 72:650, 1992.

58. Bland RD: Formation of fetal lung liquid and its removal near birth. *In* Polin RA, Fox WW (eds): Fetal and Neonatal Physiology, 2nd ed. Philadelphia, WB Saunders Company, 1998, p 1047.

59. Bland RD: Lung liquid clearance before and after birth. Semin Perinatol 12:124, 1988.

60. Bland RD, Hansen TN, Haberkern CM, et al: Lung fluid balance in lambs before and after birth. J Appl Physiol 53:992, 1982.

61. Raj JU, Bland RD: Lung luminal liquid clearance in newborn lambs. Effect of pulmonary microvascular pressure elevation. Am Rev Respir Dis 134:305, 1986.

62. Bland RD, Bressack MA, McMillan DD: Labor decreases the lung water content of newborn rabbits. Am J Obstet Gynecol 135:364, 1979.

63. Bland RD, Carlton DP, Scheerer RG, et al: Lung fluid balance in lambs before and after premature birth. J Clin Invest 84:568, 1989.

64. Jain L: Alveolar fluid clearance in developing lungs and its role in neonatal transition. Clin Perinatol 26:585, 1999.

65. Peltonen T, Hirvonen L: Experimental studies on fetal and neonatal circulation. Acta Paediatr Scand 55 (Suppl 161):8, 1965.

66. Rudolph AM: Fetal circulation and cardiovascular adjustments after birth. *In* Rudolph AM, Hoffman JIE, Rudolph CD (eds): Rudolph's Pediatrics, 20th ed. Stamford, CT, Appleton & Lange, 1996, p 1409.

67. Teitel DF: Physiologic development of the cardiovascular system in the fetus. *In* Polin RA, FOX WW (eds): Fetal and

Neonatal Physiology, 2nd ed. Philadelphia, WB Saunders Company, 1998, p 827.

68. Friedman AH, Fahey JT: The transition from fetal to neonatal circulation: normal responses and implications for infants with heart disease. Semin Perinatol 17:106, 1993.

69. Naeye RL: Arterial changes during the perinatal period. Arch Pathol Lab Med 71:121, 1961.

70. Walker AM, Ritchie BC, Adamson TM, Maloney JE: Effect of changing lung liquid volume on the pulmonary circulation of fetal lambs. J Appl Physiol 64:61, 1988.

71. Teitel DF, Iwamato HS, Rudolph AM: Changes in the pulmonary circulation during birth-related events. Pediatr Res 27:372, 1990.

72. Kinsella JP, McQueston JA, Rosenberg AA, Abman SH: Hemodynamic effects of exogenous nitric oxide in ovine transitional pulmonary circulation. Am J Physiol 263:H875, 1992.

73. Abman SH, Chatfield BA, Hall SL, McMurtry IF: Role of endothelium-derived relaxing factor during transitional pulmonary circulation at birth. Am J Physiol 259:H1921, 1990.

74. Moss AJ, Emmanoulides G, Duffie ER Jr: Closure of the ductus arteriosus in the newborn infant. Pediatrics 32:25, 1963.

75. Gentile R, Stevenson G, Dooley T, et al: Pulse Doppler echocardiographic determination of time of ductal closure in normal newborn infants. J Pediatr 98:443, 1981.

76. Heymann MA, Rudolph AM: Control of the ductus arteriosus. Physiol Rev 55:62, 1975.

77. Clyman RI: Ontogeny of the ductus arteriosus response to prostaglandins and inhibitors of their synthesis. Semin Perinatol 4:115, 1980.

78. Clyman RI: Ductus arteriosus: current theories of prenatal and postnatal regulation. Semin Perinatol 11:64, 1987.

79. Behrman RE, Lees MH: Organ blood flows of the fetal, newborn and adult rhesus monkey. Biol Neonate 18:330, 1971.

80. Phibbs RH: Delivery room management. In Avery GB, Fletcher MA, MacDonald MG (eds): Neonatology: Pathophysiology and Management of the Newborn, 5th ed. Philadelphia, Lippincott Williams & Wilkins, 1999, p 279.

81. Duffy TE, Kohle SJ, Vannucci RC: Carbohydrate and energy metabolism in perinatal rat brain: relation to survival in anoxia. J Neurochem 24:271, 1975.

82. Reid DL, Parer JT, Williams K, et al: Effects of severe reduction in maternal placental blood flow on blood flow distribution in the sheep fetus. J Dev Physiol 15:183, 1991.

83. Itskovitz J Goetzman BW, Rudolph AM: The mechanism of late deceleration of the heart rate and its relationship to oxygenation in normoxemic and chronically hypoxemic fetal lambs. Am J Obstet Gynecol 142:66, 1982.

84. Gunn AJ, Parer JT, Mallard EC, et al: Cerebral histological and electrocorticographic changes after asphyxia in fetal sheep. Pediatr Res 31:486, 1992.

85. Jones CT: The development of some metabolic responses to hypoxia in the foetal sheep. J Physiol (Lond) 265:743, 1977.

86. Vintzileos AM, Fleming AD, Scorza WE, et al: Relationship between fetal biophysical activities and umbilical cord blood gas values. Am J Obstet Gynecol 165:707, 1991.

87. Holowach-Thurston J, McDougal DB Jr: Effect of ischemia on metabolism of the brain of the newborn mouse. Am J Physiol 216:348, 1969.

88. Dawes GS: Foetal and Neonatal Physiology. Chicago, Year Book, 1968.

89. Cross KW: Resuscitation of the asphyxiated infant. Br Med Bull 22:73, 1966.

90. Gupta JM, Tizard JPM: The sequence of events in neonatal apnea. Lancet 2:55, 1967.

91. American Heart Association and American Academy of Pediatrics: Neonatal Resuscitation Textbook. American Academy of Pediatrics and American Heart Association, 2000.

92. Niermeyer S: Resuscitation of the newborn infant. In Thureen PJ, Deacon J, O'Neill P, et al (eds): Assessment and Care of the Well Newborn. Philadelphia, WB Saunders Company, 1999.

93. Apgar V: A proposal for a new method of evaluation of the newborn infant. Anesth Analg 32:260, 1953.

94. Jain L, Ferre C, Vidyasagar D: Cardiopulmonary resuscitation of apparently stillborn infants: survival and longterm outcome. J Pediatr 118:778, 1991.

95. Wiswell TE, Fuloria M: Management of meconium-stained amniotic fluid. Clin Perinatol 26:659, 1999.

96. Carson BS, Losey RW, Bowes WA, Simmons MA: Combined obstetric and pediatric approach to prevent meconium aspiration syndrome. Am J Obstet Gynecol 126:712, 1976.

97. Katz VL, Bowes WA: Meconium aspiration syndrome: reflections on a murky subject. Am J Obstet Gynecol 166:171, 1992.

98. Block MF, Kallenberger DA, Kern JD, Nepveux RD: In utero meconium aspiration by the baboon fetus. Obstet Gynecol 57:37, 1981.

99. Brown BL, Gleicher N: Intrauterine meconium aspiration. Obstet Gynecol 57:26, 1981.

100. Falciglia HS: Failure to prevent meconium aspiration syndrome. Obstet Gynecol 71:349, 1988.

101. Falciglia HS, Henderschott C, Potter P, Helmchen R: Does DeLee suction at the perineum prevent meconium aspiration syndrome? Am J Obstet Gynecol 167:1243, 1992.

102. Linder N, Aranda JV, Tsur M, et al: Need for endotracheal intubation and suction in meconium-stained neonates. J Pediatr 112:613, 1988.

103. Yoder BA: Meconium-stained amniotic fluid and respiratory complications: impact of selective tracheal suction. Obstet Gynecol 83:77, 1994.

104. Wiswell TE, Gannon CM, Jacob J, et al: Delivery room management of the apparently vigorous meconium-stained neonate: Results of the multicenter international collaborative trial. Pediatrics 105:1, 2000.

105. Murphy JD, Vawter GF, Reid LM: Pulmonary vascular disease in fatal meconium aspiration. J Pediatr 104:758, 1984.

106. Jovanovic R, Nguyen HT: Experimental meconium aspiration in guinea pigs. Obstet Gynecol 73:652, 1989.

107. Pierce J, Gaudier FL, Sanchez-Ramos L: Intrapartum amnioinfusion for meconium-stained fluid: meta-analysis of prospective clinical trials. Obstet Gynecol 95:1051, 2000.

108. MacDonald HM, Mulligan JC, Allen AC, Taylor PM: Neonatal asphyxia. I. Relationship of obstetric and neonatal complications to neonatal mortality in 38,405 consecutive deliveries. J Pediatr 96:898, 1980.

109. Brown JK, Purvis RJ, Forfar JO, Cockburn F: Neurologic aspects of perinatal asphyxia. Dev Med Child Neurol 16:567, 1974.

110. Piazza AJ: Postasphyxial management of the newborn. Clin Perinatol 26:749, 1999.

111. Hall RT, Hall FK, Daily DK: High dose phenobarbital therapy in term newborn infants with severe perinatal asphyxia: a randomized prospective study with three-year follow-up. J Pediatr 132:345, 1998.

112. Vannucci RC, Perlman JM: Interventions for perinatal hypoxic-ischemic encephalopathy. Pediatrics 100:1004, 1997.

113. Gunn AJ, Gunn TR, Gunning MI, et al: Neuroprotection with prolonged head cooling started before postischemic seizures in fetal sheep. Pediatrics 102:1098, 1998.

114. Van Bel F, Shadid M, Moison RMW, et al: Effect of allopurinol on postasphyxial free radical formation, cerebral hemo-

dynamics, and electrical brain activity. Pediatrics 101:185, 1998.

115. Nelson KB, Emery ES III: Birth asphyxia and the neonatal brain: what do we know and when do we know it? Clin Perinatol 20:327, 1993.

116. Scheller JM, Nelson KB: Does cesarean delivery prevent cerebral palsy or other neurologic problems of childhood? Obstet Gynecol 83:624, 1994.

117. Grant A, Joy M-T, O'Brien N, et al: Cerebral palsy among children born during the Dublin randomised trial of intrapartum monitoring. Lancet 2:1233, 1989.

118. Nelson KB, Dambrosia JM, Ting TY, et al: Uncertain value of electronic fetal monitoring in predicting cerebral palsy. N Engl J Med 334:613, 1996.

119. Nelson KB, Ellenberg JH: Obstetric complications as risk factors for cerebral palsy or seizure disorders. JAMA 251:1843, 1984.

120. Goldaber KB, Gilstrap LC, Leveno KJ, et al: Pathologic fetal acidemia. Obstet Gynecol 78:1103, 1991.

121. Finer NN, Robertson CMT: Long-term follow-up of term neonates with perinatal asphyxia. Clin Perinatol 20:483, 1993.

122. Simon NP: Long-term neurodevelopmental outcome of asphyxiated newborns. Clin Perinatol 26:767, 1999.

123. Perlman JM, Tack ED: Renal injury in the asphyxiated newborn infant: relationship to neurologic outcome. J Pediatr 113:875, 1988.

124. Freeman JM, Nelson KB: Intrapartum asphyxia and cerebral palsy. Pediatrics 82:240, 1988.

125. Freeman JM (ed): Prenatal and Perinatal Factors Associated with Brain Disorders, Publication No. 85-1149. Bethesda, MD, NIH, 1985.

126. Nelson KB, Ellenberg JH: Antecedents of cerebral palsy: multivariate analysis of risk. N Engl J Med 315:81, 1986.

127. Schullinger JN: Birth trauma. Pediatr Clin North Am 40: 1351, 1993.

128. Zelson C, Lee SJ, Pearl M: The incidence of skull fractures underlying cephalohematomas in newborn infants. J Pediatr 85:371, 1974.

129. Volpe JJ: Neonatal intracranial hemorrhage: pathophysiology, neuropathology, and clinical features. Clin Perinatol 4:77, 1977.

130. Bager B: Perinatally acquired brachial plexus palsy—a persisting challenge. Acta Paediatr Scand 86:1214, 1997.

131. Medlock MD, Hanigan WC: Neurologic birth trauma. Intracranial, spinal cord, and brachial plexus injury. Clin Perinatol 24:735, 1997.

132. Gresham EL: Birth trauma. Pediatr Clin North Am 22:317, 1975.

133. Klaus MH, Martin RJ, Fanaroff AA: The physical environment. *In* Klaus MH, Fanaroff AA (eds): Care of the High-Risk Neonate, 4th ed. Philadelphia, WB Saunders Company, 1993, p 114.

134. Brück K: Neonatal thermal regulation. *In* Polin RA, Fox WW (eds): Fetal and Neonatal Physiology, 2nd ed. Philadelphia, WB Saunders Company, 1998, p 676.

135. Adamsons K Jr, Gandy GM, James LS: The influence of thermal factors upon oxygen consumption of the newborn human infant. J Pediatr 66:495, 1965.

136. Dawkins MJR, Hull D: Brown adipose tissue and the response of new-born rabbits to cold. J Physiol (Lond) 172:216, 1964.

137. Aherne W, Hull D: The site of heat production in the newborn infant. Proc R Soc Med 57:1172, 1962.

138. Karlberg P, Moore RE, Oliver TK Jr: The thermogenic response of the newborn infant to noradrenaline. Acta Paediatr Scand 51:284, 1962.

139. Gunn TR, Ball KT, Power GG, Gluckman PD: Factors influencing the initiation of nonshivering thermogenesis. Am J Obstet Gynecol 164:210, 1991.

140. Hey EN, Katz G, O'Connell B: The total thermal insulation of the new-born baby. J Physiol (Lond) 207:683, 1970.

141. Hey EN, Katz G: Evaporative water loss in the newborn baby. J Physiol (Lond) 200:605, 1969.

142. Hey EN, Katz G: The optimum thermal environment for naked babies. Arch Dis Child 45:328, 1970.

143. Scopes JW: Metabolic rate and temperature control in the human body. Br Med Bull 22:88, 1966.

144. Hey EN, O'Connell B: Oxygen consumption and heat balance in the cot-nursed baby. Arch Dis Child 45:335, 1970.

145. Silverman WA, Sinclair JC, Agate FJ Jr: The oxygen cost of minor changes in heat balance of small newborn infants. Acta Paediatr Scand 55:294, 1966.

146. Adamsons K Jr, Towell ME: Thermal homeostasis in the fetus and newborn. Anesthesiology 26:531, 1965.

147. Power GG: Perinatal thermal physiology. *In* Polin RA, Fox WW (eds): Fetal and Neonatal Physiology, 2nd ed. Philadelphia, WB Saunders Company, 1998, p 671.

148. Silverman WA, Fertig JW, Berger AP: The influence of the thermal environment upon the survival of newly born premature infants. Pediatrics 22:876, 1958.

149. Buetow KC, Klein SW: Effect of maintenance of "normal" skin temperature on survival of infants of low birth weight. Pediatrics 34:163, 1964.

150. Day RL, Caliguiri L, Kamenski C, Ehrlich F: Body temperature and survival of premature infants. Pediatrics 34:171, 1964.

151. Glass L, Silverman WA, Sinclair JC: Effect of the thermal environment on cold resistance and growth of small infants after the first week of life. Pediatrics 41:1033, 1968.

152. Mancini AJ, Sookdeo-Drost S, Madison KC, et al: Semipermeable dressings improve epidermal barrier function in premature infants. Pediatr Res 36:306, 1994.

153. Vobra S, Frent G, Campbell V, et al: Effect of polyethylene occlusive skin wrapping on heat loss in very low birth weight infants at delivery: a randomized trial. J Pediatr 134:547, 1999.

154. Sloan NL, Camacho LWL, Rojas EP, et al: Kangaroo mother method: randomized controlled trial of an alternative method of care for stabilized low-birth weight infants. Lancet 344: 782, 1994.

155. Bauer K, Uhrig C, Sperling P, et al: Body temperatures and oxygen consumption during skin-to-skin (kangaroo) care in stable preterm infants weighing less than 1500 grams. J Pediatr 130:240, 1997.

156. Bauer J, Sontheimer G, Fischer C, et al: Metabolic rate and energy balance in very low birth weight infants during kangaroo holding by their mothers and fathers. J Pediatr 129:608, 1996.

157. Bier JB, Ferguson AE, Morales Y, et al: Comparison of skin to skin contact with standard contact in low birth weight infants who are breast fed. Arch Pediatr Adolesc Med 150: 1265, 1996.

158. Mann TP, Elliott RIK: Neonatal cold injury due to accidental exposure to cold. Lancet 1:229, 1957.

159. Ziegler EE, O'Donnell AM, Nelson SE, Fomon SJ: Body composition of the reference fetus. Growth 40:329, 1976.

160. Friis-Hansen B: Water distribution in the foetus and newborn infant. Acta Paediatr Scand Suppl 305:7, 1983.

161. Sinclair JC, Silverman WA: Intrauterine growth in active tissue mass of the human fetus, with particular reference to the undergrown baby. Pediatrics 38:48, 1966.

162. Bell EF, Oh W: Fluid and electrolyte management. *In* Avery GB, Fletcher MA, MacDonald MG (eds): Neonatology: Path-

ophysiology and Management of the Newborn, 5th ed. Philadelphia, Lippincott Williams & Wilkins, 1999, p 345.

163. Liechty EA: Water requirements. *In* Polin RA, Fox WW (eds): Fetal and Neonatal Physiology, 2nd ed. Philadelphia, WB Saunders Company, 1998, p 305.

164. Committee on Nutrition, American Academy of Pediatrics: Nutritional needs of preterm infants. *In* Kleinman RE (ed): Pediatric Nutrition Handbook, 4th ed. Elk Grove Village, IL, American Academy of Pediatrics, 1998, p 55.

165. Räihä NCR, Heinonen K, Rassin DK, Gaull GE: Milk protein quantity and quality in low-birth-weight infants. 1. Metabolic responses and effects on growth. Pediatrics 57:659, 1976.

166. Hanning RM, Zlotkin SH: Amino acid and protein needs of the neonate: effects of excess and deficiency. Semin Perinatol 13:131, 1989.

167. Carlson SE, Cooke RJ, Rhodes PG, et al: Effect of vegetable and marine oils in preterm infant formulas on blood arachidonic and docosahexaenoic acids. J Pediatr 120:S159, 1992.

168. Fomon S (ed): Infant Nutrition, 2nd ed. Philadelphia, WB Saunders Company, 1974.

169. Auricchio S, Rubino A, Murset G: Intestinal glycosidase activities in the human embryo, fetus, and newborn. Pediatrics 35:944, 1965.

170. Ehrenkranz RA: Mineral needs of the very low birth weight infant. Semin Perinatol 13:142, 1989.

171. Greene HL, Hambidge KM, Schanler R, Tsang RC: Guidelines for the use of vitamins, trace elements, calcium, magnesium and phosphorus in infants and children receiving total parenteral nutrition. Am J Clin Nutr 48:1324, 1989.

172. American Academy of Pediatrics: Workgroup on beastfeeding: breastfeeding and the use of human milk. Pediatrics 100:1035, 1997.

173. Schanler RJ, Hurst NM, Lau C: The use of human milk and breastfeeding in premature infants. Clin Perinatol 26:379, 1999.

174. Lucas A, Cole TJ: Breast milk and necrotizing enterocolitis. Lancet 336:1519, 1990.

175. Lucas A, Morley R, Cole TJ, et al: Breast milk and subsequent intelligence quotient in children born preterm. Lancet 339:261, 1992.

176. Lucas A, Morley R, Cole TJ, Gore SM: A randomised multicenter study of human milk versus formula and later development in preterm infants. Arch Dis Child 70:F141, 1994.

177. Morley R, Lucas A: Nutrition and cognitive development. Br Med Bull 53:123, 1997.

178. Lawrence RA: Breast-Feeding: A Guide for the Medical Profession, 5th ed. St. Louis, CV Mosby, 1994.

179. McGowan J: Neonatal hypoglycemia. NeoReviews 20:e6, 1999.

180. Hawdon JM, Ward Platt MP, Aynsley-Green A: Prevention and management of neonatal hypoglycemia. Arch Dis Child 70:F60, 1994.

181. Hawdon JM, Ward Platt MP, Aynsley-Green A: Patterns of metabolic adaptation for preterm and term infants in the first neonatal week. Arch Dis Child 67:357, 1992.

182. Hawdon JM, Ward Platt MP: Metabolic adaptation in small for gestational age infants. Arch Dis Child 68:262, 1993.

183. Lucas A, Morley R, Cole TJ: Adverse neurodevelopmental outcome of moderate neonatal hypoglycemia. BMJ 297:1304, 1988.

184. Duvanel CB, Fawer C-L, Cotting J, et al: Long-term effects of neonatal hypoglycemia on brain growth and psychomotor development in small-for-gestational age preterm infants. J Pediatr 134:492, 1999.

185. Conrad PD, Sparks JW, Osberg I, et al: Clinical application of a new glucose analyzer in the neonatal intensive care unit: comparison with other methods. J Pediatr 114:281, 1989.

186. Reyes HM, Meller JL, Loeff D: Management of esophageal atresia and tracheoesophageal fistula. Clin Perinatol 16:79, 1989.

187. Kays DW: Surgical conditions of the neonatal intestinal tract. Clin Perinatol 23:353, 1996.

188. Meller JL, Reyes HN, Loeff DS: Gastroschisis and omphalocoele. Clin Perinatol 16:113, 1989.

189. Chahine AA, Ricketts RR: Resuscitation of the surgical neonate. Clin Perinatol 26:693, 1999.

190. Van Meurs K, Short BL: Congenital diaphragmatic hernia: the neonatologists perspective. NeoReviews 20:e79, 1999.

191. Benachi A, Chailley B, Delezoide A-L, et al: Lung growth and maturation after tracheal occlusion in diaphragmatic hernia. Am J Respir Crit Care Med 157:921, 1998.

192. Harrison MR, Mychaliska GB, Albanese CT, et al: Correction of congenital diaphragmatic hernia in utero: IX. Fetuses with poor prognosis (liver herniation and low lung-to-head ratio) can be saved by fetoscopic temporary tracheal occlusion. J Pediatr Surg 33:1017, 1998.

193. Stoll BJ: Epidemiology of necrotizing enterocolitis. Clin Perinatol 21:205, 1994.

194. Wiswell TE, Robertson CF, Jones TA, Tuttle DJ: Necrotizing enterocolitis in full-term infants. A case control study. Am J Dis Child 142:532, 1988.

195. Kliegman RM, Walker WA, Yolken RH: Necrotizing enterocolitis. Research agenda for a disease of unknown etiology and pathogenesis. Clin Perinatol 21:437, 1994.

196. Norton ME, Merrill J, Cooper BAB, et al: Neonatal complications after the administration of indomethacin for preterm labor. N Engl J Med 329:1602, 1993.

197. Major CA, Lewis DF, Harding JA, et al: Tocolysis with indomethacin increases the incidence of necrotizing enterocolitis in the low-birth-weight neonate. Am J Obstet Gynecol 170:102, 1994.

198. Maisels MJ: Jaundice. *In* Avery GB, Fletcher MA, MacDonald MG (eds): Neonatology: Pathophysiology and Management of the Newborn. 5th ed. Philadelphia, Lippincott Williams & Wilkins, 1999, p 765.

199. Bhutani VK, Johnson L, Sivieri EM: Predictive ability of a predischarge hour-specific serum bilirubin for subsequent significant hyperbilirubinemia in healthy term and near-term newborns. Pediatrics 103:6, 1999.

200. Auerbach KG, Gartner LM: Breast feeding and human milk: their association with jaundice in the neonate. Clin Perinatol 14:89, 1987.

201. Maisels MJ, Gifford KL: Normal serum bilirubin levels in the newborn and the effect of breast-feeding. Pediatrics 78:837, 1986.

202. Gourley GR: Pathophysiology of breast-milk jaundice. *In* Polin RA, Fox WW (eds): Fetal and Neonatal Physiology, 2nd ed. Philadelphia, WB Saunders Company, 1998, p 1499.

203. Perlstein MA: The late clinical syndrome of posticteric encephalopathy. Pediatr Clin North Am 7:665, 1960.

204. Hsia DY, Allen FH Jr, Gellis SS, Diamond LK: Erythroblastosis fetalis. VIII. Studies of serum bilirubin in relation to kernicterus. N Engl J Med 247:668, 1952.

205. Newman TB, Maisels MJ: Does hyperbilirubinemia damage the brain of healthy full-term infants? Clin Perinatol 17:331, 1990.

206. Johnson L, Bhutani VK: Guidelines for management of the jaundiced term and near-term infant. Clin Perinatol 25:555, 1998.

207. Newman TB, Maisels MJ: Evaluation and treatment of jaundice in the term newborn: a kinder, gentler approach. Pediatrics 89:809, 1992.

208. Maisels MJ, Newman TB: Kernicterus in otherwise healthy, breast-fed term newborns. Pediatrics 96:730, 1995.

209. Brown AK, Johnson L: Loss of concern about jaundice and the reemergence of kernicterus in full term infants in the era of managed care. *In* Fanaroff AA, Klaus MH (eds): Yearbook of Neonatal-Perinatal Medicine. St. Louis, CV Mosby, 1996, p xvii.

210. Watchko JF, Oski FA: Kernicterus in preterm newborns: past, present, and future. Pediatrics 90:707, 1992.

211. Yoder MC: Embryonic hematopoiesis. *In* Christensen RD (ed): Hematologic Problems of the Neonate. Philadelphia, WB Saunders Company, 2000, p 3.

212. Christensen RD: Expected hematologic values for term and preterm neonates. *In* Christensen RD (ed): Hematologic Problems of the Neonate. Philadelphia, WB Saunders Company, 2000, p 117.

213. Forestier F, Daffos F, Catherine N, et al: Developmental hematopoiesis in normal human fetal blood. Blood 77:2360, 1991.

214. Pearson HA: Anemia in the newborn: a diagnostic approach and challenge. Semin Perinatol 15(Suppl 2):2, 1991.

215. Werner EJ: Neonatal polycythemia and hyperviscosity. Clin Perinatol 22:693, 1995.

216. Black VD, Lubchenco LO: Neonatal polycythemia and hyperviscosity. Pediatr Clin North Am 29:1137, 1982.

217. Ramamurthy RS, Berlanga M: Postnatal alteration in hematocrit and viscosity in normal and polycythemic infants. J Pediatr 110:929, 1987.

218. Black VD, Camp BW, Lubchenco LO, et al: Neonatal hyperviscosity association with lower achievement and IQ scores at school age. Pediatrics 83:662, 1989.

219. Black VD, Lubchenco LO, Koops BL, et al: Neonatal hyperviscosity: randomized study of effect of partial plasma exchange on long term outcome. Pediatrics 75:1048, 1985.

220. Bada HS, Korones SB, Pourcyrous M, et al: Asymptomatic syndrome of polycythemia hyperviscosity: effect of partial exchange transfusion. J Pediatr 120:579, 1992.

221. Cines DB, Dusak B, Tomaski A, et al: Immune thrombocytopenic purpura and pregnancy. N Engl J Med 306:826, 1982.

222. Kelton JG: Management of the pregnant patient with idiopathic thrombocytopenic purpura. Ann Intern Med 99:796, 1983.

223. Al Mofada SM, Osman ME, Kides E, et al: Risk of thrombocytopenia in the infants of mothers with idiopathic thrombocytopenia. Am J Perinatol 11:423, 1994.

224. Sainio S, Jousti L, Jarvenpaa AL, et al: Idiopathic thrombocytopenic purpura in pregnancy. Acta Obstet Gynecol Scand 77: 272, 1998.

225. Cook RL, Miller RC, Katz VL, et al: Immune thrombocytopenic purpura in the pregnancy: a reappraisal of management. Obstet Gynecol 78:578, 1991.

226. Mueller-Eckhardt C, Kiefel V, Grubert A, et al: 348 cases of suspected neonatal alloimmune thrombocytopenia. Lancet 1: 363, 1989.

227. Johnson JM, Ryan G, Al-Muse A, et al: Prenatal diagnosis and management of neonatal alloimmune thrombocytopenia. Semin Perinatol 21:45, 1997.

228. Bussel JB, Zabusky MR, Berkowitz RL, et al: Fetal alloimmune thrombocytopenia. N Engl J Med 337:22, 1997.

229. Greer FR: Vitamin K deficiency and hemorrhage in infancy. Clin Perinatol 22:759, 1995.

230. Fox WW, Duara S: Persistent pulmonary hypertenson in the neonate: diagnosis and management. J Pediatr 103:505, 1983.

231. Rudolph AM: High pulmonary vascular resistance after birth. 1. Pathophysiologic considerations and etiologic classification. Clin Pediatr 19:585, 1980.

232. Walsh-Sukys MC: Persistent pulmonary hypertension of the newborn: the black box revisited. Clin Perinatol 20:127, 1993.

233. Kanto WP: A decade of experience with neonatal extracorporeal membrane oxygenation. J Pediatr 124:335, 1994.

234. Kennaugh JM, Kinsella JP, Abman S, et al: Impact of new treatments for neonatal pulmonary hypertension on extracorporeal membrane oxygenation use and outcome. J Perinatol 17:366, 1997.

235. Kinsella JP: Clinical trials of inhaled nitric oxide therapy in the newborn. NeoReviews 20:e110, 1999.

236. Kinsella JP, Truog WE, Walsh WF, et al: Randomized multicenter trial of inhaled nitric oxide and high frequency oscillatory ventilation in severe persistent pulmonary hypertension of the newborn. J Pediatr 131:55, 1997.

237. Clark RH: High frequency ventilation. J Pediatr 124:661, 1994.

238. Avery ME, Gatewood OB, Brumley G: Transient tachypnea of the newborn. Am J Dis Child 111:380, 1966.

239. St. Geme JW Jr, Murray DL, Carter J, et al: Perinatal bacterial infection after prolonged rupture of amniotic membranes: an analysis of risk and management. J Pediatr 104:608, 1984.

240. Belady PH, Parkouh LJ, Gibbs RS: Intra-amniotic infection and premature rupture of the membranes. Clin Perinatol 25: 123, 1998.

241. Weisman LE, Stoll BJ, Cruess DF, et al: Early onset group B streptococcal sepsis: a current assesment. J Pediatr 121:428, 1992.

242. Siegel JD, McCracken GH Jr: Sepsis neonatorum. N Engl J Med 304:642, 1981.

243. Ablow RC, Driscoll SG, Effman EL, et al: A comparison of early-onset group B streptococcal neonatal infection and the respiratory-distress syndrome of the newborn. N Engl J Med 294:65, 1976.

244. Whitsett JA, Pryhuber GS, Rice WR, et al: Acute respiratory disorders. *In* Avery GB, Fletcher MA, MacDonald MG (eds): Neonatology: Pathophysiology and Management of the Newborn, 5th ed. Philadelphia, Lippincott Williams & Wilkins, 1999, p 485.

245. Avery ME, Mead J: Surface properties in relation to atelectasis and hyaline membrane disease. Am J Dis Child 97:517, 1959.

246. Jobe AH: Pathophysiology of respiratory distress syndrome and surfactant metabolism. *In* Polin RA, Fox WW (eds): Fetal and Neonatal Physiology, 2nd ed. Philadelphia, WB Saunders Company, 1998, p 1299.

247. Northway WH Jr, Rosan RC, Porter DY: Pulmonary disease following respiratory therapy of hyaline membrane disease. N Engl J Med 276:357, 1967.

248. Farrell PA, Fiascone JM: Bronchopulmonary dysplasia in the 1990's: a review for the pediatrician. Curr Probl Pediatr 27: 129, 1997.

249. Bregman J, Farrell EE: Neurodevelopmental outcome in infants with bronchopulmonary dysplasia. Clin Perinatol 19: 673, 1992.

250. Jacob SV, Coates AL, Lands LC, et al: Long-term pulmonary sequelae of severe bronchopulmonary dysplasia. J Pediatr 133:193, 1998.

251. Northway WH Jr, Moss RB, Carlisle KB, et al: Late pulmonary sequelae of bronchopulmonary dysplasia. N Engl J Med 323:1793, 1990.

252. Frank L: Pathophysiology of lung injury and repair: special features of the immature lung. *In* Polin RA, Fox WW (eds): Fetal and Neonatal Physiology, 2nd ed. Philadelphia, WB Saunders Company, 1998, p 1175.

253. Kattwinkel J: Surfactant. Evolving issues. Clin Perinatol 25: 17, 1998.

254. Survanta: Multidose Study Group: Two-year follow-up of infants treated for neonatal respiratory distress syndrome with bovine surfactant. J Pediatr 124:962, 1994.

255. Philip AGS, Allan WC, Tito AM, Wheeler LR: Intraventricular hemorrhage in preterm infants: declining incidence in the 1980s. Pediatrics 84:797, 1989.

256. Batton DG, Holtrop P, DeWitte D, et al: Current gestational age related incidence of major intraventricular hemorrhage. J Pediatr 125:623, 1994.

257. Pasternak JF, Groothuis DR, Fischer JM, Fischer DP: Regional cerebral blood flow in the newborn beagle pup: the germinal matrix is a "low-flow" structure. Pediatr Res 16:499, 1982.

258. Goddard J, Lewis RM, Armstrong DL, Zeller RS: Moderate, rapidly induced hypertension as a cause of intraventricular hemorrhage in the newborn beagle model. J Pediatr 96:1057, 1980.

259. Kuban K, Sanocka U, Leviton A: White matter disorders of prematurity: association with intraventricular hemorrhage and ventriculomegaly. J Pediatr 134:539, 1999.

260. Perlman JM, Risser R, Broyles S: Bilateral cystic periventricular leukomalacia in the premature infant: associated risk factors. Pediatrics 97:822, 1996.

261. Dammann D, Leviton A: Maternal intrauterine infection, cytokines and brain damage in the preterm newborn. Pediatr Res 42:1, 1997.

262. Partridge JC, Babock DS, Steichen JJ, Han BK: Optimal timing for diagnostic cranial ultrasound in low-birth-weight infants: detection of intracranial hemorrhage and ventricular dilation. J Pediatr 102:281, 1983.

263. Papile L-A, Burstein J, Burstein R, Koffler H: Incidence and evolution of subependymal and intraventricular hemorrhage: a study of infants with birth weight less than 1500 gm. J Pediatr 92:529, 1978.

264. Ford LM, Steichen J, Steichen Asch PA, et al: Neurologic status and intracranial hemorrhage in very-low-birth-weight preterm infants: outcome at 1 and 5 years. Am J Dis Child 143:1186, 1989.

265. Lowe J, Papille LA: Neurodevelopmental performance of very-low-birth-weight infants with mild periventricular, intraventricular hemorrhage. Outcome at 5 to 6 years of age. Am J Dis Child 144:1242, 1990.

266. Guzzetta F, Shackelford GD, Volpe S, et al: Periventricular echodensities in the premature newborn: critical determinant of neurologic outcome. Pediatrics 78:995, 1986.

267. Shankaran S, Koepke T, Woldt E, et al: Outcome after posthemorrhagic ventriculomegaly in comparison with mild hemorrhage without ventriculomegaly. J Pediatr 114:109, 1989.

268. Szymonowicz W, Yu VYH, Bajuk B, Astbury J: Neurodevelopmental outcome of periventricular hemorrhage and leukomalacia in infants 1250g or less at birth. Early Hum Dev 14:1, 1986.

269. Perlman JM: White matter injury in the preterm infant: an important determination of abnormal neurodevelopmental outcome. Early Hum Dev 53:99, 1998.

270. Ment LR, Oh W, Ehrenkranz RA, et al: Low dose indomethacin and prevention of intraventricular hemorrhage; a multicenter randomized trial. Pediatrics 93:543, 1994.

271. Rosenberg AA, Galan HC: Fetal drug therapy. Pediatr Clin North Am 44:113, 1997.

272. Thorp JA, Ferrette-Smith D, Gaston LA, et al: The effect of combined antenatal vitamin K and phenobarbital therapy for preventing intracranial hemorrhage in newborns less than 34 weeks gestation. Obstet Gynecol 86:1, 1995.

273. Shankaran S, Papile L-A, Wright LL, et al: The effect of antenatal phenobarbital therapy on neonatal intracranial hemorrhage in preterm infants. N Engl J Med 337:466, 1997.

274. Ment LR, Oh W, Ehrenkranz RA, et al: Antenatal steroids, delivery mode, and intraventricular hemorrhage in preterm infants. Am J Obstet Gynecol 172:795, 1995.

275. Scher MS: Seizures in the newborn infant. Diagnosis, treatment, and outcome. Clin Perinatol 24:735, 1997.

276. Dubowitz LMS, Dubowitz V, Goldberg C: Clinical assessment of gestational age in the newborn infant. J Pediatr 77:1, 1970.

277. Ballard JL, Kazmaier K, Driver M: A simplified assessment of gestational age. Pediatr Res 11:374, 1977.

278. Ballard JL, Khoury JC, Wedig K, et al: New Ballard Score, expanded to include extremely premature infants. J Pediatr 119:417, 1991.

279. Donovan EF, Tyson JE, Ehrenkranz RA, et al: Inaccuracy of Ballard scores before 28 weeks' gestation. J Pediatr 135:147, 1999.

280. Lubchenco LO, Hansman C, Boyd E: Intrauterine growth in length and head circumference as estimated from live births at gestational ages from 26 to 42 weeks. Pediatrics 37:403, 1966.

281. Koops BL, Morgan LJ, Battaglia FC: Neonatal mortality risk in relation to birth weight and gestational age: update, J Pediatr 101:969, 1982.

282. McIntire DD, Bloom SL, Casey B, et al: Birth weight in relation to morbidity and mortality among newborn infants. N Engl J Med 340:1234, 1999.

283. Lin C-C, Santoloya-Forgas J: Current concepts of fetal growth restriction: Part I. Causes, classification, and pathophysiology. Obstet Gynecol 92:1044, 1998.

284. Khoury MJ, Erickson JD, Cordero JF, McCarthy BJ: Congenital malformations and intrauterine growth retardation: a population study. Pediatrics 82:83, 1988.

285. American Academy of Pediatrics Task Force on Newborn and Infant Hearing: Newborn and infant hearing loss: detection and intervention. Pediatrics 103:527, 1999.

286. American Academy of Pediatrics Task Force on Infant Positioning and SIDS: Positioning and sudden infant death syndrome (SIDS): update. Pediatrics 98:1216, 1996.

287. Conrad PD, Wilkening RB, Rosenberg AA: Safety of newborn discharge in less than 36 hours in an indigent population. Am J Dis Child 143:98, 1989.

288. American Academy of Pediatrics, American College of Obstetricians and Gynecologists: Guidelines for Perinatal Care, 4th ed. Elk Grove Village, IL, American Academy of Pediatrics, 1997.

289. American Academy of Pediatrics Task Force on Circumcision: Circumcision policy statement. Pediatrics 103:686, 1999.

290. Klaus MH, Kennel JH: Care of the parents. In Klaus MH, Fanaroff AA (eds): Care of the High-Risk Neonate, 4th ed. Philadelphia, WB Saunders Company, 1993, p 189.

291. Brazelton TB, Scholl ML, Robey JS: Visual responses in the newborn. Pediatrics 37:284, 1966.

292. Klaus MH, Jerauld R, Kreger NC: Maternal attachment: importance of the first post-partum days. N Engl J Med 286:460, 1972.

293. Whitelaw A: Kangaroo baby care: just a nice experience or an important advance for preterm infants? Pediatrics 85:604, 1990.

294. Als H, Lawhon G, Duffy FH: Individual developmental care for the very low-birth-weight preterm infant. Medical and neurofunctional effects. JAMA 272:853, 1994.

295. Solnit AJ, Stark MH: Mourning and the birth of a defective child. Psychoanal Study Child 16:523, 1961.

296. Cullberg J: Mental reactions of women to perinatal death. In Morris N (ed): Psychosomatic Medicines in Obstetrics and Gynecology. New York, S Karger, 1972, p 326.

297. Stevenson DK, Wright LL, Lemons JA, et al: Very low birth

weight outcomes of the National Institute of Child Health and Human Development Neonatal Research Network, January 1993 through December 1994. Am J Obstet Gynecol 179: 1632, 1998.

298. Hack M, Fanaroff AA: Outcomes of children of extremely low birthweight and gestational age in the 1990's. Early Hum Dev 53:193, 1999.

299. Piecuch RE, Leonard CH, Cooper BA, et al: Outcome of extremely low birthweight infants (500 to 999 grams) over a 12-year period. Pediatrics 100:633, 1997.

300. Bregman J: Developmental outcome in very low birthweight infants. Current status and future trends. Pediatr Clin North Am 45:673, 1998.

301. Halsey CL, Collin MF, Anderson CL: Extremely low birth weight children and their peers: a comparison of preschool performance. Pediatrics 91:807, 1993.

302. Hack M, Taylor G, Klein N, et al: School-age outcomes in children with birth weights under 750g. N Engl J Med 331: 753, 1994.

303. Bozynski MEA, Nelson MN, Matalon TAS, et al: Prolonged mechanical ventilation and intracranial hemorrhage: impact on developmental progress through 18 months in infants weighing 1,200 grams or less at birth. Pediatrics 79:670, 1987.

304. Roth SC, Baudin J, McCormick DC, et al: Relation between ultrasound appearance of the brain of very preterm infants and neurodevelopmental impairment at 8 years. Dev Med Child Neurol 35:755, 1993.

305. Hack M, Breslau N, Weissman B, et al: Effect of very low birth weight and subnormal head size on cognitive abilities at school age. N Engl J Med 325:231, 1991.

306. Ornstein M, Ohlsson A, Edmonds J, Asztalos E: Neonatal follow-up of very low birthweight/extremely low birthweight infants to school age: a critical overview. Acta Pediatr Scand 80:741, 1991.

307. Kok JH, Den Ouden AL, Verloove-Vanhornick SP, et al: Outcome of very preterm small for gestational age infants: the first nine years of life. Br J Obstet Gynaecol 105:162, 1998.

308. Vohr BR, Wright LL, Dusick AM, et al: Neurodevelopmental and functional outcomes of extremely low birth weight infants in the National Institute of Child Health and Human Development Neonatal Research Network, 1993–1994. Pediatrics 105:1216, 2000.

309. Lucey JF, Dangman B: A reexamination of the role of oxygen in retrolental fibroplasia. Pediatrics 73:82, 1984.

310. Valentine PH, Jackson JC, Kalina RE, Woodrum DE: Increased survival of low birth weight infants: impact on the incidence of retinopathy of prematurity. Pediatrics 84:442, 1989.

311. Kramer SJ, Vertes DR, Condom M: Auditory brainstem responses and clinical followup of high risk infants. Pediatrics 83:385, 1989.

Postpartum Care

WATSON A. BOWES, JR. AND VERN L. KATZ

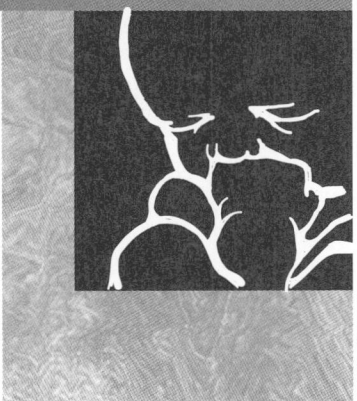

The postpartum time period, also called the puerperium, lasts from delivery of the placenta until 6 to 12 weeks after delivery. Most of the physiologic changes in pregnancy will have returned to prepregnancy physiology by 6 weeks. However, many of the cardiovascular changes and psychological changes may persist for many more months.

Much information is known about the changes and problems that can occur in the weeks after delivery. However, because the care of a new infant is so important to the survival of any family, clan, or tribe, the postpartum period is associated with as much tradition and superstition as any other time in life. In order to support the successful recovery of the mother, and the healthy transition through the neonatal period, customs, taboos, and rituals have developed in most cultures. Indeed, most of the current medical recommendations about puerperium have developed from adaptations of socially acceptable traditions, rather than science. This chapter examines the physiologic adjustments of the postpartum period, the return of the female genital tract to its prepregnancy state (involution), the major puerperal disease states, and the natural course of lactation.

Most of the postpartum traditions from non-Western cultures involve special activities and different foods for the newly delivered mother, as well as particular and unique taboos. In the rural Philippines, the mother, who works up until she goes into labor, is prohibited from working after delivery, and she is given a new name. The maternal grandmother visits daily unless she has died, in which case the visits are made by the grandmother-in-law. The grandmother does all the house work and cooking for 8 weeks. The mother is bathed by the grandmother daily. When the umbilical cord falls off the infant, a feast is prepared. The cord is blessed at the feast. The new father is prohibited from building stone walls and from driving nails for 6 months. For 2 months, the relatives tend the fields.

In parts of rural India, the new mother returns to her mother's house for 16 weeks. She is given a hot bath every day. Cold baths are taboo, as cold water is associated with disease.

Many cultures have rituals regarding treatment of the placenta. It may be dried and turned to powder for its "medical" powers. The umbilical cord was hung in a nearby tree by some eastern American Indian tribes. In European tradition, it was buried under certain corners of the house, to ensure prosperity. For many cultures, the period of rest for the mother and abstention from sexual activity was 40 days. The 40-day time period corresponds to the 6 weeks of restricted activity in American culture. Many European countries have adopted different time periods before the mother returns to her predelivery status.

POSTPARTUM INVOLUTION

The Uterus

The crude weight of the pregnant uterus at term (excluding the fetus, placenta, membranes, and amniotic fluid) is approximately 1,000 g.[1] The weight of the nonpregnant uterus is between 50 and 100 g. It is not known how rapidly this 10-fold involution in organ weight occurs, but within 2 weeks after birth the uterus has usually returned to the pelvis, and by 6 weeks it is usually normal size, as estimated by palpation. The involution of the uterus after childbirth has been studied for more than 100 years. The gross anatomic and histologic characteristics of the involutional process are based on the study of autopsy, hysterectomy, and endometrial biopsy specimens.[2-4] The decrease in the size of the uterus and cervix during the puerperium has been demonstrated with serial magnetic resonance imaging (MRI) as illustrated in Figure 21–1.[5] The findings are consistent with those of serial sonography and computed tomography (CT).[6-8]

Immediately after delivery, the decrease in endometrial surface contributes to the shearing off of the placenta at the decidual layer. The average diameter of the placenta is 18 cm; in the immediate postpartum uterus the average diameter of the site of placental attachment measures 9 cm. The placental site in the first 3 days after delivery is infiltrated with granulocytes and mononuclear cells, a reaction that extends into the endometrium and superficial myometrium. By the seventh day, there is evidence of the regeneration of endometrial glands, often appearing atypical, with irregular chroma-

tin patterns, misshapen and enlarged nuclei, pleomorphism, and increased cytoplasm. By the end of the first week, there is also evidence of the regeneration of endometrial stroma, with mitotic figures noted in gland epithelium; by postpartum day 16, the endometrium is fully restored.

Decidual necrosis begins on the first day, and by the seventh day, a well-demarcated zone can be seen between necrotic and viable tissue. An area of viable decidua remains between the necrotic slough and the deeper endomyometrium. Sharman[3] described the nonnecrotic decidual cells as participating in the reconstruction of the endometrium, a likely role, since they were originally endometrial connective tissue cells to which they ultimately revert in the involutional process. By the sixth week, it is rare to find decidual cells.

The immediate inflammatory cell infiltrate of polymorphonuclear leukocytes and lymphocytes persists for

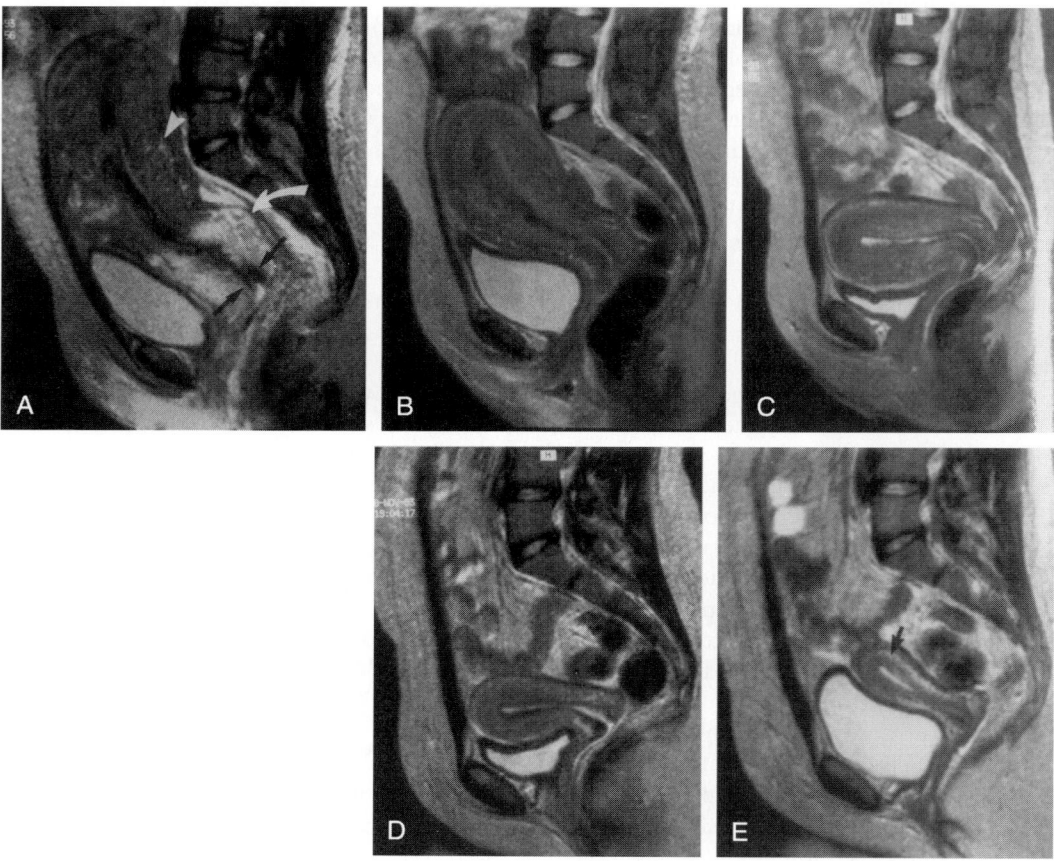

Figure 21–1. Sagittal T2-weighted fast spin echo magnetic resonance images (3/500/100) obtained serially after uncomplicated vaginal delivery. *A*, Initial image obtained less than 30 hours after delivery. Uterus and cervix are large and thick-walled. The uterine cervix is clearly distinguished from the uterine corpus by the high-signal-intensity outer cervical stroma (OCS) (*white arrow*). The low-signal-intensity inner cervical stroma (ICS) is apparent (*black arrows*). The myometrium has heterogeneous signal intensity, and prominent myometrial vessels are seen (*arrowhead*). The myometrial vessels remained prominent on images obtained 1 week (*B*) and 2 weeks (*C*) after delivery. At 1 week, the uterus and cervix have diminished substantially in size, the OCS has diminished in signal intensity, and the ICS is more clearly defined. The low signal intensity in the endometrial canal in *A* and *B* likely represents blood products. At 2 weeks (*C*), 6 weeks (*D*), and 6 months (*E*), the uterus has progressively deceased in size. At 2 weeks, the endometrium has returned to a normal high signal intensity. By 6 months, the junctional zone has been restored (*arrow* in *E*); however, it is broadened, measuring approximately 7 mm. (From Willms AB, Brown ED, Kettritz UI, et al: Anatomic changes in the pelvis after uncomplicated vaginal delivery: evaluation with serial MR imaging. Radiology 195:91, 1995, with permission.)

about 10 days, presumably serving as an antibacterial barrier. The leukocyte response diminishes rapidly after the 10th day, and plasma cells are seen for the first time. The plasma cell and lymphocyte response may last as long as several months. In fact, endometrial stromal infiltrates of plasma cells and lymphocytes are the sign (and may be the only sign) of a recent pregnancy.

Hemostasis immediately after birth is accomplished by arterial smooth muscle contraction and compression of vessels by the involuting uterine muscle. Vessels in the placental site are characterized during the first 8 days by thrombosis, hyalinization, and endophlebitis in the veins and by hyalinization and obliterative fibrinoid endarteritis in the arteries. The mechanism for hyalinization of arterial walls, which is not completely understood, may be related to the previous trophoblastic infiltration of arterial walls that occurs early in pregnancy. Many of the thrombosed and hyalinized veins are extruded with the slough of the necrotic placental site, but hyalinized arteries remain for extended periods as stigmata of the placental site.

Restoration of the endometrium in areas other than the placental site occurs rapidly, with the process being completed by day 16 after delivery. The gland epithelium does not undergo the reactivity or the pseudoneoplastic appearance noted in placental site glands.[4]

The postpartum uterine discharge or lochia begins as a flow of blood lasting several hours, rapidly diminishing to a reddish brown discharge through the third or fourth day postpartum. This is followed by a transition to a mucopurulent, somewhat malodorous discharge, lochia serosa, requiring the change of several perineal pads per day. The median duration of lochia serosa is 22 to 27 days.[9,10] However, 10 to 15 percent of women will have lochia serosa at the time of the 6-week postpartum examination. In the majority of patients, the lochia serosa is followed by a yellow-white discharge, lochia alba. Breast-feeding or the use of oral contraceptive agents does not affect the duration of lochia. Not infrequently there is a sudden but transient increase in uterine bleeding between 7 and 14 days postpartum. This corresponds to the slough of the eschar over the site of placental attachment. Myometrial vessels of greater than 5 mm in diameter are present for up to 2 weeks postpartum, which accounts for the dramatic bleeding that can occur with this phenomenon.[5] Although it can be profuse, this bleeding episode is usually self-limited, requiring nothing more than reassurance of the patient. If it does not subside within 1 or 2 hours, the patient should be evaluated for possible retained placental tissue.

Ultrasound is useful in the management of abnormal postpartum bleeding. The empty uterus with a clear midline echo is quite easy to distinguish from the uterine cavity expanded by clot (sonolucent) or retained tissue (echo dense). Serial ultrasound examinations of postpartum patients showed that in 20 to 30 percent there was some retained blood or tissue within 24 hours after delivery. By the fourth postpartum day, only about 8 percent of patients showed endometrial cavity separation, a portion of which eventually had abnormal postpartum bleeding because of retained placental tissue.[11] In cases of abnormal postpartum bleeding, ultrasound examination efficiently detects patients who have retained tissue and who will therefore benefit from uterine evacuation and curettage. Those who have an empty uterine cavity will respond to therapy with oxytocin or methylergonovine.[12]

The Cervix

During pregnancy, the cervical epithelium increases in thickness, and the cervical glands show both hyperplasia and hypertrophy. Within the stroma, a distinct decidual reaction occurs. These changes are accompanied by a substantial increase in the vascularity of the cervix.[13] Colposcopic examination performed after delivery has demonstrated ulceration, laceration, and ecchymosis of the cervix.[14] Regression of the cervical epithelium begins within the first 4 days after delivery, and by the end of the first week edema and hemorrhage within the cervix are minimal. Vascular hypertrophy and hyperplasia persist throughout the first week postpartum. By 6 weeks' postpartum, most of the antepartum changes have resolved, although round cell infiltration and some edema may persist for several months.[15]

The Fallopian Tube

The epithelium of the fallopian tube during pregnancy is characterized by a predominance of nonciliated cells, a phenomenon that is maintained by the balance between the high levels of progesterone and estrogen.[16] After delivery, in the absence of progesterone and estrogen, there is further extrusion of nuclei from nonciliated cells and diminution in height of both ciliated and nonciliated cells. Andrews[16] demonstrated that the number and height of ciliated cells can be increased in the puerperium by treatment with estrogen.

Fallopian tubes removed between postpartum days 5 and 15 demonstrate inflammatory changes of acute salpingitis in 38 percent of cases, but no bacteria are found. The specific cause of the inflammatory change is unknown.[16] Furthermore, there is no correlation between the presence of histologic inflammation in the fallopian tubes and puerperal fever or other clinical signs of salpingitis.

Ovarian Function

It has long been recognized that women who breast-feed their infants will be amenorrheic for long periods of time, often until the infant is weaned. Several studies, using a variety of methods to indicate ovulation, have demonstrated that ovulation occurs as early as 27 days after delivery, with the mean time being approximately 70 to 75 days in nonlactating women.[17,18] Among those women who are breast-feeding their infants, the mean time to ovulation is about 6 months.

Menstruation resumes by 12 weeks' postpartum in 70 percent of women who are not lactating, and the mean time to the first menstruation is 7 to 9 weeks. In one study of lactating women, it was 36 months before 70 percent began to menstruate. The duration of anovulation depends on the frequency of breast-feeding, the duration of each feed, and the proportion of supplementary feeds.[19] The risk of ovulation within the first 6 months' postpartum in a woman exclusively breast-feeding is 1 to 5 percent.

The hormonal basis for puerperal ovulation suppression in lactating women appears to be the persistence of elevated serum prolactin levels.[20] Prolactin levels fall to the normal range by the third week postpartum in nonlactating women, but remain elevated into the sixth week postpartum in lactating patients. Estrogen levels fall immediately after delivery in both lactating and nonlactating women and remain depressed in lactating patients. In those who are not lactating, estrogen levels begin to rise 2 weeks after delivery and are significantly higher than in lactating women by postpartum day 17. Follicle-stimulating hormone (FSH) levels are identical in breast-feeding and non–breast-feeding women. It is therefore assumed that the ovary does not respond to FSH stimulation in the presence of increased prolactin levels.

Weight Loss

One of the most welcomed changes for the majority of women who have recently given birth is the loss of the weight that was accumulated during pregnancy. The immediate loss of 10 to 13 lb is attributed to the delivery of the infant, placenta, and amniotic fluid and to blood loss.[21] By six weeks postpartum, 28 percent of women will have returned to their prepregnant weight. The remainder of the weight loss occurs from 6 weeks postpartum until 6 months after delivery. Women with excess weight gain in pregnancy (>35 lb) are likely to have a net gain of 11 lb.[22] Breast-feeding has relatively little effect on postpartum weight loss.[23] In a program of diet and exercise, weight loss of approximately 0.5 kg/wk between 4 and 14 weeks postpartum in overweight women did not affect the growth weight of their infants.[24] Aerobic exercise had no adverse effect on lactation.[25]

Thyroid Function

Thyroid size and function throughout pregnancy and the puerperium have been quantitated with ultrasonog-

raphy and thyroid hormone levels.[26] Thyroid volume increases approximately 30 percent during pregnancy and regresses to normal size gradually over a 12-week period. Thyroxine and triiodothyronine, which are both elevated throughout pregnancy, return to normal within 4 weeks postpartum. It is now recognized that the postpartum period is associated with an increased risk for the development of a transient autoimmune thyroiditis that may in some cases lead to permanent hypothyroidism.[27] Asymptomatic postpartum thyroid dysfunction may occur in as many as 10 percent of parturients.[28] Pedersen et al. found a relationship between subclinical thyroid dysfunction and postpartum depression,[29] although this was not confirmed by Kent et al.[28,30]

Cardiovascular System and Coagulation

Blood volume increases throughout pregnancy to levels in the third trimester about 35 percent above nonpregnant values.[31] The greatest proportion of this increase consists of an expansion in plasma volume that begins in the first trimester and amounts to an additional 1,200 ml of plasma, representing a 50 percent increase by the third trimester. Red blood cell volume increases by about 250 ml.

Immediately after delivery, plasma volume is diminished by approximately 1,000 ml because of blood loss. By the third postpartum day, plasma volume has increased by 900 to 1,200 ml because of a shift of extracellular fluid into the vascular space.[32] The total blood volume by the third postpartum day, however, declines by 16 percent of the predelivery value.[33] Ueland found that blood volume changes in the puerperium were the same regardless of the method of delivery, but patients who delivered vaginally had a 5 percent increase in hematocrit, whereas those who had a cesarean delivery had a 6 percent decrease in hematocrit.[33] The rate at which red blood cell volume returns to prepregnancy levels is unknown, but when measured at 8 weeks postpartum it is found to be within the normal range.[34] As blood volume decreases, venous tone returns to normal. Macklon and Greer examined 42 women, longitudinally, at 4 and 42 days postpartum. The investigators demonstrated significant reduction in deep vein vessel size and a concomitant increase in venous flow velocity in the lower extremities.[35]

Pulse rate increases throughout pregnancy, as does stroke volume and cardiac output. Immediately after delivery, these remain elevated or rise even higher for 30 to 60 minutes. Following delivery, there is a transient rise of approximately 5 percent in both diastolic and systolic blood pressures throughout the first 4 days postpartum.[36] In 12 percent of otherwise normotensive patients, the diastolic blood pressure will exceed 100 mm Hg. Data are scant regarding the rate at which cardiac hemodynamics return to prepregnancy levels. Early studies suggested cardiac output had returned to normal when measurements were made 8 to 10 weeks postpartum.[37] Clapp and Capeless performed longitudinal evaluations of cardiac function at bimonthly intervals in 30 healthy women using M-mode ultrasound, prior to pregnancy; during gestation; and at 12, 24, and 52 weeks postpartum. Cardiac output and left ventricular volume peaked at 24 weeks' gestation. There was a slow return to prepregnancy values over the year of study. However, even 1 year after delivery, there was a significantly higher cardiac output in both nulliparous and multiparous women than prepregnancy values. The authors suggested that this "cardiac remodeling" from pregnancy may last for an extended time in healthy women.[38] Elite athletes have tried to take advantage of this physiologic boost to cardiac function, by planning pregnancies a year prior to major sporting events.

Ygge[39] studied blood coagulation and fibrinolysis in 10 normal pregnant women during the 4 weeks before delivery, during labor and delivery, and 2 weeks postpartum. Compared with antepartum values, there was a rapid decrease in platelets in some patients and no change or an increase in others. However, 2 weeks after delivery, all patients demonstrated an increase in platelet count. Fibrinolytic activity increased in the first 1 to 4 days after delivery and returned to normal in 1 week. The greatest level of coagulability was observed immediately postpartum through 48 hours. Fibrinogen concentration gradually diminished over the 2-week postpartum period studied. The changes in the coagulation system together with vessel trauma and immobility account for the increased risk of thromboembolism noted in the puerperium, especially when operative delivery has occurred.

The Urinary Tract and Renal Function

It is generally accepted that the urinary tract becomes dilated during pregnancy, especially the renal pelves and the ureters above the pelvic brim. These findings, demonstrated 50 years ago by Baird,[40] affect the collecting system of the right kidney more than that of the left. These changes are caused by compression of the ureters by adjacent vasculature and by compression from the enlarged uterus, and by the effect of progesterone. Ureteral tone above the pelvic brim, which in pregnancy is higher than normal, diminishes in the lateral recumbent position and returns to nonpregnant levels immediately after cesarean delivery.[41]

The intravenous urography studies performed by Dure-Smith[42] suggest that subtle anatomic changes take place in the ureters that persist long after the pregnancy has ended. Ultrasound studies of the urinary tract also document the enlargement of the collecting system throughout pregnancy.[43] A study of serial ultrasound examinations of the urinary tract in 20 women throughout pregnancy included a single postpartum examination 6 weeks after delivery.[44] The overall trend was that of dilatation of the collecting system throughout pregnancy, estimated by measurements of the separation of the pelvis–calyceal echo complex, from a mean of 5.0 mm (first trimester) to 10 mm (third trimester) in the right kidney and from 3.0 to 4.0 mm in the left collecting system. Measurements in all but two patients had returned to prepregnancy status at the time of the 6-week postpartum examination. Cietak and Newton[45] performed serial nephrosonography on 24 patients throughout pregnancy and the puerperium. At 12 weeks postpartum, more than half of the patients demonstrated persistence of urinary stasis, described as a slight separation of the renal pelvis. This finding is evidence of hyperdistensibility and suggests that pregnancy has a permanent effect on the size of the upper renal tract.

Studies in which water cystometry and uroflowmetry were performed within 48 hours of delivery and again 4 weeks postpartum demonstrated a slight but significant decrease in bladder capacity (from 395.5 to 331 ml) and volume at first void (from 277 to 224 ml) in the study interval. Nevertheless, all the urodynamic values studied were within normal limits on both occasions. The results were not affected by the weight of the infant or by an episiotomy. However, prolonged labor and the use of epidural anesthesia appeared to diminish postpartum bladder function transiently.[46]

The most detailed study of renal function in normal pregnancy is that of Sims and Krantz,[47] who studied 12 patients with serial renal function tests throughout pregnancy and for up to 1 year after delivery. Glomerular filtration, which increased by 50 percent early in pregnancy and remained elevated until delivery, returned to normal nonpregnant levels by postpartum week 8. Endogenous creatinine clearance, similarly elevated throughout pregnancy, also returned to normal by the eighth postpartum week. Renal plasma flow increased by 25 percent early in pregnancy, gradually diminished in the third trimester (even when measured in the lateral recumbent position), and continued to decrease to below-normal values in the postpartum period for up to 24 weeks.[48] Normal values were finally established by 50 to 60 weeks after delivery. The reason for the prolonged postpartum depression of renal plasma flow is not clear.

Other Changes

Hair growth slows in the puerperium. Often, women will experience hair loss, as temporarily more hair is lost than is regrown. This is a transient phenomenon, and the patient may be reassured that hair patterns return to normal within a few months.

Several investigators have reported on bone mineral changes with lactation and the associated amenorrhea. After delivery, there is a generalized decrease in bone mineralization that is most always temporary and resolves by 18 months postpartum in most women.[49] Bone loss appears to be greatest in the femoral neck than in other areas of the skeleton.[50,51] Calcium supplementation does not seem to ameliorate the bone loss, since it is not a problem of inadequate calcium stores. Exercise does not prevent this bone loss.[52]

Management of the Puerperium

For most parturients, the immediate puerperium is spent in the hospital or birthing center. The ideal duration of hospitalization for patients with uncomplicated vaginal births has been controversial, with most authorities recommending a 2-day stay for first-time mothers. For patients with an uncomplicated postoperative course following cesarean delivery, the postpartum stay is 3 or 4 days. Approximately 3 percent of women who have vaginal deliveries and 9 percent of women who have cesareans have at least one childbirth-related complication requiring prolonged hospitalization after delivery or readmission to the hospital.[53]

In a recent study, 1,249 randomly selected patients were questioned 8 weeks following delivery about health problems that occurred during the puerperium.[54] Eighty-five percent reported at least one problem during their hospitalization, and 76 percent noted at least one problem that persisted for 8 weeks. A wide range of problems were reported by the patients, including a painful perineum, difficulties with breast-feeding, urinary infections, urinary and fecal incontinence, and headache. Three percent of the patients had been rehospitalized, most commonly for abnormal bleeding or infection. This study draws attention to a substantial amount of symptomatic morbidity that occurs during the puerperium.

If a patient has adequate support at home (i.e., help with housekeeping and meal preparation), there is little value in an extended hospital stay, provided the mother is adequately educated about infant care and feeding, family planning, and identification of danger signs in either the infant or herself. Except for an increased incidence of rehospitalization of some neonates for hyperbilirubinemia, there are few disadvantages to postpartum hospitalization of less than 48 hours for many patients.[55-58] For mothers who do not have adequate support at home and who are insecure about infant care and feeding, extending the hospital stay will provide time for mothers to gain adequate education and some measure of self-confidence.[59] Video presentations are an efficient means of patient education. Also, home nursing visits can be helpful in providing support, education, and advice to mothers.

In addition to the video presentation, patients should be given ample opportunity to discuss specific questions or concerns with a nurse or physician. It is also important to provide a new mother time and a sympathetic listener so that she can express her feelings and ask questions about her labor and delivery experience.

The time from delivery until complete physiologic involution and psychological adjustment has been called "the fourth trimester."[60] Patients should understand that lochia will persist for 3 to 8 weeks and that on days 7 to 14 there is likely to be an episode of heavy vaginal bleeding, which occurs when the placental eschar sloughs. Tampons are permissible if they are comfortable upon insertion and are changed frequently and if there are no perineal, vaginal, or cervical lacerations, which preclude insertion of a tampon until healing has occurred.

Physical activity, including walking up and down stairs, lifting heavy objects, riding in or driving a car, and performing muscle-toning exercises, can be resumed without delay if the delivery has been uncomplicated. Instructions regarding exercise are patient specific. Recent studies have found that exercise postpartum does not affect lactation, and may decrease anxiety levels.[61,62] As such, exercise may have benefits beyond the mother's desire to "get back into shape." The most troublesome complaint is lethargy and fatigue. Consequently, every task or activity should be a brief one in the first few days of the puerperium. Mothers whose lethargy persists beyond several weeks must be evaluated, especially as regards thyroid dysfunction. Transient postpartum thyrotoxicosis may occur followed by hypothyroidism. These episodes are characterized by goiter formation, the presence of antithyroid antibodies, and eventual resolution.[63,64]

Sexual activity may be resumed when the perineum is comfortable and when bleeding has diminished. The desire and willingness to resume sexual activity in the puerperium varies greatly among women, depending on the site and state of healing of perineal or vaginal incisions and lacerations, the amount of vaginal atrophy secondary to breast-feeding, and the return of libido.[65] Although the median time to resuming intercourse after delivery is 6 weeks, approximately one half of women who do so have dyspareunia, and in a substantial number it lasts for a year or more.[66,67] Postpartum dyspareunia is not predominantly related to vulvar repair and occurs in some women who have a cesarean delivery. It is also observed in women who use oral contraceptives and do not breast-feed, suggesting that lack of estrogen effect on the vagina is not the major cause of postpartum dyspareunia. In a study of 50 parturients, Ryding[68] found that 20 percent had little desire for sexual activity 3 months after delivery, and an additional 21 percent had complete loss of desire or aversion to sexual activity. This variation in attitude, desire, and willingness must be acknowledged when counseling women about the resumption of sexual activity.

Many patients will be returning to work situations outside the home after their pregnancies. Frequently, the physician must complete insurance or employer forms to establish maternity leave for patients. Six weeks is regarded as the normal period of "disability" following delivery,[69] although some mothers return to work sooner.

A follow-up examination is frequently scheduled for 6 weeks after delivery. Several studies have shown that a routine postpartum visit to the physician at 1 or 2 weeks after delivery or a home visit by a nurse midwife does not reduce maternal or infant morbidity.[70,71] Nevertheless, for some patients, an appointment approximately 2 weeks postpartum or a home visit by a visiting nurse or nurse midwife will be more productive in detecting problems and providing support for a mother. Late puerperal infections, postpartum depression, and problems with infant care and feeding often occur before the 6-week postpartum visit.

Some women with chronic medical diseases, such as collagen vascular disease, autoimmune disorders, and neurologic conditions, should be seen at close intervals. Many patients with these disorders may experience "flares" of their symptoms after delivery. This has been theorized as a rebound of the immune system after a period of relative immune suppression during pregnancy. Prophylactic therapy is not recommended for women with systemic lupus or multiple sclerosis. However, warning patients to be attuned to signs and symptoms that reflect a flare of their illness allows for early and more effective interventions.

Perineal Care

Many women who give birth have an episiotomy or spontaneous lacerations of the perineum or vagina. In the United States, episiotomies are more often performed as midline than as mediolateral incisions. Provided that the incision or the laceration does not extend beyond the transverse perineal muscle, that there is no hematoma or extensive ecchymosis, and that a satisfactory repair has been accomplished, there is little need for perineal care beyond routine cleansing with a bath or shower. Analgesia can be accomplished in most patients with nonsteroidal anti-inflammatory drugs such as ibuprofen. These drugs have been shown to be superior to acetaminophen or propoxyphene for episiotomy pain and uterine cramping.[72] Furthermore, because of a low milk/maternal plasma drug concentration ratio, a short half-life, and transformation into glucuronide metabolites, ibuprofen is safe for nursing mothers.

A patient who has had a mediolateral episiotomy or who has a third- or fourth-degree extension of a midline episiotomy and extensive spontaneous second-degree laceration or extensive perineal bruising may experience considerable perineal pain. Occasionally, the pain and periurethral swelling will prevent the patient from voiding, making urethral catheterization necessary.

When a patient complains of inordinate perineal pain, the first and most important step is to reexamine the perineum, vagina, and rectum to detect and drain a hematoma or to identify a perineal infection. Perineal pain may be the first symptom of the rare but potentially fatal complications of angioedema, necrotizing fasciitis, or perineal cellulitis.[73-75]

In cases of moderate perineal pain, sitz baths will provide additional pain relief. Although hot sitz baths have long been customary therapy for perineal pain, Droegemueller[76] outlined the rationale for using cold or "iced" sitz baths. This therapy is similar to that for the treatment of athletic injuries, for which considerable success has been achieved with cold therapy. Cold provides immediate pain relief as a result of decreased excitability of free nerve endings and decreased nerve conduction. Further pain relief comes from local vasoconstriction, which reduces edema, inhibits hematoma formation, and decreases muscle irritability and spasm. Patients who have alternated using hot and cold sitz baths usually prefer the cold.

The technique for administering a cold sitz bath is first to have the patient sit in a tub of water at room temperature to which ice cubes are then added. This avoids the sensation of sudden immersion in ice water. The patient remains in the ice water for 20 to 30 minutes.

Frequently, what appears to be severe perineal pain is, in fact, the pain of prolapsed hemorrhoids. Witch hazel compresses, suppositories containing corticosteroids, or local anesthetic sprays or emollients may be helpful. Occasionally, a thrombus will occur in a prolapsed hemorrhoid. It is a simple task to remove the thrombus through a small scalpel incision using local anesthesia. Dramatic relief of pain usually follows this procedure.

Patients with perineal incisions or lacerations should be advised to postpone sexual intercourse for 3 weeks or until there is no perineal discomfort. Tampons may be inserted whenever the patient is comfortable doing so. However, to avoid any risk of toxic shock syndrome, the use of tampons should be confined to the daytime to prevent leaving a tampon in the vagina for prolonged periods. Urinary and anal incontinence occur in some women following delivery.[77] Approximately 15 percent of women have urinary incontinence and 5 percent have anal incontinence 3 months after giving birth.[78] Operative vaginal delivery and anal sphincter lacerations are associated with an increased risk of postpartum anal incontinence, while cesarean delivery, especially if performed prior to the second stage of labor, is associated with a decreased risk for this problem. Often, women do not complain of symptoms of incontinence because they are embarrassed or they regard the symptoms as the normal consequence of delivery. Postpartum urinary and fecal incontinence are often transient and resolve within 6 months. If the symptoms persist for more than 6 months, studies should be undertaken to define the specific neuromuscular or anatomic abnormality so that the appropriate pharmacologic, biophysical, or surgical treatment can begin.

Delayed Postpartum Hemorrhage

The causes and management of immediate postpartum hemorrhage are discussed in Chapter 17. Delayed postpartum uterine bleeding of sufficient quantity to require medical attention occurs in 1 to 2 percent of patients. One of the most common causes of postpartum hemorrhage that occurs 2 to 5 days after delivery is von Willebrand's disease. Women presenting in this time frame should be screened for this condition. Von Willebrand's factor increases in pregnancy, and thus bleeding usually does not occur in the first 48 hours after birth. Uterine atony and postpartum hemorrhage are responsible for approximately eight maternal deaths each year in the United States.[79] The bleeding occurs most frequently between days 8 and 14 of the puerperium.[80] The bleeding is usually self-limited and of short duration. The cause of most of these cases is presumed to be sloughing of the placental escar. It is helpful to warn patients about these symptoms. However, when the bleeding is of greater amount, requiring curettage, retained gestational products will be found in about 40 percent of cases. Whether small placental remnants are the cause is not known. In the management of patients with heavy delayed bleeding, ultrasound examination will usually determine if there is a significant amount of retained material, although it is sometimes difficult to distinguish between blood clot and retained placental fragments. Suction evacuation of the uterus is successful in arresting the bleeding in almost all cases whether or not there is histologic confirmation of retained gestational products. If curettage is required at this time, especially if a sharp curette is used, a course of antibiotics begun prior to surgery is advisable for its possible benefit in reducing the formation of uterine synechiae. The curettage should be performed with care, as the postpartum uterine wall is soft and easier to perforate. In those rare instances in which delayed postpartum hemorrhage does not respond to the use of oxytocic agents and curettage, selective arterial embolization is effective in controlling the bleeding.[81]

Postpartum Infection

The standard definition of postpartum febrile morbidity is a temperature of 38.0°C (100.4°F) or higher on any 2 of the first 10 days after delivery, exclusive of the first 24 hours. However, most clinicians do not wait 2 full days to begin evaluation and treatment of patients who develop a fever in the puerperium.[82] The most common cause of postpartum fever is endometritis, which occurs after vaginal delivery in approximately 2 percent of patients and after cesarean delivery in about 10 to 15 percent. The differential diagnosis includes urinary tract infection, lower genital tract infection, wound infections, pulmonary infections, thrombophlebitis, and mastitis. The diagnosis and management of postpartum infection are discussed in detail in Chapter 40.

Maternal–Infant Attachment

Klaus et al.[83] were among the first investigators to study maternal–infant attachment and to bring attention to the importance of the first few hours of maternal–infant association. Their studies as well as those of others have contributed substantially to major changes in hospital policies dealing with patients in labor and delivery and during the postpartum confinement. It is now recognized that there should be opportunities for parents to be with their newborns even from the first few moments after birth and as frequently as possible during the first days thereafter. These associations are usually characterized by fondling, kissing, cuddling, and gazing at the infant, which are manifestations of maternal commitment and protectiveness toward her infant. Separation of mother and infant in the first hours after birth has been shown to diminish or delay the development of these characteristic mothering behaviors,[84] a problem that is intensified when medical, obstetric, or newborn complications require intensive care for either the mother or her newborn infant.

Robson and Powell[85] summarized the literature on early maternal attachment and emphasized how difficult it is to accomplish good research studies about this phenomenon. While it is generally agreed that early association of the mother and infant is beneficial and should not be interfered with unnecessarily, there are still doubts about the long-term implications, if any, of a lack of early maternal–infant association. In their monograph summarizing their investigations about parent–infant attachment, Klaus and Kennel[86] warn against drawing far-reaching conclusions. Although favoring the theory of a "sensitive period" soon after birth, during which close parent–infant interaction facilitates subsequent attachment and beneficial parenting behavior, these investigators concur that humans are highly adaptable and state that "there are many failsafe routes to attachment." This appears to be the prevailing view among experts at this time.

The modern hospital maternity ward should enhance and encourage parent–infant attachment by such policies as flexible visiting hours for the father, encouragement of the infant rooming with the mother, and supportive attitudes about breast-feeding. These policies also allow the nursing staff to observe parenting behavior and to identify inept, inexperienced, or even malicious behavior toward the infant. Some situations may call for more intensive follow-up by visiting nurses, home health visitors, or social workers to provide further support for the family during the posthospital convalescence.

The role of postpartum home visits in enhancing parenting behavior is controversial. Gray et al.[87] found this approach quite beneficial. Siegel et al.[88] studied the effect of early and prolonged mother–infant contact in the hospital and a postpartum visitation program on attachment and parenting behavior. They found that early and prolonged maternal–infant contact in the hospital had a significant effect on enhancing subsequent parenting behavior, but the postpartum home visitations had no impact.

The development of the qualities associated with good parenting depends on many factors. Certainly it does not depend solely on what transpires in the few hours surrounding the birth experience. There is evidence that specific identification of an infant with its mother's voice begins in utero during the third trimester.[89] Furthermore, the parents' own experiences as children, as well as their intellectual and emotional attitudes about children, must play a large role in their own parenting behavior. Areskog et al.[90] showed that women who expressed fear of childbirth during the antenatal period had more complications and more pain in labor and also had more difficulties in attachment to their infants. Consequently, the peripartum period provides opportunities to enhance parenting behavior and to identify families for which follow-up after birth may be necessary to ensure the most favorable child development.

In summary, the postpartum ward should be an environment that provides parents ample opportunity to interact with their newborn infants. Personnel, including nurses, nurses' aides, and physicians, caring for mothers and infants should be alert to signs of abnormal parenting (e.g., refusal of the mother to care for the infant, the use of negative or abusive names in describing or referring to the infant, inordinate delay in naming the infant, or obsessive and unrealistic concerns about the infant's health). These or other signs that maternal–infant attachment is delayed or endangered are as deserving of frequent follow-up during the postpartum period as are any of the traditional medical or obstetric complications.

LACTATION AND BREAST-FEEDING

One of the important objectives of the puerperium is to enhance the maternal–infant interaction as regards nutrition of the infant. After several decades during which interest in breast-feeding languished in Western cultures, there has been renewed interest and enthusiasm for what is clearly the most reasonable means of feeding most newborn infants. In the United States, the proportion of mothers who breast-fed their infants in the early postpartum period increased from 52 percent in 1990 to 62 percent in 1997. The proportion of infants who were breast-fed for 6 months increased from 18 percent in 1990 to 26 percent in 1997.[91] Although the increase in breast-feeding is seen in all demographic groups, it is greatest in upper income and more highly educated groups. The increase in the popularity of breast-feeding is due in part to an increasing awareness of the advantages. The benefits include improved infant nutrition, increased resistance to infection, decreased expense, and increased convenience.[92] Furthermore, women who use lactation amenorrhea as a contraceptive alternative have higher rates of using other contraceptive methods and more effective delay of subsequent pregnancies than comparable women who do not breast feed.[93] Successful breast-feeding depends to a great extent on the motivation of the mother and on the support she receives from family, friends, and health care providers. Undoubtedly, the mother's experiences as a child contribute to her attitudes about childbearing and infant feeding. Nevertheless, additional knowledge about breast-feeding may be gained during prenatal care from well-informed, enthusiastic, and supportive physicians and nurses, by reading from one of several lay books on breast-feeding, and by participating in classes on prepared childbirth. A variety of hospital practices, including the use of audiovisual aids, telephone hotlines, and in-service training for personnel, have been shown to increase the incidence of successful breast-feeding.[94]

The prenatal physical examination may identify problems that will affect breast-feeding. These include inverted nipples, which can be corrected in part by wearing breast shields, or *Candida* vaginal infections, which should be treated to avoid thrush in the infant, and painful *Candida* infection of the nipples.

The Term Infant

Hospital routines should not interfere with reasonable breast-feeding practices. Allowing the infant to nurse in its wakeful period immediately after birth when the mouthing movements and rooting reflex are active will give the mother confidence and promote milk production and let-down. Furthermore, early suckling not only provides the infant with the important immunologic and anti-infective properties of colostrum, but also has been shown to enhance successful breast-feeding.

Rooming-in allows the parents to become accustomed to demand feeding and provides the mother with opportunities to seek help from the nursing staff while she enhances her breast-feeding skills. Although the rooting and suckling reflexes are intact in a healthy newborn, successful breast-feeding is a learned talent for mother and infant. Neifert and Seacat[95] recommend that the infant be allowed to suckle for 5 minutes per breast per feeding the first day, 10 minutes the second day, and 15 minutes or more per breast per feeding thereafter. If suckling is interrupted before initiation of the let-down reflex, the likelihood of breast engorgement and nipple soreness is increased.

The initial breast engorgement that occurs on the second to fourth postpartum days is caused by lymphatic and vascular congestion, interstitial edema, and increased tension in the milk ducts. It is best managed with 24-hour demand feedings and, in stubborn cases, the use of oxytocin nasal spray to promote milk letdown. Hot compresses before nursing will facilitate letdown, and cold compresses between feedings may provide additional relief.

A common problem is nipple confusion, in which an infant accepts an artificial nipple but refuses the mother's nipple. This can be avoided by not offering supplemental fluids and by informing the mother of methods to make her nipple more protractile. Breast engorgement enhances this problem, but with patience it usually resolves within 24 to 48 hours.

Nipple soreness, another common complaint during the immediate puerperium, can be relieved by rotating breasts and the infant's position every 5 minutes while nursing; using frequent, shorter feedings rather than prolonged feeding times; avoiding irritating soaps, wet nursing pads, or other applications; and exposing the nipples for air-drying followed by the application of hydrous lanolin. In cases of persistent nipple soreness or of sudden appearance of nipple soreness after lactation has been established, *Candida* infection of the nipple must be considered.[95] The infection, which often occurs in association with thrush or *Candida* diaper rash, can be documented by culture; it responds promptly to applications of nystatin cream.

An empathetic and knowledgeable nursing staff is essential to successful breast-feeding by the mother who is attempting it for the first time. In the hospital, education and patient confidence can be facilitated with a brief videotape presentation about breast-feeding, which describes some of the problems that might be encountered and offers helpful solutions. Professional lactation counselors are often available to provide education and support in prenatal classes, during the immediate puerperium, and in the home following discharge from the hospital or birthing center. In many areas, the local chapter of the La Leche League will offer valuable advice to women who encounter problems with breast-feeding. Also, there are helpful Web sites on the Internet, such as *www.breastfeeding.com*.

Maternal Nutrition During Lactation

The impact of lactation on the nutritional status of the mother is well reviewed by Casey and Hambidge[96] and in the publication by the Institute of Medicine entitled *Nutrition During Lactation*.[97] A healthy mother breast-feeding a healthy infant will produce approximately 600 to 900 ml breast milk per day and will provide her infant with approximately 520 kcal/day. This requires about 600 kcal/day (including the energy required to produce the milk), which must be made up from the mother's diet or her body stores. For this purpose, the well-nourished woman stores about 5 kg of fat throughout pregnancy, which can be called on during lactation to make up any nutritional deficit.

The daily allowances of nutrients recommended for the mother during the first 6 months of lactation by the U.S. National Research Council[98] are listed in Table 21–1.

With the exception of iron and calcium, almost all of the other nutrients are provided in a well-balanced American diet. Even in situations in which there is obvious nutritional deprivation, the quantity and quality of breast milk seem to suffer very little. The composition of breast milk, however, can be influenced to some extent by the mother's diet. The protein content of breast milk is not influenced by the mother's diet, but the fat content is quite susceptible to dietary manipulation. Women who have diets in which the fat is largely of animal origin produce milk with high stearic acid content and low linoleic acid levels, whereas women

Table 21–1. DAILY ALLOWANCES OF NUTRIENTS RECOMMENDED FOR THE MOTHER DURING THE FIRST 6 MONTHS OF LACTATION*

Nutrients	Recommended Amount
Calories	2,500
Protein	65 g
Vitamin A	1,300 μg (retinol equiv.)
Vitamin D	10 μg (400 IU)
Vitamin E	12 mg (α-tocopherol equiv.)
Thiamine	1.6 mg
Riboflavin	1.8 mg
Niacin	20 mg (niacin equiv.)
Folacin	280 μg
Vitamin B_6	2.1 mg
Vitamin B_{12}	2.6 μg
Ascorbic acid	95 mg
Calcium	1,200 mg
Phosphorus	1,200 mg
Magnesium	355 mg
Iron	15 mg
Zinc	19 mg
Iodine	200 μg

* U.S. National Research Council recommendations.

with diets high in polyunsaturated fatty acids produce milk with high levels of linoleate. The importance of these differences on the subsequent health of breast-fed infants is unknown.

Levels of some but not all vitamins in breast milk can be influenced by maternal intake, but there is little evidence that breast milk in the otherwise well-nourished mother is vitamin deficient. Consequently, the need for vitamin supplementation for the lactating woman on a normal diet is not well established. Some vegetarians may have diets deficient in vitamin B_{12}, and vitamin B_{12} deficiency has been documented in a breast-fed infant of a vegetarian mother.[99] Also, infants of dark-skinned mothers who have had inadequate exposure to sunlight may become vitamin D deficient. This can be avoided by brief daily exposure to sunlight.[100]

Frequently, women inquire about the advisability of dieting and weight loss during lactation. Because of the increased metabolic rate and the increased energy requirements of lactating women, the appetite increases, leading to an increase in caloric intake. However, a persistent weight loss can be achieved through modest dietary restrictions without an untoward effect on the health of either the mother or the infant. Whichelow[101] found that lactating mothers who were losing weight had an average daily intake of 2,509 kcal, whereas women who were not losing weight consumed 2,946 kcal.

Bone mineral density decreases, especially in the spine, in women who breast-feed compared to those who do not. This is not affected by calcium supplementation; and bone mineral density returns to normal 12 months after lactation is discontinued.[49,102]

Contraindications to Breast-Feeding

There are very few contraindications to breast-feeding. Reduction mammoplasty with autotransplantation of the nipple simply makes breast-feeding impossible.

Puerperal infections, including acute mastitis, can be managed quite successfully while the mother continues to breast-feed. There is the possibility of transmitting certain viral infections in the breast milk, including cytomegalovirus, herpes simplex, hepatitis B virus (HBV), and human immunodeficiency virus (HIV). The morbidity of cytomegalovirus infection contracted by a healthy term neonate is sufficiently low that potentially infected mothers should not be discouraged from breast-feeding. Although one possible case of viral transmission in the breast milk occurred,[103] the source of neonatal herpes infection is surface contact with the virus; consequently, instruction of the mother in proper handwashing and care of possibly contaminated articles of clothing is sufficient to protect the infant and to permit continued breast-feeding. As regards HBV infection, McGregor and Neifert[103] recommend that breast-feeding not be

encouraged in women with acute hepatitis, hepatitis B/e antigenemia (HB_eAg), or other markers of heightened infectivity such as titers of HB_eAg over 1:1,000. However, breast-feeding is permissible in women without active HBV disease and certainly in the uncommon circumstance of an HB_eAg-positive newborn. Thus, most mothers with HBV infection before or during pregnancy can be supported in their decision to breast-feed. Women with chronic hepatitis C virus (HCV) infection may breast-feed their infants. A number of studies have found no evidence of transmission of HCV in breast milk.[105] HIV is present in breast milk, and the risk of vertical transmission is doubled if an infant breast-feeds.[106] In a randomized clinical trial conducted in Nairobi, Kenya, formula feeding significantly reduced HIV transmission to infants of infected mothers.[107] Consequently, in developed countries where there is not a high risk of newborn infectious disease associated with bottle feeding, breast-feeding is contraindicated for mothers with HIV infection.

Most medications taken by the mother will enter the breast milk to a small degree (see Chapter 9). Because of the short duration for which most medications are prescribed, however, and the minimal amounts of drug that reach the breast milk (usually in concentrations similar to or less than in maternal plasma), it is usually safe to recommend that the infant continue nursing. The pharmacokinetics of most drugs ingested by breast-feeding women are such that administration of the drug at the time of or immediately after the infant nurses will result in the lowest amount of drug in the milk at the subsequent feeding. If there is any doubt about the effect of a specific drug taken by a mother and whether she should continue breast-feeding, one should consult a recent reference about the effects of drugs in the nursing infant (see Chapter 9).[108,109]

Breast Milk for the Premature Infant

There are substantial data confirming the psychological, nutritional, and immunologic advantages to using a mother's breast milk to feed her premature infant. Preterm infants fed their mothers' milk will gain weight at the same rate as when they are fed formula.[110] Metabolic disturbances (azotemia, hyperaminoacidemia, and metabolic acidosis) are more frequent in infants receiving higher intakes of protein from formulas compared with human milk. Furthermore, the immunologically active constituents of breast milk (lactoferrin, lysozyme, lactoperoxidase, complement, leukocytes, and specific immunoglobulins) undoubtedly account for the lower incidence of infectious complications found in premature infants fed breast milk[109] (see Chapter 5).

In addition to the nutritional and immunologic[111] advantages of breast milk for the premature infant, there are the important psychological benefits for the mother.

Women who give birth to preterm infants often have a sense of guilt and failure. By providing breast milk, the mother takes an active part in the infant's daily care, which gives her a renewed sense of worth and importance.

In situations in which breast milk will be used for a premature infant, the mother must be instructed in the various methods of milk expression, collection, preservation, and transport. Most intensive care nurseries and many postpartum wards provide written instructions about milk expression and collection techniques.[112] A pump is more efficient and less time consuming than hand expression. Electric pumps, which simulate the physiologic suckling action of the infant, are available in many nurseries and can be leased from surgical supply companies or rental outlets. Often, the local chapter of the La Leche League will provide information on the availability of electric pumps. Hand pumps can also be used.

Occasionally, it is difficult to maintain an adequate milk supply using artificial expression. Hopkins et al.[113] have demonstrated that in mothers who have delivered prematurely, milk volume is inversely related to the delay in initiation of milk expression. Optimal milk production is associated with five or more milk expressions per day and pumping durations that exceed 100 min/day. Breast milk can be refrigerated for 24 hours at 1° to 5°C or frozen at −18° to −23°C for up to 3 months.

Complications of Breast-Feeding

The most common complication of breast-feeding is puerperal mastitis. This condition, which is characterized by fever, myalgias, and an area of pain and redness in either breast, usually has its onset before the end of the second postpartum week, but there is also an increase in its incidence in the fifth and sixth weeks postpartum. Niebyl et al.[114] reported 20 women in whom sporadic (nonepidemic) puerperal mastitis developed. The women were treated with penicillin V, ampicillin, or dicloxacillin and allowed to continue breast-feeding their infants. No abscess developed. This experience is similar to that of others,[115] who have found that in sporadic puerperal mastitis breast-feeding need not be discontinued. In fact, the combination of a penicillinase-resistant penicillin and continued breast-feeding will promptly result in resolution of the infection in 96 percent of cases.

From time to time, a patient will report problems with inadequate milk production, sometimes called *lactation failure*. This problem is usually caused by infrequent suckling, which can be corrected by shortening the interval between feedings. If the milk supply is inadequate in spite of these measures, endogenous suppression of prolactin may be the problem, as in the unusual situation of retained placental fragments inhibiting lactogenesis as described by Neifert et al.[116] Removal of the retained placental tissue by curettage will result in prompt resumption of milk production. In the absence of any obvious source of prolactin inhibition (e.g., ergot preparation, pyridoxine, or diuretics), pharmacologic enhancement of lactation should be considered. Metoclopramide (Reglan)[117] and sulpiride[118] have both been shown to enhance milk production, presumably by blocking dopamine receptors and stimulating prolactin secretion. Given in doses of 10 mg three or four times a day, metoclopramide may be helpful in stubborn cases of lactation failure.

Lactation Suppression

For those patients who for personal or medical reasons will not breast-feed, breast support, ice packs, and analgesic medications are helpful in ameliorating the symptoms of breast engorgement. The new mother should avoid suckling or other means of milk expression, and the natural inhibition of prolactin secretion will result in breast involution. In 30 to 50 percent of patients, this will be associated with breast engorgement and pain that may last for most of the first postpartum week.[119]

Bromocriptine is no longer approved by the Food and Drug Administration (FDA) for lactation suppression. This ergot derivative is a dopamine receptor agonist with prolonged action that inhibits the release of prolactin. Twenty-three percent of patients have side effects, including symptomatic hypotension, nausea, and vomiting, and 18 to 40 percent have rebound breast secretion, congestion, or engorgement following the termination of therapy.[120] Furthermore, there have been reports of puerperal stroke, seizures, and myocardial infarctions in association with the use of bromocriptine prescribed for lactation suppression.[121-124] While these events are rare and a causal relationship with bromocriptine has not been established, the manufacturers' prescription recommendations include instructions to avoid the use of this medication in patients with hypertensive complications of pregnancy and to monitor blood pressure periodically during the time the patient is using the drug. Consequently, it can be questioned whether it is prudent to use a medication for 2 weeks that has this incidence of side effects, possibly life-threatening complications, and the requirement for blood pressure monitoring during therapy. Puerperal breast engorgement, although painful, is never fatal and in most instances resolves within the first postpartum week.

PREGNANCY PREVENTION AND BIRTH CONTROL

The immediate postpartum period is a convenient time for a discussion of family planning with patients. Ideally, these conversations begin during prenatal care. The period of anovulation infertility lasts from 5 weeks in nonlactating women to 8 weeks or more in women who breast-feed their infants without supplementation.[13] The pregnancy rate during lactational amenorrhea is 1 percent at 1 year postpartum.[125] Robson et al.[126] found that most women have resumed intercourse by 3 months, and for some resumption of an active sexual life begins much earlier. Consequently, it is important that a decision be made about pregnancy prevention before the patient leaves the hospital.

A patient should be made aware of the various options of pregnancy prevention and birth control in terms that she and her partner can understand. This may be done by individual instruction from nurses, physicians, or physician assistants or by a variety of films or videotapes. The decision about family planning methods will depend on the patient's motivation, number of children, state of health, whether she is breast-feeding, and on the religious background of the couple. It cannot be assumed because a woman has used a method of contraception effectively before the current pregnancy that she will need no counseling thereafter. Debrovner and Winikoff[127] found that more than one half of patients change contraceptive techniques between pregnancies.

Natural Methods

The natural family planning methods, which depend on predicting the time of ovulation by use of basal body temperature or assessment of cervical mucus, cannot be used until regular menstrual cycles have resumed.[128] In the first weeks or months following birth, provided there is little or no supplemental feeding for the infant, breast-feeding will provide 98 percent contraceptive protection for up to 6 months. At 6 months, or if menses return, or if breast-feeding ceases to be full or nearly full before the sixth month, the risk of pregnancy increases.[129] Once regular menses have resumed, natural family planning methods, which depend on detection of the periovulation period using changes in cervical mucus or basal body temperature or both, can be employed. These techniques are associated with pregnancy rates very close to those for barrier methods of contraception, yet they are often overlooked, poorly understood, or misrepresented by health care workers who are not well educated in their use.[130]

Barrier Methods

Barrier methods of contraception and vaginal spermicides were long used in Europe and England before they were manufactured in this country beginning in the 1920s.[131] The failure rate for the diaphragm varies from 2.4 to 19.6 per 100 woman-years. Because this method of contraception requires substantial motivation, instruction, and experience, it is more effective in older women who are familiar with the technique. Vessey and Wiggins[132] found a failure rate of 2.4 per 100 woman-years among diaphragm users who were over 25 years old and who had a minimum of 5 months' experience using it. This pregnancy rate is comparable to that reported for intrauterine device users.

The proper size of the diaphragm should be determined at the 6-week postpartum visit, even in patients who previously used this form of contraception. In women who are breast-feeding, anovulation leads to vaginal dryness and tightness, which may make the proper fitting of a diaphragm more difficult than in women who are not lactating. The diaphragm should be used with one of the spermicidal lubricants, all of which contain nonoxynol-9.

The use of condoms alone or in combination with spermicides is often advised for women who wish to postpone a decision about sterilization or oral contraceptive therapy until the postpartum visit. Pregnancy rates for the condom are reported to be from 1.6 to 21 per 100 woman-years, depending on the age and motivation of the population studied.[133]

Steroid Contraceptive Medications

The combined estrogen-progestin preparations have proved to be the most effective method of contraception, with pregnancy rates reported as less than 0.5 per 100 woman-years. Most compounds include 35 μg or less of estrogen and varying amounts of progestins. Compounds containing the progestational components desogestrel, gestodene, or norgestimate appear to be less androgenic and have less impact on carbohydrate and lipid metabolism than compounds containing levonorgestrel or norethindrone.[134] Cardiovascular complications, including hypertension, venous thrombosis, stroke, and myocardial infarction, have been substantially reduced with the reduction in estrogen content. The cardiovascular complications are found predominantly in women who smoke.[135] In nonsmoking women, the risk benefit ratio is clearly in favor of using oral contraceptive agents. This is particularly true when the additional benefits of these agents are considered, which include lowered risks of benign breast disease, ovarian and endometrial cancer, iron deficiency anemia, toxic shock syndrome, pelvic inflammatory disease, and ectopic pregnancy.[136]

In patients who are not breast-feeding, oral contraceptive agents can be taken as early as 2 to 3 weeks after delivery. The effect of oral contraceptive agents on lactation is controversial. Controlled studies of the combined-type oral contraceptive agents with doses of ethinyl estradiol or mestranol of 50 μg or more demonstrated a suppressive effect on lactation. Progestin-only medications (e.g., norethindrone 0.35 mg every day) do not diminish lactation performance and may, in fact, increase the quality and duration of lactation.[137] While there is no direct evidence that has related lactation failure to the administration of progestin-only contraceptive agents taken before the onset of lactation, it is recommended that the use of these medications be delayed until lactation has been established.[138] Also, progestin-only oral contraceptives should be avoided in Hispanic women with gestational diabetes who are breast-feeding, because of an increased risk for the subsequent development of type II diabetes.[139]

Diaz et al.[140] studied the effect of a low-dose combination oral contraceptive containing 0.03 mg ethinyl estradiol and 0.15 mg levonorgestrel. The medication was begun after all women had been nursing for 1 month. Among those women taking the oral contraceptive medications, there was a small but significant decrease in lactation performance and in the weight gain of their infants compared with controls. In women whose motivation to breast-feed is marginal, the slight inhibition of lactation induced by oral contraceptive agents may be sufficient to discourage them from continuing to nurse their infants, and so progestin-only preparations should be offered to these women. Depot medroxyprogesterone acetate (DMPA) 150 mg intramuscularly every 3 months, which has a contraceptive efficiency exceeding 99 percent, is used by many women following delivery.[141] The most annoying side effect is unpredictable spotting and bleeding. Long-term DMPA use has been associated with reversible reduction in bone density and unfavorable changes in lipid metabolism. The major advantages of this form of contraception are the ease of administration and patient convenience.

Levonorgestrel subdermal implants were approved by the FDA for contraceptive use in the United States in 1990. Each implant consists of six Silastic capsules that contain 36 mg of crystalline levonorgestrel. Although not as yet commercially available in the United States, a delivery system involving two levonorgestrel-containing rods has been tested and found to be equally effective for contraception but easier to insert and remove than the six-capsule system.[142] Pregnancy rates in women using the implants are lower than with any other reversible contraception.[143] Implants inserted 4 weeks after delivery have no effect on lactation or growth of an infant who is nursing even though small amounts of levonorgestrel are excreted in the milk. Although the usual time of insertion is 4 to 6 weeks following delivery, the implants can be inserted in the immediate puerperium or, in women who are breast-feeding, as soon as lactation is established. Irregular uterine bleeding, expense, and the occasional difficulty in removing the implants are the major drawbacks to the use of this form of contraception. Despite the proven contraceptive effectiveness of levonorgestrel implants, there has been a decline in the perceived desirability of this method of birth control in recent years.[144]

Intrauterine Devices

The copper-containing TCu 380 Ag IUD (copper-T IUD, ParaGard T380A) and the progesterone-releasing device (Progestasert) are highly effective in preventing pregnancy (2 to 3 pregnancies per 100 woman-years).[145,146] The advantage of the copper-containing IUD is that it is effective for 10 years; its disadvantage is an increase in irregular uterine bleeding. The device that releases progesterone reduces uterine bleeding, but it must be replaced annually.

The biologic action of IUDs is a matter of concern to those who might object to this method if its principal action is prevention of implantation of the blastocyst. The investigations of Alvarez et al.[147] convincingly support the concept that the principal mode of action of IUDs is by a method other than destruction of live embryos. Both the World Health Organization (WHO) and the American College of Obstetricians and Gynecologists (ACOG) have reviewed the evidence and concluded that the IUD is not an abortifacient.[148]

The pregnancy rate with an IUD is reported to be between 1 and 6 per 100 woman-years, with expulsion rates being 4 to 18 and removal for medical reasons being 12 to 16 per 100 women during the first year of use.[149] Addition of bioactive materials such as copper or progesterone to the IUD has not significantly reduced pregnancy rates but has reduced the risk of expulsion or abnormal bleeding.

The major side effects and complications are syncope and uterine perforation during insertion, abnormal uterine bleeding, uterine and pelvic infection, and ectopic pregnancy.[110] Syncope is a result of the vagal response that occurs in some women at the time of IUD insertion. Patients with a history of syncope or severe menstrual pain may be at greater risk from a complication, and the use of sedatives, analgesics, or atropine should be considered. These reactions are less common when the IUD is inserted in the puerperium, because functionally the cervix is slightly dilated.

Uterine perforation occurs in 0 to 8 per 1,000 insertions and is highest when the insertion is performed from 1 to 8 weeks after delivery. This is an important consideration when the insertion of the device is planned for the 6-week postpartum visit. If there is any doubt about adequate involution of the uterus, IUD insertion should be postponed for 2 to 3 additional weeks. However, Mishell and Roy[150] demonstrated no increase in perforation with the use of the copper-T inserted 4 to 8 weeks after delivery using a withdrawal method for insertion which appears to reduce the risk of this complication.

Bleeding and uterine cramping occur in 8 to 10 percent of women using an IUD and account for 4 to 15 removals of the device per 100 women in the first year of use. The causes of these symptoms are unknown, although they may be caused by the local production of proteolytic enzymes and prostaglandins within the endometrium adjacent to the IUD. A variety of methods have been used to treat this complication, including the use of hormones, vitamins, and prostaglandin synthetase inhibitors, but there are no data establishing the effectiveness of any of these measures.

The relative risk of pelvic infection in IUD users ranges from 1.7 to 9.3. A variety of microorganisms have been implicated, including *Actinomyces* in rare cases. Prompt removal of the device and antibiotic therapy are recommended when there is any evidence of salpingitis. However, in parous women who have used the IUD, the risk of infertility caused by pelvic infection is no greater than in patients who have never used an IUD.[151]

Although the overall risk of ectopic pregnancy is lower in women using the IUD when compared with women using no contraception, the chances that a pregnancy will be ectopic is 7 to 10 times higher in the IUD user.

There has been some enthusiasm for insertion of the IUD during the immediate postpartum period. Surprisingly, this practice is associated with fewer perforations than are insertions between 1 and 8 weeks. Not surprising, however, is the finding that much higher expulsion rates are noted (10 to 21 percent).[152]

The IUD has been found to be a satisfactory method of birth control in women who are breast-feeding. In a multicenter study, Cole et al.[153] observed that breast-feeding did not increase the risk of expulsion or other complications regardless of the time of insertion of the device.

Sterilization

Tubal sterilization is the most frequently used method of contraception in the United States.[154] The puerperium is a convenient time for tubal ligation procedures to be performed in women who desire sterilization. The procedure can be performed at the time of a cesarean delivery or within the first 24 to 48 hours after delivery. In some hospitals the operation is performed immediately after delivery in uncomplicated patients, especially when epidural anesthesia was given for labor analgesia. With the use of small paraumbilical incision, the procedure seldom prolongs the patient's hospitalization.

The 10-year failure rate of postpartum partial salpingectomy is 0.75 percent.[155] There are several modifications of this procedure: the Pomeroy, Parkland, Uchida, and Irving (see Chapter 19).[156,159] There are also reports of immediate postpartum sterilization with the laparoscope,[160] but this method lacks widespread enthusiasm. Because of the relaxed abdominal wall and the easy accessibility of the fallopian tubes, the minilaparotomy has the advantages of convenience and speed without the possible risks of visceral injury that might occur with the trocar of the laparoscope.

Perhaps more important than the type of procedure is the decision about the timing of the procedure or whether it should be performed at all. Puerperal sterilization compared with interval sterilization is associated with increased incidence of guilt and regret.[161] With increasing frequency, couples are postponing tubal ligation procedures until 6 to 8 weeks after delivery. This provides time to ensure that the infant is healthy and to review all the implications of the decision. In most patients, laparoscopic tubal ligation can be accomplished as an outpatient procedure with a minimum of morbidity or loss of time from work or family.

The risks of tubal ligation procedures, whether performed in the puerperium or as an interval procedure, include the short-term problems of anesthetic accidents, hemorrhage, injury of the viscera, and infection. These complications are infrequent, and deaths from the procedure occur in 2 to 12 per 100,000 procedures. Long-term complications are less well defined and more controversial. About 10 to 15 percent of patients will have irregular menses and increased menstrual pain after tubal sterilization. This so-called posttubal syndrome is sufficiently severe in some cases to require hysterectomy. Well-controlled prospective studies, however, have failed to provide convincing evidence that these symptoms occur more commonly after tubal sterilization than in control patients of the same age and previous menstrual history.[162,163]

There has also been concern about poststerilization depression.[164] Because depression is common in women of childbearing age and is even more common in the puerperium, it is difficult to know whether sterilization procedures are independent risk factors for depression. It is obvious, however, that the loss of fertility associated with a sterilization procedure will have important conscious and subconscious implications for many women. It is therefore not surprising that some patients manifest transient grief reactions in response to tubal ligation. The loss of libido that may occur in such situations may be frightening to some women and equally disturbing to their partners. Reassurance that such reactions are temporary and are not necessarily symptoms of a seriously disturbed psyche is an important means of support during this crisis. Both partners must be aware of the dynamics of this situation to avoid a sense of estrangement.

Obstetricians must remember that vasectomy is often a more advisable and desirable alternative for a couple considering sterilization.[165,166] It can be performed as an outpatient procedure under local anesthesia with insignificant loss of time from work or family. Furthermore, almost all the failures (about 3 to 4 per 1,000 procedures) can be detected by a postoperative semen analysis. This is a decided advantage over the tubal ligation, in which failures are discovered only when a pregnancy occurs. Furthermore, vasectomy is less expensive and overall is associated with fewer complications. In addition, women whose husbands undergo vasectomy are less likely to have hysterectomies than are women who have had tubal sterilization.[167] Studies of long-term health effects of vasectomy found no evidence of an increased risk of atherosclerotic heart disease or other chronic illnesses.[165,168]

Tubal ligation can be reversed, but a patient should not undergo sterilization if she is contemplating reversal. Success as measured by the occurrence of pregnancy following tubal reanastamosis varies from 40 to 85 percent, depending on the type of tubal ligation performed and on the length of functioning tube that remains. Success rates for vas reanastamosis vary from 37 to 90 percent, with higher success rates being associated with shorter intervals from the time of vas ligation.

Hysterectomy has been advocated as a means of sterilization that has the advantage of protecting the patient from future uterine or cervical cancer. However, the morbidity of cesarean or puerperal hysterectomy operations is sufficiently great to preclude their consideration for elective sterilization.[169]

POSTPARTUM PSYCHOLOGICAL REACTIONS

The psychological reactions experienced following childbirth include the common, relatively mild, physiologic, and transient "maternity blues" (50 to 70 percent of women). True depression occurs in 8 to 20 percent, and frank puerperal psychosis occurs in 0.14 to 0.26 percent. Although the specific etiology of these psychological disorders is unknown, they are not a continuum of progressively severe manifestations of a single underlying disorder. Although psychologic and psychiatric symptoms often fall along a continuum, the specific diseases of postpartum depression and postpartum psychosis are quite different.

Maternity Blues

Maternity blues is a common psychological manifestation of the puerperium. It is manifest by a transient state of tearfulness, anxiety, irritation, and restlessness, variously described as "maternity blues" or "postpartum blues." As it occurs in up to 70 percent of parturients,[170] it might well be considered a normal involutional phenomenon. The symptoms may appear on any day within the first week after delivery and usually have resolved by postpartum day 10. Occasional patients will note transient recurrence of the symptoms, especially weeping, for several weeks after delivery.[171] Also, as might be expected, the disruptive sleep patterns in the first weeks following delivery have been shown to contribute to an increase in dysphoric mood experienced by women during this time.[172]

Patients suffering from maternity blues manifest a wide range of symptoms, including weeping, depression, restlessness, elation, mood lability, headache, confusion, forgetfulness, irritability, depersonalization, insomnia, and negative feelings toward their infants. Not every patient experiences all these symptoms.

There appear to be no obstetric, social, economic, or personality correlates for maternity blues. While it is tempting to ascribe the symptoms of this syndrome to the changes in steroid hormone levels that occur immediately following delivery, no such correlation has been found.[173] However, lower than expected tryptophan levels have been documented in association with the depressive symptoms in the immediate postpartum period, suggesting a role for neurotransmitters in the elaboration of puerperal mood changes.[174] Hyperactivity of the hypothalamic-pituitary-adrenal axis, blunted responsiveness of the hypothalamic-pituitary-thyroid axis, and altered central neurotransmitter function characterize postpartum depression as well as nonpuerperal major depression.[175] Behavioral psychiatrists have theorized that the "blues" may represent a transient response to the rapid role changes and psychologic tasks that occur after delivery.

Because the syndrome is transient and of short duration, no therapy is indicated. Some of the symptoms may be exacerbated by sleep deprivation, and increased rest may be helpful. Anticipatory explanation and a sympathetic and understanding attitude on the part of family members and those caring for the patient are all that are required for this troublesome and common mood change.

Postpartum Depression

The incidence of postpartum major depression varies from 8 to 20 percent.[176-178] This affective disorder occurs after pregnancies of all duration, from spontaneous abortions to full-term deliveries. The depression varies from mild to a suicidal depression. It may occur anytime after delivery up to 1 year postpartum. Symptoms most commonly begin in the first 4 to 6 weeks after delivery. Pitt[178] was one of the first to document the incidence of neurotic depression in the puerperium. He found that 11 percent of the patients studied at 28 weeks' gestation and at 6 weeks after delivery developed new cases of depression during the postpartum period.

Much research has been done in an attempt to clarify the etiology of postpartum depression. Significant alterations in levels of estrogen, progesterone, prolactin, and cortisol are not different in women suffering from depression and controls. However, changes in the hypothalamic-pituitary-adrenal axis, including corticotropin-releasing hormone, may occur in women with postpartum depression.[179,180] In a study of 128 women randomly selected and interviewed on several occasions during their pregnancies and for 1 year after birth, Watson et al. found that it was unusual for postpartum depression to occur in a patient with an otherwise psychologically uncomplicated pregnancy and past history. They also confirmed a lack of association between postnatal depression and social class, marital status, or parity. Not surprisingly, several authors have found an increased incidence of postpartum depression after pregnancy loss.[182]

The signs and symptoms of postpartum depression are not different from those in nonpregnant patients, but may be difficult to differentiate from normal involutional phenomena (e.g., weight loss, sleeplessness) or from the transient "maternity blues."[183] However, in addition to the more common symptoms of depression, the postpartum patient may manifest a sense of incapability of loving her family and manifest ambivalence toward her infant.

There is a high risk of recurrence (50 to 100 percent) of postpartum depression in subsequent pregnancies and a 20 to 30 percent risk of postpartum depression in women who have had a previous depressive reaction not associated with pregnancy. Consequently, it is important to inquire about depression as well as psychiatric illness when taking the prenatal history. Importantly, a family history of depression is also a risk factor.

There are a number of questionnaires that may help to identify the antepartum patient who is at high risk for postpartum major depression.[184] Several investigators have found that one or more of the characteristics listed in the box (Characteristics of Antenatal Patients that Increase the Risk For Major Postpartum Depression) should be a cause for concern that a patient is at increased risk for postpartum major depression.[185,186] It is appropriate that questions addressing some of these risk factors as well as the simple inquiry "Are you happy?" be incorporated into the antenatal history.

In addition to a family or personal history of depression, and difficult social situations, adverse pregnancy

Characteristics of Antenatal Patients that Increase the Risk for Major Postpartum Depression

Under 20 years of age

Unmarried

Medically indigent

Comes from a family of six or more children

Separated from one or both parents in childhood or adolescence

Received poor parental support and attention in childhood

Had limited parental support in adulthood

Has poor relationship with husband or boyfriend

Has economic problem with housing or income

Is dissatisfied with amount of education

Shows evidence of emotional problem, past or present

Has low self-esteem

Data from Posner et al.[185]

outcomes are also associated with an increased incidence of postpartum depression. Behavioral psychiatrists have postulated that the increased stress associated with complications leads to a greater strain on the mother's compensatory defenses and thus depression develops. Pregnancy complications associated with postpartum depression include miscarriage, fetal demise, and neonatal death. Cesarean delivery is not associated with an increased risk.

Puerperal hypothyroidism often presents with symptoms including mild dysphoria; consequently, thyroid function studies may be useful in patients presenting with suspected postpartum depression. However, the onset associated with thyroid disease is often a few months after delivery.[187]

Early recognition of the signs and symptoms and supportive care and reassurrance from family and health care professionals are the first line of treatment. The most well-validated tool for identifying patients in the puerperium who are high risk for depression is the Edinburgh Postnatal Depression Scale (EPDS).[188] This is a short, 10-question scale. Because of the long-term effects of postpartum depression, as well as the high incidence of this disease, some authors have called for population-based screening using the EPDS.[189] Women with a score of 12 or greater are very likely to have major depression and deserve careful clinical assessment to establish the diagnosis. Also, women with risk factors such as a family history of depression, or difficult social situations, should be cautioned about symptoms

Edinburgh Postnatal Depression Scale (EPDS)

In the past 7 days:

1. I have been able to laugh and see the funny side of things:
   As much as I always could
   Not quite so much now
   Definitely not so much now
   Not at all

2. I have looked forward with enjoyment to things:
   As much as I ever did
   Rather less than I used to
   Definitely less than I used to
   Hardly at all

3. **I have blamed myself unnecessarily when things went wrong:**
   Yes, most of the time
   Yes, some of the time
   Not very often
   No, never

4. **I have been anxious or worried for no good reason:**
   No, not at all
   Hardly ever
   Yes, sometimes
   Yes, very often

5. **I have felt scared or panicky for no very good reason:**
   Yes, quite a lot
   Yes, sometimes
   No, not much
   No, not at all

6. **Things have been getting on top of me:**
   Yes, most of the time I haven't been able to cope at all
   Yes, sometimes I haven't been coping as well as usual
   No, most of the time I have coped quite well
   No, I have been coping as well as ever

7. **I have been so unhappy that I have had difficulty sleeping:**
   Yes, most of the time
   Yes, sometimes
   Not very often
   No, not at all

8. **I have felt sad or miserable:**
   Yes, most of the time
   Yes, quite often
   Not very often
   No, not at all

9. **I have been so unhappy that I have been crying:**
   Yes, most of the time
   Yes, quite often
   Only occasionally
   No, never

10. **The thought of harming myself has occurred to me:**
    Yes, quite often
    Sometimes
    Hardly ever
    Never

Response categories are scored 0, 1, 2, and 3 according to increased severity of the symptom. Items in bold type are reverse scored (3, 2, 1, 0). The total score is calculated by adding together the scores for each of the 10 items.

From Cox JL, Holden JM, Sagovsky R: Detection of postnatal depression. Development of the 10-item Edinburgh Postnatal Depression Scale. Br J Psychiatry 150:782, 1987, with permission.

of depression, and visits at 2 and or 4 weeks postpartum should be considered.

Treatment for postpartum depression should be begun early. Optimal treatment includes both counseling and medications. In the past, tricyclic antidepressants (nortriptyline or desipramine) have been noted to be helpful, but recent studies suggest that serotonin uptake inhibitors (fluoxetine, paroxetine, or sertraline) are equally effective and have fewer side effects.[190,191] These agents are considered safe for breast-feeding. Other treatments include the estrogen patch.[192] In women with a previous episode of postpartum depression, it has been suggested that prophylactic serotonin selective reuptake inhibitor (SSRI) medications be started 2 to 3 weeks prior to delivery. This approach allows these drugs to achieve an effective level by the postpartum period.[193] If there is no prompt response to general supportive measures and initial use of medication, psychiatric consultation is advisable. The prognosis for treated postpartum depression is good, although symptoms may persist for up to a year. Unfortunately, untreated postpartum depression has significant consequences. Depression may progress to frank suicidal psychosis. Less severe depression has been noted in multiple studies to have long-term effects on the infants of depressed mothers. These effects include behavioral changes, cognitive changes, and emotional reactions that are different than control infants and children.[186,194] Vandenberg[195] emphasizes the importance of the family in the therapy of postpartum depression. Being physically and emotionally drained from the stresses of pregnancy and childbirth and further burdened by the incessant demands of her infant, the postpartum patient may be unable to meet the demands of her husband and the other children. This will compound her feeling of self-worthlessness. Helping the husband and other family members to understand the nature of the patient's illness and mobilizing resources to provide the patient with help with her home chores and the care of the other children will help to prevent her sense of entrapment and isolation.

If a patient is at high risk for developing postpartum depression or if suspicious signs or symptoms develop during the immediate postpartum period, it is mandatory that the postpartum visits be scheduled sooner than the traditional 6 weeks. The moderately depressed mother will often experience such guilt and embarrassment secondary to her sense of failure in her mothering role that she will be unable to call her physician or admit the symptoms of her depression.[195] Consequently, ample time must be set aside to explore in depth even the slightest symptoms or sign of depression. Home visits in this situation may be appropriate to assess the patient. When a patient calls with a seemingly innocuous question, she should be asked two or three open-ended questions about her general status. These questions allow the patient to open up if there is an underlying depression that she is too guilty or afraid to express initially; for example:

1. How do you feel things are going?
2. How are things with the baby?
3. Are you feeling like you expected?

Because nursing staff often triage phone calls for physicians and midwives, it is important that such personnel be instructed to be alert to this protocol. Additionally, we recommend that both parents be warned prior to hospital discharge that if the maternity blues seem to be lasting longer than 2 weeks, or become "too tough" to handle, then either partner should call.

Postpartum Psychosis

Schizophrenia is seen with increased frequency in the puerperium, suggesting that there is a psychosis specific to the postpartum condition. It may occur in up to 0.1 percent of women with a past history of psychosis or a family history. Symptoms usually become manifest in the first 2 to 3 days postpartum, but may occur up to several months after delivery. In a study of all patients giving birth in 1966 and 1967 in Southamptom, England, Nott[196] documented a significant increase in psychiatric referrals for specific psychoses in the 16 weeks after delivery. This confirmed the observation by Kendall et al.,[197] who found a significant increase in admission to psychiatric hospitals during the puerperium compared with the antepartum or the nonpregnant state.

There is considerable debate as to whether the psychotic reactions that occur in the puerperium represent a unique psychiatric entity.[198] The signs and symptoms differ only slightly from those of acute, nonpuerperal psychosis. Postpartum psychosis is usually manifest by an increased degree of anxiety and a more "organic sense" of symptomatology versus nonpuerperal psychosis, which appears much more as a purer thought disorder. The frequency of symptoms differs substantially as well. Some patients with puerperal psychosis are manic-depressive. Women with bipolar disease have a higher than expected recurrence in the postpartum period. They may present with confusion and disorientation as prominent features of the clinical presentation. Furthermore, the psychotic reactions occurring in the puerperium appear to have a more favorable prognosis than the nonpuerperal psychosis. If the duration of the illness is only 2 or 3 months, and manifest by greater affective symptoms, then the prognosis is more favorable for long-term recovery.

During the immediate postpartum period, the early signs of depression may be difficult to distinguish from "maternity blues," but if suicidal thoughts or attempts occur, or if frankly delusional thoughts are expressed, the diagnosis of postpartum psychosis can be made.[195]

Clearly, all patients with puerperal psychosis require hospitalization for at least initial evaluation and institution of therapy. However, specific therapeutic management of puerperal psychotic disorders is a matter of controversy because of the lack of properly conducted treatment trials in these disorders.[198] Antipsychotic agents, eletroconvulsive therapy, antidepressants, neuroleptic, and lithium carbonate have all been recommended for specific subgroups of puerperal psychosis, but none has been proven to enhance recovery. There is recent evidence, however, that sublingual estradiol (1 mg 3–6 times daily) results in substantial improvement in patients with postpartum psychosis.[199] Whatever therapy for these conditions is instituted, it should be conducted or supervised by a psychiatrist.

Women with postpartum psychosis should be supervised at all times. These patients have a 5 percent rate of suicide, and a 5 percent rate of infanticide!

MANAGING PERINATAL GRIEVING

For the most part, perinatal events are happy ones and are occasions for rejoicing. When a patient and her family experience a loss associated with a pregnancy, special attention must be given to the grieving patient and her family.

The most obvious cases of perinatal loss are those in which a fetal or neonatal death has occurred. Other more subtle losses can be associated with a significant amount of grieving, such as the birth of a critically ill or malformed infant, an unexpected hysterectomy performed for intractable postpartum hemorrhage, or even a planned postpartum sterilization procedure. Grief will occur with any significant loss whether it is the actual death of an infant or the loss of an idealized child in the case of the birth of a handicapped infant.[200]

Mourning is as old as the human race, but the clinical signs and symptoms of grief and their psychological ramifications as they relate to loss suffered by women during their pregnancies have been given special consideration in recent years. In studying the relatives of servicemen who died in World War II, Lindemann[201] recognized five manifestations of normal grieving. These include somatic symptoms of sleeplessness, fatigue, digestive symptoms, and sighing respirations; preoccupation with the image of the deceased; feelings of guilt; feelings of hostility and anger toward others; and disruption of the normal pattern of daily life. He also described the characteristics of what is now recognized as pathologic grief, which may occur if acute mourning is suppressed or interrupted. Some of the manifestations of this so-called morbid grief reaction are overactivity without a sense of loss; appearance or exacerbations of psychosomatic illness; alterations in relationships with friends and relatives; furious hostility toward specific persons; lasting loss of patterns of social interaction; activities detrimental to personal, social, and economic existence; and agitated depression.

Kennel et al.[202] studied the reaction of 20 mothers to the loss of their newborn infants. Characteristic signs and symptoms of mourning occurred in all the patients, even in situations in which the infant was nonviable. Similar grief reactions occurred in most of the parents of 101 critically ill infants who survived after referral to a regional neonatal intensive care unit,[203] showing that separation from a seriously ill newborn is sufficient to provoke typical grief reaction.

It is important that the characteristics of the grieving patient be recognized and understood by health professionals caring for such patients; otherwise, substantial misunderstanding and mismanagement of the patient will occur. For example, if the patient's reaction of anger and hostility is not anticipated, a nurse or physician may take personally statements or actions by the patient or her family and avoid the patient at the very time she needs the most consolation and support. Because of their own discomfort with the implications of death, physicians, nurses, and others on the postpartum unit often find it uncomfortable to deal with patients whose fetus or infant has died. As a consequence, there

is a reluctance to discuss the death with the patient and a tendency to rely on the use of sedatives or tranquilizers to deal with the patient's symptoms of grief.[204-206] What is actually beneficial at such a time is a sympathetic listener and an opportunity to express and discuss feelings of guilt, anger, and hopelessness and the other symptoms of mourning.

It is not surprising that postpartum depression is more common and more severe in families that have suffered a perinatal loss. In one study, the prolonged grief response occurred more often in those women who became pregnant within 5 months of the death of the infant.[207] This finding suggests that in counseling women after the loss of an infant, one should avoid the traditional advice of encouraging the family to embark soon on another pregnancy as a "replacement" for the infant who died. Just how long the normal grief reaction lasts is not known, and surely it varies with different families. Lockwood and Lewis[208] studied 26 patients who had suffered a stillbirth; they followed several patients for as long as 2 years. Their data suggest that grief in this situation is usually resolved within 18 months, invariably with a resurgence of symptoms at the first anniversary of the loss.

Somatic symptoms of grief, such as anorexia, weakness, and fatigue, are now well recognized; other psychological manifestations are also reported. Spontaneous abortion and infertility increase among couples who attempt to conceive after the loss of an infant.[209] Schleifer et al.[210] found significant suppression of lymphocyte stimulation in the spouses of women with advanced breast carcinoma. Although the most intense suppression was noted within the month after bereavement, a modified response was noted for as long as 14 months. These investigators suggest that this may account for the increase in morbidity and mortality associated with bereavement.

The regionalization of perinatal health care has resulted in a large proportion of the perinatal deaths occurring in tertiary centers. In some of these centers teams of physicians, nurses, social workers, and pastoral counselors have evolved to aid specifically in the management of families suffering a perinatal loss.[211-214] While this approach ensures an enlightened, understanding, and consistent approach to bereaved families, it suggests that the support of a grieving patient is a highly complex endeavor, to be accomplished only by a few specially trained individuals who care for postpartum patients. Enlightened and compassionate counseling of parents who have suffered a perinatal loss may be accomplished by any of the mother's health care professionals by using the guidelines listed in the box (Guidelines for Managing Perinatal Loss).[214] Clearly, management of grief is not solely a postpartum responsibility. This is particularly true when a prenatal diagnosis is made of fetal death or fetal abnormality. A

Guidelines for Managing Perinatal Loss

Keep parents informed; be honest and forthright.

Recognize and facilitate anticipatory grieving.

Inform parents about the grieving process.

Encourage support person to remain with the mother throughout labor.

Encourage the mother to make as many choices about her care as possible.

Support parents in seeing, touching, or holding the infant.

Describe the infant in detail, especially for couples who choose not to see the infant.

Allow photographs of the infant.

Prepare the couple for hospital paperwork, such as autopsy requests.

Discuss funeral or memorial services.

Assist the couple in how to inform siblings, relatives, and friends.

Discuss subsequent pregnancy.

Liberal use of follow-up home or office visits.

Modified from Kowalski K: Managing perinatal loss. Clin Obstet Gynecol 23:1113, 1980.

continuum of support is essential as the patient moves from the prenatal setting, to labor and delivery, to the postpartum ward, and finally to her home. Relaxation of many of the traditional hospital routines may be necessary to provide the type of support these families need. For example, allowing a loved one to remain past visiting hours, providing a couple a private setting to be with their deceased infant, or allowing unusually early discharge with provisions for frequent phone calls and follow-up visits will often facilitate the resolution of grief.

It is also important to realize that the fathers of infants who die have somewhat different grief responses than do the mothers. In a study of 28 fathers who had lost infants, Mandell et al.[215] found their grief characterized by the necessity to keep busy with increased work, feelings of diminished self-worth, self-blame, and limited ability to ask for help. Stoic responses are typical of men and may obstruct the normal resolution of grief.

Postpartum Posttraumatic Stress

Posttraumatic stress disorder may occur after any physical or psychological trauma. It may lead to behavioral sequelae including flashbacks, avoidance, and inability to function. Emergency operative deliveries, both vaginal and abdominal, and severe unexpected pain have been reported to have produced posttraumatic stress. The reaction may lead to fear of a subsequent delivery that may become incapacitating, as well as generalized symptoms of this disorder. Whenever an emergency procedure is indicated, debriefing afterwards, both early and a few weeks later, may help to decrease the incidence of this problem. Women with adverse outcomes frequently will experience transference of their previous experience as the next delivery approaches.[216–219]

Key Points

➤ By 6 weeks postpartum, 28 percent of women will have returned to their prepregnant weight.

➤ Approximately 50 percent of parturients experience diminished sexual desire during the 3 months following delivery.

➤ Postpartum uterine bleeding of sufficient quantity to require medical attention occurs in 1 to 2 percent of parturients. In patients requiring curettage, 40 percent will be found to have retained placental tissue.

➤ Late-onset endometritis (after 7 days) is frequently caused by *Chlamydia trachomatis*.

➤ *Candida* infection is a common cause of persistent nipple soreness in women who are breast-feeding.

➤ Most women with puerperal mastitis can be adequately prepared with penicillin V, ampicillin, or dicloxacillin while they continue to breast-feed their infants.

➤ Breast-feeding will result in 98 percent contraceptive protection for up to 6 months following delivery, provided there is little or no supplemental feeding of the infant.

➤ Progestin-only contraceptive medication (norethindrone 0.35 mg daily) does not diminish lactation performance.

➤ Postpartum, major depression occurs in 8 to 20 percent of parturients.

➤ Puerperal hypothyroidism often presents with symptoms that include mild dysphoria; consequently, thyroid function studies are suggested in the evaluation of patients with suspected postpartum depression that occurs 2 to 3 months after delivery.

REFERENCES

1. Hytten FE, Cheyne GA: The size and composition of the human pregnant uterus. J Obstet Gynaecol Br Commonw 76: 400, 1969.
2. Williams JS: Regeneration of the uterine mucosa after delivery, with special reference to the placental site. Am J Obstet Gynecol 122:664, 1931.
3. Sharman A: Postpartum regeneration of the human endometrium. J Anat 87:1, 1953.
4. Anderson WR, Davis J: Placental site involution. Am J Obstet Gynecol 102:23, 1968.
5. Willms AB, Brown ED, Kettritz UI, et al: Anatomic changes in the pelvis after uncomplicated vaginal delivery: evaluation with serial MR imaging. Radiology 195:91, 1995.
6. Lavery JP, Shaw LA: Sonography of the puerperal uterus. J Ultrasound 8:481, 1989.
7. van Rees D, Bernstine RL, Crawford W: Involution of the postpartum uterus: an ultrasonic study. J Clin Ultrasound 9:5, 1981.
8. Garagiola DM, Tarver RD, Gibson L, et al: Anatomic changes in the pelvis after uncomplicated delivery: a CT study on 14 women. AJR Am J Roengenol 153:1239, 1989.
9. Oppenheimer LS, Sheriff EA, Goodman JDS, et al: The duration of lochia. Br J Obstet Gynaecol 93:754, 1986.
10. Visness CM, Kennedy KI, Ramos R: The duration and character of postpartum bleeding among breast-feeding women. Obstet Gynecol 89:159, 1997.
11. Lipinski JK, Adam AH: Ultrasonic prediction of complications following normal vaginal delivery. J Clin Ultrasound 9: 17, 1981.
12. Chang YL, Madrozo B, Drukker BH: Ultrasonic evaluation of the postpartum uterus in management of postpartum bleeding. Obstet Gynecol 58:227, 1981.
13. Glass M, Rosenthal AH: Cervical changes in pregnancy, labor and puerperium. Am J Obstet Gynecol 60:353, 1950.
14. Coppleson M, Reid BL: A colposcopic study of the cervix during pregnancy and the puerperium. J Obstet Gynaecol Br Commonw 73:575, 1966.
15. McLaren HC: The involution of the cervix. Br Med J 1:347, 1952.
16. Andrews MC: Epithelial changes in the puerperal fallopian tube. Am J Obstet Gynecol 62:28, 1951.
17. Cronin TJ: Influence of lactation upon ovulation. Lancet 2: 422, 1968.
18. Perex A, Uela P, Masnick GS, et al: First ovulation after childbirth: the effect of breast feeding. Am J Obstet Gynecol 114:1041, 1972.
19. Gray RH, Campbell ON, Apelo R, et al: Risk of ovulation during lactation. Lancet 335:25, 1990.
20. Bonnar J, Franklin M, Nott PN, et al: Effect of breast-feeding on pituitary-ovarian function after childbirth. Br Med J 4:82, 1975.
21. Crowell DT: Weight change in the postpartum period: a review of the literature. J Nurse Midwifery 40:418, 1995.
22. Scholl TO, Hediger ML, Schall JI, et al: Gestational weight gain, pregnancy outcome, and postpartum weight retention. Obstet Gynecol 86:423, 1995.
23. Schauberger CW, Rooney BL, Brimer LM: Factors that influence weight loss in the puerperium. Obstet Gynecol 79:424, 1992.
24. Lovelady CA, Garner KE, Thoreno KL, et al: The effect of weight loss in overweight, lactating women on the growth of their infants. N Engl J Med 342:449, 2000.
25. Dewey KG, Lovelady CA, Nommsen-Rivers LA, et al: A randomized study of the effects of aerobic exercise by lactating women on breast-milk volume and composition. N Engl J Med 330:449, 1994.
26. Rasmusen NG, Hornnes PJ, Hegedus L: Ultrasonographically determined thyroid size in pregnancy and postpartum: the goitrogenic effect of pregnancy. Am J Obstet Gynecol 160: 1216, 1989.
27. Jausson R, Dahlberg PA, Winsa B, et al: The postpartum period constitutes an important risk for the development of clinical Graves disease in young women. Acta Endocrinol 116:321, 1987.
28. Kent GN, Stuckey BGA, Allen JR, et al: Post partum thyroid dysfunction: clinical assessment and relationship to psychiatric affective morbidity. Clin Endocrinol 51:429, 1999.
29. Pedersen CA, Stern RA, Pate J, et al: Thyroid and adrenal measures during late pregnancy and the puerperium in women who have been major depressed or who become dysmorphic postpartum. J Affect Disord 29:201, 1993.
30. Terry AJ, Hague WM: Postpartum thyroiditis. Semin Perinatol 22:497, 1998.
31. Walters WAW, Limm VL: Blood volume and haemodynamics in pregnancy. Clin Obstet Gynaecol 2:301, 1975.
32. Lindesman R, Miller MM: Blood volume changes during the immediate postpartum period. Obstet Gynecol 21:40, 1963.
33. Ueland K: Maternal cardiovascular dynamics. VIII. Intrapartum blood volume changes. Am J Obstet Gynecol 126:671, 1976.
34. Paintin DB: The size of the total red cell volume in pregnancy. J Obstet Gynaecol Br Commonw 69:719, 1962.
35. Macklon NS, Greer IA: The deep venous system in the puerperium: an ultrasound study. Br J Obstet Gynaecol 104:198, 1997.
36. Walters WAW, MacGregor WG, Hills M: Cardiac output at rest during pregnancy and the puerperium. Clin Sci 30:1, 1966.
37. Walters BNJ, Thompson ME, Lea E, DeSwiet M: Blood pressure in the puerperium. Clin Sci 71:589, 1986.
38. Clapp JF III, Capeless E: Cardiovascular function before, during, and after the first and subsequent pregnancies. Am J Cardiol 80:1469, 1997.
39. Ygge J: Changes in blood coagulation and fibrinolysis during the puerperium. Am J Obstet Gynecol 104:2, 1969.
40. Baird D: The upper urinary tract in pregnancy and puerperium, with special reference to pyelitis of pregnancy. J Obstet Gynaecol Br Emp 42:733, 1935.
41. Rubi RA, Sala NC: Ureteral function in pregnant women. III. Effect of different positions and of fetal delivery upon ureteral tonus. Am J Obstet Gynecol 101:230, 1968.
42. Dure-Smith P: Pregnancy dilatation of the urinary tract. Radiology 96:545, 1970.
43. Peake SL, Roxburgh HB, Langlois SL: Ultrasonic assessment of hydronephrosis of pregnancy. Radiology 146:167, 1983.
44. Fried AM, Woodring JH, Thompson DJ: Hydronephrosis of pregnancy: a prospective sequential study of the course of dilatation. J Ultrasound Med 2:255, 1983.
45. Cietak KA, Newton JR: Serial qualitative maternal nephrosonography in pregnancy. Br J Radiol 58:399, 1985.
46. Kerr-Wilson RHJ, Thompson SW, Orr JW Jr, et al: Effect of labor on the postpartum bladder. Obstet Gynecol 64:115, 1984.
47. Sims EAH, Krantz KE: Serial studies of renal function during pregnancy and the puerperium in normal women. J Clin Invest 37:1764, 1958.
48. DeAlvarez RR: Renal glomerulotubular mechanisms during normal pregnancy. Am J Obstet Gynecol 75:931, 1958.

49. Polatti F, Capuzzo E, Viazzo F, et al: Bone mineral changes during and after lactation. Obstet Gynecol 94:52, 1999.

50. Holmberg-Marttila D, Sievanen H: Prevalence of bone mineral changes during postpartum amenorrhea and after resumption of menstruation. Am J Obstet Gynecol 180:537, 1999.

51. Lasky MA, Prentice A: Bone mineral changes during and after lactation. Obstet Gynecol 94:608, 1999.

52. Little KD, Clapp JF III: Self-selected recreational exercise has no impact on early postpartum lactation-induced bone loss. Med Sci Sports Exerc 30:831, 1998.

53. Hebert PR, Reed G, Entman SS, et al: Serious maternal morbidity after childbirth: prolonged hospital stays and readmissions. Obstet Gynecol 94:942, 1999.

54. Glazener CMA, Abdalla M, Stroud P, et al: Postnatal maternal morbidity: extent, causes, prevention and treatment. Br J Obstet Gynaecol 102:282, 1995.

55. Liu LL, Clemens CJ, Shay DK, et al: The safety of early newborn discharge: the Washington state experience. JAMA 278:293, 1997.

56. Mandl KD, Brennan TA, Wise PH, et al: Maternal and infant health: effects of moderate reductions in postpartum length of stay. Arch Pediatr Adolesc Med 151:915, 1997.

57. Britton JR, Britton HL, Gronwaldt V: Early perinatal hospital discharge and parenting during infancy. Pediatrics 104:1070, 1999.

58. Brumfield CG: Early postpartum discharge. Clin Obstet Gynecol 41:611, 1998.

59. Moran CF, Holt VL, Martin DP: What do women want to know after childbirth? Birth 24:27, 1997.

60. Jennings B, Edmundson M: The postpartum periods: after confinement: the fourth trimester. Clin Obstet Gynecol 23:1093, 1980.

61. Koltyn KF, Schultes SS: Psychological effects of an aerobic exercise session and a rest session following pregnancy. J Sports Med Phys Fitness 37:287, 1997.

62. Sampselle CM, Seng J, Yeo S, et al: Physical activity and postpartum well-being. J Obstet Gynecol Neonatal Nurs 28:41, 1999.

63. Fein J, Goldman JM, Weintraub BD: Postpartum lymphocytic thyroiditis in American women: a spectrum of thyroid dysfunction. Am J Obstet Gynecol 138:504, 1980.

64. Amino N, Mori H, Iwatani Y, et al: High prevalence of transient postpartum thyrotoxicosis and hypothyroidism. N Engl J Med 306:849, 1983.

65. Reamy K, White SE: Sexuality in pregnancy and the puerperium: a review. Obstet Gynecol Surv 40:1, 1985.

66. Glazener CMA: Sexual function after childbirth: women's experiences, persistent morbidity and lack of professional recognition. Br J Obstet Gynaecol 104:330, 1997.

67. Goetsch MF: Postpartum dysparunia. An unexplored problem. J Reprod Med 44:963, 1999.

68. Ryding E-L: Sexuality during and after pregnancy. Acta Obstet Gynecol Scand 63:679, 1984.

69. American College of Obstetricians and Gynecologists: Pregnancy, Work, and Disability. Technical Bulletin No. 58. Washington, DC, ACOG, 1980.

70. Gagnon AJ, Edgar L, Kramer MS, et al: A randomized trial of a program of early postpartum discharge with nurse visitation. Am J Obstet Gynecol 176:205, 1997.

71. Gunn J, Lumley S, Chondros P, Young D: Does an early postnatal check-up improve maternal health: results from a randomized trial in Australian general practice. Br J Obstet Gynaecol 105:991, 1998.

72. Windle ML, Booker LA, Rayburn WF: Postpartum pain after vaginal delivery: a review of comparative analgesic trials. J Reprod Med 34:891, 1989.

73. Shy KK, Eschenbach DA: Fatal perineal cellulitis from episiotomy site. Obstet Gynecol 54:929, 1979.

74. Stiller RJ, Kaplan BM, Andreoli JW Jr: Hereditary angioedema and pregnancy. Obstet Gynecol 64:133, 1984.

75. Ewing TL, Smale LE, Eliot FA: Maternal deaths associated with postpartum vulvar edema. Am J Obstet Gynecol 134:173, 1979.

76. Droegemueller W: Cold sitz baths for relief of postpartum perineal pain. Clin Obstet Gynecol 23:1039, 1980.

77. Connolly AM, Thorp JM Jr: Childbirth-related perineal trauma: clinical significance and prevention. Clin Obstet Gynecol 42:820, 1999.

78. Chaliha C, Kalia V, Stanton S, et al: Antenatal prediction of postpartum fecal incontinence. Obstet Gynecol 94:689, 1999.

79. Chichakli LO, Atrash HK, Mackay AP, et al: Pregnancy-related mortality in the United States due to hemorrhage: 1979–1992. Obstet Gynecol 94:721, 1999.

80. King PA, Duthie SJ, Dip V, et al: Secondary postpartum hemorrhage. Aust N Z J Obstet Gynaecol 29:394: 1989.

81. Pelage J-P, Phillippe S, Repiquet D, et al: Secondary postpartum hemorrhage: treatment with selective arterial embolization. Radiology 212:385, 1999.

82. Charles J, Charles D: Postpartum infection. *In* Charles D (ed): Obstetric and Perinatal Infections. St Louis, Mosby Year Book, 1993, p 60.

83. Klaus MH, Jerauld R, Kreger NC, et al: Maternal attachment: importance of the first postpartum days. N Engl J Med 286:460, 1972.

84. McClellan MS, Cabianca WC: Effects of early mother–infant contact following cesarean birth. Obstet Gynecol 56:52, 1980.

85. Robson KM, Powell E: Early maternal attachment. *In* Brickington IF, Kumar R (eds): Motherhood and Mental Illness. San Diego, Acadmic Press, 1982, p 155.

86. Klaus M, Kennel J: Parent–Infant Bonding. St Louis, CV Mosby, 1982.

87. Gray J, Butler C, Dean J, et al: Prediction and prevention of child abuse and neglect. Child Abuse Neglect 1:45, 1977.

88. Siegel E, Cauman KE, Schaefer ES, et al: Hospital and home support during infancy: impact on maternal attachment, child abuse and neglect and health care utilization. Pediatrics 66:183, 1980.

89. DeCasper AJ, Fifer W: Of human bonding: newborns prefer their mother's voices. Science 208:1174, 1980.

90. Areskog B, Uddenberg N, Kjessler B: Experience of delivery in women with and without antenatal fear of childbirth. Gynecol Obstet Invest 16:1, 1983.

91. Healthy People, Progress Review, May 5, 1999, DHHS, Public Health Service.

92. Jeliffe DB, Jeliffe EFP: "Breast is best": modern meanings. N Engl J Med 297:912, 1977.

93. Hardy E, Santos LC, Osis MJ, et al: Contraceptive use and pregnancy before and after introducing lactational amenorrhea (LAM) in a postpartum program. Contraception 14:59, 1998.

94. Winikoff B, Myers D, Laukaran VH, Stone R: Overcoming obstacles to breast-feeding in a large municipal hospital: applications of lessons learned. Pediatrics 80:423, 1987.

95. Neifert MR, Seacat JM: Medical management of successful breast-feeding. Pediatr Clin North Am 33:743, 1986.

96. Casey CE, Hambidge KM: Nutritional aspects of human lactation. *In* Neville MC, Neifert MR (eds): Lactation, Physiology, Nutrition, and Breast-Feeding. New York, Plenum Press, 1983, p 199.

97. Institute of Medicine (Subcommittee on Nutrition During Lactation): Nutrition During Lactation. Washington, DC, National Academy Press, 1991.

98. National Research Council, Food and Nutrition Board: Recommended Dietary Allowances, 10th ed. Washington, DC, National Academy of Sciences, 1989.

99. Higginbottom MC, Sweetman L, Nyhan WL: A syndrome of methylmalonic acidemia, homocystinuria, megaloblastic anemia and neurologic abnormalities in a vitamin B12 deficient breast-fed infant of a strict vegetarian. N Engl J Med 299: 317, 1978.

100. O'Connor P: Vitamin D deficiency in rickets in two breast-fed infants who were not receiving vitamin D supplementation. Clin Pediatr 16:361, 1977.

101. Whichelow MJ: Success and failure of breast-feeding in relation to energy intake. Proc Nutr Soc 35:62A, 1975.

102. Kalkwarf HJ, Specker BL: Bone mineral loss during lactation and recovery after weaning. Obstet Gynecol 86:26, 1995.

103. Dunkle LM, Schmidt RR, O'Connor DP: Neonatal herpes simplex infection possibly acquired via maternal breast milk. Pediatrics 63:250, 1979.

104. McGregor JA, Neifert MR: Maternal problems in lactation. *In* Neville MC, Neifert MR (eds): Lactation: Physiology, Nutrition and Breast-Feeding. New York, Plenum Press, 1983, p 333.

105. Hunt CM, Carson KL, Shara AI: Hepatitis C in pregnancy. Obstet Gynecol 89:883, 1997.

106. Peckham C, Gibb D: Mother-to-child transmission of the human immunodeficiency virus. N Engl J Med 333:298, 1995.

107. Nduati R, John G, Mbori-Ngacha D, et al: Effects of breast-feeding and formula feeding on transmission of HIV-1. JAMA 283:1167, 2000.

108. Briggs GC, Freeman RK, Yaffe SJ: Drugs in Pregnancy and Lactation. Baltimore, Williams & Wilkins, 1998.

109. American Academy of Pediatrics: Committee on Drugs. The transfer of drugs and other chemicals into human milk. Pediatrics 93:137, 1994.

110. Schanler RJ, Hurst NM, Lau C: The use of human milk and breast feeing in premature infants. Clin Perinatol 26:379, 1999.

111. Haywood AR: The immunology of breast milk. *In* Neville MC, Neifert MR (eds): Lactation: Physiology, Nutrition, and Breast-Feeding. New York, Plenum Press, 1983, p 249.

112. Wheeler JL, Johnson M, Collie L, et al: Promoting breastfeeding in the neonatal intensive care unit. Breastfeeding Rev 7: 15, 1999.

113. Hopkins JM, Schanler RJ, Garza C: Milk production by mothers of premature infants. Pediatrics 81:815, 1988.

114. Niebyl JR, Spence MR, Parmley TH: Sporadic (nonepidemic) puerperal mastitis. J Reprod Med 20:97, 1978.

115. Thomsen AC, Espersen T, Maigaard S: Course and treatment of milk statis, noninfectious inflammation of the breast, and infectious mastitis in nursing women. Am J Obstet Gynecol 149:492, 1984.

116. Neifert MR, McDonough SI, Neville MC: Failure of lactogenesis associated with placental retention. Am J Obstet Gynecol 140:477, 1981.

117. Sousa PSR: Meloclopramide and breast feeding. Br Med J 1: 512, 1975.

118. Aono R, Shigi T, Aki T, et al: Augmentation of puerperal lactation by oral administration of sulpifide. J Clin Endocrinol Metab 48:478, 1979.

119. Spitz AM, Lee NC, Peterson HB: Treatment for lactation suppression: little progress in one hundred years. Am J Obstet Gynecol 179:1485, 1998.

120. Sandoz Pharmaceuticals: Drug Information Brochure re. Parlodel (Bromocriptine Mesylate). East Hanover, NJ, Sandoz Pharmaceuticals, 1987.

121. Willis J (ed): Postpartum hypertension, seizures, and strokes reported with bromocriptine. FDA Drug Bull 14:3, 1984.

122. Katz M, Kroll I, Pak I, et al: Puerperal hypertension, stroke, and seizures after suppression of lactation with bromocriptine. Obstet Gynecol 66:822, 1985.

123. Iffy L, TenHove W, Frisoli G: Acute myocardial infarction in the puerperium in patients receiving bromocriptine. Am J Obstet Gynecol 155:371, 1986.

124. Ruch A, Duhring J: Postpartum myocardial infarction in a patient receiving bromocriptine. Obstet Gynecol 74:448, 1989.

125. Kazi A, Kennedy KI, Visness CM, Kahn T: Effectiveness of the lactational amenorrhea method in Pakistan. Fertil Steril 64:717, 1995.

126. Robson KM, Brant H, Kumar R: Maternal sexuality during first pregnancy after childbirth. Br J Obstet Gynaecol 88:882, 1981.

127. Debrovner CH, Winikoff B: Trends in postpartum contraceptive choice. Obstet Gynecol 63:65, 1984.

128. Flynn AM: Natural methods of family planning. Clin Obstet Gynaecol 11:661, 1984.

129. Rojnik B, Kosmelj K, Andolsek-Jeras L: Initiation of contraception postpartum. Contraception 51:75, 1995.

130. Stanford JB, Thurnau PB, Lemaire JC: Physicians' knowledge and practices regarding natural family planning. Obstet Gynecol 94:672, 1999.

131. Wortman J: The diaphragm and other intravaginal barriers—a review. Popul Rep H:58, 1979.

132. Vessey M, Wiggins P: Use-effectiveness of the diaphragm in a selected family planning clinic population in the United Kingdom. Contraception 9:15, 1974.

133. Mills A: Barrier contraception. Clin Obstet Gynaecol 11:641, 1984.

134. Speroff L, DeCherney A: Evaluation of a new generation of oral contraceptives. Obstet Gynecol 81:1034, 1993.

135. Kay CR: The Royal College of General Practitioners' oral contraceptive study: some recent observations. Clin Obstet Gynaecol 11:759, 1984.

136. Baird DT, Glasier AF: Hormonal contraception. N Engl J Med 328:1543, 1993.

137. Koetsawang S: The effects of contraceptive methods on the quality and quantity of breast milk. Int J Gynaecol Obstet 25 (Suppl):115, 1987.

138. Kennedy KI, Sort RV, Tully MR: Premature introduction of progestin-only contraceptive methods during lactation. Contraception 55:347, 1997.

139. Kjos SL, Peters RK, Xiang A, et al: Contraception and the risk of type 2 diabetes mellitus in Latina women with prior gestational diabetes mellitus. JAMA 280:533, 1998.

140. Diaz S, Peralta G, Juez C, et al: Fertility regulation in nursing women: III. Short-term influence of low-dose combined contraceptive upon lactation and infant growth. Contraception 27:1, 1983.

141. Kaunitz AM: Long-acting injectable contraception with depot medroxyprogesterone acetate. Am J Obstet Gynecol 170: 1543, 1994.

142. Sivin I, Campodonica I, Kiriwat O, et al: The performance of levonoregestrel rod and Norplant contraceptive implants: a 5 year randomized study. Hum Reprod 13:3371, 1998.

143. Darney PD: Hormonal implants: contraception for a new century. Am J Obstet Gynecol 170:1536, 1994.

144. Berenson AB, Wiemann CM, McCombs SL, Soma-Garcia A: The rise and fall of levonogestrel implants: 1992–1996. Obstet Gynecol 92:790, 1998.

145. Harlap S, Kost K, Forrest JD: Preventing Pregnancy, Protecting Health: A New Look at Birth Control Choices in the United States. New York, The Alan Guttmacher Institute, 1991.

146. Dardano KL, Burkman RT: The intrauterine contraceptive

device: an often-forgotten and maligned method of contraception. Am J Obstet Gynecol 181:1, 1999.

147. Alvarez T, Brache V, Fernandez E, et al: New insights on the mode of action of intrauterine contraceptive devices in women. Fertil Steril 49:768, 1988.

148. Rivera R, Yacobson I, Grimes D: The mechanism of action of hormonal contraceptives and intrauterine contraceptive devices. Am J Obstet Gynecol 181:1263, 1999.

149. U.S. Department of Health, Education and Welfare: Second Report on Intrauterine Contraceptive Devices, The Medical Device and Drug Advisory Committees on Obstetrics and Gynecology. Washington, DC, Food and Drug Administration, 1978.

150. Mishell DR Jr, Roy S: Copper intrauterine contraceptive device event rate following insertion 4 to 8 weeks postpartum. Am J Obstet Gynecol 143:29, 1982.

151. Daling JR, Weiss NS, Metch BJ, et al: Primary tubal infertility in relation to use of an IUD. N Engl J Med 312:937, 1985.

152. Cole LP, Edelman DA, Potts DM, et al: Postpartum insertion of modified intrauterine devices. J Reprod Med 29:677, 1984.

153. Cole LP, McCann MF, Higgins JE, et al: Effects of breast feeding on IUD performance. Am J Public Health 73:384, 1983.

154. Peterson LS: Contraceptive use in the United States: 1982–1990. Advanced Data from Vital Health Statistics. No. 260 Hyattsville, MD: National Center for Health Statistics, 1995 (DHHS publication no. PHS 95-1250).

155. Peterson HB, Xia Z, Hughes JM, et al: The risk of pregnancy after tubal sterilization: findings from The U.S. Collaborative Review of Sterilization. Am Obstet Gynecol 174:1161, 1996.

156. Cunningham FG, MacDonald PC, Leveno KJ, et al: Williams Obstetrics, 19th ed. Norwalk, CT, Appleton & Lange, 1993.

157. Uchida H: Uchida tubal sterilization. Am J Obstet Gynecol 121:153, 1975.

158. Benedetti TJ, Miller FC: Uchida tubal sterilization failure: a report of four cases. Am J Obstet Gynecol 132:116, 1978.

159. Irving FC: A new method of insuring sterility following cesarean section. Am J Obstet Gynecol 8:335, 1924.

160. Aranda C, Prada C, Broutin A, et al: Laparoscopic sterilization immediately after term delivery: preliminary report. J Reprod Med 14:171, 1963.

161. Hillis SD, Marchbanks PA, Taylor LR, Peterson HB: Poststerilization regret: findings from the United States Collaborative Review of Sterilization. Obstet Gynecol 93:889, 1999.

162. Vessy M, Huggins G, Lawless M, et al: Tubal sterilization: findings in a large prospective study. Br J Obstet Gynaecol 90:203, 1983.

163. Bhiwandiwala PP, Mumford SD, Feldblum PJ: Menstrual pattern changes following laparoscopic sterilization with different occlusion techniques: a review of 10,004 cases. Am J Obstet Gynecol 145:684, 1983.

164. Bledin KD, Brice B: Psychological conditions in pregnancy and the puerperium and their relevance to postpartum sterilization: a review. Bull WHO 61:533, 1983.

165. Peterson HB, Huber DH, Belker AM: Vasectomy: an appraisal for the obstetrician-gynecologist. Obstet Gynecol 76:568, 1990.

166. Hendrix NW, Chauhan SP, Morrison JC: Sterilization and its consequences. Obstet Gynecol Surv 54:766, 1999.

167. Hillis SD, Marchbanks PA, Taylor LR, Peterson HB: Higher hysterectomy risk for sterilized than nonsterilized women: findings from the U.S. Collaborative Review of Sterilization Working Group. Obstet Gynecol 91:241, 1998.

168. Walker MW, Jick H, Hunter JR: Vasectomy and non-fatal myocardial infarction. Lancet 1:13, 1981.

169. Haynes DM, Martin BJ: Cesarean hysterectomy: a twenty-five year review. Am J Obstet Gynecol 46:215, 1975.

170. Yalom I, Lunde D, Moos R, et al: Postpartum blues syndrome. Arch Gen Psychiatry 18:16, 1968.

171. Stein G: The maternity blues. In Brockington IF, Kumar R (eds): Motherhood and Mental Illness. London, Academic Press, 1982, p 119.

172. Swain AM, O'Hara MWS, Starr KR, Gorman LL: A prospective study of sleep, mood, and cognitive function in postpartum and non-postpartum women. Obstet Gynecol 90:381, 1997.

173. Nott PN, Franklin M, Armitage C, et al: Hormonal changes and mood in the early puerperium. Br J Psychiatry 128:379, 1976.

174. Handley SL, Sunn TL, Waldron S, et al: Tryptophan, cortisol and puerperal mood. Br J Psychiatry 136:498, 1980.

175. Stowe ZN, Nemeroff CB: Women at risk for postpartum-onset major depression. Am J Obstet Gynecol 173:639, 1995.

176. Cox JL, Murray D, Chapman G: A controlled study of the onset, duration and prevalence of postnatal depression. Br J Psychiatry 163:27, 1993.

177. Pop VJM, Essed GGM, de Geus CA, et al: Prevalence of post partum depression—or is it post-puerperium depression? Acta Obstet Gynaecol Scand 72:354, 1993.

178. Pitt B: Atypical depression following childbirth. Br J Psychiatry 114:1325, 1968.

179. Hendrick V, Altshuler LL, Suri R: Hormonal changes in the postpartum and implications for postpartum depression. Psychosomatics 39:93, 1998.

180. Magiakou M-A, Matorakos G, Rabin D, et al: Hypothalamic corticotropin-releasing hormone suppression during the postpartum period: implication for the increase in psychiatric manifestations at this time. J Clin Endocrinol 81:1912, 1996.

181. Watson JP, Elliot SA, Rugg AJ, et al: Psychiatric disorders in pregnancy and the first postnatal year. Br J Psychiatry 144:453, 1984.

182. Neugebauer R, Kline J, Shrout P, et al: Major depressive disorder in the 6 months after miscarriage. JAMA 227:383, 1997.

183. Kumar R, Robson K: Neurotic disturbance during pregnancy and the puerperium: preliminary report of a prospective survey of 119 primiparae. In Sand M (ed): Mental Illness in Pregnancy and the Puerperium. London, Oxford University Press, 1978, p 40.

184. Horowitz JA, Damato E, Solon L, et al: Postpartum depression: issues in clinical assessment. J Perinatol 15:268, 1995.

185. Posner NA, Unterman RR, Williams KN: Postpartum depression: the obstetrician's concerns. In Inwood DG (ed): Recent Advances in Postpartum Psychiatric Disorders. Washington, DC, American Psychiatric Press, Inc, 1985, p 69.

186. Beck CT: The effects of postpartum depression on child development: a meta-analysis. Arch Psychiatric Nurs 12:12, 1998.

187. Bokhari R, Bhatara VS, Bandettini F, McMillin JM: Postpartum psychosis and postpartum thyroiditis. Psychoneuroendocrinology 23:643, 1998.

188. Cox JL, Holden JM, Sagovsky R: Detection of postnatal depression. Development of the 10-item Edinburgh Postnatal Depression Scale. Br J Psychiatry 150:782, 1987.

189. Georgiopoulos AM, Bryan TL, Yawn BP, et al: Population-based screening for postpartum depression. Obstet Gynecol 93:653, 1999.

190. Altshuler LL, Hendrick V, Cohen LS: Course of mood and anxiety disorders during pregnancy and the postpartum period. J Clin Psychiatry 59(Suppl 2):21, 1998.

191. Cohen LS: Pharmacologic treatment of depression in women:

PMS, pregnancy and the postpartum period. Depress Anxiety 8:18, 1998.

192. Gregoire AJP, Kumar R, Everitt B, et al: Transdermal oestrogen for treatment of severe postnatal depression. Lancet 347: 930, 1996.

193. Wisner KL, Wheeler SB: Prevention of recurrent postpartum major depression. Hosp Commun Psychiatry 45:1191, 1994.

194. Murray L, Cooper PJ: Postpartum depression and child development. Psychol Med 27:253, 1997.

195. Vandenberg RL: Postpartum depression. Clin Obstet Gynaecol 23:1105, 1980.

196. Nott PN: Psychiatric illness following childbirth in Southampton: a case register study. Psychol Med 12:557, 1982.

197. Kendell RE, Rennie D, Clark JA, et al: The social and obstetric correlates of psychiatric admission in the puerperium. Psychol Med 11:341, 1981.

198. Brockington IF, Winokur G, Dean C: Puerperal psychosis. *In* Brockington IF, Kumar R (eds): Motherhood and Mental Illness. London, Academic Press, 1982, p 37.

199. Ahokas A, Aito M, Rimón R: Positive treatment effect of estradiol in postpartum psychosis: a pilot study. J Clin Psychiatry 61:166, 2000.

200. Drotar D, Baskiewicz A, Irvin N, et al: The adaptation of parents to the birth of an infant with a congenital malformation: a hypothetical model. Pediatrics 56:710, 1975.

201. Lindemann E: Symptomatology and management of acute grief. Am J Psychol 101:141, 1944.

202. Kennel JH, Slyter H, Claus MKH: The mourning response of parents to the death of a newborn. N Engl J Med 83:344, 1970.

203. Benfield DG, Leib SA, Reuter J: Grief response of parents after referral of the critically ill newborn to a regional center. N Engl J Med 294:975, 1976.

204. Giles PFH: reactions of women to perinatal death. Aust N Z J Obstet Gynaecol 10:207, 1970.

205. Zahourek R, Jensen J: Grieving and the loss of the newborn. Am J Nurs 73:836, 1973.

206. Seitz PM, Warrick LH: Perinatal death: the grieving mother. Am J Nurs 74:2028, 1974.

207. Rowe J, Clyman R, Green C, et al: Follow-up of families who experience perinatal death. Pediatrics 62:166, 1978.

208. Lockwood S, Lewis IC: Management of grieving after stillbirth. Med J Aust 2:308, 1980.

209. Mandell F, Wolf LC: Sudden infant death syndrome and subsequent pregnancy. Pediatrics 56:774, 1975.

210. Schleifer SJ, Keller SE, Camerimo M, et al: Suppression of lymphocyte stimulation following bereavement. JAMA 250: 374, 1983.

211. Lake M, Knuppel R, Murphy J, et al: The role of a grief support team following stillbirths. Am J Obstet Gynecol 61: 497, 1983.

212. Furlong R, Hobbins J: Grief in the perinatal period. Obstet Gynecol 61:497, 1983.

213. Condon JT: Management of established pathological grief reaction after stillbirth. Am J Psychiatry 143:987, 1986.

214. Kowalski K: Managing perinatal loss. Clin Obstet Gynecol 23:1113, 1980.

215. Mandell F, McAnulty E, Race RM: Observations of paternal response to sudden unanticipated infant deaths. Pediatrics 65: 221, 1980.

216. Saisto T, Ylikorkala O, Halmesmaki E: Factors associated with fear of delivery in second pregnancies. Obstet Gynecol 94:679, 1999.

217. Fisher J, Astbury J, Smith A: Adverse psychological impact of operative obstetric interventions: a prospective longitudinal study. Aust N Z J Psychiatry 31:728, 1997.

218. Reynolds JL: Post-traumatic stress disorder after childbirth: the phenomenon of traumatic birth. Can Med Assoc J 156: 831, 1997.

219. Ryding EL, Wijma K, Wijma B: Predisposing psychological factors for posttraumatic stress reactions after emergency cesarean section. Acta Obstet Gynecol Scand 77:351, 1998.

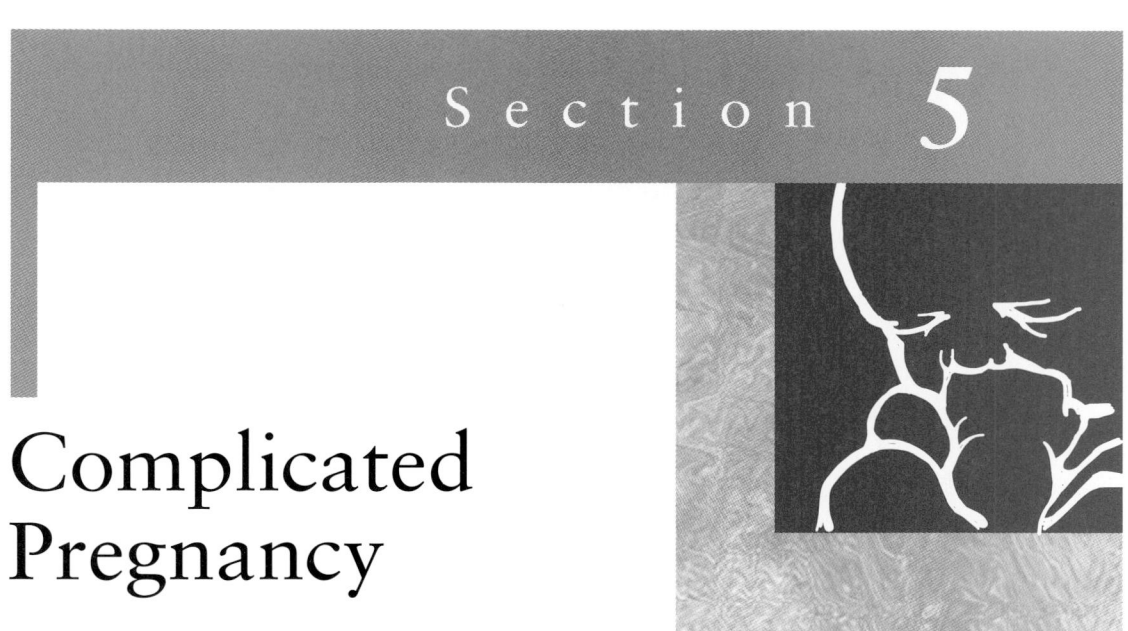

Section 5

Complicated Pregnancy

Chapter 22

Fetal Wastage

JOE LEIGH SIMPSON

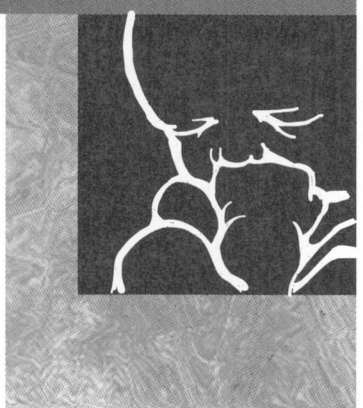

Not all conceptions result in a liveborn infant. Of clinically recognized pregnancies, 10 to 15 percent are lost. Of married women in the United States, 4 percent have experienced two fetal losses and 3 percent have experienced three or more.[1] It is accepted that a subset of women genuinely manifest repetitive spontaneous abortions as opposed to merely representing random untoward events. This chapter considers the causes of fetal wastage, the management of couples experiencing repetitive losses, and the topic of ectopic gestations.

FREQUENCY AND TIMING OF PREGNANCY LOSSES

Pregnancy is not generally recognized clinically until 5 to 6 weeks after the last menstrual period, but before this time β-human chorionic gonadotropin (β-hCG) assays can detect preclinical pregnancies. Wilcox et al.[2] performed daily urinary hCG assays beginning around the expected time of implantation (day 20 of gestation). Of pregnancies detected in this fashion, 31 percent (61 of 198) were lost; the preclinical loss rate was 22 percent (43 of 198), and the clinically recognized loss rate was 12 percent (19 of 155). These rates are consistent with data gathered by this author and colleagues[3] in a National Institute of Child Health and Human Development collaborative study in which serum β-hCG assays were performed 28 to 35 days after the previous menses. The total fetal loss rate (preclinical and clinical) for pregnancies detected at 4 to 5 weeks or approximately 10 days later than those ascertained by Wilcox et al.[2] was 16 percent.

Clinically recognized first-trimester fetal loss rates of 10 to 12 percent overall are well documented in both retrospective and prospective cohort studies.[4] The higher loss rates reported in some older studies probably reflect unwitting inclusion of surreptitious illicit abortions, a common occurrence during the era in which legal termination was proscribed. Loss rates reflect many factors that will be discussed in this chapter, but two associations are worth emphasizing here. First, maternal age greatly increases risk, a 40-year-old woman carrying twice the risk of a 20-year-old woman. Second, prior pregnancy history is pivotal. Loss rates are lowest (6 percent) among nulliparous women who have never experienced a loss[5] rising to 25 to 30 percent after three or more losses. Most recurrence risk data were derived from studying women whose losses were usually not recognized until 9 to 12 weeks' gestation. However, the same counseling figures are appropriate for couples whose pregnancies are ascertained in the fifth week of gestation.[6]

Abortion rates may be lower when conception occurs on days other than the date of ovulation or day prior (optimal interval). In couples with prior abortions, loss rates were 7 percent when conception occurred on the day of ovulation or 1 day earlier, but 23 percent when conception occurred on other (nonoptimal) days of the cycle.[7] Wilcox et al.[8] studied a cohort of 189 pregnancies of which 141 lasted beyond 6 weeks. Among the implantations leading to a clinical pregnancy, 84 percent did so on days 8, 9, or 10 after ovulation. No pregnancies occurred when implantation occurred beyond day 12. The loss rate was 13 percent if implantation occurred by day 9, increasing to 26 percent, 52 percent, and 82 percent and on the next 3 days, respectively.

Studies utilizing ultrasonography have now made it clear that fetal demise occurs before overt clinical signs are manifested. This conclusion is based on cohort studies showing that only 3 percent of viable pregnancies are lost after 8 weeks' gestation.[9] Given an accepted clinical loss rate of 10 to 12 percent, fetal viability must cease weeks before maternal symptoms appear; thus, most fetuses aborting clinically at 9 to 12 weeks must have died weeks previously. Most pregnancy losses after 8 weeks likely occur in the next 2 gestational months, as loss rates are only 1 percent in women confirmed by ultrasound to have viable pregnancies at 16 weeks. Overall, almost all losses are "missed abortions" (retained in utero for an interval prior to clinical recognition); thus, the term is archaic.

ETIOLOGY OF PRECLINICAL LOSSES

Establishing an etiology for preclinical losses is not easy, but the one proven explanation is morphologic and genetic abnormalities in the early embryo. Decades ago, Hertig and Rock[10-12] examined the fallopian tubes, uterine cavities, and endometria of women undergoing elective hysterectomy. These women were of proved fertility, with a mean age of 33.6 years. Coital times were recorded before hysterectomy. Eight preim-

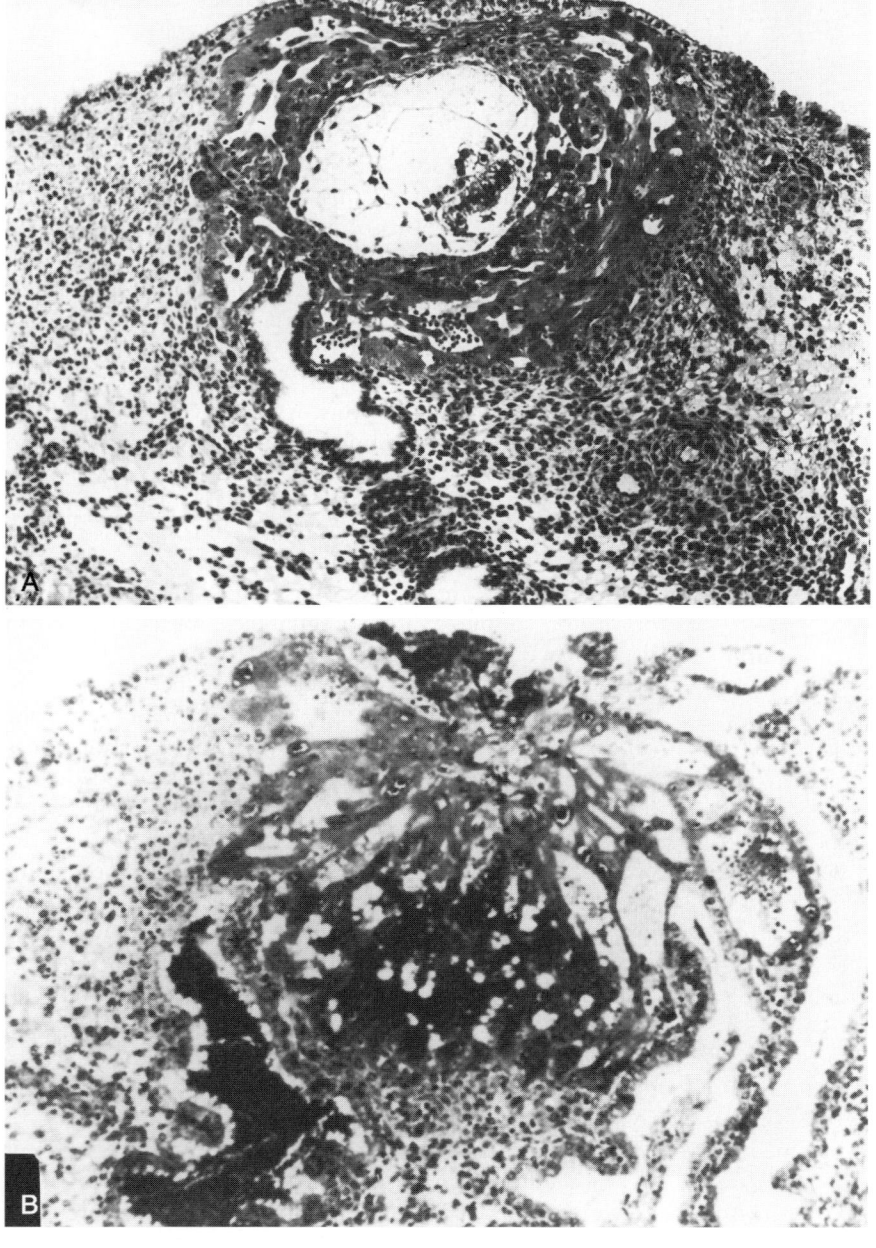

Figure 22–1. Cross section of endometrium containing an abnormal 14-day-old embryo (*A*) compared with a normal 11-day-old embryo. *B*, In the abnormal embryo no embryonic disk is present and only syncytiotrophoblasts are identifiable. (From Hertig A, Rock J: A series of potentially abortive ova recovered from fertile women prior to the first missed menstrual period. Am J Obstet Gynecol 58: 968, 1949, with permission.)

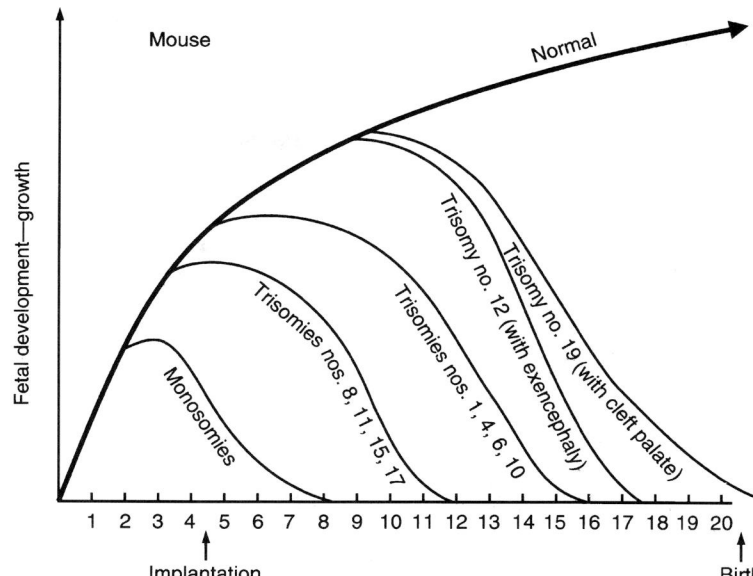

Figure 22–2. Timing for loss of murine autosomal monosomy and murine autosomal trisomy. (From Gropp A: Chromosomal animal model of human disease. Fetal trisomy and development failure. *In* Berry L, Poswillo DE [eds]: Teratology. Berlin, Springer-Verlag, 1975, p 17, with permission.)

plantation embryos (<6 days from conception) were recovered. Four of these eight embryos were morphologically abnormal. The four abnormal embryos presumably would not have implanted or, if implanted, would not have survived long thereafter. Nine of 26 implanted embryos (6 to 14 embryonic days) were morphologically abnormal (Fig. 22–1).

The frequency of chromosomal abnormalities in human preimplantation embryos normal and abnormal is very high.[13,14] Of morphologically normal embryos, 25 percent show abnormal metaphases (usually aneuploidy). This percentage is consistent with the 25 to 30 percent aneuploidy rate on the basis of studies using fluorescent in situ hybridization (FISH) using chromosome-specific probes for chromosomes 13, 18, and 21.[15] The 25 percent aneuploidy rate in morphologically normal embryos is also consistent with aneuploidy observed in 6 percent of sperm from ostensibly normal males[16] and in perhaps 20 percent of oocytes.[17,18]

Chromosomal abnormalities are even more frequent in morphologically abnormal embryos. Using metaphase analysis, Plachot et al.[13] found chromosomal abnormalities in 78 percent of fragmented embryos, compared to 12.5 percent in morphologically normal embryos. Pellestor et al.[19] reported 90 percent abnormalities in 118 poor quality embryos. Using FISH with chromosome-specific probes, abnormality rates of 50 to 75 percent are observed even with a limited number of chromosomes tested.[15] Given the above, it has been accepted for over a decade that chromosomal abnormalities would be expected to be the next frequent explanation for the morphologically abnormal embryos recovered by Hertig et al.[10–12]

Consistent with this conclusion are elegant studies in the mouse by Gropp.[20] Mice heterozygous for a variety of robertsonian translocations were mated to produce various monosomies and trisomies. By selective mating and sacrifice of pregnant animals at varying gestational ages, both survivability and phenotypic characteristics of the aberrant complements could be determined. In mice, as presumably in humans, autosomal monosomy proved inviable. Most monosomes aborted around the time of implantation (4 to 5 days after conception) (Fig. 22–2). Most trisomies survived longer, but only rarely to term. These findings are analogous to those observed in aneuploid human fetuses.

CYTOGENETIC ETIOLOGY IN CLINICALLY RECOGNIZED LOSSES

The major cause of clinically recognized pregnancy losses is chromosomal abnormalities. At least 50 percent of clinically recognized pregnancy losses result from a chromosomal abnormality.[21–23] The frequency is probably even higher. If one analyzes chorionic villi after ultrasound diagnosis of fetal demise, rather than relying on later recovery of spontaneously expelled products, the frequency of chromosomal abnormalities proves to be 75 to 90 percent.[24,25]

Among second-trimester losses, one also observes chromosomal abnormalities similar to those observed in liveborn infants: trisomies 13, 18, and 21; monosomy X; and sex chromosomal polysomies. Among third-trimester losses (stillborn infants) the frequency of chromosomal abnormalities is approximately 5 percent.[26] This frequency is less than that observed in earlier abortuses, but still higher than found among liveborns (0.6 percent).

Autosomal Trisomy

Autosomal trisomies comprise the largest (approximately 50 percent) single class of chromosomal complements in cytogenetically abnormal spontaneous abortions. Frequencies of these trisomies are listed in Table 22–1. Trisomy for every chromosome except chromosome 1 has been reported, and trisomy for that chromosome has been observed in an eight-cell embryo.[27]

Table 22–1. CHROMOSOMAL COMPLEMENTS IN SPONTANEOUS ABORTIONS: RECOGNIZED CLINICALLY IN THE FIRST TRIMESTER*

Complement	Frequency	(%)
Normal 46,XX or 46,XY		54.1
Triploidy		7.7
69,XXX	2.7	
69,XYX	0.2	
69,XXY	4.0	
Other	0.8	
Tetraploidy		2.6
92,XXX	1.5	
92,XXYY	0.55	
Not Stated	0.55	
Monosomy X		18.6
Structural abnormalities		1.5
Sex chromosomal polysomy		0.2
47,XXX	0.05	
47,XXY	0.15	
Autosomal monosomy (G)		0.1
Autosomal trisomy for chromosomes		22.3
1	0	
2	1.11	
3	0.25	
4	0.64	
5	0.04	
6	0.14	
7	0.89	
8	0.79	
9	0.72	
10	0.36	
11	0.04	
12	0.18	
13	1.07	
14	0.82	
15	1.68	
16	7.27	
17	0.18	
18	1.15	
19	0.01	
20	0.61	
21	2.11	
22	2.26	
Double trisomy		0.7
Mosaic trisomy		1.3
Other abnormalities or not specified		0.9
		100.0

* Pooled data from several series, as referenced elsewhere by Simpson and Bombard.[23]

The most common trisomy is trisomy 16. Most trisomies show a maternal age effect, but the effect is variably marked among certain chromosomes. The maternal age effect is especially impressive for double trisomies.

Various attempts have been made to correlate morphologic abnormalities with specific trisomies,[28,29] but relationships are imprecise. Trisomies incompatible with life predictably show slower growth than trisomies compatible with life (trisomies 13, 18, and 21). For example, the mean crown–rump length in abortuses shown to be trisomic (13, 18, and 21) is 20.65 mm compared with only 10.66 mm for trisomies that virtually never survive to term (e.g., trisomy 10 or 16).[28] Either the former survive longer or the latter show greater intrauterine growth retardation, or both. Potentially viable trisomies tend to show anomalies consistent with those found in full-term liveborn trisomic infants.[28,29] The malformations present have been said to be more severe than these found in induced abortuses detected after prenatal diagnosis.

Aneuploidy usually results from errors of meiosis I, specifically arising in maternal meiosis. Most trisomies are accounted for by maternal meiotic errors. In trisomy 13 and trisomy 21, 90 percent of these maternal cases arise at meiosis I; almost all trisomy 16 cases arise in maternal meiosis I.[30] A notable exception is trisomy 18, in which two thirds of the 90 percent maternal meiotic cases arise at meiosis II.[31,32]

Errors of maternal meiosis I are associated with advanced maternal age and in turn correlate with decreased to absent meiotic recombination.[31–33] The cytologic hypothesis invoked to explain this relationship generally is the product-line hypothesis, which states that oocytes ovulated earlier in life are characterized by more recombinants and, hence, less likelihood for nondisjunction.[34] The clinical significance is that adverse periconceptional events (e.g., exposure to toxins, potentially fertilization involving gametes aged in vivo) are unlikely to play a major etiologic role in human trisomies. Thus, failure to find increased frequency of Down syndrome in pregnancies conceived on days other than the day of ovulation or the day before is not surprising.[35,36]

Errors in *paternal* meiosis account for 10 percent of acrocentric (13, 14, 15, 21, and 22) trisomies.[37] In trisomy 21, paternal meiotic errors are equally likely to arise in meiosis I or II,[38] a circumstance that contrasts with the situation in maternal meiotic errors.

Among nonacrocentric chromosomes, paternal contribution to aneuploidy is even less than 10 percent.

Polyploidy

In polyploidy, more than two haploid chromosomal complements exist. Triploidy (3n = 69) and tetraploidy

(4n = 92) occur often in abortuses. Triploid abortuses are usually 69,XXY or 69,XXX, resulting from dispermy.[39,40] Pathologic findings in triploid placentas include a disproportionately large gestational sac, cystic degeneration of placental villi, intrachorial hemorrhage, and hydropic trophoblasts (pseudomolar degeneration).[28,29] Malformations include neural tube defects and omphaloceles, anomalies reminiscent of those observed in triploid conceptuses progressing to term. Facial dysmorphia and limb abnormalities have also been reported. An association exists between triploidy and hydatidiform mole, a "partial mole" said to exist if molar tissue and fetal parts coexist. The more common "complete" hydatidiform mole is 46,XX, of androgenetic origin.[40]

Tetraploidy is uncommon, rarely progressing beyond 2 to 3 weeks of embryonic life.

Monosomy X

Monosomy X is the single most common chromosomal abnormality among spontaneous abortions, accounting for 15 to 20 percent of abnormal specimens (Fig. 22–3). Monosomy X embryos usually consist of only an umbilical cord stump. Later in gestation, anomalies characteristic of the Turner syndrome may be seen, specifically cystic hygromas and generalized edema. Although liveborn 45,X individuals usually lack germ cells, 45,X abortuses show germ cells; however, these germ cells rarely develop beyond the primordial germ cell stage. The pathogenesis of 45,X germ cell failure thus involves not so much failure of germ cell development as more rapid attrition in 45,X than in 46,XX embryos.[41,42] Incidentally, this observation makes plausible the rare but well-documented pregnancies occurring in 45,X individuals.[43]

Monosomy X usually (80 percent) occurs as a result of paternal sex chromosome loss.[44] This observation is consistent with the lack of a maternal age effect in 45,X or possibly even an inverse effect.

Structural Chromosomal Rearrangement

Structural chromosomal rearrangement account for 1.5 percent of all abortuses (Table 22–1). Rearrangements (e.g., translocation) may either arise de novo during gametogenesis or be inherited from a parent carrying a "balanced" translocation or inversion. Phenotypic consequences depend on the specific duplicated or deficient chromosomal segments. Although not a common cause of sporadic losses, inherited translocations are an important cause of *repeated* fetal wastage.

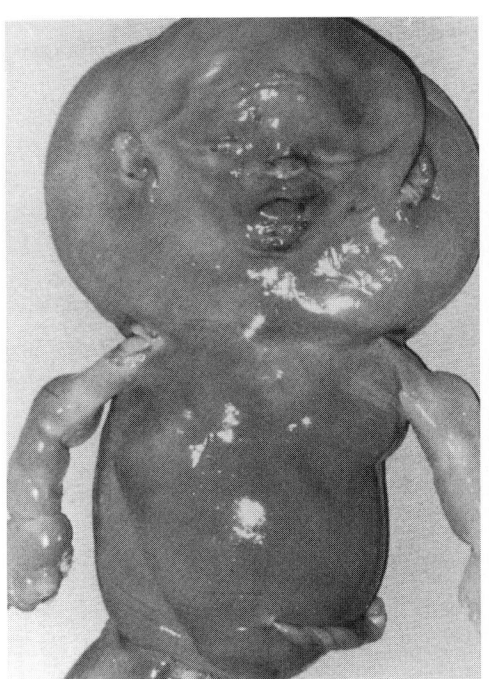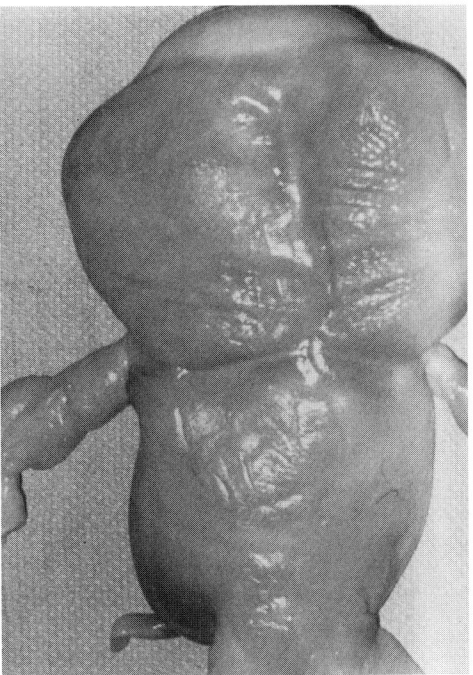

Figure 22–3. Photograph of a 45,X abortus. (From Simpson CL, Bombard AT: Chromosomal abnormalities in spontaneous abortion: frequency, pathology and genetic counseling. *In* Edmonds K, Bennett MJ [eds]: Spontaneous Abortion. London, Blackwell, 1987, p 51, with permission.)

Sex Chromosomal Polysomy (X or Y)

The complements 47,XXY and 47,XYY each occur in about 1 per 800 liveborn male births; 47,XXX occurs in 1 per 800 female births. X or Y polysomies are only slightly more common in abortuses than in liveborns.

MENDELIAN AND POLYGENIC/ MULTIFACTORIAL ETIOLOGY

The 30 to 50 percent of first-trimester abortuses that show no chromosomal abnormalities could still have undergone fetal demise as a result of other genetic etiologies. Neither mendelian nor polygenic/multifactorial disorders show chromosomal abnormalities. Many excellent anatomic studies of abortuses have demonstrated structural abnormalities, but lack of cytogenetic data on the dissected specimens makes it nearly impossible to determine the precise role of noncytogenetic mechanisms in early embryonic maldevelopment. Doubtless pivotal to early development are many mendeliam genes, mutation of which would be expected to result in embryonic death and pregnancy loss.

Novel Cytogenetic Mechanisms

Beyond the scope of this chapter are several novel cytogenetic mechanisms that have been shown to explain certain placental abnormalities and, hence, fetal losses in conceptuses with a diploid number of chromosomes.

One possibility is mosaicism restricted to the placenta, the embryo per se being normal. This phenomenon is termed "confined placental mosaicism." Losses caused by this mechanism may already be reflected in extant data because most studies have involved analysis only of villous material. Related to confined placental mosaicism (CPD) is the phenomenon of uniparental disomy (UPD). In UPD, both homologues for a given chromosome are derived from a single parent, probably as a result of expulsion of a chromosome from a trisomic zygote. The karyotype would appear normal (46,XX or 46,XY), but genes on the involved chromosome would actually lack contribution of one parent. For example, uniparental disomy for chromosome 21 has been detected in an embryonic abortus.[45]

Genes acting in novel fashion can also cause spontaneous abortions. One hypothesis is that highly skewed X-inactivation is associated with recurrent abortions. Of 48 women having two prior losses without explanation, 7 (14.6 percent) had highly skewed X-inactivation, defined as 90 percent of their X chromosomes originating from one specific parent (expected 50 percent); only 1 of 67 controls (1.5 percent) showed

skewed X-inactivation).[46] Male offspring of a woman with skewed X-inactivation might be aborted. A pedigree consistent with this hypothesis has been reported.[47]

GENETIC COUNSELING AND RECURRENT RISKS

The obstetrician faced with a couple experiencing spontaneous abortion has several immediate obligations: (1) inform the couple concerning the frequency of fetal wastage (10 to 12 percent clinically recognized pregnancies) and its likely etiology (at least 50 percent cytogenetic), (2) provide recurrence risk rates, and (3) determine the necessity of a formal clinical evaluation.

Patient Information

The responsibility of informing patients can be fulfilled by summarizing the salient facts cited in this chapter and emphasizing common etiologies responsible for fetal losses. Worth citing explicitly is the positive correlation between loss rates and both advancing maternal age and prior losses (see below). The maternal age effect is not solely the result of increased trisomic abortions, but presumably reflects endometrial factors as well.

Recurrence Risks

Loss rates are definitely increased among women who have experienced previous losses, but not nearly to the extent once thought (Table 22–2). For decades, obstetricians fervently believed in the concept of "habitual

Table 22–2. APPROXIMATE RECURRENCE RISK FIGURES USEFUL FOR COUNSELING WOMEN WITH REPEATED SPONTANEOUS ABORTIONS*

	Prior Abortions	Risk (%)
Women with liveborn infants	0	5–10
	1	20–25
	2	25
	3	30
	4	30
Women without liveborn infants	3	30–40

* Recurrence risks are slightly higher for older women and for those who smoke cigarettes or drink alcohol and for those exposed to high levels of selected chemical toxins.
Based on data from Warbuton and Fraser,[49] Poland et al.,[50] and Regan[5].

abortion." After three losses, the risk of subsequent losses was thought to rise sharply. Such beliefs were based on calculations made in 1938 by Malpas,[48] who concluded that following three abortions the likelihood of a subsequent one was 80 to 90 percent. Occurrence of three consecutive spontaneous abortions was thus said for decades to confer upon a women the designation of "habitual aborter." These risk figures not only proved incorrect but also were and unfortunately still seem subconsciously to be used as "controls" for clinical studies evaluating various treatment plans. This practice led to unwarranted acceptance of certain interventions, the most famous of which was diethylstilbestrol (DES) treatment.

In 1964, Warburton and Fraser[49] showed that the likelihood of recurrent abortion rose only to 25 to 30 percent, irrespective of whether a woman had previously experienced one, two, three, or even four spontaneous abortions. This concept has been confirmed in many subsequent studies, with the additional observation that if no previous liveborns have occurred the likelihood of fetal loss is somewhat higher.[50] Lowest risks (5 percent) are observed in nulliparous women with no prior losses.[5] Women who smoke cigarettes or drink alcohol moderately are probably at slightly higher risk.[51] Recurrence risks are higher if the abortus is cytogenetically normal than cytogenetically abnormal.[52]

Taking all the above into account, the prognosis is reasonably good even without therapy, the predicted success rate being 70 percent. Indeed, Vlaanderen and Treffers[53] reported successful pregnancies in each of 21 women having unexplained prior repetitive losses but subjected to no intervention. Other groups reached similar conclusions, including the control (placebo) group in a recent well-publicized immunotherapy study.[54,55] To be judged efficacious, therapeutic regimens must achieve successes greater than 70 percent.

Necessity of Formal Evaluation

Every couple experiencing a fetal loss should be counseled and provided recurrence risk rates, but not every couple requires formal assessment. Infertile couples who are in their fourth decade may choose to be evaluated after only two losses. After three losses, all couples should be offered formal evaluation. Once a couple enters evaluation, they should undergo all tests standard for a given practitioner. There is no scientific rationale for performing some studies after three losses but deferring others until after four losses. Any couple having a stillborn or anomalous liveborn infant should undergo cytogenetic studies unless the stillborn was known to have a normal chromosome complement. Parental chromosomal rearrangements (i.e., translocations or inversions) should be excluded.

ETIOLOGY AND CLINICAL EVALUATION OR REPETITIVE ABORTIONS

Translocations

Structural chromosomal abnormalities are generally accepted as one explanation for repetitive abortions. The most common structural rearrangement encountered is a translocation, found in about 5 percent of couples experiencing repeated losses.[56–58] Individuals with balanced translocations are phenotypically normal, but abortuses or abnormal liveborns may show chromosomal duplications or deficiencies as a result of normal meiotic segregation. About 60 percent of the translocations detected are reciprocal, and 40 percent are robertsonian. Females are about twice as likely as males to show a balanced translocation.[56]

The clinical significance of translocations is illustrated in Figure 22–4. If a child has Down syndrome as a result of such a translocation, the rearrangement will prove to have originated de novo in 50 to 75 percent of cases. That is, a balanced translocation will not exist in either parent. The likelihood of Down syndrome recurring in subsequent offspring is minimal. On the other hand, the risk is significant in the 25 to 50 percent of families in which individuals have Down syndrome as the result of a balanced parental translocation (e.g., parental complement $45,XX,-14,-21,+t[14q;21q]$). The theoretical risk of having a child with Down syndrome is 33 percent, but empirical risks are considerably less. The likelihood is only 2 percent if the father carries the translocation and 10 percent if the mother carries the translocation.[59,60] If robertsonian (centric-fusion) translocations involve other chromosomes, empirical risks are lower. In t(13q;14q), the risk for liveborn trisomy 13 is 1 percent or less.

Reciprocal translocations are those that do not involve centromeric fusion. Empirical data for specific translocations are usually not available, but useful generalizations can be made on the basis of pooled data derived from many different translocations. Studies of sperm chromosomes[61] theoretically might provide data specific for a given translocation in a specific individual, but this is not readily available. Of interest is that sperm of fathers experiencing repeated losses show no more than the expected 10 percent of cytogenetic abnormalities.[62]

Irrespective, theoretical risks for abnormal offspring (unbalanced reciprocal translocations) are far greater than empirical risks. Overall, the risk is 12 percent for offspring of either female heterozygotes or male heterozygotes.[59,60] Detecting a parental chromosomal rearrangement thus profoundly affects subsequent preg-

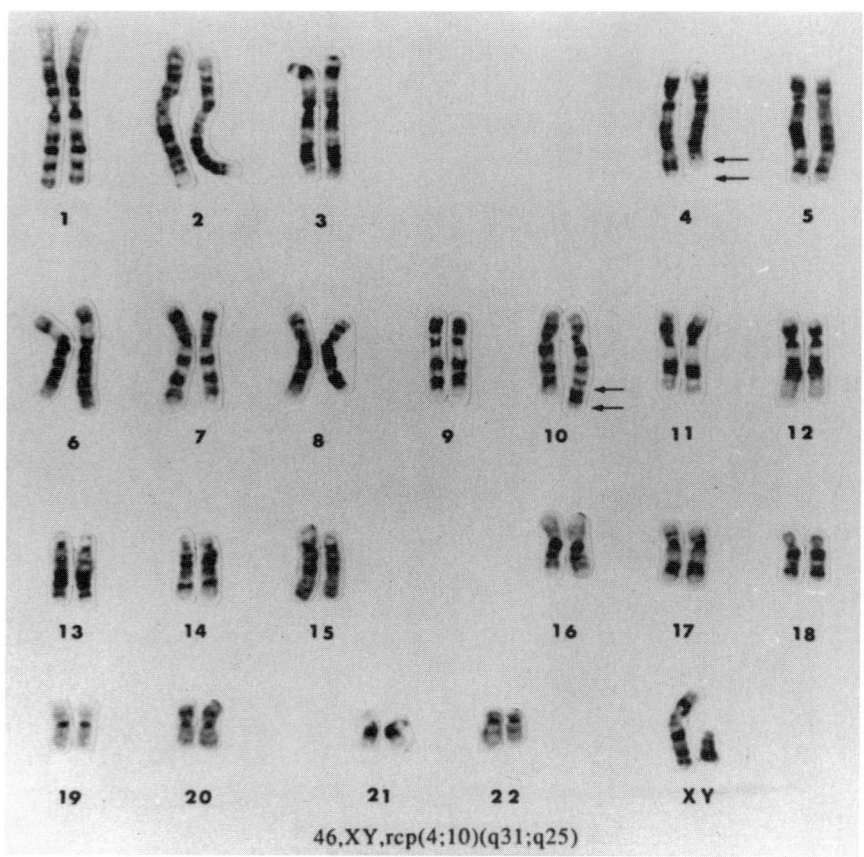

46,XY,rcp(4:10)(q31;q25)

Figure 22–4. Balanced translocation detected in a woman experiencing multiple abortions. (From Simpson JL, Tharapel AT: Principles of cytogenetics. *In* Philip E, Barnes J [eds]: Scientific Foundations of Obstetrics and Gynaecology, 4th ed. London, Heinemann Medical Books, 1991, p 27, with permission.)

nancy management. Antenatal cytogenetic studies should be offered in subsequent pregnancies. The frequency of unbalanced fetuses is lower if parental balanced translocations are ascertained through repetitive abortions (3 percent) than through anomalous liveborns (nearly 20 percent).[59]

A few translocations preclude the possibility of normal liveborn infants, namely, translocations involving homologous chromosomes (e.g., t[13q13q] or t[21q21q]). If the father carries such a structural rearrangement, artificial insemination may be appropriate. If the mother carries the rearrangement, donor oocytes or donor embryos (assisted reproductive technologies) should be considered.

Inversions

A less common parental chromosomal rearrangement responsible for repetitive pregnancy losses is an inversion. In inversions the order of genes is reversed. Analogous to translocations, individuals heterozygous for an inversion should be normal if their genes are merely rearranged. However, individuals with inversions suffer abnormal reproductive consequences as a result of normal meiotic phenomena, namely, crossing-over in their

gametes, yielding unbalanced gametes. Pericentric inversions (see Chapter 9) are present in perhaps 0.1 percent of females and 0.1 percent of males experiencing repeated spontaneous abortions. Paracentric inversions are even rarer.

Counseling a couple having an inversion is complex. Inversions involving only a small portion of the total chromosomal length paradoxically may be less significant clinically because the large duplications or large deficiencies that follow crossing-over are usually lethal. By contrast, inversions involving only 30 to 60 percent of the total chromosomal length are relatively more likely to be characterized by duplications or deficiencies compatible with survival.[63]

Overall, females with a *pericentric* inversion have a 7 percent risk of abnormal liveborns; males carry a 5 percent risk. Pericentric inversions ascertained through phenotypically normal probands are less likely to result in abnormal liveborns.

Few data are available on recurrence risks for *paracentric* inversions. Theoretically, there should be less risk for detecting unbalanced products at chorionic villus sampling (CVS) or amniocentesis than with pericentric inversions because paracentric recombinants are usually lethal. On the other hand, abortions and abnormal liveborns have been observed within the same kindred, and the risk for unbalanced viable offsprings has been tabulated at 4 percent.[64] Antenatal cytogenetic studies should be offered.

Recurrent Aneuploidy

Already discussed at length as the most common overall cause for sporadic abortions, numerical chromosomal abnormalities (aneuploidy) may be responsible for both recurrent as well as sporadic losses. This reasoning is made on the basis of observations that the complements of successive abortuses in a given family are more likely to be either recurrently normal or recurrently abnormal (Table 22–3). If the complement of the first abortus is abnormal, the likelihood is 80 percent that the complement of the second abortus also will be abnormal.[65] The recurrent abnormality usually is trisomy.

These data suggest that certain couples are predisposed toward chromosomally abnormal conceptions. Although it can be argued that corrections for maternal age render the ostensible nonrandom distribution nonsignificant, this author counsels increased risks compared with normal women of comparable age. If couples are predisposed to recurrent aneuploidy, they might logically be at increased risk not only for aneuploid abortuses but also for aneuploid liveborns. The trisomic autosome in a subsequent pregnancy might not always confer lethality, but rather might be compatible with life (e.g., trisomy 21). Indeed, the risk of liveborn trisomy 21 following an aneuploid abortus is about 1 percent.[66]

Information concerning fetal chromosomal status may be lacking for couples having repetitive abortions. Antenatal diagnosis then may or may not be appropriate. Risks for abnormal offspring are probably increased, but the risk of amniocentesis or CVS is especially troublesome to couples who have had difficulty achieving pregnancy. Finally, there is some evidence that abortion rates are *lowest* in couples with prior losses when conception occurred in midcycle.[52] Midcycle fertilization is recommended in subsequent pregnancies.

Luteal Phase Defects

Implantation in an inhospitable endometrium is a plausible explanation for spontaneous abortion. The hormone usually hypothesized to be deficient is progesterone, a deficiency of which might fail to prepare the estrogen-primed endometrium for implantation. Luteal phase defects (LPDs) is the term used to describe the endometrium manifesting an inadequate progesterone effect. Progesterone secreted by the corpus luteum is necessary to support the endometrium until the trophoblast produces sufficient progesterone to maintain pregnancy, an event occurring around 7 gestational (menstrual) weeks or 5 weeks after conception. Plausible pathogenic mechanisms underlying LPD include decreased gonadotropin-releasing hormone (GnRH), decreased follicle-stimulating hormone (FSH), inadequate luteinizing hormone (LH), inadequate ovarian steroidogenesis, or endometrial receptor defects.

Once almost universally accepted as a common cause for fetal wastage, LPD now seems to be considered an uncommon cause. Although plausible clinically, there are no randomized studies verifying efficacy of treatment. Moreover, histology identical to that observed with luteal phase "defects" exists in fertile women. When regularly menstruating fertile women with no history of abortions were biopsied in serial cycles, the frequency of LPD was 51.4 percent in any single cycle and 26.7 percent in sequential cycles.[67]

A major difficulty in determining the frequency as well as validity of LPD is lack of standard diagnostic criteria. LPD was originally defined on the basis of an endometrial biopsy lagging at least 2 days behind the actual postovulation date. This was determined by counting backward from the next menstrual period, as-

Table 22–3. RECURRENT ANEUPLOIDY: THE RELATIONSHIP BETWEEN KARYOTYPES OF SUCCESSIVE ABORTUSES*

Complement of First Abortus	Complement of Second Abortus					De Novo Rearrangement
	Normal	Trisomy	Monosomy	Triploidy	Tetraploid	
Normal	142	18	5	7	3	2
Trisomy	31	30	1	4	3	1
Monosomy X	7	5	3	3	0	0
Triploidy	7	4	1	4	0	0
Tetraploidy	3	1	0	2	0	0
De novo rearrangement	1	3	0	0	0	0

* Tabulation by Warburton et al.[65]

suming 14 days from the date of ovulation to menses. However, the original reports of Noyes et al.[68] showed a mean error of 1.81 days in dating, suggesting that an endometrial biopsy should be designated "out-of-phase" only if it lags 3 or more days behind the actual postovulation date. Not surprisingly, interobserver variation is considerable. Endometrial biopsies (n = 62) read by five different pathologists resulted in differences in interpretation that would have altered management in approximately one third of patients.[69] Reading coded endometrial biopsy slides a second time, the same pathologist agreed with his or her initial diagnosis in only 25 percent of samples.[70] At a minimum, at least two out-of-phase biopsies are necessary to make the diagnosis of LPD. Other diagnostic criteria have been proposed, such as integrated serum progesterone (three values) levels.[71] However, most investigators believe hormone levels are no better than endometrial biopsy. (Indeed, in patients with two or more spontaneous abortions, a low serum progesterone in the luteal phase is only 71 percent predictive of an LPD as defined on the basis of an abnormal endometrial biopsy.[72])

Attempting to characterize gonadotropin and progesterone secretion in LPD, Soules et al.[73,74] concluded that diagnosis is best made on the basis of a single assay of three pooled blood samples; a level of ≤ 10 ng/ml connotes LPD.[75]

A major shortcoming is that no randomized studies have proved LPD to be a genuine entity. Efficacy of treatment is even less well established. Studies by Tho et al.[76] and Daya and Ward[77] are among those cited as evidence of efficacy, but actually their experimental designs are not optimal,[78] because concurrent control groups were not recruited. Meta-analysis by Karamardian and Grimes[79] showed no beneficial effect of progesterone treatment. Thus, LPD is an arguable entity, and if valid, may or may not be treated successfully with progesterone or progestational agents.

Of interest are observations suggesting a relationship between fetal loss and either oligomenorrhea[80] or clinically evident polycystic ovary disease.[81] These observations could be consistent with the studies described above showing pregnancy loss is lowest when conceptions occur in midcycle.[7] The pathogenesis could be endometrial dyssynchrony mediated through perturbations of LH. Regan et al.[82] reported increased pregnancy loss in 20 women with elevated LH; however, treatment to lower LH failed to decrease pregnancy loss rate.[83] Neither Carp et al.,[84] nor Tulppala et al.,[85] nor Bussen et al.[86] observed elevated LH.

Thyroid Abnormalities

Decreased conception rates and increased fetal losses are associated with overt hypothyroidism or hyperthyroidism. Subclinical thyroid dysfunction has generally not been considered an explanation for repeated losses,[87] but the situation may be more complex. Bussen and Steck[88] studied 22 habitual aborters and like numbers of nulligravid and multigravid controls. Thyroid antibodies were increased in the former. Stagnaro-Green et al.[89] and Glinoer et al.[90] concluded that antithyroid antibodies and mild thyroid disease were associated with spontaneous abortions, whereas Singh et al.[91] thought that thyroid antibodies were a useful marker for clinical losses in the ART population. Pratt et al.[92] reported increased antithyroid antibodies in euthyroid women experiencing first trimester losses, but the same group[93] also concluded that the ostensible association was secondary to nonspecific organ antibodies. Rushworth et al.[94] followed women in a repetitive abortion clinic who had antibodies against thyroglobulin or thyroid microsomal factors. The overall prevalence of antibodies in 164 women was 19 percent. However, subsequent outcomes were not significant difference whether thyroid antibody-positive or -negative.

Overall, asymptomatic thyroid antibodies would still not seem to be a major cause of early pregnancy loss.

Diabetes Mellitus

Women whose diabetes mellitus is poorly controlled are at increased risk for fetal loss.[3] In one study, women whose glycosylated hemoglobin level was greater than 4 SD above the mean showed higher pregnancy loss rates than women with lower glycosylated hemoglobin levels. This finding was also found in retrospective studies.[95] Poorly controlled diabetes mellitus should be considered one cause for early pregnancy loss, but well-controlled or subclinical diabetes is probably not a cause of early miscarriage.

Intrauterine Adhesions (Synechiae)

Intrauterine adhesions could interfere with implantation or early embryonic development. Adhesions may follow overzealous uterine curettage during the postpartum period, intrauterine surgery (e.g., myomectomy), or endometritis. Curettage is the usual explanation, with adhesions most likely to develop if curettage is performed 3 or 4 weeks after delivery. Individuals with uterine synechiae usually manifest hypomenorrhea or amenorrhea, but 15 to 30 percent show repeated abortions. If adhesions are detected in a woman experiencing repetitive losses, lysis under direct hyperoscopic visualization should be performed. Postoperatively, an intrauterine device or inflated Foley catheter may be inserted in the uterus to discourage reapposition of healing uterine surfaces. Estrogen administration should also be initiated. Approximately 50 percent of patients conceive after surgery, but the frequency of abortions remains high.

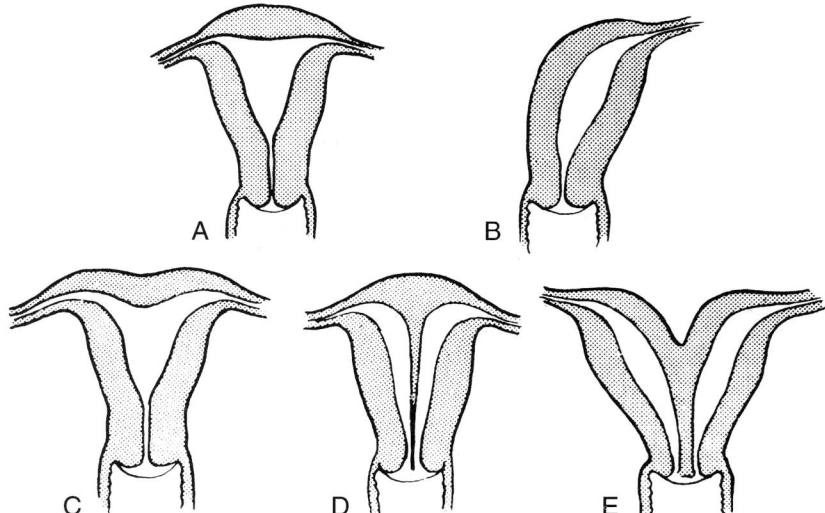

Figure 22–5. Diagrammatic representation of some müllerian fusion anomalies. *A,* Normal uterus, fallopian tubes, and cervix. *B,* Uterus unicornis (absence of one uterine horn). *C,* Uterus arcuatus (broadening and medial depression of a portion of the uterine septum). *D,* Uterus septus (persistence of a complete uterine septum). *E,* Uterus bicornis unicollis (two hemiuteri, each leading to same cervix). (From Simpson JL: Disorders of Sexual Differentiation, Etiology and Clinical Delineation. San Diego, Academic Press, 1976, with permission.)

Incomplete Müllerian Fusion

Müllerian fusion defects (Fig. 22–5) are an accepted cause of *second*-trimester losses and pregnancy complications. Low birth weight, breech presentation, and uterine bleeding are other abnormalities associated with müllerian fusion defects. Ben Rafael et al.[96] confirmed these conclusions after comparison with women with hysterosalpingogram-proven normal uteri; however, most other reports lack controls.[97–103] A few studies claim that the worst outcomes are associated with either septate uteri[99] or T-shaped uteri,[98] but others discern few differences among various anomalies.[102] Some authors[104] believe that minor structural defects may be just as deleterious as overt defects, but this does not seem completely plausible.

The major problem in attributing cause and effect for second-trimester complications and uterine anomalies is that the latter are so frequent that adverse outcomes could often be coincidental. For example, Stampe-Sorensen[105] found unsuspected bicornuate uteri in 1.2 percent of 167 women undergoing laparoscopic sterilization; 3.6 percent had a severely septate uterus, and 15.3 percent had fundal anomalies. Simon et al.[106] found müllerian defects in 3.2 percent (22 of 679) of fertile women; 20 of the 22 defects were septate. Treatment has traditionally involved surgical correction, such as metroplasty. Ludmire et al.[107] wondered if conservative treatment might not be just as efficacious as surgical correction, following 101 women with an uncorrected malformation through a standardized protocol to decrease physical activity. Fetal survival rates in both bicornuate and septate groups (58 and 65 percent, respectively) did not differ significantly from rates in the same patients prior to institution of the protocol (52 and 53 percent, respectively).

First-trimester abortions might also be caused by müllerian fusion defects. Septate uteri might raise the risk of poor implantation on a poorly vascularized and inhospitable surface. Abortions occurring after ultrasonographic confirmation of a viable pregnancy at 8 or 9 weeks may properly be attributed to uterine fusion defects if the latter is present; however, losses having no confirmation of fetal viability at that time are statistically more likely to represent missed abortions in which fetal demise occurred prior to 8 weeks. Women experiencing second-trimester abortions can be assumed to benefit from uterine reconstruction, but reconstructive surgery is not necessarily advisable if losses are restricted to the first trimester.

Leiomyomas

Although leiomyomas are very frequent, relatively few affected women with leiomyomas develop symptoms requiring medical or surgical therapy. That leiomyomas cause pregnancy wastage per se rather than obstetric complications like prematurity is thus plausible but probably rare. Analogous to uterine anomalies, the coexistence of uterine leiomyomas and reproductive losses need not necessarily imply a causal relationship. Location of leiomyomas is probably more important than size, submucous leiomyomas being most likely to cause abortion. Postulated mechanisms leading to pregnancy loss include (1) thinning of the endometrium over the surface of a submucous leiomyoma, predisposing to implantation in a poorly decidualized site; (2) rapid growth caused by the hormonal milieu of pregnancy, compromising the blood supply of the leiomyoma and resulting in necrosis ("red degeneration") that in turn leads to uterine contractions and eventually fetal expulsion; and (3) encroachment of leiomyomas upon the space required by the developing fetus, leading to premature delivery through mechanisms presumably analogous to those operative in incomplete müllerian fusion. Relative lack of space can also lead to fetal deformations (i.e., positional abnormalities arising in a genetically normal fetus).

Surgical procedures to reduce leiomyomata may occasionally be warranted for women experiencing repetitive second-trimester abortions, but more often leiomyomata will have no etiologic relationship to pregnancy loss. Surgery should be reserved for women whose abortuses were both phenotypically and karyotypically normal and in which viability until at least 9 to 10 weeks was documented.

Incompetent Internal Cervical Os

A functionally intact cervix and lower uterine cavity are obvious prerequisites for a successful intrauterine pregnancy. Characterized by painless dilation and effacement, cervical incompetence usually occurs during the middle second or early third trimester. This condition frequently follows traumatic events like cervical amputation, cervical lacerations, forceful cervical dilatation, or conization. A relationship to various connective tissue disorders is plausible but yet unproved. The various surgical techniques to correct cervical incompetence are discussed in Chapter 23.

Infections

Infections are accepted causes of late fetal wastage and logically could be responsible for early fetal loss as well. Microorganisms and conditions reported to be associated with spontaneous abortion include variola, vaccinia, *Salmonella typhi*, *Vibrio fetus*, malaria, Cytomegalovirus, *Brucella, Toxoplasma, Mycoplasma hominis, Chlamydia trachomatis,* and *Ureaplasma urealyticum.* Transplacental infection doubtless occurs with each of these microorganisms, and sporadic losses could logically be caused by any. However, verification at these logical deductions has not been forthcoming. Other studies have found no difference in outcome between women treated and not treated with antibiotics. Unanswered also is whether the infectious agents were causative in the fetal losses or merely arose secondarily after demise caused by a noninfectious etiology. Confounding variables (e.g., maternal age, prior pregnancy history) are also rarely taken into account. Overall, a purported association between a common microorganism and pregnancy loss could easily reflect chance findings or be explained by other factors.

Of all organisms mentioned, *Ureaplasma* and *Chlamydia* are not only the most commonly implicated in *repetitive* abortion but also fulfill certain prerequisites necessary to assume a causal relationship. Both can exist in an asymptomatic state, and neither necessarily is so severe as to cause infertility. From 46 women with histories of three or more consecutive losses of unknown etiology, Stray-Pedersen et al.[108] recovered *Ureaplasma* significantly more often among women with repetitive abortions (28 percent) than among female controls (7 percent). Infected women and their husbands ($n = 43$) were then treated with doxycycline, with subsequent cultures confirming eradication of *Ureaplasma.* Nineteen of the 43 women became pregnant; of the 19, three experienced another spontaneous abortion and 16 had normal full-term infants. Among 18 women with untreated *Ureaplasma*, only 5 full-term pregnancies occurred.

Because of the presence of chlamydial antibodies in the sera of women who experienced repeated losses, an association has been claimed on the basis of presence of high titers.[109,110] However, other data show no relationship.[111,112] An immunohistochemical study found no difference in the frequency of cytomegalovirus antigen in karyotypically normal and abnormal abortuses, suggesting no causal association.[113] Paukku et al.[114] found no differences in the frequencies of IgG-IgA antibodies to *C. trachomatis* in a study of 70 Finnish women with multiple losses. Toxoplasmosis antibodies have been observed in Mexican and in Egyptian women having repetitive losses,[115,116] but whether frequencies are higher in those general populations is unclear. The most recent studies have not concluded that toxoplasmosis is not a significant cause of pregnancy loss.[117]

A key question is whether infectious agents *cause* fetal losses or merely arise following fetal demise for a host of other etiologies. Cohort surveillance for infections beginning in early pregnancy is necessary in order to determine the etiologic role of infections in pregnancy loss. To this end, Simpson et al.[118] analyzed data collected prospectively on clinical infections in 818 women followed frequently from early in the first trimester. No clinical evidence was found that infection occurred more often in the 112 subjects experiencing pregnancy loss compared to the 706 having successful pregnancies. This observation held both for the 2-week interval in which a given loss was recognized clinically as well as in the prior 2-week interval. These data suggest that the attributable risk of infection in first-trimester spontaneous abortion is low.

What evaluation and management is recommended? Culturing the endometrium for *U. urealyticum* seems reasonable, with culture-positive women having such infections treated. Alternatively, tetracycline therapy can be reasoned to be so innocuous that empiric treatment with doxycycline (100 mg orally twice a day for 10 days, both husband and nonpregnant wife) could be recommended.

Antifetal Antibodies

Perturbations of the immune system can be responsible for fetal wastage. However, the nature of the immunologic process responsible for maintaining pregnancy has proved to be complex. Several different immunologic processes may play a role.

In one immunologic process, an otherwise normal mother produces antibodies against her fetus on the basis of genetic dissimilarities. Fetal loss is well documented in Rh-negative (D-negative) women having anti-D antibodies. More apropos for early pregnancy loss is the presence of anti-P antibodies. Most individuals are genotype Pp or PP, but one may be homozygous for p (pp). If a woman of genotype pp has a Pp or PP mate, resulting offspring may or must be Pp. If the mother develops anti-P antibodies, Pp fetuses will be rejected (aborted) early in gestation. Plasmapheresis and other modalities may be therapeutically efficacious.[119,120]

Hill and colleagues[121] proposed that perturbations of cytokines cause repetitive abortions in women through T-helper cell abnormalities. The rationale is based on T-helper 1 (Th1) cytokines being deleterious, but Th2 cytokines not. The former includes tumor necrosis factor (TNF), interleukin (IL) -2, and interferon (IFN)-γ; the latter includes IL-4, IL-5, IL-6, and IL-10, all secreted by activated T cells expressing the CD4 phenotype. Natural killer cells expressing CD56 also produce salutary cytokines. In women with recurrent loss, immune cell responsiveness becomes activated to produce increased IFN-γ and TNF.[122] Supporting the hypothesis that Th1 cytokines are deleterious, down-regulation of Th1 cytokines in certain mammalian species improves pregnancy outcome.[123,124] Progesterone therapy is said by some to mitigate against the deleterious effects.

Autoimmune Disease

An association between second-trimester pregnancy loss and certain autoimmune disease is generally accepted.[125,126] Antibodies found in women with pregnancy loss encompass nonspecific antinuclear antibodies (ANAs) as well as antibodies against such cellular components as phospholipids, histones, and double- or single-stranded DNA. Antiphospholipid antibodies in turn represent a broad category that encompasses lupus anticoagulant (LAC) antibodies and anticardiolipin antibodies (aCL). Most investigators[127] agree that midtrimester fetal death is increased in women with LAC or aCL; in fact, dramatically so. Controversy centers on the role of these antibodies in first-trimester losses.

Descriptive studies initially seemed to show increased anticardiolipin antibodies in women with first-trimester pregnancy losses. However, frequencies of various antiphospholipid antibodies (LAC, aCL, aPL) soon were shown to be similar in women who experience and who do not experience first-trimester abortions.[128–131] A major pitfall in assessing the role of these antibodies in first-trimester losses is the unavoidable selection bias in studying couples only after they have presented with spontaneous abortions. That antibodies did not arise until *after* the pregnancy loss can not be excluded in most experimental designs. To address this pitfall, Simpson et al.[132] analyzed sera prospectively obtained from women within 21 days of conception. A total of 93 women who later experienced pregnancy loss were matched 2:1 with 190 controls who subsequently had a normal liveborn offspring.[132] No association was observed between pregnancy loss and presence of either aPL or aCL.

Although neither aCL nor aPL would seem to contribute greatly, if at all, to first-trimester pregnancy loss in the general population, the issue remains open in the opinion of some. For example, some believe that results would be different if more specific assays were performed, such as antiphophatidylethanolamine.[133] Another pitfall is that marked variation in antiphospholipid antibodies occurs during pregnancy.[134] Another subset consists of women successfully achieving pregnancy by in vitro fertilization, who in some reports show increased prevalences of aCL.[135] Power calculations are also inadequate to exclude an effect limited to selected subsets, like the 3 to 4 percent of women with three or more repetitive losses; however, one third of women in the cohort study of Simpson et al.[132] experienced at least one prior loss, and in that group the frequency of aCL and aPL was not increased compared to those of women without prior losses.[136]

It has also been claimed that even if aCL and aPL are not present, antibodies b2 glycoprotein (aβ2GP-1) might still be increased in repetitive aborters. However, Balasch et al.[137] found no increase. Only 1 of 100 women having repetitive abortions and not having LAC or aCL showed elevated aβ2GP-1. No relationship is likely to exist between aβ2GP-1 and failure of implantation in the in vitro fertilization population, despite earlier claims of Stern et al.[138]

In conclusion, a relationship between first-trimester loss and aPL and aCL seems unlikely to be applicable to more than a small subset of cases. Given this, treatment regimens should be offered hesitantly and only with nontoxic agents (e.g., aspirin and heparin, but not steroids). Similarly, treating aborters with intravenous immunoglobulin is not recommended.[139]

Alloimmune Disease (Shared Parental Antigens)

If fetal rejection occurs as a result of diminished fetal–maternal immunologic interaction (alloimmune factors), immunotherapy might be beneficial to stimulate beneficial blocking antibodies generated at the few loci differing from father and mother and, hence, potentially fetus. The first prospective randomized trial produced impressive results,[140] but later studies have been far less so. In 1994 a multicenter U.S. effort pooling results of immunotherapy by injection of paternal leukocytes into the mother reported a scant 11 percent increased pregnancy rate in the immunized group.[141] Meta-analysis by Fraser et al.[142] found the odds ratio to be only 1.3 in favor of a beneficial effect. In 1999, Ober et al.[143] definitively reported a NICHD collaborative effort involving six U.S. and Canadian centers. Women with three or more spontaneous abortions of unknown cause were randomized into one arm (*n* = 91) that underwent immunization with paternal mononuclear cells; women in the other arm were given saline (controls) (*n* = 92). Pregnancy beyond 28 weeks occurred in 46 percent (31 of 68) of the immunized group versus 65 percent (41 of 63) in the nonimmunized group. These findings were the opposite of expectation if immunotherapy were salutary.

In conclusion, parental human leukocyte antigen (HLA) sharing leading to fetal rejection seems to be valid, with HLA-B the locus showing the strongest association. However, the attributable role of HLA sharing in pregnancy losses in the general population must be low, and immunotherapy is clearly not useful.

Drugs, Chemicals, and Noxious Agents

Various exogenous agents have been implicated in fetal losses. Indeed, women are exposed frequently to relatively low doses of ubiquitous agents. However, few agents can be implicated with confidence. Rarely are data adequate to determine the true role of these exogenous factors in early pregnancy losses.

Outcomes following exposures to exogenous agents are usually deduced on the basis of case-control studies. In such studies, women who aborted claimed exposure to the agent in question more often than controls. However, case-control studies suffer certain inherent biases, as reviewed in Chapter 8. The primary bias is that controls have less incentive to recall antecedent events than subjects experiencing an abnormal outcome (recall bias). Employers attempt to limit exposure of women in the reproductive age group; thus, exposures to potentially dangerous chemicals are usually unwitting and, hence, poorly documented. Moreover, pregnant women usually are exposed to many agents concurrently, making it nearly impossible to attribute adverse effects to a single agent. Given these caveats, physicians should be cautious about attributing pregnancy loss to exogenous agents. On the other hand, common sense dictates that exposure to potentially noxious agents be minimized.

X-Irradiation

Irradiation and antineoplastic agents in high doses are acknowledged abortifacients. Of course, therapeutic x-rays or chemotherapeutic drugs are administered during pregnancy only to seriously ill women whose pregnancies often must be terminated for maternal indications. On the other hand, pelvic x-ray exposure of up to perhaps 10 rad places a woman at little to no increased risk. Exposure doses are usually far less (1 to 2 rad). Still, it is prudent for pregnant hospital workers to avoid handling chemotherapeutic agents and minimize potential exposures during diagnostic x-ray procedures.

Cigarette Smoking

Smoking during pregnancy is accepted as associated with spontaneous abortion, but this could be explained partly on the basis of confounding variables. Kline et al.[144] found increased abortion rates in smokers, independent of maternal age and independent of alcohol consumption. Ness et al.[145] studied the relationship between pregnancy loss and tobacco use, as assessed by urinary cotinine levels. Four hundred women with spontaneous abortions were compared with 570 who experienced ongoing pregnancies. Women with urinary cotinine had increased risk of abortion, but the odds ratio only reached 1.8 (95 percent confidence interval [CI] 1.3 to 2.6).

Caffeine

The consensus has long been that no deleterious effects of caffeine exist, whereas most studies were retrospective and case-control in design. Data gathered in cohort fashion by Mills et al.[146] are reassuring. The odds ratio for an association between caffeine (coffee and other dietary forms) was only 1.15 (95 percent CI 0.89 to 1.49).[146] Additional data from women exposed to very high levels (>300 mg caffeine daily) would be useful, as shown by the reports of Klebanoff et al.[147] showing an association between pregnancy losses and caffeine ingestion, 7 mg daily and by Cnattinguis et al.[147a] A problem with the latter studies is difficulty in being able to separate the effects of nausea, which typically is more common in successful pregnancies. However, in general reassurance can be given concerning moderate caffeine exposure and pregnancy loss.

Alcohol

An association between alcohol consumption and fetal loss once seemed generally accepted. In one study,[144] 616 women suffering spontaneous abortions were compared with 632 women delivering at 28 gestational weeks or more. Among women whose pregnancies ended in spontaneous abortion, 17 percent drank at least twice per week; only 8.1 percent of controls drank similar quantities of alcohol. Harlap and Shiono[148] also found a slightly increased risk for abortion in women who drank in the first trimester. More recent studies have not reported a relationship in moderate drinkers. Halmesmärki et al.[149] found that alcohol consumption was nearly identical in women who did and did not experience an abortion; 13 percent of aborters and 11 percent of control women drank on average three to four drinks per week; other investigations have reached a similar conclusion.[145,150]

Alcohol consumption should be avoided or minimized during pregnancy for many reasons, but abstinence may only minimally if at all decrease pregnancy loss rate. Avoidance has other benefits that can be better substantiated.

Contraceptive Agents

Conception with an intrauterine device in place clearly increases the risk of fetal loss. However, if the device is removed prior to pregnancy, there is no increased risk of spontaneous abortions. Use of oral contraceptives before or during pregnancy is not associated with fetal loss, nor is spermicide exposure either prior to or after conception (see Chapter 9).

Environmental Chemicals

Limiting exposure to potential toxins in the workplace is recognized as prudent for pregnant women. The difficulty lies in defining the precise effect of lower exposures and attributing a specific risk. False alarms concerning potential toxins are frequent. Among the many chemical agents variously claimed to be associated with fetal losses, consensus seems to be evolving around a selected few.[151] These include anesthetic gases, arsenic, aniline dyes, benzene, solvents, ethylene oxide, formaldehyde, pesticides, and certain divalent cations (lead, mercury, cadmium). Workers in rubber industries, battery factories, and chemical production plants are among those at potential risk (see Chapter 7).

Trauma

Women commonly attribute pregnancy losses to trauma, such as a fall or blow to the abdomen. However, fetuses are actually well protected from external trauma by intervening maternal structures and amniotic fluid. The temptation to attribute a loss to minor traumatic events should be avoided.

Psychological Factors

That impaired psychological well-being predisposes to early fetal losses has been claimed but never proved. Certainly, neurotic or mentally ill women experience losses just like normal women. Whether the frequency of losses is higher in the former is less certain because potential confounding variables have not been taken into account.

Investigations cited as proving a benefit of psychological well-being are those of Stray-Pedersen et al.[152] Pregnant women who previously experienced repetitive abortions received increased attention but no specific medical therapy ("tender loving care"). These women ($n = 16$) proved more likely (85 percent) to complete their pregnancy than 42 women not offered such close attention (36 percent successful outcome). One potential pitfall was that only women living "close" to the university were eligible to be placed in the increased-attention group. Women living farther away served as "controls"; however, these women may have differed from the experimental group in other ways as well.

Other studies have also reported a beneficial effect of psychological well-being.[153–156] However, the biologic explanation for this effect remains obscure.

Severe Maternal Illness

Many debilitating maternal diseases have been implicated in early abortion. Pathogenesis is not necessarily independent of mechanisms discussed previously, specifically endocrinologic or immunologic. Symptomatic maternal diseases established as causes of fetal wastage include Wilson's disease, maternal phenylketonuria, cyanotic heart disease, hemoglobinopathies, and inflammatory bowel disease. Actually, any life-threatening disease would be expected to be associated with an increased abortion rate. Seriously ill women rarely become pregnant, but the disease process may deteriorate after the onset of pregnancy. Overall, relatively few fetal losses will be the result of severe maternal disease, with the same even more applicable for repetitive losses.

ECTOPIC PREGNANCY

In ectopic pregnancy, implantation occupies at a site other than the endometrium. Ectopic pregnancies are responsible for approximately 10 percent of all maternal mortality.[157] Moreover, the prognosis for future reproduction is poor. Only one half of women having an ectopic pregnancy are eventually delivered of a liveborn infant. Most of these never become pregnant, and up to 25 percent of those who do suffer a repeat ectopic pregnancy.[158] Various factors contribute to ectopic pregnancies, the most common being infection. Unlike intrauterine spontaneous abortions, genetic factors are not paramount in the etiology of ectopic pregnancy. Ectopic embryos show chromosomal abnormalities no more often than predicted on the basis of embryonic age.[159]

Incidence

The incidence of recorded ectopic gestation is increasing. Some of this increase seems real and some spurious. A true increase can be hypothesized as a result of

(1) improved treatment for pelvic inflammatory disease, a condition that in the past would have conferred sterility; (2) an increase in surgical corrections of fallopian tube occlusion; and (3) a greater number of elective sterilizations, some of which are later reversed surgically. However, there is also an artificial increase related to improved diagnostic techniques. Ectopic pregnancies that in the past would have been mislabeled as unexplained abdominal pain or bleeding are readily recognized today because pregnancy tests have become very sensitive.

Most ectopic pregnancies (96 percent) are tubal. The remainder are interstitial uterine ectopic pregnancies and, rarely, cervical, abdominal, or ovarian pregnancies.[160] Most tubal pregnancies are located in the distal (ampullary) two thirds of the tube. A few ectopic pregnancies are isthmic, located in the proximal portion of the extrauterine part of the tube. On rare occasions both intrauterine and extrauterine gestations can coexist (heterotopic pregnancy).

Signs and Symptoms

Abdominal pain and irregular vaginal bleeding are the most common presenting symptoms in ectopic pregnancy.[161,162] In a 1983 report of 328 patients presenting with ectopic pregnancy, 94 percent had pain, 89 percent had a missed menstrual period, 80 percent had vaginal bleeding, and 20 percent had hypotension.[163] An abdominal mass is palpable in only one half of patients with an ectopic pregnancy. Of course, passage of a decidual cast in association with vaginal bleeding nearly unequivocally indicates ectopic pregnancy, but this is uncommon. The Arias-Stella phenomenon is frequently found in the endometrium in association with ectopic pregnancies; however, this phenomenon is also seen in 70 to 80 percent of therapeutic and spontaneous abortions,[164] so it is not specific for ectopic gestation.

Ectopic pregnancies should be diagnosed before the onset of hypotension, bleeding, pain, and overt rupture. Patients with a history of tubal surgery, pelvic inflammatory disease, tubal disease, or previous ectopic pregnancy are at special risk for ectopic pregnancy and would benefit not only from their physicians' vigilance but also from routine hormone screening of the type discussed below. Fortunately, *early* diagnosis of ectopic gestation is now quite feasible. Ectopic pregnancy can be detected by 6 weeks' gestation, often as early as at 4½ gestational weeks.

Chronic ectopic pregnancy is a distinct entity. Diagnosis may be difficult because normal anatomic landmarks are distorted by the formation of adhesions resulting from chronic inflammatory processes. Chronic ectopic pregnancies present a management quandary because the significance of the associated declining

β-hCG levels is difficult to determine. The dilemma is whether resolution will occur spontaneously or require surgical intervention to prevent catastrophic hemorrhage and permanent adhesion formation resulting in tubal damage.

Diagnosis

Direct vision by laparoscopy has been the diagnostic standard for ectopic pregnancy. However, if the pregnancy is early and the gestational sac small, the gestation may not be visualized. Thus, algorithms incorporating a single measurement of serum progesterone, serial measurement of the β-subunit of hCG, pelvic ultrasonography, and uterine curettage are accepted.[164] Figure 22–6 shows a useful approach.

Single Measurement of Serum Progesterone

Serum progesterone reflects production of progesterone by the corpus luteum, which is stimulated by a viable pregnancy. Measurement of progesterone is an inexpensive screening test that can identify patients who need to undergo further testing. Ectopic pregnancy can be excluded and viable intrauterine pregnancy diagnosed with 97.5 percent sensitivity if serum progesterone levels are 25 ng/ml (≥79.5 nmol/L) or higher, obviating the need for further testing. Conversely, serum progesterone can identify nonviable pregnancies with 100 percent sensitivity if progesterone levels are 5 ng/ml (≤15.9 nmol/L) or lower.[165-168] If a single progesterone level is 5 ng/ml or lower, diagnostic uterine evacuation can be performed even if ectopic pregnancy cannot otherwise be distinguished from a spontaneous intrauterine abortion. Progesterone values above 5 but below 25 ng/ml necessitate establishing viability by ultrasonography.

Serial Serum β-hCG Measurements

β-hCG is produced by trophoblastic cells. In normal pregnancies, β-hCG concentration increases 67 percent over a 2-day interval.[169] Abnormal intrauterine or ectopic pregnancies have impaired β-hCG production and, hence, a prolonged hCG doubling time. Thus, serial β-hCG measurements can be used to assess the viability of pregnancy, signal the optimal time for ultrasonography, and document the effectiveness of diagnostic curettage.

Transvaginal Ultrasound

If β-hCG is greater than 1,500 mIU/ml and the pregnancy is intrauterine, a gestational sac should be visual-

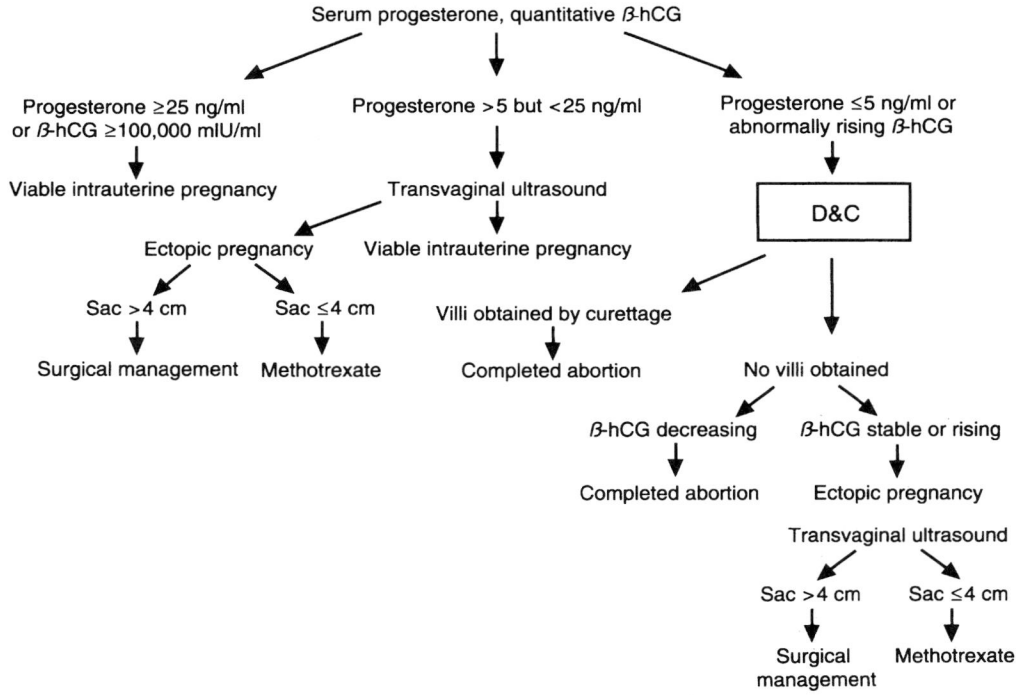

Figure 22–6. Algorithm for the diagnosis of unruptured ectopic pregnancy without laparoscopy. Progesterone measurements increase the sensitivity of the algorithm by inexpensively screening large numbers of patients during the first trimester of pregnancy. The definitive diagnosis is made by transvaginal ultrasound or uterine curettage and does not depend on the serum progesterone concentrations obtained during screening. (From Carson SA, Buster JE: The ectopic pregnancy: new advances in diagnosis and treatment. N Engl J Med 329:1174, 1993, with permission.)

ized by transvaginal ultrasound. By transabdominal ultrasound the gestational sac may not be identified until β-hCG reaches 6,000 mIU/ml. If β-hCG is greater than these levels but the gestational sac cannot be visualized, an ectopic location should be assumed. Conversely, intrauterine pregnancies may also be confirmed by ultrasound, specifically excluding ectopic pregnancy.[165–168]

Widely available in gynecologic offices and emergency rooms, ultrasonography with a 5-mHz transvaginal ultrasound probe can document intrauterine gestation earlier than transabdominal ultrasonography. Transvaginal color Doppler sonography may further enhance early diagnostic sensitivity and specificity through the identification of characteristic uterine and adnexal flow patterns.[170]

Uterine Curettage

Villi float in saline, a characteristic permitting identification of tissue obtained by curettage. If no villi are recognized and a decrease in the β-hCG level of 15 percent or more 8 to 12 hours occurs after curettage, a completed abortion can be assumed to exist. If villi are not visualized and β-hCG titers plateau or rise, trophoblasts can be assumed *not* to have been removed by the uterine curettage; thus, an ectopic pregnancy can be presumed to be present.

Surgical Treatment

Salpingectomy by laparotomy has long offered almost a 100 percent cure. However, current emphasis is not just to prevent death but also to facilitate rapid recovery, preserve fertility, and reduce costs. Laparoscopic salpingostomy and partial salpingectomy are thus rapidly replacing laparotomy. Laparotomy should be performed only when a laparoscopic approach is too difficult, the surgeon is not trained in operative laparoscopy, or the patient is hemodynamically unstable.

Linear salpingostomy is the standard laparoscopic operation when an ectopic mass is unruptured yet more than 4 cm in length by ultrasound.[165,171–175] Over the bulging antimesenteric border of the implantation site, a longitudinal incision is made by electrocautery, scissors, or laser. The products of conception are removed by forceps or suction. After hemostasis is achieved, the incision is allowed to heal by secondary intention. Alternatively, sutures can be placed. Approximately 95 percent of laparoscopic salpingostomies are successful (i.e., no additional procedures are needed).[165] Of the 93 women evaluated in one study, 86 percent were later shown to have patent oviducts; 66 percent of 430 women who were followed subsequently became pregnant, with 23 percent of those pregnancies being ectopic.[176]

Segmental resection is necessary if ectopic pregnancies are located in the isthmus (the midportion of the oviduct). Subsequent laparotomy is then necessary for reanastomosis of the surgically divided oviduct. Laparoscopic salpingectomy is also desirable for patients who do not wish to become pregnant again.

Postoperative bleeding, elevated β-hCG levels indicative of persistent viable trophoblastic tissue, and other symptoms occur in up to 20 percent of cases after conservative laparoscopic surgery. Excision of the involved oviduct or medical therapy may then be necessary.

Medical Treatment

Although operative laparoscopy has substantially fewer complications than laparotomy, there remains irreducible morbidity intrinsic to surgery and anesthesia. Medical treatments can greatly reduce this morbidity. To supplant surgery, however, medical therapies must match the high success rates, low complication rates, and good reproductive potential achieved with laparoscopic operations. This appears to be true.[165,177] The agent used is the folic acid antagonist methotrexate, which inhibits synthesis of purines and pyrimidines and thus interferes with DNA synthesis and cell multiplication. Actively proliferating trophoblasts have long been known to be vulnerable to methotrexate, as illustrated by its successful use in the treatment of gestational trophoblastic disease.

Hemodynamically stable patients with ectopic pregnancies are eligible for treatment with methotrexate if the mass is unruptured and measures 4 cm or less in diameter by ultrasound.[165] Patients with larger ectopic masses, embryonic cardiac activity, or evidence of acute intra-abdominal bleeding (acute abdomen, hypotension, or falling hematocrit) are not eligible for methotrexate therapy.[165] Outcome of treatment with systemic methotrexate (Table 22–4)[165,178] compares favorably with that of laparoscopic salpingostomy; 94 percent of women successfully treated with systemic methotrexate needed no subsequent therapy. Of women tested, 81 percent had patent oviducts; 71 percent subsequently became pregnant, with 11 percent of those being ectopic.

High doses of methotrexate can cause bone marrow suppression, acute and chronic hepatotoxicity, stomatitis, pulmonary fibrosis, alopecia, and photosensitivity. Fortunately, these side effects are not only infrequent with the shorter treatment schedules used for an ectopic pregnancy but can be mitigated against by the administration of leucovorin (citrovorum factor). Experience with methotrexate in gestational trophoblastic disease provides little reason for concern about the risks of subsequent neoplasia or congenital anomalies in later pregnancies.[179]

Safeguards are necessary to enhance the success and

Table 22–4. SUMMARY OF THE METHOTREXATE REGIMENS USED

Regimen	Monitor

Multiple dose
  Methotrexate, 1 mg/kg of body weight intramuscularly every other day (days 1, 3, and so on)
  Leucovorin, 0.1 mg/kg intramuscularly every other day (days 2, 4, and so on)
  Continue treatment until β-hCG drops ≥15% in 48 hours or 4 doses of methotrexate have been given
	Serum β-hCG weekly until undetectable; blood count, platelet count, liver enzyme levels

Single dose
  Methotrexate, 50 mg/m² of body surface area intramuscularly
  No leucovorin
	Serum β-hCG level days 4 and 7, then weekly until undetectable; initial blood count, platelet count, liver enzyme levels

From Carson SA, Buster JE: The ectopic pregnancy: new advances in diagnosis and treatment. N Engl J Med 329:1174, 1993, with permission.

minimize the toxicity of systemic methotrexate. First, the patient should undergo a pelvic examination by only a single examiner and then only once. Self-control concerning this part of management should be similar to that employed with placenta previa. Second, both physician and patient must recognize that transient pain is common, usually occurring 3 to 7 days after initiation of methotrexate therapy. The pain, presumably caused by tubal abortion, normally lasts 4 to 12 hours. Perhaps the most difficult aspect of methotrexate therapy is distinguishing the transient abdominal pain associated with successful therapy from that of rupturing ectopic pregnancy. Surgical intervention becomes necessary only when pain is accompanied by orthostatic tachycardia, hypotension, or a falling hematocrit. If uncertainty exists concerning the patient's hemodynamic stability, physicians may prefer to hospitalize the patient with pain for observation. Because colicky abdominal pain is common during the first 2 or 3 days of methotrexate therapy, patients should also be warned to avoid gas-producing foods such as leeks and cabbage. Patients should also avoid exposure to the sun because of the photosensitivity methotrexate produces.

Intramuscular methotrexate is not the only route of therapy, but less experience exists with other methods. These include the direct injection of methotrexate into the ectopic, methotrexate administered by tubal cannulation, or prostaglandins by direct injection.

Finally, few medical advances evolve without negative consequences. As ectopic pregnancy is detected earlier and more efficiently, some pregnancies that would otherwise have been spontaneously absorbed are now treated, in retrospect, needlessly. Identifying early ectopic pregnancies that are destined for spontaneous remission would thus be useful, although efforts to do so have so far been unsuccessful. "Overtreatment" of ectopic pregnancy will thus be the inevitable corollary of early intervention.

Relative Benefits of Surgical Versus Medical Therapy

Conservative laparoscopic surgery is very efficacious, as is that of systemic methotrexate therapy. Systemic methotrexate therapy is less expensive than operative laparoscopy, and patients lose less time from work. On the other hand, some patients prefer surgical therapy because they wish to avoid the possible side effects of systemic chemotherapy and a more protracted counsel of treatment. However, even after laparoscopic removal of ectopic tissue, residual tissue remains to cause hemorrhage and other complications in 20 percent of cases. With either surgical or medical treatment, weekly blood tests are thus necessary until β-hCG becomes undetectable. Only a small subgroup of patients treated with either medical or surgical therapy have been followed to determine subsequent reproductive capabilities; thus, it is difficult to state conclusively whether the rates of pregnancy, tubal patency, and recurrent ectopic pregnancy differ between medical and surgical treatment. Not until a prospective randomized study is conducted will the optimal choice of the therapy for each patient be known.

In conclusion, removal of the ectopic pregnancy by salpingostomy is recommended when laparoscopy is needed for diagnosis. We recommend systemic methotrexate when laparoscopy is not required for diagnosis. Laparoscopic surgery is also preferable when the ectopic mass is larger than 4.0 cm. A laparotomy is performed only for catastrophic hemorrhage or hemodynamic instability.

RECOMMENDED EVALUATION FOR RECURRENT PREGNANCY LOSSES

1. Couples experiencing only one first-trimester abortion should receive pertinent information, but not necessarily be evaluated formally. Mention the relatively high (10 to 15 percent) pregnancy loss rate in the general population and the beneficial effects of abortion in eliminating abnormal conceptuses. Provide the relevant recurrence risks, usually 20 to 25 percent subsequent loss in the presence of a prior liveborn and somewhat higher in the absence of a prior liveborn. Risks are higher for older women. If a specific medical illness exists, treatment is obviously necessary. Intrauterine adhesions should be lysed. Otherwise, no further evaluation need be undertaken, even if uterine anomalies or leiomyomas are detected. On the other hand, occurrence of an anomalous stillborn or liveborn warrants genetic evaluation irrespective of the number of pregnancy losses.

2. Investigation may or may not be necessary after two spontaneous abortions, depending on the patient's age and personal desires. After three spontaneous abortions, evaluation is usually indicated. One should then (a) obtain a detailed family history, (b) perform a complete physical examination, (c) discuss recurrence risks, and (d) order the selected tests cited below.

3. Parental chromosomal studies should be performed on all couples having repetitive losses. Antenatal chromosomal studies should be offered if a balanced chromosomal rearrangement is detected in either parent or if autosomal trisomy occurred in any previous abortus.

4. Although it is impractical to karyotype all abortuses, cytogenetic information on abortuses may exist. Detection of a trisomic abortus suggests the phenomenon of recurrent aneuploidy, justifying prenatal cytogenetic studies in future pregnancies. Performing prenatal cytogenetic studies solely on the basis of repeated losses is more arguable, but not unreasonable among women aged 30 to 34 years.

5. The validity of LPD as a discrete entity increasingly seems arguable. To detect LPD, timed endometrial biopsies should be performed late in the luteal phase in two or more cycles. Results should be correlated with the date of ovulation. If histologic dating reveals an endometrium 2 or more days less than expected, the diagnosis can be made. Diagnosis on the basis of progesterone levels is preferred by some. Progesterone therapy has been proposed, but its efficacy has not been proved.

6. Other endocrine causes for repeated fetal losses include poorly controlled diabetes mellitus (hyperglycemia) and possibly thyroid dysfunction.

7. To determine the role of infectious agents, the endometrium may be cultured for *Ureaplasma urealyticum*. Alternatively, a couple could be treated empirically with doxycycline (100 mg two times per day for 10 days) before pregnancy. Of other infections agents, only *Chlamydia trachomatis* seems plausible. These agents are more likely to cause sporadic than repetitive losses.

8. If an abortion occurs after 8 to 10 weeks' gestation, a uterine anomaly or submucous leiomyoma should be considered. The uterine cavity should be

explored by hysteroscopy or hysterosalpingography. If a müllerian fusion defect (septate or bicornuate uterus) is detected in a woman experiencing one or more second-trimester spontaneous abortions, surgical correction may be warranted. A large submucous leiomyoma may also justify myomectomy or reduction. However, the same statements do not necessarily apply following *first*-trimester losses. Cervical incompetence should be managed by surgical cerclage during the next pregnancy.

9. To exclude autoimmune disease involving antiphospholipid antibodies, assessment should include aPL and aCL. Women with antibodies who experience midtrimester losses may benefit from treatment with heparin and aspirin, but the same does not necessarily hold when these antibodies are detected in asymptomatic women having first-trimester pregnancy losses. This recommendation also holds for women undergoing assisted reproductive technologies (ART). Testing for other autoantibodies (e.g., DNA) is not indicated.

10. There is some deleterious effect of HLA sharing (HLA-β), but not enough to alter clinical approach. Determining parental HLA types in the absence of other immunologic testing is not recommended. Immunotherapy (by inoculation of the mother with her husband's leukocytes) has been unequivocally shown to be ineffective.

11. One should discourage exposure to cigarettes and alcohol, yet remain cautious in ascribing cause and effect in individual cases. Similar counsel should apply for exposures to other potential toxins.

Key Points

➤ Approximately 22 percent of all pregnancies detected on the basis of urinary hCG assays are lost, usually before clinical recognition.

➤ The clinical loss rate is 10 to 12 percent. Most of these pregnancies are lost before 8 weeks' gestation. Only 3 percent of pregnancies are lost after an ultrasonographically viable pregnancy at 8 to 9 weeks, and only 1 percent are lost after 16 weeks' gestation.

➤ Pregnancy losses may be recurrent, 4 percent of U.S. women experiencing two losses and 3 percent three or more losses. Although increasing after one loss, the recurrence risk generally reaches no more than 25 percent after three or four losses. Loss rates for 40-year-old women are approximately twice that of 20-year-old women.

➤ By far the most common causes of pregnancy losses are chromosomal abnormalities. At least 50 percent of clinically recognized pregnancy losses show a chromosomal abnormality. The types of chromosomal abnormalities differ from those found in liveborns, but autosomal trisomy still accounts for 50 percent of abnormalities. A balanced translocation is present in about 5 percent of couples having repeated spontaneous abortions.

➤ Many nongenetic causes of repetitive abortions have been proposed, but few are proved. It is reasonable to evaluate couples for these conditions, but efficacy of treatment remains uncertain and relatively few pregnancy losses are caused by these factors.

➤ Uterine anomalies are accepted causes of second-trimester pregnancies. Couples experiencing such losses may benefit from metroplasty or hysteroscopic resection of a uterine septum. Uterine anomalies are less common causes of first-trimester losses.

➤ Drugs, toxins, and physical agents are associated with spontaneous abortion, but usually not in repetitive pregnancies. Avoiding potential toxins is obviously desirable, but one should not assume that such exposures explain repetitive losses.

➤ LAC antibodies, aPL, and aCL are clearly associated with second-trimester losses, but their role in first-trimester losses is more arguable. Immunotherapy for couples sharing HLA antigens or otherwise showing blunted maternal response to paternal antigens (alloimmune disease) is not recommended. Determining parental HLA types in the absence of other immunologic evaluations is not recommended.

➤ Management of ectopic pregnancy has undergone significant modification over recent years. The condition is less commonly an acute emergency and more easily diagnosed early in gestation on the basis of maternal serum progesterone, maternal β-hCG, transvaginal ultrasound, and uterine curettage. The earlier detection of an unruptured ectopic pregnancy has greatly modified treatment. Laparotomy is now rarely necessary. Laparoscopic procedures (linear salpingostomy) are commonly used, with an increase in subsequent pregnancy rates and a decrease in repeat ectopic gestations. About one third of women with ectopic pregnancies prove eligible for medical treatment (methotrexate). Patients at high risk for ectopic pregnancy may benefit from a screening serum progesterone determination at the time of initial pregnancy test.

REFERENCES

1. U.S. Department of Health and Human Services: Reproductive impairments among married couples. *In* U.S. Vital and Health Statistics Series 23, No. 11. Hyattsville, MD, National Center for Health Statistics, 1982, p 5.

2. Wilcox AJ, Weinberg CR, O'Connor JF, et al: Incidence of early pregnancy loss. N Engl J Med 319:189, 1988.

3. Mills JL, Simpson JL, Driscoll SG, et al: NICHD-DIEP Study: incidence of spontaneous abortion among normal women with insulin-dependent diabetic women whose pregnancies were identified within 21 days of conception. N Engl J Med 319:1617, 1988.

4. Simpson JL, Carson SA: Genetic and non-genetic causes of spontaneous abortions. *In* Sciarra JJ (ed): Gynecology and Obstetrics, Vol 3. Philadelphia, JB Lippincott, 1995.

5. Regan L: A prospective study on spontaneous abortion. *In* Beard RW, Sharp F (eds): Early Pregnancy Loss: Mechanisms and Treatment. London, The Royal College of Obstetricians and Gynaecologists, 1988, p 22.

6. Simpson JL, Gray RH, Queenan JT, et al: Risk of recurrent spontaneous abortion for pregnancies discovered in the fifth week of gestation. Lancet 344:964, 1994.

7. Gray RH, Simpson JL, Kambic RT, et al: Timing of conception and the risk of spontaneous abortion among pregnancies occurring during the use of natural family planning. Am J Obstet Gynecol 172:1567, 1995.

8. Wilcox AJ, Baird DD, Weinberg CR: Time of implantation of the conceptus and loss of pregnancy. N Engl J Med 340:1796, 1999.

9. Simpson JL, Mills JL, Holmes LB, et al: Low fetal loss rates after demonstration of a live fetus in the first trimester. JAMA 258:2555, 1987.

10. Hertig AT, Rock J, Adams EC: Description of human ova within the first 17 days of development. Am J Anat 98:435, 1956.

11. Hertig AT, Rock J, Adams EC, Menkin MC: Thirty-four fertilized human ova, good, bad and indifferent, recovered from 210 women of known fertility. A study of biologic wastage in early human pregnancy. Pediatrics 25:202, 1959.

12. Hertig AT, Rock J: Searching for early human ova. Gynecol Invest 4:121, 1973.

13. Plachot M, Junca AM, Mandelbaum J, et al: Chromosome investigations in early life. Human preimplantation embryos. Hum Reprod 2:29, 1987.

14. Papadopoulos G, Templeton AA, Fisk N, Randall J: The frequency of chromosome anomalies in human preimplantation embryos after in-vitro fertilization. Hum Reprod 4:91, 1989.

15. Munné S, Alikani M, Tomkin G, et al: Embryo morphology, developmental rates, and maternal age are correlated with chromosome abnormalities. Fertil Steril 64:382, 1995.

16. Egozcue J, Blanco J, Vidal F: Chromosome studies in human sperm nuclei using fluorescence in-situ hybridization (FISH). Hum Reprod Update 3:441, 1997.

17. Plachot M: Genetics of human oocytes. *In* Boutaleb Y, Gzouli A (eds): New Concepts in Reproduction. Vol 88. Lanes, England, Parthenon, 1992, p 367.

18. Martin R: Chromosomal analysis of human spermatozoa. *In* Verlinsky Y, Kuliev A (eds): Preimplantation Genetics. New York, Plenum Press, 1991, p 91.

19. Pellestor F, Dufour MC, Arnal F, et al: Direct assessment of the rate of chromosomal abnormalities in grade IV human embryos produced by in-vitro fertilization procedure. Hum Reprod 9:293, 1994.

20. Gropp A: Chromosomal animal model of human disease. Fetal trisomy and development failure. *In* Berry L, Poswillo DE (eds): Teratology. Berlin, Springer-Verlag, 1975, p 17.

21. Boué J, Boué A, Lazar P: Retrospective and prospective epidemiological studies of 1500 karyotyped spontaneous human abortions. Teratology 12:11, 1975.

22. Hassold T: A cytogenetic study of repeated spontaneous abortions. Am J Hum Genet 32:723, 1980.

23. Simpson JL, Bombard AT: Chromosomal abnormalities in spontaneous abortion: frequency, pathology and genetic counseling. *In* Edmonds K, Bennett MJ (eds): Spontaneous Abortion. London, Blackwell, 1987, p 51.

24. Sorokin Y, Johnson MP, Zadoe IE, et al: Postmortem chorionic villus sampling: correlation of cytogenetic and ultrasound findings. Am J Med Genet 39:314, 1991.

25. Strom C, Ginsberg N, Applebaum M, et al: Analyses of 95 first trimester spontaneous abortions by chorionic villus sampling and karyotype. J Assist Reprod Genet 9:458, 1992.

26. Kuleshov NP: Chromosome anomalies of infants dying during the perinatal period and premature newborn. Hum Genet 34:151, 1976.

27. Watt JL, Templeton AA, Messinis I, et al: Trisomy 1 in an eight cell human pre-embryo. J Med Genet 24:60, 1987.

28. Warburton D, Byrne J, Canik N: Chromosome Anomalies and Prenatal Development: An Atlas. New York, Oxford University Press, 1991.

29. Kalousek DK: Pathology of abortion: chromosomal and genetic correlations. *In* Kraus FT, Damjanov I, Kaufman N (eds): Pathology of Reproductive Failure. Baltimore, Williams & Wilkins, 1991, p 228.

30. Hassold T, Merrill M, Adkins K, et al: Recombination and maternal age-dependent nondisjunction: molecular studies of trisomy 16. Am J Hum Genet 57:867, 1995.

31. Fisher JM, Harvey JF, Morton NE, et al: Trisomy 18: studies of the parent and cell division of origin and the effect of aberrant recombination on nondisjunction. Am J Hum Genet 56:669, 1995.

32. Bugge M, Collins A, Petersen MB, et al: Non-disjunction of chromosome 18. Hum Mol Genet 7:661, 1998.

33. Hassold TJ: Nondisjunction in the human male. Curr Top Dev Biol 37:383, 1998.

34. Henderson SA, Edwards RG: Chiasma frequency and maternal age in mammals. Nature 217:22, 1968.

35. Castilla EE, Simpson JL, Queenan JT: Down syndrome is not increased in offspring of natural family planning users (case control analysis) [letter]. Am J Med Genet 59:525, 1995.

36. Simpson JL, Gray RH, Queenan JT, et al: Pregnancy outcome associated with natural family planning (NFP): scientific basis and experimental design for an international cohort study. Adv Contracept 4:247, 1988.

37. Hassold T, Abruzzo M, Adkins K, et al: Human aneuploidy: incidence, origin, and etiology. Environ Mol Mutagen 28:167, 1996.

38. Savage AR, Petersen MB, Pettay D, et al: Elucidating the

mechanisms of paternal non-disjunction of chromosome 21 in humans. Hum Mol Genet 7:1221, 1998.

39. Jacobs PA, Angell RR, Buchanan IM, et al: The origin of human triploids. Ann Hum Genet 42:49, 1978.

40. Beatty RA: The origin of human triploidy: an integration of qualitative and quantitative evidence. Ann Hum Genet 41:299, 1978.

41. Singh RJ, Carr DH: The anatomy and histology of XO embryos and fetuses. Anat Rec 155:369, 1966.

42. Jirásek JE: Principles of reproductive embryology. In Simpson JL (ed): Disorders of Sex Differentiation: Etiology and Clinical Delineation. San Diego, Academic Press, 1976, p 51.

43. Simpson JL: Pregnancies in women with chromosomal abnormalities. In Shulman JD, Simpson JL (eds): Genetic Diseases in Pregnancy. San Diego, Academic Press, 1981, p 439.

44. Chandley AC: The origin of chromosome aberrations in man and their potential for survival and reproduction in the adult human populations. Ann Genet 24:5, 1981.

45. Henderson DJ, Sherman LS, Loughna SC, et al: Early embryonic failure associated with uniparental disomy for human chromosome 21. Hum Mol Genet 3:1373, 1994.

46. Lanasa MC, Hogge WA, Kubik C, et al: Highly skewed X-chromosome inactivation is associated with idiopathic recurrent spontaneous abortion. Am J Hum Genet 65:252, 1999.

47. Pegoraro E, Whitaker J, Mowery-Rushton P, et al: Familial skewed X inactivation: a molecular trait associated with high spontaneous-abortion rate maps to Xq28. Am J Hum Genet 61:160, 1997.

48. Malpas P: A study of abortion sequences. J Obstet Gynaecol Br Emp 45:932, 1938.

49. Warburton D, Fraser FC: Spontaneous abortion risks in man: data from reproductive histories collected in a medical genetics units. Am J Human Genet 16:1, 1964.

50. Poland BJ, Miller JR, Jones DC, et al: Reproductive counseling in patients who have had a spontaneous abortion. Am J Obstet Gynecol 127:685, 1977.

51. Kline J, Stein ZA, Susser M, Warburton D: Smoking: a risk factor for spontaneous abortion. N Engl J Med 297:793, 1977.

52. Boué J, Boué A: Chromosomal analysis of 2 consecutive abortions in each of 43 women. Humangenetik 19:275, 1973.

53. Vlaanderen W, Treffers PE: Prognosis of subsequent pregnancies after recurrent spontaneous abortion in first trimester. BMJ 295:92, 1987.

54. Liddell HS, Pattison NS, Zanderigo A: Recurrent miscarriage—outcome after supportive care in early pregnancy. Aust N Z J Obstet Gynaecol 31:320, 1991.

55. Houwert DE, Jong MH, Termijtelen A, et al: The natural course of habitual abortion. Eur J Obstet Gynecol Reprod Biol 33:221, 1989.

56. Simpson JL, Elias S, Martin AO: Parental chromosomal rearrangements associated with repetitive spontaneous abortion. Fertil Steril 24:1023, 1981.

57. Simpson JL, Meyers CM, Martin AO, et al: Translocations are infrequent among couples having repeated spontaneous abortions but no other abnormal pregnancies. Fertil Steril 51:811, 1989.

58. De Braekeleer M, Dao TN: Cytogenetic studies in couples experiencing repeated pregnancy losses. Hum Reprod 5:519, 1990.

59. Boué A, Gallano P: A collaborative study of the segregation of inherited chromosome structural arrangements in 1356 prenatal diagnoses. Prenat Diagn 4:45, 1973.

60. Daniel A, Hook EB, Wulf G: Risks of unbalanced progeny at amniocentesis to carriers of chromosome rearrangements: data from United States and Canadian laboratories. Am J Med Genet 31:14, 1989.

61. Martin RH: Segregation analysis of translocations by the study of human sperm chromosome complements. Am J Hum Genet 44:461, 1989.

62. Rosenbusch B, Sterzik K, Lauritzen C: Cytogenetic analysis of sperm chromosomes in couples with habitual abortion. Geburtsh Frauenheilk 51:369, 1991.

63. Sutherland GR, Gardiner AJ, Carter RF: Familial pericentric inversion of chromosome 19 inv (19) (p13q13) with a note on genetic counseling of pericentric inversion carries. Clin Genet 10:53, 1976.

64. Schwartz S, VanDyke DL, Palmer CG: Paracentric inversions in humans: a review of 446 paracentric inversions with presentation of 120 new cases. Am J Med Genet 55:171, 1995.

65. Warburton D, Kline J, Stein Z, et al: Does the karyotype of a spontaneous abortion predict the karyotype of a subsequent abortion? Evidence from 273 women with two karyotyped spontaneous abortions. Am J Hum Genet 41:465, 1987.

66. Alberman ED: The abortus as a predictor of future trisomy 21. In De la Cruz FF, Gerald PS (eds): Trisomy 21 (Down syndrome). Baltimore, University Park Press, 1981, p 69.

67. Davis OK, Berkley AS, Cholst IN, et al: The incidence of luteal phase defect in normal, fertile women, determined by serial endometrial biopsy. Fertil Steril 51:582, 1989.

68. Noyes RW, Hertig ATR, Rock J: Dating the endometrial biopsy. Fertil Steril 1:3, 1950.

69. Scott RT, Synder RR, Strickland DM, et al: The effect of interobserver variation in dating endometrial history on the diagnosis of luteal phase defects. Fertil Steril 50:888, 1988.

70. Li TC, Dockery P, Rogers AW, Cooke ID: How precise is histologic dating of endometrium using the standard dating criteria. Fertil Steril 759:51, 1989.

71. Jordan J, Craig K, Clifton DK, Soules MR: Luteal phase defect: the sensitivity and specificity of diagnostic methods in common clinical use. Fertil Steril 62:54, 1994.

72. Daya S, Ward S, Burrows E: Progesterone profiles in luteal phase defect cycles and outcome of progesterone treatment in patients with recurrent spontaneous abortions. Am J Obstet Gynecol 158:225, 1988.

73. Soules MR, Clifton DK, Cohen NL, et al: Luteal phase deficiency: abnormal gonadotropin and progesterone secretion patterns. J Clin Endocrinol Metab 69:813, 1989.

74. Soules MR, McLachlan RI, Ek M, et al: Luteal phase deficiency: characterization of reproductive hormones over the menstrual cycle. J Clin Endocrinol Metal 69:804, 1989.

75. Soules M, Wiebe RN, Aksel S, et al: The diagnosis and therapy of luteal phase deficiency. Fertil Steril 28:1033, 1997.

76. Tho PT, Byrd JR, McDonough PC: Etiologies and subsequent reproductive performance of 100 couples with recurrent abortions. Fertil Steril 32:389, 1979.

77. Daya S, Ward S: Diagnostic test properties of serum progesterone in the evaluation of luteal phase defects. Fertil Steril 49:168, 1988.

78. Simpson JL: Fetal Wastage. In Gabbe SG, Niebyl JR, Simpson JL (eds): Obstetrics: Normal and Problem Pregnancies, 3rd ed. New York, Churchill Livingstone, 1996.

79. Karamardian LM, Grimes DA: Luteal phase deficiency: effect of treatment on pregnancy rates. Am J Obstet Gynecol 167:1391, 1992.

80. Quenby SM, Farquharson RG: Predicting recurring miscarriage: what is important? Obstet Gynecol 82:132, 1993.

81. Sagle M, Bishop K, Ridley N, et al: Recurrent early miscarriage and polycystic ovaries. BMJ 297:1027, 1988.

82. Regan L, Owen EJ, Jacobs HS: Hypersecretion of lutenising hormone, infertility, and miscarriage. Lancet 336:1141, 1990.

83. Clifford K, Rai R, Watson H, et al: Does suppressing luteinizing hormone secretion reduce the miscarriage rate? Results of a randomized controlled trial. BMJ 312:1508, 1996.

84. Carp HJ, Hass Y, Dolicky M, et al: The effect of serum follicular phase luteinizing hormone concentrations in habitual abortion: correlation with results of paternal leukocyte immunization. Hum Reprod 10:1702, 1995.

85. Tulppala M, Stenman UH, Cacciatore B, et al: Polycystic ovaries and levels of gonadotrophins and androgens in recurrent miscarriage: prospective study in 50 women. Br J Obstet Gynaecol 100:348, 1993.

86. Bussen S, Sutterlin M, Steck T: Endocrine abnormalities during the follicular phase in women with recurrent spontaneous abortion. Hum Reprod 14:18, 1999.

87. Montero M, Collea JV, Frasier D, Mestman J: Successful outcome of pregnancy in women with hypothyroidism. Ann Intern Med 94:31, 1981.

88. Bussen S, Steck T: Thyroid autoantibodies in euthyroid nonpregnant women with recurrent spontaneous abortions. Hum Reprod 10:2938, 1995.

89. Stagnaro-Green A, Roman SH, Cobin RH, et al: Detection of at-risk pregnancy by means of highly sensitive assays for thyroid autoantibodies. JAMA 264:1422, 1990.

90. Glinoer D, Soto MF, Bourdoux P, et al: Pregnancy in patients with mild thyroid abnormalities: maternal and neonatal repercussions. J Clin Endocrinol Metab 73:421, 1991.

91. Singh J, Hunt P, Eggo MC, et al: Thyroid-stimulating hormone rapidly stimulates inositol polyphosphate formation in FRTL-5 thyrocytes without activating phosphoinositidase C. Biochem J 316:175, 1996.

92. Pratt DE, Kaberlein G, Dudkiewicz A, et al: The association of antithyroid antibodies in euthyroid nonpregnant women with recurrent first trimester abortions in the next pregnancy. Fertil Steril 60:1001, 1993.

93. Pratt DE, Novotny M, Kaberlein G, et al: Antithyroid antibodies and the association with non-organ-specific antibodies in recurrent pregnancy loss. Am J Obstet Gynecol 168:837, 1993.

94. Rushworth FH, Tulppala M, Rai R, et al: Prospective pregnancy outcome in untreated recurrent miscarries with thyroid autoantibodies [abstract P-169]. Hum Reprod 14:225, 1999.

95. Miodovnik M, Mimouni F, Tsang RL, et al: Glycemic control and spontaneous abortion in insulin dependent diabetic women. Obstet Gynecol 68:366, 1986.

96. Ben Rafael Z, Seidman DS, Recabi K, et al: Uterine anomalies. A retrospective, matched control study. J Reprod Med 36:723, 1991.

97. Michalas SP: Outcome of pregnancy in women with uterine malformation: evaluation of 62 cases. Int J Gynaecol Obstet 35:215, 1991.

98. Makino T, Sakai A, Sugi T, et al: Current comprehensive therapy of habitual abortion. Ann N Y Acad Sci 626:597, 1991.

99. Mouton DM, Damewood MD, Schlaff WD, Rock JA: A comparison of the reproductive outcome between women with a unicornuate uterus and women with a didelphic uterus. Fertil Steril 58:88, 1992.

100. Golan A, Langer R, Neuman M, et al: Obstetric outcome in women with congenital uterine malformations. J Reprod Med 37:233, 1992.

101. Candiani GB, Fedele L, Parazzini F, Zamberletti D: Reproductive prognosis after abdominal metroplasty in bicornuate or septate uterus: a life table analysis. Br J Obstet Gynaecol 97:613, 1990.

102. Stein AL, March CM: Pregnancy outcome in women with müllerian duct anomalies. J Reprod Med 35:411, 1990.

103. Makino T: Management of uterine congenital malformations: evaluation of outcome. In Hedon B, Springer J, Mores P (eds): Proceedings of the 15th World Congress on Fertility and Sterility, Montpellier, France, 17–22 September, 1995. New York, Parthenon, 1995.

104. Makino T, Umeuchi M, Nakada K, et al: Incidence of congenital uterine anomalies in repeated reproductive wastage and prognosis for pregnancy after metroplasty. Int J Fertil 37:167, 1992.

105. Stampe-Sorensen S: Estimated prevalence of müllerian anomalies. Acta Obstet Gynecol Scand 67:441, 1988.

106. Simon C, Marinex L, Pardo F, et al: Müllerian defects in women with normal reproductive outcome. Fertil Steril 56:1192, 1991.

107. Ludmire J, Samuels P, Brooks S, Mennuti MT: Pregnancy outcome of patients with uncorrected uterine anomalies managed in a high-risk obstetric setting. Obstet Gynecol 75:906, 1990.

108. Stray-Pedersen B, Eng J, Reikvan TM: Uterine T-mycoplasma colonization in reproductive failure. Am J Obstet Gynecol 130:307, 1978.

109. Quinn PA, Petric M, Barkin M, et al: Prevalence of antibody to Chlamydia trachomatis in spontaneous abortion and infertility. Am J Obstet Gynecol 156:291, 1987.

110. Witkin SS, Ledger WJ: Antibodies to chlamydia trachomatis in sera of women with recurrent spontaneous abortions. Am J Obstet Gynecol 167:135, 1992.

111. Rae R, Smith IW, Liston WA, Kilpatrick DC: Chlamydial serologic studies and recurrent spontaneous abortion. Am J Obstet Gynecol 170:782, 1994.

112. Olliaro R, Regazzetti A, Gorini G, et al: Chlamydia trachomatis infection in "sine causa" recurrent abortion. Bol 1st Sieroter Milan 70:467, 1991.

113. van Lijnschoten G, Stals F, Evers JLH, et al: The presence of cytomegalovirus antigens in karyotyped abortions. In van Lijnschoten G (ed): Morphology and Karyotype in Early Abortion. Amsterdam, University Press Maastricht, 1993, p 79.

114. Paukku M, Tulppala M, Puolakkainen M, et al: Lack of association between serum antibodies to Chlamydia trachomatis and a history of recurrent pregnancy loss. Fertil Steril 72:427, 1999.

115. Zavala-Vlazquez J, Guzman-Marin E, Barrera-Perez M, Rodriguez-Feliz ME: Toxoplasmosis and abortion in patients at the O'Horan Hospital of Merida, Yucatan. Salud Publica Mex 31:664, 1989.

116. el Ridi AM, Nada SM, Aly AS, et al: Toxoplasmosis and pregnancy: an analytical study in Zagazig, Egypt. J Egypt Soc Parasitol 21:81, 1991.

117. Sahwi SY, Zaki MS, Haiba NY, et al: Toxoplasmosis as a cause of repeated abortion. Obstet Gynaecol 21:145, 1995.

118. Simpson JL, Mills JL, Kim H, et al: Infectious processes: an infrequent cause of first trimester spontaneous abortions. Hum Reprod 11:668, 1996.

119. Rock JA, Shirey RS, Braine HG, et al: Plasmapheresis for the treatment of repeated early pregnancy wastage associated with anti-P. Obstet Gynecol 66:57S, 1985.

120. Strowitzki T, Wiedemann R, Heim MU, et al: Pregnancy with an extremely rare P blood group with anti-PP1Pk. Geburtsh Frauenheilk 51:710, 1991.

121. Hill JA, Polgar K, Anderson DJ: T-helper 1-type immunity to trophoblast in women with recurrent spontaneous abortion. JAMA 273:1933, 1995.

122. Mills JL, Holmes L, Aaron JH, et al: Moderate caffeine use and the risk of spontaneous abortion and intrauterine growth retardation. JAMA 269:593, 1993.

123. Raghupathy R: Th1-type immunity is incompatible with successful pregnancy. Immunol Today 18:478, 1997.

124. Wegmann TG, Lin H, Guilbert L, et al: Bidirectional cytokine interactions in the maternal-fetal relationship: is successful pregnancy a Th2 phenomenon? Immunol Today 14:353, 1993.

125. Cowchock S: Autoantibodies and pregnancy wastage. Am J Reprod Immun 26:38, 1991.

126. Branch DW, Ward K: Autoimmunity and pregnancy loss. Semin Reprod Endocrinol 7:168, 1989.

127. Scott JR, Rote NS, Branch DW: Immunologic aspects of recurrent abortions and fetal death. Obstet Gynecol 70:645, 1987.

128. Petri M, Golbus M, Anderson R, et al: Antinuclear antibody, lupus anticoagulant, and anticardiolipin antibody in women with idiopathic habitual abortion. Arthritis Rheum 30:601, 1987.

129. Carp HJ, Menashe Y, Frenkel Y, et al: Lupus anticoagulant. Significance in habitual first-trimester abortion. J Reprod Med 38:549, 1993.

130. Mishall DR Jr: Recurrent abortion. J Reprod Med 38:250, 1993.

131. Eroglu GE, Scopelitis E: Antinuclear and antiphospholipid antibodies in healthy women with recurrent spontaneous abortion. Am J Reprod Immunol 31:1, 1994.

132. Simpson JL, Gray RH, Perez A, et al: Pregnancy outcome in natural family planning users: cohort and case-control studies evaluating safety. Adv Contracept 13:201, 1997.

133. Sugi T, Katsunuma J, Izumi S, et al: Prevalence and heterogeneity of antiphosphatidylethanolamine antibodies in patients with recurrent early pregnancy losses. Fertil Steril 71:1060, 1999.

134. Topping J, Quenby S, Farquharson R, et al: Marked variation in antiphospholipid antibodies during pregnancy: relationships to pregnancy outcome. Hum Reprod 14:224, 1999.

135. Egbase PE, Al Sharhan M, Diejomaoh M, et al: Antiphospholipid antibodies in infertile couples with two consecutive miscarriages after in-vitro fertilization and embryo transfer. Hum Reprod 14:1483, 1999.

136. Simpson JL, Carson SA, Chesney C, et al: Lack of association between antiphospholipid antibodies and first-trimester spontaneous abortion: prospective study of pregnancies detected within 21 days of conception. Fertil Steril 69:814, 1998.

137. Balasch J, Reverter JC, Creus M, et al: Human reproductive failure is not a clinical feature associated with beta(2) glycoprotein-I antibodies in anticardiolipin and lupus anticoagulant seronegative patients. Hum Reprod 14:1956, 1999.

138. Stern C, Chamley L, Hale L, et al: Antibodies to beta2 glycoprotein I are associated with in vitro fertilization implantation failure as well as recurrent miscarriage: results of a prevalence study. Fertil Steril 70:938, 1998.

139. ASRM Practice Committee Report, 1998. 31:1, 1994.

140. Mowbray JF, Gibbings C, Liddell H, et al: Controlled trial of treatment of recurrent spontaneous abortion by immunization with paternal cells. Lancet 1:941, 1985.

141. Recurrent Miscarriage Immunotherapy Trials Group: Worldwide collaborative observational study and meta-analysis on allogenic leukocyte immunotherapy for recurrent spontaneous abortion. Am J Reprod Immunol 32:55, 1990.

142. Fraser EJ, Grimes DA, Schultz KF: Immunization as therapy for recurrent spontaneous abortion: a review and meta-analysis. Obstet Gynecol 82:854, 1993.

143. Ober C, Karrison T, Odem RR, et al: Mononuclear-cell immunosation in prevention of recurrent miscarriages: a randomized trial. Lancet 354:365, 1999.

144. Kline J, Shrout P, Stein ZA, et al: Drinking during pregnancy and spontaneous abortion. Lancet 2:176, 1980.

145. Ness RB, Grisso JA, Hirschinger N, et al: Cocaine and tobacco use and the risk of spontaneous abortion. N Engl J Med 340:333, 1999.

146. Mills JL, Holmes L, Aarons JH, et al: Moderate caffeine use and the risk of spontaneous abortion and intrauterine growth retardation. JAMA 269:593, 1993.

147. Klebanoff MA, Levine RJ, DerSimonian R, et al: Maternal serum paraxanthine, a caffeine metabolite, and the risk of spontaneous abortion. N Engl J Med 341:1639, 1999.

147a. Cnattinguis S, Signorello LB, Annerén G, et al: Caffeine intake and the risk of first-trimester spontaneous abortion. N Engl J Med 343:1839, 2000.

148. Harlap S, Shiono PH: Alcohol, smoking and incidence of spontaneous abortions in the first and second trimester. Lancet 2:173, 1980.

149. Halmesmärki E, Valimaki M, Roine R, et al: Maternal and paternal alcohol consumption and miscarriage. Br J Obstet Gynaecol 96:188, 1989.

150. Parazzini F, Bocciolone L, LaVecchia C, et al: Maternal and paternal moderate daily alcohol consumption and unexplained miscarriages. Br J Obstet Gynaecol 97:618, 1990.

151. Savitz DA, Sonnenfeld NL, Olshan AF: Review of epidemiologic studies of paternal occupational exposure and spontaneous abortion. Am J Ind Med 25:361, 1994.

152. Stray-Pedersen B, Stray-Pedersen S: Recurrent abortion: the role of psychotherapy. In Beard RW, Sharp F (eds): Early Pregnancy Loss: Mechanism and Treatment. London, Royal College of Obstetricians and Gynaecologists, 1988, p 433.

153. Liddell HS, Pattison NS, Zanderigo A: Recurrent miscarriage—outcome after supportive care in early pregnancy. Aust N Z J Obstet Gynaecol 31:320, 1991.

154. Houwert-de Jong MH, Termijtelen A, Eskes TK, et al: The natural course of habitual abortion. Eur J Obstet Gynecol Reprod Biol 33:221, 1989.

155. Clifford K, Rai CK, Regan L: Future pregnancy outcome in unexplained recurrent first trimester miscarriage. Hum Reprod 12:387, 1997.

156. Bergant AM, Reinstadler K, Moncayo HE, et al: Spontaneous abortion and psychosomatic. A prospective study on the impact of psychological factors as a cause for recurrent spontaneous abortion. Hum Reprod 12:1106, 1997.

157. Dorfman SF: Deaths from ectopic pregnancy, United States, 1979 to 1980. Obstet Gynecol 62:334, 1983.

158. Thorburn J, Philipson M, Lindblom B: Fertility after ectopic pregnancy in relation to background factors and surgical treatment. Fertil Steril 49:595, 1988.

159. Elias S, LeBeau M, Simpson JL, Martin AO: Chromosome analysis of ectopic human conceptuses. Am J Obstet Gynecol 141:698, 1981.

160. Breen JL: A 21 year study of 654 ectopic pregnancies. J Obstet Gynecol 106:1004, 1970.

161. Brenner PF, Roy S, Mishell DR Jr: Ectopic pregnancy: a study of 300 consecutive surgically treated cases. JAMA 243:673, 1980.

162. DeCherney AH, Maheux R: Modern management of tubal pregnancy. In Leventhal JM, et al: Current Problems in Obstetrics and Gynecology. Chicago, Year Book, 1983, p 61.

163. Thornburn JEK, Janson PO, Lindstedt G: Early diagnosis of ectopic pregnancy. Acta Obstet Gynecol Scand 62:543, 1983.

164. Silverberg SG: Arias-Stella phenomenon in spontaneous and therapeutic abortion. Am J Obstet Gynecol 112:777, 1972.

165. Carson SA, Buster JE: The ectopic pregnancy: new advances in diagnosis and treatment. N Engl J Med 329:1174, 1993.

166. Stovall TG, Ling FW, Carson SA, Buster JE: Nonsurgical diagnosis and treatment of tubal pregnancy. Fertil Steril 54:537, 1990.

167. Stoval TG, Ling FW, Gray LA, et al: Methotrexate treatment

of unruptured ectopic pregnancy: a report of 100 cases. Obstet Gynecol 77:749, 1991.

168. Stovall TG, Ling FW, Carson SA, Buster JE: Serum progesterone and uterine curettage in differential diagnosis of ectopic pregnancy. Fertil Steril 57:456, 1992.

169. Lenton EA, Neal LM, Sulaiman R: Plasma concentrations of human chorionic gonadotropin from the time of implantation until the second week of pregnancy. Fertil Steril 37:773, 1982.

170. Emerson DS, Carier MS, Altieri LA, et al: Diagnostic efficacy of endovaginal color Doppler flow imaging in an ectopic pregnancy screening program. Radiology 183:413, 1992.

171. DeCherney AH, Diamond MP: Laparoscopic salpingostomy for ectopic pregnancy. Obstet Gynecol 70:948, 1987.

172. Lindblom B: Ectopic pregnancy: laparoscopic and medical treatment. Curr Opin Obstet Gynecol 4:400, 1992.

173. Chapron C, Querleu D, Crepin G: Laparoscopic treatment of ectopic pregnancies: a one hundred cases study. Eur J Obstet Gynecol Reprod Biol 41:187, 1991.

174. Vermesh M, Silva PD, Rosen GF, et al: Management of unruptured ectopic gestation by lineal salpingostomy: a prospective, randomized clinical trial of laparoscopy versus laparotomy. Obstet Gynecol 73:400, 1989.

175. Brumsted J, Kessler C, Gibson C, et al: A comparison of laparoscopy and laparotomy for the treatment of ectopic pregnancy. Obstet Gynecol 71:889, 1988.

176. Seifer DB, Gutmann JN, Doyle MB, et al: Persistent ectopic pregnancy following laparoscopic linear salpingostomy. Obstet Gynecol 76:1121, 1990.

177. Stovall TG, Ling FW, Gray LA: Single-dose methotrexate for treatment of ectopic pregnancy. Obstet Gynecol 77:754, 1991.

178. Ory SJ, Villanueva AL, Sand PK, Tamura RK: Conservative treatment of ectopic pregnancy with methotrexate. Am J Obstet Gynecol 154:1299, 1986.

179. Ross GT: Congenital anomalies among children born of mothers receiving chemotherapy for gestational trophoblastic neoplasms. Cancer Suppl 37:1043, 1976.

Preterm Birth

JAY D. IAMS

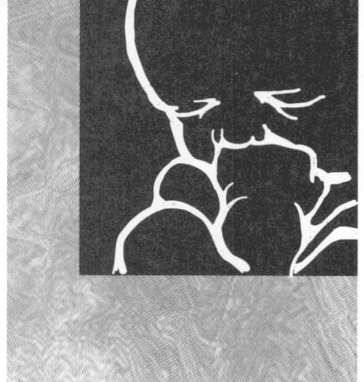

In developed nations, complications of prematurity account for the majority of perinatal mortality and morbidity in nonanomalous infants. In the United States, prematurity-related disorders cause more than 70 percent of fetal and neonatal deaths.[1] Long-term sequelae of prematurity disproportionately contribute to developmental delay, visual and hearing impairment, chronic lung disease, and cerebral palsy.[2]

Advances in neonatal care have led to increased survival and reduced short- and long-term morbidity for infants born before 37 weeks of pregnancy, but the rate of low-birth-weight deliveries actually increased between 1989 and 1997[3] (Fig. 23–1). In 1997, 11.4 percent of births occurred before 37 weeks, up from 11.0 percent in 1996. These rates represent increases of 8 percent since 1990 and 20 percent since 1981. There are two notable trends in the data. The first is the racial difference in the rate of preterm birth before 37 and 32 weeks' gestation: 9.9 and 1.49 percent for white; 11.2 and 1.68 percent for Hispanic; and 17.6 and 4.19 percent for black women, respectively.[3] The rate of preterm birth has been falling slowly among blacks, rising slowly among whites, and stable in the Hispanic population, but the black–white differences are persistent and largely unexplained. The second major trend is the increased number and rate of preterm births among multiple gestations. The rate of twins has increased 11 percent since 1990, from 22.6 to 26.8 per 1,000 births. The rate of higher order (more than two fetuses) multiple gestations has more than doubled since 1991, from 81.4 to 173.6 per 100,000, and has quadrupled since 1980, from a rate of 37.0 per 100,000.[3] These increased rates of multiple gestation have fueled the rise in preterm births in both the United States and Canada.[4] In the United States, the rate of preterm birth in 1997 was 10.0 percent for singletons, 54.9 percent for twins, and 93.6 percent for higher order multiples.[3]

Three other factors may also explain the rise in preterm birth: (1) greater willingness to deliver preterm infants when maternal complications occur; (2) increased use of ultrasound to date pregnancy, which tends to correct menstrual dates in most cases by reducing gestational age; and (3) increased registration of extremely immature deliveries before 20 to 22 weeks.[5] Efforts to identify and treat the conditions leading to prematurity have been largely disappointing, fulfilling the prophetic words of Nicholson Eastman in 1947: "Only when the factors underlying prematurity are completely understood can any intelligent attempt at prevention be made."[6] Significant progress has been made toward understanding the factors that underlie preterm birth, but the goal remains elusive.

THE PROBLEM OF PREMATURITY

Definitions

Discussion of the problems of premature and low-birth-weight infants are complicated by use of data that incorrectly interchange the definitions of *prematurity,* defined by the duration of pregnancy, and *low birth weight,* defined by the size of the infant at birth.

- *Preterm or premature:* Infants born before 37 weeks' gestation (259 days from the first day of the mother's last menstrual period, or 245 days after conception).
- *Low birth weight (LBW):* Infants who weigh less than 2,500 g at birth, regardless of gestational age.

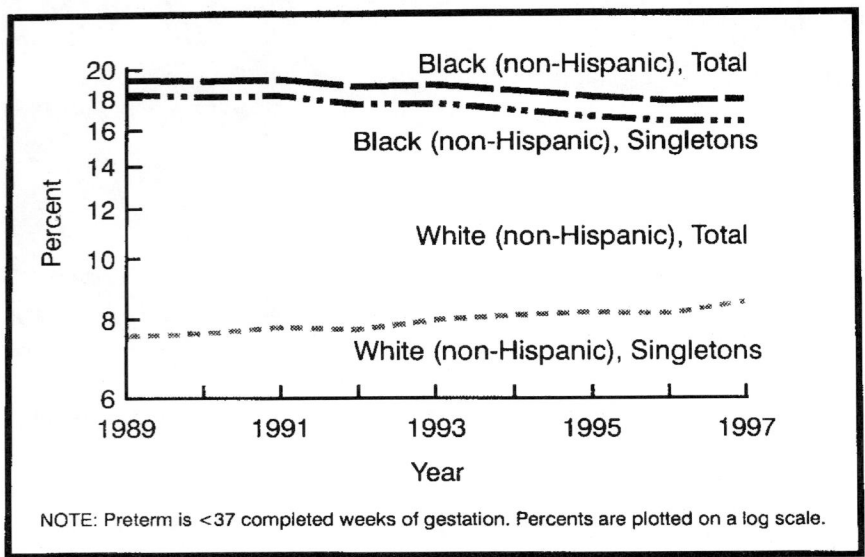

Figure 23–1. Rate of preterm birth by plurality and race/Hispanic origin of mother: United States, 1989–1997. (From Ventura SJ, Martin JA, Curtin SC, Mathews TJ: Births: Final data for 1997. Natl Vital Stat Rep 47:1, 1999.)

- *Very low birth weight (VLBW):* Infants who weigh less than 1,500 g at birth.
- *Extremely low birth weight (ELBW):* Infants who weigh less than 1,000 g at birth

Obviously, age does not equal size. For example, infants born after 37 weeks whose birth weight is below 2,500 g are low birth weight but not preterm. The confusion first occurred because gestational age could not be determined with confidence prior to the availability of sensitive serologic and ultrasonographic means of pregnancy dating. It is now possible to determine gestational age very accurately by correlation of menstrual history with sensitive pregnancy tests and by measurements of fetal size with ultrasound in the first half of pregnancy. Unfortunately, these methods of pregnancy dating are not available for some pregnancies. Because gestational age and birth weight are directly correlated throughout most of gestation, birth weight has been used as an indirect indicator of gestational age in many studies, especially when gestational age is determined retrospectively. Interchanging the two measures may lead to erroneous interpretation of clinical and epidemiologic data because the problems of LBW infants may be the result of prematurity in some instances, of poor intrauterine growth in others, and of both in still others. Similarly, problems due to prematurity in preterm infants whose birth weight exceeds 2,500 g may go unrecognized because of their apparently "full-term" appearance.

The proportion of LBW infants who are preterm versus term varies widely between developed and underdeveloped nations. In underdeveloped areas, most LBW infants are born after 37 weeks, their low birth weight the result of poor intrauterine nutrition and chronic maternal illness and/or malnutrition. In developed nations, most LBW infants are premature, although there are wide variations within the United States according to race, parity, fetal sex, and environmental factors such as maternal cigarette smoking and altitude. The birth weight data in Figure 23–2 from Brenner[7] is based on a racially mixed population near sea level. Ideally, each region or state should generate a birth weight versus gestational age chart for its own population. In the absence of such data, a published chart based on a similar population can be used.

The incidences of LBW and VLBW deliveries have changed little since 1970.[3] The LBW rate was 6.00 percent of liveborn infants in 1989, 5.93 percent in 1992, and 6.08 percent in 1997. The rate of VLBW (<1,500 g) was 1.15 percent in 1980 and increased slowly to 1.42 percent in 1997. This small increase is more important than it may seem. In 1996, VLBW infants accounted for slightly more than 1 percent of all births, but 50 percent of all infant deaths. Rates of LBW and VLBW newborns in blacks are consistently about twice as high as corresponding rates in nonblacks (Fig. 23–3). Even when corrected for age and educational level, black women continue to deliver more LBW infants than do white women.

Perinatal Mortality and Morbidity

Analysis of perinatal mortality and morbidity statistics has long been confounded by the various definitions of fetal, perinatal, neonatal, and infant time periods that have been used across the United States and around the world. The definitions endorsed by the American College of Obstetricians and Gynecologists (ACOG) are used here.[8] A *perinatal death* is one that occurs be-

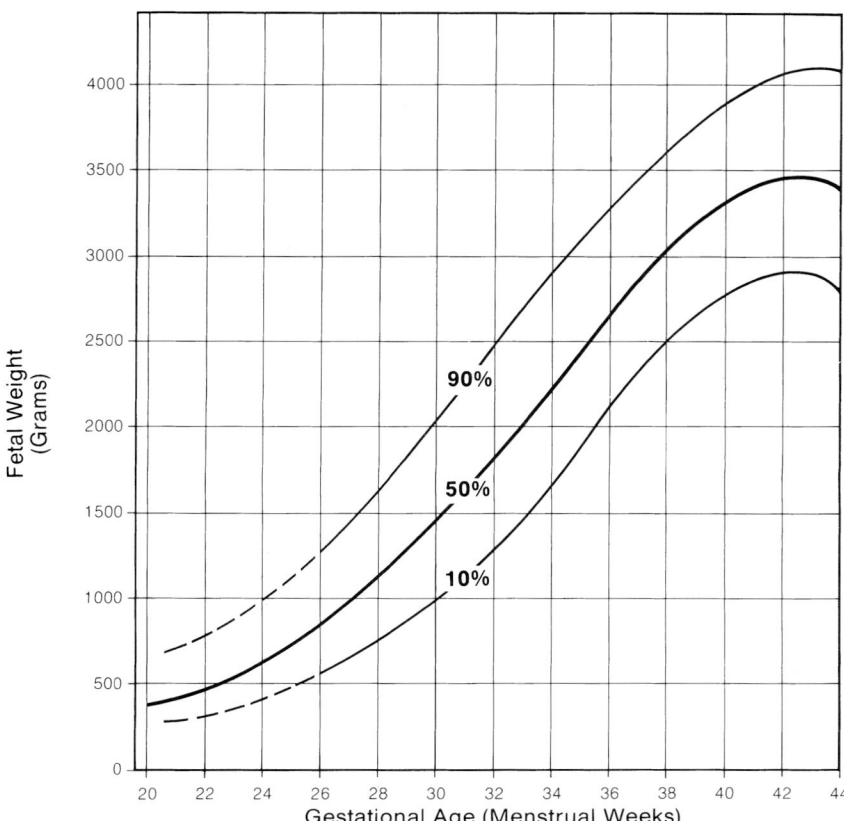

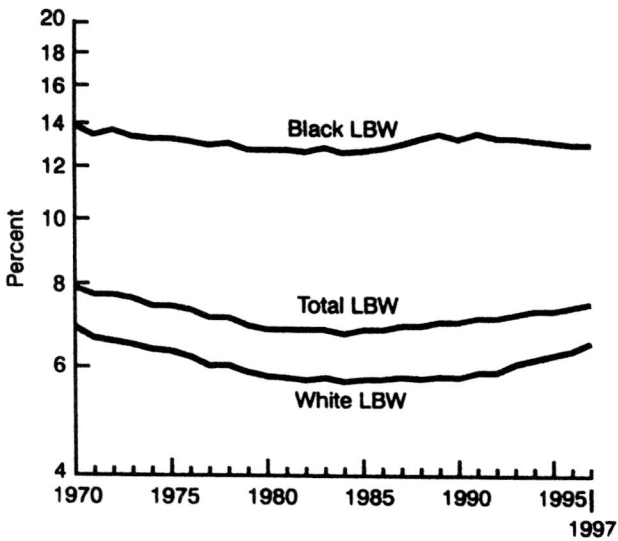

Figure 23–2. Percentage of low birth weight infants by race: 1975–1992. (From Brenner WE, Edelman DA, Hendricks CH: A standard of fetal growth for the United States of America. Am J Obstet Gynecol 126:555, 1976, with permission.)

NOTE: Low birthweight (LBW) is less than 2,500 grams. Percents are plotted on a log scale.

Figure 23–3. Percent low birth weight by race: United States, 1970–1997. (From Ventura SJ, Martin JA, Curtin SC, Mathews TJ: Births: Final data for 1997. National Vital Stat Rep 47:1, 1999.)

tween 22 weeks, or 500 g if gestational age is not known, and 28 days following delivery, and includes both deaths in utero before delivery (fetal deaths) and deaths from birth through 28 days of neonatal life. An early neonatal death occurs between birth and 7 days of life; a late neonatal death occurs between 8 and 28 days of life. Infant mortality occurs between 28 days of life and 1 year of age.

Perinatal mortality and morbidity for preterm infants are inversely related to both gestational age and birth weight: the greater the gestational age and birth weight, the lower the perinatal mortality and morbidity. Because the goals of prenatal care are maintenance of maternal well being and delivery of an infant with the lowest possible chance of mortality and morbidity, obstetricians frequently weigh the risks of preterm birth for the infant against the potential risks of prolonging the pregnancy for the mother. Knowledge of the gestational age-related risks for the baby of preterm birth is therefore an important part of obstetric practice.

Significant improvements in survival rates for all preterm infants have been documented for the past 40 years, and have been especially important for infants born before 28 weeks. In 1970, most hospitals did not expect infants born at or before 28 weeks or who weighed less than 1 kg to survive. Major improvements in the survival of extremely preterm (<26 weeks) in-

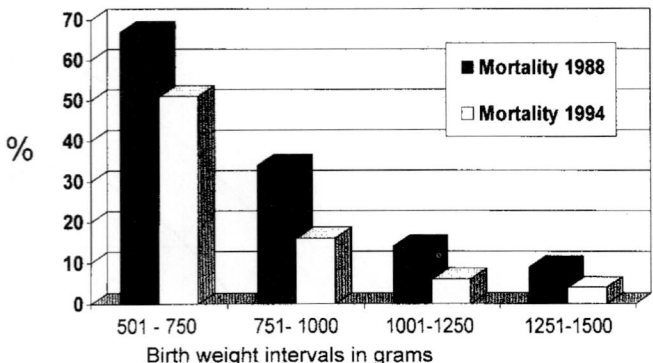

Figure 23–4. Mortality and very low birth weight infants born in 1988 and 1994 in the NICHD NICU Network. (Data from Stevenson DK, Wright LL, Lemons JA, et al: Very low birth weight outcomes of the National Institute of Child Health and Human Development Neonatal Research Network, January 1993 through December 1994. Am J Obstet Gynecol 179:1632, 1998.)

fants weighing less than 1,000 g have occurred over the last three decades. Data from 1982 to 1986, before the introduction of neonatal artificial surfactant, show survival rates of only 1.8 percent at 23 weeks', 9.9 percent at 24 weeks', 15.5 percent at 25 weeks', and 54.7 percent at 26 weeks' gestation.[9] After the introduction

of neonatal surfactant therapy, recent data show survival to hospital discharge rates of greater than 20 percent for infants born at 23 weeks', 50 percent at 24 weeks', 60 percent at 25 weeks', and 80 percent at 26 weeks' gestation for infants born in 1993 to 1994[10] (Figs. 23–4 to 23–6). Neonatal reports do not include data from all fetuses who were alive at the time of maternal hospital admission, and may therefore be more optimistic than obstetric reports. However, obstetric series have also shown similar trends of improved survival. A report of neonatal outcomes among 799 nonanomalous infants born in 1992 to 1993 at 22 to 26 weeks in 11 American tertiary perinatal centers found that survival to 120 days was 2 percent at 21 weeks', 14 percent at 22 weeks', 26 percent at 23 weeks', 33 percent at 24 weeks', and 68 percent at 25 weeks' gestation.[11] However, this study followed infants only until hospital discharge or 120 days of life, as shown in Table 23–1. Long-term follow-up was performed for a cohort of 138 nonanomalous infants born at 24 to 26 weeks' gestation between 1990 and 1994; 94 infants (68 percent) survived to hospital discharge. The increase in survival by week of gestation was dramatic, from 43 percent at 24 weeks to 74 percent at 25 weeks and 83 percent at 26 weeks[12] (Table 23–2).

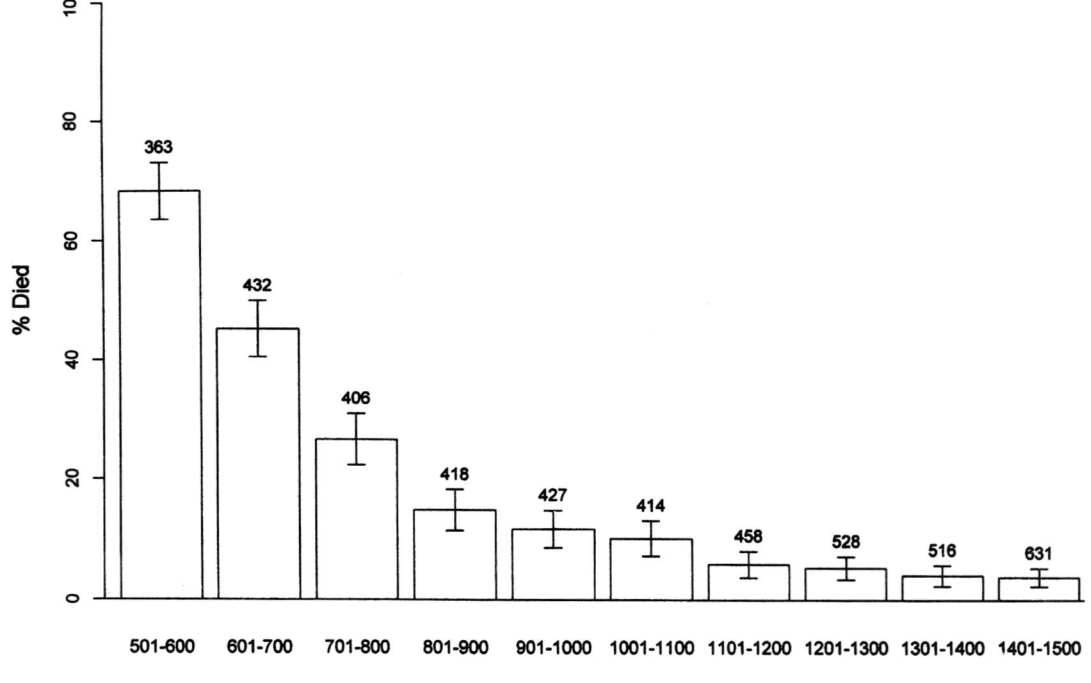

Figure 23–5. Mortality rate before discharge by birth weight among infants born in the NICHD NICU Network Centers between January 1, 1993, and December 21, 1994. Data expressed as number, percentage who died, and 95 percent confidence interval for each 100-g birth weight interval. (From Stevenson DK, Wright LL, Lemons JA, et al: Very low birth weight outcomes of the National Institute of Child Health and Human Development Neonatal Research Network, January 1993 through December 1994. Am J Obstet Gynecol 179:1632, 1998.)

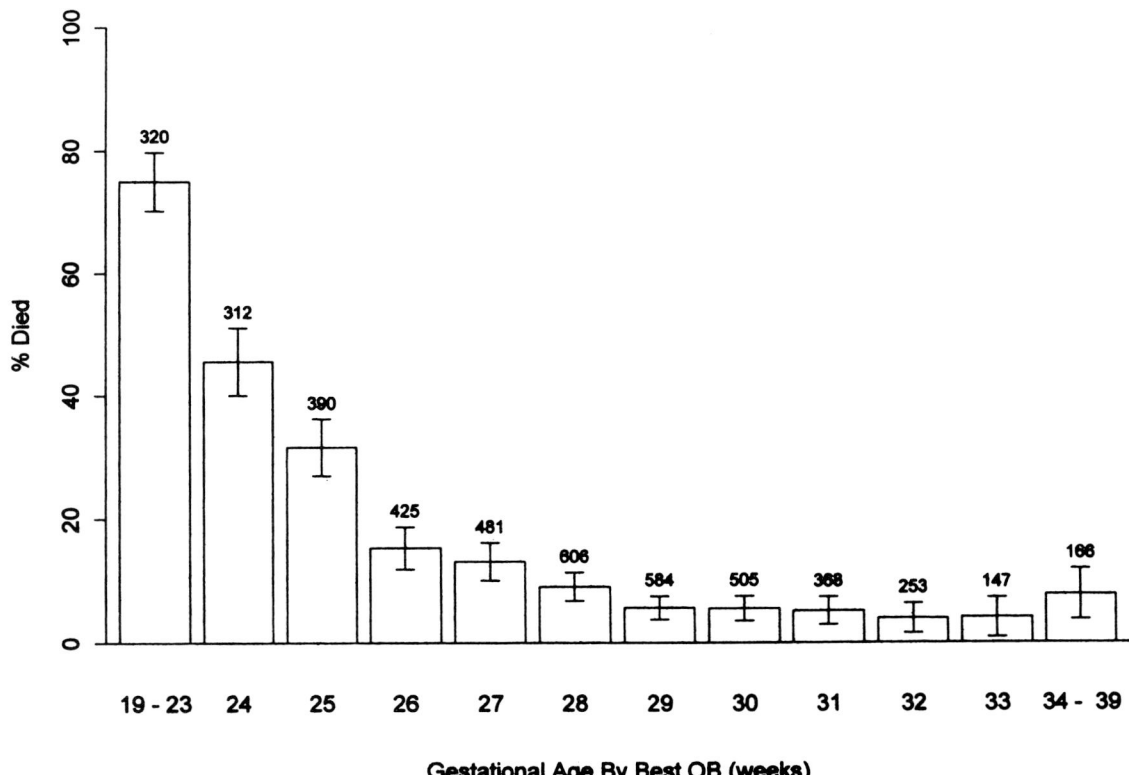

Figure 23–6. Mortality rate before discharge by gestational age, as estimated by best obstetric estimate among infants born in the NICHD NICU Network Centers between January 1, 1993, and December 21, 1994. Data expressed as number, percentage who died, and 95 percent confidence interval for each gestational age group. Thirty-six babies had missing gestational age data. (From Stevenson DK, Wright LL, Lemons JA, et al: Very low birth weight outcomes of the National Institute of Child Health and Human Development Neonatal Research Network, January 1993 through December 1994. Am J Obstet Gynecol 179:1632, 1998.)

When these infants were examined at a mean age of 32 months, developmental outcomes other than cerebral palsy were also related to gestational age at birth. The percentage who survived without neurologic deficit rose from 28 percent at 24 weeks' to 47 percent at 25 weeks' and 63 percent at 26 weeks' gestation[13] (Table 23–3). When data from the initial cohort of 138 fetuses are combined (Table 23–4), the same trends are evident. However, the percentage of intact survivors falls as a result of the inclusion of fetal, perinatal, and infant deaths. Because they include fetal and neonatal outcomes, these data may be the most appropriate for perinatal decision making before delivery (see last section of chapter). The survival rates cited in these studies

Table 23–1. OUTCOME AT 120 DAYS FOR INFANTS BORN WEIGHING LESS THAN 1,000 g ACCORDING TO GESTATIONAL AGE AT BIRTH

Outcome	OB Gestational Age at Birth (weeks)					
	21	22	23	24	25	26
Number	41	69	91	118	124	102
Stillborn (%)	20	15	12	17	1	0
Neonatal death (%)	78	71	62	50	31	26
Major morbidity (%)	2	12	17	33	35	34
"Intact" at 120 days (%)	0	3	10	15	34	40

From Bottoms SF, Paul RH, Iams JD, et al: Obstetric determinants of neonatal survival: Influence of willingness to perform cesarean delivery on survival of extremely low birth weight infants. Am J Obstet Gynecol 176:960, 1997, with permission.

Table 23–2. IMMEDIATE PERINATAL OUTCOME FOR INFANTS BORN AT 24–26 WEEKS IN 1991–1994

Outcome	Gestational Age		
	24 wk	25 wk	26 wk
Stillbirth (%)	12	5	0
No resuscitation (%)	7	0	0
Died in hosptial (%)	38	21	17
Discharged alive (%)	43	74	83

From Kilpatrick SJ, Schleuter MA, Piecuch R, et al: Outcome of infants born at 24–26 weeks' gestation: I. Survival and cost. Obstet Gynecol 90:803, 1997; American College of Obstetricians and Gynecologists, with permission.

Table 23–3. NEURODEVELOPMENTAL OUTCOME AT 32 MONTHS OF AGE FOR INFANTS BORN AT 24–26 WEEKS IN 1991–1994

Outcome	Gestational Age at Birth		
	24 wk	25 wk	26 wk
No. alive at discharge	18	31	45
No. followed	18	30	38
Normal neuro exam (%)	67	73	89
Cerebral palsy (%)	11	20	11
NL cognitive (%)	28	47	71
No deficit (%)	28	47	63

From Piecuch RE, Leonard CH, Cooper BA, et al: Outcome of infants born at 24–26 weeks' gestation: II. Neurodevelopmental outcome. Obstet Gynecol 90: 809, 1997. Copyright 1997 American College of Obstetricians and Gynecologists, with permission.

come from tertiary perinatal care centers, and do not necessarily reflect the experience in the general population. For example, a population-based study from the north of England described the outcome for births before 28 weeks between 1983 and 1994.[14] As in the United States, survival increased over time, but the survival rates are much lower at the margins of viability. This is a reflection more of the broadly inclusive dataset (all births in a region of the country vs. selected births at regional centers) than of any differences in perinatal care between the United Kingdom and the United States. Data from the last 2 years of this report are shown in Table 23–5.

Perinatal care can clearly influence mortality statistics. A study of 1126 infants who weighed between 501 and 800 grams at birth[15] confirmed earlier observations,[16] that in addition to birth weight (odds ratio [OR], 0.38; 95 percent confidence interval [CI], 0.29 to 0.49), variables such as female gender (OR, 0.42; 95 percent CI, 0.29 to 0.61), small for gestational age (OR, 0.58; 95 percent CI, 0.38 to 0.88), and antenatal

Table 23–4. OUTCOME AT 2 TO 3 YEARS OF AGE FOR INFANTS BORN AT 24–26 WEEKS

Outcome	Gestational Age at Birth		
	24 wk	25 wk	26 wk
Died <1 year (%)	57	26	17
Alive (%)	43	74	83
Alive w/cerebral palsy (%)	5	15	5
Normal cognitive (%)	12	35	59
No deficit (%)	12	35	52

% = percentage of original number of fetuses, not percentage of survivors.
Data from Kilpatrick SJ, Schleuter MA, Piecuch R, et al: Outcome of infants born at 24–26 weeks' gestation: I. Survival and cost. Obstet Gynecol 90:803, 1997; and Piecuch RE, Leonard CH, Cooper BA, et al: Outcome of infants born at 24–26 weeks' gestation: II. Neurodevelopmental outcome. Obstet Gynecol 90:809, 1997.

Table 23–5. SURVIVAL AT 22 TO 27 WEEKS

Outcome	Gestational Age (wk)					
	22	23	24	25	26	27
Antepartum death (%)	40	35	25	19	23	20
Intrapartum death (%)	40	27	17	10	7	5
Neonatal death (%)	20	36	45	41	27	20
Infant death (%)	0	1	3	6	57	3
Survived to 1 year (%)	0	0.8	10	25	37	54

Data from Tin W, Wariyar U, Hey E, et al: Changing prognosis for babies of less than 28 weeks' gestation in the north of England between 1983 and 1994. BMJ 314:107, 1997.

treatment with corticosteroids (OR, 0.52; 95 percent CI, 0.36 to 0.76) have a favorable effect on mortality (Fig. 23–7). Neonatal treatment with surfactant (favorable effect) and intrauterine infection (unfavorable effect) also influence survival significantly.[17]

Twins have in the past been thought to have higher rates of mortality than singletons born at the same gestational age, but recent reports from single institutions[18] and from multicenter studies[19] indicate rates of neonatal mortality and morbidity for liveborn twins that do not differ significantly from singletons born at the same gestational age.

There are significant but unexplained differences in survival and morbidity rates for LBW babies reported

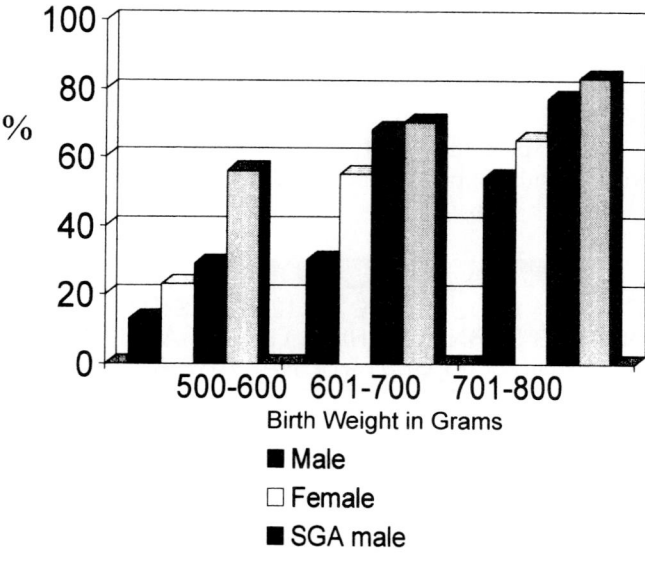

Figure 23–7. Intact survival by birth weight, SGA, and gender in extremely low birth weight infants. (Redrawn from Tyson JE, Younes N, Verter J, et al: Viability, morbidity, and resource use among newborns of 501- to 800-g birth weight. JAMA 276:1645, 1996. Copyright 1997 American College of Obstetricians and Gynecologists.)

by apparently similar neonatal intensive care units.[20] Thus, when available, it is best to use local statistics when counseling patients.

Despite marked improvements in neonatal survival, the United States compares relatively unfavorably with other developed countries with respect to neonatal mortality. In the past, this poor international ranking was blamed on an excess of LBW infants at all gestational ages in the United States. However, a study[21] of linked birth and perinatal death records from 105,084 Norwegian and 7,445,914 American births found that the higher rate of perinatal death in the United States is due almost entirely to a small excess of preterm births in the United States (2.9 percent) versus Norway (2.1 percent). The authors noted that a reduction in preterm delivery in the United States to the rate observed in Norway would produce the same perinatal mortality rate in both countries. They concluded that prevention of perinatal mortality in the United States depends more on prevention of prematurity, especially extreme prematurity, than of low birth weight.

Preterm infants are at risk for specific diseases related to the immaturity of various organ systems. Common complications in these very premature infants include respiratory distress syndrome (RDS); intraventricular hemorrhage (IVH); bronchopulmonary dysplasia (BPD); patent ductus arteriosus (PDA); necrotizing enterocolitis (NEC); and sepsis, apnea, and retinopathy of prematurity (ROP). Extremely preterm infants are at greatest risk. There is wide geographic variation in the frequency of these sequelae, which may reflect differences in definitions as well as clinical practices.[20] Robertson et al.[22] reported gestational age-specific morbidities for 20,662 infants born from well-dated pregnancies, 1,539 of whom were born before 36 weeks. Rates of neonatal morbidities by gestational age are shown in Figure 23–8.[22]

Long-Term Morbidity

During the 1950s, preterm infants were found to be at increased risk for neurodevelopmental handicaps such as severe mental retardation (IQ or DQ [developmental quotient] <70), cerebral palsy, seizure disorders, blindness, and deafness. Since then, concern about long-term neurologic sequelae has focused on smaller and smaller infants of increasingly earlier gestational age. The rate of intact survival has steadily increased for VLBW and ELBW infants (Fig. 23–9). Despite fears to the contrary, the proportion of survivors within each birth weight group who have serious handicaps has not increased since the introduction of neonatal intensive care. However, the increased number of survivors has increased the absolute number of individuals who survive with long-term morbidities of prematurity.[23–25]

Long-term outcomes for infants with birth weights below 1,000 g have been reported as these children have reached adolescence. A 1994 study of school-age outcomes found higher rates of cerebral palsy, severe visual impairment, and reduced head size and height for children with birth weights under 750 g when compared with children with birth weights 750 to 1,499 g and children born at term (Fig. 23–10).[2] Abnormal cognitive, academic, visual motor, gross motor, and adaptive performance was also more frequent among children with birth weights below 750 g (Fig. 23–11). A study of 141 adolescents who weighed less than 1,000 g at birth reported significantly more self-perceived limitations in cognition, sensation, self-care, and pain at 12 to 16 years of age compared with controls. However, the median self-perceived health scores for subjects and controls were similar.[26] Among 72 adolescents born before 33 weeks and studied at 14 to 15 years of age, researchers found neurologic magnetic resonance imaging (MRI) abnormalities in 40. Abnormal MRI findings were significantly related to reading, adjustment, and neurologic impairment.[27] These reports describe children who were born before the introduction of surfactant and before the aggressive use of antenatal corticosteroids. A recent report described outcomes for ELBW infants born in 1993 to 1994 when surfactant was more commonly used. Factors significantly associated with neurodevelopmental disability among survivors at 18 to 22 months include chronic lung disease, grades 3 to 4 intraventricular hemorrhage and periventricular leukomalacia, necrotizing enterocolitis, male gender, lower maternal education, and nonwhite race.[28]

The relationship between prematurity and long-term morbidity is apparently more complex than can be explained only by immature organ systems. Recent clinical and pathologic studies have linked chorioamnionitis to neonatal morbidities other than neonatal infections, especially including cerebral palsy and bronchopulmonary dysplasia.[29–39] These investigations indicate that a chronic intrauterine inflammatory process is responsible not only for much of the neonatal morbidity traditionally attributed simply to prematurity, but for the occurrence of preterm birth itself in many cases.[30] Amniotic fluid cytokines have been related to neonatal brain lesions (e.g., IVH and periventricular leukomalacia) thought to be precursors for cerebral palsy,[29,36] to the development of cerebral palsy,[39] and to bronchopulmonary dysplasia.[31,32] Umbilical cord blood levels of interleukin-6 (IL-6) obtained at delivery have been found to predict neonatal brain lesions and subsequent cerebral palsy.[34]

In addition to prolonged hospitalization at birth, many VLBW infants are rehospitalized during the first year of life.[40] Although less well studied, there is concern that preterm birth disrupts maternal–infant bonding, which can have a major impact on family function,

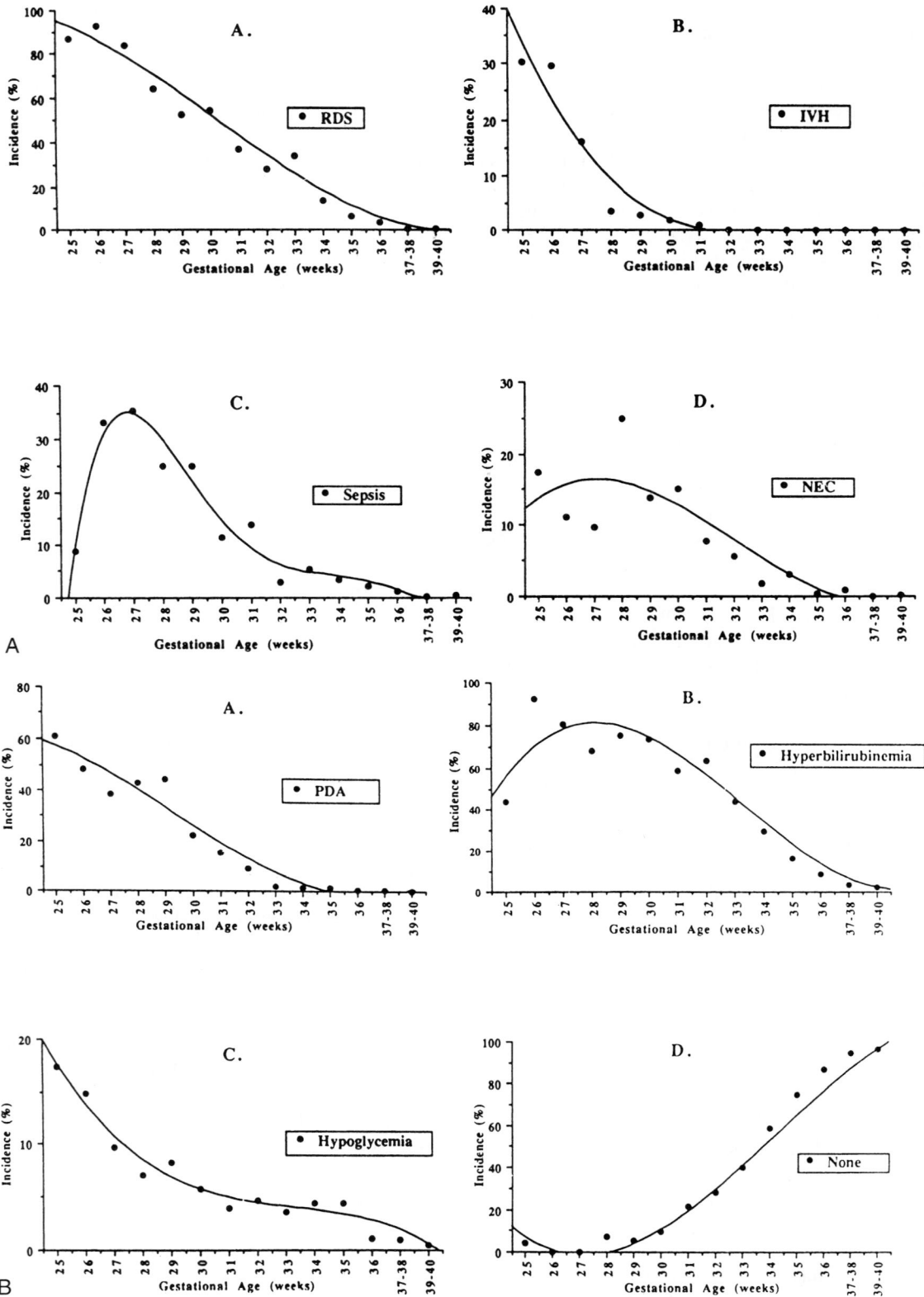

Figure 23–8. Incidence of various neonatal morbidities by gestational age at birth in infants born between 1982 and 1986 in a five-center prospective trial. *A,* Rates of respiratory distress syndrome (RDS; *A*), intraventricular hemorrhage (IVH; *B*), sepsis (*C*), and necrotizing enterocolitis (NEC; *D*). *B,* Rates of patent ductus arteriosus (PDA; *A*), hyperbilirubinemia (*B*), hypoglycemia (*C*), and of no morbidity (*D*). (From Robertson PA, Sniderman SH, Laros RK, et al: Neonatal morbidity according to gestational age and birth weight from five tertiary care centers in the United States 1983 through 1986. Am J Obstet Gyencol 166:1629, 1992, with permission.)

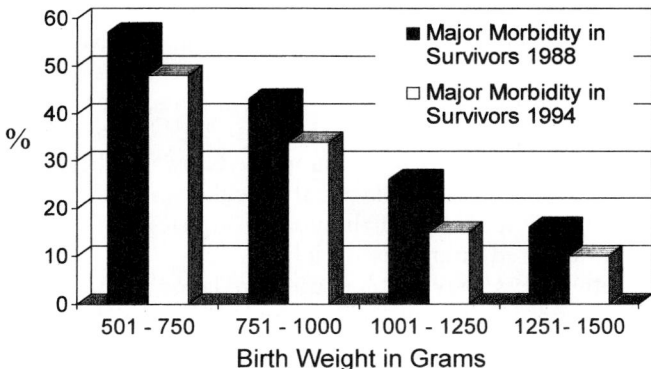

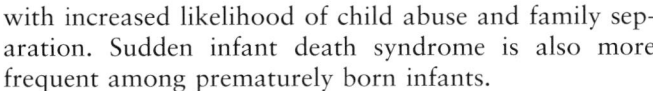

Figure 23–9. Major morbidity among survivors for very low birth weight infants born in 1988 and 1994 in the NICHD NICU Network. (Data from Stevenson DK, Wright LL, Lemons JA, et al: Very low birth weight outcomes of the National Institute of Child Health and Human Development Neonatal Research Network, January 1993 through December 1994. Am J Obstet Gynecol 179:1632, 1998.)

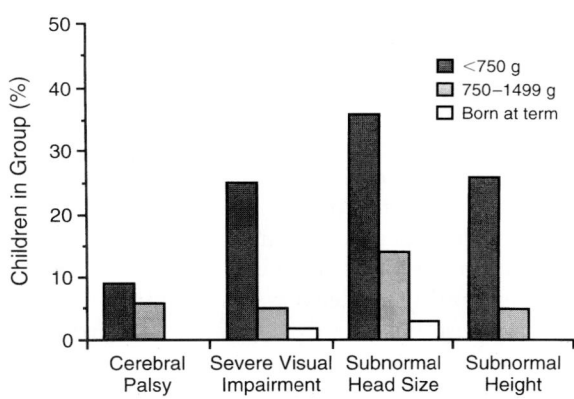

Figure 23–10. Percentage of children with cerebral palsy, severe visual impairment, subnormal head size, and subnormal height in infants born less than 750 g birth weight, 750 to 1499 g birth weight, and at term. (From Hack M, Taylor HG, Klein N, et al: School-age outcomes in children with birth weights under 750 g. N Engl J Med 331:756, 1994, with permission.)

with increased likelihood of child abuse and family separation. Sudden infant death syndrome is also more frequent among prematurely born infants.

OVERVIEW OF THE PATHOGENESIS OF PREMATURITY

The Epidemiology of Preterm Birth

The list of maternal and fetal diagnoses antecedent to preterm deliveries is both long and diverse. Preterm labor, preterm ruptured membranes, preeclampsia, abruptio placentae, multiple gestation, placenta previa, fetal growth restriction, excessive or inadequate amniotic fluid volume, fetal anomalies, amnionitis, incompetent cervix, as well as maternal medical problems such as diabetes mellitus, asthma, drug abuse, and pyelonephritis may all lead to preterm delivery. Maternal char-

acteristics associated with preterm delivery are equally numerous: maternal race (black greater than nonblack), a history of previous preterm birth, low socioeconomic status, poor nutrition, low prepregnancy weight, absent or inadequate prenatal care, age less than 18 or over 40, strenuous work, high personal stress, anemia, cigarette smoking, bacteriuria, genital colonization or infection (e.g., bacterial vaginosis, *Neisseria gonorrhoeae, Chlamydia trachomatis, Mycoplasma,* and *Ureaplasma*), cervical injury or abnormality (e.g., in utero exposure to diethylstilbestrol, a history of cervical conization, or second-trimester induced abortion), uterine anomaly or fibroids, excessive uterine contractility, and premature cervical dilation of more than 1 cm or effacement greater than 80 percent. The list of risk factors is so long that it is hard to see any common thread.

The multitude of clinical disorders and risk factors has been usefully organized into two broad categories, called *spontaneous* and *indicated* preterm births, based upon the clinical presentation, the health of the mother

Figure 23–11. Percentage of children with subnormal cognitive function, academic skills, visual and gross motor function, and adaptive function in infants born less than 750 g birth weight, 750 to 1499 g birth weight, and at term. (From Hack M, Taylor HG, Klein N, et al: School-age outcomes in children with birth weights under 750 g. N Engl J Med 331:756, 1994, with permission.)

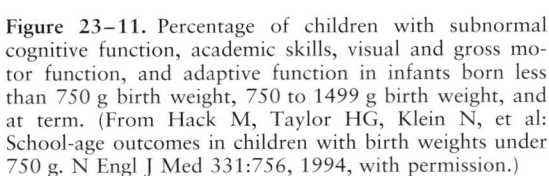

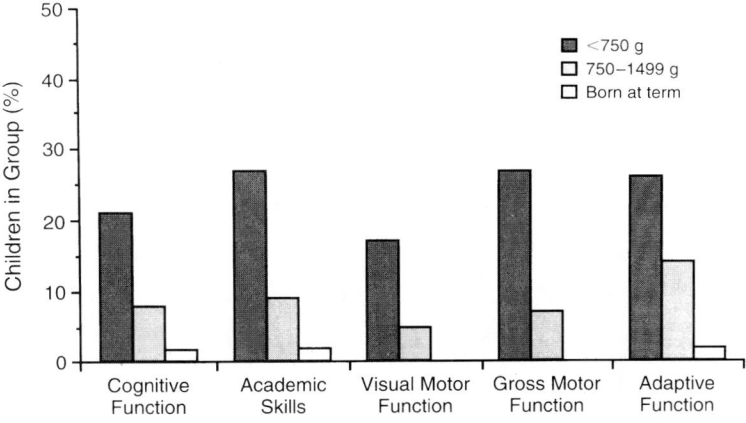

and fetus, and the epidemiologic profile of affected pregnant women.[41-44] Approximately 75 percent of preterm births occur "spontaneously" after preterm labor (PTL), preterm premature rupture of membranes (preterm PROM), or related diagnoses such as amnionitis and incompetent cervix (PROM refers to rupture of membranes before the onset of labor at any gestational age, hence the apparently redundant "preterm PROM"). Complications of PTL and preterm PROM may lead to an "indication" for delivery (e.g., intrauterine infection), but these births are nevertheless termed "spontaneous" because they follow spontaneous preterm labor or preterm PROM. Risk factors for PTL and preterm PROM are similar, with a few exceptions. Women with preterm PROM are more likely to be indigent,[41] to smoke,[45] and to have experienced bleeding in the current pregnancy[46] than are women who present with preterm labor.

Indicated preterm births follow medical or obstetric disorders that place the fetus at risk (e.g., acute or chronic maternal hypertension, diabetes mellitus, placenta previa or abruption, and intrauterine growth restriction). Indicated preterm births account for 20 to 30 percent of births before 37 weeks in most series.[42,43] Some risk factors are associated with both spontaneous and indicated prematurity (e.g., multiple gestation, prepregnancy weight <55 kg, nulliparity, black race, and bleeding in the first or second trimester), and some clinical risk factors are primarily related to one or the other (Table 23–6).

The distinction between spontaneous and indicated preterm births rests on an assumption that fetal growth and well-being have been satisfactory before the spontaneous occurrence of preterm labor or PROM. Most data support this premise, but poor intrauterine growth may be more common in preterm infants, even in the absence of apparent maternal disease.[47-49] These clinical observations have been supported by studies that showed decidual and placental vascular lesions[50-52] and increased impedance in the uterine arteries[53] of women who delivered after preterm labor.

Fetal stress may initiate preterm labor by uteroplacental production of corticotropin-releasing hormone (CRH), a peptide produced by the placenta, amniochorion, and decidua and known to enhance prostanoid production in these same cells.[54] These reports provide a biologically plausible mechanism by which abnormalities of the placenta and uteroplacental blood flow may lead to spontaneous preterm birth, either directly, through decidual and/or membrane injury, or indirectly by inducing fetal stress.

The Epidemiology and Pathogenesis of Spontaneous Preterm Birth

Just as epidemiologic observations provide clues to the distinction between the causes of spontaneous and indicated preterm births, so also does epidemiology provide clues to pathogenesis of spontaneous prematurity. Ultimately, the final steps of the parturitional process are the same at any gestational age, regardless of the initiating cause. Whether preterm parturition is just normal labor that is initiated too soon, or follows a distinctly different pathway until the final stages of labor, has been the subject of great debate. Increasingly, the evidence favors the latter interpretation, with several pathologic processes capable of initiating the process.

The epidemiology of preterm birth reveals several major trends. The first is that early preterm birth (<32 weeks) and late preterm birth (>32 weeks) have a different epidemiology. Another is that some risk factors are associated with recurrent preterm birth, while others appear to be unique to the affected pregnancy.[44] Risk factors for recurrent and nonrecurrent preterm birth are similar but not identical to those for early and later prematurity, respectively, suggesting at least two general pathways. Early preterm birth is more likely to recur, is more strongly associated with a short cervix and the presence of fetal fibronectin in cervicovaginal secretions, and is more often accompanied by clinical or subclinical evidence of infection and by long-term morbidity for the infant.[44] Later preterm birth is more likely to be associated with increased uterine contraction frequency and with a rise in maternal excretion of estriol (an indicator of increasing maturation of the fetal hypothalamic-pituitary-adrenal axis), and thus to mimic normal labor at term.[55]

Table 23–6. COMPARISON OF CLINICAL RISK FACTORS FOR SPONTANEOUS AND INDICATED PRETERM BIRTH

Spontaneous Preterm Birth	OR	Indicated Preterm Birth	OR
Prior preterm birth	4	Müllerian duct anomaly	7
Bleeding in second trimester	2	Proteinuria	5
		Hypertension	4
Genitourinary infections	2	Prior stillbirth	3.5
Black race	2	Lung disease	2.5
Low prepregnancy weight	2	Age >30 years	2.4
		Bacteriuria	2
Age <18 years	2		
Smoking	1.5		
Frequent contractions	1.5		

OR, odds ratio.
Data from Meis PJ, Michielutte R, Peters TJ, et al: Factors associated with preterm birth in Cardiff Wales: II. Indicated and spontaneous preterm birth. Am J Obstet Gynecol 173:597, 1995; Meis PJ, Goldenberg RL, Mercer BM, et al: The preterm prediction study: Risk factors for indicated preterm birth. Am J Obstet Gynecol 178:562, 1998; Goldenberg RL, Iams JD, Mercer BM, et al: The preterm prediction study: The value of new vs. standard risk factors predicting early and all spontaneous preterm births. Am J Public Health 88:233, 1998.

Nonrecurrent Preterm Birth

Risk factors for nonrecurrent spontaneous preterm birth include second-trimester bleeding, abnormal amniotic fluid volume, multiple gestation, substance abuse, and trauma. These events have in common that they may lead to ischemia, injury, or disruption to the junction of the maternal decidua with the fetal chorion. Premature contractions or membrane rupture may result from decidual hemorrhage with thrombin generation, which in turn may stimulate uterine contractions and proteases that affect membrane integrity (see the section Preterm Premature Rupture of the Membranes, below).

Excessive uterine volume, as may occur with polyhydramnios or multiple gestation, is another pathway to increased uterine activity via increased formation of gap junctions, oxytocin receptors, and prostaglandin and collagenase production.

There is increasing evidence, however, that preterm birth in multiple gestation is more complex than can be explained simply by uterine distention. Women who carry a multifetal gestation beyond 34 weeks are more likely to have conceived spontaneously (without assisted reproductive technology)[56] and to have a cervical length above the 50th centile at 24 to 26 weeks' gestation.[57] Increased levels of maternal serum relaxin following superovulation[58] and the potential for intrauterine inoculation with vaginal microorganisms during cervical instrumentation are potential mechanisms under investigation.[59] Also, spontaneous or induced fetal loss in higher order multiple gestation has been associated with an increased risk of preterm birth, perhaps mediated by decidual hemorrhage or necrosis.

Recurrent Preterm Birth

Recurrent spontaneous preterm birth is associated with prior preterm births, especially before 32 weeks, African-American race, maternal genital tract infection, maternal cervical length less than the 10th percentile, and the presence of fetal fibronectin in cervicovaginal mucus.[44,60–63] The interrelationship of these risk factors has begun to explain some of the mechanisms of preterm delivery.

Obstetric History and Preterm Birth

The risk of spontaneous preterm birth is increased by a history of prior preterm delivery. The recurrence risk rises as the number of prior preterm births increases.[64] As can be seen in Table 23–7, the most recent birth is the most predictive. The likelihood of recurrent preterm birth also increases as the gestational age of the prior preterm birth decreases. The earlier the prior preterm birth, the greater the recurrence risk.[62] A population-

Table 23–7. RISK OF PRETERM BIRTH ACCORDING TO OBSTETRIC HISTORY

First Birth	Second Birth	N	Subsequent Preterm Birth	
			Percentage	Relative Risk
Term	—	25,817	4.4%	1.0
Preterm	—	1,860	17.2%	3.9
Term	Term	24,689	2.6%	0.6
Preterm	Term	1,540	5.7%	1.3
Term	Preterm	1,128	11.1%	2.5
Preterm	Preterm	320	28.4%	6.5

From Bakketeig LS, Hoffman HJ: Epidemiology of preterm birth: Results from a longitudinal study of births in Norway. *In* Elder MG, Hendricks CH (eds): Preterm Labor. London and Boston, Butterworths, 1981, p 17, with permission.

based cohort study of births over 15 years in Georgia found that, of second deliveries between 20 and 31 weeks' gestation, 29.4 percent for white and 37.8 percent for black women were preceded by a preterm delivery.[63]

The biologic variable most consistently related to recurrent spontaneous preterm birth is cervical length when measured by transvaginal sonography.[44,60,61] These reports suggest that cervical function is at least in part a constitutional factor that influences preterm birth risk in successive pregnancies.

Maternal Race and Preterm Birth

African-American women have a rate of preterm delivery that is approximately twice that of women of other races. In 1996, 16.3 percent of non-Hispanic black women delivered before 37 completed weeks' gestation, compared with 10.1 percent for Hispanic women and 8.1 percent of non-Hispanic white women.[65] Although the rate of preterm birth declines with advancing education among African-Americans, it is higher than the rate among nonblack women at all educational levels. In fact, the ratio of black to white preterm birth rates in 1995 was 1.95 for women with some college education and 1.74 for women who did not finish high school.[66] Black women born outside the United States do not share this increased risk of preterm delivery.[67]

Sociodemographic factors also do not explain the higher rate of preterm birth in U.S.-born African-American women. A study of 1,029 black and 462 white parous indigent women in Alabama found that black women delivered preterm and low-birth-weight infants more frequently than white women, even though white indigent women in the population studied had greater sociodemographic risk.[68] One small study of 125 women suggested that cervical length might be an explanation for the observed racial differences.[69] However, among 2,929 women in the Preterm Prediction

Table 23–8. COMPARISON OF BISHOP SCORE TO CERVICAL ULTRASOUND AT 22 TO 24 WEEKS TO PREDICT PRETERM BIRTH <35 WEEKS' GESTATION

	Bishop Score ≥4	Cervical Ultrasound Examination			
		≤20 mm	≤25 mm	≤30 mm	Funneling
Sensitivity (%)	28	23	37	54	25
Specificity (%)	91	97	92	76	95
PPV (%)	12	26	18	9	17
NPV (%)	97	96	97	97	97

PPV, positive predictive power; NPV, negative predictive power.

Data from Iams JD, Goldenberg RL, Meis PJ, et al: The length of the cervix and the risk of spontaneous premature delivery. N Engl J Med 334:567, 1996.

Study, cervical length was related to preterm birth but not to race[70] (Table 23–8). This study controlled for bacterial vaginosis in relating cervical length to preterm birth, an important consideration because bacterial vaginosis is itself related to risk of preterm birth[44] and to cervical length.[71]

The higher prevalence of bacterial vaginosis among African-American women is a potential explanation for racial differences in preterm birth rates. A series of studies have linked bacterial vaginosis to preterm birth, particularly among African-Americans. The Vaginal Infections in Pregnancy (VIP) Study, a large observational study of vaginal microflora in pregnancy, found organisms associated with bacterial vaginosis more often in black women, even when differences in health behaviors were controlled.[72] The Preterm Prediction Study[44] revealed that the relationships between preterm birth, black race, and bacterial vaginosis (BV) were mediated by fetal fibronectin. The relation between preterm birth before 32 weeks and bacterial vaginosis was significant only in black women, where the population-attributable risk for BV was 40 percent for births before 32 weeks. In contrast, for nonblack women, a low body mass index (<19.8 kg/m²) had the strongest association with early preterm birth.[44]

Infection and Prematurity

The association between preterm birth and infection has been reported for more than 50 years.[73,74] Evidence relating infection to preterm labor and birth comes from multiple sources: epidemiologic, microbiologic, histologic, and clinical. Maternal and neonatal infections occur more frequently after preterm than term birth. Numerous microorganisms, including *Ureaplasma urealyticum, Mycoplasma* species, *Chlamydia trachomatis, Trichomonas, Escherichia coli,* group B *Streptococcus,* and especially anaerobes such as *Fusobacterium, Bacteroides,* anaerobic streptococci, and *Mobiluncus,* have been recovered from the lower and upper genital tract and amniotic fluid of women with preterm labor and preterm ruptured membranes.[75–83]

The strength of the association between both clinical infection and histologic amnionitis increases as the gestational age at delivery decreases, especially before 30 to 32 weeks. A study of placental histology revealed that membrane inflammation was nearly universal at 21 to 24 weeks and declined as gestational age advanced to a rate of 10 percent at term.[78] In a study that related cultures of the fetal membranes to gestational age at delivery, positive cultures were found in more than 70 percent of births before 30 weeks compared with 20 percent at term.[79] Positive amniotic fluid cultures have been reported in 20 to 30 percent of women with preterm labor, especially before 30 weeks' gestation and when the labor is refractory to tocolytic drugs.[75–77,83] The same inverse relationship between gestational age and positive amniotic fluid cultures was reported in study of amniotic fluid cultures obtained from women with preterm labor who did not have overt clinical chorioamnionitis[83] as shown in Figure 23–12. The most common organisms recovered were *Fusobacterium nucleatum, Bacteroides* species, and *Ureaplasma urealyticum.* Another study (Fig. 23–13)[84] found that both positive membrane cultures and increased amniotic fluid

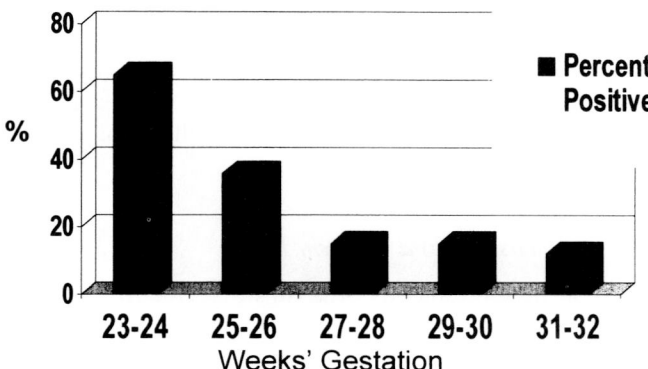

Figure 23–12. Gestational age and amniotic fluid cultures in preterm labor. (Redrawn from Watts DH, Krohn MA, Hillier SL, et al: The association of occult amniotic fluid infection with gestational age and neonatal outcome among women in preterm labor. Obstet Gynecol 79:351, 1992. Copyright 1992 American College of Obstetricians and Gynecologists, with permission.)

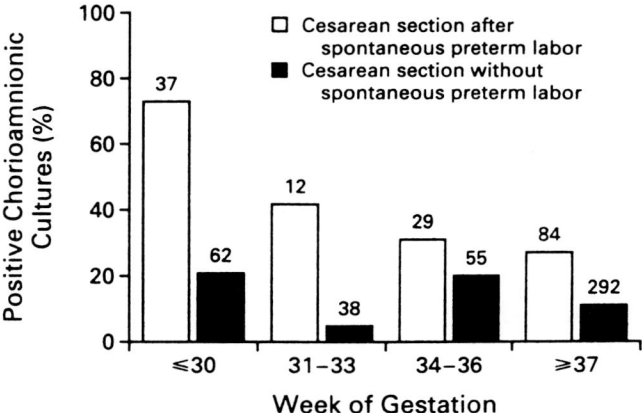

Figure 23–13. Chorioamnion colonization in spontaneous and indicated preterm births. (Redrawn from Goldenberg RL, Hauth JC, Andrews WW: Intrauterine infection and preterm delivery. N Engl J Med 342:1500, 2000, with permission.)

IL-6 levels occurred more frequently in spontaneous than indicated preterm births.[84]

Infections outside the genital tract have also been related to preterm birth, most commonly urinary tract and intra-abdominal infections (e.g., pyelonephritis and appendicitis). Recently, maternal periodontal infections have been associated with increased risk of spontaneous preterm birth.[85]

Pregnant women treated with antimicrobial drugs effective against *Ureaplasma*, *Mycoplasma*, and *Chlamydia* had reduced rates of preterm birth in some studies.[86–88] However, prospective trials of the same antibiotics to prevent preterm birth in women colonized with *Ureaplasma* and *Chlamydia* found no difference in the incidence of premature delivery[89,90] (Table 23–9). The failure of these trials fostered reconsideration of

the relationship between infection and prematurity, and particularly of the association between maternal BV and spontaneous preterm birth.[79–81,91,92] Rather than a specific infection caused by a single organism, BV is an alteration of the maternal vaginal flora in which gram-negative anaerobic bacteria and *Mycoplasma* species largely replace the normally predominant lactobacilli. The association between BV and prematurity has been noted in microbiological, histological, and clinical studies. In a report from the Vaginal Infections and Prematurity Study, maternal bacterial vaginosis with mycoplasma and bacteroides colonization was significantly related to low birth weight (OR, 2.1; 95 percent CI, 1.5 to 3.0) but neither organism was related to low birth weight when BV was not present.[92] The authors cited other work showing an association between BV and elevated levels of endotoxin, IL-1α, mucinase, and sialidase, and suggested that BV may result in the production of cytokines with biologic effects on the uterus, cervix, and membranes.

Two prospective trials of antibiotic treatment reported reduced rates of preterm birth in women who had a history of preterm birth and BV, but there was no benefit for women who had either risk factor alone.[93,94] However, the rate of preterm birth was not affected by treatment with metronidazole in a placebo-controlled trial that enrolled 1,900 women with asymptomatic bacterial vaginosis.[95] The rates of birth before 37, 35, and 32 weeks were not reduced by treatment, nor were the rates of LBW or VLBW infants. Analysis of subsets of women according to their obstetric history of preterm birth, race, gestational age at initiation of treatment, eradication of BV, and prepregnancy weight did not reveal any subgroup for whom the antibiotic produced a reduced preterm birth rate. Remarkably, a

Table 23–9. RANDOMIZED TRIALS OF ANTIBIOTICS TO PREVENT PRETERM BIRTH

First Author	Year	Entry Criteria	Antibiotic(s)	Outcome
Elder	1971	Bacteriuria	Oral tetracycline	Decreased LBW
Eschenbach	1991	*Ureaplasma urealyticum*	Oral erythromycin	No effect
Kelbanoff	1995	Group B streptococcus	Oral erythromycin	No effect
Hauth	1995	Prior PTD or maternal weight <50 kg	Oral metronidazole & erythromycin	No effect if BV-negative, reduced PTD if BV-positive
Joesoef	1995	Bacterial vaginosis	Vaginal clindamycin	No effect
McDonald	1997	Bacterial vaginosis	Oral metronidazole	No effect if no Hx PTD, benefit if Hx prior PTD
Gichangi	1997	Poor obstetric Hx*	Cefetamet-pivoxil	Reduced LBW
Carey	2000	Bacterial vaginosis	Metronidazole	No effect, regardless of prior obstetric Hx history
Carey	2000	Trichomonas	Metronidazole	Increased PTD

PTD, preterm delivery; LBW, low birth weight; Hx, history; HIV, human immunodeficiency virus; BV, bacterial vaginosis.
*18% of subjects were HIV-positive, 10% had had syphilis, 45% had prior preterm birth, and 30% had a prior perinatal death.
Data from citations listed, plus these references not cited in text: Gichangi PB, Ndinya-Achola O, Ombete J, et al: Antimicrobial prophylaxis in pregnancy: a randomized, placebo-controlled trial with cefetamet-pivoxil in pregnant women with a poor obstetric history. Am J Obstet Gynecol 177:680, 1997; and Joesoef MR, Hillier SL, Winkjosastro G, et al: Intravaginal clindamycin treatment for bacterial vaginosis: Effects on preterm delivery and low birth weight. Am J Obstet Gynecol 173:1527, 1995.

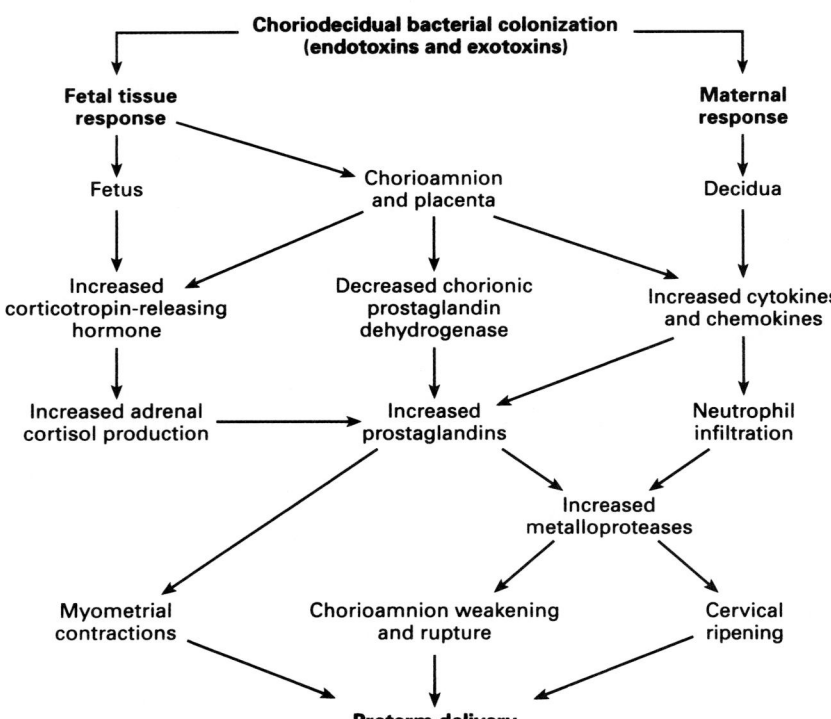

Figure 23–14. Potential pathways from choriodecidual bacterial colonization to preterm delivery. (From Goldenberg RL, Hauth JC, Andrews WW: Intrauterine infection and preterm delivery. N Engl J Med 342:1500, 2000, with permission.)

companion study conducted simultaneously in women with *Trichomonas vaginalis* reported an increase in the rate of preterm birth in those randomized to receive metronidazole.[96]

These trials indicate that the relationship between infection and prematurity is more complex than can be explained by the ascent of organisms from the lower to the upper genital tract during pregnancy. Recent research has examined the roles played by host defense, including the cervix and the maternal and fetal immune response, in the occurrence of preterm birth. Andrews and Goldenberg have argued that microorganisms responsible for preterm birth, especially early, recurrent preterm birth, are actually present in the endometrium before conception, and become clinically manifest as preterm labor, PROM, or even incompetent cervix only in the second and early third trimester.[97] The pathways by which intrauterine infection may lead to spontaneous preterm birth are indicated in Figure 23–14.[98]

Cervical Length

The length of the uterine cervix as measured by transvaginal ultrasonography is inversely and continuously related to the risk of preterm birth in both singleton[99] and multiple gestation.[100] The shorter the cervical length at 18 to 28 weeks' gestation, the greater the risk of spontaneous prematurity[99,101,102] (Fig. 23–15). This relationship has been observed throughout the entire range of cervical length, not only for cervical length below the 10th percentile (Fig. 23–16). Cervical length is also strongly related to a history of spontaneous preterm birth, especially before 32 weeks' gestation. In one study, the gestational age at delivery in prior pregnancies was related to cervical length in a subsequent

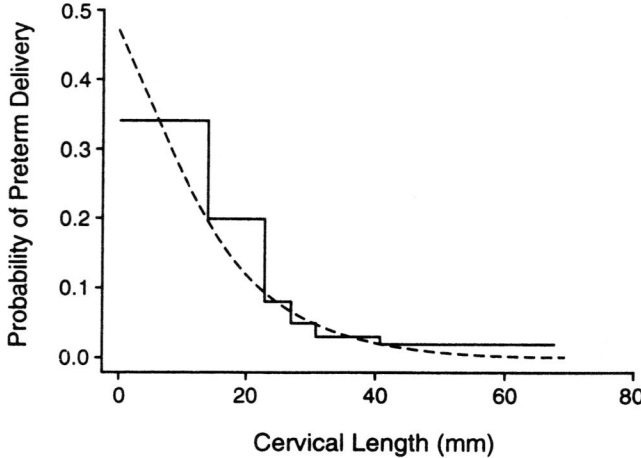

Figure 23–15. Estimated probability of spontaneous preterm delivery before 35 weeks' gestation from the logistic regression analysis (*dashed line*) and observed frequency of spontaneous preterm delivery (*solid line*) according to cervical length measured by transvaginal ultrasonography at 24 weeks. (From Iams JD, Goldenberg RL, Meis PJ, et al: The length of the cervix and the risk of spontaneous premature delivery. N Engl J Med 334:567, 1996, with permission.)

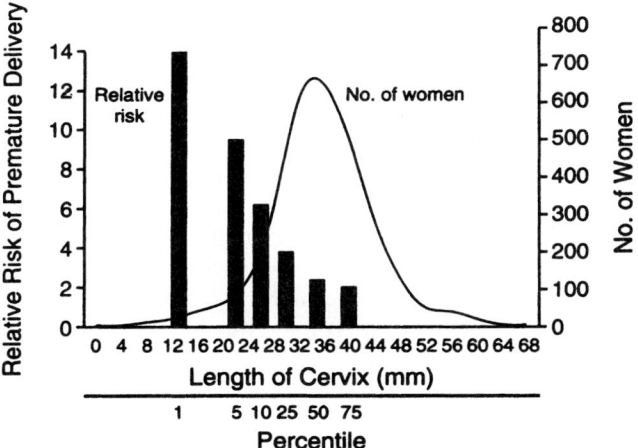

Figure 23-16. Distribution of subjects by percentile of cervical length measured by transvaginal sonography at 24 weeks (*solid line*) and relative risk of spontaneous preterm birth before 35 weeks according to percentiles of cervical length (*bars*). Relative risk of spontaneous preterm delivery for women at the 1st, 5th, 10th, 25th, 50th, and 75th percentiles are compared with the risks among women with cervical lengths above the 75th percentile. (From Iams JD, Goldenberg RL, Meis PJ, et al: The length of the cervix and the risk of spontaneous premature delivery. N Engl J Med 334:567, 1996, with permission.)

pregnancy: the earlier the gestational age at delivery, the shorter the cervix in the next pregnancy.[60] Cervical length is also related to the risk of recurrent preterm birth.[61,103] For women with a prior preterm birth, the likelihood of recurrent preterm birth before 35 weeks fell from 31 percent when the cervical length at 24 weeks was 25 mm or less to 16 percent when the cervical length was 26 to 35 mm, and to 8 percent when the cervical length was 36 mm or more (>50th centile). In contrast, among women whose only prior birth(s) were at term, the rate of birth less than 35 weeks was 8 percent when the cervix was 25 mm or less, 4 percent when it was 26 to 35 mm, and 2 percent when it was 36 mm or more.[61]

The correlation between cervical length and preterm birth risk may be explained by the physical strength or resistance of the cervix to factors such as intrauterine weight or volume, biochemical influences arising from infectious or other inflammatory stimuli,[71,105,106] or biophysical effects of uterine activity. Whatever the explanation, these investigations indicate that cervical length is a marker for cervical competence, and that cervical competence operates as a continuum. These data contradict the previous understanding of the cervix as a categorical rather than a continuous variable (i.e., either competent or incompetent). If the cervix has degrees of "competence," then cervical incompetence is simply the lowermost end of a spectrum.[60] That cervical length is related to gestational age at delivery in both previous and future pregnancies indicates that cer-

vical length is an independent risk factor for prematurity.[104]

Fibronectin

Fibronectin is an extracellular matrix protein that is best described as the "glue" that attaches the fetal membranes to the underlying uterine decidua.[107] Fibronectin is normally found in the cervicovaginal secretions before 20 to 22 weeks of pregnancy, and again at the end of normal pregnancy as labor approaches. It is not normally present in cervicovaginal secretions between 22 and 37 weeks. The presence of fibronectin in cervicovaginal secretions after 22 weeks is a marker of disruption of the decidual–chorionic interface. In the NICHD Preterm Prediction Study, multivariate analysis revealed that the strongest predictors of spontaneous preterm birth (SPTB) were cervicovaginal fibronectin,[108] transvaginal sonographic cervical length,[99] an obstetric history of previous preterm birth,[109] and presence of BV,[91] respectively. Fibronectin status at 22 to 24 weeks was strongly correlated with the presence of BV and with subsequent histologic chorioamnionitis, postpartum endometritis, and neonatal sepsis.[110] Almost all BV-positive women who delivered before 32 weeks were fibronectin positive at 22 to 24 weeks, suggesting that BV either causes or is a marker for disruption of the choriodecidual interface.[44] The relative risk of preterm birth before 32 weeks was 14.1 (CI 9.3, 21.4) for fibronectin-positive versus -negative women, compared with 2.7 (CI 1.6, 4.6) for BV-positive versus -negative women. Among women with lower tract BV, the presence of fibronectin in cervical and vaginal fluid therefore distinguishes women with upper tract infection from those with only lower tract colonization, and thus to identify those with the highest risk of early preterm birth. Why do some women with BV have upper tract involvement while others do not? The difference may lie in the timing of upper tract colonization, in the maternal and fetal immune response to the presence of organisms in the uterus, or both.

Clear linkages between the most consistent risk factors for preterm birth have emerged from recent research and produced alternate explanations for prematurity that begin with the observation that maternal lower genital tract colonization is much more common than upper tract colonization, and both are more common than preterm birth. Older hypotheses to explain the presence in the upper genital tract of microorganisms from the lower tract have had to be reexamined. Theories that begin either with idiopathic uterine contractions that open the cervix to allow ascent of organisms into the uterus[111] or with cytokines produced in the decidua that initiate prostaglandin production leading to cervical ripening and uterine contractions have been challenged by reports that suggest an indolent role for microorganisms in the pathogenesis of preterm birth. An ascending route from the vagina through the cervix is consistent with reported relationships between spontaneous preterm birth and cervical dilation.[112-114] and length.[99,101] However, reports indicating that intrauterine colonization and infection precede cervical effacement and dilation suggest another explanation for the presence of microorganisms within the uterus, based in part on a report of chronic plasma cell endometritis in endometrial biopsy specimens from 10 of 22 women with BV, compared to only 1 of 19 controls (OR, 15; 95 percent CI, 2 to 686).[115] Chronic intrauterine colonization of the endometrium with BV before conception, with subsequent proliferation of these low-virulence organisms within the uterus in the altered immune environment of pregnancy is an attractive theory to explain the above reports that relate BV and fibronectin to preterm birth risk. This pathway is further supported by observations of increased levels of cytokines released in response to infection[116,117] or ischemia[118] in amniotic fluid samples obtained at midtrimester genetic amniocentesis from women who experienced spontaneous preterm labor weeks later.

The Spontaneous Preterm Birth Syndrome

When information about fibronectin, cervical length, maternal infection, and second-trimester amniotic fluid cytokines are considered together with data presented earlier in the chapter about intrauterine infection and neonatal morbidity, a model of early preterm birth as an indolent rather than acute process emerges.[119] Romero et al. have termed this the "preterm labor syndrome".[120] In response to a chronic intrauterine inflammatory insult (usually infectious or ischemic), and influenced by both the maternal and fetal immune response,[30] the fetal membranes and decidua produce cytokines (tumor necrosis factor-α [TNF-α], IL-1, and IL-6). This cytokine-mediated process ultimately leads to one or more of the following: (1) continued leakage of fetal fibronectin from the decidua–membrane interface, (2) elaboration of uterotonic bioactive lipids (prostaglandin E_2 [PGE_2], prostaglandin $F_{2\alpha}$ [$PGF_{2\alpha}$], thromboxane A_2, leukotrienes B_4 and C_4,[121] hydroperoxyeicosatetraenoic acid [5-HETE] and others) that (3) stimulate myometrial contractions and (4) initiate release of proteases that are capable of injuring the membranes and underlying decidua that (5) incites prostaglandin stimulation that results in (6) cervical ripening, dilation, and/or membrane rupture, and (7) in utero injury to the fetal brain, lung, or gut.

In this model, most women with microorganisms in the lower or upper tract or other sources of inflammation experience neither preterm birth nor neonatal morbidity. That some do while most do not may be attributed to differences in behavioral (physical or sexual activity, smoking) and/or genetic (e.g., cervical length, immune response) factors or both.

Other potential initiators of the process may include premature activation of the maternal–fetal hypothalamic-pituitary axis and/or pathologic uterine distention (as shown in Fig. 23–17),[122] both of which are more likely to cause later preterm births and less likely to cause major neonatal neurologic morbidity.

PREVENTION AND TREATMENT OF PRETERM BIRTH

Prevention and treatment strategies for prematurity may be described according to the public health concepts of primary, secondary, and tertiary care.[119,123] *Primary* care or prevention is the elimination or reduction of risk in an entire population. Effective primary care requires a good understanding of the pathophysiology of the disease, and public health educational efforts to modify behaviors and eliminate risk factors. For preterm birth, the target population is clear (preteens and women of childbearing age), but effective primary interventions have not been demonstrated. A primary program to reduce the incidence of prematurity might include efforts to prevent smoking and sexually transmitted diseases, to avoid unplanned pregnancies through use of birth control, to plan pregnancy to reduce stress and improve nutrition, to avoid higher order multifetal gestation, and to foster employment policies that promote the needs of pregnancy over the workplace.[124,125] *Secondary* care selects individuals with increased risk for surveillance and/or prophylactic treatment. Effective secondary care requires both accurate screening tests and effective interventions to prevent or reduce risk. Examples of secondary care for preterm birth are screening for preterm birth risk, early diagnosis and patient education programs, prophylactic medications (e.g., tocolytic drugs, progesterone supplementation, or antibiotics) and lifestyle changes such as reduced physical or sexual activity. Unfortunately, none of these has led to a decline in prematurity.[126] *Tertiary* care is treatment of an individual patient after an index illness has occurred. Tertiary care has no effect on the incidence of the disease, but rather is aimed at reducing morbidity and mortality after the diagnosis has been made. For preterm birth, tertiary care includes prompt and accurate diagnosis, referral to an appropriate care site, and specific treatment (e.g., tocolytic drugs to arrest preterm labor, antibiotics for group B β-hemolytic streptococcal

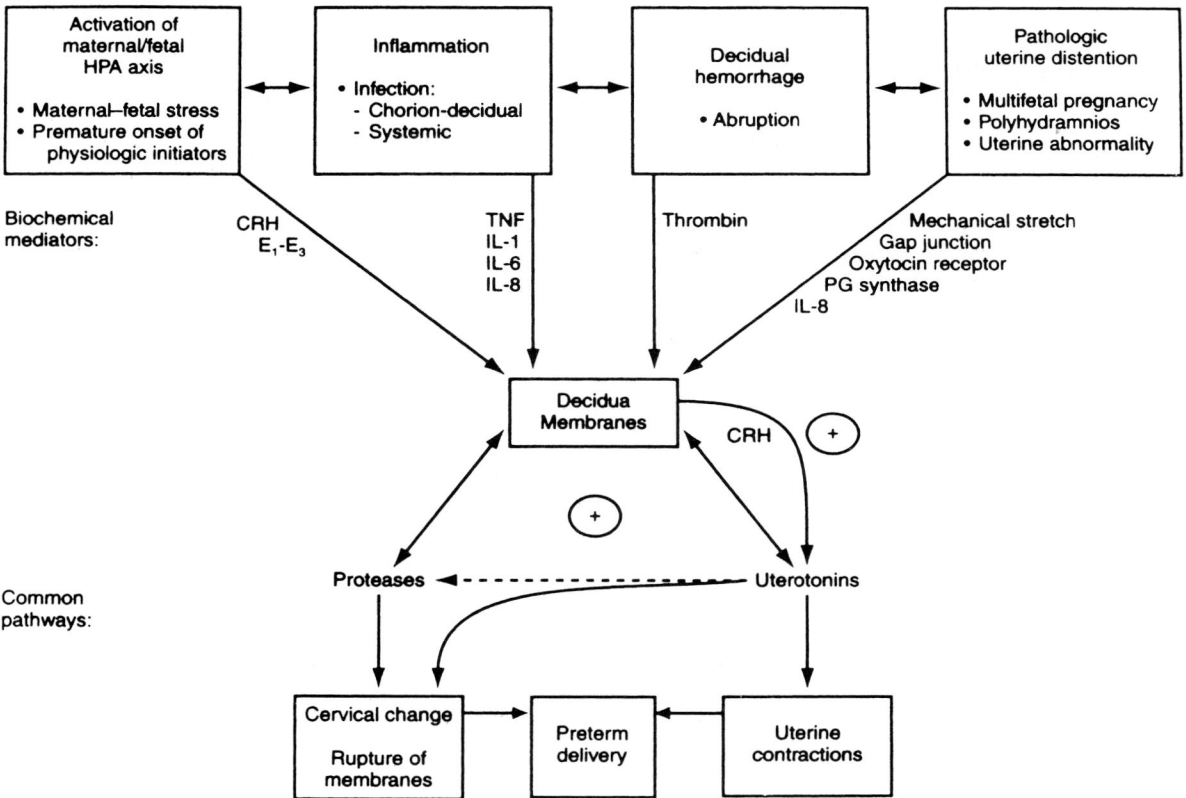

Figure 23–17. Major pathogenic pathways of preterm delivery resulting in preterm rupture of membranes, preterm labor, or both. HPA, hypothalamic-pituitary-adrenal; CRH, corticotropin-releasing hormone; E_1, estrone; E_3, estriol; TNF, tumor necrosis factor; IL-1, IL-6, and IL-8, interleukins-1β, -6, and -8, respectively; PG, prostaglandin. *Activation of the maternal and/or fetal HPA axis:* Maternal and fetal stress lead to increased expression of placental-amniochorion-decidual CRH and placental estrogen expression. CRH enhances PG production in placental-amniochorion-decidual cells, while estrogens activate the myometrium. *Inflammation:* Ascending genital tract and severe systemic infections lead to activation of genital tract cytokine networks generating IL-1 and TNF-1, which enhance production of myometrial-decidual-amniochorionic-cervical uterotonins (i.e., prostaglandins, endothelins, leukotrienes) and proteases (e.g., matrix metalloproteinases-collagenases, plasmin). These proparturition effects are amplified by IL-1–TNF-mediated induction of (a) IL-6, which further enhances PG production; and (b) IL-8, a granulocyte chemotactant and activator, which causes the release of elastases and collagenases. *Decidual hemorrhage:* Abruptions lead to local generation of thrombin, which binds to cellular receptors in the decidua to enhance local protease and PG production. *Pathologic uterine distention:* Multifetal gestation, hydramnios, and uterine abnormalities resulting from diethylstilbestrol exposure and congenital müllerian duct defects promote excessive stretching of the fetal membranes, the myometrium, or both, which causes myometrial activation (enhanced gap junctions, oxytocin receptors, $PGF_{2\alpha}$, synthase) and fetal membrane cytokine (IL-8) production. *Final common pathway:* Each of these four pathogenic mechanisms has a unique set of biochemical initiators but shares a final common pathway: enhanced expression of fetal membrane, decidual, and cervical proteases and uterotonins (e.g., prostaglandins). This leads to membrane rupture, cervical change and progressive uterine contractions, and preterm delivery. (From The American College of Obstetricians and Gynecologists. Preterm labor and delivery. Precis: Obstetrics, 2nd ed. Washington, DC, 1999. Copyright ACOG, 1999, with permission.)

sepsis prophylaxis or amnionitis, and corticosteroids to reduce neonatal mortality and morbidity).

Prevention: Secondary Care of Preterm Birth

Secondary care strategies require identification of pregnancies at risk and effective interventions to prevent or reduce the morbidity of preterm birth. There has been more progress on the former than the latter. Care of prematurity as a clinical problem to be solved has been described either as a pointless exercise: "Only when the factors causing prematurity are clearly understood can any intelligent attempt at prevention be made"[6]; or as a social problem beyond the purview of obstetricians: "I do not think that . . . prematurity can be reduced . . . by better obstetrics . . . . These problems are social, not obstetric."[127] These sentiments were challenged as unduly nihilistic by some[128,129] who argued that premature birth could be addressed proactively, even though the pathophysiology is not entirely clear, and despite the frustrating social correlates that so often accompany preterm birth. Although screening and intervention programs have not been effective in reducing preterm birth in this country,[126] researchers have continued to look for tests that can identify women with increased risk and for therapies to reduce that risk.[130–132]

Clinical Risk Factors for Preterm Birth

Because clinical risk factors for spontaneous preterm birth have relatively high prevalence but low sensitivity and positive predictive value, efforts to create scoring systems to identify pregnancies at risk have faltered.[133–136] Scoring systems for preterm birth risk have been abandoned by most centers as insensitive. Nevertheless, women with these major risk factors should be considered to be at risk of preterm birth:

1. *Prior preterm delivery.* A history of prior preterm birth between 16 and 36 weeks carries a three- to fourfold increase in risk of recurrent preterm birth. The magnitude of risk increases as the gestational age of the previous preterm birth decreases.[63,109]
2. *Multiple gestation.* Twin pregnancies are five to six times more likely than singletons to deliver preterm. Higher order multiples have even higher risk of prematurity. Twins account for 2 to 3 percent of births, but 12 percent of preterm births and 15 percent of neonatal mortality.[137] The increased number of pregnancies achieved with assisted reproductive technologies has produced a significant increase in twin and higher order multiple gestations.[3,4]
3. *Low prepregnancy weight* manifested by a body mass index below 19.8 kg/m² has been consistently associated with preterm delivery, particularly in white women.[44,136,138]
4. *Vaginal bleeding in the second or third trimester* has been reported to have a relative risk for preterm birth ranging from 1.6[136] to as much as 15,[46] especially for preterm prematurely ruptured membranes.

These historical risk factors are easily elicited, but identify less than half of women who will deliver prematurely. Just as screening for preeclampsia is part of routine prenatal care, all pregnant women should receive care and education aimed at the problem of prematurity. Other possible risk factors that have been studied as screening tests for preterm birth risk include uterine contraction frequency, digital and ultrasound examination of the cervix, vaginal microbiology, serologic markers, and the presence of fetal fibronectin in cervicovaginal secretions.

Uterine Contractions

Uterine activity increases as pregnancy progresses[139,140] and is slightly more frequent in women destined to deliver prematurely.[139,141] A cross-sectional study of uterine activity recorded during antenatal fetal heart rate testing in 2,446 women after 30 weeks found that uterine activity increased by 4.7 percent per week.[139] Women who delivered preterm had more and those who delivered postterm had fewer contractions per 10-minute window of observation. A longitudinal study[140] of 109 normal women who recorded 24-hour uterine activity profiles twice a week between 24 weeks and delivery found that no contractions were recorded in 73 percent of monitored hours; 96 percent of hours had fewer than four contractions per hour (Fig. 23–18). Contraction frequency was similar in nulliparous and parous subjects. Contraction frequency was increased at night and with gestational age. The 95th percentile of uterine activity was 1.3 ± 0.5 (SD) contractions per hour at 21 to 24 weeks, 2.9 ± 1.0 at 28 to 32 weeks, and 4.9 ± 1.7 at 38 to 40 weeks ($p < 0.0001$). The night/day ratio of contractions per hour was 1.8:1 at 21 to 24 weeks, 2.3:1 at 28 to 32 weeks, and 2.0:1 at 38 to 40 weeks ($p < 0.001$). A few women recorded more than 15 contractions per hour, yet delivered at term without intervention. Contraction frequency decreased after recumbency and increased after coitus.

Another longitudinal study compared uterine activity in 254 women with historical risk factors for preterm birth and 52 low-risk women.[141] Contraction frequency did not differ according to risk status, but women destined to deliver preterm had more contractions than did women delivered at term. Although statistically significant, the difference was too small to be clinically valuable. The sensitivity and positive predictive value of contraction frequency to predict preterm birth before 35 weeks were both less than 25 percent. Sensitivity for and prediction of birth before 32 weeks were even lower.

Initial hopes that ambulatory monitoring of contractions could select women with increased risk of preterm

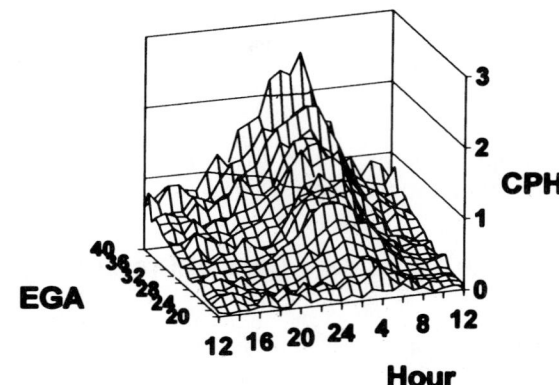

Figure 23–18. Mean hourly frequency of monitored uterine contractions by gestational age and time of day in 109 normal pregnant women who delivered at term after uncomplicated pregnancies. (From Moore TR, Iams JD, Creasy RK, et al: Diurnal and gestational patterns of uterine activity in normal human pregnancy. Obstet Gynecol 83:517, 1994, with permission.)

birth for further diagnostic assessment or treatment to reduce the incidence of preterm birth have not been fulfilled, perhaps because of the low sensitivity and predictive value of contraction frequency. Numerous studies[142–149] and analyses[150–154] of this strategy have been performed with variable results. The definitive assessment of ambulatory contraction monitoring was provided by a large trial published in 1998. Dyson et al.[155] enrolled 2,422 women with risk factors for preterm birth. Subjects were assigned randomly to receive weekly contact with a nurse, daily contact with a nurse, or daily contact with a nurse together with uterine contraction monitoring. There were no differences in the occurrence of preterm birth before 35 weeks, in cervical dilation at the diagnosis of preterm labor, or in any neonatal outcomes. The failure of the contraction detection and suppression strategy to reduce the rate of preterm delivery is instructive. First, although contraction frequency is increased in women destined for preterm birth, this association did not translate into an effective screening test. Second, the theory behind this strategy may be false. If premature labor begins with excessive uterine contractile activity, then early detection and suppression of contractions should have been an effective strategy. The inability to demonstrate benefit for contraction detection and suppression indicates either that this theory is incorrect, or that it is applicable to relatively few cases of preterm labor. As will become evident in the following paragraphs, these same observations may be made about other prematurity prevention strategies.

Cervical Examination

An association between preterm delivery and cervical dilation of 2 cm or more and/or effacement of 80 percent or more has been reported in several studies.[112–114,136] As with uterine contractions, however, the observation of an association has not led to a reduced incidence of preterm delivery. A randomized study[156] found no difference in rates of preterm birth among 2,803 women who were followed with serial cervical exams as compared with 2,799 women in whom examination was not routinely performed.

Digital examination of the cervix is reasonably accurate in active labor, but is subject to great interexaminer variation when dilation is less than 3 cm and/or effacement is less than 80 percent.[157] Endosonographic measurement of the cervix is more reproducible than digital or transabdominal examination.[158,159] Moreover, this technique has provided information not previously available about the nature and timing of cervical changes preceding delivery (see also later section regarding cervical competence). The cervix effaces or thins from the internal os caudad toward the external os. The length of the cervix varies normally in the

second trimester from less than 1 cm (below the first percentile) to values in excess of 4.5 cm, above the 95th percentile, with a median value of about 3.5 cm.[70] The risk of preterm birth increases as cervical length decreases throughout the entire range[70,101] (Figs. 23–15 and 23–16). Not only do women with the shortest cervical length have the greatest risk of preterm birth, but those whose cervical length is at the 50th percentile have more risk than do women whose cervical length is above the 75th percentile.[70] A comparison of digital and ultrasonographic assessment of the cervix at 24 weeks to predict spontaneous preterm birth before 35 weeks is shown in the Table 23–8, using data from the NICHD MFMU Preterm Prediction Study.[70] The data in the table indicate that neither test is an especially sensitive predictor of preterm birth, nor is sonography superior to a carefully performed Bishop score to predict risk. However, sonographic cervical length was significantly more reproducible than either Bishop score or funneling in this study. As expected, the positive predictive values rise as the cervical length threshold declines, accompanied by a corresponding decline in sensitivity.

Although cervical sonography has been useful in redefining the contribution of cervical factors to the pathogenesis of early preterm birth, there is no evidence that interventions such as maternal rest or cerclage based on a finding of a short cervix can be translated into a reduced rate of preterm birth. One nonrandomized study found fewer births after 32 weeks among 42 women with cervical length less than or equal to 1.5 cm at 23 weeks who were treated with cerclage compared with expectant management, but there was no significant difference in neonatal survival.[160] In another study of endovaginal sonography conducted in 97 women with a history of preterm birth, both a cervical length less than 25 mm and a funneling of the internal os were strongly correlated with preterm birth (relative risk, 4.8; 95 percent CI, 2.3 to 10.1).[161] The incidence of preterm birth and interval from detection of cervical changes to delivery was not different for those treated by cerclage compared with expectant management. Finally, neither of two recent randomized trials of cerclage in women treated on the basis of obstetric history and cervical sonography found an advantage for the cerclage group.[162,163]

Genital Colonization with Microorganisms

The association of maternal colonization with various genital microorganisms and risk of preterm birth has led to investigations of screening tests to identify and treat women at risk. In the VIP Study,[89,164] parturients who were culture positive for various microorganisms were randomly assigned to receive placebo or antibiotic treatment (Table 23–9). No reduction in preterm birth was associated with screening and treatment for *Chla-*

mydia trachomatis, Ureaplasma urealyticum or group B *Streptococcus* (GBS), despite preliminary data suggesting an association of these organisms with increased risk of preterm birth for *Ureaplasma*[89] and for GBS.[164] Antibiotic treatment was employed after 25 weeks in this trial; the authors speculated that earlier treatment might have been more successful. Another randomized trial of antibiotic treatment in women with a history of preterm birth found benefit, but only for women who also had bacterial vaginosis.[93] Treatment with metronidazole and erythromycin resulted in a significantly reduced rate of spontaneous preterm birth, from 49 percent in the placebo group to 31 percent in the antibiotic group. Unlike the VIP Study, in which all colonized subjects were eligible for randomization, the trial of BV treatment was limited to women with a history of prior preterm birth. The epidemiologic association of BV with preterm delivery (PTD) in multiple regression analyses[91] together with reports of reduced preterm birth following treatment of BV-positive women at risk[93] has led some to recommend routine screening and treatment, at least for high-risk women. However, this conclusion was not supported by a larger, multicenter trial of metronidazole treatment for women with BV.[95] At present, the American College of Obstetricians and Gynecologists suggests that physicians "consider" BV screening and treatment only in women with a history of preterm birth.[165] The value of microbiologic screening and treatment to reduce preterm birth remains unsettled.

Biochemical Markers

Maternal blood assays for progesterone, prolactin, relaxin, major basic protein, C-reactive protein, interleukins, and collagenase have all been tested in attempts to identify pregnancies with increased risk. In each, a biologic correlation has been observed, but correlation does not translate into prediction. Among the serum assays collected in the Preterm Prediction Study, three were found to correlate with preterm birth before 32 weeks: α-fetoprotein greater than the 90th percentile,

alkaline phosphatase greater than the 90th percentile, and granulocyte-colony stimulating factor greater than the 75th percentile.[166] Increased levels of estriol in maternal saliva have also been reported to correlate with the risk of preterm birth after 32 weeks' gestation.[167] IL-6 has been associated with preterm birth and intraamniotic infection.[168]

Assays of cervical fluid for fetal fibronectin have shown promise as markers for preterm birth, particularly for births before 30 weeks. Data from 2,929 women enrolled in the NICHD Preterm Prediction Study revealed that a single positive fibronectin assay performed at 24 to 26 weeks may identify up to 60 percent of women destined to deliver before 30 weeks' gestation.[44,108] However, the sensitivity of the 24- to 26-week fibronectin assay to predict spontaneous preterm birth before 35 weeks was just 25 percent. Once again, there are no studies in which treatment of fibronectin-positive women has led to decreased prematurity. Based on the reported association of fibronectin and BV,[110] randomized trials of antibiotic prophylaxis in fibronectin-positive women are ongoing.

A study that compared multiple tests, including maternal symptoms, contraction frequency, Bishop score, cervical ultrasound, and fibronectin, to predict preterm birth enrolled 254 high-risk and 52 low-risk pregnant women at 11 sites.[141] Although each variable was significantly and independently related to risk of preterm birth, none performed well as an efficient screening test for preterm birth before 32, 35, or 37 weeks (Table 23–10 shows results for data collected at 22 to 24 weeks).

The low sensitivity of individual tests for spontaneous preterm birth prompted a search for a combination of tests that could improve both sensitivity and positive predictive value. Among the 28 different tests evaluated as potential markers in the Preterm Prediction Study, seven were available at 24 weeks and identified by multiple regression as significantly related to spontaneous birth before 35 weeks (listed in descending order of the strength of the odds ratio between cases and controls): fetal fibronectin (OR, 6.6), alkaline phosphatase above

Table 23–10. PREDICTION AT 22 TO 24 WEEKS OF SPONTANEOUS PRETERM BIRTH BEFORE 35 WEEKS

Test	Sensitivity	Specificity	Predictive Value	
			Positive	Negative
Multiple PTL symptoms	50.0%	63.5%	21.4%	86.4%
Uterine contractions ≥4/hr	6.7%	92.3%	25.0%	84.7%
Bishop Score ≥4	32.0%	91.4%	42.1%	87.4%
Cervical length ≤25 mm	40.8%	89.5%	42.6%	88.8%
Fibronectin ≥50 ng/ml	18.0%	95.3%	42.9%	85.6%

Data from Iams JD, for the NICHD MFMU Network: Home uterine monitoring to predict preterm birth. Uterine contraction frequency and preterm birth [abstracts 2 and 670]. Am J Obstet Gynecol 178:S2 and S188, 1998; and Self perceived symptoms to predict preterm birth [abstract 47]. Am J Obstet Gynecol 182:S32, 2000.

the 90th percentile (4.0), a prior spontaneous preterm birth (4.0), cervical length less than or equal to 25 mm (3.9), α-fetoprotein above the 90th percentile (3.9), granulocyte colony-stimulating factor above the 75th percentile (3.1), and vaginal bleeding (2.2).[166] Individually, these tests suffer from the same low sensitivity and positive predictive value as the other markers previously described. Because few women were positive for more than one of the listed markers, it is possible that a combination or "multiple marker" test could be applied at 24 weeks that might have sufficient collective sensitivity to be clinically useful. It is unlikely, however, that a single interventional strategy will be effective for women identified by such disparate tests.

Interventions to Prevent Preterm Birth

Attempts to prevent prematurity have been based on a traditional medical model of identifying and correcting a potential "cause" of preterm birth, with the expectation that the rate of preterm birth would decline. Intervention trials have addressed early identification of preterm labor through patient education, pharmacologic suppression of uterine contractions, antimicrobial therapy of vaginal microorganisms, cerclage sutures to bolster the cervix, reduction of maternal stress, improved access to prenatal care, and reduced physical activity. Some trials have enrolled women with the risk factor in question without regard to obstetric history (e.g., the VIP Studies[89,164]), while others have been limited to women with a prior preterm delivery (e.g., the European cerclage trials[169–171]). In no case has a study that focused on elimination of a single risk factor led to a decrease in preterm birth, but there have been hopeful trends identified in some of them. In virtually every trial, reports of an association between a risk factor and SPTB have been followed by small trials, usually observational in design, that describe promising early results, only to find minimal if any benefit when carried out in larger populations.

Education of At-Risk Women About the Signs and Symptoms of Preterm Labor

Initial studies[133] described reductions in SPTB, but subsequent reports showed inconsistent results.[134,135,172] In a multicenter investigation, the March of Dimes Collaborative Trial found significant benefit in two centers, but no benefit at three other sites.[135]

Antibiotics to Prevent Preterm Birth

The serendipitous observation[173] of a reduced frequency of preterm birth in women who received tetracycline as prophylaxis for urinary tract infection has been followed by a mixed literature of success and failure

(Table 23–9). Clearly, there is a relationship between genital microorganisms and preterm birth, but the results of these trials just as clearly indicate that infection does not operate independently as a cause of preterm birth.

Social Support and Improved Access to Prenatal Care

Prenatal care is correlated with the rate of SPTB in both black and white women but the reason is not clear. Prospective interventions designed to reduce preterm birth through better access to care, reduced stress, and the like, have been unsuccessful,[174,175] but one trial found reduced preterm births for indigent black women age 19 and older.[176]

Prophylactic Cerclage for Women with a Prior Preterm Birth

A historical study[177] described significant improvements in pregnancy outcome for women with a history of early preterm birth, but subsequent attempts to reduce the incidence of preterm birth with cerclage have been mixed. Two studies[170,171] found no benefit, while another[169] reported a reduction in the incidence of early preterm births, but no effect on the overall rate of SPTB. More recent reports of cerclage for women with a history of preterm birth who also had ultrasound evidence of a short or funneled cervix have been mixed.[160–163]

Prophylactic Medications

Tocolytic agents have been widely used as prophylaxis, but this has not been associated with either a reduction in preterm or low-birth-weight deliveries.[132] Parenteral progesterone (17α-hydroxprogesterone caproate) was used for prophylaxis against preterm labor after reports[178] suggested a decreased incidence of preterm births in treated women. Another study in an active-duty military population failed to demonstrate any reduction in preterm delivery rates compared with a placebo group.[179]

Bed Rest/Activity Modification

Although there is a modest relationship between maternal physical activity and preterm birth risk,[180,181] there is no evidence from properly conducted trials that bed rest offers any benefit for pregnant women.[182]

TERTIARY CARE

Diagnosis and Treatment of Spontaneous Preterm Birth

Clinical Assessment of Spontaneous Versus Indicated Preterm Delivery

The distinction between indicated and spontaneous prematurity, although helpful to understand the pathogenesis of prematurity, can be difficult to apply in practice. Evaluation of a woman with apparent preterm labor or ruptured membranes begins with a search for the underlying cause and an assessment of fetal well-being. The reason for preterm labor and the well-being of the fetus are always considered simultaneously, because they are interrelated in both diagnosis and treatment. The factor(s) that led to preterm labor may also lead to fetal compromise, as might occur in a patient with placental abruption or oligohydramnios. Conversely, a decision to treat the mother with drugs to arrest labor implies that further intrauterine growth and maturity will occur in a safe intrauterine environment. Preterm labor associated with infection or ischemia is more likely to result in perinatal morbidity than preterm labor for which no cause is found.[183] There is evidence that restriction of fetal growth occurs more commonly among infants delivered after preterm labor or preterm PROM, even in apparently otherwise uncomplicated pregnancies.[184] Therefore, a careful evaluation of fetal growth and well-being must precede and accompany any treatment to prolong pregnancy. For example, preterm labor and preterm PROM may be accompanied by abnormal amniotic fluid volume and/or bleeding. A patient with light bleeding and oligohydramnios may have spontaneously ruptured membranes, a growth-restricted fetus and occult preeclampsia, or a fetal renal anomaly. In a patient with polyhydramnios, preterm labor may be the result of fetal anomaly, maternal diabetes, or an intrauterine viral infection. In summary, clinical management of preterm labor is based on a careful assessment of the risks for mother and infant of continuing the pregnancy versus delivery.

After causes of preterm labor have been evaluated, the gestational age must be considered. The intensity of treatment to delay delivery is inversely related to the expected neonatal morbidity and mortality: the earlier the gestational age, the greater the risk of prematurity-related problems for the newborn. This assessment in turn determines the degree of risk and discomfort the mother may be asked to accept on behalf of her fetus. Decisions made prior to spontaneous preterm birth typically focus on assessment of risks for the infant, but maternal interests must always be considered.

Diagnosis of Preterm Labor

The diagnosis of preterm labor is traditionally made when persistent uterine contractions are accompanied by dilation and/or effacement of the cervix detected by digital examination.[185] Symptoms of preterm labor are nonspecific and are not necessarily those of labor at term. Women treated for preterm labor report symptoms of pelvic pressure, increased vaginal discharge, backache, and menstrual-like cramps, all of which may occur in normal pregnancy. Contractions may be painful or painless, and are distinguished from the benign contractions of normal pregnancy (called Braxton-Hicks contractions) only by their persistence. The accuracy of these criteria has been questioned by studies suggesting poor sensitivity and specificity. In placebo-controlled trials of drugs to arrest preterm labor, 40 percent of subjects treated with placebo delivered at term.[186] Conversely, other studies have found rates of preterm birth of 20 percent in women who were sent home without treatment after evaluation for possible preterm labor.[187] Difficulty in accurate diagnosis is the product of the high prevalence of the symptoms and signs of early preterm labor among normal healthy women, and the imprecision of the digital examination of the cervix. Observational studies of ambulatory women with risk factors for preterm birth have found that symptoms are poorly predictive because of the common occurrence of the same symptoms in women who do not develop preterm labor.[114,141,188] Uterine contraction frequency varies considerably in normal pregnancy according to gestational age, time of day, and maternal activity[140] (Fig. 23–18). Contraction frequency alone is therefore insufficient to establish the diagnosis of preterm labor. The practice of initiating tocolytic drugs for contraction frequency without additional diagnostic criteria results in unnecessary treatment of women who do not actually have preterm labor.[189] Overdiagnosis might be acceptable if treatment were clearly effective, but that is not the case (see paragraphs to follow on the efficacy of each tocolytic drug). Although digital assessment of cervical dilation of 3 cm or more is straightforward, the reproducibility of digital examination when dilation is less than 3 cm and/or effacement is less than 80 percent is low.[190] Despite their imprecision, these symptoms and subtle changes in the cervix remain the basis of the early diagnosis of preterm labor.[185]

Among symptomatic women, the best clinical predictors of preterm delivery within 24 hours to 7 days include initial cervical dilation greater than 3 cm or effacement of 80 percent or more, vaginal bleeding, and ruptured membranes.[189,191,192] Surprisingly, contraction frequency of 4 or more per hour has low positive predictive value for preterm birth within 7 to 14 days of presentation.[193,194] For this reason, symptomatic

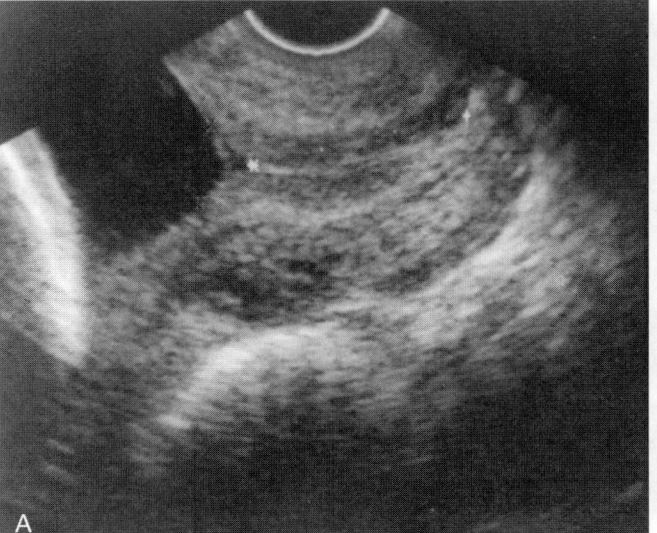
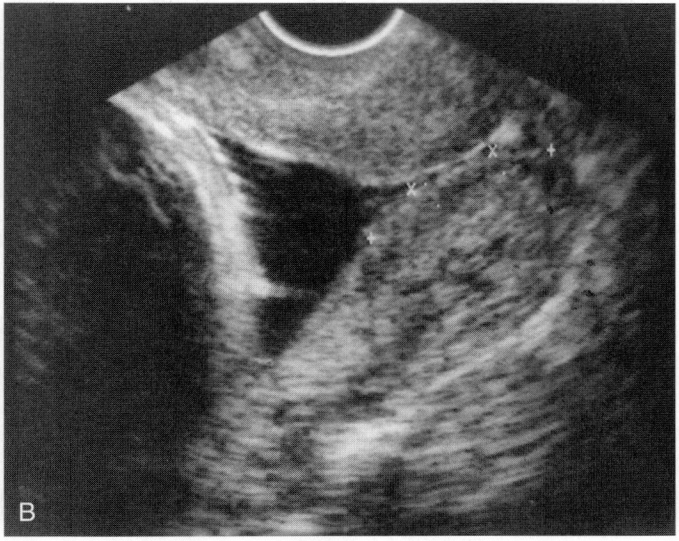

Figure 23–19. *A,* Transvaginal ultrasound image of the cervix at 28 weeks in a normal pregnancy. Calipers (+) are placed at the notches marking the internal and external os where the anterior and posterior walls of the cervical canal touch. *B,* Transvaginal ultrasound image of the cervix at 28 weeks in a patient with preterm labor. The (X) calipers mark the length of the cervical canal that is used for clinical evaluation. The (+) calipers are placed at the outer edges of the cervix; this length is not useful clinically because of wide variation among patients.

women whose cervical dilation is less than 2 cm and/or whose effacement is less than 80 percent present a diagnostic challenge. Diagnostic accuracy may be improved in these patients with transvaginal sonographic measurement of cervical length,[195–200] and/or testing for fetal fibronectin in cervicovaginal fluid.[193,194,201] Cervical sonography is useful to exclude preterm labor in some patients, and may add sensitivity to the diagnosis in others. In a review of cervical sonography as a marker for preterm birth, a sonographic cervical length of 18 mm had the optimal positive predictive value, and 30 mm the optimal negative predictive value for the diagnosis of preterm labor in symptomatic women.[200] These studies were performed with transvaginal sonography. Transabdominal sonography has poor reproducibility for cervical measurement and should not be used clinically without confirmation by a transvaginal ultrasound[159,202] (Fig. 23–19). Cervical sonography may also be useful to evaluate patients whose contractions are accompanied by vaginal bleeding of uncertain origin (Fig. 23–20). Fetal fibronectin is described earlier in the chapter. As the gestational sac implants and attaches to decidua in the first half of pregnancy, fibronectin is normally present in cervicovaginal fluid. The presence of fibronectin in the cervix or vagina after the 22nd week is uncommon (<5 percent of pregnancies),[108] and indicates disruption of the attachment of the membranes to the decidua. Fibronectin commonly reappears in cervicovaginal secretions as labor approaches at term. A positive fibronectin test between 22 and 37 weeks is associated with an increased

risk of preterm birth, especially in symptomatic women.[193,194,203] A positive test result in a patient with persistent contractions and cervical dilation of less than 3 cm has better sensitivity (90 percent) and positive predictive value for delivery less than 7 to 14 days than standard clinical markers, but the positive predictive value is just 18 percent in accumulated series, depending on the population studied (Tables 23–11 and 23–12).[193,194,203–206] The clinical value of the test in symptomatic women is primarily its high negative predictive value, as a test to avoid overdiagnosis and unnecessary treatment, (e.g., similar to cardiac enzymes in the evaluation of chest pain).

Two studies have evaluated the effect of introduction of the fibronectin test into clinical care algorithms. In one, admissions for preterm labor, duration of hospitalization, and use of tocolytic medication were reduced without affecting neonatal outcome.[207] In the other, the test had no benefit for women whose cervical dilation was greater than or equal to 3 cm, but a negative test in women without significant dilation allowed a 90 percent reduction in maternal transfer to a tertiary care facility.[208] Both reports indicate that to be clinically useful in the acute management of preterm labor, the test must be rapidly available, and the clinician must be willing to act on a negative test result by not initiating treatment. The results of a trial conducted in 200 symptomatic women at a center in which tocolysis was not employed may therefore be reassuring.[209] The sensitivity, specificity, and positive and negative predictive values for delivery at less than or equal to 7 days were

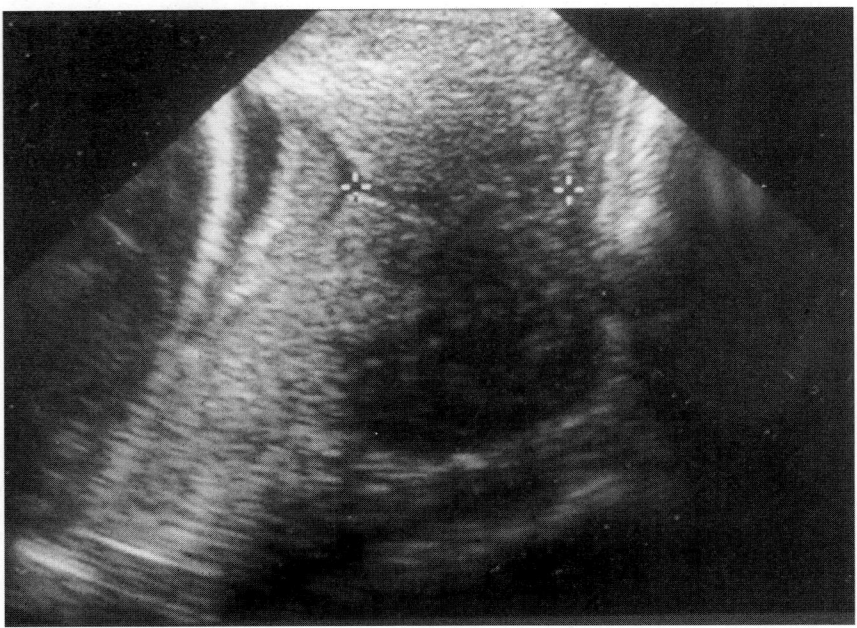

Figure 23–20. Midline sagittal image from transvaginal ultrasound showing a blood clot at the internal cervical os in a patient with contractions and vaginal bleeding.

62.5, 87.0, 16.7, and 98.2 percent, respectively. Three of 170 fibronectin-negative women (1.8 percent) delivered at 7 days or earlier at this center. Although the studies cited above suggest that overdiagnosis can be reduced with this test, fibronectin is not helpful when the patient has overt symptoms of preterm labor accompanied by cervical dilation greater than 3m.[208] It is also not clear how a positive result should influence clinical management protocols. It may on occasion improve sensitivity by identifying women at risk who did not meet traditional criteria for tocolysis and/or steroids.

Fibronectin has been compared to contraction frequency, cervical dilation greater than 1 cm, and vaginal bleeding (Table 23–12) and to the clinician's diagnosis of preterm labor (Table 23–13) in data drawn from two U.S. studies.[193,194] When masked fibronectin results were compared to the clinician's decision to use tocolysis (Table 23–13) in symptomatic women with cervical dilation less than 3 cm, the fibronectin assay improved both sensitivity and specificity. Sixteen of 68 women (23.5 percent) treated with tocolysis and who had a positive fibronectin delivered within 7 days. Of 146 women treated for preterm labor who had a negative fibronectin, four (2.7 percent) delivered within 7 days, a rate similar to that seen in untreated women. This suggests that treatment might have been safely withheld in 142 patients. Interestingly, 16 women not deemed to be in labor by clinical criteria were identified with fibronectin testing.[210]

Combined use of fibronectin and cervical sonography in the evaluation of symptomatic women has been evaluated in two studies. One found the tests to be complementary in improving the accuracy of diagnosis[211]; the

Table 23–11. FETAL FIBRONECTIN AND PREDICTION OF PRETERM BIRTH WITHIN 7 DAYS IN SYMPTOMATIC WOMEN*

Fibronectin	Delivery ≤7 Days	Delivery >7 Days	Total
Positive	46	207	253
Negative	6	945	951
Total	52	1,152	1,204

* Sensitivity, 88.5%; specificity, 82.0%; positive predictive value, 18.2%; negative predictive value, 99.3%.

Summary of six studies in symptomatic women with cervix dilation <3 cm: Lockwood et al.,[203] Iams et al.,[193] Senden and Owen,[206] Bartnicki et al.,[204] Malak et al.,[205] and Peaceman et al.[194]

Table 23–12. SENSITIVITY OF TESTS TO PREDICT DELIVERY WITHIN 7 DAYS

Characteristic	Sensitivity
Fibronectin positive	90%
Cervix > 1 cm dilated	35%
Contractions > 4/hr	55%
Bleeding	40%

Combined data from Iams JD, Casal D, McGregor JA, et al: Fetal fibronectin improves the accuracy of diagnosis of preterm labor. Am J Obstet Gynecol 173: 141, 1995; and Peaceman AM, Andrews WW, Thorp JM, et al: Fetal fibronectin as a predictor of preterm birth in patients with symptoms: A multicenter trial. Am J Obstet Gynecol 177:13, 1997.

Table 23–13. FIBRONECTIN VERSUS CLINICAL DIAGNOSIS TO PREDICT DELIVERY WITHIN 7 DAYS IN SYMPTOMATIC WOMEN: CLINICIAN'S DIAGNOSIS OF PRETERM LABOR*

	Yes = tocolysis	No = no tocolysis
Fibronectin-positive	16/68	16/127
	23.5%	12.6%
Fibronectin-negative	4/146	0/614
	2.7%	0%

* Each cell shows the number of women delivered within 7 days/the number treated or not.
Data from Iams JD: Reply to a letter from M. Plaut. Am J Obstet Gynecol 172: 79, 1996.

other found that the combination was not superior to either one alone.[212]

The suggested protocol for evaluation and treatment of women with possible preterm labor in the box incorporates fibronectin into current clinical care patterns, and should always be preceded by an evaluation of the etiology of SPTD. Transvaginal sonography can be used as an adjunctive test in patients with persistent contractions and cervical dilation of 2 cm or less. Because of

---

Clinical Evaluation of Patients with Possible Preterm Labor

1. **Patient presents with signs/symptoms of preterm labor:**
   - Persistent contractions (painful or painless)
   - Intermittent abdominal cramping, pelvic pressure, or backache
   - Increase or change in vaginal discharge
   - Vaginal spotting or bleeding
2. **General physical examination:**
   - Sitting pulse and blood pressure
   - Temperature
   - External fetal heart rate and contraction monitor
3. **Sterile speculum examination**
   - pH
   - Fern
   - Pooled fluid
   - Fibronectin swab (posterior fornix or external cervical os, avoiding areas with bleeding)
   - Cultures for *Chlamydia* (cervix), and *N. gonorrhoeae* (cervix), and group B *Streptococcus* (outer one third of vagina and perineum)
4. **Transabdominal ultrasound examination:**
   - Placental location
   - Amniotic fluid volume
   - Estimated fetal weight and presentation
   - Fetal well-being
5. **Cervical examination (after ruptured membranes excluded):**
   - Cervix ≥3 cm dilation / 80 percent effaced—Preterm labor diagnosis confirmed. Evaluate for tocolysis
   - Cervix 2 to 3 cm dilation and <80 percent effaced—Preterm labor likely but not established. Monitor contraction frequency and repeat digital examination in 30 to 60 minutes. Preterm labor diagnosis if cervical change. If not, send fibronectin or obtain transvaginal cervical ultrasound. Evaluate for tocolysis if any cervical change, cervical length <20 mm or positive fibronectin.
   - Cervix <2 cm dilation and <80 percent effaced—Preterm labor diagnosis uncertain. Monitor contraction frequency, send fibronectin and/or obtain cervical sonography, and repeat digital examination in 1 to 2 hours. Evaluate for tocolysis if there is a 1-cm change in cervical dilation, effacement >80 percent, cervical length <20 mm or positive fibronectin.
6. **Use of Cervical Ultrasound:**
   - Cervical length <20 mm and contraction criteria met = preterm labor
   - Cervical length 20 to 30 mm and contraction criteria met = probable preterm labor
   - Cervical length >30 mm = preterm labor very unlikely regardless of contraction frequency
7. **Treatment of Symptomatic Fibronectin-Positive Patients:**
   - Parenteral tocolysis
   - Steroids
   - Maternal transfer if appropriate
   - Group B *Streptococcus* prophylaxis
8. **Care for Symptomatic Fibronectin-Negative Patients:**
   - When tocolysis initiated before fibronectin returned (risk of delivery ≤7 days = 1.7 to 3.5 percent)
     Conclude course of tocolysis
     Reduce hospital stay
   - When tocolysis not initiated (risk of delivery ≤7 days = 0 to 1.8 percent)
     Observe in outpatient setting
   - Cervical sonography should be considered in these patients to assess risk of SPTD

variation introduced by maternal bladder filling, transabdominal sonography is not sufficiently reproducible to be useful.[202]

To summarize, the diagnosis of preterm labor is often uncertain, and as can be seen in the next section, the treatment is not always benign. In order to increase the sensitivity of diagnosis without treating unnecessarily, it is best to be *liberal* in looking for preterm labor, but *conservative* in diagnosis and treatment. The goal of first contact with a patient who may have preterm labor should be sensitivity, while the goal of evaluation in labor and delivery should be specificity. We recommend the following maxims:

1. Invite any patient complaining of possible symptoms of preterm labor to come in for contraction monitoring and cervical exam. Severity of symptoms bears little relation to their clinical significance.
2. Wait for cervical change of at least 1 cm in dilation, dilation of 2 cm or more, or a positive fibronectin before accepting the diagnosis of preterm labor in a patient with persistent contractions.
3. Use cervical sonography (cervix $\geq$30 mm) as a test to support continued observation.
4. Be wary of "incidental" diagnosis of preterm labor, especially in the afternoon and early evening. Remember the wide range of contraction frequency and the normal increase in contractions in the late afternoon and evening in normal pregnancy.

Premature Birth and Assessment of Fetal Maturity

The goal of care for preterm labor and PROM is to reduce perinatal morbidity and mortality, most of which is caused by immaturity of the respiratory, gastrointestinal, coagulation, and central nervous systems of the premature infant. Fetal pulmonary immaturity is the most frequent cause of serious newborn illness, and is the only organ system whose function is directly testable before delivery. If the quality of obstetric dating is good and intrauterine fetal well-being is not compromised, the likelihood of neonatal respiratory distress syndrome can often be satisfactorily estimated from the gestational age (Fig. 23–8).

Amniotic fluid studies of fetal pulmonary maturity are important in two settings: (1) when dates are uncertain (e.g., fetal size larger than expected for dates, suggesting a more advanced gestation or maternal glucose intolerance, or size less than expected, suggesting fetal growth restriction); and (2) when fetal jeopardy is not now present (prompt delivery would be indicated) but may occur during the remaining days or weeks of pregnancy (e.g., when membranes have ruptured, fetal heart patterns are nonreassuring, or growth restriction is sus-

pected). Occasionally, amniocentesis may be indicated for other studies such as fetal karyotype in patients with polyhydramnios, or culture, glucose, and Gram stain when amnionitis is suspected.

Treatment of Preterm Labor: Goals and Efficacy of Treatment

The ultimate goal for pregnancies complicated by preterm labor is delivery of an infant who suffers none of the sequelae of prematurity. Given the uncertain accuracy of the diagnosis, the treatment of women without true preterm labor in studies of tocolysis, and the relative infrequency of serious neonatal morbidity after 32 to 34 weeks, it has been difficult to demonstrate that treatment of preterm labor achieves this end point. The surrogate end point for neonatal outcome in clinical trials is usually prolongation of gestation to 32, 34, 35, 36, or 37 weeks. Other surrogate end points studied include respiratory distress syndrome, days and/or cost of neonatal intensive care, or more recently, composite or combined morbidities. Putting issues of accurate diagnosis aside, the efficacy of tocolytic drugs has been addressed through studies that compare one tocolytic drug to another, or less commonly, to a placebo. Most studies have been too small to allow firm conclusions. That in turn has led to reviews or meta-analyses wherein several studies of similar design are combined in an attempt to reach a definitive conclusion.[186,213] These studies indicate that tocolytics do not prevent preterm birth but can delay delivery for at least 48 hours, an important interval during which effective antenatal interventions to reduce neonatal morbidity and mortality may be accomplished:

1. Antepartum transfer of the mother and fetus to the most appropriate hospital, especially when the estimated birth weight is expected to be less than 1,500 g.[214,215]
2. Antibiotic prophylaxis of neonatal group B streptococcal infection.[216]
3. Antepartum administration of corticosteroids to the mother to reduce the risk of death, respiratory distress syndrome, and intraventricular hemorrhage in the preterm neonate.[217]

A recent meta-analysis of the effect of acute treatment of preterm labor[213] evaluated the results of 16 randomized controlled trials that enrolled women with intact membranes and focused on three outcome measures: prolongation of pregnancy in days, gestational age at delivery, and birth weight. Studies of agents from each major class of tocolytic drugs (β-mimetics, calcium channel blockers, magnesium sulfate, and the nonsteroidal anti-inflammatory drugs [NSAIDs]) were

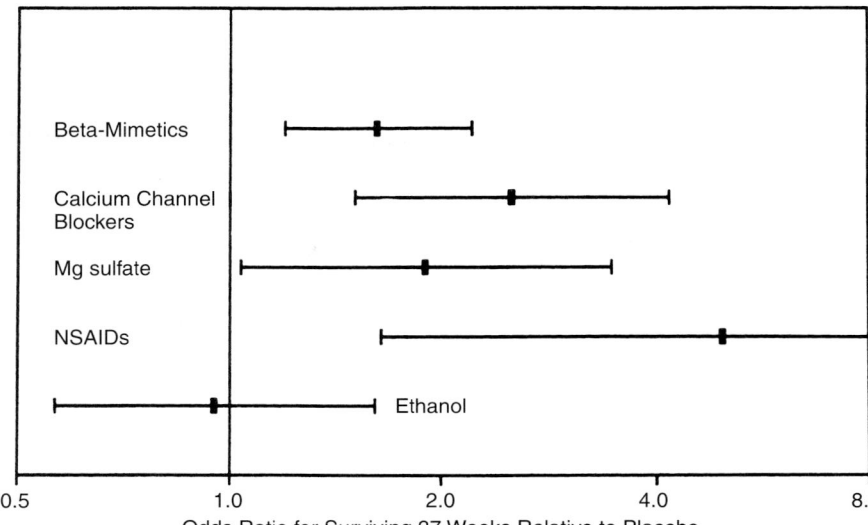

Figure 23–21. Meta-analysis of 16 randomized controlled trials of the effect of acute tocolytic treatment on delivery ≥37 weeks' gestation in women with preterm labor, analyzed by type of tocolytic drug. NSAIDs = Non-steroidal anti-inflammatory drugs. (From Evidence Report/Technology Assessment No. 18: Management of Preterm Labor [AHRQ Publication No. 01-E021]). October 2000. Access at www.ahrq.gov/clinic/epcix.htm.)

combined in a meta-analysis suggesting that all four are associated with a decline in the occurrence of birth before 37 weeks. For each type of tocolytic drug, the odds ratios were greater than 1, with 95 percent confidence intervals that did not cross unity (Fig. 23–21). The authors cautioned that the number of subjects in the NSAID trials is small, and confidence limits, although significant, are wide. This analysis of acute use of tocolytic drugs was not able to address directly whether the observed prolongation of pregnancy was accompanied by reduced neonatal mortality.

Initial Evaluation of Preterm Labor

The initial evaluation of the patient in preterm labor is focused on the risks and benefits of continuing the pregnancy for both mother and fetus. Common maternal contraindications to tocolysis include hypertension, bleeding, and cardiac disease (see the box "Contraindications to Tocolysis"). Preterm labor accompanied by maternal hypertension places both mother and fetus at risk of acute hypertensive crises, and may occur in response to fetal stress or distress, uterine ischemia, or occult placental abruption. Although vaginal spotting may occur in women with preterm labor because of cervical effacement or dilation, any bleeding beyond light spotting is rarely due to labor alone. Placenta previa and abruption must be considered, because both may be accompanied by uterine contractions. In general, both diagnoses contraindicate tocolytic treatment. However, in rare instances prophylactic use of tocolysis in women with these dangerous diagnoses may be considered to achieve time for corticosteroids in the setting of extreme prematurity when the bleeding is believed to occur in response to contractions. Such treatment is

fraught with difficulty, because even low doses of some tocolytic agents can be hazardous in a patient with bleeding. β-Mimetic agents and calcium channel blockers may hamper maternal cardiovascular response to hypotension, and prostaglandin inhibitors are known to impair maternal platelet function. Cardiac disease is a contraindication because of the risks of tocolytic drug treatment in these patients.

Potential causes of preterm labor should be sought in the initial evaluation and reassessed during the course of treatment. An underlying cause of preterm labor may be found that requires delivery (e.g., abruptio placentae or chorioamnionitis), that may affect the choice of tocolytic (e.g., a degenerating myoma often

---

Contraindications to Tocolysis

Maternal Contraindications to Tocolysis
- Significant hypertension (eclampsia, severe preeclampsia, chronic hypertension)
- Antepartum hemorrhage
- Cardiac disease
- Any medical or obstetric condition that contraindicates prolongation of pregnancy
- Hypersensitivity to a specific tocolytic agent

Fetal Contraindications to Tocolysis
- Gestational age <37 weeks
- Advanced dilation effacement
- Demise or lethal anomaly
- Chorioamnionitis
- In utero fetal compromise
  Acute: fetal distress
  Chronic: IUGR or substance abuse

responds best to a prostaglandin synthetase inhibitor), or that requires adjunctive treatment (e.g., antibiotics for pyelonephritis or therapeutic amniocentesis for polyhydramnios).

Myometrial Contractility and Tocolytic Action

A brief review of myometrial activity (see the box "Uterine Muscle Physiology") and the site(s) of action of the various tocolytic agents is appropriate. Figure 23–22 summarizes the current knowledge of the regulatory mechanisms of uterine smooth muscle contractility. The key process in actin–myosin interaction, and thus contraction, is myosin light-chain phosphorylation. This reaction is controlled by myosin light-chain kinase (MLCK). The activity of tocolytic agents can be explained by their effect on the factors regulating the activity of this enzyme, notably calcium and cyclic adenosine monophosphate (cAMP) (Fig. 23–22). Calcium is essential for the activation of MLCK and binds to the kinase as calmodulin–calcium complex. Intracellular calcium levels are regulated by two general mechanisms: (1) influx across the cell membrane and (2) release from intracellular storage sites. Entry of calcium into cells occurs by at least two mechanisms. Depolarization leads to calcium influx through specific calcium channels that are voltage dependent. This is the site of action of the calcium channel blockers. Calcium can also enter through voltage-independent mechanisms, most notably the calcium-magnesium-adenosine triphospatase (ATPase) system. Magnesium ions may interact here and also may compete with calcium for the voltage-dependent channels. Calcium is stored within cells in the sarcoplasmic reticulum and in mitochondria. Progesterone and cAMP promote calcium storage at these sites, while $PGF_{2\alpha}$ and oxytocin stimulate its release (Fig. 23–22) MLCK is also regulated by cAMP, which directly inhibits MLCK function via phosphorylation. Levels of cAMP are increased by the action of adenylate cyclase, which in turn is stimulated by β-adrenergic agents. Therefore, β-mimetic tocolytics act through adenylate cyclase to increase cAMP, which inhibits MLCK activity both by direct phosphorylation and by reducing intracellular free calcium (by inhibiting calcium release from storage vesicles) (Fig. 23–22). β-Mimetics also interact with surface receptors on the trophoblast, leading to increased cAMP, which in this tissue increases production of progesterone.[218] Hormonal production is a lengthy process, and significant production is not seen for at least 18 hours. For the myometrium to contract in a coordinated and effective manner (i.e., labor, whether term or preterm), individual smooth muscle cells must be functionally interconnected and able to communicate with adjacent cells. The key element of intercellular coordination of effective labor contractions is the gap junction. Estrogens and progesterone regulate formation of gap junctions and the concentration of oxytocin receptors.[218]

Choosing a Tocolytic Agent

Tocolytic drugs are reasonably safe when used according to standard protocols. However, their apparent safety is due more to the youth and general good health of the patients treated than to the inherent safety of the drugs. The choice of tocolytic requires consideration of the efficacy, risks, and side effects for each individual patient.

Magnesium Sulfate

Intravenous magnesium sulfate has been used for seizure prophylaxis in preeclampsia for decades, but was not used for the inhibition of preterm labor until the 1970s.[219] Because of its safety and familiarity, magnesium has displaced the β-mimetic drugs ritodrine and terbutaline to become the most commonly used tocolytic. The mechanism of tocolytic activity of magnesium is unclear. In vitro studies of uterine muscle strips show reduced contractility in the presence of magnesium ion. It has been suggested that magnesium acts by competition with calcium either at the motor end plate, reducing excitation, or at the cell membrane, reducing calcium influx into the cell at depolarization.

Efficacy of Magnesium Sulfate

The efficacy of magnesium to arrest labor has been studied in small clinical trials. In one study, 24 of 31 women treated with magnesium sulfate remained undelivered 24 hours after beginning therapy, compared to 14 of 31 treated with intravenous ethanol.[219] In an observational study of magnesium-treated women with singleton pregnancies with intact membranes and cervical dilation of 3 to 4 cm, 64 percent of subjects were undelivered at 48 hours and 56 percent were undelivered at 7 days.[220] A study in which 120 subjects with preterm labor were randomly assigned to receive either

---

Uterine Muscle Physiology

- Actin plus myosin $\longrightarrow$ (myosin light chain kinase [MLCK]) $\longrightarrow$ contraction
- MLCK becomes active in presence of free intracellular calcium
- Increased free intracellular calcium $\longrightarrow$ Increased MLCK $\longrightarrow$ contractions
- Decreased free intracellular calcium $\longrightarrow$ decreased contractions

Control of Myometrial Contractility:
Myosin Light-Chain Kinase (MLK) is the key enzyme

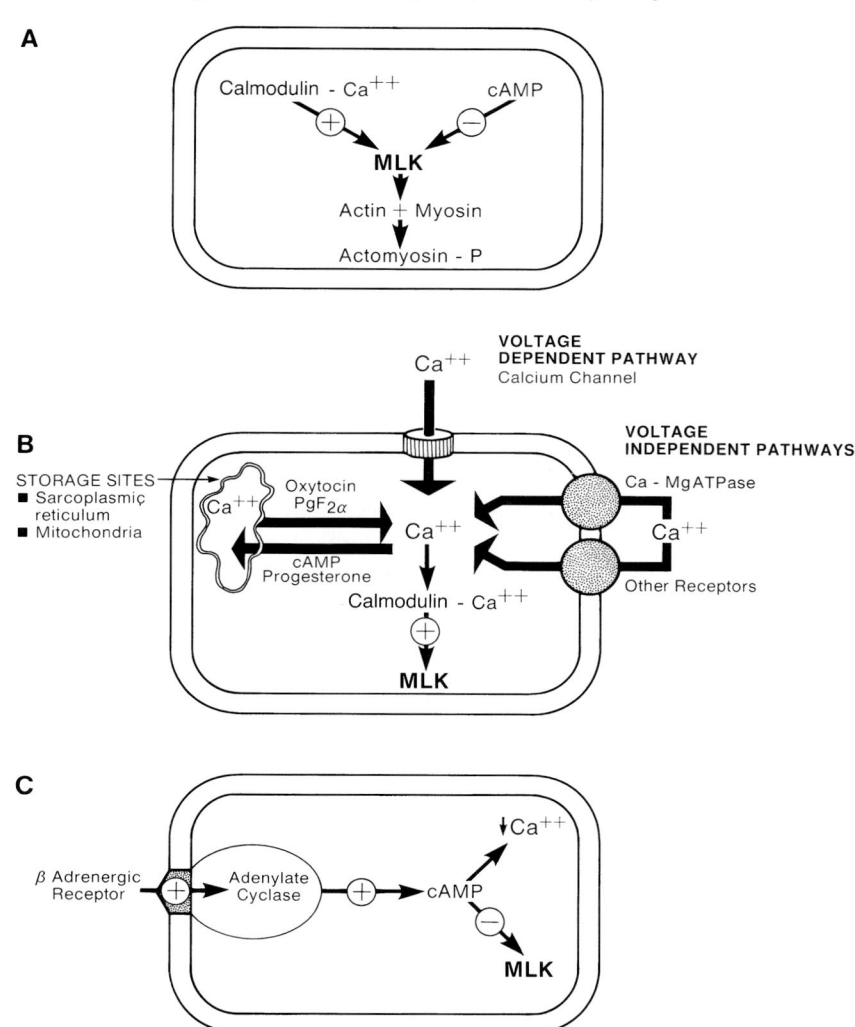

Figure 23–22. Control of myometrial contractility; myosin light-chain kinase (MLK) is the key enzyme. See text for details.

ritodrine or magnesium reported that only 4 percent and 8 percent of subjects, respectively, were delivered within 48 hours; and only 17 percent and 20 percent of ritodrine- and magnesium-treated subjects had delivered at 7 days.[221] More than 45 percent of subjects in each group remained undelivered at 37 weeks, suggesting that many enrolled subjects did not have true preterm labor. In the only trial that compared magnesium to no therapy,[222] 156 women between 24 and 34 weeks' gestation were randomly assigned to receive either magnesium or no tocolysis. There was no difference in duration of pregnancy, birth weight, neonatal morbidity, or perinatal mortality. The rate of delivery within 24 hours of enrollment was about 30 percent in each group. Delivery within 7 days of enrollment occurred in 47 percent of magnesium-treated subjects compared to 37 percent of controls. About 35 percent of subjects in each group delivered more than 28 days after enroll-

ment, again suggesting overdiagnosis of preterm labor in one third of subjects. One review of tocolytic agents concluded that there was insufficient evidence to support magnesium as an effective tocolytic,[223] but a meta-analysis[213] reached a favorable conclusion. Magnesium has become the first choice for tocolysis more because of its relative safety than for its efficacy.

Maternal Side Effects

Magnesium has a low rate of serious side effects compared with other tocolytic drugs.[224] However, flushing, nausea, vomiting, headache, generalized muscle weakness, diplopia, and shortness of breath are not rare. Major and life-threatening complications, including chest pain and pulmonary edema, also occur rarely. Side effects were noted in 7 percent of 355 patients treated with magnesium.[220] Four patients (1.1 percent) developed pulmonary edema, a rate similar to that seen with β-mimetics. Side effects are significantly more common when magnesium and β-mimetics are administered simultaneously.[221] Most centers avoid combined use for this reason.

Neonatal Side Effects

Although magnesium crosses the placenta and achieves serum levels comparable to maternal levels, serious neonatal complications are uncommon. Lethargy, hypotonia, and even respiratory depression may occur. Neonatal bony anomalies were reported in 6 of 11 infants who were exposed to magnesium for more than 7 days, but the clinical significance of this phenomenon is unknown.[225]

For reasons that remain unclear, antenatal maternal magnesium treatment has also been related to improved neonatal outcome in several recent studies. A case-control study found that maternal magnesium treatment for either preeclampsia or preterm labor was associated with lower rates of cerebral palsy (CP).[226] Only 7.1 percent of 42 children with cerebral palsy had been exposed to antenatal magnesium, compared to 36 percent of 75 controls without CP (OR, 0.14; 95 percent CI, 0.05 to 0.51). Another cohort study followed 519 infants whose birth weight was less than 1,500 g. The relationship of in utero magnesium exposure was related to CP at 1 year of age. At 3 to 5 years of age, none of 52 infants exposed to magnesium had CP and one was mentally retarded, compared to 29 with CP and 21 with mental retardation born to 337 mothers who did not receive magnesium.[227] The odds ratios and 95% confidence intervals were 0.00 (0.00 to 0.92) for cerebral palsy and 0.31 (0.04 to 2.34) for mental retardation. However, there has also been a report of increased perinatal mortality and morbidity associated with antenatal magnesium.[228] Prospective studies to evaluate the possible benefits of perinatal magnesium are ongoing.

Dosage of Magnesium Sulfate

Magnesium sulfate must be given parenterally to elevate serum levels above the normal range. Therapeutic dosage and serum levels have not been formally established but empirically are similar to those used for intravenous treatment of preeclampsia. A loading dose of 4 to 6 g is given over 20 to 30 minutes, followed by an infusion of 2 to 4 g/hr.[220] The relationship of serum magnesium levels to therapeutic effect is controversial. A review of 101 episodes of preterm labor treated with magnesium sulfate found no difference in the rate of tocolytic success when serum levels were less than 6 mg/dl, compared with levels of greater than 6 mg/dl.[229]

Mean serum magnesium levels in patients with successful tocolysis were similar to those in patients in whom tocolysis failed. The investigators concluded that serum magnesium levels alone should not serve as the end point of therapy and that the drug should be titrated on the basis of clinical efficacy and toxicity.

Provided renal function is normal, the kidney rapidly excretes excess magnesium. In patients with evidence of renal impairment (e.g., oliguria or serum creatinine levels >0.9 mg/dl), magnesium therapy should be approached cautiously, and the patient should be followed with serum levels, and doses adjusted accordingly. Magnesium sulfate should not be used in patients with myasthenia gravis because the magnesium ion competes with calcium.

A clinical protocol for magnesium sulfate as a tocolytic is shown in the box.

Summary of Magnesium

Magnesium sulfate is a safe agent with limited tocolytic effectiveness. Because of its favorable safety profile, magnesium may be an especially useful choice when the diagnosis of preterm labor is early and uncertain, and in patients for whom other agents are contraindicated (e.g., type 1 diabetes mellitus).

Indomethacin

Prostaglandins are mediators of the final pathways of uterine muscle contraction. Labor at term is associated with increased concentrations of arachidonic acid, and PGE_2 and $PGF_{2\alpha}$ in amniotic fluid. Prostaglandins given to pregnant women can ripen the cervix and/or induce labor, depending on the dosage and route of administration. Prostaglandins cause an increase in free intracellular calcium levels in myometrial cells and increased activation of MLCK, resulting in uterine contractions. Myometrial gap junction formation, an important step in synchronized uterine activity, is enhanced by prostaglandins. Prostaglandin synthetase, also known as cyclo-oxygenase (COX), is the enzyme that converts arachidonic acid to PGG_2. Prostaglandin synthesis is increased when the COX-2 form of this enzyme is induced by cytokines, bacterial products such as phospholipases and endotoxins, and corticosteroids. Inhibition of prostaglandin synthetase by NSAIDs leads to reduced synthesis of prostaglandins. The NSAID agents vary in their activity, potency, and side-effect profile. Indomethacin is the most widely used agent in this class, which also includes sulindac, naproxen, aspirin, and fenoprofen.

The potential for clinical use of these agents was noted in studies showing prolonged pregnancy and

Protocol for Magnesium Sulfate Tocolysis

1. Administer loading dose of 6 g magnesium sulfate in 10 to 20 percent solution over 20 to 30 minutes.
2. Maintenance dose of 2 g/hr (40 g of magnesium sulfate added to 1 L D5 0.9 normal saline or lactated Ringer's at 50 ml/hr.
3. Increase magnesium sulfate by 1 g/hr until the patient has one or less contraction per 10 minutes or a maximum dose of 4 to 5 g/hr is reached.
4. Limit intravenous fluid to 125 ml/hr. Follow fluid status closely with an indwelling urinary catheter if needed.
5. Maintain magnesium sulfate tocolysis for 12 hours after contractions have stopped or decreased to less than one per 15 minutes. Therapy may be stopped without tapering the dose.
6. Recurrent contractions require reevaluation to look for an underlying cause of the preterm labor such as amnionitis or occult abruption. Amniocentesis should be considered. The accuracy of the original diagnosis of preterm labor should be reconsidered with cervical sonography or fibronectin.
7. Patients treated with magnesium sulfate should be followed with
   a. Deep tendon reflexes and vital signs hourly.
   b. Intake and output every 2 to 4 hours.
   c. Magnesium levels if infusion exceeds 4 g/hr or if clinical concern about toxicity.

longer mean duration of labor in women taking therapeutic doses of salicylates.[230]

Efficacy of Indomethacin

Indomethacin was first reported to delay delivery by more than 7 days in 80 percent of treated subjects.[231] In randomized, placebo-controlled trials, indomethacin was superior to placebo in delaying delivery for 48 hours (80 percent vs. 33 percent in one trial[232] and 95 percent vs. 23 percent in the other).[233,234] After 7 days, 83 percent of the indomethacin-treated subjects were undelivered, compared with 16 percent for the placebo group.[233,234] Additional randomized trials have produced mixed results. A randomized comparison of indomethacin to ritodrine[235] found no difference in pro-

longation of pregnancy, but the indomethacin group had significantly fewer maternal side effects. In a randomized, placebo-controlled trial of indomethacin, pregnancy was prolonged beyond 48 hours in 13 of 16 (81 percent) of the indomethacin-treated subjects versus 10 of 18 (56 percent) in the placebo arm.[236] However, serious neonatal morbidity occurred in twice as many of the indomethacin-treated infants. An observational study compared neonatal outcome among infants born after maternal treatment with ritodrine with infants born after combined treatment with ritodrine and indomethacin.[237] Gestation was not significantly prolonged, but neonatal respiratory complications were increased in the indomethacin group. Because indomethacin was used in this trial only for patients with persistent contractions, the complications observed may relate more to the underlying cause of preterm labor than to the medication.

Maternal Side Effects of Indomethacin

Prostaglandin inhibition may have multiple and diverse side effects because of the abundance of prostaglandin-mediated physiologic functions. Nevertheless, the principal advantage of this agent is the relative infrequency of serious maternal side effects when the agent is used in a brief course of tocolysis. As with any NSAID, gastrointestinal side effects such as nausea, heartburn, and vomiting are the most common, but usually mild. More serious complications include gastrointestinal bleeding, alterations in coagulation, thrombocytopenia, and asthma in aspirin-sensitive patients. Lunt et al.[238] reported normal prothrombin and activated partial thromboplastin times, but found abnormal prolonged bleeding times in 65 percent of women treated for 48 hours. Prolonged treatment can lead to renal injury, especially when other nephrotoxic drugs are employed. Hypertensive women may rarely experience acute increased blood pressure after indomethacin treatment. Drugs of this class are antipyretic agents and may obscure a clinically significant fever. Maternal contraindications to indomethacin tocolysis include renal or hepatic disease, active peptic ulcer disease, poorly controlled hypertension, asthma, and coagulation disorders.

Fetal and Neonatal Side Effects

In contrast to the generally favorable maternal side-effect profile, the potential for fetal and neonatal complications of indomethacin tocolysis is worrisome. In actual practice, serious complications have been rare, but there is potential for injury to the fetus if treatment protocols are not followed carefully. Before the pathologic mechanisms of fetal injury were recognized, there were case reports of neonatal death following maternal indomethacin tocolysis. Three principal side effects of indomethacin have been of concern: constriction of the ductus arteriosus, oligohydramnios, and neonatal pulmonary hypertension. The ductal constriction occurs because formation of prostacyclin and PGE_2, which maintain ductal vasodilation, is inhibited by indomethacin.[239] Doppler evidence of ductal constriction was found in 7 of 14 fetuses of women treated with indomethacin between 27 and 31 weeks of pregnancy.[240] Tricuspid regurgitation occurred in three fetuses; all ductal abnormalities resolved within 24 hours after the medication was discontinued. The likelihood of ductal constriction increased after 32 weeks of pregnancy.[239] Prior to 32 weeks, the incidence of ductal constriction was 5 to 10 percent. At 32 to 35 weeks, the incidence increased to 50 percent after 48 hours of indomethacin exposure. Although potentially serious, ductal constriction is usually transient, and responds to discontinuation of the drug. However, persistent ductal constriction and irreversible right heart failure have been reported.[241] A review of fetal echocardiographs obtained from 61 women treated with indomethacin for preterm labor found evidence of ductal constriction in 50 percent of fetuses.[242] Constriction was detected at an average of 30.9 ± 2.3 weeks after an average of 5.1 ± 6.0 days of indomethacin therapy, and reversed in all fetuses after cessation of medication.

Oligohydramnios associated with indomethacin tocolysis is common, dose related, and reversible, but there is a report of neonatal renal insufficiency and death after prolonged administration.[243] Oligohydramnios is a consequence of reduced fetal urine production, due in turn to reduction by indomethacin of the normal prostaglandin inhibition of antidiuretic hormone, and by direct effects on fetal renal blood flow.

Primary pulmonary hypertension in the neonate is a potentially fatal illness that has also been associated with prolonged (>48 hours) indomethacin therapy.[244,245] Primary neonatal pulmonary hypertension has not been reported with 24 to 48 hours of therapy, but the incidence may be as high as 5 to 10 percent with long-term therapy.[235]

Other complications, including necrotizing enterocolitis, small bowel perforation, patent ductus arteriosus, jaundice, and intraventricular hemorrhage, have been observed when indomethacin was outside of standardized protocols that did not limit the duration of treatment and/or employed the drug after 32 weeks.[246] Fetuses treated in utero with indomethacin have been followed in childhood without evidence of significant long-term effects.[247–249]

Sulindac is an alternate NSAID that has been favorably compared to indomethacin as a tocolytic. Placental transfer of this drug is less than with indomethacin, but the tocolytic efficacy of sulindac has not been studied in large numbers.[250] One study[251] found fewer fetal cardiovascular effects detected by Doppler ultrasound with sulindac than with indomethacin.

Because of the effect on fetal urine production and amniotic fluid volume, indomethacin may be an appropriate tocolytic when preterm labor is associated with polyhydramnios. Indomethacin has been used successfully to treat preterm labor in women with polyhydramnios,[252] and for polyhydramnios without labor.[253,254] Uterine activity and pain associated with degenerating uterine fibroids in pregnancy also respond well to indomethacin.

Dosage of Indomethacin

Indomethacin is well absorbed orally or per rectum. The usual dose is a 50-mg loading dose by mouth or 50 to 100 mg per rectum. Subsequently, 25 to 50 mg is administered orally every 6 hours, depending on the response. Therapy is usually limited to 2 to 4 days because of concern about side effects of oligohydramnios and neonatal pulmonary hypertension (see the box "A Protocol For Indomethacin Tocolysis").

Summary of Indomethacin

Indomethacin is an effective tocolytic agent that is well tolerated by the mother. Concern about fetal side ef-

---

A Protocol for Indomethacin Tocolysis

1. Limit use to preterm labor before 32 weeks' gestation in subjects with normal amniotic fluid volume and normal renal function.
2. Loading dose of 50 mg rectally or orally; repeated in 1 hour if no decrease in contractions.
3. Give 25 to 50 mg every 6 hours for 48 hours.
4. Check amniotic fluid volume prior to initiation and at 48 to 72 hours. If oligohydramnios is present, the drug should be discontinued.
5. Use the drug for no longer than 48 to 72 consecutive hours. Treatment for >48 hours requires extraordinary circumstances. Ductal flow should be evaluated with Doppler echocardiography.
6. Discontinue therapy promptly if delivery seems imminent.
7. Fetal contraindications to use of indomethacin include growth restriction, renal anomalies, chorioamnionitis, oligohydramnios, ductal dependent cardiac defects, and twin–twin transfusion syndrome.

fects has appropriately limited use of indomethacin to brief courses of therapy in patients experiencing preterm labor before 32 weeks. A review of tocolytic efficacy and safety concluded that indomethacin was the only tocolytic for which there was convincing evidence of effectiveness, and that there was little risk to the fetus when used before 32 weeks according to published protocols.[223] However, indiscriminate use of prostaglandin inhibitors (e.g., for patients beyond 32 weeks or who have frequent contractions in the absence of a positive fibronectin or cervical dilation >2 cm) does not have a favorable risk/benefit ratio for the fetus.

The β-Mimetic Tocolytics

The β-mimetic tocolytic drugs have been widely used for 30 years. They are structurally related to epinephrine and norepinephrine, and include ritodrine, terbutaline (marketed in the United States only as a drug for asthma but often used as a tocolytic), albuterol, fenoterol, hexoprenaline, isoxuprine, metaproterenol, nylidrin, orciprenaline, and salbutamol. The U.S. Food and Drug Adminitration (FDA) approved ritodrine as a parenteral tocolytic in 1980, but it is used less often than terbutaline because of a perceived higher rate of maternal side effects. Terbutaline use continues despite not only the lack of FDA approval but also the specific FDA disapproval of its use as a tocolytic.[255]

Efficacy of β-Mimetics

There is evidence that the β-mimetic agents are successful in prolonging pregnancy for at least 48 hours and perhaps longer. A meta-analysis[186] of the randomized trials of β-mimetic drugs found that treated subjects were less likely to deliver within 24 (OR, 0.29; 95 percent CI, 0.21 to 0.41), and 48 (OR, 0.59; 95 percent CI, 0.42 to 0.83) hours of admission. There was a reduction in preterm births less than 37 weeks in treated subjects in 3 of 15 studies (OR, 0.71; 95 percent CI, 0.53 to 0.96). There was no advantage for the treated group compared to placebo controls in the frequency of low birth weight below 2,500 g (OR, 0.75; 95 percent CI, 0.55 to 1.02), severe RDS (OR, 1.07; 95 percent CI, 0.71 to 1.61), or perinatal death (OR, 0.96; 95 percent CI, 0.55 to 1.68). A Canadian prospective randomized trial of ritodrine compared with placebo reported similar results.[256] A reduction in deliveries within 2 to 7 days of diagnosis was noted, but there was no significant difference in births before 37 weeks. A trend toward fewer deliveries before 32 weeks did not achieve statistical significance. Any benefit of tocolysis evident in these analyses would seem to be conferred by the opportunity to administer steroids, antibiotics, and the like, and not by prolongation of

pregnancy to allow further intrauterine growth and maturation of the fetus.

Long-term use of β-mimetic drugs, given by mouth or subcutaneous infusion, has been championed by investigators whose approach to prematurity prevention is based on detection and suppression of contractions. This approach is supported by observational studies[257] that have not been confirmed in randomized placebo-controlled trials.[258–260] These and other studies[186] support the use of β-mimetic agents only for the acute suppression of contractions. The concern expressed by the FDA Advisory relates specifically to subcutaneous infusion for prevention and treatment of preterm labor:

> Published studies on the safety of this use (subcutaneous infusion) are seriously limited by methodologic inadequacies. In the absence of data establishing the effectiveness and safety of the drug/device (for subcutaneous infusion) the FDA is alerting practitioners . . . and others that continuous administration of subcutaneous terbutaline sulfate has not been demonstrated to be effective and is potentially dangerous.[255]

The agency was responding to reports of maternal cardiac symptoms and one reported maternal death that occurred during outpatient use of terbutaline infusion. It should be noted that the incidence of such serious side effects is low. In a report of 8,709 women treated with a continuous subcutaneous infusion, only 0.54 percent had cardiopulmonary symptoms.[261] However, any risk is unacceptable in the absence of benefit.

The remaining value for terbutaline in the care of preterm labor may lie in its rapid onset of action and ease of administration via a single subcutaneous injection. This use has been helpful to reduce contractions during transfer to a regional facility or in a protocol for triage evaluation of women with possible preterm labor.[262] The subject of long-term suppression of contractions is reviewed further for all tocolytics later in the chapter.

Pharmacology of β-Mimetics

Sympathomimetic drugs act through either α- or β-receptors. Stimulation of α-receptors leads to contraction of smooth muscles, while β-receptor stimulation carries the opposite effect, leading to smooth muscle relaxation at all sites: vascular, gastrointestinal, and uterine. The presence of β-receptors in other tissues (e.g., the heart) accounts for the side effects of β-mimetics. β-Receptors are divided into β_1- and β_2-subtypes. The β_1-receptors are largely responsible for the cardiac effects, while β_2-receptors mediate the smooth muscle relaxation as well as hepatic glycogen production and islet cell release of insulin. All β-mimetics are structurally related to epinephrine, with two carbons separating a benzene ring from an amino group. Relative β_2 activity appears to be associated with large alkyl substitutions on the amino group while maintaining hydroxyl groups at the 3 or 5 position on the benzene ring.[263] It should be noted that when drugs are referred to as β_2-selective or β_2-specific, the selectivity is relative, not absolute. β-Receptors are not distributed on an all-or-none basis; variable ratios of β_2- to β_1-receptors occur in various tissues. For example, the heart is primarily stimulated by β_1-agonists, but 14 percent of its β-receptors are β_2. In addition, not all β_2-specific drugs are perfectly selective and will stimulate β_1-receptors to some degree, especially when serum concentrations are elevated.

Pharmacokinetics

Ritodrine is conjugated in the liver to inactive glucuronic and sulfuric esters. Both unconjugated and conjugated drugs are then excreted in the urine. Actual serum ritodrine levels vary greatly at a given infusion rate.[264] The variability in serum levels among individuals at the same infusion rates appears to be related to differences in hepatic blood flow or serum concentrations of protein rather than maternal weight.[265] Concentrations of 80 ng/ml or more are commonly required initially to inhibit preterm labor. Ritodrine crosses the placenta readily. Fetal concentrations average 30 percent of maternal levels after a 2-hour infusion and are equal to those of the mother after longer infusions. In kinetics studies, serum ritodrine levels reach 75 percent of maximum levels within 20 minutes of a constant intravenous infusion.[265] The manufacturer's recommended protocol for intravenous therapy starts at 0.1 mg (100 μg)/min and is increased by 0.05 mg (50 μg) every 10 minutes until contractions cease, side effects occur, or the maximum rate (0.35 mg (350 μg)/min) is reached. The infusion is then maintained at the effective level for 12 hours after contractions cease. Side effects occur most often when the infusion rate and concentration of ritodrine are increasing.[264] The rate of change in the infusion rate or drug concentration is more important than absolute drug level in causing side effects.[265] An alternative protocol with equal efficacy and fewer side effects begins with an initial infusion of 50 μg/min, increasing by 50 μg/min every 20 minutes only if contractions are more frequent than every 10 minutes. Once labor is stopped, the infusion rate is maintained for 1 hour and then reduced every 20 minutes to the lowest rate that inhibits contractions adequately. This rate is then maintained for 12 hours.

Terbutaline has a longer half-life than ritodrine, and as a result has been associated with fewer side effects. Terbutaline levels are 30 percent lower in pregnant patients than in nonpregnant volunteers given the same dose. The onset of action is rapid with both intravenous bolus (1 to 2 minutes) and subcutaneous administration (3 to 5 minutes). Because terbutaline is not FDA approved, there is no manufacturer's protocol for preterm labor. Nevertheless, there is abundant clinical and published information about tocolytic use of terbutaline. Currently published protocols often employ subcutaneous administration, with a usual dose of 0.25 mg (250 μg) every 3 to 4 hours.[266] A single subcutaneous dose of terbutaline to arrest contractions during the initial evaluation of preterm contractions was found in one report to be an efficient method of evaluating women presenting with possible preterm labor.[262] None of three options studied affected pregnancy outcome, but women treated with a single subcutaneous dose of terbutaline had shorter, less expensive triage visits than women who received either intravenous or oral hydration. Intravenous administration of terbutaline has been employed in some centers, beginning at 2.5 μg/min and increasing by 2.5 μg/min every 20 minutes in a manner similar to ritodrine until a maximum of 17.5 to 20 μg/min is reached.[267]

Tachyphylaxis with β-Mimetic Drugs

Tachyphylaxis or desensitization of the adrenergic receptor occurs throughout the body after prolonged exposure to β-agonists, and affects the clinical use as tocolytics. Animal studies suggest that contractions resume after only several hours of *continuous* intravenous therapy with high-dose β-mimetic therapy; the myometrium remains quiescent longer with *pulsatile* administration of lower doses of the same tocolytic agent.[268] Caritis et al. observed reduced β-receptor sensitivity to continuous versus intermittent administration of ritodrine[269,270] and showed that the mechanism of this altered sensitivity occurs via reduced receptor density and adenyl cyclase activity. Interestingly, dexamethasone treatment ameliorated these effects and preserved the tocolytic effect. These observations led to studies of intermittent administration of β-mimetic agents.

Side Effects and Complications of Parenteral β-Mimetic Tocolysis

Maternal side effects of the β-mimetic drugs are common and diverse, as shown in Table 23–14. Most side effects are mild and of limited duration, but serious maternal cardiopulmonary and metabolic complications have been reported, including maternal death when β-adrenergic agents were given to mothers with unrecognized or occult cardiac disease. A thorough history and review of possible cardiac symptoms before initiating treatment should be performed. Prompt attention to any patient with persistent symptoms during treatment is important to prevent complications. Some centers ob-

Table 23–14. SIDE EFFECTS AND COMPLICATIONS OF β-MIMETIC TOCOLYSIS

Maternal	Fetal and Neonatal
Physiologic	*Fetal*
Apprehension	Tachycardia
Jitteriness	Cardiac arrhythmia
Headache	Myocardial and
Nausea and vomiting	septal
Fever	hypertrophy
Hallucinations	Myocardial ischemia
Metabolic	Heart failure
Hyperglycemia	Hyperglycemia
Hyperinsulinemia	Hyperinsulinemia
Hyperlactacidemia	Death
Hypokalemia	*Neonatal*
Hypocalcemia	Tachycardia
Antidiuresis, water retention	Hypoglycemia
Altered thyroid function	Hypocalcemia
Elevated transaminases	Hyperbilirubinemia
Cardiac	Tachycardia
Tachycardia	Myocardial ischemia
Pulmonary edema	Hypotension
Hypotension	Intraventricular
Arrhythmias/palpitations	hemorrhage
Heart failure	Decreased
Myocardial ischemia,	myocardial
altered ECG and chest	contractility
pain	
Shortness of breath	
Other	
Skin rash	
Pruritis	
Ileus	
Death (cardiac)	

Data from Hill WC: Risks and complications of tocolysis. Clin Obstet Gynecol 38:725, 1995.

tain routine electrocardiograms before beginning treatment with β-mimetic agents, but a normal electrocardiogram (ECG) does not exclude underlying cardiac disease and is probably not cost-effective in women without a worrisome history or persistent symptoms.

Cardiopulmonary Complications

The β-mimetic drugs have the potential for serious complications, but have an acceptable margin of safety if used with care and contraindications are strictly observed. Side effects are frequent with high-dose therapy. About 20 to 30 percent of patients experience nausea, and more than 50 percent of patients develop tachycardia greater than 120 bpm.[267,271] Pulmonary edema is serious but can often be prevented.[272] Pulmonary edema in association with tocolysis was once thought to be secondary to volume overload with left heart failure. However, evaluation of cardiac function with Swan-Ganz catheters and echocardiography has failed to demonstrate left ventricular failure in all but a few cases of pulmonary edema, most of which were associated with underlying hypertension.[273] Noncardiogenic contributing causes include decreased colloid oncotic pressure and increased pulmonary vascular permeability, especially when premature labor is associated with amnionitis.[274] Most patients with pulmonary edema have received either physiologic saline solutions or lactated Ringer's solution, which further decreases colloid oncotic pressure and expands vascular volume. A patient treated with β-mimetics should be considered as having a compromised cardiovascular system and should not receive large amounts of saline or lactated Ringer's solution.

It is uncommon for pulmonary edema to develop in the first 24 hours of β-mimetic therapy unless one of the predisposing factors (see the box "Contraindications and Relative Contraindications to β-Mimetic Tocolytics") is present. In fact, more than 90 percent of reported cases of pulmonary edema occur after 24 hours of β-mimetic therapy. Glucocorticoids have been suggested to be a predisposing factor, but neither betamethasone nor dexamethasone have mineralocorticoid activity. Their association with maternal pulmonary edema is probably coincidental. Pulmonary edema has been reported without concomitant use of corticosteroids, and with tocolytics other than the β-mimetics.

Symptomatic cardiac arrhythmias and myocardial ischemia have occurred during β-agonist tocolytic therapy. Myocardial infarction with resultant maternal death has also been reported.[271] Ischemia appears to be localized to the subendocardial region. The subendocardial ratio of oxygen supply to demand can be reduced

---

Contraindications and Relative Contraindications to β-Mimetic Tocolytics

Contraindications to β-Mimetic Tocolytics
- Maternal cardiac disease (structural, ischemia, or dysrhythmia)
- Eclampsia, severe preeclampsia, or other significant hypertensive disease
- Significant antepartum hemorrhage
- Uncontrolled diabetes mellitus
- Maternal hyperthyroidism

Relative Contraindications to β-Mimetic Tocolytics
- Diabetes, both diet and insulin controlled
- Hypertension
- History of severe migraine headaches
- Fever
- Increased risk of pulmonary edema

by two factors that are known to be operative during pregnancy and β-mimetic therapy: the normal placental arteriovenous shunt that diminishes aortic diastolic blood pressure, and the drug-induced tachycardia that shortens diastole, the time for myocardial perfusion.

If a patient develops chest pain during tocolytic therapy, tocolysis should be discontinued and oxygen administered. With severe pain, treatment with nitrates may be necessary. Premature ventricular contraction, premature nodal contractions, and atrial fibrillation have been noted in association with β-mimetic therapy.[271] These usually respond well to discontinuation of the drug and oxygen administration. The most important steps to prevent these cardiac complications are (1) excluding patients with prior cardiac disease and (2) limiting infusion rates so that maternal pulse does not exceed 130 bpm. Baseline or routine electrocardiograms before or during treatment are not helpful. There is a very poor correlation between symptoms of myocardial ischemia and electrocardiographic changes in these patients.[275] Nonetheless, an electrocardiogram is indicated if there is no response to oxygen and cessation of β-mimetic therapy.

The β-mimetic agents produce a mild (5 to 10 mm Hg) fall in diastolic blood pressure, and the extensive peripheral vasodilatation makes it difficult for the patient to mount a normal response to hypovolemia. This is one of the reasons β-mimetics may be dangerous in women with antepartum hemorrhage. Another is that the important early signs of excessive blood loss (e.g., maternal and fetal tachycardia) are masked by these drugs.[271]

Metabolic Complications

β-Mimetic agents may induce transient mild hyperglycemia in nondiabetic pregnant women,[267] lead to gestational diabetes with prolonged oral use,[276,277] elevate blood glucose sufficiently to require insulin patients with diet-controlled gestational diabetes, and seriously compromise glucose control in type 1 and type 2 maternal diabetes. Increased glycogenolysis with resultant hyperglycemia, increased lactic acid release from skeletal muscles, and ketone formation from fat stores, as well as a fall in bicarbonate, markedly increase the risk of ketoacidosis. These drugs should in general be avoided in women with diabetes. If it is absolutely necessary to use β-mimetics, a simultaneous intravenous insulin infusion should be employed to avoid ketoacidosis. β-Mimetics also lead to potassium flux from plasma into cells, thereby causing a fall in serum measurements without a change in excretion. Hence, there is no change in total body potassium. Measurement of glucose and potassium before initiating therapy and on occasion during the first 24 hours of treatment is appropriate. This surveillance will ensure that the patient

with unrecognized gestational diabetes and the occasional normal patient in whom significant hyperglycemia (>180 mg/dl) develops will not be missed. After 24 hours of therapy, both the serum glucose and potassium levels will have begun to return to baseline even without specific therapy.[278] No potassium replacement is needed unless the serum potassium level falls below 2.5 mEq/L.

In most women treated for 24 to 48 hours with β-agonist tocolytics, these metabolic changes are mild and transient. Prolonged treatment, however, has the potential to induce significant alterations in maternal blood glucose, insulin levels, and energy expenditure.[279] The risk of abnormal glucose metabolism is further increased by simultaneous treatment with corticosteroids,[280] a common combination for threatened preterm labor. Subcutaneous infusion has been found to induce fewer new cases of gestational diabetes than oral terbutaline.[281] However, the same study found that 100 percent of women who already had gestational diabetes required insulin to maintain euglycemia during treatment with subcutaneous terbutaline infusion.

Neonatal Side Effects of β-Mimetics

β-Mimetic tocolysis has been linked to an increased risk of neonatal intraventricular hemorrhage.[282] This and the other maternal complications cited above led many centers to replace the β-mimetic drugs with magnesium, nifedipine, or indomethacin as the tocolytic agent of first choice. Neonatal hypoglycemia and ileus have also been reported with β-mimetics, and can be clinically significant if the maternal infusion is not discontinued more than 2 hours before delivery.[283] Neonatal hypocalcemia may also occur. With all tocolytic drugs, and particularly β-mimetics and magnesium sulfate, adverse neonatal effects are greatest when the fetus is born close to a period of high-dose parenteral therapy. These drugs must be used with great caution if at all when there is advanced cervical dilatation and delivery appears inevitable. Situations in which the patient is at increased risk for β-mimetic complications (relative contraindications) are listed in box above. Careful risk/benefit evaluation needs to be performed on an individual basis in these cases.

Summary of β-Mimetic Tocolysis

β-Mimetic drugs were the tocolytics of first choice for a long time, but have been replaced by other drugs with better safety and side-effect profiles. Although ritodrine is still the only FDA-approved tocolytic agent, it is not commonly used in the United States. Terbutaline is a familiar choice that, when used as a single subcutaneous injection of 0.25 mg to facilitate maternal transfer or to initiate tocolysis while another agent with a slower onset of action is being given, has relatively few serious side effects. Long-term oral or subcutaneous treatment has not been shown to reduce either prematurity or neonatal morbidity in controlled trials.

Calcium Channel Blockers

Inhibitors of intracellular calcium entry affect the contraction of smooth muscle, and thus have potential use as tocolytics. Calcium channel blockers are marketed for treatment of hypertension, angina, and arrhythmias, but have been used off-label as tocolytic drugs. The pharmacologic effect is believed to occur via inhibition of the voltage-dependent channels of calcium entry into smooth muscle cells, resulting in a direct decrease in intracellular calcium as well as decreased release of calcium from intracellular storage sites. Nifedipine and nicardipine have been studied as tocolytic agents because they selectively inhibit uterine contractions compared to others such as verapamil. Unlike other tocolytics, calcium channel blockers are rapidly absorbed after oral administration. The pharmacokinetics in pregnancy are apparently similar to that seen in nonpregnant individuals, with appearance of nifedipine within plasma within just a few minutes, peak concentrations at 15 to 90 minutes, and a half-life of 81 minutes after oral administration.[284] Placental transfer of nifedipine was documented in this study in two patients who delivered 2 to 3 hours after receiving nifedipine. The duration of action of a single dose can be as long as 6 hours.

Efficacy

Nifedipine was reported in a small observational study[285] to be effective in suppressing contractions and well tolerated by mother and fetus. There are no placebo-controlled trials of calcium channel blockers. When nifedipine has been compared with β-mimetics,[286-289] its efficacy has been comparable or superior, and side effects lower than with β-mimetics. In a comparison with magnesium, nifedipine was equally effective in delaying delivery for 72 hours.[290] Hypotension was common (almost 40 percent) with nifedipine, but all other side effects occurred more often with magnesium. Another calcium channel blocker, nicardipine, was compared with magnesium in a randomized trial of 122 subjects.[291] There were no differences in neonatal outcomes, gestational age at delivery, or delay in delivery, but side effects were more common with magnesium.

Side Effects

As noted above, maternal side effects are less common with nifedipine and nicardipine than β-mimetics. A de-

crease in blood pressure and rise in pulse have been noted by most authors, with occasional cases of significant hypotension.[286] Unlike the β-mimetics, nifedipine is not associated with a decrease in serum potassium, although modest increases in glucose have been noted. Maternal symptoms are often related to hypotension and include headache (20 percent), flushing (8 percent), dizziness, and nausea (6 percent). Pretreatment with fluids may reduce their incidence. Most effects have been mild, but there are reports of serious complications. A 29-year-old healthy woman treated with intravenous ritodrine followed by oral nifedipine had a documented myocardial infarction 45 minutes after her second dose of nifedipine.[292] Whether her illness was due solely to the nifedipine or to the sequential use of a β-mimetic and calcium channel blocker is not known, but simultaneous or immediately sequential use of calcium channel blockers and β-mimetics is not recommended. Two reports describe skeletal muscle blockade when used in conjunction with magnesium sulfate,[293,294] so this combination therapy should be avoided. Both reports describe a prompt response to cessation of magnesium and/or treatment with calcium gluconate. A case of hepatotoxicity requiring discontinuation of the drug has also been reported.

Widespread acceptance of nifedipine as a tocolytic was limited by initial animal studies that reported reduction in uteroplacental blood flow, fetal bradycardia, and hypoxic myocardial depression with other calcium channel blockers, including verapamil, nicardipine, and diltiazem. However, animal studies of nifedipine have not shown such effects unless large doses were infused. Reports of Doppler ultrasound assessment of fetal and uteroplacental circulation during nifedipine use in women for treatment of preterm labor have also been reassuring.[295] No changes in the fetal middle cerebral artery, renal artery, ductus arteriosus, umbilical artery, or maternal vessels were noted in one study of 11 women treated with nifedipine for preterm labor. In an observational series of 102 mothers and 120 neonates treated with nifedipine, fetal well-being and neonatal complications such as low Apgar scores and cord pH less than 7.20 were typical for premature infants.[296] Ray et al.[297] found no significant differences in Apgar scores or umbilical venous blood gas values in infants exposed to nifedipine compared with infants not exposed to any tocolytic medicines. These human studies have provided sufficient reassurance, and some centers now use nifedipine as the tocolytic of first choice.[298]

Dosage

Nifedipine is usually given as a 10- to 20-mg dose every 6 to 8 hours by mouth (see the box "Nifedipine Tocolysis"). *Sublingual administration is not recommended* for general medical or obstetric patients because of re-

---

Nifedipine Tocolysis

10 to 20 mg *orally* as initial dose, then 20 mg orally every 6 hours for 24 hours, then 20 mg orally every 8 hours (*do not use sublingual route*)

---

ports of profound hypotension and myocardial ischemia.[292, 299]

Summary of Calcium Channel Blockers

Nifedipine has become the tocolytic agent of choice at some hospitals because of the low incidence of significant maternal side effects and ease of administration. There are few remaining concerns about fetal side effects because animal studies suggesting fetal compromise were performed with agents other than nifedipine, and because of an increasing number of reports of safe use in humans. Nifedipine should not be combined with magnesium or β-mimetics. Use should follow published dosage schedules closely until more extensive clinical experience has been reported.

New Tocolytic Agents

The oxytocin antagonist atosiban has been investigated in a randomized, placebo-controlled trial in which 501 subjects with acute preterm labor were randomized to receive either intravenous and subcutaneous atosiban or intravenous and subcutaneous placebo. Subjects who continued to exhibit contractions and progressive cervical change after 1 hour of initial treatment in either the placebo or atosiban arms were treated with an open-label "rescue" tocolytic agent of the clinician's choice, thus confounding any direct comparison of efficacy.[300] A significantly greater number of subjects remained undelivered without an alternate tocolytic at 24 hours (73 percent vs. 58 percent; OR, 1.93; 95 percent CI, 1.30 to 2.86), at 48 hours (67 percent vs. 56 percent; OR, 1.62; 95 percent CI, 1.62 to 2.37), and at 7 days (62 percent vs. 49 percent; OR, 1.70; 95 percent CI, 1.17 to 2.46). These differences were confined to subjects enrolled after 28 weeks; there were no advantages over placebo for subjects enrolled between 20 and 28 weeks. Unexpectedly, a significantly greater number of babies born to subjects enrolled into the atosiban arm died. The explanation for this observation is unclear, but the excess perinatal deaths all occurred among infants enrolled before 26 weeks. This suggests that enrollment may have been biased toward enrollment of early preterm labor subjects into the treatment arm. Maternal side effects of atosiban were few except for injection site inflammation. Although the differences in pregnancy prolongation were significant, the FDA did not approve atosiban. As in other placebo-controlled tocolytic trials, the rate of "successful" treatment in the placebo group was 50 percent or more, confirming the high rate of false-positive diagnosis of preterm labor based on contraction frequency and digital examination of the cervix. A companion trial compared subcutaneous infusions of atosiban to placebo.[301] The interval from the start of maintenance infusion therapy to the first recurrence of preterm labor was longer for the atosiban group, but there were no differences in the rate of preterm birth before 28, 32, or 37 weeks' gestation. An international study group compared the efficacy and side-effect profile of atosiban with ritodrine.[302] Efficacy to delay delivery for 48 hours (about 85 percent for both drugs) and 7 days (about 75 percent for both drugs) was similar, but cardiovascular side effects were much less common for atosiban (4 percent) than for ritodrine therapy (84 percent).

The nitric oxide donor glyceryl trinitrate has been studied in a trial in which 245 women with acute preterm labor were randomly assigned to receive either transdermal glyceryl trinitrate or standard ritodrine tocolysis.[303] The rate of prolongation to 37 weeks was 74 percent in both treatment arms. Headache occurred in 30 percent of the patients who received glyceryl trinitate.

Clinical Use of Tocolytic Drugs

Tocolytic therapy is employed in several clinical circumstances. In a patient who presents in active labor with advanced cervical effacement, the diagnosis is not in question, and the goal is prompt treatment to allow maternal transfer and time for corticosteroids and GBS prophylaxis. In this setting, oral nifedipine or subcutaneous terbutaline may be the best initial choice to stop contractions promptly, with either additional nifedipine or magnesium to suppress contractions for 8 to 24 hours. When the clinical presentation is more indolent, with persistent contractions and cervical effacement less than 80 percent, a slower acting agent such as magnesium is often chosen as the initial drug. Acute treatment for preterm labor is typically continued for some period of time, usually 6 to 12 hours, after contractions have stopped, or occur less than four times per hour without additional cervical change. When labor has been difficult to stop in a patient with complete cervical effacement, acute treatment is sometimes continued until a full course of steroid therapy is completed (48 hours).

If contractions persist despite therapy, the wisdom of tocolytic treatment should be reconsidered. The cervix should be reexamined; if cervical dilation has progressed beyond 4 cm, tocolytic therapy in most cases should be discontinued. Fetal well-being and the possibility of placental abruption or intra-amniotic infection should be reevaluated. If these concerns can be excluded, the accuracy of the original diagnosis should be reevaluated, remembering that significant effacement and development of the lower uterine segment are the features of the digital exam that most reliably indicate preterm labor. If a fibronectin swab was collected before therapy was begun, it should be sent for analysis. A positive result is not confirmatory, but a negative fibronectin, if collected before performance of a digital examination, provides evidence that the patient's contractions are benign.[201] Alternately, a transvaginal cervical ultrasound examination may be performed. A length of 30 mm or more essentially excludes the diagnosis.[200]

It should also be remembered that the definition of "successful" tocolysis does not necessarily require that *no* contractions occur, only that the frequency be reduced to less than 4 to 6 per hour without further cervical change. If these issues can be resolved, the adequacy of the tocolytic medication may be an issue. Unlike other drugs, serum levels are not clinically helpful to adjust the dose of tocolytics. A change to a second agent, or combination therapy with multiple agents, may improve efficacy, but often result in increased side effects as well. If magnesium was the initial agent, a supplemental dose of subcutaneous terbutaline 0.25 mg is appropriate for patients with active preterm labor. This combination is reasonably effective and is safe if supplemental terbutaline is given only once or twice. Sustained treatment with both magnesium and a β-mimetic has been found to increase the risk of significant side effects and should be avoided.[304,305] Both β-mimetics and magnesium sulfate cause increased cardiac output and decreased peripheral vascular resistance, so the high rate of side effects is not surprising.

Combined use of either β-mimetics or magnesium sulfate with calcium channel blockers should be avoided. Although many centers employ indomethacin as a second-line agent when magnesium fails, a recent trial found no additional neonatal benefit when indomethacin was added to ritodrine.[237] Such reports at first suggest ineffective treatment, but there is increasing evidence that occult chorioamnionitis may be responsible not only for persistent contractions but also for short- and long-term neurologic morbidity reported after combination tocolytic drug therapy.[306,307] These findings emphasize the importance of careful evaluation of the preterm labor patient whose contractions do not respond promptly to tocolysis, especially before 30 weeks' gestation (see the box "Management of Persistent Contractions Despite 12 to 24 Hours of Tocolysis").

Amniocentesis can be helpful in the management of some women with preterm labor. In addition to evaluation for infection, amniotic fluid studies for fetal pulmonary maturity may be helpful in the following circumstances:

Management of Persistent Contractions Despite 12 to 24 Hours of Tocolysis

1. Is the patient infected? Repeat clinical exam, white blood cell counts, and fetal assessment. Consider amniocentesis for glucose, Gram stain, and culture.
2. Is the fetal compromised? Review the fetal heart tracings and do a biophysical assessment.
3. Is there evidence of abruption? Is there a suspicion of uterine anomaly with implantation of the placenta on the septum? Repeat hemoglobin, hematocrit, and coagulation profile, and abdominal sonography for placental implantation site.
4. Is the diagnosis of preterm labor correct? Is the cervix changing? Perform a transvaginal cervical ultrasound to measure cervical length and look for funneling or separation of the membranes from the lower segment. Send a fibronectin swab.
5. If infection, fetal compromise, and abruption can be excluded, stop parenteral tocolysis for 24 hours and observe. Most patients will stop contracting spontaneously.

1. When the gestational age is in doubt.
2. When the size of the fetus suggests poor or excessive intrauterine growth.
3. When there is any question of a chronic hostile intrauterine environment (e.g., maternal hypertension, decreased amniotic fluid volume, substance abuse).
4. When the gestational age is between 34 and 37 weeks.[307,308]

Routine use of amniocentesis to assess pulmonary maturity in all patients with preterm labor is not practiced in most hospitals, but may be justified in centers that care for populations with poor dates, high rates of maternal substance abuse, or fetal growth restriction.

Maintenance Tocolytic Treatment

Continued suppression of contractions after acute tocolysis has been studied in multiple placebo-controlled trials[310-314] (see Table 23-15), none of which found a significant reduction in the rate of preterm birth. Other studies that compared oral medications to no treatment also found no reduction in preterm birth.[315-318] Because many of the trials are small, several meta-analyses have been performed.[213,260,319] All have found no benefit in any outcome studied, including prolongation of pregnancy, frequency of preterm birth, and reduction in

Table 23–15. PLACEBO-CONTROLLED TRIALS OF ORAL TOCOLYSIS AFTER ACUTE TREATMENT OF PRETERM LABOR

First Author	Year	N	Drug(s)	Preterm Birth (%)		OR (95% CI)
				Rx	Placebo	
Creasy	1980	55	Ritodrine	40.2	46.4	0.51 (0.19–1.40)
Carlan	1995	69	Sulindac	39.4	47.1	0.73 (0.28–1.93)
Holleboom	1996	95	Ritodrine	32.0	28.9	1.16 (0.48–2.78)
Lewis	1996	200	Terbutaline	63.0	63.0	1.00 (0.56–1.78)*
Rust	1996	205	Terb/Mag Cl	56.9	57.3	0.98 (0.55–1.77)

* Some benefit limited to subjects enrolled before 32 weeks.

recurrent preterm labor associated with oral medication to suppress contractions. The evidence showing no benefit is important because oral terbutaline continues to be prescribed, and because chronic administration of β-mimetic tocolytics can have significant side effects, both fetal and maternal. One case report[320] describes a woman whose fetus developed hypertrophy of the myocardial septum, apparently as a result of prolonged β-mimetic–induced fetal tachycardia. Other studies have documented a clear deterioration in glucose tolerance after more than 5 days of oral β-mimetics.[276,277] Continuous administration of terbutaline via a subcutaneous infusion pump has been proposed to reduce the occurrence of tachyphylaxis[321] and side effects. Descriptive studies have found fewer side effects than with oral terbutaline,[257] but these studies lack control groups and cannot be used to judge efficacy. Two randomized placebo-controlled trials of subcutaneous terbutaline to prolong pregnancy after acute treatment of preterm labor found no benefit to this treatment.[258,259]

There are several possible reasons for the inability of maintenance tocolytics to improve outcome. First, oral β-mimetics and magnesium do not achieve levels in the blood comparable to levels produced by parenteral therapy.[322] The Canadian ritodrine study[256] reported prolongation of pregnancy for 2 to 5 days while the drug was given parenterally, but there was no additional prolongation of pregnancy when the medication was administered orally. The dose was insufficient to achieve therapeutic blood levels. Another explanation of the failure of maintenance tocolysis is the evidence cited previously that preterm labor is a usually chronic process that develops over weeks or months, not days. This conclusion is also consistent with studies that found no decrease in prematurity for women followed with ambulatory or home uterine contraction monitoring, a strategy based on detection and suppression of uterine contractions. None of three randomized trials of home contraction monitoring after acute treatment of preterm labor found a benefit for the monitored group.[323–325] A meta-analysis of these three trials found no advantage to home monitoring for delivery before 37 weeks, birth weight, or gestational age at delivery.[213] A multicenter randomized trial in which uterine activity was monitored but the data were ignored in one group also found no improvement in preterm birth rate when contraction data were used.[149]

The duration of hospitalization for an episode of preterm labor will vary according to several factors including the dilation, effacement, and sonographic length of the cervix; ease of tocolysis; gestational age, obstetric history; distance from hospital; and the availability of home care and family support. Women with complete cervical effacement at a gestational age at the margins of perinatal viability are more likely to benefit from prolonged hospital care. Associated risk factors that may complicate or increase the risk of recurrent preterm labor, such as a positive genital culture for GBS, chlamydia, or gonorrhea; urinary tract infection; or anemia should be controlled before discharge from hospital care. Social issues such as homelessness, availability of child care, or protection from an abusive partner are important determinants of a patient's ability to comply with medical care, and must be considered before the patient is discharged from the hospital.

Adjunctive Treatment for Women with Preterm Labor

The initial goal of treatment of women with preterm labor is to delay delivery long enough to allow three adjunctive interventions that have been shown to reduce the neonatal morbidity and mortality related to prematurity:

1. Transfer of mother and fetus to a hospital equipped to care for a premature infant.[214,215]
2. Administration of glucocorticoids to decrease neonatal morbidity and mortality.[217,326]
3. Administration of antibiotic prophylaxis to prevent neonatal GBS infection.[216,327]

These three interventions are effective. The only questions about their use relate to selection of the appropriate women for treatment. Other potential interventions currently being investigated include antibiotics to enhance the effectiveness of tocolysis and antenatal magnesium to reduce neonatal neurological morbidity.

Maternal and Neonatal Transfer

Regionalized neonatal and maternal care has been shown to improve the rates of morbidity and mortality for LBW and especially for VLBW infants. Neonatal transfer of the LBW infant led to marked improvements in neonatal outcome. When it was recognized that some VLBW infants died before a regional center's neonatal care team could arrive, transfer of the mother with the fetus in utero became the preferred alternative whenever possible. In recognition of the advantages of concentrating care for VLBW infants in special centers, most states have adopted systems of regionalized perinatal care. Hospitals and birth centers caring for normal mothers and infants are designated as Level I. Larger urban hospitals that care for the majority of maternal and infant complications are designated as Level II centers; these hospitals have neonatal intensive care units staffed and equipped to care for most infants with birth weights above 1,000 to 1,250 g. Level III centers typically provide care for the sickest and smallest infants, and for maternal complications requiring intensive care.

Antenatal Corticosteroids

In 1972, Liggins and Howie[328] reported a reduction in hyaline membrane disease or RDS in infants born to women treated with antenatal corticosteroids. Since then, many studies have confirmed the benefit of maternal steroid treatment to reduce the incidence and severity of RDS and other neonatal morbidity including intraventricular hemorrhage, necrotizing enterocolitis, and patent ductus arteriosus. Most important, meta-analyses indicate that antenatal glucocorticoid treatment has led to decreased perinatal mortality, with odds ratios ranging from 0.32 to 0.9[217,329] (Fig. 23–23).

Physiologic Effects of Antenatal Corticosteroids

Antenatal steroids influence the synthesis of fetal proteins and peptides. In general, glucocorticoids act to enhance cell differentiation and maturation rather than cell growth. In the fetal lung, steroids induce several changes that favorably affect neonatal pulmonary performance. Production of surfactant is enhanced by the effect of glucocorticoids on enzymes important in the synthesis of phosphatidylcholine, a major component of surfactant; neonatal lung compliance is increased; production of proteins that enhance surfactant activity is increased; and alveolar protein leakage is decreased. Steroids also affect other organ systems, inducing maturation in the fetal brain, skin, and gastrointestinal tract. Animal studies have suggested that steroids promote maturation of the germinal matrix and thereby reduce the occurrence of perinatal intraventricular hemorrhage.[330]

Therapeutic Effects of Antenatal Corticosteroids

PERINATAL MORTALITY. Perinatal mortality has been reduced in infants born to steroid-treated mothers in

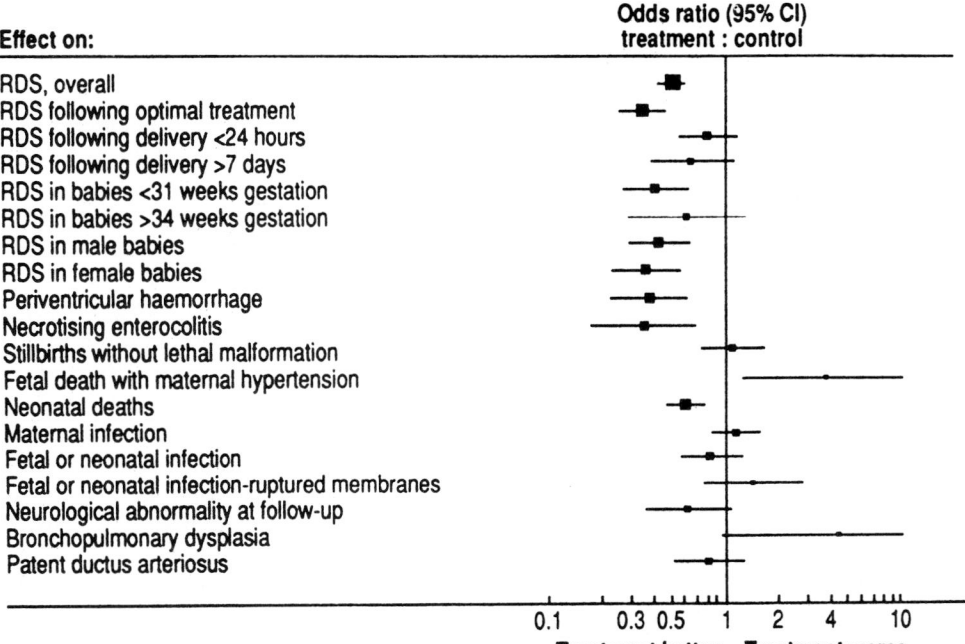

Figure 23–23. Summary of meta-analysis of 15 trials of the effect of corticosteroid use before preterm delivery on maternal and newborn outcome. RDS, respiratory distress syndrome. (From Crowley PA: Antenatal corticosteroid therapy. A meta-analysis of the randomized trials. Am J Obstet Gynecol 173:322, 1995, with permission.)

Effect on:

Odds ratio (95% CI)
treatment : control

RDS, overall
RDS following optimal treatment
RDS following delivery <24 hours
RDS following delivery >7 days
RDS in babies <31 weeks gestation
RDS in babies >34 weeks gestation
RDS in male babies
RDS in female babies
Periventricular haemorrhage
Necrotising enterocolitis
Stillbirths without lethal malformation
Fetal death with maternal hypertension
Neonatal deaths
Maternal infection
Fetal or neonatal infection
Fetal or neonatal infection-ruptured membranes
Neurological abnormality at follow-up
Bronchopulmonary dysplasia
Patent ductus arteriosus

0.1   0.3 0.5   1   2   4   10

Treatment better   Treatment worse

most reported trials. In a meta-analysis of multiple studies,[217] the odds ratio for neonatal mortality after antenatal steroid treatment was 0.61 (95 percent CI, 0.49 to 0.78). This figure is consistent with the original report[328] and subsequent analyses[329] showing a 40 percent reduction in neonatal mortality after steroid treatment.

Pulmonary Function

The original study reported a 50 percent reduction in RDS in steroid-treated neonates.[328] A meta-analysis[217] of 15 trials found an odds ratio of 0.51 (95 percent CI, 0.42 to 0.61) in the cumulative data for the occurrence of RDS in infants born to mothers treated with antepartum steroids compared with placebo-treated controls (Fig. 23–23). Questions remain about the efficacy of steroids in reducing RDS in patients with preterm PROM, but the magnitude and the consistency of the benefit across multiple trials have eliminated any doubt of reduced RDS in patients with intact membranes. Questions raised by earlier trials[331] that the effectiveness of steroids might be limited to certain subgroups (e.g., female and/or black infants, or infants only between 28 and 32 weeks) have been answered by the larger numbers accumulated in meta-analyses. Reduction in RDS occurs for male and female and for black and nonblack infants across a wide range of gestational ages from 24 through 34 weeks. Earlier questions about efficacy in subgroups were the result of inadequate statistical power due to small sample sizes for subgroup analysis in the initial trials. However, two principal unresolved issues about clinical use of antenatal steroids remain: (1) appropriate use of multiple courses of steroids, and (2) use in women with preterm PROM.

Maternal steroid treatment is not uniformly effective in eliminating RDS, but has been shown to ameliorate the severity of RDS when it does occur, manifested by reduced ventilator pressure settings and fewer neonatal intensive care unit (NICU) days.[332] Exogenous surfactant, an effective *postnatal* treatment for RDS, does not replace the respiratory benefits of antenatal steroid treatment. Rather, the effects of antenatal steroids and postnatal surfactant have been found to be additive for infants who receive both treatments, including significant reduction in mortality compared with those who received either therapy alone.[333–336] Despite the clear effect on RDS, the impact of antenatal steroids on the incidence of bronchopulmonary dysplasia is uncertain.[217]

INTRAVENTRICULAR HEMORRHAGE. Placebo-controlled trials have shown that antenatal steroid treatment is associated with a 50 percent reduction in the incidence of intraventricular hemorrhage[217,329,337,338] (Fig. 23–23). The mechanism by which steroids produce this benefit was originally attributed entirely to the reduced frequency and severity of RDS, but effects independent of RDS have been postulated based on studies that controlled for RDS severity[339] and cranial ultrasound studies of neonates performed shortly after birth.[340] A study confined to patients treated between 24 and 28 weeks[332] in which the severity but not the incidence of RDS was reduced nevertheless found a reduction in IVH from 25 percent in untreated to 3 percent (p = 0.012) in treated infants. A reduction in the size of cerebral infarction has been shown in animals treated with dexamethasone prior to but not after an experimental hypoxic brain injury.[330] The neurologic benefits of antenatal corticosteroids for VLBW were supported by a retrospective cohort analysis of 1,604 infants who weighed between 500 and 1,500 g at birth.[341] The rate of postnatal ventriculomegaly when examined at mean intervals of 1, 7, and 22 days of life was reduced by half in infants who had received either a full or partial course of antenatal corticosteroids compared with those who had not received steroids. One report found that betamethasone was more effective than dexamethasone in reducing the occurrence of periventricular leukomalacia.[342]

OTHER BENEFITS. Antenatal steroid treatment has been associated with other favorable effects on neonatal outcome, including a 65 percent reduction in the incidence of necrotizing enterocolitis (OR, 0.35; 95 percent CI, 0.18 to 0.68).[217] Reductions in the incidence of patent ductus arteriosus and circulatory instability, and improved Apgar scores[343] have also been reported.

DOSAGE OF CORTICOSTEROIDS. Two glucocorticoid regimens have been found effective: *betamethasone,* given as a mixture of 6 mg each of betamethasone phosphate and betamethasone acetate (Celestone) 12 mg intramuscularly every 24 hours for 2 doses, and *dexamethasone* (Decadron) 6 mg, also given intramuscularly, every 12 hours for 4 doses. The oral preparation of dexamethasone should not be used. A randomized trial of oral versus intramuscular dexamethasone was halted after a blinded review found an unexplained increase in intraventricular hemorrhage and neonatal sepsis in babies whose mothers were in the oral treatment arm.[344] Other steroid preparations (e.g., prednisone) are not effective because of poor placental transfer and should not be used. In studies of neonatal respiratory morbidity, betamethasone and dexamethasone produce similar clinical benefits. However, there may be important differences. Dexamethasone, but not betamethasone, was associated with altered neurobehavioral development in mice.[345] In another study that evaluated the occurrence of cystic periventricular leukomalacia among infants born between 24 and 31 weeks' gestation, the rate of periventricular leukomalacia was 4.4 percent among 361 infants who were treated antenatally with betamethasone, 11.0 percent among 165 infants who received dexamethasone, and 8.4 percent among 357 infants who were not treated with antenatal glucocorticoids.[342] Betamethasone, but not dexamethasone, transiently alters the fetal biophysical profile, inducing absent fetal heart variability and decreased tone and breathing movements for 48 to 72 hours.[346,347]

Several issues about the appropriate dosage schedules remain unresolved. It is not known whether steroids accelerate the normal maturational process transiently or permanently. The issue is difficult to study because the interval between treatment and delivery in clinical trials is variable, and because some effects may be transient while others are permanent. Neonatal benefit has been most easily observed when the interval between the first dose and delivery exceeds 48 hours, but benefit also accrues for babies born after a partial or incomplete course. The initial studies[348] seemed to indicate that the respiratory benefits were limited to the first week after treatment. However, there were very few cases of RDS among infants delivered more than 7 days after treatment, limiting the power of this observation. In contrast, a large multicenter trial[349] found evidence of benefit for as long as 18 days after the initial course of antenatal steroids.

RISKS OF ANTENATAL CORTICOSTEROID TREATMENT. Concerns about both short- and long-term adverse effects of corticosteroids have arisen as the frequency of antenatal therapy increased after the 1994 NICHD Consensus Conference.[350] Short-term concerns include possible reduced resistance to infection for both the mother and infant, impaired glucose tolerance, suppression of maternal or neonatal adrenal function, and alteration of the fetal biophysical profile following steroid treatment. The largest studies[331,351,352] did not find any increased incidence of neonatal or maternal infections. Infection is a greater concern when steroids are given to women with preterm PROM, but even in that subgroup, an increase in infectious morbidity has not been definitively shown. Increased fetal jeopardy in pregnancies complicated by proteinuric hypertension was suggested by the original[335] study, but was not confirmed in subsequent series.[353,354]

In women with insulin-dependent diabetes mellitus, steroid treatment virtually always results in 48 to 96 hours of increased blood glucose that can be difficult to control with standard insulin regimens. Intravenous infusion of insulin is often necessary. In women without diabetes, impairment of maternal glucose tolerance may also occur, especially in women treated with β-mimetic drugs[280] or when traditional risk factors for gestational diabetes such as maternal age, obesity, or family history are present. Therefore, maternal glucose testing should be considered when repeated courses of glucocorticoids are administered.

Whether antenatal steroids inhibit adrenal response in the mother or newborn in a clinically relevant manner is uncertain. Transient suppression of neonatal cortisol levels has been reported.[361] The doses given produce levels of corticoids comparable to those endogenously produced by the neonatal adrenal gland in response to the stress of RDS. Women treated with multiple courses of steroids during pregnancy were found to have a blunted response to adrenocorticotropic hormone (ACTH) stimulation later in pregnancy or during the puerperium.[356]

Maternal treatment with betamethasone[357] but not dexamethasone[346,347] has been associated with transient reduction in fetal heart rate variability and body and breathing movements in several studies. When it occurs, typically between 48 and 72 hours after the first dose, the alteration in fetal biophysical behavior is striking. Both short- and long-term heart rate variability is reduced, and fetal body and breathing motion may be absent or significantly reduced. The effects resolve spontaneously by the 4th day. Doppler ultrasound studies are unaffected by corticosteroid administration and may therefore provide reassurance about fetal well being.[358]

Concern about long-term fetal effects is founded upon the observation that corticosteroids act to accelerate fetal cellular and organ maturation at the expense of cell and organ growth.[359] Data about long-term risks are mostly but not wholly reassuring, and must be viewed against the overwhelming evidence of neonatal benefit. Studies in mice[360] and sheep[361] have reported decreased fetal size after repeated doses of steroids. Antenatal steroid therapy given in a rodent model at a gestational age analogous to the early third trimester in humans was associated with reduced brain cell number and decreased brain DNA content.[362] In the sheep, repeated injections of corticosteroids were associated with a significant delay in myelination of the optic nerve.[363] Slotkin[364] cautioned that "therapeutic use of antenatal steroids . . . occupies precisely the timeframe of maximum vulnerability of the central nervous system (CNS) . . . (and) . . . low doses of glucocorticoids that lie at or below the threshold for eliciting changes in lung surfactant production are capable of altering CNS development." He also noted that steroids could possibly affect tissue response to hypoxia in organ systems other than the CNS. Additional concern about repeated courses has been raised by reports in humans of reduced growth associated with multiple courses of antenatal steroids. An Australian study found that 17 percent of infants who received a single in utero course of antenatal steroids had birth weights below the 10th percentile, compared with 35 percent of infants exposed to more than three antenatal courses.[365] There was also a significant association between multiple courses and reduced head circumference in this study. In view of these concerns, it is reassuring to note that the original cohorts of infants treated with a single course of antenatal steroids have displayed no differences when compared with gestational age-matched controls in physical or mental function.[352,366]

Clinical Use of Antenatal Corticosteroids

Despite the impressive evidence of both medical and economic benefit,[367,368] maternal steroid treatment preceded only 26 percent of low-birth-weight deliveries in a 1990 survey.[369] Fewer than half of treated infants in this review had received a full course of treatment. The underutilization apparently occurred for diverse reasons. Some did not receive treatment for unavoidable causes such as presentation in advanced labor or maternal illness requiring immediate delivery (e.g., eclampsia or significant obstetric hemorrhage). Others were not treated because of underestimation of neonatal survival rates for ELBW babies, concern about maternal or neonatal risks of infectious morbidity, or questions about the effectiveness of partial treatment or of population subsets such as white male fetuses.

In response to these concerns, the NICHD convened a Consensus Development Conference on Antenatal Steroids in 1994.[370] The recommendations of this conference were reviewed by the Committee on Obstetric Practice Opinion (No. 210) of the American College of Obstetricians (ACOG) and Gynecologists.[326] Both NICHD and ACOG recommend antenatal steroids for mothers expected to deliver before 32 weeks' gestation to reduce mortality and the incidence of RDS and IVH, regardless of the status of the fetal membranes. At 32 to 34 weeks, both recommend antenatal steroid treatment for mothers with intact membranes who were likely to deliver within 7 days, but noted that the benefit for infants born to women with ruptured membranes after 32 weeks is still controversial. The controversy centers on whether a large trial[371] that found a substantial benefit of steroids should be included in meta-analyses. The results of this trial may have been confounded by concomitant treatments and by a remarkably high rate of RDS in the control group. When meta-analyses of steroid trials in patients with PPROM exclude the data from this trial, the beneficial effect of steroids on the incidence of RDS is lost, but the effect on intraventricular hemorrhage is retained.

In addition to the preterm PROM issues, questions regarding the need for and risk of repeated courses of steroids remain unanswered. The opportunity for long-term risk would seem to be greater with repeated dosing. The 1994 NICHD Consensus Panel reconvened in August 2000. The Panel recommended that repeat dosing not be used in clinical practice pending data from ongoing research studies. The risk and consequences of imminent preterm birth, in contrast, are immediate and real, and will vary in individual ways as the pregnancy continues. A weekly reassessment of the need for steroids, rather than a policy of routinely administering

steroids each week to high-risk patients, is probably the wisest course.

The NICHD Consensus Panel's successful campaign to increase the use of steroids has also led to new unanswered questions about the indications for steroid treatment of high-risk patients. What risk of imminent preterm delivery is sufficient to treat the patient with antenatal corticoids? Is actual preterm labor or preterm PROM required, or is a history of a previous preterm delivery and/or a dilated or effaced cervix enough? At our center, we have used admission to the hospital as the principal criterion for steroid treatment. Asymptomatic women with historical risk factors who inquire about receiving prophylactic corticosteroids may be reassured by a negative fibronectin test or cervical ultrasound examination, thus avoiding indiscriminate use of steroids.

Antibiotics for Women with Preterm Labor

There are two potential uses for antibiotics in women with preterm labor. The first is prophylaxis of neonatal GBS infection, an intervention that is clearly effective (see Chapter 40). The second is antibiotic therapy aimed at prolonging gestation in women with preterm labor by targeting a broad range of microorganisms that have been implicated in the pathogenesis of spontaneous preterm birth. Administration of antibiotics to women being treated for preterm labor has been studied extensively with disappointing results.[372-377] Results from the largest trial[375] are shown in Table 23–16.

Given the extensive and persuasive literature that links genital tract colonization and infection with spontaneous prematurity,[98] what can be the reasons for the failure of supplemental prophylactic antibiotics to enhance tocolysis? The first is the problem that has hampered all studies of preterm labor, the overdiagnosis of preterm labor. The inclusion of women who do not actually have preterm labor in trials of interventions for preterm labor confounds interpretation of the results.

Table 23–16. SUPPLEMENTAL ANTIBIOTIC TREATMENT IN WOMEN WITH PRETERM LABOR*

Outcome	Antibiotic Rx ($n = 131$)	Placebo ($n = 144$)
Delivery <37 weeks (%)	53	52
Entry to delivery (days)	35	32
Mean birth weight (g)	2,535	2,883
Preterm PROM (%)	19	15
Amnionitis (%)	2	5

* Prospective, randomized trial by NICHD MFMU network; ampicillin + erythromycin vs. placebo; 277 subjects with PTL at 24–34 wk, intact membrane.

Data from Romero R, Sibai B, Caritis S, et al: Antibiotic treatment of preterm labor with intact membranes: a multicenter, randomized, double-blinded, placebo-controlled trial. Am J Obstet Gynecol 169:764, 1993.

Antibiotic trials limited to subjects who are fibronectin-positive might produce different results. The second reason is that the clinical diagnosis of preterm labor, even when accurate, may occur so late in the pathologic sequence that it is simply too late for antibiotics to exert any favorable effect. Regardless of the explanation, it is clear that supplemental antimicrobial therapy for reasons other than treatment of a specific pathogen such as gonorrhea or prophylaxis of GBS is not justified at present for women with preterm labor.

Other Adjunctive Antenatal Treatment to Reduce Fetal Morbidity

The persistence of cases of RDS among infants born to women treated with steroid therapy has led to investigation of alternative treatment approaches to further enhance pulmonary maturation. Neonatal treatment with surfactant is an effective adjunctive therapy that adds independently and synergistically to the benefit of corticosteroids in reducing RDS-related morbidity. Three large randomized, placebo-controlled trials of maternal treatment with antenatal thyrotropin-releasing hormone (TRH) to reduce neonatal lung disease have found no benefit over corticosteroids alone.[378–380] Together, these trials enrolled 1,771 subjects.

Studies of other agents given to the mother before delivery to reduce or prevent neonatal neurologic morbidity have been reported for phenobarbital and vitamin K. Initial studies of both agents appeared promising but larger placebo-controlled trials have found no benefit to treatment with these agents. Rates of grade III and IV intraventricular hemorrhage, of any IVH, and of neonatal mortality did not differ between 181 infants born to mothers who received placebo and 191 whose mothers received both vitamin K and phenobarbital.[381] Another randomized trial found no difference between antenatal phenobarbital and placebo in either intracranial hemorrhage or early death in 610 preterm infants.[382]

A reduced incidence of intraventricular hemorrhage and cerebral palsy in premature infants exposed to antepartum maternal magnesium sulfate treatment for both preterm labor tocolysis and seizure prophylaxis has been noted in retrospective analyses.[226,227] This association is unexplained, and is currently being tested in randomized trials.

ABNORMAL CERVICAL COMPETENCE

Definition

Few topics in obstetrics have been the subject of greater controversy than has cervical incompetence. The diagnosis of incompetent cervix has traditionally been made and is still most confidently established by an obstetric history of passive and painless dilation of the cervix in the second trimester. The controversy has centered on whether this classic picture is the only true presentation for this disorder, or whether there are other clinical presentations. A history of the amniotic sac found bulging through a well-effaced and partially dilated cervix in the absence of contractions, bleeding, infection, or amniorrhexis is classic but is not common.

Arguments about the presentation and incidence of incompetent cervix derive from two different theories. According to the traditional view, the cervix operates as a categorical variable in which it is either fully functional (competent), or nonfunctional (incompetent). Preterm labor, ruptured membranes, bleeding, or intra-amniotic infection in women presenting at 16 to 26 weeks are assumed to be primary etiologic diagnoses in which a competent cervix changes only in response to uterine activity, whether overt or occult. This understanding of cervical competence as either categorically competent or incompetent is based on studies of the cervix in which digital examination was used to assess cervical dilation and length. The authors of a 1961 study " . . . wondered whether there can be any degrees in the incompetence of the internal os. If an incompetent os can cause abortion, is it possible that a lesser degree of incompetency . . . can lead to premature labour?"[383] They performed digital examination of the cervix in 655 subjects and concluded that "A degree of incompetence of the internal os that would lead to a premature labour does not seem to exist." This once dominant conclusion was challenged by studies suggesting that women with a history of second-trimester delivery might benefit from prophylactic cerclage.[169,177] These investigations indicated that the traditional clinical presentation of incompetent cervix may be simply fortuitous (i.e., that some women with a passively dilated cervix and bulging amniotic sac might develop contractions, infection, or membrane rupture as the consequence of incompetent cervix).

Subsequent studies of the cervix with ultrasound have revealed that the cervix functions along a continuum of "competence."[101] One study used transvaginal ultrasound to measure cervical length in three groups of pregnant women: (1) women with an obstetric history typical of incompetent cervix, (2) women with a history of a prior spontaneous preterm birth, and (3) women who had normal obstetric histories and normal current pregnancies.[60] The hypothesis was that if cervical function were categorical, cervical length would be short in women with incompetent cervix but would be similar in both normal pregnancies and in the women who delivered preterm. Alternately, if cervical function were continuous, cervical length would decrease as the gestational age at delivery in the previous pregnancy decreased. The results were consistent with the latter hypothesis: the earlier the gestational age at delivery in the prior pregnancy, the shorter the cervix in the current pregnancy. Two prospective studies correlated transvaginal sonographic measurements of the cervix in the late second and early third trimesters with risk of preterm delivery. In a cross-sectional study of 178 women,[101] the risk of preterm delivery increased as cervical length decreased. A multicenter observational study[70] of 2,915 pregnant women found that the risk of preterm birth increased as cervical length decreased across the whole range of cervical length (Figs. 23–15 and 23–16).

The same cervical changes (shortened cervix, funneled internal os) that are associated with increased risk of spontaneous preterm birth have been described in women who present with typical cervical incompetence.[384] The only difference is the duration of pregnancy at the time of examination. The same changes have been noted as early as 16 weeks.[385] However, although the risk of preterm birth is increased approximately six fold in women whose cervical length is below the 10th percentile (25 mm), the majority of women in whom these changes are observed do not present with typical incompetent cervix, or even deliver preterm.[70,102]

These studies have changed our understanding of the cervix from a categorical concept of cervical "incompetence" versus "competence" to one of variable competence, wherein cervical function is described by a bell-shaped curve that roughly corresponds to length. The risk of spontaneous preterm birth increases as cervical length decreases. Women whose cervical length lies below the 5th or 10th centile clearly have the greatest risk for spontaneous preterm birth (Fig. 23–16), but the clinical presentation is not uniform. Some will present with preterm labor, others with PPROM, and still others with the classic picture of incompetent cervix.

If cervical length correlates with risk of preterm birth, is it possible to define reduced cervical competence according to a cervical length below, for example, the 5th percentile? The answer is no. Cervical length is influenced by several factors, including biologic or inherent differences (the ratio of muscle to collagen is increased in women with incompetent cervix),[386] by the duration of pregnancy (the cervix elongates in the first and early second trimesters and shortens slowly thereafter as the volume of the uterus increases), by the action of cytokines and prostaglandins,[71,387] and finally by uterine contractions. The contribution of each of these to any individual cervical length measurement is uncertain.

Despite the unanswered questions, this much is clear: cervical competence is variable, and so is the clinical presentation. The only clearly diagnostic presentation is still a history of painless dilation, but any patient with a history of early preterm birth before 26 weeks may have reduced cervical competence, a term that more accurately reflects the data described above.

Etiology

Reduced cervical competence may be congenital or acquired. Some women have typical histories of painless dilation in the first and every subsequent pregnancy, while others experience progressively earlier delivery with each pregnancy until a typical "incompetent" history occurs. Still others have several term births before an obstetric injury in the penultimate pregnancy creates a damaged cervix. The concept of percentiles of competence suggests that women with cervical lengths below the 25th to 50th percentiles may suffer clinically meaningful injury to the cervix as a result of obstetric or gynecologic trauma that would not have clinical consequences had the initial cervical length been longer.

Cervical trauma may occur in the course of either vaginal or cesarean delivery. The cervix may be lacerated and heal poorly, or may be stretched beyond tolerance. It is not uncommon to care for women whose typical presentation of incompetent cervix followed a prior cesarean delivery performed for disproportion after prolonged pushing in the second stage of labor. Obstetric trauma may rarely accompany dilation and curettage. Insertion of laminaria to soften the cervix before dilatation and extraction or dilatation and curettage may reduce cervical trauma. A history of prior first-trimester elective abortion carries a risk of injury so small as to be insignificant if it was performed by an experienced operator using local anesthesia only, and if laminaria were used in nulliparas.[388] Depending on the amount of tissue removed, cervical cone biopsy may lead to reduced cervical competence, but has less risk than is commonly thought.[389] Patients with a higher concentration of smooth muscle relative to collagen fibers in the cervix may be at increased risk for cervical incompetence.[386] Congenital structural changes in the cervix can occur in association with Müllerian uterine malformations or after diethylstilbestrol (DES) exposure. We have followed women with prior conization, Müllerian anomalies, and in utero DES exposure with serial transvaginal sonography, and have had success in selecting candidates for cerclage when funneling or shortening below 20 mm occurs, thus limiting cerclage to relatively few patients with these risk factors.

Diagnosis

Reduced cervical competence is a clinical diagnosis marked by gradual, painless dilatation and effacement of the cervix with membranes visible through the cervix. This history establishes the diagnosis, but is probably a fortuitous presentation; eventually, women with this cervical status may develop membrane rupture, labor, or even amnionitis with intact membranes. Short labors with the delivery of an immature fetus or loss of the pregnancy at progressively earlier gestational ages in successive pregnancies is characteristic of reduced competence. Until recently, objective criteria in the absence of the typical history have been lacking. Dilators or balloons to determine cervical resistance and/or hysterosalpingograms to measure the width of the cervical canal between pregnancies are neither sensitive nor specific, and digital examination of the cervix is highly subjective.[157,390] Sonography has provided a reproducible method of evaluating the cervix.[158,391] The sonographic characteristics of reduced competence are a short cervix, with a length of less than 20 mm, before 24 weeks' gestation often but not always accompanied by funneling of the internal os. Funneling may be thought of as "effacement in progress": The process proceeds from the inside out, beginning at the internal os and moving caudad. It may be first identified on digital exam by a subtle softening of the lower segment and on ultrasound examination by a narrow funnel or echolucent proximal third of the endocervical canal (Fig. 23–24A). As the process continues, the opening of the internal os becomes broader and the shoulders of the funnel more pronounced (Fig. 23–24B). Eventually, the shoulders disappear, leaving only a short cervical length. Remarkably, the process is dynamic, with the internal os opening and closing in response to fundal or suprapubic pressure or assumption of the standing position. Local or coordinated uterine activity may accompany the funneling of the internal os, but more commonly there is no palpable or measurable uterine contraction. Note that these criteria are essentially identical to those seen in preterm labor, differing only in the absence of contractions and the earlier gestational age at which the reduced competence phenomenon occurs. Zilianti et al.[392] have suggested a useful acronym to describe the process of effacement as seen by transvaginal sonography: TYVU. These letters form, in chronologic sequence, the sonographic appearance of the cervical canal and lower segment as it changes from the uneffaced T to the beginning funnel Y, with further shortening to V, and finally to a fully developed lower uterine segment, U. Because of the variation of the appearance of the upper funneled portion of the cervix, we have concentrated on accurate measurement of the residual lower cervical length as the most consistent measurement, both serially for each woman and for comparison with other centers.

A diagnosis of reduced cervical competence may be made prior to pregnancy or in the first trimester, if a typical history of painless dilatation and effacement of the cervix in a prior pregnancy can be documented. Women with a history of a previous second-trimester loss in which cervical sonography documented the classic picture of funneling and shortened cervical length are also candidates for prophylactic cerclage sutures. However, when the history is atypical or uncertain, it is more appropriate to follow the patient closely with frequent transvaginal ultrasound examinations beginning at 16 to 18 weeks' gestation, looking for the criteria noted above, and for funneling in response to fundal pressure. Funneling did not occur in response to fundal pressure in 150 normal pregnancies, but was seen in 14 of 31 women with a history suggestive of abnormal competence.[393] Without a history of early preterm birth, the appearance of spontaneous or induced funneling after 24 weeks of pregnancy does not establish a diagnosis of cervical incompetence, nor does it require a cerclage. The obstetric history and the cervical length exclusive of any funneling are the most predictive. The appearance of a funnel with a normal residual length has little import.

When reduced cervical competence presents unexpectedly in a patient without a worrisome history, the initial symptoms may include a sense of pelvic pressure, low backache, or premenstrual molimina accompanied by an increase in vaginal discharge that may be light tan or blood streaked. Sonography at this point will usually reveal a large funnel and substantial shortening, with or without dilation of the external os. Later, overt fluid leakage or contractions may ensue.

Cerclage Technique

Prophylactic Cerclage

In 1955, Shirodkar[394] reported successful management of cervical incompetence with a submucosal band of Mersilene tape, placed at the level of the internal os. This procedure requires anterior displacement of the bladder and submucosal dissection. The Shirodkar cerclage may be difficult to remove so that successful pregnancies may require delivery via cesarean section. Several years later, McDonald[395] described the use of a purse-string technique that could easily be performed during pregnancy. This approach involves either four or five "bites" as high on the cervix as possible. A metal catheter may be used to help identify the margin of the bladder. The knot is placed anteriorly to facilitate removal. This operative technique is illustrated in Figure 23–25. We use two purse-string stitches of 5 Ethibond, but there are many suitable variations. The McDonald procedure has proved to be as effective as the Shirodkar technique[396] and requires considerably less dissection. Prophylactic cerclage sutures may be placed at 10 to 15 weeks' gestation. We do not use tocolytics at the time of prophylactic cerclage, but do give perioperative antibiotics. Intercourse, prolonged (>90 minutes) standing, and heavy lifting are omitted following cerclage. We follow these patients with periodic vaginal sonography to assess stitch location and funneling.[397] No addi-

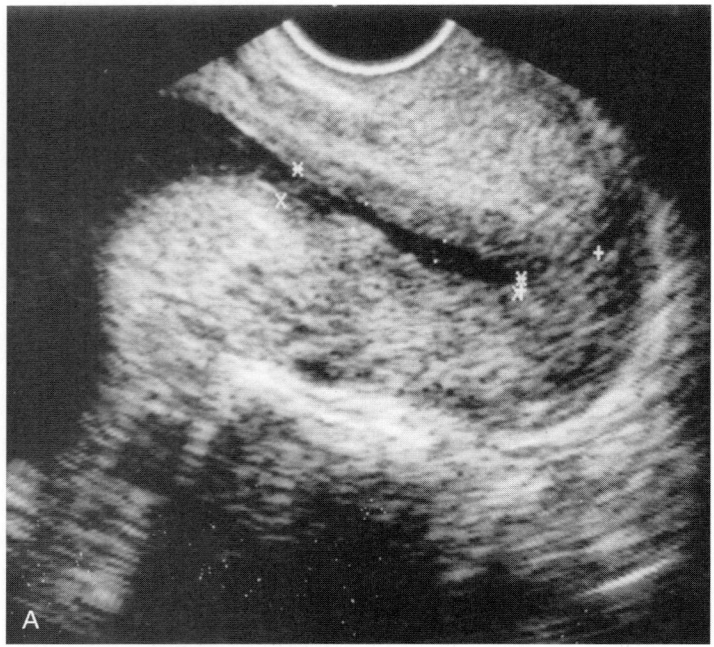

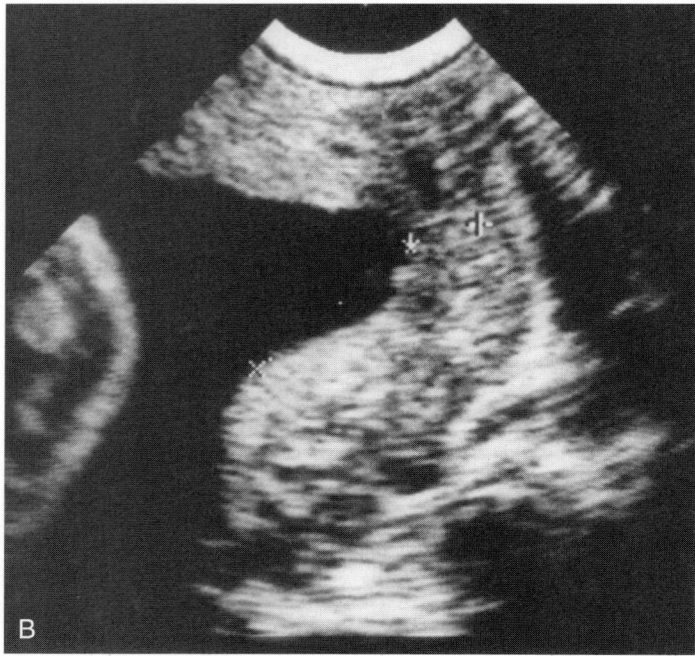

Figure 23–24. *A,* Transvaginal ultrasound image of the cervix in a woman with abnormal cervical competence showing mild separation of the canal or early evidence of funneling. Cervical length is marked by the (+) caliper; the other calipers define the funnel. *B,* Transvaginal ultrasound image of the cervix in a woman with abnormal cervical competence showing a marked funnel. The (−) caliper shows the length of the remaining cervix and the (×) caliper the length of the funnel.

tional restrictions are recommended as long as the stitches remain within the middle or upper third of the cervix without the development of a funnel, and the length of the cervix is greater than 25 mm. Some shortening of the cervix should be expected after 20 weeks. In fact, if the cervical length remains greater than 35 mm throughout the second trimester, the accuracy of the original diagnosis may be questioned.[398] For patients who have not been successful with a vaginal su-

ture despite aggressive ancillary care and sonographic surveillance, a transabdominal cerclage may be appropriate.[399]

Emergency Cerclage

Care of the patient with newly detected reduced cervical competence in the second trimester is both difficult and controversial. The introduction of sonography has

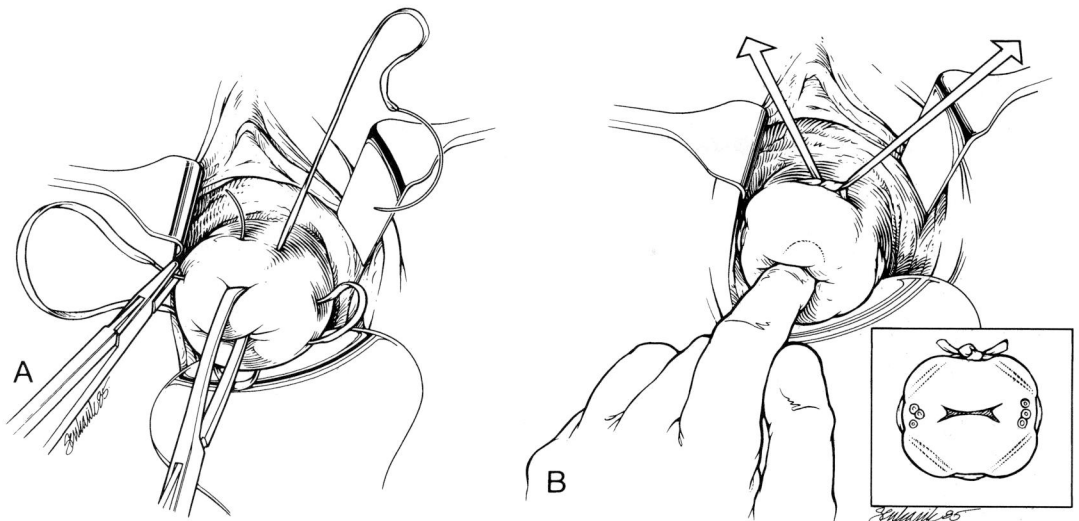

Figure 23–25. Placement of sutures for McDonald cervical cerclage. *A,* We use a double-headed Mersilene band with four "bites" in the cervix, avoiding the vessels. *B,* The suture is placed high upon the cervix close to the cervical-vaginal junction, approximately the level of the internal os.

been helpful in making early diagnoses and avoiding the complications that accompany advanced dilation and effacement. When the diagnosis is made before cervical dilation has occurred and when there is still 10 to 15 mm or more of cervical length, we admit the patient for 24 hours of treatment with perioperative indomethacin and broad-spectrum antibiotics before placing the cerclage sutures, and observe the patient for 48 to 96 hours postoperatively. However, if the cervix has dilated to allow visualization of the membranes, the patient may remain hospitalized for several days after cerclage placement. The prognosis for these patients is better than generally expected, with many women delivering a "viable" (usually defined as >1,000 g) infant, but aggressive therapy may be required to achieve these results. The prognosis is influenced by the gestational age at the time the heroic suture is placed.[400] If the sutures appear tenuous, prolonged hospitalization with Trendelenburg position may be required.

In the setting of advanced dilatation with bulging membranes, several techniques may be helpful. First, careful inspection of the membranes to identify separation or loss of the chorion from the intact amnion should be performed. If only the amnion remains, prolongation of pregnancy beyond a few days is unlikely. Precerclage amniocentesis to remove sufficient fluid to reduce the bulging membranes can be helpful. Overfilling the bladder with 1,000 ml of saline may help by elevating the membranes out of the operative field, but may also obstruct the surgeon's view.[401] We often place a Foley catheter balloon inside the cervix, and overfill it with at least 50 ml of saline to gently push the membranes out of the lower segment. The cerclage can then

be placed and tied as the balloon fluid is evacuated. Cerclage is rarely performed after 24 to 25 weeks of pregnancy. The great risk of inducing PROM or preterm labor and the ability to prolong gestation with bed rest and suppressive medications argue against surgical intervention in such cases.

The cerclage is removed at 37 weeks' gestation or at the onset of labor.

Risks of Cerclage

Cervical injury at the time of delivery is the most commonly reported morbidity from a McDonald cerclage. While fibrous scar tissue may form at the site of the stitch, producing an abnormal labor curve, most patients will have a normal labor curve after cerclage.[402] A fibrous "band" may rupture, leading to a cervical laceration (1 to 13 percent), or never dilate (cervical dystocia, 2 to 5 percent), requiring cesarean birth.[403] Rarely, a laceration may extend to the broad ligament or corpus of the uterus, requiring extensive repair or even hysterectomy.

For elective cerclage at the beginning of the second trimester, the risk of infection is small, estimated at less than 1 percent. Later in the pregnancy, displacement of the suture also can occur (3 to 12 percent). A second cerclage has a much lower success rate. Late complications of cerclage include PROM or preterm labor and chorioamnionitis; the risk varies with the duration of gestation and the presence of cervical dilation. When fluid leakage occurs in a patient with a cerclage, removal of the suture[404,405] to reduce the risk of infection is controversial.

Efficacy of Cervical Cerclage

There has never been a randomized prospective study documenting the benefit of cerclage for women with a "classic" history of cervical incompetence, but 80 to 90 percent of reported pregnancies in observational studies have resulted in live births of viable infants.[403]

Three prospective randomized trials of cerclage[169–171] have been conducted in patients with increased risk of preterm birth, *excluding* women with classic indications for cerclage. Two trials[170,171] found no benefit from cervical cerclage in this patient population, and one noted an increase in the need for antepartum hospitalization.[171] The third, a prospective randomized study that enrolled 905 women for whom the obstetrician was uncertain about the need for cerclage, found a small decrease in the occurrence of preterm births before 33 weeks in women treated with a cerclage compared with controls (13 percent vs. 18 percent, $p = 0.03$).[169] There were similar statistically significant reductions in birth weight under 1,500 g and in neonatal death.

PRETERM PREMATURE RUPTURE OF THE MEMBRANES

The fetal membranes normally rupture spontaneously during labor, presumably due to the physical effects of repetitive uterine contractions. Spontaneous rupture of the fetal membranes before the onset of labor is called premature rupture of the membranes (PROM) regardless of gestational age. Preterm PROM is defined as PROM that occurs before 37 weeks' gestation.

Etiology

The fetal membranes are made up of a thin layer of amnion and a thicker outer layer of chorion that is directly apposed to maternal decidual tissue. Interspersed between the amnion and chorion is a collagen-rich connective tissue zone that serves in part to replenish the amnion. By 26 weeks' gestation, the amnion is composed of a single layer of cuboidal cells. The chorion is four to six cell layers in thickness. The amnion has greater tensile strength than the chorion, although both membrane layers together withstand greater bursting pressures than they do separately. The amount of physical stress tolerated by the membranes decreases as pregnancy progresses. Membranes supported by a closed cervix require much greater pressures to rupture than do membranes covering an open area of 3 to 4 cm in diameter.[406] As gestational age advances, the relative concentration of collagen decreases as well.[407] These

factors help to maintain integrity of the membranes throughout pregnancy, yet allow rupture of membranes in labor at term.

Collagen maintenance and degradation are regulated in fetal membranes by the interaction of matrix metalloproteinases (MMPs) and specific tissue inhibitors (tissue inhibitor of matrix metalloproteinases [TIMPs]), so imbalances in the action of this system may be associated with preterm rupture.[408] Both collagenase and protease activity are increased in women with premature ruptured membranes.[409] These mechanisms of collagen maintenance and degradation may be altered in the presence of clinical risk factors that have been linked to the occurrence of preterm PROM, such as maternal gene expression,[410,411] connective tissue disorders (e.g., Ehlers-Danlos syndrome), genital tract infection or colonization with various microorganisms,[412] coitus,[413] low socioeconomic status,[41] uterine overdistention,[414] second- and third-trimester bleeding,[46] nutritional deficiencies of copper and ascorbic acid,[409] and maternal smoking.[46,409,415] One study[416] found that a short cervical length (≤ 25 mm) at 24 weeks was associated with preterm PROM that occurred weeks later. This suggests that the process leading to preterm PROM is chronic rather than acute in many cases.

Evidence of the association of infection with preterm PROM is abundant.[417] Naeye[413] observed an association between preterm PROM, recent coitus, and histologic chorioamnionitis. Histologic studies of the membranes after preterm PROM often demonstrate significant bacterial contamination along the choriodecidual interface with minimal involvement of the amnion. This suggests spread of the organisms along the maternal–fetal surfaces *before* membrane rupture.[418]

Specific genital tract pathogens have also been correlated with the occurrence of PROM. The organisms include *B. fragilis* and other anaerobes, *N. gonorrhoeae*, *C. trachomatis*, *T. vaginalis*, and group B β-hemolytic streptococci.[418] Group B streptococcal colonization was not associated with PROM in the Preterm Prediction Study.[416] A consistent association has been found between bacterial vaginosis and spontaneous preterm births, including those following preterm PROM (see earlier section of this chapter).

Diagnosis

The most common presentation is a gush of fluid from the vagina followed by persistent, uncontrolled leakage, but some patients report only intermittent leakage or perineal wetness. Any history of passing fluid through the vagina should be evaluated by a sterile speculum examination to collect fluid for confirmatory tests. Digital examination of the cervix in women with possible preterm labor or preterm PROM should be avoided until the diagnosis of ruptured membranes has been excluded. Because of the risk of introducing bacteria into the endocervix, digital examination for women with preterm PROM should be avoided until labor occurs or delivery is anticipated within 24 hours. Increased neonatal infection and mortality were observed when a digital examination precedes delivery by more than 24 hours in the presence of PROM.[419] Mean interval from rupture to delivery was much shorter (2.1 days vs. 11.3 days) in 121 women who had a digital examination compared with 144 women who had only a sterile speculum examination.[420] However, a study of 794 women with preterm PROM has challenged these traditional maxims, at least when the number of exams is less than or equal to 2.[421] In this study of a predominantly indigent population, 161 women had one, 27 had two, and 606 had no digital exams. There were no differences in the rates of chorioamnionitis, endometritis, early neonatal sepsis, or composite neonatal morbidity according to the number of exams. To avoid a digital exam, a visual estimate at the time of sterile speculum examination can sometimes identify women with advanced dilation.[422] The sterile speculum examination may also reveal a collection or "pool" of fluid that can be tested for pH with nitrazine paper. Since amniotic fluid is slightly alkaline (the pH is about 7.15), vaginal secretions containing amniotic fluid will usually result in pH changes in the blue-green range, 6.5 to 7.5. Nitrazine testing is accurate in 90 to 98 percent of cases.[423] False-positive values can result from infections that raise vaginal pH (e.g., *T. vaginalis*), the presence of blood, or rarely, cervical mucus. False-negative reactions are frequent when only a scant amount of fluid is present.

When placed on a clean slide and allowed to air dry, amniotic fluid produces a microscopic crystallization in

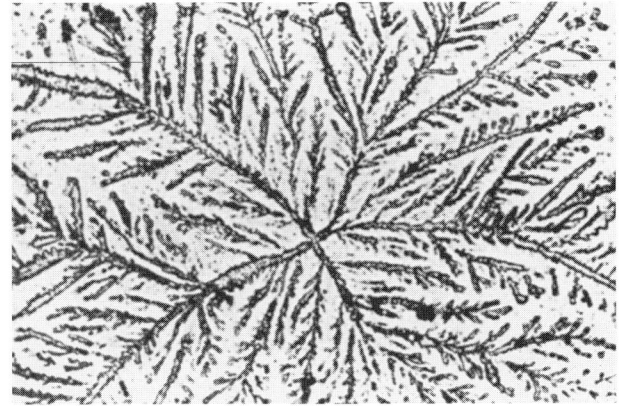

Figure 23–26. Demonstration of amniotic fluid arborization pattern. (From Reece EA, Chervenak F, Moya F, et al: Amniotic fluid arborization: Effect of blood, meconium, and pH alterations. Obstet Gynecol 64:248, 1984, with permission.)

a "fern" pattern. Figure 23–26 demonstrates the typical appearance. This phenomenon is due to the interaction of amniotic fluid proteins and salts and accurately confirms PROM in 85 to 98 percent of cases. False-positive tests can result from the collection of cervical mucus, which also "ferns," but usually in a more floral pattern. The fern test is unaffected by meconium, changes in vaginal pH, and blood/amniotic fluid ratios of up to 1:5. The fern pattern in samples heavily contaminated with blood is atypical and appears more "skeletonized."[424,425]

An ultrasound evaluation for amniotic fluid volume should be performed in women with preterm PROM to determine fetal presentation, fetal weight, and gestational age. If the diagnosis of membrane rupture is equivocal, a finding of decreased or absent fluid by ultrasound supports a diagnosis of ruptured membranes. When abundant residual fluid is observed in women after a confirmed diagnosis of PROM, the possibility of polyhydramnios prior to rupture should be considered. In uncertain cases, a repeat sterile speculum examination after the patient has rested in a semiupright position for approximately 1 hour to allow the pooling of secretions in the posterior vagina may be helpful. During this time, the woman may be monitored to evaluate fetal well-being and uterine contractions. Variable decelerations suggest umbilical cord compression secondary to reduced amniotic fluid volume. When all other tests are equivocal in a patient with reduced fluid and a good history, a vaginal swab for fetal fibronectin (fibronectin is abundant in amniotic fluid) may be helpful to exclude the diagnosis. In rare instances, an amniocentesis to inject a dilute solution of indigo carmine dye to look for transcervical leakage onto a tampon can be used to make an absolute diagnosis. Methylene blue dye has been associated with hemolytic anemia and hyperbilirubinemia in the infant and should not be used. Amniocentesis is seldom indicated, but its use underscores the importance of making an accurate diagnosis of ruptured membranes. Careful evaluation is required whenever PROM is suspected at any gestational age. Preterm PROM is not a diagnosis that can be made casually and should never be entirely excluded in any patient with either oligohydramnios or symptoms of persistent leakage.

Natural History

Care of women with preterm PROM is determined by estimation of the likely course of pregnancy in the absence of medical intervention. For women with preterm PROM between 20 and 34 weeks, the duration of pregnancy after PROM is inversely related to the gestational age at time of membrane rupture. When PROM occurs prior to 26 weeks' gestation, 30 to 40 percent of cases will gain at least 1 additional week before delivery and 20 percent will gain over 4 weeks.[426] By contrast, 70 to 80 percent of patients who experience PROM between 28 and 36 weeks' gestation deliver within the first week after PROM and more than one half of these within the first 4 days.[427] Between 32 and 34 weeks, the mean interval between rupture and delivery is 4 days.[428] At term, 80 percent enter labor within 24 hours after rupture of the membranes. These data describe the aggregate experience for women with preterm PROM, but it is difficult to predict the clinical course of an individual patient. Some reports have linked socioeconomic status to the likelihood of delivery and infection after preterm PROM. For example, a study of 298 indigent women with preterm PROM before 34 weeks found that 93 percent were in labor within 48 hours after membrane rupture.[429] The rate of chorioamnionitis in those managed expectantly was 16 percent. However, a study that compared 317 indigent women with 194 insured women found no difference in either the interval from rupture to delivery or the rate of chorioamnionitis.[430]

Maternal Risks

Whether a cause or result of preterm PROM, intrauterine infection is a potentially serous complication to the mother. Clinical chorioamnionitis accompanies preterm PROM in approximately 10 percent of cases (range, 3 to 30 percent).[418] Regardless of clinical signs of infection, as many as 25 to 30 percent of women with preterm PROM (range, 15 to 45 percent) will have a positive amniotic fluid culture. Most instances of amnionitis respond well to antibiotic treatment and delivery, but maternal deaths from sepsis can occur.[431] Amnionitis is more common when PROM occurs before 30–32 weeks.

Fetal and Neonatal Risks

Infection is a major potential complication for the fetus and neonate. The same organisms responsible for maternal infection can result in congenital pneumonia, sepsis, or meningitis. However, the majority of women with clinically overt amnionitis do not deliver infants who experience serious neonatal infection. In published series, the range of neonatal sepsis in cases of preterm PROM with or without clinical amnionitis is 2 to 19 percent. Neonatal deaths caused by infection are reported in 1 to 7 percent of infants born to women with chorioamnionitis. The frequency of neonatal infection varies considerably with gestational age, race, and maternal antepartum course, as well as the criteria for infection chosen. Studies requiring positive cultures for diagnosis tend to detect lower sepsis rates than those

---

Infectious Risks after Preterm PROM

Cord prolapse
  More common in non vertex presentations
Cesarean delivery
  Failed induction—44 percent cesarean births, all for failed induction
Abruption: 3 studies associated prolonged PROM with abruption
  5 to 6 percent of preterm PROMs; abruption rate = 25 percent if bleeding after PROM
Pulmonary hypoplasia
  Correlates with gestational age at time of rupture[436]
    19 wk: 50 percent
    22 wk: 25 percent
    26 wk: <10 percent
Respiratory distress syndrome
  Reduced rates of respiratory distress after preterm PROM have been inconsistently observed

---

combining clinical course, radiographic findings, and neonatal bacterial colonization for diagnosis.

Other noninfectious fetal complications that may occur after preterm PROM shown in the box.

There is a higher risk of frank or occult cord prolapse, particularly if the fetus is not in a cephalic presentation. Regardless of presentation, the risks of fetal distress in labor leading to cesarean delivery are significantly higher with preterm PROM than with isolated preterm labor (7.9 vs. 1.5 percent).[432] The most common fetal heart rate tracing leading to operative delivery is severe variable decelerations due to cord compression. Amnioinfusion may be used to prevent or reduce cord compression secondary to oligohydramnios (see Chapter 14).

Placental abruption occurs in 4 to 6 percent of cases of preterm PROM, especially when PROM is accompanied by bleeding.[433,434] A 15 percent rate of abruption has been observed when patients with prolonged preterm PROM manifest vaginal bleeding in addition to fluid leakage. When abruption occurs after PROM, the rate of acute intrapartum fetal distress approaches 50 percent.[435]

Pulmonary hypoplasia is a particular concern when fetal membranes are ruptured prior to 26 weeks' gestation. About 25 percent of babies delivered after 26 weeks' gestation following PROM that occurred before 26 weeks' gestation were found to have pulmonary hypoplasia following birth.[426] The duration and degree of oligohydramnios are associated with the chance of pulmonary hypoplasia. The frequency of pulmonary hypo-

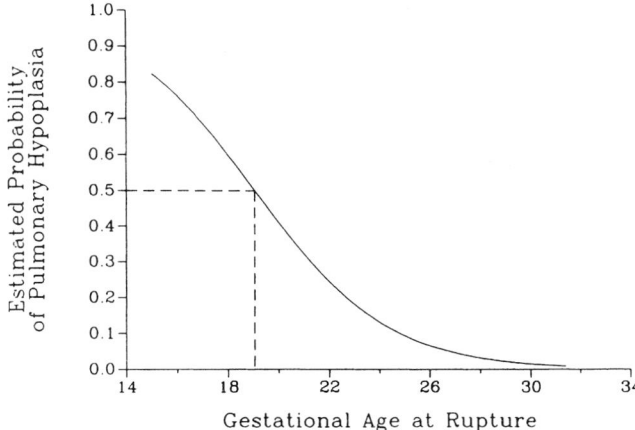

Figure 23–27. Curve relating probability of pulmonary hyperplasia to gestational age at time of rupture of membranes. (From Rotschild A, Ling EW, Peterman ML, Farquharson D: Neonatal outcome after prolonged preterm rupture of the membranes. Am J Obstet Gynecol 162:46, 1990, with permission.)

plasia is most consistently correlated with gestational age at rupture.[436,437] When rupture occurs before 19 weeks, approximately 50 percent of infants will have hypoplastic lungs (Fig. 23–27). The rate falls to 25 percent for infants born at 22 weeks, and to less than 10 percent at 26 weeks or later.

Prediction of pulmonary hypoplasia has been attempted by measuring residual fluid volume, lung length, comparison of the thoracic and abdominal circumferences, assessment of fetal breathing, and Doppler studies of perinasal amniotic fluid motion. None have added significantly to estimates of risk based upon the gestational age at the time of rupture.

Skeletal deformities may occur due to compression but usually resolve within 12 months. In one series, 27 percent of fetuses born after prolonged PROM before 26 weeks developed skeletal deformations.[438]

Initial Evaluation and Management

After the diagnosis of preterm PROM has been confirmed, maternal and fetal indications for immediate delivery should be ruled out before considering other management options. The most dangerous fetal complications of PROM at any gestational age are prolapse of the umbilical cord, and fetal bradycardia caused by cord compression. The principal maternal indication for delivery is chorioamnionitis. If a firm diagnosis of chorioamnionitis can be made by the presence of maternal fever greater than or equal to 101°F, uterine tenderness, and leukocytosis greater than or equal to 20,000/mm³, delivery should be undertaken promptly regardless of the gestational age. In the absence of indications for immediate delivery, gestational age should be carefully assessed to estimate the relative risks for the fetus of

delivery versus expectant management (see below). All clinical and ultrasound dating criteria should be reviewed. Because oligohydramnios may flatten the fetal head, biparietal diameter measurements to estimate fetal weight by ultrasound may be inaccurate in women with preterm PROM.[439] Fetal tables based on head circumference, femur length, or cerebellar diameter are more reliable indicators of gestational age and fetal weight in these situations.

Before 30 to 32 weeks' gestation, the neonatal risks of prematurity will usually outweigh the in utero risks of infection and fetal compromise caused by oligohydramnios, while the reverse is usually the case after 34 to 35 weeks' gestation.[440] A randomized trial of expectant management versus immediate delivery in 120 women with preterm PROM between 34 and 37 weeks at a university center found that both chorioamnionitis (16 percent vs. 2 percent) and the duration of maternal hospitalization (5.2 ± 6.8 vs. 2.6 ± 1.6 days) were greater in the expectantly managed group.[441] A retrospective observational report from a private hospital of 236 women with preterm PROM between 32 and 36 weeks found no advantage to expectant management after 34 weeks. Before 34 weeks, modest benefits in neonatal hospital days and hyperbilirubinemia were observed.[442] Consideration of individual risks forms the basis for management for women with preterm PROM and is among the most challenging tasks in obstetrics. The relative risks of prematurity, infection, and fetal well-being must be repeatedly evaluated for expectantly managed patients with preterm PROM. As will be evident in the following paragraphs, the methods of risk assessment are not uniformly satisfactory.

Amniocentesis for Women with Preterm PROM

Assessment of amniotic fluid for infection and maturity studies should always be considered in women with preterm PROM. Expectant management requires repeated assessment of mother and fetus for evidence of maternal and fetal infection, cord prolapse, and abruption. Demonstration of either fetal pulmonary maturity or intra-amniotic bacteria may allow a decision for delivery, thus obviating the difficulties of fetal and maternal surveillance. Amniotic fluid may be obtained from either free-flowing vaginal fluid or amniocentesis for studies of fetal maturity, but amniocentesis is required to obtain fluid for culture, Gram stain, and glucose tests for infection. Placing the patient in the Trendelenburg position prior to the amniocentesis may facilitate the procedure by favoring intrauterine retention of fluid. Amniocentesis has been successfully accomplished in 50[427] to 96 percent[443] of reported series of patients with preterm PROM. The success rate is apparently influenced primarily by the aggressiveness of the investigators. Although the amniotic fluid pocket may be small, amniocentesis is reasonably safe when performed with ultrasound guidance. A literature review reported the risk of fetal injury to be between 0.6 and 2.0 percent and that of placenta and cord injury to be 0.3 to 1.1 percent.[444] If there is free-flowing amniotic fluid in the vaginal vault at the time of sterile speculum examination, it may be used for lung maturity testing, but is not reliable for infection studies.[445] Bacterial contaminants in vaginally collected fluid have been reported to produce phosphatidylglycerol, creating a false impression of fetal lung maturity with this test.[446]

In a study[427] of amniocentesis in women with PROM between 28 and 34 weeks, none of the 98 patients who had an amniocentesis demonstrated signs of clinical amnionitis, and none were in labor. A mature lecithin/sphingomyelin (L/S) ratio of at least 1.8:1 was found in 39 percent of samples. An additional 13 percent had Gram stains of unspun amniotic fluid that demonstrated the presence of bacteria. Thus, 52 percent of these asymptomatic women were delivered expeditiously because of amniotic fluid findings. In another study of amniotic fluid results between 32 and 36 weeks' gestation in 164 women with preterm PROM, there were 13 (7.9 percent) with immature lung studies, 12 (7.3 percent) in whom fluid could not be obtained, and 4 (2.4 percent) with chorioamnionitis.[447] Ninety-three subjects with mature amniotic fluid studies and reassuring fetal heart rate testing consented to be randomized to either induction of labor or expectant management. Women in whom labor was induced had a lower rate of chorioamnionitis (10.9 percent vs. 27.7 percent) and shorter hospital stays (2.3 vs. 3.5 days). There was no difference in the cesarean section rate. Infants born after expectant management were treated more often for suspected sepsis, but there was no difference in neonatal survival or significant morbidity. These trials support the value of obtaining amniotic fluid maturity testing in women with preterm PROM after 32 weeks' gestation.

Tests for Infection in Patients with Preterm PROM

Expectant management of preterm PROM requires initial and continued surveillance for infection. Ultimately, the end point for tests of "infection" in this clinical setting should be clinically important maternal or fetal/neonatal infection. Intermediate end points (e.g., amniotic fluid bacteria, white blood cells, glucose, and even culture), while associated with perinatal infection, do not equate uniformly with clinical infectious morbidity or mortality. The incidence of clinical amnionitis approximates 10 percent (range, 3 to 30 percent) in women with preterm PROM. Of infants born to mothers with clinical amnionitis, only 1 to 15 percent will have positive cultures that confirm a diagnosis of neonatal sepsis. Finally, the rate of perinatal mortality caused by infection has ranged from 0 to 13 percent in studies of infants born after preterm PROM. The principal causes of perinatal morbidity and mortality after preterm PROM are still more often related to prematurity (e.g., respiratory distress syndrome, intraventricular hemorrhage) than to infection. Nevertheless, when it occurs, neonatal infection can be devastating. It is important to make an early diagnosis of infection because a two- to fourfold increase in perinatal mortality, intraventricular hemorrhage, and neonatal sepsis has been reported in infants born after amnionitis compared with gestational age-matched controls born to noninfected mothers.[448] Importantly, antepartum treatment of maternal amnionitis clearly decreases the incidence of neonatal sepsis (Table 23–17).[449–451]

Clinical surveillance of expectantly managed patients with preterm PROM includes frequent examinations for maternal heart rate, contractions, uterine tenderness, fever greater than or equal to 38°C, and biophysical profile or nonstress testing, looking for variable decelerations, tachycardia, and absent movement. An extensive review of laboratory tests to detect intrauterine infection concluded that none was wholly satisfactory.[452] White blood cell counts are customary in patients with preterm PROM, but are not always predictive of the presence or absence of chorioamnionitis. An elevated maternal leukocyte count has a reported sensitivity of 23 to 80 percent, a specificity of 60 to 95 percent, a positive predictive value of 50 to 75 percent, and a negative predictive value of 40 to 90 percent to predict clinical or histologic amnionitis.[453]

Nonstress testing (NST) for patients with preterm PROM is appropriate to look for evidence of cord compression, but may not be a reliable test for incipient or occult infection. A biophysical profile score of less than 6 has been related to subsequent maternal or neonatal infection.[454] However, when compared in a randomized clinical trial, both daily nonstress and biophysical profile testing had low sensitivity (39 percent vs. 25 percent, respectively) to predict subsequent infectious

Table 23–17. IMPORTANCE OF ANTEPARTUM DIAGNOSIS AND TREATMENT OF AMNIONITIS

| First Author | Ref | N | Neonatal Sepsis | |
			If Treated Antepartum	If Treated Postpartum
Sperling	449	257	2.8%	19.6%
Gilstrap	451	273	1.5%	5.7%
Gibbs	450	45	0	21.0%

morbidity in 135 women with preterm PROM, all of whom received antibiotics for group B streptococcal prophylaxis.[455] Specificity was 85 percent for the NST and 93 percent for the biophysical profile. Clinical, laboratory, and biophysical surveillance each contribute to management, but all have suboptimal sensitivity and must be repeated frequently. Amniotic fluid obtained by amniocentesis can be used to detect amnionitis, based on demonstration of bacteria on a Gram stain of unspun fluid, amniotic fluid glucose levels, or the presence of IL-6. Approximately 10^5 organisms/ml are needed before a Gram stain will be positive. Thus, not all culture-positive fluids have positive Gram stains, though virtually all positive Gram stains result from culture-positive fluids. The Gram stain for bacteria has reported sensitivity ranging from 36 to 80 percent, and a specificity of 80 to 97 percent to predict a subsequent positive culture. Amniotic fluid culture has a reported sensitivity of 65 to 85 percent and a specificity of 85 percent to predict clinical chorioamnionitis. The presence of white blood cells in amniotic fluid has not proven helpful in predicting infection, but a low amniotic fluid glucose (≤ 16 to 20 mg/dl) has been found to correlate well with a positive fluid culture, with sensitivity and specificity of approximately 80 to 90 percent. The amniotic fluid glucose is simple, rapid, and available around the clock. A study of 108 women with preterm PROM to identify clinical characteristics that were associated with a positive Gram stain found associations with earlier gestational age, maternal temperature, and white blood cell count, and for fetal tachycardia and nonreactive fetal heart rate tracings.[453] Evaluation of amniotic fluid from 127 women with preterm labor and 26 with preterm PROM revealed that the combination of Gram stain and amniotic fluid glucose were superior to either test alone to predict a positive culture.[456] Interleukin-6 in amniotic fluid is also a good marker for intra-amniotic fluid infection.[457]

Management Strategies

When a thorough assessment reveals no evidence of fetal distress or infection, and fetal pulmonary maturity cannot be confirmed, three management options remain. The first is conservative or expectant management, in which the patient is hospitalized for intensive surveillance for signs of fetal compromise or infection, at which time labor is allowed or induced if necessary. This approach is associated with a low rate of cesarean delivery, but relies upon methods of fetal assessment that must be performed at least daily and, as noted, are not always accurate. An alternate choice is immediate delivery for pregnancies beyond a certain gestational age (e.g., ≥ 32 weeks) or estimated fetal weight (e.g., $\geq 1,500$ to 1,800 g). This strategy avoids the need for ongoing surveillance for fetal well-being and infection,

but commits to delivery some women who might have continued the pregnancy long enough to allow additional fetal development and reduced neonatal morbidity. This strategy has a high rate of cesarean delivery for failed induction. The third strategy is an attempt to delay delivery in order to influence the relative risks of prematurity and infection. For example, antibiotics have been found to reduce morbidity and prolong pregnancy[458] and corticosteroids are effective for reducing fetal morbidity, (especially intraventricular hemorrhage) and mortality, when given to women with PROM before 32 weeks. Any of the three strategies may be an appropriate choice, depending on the gestational age and individual assessments of the risk of infection and prematurity. For example, expectant management is often chosen for women who present before 26 to 28 weeks, immediate delivery for women after 32 to 34 weeks, with interventionist strategies employed between 26 and 34 weeks. Adherence to a single strategy for all women with preterm PROM ignores the important individual differences among patients' risk of infection and immaturity.

Corticosteroids and Antibiotics

Antenatal corticosteroids appear to reduce the risk of intraventricular hemorrhage for infants born before 32 weeks, regardless of the status of the membranes before delivery. Because grades III and IV intraventricular hemorrhages are rare after 32 weeks, the decision to use steroids after 32 weeks depends on analyses of the effect of steroids on morbidity other than IVH. As noted above, randomized trials of the effect of corticosteroids on RDS in the presence of PROM have revealed conflicting results.

It is not clear whether women with preterm PROM should receive more than one course of antenatal steroids. A significant increase in early-onset neonatal sepsis was observed in 72 infants born to women with preterm PROM who had received multiple courses of steroids when compared with 99 who received one course, and 203 who did not receive steroids.[460] Multiple courses were also significantly related to chorioamnionitis and postpartum endometritis. The 1994 NICHD Consensus Conference encouraged more study of steroids for reduction of RDS in preterm PROM after 32 weeks.[370] The ACOG also advocates caution in using steroids for preterm PROM after 32 weeks.[326] At our center, we currently administer a single course of antenatal steroids to expectantly managed patients with preterm PROM up to 34 weeks.

Because the risk of perinatal group B streptococcal infection is associated with both premature birth and duration of membrane rupture before delivery, women with preterm PROM prior to 37 weeks should be treated presumptively with an appropriate antibiotic.

The importance of maternal antibiotics for group B streptococcal prophylaxis in preterm PROM has been well established and is endorsed by both the ACOG[327] and by the American Academy of Pediatrics.[461]

Antibiotic prophylaxis has also been studied as a method of prolonging the interval from rupture to delivery in an effort to reduce perinatal morbidity and mortality due to infection and prematurity. A multicenter trial enrolled 614 women with preterm PROM between 24 and 32 weeks in a study that compared combined neonatal morbidity and mortality in subjects randomly assigned to receive treatment with either antibiotics or placebo within 72 hours of amniorrhexis[458] (Table 23–18). The antibiotic group received 48 hours of intravenous ampicillin and erythromycin, followed by oral amoxicillin and erythromycin for 5 days or until delivery. Erythromycin was combined with ampicillin to treat *Mycoplasma* and *Ureaplasma urealyticum*. None of the subjects in this trial received antenatal corticosteroids. Women in both groups who were colonized with group B streptococcus were treated with open-label ampicillin or erythromycin in addition to their assigned study regimen; these 118 subjects were analyzed separately. The primary outcome was composite mortality and morbidity including sepsis within 72 hours of birth, RDS, grade III to IV intraventricular hemorrhage, and stage 2 to 3 necrotizing enterocolitis. The mortality rate was 5 percent in both groups, but the antibiotic group had significantly less morbidity as shown in Table 23–18. Latency was prolonged in the antibiotic group. Infants born to women who were treated for positive group B streptococcus cultures did as well as the antibiotic study group. As might be expected in a study that enrolled a largely indigent population, chorioamnionitis was relatively common in both groups.

The combined use of antibiotics and corticosteroids appears to confer greater benefit than either treatment alone for women with preterm PROM. One study randomized women with preterm PROM who were expec-tantly managed and treated with ampicillin-sulbactam to receive either betamathasone or no steroids.[462] There were no differences in neonatal or maternal infectious morbidity, but the group that received steroids had fewer cases of respiratory distress, 18.4 percent vs. 43.6 percent, than the no-steroid group. However, this trial had a small sample size ($n = 77$), did not employ a placebo, and observed a relatively high rate of RDS in the control group. Another trial enrolled and randomly assigned 112 women with preterm PROM, all of whom were treated with corticosteroids, to treatment with one of two antibiotic regimens or placebo.[463] Neonatal mortality, sepsis, and respiratory morbidity were less common in the combined antibiotic groups compared with the placebo group.

In summary, prophylactic antibiotics should be given to all women with preterm PROM to reduce the risk of neonatal group B streptococcal infection. Significant reductions in composite neonatal morbidity can also be achieved with broad-spectrum antibiotic treatment, especially in populations with a high prevalence of chorioamnionitis. Furthermore, combined treatment with corticosteroids benefits infants born after preterm PROM before 32 weeks of pregnancy.

Use of Tocolytics

There is currently little evidence to support routine use of tocolytic agents in women with preterm PROM. A report from the National Institutes of Health Collaborative Study on Antenatal Steroids noted an association between tocolytic use in PROM and a higher rate of RDS.[464] Prospective randomized trials of prophylactic tocolysis revealed no consistent benefit to adjunctive tocolytics for these patients.[465,466] However, the studies cited above that suggest benefit for adjunctive antibiotics and steroids have raised anew the question of short-term tocolysis in order to allow a course of steroids and antibiotics.

Table 23–18. EFFECT OF PROPHYLACTIC ANTIBIOTICS ON PERINATAL MORBIDITY IN INFANTS BORN TO WOMEN WITH PRETERM PROM

	Ampicillin + Erythromycin (n = 239)	Placebo (n = 257)	RR	95% CI
All morbidity	45%	55%	0.82	0.69–0.98
RDS	41%	51%	0.80	0.66–0.97
Sepsis	8%	15%	0.54	0.33–0.88
Pneumonia	3%	7%	0.42	0.18–0.96
Chronic lung disease	14%	21%	0.68	0.46–1.00
Amnionitis	24%	34%	0.70	0.53–0.93

Data from Mercer BM, Miodovnik M, Thurnau GR, et al: Antibiotic therapy for reduction of infant morbidity after preterm premature rupture of the membranes. JAMA 278:989, 1997.

Preterm PROM in Special Circumstances

Preterm PROM before 26 weeks of pregnancy has diverse etiologies that may alter management. For instance, PROM may occur following amniocentesis. If the amniocentesis was performed for genetic studies or evaluation of rhesus disease, a good outcome should be expected. A brief course of bed rest and expectant management until the leakage stops and does not resume is usually all that is required. However, infection and/or delivery are likely if the amniocentesis was performed to evaluate a patient with advanced cervical dilation or preterm labor. When preterm PROM occurs in a woman who has experienced persistent second-trimester bleeding, especially when accompanied as well by a history of prerupture oligohydramnios and/or an elevated maternal serum α-fetoprotein, the prognosis for a surviving infant is poor. These patients often have had abnormal placental implantation noted on ultrasound evaluation. Management of these patients should include a thorough history and placental evaluation, to detect placental trauma or loss of a blighted twin, and an attempt to obtain both placental and fetal samples for karyotype. Other possible diagnoses for second-trimester losses (e.g., fetal anomaly or aneuploidy, uterine anomalies, DES, incompetent cervix, and maternal trauma), both exogenous and self induced, should all be considered.

When preterm PROM occurs before 26 weeks, risks for both mother and fetus are higher than for PROM later in pregnancy and decisions are more difficult. Because neonatal outcome for infants born before 24 to 25 weeks is poor, immediate delivery is not an easy choice. On the other hand, expectant management carries concern about maternal risks and an uncertain outcome for the fetus. Maternal risk is the first concern. A review[467] of 898 women with early preterm PROM reported in 11 observational studies found that only six women (0.7 percent) developed sepsis; however, there was a single maternal death. Other maternal risks of expectant management include the consequences of activity restriction: muscle wasting, bone demineralization, venous thromboembolism, and its prophylaxis (e.g., heparin-induced thrombocytopenia). In the collected series cited above, 15 percent of infants were stillborn, 39 percent died before 28 days of life, and 46 percent (417 of 914) survived the neonatal period. Among 195 infants who were followed for 3 to 36 months, 119 (61 percent) had normal neurologic examinations.[467]

A 1990 report found that the strongest determinant of survival was the occurrence of pulmonary hypoplasia, which in turn was related principally to gestational age at the time of rupture.[436] Only 8 of 74 infants without pulmonary hypoplasia (11 percent) died, compared with 10 of 14 (71 percent) of infants with evidence of pulmonary hypoplasia. Improved neonatal and

2-year outcomes for infants born after extremely preterm PROM were reported from Sweden in 1998.[468] Among 53 pregnancies complicated by PROM at 14 to 28 weeks, neonatal survival rates were 40 percent ($n = 10$) when rupture occurred between 14 and 19 weeks and 88 percent when rupture occurred between 20 and 25 weeks ($n = 24$). At 2 years of age, three of four surviving infants born after PROM at 14 to 19 weeks, and 13 of 20 survivors born after PROM at 20 to 25 weeks had no neurologic impairment. The mean age at delivery in both groups was 27 weeks, with mean latent periods of 70 and 19 days. This encouraging report may not apply to many North American populations. Given the data cited here, it is easy to see why decisions about management in this setting are so complex. Fortunately, the literature supports the maternal safety of a period of observation for these women to allow time for an informed decision.

An observational study of 18 women with preterm PROM complicated by a history of maternal genital herpes simplex infection estimated that the theoretical maximum risk of neonatal HSV was no greater than 19 percent.[469] Prophylactic treatment with an antiviral agent such as acyclovir may be appropriate for these patients.

The question of whether to retain or remove a cerclage suture in women who later develop preterm PROM is controversial. One report favored removal,[404] but latency and perinatal outcome were not related to retention or removal of the cerclage suture in another study of 81 women with preterm PROM before 34 weeks.[405]

CONDUCT OF LABOR AND DELIVERY FOR THE PRETERM INFANT

Intrapartum care for women in labor before term is often accompanied by concerns unique to the preterm mother and her fetus. Many relate to the underlying reason(s) for preterm delivery. Complications such as maternal hypertension or fetal growth restriction may increase the chance of intrapartum fetal compromise because of poor placental function. Reduced or absent amniotic fluid may lead to umbilical cord compression during labor after preterm PROM, or when oligohydramnios occurs with intrauterine growth restriction (IUGR) or preeclampsia. When labor is induced preterm for maternal or fetal indications, the lower uterine segment and cervix may not be well prepared for labor, leading to a prolonged latent phase. When the cause of preterm labor is unclear, the possibility of occult abruption must be considered. Labor in women with amnionitis may be complicated by fever, fetal tachycardia, or inefficient contractions, any of which may lead to fetal compromise. Because digital examination of the cervix is avoided in women with expectantly managed preterm PROM, labor may not be recognized in these patients until it is well established. This recurrent problem can never be entirely avoided and requires constant vigilance by both nurses and physicians. Spontaneous preterm labor that begins at home may not be easily recognized by the woman, her family, or the medical care team. Finally, labor in women with reduced cervical competence may be relatively painless, again leading to delayed intrapartum surveillance of the preterm fetus.

Estimation of Gestational Age-Specific Neonatal Mortality and Morbidity

Infants born after 26 weeks experience intact survival rates in excess of 60 percent, but concerns about both the likelihood and quality of survival are important in the conduct of labor before 26 weeks. As neonatal and perinatal care has improved, the lower limit of "viability" has been a progressively earlier gestational age. Regionalized perinatal care, broader use of antenatal corticosteroids, and advances in neonatal care (e.g., surfactant treatment) have led to steady improvements in perinatal, neonatal, and infant morbidity and mortality. As many as 15 percent of infants born at 23 weeks, 56 percent at 24 weeks, and 80 percent at 25 weeks may now survive to hospital discharge in the postsurfactant era.[470] Several studies have reported that the expectation by the medical team of survival for the ELBW infant actually influences the likelihood of survival. A study of 66 infants with birth weights between 500 and 749 g found that after controlling for birth weight and gestational age, fetuses who were considered "viable" (i.e., likely to survive) were 18 times more likely to survive than fetuses who were deemed previable.[471] Another study of 713 infants with birth weights below 1,000 g found that, although cesarean delivery did not itself influence the rate of neonatal survival, the *willingness* to perform cesarean delivery was associated with higher rates of both intact and morbid survival for ELBW infants.[11] Parents and medical professionals often do not share the same beliefs about the quality of life[472] or the potential for intact survival in premature infants. The likelihood of survival is often underestimated by medical personnel[473] but, due to well-publicized but uncommon cases of intact survival among ELBW infants, may be overestimated by the patient and her family. Health care providers also may not invite parental and family participation in the decisions surrounding the birth of an extremely preterm infant.[474]

These observations underscore the importance of accurate information about neonatal outcome during labor management before 26 weeks of pregnancy. The "best obstetric estimate of gestational age," combining menstrual history and laboratory confirmation of pregnancy with earliest ultrasound biometry, is a more reliable antenatal predictor of neonatal survival than either estimated fetal weight or biparietal diameter (BPD).[475,476] One study identified ultrasound biometric thresholds (femur length <40 mm, BPD <54 mm, estimated weight <382 g, or estimated gestational age <22 weeks) below which there were no survivors, regardless of gestational age.[476] Unfortunately, infants who survived to 120 days with markers of serious long-term morbidity could not be distinguished before delivery from those who survived without morbidity markers by any antenatal information. Each patient's situation is unique. Kilpatrick and Piecuch developed a useful algorithm based on both literature and experience to begin discussions of intrapartum care and neonatal resuscitation, as shown in Table 23–19.[12,13] Information available after delivery (e.g., actual birth weight) more accurately predicts outcome than information before birth, so it is always important to remind parents that a neonatal reassessment of the very preterm infant's prognosis is appropriate.

Intrapartum Fetal Assessment

Fetal monitoring is especially important when the fetus is premature. The preterm fetus may tolerate labor poorly, and the cause of the preterm birth may create additional intrapartum risk. Careful fetal surveillance has been associated with significantly improved outcome. One study showed that attentive nursing care (one on one) for preterm fetuses with auscultation every 15 minutes gives perinatal mortality results equal to those with electronic fetal heart rate monitoring.[477] However, the same authors subsequently found that electronic monitoring provides better information about fetal and neonatal well-being.[478] Ominous heart rate

Table 23–19. INTRAPARTUM CARE AND NEONATAL RESUSCITATION AT 23 TO 25 WEEKS

Gestational Age	Cesarean for Distress?	Pediatrics at Delivery?
≤23 w, 6 d	No	No
24 to 24 w + 6 d	Advise against, but OK if family insists	Yes
≥25 w, 0 d	Yes	Weigh in delivery room

Data from Kilpatrick SJ, Schleuter MA, Piecuch R, et al: Outcome of infants born at 24–26 weeks' gestation: I. Survival and cost. Obstet Gynecol 90:803, 1997.

tracings have the same associations with fetal acidosis as they do later in gestation. Prompt intervention can minimize their effect on perinatal morbidity and mortality.[479,480] Mean fetal heart rate falls continuously, from 160 bpm at 22 weeks' gestation, to 140 bpm at term. This is apparently due to a gradual increase in parasympathetic tone. At no age after 26 to 28 weeks should the normal baseline heart rate be above 170 bpm. Changes in fetal heart rate variability in the preterm fetus carry the same or greater significance for risk of acidosis as in term infants. Although the concept that the preterm fetus may tolerate hypoxia in utero and after delivery may have some validity, particularly in considering prognosis, it should not affect management of preterm labor. Premature infants may sustain hypoxic-ischemic insults. Ominous patterns should be viewed with the same or greater level of concern as in term labor.

Anesthesia and Analgesia

There is no one method of anesthesia or analgesia in labor with a preterm fetus that is superior for all conditions. The goal of intrapartum care is to provide the neonatologist with the least traumatized, least depressed, and least acidotic fetus consistent with maternal health. Epidural anesthesia offers the advantage of pelvic floor and outlet muscle relaxation, minimizing an important source of resistance to the soft premature fetal head. Hypotension sometimes associated with this method can largely be avoided by adequate preloading with a crystalloid and more gradual onset of the block. Paracervical block is undesirable because of the risk of fetal bradycardia secondary either to transplacental passage of the anesthetic agent causing direct myocardial depression or to local uterine vascular vasospasm with diminished uteroplacental perfusion. The use of parenteral narcotics, even early in labor, is generally minimized because of concern for respiratory depression and because of the uncertain duration of preterm labor. Analgesia that allows maternal self-control is particularly helpful in the second stage of labor.

Anesthesia for cesarean delivery creates special concerns for each potential method when the fetus is preterm. The epidural technique requires a deeper, more intense block, involving more spinal segments than vaginal delivery. This may increase the chance of hypotension. General anesthesia is quicker to administer in an emergency situation and usually involves fewer changes in uteroplacental perfusion. However, it does entail greater risks to the mother, can lead to fetal depression if the surgery is difficult, and deprives the mother of perhaps her only chance to see and bond with a sick premature infant during its first hours of life.

Labor

The course of labor in a preterm gestation is often significantly shorter than that of term pregnancy. Of particular importance are the rapidity of the active phase and the short second stage of labor. Care should be taken to ensure that the fetus does not have a precipitous delivery without control of the fetal head.

Delivery

The principal goals of intrapartum management of the preterm infant are avoidance of perinatal acidosis and birth trauma. The role of perinatal acidosis was demonstrated by a study[481] of 136 neonates of less than 32 weeks' gestation in which the 1-minute Apgar score was highly correlated with survival. Preterm babies with 1-minute Apgar scores of 4 or more had a 95 percent survival, while infants with a score or 3 or less had only a 56 percent survival rate. The authors concluded that initial condition at birth affects survival. Although a generous episiotomy has been recommended to minimize the effect of perineal resistance on the small soft fetal head, data that demonstrate improved outcome associated with the use of episiotomy are difficult to find.[482] When delivering a VLBW infant, an early episiotomy is appropriate if there is perineal resistance. Few multiparous women will be in this group. Forceps may be employed for premature infants for the customary indications, but should not be used prophylactically. Studies of prophylactic forceps to protect the preterm infant's head from pressure during delivery have not shown benefit.[482]

Cesarean Delivery

Routine cesarean delivery of all preterm or VLBW infants is not justified by current literature.[483,484,485] Several large studies have failed to note improvement in perinatal morbidity or mortality with cesarean birth for indications other than classic obstetric ones.[483,485] Trends favoring cesarean delivery disappear after adjustment for confounding factors.[483] Kitchen et al.[485] found that the only antenatal intervention that was associated with improved outcome at 2 years of age was antenatal treatment with corticosteroids. Grant et al. reviewed six trials that addressed immediate neonatal and maternal morbidities after vaginal versus cesarean delivery for infants born between 24 and 36 weeks.[486] This review found increased risk of maternal morbidity with cesarean section without clear benefit for the infant. Neonatal intracranial hemorrhage appears to occur as often before and after cesarean as it does during labor and vaginal delivery.

For infants in breech presentation, there are intuitive reasons for cesarean birth, particularly to avoid trapping of the aftercoming head and other manipulations that could lead to trauma or hypoxia. Older retrospective studies that suggested a benefit for cesarean delivery led to the current custom of cesarean delivery for preterm breech fetuses, but support for this practice remains weak. Wolf et al. compared rates of survival without disability at 2 years for two cohorts of preterm (26 to 31 weeks) infants born between 1984 and 1989. At one hospital, the custom was vaginal delivery ($n = 101$), while the other preferred abdominal birth ($n = 46$). Multivariate analysis found that footling presentation was associated with a greater likelihood of poor outcome (OR, 0.4; 95 percent CI, 0.2 to 0.9) and antenatal steroid treatment more than 24 hours before birth with improved outcome (OR, 2.7; 95 percent CI, 1.1 to 6.8) but no effect of mode of delivery.[487]

When cesarean delivery for the preterm breech is chosen, it is illogical to avoid a traumatic vaginal delivery only to encounter a difficult cesarean birth because of an undeveloped lower uterine segment or an inadequate incision. Clearly, the operation must be carried out in a way that will fulfill its purpose: atraumatic delivery through a generous incision. While some have recommended routine use of a low vertical or classic incision, the exact uterine incision can depend on the fetal position and on the anatomy of the individual patient. If the lower uterine segment is well developed and the fetus is in the lower one third of the uterus, a transverse incision is reasonable.

In a study that carefully separated out "high-risk" VLBW labor (e.g., preeclampsia, vaginal bleeding, abnormal heart rate tracing) from "low-risk" VLBW (e.g., preterm labor, incompetent cervix), cesarean delivery was of no value in the low-risk group, but was associated with significantly improved survival rates in the high-risk group.[488] Thus there are situations requiring delivery in the face of a long closed cervix that may lead to a decision to cesarean delivery for VLBW fetuses rather than a long and potentially morbid induction of labor.

CONCLUSION

Only when the factors underlying preterm birth are understood will prevention occur. Tocolytics, glucocorticoids, and antibiotics are effective tertiary therapies, but can never be wholly effective in eliminating the morbidity and mortality due to prematurity. Inaccurate diagnosis of preterm labor is a major impediment to appropriate care for premature labor.

Key Points

➤ Preterm birth is the single greatest cause of perinatal morbidity and mortality in nonanomalous infants, responsible for 70 percent of fetal, neonatal, and infant deaths.

➤ The outcome for premature and low-birth-weight infants is better than most medical professionals believe it to be.

➤ Spontaneous preterm birth is a syndrome in which multiple risk factors operate collaboratively via injury to the maternal–fetal interface to produce several related clinical disorders.

➤ Preterm labor may be initiated by infection, ischemia/hemorrhage, uterine distention, or endocrine factors.

➤ Major risk factors for preterm birth are a prior history of preterm delivery, multifetal gestation, bleeding after the first trimester of pregnancy, and a low maternal body mass index (BMI), but these factors precede no more than 50 percent of preterm births. Every pregnancy is potentially at risk.

➤ Cervical "competence" is not an absolute or categorical property of the cervix, but rather is a continuum. The risk of spontaneous preterm birth increases as the length of the cervix decreases.

➤ Accurate early diagnosis of preterm labor is a major problem. Up to 50 percent of patients diagnosed with preterm labor do not actually have preterm labor, yet as many as 20 percent of symptomatic patients diagnosed as not being in labor will deliver prematurely.

➤ Effective therapies that can reduce perinatal morbidity and mortality are (1) transfer of the mother and fetus to an appropriate hospital, (2) administration of antibiotics to prevent neonatal group B streptococcus infection, (3) administration of corticosteroids to reduce neonatal respiratory distress syndrome and intraventricular hemorrhage, a treatment that has been underutilized in the past, and (4) administration of labor-arresting (tocolytic) medications to allow the above to occur.

➤ There is no truly reliable test for fetal well-being or infection in women with preterm PROM.

➤ Prevention of preterm birth will require prevention of risk in the population.

REFERENCES

1. Guyer B, Strobino DM, Ventura SJ, et al: Annual summary of vital statistics—1994. Pediatrics 96:1029, 1995.
2. Hack M, Taylor HG, Klein N, et al: School-age outcomes in children with birth weights under 750 g. N Engl J Med 331:756, 1994.
3. Ventura SJ, Martin JA, Curtin SC, Mathews TJ: Births: Final data for 1997. National Vital Stat Rep 47:1, 1999.
4. Joseph KS, Kramer MS, Marcoux S, et al: Determinants of preterm birth rates in Canada from 1981 through 1983 and from 1992 through 1994. N Engl J Med 339:1434, 1998.
5. Kramer MS: Preventing preterm birth: Are we making progress? Prenat Neonat Med 3:10, 1998.
6. Eastman NT: Prematurity from the viewpoint of the obstetrician. Am Pract 1:343, 1947.
7. Brenner WE, Edelman DA, Hendricks CH: A standard of fetal growth for the United States of America. Am J Obstet Gynecol 126:555, 1976.
8. Committee on Obstetric Practice: Perinatal and infant mortality statistics. Committee Opinion No. 167. Washington, DC, The American College of Obstetricians and Gynecologists, December 1995.
9. Copper RL, Creasy RK, Goldenberg RL, et al: A multicenter study of preterm birth weight and gestational age specific neonatal mortality. Am J Obstet Gynecol 168:78, 1993.
10. Stevenson DK, Wright LL, Lemons JA, et al: Very low birth weight outcomes of the National Institute of Child Health and Human Development Neonatal Research Network, January 1993 through December 1994. Am J Obstet Gynecol 179:1632, 1998.
11. Bottoms SF, Paul RH, Iams JD, et al: Obstetric determinants of neonatal survival: Influence of willingness to perform cesarean delivery on survival of extremely low birth weight infants. Am J Obstet Gynecol 176:960, 1997.
12. Kilpatrick SJ, Schleuter MA, Piecuch R, et al: Outcome of infants born at 24–26 weeks' gestation: I. Survival and cost. Obstet Gynecol 90:803, 1997.
13. Piecuch RE, Leonard CH, Cooper BA, et al: Outcome of infants born at 24–26 weeks gestation: II. Neurodevelopmental outcome. Obstet Gynecol 90:809, 1997.
14. Tin W, Wariyar U, Hey E, et al: Changing prognosis for babies of less than 28 weeks' gestation in the north of England between 1983 and 1994. BMJ 314:107, 1997.
15. Tyson JE, Younes N, Verter J, et al: Viability, morbidity, and resource use among newborns of 501- to 800-g birth weight. JAMA 276:1645, 1996.
16. Atkinson MW, Goldenberg RL, Gaudier FL, et al: Maternal corticosteroid and tocolytic treatment and morbidity and mortality in very low birth weight infants. Am J Obstet Gynecol 173:299, 1995.
17. Barton L, Hodgman JE, Pavlova Z: Causes of death in the extremely low birth weight infant. Pediatrics 102:446, 1999.
18. Nielsen HC, Harvey-Wilkes K, MacKinnon B, et al: Neonatal outcome of very premature infants from multiple and singleton gestations. Am J Obstet Gynecol 177:653, 1997.
19. Donovan EF, Ehrenkranz RA, Shankaran S, et al: Outcomes of very low birth weight twins cared for in the National Institute of Child Health and Human Development Neonatal Research Network's intensive care units. Am J Obstet Gynecol 179:742, 1998.
20. Horbar JD, McAuliffe TL, Adler SM, et al: Variability in 28-day outcomes for very low birth weight infants: An analysis of 11 neonatal intensive care units. Pediatrics 82:554, 1988.
21. Wilcox A, Buekens P, Kiely J: Birth weight and perinatal mortality: A comparison of the United States and Norway. JAMA 273:709, 1995.
22. Robertson PA, Sniderman SH, Laros RK, et al: Neonatal morbidity according to gestational age and birthweight from five tertiary care centers in the United States 1983 through 1986. Am J Obstet Gyencol 166:1629, 1992.
23. Katz VL, Bose CL: Improving survival of the very premature infant. J Perinatol 13:261, 1993.
24. Cooke RWI: Factors affecting survival and outcome at 3 years in extremely preterm infants. Arch Dis Child 71:F28, 1994.
25. LeFebvre F, Glorieux J, St-Laurent-Gagnon T: Neonatal survival and disability rate at age 18 months for infants born between 23 and 28 weeks of gestation. Am J Obstet 174:833, 1996.
26. Saigal S, Feeny D, Rosenbaum P, et al: Self-perceived health status and health-related quality of life of extremely low-birth-weight infants at adolescence. JAMA 276:453, 1996.
27. Stewart AL, Rifkin L, Amess PN, et al: Brain structure and neurocognitive and behavioral function in adolescents who were born very preterm. Lancet 353:1653, 1999.
28. Vohr BR, Wright LL, Dusick AM, et al: Neurodevelopmental and functional outcomes of extremely low birth weight infants in the National Institutes of Child Health and Human Development Neonatal Research Network, 1993–94. Pediatrics 105:1216, 2000.
29. Yoon BH, Romero R, Kim CJ, et al: Amniotic fluid interleukin-6; a sensitive test for antenatal diagnosis of acute inflammatory lesions of preterm placenta and prediction of perinatal morbidity. Am J Obstet Gynecol 172:9960, 1995.
30. Gomez R, Romero R, Ghezzi F, et al: The fetal inflammatory response syndrome. Am J Obstet Gynecol 179:194, 1998.
31. Yoon BH, Romero R, Jun JK, et al: Amniotic fluid cytokines (interleukin-6, tumor necrosis factor-α, interleukin 1-β) and the risk for the development of bronchopulmonary dysplasia. Am J Obstet Gynecol 177:825, 1997.
32. Yoon BH, Romero R, Kim KS, et al: A systemic fetal inflammatory response and the development of bronchopulmonary dysplasia. Am J Obstet Gynecol 181:773, 1999.
33. O'Shea TM, Klinepeter KL, Dillard RG: Prenatal events and the risk of cerebral palsy in very low birth weight infants. Am J Epidemiol 146:362, 1998.
34. Yoon BH, Romero R, Yang SH, et al: Interleukin-6 concentrations in umbilical cord plasma are elevated in neonates with white matter lesions associated with periventricular leukomalacia. Am J Obstet Gynecol 177:19, 1997.
35. Verma U, Tejani N, Klein S, et al: Obstetric antecedents of intraventricular hemorrhage and periventricular leukomalacia in the low birth weight neonate. Am J Obstet Gynecol 176:275, 1997.
36. Yoon BH, Jun JK, Romero R, et al: Amniotic fluid inflammatory cytokines (interleukin-6, interleukin 1-β, tumor necrosis factor-α), neonatal brain white matter lesions, and cerebral palsy. Am J Obstet Gynecol 177:19, 1997.
37. Alexander JM, Gilstrap LC, Cox SM, et al: Clinical chorioamnionitis and the prognosis for very low birth weight infants. Obstet Gynecol 91:725, 1998.
38. The Developmental Epidemiology Network Investigators: The correlation between placental pathology and intraventricular hemorrhage in the preterm infant. Pediatr Res 43:15, 1998.
39. Yoon BH, Park JS, Romero R, et al: Intra-amniotic inflammation and the development of cerebral palsy at three years of age [abstract 2]. Am J Obstet Gynecol 180:S2, 1999.
40. McCormick MC, Shapiro S, Starfield BH: Rehospitalization during the first year of life for high risk survivors. Pediatrics 66:991, 1980.

41. Meis PJ, Ernest JM, Moore ML: Causes of low birth-weight births in public and private patients. Am J Obstet Gynecol 156:1165, 1987.

42. Meis PJ, Michielutte R, Peters TJ, et al: Factors associated with preterm birth in Cardiff Wales: II. Indicated and spontaneous preterm birth. Am J Obstet Gynecol 173:597, 1995.

43. Meis PJ, Goldenberg RL, Mercer BM, et al: The preterm prediction study: Risk factors for indicated preterm birth. Am J Obstet Gynecol 178:562, 1998.

44. Goldenberg RL, Iams JD, Mercer BM, et al: The preterm prediction study: The value of new vs. standard risk factors predicting early and all spontaneous preterm births. Am J Public Health 88:233, 1998.

45. Hadley CB, Main DM, Gabbe SG, et al: Risk factors for preterm premature rupture of the fetal membranes. Am J Perinatol 7:374, 1990.

46. Ekwo EE, Gosselink CA, Moawad A: Unfavorable outcome in penultimate pregnancy and premature rupture of membranes in successive pregnancy. Obstet Gynecol 80:166, 1992.

47. MacGregor SN, Sabbagha RE, Tamura RK, et al: Differing fetal growth patterns in pregnancies complicated by preterm labor. Obstet Gynecol 72:834, 1988.

48. Ott WJ: Intrauterine growth retardation and preterm delivery. Am J Obstet Gynecol 168:1710, 1993.

49. Hediger ML, Scholl TO, Schall JI, Fischer RL: Fetal growth and the etiology of preterm delivery. Obstet Gynecol 85:175, 1995.

50. Salafia CM, Vogel CA, Vintzeleos AM, et al: Placental pathologic findings in preterm birth. Am J Obstet Gynecol 165:934, 1991.

51. Arias F, Rodriguez L, Rayne SC, Kraus FT: Maternal placental vasculopathy and infection: Two distinct subgroups among patients with preterm labor and preterm ruptured membranes. Am J Obstet Gynecol 168:585, 1993.

52. Arias F, Victoria A, Cho K, et al: There are different histologic groups with distinct clinical characteristics among patients with preterm premature rupture of membranes [abstract]. Am J Obstet Gynecol 174:464, 1996.

53. Strigini FA, Lencioni G, DeLuca G, et al: Uterine artery velocimetry and spontaneous preterm delivery. Obstet Gynecol 85:374, 1995.

54. Lockwood CJ: The diagnosis of preterm labor and the prediction of preterm delivery. Clin Obstet Gynecol 38:675, 1995.

55. Darne J, McGarrigle HHG, Lachelin GCL: Saliva oestriol, oestradiol, oestrone, and progesterone levels in pregnancy: Spontaneous labour at term is preceded by a rise in the saliva oestriol: progesterone ratio. Br J Obstet Gynaecol 94:227, 1987.

56. Tallo CO, Vohr B, Oh W, et al: Maternal and neonatal morbidity associated with in vitro fertilization. J Pediatr 127:794, 1995.

57. Imseis HM, Albert TA, Iams JD: Identifying twin gestations at low risk for preterm birth with a transvaginal cervical measurement at 24–26 weeks gestation. Am J Obstet Gynecol 177:1149, 1997.

58. Weiss G, Goldsmith LT, Sachdev R, et al: Elevated first trimester serum relaxin concentrations in pregnant women following ovarian stimulation predict prematurity. Obstet Gynecol 82:821, 1993.

59. Lumley J: The association between prior spontaneous abortion, prior induced abortion and preterm birth in first singleton births. Prenat Neonat Med 3:21, 1998.

60. Iams JD, Johnson F, Sonek J, et al: Cervical competence as a continuum: A study of sonographic cervical length and obstetrical performance. Am J Obstet Gynecol 172:1097, 1995.

61. Iams JD, Goldenberg RL, Mercer BM, et al: The preterm prediction study: Recurrence risk of spontaneous preterm birth. Am J Obstet Gynecol 178:1035, 1998.

62. Mercer BM, Goldenberg RL, Moawad A, et al: The preterm prediction study: Effect of gestational age and cause of preterm birth on subsequent obstetric outcome. Am J Obstet Gynecol 181:1216, 1999.

63. Adams MM, Elam-Evans LD, Wilson HG, Gilbertz DA: Rates of and factors associated with recurrence of preterm delivery. JAMA 283:1591, 2000.

64. Bakketeig LS, Hoffman HJ: Epidemiology of preterm birth: Results from a longitudinal study of births in Norway. In Elder LS, Hendricks CH (eds): Preterm Labor. London/Boston, Butterworths, 1981, p 17.

65. DIV Reproductive Health, et al, National Center for Health Statistics, and CDC. Preterm singleton births—United States, 1989–96. MMWR 48:185, 1999.

66. Kogan MD, Alexander GR: Social and behavioral factors in preterm birth. Prenat Neonat Med 3:29, 1998.

67. Cabral H, Fried LE, Levenson S, et al: Foreign-born and US-born black women: Differences in health behaviors and birth outcomes. Am J Public Health 80:70, 1990.

68. Goldenberg RL, Cliver SP, Mulvihill XP, et al: Medical, psychosocial, and behavioral risk factors do not explain the increased risk for low birthweight among black women. Am J Obstet Gynecol 175:1317, 1996.

69. Dijkstra K, Janssen CJP, Kuczynski E, et al: Cervical length in uncomplicated pregnancy: A study of sociodemographic predictors of cervical changes across gestation. Am J Obstet Gynecol 180:639, 1999.

70. Iams JD, Goldenberg RL, Meis PJ, et al: The length of the cervix and the risk of spontaneous premature delivery. N Engl J Med 334:567, 1996.

71. Surbek DV, Hoesli LM, Holzgreve W: Morphology assessed by transvaginal sonography differs in patients in preterm labor with vs. without bacterial vaginosis. Ultrasound Obstet Gynecol 15:242, 2000.

72. Goldenberg RL, Klebanoff MA, Nugent R, et al, for the Vaginal Infections in Pregnancy Study Group: Bacterial colonization of the vagina in four ethnic groups. Am J Obstet Gynecol 174:1618, 1996.

73. Knox IC, Hoerner JK: The role of infection in premature rupture of the membranes. Am J Obstet Gynecol 59:190, 1950.

74. Gibbs RS, Romero R, Hillier SL, et al: A review of premature birth and subclinical infection. Am J Obstet Gynecol 166:127, 1992.

75. Wahbeh CJ, Hill GB, Eden RD, et al: Intraamniotic bacterial colonization in premature labor. Am J Obstet Gynecol 148:739, 1984.

76. Romero R, Sirtori M, Oyarzun E, et al: Infection and labor V: prevalence, microbiology, and clinical significance of intraamniotic infection in women with preterm labor and intact membranes. Am J Obstet Gynecol 161:817, 1989.

77. Duff P, Kopelman JN: Subclinical intra-amniotic infection in asymptomatic patients with refractory preterm labor. Obstet Gynecol 69:756, 1987.

78. Russell P: Inflammatory lesions of the human placenta I. Clinical significance of acute chorioamniotis. Am J Diagn Gynecol Obstet 1:127, 1979.

79. Hillier SL, Martius J, Krohn M, et al: A case control study of chorioamniotic infection and histologic chorioamnionitis in prematurity. N Engl J Med 319:972, 1988.

80. Martius J, Krohn M, Hillier SL, et al: Relationships of vaginal *Lactobacillus* species, cervical *Chlamydia trachomatis,* and

bacterial vaginosis to preterm birth. Obstet Gynecol 71:89, 1988.

81. Krohn MA, Hillier SL, Lee ML, et al: Vaginal *Bacteroides* are associated with an increased rate of preterm delivery among women in preterm labor. J Infect Dis 164:88, 1991.

82. Gravett MG, Nelson HP, DeRouen T, et al: Independent associations of bacterial vaginosis and *Chlamydia trachomatis* infection with adverse pregnancy outcome. JAMA 256:1899, 1986.

83. Watts DH, Krohn MA, Hillier SL, et al: The association of occult amniotic fluid infection with gestational age and neonatal outcome among women in preterm labor. Obstet Gynecol 79:351, 1992.

84. Hauth JC, Andrews WW, Goldenberg RL, et al: Infection-related risk factors predictive of spontaneous preterm labor and birth. Prenat Neonat Med 3:86, 1998.

85. Offenbacher S, Lieff S, Beck JD: Periodontitis-associated pregnancy complications. Prenat Neonat Med 3:82, 1998.

86. Elder HA, Santamarina BAG, Smith S, et al: The natural history of asymptomatic bacteriuria during pregnancy: The effect of tetracycline on the clinical course and the outcome of pregnancy. Am J Obstet Gynecol 111:441, 1971.

87. McCormack WM, Rosner B, Lee Y-H, et al: Effect on birth weight of erythromycin treatment of pregnant women. Obstet Gynecol 69:202, 1987.

88. Cohen I, Veille JC, Calkins BM: Improved pregnancy outcome following successful treatment of chlamydial infection. JAMA 263:3160, 1990.

89. Eschenbach DA, Nugent RP, Rao AV, et al: A randomized placebo-controlled trial of erythromycin for the treatment of *Ureaplasma urealyticum* to prevent premature delivery. Am J Obstet Gynecol 164:734, 1991.

90. Carey JC, Yaffe SJ, Catz C, for the VIP Study Group: The vaginal infections and prematurity study: An overview. Clin Obstet Gynecol 36:809, 1993.

91. Meis PJ, Goldenberg RL, Mercer B, et al: The preterm prediction study: significance of vaginal infections. Am J Obstet Gynecol 173:1231, 1995.

92. Hillier SL, Nugent RP, Eschenbach DA, et al, for the Vaginal Infections and Prematurity Study Group: Association between bacterial vaginosis and preterm delivery of a low-birth-weight infant. N Engl J Med 333:1737, 1995.

93. Hauth JC, Goldenberg RL, Andrews WW, et al: Reduced incidence of preterm delivery with metronidazole and erythromycin in women with bacterial vaginosis. N Engl J Med 333:1732, 1995.

94. McDonald HM, O'Loughlin JA, Vigneswaran R, et al: Impact of metronidazole treatment in women with bacterial vaginosis flora (*Gardnerella vaginalis*): a randomised, placebo controlled trial. Br J Obstet Gynaecol 104:1391, 1997.

95. Carey JC, Klebanoff MA, Hauth JC, et al: Metronidazole to prevent preterm delivery in pregnant women with asymptomatic bacterial vaginosis. N Engl J Med 342:534, 2000.

96. Carey JC, Klebanoff MA, for the NICHD MFMU Network: Metronidazole treatment increased the risk of preterm birth in asymptomatic women with trichomonas [abstract 7]. Am J Obstet Gynecol 182:S13, 2000.

97. Goldenberg RL, Andrews WW: Intrauterine infection and why preterm prevention programs have failed. Am J Public Health 86:781, 1996.

98. Goldenberg RL, Hauth JC, Andrews WW: Intrauterine infection and preterm delivery. N Engl J Med 342:1500, 2000.

99. Iams JD, Goldenberg RL, Meis PJ, et al: The length of the cervix and the risk of spontaneous premature delivery. N Engl J Med 334:567, 1996.

100. Goldenberg RL, Iams JD, Miodovnik M, et al: The preterm prediction study: Risk factors in twin gestations. Am J Obstet Gynecol 175:1047, 1996.

101. Anderson HF, Nugent CE, Wanty SD, et al: Prediction for preterm delivery by ultrasonographic measurement of cervical length. Am J Obstet Gynecol 163:859, 1990.

102. Taipale P, Hiilesmaa V: Sonographic measurement of the uterine cervix at 18–22 weeks gestation and the risk of preterm delivery. Obstet Gynecol 92:902, 1998.

103. Andrews WW, Copper R, Hauth JC, et al: Second trimester cervical ultrasound: Associations with increased risk for recurrent early spontaneous delivery. Obstet Gynecol 95:222, 2000.

104. Iams JD, for the NICHD MFMU Network: The preterm prediction study: Cervical length and perinatal infection [abstract]. Am J Obstet Gynecol 176:S6 1997.

105. Iams JD: The cervix: An independent risk factor for preterm birth. Prenat Neonat Med 3:106, 1998.

106. Guzman ER, Schen-Schwarz S, Benito C, et al: The relationship between placental histology and cervical ultrasonography in women at risk for pregnancy loss and spontaneous preterm birth. Am J Obstet Gynecol 181:793, 1999.

107. Feinberg RF, Kleiman HJ, Lockwood CJ: Is oncofetal fibronectin a trophoblast glue for human implantation? Am J Pathol 138:537, 1991.

108. Goldenberg RL, Mercer BM, Meis PJ, et al: The preterm prediction study: Fetal fibronectin testing and spontaneous preterm birth. Obstet Gynecol 87:643, 1996.

109. Mercer BM, Goldenberg RL, Moawad AH, et al: The preterm prediction study: Effect of gestational age and cause of preterm birth on subsequent obstetric outcome. Am J Obstet Gynecol 181:1216, 1999.

110. Goldenberg RL, Thom E, Moawad AH, et al: The preterm prediction study: Fetal fibronectin, bacterial vaginosis, and peripartum infection. Obstet Gynecol 87:656, 1996.

111. MacDonald PC, Casey ML: The accumulation of prostglandins in amniotic fluiud is an after effect of labor and not indicative of a role for PGE2 or PGF2 alpha in the initiation of human parturition. J Clin Endocrinol Metab 76:1332, 1993.

112. Leveno KJ, Cox K, Roark M: Cervical dilatation and prematurity revisited. Obstet Gynecol 68:434, 1986.

113. Papiernik E, Bouyer J, Collin D, et al: Precocious cervical ripening and preterm labor. Obstet Gynecol 67:238, 1986.

114. Copper R, Goldenberg RL, Davis RO, et al: Warning symptoms, uterine contractions and cervical examination findings in women at risk of preterm delivery. Obstet Gynecol 162:748, 1990.

115. Korn AP, Bolan G, Padian N, et al: Plasma cell endometritis in women with symptomatic bacterial vaginosis. Obstet Gynecol 85:387, 1995.

116. Ghidini A, Jenkins CB, Spong CY, et al: Elevated amniotic fluid interleukin-6 levels during the early second trimester are associated with greater risk of subsequent preterm delivery. Am J Reprod Immunol 37:227, 1997.

117. Wenstrom KD, Andrews WW, Hauth JC, et al: Elevated second trimester amniotic fluid interleukin 6 levels predict preterm delivery. Am J Obstet Gynecol 178:546, 1998.

118. Spong CY, Ghidini A, Sherer DM, et al: Angiogenin: A marker for preterm delivery in midtrimester amniotic fluid. Am J Obstet Gynecol 176:415, 1997.

119. Iams JD: Prevention of preterm birth. N Engl J Med 338:54, 1998.

120. Romero R, Mazor M, Munoz H, et al: The preterm labor syndrome. Ann N Y Acad Sci 734:414, 1994.

121. Feinberg BB, Stellar MA, Walsh SW: Cytokine regulation of

trophoblast steroidogenesis [abstract 479]. Soc Gynecol Invest 1992.

122. The American College of Obstetricians and Gynecologists: Preterm labor and delivery. Precis: Obstetrics. Washington, DC, ACOG, 1999.

123. Thompson RS, Taplin SH, McAfee TA, et al: Primary and secondary prevention services in clinical practice. Twenty years' experience in development, implementation, and evaluation. JAMA 273:1130, 1995.

124. Hall RT: Prevention of premature birth: Do pediatricians have a role? Pediatrics 105:1137, 2000.

125. Gleicher N, Oleske DM, Tur-Kaspa I, et al: Reducing the risk of higher-order multiple pregnancy after ovarian stimulation with gonadotropins. N Engl J Med 343:2, 2000.

126. Goldenberg RL, Rouse DJ: Prevention of premature birth. N Engl J Med 339:313, 1998.

127. Taylor ES: Discussion of Main DM, Gabbe SG, Richardson D, et al: Am J Obstet Gynecol 151:892, 1985.

128. Iams JD: Obstetric inertia: An obstacle to the prevention of prematurity. Am J Obstet Gynecol 159:796, 1988.

129. Creasy RK: Preventing preterm birth. N Engl J Med 325:727, 1991.

130. Fangman JJ, Mark PM, Pratt L, et al: Prematurity prevention programs: An analysis of successes and failures. Am J Obstet Gynecol 170:744, 1994.

131. Hueston WJ, Knox MA, Eilers G, et al: The effectiveness of preterm birth education programs for high risk women: A meta-analysis. Obstet Gynecol 86:705, 1995.

132. Keirse MJNC: New perspectives for the effective treatment of preterm labor. Am J Obstet Gynecol 173:618, 1995.

133. Herron M, Katz M, Creasy RK: Evaluation of a preterm birth prevention program: Preliminary report. Obstet Gynecol 59:452, 1982.

134. Main DM, Gabbe SG, Richardson D, et al: Can preterm deliveries be prevented? Am J Obstet Gynecol 151:892, 1985.

135. Collaborative Group on Preterm Birth Prevention: Multicenter randomized, controlled trial of a preterm birth prevention program. Am J Obstet Gynecol 169:352, 1993.

136. Mercer BM, Goldenberg RL, Das A, et al: The preterm prediction study: A clinical risk assessment system. Am J Obstet Gynecol 174:1885, 1996.

137. Gardner MO, Goldenberg RL, Cliver SP, et al: The origin and outcome of preterm twin pregnancies. Obstet Gynecol 85:553, 1995.

138. Kramer MS, Coates AL, Michoud MC, et al: Maternal anthropometry and idiopathic preterm labor. Obstet Gynecol 86:744, 1995.

139. Nageotte MP, Dorchester W, Porto M, et al: Quantitation of uterine activity in preceding preterm, term, and postterm labor. Am J Obstet Gynecol 158:1254, 1988.

140. Moore TR, Iams JD, Creasy RK, et al: Diurnal and gestational patterns of uterine activity in normal human pregnancy. Obstet Gynecol 83:517, 1994.

141. Iams JD, for the NICHD MFMU Network: Home uterine monitoring to predict preterm birth. Uterine contraction frequency and preterm birth [abstracts 2 and 670] Am J Obstet Gynecol 178:S2 and S188, 1998; and Self perceived symptoms to predict preterm birth [abstract 47]. Am J Obstet Gynecol 182:S32, 2000.

142. Katz M, Gill PJ, Newman RB: Detection of preterm labor by ambulatory monitoring of uterine activity: A preliminary report. Obstet Gynecol 68:773, 1986.

143. Morrison JC, Martin JN Jr, Martin RW, et al: Prevention of preterm birth by ambulatory assessment of uterine activity: A randomized study. Am J Obstet Gynecol 156:536, 1987.

144. Iams JD, Johnson FF, O'Shaughnessy RW: A prospective random trial of home uterine activity monitoring in pregnancies at increased risk of preterm labor II. Am J Obstet Gynecol 159:595, 1988.

145. Hill WC, Flemming AD, Martin RW, et al: Home uterine activity monitoring is associated with a reduction in preterm birth. Obstet Gynecol 76:13S, 1990.

146. Dyson DC, Crites YM, Ray DA, Armstrong MA: Prevention of preterm birth in high risk patients: The role of education and provider contact versus home uterine monitoring. Am J Obstet Gynecol 164:756, 1991.

147. Mou SM, Sunderji SG, Gall S, et al: Multicenter randomized clinical trial of home uterine monitoring for detection of preterm labor. Am J Obstet Gynecol 165:858, 1991.

148. Wapner RJ, Cotton DB, Artal R, et al: A randomized multicenter trial assessing a home uterine activity monitoring device used in the absence of daily nursing contact. Am J Obstet Gynecol 172:1026, 1995.

149. Collaborative Home Uterine Monitoring Study (CHUMS) Group: A multicenter randomized controlled trial of home uterine monitoring: Active versus sham device. Am J Obstet Gynecol 173:1120, 1995.

150. Grimes DA, Schultz KF: Randomized controlled trials of home uterine activity monitoring: A review and critique. Obstet Gynecol 79:137, 1992.

151. United States Preventive Services Task Force: Home uterine activity monitoring for preterm labor. JAMA 270:369, 1992.

152. Sachs BP, Hellerstein S, Freeman R, et al: Home monitoring of uterine activity: Does it prevent prematurity? N Engl J Med 325:1374, 1991.

153. Rhoads GG, McNellis DC, Kessel SS: Home monitoring of uterine activity. Am J Obstet Gynecol 165:2, 1991.

154. Colton T, Kayne HL, Zhang Y, Heeron T: A metaanalysis of home uterine activity monitoring. Am J Obstet Gynecol 173:1499, 1995.

155. Dyson DC, Danbe KH, Bamber JA, et al: Monitoring women at risk for preterm birth. N Engl J Med 338:15 1998.

156. Buekens P, Alexander S, Boutsen M, et al: Randomized controlled trial of routine cervical examinations in pregnancy. Lancet 344:841, 1994.

157. Holcomb WL, Smeltzer JS: Cervical effacement: Variation in belief among clinicians. Obstet Gynecol 78:43, 1991.

158. Sonek JD, Iams JD, Blumenfeld M, et al: Measurement of cervical length in pregnancy: Comparison between vaginal ultrasonography and digital examination. Obstet Gynecol 76:172, 1990.

159. Anderson HF: Transvaginal and transabdominal ultrasonography of the uterine cervix during pregnancy. J Clin Ultrasound 19:77, 1991.

160. Heath VCF, Souka AP, Erasmus I, et al: Cervical length at 23 weeks of gestation: The value of Shirodkar suture for the short cervix. Ultrasound Obstet Gynecol 12:318, 1998.

161. Berghella V, Daly S, Tolosa J, et al: Prediction of preterm delivery with transvaginal ultrasonography of the cervix in high risk-pregnancies: Does cerclage prevent prematurity? Am J Obstet Gynecol 181:809, 1999.

162. Althuisius SM, Dekker GA, van Geijn HP, et al: Cervical incompetence prevention randomized cerclage trial [abstract 19]. Am J Obstet Gynecol 182:S20, 2000.

163. Rust O, Atlas R, Jones K, et al: A randomized trial of cerclage vs. no cerclage in patients with sonographically detected 2nd trimester premature dilation of the internal os [abstract 8]. Am J Obstet Gynecol 182:S13, 2000.

164. Klebanoff MA, Regan JA, Rao AV, et al: Outcome of the Vaginal Infections and Prematurity Study: Results of a clinical trial of erythromycin among pregnant women colonized with group B streptococci. Am J Obstet Gynecol 172:1540, 1995.

165. Committee on Obstetric Practice: Bacterial vaginosis screening for prevention of preterm delivery. Committee Opinion 198.

Washington, DC, American College of Obstetricians and Gynecologists, 1998.

166. Goldenberg RL, for the NICHD MFMU Network: Toward a multiple marker test for spontaneous preterm birth [abstract 2]. Am J Obstet Gynecol 182:S12, 2000.

167. McGregor JA, Jackson GM, Lachelin GC, et al: Salivary estriol as risk assessment for preterm labor: A prospective trial. Am J Obstet Gynecol 173:1337, 1995.

168. Murtha AP, Greig PC, Jimmerson CE, et al: Maternal serum interleukin-6 concentration as a marker for impending preterm delivery. Obstet Gynecol 91:161, 1998.

169. MRC/RCOG Working Party on Cervical Cerclage: Final report of the Medical Research Council/Royal College of Obstetricians and Gynaecologists multicentre randomised trial of cervical cerclage. Br J Obstet Gynaecol 100:516, 1993.

170. Rush RW, Issacs S, McPherson K, et al: A randomized controlled trial of cervical cerclage in women at high risk of spontaneous preterm delivery. Br J Obstet Gynaecol 91:724, 1984.

171. Lazar P, Gueguen S, Dreyfus J, et al: Multicentred controlled trial of cervical cerclage in women at moderate risk of preterm delivery. Br J Obstet Gynaecol 91:731, 1984.

172. Meis PJ, Ernest JM, Moore ML, et al: Regional program for prevention of premature birth in northwestern North Carolina. Am J Obstet Gynecol 157:550, 1987.

173. Elder HA, Santamaria BAG, Smith S, et al: The natural history of asymptomatic bacteriuria during pregnancy: The effect of tetracycline on the clinical course and the outcome of pregnancy. Am J Obstet Gynecol 111:441, 1971.

174. Olds DL, Henderson CR, Tatelbaum R, Chamberlain R: Improving the delivery of prenatal care and outcomes of pregnancy: A randomized trial of nurse home visitation. Pediatrics 77:16, 1986.

175. Spencer B, Thomas H, Morris J: A randomized controlled trial of the provision of a social support service during pregnancy: The South Manchester Family Worker Project. Br J Obstet Gynaecol 96:281, 1989.

176. Moore ML, Meis PJ, Ernest JM, et al: A randomized trial of nurse intervention to reduce preterm and low birth weight births. Obstet Gynecol 91:656, 1998.

177. Crombleholme W, Minkoff H, Delke I, et al: Cervical cerclage: An aggressive approach to threatened or recurrent pregnancy wastage. Am J Obstet Gynecol 146:168, 1983.

178. Johnson J, Lee P, Zachary A, et al: High-risk prematurity—progestin treatment and steroid studies. Obstet Gynecol 54:412, 1979.

179. Hauth J, Gilstrap L, Brekken A, et al: The effect of 17 alpha-hydroxyprogesterone caproate on pregnancy outcome in an active-duty military population. Am J Obstet Gynecol 146:187, 1983.

180. Dye TD, Oldenettel D: Physical activity and the risk of preterm labor. An epidemiological review and synthesis of recent literature. Semin Perinatol 20:334, 1996.

181. Mozuekewich EL, Luke B, Avni M, et al: Working conditions and adverse pregnancy outcome: A meta analysis. Obstet Gynecol 95:623, 2000.

182. Goldenberg RL, Cliver SP, Bronstein J, et al: Bedrest in pregnancy. Obstet Gynecol 84:131, 1994.

183. Germain AM, Carvajal J, Sanchez M, et al: Preterm labor: Placental pathology and clinical correlation. Obstet Gynecol 94:284, 1999.

184. Hediger ML, Scholl TO, Schall JI, et al: Fetal growth and the etiology of preterm labor. Obstet Gynecol 85:175, 1995.

185. Gonik B, Creasy RK: Preterm labor: Its diagnosis and management. Am J Obstet Gynecol 154:3, 1986.

186. King JF, Grant A, Keirse MJNC, et al: Beta mimetics in preterm labour; an overview of the randomized controlled trials. Br J Obstet Gynaecol 95:211, 1988.

187. Pircon RA, Strassner HT, Kirz DS, et al: Controlled trial of hydration and bed rest versus rest alone in the evaluation of preterm uterine contractions. Am J Obstet Gynecol 161:775, 1989.

188. Iams JD, Johnson FF, Parker M: A prospective evaluation of the signs and symptoms of preterm labor. Obstet Gynecol 84:227, 1994.

189. Hueston WJ: Preterm contractions in community settings: I. Treatment of preterm contractions. Obstet Gynecol 92:38, 1998.

190. Jackson GM, Ludmir J, Bader TJ: The accuracy of digital examination and ultrasound in the evaluation of cervical length. Obstet Gynecol 79:214, 1992.

191. Macones GA, Segel SY, Stamilo DM, Morgan MA: Predicting delivery within 48 hours in women treated with parenteral tocolysis. Obstet Gynecol 93:432, 1999.

192. Macones GA, Segel SY, Stamilo DM, Morgan MA: Prediction of delivery among women with early preterm labor by means of clinical characteristics alone. Am J Obstet Gynecol 181:1414, 1999.

193. Iams JD, Casal D, McGregor JA, et al: Fetal fibronectin improves the accuracy of diagnosis of preterm labor. Am J Obstet Gynecol 173:141, 1995.

194. Peaceman AM, Andrews WW, Thorp JM, et al: Fetal fibronectin as a predictor of preterm birth in patients with symptoms: A multicenter trial. Am J Obstet Gynecol 177:13, 1997.

195. Murakawa H, Utumi T, Hasegawa I, et al: Evaluation of threatened preterm delivery by transvaginal ultrasonographic measurement of cervical length. Obstet Gynecol 82:829, 1993.

196. Iams JD, Paraskos J, Landon MB, et al: Cervical sonography in preterm labor. Obstet Gynecol 84:40, 1994.

197. Gomez R, Galasso M, Romero R, et al: Ultrasonographic examination of the uterine cervix is better than cervical digital examinations as a predictor of the likelihood of premature delivery in patients with preterm labor and intact membranes. Am J Obstet Gynecol 171:956, 1994.

198. Timor-Tritsch I, Boozarjomehri F, Masakowski Y, et al: Can a snapshot sagittal view of the cervix by transvaginal ultrasonography predict active prterm labor? Am J Obstet Gynecol 174:990, 1996.

199. Crane JMG, Van den Hof M, Armson BA, Liston R: Transvaginal ultrasound in the prediction of preterm delivery: Singleton and twin gestations. Obstet Gynecol 90:357, 1997.

200. Leitich H, Brumbauer M, Kaider A, et al: Cervical length and dilation of the internal os detected by vaginal ultrasonography as markers for preterm delivery: A systematic review. Am J Obstet Gynecol 181:1465, 1999.

201. Leitich H, Egarter C, Kaider A, et al: Cervicovaginal fetal fibronectin as a marker for preterm delivery: A meta-analysis. Am J Obstet Gynecol 180:1169, 1999.

202. Mason GC, Maresh MJA: Alterations in bladder volume and the ultrasound appearance of the cervix. Br J Obstet Gynaecol 97:457, 1990.

203. Lockwood CJ, Senyei AE, Dische MR, et al: Fetal fibronectin in cervical and vaginal secretions as a predictor of preterm delivery. N Engl J Med 325:669, 1991.

204. Bartnicki J, Casal D, Kreaden US, et al: Fetal fibronectin in vaginal specimens predicts preterm delivery and very-low-birth-weight infants. Am J Obstet Gynecol 174:971, 1996.

205. Malak TM, Sizmur F, Bell SC, et al: Fetal fibronectin in cervicovaginal secretions as a predictor of preterm birth. Br J Obstet Gynaecol 103:648, 1996.

206. Senden IP, Owen P: Comparison of cervical assessment, fetal fibronectin and fetal breathing in the diagnosis of preterm labor. Clin Exp Obstet Gynecol 23:5, 1996.

207. Joffe GM, Jacques D, Bemis-Hayes R, et al: Impact of the

fetal fibronectin assay on admissions for preterm labor. Am J Obstet Gynecol 180:581, 1999.

208. Giles W, Bisits A, Knox M, et al: The effect of fetal fibronectin testing on admissions to a tertiary maternal-fetal medicine unit and cost savings. Am J Obstet Gynecol 182:439, 2000.

209. Adeza Biomedical: Data presented to the United States Food and Drug Administration, Bethesda, MD, April 6, 1995.

210. Iams JD: Reply to a letter from M. Plaut. Am J Obstet Gynecol 172:79, 1996.

211. Rizzo G, Capponi A, Arduini D, et al: The value of fetal fibronectin in cervical and vaginal secretions and of ultrasonographic examination of the uterine cervix in predicting premature delivery in patients with preterm labor and intact membranes. Am J Obstet Gynecol 176:1146, 1996.

212. Rozenberg P, Goffinet F, Malagrida L, et al: Evaluating the risk of preterm delivery: A comparison of fetal fibronectin and transvaginal ultrasonographic measurement of cervical length. Am J Obstet Gynecol 176:196, 1997.

213. Evidence Report/Technology Assessment No. 18: Management of Preterm Labor (AHRQ Publication No. 01-E021). October 2000. Access at www.ahrq.gov/clinic/epcix.htm.

214. Yeast JD, Poskin M, Stockbauer JW, et al: Changing patterns of regionalization of perinatal care and the impact on neonatal mortality. Am J Obstet Gynecol 178:131, 1998.

215. Towers CV, Bonebrake R, Padilla G, et al: The effect of transport on the rate of severe intraventricular hemorrhage in very low birth weight infants. Obstet Gynecol 95:291, 2000.

216. Schrag SJ, Zywicki S, Farley MM, et al: Group B streptococcal disease in the era of intrapartum antibiotic prophylaxis. N Engl J Med 342:15, 2000.

217. Crowley PA: Antenatal corticosteroid therapy. A meta-analysis of the randomized trials. Am J Obstet Gynecol 173:322, 1995.

218. Huszar G, Naftolin F: The myometrium and uterine cervix in normal and preterm labor. N Engl J Med 311:571, 1984.

219. Steer C, Petrie R: A comparison of magnesium sulfate and alcohol for the prevention of premature labor. Am J Obstet Gynecol 129:1, 1977.

220. Elliott J: Magnesium sulfate as a tocolytic agent. Am J Obstet Gynecol 147:277, 1983.

221. Wilkens IA, Lynch L, Mehaleb KE, et al: Efficacy and side effects of magnesium sulphate and ritodrine as tocolytic agents. Am J Obstet Gynecol 159:685, 1988.

222. Cox SM, Sherman LM, Leveno KJ: Randomized investigation of magnesium sulfate for prevention of preterm birth. Am J Obstet Gynecol 163:767, 1990.

223. Higby K, Xenakis EM, Paverstein CJ: Do tocolytic agents stop preterm labor? A critical and comprehensive review of safety and efficacy. Am J Obstet Gynecol 168:1247, 1993.

224. Beall MH, Edgar BW, Paril RH, et al: A comparison of ritodrine, terbutaline, and magnesium sulfate for the suppression of preterm labor. Am J Obstet Gynecol 153:854, 1985.

225. Holcomb WL, Shackelford GD, Petrie RH: Magnesium tocolysis and neonatal bone abnormalities: A controlled study. Obstet Gynecol 78:611, 1991.

226. Nelson KB, Grether J: Effect of MgSO$_4$ therapy on cerebral palsy rates in infants < 1500 grams. J Pediatr 95:263, 1995.

227. Schendel DE, Berg CJ, Yeargin-Allsopp M, et al: Prenatal magnesium sulfate exposure and the risk for cerebral palsy or mental retardation among very low birth weight children aged 3 to 5 years. JAMA 276:1805, 1996.

228. Mittendorf R, Covert R, Boman J, et al: Is tocolytic magnesium sulphate associated with increased total paediatric mortality? Lancet 350:1517, 1997.

229. Madden C, Owen J, Hauth JC: Magnesium tocolysis: serum levels versus success. Am J Obstet Gynecol 162:1177, 1990.

230. Lewis RB, Schulman JD: Influence of acetylsalicylic acid, an inhibitor of prostaglandin synthesis, on the duration of human gestation and labour. Lancet 2:1159, 1973.

231. Zuckerman H, Reiss U, Rubenstein I: Inhibition of human premature labor with indomethacin. Obstet Gynecol 44:787, 1974.

232. Niebyl J, Blake D, White R, et al: The inhibition of premature labor with indomethacin. Am J Obstet Gynecol 136:1014, 1980.

233. Zuckerman H, Shalev E, Gilad G, et al: Further study of the inhibition of premature labor by indomethacin. Part I. J Perinat Med 12:19, 1984.

234. Zuckerman H, Shalev E, Gilad G, et al: Further study of the inhibition of premature labor by indomethacin. Part II. J Perinat Med 12:25, 1984.

235. Besinger RE, Niebyl JR, Keyes WG, et al: A randomized comparative trial of indomethacin and ritodrine for the long-term treatment of preterm labor. Am J Obstet Gynecol 164:981, 1991.

236. Panter KR, Hannah ME, Amankwah KS, et al: The effect of indomethacin tocolysis in preterm labour on perinatal outcome: A randomised placebo-controlled trial. Br J Obstet Gynaecol 106:467, 1999.

237. Van Overmeire B, Slootmaekers V, De Loor J, et al: The addition of indomethacin to betamimetics for tocolysis: Any benefit for the neonate? Eur J Obstet Gynecol Reprod Biol 77:41, 1998.

238. Lunt CC, Satin AJ, Barth WH, et al: The effect of indomethacin tocolysis on maternal coagulation status. Obstet Gynecol 84:820, 1994.

239. Moise K: Effect of advancing gestational age on the frequency of fetal ductal constriction in association with maternal indomethacin use. Am J Obstet Gynecol 168:1350, 1994.

240. Moise KJ, Huhta JC, Sharif DS, et al: Indomethacin in the treatment of premature labor: Effects on the fetal ductus arteriosus. N Engl J Med 319:327, 1988.

241. Mohen D, Newnharn JP, Orsogna LD: Indomethacin for the treatment of polyhydramnios: A case of constriction of the ductus arteriosus. Aust N Z J Obstet Gynecol 32:243, 1992.

242. Vermillion ST, Scardo JA, Lashus AG, et al: The effect of indomethacin tocolysis on fetal ductus arteriosus constriction with advancing gestational age. Am J Obstet Gynecol 177:256, 1997.

243. van der Heijden BJ, Carlus C, Nancy F, et al: Persistent anuria, neonatal death, and renal microcystic lesions after prenatal exposure to indomethacin. Am J Obstet Gynecol 171:617, 1994.

244. Manchester D, Margolis H, Sheldon R: Possible association between maternal indomethacin therapy and primary pulmonary hypertension of the newborn. Am J Obstet Gynecol 126:467, 1976.

245. Csaba I, Sulyok E, Ertl T: Relationship of maternal treatment with indomethacin to persistence of fetal circulation syndrome. J Pediatr 92:484, 1978.

246. Norton ME, Merrill J, Cooper BAB, et al: Neonatal complications after the administration of indomethacin for preterm labor. N Engl J Med 329:1602, 1993.

247. Niebyl JR, Witter FR: Neonatal outcome after indomethacin treatment for preterm labor. Am J Obstet Gynecol 155:747, 1986.

248. Dudley DKL, Hardie MJ: Fetal and neonatal effects of indomethacin used as a tocolytic agent. Am J Obstet Gynecol 151:181, 1985.

249. Gardner M, Skelly S, Owen J, et al: Neonatal complications associated with prenatal use of indomethacin [abstract]. Am J Obstet Gynecol 172:414, 1995.

250. Carlan SJ, O'Brien WF, O'Leary TD, Mastrogiannis D: Randomized comparative trial of indomethacin and sulindac for

the treatment of refractory preterm labor. Obstet Gynecol 79: 223, 1992.

251. Rasanen J, Jouppila P: Fetal cardiac function and ductus arteriosus during indomethacin and sulindac therapy for threatened preterm labor: A randomized study. Am J Obstet Gynecol 173:20, 1995.

252. Mamopoulos M, Assimakopoulos E, Reece AE, et al: Maternal indomethacin therapy in the treatment of polyhydramnios. Am J Obstet Gynecol 162:1225, 1990.

253. Kirshon B, Mari G, Moise KJ: Indomethacin therapy in the treatment of symptomatic polyhydramnios. Obstet Gynecol 75:202, 1990.

254. Moise KJ: Indomethacin as treatment for symptomatic polyhydramnios. Contemp Obstet Gynecol 40:53, 1995.

255. US Food and Drug Administration: Warning on use of terbutaline sulfate for preterm labor. JAMA 279:9, 1998.

256. Canadian Preterm Labor Investigators Group: Treatment of preterm labor with the beta1-agonist ritodrine. N Engl J Med 327:308, 1992.

257. Lam F, Elliott J, Jones JS, et al: Clinical issues surrounding the use of terbutaline sulfate for preterm labor. Obstet Gynecol Surv 53 (Suppl):S85, 1998.

258. Wenstrom KD, Weiner CP, Merrill D, et al: A placebo controlled randomized trial of the terbutaline pump for prevention of preterm delivery. Am J Perinatol 14:87, 1997.

259. Guinn DA, Goepfert AR, Owen J, et al: Terbutaline pump maintenance therapy for prevention of preterm delivery: A double blind trial. Am J Obstet Gynecol 179:874, 1998.

260. Macones GA, Berlin M, Berlin J: Efficacy of oral beta-agonist maintenance therapy in preterm labor: A meta-analysis. Obstet Gynecol 85:313, 1995.

261. Perry KG, Morrison JC, Rust OA, et al: Incidence of adverse cardiopulmonary effects with low-dose continuous terbutaline infusion. Am J Obstet Gynecol 173:1273, 1995.

262. Guinn DA, Goepfert AR, Owen J, et al: Management options in women with preterm contractions: A randomized clinical trial. Am J Obstet Gynecol 177:814, 1997.

263. Weiner N: Norepinephrine, epinephrine and the sympathomimetic amines. *In* Gilman AG, Goodman LS, Gilman A (eds): The Pharmacological Basis of Therapeutics, 6th ed. New York, Macmillan, 1980, p 143.

264. Caritis S, Lin LS, Toig G, et al: Pharmacodynamics of ritodrine in pregnant women during preterm labor. Am J Obstet Gynecol 147:752, 1983.

265. Caritis SN, Venkataramanan R, Darby MJ, et al: Pharmacokinetics of ritodrine administered intravenously: recommendations for changes in the current regimen. Am J Obstet Gynecol 162:429, 1990.

266. Stubblefield P, Heyl P: Treatment of premature labor with subcutaneous terbutaline. Obstet Gynecol 59:457, 1982.

267. Caritis S, Toig G, Heddinger L, et al: A double blind study comparing ritodrine and terbutaline in the treatment of preterm labor. Am J Obstet Gynecol 150:7, 1984.

268. Casper RF, Lye SJ: Myometrial desensitization to continuous but not to intermittent β-adrenergic agonist infusion in the sheep. Am J Obstet Gynecol 154:301, 1986.

269. Caritis SN, Chiao JP, Moore JJ, Ward SM: Myometrial desensitization after ritodrine infusion. Am J Physiol 253:410, 1987.

270. Caritis SN, Chiao JP, Kridgen P: Comparison of pulsatile and continuous ritodrine administration: effects on uterine contractility and beta-adrenergic receptor cascade. Am J Obstet Gynecol 164:1005, 1991.

271. Benedetti T: Maternal complications of parenteral beta-sympathomimetic therapy for premature labor. Am J Obstet Gynecol 145:1, 1983.

272. Lamont RF: The contemporary use of beta-agonists. Br J Obstet Gynaecol 100:890, 1993.

273. Philipsen T, Eriksen PS, Lynggard F: Pulmonary edema following ritodrine-saline infusion in prmature labor. Obstet Gynecol 58:304, 1981.

274. Hatjis CG, Swain M: Systemic tocolysis for premature labor is associated with an increased incidence of pulmonary edema in the presence of maternal infection. Am J Obstet Gynecol 159:723, 1988.

275. Hendricks SK, Keroes J, Katz M: Electrocardiographic changes associated with ritodrine-induced maternal tachycardia and hypokalemia. Am J Obstet Gynecol 154:921, 1986.

276. Main EK, Main DM, Gabbe SG: Chronic oral terbutaline tocolytic therapy is associated with maternal glucose intolerance. Am J Obstet Gynecol 157:644, 1987.

277. Foley MR, Landon MB, Gabbe SG, et al: Effect of prolonged oral terbutaline therapy on glucose tolerance in pregnancy. Am J Obstet Gynecol 168:100, 1993.

278. Young D, Toofanian A, Leveno K: Potassium and glucose concentrations without treatment during ritodrine tocolysis. Am J Obstet Gynecol 98:105, 1983.

279. Smigaj D, Roman-Drago NM, Amini SB, et al: The effect of oral terbutaline on maternal glucose metabolisma and energy expenditure in pregnancy. Am J Obstet Gynecol 178:1041, 1998.

280. Fisher JE, Smith RS, Lagrandeur R, et al: Gestational diabetes mellitus in women receiving beta-adrenergics and corticosteroids for threatened preterm delivery. Obstet Gynecol 90:880, 1997.

281. Lindenbaum C, Ludmir J, Teplick FB, et al: Maternal glucose intolerance and the subcutaneous terbutaline pump. Am J Obstet Gynecol 166:925, 1992.

282. Groome LJ, Goldenberg RL, Cliver SP, et al: Neonatal periventricular-intraventricular hemorrhage after maternal beta-sympathomimetic tocolysis. The March of Dimes Multicenter Study Group. Am J Obstet Gynecol 167:873, 1992.

283. Epstein M, Nicholls E, Stubblefield P: Neonatal hypoglycemia after beta-sympathomimetic tocolytic therapy. Pediatrics 94: 449, 1979.

284. Ferguson JE, Schutz T, Pershe R, et al: Nifedipine pharmocokinetics during preterm labor tocolysis. Am J Obstet Gynecol 161:1485, 1989.

285. Ulmsten U, Andersson KE, Wingerup L: Treatment of preterm labor with the calcium antagonist nifedipine. Arch Gynecol 229:1, 1980.

286. Ferguson JE, Dyson DC, Holbrook H, et al: Cardiovascular and metabolic effects associated with nifedipine and ritodrine tocolysis. Am J Obstet Gynecol 161:788, 1989.

287. Ferguson JE II, Dyson DC, Schutz T, et al: A comparison of tocolysis with nifedipine or ritodrine: Analysis of efficacy and maternal, fetal and neonatal outcome. Am J Obstet Gynecol 163:105, 1990.

288. Kupfermine M, Lessing JB, Yaron Y, et al: Nifedipine vs ritodrine for suppression of preterm labour. Br J Obstet Gynaecol 100:1090, 1993.

289. Papatsonis DNM, van Geijn HP, Ader HJ, et al: Nifedipine and ritodrine in the management of preterm labor: A randomized multicenter trial. Obstet Gynecol 90:230, 1997.

290. Glock JL, Morales WJ: Efficacy and safety of nifedipine vs magnesium sulfate in the management of preterm labor: A randomized study. Am J Obstet Gynecol 169:960, 1993.

291. Larmon JE, Ross BS, May WL, et al: Oral nicardipine vs intravenous magnesium for the treatment of preterm labor. Am J Obstet Gynecol 181:1432, 1999.

292. Oei SG, Oei SK, Brolmann HAM: Myocardial infarction during nifedipine therapy for preterm labor. N Engl J Med 340: 154, 1999.

293. Snyder SW, Cardwell MS: Neuromuscular blockade with magnesium sulfate and nifedipine. Am J Obstet Gynecol 161: 35, 1989.

294. Ben-Ami M, Giladi Y, Shalev E: The combination of magnesium sulphate and nifedipine: A cause of neuromuscular blockade. Br J Obstet Gynaecol 101:262, 1944.

295. Mari G, Kirshon B, Moise KJ, et al: Doppler assessment of the fetal and uteroplacental circulation during nifedipine therapy for preterm labor. Am J Obstet Gynecol 161:1514, 1989.

296. Murray C, Haverkamp AD, Orleans M, et al: Nifedipine for the treatment of preterm labor. Am J Obstet Gynecol 167:52, 1992.

297. Ray D, Dyson D, Crites Y: Nifedipine tocolysis and neonatal acid base status at delivery. Am J Obstet Gynecol 170:387, 1994.

298. Lockwood CJ: Calcium channel blockers in the management of preterm labour. Lancet 350:1339, 1997.

299. Grossman E, Messerli FH, Grodzicki T, et al: Should a moratorium be placed on sublingual nifedipine capsules given for hypertensive emergencies and pseudoemergencies. JAMA 276:1328, 1996.

300. Romero R, Sibai BM, Sanchez-Ramos L, et al: An oxytocin-receptor antagonist (atosiban) in the treatment of preterm labor: A randomized double blind, placebo controlled trial with tocolytic rescue. Am J Obstet Gynecol 182:1171, 2000.

301. Valenzuela GJ, Sanchez-Ramos L, Romero R, et al: Maintenance treatment of preterm labor with the oxytocin antagonist atosiban. Am J Obstet Gynecol 182:1184, 2000.

302. Moutquin JM, Sherman D, Cohen H, et al: Double-blind, randomized, controlled trial of atosiban and ritodrine in the treatment of preterm labor: A multicenter effectiveness and safety study. Am J Obstet Gynecol 182:1191, 2000.

303. Lees CC, Lojacono A, Thompson C, et al: Glyceryl trinitrate and ritodrine in tocolysis: An international multicenter randomized trial. Obstet Gynecol 94:403, 1999.

304. Ferguson JE, Hensleigh PA, Kredenster D: Adjunctive use of magnesium sulfate with ritodrine for preterm labor tocolysis. Am J Obstet Gynecol 148:166, 1984.

305. Hatjis CG, Swain M, Nelson LH: Efficacy of combined administration of magnesium sulfate and ritodrine in the treatment of premature labor. Obstet Gynecol 69:317, 1987.

306. Alexander JM, Gilstrap LC, Cox SM, et al: Clinical chorioamnionitis and the prognosis for very low birth weight infants. Obstet Gynecol 91:725, 1998.

307. The Developmental Epidemiology Network Investigators: The correlation between placental pathology and intraventricular hemorrhage in the preterm infant. Pediatr Res 43:15, 1998.

308. Lewis DF, Futayyeh S, Towers CV, et al: Preterm delivery from 34 to 37 weeks of gestation: Is respiratory distress a problem? Am J Obstet Gynecol 174:525, 1996.

309. Myers ER, Alvarez JG, Richardson DK, et al: Cost-effectiveness of fetal lung maturity testing in preterm labor. Obstet Gynecol 90:824, 1997.

310. Creasy RK, Golbus M, Laros R, et al: Oral ritodrine maintenance in the treatment of preterm labor. Am J Obstet Gynecol 137:212, 1980.

311. Carlan SJ, O'Brien WF, Jones MH, et al: Outpatient oral sulindac to prevent recurrence of preterm labor. Obstet Gynecol 85:769, 1995.

312. Holleboom CAG, Merkus JMWM, van Elferen LWM, et al: Double blind evaluation of ritodrine sustained release for oral maintenance of tocolysis after active preterm labour. Br J Obstet Gynaecol 103:702, 1996.

313. Lewis R, Mercer BM, Salama M, et al: Oral terbutaline after parenteral tocolysis: A randomized, double blind, placebo controlled trial. Am J Obstet Gynecol 175:834, 1996.

314. Rust OA, Bofill JA, Arriola RM, et al: The clinical efficacy of oral tocolytic therapy. Am J Obstet Gynecol 175:838, 1996.

315. Ricci JM, Hariharan S, Helfgott A, et al: Oral tocolysis with magnesium chloride. Am J Obstet Gynecol 165:603, 1991.

316. Parilla BV, Dooley SL, Minogue JP, et al: The efficay of oral terbutaline after intraveneous tocolysis. Am J Obstet Gynecol 169:965, 1993.

317. How HY, Hughes SA, Vogel RL, et al: Oral terbutaline in the outpatient management of preterm labor. Am J Obstet Gynecol 173:1518, 1995.

318. Carr DB, Clark AL, Kernek K, et al: Maintenance oral nifedipine for preterm labor. A randomized clinical trial. Am J Obstet Gynecol 181:822, 1999.

319. Sanchez-Ramos L, Kaunitz AM, Gaudier FL, et al: Efficacy of maintenance therapy after acute tocolysis: A meta-analysis. Am J Obstet Gynecol 181:484, 1999.

320. Fletcher SE, Fyfe DA, Case CL, et al: Myocardial necrosis after long-term maternal subcutaneous terbutaline infusion for suppression of preterm labor. Am J Obstet Gynecol 165:1401, 1991.

321. Lam F, Gill P, Smith M, et al: Use of subcutaneous terbutaline pump for long-term tocolysis. Obstet Gynecol 72:810, 1988.

322. Caritis SN, Venkataramanan R, Cotroneo M, et al: Pharmacokinetics of orally administered ritodrine. Am J Obstet Gynecol 161:32, 1989.

323. Iams JD, Johnson FF, O'Shaughnessy RW: Ambulatory uterine activity monitoring in the posthospital care of patients with preterm labor. Am J Perinatol 7:170, 1990.

324. Nagey DA, Bailey-Jones C, Herman AA: Randomized comparison of home uterine activity monitoring and routine care in patients discharged after treatment for preterm labor. Obstet Gynecol 82:319, 1993.

325. Brown HL, Britton KA, Brizendine EJ, et al: A random comparison of home uterine activity monitoring in the outpatient management of women treated for preterm labor. Am J Obstet Gynecol 180:798, 1999.

326. American College of Obstetricians and Gynecologists Committee on Obstetric Practice: Antenatal corticosteroid therapy for fetal maturation. ACOG Committee Opinion 210. Washington, DC, 1998.

327. American College of Obstetricians and Gynecologists Committee on Obstetric Practice: Prevention of early-onset group B streptococcal disease in newborns. ACOG Committee Opinion 173. Washington, DC, 1996.

328. Liggins GC, Howie RN: A controlled trial of antepartum glucocorticoid treatment for prevention of the respiratory distress syndrome in premature infants. Pediatrics 50:515, 1972.

329. Wright L, Verter J, Younes N, et al: Antenatal corticosteroid administration and neonatal outcome in very low birth weight infants: The NICHD Neonatal Research Network. Am J Obstet Gynecol 173:269, 1995.

330. Barks JDE, Post M, Tuor UI: Dexamethasone prevents hypoxic-ischemic brain damage in the neonatal rat. Pediatr Res 29:558, 1991.

331. Collaborative Group on Antenatal Steroid Therapy: Effect of antenatal dexamethasone administration on the prevention of respiratory distress syndrome. Am J Obstet Gynecol 141:276, 1981.

332. Garite TJ, Rumney PJ, Briggs GG, et al: A randomized, placebo-controlled trial of betamethasone for the prevention of respiratory distress syndrome at 24 to 28 weeks gestation. Am J Obstet Gynecol 166:646, 1992.

333. Kari MA, Hallman M: Prenatal dexamethasone treatment in conjunction with rescue therapy of human surfactant: A randomized placebo-controlled multicenter study. Pediatrics 93:730, 1994.

334. Jobe AH, Mitchell BR, Gunkel JH: Beneficial effects of the combined use of prenatal corticosteroids and postnatal surfactant on preterm infants. Am J Obstet Gynecol 168:508, 1993.

335. Andrews EB, Marcucci G, White A, et al: Associations be-

tween use of antenatal corticosteroids and neonatal outcomes within the Exosurf Neonatal Treatment Investigational New Drug Study Group. Am J Obstet Gynecol 173:290, 1995.

336. Farrell EE, Silver RK, Kimberlin LV, et al: Impact of antenatal dexamethasone administration on respiratory distress syndrome in surfactant-treated infants. Am J Obstet Gynecol 161:628, 1989.

337. Shankaran S, Bauer CR, Bain R, et al: Relationship between antenatal steroid administration and grades III and IV intracranial hemorrhage in low birth weight infants. Am J Obstet Gynecol 173:305, 1995.

338. Howie RN, Liggins GC: Clinical trial of antepartum betamethasone for prevention of respiratory distress in preterm infants. *In* Anderson AB, et al (eds): Preterm Labor. Proceedings of the 5th Study Group of the Royal College of Obstetricians and Gynecologists, London, 1977. London, Royal College of Obstetricians and Gynecologists, 1977, p 281.

339. Leviton A, Kuban KC, Pagano M, et al: Antenatal corticosteroids appear to reduce the risk of postnatal germinal matrix hemorrhage in preterm infants. Pediatrics 91:1083, 1993.

340. Ment LR, Oh W, Ehrenkrantz RA, et al: Antenatal steroids, delivery mode, and intraventricular hemorrhage in preterm infants. Am J Obstet Gynecol 172:795, 1995.

341. Leviton A, Dammann O, Allred EN, et al: Antenatal corticosteroids and cranial ultrasonographic abnormalities. Am J Obstet Gynecol 181:1007, 1999.

342. Baud O, Foix-L'Helias L, Kaminski M, et al: Antenatal glucocorticoid treatment and cystic periventricular leukomalacia in very premature infants. N Engl J Med 341:1190, 1999.

343. Gardner MO, Goldenberg RL, Gaudier FL, et al: Predicting low Apgar scores of infants weighing less than 1000 grams: The effect of corticosteroids. Obstet Gynecol 85:170, 1995.

344. Egerman RS, Mercer BM, Doss JL, et al: A randomized, controlled trial of oral and intramuscular dexamethasone in the prevention of neonatal respiratory distress syndrome. Am J Obstet Gynecol 179:1120, 1998.

345. Rayburn WF, Christensen HD, Gonzalez CL: A placebo-controlled comparison between betamethasone and dexamethasone for fetal maturation: differences in neurobehavioral development of mice offspring. Am J Obstet Gynecol 176:842, 1997.

346. Mulder EJH, Derks JB, Visser GHA, et al: Antenatal corticosteroid therapy and fetal behaviour: a randomised study of the effects of betamethasone and dexamethasone. Br J Obstet Gynaecol 104:1239, 1997.

347. Senat MV, Minoui S, Multon O, et al: Effect of dexamethasone and betamethasone on fetal heart rate variability in preterm labour: A randomized study. Br J Obstet Gynaecol 105:749, 1998.

348. Howie RN, Liggins GC: The New Zealand study of antepartum glucocorticoid treatment. Lung Dev Biol Clin Perspect II: 255, 1982.

349. Gamsu H, Mullinger B, Donnai P, et al: Antenatal administration of betamethasone to prevent respiratory distress syndrome in preterm infants: Report of a UK multicentre trial. Br J Obstet Gynaecol 96:401, 1989.

350. Leviton LC, Goldenberg RL, Baker CS, et al: Methods to encourage the use of antenatal corticosteroid therapy for fetal maturation. JAMA 281:46, 1999.

351. Liggins GC: The prevention of RDS by maternal beta-methasone administration. *In* Moore TD (ed): Lung Maturation and the Prevention of Hyaline Membrane Disease. Report of the Seventieth Ross Conference on Pediatric Research. Columbus, OH, Ross Laboratories, 1976, p 97.

352. Collaborative Group on Antenatal Steroid Therapy: Effects of antenatal dexamethasone administration in the infant: long-term follow-up. J Pediatr 104:259, 1984.

353. Nochimson D, Petrie R: Glucocorticoid therapy for the induction of pulmonary maturity in severely hypertensive gravid women. Am J Obstet Gynecol 133:449, 1979.

354. Ricke PS, Elliott JP, Freeman R: Use of corticosteroids in pregnancy-induced hypertension. Obstet Gynecol 55:206, 1980.

355. Teramo DA, Hallman M, Raivo KO, et al: Neonatal effects and serum cortisol levels after multiple courses of maternal corticosteroids. Obstet Gynecol 90:819, 1997.

356. McKenna DS, Wittber GM, Samuels P: The effects of repeated doses of antenatal corticosteroids on maternal adrenal function [abstract 35]. Am J Obstet Gynecol 180:S15, 1999.

357. Derks JB, Mulder EJH, Visser GHA: The effects of maternal betamethasone administration on the fetus. Br J Obstet Gynaecol 102:40, 1995.

358. Cohlen BJ, Stigter RH, Derks JB, et al: Absence of significant hemodynamic changes in the fetus following maternal betamethasone administration. Ultrasound Obstet Gynecol 8:252, 1996.

359. Loeb JN: Corticosteroids and growth. N Engl J Med 295:547, 1976.

360. Stewart JD, Gonzalez CL, Christensen HD, et al: Impact of multiple antenatal doses of betamethasone on growth and development of mice offspring. Am J Obstet Gynecol 177:1138, 1997.

361. Jobe AH, Wada N, Berry LM, et al: Single and repetitive maternal glucocorticoid exposures reduce fetal growth in sheep. Am J Obstet Gynecol 178:880, 1998.

362. Cotterrell M, Balazs R, Johnson AL: Effects of corticosteroids on the biochemical maturation of rat brain. Postnatal cell formation. J Neurochem 19:2151, 1972.

363. Dunlop SA, Archer MA, Quinlivan JA, et al: Repeated prenatal corticosteroids delay myelination in the ovine central nervous system. J Maternal Fetal Med 6:309, 1997.

364. Slotkin TA: Adverse effects of antenatal steroids on nervous system development: Animal models. National Institute of Health Consensus Development Conference on Effect of Corticosteroids for Fetal Maturation on Perinatal Outcomes, February 28–March 2, 1994.

365. French NP, Hagan R, Evans SF, et al: Repeated antenatal corticosteroids: Size at birth and subsequent development. Am J Obstet Gynecol 180:114, 1999.

366. Dessens AB, Smolders-de Haas R, Koppe JG, et al: Twenty year follow up of antenatal corticosteroid treatment [abstract]. Pediatrics 105:e77, 2000.

367. Mugford M, Piercy J, Chalmers I: Cost implications of different approaches to the prevention of respiratory distress syndrome. Arch Dis Child 66:757, 1991.

368. Simpson KN, Lynch SR: Cost savings from the use of antenatal steroids to prevent respiratory distress syndrome and related conditions in premature infants. Am J Obstet Gynecol 173:316, 1995.

369. Vermont-Oxford Trials Network: Very low birthweight outcomes for 1990. Pediatrics 91:540, 1993.

370. Effect of corticosteroids for fetal maturation on perinatal outcomes: National Institutes of Health Consensus Statement 1994, Feb 28–Mar 2; 12(2):1–24. (also reprinted in Am J Obstet Gynecol 173:246, 1995.)

371. Morales WJ, Deibel ND, Lazar AJ, Zadrozny D: The effect of antenatal dexamethasone on the prevention of respiratory distress syndrome in preterm gestation with premature rupture of the membranes. Am J Obstet Gynecol 154:591, 1986.

372. McGregor JA, French JI, Reller LB, et al: Adjunctive erythromycin treatment for idiopathic preterm labor. Am J Obstet Gynecol 154:498, 1986.

373. Newton ER, Dinsmoor MJ, Gibbs RS: A randomized,

blinded, placebo-controlled trial of antibiotics in idiopathic term labor. Obstet Gynecol 74:562, 1989.

374. Newton ER, Shields L, Ridgway LE, et al: Combination antibiotics and indomethacin in idiopathic preterm labor: a randomized double blind clinical trial. Am J Obstet Gynecol 165:1753, 1991.

375. Romero R, Sibai B, Caritis S, et al: Antibiotic treatment of preterm labor with intact membranes: a multicenter, randomized, double-blinded, placebo-controlled trial. Am J Obstet Gynecol 169:764, 1993.

376. Norman K, Pattinson RC, de Souza J, et al: Ampicillin and metronidazole treatment in preterm labour: a multicentre, randomised controlled trial. Br J Obstet Gynaecol 101:404, 1994.

377. Gordon M, Samuels P, Shubert P, et al: A randomized, prospective study of adjunctive ceftizoxime in preterm labor. Am J Obstet Gynecol 172:1546, 1995.

378. Knight DB, Liggins GC, Wealthall SR: A randomized, controlled trial of antepartum thyrotropin-releasing hormone and betamethasone in the prevention of respiratory disease in preterm infants. Am J Obstet Gynecol 171:11, 1994.

379. Collaborative Santiago Surfactant Group: Collaborative trial of prenatal thyrotropin-releasing hormone and corticosteroids for prevention of respiratory distress syndrome. Am J Obstet Gynecol 178:33, 1998.

380. Ballard RA, Ballard PL, Cnaan A, et al: Antenatal thyrotropin-releasing hormone to prevent lung disease in preterm infants. N Engl J Med 338:493, 1998.

381. Thorp JA, Ferrette-Smith D, Gaston LA, et al: Combined antenatal vitamin K and phenobarbital for preventing intracranial hemorrhage in newborns less than 34 weeks gestation. Obstet Gynecol 86:1, 1995.

382. Shankaran S, Papile LA, Wright LL, et al: The effect of antenatal phenobarbital therapy on neonatal intracranial hemorrhage in preterm infants. N Engl J Med 337:466, 1997.

383. Parikh MN, Mehta AC: Internal cervical os during the second half of pregnancy. J Obstet Gynaecol Br Commonw 68:818, 1961.

384. Brook I, Feingold M, Schwartz A, et al: Ultrasonography in the diagnosis of cervical incompetence in pregnancy—a new diagnostic approach. Br J Obstet Gynaecol 88:640, 1981.

385. Andrews WW, Copper R, Hauth JC, et al: Second-trimester cervical ultrasound: Associations with increased risk for recurrent early spontaneous preterm delivery. Obstet Gynecol 95:222, 2000.

386. Buckingham JC, Buethe RA, Danforth DN: Collagen–muscle ratio in clinically normal and clinically incompetent cervices. Am J Obstet Gynecol 91:231, 1965.

387. Ugwumadu AHN: Cervical morphology in pregnancy, bacterial vaginosis, and the risk of preterm delivery. Ultrasound Obstet Gynecol 15:174, 2000.

388. Schuly KF, Grimes DA, Cates W Jr: Measures to prevent cervical injury during suction curettage abortion. Lancet 1:1182, 1983.

389. Jones JM, Sweetnam P, Hibbard BM: The outcome of pregnancy after cone biopsy of the cervix: A case control study. Br J Obstet Gynaecol 86:913, 1979.

390. Phellps JY, Higby K, Smyth MH, et al: Accuracy and intraobserver variability of simulated cervical dilation measurements. Am J Obstet Gynecol 173:942, 1995.

391. Jackson GM, Ludmir J, Bader TJ: The accuracy of digital examination and ultrasound in the evaluation of cervical length. Obstet Gynecol 79:214, 1992.

392. Zilianti M, Azuaga A, Calderon F, et al: Monitoring the effacement of the uterine cervix by transperineal sonography: A new perspective. J Ultrasound Med 14:719, 1995.

393. Guzman ER, Rosenberg JC, Houlihan C, et al: A new method using ultrasound and transfundal pressure to evaluate the asymptomatic incompetent cervix. Obstet Gynecol 83:248, 1994.

394. Shirodkar VN: A method of operative treatment for habitual abortions in the second trimester of pregnancy. Antiseptic 52:299, 1955.

395. McDonald IA: Suture of the cervix for inevitable abortion. J Obstet Gynaecol Br Emp 64:346, 1957.

396. Harger J: Comparison of success and morbidity in cervical cerclage procedures. Obstet Gynecol 56:543, 1980.

397. Andersen HF, Karimi A, Sakala EP, Kalugdan R: Prediction of cervical cerclage outcome by endovaginal ultrasonography. Am J Obstet Gynecol 171:1102, 1994.

398. Quinn MJ: Vaginal ultrasound and cervical cerclage: a prospective study. Ultrasound Obstet Gynecol 2:410, 1992.

399. Novy MJ: Transabdominal cervicoisthmic cerclage: A reappraisal 25 years after its introduction. Am J Obstet Gynecol 164:163, 1991.

400. Aarts JM, Brons JT, Bruinse HW, et al: Emergency cerclage: A review. Obstet Gynecol Surv 50:459, 1995.

401. Scheerer LJ, Lam F, Bartolucci L, et al: A new technique for reduction of prolapsed fetal membranes for emergency cervical cerclage. Obstet Gynecol 74:408, 1989.

402. Weissman A, Jakobi P, Zahi S, Zimmer EZ: The effect of cervical cerclage on the course of labor. Obstet Gynecol 76:168, 1990.

403. Harger JH: Cervical cerclage: Patient selection, morbidity, and success rates. Clin Perinatol 10:321, 1983.

404. Ludmir J, Bader T, Chen L, et al: Poor perinatal outcome associated with retained cerclage in patients with premature rupture of membranes. Obstet Gynecol 84:823, 1994.

405. McElrath TF, Norwitz ER, Lieberman ES, et al: Cervical cerclage and preterm premature rupture of the membranes: Should the stitch be removed? [abstract]. Am J Obstet Gynecol 182:S155, 2000.

406. Kitzmiller J: Preterm premature rupture of the membranes. In Fuchs F, Stubblefield PG (eds): Preterm Birth Causes, Prevention and Management. New York, Macmillan, 1984, p 298.

407. Skinner S, Campos G, Liggins G: Collagen content of human amniotic membranes: Effect of gestation length and premature rupture. Obstet Gynecol 57:487, 1981.

408. Athayde N, Edwin SS, Romero R, et al: A role for matrix metalloproteinase-9 in spontaneous rupture of the fetal membranes. Am J Obstet Gynecol 179:1248, 1998.

409. Parry S, Strauss JF: Premature rupture of the fetal membranes. N Engl J Med 338:663, 1998.

410. Roberts AK, Monzon-Bordonaba F, Van Deerlin PG, et al: Association of polymorphism within the promoter of the tumor necrosis factor α gene with increased risk of preterm premature rupture of the fetal membranes. Am J Obstet Gynecol 180:1297, 1999.

411. Millar LK, Boesche MH, Yamamoto SY, et al: A relaxin mediated pathway to preterm premature rupture of the fetal membranes that is independent of infection. Am J Obstet Gynecol 179:126, 1998.

412. Minkoff H, Grunebaum AN, Schwartz RH, et al: Risk factors for prematurity and premature rupture of membranes: A prospective study of the vaginal flora in pregnancy. Am J Obstet Gynecol 150:965, 1984.

413. Naeye R: Factors that predispose to premature rupture of the fetal membranes. Obstet Gynecol 60:93, 1982.

414. Maradny EE, Kanayama N, Halim A, et al: Stretching of fetal membranes increases the concentration of interleukin-8 and collagenase activity. Am J Obstet Gynecol 174:843, 1996.

415. Harger JH, Hsing AW, Tuomala RE, et al: Risk factors for preterm premature rupture of fetal membranes: A multicenter case-control study. Am J Obstet Gynecol 163:130, 1990.

416. Mercer BM, Goldenberg RL, Iams JD, et al: The Preterm Prediction Study: Analysis of risk factors for preterm premature rupture of the membranes. J Soc Gynecol Invest 3:350A, 1996.

417. Lonky NM, Hayashi RH: A proposed mechanism for premature rupture of membranes. Obstet Gynecol Surv 43:22, 1988.

418. Romero R, Mazor M: Infection and preterm labor. Clin Obstet Gynecol 31:553, 1988.

419. Schutte M, Treffers P, Kloosterman G, et al: Management of premature rupture of membranes: The risk of vaginal examination to the infant. Am J Obstet Gynecol 146:395, 1983.

420. Lewis DF, Major CA, Towers CV, et al: Effects of digital vaginal examinations on latency period in preterm premature rupture of membranes. Obstet Gynecol 80:630, 1992.

421. Alexander JM, Mercer BM, Miodovnik M, et al: The impact of digital cervical examination on expectantly managed preterm ruptured membranes. Am J Obstet Gynecol 183:1003, 2000.

422. Brown CL, Ludwiczak MH, Blanco JD, et al: Cervical dilation: Accuracy of visual and digital examinations. Obstet Gynecol 81:215, 1993.

423. Smith R: A technic for the detection of rupture of the membranes: A review and preliminary report. Obstet Gynecol 48:172, 1976.

424. Reece EA, Chervenak F, Moya F, et al: Amniotic fluid arborization: Effect of blood, meconium, and pH alterations. Obstet Gynecol 64:248, 1984.

425. Rosemond RL, Lombardi SJ, Boehm FH: Ferning of amniotic fluid contaminated with blood. Obstet Gynecol 75:338, 1990.

426. Taylor J, Garite T: Premature rupture of membranes before fetal viability. Obstet Gynecol 64:615, 1984.

427. Garite T, Freeman R, Linzey E, et al: Prospective randomized study of corticosteroids in the management of premature rupture of the membranes and the premature gestation. Am J Obstet Gynecol 141:508, 1981.

428. Dale PO, Tanbo T, Bendvold E, Moe N: Duration of the latency period in preterm premature rupture of the membranes. Eur J Obstet Gynecol Reprod Biol 30:257, 1989.

429. Cox SM, Williams ML, Leveno KJ: The natural history of preterm ruptured membranes: What to expect of expectant management. Obstet Gynecol 71:558, 1988.

430. Nelson LH, Anderson RL, O'Shea TM, Swain M: Expectant management of preterm premature rupture of the membranes. Am J Obstet Gynecol 171:350, 1994.

431. Moretti M, Sibai BM: Maternal and perinatal outcome of expectant management of premature rupture of membranes in the midtrimester. Am J Obstet Gynecol 159:390, 1988.

432. Moberg L, Garite T, Freeman R: Fetal heart rate patterns and fetal distress in patients with preterm premature rupture of membranes. Obstet Gynecol 64:60, 1984.

433. Nelson DM, Stempel LE, Zuspan FP, et al: Association of prolonged preterm premature rupture of the membranes and abruptio placentae. J Reprod Med 31:249, 1986.

434. Vintzileos AM, Campbell WA, Nochimson DJ, et al: Preterm premature rupture of the membranes: A risk factor for the development of abruptio placentae. Am J Obstet Gynecol 156:1235, 1987.

435. Major CA, de Veciana M, Lewis DF, Morgan MA: Preterm premature rupture of the membranes and abruptio placentae: Is there an association between these pregnancy complications? Am J Obstet Gynecol 172:672, 1995.

436. Rotschild A, Ling EW, Peterman ML, Farquharson D: Neonatal outcome after prolonged preterm rupture of the membranes. Am J Obstet Gynecol 162:46, 1990.

437. Carroll SG, Blott M, Nicolaides KH: Preterm prelabor amniorrhexis: Outcome of live births. Obstet Gynecol 86:18, 1995.

438. Nimrod C, Varela-Gittings F, Machin G, et al: The effect of very prolonged membrane rupture on fetal development. Am J Obstet Gynecol 148:540, 1984.

439. Bottoms SF, Welch RA, Zador IE, et al: Clinical interpretation of ultrasound measurements in preterm pregnancies with premature rupture of membranes. Obstet Gynecol 69:358, 1987.

440. Garite T: Premature rupture of the membranes: The enigma of the obstetrician. Am J Obstet Gynecol 151:1001, 1985.

441. Naef RW, Allbert JR, Ross EL, et al: Premature rupture of membranes at 34 to 37 weeks' gestation: Aggressive vs conservative management. Am J Obstet Gynecol 178:126, 1998.

442. Neerhoff MG, Cravello C, Haney EI, et al: Timing of labor induction after premature rupture of membranes between 32 and 36 weeks gestation. Am J Obstet Gynecol 180:349, 1999.

443. Romero R, Quintero R, Oyarzun E, et al: Intraamniotic infection and the onset of labor in preterm premature rupture of the membranes. Am J Obstet Gynecol 159:661, 1988.

444. Galle P, Meis P: Complications of amniocentesis. J Reprod Med 27:149, 1982.

445. Shaver DC, Spinnato JA, Whybrew D, et al: Comparison of phospholipids in vaginal and amniocentesis specimens of patients with premature rupture of membranes. Am J Obstet Gynecol 156:454, 1987.

446. Schumacher RE, Parisi VM, Steady HM, et al: Bacteria causing false positive test for phosphatidylglycerol in amniotic fluid. Am J Obstet Gynecol 151:1067, 1985.

447. Mercer BM, Crocker LG, Boe NM, et al: Induction versus expectant management in prematurity of the membranes with mature amniotic fluid at 32–36 weeks: A randomized trial. Am J Obstet Gynecol 1679:775, 1993.

448. Garite TJ, Freeman RK: Chorioamnionitis in the preterm gestation. Obstet Gynecol 59:539, 1982.

449. Sperling RS, Ramamurthy RS, Gibbs RS: A comparison of intrapartum versus immediate postpartum treatment of intraamniotic infection. Obstet Gynecol 70:861, 1987.

450. Gibbs RS, Dinsmoor MJ, Newton ER, Ramamurthy RS: A randomized trial of intrapartum versus immediate postpartum treatment of women with intra-amniotic infection. Obstet Gynecol 72:823, 1988.

451. Gilstrap LC, Leveno KJ, Cox SM, et al: Intrapartum treatment of acute chorioamnionitis: Impact on neonatal sepsis. Am J Obstet Gynecol 159:579, 1988.

452. Ohlsson A, Wang E: An analysis of antenatal tests to detect infection in preterm premature rupture of the membranes. Am J Obstet Gynecol 162:809, 1990.

453. Asrat T, Nageotte MP, Garite SE, Dorchester W: Gram stain results from amniocentesis in patients with preterm premature rupture of the membranes—comparison of maternal and fetal characteristics. Am J Obstet Gynecol 163:887, 1990.

454. Hanley ML, Vintzeleos AM: Biophysical testing in premature rupture of the membranes. Semin Perinatol 20:418, 1996.

455. Lewis DF, Adair CD, Weeks JW, et al: A randomized clinical trial of daily nonstress testing vs biophysical profile in the management of preterm premature rupture of membranes. Am J Obstet Gynecol 181:1495, 1999.

456. Hussey MJ, Levy ES, Pombar X, et al: Evaluating rapid diagnostic tests of intra-amniotic infection: Gram stain, amniotic fluid glucose level, and amniotic fluid to serum glucose level ratio. Am J Obstet Gynecol 179:650, 1998.

457. Romero R, Yoon BH, Mazor M, et al: A comparative study of the diagnostic performance of amniotic fluid glucose, white blood cell count, interleukin-6, and Gram stain in the detection of microbial invasion in patients with preterm premature rupture of membranes. Am J Obstet Gynecol 169:839, 1993.

458. Mercer BM, Miodovnik M, Thurnau GR, et al: Antibiotic

therapy for reduction of infant morbidity after preterm premature rupture of the membranes. JAMA 278:989, 1997.

459. Ohlsson A: Treatments of preterm premature rupture of the membranes: A meta-analysis. Am J Obstet Gynecol 160:890, 1989.

460. Vermillion ST, Soper DE, Chasedunn-Roark J: Neonatal sepsis after betamethasone administration to patients with preterm premature rupture of membranes. Am J Obstet Gynecol 181:320, 1999.

461. American Academy of Pediatrics (Committee on Infectious Diseases and Committee on Fetus and Newborn of the American Academy of Pediatrics): Guidelines for the prevention of group B streptococcal (GBS) infection by chemoprophylaxis. Pediatrics 90:775, 1992.

462. Lewis DF, Brody K, Edwards MS, et al: Preterm premature ruptured membranes: A randomized trial of steroids after treatment with antibiotics. Obstet Gynecol 88:801, 1996.

463. Lovett SM, Weiss JD, Diogo MJ, et al: A prospective, double blind randomized, controlled clinical trial of ampicillin-sulbactam for preterm premature rupture of membranes in women receiving antenatal corticosteroid therapy. Am J Obstet Gynecol 176:1030, 1997.

464. Curet L, Rao V, Zachman R, et al: Association between ruptured membranes, tocolytic therapy, and respiratory distress syndrome. Am J Obstet Gynecol 148:263, 1984.

465. Garite TJ, Keegan KA, Freeman RK, et al: A randomized trial of ritodrine tocolysis versus expectant management in patients with premature rupture of membranes at 25 to 30 weeks of gestation. Am J Obstet Gynecol 157:388, 1987.

466. Weiner CP, Renk K, Klugman M: The therapeutic efficacy and cost-effectiveness of aggressive tocolysis for premature labor associated with premature rupture of the membranes. Am J Obstet Gynecol 159:216, 1988.

467. Ghidini A, Romero R: Premature rupture of the membranes: When it occurs in the second trimester. Contemp Ob Gyn 39:66, 1994.

468. Farooqi A, Holmgren PA, Engberg S, Serenius F: Survival and 2-year outcome with expectant management of second trimester rupture of membranes. Obstet Gynecol 92:895, 1998.

469. Major CA, Towers CV, Lewis DF, Asrat T: Expectant management of patients with both preterm premature rupture of the membranes and genital herpes. Am J Obstet Gynecol 164:248, 1991.

470. Allen MC, Donohue PK, Dusman AE, et al: The limit of viability neonatal outcome infants born at 22–25 weeks gestation. N Engl J Med 329:1597, 1993.

471. Reuss ML, Gordon HR: Obstetrical judgments of viability and perinatal survival of extremely low birth weight infants. Am J Public Health 85:362, 1995.

472. Saigal S, Stoskopf BL, Feeny D, et al: Differences in preferences for neonatal outcomes among health care professionals, parents and adolescents. JAMA 281:1991, 1999.

473. Haywood JL, Goldenberg RL, Bronstein J, et al: Comparison of perceived and actual rates of survival and freedom from handicap in premature infants. Am J Obstet Gynecol 171:432, 1994.

474. Martinez AM, Weiss E, Partridge JC, et al: Management of extremely low birth weight infants: Perceptions of viability and parental counseling practices. Obstet Gynecol 92:250, 1998.

475. Bahado-Singh RO, Dashe J, Deren O, et al: Prenatal prediction of neonatal outcome in the extremely low birth weight infant. Am J Obstet Gynecol 178:462, 1998.

476. Bottoms SF, Paul RH, Mercer BM, et al: Obstetric determinants of neonatal survival: Antenatal predictors of neonatal survival and morbidity in extremely low birth weight infants. Am J Obstet Gynecol 180:665, 1999.

477. Luthy DA, Shy KK, van Belle G, et al: A randomized trial of electronic fetal monitoring in preterm labor. Obstet Gynecol 69:687, 1987.

478. Larson EB, van Belle G, Shy KK, et al: Fetal monitoring and predictions by clinicians: Observations during a randomized clinical trial in very low birth weight infants. Obstet Gynecol 74:584, 1989.

479. Zanini B, Paul R, Huey J: Intrapartum fetal heart rate: Correlation with scalp pH in the preterm fetus. Am J Obstet Gynecol 136:43, 1980.

480. Bowes W, Gabbe S, Bowes C: Fetal heart rate monitoring in premature infants weighing 1,500 gm or less. Am J Obstet Gynecol 137:791, 1980.

481. Myers S, Paton J, Fisher D: Neonatal survival of the tiny infant: The challenge. Presented at the Annual Meeting, Society of Perinatal Obstetricians, 1985.

482. Barrett J, Boehm F, Vaughn W: The effect of type of delivery on neonatal outcome in singleton infants of birth weight of 1,000 g or less. JAMA 250:625, 1983.

483. Malloy MH, Onstad L, Wright E, et al: The effect of cesarean delivery on birth outcome in very low birth weight infants. Obstet Gynecol 77:498, 1991.

484. Hack M, Fanarof AA: Outcomes of extremely low birth weight infants between 1982 and 1988. N Engl J Med 321:1642, 1989.

485. Kitchen WH, Permezel MJ, Doyle LW, et al: Changing obstetric practice and 2-year outcome of the fetus of birth weight under 1000g. Obstet Gynecol 79:268, 1992.

486. Grant A, Penn ZJ, Steer PJ: Elective or selective caesarean delivery of the small baby? A systematic review of the controlled trials. Br J Obstet Gynaecol 103:1197, 1996.

487. Wolf H, Schaap AHP, Bruinse HW, et al: Vaginal delivery compared with caesarean section in early preterm breech delivery: A comparison of long term outcome. Br J Obstet Gynaecol 106:486, 1999.

488. Dietl J, Arnold H, Mentzel H, et al: Effect of cesarean section on outcome in high- and low-risk very preterm infants. Arch Gynecol Obstet 246:91, 1989.

Chapter 24

Multiple Gestations

USHA CHITKARA AND RICHARD L. BERKOWITZ

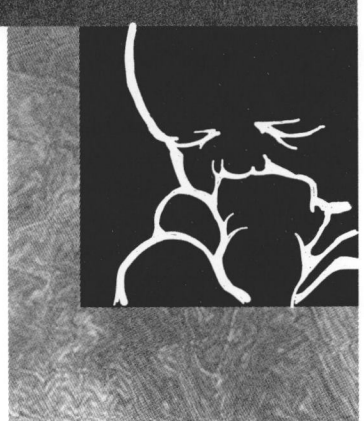

The phenomenon of twinning has fascinated mankind throughout its recorded history. Twins have often been regarded as being inherently "different" from singletons, and societal responses to their birth have ranged from awe to fear. Researchers have been interested in exploiting their uniqueness in an attempt to separate the influences of genetic and environmental factors on both fetal and postpartum development.[1] Obstetricians have long been aware that pregnancies complicated by twinning are by their very nature at higher risk than those of most singletons. Finally, parents and future siblings are often overjoyed or overwhelmed when they are told that twins are expected but are virtually never neutral in their response.

Twins are either monozygotic (MZ) or dizygotic (DZ). In the former case, a single fertilized ovum splits into two distinct individuals after a variable number of divisions. Such twins are almost always genetically identical and therefore of the same sex. On rare occasions, mutations can cause genetic discordance resulting in phenotypic and chromosomal dissimilarities between MZ twins. On the other hand, when two separate ova are fertilized, DZ twins result. These individuals are as genetically distinct as any other children born to the same couple. Sets of DZ twins may have the same or opposite sex. DZ half-siblings have been reported in which two ova were fertilized by different fathers, and it has been hypothesized that monovular dispermic fertilization may occur. These latter situations are very uncommon, however. In most cases, DZ twins are genetically dissimilar true siblings, while MZ twins are genetically identical.

The frequency of MZ twins is fairly constant throughout the world at a rate of approximately 4 per 1,000 births. This rate does not seem to vary with maternal characteristics such as age or parity. DZ twinning, however, is associated with multiple ovulation, and its frequency varies between races and within countries and is affected by several identifiable factors. In general, the frequency of DZ twins is low in Asians, intermediate in whites, and high in blacks. The Yorubas of western Nigeria have a frequency of 45 twins per 1,000 births, and about 90 percent are DZ.[2]

The frequency of DZ births is affected by maternal age, increasing from a rate of 3 in 1,000 in women under age 20, to 14 in 1,000 at ages 35 to 40. Between 1980 to 1987, the greatest increase in U.S. birth rates of triplets and higher order multiple pregnancies occurred in women aged 30 to 39—an almost sevenfold increase in that time period.[3] Above age 40, the rate declines. The frequency of DZ twinning also increases with parity independent of maternal age.[1]

The different rates of DZ twinning may be due to racial or individual variations in pituitary gonadotropin production. Infertility patients treated with menopausal urinary gonadotropins (Pergonal) or clomiphene citrate are well known to have a dose-dependent increase in multiple births when compared with women who conceive without these agents. While DZ twins predominate in these patients, triplets and higher numbers of conceptuses may also occur. The use of in vitro fertilization (IVF) and embryo transfer has further increased the incidence of multiple pregnancies, and reports suggest that the incidence of multiple gestations in IVF patients may be as high as 22 percent.[4,5] In early 1980, the reported incidence of twins in the United States was 12 per 1,000 births, with two thirds of these being DZ.[1] Current data suggest that since 1980, twin births have risen 52 percent and that triplet and higher order births have quadrupled. This dramatic rise in multiple births is mainly attributed to the growing popularity of IVF and other methods of assisted reproductive technology (ART).[3]

The cause of MZ twinning is unclear. Benirschke and

Kim[6] state that it is probably an uncommon occurrence among other mammals. In two species of armadillo, however, polyembryony regularly follows implantation of a single blastocyst. Oxygen deprivation has been experimentally shown to enhance fission in fish embryos, and some teratogens have been associated with increased MZ twinning rates in laboratory animals, but there is currently no satisfactory explanation for the fact that MZ twins occur in humans with such a constant frequency around the world. The majority of multiple pregnancies that occur after fertility treatment result from fertilization and implantation of multiple embryos, yielding polyzygotic gestations. However, MZ twinning is also increased by ovulation induction and other modern ART methods. Against a spontaneous rate of 0.4 percent MZ twinning in the general population, some studies have reported an increased incidence of MZ twins to 1.2 percent with conventional ovulation induction methods[7] and a 3.2 percent incidence

with use of other ART methods.[8] In these cases, it is believed that alterations in either the structure or physical properties of the zona pellucida surrounding the early embryo are responsible for the increased tendency toward iatrogenic zygote splitting and resultant MZ twins.

PLACENTATION

Twin placentas are described in terms of their membranes (Fig. 24–1). The sac of a singleton pregnancy consists of an outer chorion and an inner amnion. Each DZ twin develops within a similar sac because both blastocysts generate their own placentas. If implantation of these blastocysts is not proximal to each other, two separate placentas will result, each of which will

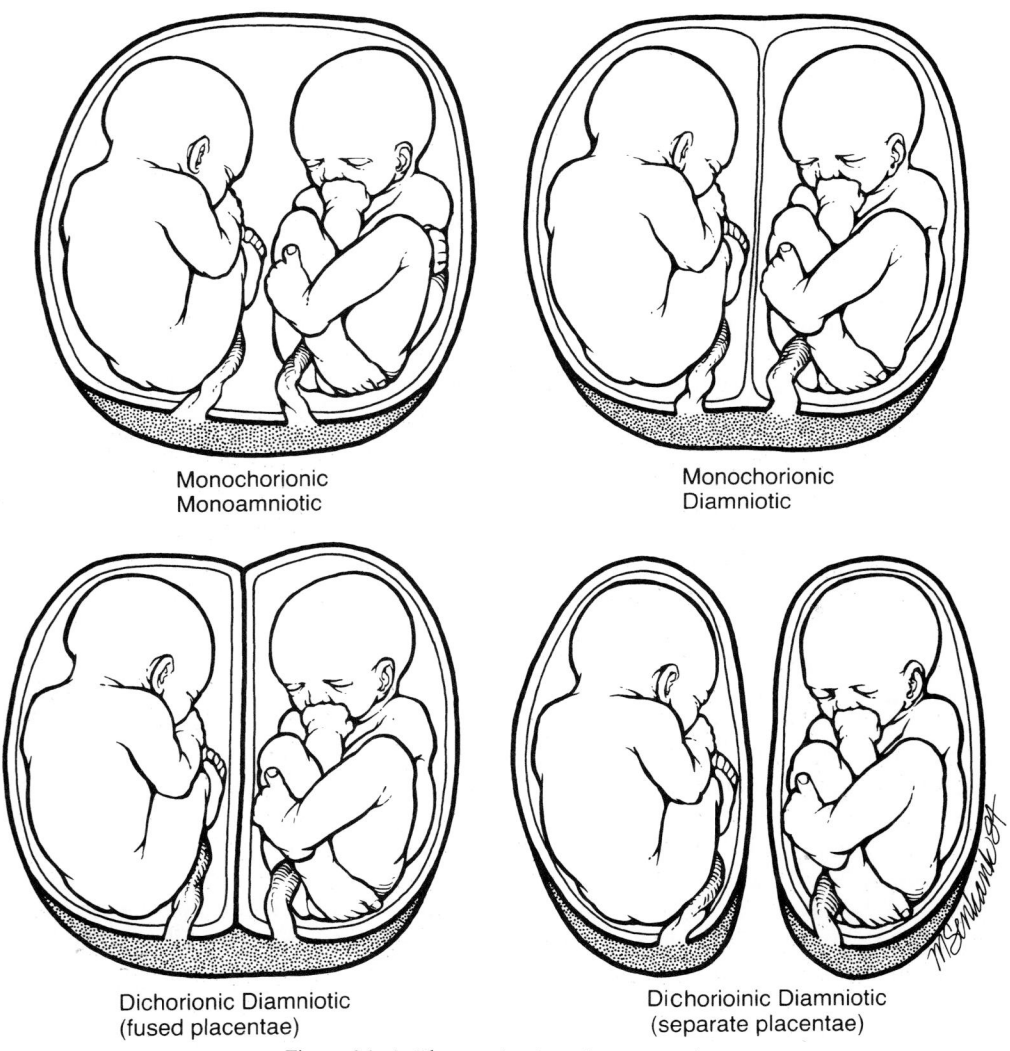

Monochorionic
Monoamniotic

Monochorionic
Diamniotic

Dichorionic Diamniotic
(fused placentae)

Dichorioinic Diamniotic
(separate placentae)

Figure 24–1. Placentation in twin pregnancies.

have a chorion and an amnion. Should they implant side by side, intimate fusion of the placental disks will occur, but these placentas are always diamniotic and dichorionic, and vascular anastomoses rarely occur. While MZ twins may also have placentas with two amnions and two chorions, this generally is not the case. Monochorionic placentas have a single chorion that usually surrounds two amnions, but occasionally there is only a single amnion. Regardless of whether these monochorial placentas are diamniotic or monoamniotic, they are always a single disk and only occur in MZ twins. Triplets and quadruplets have also been delivered with monochorial placentas and shown to be MZ. Almost all monochorial placentas have blood vessel communications between the fetal circulations.

The type of placenta that develops in an MZ pregnancy is determined by the timing of cleavage of the fertilized ovum. If twinning is accomplished during the first 2 to 3 days, it precedes the setting aside of cells that eventually become the chorion. In that case, two chorions and two amnions will be formed. After approximately 3 days, however, twinning cannot split the chorionic cavity, and from that time on a monochorial placenta must result. If the split occurs between the third and eighth days, a diamniotic monochorial placenta will develop. Between the 8th and 13th days, the amnion has already formed, and the placenta will therefore be monoamniotic and monochorionic. Embryonic cleavage between the 13th and 15th days will result in conjoined twins within a single amnion and chorion; beyond that point, the process of twinning cannot occur.

The frequency of placental types within a population is influenced by the rate of DZ twinning. In the United States, approximately 80 percent of twin placentas are dichorionic, and 20 percent are monochorionic. In Nigeria, where DZ twinning is much more common, the frequency of dichorionic placentas approaches 95 percent.[6] With triplets, quadruplets, and higher orders of multiple gestation, monochorionic and dichorionic placentations may coexist.

Because monochorial placentas can only occur in MZ pregnancies, study of the membranes will establish zygosity in 20 percent of cases in the United States. In approximately 35 percent of cases the twins will be of opposite sex and therefore necessarily DZ. This leaves only 45 percent of cases (twins of like sex having dichorionic placentas) in which further studies are necessary in order to determine zygosity. Cameron[9] found that this 45 percent breaks down into 8 percent MZ and 37 percent DZ. He states that "the percentage of monozygotic dichorionic pairs is inversely proportional to the completeness of the genotyping." In other words, the more genotypic markers that are studied, the greater the likelihood of demonstrating dizygosity. Cameron used six blood group markers, four red blood cell (RBC) enzymes, and placental alkaline phosphatase in order to determine zygosity. However, at present, the most accurate method for determination of twin zygosity is by analysis of DNA polymorphism.[10,11] The often-cited Weinberg rule states that in a population of twins the estimated number of MZ pairs is almost exactly equal to the total minus twice the number of twins of unlike sex. The assumption underlying this rule is that among DZ pairs the sex of one twin is independent of that of the other, resulting in almost exactly equal numbers of like and unlike sexed pairs. The small difference anticipated from exact equality is due to the fact that the sex ratio is not precisely 0.5. This rule has been questioned by several authorities who present evidence that in DZ populations there seems to be a higher frequency of like-sex than opposite-sex twins at birth.[12] Cameron's data[9] would favor the latter view.

PERINATAL MORBIDITY AND MORTALITY

Numerous reports have documented that perinatal morbidity and mortality are greater in twins than in singletons. A collaborative study was published by Kohl and Casey regarding 6,503 sets of twins delivered at 32 different hospitals between 1961 and 1972.[13] The overall perinatal mortality in this series was 124 per 1,000 births. When only those twins weighing more than 1,000 g were considered, the perinatal loss was 62 per 1,000 births, which was approximately three times greater than that of comparable singletons at the same institutions.

A high incidence of low-birth-weight infants is the major cause of the increased perinatal mortality in twins. Both preterm delivery and intrauterine growth restriction (IUGR) contribute to this problem. In addition to prematurity and growth restriction, twins have an increased frequency of congenital anomalies, placenta previa, abruptio placentae, preeclampsia, cord accidents, and malpresentations.

Because of advances in both maternal–fetal medicine and neonatal care, a general decline in perinatal mortality has been reported over the past two decades from centers around the world. In general, this overall trend has also been noted for multiple gestations. Desgranges et al.[14] reported a perinatal mortality rate of 95 per 1,000 in 213 twins delivered between 1969 and 1973 compared with 56 per 1,000 in 221 twins delivered between 1974 and 1979 at the Hopital Notre-Dame in Montreal. During these periods, there was essentially no change in the fetal death rates (28 per 1,000 vs. 32 per 1,000), but the neonatal mortality fell from 68 per 1,000 to 24 per 1,000. The frequency of anomalies during the entire period was 23 per 1,000, and these accounted for 18 percent of all deaths. The average length of pregnancy in both study periods was identical, and the improved neonatal outcome was found to be due to increased survival rates in neonates weighing 1,000 to 1,500 g at birth.

With the routine use of antenatal fetal heart rate testing, Rattan and colleagues[15] noted a marked reduction in fetal mortality after 32 weeks when 153 twins delivered between 1975 and 1979 were compared with 160 twins delivered between 1980 and 1983. The rate of stillbirths fell from 23 per 1,000 in the former period to 0 per 1,000 in the latter.

Despite these encouraging trends, the problems associated with multiple gestations continue to place these infants at higher risk than their singleton counterparts. Hawrylyshyn et al.[16] reported an overall perinatal mortality rate of 91 per 1,000 births in 177 twin pairs delivered between 1975 and 1979 in Toronto. The number of cases in each year was fairly small, but there was no demonstrable decline in perinatal mortality during the study period. In this series, more than 70 percent of the deaths occurred before 30 weeks' gestation. Those deaths either took place in utero or during the neonatal period in association with respiratory distress syndrome, intracerebral hemorrhage, or necrotizing enterocolitis. These workers concluded that if obstetricians are to have a major impact on the perinatal survival of twins, they must concentrate on the period between 25 and 30 weeks' gestation.

In multifetal gestations with three or more fetuses, the most important complication again is premature delivery with its concomitant increase in perinatal morbidity and mortality. In general, delivery of multiple gestations occurs much earlier than singletons. The cumulative distribution of gestational age for singletons, twins, and triplets born in the United States during 1980 to 1994 indicated that 1.2 percent of singletons, 11 percent of twins, and 31 percent of triplets were born before 32 weeks of gestation. In the same years, infants born before 35 weeks' gestation constituted 3.1 percent singletons, 25 percent twins, and 67 percent triplets. However, when considered by the usually accepted definition of preterm as less than 37 weeks' gestation, 8.5 percent of singletons, 50 percent of twins, and 90 percent of triplets were born preterm.[17] Accurate knowledge regarding outcome of these pregnancies remains limited because of the relatively small numbers in any reported series, especially for quadruplets and higher order births. Among three fairly large series published before 1983, Holcberg et al.[18] reported a perinatal mortality rate of 312 per 1,000 among 31 triplet pregnancies managed in their institution between 1960 and 1979. Ron-El et al.[19] reported a perinatal mortality of 185 per 1,000 in their series of 29 triplet and 6 quadruplet gestations managed between 1970 and

1978. Loucopoulos and Jewelewicz,[20] in a series of 27 triplets, 7 quadruplets, and 1 quintuplet cared for from 1965 to 1981, noted a perinatal mortality rate of 148 per 1,000. Major improvements in perinatal and neonatal care over the past two decades have resulted in significantly better survival rates for triplets and perhaps higher order pregnancies. This is reflected in the results of some of the more recent published reports on multiple gestations. Lipitz et al.[21] reported a perinatal mortality of 93 per 1,000 among 78 triplet gestations managed in their institution between 1975 and 1988. Gonen et al.,[22] presenting their data on 30 multiple gestations (24 triplets, 5 quadruplets, and 1 quintuplet) from 1978 to 1988, reported a perinatal mortality rate of 51.5 per 1,000; and the experience of Newman et al.[23] with 198 triplet pregnancies delivered between 1985 and 1988 was similar. Three recent publications from Britain, Switzerland, and Australia report outcome data on multiple gestations conceived spontaneously or by assisted reproductive technology. The British report[24] contained 143 sets of triplets and 12 sets of quadruplets with perinatal mortality rates of 70 per 1,000 and 104 per 1,000, respectively. The Swiss data[25] included 77 sets of triplets with a perinatal mortality of 89 per 1,000 and 9 quadruplet sets with a perinatal mortality of 147 per 1,000; whereas the Australian series, including 133 sets of triplets and 6 sets of quadruplets, reported perinatal mortality of 108 per 1,000 and 250 per 1,000, respectively.[26]

A review of the subject by Alvarez and Berkowitz[27] in 1990 concluded that although perinatal mortality rates had decreased, the risk of prematurity in multifetal gestations had not changed significantly over the past 20 to 30 years. The average gestational age at delivery for triplets consistently seems to be 33 to 35 weeks. Approximately 75 percent of these patients deliver prior to 37 weeks, and at least 20 percent deliver prior to 32 weeks. The number of reported patients with four or more fetuses remains too small for a meaningful analysis of perinatal morbidity and mortality rates. However, one can assume that at best the outcome in those pregnancies is the same as with triplets, and it probably is worse.

The infant mortality rate for multiple births is also high. Luke and Keith[28] analyzed the National Infant Mortality Surveillance (NIMS) Project based on the 1980 U.S. birth cohort and reported an overall infant mortality rate of 8.6 per 1,000 for singletons, 56.6 per 1,000 for twins, and 166.7 per 1,000 for triplets. This represents a 6.6-fold and 19.4-fold higher mortality in twins and triplets, respectively, compared with singletons. Likewise, among survivors, the incidence of severe handicap was significantly higher among multiple births, being 19.7, 34.0, and 57.5 per 1,000 postneonatal survivors in singletons, twins, and triplets, respectively, and representing a 1.7-fold and 2.9-fold higher rate among twins and triplets compared with singletons. Interestingly, however, the risk of death or morbidity from chronic lung disease or grade III or IV intracranial hemorrhage was found to be similar for twins and singletons that were below 28 weeks' gestation and very low birth weight (i.e., between 401 and 1,500 g).[29]

DIAGNOSIS

It is obviously impossible to offer specialized antepartum care if multiple gestation remains undiagnosed until the intrapartum period. An often-quoted statistic in the older literature is that 50 percent of twins remain undiagnosed until the time of delivery.[30] Because of the current widespread use of diagnostic ultrasound, this is certainly no longer true. The number of twins in the United States diagnosed during the antenatal period is currently unknown, but there must be substantial variations from one institution to another, depending on the degree to which ultrasound is used. In a report from Yale-New Haven Hospital,[31] 91 percent of 385 twin sets delivered between 1977 and 1981 were diagnosed before the onset of labor.

Multiple gestations should be suspected whenever (1) the uterus seems to be larger than dates, (2) hydramnios or unexplained maternal anemia develops, (3) auscultation of more than one fetal heart is suspected, or (4) the pregnancy has occurred following ovulation induction or in vitro fertilization. Multiple gestation may also be diagnosed serendipitously at the time of ultrasound scanning before a genetic amniocentesis or as a result of an elevated serum α-fetoprotein (AFP) level in mass-screening programs.

An argument often used in support of universal ultrasound screening for all pregnant women during the second trimester is that it would result in the early diagnosis of multiple pregnancies with almost 100 percent accuracy.[32] Persson and Kullander[33] reported the results of this type of screening program, which has been in effect at the Malmo General Hospital in Sweden since 1973. Originally, the program began with a single scan performed in the 30th week, but subsequently all women were offered examinations at both 17 and 33 weeks. Between 1974 and 1982, 98 percent of 254 multiple gestations were detected by ultrasound screening. There were no false-positive diagnoses, but 2 percent of multiple gestations were missed on the first examination. These authors also reported a reduction in perinatal mortality from 107 per 1,000 to 34 per 1,000 when similar numbers of twins delivered between 1970 and 1974 were compared with those delivered from 1975 to 1982. Major morbidity (e.g., cerebral palsy, mental retardation, late motor development, and hearing defects) decreased from 9.6 to 3.6 percent, and the frequency of delivery prior to 38 weeks dropped from 34 to 15.8 percent. The marked improvement in these figures was obviously due to multiple factors, but early diagnosis was among them. Results of the Routine Antenatal Diagnostic Imaging with Ultrasound (RADIUS) study from the United States indicate a similar experience.[34] This study compared a group of low-risk pregnant women who underwent routine ultrasound screening in the second and third trimesters of pregnancy with a control group who had an ultrasound examination only when medically indicated. The diagnosis of multiple gestation, when present, was made before 26 weeks' gestation in all women who had the screening ultrasound examination. In contrast, among women in the control group, 37 percent of multiple gestations were not identified until after 26 weeks' gestation, and in 13 percent the diagnosis was not made until the delivery admission.

Separate gestational sacs can be identified ultrasonically as early as 6 weeks from the first day of the last menstrual period. With transabdominal scanning, an embryo within each sac should be visible by 7 weeks, and beating fetal hearts should be seen by 7.5 to 8 weeks.[35] With good equipment, the fetal cranial pole is also identifiable during this period, but the intracranial landmarks used for accurate biparietal diameter measurements are usually not seen until 14 to 16 weeks. Increasing sophistication in the development and use of endovaginal scanning has made it possible to visualize these developmental landmarks 1 to 2 weeks earlier than with abdominal scanning techniques so that the embryonic pole and fetal heart can be seen by 6 weeks and the intracranial landmarks are visible by 10 to 12 weeks' gestation.[36]

In general, the ultrasonic diagnosis of multiple gestations within the first trimester is relatively straightforward. It is mandatory, however, to visualize separate fetuses (Fig. 24–2). Retromembranous collections of blood or fluid or a prominent fetal yolk sac should not be confused with a twin gestation. Demonstration of the viability of each fetus at the time of the examination requires visualization of independent cardiac activity. Unfortunately, mistakes can be made regarding the number of fetuses present when scans are hastily interpreted. This is particularly true in the third trimester, but may also occur in the first and second trimesters, especially with four or more fetuses. It must be remembered that an ultrasound image, unlike a flat plate of the abdomen, does not provide a composite overview. The image displayed is only a tomographic slice through the area being studied. It is therefore possible to display two circular structures that may represent different fetal heads or, alternatively, the head and thorax of the same fetus in a tucked position. Misinterpre-

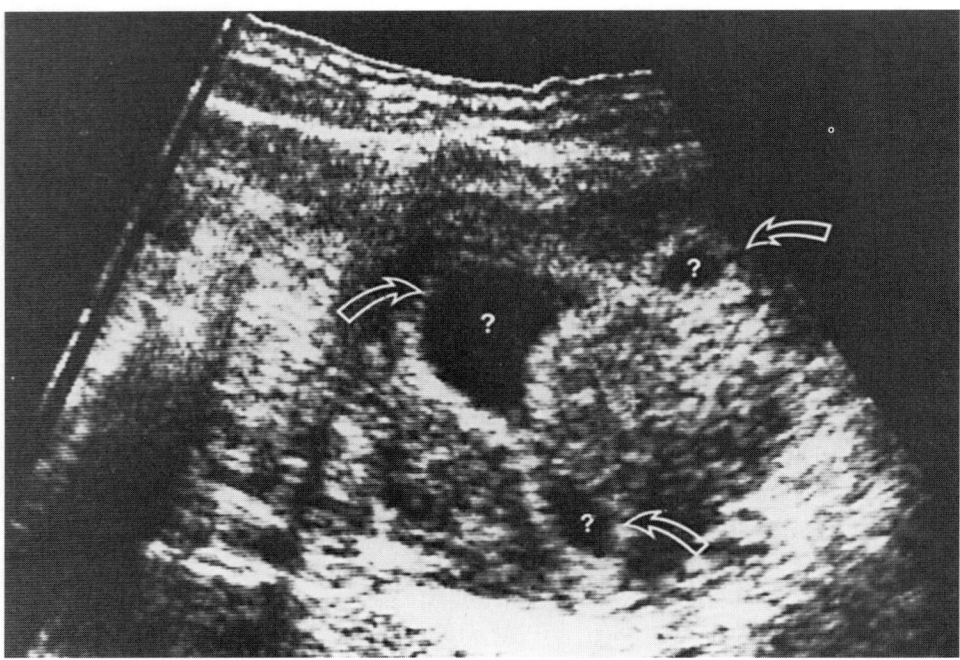

Figure 24–2. The scanning plane may artifactually transect a sac in such a fashion as to give the impression of multiple sacs. In this case, the three gestational sacs were all part of the single normal larger one. (From Jeanty P, Romero R: What does an early gestation look like? *In* Obstetrical Ultrasound. New York, McGraw-Hill, 1984, p 34, with permission.)

tation in this setting has resulted in the incorrect diagnosis of twins when only one fetus was present. On the other hand, rapid and careless scanning may result in failure to detect a second fetus whose head is deeply engaged in the pelvis or pushed up under the ribs. If a multiple gestation is suspected, the ultrasonologist must be compulsive in examining the entire uterine cavity. A scan should not be completed until the orientation of all the visualized fetal parts is understood.[37]

EARLY WASTAGE IN MULTIPLE GESTATIONS

As a result of ultrasound studies performed during the first trimester, there is evidence to suggest that the incidence of multiple gestations in humans is higher than is usually appreciated and that a significant amount of early wastage occurs in these pregnancies. This has led

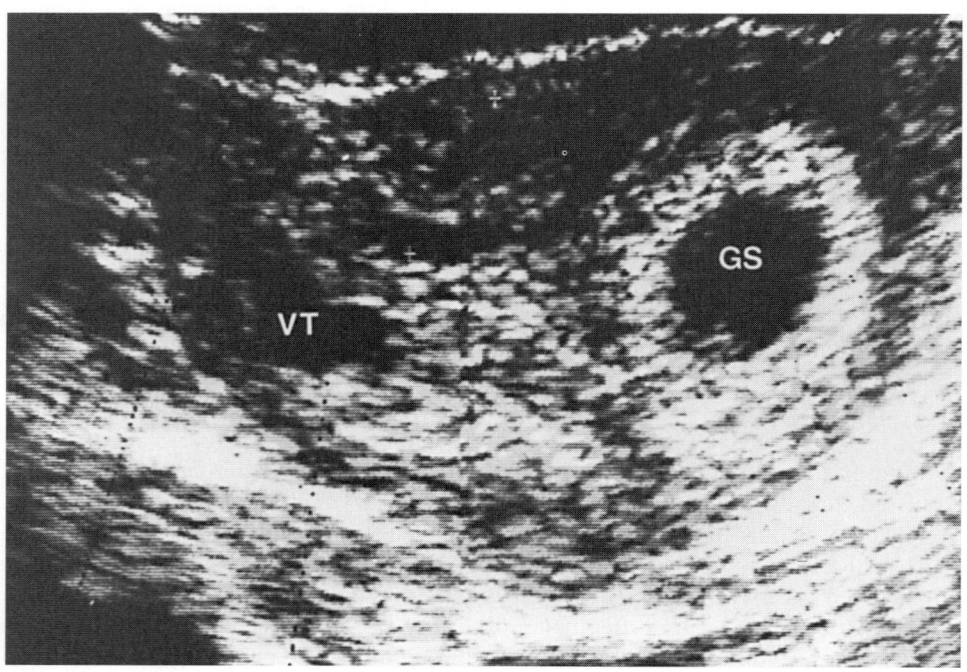

Figure 24–3. This scan shows an early gestational sac (GS) with a well-formed trophoblastic rim and an adjacent vanishing twin (VT). (From Jeanty P, Romero R: What does an early gestation look like? *In* Obstetrical Ultrasound. New York, McGraw-Hill, 1984, p 34, with permission.)

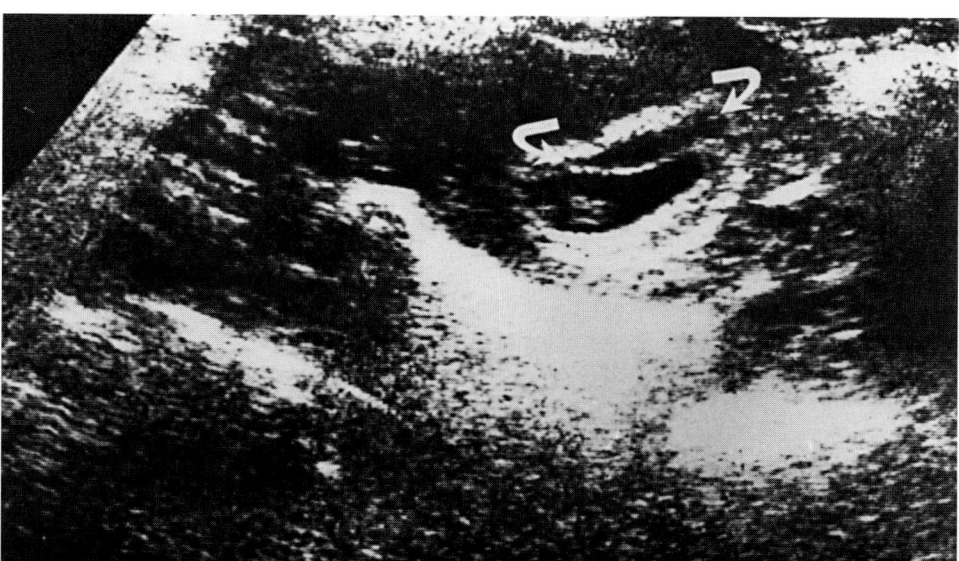

Figure 24–4. Vanishing twin with an incomplete trophoblastic rim (*arrows*) (From Jeanty P, Romero R: What does an early gestation look like? *In* Obstetrical Ultrasound. New York, McGraw-Hill, 1984, p 34, with permission.)

to the concept of the "vanishing twin" (Figs. 24–3 and 24–4). Landy et al.[38] reviewed nine series that have addressed this phenomenon. The series vary in regard to the populations studied, timing of the ultrasonography, and number of scans performed. Frequencies of twin "disappearance" in patients scanned before 14 weeks' gestation reportedly range from 13 to 78 percent. The higher rates were found in studies performed before 10 weeks' gestation.

One explanation for the disappearance of a gestational sac is resorption, which has been documented to occur in both human singleton pregnancies and lower animals (Fig. 24–5). This phenomenon has been ultrasonically described in human multiple gestations between 7 and 12 weeks. The true incidence of resorption of one or more gestational sacs is unknown, but it can occur without adverse effects on a coexisting fetus. Another explanation for sac disappearance is the presence of a blighted ovum or anembryonic pregnancy. Robinson and Caines[39] define a blighted ovum as a gestational sac having a volume of 2.5 ml or more in which no fetus can be identified on ultrasound examination. It should be noted that the sac need not be totally anechoic, because disorganized echoes may be present in some cases. Several studies have reported that the only apparent complication of regression of a blighted ovum is slight vaginal bleeding. Regardless of whether vaginal bleeding accompanies regression of a blighted ovum, a coexisting normal pregnancy has a good prognosis for carrying to term. Furthermore, experience with patients undergoing elective first-trimester reduction of multifetal pregnancies suggests that the clinical course and outcome of these pregnancies is similar to that observed with the naturally occurring phenomenon of a blighted or "disappearing" co-twin.[40–42]

Landy et al.[38] point out that pathologic evidence to confirm "disappearance" rates as high as 78 percent is lacking. Examination of the placenta and membranes after delivery of a singleton thought to be a surviving twin rarely shows evidence of the one that disappeared. It is also true that examination of the products of an abortion is usually not helpful in verifying the presence of a sac that has "vanished." The difficulty encountered in obtaining positive pathologic confirmation of the diagnosis, however, does not mean that it is incorrect. On the other hand, false diagnoses are certainly possible as a result of poor ultrasound studies. If equipment with inferior resolution is used, or if the types of artifacts described earlier are misread as being second sacs, the presence of multiple gestations may be overdiagnosed. Particular attention should be paid to the fact that pressure from the scanning transducer can create an hourglass appearance in a normal single sac that may be incorrectly interpreted as demonstrating two separate sacs.

Aside from first-trimester bleeding, there are no reported maternal complications associated with the early disappearance of a fetus.[38] The associated overall abortion rates in reported series range from 7 to 37 percent. However, in two studies when a vanished sac was associated with vaginal bleeding during the first trimester, spontaneous abortions occurred in 26 percent[43] and 92 percent[44] of cases. In a retrospective review of the first-trimester ultrasound data for 260 twin pregnancies in which one or both fetuses delivered at term, Dickey et al.[45] found that disparities in gestational sac diameter and crown-rump length (CRL) were good predictors of eventual outcome. When disparities of 3 mm or more were observed either between the twin gestational sac diameters (at ≤49 days gestation) or between the twin

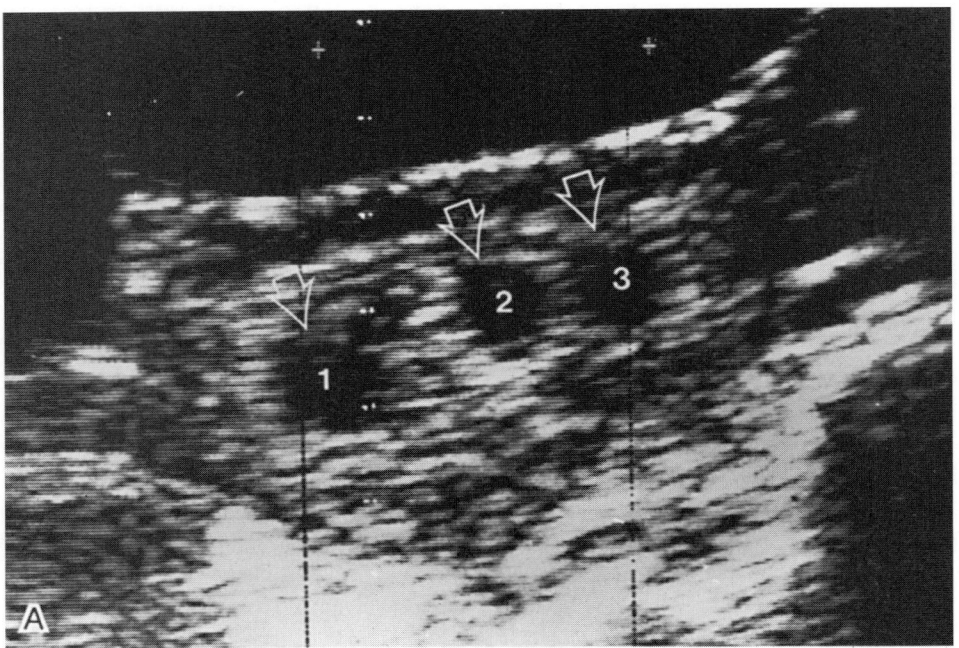

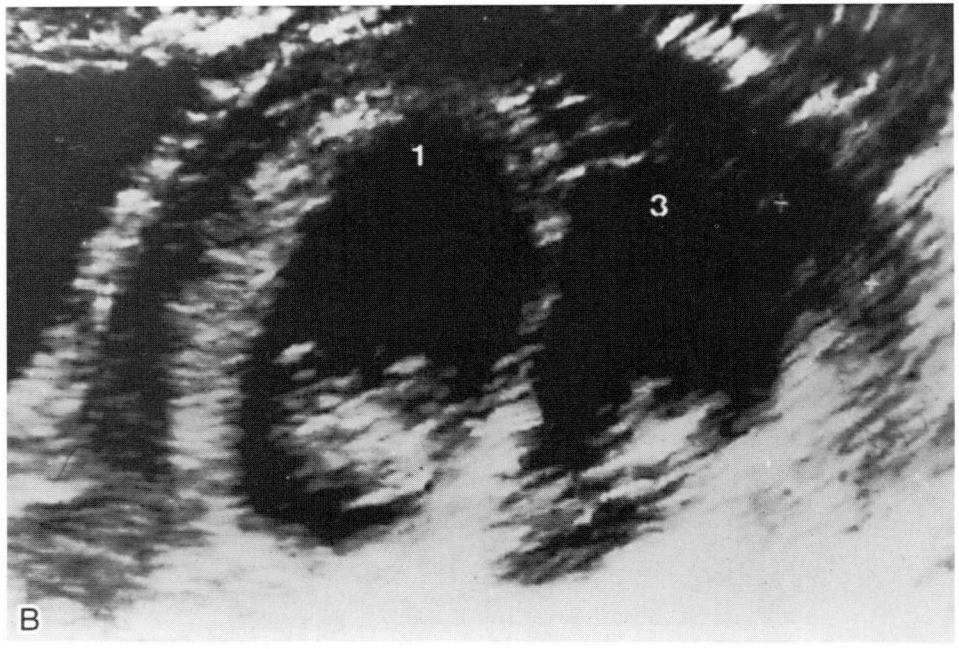

Figure 24–5. *A,* Three gestational sacs seen early in the first trimester. *B,* Two weeks later, the second sac has disappeared, and only the two lateral ones remain. (From Jeanty P, Romero R: What does an early gestation look like? *In* Obstetrical Ultrasound. New York, McGraw-Hill, 1984, p 34, with permission.)

CRL measurements (at ≤ 63 days gestation), these were associated with an embryo loss rate of 50 percent or more. The incidence of these disparities was lower in pregnancies resulting from assisted reproductive technologies than spontaneous conceptions and was unrelated to differences in birth weight, length, or gender of the neonate.

Landy et al.[38] conclude that the phenomenon of the vanishing twin seems to truly exist. While on the basis of current information it is impossible to determine the exact prevalence of this occurrence, their data suggest that a reasonable figure for its incidence may be as high as 21 percent.[46] These authors caution, however, that it is necessary to make "an accurate, faultless diagnosis" of multiple gestation in the first trimester before sharing this information with the mother because of its inevitable emotional and social impact.

GROWTH AND DEVELOPMENT

Normal individual twins grow at the same rate as singletons up to 30 to 32 weeks' gestation. After that time, they do not gain weight as rapidly as singletons of the same gestational age.[47] Daw and Walker[48] stated that after 32 weeks the combined weight gain of both twins is approximately equivalent to that gained by a singleton for the remaining portion of the pregnancy. The restriction in each twin's somatic growth is thought to be related to "crowding" in utero. The implication of this concept is that at some point in the third trimester the placenta can no longer keep pace with the nutrient requirements of both developing fetuses. This process occurs even earlier than 30 weeks when more than two fetuses are present.

A study of specimens obtained by induced abortion performed between 8.5 and 21 weeks showed the relationship between body weight and length in twins to be the same as that for singletons.[49] This finding supports the concept that twins are not growth restricted during the first half of pregnancy. Fenner et al.[50] have provided some insight into the other end of the gestational age spectrum by studying 146 twins admitted to their neonatal unit with gestational ages at birth ranging from 30 weeks to term. When data from these infants were plotted on Lubchenco's growth charts for singletons, these workers found that the twins' birth weights dropped below the mean for singletons by 32 weeks but remained within the low normal range until the 36th week, after which time they fell progressively below the tenth percentile. Twin birth lengths and head circumferences, however, remained within the low normal range for singletons throughout the entire pregnancy. The disparity between relatively normal head size and body length in association with somatic deprivation is compatible with the concept of asymmetric growth restriction. The latter is a mechanism whereby growth-restricted fetuses preferentially favor head growth at the expense of increases in body weight.[51] These studies suggest that alterations in twin growth occur primarily in the third trimester, worsen as gestational age progresses, and are usually asymmetric in nature. In the large collaborative study conducted by Kohl and Casey,[13] birth weights differed between 500 and 999 g in 18 percent of the twin sets and were in excess of 1,000 g in 3 percent. Obviously these discrepancies in birth weight could be due, in part, to constitutional factors. Because DZ twins are genetically distinct individuals, it is not surprising that they should be programmed to have very different weights at birth. There are, however, several pathologic situations in which twins may be born with substantial weight differences. These include the twin-to-twin transfusion syndrome, the combination of an anomalous fetus with a normal co-twin, and growth restriction, affecting only one twin because of local placental factors.[37] IUGR, on the other hand, can affect both twins relatively equally, in which case they would both be small, but not discordant in size. Detection of differences in size in utero therefore suggests that IUGR may be present but is not diagnostic of that condition. Conversely, the demonstration that twin fetuses have similar sizes does not rule out abnormal growth. It therefore is necessary to assess each twin individually if abnormal growth in utero is to be detected.

ASSESSING FETAL GROWTH WITH ULTRASOUND

Ultrasound is the most accurate method for assessing fetal growth (see Chapter 10). Regular ultrasonic scanning permits ongoing assessment of individual growth.

Are Singleton Nomograms Applicable to Twins?

The first question to be asked is whether ultrasound nomograms devised for singletons can be used to follow twins. Conflicting data exist in the published literature regarding this issue. Some investigators have found twins to have smaller biparietal diameters (BPDs) than those of singletons at all gestational ages,[52] while others have found mean BPD values corresponding to those of singletons until the third trimester but demonstrate progressive slowing in growth of the twin BPDs thereafter.[53-57] When, however, 18 sets of concordant twins with verified menstrual dates were compared with values from singletons that were appropriate for gestational age (AGA) at birth, Crane et al.[58] found the two groups to have mean BPD values that were essentially identical throughout gestation. These authors conclude that normal twin BPD growth is similar to that of AGA singletons at all stages of gestation, and the conflicting results of earlier studies are due to the inclusion of discordant twins with IUGR in the study group. A similar conclusion was reached by Graham et al.,[59] who studied 104 twins with concordant growth, excellent gestational age assessment, and delivery after 36 weeks; they found almost identical results when BPD and femur length values were compared with those from a selected population of singletons. Other investigators[57,60] also found no significant difference in BPD between uncomplicated singleton and twin pregnancies, suggesting that charts derived from singleton pregnancies may be reliably used to estimate gestational age of twins.

Neonatal anthropometric data obtained from concordant twins suggests that although there is significant reduction of birth weights of twins in late pregnancy, head circumference and body lengths are generally similar to those of normal singletons at corresponding gestational age.[56,58] These findings are consistent with ultrasound observations showing twin femur length growth patterns similar to singletons throughout gestation,[55,59,61] but a reduction in the abdominal circumference growth in twins after 32 weeks.[55,56]

The Significance of Divergent Biparietal Diameters

In 1976, Dorros[62] reported a case in which BPD values in a set of twins were discordant by 7 to 10 mm on three examinations performed between 38 and 41 weeks. At delivery, one infant was found to be severely growth restricted, while the other was AGA. The placenta had an infarct covering approximately 20 percent of the total surface area and was located near the origin of the growth-restricted twin's umbilical cord. Several series have subsequently shown that as the difference between twin BPDs increases, the likelihood that the smaller fetus will be growth restricted increases. Leveno et al.[63] reported that a comparison of BPD differences of 4 mm or less with those of 5 mm or greater was associated with an increase from 7 to 22 percent in the number of twin pairs with one growth-restricted infant. Houlton[64] noted an overall increase in small-for-gestational-age (SGA) infants from 40 to 71 percent in a comparison of BPD differentials below 6 mm with those of 6 mm or greater.

Crane et al.[58] defined discordance in utero as an intrapair difference in BPD of 5 mm or more and a fall in BPD below 2 SD for gestational age on their normal twin curve. Twelve sets of twins met this criterion for discordancy, nine of whom were subsequently shown to have a difference in birth weight of more than 25 percent. They suggested that head circumference (HC) be measured if BPD intrapair differences exceed 5 mm. Since HC is less likely to be affected by molding in utero, an intrapair HC difference of less than 5 percent suggests that true discrepancy does not exist. Chitkara et al.[65] also found that BPD intrapair differentials of 5 mm or greater correlated with an increased incidence of significant birth weight differences. However, estimated fetal weight and abdominal circumference measurements were found to be better predictors of discordant size. Other investigators have corroborated these observations.[66]

This compilation of confusing and seemingly conflicting data can probably be summarized as follows. Significant differences in twin BPDs may indicate that one twin is growth restricted. However, the finding could be purely artifactual because of flattening of the head in association with malpresentation or in utero crowding. Measurements of several parameters, along with serial examinations, will help distinguish fetal growth abnormalities in most cases. Nevertheless, while major intrapair BPD differences may reflect IUGR in one fetus, it is not the only criterion that should be used to look for abnormal development in utero because it will not be present when both twins are growth restricted.

The Use of Multiple Parameters to Assess for IUGR and Growth Discordance

How then should growth in utero be followed in multiple pregnancies? BPD alone, as an isolated variable, is a poor predictor of IUGR in twins. Neilson[67] retrospectively analyzed 66 twin pregnancies with good dates by plotting BPD values on a singleton nomogram. Only 56 percent of the 43 SGA neonates were found to have abnormal BPD growth, while 49 percent of the fetuses with abnormal BPD curves were found not to be growth restricted at delivery. Our experience[65] and that of others[56,68,70] suggest that a survey of multiple parameters on serial ultrasound examinations provides the most accurate assessment of the size of each individual fetus in twin gestations. The highest accuracy for predicting either appropriate or restricted growth is obtained by estimating the fetal weight. Among individual parameters, abdominal circumference is the single most sensitive measurement in predicting both IUGR and growth discordance.[65,66,69,70] Recent studies suggest that an intrapair difference in abdominal circumference measurement of 2 cm or more can be effectively used as a screening test for discordant fetal growth and IUGR in the smaller twin.[66,69,70] On the other hand, individual measurements of BPD, HC, or femur length are relatively poor predictors for either IUGR or growth discordance.[65,69,70]

Probably the most important conclusions that can be drawn from these various studies are that it is technically feasible to measure multiple ultrasound parameters in twin pregnancies and that a consideration of as many variables as possible will maximize the effectiveness of an ultrasonic assessment of fetal size. The same general principles can be applied to the assessment of growth in triplets and higher order multiple gestations. Another point that should be stressed is that growth is a dynamic process and therefore patients with multiple gestations should be followed with serial scans. Since growth restriction is a process that usually occurs during the third trimester and the predictive accuracy of any fetal measurement in utero is inversely proportional to the scan–delivery interval, we recommend that women with twins be scanned every 3 to 4 weeks after the 26th week and more frequently than that if IUGR or growth discordance is suspected.

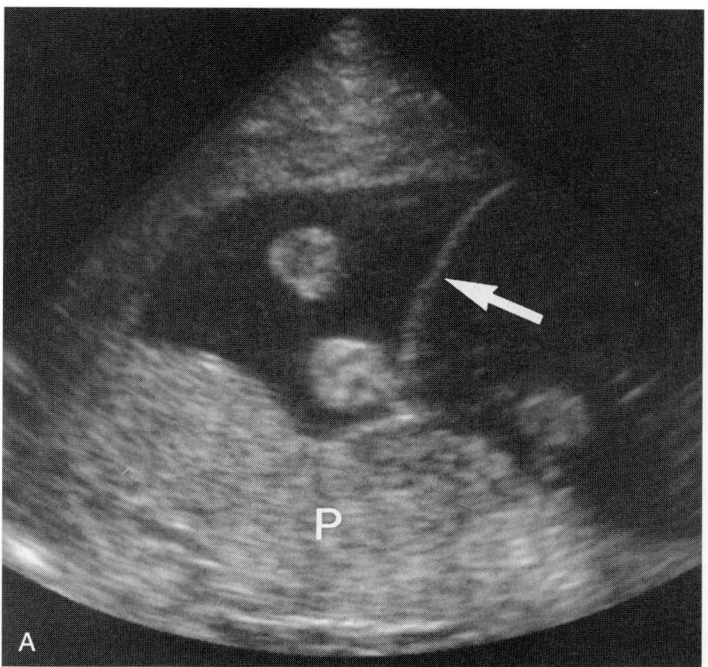
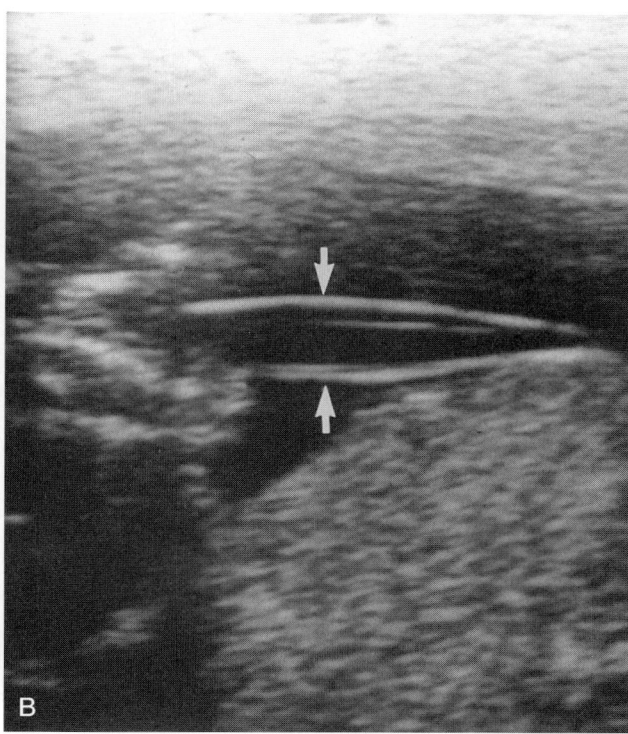

Figure 24–6. *A,* The dividing membrane *(arrow)* is thick, suggestive of a DC/DA placentation. *B,* Visualization of four layers in the dividing membrane suggests DC/DA placentation.

Ultrasonographic Prediction of Amnionicity and Chorionicity

The risk for many of the complications occurring in multiple gestation depends on whether the placentation is monochorionic (MC) or dichorionic (DC). The incidences of IUGR and fetal death are higher in monochorionic than dichorionic twins, and the twin-to-twin transfusion syndrome (TTS) occurs only in monochorionic twins. Antenatal knowledge of the type of placentation and chorionicity is not only helpful but in some cases is critical for determining optimal management. This is true when deciding whether IUGR in one fetus of a twin gestation is due to TTS or uteroplacental insufficiency, when contemplating the selective termination of one abnormal twin, or when performing an elective first-trimester multifetal pregnancy reduction procedure. In these latter situations, if the gestation is monochorionic, a shared placental circulation could result in death or damage to a surviving fetus.

The sonographic prediction of chorionicity and amnionicity should be systematically approached by determining the number of placentas visualized and the sex of each fetus and then by assessing the membranes that divide the sacs. The pregnancy is clearly dichorionic if two separate placental disks are seen or if the twins are of different sex. When a single placenta is present and the twins are of the same sex, careful sonographic examination of the dividing membrane will usually result

in a correct diagnosis. Evaluation of three features in the intertwin membrane will provide an almost certain diagnosis about the mono- or dichorionicity of a twin pregnancy. These three features are (1) thickness of the intertwin membrane, (2) the number of layers visualized in the membrane, and (3) assessment of the junction of the membrane with the placental site for what has been described as the "twin peak" sign.[71] In dichorionic diamniotic pregnancies, the dividing membrane appears "thick"[72–74] and has a measured diameter of greater than or equal to 2 mm,[75] and either three or four layers can often be identified (Fig. 24–6).[76,77] With a monochorionic diamniotic pregnancy, only two layers of membranes will be identified, and the membrane appears to be "thin and hairlike"[76] (Fig. 24–7). D'Alton and Dudley[77] caution that a floating monochorionic diamniotic membrane may fold back upon itself and give a false impression of having four layers. These authors suggest that inspection of the membranes near their placental insertion will reduce this artifact. It should be mentioned that significant magnification of the image is helpful in counting the number of layers. Determination of membrane thickness allows correct identification of di- or monochorionic gestation in 80 to 90 percent of cases.[71–73] Counting the number of layers adds a few extra minutes to the total scanning time but can increase the predictive accuracy to almost 100 percent.[76,77]

Initially described as the *lambda sign* by Bessis and

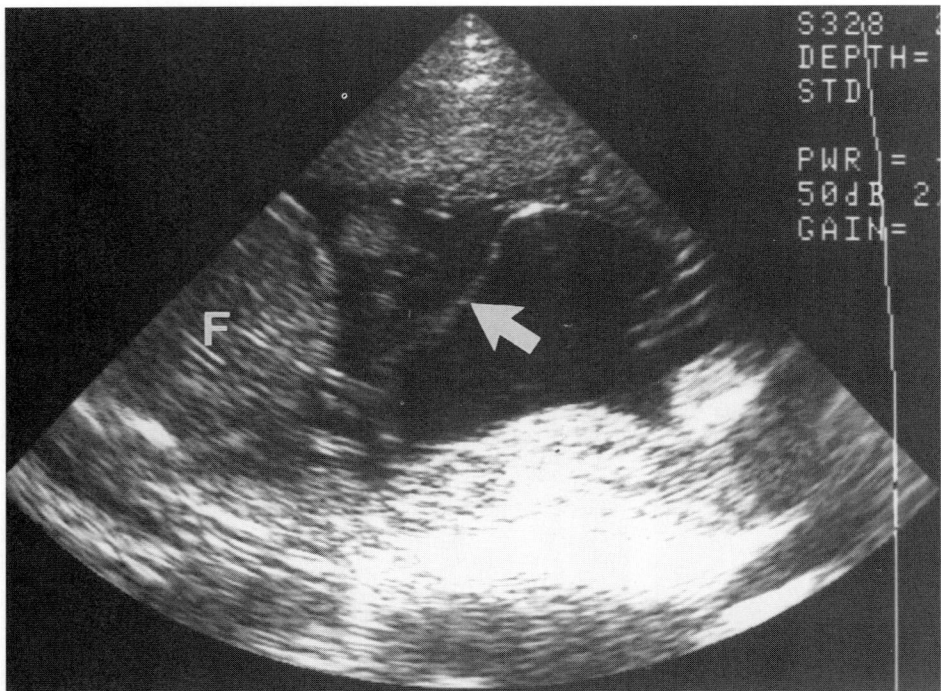

Figure 24–7. The dividing membrane (*arrow*) is thin and hair-like, suggestive of MC/DA placentation.

Papiernik[78] in 1981, the twin peak sign was identified by Finberg[79] in 15 twin and 5 triplet pregnancies undergoing ultrasound studies during the second and third trimesters. All twin pregnancies were proven to be dichorionic and all triplet pregnancies were proven to be trichorionic by placental pathology. They described the twin peak sign as a triangular projection of tissue with the same echogenicity as the placenta extending beyond the chorionic surface of the placenta. This tissue is insinuated between the layers of the intertwin membrane,

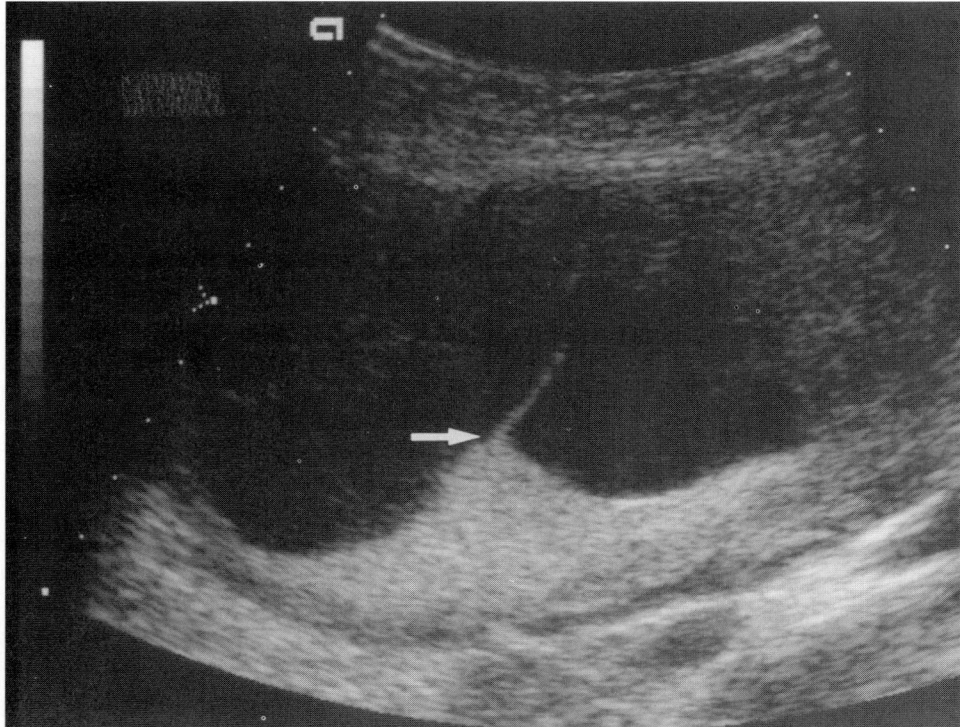

Figure 24–8. "Twin peak" sign appears as a triangular extension of placental tissue, wide at the placental surface and tapering to a point at its junction with the intertwin membrane (*arrow*).

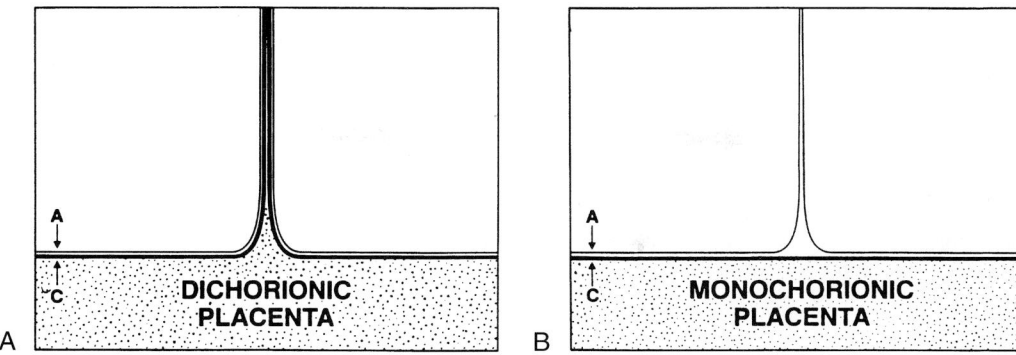

Figure 24–9. *A,* In a dichorionic pregnancy with fused placentas, both the amnions (A) and the chorions (C) reflect away from the placental surface at the point of origin of the septum. This creates a potential space in direct continuity with the chorionic villi and into which they can extend. *B,* In a monochorionic twin pregnancy, the septum is formed by reflection of the two amnions away from the placenta. There is a continuous single chorion, which provides an intact barrier, preventing extension of placental villi into the potential interamniotic space.

wider at the chorionic surface and tapering to a point at some distance inward from that surface (Fig. 24–8). This finding is produced by extension of chorionic villi into the potential interchorionic space of the twin membrane. This space exists only in a dichorionic pregnancy and is produced by reflection of each chorion away from its placenta at the place where it encounters the chorion and placenta of the co-twin (Fig. 24–9A). The twin peak sign cannot occur in monochorionic placentation because the single continuous chorion does not extend into the potential interamniotic space of the monochorionic diamniotic twin membrane (Fig. 24–9B). In assessing the twin peak sign with ultrasonography, it is important that the zone of intersection of the membrane with the placenta be carefully scrutinized over as much length as can be detected. It should be mentioned that the absence of the twin peak sign alone does not guarantee that the pregnancy is monochorionic. Under these circumstances, evaluation of other features of the membrane previously described (i.e., thickness and number of layers) will give additional diagnostic clues regarding chorionicity and amnionicity. Chorionicity can best be determined by ultrasound examination at 6 to 9 weeks' gestation, when in dichorionic twins there is a thick septum between the chorionic sacs. After 9 weeks, this septum becomes progressively thinner to form the chorionic component of the intertwin membrane, but it remains thick and easy to identify at the base of the membrane as a triangular projection, the lambda or twin peak sign.[78–82] At 11 to 14 weeks' gestation, sonographic examination of the base of the intertwin membrane for the presence or absence of the lambda sign provides reliable distinction between DC and MC pregnancies.[83]

In some pregnancies with monochorionic diamniotic placentation, the dividing membranes may not be sonographically visualized because they are very thin. In other cases they may not be seen because severe oligo-

hydramnios causes them to be closely apposed to the fetus in that sac. This results in a "stuck twin" appearance, where the trapped fetus remains firmly held against the uterine wall despite changes in maternal position (Fig. 24–10).[71] Diagnosis of this condition confirms the presence of a diamniotic gestation, which should be distinguished from a monoamniotic gestation where dividing membranes are absent. In the latter situation, free movement of both twins, and occasionally entanglement of their umbilical cords, can be demonstrated.[84]

Doppler Studies in Multiple Gestation

Advances in Doppler ultrasound technology within the past decade have made it possible to evaluate fetoplacental hemodynamics in normal and abnormal pregnancies (see Chapters 12 and 25). Several studies in singleton pregnancies have demonstrated that abnormal Doppler velocimetry in the umbilical artery (UA) and other fetal vessels is often associated with fetal IUGR, pregnancy complications, and adverse perinatal outcome.[85–88] Although some investigators favor continuous wave systems, we think that Doppler studies in multiple gestations are best performed using a pulsed Doppler duplex system to be certain that the vessel being studied belongs to a targeted fetus.

In 32 uncomplicated twin pregnancies where both fetuses were AGA, Giles et al.[89] found that the umbilical artery systolic/diastolic (S/D) ratios were similar to those of normal singleton AGA fetuses. Their findings were confirmed by Gerson et al.,[90] who prospectively studied 65 normal twin pregnancies between 20 and 39 weeks' gestation. These authors reported that umbilical artery S/D ratios in normal twins decrease with advancing gestation and that the relationship between S/D ratio and gestational age is the same in singleton and normal AGA twins. These studies, and our own obser-

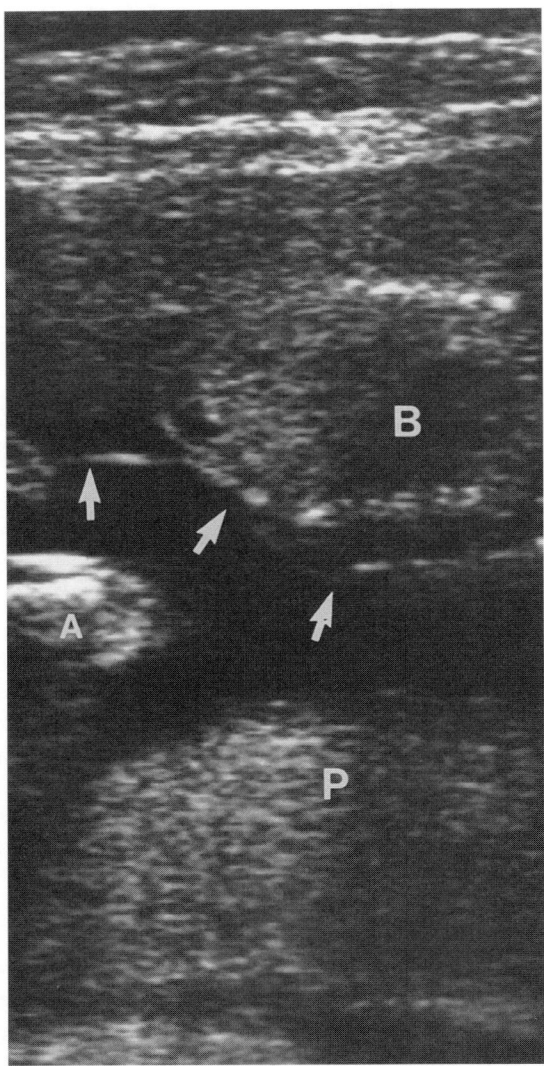

Figure 24–10. Twin gestation with severe oligohydramnios in sac of twin B. The separating membrane (*arrows*) is closely apposed to this fetus and was visualized with difficulty. Sac of twin A showed severe polyhydramnios. P, placenta.

vations, suggest that the umbilical artery S/D ratios in fetuses of a twin gestation can be evaluated as if two singleton fetuses were being assessed.

Fetal growth restriction in singleton pregnancies is often associated with abnormal Doppler studies, which may precede documentation of the IUGR by sonographic biometry or abnormalities in other tests of fetal well-being.[88] These observations are consistent with histologic evidence that abnormal umbilical artery waveforms may reflect vascular lesions in the placenta, which can be presumed to increase resistance to blood flow through the umbilical arteries.[91] Similar alterations in umbilical artery S/D ratios have been documented in some growth-restricted twins. In their study of 76 twin pregnancies, Giles et al.[89] had 33 patients in whom one

or both twins were SGA; in 78 percent of these pregnancies at least one fetus had an elevated S/D ratio. Farmakides et al.[92] performed Doppler studies in 43 twin pregnancies and tried to predict growth discordancy by examining S/D ratio differences in each twin pair. They found that a ratio difference of 0.4 or more between the twins was predictive of a weight difference of more than 349 g, with a sensitivity of 73 percent and specificity of 82 percent. Similar observations were reported by Saldana et al.[93] These investigators found that an S/D ratio difference of 0.4 or more was a better predictor than ultrasound for birth weight discordancy in the SGA/AGA twin pairs, but was poor in predicting discordant weight in the SGA/SGA, AGA/AGA, or AGA/LGA twin pairs. They also suggested that in order to obtain maximal information, the absolute S/D ratios as well as differences in these ratios must be carefully evaluated in all cases.

Opinions vary regarding the usefulness of routinely performing Doppler studies in all twin pregnancies. Two studies illustrate this controversy. The first, by Giles et al.,[94] described the clinical management and pregnancy outcome in a study group of 112 women with twin gestations in whom results of two or more Doppler studies were made available to the patients' obstetricians. These results were compared with a group of 95 patients in whom Doppler studies were performed but not reported to the clinicians. In the study group, the first test was performed at 28 to 32 weeks' gestation, and this was repeated 4 to 5 weeks later if the initial study was normal. If, however, a Doppler evaluation was abnormal, further studies were repeated as often as once a week, along with nonstress tests and sonographic studies. Patients were delivered if their nonstress tests were persistently abnormal or serial sonographic studies showed failure of fetal growth. In this series, a significant reduction in perinatal mortality and morbidity was noted in the study group. It is interesting that the improvement in outcome was achieved without any appreciable differences in gestational age at delivery or mode of delivery between the two study groups. The second study[95] was a prospective evaluation of 89 twin pregnancies in which an attempt was made to determine the predictive value of umbilical artery Doppler studies in identifying twin fetuses destined to be SGA at birth. Serial Doppler recordings were made from each twin once a month from 22 weeks' gestation until delivery, but the results were not made available to the patients' clinicians. Thirty-two of the 178 infants in this series were SGA at birth, but only 24 of the 82 Doppler studies performed in the growth-restricted fetuses were abnormal, giving an overall sensitivity of 29 percent and a positive predictive value of 34 percent. This study, therefore, did not confirm the relatively high predictive value of Doppler studies for SGA twins reported by other investigators.[89,92]

A few more recent studies have also attempted to evaluate the usefulness of Doppler velocimetry in predicting twin fetuses that are small for gestational age, those with TTS, and those with discordant growth.[91-94] In a longitudinal prospective study by Degani et al.,[97] serial ultrasound biometry and Doppler studies were performed at monthly intervals in 37 twin pregnancies. While the overall sensitivity of Doppler alone for predicting an SGA fetus was only 58 percent, abnormal Doppler findings preceded sonographic diagnosis of SGA by about 3.7 weeks. A combination of sonographic and Doppler parameters improved the sensitivity to 84 percent, suggesting that Doppler velocimetry complements real-time ultrasonography in the early detection of abnormal growth in twin pregnancies. Gaziano et al.[96] found an increased incidence of SGA infants in patients with abnormal Doppler studies, and the incidence of other adverse pregnancy complications, including stillbirth and major anomalies, was also found to be high in this group.

From our review of the current literature, we are not convinced that Doppler studies need to be routinely performed as part of the antepartum surveillance of women with multiple gestations. However, when IUGR is suspected in one or more fetuses, Doppler velocimetry is a useful adjunct in assessing and following these pregnancies. Our routine for the surveillance of patients with multiple gestations is as follows:

1. Ideally, an initial ultrasound is performed at 10 to 14 weeks' gestation to determine the number of fetuses and the amnionicity/chorionicity in order to differentiate monochorionic and dichorionic gestations.
2. The second ultrasound evaluation is scheduled at 18 to 20 weeks' gestation. This includes standard biometry to confirm gestational age and the size of each fetus, assessment of amniotic fluid volume in each sac, and an anatomic survey of each fetus to rule out morphologic anomalies. If the patient did not have a first-trimester ultrasound, an attempt is made to determine chorionicity by examining fetal gender, the number of placentas, the thickness as well as number of layers in the membrane separating the sacs, and the presence or absence of the lambda or twin peak sign.
3. If the first two scans are normal and suggestive of a DC/DA twinning, subsequent scans for fetal growth are performed at 24 to 26 weeks and every 3 to 4 weeks thereafter as long as fetal growth and amniotic fluid volume in each sac remains normal.
4. If the initial ultrasound is suggestive of a MC/DA placentation, and therefore a potential risk for developing TTS, subsequent scans are repeated at a minimum of 2-week intervals. Furthermore, NST's should be performed frequently after viability has been reached in patients with MC/MA placentation.
5. If there is evidence of IUGR, discordant fetal growth, or discordant fluid volumes, fetal surveillance is intensified and includes frequent nonstress testing along with biophysical profile and Doppler velocimetry studies. Because absent end-diastolic or reversed diastolic flow can be a predictor of poor outcome or imminent death in utero, serious consideration is given to delivering patients with these findings if the healthy fetus is mature enough for an elective delivery.

ABNORMALITIES ASSOCIATED WITH MULTIPLE GESTATION

Twin-to-Twin Transfusion Syndrome

Benirschke and Kim[6] state that, as a group, MZ monochorial twins have greater disparity in weight than do dichorial twins. A comparison of dichorial MZ and DZ twins with MZ twins having a monochorial placenta shows this effect on birth weight to be due entirely to the type of placentation and not zygosity. This finding is best explained by the twin-to-twin transfusion syndrome.

To our knowledge, TTS in humans has only been reported in association with monochorionic placentas. On very rare occasions, vascular communications may exist between dichorial placentas, even in the case of DZ twins as evidenced by the occurrence of blood group chimeras,[6] but among monochorionic twins these anastomoses are the rule rather than the unusual exception. The potential for the transfusion syndrome occurs when the arterial circulation of one twin is in communication with the venous circulation of the other through arteriovenous shunts in a "common villous district" (Fig. 24–11).[6] In this situation, one fetus becomes a donor that transfuses its co-twin. The donor becomes anemic and growth restricted. Although occasionally it may become hydropic as a result of high-output failure, more frequently this twin is significantly smaller than the other. The recipient twin, on the other hand, becomes polycythemic and can suffer from congestive heart failure as a result of circulatory overload (Fig. 24–12). Thromboses of peripheral vessels may also develop in association with its hypertransfused state. The perinatal mortality associated with TTS may be as high as 70 percent. Several studies have shown antenatal factors that predict a poor outcome in these pregnancies, including (1) an early gestational age at

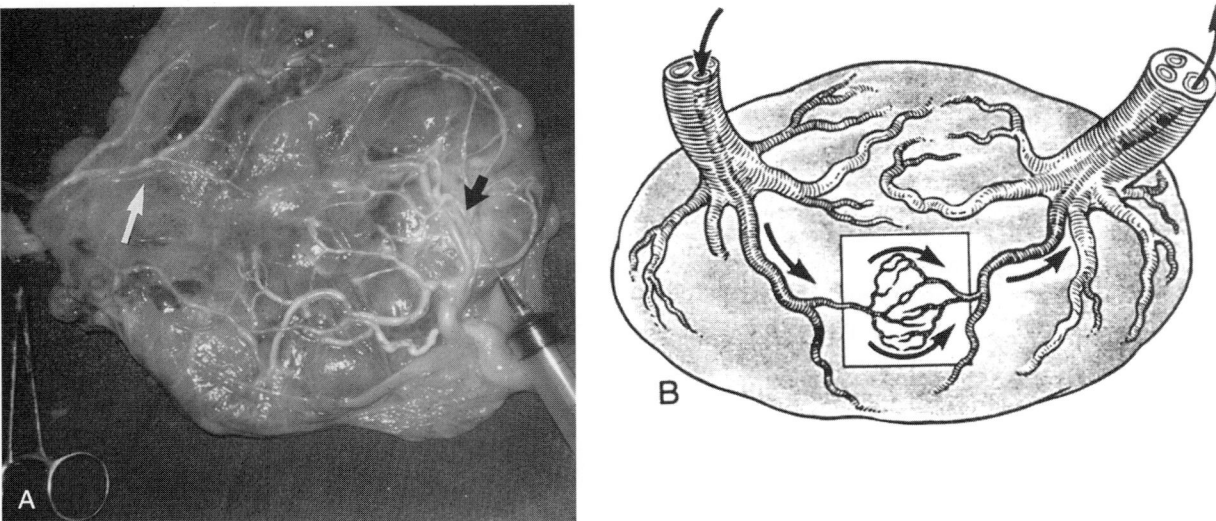

Figure 24–11. *A,* The placenta of a pregnancy complicated by the TTS. Milk has been injected into an artery on the "donor" side of the placenta (*black arrow*). It can be seen returning through the venous circulation on that side but is also evident in the venous circulation of the "recipient" (*white arrow*). *B,* The arteriovenous shunt shown in *A.*

diagnosis with delivery before 28 weeks, (2) severe polyhydramnios requiring multiple therapeutic amniocenteses, (3) fetal hydrops, and (4) absent or reversed diastolic flow on umbilical artery Doppler studies. If hydramnios develops early, premature labor often occurs before the third trimester.[100-102] If the birth

weights of MZ twins differ by less than 20 percent, the difference will usually not persist during later development. However, if the weights are discrepant by more than 25 percent, differences in height, and in some cases developmental delay, may persist into adult life.[103]

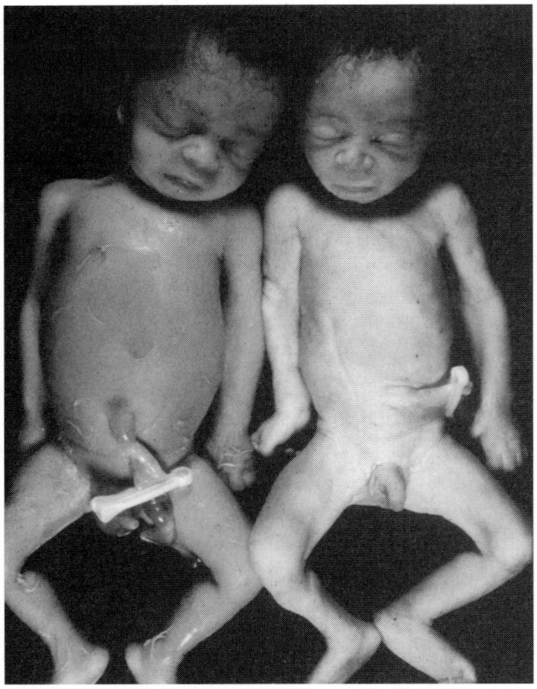

TTS can be ultrasonically detected in utero.[104] When severe, the syndrome usually manifests itself clinically as a result of polyhydramnios that is almost always found to exist in the sac of the larger twin. Sonographic criteria that provide an almost unequivocal antenatal diagnosis of TTS include (1) the presence of same-sex twins with a single placenta; (2) thin (two-layer) separating membrane between the sacs; (3) significant discordance in fetal growth (although this is not invariably present); (4) discordant amniotic fluid volume with polyhydramnios in the sac of the larger recipient twin and often a "stuck twin" appearance as a result of oligohydramnios in the sac of the donor twin; and (5) signs of hydrops or cardiac failure in either fetus, but this occurs more frequently in the larger twin.

When twins of unequal size are discovered on ultrasound examination, it is important to distinguish TTS from a pregnancy in which one fetus is growth restricted but the other is developing normally. In the latter situation the normal twin is usually surrounded by an appropriate quantity of amniotic fluid, and oligohydramnios may or may not be present in the other sac. In TTS, however, polyhydramnios and sonographic evidence of hydrops are often seen in association with the larger twin, while the donor is smaller than it should be and not simply smaller than its larger sibling.

Figure 24–12. Stillborn male twins at 31 weeks' gestation, secondary to the TTS. The plethoric twin on the left weighed 1,670 g and the anemic growth-restricted twin on the right weighed 1,300 g.

This latter point may be useful in ruling out a third uncommon situation, namely, that of a normal fetus and a larger hydropic co-twin that is anomalous or erythroblastotic.

In addition to the usual fetal biometry and amniotic fluid volume assessment by ultrasonography, several investigators have attempted to evaluate the role of Doppler velocimetry studies in making or confirming a diagnosis of TTS. To date, these studies have only provided conflicting data. Farmakides et al.[92] reported two cases in which umbilical artery waveforms of the twins were discordant and concluded that a simultaneous observation of high- and low-resistance S/D ratios was highly suggestive of this diagnosis. On the other hand, in eight cases where the diagnosis was documented or strongly suspected, Giles et al.[89] found no difference in interpair S/D ratios. Pretorius et al.[105] also reported eight cases of TTS and found no consistent pattern of umbilical artery Doppler S/D ratios. Other studies have reported similar observations on umbilical Doppler velocimetry in twin pregnancies with TTS.[96,97,99] The mortality rate in the study by Pretorius et al.[105] was very high, with five of eight pregnancies ending in fetal or neonatal death of both twins. In all five instances of perinatal loss, one or both of the twins had either absent or reversed diastolic flow. The authors concluded that, although evidence of greatly increased placental resistance (i.e., absent or reversed diastolic flow) is not helpful in identifying the donor from the recipient twin, it invariably predicts a poor outcome. Recent data from the Australian and New Zealand TTS Registry[102] supports the observations of Pretorius et al.[105] In their study of umbilical artery blood flow velocity waveforms, Ishimatsu et al.[106] were also unable to identify any distinctive findings in patients with TTS. However, the presence of cardiomegaly in five recipient twins, with tricuspid regurgitation and a biphasic umbilical vein waveform in three others, led them to suggest that these findings may be more diagnostic than umbilical artery Doppler velocimetry and representative of the hemodynamic changes that occur in TTS.

Other investigators have utilized much more invasive techniques in an attempt to make a definitive prenatal diagnosis of TTS. Bruner and Rosemund[107] performed cordocentesis on both twins and were unable to demonstrate consistently a hemoglobin difference of 5 g or more between the recipient and donor twins. Tanaka et al.[108] suggested the "pancuronium test," which involves cordocentesis and intravascular injection of pancuronium bromide, a nondepolarizing neuromuscular blocking agent, into one twin. Paralysis of both twins under these circumstances would confirm transplacental vascular communications and a diagnosis of TTS. The role of such invasive methods for the diagnosis of this condition is unclear and, in our opinion, the potential risks from a cordocentesis probably outweigh the benefits of definitively establishing the diagnosis.

The pathophysiology of polyhydramnios in TTS is poorly understood. Based on their observation of significantly increased concentrations of atrial natriuretic factor (ANF) in the cord blood of recipient twins compared with donor twins in three cases of TTS, Wieacker et al.[109] suggested that chronic overload of circulatory volume in the recipient twin causes increased release of ANF from the fetal heart. This in turn results in increased fetal urine production, leading to polyhydramnios. Fries et al.,[110] on the other hand, proposed a more mechanical explanation for the presence of polyhydramnios in TTS. These authors found a high prevalence of velamentous cord insertion associated with this syndrome. They concluded that this might contribute to the development of profound disparity in amniotic fluid volume because the easy compressibility of the membranously inserted cord could result in reduced blood flow to one twin. They also suggested that removal of a large volume of amniotic fluid by amniocentesis may help reduce this compressive force on the cord insertion site, thereby leading to a reversal of the fluid imbalance.

Pregnancy outcome in patients with TTS appears to depend on the number and type of vascular anastomoses between the placentas, the pressures and directions of blood flow, and the timing of the imbalanced transfusion during the pregnancy. Even though the majority of monozygotic twins have monochorial placentas and communicating vessels, only 5 to 17 percent are reported to develop a significant transfusion syndrome.[111–113] Machin and Keith[114] suggest that intertwin vascular communications are of two main types—superficial and deep. Superficial connections form between vessels of like type (i.e., arterioarterial and venovenous). These are end-to-end anastomoses and usually not the structural basis for antenatal TTS. In fact, they usually act to protect twin pairs who might otherwise develop TTS. This is true more for the arterioarterial anastomosis, since venovenous connections operate at lower pressures and can be associated with poor outcomes. Vascular anastomoses deep in the parenchyma are arteriovenous and represent a zone of placental parenchyma supplied with arterial blood from one twin (the donor), but from which venous blood is returned to the other twin (the recipient). Indeed, when this is the only placental circulatory connection between twins, the onset of antenatal TTS is inevitable.[114]

The actual incidence of TTS is very likely underestimated either because of the selection bias of studying liveborn twins or because the majority of dead monochorionic twins escape diagnosis at their co-twin's birth.[113] Clinical manifestations of TTS are usually characterized by the onset of acute polyhydramnios with or without associated preterm labor. Mortality rates associated with this presentation can range from 60 to 100 percent, the highest rates occurring in cases where the manifestation of this syndrome appears before 24 weeks' gestation.[6,113,115–118]

Various therapeutic maneuvers have been attempted in an effort to improve pregnancy outcome in severe cases of TTS. These approaches include therapeutic amniocenteses,[102,119–122] laser ablation of vascular anastomoses,[123–125] selective feticide,[126,127] and maternal treatment with digoxin or indomethacin.[128–130] In a review of the subject in 1990, Blickstein[131] concluded that therapeutic amniocenteses had poor efficacy in these cases. However, other reports have suggested that a much better pregnancy outcome can be achieved with the use of serial therapeutic amniocenteses.[102,119–121] The overall survival of one or both twins in most series ranges from 74 to 83 percent.[122] A recent study compared endoscopic laser surgery with serial amniocenteses, and concluded that laser coagulation of placental vascular anastomoses offers a more effective alternative to serial amniocenteses, with a higher fetal survival rate and lower incidence of sonographic abnormalities in the brain of surviving infants.[132] Another study has proposed the use of amniotic septostomy (intentional puncture of the intertwin membrane) for the treatment of TTS.[133] Excellent survival rates of 83 percent were reported in this small study consisting of 12 patients. It must be pointed out that this method, while promising, should at present be considered experimental until further studies confirm its efficacy and safety. It should also be noted that iatrogenic or spontaneous disruption of the intertwin membrane has been reported in some cases to result in subsequent cord entanglement and fetal death.[134–136] Therefore, if a rent of the intertwin membrane is suspected, it is recommended that the pregnancy be managed as if it were a true monoamniotic twin pregnancy.[134–136]

Isolated maternal treatment with either digoxin or indomethacin for TTS has not proven beneficial in improving fetal outcome.[128–130] Selective feticide of one twin in the presence of the placental vascular communications expected in TTS can have devastating consequences, including death of the co-twin or survival with permanent damage.[137] Fetoscopically directed Yttrium-aluminum-garnet (YAG) laser occlusion of placental vascular communications as suggested and reported by a few centers[124,125,132] has tremendous appeal, since it aims to address the problem at its source. However, the technical expertise and special equipment required for this procedure limit its use to a very few specialized centers.

The weight of evidence from clinical reports and ease of performing the procedure suggest that at the present time, repeated therapeutic amniocenteses provide the best option for treatment until delivery is possible.[119–121]

The total number and frequency of amniocenteses must be individualized, since some patients show improvement following one or two procedures, whereas others may require that it be performed far more frequently. The volume of fluid aspirated at any one time should again be individualized, with an aim to removing as much fluid as possible from the polyhydramniotic sac and attaining a relatively "normal" fluid volume or a maximum vertical fluid pocket of about 7 cm at the end of the procedure. The role of prophylactic tocolysis in these cases remains unproven. However, our clinical observations suggest that a brief period of tocolysis at the time of amniocentesis may be helpful in reducing uterine irritability and contractions during the procedure.

CONGENITAL ANOMALIES IN MULTIPLE GESTATIONS

There is general agreement that anomalies occur more frequently in twins than in singletons, but controversy exists regarding the degree of difference. A large series from Czechoslovakia[138] reported a rate of anomalies of 1.4 percent for singletons, 2.7 percent for twins, and 6.1 percent for triplets. Among cases of twins in which anomalies were detected, both twins were affected in 14.8 percent. There were no cases of triplets in which all three infants were affected. Hendricks[139] found the frequency of anomalies to be more than three times higher in twins than in singletons, while in Kohl and Casey's series[13] the frequency was 1.5 to 2 times higher. Other studies cited by Benirschke and Kim[6] report smaller increases.

The diagnosis of a variety of morphologic abnormalities in multiple gestations has been made in utero with ultrasound. It is possible to detect anomalies of one or both fetuses or conversely to rule out specific disorders in twins who are known to be at increased risk for them. As is true for singletons, however, an ultrasonic diagnosis can only be made when a potentially detectable anatomic abnormality has become manifest at the time the fetus is studied. Neilson et al.[140] describe four cases in which anomalies in one or both twins were heralded by elevated serum AFP values. In all these patients, the abnormalities were detected by ultrasound.

Anomalies Related to Twinning

Some anomalies such as acardia and conjoined twins are directly related to the twinning process. *Acardia* is a malformation that occurs in one of MZ twins, triplets, or even quintuplets with a frequency of approximately 1 per 30,000 deliveries.[6] These extremely malformed

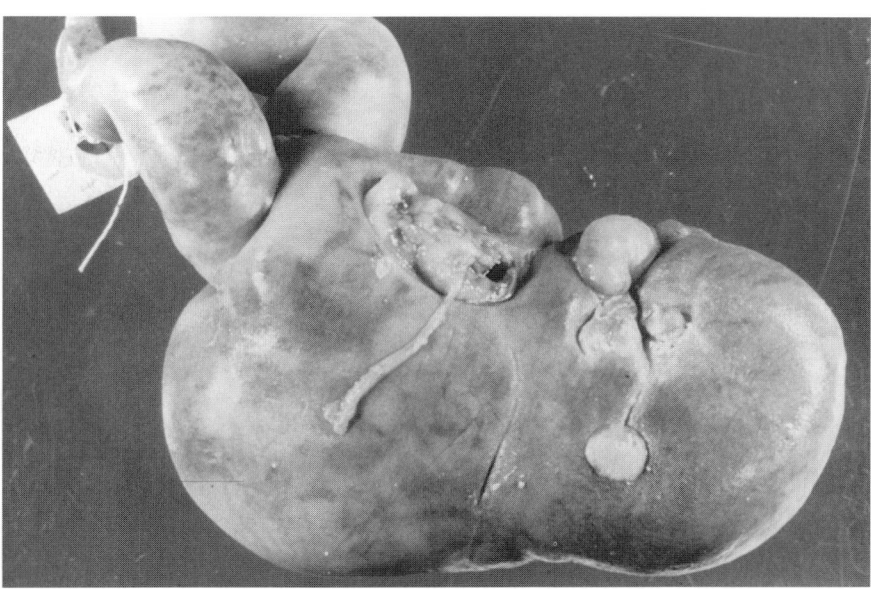

Figure 24–13. Acardiac twin. (Courtesy of Dr. James Wheeler, Department of Surgical Pathology, Hospital of the University of Pennsylvania, Philadelphia, PA.)

fetuses either have no heart at all (holoacardia) or only some rudimentary cardiac tissue (pseudoacardia) in association with other multiple developmental abnormalities (Fig. 24–13). These patients always have monochorial placentas and vascular anastomoses that sustain the life of the acardiac twin. Because of their isosexual status and monochorial relationship, they are considered to be MZ and therefore represent the ultimate of discordance in the development of genetically identical individuals. Controversy exists regarding the etiology of this condition. Kaplan and Benirschke[141] believe that reversal of flow through the acardiac twin secondary to at least one artery-to-artery and one vein-to-vein connection in the placenta leads to the anomaly of twin reversed arterial perfusion (TRAP) sequence. Retrograde fetal perfusion has been documented to occur by Doppler studies in two cases.[142,143] Other authors,[103] however, believe that acardia is a primary defect in cardiac development, and, while the placental vascular anastomoses are necessary for survival of the affected twin, these are not responsible for the abnormalities.

There is also a high incidence of chromosomal abnormalities in these pregnancies. In 6 of the 12 acardiac cases reported by Van Allen et al.,[144] an abnormal karyotype was found in the perfused twin, while the karyotype of the pump twin was normal. The remaining six perfused twins were chromosomally normal.

Antenatal diagnosis by ultrasound of an acardiac fetus coexisting with a normal co-twin is fairly straightforward. The anomalous twin may appear to be an amorphous mass or may show a wide range of abnormalities that depend on which organ system has failed to develop. The lower extremities and body are typically more completely developed, while the most severe abnormalities involve the upper body. The heart is fre-

quently absent or rudimentary, and a single umbilical artery is present in approximately half the cases. A retrograde pattern of fetal perfusion can be demonstrated to occur through the umbilical arteries by Doppler studies.[142,143]

The pump twin, although structurally normal, is at increased risk for in utero cardiac failure, and mortality rates of 50 percent or higher have been reported.[145] When the size ratio of the acardiac to that of the pump twin is less than 25 percent, the mortality rate is diminished. However, the prognosis worsens when polyhydramnios, preterm labor, or cardiac decompensation of the pump twin are present.[145] Various techniques have been used to interrupt the vascular communication between the twins in an effort to improve outcome of the normal pump twin. These methods have included hysterotomy with physical removal of the acardiac twin,[146-148] ultrasound-guided injection of thrombogenic materials into the umbilical circulation of the acardiac twin,[149-151] and, more recently, ligation of the umbilical cord of the acardiac twin under fetoscopic guidance.[153]

Nance[103] presents evidence to suggest that a group of birth defects involving midline structures, including symmelia, extrophy of the cloaca, and midline neural tube defects, may be associated in some way with the twinning process. Symmelia is a rare severe defect that results from fusion of the preaxial halves of the developing hindlimb buds. This produces a single lower extremity with a knee that flexes in the opposite direction from normal. The incidence of this condition is 100 times higher in MZ births than in singletons. MZ twins have also been shown to have a higher frequency of neural tube defects than singletons,[154] and they are often discordant for the abnormality. Nance[103] suggests that the MZ twinning process, with its attendant opportunities for asymmetry, cytoplasmic deficiency, and competition in utero, may favor the discordant expression of midline neurologic defects in these twins. He also cites evidence that 10 percent of all cases of extrophy of the cloaca occur in like-sex twins. In each of these instances, it is unclear whether the occurrence of a malformation somehow initiates the twinning process or whether a common factor predisposes to both events. Discordance is often, but not always, a feature of these midline defects in MZ twins.

Conjoined twins occur with a frequency of about 1 per 50,000 deliveries and in approximately 1 per 600 twin births.[155-157] The most famous conjoined twins were Chang and Eng Bunker, who were born in Siam in 1811. These xiphopagus twins (i.e., joined by a band of tissue extending from the umbilicus to the xiphoid cartilage) lived unseparated for 63 years. P.T. Barnum exhibited them extensively for a number of years. At the age of 31, they married two sisters who bore them a total of 26 children. They died within hours of each other.[155-157]

The precise etiology of conjoined twinning is unknown, but the most widely accepted theory is that incomplete division of an MZ embryo occurs at approximately 13 to 15 days postovulation. Most conjoined twins are female, with the ratio of females to males being reported as 2:1 or 3:1. The majority of these infants are delivered prematurely and are stillborn.[156] They are classified according to their site of union. The most common location is the chest (thoracopagus) (Fig. 24–14), followed by the anterior abdominal wall from the xiphoid to the umbilicus (xiphopagus), the buttocks (pygopagus), the ischium (ischiopagus), and the head (craniopagus).[156] Organs may be shared to varying degrees in different sets of twins. Major congenital anomalies of one or both twins are not uncommon and must be carefully searched for before definitive therapy is attempted. The success of surgical separation depends on the degree of union, the absence of major anomalies, and the presence of separate hearts.

In 1950, Gray et al.[158] proposed a set of radiographic criteria for diagnosing ventrally fused twins. These include the twins facing each other with their heads at the same level and thoracic cages in close proximity, loss of the usual flexion of the fetal spines and occasionally hyperextension of the cervical spines, and no change in position of the twins relative to each other in response to external manipulations or spontaneous fetal movement. Polyhydramnios is said to be present in almost one half the reported cases of conjoined twins. Amniography or fetography and even contrast magnetic resonance has been used in establishing the diagnosis radiographically because these procedures outline the fetal body contours and can demonstrate a shared gas-

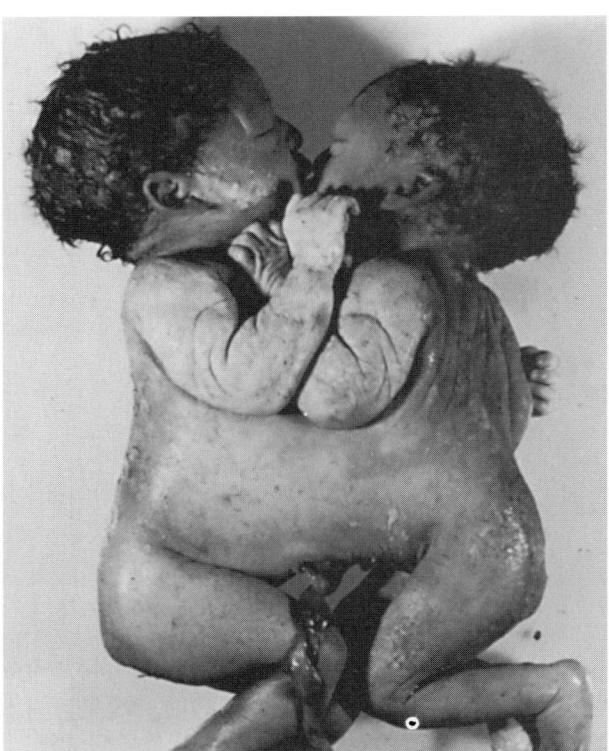

Figure 24–14. Conjoined twins attached at the chest or thoracopagus, the most common form of conjoined twins. They originate at the primitive streak stage of the embryonic plate (13 to 15 days). (Courtesy of Dr. James Wheeler, Department of Surgical Pathology, Hospital of the University of Pennsylvania, Philadelphia, PA.)

trointestinal tract.[159] Ultrasound, however, has become the safest and most reliable way to make this diagnosis in utero. Several reports have been published in which sonographic detection of this condition has been made antenatally.[159-167] In some cases the diagnosis has been made as early as the first trimester of pregnancy by transvaginal ultrasound.[168,169] Recent reports have also demonstrated that color Doppler and three-dimensional ultrasound can be effectively used to complement two-dimensional imaging, to confirm the diagnosis as well as determine the extent of organ sharing and definitive classification of conjoined twinning.[170,171] Since fetal soft tissues are so well visualized with today's sonographic equipment, invasive imaging procedures such as amniography should no longer be necessary.

Once antenatal diagnosis has been established, the mode of delivery can be planned. Vaughn and Powell[156] point out that dystocia, previously thought to be rare, since the union between conjoined twins is usually soft and pliable, may be a frequent and serious complication if vaginal delivery is attempted at term. When dystocia occurs in this setting, intrauterine surgical separation may be required that could result in devastating consequences for the fetuses and significant trauma to the mother. Craniopagus twins will not develop this type of dystocia, since it can be anticipated that they will deliver "in series" rather than "in parallel." It is therefore recommended that most conjoined twins be delivered by cesarean section at term or if they present in premature labor and are potentially salvageable.[156] If they are considered to have a poor chance of surviving and are small enough to pass through the birth canal without damaging the mother, vaginal delivery might be the preferable option. Compton[172] states that with near-term-sized twins, cesarean delivery seems indicated even if the fetuses are dead. This is based on the premise that maternal morbidity from elective cesarean delivery is predictably lower than that associated with failed partial vaginal delivery necessitating an emergency operative delivery.

Chromosomal Anomalies in Twins

Most known chromosomal anomalies have been reported in twins.[173] DZ twins are usually discordant for these anomalies and, surprisingly, MZ twins may be as well. In dizygotic pregnancies, the maternal age-related risk for chromosomal abnormalities for each twin may be the same as in singleton pregnancies. Therefore, it has been suggested that the chance of at least one fetus being affected by a chromosomal defect is twice as high as in singleton pregnancies. Furthermore, since the rate of dyzygotic twinning increases with maternal age, the proportion of twin pregnancies with chromosomal defects may be higher than in singleton pregnancies.[174] In monozygotic twins, the risk for chromosomal abnormalities is the same as in singleton pregnancies, and in the vast majority of cases, both fetuses are affected. There are, however, occasional case reports of monozygotic twins discordant for abnormalities of autosomal or sex chromosomes, most commonly with one fetus having Turner syndrome and the other fetus either a normal male or female phenotype, but usually with a mosaic karyotype.[175–177]

DEATH OF ONE TWIN IN UTERO

The death of one twin in utero is not an exceptionally rare event. Hanna and Hill[178] report a frequency of 2.2 percent over an 8-year period at their institution and cite a Swiss study in which the frequency was 6.8 percent over a period of almost 10 years. When only one twin dies in utero, it may become a fetus papyraceous. In that condition, the fluid is resorbed from the dead twin's body, and it is compressed into the adjacent membranes by the growth of the living fetus. Benirschke and Kim[6] observed that this process can occur with any kind of placentation and that it is occasionally seen as a result of TTS.

When a dead twin remains undelivered, a legitimate medical concern is the potential for disseminated intravascular coagulation (DIC) in the mother. DIC is well known to complicate some cases of retained dead fetuses in singleton pregnancies.[179] This is usually a chronic process that develops slowly in response to the release of thromboplastic material from the degenerating fetus into the maternal circulation. Although most cases of this type of DIC have been reported in the setting of a singleton gestation, it can occur after the death of one fetus in a multiple gestation.[180] Romero and colleagues[181] have reported a case in which death of one twin in utero was detected at 26 weeks' gestation (Fig. 24–15). Three and a half weeks later, the

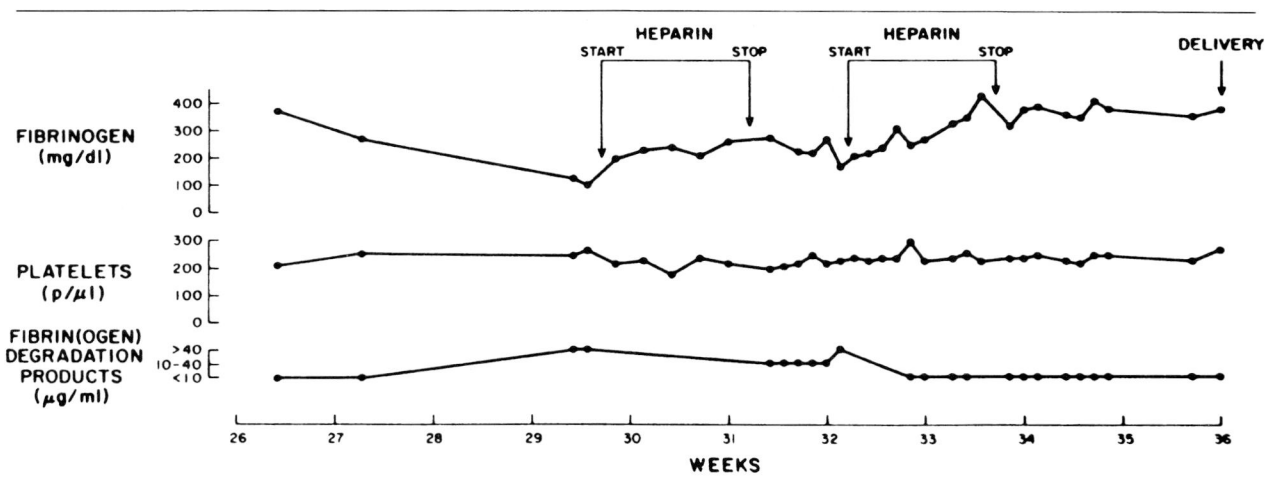

Figure 24–15. Effect of heparin therapy after 26 weeks' gestation on the platelet count and the plasma concentrations of fibrinogen and fibrin/fibrinogen degradation products in a pregnancy complicated by the death of one twin in utero. (From Romero R, Duffy TP, Berkowitz RL, et al: Prolongation of a preterm pregnancy complicated by death of a single twin in utero and disseminated intravascular coagulation. N Engl J Med 310:772, 1984, with permission.)

patient's fibrinogen level had fallen from an initial value of 370 mg/dl to 95 mg/dl. In response to an intravenous infusion of heparin, the hypofibrinogenemia was reversed. After a total of 25 days of therapy, the heparin was stopped and the patient went on to vaginally deliver a 2,040-g infant with Apgar scores of 9 and 9 and a macerated 350-g stillborn at 36 weeks. Successful reversal of maternal antepartum DIC with the use of heparin has been documented in two other patients. In each case, the pregnancy was prolonged by 10 weeks, with a normal outcome of the surviving twin.[180,182] These cases demonstrate that in selected situations it may be possible to treat the chronic maternal coagulopathy associated with a retained dead twin in order to allow a premature living co-twin to continue to develop in utero. Fortunately, however, this is usually not necessary because the incidence of this complication must be very low. In our experience with several cases in which death of an anomalous twin fetus was selectively induced during the second trimester, none of the patients developed evidence of clinical DIC. Similar experiences have been reported by other groups.[137,183–185] Therefore, as Hanna and Hill[178] have suggested, when death in utero of one twin is detected before 34 weeks, conservative management is the wisest course. This should include weekly maternal clotting profiles and serial assessments of fetal growth and well-being. Since no coagulation disorders have been observed after spontaneous or induced first-trimester death of one or more fetuses in a multiple gestation, monitoring of coagulation factors is not necessary when fetal loss occurs prior to 13 weeks' gestation.

It should be noted that normal maternal fibrinogen levels or successful reversal of a consumption coagulopathy within the maternal circulation does not ensure that the surviving fetus will be unaffected by the process. If vascular anastomoses exist within a monochorial placenta, the shared circulation may permit embolization of thromboplastic material from the dead fetus directly into its living sibling. This phenomenon has been cited as the cause of intrauterine DIC and bilateral cortical necrosis,[186] multicystic encephalomalacia,[187] and other structural abnormalities[188,190] in liveborn MZ twins with stillborn macerated co-twins. Another mechanism that may lead to death or damage of the living twin could be massive loss of blood from the survivor into the circulation of the other twin because of the lowered resistance that results from its death.[191] By contrast, because of the virtual absence of shared circulations, damage to the survivor should occur far less frequently in the case of DZ twins or MZ twins with dichorionic placentas. Carlson and Towers[192] presented a series of 17 multiple gestations in which one fetus had died and also reviewed the literature on this subject. They concluded that there is a 17 percent chance that the "surviving twin" in a monochorionic gestation will either die or suffer major morbidity, whereas these possibilities are unlikely to occur in the surviving twin in a dichorionic gestation. In a series of 43 twin pregnancies with single fetal death occurring at various times during pregnancy, Prompeler et al.[193] observed that the loss of one of the twins in the first trimester did not impair the development of the surviving twin. If, however, fetal death occurred after 17 weeks' gestation, there was an increased risk of IUGR, preterm labor, and perinatal mortality. These authors and others also observed a high incidence of other morbidities (i.e., an increased incidence of IUGR, preterm delivery, and preeclampsia) in these pregnancies.[194,195]

SELECTIVE TERMINATION OF AN ANOMALOUS FETUS

The diagnosis of discordancy for a major genetic disease before the time limit for legal termination of pregnancy in the second trimester places the parents in an extremely difficult position. Traditional choices in this setting are to terminate the pregnancy and sacrifice one normal child or to continue the pregnancy with the certain knowledge that one child will be afflicted with a devastating condition. A third choice is to perform selective termination of the affected fetus, anticipating healthy survival of the normal twin. Technical difficulties associated with this latter procedure in DZ twin gestations have, to a large extent, been resolved since its first description over a decade ago.[196] However, several issues pertaining to technical, medical, ethical, and psychological problems related to this procedure must be carefully considered and discussed with the parents.

Several techniques that have been successfully used to perform selective terminations in the second trimester include cardiac puncture with exsanguination,[196,197] removal of the affected twin at hysterotomy,[198] cardiac puncture with intracardiac injection of calcium gluconate,[184] air embolization through the umbilical vessels with fetoscopic guidance,[183] and intracardiac injection of potassium chloride.[199] The latter approach has gained acceptance because of its safety and is currently preferred both for selective termination procedures in the second trimester and for elective reduction of fetal numbers in the first trimester.[40–42,139,185,198]

Immediate problems and complications associated with selective termination procedures include selecting the wrong fetus, technical inability to accomplish the objective of the procedure, premature rupture of the membranes, infection, and loss of the entire pregnancy. Before initiating the procedure, it is critical that the abnormal fetus be correctly identified. When the indication for selective termination is an abnormal karyotype diagnosed by amniocentesis or chorionic villus sampling, a sonographically identifiable marker may or may not be present. If the gender of the twins is different, or the affected fetus has a gross morphologic anomaly such as hydrocephaly or omphalocele, the abnormal twin can be easily identified by sonography. However, in the absence of such visible signs, one must rely on the information provided from the original diagnostic procedure, which frequently has been performed elsewhere and several days or weeks before the patient presents herself to undergo the termination. In those cases where accurate localizing information is lacking, fetal blood sampling and rapid karyotype determination should be performed to reidentify the abnormal fetus before selective termination is attempted. Furthermore, in all cases a sample of fetal tissue must be obtained from the terminated twin to confirm that the correct fetus has been selected.

Since the procedure of second-trimester selective termination was first described over two decades ago,[196] it has been utilized in many centers around the world. Evans et al.[200] recently reported the experience and outcome of 402 cases from eight centers in four countries. Potassium chloride was the drug used in all cases. The overall results were excellent, with delivery of a viable infant or infants in over 90 percent of cases. There were no cases of DIC or serious maternal complications.

In considering selective termination of an abnormal twin, particular caution must be exercised to exclude the possibility of a monochorionic gestation. Vascular connections between fetal circulations occur in approximately 70 percent of MZ twins. In this situation, a lethal agent injected into the anomalous twin could enter the circulation of its normal sibling and result in death or permanent damage.[137] To avoid this possibility, it has been suggested that pericardial tamponade with an innocuous agent such as normal saline might be attempted.[201] However, even if this were technically successful, it is possible that the living normal twin could exsanguinate into the vasculature of its dead co-twin because of marked decrease in peripheral resistance of the shared circulations.[137] To date, most reported attempts at selective termination in monochorionic pregnancies have been followed by death of the second twin within a short time. This has led perinatologists to attempt to occlude completely the circulation of the anomalous monochorionic twin at the time of the procedure by performing cord ligation with surgical removal of the fetus by hysterotomy[137,202,203] or cord ligation by fetoscopy[140] or use of a helical metal coil,[151] or surgical silk suture soaked in 96 percent ethanol[204] to induce thrombosis.

In summary, the therapeutic option of selective termination requires extensive counseling, the need to establish placental chorionicity prior to the procedure, signif-

icant technical competence, and verification of the diagnosis on the fetus that is terminated. When everything has been considered, selective termination may be the best choice for a particular set of parents in this unenviable predicament, but detailed and truly informed consent is mandatory.

FIRST-TRIMESTER MULTIFETAL PREGNANCY REDUCTION

The increasingly successful use of ovulatory drugs, in vitro fertilization, and related therapies has resulted in a growing incidence of multifetal pregnancies with three or more fetuses. Because of a high risk of perinatal morbidity and mortality from premature delivery in these pregnancies, first-trimester reduction[36-38] of the number of fetuses has been advocated as a method to improve outcome. The original method of transcervical aspiration of gestational sacs described by Dumez and Oury[205] has largely been abandoned. Currently, the method of choice consists of injecting a small dose of potassium chloride into the fetal thorax under real-time sonographic guidance using either a transabdominal[185,191,192,206-208] or transvaginal[209,210] approach.

Our experience,[206] as well as that reported from several other centers,[185,207-209] indicates that first-trimester pregnancy reduction is technically feasible and results in the delivery of healthy infants close to term in the majority of cases. The largest series has been reported by Evans et al.[208] These authors combined data from 11 centers in 5 countries around the world that included 3,513 completed cases which were analyzed by the time period in which the procedures were performed, starting and finishing number of embryos/fetuses and pregnancy outcomes. With increasing experience over more than a decade the overall series loss rate was 9.6 percent, with early premature deliveries (25–28 weeks) occurring in 3.7 percent. The miscarriage and severe preterm delivery rates were related to both the starting and finishing numbers of fetuses. The most recent collaborative overall loss rates (1995–1998) were 4.5 percent for patients starting with triplets, 7.3 percent for quadruplets, 11.4 percent for quintuplets, and 15.4 percent for sextuplets or higher. The data on finishing numbers confirm that reducing to twins had the lowest loss rate (6.0%), although the gap with singletons had decreased considerably from older data (6.7%). The loss rate for patients who reduced to triplets (18.4%) was considerably higher. The rates of prematurity, however, correlated directly with the finishing number. This paper, which analyzed the experience of the same operators over an extended period of time, clearly indicates that the outcome of the procedure improves substantially with increased operator experience.

While most people would agree that perinatal morbidity and mortality are likely to improve when pregnancies with four or more fetuses are reduced to smaller numbers, the advantages of reducing triplets to twins remains far more controversial. In the absence of special circumstances, we do not believe that a first-trimester reduction from three to two fetuses can be justified on the basis of improving perinatal mortality. However, since three recently published series containing data on 198, 133, and 106 sets of triplets[23,212,213] indicated that 20, 32, and 24 percent, respectively, delivered at 32 weeks or earlier, a reduction in the morbidity associated with severe prematurity may result from reducing triplets to twins. Until more detailed data are available from triplet pregnancies managed conservatively under modern circumstances, it is not possible to know whether multifetal pregnancy reduction does truly reduce perinatal morbidity in these cases.

PROBLEMS RELATED TO PLACENTATION

Benirschke and Kim[6] note that prolapse of the cord and rupture of a vasa previa with fetal exsanguination are more common in twins than in singletons. They attribute the latter to the fact that a velamentous cord insertion occurs in 7 percent of twin placentas as op-posed to 1 percent in singletons. Robinson et al.[214] found that 7.1 percent of 72 pregnancies having a velamentous insertion of the cord had associated deformational defects of the neonate. This is defined as an alteration in shape and/or structure of a part of the fetus that has differentiated normally (e.g., clubfoot). These investigators speculate that competition for space between the developing fetus and the placenta due to mechanical factors that cause crowding in utero leads to fetal structural defects of a deformational nature and also alters the direction in which the placenta can grow. The latter situation secondarily causes velamentous insertion to occur when the bulk of the placental tissue is forced to grow laterally leaving the umbilical cord, which initially was located centrally, in an area that eventually becomes atrophic chorion laeve. The increased incidence of velamentous cord insertions in twin pregnancies may result from competition for space when two blastocysts happen to implant in close proximity. In support of this theory is the observation that velamentous insertions are more common in the most closely approximated twin placentas.

Monoamniotic twins are rare and have a high risk of fetal mortality. In a study from 1935, the survival rate of both twins was only 16 percent, while more recent series report double survival rates of 40 percent.[215] The high fetal mortality associated with a single amniotic sac is due to prematurity, vascular anastomoses in the placenta and, most commonly, entanglement of the umbilical cords (Fig. 24–16). The latter is said to occur in as many as 70 percent of monoamniotic twins. Cord entanglement has been detected ultrasonically at 19

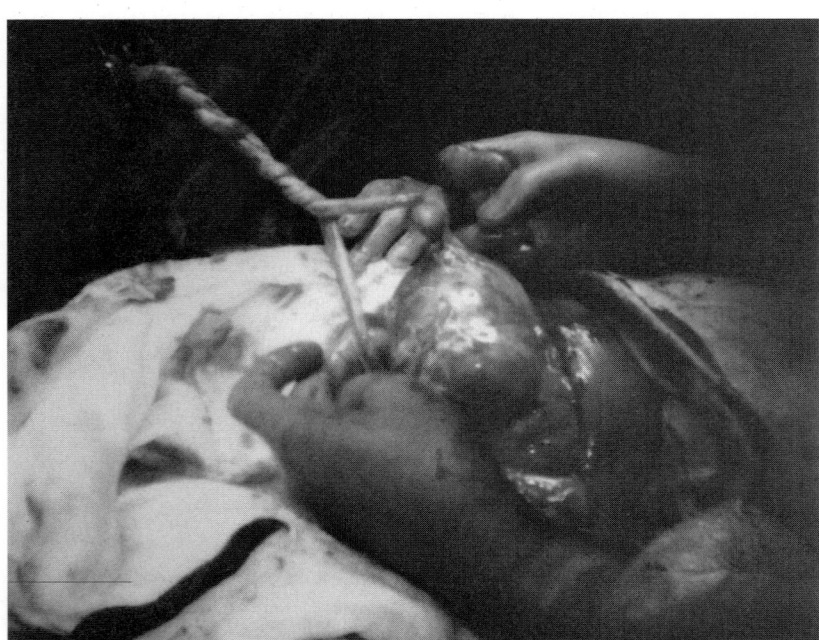

Figure 24–16. Entangled cords found during cesarean delivery in a case of MC/MA twins.

weeks in a case of monoamniotic twins discordant for an open neural tube defect.[216] Inability to visualize a membrane separating two sacs in a twin gestation is suggestive of a monoamniotic pregnancy but is not diagnostic because occasionally the membrane can remain undetected even though it is present. Townsend and Filly[217] suggest that the observation of entangled umbilical cords in the absence of a membrane separating twin fetuses provides a reliable sign for the sonographic diagnosis of monoamniotic twin gestation. They point out, though, that it is essential to trace both cords into the entangled mass before making this diagnosis. Another uncommon mishap that can result from this type of placentation is inadvertent clamping of the undelivered twin's cord after delivery of the first twin. McLeod and McCoy[218] present just such a case in which a tight cord around the neck of twin A was clamped and divided and then found to belong to twin B. After abdominal manipulation, the second twin was rapidly delivered by forceps, and both neonates survived. These workers suggest that, whenever possible, division of a cord around the first twin's neck should be avoided. They end their paper with the reminder that if the wrong cord has been severed, "immediate extraction of the second twin is essential."

The optimal management of monoamniotic twin pregnancies with respect to timing and route of delivery remains controversial. Because of an impression of increasing morbidity and mortality rates in monoamniotic twins with advancing gestations, prophylactic preterm delivery by 30 to 32 weeks has been advocated to prevent cord-related deaths late in pregnancy.[219] However, two recent retrospective studies[220,221] reviewing the outcome of 45 monoamniotic twin pregnancies found only one fetal death after 30 to 32 weeks' gestation. It occurred at 35 weeks' gestation. The authors of the latter study[221] suggested that the decreased intrauterine space available in the third trimester may prevent extensive fetal movements and therefore cord entanglement. The investigators of both studies concluded that their data did not support any particular advantage to elective delivery of these pregnancies at 30 to 32 weeks' gestation. We believe that demonstration of fetal pulmonary maturity should be taken into account as an important determinant for timing of delivery and generally target a gestational age of 32 to 34 weeks for delivering monoamniotic twins. There is less controversy regarding the mode of delivery of these patients. Although anecdotal cases of a successful monoamniotic twin vaginal delivery may be mentioned, the potential for a disastrous outcome either from complications of cord entanglement or from fetal interlocking is substantial and makes vaginal delivery in these cases less than ideal. Therefore, cesarean delivery is recommended in all viable monoamniotic twin pregnancies.

AMNIOCENTESIS IN MULTIPLE GESTATIONS

When Should Both Sacs Be Tapped?

In some situations, it is obviously necessary to perform amniocentesis on each twin sac. Genetic studies must be performed on fluid surrounding each twin because, if DZ, they are genetically distinct individuals. Twins at risk of erythroblastosis fetalis must also have each sac tapped for optical density determinations, since one twin may be Rh-positive and the other Rh-negative.[222] It should be noted that twins in Rh-sensitized pregnancies have been successfully transfused in utero.[223]

The issue of pulmonary maturity studies in twins is more complex. Two series have found a close correlation between lecithin/sphingomyelin (L/S) ratios in amniotic fluid samples from twin sets. Spellacy et al.[224] found no significant difference in fluids obtained from both sacs when L/S ratios were studied in 14 pregnancies. Sims and colleagues[225] also found the L/S ratios of both sacs to be closely related in 20 sets of twins. Obladen and Gluck,[226] however, noted significant discrepancies in postnatal phospholipid profiles of tracheal effluent in eight pairs of twins, six of whom were delivered vaginally.

Wilkinson et al.[227] reported a case of quadruplets delivered by cesarean section at 30 weeks in which the presenting baby had amniotic fluid and pharyngeal aspirate L/S ratio values that were on the borderline of maturity, while those of the other three infants were clearly immature and almost identical to each other. The firstborn infant had mild respiratory distress, while the other three developed severe hyaline membrane disease. None of the neonates experienced birth asphyxia or postnatal hypothermia, and all the pharyngeal aspirates were collected within 10 minutes of birth. These investigators cite an earlier publication from their group in which the firstborn of triplets and quadruplets had also been found to have higher pharyngeal L/S ratios and less severe respiratory distress than those of their siblings delivered subsequently. This relationship was found regardless of whether the firstborn was delivered vaginally following spontaneous labor or was the presenting fetus in a cesarean delivery.

Norman et al.[228] studied 30 African women with twins, all of whom had both sacs tapped immediately before cesarean delivery. Twenty-four of these patients were not in labor at the time of their delivery, and no significant intrapair differences in L/S ratio were found in this group. Six women who were in labor, however, were found to have a significant increase in the L/S ratio of their presenting twin when compared with its sibling. In addition, both free and unconjugated glucocorticoids were found to be increased in the amniotic fluid of the presenting twin after labor had begun, but no significant difference was noted within twin sets when labor had not commenced. These latter reports suggest that the onset of labor in a multiple pregnancy may be determined by the fetus with the most mature lungs, which apparently is often the one presenting. It is possible that one twin may be significantly more stressed in utero than the other. The concept of accelerated lung maturation in response to antenatal stress has become widely accepted.[229] It is therefore certainly conceivable that one twin may be pulmonically mature, while the other is not. Leveno et al.[230] presented a series of 42 twin pregnancies delivered by cesarean section in which amniocentesis on each sac was performed immediately before delivery. The cesarean deliveries were done for a variety of indications, and no mention was made of the presence or absence of labor. In this group of patients, there were four instances in which one twin had an L/S ratio less than 2, while the sibling's value was 2 or greater. The pair with the greatest difference had L/S ratios of 0.7 and 3.5. However, only one of these eight neonates developed hyaline membrane disease and that was a twin whose L/S ratio was 1.4 while the sibling's was 2.2. Interestingly, in this series there were seven pairs in which only one fetus was growth restricted; IUGR was not found to increase the L/S ratio significantly in these cases. Similarly, Norman et al.[228] compared the L/S ratios from each sac before the onset of labor in eight sets of twins with only one growth-restricted fetus and were unable to find significant differences.

It appears that the stress associated with IUGR may not be sufficient to cause a significant difference in lung maturity when only one twin is affected. There has been one case report,[231] however, that raises the possibility that the stress associated with premature rupture of membranes for more than 16 hours in a presenting fetus may give it a pulmonary advantage over its co-twin with intact membranes. It is likely that other stressful processes could affect twins unequally and result in major differences regarding pulmonary surfactant production.

We believe it is reasonable to assume that in most cases of nonlaboring patients with twins, an L/S ratio from one sac will accurately reflect the status of both fetuses. If one twin appears to be abnormal for any reason, however, or if the patient is in premature labor, both sacs should be tapped to assess pulmonary maturity. Should the operator elect to tap only one sac in these situations, it should be that of the twin who appears to be normal in the former case and that of the second twin in the latter. The stressed twin, or the presenting twin in these two instances, can be assumed to have an L/S ratio at least as mature as that of its sibling, and probably more so.

The Technique of Tapping Multiple Sacs

Elias et al.[232] reported that they were successful in obtaining fluid from both amniotic sacs in 19 of 20 pregnancies during the second trimester. These workers used ultrasound to identify the lie of each fetus and then introduced an amniocentesis needle into one sac using a standard insertion technique. After aspirating some fluid, they introduced a blue dye, to serve as a marker, and then removed the needle. A different needle was then inserted and the aspiration of untinged fluid indicated that the second sac had been successfully entered.

Several points should be stressed:

1. The usual precautions applying to all cases of amniocentesis must certainly be followed when multiple sacs are to be tapped. A thorough ultrasound examination should precede the amniocentesis, at which time the viability of all fetuses should be verified and their gestational ages and relative sizes assessed. The position of the placenta(s) and dividing membranes should be noted (Figs. 24-17 and 24-18) and a search for gross fetal, uterine, and adnexal pathology performed. It is particularly important to note the position of one fetus relative to the other(s) and to label the aspirated fluids appropriately, as well as placing a drawing in the patient's chart so that at a later date it is possible to correlate a particular fetus with its fluid specimen. This becomes even more critically important in the case of genetic studies if at a later date selective termination of one fetus is to be considered.

2. Direct ultrasonic visualization of the needle tip during its insertion allows for much greater precision in guiding the needle to an optimal sampling site. It also reduces the potential for traumatizing the fetus. Jeanty et al.[233] published a description of how this can easily be accomplished.

3. Use of a marker dye is very helpful in performing amniocentesis on more than one sac, but methylene blue has been associated with fetal hemolysis when injected intra-amniotically.[234] Furthermore, multiple ileal obstructions[235] or jejunal atresia[236,237] have been reported in twins whose sacs have been injected with 1 percent methylene blue at the time of a diagnostic tap in the second trimester. It is therefore recommended that either indigo carmine or Evan's blue be used rather than methylene blue. Whatever dye is used, it should not be red so as to avoid confusion in the event of a bloody tap.

4. When failure to see a separating membrane between the sacs suggests the possibility of a monoamniotic twin gestation, use of a marker dye alone may not definitively rule out this diagnosis, since aspiration of colored fluid on a second needle insertion may

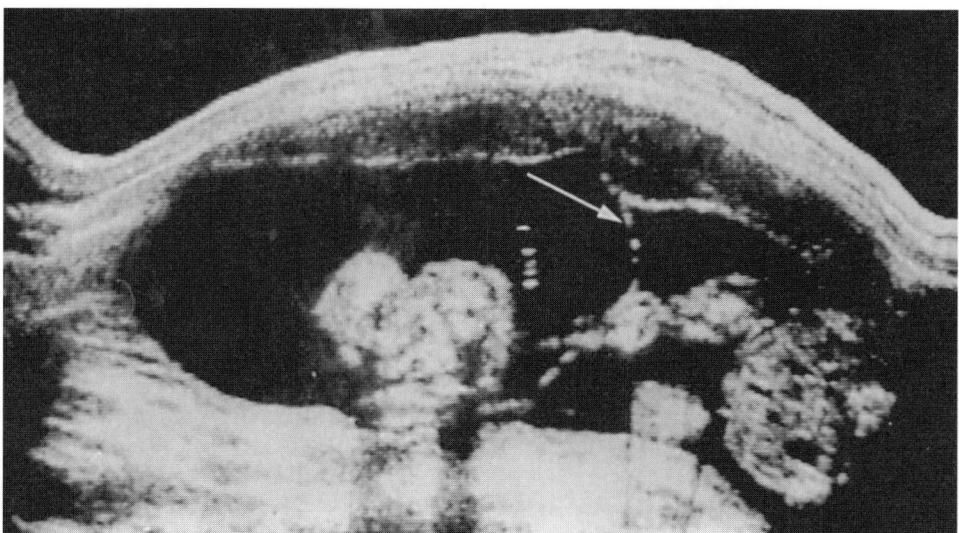

Figure 24–17. Sagittal scan with a single anterior placenta demonstrating a vertical membrane (*arrow*) separating the two sacs.

represent reentry into the first sac. Under these circumstances, a technique described by Tabsh[238] may be useful in differentiating a single monoamniotic sac from separate diamniotic sacs where the membrane is simply not being visualized. Leaving the needle in place after an initial sample of fluid is withdrawn, 0.1 ml of air drawn into the syringe through a micropore filter is mixed with 0.5 ml of marker dye and 5 ml of aspirated amniotic fluid. This mixture is then injected back into the sac under firm, gentle pressure in order to create microbubbles within the amniotic fluid. The microbubbles serve as ultrasonic contrast agents within the first sac and should demarcate it from a second sac if one is present. A site for needle insertion into the second sac can then be selected. Aspiration of colorless fluid confirms that a second sac has been entered, whereas fluid colored with dye indicates that the original sac has been reentered. If the microbubbles are seen around both fetuses, a diagnosis of monoamniotic twins can be confirmed.

Sebire et al., in 1996, described a technique utilizing single uterine entry for genetic amniocentesis in 176 twin pregnancies.[239] After amniotic fluid is aspirated from the sac of one twin, the syringe is removed, the stylet replaced, and the needle advanced through the intertwin membrane under continuous ultrasound guidance into the sac of the second twin. When aspirating fluid from the second sac, they recommend discarding the first 1 ml in order to avoid possible contamination from amniotic fluid of the first sac.[239] While the method described by these investigators is technically feasible, we would continue to recommend the technique described earlier, using a separate needle insertion for each sac, thus eliminating any chances of contamination of fluid samples obtained from each sac. Also, it is possible that the puncture site in the membrane separating the two sacs may enlarge and lead to a cord accident later in pregnancy as has been reported when this occurred inadvertently in cases of septostomy for TTS.[134,136]

Although second-trimester amniocentesis for genetic indications has become a well-accepted procedure, some studies have suggested a higher postprocedural fetal loss rate in twin pregnancies than in those with singletons.[240–242] Loss rates as high as 4.9 percent[241] to 16.7 percent[240] have been reported. These studies, however, did not address the question of whether the increased fetal wastage following amniocentesis is attributable to

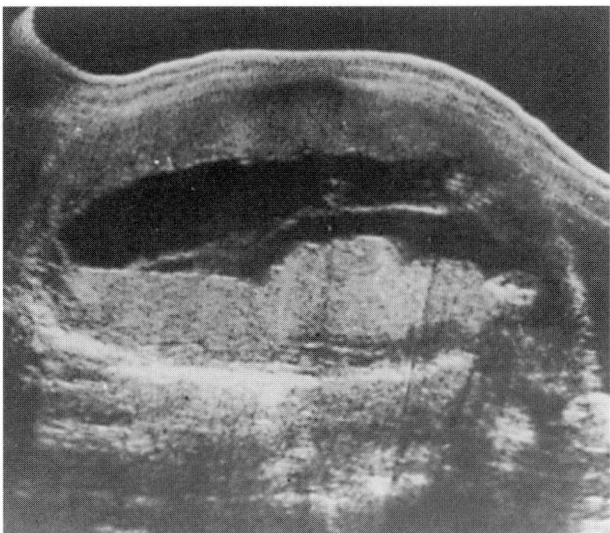

Figure 24–18. Sagittal scan revealing individual anterior and posterior placentas with the membranes running horizontally between the two sacs.

the procedure or to the twin gestation itself. In a recent case-controlled study, Ghidini et al.[243] concluded that second-trimester amniocentesis in twin pregnancies was not associated with excess pregnancy loss and that the likelihood of fetal loss secondary to this procedure is probably of the same order of magnitude as that in singletons.

MANAGEMENT OF MULTIPLE GESTATIONS

The Antepartum Period

Specialized antenatal care cannot be offered to women with multiple gestations unless they are known to be carrying more than one fetus. In areas in which universal ultrasound screening is not performed, the early diagnosis of twins depends on maintaining a high index of suspicion whenever uterine size appears to be larger than dates. Once suspected, twins can be easily diagnosed by performing a thorough ultrasound examination. After confirmation of a multiple gestation, the issue arises as to which, if any, of the various methods used in an attempt to improve perinatal outcome in these patients is worthy of consideration.

The value of bed rest in the hospital for a patient carrying twins is controversial. Marivate and Norman[2] cite five studies that reported a reduction in perinatal mortality and prematurity rates and two others that found no difference in those variables when patients with twins routinely admitted to the hospital were compared with those treated on an outpatient basis. Two prospective randomized trials published in 1984 and 1985 found no benefit from late hospital admission,[244,245] and in the latter study preterm delivery was more common among the hospitalized group.

Hawrylyshyn et al.[16] reported that in their series of 175 consecutive twin deliveries bed rest after 30 weeks had no effect on perinatal mortality. Since 70 percent of the perinatal deaths in their study occurred before the 30th week, these workers concluded that elective hospitalization must include the period from 25 to 30 weeks in order to exert any significant impact on both the survival and the quality of survival of twins. In support of this concept, it should be noted that Chervenak et al.[31] found that 81 percent of the perinatal mortality in their series of 385 twin pregnancies occurred before the 29th week of gestation.

Two other studies evaluated the role of early routine hospital admission for twin gestations and came to similar conclusions. The first was a multicenter randomized study from Australia in which 11 hospitals participated.[246] Of 141 women with twins in the study, 72 were assigned to outpatient care and 69 were hospital-ized from 26 to 30 weeks' gestation. No differences between the groups could be demonstrated in the frequencies of major maternal complications, preterm delivery, or mean birth weights at delivery.

Surprisingly, in fact, there was a trend toward greater frequency of preterm delivery and admission of neonates to the neonatal intensive care unit (NICU) in the group admitted to the hospital. Leveno et al.[247] similarly observed no differences in pregnancy outcome between 134 patients with twin gestations that were hospitalized from 24 to 32 weeks versus 177 patients who were not routinely hospitalized.

Bed rest in the hospital is expensive and disrupts normal family life. Since there is no evidence to suggest that elective hospitalization is universally beneficial for patients with twins, we feel that these women should only be hospitalized for the same indications that would be used to admit women with singletons.

Prophylactic administration of tocolytic agents to women with twins has been tried with varying degrees of success. Marivate and Norman[2] cite one report in which pregnancy prolongation and increased birth weight was associated with this approach and three other series that found no improvement in these variables when prophylactic tocolysis was administered to patients with twins. Since an increased incidence of maternal cardiovascular complications has been reported in women with multiple gestations who have been treated with β-agonists,[248] it seems prudent to restrict the use of these agents to women who are confirmed to be in preterm labor.

Results of studies using prophylactic cervical cerclage in women with multiple gestations have been disappointing.[2] Since this surgical procedure may be associated with adverse sequelae for both the mother and her fetuses, it is recommended that cerclage placement be limited to women with either a strong suggestive history or with objectively documented cervical incompetence.

In an attempt to predict the onset of labor in a series of women with twins, Houlton et al.[249] evaluated the effectiveness of a cervical assessment score based on the length of the cervical canal in centimeters minus the dilatation of the internal os in centimeters. These workers found a significant relationship between a cervical score of 0, or a decrease in cervical score, and the onset of labor within the subsequent 14 days. Similar effectiveness of this scoring system was reported by Neilson et al.[250] On the other hand, O'Connor et al.[251] found that routine cervical assessment and uterine activity measurements were not helpful in predicting preterm delivery. Recent studies have validated the utility of two other tests—ultrasonographic assessment of cervical length, and fetal fibronectin (FFN)—as useful adjuvant tests in the prediction of preterm labor in multiple gestations.[252–255]

Premature cervical shortening and cervical funneling on ultrasound have good predictive ability for preterm labor and delivery in patients with multiple gestations. These studies suggest that a cervical length measurement of greater than or equal to 35 mm by transvaginal ultrasound at 24 to 26 weeks in twin gestation will identify patients who are at low risk for delivery prior to 34 weeks' gestation. On the other hand, a cervical length of 25 mm or less with or without funneling at 24 to 26 weeks' gestation predicts a high risk for preterm labor and delivery.[253–255] The study reported by Goldenberg et al.[252] also found that a positive FFN test at 28 weeks is a significant predictor of spontaneous preterm labor prior to 32 weeks' gestation. Based on these studies, it would be reasonable to incorporate these two tests (i.e., FFN test and vaginal ultrasound for cervical length at 24 to 28 gestational weeks), as a screening test for all multiple gestations in order to identify those at high risk for preterm delivery before 34 weeks' gestation (see Chapter 23).

Another concept regarding early detection of preterm labor involves ambulatory home monitoring of uterine contractions with a mobile tocodynamometer. Although the efficacy of this method for detecting preterm labor in multiple gestations has not yet been evaluated with prospective randomized trials, clinical studies suggest that this may be a useful adjunct in the intensified antepartum surveillance of these patients.[23] It has been suggested that these women might benefit maximally from prophylactic bed rest in the hospital and aggressive early tocolysis for documented preterm labor. A randomized prospective study would shed some light on the efficacy of this approach, but to our knowledge this has not yet been performed.

The value of special twin clinics has been described by several investigators.[2,251] In these clinics, where all women known to be carrying twins are seen at regular intervals by the same medical team, several advantages accrue. Patients have the opportunity in this type of clinical setting to develop rapport with a small group of caregivers. This should result in an increased awareness of their special problems and may increase compliance with therapeutic directives. The patients can also talk with other women who are expecting twins and learn that their antenatal experiences are not unique. Furthermore, the medical personnel become more adept at detecting early signs of the special problems associated with twin pregnancies. Finally, and perhaps most importantly, the team of caregivers has the opportunity to develop an antenatal management protocol that is maximally effective for their population of patients. The value of performing serial ultrasound studies to evaluate the growth and development of each fetus in a multiple gestation has been mentioned earlier in this chapter. It should also be noted that assessment of fetal well-being by simultaneous nonstress heart rate testing

in twin pregnancies seems both feasible and efficacious. DeVoe and Azor[256] reported 24 sets of twins who underwent 120 simultaneously recorded nonstress tests in the third trimester. Technical problems in obtaining readable tracings were encountered in only 15 percent of cases. Reactive nonstress tests were found to be associated with a good prognosis if delivery occurred within 1 week, while nonreactive nonstress tests were less specific but in some cases reflected significant distress in utero. These authors concluded that nonstress tests in twins, whether reactive or nonreactive, appear to be prognostically comparable to those previously reported in singleton third-trimester pregnancies. The study of Blake et al.[257] in 94 patients with multiple gestations confirmed that antepartum nonstress testing is a highly reliable and predictive test in assessment of multiple gestations.

Before 1983, three relatively large series were published describing the management of pregnancies in which three or more fetuses were involved. Ron-El et al.[19] reported their experience with 29 triplet and 6 quadruplet pregnancies in Tel Aviv between 1970 and 1978. Seven of these pregnancies were conceived spontaneously, and the other 19 followed the administration of fertility drugs. The cesarean delivery rate was 44 percent and the mean birth weight was 1,830 ± 536 g. The overall perinatal mortality rate was 185 per 1,000.

In another series from Israel, Holcberg et al.[18] described the outcome of 31 triplet pregnancies managed between 1960 and 1979 at their institution in Beersheba. Twenty-one of these pregnancies were conceived spontaneously, and 10 followed the induction of ovulation. Triplet gestation was diagnosed earlier in the group with induced ovulation, and their period of hospitalization before delivery was longer than the group that conceived spontaneously. The most frequent antenatal complications for the entire group were preterm delivery (97 percent), pregnancy-induced hypertension (46 percent), and anemia (29 percent). Thirteen percent of patients required postpartum blood transfusions for excessive bleeding from an atonic uterus. The overall perinatal mortality rate was 312 per 1,000. The only neonatal death occurring in an infant born after 31 weeks was due to congenital malformations incompatible with life. The incidence of cesarean delivery was 32 percent.

Loucopoulos and Jewelewicz[20] reported the outcome of 35 pregnancies involving 27 sets of triplets, 7 sets of quadruplets, and 1 set of quintuplets at the Sloane Hospital for Women in New York between 1965 and 1981. Six patients conceived triplets spontaneously, and the remainder became pregnant after the use of ovulatory agents. The cesarean delivery rate was 42 percent, and the mean birth weight was 1,815 ± 628 g. The overall perinatal mortality rate was 148 per 1,000.

Four studies evaluated various management protocols

in multiple gestations involving three or more fetuses, Goldman et al.[258] assessed the efficacy of elective cerclage. Of 27 multiple pregnancies, 12 with triplets and 3 with quadruplets received elective cerclage, whereas 10 triplet and 2 quadruplet gestations did not. These investigators found that the cerclage group achieved a significantly longer mean gestation, higher birth weights, higher Apgar scores, lower rates of respiratory distress syndrome, and a significantly lower perinatal mortality rate. Lipitz et al.,[21] however, reporting their experience with 78 triplets managed between 1975 and 1988, concluded that there was no benefit of elective cervical cerclage either in prolonging gestation or decreasing fetal loss. Their observations are supported by a recent study also evaluating the role of elective cerclage in triplet pregnancies.[259] In the report of Lipitz et al.,[21] 86 percent of the patients delivered prematurely, with the mean gestational age at delivery being 33.2 weeks. The perinatal and neonatal mortality rates were 93 per 1,000 and 51 per 1,000 livebirths, respectively. A higher proportion of low Apgar scores and respiratory disorders occurred in the third infant in patients delivered vaginally. These authors recommend cesarean delivery for triplet pregnancies.

Gonen et al.[22] reported the outcome and follow-up data of 30 multiple gestations (24 triplets, 5 quadruplets, and 1 quintuplet) managed over a 10-year period from 1978 to 1988. In their study, the early neonatal mortality rate was 31.6 per 1,000, late neonatal mortality was 21 per 1,000, and the perinatal mortality was 51.5 per 1,000 live births. The incidence of respiratory distress syndrome was 43 percent, bronchopulmonary dysplasia 6 percent, retinopathy of prematurity 3 percent, intraventricular hemorrhage 4 percent, and cerebral palsy 2 percent. Follow-up of 84 infants for a period of 1 to 10 years showed 75 percent of them to be free from any neurologic or developmental handicap, 22 percent had mild functional delay, one infant was mildly handicapped, and one was moderately handicapped. Although all patients were not managed with the same protocol, the authors concluded that the most likely determinants of the excellent outcome in this series were early diagnosis, meticulous antenatal care, frequent evaluation of fetal well-being, cesarean delivery, presence of a trained neonatologist for each neonate at the time of delivery, and the resources of a highly skilled NICU.

Newman et al.[23] evaluated outpatient antepartum management and pregnancy outcome of 198 women who delivered triplets between 1985 and 1988. The study involved 24 centers, with individual patients managed at the discretion of obstetricians in both private and academic practices. All patients were managed with the assistance of ambulatory perinatal nursing to provide outpatient surveillance. Uterine activity was monitored twice a day with a portable tocodynamometer, and daily telephone contact along with around-the-clock availability of the nursing staff provided a liaison between the patient and her physician. Modified bed rest was prescribed for almost all patients, but prophylactic tocolytic agents or betamethasone were used at the discretion of the individual physician. Although patients were hospitalized for either preterm labor or other medical complications, the average stay for antepartum hospitalization was only 15 days in this series. The mean gestational age and birth weight at delivery were 33.6 ± 3 weeks and $1,871 \pm 555$ g, respectively. The corrected perinatal survival was 95 percent, leading the authors to conclude that routine hospitalization is unnecessary for patients with triplets, and intensive outpatient surveillance is justifiable and is associated with excellent outcomes in these pregnancies.

In a recent report, 10 cases of quadruplet pregnancies managed over a 5-year period were reported by Elliott and Radin,[260] with unusually excellent outcomes, including a perinatal mortality rate of zero. Their protocol involved prophylactic use of low-dose aspirin, home contraction monitoring, terbutaline pump tocolysis, and bed rest at home starting at 16 weeks' gestation. The superb results obtained by this group of clinicians merit further assessment of their management approach in a larger group of patients with higher order multiple gestations.

Based on a review of the published studies and our own clinical experience, we believe that management of multifetal gestations with three or more fetuses can be achieved on an outpatient basis in most cases, but must include intensified surveillance of the mother and fetuses. Our protocol includes (1) modified bed rest at home initiated at 16 weeks' gestation; (2) frequent prenatal visits with cervical assessment for evidence of effacement or dilatation and measurement of cervical length by ultrasound (routine cerclage is not recommended, but is offered to patients with clinical documentation or historical evidence of cervical incompetence); (3) contraction monitoring for evidence of increased uterine activity or signs of preterm labor beginning at 20 weeks' gestation; (4) serial ultrasound studies for evaluation of fetal growth; (5) early initiation of weekly nonstress tests at 26 to 28 weeks' gestation; (6) hospitalization for any evidence of preterm labor or other obstetric/medical complications; (7) tocolytic agents and betamethasome restricted to patients with documented preterm labor; and (8) elective cesarean delivery recommended in all cases either at onset of labor near term or at 36 completed weeks' gestation following documentation of lung maturity.

The Intrapartum Period

A number of factors must be considered when evaluating a laboring patient with twins or reviewing series that present delivery outcomes in women with multiple gestations. These variables include the gestational age and estimated weights of fetuses, their positions relative to each other, the availability of real-time ultrasound on the labor floor and in the delivery room, and the capability of monitoring each twin independently during the entire intrapartum period. Older series may not be applicable to current practice because our ability to monitor both twins closely during labor and delivery has increased considerably in recent years.

All combinations of intrapartum twin presentations can be classified into three groups: twin A vertex, twin B vertex; twin A vertex, twin B nonvertex; and twin A nonvertex, twin B either vertex or nonvertex. In a series of 362 twin deliveries presented by Chervenak et al.,[261] these presentations were found in 42.5, 38.4, and 19.1 percent of cases, respectively. These data were similar to the findings of other investigators.[13,30] In the series by Chervenak et al.,[261] 81.2 percent of the vertex-vertex twin gestations were delivered vaginally. These investigators, and several others cited in their article, believe that when both twins are in vertex presentation, a cesarean delivery should only be performed for the same indications applied to singletons. This recommendation holds true for any gestational age and implies that both twins can be monitored during labor. Currently, cesarean delivery seems to be the method of choice when the presenting twin is in a nonvertex position, as there are no studies documenting the safety of vaginal delivery for this group. External cephalic version of the presenting twin would be difficult, if not impossible, in these patients. Furthermore, if the second twin is in a vertex presentation and faces its sibling, the potential for locking exists. Khunda[262] states that frequency of locking is approximately 1 per 1,000 twin deliveries, with an associated fetal mortality of 31 percent. This condition occurs most commonly in breech-vertex presentations when the fetal chins overlie each other. It is usually not recognized until the body of the presenting twin is out of the vagina and the aftercoming head cannot be delivered. Eventually it becomes clear that entry of the first twin's head into the pelvis is being obstructed by that of the second twin. Sevitz and Merrell[263] published a case in which a vaginal delivery was accomplished and one twin survived after intravenous administration of a β-mimetic agent to a woman whose twins had locked during delivery. The more devastating consequences of this disorder, however, have been aptly described by Nissen.[264] Finally, it is possible that the second twin could complicate the delivery of the first twin in more subtle ways, such as by deflexing its head. It may eventually be shown that in some circumstances fears regarding a vaginal delivery when the leading twin presents in a nonvertex position are unwarranted, but this has not yet been convincingly demonstrated.

The management of that subset of women whose twins are in a vertex-breech or vertex-transverse lie is particularly controversial. Chervenak et al.[261] cite 11 references in which depressed Apgar scores and increased perinatal mortality rates associated with vaginal breech delivery of the second twin have led some of the investigators to recommend cesarean delivery whenever twin B is in a nonvertex lie. Conflicting data have been reported, however. Acker et al.[265] found no perinatal deaths when 74 nonvertex first or second twins weighing more than 1,499 g were delivered by cesarean section or when 76 nonvertex second twins with similar birth weights were delivered vaginally. Furthermore, no statistically significant difference was found in low 5-minute Apgar scores when these two groups were compared.

Chervenak and colleagues[266] presented the intrapartum management of 93 vertex-breech and 42 vertex-transverse twin sets. Seventy-eight percent of the vertex-breech group and 53 percent of the vertex-transverse group were delivered vaginally. Seventy-six second twins were delivered vaginally by breech extraction, 16 of whom had birth weights of less than 1,500 g. Within that group there were six neonatal deaths, four intraventricular hemorrhages, and a 67 percent occurrence of depressed 5-minute Apgar scores. It should be noted, however, that there were also seven neonatal deaths and four intraventricular hemorrhages in the firstborn fetuses of the same pregnancies, all of whom were delivered in vertex presentation. At birth weights above 1,500 g, there were no neonatal deaths or documented intraventricular hemorrhages and only three cases (5 percent) of 5-minute Apgar scores of less than 7 in the group of second twins delivered vaginally by breech extraction. Chervenak et al.[266] state that their data do not prove vaginal breech delivery of the low-birth-weight second twin to be more damaging than cesarean delivery. Nevertheless, because of the documented ill effects of vaginal delivery on low-birth-weight singleton breech infants[267,268] and the absence of evidence that being a second twin gives these infants an advantage relative to their singleton counterparts, vaginal breech delivery was not advised for second twins weighing less than 1,500 g. On the other hand, if a second twin weighs between 1,500 and 3,500 g and the criteria for vaginal delivery of a singleton breech are met, this series suggests that vaginal breech delivery is an acceptable option.

The same group has also reported their experience with 25 external cephalic versions performed on 14 transverse and 11 breech malpositioned second twins.[269] Version-to-vertex presentation was successful in 71 and 73 percent of cases, respectively. Among the 25 attempted cases, only 2 neonates had 5-minute Apgar scores below 7. However, in a study reported by Gocke et al.,[270] the success rate for external cephalic version of the second twin was only 46 percent. Their study analyzed 136 sets of vertex-nonvertex twins with birth weights above 1,500 g in whom delivery of the second twin was managed by primary cesarean delivery, external version, or primary breech extraction. A primary attempt at delivery of the second twin by external version was performed on 41 twins, 55 underwent attempted breech extraction, and 40 patients had a primary cesarean delivery. No differences were noted in the incidence of neonatal mortality or morbidity among the three modes of delivery. External version was associated not only with a higher failure rate than breech extraction, but also a higher rate of fetal distress, cord prolapse, and compound presentation. The authors, therefore, suggest that primary breech extraction of the second nonvertex twin weighing more than 1,500 g is a reasonable alternative to either cesarean delivery or external version. Analyzing their own extensive experience along with a review of the published literature, Chervenak et al.[261] have made the following recommendations for patients presenting with twins in vertex-nonvertex presentation. During the intrapartum period, a sonographic estimation of fetal weight (EFW) for twin B should be determined. With current methods,[271] there is a 10 percent SD in the sonographic EFW so that 95 percent of the time estimates are accurate to within ±20 percent. Therefore, using a cutoff for EFW of 2,000 g is unlikely to result in the birth of a neonate weighing less than 1,500 g. On the basis of the arguments cited above, the investigators believe that a birth weight in excess of 1,500 g is sufficient for a vaginal breech delivery, but a lesser weight is not. Regardless of the estimated weight, they suggest that an attempt be made to convert the second twin to a vertex presentation by performing an external version after the first twin has been delivered. If this proves successful, a vaginal delivery can be anticipated. If the attempted version is unsuccessful and the EFW is between 2,000 and 3,500 g, a breech extraction can be performed unless the other criteria for a singleton vaginal breech delivery are not satisfied. Recent reports support these recommendations and have documented the efficacy and safety of either external cephalic version[272] or total breech extraction[273,274] for the delivery of second nonvertex twins weighing more than 1,500 g. However, if the EFW of the second twin is less than 2,000 g, or the criteria for a singleton vaginal breech delivery are not met, a cesarean delivery should be performed following a failed external version. Evrard and Gold[275] discuss the reluctance of some obstetricians to ever consider a combined vaginal-abdominal approach to delivering twins but point out that there are some situations in which it is appropriate. Other workers have made reference to this form of delivery in a small number of patients in their twin series.[261,276]

In commenting on their series of triplets, quadruplets, and quintuplets, Loucopoulos and Jewelewicz[20] state that "the mode of delivery does not seem to play any particular role insofar as outcome is concerned." Several studies prior to 1990 suggested low neonatal morbidity and mortality rates with cesarean section delivery of patients with triplet pregnancies, and therefore recommended cesarean delivery in all these patients.[19,278-281] More recent studies, however, suggest that in selected cases vaginal delivery of triplets can be accomplished without increased neonatal or maternal morbidity and mortality. Furthermore, successful vaginal delivery in these patients would decrease maternal hospital stay and postoperative morbidity.[282-285] Loucopoulos and Jewelewicz[20] suggest that "continuous fetal surveillance, speed, and atraumatic delivery are the hallmarks of successful intrapartum management. In experienced hands, vaginal delivery should be attempted unless there is a medical indication for cesarean section." They caution, however, that general anesthesia should be used if one is contemplating vaginal delivery, since the absence of adequate uterine relaxation could make an internal version or extraction impossible and thereby increase the risk of neonatal injury. It is fair to point out that great skill with external versions and/or breech deliveries might be required in order to achieve the atraumatic but speedy delivery called for by these authors. In our opinion, only an experienced obstetrician with demonstrated expertise in these maneuvers should even consider attempting the vaginal delivery of a patient who is known to have three or more viable fetuses. We currently feel that elective cesarean delivery is the safest mode for these pregnancies.

TIME INTERVAL BETWEEN DELIVERIES

Another variable that many investigators have considered important in the outcome of twin pregnancies is the time interval between their deliveries. After delivery of the first twin, uterine inertia may develop, the second twin's cord can prolapse, and partial separation of its placenta may render the second twin hypoxic. In addition, the cervix can clamp down, making rapid delivery of the second twin extremely difficult if fetal distress develops. Many reports have suggested that the interval between deliveries should ideally be within 15 minutes and certainly not more than 30 minutes.[6,13,30,285,286] Most of the data in support of this view, however, were obtained before the advent of intrapartum fetal monitoring.

There are obviously situations in which expeditious

delivery of the second twin is desirable shortly after the birth of the first, but this is not always the case. Several extraordinary examples attest to this fact. Mashiach et al.[287] reported a case of a woman with a triplet pregnancy in a uterus didelphys, with fetuses A and B in the right uterine horn and fetus C in the left horn. A missed abortion of fetus A was noted at 22 weeks. At 27 weeks the right horn began to contract and a macerated fetus A was delivered vaginally, but the passage of fetus B was obstructed by the vertex of fetus C. A cesarean section was then performed on the right uterine horn and a 1,080-g infant was delivered who died in 2 weeks.

Since the left horn was not contracting, it was left intact. At 37 weeks, 72 days after the first two deliveries, an elective cesarean delivery was performed, and a 2,490-g healthy infant was delivered who went home with the mother on the seventh postpartum day. These workers cite several other examples of significant delays in the delivery of twins who were located in separate uterine horns.

Woolfson et al.[288] reported the case of a woman with a single normally shaped uterus who delivered a 570-g first twin vaginally as a breech at 25 weeks. This infant died of respiratory distress in 5 days. The first twin's placenta was retained within the uterus, and the cervical os closed to less than 3 cm after delivery. The cord was cut at the level of the cervix, and prophylactic antibiotics were administered. The patient was followed with serial maternal clotting profiles and ultrasound examinations of the remaining fetus. At 32 weeks, after 53 days in the hospital following delivery of the first twin, labor resumed and spontaneous rupture of the membranes occurred. A cesarean delivery was performed and a 1,600-g infant with Apgar scores of 7 and 9 was delivered. The placentas weighed 310 and 110 g, and the patient's postoperative course was uneventful. These authors cite four other reports in which intervals varying from 14 to 84 days were reported in twin deliveries wherein tocolytics, cervical cerclage, or simple observation were the mainstays of management.

Another such case reported by Feichtinger et al.[289] achieved 12 additional weeks and delivery of a healthy second twin, following delivery and death of the first twin at 21 weeks' gestation. This patient presented with preterm labor and ruptured membranes at 21 weeks. A cerclage suture that had been prophylactically placed at 12 weeks gestation was removed to allow delivery of a nonviable twin A. There was no evidence of placental separation, the sac of twin B was intact, and its heart rate monitoring was normal. A Shirodkar type of cerclage was then placed, and the patient was treated with tocolytics, intravenous antibiotics, and vaginal antiseptic suppositories. Her subsequent antepartum course after discharge from the hospital at 24 weeks was apparently unremarkable, until readmission for preterm labor and uneventful delivery at 33 weeks' gestation. The infant weighed 1,750 g and had an uncomplicated neonatal course.

The total number of reported cases in which delayed delivery of the retained twin, triplets, or quadruplets has been attempted are limited. Four publications report the authors' experience and a review of the literature on this subject.[290–293] These reports suggest general agreement on a management protocol for these patients, which should include high ligation of the umbilical cord of the delivered twin with an absorbable suture, prophylactic use of tocolytics, bed rest, ongoing monitoring of the patient for evidence of infection and/or coagulation disorders, and serial monitoring for growth and well-being of the viable fetus(es). In the management of these pregnancies, three areas that still remain controversial are the routine use of cervical cerclage, prophylactic antibiotics, and corticosteriods for enhancement of fetal lung maturity of the viable fetus(es).

It must be recognized that most of the reported cases represent spectacular successes. This type of management, however, should not be considered "standard of care." If an individual case is considered for such a treatment protocol, the potential risks, which may be considerable, along with the benefits must be discussed in detail and a fully informed consent obtained from the patient and her partner.

Rayburn et al.[276] reported the outcome of 115 second twins delivered vaginally at or beyond 34 weeks' gestation after the vertex delivery of their siblings. The second twin was visually monitored ultrasonically on some occasions, and continuous monitoring of the fetal heart was performed in all cases. Oxytocin was used if uterine contractions subsided within 10 minutes after delivery of the first twin. In this series, 70 second twins delivered within 15 minutes of the first twin, 28 within 16 and 30 minutes, and 17 more than 30 minutes later. The longest interdelivery interval was 134 minutes. All these infants survived, and none of them had traumatic deliveries. All 17 of the neonates delivering beyond 30 minutes had 5-minute Apgar scores of 8 and 10. In those cases with delivery intervals in excess of 15 minutes, the birth weight differential was not in excess of ±200 g when first and second twins were compared. In the series reported by Chervenak et al.,[269] the fetal heart of the second twin was monitored with ultrasound visualization throughout the period between twin deliveries, and no difference in the occurrence of low 5-minute Apgar scores was noted in relationship to the length of the interdelivery interval.

It therefore seems apparent that while some second twins may require rapid delivery, others can be safely followed with fetal heart rate surveillance and remain undelivered for substantial periods of time. This less hurried approach when twin B is not in distress may reduce the incidence of both maternal and fetal trauma associated with difficult deliveries performed to meet arbitrary deadlines.

ULTRASOUND AND THE INTRAPARTUM MANAGEMENT OF MULTIPLE GESTATIONS

Ultrasound can also be useful during labor and delivery. On admission to the delivery floor, the position of each twin can be quickly and accurately assessed and viability of both fetuses confirmed by direct visualization of their hearts. Knowledge of the presentation of each twin permits the establishment of a management protocol regarding the anticipated route of delivery. If a vaginal delivery is to be attempted, the weights of both twins can be rapidly estimated. This information is particularly important for the second twin because if it is thought to weigh less than 1,500 g or more than 3,500 g, a vaginal breech delivery might not be attempted. It is also possible to rule out extension of the head when a fetus is in breech presentation by using the method described by Berkowitz and Hobbins.[294] Ballas et al.[295] cited an incidence of more than 70 percent for spinal cord transection when 11 breeches with extended heads were delivered vaginally compared with no cord injuries when nine infants with deflexed heads were delivered by cesarean section. Although these data were derived from singleton breeches, there is no reason to believe that they could not apply to twins as well.

Both fetuses must be monitored electronically throughout labor in order to ensure their well-being. When membranes are already ruptured, a scalp electrode can easily be attached to the presenting part of twin A, and the second twin can be monitored with an external Doppler transducer. In practice, however, it is sometimes difficult to find the optimal spot from which to monitor the second twin. By using real-time ultrasound, the heart of twin B can be precisely located and the Doppler transducer placed accordingly. If movement of the second twin results in loss of a readable tracing, the transducer can be repositioned after real-time ultrasound has revealed the new position of twin B's heart. When a patient with twins or triplets is taken to the delivery room, the real-time scanner should accompany her. After delivery of the first infant, real-time examination immediately and precisely establishes the position of the second fetus. Visualization of the fetal heart allows the second fetus to be monitored for evidence of bradycardia until one fetal pole settles into the pelvis, membranes are ruptured, and a scalp electrode is applied. While visual monitoring of the heart does not provide subtle information such as a loss of baseline variability, it does permit early detection of significant deviations from the normal fetal heart rate range.

In addition to monitoring heart rate, visualization of the second twin permits both external and internal manipulations to be performed in a more controlled fashion. Externally, it is often possible to guide the vertex over the inlet by directing pressure from the ultrasound transducer over the fetal head while pushing the buttocks toward the fundus with the other hand.[294] If this is unsuccessful, an internal version can be made less difficult by visualizing the operator's hand within the uterus and directing it toward the fetal feet. This technique can reduce the confusion often experienced when a small fetal part is blindly caught, and it is unclear whether it belongs to an upper or a lower extremity.

CONCLUSION

The patient carrying more than one fetus presents a formidable challenge to the obstetrician. The high perinatal morbidity and mortality rates traditionally associated with multiple gestations are due to many factors, some of which can still not be altered. The extraordinary advances in technology during the past 25 years, however, have given us new insights into some problems peculiar to multifetal pregnancies as well as some tools with which to detect those problems. Early diagnosis of multiple gestations and follow-up with serial studies hold the potential for administering specialized regimens to selected patients, and this should have a beneficial impact on the outcome of those pregnancies.

Key Points

➤ Perinatal/neonatal morbidity and mortality are significantly higher in multiple gestations than singleton pregnancies.

➤ Any patient with a multiple gestation should be clinically managed as a high-risk pregnancy.

➤ The incidence of congenital structural malformations is two to three times higher in fetuses of multiple gestations when compared with those of singleton gestations.

➤ Ultrasound evaluation is the single most important diagnostic test in multiple gestations.

➤ All patients with multiple gestations should have a thorough first- and second-trimester ultrasound examination to assess for chorionicity, amnionicity, individual fetal growth, and congenital malformations.

➤ Twin-to-twin transfusion syndrome is a serious potential complication in monozygotic twins, with a high fetal mortality rate.

➤ Prophylactic cerclage, tocolytics, or hospitalization for bed rest do not have any proven advantage in the management of multiple gestations.

➤ In twin pregnancies with discordant growth, fetal lung maturity studies obtained from amniotic fluid of the larger twin will usually also represent similar or greater lung maturity of the smaller twin.

➤ The presentation of each fetus must be sonographically verified as soon as a patient with twin pregnancy presents in labor.

➤ As a general rule, mode of delivery should be vaginal when both twins are vertex, individualized for vertex-nonvertex twins, and cesarean section when the first twin is nonvertex. For triplets or more, the safest mode of delivery is by cesarean section.

REFERENCES

1. Hrubec Z, Robinette CD: The study of human twins in medical research. N Engl J Med 310:435, 1984.
2. Marivate M, Norman RJ: Twins. Clin Obstet Gynaecol 9:723, 1982.
3. Martin JA, Park MM: Trends in twin and triplet births. 1980–97. National Vital Statistics Reports, Vol. 47, No. 24, DHHS Publication No. (PHS) 99-1120. Hyattsville, MD, National Center for Health Services, Department of Health and Human Services, 1999.
4. Kurachi K, Aono T, Susuki M, et al: Results of HMG (Hurregon)–HCG therapy in 6,096 treatment cycles of 2,166 Japanese women with anovulatory infertility. Eur J Obstet Gynecol Reprod Biol 19:43, 1985.
5. Australian In-Vitro Fertilization Collaborative Group: In-vitro fertilization pregnancies in Australia and New Zealand. Med J Aust 148:429, 1988.
6. Benirschke K, Kim CK: Multiple pregnancy [first of two parts]. N Engl J Med 288:1276, 1973.
7. Derom C, Derom R, Vlietnik R, et al: Increased monozygotic twinning rate after ovulation induction. Lancet 2:1236, 1987.
8. Wenstrom KD, Syrop CH, Hammitt DG, et al: Increased risk of monochorionic twinning associated with assisted reproduction. Fertil Steril 60:510, 1993.
9. Cameron AH: The Birmingham twin survey. Proc R Soc Med 61:229, 1968.
10. Derom C, Bakker E, Vlietnick R, et al: Zygosity determination in newborn twins using DNA variants. J Med Genet 22:279, 1985.
11. Hill AVS, Jeffreys AJ: Use of minisatellite DNA probes for determination of twin zygosity at birth. Lancet 2:1394, 1985.
12. James WH: Is Weinberg's differential rule valid? Acta Genet Med Gemellol 28:69, 1979.
13. Kohl SG, Casey G: Twin gestation. Mt Sinai J Med 42:523, 1975.
14. Desgranges MF, De Muylder X, Moutquin JM, et al: Perinatal profile of twin pregnancies: A retrospective review of 11 years (1969–1979) at Hopital Notre-Dame, Montreal, Canada. Acta Genet Med Gemollol 31:157, 1982.
15. Rattan PK, Knuppel RA, O'Brien WF: Intrauterine fetal death in twins after thirty-two weeks of gestation [abstract 132]. Society of Perinatal Obstetricians. Annual Meeting, February 1984.
16. Hawrylyshyn PA, Barkin M, Bernstein A, Papsin FR: Twin pregnancies—a continuing perinatal challenge. Obstet Gynecol 59:463, 1982.
17. Kiely JL: What is the population based risk of preterm birth among twins and other multiples? Clin Obstet Gynecol 41:3, 1998.
18. Holcberg G, Biele Y, Jewenthal H, Insler V: Outcome of pregnancy in 31 triplet gestations. Obstet Gynecol 59:472, 1982.
19. Ron-El R, Caspi E, Schreyers P, et al: Triplet and quadruplet pregnancies and management. Obstet Gynecol 57:458, 1981.
20. Loucopoulos A, Jewelewicz R: Management of multifetal pregnancies: Sixteen years' experience at the Sloane Hospital for Women. Am J Obstet Gynecol 143:902, 1982.
21. Lipitz S, Reichman B, Paret G, et al: The improving outcome of triplet pregnancies. Am J Obstet Gynecol 161:1279, 1989.
22. Gonen R, Heyman E, Asztalos EV, et al: The outcome of triplet, quadruplet, and quintuplet pregnancies managed in a perinatal unit: Obstetric, neonatal, and follow-up data. Am J Obstet Gynecol 162:454, 1990.
23. Newman RB, Hamer C, Clinton Miller M: Outpatient triplet management: A contemporary review. Am J Obstet Gynecol 161:547, 1989.
24. Levene MI, Wild J, Steer P: Higher multiple births and the modern management of infertility in Britain. Br J Obstet Gynaecol 99:607, 1992.
25. Arlettaz R, Duc G: Triplets and quadruplets in Switzerland, 1985–88. Schweiz Med Wochenschr 122:511, 1992.
26. Jones HA, Lumley J: Triplets and quadruplets born in Victoria between 1982 and 1990. The impact of IVF and GIFT on rising birthrates. Med J Aust 158:659, 1993.
27. Alvarez M, Berkowitz RL: Multifetal gestation. Clin Obstet Gynecol 33:79, 1990.
28. Luke B, Keith LG: The contribution of singletons, twins and triplets to low birth weight, infant mortality and handicap in the United States. J Reprod Med 37:661, 1992.
29. Donovan EF, Ehrenkrang RA, Shankaran S, et al: Outcomes of very low birth weight twins cared for in the National Institute of Child Health and Human Development Neonatal Research Network's intensive care units. Am J Obstet Gynecol 179:742, 1998.
30. Farooqui MO, Grossman JH, Shannon RA: A review of twin pregnancy and perinatal mortality. Obstet Gynecol Surv 28:144, 1973.
31. Chervenak FA, Youcha S, Johnson RE, et al: Antenatal diag-

nosis and perinatal outcome in a series of 385 consecutive twin pregnancies. J Reprod Med 29:727, 1984.

32. Cetrulo CL, Ingardia CJ, Sbarra AJ: Management of multiple gestation. Clin Obstet Gynecol 23:533, 1980.

33. Persson PH, Kullander S: Long-term experience of general ultrasound screening in pregnancy. Am J Obstet Gynecol 146:942, 1983.

34. LeFevre ML, Bain RP, Ewigman BG, et al: A randomized trial of prenatal ultrasonographic screening: Impact on maternal management and outcome. Am J Obstet Gynecol 169:483, 1993.

35. Jeanty P, Romero R: What does an early gestation look like? *In* Obstetrical Ultrasound. New York, McGraw-Hill, 1984, p 34.

36. Timor-Tritsch IE, Blumenfeld Z, et al: Sonoembryology. *In* Timor-Tritsch IE, Rottem S (eds): Transvaginal Sonography. New York, Elsevier, 1991, p 225.

37. Berkowitz RL: Ultrasound in the antenatal management of multiple gestations. *In* Hobbins JC (ed): Diagnostic Ultrasound in Obstetrics. Vol. 3. New York, Churchill Livingstone, 1979, p 69.

38. Landy HJ, Keith L, Keith D: The vanishing twin. Acta Genet Med Gemellol 31:179, 1982.

39. Robinson HP, Caines JS: Sonar evidence of early pregnancy failure in patients with twin conceptions. Br J Obstet Gynaecol 84:22, 1977.

40. Berkowitz RL, Lynch L, Chitkara U, et al: Selective reduction of multifetal pregnancies in the first trimester. N Engl J Med 318:1043, 1988.

41. Khalil M, Tabsh A: Transabdominal multifetal pregnancy reduction: Report of 40 cases. Obstet Gynecol 75:739, 1990.

42. Lynch L, Berkowitz RL, Chitkara U, Alvarez M: First-trimester transabdominal multifetal pregnancy reduction: A report of 85 cases. Obstet Gynecol 75:735, 1990.

43. Finberg HJ, Birnholz JC: Ultrasound observations in multiple gestation with first trimester bleeding. The blighted twin. Radiology 132:137, 1979.

44. Varma TR: Ultrasound evidence of early pregnancy failure in patients with multiple conceptions. Br J Obstet Gynaecol 86:290, 1979.

45. Dickey RP, Olar TT, Taylor SN, et al: Incidence and significance of unequal gestational sac diameter or embryo crown-rump length in twin pregnancy. Hum Reprod 7:1170, 1992.

46. Landy HJ, Weiner S, Corson SL, et al: The "vanishing twin": Ultrasonographic assessment of fetal disappearance in the first trimester. Am J Obstet Gynecol 155:14, 1986.

47. McKeown T, Record RG: Observations on foetal growth in multiple pregnancy in man. J Endocrinol 8:386, 1952.

48. Daw E, Walker J: Growth differences in twin pregnancy. Br J Clin Pract 29:150, 1975.

49. Iffy L, Lavenhar MA, Jakobovits A, Kaminetzky HA: The rate of early intrauterine growth in twin gestation. Am J Obstet Gynecol 146:970, 1983.

50. Fenner A, Malm T, Kusserow U: Intrauterine growth of twins. Eur J Pediatr 133:119, 1980.

51. Winick M, Brasel JA, Velasco EG: Effects of prenatal nutrition upon pregnancy risk. Clin Obstet Gynecol 16:184, 1973.

52. Leveno KJ, Santos-Ramos R, Duenhoelter JH, et al: Sonar cephalometry in twins: A table of biparietal diameters for normal twin fetuses and a comparison with singletons. Am J Obstet Gynecol 135:727, 1979.

53. Bleker OP, Kloosterman GJ, Huidekoper BL, Breur W: Intrauterine growth of twins as estimated from birthweight and the fetal biparietal diameter. Eur J Obstet Reprod Biol 7:85, 1977.

54. Schneider L, Bessis R, Tabaste JL, et al: Echographic survey of twin foetal growth: A plea for specific charts for twins. *In*

WE Nance (ed): Twin Research: Clinical Studies. New York, Alan R Liss, 1977, p 137.

55. Grumbach K, Coleman BG, Arger PH, et al: Twin and singleton growth patterns compared using ultrasound. Radiology 158:237, 1986.

56. Socol ML, Tamura RK, Sabbagha RE, et al: Diminished biparietal diameter and abdominal circumference growth in twins. Obstet Gynecol 64:235, 1984.

57. Scheer K: Ultrasound in twin gestations. J Clin Ultrasound 2:197, 1975.

58. Crane JP, Tomich PG, Kopta M: Ultrasonic growth patterns in normal and discordant twins. Obstet Gynecol 55:678, 1980.

59. Graham D, Shah Y, Moodley S, et al: Biparietal diameter femoral length growth in normal twin pregnancies [abstract 112]. Society of Perinatal Obstetricians. Annual Meeting, February 1984.

60. Shah YG, Graham D, Stinson SK, et al: Biparietal diameter growth in uncomplicated twin gestation. Am J Perinatol 4:229, 1987.

61. Haines CJ, Langlois SL, Jones WR: Ultrasonic measurement of fetal femoral length in singleton and twin pregnancies. Am J Obstet Gynecol 155:838, 1986.

62. Dorros G: The prenatal diagnosis of intrauterine growth retardation in one fetus of a twin gestation. Obstet Gynecol 48(Suppl):46, 1976.

63. Leveno KJ, Santos-Ramos R, Duenhoelter JH, et al: Sonar cephalometry in twin pregnancy: Discordancy of the biparietal diameter after 28 weeks' gestation. Am J Obstet Gynecol 138:615, 1980.

64. Houlton MCC: Divergent biparietal diameter growth rates in twin pregnancies. Obstet Gynecol 49:542, 1977.

65. Chitkara U, Berkowitz GS, Levine R, et al: Twin pregnancy: Routine use of ultrasound examinations in the prenatal diagnosis of IUGR and discordant growth. Am J Perinatol 2:49, 1985.

66. Hill LM, Guzick D, Chenevey P, et al: The sonographic assessment of twin growth discordancy. Obstet Gynecol 84:501, 1994.

67. Neilson JP: Detection of the small-for dates twin fetus by ultrasound. Br J Obstet Gynaecol 88:27, 1981.

68. Yarkouni S, Reece EA, Holford T, et al: Estimated fetal weight in the evaluation of growth in twin gestations: a prospective longitudinal study. Obstet Gynecol 69:636, 1987.

69. Storlazzi E, Vintzileos AM, Campbell WA, et al: Ultrasonic diagnosis of discordant fetal growth in twin gestations. Obstet Gynecol 69:363, 1987.

70. Brown CEL, Guzick DS, Leveno KJ, et al: Prediction of discordant twins using ultrasound measurement of biparietal diameter and abdominal perimeter. Obstet Gynecol 70:677, 1987.

71. Barss VA, Benacerraf BR, Frigoletto FD: Ultrasonographic determination of chorion type in twin gestation. Obstet Gynecol 66:779, 1985.

72. Mahony BS, Filly RA, Callen PW: Amnionicity and chorionicity in twin pregnancies: Prediction using ultrasound. Radiology 155:205, 1985.

73. Hertzberg BS, Kurtz AB, Choi HY, et al: Significance of membrane thickness in the sonographic evaluation of twin gestations. AJR Am J Roentgenol 148:151, 1987.

74. Townsend RR, Simpson GF, Filly RA: Membrane thickness in ultrasound prediction of chorionicity of twin gestations. J Ultrasound Med 7:327, 1988.

75. Winn HN, Gabrielli S, Reece EA, et al: Ultrasonographic criteria for the prenatal diagnosis of placental chorionicity in twin gestations. Am J Obstet Gynecol 161:1540, 1989.

76. D'Alton ME, Dudley DKL: Ultrasound in the antenatal management of twin gestation. Semin Perinatol 10:30, 1986.

77. D'Alton ME, Dudley DK: The ultrasonographic prediction of chorionicity in twin gestation. Am J Obstet Gynecol 160:557, 1989.

78. Bessis R, Papiernik E: Echographic imagery of amniotic membranes in twin pregnancies. *In* Twin Research 3: Twin Biology and Multiple Pregnancy. New York, Alan R Liss, 1981, p 183.

79. Finberg HJ: The "twin peak" sign: Reliable evidence of dichorionic twinning. J Ultrasound Med 11:571, 1992.

80. Kurtz AB, Wopner RJ, Mata J, et al: Twin pregnancies: Accuracy of first trimester abdominal US in predicting chorionicity and amnionicity. Radiology 185:759, 1992.

81. Monteagudo A, Timor-Tritsch IE, Sharma S: Early and simple determination of chorionic and amniotic type in multifetal gestations in the first fourteen weeks by high-frequency transvaginal ultrasonography. Am J Obstet Gynecol 170:824, 1994.

82. Hill LM, Chenevey P, Hecker J, et al: Sonographic determination of first trimester twin chorionicity and amnionicity. J Clin Ultrasound 24:305, 1996.

83. Sepulveda W, Seibre NJ, Hughes K, et al: The lambda sign at 10–14 weeks of gestation as a predictor of chorionicity in twin pregnancies. Ultrasound Obstet Gynecol 7:421, 1996.

84. Nyberg DA, Filly RA, Golbus MS, et al: Entangled umbilical cords: a sign of monoamniotic twins. J Ultrasound Med 3:29, 1984.

85. Trudinger BJ, Giles WB, Cook CM: Flow velocity waveforms in the maternal uteroplacental and fetal umbilical placental circulations. Am J Obstet Gynecol 152:155, 1985.

86. Campbell S, Pearce JMF, Hackett G, et al: Qualitative assessment of uteroplacental blood flow: Early screening test for high-risk pregnancies. Obstet Gynecol 68:649, 1986.

87. Fleischer A, Schulman H, Farmakides G, et al: Uterine artery Doppler velocimetry in pregnant women with hypertension. Am J Obstet Gynecol 154:806, 1986.

88. Berkowitz GS, Chitkara U, Rosenberg J, et al: Sonographic estimation of fetal weight and Doppler analysis of umbilical artery velocimetry in the prediction of intrauterine growth retardation: A prospective study. Am J Obstet Gynecol 158:1149, 1988.

89. Giles WB, Trudinger BJ, Cook CM: Fetal umbilical artery flow velocity-time waveforms in twin pregnancies. Br J Obstet Gynaecol 92:490, 1985.

90. Gerson A, Johnson A, Wallace D, et al: Umbilical arterial systolic/diastolic values in normal twin gestation. Obstet Gynecol 72:205, 1988.

91. Giles WB, Trudinger BJ, Baird PJ: Fetal umbilical artery flow velocity waveforms and placental resistance: Pathological correlation. Br J Obstet Gynaecol 92:31, 1985.

92. Farmakides G, Schulman H, Saldana LR, et al: Surveillance of twin pregnancy with umbilical arterial velocimetry. Am J Obstet Gynecol 153:789, 1985.

93. Saldana LR, Eads MC, Schaefer TR: Umbilical blood waveforms in fetal surveillance of twins. Am J Obstet Gynecol 157:712, 1987.

94. Giles WB, Trudinger BJ, Cook CM, Connelly A: Umbilical artery flow velocity waveforms and twin pregnancy outcome. Obstet Gynecol 72:894, 1988.

95. Hastie SJ, Danskin F, Neilson JP, Whittle MJ: Prediction of the small for gestational age twin fetus by Doppler umbilical artery waveform analysis. Obstet Gynecol 74:730, 1989.

96. Gaziano E, Knox E, Bendel R, et al: Is pulsed Doppler velocimetry useful in the management of multiple gestation pregnancies? Am J Obstet Gynecol 164:1426, 1991.

97. Degani S, Gonen R, Shapiro I, et al: Doppler flow velocimetry waveforms in fetal surveillance of twins: a prospective longitudinal study. J Ultrasound Med 11:537, 1992.

98. Kurmanavicius J, Hebisch G, Huch R, et al: Umbilical artery blood flow velocity waveforms in twin pregnancies. J Perinat Med 20:307, 1992.

99. Shah Y, Gragg L, Moodley S, et al: Doppler velocimetry in concordant and discordant twin gestations. Obstet Gynecol 80:272, 1992.

100. Bebbington MW, Wittmann BK: Fetal transfusion syndrome: Antenatal factors predicting outcome. Am J Obstet Gynecol 160:913, 1989.

101. Gonsoulin W, Moise KJ, Kirshon B, et al: Outcome of twin-twin transfusion diagnosed before 28 weeks of gestation. Obstet Gynecol 75:214, 1990.

102. Dickinson JE, Evans SF: Obstetrics and perinatal outcomes from The Australian and New Zealand Twin-Twin Transfusion Syndrome Registry. Am J Obstet Gynecol 182:706, 2000.

103. Nance WE: Malformations unique to the twinning process. Prog Clin Biol Res 69A:123, 1981.

104. Wittman BK, Baldwin VJ, Nichol B: Antenatal diagnosis of twin transfusion syndrome by ultrasound. Obstet Gynecol 58:123, 1981.

105. Pretorius DH, Manchester D, Barkin S, et al: Doppler ultrasound of twin transfusion syndrome. J Ultrasound Med 7:117, 1988.

106. Ishimatsu J, Yoshimura O, Manabe A, et al: Ultrasonography and Doppler studies in twin-to-twin transfusion syndrome. Asia Oceania J Obstet Gynecol 18:325, 1992.

107. Bruner JP, Rosemund RL: Twin-to-twin transfusion syndrome: A subset of the twin oligohydramnios-polyhydramnios sequence. Am J Obstet Gynecol 169:925, 1993.

108. Tanaka M, Natori M, Ishimoto H, et al: Intravascular pancuronium bromide infusion for prenatal diagnosis of twin-twin transfusion syndrome. Fetal Diagn Ther 7:36, 1992.

109. Wieacker P, Wilhelm C, Prompeler H, et al: Pathophysiology of polyhydramnios in twin transfusion syndrome. Fetal Diagn Ther 7:87, 1992.

110. Fries MH, Goldstern RB, Kilpatrick SJ, et al: The role of velamentous cord insertion in the etiology of twin-twin transfusion syndrome. Obstet Gynecol 81:569, 1993.

111. Robertson EG, Neer KJ: Placental injection studies in twin gestation. Am J Obstet Gynecol 147:170, 1983.

112. Naeye RL: Functionally important disorders of the placenta, umbilical cord, and fetal membranes. Hum Pathol 18:680, 1985.

113. Rausen AR, Seki M, Strauss L: Twin transfusion syndrome. A review of 19 cases studied at one institution. J Pediatr 66:613, 1965.

114. Machin GA, Keith LG: Can twin-to-twin transfusion syndrome be explained, and how is it treated? Clin Obstet Gynecol 41:105, 1998.

115. Hoyme HE, Higginbottom MC, Jones KL: Vascular etiology of disruptive structural defects in monozygotic twins. Pediatrics 67:288, 1981.

116. Brown DL, Benson DL, Driscoll SG, et al: Twin-twin transfusion syndrome: Sonographic findings. Radiology 170:761, 1989.

117. Chescheir NC, Seeds JW: Polyhydramnios and oligohydramnios in twin gestations. Obstet Gynecol 71:882, 1987.

118. Bebbington MW, Wittmann BK: Fetal transfusion syndrome: Antenatal factors predicting outcome. Am J Obstet Gynecol 160:913, 1989.

119. Elliott JP, Urig MA, Clewell WH: Aggressive therapeutic amniocentesis for treatment of twin-twin transfusion syndrome. Obstet Gynecol 77:537, 1991.

120. Pinette MG, Pan Y, Pinette SG, et al: Treatment of twin-twin transfusion syndrome. Obstet Gynecol 82:841, 1993.

121. Reisner DP, Mahony BS, Petty CN, et al: Stuck twin syndrome: Outcome in thirty-seven consecutive cases. Am J Obstet Gynecol 169:991, 1993.

122. Saunders NJ, Snijders RJ, Nicolaides KH: Therapeutic amniocentesis in twin-twin transfusion syndrome appearing in the second trimester of pregnancy. Am J Obstet Gynecol 166:820, 1992.

123. De Lia JE, Cruikshank DP, Keye WR: Fetoscopic neodymium: YAG laser occlusion of placental vessels in severe twin-twin transfusion syndrome. Obstet Gynecol 75:1046, 1990.

124. Ville Y, Hecher K, Gagnon A, et al: Endoscopic laser coagulation in the management of severe twin-to-twin transfusion syndrome. Br J Obstet Gynaecol 105:446, 1998.

125. De Lia JE, Kuhlman RS, Lopez KP: Treating previable twin-twin transfusion syndrome with fetoscopic laser surgery: Outcomes following the learning curve. J Perinat Med 27:61, 1999.

126. Wittmann BK, Farquharson DF, Thomas WD, et al: The role of fetocide in the management of severe twin transfusion syndrome. Am J Obstet Gynecol 155:1023, 1986.

127. Weiner CP: Diagnosis and treatment of twin to twin transfusion in the mid-second trimester of pregnancy. Fetal Ther 2:71, 1987.

128. De Lia JR, Emery MG, Sheafor SA, et al: Twin transfusion syndrome: Successful in utero treatment with digoxin. Int J Gynecol Obstet 23:197, 1985.

129. Simpson PC, Trudinger BJ, Walker A, et al: The intrauterine treatment of fetal cardiac failure in a twin pregnancy with an acardiac, acephalic monster. Am J Obstet Gynecol 147:842, 1983.

130. Jones JM, Sbarra AJ, Dilillo L, et al: Indomethacin in severe twin-to-twin transfusion syndrome. Am J Perinatol 10:24, 1993.

131. Blickstein I: The twin-twin transfusion syndrome. Obstet Gynecol 76:714, 1990.

132. Hecher K, Plath H, Bregenzer T, et al: Endoscopic laser surgery versus serial amniocentesis in the treatment of severe twin-twin transfusion syndrome. Am J Obstet Gynecol 180:717, 1999.

133. Saade GR, Belfort MA, Berry DL, et al: Amniotic septostomy for the treatment of twin oligohydramnios-polyhydramnios sequence. Fetal Diagn Ther 13:86, 1998.

134. Cook TL, O'Shaughnessy R: Iatrogenic creation of a monoanniotic twin gestation in severe twin-twin transfusion syndrome. J Ultrasound Med 16:853, 1997.

135. Bruner JP, Crean DM: Equalization of amniotic fluid volumes after decompression amniocentesis for treatment of the twin oligohydramnios-polyhydramnios sequence. Fetal Diagn Ther 14:80, 1999.

136. Suzuki S, Ishikawa G, Sawa R, et al: Iatrogenic monoamniotic twin gestation with progressive twin-twin transfusion syndrome. Fetal Diagn Ther 14:98, 1999.

137. Golbus MS, Cunningham N, Goldberg JD, et al: Selective termination of multiple gestations. Am J Med Genet 34:339, 1988.

138. Onyskowova A, Dolezal A, Jedlicka V: The frequency and the character of malformations in multiple birth (a preliminary report). Teratology 4:496, 1971.

139. Hendricks CH: Twinning in relation to birth weight, mortality, and congenital anomalies. Obstet Gynecol 27:47, 1966.

140. Neilson JP, Hood VD, Cupples W: Ultrasonic evaluation of twin pregnancies associated with raised serum alpha-fetoprotein levels. Acta Genet Med Gemellol 31:229, 1982.

141. Kaplan C, Benirschke K: The acardiac anomaly: New case reports and current status. Acta Genet Med Gemellol 28:51, 1979.

142. Pretorius DH, Leopold GR, Moore TR, et al: Acardiac twin: Report of Doppler sonography. J Ultrasound Med 7:413, 1988.

143. Benson CB, Bieber FR, Genest DR, Doubilet PM: Doppler demonstration of reversed umbilical blood flow in an acardiac twin. J Clin Ultrasound 17:291, 1989.

144. Van Allen MI, Smith DW, Shepard TH: Twin reversed arterial perfusion (TRAP) sequence: A study of 14 twin pregnancies with acardius. Semin Perinatol 7:285, 1983.

145. Moore TR, Gale S, Benirschke K: Perinatal outcome of forty-nine pregnancies complicated by acardiac twinning. Am J Obstet Gynecol 163:907, 1990.

146. Robie GF, Payne GG Jr, Morgan MA: Selective delivery of an acardiac, acephalic twin. N Engl J Med 320:512, 1989.

147. Fries MH, Goldberg JD, Golbus MS: Treatment of acardiac-acephalus twin gestations by hysterotomy and selective delivery. Obstet Gynecol 79:601, 1992.

148. Ginsberg NA, Applebaum M, Rabin SA, et al: Term birth after midtrimester hysterotomy and selective delivery of an acardiac twin. Am J Obstet Gynecol 167:33, 1992.

149. Hamada H, Okane M, Koresawa M, et al: Fetal therapy in utero by blockage of the umbilical blood flow of acardiac monster in twin pregnancy. Nippon Sanka Fujinka Gakkai Zasshi 41:1803, 1989.

150. Roberts RM, Shah DM, Jeanty P, Beattie JF: Twin, acardiac, ultrasound-guided embolization. Fetus 1:5, 1991.

151. Porreco RP, Barton SM, Haverkamp AD: Occlusion of umbilical artery in acardiac, acephalic twin. Lancet 337:326, 1991.

152. Grab D, Schneider V, Keckstein J, Terinde R: Twin, acardiac, outcome. Fetus 2:11, 1992.

153. Quintero RA, Romero R, Reich H, et al: In utero percutaneous umbilical-cord ligation in the management of complicated monochorionic multiple gestations. Ultrasound Obstet Gynecol 8:16, 1996.

154. Windham GC, Bjerkedal T, Sever LE: The association of twinning and neural tube defects: Studies in Los Angeles, California, and Norway. Acta Genet Med Gemellol 31:165, 1982.

155. Harper RG, Kenigsberg K, Sia CG: Xiphopagus conjoined twins: A 300-year review of the obstetric, morphopathologic, neonatal and surgical parameters. Am J Obstet 137:617, 1980.

156. Vaughn TC, Powell C: The obstetrical management of conjoined twins. Obstet Gynecol 53(Suppl):67, 1979.

157. Wedberg R, Kaplan C, Leopold G, et al: Cephalothoracopagus (Janiceps) twinning. Obstet Gynecol 54:392, 1979.

158. Gray CM, Nix HG, Wallace AJ: Thoracopagus twins: Prenatal diagnosis. Radiology 54:398, 1950.

159. Apuzzio JJ, Ganesh V, Landau I, Pelosi M: Prenatal diagnosis of conjoined twins. Am J Obstet Gynecol 148:343, 1984.

160. Zoppini C, Vanzulli A, Kustermann A, et al: Prenatal diagnosis of anatomical connections in conjoined twins by use of contrast magnetic resonance imaging. Prenat Diagn 13:995, 1993.

161. Austin E, Schifrin BS, Pomerance JJ, et al: The antepartum diagnosis of conjoined twins. J Pediatr Surg 15:332, 1980.

162. Fagan CJ: Antepartum diagnosis of conjoined twins by ultrasonography. AJR Am J Roentgenol 129:921, 1977.

163. Gore RM, Filly RA, Parer JT: Sonographic antepartum diagnosis of conjoined twins. JAMA 247:3351, 1982.

164. Morgan CL, Trought WS, Sheldon G, et al: B-scan and real time ultrasound in the antepartum diagnosis of conjoined twins and pericardial effusion. AJR Am J Roentgenol 130:578, 1978.

165. Schmidt W, Herberling D, Kubli F: Antepartum ultrasonographic diagnosis of conjoined twins in early pregnancy. Am J Obstet Gynecol 139:961, 1981.

166. Wilson RL, Shaub MS, Cetrulo CJ: The antepartum findings of conjoined twins. J Clin Ultrasound 5:35, 1977.

167. Wood MJ, Thompson HE, Roberson FM: Real-time ultrasound diagnosis of conjoined twins. J Clin Ultrasound 9:195, 1981.

168. Fontanarosa M, Bagnoli G, Ciolini P, et al: First trimester sonographic diagnosis of diprosus twins with craniorachischisis. J Clin Ultrasound 20:69, 1992.

169. Meizner I, Levy A, Katz M, et al: Early ultrasonic diagnosis of conjoined twins. Harefuah 124:741, 1993.

170. Bonilla-Musoles F, Raga F, Bonilla F Jr, et al: Early diagnosis of conjoined twins using two-dimensional color Doppler and three-dimensional ultrasound. J Natl Med Assoc 90:552, 1998.

171. Maymon R, Halperin R, Weintraub Z, et al: Three-dimensional transvaginal sonography of conjoined twins at 10 weeks: A case report. Ultrasound Obstet Gynecol 11:292, 1998.

172. Compton HL: Conjoined twins. Obstet Gynecol 37:27, 1971.

173. Benirschke K, Kim CK: Multiple pregnancy [second of two parts]. N Engl J Med 288:1329, 1973.

174. Nicolaides KH, Sebire NJ, Snijders RJM (eds): The 11-14-Week Scan. The Diagnosis of Fetal Abnormalities. New York, Parthenon Publishing, 1999, p 168.

175. Rogers JG, Voullaire L, Gold H: Monozygotic twins discordant for trisomy 21. Am J Med Genet 11:143, 1982.

176. Dallapiccola B, Stomeo C, Ferranti B, et al: Discordant sex in one of three monozygotic triplets. J Med Genet 22:6, 1985.

177. Perlman EJ, Stetten G, Tuck-Muller CM, et al: Sexual discordance in monozygotic twins. Am J Obstet Gynecol 37:551, 1990.

178. Hanna JH, Hill JM: Single intrauterine fetal demise in multiple gestation. Obstet Gynecol 63:126, 1984.

179. Pritchard JA, Ratnoff OD: Studies of fibrinogen and other hemostatic factors in women with intrauterine death and delayed delivery. Surg Obstet Gynecol 101:467, 1955.

180. Skelly H, Marivate M, Norman R, et al: Consumptive coagulopathy following fetal death in a triplet pregnancy. Am J Obstet Gynecol 142:595, 1982.

181. Romero R, Duffy TP, Berkowitz RL, et al: Prolongation of a preterm pregnancy complicated by death of a single twin in utero and disseminated intravascular coagulation. N Engl J Med 310:772, 1984.

182. Angel JL, O'Brien WF: Management of the dead fetus syndrome with a surviving twin. Clin Decisions Obstet Gynecol 1:6, 1987.

183. Rodeck CH, Mibeshan RS, Abramowicz J, Campbell S: Selective fetocide of the affected twin by fetoscopic air embolism. Prenat Diagn 2:189, 1982.

184. Antsaklis A, Politis J, Karagiannopoulos C, Kaskarelis D: Selective survival of only the healthy fetus following prenatal diagnosis of thalassaemia major in binovular twin gestation. Prenat Diagn 4:289, 1984.

185. Wapner RJ, Davis G, Johnson A, et al: Selective reduction of multifetal pregnancies. Lancet 335:90, 1990.

186. Moore CM, McAdams AJ, Sutherland J: Intrauterine disseminated intravascular coagulation: A syndrome of multiple pregnancy with a dead twin fetus. J Pediatr 74:523, 1969.

187. Yoshioka H, Kadomoto Y, Mino M, et al: Multicystic encephalomalacia in liveborn twin with a stillborn macerated co-twin. J Pediatr 95:798, 1979.

188. Benirschke K: Twin placenta in perinatal mortality. N Y State J Med 61:1499, 1961.

189. Hoyme HE, Higginbottom MC, Jones KL: Vascular etiology of disruptive structural defects in monozygotic twins. Pediatrics 67:288, 1981.

190. Schinzel AAGL, Smith DW, Miller JR: Monozygotic twinning and structural defects. J Pediatr 95:921, 1979.

191. Benirschke K: Intrauterine death of a twin: Mechanisms, implications for surviving twin, and placental pathology. Semin Diagn Pathol 10:222, 1993.

192. Carlson NJ, Towers CV: Multiple gestation complicated by the death of one fetus. Obstet Gynecol 73:685, 1989.

193. Prompeler HJ, Madjar H, Klosa W, et al: Twin pregnancies with single fetal death. Acta Obstet Gynecol Scand 73:205, 1994.

194. Axt R, Mink D, Hendrik J, et al: Maternal and neonatal outcome of twin pregnancies complicated by single fetal death. J Perinat Med 27:221, 1999.

195. Peterson IR, Nyholm HC: Multiple pregnancies with single intrauterine demise. Description of twenty-eight pregnancies. Acta Obstet Gynecol Scand 78:202, 1999.

196. Aberg A, Mitelman F, Cantz M, Gehler J: Cardiac puncture of fetus with Hurler's disease avoiding abortion of unaffected co-twin. Lancet 2:990, 1978.

197. Kerenyi TD, Chitkara U: Selective birth in twin pregnancy with discordancy for Down's syndrome. N Engl J Med 304:1525, 1981.

198. Beck L, Terinde R, Rohrborn G, et al: Twin pregnancy, abortion of one fetus with Down's syndrome by sectioparva, the other delivered mature and healthy. Eur J Obstet Gynaecol Reprod Biol 12:267, 1981.

199. Chitkara U, Berkowitz RL, Wilkins IA, et al: Selective second-trimester termination of the anomalous fetus in twin pregnancies. Obstet Gynecol 73:690, 1989.

200. Evans MI, Goldberg JD, Horenstein J, et al: Selective termination for structural, chromosomal, and mendelian anomalies: International experience. Am J Obstet Gynecol 181:893, 1999.

201. Wittman BK, Farquharson DF, Thomas WDS: The role of feticide in the management of severe twin transfusion syndrome. Am J Obstet Gynecol 155:1023, 1986.

202. Robie GF, Payne GG, Morgan MA: Selective delivery of an acardiac acephalic twin. N Engl J Med 320:512, 1989.

203. Urig MA, Simpson GF, Elliott JP, Clewell WH: Twin-twin transfusion syndrome: The surgical removal of one twin as a treatment option. Fetal Ther 3:185, 1988.

204. Holzgreve W, Tercanli S, Krings W, et al: Letter to the Editor. N Engl J Med 331:56, 1994.

205. Dumez Y, Oury JF: Method for first trimester selective abortion in multiple pregnancy. Contrib Gynecol Obstet 15:50, 1986.

206. Berkowitz RL, Lynch L, Lapinski R, Bergh P: First-trimester transabdominal multifetal pregnancy reduction: A report of two hundred completed cases. Am J Obstet Gynecol 169:17, 1993.

207. Khalil MA, Tabsh A: A report of 131 cases of multifetal pregnancy reduction. Obstet Gynecol 82:57, 1993.

208. Evans MI, Berkowitz RL, Wapner RJ, et al: Multifetal Pregnancy Reduction (MPR): Improved outcomes with increased experience. Am J Obstet Gynecol (in press).

209. Timor-Tritsch IE, Peisner DB, Monteagudo A, et al: Multifetal pregnancy reduction by transvaginal puncture: Evaluation of the technique used in 134 cases. Am J Obstet Gynecol 168:799, 1993.

210. Gonen Y, Blankier J, Casper RF: Transvaginal ultrasound in selective embryo reduction for multiple pregnancy. Obstet Gynecol 75:720, 1990.

211. Evans MI, Dommergues M, Wapner RJ, et al: International, collaborative experience of 1789 patients having multifetal

pregnancy reduction: A plateauing of risks and outcome. J Soc Gynecol Investig 3:23, 1996.

212. Lipitz S, Reichman BN, Uval J, et al: A prospective comparison of the outcome of triplet pregnancies managed expectantly or by multifetal reduction to twins. Am J Obstet Gynecol 170:874, 1994.

213. Jonas HA, Lumley J: Triplets and quadruplets born in Victoria between 1982 and 1990: The impact of IVF and GIFT on rising birthrates. Med J Aust 158:659, 1993.

214. Robinson LK, Jones KL, Benirschke K: The nature of structural defects associated with velamentous and marginal insertion of the umbilical cord. Am J Obstet Gynecol 146:191, 1983.

215. Colburn DW, Pasquale SA: Monoamniotic twin pregnancy. J Reprod Med 27:165, 1982.

216. Nyberg DA, Filly RA, Golbus MS, Stephens JD: Entangled umbilical cords: A sign of monoamniotic twins. J Ultrasound Med 3:29, 1984.

217. Townsend RR, Filly RA: Sonography of nonconjoined monoamniotic twin pregnancies. J Ultrasound Med 7:665, 1988.

218. McLeod FN, McCoy DR: Monoamniotic twins with an unusual cord complication. Br J Obstet Gynaecol 88:774, 1981.

219. Rodis JF, Vintzeleos AM, Campbell WA, et al: Antenatal diagnosis and management of monoamniotic twins. Am J Obstet Gynecol 157:1255, 1987.

220. Carr SR, Aronson MP, Coustan DR: Survival rates of monoamniotic twins do not decrease after 30 weeks' gestation. Am J Obstet Gynecol 163:719, 1990.

221. Tessen JA, Zlatnik FJ: Monoamniotic twins: A retrospective controlled study. Obstet Gynecol 77:832, 1991.

222. Beischer NA, Pepperell RJ, Barrie JU: Twin pregnancy and erythroblastosis. Obstet Gynecol 34:22, 1969.

223. Ellis MI, Coxon A, Noble C: Intrauterine transfusion of twins. BMJ 1:609, 1970.

224. Spellacy WN, Cruz AC, Buhi WC, Birk SA: Amniotic fluid L/S ratio in twin gestation. Obstet Gynecol 50:68, 1977.

225. Sims CD, Cowan DB, Parkinson CE: The lecithin sphingomyelin (L/S) ratio in twin pregnancies. Br J Obstet Gynaecol 83:447, 1976.

226. Obladen M, Gluck L: RDS and tracheal phospholipid composition in twins: Independent of gestational age. J Pediatr 90:799, 1977.

227. Wilkinson AR, Jenkins PA, Baum JD: Uterine position and fetal lung maturity in triplet and quadruplet pregnancy. Lancet 2:663, 1982.

228. Norman RJ, Joubert SM, Marivate M: Amniotic fluid phospholipids and glucocorticoids in multiple pregnancy. Br J Obstet Gynaecol 90:51, 1983.

229. Gluck L, Kulovich MV: Maturation of the fetal lung, RDS, and amniotic fluid. *In* Villee CA, Villee DB, Zuckerman J (eds): Respiratory Distress Syndrome. New York, Academic Press, 1973.

230. Leveno KJ, Quirk JG, Whalley PJ, et al: Fetal lung maturation in twin gestation. Am J Obstet Gynecol 148:405, 1984.

231. Wender DF, Kandall C, Leppert PC, Berkowitz RL: Hyaline membrane disease in twin B following prolonged rupture of membranes for twin A. Conn Med 45:83, 1981.

232. Elias S, Gerbie AB, Simpson JL, et al: Genetic amniocentesis in twin gestations. Am J Obstet Gynecol 138:169, 1980.

233. Jeanty P, Rodesch F, Romero R, et al: How to improve your amniocentesis technique. Am J Obstet Gynecol 146:593, 1983.

234. McEnerney JK, McEnerney LN: Unfavorable neonatal outcome after intraamniotic injection of methylene blue. Obstet Gynecol 61(Suppl):35, 1983.

235. Nicolini U, Monni G: Intestinal obstruction in babies exposed in utero to methylene blue. Lancet 336:1258, 1990.

236. Van Der Pol JG, Wolf H, Boer K, et al: Jejunal atresia related to the use of methylene blue in genetic amniocentesis in twins. Br J Obstet Gynaecol 99:141, 1992.

237. McFadyen I: The dangers of intraamniotic methylene blue. Br J Obstet Gynaecol 99:89, 1992.

238. Tabsh K: Genetic amniocentesis in multiple gestation. A new technique to diagnose monoamniotic twins. Obstet Gynecol 75:296, 1990.

239. Sebire NJ, Noble PL, Odibo A, et al: Single uterine entry for genetic amniocentesis in twin pregnancies. Ultrasound Obstet Gynecol 7:26, 1996.

240. Palle C, Andersen JW, Tabor A, et al: Increased risk of abortion after genetic amniocentesis in twin pregnancies. Prenat Diagn 3:83, 1983.

241. Pijpers L, Jahoda MGJ, Vosters RPL, et al: Genetic amniocentesis in twin pregnancies. Br J Obstet Gynaecol 95:323, 1988.

242. Anderson RL, Goldberg JD, Golbus MS: Prenatal diagnosis in multiple gestation: 20 years' experience with amniocentesis. Prenat Diagn 11:263, 1991.

243. Ghidini A, Lynch L, Hicks C, et al: The risk of second-trimester amniocentesis in twin gestations: A case-control study. Am J Obstet Gynecol 169:1013, 1994.

244. Hartikainen-Sorri AL, Jouppila P: Is routine hospitalization needed in antenatal care of twin pregnancy? J Perinat Med 12:31, 1984.

245. Saunders MC, Dick JS, Brown IM: The effects of hospital admission for bed rest on the duration of twin pregnancy: A randomized trial. Lancet 2:793, 1985.

246. MacLennan AH, Green RC, O'Shea R, et al: Routine hospital admission in twin pregnancy between 26 and 30 weeks' gestation. Lancet 335:267, 1990.

247. Leveno KJ, Andrews WW, Gilstrap LC, et al: Impact of elective hospitalization on outcome of twin pregnancy. Presented at the Tenth Annual Meeting, Society of Perinatal Obstetricians, Houston, Texas, January 1990.

248. Katz M, Robertson PA, Creasy RK: Cardiovascular complications associated with terbutaline treatment for preterm labor. Am J Obstet Gynecol 139:605, 1981.

249. Houlton MCC, Marivate M, Philpott RH: Factors associated with preterm labour and changes in the cervix before labour in twin pregnancy. Br J Obstet Gynaecol 89:190, 1982.

250. Neilson JP, Verkuyl AA, Crowther CA, Bannerman C: Preterm labor in twin pregnancies: Prediction by cervical assessment. Obstet Gynecol 72:719, 1988.

251. O'Connor MC, Arias E, Royston JP, Dalrymple IJ: The merits of special antenatal care for twin pregnancies. Br J Obstet Gynaecol 88:222, 1981.

252. Goldenberg RL, Iams JD, Miodovnik M, et al: The preterm prediction study: Risk factors in twin gestations. National Institute of Child Health and Human Development Maternal-Fetal Medicine Units Network. Am J Obstet Gynecol 175:1047, 1996.

253. Crane JM, Van den Hof M, Armson BA, et al: Transvaginal ultrasound in the prediction of preterm delivery: Singleton and twin gestations. Obstet Gynecol 90:357, 1997.

254. Imseis HM, Albert TA, Iams JD: Identifying twin gestations at low risk for preterm birth with a transvaginal ultrasonographic cervical measurement at 24 to 26 weeks' gestation. Am J Obstet Gynecol 177:1149, 1997.

255. Ramin KD, Ogburn PL Jr, Mulholland TA, et al: Ultrasonographic assessment of cervical length in triplet pregnancies. Am J Obstet Gynecol 180:1442, 1999.

256. DeVoe LD, Azor H: Simultaneous nonstress fetal heart rate testing in twin pregnancy. Obstet Gynecol 58:450, 1981.

257. Blake GD, Knuppel RA, Ingardia CJ, et al: Evaluation of nonstress fetal heart rate testing in multiple gestations. Obstet Gynecol 63:528, 1984.

258. Goldman GA, Dicker D, Peleg A, Goldman JA: Is elective cerclage justified in the management of triplet and quadruplet pregnancy? Aust N Z J Obstet Gynaecol 29:9, 1989.

259. Mordel N, Zajicek G, Benshushan A, et al: Elective suture of uterine cervix in triplets. Am J Perinatol 10:14, 1993.

260. Elliott JP, Radin TG: Quadruplet pregnancy: Contemporary management and outcome. Obstet Gynecol 80:421, 1992.

261. Chervenak FA, Johnson RE, Youcha S: Intrapartum management of twin gestation. Obstet Gynecol 65:119, 1985.

262. Khunda S: Locked twins. Obstet Gynecol 39:453, 1972.

263. Sevitz H, Merrell DA: The use of a beta-sympathomimetic drug in locked twins. Br J Obstet Gynaecol 88:76, 1981.

264. Nissen ED: Twins: collision, impaction, compaction, and interlocking. Obstet Gynecol 11:514, 1958.

265. Acker D, Lieberman M, Holbrook H, et al: Delivery of the second twin. Obstet Gynecol 59:710, 1982.

266. Chervenak FA, Johnson RE, Berkowitz RI, et al: Is routine cesarean section necessary for vertex-breech and vertex-transverse twin gestations? Am J Obstet Gynecol 148:1, 1984.

267. Duenhoelter JH, Wells CE, Reisch JS: A paired controlled study of vaginal and abdominal delivery of the low birth weight breech fetus. Obstet Gynecol 54:310, 1979.

268. Goldenberg RL, Nelson KG: The premature breech. Am J Obstet Gynecol 127:240, 1977.

269. Chervenak FA, Johnson RE, Berkowitz RL, Hobbins JC: Intrapartum external version of the second twin. Obstet Gynecol 62:160, 1983.

270. Gocke SE, Nageotte MP, Garite T, et al: Management of the nonvertex second twin: Primary cesarean section, external version, or primary breech extraction. Am J Obstet Gynecol 161:111, 1989.

271. Shepard MJ, Richards VA, Berkowitz RL, et al: An evaluation of the two equations for predicting fetal weight by ultrasound. Am J Obstet Gynecol 142:47, 1982.

272. Tchabo JG, Tomai T: Selected intrapartum external cephalic version of the second twin. Obstet Gynecol 79:421, 1992.

273. Fishman A, Grubb DK, Kovacs BW: Vaginal delivery of the nonvertex second twin. Am J Obstet Gynecol 168:861, 1993.

274. Greig PC, Veille JC, Morgan T, et al: The effect of presentation and mode of delivery on neonatal outcome in the second twin. Am J Obstet Gynecol 167:901, 1992.

275. Evrard JR, Gold EM: Cesarean section for delivery of the second twin. Obstet Gynecol 57:581, 1981.

276. Rayburn WF, Lavin JP, Miodovnik M, Varner MW: Multiple gestation: Time interval between delivery of the first and second twins. Obstet Gynecol 63:502, 1984.

277. Pheiffer EL, Golan A: Triplet pregnancy. A 10-year review of cases at Baragwanath Hospital. S Afr Med J 19:843, 1979.

278. Deale CJ, Cronje HS: A review of 367 triplet pregnancies. S Afr Med J 66:92, 1984.

279. Collins JW, Merrick D, David RJ, et al: The Northwestern University triplet study III: Neonatal outcome. Acta Genet Med Gemellol (Roma) 37:77, 1988.

280. Crowther CA, Hamilton RA: Triplet pregnancy: A 10 year review of 105 cases at Harare Maternity Hospital, Zimbabwe. Acta Genet Medal Gemellol (Roma) 38:271, 1989.

281. Dommergues M, Mahieu-Caputo D, Mandelbrot L, et al: Delivery of uncomplicated triplet pregnancies: Is the vaginal route safer? A case control study. Am J Obstet Gynecol 172:513, 1995.

282. Wildshut HI, van Roosmalen J, van Leeuwen E, et al: Planned abdominal compared with planned vaginal birth in triplet pregnancies. Br J Obstet Gynaecol 102:292, 1995.

283. Grobman WA, Peaceman AM, Haney EI, et al: Neonatal outcomes in triplet gestations after a trial of labor. Am J Obstet Gynecol 179:942, 1998.

284. Alamia V Jr, Royck AB, Jackle RK, et al: Preliminary experience with a prospective protocol for planned vaginal delivery of triplet gestations. Am J Obstet Gynecol 179:1133, 1998.

285. Ferguson WF: Perinatal mortality in multiple gestations. A review of perinatal deaths from 1609 multiple gestations. Obstet Gynecol 23:861, 1964.

286. Spurway JH: The fate and management of the second twin. Am J Obstet Gynecol 83:1377, 1962.

287. Mashiach S, Ben-Rafael Z, Dor J, Serr DM: Triplet pregnancy in uterus didelphys with delivery interval of 72 days. Obstet Gynecol 58:519, 1981.

288. Woolfson J, Fay T, Bates A: Twins with 54 days between deliveries. Case report. Br J Obstet Gynaecol 90:685, 1983.

289. Feichtinger W, Breitenecker G, Frohlich H: Prolongation of pregnancy and survival of twin B after loss of twin A at 21 weeks' gestation. Am J Obstet Gynecol 161:891, 1989.

290. Wittmann BK, Farquharson D, Wong GP, et al: Delayed delivery of second twin: Report of four cases and review of the literature. Obstet Gynecol 79:260, 1992.

291. Poeschmann PP, Van Oppen CAC, Bruinse HW: Delayed interval delivery in multiple pregnancies: Report of three cases and review of the literature. Obstet Gynecol Surv 47:139, 1992.

292. Arias F: Delayed delivery of multifetal pregnancies with premature rupture of membranes in the second trimester. Am J Obstet Gynecol 170:1233, 1994.

293. Porreco RP, Sabin ED, Heyborne KD, et al: Delayed interval delivery in multifetal pregnancy. Am J Obstet Gynecol 178:20, 1998.

294. Berkowitz RL, Hobbins JC: Delivering twins with the help of ultrasound. Contemp Obstet Gynecol 19:128, 1982.

295. Ballas S, Toaff R, Jaffa AJ: Deflexion of the fetal head in breech presentation. Obstet Gynecol 52:653, 1978.

Chapter 25

Intrauterine Growth Restriction

IRA BERNSTEIN, STEVEN G. GABBE, AND
KATHRYN L. REED

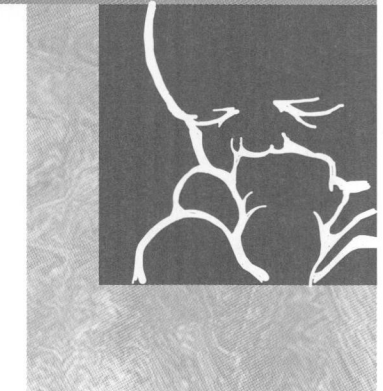

The identification of pregnancies at risk for preventable perinatal morbidity and mortality is a primary goal of the obstetric care provider. Intrauterine growth restriction (IUGR) is the second leading contributor to the perinatal mortality rate.[1] The perinatal mortality rate for these infants is 6 to 10 times greater than that for a normally grown population, 120 per 1,000 for all cases of growth restriction and 60 to 80 per 1,000 if anomalous infants are excluded. As many as 40 percent of all stillborns are growth restricted.[63] This includes 53 percent of preterm stillbirths and 26 percent of term stillbirths. The incidence of intrapartum asphyxia in cases complicated by IUGR has been reported to be 50 percent.[2] A portion of these perinatal complications are preventable. If the growth-restricted fetus is appropriately identified and managed, the perinatal mortality can be lowered. This chapter presents the varied etiologies of the growth restriction syndromes, recent advances in the detection and management of this problem, and the available information on the long-term prognosis for infants who have suffered from impaired intrauterine growth.

NOMENCLATURE

A variety of terms have been used to identify the fetus who is small relative to its peers. They include "premature," "low birth weight," "small for gestational age," "fetal growth retarded," "small for dates," and "intrauterine growth restricted." All represent the small fetus and have intentional distinctions based on their origins, found primarily in the pediatric literature.

The evolution of terms used to classify the small newborn is illustrative of the difficulty in identifying the

appropriate descriptive term for the growth-restricted fetus. The recognition and identification of the small neonate has its modern origin in 1919. Ylppo[3] suggested that all children with birth weights under 2,500 g be labeled "premature," while recognizing that many small children were the products of normal length gestations. This label persisted until 1961, when the WHO Expert Committee on Maternal and Child Health acknowledged that many babies defined as premature were not born prematurely and reclassified birth weight below 2,500 g as "low birth weight."[4] As early as 1946, McBurney[5] reported cases of "undernourished full-term infants," and this phenomenon was further highlighted in 1963 by Gruenwald,[6] who noted the important differences between the neonate with low birth weight secondary to prematurity, the infant born too soon, and the infant who was small compared with other newborns of the same gestational age. Lubchenco et al.,[7] Usher and McLean,[8] and others throughout the 1960s laid the groundwork for the classification of the growth-deficient infant through population studies that established the relationship between gestational age and weight. In 1974, at the WHO Scientific Meeting in Geneva, the concepts of "light" and "heavy" for dates emerged.[9] These concepts correlate most closely with the current classification of the growth-restricted neonate. However, the definition used to define "light for dates" (either by percentile rank or standard deviations [SD]) was not established. A commonly used subclassification has developed that reserves the obstetric label of IUGR for the fetus who suffers morbidity and/or mortality associated with the failure to reach growth potential (Fig. 25–1) and the pediatric term "small for gestational age" as the more general term for the small fetus for whom no pathology is identified. For the purposes of this chapter, we have chosen the terms "fetal" or "intrauterine growth restriction" and apply the label

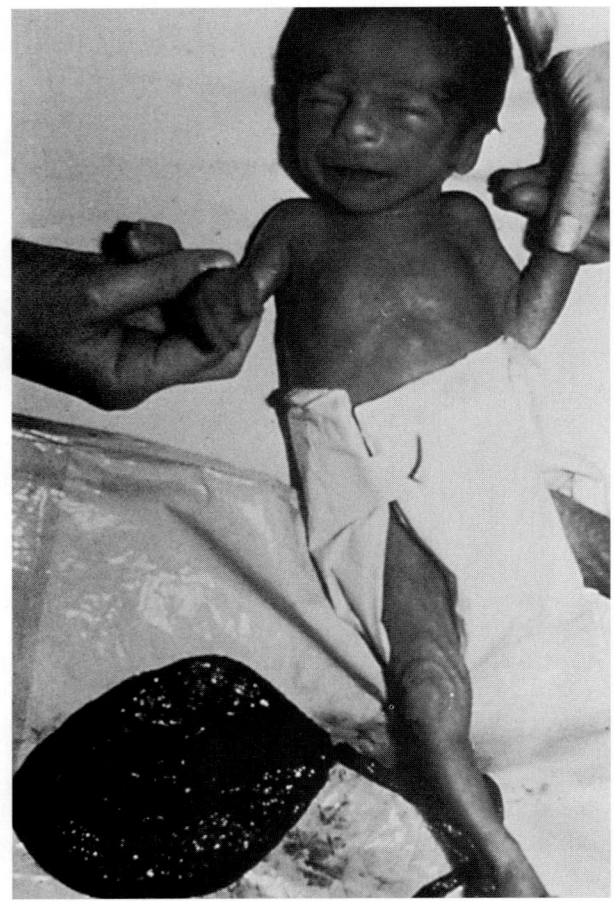

Figure 25–1. A growth-restricted infant exhibiting subcutaneous wasting.

in the prenatal period based on estimates of fetal size alone. We believe that this term appropriately characterizes the syndrome and eliminates the negative cognitive associations of the term "retardation."

DEFINITION

Neonatal growth restriction is recognized as a syndrome encompassing small size as well as specific metabolic abnormalities including hypoglycemia, hypothermia, and polycythemia. In contrast, IUGR is currently characterized as a syndrome marked by failure to reach growth potential. Additional prenatal diagnostic criteria that support the diagnosis of fetal growth restriction exist but are generally not required for the diagnosis to be applied. Small size is therefore the hallmark of the syndrome, and varying criteria have been used to identify the growth-restricted fetus.

Whereas failure to reach growth potential is the ab-

normality recognized in this disorder, individual growth capacity is not routinely established, and as a result, fetal size is most often compared with appropriate population-based "growth curves." On occasion, individual growth projections may be available, and this allows for a more direct examination of a failure to achieve growth potential.

Ultrasound criteria have emerged as the diagnostic standard used in the identification of fetal growth restriction. Wilcocks et al.[10] in 1964 first demonstrated the correlation between ultrasound measurement of the fetal head and birth weight. Campbell and Dewhurst[11] published the first sonographic descriptions of fetal growth restriction with their analysis of the changes in biparietal diameter over time. Two patterns of altered head growth were described. In "late flattening," which represents approximately two thirds of all cases of IUGR, the biparietal diameter (BPD) increases normally until late pregnancy and then lags behind. In the "low-profile" or symmetric type, impaired head growth occurs much earlier in gestation. These abnormal growth patterns were later labeled types 1 (late flattening) and 2 (low profile), and these concepts would become generalized to describe asymmetric and symmetric growth deficiencies, respectively.

As an individual parameter, abdominal circumference (AC) has demonstrated the greatest sensitivity in the identification of the small child. The use of AC, a directly measurable fetal parameter, in combination with head circumference has been widely adopted for the identification of growth restriction by many clinicians.

The most common assessment of fetal size in the United States is the estimation of fetal weight. This was first described by Campbell and Wilkin[12] using a combination of BPD and abdominal circumference. Since that report, numerous investigators have identified distinct fetal parameters identifiable by ultrasound that are useful in the estimation of fetal size.[13–15] All of the techniques incorporate an index of abdominal size as a variable contributing to the estimation of fetal weight. These techniques generally have 95 percent confidence limits that deviate approximately 15 percent around the actual value. Numerous population-specific formulas have been derived.[16]

An absolute threshold used for the definition of growth restriction can be applied to any of the parameters evaluated (BPD, AC, or estimated fetal weight [EFW]). These criteria have been statistically defined rather than outcome based and use either a threshold percentile ranking (nonnormative data) or a number of standard deviations below the mean (normative data) for the definition to be fulfilled. Birth weight below the population 10th percentile, corrected for gestational age, has been the most widely used criterion for defining growth restriction at birth, and this has been generalized to imply a sonographically estimated fetal weight below the 10th percentile for appropriate population-based cross-sectional growth charts.

Although ultrasound estimation of fetal size is independently capable of fulfilling the diagnostic criteria for growth restriction, the identification of small fetal size serves as a screen for the identification of the fetus at risk. It woud be logical, therefore, for the major aim of identifying growth restriction sonographically to be sensitivity in the identification of a group of fetuses at increased risk for perinatal morbidity and mortality. Using the birth weight 10th percentile cutoff, approximately 70 percent of the infants thus identified as growth restricted are normally or constitutionally small, so-called light for gestational age or small for gestational age (SGA).[17] These neonates are *not* at increased risk for poor outcome, but represent one end of the spectrum of normal neonatal size. This group, however, does include infants who are truly growth restricted and who are at risk for increased perinatal morbidity and mortality. Usher and McLean[8] have pointed out that, when restricting the cutoff weight for IUGR to 2 SD below the mean, only infants below the 3rd percentile are considered growth restricted. The exact thresholds are a matter of debate. Using the 3rd percentile overlooks an increased number of growth-restricted infants, whereas the 10th percentile cutoff includes normal infants who will be monitored unnecessarily. Others have suggested a cutoff of the 5th percentile based on the distribution of short-term morbidity in their population. More recently, Seeds and Peng have demonstrated increased mortality for birth weights through the 15th percentile with an odds ratio of 1.9 for mortality in newborns with birth weights between the 10th and 15th percentiles.[18]

The biologic significance of any definition of IUGR can only be measured by discovering which parameters most accurately predict infants at risk for both short- and long-term impairment. The broad prognostic significance of the 3rd, 5th, 10th, or 15th percentiles still remains to be clinically validated. It is this information that will allow us to uniformly apply appropriate population-specific growth curves. Only then will we be able to determine how effectively we have detected and treated IUGR.

ETIOLOGY

When considering the definition and detection of IUGR, it is important to review the etiologies of IUGR and possible therapies. Etiologies for fetal growth restriction can be crudely separated into fetoplacental and mater-

Fetoplacental Etiologies of Fetal Growth Retardation

Chromosomal abnormalities
  Trisomies (13, 18, 21)
  Trisomy 9 mosaicism
  Trisomy 4p
  4p–, 5p–, 11p–, 13q– syndromes
  Partial trisomy 10q
Genetic syndromes
  Cretinism (hypothyroidism)
  Russell-Silver
  Bloom's
  Lowe's
  De Lange's
  Progeria
  Leprechaunism
Congenital malformations
Infectious diseases
  Cytomegalovirus
  Toxoplasmosis
  Rubella
Placental pathology
  Previa
  Abruption
  Circumvallate
  Mosaicism
  Infarctions
  Twins

nal in origin (see the boxes "Fetoplacental Etiologies of Fetal Growth Retardation" and "Risk Factors for Fetal Growth Restriction"). The fetoplacental origins of growth restriction include those etiologies that have been traditionally ascribed to the fetus, including the chromosomal abnormalities, the genetic syndromes, and the infectious etiologies, as well as those secondary to placental abnormalities.

Fetoplacental Origins

Intrauterine infection, though long recognized as a cause of growth restriction, accounts for less than 10 percent of all cases. Herpes, cytomegalovirus, rubella, and toxoplasmosis are well documented, and other intrauterine infections are strongly suspected (see Chapter 40). The infectious process produces early disruption of fetal growth during the stage of cell hyperplasia and is, therefore, associated with a poor prognosis for normal development. For the agents associated with IUGR, prevention of the infection is the most important therapy.

> ### Risk Factors for Fetal Growth Restriction: Indications for Ultrasound
>
> History of fetal growth restriction
> Hypertension
> Diabetes mellitus
> Elevated MSAFP/hCG
> Antiphospholipid syndrome
> Chronic medical illnesses
> Low maternal prepregnancy weight (<90% IBW)
> Poor maternal weight gain
> Twin gestation
> Substance abuse (tobacco, alcohol, drugs)
> Preterm labor
> Abnormalities of placentation
> Vaginal bleeding
> Maternal anemia (Hgb < 10)
> Maternal hypoxia (cyanotic cardiac or pulmonary disease, altitude)
> Maternal hemoglobinopathies
> Drug ingestion (hydantoin, coumarin)

Chromosomal abnormalities, congenital malformations, and genetic syndromes have been associated with less than 10 percent of cases of IUGR. Abnormalities in cell replication and reduced cell number produce a pattern of impaired growth that is early in onset and symmetric. Neonatal prognosis in these cases is determined by the specific abnormality identified. Growth restriction has been observed in 53 percent of cases of trisomy 13, and 64 percent of cases of trisomy 18.[19] This growth abnormality may manifest as early as the first trimester.[20] Congenital anomalies such as renal agenesis represent a related situation.

Placental abnormalities can be a cause of fetal growth restriction. An absolute or relative decrease in placental mass affects the quantity of substrate the fetus receives and has been recognized ultrasonographically to antedate fetal growth restriction. Thus, a circumvallate placenta, partial placental abruption, placenta accreta, placental infarction, or hemangioma may result in growth restriction. An elevated maternal serum α-fetoprotein (MSAFP) or human chorionic gonadotropin (hCG) level in the second trimester has been associated with an increased risk for IUGR and may result from abnormal placentation.[21–24] Davis has suggested that elevated MSAFP precedes an increased risk of preterm birth, but not growth restriction.[25] However, the strong association of preterm birth with fetal growth restric-

tion discussed in detail later in this chapter suggests that when live birth criteria are used to evaluate newborn size, a stability in birth weight percentile in preterm neonates reflects an increased frequency of fetal growth restriction. Intrinsic placental pathology has been identified in some cases of growth restriction, including the presence of a single umbilical artery or the presence of placental mosaicism, either of which may act to impair normal fetoplacental exchange mechanisms.[26] Placental location has also been linked to growth restriction. Placenta previa without bleeding has been suggested as a risk factor, because the low implantation site may not be optimal for nutrient transfer.[27]

Twin gestation is often associated with IUGR (see Chapter 24). In 1966, Gruenwald[28] observed that the growth curve of twins deviated from that of singletons with a progressive fall of growth after 32 weeks. This finding implies relative placental insufficiency as opposed to intrinsic fetal compromise and suggests that the longer the twin pregnancy continues, the greater the delay in intrauterine growth, with "catch-up" growth observed after birth. Thus, twins represent a group of fetuses at high risk for IUGR, as confirmed by an incidence of 17.5 percent in one study.[29] The appropriate growth standard to apply to twin fetuses would appear to be the same as that for singletons. Two trials demonstrate that the morbidity and mortality of fetuses from twin gestations are equivalent, or elevated when the twins are monochorionic, when compared with birth weight and gestational age-matched singletons.[30,31]

Maternal Origins

Decreased uteroplacental blood flow with its associated reduction in transfer of nutrients to the fetus is responsible for the majority of clinically recognized cases of IUGR. Maternal vascular disease, whether chronic hypertension, preeclampsia, or diabetes with vasculopathy, has been associated with impaired fetal growth. In preeclampsia, failure of trophoblastic influenced modification of maternal spiral arterioles by 20 to 22 weeks' gestation and intimal thickening accompanied by fibrinoid degeneration of the media of these arterioles result in luminal narrowing and, therefore, decreased blood flow through the placental bed.[32] Such cases are generally marked by asymmetric IUGR with maintenance of normal fetal head growth and reduction in the size of the fetal liver, heart, thymus, spleen, pancreas, and adrenal glands. Ward et al.[33] have demonstrated that mutations in the angiotensinogen gene contribute to the development of both preeclampsia and the associated incidence of fetal growth restriction. Thus, a portion of this compromised maternal vascular expansion may be explained by specific genetic deficiencies. Decreased placental blood flow from postural maternal hypotension and maternal hyperviscosity with sludging has also been reported to cause IUGR. Some patients with, or at risk for, pregnancy-associated hypertension have either a reduction in the expansion of blood volume in pregnancy, or have a baseline reduction in circulating volume.[34-36] This contracted circulating blood volume has been correlated with IUGR.[37] A reduction in circulating volume or maternal oxygenation in women living at high altitude or those with cyanotic heart disease or parenchymal lung disease may be responsible for the IUGR observed with these conditions. Those hemoglobinopathies and anemias that impair maternal and fetal oxygenation have also been linked to limited fetal growth.

Poor maternal weight gain has long been recognized as a risk factor for growth restriction. Controversy still exists about the contribution maternal malnutrition can make to IUGR. Studies of the offspring of women pregnant during the siege of Leningrad in 1942 and the Dutch famine in 1945 indicate little effect on fetal growth by such dietary restriction.[38] In Holland, despite a maternal intake of 600 to 900 calories daily for 6 months, the average birth weight fell only 240 g in women with good prepregnancy nutritional status. However, investigation of Guatemalan Indian tribes has indicated that protein malnutrition before 26 weeks can result in symmetric growth restriction.[39] Protein restriction after 26 weeks did not limit fetal growth. The degree of malnourishment observed in Guatemala or during the Dutch famine would not ordinarily be found in the United States. Nevertheless, maternal prepregnancy weight and weight gain in pregnancy are two of the most important variables contributing to birth weight.

Pregnant women may be subject to poor nutrition through limited gastrointestinal absorption imposed by Crohn's disease or ulcerative colitis. These conditions have not been generally associated with increased numbers of growth-restricted infants. Massively obese women who have undergone iliojejunal bypass are reported to have smaller infants than average, but they usually fall above the 10th percentile in birth weight.

Glucose is a critical fetal nutrient, and if its supply is reduced growth restriction may result. Using cord blood sampling, Economides and Nicolaides[40] observed significantly lower maternal and fetal glucose levels in cases of growth restriction and speculated that the major cause of fetal hypoglycemia in these cases was reduced glucose supply from the mother caused by impaired placental perfusion. Khouzami et al.[41] documented a significant association between maternal hypoglycemia on a 3-hour oral glucose tolerance test (GTT) and subsequent birth of non–low-birth-weight but growth-restricted babies. Sokol et al.[42] and Langer et al.[43] have confirmed that a flat maternal response to glucose loading is associated with an increased risk for fetal growth restriction. Langer et al.[43] demonstrated

that a "flat" GTT was associated with a 20-fold increase in IUGR in normotensive patients. This relationship is further strengthened by the data of Caruso et al., who have demonstrated heightened maternal insulin sensitivity in association with otherwise unexplained fetal growth restriction.[44]

Maternal drug ingestion may result in IUGR by a direct effect on fetal growth as well as through inadequate dietary intake. Smoking produces a symmetrically smaller fetus through reduced uterine blood flow and impaired fetal oxygenation and is a major cause of growth restriction in developed countries. The consumption of alcohol and the use of coumarin or hydantoin derivatives are now well known to produce particular dysmorphic features in association with impaired fetal growth. Mills et al.[45] have demonstrated a significant increase in the risk of IUGR with the consumption of one to two drinks daily, in the absence of fetal alcohol syndrome. Maternal use of cocaine has been associated with not only IUGR but also reduced head circumference growth.[46]

In 1971, Lobi et al.[47] reported that advanced maternal age was a factor in the etiology of IUGR. Berkowitz et al.[48] found no evidence that the first births of women between 30 and 34 years or those over 35 years were at increased risk for growth restriction. In summary, if one controls for underlying medical complications, maternal age is not related to restricted fetal growth.

A history of poor pregnancy outcome is clearly correlated with the subsequent delivery of a growth-restricted infant. Galbraith et al.[49] and Tejani[50] have shown that prior birth of an IUGR infant is the obstetric factor most often associated with the subsequent birth of a growth-restricted infant. These study populations did include women with underlying medical problems. Tejani and Mann[51] in a retrospective study of 83 multigravidas who had delivered IUGR infants noted that the perinatal wastage from their 200 prior pregnancies was 41 percent. This striking figure, which includes spontaneous abortions as well as neonatal and intrauterine deaths, points to the significance of poor obstetric history as a risk factor for IUGR. Women whose first pregnancy results in a growth-restricted infant have a one in four risk of delivering a second infant below the 10th percentile. After two pregnancies complicated by IUGR, there is a fourfold increase in the risk of a subsequent growth-restricted infant.[52] When all indices of risk have been applied, the one third of the population considered at highest risk accounts for two thirds of the infants identified as growth restricted. Two thirds of pregnancies, although not judged to be "at risk" for IUGR, yield one third of neonates below the 10th percentile.[49] Most of these babies are constitutionally small.

In summary, a framework does exist for considering

the causes of growth restriction. Is the fetus abnormal? Is the delivery system disrupted? Is the maternal supply line compromised? These questions categorize the source of the problem without explaining the mechanism by which the growth process is disturbed. Even when one is aware of these clinical associations, the sum of the many factors affecting the growth of an individual fetus is unpredictable.

DIAGNOSIS

Significant improvements have been made in detecting and characterizing the growth-restricted fetus. These improvements have served as the basis for plans designed to reduce the associated perinatal morbidity and mortality. In the past, clinical parameters such as maternal weight gain and measurement of fundal height were used to reflect fetal growth. Belizan et al.[53] observed that curvilinear fundal height measurements in centimeters from the symphysis pubis could be closely correlated with gestational age: a lag of 4 cm or more suggests growth restriction. Persson et al.[54] reported a sensitivity of only 27 percent and a positive predictive value of 18 percent using carefully performed fundal height measurements to detect IUGR. Additional studies have confirmed the lack of sensitivity of fundal height measurements for detecting fetal growth restriction. The presence of risk factors should therefore prompt ultrasound estimation of fetal size independent of maternal weight gain or fundal height growth.

Fetal Measurements

The use of fetal weight has been the most common method for characterizing fetal size and thereby growth abnormalities. This requires that an accurate sonographic estimate of fetal weight can be performed to detect and follow patients suspected of having a growth-restricted infant.[55] Using a multifactorial equation and a measurement of abdominal size, a weight can be predicted and related to BPD. Formulas that incorporate the femur length (FL) may increase the accuracy of in utero weight estimation for the fetus with IUGR.

A significant limitation of using estimated fetal weight to measure fetal size is that it cannot be measured directly, but must be calculated from a combination of directly measured parameters. This results in an increased error in the estimate. In addition, the lack of directly measured normative data creates difficulty in establishing normal growth curves. Commonly, cross-sectional birth weight data have been used to characterize ultrasound-estimated fetal weight. These live birth-weight criteria, however, do not appropriately describe

sonographic estimated fetal weights, as there is a significant association of preterm birth with fetal growth restriction.[56] Thus, the weights of preterm infants are not normally distributed as they are at term. This association has been highlighted by several investigators who have identified the discrepancy between birth-weight–defined growth curves and sonographically estimated fetal weight–defined growth curves in preterm gestation.[57–59] Ultrasound-generated estimated fetal weight growth curves consistently demonstrate higher fetal weights over the range of preterm gestation than do birth-weight–generated growth curves. This discrepancy results from the fact that ultrasound examinations represent a larger breadth of the entire population at any gestational age. Preterm birth weight reflects only those individuals who have delivered under abnormal circumstances. It is therefore most appropriate to compare estimated fetal weights by ultrasound with ultrasound-derived growth curves in order to characterize preterm estimated fetal weight appropriately. The utility of this approach has been confirmed in preterm gestation by Lackman et al., who demonstrated that the use of fetal growth curves, rather than live birth curves, was associated with an improved ability to identify perinatal mortality risk.[60]

The use of the individualized growth model has been supported by several investigators.[61,62] The obvious advantage is the lack of dependency on population-based normative data and the ability to detect a true personal growth restriction. This can be done even when the estimated fetal weight is greater than the 10th percentile for the population. The disadvantages of these models are that they require baseline ultrasound morphometric data in the second trimester as well as an additional later scan to establish growth potential for an individual morphometric parameter. A third scan is then necessary to identify that a growth abnormality exists. This volume of information is frequently not available, limiting the practical application of this type of individual growth model. An alternative approach using individualized growth modeling is to account for the variables that contribute the majority of the variance to newborn size. These include early pregnancy weight, maternal height, ethnic group, parity, and sex.[63] Using these variables and fetal growth patterns, the estimated size of a fetus of a given mother can be projected at term and estimated at any specific point in gestation. Deviations from this projected growth pattern can then be recognized. Overall, the diagnostic advantages of these individualized growth models has been questioned when compared with the sequential comparison of the percentile ranking of individual or composite growth parameters to population-based growth curves.[64]

Fetal growth as opposed to fetal size is a dynamic process and requires more than a single evaluation for its estimation. The absence of fetal growth over a sus-

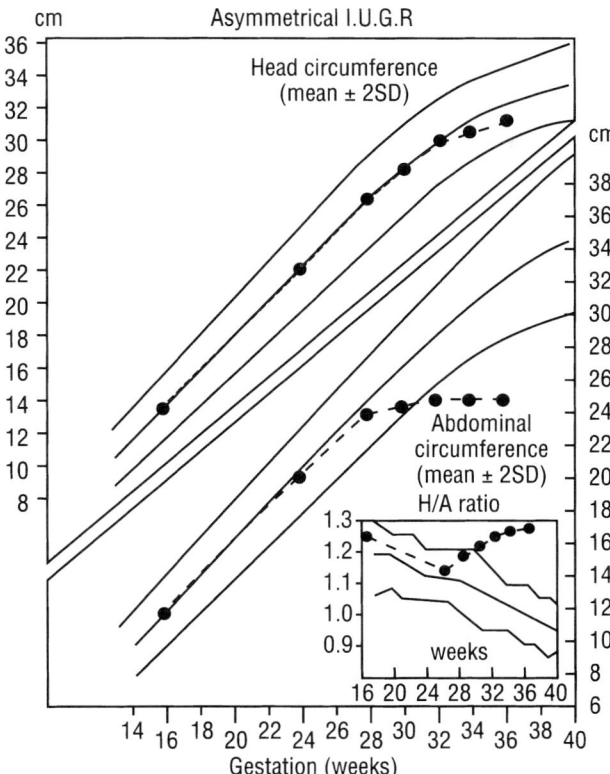

Figure 25–2. Growth chart in a case of asymmetric IUGR. Although head circumference is preserved, AC growth falls off early in the third trimester. For this reason, the H/A ratio shown in the lower right corner of the graph becomes elevated. IUGR, intrauterine growth restriction. (From Chudleigh P, Pearce JM: Obstetric Ultrasound. Edinburgh, Churchill Livingstone, 1986, with permission.)

tained period is a concern. The routine clinical evaluation of fetal growth is based on fundal height enlargement during the course of pregnancy. In pregnancies at risk or in those in whom fetal size is already estimated to be below the 10th percentile, serial ultrasound estimations of fetal size are performed. The appropriate observation interval for the evaluation of fetal growth has been based on two assumptions: (1) growth is continuous rather than sporadic and (2) the identification of growth is limited by the technical capability of the ultrasound equipment used to measure the fetus.[3] The recommended interval between evaluations is 3 weeks, as shorter intervals increase the likelihood of a false-positive diagnosis.[65,66] Recent data have demonstrated that early childhood growth, up to 21 months of age, is characterized by sporadic growth pulses that punctuate prolonged periods of growth stasis.[67] Whereas the fetal growth rate of the third trimester is greater than the early childhood growth rate, it may be that fetal growth is also saltatory and that the detection of growth is limited by the physiologic interval of growth pulses rather than by the technical limitations of the measuring tool.[68]

In an attempt to increase detection of the fetus with asymmetric growth restriction, head circumference

(HC)/AC ratios can be assessed (Figs. 25–2 and 25–3).[69,70] In the normally growing fetus, the HC/AC ratio exceeds 1.0 before 32 weeks' gestation, is approximately 1.0 at 32 to 34 weeks' gestation, and falls below 1.0 after 34 weeks' gestation. In fetuses affected by asymmetric growth restriction, the HC remains larger than that of the body (Fig. 25–2). The HC/AC ratio is then elevated. In symmetric IUGR, both the HC and the AC are reduced, and the HC/AC ratio remains normal (Fig. 25–3). Using the HC/AC ratio, 85 percent of growth-restricted fetuses are detected, with a reduction in false-negative diagnoses. Thus, a single set of measurements, even when determined in the latter part of pregnancy, can be very helpful in evaluating the status of intrauterine growth.

In some cases, measurement of the HC may be difficult as a result of fetal position. One can then compare the FL, which is relatively spared in asymmetric IUGR, to the AC.[71] The FL/AC is 22 at all gestational ages from 21 weeks to term and so can be applied without knowledge of the number of weeks gestation. An FL/AC ratio greater than 23.5 suggests IUGR.

In summary, the ability to determine appropriate fetal growth using fundal height measurements in a nor-

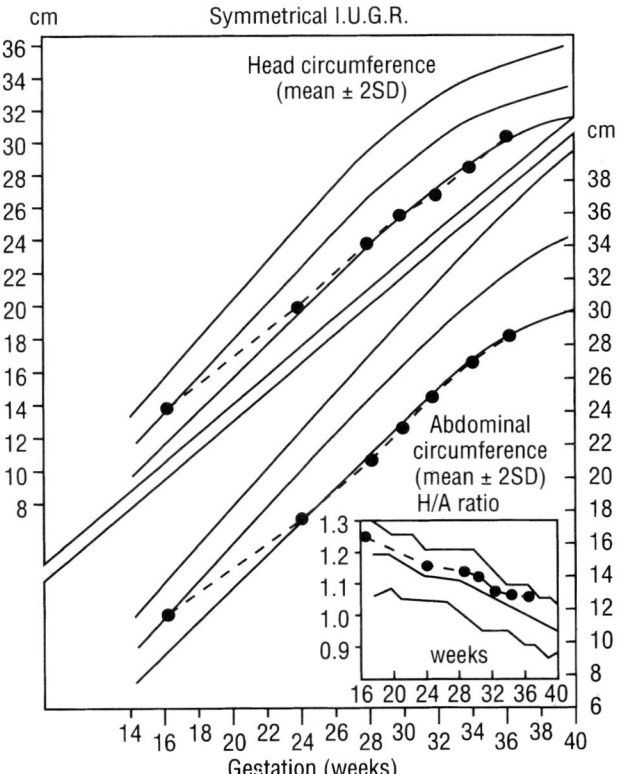

Figure 25–3. Growth chart in a case of symmetric IUGR. Note the early onset of both HC and AC growth restriction. For this reason, the H/A ratio shown in the lower right corner remains normal. IUGR, intrauterine growth restriction. (From Chudleigh P, Pearce JM: Obstetric Ultrasound. Edinburgh, Churchill Livingstone, 1986, with permission.)

mal population is limited. Fundal height measurements lack both sensitivity and specificity in the identification of the small fetus. It is therefore reasonable to use a better tool (ultrasound) whenever clinical circumstances point to an increased risk for a growth-restricted fetus. A number of clinical conditions that increase the risk for a small child were listed earlier. In the absence of routine clinical indications, ultrasound screening of these high-risk pregnancies should be performed at 16 to 18 weeks for dating (if not otherwise established) and again at 32 to 34 weeks.

Oligohydramnios

Decreased amniotic fluid volume has been associated clinically with IUGR and may be the earliest sign detected on ultrasonography, preceding an elevation in HC/AC ratio and lagging fetal growth (Fig. 25–4). Decreased perfusion of the fetal kidneys and reduced urine production explain this observation.[72] In an early study, Manning et al.[73] reported that a vertical pocket of amniotic fluid measuring 1 cm or more reflected an adequate fluid volume. Of fetuses with fluid pockets less than 1 cm, 96 percent were actually growth restricted. Only 5 of 91 cases with an adequate amount of amniotic fluid exhibited IUGR. The patient with an uncertain gestational age who presents late in pregnancy poses a difficult diagnostic dilemma because interpretation of BPD and HC/AC ratios must be related to accurate gestational age. Under these conditions, measuring an amniotic fluid pocket, or an FL/AC ratio, may be helpful, as these do not rely on knowledge of the gestational age. Manning and his colleagues[74] later broadened their criteria. A 2-cm vertical pocket was considered normal, 1 to 2 cm marginal, and less than 1 cm decreased. Using this definition, they observed a 6 percent incidence of IUGR with a pocket 2 cm or larger, 20 percent with a pocket 1 to 2 cm, and 39 percent with a pocket less than 1 cm. One may also use the amniotic fluid index to quantitate amniotic fluid volume (see Chapter 10), although this technique requires a knowledge of gestational age. The overall clinical impression of reduced amniotic fluid on ultrasonography may be most important. The volume of amniotic fluid also has prognostic significance for the course of labor. Groome et al.[75] demonstrated that oligohydramnios associated with fetal oliguria is associated with a higher rate of intrapartum complications that may be attributed to reduced placental reserve.

Maternal Doppler Velocimetry

Doppler velocimetry of the maternal uterine artery has been examined to establish its usefulness in the prediction of pregnancies destined to produce a growth-restricted newborn. Schulman[76] found that women with hypertensive disorders who had an elevated uterine artery systolic/diastolic (S/D) ratio (>2.6) and/or diastolic notching were more likely to have pregnancies complicated by IUGR and intrauterine fetal death. He noted that the changes in uterine artery flow patterns might precede those observed in the umbilical artery and antedate fetal growth restriction. Jacobson et al.[77] observed that an elevated uteroplacental artery resistance index (RI) predicted fetal growth restriction with a sensitivity of 70.6 percent and had a positive predictive value of 33.3 percent in women at high risk for either preeclampsia or growth restriction. In low-risk patients, the examination of second-trimester maternal uterine artery waveforms has produced sensitivities and positive predictive values for fetal growth restriction as high as 72 percent and 35 percent, respectively; values slightly better than routine clinical indicators of fetal growth.[78–82] Valensise and Romanini[83] have demonstrated that the combination of abnormal second-trimester maternal uterine artery Doppler velocimetry and maternal glucose tolerance testing demonstrating a "flat" response results in a positive predictive value of 94 percent and a sensitivity of 54 percent for the detection of fetal growth restriction.

In summary, the overall value of second-trimester maternal uterine artery Doppler waveforms in screening of pregnancies at risk for growth restriction is unclear. At present, there are no data suggesting that sensitivity is improved beyond that achieved with standard clinical assessment. The availability of second-trimester stratification of risk for fetal growth restriction has not yet demonstrated an impact on perinatal morbidity or mortality.

Fetal Body Composition

The ponderal index was first described by Rohrer[84] in 1921 as an index of corpulence. This index of neonatal size (weight/length[3]) that is normally distributed accurately described the nutritional state of the neonate. When compared with birth weight percentile, the ponderal index demonstrates an improved ability to predict neonatal asphyxia, acidosis, hypoglycemia, and hypothermia.[85] The ponderal index also correlates with direct measures of neonatal fat as estimated by skinfold thickness.[86] Attempts to translate the ponderal index directly to the fetus have been hampered by the difficulty in accurately assessing fetal length. Attempts to modify the ponderal index for fetal sonographic estimation have been made. Yagel et al.[87] demonstrated that the addition of a fetal ponderal index improved the prediction of perinatal morbidity in fetuses already suspected of having IUGR. Alternative methods for the characterization of fetal growth by physiologic compartments have recently been attempted. Several studies have examined fetal subcutaneous fat content using

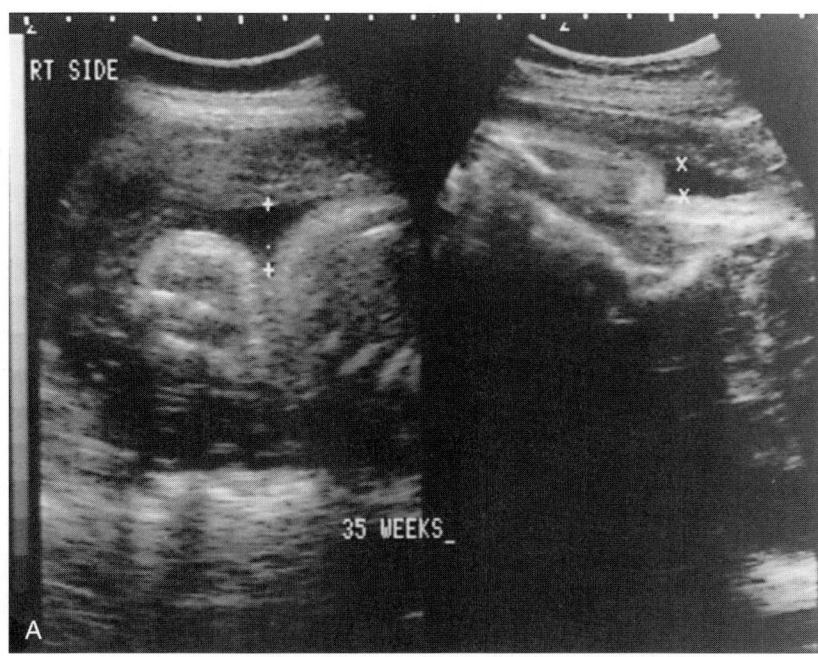

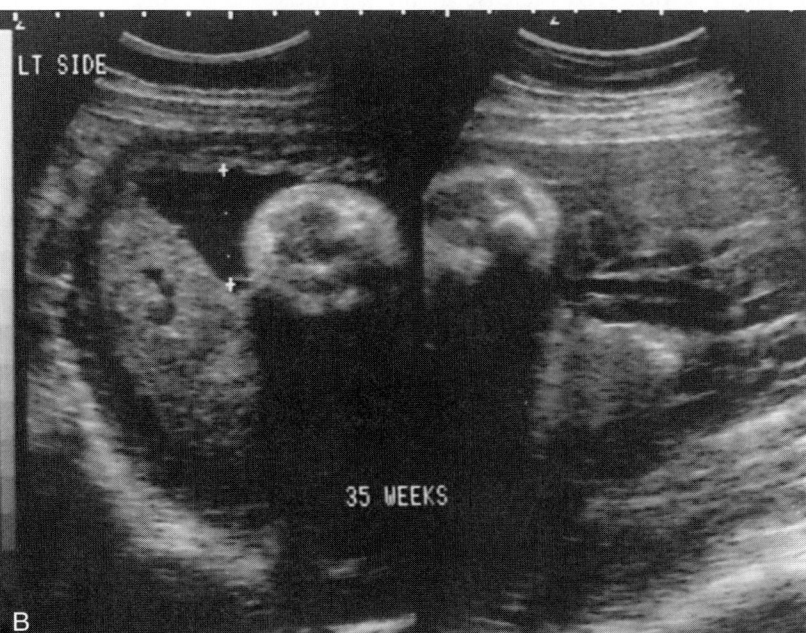

Figure 25–4. *A* and *B,* Amniotic fluid index (AFI) performed at 35 weeks on a patient whose fundal height measured 30 cm. Findings consistent with asymmetric growth restriction were observed, including estimated fetal weight of 1,500 g, HC/AC ratio of 1.15, and AFI of 5.0 cm, as illustrated. At 35 weeks, the 50th percentile for the AFI is 14.0 cm; the 5th percentile is 7.9 cm. Note that one amniotic fluid pocket greater than 2.0 cm was found.

ultrasound examination. Subcutaneous fat deposition has been examined in the face, abdomen, arm, and thigh.[88–92] Reduction in facial fat stores has been strongly associated with being SGA. This reduction in fat content is consistent with observations made in the growth-restricted neonate and may prove to be a sensitive indicator of the small fetus at increased risk for perinatal complications. The optimal method of in utero assessment for fetal fat has not yet been determined.

Biochemical Markers

Biochemical markers have been used to assist in the identification of the small fetus who is at increased risk for the morbidity and mortality associated with fetal growth restriction. The most widely examined include fetal erythropoietin and amino acid concentrations.

Erythropoietin production in the fetus, as in the adult, is stimulated by the presence of anemia or hypoxia.[93,94] Numerous studies have demonstrated the ability of the fetus to respond to hypoxic conditions with the production of erythropoietin. This increase in erythropoietin may or may not lead to increased red cell production, depending on erythropoietic reserve.[93,95] Erythropoietin, identified in the cord blood of growth-restricted fetuses by cordocentesis, amniotic fluid, or cord blood at delivery, may prove to be of benefit in the identification of the child at risk for long-term morbidity.[95-98] Ruth et al.[99] identified an association between cord blood erythropoietin levels and developmental outcome (including cerebral palsy and death) at 2 years in nonpreeclamptic patients with evidence of acute asphyxia at birth. Neonates from pregnancies complicated by preeclampsia had elevated cord erythropoietin levels regardless of outcome.[99]

Altered amino acid concentrations, particularly the relationship between the branched chain amino acids such as valine and the gluconeogenic amino acids like glycine, have been identified in the growth-restricted fetus and newborn. These changes reflect a specific fetal response that is independent of maternal amino acid levels. The observed increase in the glycine/valine ratio appears to result from a reduction in phosphoenolpyruvate carboxykinase activity, a rate-limiting enzyme for gluconeogenesis.[100] Studies have demonstrated that cord blood samples from growth-restricted neonates demonstrate an increased glycine/valine ratio within the first few hours of life.[101] This profile of amino acids parallels the aminogram observed in children who suffer from protein calorie malnutrition.[102] In the growth-restricted neonate, the glycine/valine ratio of umbilical cord blood has been correlated with specific neonatal risk, including hypoglycemia and death.[103] Amino acid data from umbilical venous plasma obtained by percutaneous umbilical blood sampling and amniotic fluid confirms that the elevation in glycine/valine ratio precedes parturition in the growth-restricted fetus.[104-107] Fetal cord blood glycine/valine ratios have been shown to be inversely proportional to fetal arterial oxygen content.[105] No relationship with short-term or long-term morbidity has been established. Elevated amniotic fluid glycine/valine ratios in growth-restricted fetuses have not been found to predict neonatal hypoglycemia or cord blood gas abnormalities.[108]

MANAGEMENT

In developing a plan for the management of suspected growth restriction, it is important to remember the major etiologic groups. Most infants thought to be growth restricted are constitutionally small and require no intervention. Approximately 15 percent exhibit symmetric growth restriction attributable to an early fetal insult

for which there is no effective therapy. Here, an accurate diagnosis is essential. Finally, approximately 15 percent have growth restriction or extrinsic growth failure because of placental disease or reduced uteroplacental blood flow. In such cases, antepartum fetal monitoring and carefully timed delivery may be critical.

Once growth restriction is suspected, a well-organized approach to management should be undertaken. The clinician should evaluate and treat problems that may be contributing to growth restriction. Therapy of growth restriction is often nonspecific but should be directed at the underlying cause of poor fetal growth if one can be determined. When a maternal medical problem such as inflammatory bowel disease is contributing to poor growth, specific therapy should be instituted. Alleviation of hypoxia, therapy of high blood pressure and anemia, and hyperalimentation are three examples.

When placental infarction was implicated as the underlying etiology, Moe[109] reported subcutaneous heparin therapy to have a favorable influence on pregnancy outcome. Certainly, mothers should be counseled to stop smoking and ingesting alcohol. Nonspecific therapies include bed rest in the left lateral decubitus position to increase placental blood flow. Although an inadequate diet has not been clearly established as a cause of growth restriction in this country, dietary supplementation may be helpful in those with poor weight gain or low prepregnancy weight.

Antepartum Evaluation

Fetal Growth

Serial evaluations of fetal growth should be instituted as soon as the diagnosis of growth restriction is confirmed or for patients in whom the suspicion for growth restriction is high. Ultrasound examinations should be scheduled every 3 to 4 weeks and should include determinations of the BPD, HC/AC, fetal weight, and amniotic fluid volume (Table 25-1). Arrested head growth is of great concern, especially in light of the most recent data available on ultimate developmental potential for the growth-restricted infant. Clear documentation of arrested head growth over a 4-week period is alarming, and the feasibility and safety of delivery should be reviewed.[110]

Ultrasound should be used not only to document abnormal growth but also to detect lethal congenital malformations such as renal agenesis (see Chapter 10). In cases of severe symmetric growth restriction, amniocentesis, placental biopsy, or cordocentesis should be considered to rule out a chromosomal abnormality such as trisomy 13, 18, or 21 (Table 25-2).[19] Trisomy 18 may present with the unusual combination of growth restriction and polyhydramnios. If the diagnosis of a lethal anomaly can be made with certainty, an unneces-

Table 25-1. UTILIZATION OF ULTRASONOGRAPHY IN THE DIAGNOSIS AND EVALUATION OF IUGR

Parameter	Results	Diagnosis	Plan
BPD	Appropriate for dates (within 2 weeks of dates)	No IUGR	Repeat only if indicated by clinical parameters (e.g., lagging fundal growth)
EFW	Above 10th percentile		
HC/AC ratio	In normal range		
Amniotic fluid volume	Normal		
BPD	Appropriate for dates (within 2 weeks of dates)	Probable asymmetric IUGR	Repeat ultrasound examination every 3 weeks if not delivered
EFW	Below 10th percentile		Start antepartum surveillance and continue until delivery
HC/AC ratio	Above 95th percentile		
Amniotic fluid volume	Low		
BPD	2 weeks or more; smaller than expected for menstrual dates	Probable symmetric IUGR	Repeat ultrasound examination every 3 weeks if not delivered
EFW	Below 10th percentile		Start antepartum surveillance and continue until delivery
HC/AC ratio	In normal range		If IUGR present before 20 weeks, scan for anomalies and
Amniotic fluid volume	Normal or low		consider fetal karyotype

Modified from Grannum PAT: Ultrasonic measurements for diagnosis. *In* Gross TM, Sokol RJ (eds): Intrauterine Growth Retardation. Chicago, Year Book Medical Publishers, 1989, p 123.

sary cesarean delivery for fetal distress may be prevented.

Fetal Well-Being

Fetal well-being should also be assessed regularly once the diagnosis of growth restriction is entertained. These infants have an increased incidence of intrauterine demise, presumably from cord compression as well as placental insufficiency. Monitoring these infants decreases the stillbirth rate by detecting the compromised fetus and allowing timely intervention. Experience with the nonstress test (NST) in cases of growth restriction has confirmed that a reactive NST correlates highly with a fetus that is not in immediate danger of intrauterine demise. Twice-weekly nonstress testing is an appropriate interval.[111] Visser and associates[112] performed antepartum fetal heart rate monitoring immediately before cordocentesis in 58 growth-restricted and 29 appropriately grown fetuses. In the appropriately grown fetuses, blood PO_2 and pH values were within the normal range for gestation in 27 cases, demonstrating a reactive heart rate pattern and in 2 in which the tracing was nonreactive. In contrast, abnormal antepartum heart rate patterns were found in 15 of the 19 growth-restricted fetuses with hypoxemia, acidemia, or both. The best heart rate marker for fetal hypoxemia was a pattern characterized by repetitive decelerations. In that group, only two fetuses demonstrated normal PO_2 and pH values. In none of the cases with a reactive heart rate pattern was the growth-restricted fetus acidemic. However, many growth-restricted fetuses with a normal heart rate pattern were found to have fetal PO_2 values in the lower range of normal. Overall, antepartum fetal heart rate patterns in both normal and growth-restricted fetuses were found to correlate well with fetal oxygenation. The appearance of spontaneous decelerations during the NST may reflect oligohydramnios and cord compression and has been associated with a high perinatal mortality rate.[113] The addition of a measure of amniotic fluid volume to the NST has been called a "modified biophysical profile." When compared with a weekly contraction stress test, the twice-weekly modified biophysical profile results in similar perinatal outcome.[114] An assessment of amniotic fluid volume at least weekly is advised in cases of suspected IUGR.

Table 25-2. CHROMOSOMAL ABNORMALITIES AND IUGR

IUGR	Anomaly	Hydramnios	Abnormal Karyotype
Ultrasound Findings Present			
X			12/180 (7%)
X	X		18/57 (32%)
X		X	6/22 (27%)
X	X	X	7/15 (47%)

From Eydoux P, Choiset A, LePorrier N, et al: Chromosomal prenatal diagnosis: study of 936 cases of intrauterine abnormalities after ultrasound assessment. Prenat Diagn 9:255, 1989, with permission.

Nonreactive NST results are often falsely positive and should be further evaluated before any management decision is made. Contraction stress testing (CST) is one option for additional testing. A negative CST result, even when the CST is performed early in the third trimester, is an indication of adequate placental respiratory reserve.[115] Conversely, positive CST results occur in 30 percent of the pregnancies complicated by proven growth restriction. In a study by Lin et al.,[116] 30 percent of growth-restricted infants had nonreactive NST results and 40 percent had positive CST results. Ninety-two percent of IUGR infants with a nonreactive positive pattern exhibited perinatal morbidity. However, a 25 to 50 percent false-positive rate has been associated with the CST by some investigators.[115] Therefore, information from antepartum fetal heart rate testing must always be reviewed in concert with the gestational age of the fetus, as well as other indices of fetal well-being and fetal growth.

The fetal biophysical profile score developed by Manning et al.[117] can provide appropriate follow-up to nonreassuring fetal heart rate testing or can be used as an alternative method for primary antenatal surveillance. Several studies have demonstrated good correlation between these test results and the level of fetal acidemia as determined by percutaneous umbilical blood sampling in the growth-restricted fetus without anomalies.[118,119] Vintzileos et al.[120] have demonstrated that the components of the biophysical score are affected at different levels of hypoxemia and acidemia, the earliest manifestations of abnormal fetal biophysical activity being the loss of reactivity in the NST along with the absence of fetal breathing. This is followed by decreased fetal tone and movement in association with more advanced acidemia, hypoxemia, and hypercapnia. As a backup test for nonreassuring fetal heart rate testing the biophysical profile leads to lower rates of intervention when compared with the CST, with no impact on perinatal outcome.[121]

Maternal monitoring of fetal activity has been used extensively in Great Britain, Scandinavia, and Israel for the assessment of pregnancies complicated by IUGR. In a study of 50 cases, Matthews[122] clearly showed the predictive value of fetal activity charting for growth-restricted fetuses subsequently demonstrating distress in labor. The techniques available for monitoring fetal movement are reviewed in Chapter 12.

Doppler flow studies of the fetal circulation have been used to identify and manage the fetus with suspected growth restriction. These studies have also contributed to our understanding of the pathophysiology of IUGR. Doppler studies of fetal internal carotid and intracerebral arterial blood flow have shown a decrease in pulsatility index in these vessels in fetuses with IUGR.[123,124] The mechanism would be consistent with an increase in blood flow that results from vasodilation in response to hypoxia. Renal and aortic blood flow velocity waveforms show evidence of increased pulsatility indices, consistent with increases in resistance.[125,126] These findings and others have confirmed some of the basic fetal responses to growth restriction, including the preservation of brain growth and oligohydramnios observed in asymmetric IUGR.

The major focus of Doppler studies for the assessment of fetal health has been the umbilical circulation. The association between an increase in Doppler blood flow indices in the umbilical artery and increased resistance in the placental circulation has been demonstrated by many investigators. Trudinger embolized the umbilical arterial circulation in fetal lambs and found an increase in the umbilical arterial S/D velocity ratio along with an increase in arterial resistance.[127] In a similar model, Morrow and Ritchie demonstrated progression from normal to increased S/D ratios and the eventual development of reversed end-diastolic velocities, even in the absence of hypoxia.[128] Studies by Giles et al.[129] demonstrated that the small arterial vessel count in the tertiary stem villi of the placenta is significantly lower in patients with high umbilical artery S/D ratios than in those with normal S/D ratios. Rochelson et al.[130] also confirmed a significant reduction in the small muscular artery count and the small muscular artery/villus ratio in the placentas of trisomic fetuses. This study suggests that growth restriction in the fetus with a chromosomal abnormality may be attributable not only to poor intrinsic growth potential but also to abnormalities in placental morphology and fetoplacental blood flow. Based on these observations, it is suggested that the increased resistance to flow indicated by a high S/D ratio is associated with a failure to develop, or an obliteration, of the small muscular arteries in the tertiary stem villi.

Randomized prospective trials have been performed to examine the impact of Doppler velocimetry on perinatal outcome. Divon and Ferber summarized three meta-analyses on the association of the use of umbilical artery Doppler studies and perinatal outcome.[131] In these studies, the use of umbilical artery Doppler was associated with a decrease in perinatal mortality, antenatal admissions, inductions of labor, and cesarean deliveries for fetal distress in labor in women considered at high risk.[132–134] No improvement in outcome was demonstrated with the use of Doppler in screening normal pregnancies.[135]

Absent or reversed end-diastolic velocity in the umbilical artery has repeatedly been associated with poor perinatal outcome (Fig. 25–5). Farine summarized 31 reports of 904 fetuses with absent or reversed end-diastolic flow velocities in the umbilical artery.[136] Eighty percent of the fetuses were growth-restricted. The perinatal mortality was 36 percent. The time between the discovery of the absence of end-diastolic

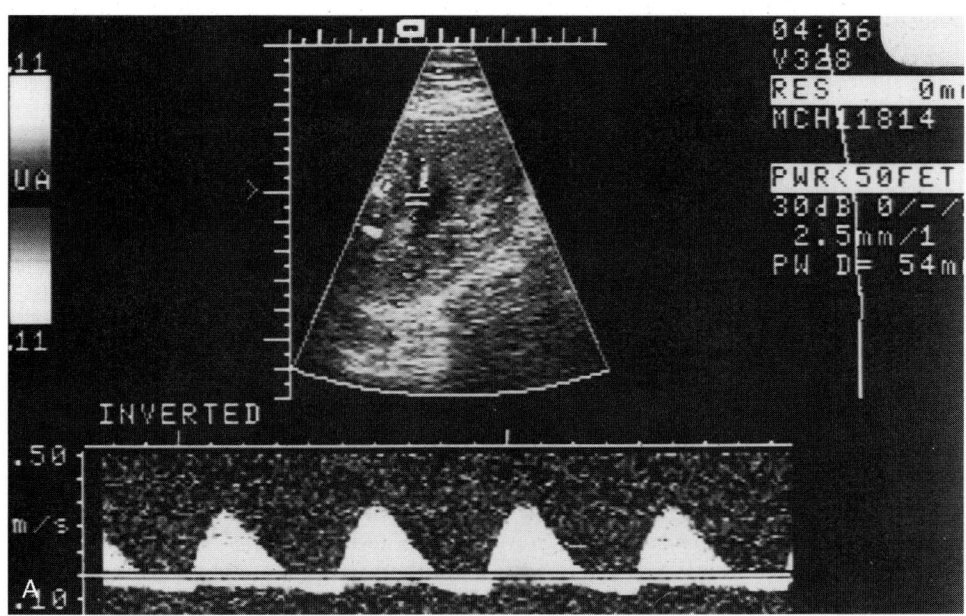

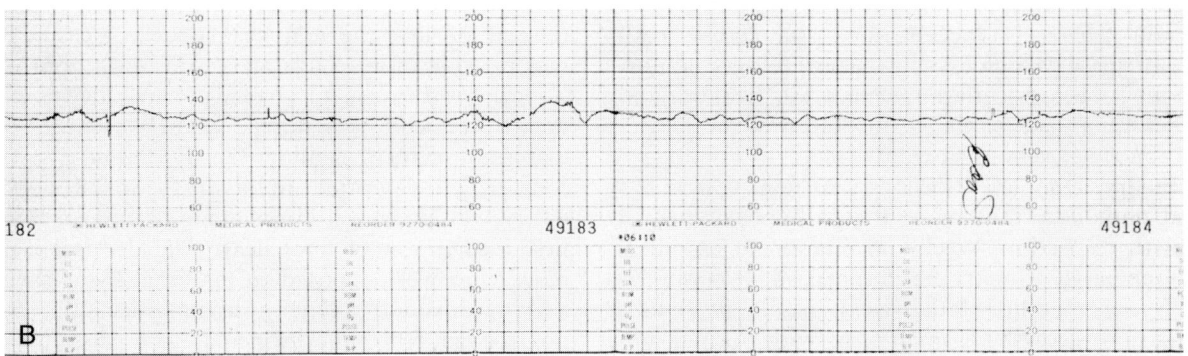

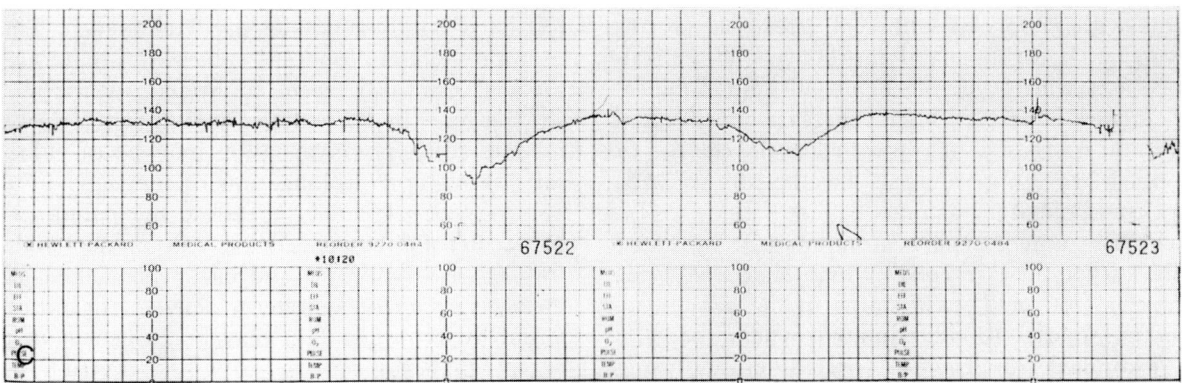

Figure 25–5. A 30-year-old G1P0 at 28³/₇ weeks' gestation who was found to have an estimated fetal weight below the 10th percentile for population-based norms. Doppler flow studies (*A*) demonstrated reversed end-diastolic flow in the umbilical artery. The patient was taken to labor and delivery, where she was placed on face mask oxygen and betamethasone was administered. The fetal heart heart tracing (*B*) was considered reassuring. Within 24 hours, the fetal heart rate tracing deteriorated (*C*) and the patient was taken for primary cesarean delivery. A viable male infant weighing 480 g was delivered and received Apgar scores of 3 and 8.

blood flow in the umbilical artery and an indication for delivery, such as abnormal fetal heart rate testing, averaged 6 to 8 days and ranged from 0 to 49 days.

Fetuses with absent end-diastolic umbilical flow velocity should undergo intensive antenatal surveillance at a level greater than that usually provided for the small fetus. Reversed end-diastolic flow in the umbilical artery reflects severe fetal compromise and is an ominous finding. Fetuses with this finding should be monitored immediately, and delivery should be considered.

In several studies, the umbilical venous circulation of fetuses with abnormal Doppler umbilical arterial velocities has been examined. Indik reported a 54 percent mortality in fetuses with absent end-diastolic velocities in the umbilical artery and umbilical venous pulsations compared with a 10 percent mortality in fetuses with similar arterial velocities and normal (monophasic) venous velocities.[137] Arduini studied fetuses from the time of onset of absent end-diastolic velocities in the umbilical artery until the onset of abnormal heart rate testing or delivery. He found that gestational age at onset, maternal hypertension, and the development of pulsations in the umbilical venous velocities were significantly correlated with the interval of time between diagnosis and delivery.[138] Hecher noted that fetuses with abnormal arterial velocities who also developed abnormal venous velocities (inferior vena cava, hepatic, and ductus venosus) had a higher morbidity than fetuses without abnormal venous flow.[139]

In summary, Doppler velocimetry of fetal vessels has improved our understanding of the pathophysiology of fetal growth restriction. Weekly evaluation of umbilical artery Doppler velocimetry has been used in combination with the modified biophysical profile in fetuses exhibiting poor growth. A small fetus with normal umbilical artery Doppler studies is probably constitutionally small and is at low risk for morbidity. However, a small fetus with abnormal umbilical artery waveforms is at greater risk for neonatal morbidity and mortality.[66,140] Fetuses with development of pulsatile umbilical venous velocities have even higher increases in neonatal morbidity and mortality. In controlled trials, the use of fetal Doppler waveform analysis has been associated with improved perinatal outcome.

As previously noted, cordocentesis may be indicated to rapidly karyotype a severely growth-restricted fetus. Evaluation of fetal acid–base status in the growth-restricted fetus appears to offer limited benefit. Nicolini et al.[141] examined 58 growth-restricted fetuses, using cordocentesis for acid–base evaluation in addition to karyotyping. They found significant differences in pH, PCO_2, PO_2, and base equivalents in fetuses who had no evidence of end-diastolic flow by umbilical artery Doppler velocimetry. However, they observed no relationship between acid–base determination and perinatal outcome. Pardi et al.[142] examined umbilical blood

acid–base status in 56 growth-restricted fetuses and demonstrated an association between acid–base status and the results of cardiotocographic and umbilical artery Doppler waveform analysis. If both fetal heart rate and Doppler studies were normal, neither hypoxemia nor acidemia was noted. When both tests were abnormal, 64 percent of the growth-restricted fetuses demonstrated abnormal acid–base analysis. Unfortunately, the prognostic significance of these abnormalities is uncertain. In summary, there would appear to be no direct fetal benefit from the use of percutaneous umbilical blood sampling in the setting of fetal growth restriction.

Therapy

Several studies have examined the potential benefits of maternal hyperoxygenation in the treatment of the compromised growth-restricted fetus. Nicolaides et al.[143] administered 55 percent oxygen by face mask to mothers whose pregnancies were complicated by severe growth restriction, oligohydramnios, and decreased blood flow in the fetal descending aorta. Ten minutes of maternal hyperoxygenation raised the fetal PO_2, to normal or near normal in five of six cases. Therapy was provided for an average duration of approximately 5 weeks in the five survivors. No improvement in fetal growth velocity was noted. Ribbert et al.[144] provided maternal oxygen therapy (2.5 L/min nasal prong) to four growth-restricted infants at 27 to 28 weeks. Pregnancy was prolonged an average of 9 days beyond the first recognition of fetal heart rate decelerations. Neonates who were exposed to maternal hyperoxygenation had improved blood gas measurements but more hypoglycemia, thrombocytopenia, and disseminated intravascular coagulation compared with concordant gestational age and fetal heart rate–matched growth-restricted controls not exposed to oxygen. The ability to improve fetal blood gas values with maternal oxygen therapy has also been confirmed in the growth-restricted fetus by Battaglia et al.[145]

Maternal hyperoxygenation may be of value for the safe, short-term prolongation of pregnancy. Such therapy may be of benefit to allow the administration of corticosteroids to reduce the risk of neonatal respiratory distress syndrome and intraventricular hemorrhage in anticipation of a preterm delivery. In addition, maternal hyperoxygenation may be of benefit in prolonging pregnancy when the growth-restricted fetus is too immature to survive. Although maternal hyperoxygenation may reduce fetal hypoxia, overall neonatal outcome may not be improved with prolonged therapy, since the deleterious effects of continued intrauterine substrate deprivation may extend beyond the benefits of improved fetal oxygen tension.

In 1987, Wallenburg and Rotmans[146] significantly reduced the incidence of fetal growth restriction in women with a history of recurrent IUGR using low-dose aspirin and dipyridamole beginning at 16 weeks' gestation. Women receiving therapy had a rate of fetal growth restriction of 13 percent compared with 61 percent in an untreated control group. No treated woman had a child with severe growth restriction (birth weight <2.3 percentile) compared with 27 percent in the untreated group. Recently, a meta-analysis of the efficacy of low-dose aspirin (50 to 100 mg/day) has demonstrated a significant reduction in the frequency of IUGR when low-dose aspirin is used.[147] There is a dose-dependent relationship in that higher doses (100 to 150 mg/day) were significantly more effective in preventing IUGR than were lower doses (50 to 80 mg/day). The authors concluded that low dose aspirin should not be used routinely in pregnant women. We agree and restrict its usage, at the higher dose level, to women who have previously experienced early-onset IUGR associated with significant preterm delivery (<32 weeks).

Timing of Delivery

Proper timing of delivery is often the critical management issue when dealing with the growth-restricted fetus. Frigoletto[148] has emphasized, "The majority of fetal deaths occur after the 36th week of gestation and before labor which leads to the conclusion that many deaths could be prevented by accurate recognition of growth restriction and appropriately timed and conducted intervention." The crux of management is to balance the hazards of prematurity with the threat of intrauterine demise. Careful consideration should be given to the reliability of the information on which the gestational age of the fetus has been established, the fetal growth curve, and the results of antepartum fetal monitoring.

Amniocentesis may be an important adjunct to this decision-making process. The lecithin/sphingomyelin (L/S) ratio may also provide information that allows more accurate dating of the pregnancy. A surprisingly low L/S ratio would suggest an earlier gestational age rather than fetal growth restriction. In cases of symmetric growth restriction, a late amniocentesis may also be used to obtain amniotic fluid for a fetal karyotype.

To review, if growth restriction is suspected or anticipated, appropriate fetal testing and daily maternal assessment of fetal activity should be instituted. Ultrasound examinations to assess fetal growth should be scheduled every 3 to 4 weeks. As long as studies show continued fetal head growth and test results remain reassuring, no intervention is required. If the patient fails a primary surveillance tool such as the NST or fetal Doppler surveillance, follow-up evaluation may be appropriate. If the CST result is positive, or the fetal biophysical profile score is either 6 with oligohydram-

nios or 4 or less or reversed end-diastolic flow is observed, delivery should be considered. An assessment of fetal lung maturity should be made if possible. In the face of a mature L/S ratio and ominous antepartum test results, delivery should be effected. If the patient has an immature L/S ratio and abnormal test findings, then consideration can be given to steroid administration with continuous heart rate monitoring and oxygen supplementation until delivery or until antepartum test results improve. If amniotic fluid cannot be obtained for an L/S ratio as a result of oligohydramnios and the clinical picture supports the diagnosis of severe IUGR, early delivery should be considered.

Because a large proportion of growth-restricted infants suffer intrapartum asphyxia, intrapartum management demands continuous fetal heart rate monitoring. Cord blood sampling has demonstrated that these fetuses may exhibit increased lactic acid levels, polycythemia, hypoglycemia, and acidosis before labor.[149] During labor, a tracing without late decelerations is predictive of a good outcome in cases complicated by IUGR. However, with late decelerations, the incidence of asphyxia in growth-restricted infants is far greater than in normally grown infants. Therefore, earlier intervention may be indicated.[150] As many growth-restricted fetuses require preterm delivery, an unfavorable cervix is not uncommon. The presence of IUGR has been considered a relative contraindication to the use of prostaglandin for cervical preparation by some authors.[151] An unfavorable cervix may also preclude internal fetal heart rate monitoring. In the face of an inadequate external tracing, cesarean delivery may be necessary.

NEONATAL OUTCOME

Immediate Morbidity

The association of selected neonatal morbidity with fetal growth restriction is a complex one (see the box "Early Neonatal Morbidities in IUGR"). Initial reports suggested the possibility of a protective effect of IUGR with reduced occurrence of respiratory distress syndrome (RDS) and intraventricular hemorrhage (IVH).[152] In contrast, Piper and Langer[153] found no difference in indices of fetal lung maturity comparing gestational age-matched SGA and appropriate-for-gestational-age (AGA) fetuses. Similarly, Thompson et al.[154] found no difference in the frequency of ventilatory support when growth-restricted and AGA infants were matched for gestational age and mode of delivery. Most recently, several large trials suggest that RDS is significantly more likely to occur in growth-restricted neonates.[155,156] Bernstein has also demonstrated a significant increase in

Early Neonatal Morbidities in IUGR

Birth asphyxia
Meconium aspiration
Hypoglycemia
Hypocalcemia
Hypothermia
Polycythemia, hyperviscosity, hyperbilirubinemia
Thrombocytopenia
Pulmonary hemorrhage
Malformations
Sepsis
Respiratory distress syndrome
Necrotizing enterocolitis

the risk for necrotizing enterocolitis and no difference in the rates of intraventricular hemorrhage when growth-restricted newborns are evaluated. Dashe noted a significant increase in RDS in infants with asymmetric IUGR when compared with neonates with symmetric IUGR (9 percent vs. 4 percent).[157] Mortality rates are uniformly higher when IUGR is present. These data should put to rest the notion that fetal growth restriction is associated with any reduction in newborn illness.

The impact of prenatal glucocorticoid administration on illness in the growth-restricted newborn has recently been examined. Elimian et al. studied 1,148 newborns with birth weights less than 1,750 g and demonstrated no benefits to neonatal outcome when perinatal glucocorticoids were used.[158] Bernstein et al., in a study of 19,759 newborns between 500 and 1,500 g, controlled for a different set of confounding variables, and demonstrated a significant reduction in neonatal RDS, IVH, and death when prenatal glucocorticoids were administered. These benefits were not qualitatively different from those observed in appropriately sized newborns.[156] The potential benefits of prenatal glucocorticoid administration on neonatal morbidity and mortality in the growth-restricted newborn would appear to be an area worthy of prospective evaluation.

Additional neonatal morbidity must be anticipated when the growth-restricted fetus is delivered. These infants suffer more frequently from meconium aspiration than do appropriately grown infants. Gasping in utero in response to asphyxia appears to contribute to this problem. Meconium aspiration is rarely seen before 34 weeks' gestation and is, therefore, largely a problem of the mature growth-restricted infant. At delivery, careful suctioning of the nasopharynx and oropharynx with the DeLee catheter decreases the incidence of this complication.[159] Further clearing of the airway can be ac-

complished at delivery by direct laryngoscopy and aspiration by an experienced pediatrician. Because immediate attention to the many neonatal problems experienced by these infants is essential, appropriate pediatric support should be present in the delivery room when an infant suspected of being growth restricted is to be delivered.

Hypoglycemia is a frequent problem in growth-restricted infants, a result of both inadequate glycogen reserves secondary to intrauterine malnutrition and a gluconeogenic pathway that is less responsive to hypoglycemia than that of the normally grown infant.[160] Hypoglycemia should be anticipated in all growth-restricted infants and frequent blood glucose monitoring instituted. Hypocalcemia, another well-recognized problem in growth-restricted babies, may be caused by relative hypoparathyroidism, a result of acidosis associated with intrauterine asphyxia.[161] Hyperphosphatemia secondary to tissue breakdown may also contribute. Frequent calcium monitoring is essential, as symptoms are nonspecific and similar to those associated with hypoglycemia.

Polycythemia is observed three to four times more frequently in the growth-restricted infant than in weight-matched controls. Polycythemia results from hypoxia, which leads to increased production of red blood cells, and from transfer of blood volume from the placental circulation to the fetal circulation in the face of intrauterine asphyxia.[160] Thus, these infants produce more red blood cells that are shunted to them if hypoxia occurs during labor. Polycythemia leads to increased red blood cell breakdown, accounting in part for the high incidence of hyperbilirubinemia in these infants. Polycythemia is a criterion for, but does not necessarily lead to, hyperviscosity, which can result in capillary bed sludging and thrombosis. Multiple organ systems can be affected, leading to pulmonary hypertension, cerebral infarction, and necrotizing enterocolitis.

Hyponatremia resulting from impaired renal function is also frequently reported in growth-restricted infants. The renal complications associated with IUGR may be attributed to asphyxia, which can produce central nervous system injury leading to inappropriate antidiuretic hormone (ADH) secretion.[160]

Hypothermia is another common problem for the growth-restricted infant and results from decreased body fat stores secondary to intrauterine malnourishment.[160] Hypothermia, if unrecognized and untreated, can contribute to the metabolic deterioration of an already unstable growth-restricted infant.

Long-Term Morbidity

The past two decades have seen tremendous advances in the overall management of the low-birth-weight infant. Obstetricians are more aware of the syndrome of IUGR, and improved techniques for the detection of impaired intrauterine growth and the assessment of well-being are now available. Technology required for the neonatal care of these infants advances each year. Have improvements in obstetric and pediatric care favorably affected the outcome of the growth-restricted infant? The perinatal mortality rate for those infants who receive optimal intrapartum and neonatal management is decreased when compared with that for age-matched controls who did not have intensive care.[162]

The ultimate growth potential for growth-restricted infants appears to be good. The degree of catch-up growth observed in several longitudinal studies suggests that these infants can be expected to have normal growth curves and normal albeit slightly reduced size as adults. In an 8-year follow-up of children weighing less than 1,500 g at birth by Kitchen et al.,[163] 75 percent of growth-restricted infants achieved a height and weight above the 10th percentile. Of infants whose birth weight fell below the 3rd percentile, 60 percent had reached the 25th percentile for weight at 8 years. In Kitchen and associates' study,[163] however, 50 percent of the children with small head circumferences still had head circumferences below the 10th percentile at the 8-year follow-up visit in spite of their growth in height and weight. Hediger observed that growth-restricted infants experienced a period of catch-up growth in early infancy but remained near the 25th percentile through age 47 months.[164] Kumar et al.[165] noted that in infants whose birth weights were less than 1,250 g, at 1 year 46 percent of the growth-restricted infants remained less than the 3rd percentile for weight and 38 percent remained less than the 3rd percentile for height. In general, those infants suffering growth restriction near the time of delivery do tend to catch up. However, those neonates with earlier onset and more longstanding growth restriction in utero continue to lag behind.

The issue of long-term neurologic sequelae remains unresolved. In 1972, Fitzhardinge and Steven,[166] evaluating a group of 96 growth-restricted infants, noted that 50 percent of males and 36 percent of females had poor school performance and, overall, 25 percent had minimal cerebral dysfunction. Major neurologic deficits were much less frequent. Other studies have shown low birth weight and short gestation to be risk factors for cerebral palsy. However, the vast majority of children with cerebral palsy are not growth restricted.

The positive effect of intrapartum surveillance for the growth-restricted fetus is reflected in the data of Low et al.[167] In a study of 88 growth-restricted infants, they reported no severe neurologic sequelae. They did detect a lag in mental development that was significant in the growth-restricted babies when compared with appropriately grown controls, especially in the group with birth weights less than 2,300 g. This study correlates well with the data of Lipper et al.[167] on low-birth-weight babies. They observed that growth-restricted infants with a head circumference below the 10th percentile have two to three times the number of serious neurologic sequelae of their normocephalic counterparts. Strauss and Dietz found that term infants with IUGR and a head circumference less than 2 SD below the mean had significantly poorer performance on intelligence and visual motor development testing at age 7 when compared with their control siblings.[168] Walther,[169] in an examination of 7-year-olds who suffered no perinatal complications despite IUGR and who were matched for social class with a control group, showed an increase in teacher-identified hyperactivity, poor concentration, and clumsiness. In a study of school performance in 8-year-olds matched for socioeconomic status, Robertson et al.[170] demonstrated a tendency toward hyperactivity in preterm growth-restricted children compared with control groups. Low et al.[171] have shown that in 9- to 11-year-olds only fetal growth restriction and socioeconomic status contributed independently to the presence of learning deficits. Intrapartum fetal asphyxia, assessed by umbilical artery base deficit, was not associated with learning deficits in this group of children.

The pattern that emerges from evaluation of these data emphasizes that neurologic outcome depends on the degree of growth restriction, especially the impact on head growth, its time of onset, the gestational age of the infant at birth, and the postnatal environment. An early intrauterine insult, between 10 and 17 weeks' gestation, could limit neuronal cellular multiplication and would obviously have a profound effect on neurologic function.[172] In the third trimester, brain development is characterized by glial multiplication, dendritic arborization, establishment of synaptic connections, and myelinization, all of which continue during the first 2 years of life. Recovery after a period of impaired growth in the third trimester is, therefore, more likely to occur. Thus, the preterm appropriately grown infant has more normal neurologic development and fewer severe neurologic deficits than its preterm growth-restricted counterpart. Developmental milestones and neurologic development of mature infants with IUGR and mature infants of normal birth weight are similar. Presumably, this also reflects heightened physician awareness of the growth-restricted infant that allows detection, appropriate antepartum management, intrapartum therapy, and early pediatric intervention. The premature growth-restricted infant suffers from increased susceptibility to intrauterine asphyxia and all of the neonatal complications of the premature, as well as those of the infant with IUGR. If growth restriction is associated with lagging head growth before 26 weeks, even mature infants have significant developmental delay at 4 years of age.[173]

There has been significant interest in the hypothesis that diseases commonly associated with adulthood may have their origins during fetal life, the "Barker Hypothesis." Dr. David Barker, an epidemiologist from Southampton, England, first proposed that intrauterine conditions could program the development of the cardiovascular system later in life.[174] He and his colleagues took advantage of meticulous birth records maintained in England and Wales. Those areas in which infant mortality was highest in 1901 to 1910 correlated with areas in which there was also an increased risk for coronary artery disease in men ages 35 to 74 during the 1960s and 1970s.[175] Barker realized that the infant mortality was highest in low-birth-weight infants and proposed that low-birth-weight survivors might be at greater risk for coronary artery disease. Examining birth records that included not only the infant's birth weight but its birth length, abdominal and head circumference measurements, and placental weight, these investigators found that infants with a birth weight of less than 5.5 lb had a threefold increase in death attributable to coronary artery disease later in life.[175] The risks for stroke and hypertension were also greater. The infants at greatest risk were those who not only were low birth weight but had a smaller head circumference, were shorter, and had an increased placenta/birth weight ratio.

Epidemiologic data support a link between IUGR, low birth weight and an increased risk of developing cardiovascular disease, abdominal obesity, type 2 diabetes mellitus, and hyperlipidemia.[176–179] Proposed mechanisms for this association include congenital pancreatic deficiency, which manifests in later life as insulin resistance,[180,181] as well as alterations in sympathetic nervous activity[182] or adrenocortical function.[183–185]

In summary, there is increasing evidence to support the observed epidemiologic association between low birth weight, fetal growth restriction, and adult diseases.

SUMMARY

Overall, increased awareness of the IUGR syndrome and an improved ability to observe intrauterine growth and evaluate fetal well-being in utero have improved along with our understanding of this disease. Continued assessment of the underlying physiology, the efficacy of therapy, and the relationship of fetal status to specific short- and long-term developmental outcome are necessary if overall morbidity and mortality are to be decreased.

Key Points

➤ Fetal growth restriction is a major cause of perinatal morbidity and mortality. Intrauterine growth restriction is currently defined by fetal size alone.

➤ Characterization of fetal size should be performed using growth curves that are population specific and appropriate.

➤ The definition of fetal growth restriction has not been based on correlations with short- and long-term morbidity.

➤ Preterm delivery is associated with an increased incidence of fetal growth restriction.

➤ Fundal height measurements have low sensitivity in the identification of fetal growth restriction.

➤ Mortality resulting from fetal growth restriction can be reduced with appropriate antenatal surveillance strategies, which may include early delivery.

➤ Low-dose aspirin therapy can prevent recurrent IUGR.

➤ The use of fetal umbilical Doppler flow studies in the management of the growth-restricted fetus reduces perinatal morbidity and mortality.

➤ Fetal growth restriction is associated with high rates of intrapartum asphyxia.

➤ Intrauterine growth restriction can result in both short-term and lifelong morbidities.

REFERENCES

1. Wolfe HM, Gross TL: Increased risk to the growth retarded fetus. *In* Gross TM, Sokol RJ (eds): Intrauterine Growth Retardation. Chicago, Year Book Medical Publishers, 1989, p 111.
2. Low JA, Boston RW, Pancham SR: Fetal asphyxia during the intrapartum period in intrauterine growth-retarded infants. Am J Obstet Gynecol 113:351, 1972.
3. Ylppo A: Zur Physiologie, Klinik und zum Schicksal der Fruhgeborenen. Ztschr Kinderh 24:1 1920.
4. Dunn PM: The search for perinatal definitions and standards. Acta Paediatr Scand 319:7, 1985.
5. McBurney RD: The undernourished fullterm infant. West J Surg 55:363, 1946.
6. Gruenwald P: Chronic fetal distress and placental insufficiency. Biol Neonate 5:215, 1963.

7. Lubchenco LO, Hansman C, Boyd E: Intrauterine growth in length and head circumference as estimated from live births at gestational ages from 26 to 42 weeks. Pediatrics 37:403, 1966.

8. Usher R, McLean F: Intrauterine growth of live-born Caucasian infants at sea level: standards obtained from measurements in 7 dimensions of infants born between 25 and 44 weeks of gestation. J Pediatr 74:901, 1969.

9. World Health Organization: Report of a Scientific Group on Health Statistics Methodology Related to Perinatal Events, Document ICD/PE/74.4:1, 1974.

10. Wilcocks J, Donald J, Duggan TC, Day N: Fetal cephalometry by ultrasound. J Obstet Gynaecol Br Commonw 71:11, 1964.

11. Campbell S, Dewhurst CJ: Diagnosis of the small-for-dates fetus by serial ultrasonic cephalometry. Lancet 2:1002, 1971.

12. Campbell S, Wilkin D: Ultrasonic measurement of fetal abdomen circumference in the estimation of fetal weight. Br J Obstet Gynaecol 82:689, 1975.

13. Hadlock FP, Harrist RB, Sharman RS, et al: Estimation of fetal weight with the use of head, body, and femur measurements—a prospective study. Am J Obstet Gynecol 151:333, 1985.

14. Vintzileos AM, Campbell WA, Rodis JF, et al: Fetal weight estimation formulas with head, abdominal, femur and thigh circumference measurements. Am J Obstet Gynecol 157:410, 1987.

15. Combs CA, Jaekle RK, Rosenn B, et al: Sonographic estimation of fetal weight based on a model of fetal volume. Obstet Gynecol 82:365, 1993.

16. Sabbagha RE, Minogue J, Tamura RK, Hungerford SA: Estimation of birth weight by use of ultrasonographic formulas targeted to large-, appropriate-, and small-for-gestational age fetuses. Am J Obstet Gynecol 160:854, 1989.

17. Ott WJ: The diagnosis of altered fetal growth. Obstet Gynecol Clin North Am 15:237, 1988.

18. Seeds JW, Peng T: Impaired fetal growth and risk of fetal death: is the tenth percentile the appropriate standard. Am J Obstet Gynecol 178:658, 1998.

19. Eydoux P, Choiset A, LePorrier N, et al: Chromosomal prenatal diagnosis: study of 936 cases of intrauterine abnormalities after ultrasound assessment. Prenat Diagn 9:255, 1989.

20. Dugan A, Johnnson MP, Isada I, et al: The smaller than expected first trimester fetus is at increased risk for chromosomal anomalies. Am J Obstet Gynecol 167:1525, 1992.

21. Yaron Y, Cherry M, Kramer RL, et al: Second-trimester maternal serum marker screening: maternal serum alpha-fetoprotein, beta-human chorionic gonadotropin, estriol, and their various combinations as predictors for pregnancy outcome. Am J Obstet Gynecol 181:968, 1999.

22. Onderoglu LS, Kabukcu A: Elevated second trimester human chorionic gonadotropin level associated with adverse pregnancy outcome. Int J Gynaecol Obstet 56:245, 1997.

23. Cusick W, Rodis JF, Vintzileos AM, et al: Predicting pregnancy outcome from the degree of maternal serum alpha-fetoprotein elevation. J Reprod Med 5:327, 1996.

24. Waller DK, Lustig LS, Cunningham GC, et al: The association between maternal serum alpha-fetoprotein and preterm birth, small for gestational age infants, preeclampsia, and placental complication. Obstet Gynecol 88:816, 1996.

25. Davis RO, Goldenberg RL, Boots L, et al: Elevated levels of midtrimester maternal serum alpha-fetoprotein are associated with preterm delivery but not with fetal growth retardation. Am J Obstet Gynecol 167:596, 1992.

26. Cowles T, Tatlor S, Zneimer S, Elder F: Association of confined placental mosaicism with intrauterine growth restriction [abstract]. Am J Obstet Gynecol 170:273, 1994.

27. Chapman MG, Furness ET, Jones WR, et al: Significance of the ultrasound location of placental site in early pregnancy. Br J Obstet Gynaecol 86:846, 1979.

28. Gruenwald P: Growth of the human fetus. II: Abnormal growth in twins and infants of mothers with diabetes, hypertension, or isoimmunization. Am J Obstet Gynecol 94:1120, 1966.

29. Houlton MCC, Marivate M, Philpott RH: The prediction of fetal growth retardation in twin pregnancy. Br J Obstet Gynaecol 88:264, 1981.

30. Baker ER, Beach ML, Craigo SD, et al: A comparison of neonatal outcomes of age-matched, growth restricted twins and growth restricted singletons. Am J Perinatol 14:499, 1997.

31. Hamilton EF, Platt RW, Morin L, et al: How small is too small in a twin pregnancy? Am J Obstet Gynecol 179:682, 1998.

32. DeWolf F, Brosens I, Renaer M: Fetal growth retardation and the maternal arterial supply of the human placenta in the absence of sustained hypertension. Br J Obstet Gynaecol 87: 678, 1980.

33. Ward K, Hata A, Jeunemaitre X, et al: A molecular variant of angiotensinogen associated with preeclampsia. Nat Genet 4:59, 1993.

34. Silver HM, Seebeck M, Carlson R: Comparison of total blood volume in normal, preeclamptic and nonproteinuric gestational hypertensive pregnancy by simultaneous measurement of red blood cell and plasma volumes. Am J Obstet Gynecol 179:87, 1998.

35. Bernstein IM, Ziegler W, Stirewalt WS, et al: Angiotensinogen genotype and plasma volume in nulligravid women. Obstet Gynecol 92:171, 1998.

36. Croall J, Sherrif S, Matthews J: Non-pregnant plasma volume and fetal growth retardation. Br J Obstet Gynaecol 85:90, 1978.

37. Duvekot JJ, Cheriex EC, Pieters FAA, et al: Maternal volume homeostasis in early pregnancy in relation to fetal growth restriction. Obstet Gynecol 85:361, 1995.

38. Smith CA: Effects of maternal undernutrition upon the newborn infant in Holland (1944–1945). Am J Obstet Gynecol 30:229, 1947.

39. Lechtig A, Yarbrough C, Delgado H, et al: Effect of moderate maternal malnutrition on the placenta. Am J Obstet Gynecol 123:191, 1975.

40. Economides DL, Nicolaides KH: Blood glucose and oxygen tension levels in small-for-gestational-age fetuses. Am J Obstet Gynecol 160:385, 1989.

41. Khouzami VA, Ginsburg DS, Daikoku NH, et al: The glucose tolerance test as a means of identifying intrauterine growth retardation. Am J Obstet Gynecol 139:423, 1981.

42. Sokol RJ, Kazzi GM, Kalhan SC, Pillay SK: Identifying the pregnancy at risk for intrauterine growth retardation: possible usefulness of the intravenous glucose tolerance test. Am J Obstet Gynecol 143:220, 1983.

43. Langer O, Damus K, Maiman M, et al: A link between relative hypoglycemia-hypoinsulinemia during oral glucose tolerance tests and intrauterine growth retardation. Am J Obstet Gynecol 155:711, 1986.

44. Caruso A, Paradisi G, Ferrazzani S, et al: Effect of maternal carbohydrate metabolism on fetal growth. Obstet Gynecol 92: 8, 1998.

45. Mills JL, Graubard BI, Harley EE, et al: Maternal alcohol consumption and birth weight. How much drinking during pregnancy is safe? JAMA 252:1875, 1984.

46. Little BB, Snell LM, Klein VR, et al: Cocaine abuse during pregnancy: maternal and fetal implications. Obstet Gynecol 74:157, 1989.

47. Lobi M, Welcher DW, Mellits ED: Maternal age and intellectual function of offspring. Johns Hopkins Med J 128:347, 1971.

48. Berkowitz GS, Skovron ML, Lapinski RH, et al: Delayed childbearing and the outcome of pregnancy. N Engl J Med 322:659, 1990.

49. Galbraith RS, Karchman EJ, Piercy WN, et al: The clinical prediction of intrauterine growth retardation. Am J Obstet Gynecol 133:231, 1979.

50. Tejani NA: Recurrence of intrauterine growth retardation. Obstet Gynecol 59:329, 1982.

51. Tejani N, Mann LI: Diagnosis and management of the small for gestational age fetus. *In* Frigoletto FD (ed): Clinical Obstetrics and Gynecology. Hagerstown, MD, Harper & Row, 1977, p 943.

52. Wolfe HM, Gross TL, Sokol RJ: Recurrent small for gestational age birth: perinatal risks and outcomes. Am J Obstet Gynecol 157:288, 1987.

53. Belizan JM, Villar J, Nardin JC, et al: Diagnosis of intrauterine growth retardation by a simple clinical method: measurement of uterine height. Am J Obstet Gynecol 131:643, 1978.

54. Persson B, Stangenberg M, Lunell NO, et al: Prediction of size of infants at birth by measurement of symphysis fundus height. Br J Obstet Gynaecol 93:206, 1986.

55. Sabbagha RE, Minogue J, Tamura RK, et al: Estimation of birth weight by use of ultrasonographic formulas targeted to large-, appropriate-, and small-for-gestational-age fetuses. Am J Obstet Gynecol 160:854, 1989.

56. Weiner CP, Sabbagha RE, Vaisrub N, Depp R: A hypothetical model suggesting suboptimal intra-uterine growth in infants delivered preterm. Obstet Gynecol 65:323, 1985.

57. Ott WJ: Intrauterine growth retardation and preterm delivery. Am J Obstet Gynecol 168:1710, 1993.

58. Bernstein IM, Meyer MC, Capeless EL: "Fetal growth charts": comparison of cross-sectional ultrasound examinations with birthweight. Maternal Fetal Med 3:182, 1994.

59. Hadlock FP, Harrist RB, Martinez-Poyer J: In utero analysis of fetal growth: a sonographic weight standard. Radiology 181:129, 1991.

60. Lackman F, Capewell V, Richardson B, et al: Fetal or neonatal growth curve: which is more appropriate in predicting the impact of fetal growth on the risk of perinatal mortality. Am J Obstet Gynecol 180:S145, 1999.

61. Eik-Nes SH, Grottum P, Persson PH, Marsal K: Prediction of fetal growth by ultrasound biometry. I. Methodology. Acta Obstet Gynecol Scand 61:53, 1982.

62. Rossavik IK, Deter RL: Mathematical modeling of fetal growth. I. Basic principles. J Clin Ultrasound 12:529, 1984.

63. Gardosi J, Mul T, Mongelli M, Fagan D: Analysis of birthweight and gestational age in antepartum stillbirths. Br J Obstet Gynaecol 105:524, 1998.

64. Shields LE, Huff RW, Jackson GM, et al: Fetal growth: a comparison of growth curves with mathematical modeling. J Ultrasound Med 5:271, 1993.

65. Mongelli M, Sverker EK, Tambyrajia R: Screening for fetal growth restriction: a mathematical model of the effect of time interval and ultrasound error. Obstet Gynecol 92:908, 1998.

66. Bobrow CS, Soothill P: Fetal growth velocity: a cautionary tale. Lancet 353:1460, 1999.

67. Lampl M, Veldhuis JD, Johnson ML: Saltation and stasis: a model of human growth. Science 258:801, 1992.

68. Bernstein IM, Blake K: Evidence that normal fetal growth is not continuous [abstract]. Maternal Fetal Med 4:197, 1995.

69. Crane JP, Kopta MM: Prediction of intrauterine growth retardation via ultrasonically measured head/abdominal circumference ratios. Obstet Gynecol 54:597, 1979.

70. Seeds JW: Impaired fetal growth: ultrasonic evaluation and clinical management. Obstet Gynecol 64:577, 1984.

71. Hadlock FP, Deter RL, Harrist RB, et al: A date-independent predictor of intrauterine growth retardation: femur length/ abdominal circumference ratio. AJR Am J Roentgenol 141: 979, 1983.

72. Veille JC, Kanaan C: Duplex Doppler ultrasonographic evaluation of the fetal renal artery in normal and abnormal fetuses. Am J Obstet Gynecol 161:1502, 1989.

73. Manning FA, Hill LM, Platt LD: Qualitative amniotic fluid volume determination by ultrasound: antepartum detection of intrauterine growth retardation. Am J Obstet Gynecol 193: 254, 1981.

74. Manning FA, Lange IR, Morrison I, Harman CR: Determination of fetal health: methods for antepartum and intrapartum fetal assessment. Curr Probl Obstet Gynecol 7:1, 1983.

75. Groome LJ, Owen J, Neely CL, Hauth JC: Oligohydramics: antepartum fetal urine production and intrapertum fetal distress. Am J Obstet Gynecol 165:1077, 1991.

76. Schulman H: The clinical implications of Doppler ultrasound analysis of the uterine and umbilical arteries. Am J Obstet Gynecol 157:889, 1987.

77. Jacobsen S-L, Imhof R, Manning N, et al: The value of Doppler assessment of the uteroplacental circulation in predicting preeclampsia or intrauterine growth retardation. Am J Obstet Gynecol 162:110, 1990.

78. North RA, Ferrier C, Long D, et al: Uterine artery Doppler velocity waveforms in the second trimester for the prediction of preeclampsia and fetal growth retardation. Obstet Gynecol 83:378, 1994.

79. Bewley S, Cooper D, Campbell S: Doppler investigation of uteroplacental blood flow resistance in the second trimester: a screening study for preeclampsia and intrauterine growth retardation. Br J Obstet Gynaecol 98:871, 1991.

80. Steele SA, Pearce JM, McParland PM, Chamberlain GVP: Early Doppler ultrasound screening in prediction of hypertensive disorders of pregnancy. Lancet 335:1548, 1990.

81. Bower S, Schuchter K, Campbell S: Doppler ultrasound screening as part of routine antenatal scanning: prediction of preeclampsia and intrauterine growth retardation. Br J Obstet Gynaecol 100:989, 1993.

82. Harrington K, Goldfrad C, Carpenter RG, Campbell S: Transvaginal uterine and umbilical artery Doppler examination of 12–16 weeks and the subsequent development of preeclampsia and intrauterine growth retardation. Ultrasound Obstet Gynecol 9:94, 1997.

83. Valensise H, Romanini C: Second-trimester uterine artery flow velocity waveform and oral glucose tolerance test as a means of predicting intrauterine growth retardation. Ultrasound Obstet Gynecol 3:412, 1993.

84. Rohrer VF: Der index der korperfulle als mass des ernahrungszustandes. Munch Med Wochenschr 19:580, 1921.

85. Walther FJ, Ramaekers LHJ: The ponderal index as a measure of the nutritional status at birth and its relation to some aspects of neonatal morbidity. J Perinat Med 10:42, 1982.

86. Miller HC, Hassanein K: Diagnosis of impaired fetal growth in newborn infants. Pediatrics 48:511, 1971.

87. Yagel S, Zacut D, Igelstein S, et al: In utero ponderal index as a prognostic factor in the evaluation of intrauterine growth retardation. Am J Obstet Gynecol 157:415, 1987.

88. Bernstein IM, Catalano PM: Ultrasonographic estimation of fetal body composition for children of diabetic mothers. Invest Radiol 26:722, 1991.

89. Landon MB, Sonek J, Foy P, et al: Sonographic measurement of fetal humeral soft tissue thickness in pregnancy complicated by GDM. Diabetes 40 (Suppl 2):66, 1991.

90. Abramowicz JS, Sherer DM, Woods JR: Ultrasonographic measurement of cheek-to-cheek diameter in fetal growth disturbances. Am J Obstet Gynecol 169:405, 1993.

91. Gardeil F, Greene R, Stuart B, Turner MJ: Subcutaneous fat in the fetal abdomen as a predictor of growth restriction. Obstet Gynecol 94:209, 1999.

92. Chauhan S, West DJ, Scardo JA, et al: Antepartum detection of macrosomic fetus: clinical versus sonographic, including soft-tissue measurements. Obstet Gynecol 95:639, 2000.

93. Cox WL, Daffos F, Forestier F, et al: Physiology and management of intrauterine growth retardation. A biologic approach with fetal blood sampling. Am J Obstet Gynecol 159:36, 1988.

94. Fisher JW: Control of erythropoietin production. Proc Soc Exp Biol Med 173:289, 1983.

95. Finne PH: Erythropoietin levels in cord blood as an indicator of intrauterine hypoxia. Acta Pediatr Scand 55:478, 1966.

96. Maier RF, Bohme K, Dudenhausen JW, Obladen M: Cord blood erythropoietin in relation to different markers of fetal hypoxia. Obstet Gynecol 81:575, 1993.

97. Snijders RJM, Abbas A, Melby O, et al: Fetal plasma erythropoietin concentration in severe growth retardation. Am J Obstet Gynecol 168:615, 1993.

98. Teramo KA, Widness JA, Clemons GK, et al: Amniotic fluid eyrthropoietin correlates with umbilical plasma erythropoietin in normal and abnormal pregnancy. Obstet Gynecol 69:710, 1987.

99. Ruth V, Autti-Ramo I, Granstrom ML, et al: Prediction of perinatal brain damage by cord plasma vasopressin, erythropoietin, and hypoxanthine values. J Pediatr 113:880, 1988.

100. Pollack A, Susa JB, Stonestreet BS, et al: Phosphoenolpyruvate carboxykinase in experimental intrauterine growth retardation in rats. Pediatr Res 13:175, 1979.

101. Haymond MW, Karl IE, Pagliara AS: Increased gluconeogenic substrates in the small for gestational age infant. N Engl J Med 291:322, 1974.

102. Edozien JC, Phillips EJ, Collis WRF: The free aminoacids of plasma and urine in kwashiorkor. Lancet 1:615, 1960.

103. Mestyan J, Soltesz G, Schultz K, Horvath M: Hyperaminoacidemia due to the accumulation of gluconeogenic amino acid precursors in hypoglycemic small for gestational age infants. J Pediatr 87:409, 1975.

104. Cetin I, Corbetta C, Sereni LP, et al: Umbilical amino acid concentrations in normal and growth retarded fetuses sampled in utero by cordocentesis. Am J Obstet Gynecol 162:253, 1990.

105. Economides DL, Nicolaides KH, Gahl WA, et al: Cordocentesis in the diagnosis of intrauterine starvation. Am J Obstet Gynecol 161:1004, 1989.

106. Economides DL, Nicolaides KH, Gahl WA, et al: Plasma amino acids in appropriate and small for gestational age fetuses. Am J Obstet Gynecol 161:1219, 1989.

107. Bernstein IM, Rhodes S, Stirewalt WS: Amniotic fluid glycine/valine ratio is elevated in fetuses with growth retardation. Maternal Fetal Med 3:251, 1994.

108. Bernstein IM, Silver R, Nair KS, Stirewalt WS: Amniotic fluid glycine-valine ratio and neonatal morbidity in fetal growth restriction. Obstet Gynecol 90:933, 1997.

109. Moe N: Anticoagulant therapy in the prevention of placental infarction and perinatal death. Obstet Gynecol 58:481, 1981.

110. Grannum PAT: Ultrasonic measurements for diagnosis. *In* Gross TM, Sokol RJ (eds): Intrauterine Growth Retardation. Chicago, Year Book Medical Publishers, 1989, p 123.

111. Flynn AM, Kelly J, O'Connor M: Unstressed antepartum cardiotocography in the management of the fetus suspected of growth retardation. Br J Obstet Gynaecol 86:106, 1979.

112. Visser GHA, Sadovsky G, Nicolaides KH: Antepartum heart rate patterns in small-for-gestational-age third-trimester fetuses: correlations with blood gas values obtained at cordocentesis. Am J Obstet Gynecol 162:698, 1990.

113. Pazos R, Vuolo K, Aladjem S, et al: Association of spontaneous fetal heart rate decelerations during antepartum nonstress testing and intrauterine growth retardation. Am J Obstet Gynecol 144:574, 1982.

114. Nageotte MP, Towers CV, Asrat T, et al: The value of a negative antepartum test: contraction stress test and modified biophysical profile. Obstet Gynecol 84:231, 1994.

115. Gabbe SG, Freeman RD, Goebelsmann U: Evaluation of the contraction stress test before 33 weeks' gestation. Obstet Gynecol 52:649, 1978.

116. Lin CC, Devoe LD, River P, et al: Oxytocin challenge test and intrauterine growth retardation. Am J Obstet Gynecol 140:282, 1981.

117. Manning FA, Platt FA, Sipos L: Antepartum fetal evaluation: development of a fetal biophysical profile. Am J Obstet Gynecol 136:787, 1980.

118. Manning FA, Snijders R, Harman CR, et al: Fetal biophysical profile score: VI. Correlation with antepartum umbilical venous fetal pH. Am J Obstet Gynecol 169:755, 1993.

119. Ribbert LSM, Snijders RFM, Nicolaides KH, Visser GHA: Relationship of fetal biophysical profile and blood gas values at cordocentesis in severely growth-retarded fetuses. Am J Obstet Gynecol 163:569, 1990.

120. Vintzileos AM, Fleming AD, Scorza WE, et al: Relationship between fetal biophysical activities and umbilical cord blood gas values. Am J Obstet Gynecol 165:707, 1991.

121. Nageotte MP, Towers CV, Asrat A, Freeman RK: Perinatal outcome with the modified biophysical profile. Am J Obstet Gynecol 170:1672, 1994.

122. Matthews DD: Maternal assessment of fetal activity in small-for-dates infants. Obstet Gynecol 45:488, 1975.

123. Wladimiroff JW, Wijngaard JAGW, Degani S, et al: Cerebral and umbilical arterial blood flow velocity waveforms in normal and growth-retarded pregnancies. Obstet Gynecol 69:705, 1987.

124. Arbeille P, Leguyader P, Fignon A, et al: Fetal hemodynamics and flow velocity indices. *In* Copel JA, Reed KL (eds): Doppler Ultrasound in Obstetrics and Gynecology. New York, Raven Press, 1995, p 19.

125. Hackett GA, Campbell S, Gamsu H, et al: Doppler studies in the growth retarded fetus and prediction of neonatal necrotizing enterocolitis, haemorrhage, and neonatal morbidity. BMJ 294:13, 1987.

126. Veille JC, Kanaan C: Duplex Doppler ultrasonographic evaluation of the fetal renal artery in normal and abnormal fetuses. Am J Obstet Gynecol 161:1502, 1989.

127. Trudinger BJ, Stevens D, Connelly A, et al: Umbilical artery flow velocity waveforms and placental resistance: the effects of embolization of the umbilical circulation. Am J Obstet Gynecol 157:1443, 1987.

128. Morrow RJ, Hill AA, Adamson SL: Experimental models used to investigate the diagnostic potential of Doppler ultrasound in the umbilical circulation. *In* Copel JA, Reed KL (eds): Doppler Ultrasound in Obstetrics and Gynecology. New York, Raven Press, 1995, p 5.

129. Giles WB, Trudinger BJ, Bard PJ: Fetal umbilical artery flow velocity waveforms and placental resistance: pathological correlation. Br J Obstet Gynaecol 92:31, 1985.

130. Rochelson B, Kaplan C, Guzman E, et al: A quantitative

analysis of placental vasculature in the third-trimester fetus with autosomal trisomy. Obstet Gynecol 75:59, 1990.

131. Divon MY, Ferber A: Evidence-based antepartum fetal testing. Perinat Neonat Med 5:3, 2000.

132. Giles WB, Bisits A: Clinical use of Doppler in pregnancy: information from six randomized trials. Fetal Diagn Ther 8: 247, 1993.

133. Alfirevic Z, Neilson JP: Doppler ultrasonography in high-risk pregnancies: systematic review with meta-analysis. Am J Obstet Gynecol 172:1379, 1995.

134. Neilson JP, Alfirevic Z: Doppler ultrasound in high-risk pregnancies (Cochrane Review). *In* The Cochrane Library, Issue 4. Oxford: Update Software, 1999.

135. Goffinet F, Paris-Llado J, Nisand I, Breart G: Umbilical artery Doppler velocimetry in unselected and low risk pregnancies: a review of randomized controlled trials. Br J Obstet Gynaecol 104:425, 1997.

136. Farine D, Kelly EN, Ryan G, et al: Absent and reversed umbilical artery end-diastolic velocity. *In* Copel JA, Reed KL (eds): Doppler Ultrasound in Obstetrics and Gynecology. New York, Raven Press, 1995, p 187.

137. Indik JH, Chen V, Reed KL: Association of umbilical venous with inferior vena cava blood flow velocities. Obstet Gynecol 77:551, 1991.

138. Arduini D, Rizzo G, Romanini C: The development of abnormal heart rate patterns after absent end-diastolic velocity in umbilical artery: Analysis of risk factors. Am J Obstet Gynecol 168:50, 1993.

139. Hecher K, Campbell S, Doyle P, et al: Assessment of fetal compromise by Doppler investigation of the fetal circulation. Circulation 91:129, 1995.

140. Ott WJ: Intrauterine growth restriction and Doppler ultrasonography. J Ultrasound Med 19:661, 2000.

141. Nicolini U, Nicolaidis P, Fisk NM, et al: Limited role of fetal blood sampling in prediction of outcome in intrauterine growth retardation. Lancet 336:768, 1990.

142. Pardi G, Cetin I, Marconi AM, et al: Diagnostic value of blood sampling in fetuses with growth retardation. N Engl J Med 328:692, 1993.

143. Nicolaides KH, Bradley RJ, Soothill PW, et al: Maternal oxygen therapy for intrauterine growth retardation. Lancet 1:942, 1987.

144. Ribbert LSM, van Lingen RA, Visser GHA: Continuous maternal hyperoxygenation in the treatment of early fetal growth retardation. Ultrasound Obstet Gynecol 1:331, 1991.

145. Battaglia C, Artini PG, D'Ambrogio G, et al: Maternal hyperoxygenation in the treatment of intrauterine growth retardation. Am J Obstet Gynecol 167:430, 1992.

146. Wallenburg HCS, Rotmans N: Prevention of recurrent idiopathic fetal growth retardation by low-dose aspirin and dipyridamole. Am J Obstet Gynecol 157:1230, 1987.

147. Leitich H, Egarter C, Husslein P, et al: A meta-analysis of low dose aspirin for the prevention of intrauterine growth retardation. Br J Obstet Gynaecol 104:450, 1997.

148. Frigoletto FD: Evaluation and management of deferred-fetal growth. *In* Frigoletto FD (ed): Clinical Obstetrics and Gynecology. Hagerstown, MD, Harper & Row, 1977, p 922.

149. Soothill PW, Nicolaides KH, Campbell S: Prenatal asphyxia, hyperlacticaemia, hypoglycaemia, and erythroblastosis in growth retarded fetuses. BMJ 294:1051, 1987.

150. Lin CC, Moawad AH, Rosenow PJ, et al: Acid-base characteristics of fetuses with intrauterine growth retardation during labor and delivery. Am J Obstet Gynecol 137:553, 1980.

151. Sawai SK, Williams MC, O'Brien WF, et al: Sequential outpatient application of intravaginal prostaglandin E$_2$ gel in the management of postdates pregnancies. Obstet Gynecol 78:19, 1991.

152. Procianoy RS, Garcia-Prats FA, Adams JM, et al: Hyaline membrane disease and intraventricular haemorrhage in small for gestational age infants. Arch Dis Child 55:502, 1980.

153. Piper JM, Langer O: Is lung maturation related to fetal growth in diabetic or hypertensive pregnancies? Eur J Obstet Gynecol Reprod Biol 51:15, 1993.

154. Thompson PJ, Greenough A, Gamsu HR, Nicolaides KH: Ventilatory requirements for respiratory distress syndrome in small-for-gestational-age infants. Eur J Pediatr 151:528, 1992.

155. McIntire DD, Bloom SL, Casey BM, Leveno MJ: Birth weight in relation to morbidity and mortality among newborn infants. N Engl J Med 340:1234, 1999.

156. Bernstein IM, Horbar JD, Badger GJ, et al: Morbidity and mortality in growth restricted very low birth weight newborns. Am J Obstet Gynecol 182:198, 2000.

157. Dashe JS, McIntire DD, Lucas MJ, Leveno KJ: Effects of symmetric and asymmetric fetal growth on pregnancy outcomes. Obstet Gynecol 96:321, 2000.

158. Elimian A, Verma U, Canterino J, et al: Effectiveness of antenatal steroids in obstetric subgroups. Obstet Gynecol 93:174, 1999.

159. Carson BS, Losey RW, Bowes WA Jr, et al: Combined obstetric and pediatric approach to prevent meconium aspiration syndrome. Am J Obstet Gynecol 126:712, 1976.

160. Oh W: Considerations in neonates with intrauterine growth retardation. *In* Frigoletto FD (ed): Clinical Obstetrics and Gynecology. Hagerstown, MD, Harper & Row, 1977, p 989.

161. Tsang RC, Oh W: Neonatal hypocalcemia in low birthweight infants. Pediatrics 45:773, 1970.

162. Kitchen WH, Richards A, Ryan MM, et al: A longitudinal study of very low-birthweight infants. II: Results of controlled trial of intensive care and incidence of handicaps. Dev Med Child Neurol 21:582, 1979.

163. Kitchen WH, McDougass AB, Naylor FD: A longitudinal study of very low-birthweight infants. III: Distance growth at eight years of age. Dev Med Child Neurol 22:1633, 1980.

164. Hediger ML, Overpeck MD, Maurer KR, et al: Growth of infants and young children born small or large for gestational age: findings from the Third National Health and Nutrition Examination Survey. Arch Pediatr Adolesc Med 152:1225, 1998.

165. Kumar SP, Anday EK, Sacks LM, et al: Follow-up studies of very low birthweight infants (1,250 grams or less) born and treated within a perinatal center. Pediatrics 66:438, 1980.

166. Fitzhardinge PM, Steven EM: The small-for-dates infant. II: Neurological and intellectual sequelae. Pediatrics 50:50, 1972.

167. Low JA, Galbraith RS, Muir D, et al: Intrauterine growth retardation: a preliminary report of long-term morbidity. Am J Obstet Gynecol 130:534, 1978.

168. Lipper E, Lee K-S, Gartner LM, et al: Determinants of neurobehavioral outcome in low birthweight infants. Pediatrics 67: 502, 1981.

169. Strauss R, Dietz WH: Growth and development of term children born with low birth weight: effects of genetic and environmental factors. J Pediatr 133:67, 1998.

170. Walther FJ: Growth and development of term disproportionate small-for-gestational age infants at the age of 7 years. Early Hum Dev 18:1, 1988.

171. Robertson CMT, Etches PC, Kyle JM: Eight-year school performance and growth of preterm, small for gestational age infants: a comparative study with subjects matched for birth weight or for gestational age. J Pediatr 116:19, 1990.

172. Low JA, Handley-Derry MH, Burke SO, et al: Association of intrauterine fetal growth retardation and learning deficits at age 9 to 11 years. Am J Obstet Gynecol 167:1499, 1992.

173. Dobbing J: The later development of the brain and its vulnerability. *In* Davis JA, Dobbing J (eds): Scientific Foundations

of Paediatrics. Philadelphia, WB Saunders Company, 1974, p 565.

174. Fancourt R, Campbell S, Harvey D, et al: Follow-up study of small-for-dates babies. BMJ 1:1435, 1976.

175. Law CM, Barker DJP, Osmond C, et al: Early growth and abdominal fatness in adult life. J Epidemiol Community Health 46:184, 1992.

176. Nathanielsz PW: Life in the Womb: The Origin of Health and Disease. Ithaca, NY, Promethian Press, 1999, p 59.

177. Barker DJP, Osmond C: Infant mortality, childhood nutrition and ischaemic heart disease in England and Wales. Lancet 1: 1077, 1986.

178. Phipps K, Barker DJP, Hales CHD, et al: Fetal growth and impaired glucose tolerance in men and women. Diabetologia 36:225, 1993.

179. Barker DJP, Hales CN, Fall CHD, et al: Type 2 diabetes mellitus, hypertension and hyperlipidemia (syndrome X): relation to reduced fetal growth. Diabetologia 36:62, 1993.

180. Barker DJP, Gluckman PD, Godfrey KM, et al: Fetal nutri-

tion and cardiovascular disease in adult life. Lancet 341:938, 1993.

181. Hubinont C, Nicolini U, Fisk NM, et al: Endocrine pancreatic function in growth retarded fetuses. Obstet Gynecol 77:541, 1991.

182. Van Assche FA, Aerts L, Holemans K: Fetal growth retardation is associated with a reduced function of insulin producing B cells and may explain insulin resistance in later life [abstract]. Am J Obstet Gynecol 170:315, 1994.

183. Phillips DI, Barker DJ: Association between low birthweight and high resting pulse in adult life: is the sympathetic nervous system involved in programming the insulin resistance syndrome? Diabet Med 14:673, 1997.

184. Clark PM, Hindmarsh PC, Shiell AW, et al: Size at birth and adrenocortical function in childhood. Clin Endocrinol 45:721, 1996.

185. Phillips DI, Barker DJ, Fall CH, et al: Elevated plasma cortisol concentrations: a link between low birth weight and the insulin resistance syndrome. J Clin Endocrinol Metab 83:757, 1998.

Alloimmunization in Pregnancy

MARC JACKSON AND D. WARE BRANCH

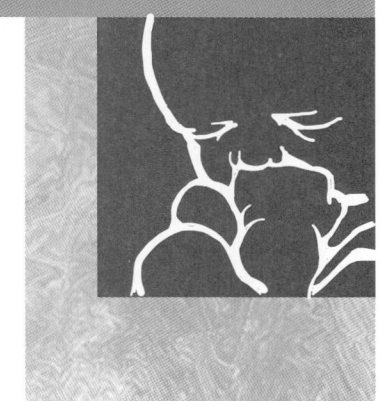

This chapter reviews the causes and management of alloimmunization in pregnancy. Topics included are Rh alloimmunization, sensitization caused by other erythrocyte antigens, and platelet alloimmunization. Rh alloimmunization is emphasized because it remains a leading cause of perinatal death from hemolytic disease. Also, to a great degree, the principles of pathophysiology and management discussed under Rh alloimmunization apply to the other causes of alloimmunization. With regard to Rh alloimmunization, the following are discussed: the genetics and biochemistry of the Rh antigen, the causes of Rh alloimmunization, the use of Rh-immune globulin, and the assessment and management of the Rh-alloimmunized pregnancy. Throughout this chapter, the traditional term *sensitization* is used interchangeably with *alloimmunization*.

and passed into the maternal circulation, causing her to develop the agglutinin. This was the first suggestion that erythroblastosis fetalis was an alloimmune disorder, and within 3 years the role of alloimmunization in the pathogenesis of erythroblastosis was established.[4]

Although many erythocyte antigens have subsequently been described, only a few are clinically important causes of maternal alloimmunization leading to hemolysis of fetal and neonatal cells. Fortunately, the number of cases of fetal and neonatal hemolytic disease resulting from Rh antigen incompatibility has greatly decreased because of the widespread use of Rh-immunoglobulin prophylaxis. This has led to an increase in the importance of the "minor antigens" of the erythrocyte membrane as a cause of alloimmunization.

HISTORY OF ERYTHROBLASTOSIS FETALIS

In 1932, Diamond et al.[1] observed that erythroblastosis fetalis was associated with fetal edema, neonatal hyperbilirubinemia, and neonatal anemia. Later, Darrow[2] proposed that these related conditions were caused by the passage of maternal antibodies across the placenta and that it was the antibodies that caused the destruction of the fetal erythrocytes. In 1939, Levine and Stetson[3] observed the presence of atypical agglutinins in the serum of a woman who had just delivered a hydropic stillborn infant; these agglutinins were found to be active against her husband's erythrocytes even though he was of the same ABO blood group. Levine and Stetson suggested that an immunizing property in the blood or tissues of the fetus had been inherited from the father

GENETICS AND BIOCHEMISTRY OF THE Rh ANTIGEN

Nomenclature

In 1940, Landsteiner and Wiener[5] announced that they had produced rabbit immune sera to rhesus monkey erythrocytes that, even after adsorption, agglutinated the majority (85 percent) of human erythrocytes; they designated this newly discovered property of serum the *Rh factor*. Agglutinated cells were called *Rh-positive*. It is now recognized that the "Rh factor" is an antibody directed against an erythrocyte surface antigen of the rhesus blood group system.

Since its discovery, the development of an adequate nomenclature for the Rh blood group system has been hampered by its high degree of polymorphism. Five major antigens can be identified with known typing sera, and there are many variant antigens. Unfortunately, three different systems of nomenclature have been suggested since the discovery of the Rh antigen. Two of these, the Fisher-Race system and the Wiener system, were established during the 1940s and are the ones most frequently used in the literature. The HLA-like system of Rosenfield and colleagues[6] was proposed in 1962.

In obstetrics, the Fisher-Race nomenclature is best known. Although this system has some limitations in terms of our current understanding of genetics and in its classification of the numerous variant antigens, it is well suited to understanding the inheritance of the Rh antigen and the clinical management of Rh alloimmunization.[7]

The Fisher-Race nomenclature assumes the presence of three genetic loci, each with two major alleles. The antigens produced by these alleles were originally identified by specific antisera and have been lettered C, c, D, E, and e. No antiserum specific for a "d" antigen has been found, and use of the letter "d" indicates the absence of a discernible allelic product. Anti-C, anti-c, anti-D, anti-E, and anti-e designate specific antibodies directed against the respective antigens.

An Rh gene complex is described by the three appropriate letters; thus eight gene complexes could exist (listed in decreasing order of frequency in the white population): CDe, cde, cDE, cDe, Cde, cdE, CDE, and CdE. Genotypes ere indicated as pairs of gene complexes, such as CDe/cde. Certain genotypes, and thus certain phenotypes, are more prevalent than others. The genotypes CDe/cde and CDe/CDe are the most common, with approximately 55 percent of all whites having the CcDe or CDe phenotype (Table 26–1).[8] The genotype CdE has actually never been demonstrated.[7] Although the alleles are always written in the order C(c), D, E(e), the actual order for the genes on chromosome 1 coding for the antigens is D, C(c), E(e).

According to the Fisher-Race concept, the Rh antigen complex is the final expression of a group of at least five possible antigens (C, D, E, c, e). The vast majority of Rh alloimmunization causing transfusion reactions or serious hemolytic disease of the fetus and newborn is the result of incompatibility with respect to the D antigen. For this reason, common convention holds that *Rh-positive* indicates the presence of the D antigen and *Rh-negative* indicates the absence of D antigen on erythrocytes.

Working at the same time as Fisher and Race, Wiener[9] developed a system of nomenclature based on the assumption of only one genetic locus. In the Wiener system, the eight genotypes are designated (in decreasing order of frequency in the white population) R^1, r, R^2, R^0, r', r", R^z, and r^v (Table 26–1).

In the 1970s, Rosenfield and co-workers[6,10] suggested that none of the previously described models could explain the vast quantitative differences observed in the

Table 26–1. FREQUENCY OF Rh PHENOTYPES AND GENOTYPES AMONG WHITES

Phenotype	Population Frequency (%)	Frequency Within Genotype	(%)
CcDe	35	CDe/cde (R^1/r)	94
		CDe/cDe (R^1/R^0)	6
		cDe/Cde (R^0/r')	<1
CDe	20	CDe/CDe (R^1/R^1)	95
		CDe/Cde (R^1/r')	5
ce	16	cde/cde (r/r)	100
CcDEe	13	CDe/cDE (R^1/R^2)	89
		CDe/cdE (R^1/r")	7
		cDE/Cde (R^2/r')	2
		CDE/cde (R^z/r)	1
		CDE/cDe (R^z/R^0)	<1
cDEe	10	cDE/cde (R^2/r)	93
		cDE/cDe (R^2/R^0)	6
		cDe/cdE (R^0/r")	1
cDE	3	cDE/cDE (R^2/R^2)	86
		cDE/cdE (R^2/r")	14
cDe	2	cDe/cde (R^0/r)	97
		cDe/cDe (R^0/R^0)	3
Cce	1	Cde/cde (r'/r)	100

expression of Rh antigens. Furthermore, they pointed out that genetic concepts such as the operon model of gene function with nonlinked regulator genes were poorly accommodated by the simple mendelian model of Fisher and Race. Rosenfield therefore proposed an updated system of nomenclature that numbered the antigens, designated Rh1 through Rh48.

Unique Rh antibodies have been used to identify more than 30 antigenic variants in the Rh blood group system. Two of the most common (albeit infrequent in absolute terms) are the C^w antigen and the D^u antigen, which is now referred to as *weak D*. The latter is a heterogeneous group of clinically important D antigen variants most often found in blacks. The erythrocytes of most weak D–positive individuals appear to have a quantitative decrease in expression of the normal D antigen, although some weak D variants are significantly different, antigenically speaking, from D. Thus, it appears that there are at least two cellular expressions responsible for the weak D phenotype, including a reduction in the number of D antigen sites with all epitopes represented, and expression of only some of the various D antigen epitopes with some epitopes missing. Weak D–positive erythrocytes can bind anti-D typing sera, but in some cases only by sensitive indirect antiglobulin methods. At least some weak D–positive patients are capable of producing anti-D, presumably by sensitization to missing D epitopes. This could result in a weak D–positive mother becoming sensitized to her D–positive fetus, but such an occurrence is exceedingly rare.

Genetic Expression

The genetic locus for the Rh antigen complex is on the short arm of chromosome 1.[11,12] Within the Rh locus are two distinct structural genes adjacent to one another, RhCcEe and RhD. These two genes likely share a single genetic ancestor, as they are identical in more than 95 percent of their coding sequences.[13] The first gene codes for the C/c and E/e antigens, and the second gene codes for the D antigen.

Expression of the D antigen occurs if one (heterozygous) or both (homozygous) chromosome 1 contains a normal RhD gene sequence. Patients who are D-negative lack the normal RhD gene sequence on both their chromosomes. Therefore, they cannot transcribe this region, which is responsible for producing the D antigen.

The expression of the Rh antigen on the erythrocyte membrane is genetically based, not only in terms of the structure of the antigen but also in terms of the number of specific Rh-antigen sites (e.g., D, E, C, c, or e). Several genetic factors have been shown to alter the number of specific Rh-antigen sites; these include the gene dose, the relative position of the alleles, and the presence or absence of regulator genes.

There is a relatively constant number of Rh antigen sites available on the erythrocyte surface, totaling about 100,000 sites per cell; these sites appear to be approximately evenly divided between C(c), D, and E(e) antigens.[14,15]

Gene dosage has an effect on the number of specific Rh antigen sites that express antigen; individuals who are homozygous for a particular genotype have more antigen sites than individuals who are heterozygous.[16] For example, the erythrocytes of individuals who are homozygous for the c allele have twice as many c antigen sites expressed as are found on the erythrocytes of heterozygotes. Similar observations have been made with regard to the other alleles (E, e, and C).[16,17]

An effect of allelic interaction on Rh antigen sites has been described: erythrocytes of genotype CDe/cde express less D antigen than do the erythrocytes of genotype cDE/cde.[18] Thus, the presence of the C antigen seems to affect the expression of the D antigen. Similarly, individuals of genotype CDe/cDE express less C antigen than individuals of genotype CDe/cde.[8] In addition, genes other than those coding for the Rh antigen may affect the final antigenic expression; two independently segregating regulator genes have been described.[10]

Biochemistry and Immunology

The Rh antigens on human erythrocytes are polypeptides embedded in the lipid phase of the erythrocyte membrane, distributed throughout the membrane in a nonrandom fashion. D antigen sites are spaced in a lattice-like pattern across the red cell membrane, at a mean distance of 92 nm in RhD heterozygotes and 64 nm in homozygotes.[19,20] The Rh polypeptides are polymorphic, with the molecular weight of the D antigen being approximately 31,900 daltons and the C(c) and E(e) polypeptides having a molecular weight of about 33,100 daltons.[21] The final tertiary structure and antigenic expression of the protein are dependent on its association with lipids in the membrane, and in this context it may be thought of as a protein–lipid complex, or proteolipid.[22,23] It appears that most of the Rh polypeptide lies within the phospholipid bilayer of the erythrocyte membrane, spanning the membrane 13 times, with short segments extending outside the red cell and extruding into the cytoplasm.[24,25]

The D antigen appears very early in embryonic life and has been demonstrated on the red blood cells of a 38-day-old fetus.[26] The antigen is also expressed early in the erythroid cell series; with ^{125}I-labeled anti-D, pronormoblasts have been shown to contain D antigen.[27]

Ten different D antigen epitopes have been identified or deduced using human monoclonal anti-D antibodies, and as many as 30 may exist.[28,29] One hypothesis suggests that these different epitopes are part of the same protein–lipid complex, but are more or less expressed according to the depth that the polypeptide portion is embedded in the red cell membrane lipid bilayer.[30] It is possible that some of the immunologic variation in the Rh blood group system (and fetal hemolytic disease) is explained by the variable expression of the D antigen epitopes and the specificity of the antibodies formed against them.

The precise function of the Rh antigens is unknown, although they probably have a role in maintaining red cell membrane integrity. Rh_{null} erythrocytes, which lack all of the Rh antigens, manifest several membrane defects. The Rh antigens may interact with a membrane adenosine triphosphatase,[23] possibly functioning as part of a proton or cation pump that controls volume or electrolyte flux across the erythrocyte membrane. Supporting this hypothesis, Rh_{null} erythrocytes have increased osmotic fragility and abnormal shapes.[31] It has also been proposed that Rh antigens regulate the asymmetric distribution of different phospholipids through the red cell membrane as a component of the enzyme phosphatidyl flippase.[32,33]

CAUSES OF Rh ALLOIMMUNIZATION

For Rh alloimmunization to occur in a pregnancy, at least three circumstances must exist:

1. The fetus must have Rh-positive erythrocytes, and the mother must have Rh-negative erythrocytes.
2. A sufficient number of fetal erythrocytes must gain access to the maternal circulation.
3. The mother must have the immunogenic capacity to produce antibody directed against the D antigen.

Incidence of Rh-Incompatible Pregnancy

About 15 percent of whites of European extraction are Rh-negative; only 5 to 8 percent of American blacks and 1 to 2 percent of Asians and Native Americans are Rh-negative. In the white population, an Rh-negative woman has about an 85 percent chance of mating with an Rh-positive man. About 60 percent of Rh-positive men are heterozygous and 40 percent are homozygous at the D locus. Given that one half of conceptions due to heterozygous men will be Rh-positive, the overall chance of an Rh-positive man producing an Rh-positive fetus is about 70 percent. Thus, without knowing the father's blood type, an Rh-negative woman has about a 60 percent chance of bearing an Rh-positive fetus (0.85 × 0.70). Among whites, the net result is that about 10 percent of pregnancies are Rh incompatible (0.15 × 0.60). However, because sufficient fetomaternal hemorrhage and a subsequent maternal antibody response do not occur in every case, less than 20 percent of incompatible pregnancies eventuate in maternal sensitization. Thus, in the era before Rh-immune globulin prophylaxis, about 1 percent of pregnant women had anti-D antibody.

Fetomaternal Hemorrhage

Although transplacental passage of fetal erythrocytes was proposed to be the cause of maternal alloimmunization in the 1940s,[4] it was not until the mid-1950s that fetal erythrocytes were first demonstrated in the maternal circulation.[34] Since then, numerous studies have confirmed that fetal red cells gain access to the maternal circulation during pregnancy and the immediate postpartum period. Fetomaternal hemorrhage in a volume sufficient to cause alloimmunization is most common at delivery, occurring in about 15 to 50 percent of births.[34-37] In more than half of these intrapartum fetomaternal bleeds, the amount of fetal blood entering the maternal circulation is 0.1 ml or less.[37,38] However, in 0.2 to 1 percent of cases, the estimated volume of fetomaternal hemorrhage is 30 ml or more.[35, 39, 40] Clinical factors such as cesarean delivery, multiple gestation, bleeding placenta previa or abruption, manual removal of the placenta, and intrauterine manipulation may increase the chance of substantial hemorrhage. However, the majority of excessive fetomaternal hemorrhages occur in patients without risk factors who have an uncomplicated vaginal delivery.[40,41]

The amount of fetomaternal hemorrhage necessary to cause alloimmunization varies from patient to patient, probably due to the immunogenic capacity of the Rh-positive erythrocytes and the immune responsiveness of the mother. As little as 0.1 ml of Rh-positive red blood cells has been shown to sensitize some Rh-negative volunteers, and about 3 percent of women found to have 0.1 ml of fetal erythrocytes in their circulation after an Rh-incompatible delivery develop anti-D antibodies within 6 to 12 months.[37]

Overall, about 16 percent of Rh-negative women will become alloimmunized by their first Rh-incompatible (ABO-compatible) pregnancy if not treated with Rh-immune globulin.[38] Half of these women respond with the production of sufficient anti-D antibody to be detectable within the first 6 months after delivery; in the remainder, anti-D is not detected until early in the next incompatible pregnancy. In this latter group, sensitization likely occurred during the first pregnancy, but the primary immune response was too slight for detectable antibody levels to develop. Though not all Rh-negative women bearing Rh-positive infants will become sensitized, the risk of sensitization approaches 50 percent after several incompatible pregnancies.

Even without labor or obvious disruption of the choriodecidual junction, antepartum fetomaternal hemorrhage occurs in sufficient volume to result in alloimmunization in a small percentage of cases. In one large series, fetomaternal hemorrhage was detected in the first trimester in 7 percent of patients, in 16 percent of patients during the second trimester, and in 29 percent of the third-trimester determinations.[34] The result of this antepartum fetomaternal hemorrhage is an overall rate of Rh sensitization of about 1 to 2 percent before delivery.[42] However, antepartum sensitization rarely occurs before the third trimester.

Fetomaternal hemorrhage leading to alloimmunization has also been described with abortion and tubal pregnancy.[43-46] As mentioned above, fetal Rh antigens are present at least by the 38th day after conception and, assuming that as little as 0.1 ml of fetal blood can cause alloimmunization, a fetomaternal hemorrhage leading to sensitization could occur by the seventh week after the last menses.[47] In one case, a significant number of fetal red blood cells was demonstrated in the maternal circulation after an elective termination of pregnancy at 6 weeks after the last menses.[48]

Estimates of the incidence and the amount of fetomaternal hemorrhage after spontaneous abortion have varied, but review of the literature suggests that between 5 and 25 percent of spontaneous abortions result in detectable fetomaternal hemorrhage.[36] For the unsensitized Rh-negative woman, a spontaneous first-trimester abortion carries a 3 to 4 percent risk of alloimmunization.[49] Induced abortions are also likely to produce detectable fetomaternal hemorrhage (in 7 to 27 percent of cases); the overall risk of sensitization is about 5 percent.[46] In the second trimester, pregnancy termination by either saline injection or hysterotomy is associated with significant fetomaternal hemorrhage.[45,46]

Threatened abortion in the first trimester may also increase the risk of sensitization. Fetomaternal hemorrhage can be demonstrated in 11 to 45 percent of such patients,[50,51] and a case of apparent sensitization following threatened first-trimester miscarriage has been reported.[52]

As discussed below, all Rh-negative unsensitized women should received 50 μg of Rh-immune globulin within 72 hours of induced or spontaneous first-trimester abortion. Patients in the second trimester, 13 weeks or more, are routinely given a full dose, 300 μg.

Ectopic pregnancy can result in alloimmunization in a susceptible woman.[43] The risk of significant fetomaternal hemorrhage may be greater in cases of ruptured tubal pregnancy, presumably because of the absorption of fetal erythrocytes into the maternal circulation across the peritoneum.[53]

Amniocentesis in the second and third trimesters is associated with fetomaternal hemorrhage in 15 to 25 percent of cases, even when ultrasound is used to identify placental location.[54,55] Alloimmunization occurring after amniocentesis has been reported.[56]

Maternal Immunologic Response

At least two characteristics affect whether alloimmunization will occur in a susceptible Rh-negative woman. First, as many as 30 percent of Rh-negative individuals appear to be immunologic "nonresponders" who will not become sensitized, even when challenged with large volumes of Rh-positive blood.[57,58] Second, ABO incompatibility exerts a protective effect against the development of Rh sensitization.[59] Levine and Stetson[3] are credited with first recognizing the association between ABO incompatibility and a lower than expected incidence of Rh sensitization, and fetomaternal ABO incompatibility is now well accepted as being partially protective.[59,60]

Two mechanisms explaining the protective effect of ABO incompatibility have been proposed. The first suggests that the ABO-incompatible fetal cells are more rapidly cleared from the maternal circulation so that trapping of the antigen in the spleen, where sensitization can be initiated, does not occur. Although the incidence of fetomaternal hemorrhage is no different in ABO-incompatible pregnancies, the number of fetal cells in the maternal circulation is less than in ABO-compatible pregnancies, suggesting an increased clearance rate.[35,36] A second mechanism for the protective effect of ABO incompatibility proposes that maternal anti-A or anti-B antibodies damage or alter the fetal Rh antigen so that it is no longer immunogenic.[60]

Whatever the mechanism, ABO incompatibility diminishes the risk of alloimmunization to about 1.5 to 2 percent after the delivery of an Rh-positive fetus.[61] This effect is most pronounced in matings in which the mother is type O and the father is type A, type B, or type AB.[62]

THE USE OF Rh-IMMUNE GLOBULIN

The principle that a passively administered antibody will prevent active immunization by its specific antigen is termed *antibody-mediated immune suppression* (AMIS) and was well known to immunologists for decades before being applied to the prevention of Rh disease. During the early 1960s, Freda et al.[63] in the United States and Clarke et al.[64] in Great Britain simultaneously undertook to evaluate AMIS in humans. Both groups achieved a high degree of protection from alloimmunization by administering anti-D immune globulin (Rh-immune globulin) to Rh-negative male volunteers who had been infused with Rh-positive red cells.[63,64] In 1963, Pollack et al.[65] established that 300 μg of Rh-immune globulin would reliably prevent alloimmunization in male volunteers who had received 10 ml of Rh-positive cells. By extrapolation of the data, Pollack et al. showed that 20 μg of Rh-immune globulin per milliliter of fetal erythrocytes or 10 μg/ml of whole fetal blood was required to prevent alloimmunization. Thus, the rule was established that 10 μg Rh-immune globulin should be given for every 1 ml of fetal blood in the maternal circulation.

The early trials using AMIS to prevent alloimmunization in Rh-negative women delivering Rh-positive infants were excitingly successful.[66-68] The administration of Rh-immune globulin within 72 hours of delivery reduced alloimmunization to less than 1.5 percent in the Rh-negative women who were followed through a subsequent incompatible pregnancy. This represented a 7- to 10-fold decrease in alloimmunization compared with untreated controls. Although 300 μg or more of Rh-immune globulin was used, it has subsequently been shown that a dose of 100 to 150 μg is probably adequate for routine use.[68,69] Nonetheless, the standard approved dose for Rh prophylaxis in the United States remains 300 μg.

The 72-hour time limit set for the postpartum administration of Rh-immune globulin is an artifact of the design of the early male prisoner volunteer studies. Prison officials would only allow the investigators to visit the volunteers at 3-day intervals[70]; thus, the use of Rh-immune globulin at intervals of more than 3 days after a challenge with Rh-positive cells was never extensively evaluated. However, to be effective, Rh-immune globulin must be given before the primary immune response is established. The time required to mount a primary immune response doubtlessly varies from case to case, and it is prudent to administer Rh-immune globulin to appropriate mothers as soon as possible after delivery. If for some reason the neonatal Rh status is unknown by the third day after delivery, it is preferable to administer Rh-immune globulin to an Rh-negative mother rather than to continue to await the neonatal results. Finally, if an Rh-negative mother who is a candidate for Rh-immune prophylaxis is mistakenly not treated within the recommended 72 hours following delivery, she may be given Rh-immune globulin up to 14 to 28 days after delivery in an effort to avoid sensitization.[71]

Antepartum Prophylaxis

Early trials showed that 1 to 2 percent of susceptible women became sensitized in spite of postpartum Rh-immune prophylaxis. The majority of these "prophylaxis failures" resulted from antepartum fetomaternal hemorrhage. In an effort to address this problem, Bowman and colleagues[72] in Canada conducted an antepartum Rh prophylaxis trial in which 300 μg of Rh-immune globulin was given at 28 and 34 weeks' gestation. Antenatal sensitization was reduced from 1.8 to 0.1 percent. Subsequently, it was shown that 300 μg of Rh-immune globulin given only at 28 weeks' gestation is nearly as effective.[73] Reviewing several large studies, the 1979 McMaster University Conference on the prevention of Rh disease confirmed that the antepartum administration of Rh-immune globulin could reduce the risk of antepartum alloimmunization by more than half.[42] In more than 18,000 control cases, the incidence of antepartum sensitization was 1.05 percent, whereas in the 10,000 treated cases it was only 0.17 percent.

Despite these results, antepartum Rh prophylaxis remains somewhat controversial. From a safety perspective, there is a risk of infection (although exceedingly small) to the donors who provide plasma for human anti-D immunoglobulin, which is produced by immunization and antibody boosting by injecting incompatible Rh-positive red cells into Rh-negative volunteers. Also, Hensleigh[74] has argued that the safety of Rh-immune globulin prophylaxis to the recipient mother and fetus has not been convincingly demonstrated. However, decades of experience with Rh-immune globulin have not produced any suspicion of detrimental effects, and a systematic evaluation of a large cohort of women receiving Rh-immune globulin failed to detect any untoward side effects.[75]

The cost-effectiveness of antepartum prophylaxis has also been addressed. Setting aside the ethical issues of withholding Rh-immune globulin prophylaxis because of financial concerns, it nonetheless appears that routine antepartum prophylaxis is much less expensive than managing later sensitized pregnancies.[71,76] Baskett and Parsons[77] calculated that the cost per case of Rh alloimmunization prevented was less than half of the cost per case treated, with 80 percent of treatment costs being accounted for by neonatal intensive care.

More recently, monoclonal antibody techniques have been used to produce human anti-D.[78] This technology has the potential to produce a standardized antibody in essentially unlimited supply. Human donor risk will be eliminated, and production costs seem certain to decrease, improving the cost/benefit ratio even further. Initial in vitro testing of monoclonal anti-D has been favorable,[79] and preliminary human trials to determine effectiveness in blocking endogenous anti-D production are underway.[80] At this point, though, it is uncertain whether monoclonal anti-D will be as effective as human-derived polyclonal Rh-immune globulin, and routine clinical use of monoclonal anti-D is likely years away.

Mechanism of Action

The precise mechanism of AMIS is not clearly understood. There are three theories: (1) antigen deviation, (2) antigen blocking–competitive inhibition, and (3) central inhibition. The hypothesis that AMIS works by deviation of the antigen away from the immunologic apparatus that is responsible for the formation of antibody was first suggested by Race and Sanger.[7] Support for this theory came from the observation of an increased clearance of ^{51}Cr-labeled Rh-positive red cells in Rh-negative volunteers who were treated with Rh-immune globulin. This increase in clearance was presumed to be caused by intravascular hemolysis that resulted in the destruction or alteration of the Rh antigen so that it did not incite the production of anti-D antibody. However, it is now known that IgG anti-D does not cause intravascular hemolysis of Rh-positive cells; instead, the intact, antibody-coated cells are removed from the circulation by the spleen or lymph nodes,[81] the very site of antibody formation.

Antigen deviation could also occur by the phagocytosis of the antibody-coated Rh-positive cells; this could, and presumably does, occur in the spleen and lymph nodes. However, macrophage ingestion and processing of antigen are essential for immunization to occur, and passive immunization that is directed against red cell antigens has been shown to be specific.[82] Also, if antigen deviation through phagocytosis was the primary mechanism of AMIS, it seems likely that all red cell antigens would be destroyed. For these reasons, antigen deviation is probably not the mechanism of AMIS.

Antigen blocking by anti-D antibody is also not the probable mechanism for AMIS: antibody preparations that lack the Fc portion have been shown to bind avidly to antigen, yet they do not suppress the immune response.[83] In addition, with the usual doses of anti-D used to effect immune suppression, less than 20 percent of the Rh antigen is bound.[82]

The most likely mechanism for AMIS is that of central inhibition, as proposed by Gorman and elaborated upon by Pollack.[82] In this hypothesis, fetal erythrocytes coated with exogenously administered anti-D are filtered out of the circulation by the spleen and lymph nodes. The increase in the local concentrations of anti-D bound to the D antigen appears to "suppress" the primary immune response by interrupting the commitment of B cells to IgG-producing plasma cell clones. Exactly how this suppression is effected is poorly understood, but the binding of antibody–antigen complexes (anti-D–D antigen complexes) by immune effector cells results in the release of cytokines that inhibit the proliferation of B cells specific for the antigen. The process appears to be dependent on the presence of the Fc receptor on IgG, as Fab fragments do not inhibit AMIS.

MANAGEMENT OF THE UNSENSITIZED Rh-NEGATIVE PREGNANT WOMAN

At the first prenatal visit of each pregnancy, every patient should have her ABO blood group, Rh type, and antibody screen checked (Fig. 26–1). It is essential that these determinations are made in each subsequent pregnancy, as previous maternal antibody screening is not an adequate assessment.

If the patient is Rh-negative, weak D-negative, and has no demonstrable antibody, she is a candidate for 300 μg Rh-immune globulin as prophylaxis at 28 weeks' gestation and again immediately after birth. It is the recommendation of the American Association of Blood Banks that a second antibody screen be obtained before administration of Rh-immune globulin at the beginning of the third trimester,[84] to ensure that the patient is not already sensitized and producing anti-D, but this second screen is probably clinically unnecessary.[85] Similarly, a repeat antepartum antibody screen at 35 to 36 weeks' gestation is unnecessary. Routine screening of Rh-positive patients for irregular antibodies at the beginning of the third trimester is not warranted.[86]

When the Rh-negative, unsensitized patient is admit-

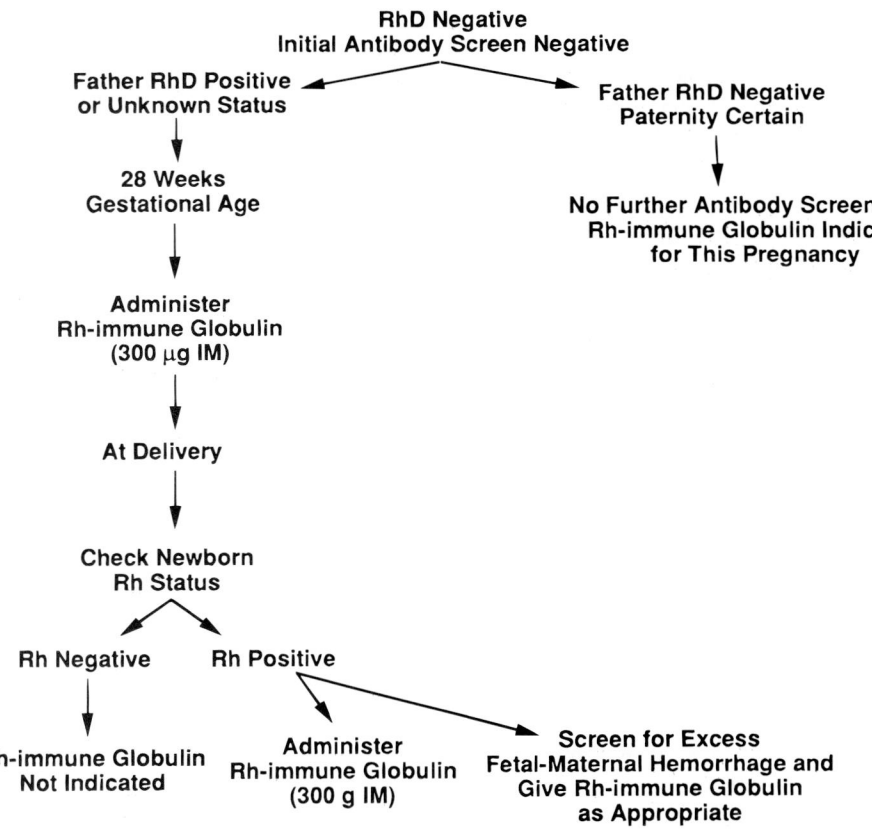

Figure 26–1. Flow diagram outlining the management of Rh-negative, non-immunized pregnancies.

ted for delivery, an antibody screen is routinely done. If the antibody screen is negative and the newborn is Rh-positive or weak D-positive, the patient should again be given Rh-immune globulin.

Because up to 1 percent of deliveries result in a fetomaternal hemorrhage of greater than 30 ml (the largest volume of fetal blood adequately covered by a standard 300 μg dose of Rh-immune globulin), Rh-negative patients with an Rh-positive or weak D–positive newborn should be screened for "excessive" fetomaternal hemorrhage immediately postpartum.[84] An erythrocyte rosette test has been shown to be a simple and sensitive method for detecting excessive fetomaternal bleeding,[40] and most laboratories use one of the commercially available versions of the erythrocyte rosette test as a screening test. For patients with a positive screen, Kleihauer-Betke testing can be used to quantitate the volume of fetal red cells in the maternal circulation. In this way, the appropriate dose of Rh-immune globulin can be calculated. If the volume of hemorrhage is estimated to be greater than 30 ml whole blood, a dose of Rh-immune globulin calculated at 10 μg/ml of whole fetal blood should be administered.

Management of the weak D–positive patient is sometimes confusing. A weak D–positive mother who delivers an Rh-positive infant is not at significant risk of Rh sensitization, probably because the weak D antigen is actually an incompletely expressed D antigen. Thus, weak D–positive mothers are clinically treated as if they were Rh-positive, and they do not require Rh-immune globulin. However, occasionally a woman previously typed as Rh-negative is unexpectedly found to be weak D–positive during pregnancy or after delivery. In this situation, the clinician should be suspicious that the patient's "new" weak D–positive status is actually due to a large number of Rh-positive fetal cells in the maternal circulation. Appropriate diagnostic studies should be performed, and if fetomaternal hemorrhage is found, the mother should be treated with Rh-immune globulin.

Because of the risk of significant fetomaternal hemorrhage with abortion or ectopic pregnancy, Rh-immune globulin prophylaxis is indicated if the patient is Rh-negative and unsensitized. If the pregnancy loss occurs at 12 weeks' gestation or less, a 50-μg dose of Rh-immune globulin is adequate to cover the entire fetal blood volume[87] (Table 26–2). If the gestational age is unknown or beyond 12 weeks, a full 300 μg dose of Rh-immune globulin is indicated.

Management of the Rh-negative patient with threatened miscarriage in the first trimester is controversial, and there is no clear consensus or evidence-based recommendation on use of Rh-immune globulin.[85] Even though fetal–maternal hemorrhage can occur with threatened abortion before 12 weeks,[51] documented sensitization is extremely uncommon. In the United

Table 26–2. RECOMMENDED DOSES OF Rh-IMMUNE GLOBULIN

Indication	Dose (μg) of Rh-Immune Globulin
First-trimester spontaneous or induced abortion	50
First-trimester chorionic villus sampling	50
Ectopic pregnancy	
Prior to 12 weeks' gestation	50
After 12 weeks' gestation	300
Amniocentesis, second-trimester chorionic villus sampling, or other intrauterine procedures	300
Abdominal trauma or fetal death in the second or third trimester	300
Fetomaternal hemorrhage	10 per estimated ml of whole fetal blood

From American College of Obstetricians and Gynecologists: Prevention of RhD alloimmunization. ACOG Practice Bulletin 4. Washington, DC, American College of Obstetricians and Gynecologists, 1999.

Kingdom, current recommendations are that Rh-immune globulin is unnecessary with threatened miscarriage before 12 weeks, although anti-D can be considered for patients with heavy or repeated bleeding late in the first trimester.[88]

An Rh-negative, unsensitized patient who has antepartum bleeding or suffers an unexplained second- or third-trimester fetal death should receive 300 μg Rh-immune globulin and be evaluated for the possibility of massive fetomaternal hemorrhage. If fetal cells are found in the maternal circulation, Rh-immune globulin is indicated at a dose of 10 μg per estimated milliliter of whole fetal blood (Table 26–2).

Antenatal Rh-immune globulin is indicated at the time of chorionic villus sampling or amniocentesis in an Rh-negative, unsensitized patient. For first-trimester procedures, 50 μg of Rh-immune globulin is protective. However, for second- or third-trimester procedures, a full 300-μg dose is indicated even if the procedure is not associated with detectable hemorrhage (Table 26–2). When amniocentesis is performed within 72 hours of delivery, such as for the determination of fetal pulmonary maturity, Rh-immune globulin may be withheld and administered immediately postpartum if the infant is found to be Rh-positive or D[u] positive; if delivery is to be delayed for more than 72 hours, Rh-immune globulin should be given.

Since Rh-immune globulin became available in the United States in the late 1960s, the incidence of Rh alloimmunization has been drastically reduced. Antepartum sensitizations have markedly declined with the now widespread practice of antepartum prophylaxis; however, postpartum prophylaxis failures still represent a significant problem.[89] The routine use of postpartum screening programs to detect "excessive" fetomaternal hemorrhage will likely avoid the majority of these postpartum sensitizations.

Failure to administer Rh-immune globulin when it is indicated also remains a problem.[89] In one study, nearly one fourth of the cases of new sensitization were due to this inexcusable oversight.[90] It is imperative that the physician be responsible for determining the Rh type in every patient who undergoes abortion, chorionic villus sampling, amniocentesis, blood transfusion, or pregnancy.

THE Rh-ALLOIMMUNIZED PREGNANCY: ASSESSMENT OF THE FETUS

Any patient with an anti-D antibody titer of greater than 1:4 should be considered Rh sensitized and her pregnancies managed accordingly. The eventual goal of management is to minimize fetal and neonatal morbidity and mortality. Patients (fetuses) can be roughly categorized as (1) those who are unlikely to require intrauterine intervention and who can be delivered when they achieve pulmonary maturity and (2) those who will likely have moderate to severe hemolytic disease and require intrauterine transfusion and early delivery. An accurate assignment of gestational age using menstrual dates and early ultrasound is crucial in management of the Rh-alloimmunized pregnancy, as the timing of amniocentesis, umbilical cord blood sampling, in utero treatment, and delivery will depend on it.

Determination of the Fetal Antigen Status

When first confronted with an Rh-immunized pregnancy, the possibility that the fetus might be Rh-negative and therefore not need expensive and potentially hazardous procedures should be considered. If the woman might have become sensitized during a pregnancy fathered by another partner or by a mismatched blood transfusion, determining the paternal Rh antigen status is reasonable, since the father of the current pregnancy might be Rh-negative. If he is Rh-negative (and it is certain that he is the father of the fetus), further assessment and intervention are unnecessary. If the father is Rh-positive, the blood bank laboratory can reliably estimate the probability that he is heterozygous for the D antigen by using Rh antisera to determine his most likely genotype (Table 26–1). Alternatively, DNA analysis can be used to determine his zygosity with a high degree of certainty.[91] Of course, if the man has

fathered Rh-negative children, he is a known heterozygote.

If the father is homozygous for the D antigen, all his children will be Rh-positive; if he is heterozygous, there is a 50 percent likelihood that each pregnancy will have an Rh-negative fetus who is at no risk of anemia and does not require further assessment or treatment.

In the past, cordocentesis with analysis of fetal red blood cells was required to determine fetal antigen status. Some authors advocated routine umbilical cord blood sampling for fetal Rh antigen status at 18 to 20 weeks' gestation in all Rh-immunized pregnancies with a heterozygous father.[92] However, this approach never gained widespread acceptance, at least in part because of the increased risks of fetal loss and fetomaternal hemorrhage associated with cordocentesis.[93]

More recently, advances in molecular genetics have made it possible to determine fetal Rh status without direct analysis of fetal red blood cells. The Rh locus on chromosome 1p34-p36 has been cloned,[94] and polymerase chain reaction (PCR) now allows determination of fetal Rh status from the uncultured amniocytes in 2 ml of amniotic fluid or as little as 5 mg of chorionic villi.[95,96]

Several PCR techniques using different primers have been developed.[95,97–99] Initial reports of fetal Rh genotyping used a single primer set to identify the RhD locus, with a second primer specific for the CcEe locus used as a control.[95,96] Using a single set of primers, error rates of 0.3 to 2.5 percent were reported.[97,100,101] In an effort to reduce error, PCR was performed using two independent sets of primers specific for different regions of the RhD gene. Simsek et al.,[97] using blood, and Spence et al.,[102] using amniotic fluid and chorionic villi, both reported complete concordance between two-primer PCR results and serologic testing.

Because of the possibility of severe fetal anemia and death, it is most important that an Rh-positive fetus not be misidentified as Rh-negative. Van den Veyver et al.[103] pointed out that such a misdiagnosis can occur when an Rh-positive father carries a gene rearrangement near the RhD locus which would prevent binding of the primer and yield a negative result with PCR. They recommended that paternal blood be analyzed simultaneously with amniotic fluid, using the same primers and PCR technique.

Although DNA testing for fetal Rh status has proven to be highly accurate, errors do not happen in clinical practice. Although estimates vary, misdiagnosis is thought to occur in about 1 percent of cases.

At most centers in the United States, DNA analysis of fetal cells is routinely included in the Rh assessment protocol. If an Rh-sensitized patient (with a partner who is heterozygous or whose status is unknown) is having a chorionic villus sampling or second-trimester amniocentesis for another, unrelated indication, fetal

RhD typing is performed at that time. In other cases, fetal Rh typing is performed at the time of the first amniocentesis for amniotic fluid bilirubin analysis. When PCR results indicate an Rh-negative fetus, patients are offered surveillance with fetal kick counts and serial ultrasounds, after a full discussion and explanation of the small likelihood of a misdiagnosis.

Because of the added risk and expense, chorionic villus sampling or early amniocentesis are not warranted solely for Rh typing, except for patients with severe Rh sensitization who would consider termination of an Rh-positive pregnancy. In the future, it seems likely that fetal Rh status may be routinely available from analysis of maternal blood. Favorable early experience with prenatal diagnosis of fetal antigen status has been reported using maternal blood,[104] fetal DNA extracted from maternal plasma,[105] and fetal mRNA in maternal blood.[106] Preimplantation genetic diagnosis of RhD type on single blastomeres has also been described.[99]

Antibody Titer

In the first sensitized pregnancy, the level of the anti-D antibody titer determines the need for amniocentesis. A number of authors have noted that severe erythroblastosis or perinatal death does not occur when the antibody levels remain below a certain "critical titer."[60,107,108] This titer varies between laboratories but is usually 1:16 or 1:32. For instance, Freda[108] found no perinatal deaths caused by hemolytic disease when the anti-D titer within 1 week of delivery was 1:16 or less. Queenan[60] reported no intrauterine deaths with a maternal anti-D titer of 1:16 or less and only one fetal death with an anti-D titer of 1:32. Gottvall et al.[109] found that no newborns in their series needed exchange transfusion if the maternal anti-D titer was 1:32 or less within 2 weeks of delivery.

Unfortunately, the reliability and method of antibody titration vary greatly between laboratories. As the number of sensitized pregnancies diminishes, the familiarity of laboratory personnel with titration techniques also decreases. Because of this potential difficulty, an anti-D titer of 1:8 or greater is considered at many centers to be an indication for amniocentesis to manage the sensitized pregnancy (Fig. 26–2). If the initial anti-D titer is less than 1:8, and if the patient does not have a history of a previously affected infant, the pregnancy may be followed with anti-D titers every 2 to 4 weeks and serial ultrasound assessment of the fetus.

Measurement of serial antibody titers has not been commonly used in Rh-sensitized pregnancies other than for determining the need for amniocentesis in first sensitized pregnancies. However, when anti-D levels are above the critical titer, a substantial proportion of fetuses are not significantly anemic. A number of investigators have sought to determine whether serial antibody titers might reduce the need for amniocentesis. MacGregor et al.[110] reported a small series of patients in which amniocentesis results were poorly predictive of fetal anemia. However, a three-fold rise in anti-D titer identified all five fetuses with anemia, while none of those with an anti-D rise of two-fold or less were anemic.

In Europe, anti-D is generally measured with an AutoAnalyzer (using one of several reference standards) and reported as a concentration, rather than as a dilutional titer. A number of authors have suggested that anti-D concentrations have better predictive value than titers.[109,111] Nicolaides and Rodeck[112] showed a close association between anti-D concentration and degree of fetal anemia at cord blood sampling, and no fetuses had moderate or severe anemia if the maternal anti-D concentration was less than 15 IU/ml. Similar findings were reported by Economides et al.[113]

Gottvall et al.[109] measured anti-D titers and concentrations in 93 Rh-sensitized pregnancies. They found that anti-D titers less than 1:32 or greater than 1:1,000 were strong predictors of mild and severe disease, respectively. In the group with intermediate titer levels,

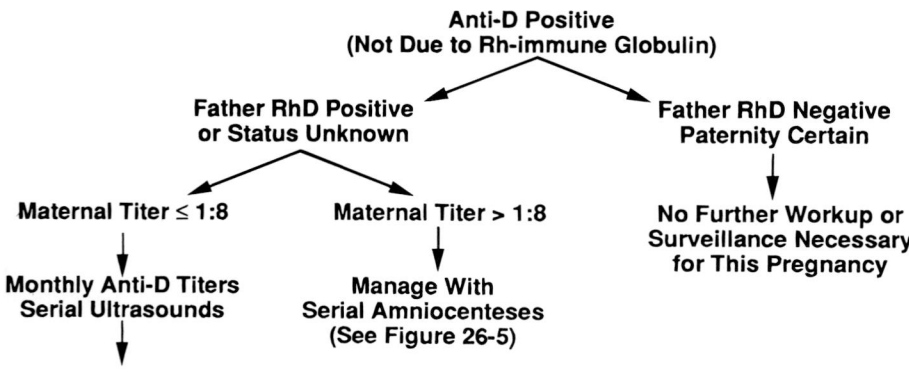

Figure 26–2. Flow diagram outlining the management of a first Rh-sensitized pregnancy.

however, anti-D concentration was a superior predictor, as 72 percent of patients with levels above their cutoff had moderate or severe disease, while 78 percent of patients below that cutoff had mild disease. They concluded that measurement of serial anti-D concentrations may decrease the need for amniocentesis in patients with Rh disease.

Even though anti-D concentrations were more predictive of anemia in the middle range of titers, Gottvall et al.[109] failed to identify 20 percent of fetuses with moderate to severe anemia by following anti-D concentrations, and 28 percent of patients above the cutoff did not have significant neonatal anemia. Bowell et al.[114] reported similar results, finding that less than a quarter of patients with concentrations above their cutoff had newborn hemoglobin levels less than 10 g/dl.

Currently, maternal serum anti-D titers are not particularly useful in the management of most Rh-alloimmunized pregnancies, except for using the "critical titer" to establish the need for amniocentesis in the first sensitized pregnancy. Indeed, titers may remain stable throughout gestation in as many as 80 percent of severely affected pregnancies.[104] Variability between maternal antibody levels and severity of fetal disease is explained by the fact that antibody concentration is only one factor influencing the degree of anemia. Other factors, which vary between individuals, include antibody subclass and degree of glycosylation, placental transfer of antibody, antigen expression on fetal erythrocytes, functional maturity of the fetal reticuloendothelial system, and the presence of HLA-related antibodies that inhibit fetal erythrocyte destruction.[30,111]

Obstetric History

A well-documented obstetric history can be an important management guide for the Rh-alloimmunized patient. Fetal hemolytic disease tends to be either as severe, or more severe, in subsequent pregnancies. A history of previous intrauterine or neonatal death from hemolytic disease carries a particularly grave prognosis.[107,115] As a general rule of thumb, if a mother has had a hydropic fetus, the chance that the next Rh-incompatible fetus will become hydropic (if left untreated) is more than 80 percent. Only occasionally will an Rh-incompatible fetus be less severely affected than its previous sibling.

In general, hemolysis and hydrops develop at about the same time or somewhat earlier in subsequent pregnancies; this can be used as a rough guide for timing initial fetal studies and transfusions. However, the history is not particularly helpful if the previous pregnancy was the first sensitized pregnancy, since relatively few fetuses develop hydrops in a first sensitized pregnancy.

Amniotic Fluid Analysis

Assessment of amniotic fluid in Rh immunization is based on the original observations of Bevis[116] that spectrophotometric determinations of amniotic fluid bilirubin correlated with the severity of fetal hemolysis. The bilirubin in amniotic fluid is a by-product of fetal hemolysis that reaches the amniotic fluid primarily by excretion into fetal pulmonary and tracheal secretions and diffusion across the fetal membranes and the umbilical cord. Using a semilogarithmic plot, the curve of optical density of normal amniotic fluid is approximately linear between wavelengths of 525 and 375 nm. Bilirubin causes a shift in the spectrophotometric density with a peak at a wavelength of 450 nm. The amount of shift in optical density from linearity at 450 nm (the ΔOD_{450}) is used to estimate the degree of fetal red cell hemolysis (Fig. 26–3).

Liley[117] provided a framework for the management of Rh-immunized pregnancies on the basis of ΔOD_{450} values in the third trimester. Retrospectively, he correlated amniotic fluid ΔOD_{450} values with newborn outcome by dividing a semilogarithmic graph of gestational age versus ΔOD_{450} into three zones. Unaffected fetuses and those with mild anemia had ΔOD_{450} values in zone I (the lowest zone), whereas severely affected

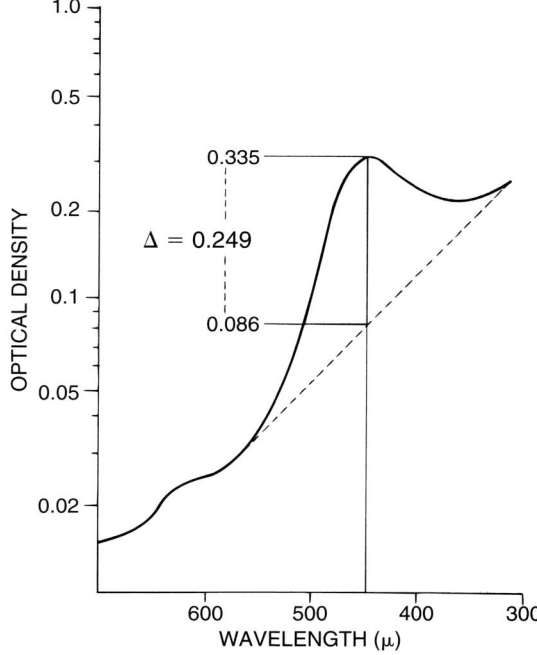

Figure 26–3. Graph of spectrophotometric analysis of amniotic fluid taken from an Rh-sensitized pregnancy with fetal hydrops. The *solid line* is the plot of the optical density of the bilirubin-containing fluid across the wavelengths on the x-axis. The interrupted line represents the curve expected from amniotic fluid without increased bilirubin. The difference between the optical density of the *solid line* and the *interrupted line* at 450 nm is the ΔOD_{450} value.

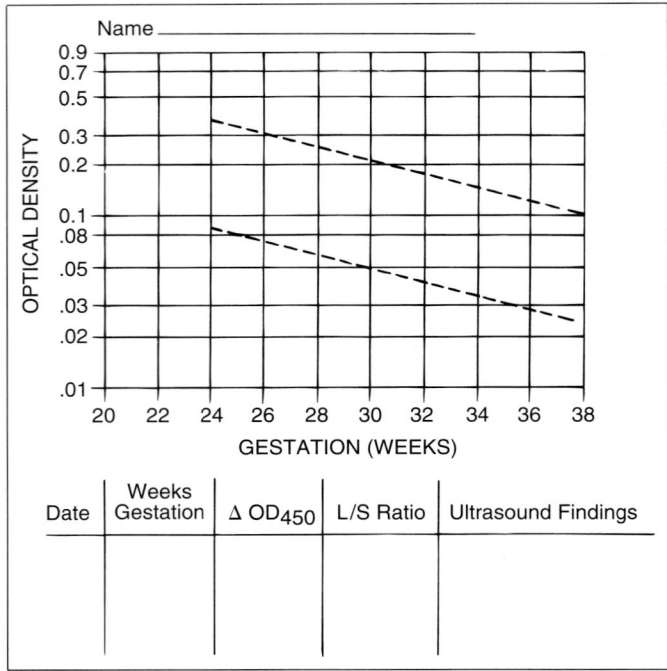

Figure 26–4. Liley graph with linear extrapolation of boundaries to 24 weeks' gestation.

Date	Weeks Gestation	Δ OD₄₅₀	L/S Ratio	Ultrasound Findings

fetuses had ΔOD_{450} values in zone III (the highest zone). Fetuses with zone II values (the middle zone) had disease ranging from mild to severe, indicated primarily by the trend of the amniotic fluid bilirubin determinations. There is a normal tendency for amniotic fluid bilirubin to decrease as pregnancy advances; thus, the boundaries of the zones slope downward as gestational age increases (Fig. 26–4).

Management prior to this time consisted primarily of early induced delivery, but Liley's method identified pregnancies that could be safely allowed to continue without great risk of hydrops and stillbirth. In this way, iatrogenic prematurity was avoided in many cases, with a reduction in perinatal mortality from 22 percent to 9 percent over a 5-year period.[117]

It became clear with further study that a single measurement of ΔOD_{450} was poorly predictive of fetal condition unless it was very high or very low.[11] Also, because of the wide range of severity of disease in the middle zone, Liley emphasized the need for repeating the amniotic fluid analyses to establish the ΔOD_{450} trend. Queenan[119] subsequently analyzed serial amniotic fluid ΔOD_{450} values in patients delivering unaffected (Rh-negative), mildly affected (cord hemoglobin > 14 g/dl), severely affected (cord blood hemoglobin < 10 g/dl), and stillborn infants. There was a clear downward trend in the ΔOD_{450} values in unaffected and mildly affected infants, and values from the severely affected fetuses showed a mixed pattern of higher values. The amniotic fluid ΔOD_{450} values from infants who died in utero from erythroblastosis showed upward trends except in a single case that was complicated by polyhydramnios. Thus, a horizontal or rising trend is ominous and indicates the need for intervention either by intrauterine transfusion or delivery. Clinical management now includes serial amniocenteses to determine the trend of ΔOD_{450} values over time.[119,120]

The usefulness of the late second- and early third-trimester amniotic fluid ΔOD_{450} determinations for the management of Rh-immunized pregnancies has been confirmed by decades of experience in many centers. However, several practical caveats deserve emphasis. First, a single ΔOD_{450} value is often insufficient for management purposes; the ΔOD_{450} trend, as established by serial amniocenteses, provides more reliable information about the fetal status. Second, amniotic fluid bilirubin levels are an indirect measure of fetal anemia, and relying solely on the ΔOD_{450} values occasionally leads to the false impression that a mildly or moderately involved fetus is severely anemic or vice versa. Finally, the fairly common practice of extrapolating Liley's original graph for use prior to 27 weeks' gestation is controversial.

Data for ΔOD_{450} analysis were originally obtained from third-trimester pregnancies, and several investigators have arbitrarily extrapolated the Liley graph backward and interpreted the results as for third-trimester fetuses.[121] Nicolaides and colleagues[122] questioned this approach. They obtained amniotic fluid and umbilical cord blood samples from 59 fetuses with Rh immunization between 18 and 25 weeks' gestation and correlated ΔOD_{450} values with fetal hemoglobin. Whereas, the ΔOD_{450} roughly correlated with the degree of fetal anemia, the ΔOD_{450} values were widely scattered and did not accurately predict the hematocrit in an individual fetus. Also, two thirds of severely affected fetuses (hemoglobin < 6 g/dl) had ΔOD_{450} values in the middle or lower zone, incorrectly suggesting only mild to moderate anemia. The authors concluded that second-trimester amniotic fluid bilirubin analysis is unreliable and that umbilical cord blood sampling is the only accurate method of assessing fetal anemia.[122] These results were widely accepted, and standard recommendations for second-trimester fetal assessment were modified to include fetal blood sampling instead of amniocentesis.[123]

However, some authors disagreed with these conclusions. Spinnato and co-workers[124] suggested that the ΔOD_{450} results of Nicolaides et al.[122] were misleading because no correction for amniotic fluid contamination was utilized. They showed that chloroform extraction of amniotic fluid in Rh-immunized pregnancies (to recover bilirubin and remove contaminants such as blood and meconium) resulted in a decrease in ΔOD_{450} values in 90 percent of samples by a mean of 20 percent and allowed accurate clinical categorization of each patient tested. Nicolaides' group also included hydropic fetuses in their analysis, relied more on single ΔOD_{450} values than on trends, and did not address the risk/benefit ratio for routine umbilical cord blood sampling. Spinnato et al.[124] concluded that second-trimester chloroform-extracted amniotic fluid bilirubin analysis permits accurate fetal assessment and avoids umbilical cord blood sampling in all but about 15 percent of patients.

Others have found amniotic fluid bilirubin analysis before 28 weeks to be valuable as well. Ananth and Queenan[125] studied ΔOD_{450} values and trends in 32 Rh-sensitized pregnancies between 16 and 20 weeks' gestation. They found that ΔOD_{450} values greater than or trending above 0.15 predicted severe alloimmunization, whereas ΔOD_{450} values below 0.09 indicated mild or absent disease. They concluded that umbilical blood sampling is necessary only in second-trimester pregnancies with ΔOD_{450} values greater than 0.15; fetuses with ΔOD_{450} values below 0.15 can be managed with serial amniocenteses to determine whether the trend indicates severe disease.

In a subsequent analysis of amniotic fluid bilirubin levels obtained between 14 and 40 weeks' gestation, Queenan et al.[126] plotted 520 ΔOD_{450} values from unaffected fetuses and 163 ΔOD_{450} values from Rh-immunized pregnancies, using a nonlogarithmic graph. In unaffected pregnancies, normal amniotic fluid ΔOD_{450} values trended upward between 14 and 22 weeks, leveled off until 26 weeks, then declined steadily until term. Using the mean and standard deviation of values across the gestational age range, these authors proposed a new graphic framework for assessment of ΔOD_{450} values in Rh-sensitized pregnancies, with four zones instead of Liley's three. Queenan et al. then proposed a management scheme based on their review of data, with timing of repeat amniocentesis or cordocentesis based on the ΔOD_{450} results.

To evaluate the accuracy of Queenan's chart, Spinnato et al.[127] compared ΔOD_{450} results using both Queenan's graph and a Liley curve extrapolated linearly back to 20 weeks. They plotted 231 ΔOD_{450} values from 73 alloimmunized patients using both methods and found that Queenan's graph was twice as likely to overestimate risk both before and after 28 weeks, and placed patients' highest ΔOD_{450} value in the upper zone three times as often. Queenan's standards were more accurate for only two patients, both at 21 to 22 weeks' gestation. Using the extended Liley curve for clinical management, only 16 percent of patients required cordocentesis or transfusion, and no fetuses developed hydrops. Spinnato et al.[127] concluded that a linearly extended Liley curve is safe and accurate for second- and third-trimester assessment, and that Queenan's chart overestimates risk of fetal anemia.

Others have reported similar findings. Scott and Chan[128] superimposed Queenan's graph and the Liley curve, and showed that Queenan's cutoff levels are lower than those of Liley, especially before 32 weeks. Although they concluded that Queenan's chart is a suitable alternative to the Liley curve, Scott and Chan found that 11 of 13 ΔOD_{450} values from fetuses with moderate anemia fell in Queenan's intrauterine death risk zone, and only 2 of 18 values from unaffected fetuses were in the lowest zone.[128]

Recognizing that this issue is not completely settled, we currently use a standard semilogarithmic Liley curve for amniotic fluid assessment, extrapolated linearly back to 24 weeks' gestational age (Fig. 26-4). As mentioned above, we emphasize trends rather than single ΔOD_{450} values, especially before the third trimester, taking history and gestational age into consideration in clinical management.

Fetal Blood Analysis

Direct fetal vascular access with fetoscopy and ultrasound-guided umbilical vein puncture was developed in the 1980s, thus enabling accurate assessment of the degree of fetal anemia and fetal intravascular transfusion.[129-131] At that time, fetal blood sampling was also the only method to reliably determine fetal antigen status when the zygosity of the father was unknown or uncertain. As a result, fetal blood sampling was considered by many to be the first step in the assessment of the fetus at risk for severe hemolytic disease.

MacKenzie and colleagues[132] confirmed the utility of fetal blood sampling in the management of Rh-alloimmunized pregnancies. In 51 consecutive sensitized pregnancies, 11 fetuses were found by blood sampling to be Rh-negative and thus required no further evaluation. Of the continuing pregnancies, the fetal hematocrit and the amniotic fluid ΔOD_{450} values were in agreement in 79 percent of instances. However, the amniotic fluid ΔOD_{450} value underestimated the degree of fetal anemia in 11 percent of comparisons and overestimated the degree of fetal anemia in 10 percent.

Adoption of routine umbilical cord blood sampling has not been universal because of concern for potential fetal and maternal morbidity. The procedure is successful in greater than 95 percent of cases, but attributable fetal loss rates between 0.5 and 2 percent per procedure have been reported by experienced investigators.[133-135] In approximately 5 percent of patients, other morbidity occurs; complications such as acute refractory fetal distress, umbilical cord hematoma, amnionitis with maternal adult respiratory distress syndrome, and placental abruption have been described.[136-138]

Additionally, there appears to be a significant risk of fetomaternal bleeding with umbilical cord blood sampling, with the potential for worsened maternal sensitization and fetal involvement.[139-141] Although most studies of this issue have described patients undergoing cordocentesis with intravascular transfusion rather than umbilical blood sampling alone, it appears that significant fetomaternal hemorrhage occurs in 25 to 50 percent of procedures.

Traversing an anterior placenta with the sampling needle is generally thought to increase the likelihood of fetomaternal hemorrhage. In the series of Nicolini et al.,[93] 65 percent of patients with an anterior placenta had significant increases in maternal serum α-fetoprotein (used as a marker for fetomaternal bleeding) compared with 17 percent of patients with a posterior placenta. However, Bowman et al.[141] found little effect of placental location on the incidence of fetomaternal hemorrhage. Using Kleihauer-Betke testing for the presence of fetal cells in the maternal circulation, they identified transplacental hemorrhage greater than 0.05 ml in 61 percent of those with an anterior placenta and 48 percent with a posterior placenta. Similarly, they found a significant increase in maternal antibody levels in approximately one half of the patients, regardless of placental location. Also, they reported that 56 percent of patients having a cordocentesis without transfusion had significant transplacental hemorrhage.

Although concern for worsened maternal sensitization as a consequence of fetal blood sampling has been raised, there are no longitudinal data available with which to determine whether cordocentesis with fetomaternal bleeding and increased antibody titers worsen the prognosis for subsequent pregnancies.

Currently, the need for cordocentesis to determine fetal antigen status has been obviated by the availability of DNA analysis of amniotic fluid. Thus, the role of umbilical cord blood sampling in the management of alloimmunization is limited to assessment of those fetuses already known to be antigen-positive and who are suspected of having moderate to severe anemia. Because of the technical difficulty and increased hazard (both immediate and remote) associated with the procedure, umbilical cord blood sampling should be used with caution and performed only by properly trained personnel.

Ultrasound and Doppler Studies

Ultrasonographic examination of the fetus has become an extremely important adjunct in the management of the Rh-sensitized pregnancy, primarily as a guide to amniocentesis, fetal blood sampling, and intrauterine transfusion. Ultrasound has also been studied in an effort to identify sonographic findings that might predict the severity of erythroblastosis fetalis and reduce the need for invasive assessments. Polyhydramnios, placental thickness greater than 4 cm, pericardial effusion, dilation of the cardiac chambers, chronic enlargement of the spleen and liver, visualization of both sides of the fetal bowel wall, and dilation of the umbilical vein have all been proposed as indicators of significant pre-hydropic fetal anemia.[142-151]

In an effort to determine which, if any, ultrasound parameters are most predictive, Chitkara et al.[146] reviewed the ultrasound findings just prior to umbilical cord blood sampling on 35 occasions between 21 and 33.5 weeks' gestation in 15 severely sensitized pregnancies. The relationship between fetal hematocrit and the sonographic findings of polyhydramnios, increased placental thickness, increased umbilical vein diameter, and hydrops was studied. All fetuses with hydrops had a hematocrit less than 15 percent, but two of eight fetuses with a hematocrit below 15 percent had a normal sonogram and another had only moderate polyhydramnios. Of 19 fetuses with a hematocrit between 16 and 29 percent, more than half had a normal sonogram, 42 percent had mild to moderate polyhydramnios, and 17 percent had placental thickening. Polyhydramnios was the first and only sonographic sign before fetal anemia (hematocrit < 26 percent) in 6 of 10 patients studied serially. Although polyhydramnios may be an early indication of significant hemolysis and fetal anemia, the absence of this sonographic finding did not preclude significant anemia; half of fetuses with normal ultrasound examinations had hematocrits below 30 percent. Although these results indicate that ultrasound is insensitive for detection of fetal anemia, it is important to note that there was no normal control group for comparison, and many of these sonograms were performed when fetuses had already undergone at least one transfusion.

Nicolaides et al.[147] measured fetal head circumference, abdominal circumference, head/abdomen ratio, estimated intraperitoneal volume, placental thickness, and extrahepatic and intrahepatic umbilical vein diameters in 50 patients prior to umbilical cord blood sampling for severe Rh disease. No fetus had been transfused, and the measurements were compared with those from 410 healthy women with normal singleton pregnancies. The presence of hydrops predicted a fetal hemoglobin less than 5 g/dl in all 12 cases so affected. In the absence of hydropic changes on ultrasound, none of the other ultrasonographic parameters differentiated mild from severe anemia. Half of the fetuses with a hemoglobin less than 5 g/dl had no sonographic abnormality, and no consistent pattern was apparent in those with abnormal ultrasound findings. Of the fetuses with a hemoglobin level of 5 to 10 g/dl, two thirds had a normal ultrasound examination.

Taken together, these data suggest that sonographic findings other than hydrops are not sufficiently reliable in distinguishing mild from severe hemolytic disease, even in experienced hands, and the role of ultrasound in the monitoring of fetuses with severe Rh immunization is still limited to the establishment of gestational age; monitoring for hydropic changes; and guidance for amniocentesis, umbilical cord blood sampling, and transfusion.

Doppler flow velocity waveforms have also been extensively investigated as noninvasive predictors of fetal anemia[152-161] and acidosis.[162,163] Fetal cardiac output and blood velocities in the umbilical artery, umbilical vein, fetal descending aorta, fetal ductus venosus, fetal splenic artery, and fetal middle cerebral artery have all been studied in alloimmunized pregnancies.

Nicolaides et al.[154] compared fetal aorta Doppler blood velocities in 68 severely immunized fetuses and 218 normal controls. In nonhydropic fetuses, an aortic mean velocity above the normal range suggested fetal anemia, and a normal mean velocity made significant anemia unlikely. However, the authors concluded that because of the large overlap in values between anemic and nonanemic fetuses, Doppler measurements of the aortic blood flow cannot accurately predict the degree of fetal anemia.

In a similar study, Copel et al.[155] retrospectively found that a calculation based on the peak velocity in the descending aorta was predictive of a fetal hematocrit above or below 25 percent with a high degree of sensitivity. However, their formula and its modifications were not useful in predicting the hematocrit after fetal transfusion. Most importantly, this group was unable to predict the degree of fetal anemia in a prospective evaluation of their method.[156]

Legarth and colleagues[159] compared Doppler blood flow velocities to umbilical vein hematocrit during 49 fetal blood sampling or transfusion procedures. Using the S/D ratio, the pulsatility index, and the resistance index, they found no correlation between umbilical artery Doppler indices and fetal hematocrit at the time of blood sampling, and the blood flow velocity indices did not predict fetal hematocrit.

Most recently, Mari and colleagues[160] measured the peak systolic velocity of the middle cerebral artery in 111 fetuses undergoing cordocentesis for red cell alloimmunization. They found that all fetuses with moderate or severe anemia had peak velocity greater than 1.5 times the median of values derived from normal controls, with the same cutoff having a false-positive rate of 12 percent. Although the study population was relatively large, patients were sensitized to a number of different antigens, and Mari et al. used definitions of anemia not commonly employed in clinical management. Although encouraging, these data await confirmation by others and comparison with standard screening techniques.

In general, fetal blood flow velocity waveforms have not been predictive of acid–base status in Rh-alloimmunized pregnancies. Similarly, although many studies have found statistically significant differences in blood flow indices between groups of anemic and nonanemic fetuses, the wide range and overlap of values in both groups of patients have limited the clinical utility of Doppler technology.

Ultrasound and Doppler ultrasound technology continue to advance rapidly. It seems likely that these noninvasive tools may one day be used to reliably determine the degree of fetal anemia and, thus, to direct fetal management. However, at present, neither ultrasound nor Doppler blood flow analysis can be recommended in lieu of amniotic fluid ΔOD_{450} determinations or fetal blood sampling for determining the need for intrauterine transfusion or delivery in Rh-immunized pregnancies.

Determining the Need for Intrauterine Transfusion

About one half of susceptible infants of Rh-immunized pregnancies do not require intrauterine transfusion or extensive extrauterine therapy. Such fetuses are considered to have mild to moderate hemolytic disease. In general, mild to moderate fetal hemolysis is expected when (1) the involved pregnancy is the first sensitized pregnancy or (2) previously delivered Rh-positive infants have been mildly to moderately affected (mild to moderate anemia without hydrops). In such cases, we perform ultrasound examinations of the fetus every 2 to 4 weeks from 20 weeks' gestation until delivery. If the fetus shows no signs of hydrops, we use amniotic fluid ΔOD_{450} determinations for the initial management, performing the first amniocentesis at 24 to 28 weeks' gestation. The timing of repeat amniocenteses and determination of the need for intrauterine transfusion or delivery are based on the ΔOD_{450} values and trend (Fig. 26–5). If the values fall within the low zone or the lower half of the middle zone on the Liley graph, amniocentesis is repeated every 2 to 4 weeks, depending on the ΔOD_{450} trend. Severe anemia requiring intrauterine transfusion is suspected when the ΔOD_{450} values rise into the upper quarter of the middle zone or into zone III, especially before 30 weeks' gestation. Depending on the clinical situation, a single ΔOD_{450} value in zone III also may be taken as an indication of severe anemia. If at any time the fetus has evidence of hydrops by ultrasound, one can assume a fetal hematocrit less than about 15 percent,[146,147] and fetal blood sampling and transfusion should be arranged immediately.

The need for cordocentesis in the management of nonhydropic fetuses with ΔOD_{450} values indicative of severe anemia (and requiring intrauterine transfusion) is controversial. As discussed below, there is no proven advantage to cordocentesis and intravascular transfusion in nonhydropic fetuses, and experienced practition-

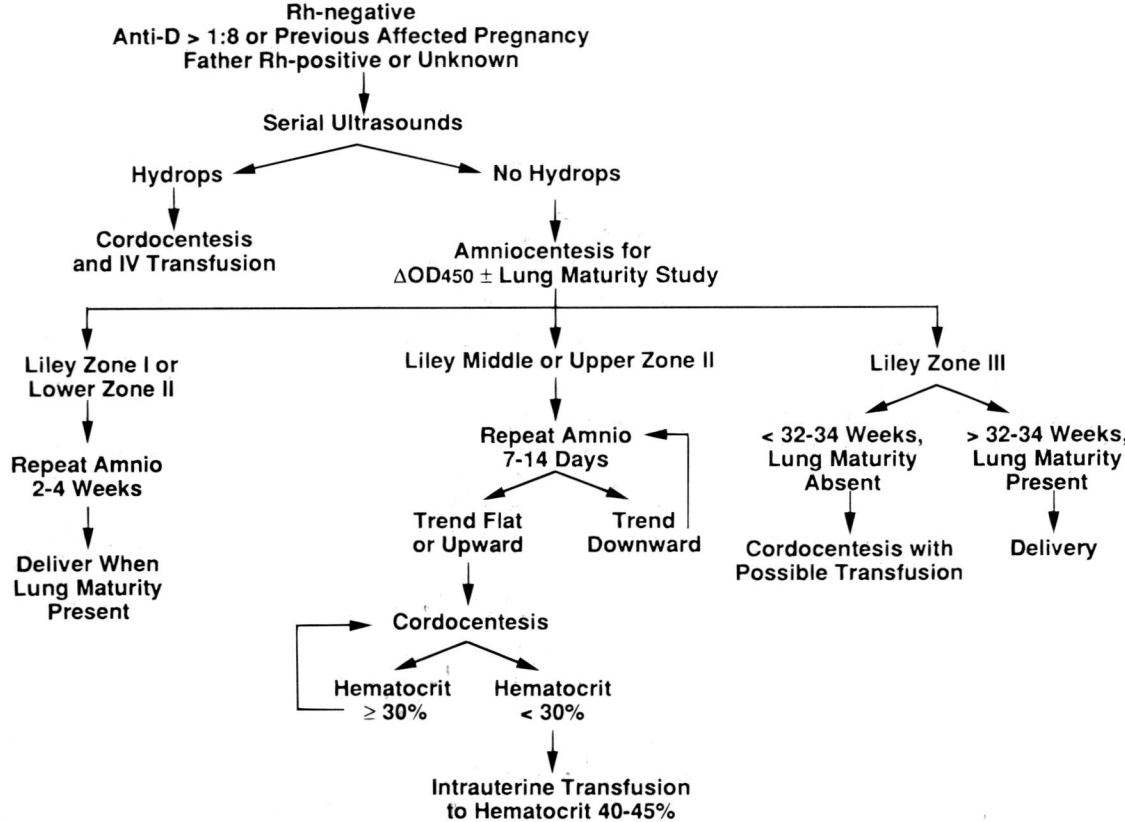

Figure 26–5. Flow diagram outlining the management of an Rh-sensitized pregnancy. The timing of the first amniocentesis is based on the history, maternal titer, and gestational age. At the first amniocentesis, fluid should be sent for determination of fetal antigen status, and if negative, a noninvasive surveillance protocol is continued. In incompatible pregnancies, all patients monitor fetal movements on a daily basis after 26 to 28 weeks and have nonstress tests one to two times weekly and ultrasound exams every 1 to 2 weeks, in addition to assessment of amniotic fluid bilirubin or umbilical cord hematocrit.

ers have described excellent perinatal outcomes using amniotic fluid ΔOD_{450} values with intraperitoneal transfusions.[164–166] However, because of the morbidity associated with fetal transfusion regardless of route, it seems appropriate to obtain umbilical cord blood when practical to confirm anemia prior to transfusion. The optimum management in any individual case will be determined by the clinical presentation and the experience and expertise of the physicians involved.

When the obstetric history suggests that the fetus is at risk for moderate to severe hemolysis and hydrops, we are more likely to begin the search for fetal anemia earlier in the pregnancy. In this situation, we usually follow the trend of ΔOD_{450} values, using an extrapolation of the Liley curve, with the understanding that interpretation of ΔOD_{450} values before 24 weeks is difficult. Between 18 and 24 weeks, we stress ΔOD_{450} trends over single values and typically use Queenan's horizontal zones,[125] with ΔOD_{450} values below 0.09 suggesting an unaffected or mildly affected infant and ΔOD_{450} values above 0.15 suggesting fetal anemia. In some cases, especially those with a history of severe

second-trimester disease or previous severe disease with misleading ΔOD_{450} values, cordocentesis to determine the fetal hematocrit is a reasonable first step. Again, the optimum management in an individual case will be determined by history, clinical findings, and the experience and expertise of the management team.

At any gestational age, the presence of fetal hydrops should be taken as evidence of severe fetal anemia, and cordocentesis with immediate intravascular transfusion is indicated.

INTRAUTERINE TRANSFUSION IN THE Rh-ALLOIMMUNIZED PREGNANCY

When Liley[167] reported the first successful intrauterine transfusion in 1963, a new therapy was created that provided obstetricians with a much-needed alternative to preterm delivery in severe erythroblastosis fetalis.

The administration of erythrocytes to the anemic fetus accomplishes two goals: (1) it corrects fetal anemia and consequently improves fetal oxygenation, and (2) it reduces extramedullary hematopoietic demand, leading to a fall in portal venous pressure and improved hepatic function.

Originally, intrauterine transfusions were done by the intraperitoneal route, and this approach was the mainstay of transfusion therapy until the mid-1980s. In 1981, Rodeck et al.[129] reported the successful intravenous transfusion of two erythroblastotic fetuses using a fetoscopic technique. Although successful,[130] the fetoscopic approach is complicated and introduction of the transfusion needle by ultrasound guidance (without the fetoscope) has become the standard technique.[168–176] The umbilical vein is the most commonly used vessel, usually at its insertion into the placenta.

Intrauterine Intraperitoneal Transfusion

Placement of erythrocytes in the fetal peritoneal cavity reverses fetal anemia by gradual uptake of the transfused red cells into the fetal circulatory system via subdiaphragmatic lymphatics. Perinatal survival following intraperitoneal transfusion is related to gestational age at delivery and the severity of fetal disease, particularly with regard to whether hydrops develops. When transfusions were performed with radiographic guidance, overall neonatal survival was approximately 60 percent, survival of nonhydropic infants was near 70 percent, and less than 40 percent of those developing hydrops survived.[38] The routine use of ultrasound for transfusion and monitoring, improvements in transfusion technique, and advances in neonatal care have led to more favorable outcomes (Table 26–3).

Prior to intraperitoneal transfusion, an intravenous line is placed in the mother, and she is often sedated with an intravenous narcotic or short-acting benzodiazepine. Many practitioners also administer an antiemetic and a prophylactic antibiotic. Using real-time ultrasound, fetal size, position, and condition; placental location; and amniotic fluid volume are determined. Intraperitoneal access is best accomplished with the fetus on its side or back, and some authors have suggested external manipulation of the fetus for positioning.[121,177] Peritoneal access is ideally accomplished through the lateral or anterolateral abdominal wall, with the fetal bladder and pelvic bones serving as landmarks. Care should be taken to avoid the umbilical cord and its insertion into the fetal abdomen.

After a site for needle insertion is chosen on the maternal abdomen, the area is prepared and draped in sterile fashion, and a local anesthetic is injected. Using a sterile technique, an 18- or 20-gauge needle is directed under continuous real-time ultrasound guidance into the fetal peritoneum, ideally just cephalad and lateral to the fetal bladder. When it appears that the needle tip has entered the fetal peritoneal cavity, saline or a small air bubble is introduced through the needle to verify its location (Fig. 26–6). Although we prefer to infuse the blood through the needle, Bowman[120] suggests using an epidural catheter passed through a 16-gauge Tuohy needle for the actual transfusion. When the catheter is clearly seen in the fetal peritoneal cavity, the needle is then withdrawn from the maternal abdomen, leaving the catheter threaded for transfusion.

After confirmation that the needle tip or catheter is in the fetal peritoneal cavity, the transfusion is performed at a rate no faster than 5 to 10 ml/min. With real-time ultrasound, the flow of red cells into the peritoneum can usually be visualized. Type O-negative, leukocyte-poor, packed erythrocytes cross-matched with

Table 26–3. PERINATAL SURVIVAL RATES WITH INTRAUTERINE TRANSFUSION

	Nonhydropic	Hydropic	Overall
Intraperitoneal transfusion: neonatal survival			
Bowman and Manning[164]	16/16 (100%)	6/8 (75%)	2/24 (92%)
Scott et al.[165]	12/14 (86%)	4/6 (67%)	16/20 (80%)
Watts et al.[166]	26/26 (100%)	4/9 (44%)	30/35 (86%)
Harman et al.[175]	19/23 (83%)	10/21 (48%)	29/44 (66%)
Total	73/79 (92%)	24/44 (55%)	97/123 (79%)
Intravascular transfusion: neonatal survival			
Grannum et al.[171]	5/6 (83%)	16/20 (80%)	21/26 (81%)
Nicolaides et al.[172]	8/8 (100%)	9/10 (90%)	17/18 (94%)
Berkowitz et al.[173]	13/16 (81%)	0/1 (0%)	13/17 (76%)
Poissonnier et al.[174]	55/60 (92%)	29/47 (62%)	84/107 (79%)
Harman et al.[175]	22/23 (96%)	18/21 (86%)	40/44 (91%)
Weiner et al.[176]	35/35 (100%)	11/13 (85%)	46/48 (92%)
Total	138/148 (93%)	83/112 (74%)	221/260 (85%)

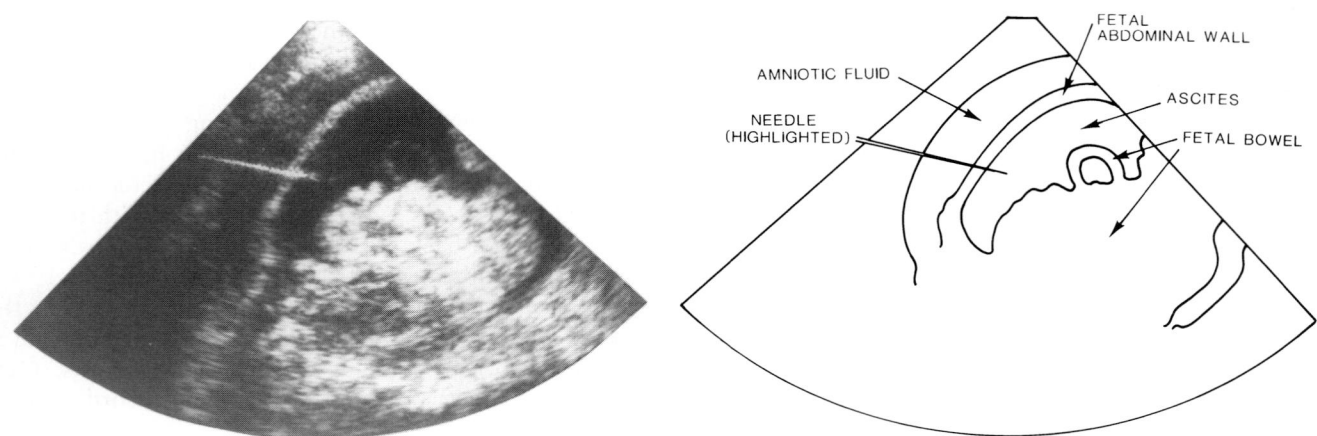

Figure 26–6. Sonogram showing intrauterine transfusion needle in the fetal peritoneal cavity.

the maternal serum are used; the desired hematocrit for the packed cells is 75 to 85 percent. The transfusion is carried out manually with a 20- or 30-ml syringe connected to the transfusion line with a three-way stopcock.

The volume of blood in milliliters for intraperitoneal transfusion is calculated by subtracting 20 from the gestational age in weeks and then multiplying by 10. Thus, a 28-week fetus would receive 80 ml of blood. This simple formula is intended to provide a reasonable amount of blood to the fetus without creating undue intraperitoneal pressure. When fetal ascites is present, some of this fluid should be gently aspirated before transfusion. Bowman[38] has suggested that no more than twice the volume of the proposed transfusion should be removed, with a maximum being 150 ml. The rate of absorption of the transfused blood from the peritoneal cavity into the bloodstream is said to be about 12 percent per day in the nonhydropic fetus. In our experience, little or none of the transfused blood is detectable by ultrasonographic examination 3 to 5 days after transfusion in cases in which the fetus was not hydropic. If the fetus is hydropic, red cell uptake is variable and unpredictable; in some cases it is adequate,[38] but in others absorption is quite poor.

It is important that the fetal heart rate be monitored periodically during the transfusion in case fetal bradycardia occurs. Bradycardia early in the procedure presages fetal death.[120] Late in the procedure, a fall in the fetal heart rate may indicate compression of the vena cava by increased intraperitoneal pressure. Measurement of fetal heart rate during the transfusion can easily be done with ultrasound.

Bowman[120] developed a formula for estimating the residual donor hemoglobin in the fetus following transfusion. With a goal of keeping the hemoglobin in the fetus above 10 g/dl, the first and second transfusions are performed about 10 days apart. The timing of subsequent transfusions can then be calculated using the donor hemoglobin and estimated fetal weight, and assuming that 55 percent of the transfusion hemoglobin enters the fetal circulation after intraperitoneal instillation and that the daily red cell loss is about 1/120th of the total. According to Bowman's formula, the basic intraperitoneal transfusion schedule puts the second transfusion about 10 days after the first, and repeat transfusions every 4 weeks thereafter.

The routine use of ultrasound for needle guidance has dramatically reduced the procedure-related morbidity and mortality associated with intraperitoneal transfusion. Confirmation of appropriate needle placement is usually straightforward, but inadvertent transfusion into the bowel, liver, abdominal wall, and retroperitoneum may occur. Infection, premature rupture of the membranes, refractory preterm labor, and fetal distress necessitating immediate delivery continue to be hazards. Bowman and Manning[164] reported 5 traumatic deaths in 53 transfusions (9.4 percent) during the 2 years prior to instituting ultrasound guidance; there were no deaths in the 64 transfusions after ultrasound was introduced. In a similar analysis, Scott et al.[165] observed a reduction in traumatic death rate from 8.0 percent to 2.3 percent per transfusion. Most recently, Harman et al.[175] have reported a traumatic death rate of 7.6 percent per procedure; nearly three fourths of the fetal and neonatal deaths in this series were due to trauma or complications of prematurity and not to Rh disease. Thus, while intraperitoneal transfusion has evolved into a relatively safe procedure, it is not without risk for fetal loss.

Intrauterine Intravascular Transfusion

First described by Rodeck et al.[129] with fetoscopy, intravascular fetal transfusion has been widely adopted in modified form using ultrasound to guide placement of a needle into the umbilical vein. Direct access to the fetal circulation for transfusion offers several advantages over the intraperitoneal approach: (1) the initial fetal hematocrit can be measured, allowing a more precise calculation of the volume of blood required for transfusion; (2) in some cases, the fetus will have a higher hematocrit than expected and transfusion can be delayed; and (3) a post-transfusion hematocrit can be used to determine whether the transfusion was adequate and when the next one should be scheduled. Also, transfusion into the fetal vascular system ensures complete uptake of the intended red blood cell mass with a more rapid correction of fetal anemia. This is especially important for hydropic fetuses who often do not adequately absorb intraperitoneally transfused erythrocytes. Potential disadvantages of intravascular fetal transfusion include the rare possibility of volume overload in the compromised fetus, procedure-related complications, and the risk of increasing the severity of maternal sensitization due to fetomaternal hemorrhage.

Despite the recent popularity of intravascular over intraperitoneal transfusion, perinatal survival in pregnancies managed with intravascular transfusion is convincingly improved only for hydropic fetuses. Reported overall survival rates range from 76 to 94 percent (Table 26–3). The perinatal survival of nonhydropic fetuses exceeds 90 percent, and approximately 75 percent of hydropic fetuses survive with intravascular transfusion.

Preparation of the patient is the same as for fetal intraperitoneal transfusion, and the approach to the umbilical cord is defined with real-time ultrasound. A 20- or 22-gauge needle is used, and the progress of the needle tip is guided with continuous ultrasound. When the placenta is anterior, we prefer to use the transplacental approach into the umbilical vein (Fig. 26–7). Otherwise, we attempt to enter the vessel by traversing the amniotic sac and puncturing the cord near its insertion into the placenta. If the fetus is particularly active (in spite of sedation administered to the mother) or if the needle passes near the fetal extremities, the fetus can be paralyzed immediately upon entry into the vein by injecting pancuronium bromide, 0.1 to 0.3 mg/kg of estimated fetal weight.[178,179] As with intraperitoneal transfusion, O-negative, leukocyte-poor, packed erythrocytes cross-matched with the maternal serum are used.

When vascular access is attained, a small amount of blood is withdrawn into one to three heparinized 1-ml syringes and the initial fetal hematocrit immediately determined. With adequate visualization using ultrasound, there is usually little doubt about the proper placement of the needle tip in the fetal circulation. Comparison of the red cell indices to those of a maternal sample can help confirm that the blood sample is of fetal origin; in addition to the expected difference in hematocrit, fetal red cells have a higher mean corpuscular volume than

ANTERIOR or FUNDAL PLACENTA
Needle (highlighted)

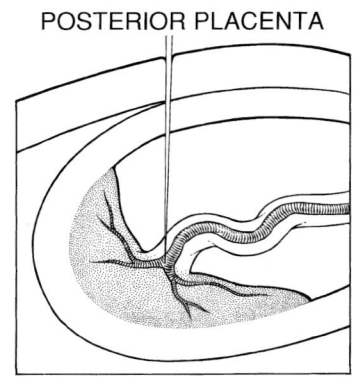

POSTERIOR PLACENTA

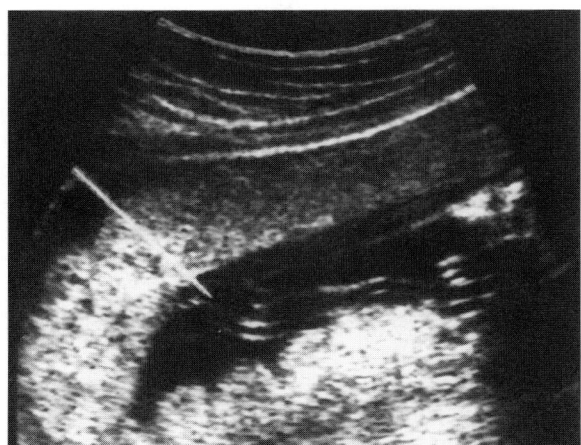

Figure 26–7. Needle placement for intravascular fetal transfusion.

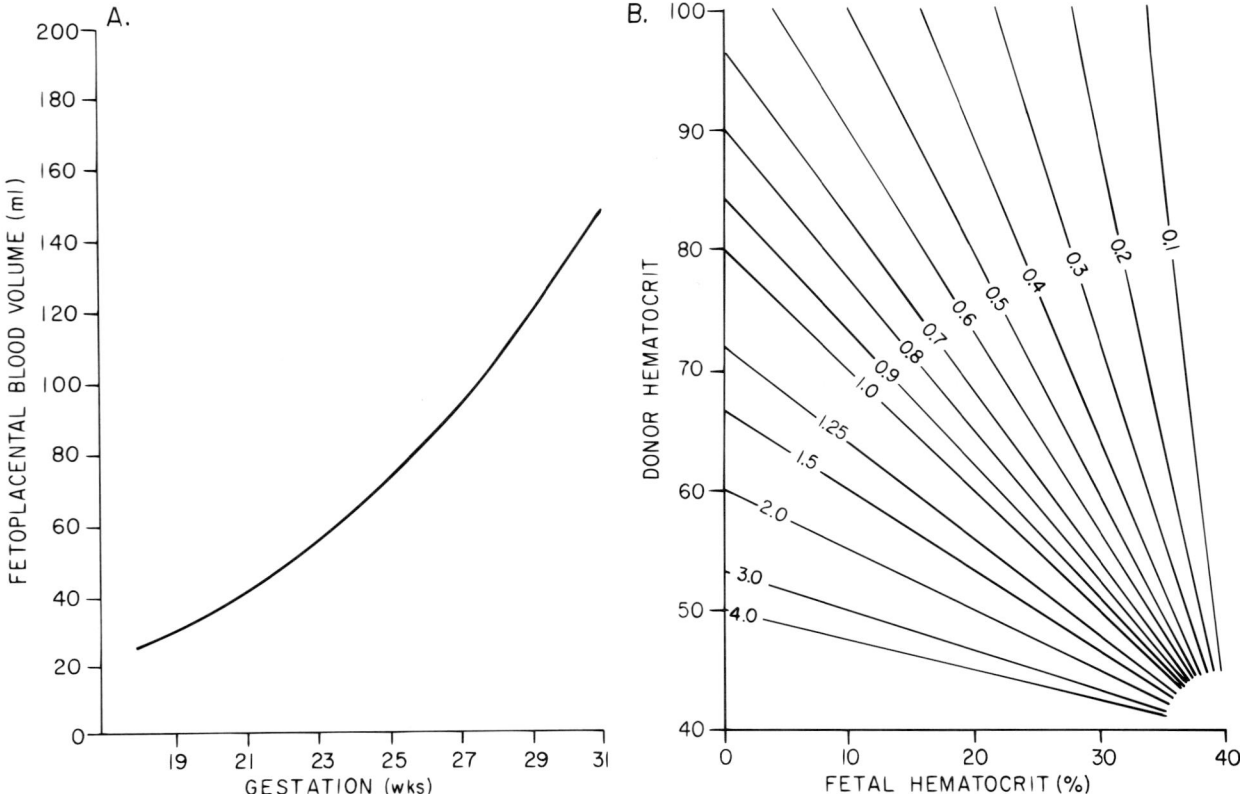

Figure 26–8. Graphs used to rapidly determine the volume of blood to be transfused intravascularly to achieve a posttransfusion hematocrit of 40 to 45 percent. First, the estimated fetoplacental blood volume (EFBV) is determined using the gestational age and *A*. Second, the pretransfusion fetal hematocrit and the donor blood hematocrit are used in conjunction with *B* to derive the multiplying factor. This factor is then multiplied by the EFBV to determine the amount of blood to be transfused. For example, at 26 weeks' gestation, the EFBV is found on the abscissa of *A* to be 85 ml. If the pretransfusion hematocrit is 20 percent and the donor blood hematocrit is 80 percent, the multiplying factor derived from *B* is 0.5. Multiplying this number by the EFBV (0.5 × 85 ml) shows that about 42 ml should be transfused. (Adapted from Nicolaides KH, Clewell WH, Mibashan RS, et al: Fetal haemoglobin measurement in the assessment of red cell isoimmunization. Lancet 1:1073, 1988.)

adult erythrocytes. One sample should be used to determine the fetal antigen status if it is still uncertain.

Several different methods of estimating the volume of blood needed for transfusion have been reported.[181–184] A posttransfusion hematocrit of around 40 percent is generally the target of these formulae, although some have suggested that transfusion of larger volumes to a hematocrit of 45 to 55 percent is superior.[185]

We calculate the volume of blood to be transfused according to the method described by Nicolaides et al.,[180] with a posttransfusion hematocrit of 40 to 45 percent as the usual goal. The initial fetal hematocrit, the hematocrit of the donor blood, and the gestational age are used in conjunction with the graphs shown in Figure 26–8 to determine the amount of blood to be infused. When the infusion is started, streaming or turbulence can be seen within the vessel, confirming that the needle tip is still within the vein. We infuse the blood at a rate of about 10 ml/min. At the end of the transfusion and before withdrawing the needle, a minute or so of circulation time is allowed; then a post-

transfusion sample is drawn for measurement of the final hematocrit.

Following intravascular transfusion, the decline in the donor hematocrit is most dependent on the life span of the donor erythrocytes, the rate of fetal growth (and increased vascular volume), and the ratio of fetal to donor erythrocytes (since the fetal erythrocytes are subject to continued hemolysis). The latter is most influential between the first and second intravascular transfusions, when the ratio of fetal cells to donor cells is greatest. MacGregor and colleagues[186] have used the following equations to predict the fetal hematocrit after transfusion:

Predicted Hct after first transfusion
$$= [(Hct_f - Hct_i) \times (EFW1/EFW2) \times (120 - \text{days elapsed})] \div 120$$

Predicted Hct after subsequent transfusions
$$= [Hct_f \times (EFW1/EFW2) \times (120 - \text{days elapsed})] \div 120$$

where Hct$_f$ is the post-transfusion hematocrit, Hct$_i$ is the initial (pretransfusion) hematocrit. EFW1 is the estimated fetal weight at the index transfusion, and EFW2 is the estimated fetal weight at the subsequent transfusion. Using different methods, other authors have predicted similar hematocrit changes.[187]

On average, the decline in the fetal hematocrit following the first transfusion is about 1.5 percent per day; following subsequent transfusions, the decline in fetal hematocrit is about 1.0 to 1.2 percent per day. Using intravascular transfusions for the management of severe fetal hemolysis, repeat transfusions are scheduled to keep the fetal hematocrit above 20 to 25 percent.

Although most authors recommend simple transfusion, some perform intravascular exchange transfusions, feeling that exchange transfusion may allow a longer interval between intravascular transfusions by replacing a greater volume of the fetal cells with donor cells.[171] Also, exchange transfusion is preferred in some centers because of the fear that the increase in blood volume with simple transfusion might compromise fetal cardiac capacity.[171,174] These fears are probably unfounded, as it seems that even a hydropic fetus can tolerate a bolus infusion of red cells without further compromise.[188]

Morbidity and mortality related to the technique of vascular access and transfusion are similar to those with intraperitoneal transfusion.[136,172,174,176] Fetal bradycardia is the most common problem, occurring in 8 to 12 percent of cases, although it is usually transient and only rarely requires immediate delivery. Postprocedure infection and premature rupture of the membranes have also been reported. The reported fetal death rate ranges between 0.6 percent[175] and 4.7 percent[136] per procedure, with hydropic fetuses being at greatest risk. Overall, it appears that intravascular transfusion in experienced hands seems to have a procedure-related complication rate of around 10 to 15 percent and a perinatal mortality rate of between 1 and 5 percent.

Using intravascular transfusions alone probably increases the total number of procedures required for each pregnancy because the volume of blood transfused at each procedure is smaller than that given via the intraperitoneal route. Also, up to 80 percent of blood transfused into the peritoneal cavity of nonhydropic fetuses appears in the fetal circulation,[189] a figure considerably higher than originally thought. Finally, as mentioned above, concern has been raised that intravascular procedures may increase maternal sensitization and iatrogenically worsen the disease.[93,139,141] It appears that umbilical cord blood sampling and intravascular transfusion can be associated with significant fetomaternal bleeding and a heightened maternal immune response, but actual clinical data from subsequent pregnancies are not available. Additionally, comparative data from intraperitoneal procedures are not available,

and it is not certain whether increases in α-fetoprotein and anti-D are greater following intravascular transfusion than following intraperitoneal transfusion.

Intraperitoneal versus Intravascular Transfusion

For the hydropic fetus, analysis of the collective experience of the last 15 years definitely shows an improved survival rate using intravascular transfusion when compared with treatment with intraperitoneal transfusion. However, the difference in outcome between the two techniques is much less clear in nonhydropic fetuses. In the absence of hydrops, survival rates of 80 to 100 percent have been documented for both methods, with near-identical rates of survival when the large published series are combined (Table 26–3). Unfortunately, a prospective, randomized clinical trial designed to determine the superior technique for the nonhydropic fetus has not been performed.

In an attempt to compare the two methods, Harman et al.[175] analyzed results from patients who underwent intravascular and intraperitoneal transfusions for severe fetal anemia. Forty-four patients undergoing 173 intravascular transfusions were compared retrospectively to 44 fetuses treated with 104 intraperitoneal transfusions in the same institution and matched for severity of disease, placental location, and gestational age. The authors concluded that intravascular transfusion was superior, based on a higher survival rate, a greater gestational age at delivery, and significant reductions in low Apgar scores, cesarean delivery rate, the need for and number of neonatal exchange transfusions, and intensive care nursery admissions and duration of stay. Additionally, the intraperitoneal group had a higher procedure-related mortality (7.7 percent vs. 0.6 percent per transfusion) and a greater overall rate of maternal complication (12.5 percent vs. 3 percent). However, the survival of nonhydropic fetuses was not significantly different between the two treatment groups, and the morbidity data were not analyzed separately for hydropic and nonhydropic fetuses. Acknowledging that the difference in survival for nonhydropic fetuses was statistically unconvincing, the authors nonetheless argued that the lower procedure-related loss rate with intravascular treatment was clinically significant and that intraperitoneal transfusion should be reserved for those situations where intravascular transfusion is impossible due to position of the fetus and cord.

Combined Intravascular Intraperitoneal Transfusion

In an effort to reduce the number of transfusions necessary during treatment of a severely involved pregnancy, Nicolini et al.[190] have combined intravascular and intraperitoneal transfusions. After intravascular transfusion to a fetal hematocrit of approximately 40 percent, additional blood calculated to raise the intravascular hematocrit to 60 percent was then transfused intraperitoneally. Using the estimated decline in fetal hematocrit and clinical parameters to decide upon the timing of the next transfusion, the authors performed only 3.2 procedures per patient, and the mean fall in hematocrit was slightly less than 1 percent per day. Comparison of 32 patients who had combined procedures to another 17 who received only intravascular transfusions revealed a slightly increased mean interval between transfusions (24.2 vs. 21.6 days) and a higher fetal hematocrit at the time of the subsequent procedure (27.0 vs. 23.2 percent). Although these differences achieved statistical significance, their clinical importance is unclear. While some authors have advocated routinely combining intravascular and intraperitoneal transfusion,[191] it is unknown whether the addition of intraperitoneal erythrocytes can reduce the number of transfusions per pregnancy or improve the outcomes achieved with intravascular transfusion alone. Because the increased morbidity associated with intraperitoneal transfusion likely offsets any benefits of the combined procedure, we do not routinely perform combined intravascular and intraperitoneal transfusions.

Other Therapies

A number of noninvasive alternatives to intrauterine transfusion have been investigated for the treatment of fetal hemolysis. Most of these alternative therapies have been aimed at modifying the maternal immune response so as to decrease the severity of erythroblastosis. Two of these, promethazine and oral ingestion of Rh-positive erythrocytes, are of historical interest only and were never proven to be of benefit.[192-195]

Plasmapheresis to reduce the level of maternal anti-D has been used in the treatment of severe Rh alloimmunization. Although the removal of several liters of plasma per week will result in a transient reduction in the anti-D titer during or immediately after treatment, a chronic, significant reduction in antibody titer is difficult, if not impossible, to achieve by this technique.[196-198] Some studies have suggested a benefit from plasmapheresis, but these results are difficult to interpret because of the concurrent use of other treatments and the lack of controls.[199,200] Furthermore, all studies of plasmapheresis in which several or more liters of plasma were removed weekly demonstrated an increase in anti-D titers or concentration soon after plasmapheresis was stopped. This "rebound" phenomenon has been attributed to the removal of the negative feedback influence on further anti-D production by high circulating titers of anti-D antibody.[201] Repeated, "small-volume" plasmapheresis may avoid antibody rebound.[201] The potential usefulness of plasmapheresis must be tempered by its potential for serious consequences for the mother and fetus, including sepsis.[197,199] Lacking a clearly documented benefit, plasmapheresis is not currently used at most centers in the treatment of severe Rh sensitization.

Plasmapheresis in combination with immunosuppression to prevent antibody rebound has also been used to treat severe Rh alloimmunization. Odendaal et al.[202] reported their experience with nine patients, seven of whom had a previous pregnancy loss or neonatal death directly or indirectly due to alloimmunization. Using plasmapheresis three to seven times a week and immunosuppression with azathioprine and prednisone, eight patients delivered liveborns between 28 and 33 weeks' gestation, with the single fetal death being associated with a placental abruption. Again, because of the potential for morbidity with plasmapheresis and immunosuppression, and because benefit has not yet been demonstrated in adequate numbers of patients, such therapy is not commonly used.

The successful use of high-dose intravenous immunoglobulin (IVIG) in platelet alloimmunization has led to its use in the treatment of severe Rh alloimmunization.[203-209] The mechanism of action is uncertain, but is thought to be via blockade of Fc-mediated antibody placental transport (limiting the transplacental passage of anti-D to the fetus), by blockade of Fc receptors in the fetal reticluoendothelial system (inhibiting the removal and destruction of anti-D–coated erythrocytes in the fetal spleen and liver), or by feedback inhibition of maternal anti-D production. It is most likely that the effect of IVIG is at the maternal or placental level, since anecdotal evidence suggests that administration of IgG directly to the fetus is not reliably effective in either Rh disease[210] or platelet alloimmunization.[211,212] Also, placental transport of exogenous IgG may be limited before 32 weeks' gestation.[213]

Unfortunately, data regarding IVIG use are mostly case reports and small case series using very different doses and schedules, and no sizable randomized trials are available. For instance, Marguiles et al.[204] administered IVIG to 24 Rh-sensitized women at a dose of 400 mg/kg for 5 consecutive days, every 2 weeks. All patients had either ΔOD_{450} results suggesting severe anemia, or a severely affected fetus in a previous pregnancy. None of the treated fetuses developed hydrops or required transfusion in utero or as neonates. Porter et al.[205] reported a patient with severe Rh disease whose clinical course was improved by weekly administration of IVIG, given at 1,000 mg/kg.

Deka et al.[206] treated six patients with severe Rh sensitization who had previous pregnancies complicated by hydrops at 28 to 34 weeks, four with stillbirths. Beginning at 14 to 18 weeks, they infused 100 mg/kg

IVIG every 3 to 4 weeks until fetal transfusion or delivery was necessary. Four patients delivered after 34 weeks without fetal treatment, and although the others required intrauterine transfusion, both delivered after 32 weeks.

Other groups have used IVIG but with less success. Voto et al.[207] reported a higher survival rate in selected Rh-sensitized patients who received IVIG, but found no improvement in the number of intrauterine transfusions necessary, the incidence of severe fetal anemia, or neonatal morbidity. Similar unimpressive findings have been reported elsewhere,[208] and a publication bias favoring positive outcomes is likely.

The success of IVIG therapy in ameliorating some cases of severe Rh disease presents exciting possibilities. Currently, use of IVIG should be reserved for the most severe cases that are refractory to traditional treatment. Further study and experience with more patients will be necessary before IVIG therapy has a place in the routine management of severe Rh immunization.

Timing of Delivery

During the early 1960s, liberalized use of preterm delivery markedly reduced the incidence of perinatal death in Rh-sensitized pregnancies, primarily by decreasing the incidence of intrauterine death.[114,214] However, severely affected fetuses continued to die in utero or from complications of prematurity. Fortunately, refinements in the technique of intrauterine transfusion have made possible the prolongation of pregnancy until a gestational age compatible with neonatal survival is reached. Also, the analysis of the phospholipid content of amniotic fluid to determine fetal pulmonary maturity has greatly clarified neonatal risk in relation to the timing of delivery. Finally, the tremendous improvements in neonatal care over the past three decades have led to excellent survival rates, with acceptable morbidity rates, for even the very preterm infant.

If the history and antenatal studies indicate only mild fetal hemolysis, we undertake delivery by induction of labor at 37 to 38 weeks' gestation, unless fetal pulmonary maturity is documented earlier by amniocentesis. In these cases, fetal pulmonary maturation does not seem to be either delayed or accelerated by disease, and amniotic fluid studies accurately reflect fetal maturity.[215,216] If the cervix is not ripe, we typically use intracervical prostaglandin gel prior to oxytocin induction.

With severely sensitized pregnancies, the risks of continued cord blood sampling and transfusions must be weighed against the expected neonatal morbidity and mortality associated with early delivery. Because the overall neonatal survival rate in most neonatal intensive care nurseries is greater than 95 percent after 32 weeks,

procedures have generally been timed so that the last transfusion is performed at around 30 to 32 weeks' gestation, with patients then delivered at 32 to 34 weeks after maternal steroid administration to enhance fetal pulmonary maturity.

A number of authors, in the interest of limiting neonatal morbidity, now recommend intrauterine transfusion up to 36 weeks' gestation when intravascular transfusion is feasible.[217] Delivery can then be accomplished between 37 and 38 weeks. Because the procedure-related death rate likely decreases with advancing gastational age, others have proposed performing transfusion as late as 37 weeks in selected cases, in order to decrease neonatal morbidity and cost.[218]

Rather than subject the fetus to the risk of repeated intrauterine transfusions, we generally time the last procedure so that delivery can be carried out at about 34 to 36 weeks. Overall neonatal survival approaches 100 percent at this gestational age and long-term morbidity from prematurity is exceedingly low. Regardless of the usual institutional practices, individual case circumstances need to be carefully weighed when making the decision as to when the fetus should be delivered.

SENSITIZATION CAUSED BY MINOR ANTIGENS

In addition to the D antigen, hundreds of other distinct antigens exist on the red blood cell surface. Known as "minor," "atypical," or "irregular" antigens, they have different frequencies in different ethnic populations. For instance, about 30 percent of blacks are positive for the Duffy antigen, whereas less than 5 percent of whites are Duffy positive.

In the past, minor antigens were a relatively infrequent cause of maternal sensitization and fetal or neonatal hemolytic disease. Because of the reduction in Rh disease brought about by Rh-immune globulin prophylaxis, minor antigen sensitization has become relatively more frequent in pregnancy. In fact, antibodies to minor antigens are much more common in the general population than antibodies to the D antigen.[90]

The large majority of cases of minor antigen sensitization are caused by incompatible blood transfusion. Although some authors have argued for adoption of routine screening of Kell status, most blood banks do not routinely assess donor–recipient compatibility for antigens other than ABO and RhD. Overall, antibodies to minor antigens occur in about 1.5 to 2.5 percent of obstetric patients.[219,220] Fortunately, some of the most common atypical antibodies, such as anti-Le[a], anti-Le[b], and anti-I, do not cause fetal or neonatal hemolysis. Le[a] and Le[b], the Lewis antigens are not true erythrocyte antigens, but are secreted by other tissues and then adsorbed onto the red cell surface.[221] Fetal erythrocytes acquire very little antigen in utero and thus react only weakly to anti-Lewis.

However, antibodies to a number of the minor antigens can result in fetal anemia and hydrops. Of the potentially serious antibodies, anti-E, anti-Kell, anti-c, anti-c + E, and anti-Fy[a] (Duffy) are the most common.[90] A complete listing of the irregular antigens and antibodies as compiled by Weinstein[222] is shown in Table 26–4, with the potential severity of fetal involvement and proposed management listed.

As with RhD, the genes coding for a number of the minor antigens have been identified and DNA-based diagnosis is commercially available.[223–228] The C, c, E, and e genes have been identified together on chromosome 1, Duffy is elsewhere on chromosome 1, Kell is on the long arm of chromosome 7, and Kidd (Jk[a]) is found on chromosome 18. Using PCR techniques to amplify fetal DNA, fetal antigen status can be reliably determined from fetal cells in uncultured amniotic fluid. At the time of the first amniocentesis, an additional 5 ml of amniotic fluid should be withdrawn and sent for fetal genotyping, if available.

In general, management of the pregnant patient with antibody to one of the significant minor antigens has been much the same as for RhD immunization. Pregnancies are followed using previous history as a guide, paternal antigen and zygosity testing to determine risk, frequent measurement of maternal antibody levels until a critical titer is reached, then serial amniocenteses with assessment of fetal antigen status and amniotic fluid bilirubin levels, and transfusion or delivery based on the ΔOD_{450} values and trends.[120,222] However, few centers have a large number of pregnancies affected by minor antigen sensitization; thus, establishment of a critical maternal titer is difficult, and it is uncertain whether amniotic fluid bilirubin studies are as reliable as with RhD alloimmunization.

Several of the minor antigens deserve special mention. The M antigen is part of the MNSs blood group system and is one of the commonly encountered minor antigens, since approximately 20 to 25 percent of the population is M negative. Improvements in antibody screening techniques have improved the sensitivity of detection of anti-M, and the frequency of identification of maternal anti-M is apparently increasing. De Young-Owens et al.[229] reported on 115 pregnancies complicated by M alloimmunization over more than 25 years. Of the 70 incompatible fetuses, none had severe fetal or neonatal anemia, and only 9 (13 percent) required phototherapy. Also, 104 of the 115 pregnancies (90 percent) had an initial anti-M titer of 1:4 or less, and only one of these patients had a titer rise to greater then 1:32. The authors concluded that there is limited benefit

to following serial anti-M titers, and if there is no previous history of an affected fetus and the initial titer is 1:4 or less, no further assessment of anti-M titers is necessary.

However, there are a number of case reports of severe fetal and neonatal hemolytic disease due to M sensitization.[230,231] It has been suggested that although most anti-M is an IgM antibody with no implications for the fetus, some sensitized women produce a potent anti-M IgG which can cross the placenta and result in fetal anemia and hydrops.

Despite the favorable experience of De Young-Owens et al.,[229] we assess paternal M antigen status and perform serial anti-M titers in sensitized pregnancies without a history of an affected fetus. If the titer rises unexpectedly, amniocentesis is performed for amniotic fluid bilirubin studies and determination of fetal M status. Because anti-M does not seem to be as aggressive or as serious as most of the other antigens, our threshold for amniocentesis is generally higher than for the other serious antigens, although we consider each case on an individual basis.

The Kell antigen also requires additional discussion. Pregnancy with Kell sensitization can result in severe fetal anemia, hydrops, and fetal death. In common usage, "Kell" refers to the K or K1 antigen of the Kell blood group system. Only about 9 percent of whites are positive for the Kell antigen; the population frequency of kk (Kell negative) is 91.1 percent, Kk (heterozygous positive) 8.7 percent, and KK (homozygous positive) 0.2 percent.[7] About 0.2 percent of pregnant women are positive for anti-Kell and, as mentioned above, most cases of immunization are the result of Kell-incompatible transfusion.

A number of investigators have suggested that the fetal anemia associated with Kell sensitization is qualitatively different from that of Rh disease and requires a different management protocol.[232,238] Specifically, maternal titers and amniotic fluid ΔOD_{450} values may not be as predictive of the degree of fetal anemia as with RhD sensitization. For example, Berkowitz et al.[232] reported a case of fetal hydrops and death due to Kell sensitization despite amniotic fluid ΔOD_{450} values trending downward in the lower third of the Liley midzone. Similarly, Parilla et al.[233] reported a Kell-positive fetus that developed hydrops despite declining values in zone II of the modified Liley curve. Copel et al.[234] reported a case of fetal hydrops with a maternal anti-Kell titer of 1:4; in another patient, the anti-Kell titer spontaneously rose from 1:32 to 1:2,048 even though the fetus was Kell negative.

It has been proposed that the mechanism of anemia in Kell sensitization is different than with RhD disease. Although hemolysis is important and Kell antibody can activate the complement cascade to attach C3 to red cell membranes,[238] it also appears that suppression of

Table 26-4. ATYPICAL ANTIBODIES AND THEIR RELATIONSHIP TO FETAL HEMOLYTIC DISEASE

Blood Group System	Antigens Related to Hemolytic Disease	Hemolytic Disease Severity	Proposed Management
Lewis	Not a proven cause of hemolytic disease of the newborn		
I	Not a proven cause of hemolytic disease of the newborn		
Kell	K	Mild to severe with hydrops fetalis	Amniotic fluid bilirubin studies
	k	Mild	Expectant
	Ko	Mild	Expectant
	Kp^a	Mild	Expectant
	Kp^b	Mild	Expectant
	Js^a	Mild	Expectant
	Js^b	Mild	Expectant
Rh (non-D)	E	Mild to severe with hydrops fetalis	Amniotic fluid bilirubin studies
	C	Mild to severe with hydrops fetalis	Amniotic fluid bilirubin studies
	c	Mild to severe with hydrops fetalis	Amniotic fluid bilirubin studies
Duffy	Fy^a	Mild to severe with hydrops fetalis	Amniotic fluid bilirubin studies
	Fy^b	Not a cause of hemolytic disease in the newborn	
	By^3	Mild	Expectant
Kidd	Jk^a	Mild to severe	Amniotic fluid bilirubin
	Jk^b	Mild	Expectant
	Jk^3	Mild	Expectant
MNSs	M	Mild to severe	Amniotic fluid bilirubin studies
	N	Mild	Expectant
	S	Mild to severe	Amniotic fluid bilirubin studies
	s	Mild to severe	Amniotic fluid bilirubin studies
	U	Mild to severe	Amniotic fluid bilirubin studies
	Mi^a	Moderate	Amniotic fluid
MSSs	Mt^a	Moderate	Amniotic fluid bilirubin studies
	Vw	Mild	Expectant
	Mur	Mild	Expectant
	Hil	Mild	Expectant
	Hut	Mild	Expectant
Lutheran	Lu^a	Mild	Expectant
	Lu^b	Mild	Expectant
Diego	D1^a	Mild to severe	Amniotic fluid bilirubin studies
	Di^b	Mild to severe	Amniotic fluid bilirubin studies
Xg	Xg^a	Mild	Expectant
P	PP$_{1pk}$(Tj^a)	Mild to severe	Amniotic fluid bilirubin studies
Public antigens	Yt^a	Moderate to severe	Amniotic fluid bilirubin studies
	Yt^b	Mild	Expectant
	Lan	Mild	Expectant
	En^a	Moderate	Amniotic fluid bilirubin studies
	Ge	Mild	Expectant
	Jr^a	Mild	Expectant
	Co^a	Severe	Amniotic fluid bilirubin studies
	Co^{1-b-}	Mild	Expectant
Private antigens	Batty	Mild	Expectant
	Becker	Mild	Expectant
	Berrens	Mild	Expectant
	Biles	Moderate	Amniotic fluid bilirubin studies
	Evans	Mild	Expectant
	Gonzales	Mild	Expectant
	Good	Severe	Amniotic fluid bilirubin studies
	Heibel	Moderate	Amniotic fluid
	Hunt	Mild	Expectant
	Jobbins	Mild	Expectant
	Radin	Moderate	Amniotic fluid bilirubin studies
	Rm	Mild	Expectant
	Ven	Mild	Expectant
	Wright^a	Severe	Amniotic fluid bilirubin studies
	Wright^b	Mild	Expectant
	Zd	Moderate	Amniotic fluid bilirubin studies

Modified from Weinstein L: Irregular antibodies causing hemolytic disease of the newborn: a continuing problem. Clin Obstet Gynecol 25:321, 1982.

fetal erythropoiesis plays a role in the development of fetal anemia due to anti-Kell.[239–241]

Vaughn et al.[239] compared amniotic fluid bilirubin concentrations and nucleated red blood cell and reticulocyte counts in fetuses with Kell and RhD alloimmunization. Kell-sensitized pregnancies had lower levels of all three parameters and no relation between fetal hematocrit and reticulocytosis, in contrast to Rh-sensitized pregnancies. Similar findings were reported by Weiner et al.,[240] who also showed that fetal erythropoeitin levels in both groups rose significantly as hematocrit declined. Weiner and colleagues speculated that the anemia of Kell sensitization is associated with greater hemolysis of nonhemoglobinized or incompletely hemoglobinized erythroid precursors.

To test the effect of Kell sensitization on fetal erythropoiesis, Vaughn et al.[241] compared the growth in vitro of immature Kell-positive and Kell-negative red cells in the presence of anti-Kell IgG antibody. They found that anti-Kell antibody inhibited Kell-positive erythroid progenitor cell growth in a dose-dependent fashion, with the more immature progenitor cells being affected the most. There was no inhibition of Kell-negative cells, and anti-D did not impair the growth of immature RhD-positive erythrocytes.

Caine and Mueller-Heubach[235] described their clinical experience with 127 Kell-sensitized pregnancies. Thirteen (10 percent) had an affected Kell-positive fetus, and five (38 percent of those affected) had severe disease. Only 3 percent of pregnancies with a maternal titer of less than or equal to 1:16 had a Kell-positive fetus compared with 29 percent of those with a titer greater than 1:16. No patient with a titer less than or equal to 1:16 had a fetal death, and all patients with a poor perinatal outcome had a titer greater than or equal to 1:128 at delivery. Importantly, no patient with a poor outcome had an amniotic fluid ΔOD_{450} value in the highest Liley zone, suggesting that serious hemolytic disease develops at lower ΔOD_{450} values than with Rh sensitization.

Leggat and co-workers[236] described 194 pregnancies over 25 years in which anti-Kell was the only antibody identified. Of the 178 unaffected babies, 106 (60 percent) had maternal titers greater than or equal to 1:16. There were 16 affected infants (9 percent of the total), 10 with mild disease and 6 with moderate or severe anemia. Of the six mothers who delivered affected infants, four had titers greater than or equal to 1:16, while two had titers less than or equal to 1:8. Amniotic fluid analysis was also performed in pregnancies that resulted in 16 unaffected and five affected newborns; fetuses with disease of moderate or greater severity had ΔOD_{450} values trending upward or in the upper part of the Liley midzone, but four unaffected fetuses had ΔOD_{450} values that would be associated with moderate to severe hemolysis in Rh disease. The authors concluded that neither maternal antibody titer or amniotic fluid analysis was a satisfactory predictor of fetal status.

Bowman and colleagues,[242] on the other hand, found that amniotic fluid ΔOD_{450} measurements were accurate in predicting fetal status in 16 of 18 Kell-negative pregnancies. In 10 of 12 Kell-positive fetuses, ΔOD_{450} values appropriately predicted disease severity, although the ΔOD_{450} level of one fetus with a hydropic death was in the lower half of zone II, and those of another fetus with only moderate disease reached the line between zones II and III.

McKenna et al.[243] reported their experience with 21 pregnancies affected with Kell alloimmunization. Eight (38 percent) were severely affected, and all of these had maternal anti-Kell titers of 1:32 or greater. Using a Liley curve extrapolated back to 20 weeks, the authors also showed that ΔOD_{450} values which remained in zone I excluded severe disease. Similar to others' experience (and to that with Rh disease), values in zone III nearly always indicated severe involvement, whereas values in zone II were difficult to characterize, being a mix of severe, mild, and unaffected fetuses.

Because of concern for misleading amniotic fluid results, several authors suggested a management scheme for Kell-sensitized pregnancies that includes umbilical cord blood sampling at 20 weeks' gestation when the father is either Kell positive or of uncertain status.[237,244] With this protocol, more than half of the fetuses will be found to be Kell negative, and no further testing will be necessary; rarely, a fetus will be found to be significantly anemic and can be promptly transfused. However, management after 20 weeks' gestation of the approximately 80 percent of Kell-positive fetuses destined to have mild or moderate disease is not addressed by this cord sampling protocol. Also, the more recent advances in diagnosis of antigen status from amniotic fluid obviate the need for cordocentesis for determining fetal blood type.

Recognizing that amniotic fluid bilirubin studies may be misleading in some pregnancies and that more liberal use of umbilical cord blood sampling is appropriate, we agree with Bowman et al.,[242] and McKenna et al.[243] that serial ΔOD_{450} measurements are still of value. When the father is known to be Kell negative, the fetus will also be Kell negative, and no surveillance or testing is necessary. When the father is Kell positive or of uncertain status and there is no history of severe fetal involvement, we follow maternal anti-Kell titers, track fetal movements, and perform serial ultrasounds as long as the maternal titer remains below 1:8. For patients whose titers rise above 1:8 or who have a history of fetal involvement, we perform serial amniocenteses every 1 to 4 weeks unless the fetus is known to be Kell negative, beginning at 20 to 28 weeks depending on history, maternal titer, and previous

ΔOD_{450} value. At the first amniocentesis, we also determine fetal Kell antigen status by DNA testing. As with RhD disease, we use a modified Liley curve extrapolated back to 24 weeks (Fig. 26–4); before 24 weeks' gestation, we typically use Queenan's boundaries[125] with an emphasis on ΔOD_{450} trends. If ΔOD_{450} levels rise into or above the middle of zone II, we recommend umbilical cord blood sampling for hematocrit, with blood ready for transfusion if necessary. Between amniocenteses and/or fetal blood samplings, we perform nonstress tests and frequent ultrasounds, watching for any signs of developing hydrops.

PLATELET ALLOIMMUNIZATION

Like erythrocytes, platelets contain specific surface antigens, and maternal sensitization to platelet antigens can occur when there is an incompatibility between fetus and mother. In a situation analogous to Rh disease, alloimmune thrombocytopenia is the result of maternal sensitization to incompatible fetal platelets with transfer of antiplatelet antibody to the fetus and subsequent sequestration of platelets in the reticuloendothelial system.[245] In affected cases, the maternal platelet count is normal, and fetal–neonatal thrombocytopenia ranges from mild to profound.

Five major biallelic systems of platelet-specific antigens have been well described. Formerly known as Pl[A1]/Pl[A2], Ko[b]/Ko[a], Bak[a]/Bak[b] (Lek[a]/Lek[b]), Pen[a]/Pen[b] (Yuk[b]/Yuk[a]), and Br[b]/Br[a], a new and simplified system of nomenclature for the human platelet antigens has been proposed (Table 26–5).[246] The major platelet antigen families are now numbered in chronologic order of discovery (HPA-1 through HPA-5), and the older naming system is gradually being replaced. Platelets also express HLA class I antigens but not those of class II.[247,248]

Table 26–5. PLATELET-SPECIFIC ALLOANTIGENS

Old Nomenclature	New Nomenclature	Gene Frequency
Pl[A1]	HPA-1a	0.85
Pl[A2]	HPA-1b	0.15
Ko[b]	HPA-2a	0.93
Ko[a]	HPA-2b	0.07
Bak[a] (Lek[a])	HPA-3a	0.61
Bak[b] (Lek[b])	HPA-3b	0.39
Pen[a] (Yuk[b])	HPA-4a	0.99
Pen[b] (Yuk[a])	HPA-4b	0.01
Br[b]	HPA-5a	0.89
Br[a]	HPA-5b	0.11

Sensitization to the HPA-1a (Pl[A1]) antigen is the etiology in about three fourths of cases of neonatal alloimmune thrombocytopenia. Approximately 2 percent of whites, 0.4 percent of blacks, and less than 0.1 percent of Asians are negative for HPA-1a. Sensitization to HPA-5b (Br[a]) and HPA-3a (Bak[a]) account for most of the remainder of cases of neonatal alloimmune thrombocytopenia; about 15 percent of whites are negative for HPA-3a, and less than 1 percent of whites are negative for HPA-5b.[247,248] Although HLA antigens are less immunogenic on platelets than on other cells, anti-HLA antibodies can rarely cause neonatal alloimmune thrombocytopenia.[249]

Neonatal alloimmune thrombocytopenia occurs in about 1 in 1,000 to 1 in 2,000 births and is probably the most common reason for severe thrombocytopenia in the newborn.[245,250,252] Even though fetal–maternal incompatibility to platelet antigens is relatively common, only a small fraction of gravidas become sensitized. For instance, around 2 percent of all pregnancies are complicated by HPA-1a incompatibility, and as many as 60 percent of pregnancies are mismatched for HPA-3a. The reasons for the infrequent occurrence of alloimmunization are not completely clear, but in addition to platelet antigen incompatibility, maternal HLA class II type appears to influence susceptibility to platelet alloimmunization; HLA-DRw52 is associated with HPA-1a alloimmunization, and HLA-DRw6 is associated with sensitization to HPA-5b.[253]

The clinical severity of neonatal alloimmune thrombocytopenia varies widely. Approximately 90 percent of affected newborns have diffuse petechiae, and 9 to 12 percent suffer intracranial bleeding, with a neonatal mortality of 5 to 13 percent.[247,250] About 45 percent of cases of central nervous system hemorrhage are thought to occur before birth, often resulting in porencephalic cysts that can be identified with ultrasound.[254] Fetal thrombocytopenia appears to be most common in the third trimester, but has been detected as early as 20 weeks' gestation.[134,255]

Unlike Rh alloimmunization, maternal titers of antibody to the platelet antigen are not predictive of clinical outcome, antiplatelet IgG production can occur in the first pregnancy, and firstborn children are often affected. Primiparas account for between 20 and 60 percent of identified cases,[247,256] and mothers at risk are usually identified only after the birth of an affected newborn.

Although routine testing of pregnant women for HPA status has been proposed,[257] there are several reasons why all pregnant women are not screened for antigen status or the presence of antiplatelet antibodies. First, perhaps one fourth of cases of alloimmune neonatal thrombocytopenia are not due to the most commonly involved antigen. Second, the maternal immune response seems to be influenced by other factors such as HLA type, and only a minority of infants of mothers negative for the platelet antigen will develop significant thrombocytopenia. Finally, adequate analyses of risk/benefit ratio and cost effectiveness have not been performed.

Recognizing the possibility of ascertainment bias, the incidence of recurrent fetal–neonatal thrombocytopenia following delivery of an affected newborn is thought to be 90 to 95 percent, generally of equal or greater severity.[247,248] Bussel and colleagues[258] described the natural history of alloimmune thrombocytopenia in 107 untreated fetuses; nearly all cases were identified because of thrombocytopenia in an older sibling. With cordocentesis at a mean gestational age of 25 weeks, 42 percent had a platelet count less than the newborn count of their older sibling, 70 percent had a platelet count less than 50,000 cells/μl, and 50 percent had platelet counts less than 20,000 cells/μl. Seven fetuses had an initial platelet count greater than 80,000/μl and were not treated; follow-up sampling showed decreases in platelet count of at least 10,000 cells/μl per week in these fetuses.

Bussel et al.[258] found no correlation between the platelet count at cordocentesis and the degree of thrombocytopenia in the previously affected sibling. However, patients with HPA-1a incompatibility had lower cord blood platelet counts than those sensitized to other antigens, and a past history of antenatal intracranial hemorrhage predicted a more severe thrombocytopenia.

The management of patients at risk for neonatal alloimmune thrombocytopenia is directed at preventing hemorrhage in the fetus and neonate. Before the availability of umbilical cord blood sampling, the management strategy for these pregnancies was to avoid fetal trauma with bed rest during the pregnancy and cesarean delivery before labor.[259,260] However, since approximately half of fetuses who suffer intracranial bleeding do so before labor, avoidance of labor and vaginal delivery only partially reduces the associated morbidity and mortality. As mentioned, maternal platelet counts are normal, and maternal antibody levels are not predictive of fetal platelet count. Umbilical cord blood sampling and direct measurement of fetal platelet count is currently the only method to accurately assess disease severity.

Several strategies have been proposed for the management of pregnancies at risk for alloimmune thrombocytopenia. One group has suggested that the diagnosis of fetal thrombocytopenia be made by cordocentesis at 20 to 22 weeks' gestation, and patients with an affected fetus should be advised to rest carefully and avoid abdominal trauma.[261,262] At 37 weeks' gestation, umbilical cord blood sampling can be repeated, and if the fetal platelet count is normal, labor can be induced; if the platelet count is less than 50,000 cells/μl, maternal platelets are transfused into the fetal circulation using the following formula, allowing safe induction of labor and vaginal delivery:

$$V = \frac{EFBV \times (\text{desired FPC} - \text{pretransfusion FPC})}{\text{Platelet count of infusate}}$$

where V is volume of platelet concentrate to be transfused, EFBV is estimated fetal blood volume, and FPC is fetal platelet count.[262] This approach, with a single fetal platelet transfusion immediately before delivery, does not address the possibility of spontaneous hemorrhage in utero, but may be the most reasonable management plan for fetuses considered to be at low risk for antepartum bleeding.

In an effort to prevent antepartum intracranial bleeding, Nicolini et al.[263] and Murphy et al.[264] reported the use of serial platelet transfusions throughout the third trimester. Both patients described had previous infants with HPA-1a alloimmune thrombocytopenia leading to severe antepartum intracranial hemorrhage with neurologic sequelae. Fetal thrombocytopenia was documented with cordocentesis, and weekly platelet transfusions were begun at 26 to 29 weeks. Platelets transfused in utero have a short life span (even HPA-1a–negative platelets), and counts dropped from posttransfusion levels of over 150,000 cells/μl to less than 50,000 cells/μl at the next weekly transfusion. The pregnancies were carried to 32 and 35 weeks, respectively, and delivered by cesarean section. Neonatal platelet counts were greater than 44,000 cells/μl, and neither infant suffered intracranial bleeding. Because of the potentially high fetal morbidity and mortality associated with frequent cordocentesis in alloimmune thrombocytopenia[265] and because of the difficulty and risks of repeated maternal platelet pheresis, this management scheme has not been widely adopted. Fetal intracranial hemorrhage is rare before the third trimester, and it has been suggested that the weekly intrauterine platelet transfusion might be limited to the third trimester, with delivery as soon as pulmonary maturity is documented.[266,267]

The most widely used management for fetal thrombocytopenia involves the maternal administration of high-dose IgG.[258,269] This treatment is based on the well-established observation that most cases of neonatal alloimmune thrombocytopenia are effectively treated by giving the neonate IVIG.[270-272] The mechanism of action in pregnancy is uncertain but may involve Fc-receptor blockade in the fetal reticuloendothelial system and inhibition of uptake of IgG-coated platelets by reticuloendothelial cells, or Fc-receptor saturation in the placenta, inhibiting the transplacental transfer of specific antiplatelet antibody. A maternal or placental mechanism of effect seems more likely, since maternally administered IgG does not appear to cross the placenta effectively prior to 32 weeks' gestation.[213] Reports of umbilical cord infusion of IgG failing to improve fetal platelet count, and a lack of correlation between fetal IgG levels and response to treatment also suggest that any beneficial effect of maternal immunoglobulin infusion is likely attributable to maternal or placental factors.[211,212] Finally, immunoglobulin has been shown in vitro to block transport of anti–HPA-1a in a human placental perfusion model.[273]

Expanding on an earlier report,[255] Lynch and coworkers[268] administered IVIG (maternal) and serially measured fetal platelet counts in 18 women who had previously delivered an infant with severe alloimmune thrombocytopenia. After confirming thrombocytopenia at 20 to 22 weeks' gestation or at referral, weekly infusions of IVIG (1.0 g/kg body weight) were initiated. Umbilical cord blood sampling was repeated 4 to 6 weeks later to assess the effect of the therapy and then again at term to determine the mode of delivery. Nine of the 18 patients also received corticosteroids. The median platelet count rose from 32,000 cells/μl before treatment to 60,000 cells/μl at birth. Only three infants had a fetal platelet count less than 30,000 cells/μl at term, and there were no cases of intracranial hemorrhage (compared with 7 of the 18 previous, untreated siblings). In this series, steroid treatment did not appear to have a beneficial effect on fetal platelet count.

Bussel and colleagues[269] then studied the effect of maternal IVIG and steroids in 54 pregnancies complicated by alloimmune thrombocytopenia; 52 cases were due to HPA-1a alloimmunization, and all fetuses had platelet counts less than 100,000 cells/μl at first cordocentesis. Forty-seven patients had a second cordocentesis after weekly IVIG (1.0 g/kg), either with or without additional dexamethasone (1.5 mg/day). Seventy-four percent of these patients demonstrated a favorable response to treatment, defined as either (1) an increased platelet count, with a level of at least 20,000 cells/μl; or (2) a decrease of no more than 10,000 cells/μl while maintaining a count greater than 40,000 platelets/μl. Addition of steroids did not influence the response.

Nine patients who failed initial treatment (and another with late presentation who was not previously treated) were then given "salvage" therapy with prednisone (60 mg/day) added to their IVIG regimen.[269] Five patients had a favorable response, increasing their platelet count to a mean of 77,600 cells/μl at birth, and all newborns had a platelet count greater than 30,000 cells/μl. Thus, Bussel and colleagues found that around 75% of patients with alloimmune thrombocytopenia responded adequately to weekly maternal IVIG, and half of the nonresponders improved with addition of high-dose prednisone. There were no cases of intracranial hemorrhage in their series.

Similar results have been reported by others. Kaplan et al.[274] had 67 percent of patients respond with either an improvement or plateau in fetal platelet counts with use of maternal IVIG; only about a third of patients treated with prednisone alone showed a favorable effect. Silver et al.[212] reported that six of eight patients treated with IVIG had an increase in fetal platelet count, with five of the six having a neonatal platelet count greater than 50,000 cells/μl.

Although these results are encouraging, fetal platelet count is not always increased with maternal high-dose immunoglobulin infusion, even with a documented increase in fetal immunoglobulin levels.[212,262,275–277] Also, IVIG is quite expensive ($> \$1,000$ per weekly infusion), occasional shortages in supply have occurred, and although the infectious risk of blood product infusion is low, sporadic outbreaks of acute hepatitis C associated with use of IVIG have been reported.[278]

Determination of platelet antigen genotypes using PCR has been described,[279,280] and confirmation of paternal zygosity is straightforward. In cases of alloimmunization where the father is homozygous for the antigen and paternity is certain, the fetus will always be heterozygous and at significant risk for thrombocytopenia. On the other hand, if the father is heterozygous, there is a 50 percent likelihood that the fetus will not inherit the platelet incompatibility. About 25 percent of whites are heterozygous HPA-1a/HPA-1b, around 50 percent are heterozygous HPA-3a/HPA-3b, and 20 percent are heterozygous HPA-5a/HPA-5b. Thus, a significant proportion of the fetuses of alloimmunized women will not be at risk for thrombocytopenia.

As with Rh disease, determination of fetal antigen status (and risk of thrombocytopenia) in sensitized pregnancies is routinely available from uncultured amniocytes, and diagnosis of fetal platelet antigen status is possible without umbilical cord blood sampling.[281,282]

In the management of patients at risk for alloimmune thrombocytopenia, we first determine paternal genotype. If the father is heterozygous for the particular antigen, we recommend amniocentesis at 16 to 20 weeks to assess fetal antigen status. If the fetus is antigen-negative, there is no significant risk of thrombocytopenia or intracranial hemorrhage and no fetal blood sampling is performed.

If the fetus is antigen-positive, we offer cordocentesis at 22 to 26 weeks to determine fetal platelet count. If the platelet count is normal, or if the patient declines cordocentesis and treatment, we advocate modified bed rest with avoidance of abdominal trauma. In cases where the fetal platelet count is less than about 100,000 cells/μl, weekly infusions of IgG are initiated.

In agreement with the protocol of Bussel et al.[269] we then recommend a second cordocentesis about 6 weeks later, regardless of initial platelet count. If an untreated patient manifests thrombocytopenia at the second sampling, weekly infusions of IgG are begun. If a treated patient demonstrates a favorable response, IVIG is continued. On the other hand, if a treated patient has a further decline in platelet count or if their count is unacceptably low, we add daily prednisone to their IgG regimen.

If vaginal delivery is anticipated, a third cordocentesis is performed at about 37 weeks. If the platelet count is greater than 50,000 cells/μl, labor is induced. If the platelet count is less than 50,000 cells/μl, platelet transfusion into the umbilical vein, with documentation of an adequate posttransfusion platelet count, is followed by induction of labor. If cesarean delivery is planned, this final cordocentesis is omitted from the management scheme.

Patients thought to be at relatively lower risk for intracranial hemorrhage may begin their assessment somewhat later than outlined above. Conversely, patients with a previous severely thrombocytopenic fetus and significant antepartum morbidity are generally offered surveillance at an earlier gestational age, but the risks of repeated umbilical blood sampling and serial platelet transfusions do not seem to be warranted except in extreme cases. If the fetus remains severely thrombocytopenic (<50,000 platelets/μl) in spite of attempts to raise the platelet count, cesarean delivery is preferred.

The risks of umbilical cord blood sampling have been described, with reported fetal death rates of around 0.5 to 2 percent.[133–138] The fetus with thrombocytopenia is perhaps at greatest risk from cordocentesis, because of the possibility of uncontrolled bleeding at the puncture site. Paidas et al.[265] described five fetuses who died following cordocentesis for alloimmune thrombocytopenia. The group had a mean platelet count of only 5,000 cells/μl, and all five had levels less than 20,000 platelets/μl. Four of the five had a previous sibling with antenatal intracranial hemorrhage, a significantly greater proportion than in a comparison group without fetal loss.

To reduce the risk of exsanguination, concentrated maternal (antigen-negative) platelets, obtained by pheresis a day or two prior to cordocentesis, should be infused after sampling and before needle removal. The volume to be infused can be calculated using the formula above, aiming for a target of at least 50,000 cells/μl, and is generally in the range of 3 to 10 ml, depending on gestational age and concentration of the infusate. Despite use of maternal platelets, postprocedure hemorrhage is still a risk; one patient in the series of Silver et al. bled after an apparently uneventful cordocentesis with prophylactic platelet infusion.[212] Because of the risk of emergent delivery after cordocentesis, we generally administer corticosteroids for enhancement of fetal pulmonary maturity prior to the procedure.

In all cases of documented fetal–neonatal alloimmune thrombocytopenia, maternal platelets should be available for transfusion after delivery, regardless of the treatment protocol used or the antepartum fetal platelet count.

Key Points

➤ To reduce the incidence of Rh sensitization, Rh-immune globulin should be given to Rh-negative unsensitized women at 28 weeks' gestational age and again after delivery if the newborn is Rh-positive. Rh-immune globulin is also indicated for these patients in cases of miscarriage; ectopic pregnancy; chorionic villus sampling, amniocentesis, or other intrauterine procedures; abdominal trauma or fetal death in the second or third trimester; or fetomaternal hemorrhage.

➤ The gene coding for the D antigen has been identified, and prenatal determination of fetal Rh status is routinely available from uncultured amniocytes obtained at amniocentesis.

➤ Measurement of amniotic fluid bilirubin remains the standard for assessment of pregnancies at risk for significant fetal anemia. Neither ultrasound alone nor Doppler studies are adequately sensitive to identify anemic fetuses.

➤ The timing of the first amniocentesis is based on history, maternal anti-D titers, gestational age, and ultrasound findings. The timing of subsequent amniocenteses is based on the ΔOD_{450} values and trends.

➤ Analysis of amniotic fluid bilirubin before 26 weeks is controversial. Although most data suggest that ΔOD_{450} values and trends are accurate before the third trimester, more liberal use of cordocentesis may be appropriate.

➤ Fetal transfusion can be performed using either the intraperitoneal or intravascular route. For hydropic fetuses, intravascular transfusion is clearly superior. For nonhydropic fetuses, perinatal survival rates are similar with either method. Despite this, the intravascular route is generally preferred because of its directness and precision in correcting anemia, and because of the greater morbidity of intraperitoneal transfusion.

➤ With the reduction in Rh disease brought about by widespread use of Rh-immune globulin prophylaxis, sensitization to the minor or atypical antigens has become relatively more common. A number of these minor antigens can cause several fetal anemia.

➤ Management of pregnancies complicated by sensitization to one of the serious minor antigens (such as Kell) is based on the experience with Rh disease, and determination of fetal antigen status from uncultured amniocytes is available for the most common antigens. However, amniotic fluid bilirubin analysis may not be as accurate an indicator of fetal anemia with Kell sensitization as with Rh disease, and a more frequent use of cordocentesis is probably appropriate.

➤ Platelets also carry distinct antigens and, in a process similar to Rh sensitization, platelet alloimmunization can occur. Unlike Rh disease, firstborn fetuses can be affected, and maternal antibody titers do not predict fetal platelet count.

➤ The optimal management scheme for pregnancies affected with platelet alloimmunization is unclear. A protocol has been proposed that involves (1) cordocentesis at 22 to 26 weeks for documentation of thrombocytopenia, (2) weekly maternal administration of IVIG, (3) a second cordocentesis later to assess response, and (4) addition of prednisone to the regimen for patients who fail initial treatment. A third cordocentesis is then performed at term to determine platelet count before delivery, unless cesarean section is planned.

REFERENCES

1. Diamond LK, Blackfan KD, Baty JM: Erythroblastosis fetalis and its association with universal edema of the fetus, icterus gravis neonatorum and anemia of the newborn. J Pediatr 1:269, 1932.
2. Darrow RR: Icterus gravis (erythroblastosis) neonatorum: examination of etiologic considerations. Arch Pathol Lab Med 25:378, 1938.
3. Levine P, Stetson RE: An unusual case of intragroup agglutination. JAMA 113:126, 1939.
4. Levin P, Burnham L, Katzin EM, et al: The role of isoimmunization in the pathogenesis of erythroblastosis fetalis. Am J Obstet Gynecol 42:925, 1941.
5. Landsteiner K, Wiener AS: An agglutinable factor in human blood recognized by immune sera for rhesus blood. Proc Soc Exp Biol Med 43:223, 1940.
6. Rosenfield RE, Allen FH Jr, Swisher SN, Kochwa S: A review of Rh serology and presentation of a new terminology. Transfusion 2:287, 1962.
7. Race RR, Sanger R: Blood Groups in Man. 6th ed. Blackwell, Oxford, 1975.
8. Rote NS: Pathophysiology of Rh isoimmunization. Clin Obstet Gynecol 25:243, 1982.
9. Wiener AS: The Rh series of allelic genes. Science 100:595, 1944.
10. Rosenfield RE, Allen FH, Rubenstein P: Genetic model for the Rh blood-group system. Proc Natl Acad Sci U S A 70:1303, 1973.
11. Marsh WL, Chaganti RSK, Mayer K, et al: Mapping human autosomes: evidence supporting assignment of rhesus to the short arm of chromosome number 1. Science 183:966, 1974.
12. Marsh W, Kimball LF: Mapping assignment of the Rh and Duffy blood group genes to chromosome 1. Mayo Clin Proc 52:145, 1977.
13. Colin Y, Cherif-Zahar B, Le Van Kim C, et al: Genetic basis of the RhD-positive and RhD-negative blood group polymorphism as determined by Southern analysis. Blood 80:1074, 1991.
14. Merry AH, Thomson EE, Anstee DJ, et al: The quantification of erythrocyte antigen sites with monoclonal antibodies. Immunology 51:793, 1984.
15. Bloy C, Blanchard D, Lambin P, et al: Characterization of the C, c, E, and G antigens of the Rh blood group system with human monoclonal antibodies. Mol Immunol 225:925, 1988.
16. Hughes-Jones NC, Gardner B, Lincoln PJ: Observations on the number of available c, D, and E antigen sites on red cells. Vox Sang 21:210, 1971.
17. Skov F, Hughes-Jones NC: Observations on the number of available C antigen sites on red cells. Vox Sang 33:170, 1977.
18. Masouredis SP: Relationship between Rho(D) genotype and quantity of I^{131} anti-Rho(D) bound to red cells. J Clin Invest 39:1450, 1960.
19. James NT, James V: Nearest neighbor analysis on the distribution of Rh antigens on erythrocyte membranes. Br J Haematol 40:657, 1978.
20. Masouredis SP, Sudora EJ, Mahan L, Victoria EJ: Antigen site densities and ultrastructural distribution patterns of red cell Rh antigens. Transfusion 16:94, 1976.
21. Moore S, Green C: The identification of specific Rhesus polypeptide blood group ABH active glycoprotein complexes in the human red cell membrane. Biochem J 244:735, 1987.
22. Bloy C, Blanchard D, Lambin P, et al: Human monoclonal antibody against Rh(D) antigen: partial characterization of the Rh(D) polypeptide from human erythrocytes. Blood 69:1491, 1987.
23. Brown PJ, Evans JP, Sinor LT, et al: The rhesus antigen. A dicyclohexylcarbodiimide-binding proteolipid. Am J Pathol 110:127, 1983.
24. Avent ND, Ridgwell K, Tanner MJA: cDNA cloning of a 30 kDA erythrocyte membrane protein associated with Rh (Rhesus)-blood-group-antigen expression. Biochem J 271:821, 1990.
25. Cherif-Zahar B, Bloy C, Le Van Kim, et al: Molecular cloning and protein structure of a human blood group Rh polypeptide. Proc Natl Acad Sci U S A 87:6243, 1990.
26. Bergstrom H, Nilsson LA, Nilsson L, et al: Demonstration of Rh antigens in a 38-day-old fetus. Am J Obstet Gynecol 99:130, 1967.
27. Reardon A, Masouredis SP: Blood group D antigen content of nucleated red cell precursors. Blood 50:981, 1977.
28. Tippett P, Lomas-Francis C, Wallace M: The Rh antigen D: Partial D antigens and associated low-density antigens. Vox Sang 70:121, 1996.

29. Jones J, Scott ML, Voak D: Monoclonal anti-D specificity and RhD structure: criteria for selection of monoclonal anti-D reagents for routine typing of patients and donors. Transfus Med 5:171, 1995.

30. Gorick BD, Thompson KM, Melamed MD, Hughes-Jones NC: Three epitopes on the human Rh antigen D recognized by ^{125}I-labelled human monoclonal IgG antibodies. Vox Sang 55:165, 1988.

31. Lauf PK, Clinton HJ: Increased potassium transport and ouabain binding in human Rh null red blood cells. Blood 48:457, 1976.

32. Kuypers F, van Linde-Sibenius-Trip M, Roelofsen B, et al: Rh$_{null}$ human erythrocytes have an abnormal membrane phospholipid organization. Biochem J 221:931, 1984.

33. Issitt PD: The Rh blood groups. In Garrity G (ed): Immunobiology of Transfusion Medicine. New York, Marcel Dekker, 1994, p 111.

34. Cohen F, Zuelzer WW, Gustafson DC, et al: Mechanisms of isoimmunization. I. The transplacental passage of fetal erythrocytes in homospecific pregnancies. Blood 23:621, 1964.

35. Lloyd LK, Miya F, Hebertson RM, et al: Intrapartum fetomaternal bleeding in Rh-negative women. Obstet Gynecol 56:285, 1980.

36. Woodrow JC: Transplacental hemorrhage. Ser Haematol 111:15, 1970.

37. Zipursky A, Israels LG: The pathogenesis and prevention of Rh immunization. Can Med Assoc J 97:1245, 1967.

38. Bowman JM: The management of Rh-isoimmunization. Obstet Gynecol 52:1, 1978.

39. Sebring ES, Polesky HF: Detection of fetal maternal hemorrhage in Rh immune globulin candidates: a rosetting technique using enzyme-treated Rh$_2$Rh$_2$ indicator erythrocytes. Transfusion 22:486, 1982.

40. Stedman CM, Baudin JC, White CA, Cooper ES: Use of the erythrocyte rosette test to screen for excessive fetomaternal hemorrhage in Rh-negative women. Am J Obstet Gynecol 154:1363, 1986.

41. Ness PM, Baldwin ML, Niebyl JR: Clinical high-risk designation does not predict excess fetal-maternal hemorrhage. Am J Obstet Gynecol 156:154, 1987.

42. Davey MG, Zipursky A: McMaster conference on prevention of Rh immunization. Vox Sang 36:50, 1979.

43. Aborjaily AN: Rh sensitization after tubal pregnancy. N Engl J Med 281:1076, 1969.

44. Litwak O, Taswell HF, Banner EA, et al: Fetal erythrocytes in maternal circulation after spontaneous abortion. JAMA 214:531, 1970.

45. Matthews CD, Matthews AEB, Gilbey BE: Antibody development in rhesus-negative patients following abortion. Lancet 2:318, 1969.

46. Queenan JT, Shah S, Kubarych SF, et al: Role of induced abortion in Rhesus immunization. Lancet 1:815, 1971.

47. Ascari WQ: Abortion and maternal Rh immunization. Clin Obstet Gynecol 14:625, 1971.

48. Leong M, Duby S, Kinch RA: Fetal-maternal transfusion following early abortion. Obstet Gynecol 54:424, 1979.

49. Freda VJ, Gorman JG, Galen RS, et al: The threat of Rh immunization from abortion. Lancet 2:147, 1970.

50. Litwalk O, Taswell H, Banner E, Keith L: Fetal erythrocytes in maternal circulation after spontaneous abortion. JAMA 215:521, 1970.

51. Von Stein GA, Munsick RA, Stiver K, Ryder K: Fetomaternal hemorrhage in threatened abortion. Obstet Gynecol 79:383, 1992.

52. Dayton VD, Anderson DS, Crosson FT, Cruikshank SH: A case of Rh isoimmunization: should threatened first-trimester abortion be an indication for Rh immune globulin prophylaxis? Am J Obstet Gynecol 163:63, 1990.

53. Katz J, Marcus RG: The risk of Rh isoimmunization in ruptured tubal pregnancy. BMJ 3:667, 1972.

54. Harrison R, Campbell S, Craft I: Risks of fetomaternal hemorrhage resulting from amniocentesis with and without ultrasound placental localization. Obstet Gynecol 48:557, 1976.

55. Mennuti MT, Brummond W, Crombleholme WR, et al: Fetal maternal bleeding associated with genetic amniocentesis. Obstet Gynecol 55:48, 1980.

56. Henry G, Wexler P, Robinson A: Rh-immune globulin after amniocentesis for genetic diagnosis. Obstet Gynecol 48:557, 1976.

57. Pollack W, Ascari WQ, Crispen JF, et al: Studies on Rh prophylaxis after transfusion with Rh-positive blood. Transfusion 11:340, 1971.

58. Pollack W, Ascari WQ, Kochesky RJ, et al: Studies on Rh prophylaxis. I. Relationship between doses of anti-Rh and size of antigenic stimulus. Transfusion 11:333, 1971.

59. Nevanlinna HR, Vainio T: The influence of mother-child ABO incompatibility on Rh immunization. Vox Sang 1:26, 1956.

60. Queenan JT: Modern Management of the Rh Problem. 2nd ed. Hagerstown, MD, Harper & Row, 1977.

61. Woodrow JC: Rh Immunization and Its Prevention. Series Hematologica, Vol. 3. Copenhagen, Munksgaard, 1970.

62. Ascari WQ, Levin P, Pollack W: Incidence of maternal Rh immunization by ABO compatible and incompatible pregnancies. BMJ 1:399, 1969.

63. Freda VJ, Gorman JG, Pollack W: Successful prevention of experimental Rh sensitization in man with anti-Rh gamma 2-globulin antibody preparation. Transfusion 4:26, 1964.

64. Clarke CA, Donohoe WTA, Finn R, et al: Further extraperitoneal studies on the prevention of Rh haemolytic disease. BMJ 1:979, 1963.

65. Pollack W, Gorman JG, Freda VJ: Rh immune suppression: past, present, and future. In Frigoletto FD, Jewett JR, Konugres AD (eds): Rh Hemolytic Disease: New Strategy for Eradication. Boston, GK Hall, 1982, p 9.

66. Hamilton EG: Prevention of Rh isoimmunization by injection of anti-D antibody. Obstet Gynecol 30:812, 1967.

67. Pollack W, Singer HO, Gorman JG, et al: The prevention of isoimmunization to the Rh factor by passive immunization with Rh D immune globulin. Haematology 2:1, 1968.

68. Chown B, Duff AM, James J, et al: Prevention of primary Rh immunization: first report of the Western Canadian Trial. Can Med Assoc J 100:1021, 1969.

69. Mollison PL, Barron SL, Bowley C, et al: Controlled trial of various anti-D dosages in suppression of Rh sensitization following pregnancy. BMJ 2:75, 1974.

70. Freda VJ, Gorman JG, Pollack W, et al: Prevention of Rh hemolytic disease—ten years clinical experience with Rh immune globulin. N Engl J Med 292:1014, 1975.

71. Bowman JM: Controversies in Rh prophylaxis. Who needs Rh immune globulin and when should it be used? Am J Obstet Gynecol 151:289, 1985.

72. Bowman JM, Chown B, Lewis M, Pollack JM: Rho-isoimmunization during pregnancy. Can Med Assoc J 118:623, 1978.

73. Bowman JM, Pollock JM: Antenatal Rh prophylaxis: 28 weeks' gestation service program. Can Med Assoc J 118:627, 1978.

74. Hensleigh PA: Preventing rhesus isoimmunization. Antepartum Rh immune globulin prophylaxis versus a sensitive test for risk identification. Am J Obstet Gynecol 146:749, 1983.

75. Thornton JG, Page C, Foote G, et al: Efficacy and long term effects of antenatal prophylaxis with anti-D immunoglobulin. BMJ 298:1671, 1989.

76. Kochenour NK, Beeson JH: The use of Rh-immune globulin. Clin Obstet Gynecol 25:283, 1982.

77. Baskett TF, Parsons ML: Prevention of Rh(D) alloimmunization: a cost-benefit analysis. Can Med Assoc J 142:337, 1990.

78. Kumpel BM, Poole D, Bradley BA: Human monoclonal antibodies. Their production, serology, quantitation, and potential use as blood grouping reagents. Br J Haematol 71:125, 1989.

79. Thomson A, Contreras M, Gorick B, et al: Clearance of Rh D-positive cells with monoclonal anti-D. Lancet 336:1147, 1990.

80. Selinger M: Immunoprophylaxis for rhesus disease—expensive but worth it? Br J Obstet Gynaecol 98:509, 1991.

81. Mollison PL: The reticulo-endothelial system and red cell destruction. Proc R Soc Med 55:915, 1962.

82. Pollack W: Recent understanding for the mechanism by which passively administered antibody suppresses the immune response to Rh antigen in unimmunized Rh-negative women. Clin Obstet Gynecol 25:255, 1982.

83. Chan PL, Sinclair NR: Regulation of the immune response. VI. Inability of F(ab)2 antibody to terminate established immune responses and its ability to interfere with IgG antibody-mediated immunosuppression. Immunology 24:289, 1973.

84. Standards Committee, American Association of Blood Banks: Standards for Blood Banks and Transfusion Services. 19th ed. Washington, DC, American Association of Blood Banks, 1999.

85. American College of Obstetricians and Gynecologists: Prevention of RhD alloimmunization. ACOG Practice Bulletin 4. Washington, DC, American College of Obstetricians and Gynecologists, 1999.

86. Barss VA, Frigoletto FD, Konugres A: The cost of irregular antibody screening. Am J Obstet Gynecol 159:428, 1988.

87. Keith LG, Berger GS: The risk of Rh immunization associated with abortion, spontaneous and induced. In Frigoletto FD, Jewett JF, Konugres AA (eds): Rh Hemolytic Disease: New Strategy for Eradication. Boston, GK Hall, 1982, p. 111.

88. Robson SC, Lee K, Urbaniak S: Anti-D immunoglobulin in RhD prophylaxis. Br J Obstet Gynaecol 105:129, 1998.

89. Baskett TF, Parsons ML, Peddle LJ: The experience and effectiveness of the Nova Scotia Rh Program, 1964–84. Can Med Assoc J 134:1259, 1986.

90. Tovey LAD: Haemolytic disease of the newborn—the changing scene. Br J Obstet Gynecol 93:960, 1986.

91. Kanter MH: Derivation of new mathematic formulas for determining whether a D-positive father is heterozygous or homozygous for the D antigen. Am J Obstet Gynecol 166:61, 1992.

92. Reece EA, Copel JA, Scioscia AL, et al: Diagnostic fetal umbilical blood sampling in the management of isoimmunization. Am J Obstet Gynecol 159:1057, 1988.

93. Nicolini U, Kochenour NK, Greco P, et al: Consequences of fetomaternal hemorrhage after intrauterine transfusion. BMJ 297:1379, 1988.

94. Le Van Kim C, Mouro I, Cherif-Zachar B, et al: Molecular cloning and primary structure of the human blood group RhD polypeptide. Proc Natl Acad Sci U S A 89:10,900, 1992.

95. Bennett PR, Warwick R, Vaughan JV, et al: Prenatal determination of fetal RhD type by DNA amplification. N Engl J Med 329:607, 1993.

96. Fisk NM, Bennett P, Warwick RB, et al: Clinical utility of fetal RhD typing in alloimmunized pregnancies by means of polymerase chain reaction on amniocytes or chorionic villi. Am J Obstet Gynecol 171:50, 1994.

97. Simsek S, Bleker PMM, von dem Borne AEGK: Prenatal determination of fetal Rh type. N Engl J Med 330:795, 1994.

98. Rossiter JP, Blakemore KJ, Kickler TS, et al: The use of polymerase chain reaction to determine fetal RhD status. Am J Obstet Gynecol 171:1047, 1994.

99. Van den Veyver IB, Chong SS, Cota J, et al: Single-cell analysis of the RhD blood type for use in preimplantation diagnosis in the prevention of severe hemolytic disease of the newborn. Am J Obstet Gynecol 172:533, 1995.

100. Dildy GA, Jackson GM, Ward K: Determination of fetal RhD status from uncultured amniocytes. Obstet Gynecol 8:207, 1996.

101. Lighten AD, Overton TG, Sepulveda W, et al: Accuracy of prenatal determination of RhD type status by polymerase chain reaction with amniotic cells. Am J Obstet Gynecol 173:1182, 1995.

102. Spence WC, Maddalena A, Demers DB, Bick DP: Molecular analysis of the RhD genotype in fetuses at risk for RhD hemolytic disease. Obstet Gynecol 85:296, 1995.

103. Van den Veyver IB, Subramanian SB, Hudson KM, et al: Prenatal diagnosis of the RhD fetal blood type on amniotic fluid by polymerase chain reaction. Obstet Gynecol 87:419, 1996.

104. Lo Y-MD, Bowell PJ, Selinger M, et al: Prenatal determination of fetal RhD status by analysis of peripheral blood of rhesus negative mothers. Lancet 341:1147, 1993.

105. Lo YMD, Hjelm NM, Fidler C, et al: Prenatal diagnosis of fetal RhD status by molecular analysis of maternal plasma. N Engl J Med 339:1734, 1998.

106. Al-Mufti R, Howard C, Overton T, et al: Detection of fetal messenger ribonucleic acid in maternal blood to determine fetal RhD status as a strategy for noninvasive prenatal diagnosis. Am J Obstet Gynecol 179:210, 1998.

107. Allen H, Diamond LK, Jones AR: Erythroblastosis fetalis. IX. Problems of stillbirth. N Engl J Med 251:453, 1954.

108. Freda VJ: The Rh problem in obstetrics and a new concept of its management using amniocenteses and spectrophotometric scanning of amniotic fluid. Am J Obstet Gynecol 92:341, 1965.

109. Gottvall T, Hilden J-O: Concentration of anti-D antibodies in Rh(D) alloimmunized pregnant women, as a predictor of anemia and/or hyperbilirubinemia in their newborn infants. Acta Obstet Gynecol Scand 76:733, 1997.

110. MacGregor SN, Silver RK, Gupta A, et al: Prediction of fetal anemia in red blood cell alloimmunization not receiving in utero transfusion using serial maternal antibody titers. Am J Obstet Gynecol 172:336, 1995.

111. Hadley AG: A comparison of in vitro tests for predicting the severity of haemolytic disease of the fetus and newborn. Vox Sang 74:375, 1998.

112. Nicolaides KH, Rodeck CH: Maternal serum anti-D antibody concentration and assessment of rhesus isoimmunisation. BMJ 304:1155, 1992.

113. Economides DL, Bowell PF, Selinger M, et al: Anti-D concentrations in fetal and maternal serum and amniotic fluid in rhesus allo-immunised pregnancies. Br J Obstet Gynaecol 100:923, 1993.

114. Bowell P, Wainscoat JS, Peto TEA, et al: Maternal anti-D concentrations and outcome in rhesus haemolytic disease of the newborn, BMJ 285:327, 1982.

115. McElin TW, Buckingham JC, Danforth DN: The outcome and treatment of Rh-sensitized pregnancies. Am J Obstet Gynecol 84:4678, 1962.

116. Bevis DCA: Blood pigments in haemolytic disease of the newborn. J Obstet Gynaecol Br Emp 63:65, 1956.

117. Liley AW: Liquor amnii analysis in the management of pregnancy complicated by rhesus sensitization. Am J Obstet Gynecol 82:1359, 1961.

118. Liley AW: Errors in the assessment of hemolytic disease from amniotic fluid. Am J Obstet Gynecol 86:485, 1963.

119. Queenan JT: Current management of the Rh-sensitized patient. Clin Obstet Gynecol 25:293, 1982.

120. Bowman JM: Hemolytic disease (erythroblastosis fetalis). *In* Creasy RK, Resnik R (eds): Maternal Fetal Medicine: Principles of Practice. 4th ed. Philadelphia, WB Saunders Company, 1999, p 736.

121. Berkowitz RL, Hobbins JC: Intrauterine transfusion utilizing ultrasound. Obstet Gynecol 57:33, 1981.

122. Nicolaides KH, Rodeck CH, Mibashan RS, Kemp JR: Have Liley charts outlived their usefulness? Am J Obstet Gynecol 155:90, 1986.

123. American College of Obstetricians and Gynecologists: Management of D isoimmunization in pregnancy. ACOG Technical Bulletin 148. Washington, DC, American College of Obstetricians and Gynecologists, 1990.

124. Spinnato JA, Ralston KK, Greenwell ER, et al: Amniotic fluid bilirubin and fetal hemolytic disease. Am J Obstet Gynecol 165:1030, 1991.

125. Ananth U, Queenan JT: Does midtrimester ΔOD_{450} of amniotic fluid reflect the severity of Rh disease? Am J Obstet Gynecol 161:47, 1989.

126. Queenan JT, Tomai TP, Ural SH, King JC: Deviation in amniotic fluid optical density at a wavelength of 450 nm in Rh-immunized pregnancies from 14 to 40 weeks' gestation: a proposal for clinical management. Am J Obstet Gynecol 168:1370, 1993.

127. Spinnato JA, Clark AL, Ralston KK, et al: Hemolytic disease of the fetus: a comparison of the Queenan and extended Liley methods. Obstet Gynecol 92:441, 1998.

128. Scott F, Chan FY: Assessment of the clinical usefulness of the 'Queenan' chart versus the 'Liley' chart in predicting severity of rhesus iso-immunization. Prenat Diagn 18:1143, 1998.

129. Rodeck CH, Holman CA, Karnicki J, et al: Direct intravascular fetal blood transfusion by fetoscopy in severe rhesus isoimmunization. Lancet 1:625, 1981.

130. Rodeck CH, Nicolaides KH, Warsof SL, et al: The management of severe rhesus isoimmunization by fetoscopic intravascular transfusion. Am J Obstet Gynecol 150:749, 1984.

131. Nicolaides KH, Rodeck CH, Millar DS, Mibashan RS: Fetal haematology in rhesus isoimmunization. BMJ 290:661, 1985.

132. MacKenzie IA, Bowell PF, Castle BM, et al: Serial fetal blood sampling for the management of pregnancies complicated by severe rhesus (D) isoimmunization. Br J Obstet Gynecol 95:735, 1988.

133. Daffos F, Capella-Pavlovsky M, Forestier F: Fetal blood sampling during pregnancy with use of a needle guided by ultrasound: a study of 606 consecutive cases. Am J Obstet Gynecol 153:655, 1985.

134. Daffos F, Forestier F, Kaplan C, Cox W: Prenatal diagnosis and management of bleeding disorders with fetal blood sampling. Am J Obstet Gynecol 158:939, 1988.

135. Ghidini A, Sepulveda W, Lockwood CJ, Romero R: Complications of fetal blood sampling. Am J Obstet Gynecol 168:1339, 1993.

136. Pielet BW, Socol ML, MacGregor SN, et al: Cordocentesis: an appraisal of risks. Am J Obstet Gynecol 159:1497, 1988.

137. Wilkins I, Mezrow G, Lynch L, et al: Amnionitis and life-threatening respiratory distress after percutaneous umbilical blood sampling. Am J Obstet Gynecol 160:427, 1989.

138. Feinkind L, Nanda D, Delke I, Minkoff H: Abruptio placentae after percutaneous umbilical cord sampling: a case report. Am J Obstet Gynecol 162:1203, 1990.

139. Bowell PJ, Selinger M, Ferguson J, et al: Antenatal fetal blood sampling for the management of alloimmunized pregnancies: effect upon maternal anti-D potency levels. Br J Obstet Gynaecol 95:759, 1988.

140. MacGregor SN, Silver RK, Sholl JS: Enhanced sensitization after cordocentesis in a rhesus-isoimmunized pregnancy. Am J Obstet Gynecol 165:382, 1991.

141. Bowman JM, Pollock LM, Peterson LE, et al: Fetomaternal hemorrhage following funipuncture: increase in severity of maternal red-cell alloimmunization. Obstet Gynecol 84:839, 1994.

142. Frigoletto FD, Greene MF, Benacerraf BR, et al: Ultrasonographic fetal surveillance in the management of the immunized pregnancy. N Engl J Med 315:430, 1986.

143. Benacerraf BR, Frigoletto FD: Sonographic sign for the detection of early fetal ascites in the management of severe isoimmune disease without intrauterine transfusion. Am J Obstet Gynecol 152:1039, 1985.

144. DeVore GR, Mayden K, Tortora M, et al: Dilatation of the umbilical vein in rhesus hemolytic anemia: a predictor of severe disease. Am J Obstet Gynecol 141:464, 1981.

145. Witter FR, Graham D: The utility of ultrasonically measured umbilical vein diameters in isoimmunized pregnancies. Am J Obstet Gynecol 146:225, 1983.

146. Chitkara U, Wilkins I, Lynch L, et al: The role of sonography in assessing severity of fetal anemia in Rh and Kell-isoimmunized pregnancies. Obstet Gynecol 71:393, 1988.

147. Nicolaides KH, Fontanarosa M, Gabbe SG, Rodeck CH: Failure of ultrasonographic parameters to predict the severity of fetal anemia in rhesus isoimmunization. Am J Obstet Gynecol 158:920, 1988.

148. Vintzileos AM, Campbell WA, Storlazzi E, et al: Fetal liver ultrasound measurements in isoimmunized pregnancies. Obstet Gynecol 68:162, 1986.

149. Roberts AB, Mitchell JM, Pattison NS: Fetal liver length in normal and isoimmunized pregnancies. Am J Obstet Gynecol 161:42, 1989.

150. Bahado-Singh R, Oz U, Mari G, et al: Fetal splenic size in anemia due to Rh-alloimmunization. Obstet Gynecol 92:828, 1998.

151. Ouzounian JG, Monteiro HA, Alsulyman OM, Songster GS: Ultrasonographic fetal cardiac measurement in isoimmunized pregnancies. J Reprod Med 42:342, 1997.

152. Kirkinen P, Jouppila P: Umbilical vein blood flow in rhesus isoimmunization. Br J Obstet Gynaecol 90:640, 1983.

153. Rightmire DA, Nicolaides KH, Rodeck CH, Campbell S: Fetal blood velocities in Rh isoimmunization: relationship to gestational age and to fetal hematocrit. Obstet Gynecol 68:233, 1986.

154. Nicolaides KH, Bilardo CM, Campbell S: Prediction of fetal anemia by measurement of the mean blood velocity in the fetal aorta. Am J Obstet Gynecol 162:209, 1990.

155. Copel JA, Grannum PA, Belanger K, et al: Pulsed Doppler flow-velocity waveforms before and after intrauterine intravascular transfusion for severe erythroblastosis fetalis. Am J Obstet Gynecol 158:768, 1988.

156. Copel JA, Grannum PA, Green JJ, et al: Pulsed Doppler flow-velocity waveforms in the prediction of fetal hematocrit of the severely isoimmunized pregnancy. Am J Obstet Gynecol 161:341, 1989.

157. Copel JA, Grannum PA, Green JJ, et al: Fetal cardiac output in the isoimmunized pregnancy: a pulsed Doppler-echocardiographic study of patients undergoing intravascular intrauterine transfusion. Am J Obstet Gynecol 161:361, 1989.

158. Oepkes D, Vandenbussche FP, Van Bel F, Kanhai HHH: Fetal ductus venosus blood flow velocities before and after transfusion in red-cell alloimmunized pregnancies. Obstet Gynecol 82:237, 1993.

159. Legarth J, Lingman G, Stangenberg M, Rahman F: Umbilical artery Doppler flow-velocity waveforms in rhesus-isoimmunized fetuses before and after fetal blood sampling or transfusion. J Clin Ultrasound 22:43, 1994.

160. Mari G: Noninvasive diagnosis by Doppler ultrasonography

of fetal anemia due to maternal red-cell alloimmunization. N Engl J Med 342:9, 2000.

161. Bahado-Singh R, Oz U, Derren O, et al: Splenic artery Doppler peak systolic velocity predicts severe fetal anemia in rhesus disease. Am J Obstet Gynecol 182:1222, 2000.

162. Legarth J, Lingman G, Stangenberg M, Rahman F: Lack of relation between fetal blood gases and fetal blood flow velocity waveform indices found in rhesus isoimmunised pregnancies. Br J Obstet Gynaecol 99:813, 1992.

163. Legarth J, Lingman G, Stangenberg M, Rahman F: Umbilical artery Doppler flow-velocity waveforms and fetal acid-base balance in rhesus-isoimmunized pregnancies. J Clin Ultrasound 22:37, 1994.

164. Bowman JM, Manning FA: Intrauterine fetal transfusions: Winnipeg, 1982. Obstet Gynecol 61:201, 1983.

165. Scott JR, Kochenour NK, Larkin RM, et al: Changes in the management of severely Rh-immunized patients. Am J Obstet Gynecol 149:336, 1984.

166. Watts DH, Luthy DA, Benedetti TJ, et al: Intraperitoneal fetal transfusion under direct ultrasound guidance. Obstet Gynecol 71:84, 1988.

167. Liley AW: Intrauterine transfusion of foetus in haemolytic disease. BMJ 2:1107, 1963.

168. Bang J, Bock J, Trolle D: Ultrasound guided fetal intravenous transfusion for severe rhesus haemolytic disease. BMJ 284:373, 1982.

169. Berkowitz RL, Chitkara U, Goldberg JD, et al: Intrauterine intravascular transfusions for severe red blood cell isoimmunization: ultrasound-guided percutaneous approach. Am J Obstet Gynecol 155:574, 1986.

170. Seeds JW, Bowes WA: Ultrasound-guided fetal intravascular transfusion in severe rhesus isoimmunization. Am J Obstet Gynecol 154:1105, 1986.

171. Grannum PA, Copel JA, Plaxe SC, et al: In utero exchange transfusion by direct intravascular injection in severe erythroblastosis fetalis. N Engl J Med 314:1431, 1986.

172. Nicolaides KH, Soothill PW, Rodeck CH, et al: Rh disease: intravascular blood transfusion by cordocentesis. Fetal Ther 1:185, 1986.

173. Berkowitz RL, Chitkara U, Wilkins IA, et al: Intravascular monitoring and management of erythroblastosis fetalis. Am J Obstet Gynecol 158:83, 1988.

174. Poissonnier H-M, Brossard Y, Demedeiros N, et al: Two hundred intrauterine exchange transfusions in severe blood incompatibilities. Am J Obstet Gynecol 161:709, 1989.

175. Harman CR, Bowman JM, Manning FA, Menticoglou SM: Intrauterine transfusion—intraperitoneal versus intravascular approach: a case-control comparison. Am J Obstet Gynecol 162:1053, 1990.

176. Weiner CP, Williamson RA, Wenstrom KD, et al: Management of fetal hemolytic disease by cordocentesis. II. Outcome of treatment. Am J Obstet Gynecol 165:1302, 1991.

177. Clewell WH, Dunne MG, Johnson ML, Bowes WA: Fetal transfusion with real-time ultrasound guidance. Obstet Gynecol 57:516, 1981.

178. Copel JA, Grannum PA, Harrison D, Hobbins J: The use of intravenous pancuronium bromide to produce fetal paralysis during intravascular transfusion. Am J Obstet Gynecol 158:170, 1988.

179. Moise KJ, Deter R, Kirshon B, et al: Intravenous pancuronium bromide for fetal neuromuscular blockade during intrauterine transfusion for red-cell alloimmunization. Obstet Gynecol 74:905, 1989.

180. Nicolaides KH, Clewell WH, Mibashan RS, et al: Fetal haemoglobin measurement in the assessment of red cell isoimmunization. Lancet 1:1073, 1988.

181. Christmas JT, Little BB, Johnston WL, et al: Nomograms for rapid estimation of intravascular intrauterine exchange transfusion. Obstet Gynecol 75:887, 1990.

182. Mandelbrodt L, Daffos F, Forestier F, et al: Assessment of fetal blood volume for computer-assisted management of in utero transfusion. Fetal Ther 3:60, 1998.

183. Plecas DV, Chitkara U, Berkowitz GS, et al: Intrauterine intravascular transfusion for severe erythroblastosis fetalis: how much to transfuse? Obstet Gynecol 75:965, 1990.

184. Giannina G, Moise KJ, Dorman K: A simple method to estimate volume for fetal intravascular transfusions. Fetal Diagn Ther 13:94, 1998.

185. Inglis SR, Lysikiewicz A, Sonnenblick AL, et al: Advantages of larger volume, less frequent intrauterine red blood cell transfusions for maternal red cell alloimmunization. Am J Perinatol 13:27, 1996.

186. MacGregor SN, Socol ML, Pielet BW, et al: Prediction of hematocrit decline after intravascular fetal transfusion. Am J Obstet Gynecol 161:1491, 1989.

187. Egberts J, van Kamp IL, Kanhai HHH, et al: The disappearance of fetal and donor red blood cells in alloimmunised pregnancies: a reappraisal. Br J Obstet Gynaecol 104:818, 1997.

188. Rodeck CH, Letsky E: How the management of erythroblastosis fetalis has changed. Br J Obstet Gynaecol 96:759, 1989.

189. Pattison N, Roberts A: The management of severe erythroblastosis fetalis by fetal transfusion: survival of transfused adult erythrocytes in the fetus. Obstet Gynecol 74:901, 1989.

190. Nicolini U, Kochenour NK, Greco P, et al: When to perform the next intrauterine transfusion in patients with Rh alloimmunization: combined intravascular and intraperitoneal transfusion allows longer intervals. Fetal Ther 4:14, 1990.

191. Lenke RR, Persutte WH, Nemes JM: Combined intravascular and intraperitoneal transfusions for erythroblastosis fetalis. A report of two cases. J Reprod Med 35:425, 1990.

192. Gusdon JP, Moore V, Myrvik QN, et al: Promethazine HCl as an immunosuppressant. J Immunol 108:1340, 1972.

193. Gusdon JP: The treatment of erythroblastosis with promethazine hydrochloride. J Reprod Med 26:454, 1981.

194. Bierme SJ, Blanc M, Abbal M, Fournie A: Oral Rh treatment for severely immunized mothers. Lancet 1:604, 1979.

195. Bierme SJ, Blanc M, Fournie A, et al: Desensitization by oral antigen. In Frigoletto FD, Jewett JF, Konugres AA (eds): Rh Hemolytic Disease: New Strategy for Eradication. Boston, GK Hall, 1982, p 249.

196. Bowman JM, Peddle LJ, Anderson C: Plasmapheresis in severe Rh isoimmunization. Vox Sang 15:272, 1968.

197. Clarke CA, Bradley J, Elson CJ, et al: Intensive plasmapheresis as a therapeutic measure in rhesus-immunized women. Lancet 1:793, 1970.

198. Powell LC: Intense plasmapheresis in the pregnant Rb-sensitized woman. Am J Obstet Gynecol 101:153, 1968.

199. Fraser ID, Bennett MO, Bothamley JE, et al: Intensive antenatal plasmapheresis in severe rhesus isoimmunization. Lancet 1:6, 1976.

200. Graham-Pole J, Barr W, Willoughby MLN: Continuous-flow plasmapheresis in management of severe rhesus disease. BMJ 1:1185, 1974.

201. Rubinstein P: Repeated small volume plasmapheresis in the management of hemolytic disease of the newborn. In Frigoletto FD, Jewett JF, Konugres AA (eds): Rh Hemolytic Disease: New Strategy for Eradication. Boston, GK Hall, 1982, p 211.

202. Odendaal HJ, Tribe R, Kriel CJ, et al: Successful treatment of severe Rh isoimmunization with immunosuppression and plasmapheresis. Vox Sang 60:169, 1991.

203. Berlin G, Selbing A, Ryden G: Rhesus haemolytic disease

treated with high-dose intravenous immunoglobulin. Lancet 1: 1153, 1985.

204. Marguiles M, Voto LS, Mathet ER, et al: High-dose intravenous IgG for the treatment of severe rhesus alloimmunization. Vox Sang 61:181, 1991.

205. Porter TF, Silver RM, Jackson GM, et al: Intravenous immune globulin in the management of severe Rh D hemolytic disease. Obstet Gynecol Surv 2:193, 1997.

206. Deka D, Buckshee K, Kinra G: Intravenous immunoglobulin as primary therapy or adjuvant therapy to intrauterine fetal blood transfusion: a new approach in the management of severe Rh-immunization. J Obstet Gynaecol Res 22:561, 1996.

207. Voto LS, Mathet ER, Zapaterio JL, et al: High-dose gammaglobulin (IVIG) followed by intrauterine transfusions (IUTs): a new alternative for the treatment of severe fetal hemolytic disease. J Perinat Med 25:85, 1997.

208. Chitkara U, Bussel J, Alvarez M, et al: High-dose intravenous gamma globulin: does it have a role in the treatment of severe erythroblastosis fetalis? Obstet Gynecol 76:703, 1990.

209. de la Camara C, Arrieta R, Gonzalez A, et al: High-dose intravenous immunoglobulin as the sole prenatal treatment for severe Rh immunization. N Engl J Med 318:519, 1988.

210. Scott JR, Branch DW, Kochenour NK, Ward K: Intravenous immunoglobulin treatment of pregnant patients with recurrent pregnancy loss caused by antiphospholipid antibodies and Rh immunization. Am J Obstet Gynecol 159:1055, 1988.

211. Marzuch K, Wiest E, Pfeiffer KH, et al: Antenatal fetal therapy for neonatal alloimmune thrombocytopenia with high dose immune globulin. Br J Obstet Gynaecol 101:1011, 1994.

212. Silver RM, Porter TF, Branch DW, et al: Neonatal alloimmune thrombocytopenia: antenatal management. Am J Obstet Gynecol 182:1233, 2000.

213. Sidiropoulos D, Herrmann U, Morell A, et al: Transplacental passage of intravenous immunoglobulin in the last trimester of pregnancy. J Pediatr 109:505, 1986.

214. Boggs TR: Survival rates in Rh sensitizations. Pediatrics 33: 758, 1964.

215. Quinlan RW, Buhi WC, Cruz A: Fetal pulmonary maturity in isoimmunized pregnancies. Am J Obstet Gynecol 148:787, 1984.

216. Horenstein J, Golde S, Platt LD: Lung profiles in the isoimmunized pregnancy. Am J Obstet Gynecol 153:443, 1985.

217. Bowman JM: Maternal alloimmunization and fetal hemolytic disease. *In* Reece EA, Hobbins JC (eds): Medicine of the Fetus and Mother, 2nd ed. Philadelphia, Lippincott-Raven Publishers, 1999, p 1241.

218. Manning FA: The alloimmune pregnancy. *In* Fetal Medicine Principles and Practice. Norwalk, CT, Appleton Lange, 1995, p 395.

219. Queenan JT, Smith BD, Haber JM, et al: Irregular antibodies in the obstetric patient. Obstet Gynecol 34:767, 1969.

220. Polesky HF: Blood group antibodies in prenatal sera. Minn Med 50:601, 1967.

221. Giblett ER: Blood group antibodies causing hemolytic disease of the newborn. Obstet Gynecol 7:1044, 1964.

222. Weinstein L: Irregular antibodies causing hemolytic disease of the newborn: a continuing problem. Clin Obstet Gynecol 25: 321, 1982.

223. Murphy MT, Morrison N, Miles JS, et al: Regional chromosomal assignment of the Kell blood group locus (KEL) to chromosome 7q33-q35 by fluorescence in situ hybridization: evidence for the polypeptide nature of antigenic variation. Hum Genet 91:585, 1993.

224. Lee S, Zambas ED, Marsh WL, Redman CM: The human Kell blood group gene maps to chromosome 7q33 and its expression is restricted to erythroid cells. Blood 81:2804, 1993.

225. Hessner MJ, Pircon RA, Johnson ST, Luhm RA: Prenatal genotyping of Jk^a and Jk^b of the human Kidd blood group system by allele-specific polymerase chain reaction. Prenat Diagn 18:1225, 1998.

226. Hessner MJ, Pircon RA, Johnson ST, Luhm RA: Prenatal genotyping of the Duffy blood group system by allele-specific polymerase chain reaction. Prenat Diagn 19:41, 1999.

227. Goodrick MJ, Hadley AG, Poole G: Haemolytic disease of the fetus and newborn due to anti-Fy^a and the potential clinical value of Duffy genotyping in pregnancies at risk. Transfus Med 7:301, 1997.

228. Cornfield VA, Moolman JC, Martell R, Brink PA: Polymerase chain reaction-based detection of *MN* blood group-specific sequences in the human genome. Transfusion 33:119, 1993.

229. De Young-Owens A, Kennedy M, Rose RL, et al: Anti-M alloimmunization: management and outcome at the Ohio State University from 1969 to 1995. Obstet Gynecol 90:962, 1997.

230. Kanra T, Yuce K, Ozcebe OI: Hydrops fetalis and intrauterine deaths due to anti-M. Acta Obstet Gynecol Scand 75:415, 1996.

231. Kanra T, Erdem G, Tekinalp G, et al: Further hemolytic disease of the newborn caused by anti-M. Am J Hematol 53: 280, 1996.

232. Berkowitz RL, Beyta Y, Sadovsky E: Death in utero due to Kell sensitization without excessive elevation of the ΔOD_{450} value in amniotic fluid. Obstet Gynecol 60:746, 1982.

233. Parilla BV, Socol ML: Hydrops fetalis with Kell alloimmunization. Obstet Gynecol 88:730, 1996.

234. Copel JA, Scioscia A, Grannum PA, et al: Percutaneous umbilical blood sampling in the management of Kell isoimmunization. Am J Obstet Gynecol 67:288, 1986.

235. Caine ME, Mueller-Heubach E: Kell sensitization in pregnancy. Am J Obstet Gynecol 154:85, 1986.

236. Leggat JM, Gibson JM, Barron SL, Reid MM: Anti-Kell in pregnancy. Br J Obstet Gynaecol 98:162, 1991.

237. Goh JTW, Kretowicz EM, Weinstein S, Ramsden GH: Anti-Kell in pregnancy and hydrops fetalis. Aust N Z J Obstet Gynaecol 33:210, 1993.

238. Marsh WL, Redman CM: The Kell blood group system: a review. Transfusion 30:158, 1990.

239. Vaughan JI, Warwick R, Letsky E, et al: Erythropoietic suppression in fetal anemia because of Kell alloimmunization. Am J Obstet Gynecol 171:247, 1994.

240. Weiner CP, Widness JA: Decreased fetal erythropoiesis and hemolysis in Kell hemolytic anemia. Am J Obstet Gynecol 174:547, 1996.

241. Vaughn JI, Manning M, Warwick RM, et al: Inhibition of erythroid progenitor cells by anti-Kell antibodies in fetal alloimmune anemia. N Engl J Med 338:798, 1998.

242. Bowman JM, Pollock JT, Manning FA, et al: Maternal Kell blood group alloimmunization. Obstet Gynecol 79:239, 1992.

243. McKenna DS, Nagaraja HN, O'Shaughnessy R: Management of pregnancies complicated by anti-Kell alloimmunization. Obstet Gynecol 93:667, 1999.

244. Constantine G, Fitzgibbon N, Weaver JB: Anti-Kell in pregnancy. Br J Obstet Gynaecol 98:943, 1991.

245. Resnikoff-Etievant MF: Management of alloimmune neonatal and antenatal thrombocytopenia. Vox Sang 55:193, 1988.

246. von dem Borne AE, Decary F: Nomenclature of platelet-specific antigens. Transfusion 30:477, 1990.

247. Shulman NR, Reid DM: Platelet immunology. *In* Colman RW, Hirsh J, Marder VJ, Salzman EW (eds): Hemostasis and Thrombosis: Basic Principles and Clinical Practice. 3rd ed. Philadelphia, JB Lippincott, 1994, p 414.

248. von dem Borne AE, Simsek S, van der Schoot CE, Goldschmeding R: Platelet and neutrophil alloantigens: their nature and role in immune-mediated cytopenias. *In* Garrity G (ed): Immunobiology of Transfusion Medicine. New York, Marcel Dekker, 1994, p 149.

249. Sternbach MS, Malette M, Nadon F, Guevin RM: Severe alloimmune neonatal thrombocytopenia due to specific HLA antibodies. Curr Stud Hematol Blood Transfus 52:97, 1986.

250. Mueller-Eckhardt C, Grubert A, Weisheit M, et al: 384 cases of suspected neonatal alloimmune thrombocytopenia. Lancet 1:363, 1989.

251. Burrows RF, Kelton JG: Incidentally detected thrombocytopenia in healthy mothers and their infants. N Engl J Med 319:142, 1988.

252. Blanchette VS, Chen L, Salomon de Friedberg Z, et al: Alloimmunization to the PL^{A1} antigen: results of a prospective study. Br J Haematol 74:209, 1990.

253. Mueller-Eckhardt C: Platelet allo- and autoantigens and their clinical implications. *In* Nance SJ (ed): Transfusion Medicine in the 1990's. Arlington, VA, American Association of Blood Banks, 1990, p 63.

254. Herman JH, Jumbelic MI, Ancona RJ, Kickler TS: In utero cerebral hemorrhage in alloimmune thrombocytopenia. Am J Pediatr Hematol Oncol 8:312, 1986.

255. Bussel JB, Berkowitz RL, McFarland JH, et al: Antenatal treatment of neonatal alloimmune thrombocytopenia. N Engl J Med 319:1374, 1988.

256. Pearson HA, Shulman NR, Marder VJ, Cone TE: Isoimmune neonatal thrombocytopenic purpura: clinical and therapeutic considerations. Blood 23:154, 1964.

257. Flug F, Karpatkin M, Karpatkin S: Should all pregnant women be tested for their platelet PLA (Zw, HPA-1) phenotype? Br J Haematol 86:1, 1994.

258. Bussel JB, Zabusky MR, Berkowitz RL, McFarland JG: Fetal alloimmune thrombocytopenia. N Engl J Med 337:22, 1997.

259. Mennuti M, Schwarz RH, Gill F: Obstetric management of isoimmune thrombocytopenia. Am J Obstet Gynecol 118:565, 1974.

260. Sitarz AL, Driscoll JM Jr, Wolff JA: Management of isoimmune neonatal thrombocytopenia. Am J Obstet Gynecol 124:39, 1976.

261. Daffos F, Forestier F, Muller JY, et al: Prenatal treatment of alloimmune thrombocytopenia. Lancet 2:632, 1984.

262. Kaplan C, Daffos F, Forestier F, et al: Management of alloimmune thrombocytopenia: antenatal diagnosis and in utero transfusion of maternal platelets. Blood 72:340, 1988.

263. Nicolini U, Rodeck CH, Kochenour NK, et al: In-utero platelet transfusions for alloimmune thrombocytopenia. Lancet 2:506, 1988.

264. Murphy MF, Pullon HWH, Metcalfe P, et al: Management of fetal alloimmune thrombocytopenia by weekly in utero platelet transfusions. Vox Sang 58:45, 1990.

265. Paidas JM, Berkowitz RL, Lynch L, et al: Alloimmune thrombocytopenia: fetal and neonatal losses related to cordocentesis. Am J Obstet Gynecol 172:475, 1995.

266. Mueller-Eckhardt C, Kiefel V, Jovanovic V, et al: Prenatal treatment of fetal alloimmune thrombocytopenia. Lancet 2:910, 1988.

267. Management of alloimmune neonatal thrombocytopenia. Editorial. Lancet 1:137, 1989.

268. Lynch L, Bussel JB, McFarland JG, et al: Antenatal treatment of alloimmune thrombocytopenia. Obstet Gynecol 80:67, 1992.

269. Bussel JB, Berkowitz RL, Lynch L, et al: Antenatal management of alloimmune thrombocytopenia with intravenous gamma-globulin: A randomized trial of the addition of low-dose steroid to intravenous gamma-globulin. Am J Obstet Gynecol 174:1414, 1996.

270. Derycke M, Drysus M, Ropert JC, Tchernia G: Intravenous immunoglobulin for neonatal isoimmune thrombocytopenia. Arch Dis Child 60:667, 1985.

271. Sidiropoulos D, Straume B: Treatment of neonatal isoimmune thrombocytopenia with intravenous immunoglobulin. Blut 48:383, 1984.

272. Massey GV, McWilliams NB, Mueller DG, et al: Intravenous immunoglobulin in treatment of neonatal isoimmune thrombocytopenia. Pediatrics 111:133, 1987.

273. Morgan CL, Cannell GR, Addison RS, Minchinton RM: The effect of intravenous immunoglobulin on placental transfer of platelet-specific antibody: anti Pl^{A1}. Transfus Med 1:209, 1991.

274. Kaplan C, Murphy MF, Kroll H, Waters AH: Feto-maternal alloimmune thrombocytopenia: antenatal therapy with IvIgG and steroids-more questions than answers. Br J Haematol 100:62, 1998.

275. Water AH, Ireland R, Mibashan RS, et al: Fetal platelet transfusions in the management of alloimmune thrombocytopenia. Thromb Haemost 58:323, 1987.

276. Mir N, Samson D, House MJ, Kovar IZ: Failure of antenatal high-dose immunoglobulin to improve fetal platelet count in neonatal alloimmune thrombocytopenia. Vox Sang 55:188, 1988.

277. Nicolini U, Tannirandorn Y, Gonzalez P, et al: Continuing controversy in alloimmune thrombocytopenia: fetal hyperimmunoglobulinemia fails to prevent thrombocytopenia. Am J Obstet Gynecol 163:1144, 1990.

278. Outbreak of hepatitis C associated with intravenous immunoglobulin administration—United States, October 1993–June 1994. MMWR Morb Mortal Wkly Rep 43:505, 1994.

279. Skogen B, Bellissimo DB, Hessner MJ, et al: Rapid determination of platelet alloantigen genotypes by polymerase chain reaction using allele-specific primers. Transfusion 34:955, 1994.

280. Bray PF, Jin Y, Kickler T: Rapid genotyping of the five major platelet alloantigens by reverse dot-blot hybridization. Blood 84:4361, 1994.

281. McFarland JG, Aster RH, Bussel JB, et al: Prenatal diagnosis of neonatal alloimmune thrombocytopenia using allele-specific oligonucleotide probes. Blood 78:2276, 1991.

282. Khouzami AN, Kickler TS, Bray PF, et al: Molecular genotyping of fetal platelet antigens with uncultured amniocytes. Am J Obstet Gynecol 173:1202, 1995.

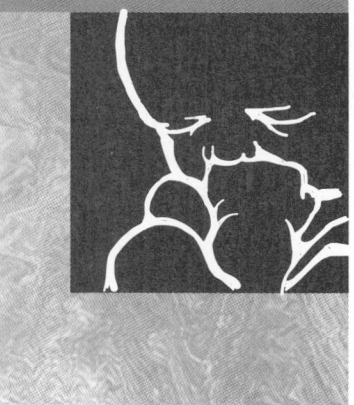

Chapter 27

Prolonged Pregnancy

MICHAEL Y. DIVON

In 1902, Ballantyne questioned the ability of the placenta to support the fetus that "has stayed too long in intrauterine surroundings."[1] Ballantyne further stated that the postmature infant "has remained so long in utero that his difficulty is to be born with safety to himself and his mother." For the better part of the 20th century most authors recognized that prolonged pregnancy was associated with an increased risk for fetal macrosomia and its related morbidity, but felt that the risk of adverse perinatal outcome was small relative to the risks related to induction of labor in the presence of an unfavorable uterine cervix. In 1954, Clifford recognized that prolonged pregnancy could result in fetal growth restriction when he described the "postmaturity with placental dysfunction syndrome."[2] Clifford suggested that these neonates appeared malnourished due to recent weight loss with loose, peeling skin and meconium staining. Birth asphyxia, meconium aspiration, and perinatal death were reported in severe cases.

It was only in the 1970s that it became apparent that perinatal mortality was significantly increased in prolonged pregnancies, and that fetal surveillance combined with selective use of induction of labor might result in improved perinatal outcome.

DEFINITION

Different terms are used loosely to describe pregnancies whose duration has exceeded the upper limit of a normal term gestation. The lack of consensus regarding definitions of terms such as "postmaturity," "postdates," "postterm" or "prolonged pregnancy," combined with the absence of a precise definition of the upper limit of a normal term gestation, result in a wide range of pregnancies reported as "prolonged pregnancy."

The definition of the upper limit of a normal pregnancy is somewhat arbitrary and certainly imprecise. The standard definition of a prolonged pregnancy is 42 completed weeks of gestation (i.e., 294 days after the first day of the last menstrual period [LMP] or more). This definition is endorsed by the American College of Obstetricians and Gynecologists (ACOG), The World Health Organization (WHO), and the International Federation of Gynecology and Obstetrics (FIGO).[3-5] It is based on data derived prior to the widespread use of fetal surveillance modalities and the use of ultrasound for pregnancy dating. In view of more recent perinatal mortality data that were derived from accurately dated pregnancies, it would be reasonable to conclude that prolonged pregnancy should be defined as a gestational age at birth of greater than or equal to 41 weeks of gestation (see section Perinatal Morbidity and Mortality, below).

The incidence of prolonged pregnancy varies depending on the criteria used to define gestational age at birth. It is estimated that 4 to 19 percent of pregnancies reach or exceed 42 weeks' gestation and 2 to 7 percent complete 43 weeks of gestation. Ventura and colleagues estimated that approximately 520,000 of the 4 million neonates born in the United States during 1993 were born at 41 weeks' gestation, whereas approximately 360,000 were born at or beyond 42 weeks' gestation.[6]

ETIOLOGY

Labor is a poorly defined biologic process involving fetal, placental, and maternal signals.[7,8] Recent data

Clinical Features Associated with Prolonged Pregnancy

1. Incorrect dates
2. Biologic variability
3. Maternal factors: previous prolonged pregnancy, primiparity
4. Fetal factors: congenital anomalies (e.g., adrenal hypoplasia, anencephaly)
5. Placental factors: sulfatase deficiency

suggest that human parturition is determined by placental release of corticotropin-releasing hormone (CRH) and that women who have low levels of this hormone are more likely to deliver beyond their due date.[9] While the details of these physiologic processes await further definition, it is clear that the most common cause of prolonged gestation is an error in determining the patient's due date. Using the LMP for the determination of gestational age is fraught with inaccuracy. Patients' failure to recall accurately the date of the first day of their LMP combined with the varying duration of the luteal and follicular phases of the menstrual cycle may result in an overestimation of gestational age. When prolongation of pregnancy is adequately documented, its cause is often undetermined and the most likely etiology is biologic variability of the duration of pregnancy.

Various fetal and placental abnormalities may predispose to prolongation of pregnancy. The increase in the incidence of fetal anomalies among women who deliver beyond their due date is generally explained by abnormalities of the fetal hypothalamic-pituitary-adrenal axis.[8] Indeed, major central nervous system (CNS) abnormalities (such as anencephaly) have long been associated with loss of the normal mechanisms that initiate labor at term. The role of the fetal adrenal gland in the initiation of labor was highlighted by Naeye, who documented marked adrenal hypoplasia in 10 of 19 postterm fetuses with lethal congenital anomalies.[10]

Additional evidence regarding the complexity of the mechanisms involved with initiation of labor is provided by the X-linked recessive deficiency of placental sulfatase, which leads to abnormally low estrogen production in affected male fetuses with a subsequent prolongation of pregnancy and difficulties in both cervical ripening and labor induction.[11]

The role of primary prostaglandins (such as PGE_2 and PGF_2) as uterine stimulants is well established. Nonsteroidal anti-inflammatory drugs inhibit the synthesis of these prostaglandins and, therefore, their use is thought to possibly prolong gestation. Nonetheless, the extent to which the chronic use of these drugs (such as aspirin) results in actual prolongation of pregnancy is unknown.

Various maternal conditions have been suggested as risk factors for the development of prolonged pregnancy. A recent regression analysis performed on a large data set evaluated maternal age, parity, and marital status as well as maternal health before and during pregnancy. Primiparity was identified as the only maternal variable, which had a small but significant association with prolonged pregnancies of greater than or equal to 294 days (relative risk [RR] of 1.06 and 95 percent confidence interval [CI], 1.05 to 1.07).[12] Interestingly, maternal age of 35 years or older and the use of medicines during pregnancy were associated with a small but significant protective effect (odds ratios [OR] of 0.93 and 0.93, respectively), probably suggesting that older women and those on chronic medications were induced prior to 42 weeks' gestation. Zweidling suggested that women who have previously delivered beyond term have a 50 percent chance of experiencing a subsequent prolonged pregnancy.[13] Thus, history of a previous delivery beyond term is a strong predictor of a subsequent late delivery.

The significance of overestimation of the duration of gestation with the use of the LMP should not be overlooked. Congenital anomalies such as anencephaly are easily diagnosed by ultrasound and their presence mandates management options that may not be related to the gestational age at the time of delivery. The contributions attributable to primiparity or to the presence of a male fetus are so minimal that they are unlikely to result in any clinically useful information. In contrast, the fact that 50 percent of women who previously had a prolonged pregnancy would have a similar occurrence with their subsequent pregnancy could be used in counseling the patient and outlining potential management schemes long before the patient reaches her estimated due date.

DIAGNOSIS

The term "prolonged pregnancy" represents a diagnosis that is based on the best available estimation of the duration of gestation at the time of delivery. Optimal diagnosis of gestational age at the time of delivery is hindered by inaccuracy in pregnancy dating. Recently, it has become apparent that clinical methods for estimation of gestational age are inferior to sonographic measurements obtained early in pregnancy.[14] Several studies have demonstrated that the use of more accurate estimates of gestational age based on early ultrasound or known conception dates results in a significantly lower frequency of prolonged pregnancies. Boyd et al. showed that the incidence of patients whose pregnancy exceeded 293 days was 7.5 percent by menstrual dating and fell to 2.6 percent when dates were based on early sonographic examination. This incidence fell to 1.1 percent when the diagnosis was limited to patients whose gestational age exceeded 293 days by both menstrual dates and sonographic dates.[15] A similar conclusion was reached by Gardosi et al., who evaluated 24,675 spontaneous, singleton, nonanomalous deliveries and showed a drop in the postterm (>294 days) pregnancy rate from 7.5 percent when these pregnancies were dated by LMP to 1.5 percent when ultrasound dating was used.[14] These authors also found that 71.5 percent of routine labor inductions at 42 weeks' gestation were actually not indicated because they were performed before the patients reached 42 weeks by scan dates. Recently, Nguyen et al. evaluated 14,805 spontaneous deliveries with a reliable LMP and showed that ultrasound dating reduced the proportion of deliveries beyond 294 days of gestation by 39 percent (from 7.9 percent to 5.2 percent).[16] Furthermore, when scan and LMP dates were compared to known dates in patients who had undergone assisted reproduction, it was shown that the 95 percent CI for scan dates was ±8.3 days. In contrast, the 95 percent CI of menstrual dating was −9 to +27 days.[17,18] These results suggest that the LMP is more likely to overestimate, rather than underestimate, the gestational age at delivery.

The error in gestational dating by the LMP is mainly due to poor recall by the patient. It is, however, important to recognize that even when the LMP is recalled with certainty, it is not a good predictor of ovulation and that physiologic variations in the duration of the follicular phase result in an error that favors an overestimation of the true gestational age. In fact, similar considerations have led to the conclusion that even when both early ultrasound and a reliable LMP are available, gestational dating should be based solely on the ultrasound measurements.[19]

Since the true date of conception is seldom known, there is a possibility that any adjustment of gestational age may increase the risk of adverse perinatal outcome by failing to identify pregnancies that are actually beyond term but are misclassified as being at term. Therefore, Tunon et al. have evaluated fetal outcome in pregnancies defined as postterm according to the LMP but whose scan dates indicated that they were less than 295 days at the time of delivery.[20] A total of 11,510 singleton pregnancies with reliable LMP were studied. Apgar score of less than 7 at 5 minutes and admission to the neonatal intensive care unit (NICU) were used as outcome variables. The authors concluded that there was no increase in perinatal morbidity when scan dates were used as the sole predictor of gestational age at delivery.

PERINATAL MORTALITY AND MORBIDITY

Recent studies that have used very large computerized databases of well-dated pregnancies provide new insights into the true incidence and nature of adverse perinatal outcome in prolonged pregnancy. Divon et al. evaluated fetal and neonatal mortality rates in 181,524 accurately dated term and prolonged pregnancies.[21] A significant increase in fetal mortality was detected from 41 weeks' gestation onward (OR of 1.5, 1.8, and 2.9 at 41, 42, and 43 weeks, respectively). The odds ratios for neonatal mortality did not demonstrate a significant gestational age dependency. Fetal growth restriction (i.e., birthweight of <2 SD below the mean for gestational age) was associated with significantly higher odds ratios for both fetal and neonatal mortality rates at every gestational age examined with odds ratios ranging from 7.1 to 10.0 for fetal death and from 3.4 to 9.4 for neonatal death. Thus, this study documented a small but significant increase in fetal mortality in accurately dated pregnancies that extend beyond 41 weeks' gestation and demonstrated that fetal growth restriction is independently associated with a large increase in perinatal mortality in these pregnancies. These results were confirmed by other investigators.[22,23] Clausson et al. studied perinatal mortality rates among 458,744 term appropriate-for-gestational-age (AGA) infants, 10,312 term small-for-gestational-age (SGA) infants, 39,415 postterm (≥294 days) AGA infants and 1,558 postterm SGA infants.[23] Odds ratios for perinatal death in the postterm AGA infant were not significantly different when compared to AGA term deliveries. In contrast, SGA fetuses had an OR of 10.5 (95 percent CI, 6.9 to 16.0) and 5.0 (95 percent CI, 3.0 to 8.2) for stillbirth and neonatal death, respectively. The stillbirth rate did not change significantly when fetuses with congenital malformations were excluded. However, an 80 percent drop in neonatal deaths occurred when malformed neonates were excluded from the analysis. Further support for the concept that the "small and old" fetus suffers from increased perinatal mortality was provided by Campbell et al., who performed a multivariate analysis of factors associated with perinatal death among 65,796 singleton postterm (≥294 days) births.[12] Three variables were identified as independent predictors of perinatal mortality: (1) SGA status (i.e., birthweight <10th percentile for gestational age) had a RR of 5.7 and 95 percent CI, 4.4 to 7.4; (2) maternal age equal or greater than 35 years had a RR of 1.88 and 95 percent CI, 1.2 to 2.9; (3) interestingly, LGA status (i.e., birthweight ≥90th percentile for gestational age) was associated with a modest protective effect for perinatal death (RR of 0.51 with 95 percent CI, 0.26 to 1.0). The independent impact of an increasing gestational age on these mortality rates was minimal.

An interesting concept was recently proposed by Hilder et al., who argued that the risk of stillbirth should be expressed by fetal losses per 1,000 ongoing pregnancies rather than by the traditional mortality rates, which reflect the number of stillbirths per 1,000 live births.[24] Using this methodology, the authors demonstrated an eightfold increase in perinatal mortality from 37 weeks' to 43 weeks' gestation (0.7 per 1,000 ongoing pregnancies at 37 weeks to 5.8 per 1,000 ongoing pregnancies at 43 weeks).

Several recent studies evaluated the association of perinatal morbidity with prolonged pregnancy. Campbell et al. compared 65,796 Norwegian pregnancies at greater than or equal to 42 weeks with 379,445 term births (37 to 41 weeks) and concluded that prolongation of pregnancy was associated with a significant increase in adverse outcome (Table 27–1).[12] Fetal compromise was more common in the SGA fetuses, whereas shoulder dystocia, labor dysfunction, obstetric trauma, and maternal hemorrhage were more common in the LGA fetus.

Clausson et al. evaluated a large Swedish database of term and postterm (defined as ≥294 days) singleton, normally formed neonates, and showed that prolonged pregnancies were associated with an increased frequency of neonatal convulsions, meconium aspiration syndrome, and Apgar scores of less than 4 at 5 minutes (Table 27–2).[23] Again, morbidity in postterm SGA infants was higher than in postterm AGA infants.

Tunon et al. compared NICU admission rates among 10,048 term pregnancies and 246 prolonged pregnancies (≥296 days by both scan and LMP dates).[20] Prolonged pregnancy was associated with a significant increase in NICU admissions (OR of 2.05, 95 percent CI, 1.35 to 3.12).

Table 27–1. COMPLICATION RATES IN TERM AND POSTTERM BIRTHS

Complication	Prevalence (%)		Relative Risk (95% CI) Postterm vs. Term
	In Term Births	In Postterm Births	
Fetal distress	5.0	8.4	1.68 (1.62–1.72)
Shoulder dystocia	0.5	0.7	1.31 (1.21–1.42)
Labor dysfunction	9.4	11.9	1.26 (1.23–1.29)
Obstetric trauma	2.6	3.3	1.25 (1.20–1.31)
Hemorrhage	9.1	10.0	1.09 (1.06–1.12)

Adapted from Campbell MK, Ostbye T, Irgens LM: Post-term birth: risk factors and outcomes in a 10-year cohort of Norwegian births. Obstet Gynecol 89:543, 1997. Copyright 1997 American College of Obstetricians and Gynecologists, with permission.

Table 27–2. NEONATAL MORBIDITY IN POSTTERM AGA AND SGA INFANTS

Complications	Odds Ratios and 95% CI vs. Term AGA Neonates	
Convulsions		
Term SGA	2.3	(1.6–3.4)
Postterm AGA	1.5	(1.2–2.0)
Postterm SGA	3.4	(1.5–7.6)
Meconium aspiration		
Term SGA	2.4	(1.6–3.4)
Postterm AGA	3.0	(2.6–3.7)
Postterm SGA	1.6	(0.5–5.0)
Apgar score <4 at 5 min		
Term SGA	2.2	(1.4–3.4)
Postterm AGA	2.0	(1.5–2.5)
Postterm SGA	3.6	(1.5–8.7)

SGA, small for gestational age; AGA, appropriate for gestational age.
Adapted from Clausson B, Cnattinguis S, Axelsson O: Outcomes of post-term births: the role of fetal growth restriction and malformations. Obstet Gynecol 94:758, 1999. Copyright 1999 American College of Obstetricians and Gynecologists, with permission.

LONG-TERM OUTCOME

Small study populations and the lack of appropriate controls hinder evaluation of long-term developmental outcome in children born after a prolonged gestation. Additional difficulties are introduced by inconsistent definitions of prolonged pregnancy, inaccuracy in pregnancy dating, and the fact that these studies do not differentiate between the apparently normal newborn and those suffering from perinatal asphyxia, severe growth restriction, or meconium aspiration. An uncontrolled study of 106 infants revealed a relatively large frequency of abnormal neurologic signs, sleep disorders, and inadequate social competence during the first year of life.[25] In contrast, Ting et al. suggested that there are no physical or mental deficiencies in surviving dysmature infants.[26] These results were confirmed by a prospective study of 129 well-dated children born after a prolonged pregnancy and 184 controls. This report did not demonstrate any significant differences in either intelligence scores or physical milestones at 1 and 2 years of age.[27] Thus, until large-scale prospective studies are available, it is reasonable to conclude that in the absence of perinatal asphyxia, growth restriction, or meconium aspiration, prolonged pregnancy is associated with normal, long-term neonatal developmental outcome.

ABERRANT FETAL GROWTH

In 1954, Clifford pointed out that prolongation of pregnancy is associated with placental dysfunction and neonatal dysmaturity.[2] Typically, the affected neonates would appear malnourished with wasting of subcutaneous tissue, meconium staining, and peeling of skin. More recently, Campbell et al. identified birthweight less than or equal to the 10th percentile for gestational age as the risk factor with the largest effect on perinatal mortality (RR of 5.68; 95 percent CI, 4.37 to 7.38) in patients at greater than or equal to 42 weeks' gestation.[12] These authors also showed that macrosomia was associated with a protective effect. The relative risk for perinatal death in the presence of fetal macrosomia was only 0.51 (95 percent CI, 0.26 to 1.00). However, macrosomia was associated with a higher incidence of labor dysfunction, obstetric trauma, shoulder dystocia, and maternal hemorrhage.

The incidence of fetal macrosomia increases with advancing gestational age.[28] For example, a gradual increase in both birthweight and head circumference was documented by McLean et al., who studied 7,000 pregnancies between 39 and 43 weeks' gestation.[29] Similarly, Nahum et al. showed that fetal growth is a linear function of gestational age between 37 and 42 weeks' gestation with a daily fetal weight gain of 12.7 ± 1.4 g (mean $\pm$ SD).[30] Thus, it should come as no surprise that Pollack et al. who evaluated 519 singleton pregnancies at greater than or equal to 41 weeks' gestation, detected a 23 percent incidence of infants whose birthweight was greater than 4,000 g and a 4 percent incidence of birthweights greater than 4,500 g.[31] Chervenak et al. have shown that prolonged pregnancy is not only associated with an increased incidence of macrosomia, but that this increase also results in doubling the cesarean delivery rate for protraction or descent disorders.[32]

The accurate and timely prediction of macrosomia may well influence delivery management decisions. However, one should note that the accurate estimation of fetal weight must be viewed in its broad clinical context of fetopelvic disproportion. Thus, the crucial factor is the relationship of the fetal size to the maternal pelvis rather than the common clinical preoccupation with macrosomia alone. Focusing on either one of these factors in isolation represents a conceptual error.[33] For example, despite an increase in the relative risk of birth trauma in infants weighing more than 4,000 g, most are delivered vaginally without complications. Likewise, a birth weight of less than 4,000 g does not preclude the possibility of shoulder dystocia. In fact, most infants with brachial plexus injury weigh less than 4,000 g at birth.

Traditionally, obstetricians have predicted fetal weight by abdominal palpation or symphysial-fundal height measurement. When ultrasound was first utilized to estimate fetal weight, there was widespread expectation that it would provide a more useful tool than the traditional clinical methods. Chervenak et al. evaluated

317 patients at greater than or equal to 41 weeks' gestation and reported that a sonographic estimate of fetal weight (EFW) of greater than 4,000 g had a sensitivity, specificity, positive predictive value, and negative predictive value of 61, 91, 70, and 87 percent, respectively, in the diagnosis of a birthweight greater than 4,000 g.[32] In a subsequent study of 519 pregnancies of greater than or equal to 41 weeks' gestation, Pollack et al. reported that sonographic estimates of fetal weight that were obtained within 1 week of delivery in pregnancies of greater than or equal to 41 weeks were associated with a mean absolute error of 7.7 percent and a wide range of actual birth weights.[31] For example, the 95 percent CI of an EFW of 4,000 g ranged from 3,142 g to 4,665 g, and the 95 percent CI for an EFW of 4,500 g ranged from 3,465 g to 4,993 g. The positive predictive value of an EFW greater than or equal to 4,000 g in the prediction of a birth weight greater than or equal to 4,000 g was only 64 percent and, therefore, the authors concluded that routine sonographic screening for macrosomia in prolonged pregnancies is associated with relatively low accuracy.

In an attempt to improve the accuracy of sonographic estimates of fetal weight, O'Reilly-Green and Divon used receiver operating characteristic curve analysis to identify optimal cut-off values of EFW in the prediction of macrosomia in prolonged pregnancies.[34] At the inflection point cut-off level of 3,711 g, sensitivity, specificity, and positive and negative predictive values for predicting birthweight of greater than or equal to 4,000 g were 85, 72, 49, and 94 percent, respectively. At the inflection point cut-off level of 4,192 g for predicting birthweight of greater than or equal to 4,500 g, these values were 83, 92, 30, and 99 percent. The authors concluded that cut-off values derived from their analysis resulted in reasonable sensitivities but disappointingly low positive predictive values.

The practical implications of the low predictive value of ultrasonography have been recently highlighted by Rouse et al.[35,36] These authors have shown that in non-diabetic pregnancies, the level of intervention and the economic costs of prophylactic cesarean delivery for fetal macrosomia diagnosed by means of ultrasonography would be excessive. The inaccuracy of sonographic estimates of fetal weight combined with the rarity of permanent brachial plexus injury led these authors to conclude that "a prophylactic cesarean policy with either a 4,000 g or 4,500 g macrosomia threshold would require more than 1,000 cesarean deliveries and millions of dollars to avert a single permanent brachial plexus injury." Even more striking is their suggestion that a policy of prophylactic cesarean would result in one maternal death for every 3.2 brachial plexus injuries that would be prevented.

Despite many years of research and debate, the management of suspected fetal macrosomia is still controversial. The increased incidence of maternal and fetal morbidity associated with macrosomia has prompted some authors to recommend a proactive approach including either a cesarean delivery for cases of "established" macrosomia or a prophylactic induction of labor for "impending" macrosomia. It would seem reasonable that as fetal weight continues to increase with advancing gestational age, delivery of those pregnancies with a potential for macrosomia might prevent some cases of shoulder dystocia and a subsequent brachial plexus injury. However, this intervention could be achieved only by increasing the rate of inductions of labor or by an increased use of cesarean deliveries, both of which would subject the patient to added morbidity or even unnecessary mortality. Furthermore, preliminary evidence suggesting that such interventions would be beneficial is lacking.

Leaphart et al. evaluated the practice of labor induction when fetal macrosomia is suspected.[37] Similar to many other studies, they showed that induction of labor resulted in doubling of their baseline cesarean section rate (from 17 percent to 36 percent), a more frequent use of regional analgesia (from 53 percent to 83 percent), and no difference in the incidence of shoulder dystocia relative to matched controls who were managed by awaiting spontaneous onset of labor. The authors concluded that induction of labor following a prenatal diagnosis of macrosomia results in unnecessary cesarean deliveries and emphasized that their data support a plan of expectant management when fetal macrosomia is suspected. In a prospective randomized study of 273 patients with suspected macrosomia at term, Gonen et al. could not demonstrate that induction of labor resulted in reduced neonatal morbidity.[38] The authors concluded that "ultrasonic estimation of fetal weight between 4,000 g and 4,500 g should not be considered an indication for induction of labor."

Some authors have gone as far as suggesting that the availability of a sonographic EFW indicating macrosomia is in and of itself responsible for an increased cesarean delivery rate and have questioned the logic of obtaining these EFWs if their availability does not improve perinatal outcome.[39] Although the recommendation for proactive management of the macrosomic fetus is well intentioned, evidence-based research does not support the practice of either induction of labor or a cesarean delivery for fetal macrosomia in the absence of other indications for these interventions. A more reasonable policy for management of macrosomia would entail a conservative approach awaiting the onset of spontaneous labor in the absence of a favorable uterine cervix, adequate intrapartum management such as assessment of the adequacy of the maternal pelvis, assessment of the progress of labor and careful use of oxytocin, avoidance of vaginal operative deliveries, and avoidance of excessive traction on the impacted shoulder in favor of the maneuvers described for the management of shoulder dystocia (see Chapter 16).

FETAL SURVEILLANCE

Fetal surveillance may be used in an attempt to observe the prolonged pregnancy safely while awaiting the onset of labor or spontaneous ripening of the cervix prior to elective induction. The pitfalls of the use of antenatal testing in this setting are twofold. On the one hand, false-positive tests commonly lead to unnecessary interventions that are potentially hazardous to the gravida. On the other hand, to date, no program of fetal testing has been shown to completely eliminate the risk of stillbirth. Current research on the use of fetal testing has focused on the refinement of testing protocols and the application of new technology to address these issues.

The optimal gestational age for the initiation of fetal testing has not been established. Data presented earlier in this chapter indicate that perinatal mortality is significantly increased as early as 41 weeks' gestation. Additional support for this concept was provided by Guidetti et al., who reported an increased incidence of perinatal morbidity at greater than or equal to 41 weeks' gestation and by Jazayeri et al., who demonstrated elevated plasma erythropoietin levels, indicating altered fetal oxygenation, in patients at greater than or equal to 41 weeks.[40,41] Thus, it would seem prudent to initiate fetal testing at 41 weeks of gestation.

Extensive experience with biophysical profile testing in high-risk populations indicates a perinatal mortality rate of 0.73 per 1,000 tested pregnancies within 1 week of a normal test, provided that the amniotic fluid volume is normal.[42] Twice-weekly testing with the biophysical profile in a series of 293 patients followed beyond 42 weeks of gestation has been reported. No stillbirths were observed in this small series.[43]

The primary disadvantages of biophysical profile scoring are the time required to perform the test and the need for an experienced sonographer. Recently, investigators have examined the efficacy of using the nonstress test as a primary testing modality with the addition of a sonographic assessment of amniotic fluid volume. Measurement of the amniotic fluid index (AFI) requires minimal sonographic experience,[44] and vibroacoustic stimulation may be used to shorten the duration of the nonstress test.[45] Results of the use of such a protocol in the antepartum management of 5,973 high-risk pregnancies have been described by Clark et al.[46] Amniotic fluid volume assessment was performed by measurement of the AFI, with induction of labor reserved for an AFI of 5 cm or less. Twice-weekly testing was performed in a subset of 279 prolonged pregnancies. No stillbirths were recorded.

More recently, Miller et al. reported the use of a similar protocol in 15,482 high-risk pregnancies for which 54,617 tests were performed.[47] The false-negative rate of this test was 0.8 per 1,000 women tested—a rate that favorably compares with those reported for the contraction stress test or the complete biophysical profile.[42,48] Of note, 6,390 patients were assessed in this study for prolonged pregnancy. These patients were first evaluated in the 41st week of gestation and twice-weekly testing was initiated after 42 weeks of gestation. Five stillbirths were reported in this subpopulation. An analysis of all false-positive tests showed that the routine use of nonstress testing combined with the AFI resulted in a 60 percent false-positive rate in the prediction of intrapartum fetal compromise compared with a 40 percent false-positive rate using the complete biophysical profile. This increase in false-positive tests was felt to be partly a result of poor specificity of the AFI in predicting fetal compromise.

Oligohydramnios

The formation of amniotic fluid is a complex and poorly understood process. Many authors have demonstrated that amniotic fluid volume decreases as gestational age advances beyond 32 or 34 weeks' gestation. Marks and Divon evaluated the AFI in 511 well-dated prolonged pregnancies.[49] Gestational age at the time of the study ranged from 41 weeks to 43 weeks and 6 days. AFI measurements ranged from 1.7 to 24.6 cm with a mean and standard deviation of 12.4 cm $\pm$ 4.2 cm at 41 weeks. Oligohydramnios (AFI <5.0 cm) was detected in 11.5 percent of the study population. Longitudinal data were available from 121 patients. These patients demonstrated a mean decrease in AFI of 25 percent per week. Thus, the authors concluded that the majority of pregnancies at greater than or equal to 41 weeks' gestation have a normal volume of amniotic fluid.

Numerous hypotheses have been offered to explain the pathophysiology of oligohydramnios. Oligohydramnios, when defined as an AFI less than or equal to 5.0 cm, has an incidence of 8.5 to 15.5 percent. In the absence of ruptured membranes or fetal urinary tract abnormalities, diminishing levels of amniotic fluid volume may be related to poor placental function.[50] Nicolaides et al. hypothesized that fetal hypoxemia may result in redistribution of blood flow with decreased renal perfusion and diminished urine production, which in turn may cause oligohydramnios.[51] A vicious cycle could develop with oligohydramnios causing cord compression, resulting in further hypoxemia, oligohydramnios, and fetal heart rate (FHR) abnormalities. Under these circumstances, fetal hypoxemia may induce relax-

ation of the rectal sphincters and hence meconium staining resulting in meconium aspiration syndrome. In fact, meconium-stained amniotic fluid is found in up to 50 percent of pregnancies at 42 weeks' gestation upon rupture of the membranes. Trimmer et al. detected diminished urine production in pregnancies of 42 weeks or more with oligohydramnios and suggested that decreased fetal urine production was the result of preexisting oligohydramnios, which limited fetal swallowing of amniotic fluid rather than a decrease in renal perfusion.[52] Bar-Hava et al. used pulsed wave Doppler to evaluate resistance index values in the fetal middle cerebral artery, renal, and umbilical arteries in 57 pregnancies at greater than or equal to 41 weeks' gestation.[53] Oligohydramnios (AFI <5 cm) was detected in 15 patients. The various resistance index values and the ratios among them were not significantly different in patients with or without oligohydramnios. Interestingly, the mean birthweight in patients with oligohydramnios was significantly lower than the mean birthweight in patients with a normal AFI (3,297 $\pm$ 438 g vs. 3,742 $\pm$ 448 g, respectively). The author concluded that oligohydramnios in these patients is not associated with a noticeable redistribution of blood flow and suggested that the cause of oligohydramnios is probably unrelated to renal perfusion.

The fact that oligohydramnios was found more often in the smaller fetuses is intriguing. It suggests that the appearance of oligohydramnios is a pathologic rather than a physiologic process. It may indicate that the pathophysiology of oligohydramnios in prolonged pregnancy is similar to that involved with the formation of oligohydramnios in the growth-restricted fetus, and overall, it is consistent with the concept that it is the small and "older" fetus who is more prone to complications arising from asphyxia. Other causes of oligohydramnios include spontaneous rupture of membranes, genitourinary anomalies, and an abnormal karyotype. It is important to rule out these other causes of oligohydramnios before attributing reduced amniotic fluid levels to fetal hypoxemia.

Regardless of the exact cause of oligohydramnios, its presence has been used by Leveno et al. to explain the increased incidence of abnormal antepartum and intrapartum FHR abnormalities seen in prolonged pregnancies.[54] These authors suggested that prolonged FHR decelerations representing cord compression preceded 75 percent of cesarean deliveries for fetal jeopardy. The association between a reduced AFI and variable decelerations is well documented.[55,56] As suggested by Gabbe et al. and Lee and Hon, variable FHR decelerations detected in patients with oligohydramnios are probably related to increased umbilical cord compression.[55,57] This concept is further supported by reports of intrapartum amnioinfusion in mothers with oligohydramnios. This procedure was shown to reduce the incidence of variable FHR decelerations, meconium staining below the vocal cords, and operative delivery for fetal distress.[58,59] A similar mechanism is probably functional in the antepartum period. Both Phelan et al. and Divon et al. found that the frequency of nonstress tests demonstrating FHR decelerations or bradycardia increased as the ultrasonographic estimates of the amniotic fluid declined.[60–63]

Quantifying amniotic fluid volume presents significant problems. Various sonographic semiquantitative estimates such as the 1-cm pocket, the 2-cm pocket, or the 3-cm pocket have been proposed as definitions of oligohydramnios.[64–66] The use of an AFI of less than or equal to 5.0 cm to define oligohydramnios was first suggested by Phelan et al. in 1987, as an arbitrary cut-off value based on retrospective studies. Nevertheless, it has since gained popular appeal.[60,62] A recent meta-analysis evaluated the risk of cesarean delivery for fetal distress, 5-minute Apgar score of less than 7, and umbilical artery pH less than 7.00 in patients with antepartum or intrapartum AFI or less than 5.0 cm.[67] Eighteen reports describing 10,551 patients at various gestational ages were included in the analysis. The overall incidence of oligohydramnios was 15.2 percent. The authors concluded that an AFI of less than or equal to 5.0 cm is associated with an increased risk of cesarean delivery for fetal distress (RR of 2.2; 95 percent CI, 1.5 to 3.4) and an Apgar score of less than 7 at 5 minutes (RR of 5.2; 95 percent CI, 2.4 to 11.3). However, no association was demonstrated between oligohydramnios and severe fetal acidosis.

The presence of sonographically diagnosed oligohydramnios is often used as an indication for delivery of pregnancies that reach term gestation or extend beyond term. One should realize, however, that up to 50 percent of patients who are diagnosed as having oligohydramnios by ultrasound will have a normal volume of amniotic fluid upon artificial rupture of the membranes.[68] In addition, there are no large-scale, prospective, randomized studies documenting the benefits of delivery once oligohydramnios has been detected. In the absence of such studies, it would seem prudent to deliver patients at or beyond 41 weeks' gestation who demonstrate oligohydramnios primarily because of the large body of data that documents an association between diminished amniotic fluid volume and adverse perinatal outcome.

Doppler Ultrasound

Umbilical artery Doppler velocimetry has not been able to improve the positive predictive value of fetal testing in prolonged pregnancy.[69–71] Recently, Doppler ultrasound has been applied to investigations of the fetal circulation in an attempt to identify perturbations that might be associated with adverse outcomes. Bar-Hava

et al. analyzed renal artery and middle cerebral blood velocity waveforms in 57 pregnancies prolonged beyond 287 days' gestation.[53] Findings in pregnancies complicated by oligohydramnios were compared with those found in pregnancies with normal amniotic fluid volume. It was expected that, with hypoxia, impedance in the cerebral circulation might decrease as impedance increased in the renal circulation. However, no differences were seen. These results were confirmed in a larger, prospective investigation undertaken by Zimmermann et al.[72] In this cross-sectional, prospective study, 153 pregnancies were examined beyond 287 days of gestation and 36 percent were followed beyond 42 weeks of gestation. The resistance indices of umbilical artery and middle cerebral artery waveforms were studied every 2 days until delivery. All velocities fell within the known 95 percent CIs for normal term fetuses. Doppler measurements were unable to predict adverse fetal outcomes, such as abnormal fetal heart rate tracings, thick meconium, the need for urgent operative delivery, acidemia at delivery, or neonatal encephalopathy.

Weiner et al. used Doppler ultrasound to study fetal cardiac function in prolonged pregnancy. The velocity time integral of blood flow across each valve was multiplied by the fetal heart rate to obtain a measure of fetal ventricular function.[73] Results were compared with measurements obtained from a control group of patients studied between 38 and 41 weeks of gestation. No differences were seen between controls and prolonged pregnancies with an AFI of 6 cm or greater. Prolonged pregnancies with abnormal amniotic fluid volumes had statistically significant differences in fetal left cardiac function. The authors concluded that an abnormality of cardiac function may be present prior to or coincident with the development of oligohydramnios.

MANAGEMENT

In spite of many years of research, the optimal management of the prolonged pregnancy is still controversial. These pregnancies have traditionally been considered to be at elevated risk for adverse perinatal outcome. Thus, it is generally accepted that these patients should undergo some form of fetal testing. Although most authors agree that induction of labor is indicated in women with an "inducible" uterine cervix, there is lack of agreement as to the management of the patient whose cervix is deemed "unfavorable." Antenatal testing may be used in an attempt to observe the prolonged pregnancy safely while awaiting the spontaneous onset of labor or for ripening of the cervix prior to labor induction. Other opinions argue in favor of induction of labor regardless of the cervical status.

Fibronectin

Approximately 50 percent of patients who are undelivered by 41 weeks' gestation will present in spontaneous labor within 7 days, and over 90 percent will do so by 44 weeks.[74] Attempts to evaluate the role of fetal fibronectin in cervical secretions as a predictor of the onset of spontaneous labor have been inconclusive. Goffeng et al. studied 80 women at 42 weeks' gestation and found that the presence of fetal fibronectin was not significantly correlated with either the Bishop score or the time interval between cervical sampling and delivery.[75] In contrast, Mouw et al. concluded that the sensitivity and specificity of fetal fibronectin concentration of at least 50 ng/ml in the prediction of spontaneous onset of labor within 3 days of examination were 71 and 64 percent, respectively.[76] With a sensitivity of only 71 percent and a relatively low specificity, it is unlikely that this test would have any practical clinical application in the management of the prolonged pregnancy.

Sweeping the Membranes

Membrane sweeping or stripping is an age-old method of inducing labor that is still in common use. This intervention results in a local increase in prostaglandin production and is believed to hasten the onset of labor. A meta-analysis of the use of sweeping of the membranes to induce labor or to prevent prolonged pregnancy has recently been published.[77] The analysis showed that sweeping of the membranes in term pregnancies shortens the duration of pregnancy by a mean of 4 days. Consequently, it decreases the frequency of patients reaching 41 or 42 weeks' gestation. Eight women need to be treated at term in order to avoid one pregnancy continuing beyond 41 weeks, and 25 women need to be treated to avoid one pregnancy continuing beyond 42 weeks' gestation. The intervention had no significant impact on mode of delivery or the incidence of maternal or neonatal infections. Vaginal bleeding, painful uterine contractions not leading to delivery, and discomfort during vaginal examination were significantly more common in women allocated to sweeping of the membranes.

Induction of Labor

A major concern in the management of the prolonged pregnancy is the balance between the likelihood of a successful induction of labor and the risks of expectant management. The October 1997 ACOG Practice Patterns states that there is insufficient information to determine whether either labor induction or expectant management result in the best outcome in women with a prolonged pregnancy and a favorable cervix.[3] This publication does state that "according to current obstetric practice, labor is induced in most of these women." Accordingly, most practitioners feel that if the likelihood of a successful vaginal delivery is sufficiently high, there is no reason to expose the patient to the added risks associated with prolongation of pregnancy. Thus, in the absence of randomized controlled trials, induction of labor in women with prolonged pregnancy and a favorable cervix is a reasonable approach.

The management of the patient who presents with an unfavorable cervix is much more controversial. It consists of either expectant management (i.e., antenatal surveillance until there are signs of fetal jeopardy, or until the patient presents in either spontaneous labor or with a favorable cervix) or induction of labor any time after 41 weeks' gestation.

Magann et al. showed that daily membrane stripping or daily placement of prostaglandin gel (0.15 mg of PGE_2) beginning at 41 weeks resulted in fewer inductions at 42 weeks.[78] Other attempts at outpatient management have been inconclusive. Lien et al. randomized patients to either PGE_2 gel or placebo gel at the time of scheduled nonstress testing and showed that there was no decrease in the induction rate or cesarean delivery rate in patients with prolonged pregnancy who received intracervical PGE_2 gel.[79] In contrast, Ohel et al. randomized patients at 40 to 41 weeks into either outpatient administration of 3 mg of vaginal PGE_2 or expectant management, and observed that the average number of days to delivery was significantly lower in the induction group (1.6 vs. 5.2 days), with no difference in the cesarean section rates between groups.[80]

Several other investigators have evaluated the use of PGE_2 gel for inducing labor in patients with a prolonged pregnancy and an unfavorable cervix. Shaw et al. studied PGE_2 gel in a double-blind, placebo-controlled trial and showed that it was associated with an improvement in cervical ripeness, shorter duration of labor, reduced need for high-dose oxytocin, and a lower rate of cesarean deliveries.[81] A study by Papageorgiou et al.[82] confirmed these findings, as PGE_2 gel was associated with a higher success rate and a lower cesarean delivery rate when compared to oxytocin. In contrast, a large and well-designed multicenter, randomized, controlled trial of expectant management versus induction of labor reported no reduction in the induction–delivery interval or in the cesarean delivery rate in the PGE_2 group relative to placebo.[83]

Other medical and mechanical methods for induction of labor have been described such as misoprostol, relaxin, balloon catheters, nipple stimulation, and hygroscopic tents.[84] Unfortunately, the ideal mode of induction of labor has yet to be determined. Oxytocin in combination with amniotomy remains the method of choice for inducing labor in women with a favorable cervix. The use of cervical ripening agents in patients with an unfavorable cervix certainly results in a significant increase in cervical dilation and effacement. However, the use of these agents is still associated with a high cesarean delivery rate subsequent to a failed induction of labor. Relative to women who present in spontaneous labor, the cesarean delivery rate is approximately doubled when induction of labor is attempted in nulliparous women at term.[85]

Induction of Labor versus Expectant Management

Although most authors agree that induction of labor is indicated in women with an "inducible" uterine cervix, there is lack of agreement as to the management of the patient whose cervix is deemed "unfavorable." Induction of labor in all women at 42 weeks' gestation is one option. Another option is serial fetal surveillance to assess well-being in women with an unfavorable cervix. These surveillance programs have focused on the detection of fetal hypoxia associated with uteroplacental insufficiency. To this end, fetal heart rate monitoring, biophysical profile, and ultrasonographic assessment of amniotic fluid volume have been utilized. Delivery is undertaken when signs of fetal or maternal compromise are detected. In a recent study, Hanna et al. randomized 3,407 women with uncomplicated pregnancies of 41 or more weeks' gestation to two management protocols: induction of labor or serial fetal monitoring.[86] They concluded that the rates of perinatal morbidity and mortality were the same with the two approaches; however, the cesarean section rate was lower in the induction group. In contrast, Almstrom et al., who also randomized patients into active and conservative management protocols, concluded that serial fetal monitoring resulted in a lower cesarean section rate.[87] A recent meta-analysis of 11 prospective studies demonstrated that induction of labor resulted in a slightly lower cesarean section rate compared with expectant management.[88] The randomized controlled trial ($n = 440$) conducted by the National Institute of Child Health and Human Development Network of Maternal-Fetal Medicine Units reported no fetal or maternal advantages to elective induction of labor at 41 weeks of gestation relative to serial fetal monitoring and indicated that either management approach was acceptable.[83] Adverse fetal outcome was defined by the presence of neonatal seizures, intracranial hemorrhage, need for mechanical ventilation, or nerve injury. The incidence of adverse fetal outcome was 1.5 percent in the induction group and 1 percent in the expectant management group. The cesarean delivery rate was 18 percent in the expectant group, 23 percent in the PGE$_2$ gel group, and 18 percent in the placebo gel group. The authors concluded

that there is good evidence that no approach is superior, thus suggesting that either induction of labor or serial monitoring would be equally reasonable.

SUMMARY AND RECOMMENDATION

Management of the prolonged pregnancy is primarily determined by the interplay of three factors: certainty of gestational dating, the risks associated with expectant management, and the likelihood of spontaneous vaginal delivery following an induction of labor.

Key Points

➤ Whenever possible, gestational age should be established by a first- or an early second-trimester ultrasound examination.

➤ Sweeping of the membranes at term decreases slightly the number of pregnancies reaching either 41 or 42 weeks' gestation.

➤ Consider induction of labor at or beyond 41 weeks' gestation in patients with a favorable cervix.

➤ Initiate semiweekly fetal testing (nonstress test and AFI) at 41 weeks' gestation.

➤ Conservative management (i.e., semiweekly fetal testing) or active management (i.e., induction of labor) are equally reasonable options for patients with an unfavorable cervix.

➤ Perinatal morbidity and mortality are significantly increased when gestational age at birth is 41 weeks or more.

REFERENCES

1. Ballantyne JW: The problem of the postmature infant. J Obstet Gynaecol Br Emp 2:521, 1902.
2. Clifford SH: Postmaturity with placental dysfunction, clinical syndrome and pathologic findings. J Pediatr 44:1, 1954.
3. American College of Obstetricians and Gynecologists: Management of post term pregnancy. Practice Patterns No 6, October 1997.
4. World Health Organization (WHO): Recommended definition terminology and format for statistical tables related to the perinatal period and rise of a new certification for cause of perina-

tal deaths. Modifications recommended by FIGO as amended, October 14, 1976. Acta Obstet Gynecol Scand 56:347, 1977.

5. Federation of Gynecology and Obstetrics (FIGO): Report of the FIGO subcommittee on Perinatal Epidemiology and Health Statistics following a workshop in Cairo, November 11–18, 1984. London, International Federation of Gynecology and Obstetrics, 1986, p 54.

6. Ventura SJ, Martin JA, Taffel M: Advance report of final mortality statistics, 1993. Monthly Vital Statistics Report (Suppl). Vol 44, No 3. Hyattsville, MD, National Center for Health Statistics, 1995.

7. Norwitz ER, Robinson JN, Challis JR: The control of labor. N Engl J Med 341:660, 1999.

8. Liggins GC: The role of the hypothalamic-pituitary-adrenal axis in preparing the fetus for birth. Am J Obstet Gynecol 182:475, 2000.

9. Smith R: The timing of birth. Sci Am 280:68, 1999.

10. Naeye RL: Causes of perinatal mortality excess in prolonged gestation. Am J Epidemiol 108:429, 1978.

11. Rabe T, Hosch R, Runnebaum B: Sulfatase deficiency in the human placenta: clinical findings. Biol Res Pregnancy Perinatol 4:95, 1983.

12. Campbell MK, Ostbye T, Irgens LM: Post-term birth: risk factors and outcomes in a 10-year cohort of Norwegian births. Obstet Gynecol 89:543, 1997.

13. Zweidling MA: Factors pertaining to prolonged pregnancy and its outcome. Pediatrics 40:202, 1967.

14. Gardosi J, Vanner T, Francis A: Gestational age and induction of labor for prolonged pregnancy. Br J Obstet Gynaecol 104:792, 1997.

15. Boyd ME, Usher RH, McLean FH, Kramer MS: Obstetric consequences of postmaturity. Am J Obstet Gynecol 158:334, 1988.

16. Nguyen TH, Larsen T, Engholm G, Moller H: Evaluation of ultrasound-estimated date of delivery in 17,450 spontaneous singleton births: do we need to modify Naegele's rule? Ultrasound Obstet Gynecol 14:23, 1999.

17. Mul T, Mongelli M, Gardosi J: A comparative analysis of second-trimester ultrasound dating formulae in pregnancies conceived with artificial reproductive techniques. Ultrasound Obstet Gynecol 8:397, 1996.

18. Gardosi J, Mongelli M: Risk assessment adjusted for gestational age in maternal serum screening for Down's syndrome. BMJ 306:1509, 1993.

19. Gardosi J: Dating of pregnancy: time to forget the last menstrual period. Ultrasound Obstet Gynecol 9:367, 1997.

20. Tunon K, Eik-Nes SH, Grottum P: Fetal outcome in pregnancies defined as post-term according to the last menstrual period estimate, but not according to the ultrasound estimate. Ultrasound Obstet Gynecol 14:12, 1999.

21. Divon MY, Haglund B, Nisell H, et al: Fetal and neonatal mortality in the post-term pregnancy: the impact of gestational age and fetal growth restriction. Am J Obstet Gynecol 178:726, 1998.

22. Ingemarsson I, Kallen K: Stillbirths and rate of neonatal deaths in 76,761 postterm pregnancies in Sweden, 1982–1991: a register study. Acta Obstet Gynecol Scand 76:658, 1997.

23. Clausson B, Cnattingius S, Axelsson O: Outcomes of post-term births: the role of fetal growth restriction and malformations. Obstet Gynecol 94:758, 1999.

24. Hilder L, Costeloe K, Thilaganathan B: Prolonged pregnancy: evaluating gestation-specific risks of fetal and infant mortality. Br J Obstet Gynaecol 105:169, 1998.

25. Lovell KE: The effect of postmaturity on the developing child. Med J Aust 1:131, 1973.

26. Ting RV, Wang MH, Scott TF: The dysmature infant. Associated factors and outcome at 7 years of age. J Pediatr 90:943, 1977.

27. Shime J, Librach CL, Gare DJ, Cook CJ: The influence of prolonged pregnancy on infant development at one and two years of age: a prospective controlled study. Am J Obstet Gynecol 154:341, 1986.

28. Boyd ME, Usher RH, McLean FH: Fetal macrosomia: prediction, risks, proposed management. Obstet Gynecol 61:715, 1983.

29. McLean FH, Boyd ME, Usher RH, Kramer MS: Post-term infants: too big or too small? Am J Obstet Gynecol 164:619, 1991.

30. Nahum GG, Stanislaw H, Huffaker BJ: Fetal weight gain at term: linear with minimal dependence on maternal obesity. Am J Obstet Gynecol 172:1387, 1995.

31. Pollack RN, Hauer-Pollack G, Divon MY: Macrosomia in postdates pregnancies: the accuracy of routine ultrasonographic screening. Am J Obstet Gynecol 167:7, 1992.

32. Chervenak LJ, Divon MY, Hirsch J, et al: Macrosomia in the post-date pregnancy: is routine sonography screening indicated? Am J Obstet Gynecol 161:753, 1989.

33. Pollack RN, Divon MY: Problems in detecting fetal macrosomia. Contemp Ob/Gyn, October 1991.

34. O'Reilly-Green CP, Divon MY: Receiver operating characteristic curves of sonographic estimated fetal weight for prediction macrosomia in prolonged pregnancies. Ultrasound Obstet Gynecol 9:403, 1997.

35. Rouse DJ, Owen J: Prophylactic cesarean delivery for fetal macrosomia diagnosed by means of ultrasonography—a faustian bargain? Am J Obstet Gynecol 181:332, 1999.

36. Rouse DJ, Owen J, Goldenberg RL, Cliver SP: The effectiveness and costs of elective cesarean delivery for fetal macrosomia diagnosed by ultrasound. JAMA 276:1480, 1996.

37. Leaphart WL, Meyer MC, Capeless EL: Labor induction with a prenatal diagnosis of fetal macrosomia. J Matern Fetal Med 6:99, 1997.

38. Gonen O, Rosen DJ, Dolfin Z, et al: Induction of labor versus expectant management in macrosomia: a randomized study. Obstet Gynecol 89:913, 1997.

39. Levine AB, Lockwood CJ, Brown B, et al: Sonographic diagnosis of the large for gestational age fetus at term: does it make a difference? Obstet Gynecol 79:55, 1992.

40. Guidetti DA, Divon MY, Langer O: Postdate fetal surveillance: is 41 weeks too early? Am J Obstet Gynecol 161:91, 1989.

41. Jazayeri A, Tsibris JCM, Spellacy WN: Elevated umbilical cord plasma erythropoietin levels in prolonged pregnancies. Obstet Gynecol 92:63, 1998.

42. Manning FA, Morrison I, Harman CR, et al: Fetal assessment based on fetal biophysical profile scoring: experience in 19,221 referred high-risk pregnancies. II. An analysis of false-negative fetal deaths. Am J Obstet Gynecol 157:880, 1987.

43. John JM, Harman CR, Lange IR, Manning FA: Biophysical profile scoring in the management of the post term pregnancy: an analysis of 307 patients. Am J Obstet Gynecol 154:269, 1986.

44. Phelan JP, Ahn MO, Smith CV, et al: Amniotic fluid index measurements during pregnancy. J Reprod Med 32:601, 1987.

45. Smith CV, Phelan JP, Platt LD, et al: Fetal acoustic stimulation testing (the Fas test). II. A randomized clinical comparison with the nonstress test. Am J Obstet Gynecol 155:131, 1986.

46. Clark SL, Sabey P, Jolley K: Nonstress testing with acoustic stimulation and amniotic fluid volume assessment: 5973 tests without unexpected fetal death Am J Obstet Gynecol 160:694, 1989.

47. Miller DA, Rabello YA, Paul RH: The modified biophysical profile: antepartum testing in the 1990's. Am J Obstet Gynecol 174:812, 1996.

48. Freeman RK, Anderson G, Dorcester W: A prospective multicenter multiinstitutional study of antepartum fetal heart rate monitoring. II. Contraction stress test versus nonstress test for primary surveillance. Am J Obstet Gynecol 143:778, 1982.

49. Marks AD, Divon MY: Longitudinal study of the amniotic fluid index in postdates pregnancy. Obstet Gynecol 79:229, 1992.

50. Gresham EL, Rankin JHG, Makowski EL, et al: An evaluation of fetal renal function in chronic sheep preparation. J Clin Invest 51:149, 1972.

51. Nicolaides KH, Peters MT, Vyas S, et al: Relation of rate of urine production to oxygen tension in small for gestational age fetuses. Am J Obstet Gynecol 162:387, 1990.

52. Trimmer KJ, Leveno KJ, Peters MT, Kelly MA: Observation on the cause of oligohydramnios in prolonged pregnancy. Am J Obstet Gynecol 163:1900, 1990.

53. Bar-Hava I, Divon MY, Sardo M, Barnhard Y: Is oligohydramnios in post-term pregnancy associated with redistribution of fetal blood flow? Am J Obstet Gynecol 173:519, 1995.

54. Leveno KJ, Quirk JG Jr, Cunningham FG, et al: Prolonged pregnancy observations concerning the causes of fetal distress. Am J Obstet Gynecol 150:465, 1984.

55. Gabbe SG, Ettinger BB, Freeman RK, Martin CB: Umbilical cord compression associated with amniotomy: laboratory observations. Am J Obstet Gynecol 126:353, 1976.

56. Miyazaki FS, Taylor NA: Saline amnioinfusion for relief of variable or prolonged decelerations. A preliminary report. Am J Obstet Gynecol 146:670, 1983.

57. Lee ST, Hon EH: Fetal hemodynamic response to umbilical cord compression. Obstet Gynecol 22:553, 1963.

58. Strong TH, Hetzler G, Sarno AP, Paul RH: Prophylactic intrapartum amnioinfusion: a randomized clinical trial. Am J Obstet Gynecol 162:1370, 1990.

59. Wenstrom KD, Parsons MT: The prevention of meconium aspiration in labor using amnioinfusion Obstet Gynecol 73:647, 1989.

60. Phelan JP, Smith CV, Broussard P, Small M: Amniotic fluid volume assessment with the four-quadrant technique at 36–42 weeks' gestation. J Reprod Med 32:540, 1987.

61. Phelan JP, Platt LD, Yeh SY, et al: The role of ultrasound assessment of amniotic fluid volume in the management of the postdate pregnancy. Am J Obstet Gynecol 151:304, 1985.

62. Phelan JP, Ahn MO, Smith CV, et al: Amniotic fluid index measurements during pregnancy. J Reprod Med 32:601, 1987.

63. Divon MY, Marks AD, Henderson CE: Longitudinal measurement of amniotic fluid index in postterm pregnancies and its association with fetal outcome. Am J Obstet Gynecol 172:142, 1995.

64. Manning FA, Platt LD, Sipos L: Antepartum fetal evaluation: development of a fetal biophysical profile. Am J Obstet Gynecol 136;787, 1980.

65. Chamberlain PF, Manning FA, Morrison I, et al: Ultrasound evaluation of amniotic fluid volume. I. The relationship of marginal and decreased amniotic fluid volumes to perinatal outcome. Am J Obstet Gynecol 150:245, 1984.

66. Crowley P, O'Herlihey C, Boylan P: The value of ultrasound measurement of amniotic fluid volume on the management of prolonged pregnancies. Br J Obstet Gynaecol 91:444, 1984.

67. Chauhan SP, Sanderson M, Hendrix N, et al: Perinatal outcome and amniotic fluid index in the antepartum and intrapartum periods: a meta-analysis. Am J Obstet Gynecol 181:1473, 1999.

68. O'Reilly-Green CP, Divon MY: Predictive value of amniotic fluid index for oligohydramnios in patients with prolonged pregnancies. J Matern Fetal Med 5:218, 1996.

69. Strokes HJ, Roberts RV, Newnham JP: Doppler flow velocity waveform analysis in postdate pregnancies. Aust N Z J Obstet Gynecol 31:27, 1991.

70. Guidetti DA, Divon MY, Cavalieri RL, et al: Fetal umbilical artery flow velocimetry in postdate pregnancies. Am J Obstet Gynecol 157:1521, 1987.

71. Farmakides G, Schulman H, Ducey J, et al: Uterine and umbilical Doppler velocimetry in post term pregnancy. J Reprod Med 33:259, 1988.

72. Zimmermann P, Albck T, Koskinen J, et al: Doppler flow velocimetry of the umbilical artery, uteroplacental arteries and fetal middle cerebral artery in prolonged pregnancy. Ultrasound Obstet Gynecol 5:189, 1995.

73. Weiner Z, Farmakides G, Schulman H, et al: Central and peripheral haemodynamic changes in post-term fetuses: correlation with oligohydramnios and abnormal fetal heart rate pattern. Br J Obstet Gynaecol 103:541, 1996.

74. Roach VJ, Rogers MS: Pregnancy outcome beyond 41 weeks' gestation. Int J Gynaecol Obstet 59:19, 1997.

75. Goffeng AR, Milsom I, Lindstedt G, et al: Fetal fibronectin in vaginal fluid of women in prolonged pregnancy. Gynecol Obstet Invest 44:224, 1997.

76. Mouw RJ, Egberts J, Kragt H, van Roosmalen J: Cervicovaginal fetal fibronectin concentrations: predictive value of impending birth in post-term pregnancies. Eur J Obstet Gynecol Reprod Biol 80:67, 1998.

77. Boulvain M, Irion O: Stripping/sweeping of the membranes to induce labour or to prevent post-term pregnancy (Cochrane Review). *In* The Cochrane Library, Issue 4. Oxford, Update Software, 1998

78. Magann EF, Chauhan SP, Nevils BG, et al: Management of pregnancies beyond forty-one weeks' gestation with an unfavorable cervix. Am J Obstet Gynecol 178:1279, 1998.

79. Lien JM, Morgan MA, Garite TJ, et al: Antepartum cervical ripening: applying prostaglandin E2 gel in conjunction with scheduled non-stress tests in postdates pregnancies. Am J Obstet Gynecol 79:453, 1998.

80. Ohel G, Rahav D, Rothbard H, Rauch M: Randomized trial of outpatient induction of labor with vaginal PGE_2 at 40–41 weeks of gestation versus expectant management. Arch Gynecol Obstet 258:109, 1996.

81. Shaw KJ, Medearis AL, Horenstein J, et al: Selective labor induction in post-term patients. Observations and outcomes. J Reprod Med 37:157, 1992.

82. Papageorgiou I, Tsionou C, Minaretzis D, et al: Labor characteristics of uncomplicated prolonged pregnancies after induction with intracervical prostaglandin E_2 gel versus intravenous oxytocin. Gynecol Obstet Invest 34:92, 1992.

83. The National Institute of Child Health and Human Development Network of Maternal Fetal Medicine Units: A clinical trial of induction of labor versus expectant management in post term pregnancy. Am J Obstet Gynecol 170:716, 1994.

84. Reichler A, Romem Y, Divon MY: Induction of labor. Curr Opin Obstet Gynecol 7:432, 1995.

85. Seyb ST, Berka RJ, Socol ML, Dooley SL: Risk of cesarean delivery with elective induction of labor at term in nulliparous women. Obstet Gynecol 94:600, 1999.

86. Hannah ME, Hannah WJ, Hellman J, et al: Induction of labor as compared with serial antenatal monitoring in post-term pregnancies. A randomized controlled trial. The Canadian Multicenter Post-term Pregnancy Trial Group. N Engl J Med 327:1587, 1992.

87. Almstrom H, Granstrom L, Ekman G: Serial antenatal monitoring compared with labor induction in post-term pregnancies. Acta Obstet Gynecol Scand 74:599, 1995.

88. Grant JM: Induction of labour confers benefits in prolonged pregnancy. Br J Obstet Gynaecol 101:99, 1994.

Pregnancy and Coexisting Disease

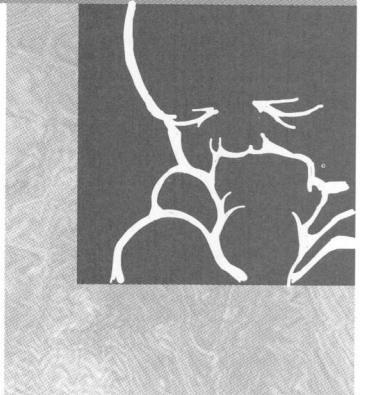

C h a p t e r 28

Hypertension

BAHA M. SIBAI

Hypertensive disorders are the most common medical complications of pregnancy, with a reported incidence between 5 and 10 percent.[1] The incidence varies among different hospitals, regions, and countries. In addition, these disorders are a major cause of maternal and perinatal mortality and morbidity worldwide.[2] The term *hypertension in pregnancy* is usually used to describe a wide spectrum of patients who may have only mild elevations in blood pressure or severe hypertension with various organ dysfunctions. The manifestations in these patients may be clinically similar (e.g., hypertension, proteinuria); however, they may result from different underlying causes such as chronic hypertension, renal disease, or pure preeclampsia. The three most common forms of hypertension are acute gestational hypertension, preeclampsia, and chronic essential hypertension.

The terminology used to classify the hypertensive disorders of pregnancy has been confusing and inconsistent, making comparison of studies difficult and often impossible. For many years, the hypertensive disorders of gestation were labeled *toxemia of pregnancy*. This term was used because it was felt that this wide variety of disorders had as a common etiologic agent a circulating toxin. We now know this to be untrue.

DEFINITIONS

Hypertension may be present before pregnancy, or it may be diagnosed for the first time during pregnancy. In addition, in some women hypertension may become evident only intrapartum or postpartum. For clinical purposes, women with hypertension may be classified into one of three categories (Table 28–1).[2]

Gestational Hypertension

Gestational hypertension is the development of an elevated blood pressure during pregnancy or in the first 24 hours postpartum without other signs or symptoms of preeclampsia or preexisting hypertension. The blood pressure must return to normal within 6 weeks after delivery. Hypertension is defined as a blood pressure greater than or equal to 140 mm Hg systolic or 90 mm Hg diastolic. The hypertension should be present on at least two occasions, at least 4 hours apart, but within a maximum of a 1-week period.[3] Some women with gestational hypertension may have undiagnosed chronic hypertension, whereas others will subsequently progress to develop the clinical syndrome of preeclampsia.[4] In general, the rate of progression to preeclampsia will depend on gestational age at time of diagnosis, with higher rates if onset of hypertension is before 35 weeks' gestation.[4]

Preeclampsia and Eclampsia

The so-called classic triad of preeclampsia includes hypertension, proteinuria, and edema. However, there is now universal agreement that edema should not be considered as part of the diagnosis of preeclampsia.[5–7] Indeed, edema is neither sufficient nor necessary to confirm the diagnosis of preeclampsia, since edema is a common finding in normal pregnancy and approximately one third of eclamptic women never demonstrate the presence of edema.[8] At present, preeclampsia is primarily defined as gestational hypertension plus proteinuria. Proteinuria is defined as a concentration of 0.1 g/L or more in at least two random urine specimens collected 4 hours or more apart or 0.3 g in a 24-hour period. In the absence of proteinuria, the syndrome of preeclampsia should be considered when gestational hy-

Table 28–1. HYPERTENSIVE DISORDERS OF PREGNANCY

Clinical Findings	Chronic Hypertension	Gestational Hypertension*	Preeclampsia
Time of onset of hypertension	<20 weeks	Usually in third trimester	≥20 weeks
Degree of hypertension	Mild or severe	Mild	Mild or severe
Proteinuria*	Absent	Absent	Usually present
Serum urate >5.5 mg/dl (0.33 mmol/L)	Rare	Absent	Present in almost all cases
Hemoconcentration	Absent	Absent	Severe disease
Thrombocytopenia	Absent	Absent	Severe disease
Hepatic dysfunction	Absent	Absent	Severe disease

* Defined as ≥1+ by dipstick testing on two occasions or ≥300 mg in a 24-hour urine collection.
From Sibai BM: Drug therapy: treatment of hypertension in pregnant women. Drug Therapy Series. N Engl J Med 335:257, 1996. Copyright 1996 Massachusetts Medical Society, with permission.

pertension is present in association with persistent cerebral symptoms, epigastric or right upper quadrant pain plus nausea or vomiting, fetal growth restriction, or with abnormal laboratory tests such as thrombocytopenia and abnormal liver enzymes.[3,9] In mild preeclampsia, the diastolic blood pressure remains below 110 mm Hg and the systolic blood pressure remains below 160 mm Hg (see the box "Criteria for Severe Preeclampsia"). Eclampsia is the occurrence of seizures not attributable to other causes.

Chronic Hypertension

Chronic hypertension is defined as hypertension present before the pregnancy or that diagnosed before the 20th week of gestation. Hypertension that persists for more than 42 days postpartum is also classified as chronic hypertension.

Chronic Hypertension with Superimposed Preeclampsia

Women with chronic hypertension may develop superimposed preeclampsia, which increases morbidity for both the mother and fetus. The diagnosis of superimposed preeclampsia is based on one or more of the following findings. In women with hypertension and no proteinuria prior to 20 weeks' gestation, development of new-onset proteinuria is defined as the urinary excretion of 0.5 g protein or greater in a 24-hour specimen. In women with hypertension and proteinuria before 20 weeks, the diagnosis requires severe exacerbation in hypertension plus development of symptoms and/or thrombocytopenia and abnormal liver enzymes.[10]

Gestational Hypertension

Gestational hypertension is the most frequent cause of hypertension during pregnancy. The incidence ranges between 6 and 18 percent in nulliparous women[3,11–13] and between 6 and 8 percent in multiparous women.[12] The incidence is markedly increased in patients with twin pregnancies.[12,13] In general, the majority of cases of gestational hypertension develop at or beyond 37 weeks' gestation, and thus the overall pregnancy outcome is usually similar or superior to that seen in women with normotensive pregnancies.[3,12,13] Both gestational age at delivery and birth weight in these pregnancies are significantly higher than that in normotensive pregnancies.[3,11,12] However, women with gestational hypertension have higher rates of induction of labor for maternal reasons and higher rates of cesarean delivery as compared to women with normotensive gestation.[3,13]

Management

Women with gestational hypertension are at risk for progression to either severe hypertension, preeclampsia, or eclampsia.[4] The risks are increased with lower gestational age at time of diagnosis. Therefore, these patients require close observation of maternal and fetal conditions. Maternal evaluations require weekly prenatal visits, education about reporting preeclamptic symptoms,

---

Criteria for Severe Preeclampsia

1. Blood pressure of ≥160 mm Hg systolic or ≥110 mm Hg diastolic, recorded on at least two occasions at least 6 hours apart with patient at bed rest
2. Proteinuria of ≥5 g in 24 hours
3. Oliguria (≤400 ml in 24 hours)
4. Cerebral visual disturbances
5. Epigastric pain, nausea, and vomiting
6. Pulmonary edema
7. Impaired liver function of unclear etiology
8. Thrombocytopenia

evaluation of complete blood count, platelet count, and liver enzymes.[14] Fetal evaluation includes ultrasound examination of fluid and estimated fetal weight at time of diagnosis and weekly nonstress testing.[15] Restriction of neither dietary salt nor activity has been proven beneficial in the management of these patients.[16] Additionally, the results of several randomized trials reveal that control of maternal blood pressure with antihypertensive drugs does not improve pregnancy outcome in women with gestational hypertension.[2,16,17]

In the absence of progression to severe hypertension and/or preeclampsia, women with gestational hypertension can continue pregnancy until term. During labor and immediately postpartum, they do not require any prophylaxis against seizures, since the rate of eclampsia in these women is less than 1 in 500.[18]

PREECLAMPSIA

Preeclampsia is a form of hypertension that is unique to human pregnancy. Very rarely, it has been reported in subhuman primates.[19] Incidence ranges between 3 and 7 percent in nulliparas[3,11-13] and between 0.8 and 5.0 percent in multiparas.[12,20] The incidence is significantly increased in patients with twin pregnancies, where both the rates and severity are higher than singleton pregnancies[12,13] (see the box "Risk Factors for Preeclampsia").

The etiology of preeclampsia is unknown. Many theories have been suggested, but most of them have not withstood the test of time. Some of the theories that are

---

Risk Factors for Preeclampsia

Nulliparity
Family history of preeclampsia
Obesity
Multifetal gestation
Preeclampsia in previous pregnancy
Poor outcome in previous pregnancy
   Intrauterine growth retardation, abruptio, fetal
    death
Preexisting medical—genetic conditions
   Chronic hypertension
   Renal disease
   Type 1 (insulin-dependent) diabetes mellitus
   Thrombophilias
      Antiphospholipid antibody syndrome
      Protein C, S, antithrombin deficiency
Factor V Leiden

Theories Associated with the Etiology of Preeclampsia

Abnormal trophoblast invasion
Coagulation abnormalities
Vascular endothelial damage
Cardiovascular maladaptation
Immunologic phenomena
Genetic predisposition
Dietary deficiencies or excesses

---

still under consideration are listed in the box "Theories Associated with the Etiology of Preeclampsia."

Pathophysiology

During normal pregnancy, impressive physiologic changes occur in the uteroplacental vasculature in general, and in the cardiovascular system in particular. These changes are most likely induced by the interaction of the fetal (parental) allograft with maternal tissue. The development of mutual immunologic tolerance in the first trimester is thought to lead to important morphologic and biochemical changes in the systemic and uteroplacental maternal circulation.

Uterine Vascular Changes

The human placenta receives its blood supply from numerous uteroplacental arteries that are developed by the action of migratory interstitial and endovascular trophoblast into the walls of the spiral arterioles. This transforms the uteroplacental arterial bed into a low-resistance, low-pressure, high-flow system. The conversion of the spiral arterioles of the nonpregnant uterus into the uteroplacental arteries has been termed *physiologic changes* by Brosens.[22] In a normal pregnancy, these trophoblast-induced vascular changes extend all the way from the intervillous space to the origin of the spiral arterioles from the radial arteries in the inner one third of the myometrium. It is suggested that these vascular changes are effected in two stages: "the conversion of the decidual segments of the spiral arterioles by a wave of endovascular trophoblast migration in the first trimester and the myometrial segments by a subsequent wave in the second trimester."[22] This process was reportedly associated with extensive fibrinoid formation and degeneration of the muscular layer in the arterial wall. These vascular changes result in the conversion of approximately 100 to 150 spiral arterioles into distended, tortuous, and funnel-shaped vessels that communicate through multiple openings into the intervillous space.

In contrast, pregnancies complicated by preeclampsia and/or by fetal growth restriction demonstrate inadequate maternal vascular response to placentation. In these pregnancies, the above vascular changes are usually found only in the decidual segments of the uteroplacental arteries. Hence, the myometrial segments of the spiral arterioles are left with their musculoelastic architecture, thereby rendering them responsive to hormonal influences.[23] Additionally, the number of well-developed arterioles is smaller than that found in normotensive pregnancies. The authors postulated that this defective vascular response to placentation is due to inhibition of the second wave of endovascular trophoblast migration that normally occurs from about 16 weeks' gestation onward. These pathologic changes may have the effect of curtailing the increased blood supply required by the fetoplacental unit in the later stages of pregnancy, and they may be responsible for the decreased uteroplacental blood flow seen in most cases of preeclampsia. These conclusions were recently supported by Frusca and associates.[24] These authors studied placental bed biopsies obtained during cesarean delivery from normal pregnancies (*n* = 14), preeclamptic pregnancies (*n* = 24), and chronic hypertensive pregnancies only (*n* = 5). Biopsies from the preeclamptic group demonstrated abnormal vascular changes in every case, with 18 having acute atherosclerotic changes. On the other hand, 13 of the 14 biopsies from normotensive pregnancies had normal vascular physiologic changes, while the biopsies from the hypertensive patients showed all three types of physiologic changes. In addition, they found that the mean birth weight was significantly lower in the group with atherosclerosis than it was in the other group without such findings. However, it is important to note that these vascular changes are not a consistent finding in spiral arterioles of hypertensive pregnancies and were demonstrated in a significant proportion of normotensive pregnancies complicated by fetal growth restriction.[23,25] Furthermore, a recent investigation by Meekins and associates[26] found that endovascular trophoblast invasion was not an all-or-none phenomenon in normal and preeclamptic pregnancies. They also observed that morphologic features in one spiral artery may not be representative of all vessels in a placental bed.

Using electron microscopy, Shanklin and Sibai[27] studied the ultrastructural changes in placental bed and uterine boundary vessels in 33 preeclamptic and 12 normotensive pregnancies. They found extensive ultrastructural endothelial injury in both placental site and nonplacental site in all the specimens from preeclamptic women, but not in the normotensive women. The injury appeared to affect the endothelial mitochondria, which suggests a possible metabolic link in the pathophysiology. The endothelial injury ranged from swelling to complete erosion, and the swelling was associated

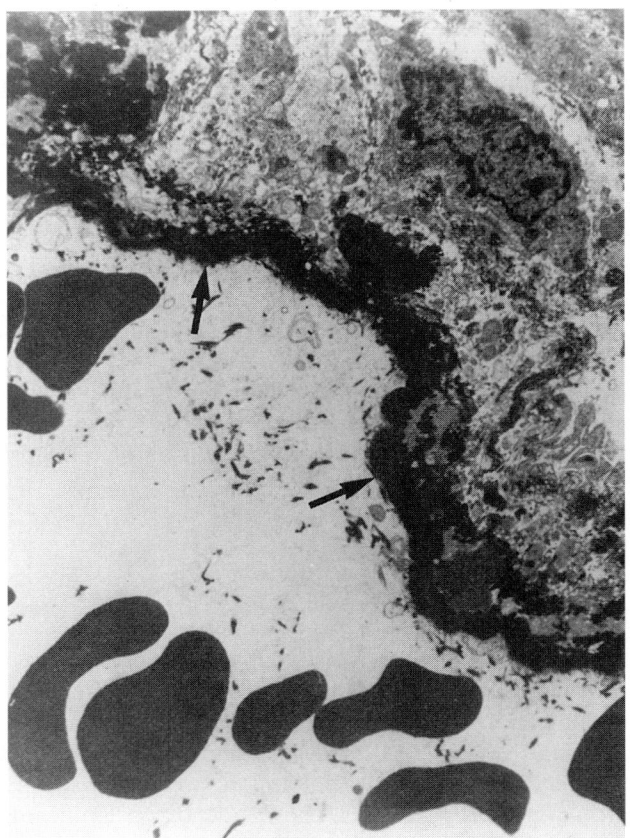

Figure 28–1. Compacted heavy fibrin deposition (*arrows*) and loose lamina fibrin replacing extensively eroded endothelium, nonplacental site region, uterine boundary zone, preeclampsia. (Original electron microscopic magnification, × 2,500). (From Shanklin DR, Sibai BM: Ultrastructural aspects of preeclampsia. I. Placental bed and uterine boundary vessels. Am J Obstet Gynecol 161:735, 1989, with permission.)

with enlargement of endothelial nuclei resulting in reduction of the lumen. In some cases, the erosion was complete with associated deposition of heavy fibrin (Fig. 28–1). In addition, there was no correlation between the type or degree of endothelial damage and the level of maternal hypertension.

Hemostatic Changes

Preeclampsia is associated with vasospasm, activation of the coagulation system, and abnormal hemostasis. There is good evidence from several studies that preeclampsia is accompanied by endothelial injury, increased platelet activation with platelet consumption in the microvasculature, and excessive clotting activity.[28,29] Saleh et al.[28] evaluated the hemostatic system before and 24 to 48 hours after delivery in 26 control pregnancies, 15 with mild preeclampsia and 18 with severe preeclampsia. They found that preeclampsia was associated with high fibronectin, low antithrombin III, and low α_2-antiplasmin levels, reflecting endothelial injury (high fibronectin), clotting (low antithrombin III), and fibrinolysis (low α_2-antiplasmin). In addition, they noted that, after delivery, fibronectin levels decreased in the preeclamptic group, while α_2-antiplasmin levels increased in all groups. They concluded that "vascular endothelial injury plays a central role in the hemostatic changes associated with preeclampsia." In a subsequent report,[29] the authors evaluated hemostasis in various hypertensive disorders of pregnancies. They found elevated fibronectin, low antithrombin III, and reduced α_2-antiplasmin in patients with pure preeclampsia as well as chronic hypertension with superimposed preeclampsia. In addition, they observed that fibronectin levels had better correlation with preeclampsia than either antithrombin III or α_2-antiplasmin. They suggested that fibronectin might be useful for diagnosing superimposed preeclampsia in women with chronic hypertension.

In recent reports, elevated fibronectin values were identified in some patients prior to the development of preeclampsia.[30,31] Taylor and colleagues[30] measured cellular fibronectin levels in plasma of women who ultimately had preeclampsia, hypertension only, or normotensive pregnancies. They found elevated cellular fibronectin levels during the second and third trimesters only in women destined to develop preeclampsia. Halligan et al. reported that increased fibronectin levels are evident as early as 9 weeks' gestation in women who ultimately develop preeclampsia.[31] Platelet consumption is a late finding in preeclampsia, but increased platelet turnover may be an early marker of preeclampsia. A mean platelet volume greater than or equal to 11 Fl at 28 weeks' gestation was found to be associated with subsequent preeclampsia by some authors.[32]

The enzyme thrombin converts fibrinogen to fibrin and is inactivated by antithrombin III, resulting in generation of thrombin–antithrombin III complexes. An increased level of these complexes suggests enhancement of thrombin generation. DeBoer et al.[33] investigated plasma levels of the coagulation inhibitors antithrombin III, protein C, protein S, and thrombin–antithrombin III complexes. They observed reduced protein C levels, but normal protein S levels, in preeclampsia compared with normotensive pregnancies. In addition, they observed an increased thrombin–antithrombin III complex level in the preeclamptic group. The level of these complexes correlated with platelet count and antithrombin III levels. Thus, they suggested that enhanced thrombin generation in preeclampsia may result from increased platelet activation and consumption. Gilabert et al.[34] evaluated protein C, protein S, and antithrombin III in normal pregnancy and severe preeclamptic states. They found reduced protein C and antithrombin III levels, but normal protein S in severe preeclampsia.

Changes In Prostanoids

Several investigators have described the various prostaglandins and their metabolites throughout pregnancy. They have measured the concentrations of these substances in plasma, serum, amniotic fluid, placental tissues, urine, or cord blood. The data have been inconsistent, reflecting differences in methodology.

During pregnancy, prostanoid production increases in both maternal and fetoplacental tissues.[35] Prostacyclin is produced by the vascular endothelium as well as in the renal cortex. It is a potent vasodilator and inhibitor of platelet aggregation. Thromboxane A_2 (TXA_2) is produced by the platelets and trophoblasts. It is a potent vasoconstrictor and platelet aggregator. Hence, these eicosanoids have opposite effects and play a major role in regulating vascular tone and vascular blood flow (Fig. 28–2).

Changes in prostaglandin production and/or catabolism in uteroplacental and umbilical tissues have been reportedly associated with the development of preeclampsia, although the reports have been inconsistent.[36-38] These discrepancies may reflect some of the inherent problems in the measurement of prostaglandins and the diagnosis of preeclampsia. An imbalance in prostanoid production or catabolism has been suggested as responsible for the pathophysiologic changes in preeclampsia.[35] However, the role of prostaglandins in the etiology of preeclampsia remains unclear.[38]

Recently, Mills and associates[38] investigated the excretion of urinary metabolites of prostaglandin I_2 (PGI_2) and TXA_2 as measured prospectively before 22 weeks', between 26 and 29 weeks', and at 36 weeks' gestation among 134 women who ultimately developed preeclampsia and 134 matched women who remained normotensive. The authors found that reduced PGI_2 production, but no increase in TXA_2 production, occurs as early as 13 to 16 weeks in women who ultimately developed preeclampsia. In addition, the ratio of TXA_2 metabolite to PGI_2 metabolite was 24 percent higher throughout pregnancy in preeclamptic women.[38]

Changes in Endothelium-Derived Factors

Recent data indicate that endothelium-derived substances such as endothelium-derived relaxing factor (EDRF) and endothelin may play a central role in the pathophysiology of preeclampsia.[39] After its discovery, EDRF was found to be nitric oxide, an extremely potent vasodilator. In contrast, endothelin is an extremely potent vasoconstrictor. Pinto and associates[40] reported a significant reduction in EDRF release from the endothelium of human umbilical blood vessels collected from patients with pregnancy-induced hypertension (PIH). In addition, Fickling et al.[41] found higher concentrations of an endogenous inhibitor of nitric oxide

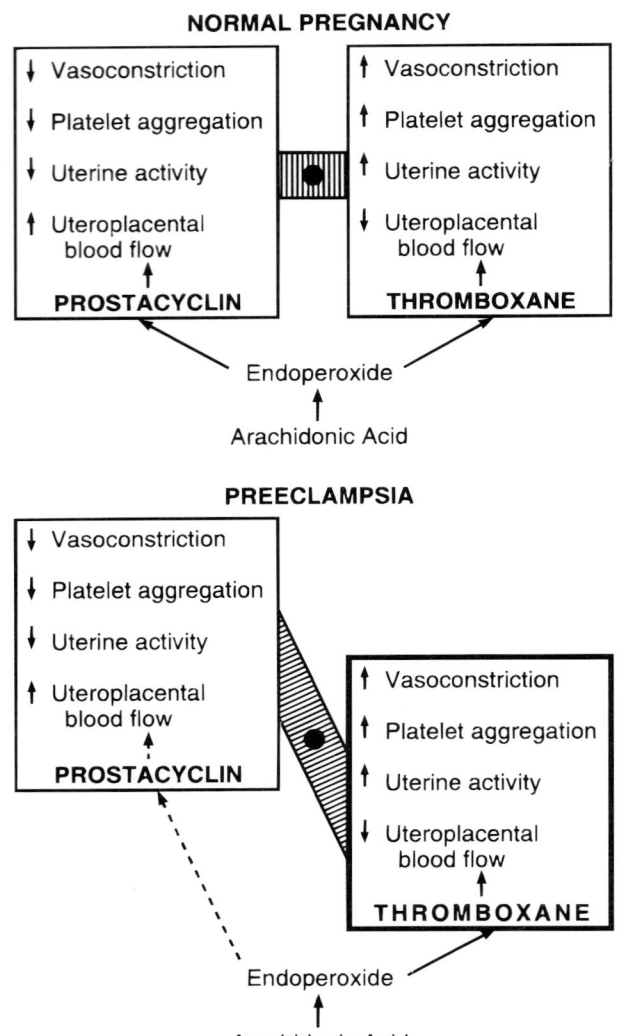

NORMAL PREGNANCY

↓ Vasoconstriction		↑ Vasoconstriction
↓ Platelet aggregation		↑ Platelet aggregation
↓ Uterine activity	●	↑ Uterine activity
↑ Uteroplacental blood flow		↓ Uteroplacental blood flow
PROSTACYCLIN		**THROMBOXANE**

Endoperoxide

Arachidonic Acid

PREECLAMPSIA

Figure 28–2. Comparison of the balance in the biologic actions of prostacyclin and thromboxane in normal pregnancy with the imbalance of increased thromboxane and decreased prostacyclin in preeclamptic pregnancy. The heavy type and box for thromboxane suggest an exacerbation of its actions in preeclampsia, whereas the lighter type and box for prostacyclin suggest a diminution of its actions. (From Walsh SW: Preeclampsia: an imbalance in placenta prostacyclin and thromboxane production. Am J Obstet Gynecol 152: 335, 1985, with permission.)

synthesis in eight third-trimester patients with preeclampsia than in nine patients with PIH and 10 women with normotensive pregnancies. Recently, numerous studies described the role of nitric oxide metabolism in the pathogenesis of preeclampsia. These findings were the subject of two reviews by Seligman et al.[42] and Baylis et al.[43] There are several reports describing plasma levels of endothelin in patients with preeclampsia. While the majority of these studies report elevated levels in preeclamptic pregnancies compared with normotensive pregnancies,[44-46] a recent study did not find higher levels of endothelin in patients with preeclamp-

sia.[47] These data suggest that levels are increased only in women with severe disease.[37]

Lipid Peroxide, Free Radicals, and Antioxidants

Evidence is accumulating that lipid peroxides and free radicals may be important in the pathogenesis of preeclampsia.[48-51] Superoxide ions may be cytotoxic to the cell by changing the characteristics of cellular membrane and producing membrane lipid peroxidation. Elevated plasma concentrations of free radical oxidation products precede the development of preeclampsia.[52] Uotila et al.[53] demonstrated that lipid peroxidation was significantly higher in 56 women with hypertension in pregnancy than in control subjects. Lipid peroxidation products had a high correlation with the level of hypertension but failed to show a significant relation to perinatal outcome. In contrast, high levels of plasma and platelet glutathione peroxidase, an antioxidant, were found to have an association with fetal growth restriction and asphyxia. In addition, several studies reported lower serum antioxidant activity in patients with preeclampsia than in normotensive pregnancies.[53-59]

Placental Peptide Hormones, Cytokines

Several investigators have studied changes in placental peptide or cytokines in maternal plasma in women with preeclampsia. These studies were the subject of two recent reviews.[21,60]

Genetic Factors in Preeclampsia

Because a family history of preeclampsia increases the risk of preeclampsia, numerous investigations during the past decade have evaluated a possible link between preeclampsia and specific genetic mutations or thrombophilia.[61-69] Some of the genetic mutations studied include a molecular variant of angiotensinogen (T_{235}), factor V Leiden mutation, which causes resistance to activated protein C, and mutations in methyltetrahydrofolate reductase, and the prothrombin gene, the presence of anticardiolipin antibodies, and inherited deficiencies in antithrombin III, protein S, and protein C. Unfortunately, the findings of these studies have been highly inconsistent.[61-69]

Diagnosis

Preeclampsia is a clinical syndrome that embraces a wide spectrum of signs and symptoms that have been clinically observed to develop alone or in combination. Elevated blood pressure is the traditional hallmark for diagnosis of the disease. However, recent evidence suggests that in some patients the disease may manifest itself in the form of either a capillary leak (edema, proteinuria) or a spectrum of abnormal hemostasis with multiple organ dysfunction. These latter patients usually present with clinical manifestations that are not typical of preeclampsia (i.e., hypertension is absent).

The diagnosis of preeclampsia and the severity of the disease process are generally based on maternal blood pressure measurements as ascertained by a variety of medical personnel who regularly measure blood pressure in prenatal clinics, local physicians' offices, and in-hospital units. There are many factors that may influence measurement of the blood pressure with a sphygmomanometer, including the accuracy of the equipment used, size of the cuff, duration of the rest period before recording, the posture of the patient, and the Korotkoff phase used (phase IV or phase V) for diastolic blood pressure measurement. Reports on effects of these factors on measurements of blood pressure have been summarized by Steer.[70] In these reports, the authors recommend that all blood pressure values be recorded with the woman in a sitting position for ambulatory patients or in a semireclining position for hospitalized patients. The right arm should be used consistently, with the arm being in a roughly horizontal position at heart level. For diastolic blood pressure measurements, both phases (muffling sound and disappearance sound) should be recorded. This is very important, since the level measured at phase IV is about 5 to 10 mm Hg higher than that measured at phase V.[71] Lopez et al.[71] compared Korotkoff phases IV and V in a cohort of 1,194 nulliparous pregnant women who were followed prospectively from the 20th week of pregnancy until delivery. Blood pressure measurements were obtained with random-zero sphygmomanometers and were recorded in supine, lateral, and seated positions. Lopez et al.[71] found that the prevalence of hypertension (diastolic blood pressure [BP] 90 mm Hg or higher occasions 6 hours apart) when phase IV was used was double the prevalence when phase V was used. However, phase IV had a better sensitivity in the prediction of complications associated with hypertension (proteinuria, hyperuricemia, and intrauterine growth restriction), but a lower specificity. In addition, the authors found that phase V was easy to obtain during pregnancy. Blank et al.[72] compared diastolic blood pressure values using Korotkoff phases IV and V in 58 pregnant women (42 hypertensive and 16 normotensive) at various stages of pregnancy. They concluded that phase V is a more accurate, reliable, and less variable measurement of diastolic blood pressure in pregnancy than muffling (phase IV). The literature in this area was recently reviewed by Johenning and Barron.[73]

A rise in blood pressure has been used by several authors as a criterion for the diagnosis of hypertension in pregnancy. This definition is usually unreliable, since a gradual increase in blood pressure from second to third trimester is seen in most normotensive pregnancies. MacGillivray et al.[74] reported that 73 percent of primigravid patients with normotensive pregnancies demonstrate a rise in diastolic blood pressure of more than 15 mm Hg at some stage during the course of their pregnancies. In a study of 16,211 singleton pregnancies, Redman and Jeffries[75] analyzed different cut-offs for diastolic blood pressure used in the diagnosis of preeclampsia. They found that an elevation in diastolic blood pressure of at least 25 mm Hg and a reading of at least 90 mm Hg were the best criteria. Similar findings were recently reported by Perry and Beevers.[76]

Villar and Sibai[77] prospectively studied blood pressure changes during the course of pregnancy in 700 young primigravidas. One hundred thirty-seven patients (19.6 percent) had preeclampsia. The pregnancy outcome according to blood pressure findings is summarized in Table 28–2. The sensitivity and positive predictive values for preeclampsia of a threshold increase in diastolic blood pressure of at least 15 mm Hg on two occasions were 39 and 32 percent, respectively. The respective values for a threshold increase in systolic pressures were 22 and 33 percent. Two recent studies, one from Australia and another from the United States, investigated pregnancy outcome in women with a rise in diastolic blood pressure of more than 15 mm Hg but an absolute diastolic level below 90 mm Hg as compared with gravidas who remained normotensive.[78,79] The Australian report[78] included women with elevated blood pressures without proteinuria, whereas the American investigation[79] included women with an increased diastolic pressure 15 mm Hg or more plus proteinuria ($\geq$ 300 mg/24 h). Both found that overall pregnancy outcomes were similar among women who remained

Table 28–2. PREGNANCY OUTCOME ACCORDING TO THRESHOLD INCREASE IN SYSTOLIC OR DIASTOLIC PRESSURES ON TWO OCCASIONS DURING THE THIRD TRIMESTER

Blood Pressure Criteria	Normotensive No. (%)	Preeclampsia No. (%)
Increase in diastolic $\geq$ 15 mm Hg	113 (68)	53 (32)
Increase in systolic $\geq$ 30 mm Hg	60 (67)	30 (33)
Threshold increase in both	32 (58)	23 (42)

Adapted from Villar MA, Sibai BM: Clinical significance of elevated mean arterial blood in second trimester and threshold increase in systolic or diastolic pressure during third trimester. Am J Obstet Gynecol 60:419, 1989.

normotensive and those who demonstrated a rise in diastolic pressure of 15 mm Hg or higher but did not reach 90 mm Hg.[78,79] The use of an increase in blood pressure as a diagnostic criterion is dependent on at least two observations during the course of pregnancy that will be influenced by at least three factors: gestational age at time of first observation, frequency of blood pressure measurements, and the two observations to be selected. Thus, these criteria are inadequate to diagnose preeclampsia as such. However, they may be useful if used in association with the presence of proteinuria, or other associated symptoms of preeclampsia such as a persistent headache, visual symptoms, or epigastric pain. It should be emphasized that the presence of these symptoms is more important than the absolute level of blood pressure in establishing the diagnosis of preeclampsia. Indeed, there is more to preeclampsia than the presence of hypertension.[80]

The diagnosis of preeclampsia requires the presence of an elevated blood pressure with proteinuria. Poor perinatal outcome is usually seen in patients who have hypertension plus proteinuria.[3,81] The presence of proteinuria is usually determined by the use of either dipstick or protein/creatinine ratio in random urine samples. The concentration of urinary protein is highly variable.[82] It is influenced by several factors, including contamination, urine-specific gravity, pH, exercise, and posture.[83] In addition, urinary protein/creatinine excretion is highly variable in patients with preeclampsia.[84,85] Moreover, recent studies found that urinary dipstick determinations correlate poorly with the amount of proteinuria found in 24-hour urine determinations.[86-89] Therefore, the definitive test for diagnosing proteinuria should be quantitative measurement of total protein excretion over a 24-hour period. The diagnosis of severe preeclampsia requires that proteinuria of more than 5 g/24 h be documented. Using urine dipstick measurements ($\geq$3+) is not adequate (Table 28–3).[87]

Prediction of Preeclampsia

A review of the world literature reveals that more than 100 clinical, biophysical, and biochemical tests have been recommended to predict or identify the patient at risk for the future development of the disease[60,90,91] (see

Clinical Tests Used to Predict Preeclampsia
Average mean arterial pressure (MAP) in the second trimester $\geq$85–90 mm Hg
MAP at 20 weeks $\geq$90 mm Hg
Rollover test at 28–32 weeks
Isometric exercise test
Angiotensin infusion test at 26–30 weeks
Doppler velocimetry of uterine and umbilical vessels at 18–26 weeks

the box "Clinical Tests Used to Predict Preeclampsia"). The results of the pooled data for the various tests and the lack of agreement between serial tests suggest that none of these clinical tests is sufficiently reliable for use as a screening test in clinical practice.[90,91] We do not use any of them for screening purposes.

There are reports describing the predictive value of a variety of substances measured in maternal plasma, serum, or urine, including cations, hormones, prostaglandins, metabolites, various parameters of coagulation and hemostasis, and uric acid.[60,90,91] These studies differ in their methodologies and have included a heterogeneous group of patients with all forms of hypertension, parity, and gestational ages at time of sampling. Comparison and evaluation is, therefore, limited, which explains the wide scatter of results and lack of agreement among these findings.

Prevention of Preeclampsia

There are numerous reports and clinical trials describing the use of various methods to prevent or reduce the incidence of preeclampsia. Since the etiology of the disease is unknown, these methods were used in an attempt to correct theoretical abnormalities in preeclampsia. Some of the methods used are summarized in the box "Methods Used to Prevent Preeclampsia."[92] No efficacy of high-protein or low-salt diets has ever been documented.

Table 28–3. VALUE OF DIPSTICK PROTEIN IN PREDICTING 24–HOUR URINARY PROTEIN EXCRETION

Urinary Dipstick	Protein Excretion (mg/24 h)	Sensitivity (%)	Specificity (%)	Positive Predictive Value (%)	Negative Predictive Value (%)
$\geq$1+	$\geq$300	67	74	92	34
$\geq$3+	$\geq$500	75	81	36	96

Methods Used to Prevent Preeclampsia

High-protein and low-salt diet
Nutritional supplementation (protein)
Calcium
Magnesium
Zinc
Fish and evening primrose oil
Antihypertensive drugs including diuretics
Antithrombotic agents
Low-dose aspirin
Dipyridamole
Heparin
Vitamins E and C

Calcium Supplementation

The relationship between dietary calcium intake and hypertension has been the subject of several experimental and observational studies.[93] Several authors reported reduced urinary excretion of calcium at the time of preeclampsia, as well as several weeks prior to the onset of PIH or preeclampsia.[94-96]

Epidemiologic studies have documented an inverse association between calcium intake and maternal blood pressure and the incidences of preeclampsia and eclampsia. These findings were recently reviewed by Belizan and associates.[97] The BP-lowering effect of calcium was thought to be mediated by alterations in plasma renin activity and parathyroid hormone. In addition, calcium supplementation during pregnancy was shown to reduce vascular sensitivity to angiotensin II.[98]

There are nine clinical studies comparing the use of calcium versus no treatment or a placebo in preg-

nancy.[98-107] These trials differ in the populations studied (low-risk or high-risk for hypertensive disorders of pregnancy), study design (randomization, double-blind, or use of a placebo), gestational age at enrollment (20 to 32 weeks' gestation), sample size in each group (range, 22 to 588), dose of elemental calcium used (156 to 2,000 mg/day), and the definition of hypertensive disorders of pregnancy used.

Eight of the studies were randomized and placebo-controlled.[94-106] The dose of elemental calcium used was 600 to 2,000 mg/day. Five of these trials studied healthy pregnant women (low risk), and the other three studied pregnant women who had either a positive rollover test or both a positive rollover test and increased sensitivity to angiotensin II infusion.[98] Results of the nine studies are summarized in Table 28–4.

The largest of these trials is the National Institute of Child Health and Human Development (NICHD) trial in healthy nulliparous women reported by Levine and associates.[104] This trial revealed no beneficial effects from calcium supplementation on the rates of preeclampsia and preterm delivery. In contrast, a recent Australian multicenter trial in nulliparous women revealed beneficial effects.[106] In summary, calcium supplementation may be beneficial in a select group of women considered at extremely high risk for preeclampsia.

Magnesium Supplementation

Serum magnesium levels are usually lower in pregnancy and rapidly return to prepregnancy concentrations after delivery. The relationship between dietary magnesium deficiency and hypertension has been the subject of several experimental and observational studies.[108] Dietary magnesium deficiency during pregnancy has been implicated in the pathogenesis of preeclampsia, fetal growth restriction, and preterm delivery.[109,110] In patients with

Table 28–4. RANDOMIZED TRIALS OF CALCIUM SUPPLEMENTATION TO PREVENT PREECLAMPSIA

Study	Enrollment GA (wk)	No. of Patients Calcium	No. of Patients Placebo	Preeclampsia (%) Calcium	Preeclampsia (%) Placebo
Lopez-Jaramillo et al.[99]*	124	55	51	3.6	23.5
Lopez-Jaramillo et al.[102]†	24–32	22	34	0.0	23.5
Villar and Repke[100]*	24	90	88	0.0	3.4
Belizan et al.[101]*	20	579	588	2.6	3.9
Sanchez-Ramos et al.[98]†	24–28	29	34	13.8	44.1
Levine et al.[104]*	13–21	2,296	2,294	6.9	7.3
Lopez-Jaramillo et al.[103]*	20	125	135	3.2	15.5
Hererra et al.[105]†	28–32	43	43	9.4	37.2
Crowther et al.[106]*	13–24	227	224	4.4	10.0
Rogers et al.[107]	22–32	144	75	5.6	9.3

* Nulliparas.
† Positive rollover test or angiotensin II.

preeclampsia, magnesium levels were reported to be lower or similar to those in normotensive pregnancies. Since parenteral magnesium sulfate is the drug of choice in the treatment of preeclampsia, some authors have suggested an etiologic relationship between magnesium deficiency and preeclampsia.[109,110]

In a retrospective study, Conradt et al.[110] compared pregnancy outcomes in 4,023 low-risk pregnancies with those in 882 high-risk pregnancies. The high-risk group was treated with β-sympathomimetic agents in combination with various doses of magnesium aspartate hydrochloride. Preeclampsia was not observed in the high-risk treated group, while the incidence was 2 percent in the control group. In addition, the incidence of fetal growth restriction was significantly reduced in the treated group. The authors concluded that routine supplementation with magnesium during pregnancy prevents preeclampsia and fetal growth restriction.

Spatling and Spatling[111] reported a double-blind study involving 568 women who were randomized to receive either 14 mmol magnesium aspartate hydrochloride ($n = 278$) or aspartic acid as a placebo ($n = 290$). The supplementation was given daily starting at or before 16 weeks' gestation and was continued throughout pregnancy. The rates of preeclampsia were similar in the two groups; however, the magnesium-supplemented group had a lower incidence of both preterm delivery and the number of newborns admitted to the intensive care unit.

Sibai et al.[108] studied 400 young primigravidas who were enrolled at 13 to 24 weeks' gestation to receive either 365 mg of elemental magnesium as magnesium aspartate hydrochloride or an aspartic acid placebo. The magnesium-supplemented group had significantly higher serum magnesium levels. However, there were no significant differences between the two groups regarding the rates of preeclampsia, fetal growth restriction, or preterm delivery. In addition, magnesium supplementation did not influence systolic or diastolic blood pressure during the course of pregnancy.

Zinc Supplementation

Dietary zinc deficiency has been associated with poor pregnancy outcome. In addition, reduced plasma zinc levels as well as lowered placental zinc levels have been reported in pregnancies complicated by preeclampsia.[112] Hunt et al.[113] studied the effects of zinc supplementation on the outcomes of pregnancy in 213 low-income Mexican women. The patients were randomly allocated in a double-blind fashion to receive either a placebo or capsules containing 20 mg zinc per day. The incidence of pregnancy-induced hypertension was significantly reduced in the zinc-supplemented group (2 vs. 16 per-

cent). There were no other differences in pregnancy outcome between the two groups.

Mohamed and associates[114] studied pregnancy outcome in 494 women who were enrolled in a zinc supplementation trial; 246 patients were given 20 mg zinc daily, while 248 received a placebo. They found no differences between the two groups regarding weight gain, blood pressure, or the incidence of preeclampsia (4.6 percent in the zinc group vs. 1.3 percent in the control group). In addition, they found no differences regarding neonatal birth weight, fetal growth restriction, or the incidence of preterm delivery.

At the present time, there are inadequate data to prove a strong association between the prevention of preeclampsia and any nutritional supplementation. For this reason, routine supplementation with these nutrients is not recommended.

Antithrombic Agents

Preeclampsia is associated with vasospasm and activation of the coagulation-hemostasis systems. Enhanced platelet activation plays a central role in the above process with resultant abnormality in the thromboxane/prostacyclin balance. Hence, several authors have used pharmacologic manipulation to alter the above ratio in an attempt to prevent or ameliorate the course of preeclampsia.

Aspirin inhibits the synthesis of prostaglandins by irreversibly acetylating and inactivating cyclooxygenase. In vitro, platelet cyclooxygenase is more sensitive to inhibition by low doses of aspirin (<80 mg) than vascular endothelial cyclooxygenase. Therefore, treatment with low-dose aspirin could alter the balance between prostacyclin and thromboxane.[115] This biochemical selectivity of low-dose aspirin appears to be related to its unusual kinetics that result in presystemic acetylation of platelets exposed to higher concentrations of aspirin in the portal circulation. Sibai et al.[116] found that effective inhibition of thromboxane generation by platelets, 98 percent decrease from baseline, can be achieved after 1 week of therapy with 80 mg of daily aspirin during pregnancy. In addition, they observed that a 60-mg dose resulted in a 60 percent decrease in platelet thromboxane generation after 1 week and a 97 percent decrease after 2 weeks of therapy.

Several studies have described the effects of low-dose aspirin (60 to 81 mg/day) on angiotensin II sensitivity during pregnancy.[117] These data suggest that enhanced vascular responsiveness to angiotensin II infusions may be mediated by an imbalance in thromboxane/PGI_2 production that may be corrected in some women by the use of low-dose aspirin. In addition, several prospective studies suggest that the administration of aspirin in women at high risk for preeclampsia might

Table 28–5. RANDOMIZED TRIALS OF LOW-DOSE ASPIRIN TO PREVENT PREECLAMPSIA

Series	Risk Factors	Enrollment GA (wk)	No. of Patients		Preeclampsia (%)	
			Aspirin	Placebo	Aspirin	Placebo
Hauth et al.[118]	Nulliparas	24	302	302	1.7	5.6*
Sibai et al.[9]	Nulliparas	13–26	1,485	1,500	4.6	6.3
Italian study[119]†	Obstetric Hx	16–32	565	477*	2.9	2.7
CLASP[120]	Obstetric Hx	12–32	4,659	4,650	6.7	7.6
ECPPA[121]	Obstetric Hx	12–32	476	494	6.7	6.1
JAMAICA[122]	Nulliparas	12–32	3,022	3,024	7.1	6.3
Caritis et al.[123]	High-risk	13–26	1,254	1,249	18.4	20.3
BLASP[124]	None	12–32	1,819	1,822	2.2	2.5

* $p = 0.009$.
† No treatment.

reduce the incidence of hypertensive disorders of pregnancy, fetal growth restriction, and preterm delivery. These studies included a limited number of patients who were identified to be at high risk for preeclampsia on the basis of a poor obstetric history, chronic hypertension, positive rollover test, increased sensitivity to angiotensin II infusions, or abnormal Doppler studies of the uterine vessels. In general, these studies[117] suggested that low-dose aspirin was highly effective in the prevention of preeclampsia and fetal growth restriction in women considered at risk for these complications.

Recently, several multicenter, randomized, prospective trials have been reported from centers around the world. Some of these studies were conducted in healthy nulliparous women,[91] whereas others included patients with a variety of obstetric and medical complications.[9,118–124] In general, about 75 percent of all preeclampsia occurs in nulliparous women. Therefore, prevention of preeclampsia in these women has major clinical implications. There are four randomized, placebo-controlled trials describing the use of 60 mg/day of aspirin in healthy nulliparous women (Table 28–5). The results reveal no reduction in the rates of preeclampsia with low-dose aspirin. In addition, four trials included women at risk for preeclampsia, but none revealed a reduction in rates of preeclampsia. The largest of these trials was conducted by the NICHD Maternal-Fetal Network Units in women with pregestational diabetes, chronic hypertension, previous preeclampsia-eclampsia, and multifetal gestation. Reduction of preeclampsia was not achieved in any of the groups studied (Table 28–6).[123]

In summary, the use of low-dose aspirin in healthy nulliparous women does not improve pregnancy outcome even when the rate of preeclampsia is reduced. The role of low-dose aspirin in women at high risk for preeclampsia—particularly those with previous severe preeclampsia before 28 weeks and those with marked abnormalities in uterine Doppler studies at both 18 to 20 weeks' and 24 weeks' gestation—remains controversial.[125–127]

Fish Oil

Researchers have evaluated the effects of N-3 fatty acid supplementation during pregnancy on the rates of preeclampsia in high-risk women.[92] Overall, no reduction in the rate of preeclampsia was observed with N-3 fatty acid supplementation in a recent randomized trial.[128]

One recent study has suggested a beneficial effect from pharmacologic doses of vitamins E and C in women identified at-risk for preeclampsia by means of abnormal uterine Doppler flow velocimetry.[59] However,

Table 28–6. LOW-DOSE ASPIRIN IN HIGH-RISK WOMEN: NICHD TRIAL

Entry Criteria	Number of Women	Preeclampsia (%)	
		Aspirin*	Placebo*
Normotensive and no proteinuria	1,613	14.5	17.7
Proteinuria and hypertension	119	31.7	22.0
Proteinuria only	48	25.0	33.3
Hypertension only	723	24.8	25.0
Insulin-dependent diabetes	462	18.3	21.6
Chronic hypertension	763	26.0	24.6
Multifetal gestation	678	11.5	15.9
Previous preeclampsia	600	16.7	19.0

* No difference for any of the groups.
Data from Caritis SN, Sibai BM, Hauth J, et al, for the National Institute of Child Health and Human Development: Low-dose aspirin therapy to prevent preeclampsia in women at high risk. N Engl J Med 338:701, 1998.

the study had limited sample size and must be confirmed in other populations.

Finally, it is important to emphasize that most of the positive trials found a benefit in the prevention of a "definition of preeclampsia," but not in pregnancy outcome.

Laboratory Abnormalities in Preeclampsia

Women with preeclampsia may exhibit a symptom complex ranging from minimal blood pressure elevation to derangements of multiple organ systems. The renal, hematologic, and hepatic systems are most likely to be involved.

Renal Function

Renal plasma flow and glomerular filtration rate (GFR) increase during normal pregnancy. These changes are responsible for a fall in serum creatinine, urea, and uric acid concentrations. In preeclampsia, vasospasm and glomerular capillary endothelial swelling (glomerular endotheliosis) lead to an average reduction in GFR of 25 percent below the rate for normal pregnancy.[129] Serum creatinine is rarely elevated in preeclampsia, but uric acid is commonly increased.[130] In a study of 200 women with mild preeclampsia remote from term, Sibai et al.[130] found the mean serum creatinine to be 0.80 mg/dl, mean uric acid 6.1 mg/dl, and mean creatinine clearance 112 ml/min. In a subsequent study of 95 women with severe preeclampsia, Sibai and associates[131] reported a mean serum creatinine of 0.91 mg/dl, a mean uric acid of 6.6 mg/dl, and a mean creatinine clearance of 100 ml/min.

The clinical significance of elevated uric acid levels in preeclampsia/eclampsia has been confusing. In a study of 332 women with preexisting hypertension, plasma urate levels were found to be a better indicator of fetal prognosis than blood pressure. Uric acid levels above 5 mg/dl were associated with poor perinatal outcome.[132] However, in a comparison of 69 eclamptic women who had uric acid levels of less than 6.0 mg/dl with those who had values above 10.0 mg/dl, Pritchard and Stone[133] found no significant difference between the two groups in blood pressure, perinatal outcome, or the incidence of hypertension in subsequent pregnancies.

Hepatic Function

The liver is not primarily involved in preeclampsia, and hepatic involvement is observed in only 10 percent of women with severe preeclampsia.[134] Fibrinogen deposition has been found along the walls of hepatic sinu-soids in preeclamptic patients with no laboratory or histologic evidence of liver involvement.[135] When liver dysfunction does occur in preeclampsia, mild elevation of serum transaminase is most common.[136] Bilirubin is rarely increased in preeclampsia but, when elevated, the indirect fraction predominates. Elevated liver enzymes are part of the syndrome of hemolysis, elevated liver enzymes, and low platelets (HELLP), a variant of severe preeclampsia.

Hematologic Changes

Many studies have evaluated the hematologic abnormalities in women with preeclampsia.[137,138] Plasma fibrinopeptide-A, D-dimer levels, and circulating thrombin–antithrombin complexes are higher in women with preeclampsia than in normotensive gravidas. In contrast, plasma antithrombin III activity is decreased. These findings indicate enhanced thrombin generation.[137,138]

Plasma fibrinogen rises progressively during normal pregnancy. When a group of 50 severe preeclamptic women were compared with 50 normotensive women matched by gestational age, no differences in mean plasma fibrinogen levels were found between the two groups.[139] In general, plasma fibrinogen levels are rarely reduced in women with preeclampsia in the absence of abruptio placentae.

Thrombocytopenia is the most common hematologic abnormality in women with preeclampsia. Its incidence will depend on the severity of the disease process, definition, and the presence or absence of abruptio placentae. A platelet count of less than 150,000/mm³ was reported in 32 to 50 percent of women with severe preeclampsia.[139,140] In a study of 1,414 women with hypertension during pregnancy, Burrows and Kelton[141] found a platelet count of less than 150,000/mm³ in 15 percent.

Leduc and associates[140] studied the coagulation profile (platelet count, fibrinogen, prothrombin time, and partial thromboplastin time) in 100 consecutive women with severe preeclampsia. A platelet count less than 150,000/mm³ was found in 50 percent and a count of less than 100,000/mm³ in 36 percent of the women. Thirteen women had a fibrinogen level of less than 300 mg/dl, and two had prolonged prothrombin and partial thromboplastin times, as well as thrombocytopenia on admission. They found the admission platelet count to be an excellent predictor of subsequent thrombocytopenia, and concluded that fibrinogen levels, prothrombin time, and partial thromboplastin time should be obtained only in women with a platelet count of less than 100,000/mm³. A recent study by Barron et al. reported similar results in over 800 women with hypertension in pregnancy.[142]

The HELLP Syndrome

Recent reports have described the HELLP syndrome in severe preeclampsia. There is considerable debate regarding the definition, diagnosis, incidence, etiology, and management of this syndrome.[143] Patients with such findings were previously described by many investigators. Goodlin[144] labeled this syndrome "EPH gestosis type B"; he claimed that this clinical presentation had been reported in the obstetric literature a century earlier. Weinstein[134] considered it a unique variant of preeclampsia and coined the term "HELLP syndrome" for this entity, while MacKenna and colleagues[145] considered it to be misdiagnosed preeclampsia.

A review of the literature highlights the differences regarding the degree of abnormal laboratory findings and the criteria used to diagnose HELLP syndrome. Thrombocytopenia, a platelet count less than 100,000/mm³, has been the most consistent finding among the various reports. However, some investigators have included only those values determined before delivery, while others have reported platelet counts obtained both antepartum and postpartum. In addition, there are considerable differences regarding what constitutes an abnormal level of serum glutamic-oxaloacetic transaminase (SGOT) or bilirubin. Several reports have not even included these data.[146] Barton and associates[147] performed liver biopsies in patients with preeclampsia and HELLP syndrome. Periportal necrosis and hemorrhage were the most common histopathologic findings. In addition, they found that the extent of the laboratory abnormalities in HELLP syndrome including the platelet count and liver enzymes did not correlate with hepatic histopathologic findings.

Based on a retrospective review of 302 cases of HELLP syndrome, Martin et al.[148] devised the following classification based on platelet count nadir. Class I HELLP syndrome was defined as a platelet nadir below 50,000/mm³, class 2 platelet nadirs between 50,000 and 100,000/mm³, and class 3 a platelet nadir between 100,000 and 150,000/mm³. These classes have been used to predict the rapidity of recovery postpartum, maternal–perinatal outcome, and the need for plasmapheresis.[149] Miles et al.[150] reported a strong association between the presence of HELLP syndrome and eclampsia. In that study, the HELLP syndrome was present in 30 percent of patients with postpartum eclampsia and in 28 percent of patients having eclampsia prior to delivery.

Hemolysis, defined as the presence of microangiopathic hemolytic anemia, is the hallmark of the HELLP syndrome. The role of disseminated intravascular coagulation (DIC) in preeclampsia is controversial. Most authors do not regard HELLP syndrome to be a variant of DIC, since coagulation parameters such as pro-

thrombin time, partial thromboplastin time, and serum fibrinogen are normal. However, the diagnosis of DIC in clinical practice is difficult. When sensitive determinants of this condition are used such as antithrombin III, fibrinopeptide-A, fibrin monomer, D-dimer, α_2-antiplasmin, plasminogen, prekallikrein, and fibronectin, many patients have laboratory values consistent with DIC.[151,152] Unfortunately, these tests are time consuming and not suitable for routine monitoring. Consequently, less sensitive parameters are often used in clinical practice. Sibai et al.[143] defined DIC as the presence of thrombocytopenia, low fibrinogen levels (plasma fibrinogen <300 mg/dl), and fibrin split products above 40 mg/ml. These authors observed DIC in 38 percent of the 112 patients with HELLP syndrome. In a subsequent report, Sibai et al.[153] noted the present of DIC in 21 percent of 442 patients with HELLP syndrome. They also found that the majority of cases occurred in women who had antecedent abruptio placentae or peripartum hemorrhage and in all four women who had subcapsular liver hematomas. In the absence of these complications, the frequency of DIC was only 5 percent.[153] Aarnoudse et al.[154] diagnosed DIC in HELLP syndrome by light microscopic and immunofluorescence findings in tissue biopsies and laboratory findings of thrombocytopenia, elevated fibrinogen degradation products, reduced antithrombin III levels, and fragmented red blood cells.

In view of the above diagnostic problems, Sibai[146] recommended that uniform and standardized laboratory values be used to diagnose this syndrome. He suggested that low-density lipoprotein and bilirubin values be included in the diagnosis of hemolysis. In addition, the degree of abnormality of liver enzymes should be defined as a certain number of standard deviations from the normal value for each hospital population. Furthermore, the rate of change in either liver enzymes or platelet count may be as important as the absolute value in establishing the diagnosis. Our laboratory criteria to establish the diagnosis are presented in the box "Criteria to Establish the Diagnosis of HELLP Syndrome."

The reported incidence of HELLP syndrome in preeclampsia has ranged from 2 to 12 percent,[146] reflecting the differences in diagnostic criteria used. The syndrome appears to be most common in Caucasian patients. The incidence of HELLP syndrome is also higher in preeclamptic patients who have been managed conservatively.

The patient is usually seen remote from term complaining of epigastric or right upper quadrant pain (65 percent), some will have nausea or vomiting (50 percent), and others will have nonspecific viral syndrome-like symptoms. The majority of patients (90 percent) will give a history of malaise for the past few days

---

Criteria to Establish the Diagnosis of HELLP Syndrome

Hemolysis
    Abnormal peripheral blood smear
    Increased bilirubin <1.2 mg/dl
    Increased lactic dehydrogenase >600 IU/L
Elevated liver enzymes
    Increased SGOT ≥72 IU/L
    Increased lactic dehydrogenase >600 IU/L
Thrombocytopenia
    Platelet count <100,000/mm³

---

before presentation; some may present with hematuria or gastrointestinal bleeding. Hypertension and proteinuria may be absent or slightly abnormal.[153-155] Physical examination will demonstrate right upper quadrant tenderness and significant weight gain with edema.

It is important to remember that severe hypertension is not a constant or even a frequent finding in HELLP syndrome. Although 66 percent of the 112 patients studied by Sibai and associates[143] had a diastolic blood pressure of at least 110 mm Hg, 14.5 percent had a diastolic blood pressure of leas than 90 mm Hg. Aarnoudse and colleagues[154] described six women presenting with severe epigastric pain in the third trimester who had significantly elevated liver enzymes, low platelets, and evidence of hemolysis. None of these patients had a blood pressure higher than 140/90 mm Hg pro-

teinuria. As a result, they are often misdiagnosed as having various medical and surgical disorders (see the box "Medical and Surgical Disorders Confused with the HELLP Syndrome"). Occasionally the presence of this syndrome is associated with hypoglycemia leading to coma, severe hyponatremia, and cortical blindness. A rare but interesting complication of HELLP syndrome is transient nephrogenic diabetes insipidus. Unlike central diabetes insipidus, which occurs due to the diminished or absent secretion of arginine vasopressin by the hypothalamus, transient nephrogenic diabetes insipidus is characterized by a resistance to arginine vasopressin mediated by excessive vasopressinase. It is postulated that elevated circulating vasopressinase may result from impaired hepatic metabolism of the enzyme.

It is important to emphasize that these patients may have a variety of unusual signs and symptoms, none of which are diagnostic of severe preeclampsia. Pregnant women with probable preeclampsia presenting with atypical symptoms should have a complete blood count, a platelet count, and liver enzyme determinations irrespective of maternal blood pressure.[146]

Management of preeclamptic patients presenting with the HELLP syndrome is highly controversial.[146] Consequently, there are several therapeutic modalities described in the literature to treat or reverse the HELLP, syndrome. Most of these modalities are similar to those used in the management of severe preeclampsia remote from term (see the box "Therapeutic Modalities Used to Treat or Reverse HELLP Syndrome").[146]

Medical and Surgical Disorders Confused with the HELLP Syndrome

Acute fatty liver of pregnancy
Appendicitis
Diabetes mellitus
Gallbladder disease
Gastroenteritis
Glomerulonephritis
Hemolytic uremic syndrome
Hepatic encephalopathy
Hyperemesis gravidarum
Idiopathic thrombocytopenia
Kidney stones
Peptic ulcer
Pyelonephritis
Systemic lupus erythematosus
Thrombotic thrombocytopenic purpura
Viral hepatitis

Therapeutic Modalities Used to Treat or Reverse HELLP Syndrome

Plasma volume expansion
    Bed rest
    Crystalloids
    Albumin 5 to 25 percent
Antithrombotic agents
    Low-dose aspirin
    Dipyridamole
    Heparin
    Antithrombin III
    Prostacyclin infusions
Immunosuppressive agents
    Steroids
Miscellaneous
    Fresh frozen plasma infusions
    Exchange plasmapheresis
    Dialysis

From Sibai BM: The HELLP Syndrome (hemolysis, elevated liver enzymes, and low platelets): much ado about nothing? Am J Obstet Gynecol 162:311, 1990, with permission.

Goodlin[156] described five patients with features of HELLP syndrome who were treated conservatively with bed rest in an attempt to increase plasma volume. Three women also received intravenous infusions of 5 or 25 percent albumin. Goodlin felt that the efforts at plasma volume expansion were in part beneficial as measured by a fall in hemoglobin concentration, a rise in platelet count, and resolution of some of the symptoms of "severe toxemia." Thiagarajah et al.[157] treated five patients with prednisone or betamethasone and observed an improvement in platelet count and liver enzymes.

Heyborne[158] reported five cases where temporary reversal of the HELLP syndrome was achieved using low-dose aspirin (81 mg/day) and corticosteroids. The average prolongation of pregnancy was 4 weeks; however, three pregnancies beginning at 25 weeks or earlier were prolonged for an average of 5.5 weeks. No long-term maternal morbidity occurred, although one patient developed DIC and eclampsia. Critics of this study note that three patients had platelet counts above 100,000 mm³ at initial diagnosis, and hemolysis was not documented in three patients.

Clark and associates[159] reported three cases in which temporary reversal of the HELLP syndrome was achieved using bed rest and corticosteroids. Pregnancy was prolonged 4 to 10 days, and all patients had a live birth. It is important to note that two of the patients had a platelet count of more than 100,000/mm³, and one had normal liver enzymes.

Van Assche and Spitz[160] treated a patient who developed preeclampsia and HELLP syndrome at 32 weeks' gestation with bed rest, albumin infusion, and dazoxiben, a thromboxane synthetase inhibitor. All maternal laboratory values returned to normal after 4 days of treatment with dazoxiben. The patient had a cesarean delivery 1 week later, delivering a small-for-gestational-age infant. The authors suggested that dazoxiben might have beneficial effects in the management of such patients.

Two reports by Magann and associates from the University of Mississippi[161,162] suggested that the use of corticosteroids either antepartum or postpartum results in transient improvement in laboratory values and urine output in some patients diagnosed with HELLP syndrome. It is important to note that in the antepartum group delivery was delayed by an average of only 41 hours and the study was not placebo controlled.[161] Recently, authors from the same institution expanded on their experience with the use of high-dose dexamethasone in the management of women with HELLP syndrome. They observed improved outcomes, shorter hospital stays, and fewer blood transfusions.[163] A transient beneficial effect on hematologic findings with steroids was also reported by Tompkins and Thiagarajah.[164] However, these recommendations require testing in a randomized trial and their use should be considered experimental.

Recently, investigators from the Netherlands reported that expectant management is possible in women with HELLP syndrome below 34 weeks' gestation.[165,166] Visser and Wallenburg reported the use of plasma volume expansion in 128 women with HELLP syndrome before 34 weeks' gestation. They noted complete reversal of HELLP in 43 percent of their patients. Pregnancy was prolonged a median of 10 days (range, 0 to 62). Overall perinatal mortality was 14.1 percent, and no maternal complications occurred.[165] Similar management was reported to improve outcome in women with preterm HELLP by Van Pampus et al.[166]

Confounding variables make it difficult to evaluate any treatment modality proposed for this syndrome. Occasionally, some patients without true HELLP syndrome may demonstrate antepartum reversal of hematologic abnormalities following bed rest, the use of steroids, or plasma volume expansion. However, the majority of these patients will experience deterioration in either maternal or fetal condition within 1 to 10 days after conservative management. It is doubtful that such limited pregnancy prolongation will result in improved perinatal outcome, and maternal and fetal risks are substantial.

There is general agreement that pregnancies complicated by preeclampsia and the HELLP syndrome are associated with poor maternal and perinatal outcomes.[4,16,153] The reported perinatal mortality has ranged from 7.7 to 60 percent and maternal mortality from 0 to 24 percent. Maternal morbidity is common. Most of these patients have required transfusions of blood and blood products and are at increased risk for the development of acute renal failure, pulmonary edema, ascites, pleural effusions, and hepatic rupture.[151,153,164,167–170] Moreover, these pregnancies are associated with high incidences of abruptio placentae and DIC (Table 28–7).[170]

The HELLP syndrome may develop antepartum or postpartum. Analysis of 442 cases studied by Sibai and associates[153] revealed that 309 (70 percent) had evidence of the syndrome antepartum, and 133 (30 percent) developed the manifestations postpartum. There were four maternal deaths, and morbidity was frequent (Table 28–8).

In the postpartum period, the time of onset of the manifestations may range from a few hours to 7 days, the majority developing within 48 hours postpartum. Eighty percent of the postpartum patients had preeclampsia prior to delivery, whereas 20 percent had no evidence of either preeclampsia either antepartum or intrapartum. It is the author's experience that patients in this group are at increased risk for the development of pulmonary edema and acute renal failure (Table 28–9). The differential diagnosis should include exacerba-

Table 28–7. MATERNAL COMPLICATIONS IN 316 PREGNANCIES WITH HELLP SYNDROME, PARTIAL HELLP SYNDROME, OR SEVERE PREECLAMPSIA WITH NORMAL LABORATORY VALUES

	HELLP (*n* = 67)	Partial HELLP (*n* = 71)	Severe (*n* = 178)
Blood products transfusion (%)	25*	4	3
DIC (%)	15*	0	0
Wound hematoma/ infection (%)†	14‡	11§	2§
Pleural effusion (%)	6‡	0	1
Acute renal failure (%)	3‡	0	0
Eclampsia (%)	9	7	9
Abruptio placentae (%)	9	4	5
Pulmonary edema (%)	8	4	3
Subcapsular liver hematoma (%)	1.5	0	0
Intracerebral hemorrhage (%)	1.5	0	0
Death (%)	1.5	0	0

* $p < 0.001$, HELLP vs. partial HELLP and severe.
† Percentages of women who had cesarean delivery.
‡ $p < 0.05$, HELLP vs. severe.
§ $p < 0.05$, partial HELLP vs. severe.
From Audibert F, Friedman SA, Frangieh AY, Sibai BM: Clinical utility of strict diagnostic criteria for the HELLP (hemolysis, elevated liver enzymes, and low platelets) syndrome. Am J Obstet Gynecol 175:460, 1996, with permission.

tion of systemic lupus erythematosus, thrombotic thrombocytopenic purpura, and hemolytic uremic syndrome.

Patients with the HELLP syndrome who are remote from term should be referred to a tertiary care center, and their initial management should be the same as that for any patient with severe preeclampsia. The first priority is to assess and stabilize maternal condition, particularly coagulation abnormalities. The next step is to evaluate fetal well-being using the nonstress test and biophysical profile. Then, a decision must be made as to whether immediate delivery is indicated. Amniocentesis may be performed in patients at less than 34 weeks' gestation. In the absence of laboratory evidence of DIC and fetal lung maturity, the patient may be given two doses of steroids to accelerate fetal lung maturity and then delivered 24 hours after the last dose. During this time, both maternal and fetal conditions should be monitored closely. This syndrome is not an indication for immediate cesarean delivery. It is the author's opinion that such an approach might prove detrimental for both mother and fetus. Patients presenting with well-established labor should be allowed to deliver vaginally as indicated. In addition, labor may be initiated with oxytocin in those with a favorable cervix.

Patients with delayed resolution of HELLP syndrome including persistent severe thrombocytopenia represent a management dilemma. Exchange plasmapheresis with fresh frozen plasma has been advocated as a treatment by some authors.[149,171] Since the majority of these patients will have spontaneous resolution of their disease, however, early initiation of plasmapheresis may be an unnecessary intervention. Schwartz[171] suggested that serial studies indicating a progressive elevation of bilirubin or creatinine associated with hemolysis and thrombocytopenia be considered an indication for plasmapheresis. Martin et al.[149] reported the use of plasma exchange with fresh frozen plasma in seven women in the postpartum period with HELLP syndrome that persisted for more than 72 hours following delivery. All patients had persistent thrombocytopenia, rising lactic dehydrogenase, and evidence of multiorgan dysfunction. Sustained increases in mean platelet count and decreases in LDH concentrations were associated with plasma exchange. The authors recommended that a trial of plasma exchange with fresh frozen plasma be considered in HELLP syndrome that persists past 72 hours postpartum and in which there is evidence of a life-threatening microangiopathy. Potential adverse effects of this technique are numerous. Ultimately, the question remains how many patients would spontaneously improve without benefit of plasmapheresis. It is the author's experience that plasmapheresis is not needed in the management of such patients.[153,170]

Subcapsular Hematoma of the Liver in HELLP Syndrome

Because it occurs so rarely, the diagnosis of a subcapsular hematoma of the liver in pregnancy is often overlooked. Indeed, in four recent cases managed at our institution, our initial clinical impression was placental abruption with DIC in three cases and a complication

Table 28–8. SERIOUS MATERNAL COMPLICATIONS IN 442 PATIENTS WITH HELLP SYNDROME

Complication	No.	%
Disseminated intravascular coagulopathy	92	21
Abruptio placentae	69	16
Acute renal failure	33	8
Severe ascites	32	8
Pulmonary edema	26	6
Pleural effusions	26	6
Cerebral edema	4	1
Retinal detachment	4	1
Laryngeal edema	4	1
Subcapsular liver hematoma	4	1
Adult respiratory distress syndrome	3	1
Death, maternal	4	1

From Sibai BM, Ramadan MK, Usta I, et al: Maternal morbidity and mortality in 442 pregnancies with hemolysis, elevated liver enzymes, and low platelets (HELLP syndrome). Am J Obstet Gynecol 169:1000, 1993, with permission.

Table 28–9. OUTCOME AND COMPLICATIONS OF HELLP SYNDROME IN RELATION TO TIME OF ONSET

	Antepartum Onset (n = 309) (%)	Postpartum Onset (n = 133) (%)	Relative Risk	95% Confidence Interval
Delivery at <27 weeks*	15	3	4.84	2.0–11.6
Delivery at 37–42 weeks†	15	25	0.61	0.41–0.91
Pulmonary edema	5	9	0.50	0.24–1.05
Acute renal failure†	5	12	0.46	0.24–0.87
Eclampsia	7	10	0.73	0.38–1.40
Abruptio placentae	16	15	1.05	0.65–1.70
DIC	21	20	1.09	0.73–1.64

* $p < 0.0007$.
† $p < 0.002$.
DIC, disseminated intravascular coagulopathy.
From Sibai BM, Ramadan MK, Usta I, et al: Maternal morbidity and mortality in 442 pregnancies with hemolysis, elevated liver enzymes, and low platelets (HELLP syndrome). Am J Obstet Gynecol 169:1000, 1993, with permission.

of a postpartum tubal ligation in the fourth patient.[153] The differential diagnosis of an unruptured subcapsular hematoma of the liver in pregnancy should include acute cholecystitis with sepsis, acute fatty liver of pregnancy, ruptured uterus, placental abruption with DIC, and thrombotic thrombocytopenia purpura (TTP). Most patients present in the third or late second trimester of pregnancy, although cases have been reported in the immediate postpartum period. In addition to the signs and symptoms of preeclampsia, physical findings consistent with peritoneal irritation and hepatomegaly may be present. Profound hypovolemic shock with hypotension in a previously hypertensive patient is a hallmark of rupture of the hematoma.

Laboratory evaluation is often consistent with DIC, including low platelet count, low fibrinogen, and prolonged prothrombin and partial thromboplastin times. As a result of hemolysis, total bilirubin and serum lactate dehydrogenase are markedly elevated. Other liver function tests such as aspartate and alanine aminotransferase are also significantly elevated.[153,172]

Rupture of a subcapsular hematoma of the liver is a life-threatening complication of HELLP syndrome. In most instances, rupture involves the right lobe and is preceded by the development of a parenchymal hematoma. The condition usually presents with severe epigastric pain that may persist for several hours prior to circulatory collapse. Patients frequently present with shoulder pain, shock, or evidence of massive ascites, respiratory difficulty, or pleural effusions, and often with a dead fetus. An ultrasound or computed axial tomographic (CAT) scan of the liver should be performed to rule out subcapsular hematoma and detect the presence of intraperitoneal bleeding.[172] Paracentesis can confirm intraperitoneal hemorrhage suspected by radiographic imaging.

The presence of a ruptured subcapsular liver hematoma resulting in shock is a surgical emergency requiring acute multidisciplinary treatment. Resuscitation should consist of massive transfusions of blood, correction of the coagulopathy with fresh frozen plasma and platelets, and immediate laparotomy. Options at laparotomy include packing and drainage, the preferred approach, surgical ligation of the hemorrhaging hepatic segments, embolization of the hepatic artery to the involved liver segment, and loosely suturing omentum or surgical mesh to the liver to improve integrity. Even with appropriate treatment, maternal and fetal mortality is over 50 percent. Mortality is most commonly associated with exsanguination and coagulopathy. Initial survivors are at increased risk for developing adult respiratory distress syndrome, pulmonary edema, and acute renal failure in the postoperative period.[153,168]

Surgical repair has been recommended for hepatic hemorrhage without liver rupture. More recent experience suggests, however, that this complication can be managed conservatively in patients who remain hemodynamically stable.[172–174] Management should include close monitoring of hemodynamics and coagulation status. Serial assessment of the subcapsular hematoma with ultrasound or computed tomographic (CT) scan is necessary with immediate intervention for rupture or worsening maternal status. It is important with conservative management to avoid exogenous sources of trauma to the liver such as abdominal palpation, convulsions, or emesis and to use care in transportation of the patient. Indeed, any sudden increase in intra-abdominal pressure could potentially lead to rupture of the subcapsular hematoma.[175]

Smith et al.[176] reviewed their management of seven cases of spontaneous rupture of the liver occurring during pregnancy. Of the four survivors, the mean gestational age was 32.8 weeks and the mean duration of hospitalization was 16 days. All the survivors were managed with packing and drainage of the liver, whereas the three patients treated with hepatic lobectomy died. The authors also extracted 28 cases from the literature reported since 1976. In 35 cases, there was an 82 percent overall survival for the 27 patients managed by packing and drainage, whereas only 25 percent of eight gravidas undergoing hepatic lobectomy survived. The authors emphasized that hepatic hemorrhage with persistent hypotension unresponsive to transfusion of blood products may be managed surgically with laparotomy, evaluation of the hematoma, packing the damaged liver, and draining the operative site. In certain cases where the patient is stable enough to undergo angiography, transcatheter embolotherapy is a reasonable alternative to surgery.[177]

At the University of Tennessee, Memphis, we have managed four patients with HELLP syndrome complicated by ruptured subcapsular hematoma in 14 years. Three cases required transfusion of 22 to 40 units of packed red blood cells and multiple units of platelets and fresh frozen plasma. Two of these three cases were complicated by pulmonary edema and acute renal failure, but all survived without any residual deficiency. The fourth case was a patient who presented in profound shock and with DIC. This patient subsequently died secondary to a ruptured pulmonary emphysematous bleb during management of adult respiratory distress syndrome.[153]

Any algorithm for the management of a subcapsular hematoma of the liver in pregnancy must emphasize the potential need for large amounts of blood products and the need for aggressive intervention if rupture of the hematoma is suspected. Our algorithm, employed at the University of Tennessee, Memphis, is presented in Figure 28–3. Our experience is in agreement with the recent observations of Smith et al.[176] in that a stable patient with an unruptured subcapsular hematoma may be managed conservatively. Constant monitoring must

continue during this management, however, as patients can rapidly become unstable following rupture of the hematoma.

Survival depends on rapid diagnosis and medical and surgical stabilization. The coagulopathy must be aggressively reversed, as failure to do so is associated with an increased incidence of renal failure. In addition, these patients should be managed in an intensive care unit with close hemodynamic monitoring to avoid pulmonary edema, respiratory compromise, or both.

Postpartum follow-up for patients with subcapsular hematoma of the liver should include serial computed tomography or ultrasound until the defect resolves.[172]

Hemodynamic Changes in Preeclampsia

The cardiovascular hemodynamics of preeclampsia have been investigated over the years by many authors using various techniques for measurements of blood pressure, cardiac output, pulmonary capillary wedge pressure (PCWP), and central venous pressure (CVP).[178]

The true hemodynamic findings in patients with preeclampsia are controversial. A review of the English literature demonstrates considerable disagreement regarding one or more of the hemodynamic parameters studied. This lack of agreement has been attributed to differences in the definition of preeclampsia, variable severity and duration of the disease process, presence of underlying cardiac or renal disease, the techniques used to measure cardiac output and blood pressure, and the therapeutic interventions applied before obtaining the various measurements. In addition, the dynamic minute-to-minute fluctuation of the various cardiovascular parameters studied makes it difficult to standardize the conditions under which these observations are made, limiting the value of a single measurement.

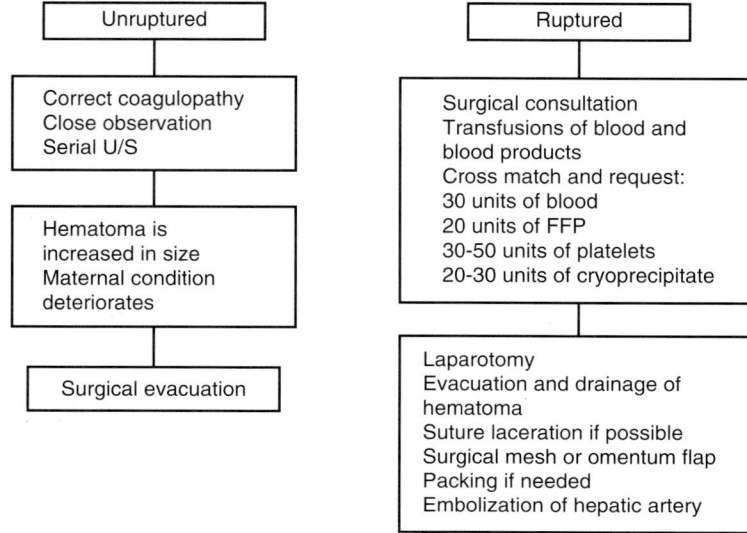

Figure 28–3. An algorithm for the management of a subcapsular hematoma at the University of Tennessee, Memphis.

Invasive techniques have been used by many authors to study the hemodynamic findings in untreated women with severe preeclampsia.[179-183] The reported cardiac index ranged from a low of 2.8 to a high of 4.8 L/min/m², and the reported PCWP from a low of 3.3 to a high of 12 mm Hg. The findings suggest that cardiac index and PCWP are either low or normal in severe preeclampsia. The reported CVP values also ranged from 2 to 6 mm Hg.

Table 28–10 compares the invasive hemodynamic findings in treated patients with severe preeclampsia.[181,184,185] The data for the various parameters are similar among the three studies. The findings demonstrate that treated patients with preeclampsia have normal to high cardiac index, normal to high systemic vascular resistance index, and normal to high PCWP.

In summary, the true hemodynamic findings of preeclampsia remain unknown. The majority of the data indicate that both cardiac output and systemic vascular resistance appear to be elevated in women with severe preeclampsia. This finding suggests that the problem in preeclampsia is a systemic vascular resistance that is inappropriately high for the level of cardiac output. Both the PCWP and the CVP appear to be in the low to normal range; however, there is no correlation between the two values.

Doppler Velocimetry Studies

There are numerous reports describing the use of uteroplacental and umbilical arterial flow velocity waveforms (FVWs) in the prediction, diagnosis, and management of preeclampsia (see Chapters 12 and 25).[186] Early studies suggested that Doppler ultrasound held great promise as a noninvasive, repeatable, and simple method of predicting hypertension in pregnancy and identifying those hypertensive pregnancies at high risk for maternal and fetal complications.[187-190] However, subsequent studies have emphasized the multiplicity of factors that may influence the Doppler waveform pattern.[186]

Steel et al.[191] screened 1,014 nulliparous women with Doppler waveforms from the uteroplacental circulation at 18 to 20 weeks. One hundred eighteen (12 percent) had persistently abnormal tests at both 18 and 24 weeks' gestation. The incidence of hypertension among these 118 women was 25 percent. The sensitivity was high for hypertension associated with proteinuria (63 percent) or intrauterine growth restriction (100 percent).

Bower and associates[192] screened 2,430 women with continuous wave Doppler ultrasound of both uterine arteries at 18 to 20 weeks' gestation. An abnormal FVW in either uterine artery was used to predict preeclampsia and poor perinatal outcome. Including an early diastolic notch in the definition of an abnormal FVW increased the sensitivity for moderate and severe preeclampsia to 79 to 88 percent and the specificity to 85 percent. However, the positive predictive value was only 4.3 to 6.9 percent. Another study was less encouraging.[193,194]

Trudinger and Cook[195] studied Doppler umbilical and uterine FVW in women with severe hypertension in pregnancy. They found that perinatal complications correlated more closely with umbilical artery indices than uteroplacental indices. More recently, Yoon and associates[196] examined umbilical artery waveforms in 72 women with preeclampsia. The Doppler studies were performed within 7 days of delivery. They found that an abnormal umbilical artery waveform was a strong and independent predictor of adverse perinatal outcome in patients with preeclampsia.

Pattinson and associates[197] reported on a randomized controlled trial evaluating the role of umbilical artery Doppler velocimetry in the management of patients with hypertensive diseases or suspected fetal growth re-

Table 28–10. INVASIVE HEMODYNAMIC FINDINGS IN TREATED PATIENTS WITH SEVERE PREECLAMPSIA/ECLAMPSIA: COMPARISON OF THREE LARGE SERIES

	Wallenburg[181] (n = 22)*	Cotton et al.[184] (n = 45)†	Mabie et al.[185] (n = 41)‡
Diastolic pressure (mm Hg)	110	110 ± 2	106 ± 2
Pulmonary artery pressure (mm Hg)	19	17 ± 1	15 ± 0.5
Cardiac index (L/min/m²)	3.8	4.1 ± 0.1	4.4 ± 0.1
SVRI (dynes·sec·cm⁻⁵, m²)	2,475	2,726 ± 1	2,293 ± 65
PWCP (mm Hg)	8	10 ± 1	8.3 ± 0.3
Central venous pressure (mm Hg)	2	4 ± 1	4.8 ± 0.4

* Values expressed as median.
† Values as mean ± SEM; includes two patients with pulmonary edema.
‡ Values as mean ± SEM; excludes eight patients with pulmonary edema.
SVRI, systemic vascular resistance index; PWCP, pulmonary capillary wedge pressure; SEM, standard error of the mean.

striction. The Doppler findings were revealed to the managing physicians of 108 patients, but blinded in another 104 patients. Knowledge of Doppler velocimetry results was beneficial only in the subset of patients with absent end-diastolic velocities.

In summary, the data regarding examination of the uteroplacental circulation for the prediction of preeclampsia indicate that the presence of abnormal tests at 18 to 20 weeks' and at 24 weeks' gestation, particularly the presence of a diastolic notch, may be helpful as a screening test in selected, high-risk populations. On the other hand, evaluation of the umbilical artery is valuable in identifying those pregnancies that might require frequent monitoring with traditional tests of fetal well-being such as the nonstress test and biophysical profile. In general, the presence or absence of end-diastolic frequencies or reverse flow patterns in the umbilical artery is usually associated with poor perinatal outcome.[198]

The Management of Preeclampsia

Once the diagnosis of preeclampsia has been made, definitive therapy in the form of delivery is the only cure. The primary considerations of therapy must always be the safety of the mother and then the delivery of a live, mature newborn who will not require intensive and prolonged neonatal care. However, in some cases such an approach is not in the best interest of the fetus. As a result, the decision between immediate delivery and expectant management will depend on one or more of the following: the severity of the disease process, maternal and fetal status at the time of initial evaluation, fetal gestational age, presence of labor, the Bishop score, and the wishes of the mother.

Mild Preeclampsia

Patients with diagnosed preeclampsia should ideally be hospitalized at the time of diagnosis for evaluation of maternal and fetal conditions. These pregnancies may be associated with reduced uteroplacental blood flow jeopardizing the fetus. In addition, the mother is at a slightly increased risk for the development of abruptio placentae or convulsions, particularly in cases remote from term. Thus, women with mild disease who have a favorable cervix at or near term should undergo induction of labor for delivery. The pregnancy should not continue past 40 weeks' gestation, even if conditions for induction of labor are unfavorable.

The optimal management of mild preeclampsia remote from term (<37 weeks' gestation) is controversial. There is considerable disagreement regarding the need for hospitalization versus ambulatory management, the use of antihypertensive drugs, and the use of sedatives.[14,15]

In the past, management of these patients has involved bed rest in the hospital for the duration of pregnancy because this approach enhanced fetal survival and diminished the frequency of progression to severe disease.[199,200] On the other hand, the benefits of prolonged antepartum hospitalization for women with mild gestational hypertension without proteinuria were challenged by several European investigators who reported that most of these patients can be safely managed on an ambulatory basis or in a day-care facility.

Two studies reported on pregnancy outcome in women with mild hypertension without proteinuria remote from term who were randomized to either bed rest in the hospital or normal activity at home.[201,202] Both studies questioned the value of hospitalization and came to the conclusion that management at home was safe and cost effective. Two other studies reported that management of these women can be done safely and efficiently in day-care units, thereby diminishing the number of hospitalization days.[203,204] Finally, a recent review analyzing the value of bed rest in obstetrics including mild hypertension suggested that this approach is not cost effective and might be potentially harmful.[205]

There are numerous clinical reports, both controlled and uncontrolled, describing the use of various drugs in an attempt to prolong gestation and improve perinatal outcome in women with mild preeclampsia remote from term. However, it is almost impossible to evaluate and compare the results because of the heterogeneous populations studied, and the absence of a placebo group in most reports.[2,16] Overall, these studies have revealed lower rates of progression to severe disease with no impact on perinatal outcome.[130,200] Of note, the sample size was inadequate in any of these studies to evaluate small differences in adverse perinatal outcome.[2,16]

In a prospective, randomized trial, Sibai et al.[130] compared no therapy to the use of nifedipine in the management of mild preeclampsia remote from term (Table 28–11). They found that nifedipine was effective in reducing maternal systolic and diastolic blood pressures in women with mild preeclampsia. However, this reduction in maternal blood pressure was not associated with a reduction in antepartum hospital days in the nifedipine group. In addition, while the use of nifedipine led to a lower incidence of delivery for severe hypertension (9 percent vs. 18 percent), there was no difference in the gestational age at delivery.

Our management plan at the University of Tennessee, Memphis, for women with mild preeclampsia is summarized in Figure 28–4. Patients who are unreliable are hospitalized at the time of their diagnosis. During hospitalization, patients receive a regular diet with no salt restriction and no activity limits. Diuretics and antihypertensive drugs are not prescribed, and sedatives

Table 28–11. RANDOMIZED TRIALS OF ANTIHYPERTENSIVE DRUGS OR NO TREATMENT IN MILD PREECLAMPSIA

Authors	Patients (No.)	GA at Entry	GA at Delivery	Birth Weight (g)	SGA, No. (%)	Perinatal Deaths, No. (%)
Sibai et al.[130]						
Nifedipine	100	32.8	36.1	2,403	15 (15)	0
No treatment	100	33.4	36.7	2,509	13 (13)	0
Mabie et al.[200]						
Labetalol	92	32.6	35.4	2,204	18 (19.1)	1 (1.1)
No treatment	94	32.4	35.5	2,258	9 (9.3)	0

GA, gestational age; SGA, small for gestational age.

are not used. Patients initially undergo evaluation of maternal and fetal well-being. The frequency of subsequent testing usually depends on the gestational age and maternal response following hospitalization. Subsequent fetal evaluation includes serial ultrasonography for fetal growth every 3 weeks, daily fetal movement count, nonstress testing every week, and a biophysical profile if needed. Maternal evaluation includes blood pressure monitoring (every 4 hours during the day) and daily assessment of maternal weight to detect excessive weight gain. In addition, women are questioned regarding symptoms of impending eclampsia (persistent headache, visual disturbances, or epigastric pain). Laboratory evaluation includes measurements of urine protein, hematocrit, platelet count, and liver function tests once or twice weekly. This evaluation is extremely important because patients may develop thrombocytopenia and

elevated liver enzymes with minimal blood pressure elevation.[155]

If the patient's blood pressure remains stable in the absence of either significant proteinuria (<1,000 mg/ 24 h) or maternal symptoms (headaches, visual disturbances, or epigastric pain), then outpatient observation may be considered on a selective basis. This form of management is appropriate in a reliable patient only during the early stages of the disease and in the absence of fetal jeopardy (abnormal testing or abnormal fetal growth).[15] Patients are instructed to rest at home and have daily urine dipstick measurements of proteinuria and blood pressure monitoring they perform or by a nurse. The patient is also instructed to keep fetal movement counts and to report any symptoms of impending eclampsia. The patient is then evaluated in the antepartum testing area for maternal and fetal well-being at

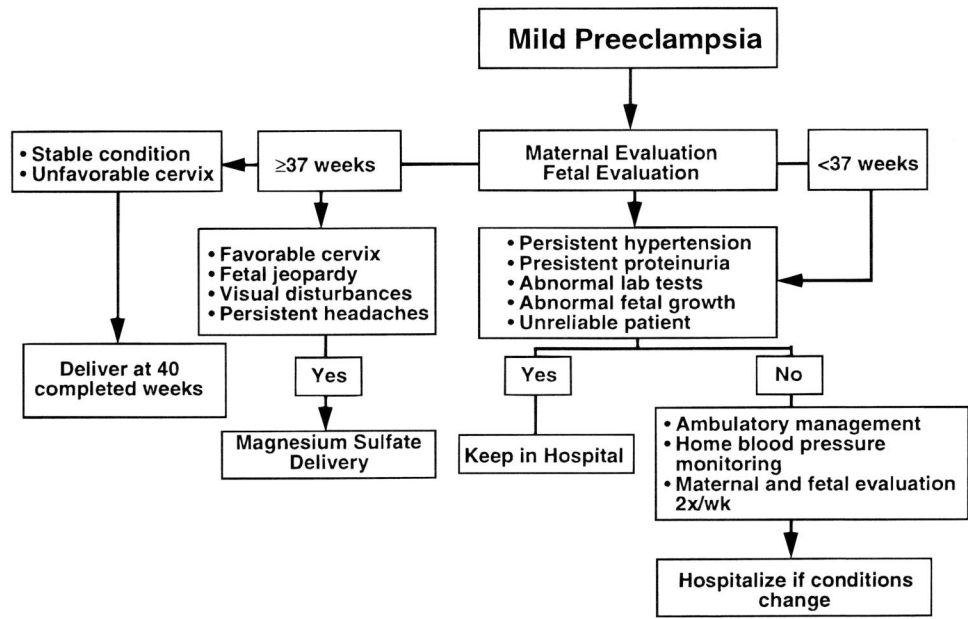

Figure 28–4. University of Tennessee, Memphis, management plan for patients with mild preeclampsia.

least two times per week. If there is any evidence that her condition is worsening such as acute hypertension or substantial proteinuria, then prompt hospitalization is indicated.

The success rate of outpatient management will depend on the gestational age and maternal status at time of diagnosis. Patients diagnosed with mild hypertension only (diastolic pressure <100 mm Hg, absent proteinuria) will have a longer duration of pregnancy prolongation than those diagnosed with moderate elevations of hypertension (diastolic >100 mm Hg) and significant proteinuria.[206] After 37 weeks gestation, labor should be induced as soon as the cervix is favorable (Bishop score ≥6).

The prophylactic use of magnesium sulfate in women with mild gestational hypertension or mild preeclampsia to prevent eclamptic convulsions remains controversial. There are few retrospective studies evaluating the frequency of eclampsia in women not receiving seizure prophylaxis.[18] There is only one randomized, placebo-controlled study in a limited number of women with mild preeclampsia ($n = 135$).[207] A large trial compared the use of phenytoin to magnesium sulfate in a heterogenous group of women ranging from mild gestational hypertension to severe preeclampsia.[208] This trial revealed magnesium sulfate to be superior to phenytoin for the prevention of eclamptic convulsions.[208] Women with mild preeclampsia should be considered for prophylactic therapy if they have symptoms. At present, there is a need for a large randomized, placebo-controlled trial to investigate the efficacy of magnesium sulfate seizure prophylaxis in women with mild preeclampsia.[18]

Severe Preeclampsia

The clinical course of severe preeclampsia may be characterized by progressive deterioration in both maternal and fetal conditions. Because these pregnancies have been associated with increased rates of perinatal mortality and significant risks for maternal morbidity and mortality, there is universal agreement that all such patients should be delivered if the disease develops after 34 weeks' gestation or prior to that time if there is evidence of maternal or fetal distress.[209] There is also agreement on delivery of such patients prior to 35 weeks' gestation in the presence of any of the following: premature rupture of membranes, labor, or severe fetal growth restriction (<5th percentile for age). In this situation, appropriate management consists of parenteral medications to prevent convulsions, control of maternal blood pressure within a relatively safe range, and then induction of labor to achieve delivery.[131] If delivery of a preterm infant less than 34 weeks' gestation is anticipated at a Level I or Level II hospital, the

mother should be transferred to a tertiary care center with adequate neonatal intensive care facilities.

On the other hand, there is considerable disagreement about management of patients with severe disease prior to 34 weeks' gestation. Some authors consider delivery as the definitive therapy for all cases, regardless of gestational age, whereas others recommend prolonging pregnancy in all severe preeclamptic gestations remote from term until development of fetal lung maturity, fetal or maternal distress, or a gestational age of 34 to 36 weeks is achieved.[169,170,209–213] Some of the measures used in these latter cases have included one or more of the following: antihypertensive agents, diuretics, sedatives, chronic parenteral magnesium sulfate, plasma volume expanders, and antithrombotic agents.

Severe Preeclampsia at 28 to 32 Weeks' Gestation

There are several retrospective studies describing expectant management of women with severe preeclampsia at 28 to 32 weeks' gestation.[209] In general, these studies suggest that expectant management can improve outcome in selected patients.[209]

There are three randomized trials describing expectant management in patients with severe preeclampsia. In the first study, the results of individualized management were reported in 58 women with severe preeclampsia at 28 to 34 weeks' gestation.[214] These patients were treated initially with magnesium sulfate, hydralazine, and corticosteroids to accelerate fetal lung immaturity. All received intensive maternal and fetal care in a high-risk obstetric ward. Nonstress tests were done at least three times daily, and laboratory tests were evaluated at least twice weekly. Twenty of the 58 women were delivered because of maternal or fetal reasons within 48 hours after hospitalization. The remaining 38 were then randomized to either aggressive or expectant management ($n = 20$). Patients assigned to the aggressive management group received steroids and were delivered within 72 hours. Patients assigned to the expectant management group were treated with hydralazine to maintain blood pressure between 140/90 and 150/100 mm Hg. In addition, they received frequent evaluations for maternal and fetal well-being. These patients were delivered at 34 weeks' gestation or before in the presence of maternal or fetal distress. The authors found lower neonatal complications and lower number of days spent in the neonatal intensive care unit in the expectant-management group.[214]

In a second study,[215] a randomized clinical trial was conducted in which patients with severe preeclampsia between 26 and 36 weeks' gestation were assigned to be treated with either nifedipine ($n = 24$) or hydralazine ($n = 25$). Patients assigned to the nifedipine group

Table 28–12. PREGNANCY OUTCOME

	Aggressive Management (n = 46)	Expectant Management (n = 49)	Significance
Gestational age at delivery (wk)	30.8 ± 1.7	32.9 ± 1.5	$p < 0.0001$
Placental weight (g)	355 ± 88	435 ± 117	$p < 0.01$
Birth weight (g)	1,233 ± 287	1,622 ± 360	$p = 0.0004$
Cesarean delivery, No. (%)	39 (85)	36 (73)	NS
Abruptio placentae, No. (%)	2 (4.3)	2 (4.1)	NS
HELLP syndrome, No. (%)	1 (2.1)	2 (4.1)	NS
Postpartum stay (days)	5.3 ± 2.1	5.1 ± 1.9	NS

NS, not significant; HELLP, hemolysis, elevated liver enzymes, low platelets.
From Sibai BM, Mercer BM, Schiff E, Friedman SA: Aggressive versus expectant management of severe preeclampsia at 28 to 32 weeks' gestation: a randomized controlled trial. Am J Obstet Gynecol 171:818, 1994.

received 10 to 30 mg sublingually initially, then 40 to 120 mg/day orally. Those assigned to the hydralazine group received 6.25 to 12.5 mg intravenously initially. Maternal evaluation included frequent measurements of blood pressure, heart rate, patellar reflexes, urine output, and laboratory tests. Fetal evaluation included daily fetal heart rate monitoring, biophysical profile three times a week, and weekly ultrasonographic assessment of fetal growth. The authors found better control of blood pressure and a lower incidence of nonreassuring fetal testing in the group managed with nifedipine.[215] In addition, the group receiving nifedipine had a better perinatal outcome than those receiving hydralazine. They concluded that nifedipine is a safe and effective drug in the management of patients with severe preeclampsia remote from term.[215]

Sibai et al.[131] studied 95 women with severe preeclampsia at 28 to 32 weeks' gestation who were randomly assigned to either aggressive management (AM) (n = 46) or expectant management (EM) (n = 49). The two groups were similar at the time of randomization with respect to several clinical and laboratory findings.

The average pregnancy prolongation in the EM group was 15.4 ± 6.6 days (range, 4 to 36 days), which was significantly higher than the average in the AM group of 2.6 days ($p < 0.0001$; range, 2 to 3 days). In the EM group, the average pregnancy prolongation period was not affected by the amount of proteinuria at randomization. Indications for delivery in the EM group were worsening maternal status (n = 16), fetal compromise (n = 13), attainment of 34 weeks' gestation (n = 10), preterm labor or rupture of membranes (n = 7), or vaginal bleeding (n = 3). The maternal indications for delivery were thrombocytopenia (n = 5), uncontrolled severe hypertension (n = 3), headache/blurred vision (n = 3), epigastric pain (n = 2), severe ascites (n = 1), and maternal demand (n = 2).

Table 28–12 compares the pregnancy outcomes in the two groups. Gestational age at delivery, placental weight, and birth weight were significantly higher in the EM group. The two cases of abruptio placentae in the AM group were found at the time of cesarean delivery, whereas the two cases in the EM group were suspected because of abnormal fetal heart rate testing and vaginal bleeding. There were no cases of eclampsia, pulmonary edema, renal failure, or disseminated coagulopathy in either group.

No fetal or neonatal deaths occurred in either group. The number of infants admitted to a neonatal intensive care unit (37 vs. 46 percent), average duration of stay in that unit (20 vs. 37 percent), and the frequency of respiratory distress syndrome (22 vs. 50 percent) and necrotizing enterocolitis (0 vs. 11 percent) were significantly lower in the EM group.[131]

Mid-Trimester Severe Preeclampsia

Severe preeclampsia developing in the mid-trimester is associated with high perinatal mortality and morbidity.[216,217] Aggressive management with immediate delivery will result in high neonatal mortality. In addition, all surviving neonates will develop significant neonatal complications and will require prolonged hospitalization in neonatal intensive care units. On the other hand, attempts to prolong pregnancy may result in fetal demise or asphyxial damage in utero. Moreover, this management may expose the mother to severe morbidity and even mortality. The perinatal survival rate is usually poor when the disease develops before 24 weeks' gestation (2 percent); however, it is better when the disease occurs at or beyond 25 weeks' gestation.[216-218]

Initially, Sibai et al.[217] reviewed pregnancy outcome in 60 such patients who had had conservative management over a 7-year period. The mean gestational age at time of management was 24.8 weeks (range, 17 to 27), and average days of pregnancy prolongation was 11.4 days (range, 2 to 40). The perinatal outcomes of these pregnancies were poor, with 31 of the 60 resulting in fetal demise and 21 ending in neonatal death, for a total perinatal mortality of 87 percent. In addition, maternal morbidity was significantly high. This study was retrospective, most patients were managed at Level I hospitals, and few of these pregnancies had antepartum fetal evaluation.

Pattinson et al.[216] described the results of conservative management in 34 patients who had severe preeclampsia before 28 weeks. The patients were managed by bed rest, antihypertensive drugs, and intensive fetal and maternal monitoring. Eleven patients presented before 24 weeks, all of them resulting in perinatal deaths, and the remaining 34 were between 24 and 37 weeks' gestation, with 13 (38 percent) resulting in a surviving infant. Maternal complications included three cases (9 percent) of pulmonary edema and one case (3 percent) with pleural effusion.

More recently, Sibai et al.[218] described a new protocol for managing severe preeclampsia in the mid-trimester. The study included 109 patients with severe preeclampsia at 19 to 27 weeks' gestation. All patients were first admitted to labor and delivery and were evaluated carefully for the presence of either maternal or fetal compromise. Pregnancy termination was recommended for patients with gestational ages of 24 weeks or less (n = 25), whereas expectant management was recommended for patients with gestational age over 24 weeks (n = 84). Of the 25 patients with gestational age 24 weeks or less, 10 accepted termination and the other 15 elected to continue with their pregnancies. The latter patients were managed with bed rest, antihypertensive drugs, and frequent evaluation of maternal and fetal well-being. The average days of pregnancy prolongation in these 15 pregnancies was 19.4 days; 11 ended in stillbirths, and 3 resulted in neonatal deaths, for an overall perinatal survival of 6.7 percent. Of the 84 patients with gestational ages more than 24 weeks, 30 had immediate delivery either because of patient's desire or because of attending staff decision. These patients received magnesium sulfate, antihypertensive drugs, and steroids and then were delivered within 48 hours. The other 54 patients were managed conservatively with antihypertensive drugs and daily evaluation of maternal and fetal well-being. The conservative management group had significantly higher perinatal survival (64.5 vs. 23.6 percent) and lower neonatal complications. In addition, the two groups had similar frequencies of maternal complications. They concluded that expectant management for women with severe preeclampsia should be selective and done only in a tertiary care center with adequate intensive care facilities.[218]

At the University of Tennessee, Memphis, patients with severe preeclampsia remote from term are admitted initially to the labor and delivery area for continuous evaluation of maternal and fetal conditions for at least 24 hours. Subsequent management is based on gestational age (Fig. 28–5). During observation, they receive continuous infusion of magnesium sulfate to

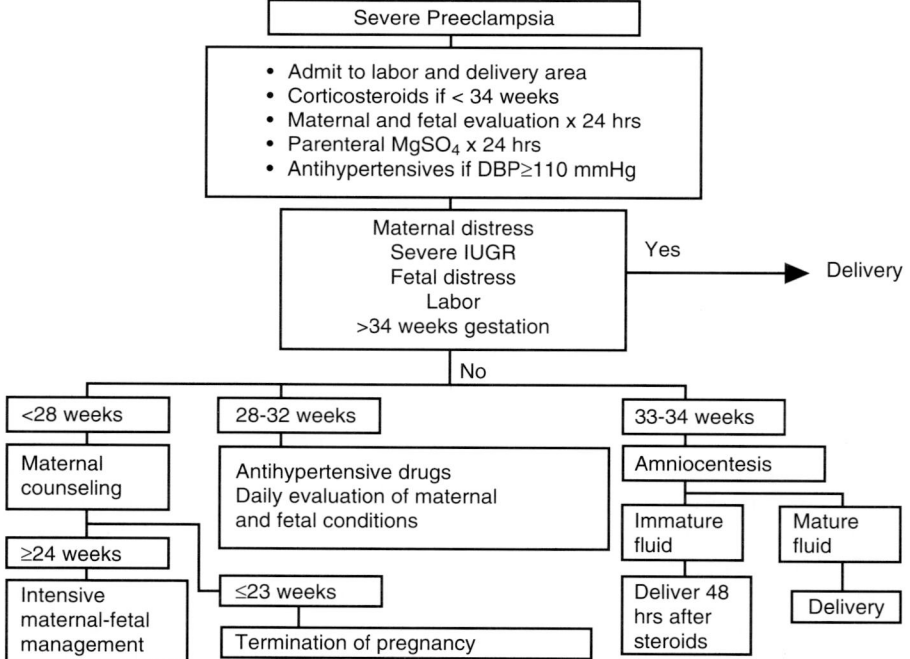

Figure 28–5. University of Tennessee, Memphis, management plan for patients with severe preeclampsia.

prevent convulsions and bolus doses of hydralazine (5 to 10 mg), labetalol (20 to 40 mg), or oral nifedipine (10 mg) as needed to keep diastolic blood pressure below 110 mm Hg. Patients at gestational age less than 34 weeks' gestation are given corticosteroids to accelerate fetal lung maturity. Maternal evaluation includes continuous monitoring of blood pressure, heart rate, urine output, cerebral status, and the presence of epigastric pain. Laboratory evaluation includes a platelet count and liver enzymes. Fetal evaluation includes continuous fetal heart monitoring, a biophysical profile, and ultrasonographic assessment of fetal growth. Patients with resistant severe hypertension or other signs of maternal or fetal deterioration are delivered within 24 hours, irrespective of gestational age or fetal lung maturity.[209] In addition, patients in labor, or those with fetuses with a gestational age greater than 35 weeks, and those with evidence of fetal lung maturity by amniocentesis at 33 to 35 weeks also are delivered within 24 hours.[209] Patients at 33 to 35 weeks' gestation with immature fluid receive steroids to accelerate fetal lung maturity and are delivered 24 hours after the last dose of steroids in the absence of any change in maternal or fetal condition.

It is a commonly held clinical impression that fetuses of preeclamptic women have accelerated lung maturation as a result of stress in utero. This phenomenon, however, has never been documented in a well-controlled study. The effect of hypertension during pregnancy on the incidence of neonatal respiratory distress syndrome is highly controversial.[219] Schiff and associates[219] compared fetal lung maturity indices in 127 preterm patients with preeclampsia and 127 normotensive controls matched by gestational age, race, and fetal gender. They found no differences in the incidences of immature results between the two groups. They concluded that fetuses of preeclamptic women do not exhibit accelerated lung maturation.[219] Similar findings were also reported by Piazze et al. from Italy.[220]

Corticosteroids have been suggested as safe and effective drugs for preventing respiratory distress syndrome, treating thrombocytopenia, and improving perinatal outcome in severe preeclampsia. A review of the literature reveals substantial differences in methodology and drug selection among investigators who advocate the use of steroids for preeclampsia.[221] A patient may be considered suitable for steroid therapy if there is no evidence of maternal or fetal jeopardy and if delivery is not expected to occur within 48 hours. Maximum benefit is achieved when steroid therapy is given in appropriate doses and the last dose is given at least 24 hours before delivery. Different regimens of steroids have been suggested for preventing respiratory distress syndrome, but we prefer betamethasone given as 12 mg as soon as possible and the dose repeated 24 hours later.

Patients at 28 to 32 weeks' gestation receive individualized management based on their clinical response during the observation period. All of these patients receive steroids to accelerate fetal lung maturity, as there is still benefit even if the delivery occurs in less than 24 hours or more than 1 week later. Some demonstrate marked diuresis and improvement in blood pressure during the observation period. If the blood pressure remains below 100 mm Hg diastolic without antihypertensive therapy after the observation period, magnesium sulfate is discontinued, and the patients are followed closely on the antepartum high-risk ward until fetal maturity is achieved. During hospitalization, they receive antihypertensive drugs, usually oral nifedipine 40 to 120 mg/day, to keep their diastolic blood pressure between 90 and 100 mm Hg, with daily evaluation of maternal and fetal well-being. In general, most of these patients will require delivery within 2 weeks.[131] However, some patients may continue their pregnancies for several weeks. It is important to note that such pregnancies should be managed at tertiary care centers because their courses are unpredictable.

There is one placebo-controlled trial evaluating the use of magnesium sulfate in women with severe preeclampsia.[222] The trial revealed a significant reduction in eclampsia in the treated group (1 of 345 vs. 11 of 340; relative risk, 0.09; confidence interval, 0.01 to 0.69). Therefore, all women with severe preeclampsia should receive magnesium sulfate during labor and for 24 hours postpartum. Magnesium sulfate is administered by a controlled continuous intravenous infusion with a loading dose of 6 g in 100 ml over 15 to 20 minutes. We believe that the intravenous route for magnesium therapy permits more precise control of the patient's blood level and avoids the pain of intramuscular injections. Maintenance therapy is given at a rate of 2 g in 100 ml of fluid per hour. Treatment is continued for 12 to 24 hours after delivery.

The magnesium ion goes beyond extracellular fluid and enters bones and cells as well.[223] Magnesium circulates largely unbound to protein and is excreted in the urine. Therefore, an accurate record of maternal urine output must be maintained. In patients with normal renal function, the half-life for magnesium excretion is about 4 hours. In the therapeutic range (4.8 to 9.6 mg/dl), magnesium sulfate slows neuromuscular conduction and depresses central nervous system irritability. For this reason, maternal respiratory rate, deep tendon reflexes, and state of consciousness must be frequently monitored to detect magnesium toxicity. An ampule of calcium gluconate, 1 g (10 ml of 10 percent solution) should be drawn up in a syringe, clearly labeled, and kept at the bedside in case of magnesium toxicity. If magnesium toxicity is suspected, the infusion of magnesium sulfate should be discontinued. If respiratory depression occurs, the calcium gluconate should be given intravenously over 3 minutes. If respi-

Magnesium Toxicity	
Loss of patellar reflex	8–12 mg/dl
Feelings of warmth, flushing	9–12 mg/dl
Somnolence	10–12 mg/dl
Slurred speech	10–12 mg/dl
Muscular paralysis	15–17 mg/dl
Respiratory difficulty	15–17 mg/dl
Cardiac arrest	30–35 mg/dl

ratory arrest develops, the patient should receive mechanical ventilatory support as needed (see the box "Magnesium Toxicity").

We carefully monitor the volume of intravenous fluids used in women with preeclampsia or eclampsia. Intake and output should be assessed hourly. We give a 5 percent dextrose in lactated Ringer's solution at 100 to 125 ml/h. A Foley catheter should be inserted to permit accurate evaluation of urine output. We are particularly cautious when treating women with chronic hypertension or renal disease. Frequently, in the active phase of labor, urine output may drop below 30 ml/h. In those cases, in which the cervix is continuing to dilate, we have not given a fluid challenge or diuretics. Typically in these women, urine output will increase to 30 ml/h after 2 to 3 hours. Our goal is to maintain the urine output at 30 ml/h. If urine output drops below 100 ml in 4 hours, the dose of magnesium sulfate and intravenous fluids should be reduced accordingly. Another cause of decreased urine output is a drop in maternal blood pressure due to repeated injections of hydralazine. Hydralazine has a relatively long duration of action and, when multiple bolus injections of hydralazine are used to control blood pressure, the diastolic blood pressure may be reduced more than intended, that is, below 90 mm Hg. This action will frequently reduce urine output for 2 to 3 hours. One of the potential problems when attempting to limit intravenous fluids to 125 ml/h is that high concentrations of drugs must be used if the woman is receiving intravenous magnesium sulfate, oxytocin, and hydralazine.

To control severe maternal hypertension intrapartum, we use bolus injections of hydralazine 5 to 10 mg every 20 to 30 minutes to lower the diastolic blood pressure to the 90 to 100 mm Hg range. This requires monitoring of blood pressure every 5 minutes for at least 30 minutes after the drug is given. Recently, Patterson-Brown and associates described 70 women with severe preeclampsia who received bolus injections of hydralazine for the treatment of sustained severe hypertension (mean arterial pressure >125 mm Hg for 45 minutes or >140 mm Hg for 15 minutes).[224] Each treatment episode consisted of hydralazine 5 mg given as an intravenous bolus dose, repeated after 15-minute intervals until the mean arterial pressure fell below 125 mm Hg, up to a maximum of three boluses. All women received a 400- to 500-ml albumin solution (5 percent) over 20 minutes prior to hydralazine. They found that this protocol was effective in lowering maternal blood pressure in 89 percent of the cases. In addition, they observed no significant maternal or fetal side effects from such therapy. They concluded that hydralazine given in 5-mg boluses is a safe and effective method for treating severe hypertension in preeclampsia.[224] An alternative regimen is to use bolus injections of labetalol hydrochloride, 20 to 80 mg. Unlike hydralazine, labetalol does not cause maternal tachycardia, flushing, or headaches. We have found this drug to be safe and effective in the management of these patients.[225] Oral nifedipine in doses of 10 to 20 mg every 4 to 6 hours may also be used (Table 28–13).[226,227] Other potent antihypertensive medications such as sodium nitroprusside, or nitroglycerin are rarely needed in managing these patients. Diuretics such as furosemide are not used except in the presence of pulmonary edema.[228]

Anesthesia in Severe Preeclampsia

Maternal analgesia can be provided by the intermittent use of small doses (25 to 50 mg) of intravenous meperidine or segmental epidural analgesia. Local infiltration anesthesia with or without pudendal block or epidural can be used for all cases of vaginal delivery for patients with mild disease. In addition, continuous epidural anesthesia or balanced general anesthesia can be used for all cesarean deliveries. The use of epidural anesthesia for patients with severe preeclampsia/eclampsia is controversial. It is important to emphasize that the administration of epidural requires the availability of personnel with special expertise in obstetric anesthesia. In addition, in selected cases it requires the availability of central hemodynamic monitoring, since infusions of large amounts of crystalloids or colloids are usually used as precautionary measures before its administration. Moreover, the use of conduction anesthesia is contraindicated in the presence of coagulopathy.

On the other hand, significant hypertension and tachycardia are frequently observed after laryngoscopy and endotracheal intubation as well as during extubation in patients undergoing general anesthesia. Transient but severe hypertension after tracheal intubation can result in a significant increase in maternal intracranial pressures with the dangers of cerebral edema and hemorrhage and increased afterload with the dangers of pulmonary edema. These responses can be prevented or attenuated by the use of labetalol prior to endotracheal intubation. Labetalol should be used in a dose of 20 mg intravenously followed by 10-mg increments up to a total dose of 1 mg/kg.[229] In addition, endotracheal

Table 28–13. PARENTERAL AND ORAL DRUGS FOR TREATMENT OF SEVERE HYPERTENSION IN PREGNANCY

Drug	Dose	Onset of Action	Duration of Action	Adverse Effects
Hydralazine	5–10 mg IV q 20 min	10–20 min	3–6 h	Tachycardia, headache, flushing, aggravation of angina
Labetalol	20–40 mg IV q 10 min 1 mg/kg as needed	10–20 min	3–6 h	Scalp tingling, vomiting, heart block
Nifedipine	10–20 mg PO q 20–30 min	10–15 min	4–5 h	Headache, tachycardia, synergistic interaction with magnesium sulfate
Nicardipine	5–15 mg/h IV	5–10 min	1–4 h	Tachycardia, headache, phlebitis
Sodium nitroprusside	0.25–5 μg/kg/min IV	Immediate	1–2 min	Nausea, vomiting, muscle twitching, thiocyanate and cyanide intoxication
Nitroglycerin	5–100 μg/min IV	2–5 min	3–5 min	Headache, methemoglobinemia, tachyphylaxis

intubation increases the risk of aspiration, and there is the potential for failed intubation in the presence of airway edema, morbid obesity, and a short neck.[230] In such situations, it is preferable to perform awake intubation using fiberoptic guidance.

Ramanathan and associates[231] conducted a prospective evaluation of the hemodynamic and neuroendocrine stress responses at the time of cesarean delivery in 21 women with severe preeclampsia. Eleven received epidural anesthesia and 10 general anesthesia. The authors found that epidural anesthesia caused blunting of the hemodynamic and neuroendocrine stress responses to cesarean delivery in women with severe preeclampsia. The findings support the concept that epidural anesthesia should be the method of choice in these patients.

Recent data also suggest that epidural, spinal, and combined spinal-epidural techniques offer many advantages for labor analgesia and for cesarean delivery in women with preeclampsia/eclampsia.[232–234] Hypotension can usually be avoided by meticulous attention to technique and proper volume expansion. In addition, a recent study indicates that epidural appears to be a safe and effective technique in women with severe hypertension in pregnnacy.[234] It must be emphasized, however, that there are no randomized studies comparing the safety of conduction to general anesthesia for cesarean delivery in women with severe preeclampsia/eclampsia.

For patients with the HELLP syndrome, the use of pudendal block or epidural anesthesia is contraindicated, since these patients are at risk of bleeding into these areas. In case of cesarean delivery, platelet transfusions are usually indicated to correct severe thrombocytopenia. Our policy is to transfuse 6 to 10 units of platelets in all patients with a platelet count less than

50,000/mm³ prior to intubation. Generalized oozing from the operative site is common, and, to minimize the risk of hematoma formation, we recommend that a subfascial drain be used, the bladder flap be left open, and the wound be left open with sutures in situ above the fascia. These wounds can be successfully closed within 72 hours. Failure to adhere to these recommendations may result in a 25 percent incidence of hematoma formation.

Some investigators recommended the use of invasive hemodynamic monitoring in managing patients with severe preeclampsia. Clark and Cotton[235] reported that indications for such monitoring should include pulmonary edema, persistent oliguria unresponsive to a fluid challenge, intractable severe hypertension and, in some patients, epidural anesthesia. Others have recommended using Swan-Ganz catheters to monitor fluid therapy and response to antihypertensive drugs. These authors utilize plasma volume expansion with colloid plasma substitute to increase cardiac index and pulmonary capillary wedge pressure prior to the use of epidural or vasodilator drugs in an attempt to avoid the potential of severe hypotension.

We believe that the use of invasive hemodynamic monitoring is rarely indicated in managing these patients. Its use for the above indications is empiric, and its benefit has not been conclusively proven. We believe that only a select group of women with pulmonary edema may benefit from invasive hemodynamic monitoring.[236]

Management

If the patient is already in spontaneous labor, continuous electronic fetal heart rate and uterine activity monitoring should be instituted in all cases. If labor is not well established, and in the absence of fetal malpresentation or a nonreassuring fetal heart rate tracing, intravenous oxytocin can be administered to induce labor. This approach is used in patients with a favorable cervix and with a gestational age of 30 weeks or more irrespective of cervical status. In patients with an unripe cervix and a gestational age of less than 30 weeks, either cervical ripening agents or elective cesarean delivery may be used for patients with severe preeclampsia or eclampsia. This approach is based on our experience of a high incidence of intrapartum complications such as abruptio placentae and nonreassuring fetal heart rate tracings in these patients.

At delivery, blood loss may be increased above that expected in normal patients. Magnesium sulfate may impair uterine contractility after delivery. The woman with severe preeclampsia or eclampsia has a contracted blood volume and tolerates blood loss poorly. For these reasons, these patients should have blood typed and cross-matched and available in the delivery area. A sudden drop in blood pressure following delivery may be due to hypovolemia and require prompt transfusion.

Following delivery, the patient should be kept in the recovery room under close observation for about 24 hours, during which magnesium sulfate should be continued. Most patients will show evidence of resolution of the disease process within 24 hours. However, some patients, especially those with the HELLP syndrome or severe disease in the mid-trimester, may require intensive monitoring for several days. Such patients will require magnesium sulfate administration for more than 24 hours. These patients are at increased risk for the development of pulmonary edema from fluid overload, fluid mobilization, and compromised renal function.

Maternal and Perinatal Outcome with Preeclampsia

Perinatal outcome in preeclampsia is usually dependent on one or more of the following factors: gestational age at the onset of preeclampsia and at the time of delivery, the severity of the disease process, the presence of multiple gestation, and the presence of underlying hypertensive or renal disease. For patients with mild disease at term, the perinatal mortality, incidence of fetal growth restriction, and neonatal morbidity are similar to those of normotensive pregnancies. At the E.H. Crump Women's Hospital in Memphis, the perinatal mortality rate in these pregnancies is 1 in 1,000, and the incidence of fetal growth restriction is only 4 percent.

In contrast, in women with severe preeclampsia remote from term, perinatal outcome will depend on gestational age at the time of delivery (Table 28–14). Overall, perinatal outcome is good if disease develops beyond 32 weeks' gestation, whereas it is less favorable for women requiring delivery at less than or equal to 28 weeks.[237]

Severe preeclampsia is a major cause of maternal mortality and morbidity. Complicated or mismanaged cases are responsible for most deaths. Patients with onset in the mid-trimester and those with the HELLP syndrome and pulmonary edema are at significant risk for maternal mortality and morbidity.[170]

Counseling Women Who Have Had Preeclampsia in Prior Pregnancies

There appears to be a strong familial predisposition for preeclampsia. The incidence of severe preeclampsia was compared in the first pregnancies of sisters of primi-

Table 28–14. PREGNANCY OUTCOMES OF 269 WOMEN WITH HELLP SYNDROME, PARTIAL HELLP SYNDROME, AND SEVERE PREECLAMPSIA WITH NORMAL LABORATORY VALUES

	HELLP (n = 68)	pHELLP (n = 65)	Severe (n = 136)
Gestational age at delivery (wk)*	30.7 ± 3.2*	31.2 ± 3.3†	32.7 ± 2.8
5-minute Apgar ≤6 (%)	29	23	13
Birth weight (g)*	1,340 ± 562*	1,552 ± 731†	1,795 ± 706
IUGR (%)	28	31	22
Neonatal death			
≤28 wk	4/18 (22)	4/15 (27)	3/14 (21)
29–33 wk	0/30 (0)	1/26 (4)	2/40 (5)
33–36 wk	1/20 (5)	0/24 (0)	0/82 (0)

* $p < 0.005$ compared with severe.
† $p < 0.05$ compared with severe.
HELLP, hemolysis, elevated liver enzymes, low platelets; pHELLP, partial HELLP; IUGR, intrauterine growth restriction.
Adapted from Abramovici D, Friedman SA, Mercer BM, et al: Neonatal outcome in severe preeclampsia at 24 to 36 weeks' gestation: does the HELLP (hemolysis, elevated liver enzymes, and low platelet count) syndrome matter? Am J Obstet Gynecol 180:221, 1999, with permission.

gravidas with and without preeclampsia.[238] In 273 primigravidas whose sisters did not have preeclampsia, the incidence of severe preeclampsia was 4.5 percent. However, the incidence of severe preeclampsia was 13.8 percent for women whose sisters had severe preeclampsia during their first pregnancies. The frequency of severe preeclampsia in the mothers and mothers-in-law of women in whom preeclampsia developed during their first pregnancies has been examined as well. The incidence of severe preeclampsia was 15.9 percent in the 126 mothers of primigravidas who had severe preeclampsia compared with 4.4 percent in the 136 mothers-in-law. The incidence of severe preeclampsia in a control group of primigravidas was 3.1 percent. The incidence of mild preeclampsia was higher in the mothers than in the mothers-in-law of these women, but this difference was not significant.

We have examined the pregnancy outcomes and incidences of preeclampsia in subsequent pregnancies, as well as the frequency of chronic hypertension and diabetes mellitus in women who had severe preeclampsia (287 women) or eclampsia (119 women) in their first pregnancies (aged 11 to 25 years) compared with 409 women (aged 12 to 25 years) who remained normotensive during their first pregnancies. Each woman had at least one subsequent pregnancy (range, 1 to 11) and was followed for a minimum of 2 years (range, 2 to 24). There was no significant difference in the incidences of diabetes mellitus in the two groups (1.3 vs. 1.5 percent). The incidence of chronic hypertension was significantly higher in the preeclampsia patients (14.8 vs. 5.6 percent; $p < 0.001$). This difference became even greater for those women followed for more than 10 years (51 vs. 14 percent; $p < 0.001$). The incidence of severe preeclampsia was also significantly higher in the second pregnancies (25.9 to 4.6 percent) as well as in the subsequent pregnancies (12.2 to 5.0 percent) of women with preeclampsia.[239]

In a later report, subsequent pregnancy outcome and long-term prognosis were studied in 108 women who had severe preeclampsia in the second trimester.[240] These women were followed for a minimum of 2 years (range, 2 to 12 years) and had a total of 169 subsequent pregnancies. Fifty-nine (35 percent) subsequent pregnancies were normotensive, and 110 (65 percent) were complicated by preeclampsia. Overall, 21 percent of all subsequent pregnancies were complicated by severe preeclampsia in the second trimester. In addition, these women had a high rate of chronic hypertension on follow-up, with the highest incidence being in those who had recurrent severe preeclampsia in the second trimester (55 percent).

Some women with preeclampsia remote from term may have abruptio placentae. The risk of this complication is increased significantly in those with severe preeclampsia before 34 weeks' gestation and particularly in those who have severe preeclampsia in the second trimester.[241] For patients with preeclampsia complicated by abruptio placentae, the risk of subsequent abruptio ranges from 5 to 20 percent. In addition, these women are at increased risk for subsequent chronic hypertension.[241]

Pregnancy outcome and long-term prognosis were studied in 37 women with severe preeclampsia complicated by pulmonary edema, and 18 of these women had subsequent pregnancies.[226] Ten of the 18 were normotensive, four were complicated by chronic hypertension, and four by preeclampsia; one of the latter women also had pulmonary edema.

Pregnancy outcome and remote prognosis were also studied in 18 women with severe preeclampsia complicated by acute renal failure.[242] All 18 had acute tubular necrosis, 9 required dialysis, and 2 died within 8 weeks after birth. All patients had serial evaluation of renal function, urine microscopic testing, and electrolyte studies at the onset of acute renal failure and during follow-up. All 16 surviving patients had normal renal function on long-term follow-up (average, 4 years). Four of the 16 women had seven subsequent pregnancies: one ended in miscarriage, one was complicated by preeclampsia at 35 weeks, and five were term pregnancies without complications.[242]

Patients with preeclampsia and the HELLP syndrome can receive oral contraceptives without any risk of developing the syndrome again. In addition, the recurrence risk for this syndrome in subsequent pregnancies is low. Sibai and associates[243] followed 152 patients with previous HELLP syndrome through their subsequent pregnancies. Thirteen patients with preexisting chronic hypertension had 20 subsequent pregnancies, whereas 139 normotensive women had 192 subsequent pregnancies following HELLP. The outcomes of these pregnancies are listed in Table 28–15. Overall, the risk for recurrent HELLP syndrome was 5 percent in women with preexisting chronic hypertension and 3 percent in normotensive women.[243] Two women with previous ruptured liver hematomas were followed through three subsequent pregnancies without complications. Two other case reports described successful pregnancy outcomes in women with previous ruptured liver hematomas.[244,245]

Patients with preeclampsia remote from term are reportedly at increased risk for undiagnosed renal disease. In one report, renal function was studied 6 weeks to 6 months postpartum in 84 women who had severe preeclampsia at 24 to 36 weeks' gestation.[248] Maternal evaluation included a 24-hour urine collection, urine microscopic testing, intravenous pyelography, and renal biopsy when appropriate. The authors found a high incidence of renal disease and essential chronic hypertension (90 percent) in these women. In two thirds, the renal lesion was glomerulonephritis, mostly of the im-

Table 28–15. SUBSEQUENT PREGNANCY OUTCOME AFTER HELLP SYNDROME IN THE INDEX PREGNANCY

	Normotensive ($n = 139$)	Hypertensive ($n = 13$)	Significance
Pregnancies (No.)	192	20	
Normotensive (%)*	73	—	
Hypertension only (%)	8	25	$p = 0.09$
Preeclampsia (%)	19	75	$p < 0.001$
Mild (%)	11	15	$p = 0.48$
Severe (%)	6	55	$p < 0.001$
HELLP (%)	3	5	$p = 0.45$
Delivery <37 weeks (%)	21	80	$p < 0.001$
IUGR (<10th percentile) (%)	12	45	$p < 0.001$
Abruptio placentae (%)	2	20	$p = 0.002$
Perinatal death (%)	4	40	$p < 0.001$

HELLP, hemolysis, elevated liver enzymes, low platelets; IUGR, intrauterine growth restriction.
* Percentage of pregnancies.
From Sibai BM, Ramadan MK, Chari RS, Friedman SA: Pregnancies complicated by hemolysis, elevated liver enzymes, and low platelets (HELLP): subsequent pregnancy outcome and long–term prognosis. Am J Obstet Gynecol 172:125, 1995, with permission.

munoglobulin A variety. They concluded that women with severe preeclampsia remote from term may have underlying renal disease for which they should be evaluated after delivery.

Recently, several studies have suggested evaluating women with severe preeclampsia before 34 weeks' gestation for the presence of thrombophilias.[61–69] However, subsequent reports did not confirm a high rate of association between thrombophilias and severe early onset of preeclampsia. At present, more data are needed before such screening is recommended for all women with previous severe preeclampsia.[69]

ECLAMPSIA

Eclampsia is the occurrence of convulsions or coma unrelated to other cerebral conditions with signs and symptoms of preeclampsia. Early writings of both the Egyptians and Chinese warned of the dangers of convulsions encountered during pregnancy.[247] Hippocrates noted that headaches, convulsions, and drowsiness were ominous signs associated with pregnancy. The term *eclampsia* appeared in a treatise on gynecology written by Varandaeus in 1619. Clonic spasms in association with pregnancy were described by Pew in 1694. In 1772, De la Motte recognized that prompt delivery of pregnant women with convulsions favored their recovery. Stroganoff, in 1900, reported a 5.4 percent maternal mortality rate compared with 17 to 29 percent for European clinics and 21 to 49 percent for American clinics of the same period.[248] Stroganoff placed his patients in a darkened room and administered chloro-

form, chloral hydrate, and morphine to produce profound sedation and narcosis. Modifications were made in this regimen; eventually, magnesium sulfate was popularized by Pritchard and Zuspan as the drug of choice for eclampsia.

Pathophysiology

Although great advances have been made in treating eclampsia, the pathophysiologic events leading to convulsions remain unknown. Several theories have been advanced but are unproven. There is a functional derangement of multiple organ systems, such as the central nervous system and hematologic, hepatic, renal, and cardiovascular systems.[249] The degree of dysfunction depends not only on other medical or obstetric factors that may be present but on whether there has been a delay in the treatment of preeclampsia or iatrogenic complicating factors as well (see the box "Organ System Derangements in Eclampsia").

Women in whom eclampsia develops exhibit a wide spectrum of signs and symptoms, ranging from extremely high blood pressure, 4+ proteinuria, generalized edema, and 4+ patellar reflexes to minimal blood pressure elevation, no proteinuria or edema, and normal reflexes.

Eclampsia usually begins as a gradual process, starting with rapid weight gain and ending with the onset of generalized convulsions or coma. Excess weight gain (with or without clinical edema) of more than 2 pounds per week during the last trimester may be the first warning sign. Hypertension is the hallmark of eclampsia and excess weight gain or edema are not necessary for the diagnosis.[8] In about 16 percent of

Organ System Derangements in Eclampsia

Cardiovascular
  Generalized vasospasm
  Increased peripheral vascular resistance
  Increased left ventricular stroke work index
  Decreased central venous pressure
  Decreased pulmonary wedge pressure
Hematologic
  Decreased plasma volume
  Increased blood viscosity
  Hemoconcentration
  Coagulopathy
Renal
  Decreased glomerular filtration rate
  Decreased renal plasma flow
  Decreased uric acid clearance
Hepatic (at autopsy)
  Periportal necrosis
  Hepatocellular damage
  Subcapsular hematoma
Central nervous system (at autopsy)
  Cerebral edema
  Cerebral hemorrhage

Table 28–16. GESTATIONAL AGE AT ONSET OF CONVULSIONS ($n = 399$)

Weeks' Gestation	Total Cases No.	Total Cases %	Postpartum Cases (n)
≤20	6	1.5	0
21–27	31	7.8	3
28–31	55	14.0	3
≥32	305	78.2	104

From Mattar F, Sibai BM: Eclampsia VIII. Risk factors for maternal morbidity. Am J Obstet Gynecol 182:307, 2000.

population and the number of maternal referrals to the hospital. At the University of Mississippi Medical Center, the incidence of eclampsia was 1 in 147 from 1955 to 1960 and 1 in 254 from 1971 to mid-1973.[250] Of interest, only 7.2 percent of these patients received prenatal care in the medical center's prenatal clinics. The incidence of eclampsia at the E. H. Crump Women's Hospital is now 1 in 337 deliveries; however, the hospital has a large number of referrals (approximately 2,000 women annually). Table 28–17 shows the incidences of eclampsia reported from several institutions.

Cerebral Pathology of Eclampsia

Autoregulation of the cerebral circulation is a mechanism for the maintenance of constant cerebral blood flow during changes in blood pressure and may be altered in eclampsia. Through active changes in cerebrovascular resistance at the arteriolar level, cerebral blood flow normally remains relatively constant when cerebral perfusion pressure ranges between 60 and 120 mm Hg. In this normal range, vasoconstriction of cerebral vessels occurs in response to elevations in blood pressure,

cases, hypertension may be "relative" (130 to 140/80 to 90 mm Hg), signified by a rise in blood pressure that is 25 mm Hg diastolic above the nonpregnant blood pressure reading. Eclampsia is usually associated with significant proteinuria (>2+ on dipstick). In eclamptic women, headache, visual disturbances, and right upper quadrant/epigastric pain are the most common premonitory symptoms before convulsions. Of interest was the absence of edema (26 percent) and proteinuria (14 percent) in 399 eclamptic women studied by the author.[8]

Convulsions may occur antepartum, intrapartum, or postpartum. Half of all cases of eclampsia usually occur before the onset of labor, with the other 50 percent equally divided between the intrapartum and postpartum periods. Analysis of 399 cases of eclampsia managed at our institution revealed that eclampsia developed before delivery in 289 patients (72 percent) and postpartum in 110 (28 percent).[8] Although rare, atypical eclampsia may occur before the 20th week of gestation and more than 48 hours after delivery.[250,251] Table 28–16 summarizes the time of onset of eclampsia among 399 eclamptic women studied by the author.[8]

Eclampsia is primarily a disease of the young primigravida. The incidence of eclampsia has ranged from 1 in 147 for 1 in 3,448 pregnancies,[252,253] with an incidence of 3.6 percent in twin gestations. The incidence depends on the socioeconomic status of the patient

Table 28–17. INCIDENCE OF ECLAMPSIA

Institution	Patient Population	Incidence
University of Tennessee (Memphis)		
1960–1970	All	1 in 300
1977–1992	All	1 in 337
University of Mississippi		
1955–1960	All	1 in 147
1971–mid-1973	All	1 in 254
University of Virginia		
1938–1963	All	1 in 235
1970–1976	All	1 in 623
Parkland Memorial Hospital		
1955–1975	All	1 in 766
Athens General (Athens, GA)		
1966–1975	All	1 in 1,228

while vasodilation occurs as blood pressure is lowered. Once cerebral perfusion pressure exceeds 130 to 150 mm Hg, however, the autoregulatory mechanism fails. In extreme hypertension, the normal compensatory vasoconstriction may become defective and cerebral blood flow increases. As a result, segments of the vessels become dilated, ischemic, and increasingly permeable. Thus, exudation of plasma occurs, giving rise to focal cerebral edema and compression of vessels, resulting in a decreased cerebral blood flow.[254] Hypertensive encephalopathy, a possible model for eclampsia, is an acute clinical condition that results from abrupt severe hypertension and subsequent severe increases in intracranial pressure. Since this is an acute disturbance in the hemodynamics of cerebral arterioles, morphologic changes in anatomy may not be uniformly evident in pathology material. Several autopsy findings that are relatively constant include cerebral swelling and fibrinoid necrosis of vessel walls. Petechial hemorrhages and microinfarcts may appear in some cases, not dissimilar to those noted in eclampsia.

The mechanisms leading to the development of convulsions or coma in eclamptic patients may include cerebral edema, ischemia, hemorrhage, or transient vasospasm. However, none of these mechanisms has been conclusively proven.

Computerized Axial Tomography

The introduction of the CAT scan has provided an opportunity to investigate the nature of cerebral abnormalities in eclamptic patients, although CAT scan and other imaging studies have not proven helpful in patient care. This technique is considered safe in pregnancy when performed beyond the first trimester. There are several reports describing the CAT scan findings in complicated cases of eclampsia (see the box "Reported Abnormal CAT Scan Findings in Complicated Eclampsia").[255,256]

Cerebral hemorrhage is a common autopsy finding in patients dying from eclampsia; however, it is an unusual finding on CAT scanning. Beck and Menezes[256] reported a case of eclampsia in which CAT scan evaluation demonstrated the presence of periventricular subependymal hemorrhage. Colosimo et al.[257] reported abnormal CAT scan findings in five eclamptic women, one of whom demonstrated the presence of intracerebral hemorrhage. Will et al.[258] reported on three patients with eclampsia who developed acute neurologic deterioration in the postpartum period. Two patients had subarachnoid hemorrhage, and one of them had a residual neurologic deficit. CAT scan demonstrated the presence of infarcts in two cases and intracerebral hemorrhage in the third case. In all three cases, cerebral angiography revealed widespread arterial vasoconstriction. In one case demonstrating hemorrhage on CAT

Reported CT Scan Findings in Complicated Eclampsia

Cerebral edema
   Diffuse white matter low-density areas
   Patchy areas of low density
   Occipital white matter edema
   Loss of normal cortical sulci
   Reduced ventricular size
   Acute hydrocephalus
Cerebral hemorrhage
   Intraventricular hemorrhage
   Parenchymal hemorrhage (high density)
Cerebral infarction
   Low-attenuation areas
   Basal ganglia infarctions

From Barton JR, Sibai BM: Cerebral pathology in eclampsia. *In* Sibai BM (ed): Clinics Perinatology, Vol. 18. Philadelphia, WB Saunders Company, 1991, p 891, with permission.

---

scan, a magnetic resonance imaging (MRI) examination performed 1 week later was reported normal.

Richards et al.[259] described the cranial CAT scan findings in 20 patients remaining in a coma for 6 hours or more after delivery. Scan appearance was normal in five patients (25 percent), while the remaining 15 patients (75 percent) had scans demonstrating low-density areas consistent with cerebral edema of varying degrees. A low-density pattern diffusely distributed throughout the white matter was regarded as the most severe form of edema. Three of four patients with this specific finding had significantly elevated intracranial pressure during monitoring.

Four large series presenting the CAT scan findings in eclampsia were reported. Abnormal CAT scan findings were found in 14 (29 percent) of 49 eclamptic patients studied by Brown and associates.[260] These authors noted that the incidence of abnormal CAT scan findings significantly increased with the recent use of high-resolution CAT scan equipment. The CAT scans were performed over a 6-year period, with the highest incidence of abnormal findings (50 percent) being present during the final year of the study. This increased sensitivity was attributed to improved "fourth-generation" imaging equipment. Furthermore, they noted that 50 to 60 percent of scans performed within 2 days of a seizure were normal, implying rapid reversal of abnormalities detected by CAT scan. The authors noted, however, that CAT scan findings altered the clinical management in only one patient. Milliez et al.[261] described cranial CAT scans in 44 women with eclampsia performed within 24 hours of seizure. Twenty-six scans (59 percent) were considered normal, while three (7 percent) had evidence of cerebral hemorrhage or thrombosis and six (14 percent) revealed areas of localized hypodensity located in the cortical lobes and the subcortical white matter. Of the remaining nine scans (20 percent), the interpretation was of minimal cerebral atrophy with enlarging cerebral ventricles. Moodley and associates[262] documented cranial CAT scan findings in 31 women with eclampsia. Ten of these women also had focal neurologic findings. Fourteen (45 percent) of the scans were considered abnormal. Lesions consistent with cerebral edema and multifocal hemorrhages have been described in CAT scans reported by Drislane and Wang.[263]

Magnetic Resonance Imaging and Eclampsia

MRI is a recently developed noninvasive technique that appears superior to other processes for defining intracranial anatomy and pathophysiology. The technique provides images in multiple planes, avoids the use of ionizing radiation, and, except for selected contraindications (some aneurysm clips, pacemakers), there are no significant health risks associated with MRI when used at present operating conditions.

There are several case reports and three large series describing abnormal MRI findings in eclampsia.[264,265] Sanders et al.[266] studied MRI findings in eight women with eclampsia. Abnormal findings were reported in seven of the eight women. Digre and associates[265] documented MRI findings in 16 women with severe preeclampsia and 10 women with eclampsia. They found that half of the women with severe preeclampsia had abnormal scans with nonspecific foci of increased signal in the deep cerebral white matter on T2-weighted images. In contrast, nine women with eclampsia had abnormal findings in the form of either a multifocal area of increased signal at the gray-white matter junction on T2-weighted images or cortical edema and hemorrhage. Dahmus et al.[255] compared MRI and CAT scan findings in 24 women with eclampsia. Forty-six percent of the MRIs were abnormal and 33 percent of the CAT scans were abnormal. The authors concluded that cerebral imaging is not necessary in women with uncomplicated eclampsia.[255] Hemorrhages and cerebral edema, particularly in the posterior hemispheres or in the watershed areas, were reported on MRI studies in women with eclampsia.[267] These findings are consistent with global ischemias probably induced by vasospasm.[267]

Angiography and Eclampsia

The use of cerebral angiography in the evaluation of eclampsia is limited.[264] Will et al.[258] described the cerebral angiographic findings in three patients with preeclampsia/eclampsia. All were significant for widespread arterial vasoconstriction of the intracranial vessels. Trommer et al.[268] reported cerebral angiography find-

ings in a single eclamptic patient. Similarly, they reported diffuse vasospasm of large- and medium-caliber cerebral vessels. Cranial CAT scan obtained following the angiography revealed diffuse hypodensity throughout the brain stem, thalamus, and internal capsules bilaterally. These few studies support cerebral vasoconstriction as an important cause of neurologic complications in preeclampsia. Similar findings were also reported with the use of cerebral and retinal vascular Doppler flow studies.

Doppler Studies and Eclampsia

The use of ultrasonographic Doppler techniques to study cerebral vasoconstriction in women with severe preeclampsia-eclampsia suggests that this process plays an important role in the etiology of cerebral manifestations in women with preeclampsia/eclampsia.[269–271]

Electroencephalographic Findings

Abnormal electroencephalograms (EEGs) have been reported in women with eclampsia.[254] Most common were changes compatible with a recent convulsive state. We performed EEGs on 65 women with eclampsia.[272] Initial EEGs were obtained within 48 hours of hospitalization and then serially during the next 6 months. Three women also had normal cerebral arteriograms. Forty-nine of the 65 patients with eclampsia (75 percent) had abnormal findings. All patients had adequate serum magnesium levels (4.5 to 11 mg/dl). Five of the 65 women demonstrated seizure activity on EEG with serum magnesium levels in the therapeutic range. It appears that magnesium suppresses seizure activity by a mechanism that does not alter the EEG. All the abnormalities noted on EEG are nonspecific and have been reported in other conditions such as polycythemia, hypoxia, renal disease, hypocalcemia, hypercalcemia, and water intoxication.[273]

Abnormal EEG findings were confirmed in 90 percent of eclamptic women studied by Moodley and associates.[262] EEG abnormalities were directly related to the severity of maternal hypertension, with some abnormal EEGs becoming normal after lowering blood pressure to the normotensive range. We found no correlation between the degree of blood pressure elevation and EEG abnormalities and consider it unlikely that these abnormal EEG changes were due to hypertensive encephalopathy alone.[273]

Management of Labor and Delivery in Eclampsia

The woman with eclampsia should undergo continuous intensive monitoring. She should not be left alone in a darkened room. The guard rails should be up on the bed and a padded tongue blade kept at the bedside. A large-bore peripheral intravenous line should be in place. No other anticonvulsants should be left at the bedside except for a syringe containing 2 to 4 g magnesium sulfate. Control of convulsions with magnesium sulfate is outlined below. We agree with Pritchard et al.[274] that no more than 8 g magnesium sulfate should be given over a short period of time to control convulsions.

No single test or set of laboratory determinations is useful in predicting maternal or neonatal outcome in women with eclampsia. Alterations in renal or hepatic function occur frequently. There is unlikely to be a significant disturbance in the integrity of the coagulation system. We previously recommended only a complete blood count including blood smear and platelet count, clot observation, and serum creatinine in women with eclampsia.[275] Liver function tests were obtained only in women with upper abdominal pain. However, because of an increase in the number of women with HELLP syndrome and eclampsia as well as those with serious medical problems, we have expanded the laboratory tests ordered in eclamptic women to include fibrinogen, electrolytes, and arterial blood gases.

Once convulsions have been controlled and the woman has regained consciousness, her general medical condition is assessed. When she is stable, induction of labor with oxytocin is initiated. Delivery is the treatment for eclampsia. Fetal heart rate and intensity of uterine contractions should be closely monitored. If labor is not well established, and in the absence of fetal malpresentation or fetal compromise, oxytocin may be used to induce labor in all patients beyond 30 weeks' gestation irrespective of cervical dilatation or effacement. The same approach is used for patients with a gestational age below 30 weeks if the cervix is favorable for induction. However, women with an unfavorable cervix and a gestational age of 30 weeks or less are stabilized with magnesium sulfate and are then delivered electively by cesarean section. This approach is based on our previous experience with high intrapartum complication rates in eclampsia that develops before 30 weeks' gestation.[276] These complications include a high incidence of fetal growth restriction (30 percent), abruption (23 percent), and fetal distress during labor (65 percent).

In a review of 10 women who had undergone electronic internal fetal monitoring during an eclamptic convulsion, 6 had fetal bradycardia (fetal heart rate <120 beats/min) that varied in duration from 30 seconds to 9 minutes.[277] The interval from onset of the seizure to the fall in fetal heart rate was 5 minutes. Transitory fetal tachycardia occurred frequently after the prolonged bradycardia. In addition, loss of beat-to-beat variability with transitory late decelerations occurred during the recovery phase. Uterine hyperactivity

demonstrated by both increased uterine tone and increased frequency of uterine contractions occurs during an eclamptic seizure. The duration of the increased uterine activity varies from 2 to 14 minutes.

Fetal outcome is generally good after an eclamptic convulsion. The mechanism for the transitory fetal bradycardia may be a decrease in uterine blood flow caused by intense vasospasm and uterine hyperactivity. The absence of maternal respiration during the convulsion may also be a contributing factor to these fetal heart rate changes. Since the fetal heart rate pattern usually returns to normal after a convulsion, other conditions should be considered if an abnormal pattern persists. It may take longer for the heart rate pattern to return to baseline in an eclamptic woman whose fetus is preterm with growth restriction. Placental abruption may occur after the convulsion and should be considered if uterine hyperactivity remains or the bradycardia persists.

Treatment of Eclamptic Convulsions

Eclamptic convulsions are a life-threatening emergency and require proper care in order to minimize morbidity and mortality. The development of an eclamptic convulsion is frightening to observe. Initially, the patient's face becomes distorted with protrusion of the eyes. This is followed by a congested facial expression. Foam often exudes from the mouth. The woman usually bites her tongue unless it is protected. Respirations are absent throughout the seizure. Typically, the convulsion, which can be divided into two phases, will continue for 60 to 75 seconds. The first phase, which lasts 15 to 20 seconds, begins with facial twitching, proceeding to the body becoming rigid with generalized muscular contractions. The second phase lasts approximately 60 seconds and consists of the muscles of the body alternately contracting and relaxing in rapid succession. This phase begins with the muscles of the jaw and rapidly involves the eyelids, other facial muscles, and then all the muscles of the body. Coma follows the convulsion, and the woman usually remembers nothing of the recent events. If she has repeated convulsions, some degree of consciousness returns after each convulsion. She may enter a combative state and be agitated and difficult to control. Rapid and deep respirations usually begin as soon as the convulsions end. Maintenance of oxygenation is usually not a problem after a single convulsion; the risk of aspiration is low in the well-managed patient.

Several steps should be taken in managing an eclamptic convulsion:

1. *Do not attempt to shorten or abolish the initial convulsion:* Because eclampsia is so frightening, the natural tendency is to do something to abolish the convulsion. Drugs such as diazepam should not be

given in an attempt to stop or shorten the convulsion, especially if the patient does not have an intravenous line in place and someone skilled in intubation is not immediately available. Diazepam causes phlebitis and venous thrombosis and should not be given without secure intravenous access. In addition, no more than 5 mg should be given over a 60-second period. Rapid administration of diazepam may lead to apnea or cardiac arrest, or both.[278]

2. *Prevent maternal injury during the convulsion:* A padded tongue blade should be inserted between the patient's teeth to prevent biting of the tongue. Care should be taken to avoid stimulating the gag reflex with the blade. Its only purpose is to prevent the patient from biting her tongue. Place the woman on her left side and then suction the foam and secretions from her mouth. That serious maternal injuries may occur during eclamptic seizures is well demonstrated in the report from Magee-Women's Hospital.[279] Among the 52 women with eclampsia, one had a dislocated shoulder, fractured humerus, and multiple facial contusions from a fall in the emergency room following a convulsion. Two other women had severe airway obstruction.

3. *Maintain adequate oxygenation:* After the convulsion has ceased, the patient begins to breathe again and oxygenation is rarely a problem. Difficulty with oxygenation may occur in women who have had repetitive convulsions or who have received drugs in an attempt to abolish the convulsions. Such women should have a chest radiograph to rule out aspiration pneumonia.

4. *Minimize the risk of aspiration:* Aspiration should be a rare occurrence with eclamptic convulsions. It may be caused by forcing the padded tongue blade to the back of the throat, stimulating the gag reflex with resultant vomiting and aspiration. At our hospital, all the women who have had aspiration as a result of eclamptic convulsions had received many drugs in an attempt to control their convulsions. The lungs should always be auscultated after the convulsion has ended to ensure they are clear.

5. *Give adequate magnesium sulfate to control the convulsions:* As soon as the convulsion has ended, a large secure intravenous (IV) line should be inserted and a loading dose of magnesium sulfate given intravenously. In our institution, we use a 6-g intravenous loading dose given over *15 to 20 minutes*. In addition to providing a good initial serum magnesium level, the serum magnesium level does not fall below the therapeutic range for several hours after the initial 6-g loading dose as often happens when using a 4-g loading dose. If the patient has a convulsion after the loading dose, another bolus of 2 g magnesium sulfate can be given intravenously over 3 to 5 minutes. Approximately 10 to 15 percent of

women will have a second convulsion after receiving the intravenous loading dose of magnesium sulfate. Pritchard et al.[274] reported that 10 of 83 women who had eclampsia treated before delivery again suffered convulsions shortly after an initial injection of magnesium sulfate, 4 g IV and 10 g intramuscularly (IM). However, most remained free of seizures after an additional 2 g magnesium sulfate IV.

We use serum magnesium levels in the clinical management of the eclamptic woman. If the initial level, obtained 4 hours after the loading dose, is high, over 10 mg/dl, we reduce the 2-g maintenance dose of magnesium sulfate. This will occasionally occur in women with renal compromise. Similarly, in the rare patient with a brisk urine output, we give a maintenance dose of 3 g to keep levels in the therapeutic range.

In my series of 262 eclamptic women, 36 (14 percent) had an additional convulsion after receiving magnesium sulfate.[280] An occasional patient will have recurrent convulsions while receiving therapeutic doses of magnesium sulfate. In these cases, a short-acting barbiturate such as sodium amobarbital can be given in a dose of up to 250 mg IV over 3 to 5 minutes. We treated one patient who had recurrent convulsions with a serum magnesium level of 9.4 mg/dl and who had also received sodium amobarbital. She was given an intravenous sodium pentothal drip and experienced no further seizures.

Magnesium toxicity was responsible for the only death in the Pritchard et al.[274] series of eclamptic women and nearly led to a maternal death at the University of Tennessee, Memphis.[281] In both cases, the patients were supposed to have received a loading dose of 4 g magnesium sulfate but, because of an error in preparing the drug, received 20 g magnesium sulfate over a few minutes.

Rarely, a woman may have an eclamptic seizure, lapse into a coma, and die. Magnesium toxicity should be considered in those women who do not regain consciousness. A case report of magnesium sulfate toxicity details the features of this serious complication.[281] Within a few minutes of starting what was supposed to be a magnesium loading dose, 4 g magnesium sulfate in 250 ml saline, the patient went into cardiorespiratory arrest. Immediate resuscitation including intubation was performed. Approximately one half of the loading dose had been given. An intracerebral accident or eclampsia was thought to be the cause of the coma; the loading dose was continued and maintenance therapy started. Initial blood gases were normal, and the electrocardiogram (ECG) was normal 15 minutes after the arrest. Mechanical ventilatory support was required. The patient's vital signs were stable, but her pupils were nonreactive. Serum electrolytes, glucose, blood urea nitrogen, and creatinine were normal. Computed tomographic scan of the head and cerebral angiograms were normal. A magnesium level of 35 mg/dl was reported 3.5 hours later from a blood sample taken via femoral venipuncture at the time of arrest. The magnesium sulfate infusion was stopped immediately. During the first 5 hours after the cardiorespiratory arrest, 1,344 mg of magnesium were excreted in the urine. Twelve hours after the arrest, an uncomplicated low vertical cesarean delivery was done for a breech presentation. The 3,160-g male infant had Apgar scores of 8 and 9 at 1 and 5 minutes, respectively. Maternal and cord blood magnesium levels at delivery were 5.8 mg/dl. Both mother and baby were discharged from the hospital with no apparent residual effects. Of interest, the patient reported she could hear and see what was occurring around her, but she could not make any movements while she had the endotracheal tube in place. Figure 28–6 presents the maternal magnesium levels in this case.[281]

6. *Maternal acidemia should be corrected:* We obtain a blood gas reading on every patient who has had an eclamptic convulsion. Blood oxygenation and pH should be in the normal range. Patients who have had repeated convulsions may be acidotic and a low PO$_2$ may indicate aspiration pneumonitis. Sodium bi-

carbonate is not given unless the pH is below 7.10. Abnormal blood gases may be the result of respiratory depression.

7. *Avoid polypharmacy:* Polypharmacy is extremely hazardous in the woman with eclampsia, as addition of diazepam or phenytoin may lead to respiratory depression or respiratory arrest.

During the past 60 years, numerous anticonvulsive drugs have been introduced and replaced due to the dissatisfaction with the results obtained with the use of these agents. These drugs have included bromethol, chloral hydrate, paraldehyde, phenothiazines, lytic cocktails, barbiturates, diazepam, chlordiazepoxide, and clonazepam. The overzealous use of these drugs in eclampsia can lead to significant maternal–neonatal central nervous system (CNS) and respiratory depression.[282] The use of large doses of diazepam (>30 mg) during labor is associated with loss of beat-to-beat fetal heart rate variability and significant neonatal morbidity including respiratory depression, apnea, hypotonia, cold stress, and poor sucking. The use of the barbiturate chlormethiozole, commonly used in Europe and Australia in anticonvulsive doses, may depress maternal laryngeal reflexes, thus increasing the likelihood of aspiration during convulsion. In addition, the use of intravenous phenobarbital has the potential of producing laryngospasm and circulatory and respiratory depression. Moreover, none of these drugs has been proven to be superior to or as effective as magnesium sulfate in treating eclamptic convulsions.[18]

There are five randomized studies comparing the use of magnesium sulfate to phenytoin or diazepam in eclampsia.[283–287] Dommisse[283] reported 22 patients with eclampsia who were randomly allocated to receive intravenous phenytoin or intravenous magnesium sulfate. None of 11 patients managed with magnesium sulfate had further convulsions, while 4 of 11 patients treated with phenytoin had another seizure. All four patients who failed phenytoin therapy were then effectively treated with magnesium sulfate, and the author suggested that magnesium sulfate is a more effective agent in eclampsia. Crowther,[284] in a randomized controlled trial, compared the use of magnesium sulfate and diazepam as an anticonvulsant in 51 eclamptic patients. She noted that the use of magnesium sulfate was associated with less serious morbidity, but the difference was not statistically significant. Balla et al.[285] compared magnesium sulfate to a lytic cocktail in 90 women with eclampsia, whereas Friedman et al.[286] compared magnesium sulfate to phenytoin in 24 eclamptic women. Both studies revealed magnesium sulfate to be superior for the prevention of eclamptic convulsion. The Eclampsia Trial Collaborative Group studied 1,680 women randomized to receive magnesium sulfate, diazepam, or phenytoin after convulsions. Magnesium sulfate proved

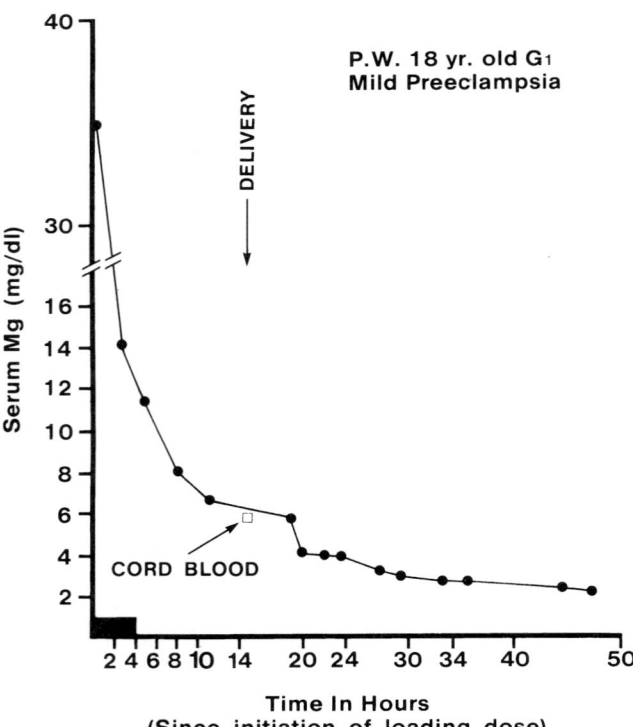

Figure 28–6. A patient with magnesium toxicity. (From McCubbin JH, Sibai BM, Abdella TN, et al: Cardiopulmonary arrest due to acute maternal hypermagnesemia, letter. Lancet 1:1058, 1981, with permission.)

Table 28–18. RANDOMIZED TRIALS COMPARING MAGNESIUM SULFATE VERSUS OTHER ANTICONVULSANTS IN ECLAMPSIA

Authors	Antihypertensive Therapy	Recurrent Seizures		RR (95% CI)
		MgSO$_4$, No. (%)	Other, No. (%)	
Dommisse[283]	Dihydralazine	0.11 (0)	4/11 (36.7)*	
Crowther[284]	Dihydralazine	5/24 (20.8)	7/27 (26)†	0.8 (0.29–2.2)
Bhalla et al.[285]	Nifedipine	1/45 (2.2)	11/45 (24.4)‡	0.09 (0.01–0.68)
Friedman et al.[286]	Nifedipine, labetalol	0/11 (0)	2/13 (15.4)*	
Collaborative Trial[287]	NR	60/453 (13.2)	126/452 (27.9)†	0.48 (0.36–0.63)
Collaborative Trial[287]	NR	22/388 (5.7)	66/387 (17.1)*	0.33 (0.21–0.53)
All studies		88/922 (9.4)	216/935 (23.1)	0.41 (0.32–0.51)

* Phenytoin.
† Diazepam.
‡ Lytic cocktail.
NR, not reported; MgSO$_4$, magnesium sulfate; RR, relative risk; CI, confidence interval.

superior in preventing recurrent seizures (Table 28–18).[287]

Atypical Eclampsia

Eclampsia occurring before the 20th week of gestation or more than 48 hours postpartum is exceedingly rare and, for lack of a better term, has been called *atypical eclampsia*. Eclampsia occurring before the 20th week of gestation has usually been reported with molar or hydropic degeneration of the placenta. Chesley et al.[288] observed 35 cases of probable eclampsia associated with molar degeneration of the placenta in a review of the literature through 1944. In 26 of these patients, eclampsia occurred during the first half of gestation. Six of the women had a coexistent fetus. A case report and a review of the literature was recently reported by Newman and Eddy.[289] Two cases of eclampsia have been reported without molar degeneration of the placenta during the first half of gestation.[290,291] In one woman who had Rh isoimmunization, eclampsia developed at 16 weeks' gestation. The placenta revealed cystic hydropic degeneration of the villi but no molar changes.

Although rare, eclampsia can occur during the first half of gestation.[8] These women may be misdiagnosed as having hypertensive encephalopathy or a seizure disorder. Women in whom convulsions develop in association with hypertension and proteinuria during the first half of pregnancy should be considered to have eclampsia. They should be treated with parenteral magnesium sulfate to control convulsions, with termination of pregnancy as the definitive goal.

Late postpartum eclampsia is eclampsia that occurs more than 48 hours after delivery. Of the women we have treated for eclampsia during the past 15 years, eclampsia developed in 54 patients more than 48 hours postpartum (16 percent). A review of the clinical course of late postpartum eclampsia has been reported.[251] Thirty of the 54 women described in that report had been treated for preeclampsia and received standard intravenous magnesium sulfate therapy. The mean duration of magnesium sulfate therapy was 32 hours (range, 24 to 72 hours). Several women were at home when the convulsions developed. Forty-five had experienced headaches or visual disturbances, blurred vision, and scotomas from 2 to 72 hours before the onset of convulsions.[251] The most striking finding in these women was the brisk diuresis that occurred immediately after the convulsion. Urinary outputs of 500 to 1,000 ml during the first hour after the seizure were common. Because of the unusual time of occurrence of eclampsia in these women, neurologic consultations are recommended to rule out abnormalities.[251]

Of interest is the high rate of occurrence of late postpartum eclampsia in Nigerian women. In a report of 25 cases of postpartum eclampsia, 17 (68 percent) occurred more than 48 hours postpartum.[292] Uric acid levels were elevated in these women with eclampsia before delivery or during the immediate postpartum period.

Maternity Morbidity and Mortality in Eclampsia

Pritchard et al.[274] reported only 1 maternal death in 245 women treated for eclampsia at Parkland Hospital (Dallas, TX) from 1955 to 1983, a maternal mortality rate of 0.4 percent. This death was caused by magnesium toxicity. Endotracheal intubation was not accomplished promptly in this short, obese woman; as a result, respiratory arrest, cardiorespiratory arrest, and death ensued. Three other women had respiratory depression.

Two maternal deaths occurred in our series of 399 patients with eclampsia.[8] One patient had five convulsions before arriving at our hospital and went into cardiorespiratory arrest in the parking lot. The patient was resuscitated, and her seizures were controlled with magnesium sulfate. However, the patient did not regain consciousness after cardiac arrest. She underwent a cesarean delivery for fetal distress and had a 3,090-g infant with normal Apgar scores. The child had no serious problems in the nursery and was discharged in good condition. DIC developed after the operation. The postoperative course was complicated by sepsis, continuing convulsions, and pulmonary insufficiency. An EEG on the second postoperative day demonstrated absent cortical activity. A CAT scan failed to demonstrate either intracerebral hemorrhage or cerebral edema. The patient remained comatose and died 8 weeks postpartum. The second patient also arrived with severe encephalopathy with cerebral herniation and subsequently died within 1 week postpartum from adult respiratory distress syndrome and multiorgan failure.[8]

Harbert et al.[293] reported 168 women treated for eclampsia between 1939 and 1963. Delivery within an arbitrary time limit after control of the convulsion was not an essential part of therapy. Forty-seven of the 83 patients in whom eclampsia occurred before the spontaneous onset of labor were delivered within 48 hours of the first convulsive episode. In the other 36 patients with eclampsia before delivery, the interval between occurrence of the convulsion and spontaneous onset of labor ranged from 93 hours to 43 days. During the first 6 years of the study, eight maternal deaths occurred. From December 1944 to termination of the study in 1963, 108 women with eclampsia were managed without another maternal death. The uncorrected perinatal mortality rate was 216 of 1,000, and 28 percent (14 fetal deaths and three neonatal deaths) in 60 patients delivered 72 hours or longer after admission.

Lopez-Llera[294] reviewed 990 cases of eclampsia in Mexican women during a 22-year period ending in 1985. There were 138 deaths, for a mortality rate of 14 percent. Several factors were found to increase the risk of maternal death: eclampsia at an earlier gestational age, maternal age, underlying disease, and multiple gestation. In addition, Douglas and Redman reported on maternal mortality and morbidity among women with eclampsia from the United Kingdom.[295] They found that antepartum onset and onset before 37 weeks' gestation was associated with high maternal morbidity. We found similar results when eclampsia develops before 32 weeks' gestation.[8]

In our experience, primigravid women with eclampsia have a lower incidence of serious complications than multigravid women. This is probably attributable to the higher incidence of chronic hypertension and underlying renal disease in the multigravid patients rather than to any effect of eclampsia per se. In particular, we believe that careful attention should be given to intravenous fluid therapy in multigravid women with eclampsia. In our experience, pulmonary edema is much more likely to develop in this group. Likewise, the incidence of renal failure is much higher in multigravid patients with eclampsia.

In our series, maternal transfers and patients who had received no prenatal care had higher complication rates. More than 90 percent of women with eclampsia who had no prenatal care were first seen in the emergency room of another hospital. Many were treated by a physician who was seeing his or her first case of eclampsia. Referral often occurred before the women had received adequate treatment with magnesium sulfate.

Perinatal Outcome in Eclampsia

The main risks to the fetus of the eclamptic woman are abruptio placentae, prematurity, intrauterine growth restriction, and hypoxic episodes during the convulsions.[8,274,294,295]

Sibai et al.[296] followed 28 premature infants and 14 full-term infants of eclamptic mothers for up to 50 months. Eight of the 12 infants who were small for gestational age by weight at birth showed catch-up growth at an average of 20.6 months (range, 2 to 48 months). In all, only two of the infants remained growth restricted by weight, height, and head circumference; both were mentally retarded. A total of three infants had major neurologic deficits resulting in cerebral palsy and mental retardation on follow-up evaluation. General health continued to be a problem for the premature infants during the first year of life. Several had multiple hospitalizations for either pulmonary or neurologic complications.

Maternal Transport of the Eclamptic Patient

During the past 20 years, there has been a marked reduction in the number of eclamptic patients. Consequently, most obstetricians have little or no experience in the management of eclampsia. A recent survey of a random sample of obstetricians from all 50 states indicated that about 50 percent of obstetricians in private practice had not seen an eclamptic patient during the past year.

Because management of the eclamptic patient requires the availability of neonatal and obstetric intensive care units and personnel with special expertise, we believe that eclamptic patients should not be managed at Level I hospitals. We recommend that eclamptic patients with term gestations be cared for only at Level II or III hospitals with adequate facilities and with consultants from other specialties, if needed. For those eclamptic patients who are remote from term, referral should be made to a tertiary care center. We recommend that the following steps be taken before transfer of these critically ill patients:

1. The referring physician or nurse should consult with the physician at the perinatal center regarding the referral and appropriate treatment. All maternal records including prenatal data and a detailed summary of the patient's condition should be sent with the patient.
2. Blood pressure should be stabilized and convulsions controlled.
3. Adequate prophylactic anticonvulsive medications should be given. An accepted regimen is 4 g intravenous magnesium sulfate as a loading dose, with a simultaneous intramuscular dose of 10 g.
4. Such patients should be sent in an ambulance with medical personnel in attendance for proper management in case of subsequent convulsions.

Can Eclampsia Be Prevented?

Eclampsia is generally considered a preventable complication of pregnancy. Zuspan[295] believes that the severe forms of preeclampsia should be preventable by appropriate prenatal care. He also contends that convulsions should not occur once the woman with preeclampsia is admitted to the hospital.

We recently reviewed 254 cases of eclampsia treated at the University of Tennessee in an attempt to determine the number of cases of preventable eclampsia.[296] All factors that may have been involved in the development of eclampsia were reviewed. Patients were then grouped into categories of physician error, patient failure, and failure of magnesium sulfate therapy. We found that about 30 percent of cases were nonpreventable.

These findings are in agreement with those of Campbell and Templeton,[297] who studied factors leading to the development of eclampsia in 66 patients. These workers found that in 28 patients (42.4 percent), eclampsia was not preventable.

Counseling Women with Eclampsia and Their Relatives

Bryans et al.,[298] in their long-term follow-up study of women who had eclampsia treated at the Medical College of Georgia, found no increase in hypertension in these patients above that expected in the general female population. They concluded that preeclampsia/eclampsia did not cause hypertensive disease and was not a manifestation of subsequent essential hypertension in pregnant women. Chesley et al.[299] followed women who developed eclampsia at the Margaret Hague Hospital from its opening in 1931 through 1951. They traced all but three of the women who survived to 1974. Chesley et al. also concluded that eclampsia does not cause hypertension. The average annual death rate was 5.11 per 1,000, with 31 deaths in the 187 Caucasian women who had eclampsia during their pregnancies. This was not significantly different from the number of deaths expected. However, 33 of 59 Caucasian women who had eclampsia as multiparas had died at an average rate of 21.3 per 1,000, which was significantly higher than the expected mortality rate. Eighty-two percent of the remote deaths were due to cardiovascular/renal disease in the multiparous group.

Chesley et al.[300] reported that the prognosis for future pregnancies after eclampsia was good. Another 409 pregnancies occurred in the 158 women with eclampsia during their first pregnancy. Preeclampsia/eclampsia recurred in 34.5 percent of the women and in 20.6 percent of their subsequent pregnancies. When hypertension occurred in a future pregnancy, it was usually mild. Eclampsia developed in three women, for an incidence of 0.9 percent in pregnancies beyond 20 weeks' gestation.

The sisters and daughters of eclamptic women are at increased risk for the development of preeclampsia and eclampsia.[301] Chesley et al.[302] reviewed the incidence of preeclampsia in the first pregnancies of daughters of eclamptic mothers. Preeclampsia occurred in 63 of the 257 first pregnancies (24.9 percent), and eclampsia in seven pregnancies (2.7 percent). The outcomes of the first pregnancies carried to viability by sisters of eclamptic women were also studied. Preeclampsia was observed in 54 (37 percent) of first pregnancies, and eclampsia developed in six women (4.1 percent). Because of the increased risk of preeclampsia/eclampsia in these siblings, their pregnancies should be closely monitored.

During the past 20 years, four studies have described pregnancy outcomes after eclampsia.[302–304] The incidence of preeclampsia is much higher in future pregnancies in women who have had eclampsia remote from term.

Sibai and associates[305] studied the long-term effects of eclampsia on maternal blood pressure in 210 women who were normotensive prior to the eclamptic pregnancy. The average duration of follow-up in these women was 7.2 years (range, 2 to 13 years). The overall incidence of chronic hypertension on follow-up was only 9.5 percent.

CHRONIC HYPERTENSION

Pathophysiology of Chronic Hypertension

Patients with labile or borderline hypertension have several pathophysiologic alterations with elevated cardiac output, central redistribution of blood volume, enhanced activity of the autonomic nervous system, increased left ventricular ejection rate, and a normal total peripheral resistance.[306] However, patients with mild to moderate hypertension have a normal cardiac output. In these cases, the increase in blood pressure is due to an increase in total peripheral resistance. Because vascular resistance and arterial pressure are elevated, ventricular workload is increased. The heart rate may be increased, while stroke volume and left ventricular ejection rate are normal. Over time, the patient with moderate essential hypertension will show evidence of cardiac strain. Stroke volume remains normal or may start to fall. Myocardial contractility remains normal, while ECG studies frequently show an increased thickness of the left ventricular wall. In the absence of renal disease, plasma volume contraction is proportionate to the increase in diastolic blood pressure. When the diastolic blood pressure equals or exceeds 105 mm Hg, a decrease in plasma volume becomes more apparent.

Clinical evidence of end organ damage characterizes severe essential hypertension. Cardiac enlargement is evident on chest radiograph and ECG. Total peripheral resistance becomes even higher, and cardiac output may begin to fall. Stroke volume decreases, and intravascular volume decreases still further. With the decrease in cardiac output and intravascular volume, plasma renin activity rises. These changes lead to a great increase in left ventricular tension, making myocardial contractions increasingly difficult. Pulmonary edema will occur if the patient is not treated.

Diagnosis of Chronic Hypertension

The diagnosis of chronic hypertension in pregnancy is usually made on the basis of either of the following:

1. Documented history of high blood pressure antedating pregnancy
2. Persistent elevation of blood pressure (at least 140/90 mm Hg) on two occasions more than 24 hours apart before the 20th week of gestation

When a firm diagnosis, by both or either of the above findings, cannot be made, other findings might be suggestive of the presence of chronic hypertension:

1. Retinal changes on funduscopic examination
2. Cardiac enlargement on chest radiograph and ECG
3. Compromised renal function or associated renal disease
4. Presence of medical disorders known to lead to hypertension
5. Multiparity with previous history of hypertensive pregnancies
6. Evidence of persistent hypertension beyond the 42nd day postpartum

Sometimes the diagnosis is difficult to make because of the marked and variable changes seen with blood pressure during midpregnancy. This becomes problematic in patients with no prior medical care and who are first seen in early third trimester. Chesley and Annitto[307] observed that women with chronic hypertension show greater decreases in their blood pressure during pregnancy than do normotensive patients. They reported a marked decrease in 39 percent of 301 pregnancies studied. They also noted that during midpregnancy the blood pressure was in the normal range in women who were severely hypertensive prior to pregnancy. Similar findings were observed at our institution in the course of pregnancy in 211 patients with mild chronic hypertension.[308]

Etiology and Classification of Chronic Hypertension

Essential hypertension is by far the most common cause of chronic hypertension during pregnancy. Chronic hypertension in pregnancy is classified as mild or severe depending on the systolic or diastolic blood pressure reading. The hypertension is classified as mild if systolic blood pressure is less than 160 mm Hg and the diastolic is less than 110 mm Hg. Hypertension is severe if either systolic pressure is more than 160 mm Hg or diastolic pressure is above 110 mm Hg.

Superimposed preeclampsia is defined as exacerbation of hypertension of at least 30 mm Hg in systolic or at least 15 mm Hg in diastolic blood pressure, together with the development of proteinuria during the course of the pregnancy (at least 500 mg/24 h), or exacerbation of preexisting proteinuria (at least 5 g/24 h), and elevation of serum liver enzymes, low platelets, or development of symptoms.[10]

Maternal and Fetal Risks of Chronic Hypertension

Pregnancies complicated by chronic hypertension are at increased risk for the development of superimposed preeclampsia, abruptio placentae, and poor perinatal outcome. The reported incidence of superimposed preeclampsia ranges from 4.7 to 52 percent depending on the severity of hypertension at the onset of pregnancy and on the criteria used to make the diagnosis.[307-310] As for the severity of hypertension in the first trimester, the reported incidence of superimposed preeclampsia ranged from 28.2 to 52 percent in severe chronic hypertension, and this rate was unaffected by the use of antihypertensive medication.[310,311] On the other hand, the reported incidence for patients with mild hypertension in pregnancy was as low as 4.7 percent.[312] Three large observational studies have recently described the fetal risks in women with chronic hypertension.[8,313,314] The rates of superimposed preeclampsia in these studies ranged from 17 to 25 percent. In addition, the risks of growth-restricted infants and perinatal deaths were increased, particularly in the presence of superimposed preeclampsia.

The criteria used to diagnose superimposed preeclampsia have included one or more of the following: exacerbation of hypertension, development of edema, appearance of proteinuria, and elevation of serum uric acid levels (>6 mg/dl). In general, the incidence of this complication will be high if only exacerbation of blood pressure is used in the diagnosis, whereas this incidence will be lower if significant proteinuria (>1 g/24 h) is added. This incidence is increased in severe disease (25 to 52 percent).[310] Some pregnant chronic hypertensives may have silent undiagnosed chronic renal disease and may experience urinary protein excretion that increases with advancing gestation, particularly in the third trimester (usually >300 mg, but <1 g/24 h); many of these women will also demonstrate an increase in either their systolic (>30 mm Hg) or diastolic (>15 mm Hg) blood pressure with advancing gestation.[315] Therefore, it is recommended that superimposed preeclampsia be diagnosed on the basis of exacerbated hypertension *plus* the development of either substantial proteinuria (>1 g/24 h) or elevated serum uric acid levels. In women on antihypertensive medications where exacerbation of blood pressure is less common, the diagnosis should be based on the development of substantial proteinuria and abnormal laboratory tests or symptoms.[10]

In general, pregnancies complicated only by exacerbation of blood pressure have a perinatal outcome similar to those in normotensive women, while the appearance of proteinuria is more significant for fetal prognosis since most of the poor perinatal outcomes are associated with proteinuria. Because many obstetricians consider superimposed preeclampsia an indication for delivery, it is important to use strict criteria to avoid unnecessary preterm delivery.

The incidence of abruptio placentae is reportedly increased in chronic hypertension and ranges between 0.45 and 10 percent depending on the duration and the severity of hypertension. For those with mild uncomplicated disease, the incidence has ranged from 0.45 to 2.0 percent,[313-317] while in cases with severe hypertension the incidence was markedly increased from 2.3 to 10 percent.[307,310] This incidence is not influenced by the use of antihypertensive medications.[317] In cases complicated by abruptio placentae, superimposed preeclampsia is associated with a higher perinatal mortality. This incidence is substantially increased in those with a history of abruption in previous pregnancies.[318]

The above-mentioned complications are responsible for most for the perinatal deaths as well as the increased incidence of fetal growth restriction and premature delivery in such pregnancies. In addition, these pregnancies are reportedly associated with increased frequency of midtrimester losses, particularly in those not receiving antihypertensive therapy.[313,319,320] In general, perinatal mortality and morbidity are not increased in patients with uncomplicated mild chronic hypertension, whereas they are markedly increased in patients with severe disease, in those with renal disease, and in those complicated by superimposed preeclampsia.[2,309]

Pregnancy Outcome in Relation to Treatment of Chronic Hypertension

There is general agreement that chronic antihypertensive therapy will decrease the incidence of cardiovascular complications and cerebrovascular accidents in nonpregnant patients with diastolic blood pressures exceeding 105 mm Hg. In addition, since maternal mortality and morbidity are increased in pregnant women with diastolic blood pressures of 110 mm Hg or higher,[309,310] there are potential maternal and fetal benefits from treating severe chronic hypertension during pregnancy.[321] However, it is not clear if antihypertensives are equally beneficial in pregnancies with mild uncomplicated hypertension, which is seen in about 95 percent of all pregnant women with chronic hypertension. In addition, neither controlled nor uncontrolled studies showed any reduction in the incidence of superimposed preeclampsia or abruptio placentae when antihypertensives were used.[2,310]

Severe Chronic Hypertension in Pregnancy

There are few reports describing pregnancy outcomes in women with severe chronic hypertension. Three retrospective studies described pregnancy outcomes in untreated women with severe chronic hypertension early in pregnancy.[307,311,322] These studies were conducted during 1931 to 1953, before modern advances in obstetric and neonatal practices. The reported perinatal survival ranged from 19 to 50 percent, and most of the fetal losses occurred in women with superimposed preeclampsia. In addition, the studies reported an increased frequency of maternal mortality and morbidity, both acute and long term. As a result, the reported maternal and perinatal outcome was invariably poor. Hence, concerns about the risk of acute renal failure and cerebrovascular accidents have led many obstetricians to recommend early termination of such pregnancies. A recent survey of American obstetricians (B.M. Sibai and D.L. Watson, unpublished data) found that 20 percent of the respondents recommended termination of such pregnancies regardless of renal function, while 45 percent did so only in the presence of impaired renal function.

In 1966, Kincaid-Smith et al.[321] reported pregnancy outcomes in 32 patients with severe hypertension who were treated with methyldopa during their pregnancy. The perinatal survival was 90.7 percent, and there were no maternal complications. The authors attributed this good outcome to the control of maternal blood pressure with methyldopa. However, only five subjects were started on treatment during the first trimester, while 27 received treatment during the second or third trimester. Recently, Sibai et al.[310] documented pregnancy outcomes in 44 patients with severe hypertension who were seen during the first trimester. Each was treated with methyldopa and oral hydralazine as needed to keep diastolic blood pressure below 110 mm Hg. The patients were observed closely throughout pregnancy, with frequent prenatal visits and intensive monitoring of the clinical status of both mother and fetus. Twenty-three women (52 percent) developed superimposed preeclampsia; there were no maternal deaths. The total perinatal survival was 75 percent; 31 infants (70 percent) were delivered preterm and 19 (43 percent) were small for gestational age (Table 28–19). However, among the subjects without superimposed preeclampsia, there were no perinatal deaths and only one infant (5 percent) was small for gestational age. These findings argue against the practice of recommending termination of pregnancy for severe hypertension in the first trimester. However, such women should be counseled regarding the potential maternal risks, and they must be observed and managed at a tertiary care center with adequate maternal–neonatal care facilities.

Mild Chronic Hypertension in Pregnancy

There are many reports, both retrospective and prospective, describing pregnancy outcome in women with mild to moderate hypertension. It is, however, difficult to evaluate or compare the benefits of antihypertensive therapy in the management of these pregnancies because of differences in definition, populations studied, and treatments used. Some of these studies were controlled, and others were selective; some studied chronic hypertension only, yet others included all forms of hypertension. Some compared treatment with no treatment or with placebo, others compared two different antihypertensive drugs, and still others used a combination of drugs. In addition, the gestational ages at treatment and the durations of therapy were highly variable.[2,309]

Methyldopa is the drug most commonly used to treat chronic hypertension during pregnancy.[2,309] As a result, most clinical trials have compared methyldopa with either no medication or β-blockers. To evaluate the effects of antihypertensive drugs in pregnancy, we will describe only randomized trials in which adequate pregnancy data were available.[312,317,319,323–325]

Six prospective controlled trials compared methyldopa with either no medication or a placebo for the management of mild chronic hypertension in pregnancy, while in the sixth study atenolol was used (Table 28–20). Only two studies included a placebo in a double-blind fashion,[324,325] but the sample size was limited in both trials and the diagnosis of chronic hypertension in one of them was based on an increased blood pressure before 34 weeks' gestation. The other four studies were not placebo controlled, and only one included subjects who were randomized in the first trimester.[317] It is evident from Table 28–20 that the use of antihypertensive medications did not affect perinatal outcome except for reducing second-trimester abortions. There were three second-trimester abortions in the control group of Leather et al.[319]; however, it was unclear whether these losses were the result of severe hypertension or were spontaneous abortions. Of the four second-trimester abortions in the control group in the study reported by Redman et al.,[312] none were directly related to hypertension, and none had evidence of preeclampsia. These losses might have been due to preterm labor or incompetent cervix. On the other hand, Sibai et al.[317] noted only one second-trimester loss, which occurred in the methyldopa group. Also in the study of Butters et al.,[325] the only stillbirth was in the atenolol group. In the six trials summarized in Table 28–20, there were no maternal benefits from antihypertensive therapy except for a reduction in the fre-

Table 28–19. PREGNANCY OUTCOME IN 44 WOMEN WITH SEVERE HYPERTENSION IN THE FIRST TRIMESTER

	With Preeclampsia ($n = 23$)	Without Preeclampsia ($n = 21$)
Gestational age (wk)	28.6 ± 2.4	36.5 ± 2.9
<37 weeks	23 (100%)	8 (38%)
Birth weight (g)	827 ± 314	2632 ± 743
SGA	18 (78%)	1 (5%)
Perinatal deaths	11 (48%)	0
Abruptio placentae	2 (8.7%)	0
Deterioration in renal function	15 (65%)	5 (24%)

Table 28–20. PREGNANCY OUTCOME IN RANDOMIZED CONTROLLED TRIALS OF CHRONIC HYPERTENSION*

Author(s)	Gestation at Entry (wk)	Gestation at Delivery (wk)	Birth Weight (g)	IUGR (%)	Preeclampsia (%)	Perinatal Death (%)
Leather et al.[319]						
Control (n = 24)	<28	36.5	2,520		N/A	8.3[†]
Treated (n = 23)		38.0	2,840	N/A	N/A	0
Redman et al.[312]						
Control (n = 107)	20.6 ± 0.5	38.1 ± 0.2	3,130 ± 49		4.7	1.9[†]
Treated (n = 101)	21.9 ± 0.5	38.1 ± 0.2	3,090 ± 60	N/A	6.7	1.0
Arias and Zamora[323]						
Control (n = 29)	16.4 ± 1.1	38.3 ± 0.4	3,011 ± 103	14.2	10.3	3.4
Treated (n = 29)	14.7 ± 1.0	38.1 ± 0.5	2,926 ± 131	14.2	3.4	0
Weitz et al.[324]						
Control (n = 12)	<34	37.6 ± 0.5	2,820	25	33.3	0
Treated (n = 13)		39.0 ± 0.4	3,140	0	38.4	0
Sibai et al.[317]						
Control (n = 90)	11.3 ± 0.2	39.0 ± 0.2	3,123 ± 69	8.9	15.6	1.1
Treated (n = 173)	11.2 ± 0.2	38.7 ± 0.2	3,060 ± 72	7.5	17.3	1.2
Butters et al.[325]						
Control (n = 14)	15.9	39.5	3,530	0	N/A	0
Treated (n = 15)	15.8	38.5	2,620	66	N/A	6

* Data are presented as mean ± SEM where available.
† Excludes second-trimester losses.
IUGR, intrauterine growth retardation; preeclampsia, increased blood pressure plus proteinuria; N/A, not available.

quency of exacerbation of hypertension. The incidence of perinatal death among the controls ranged from 0 to 8.3 percent; this incidence was particularly low (<2 percent) in the two studies with the largest number of subjects. None of these trials had a sample size sufficient enough to permit direct assessment of the effects of antihypertensive drugs on perinatal death rate.

Recently, a double-blind, placebo-controlled trial compared the use of low-dose aspirin (n = 69) to aspirin plus ketanserin (n = 69) in women with mild chronic hypertension in pregnancy.[326] The rate of preeclampsia was significantly lower in the ketanserin group (3 percent vs. 19 percent). In addition, the rate of abruptio placentae was reduced in the ketanserin group as compared to placebo (1 percent vs. 8 percent). The authors concluded that ketanserin improves pregnancy outcome in women with mild chronic hypertension.[326]

Three prospective controlled trials have compared methyldopa with a β-blocker for mild hypertension in pregnancy (Table 28–21).[327–329] Gallery et al.[327] found

Table 28–21. METHYLDOPA VERSUS β–BLOCKERS FOR MILD HYPERTENSION IN PREGNANCY*†

	Gallery et al.		Fidler et al.‡		Plouin et al.	
	Methyldopa	Oxprenolol	Methyldopa	Oxprenolol	Methyldopa	Labetalol
No.	27	26	22	24	85	91
Initial systolic pressure (mm Hg)	151 ± 12	147 ± 14	146 ± 9	151 ± 9	148 ± 13	146 ± 13
Initial diastolic pressure (mm Hg)	102 ± 10	102 ± 12	99 ± 3	99 ± 4	96 ± 9	94 ± 8
Initial gestational age (wk)	32 ± 4.2	31 ± 9.1	23.9 ± 6.7	22.5 ± 7.2	26.2 ± 6.8	25.8 ± 7.5
Birth weight (g)	2,654 ± 821	3,051 ± 663	2,992 ± 732	2,715 ± 919	2,897 ± 727	2,860 ± 728
Preeclampsia (%)	7.4	7.6	9.1	8.3	9.4	8.8
Perinatal death (%)	7.4	0	4.5	4.2	4.7	1.1

* Data are presented as mean ± SD.
† Includes patients with all forms of mild hypertension (diastolic pressure <110 mm Hg).
‡ Excludes patients enrolled beyond 32 weeks' gestation.
Adapted from Sibai BM: Diagnosis and management of chronic hypertension in pregnancy. Obstet Gynecol 78:451, 1991. Copyright 1991 American College of Obstetricians and Gynecologists, with permission.

greater plasma volume expansion, higher neonatal birth weights, and no perinatal deaths among 26 oxprenolol-treated patients. In contrast, Fidler et al.[328] found no difference in pregnancy outcome and neonatal birth weight between 24 women treated with oxprenolol and 22 treated with methyldopa. They also found that the oxprenolol-treated group had a higher incidence of abnormal fetal heart tracings during labor. Plouin et al.[329] found no difference in neonatal heart rate, blood pressure, and respiratory rate between the two treatment groups and concluded that labetalol is as safe as methyldopa for the fetus and newborn. However, all three studies included patients with all forms of hypertension; less than one third of the subjects had chronic hypertension, and few were enrolled during the first trimester.[2] In addition, none of these trials had an adequate number of subjects to demonstrate a difference in either preeclampsia or perinatal death. In summary, superimposed preeclampsia and abruptio placentae are responsible for most of the poor perinatal outcome in women with mild chronic hypertension. Antihypertensive drugs do not reduce the frequency of either of these complications. Most patients with mild chronic hypertension will have a good outcome with proper obstetric follow-up without the use of antihypertensive agents.[2]

Antihypertensive Drugs in Pregnancy

Many drugs are available for treating hypertension in pregnancy. Some have been studied extensively (methyldopa, β-blockers); others have been used infrequently or are still under clinical trial (calcium channel blockers, prazosin). The drugs used most often in pregnancy are adrenoreceptor-blocking agents, thiazide diuretics, hydralazine, and recently, calcium channel blockers. There are potential adverse effects from the chronic use of any drug during pregnancy. When using antihypertensives, one must weigh the benefits of such treatment against the potential adverse effects on the mother, fetus, and neonate.

Methyldopa

Methyldopa is the only antihypertensive drug whose long-term safety for the mother and the fetus has been adequately assessed. It is the drug most commonly used to treat hypertension during pregnancy and is the standard against which other agents are compared. It lowers blood pressure by stimulation of central α_2-receptors via α-methylnorepinephrine, which is the active form of α-methyldopa. In addition, it might act as an α_2-peripheral blocker via a false neurotransmitter effect. It reduces systemic vascular resistance without causing physiologically significant changes in heart rate or cardiac output, while renal blood flow is maintained. Maternal side effects include dry mouth, lethargy, and drowsiness. Other side effects include liver function abnormalities, postural hypotension, hemolytic anemia, and a positive Coombs' test. The usual oral dosage in women with severe hypertension is an initial loading dose of 1 g followed by a maintenance dose of 1 to 2 g/day given in four divided doses, which can be increased to 4 g as needed. If used in mild hypertension, however, the usual dose is 250 mg three times daily. The plasma half-life is about 2 hours, and peak plasma levels occur within 2 hours after oral administration. The fall in blood pressure is maximal about 4 hours after an oral dose. Most of the drug is excreted via the kidney. It is considered a weak antihypertensive best suited for cases with mild hypertension, and if adequate blood pressure control is not achieved with the maximum dosage, additional antihypertensive agents, such as hydralazine, β-blockers, or nifedipine may be added.

Clonidine

Clonidine is a potent α_2-adrenoceptor central stimulant, used primarily for treatment of mild to moderate hypertension. Approximately 40 to 60 percent of the oral dose is excreted in unaltered form in the urine. Its potential side effects include sedation, dry mouth, and rebound hypertension following abrupt discontinuation. The usual oral dose in pregnancy is 0.1 to 0.3 mg/day given in two divided doses, which can be increased up to 1.2 mg/day as needed. Its safety and efficacy during pregnancy are unknown. Horvath et al.[330] reported a randomized study in 100 pregnant hypertensive women comparing clonidine to methyldopa. They found no significant difference in blood pressure control or maternal and fetal outcome. The authors concluded that clonidine was a safe and effective antihypertensive agent to use in pregnancy.

Prazosin

Prazosin is a selective α_1-postsynaptic blocker. It reduces both systolic and diastolic blood pressures, while producing significantly less tachycardia and sodium retention than methyldopa. It causes vasodilation of both the resistance and capacitance vessels, thereby reducing cardiac preload and afterload without reducing renal blood flow or glomerular filtration rate. In addition, it produces a decrease in plasma renin activity and is probably the drug of choice for treatment of hypertension characterized by high plasma renin levels. It is metabolized in the liver and excreted almost completely in the bile. The usual dose of prazosin is 1 mg twice daily; however, the drug has been used in doses as high as 20 mg/day. The first dose in some individuals can produce syncope due to exaggerated hypotension. This can be avoided by decreasing the first dose. The median time to peak concentration in nonpregnant individuals is 2 hours, and the mean elimination half-life is 2 to 3 hours. Side effects include fluid retention, orthostatic hypotension, and nasal congestion. Lubbe et al.[331] assessed the pregnancy outcomes in 14 women receiving prazosin and oxprenolol. They reported no superimposed preeclampsia, and infant birth weights were higher than those receiving either methyldopa or no medication. Sibai and Tabb (unpublished data, 1984) compared pregnancy outcomes in 80 women with chronic hypertension who were treated with either prazosin ($n = 40$) or methyldopa ($n = 40$). Both drugs were effective in controlling hypertension, and the incidence of superimposed preeclampsia was similar. There were no differences in perinatal outcome between the two groups. However, patients receiving prazosin had higher plasma volume findings at term than those receiving methyldopa.

Calcium Channel Blockers

Calcium channel blockers act by inhibiting transmembrane calcium ion influx from the extracellular space into the cytoplasm, thus blocking excitation-contraction coupling in smooth muscle fibers and thereby causing vasodilation and reduction in the peripheral resistance. They also have mild tocolytic properties. They have been used extensively in the treatment of hypertensive emergencies as monotherapy or as a part of combination therapy. They have rapid onset of action following oral administration. Nifedipine has potent vasodilating properties without reduction in cardiac output. Few reports have described the use of nifedipine in a limited number of women with acute hypertension during pregnancy.[2,130,131,213,226,227,332,333] The drug was effective in controlling maternal blood pressure, and no adverse fetal or neonatal effects were noted. However, there is limited experience with nifedipine treatment of chronic hypertension. Common side effects include headache, flushing, tachycardia, and fatigue. Care should be exercised when using nifedipine with magnesium sulfate, which is a calcium channel blocker itself, since the use of both agents together could potentiate the antihypertensive action. There are a few recent reports that have described the use of other calcium channel blockers such as nicardipine[334] and isradipine[335] in women with hypertension. In addition, one report described the use of long-acting nifedipine.[17]

Angiotensin-Converting Enzyme Inhibitors

Three angiotensin-converting enzyme (ACE) inhibitors are available in the United States: captopril, enalapril, and lisinopril. They induce vasodilation by inhibiting the enzyme that converts angiotensin I to angiotensin II, a potent vasoconstrictor, without reflex increase in the cardiac output. In addition, they increase the synthesis of vasodilating prostaglandins and diminish the rate of bradykinin inactivation. Because of their efficacy and low side effects, these agents are becoming widely used as first-line therapy for chronic hypertension in the nonpregnant state. In the experimental animal model, captopril causes abortion and fetal death, apparently by reducing the uteroplacental perfusion. In human pregnancy, the chronic use of ACE inhibitors has reportedly been associated with several fetal and neonatal complications: neonatal hypotension, fetal growth retardation, oligohydramnios, neonatal anuria and renal failure, and neonatal death.[336–339] Thus, it is recommended that the use of these agents in pregnancy be avoided.[337] Similar recommendations apply to the use of angiotensin receptor blockers.

Hydralazine

Hydralazine is a potent vasodilator that acts directly on the vascular smooth muscle. It is the agent most commonly used to control severe hypertension in preeclampsia, where it is given intravenously in bolus injections. After its intravenous use, the hypotensive effect of this drug develops gradually over 15 to 30 minutes, peaking at 20 minutes. The elimination half-life is about 3 hours. The usual bolus dose is 5 to 10 mg to be repeated every 20 to 30 minutes as needed. Its main side effects are fluid retention, tachycardia, palpitation, headache, and a lupus-like syndrome, as well as neonatal thrombocytopenia. About 50 percent of the U.S. population are genetically determined slow acetylators and thus are at higher risk for hypotension. Many of these side effects are common with high chronic doses and are usually minimized when it is used in combination with other antihypertensives. Because oral hydralazine when used as a monotherapy is a weak antihypertensive, it is usually combined with diuretics, methyldopa, or β-blockers; however, the use of multiple agents is discouraged in pregnancy. The usual oral dose is 10 mg given four times daily, but this can be increased up to 300 mg/day.

β-Blockers

The drugs in this category have different hemodynamic effects that depend on their receptor selectivity, the presence of intrinsic sympathomimetic activity (ISA), and their lipid solubility. The mechanisms of action of these drugs are complex and highly controversial.[340–342] Drugs without ISA reduce both cardiac output and heart rate in association with their antihypertensive effects. On the other hand, drugs with ISA reduce mean arterial blood pressure without influencing either cardiac output or heart rate. β-blockers have been used extensively to treat thyroid disease, mitral valve prolapse, migraine headache, glaucoma, and chronic hypertension. Side effects in the nonpregnant state include bronchial spasm, hypoglycemia, cold extremities, as well as disturbances in the lipid metabolism. Their use in pregnancy has been reportedly associated with neonatal bradycardia, hypoglycemia, fetal growth restriction, altered adaptation to perinatal asphyxia, and neonatal respiratory depression.[343] However, most of these neonatal effects could be attributed to maternal disease as well.

There are numerous reports describing the management of hypertension during pregnancy with various β-blockers, but only a few are well controlled. This subject was recently reviewed by Rubin,[343] who concluded that these drugs are safe when used in pregnancy. In addition, he reported that their use was associated with better perinatal outcome than that achieved with either methyldopa or hydralazine. However, we believe it is difficult to draw any conclusions regarding the safety and efficacy of these drugs from such studies because (1) they involved heterogeneous groups of patients with chronic hypertension, preeclampsia, and chronic hypertension with superimposed preeclampsia; (2) the β-blockers were used in association with other antihypertensive agents such as diuretics, hydralazine, methyldopa, or prazosin; and (3) the blood pressure values at the time of initiating therapy and the duration of treatment were highly variable. It is important to note that the chronic use of atenolol during pregnancy has been consistently associated with reduced fetal weights as well as placental function.[325,344-347] Therefore, its use for control of maternal blood pressure in women with chronic hypertension should be avoided.

Thiazide Diuretics

Thiazide diuretics are generally the first drugs selected in the treatment of nonpregnant hypertensive patients. Consequently, most women with chronic hypertension become pregnant while on diuretics. Initially, in the first 3 to 5 days of treatment, these drugs result in a 5 to 10 percent reduction in both plasma and extracellular fluid volumes with a concomitant decrease in the cardiac output and lowering of the blood pressure. However, these changes tend to return to pretreatment levels within 4 to 6 weeks. These effects are followed by a long-term reduction in peripheral resistance, which is thought to be related to reduced intracellular sodium concentration in vascular smooth muscle cells. A single 25-mg dose is usually given in the morning. Adverse maternal effects reported with diuretics during pregnancy include hypokalemia, hyponatremia, hyperglycemia, hyperuricemia, hyperlipidemia, hemorrhagic pancreatitis, and even death. Neonatal adverse effects are electrolyte imbalance, thrombocytopenia, and small size for gestational age.

Other harmful maternal and fetal effects reported with the use of diuretics during pregnancy include significant plasma volume depletion that may be detrimental to fetal growth.[348-350] Sibai et al.[351] noted that pregnant patients with chronic hypertension treated with diuretics have a marked reduction in plasma volume compared with a control group not receiving these medications. However, plasma volume expansion was normal after the discontinuation of diuretics. In a subsequent report, Sibai et al.[351] measured the plasma volume in 20 hypertensive women who received diuretics before and early in pregnancy. Diuretics were continued in 10 of these subjects but were stopped in the remainder. In the group whose diuretics were continued, subsequent plasma volumes at various stages of gestation were markedly reduced compared with findings in the others. Collins et al.[352] reviewed nine randomized trials of diuretics in pregnancy involving nearly 7,000 women and concluded that prophylactic thiazide therapy does not reduce the incidence of preeclampsia. Similar findings were reported by MacGillivray,[353] who found that patients receiving diuretics delivered infants who weighed less than those born to control pregnant women.

Because the initiation of diuretic therapy causes a decrease in blood volume and cardiac output, adding a diuretic late in pregnancy is probably contraindicated unless it is needed for the treatment of pulmonary edema. On the other hand, continuing a diuretic as a part of therapeutic program in patients with chronic hypertension who become pregnant remains an unresolved issue. Our policy is to discontinue thiazide diuretics in such patients at the time of first visit. Since plasma volume depletion is associated with poor perinatal outcome, we have cautioned against the use of diuretics in pregnancies complicated by chronic hypertension. Furthermore, when diuretics are discontinued, few patients require additional medications during the remainder of the pregnancy.[351]

Management of Chronic Hypertension

The primary objective in the management of pregnancies complicated with chronic hypertension is to reduce maternal risks and achieve optimal perinatal survival. This objective can be achieved by formulating a rational approach that includes preconceptional evaluation and counseling, early antenatal care, frequent antepartum visits to monitor both maternal and fetal well-being, timely delivery with intensive intrapartum monitoring, and proper postpartum management.

Preconceptional Evaluation of Chronic Hypertension

Management of patients with chronic hypertension should ideally begin before pregnancy, when extensive evaluation is undertaken to assess the etiology and the severity of the hypertension, as well as the presence of other medical illnesses, and to rule out the presence of target organ damage of long-standing hypertension.[309] An in-depth history should delineate in particular the duration of hypertension, the use of antihypertensive medications, their type, and the response to these medications. As some medications that have potentially harmful effects on the fetus are frequently used in the nonpregnant state (ACE inhibitors, ganglion blockers, atenolol), it is prudent to change these drugs to others with well-documented safety and to monitor the responses of the patients to these medications. Attention should also be given to the presence of cardiac or renal disease, diabetes mellitus, thyroid disease, and a history of a cerebrovascular accident or congestive heart failure. A detailed obstetric history should include maternal as well as neonatal outcome of previous pregnancies with emphasis on the history of development of abruptio placentae, superimposed preeclampsia, preterm delivery, small-for-gestational-age infants, intrauterine fetal death, and neonatal morbidity and mortality. A detailed physical examination should include the following: general physical examination, Funduscopic examination, measurement of blood pressure in the four extremities, measurement of blood pressure with changes in posture and after rest, detailed auscultation of chest and flanks, and checking of pulses in the four extremities.

Laboratory evaluation is obtained to assess the functions of different organ systems that are likely to be affected by chronic hypertension, and as a baseline for future assessments; these should include:

1. For all patients
   a. Urinalysis
   b. Urine culture and sensitivity
   c. 24-hour urine evaluation for protein, sodium, potassium, and creatinine clearance
   d. SMAC-20
   e. CBC
   f. Glucose tolerance test
2. Selectively
   a. If hyperglycemia or wide blood pressure swings are evident, a 24-hour urine evaluation for vanillylmandelic acid (VMA) and metanephrines is recommended to rule out pheochromocytoma.
   b. For patients with severe hypertension or significant proteinuria, chest x-ray, ECG, antinuclear antibody, and serum complement studies are indicated.
   c. For patients with severe long-standing hypertension, or if there is a suspicion of heart disease, an echocardiogram is recommended.
   d. Women with a history of poor pregnancy outcome (repetitive midpregnancy losses), and those with recent thromboembolic disease,

should be evaluated for the presence of lupus anticoagulant, anticardiolipin antibodies, and other thrombophilias.

Pregnancies in women with chronic hypertension and renal insufficiency are associated with increased perinatal loss and a higher incidence of superimposed preeclampsia, preterm delivery, and fetal growth restriction.[354–357] These risks rise in proportion to the severity of the renal insufficiency; women with severe renal insufficiency, particularly primary glomerular disease, risk rapid progression to end-stage renal disease during pregnancy or postpartum.[354–357] Thus, women with renal disease desiring pregnancy should be counseled to conceive before renal insufficiency becomes severe. For women with hypertension and severe renal insufficiency in the first trimester, the decision to continue pregnancy should not be made without extensive counseling regarding the potential maternal and fetal risks, particularly the potential need for dialysis during pregnancy.[357] Women who elect to continue their pregnancies must be observed and managed at a tertiary care center with adequate maternal–neonatal care facilities.

Initial and Subsequent Prenatal Visits for Patients with Chronic Hypertension

Early prenatal care will ensure accurate determination of gestational age as well as an assessment of the severity of hypertension in the first trimester, which have prognostic values for the outcome of such pregnancies. At the time of initial and subsequent visits, the patient should be counseled regarding the following aspects as they pertain to her pregnancy:

1. Instruction by a nutritionist regarding nutritional requirements, weight gain, and sodium intake
2. Instruction regarding the negative impact of maternal anxiety, smoking, and caffeine, as well as drugs, on maternal blood pressure and perinatal outcome
3. Counsel regarding the possible adverse effects and complications of hypertension during pregnancy
4. Counsel regarding the importance of frequent prenatal visits and their impact on preventing or minimizing the above adverse effects

If the patient is well motivated, she can be instructed in self-determination of blood pressure, as recommended by Zuspan and Rayburn.[358] This approach avoids the phenomenon of "white coat hypertension," which is associated with a visit to the physician's office, and avoids the need to start or increase the dose of antihypertensive medications. It is recommended that patient-recorded measurements of blood pressure be used to supplement those recorded in the doctor's office.

During the course of pregnancy, the patient should

be seen once every 2 to 3 weeks in the first two trimesters and thereafter adjusted based on maternal and fetal conditions. Systolic and diastolic blood pressure readings should be carefully measured at each visit. At each visit, the urine should be checked for protein. Maternal evaluation should include serial measurements of hematocrit, serum creatinine, uric acid, and 24-hour urinary excretion of protein once every trimester. Other tests are obtained as needed. The occurrence of one or more of the following may be an indication for hospitalization:

1. Pyelonephritis
2. Significant elevations in blood pressure with levels in the range of severe hypertension
3. Severe fetal growth restriction

Based on the initial assessment, the patient is then classified as having low-risk or high-risk chronic hypertension depending on duration of hypertension, severity of hypertension early in pregnancy, and the extent of cardiovascular and renal involvement at the onset of pregnancy and other factors.

Managing Low-Risk Chronic Hypertension

As stated previously, most patients with uncomplicated mild chronic hypertension will have a good perinatal outcome irrespective of the use of antihypertensive drugs. A recent analysis of pregnancy outcome in 211 patients with mild chronic hypertension managed at our institution[308] suggests that the use of antihypertensive drugs is not necessary to achieve a good pregnancy outcome. The changes in average mean arterial pressure (MAP) throughout the course of pregnancy is summarized in Figure 28–7. It is of interest to note that 49 percent of patients will demonstrate a decrease in MAP and an additional 34 percent will demonstrate no change in MAP at 20 to 26 weeks' gestation without the use of antihypertensive medications. Furthermore, only 13 percent of patients will require antihypertensive medications for exacerbation of hypertension during the third trimester. In the same study, we found that most poor outcomes were related to the development of superimposed preeclampsia in such pregnancies. In addition, in the absence of superimposed preeclampsia, the perinatal outcome in patients with mild chronic hypertension was similar to that in the general obstetric population. We attribute the good perinatal outcome in these pregnancies to early onset of prenatal care, intensive antepartum and intrapartum monitoring, and timely delivery. Thus, it is our policy to discontinue all antihypertensive medications in all such patients at the time of first prenatal visit. Antihypertensive therapy is subsequently started only if the blood pressure exceeds 160 mm Hg systolic or 110 mm Hg diastolic. These patients are usually treated with methyldopa (750 mg to 4 g/day) given as needed to keep diastolic blood

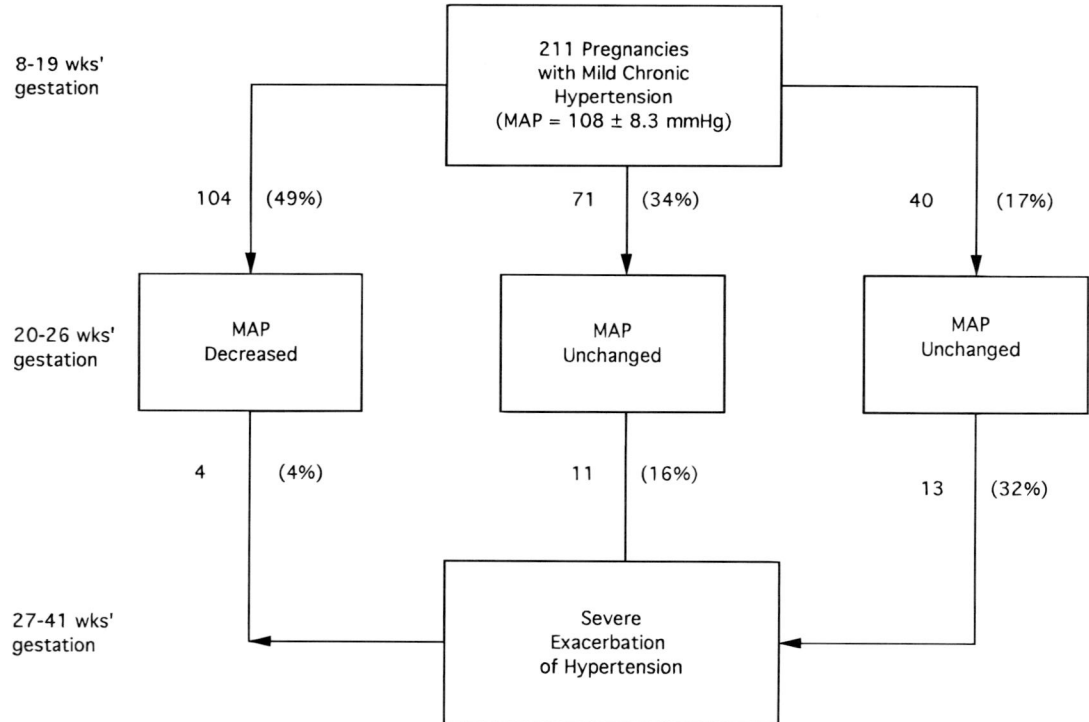

Figure 28–7. Mean arterial blood pressure (MAP) during pregnancy. (Modified from Sibai BM, Abdella TN, Anderson GD: Pregnancy outcome in 211 patients with mild chronic hypertension. Obstet Gynecol 61:571, 1983.)

pressure consistently at or below 105 mm Hg. It is important to emphasize that the development of exacerbated hypertension alone is not an indication for delivery. Pregnancy in these patients may be continued until term or the onset of superimposed preeclampsia. In the absence of superimposed preeclampsia or fetal jeopardy, routine induction before 41 weeks' gestation is not warranted. Superimposed preeclampsia or suspected fetal growth restriction is an indication for close evaluation of maternal and fetal well-being. Subsequent management is similar to that in the high-risk group and will depend on gestational age and the result of antepartum fetal testing. Mild superimposed preeclampsia is an indication for delivery if the gestational age is at least 37 weeks. Otherwise, the pregnancy can be managed conservatively until the cervix is ripe for induction, onset of labor, or completion of 40 weeks' gestation.

Managing High-Risk Chronic Hypertension

Pregnancies in women at high risk are associated with increased maternal and perinatal complications (see the box "High Risk Characteristics").[310] As a result, these patients should be managed in consultation with a maternal–fetal medicine specialist. Furthermore, patients with chronic renal disease—particularly those with primary glomerular diseases and significant renal impairment (serum creatinine >2.5 mg/dl)—should be managed in consultation with a nephrologist. All these patients should be hospitalized at the time of first prenatal visit for evaluation of cardiovascular and renal status and for regulation of antihypertensive treatment, as well as other prescribed medications (insulin, thyroid drugs, cardiac drugs). Antihypertensive agents should be used to keep systolic blood pressure between 140 and 160 mm Hg and diastolic blood pressure between 90 and 105 mm Hg. Maternal blood pressure can be controlled with methyldopa (1 to 4 g/day), labetalol

(600 mg to 2.4 g/day), or nifedipine (40 to 120 mg/day). In some patients, blood pressure may be difficult to control, demanding the use of multiple oral drugs as well as intravenous therapy. Antihypertensives must be used in all women with severe hypertension. In addition, there are short-term maternal benefits from treating women with mild hypertension and target organ damage such as diabetes mellitus, renal disease, and cardiac dysfunction. As a result, we recommend treating mild chronic hypertension in pregnant women with these complications, keeping diastolic blood pressure below 90 mm Hg. For patients with significant proteinuria in the first trimester, antinuclear antibody and serum complement are performed to rule out the presence of lupus nephritis. Early and frequent prenatal care is the key to a successful outcome for patients with high-risk characteristics. These women need close monitoring throughout pregnancy and may require multiple hospital admissions for control of blood pressure or associated medical complications. Fetal evaluation should be started as early as 26 weeks and repeated as needed. Superimposed preeclampsia is an indication for immediate hospitalization. Subsequent management will depend on the severity of preeclampsia and fetal gestational age. Severe superimposed preeclampsia is an indication for delivery in all patients with a gestational age beyond 34 weeks. If preeclampsia develops before this time, the pregnancy may be followed conservatively with daily evaluation of maternal and fetal well-being.

Hypertensive Emergencies in Chronic Hypertension

On rare occasions, pregnant women may present with life-threatening clinical conditions that require immediate control of blood pressure, such as hypertensive encephalopathy, acute left ventricular failure, acute aortic dissection, or increased circulating catecholamines (pheochromocytoma, clonidine withdrawal, cocaine ingestion). Patients at highest risk for these complications include those with underlying cardiac disease, chronic glomerular renal disease, multiple drugs to control their hypertension, superimposed preeclampsia in the second trimester, and abruptio placentae complicated by DIC. Although a diastolic blood pressure of 115 mm Hg or greater is usually considered a hypertensive emergency, this level is actually arbitrary, and the rate of change of blood pressure may be more important than absolute level.[359] The association of elevated blood pressure with evidence of new or progressive end-organ damage determines the seriousness of the clinical situation.[360]

Hypertensive Encephalopathy

Untreated essential hypertension progresses to a hypertensive crisis in up to 1 to 2 percent of cases for un-

---

High-Risk Characteristics

- Maternal age >40 years
- Duration of hypertension >15 years
- Blood pressure ≥160/110 mm Hg early in pregnancy
- Diabetes mellitus (White classes B–F)
- Renal disease (all causes)
- Cardiomyopathy
- Connective tissue disease
- Coarctation of the aorta
- Presence of thrombophilias
- Previous pregnancy with perinatal loss

known reasons. Hypertensive encephalopathy is usually seen in patients with systolic blood pressure above 250 mm Hg or diastolic blood pressure above 150 mm Hg.[360] Patients with acute onset of hypertension may develop encephalopathy at pressure levels that are generally tolerated by those with chronic hypertension. Normally, cerebral blood flow is approximately 50 ml/100 g tissue per minute. When the blood pressure falls, cerebral arterioles normally dilate, whereas when blood pressure increases, they constrict to maintain constant cerebral blood flow.[361] This mechanism usually remains operative between 60 and 120 mm Hg diastolic blood pressure. Hypertensive encephalopathy is currently considered to be a derangement of the autoregulation of cerebral arterioles, which occurs when the upper limit of autoregulation is exceeded.[359] With severe hypertension (130 to 150 mm Hg cerebral perfusion pressure), cerebral blood vessels constrict as much as possible and then reflex cerebral vasodilatation occurs. This results in overperfusion, damage to small blood vessels, cerebral edema, and increased intracranial pressure (breakthrough theory). Others believe that hypertensive encephalopathy results from an exaggerated vasoconstrictive response of the arterioles resulting in cerebral ischemia (overregulation theory). Patients who have impaired autoregulation involving the cerebral arterioles may experience necrotizing arteriolitis, microinfarcts, petechial hemorrhages, multiple small thrombi, or cerebral edema.[360] Typically, hypertensive encephalopathy has a subacute onset over 24 to 72 hours.[361]

During a hypertensive crisis, other evidence for end-organ damage may be present: cardiac, renal, or retinal dysfunction secondary to impaired organ perfusion and loss of autoregulation of blood flow.[360] Ischemia of the retina (with flame-shaped retinal hemorrhages, retinal infarcts, or papilledema) may occur—causing decreased visual acuity. Impaired regulation of coronary blood flow and marked increase in ventricular wall stress may result in angina, myocardial infarction, congestive heart failure, malignant ventricular arrhythmia, pulmonary edema, or dissecting aortic aneurysm. Necrosis of the afferent arterioles of the glomerulus results in hemorrhages of the cortex and medulla, fibrinoid necrosis, and proliferative endarteritis resulting in elevated serum creatinine (>3 mg/dl), proteinuria, oliguria, hematuria, hyaline or red blood cell casts, and progressive azotemia.[359] Severe hypertension may result in abruptio placentae with resultant DIC. In addition, high levels of angiotensin II, norepinephrine, and vasopressin accompany ongoing vascular damage. These circulating hormones increase relative efferent arteriolar tone, resulting in sodium diuresis and hypovolemia. Because levels of renin and angiotensin II are increased, the aldosterone level is also elevated. The impact of these endocrine changes may be important in maintaining the hypertensive crisis.

Treatment of Hypertensive Encephalopathy

The ultimate goal of therapy is to prevent the occurrence of a hypertensive emergency. Patients at risk for hypertensive crisis should receive intensive management during labor and for a minimum of 48 hours after delivery. Although pregnancy may complicate the diagnosis, once the life-threatening conditions are recognized, pregnancy should not in any way slow or alter the mode of therapy. The only reliable clinical criterion to confirm the diagnosis of hypertensive encephalopathy is prompt response of the patient to antihypertensive therapy. The headache and sensorium often clear dramatically—sometimes within 1 to 2 hours after the treatment. The overall recovery may be somewhat slower in patients with uremia and in whom the symptoms have been present for a prolonged period before the therapy is given. Sustained cerebrovascular deficits should suggest other diagnoses.[361]

Patients with hypertensive encephalopathy or other hypertensive crisis should be hospitalized for bed rest. Intravenous lines should be inserted for fluids and medications. Although there is a tendency to restrict sodium intake in patients with a hypertensive emergency, volume contraction from sodium diuresis may be present. A marked drop in diastolic blood pressure with a rise in heart rate on standing from the supine position is evidence of volume contraction. Infusion of normal saline solution during the first 24 to 48 hours to achieve volume expansion should be considered. Saline infusion may help decrease the activity of the renin-angiotensin-aldosterone axis and result in better blood pressure control. Simultaneous repletion of potassium losses and continuous monitoring of blood pressure, volume status, urinary output, electrocardiographic readings, and mental status is mandatory. An intra-arterial line may provide the most accurate blood pressure information. Laboratory studies include complete blood count, differential, reticulocyte count, platelets, and blood chemistries. A urinalysis should be obtained for protein, glucose, blood, cells, casts, and bacteria. Assessment for end-organ damage in the central nervous system, retina, kidneys, and cardiovascular system should be done periodically. Antepartum patients should have continuous fetal monitoring.[359,362]

Lowering Blood Pressure

There are risks associated with too rapid or excessive reduction of elevated blood pressure. The aim of therapy is to lower mean blood pressure by no more than 15 to 25 percent. Small reductions in blood pressure in the first 60 minutes, working toward a diastolic level of 100 to 110 mm Hg, have been recommended.[359,360] Although cerebral blood flow is maintained constantly over a wide range of blood pressures, there is a lower as well as an upper limit to autoregulation. In chronic hypertensive women who have a rightward shift of the cerebral autoregulation curve secondary to medial hypertrophy of the cerebral vasculature, lowering blood pressure too rapidly may produce cerebral ischemia, stroke, or coma. Coronary blood flow, renal perfusion, and uteroplacental blood flow also may deteriorate, resulting in acute renal failure, myocardial infarction, fetal distress, or death. Hypertension that proves increasingly difficult to control is an indication to end the pregnancy. If the patient's outcome appears to be grave, consideration of perimortem cesarean delivery should be made.[359]

The drug of choice in hypertensive crisis is sodium nitroprusside. Other drugs such as nitroglycerin, nifedipine, trimetaphan, labetalol, and hydralazine can also be used.

Sodium Nitroprusside

Sodium nitroprusside causes arterial and venous relaxation by interfering with both influx and the intracellular activation of calcium. It is given as an intravenous infusion of 0.25 to 8.0 μg/kg/min. The onset of action is immediate, and its effect may last 3 to 5 minutes after discontinuing the infusion. Hypotension caused by nitroprusside should resolve within a few minutes of stopping the infusion, because the drug's half-life is so short. If it does not resolve, other causes for hypotension should be suspected. The effect of nitroprusside on uterine blood flow is controversial. Nitroprusside is metabolized into thiocyanate, which is excreted in the urine. Cyanide can accumulate if there is either increased production due to large doses (>10 μg/kg/min) or prolonged administration (>48 hours), or if there is renal insufficiency or decreased metabolism in the liver. Signs of toxicity include anorexia, disorientation, headache, fatigue, restlessness, tinnitus, delirium, hallucinations, nausea, vomiting, and metabolic acidosis. When it is infused at less than 2 μg/kg/min, cyanide toxicity is unlikely. At a maximum dose rate of 10 μg/kg/min, infusion should never last more than 10 minutes. Animal experiments and the few reported cases of nitroprusside use in pregnancy have revealed that thiocyanate toxicity to mother and fetus rarely occur if it is used in a regular pharmacologic dose. Tachyphylaxis to nitroprusside usually develops before toxicity occurs. Whenever toxicity is suspected, therapy should be initiated with 3 percent sodium nitrite at a rate not exceeding 5 ml/min, up to a total dose of 15 ml. Then, infusion of 12.5 g of sodium thiosulfate in 50 ml of 5 percent dextrose in water over a 10-minute period should be started.[363]

Nitroglycerin

Nitroglycerin is an arterial but mostly venous dilator. It is given as an intravenous infusion of 5 μg/min that is gradually increased every 3 to 5 minutes to titrate blood pressure up to a maximum dose of 100 μg/min. It is the drug of choice in preeclampsia associated with pulmonary edema and for control of hypertension associated with tracheal manipulation. Side effects such as headache, tachycardia, and methemoglobinemia may develop. It is contraindicated in hypertensive encephalopathy because it increases cerebral blood flow and intracranial pressure.[360]

Postpartum Management of Hypertension

High-risk chronic hypertensive patients can develop hypertensive encephalopathy, pulmonary edema, and renal failure in the postpartum period. These risks are particularly increased in women with underlying cardiac disease, chronic glomerular renal disease, superimposed preeclampsia in the second trimester, abruptio placentae complicated by DIC, and those requiring multiple hypertensive agents.[310] Patients with these complications should receive intensive management for a minimum of 48 hours after delivery and intravenous hydralazine or labetalol for control of severe hypertension as needed. Moreover, diuretic therapy should be used in women who are at risk for delayed onset of postpartum circulatory congestion and pulmonary edema, including massively obese older women with long-standing hypertension and those with previous antepartum congestive heart failure.

Oral antihypertensive drugs may be needed to control maternal blood pressure after delivery. Some women may wish to breast-feed their infants while receiving these agents (see also Chapter 9). Unfortunately, data are limited concerning the excretion of these drugs into human breast milk and their effects on the infant.[364,365] In addition, there are no published reports describing the long-term effects of antihypertensive agents on infants exposed to these drugs through breast-feeding. Most of the published data have described the milk/plasma ratio after a single measurement of the drug concentration.[364-366] The data in the literature indicate that all studied antihypertensive agents are excreted into human breast milk, although there are differences among these drugs in the milk/plasma ratio.[365] The available data also show that there are no short-term adverse effects on the breast-feeding infant exposed to methyldopa, hydralazine, or β-blockers.

Key Points

➤ Hypertension is the most common medical complication during pregnancy.

➤ Preeclampsia is a leading cause of maternal mortality and morbidity worldwide.

➤ The pathophysiologic abnormalities of preeclampsia are numerous, but the etiology is unknown.

➤ At present, there is no proven method to prevent preeclampsia.

➤ The HELLP syndrome may develop in the absence of maternal hypertension.

➤ Expectant management improves perinatal outcome in a select group of women with severe preeclampsia before 32 weeks' gestation.

➤ Magnesium sulfate is the ideal agent to prevent or treat eclamptic convulsions.

➤ Rare cases of eclampsia can develop before 20 weeks' gestation and beyond 48 hours postpartum.

➤ Antihypertensive agents do not improve pregnancy outcome in women with mild uncomplicated chronic hypertension.

➤ Methyldopa is the drug of choice for the treatment of chronic hypertension; ACE inhibitors should be avoided.

REFERENCES

1. Samadi AR, Mayberry RM, Zaidi AA, et al: Maternal hypertension and associated pregnancy complications among African-American and other women in the United States. Obstet Gynecol 87:557, 1996.
2. Sibai BM: Drug therapy: treatment of hypertension in pregnant women. *Drug therapy series*. N Engl J Med 335:257, 1996.
3. Hauth JC, Ewell MG, Levine RJ, et al: Pregnancy outcomes in healthy nulliparas who developed hypertension. Calcium for Preeclampsia Prevention Study Group. Obstet Gynecol 95:24, 2000.
4. Saudan P, Brown MA, Buddle ML, Jones M: Does gestational hypertension become pre-eclampsia? Br J Obstet Gynaecol 105:1177, 1998.
5. Helewa ME, Burrows RF, Smith J, et al: Report of the Canadian Hypertension Society Consensus Conference: 1. Definitions, evaluation and classification of hypertensive disorders in pregnancy. Can Med Assoc J 157:715, 1997.
6. Brown MA, Hague WM, Higgins J, et al: The detection, investigation, and management of hypertension in pregnancy. Full consensus statement of recommendations from the Council of the Australian Society for the Study of Hypertension in pregnancy. Aust N Z J Obstet Gynaecol 40:139, 2000.
7. American College of Obstetricians and Gynecologists: Hypertension in pregnancy. ACOG Tech Bull 219:1, 1996.
8. Mattar F, Sibai BM: Eclampsia VIII Risk factors for maternal morbidity. Am J Obstet Gynecol 182:307, 2000.
9. Sibai BM, Caritis SN, Thom E, et al, and the National Institute of Child Health and Human Development Network of Maternal-Fetal Medicine Units: Prevention of preeclampsia with low-dose aspirin in healthy nulliparous pregnant women. N Engl J Med 329:1213, 1993.
10. Sibai BM, Lindheimer M, Hauth J, et al, and the National Institute of Child Health and Human Development Network of Maternal-Fetal Medicine Units: Risk factors for preeclampsia, abruptio, and adverse neonatal outcome in women with chronic hypertension. N Engl J Med 339:667, 1998.
11. Knuist M, Bonsel GJ, Zondervan HA, Treffers PE: Intensification of fetal and maternal surveillance in pregnant women with hypertensive disorders. Int J Gynecol Obstet 61:127, 1998.
12. Campbell DM, MacGillivray I: Preeclampsia in twin pregnancies: Incidence and outcome. Hypertens Pregnancy 18:197, 1999.
13. Sibai BM, Hauth J, Caritis S, et al, for the Network of Maternal-Fetal Medicine Units of the National Institute of Child Health and Human Development: Hypertensive disorders in twin versus singleton pregnancies. Am J Obstet Gynecol 182:938, 2000.
14. Witlin AG, Sibai BM: Hypertension. Clin Obstet Gynecol 41:533, 1998.
15. Barton JR, Witlin AG, Sibai BM: Management of mild preeclampsia. Clin Obstet Gynecol 42:455, 1999.
16. Magee LA, Ornstein MP, von Dadelzsen P: Management of hypertension in pregnancy. BMJ 318:1332, 1999.
17. Parazzini F and Gruppo di Studio Ipertnesiont in Gravidanza: Nifedipine versus expectant management in mild to moderate hypertension in pregnancy. Br J Obstet Gynaecol 105:718, 1998.
18. Witlin AG, Sibai BM: Magnesium sulfate therapy in preeclampsia and eclampsia. Obstet Gynecol 92:883, 1998.
19. Beurel JN Jr: Eclampsia in lowland gorilla. Am J Obstet Gynecol 141:345, 1981.
20. Long PA, Abell DA, Beischer NA: Parity and preeclampsia. Aust N Z J Obstet Gynaecol 19:203, 1979.
21. Dekker GA, Sibai BM: Pathogenesis and etiology of preeclampsia. Am J Obstet Gynecology 179:1359, 1998.
22. Brosens IA: Morphological changes in the uteroplacental bed in pregnancy hypertension. Clin Obstet Gynaecol 4:583, 1977.
23. Kong TY, DeWolf F, Robertson WB, Brosens I: Inadequate maternal vascular response to placentation in pregnancies complicated by preeclampsia and by small-for-gestational age infants. Br J Obstet Gynaecol 93:1049, 1986.
24. Frusca T, Morassi L, Pecorell S, et al: Histological features of uteroplacental vessels in normal and hypertensive patients in relation to birthweight. Br J Obstet Gynaecol 96:835, 1989.
25. Sheppard BL, Bonnar J: An ultrastructural study of uteroplacental spiral arteries in hypertensive and normotensive pregnancy and fetal growth retardation. Br J Obstet Gynaecol 88:695, 1981.
26. Meekins JW, Pijneborg R, Hanssens M, et al: A study of placental bed spiral arteries and trophoblast invasion in normal and severe preeclamptic pregnancies. Br J Obstet Gynaecol 101:669, 1994.

27. Shanklin DR, Sibai BM: Ultrastructural aspects of preeclampsia. I. Placental bed and uterine boundary vessels. Am J Obstet Gynecol 161:735, 1989.

28. Saleh AA, Bottoms SF, Welch RA, et al: Preeclampsia, delivery, and the hemostatic system. Am J Obstet Gynecol 157: 331, 1987.

29. Saleh AA, Bottoms SF, Faragam G, et al: Markers for endothelial injury, clotting and platelet activation in preeclampsia. Arch Gynecol Obstet 251:105, 1992.

30. Taylor RM, Crombleholme WR, Friedman SA, et al: High plasma cellular fibronectin levels correlate with biochemical and clinical features of preeclampsia but cannot be attributed to hypertension alone. Am J Obstet Gynecol 165:895, 1991.

31. Halligan A, Bonnar J, Sheppard B, et al: Haemostatic, fibrinolytic and endothelial variables in normal pregnancy and preeclampsia. Br J Obstet Gynaecol 101:488, 1994.

32. Hutt R, Ogunniyi SO, Sullivan MHF, et al: Increased platelet volume and aggregation precede the onset of preeclampsia. Obstet Gynecol 83:146, 1994.

33. de Boer K, tenCate JW, Sturk A, et al: Enhanced thrombin generation in normal and hypertensive pregnancy. Am J Obstet Gynecol 160:96, 1989.

34. Gilabert J, Fernandez JA, Espana F, et al: Physiological coagulation inhibitors (protein S, protein C and antithrombin III) in severe preeclamptic states and in users of oral contraceptives. Thromb Res 49:319, 1988.

35. Walsh SW, Parisi VM: The role of arachidonic acid metabolites in preeclampsia. Semin Perinatol 10:335, 1986.

36. Paarlberg KM, deJong CLD, Van Geijn HP, et al: Vasoactive mediators in pregnancy-induced hypertensive disorders: a longitudinal study. Am J Obstet Gynecol 179:1559, 1998.

37. Smith AJ, Waiters WA, Buckley NA, et al: Hypertensive and normal pregnancy: a longitudinal study of blood pressure, distensibility of dorsal hand veins and the ratio of the stable metabolites of thromboxane A_2 and prostacyclin in plasma. Br J Obstet Gynaecol 102:900, 1995.

38. Mills JL, DerSimonian R, Raymond E, et al: Prostacyclin and thromboxane changes predating clinical onset of preeclampsia: a multicenter prospective study. JAMA 282:356, 1999.

39. Zeeman GG, Dekker GA: Pathogenesis of preeclampsia: a hypothesis. Clin Obstet Gynecol 35:317, 1992.

40. Pinto A, Sorrentino R, Sorrentino P, et al: Endothelial-derived relaxing factor released by endothelial cells of human umbilical vessels and its impairment in pregnancy-induced hypertension. Am J Obstet Gynecol 164:507, 1991.

41. Fickling SA, Williams D, Vallance P, et al: Plasma concentrations of endogenous inhibitor of nitric oxide synthesis in normal pregnancy and pre-eclampsia. Lancet 342:242, 1993.

42. Seligman SP, Buyon JP, Clancy RM, et al: The role of nitric oxide in the pathogenesis of preeclampsia. Am J Obstet Gynecol 171:944, 1994.

43. Baylis C, Beinder E, Suto T, August P: Recent insights into the roles of nitric oxide and renin-angiotensin in the pathophysiology of preeclamptic pregnancy. Semin Nephrol 18:208, 1998.

44. Nova A, Sibai BM, Barton JR, et al: Maternal plasma levels of endothelin is increased in preeclampsia. Am J Obstet Gynecol 164:794, 1991.

45. Branch DW, Dudley DJ, Mitchell MD: Preliminary evidence for homeostatic mechanism regulating endothelin production in preeclampsia. Lancet 337:943, 1991.

46. Clark BA, Halvorson L, Sachs B, Epstein FH: Plasma endothelin levels in preeclampsia: elevations and correlation with uric acid and renal impairment. Am J Obstet Gynecol 166: 962, 1992.

47. Benigni A, Orisio S, Gaspari F, et al: Evidence against a pathologic role for endothelin in preeclampsia. Br J Obstet Gynaecol 99:798, 1992.

48. Walsh SW: Lipid peroxidation in pregnancy. Hypertension in pregnancy. Am J Obstet Gynecol 13:1, 1994.

49. Poranen AK, Ekblad U, Uotila P, Ahotuha M: Lipid peroxidation and antioxidants in normal and pre-eclamptic pregnancies. Placenta 17:401, 1996.

50. Hubel CA, Kagan VE, Kisin ER, et al: Increased ascorbate radical formation an ascorbate depletion in plasma from women with preeclampsia: implications for oxidative stress. Free Radic Biol Med 23:597, 1997.

51. Arborgast BW, Leeper SC, Merrick RD, et al: Plasma factors that determine endothelial cell lipid toxicity in vitro correctly identifying women with preeclampsia in early and late gestation. Hypertens Pregnancy 15:263, 1996.

52. Dekker GA, Kraayenbrink AA: Oxygen free radicals in preeclampsia. Am J Obstet Gynecol 164:273, 1991.

53. Uotila JT, Tuinaala RJ, Aarnis TM, et al: Findings on lipid peroxidation and antioxidant function in hypertensive complications of pregnancy. Br J Obstet Gynaecol 100:270, 1993.

54. Wang Y, Walsh SW, Guo J, et al: The imbalance between thromboxane and prostacyclin in preeclampsia is associated with an imbalance between lipid peroxides and vitamin E in maternal blood. Am J Obstet Gynecol 167:946, 1992.

55. Davidge ST, Hubel CA, Braden RD, et al: Sera antioxidant activity in uncomplicated and preeclamptic pregnancies. Obstet Gynecol 79:897, 1992.

56. Wisdom SJ, Wilson R, McKillop JH, Walker JJ: Antioxidant systems in normal pregnancy and in pregnancy-induced hypertension. Am J Obstet Gynecol 165:1701, 1991.

57. Mikhail MS, Anyaegbunam A, Garfinkel D, et al: Preeclampsia and antioxidant nutrients: decreased plasma levels of reduced ascorbic acid, -tocopherol, and beta-carotene in women with preeclampsia. Am J Obstet Gynecol 171:150, 1994.

58. Hubel CA, McLaughlin MK, Evans RW, et al: Fasting serum triglycerides, free fatty acids, and malondialdehyde are increased in preeclampsia, are positively correlated, and decrease within 48 hours postpartum. Am J Obstet Gynecol 174:975, 1996.

59. Chappell LC, Seed PT, Briley AL, et al: Effect of antioxidants on the occurrence of pre-eclampsia in women at increased risk. Lancet 354:810, 1999.

60. Myatt L, Miodovnik M: Prediction of preeclampsia. Semin Perinatol 23:45, 1999.

61. Dizon-Townson DS, Nelson LM, Easton K, Ward K: The factor V Leiden mutation may predispose women to severe preeclampsia. Am J Obstet Gynaecol 175:902, 1996.

62. Dekker GA, deVries JIP, Doelitzsch PM, et al: Underlying disorders associated with severe early-onset preeclampsia. Am J Obstet Gynecol 173:1042, 1995.

63. Van Pampus MG, Dekker GA, Wolf H, et al: High prevalence of hemostatic abnormalities in women with a history of severe preeclampsia. Am J Obstet Gynecol 180:1146, 1999.

64. Degroot CJM, Bloemenkamp KWM, Duvekot EJ, et al: Preeclampsia and genetic risk factors for thrombosis: a case-control study. Am J Obstet Gynecol 181:975, 1999.

65. Kupferminc MJ, Elder A, Steinman N, et al: Increased frequency of genetic thrombophilias in women with complications of pregnancy. N Engl J Med 340:9, 1999.

66. Livingston JC, Barton JR, Park V, et al: Maternal and fetal genetic thrombophilias are not associated with severe preeclampsia [abstract 34]. Am J Obstet Gynecol 182:S-25, 2000.

67. Powers RW, Minich LA, Lykins DA, et al: Methylene tetrahydrofolate reductase polymorphism, folate, and susceptibility to preeclampsia. J Soc Gynecol Invest 6:74, 1999.

68. O'Shaughnessy KM, Fu B, Ferraro F, et al: Factor V Leiden

and thermolalule metheylene tetrahydrofolate reductase gene variants in an East Anglian preeclampsia cohort. Hypertension 33:1338, 1999.

69. Sibai BM: Thrombophilias and adverse outcome of pregnancy—what should a clinician do? N Engl J Med 340:50, 1999.

70. Steer PJ: The definition of pre-eclampsia. Br J Obstet Gynaecol 106:753, 1999.

71. Lopez MC, Belizan JM, Villar J, Bergel E: The measurement of diastolic blood pressure during pregnancy: which Korotkoff phase should be used? Am J Obstet Gynecol 170:574, 1992.

72. Blank SG, Heleth G, Pickering TG, et al: How should diastolic blood pressure be defined during pregnancy. Hypertension 24:234, 1994.

73. Johenning AR, Barron WM: Indirect blood pressure measurement in pregnancy: Korotkoff phase 4 versus phase 5. Am J Obstet Gynecol 167:577, 1992.

74. MacGillivray I, Rose GA, Rowe D: Blood pressure survey in pregnancy. Clin Sci 72:395, 1969.

75. Redman CWG, Jeffries M: Revised definition of preeclampsia. Lancet 1:809, 1988.

76. Perry IJ, Beevers DG: The definition of pre-eclampsia. Br J Obstet Gynaecol 101:587, 1994.

77. Villar MA, Sibai BM: Clinical significance of elevated mean arterial blood in second trimester and threshold increase in systolic or diastolic pressure during third trimester. Am J Obstet Gynecol 60:419, 1989.

78. North RA, Taylor RS, Schellenberg J-C: Evaluation of a definition of pre-eclampsia. Br J Obstet Gynaecol 106:767, 1999.

79. Levine RJ, Ewell MG, Hauth JC, et al: Should the definition of preeclampsia include a rise in diastolic blood pressure of ≥15 mmHg to a level <90 mmHg in association with proteinuria? Am J Obstet Gynecol 183:787, 2000.

80. Roberts JM, Redman CWE: Pre-eclampsia is more than pregnancy-induced hypertension. Lancet 341:1447, 1993.

81. Ferrazani S, Caruso A, Carolis S, et al: Proteinuria and outcome of 444 pregnancies complicated by hypertension. Am J Obstet Gynecol 162:366, 1990.

82. Halligan AWF, Bell SC, Taylor DJ: Dipstick proteinuria: caveat emptor. Br J Obstet Gynaecol 106:1113, 1999.

83. Bell SC, Halligan AWF, Martin J, et al: The role of observer error in antenatal dipstick proteinuria analysis. Br J Obstet Gynaecol 106:1177, 1999.

84. Lindow SW, Davey DA: The variability of urinary protein and creatinine excretion in patients with gestational proteinuric hypertension. Br J Obstet Gynaecol 99:869, 1992.

85. Lopez-Ramos JG, Martins-Costa SH, Mathias MM, et al: Urinary protein/creatinine ratio in hypertensive pregnant women. Hypertens Pregnancy 18:209, 1999.

86. Kuo VS, Koumantakis G, Gallery EDM: Proteinuria and its assessment in normal and hypertensive pregnancy. Am J Obstet Gynecol 167:723, 1992.

87. Meyer NL, Mercer BM, Friedman SA, Sibai BM: Urinary dipstick protein: a poor predictor of absent or severe proteinuria. Am J Obstet Gynecol 170:137, 1994.

88. Brown MA, Buddle ML: Inadequacy of dipstick proteinuria in hypertensive pregnancy. Aust N Z J Obstet Gynaecol 35:366, 1995.

89. Saudan PJ, Brown MA, Farrell T, Shaw L: Improved methods in assessing proteinuria in hypertensive pregnancy. Br J Obstet Gynaecol 104:1159, 1997.

90. Dekker GA, Sibai BM: Early detection of preeclampsia. Am J Obstet Gynecol 165:160, 1991.

91. Friedman SA, Lindheimer MD: Prediction and differential diagnosis. *In* Lindheimer MD, Roberts JM, Cunningham GF

(eds): Chesley's hypertensive disorders in pregnancy. Stamford, CT, Appleton & Lange, 1999, p 201.

92. Sibai BM: Prevention of preeclampsia: a big disappointment. Clinical opinion. Am J Obstet Gynecol 179:1275, 1998.

93. Hatton DC, McCarron DA: Dietary calcium and blood pressure in experimental models of hypertension: a review. Hypertension 23:513, 1994.

94. Taufield PA, Ales KL, Resnick LM, et al: Hypocalciuria in preeclampsia. N Engl J Med 316:715, 1987.

95. Sanchez-Ramos L, Sandroni S, Andres FL, Kaunitz AM: Calcium excretion in preeclampsia. Obstet Gynecol 77:510, 1991.

96. Sanchez-Ramos L, Jones DC, Cullen MT: Urinary calcium as an early marker for preeclampsia. Obstet Gynecol 77:685, 1991.

97. Belizan JM, Villar J, Repke J: The relationship between calcium intake and pregnancy induced hypertension: up to date evidence. Am J Obstet Gynecol 158:898, 1988.

98. Sanchez-Ramos L, Briones DK, Kaunitz AM, et al: Prevention of pregnancy-induced hypertension by calcium supplementation in angiotensin-II sensitive patients. Obstet Gynecol 84:349, 1994.

99. Lopez-Jaramillo P, Narvaez M, Weigel RM, et al: Calcium supplementation reduces the risk of pregnancy-induced hypertension in an Andes population. Br J Obstet Gynaecol 96:648, 1987.

100. Villar J, Repke JT: Calcium supplementation during pregnancy may reduce preterm delivery in high-risk populations. Am J Obstet Gynecol 163:1124, 1990.

101. Belizan JM, Villar J, Gonzalez L, et al: Calcium supplementation to prevent hypertensive disorders of pregnancy. N Engl J Med 325:1399, 1991.

102. Lopez-Jaramillo P, Narvaez M, Felix C, Lopez A: Dietary calcium supplementation and prevention of pregnancy hypertension. Lancet 335:293, 1990.

103. Lopez-Jaramillo P, Delgado F, Jacoine P, et al: Calcium supplementation and the risk of preeclampsia in Ecuadorian pregnant teenagers. Obstet Gynecol 90:162, 1997.

104. Levine RJ, Hauth JC, Curet LB, et al: Trial of calcium to prevent preeclampsia. N Engl J Med 337:69 1997.

105. Herrera JA, Arevalo-Herrara M, Herrara S: Prevention of preeclampsia by linoleic acid and calcium supplementation: a randomized controlled trial. Obstet Gynecol 91:585, 1998.

106. Crowther CA, Hiller JE, Pridmore B, et al: Calcium supplementation in nulliparous women for the prevention of pregnancy-induced hypertension, preeclampsia and preterm birth: an Australian randomized trial. Aust N Z J Obstet Gynaecol 39:12, 1999.

107. Rogers MS, Fung HYM, Hung CY: Calcium and low-dose aspirin prophylaxis in women at high risk of pregnancy-induced hypertension. Hypertens Pregnancy 18:165, 1999.

108. Sibai BM, Villar MA, Bray E: Magnesium supplementation during pregnancy: a double-blind randomized controlled clinical trial. Am J Obstet Gynecol 161:115, 1989.

109. Altura BM, Altura BT, Carella A: Magnesium deficiency induced spasm of umbilical vessels: relation to preeclampsia, hypertension, growth retardation. Science 221:376, 1983.

110. Conradt A, Weidinger H, Algayer H: On the role of magnesium in fetal hypotrophy, pregnancy-induced hypertension and preeclampsia. Mag Bull 6:68, 1984.

111. Spatling L, Spatling G: Magnesium supplementation in pregnancy. A double-blind study. Br J Obstet Gynaecol 95:120, 1988.

112. Lazebnik N, Kuhnert BR, Kuhnert BM, Thompson KL: Zinc status, pregnancy complications and labor abnormalities. Am J Obstet Gynecol 158:161, 1988.

113. Hunt IF, Murphy NJ, Cleaver AE, et al: Zinc supplementa-

tion during pregnancy: effects on selected blood constituents and on progress and outcome of pregnancy in low-income women of Mexican descent. Am J Clin Nutr 40:508, 1984.

114. Mohamed K, James DK, Golding J, McCabe R: Zinc supplementation during pregnancy: a double-blind randomized controlled trial. BMJ 299:826, 1989.

115. Spitz B, Magness RR, Cox SM, et al: Low-dose aspirin. I. Effect on angiotensin II pressor responses and blood prostaglandin concentration in pregnant women sensitive to angiotensin II. Am J Obstet Gyneco1159:1035, 1988.

116. Sibai BM, Mirro R, Chesney CM, Leffer C: Low dose aspirin in pregnancy. Obstet Gynecol 74:551, 1989.

117. Dekker GA, Sibai BM: Low-dose aspirin: the prevention of preeclampsia and fetal growth retardation: rationale, mechanisms, and clinical trials. Am J Obstet Gynecol 168:214, 1993.

118. Hauth JC, Goldenberg RL, Parker R Jr, et al: Low-dose aspirin therapy to prevent preeclampsia. Am J Obstet Gynecol 168:1083, 1993.

119. Italian Study of Aspirin in Pregnancy: Low-dose aspirin in prevention and treatment of intrauterine growth retardation and pregnancy-induced hypertension. Lancet 341:396, 1993.

120. CLASP: A randomized trial of low-dose aspirin for the prevention and treatment of pre-eclampsia among 9364 pregnant women. Lancet 343:619, 1994.

121. ECPPA (Estudo Colaborativo para Prevencao da Pre-eclampsia com Asprina) Collaborative Group: ECPPA: randomised trial of low dose aspirin for the prevention of maternal and fetal complications in high risk pregnant women. Br J Obstet Gynaecol 103:39, 1996.

122. Golding J: A randomised trial of low dose aspirin for primiparae in pregnancy. The Jamaica Low-Dose Aspirin Study Group. Br J Obstet Gynaecol 105:293, 1998.

123. Caritis SN, Sibai BM, Hauth J, et al, for the National Institute of Child Health and Human Development: Low-dose aspirin therapy to prevent preeclampsia in women at high risk. N Engl J Med 338:701, 1998.

124. Rotchell YE, Cruickshank JK, Gay MP, et al: Barbados Low Dose Aspirin Study in Pregnancy (BLASP): a randomised trial for the prevention of pre-eclampsia and its complications. Br J Obstet Gynaecol 105:286, 1998.

125. McParland P, Pearce JM, Chamberlain GVP: Doppler ultrasound and aspirin in recognition and prevention of pregnancy-induced hypertension. Lancet 335:1552, 1990.

126. Morris JM, Fay RF, Ellwood DA, et al: A randomized controlled trial of aspirin in patients with abnormal uterine artery blood flow. Obstet Gynecol 87:74, 1996.

127. Bower SJ, Harrington KF, Schuchter K, et al: Prediction of preeclampsia by abnormal uterine Doppler ultrasound and modification by aspirin. Br J Obstet Gynaecol 103:625, 1996.

128. Olsen SF, Secher NJ, Talior T, et al: Randomised clinical trials of fish oil supplementation in high risk pregnancies. Br J Obstet Gynaecol 107:382, 2000.

129. Cunningham FG, Lindheimer MD: Hypertension in pregnancy. N Engl J Med 326:927, 1992.

130. Sibai BM, Barton JR, Akl S, et al: A randomized prospective comparison of nifedipine and bed rest versus bed rest alone in the management of preeclampsia remote from term. Am J Obstet Gynecol 167:879, 1992.

131. Sibai BM, Mercer BM, Schiff E, Friedman SA: Aggressive versus expectant management of severe preeclampsia at 28 to 32 weeks' gestation: a randomized controlled trial. Am J Obstet Gynecol 171:818, 1994.

132. Redman CWG, Beilin LJ, Bonnar J: Plasma urate measurement in predicting fetal death in hypertensive pregnancies. Lancet 1:1370, 1976.

133. Pritchard JA, Stone SR: Clinical and laboratory observations on eclampsia. Am J Obstet Gynecol 99:754, 1967.

134. Weinstein L: Syndrome of hemolysis, elevated liver enzymes, and low platelet count; a severe consequence of hypertension in pregnancy. Am J Obstet Gynecol 142:159, 1982.

135. Arias F, Mancill-Jimenez R: Hepatic fibringen deposits in preeclampsia-immunofluorescent evidence. N Engl J Med 11:294, 1976.

136. Romero R, Vizosa J, Emamian M, et al: Clinical significance of liver dysfunction in pregnancy-induced hypertension. Am J Perinatol 5:146, 1988.

137. Weiner C: Preeclampsia-eclampsia syndrome and coagulation. Clin Perinatol 18:713, 1992.

138. Perry KG Jr, Martin JN Jr: Abnormal hemostasis and coagulopathy in preeclampsia and eclampsia. Clin Obstet Gynecol 35:338, 1992.

139. Sibai BM, Watson DL, Hill GA, et al: Maternal-fetal correlations in patients with severe preeclampsia-eclampsia. Obstet Gynecol 62:745, 1983.

140. Leduc L, Wheeler JM, Kirshon B, et al: Coagulation profile in severe preeclampsia. Obstet Gynecol 79:14, 1992.

141. Burrows F, Kelton JG: Fetal thrombocytopenia in relation to maternal thrombocytopenia. N Engl J Med 329:1463, 1993.

142. Barron WM, Heckerling P, Hibbard JU, Fisher S: Reducing unnecessary coagulation testing in hypertensive disorders of pregnancy. Obstet Gynecol 94:364, 1999.

143. Sibai BM, Taslimi MM, El-Nazer A, et al: Maternal-perinatal outcome associated with the syndrome of hemolysis, elevated liver enzymes, and low platelets in severe preeclampsia-eclampsia. Am J Obstet Gynecol 155:501, 1986.

144. Goodlin RC: Hemolysis, elevated liver enzymes, and low platelets syndrome. Obstet Gynecol 64:449, 1984.

145. MacKenna J, Dover NL, Brame RG: Preeclampsia associated with hemolysis, elevated liver enzymes and low platelets-an obstetric emergency? Obstet Gynecol 62:751, 1983.

146. Sibai BM: The HELLP syndrome (hemolysis, elevated liver enzymes, and low platelets): much ado about nothing? Am J Obstet Gynecol 162:311, 1990.

147. Barton JR, Riely CA, Adamec TA, et al: Hepatic histopathologic condition does not correlate with laboratory abnormalities in HELLP syndrome. Am J Obstet Gynecol 167:1538, 1992.

148. Martin JN Jr, Files JC, Black PG, et al: Plasma exchange for preeclampsia. I. Postpartum use for persistently severe preeclampsia-eclampsia with HELLP syndrome. Am J Obstet Gynecol 162:126, 1990.

149. Martin JN Jr, Blake PG, Lowry SL, et al: Pregnancy complicated by preeclampsia-eclampsia with the syndrome of hemolysis, elevated liver enzymes, and low platelet count: how rapid is postpartum recovery? Obstet Gynecol 76:737, 1990.

150. Miles JF Jr, Martin JN Jr, Blake PG, et al: Postpartum eclampsia: a recurring perinatal dilemma. Obstet Gynecol 76:328, 1990.

151. Van Dam PA, Reiner M, Baeklandt M, et al: Disseminated intravascular coagulation and the syndrome of hemolysis, elevated liver enzymes, and low platelets in severe preeclampsia. Obstet Gynecol 73:97, 1989.

152. de Boer K, Buller HR, ten Cate JW, Treffers PE: Coagulation studies in the syndrome of haemolysis, elevated liver enzymes, and low platelets. Br J Obstet Gynaecol 98:42, 1991.

153. Sibai BM, Ramadan MK, Usta I, et al: Maternal morbidity and mortality in 442 pregnancies with hemolysis, elevated liver enzymes, and low platelets (HELLP syndrome). Am J Obstet Gynecol 169:1000, 1993.

154. Aarnoudse JG, Houthoff HF, Weits J, et al: A syndrome of liver damage and intravascular coagulation in the last trimes-

ter of normotensive pregnancy. A clinical and histopathological study. Br J Obstet Gynaecol 93:145, 1986.

155. Schwartz ML, Brenner WE: Pregnancy-induced hypertension presenting with life-threatening thrombocytopenia. Am J Obstet Gynecol 146:756, 1983.

156. Goodlin RC: Beware the great imitator—severe preeclampsia. Contemp Obstet Gynecol 20:215, 1982.

157. Thiagarajah S, Bourgeois FJ, Harbert GM, Caudle MR: Thrombocytopenia in preeclampsia: associated abnormalities and management principles. Am J Obstet Gynecol 150:1, 1984.

158. Heyborne KD, Burke MS, Porreco RP: Prolongation of premature gestation in women with hemolysis, elevated liver enzyme, and low platelets. A report of 5 cases. J Reprod Med 35:53, 1990.

159. O'Brien JM, Milligan DA, Barton JR: Impact of high-dose corticosteroid therapy for patients with HELLP syndrome. Am J Obstet Gynecol 183:921, 2000.

160. Van Assche FA, Spitz B: Thromboxane synthetase inhibition in pregnancy-induced hypertension. Am J Obstet Gynecol 159:1015, 1988.

161. Magann EF, Bass D, Chauhan SP, et al: Antepartum corticosteroids: disease stabilization in patients with the syndrome of hemolysis, elevated liver enzymes, and low platelets (HELLP). Am J Obstet Gynecol 171:1148, 1994.

162. Magann EF, Perry KO Jr, Meydrech EF, et al: Postpartum corticosteroids: accelerated recovery from the syndrome of hemolysis, elevated liver enzymes, and low platelets (HELLP). Am J Obstet Gynecol 171:1154, 1994.

163. Martin JN Jr, Perry KG, Blake PG, et al: Better maternal outcomes are achieved with dexamethasone therapy for postpartum HELLP syndrome. Am J Obstet Gynecol 177:1011, 1997.

164. Tompkins MJ, Thiagarajah S: HELLP syndrome: the benefit of corticosteroids. Am J Obstet Gynecol 181:304, 1999.

165. Visser W, Wallenburg HCS: Temporising management of severe pre-eclampsia with and without the HELLP syndrome. Br J Obstet Gynaecol 102:111, 1995.

166. Van Pampus MG, Wolf H, Westenberg SM, et al: Maternal and perinatal outcome after expectant management of the HELLP syndrome compared with preeclampsia without HELLP syndrome. Eur J Obstet Gynecol Reprod Biol 76: 31,1998.

167. Woods JB, Blake PG, Perry KG Jr, et al: Ascites: a portent of cardiopulmonary complications in the preeclamptic patient with the syndrome of hemolysis, elevated liver enzymes, and low platelets. Obstet Gynecol 80:87, 1992.

168. Abroug F, Boujdaria R, Nouira S, et al: HELLP syndrome: incidence and maternal-fetal outcome: a prospective study. Intensive Care Med 18:274, 1992.

169. Sibai BM, Ramadan MK: Acute renal failure in pregnancies complicated by hemolysis, elevated liver enzymes, and low platelets. Am J Obstet Gynecol 168:1682, 1993.

170. Audibert F, Friedman SA, Frangieh AY, Sibai BM: Clinical utility of strict diagnostic criteria for the HELLP (hemolysis, elevated liver enzymes, and low platelets) syndrome. Am J Obstet Gynecol 175:460, 1996.

171. Schwartz ML: Possible role for exchange plasmapheresis with fresh frozen plasma for maternal indications in selected cases of preeclampsia and eclampsia. Obstet Gynecol 68:136, 1986.

172. Barton JR, Sibai BM: Hepatic imaging findings in HELLP syndrome (hemolysis, elevated liver enzymes, and low platelet count). Am J Obstet Gynecol 174:1820, 1996.

173. Goodlin RC, Anderson JC, Hodgson PE: Conservative treatment of liver hematoma in the postpartum period. J Reprod Med 30:368, 1985.

174. Manas KJ, Welsh JD, Rankin RA: Hepatic haemorrhage without rupture in preeclampsia. N Engl J Med 312:424, 1985.

175. Barton JR, Sibai BM: Care of the pregnancy complicated by HELLP syndrome. Obstet Gynecol Clin North Am 18:165, 1991.

176. Smith JG Jr, Moise KJ Jr, Dildy GA, et al: Spontaneous rupture of the liver during pregnancy: current therapy. Obstet Gynecol 77:171, 1991.

177. Reinehart BK, Terrone DA, Magann EF, et al: Preeclampsia-associated hepatic hemorrhage and rupture: mode of management related to maternal and perinatal outcome. Obstet Gynecol Surv 54:196, 1999.

178. Sibai BM, Mabie WC: Hemodynamics of preeclampsia. Clin Perinatol 18:727, 1991.

179. Groenendijk R, Trimbos JBMJ, Wallenburg HCS: Hemodynamic measurements in preeclampsia. Preliminary observations. Am J Obstet Gynecol 150:812, 1985.

180. Cotton DB, Jones MM, Longmire S, et al: Role of intravenous nitroglycerin in the treatment of severe pregnancy-induced hypertension complicated by pulmonary edema. Am J Obstet Gynecol 143:91, 1986.

181. Wallenburg HS: Hemodynamics in hypertensive pregnancy. *In* Rubin PC (ed): Handbook of Hypertension—Hypertension in Pregnancy, Vol. 10. Elsevier, Amsterdam, 1988, p 66.

182. Belfort MA, Anthony J, Buccimmazza L, et al: Hemodynamic changes associated with intravenous infusion of the calcium antagonist verapamil in the treatment of severe gestational proteinuric hypertension. Obstet Gynecol 75:970, 1990.

183. Belfort MA, Uys P, Dommisse J, et al: Hemodynamic changes in gestational proteinuric hypertension: the effects of rapid volume expansion and vasodilator therapy. Br J Obstet Gynaecol 96:634, 1989.

184. Cotton DB, Lee W, Huhta JC, Dorman K: Hemodynamic profile of severe pregnancy-induced hypertension. Am J Obstet Gynecol 158:523, 1988.

185. Mabie WE, Ratts TE, Sibai BM: The hemodynamic profile of severe preeclamptic patients requiring delivery. Am J Obstet Gynecol 161:1443, 1989.

186. Fairlie FC: Doppler flow velocimetry in hypertension in pregnancy. Clin Perinatol 18:749, 1991.

187. Fleischer A, Schulman H, Favenakides G, et al: Uterine artery Doppler velocimetry in pregnant women with hypertension. Am J Obstet Gynecol 154:806, 1986.

188. Ducey J, Schulman H, Farmakides G, et al: A classification of hypertension in pregnancy based on Doppler velocimetry. Am J Obstet Gynecol 157:680, 1987.

189. Gudmundsson S, Marsal K: Ultrasound Doppler evaluation of uteroplacental and fetoplacental circulation in preeclampsia. Arch Gynecol Obstet 243:199, 1988.

190. Cameron AD, Nicholson SF, Nimrod CA, et al: Doppler waveforms in fetal aorta and umbilical artery in patients with hypertension in pregnancy. Am J Obstet Gynecol 158:339, 1988.

191. Steel SA, Pearce JM, McParland P, Chamberlain CVP: Early Doppler ultrasound screening in prediction of hypertensive disorders of pregnancy. Lancet 335:1548, 1990.

192. Bower S, Schuchter K, Campbell S: Doppler ultrasound screening as part of routine antenatal scanning: prediction of pre-eclampsia and intrauterine growth retardation. Br J Obstet Gynaecol 199:989, 1993.

193. Irion O, Masse J, Forest JC, et al: Prediction of preeclampsia, low birth weight for gestation, and prematurity by uterine artery flow velocity waveforms analysis in low risk nulliparous women. Br J Obstet Gynaecol 105:422, 1998.

194. Chien PFW, Arnott N, Gordon P, et al: How useful is uterine artery Doppler flow velocimetry in the prediction of preec-

lampsia, intrauterine growth retardation and perinatal death? An overview. Br J Obstet Gynaecol 107:196, 2000.

195. Trudinger BJ, Cook CM: Doppler umbilical and uterine flow waveforms in severe pregnancy hypertension. Br J Obstet Gynaecol 97:142, 1990.

196. Yoon BH, Lee CM, Kim SW: An abnormal umbilical artery waveform: a strong and independent predictor of adverse perinatal outcome in patients with preeclampsia. Am J Obstet Gynecol 171:713, 1994.

197. Pattinson RC, Norman K, Odendaal HJ: The role of Doppler velocimetry in the management of high risk pregnancies. Br J Obstet Gynaecol 101:114, 1994.

198. Fairlie FM, Moretti M, Walker JJ, Sibai BM: Umbilical artery and uteroplacental velocimetry in pregnancies complicated by idiopathic low birthweight centile. Am J Perinatol 9:250, 1992.

199. Gilstrap LC, Cunningham GR, Whalley PJ: Management of pregnancy induced hypertension in the nulliparous patient remote from term. Semin Perinatol 2:73, 1978.

200. Mabie WC, Gonzalez AR, Sibai BM, et al: A comparative trial of labetalol and hydralazine in the acute management of severe hypertension complicating pregnancy. Obstet Gynecol 70:328, 1987.

201. Mathews DD: A randomized controlled trial of bed rest and sedation or normal activity and non-sedation in the management of nonalbuminuric hypertension in late pregnancy. Br J Obstet Gynaecol 84:108, 1977.

202. Crawther CA, Boumeester AM, Ashwist HM: Does admission to hospital for bedrest prevent disease progression or improve fetal outcome in pregnancy complicated by non-proteinuric hypertension? Br J Obstet Gynaecol 99:13, 1992.

203. Soothill PW, Ajayi R, Campbell S, et al: Effect of a fetal surveillance unit on admission of antenatal patients to hospital. BMJ 303:269, 1991.

204. Tuffnell DJ, Lilford RJ, Buchan PC, et al: Randomized controlled trial of day care for hypertension in pregnancy. Lancet 339:224, 1992.

205. Goldenberg RL, Cliver SP, Bronstein J, et al: Bedrest in pregnancy. Obstet Gynecol 84:131, 1994.

206. Barton JR, Stanziano GJ, Sibai BM: Monitored outpatient management of mild gestational hypertension remote from term. Am J Obstet Gynecol 170:765, 1994.

207. Witlin AG, Friedman SA, Sibai BM: The effect of magnesium sulfate therapy on the duration of labor in women with mild preeclampsia at term. Am J Obstet Gynecol 176:623, 1997.

208. Lucas MJ, Leveno KJ, Cunningham FG: A comparison of magnesium sulfate with phenytoin for the prevention of eclampsia. N Engl J Med 333:201, 1995.

209. Schiff E, Friedman S, Sibai BM: Conservative management of severe preeclampsia remote from term. Obstet Gynecol 84:626, 1994.

210. Olah KS, Redman CWG, Gee H: Management of severe early preeclampsia: is conservative management justified? Eur J Obstet Gynaecol Reprod Biol 51:175, 1993.

211. Chua S, Redman CWG: Prognosis for preeclampsia complicated by 5 g or more of proteinuria in 24 hours. Eur J Obstet Gynecol Reprod Biol 43:9, 1992.

212. Odendaal HJ, Pattinson RC, DuToit R: Fetal and neonatal outcome in patients with severe preeclampsia delivered before 34 weeks. S Afr Med J 71:555, 1987.

213. Moodley J, Koranteng SA, Rout C: Expectant management of early onset of severe preeclampsia in Durban. S Afr Med J 83:584, 1993.

214. Odendaal HJ, Pattinson RC, Bam R, et al: Aggressive or expectant management of patients with severe preeclampsia between 28–34 weeks' gestation: a randomized controlled trial. Obstet Gynecol 76:1070, 1990.

215. Fenakel K, Fenakel E, Appleman Z, et al: Nifedipine in the treatment of severe preeclampsia. Obstet Gynecol 77:331, 1991.

216. Pattinson RC, Odendaal HJ, DuToit R: Conservative management of severe proteinuric hypertension before 28 weeks' gestation. S Afr Med J 73:516, 1988.

217. Sibai BM, Taslimi M, Abdella TN, et al: Maternal and perinatal outcome of conservative management of severe preeclampsia in midtrimester. Am J Obstet Gynecol 152:32, 1988.

218. Sibai BM, Akl S, Fairlie F, Moretti M: A protocol for managing severe preeclampsia in the second trimester. Am J Obstet Gynecol 163:733, 1990.

219. Schiff E, Friedman SA, Mercer BM, Sibai BM: Fetal lung maturity is not accelerated in preeclamptic pregnancies. Am J Obstet Gynecol 169:1096, 1993.

220. Piazze JJ, Maranghi L, Nigro G, et al: The effect of glucocorticoid therapy on fetal lung maturity indices in hypertensive pregnancies. Obstet Gynecol 92:220, 1998.

221. Sibai BM: Hypertension in pregnancy. Obstet Gynecol Clin North Am 19:615, 1992.

222. Coetzee EJ, Dommisse J, Anthony J: A randomized controlled trial of intravenous magnesium sulfate versus placebo in the management of women with severe preeclampsia. Br J Obstet Gynaecol 105:300, 1998.

223. Chesley LC: Parenteral magnesium sulfate and the distribution, plasma levels and excretion of magnesium. Am J Obstet Gynecol 133:1, 1979.

224. Patterson-Brown S, Robson SC, Redfern N, et al: Hydralazine boluses for the treatment of severe hypertension in preeclampsia. Br J Obstet Gynaecol 101:409, 1994

225. Mabie WC, Gonzalez AR, Sibai BM, et al: A comparative trial of labetalol and hydralazine in the acute management of severe hypertension complicating pregnancy. Obstet Gynecol 70:328, 1987.

226. Scardo JA, Vermillion ST, Hogg BB, Newman RB: Hemodynamic effects of oral nifedipine in preeclamptic hypertensive emergencies. Am J Obstet Gynecol 175:336, 1996.

227. Vermillion ST, Scardo JA, Newman RB, Chauhan SP: A randomized, double-blind trial of oral nifedipine and intravenous labetalol in hypertensive emergencies of pregnancy. Am J Obstet Gynecol 181:858, 1999.

228. Sibai BM, Mabie WE, Harvey CJ, Gonzalez AR: Pulmonary edema in severe preeclampsia-eclampsia: analysis of 37 consecutive cases. Am J Obstet Gynecol 159:650, 1988.

229. Ramanathan J, Sibai BM, Mabie WC, et al: The use of labetalol for attenuation of the hypertensive response to endotracheal intubation in preeclampsia. Am J Obstet Gynecol 159:650, 1988.

230. Hawkins JL, Koonin LM, Palmer SK, Gibbs CP: Anesthesia-related deaths during obstetric delivery in the United Staes, 1979–1990. Anesthesiology 86:277, 1997.

231. Ramanathan J, Coleman P, Sibai B: Anesthetic modification of hemodynamic and neuroendocrine stress responses to cesarean delivery in women with severe preeclampsia. Anesth Analg 73:772, 1991.

232. Wallace DH, Leveno KJ, Cunningham GF, et al: Randomized comparison of general and regional anesthesia for cesarean delivery in pregnancies complicated by severe preeclampsia. Obstet Gynecol 86:193, 1995.

233. Hood DD, Curry R: Spinal versus epidural anesthesia for cesarean section in severely preeclamptic patients: a retrospective survey. Anesthesiology 90:1276, 1999.

234. Hog B, Hauth JC, Caritis SN, et al: Safety of labor epidural anesthesia for women with severe hypertensive disease. Am J Obstet Gynecol 181:1096, 1999.

235. Clark SL, Cotton DB: Clinical indications for pulmonary ar-

tery catheterization in the patient with severe preeclampsia. Am J Obstet Gynecol 158:650, 1988.

236. Mabie WC, Ratts TE, Ramanathan KB, Sibai BM: Circulatory congestion in obese hypertensive women: a subset of pulmonary edema in pregnancy. Obstet Gynecol 72:553, 1988.

237. Abramovici D, Friedman SA, Mercer BM, et al: Neonatal outcome in severe preeclampsia at 24 to 36 weeks' gestation: does the HELLP (hemolysis, elevated liver enzymes, and low platelet count) syndrome matter? Am J Obstet Gynecol 180:221, 1999.

238. Sutherland A, Cooper DW, Howie PW, et al: The incidence of severe preeclampsia among mothers and mothers-in-law of preeclamptics and controls. Br J Obstet Gynaecol 88:785, 1981.

239. Sibai BM, El-Nazer A, Gonzalez-Ruiz AR: Severe preeclampsia-eclampsia in young primigravid women: subsequent pregnancy outcome and remote prognosis. Am J Obstet Gynecol 155:1011, 1986.

240. Sibai BM, Mercer B, Sarinoglu C: Severe preeclampsia in the second trimester: recurrence risk and long-term prognosis. Am J Obstet Gynecol 165:1408, 1991.

241. Sibai BM: Management and counseling of patients with preeclampsia remote from term. Clin Obstet Gynecol 2:426, 1992.

242. Sibai BM, Villar MA, Mabie BC: Acute renal failure in hypertensive disorders of pregnancy: pregnancy outcome and remote prognosis in thirty-one consecutive cases. Am J Obstet Gynecol 62:777, 1990.

243. Sibai BM, Ramadan MK, Chari RS, Friedman SA: Pregnancies complicated by hemolysis, elevated liver enzymes, and low platelets (HELLP): subsequent pregnancy outcome and long-term prognosis. Am J Obstet Gynecol 172:125, 1995.

244. Sakala EP, Moore WD: Successful term delivery after previous pregnancy with ruptured liver. Obstet Gynecol 68:124, 1986.

245. Alleman JSP, Delarue MWG, Hasaart THM: Successful delivery after hepatic rupture in previous pre-eclamptic pregnancy. Eur J Obstet Gynaecol 47:76, 1992.

246. Ihle BU, Long P, Oats J: Early onset preeclampsia: recognition of underlying renal disease. BMJ 294, 1987.

247. Chesley LC: History. In Chesley LC (ed): Hypertensive Disorders in Pregnancy, 2nd ed. New York, Appleton-Century-Crofts, 1978, p 17.

248. Walker VN, Baker WS: A comparison study of antihypertensive drug therapy and modified Stroganoff method in the management of severe toxemia of pregnancy. Am J Obstet Gynecol 181:1, 1961.

249. Sheehan HL, Lunch JB: Pathology of Toxemia of Pregnancy. Edinburgh, Churchill Livingstone, 1973.

250. Sibai BM, Abdella TN, Taylor HA: Eclampsia in the first half of pregnancy. Report of three cases and review of the literature. J Reprod Med 27:11, 1982.

251. Lubarsky SL, Barton JR, Friedman SA, et al: Late postpartum eclampsia revisited. Obstet Gynecol 83:502, 1994.

252. Ferraz EM, Sherline DM: Convulsive toxemia of pregnancy (eclampsia). South Med J 69:2, 1976.

253. Moller B, Lindmark G: Eclampsia in Sweden, 1976–1980. Acta Obstet Gynaecol Scand 65:307, 1986.

254. Barton JR, Sibai BM: Cerebral pathology in eclampsia. In Sibai BM (ed): Clinics Perinatology, Vol. 18. Philadelphia, WB Saunders Company, 1991, p 891.

255. Dahmus MA, Barton JR, Sibai BM: Cerebral imaging in eclampsia: magnetic resonance imaging versus computed tomography. Am J Obstet Gynecol 167:935, 1992.

256. Beck DW, Menezes AH: Intracerebral hemorrhage in a patient with eclampsia. JAMA 246:1442, 1981.

257. Colosimo C Jr, Fileni A, Moschini M, Guerrini P: CT findings in eclampsia. Neuroradiology 27:313, 1985.

258. Will AD, Lewis KL, Hinshaw DB Jr, et al: Cerebral vasoconstriction in toxemia. Neurology 37:1555, 1987.

259. Richards AM, Moodley J, Graham DI, Bullock MRR: Active management of the unconscious eclamptic patient. Br J Obstet Gynaecol 93:554, 1986.

260. Brown CEL, Purdy P, Cunningham FG: Head computed tomographic scans in women with eclampsia. Am J Obstet Gynecol 159:915, 1988.

261. Milliez J, Dahoun A, Boudraa M: Computed tomography of the brain in eclampsia. Obstet Gynecol 75:975, 1990.

262. Moodley J, Bobat SM, Hoffman M, Bill PLA: Electroencephalogram and computerized cerebral tomography findings in eclampsia. Br J Obstet Gynaecol 100:984, 1993.

263. Drislane FW, Wang AM: Multifocal cerebral hemorrhage in eclampsia and severe preeclampsia. J Neurol 244:194, 1997.

264. Royburt M, Seidman DS, Serr DM, Mashiach S: Neurologic involvement in hypertensive disease of pregnancy. Obstet Gynecol Surv 46:656, 1991.

265. Digre KB, Varner MW, Osborn AG, Crawford S: Cranial magnetic resonance imaging in severe preeclampsia vs. eclampsia. Arch Neurol 50:399, 1993.

266. Sanders TG, Clayman DA, Sanchez-Ramos L, et al: Brain in eclampsia: MR imaging with clinical correlation. Radiology 180:475, 1991.

267. Morriss MC, Twickler DM, Hatab MR, et al: Cerebral blood flow and cranial magnetic resonance imaging in eclampsia and severe preeclampsia. Obstet Gynecol 89:561, 1997.

268. Trommer BL, Homer D, Mikhael MA: Cerebral vasospasm and eclampsia. Stroke 19:326, 1988.

269. Williams KP, Wilson S: Persistence of cerebral hemodynamic changes in patients with eclampsia: a report of three cases. Am J Obstet Gynecol 181:1162, 1999.

270. Belfort MA, Saade GR, Grunewald C, et al: Association of cerebral perfusion pressure with headache in women with preeclampsia. Br J Obstet Gynaecol 106:814, 1999.

271. Belfort MA, Giannina G, Herd JA: Transcranial and orbital Doppler ultrasound in normal pregnancy and preeclampsia. Clin Obstet Gynecol 42:479, 1999.

272. Sibai BM, Spinnato JA, Watson DL, Anderson GD: Eclampsia. IV. Neurological findings and future outcome. Am J Obstet Gynecol 152:184, 1985.

273. Sibai BM, Spinnato JA, Watson DL, et al: Effects of magnesium sulfate on electroencephalographic findings in preeclampsia-eclampsia. Obstet Gynecol 64:261, 1984.

274. Pritchard JA, Cunningham FG, Pritchard SA: The Parkland Memorial Hospital protocol for treatment of eclampsia: evaluation of 245 cases. Am J Obstet Gynecol 148:951, 1984.

275. Sibai BM, Anderson GD, McCubbin JH: Eclampsia II. Clinical significance of laboratory findings. Obstet Gynecol 59:153, 1982.

276. Sibai BM, Anderson GD, Abdella TN, et al: Eclampsia III. Neonatal outcome, growth and development. Am J Obstet Gynecol 146:307, 1983.

277. Paul RH, Koh KS, Bernstein SG: Changes in fetal heart rate-uterine contraction patterns associated with eclampsia. Am J Obstet Gynecol 130:165, 1978.

278. Medical Economics Data: Physicians' Desk Reference 1994, 48th ed. Montvale, NJ, Medical Economics Data, 1994, p 1967.

279. Gedekoh RH, Hayashi TT, McDonald HM: Eclampsia at Maggee-Women's Hospital, 1970 to 1980. Am J Obstet Gynecol 140:860, 1981.

280. Sibai BM: Magnesium sulfate is the ideal anticonvulsant in preeclampsia-eclampsia. Am J Obstet Gynecol 162:1141, 1990.

281. McCubbin JH, Sibai BM, Abdella TN, et al: Cardiopulmonary arrest due to acute maternal hypermagnesemia [Letter]. Lancet 1:1058, 1981.

282. Ryan G, Lange IR, Naugler MA: Clinical experience with phenytoin prophylaxis in severe preeclampsia. Am J Obstet Gynecol 161:1297, 1989.

283. Dommisse J: Phenytoin sodium and magnesium sulphate in the management of eclampsia. Br J Obstet Gynaecol 94:104, 1990.

284. Crowther C: Magnesium sulphate versus diazepam in the management of eclampsia: a randomized controlled trial. Br J Obstet Gynaecol 97:110, 1990.

285. Bhalla AK, Dhall GI, Dhall K: A safer and more effective treatment regimen for eclampsia. Aust N Z J Obstet Gynecol 34:144, 1994.

286. Friedman SA, Schiff E, Kao L, Sibai BM: Phenytoin versus magnesium sulfate in patients with eclampsia: Preliminary results from a randomized trial [Abstract 452]. Poster presented at 15th Annual Meeting of the Society of Perinatal Obstetricians, Atlanta, GA, January 23–28, 1995. Am J Obstet Gynecol 172:384, 1995.

287. The Eclampsia Trial Collaborative Group: Which anticonvulsant for women with eclampsia? Evidence from the Collaborative Eclampsia Trial. Lancet 345:1455, 1995.

288. Chesley LC, Cosgrove SA, Preece J, et al: Hydatidiform mole, with special reference to recurrence and associated eclampsia. Am J Obstet Gynecol 52:311, 1946.

289. Newman RB, Eddy GL: Association of eclampsia and hydatidiform mole: case report and review of the literature. Obstet Gynecol Surv 43:185, 1988.

290. Lindheimer MD, Spargo BH, Katz AI: Eclampsia during the 16th gestational week. JAMA 230:1006, 1974.

291. Speck G: Eclampsia at the sixteenth week of gestation, with Rh isoimmunization and cystic degeneration of the placenta. Obstet Gynecol 15:70, 1960.

292. Agobe JT, Adewaze HO: Biochemical studies and delayed postpartum convulsions in Nigeria. In Bomar J, MacGillivray I, Symonds EM (eds): Pregnancy Hypertension. Baltimore, University Park Press, 1980, p 501.

293. Harbert GM, Claiborne HA, McGaughey HS, et al: Convulsive toxemia. Am J Obstet Gynecol 10:336, 1968.

294. Lopez-Llera M: Main clinical types and subtypes of eclampsia. Am J Obstet Gynecol 166:4, 1992.

295. Zuspan FP: Problems encountered in the treatment of pregnancy induced hypertension. Am J Obstet Gynecol 131:591, 1978.

296. Sibai BM: Eclampsia VI. Maternal-perinatal outcome in 254 consecutive cases. Am J Obstet Gynecol 163:1045, 1990.

297. Campbell DM, Templeton AA: Is eclampsia preventable? In Bonnar J, MacGillivray I, Symonds EM (eds): Pregnancy Hypertension. Baltimore, University Park Press, 1980, p 483.

298. Bryans CI, Southerland WL, Zuspan FP: Eclampsia: a long-term followup study. Obstet Gynecol 21:6, 1963.

299. Chesley LC, Cosgrove RA, Annitto JE: A followup study of eclamptic women. Am J Obstet Gynecol 83:1360, 1962.

300. Chesley LC, Cosgrove RA, Annitto JE: Pregnancy in the sisters and daughters of eclamptic women. Pathol Microbiol (Basel) 24:662, 1961.

301. Chesley LC, Annitto JE, Cosgrove RA: The familial factor in toxemia of pregnancy. Obstet Gynecol 32:303, 1968.

302. Lopez-Llera M, Horta JLH: Pregnancy after eclampsia. Am J Obstet Gynecol 119:193, 1974.

303. Adelusi B, Ojengbeda OA: Reproductive performance after eclampsia. Int J Gynaecol Obstet 24:183, 1986.

304. Chesley LC: Remote prognosis. In Chesley LC (ed): Hypertensive Disorders in Pregnancy. East Norwalk, CT, Appleton-Century-Crofts, 1978, p 421.

305. Sibai BM, Sarinoglu C, Mercer BM: Eclampsia VII. Pregnancy outcome after eclampsia and long-term prognosis. Am J Obstet Gynecol 166:1757, 1992.

306. Frohlich ED: Hemodynamics of hypertension. In Genest J, Koiw E, Kuchel O (eds): Hypertension. New York, McGraw-Hill, 1977.

307. Chesley LC, Annitto JE: Pregnancy in the patient with hypertensive disease. Am J Obstet Gynecol 53:372, 1947.

308. Sibai BM, Abdella TN, Anderson GD: Pregnancy outcome in 211 patients with mild chronic hypertension. Obstet Gynecol 61:571, 1983.

309. Sibai BM: Diagnosis and management of chronic hypertension in pregnancy. Obstet Gynecol 78:451, 1991.

310. Sibai BM, Anderson GD: Pregnancy outcome of intensive therapy in severe hypertension in first trimester. Obstet Gynecol 67:517, 1986.

311. Landesman R, Holze W, Scherr L: Fetal mortality in essential hypertension. Obstet Gynecol 6:354, 1955.

312. Redman CWE, Beilin LJ, Bonnar J, et al: Fetal outcome in trial of antihypertensive treatment in pregnancy. Lancet 2:753, 1976.

313. Rey E, Couturier A: The prognosis of pregnancy in women with chronic hypertension. Am J Obstet Gynecol 171:410, 1994.

314. McCowan LME, Buist RG, North RA, Gamble G: Perinatal morbidity in chronic hypertension. Br J Obstet Gynaecol 103:123, 1996.

315. Packham DK, Fairley KF, Ihle BU, et al: Comparison of pregnancy outcome between normotensive and hypertensive women with primary glomerulonephritis. Clin Exp Hypertens Pregnancy B6:387, 1987.

316. Dunlop JCH: Chronic hypertension and perinatal mortality. Proc R Soc Med 59:838, 1966.

317. Sibai BM, Mabie WC, Shamsa F, et al: A comparison of no medication versus methyldopa or labetalol in chronic hypertension during pregnancy. Am J Obstet Gynecol 162:960, 1990.

318. Abdella TN, Sibai BM, Hays JM, et al: Relationship of hypertensive disease to abruptio placentae. Obstet Gynecol 63:365, 1984.

319. Leather HM, Humphreys DM, Baker PB, et al: A controlled trial of hypertensive agents in hypertension in pregnancy. Lancet 1:488, 1968.

320. Silverstone A, Trudinger BJ, Lewis PJ, et al: Maternal hypertension and intrauterine fetal death in mid pregnancy. Br J Obstet Gynaecol 87:457, 1980.

321. Kincaid-Smith P, Bullen M, Mills J: Prolonged use of methyldopa in severe hypertension in pregnancy. BMJ 1:274, 1966.

322. Taylor HC Jr, Tillman AJB, Blanchard J: Fetal losses in hypertension and preeclampsia. Part I. Analysis of 4432 cases. Obstet Gynecol 3:225, 1954.

323. Arias F, Zamora J: Antihypertensive treatment and pregnancy outcome in patients with mild chronic hypertension. Obstet Gynecol 53:489, 1979.

324. Weitz C, Khouzami V, Maxwell K, Johnson JWC: Treatment of hypertension in pregnancy with methyldopa, randomized double-blind study. Int J Gynaecol Obstet 25:35, 1987.

325. Butters L, Kennedy S, Rubin PC: Atenolol in essential hypertension during pregnancy. BMJ 301:587, 1990.

326. Steyn DW, Odendaal HJ: Randomised controlled trial of ketanserin and aspirin in prevention of pre-eclampsia. Lancet 350:1267, 1997.

327. Gallery EDM, Saunders DM, Hunyor DN, et al: Randomized comparison of methyldopa and oxprenolol for treatment of hypertension in pregnancy. BMJ 1:1591, 1979.

328. Fidler J, Smith V, Fayers P, et al: Randomized controlled

comparative study of methyldopa and oxprenolol in treatment of hypertension in pregnancy. BMJ 286:1927, 1983.

329. Plouin PF, Breart G, Maillard F, et al: Comparison of antihypertensive efficacy and perinatal safety of labetalol and methyldopa in the treatment of hypertension in pregnancy: a randomized controlled trial. Br J Obstet Gynaecol 95:868, 1988.

330. Horvath JS, Phippard A, Korda A, et al: Clonidine hydrochloride: a safe and effective antihypertensive agent in pregnancy. Obstet Gynecol 66:634, 1985.

331. Lubbe WF, Hodge JV, Kellaway GSM: Antihypertensive treatment and fetal welfare in essential hypertension in pregnancy. N Z Med J 95:1, 1982.

332. Childress CH, Katz VL: Nifedipine and its indications in obstetrics and gynecology. Obstet Gynecol 83:616, 1994.

333. Magee LA, Schick B, Donnenfeld AE, et al: The safety of calcium channel blockers in human pregnancy: a prospective multicenter cohort study. Am J Obstet Gynecol 174:823, 1996.

334. Wide-Swensson DH, Ingemarsson I, Lunell N-O, et al: Calcium channel blockade (isradipine) in treatment of hypertension in pregnancy: a randomized placebo-controlled study. Am J Obstet Gynecol 173:872, 1995.

335. Janet D, Carliontle B, Sebban E, Milliez J: Nicardipine versus metoprolol in the treatment of hypertension during pregnancy: a randomized comparative trial. Obstet Gynecol 84: 354, 1994.

336. Kreft-Jais C, Plouin PF, Tchobroutsky C, Boutroy MJ: Angiotensin-converting enzyme inhibitors during pregnancy: a survey of 22 patients given captopril and 9 given enalapril. Br J Obstet Gynaecol 95:420, 1988.

337. Rosa FW, Bosco LA, Graham CF, et al: Neonatal anuria with maternal angiotensin-converting enzyme inhibitor. Obstet Gynecol 74: 371, 1989.

338. Lumbers ER, Burrell JH, Menzies RI, et al: The effects of a converting enzyme inhibitor (captopril) and angiotensin II on fetal renal function. Br J Pharmacol 110:821, 1993.

339. Hanssens M, Keirse MJNC, Vankelecom F, Van Assche FA: Fetal and neonatal effects of treatment with angiotensin-converting enzyme inhibitors in pregnancy. Obstet Gynecol 171: 128, 1991.

340. Veld AJM, Schalekamp MADH: Effects of 10 different beta-adrenoreceptor antagonists on hemodynamics, plasma renin activity, and plasma norepinephrine in hypertension. J Cardiovasc Pharmacol 5(suppl):1, 1983.

341. Svenden TL: Central hemodynamics of beta-adrenoreceptor blocking drugs: beta$_1$, selectivity versus intrinsic sympathomimetic activity. J Cardiovasc Pharmacol 5(suppl):1, 1983.

342. Van Zweiten PA, Timmermans PBMWM: Differential pharmacological properties of beta-adrenoreceptor blocking drugs. J Cardiovasc Pharmacol 5(suppl):1, 1983.

343. Rubin PC: Beta-blockers in pregnancy. N Engl J Med 305: 1323, 1981.

344. Lip GYH, Beevers M, Churchill D, et al: Effect of atenolol on birth weight. Am J Cardiol 79:1436, 1997.

345. Lydakis C, Lip GY, Beevers M, Beevers DG: Atenolol and fetal growth in pregnancies complicated by hypertension. Am J Hypertens 12:541, 1999.

346. Montan S, Ingermarsson I, Marsal K, Sjoberg NO: Randomised controlled trial of atenolol and pindolol in human pregnancy: effects on fetal hemodynamics. BMJ 304:946, 1992.

347. Easterling TR, Brateng D, Schmucker B, et al: Prevention of preeclampsia: a randomized trial of atenolol in hyperdynamic patients before onset of hypertension. Obstet Gynecol 93:725, 1999.

348. Schoenfeld A, Segal J, Friedman S, et al: Adverse reactions to antihypertensive drugs in pregnancy. Obstet Gynecol Surv 41: 67, 1986.

349. Sibai BM, Abdella TN, Anderson GD, et al: Plasma volume determination in pregnancies complicated by chronic hypertension and intrauterine fetal demise. Obstet Gynecol 60:174, 1982.

350. Sibai BM, Grossman RA, Grossman HE: Effects of diuretics on plasma volume in pregnancies with long-term hypertension. Am J Obstet Gynecol 150:831, 1984.

351. Sibai BM, Abdella TN, Anderson GD, et al: Plasma volume findings in pregnant women with mild hypertension. Therapeutic considerations. Am J Obstet Gynecol 145:539, 1983.

352. Collins R, Yusf S, Peto R: Overview of randomized trials of diuretics in pregnancy. BMJ 190:17, 1985.

353. MacGillivray I: Sodium and water balance in pregnancy hypertension: the role of diuretics. Clin Obstet Gynecol 4:459, 1977.

354. Cunningham FG, Cox SM, Harstad TW, et al: Chronic renal disease and pregnancy outcome. Am J Obstet Gynecol 163: 453, 1990.

355. Jones DC, Hayslett JP: Outcome of pregnancy in women with moderate or severe renal insufficiency. N Engl J Med 335: 226, 1996; (comment in N Engl J Med 335:277. Published erratum N Engl J Med 336:739, 1997).

356. Jungers P, Chauveau D, Choukroun G, et al: Pregnancy in women with impaired renal function. Clin Nephrol 47:281, 1997.

357. Hou S: Pregnancy in chronic renal insufficiency and end-stage renal disease. Am J Kidney Dis 33:235, 1999.

358. Zuspan FP, Rayburn WF: Blood pressure self-monitoring during pregnancy: practical considerations. Am J Obstet Gynecol 164:2, 1991.

359. Barton JR, Sibai BM: Acute life-threatening emergencies in preeclampsia-eclampsia. Clin Obstet Gynecol 35:402, 1992.

360. Prisant LM, Carr AA, Hawkins DW: Treating hypertensive emergencies: controlled reduction of blood pressure and protection of target organs. Postgrad Med 93:92, 1993.

361. Meese R, Ram CVS: Hypertensive cardiovascular emergencies. Compr Ther 11:28, 1985.

362. Silver HM: Acute hypertensive crisis in pregnancy. Med Clin North Am 73:623, 1989.

363. Gifford R Jr: Management of hypertensive crisis. JAMA 266: 829, 1991.

364. Committee on Drugs, American Academy of Pediatrics: The transfer of drugs and other chemicals into human milk. Pediatrics 93:137, 1994.

365. White WB: Management of hypertension during lactation. Hypertension 6:297, 1984.

366. Briggs GG, Freeman RK, Yaffee SJ: Drugs in pregnancy and lactation. *In* A Reference Guide to Fetal and Neonatal Risk, 5th ed. Baltimore, Williams & Wilkins, 1998.

Chapter 29

Heart Disease

THOMAS R. EASTERLING AND CATHERINE OTTO

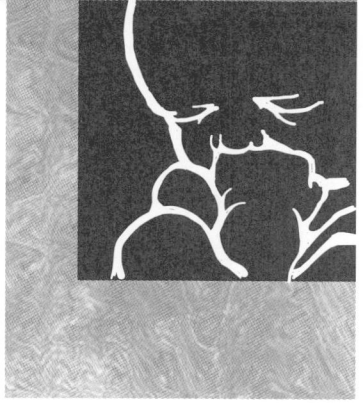

Cardiovascular adaptations to pregnancy are well tolerated by healthy young women. However, these adaptations are of such magnitude that they can significantly compromise women with abnormal or damaged hearts. Without accurate diagnosis and appropriate care, heart disease in pregnancy can be a significant cause of maternal mortality. Under more optimal conditions, many women with significant disease can experience good outcomes and should not necessarily be discouraged from becoming pregnant. This chapter develops an understanding of cardiovascular physiology as a basis for appropriate care. While published experience with more common conditions can be used to support these principles, information regarding many other conditions is limited to case reports. In general, data from case reports will be biased toward more complicated cases with more adverse outcomes. The best care for women with heart disease is usually achieved from a thorough understanding of maternal cardiovascular physiology, knowledge of existing literature, and extensive clinical experience brought by the clinical management team.

MATERNAL HEMODYNAMICS

Hemodynamics refers to the relationship between blood pressure, cardiac output, and vascular resistance. Blood pressure is measured by auscultation, use of an automated cuff, or directly with an intra-arterial catheter. Cardiac output is measured by dilutional techniques requiring central venous access, by Doppler or two-dimensional echocardiographic techniques, or by electrical impedance. Peripheral resistance is calculated using Ohm's law:

$$TPR = \frac{MAP \times 80}{CO}$$

where TPR is total peripheral resistance (dyne·sec·cm^{-5}), MAP is mean arterial pressure (mm Hg), and CO is cardiac output (L/min).

Pregnancy and events unique to pregnancy, such as labor and delivery, are associated with significant and frequently predictable changes in these parameters. The hemodynamic changes of pregnancy, while well tolerated by an otherwise healthy women, may be tolerated poorly by a woman with significant cardiac disease. Therefore, the importance of understanding these changes and placing them in the context of a specific cardiac lesion cannot be overstated.

The maternal hemodynamics of 89 nulliparous women who remained normotensive throughout pregnancy are described in Figure 29–1.[1] Mean arterial pressure falls sharply in the first trimester, reaching a nadir by midpregnancy. Thereafter, blood pressure increases slowly, reaching near nonpregnant levels by term. Cardiac output rises throughout the first and second trimesters, reaching a maximum by the middle of the third trimester. In the supine position, a pregnant woman in the third trimester may experience significant hypotension due to venocaval occlusion by the gravid uterus. In normal pregnancy, she may experience symptoms such as diaphoresis, tachycardia, or nausea but will rarely experience significant complications. Fetal heart rate decelerations may be observed but usually resolve when the mother, often spontaneously, shifts to a more comfortable position. Women with significant right or left ventricular outflow obstruction, such as aortic stenosis, may seriously decompensate in the supine position due to poor ventricular filling.

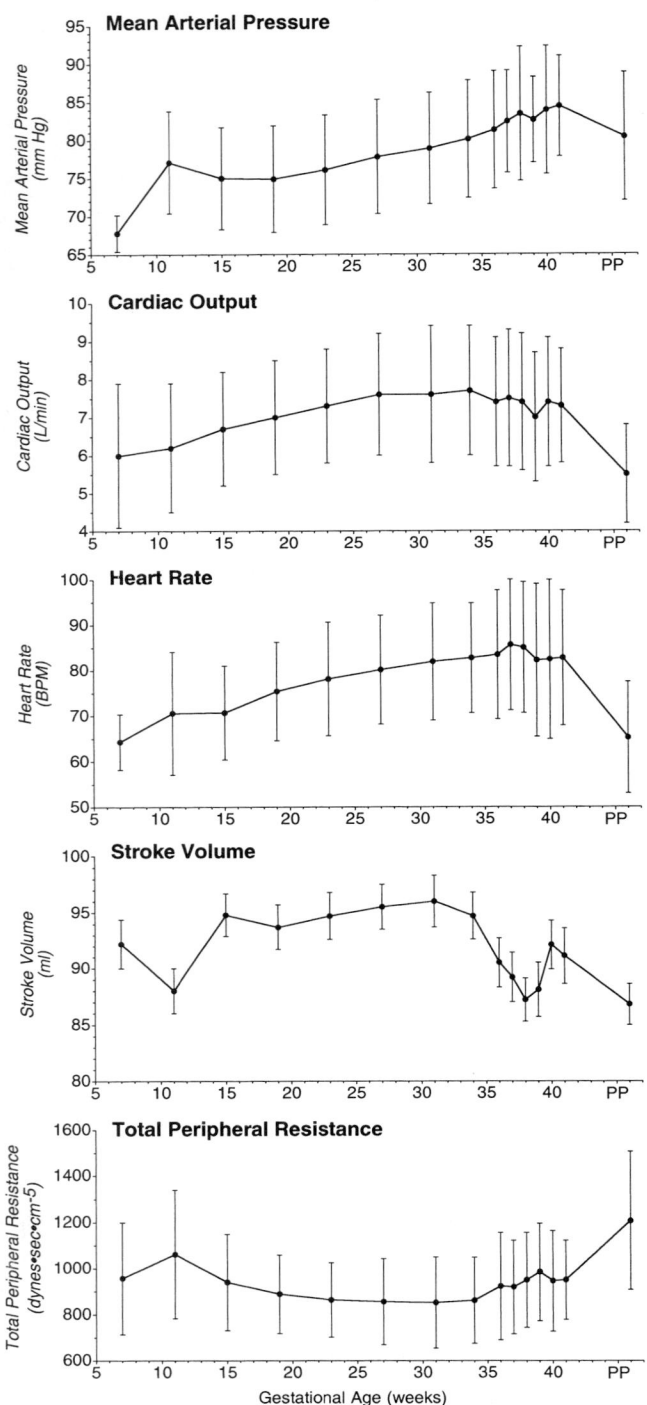

Figure 29–1. Changes in hemodynamic parameters throughout pregnancy (mean ± SD).

Cardiac output is the product of heart rate (HR) and stroke volume (SV):

$$CO = HR \times SV.$$

Heart rate and stroke volume increase as pregnancy progresses to the third trimester. After 32 weeks, stroke volume falls, with the maintenance of cardiac output becoming more and more dependent on heart rate. Vascular resistance falls in the first and early second trimesters. The magnitude of the fall is sufficient to offset the rise in cardiac output, resulting in a net decrease in blood pressure.

Labor, delivery, and the postpartum period are times of acute hemodynamic changes that may result in maternal decompensation. Labor itself is associated with pain and anxiety. Tachycardia is a normal response. Significant catecholamine release will increase afterload.

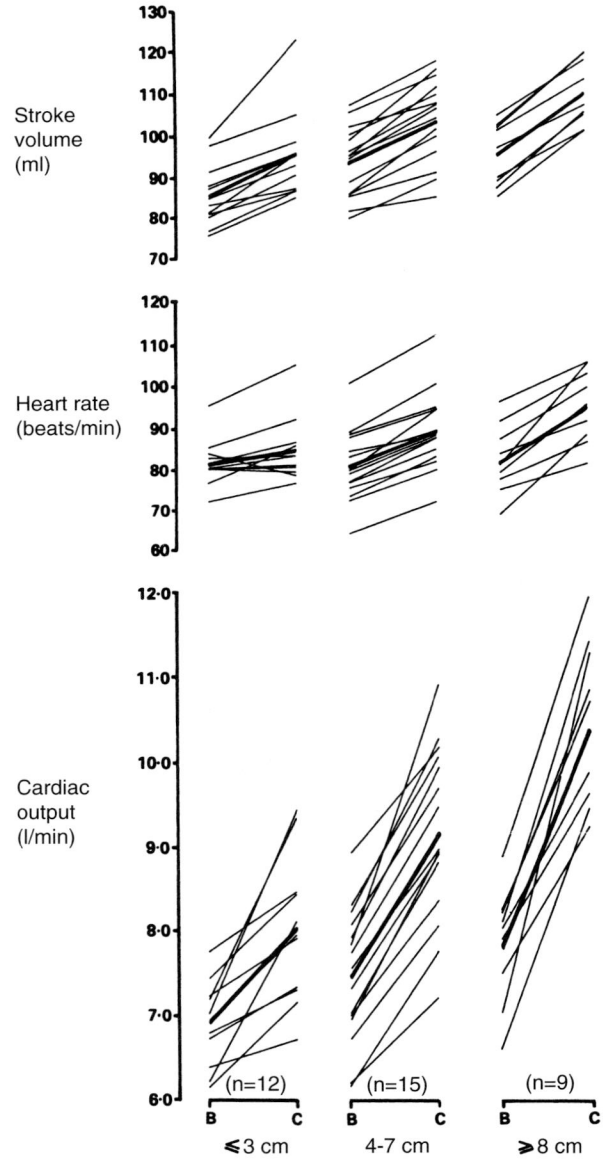

Figure 29–2. Changes in hemodynamic parameters at three different points during labor (≤3 cm, 4 to 7 cm, and ≥8 cm). Each line represents the change in an individual subject. B, before contraction; C, during contraction. (From Robson S, Dunlop W, Boys R, Hunter S: Cardiac output during labour. BMJ 295:1169, 1987, with permission.)

Each uterine contraction acutely redistributes 400 to 500 ml of blood from the uterus to the central circulation. In Figure 29–2, Robson et al. describe the hemodynamic changes associated with unmedicated labor.[2] Heart rate, blood pressure, and cardiac output all increase with uterine contractions, with the magnitude of the change increasing as labor advances. Obstructive cardiac lesions impede the flow of blood through the heart, blunting the expected rise in cardiac output at the expense of increasing pulmonary pressures and pulmonary congestion. In Figure 29–3, intrapartum hemodynamic changes of a patient with aortic stenosis and a peak gradient of 160 mm Hg are shown.[3] Note that pulmonary pressures rise in parallel with uterine contractions.

Immediately after delivery, blood from the uterus is returned to the central circulation. In normal pregnancy, this compensatory mechanism protects the parturient from the hemodynamic effects of postpartum hemorrhage. In the context of cardiac disease, this acute centralization of blood may increase pulmonary pressures and pulmonary congestion.[4] During the first 2 postpartum weeks, extravascular fluid is mobilized and diuresis ensues. Decompensation during postpartum fluid mobilization is common in women with mitral stenosis and cardiomyopathy. Unsuspected cardiac disease may be diagnosed when a woman returns to the emergency room several days postpartum with dyspnea and oxygen desaturation. Maternal cardiac output has usually normalized by 2 weeks postpartum.[5]

Three key features of the maternal hemodynamic changes in pregnancy are particularly relevant to the management of women with cardiac disease: (1) increased cardiac output, (2) increased heart rate, and (3) reduced vascular resistance. In conditions such as mitral stenosis where cardiac output is relatively fixed, the drive to achieve an elevated cardiac output may result in pulmonary congestion. If a patient has an atrial septal defect, the incremental increase in systemic flow associated with pregnancy will be magnified in the pulmonary circulation to the extent that pulmonary flow exceeds systemic flow. If, for example, a shunt ratio of 3:1 is maintained in pregnancy, pulmonary flow may be as high as 20 L/min and may be associated with increasing dyspnea and potential desaturation.

Many cardiac conditions are heart rate dependent. Flow across a stenotic mitral valve is dependent on time in diastole. Tachycardia reduces left ventricular filling and cardiac output. Coronary blood flow is also dependent on the length of diastole. Patients with aortic stenosis will have increased wall tension and therefore increased myocarial oxygen requirements. Tachycardia reduces coronary perfusion time in diastole while simultaneously further increasing myocardial oxygen require-

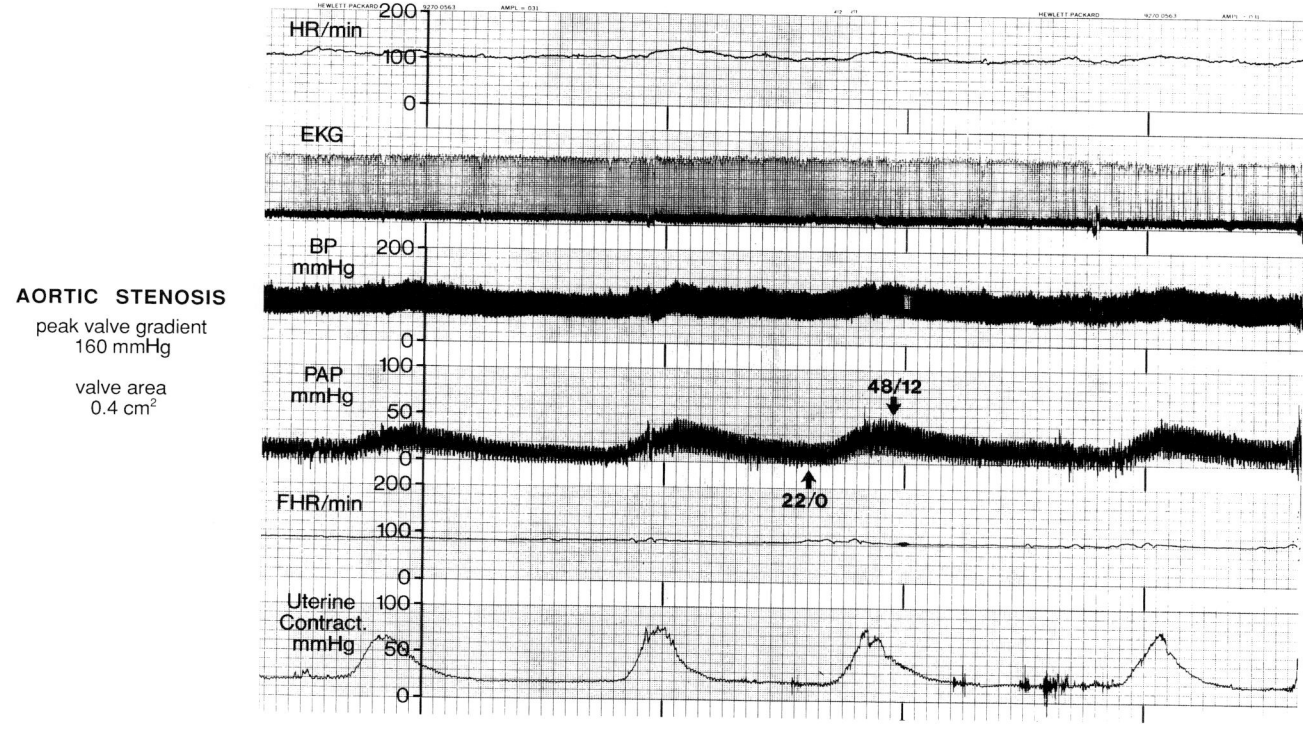

Figure 29–3. Hemodynamic monitoring of a patient with severe aortic stenosis in labor. (From Easterling T, Chadwick H, Otto C, Benedetti T: Aortic stenosis in pregnancy. Obstet Gynecol 72:113, 1988. Reprinted with permission from American College of Obstetricians and Gynecologists.)

ments. The resulting imbalance between oxygen demand and supply may precipitate myocardial ischemia. Patients with complex congenital heart disease experience significant tachyarrhythmias. The increasing heart rate in pregnancy may be associated with a worsening of tachyarrhythmias.

Reduction in vascular resistance may be beneficial to some patients; afterload reduction reduces cardiac work. Cardiomyopathy, aortic regurgitation, and mitral regurgitation benefit from reduced afterload. Alternatively, patients with intracardiac shunts, where right and left ventricular pressures are nearly equal when not pregnant, may reverse their shunt during pregnancy and desaturate.

BLOOD VOLUME

Very early in the first trimester, pregnant women experience an expansion of renal blood flow and glomerular filtration rate. Filtered sodium increases by approximately 50 percent. Despite physiologic changes that would promote loss of salt and water and contraction of blood volume, the pregnant woman will expand her blood volume by 40 to 50 percent. In part, the stimulation to retain fluid may be a response to the fall in vascular resistance and reduction in blood pressure. The renin-angiotensin system is activated, and the plasma concentration of aldosterone is elevated. While the simplicity of this explanation is attractive, the actual process is probably much more complicated.[6]

As plasma volume expands, the hematocrit falls, and hematopoiesis is stimulated. Red cell mass will expand from 18 to 25 percent depending on the status of individual iron stores. "Physiologic anemia" with a maternal hematocrit between 30 and 35 percent does not usually complicate pregnancy in the context of maternal heart disease. More significant anemia, however, may increase cardiac work and induce tachycardia. Microcytosis due to iron deficiency may impair perfusion of the microcirculation of patients who are polycythemic due to cyanotic heart disease, as microcytic red blood cells are less deformable. Iron and folate supplementation is appropriate.

In a similar fashion, serum albumin concentration falls by 22 percent despite an expansion of intravascular albumin mass by 20 percent. As a result, serum oncotic pressure falls in parallel by 20 percent to approximately 19 mm Hg.[7] In normal pregnancy, intravascular fluid balance is maintained by a fall in interstitial oncotic pressure. However, if left ventricular filling pressure becomes elevated or if pulmonary vascular integrity is disrupted, pulmonary edema will develop earlier in the disease process than in nonpregnant women.

DIAGNOSIS AND EVALUATION OF HEART DISEASE

Many women with heart disease have been diagnosed and treated prior to pregnancy. For example, in women with prior surgery for congenital heart disease, detailed historical information may be available. Others only know that they have a murmur or a "hole in my heart." Alternatively, heart disease may first be diagnosed during pregnancy due to symptoms precipitated by increased cardiac demands.

The classic symptoms of cardiac disease are palpitations, shortness of breath with exertion, and chest pain. Since these symptoms also may accompany normal pregnancy, a careful history is needed to determine if the symptoms are out of proportion to the stage of pregnancy. Symptoms are of particular concern in a patient with other reasons to suspect underlying cardiac disease, such as growing up in an area where rheumatic heart disease is prevalent.

A systolic flow murmur is present in 80 percent of pregnant women, most likely due to the increased flow volume in the aorta and pulmonary artery.[8] Typically, a flow murmur is grade 1 or 2, midsystolic, loudest at the cardiac base, and not associated with any other abnormal physical examination findings. A normal physiologic split second heart sound is heard in patients with a flow murmur. Any diastolic murmur and any systolic murmur that is loud ($\geq$ grade 3/6) or radiates to the carotids should be considered pathologic. Careful evaluation for elevation of the jugular venous pulse, for peripheral cyanosis or clubbing, and for pulmonary crackles is needed in women with suspected cardiac disease.

Indications for further cardiac diagnostic testing in pregnant women include a history of known cardiac disease, symptoms in excess of those expected in a normal pregnancy, a pathologic murmur, evidence of heart failure on physical examination, or arterial oxygen desaturation in the absence of known pulmonary disease. The most appropriate next step in evaluation of pregnant women with suspected heart disease is transthoracic echocardiography. A chest radiograph is only helpful if congestive heart failure is suspected. An electrocardiogram (ECG) is likely to be nonspecific. If symptoms are consistent with a cardiac arrhythmia, an event monitor or 24-hour ECG monitor may be indicated. Rarely, cardiac catheterization is needed for full diagnosis of valvular or congenital heart disease. The exception is an acute coronary syndrome during pregnancy where the risk of radiation exposure with cardiac catheterization is small compared to the benefit of early diagnosis and early revascularization to prevent myocardial infarction.

Echocardiography provides detailed information on

cardiac anatomy and physiology that allows optimal management of women with heart disease. Basic data obtained on echocardiography include left ventricular ejection fraction, pulmonary artery systolic pressure, qualitative evaluation of right ventricular systolic function, and evaluation of valve anatomy and function. When valvular stenosis is present, the pressure gradient (ΔP) across the valve is calculated from the Doppler-derived velocity (v) of flow across the valve: $\Delta P = 4v^2$. Similarly, pulmonary artery systolic pressure can be calculated from the maximal Doppler velocity obtained across a tricuspid regurgitant jet.

Aortic valve area is calculated using the continuity equation. Stroke volume is calculated from the product of the cross-sectional area of the left ventricular outflow tract and the time-velocity integral derived from Doppler evaluation of the outflow tract. A time-velocity integral is then derived from the stenotic valve. Since the left ventricular outflow tract and the aortic valve are in continuity, stroke volume across each are equal. Valve area can therefore be derived by dividing the stroke volume by the aortic valve time-velocity integral. Mitral valve area is measured directly by two-dimensional planimetry or by the Doppler pressure half-time method.[9] In patients with congenital disease, detailed evaluation of anatomy and previous surgical repair is possible. When complex congenital heart disease is present or when image quality is suboptimal, transesophageal imaging provides improved image quality.

GENERAL CARE

Management of cardiac disease in pregnancy is frequently complicated by unique social and psychological concerns. Children with congenital heart disease may have experienced multiple hospitalizations and be fearful of the medical environment. Some have expected never to bear children. Women with rheumatic heart disease have frequently lived outside the traditional medical care system due to conditions of poverty and cultural differences. Not uncommonly, they are recent immigrants. Care must be exercised to facilitate their access to care and their comfort with the environment of care. Their practitioner must be patient but persistent in the face of deviations from more traditional standards of compliance and medical care.

Deterioration in cardiac status during pregnancy is frequently insidious. Continuity of care with a single provider facilitates early intervention prior to overt decompensation. Regular visits should include particular attention to heart rate, weight gain, and oxygen saturation. An unexpected increase in weight may indicate the need for more aggressive outpatient therapy. A fall in

> ### Structured Review of Cardiac Symptoms
>
> "How many flights of stairs can you walk up with ease?"—"Two? One? None?"
>
> "Can you walk a level block?"
>
> "Can you sleep flat in bed?" "How many pillows?"
>
> "Does your heart race?"
>
> "Do you have chest pain?"
>   "with exercise?"
>   "when your heart races?"

oxygen saturation will often precede a clearly abnormal chest exam or radiograph. Regular use of a structured history of symptoms (see the box "Structured Review of Cardiac Symptoms") will alert the physician to a change in condition. Regular review educates the patient and reinforces their role as "partners in care."

The physiologic changes of pregnancy are usually continuous and therefore offer adequate time for maternal compensation despite cardiac disease. Intercurrent events superimposed on pregnancy in the context of maternal heart disease are usually responsible for acute decompensation. Antepartum, the most common significant "intercurrent events" are febrile episodes. Screening for bacteriuria and vaccination against influenza and pneumococcus are appropriate. Patients should be instructed to report symptoms of upper respiratory infection, particularly fever. Many patients with heart disease (adolescents, recent immigrants, and those living in poverty), will also be at risk for iron deficiency. Prophylaxis against anemia with iron and folate supplementation may decrease cardiac work.

A strategy of "standard cardiac care" for labor and delivery is described in the box. The general principles for care are similar for most cardiac diagnoses. Physiologically, the ideal labor for a woman with heart disease is short and pain free. While induction of labor facilitates organization of care and early pain control, shortening the duration of pregnancy by 1 or 2 weeks at the cost of a 2 or 3 day induction of labor is not worthwhile. Induction of labor with a favorable cervix is therefore ideal. Some patients with severe cardiac disease will benefit from invasive hemodynamic monitoring with an arterial catheter and a pulmonary artery catheter. These will be discussed in detail below. Cesarean section is usually reserved for obstetric indications. The American Heart Association does not recommend routine antibiotic prophylaxis for the prevention of endocarditis, although it is optional in high-risk patients having a vaginal delivery (Table 29–1). Because bacteremia is common at the time of vaginal delivery and

Standard Cardiac Care for Labor and Delivery

1. Accurate diagnosis
2. Mode of delivery based on obstetric indications
3. Medical management initiated early in labor
   - Prolonged labor avoided.
   - Induction with a *favorable* cervix
4. Maintenance of hemodynamic stability
   - Invasive hemodynamic monitoring when required
   - Initial, compensated hemodynamic reference point
   - Specific emphasis based on particular cardiac condition
5. Avoidance of pain and hemodynamic responses
   - Epidural analgesia with narcotic/low-dose local technique
6. Prophylactic antibiotics when at risk for endocarditis
7. Avoidance of maternal pushing
   - Caudal for dense perineal anesthesia
   - Low forceps or vacuum delivery
8. Avoidance of maternal blood loss
   - Proactive management of the third stage
   - Early but appropriate fluid replacement
9. Early volume management postpartum
   - Often careful but aggressive diuresis

cesarean section,[10,11] many practitioners will provide antibiotic prophylaxis in all patients at risk.

Women with significant heart disease should be counseled prior to pregnancy regarding the risk of pregnancy, interventions that may be required, and potential risks to the fetus. However, women with significant uncorrected disease may present with an ongoing pregnancy. In this situation, the risks and benefits of termination of pregnancy versus those of continuing a pregnancy should be addressed. The decision to become pregnant or carry a pregnancy in the context of maternal disease is a balance of two forces: (1) the objective medical risk including the uncertainty of that estimate, and (2) the value of the birth of a child to an individual woman and her partner. The first goal of counseling is to educate the patient. Only a few cardiac diseases represent an overwhelming risk of maternal mortality: Eisenmenger's syndrome, pulmonary hypertension with right ventricular dysfunction, and Marfan syndrome with significant aortic dilation. Most other conditions require aggressive management and significant disruption in lifestyle. Intercurrent events such as antepartum pneumonia or obstetric hemorrhage pose the greatest risk of initiating life-threatening events. Fastidious care can reduce but not eliminate the risk of these events. Maternal congenital heart disease increases the risk of congenital heart disease in the fetus from 1 percent to approximately 4 to 6 percent.[12,13] Marfan syndrome and some forms of hypertrophic cardiomyopathy are inherited as autosomal dominant conditions; the children of these women will carry a 50 percent chance of inheriting the disease. The second goal of counseling is to help the woman integrate the medical information into her individual value system and her

Table 29–1. PROPHYLACTIC REGIMENS FOR LABOR AND DELIVERY

Patients	Regimens
High-risk patients	
Prosthetic valves—both bioprosthetic and homografts	Ampicillin + gentamicin
Complex cyanotic congenital heart disease (CHD)	Ampicillin 2.0 g IM or IV
Surgically constructed systemic pulmonic shunts or conduits	Gentamicin 1.5 mg/kg (not to exceed 120 mg) in active labor; 6 h later,
Previous bacterial endocarditis	ampicillin 1 g IM/IV or amoxicillin 1 g PO
High-risk patients allergic to ampicillin/amoxicillin	Vancomycin + gentamicin
	Vancomycin 1.0 g IV over 1–2 h + gentamicin as above in active labor
Moderate-risk patients	
Most other CHD	Amoxicillin or ampicillin
Acquired valvular dysfunction (e.g., rheumatic heart disease)	Amoxicillin 2.0 g orally or ampicillin 2.0 g IM/IV in active labor
Hypertrophic cardiac myopathy	
Mitral valve prolapse with regurgitation	
Moderate-risk patients allergic to ampicillin/amoxicillin	Vancomycin
	Vancomycin 1.0 g IV over 1–2 h in active labor

Adapted from Dajani AS, Taubert KA, Wilson W, et al: Prevention of bacterial endocarditis: recommendations by the American Heart Association. JAMA 277:1794, 1997.

individual desire to be a mother. Many women with significant but manageable heart disease will choose to carry a pregnancy. The basis for their decisions must be individualized.

VALVULAR DISEASE

The American College of Cardiology and the American Heart Association have published guidelines for the management of valvular heart disease including some guidelines for management during pregnancy.[14] These guidelines create a general framework for preconceptional care and care during pregnancy, realizing that treatment of a specific patient must be individualized. Individualization is particularly important when one is balancing maternal and fetal risks against the desire to have children. An individual patient's value system will have a significant impact on the final direction of care.

MITRAL STENOSIS

Mitral stenosis is nearly always due to rheumatic heart disease. Valvular dysfunction progresses continuously throughout life. Deterioration may be accelerated by recurrent episodes of rheumatic fever. Rheumatic fever itself is an immunologic response to group A β-hemolytic streptococcus infections. The incidence of rheumatic fever in a population is heavily influenced by conditions of poverty and crowding. These same individuals are at risk to have reduced access and utilization of health care resources and may present undiagnosed or untreated.

Patients with asymptomatic mitral stenosis have a 10-year survival of greater than 80 percent. Once significantly symptomatic, 10-year survival without treatment is less than 15 percent. In the presence of pulmonary hypertension, mean survival is less than 3 years. Death is due to progressive pulmonary edema, right heart failure, systemic embolization, or pulmonary embolism.[14]

Stenosis of the mitral valve impedes the flow of blood from the left atrium to the left ventricle during diastole. The normal mitral valve area is 4.0 to 5.0 cm². Symptoms with exercise can be expected with valve areas less than or equal to 2.5 cm². Symptoms at rest are expected at less than or equal to 1.5 cm². The left ventricle responds with Starling mechanisms to increased venous return with increased performance, elevating cardiac output in response to demand. The left atrium is limited in its capacity to respond. Cardiac output is therefore limited by the relatively passive flow of blood through the valve during diastole; increased venous return results in pulmonary congestion rather than increased cardiac output. Thus, the drive for increased cardiac output in pregnancy cannot be achieved, resulting in increased pulmonary congestion. The relative tachycardia experienced in pregnancy shortens diastole, decreases left ventricular filling, and therefore further compromises cardiac output and increases pulmonary congestion.

The diagnosis of mitral stenosis in pregnancy prior to maternal decompensation is uncommon. Tiredness and dyspnea on exertion are characteristic symptoms of mitral stenosis but are also ubiquitous among pregnant women. While the presence of a diastolic rumble or jugular venous distention may suggest mitral stenosis, these findings are subtle and may be overlooked or not appreciated. Not uncommonly, an intercurrent event such as a febrile episode will result in exaggerated symptoms and the diagnosis of pulmonary edema or oxygen desaturation. Under these circumstances, particularly in the context of a patient from an at-risk group, an echocardiogram should be performed to rule out mitral stenosis.

Echocardiographic diagnosis of mitral stenosis is based on the characteristic appearance of the stenotic, frequently calcified valve. Calculation of valve area from pressure half-time of the Doppler wave or by two-dimensional planimetry provides an objective measure of severity. Valve areas of 1.0 cm² or less will usually require pharmacologic management during pregnancy and invasive hemodynamic monitoring during labor. Valve areas of 1.4 cm² or less usually require careful expectant management. Left atrial enlargement identifies a patient at risk for atrial fibrillation, subsequent atrial thrombus, and the potential for systemic embolization. Pulmonary hypertension, a complication of worsening mitral disease, can be diagnosed and quantified with Doppler evaluation of the regurgitant jet across the tricuspid valve. Elevated pulmonary pressures may be due to hydrostatic forces associated with elevated left atrial pressures or, in more advanced disease, due to pathologic elevations of pulmonary vascular resistance (PVR). Hydrostatic pulmonary hypertension may respond to therapy that lowers left atrial pressure. Pulmonary hypertension due to elevated PVR is life threatening in pregnancy and may precipitate right heart failure in the postpartum period.

Pregnancy itself does not negatively affect the natural history of mitral stenosis. Chesley reviewed the medical histories of 134 women with functionally severe mitral stenosis who survived pregnancies between 1931 and 1943.[15] His patients lived prior to modern management of mitral stenosis and therefore represent the natural history of the disease. By 1974, only nine of the cohort remained alive. Their death rate was exponential; during each year of follow-up, the rate for the remaining

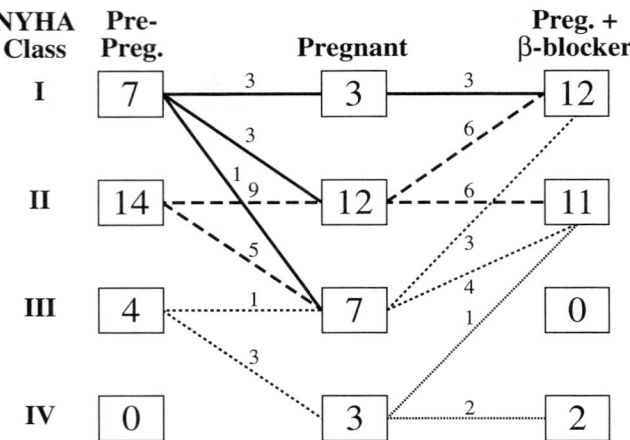

Figure 29–4. The effects of β-blockade on functional status of women with mitral stenosis. (From Al Kasab S, Sabag T, Al Zaibag M, et al: Beta-adrenergic receptor blockade in the management of pregnant women with mitral stenosis. Am J Obstet Gynecol 163:37, 1990, with permission.)

provement with treatment. Fastidious antepartum care as described above should supplement pharmacologic management.

Women with a history of rheumatic valvular disease who are at risk for contact with populations with a high prevalence of streptococcal infection should receive prophylaxis with daily oral penicillin G or monthly benzathine penicillin.[14] Most pregnant women will live in close contact with groups of children and will usually be considered at risk. Atrial fibrillation is a complication associated with mitral stenosis due to left atrial enlargement. Rapid ventricular response to atrial fibrillation may result in sudden decompensation. Digoxin, β-blockers, or calcium channel blockers can be used to control ventricular response. In the context of hemodynamic decompensation, electrical cardioversion may be necessary. Anticoagulation with heparin should be used before and after cardioversion to prevent systemic embolization. Patients with chronic atrial fibrillation and a history of an embolic event should also be anticoagulated.[14]

Labor and delivery can frequently precipitate decompensation in patients with critical mitral stenosis. Pain induces tachycardia. Uterine contractions increase venous return and therefore pulmonary congestion. Women frequently cannot tolerate the work of pushing in the second stage. Clark et al. described the abrupt elevation in pulmonary artery pressures in the immediate postpartum period associated with centralization of uterine blood (Fig. 29–5).[4] Aggressive, anticipatory diuresis will reduce pulmonary congestion and the potential for oxygen desaturation.

The hemodynamics of women with symptomatic stenosis or a valve area of 1 cm² or less should be managed with the aid of a pulmonary artery catheter. Ideally, hemodynamic parameters are assessed when the patient is well compensated, early in labor. These findings serve as a reference point to guide subsequent ther-

cohort was 6.3 percent. Women with subsequent pregnancies had comparable survival to those who did not again become pregnant, allowing the authors to conclude that pregnancy itself did not negatively affect long-term outcome.

The goal of antepartum care in the context of mitral stenosis is to achieve a balance between the drive to increase cardiac output and the limitations of flow across the stenotic valve. Most women with significant disease will require diuresis with a drug such as furosemide. In addition, β-blockade reduces heart rate, improves diastolic flow across the valve, and relieves pulmonary congestion. Kasab et al. evaluated the impact of β-blockade on 25 pregnant women with significant mitral stenosis.[16] Figure 29–4 describes the functional status of women prior to pregnancy, during pregnancy prior to β-blockade, and after β-blockade. Note the deterioration associated with pregnancy and the im-

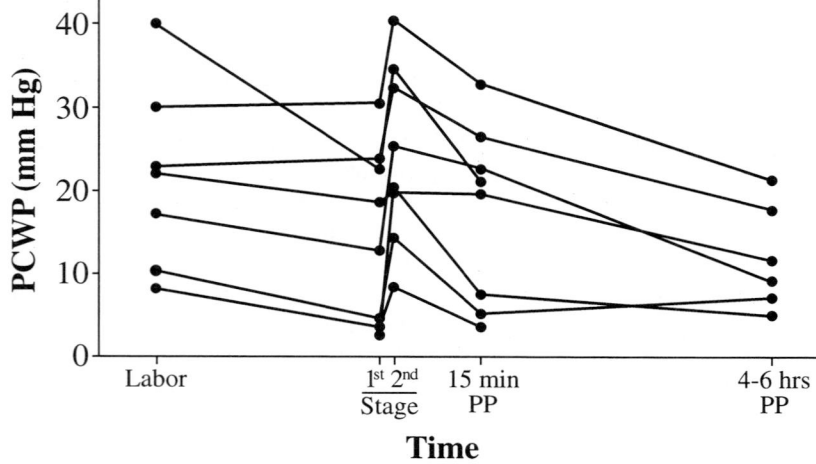

Figure 29–5. The changes in pulmonary capillary wedge pressure associated with delivery and subsequent diuresis in women with mitral stenosis. (From Clark S, Phelan J, Greenspoon J, et al: Labor and delivery in the presence of mitral stenosis: central hemodynamic observations. Am J Obstet Gynecol 152:384, 1985, with permission.)

apy. Pain control is achieved with an epidural. Heart rate control is maintained through pain control and β-blockade. To avoid pushing, the second stage is shortened with low forceps or vacuum delivery. Aggressive diuresis is initiated immediately postpartum. Cesarean section is reserved for obstetric indications.

Aggressive medical management including hospital bed rest will be sufficient to manage most women with mitral stenosis. The woman with uncommonly severe disease may require surgical intervention. While successful valve replacement and open commissurotomy have been reported in pregnancy,[17,18] they are now rarely needed. Two centers have reported successful balloon valvotomy in a series of 40 and 44 women with minimal complications.[19,20] Complications of balloon valvuloplasty outside of pregnancy occur at the following rates: mortality (0.5 percent), cerebrovascular accident (1 percent), and mitral regurgitation requiring surgery (2 percent).[14] Medical management should be clearly exhausted before assuming these risks during pregnancy, where emergent intervention such as valve replacement will be more complicated and carries a significant risk to the fetus.

Rheumatic disease can affect the aortic valve. Management of significant mitral stenosis, which limits ventricular filling, in the context of aortic stenosis that is critically dependent on ventricular filling, is particularly complicated.

MITRAL REGURGITATION

Mitral regurgitation may be due to a chronic progressive process such as rheumatic valve disease or mitral valve prolapse. As regurgitation increases over time, forward flow is maintained at the expense of left ventricular dilation with eventual impaired contractility. Left atrial enlargement may be associated with atrial fibrillation that should be managed with ventricular rate control and anticoagulation. The patient with chronic mitral regurgitation may remain asymptomatic even with exercise. Preconceptional counseling should include consideration of valve replacement in consultation with a cardiologist. In general, valve replacement is recommended for: (1) symptomatic patients, (2) atrial fibrillation, (3) ejection fraction less than 50 to 60 percent, (4) left ventricular end-diastolic dimension greater than 45 to 50 mm, or (5) pulmonary systolic pressure greater than 50 to 60 mm Hg.[14] As discussed below, the benefits of valve replacement prior to pregnancy must be balanced against the risks associated with prosthetic valve in pregnancy and the potential for prosthetic valve deterioration in pregnancy. If surgery is required,

valve repair rather than replacement is preferred to avoid the need for anticoagulation.

Acute mitral regurgitation in young patients is uncommon and may be associated with ruptured chordae tendineae due to endocarditis. Without time for left ventricular compensation, forward flow may be severely compromised. Urgent valve surgery is usually required. Inotropic left ventricular support and systemic afterload reduction can be used to stabilize the patient.

The hemodynamic changes associated with pregnancy can be expected to have mixed effects. A reduction in systemic vascular resistance will tend to promote forward flow. The drive to increase cardiac output will exacerbate left ventricular volume overload. Increased atrial dilation may initiate atrial fibrillation. Pulmonary congestion can be managed by careful diuresis with the knowledge that adequate forward flow is usually dependent on a high preload to achieve adequate left ventricular filling. Atrial fibrillation should be managed consistent with care outside pregnancy. An increase in systemic vascular resistance due to progressive hypertension secondary to preeclampsia may significantly impair forward flow and should be treated. Labor and delivery should be managed with "standard cardiac care." Catecholamine release due to pain or stress will impair forward low. Particular attention should be paid to left ventricular filling. Excessive preload will result in pulmonary congestion. Insufficient preload will not fill the enlarged left ventricle and will result in insufficient forward flow. A pulmonary artery catheter can be used to determine appropriate filling pressure in early labor or prior to induction. While a large v-wave may complicate the interpretation of pulmonary artery wedge pressure, the pulmonary artery diastolic pressure can be used as a reference point. Diuresis in the early postpartum period may be required.

Mitral valve prolapse is a common condition, affecting as many as 12 percent of young women.[21] In the absence of conditions of abnormal connective tissue such as Marfan and Ehler-Danlos syndrome and clinically significant mitral regurgitation, women with mitral prolapse can be expected to have uncomplicated pregnancies. They may experience an increase in tachyarrhythmias that can be treated with β-blockers. Prophylactic antibiotics are usually used at the time of delivery.

AORTIC STENOSIS

Most patients who develop calcific stenotic tricuspid aortic valves do so outside their childbearing years (age 70 to 80). Patients with bicuspid valves develop significant stenosis after the age of 50 to 60 years. Rheumatic disease can also affect the aortic valve, usually after the development of significant mitral disease. The majority of pregnant women with significant aortic stenosis have congenitally stenotic valves: bicuspid valves with congenitally fused leaflets, unicuspid valves, or tricuspid valves with fused leaflets.[22]

The natural history of aortic stenosis is characterized by a long, asymptomatic period. With increasing outflow obstruction, patients develop angina, syncope, and left ventricular failure. Without valve replacement, only 50 percent of patients will survive 5 years after the development of angina; 3 years after the development of syncope; and 2 years after the development of left ventricular failure.[23] While valve replacement is the only definitive treatment for calcific aortic stenosis, valvuloplasty may prove beneficial in some young adults whose valves are not calcified. Medical management of symptomatic patients is not generally efficacious. Mechanical valve replacement requires anticoagulation, complicating subsequent pregnancies.

Young women with aortic stenosis are usually asymptomatic. While they may develop increasing exercise intolerance in pregnancy, the progression is insidious and not easily distinguished from the effects of normal pregnancy. The diagnosis is usually made by the auscultation of a harsh systolic murmur. The murmur can easily be distinguished from a physiologic murmur of pregnancy by its harshness and radiation into the carotid arteries. Diagnosis is confirmed by echocardiography where the gradient across the valve can be measured by Doppler, and the valve area can be calculated with the continuity equation. Many women with significant aortic stenosis will experience the expected increase in cardiac output associated with pregnancy.[3] Increased flow across the fixed, stenotic valve will result in a proportionately increased gradient across the valve. While the pressure gradient during pregnancy may be higher than that observed postpartum, these differences are not significant.

Four series of patients with aortic stenosis in pregnancy have been reported.[3,24–26] The reports summarize experiences with wide ranges in severity of disease and management ranging from the 1960s and 1970s to the present. Arias described a series of 23 cases managed prior to 1978 with a maternal mortality of 17 percent.[24] While this report confirms the potential for maternal mortality associated with aortic stenosis in pregnancy, more recent series do not.[3,25,26] The potential for adverse outcome reported by Arias should certainly serve as an indication for intensive management. However, the rate of mortality should not necessarily be used as an indication for termination or surgical intervention. Pregnant patients have been successfully managed with aortic gradients in excess of 160 mm Hg.[3] In general, patients with a peak aortic gradient of 60 mm Hg or less had uncomplicated courses. Those with higher gradients required increasingly intensive management.

Aortic valve replacement and balloon valvotomy have been reported during pregnancy. Balloon valvotomy in a young patient without valve calcification can provide significant long-term palliation. Valvotomy prior to pregnancy may provide an interval of hemodynamic stability sufficient to complete a pregnancy without the complications associated with a prosthetic valve. Consideration for valve replacement or valvotomy during pregnancy should be reserved for patients who remain clinically symptomatic despite hospital care. In general, intervention should not be based entirely on a pressure gradient or valve area.

Aortic stenosis is a condition of excess left ventricular afterload. Ventricular hypertrophy increases cardiac oxygen requirement, while increased diastolic ventricular pressure impairs diastolic coronary perfusion. Each increases the potential for myocardial ischemia. The left ventricle requires adequate filling to generate sufficient systolic pressure to produce flow across the stenotic valve. Given a hypertrophied ventricle and some degree of diastolic dysfunction, the volume–pressure relationship will be very steep. A small loss of left ventricular filling will result in a proportionately large fall in left ventricular pressure and therefore a large fall in forward flow, cardiac output. The pregnant patient with significant aortic stenosis will be very sensitive to loss of preload associated with hemorrhage or an epidural. The window of appropriate filling pressure is narrow. Excess fluid may result in pulmonary edema; insufficient fluid may result in hypotension and coronary ischemia. In general, pulmonary edema associated with excess preload is much easier to manage than hypotension due to hypovolemia.

Appropriate antepartum care is described above. Given that most aortic stenosis in young women is congenital in origin, fetal echocardiography is indicated. While some controversy persists, cesarean section is generally reserved for obstetric indications. Pain during labor and delivery can be safely managed with regional analgesia using a low-dose bupivacaine and narcotic technique. Dense anesthesia during the second stage can be obtained with minimal hemodynamic complications using a caudal. Patients with gradients above 60 to 80 mm Hg will benefit from the use of a pulmonary artery and an arterial catheter during labor. Ideally, the woman is admitted the day before induction of labor with a favorable cervix. A prolonged induction should be avoided. Pulmonary artery and radial artery catheters as well as epidural and caudal catheters are placed. The patient should be gently hydrated overnight to achieve a pulmonary artery wedge pressure (PAWP) of 12 to 15 mm Hg. Some patients with milder disease will spontaneously diurese in the face of a volume load such that an elevation in PAWP cannot be achieved. An elevated PAWP will serve as a buffer against a loss of preload. If with bleeding or the onset of anesthesia PAWP sags, volume can be administered prior to a reduction in forward flow. In general, pushing is minimized, and the second stage is shortened with low forceps. Antibiotics are administered for the prevention of endocarditis.

Postpartum, patients should be monitored hemodynamically for 24 to 48 hours. Diuresis will usually be spontaneous; the patient can be allowed to find her predelivery compensated state. When diuresis must be induced to treat pulmonary edema, it should be done gently and carefully. Predelivery hemodynamic parameters should be used as an endpoint. Some have found that a significant delay in valve replacement after the postpartum period is associated with maternal complications.[3] These observations may be the result of accelerated valve deterioration due to pregnancy. For this reason, valve replacement within weeks of delivery may be indicated.

AORTIC REGURGITATION

Aortic regurgitation is most often due to a congenitally abnormal valve. Other causes include Marfan syndrome, endocarditis, and rheumatic disease. As with mitral regurgitation, the left ventricle compensates for a loss in forward flow with an increase in left ventricular end-diastolic volume. Afterload reduction will prevent progressive left ventricular dilation and is recommended for patients with left ventricular dysfunction or dilation. Valve replacement is generally recommended for: (1) New York Heart Association (NYHA) functional class III and class IV symptoms, (2) an ejection fraction less than 50 percent, or (3) left ventricular end-systolic dimension greater than 55 mm.[14] Acute regurgitation may be due to aortic root dissection or endocarditis and usually represents a medical emergency requiring urgent valve replacement.

The reduction in vascular resistance associated with pregnancy will tend to improve cardiac performance. If afterload reduction has been achieved with an angiotensin-converting inhibitor before pregnancy, hydralazine should be substituted. Modest elevations of heart rate should be tolerated. Bradycardia may be associated with increased regurgitation due to prolongation of diastole. Labor and delivery is managed with "standard cardiac care." Pulmonary artery catheterization is not usually required. As the hemodynamic changes associated with pregnancy resolve, a rise in vascular resistance should be anticipated and afterload reduction maintained.

PROSTHETIC VALVES

Definitive therapy for significant valvular disease requires surgical repair, or more commonly replacement. Mechanical valves are durable but require anticoagulation. Porcine tissue valves, when used in a young woman, will usually require replacement in her lifetime. Reports of pregnancies associated with prosthetic valves suggest significant variability in outcomes. Table 29–2 summarizes a review of 151 pregnancies complicated by a prosthetic valve.[27] Mechanical valves and anticoagulation were associated with a moderate increase in miscarriage and thromboembolic events. A report from France of 55 pregnancies suggests a less favorable prognosis.[28] Mechanical valves were associated with a maternal mortality rate of 3.7 percent and a thromboembolic rate of 14.8 percent. Thromboembolism was increased fourfold with heparin rather than Coumadin. Mitral valves accounted for 81 percent of thrombotic complications.

The impact of pregnancy on the life of a porcine valve has been studied.[27] Ten-year graft survival following two pregnancies was 16.7 percent compared with 54.8 percent following a single pregnancy. Pregnancy, in and of itself, seems to adversely affect the life of a porcine valve.

Decisions surrounding the timing and choice of valve replacement for a woman of reproductive age are complex. Managing a pregnancy with moderate valve disease may be less complicated than managing a pregnancy with a prosthetic valve. The durability of a mechanical valve has considerable advantages for a young person, but it is associated with more adverse outcomes in pregnancy. Delay in valve replacement until child bearing is completed is appropriate when the

Table 29–2. PREGNANCY OUTCOMES WITH PROSTHETIC VALVES

	Mechanical	Porcine
Women	31	57
Pregnancies	56	95
Fetal loss	27.7%	12.3%
Premature birth	5.9%	7.7%
Valve deterioration	5.3%	7.0%
Thromboembolic event	5.3%	—

severity of heart disease is felt to be manageable in pregnancy.

Anticoagulation is required with a mechanical valve. Oral anticoagulation in the first trimester is associated with congenital anomalies; potentially serious fetal bleeding may be encountered in the second and third trimesters. The American College of Cardiology/American Heart Association guidelines recommend consideration of subcutaneous heparin in the first trimester to avoid warfarin embryopathy, and the use of warfarin until 36 weeks, when subcutaneous heparin is substituted until after delivery.[14] These recommendations remain controversial in that they may underestimate the risk of fetal intracerebral bleeding in the absence of labor.[29] The fetus exposed to Coumadin in the second and third trimesters is at risk for developmental toxicity. Individual patients should be counseled regarding the risks of either strategy and participate actively in a final choice of therapy. If heparinization is chosen, the activated partial thromboplastin time (aPTT) should be increased to two to three times control at middosing interval. Intravenous heparin can be administered on an ambulatory basis and should be considered for mitral valves, which are more likely to clot, and for patients who may be noncompliant with subcutaneous administration. Women treated for prolonged periods with heparin should be counseled regarding the risk of osteoporosis.

Successful thrombolytic therapy of a clotted valve in pregnancy has been reported.[30,31] While significant uterine bleeding has been occasionally encountered, fibrinolysis is probably safer in pregnancy than emergent valve replacement.

CONGENITAL HEART DISEASE

Congenital heart disease is present in 0.7 to 1 percent of live births, accounting for as many as 30 percent of infants with birth anomalies. Prior to the development of corrective surgery, many children died shortly after birth or in childhood. In 1939, the first patent ductus arteriosus was ligated. In 1945, the first Blalock-Taussig shunt was performed for palliation of cyanotic heart disease. In 1953, cardiac bypass was introduced. Introduction of surgery under hypothermia in the late 1960s permitted longer and more complex repairs.[32,33] Of children who survived surgery to correct tetralogy of Fallot between 1955 and 1960, the 23-year survival is 86 percent, approaching the expected survival rate of 96 percent for normal children.[34] Prior to the 1960s, the prevalence of rheumatic heart disease in pregnancy exceeded the incidence of congenital disease by a ratio of 4:1. By the 1980s, the ratio was 1:1.[26] Currently,

congenital disease is estimated to exceed rheumatic disease by 1:4. While many will enter pregnancy with known heart disease, some women will have their disease first recognized due to the hemodynamic demands of pregnancy.

Increased survival of children with congenital disease has created a population of young women with complex medical and psychosocial conditions entering their childbearing years. Those whose congenital heart disease was diagnosed in infancy have frequently experienced multiple cardiothoracic surgeries and extended hospitalizations. They have lived with continued concerns from parents and health care professionals regarding their ongoing health. Their childhoods have been restricted. At an early age, they faced the possibility of their own death. The psychosocial impact of this experience has been described as "growing up heart sick."[35] Young women describe a childhood of overprotectiveness and "being watched." They describe a lack of information regarding childbearing and contraception. They "seemed to believe that someone else could and would decide whether they should become pregnant."[35] Body image disorders over "eternal skinniness," scars from surgery, and delayed development of secondary sex characteristics are common. Health care providers should strive to (1) objectively share information regarding reproductive health care, (2) direct decision making towards the patient rather than towards parents and health care professionals, and (3) improve self-esteem and body image. "Women with congenital heart disease want some way of being normal in their lives. Helping them to gain knowledge so that they can make responsible choices concerning contraception, pregnancy, and childbearing may be a way of assisting them to regain normalcy through feelings that they have control of their own bodies and lives."[35] When treating congenital heart disease during pregnancy, one must be willing to acknowledge and address the impact of the patient's disease on her life.

Table 29–3 summarizes the distribution of congenital heart disease in childhood and in pregnancy.[26,33]

Table 29–3. INCIDENCE OF CONGENITAL HEART DEFECTS IN CHILDHOOD AND IN PREGNANCY

	Childhood	Pregnancy
Ventricular septal defect	35%	13%
Atrial septal defect	9%	9%
Patent ductus arteriosis	8%	2.7%
Pulmonary stenosis	8%	8%
Aortic stenosis	6%	20%
Coarctation of the aorta	6%	8%
Tetralogy of Fallot	5%	12%
Transposition of the great vessels	4%	5.4%

The spontaneous closure of lesions such as ventricular septal defect and correction of patent ductus are reflected by reduced reporting in pregnancy. The increased reporting of aortic stenosis in pregnancy is probably due to a worsening of disease with age and the ease of recognition in pregnancy. The complexity and diversity of congenital heart disease confounds our ability to describe the prognosis or a management plan for the breadth of conditions. Major risks in pregnancy include (1) cyanosis, (2) left (or systemic) ventricular dysfunction, and (3) pulmonary hypertension, particularly with right ventricular dysfunction.

Outcomes have been most clearly described based on the presence or absence of maternal cyanosis. Table 29–4 is derived from a report of 482 pregnancies from 233 women with congenital heart disease who delivered between 1968 and 1982.[13] The rate of terminations was higher in the group of women with cyanotic heart disease and particularly high (42 percent) in those with uncorrected lesions. This reflects the anticipated poor neonatal outcome and maternal risks associated with uncorrected cyanotic disease. One should assume that patients with more severe disease are overly represented in the group of women who chose to terminate, which would bias the group who continued pregnancy towards a better outcome. Eighty-six to 90 percent of pregnancies without cyanosis ended in a live birth compared to 71 percent with an uncorrected lesion. Given an expected baseline rate of miscarriage, these outcomes are quite good. Corrected cyanotic disease was associated with outcomes comparable to noncyanotic disease. Table 29–5 is derived from a report of 144 pregnancies from women with congenital heart disease delivered between 1976 and 1986.[26] Adverse outcomes are again concentrated among women with uncorrected cyanotic heart disease.

Common maternal complications include congestive heart failure and pulmonary edema (4 percent), arrhythmia (4 percent), and hypertension (6 percent). Congestive heart failure and hypertension were com-

Table 29–5. NEONATAL OUTCOME WITH CONGENITAL HEART DISEASE BY SAB, SGA, PRETERM, AND BIRTH WEIGHT

	SAB	SGA	Preterm	Birth Weight
Noncyanotic	12%	6%	9%	3,300 ± 600
Cyanotic	21%	52%	35%	2,400 ± 800
Corrected	11%	25%	0%	
Uncorrected/ palliative	25%	67%	53%	

SAB, spontaneous abortion; SGA, small for gestational age; Preterm, preterm birth.

monly associated with uncorrected left ventricular outflow obstruction.[13,26] Arrhythmias were observed after surgery in and about atrial or ventricular septums. Maternal death was uncommon, 0 per 482 pregnancies in one series[13] and 1 per 144 pregnancies in a second.[26] Maternal deaths are most commonly reported in association with Eisenmenger's syndrome, discussed more fully below.

Men and women with congenital heart disease are at increased risk for having children with congenital heart disease. In a prospective study with aggressive pediatric evaluation, Whittemore estimated the incidence to be as high as 14.2 percent.[13] In a retrospective study, Rose found the risk to be 8.8 percent.[12] The rate of congenital heart disease associated with an affected mother was 2 to 3.5 times that observed with an affected father. Specific parental defects are not generally associated with the same defect in the child. The risk for cardiac maldevelopment is inherited rather than the risk for a specific defect. The risk of congenital heart disease and the character of the risk should be discussed with an affected mother. In Whittemore's report, 58 of 60 affected infants were diagnosed with relatively benign correctable lesions (atrial septal defect, ventricular septal defect, pulmonary stenosis, aortic stenosis, patent ductus arteriosis, or mitral valve prolapse). Only 2 infants from 372 pregnancies (0.5 percent) were diagnosed with complex congenital heart disease.[13] All women who have congenital heart disease should have a fetal echocardiogram performed at midpregnancy.

Contraceptive counseling should be offered to all women with congenital heart disease. Given the problems experienced growing up with heart disease, contraceptive education should probably be initiated as part of general health care education, prior to the overt need for birth control. In the context of congenital heart disease, complications associated with pregnancy are usually greater than those associated with any form of birth control. Cyanosis, pulmonary hypertension, low cardiac output, dilated cardiac chambers, sluggish venous conduits (e.g., Fontan), and atrial fibrillation

Table 29–4. NEONATAL OUTCOME WITH CONGENITAL HEART DISEASE: LIVE-BORN VERSUS TERMINATION

	Live-Born Infant	Termination
Noncyanotic	86%	5%
Cyanotic	85%	26%
Corrected	95%	17%
Palliative	87%	17%
Uncorrected	71%	42%

$$\text{Termination rate} = \frac{\text{No. of terminations}}{\text{No. of pregnancies}}$$

$$\text{Live-born rate} = \frac{\text{No. of live-born infants}}{\text{No. of pregnancies} - \text{No. of terminations}}$$

place patients at risk for thrombosis. This small group of women should probably avoid combined estrogen/progestin oral contraceptives. Progestin-only pills are not associated with risk for thrombosis but require regular dosing to achieve optimal efficacy. Parenteral progestins are safe for women with cardiac disease and are extremely effective. They do cause irregular bleeding, which may be significant if the patient is anticoagulated. The intrauterine device carries a risk for pelvic inflammatory disease and therefore a theoretical risk of bacteremia and endocarditis. The actual risk has been estimated to be 1 per 1 million patient-years.[36]

ISOLATED SEPTAL DEFECTS

Ventricular and atrial septal defects represent greater than 40 percent of congenital heart disease identified in childhood. Many defects identified in children will close with advancing age. In adulthood, 50 percent of large ventricular septal defects (>1.5 cm) lead to the development of Eisenmenger's syndrome. Ten percent of uncorrected atrial septal defects will also develop pulmonary hypertension. The management of Eisenmenger's syndrome in pregnancy is discussed below.

A harsh systolic murmur that radiates to the left sternal border but not to the carotids suggests the presence of a ventricular septal defect. The diagnosis can be confirmed by color flow Doppler echocardiography demonstrating a small, high-velocity lesion. The peak velocity of the jet across the septum can be used to assess the pressure gradient between the ventricles. A high velocity between ventricles indicates a large pressure gradient and low pressure in the right ventricle and the absence of pulmonary hypertension. In the absence of associated cardiac lesions and pulmonary hypertension, the presence of a ventricular septal defect does not usually complicate pregnancy. Small defects create loud murmurs but are not usually hemodynamically significant. The high-velocity jet of a small lesion does create a risk for endocarditis.

Atrial septal defects are more difficult to diagnose by auscultation. The characteristic finding, a split S_2 that is fixed with respiration, is subtle and usually not appreciated without specific attention. Increased right-sided flow secondary to shunting across the defect may create a flow murmur that will be augmented in pregnancy. Other endocardial cushion defects may be associated with ostium primum defects. In the absence of other anomalies, the significance of the atrial septal defect is related to its size rather than to its etiology. Hemodynamically significant defects result in significant shunting from the systemic circulation to the pulmonary circulation. As with the ventricular septal defect, Eisen-

menger's syndrome may develop, but usually at an older age. Increased pulmonary blood flow may result in dyspnea on exertion and restriction of activity. Atrial arrhythmias are commonly associated with atrial enlargement or intrinsic conduction abnormalities in the case of ostium primum defects.

The patient with a significant pulmonary/systemic shunt ratio can be expected to normally expand her cardiac output during pregnancy. However, the price of a normal systemic cardiac output is a high pulmonary flow. The pregnant patient may begin to experience symptoms at rest that she previously noted with exercise. She may also experience an increase in tachyarrhythmias. Heart rate control with a β-blocker may provide symptomatic relief. Early diuresis may benefit the patient postpartum. Elevated pulmonary blood flow associated with pregnancy could, in theory, accelerate the progression of pulmonary vascular disease. In the absence of associated anomalies, arrhythmias, and pulmonary hypertension, the presence of an atrial septal defect does not usually complicate pregnancy.

PATENT DUCTUS ARTERIOSIS

The diagnosis of a patent ductus arteriosis is suggested by the characteristic continuous murmur at the upper left sternal border. Most are identified and ligated in childhood. Of patients with an uncorrected patent ductus, as many as 50 percent will develop Eisenmenger's syndrome, the majority in childhood. In adults with a small patent ductus, the major risk is endocarditis. In the absence of Eisenmenger's syndrome, pregnancy is not usually complicated. As with the atrial septal defect, the increase in pulmonary blood flow associated with the increase in cardiac output in pregnancy may result in increased dyspnea with exertion and at rest. Early diuresis may benefit the patient postpartum.

TRANSPOSITION OF THE GREAT VESSELS

Transposition of the great vessels represents only 5 percent of pregnant women with congenital heart disease but is overrepresented in the publication of case reports and case series. The attention received in publication permits a more systematic analysis of outcomes. In transposition of the great vessels (TGV), systemic venous blood returns to the right atrium, and passes through the tricuspid valve, into the right ventricle, and directly into the transposed aorta. Although an adequate circulation for fetal life, infants decompensate at birth due to an inadequate pulmonary circulation. Some will have a sufficiently large ventricular septal defect to achieve adequate pulmonary blood flow and oxygenation; others will require an immediate palliative procedure, an atrial septotomy.

Transposition of the great vessels was first definitively corrected in 1964 with the Mustard operation.[37] A baffle is constructed through the left and right atriums so that systemic venous return is channeled through the mitral valve into the left ventricle, and pulmonary venous return is directed through the tricuspid valve into the right ventricle. With a modest surgical intervention, the right and left pumps are placed in series with physiologic flow of systemic venous return through the pulmonary circulation. The right ventricle, as the systemic ventricle, must work against systemic resistance, and the tricuspid valve is exposed to systemic pressures. Long-term complications are associated with failure of the systemic ventricle and arrhythmia. Of patients surviving the first 30 days after repair, 90 percent will be alive in 10 years and 87 percent will be alive in 20 years. After 13 years, only 5 percent suffer significant disability (NYHA class II to IV).[38] A more physiologic repair can be achieved when transposition is accompanied by a ventricular septal defect. The ventricular septum is reconstructed so that the aortic outflow tract lies within the left ventricle and a conduit is constructed to connect the right ventricle to the pulmonary artery (Rastelli repair).[39] The pulmonary conduit is prone to stenosis and deterioration of the transplanted valve. More recently, a direct surgical switch between the pulmonary artery and the aorta has been performed. Given the time when these operations were introduced, most young women entering pregnancy will have a Mustard repair. Increasing numbers will have a Rastelli repair or a great vessel switch.

The hemodynamic changes of pregnancy will have a mixed impact on a patient with a Mustard repair. Increased cardiac output will increase the volume load on the right heart. Decreased vascular resistance reduces

Pregnancy Outcomes with Congenitally Corrected Transposition of the Great Vessels

Women	41
Cyanotic	4 (10%)
Pregnancies	105
Cyanotic	13 (12%)
Live births	77 (73%)
Miscarriages*	22
Terminations	6
Fetal deaths	1
Premature birth 35 weeks*	6 (8%)
Congenital heart disease	1 (1%)
Congestive heart failure	5 (6%)
Cerebrovascular accident	1 (1%)

*Miscarriages and premature births concentrated among cyanotic mothers.

afterload on the right heart. The box "Pregnancy Outcomes with Transposition of the Great Vessels" summarizes nine papers reporting a total of 49 pregnancies in 36 women.[26,38,40-46] No maternal mortality was reported. Neonatal outcomes were good. Two women entered pregnancy with disability due to their heart disease (NYHA class III to IV). One delivered at 26 weeks due to preterm labor. The other developed severe congestive failure near term and died 19 months postpartum. Congestive heart failure was frequently associated with uncontrolled tachyarrhythmias.

Congenitally corrected transposition of the great vessels (ventricular inversion) is characterized by the passage of systemic venous blood into the right atrium, directly into the left ventricle and out through the transposed pulmonary artery. Pulmonary venous return passes directly from the left atrium into the right ventricle and out through the aorta. The right ventricle again serves as the systemic ventricle. Congenitally corrected TGV may be an isolated anomaly but may also be associated with other anomalies that result in cyanosis. See box for summary of two series of pregnancies with congenitally corrected transposition of the great vessels.[47,48] Again, maternal and neonatal outcomes are good. Consistent with outcomes associated with other cyanotic forms of congenial heart disease, miscarriage and premature birth are concentrated among the cyanotic lesions.

Young women with surgically or congenitally corrected transposition of the great vessels can be expected to successfully complete pregnancy. Women who are functionally impaired or who are cyanotic prior to pregnancy can expect more adverse outcomes and may deteriorate postpartum. Evaluation prior to pregnancy

Pregnancy Outcomes with Transposition of the Great Vessels

Women	36
Pregnancies	49
Live births	41 (84%)
Miscarriages	5
Terminations	2
Fetal deaths	1
Premature birth 35 weeks	5 (12%)
Congenital heart disease	0 (0%)
Congestive heart failure	6 (15%)
Arrhythmia	8 (20%)

should include assessment of functional status; evaluation of right, systemic, heart function; and confirmation of normal oxygenation. When the right heart is the systemic heart, pharmacologic afterload reduction should be maintained until pregnancy is confirmed. Angiotensin-converting enzyme inhibitors should be discontinued early in the first trimester.

The reported experience with transposition of the great vessels is to date the most extensive for any complex defect. The conclusions drawn from this experience are probably applicable to other less common conditions. Functional status and cyanosis are the most reliable predictors of complicated pregnancies. Arrhythmia is common and is frequently the initiator of cardiac decompensation.

FONTAN REPAIR

The Fontan repair was initially performed to achieve a physiologic correction of tricuspid atresia by connecting the right atrium directly to the pulmonary artery.[49] The Fontan repair and subsequent modifications are currently used to correct a variety of complex congenital heart conditions characterized by a single functional ventricle. The repair achieves a noncyanotic, functional flow of systemic venous return through the lungs and a functionally systemic ventricle. Without a pulmonary pump, the cardiac price for this result is elevated systemic and right atrial pressure (12 to 14 mm Hg).

Experience with pregnancy in women with the Fontan repair is limited. Young women have been discouraged from attempting pregnancy due to concerns regarding the ability of a single ventricle system to adapt to the demands of pregnancy. In a survey of 76 women of reproductive age, Canobbio et al. reported that 66 percent were counseled not to become pregnant despite a stable surgical outcome and a strong desire to have

Pregnancy Outcomes with Fontan Repair	
Women	21
Pregnancies	33
Live births	15 (45%)
Miscarriages	13
Terminations	5
Fetal deaths	0
Premature birth 35 weeks	1 (7%)
Congenital heart disease	1 (7%)
Congestive heart failure	1 (7%)
Arrhythmia	2 (15%)

children.[50] The remaining 34 percent were not counseled regarding pregnancy. Contraceptive usage, despite counseling against pregnancy, was inconsistent. The box "Pregnancy Outcomes with Fontan Repair" summarizes the outcomes of 33 pregnancies from 21 women reported by this group. While the miscarriage rate was higher than the general population, the preterm birth rate was low. Maternal complications were limited to arrhythmia, usually atrial, and congestive heart failure in the postpartum period. While not reported in these small series, sluggish flow through the right atrial and pulmonary circulation may increase the risk for thrombosis.

EISENMENGER'S SYNDROME

The pathophysiology known as Eisenmenger's syndrome was first described in 1897. Vicktor Eisenmenger described a 32-year-old patient who was short of breath and cyanotic from childhood and died from hemoptysis. Autopsy revealed a ventricular septal defect and severe pulmonary vascular disease.[51] The term is now used to describe pulmonary-to-systemic shunting associated with cyanosis and increased pulmonary pressures secondary to pulmonary vascular disease. Eisenmenger's syndrome may develop from any intracardiac shunt resulting in blood from the high-pressure systemic circulation being directed into the pulmonary circulation. Systemic pressure and excessive flow lead to microvascular injury, obliteration of pulmonary arterioles and capillaries and, in the end, elevated pulmonary vascular resistance. The time to onset of shunt reversal is variable, but most patients who have a large ventricular septal defect or large patent ductus arterosus will develop shunt reversal in infancy. Those who have an atrial septal defect will be delayed until early adulthood. Survival at 10 years from diagnosis is 80 percent; at 25 years, it is 42 percent.[51]

Patients with Eisenmenger's syndrome are at risk for congestive heart failure, hemoptysis due to pulmonary hemorrhage, sudden death due to arrhythmia, cerebrovascular accident, and hyperviscosity syndrome. The diagnosis should be considered in any cyanotic patient and is confirmed by echocardiography with the demonstration of increased pulmonary pressure and an intracardiac shunt. If the shunt is due to an atrial septal defect or a patent ductus arteriosus, transesophageal examination may be necessary. Treatment is nonspecific, and includes supportive care and avoidance of destabilizing events such as surgery and unnecessary medications. Symptomatic hyperviscosity syndrome due to an elevated hematocrit can be treated with phlebotomy. Iron deficiency, preexisting or secondary to phlebotomy, can exacerbate hyperviscosity; microcytic cells are less deformable and therefore more prone to occlude the microcirculation. Definitive therapy can only be achieved with heart/lung or lung transplantation. However, the 4-year survival with lung transplantation is less than 50 percent, a less favorable prognosis than that for many patients with Eisenmenger's syndrome.

Ventricular septal defect (VSD), atrial septal defect, and patent ductus arteriosus (PDA) are responsible for 89 percent of reported cases of Eisenmenger's syndrome in pregnancy.[52] Each lesion is initially associated with shunting from the systemic, oxygenated circulation to the pulmonary circulation. As pulmonary vascular resistance and pulmonary pressures increase over time and approach systemic pressures, the characteristic murmurs of a VSD or PDA diminish. Reversal of flow from the right to the left, the development of hypoxemia, and increasing hematocrit herald the development of Eisenmenger's syndrome. The fall in systemic vascular resistance associated with pregnancy may initiate shunt reversal in a patient not previously cyanotic.

In 1979, Gleicher reviewed published cases of Eisenmenger's syndrome in pregnancy.[53] Seventy pregnancies from 44 women were evaluated. Fifty-two percent of the women died during pregnancy. Thirty percent of the pregnancies resulted in maternal death. The risk of death associated with first, second, and third pregnancies were 36 percent, 27 percent, and 33 percent, respectively. A first successful pregnancy did not confirm the safety of subsequent pregnancies. Most deaths (70 percent) occurred at the time of delivery or within 1 week postpartum. Excessive blood loss was associated with 35 percent of deaths, while thromboembolic conditions were responsible for 44 percent. Maternal mortality associated with cesarean delivery (80 percent) exceeded that associated with vaginal delivery (34 percent). Maternal death was not reported with first-trimester termination of pregnancy. Only 26 percent of pregnancies resulted in a term birth. Fifty-five percent of newborns were delivered preterm, and thirty-two percent were small for gestational age.

A more modern review of cases in the United Kingdom between 1991 and 1995 confirms the poor prognosis for pregnant women with Eisenmenger's syndrome despite considerable advancement in the management of cardiac disease in pregnancy.[54] Mortality remains extremely high; forty percent of the women died. In addition, 85 percent of the births were preterm. A review of published cases from 1978 to 1996 again confirmed a mortality rate of 36 percent.[52] The majority of deaths (96 percent) occurred within the first 35 days postpartum. Late diagnosis (relative risk [RR], 5.4) and delayed hospitalization (RR, 1.1/wk of delay) significantly increased maternal mortality.[52]

While the risks associated with Eisenmenger's syndrome in pregnancy are clear, appropriate management is not. Decreased activity, hospital observation, and oxygen supplementation are usually employed. Reduction of pulmonary pressures and improved systemic oxygen saturation after oxygen supplementation indicates that pulmonary vascular resistance is not fixed and suggests a better prognosis. Intercurrent antepartum events such as pneumonia or urinary tract infection will be poorly tolerated. Preventing microcytosis with iron supplementation may decrease the risk of microvascular slugging.

Cesarean section is reserved for obstetric indications and is avoided whenever possible. Hemodynamic stability must be maintained during labor and the postpartum period. When pulmonary vascular resistance is not fixed, oxygen supplementation may decrease pulmonary pressures. Systemic hypotension from hemorrhage or sympathectomy from epidural analgesia will result in increased right-to-left shunting, increasing hypoxemia, increasing pulmonary vascular resistance, and worsening shunt. Volume overload or excessive systemic resistance, particularly postpartum, may further tax a failing right heart. A pulmonary artery catheter and a peripheral arterial catheter are usually used to guide hemodynamic management. Narcotic-based regional analgesia provides adequate pain relief without excessive hemodynamic instability. Anticoagulation remains controversial. If patients are anticoagulated, caution should be exercised to avoid excessive treatment and associated hemorrhage.

While use of a selective pulmonary vasodilator, inhaled nitric oxide, has been reported to reduce pulmonary pressures, increase cardiac output, and improve systemic oxygenation, maternal death was not averted.[55] Unlike many cardiac conditions in pregnancy, meticulous care will frequently fail to prevent maternal death.

COARCTATION OF THE AORTA

Coarctation of the aorta results from a constriction of the aorta at or about the level of the ductus arteriosus or left subclavian artery. Patients have a characteristic discrepancy in blood pressure between their right arm and lower extremities. Complications include dissection at the site of coarctation, cephalic hypertension, and rupture of associated berry aneurysms.

Modern reports of coarctation in pregnancy are limited. Historically, pregnancy was associated with a maternal mortality of 9 percent due to aortic rupture, congestive heart failure, cerebrovascular accidents, and endocarditis.[56] β-Blockade may serve to protect against dissection and promote diastolic flow through the aortic narrowing.

Pediatric screening identifies most significant coarctations leading to repair. After repair, systemic hypertension may persist and require treatment. In a series of 18 patients and 36 pregnancies, the prematurity rate was not elevated. Preeclampsia was diagnosed in 14 percent of all pregnancies, and 17 percent of nulliparous pregnancies. One infant in 36 was diagnosed with congenital heart disease.[57]

An increasing cohort of young women with corrected congenital heart disease will be presenting to their obstetricians pregnant and desiring to bear children. Some basic conclusions can be drawn from our experience with congenital heart disease to date. First, Eisenmenger's syndrome and pregnancy remain a lethal combination. New, effective strategies for therapy are not anticipated. Second, cyanotic heart disease in the absence of pulmonary hypertension is associated with increased rates of miscarriage and preterm birth. Third, mothers with cardiac disability (NYHA class III to IV) or with evidence of right heart dilation will have a more complicated course in pregnancy. Fourth, arrhythmias may become worse in pregnancy and precipitate cardiac decompensation. Aggressive pharmacologic treatment is appropriate. Finally, many young women who are initially well compensated and acyanotic can have successful pregnancies.

CARDIOMYOPATHY

Dilated cardiomyopathy is characterized by the development of pulmonary edema in the context of left ventricular dysfunction and dilation. Patients usually present with signs and symptoms of pulmonary edema: dyspnea, cough, orthopnea, tachycardia, and occasionally hemoptysis. These symptoms of pulmonary edema, while characteristic of heart failure, may also be due to previously undiagnosed congenital or rheumatic heart disease, preeclampsia, embolic disease, intrinsic pulmonary disease, tocolytic use, or sepsis. The diagnosis of cardiomyopathy is made in the clinical circumstances of characteristic signs and symptoms and findings of left ventricular dysfunction and dilation on echocardiographic examination. Ventricular dysfunction may be due to conditions extrinsic to the heart such as thyrotoxicosis or hypertension or due to intrinsic myocardial dysfunction. Accurate diagnosis will direct appropriate therapy and permit assessment of long-term prognosis.

Peripartum cardiomyopathy is a rare syndrome of heart failure presenting in late pregnancy or postpartum. The diagnosis is made after excluding other causes of pulmonary edema and heart failure. Failure to adhere to a rigorous definition of disease in the literature confounds conclusions regarding etiology and prognosis. A definition based on criteria for idiopathic dilated cardiomyopathy has been suggested (see the box "Diagnostic Criteria for Peripartum Cardiomyopathy").[58] The incidence is estimated to be between 1 in 1,300 and 1 in 15,000.[59] While some of the variability in reported incidence is due to regional and ethnic differences, much is due to the imprecise definition of the disease. The cause of peripartum cardiomyopathy is unknown. Nutritional and immunologic mechanisms have been proposed. The prevalence of antibodies to echovirus and coxsackievirus is not higher among women with cardiomyopathy compared to controls.[59]

> ### Diagnostic Criteria for Peripartum Cardiomyopathy
>
> 1. Heart failure within the last month of pregnancy or 5 months postpartum
> 2. Absence of prior heart disease
> 3. No determinable cause
> 4. Echocardiographic indication of left ventricular dysfunction
>   - Ejection fraction <45 percent or fractional shortening <30 percent
>   - Left ventricular end-diastolic dimension >2.7 cm/m²

The mortality rate for peripartum cardiomyopathy is reported to be 25 to 50 percent. Death is usually due to progressive congestive heart failure, arrhythmia, or thromboembolism.[59] Within 6 months, half of patients will demonstrate resolution of left ventricular dilation. Their prognosis is very good. Of those who do not, 85 percent will die within the next 4 to 5 years.[60] The magnitude of risk for subsequent pregnancies after peripartum cardiomyopathy is unclear. A recent survey of 67 pregnancies in 63 women suggests a mortality rate of 8 percent when left ventricular dysfunction has not resolved, and 2 percent in patients with normal function.[61]

Acute treatment of cardiomyopathy is directed at improving cardiac function and, when present, treating the inciting event. Diuretics are used to decrease preload and relieve pulmonary congestion. Digoxin may improve myocardial contractility and facilitate rate control when atrial fibrillation is present. Afterload reduction is achieved with angiotensin-converting enzyme inhibitors[62,63] postpartum, or hydralazine before delivery. β-Blockade has been clearly demonstrated to improve cardiac function and survival outside of pregnancy[64-66] and should not be withheld from pregnant women. Significantly dilated and hypokinetic cardiac chambers are at risk for clot formation. Anticoagulation with heparin antepartum or Coumadin postpartum should be considered. Implanted defibrillators have been used in pregnancy without significant complications.[67] Hemodynamic management during labor and delivery is frequently directed by a pulmonary artery catheter. Pain control decreases cardiac work and reduces tachycardia. A carefully dosed epidural is appropriate. Cesarean section is reserved for obstetric indications.

MYOCARDIAL INFARCTION

Myocardial infarction is a rare event among women of reproductive age. From a population base of 3.6 million women-years, Petitti et al. identified 186 cases (5.0 per 100,000 women-years).[68] The incidence was very low prior to 35 years of age, (1 per 100,000 women-years), but increased to 5.3 for ages 35 to 39 and to 18.4 for ages 40 to 44. The risk for myocardial infarction in pregnancy from this population was 1.5 per 100,000 deliveries. Based on a 9-month exposure per pregnancy, the incidence is comparable to nonpregnant women less than 35 years old.[68] Earlier estimates have been as high as 10 per 100,000 pregnancies.[69]

Due to the rarity of the event, information regarding myocardial infarction in pregnancy is derived from case reports and is therefore subject to considerable reporting bias. Routh and Elkayam have summarized information from reports of 123 pregnancies (see the box "Myocardial Infarction in Pregnancy").[70] Coronary dissection and normal coronary arteries are observed in almost 50 percent of cases. Delivery within 2 weeks of infarction may be associated with maternal mortality as high as 50 percent. Myocardial infarction has been reported in association with diabetes mellitus, pheochromocytoma, Ehlers-Danlos type IV, antiphospholipid syndrome, multiple gestation, and sickle cell anemia.[70] Medications such as ergot alkaloids given for bleeding, bromcriptine for lactation suppression, ritodrine and nifedipine for tocolysis, and prostaglandin E_2 in conjunction with severe hypertension have also been associated with myocardial infarction.[71-78]

The diagnosis of myocardial infarction in pregnancy is often delayed due to the rarity of the event and due to common symptoms of pregnancy. During normal pregnancy, most women experience some increase in exercise intolerance and dyspnea. Chest pain due to reflux is common. Electrocardiographic changes that suggest ischemia have been reported in as many as 37 percent of women having a repeat cesarean delivery.[70] The MB fraction of creatine kinase isoenzymes may be elevated at cesarean section as well.[79] Troponin I levels are not elevated during labor and delivery.[80] Given a constellation of findings suggestive of myocardial infarction, an echocardiogram can be used to confirm abnormal wall motion in the ischemic region.

Myocardial Infarction in Pregnancy	
Pregnancies	123
Mean age ± SD	32 ± 6 years
Age range	16–45 years
Anterior infarction	73%
Multiparous	84%
Hypertension	19%
Diabetes mellitus	5%
Smoking	26%
Family history of MI	8%
Hyperlipidemia	2%
Preeclampsia	11%
CHF after MI	19%
Coronary anatomy	
Stenosis	43%
Thrombus	21%
Dissection	16%
Aneurysm	4%
Spasm	1%
Normal	29%
Death	
Maternal	21%
Infant	13%*

*62% of infant deaths associated with mother's death.

Acute therapy is based on rapid coronary reperfusion. Coronary angioplasty and stinting have been reported in pregnancy and should not be withheld when appropriate for the mother's condition.[81-84] Thrombolytic therapy has also been utilized in pregnancy.[70] While effective, there may be a small but real incidence of associated maternal bleeding, preterm delivery, or fetal loss. Surgery after thrombolytic therapy is associated with significant risk for hemorrhage.

Medications commonly used in the management of myocardial infarction such as morphine, organic nitrates, lidocaine, β-blockers, aspirin, magnesium sulfate, and calcium antagonists may be used in appropriate doses in pregnancy. Care should be taken to avoid the supine position and maternal hypotension during procedures. The fetus, if viable, should be monitored.

Elective delivery within 2 weeks of infarction should be avoided. Cesarean section is reserved for obstetric indications. Labor and delivery is managed with "standard cardiac care." Pain is controlled, usually with carefully administered regional analgesia. Tachycardia is prevented with pain control and treated with β-blockers as needed. Hemodynamic stability is maintained frequently using information from pulmonary and peripheral arterial catheters. Maternal pushing is avoided, and the second stage of labor is shortened with low forceps or vacuum. Diuresis is gently initiated postpartum with diuretics.

The experience with pregnancy after a remote myocardial infarction is limited. Of 33 reported cases, recurrent infarction and significant complications have not been reported.[85]

MARFAN SYNDROME

Marfan syndrome is an autosomal dominant genetic disorder caused by an abnormal gene for fibrillin on chromosome 15.[86] Disease prevalence is estimated to be 4 to 6 per 10,000. Sporadic cases represent 15 percent of those diagnosed. The production of abnormal connective tissue results in the characteristic feature of the disease: aortic root dilation, dislocation of the optic lens, deformity of the anterior thorax, scoliosis, long limbs, joint laxity, and arachnodactyly. Diagnosis is usually based on family history, and ocular, cardiovascular, and skeletal features.

Untreated, life expectancy is reduced by a third, with the majority of deaths due to aortic dissection and rupture. Elective aortic repair is associated with a low mortality (1.5 percent), while emergent repair results in a much higher mortality (11.7 percent).[87] Elective repair has therefore been recommended when the aortic root diameter measures 5.5 to 6.0 cm. Using an absolute aortic diameter as an indication for surgery ignores relevant differences in aortic size associated with patients of different stature.[88] These considerations are particularly important when caring for young women. An aortic ratio between measured and predicted aortic diameter (AD) can be calculated. The predicted diameter for young adults can be calculated: $AD_{predicted} = 1.02 + (0.98 \times$ body surface area [BSA]). A ratio of less than 1.3 with a dilation rate of less than 5%/y suggests a low risk for a cardiovascular event.[88]

The risk for aortic dissection is associated with the rate of change of blood pressure in the aorta over time in systole. While simple reduction in blood pressure does not reduce the risk for dissection, β-blockade lowers the risk of reaching a clinical cardiac endpoint at 10 years from approximately 20 percent to 10 percent.[89]

Literature surveys of case reports suggest a maternal mortality rate associated with Marfan syndrome in pregnancy in excess of 50 percent.[90] These case reports probably represent a bias of reporting more severely affected pregnancies. Three population-based studies are summarized in the box "Marfan Syndrome in Pregnancy".[91–93] Aortic events, dissection or rapid dilation, occurred in 8 percent of cases. In seven of nine, the aortic diameter was known to be greater than 4.0 cm. Of the remaining two, one died due to aortic dissection

Marfan Syndrome in Pregnancy	
Women	84
Pregnancies	241
Live births	181 (75%)
Miscarriages	38 (16%)
Terminations	17 (7%)
Fetal deaths	2 (0.8%)
Aortic events	8 (4.3%)
Dissection	6 (3.3%)*
Rapid dilation	2 (1.1%)*
Death	2 (1.1%)*

*Observed in patients with an aortic root diameter >4 cm.

and rupture without a diagnosis and without a measurement of aortic diameter; the other had a prior graft replacement. A second death was due to endocarditis associated with mitral valve prolapse.

These studies suggest that women with mild disease, an aortic diameter less than 4.0 cm, can attempt pregnancy with only modest risk. The risk associated with more advanced disease is certainly greater. Given the data available, a precise risk of death from an aortic event cannot be quantified. Women with aortic diameters greater than 5.5 cm should certainly be counseled to have graft and valve replacement prior to pregnancy. They will then assume the risk associated with an artificial valve and the risk associated with the remaining aorta. These risks are not trivial but data do not exist to quantify the risk. Women with aortic roots greater than 4.0 cm but less than or equal to 5.5 cm are at significant risk, but aortic replacement may be premature. Fifty percent of children born to mothers with Marfan syndrome should be expected to have the disease.

Management of pregnancies affected by Marfan syndrome should begin with an accurate assessment of the aortic root. An absolute diameter or preferably an aortic ratio can be used to assess specific risk. The aortic root should be protected from hemodynamic forces with β-blockade. A resting heart rate of approximately 70 beats per minute can usually be achieved. While β-blockade may contribute to impaired fetal growth, this risk is small compared to the maternal risk without treatment.

Labor and delivery is managed with "standard cardiac care," with particular emphasis on the prevention of tachycardia. Patients with aortic roots less than 4.0 cm can certainly be delivered vaginally, reserving cesarean section for obstetric indications. Some authors have recommended cesarean delivery for women with larger roots based on concerns about increased pressure in the aorta during labor.[90] Data do not exist to confirm or to disprove this recommendation.

PULMONARY HYPERTENSION

Although pulmonary hypertension is fundamentally a pulmonary disease, the major pathologic impact is on the right heart. The incidence of primary pulmonary hypertension is 1 to 2 per 1 million, with women affected more commonly than men.[94] Secondary pulmonary hypertension may develop as a complication of cardiac disease such as mitral stenosis or secondary to intrinsic pulmonary disease. Drugs such as cocaine or appetite suppressants may also be responsible.[94] Untreated, the median survival after diagnosis is 2.5 years.[95] Pulmonary vasodilator therapy with oral nifedipine or intravenous prostacyclin have improved this prognosis. Of those who initially respond to nifedipine, the 5-year survival is 95 percent.[96] The 5-year survival for those who require treatment with prostacyclin is 54 percent.[97] The maternal mortality with severe pulmonary hypertension is reported to be as high as 50 percent.[98–100] Sudden, irreversible deterioration in the postpartum period is common.[98,99,101]

The symptoms of pulmonary hypertension are nonspecific. Increasing fatigue and shortness of breath are associated with progressive right heart failure but are also ubiquitous in pregnancy. They can easily be attributed to a presumed upper respiratory infection. Hoarseness may be present due to impingement on the laryngeal nerve by an enlarged pulmonary artery. Patients may exhibit disproportionate lower extremity edema or oxygen desaturation out of proportion for a presumed illness. The diagnosis can be confirmed with echocardiography, where the velocity of the regurgitant jet across the tricuspid valve can estimate pulmonary systolic pressure. A dilated, hypokinetic right ventricle with displacement of the intraventricular septum into the left ventricle suggests right heart failure.

Pulmonary hypertension with right ventricular dysfunction is poorly tolerated in pregnancy. A mortality rate approaching 50 percent should be expected. Should antepartum management be required, hospitalization is probably indicated. Oxygen therapy may reduce pulmonary vascular resistance and improve right ventricular performance. Pharmacologic treatment with nifedipine or intravenous prostacyclin may also be effective.[102] Anticoagulation with heparin should be considered. Worsening disease will usually be manifest by falling cardiac output rather than rising right ventricular pressure. Labor and delivery should be managed with "standard cardiac care," with particular attention to right ventricular filling as assessed by measurement of central venous pressure (CVP). While the right ventricle will require adequate filling to generate forward flow against an elevated pulmonary vascular resistance, modest elevations in CVP may precipitate increasing right ventricular dysfunction. Given fluid mobilization postpartum and the potential need to treat volume loss associated with delivery, appropriate filling may be difficult to achieve. Gentle diuresis may be required. Modest underloading or overloading of the right ventricle may result in rapid decompensation and death.

Women with pulmonary hypertension and right ventricular dysfunction should be strongly discouraged from becoming pregnant. Since pulmonary artery pressures will fall as the right ventricle fails, the condition of the right ventricle may be a more important consideration than an absolute systolic pulmonary pressure. Some women may consider pregnancy after a favorable response to treatment with nifedipine or prostacyclin. In a small series, two women whose pulmonary pressures and right ventricular function had normalized carried three pregnancies successfully while being treated with nifedipine or prostacyclin.[102] Neither experienced a deterioration in their condition over the first year postpartum.

OTHER CONDITIONS

Young women may experience malignant ventricular arrhythmias due to idiopathic ventricular fibrillation, cardiomyopathy, long-QT syndrome, congenital heart disease, or hypertrophic cardiomyopathy. Implantable defibrillators can effectively protect them from sudden death. In a report of 44 pregnancies, no women experienced generator erosion or lead fractures due to the expanding pregnancy. Twenty-five percent experienced discharges during pregnancy without complication.[67]

Hypertrophic cardiomyopathy is a genetic condition usually inherited in an autosomal dominant pattern with variable penetrance. While the condition can be subclassified, the physiologic impact of different forms is similar. Patients are at risk for failure and ischemia due to ventricular obstruction and arrhythmia. The ventricular septum hypertrophies such that the left ventricular outflow tracts is increasingly obstructed during systole. While in some regards, the impact of obstruction is similar to aortic valvular disease, the degree of obstruction is variable under different physiologic conditions. Reduced ventricular filling associated with blood loss, dehydration, or tachycardia will increase the functional obstruction. Reviews of case reports suggest a maternal mortality rate of 1 to 2 percent in these cases.[103,104] Given the biases associated with case report–derived data, this estimate probably sets an upper limit of expected mortality. In pregnancy, increased blood volume and left ventricular dimension will tend to benefit the patient. Increased heart rate will not. β-Blockers are generally used to manage tachycardia and some arrhythmias. Implantable defibrillators may also be used. Labor and delivery is managed with "standard cardiac care," with particular emphasis to ensure generous left ventricular filling. Supine hypotension must be carefully avoided. Obstetric bleeding should be treated early and aggressively with volume replacement.

CRITICAL CARE—HEMODYNAMIC MONITORING AND MANAGEMENT

Diseases unique to pregnancy, the physiologic stresses of pregnancy, and the special conditions surrounding labor and delivery operate to create circumstances where intensive care may be necessary more frequently than would be required among young nonpregnant individuals. Specialists in intensive care may not be familiar with the physiology of pregnancy and the associated unique conditions such as preeclampsia or amniotic fluid embolus. They may also be unfamiliar with maternal-fetal physiologic relationships and decision making that must balance the needs of the mother and the fetus. Therefore, obstetricians must be familiar with basic principles and techniques of critical care medicine in order to manage critically ill pregnant women themselves or to serve as valuable consultants to a critical care team.

Acute indications for invasive hemodynamic monitoring can be broadly categorized based on questions of physiology (see the box "Indications for Hemodynamic Monitoring"). Severe preeclampsia, sepsis, adult respiratory distress syndrome (ARDS), pneumonia, previously undiagnosed heart disease, and fluid management after resuscitation from obstetric hemorrhage are the most common conditions that will require hemodynamic monitoring. Certain conditions, particularly maternal heart disease as discussed above, will require a planned, prospective decision for invasive monitoring. In these cases, the therapeutic window for hemodynamic management is narrow and knowledge of the patient's baseline, compensated hemodynamic status can serve as a goal for intrapartum management.

In many cases, initial therapy can and should be made empirically based on an understanding of the patient's pathophysiology. If subsequent interventions are needed, specific data from hemodynamic monitoring may be required. Physicians with a large experience treating a particular disease will often need the benefits of invasive monitoring less and less as an improved understanding makes the clinical course more predict-

---

Indications for Hemodynamic Monitoring

1. **Why is the patient hypoxic?**
   - Are pulmonary capillary pressures high due to relative volume overload? (e.g., mitral stenosis postpartum)
   - Are pulmonary capillary pressures high due to depressed cardiac function? (e.g., cardiomyopathy)
   - Is capillary membrane integrity intact? (e.g., ARDS, pneumonia)
2. **Why is the patient persistently hypertensive?**
   - Is vascular resistance elevated?
   - Is cardiac output elevated?
3. **Why is the patient hypotensive?**
   - Is left ventricular filling pressure low? (e.g., after hemorrhage)
   - Is vascular resistance low? (e.g., septic shock)
4. **Why is the patient's urine output low?**
   - Is left ventricular filling pressure low resulting in low cardiac output?
5. **Is the patient expected to be unstable in labor?**
   - Is the window of left ventricular filling narrow? (e.g., aortic stenosis)
   - Will normal physiologic changes associated with delivery be tolerated poorly? (e.g., volume loading postpartum—mitral stenosis, pulmonary hypertension)

---

able. Physicians who find themselves in unfamiliar territory may benefit more than those who have experience. Therefore, understanding principles of management is particularly important for obstetricians who do not necessarily anticipate critically ill patients in their practice.

Hemodynamic Monitoring

The objective of hemodynamic monitoring is to provide continuous assessment of systemic and intracardiac pressures and to provide the means to determine cardiac output and, therefore, to calculate systemic and pulmonary resistances. An arterial catheter is usually placed in the radial artery to measure systemic pressure. The diastolic pressure obtained will usually correlate well with noninvasive measurements. Systolic pressure may be significantly higher than noninvasive measurements due to a very brief peak in pressure in early systole. (The spike in pressure contributes little to mean arterial pressure.) The noninvasive measurement is usually more clinically relevant to the patient's condition. The arterial catheter permits easy access to arterial blood sampling and relieves the patient from the discomfort of frequent blood draws.

Measurement of intracardiac pressures and cardiac output are obtained through the insertion of a catheter into the central venous circulation and advancement into and through the right heart. Venous access is most commonly obtained through the right internal jugular vein; a subclavian approach may also be used. Traditionally, insertion is guided by using the sternocleidomastoid muscle and the clavicle as landmarks. The higher frequency ultrasound transducer found on a vaginal probe can also be used to facilitate insertion under direct visualization. Once central venous access has been obtained and confirmed, a pulmonary artery catheter can be "floated" into the right heart and pulmonary artery. Figure 29–6 demonstrates the waveforms and normal pressure values found as the catheter passes through the heart. Success in "floating" the catheter is initially confirmed by observation of characteristic waveforms in the right ventricle, pulmonary artery, and wedged position, and subsequently with a radiograph. In experienced hands, complications from pulmonary artery catheterization are uncommon: pneumothorax (<0.1 percent), pulmonary infarction (0 to 1.3 percent), pulmonary artery rupture (<0.1 percent), and septicemia (0.5 to 2.0 percent).[105] Arrhythmias are usually transient and associated with passage of the catheter through the right ventricle. If the patient has significant pulmonary hypertension, difficulty may be encountered maintaining placement in the pulmonary artery.

Once the catheter has been successfully placed, continuous readings of central venous pressure and pulmonary artery pressures can be obtained. By inflating the balloon at the catheter tip, the catheter can be wedged in the pulmonary artery to obtain a PAWP. PAWP reflects the filling pressure, preload, in the left ventricle. CVP measured in the right atrium is a measure of right ventricular filling pressure. In pregnant women, CVP cannot be assumed to accurately reflect left ventricular filling. Right atrial pressures and systolic pulmonary pressures can be measured noninvasively by echocardiography.

Cardiac output is measured by thermodilution. A bolus of cold fluid is injected into the right atrium, and a curve of temperature change over time is recorded as the bolus passes through the pulmonary artery. From the shape of the curve, cardiac output can be calculated; when the cardiac output is higher, the dilutional curve is shorter in time and greater in maximum temperature change. More recently, catheters have been equipped with a heating element in the right atrial segment so that continuous measurement of cardiac output can be performed. Cardiac output can be measured

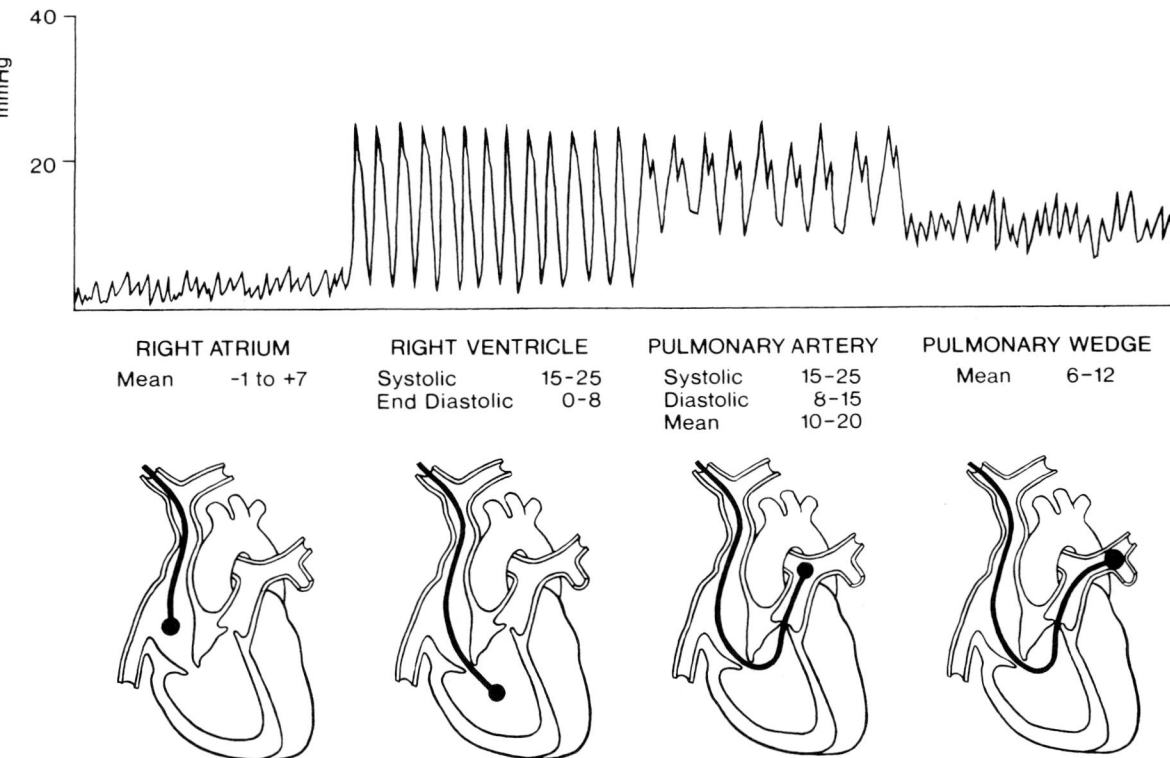

Figure 29–6. Hemodynamic waveforms and normal pressure values associated with catheter positions during advancement of a pulmonary artery catheter.

noninvasively with Doppler and impedance techniques. Doppler technique has been validated under a wide range of clinical circumstances.[106-109] Impedance technique tends to underestimate cardiac output in pregnancy but accurately reflects changes in hemodynamics in many conditions. In conditions of pathologically high flow, impedance may significantly underestimate cardiac output.[110-112] Cardiac index (CI) can be derived from cardiac output in order to adjust for maternal size: CI = CO/BSA (body surface area). However, BSA does not seem to be related to cardiac output in pregnancy; therefore, cardiac output is usually preferred.[109] When cardiac output is measured noninvasively and central venous pressure is not available, resistance is expressed as total peripheral resistance (TPR) rather than systemic vascular resistance (SVR). In most clinical conditions, the differences between the two are not important.

Table 29–6 summarizes formulas used to calculate hemodynamic parameters not directly measured. Normal values for cardiac output, mean arterial pressure, heart rate, stroke volume, and total peripheral resistance are summarized in Figure 29–1. In a study of 10 normal pregnant women at term, Clark et al. determined that central venous pressure, pulmonary artery pressure, pulmonary artery wedge pressure, and left ventricular work index were not different from nonpregnant measurements made approximately 3 months postpartum.[113] The relationship between PAWP and left ventricular work index fell within the normal range for nonpregnant individuals, suggesting normal contractility in pregnancy. Pulmonary vascular resistance was 34 percent lower, and colloid osmotic pressure was reduced by 14 percent.

Hemodynamic Management

The goal of this section is to develop strategies of hemodynamic therapy that may be applicable to a variety of clinical circumstances rather than to discuss management of specific maternal conditions. As outlined above, the use of hemodynamic monitoring should be directed at answering specific questions of maternal pathophysiology. Table 29–7 summarizes the most common clinical goals of therapy. To achieve each goal, a number of physiologic interventions are possible. Each of these interventions will precipitate a secondary or compensatory response. The secondary response, if excessive, may adversely affect the patient. The choice of intervention from available options will often be determined by the potential for and magnitude of adverse effect. Hemodynamic monitoring permits the physician to choose an intervention and subsequently assess the positive and negative impact.

Disruption of alveolar capillary fluid dynamics is frequently associated with acute oxygen desaturation due to excess alveolar fluid. Pulmonary edema is usually due to excess capillary pressure (e.g., cardiomyopathy, mitral stenosis) or to a disruption of alveolar capillary membrane integrity (e.g., pneumonia, ARDS). While a reduction in serum oncotic pressure is rarely a primary cause of pulmonary edema, the reduced serum albumin level in normal pregnancy will act in synergy with other forces, resulting in earlier or more severe pulmonary edema than would have been anticipated.

The use of pulse oximetry facilitates the early detection of maternal desaturation. Oxygen supplementation will improve maternal saturation but does not correct the underlying cause. If desaturation is progressive, further intervention will be required. In the normal heart, diuresis to reduce preload will work to decrease alveolar water in patients with elevated PAWP and in patients with capillary leak. A reduction in capillary pressure from high normal to low normal will reduce the egress of water across damaged membranes. In many circumstances, these interventions are made empirically based on a diagnosis and an understanding of maternal physiology. For example, tocolysis with β-mimetic

Table 29–6. CALCULATED HEMODYNAMIC VARIABLES

		Calculation	Units
Mean arterial pressure	MAP	$\dfrac{sBP + 2\ dBP}{3}$	mm Hg
Stroke volume	SV	$\dfrac{CO \cdot 1000}{HR}$	ml
Systemic vascular resistance	SVR	$\dfrac{(MAP-CVP) \cdot 80}{CO}$	dyne·sec·cm^{-5}
Total peripheral resistance	TPR	$\dfrac{MAP \cdot 80}{CO}$	dyne·sec·cm^{-5}
Pulmonary vascular resistance	PVR	$\dfrac{mPAP-PAWP}{CO}$	dyne·sec·cm^{-5}

sBP, systolic blood pressure; dBP, diastolic blood pressure; CO, cardiac output; CVP, central venous pressure; mPAP, mean pulmonary artery pressure; PAWP, pulmonary artery wedge pressure.

Table 29–7. HEMODYNAMIC INTERVENTIONS

Clinical Goal	Physiological Interventions	Agents	Compensatory Response
↑ Oxygenation	↑ FIO₂	O₂	
	↓ capillary pressure	Diuretic	↓ BP, ↓ CO
	↑ airway pressure	PEEP	↓ CO
	↓ resistance	Vasodilator	↑ CO
↓ Blood pressure	↓ cardiac output		
	↓ HR	β-Blocker	↓ CO
	↓ SV	Diuretic	↓ CO
	↑ resistance	α-Agonist	↓ CO
↑ Blood pressure	↑ cardiac output	Ionotropic	↑ CO
		Volume	↑ CO, ↓ O₂ saturation
	↑ cardiac output		
	↑ contractility	Ionotropic	↑ HR
↑ Perfusion	↑ preload	Volume	↓ O₂ saturation
	↓ resistance	Vasodilator	↓ BP

agents can induce pulmonary edema. Timely diagnosis, discontinuation of the offending agent, oxygen supplementation, and a single diuretic dose will usually be sufficient therapy. When initial interventions do not achieve an adequate effect, invasive monitoring may be required to direct subsequent care. Maternal diuresis to improve oxygen saturation, when excessive, may lead to a reduction in cardiac output. Fetal decompensation will usually be encountered before a significant reduction in maternal perfusion and hypotension. The maternal PAWP and cardiac output can be used to direct maternal diuresis. If desaturation continues despite hemodynamic management, intubation may be required. Positive end-expiratory pressure (PEEP) can be used to increase intra-alveolar pressure to impede the forces driving water into alveolar spaces. PEEP may impede venous return and decrease cardiac output due to the effects of the associated increase in extracardiac intrathoracic pressure. A PAWP in excess of PEEP is required for adequate ventricular filling. Only in the sickest of pregnant women will PEEP have a clinically significant impact on cardiac output.

Disorders of blood pressure and perfusion can be managed with the knowledge of maternal hemodynamics. Figure 29–7 describes the relationships between mean arterial pressure, cardiac output, and vascular resistance. Cardiac output and mean arterial pressure are represented on the x- and y-axes, respectively. Resistance is represented by diagonal isometric lines. Vasodilators or vasopressors that act on resistance produce vectors of change that run perpendicular to lines of resistance. Interventions that decrease cardiac output (β-blockers, diuresis) or increase cardiac output (dopamine, volume) produce vectors of change that run roughly parallel to lines of resistance. The region labeled "normal" represents the goal of therapy. Plotting patient data on the chart allows one to visually determine the vector or combination of vectors that could return hemodynamics to normal.

Patient A represents a patient who is hypotensive with a low cardiac output as might be expected after hemorrhage. Given a low PAWP, volume administration would be expected to create a vector that would return hemodynamics to normal. Alternatively, the patient could have a normal or high PAWP and would need an inotropic agent such as dopamine. Patient B has a normal blood pressure but a high vascular resistance and low cardiac output such as might be expected with a cardiomyopathy. Afterload reduction with a drug such as hydralazine will produce a vector of vasodilation and return hemodynamics to normal. Patient C is hypertensive with a mixed hemodynamic

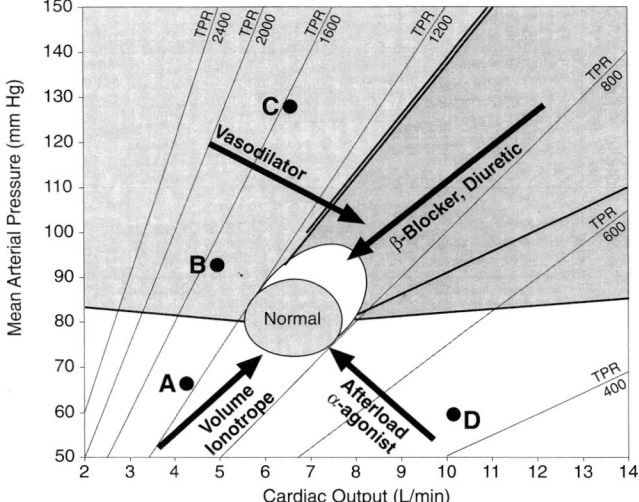

Figure 29–7. Hemodynamic flow chart. Cardiac output and mean arterial pressure are plotted on the x- and y-axes, respectively. Diagonal lines are isometric lines of vascular resistance. Anticipated vectors of change can be used to predict patient response to intervention.

pattern. She will need a combination of vectors to approach normal hemodynamics (e.g., hydralazine and β-blocker). Patient D is hypotensive and hyperdynamic with a low vascular resistance. The hemodynamics might be found in a patient with early sepsis. Treatment with volume could increase pressure but at the expense of high filling pressures and a potentially negative impact on developing ARDS. Alternatively, a small does of an α-adrenergic agent such as neosynephrine would create a vector perpendicular to lines of resistance that return hemodynamics to normal. Figure 29–7 allows one to see that vasoconstriction would achieve a normal blood pressure before adversely affecting cardiac output.

Key Points

➤ Hemodynamic changes in pregnancy may adversely affect maternal cardiac performance.

➤ Intercurrent events during pregnancy are usually the cause of decompensation.

➤ Women with heart disease in pregnancy frequently have unique psychosocial needs.

➤ Labor, delivery, and postpartum are times of hemodynamic instability.

➤ Invasive hemodynamic monitoring should be used to address specific clinical questions.

➤ Many maternal heart conditions can be medically managed during pregnancy. A few are associated with a very high risk of maternal mortality.

➤ Many patients with congenital heart disease can successfully complete a pregnancy.

➤ Preconceptual counseling is based on achieving a balance between medical information and the patient's value system.

REFERENCES

1. Easterling T, Benedetti T, Schmucker B, Millard S: Maternal hemodynamics in normal and preeclamptic pregnancies: a longitudinal study. Obstet Gynecol 76:1061, 1990.
2. Robson S, Dunlop W, Boys R, Hunter S: Cardiac output during labour. BMJ 295:1169, 1987.
3. Easterling T, Chadwick H, Otto C, Benedetti T: Aortic stenosis in pregnancy. Obstet Gynecol 72:113, 1988.
4. Clark S, Phelan J, Greenspoon J, et al: Labor and delivery in the presence of mitral stenosis: central hemodynamic observations. Am J Obstet Gynecol 152:384, 1985.
5. Robson S, Boys R, Hunter S, Dunlop W: Maternal hemodynamics after normal delivery and delivery complicated by postpartum hemorrhage. Obstet Gynecol 74:234, 1989.
6. Davison J, Lindheimer M: Volume homeostasis and osmoregulation in human pregnancy. Baillieres Clin Endocrinol Metab 3:451, 1989.
7. Whittaker P, Lind T: The intravascular mass of albumin during pregnancy: a serial study in normal and diabetic women. Br J Obstet Gynaecol 100:587, 1993.
8. Mishra M, Chambers J, Jackson G: Murmurs in pregnancy: an audit of echocardiography. BMJ 304:1413, 1989.
9. Otto C: Valvular stenosis: diagnosis, quantification, and clinical approach. In Textbook of Clinical Echocardiography. Philadelphia, WB Saunders Company, 2000, p 229.
10. Lamey J, Eschenbach D, Mitchell S, et al: Isolation of mycoplasmas and bacteria from blood of postpartum women. Am J Obstet Gynecol 143:104, 1982.
11. Boggess K, Watts D, Hillier S, et al: Bacteremia shortly after placental separation during cesarean section. Obstet Gynecol 87:779, 1996.
12. Rose V, Gold R, Lindsay G, Allen M: A possible increase in the incidence of congenital heart defects among the offspring of affected patients. J Am Coll Cardiol 6:376, 1985.
13. Whittemore R, Hobbins J, Engle M: Pregnancy and its outcome in women with and without surgical treatment of congenital heart disease. Am J Cardiol 50:641, 1982.
14. Bonow R, Carabello B, de Leon A, et al: ACC/AGA guidelines for the management of patients with valvular heart disease. Executive summary: a report of the American College of Cardiology/American Heart Association Task Force on practice guidelines (committee on management of patients with valvular heart disease). J Heart Valve Dis 7:672, 1998.
15. Chesley L: Severe rheumatic cardiac disease and pregnancy: the ultimate prognosis. Am J Obstet Gynecol 136:552, 1980.
16. Al Kasab S, Sabag T, Al Zaibag M, et al: Beta-adrenergic receptor blockade in the management of pregnant women with mitral stenosis. Am J Obstet Gynecol 163:37, 1990.
17. Becker R: Intracardiac surgery in pregnant women. Ann Thorac Surg 36:463, 1983.
18. Szekely P, Snaith L: Heart Disease and Pregnancy. Edinburgh, Churchill Livingstone, 1974.
19. Farhat M, Gamra H, Betbout F, et al: Percutaneous balloon mitral commissurotomy during pregnancy. Heart 77:564, 1997.
20. Gupta A, Lokhandwala Y, Satoskaar P, Salvi V: Balloon mitral valvotomy in pregnancy: maternal and fetal outcomes. J Am Coll Surg 187:409, 1998.
21. Devereuz R, Kramer-Fox R, Kligfield P: Mitral valve prolapse: causes, clinical manifestations, and management. Ann Intern Med 111:305, 1989.
22. Selzer A: Changing aspects of the natural history of valvular aortic stenosis. N Engl J Med 317:91, 1998.
23. Carabello B, Crawford F: Valvular heart disease. N Engl J Med 337:32, 1997.
24. Arias F, Pineda J: Aortic stenosis and pregnancy. J Reprod Med 20:229, 1978.
25. Lao T, Sermer M, MaGee L, et al: Congenital aortic stenosis and pregnancy: a reappraisal. Am J Obstet Gynecol 169:540, 1993.
26. Shime J, Mocarski E, Hastings D, et al: Congenital heart disease in pregnancy: short- and long-term implications. Am J Obstet Gynecol 156:313, 1987.
27. Lee C, Wu C, Lin P, et al: Pregnancy following cardiac prosthetic valve replacement. Obstet Gynecol 83:353, 1994.
28. Hanania G, Thomas D, Michel P, et al: Pregnancy in patients

with heart valves. A French retrospective study (155) cases. Arch Mal Coeur Vaiss 87:429, 1994.

29. Ville Y, Jenkins E, Shearer M: Fetal intraventricular haemorrhagia and maternal warfarin. Lancet 341:1211, 1993.

30. Azzano O, French P, Robin J, et al: Thrombolytic therapy with rt-PA for thrombosis of a tricuspid valve prosthesis during pregnancy. Arch Mal Coeur Vaiss 88:267, 1995.

31. Rinaldi J, Yassine M, Aboujaoude F, et al: Successful thrombolysis on an aortic valve prosthesis by plasminogen tissue activator during pregnancy. Arch Mal Coeur Vaiss 92:427, 1999.

32. Wilson N, Neutze J: Adult congenital heart disease: principles and management guidelines—part I. Aust N Z J Med 23:498, 1993.

33. Findlow D, Doyle E: Congenital heart disease in adults. Br J Anaesth 78:416, 1997.

34. Murphy J, Gersh B, Mair D, et al: Long-term outcome in patients undergoing surgical repair of tetralogy of Fallot. N Engl J Med 329:593, 1993.

35. Gantt L: Growing up heartsick: the experiences of young women with congenital heart disease. Health Care Women Int 13:241, 1992.

36. Swan L, Hillis W, Cameron A: Family planning requirements of adults with congenital heart disease. Heart 78:9, 1997.

37. Mustard W: Successful two-stage correction of transposition of the great vessels. Pediatr Surg 55:469, 1964.

38. Genoni M, Jenni R, Hoerstrup S, et al: Pregnancy after atrial repair for transposition of the great arteries. Heart 81:276, 1999.

39. Rastelli G, Wallace R, Ongley P: Complete repair of transposition of the great vessels with pulmonary stenosis: a review and report of a case corrected by using a new technique. Circulation 39:83, 1969.

40. Nwosu U: Pregnancy following Mustard operation for transposition of great arteries. J Tenn Med Assoc 85:509, 1992.

41. Neukermans K, Sullivan T, Pitlick D: Successful pregnancy after the Mustard operation for transposition of the great arteries. Am J Cardiol 57:838, 1988.

42. Megerian G, Bell E, Huhta J, et al: Pregnancy outcome following Mustard procedure for transposition of the great arteries: a report of five cases and review of the literature. Obstet Gynecol 83:512, 1994.

43. Lynch-Salamond D, Maze S, Combs C: Pregnancy after Mustard repair for transposition of the great arteries. Obstet Gynecol 82:676, 1993.

44. Lao T, Sermer M Colman J: Pregnancy following surgical correction for transposition of the great arteries. Obstet Gynecol 83:665, 1994.

45. Dellinger E, Hadi H: Maternal transposition of the great arteries in pregnancy: a case report. J Reprod Med 39:324, 1994.

46. Clarkson P, Wilson N, Neutze J, et al: Outcome of pregnancy after the Mustard operation for transposition of the great afteris with intact ventricle septum. Am Coll Cardiol 24:190, 1994.

47. Therrien J, Barnes I, Somerville J: Outcome of pregnancy in patients with congenitally corrected transposition of the great arteries. Am J Cardiol 84:820, 1999.

48. Connolly H, Grogan M, Warnes C: Pregnancy among women with congenitally corrected transposition of great arteries. J Am Coll Cardiol 33:1692, 1999.

49. Fontan F, Baudet E: Surgical repair for tricuspid atresia. Thorax 26:240, 1971.

50. Canobbio M, Mair D, Van der Velde M, Koos B: Pregnancy outcomes after the Fontan repair. J Am Coll Cardiol 28:763, 1996.

51. Vongpatanasin W, Brickner E, Hillis L, Lange R: The Eisenmenger syndrome in adults. Ann Intern Med 128:745, 1998.

52. Weiss B, Zemp L, Burkhardt S, Heiss O: Outcome of pulmonary vascular disease in pregnancy: a systematic overview from 1978 through 1996. J Am Coll Cardiol 31:1650, 1998.

53. Gleicher N, Midwall J, Hochberger D, Jaffin H: Eisenmenger's syndrome and pregnancy. Obstet Gynecol Surv 34:721, 1979.

54. Yentis S, Steer P, Plaat F: Eisenmenger's syndrome in pregnancy: maternal and fetal mortality in the 1990's. Br J Obstet Gynaecol 105:921, 1998.

55. Lust K, Boots R, Dooris M, Wilson J: Management of labor in Eisenmenger syndrome with inhaled nitric oxide. Am J Obstet Gynecol 181:419, 1999.

56. Deal K, Wooley C: Coarctation of the aorta and pregnancy. Ann Intern Med 78:706, 1973.

57. Saidi A, Bezold L, Altman C, et al: Outcome of pregnancy following intervention for coarctation of the aorta. Am J Cardiol 82:786, 1988.

58. Hibbard J, Lindheimer M, Lang R: A modified definition for peripartum cardiomyopathy and prognosis based on echocardiography. Obstet Gynecol 94:311, 1999.

59. Lampert M, Lang R: Peripartum cardiomyopathy. Am Heart J 130:860, 1995.

60. Heider A, Kuller J, Strauss R, Wells S: Peripartum cardiomyopathy: a review of the literature. Obstet Gynecol Sur 54:526, 1999.

61. Ostrzega E, Elkayam U: Risk of subsequent pregnancy in women with a history of peripartum cardiomyopathy: results of a survey. Circulation 92(suppl I):1, 1995.

62. The SOLVD Investigators: Effect of enalapril on survival in patients with reduced left ventricular ejection fractions and congestive heart failure. N Engl J Med 325:293, 1991.

63. The CONSENSUS Trial Study Group: Effects of enalapril on mortality in severe congestive heart failure. N Engl J Med 316:1429, 1987.

64. Waagstein F, Caidahl K, Wallentin I, et al: Long-term β-blockade in dilated cardiomyopathy. Circulation 80:551, 1989.

65. MERIT-HF Study Group: Effect of metoprolol CR/XL in chronic heart failure: metoprololCR/XL randomised intervention trial in congestive heart failure (MERIT-HF). Lancet 353:2001, 1999.

66. CIBIS Investigators and Committees: A randomized trial of β-blockade in heart failure. Circulation 90:1765, 1994.

67. Natale A, Davidson T, Geiger M, Newby K: Implantable cardioverter-defibrillators and pregnancy. Circulation 96:2808, 1997.

68. Petitti D, Sidney S, Queesenberry C, Bernstein A: Incidence of stroke and myocardial infarction in women of reproductive age. Stroke 28:280, 1997.

69. Ginz B: Myocardial infarction in pregnancy. J Obstet Gynaecol Br Commonw 77:610, 1970.

70. Roth A, Elkayam U: Acute myocardial infarction associated with pregnancy. Ann Intern Med 125:751, 1996.

71. Fujiwara Y, Yamanaka O, Nakamura T, et al: Acute myocardial infarction induced by ergonovine administration for artificially induced abortion. Jpn Heart J 34:803, 1993.

72. Hopp L, Weisse A, Iffy L: Acute myocardial infarction in a healthy mother using bromocriptine for milk suppression. Can J Cardiol 12:415, 1996.

73. Liao J, Cockrill B, Yurchak P: Acute myocardial infarction after ergonovine administration for uterine bleeding. Am J Cardiol 68:823, 1991.

74. Meyer W, Benton S, Hoon T, et al: Acute myocardial infarction associated with prostaglandin E2. Am J Obstet Gynecol 165:359, 1991.

75. Oei S, Oei S, Brolmann H: Myocardial infarction during nifedipine therapy for preterm labor. N Engl J Med 340:154, 1999.

76. Ottman E, Hall S: Myocardial infarction in the third trimester of pregnancy secondary to an aortic valve thrombus. Obstet Gynecol 81:804, 1993.

77. Ruch A, Duhring J: Postpartum myocardial infarction in a patient receiving bromocriptine. Obstet Gynecol 74:448, 1989.

78. Yaegashi N, Miura M, Okamura K: Acute myocardial infarction associated with postpartum ergot alkaloid administration. Int J Gynecol Obstet 64:67, 1999.

79. Tsung S: Several conditions causing elevation of serum CK-MB and C-BB. Am J Clin Pathol 75:711, 1981.

80. Shivvers S, Wians F, Keffer J, Ramin S: Maternal cardiac troponin I levels during normal labor and delivery. Am J Obstet Gynecol 180:122, 1999.

81. Sebastian C, Scherlag M, Kugelmass A, Schechter E: Primary stent implantation for acute myocardial infarction during pregnancy: use of abciximab, ticlopidine, and aspirin. Cathet Cardiovasc Diagn 45:275, 1998.

82. Giudici M, Artis A, Webel R, Alpert M: Postpartum myocardial infarction treated with percutaneous transluminal coronary angioplasty. Am Heart J 118:614, 1999.

83. Eickman F: Acute coronary artery angioplasty during pregnancy. Cathet Cardiovasc Diagn 38:369, 1996.

84. Ascarelli M, Grider A, Hsu H: Acute myocardial infarction during pregnancy managed with immediate percutaneous transluminal coronary angioplasty. Obstet Gynecol 88:655, 1996.

85. Dufour P, Occelli B, Puech F: Brief communication: pregnancy after myocardial infarction. Int J Obstet Gynecol 59:251, 1997.

86. Kainulainen K, Pulkkinin L, Savolainen A, et al: Location on chromosome 15 of the gene defect causing Marfan syndrome. N Engl J Med 323:935, 1990.

87. Gott V, Greene P, Alejo D, et al: Replacement of the aortic root in patients with Marfan's syndrome. N Engl J Med 340:1307, 1999.

88. Leggert M, Unger T, O'Sullivan C, et al: Aortic root complications in Marfan's syndrome: Indentification of a lower risk group. Heart 75:389, 1996.

89. Shores J, Berger K, Murphy E, Pyeritz R: Progression of aortic dilatation and the benefit of long-term B-adrenergic blockade in Marfan's syndrome. N Engl J Med 330:1335, 1994.

90. Elkayam U, Ostrzega E, Shotan A, Mehra A: Cardiovascular problems in pregnant women with the Marfan syndrome. Ann Intern Med 123:117, 1995.

91. Lipscomb K, Smith J, Clarke B, et al: Outcome of pregnancy in women with Marfan's syndrome. Br J Obstet Gynecol 104:201, 1997.

92. Pyeritz R: Maternal and fetal complications of pregnancy in the Marfan syndrome. Am J Med 71:784, 1981.

93. Rossiter J, Repke J, Morales A, et al: A prospective longitudinal evaluation of pregnancy in the Marfan syndrome. Am J Obstet Gynecol 173:1599, 1995.

94. Rubin L: ACCP consensus statement: primary pulmonary hypertension. Chest 104:236, 1993.

95. D'Alonzo, Barst R, Ayres S, et al: Survival in patients with primary pulmonary hypertension. Ann Intern Med 115:343, 1991.

96. Rich S, Kaufmann E, Levy P: The effect of high doses of calcium-channel blockers on survival in primary pulmonary hypertension. N Engl J Med 327:76, 1992.

97. Rubin L, Mendoza J, Hood M, et al: Treatment of primary pulmonary hypertension with continuous intravenous prostacyclin. Ann Intern Med 112:485, 1990.

98. Metcalfe J, McAnulty J, Ueland K: Pulmonary artery hypertension. In Heart Disease and Pregnancy: Physiology and Management. Boston/Toronto, Little, Brown & Co., 1986, p 265.

99. McCaffrey R, Dunn L: Primary pulmonary hypertension in pregnancy. Obstet Gynecol Surv 19:567, 1964.

100. Martinez J, Comas C, Sala X, et al: Maternal primary pulmonary hypertension associated with pregnancy. Eur J Obstet Gynaecol Reprod Biol 54:143, 1994.

101. Nelson D, Main E, Crafford W, Ahumada G: Peripartum heart failure due to primary pulmonary hypertension. Obstet Gynecol 62:58S, 1983.

102. Easterling T, Ralph D, Schmucker B: Pulmonary hypertension in pregnancy: treatment with pulmonary vasodilators. Obstet Gynecol 93:494, 1999.

103. Shah D, Sunderji S: Hypertrophic cardiomyopathy and pregnancy: report of a maternal mortality and review of the literature. Obstet Gynecol Surv 40:444, 1985.

104. Piacenza J, Kirkorian G, Audra P, Mellier G: Hypertrophic cardiomyopathy and pregnancy. Eur J Obstet Gynaecol Reprod Biol 80:17, 1998.

105. Matthay M, Chatterjee K: Bedside catheterization of the pulmonary artery: risks compared with benefits. Ann Intern Med 109:826, 1988.

106. Robson S, Dunlop W, Moore M, Hunter S: Combined Doppler and echocardiographic measurement of cardiac output: theory and application in pregnancy. Br J Obstet Gynaecol 94:1014, 1987.

107. Lee W, Rokey R, Cotton D: Noninvasive maternal stroke volume and cardiac output determinations by pulsed Doppler echocardiography. Am J Obstet Gynecol 158:505, 1988.

108. Easterling T, Carlson K, Schmucker B, et al: Measurement of cardiac output in pregnancy by Doppler technique. Am J Perinatol 7:220, 1990.

109. Easterling T, Watts D, Schmucker B, Benedetti T: Measurement of cardiac output during pregnancy: validation of Doppler technique and clinical observations in preeclampsia. Obstet Gynecol 69:845, 1987.

110. de Swiet M, Talbert D: The measurement of cardiac output by electrical impedance plethysmography in pregnancy: are the assumptions valid? Br J Obstet Gynaecol 93:721, 1986.

111. Easterling T, Benedetti T, Carlson K, Watts D: Measurement of cardiac output in pregnancy: impedance versus thermodilution techniques. Br J Obstet Gynaecol 96:67, 1989.

112. Masaki D, Greenspoon J, Ouzounian J: Measurement of cardiac output in pregnancy by thoracic electrical bioimpedance and thermodilution. Am J Obstet Gynecol 161:680, 1989.

113. Clark S, Cotton D, Lee W, et al: Central hemodynamic assessment of normal pregnancy. Am J Obstet Gynecol 161:1439, 1989.

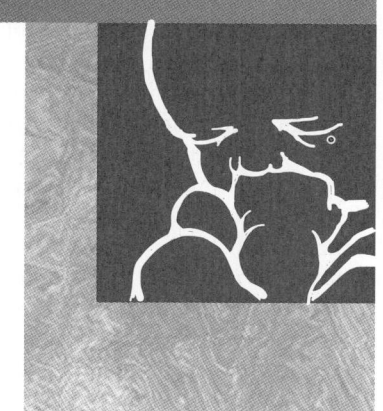

Respiratory Diseases in Pregnancy

JANICE E. WHITTY AND MITCHELL P. DOMBROWSKI

Pulmonary disease frequently complicates pregnancy. The occurrence of pulmonary disease during gestation may result in increased morbidity and/or mortality for both the mother and her fetus. Pregnancy may have an adverse or positive impact on the pulmonary function of the gravida depending on the particular complication that is being encountered. The cardiorespiratory changes that occur in pregnancy are reviewed in Chapter 3, and the obstetrician and his or her consultants would be wise to have a thorough understanding of these changes and the impact that the particular changes may have on the respiratory disease in question. It is extremely important to realize that the majority of diagnostic tests that need to be carried out to evaluate pulmonary function during gestation are not harmful to the fetus and, if indicated, should be performed. In this section, we discuss some of the respiratory complications that may be encountered during gestation, the impact of pregnancy on the disease, as well as the potential impact of the disease on pregnancy.

PNEUMONIA IN PREGNANCY

Pneumonia is a rare complication of pregnancy, complicating pregnancy in 1 per 118 deliveries to 1 per 2,288 deliveries.[1,2] However, pneumonia contributes to considerable maternal mortality and is reportedly the most common nonobstetric infection to cause maternal mortality in the peripartum period.[3] Maternal mortality was as high as 24 percent prior to the introduction of antibiotic therapy.[4] However, research reports have documented a dramatic fall in maternal mortality with modern management and antibiotic therapy, ranging

from 0 to 4 percent mortality.[2,5,6] Preterm delivery is another significant complication of pneumonia complicating pregnancy and, even with antibiotic therapy and modern management, continues to occur in 4 to 43 percent of gravidas who have pneumonia.[2,5,6]

The incidence of pneumonia in pregnancy may be increasing primarily as a reflection of the declining general health status of certain segments of the childbearing population.[6] In addition, the epidemic of human immunodeficiency virus (HIV) infection has increased the number of potential mothers who are at risk for opportunistic lung infections. HIV infection is also associated with an increased risk of invasive pneumococcal disease, with an odds ratio of 41:8, and also an increased risk for legionnaires' disease, with a ratio of 41:8.[7] HIV infection further predisposes the pregnant woman to the infectious complications of the acquired immunodeficiency syndrome (AIDS).[7,8] Women with medical conditions that increase the risk of pulmonary infection, such as cystic fibrosis, are living to childbearing age more frequently than in the past. This disorder also contributes to the increased incidence of pneumonia in pregnancy.

Pneumonia can complicate pregnancy at any time during gestation and may be associated with preterm birth, poor fetal growth, and perinatal loss. In an early report by Hopwood,[9] 17 of the 23 patients developed pneumonia between 25 and 36 weeks' gestation. In that series, seven gravidas delivered during the course of their acute illness, and there were two maternal deaths. Benedetti et al.[5] described 39 cases of pneumonia in pregnancy. Sixteen gravidas presented before 24 weeks' gestation, 15 between 25 and 36 weeks' gestation, and 8 after 36 weeks' gestation. Twenty-seven patients in this series were followed to completion of pregnancy; only two required delivery during the acute phase of pneumonia. Of these 27 patients, 3 suffered a fetal loss and 24 delivered live fetuses, although there was 1 neonatal death due to prematurity.[5] Madinger et al.[2] reported 25 cases of pneumonia occurring among 32,179 deliveries and observed that fetal and obstetric complications were much more common than in earlier studies. Preterm labor occurred in 11 of 21 patients who had complete follow-up data. Pneumonia was present at the time of delivery in 11 patients, particularly in those women who had bacteremia, needed mechanical ventilation, and had a serious underlying maternal disease. In addition to the complication of preterm labor, there were three perinatal deaths in this series. In Berkowitz and La Sala's report of 25 patients with pneumonia complicating pregnancy,[6] full-term delivery occurred in 14 women, 1 delivered preterm, 3 had a voluntary termination of pregnancy, 3 had term deliveries of growth-restricted babies, and 4 were lost to follow-up. Birth weight was significantly lower in the study group in this series (2,770 ± 224 g vs. 3,173 ± 99 g in the control group, $p < 0.01$). In this series, pneumonia complicated 1 in 367 deliveries, and Berkowitz and La Sala attributed the increase in the incidence of pneumonia in this population to a decline in general health status, including anemia, a significant incidence of cocaine use in the study group (52 percent vs. 10 percent in the general population), and HIV positivity in the study group (24 percent vs. 2 percent of the general population).

BACTERIOLOGY

Most series describing pneumonia complicating pregnancy have used incomplete methodologies to diagnose the etiologic pathogens for pneumonia, relying primarily on cultures of blood and sputum. In the majority of cases, no pathogen was identified; however, pneumococcus and *Haemophilus influenzae* remain the most common identifiable causes of pneumonia in pregnancy.[2,5,6] Because comprehensive serologic testing has rarely been done, the true incidence of viral pneumonia, *Legionella,* and *Mycoplasma* pneumonia in pregnancy is difficult to estimate. The data presented by Benedetti et al.,[5] Madinger et al.,[2] and Berkowitz and La Sala[6] all supported pneumococcus as the predominant pathogen causing pneumonia in pregnancy, with *H. influenzae* being the second most common organism. In Berkowitz and La Sala's series, one patient had *Legionella* species.[6] Several unusual pathogens have been reported to cause pneumonia in pregnancy, including mumps, infectious mononucleosis, swine influenza, influenza A, varicella, coccidioidomycosis, and other fungi.[10] Varicella pneumonia will complicate primary varicella infec-

tions in 9 percent of infections in pregnancy, as compared with 0.3 to 1.8 percent in the nonpregnant population.[11] Influenza A has a higher mortality in pregnant than in nonpregnant patients.[12] The increase in virulence of viral infections reported in pregnancy may be secondary to the alterations in maternal immune status that characterize pregnancy, including reduced lymphocyte proliferative response, reduced cell-mediated cytotoxicity by lymphocytes, and a decrease in the number of helper (T_4 T lymphocytes).[12,13] Viral pneumonias can also be complicated by superimposed bacterial infection, particularly with pneumococcus.

Chemical pneumonitis results after the aspiration of gastric contents. Chemical pneumonitis can be superinfected with pathogens present in the oropharynx and gastric juices, primarily anaerobes and gram-negative bacteria.[10]

BACTERIAL PNEUMONIA

Streptococcus pneumoniae (pneumococcus) is the most common bacterial pathogen to cause pneumonia in pregnancy, with *H. influenzae* being the next most common. These pneumonias typically present as an acute illness accompanied by fever, chills, purulent productive cough, and a lobar pattern on the chest radiograph. Streptococcal pneumonia produces a "rusty" sputum, with gram-positive diplococci on Gram stain and asymmetric consolidation with air bronchograms on chest radiograph.[13] *H. influenzae* is a gram-negative coccobacillus that produces consolidation with air bronchograms, often in the upper lobes.[13] Less frequent bacterial pathogens include *Klebsiella pneumoniae* which is a gram-negative rod that causes extensive tissue destruction, with air bronchograms, pleural effusion, and cavitation noted on chest radiograph. Patients with *Staphylococcus aureus* pneumonia present with pleuritis, chest pain, purulent sputum, and consolidation without air bronchograms noted on chest radiograph.[13]

Atypical pneumonia pathogens, such as *Mycoplasma pneumoniae, Legionella pneumophila,* and *Chlamydia pneumoniae* (TWAR agent) present with gradual onset, a lower fever, appear less ill, have a mucoid sputum, and a patchy or interstitial infiltrate on chest radiograph. The severity of the findings on chest radiograph are usually out of proportion to the mild clinical symptoms. *Mycoplasma pneumoniae* is the most common organism responsible for atypical pneumonia and is best detected by the presence of cold agglutinins in 70 percent of cases.

The normal physiologic changes in the respiratory system associated with pregnancy result in a loss of ventilatory reserve. This, coupled with the immunosuppression that accompanies pregnancy put the mother and fetus at great risk from respiratory infection. Therefore, any gravida suspected of having pneumonia should be managed aggressively. She should be admitted to the hospital and an investigation undertaken to determine the pathologic etiology. Work-up should include physical examination, arterial blood gases, chest radiograph, sputum Gram stain and culture, as well as blood cultures. Empiric antibiotic coverage should be started, usually with a third-generation cephalosporin such as ceftriaxone or cefotaxime. *Legionella* pneumonia has a high mortality and sometimes presents with consolidation, mimicking pneumococcal pneumonia. Therefore, it is recommended that a macrolide, such as azithromycin, be added to the empiric therapy. Once the results of the sputum culture, blood cultures, Gram stain, and serum studies are obtained and a pathogen has been identified, antibiotic therapy can be directed towards the identifiable pathogen. The third-generation cephalosporins are effective agents for the majority of pathogens causing a community-acquired pneumonia. They are also effective against penicillin-resistant *Streptococcus pneumoniae*. In addition to antibiotic therapy, oxygen supplementation should be given. Frequent arterial blood gas measurements should be obtained to maintain the PO_2 at 70 mm Hg, a level necessary to ensure adequate fetal oxygenation. Arterial saturation can be monitored with pulse oximetry as well. When the gravida is afebrile for 48 hours and has signs of clinical improvement, an oral cephalosporin can be started and intravenous therapy discontinued. A total of 10 to 14 days of treatment should be completed.

Pneumonia in pregnancy can be complicated by respiratory failure requiring mechanical ventilation. Should this occur, team management should include the obstetrician, maternal–fetal medicine specialist, and intensivist. In addition to meticulous management of the gravida's respiratory status, the patient should be maintained in the left lateral recumbent position to improve uteroplacental perfusion. The viable fetus should be monitored with continuous fetal monitoring. If positive end-expiratory pressure (PEEP) greater than 10 cm H_2O is required to maintain oxygenation, central monitoring with a pulmonary artery catheter should be instituted to adequately monitor volume status and maintain maternal and uteroplacental perfusion. There is no evidence that elective delivery results in an overall improvement in respiratory function.[14] Therefore, elective delivery is probably not indicated. However, if there is clear evidence of fetal compromise or profound maternal compromise and impending demise, delivery should be accomplished.

VIRAL PNEUMONIAS

Influenza Virus

There are an estimated 4 million cases of pneumonia and influenza annually in the United States, and this is the sixth leading cause of death in this country.[15] While three types of influenza virus can cause human disease, types A, B, and C, most epidemic infections are due to influenza A.[10] Influenza A typically has an acute onset after a 1- to 4-day incubation period and first manifests as high fever, coryza, headache, malaise, and cough. In uncomplicated cases, the chest examination and chest radiograph remain clear.[10] If symptoms persist longer than 5 days, especially in a pregnancy, complications should be suspected. Pneumonia may complicate influenza as the result of either secondary bacterial infection or viral infection of the lung parenchyma.[10] In the epidemic of 1957, autopsies demonstrated that pregnant women died from fulminant viral pneumonia most commonly, while nonpregnant patients died most often from secondary bacterial infection.[16] Primary influenza pneumonia is characterized by rapid progression from a unilateral infiltrate to diffuse bilateral disease. The gravida may develop fulminant respiratory failure requiring mechanical ventilation and PEEP. When pneumonia complicates influenza in pregnancy, antibiotics should be started, directed at the likely pathogens that can cause secondary infection, including *Staphylococcus aureus*, pneumococcus, *H. influenza*, and certain enteric gram-negative bacteria. Antiviral agents, such as amantadine and ribavirin, can be considered.[17] It has been recommended that the influenza vaccine be given routinely to gravidas in the second and third trimesters of pregnancy in order to prevent the occurrence of influenza and the development of pneumonia secondary to that infection.

Varicella

Varicella zoster is a DNA virus that usually causes a benign self-limited illness in children but may infect up to 2 percent of all adults.[18] Varicella infection occurs in 0.7 of every 1,000 pregnancies.[19] Pregnancy may increase the likelihood of varicella pneumonia complicating the primary infection.[11] Varicella pneumonia occurs most often in the third trimester, and the infection is likely to be severe.[11,19,20] The maternal mortality from varicella pneumonia may be as high as 35 to 40 percent as compared to 11 to 17 percent in nonpregnant individuals.[11,20] While one recent review reported a decreased mortality with only 3 deaths in 28 women with varicella pneumonia,[19] another recent study documented a maternal mortality of 35 percent.[11]

Varicella pneumonia usually presents 2 to 5 days

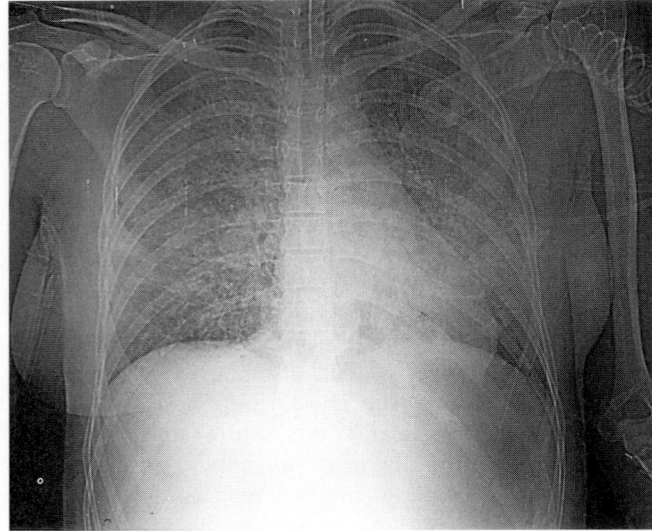

Figure 30–1. This chest x-ray demonstrates bilateral nodular and interstitial pneumonia characteristic of varicella. The patient, a 27-year-old gravida 6, para 2, abortus 3 woman, was exposed to varicella infection in her two children. Characteristic skin vesicles of varicella occurred several days before the development of pulmonary symptoms. She required endotracheal intubation and mechanical ventilation for 6 days. She was also treated with intravenous acyclovir and ceftazidime for possible superimposed infection. The patient recovered fully and delivered a healthy infant at term.

after the onset of fever, rash, and malaise and is heralded by the onset of pulmonary symptoms including cough, dyspnea, pruritic chest pain, and hemoptysis.[11] The severity of the illness may vary from asymptomatic radiographic abnormalities to fulminant pneumonitis and respiratory failure[11,21] (Fig. 30–1). All gravidas with varicella pneumonia should be aggressively treated with antiviral therapy and admitted to the intensive care unit for close observation or intubation if indicated. Acyclovir, a DNA polymerase inhibitor, should be started. The early use of acyclovir was associated with an improved hospital course after the fifth day and a lower mean temperature, lower respiratory rate, and improved oxygenation.[11] Treatment with acyclovir is safe in pregnancy. Among 312 pregnancies, there was no increase in the number of birth defects and no consistent pattern of congenital abnormalities.[22] A dose of 7.5 mg/kg intravenously every 8 hours has been recommended.[23]

TUBERCULOSIS IN PREGNANCY

The incidence of tuberculosis in the United States began to decline in the early part of the 20th century and fell steadily until 1953, when the introduction of isoniazid led to a dramatic decrease in the number of cases, from 84,000 cases in 1953 to 22,255 cases in 1984.[24] However, since 1984, there have been significant changes in tuberculosis morbidity trends. From 1985 through 1991, reported cases of tuberculosis increased by 18 percent, representing approximately 39,000 more cases than expected had the previous downward trend continued. This increase is due to many factors, including HIV epidemic, deterioration in the health care infrastructure, and more cases among immigrants.[24] The emergence of drug-resistant tuberculosis has also become a serious concern. In New York City, in 1991, 33 percent of tuberculosis cases were resistant to at least one drug, and 19 percent were resistant to both isoniazid (INH) and rifampin (RIF).[25] Between 1985 and 1992, the number of tuberculosis cases in women of childbearing age increased by 40 percent.[26] One report noted tuberculosis-complicated pregnancies in 94.8 cases per 100,000 deliveries between 1991 and 1992.[27]

Diagnosis

The majority of gravidas diagnosed with tuberculosis in pregnancy will be asymptomatic. All gravidas at high risk for tuberculosis (see the box "High-Risk Factors for Tuberculosis") should be screened with subcutaneous administration of intermediate-strength purified protein derivative (PPD). If anergy is suspected, control antigens such as candida, mumps, or tetanus toxoids should also be placed.[28] The sensitivity of the PPD is 90 to 99 percent for exposure to tuberculosis. The tine test should not be used for screening because of its low sensitivity.

The onset of the recent tuberculosis epidemic stimu-

High-Risk Factors for Tuberculosis

HIV infection

Close contact with persons known or suspected to have tuberculosis

Medical risk factors known to increase risk of disease if infected

Birth in a country with high tuberculosis prevalence

Medically underserved status

Low income

Alcohol addiction

Intravenous drug use

Residency in a long-term care facility (e.g., correctional institutions, mental institutions, nursing homes and facilities)

Health professionals working in high-risk health care facilities

lated the need for rapid diagnostic tests using molecular biology methods to detect *M. tuberculosis* in clinical specimens. Two direct amplification tests (DATs) have been approved by the Food and Drug Administration (FDA), the *Mycobacterium tuberculosis* Direct test (MTD) (Gen-Probe, San Diego, CA), and the Amplicor *Mycobacterium tuberculosis* (Amplicor MTB) test (Roche Diagnostic Systems, Inc., Branchburg, NJ). Both tests amplify and detect *M. tuberculosis* 16S ribosomal DNA.[29] When testing acid-fast stain smear-positive respiratory specimens, each test has a sensitivity of greater than 95 percent and a specificity of essentially 100 percent for detecting the *M. tuberculosis* complex.[30,31] When testing acid-fast stain smear-negative respiratory specimens, the specificity remains greater than 95 percent, but the sensitivity ranges from 40 to 77 percent.[30,31] To date, these tests are FDA-approved only for testing acid-fast stain smear-positive respiratory specimens obtained from untreated patients or those who have received no more than 7 days of antituberculosis therapy. The PPD remains the most commonly used screening test for tuberculosis.

Immigrants from areas where tuberculosis is endemic may have received the bacille Calmette-Guérin (BCG) vaccine. Such individuals will likely have a positive response to the PPD. However, this reactivity should wane over time. Therefore, the PPD should be utilized to screen these patients for tuberculosis unless their skin tests are known to be positive.[32] If the BCG vaccine was given 10 years earlier and the PPD is positive with a skin test reaction of 10 mm or more, that individual should be considered infected with tuberculosis and managed accordingly.[32]

Women with a positive PPD skin test must be evaluated for active tuberculosis with a thorough physical examination for extrapulmonary disease and a chest radiograph once they are beyond the first trimester.[13] Symptoms of active tuberculosis include cough (74 percent), weight loss (41 percent), fever (30 percent), malaise and fatigue (30 percent), and hemoptysis (19 percent).[33] Individuals with active pulmonary tuberculosis may have radiographic findings including adenopathy, multinodular infiltrates, cavitation, loss of volume in the upper lobes, and upper medial retraction of hilar markings. The finding of acid-fast bacilli in early morning sputum specimens confirms the diagnosis of pulmonary tuberculosis. At least three first-morning sputum samples should be examined for the presence of acid-fast bacilli. If sputum cannot be produced, sputum-induction, gastric washings, or diagnostic bronchoscopy may be indicated.

Extrapulmonary tuberculosis occurs in up to 16 percent of cases in the United States; however, in patients with AIDS the pattern may occur in 60 to 70 percent of all patients.[34] Extrapulmonary sites include lymph nodes, bone, kidneys, and breasts. Extrapulmonary tu-

berculosis appears to be rare in pregnancy.[35] Extrapulmonary tuberculosis that is confined to the lymph nodes has no effect on obstetric outcomes, but tuberculosis at other extrapulmonary sites does adversely affect the outcome of pregnancy.[36] Rarely, mycobacteria invade the uteroplacental circulation, and congenital tuberculosis results.[9,26,37] The diagnosis of congenital tuberculosis is based on one of the following factors: (1) demonstration of primary hepatic complex or cavitating hepatic granuloma by percutaneous liver biopsy at birth; (2) infection of the maternal genital tract or placenta; (3) lesions noted in the first week of life; and (4) exclusion of the possibility of postnatal transmission by a thorough investigation of all contacts, including attendants.[26]

Prevention

The majority of gravidas with a positive PPD in pregnancy will be asymptomatic with no evidence of active disease and therefore classified as infected without active disease. The risk of progression to active disease is highest in the first 2 years of conversion. It is important to prevent the onset of active disease while minimizing maternal and fetal risk. An algorithm for management of the positive PPD is presented in Figure 30–2.[38] In women with a known recent conversion (2 years) to a positive PPD and no evidence of active disease, the recommended prophylaxis is isoniazid, 300 mg/day, starting after the first trimester and continuing for 6 to 9 months.[13] Isoniazid should be accompanied by pyridoxine (vitamin B_6) supplementation, 50 mg/day, in order to prevent the peripheral neuropathy that is associated with isoniazid treatment. Women with an unknown or prolonged duration of PPD positivity (> 2 years) should receive isoniazid, 300 mg/day for 6 to 9 months after delivery. Isoniazid prophylaxis is not recommended for women older than 35 years of age who have an unknown or prolonged PPD positivity in the absence of active disease. The use of isoniazid is discouraged in this group because of an increased risk of hepatotoxicity. Isoniazid is associated with hepatitis in both pregnant and nonpregnant adults. However, monthly monitoring of liver function tests may prevent this adverse outcome. Among individuals receiving isoniazid, 10 to 20 percent will develop mildly elevated liver function tests. These changes resolve once the drug is discontinued.[39]

Treatment

The gravida with active tuberculosis should be treated initially with isoniazid, 300 mg/day, combined with rifampin, 600 mg/day (Table 30–1).[40] Resistant disease results from initial infection with resistant strains (33 percent) or can develop during therapy.[41] If resistance

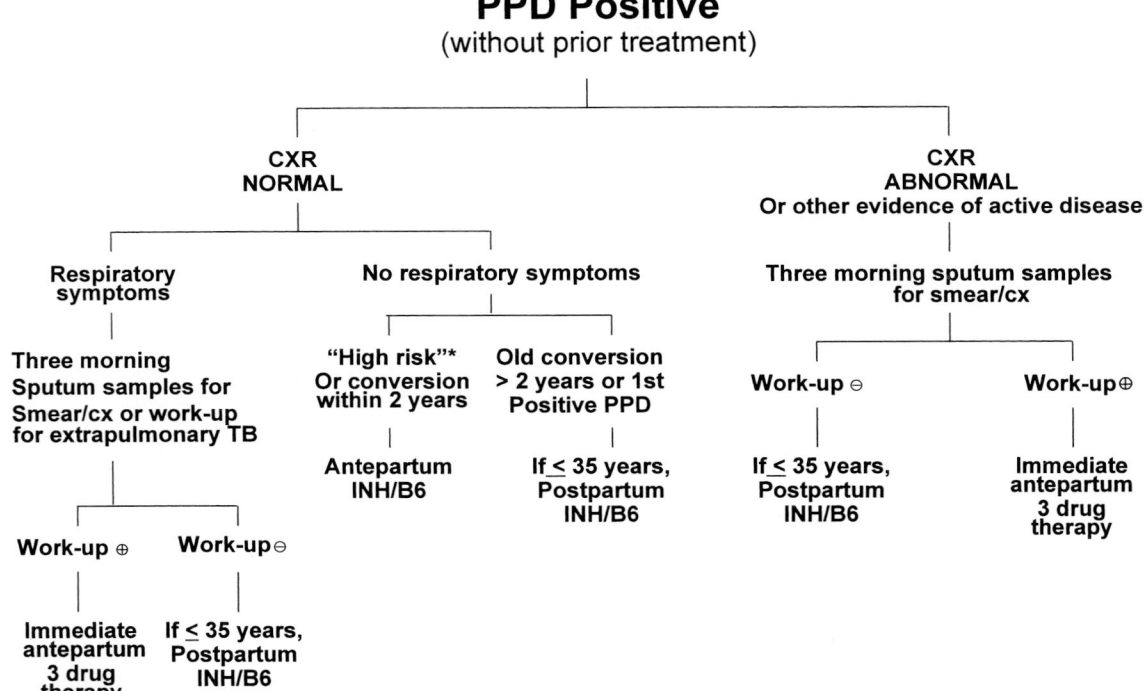

Figure 30–2. Algorithm for the management of positive PPD.

to isoniazid is identified or anticipated, ethambutol 2.5 g/day should be added and the treatment period should be extended to 18 months.[40] Ethambutol is teratogenic in animals; however, this has not been noted in humans. The most common side effect of ethambutol therapy is optic neuritis. Streptomycin should be avoided during pregnancy because it is associated with eighth nerve damage in neonates.[42] Antituberculous agents not recommended for use in pregnancy include ethionamide, streptomycin, capreomycin, kanamycin, cycloserine, and pyrazinamide.[13]

Women who are being treated with antituberculous drugs may breast-feed. Only 0.75 to 2.3 percent of INH and 0.05 percent of rifampin are excreted into breast milk. Ethambutol excretion into breast milk is also minimal. However, if the infant is concurrently taking oral antituberculous therapy, excessive drug levels may be reached in the neonate, and breast-feeding should be avoided. Breast-fed infants of women taking isoniazid therapy should receive a multivitamin supplement, including pyridoxine.[13] Neonates of women taking antituberculous therapy should have a PPD skin test at birth and again at 3 months of age. Infants born to women with active tuberculosis at the time of delivery should receive isoniazid prophylaxis (10 mg/kg/day) until maternal disease has been inactive for 3 months as evidenced by negative maternal sputum cultures.[13] Active tuberculosis in the neonate should be treated appropriately with isoniazid and rifampin immediately

upon diagnosis or with multiagent therapy should drug-resistant organisms be identified. Infants and children who are at high risk of intimate and prolonged exposure to untreated or ineffectively treated persons should receive the BCG vaccine.[43]

Summary

In summary, high-risk gravidas should be screened for tuberculosis and treated appropriately with INH prophylaxis for infection without overt disease and with dual antituberculous therapy for active disease. In addition, the newborn should be screened for evidence of tuberculosis as well. Proper screening and therapy will lead to a good outcome for mother and fetus in the majority of cases.

ASTHMA IN PREGNANCY

Asthma, which may be the most common potentially serious respiratory complication of pregnancy, is characterized by chronic airway inflammation with increased airway responsiveness to a variety of stimuli, and airway obstruction that is partially or completely reversible.[44] Approximately 4 percent of women of child-bearing age have a history of asthma, but up to

Table 30–1. ANTITUBERCULOSIS DRUGS

Drug	Dosage Forms	Daily Dose	Weekly Dose	Major Adverse Reactions
First-line drugs (for initial treatment):				
Isoniazid	PO, IM	10 mg/kg up to 300 mg	15 mg/kg up to 900 mg	Hepatic enzyme elevation, peripheral neuropathy hepatitis, hypersensitivity
Rifampin	PO	10 mg/kg up to 600 mg	10 mg/kg up to 600 mg	Orange discoloration of secretions and urine, nausea, vomiting, hepatitis, febrile reaction, purpura (rare)
Pyrazinamide	PO	15–30 mg/kg up to 2 g	50–70 mg/kg	Hepatotoxicity, hyperuricemia, arthralgias, skin rash, gastrointestinal upset
Ethambutol	PO	15 mg/kg up to 2.5 g	50 mg/kg	Optic neuritis (decreased red-green color discrimination, decreased visual acuity), skin rash
Streptomycin	IM	15 mg/kg up to 1 g	25–30 mg/kg up to 1 g	Ototoxicity, nephrotoxicity
Second-line drugs (daily therapy):				
Capreomycin	IM	15–30 mg/kg up to 1 g		Auditory, vestibular, and renal toxicity
Kanamycin	IM	15–30 mg/kg up to 1 g		Auditory and renal toxicity, rare vestibular toxicity
Ethionamide	PO	15–20 mg/kg up to 1 g		Gastrointestinal disturbance, hepatotoxicity, hypersensitivity
Para-aminosalycylic acid	PO	150 mg/kg up to 1 g		Gastrointestinal disturbance, hypersensitivity, hepatotoxicity, sodium load
Cycloserine	PO	15–20 mg/kg up to 1 g		Psychosis, convulsions, rash

10 percent of the population appears to have nonspecific airway hyperresponsiveness.[45] In general, the prevalence, morbidity, and mortality from asthma are increasing.

Insight into the pathogenesis of asthma has changed with the recognition that airway inflammation is present in nearly all cases. The effects of pregnancy on asthma are controversial. Several studies noted that over 40 percent of patients required hospitalization during pregnancy for asthma exacerbations.[46,47] In contrast, in a managed care setting with a higher socioeconomic population, Schatz et al. reported an emergency room visit rate of 12.6 percent but a hospitalization rate of only 1.1 percent for asthma exacerbations during pregnancy.[48]

Gravidas with asthma have an increased frequency of chronic hypertension[49] and maternal smoking, which may also complicate the effects of other influences.[49,50] Ethnicity may be a particularly important confounding factor in assessing the relationship between asthma and pregnancy outcomes, since African Americans (ages 15 to 44) are five times more likely to die from asthma and are twice as likely to be hospitalized from asthma compared to Caucasians.[51] A summary of possible maternal, fetal, and neonatal complications related to asthma and asthma therapy is presented in the box "Reported Effects of Asthma and Asthma Treatment Regimens."

Studies have shown that patients with more severe asthma may have the greatest risk for complications during pregnancy.[47,52] Quantitating this risk is problematic because most studies have not categorized the severity of asthma. In 1993, the National Asthma Education Program (NAEP) working group defined mild, moderate, and severe asthma according to symptomatic exacerbations (wheezing, cough, and/or dyspnea) and objective tests of pulmonary function. The most commonly used parameters are the peak expiratory flow rate (PEFR) and the forced expiratory volume in 1 second (FEV_1). The NAEP guidelines did not consider the need for regular medication to be a factor for classifying asthma severity during pregnancy. In a recent prospective observational study of 1,800 pregnant women with asthma and 900 control subjects, patients with mild asthma but who required regular medications (β-agonist, theophylline, or inhaled corticosteroids) were similar to subjects with moderate asthma in respect to asthma exacerbations.[53] It seems prudent to

Reported Effects of Asthma and Asthma Treatment Regimens

Increased maternal
  Preeclampsia
  Cesarean delivery
  Asthma exacerbations
  Preterm rupture of membranes
Increased perinatal
  Mortality
  Prematurity
  Low birth weight
  Hypoxia/asphyxia
  Hypoadrenalism
  Theophylline toxicity

consider pregnant patients requiring regular systemic corticosteroids to control asthma symptoms to have severe asthma (see the box "Modified NAEP Asthma Severity Classification").

Asthma Management

The ultimate goal of asthma therapy is maintaining adequate oxygenation of the fetus by preventing hypoxic episodes in the mother. The effective management of asthma during pregnancy relies on four integral components outlined below.

Objective Measures for Assessment and Monitoring

Subjective measures of lung function by the patient and physician provide an insensitive and inaccurate assessment of airway hyperresponsiveness, airway inflammation, and asthma severity. The FEV_1 following a maximal inspiration is the single best measure of pulmonary function. However, measurement of FEV_1 requires a spirometer. The PEFR correlates well with the FEV_1, and has the advantages that it can be measured reliably with inexpensive, disposable, portable peak flowmeters. Patient self-monitoring of PEFR provides valuable insight to the course of asthma throughout the day, assesses circadian variation in pulmonary function, and helps detect early signs of deterioration so that timely therapy can be instituted.

Avoid or Control Asthma Triggers

Limiting adverse environmental exposures during pregnancy is important for controlling asthma. Irritants and allergens that provoke acute symptoms also increase airway inflammation and hyperresponsiveness. Avoiding or controlling such triggers can reduce asthma symptoms, airway hyperresponsiveness, and the need for medical therapy. Association of asthma with allergies is common; 75 to 85 percent of patients with asthma have positive skin tests to common allergens including animal dander, house dust mites, cockroach antigens, pollens, and molds. Other common nonimmunologic triggers include tobacco smoke, strong odors, air pollutants, food additives such as sulfites, and certain drugs including aspirin and β-blockers. Another trigger can be strenuous physical activity. For some patients, exercise-induced asthma can be avoided with inhalation of a β_2-agonist 5 to 60 minutes before exercise. Specific measures for avoiding asthma triggers are listed in the box "Limiting Exposure to Asthma Triggers."

Patient Education

Patients should be made aware that controlling asthma during pregnancy is especially important for the well-being of the fetus. The patient should have a basic understanding of strategies to reduce asthma triggers and medical management during pregnancy, including self-monitoring of PEFRs and the correct use of inhalers.

Pharmacologic Therapy

The goal of asthma therapy is multiphasic: (1) relieve bronchospasm, (2) protect the airways from irritant

Modified NAEP Asthma Severity Classification

Mild asthma
  Brief (<1 hour) symptomatic exacerbations less than twice a week
  PEFR ≥80% of personal best
  FEV_1 ≥80% of predicted when asymptomatic
Moderate asthma
  Symptomatic exacerbations more than twice a week
  Exacerbations affect activity levels
  Exacerbations may last for days
  PEFR, FEV_1 range from 60 to 80% of predicted
  Regular medications necessary to control symptoms
Severe asthma
  Continuous symptoms/frequent exacerbations limit activity levels
  PEFR, FEV_1 <60% of expected, and are highly variable
  Regular oral corticosteroids necessary to control symptoms

Limiting Exposure to Asthma Triggers

Use plastic mattress and pillow covers

Weekly washing of bedding in hot water

Animal dander control
   Weekly bathing of the pet
   Keeping pets out of the bedroom
   Remove the pet from the home

Cockroach control

Avoid tobacco smoke

Inhibit mite and mold growth by reducing humidity

Do not be present when home is vacuumed

stimuli, (3) prevent the pulmonary and inflammatory response to an allergen exposure, and (4) resolve the inflammatory process in the airways leading to improved pulmonary function with reduced airway hyperresponsiveness. The therapeutic approach includes increasing the number and frequency of medications with increasing asthma severity.

Asthma Pharmacotherapy

Current medical treatment for asthma emphasizes reduction of airway inflammation to decrease airway hyperresponsiveness and prevent asthma symptoms. Although it is assumed that asthma medications are as effective in pregnant as in nonpregnant patients, differences in maternal physiology and pharmacokinetics may affect the absorption, distribution, metabolism and clearance of medications during pregnancy. Endocrinologic and immunologic changes during pregnancy include elevations in free plasma cortisol, possible tissue refractoriness to cortisol,[54] and changes in cellular immunity.[55] Although animal studies have indicated association of corticosteroids with an increased risk of cleft palate and decreased fetal survival, human studies have failed to suggest any increase in facial clefts or other birth defects.[56] However, the use of oral corticosteroids has been associated with low birth weight.[57,58] Potential adverse effects of oral or high-dose inhaled corticosteroids include adrenal suppression, weight gain, impaired fetal growth, hypertension, diabetes, cataracts, and osteoporosis.

In the United States, three classes of inhaled anti-inflammatory asthma medications are available at the present time: inhaled corticosteroids, nedocromil sodium, and cromolyn sodium. In separate controlled studies of nongravid subjects, use of inhaled corticosteroids or cromolyn sodium led to improvement in (1) asthma symptoms,[59-61] (2) pulmonary function,[59] (3) nonspecific bronchial hyperactivity,[62] (4) emergency room relapses,[61] and (5) hospitalizations[59] (see the box "Typical Dosages of Common Asthma Medications").

Inhaled Corticosteroids

Airway inflammation is present in nearly all cases; therefore, inhaled corticosteroids have even been advocated as first-line therapy for patients with mild asthma.[63] The use of inhaled corticosteroids among nonpregnant asthmatics has been associated with a marked reduction in fatal and near-fatal asthma.[64] In addition to their anti-inflammatory effect, corticosteroids increase the effectiveness of β-adrenergic drugs by inducing formation of new β_2-receptors.

Inhaled corticosteroids produce clinically important improvements in bronchial hyperresponsiveness that appear dose related,[65] can occur as early as a few weeks but take months to attain maximal effect,[66] and include prevention of increased bronchial hyperresponsiveness after seasonal exposure to an allergen.[67,68] Continued administration is also effective in reducing the immediate pulmonary response to an allergen challenge. Inhaled corticosteroids are also more effective than β-agonists, theophylline, nedocromil sodium, and cromolyn sodium in reducing airway hyperresponsiveness during maintenance treatment.[60,63,69,70] In a prospective observational study of 504 pregnant subjects with asthma, 177 patients were not initially treated with either inhaled budesonide or inhaled beclomethasone.[71] This cohort had a 17 percent acute exacerbation rate compared to only a 4 percent rate among those treated with inhaled corticosteroids from the start of pregnancy.

Several studies have found that inhaled corticoste-

Typical Dosages of Common Asthma Medications

Cromolyn sodium	2 inhalations qid
Beclomethasone	2–5 inhalations bid–qid
Triamcinolone	2 inhalations tid–qid or 4 inhalations bid
Budesonide	2–4 inhalations bid
Fluticasone	88–220 μg bid
Flunisolide	2–4 inhalations bid
Theophylline	Maintain serum levels of 8–12 μg/ml; decrease dosage by half if treated with erythromycin or cimetidine
Prednisone	1 week 40 mg/day burst for active symptoms followed by 1 week taper
Albuterol	2 inhalations q 3–4 hours

roids can cause adrenal suppression and changes in bone metabolism in nonpregnant patients.[72-77] Their potential effects on fetal adrenal function and fetal bone development are unknown. There is concern that inhaled corticosteroids impair growth in children as measured by height or lower leg growth using a kneno-meter.[78-80] Inhaled corticosteroids can cause thrush and hoarseness, problems that may be mitigated by the use of metered-dose inhalers with spacers. Only about 10 to 20 percent of the inhaled dose of corticosteroid reaches the lungs, while approximately 50 percent is deposited in the oropharynx.[81] The use of spacers can increase delivery to the lungs, and mouth rinsing after inhalation will decrease oral absorption.

In 1993, the NAEP working group recommended inhaled beclomethasone during pregnancy because most clinical studies had been conducted with beclomethasone.[45] Since then, limited data during pregnancy and data from nonpregnant subjects suggest that the other inhaled corticosteroids may have therapeutic advantages compared to beclomethasone. Therefore, it seems reasonable to recommend beclomethasone as the preferred agent when commencing inhaled corticosteroids during pregnancy, but to continue either triamcinolone acetonide, budesonide, fluticasone propionate, or flunisolide during pregnancy in a patient who is well controlled by that inhaled corticosteroid prior to pregnancy. All of the above inhaled corticosteroids are currently labeled FDA pregnancy class C.

BECLOMETHASONE DIPROPIONATE. Inhaled beclomethasone has not been associated with increased rates of fetal malformations.[82-84] A case analysis of 12,301 nonpregnant asthmatics[64] reported that use of beclomethasone for at least 1 year resulted in a significantly lower risk of fatal and near-fatal asthma compared to therapies not including inhaled corticosteroids. Inhaled beclomethasone has been associated with a reduced readmission rate for asthma exacerbations in a randomized study of 84 pregnant patients.[84] Beclomethasone is identical to betamethasone except for a chlorine at the 9-α position instead of fluorine. This is significant, since betamethasone is known to effectively cross to the fetus.

TRIAMCINOLONE ACETONIDE. Data on inhaled triamcinolone use during pregnancy are limited to a single retrospective analysis of 15 women treated with inhaled triamcinolone, 14 treated with inhaled beclomethasone, and 25 receiving oral theophylline therapy.[85] There was a significantly lower incidence of hospital admissions for asthma exacerbations among gravidas receiving inhaled triamcinolone (33 percent) compared with those treated with an inhaled beclomethasone group (79 percent; $p < 0.05$) but not compared to the theophylline group. The finding of a lower hospitalization rate among the group treated with inhaled triamcinolone

may be due to confounding factors in this small retrospective study. Triamcinolone has been shown to have minimal systemic absorption following oral administration via metered dose inhalers with spacers.[86]

BUDESONIDE. To study possible teratogenic risks, the Swedish Medical Birth Registry was utilized in 2,014 infants whose mothers had used inhaled budesonide in early pregnancy. A 3.8 percent (95 percent confidence interval [CI] 2.9 to 4.6) frequency of congenital malformations was observed, which was similar to the general population rate of 3.5 percent.[87] Budesonide and theophylline may have synergistic effects. In a double-blind, placebo-controlled trial of nongravid subjects with moderate asthma, high-dose budesonide (800 μg) was compared to low-dose budesonide (400 μg) with theophylline at serum concentrations below the recommended therapeutic range (8.7 μg/ml).[88] Compared to high-dose budesonide, the low-dose budesonide with theophylline regimen resulted in a significantly improved FEV_1. Serum cortisol concentrations were significantly reduced in the group treated with high-dose budesonide, but not the low-dose theophylline group.

FLUTICASONE PROPIONATE AND FLUNISOLIDE. Both fluticasone propionate and flunisolide are potent anti-inflammatory corticosteroids. There are no published studies of their use during human pregnancy. However, in contrast to the association of growth decelerations in adolescent children treated with inhaled beclomethasone,[78] inhaled fluticasone propionate therapy was not found to be associated with a decrease in growth velocity.[89] In a randomized double-blind study of nonpregnant adults and adolescents, inhaled fluticasone propionate was found to be significantly more effective than theophylline in the treatment of mild to moderate asthma.[90]

CROMOLYN SODIUM AND NEDOCROMIL SODIUM. Given the potential for systemic effects of inhaled corticosteroids, even at low doses, it is important to identify nonsteroidal anti-inflammatory medications. At the present time, cromolyn sodium and nedocromil sodium are the only approved medications that fit into this category. Nedocromil sodium, a pyranoquinalone, exerts a number of anti-inflammatory effects in vivo and in vitro.[91] Cromolyn sodium, which is virtually devoid of significant side effects, blocks both the early- and late-phase pulmonary response to allergen challenge as well as preventing the development of airway hyperresponsiveness.[62] Cromolyn sodium does not have any intrinsic bronchodilator or antihistaminic activity. Compared to inhaled corticosteroids, the time to maximal clinical benefit is longer for cromolyn sodium, 4 weeks versus 2 weeks. Nedocromil sodium and cromolyn sodium appear to be less effective than inhaled corticosteroids in reducing objective and subjective manifestations of asthma.

Bronchodilators

In some respects, these medications are now viewed as supplementary to nonbronchodilator antiasthma medications. An increased frequency of bronchodilator use could indicate the need for additional anti-inflammatory therapy.

THEOPHYLLINE. Theophylline has anti-inflammatory actions[92] that may be mediated by the inhibition of leukotriene production and its capacity to stimulate prostaglandin E (PGE_2) production.[93] Theophylline has been used for over 50 years, and no increased risk of developmental problems in exposed offspring has been identified. The NAEP Working Group on Asthma and Pregnancy recommended that theophylline be considered a second-line drug to be used to supplement inhaled corticosteroids when control is not achieved. High doses have been observed to cause jitteriness, tachycardia, and vomiting in both mothers and neonates.[94,95] New dosing guidelines have recommended that serum concentrations be maintained at 8 to 12 μg/ml during pregnancy.[45] Subjective symptoms of adverse theophylline effects including insomnia, heartburn, palpitations, and nausea may be difficult to differentiate from typical pregnancy symptoms. Theophylline can have significant interactions with other drugs, causing decreased clearance and resultant toxicity. Two commonly used drugs, cimetidine and erythromycin, can cause a 70 percent and a 35 percent increase, respectively, in theophylline serum levels.[96]

The main advantage of theophylline is its long duration of action, 10 to 12 hours with the use of sustained-release preparations. These are especially useful in the management of nocturnal asthma.[97] Theophylline should be added when β-agonists and inhaled anti-inflammatory agents do not adequately control symptoms. Theophylline is only indicated for chronic therapy and is not effective for the treatment of acute exacerbations during pregnancy.[84]

INHALED β-AGONISTS. β-Agonists are currently recommended for use with all degrees of asthma during pregnancy.[48,51] This group of medications has evolved from those that are relatively short acting (epinephrine, isoproterenol) to those with a longer duration of action (albuterol, terbutaline, pirbuterol), of 4 to 6 hours.[97] Their greatest advantage is a rapid onset of effect in the relief of acute bronchospasm via smooth muscle relaxation. They are also excellent bronchoprotective agents for pretreatment prior to exercise. Prior to allergen exposure, they effectively block the pulmonary response, but are of insufficient duration of action to prevent the late-phase pulmonary response unless administered in high doses.[98]

While β_2-agonists are associated with tremor, tachycardia, and palpitations, recent studies have found more serious complications including an association with an increased risk of death with chronic use.[99,100] They do not block the development of airway hyperresponsiveness.[63] Indeed, a comparison of an inhaled glucocorticoid, budesonide, with the inhaled β_2-agonist terbutaline, raised the question whether routine use of this medication could result in increased airway hyperresponsiveness.[63]

LEUKOTRIENE PATHWAY MODERATORS. Leukotrienes are arachidonic acid metabolites that have been implicated in transducing bronchospasm, mucus secretion, and increased vascular permeability.[101] Bronchoconstriction associated with aspirin ingestion can be blocked by leukotriene receptor antagonists.[102] Treatment with the leukotriene receptor antagonist montelukast has been shown to significantly improve pulmonary function as measured by FEV_1.[102] The leukotriene receptor antagonists zafirlukast (Accolate), and montelukast (Singulair) are both rated FDA pregnancy category B. The 5-lipoxygenase inhibitor zileuton (Zyflo) is rated FDA pregnancy category C because of reduced weight and skeletal variations among rats at 18 times the recommended maximum human dosage. It should be noted that there are no data regarding the efficacy or safety of these agents during human pregnancy.

Step Therapy

The step-care therapeutic approach increases the number and frequency of medications with increasing asthma severity (see the box "Step Therapy Medical Management of Asthma"). A burst of oral corticosteroids is indicated for exacerbations not responding to initial β-agonist therapy regardless of asthma severity. Additionally, patients who require increasing inhaled β_2-agonist therapy (more than 12 puffs per day) to control their symptoms may benefit from oral corticosteroids. In such cases, a short course of oral prednisone, 40 to 60 mg/day for 1 week followed by 7 to 14 days of tapering may be effective.

Antenatal Management

Patients with moderate and severe asthma should be considered to have high-risk pregnancies. Adverse outcomes can be increased by underestimation of asthma severity and under treatment of asthma exacerbations. The first prenatal visit should include a detailed medical history with attention to medical conditions that could complicate the management of asthma, including diabetes mellitus, hypertension, cardiac disease, adrenal dis-

Step Therapy Medical Management of Asthma

Mild
Inhaled β_2-agonist as needed*

Moderate
Inhaled β_2-agonist as needed*
Inhaled corticosteroids (or cromolyn)
Theophylline for nocturnal asthma or increased
symptoms

Severe
Inhaled β_2-agonist as needed*
Inhaled corticosteroids (or cromolyn)
Theophylline for nocturnal asthma or increased
symptoms
Oral systemic corticosteroids

*PEFR or FEV_1 <80 percent, asthma exacerbations, or exposure to exercise or allergens (oral corticosteroid burst if inadequate response to β_2-agonist regardless of asthma severity).

orders, hyperthyroidism, HIV, hemoglobinopathies, hepatic disease, and active pulmonary problems (cystic fibrosis, bronchiectasis, tuberculosis, sarcoidosis, recurrent sinus and pulmonary infections, bronchitis). The patient should be questioned about the presence and severity of symptoms, episodes of nocturnal asthma, the number of days of work missed due to asthma exacerbations, history of acute asthma emergency care visits, and smoking history. The type and amount of asthma medications including the number of puffs of β_2-agonists used each day should be recorded. Asthma severity should be determined (see the box "Modified NAEP Asthma Severity Classification").

Gravidas with mild, well-controlled asthma may receive routine prenatal care. Moderate and severe asthmatic women should have scheduling of prenatal visits based on clinical judgment; most will need prenatal visits at least every 2 weeks, then weekly at 36 weeks' gestation. In addition to routine care, each antenatal visit should include an evaluation of (1) asthma severity and symptom frequency, nocturnal asthma; (2) FEV_1 or PEFR; (3) medications (assessing compliance and dosage); and (4) emergency visits and hospital admissions for asthma exacerbations. Patients should be instructed on proper dosing and administration of their asthma medications. The step-care therapeutic approach includes increasing the number and frequency of medications with increasing asthma severity (see the box "Step Therapy Medical Management of Asthma"). The least number of medications needed to control asthma symptoms should be used.

Patients should be instructed on proper peak flowmeter technique; PEFR should be determined with peak flowmeters prior to medications, in the morning, and after dinner. At each of these times the patient should make the measurement while standing, to take a maximum inspiration and to note the reading on the instrument. Personal best PEFR should be determined, and personalized green, yellow, and red zones should be established and explained (see the box "Individualized PEFR Zones"). Those with moderate to severe asthma should be instructed to maintain an asthma diary containing daily assessment of asthma symptoms, including morning and evening peak flow measurements, symptoms and activity limitations, indication of any medical contacts initiated, and a record of regular and as-needed medications taken.

As previously discussed, avoidance and control of asthma triggers (see the box "Limiting Exposure to Asthma Triggers") are particularly important in pregnancy, since pharmacologic control of asthma potentially has adverse fetal effects. Specific recommendations should be made for appropriate environmental controls, based on the patient's history of exposure and, when available, demonstrated skin test reactivity.

Moderate and severe asthmatics require additional fetal surveillance in the form of ultrasound examinations and antenatal fetal testing. Because asthma has been associated with intrauterine growth restriction and preterm birth, it is critical to accurately establish pregnancy dating. Ultrasound examinations also are needed to evaluate fetal viability, anatomy, amniotic fluid volume, placental location, and interval fetal growth. Repeat ultrasound examinations are recommended for patients with suboptimally controlled asthma, and following asthma exacerbations to evaluate fetal activity, growth, and amniotic fluid volume. The intensity of antenatal fetal surveillance should be based on the severity of the asthma. All patients should be instructed to be attentive to fetal activity and keep a record of fetal kick counts. In most cases, patients with moderate and severe asthma should have fetal testing starting by 32 weeks' gestation.

HOME MANAGEMENT OF ASTHMA EXACERBATIONS

An asthma exacerbation that causes minimal problems for the mother may have severe sequelae for the fetus. Indeed, an abnormal fetal heart rate tracing may be the

Individualized PEFR Zones

Establish "personal best" PEFR, then calculate:
1. Green zone >80 percent of personal best PEFR
2. Yellow zone 50–80 percent of personal best PEFR
3. Red zone <50 percent of personal best PEFR

(Typical PEFR = 380–550 L/min)

> ## Home Management of Acute Asthma Exacerbations
>
> Use inhaled albuterol 2–4 puffs and check PEFR in 20 minutes
>
> If PEFR <50 percent predicted or symptoms are severe, obtain emergency care
>
> If PEFR is 50–70 percent predicted:
> > Repeat albuterol treatment, check PEFR in 20 minutes
> > If PEFR 50–70 percent predicted
> > > Contact care giver or go for emergency care
>
> If PEFR >70 percent predicted:
> > Continue inhaled albuterol (2–4 puffs q 3–4 h for 6–12 h as needed)
>
> If decreased fetal movement:
> > Contact care giver or go for emergency care

initial manifestation of an asthmatic exacerbation. A maternal PO_2 below 60 mm Hg or hemoglobin saturation less than 90 percent may be associated with profound fetal hypoxia. Therefore, asthma exacerbations in pregnancy must be aggressively managed. Patients should be given an individualized guide for decision making and rescue management.

Patients should be educated to recognize signs and symptoms of early asthma exacerbations such as coughing, chest tightness, dyspnea, or wheezing, or by a 20 percent decrease in their PEFR. This is important so that prompt home rescue treatment may be instituted in order to avoid maternal and fetal hypoxia. In general, patients should use inhaled albuterol 2 to 4 puffs every 20 minutes up to 1 hour. A good response is considered if symptoms are resolved or become subjectively mild, normal activities can be resumed, and the PEFR is greater than 70 percent of personal best. The patient should seek further medical attention if the response is incomplete, or if fetal activity is decreased (see the box "Home Management of Acute Asthma Exacerbations").

HOSPITAL AND CLINIC MANAGEMENT

The principal goal should be the prevention of hypoxia. Continuous electronic fetal monitoring should be initiated if gestation has advanced to the point of potential fetal viability. Albuterol should be delivered by nebulizer (2.5 mg = 0.5 ml albuterol in 2.5 ml normal saline) driven with oxygen; treatments are given every 20 minutes.[103–105] Occasionally, nebulized treatment is not effective because the patient is moving air poorly. In such cases, terbutaline 0.25 mg can be administered subcutaneously every 15 minutes for three doses. The patient should be assessed for general level of activity, color, pulse rate, use of accessory muscles, and airflow

obstruction determined by auscultation and FEV_1 and/or PEFR before and after each bronchodilator treatment. Measurement of oxygenation via pulse oximeter or arterial blood gases is essential. Arterial blood gases should be obtained if oxygen saturation remains below 95 percent. Chest x-rays are not commonly needed. Guidelines for the management of asthma exacerbations are presented in the box "Emergency Assessment and Management of Asthma Exacerbations."

LABOR AND DELIVERY MANAGEMENT

Asthma medications should not be discontinued during labor and delivery. Although asthma is usually quiescent during labor, consideration should be given to assessing PEFRs on admission and at 12-hour intervals. The patient should be kept hydrated and should receive adequate analgesia in order to decrease the risk of bronchospasm. If systemic corticosteroids have been used in the previous 4 weeks, then hydrocortisone (100 mg every 8 hours intravenously) should be administered during labor and for the 24-hour period following delivery to prevent adrenal crisis (NAEP).

It is rarely necessary to deliver a fetus via cesarean section for an acute asthma exacerbation. Usually, ma-

> ## Emergency Assessment and Management of Asthma Exacerbations
>
> 1. **Initial evaluation:**
>   History, examination, PEFR, oximetry
>   Fetal monitoring if potentially viable
>
> 2. **Initial treatment**
>   Inhaled α_2-agonist × 3 doses over 60–90 minutes
> O_2 to maintain saturation >95 percent
>   If no wheezing and PEFR or FEV_1 >70 percent baseline, discharge with follow-up
>
> 3. **If oximetry <90 percent, FEV_1 <1.0 L, or PEFR <100 L/min on presentation:**
>   Continue nebulized albuterol
>   Start intravenous corticosteroids
>   Consider intravenous aminophylline
>   Obtain arterial blood gases
>   Admit to intensive care unit
>   Possible intubation
>
> 4. **If PEFR or FEV_1 >40 percent but <70 percent baseline after β_2-agonist:**
>   Obtain arterial blood gases
>   Continue inhaled β_2-agonist every 1–4 hours
>   Start intravenous corticosteroids in most cases
>   Consider intravenous aminophylline
>   Hospital admission in most cases

ternal and fetal compromise can be managed by aggressive medical management. Occasionally, delivery may improve the respiratory status of a patient with unstable asthma who has a mature fetus. PGE_2 or PGE_1 can be used for cervical ripening, the management of spontaneous or induced abortions, or postpartum hemorrhage; however, 15-methyl $PGF_2\alpha$ and methylergonovine can cause bronchospasm. Magnesium sulfate, which is a bronchodilator, is a safe choice for treating preterm labor. Indomethacin can induce bronchospasm in the aspirin-sensitive patient. There are no reports of the use of calcium channel blockers for tocolysis among patients with asthma.

Lumbar anesthesia has the benefit of reducing oxygen consumption and minute ventilation during labor.[106] A 2 percent incidence of bronchospasm has been reported with regional anesthesia.[107] Fentanyl may be a better analgesic than meperidine, which causes histamine release, but meperidine is rarely associated with the onset of bronchospasm during labor. Ketamine is useful for the induction of general anesthesia because it can prevent bronchospasm.[108] Communication between the obstetric, anesthetic, and pediatric care givers is important for optimal care.

BREAST-FEEDING

In general, only small amounts of medications used to treat asthma enter breast milk. Prednisone, theophylline, antihistamines, beclomethasone, β-agonists, and cromolyn are not considered to be contraindications for breast-feeding.[109] However, among sensitive individuals, theophylline may cause toxic effects in the neonate including vomiting, feeding difficulties, jitteriness, and cardiac arrhythmias.

VENOUS THROMBOSIS AND PULMONARY EMBOLISM

Venous thromboembolic diseases, which include superficial and deep thrombophlebitis, pulmonary embolus, septic pelvic thrombophlebitis, and thrombosis account for almost one half of all obstetric morbidity.[110] The leading cause of pregnancy-related mortality in the United States, pulmonary embolism is responsible for 17 percent of maternal deaths.[111] Thromboembolic disease occurs more frequently during gestation, and the likelihood of venous thromboembolism in normal pregnancy and the puerperium is increased by a factor of 5 when compared with nonpregnant women of similar age.[112] An untreated deep vein thrombosis (DVT) is associated with a 15 to 25 percent incidence of pulmonary embolus, with a 12 to 15 percent mortality rate.[113]

The diagnosis of venous thromboembolism is difficult during pregnancy; however, with the recognition of thrombophilic states and the current thrust toward more accurate diagnosis of those patients who are at high risk for thromboembolic disease secondary to the hereditary thrombophilias, we may soon have better diagnostic tools with which to identify women who may be at increased risk. In this section we review the pathogenesis of thromboembolism in pregnancy, as well as the diagnosis and therapy of this dreaded condition.

Pathogenesis

Normal pregnancy is accompanied by a hypercoagulable state. The concentrations of factors XII, X, IX, VIII, VII, and V, and fibrinogen levels are increased during pregnancy, while factors XI and XIII decrease. Plasma fibrinolytic inhibitors are produced by the placenta, and there is a marked reduction in the release of tissue plasminogen activator (t-PA) in response to venous occlusion throughout pregnancy when compared with nonpregnant subjects.[114,115] There is also a rapid inhibition of released t-PA.[116,117] Protein S is markedly decreased during normal pregnancy; however, protein C is either unaltered or moderately increased.[118] These changes serve to prepare for the major hemostatic challenge of placental separation. Compression of the inferior vena cava and iliac veins by the pregnant uterus produces venous obstruction and results in increased venous capacitance and provides an element of stasis. This stasis may contribute to endothelial cell damage. In addition, local damage to pelvic veins may occur during vaginal and cesarean delivery. Therefore, all the elements of Virchow's triad are present during normal pregnancy and contribute to the increased risk of thromboembolism during pregnancy and the puerperium.[119] There are also hypercoagulable conditions that increase the risk of thromboembolism.

Hypercoagulable Conditions

Preeclampsia

Thrombin–antithrombin complex and fibrinopeptide A concentrations increase markedly in women with preeclampsia.[120–122] Antithrombin III (AT-III) levels are decreased.[123] A recent study examining the incidence of inherited thrombophilias in pregnancy complications reported a 68 percent incidence of inherited or acquired thrombophilias in women whose pregnancies were complicated by severe preeclampsia.[124] Thus, aberrations in the coagulation profile and a high incidence of thrombophilias serve to make the woman with preeclampsia at high risk for thromboembolic complications.

Inherited Thrombophilias

ANTITHROMBIN III DEFICIENCY. Six genetic defects have been identified that are associated with an increased risk of venous thrombosis. AT-III deficiency is inherited as an autosomal dominant trait with heterozygotes having an increased risk of venous thrombosis. This is a heterogeneous defect, and 79 different mutations have been identified in the antithrombin gene.[125] The incidence of AT-III deficiency in the general population is between 1 in 2,000 and 1 in 4,000, making AT-III deficiency the most common congenital clotting disorder in women.[125] Up to 70 percent of individuals with AT-III deficiency develop symptomatic thrombi, and 2 to 3 percent of patients hospitalized for recurrent thrombi will have AT-III deficiency.[126,127] Approximately two thirds of pregnant women with congenital AT-III deficiency will suffer a thrombosis, and the majority of these will occur antepartum.[128] The fetus has a 50 percent risk of inheriting AT-III deficiency and should be tested after birth. AT-III levels less than 30 percent are an indication for neonatal treatment with AT-III concentrate or fresh frozen plasma to prevent a fatal neonatal thrombosis.[113]

PROTHROMBIN 20210A ALLELE. Recently, a new genetic risk factor for venous thrombosis was identified by sequencing the prothrombin genes from families with unexplained familial thrombophilia.[129] The sequence variation observed in these subjects was a G to A transposition in position 20210 of the prothrombin gene.[129] This allele was associated with an increased risk of a first DVT (odds ratio [OR], 2.8; 95 percent CI, 1.4 to 5.6). This mutation was found in 1 to 2 percent of healthy controlled subjects, 6.2 percent of consecutive patients with a first DVT, and in 18 percent of patients that had been selected for unexplained familial thrombophilia.[129] The laboratory diagnosis for the presence of the prothrombin 20210A allele relies completely on DNA analysis.[125] In addition to increasing the risk of thromboembolic phenomena, this gene has been associated with an increased risk of pregnancy complications. The gene was found in 10 percent of women with preeclampsia, abruptio placentae, and fetal growth restriction and stillbirth, as compared with 3 percent of women without these complications.[124]

PROTEIN C DEFICIENCY. Protein C is a vitamin K–dependent protein that attaches to endothelial cells, promotes fibrinolysis, and limits coagulation by inactivation of factors Va and VIIIa.[130] Protein C deficiency is inherited as an autosomal dominant disorder. It is genetically heterogeneous, with more than 160 different mutations in the protein C gene.[125] Heterozygocity for protein C deficiency is a significant risk factor for venous thrombosis. Heterozygotes have protein C antibody levels 50 percent that of normal individuals.[131] Autosomal recessive inheritance of protein C has been observed in families from newborns with severe thrombosis resulting from homozygous or compound heterozygous protein C deficiency.[132] In normal pregnancy, protein C activity is not altered. In patients with pro-

tein C deficiency, pregnancy and delivery increase the risk of a thromboembolic event. The incidence of thromboembolism in pregnant heterozygous women is approximately 25 percent.[133] Protein C deficiency is also associated with an increased risk of pregnancy complications.[124]

PROTEIN S DEFICIENCY. Protein S is a cofactor for protein C. Protein S deficiency is inherited as an autosomal dominant disorder. Seventy different mutations in the protein S gene have been reported.[134] The prevalence of heterozygotes for a type I protein S deficiency is 6 percent in families with an inherited thrombophilia, and 1 to 2 percent in patients with a first DVT.[125] Heterozygous patients have a protein S level 50 percent that of the normal population.[113] Protein S concentration declines during normal pregnancy, and pregnancy seems to increase the risk of a thromboembolic event with women with a protein S deficiency.[113] The neonate is at risk to inherit this disorder and should be tested after birth. Protein S deficiency is associated with an increased risk of pregnancy complications as well.[124]

FACTOR V LEIDEN. Activated protein C (APC) resistance is associated with the factor V Leiden mutation. More than 80 percent of cases with APC resistance are carriers of the same mutation in a gene of factor V, a G to A transposition.[135] The factor V Leiden mutation occurs in 3 percent of healthy subjects and 19 percent of consecutive patients admitted with DVT.[125] The risk of first DVT is reportedly increased 7.9-fold in heterozygotes and 91-fold in homozygotes.[136] In addition to an increased risk of thromboembolic phenomena, the gravida with factor V Leiden mutation is also subject to an increased risk of pregnancy complications. The factor V Leiden mutation was detected in 20 percent of women with obstetric complications, as compared with 6 percent without complications.[124]

DYSFIBRINOGENEMIA. Dysfibrinogenemia is a rare disorder with a prevalence of 1 percent among selected thrombosis patients. Both autosomal dominant and recessive inheritances have been reported.[125] Although most patients with congenital dysfibrinogenemia are either asymptomatic or develop a pure bleeding diathesis, the rare patient may present with venous or arterial thromboembolism that is sometimes accompanied by mild bleeding.[137] Individuals with dysfibrinogenemia are most commonly identified by an abnormal reptilase time and/or thrombin time.[137]

HYPERHOMOCYSTEINEMIA. Hyperhomocysteinemia is a recently described condition associated with an increase of premature atherosclerosis and thromboembolism.[138,139] The inherited form of hyperhomocysteinemia is commonly the result of an abnormality in a key enzyme known as methylenetetrahydrofolate reductase. A common mutation in this enzyme is a C–T substitution at nucleotide 677. This results in a heat-labile form of the enzyme that does not efficiently convert homocysteine to methionine.[140] Hyperhomocysteinemia may also be acquired as the result of a dietary deficiency of folate. The mechanism by which homocysteine induces artherosclerosis and thrombosis is not fully understood. In vivo studies, as well as studies in animals and humans, indicate that hyperhomocysteinemia induces dysfunction of the vascular endothelium with loss of endothelium-dependent vasodilatation and endothelial antithrombotic properties as well as proliferation of vascular smooth muscle cells, all of which are key processes in current models of atherogenesis and thrombosis.[141] Studies have shown that normal antithrombotic endothelium is converted into a more prothrombotic venotype with increased factor V and factor XII activity, decreased activity of protein C, and antithrombin pathways with an accompanying inhibition of thrombomodulin expression, induction of tissue factor expression, and suppression of heparin sulfate expression.[141] All of these changes lead to facilitation of thrombin generation.

In one study, hyperhomocysteinemia was found in 31 percent of women with abruptio placentae or placental infarction as compared with 9 percent of a control group.[142] In another recent report examining the relationship between thrombophilia and adverse outcomes of pregnancy, homozygosity for the mutation in the methylenetetrahydrofolate reductase gene was found in 22 percent of women with obstetric complications as compared with 8 percent of women with normal pregnancies.[124]

Acquired Thrombophilias

LUPUS ANTICOAGULANT. The lupus anticoagulant was first identified in plasma of patients with systemic lupus erythematosus, hence the term lupus anticoagulant. The lupus anticoagulant is a monoclonal autoantibody that reacts to the phospholipid from blood platelet membrane platelet factor 3. Interference by lupus anticoagulant with platelet phospholipid causes incomplete generation of the activated prothrombin complex. Plasma from patients with the lupus anticoagulant interferes with the coagulation of normal plasma. Paradoxically, in vivo these antibodies are associated with thrombosis rather than anticoagulation. The lupus anticoagulant is associated with recurrent fetal demise, congenital heart block, and intrauterine growth restriction.[143] The antiphospholipid syndrome is associated with either recurrent embryonic pregnancy loss or death of the fetus at or beyond 10 weeks of gestation. The latter presentation may be more specific for the antiphospholipid syndrome.[144] The antiphospholipid syndrome is diagnosed when the patient tests positive for the lupus anticoagulant, or has immunoglobulin G (IgG) anticardiolipin antibody in medium to high levels (Table 30–2).[146]

Table 30–2. CLINICAL AND LABORATORY CRITERIA FOR THE DIAGNOSIS OF ANTIPHOSPHOLIPID SYNDROME

Criterion	Definition
Clinical	
Fetal loss	Three or more spontaneous abortions with no more than one live birth, or unexplained second- or third-trimester fetal death
Thrombosis	Unexplained venous or arterial thrombosis, including stroke and arterial insufficiency due to arterial thrombosis
Autoimmune thrombocytopenia	Other causes of thrombocytopenia excluded
Other features	Otherwise unexplained transient ischemic attacks or amaurosis fugax, livedo reticularis, Coombs'-positive hemolytic anemia, chorea, and chorea gravidarum
Laboratory	
Lupus anticoagulant	Detected by phospholipid-dependent clotting assays, without correction with normal plasma, and confirmed by demonstration of phospholipid dependency
Anticardiolipin antibodies	IgG isotype >15–20 GPL units (medium to high positive) detected in standardized assay using standard serum calibrators

GPL, IgG phospholipid units.

Because in many instances tests may be only transiently positive, antiphospholipid antibodies should be detected on two occasions more than 12 weeks apart.[147] The diagnosis of antiphospholipid syndrome should be considered in women with venous thrombosis in unusual sites, such as the portal, mesenteric, splenic, subclavian and cerebral veins. Antiphospholipid antibodies are detected in approximately 2 percent of patients with nontraumatic venous thrombosis.

The therapy of antiphospholipid syndrome in pregnancy will vary depending on the clinical situation (Table 30–3). The majority of women with documented antiphospholipid syndrome will require prophylactic therapy with subcutaneous heparin and low-dose aspirin daily.[146]

All of the thrombophilias are associated with an increased incidence of thromboembolic phenomena in pregnancy. They are also associated with high-risk conditions including preeclampsia, intrauterine fetal demise, intrauterine growth restriction, and abruptio placentae.[124] Therefore, any patient with a known history of a thrombophilia should be monitored closely for the above-mentioned complications of pregnancy. In particular, fetal growth should be assessed frequently and the

Table 30–3. PROPOSED MANAGEMENT FOR WOMEN WITH ANTIPHOSPHOLIPID ANTIBODIES

Feature	Management*	
	Pregnant[†]	Nonpregnant[‡]
Antiphospholipid syndrome (APS)		
APS with prior fetal death or recurrent pregnancy loss	Heparin in prophylactic doses (15,000–20,000 units of unfractionated heparin or equivalent per day) administered subcutaneously in divided doses and low-dose aspirin daily Calcium and vitamin D supplementation	Optimal management uncertain; options include no treatment or daily treatment with low-dose aspirin
APS with prior thrombosis or stroke	Heparin to achieve full anticoagulation *or* Heparin in prophylactic doses (15,000–20,000 units of unfractionated heparin or equivalent per day) administered subcutaneously in divided doses *plus* Low-dose aspirin daily Calcium and vitamin D supplementation	Warfarin administered daily in doses to maintain INR ≥3:0
APS without prior pregnancy loss or thrombosis	Optimal management uncertain; options include no treatment, daily treatment with low-dose aspirin, daily treatment with prophylactic doses of heparin and low-dose aspirin	Optimal management uncertain; options include no treatment or daily treatment with low-dose aspirin
Antiphospholipid antibodies without APS		
Lupus anticoagulant (LA) or medium to high positive IgG aCL	Optimal management uncertain; options include no treatment, daily treatment with low-dose aspirin, daily treatment with prophylactic doses of heparin and low-dose aspirin	Optimal management uncertain; options include no treatment or daily treatment with low-dose aspirin
Low levels of IgG, only IgM aCL, only IgA aCL without LA, antiphospholipid antibodies other than LA, or aCL	Optimal management uncertain; options include no treatment or daily treatment with low-dose aspirin	Optimal management uncertain; options include no treatment or daily treatment with low-dose aspirin

* The medication shown should not be used in the presence of contraindications.
† Close obstetric monitoring of mother and fetus is necessary in all cases.
‡ The patient should be counseled in all cases regarding symptoms of thrombosis and thromboembolism.

obstetrician must be alert to any signs or symptoms consistent with preeclampsia. Any signs or symptoms suspicious for a DVT or pulmonary embolus should be thoroughly investigated.

Diagnosis of Deep Vein Thrombosis

The diagnosis of a DVT during pregnancy can be challenging. Clinical suspicions are aroused by signs and symptoms including pain, tenderness to palpation, and edema. Edema of the lower extremities occurs frequently in normal pregnancy, particularly in the third trimester. However, should edema be asymmetric, that is, more than 2 cm difference in circumference between the affected and normal leg, or if there is a positive Homans' sign or Lowenberg test, an investigation to rule out a DVT should be undertaken.

Venography

Ascending contrast venography is the reference standard for the diagnosis of a DVT.[148] The technique in-

volves injection of a radiographic contrast dye into a distal, dorsal foot vein while the patient is relaxed, non–weight bearing, and in 40 percent of reversed Trendelenburg position. The diagnosis of DVT requires visualization in at least two different views of a well-defined intraluminal filling defect. False-positive studies can result from poor technique, leg muscle contraction, Baker's (popliteal) cyst, hematoma, local edema, and other conditions.[149] Pressure from the gravid uterus can cause a false-positive venogram. Therefore, uterine displacement is imperative during the procedure. False-negative results can occur if the contrast does not fill all the deep veins.[148]

If indicated during pregnancy, a limited venogram can be performed using pelvic and abdominal shielding with lead aprons. This can protect the fetus from potential hazards of radiation exposure. Visualization of the iliac veins may be compromised, and isolated iliac vein thrombosis cannot be diagnosed.[148] If complete visualization of the entire deep venous system is indicated, a complete venogram can be done. The estimated amount of radiation absorbed by the fetus with an unshielded unilateral venogram was 0.314 rad in one study.[149] This compared with less than 0.050 rad with a limited venogram. In utero exposure to radiation may be associated with a slight increase in the risk of childhood cancer following in utero exposure to radiation doses of less than 5 rad.[149] There is no increase in congenital malformations or increase in stillbirths or infant deaths following such radiation exposure. Therefore, venography is likely to be relatively safe for the fetus, particularly when pelvic shielding is used.

Fibrinogen Scanning

[125]I fibrinogen scanning is not recommended for diagnosis of deep vein thrombosis in pregnancy. It is associated with a relatively high level of radiation exposure to the fetus, estimated at approximately 2 rad.[149] In addition, radiolabeled iodine crosses the placenta, is taken up by the fetal thyroid, and is also secreted into breast milk. Therefore, ^{125}I fibrinogen scanning should also be avoided during breast-feeding.

Impedance Plethysmography

Impedance plethysmography (IPG) is a safe, inexpensive, and relatively sensitive and specific test for the detection of a proximal DVT. However, it is not sensitive for detecting proximal nonobstructive thrombi or calf DVT.[150] IPG measures electrical impedance resulting from changes in blood volume within a limb. It involves the inflation of a thigh cuff to trap blood in the leg. In the absence of venous obstruction, rapid deflation of the cuff permits a rapid outflow of blood and is associated with a concomitant sudden increase in the electrical resistance of the limb.[113] A more gradual increase in electrical resistance is observed when there is a partial or complete obstruction to venous outflow. IPG is 95 percent sensitive and 98 percent specific for the detection of proximal vein thrombi.[151] In pregnancy, compression of the inferior vena cava by the gravid uterus can produce false-positive results despite position changes.[152] Therefore, a positive IPG after 20 weeks of gestation requires confirmation by venography before initiating anticoagulant therapy.[113]

Venous Duplex Doppler Ultrasound

Venous duplex Doppler ultrasound is a safe, simple, and inexpensive method to indirectly assess the competency of the deep venous system in the lower extremities. However, this technique is subjective and requires considerable expertise.[148] A Doppler shift is recorded during changes in venous blood flow that occur within patent vessels. Changes in venous blood flow can be augmented by compressing and releasing a vein, or by observing changes in flow with breathing or the Valsalva maneuver. An occluded vein will not produce a Doppler shift. Venous Doppler assessment has a sensitivity of 76 to 94 percent and a specificity of 90 to 95 percent for a proximal DVT, but has a low sensitivity for a calf DVT.[148,153] This technique is limited by an inability to distinguish thrombotic from nonthrombotic forms of venous occlusion. In one study, venous Doppler abnormalities occurred in 25 percent of pregnant patients who were scanned in the supine position.[153] Therefore, the study should be performed with left lateral uterine displacement.

Real-time ultrasound is also useful for the diagnosis of a DVT.[113] Criteria for diagnosis of a DVT by ultrasound includes an intraluminal soft tissue mass, noncompressibility of the vein, and a dampened or absent increase in diameter during a Valsalva maneuver.[154] These criteria are useful only in the proximal veins (femoral and popliteal). In the proximal veins, the sensitivity of real-time B-mode ultrasonography has been reported to range from 94 to 100 percent with a 100 percent specificity.[113]

When there is clinical suspicion of DVT, the diagnostic approach should be such that disease can be diagnosed while minimizing potentially harmful fetal irradiation. One approach to diagnosis is to use Doppler ultrasound as the initial diagnostic test. If the test is positive, anticoagulant therapy should be given. If the ultrasound is normal, the patient's symptoms may be due to a calf DVT, which may be undetected by ultrasound. Serial ultrasound testing may then be done to assess for progression of a calf DVT into the proximal veins.[148] If repeat ultrasound identifies a newly formed proximal DVT, anticoagulation therapy should be initiated.

If isolated iliac vein thrombosis is suspected, Doppler ultrasound or IPG can be used for diagnosis. If IPG is available, this can be used as the initial test. If IPG is positive during the first or second trimester of pregnancy, then a DVT can be diagnosed and anticoagulation can be started.[148] A positive test in the third trimester may be falsely positive because of outflow obstruction caused by the gravid uterus. In this circumstance, further investigation with a limited venogram should be considered and, if a DVT is seen, treatment can be started. If limited venogram does not demonstrate a thrombus, a complete venogram should be considered, given the possibility of proximal femoral vein thrombosis or isolated iliac DVT. If the initial IPG is negative and the pretest clinical likelihood of DVT is low or moderate, then serial IPG testing should be done over a 7- to 14-day period.[148] If the repeat IPG becomes positive, then this can provide sufficient basis for diagnosing a DVT. If the initial IPG is negative and the pretest clinical likelihood for a DVT is high, a limited

Table 30–4. SIGNS AND SYMPTOMS OF PULMONARY EMBOLISM

Finding	Patients with Proven Pulmonary Embolism (%)
Tachypnea	89
Dyspnea	81
Pleuritic pain	72
Apprehension	59
Cough	54
Tachycardia	43
Hemoptysis	34
Temperature >37°C	34

venogram or Doppler ultrasound should be performed.[148] If either of these examinations is positive, therapy should be started.

Pulmonary Embolism

Pulmonary embolus (PE) contributes to significant maternal morbidity and mortality and, therefore, clinical suspicion should be high. Signs and symptoms may include dyspnea, tachypnea, cough, pleuritic chest pain, tachycardia, pleural friction rub, diaphoresis, cyanosis, hemoptysis, or a new murmur (Table 30–4). Of these, the most common sign is tachypnea.[155] Any gravida presenting with signs and symptoms consistent with a pulmonary embolus requires further evaluation. An initial evaluation should include auscultation, pulse oximetry, and an arterial blood gas. Additional tests should include a chest radiograph and electrocardiogram. A PO_2 greater than 85 mm Hg on room air is reassuring; however, it does not rule out the possibility of a PE. As many as 14 percent of patients with a pulmonary embolus have a PO_2 greater than 85 mm Hg.[155] Any patient with an oxygen saturation less than 95 percent on room air without obvious clinical conditions associated with hypoxia, such as atelectasis, pneumonia, or asthma, deserves an investigation. A chest radiograph is useful to rule out pneumonia and atelectasis; however, even the presence of an infiltrate does not rule out the possibility of PE and, again, investigation should be continued if clinical suspicion is high. The most frequent electrocardiographic finding is tachycardia; however, findings consistent with acute cor pulmonale (right axis shift and nonspecific T-wave inversions) may be seen after massive pulmonary embolism. If clinical suspicion for PE is moderate to high, the gravida should be anticoagulated while the diagnosis is pursued.

When pulmonary embolus is suspected, Doppler ultrasound or IPG may be performed to identify a DVT.

If these tests are diagnostic for DVT, one can assume the patient does indeed have a pulmonary embolus and anticoagulation therapy should be instituted. If the diagnosis of DVT has not been established, ventilation-perfusion (V/Q) lung scanning should be performed. The perfusion scan is performed by injecting ^{99m}Tc-labeled albumin. These particles are aggregated within the pulmonary precapillary arteriolar bed. A ventilation scan using ^{133}Xe isotope is done after the perfusion scan to document ventilatory defects. The V/Q scans are then examined for matching defects. These scans are interpreted as normal, indeterminate, or revealing low, moderate, or high suspicion of pulmonary embolus. If there are abnormalities on the chest radiograph that coincide with areas of perfusion defect, the scan is considered indeterminate. When there is V/Q mismatching or multiple defects, the probability of pulmonary embolism is considered high.

When the Doppler examination is negative, the V/Q scan is low probability, and the clinical suspicion of PE is low as well, the test can be considered negative, and therapy need not be initiated. If the V/Q scan is indeterminate, low or moderately suspicious for PE, and clinical suspicion is high, a pulmonary arteriogram should be performed (Fig. 30–3). If a pulmonary arteriogram is diagnostic of PE, therapy should be instituted with heparin. If the V/Q scan is consistent with high probability, the patient can be considered as having a positive test for PE, and therapy should be instituted.

Pulmonary angiography is the definitive test for pulmonary embolism. Risks of the procedure are related to the catheterization and injection of contrast dye. The morbidity rate is reportedly between 4 and 5 percent, with a 0.2 to 0.3 percent mortality rate.[113] The radiation dose to the fetus is low, and even when V/Q scanning is performed in addition to pulmonary angiography, the total radiation dose to the fetus is well below the lowest dose associated with any adverse fetal effect.[156]

When pulmonary embolus is diagnosed, therapy should be initiated immediately. Heparin is the anticoagulant of choice during pregnancy. Because of its large molecular weight (6,000 to 20,000 Da), it does not cross the placenta and is not excreted in breast milk. Heparin must be given parenterally, and intravenous therapy achieves therapeutic levels most quickly. The initial loading dose should be 70 units/kg, administered intravenously, followed by a continuous infusion of 1,000 units/h. The dose of heparin should be adjusted to keep the activated partial thromboplastin time (aPTT) approximately twice normal or the heparin level at 0.2 to 0.4 units/ml. This therapy should be continued for approximately 10 days. The patient can then be switched to subcutaneous heparin at a dose sufficient to

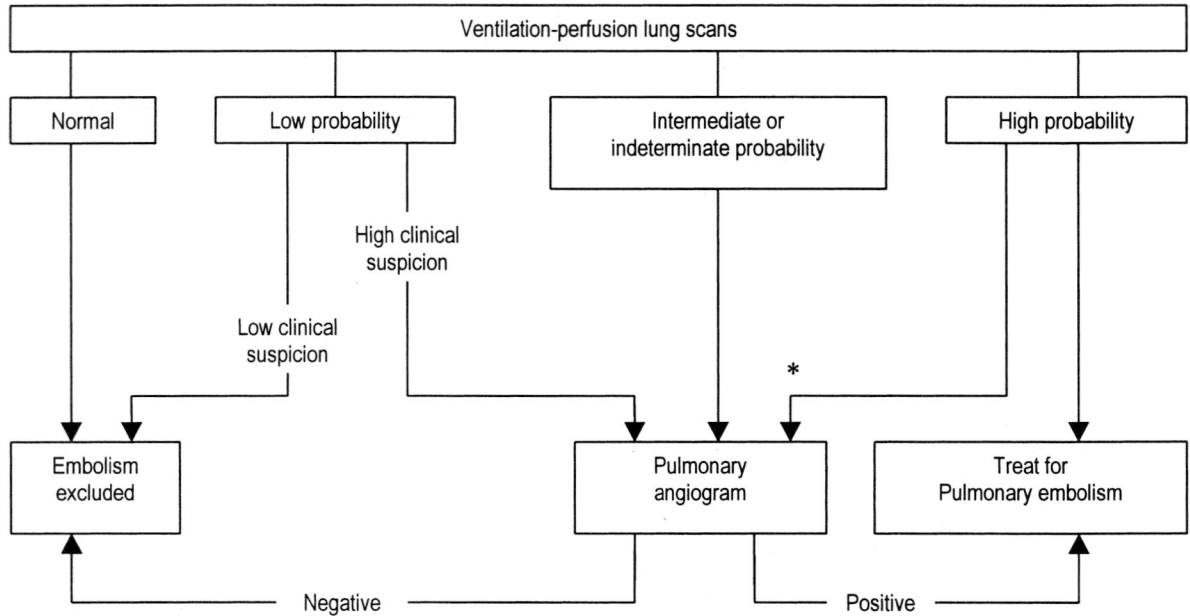

*Contraindications to anticoagulant therapy.

Figure 30–3. Diagnostic algorithm using ventilation-perfusion lung scanning in the evaluation of the patient suspected of having pulmonary embolism. (Modified from Senior RM: Pulmonary embolism. *In* Wyngaarden JB, Smith LH Jr, Bennett JC [eds]: Cecil Textbook of Medicine, 20th ed. Philadelphia, WB Saunders Company, 1996, p 425.)

keep the aPTT about $1\frac{1}{2}$ times normal and the heparin titer 0.1 to 0.2 units/ml. In general, a dose of 7,500 to 10,000 units of heparin administered every 8 to 12 hours will achieve therapeutic levels.[157] This therapy should be continued throughout gestation because the risk of a recurrent thrombus remains high. Therefore, a DVT and/or PE should be treated with full anticoagulation for at least 3 to 6 months. Subsequently, both therapeutic and prophylactic regimens of heparin have been advocated until 6 to 12 weeks postpartum.[158]

Hemorrhage is the major risk of heparin therapy. This occurs in approximately 4 percent of properly monitored nonsurgical patients receiving intravenous heparin.[159] Osteoporosis and compression fractures can occur when heparin has been administered in doses greater than 15,000 units/day for more than 6 months.[160] This side effect can be diminished by administration of adequate amounts of calcium and vitamin D and may be reversible following cessation of therapy.[158] Thrombocytopenia can also complicate heparin therapy but occurs in only 3 percent of patients treated with porcine heparin.[161] A platelet count should be obtained periodically during the first 3 weeks of therapy. Low-molecular-weight heparin has been used during gestation. Patients treated with low-molecular-weight heparin may be less likely to develop heparin-induced thrombocytopenia. Low-molecular-weight heparin has

the advantage of only single daily dosing, but is 10 times more expensive than heparin therapy.[162]

In the postpartum period, treatment can be switched to warfarin (Coumadin). This oral anticoagulant inhibits regeneration of active vitamin K in the liver. It has a molecular weight of 1,000 Da and does cross the placenta (see Chapter 9). Its use is not recommended during pregnancy. However, in the postpartum period, it can be used for anticoagulation and does not enter breast milk in significant amounts. A starting dose of 5 mg/day for the first 2 days is followed by daily dosing adjusted to the international normalized ratio (INR) of 2.0 to 3.0. An overlap of 3 to 5 days with a therapeutic INR and aPTT is recommended. Warfarin is continued for approximately 3 months or indefinitely if risk factors are still present or if thromboembolism is recurrent.[163]

Prophylaxis

Women with a previous venous thromboembolism have a 7 to 30 percent risk of recurrence during a subsequent pregnancy.[164,165] Heparin, given in a dose of 5,000 units subcutaneously twice daily has been shown to be effective for prevention of thromboembolic disease in the postoperative patient.[166] This prophylaxis has been recommended for gravidas with a history of thromboembolic phenomena; however, a recent report of 72 pregnant patients showed a 15 percent frequency of recurrent thromboembolism in patients receiving this prophylaxis, not significantly different from the 11.9 percent incidence in a control group. Therefore, the 5,000 units twice-daily dosing is considered to be inadequate, and it has been recommended that heparin prophylaxis during pregnancy be increased to 7,500 units every 12 hours, from 13 weeks of gestation, and 10,000 units every 12 hours from 30 weeks of gestation.[167]

Gravidas with known hypercoagulable states will require some prophylaxis during pregnancy. AT-III deficiency should be treated with heparin throughout gestation. The best regimen has remained controversial. The therapeutic goal for patients with AT-III deficiency is a prolongation of the partial thromboplastin time (PTT) 5 to 10 seconds above baseline, just prior to the next injection.[128] AT-III concentrate is now available in the United States and may be used to augment heparin therapy in the event of thrombosis and should be administered to gravidas with AT-III deficiency in labor.

If protein C deficiency is diagnosed, therapeutic subcutaneous heparin therapy to prolong the PTT to 1.5 to 2 times the control is recommended throughout gestation.[168] However, others have recommended low-dose heparin prophylaxis of 7,500 units subcutaneously twice daily.[169] Protein S deficiency is also associated with an increase of thromboembolic events during pregnancy and, therefore, heparin prophylaxis should be instituted once protein S deficiency is identified. For patients with protein S and protein C deficiencies, therapy should be switched to warfarin in the postpartum period.

Patients with recent pulmonary emboli or recurrent or recent ileofemoral thrombosis should continue to receive heparin intravenously during delivery. They should be converted to a regimen of continuous intravenous heparin and the dose should be adjusted to achieve a PTT of 1.5 times control during labor and delivery.[158] Continuing this regimen does not increase the incidence of postpartum hemorrhage in a normal delivery. There is a slight increase in the incidence of an episiotomy hematoma. Heparin therapy may contribute to blood loss in patients with uterine atony or a retained placenta.[158]

Alternative Therapy

Both streptokinase and urokinase produce rapid resolution of pulmonary emboli and improvement in pulmonary hemodynamics.[158] There is very limited experience with the use of these agents during pregnancy,[170,171] and they should be reserved for circumstances of significant hemodynamic instability in a patient with pulmonary embolus.[158] Postpartum hemorrhage from the pla-

cental site may be a risk when fibrinolytic agents are used during pregnancy. When pulmonary embolus is recurrent despite adequate anticoagulation, vena caval interruption is indicated. Caval interruption via ligation, plication, or insertion of an umbrella can be safely carried out during pregnancy.[172,173]

RESTRICTIVE LUNG DISEASE

Restrictive ventilatory defects occur when lung expansion is limited because of alterations in the lung parenchyma or because of abnormalities in the pleura, chest wall, or the neuromuscular apparatus.[174] These conditions are characterized by a reduction in lung volumes and an increase in the ratio of FEV_1 to forced vital capacity (FVC).[175] The interstitial lung diseases include idiopathic pulmonary fibrosis, sarcoidosis, hypersensitivity pneumonitis, pneumonicosis, drug-induced lung disease, and connective tissue disease. Additional conditions that cause a restrictive ventilatory defect include pleural and chest wall diseases, and extrathoracic conditions such as obesity, peritonitis, and ascites.[175] Restrictive lung disease in pregnancy has not been well studied. Consequently, little is known about the effects of restrictive lung disease on the outcome of pregnancy or the effects of pregnancy on the disease process itself. A recent study presented data on nine pregnant women who were prospectively managed with interstitial and restrictive lung disease.[176] Diagnoses included idiopathic pulmonary fibrosis, hypersensitivity pneumonitis, sarcoidosis, kyphoscoliosis, and multiple pulmonary emboli. Three of the gravidas presented in this paper had severe disease characterized by a vital capacity of 1.5 L or less (50 percent predicted) or a diffusing capacity less than or equal to 50 percent predicted. Five of the patients had exercise-induced oxygen desaturation, and four patients required supplemental oxygen. Of the group, one patient had an adverse outcome and was delivered at 31 weeks. She subsequently required mechanical ventilation for 72 hours. All other patients were delivered at or beyond 36 weeks with no adverse intrapartum or postpartum complications. All babies were at or above the 30th percentile for growth.[176] The authors concluded that restrictive lung disease was well tolerated in pregnancy. However, exercise intolerance was common, and patients may require early oxygen supplementations.[176]

Sarcoidosis

Sarcoidosis is a systemic granulomatosis disease of undetermined etiology that often affects young adults. Pregnancy outcome for the majority of patients with sarcoidosis is good.[177,178] In another study, 35 pregnancies in 18 patients with sarcoidosis were evaluated retrospectively.[177] In nine patients, there was no effect of the disease process during pregnancy; in six patients, improvement was demonstrated, and in three there was a worsening of the disease. During the postpartum period, no relapse was noted in 15 patients; however, in three women, a progression of the disease continued. Another retrospective study presented 15 pregnancies complicated by maternal sarcoidosis over a 10-year period.[178] Eleven of these patients remained stable, two experienced disease progression, and two died due to severe complications of severe sarcoidosis. In this group, factors indicating a poor prognosis reportedly included parenchymal lesions on chest radiograph, advanced radiographic staging, advanced maternal age, low inflammatory activity, requirement for drugs other than steroids, and the presence of extrapulmonary sarcoidosis.[178] Both of the patients who succumbed during gestation had severe disease at the onset of pregnancy. The overall cesarean section rate was 40 percent and, in addition, 4 of 15 infants (27 percent) weighed under 2,500 g. None of the patients developed preeclampsia. One possible explanation for the commonly observed improvement in sarcoidosis may be the increased concentration of circulating corticosteroids during pregnancy. However, because sarcoidosis improves spontaneously in many nonpregnant patients, the improvement may be coincident with but not due to pregnancy.

Maycock et al. reported on 16 pregnancies in 10 patients with sarcoidosis.[179] Eight of the 10 patients showed improvement in at least some of the manifestations of sarcoidosis during the antepartum period. In two patients, no effect was noted. A recurrence of the abnormal findings was observed in the postpartum period within several months after delivery in approximately half of the patients. In addition, some had new manifestations of sarcoidosis not previously noted. Another study examined 17 pregnancies in 10 patients and concluded that pregnancy had no consistent effect on the course of the disease.[180] Scadding separated patients into three categories based on characteristic patterns of their chest radiographs. When the chest radiograph had resolved before pregnancy, the normal radiograph persisted throughout gestation. In women with resolving radiographic changes before pregnancy, resolution continued throughout the prenatal period. Patients with inactive fibrotic residual disease had stable chest radiographs and those with active disease tended to have partial or complete resolution of those changes during pregnancy. Most patients in this later group, however, experienced exacerbation of the disease within 3 to 6 months after delivery.[181]

Patients with pulmonary hypertension complicating restrictive lung disease may suffer a mortality of as much as 50 percent during gestation. These patients need close monitoring during the labor, delivery, and postpartum period. Invasive monitoring with a pulmonary artery catheter may be indicated to optimize cardiorespiratory function. Gravidas with restrictive lung disease including pulmonary sarcoidosis may benefit from early institution of steroid therapy for evidence of worsening pulmonary status. Individuals with evidence of severe disease will need close monitoring and may require supplemental oxygen therapy during gestation as well.

During labor, consideration should be given to early use of epidural anesthesia if not contraindicated. The early institution of pain management in this population will minimize pain, decrease sympathetic response, and therefore decrease oxygen consumption during labor and delivery. The use of general anesthesia should be avoided if possible, as these patients may develop pulmonary complications after general anesthesia including pneumonia and difficulty weaning from the ventilator. In addition, close fetal surveillance throughout gestation is indicated, as impaired oxygenation may lead to impaired fetal growth and the development of fetal heart rate abnormalities during labor and delivery.

An additional consideration is the need to counsel all women with restrictive lung disease about the potential for continued impairment of their respiratory status during pregnancy, particularly if their respiratory status is deteriorating when they conceive. Certainly, the individual with clinical signs consistent with pulmonary hypertension and/or severe restrictive disease should be cautioned about the possibility of maternal mortality resulting from worsening pulmonary function during gestation.

In summary, although the literature on restrictive lung disease in pregnancy is limited, it supports the conclusion that the majority of patients with restrictive lung disease complicating pregnancy including those with pulmonary sarcoidosis will have a favorable pregnancy outcome. However, the clinician should keep in mind that patients with restrictive lung disease can have worsening of their clinical condition and may succumb during gestation.

CYSTIC FIBROSIS

Cystic fibrosis involves the exocrine glands and epithelial tissues of the pancreas, sweat glands, and mucous glands in the respiratory, digestive, and reproductive tracts. Chronic obstructive pulmonary disease, pancreatic exocrine insufficiency, and elevated sweat electrolytes are present in most patients with cystic fibrosis.[182] The disease is genetically transmitted with an autosomal recessive pattern of inheritance. The cystic fibrosis gene was identified and cloned in 1989. The gene is localized to chromosome 7, and the molecular defect accounting for the majority of cases has been identified.[183-185] In the United States, approximately 4 percent of the Caucasian population are heterozygous carriers of the cystic fibrosis gene. The disease occurs in 1 in 3,000 live Caucasian births.[186] Morbidity and mortality in cystic fibrosis is usually secondary to progressive chronic bronchial pulmonary disease. Pregnancy and the attendant physiologic changes can stress the pulmonary, cardiovascular, and nutritional status of women with cystic fibrosis. The purpose of this section is to familiarize the obstetrician/gynecologist with the physiologic effects of this complex disease and the impact of the disease on pregnancy and the impact of pregnancy on the disease. Additional factors that need to be addressed are the genetics of this disorder and the implications for the newborn, as well as social issues including who will raise the child should the mother succumb to her disease.

Survival for patients with cystic fibrosis has increased dramatically since 1940. According to the Cystic Fibrosis Foundation's Patient Registry, survival in 1992 had increased to 29.6 years.[182] Females had a slightly lower median age of survival (27.3 years) as compared with males (29.6 years). The reasons for sex differences in mortality are unclear. This increase in survival of patients with cystic fibrosis is likely secondary to earlier diagnosis and intervention and also to advances in antibiotic therapy and nutritional support. Therefore, more women with cystic fibrosis are entering reproductive age. In contrast to males with cystic fibrosis who, for the most part are infertile, women with cystic fibrosis are more often fertile. Infertility in women with cystic fibrosis may occasionally be due to anovulatory cycles and secondary amenorrhea, which result from significant malnutrition, associated with advanced disease. A more common reason for infertility appears to result from alteration in the physiologic properties of cervical mucus.[187]

The first case of cystic fibrosis complicating pregnancy was reported in 1960, and a total of 13 pregnancies in 10 patients with cystic fibrosis were reported in 1966.[188,189] Cohen conducted a survey of 119 cystic fibrosis centers in the United States and Canada and identified a total of 129 pregnancies in 100 women by 1976.[190] Hillman surveyed 127 cystic fibrosis centers in the United States, between 1976 and 1982.[182] A total of 191 pregnancies were reported during this period in women with cystic fibrosis, ranging in age from 16 to 36 years, with a mean age of 22.6 years.[182] The annual number of cystic fibrosis pregnancies reported to the Cystic Fibrosis Foundation's Patient Registry doubled between 1986 and 1990, with 52 pregnancies reported in 1986, compared with 111 pregnancies reported in 1990. Because the number of women with cystic fibrosis achieving pregnancy is steadily increasing, it is imperative that the obstetrician be familiar with the disease.

The Effect of Pregnancy on Cystic Fibrosis

The physiologic changes associated with pregnancy (see Chapter 3) are well tolerated by healthy gravidas; however, those with cystic fibrosis may adapt poorly. During pregnancy, there is an increase in resting minute ventilation that at term may approach 150 percent of control values.[191] This increase in minute ventilation occurs secondary to the increased oxygen consumption and increased carbon dioxide burden that occur during pregnancy. An additional impact occurs secondary to circulating progesterone, which stimulates the respiratory drive. Enlargement of the abdominal contents and upward displacement of the diaphragm leads to a decrease in functional residual volume and a decrease in residual volume.[191] Pregnancy is also accompanied by subtle alterations in gas exchange with widening of the alveolar–arterial oxygen gradient that is most pronounced in the supine position.[191] These alterations in pulmonary function are of little consequence in the normal pregnant woman. However, in the gravida with cystic fibrosis, these changes may contribute to respiratory decompensation that can lead to increase in morbidity and mortality for the mother and the fetus as well.

During normal pregnancy, blood volume increases by an average of 50 percent. Cardiac output increases as well, reaching a plateau in midpregnancy.[192] During labor, blood volume rises acutely, in large part due to the release of blood from the contracting uterus and is additionally increased after delivery, secondary to augmented venous return with the release of caval obstruction. Women with cystic fibrosis and advanced lung disease may suffer from pulmonary hypertension with high pulmonary artery pressures. Whatever the cause, pulmonary hypertension is associated with unacceptable maternal risk during pregnancy and is considered to be a contraindication to pregnancy.[192] Women with significant pulmonary hypertension may develop cardiovascular collapse at the time of labor and delivery, with a maternal mortality exceeding 25 percent.[193] Additionally, patients with pulmonary hypertension may not be able to adequately increase cardiac output during pregnancy and, therefore, suffer uteroplacental insufficiency, leading to intrauterine growth restriction and stillbirth.[186]

Nutritional requirements are increased during pregnancy, with approximately 300 kcal/day in additional fuel being needed to meet the requirements of mother and fetus.[194] Most patients with cystic fibrosis have pancreatic exocrine insufficiency. As a result, digestive enzymes and bicarbonate ions are diminished, resulting in maldigestion, malabsorption, and malnutrition.[194]

The 1966 report by Grand et al. included 13 pregnancies in 10 women with cystic fibrosis. Of these, five women had a progressive decline in their pulmonary function, two of whom died of cor pulmonale in the immediate postpartum period. In another report, pregnancy was well tolerated in 5 of 10 women, two of whom went on to have subsequent pregnancies that were similarly well tolerated.[189] In this study, the pregravid pulmonary status of the patient was the most important predictor of outcome. However, there was no quantification of pulmonary function. A case report by Novy and colleagues in 1967 described in detail the pulmonary function and gas exchange in a pregnant woman with cystic fibrosis.[195] The patient had severe disease as evidenced by a vital capacity of only 0.72 L and an arterial PO_2 of 50 mm Hg at presentation. The patient suffered a progressive increase in residual volume and decline in vital capacity that was accompanied by worsening hypoxemia and hypercapnea, resulting in respiratory distress and right-sided heart failure in the early postpartum period.[195] Based on the experience with this patient and a review of the literature, the authors recommended therapeutic abortion in any patient demonstrating progressive pulmonary deterioration and hypoxemia despite maximal medical management.[195] In 1980, Cohen et al. described 100 patients and a total of 129 pregnancies.[190] Ninety-seven of 129 (75 percent) pregnancies were completed, and 89 percent delivered viable infants. Twenty-seven percent of these fetuses were delivered preterm. There were 11 perinatal deaths and no congenital anomalies. In this study, 65 percent of patients required antibiotic therapy prior to delivery. In 1983, Palmer et al. retrospectively reviewed the prepregnancy status of eight women with cystic fibrosis who subsequently completed 11 pregnancies.[196] She found that five women tolerated pregnancy without difficulty, but three had irreversible deterioration in their clinical status. She identified four maternal factors that were predictive of outcome: clinical status (Shwachman score), nutritional status (percentage of predicted weight for height), the extent of chest radiographic abnormalities (assessed by the Brasfield chest radiograph score), and the magnitude of pulmonary function impairment. Women with good clinical studies, good nutritional status (within 15 percent of their predicted ideal body weight for height), with nearly normal chest radiographs and only mild obstructive lung disease tolerated pregnancy well without deterioration.[196]

There are several reports suggesting that patients with mild cystic fibrosis, good nutritional status, and less impairment of lung function tolerate pregnancy well. However, those with poor clinical status, malnu-

trition, hepatic dysfunction, and/or advanced lung disease are at increased risk from pregnancy.[197–199] Kent and Farquharson reviewed the literature and reported 217 pregnancies.[199] In this series, the frequency of preterm delivery was 24.3 percent, and the perinatal death rate was 7.9 percent. Poor outcomes were associated with a maternal weight gain of less than 4.5 kg and an FVC of less than 50 percent of that predicted. Edenborough et al. also reported on pregnancies in women with cystic fibrosis.[200] There were 18 live births (81.8 percent), one third of which were preterm deliveries, and 18.2 percent of patients had abortions. There were four maternal deaths within 3.2 years after delivery. In this series, lung function was available before delivery, immediately after delivery, and after pregnancy. They demonstrated a decline of 13 percent in FEV_1, and 11 percent in FVC during pregnancy. Most patients returned to baseline pulmonary function after pregnancy. While most of the women in this series tolerated pregnancy well, those with moderate to severe lung disease, an FEV_1 of less than 60 percent of predicted, more often had preterm infants and had increased loss of lung function compared to those with milder disease.[200] In two series, prepregnancy FEV_1 was found to be the most useful predictor of outcome in pregnant women with cystic fibrosis.[200,201] In addition, there was also a positive correlation of prepregnancy FEV_1 and maternal survival.

Pulmonary involvement in cystic fibrosis includes chronic infection of the airways and bronchiectasis. There is selective infection with certain microorganisms, such as *Staphylococcus aureus*, *Haemophilus influenzae*, *Pseudomonas aeruginosa*, and *Berkholderia cepacia*. *Pseudomonas aeruginosa* is the most frequent pathogen.[182] Parenteral antibiotics are the mainstays of treatment of these acute infections. However, pregnancy and cystic fibrosis–associated alterations in pharmacokinetics can have grave consequences for these patients. It is well known that pregnant subjects have lower serum levels and higher urine levels of antibiotics than nonpregnant subjects. The lower levels in plasma are attributed to the increase in volume of distribution and an increase in glomerular filtration and renal clearance of the drugs.[202] Cloxacillin, dicloxacillin, ticarcillin, and methicillin are cleared more rapidly in patients with cystic fibrosis.[203–205] Plasma ceftazidime and gentamicin levels are likewise decreased in patients with cystic fibrosis.[206,207]

Counseling Patients with Cystic Fibrosis in Pregnancy

There are several factors that must be considered when counseling a woman who has cystic fibrosis and is considering pregnancy, including the possibility that her fetus will have cystic fibrosis (see Chapter 8). Approximately 4 percent of the Caucasian population in the United States are heterozygous carriers of the cystic fibrosis gene. The disease occurs in 1 in 3,000 Caucasian births. When the mother has cystic fibrosis and the proposed father is a Caucasian of unknown genotype, the risk of the fetus having cystic fibrosis is 1 in 50, as compared with 1 in 3,000 in the general Caucasian population. If the prospective father is a known carrier of a cystic fibrosis mutation, the risk to the fetus increases to 1 in 2. If, however, DNA testing does not identify a cystic fibrosis mutation in the prospective father, it is still possible that the father is a carrier of an unidentified cystic fibrosis mutation, making the risk to the offspring 1 in 492.[208]

It is important that the woman with cystic fibrosis be advised about the potential adverse affects of pregnancy on maternal health status. Factors that may predict poor outcome include prepregnancy evidence of poor nutritional status, significant pulmonary disease with hypoxemia, and pulmonary hypertension. Liver disease and diabetes mellitus are also poor prognostic factors. Gravidas with poor nutritional status, pulmonary hypertension (cor pulmonale), and deteriorating pulmonary function early in gestation should consider therapeutic abortion, as the risk of maternal mortality may be unacceptably high.

The woman with cystic fibrosis who is considering pregnancy should also give consideration to the need for strong psychosocial and physical support after delivery. The rigors of child-rearing may add to the risk of maternal deterioration during this period. Her family should also be willing to provide physical and emotional support, and should be aware of the potential for deterioration in the mother's health and the potential for maternal mortality. In addition, the need for care of a potentially preterm growth-restricted neonate with all of its attendant morbidities and potential mortality should be discussed. Long-term, the woman and her family should also consider the fact that her life expectancy may be shortened by cystic fibrosis, and plans should be made for rearing of the child in the event of maternal death.

Management of the Pregnancy Complicated by Cystic Fibrosis

Care of the gravida with cystic fibrosis should be a coordinated, team effort. Physicians familiar with cystic fibrosis, its complications, and management should be included, as well as a maternal–fetal medicine specialist and neonatal team. The gravida should be assessed for potential risk factors such as severe lung disease, pulmonary hypertension, poor nutritional status, pancreatic failure, and liver disease, preferably prior to attempting gestation, but certainly during the early

months of pregnancy. Gravidas should be advised to be 90 percent of ideal body weight prior to conception if possible. A weight gain of 11 to 12 kg is recommended.[182] Frequent monitoring of weight, blood glucose, hemoglobin, total protein, serum albumin, prothrombin time, and fat-soluble vitamins A and E is suggested.[182] At each visit, the history of caloric intake and symptoms of maldigestion and malabsorption should be taken, and pancreatic enzymes should be adjusted if needed. Patients who are unable to achieve adequate weight gain through oral nutritional supplements may be given nocturnal enteral nasogastric tube feeding. In this situation, the risk of aspiration should be considered, especially in patients with a history of gastroesophageal reflux, which is common in cystic fibrosis.[182] If malnutrition is severe, parenteral hyperalimentation may be necessary for successful completion of the pregnancy.[209] Baseline pulmonary function should be assessed, preferably prior to conception. Assessment should include FVC, FEV_1, lung volumes, pulse oximetry, and arterial blood gases if indicated. These values should be serially monitored during gestation and deterioration in pulmonary function addressed immediately. An echocardiogram can assess the patient for pulmonary hypertension and cor pulmonale. If pulmonary hypertension (cor pulmonale) is diagnosed, the gravida should be advised of the high maternal risk.

Early recognition and prompt treatment of pulmonary infections are important in the management of the pregnant woman with cystic fibrosis. Treatment includes intravenous antibiotics in the appropriate dose, keeping in mind the increased clearance of these drugs secondary to pregnancy and cystic fibrosis. Plasma levels of aminoglycosides should be monitored and adjusted as indicated. Chest physical therapy and bronchial drainage are also important components of the management of pulmonary infections in cystic fibrosis. Because *Pseudomonas aeruginosa* is the most frequently isolated bacteria associated with chronic endobronchitis and bronchiectasis, antibiotic regimens should include coverage for this organism.

If the patient with cystic fibrosis has pancreatic insufficiency and diabetes mellitus, careful monitoring of blood glucose and insulin therapy are indicated. As previously mentioned, pancreatic enzymes may need to be replaced in order to optimize the patient's nutritional status. Because of malabsorption of fats and frequent use of antibiotics, the cystic fibrosis patient is prone to vitamin K deficiency. Therefore, prothrombin time should be checked regularly, and parenteral vitamin K should be administered if the prothrombin time is elevated.

It is imperative when managing pregnancy in a woman with cystic fibrosis to recognize that the fetus is at risk for uteroplacental insufficiency and intrauterine growth restriction. The maternal nutritional status and weight gain during pregnancy will likewise impact fetal growth. Therefore, fundal height should be measured routinely, and serial ultrasound evaluations of fetal growth and amniotic fluid volume should be made. Maternal kick counts may be useful for monitoring fetal status starting at 28 weeks. Nonstress testing should be started at 32 weeks or sooner, if there is evidence of fetal compromise. If there is evidence of severe fetal compromise such as no interval fetal growth, persistent decelerations, or poor biophysical profile scoring, delivery should be accomplished. Likewise, evidence of profound maternal deterioration such as a marked and sustained decline in pulmonary function, development of right-sided heart failure, refractory hypoxemia, and progressive hypercapnea and respiratory acidosis may be maternal indications for early delivery. If the fetus is potentially viable, the administration of betamethasone may be beneficial. Vaginal delivery should be attempted when possible.

Labor, delivery, and the postpartum period can be particularly dangerous for the patient with cystic fibrosis. The augmentation in cardiac output stresses the cardiovascular system and can lead to cardiopulmonary failure in the patient with pulmonary hypertension and cor pulmonale. These patients are also more likely to develop right-sided heart failure. Heart failure should be treated with aggressive diuresis and supplemental oxygen. Management may be optimized by insertion of a pulmonary artery catheter to monitor right- and left-sided filling pressures. Pain control will reduce the sympathetic response to labor and tachycardia. This will benefit the patient who is demonstrating pulmonary or cardiac compromise. In the patient with a normal PTT, insertion of an epidural catheter for continuous epidural analgesia may be beneficial. This is also useful in the event a cesarean delivery is indicated, as general anesthesia and its possible effects on pulmonary function can be avoided. If general anesthesia is needed, preoperative anticholinergic agents should be avoided because they tend to promote drying and inspissation of airway secretions. Close fetal surveillance is also extremely important, as the fetus who may have been suffering from uteroplacental insufficiency during gestation will be more prone to develop evidence of fetal compromise during labor. Delivery by cesarean section should be reserved for the usual obstetric indications.

In summary, more women with cystic fibrosis are living to childbearing age and are capable of conceiving. Clinical experience thus far has demonstrated that pregnancy in women with cystic fibrosis and mild disease is well tolerated. Women with severe disease have an associated increase in maternal and fetal morbidity and mortality. The potential risk to any individual with cystic fibrosis desirous of pregnancy should be assessed and discussed with the patient and her family in detail.

Key Points

➤ Pneumonia is the most common nonobstetric infection to cause maternal mortality. Preterm delivery complicates pneumonia in up to 43 percent of cases. *Streptococcus pneumoniae* is the most common bacterial pathogen to cause pneumonia. Empiric antibiotic coverage should be started, including a third-generation cephalosporin and a macrolide, such as azithromycin, to cover atypical pathogens.

➤ High-risk gravidas should be screened for tuberculosis and treated appropriately with INH prophylaxis for infection without overt disease and with dual antituberculosis therapy for active disease. If resistant tuberculosis is identified, ethambutol 2.5 g/day should be added to therapy and the treatment period should be extended to 18 months.

➤ Asthma is characterized by chronic airway inflammation with increased airway responsiveness to a variety of stimuli and airway obstruction that is partially or completely reversible. Patients with severe asthma have the greatest risk for complications during pregnancy. Complications include preeclampsia, asthma exacerbation, preterm rupture of the membranes, increased perinatal mortality, prematurity, and low birth weight. Therapy should include education, bronchodilators, and the addition of inhaled steroids.

➤ Asthma medications should be continued during labor and delivery. PEFR should be measured on admission and at 12-hour intervals. If systemic corticosteroids have been used in the previous 4 weeks, hydrocortisone (100 mg every 8 hours) should be administered during labor and for the 24-hour period following delivery to prevent adrenal crisis.

➤ Thromboembolic disease is the leading cause of pregnancy-related mortality in the United States. An untreated deep vein thrombosis (DVT) is associated with a 15 to 25 percent incidence of pulmonary embolus with a 12 to 15 percent mortality rate. Pregnancy is accompanied by a hypercoagulable state. Hypercoagulable conditions, such as AT-III deficiency, prothrombin 20210A allele, protein C deficiency, protein S deficiency, factor V Leiden, dysfibrinogenemia, hyperhomosystenemia, and the antiphospholipid syndrome may increase the risk of deep vein thrombosis and pulmonary embolus.

➤ Investigation for deep vein thrombosis in pregnancy should include impedance plethysmography, venous Doppler ultrasound, real-time ultrasound, and venography. ^{125}I fibrinogen scanning should be avoided during pregnancy because of high levels of fetal radiation exposure and concentration of the radiolabeled iodine in the fetal thyroid.

➤ A high index of suspicion for pulmonary embolus is necessary. Diagnosis should be undertaken with venous Doppler ultrasound of the extremities to identify a DVT and V/Q scanning and pulmonary arteriography if indicated.

➤ Therapy for thrombosis and pulmonary embolus in pregnancy should be accomplished with heparin. Coumadin may be used in the postpartum period. The aPTT and/or INR should be monitored closely.

➤ The interstitial lung diseases include idiopathic pulmonary fibrosis, sarcoidosis, hypersensity pneumonitis, pneumonosis, drug-induced lung disease, and connective tissue disease. Restrictive lung disease is generally well tolerated in pregnancy; however, exercise intolerance and need for oxygen supplementation may develop. Gravidas with pulmonary hypertension complicating restrictive lung disease may suffer a high mortality.

➤ An increasing number of women with cystic fibrosis are surviving to the reproductive years and usually maintain their fertility with meticulous management of pulmonary function, including pulmonary toilet and aggressive surveillance for signs of pulmonary infection and treatment of antibiotics in adequate doses. Close attention to nutrition is required secondary to maldigestion, malabsorption, and malnutrition, which can complicate cystic fibrosis. Gravidas with good clinical studies, good nutritional status, nearly normal chest radiographs, and only mild obstructive lung disease will tolerate pregnancy well. Fetal growth should be monitored closely.

REFERENCES

1. Oxorn H: The changing aspects of pneumonia complicating pregnancy. Am J Obstet Gynecol 70:1057, 1955.
2. Madinger NE, Greenspoon JS, Gray-Ellrodt A: Pneumonia during pregnancy: has modern technology improved maternal and fetal outcome? Am J Obstet Gynecol 161:657, 1989.
3. Kaunitz AM, Hughes JM, Grimes DA, et al: Causes of maternal mortality in the United States. Obstet Gynecol 65:605, 1985.
4. Finland M, Dublin TD: Pneumococcic pneumonias complicating pregnancy and the puerperium. JAMA 112:1027, 1939.
5. Benedetti TJ, Valle R, Ledger W: Antepartum pneumonia in pregnancy. Am J Obstet Gynecol 144:413, 1982.
6. Berkowitz K, LaSala A: Risk factors associated with the increasing prevalence of pneumonia during pregnancy. Am J Obstet Gynecol 163:981, 1990.
7. Koonin LM, Ellerbrock TV, Atrash HK, et al: Pregnancy-associated deaths due to AIDS in the United States. JAMA 261:1306, 1989.
8. Dinsmoor MJ: HIV infection and pregnancy. Med Clin North Am 73:701, 1989.
9. Hopwood HG: Pneumonia in pregnancy. Obstet Gynecol 25:875, 1965.
10. Rodrigues J, Niederman MS: Pneumonia complicating pregnancy. Clin Chest Med 13:679, 1992.
11. Haake DA, Zakowski PC, Haake DL, et al: Early treatment with acyclovir for varicella pneumonia in otherwise healthy adults: retrospective controlled study and review. Rev Infect Dis 12:788, 1990.
12. McKinney WP, Volkert P, Kaufman J: Fatal swine influenza pneumonia during late pregnancy. Arch Intern Med 150:213, 1990.
13. American College of Obstetricians and Gynecologists: Pulmonary disease in pregnancy. ACOG Technical Bulletin 224. Washington, DC, ACOG, 1996.
14. Tomlinson MW, Caruthers TJ, Whitty JE, Gonik B: Does delivery improve maternal condition in the respiratory-compromised gravida? Obstet Gynecol 91:108, 1998.
15. National Center for Health Statistics: National hospital discharge survey: annual summary 1990. Vital Health Stat 13:1, 1992.
16. Hollingsworth HM, Pratter MR, Irwin RS: Acute respiratory failure in pregnancy. J Intensive Care Med 4:11, 1989.
17. Kirshon B, Faro S, Zurawin RK, et al: Favorable outcome after treatment with amantadine and ribavirin in a pregnancy complicated by influenza pneumonia: a case report. J Reprod Med 33:399, 1988.
18. Cox SM, Cunningham FG, Luby J: Management of varicella pneumonia complicating pregnancy. Am J Perinatol 7:300, 1990.
19. Esmonde TG, Herdman G, Anderson G: Chickenpox pneumonia: an association with pregnancy. Thorax 44:812, 1989.
20. Smego RA, Asperilla MO: Use of acyclovir for varicella pneumonia during pregnancy. Obstet Gynecol 78:1112, 1991.
21. Harris RE, Rhades ER: Varicella pneumonia complicating pregnancy: report of a case and review of literature. Obstet Gynecol 25:734, 1965.
22. Andrews EB, Yankaskas BC, Cordero JF, et al: Acyclovir in pregnancy registry: six years' experience. Obstet Gynecol 79:7, 1992.
23. Brown ZA, Baker DA: Acyclovir therapy during pregnancy. Obstet Gynecol 73:526, 1989.
24. Centers for Disease Control and Prevention: Initial therapy for tuberculosis in the era of multidrug resistance—recommendations of the advisory council for the elimination of tuberculosis. MMWR Morb Mortal Wkly Rep 42(RR-7):1, 1993.
25. Frieden TR, Sterling T, Pablos-Mendez A, et al: The emergence of drug-resistant tuberculosis in New York City. N Engl J Med 328:521, 1993.

26. Cantwell MF, Shehab AM, Costello AM: Brief report: congenital tuberculosis. N Engl J Med 330:1051, 1994.

27. Margono F, Mroveh J, Garely A, et al: Resurgence of active tuberculosis among pregnant women. Obstet Gynecol 83:911, 1994.

28. Centers for Disease Control and Prevention: The use of preventive therapy for tuberculosis infection in the United States. MMWR 39:9, 1990.

29. Griffith DE: Mycobacteria as pathogens of respiratory infection. Infect Dis Clin North Am 12:593, 1998.

30. American Thoracic Society Workshop: Rapid diagnostic tests for tuberculosis—what is the appropriate use? Am J Respir Crit Care Med 155:1804, 1997.

31. Barnes PF: Rapid diagnostic tests for tuberculosis, progress but no gold standard. Am J Respir Crit Care Med 155:1497, 1997.

32. Centers for Disease Control and Prevention: The role of BCG vaccine in the prevention and control of tuberculosis in the United states: a joint statement by the Advisory Council for the Elimination of Tuberculosis and the Advisory Committee on Immunization Practices. MMWR Morb Mortal Wkly Rep 45:1, 1996.

33. Good JT, Iseman MD, Davidson PT, et al: Tuberculosis in association with pregnancy. Am J Obstet Gynecol 140:492, 1081.

34. American Thoracic Society: Mycobacteriosis and the acquired immunodeficiency syndrome. Am Rev Respir Dis 136:492, 1987.

35. Hamadeh MA, Glassroth J: Tuberculosis and pregnancy. Chest 101:1114, 1992.

36. Jana N, Vasishta K, Saha SC, Ghosh K: Obstetrical outcomes among women with extrapulmonary tuberculosis. N Engl J Med 341:645, 1999.

37. Vallejo JC, Starke JR: Tuberculosis and pregnancy. Clin Chest Med 13:693, 1992.

38. Riley L: Pneumonia and tuberculosis in pregnancy. Infect Dis Clin North Am 11:119, 1997.

39. Robinson CA, Rose NC: Tuberculosis: current implications and management in obstetrics. Obstet Gynecol Surv 51:115, 1999.

40. Fox CW, George RB: Current concepts in the management and prevention of tuberculosis in adults. J La State Med Soc 144:363, 1992.

41. Van Rie A, Warren R, Richardson M, et al: Classification of drug-resistant tuberculosis in an epidemic area. Lancet 356:22, 2000.

42. Robinson GC, Cambion K: Hearing loss in infants of tuberculosis mothers treated with streptomycin during pregnancy. N Engl J Med 271:949, 1964.

43. Rendig EK Jr: The place of BCG vaccine in the management of infants born to tuberculosis mothers. N Engl J Med 281:520, 1969.

44. Schatz M, Zeiger RS, Hoffman CP: Intrauterine growth is related to gestational pulmonary function in pregnant asthmatic women. Kaiser-Permanente Asthma and Pregnancy Study Grp. Chest 98:389, 1990.

45. National Asthma Education Program: Management of asthma during pregnancy. Report of the Working Group on Asthma and Pregnancy, September 1993, NIH Publication No 93-3279.

46. Mabie WC, Barton JR, Wasserstrum N, et al: Clinical observations and asthma in pregnancy. J Matern Fetal Med 1:45, 1992.

47. Perlow JH, Montgomery D, Morgan MA, et al: Severity of asthma and perinatal outcome. Am J Obstet Gynecol 167:963, 1992.

48. Schatz M, Zeiger RS, Harden KM, et al: The safety of inhaled β-agonist bronchodilators during pregnancy. J Allergy Clin Immunol 82:686, 1988.

49. Schatz M, Zeiger R, Hoffman C, et al: Perinatal outcomes in the pregnancies of asthmatic women: a prospective controlled analysis. Am J Respir Crit Care Med 151:1170, 1995.

50. Dombrowski MP, Bottoms SF, Boike GM, et al: Incidence of preeclampsia among asthmatic patients lower with theophylline. Am J Obstet Gynecol 155:265, 1986.

51. National Asthma Education Program: Guidelines for the diagnosis and management of asthma. Expert Panel Report, August 1991, NIH Publication No. 91-3042.

52. Greenberger PA, Patterson R: The outcome of pregnancy complicated by severe asthma. Allergy Proc 9:539, 1988.

53. Dombrowski MP: Should the definitions of asthma severity be modified during pregnancy? Am J Obstet Gynecol poster #541 (in press).

54. Nolten W, Rueckert P: Elevated free cortisol index in pregnancy: possible regulatory mechanisms. Am J Obstet Gynecol 139:492, 1981.

55. Bailey K, Herrod H, Younger R, et al: Functional aspects of T-lymphocyte subsets in pregnancy. Obstet Gynecol 66:211, 1985.

56. Briggs GG, Freeman RK, Yaffe SJ: In Drugs in Pregnancy and Lactation, 3rd ed. Baltimore, Williams & Wilkins, 1990, p 237, 520.

57. Reinisch JM, Simon NG, Karow WG, Gandelman R: Prenatal exposure to prednisone in humans and animals retards intrauterine growth. Science 202:436, 1978.

58. Pirson Y, Van Lierde M, Ghysen J, et al: Retardation of fetal growth in patients receiving immunosuppressive therapy [letter]. N Engl J Med 313:328, 1985.

59. Salmeron S, Guerin JC, Godard P, et al: High doses of inhaled corticosteroids in unstable chronic asthma. A multicenter, double-blind, placebo-controlled study. Am Rev Respir Dis 140:167, 1989.

60. Dutoit JI, Salome CM, Woolcock AJ: Inhaled cortocosteriods reduce the severity of bronchial hyperresponsiveness in asthma but oral theophylline does not. Am Rev Respir Dis 136:1174, 1987.

61. Shapiro GG, Konig P: Cromolyn sodium: a review. Pharmacotherapy 5:156, 1985.

62. Cockcroft DW, Murdock KY: Comparative effects of inhaled salbutamol, sodium cromoglycate, and beclomethasone dipropionate on allergen-induced early asthmatic responses, last asthmatic responses, and increased bronchial responsiveness to histamine. J Allergy Clin Immunol 79:734, 1987.

63. Haahtela T, Jarvinen M, Kava T, et al: Comparison of β-agonist, terbutalline, with an inhaled corticosteroid, budesonide, in newly detected asthma. N Engl J Med 325:338, 1991.

64. Ernst P, Spetzer WO, Suissa S, et al: Risk of fatal and near-fatal asthma in relation to inhaled coriticosteroid use. JAMA 268:3462, 1992.

65. Kraan J, Koeter GH, Van Der Mark THW, et al: Dosage and time effects of inhaled budesonide on bronchial hyperactivity. Am Rev Respir Dis 137:44, 1988.

66. Woolcock AJ, Yan K, Salome CM: Effects of therapy on bronchial hyperresponsiveness in the long-term management of asthma. Clin Allergy 18:165, 1988.

67. Lowhagen O, Rak S: Modification of bronchial hyperreactivity after treatment with sodium cromoglycate during pollen season. J Allergy Clin Immunol 75:460, 1985.

68. Woolcock AJ, Jenkins C: Corticosteroids in the modulation of bronchial hyperresponsiveness. Immunol Allergy Clin North Am 10:543, 1990.

69. Svendsen UG, Frolund L, Madsen F, et al: A comparison of

the effects of sodium cromoglycate and beclomethasone dipropionate on pulmonary function and bronchial hyperreactivity in subjects with asthma. J Allergy Clin Immunol 80:68, 1987.

70. Groot CAR, Lammers J-WJ, Molema J, et al: Effect of inhaled beclomethasone and nedocromil sodium on bronchial hyperresponsiveness to histamine and distilled water. Eur Respir J 5:1075, 1992.

71. Stenius-Aarniala BSM, Hedman J, Teramo KA: Acute asthma during pregnancy. Thorax 51:411, 1996.

72. Kerrebijn KF: Use of topical corticosteroids in the treatment of childhood asthma. Am Rev Respir Dis 141:S77, 1990.

73. Geddes DM: Inhaled corticosteroids: benefits and risks. Thorax 47:404, 1992.

74. Tabachnik E, Zadik Z: Clinical and laboratory observations: diurnal cortisol secretion during therapy with inhaled beclomethasone dipropionate in children with asthma. J Pediatr 118:294, 1991.

75. Reid DM, Nicoll JJ, Smith MA, et al: Corticosteroids and bone mass in asthma: comparisons with rheumatoid arthritis and polymyalgia rheumatica. BMJ 293:1463, 1986.

76. Puolijoki H, Liippo K, Herrala J, et al: Inhaled beclomethasone decreases serum osteocalcin in postmenopausal asthmatic women. Bone 13:285, 1992.

77. Packe GE, Douglas JG, McDonald AF, et al: Bone density in asthmatic patients taking high dose inhaled beclomethasone dipropionate and intermittent systemic corticosteroids. Thorax 47:414, 1992.

78. Tinkelman DG, Reed CE, Nelson HS, et al: Aerosol beclomethasone dipropionate compared with theophylline as primary treatment of chronic, mild to moderately severe asthma in children. Pediatrics 92:64, 1993.

79. Doull IJM, Freezer JN, Holgate ST: Growth of prepubertal children with mild asthma treated with inhaled beclomethasone dipropionate. Am J Respir Crit Care Med 151:1715, 1995.

80. Thomas BC, Stanhope R, Grant DB: Impaired growth in children with asthma during treatment with conventional doses of inhaled corticosteroids. Acta Paediatr 83:196, 1994.

81. Lipworth BJ: Airway and systemic effects of inhaled corticosteroids in asthma: dose response relationship. Pulm Pharmacol 9:19, 1996.

82. Greenberger PA, Patterson R: Beclomethasone diproprionate for severe asthma during pregnancy. Ann Intern Med 98:478, 1983.

83. Fitzsimmons R, Greenberger PA, Patterson R: Outcome of pregnancy in women requiring corticosteroids for severe asthma. J Allergy Clin Immunol 78:349, 1986.

84. Wendel PJ, Ramin SM, Barnett-Hamm C, et al: Asthma treatment in pregnancy: a randomized controlled study. Am J Obstet Gynecol 175:150, 1996.

85. Dombrowski MP, Brown CL, Berry SM: Preliminary experience with triamcinolone acetonide during pregnancy. J Matern Fetal Med 5:310, 1996.

86. Zaborny BA, Lukacsko P, Barinov-Colligaon I, Ziemniak JA: Inhaled corticosteroids in asthma: a dose-proportionality study with triamcinolone acetonide aerosol. J Clin Pharmacol 32:463, 1992.

87. Kallen B, Fydhstroem H, Aberg A: Congenital malformations after use of inhaled budesonide in early pregnancy. Obstet Gynecol 93:392, 1999.

88. Evans DJ, Taylor DA, Zetterstrom O, et al: A comparison of low-dose inhaled budesonide plus theophylline and high-dose inhaled budesonide for moderate asthma. N Engl J Med 337:1412, 1997.

89. Allen DB, Bronsky EA, LaForce CF, et al: Growth in asthmatic children treated with fluticasone propionate. Fluticasone propionate asthma study group. J Pediatr 132:472, 1999.

90. Galant SP, Lawrence M, Meltzer EO, et al: Fluticasone propionate compared with theophylline for mild-to-moderate asthma. Ann Allery Asthma Immunol 77:112, 1996.

91. Brogden RN, Sorkin EM: Nedocromil sodium: an updated review of its pharmacological properties and therapeutic efficacy in asthma. Drugs 45:693, 1993.

92. Pauwels R, Van Renterghem D, Van Der Straeten M, et al: The effect of theophylline and enprofylline on allergen-induced bronchoconstriction. J Allergy Clin Immunol 76:583, 1985.

93. Juergens UR, Degenhardt V, Stober M, Vetter H: New insights in the bronchodilatory and anti-inflammatory mechanisms of action of theophylline. Arzneimittelforschung 49:694, 1999.

94. Arwood LL, Dasta JF, Friedman C: Placental transfer of theophylline: two case reports. Pediatrics 63:844, 1979.

95. Yeh TF, Pildes RS: Transplacental aminophylline toxicity in a neonate [letter]. Lancet 1:910, 1977.

96. Hendeles L, Jenkins J, Temple R: Revised FDA labeling guideline for theophylline oral dosage forms. Pharmacotherapy 15:409, 1995.

97. Joad JP, Ahrens RC, Lindgren SD, et al: Relative efficacy of maintenance therapy with theophylline, inhaled albuterol, and the combination for chronic asthma. J Allergy Clin Immunol 79:78, 1987.

98. Twentyman OP, Finnerty JP, Holgate ST: The inhibitory effect of nebulized albuterol on the early and late asthmatic reactions and increase in airway responsiveness provoked by inhaled allergen in asthma. Am Rev Respir Dis 144:782, 1991.

99. Sears MR, Taylor DR, Print CG, et al: Regular inhaled β-agonist treatment in bronchial asthma. Lancet 336:1391, 1990.

100. Spitzer WO, Suissa S, Ernst P, et al: The use of β-agonists and the risk of death and near death from asthma. N Engl J Med 326:501, 1992.

101. Knorr B, Matz J, Bernstein JA, et al: Montelukast for chronic asthma in 6 to 14 year old children. JAMA 279:1181, 1998.

102. Wenzel SE: New approaches to anti-inflammatory therapy for asthma. Am J Med 104:287, 1998.

103. Fanta CH, Rossing TH, McFadden ER: Treatment of acute asthma: is combination therapy with sympathomimetics and methylxanthines indicated? Am J Med 80:5, 1986.

104. Nelson HS, Spector SL, Whitsett TL, et al: The bronchodilator response to inhalation of increasing doses of aerosolized albuterol. J Allergy Clin Immunol 72:371, 1983.

105. Rossing TH, Fanta CH, McFadden ER, and the Medical House Staff of the Peter Bent Brigham Hospital: A controlled trial of the use of single versus combined drug therapy in the treatment of acute episodes of asthma. Am Rev Respir Dis 123:190, 1982.

106. Hägerdal M, Morgan CW, Sumner AE, et al: Minute ventilation and oxygen consumption during labor with epidural analgesia. Anesthesiology 59:425, 1983.

107. Fung DL: Emergency anesthesia for asthma patients. Clin Rev Allergy 3:127, 1985.

108. Hirshman CA, Downes H, Farbood A, et al: Ketamine block of bronchospasm in experimental canine asthma. Br J Anaesth 51:713, 1979.

109. American Academy of Pediatrics Committee on Drugs: Transfer of drugs and other chemicals into human milk. Pediatrics 84:924, 1989.

110. Arthure M: Maternal mortality. J Obstet Gynaecol Br Commonw 75:1309, 1968.

111. Koonin LM, Atrash HK, Lawson HW, Smith JC: Maternal mortality surveillance, United States, 1979–1986. MMWR CDC Surveill Summ 40:1, 1991.

112. National Institutes of Health: Consensus Development Conference. Prevention of venous thrombosis and pulmonary embolism. JAMA 256:744,1986.

113. Rutherford SE, Phelan JP: Thromboembolic disease in pregnancy. Clin Perinatol 13:719, 1988.

114. Sipes SSL, Weiner CP: Venous thromboembolic disease in pregnancy. Semin Perinatol 14:103, 1990.

115. Uszynski M, Abildgaard U: Separation and characterization of two fibrinolytic inhibitors from human placenta. Thromb Diath Haemorr 25:580, 1971.

116. Walker JE, Gow L, Campbell DM, et al: The inhibition by plasma of urokinase and tissue activator-induced fibrinolysis in pregnancy and the puerperium. Thromb Haemost 49:21, 1983.

117. Ballegeer V, Mombaerts P, Declerck PJ, et al: Fibrinolytic response to venous occlusion and fibrin fragment D-dimer levels in normal and complicated pregnancy. Thromb Haemost 38:1030, 1987.

118. Malm J, Lurell M, Dahlback B: Changes in the plasma levels of vitamin K-dependent proteins C and S and of C4b-binding protein during pregnancy and oral contraception. Br J Haematol 68:437, 1988.

119. Virchow R: Phlogose und thrombose in gefass-system. *In* Virchow R (ed): Gesamelte Abhandlungen Zur Wissenschaflichen Medecin. Frankfurt, Von Medinger Sohn, 1856, p 458.

120. De Boer JM, ten Cate JW, Sturk A, et al: Enhanced thrombin generation in normal and hypertensive pregnancy. Am J Obstet Gynecol 160:95, 1989.

121. Weiner CP, Sabbagha RE, Vaisrub N: Distinguishing preeclampsia from chronic hypertension using antithrombin III. Proceedings of the Society for Gynecologic Investigation, Washington, DC, 1983 (abstract 29).

122. Douglas JT, Shah M, Lowe GD, et al: Plasma fibrinopeptide A and betathromboglobulin levels in preeclampsia and hypertensive pregnancy. Thromb Haemost 47:54, 1982.

123. Weiner CP, Brandt J: Plasma antithrombin III activity: an aid in the diagnosis of preeclampsia-eclampsia. Am J Obstet Gynecol 142:275, 1982.

124. Kupferminc MJ, Eldor A, Steinman N, et al: Increased frequency of genetic thrombophilia in women with complications of pregnancy. N Engl J Med 340:9, 1999.

125. Bertina RM: Factor V Leiden and other coagulation factor mutations affecting thrombotic risk. Clin Chem 43:1678, 1997.

126. Rosenberg RD: Actions and interactions of antithrombin III and heparin. N Engl J Med 292:146, 1975.

127. Lane DA, Olds RJ, Boisclair M, et al: Antithrombin mutation database: first update. Thromb Haemost 70:361, 1993.

128. Hellgren M, Tengborn L, Abildgaard U: Pregnancy in women with congenital antithrombin III deficiency: experience of treatment with heparin and antithrombin. Gynecol Obstet Invest 14:127, 1982.

129. Poort SR, Rosendaal FR, Reitsma PH, Bertina RM: A common genetic variation in the 3′-untranslated region of the prothrombin gene is associated with elevated plasma prothrombin levels and an increase in venous thrombosis. Blood 88:3698, 1996.

130. Comp PC, Esmon CT: Evidence for multiple roles of activated protein C in fibrinolysis. *In* Mann KG, Taylor FB Jr (eds): The Regulation of Coagulation. New York, Elsevier/North Holland, 1980, p 583.

131. Marlar RA, Montgomery RR, Broekmans AW, et al: Diagnosis and treatment of homozygous protein C definiency: report of the working party on homozygous protein C deficiency of the subcommittee on protein C and protein S. International Committee on Thrombosis and Haemostasis. J Pediatr 114:528, 1989.

132. Marlar RA, Montgomery R, Broekmans AW: Diagnosis and treatment of homozygous protein C deficiency. J Pediatr 114:528, 1989.

133. Conard J, Horellou MH, van Dreden P, et al: Pregnancy and congenital deficiency in antithrombin III or protein C. Thromb Haemost 58:39, 1987.

134. Alach M, Gandrille S, Emmerich J: A review of mutations causing deficiencies of antithrombin, protein C and protein S. Thromb Haemost 74:81, 1995.

135. Bertina RM, Koeleman BP, Koster T, et al: Mutation in blood coagulation factor V associated with resistance to activated protein C. Nature 369:64, 1994.

136. Rosendaal FR, Koster T, Vandenbroucke JP, Reitsma PH: High risk of thrombosis in patients homozygous for factor V Leiden (APC resistance). Blood 85:1505, 1995.

137. Mammen EF: Congenital coagulation disorders. Semin Thromb Hemost 9:1, 1983.

138. Den Heijer M, Koster T, Blom HJ, et al: Hyperhomocysteinemia as a risk factor for deep-vein thrombosis. N Engl J Med 334:759, 1996.

139. Graham IM, Daly LE, Refsum HM, et al: Plasma homocysteine as a risk factor for vascular disease: the European concerted action project. JAMA 277:1775, 1997.

140. Froost P, Blom HJ, Milos R, et al: A candidate genetic risk factor for vascular disease: a common mutation in methylene-tetrahydrofolate reductase. Nat Genet 10:111, 1995.

141. Loscalzo J: The oxidant stress of hyperhomocyst(e)inemia. J Clin Invest 98:5, 1996.

142. Goddijn-Wessel TA, Wouters MG, van de Molen EF, et al: Hyperthomucysteinemia: a risk factor for placental abruption or infarction. Eur J Obstet Gynecol Reprod Biol 66:23, 1996.

143. Reece EA, Romero R, Clyne LP, et al: Lupus-like anticoagulant in pregnancy. Lancet 1:344, 1984.

144. Rai R, Regan L: Obstetric complications of antiphospholipid antibodies. Curr Opin Obstet Gynecol 9:387, 1997.

145. Rai RS, Clifford K, Cohen H, Regan L: High prospective fetal loss rate in untreated pregnancies of women with recurrent miscarriage and antiphospholipid antibodies. Hum Reprod 10:3301, 1995.

146. American College of Obstetricians and Gynecologists: Antiphospholipid syndrome. ACOG Technical Bulletin 244. Washington, DC, ACOG, 1998.

147. Alving B: Update on recognition and management of patients with acquired or inherited hypercoagulability. Comp Ther 24:302, 1998.

148. Douketis JD, Ginsberg JS: Diagnostic problems with venous thromboembolic disease in pregnancy. Haemostasis 25:58, 1995.

149. Ginsberg JS, Hirsh J, Rainbow AJ, Coates G: Risks to the fetus of radiologic procedures used in the diagnosis of maternal venous thromboembolic disease. Thromb Haemost 61:189, 1989.

150. Napodani RJ: Deep vein thrombosis. *In* Panzer RJ, Black ER, Griner PF (eds): Diagnostic Strategies for Common Medical Problems. Philadelphia, American College of Physicians, 1991, p 84.

151. Markisz JA: Radiologic and nuclear medicine diagnosis. *In* Goldhaber SZ (ed): Pulmonary Embolism and Deep Venous Thrombosis. Philadelphia, WB Saunders Company, 1985.

152. Nicholas GG, Lorenz RP, Botti JJ, et al: The frequent occurrence of false-positive results in phleborrheography during pregnancy. Surg Gynecol Obstet 161:133, 1985.

153. Fell G, Standness DE: Diagnosis and management of acute venous thrombosis. Clin Obstet Gynecol 24:761, 1981.

154. Raghavendra BN, Rosen RJ, Lam S, et al: Deep vein thrombosis: detection by high-resolution real-time ultrasonography. Radiology 152:789, 1984.

155. Robin ED: Overdiagnosis and overtreatment of pulmonary embolism: the emperor may have no clothes. Ann Intern Med 87:775, 1977.

156. National Council on Radiation Protection and Measurements: Medical Radiation Exposure of Pregnant and Potentially Pregnant Women. Washington, DC, 1977.

157. Basu D, Gallus A, Hirsh J, et al: A prospective study of the value of monitoring heparin treatment with the activated partial thromboplastin time. N Engl J Med 287:324, 1972.

158. American College of Obstetricians and Gynecologists: Thromboembolism in pregnancy. ACOG Technical Bulletin #234. Washington, DC, ACOG, 1997.

159. Basu D, Gallus A, Hirsh J, Cade J: A prospective study of the value of monitoring heparin treatment with activated partial thromboplastin time. N Engl J Med 287:324, 1972.

160. Dahlman T, Lindvall N, Hellgren M: Osteopenia in pregnancy during long-term heparin treatment: a radiologic study post partum. Br J Obstet Gynaecol 97:221, 1990.

161. Chong BH: Heparin-induced thrombocytopenia. Br J Haematol 89:431, 1995.

162. Sturridge F, deSwiet M, Letsky E: The use of low molecular weight heparin for thromboprophylaxis in pregnancy. Br J Obstet Gynaecol 101:69, 1994.

163. Schulman S, Rhedin AS, Lindmarker P, et al: A comparison of six weeks with six months of oral anticoagulant therapy after a first episode of venous thromboembolism. N Engl J Med 332:1661, 1995.

164. Hellgren M: Thromboembolism and pregnancy. Studies on blood coagulation, fibrinolysis, and treatment with heparin and antithrombin. Stockholm, Karolinska Institute, 1981 (thesis).

165. Bonnar J: Venous thromboembolism and pregnancy. *In* Stallworthy J, Bourne G (eds): Recent Advances in Obstetrics and Gynaecology. London, Churchill Livingstone, 1979, p 173.

166. Sherry S: Low dose heparin and prophylaxis for postoperative venous thromboembolism. N Engl J Med 293:300, 1975.

167. Weiner CP: The treatment of clotting disorders during pregnancy. *In* Sciarra JJ (ed): Gynecology and Obstetrics, Vol 3. Philadelphia, JB Lippincott, 1988, p 1.

168. Vogel JJ, de Moerloose PA, Bounameaux H: Protein C deficiency and pregnancy: a case report. Obstet Gynecol 73:455, 1989.

169. Brenner B, Shapira A, Bahari C, et al: Hereditary protein C deficiency during pregnancy. Am J Obstet Gynecol 157:1160, 1987.

170. Delclos GL, Davila F: Thrombolytic therapy for pulmonary embolism in pregnancy: a case report. Am J Obstet Gynecol 155:375, 1986.

171. Kramer WB, Belfort M, Saade GR, et al: Successful urokinase treatment of massive pulmonary embolism in pregnancy. Obstet Gynecol 86:660, 1995.

172. Kempczinski RF: Surgical prophylaxis of pulmonary embolism. Chest 89:384S, 1986.

173. Hux CH, Wapner RJ, Chayen B, et al: Use of the Greenfield filter for thromboembolic disease in pregnancy. Am J Obstet Gynecol 155:734, 1986.

174. West JB: Pulmonary pathophysiology. *In* Pulmonary Pathophysiology. Baltimore, Williams & Wilkins, 1978, p 92.

175. King TE Jr: Restrictive lung disease in pregnancy. Clin Chest Med 13:607, 1992.

176. Boggess KA, Easterling TR, Raghu G: Management and outcome of pregnant women with interstitial and restrictive lung disease. Am J Obstet Gynecol 173:1007, 1995.

177. Agha FP, Vade A, Amendola MA, Cooper RF: Effects of pregnancy on sarcoidosis. Surg Gynecol Obstet 155:817, 1982.

178. Haynes de Regt R: Sarcoidosis and pregnancy. Obstet Gynecol 70:369, 1987.

179. Maycock RL, Sullivan RD, Greening RR, et al: Sarcoidosis and pregnancy. JAMA 164:158, 1957.

180. Reisfield DR: Boeck's sarcoid and pregnancy. Am J Obstet Gynecol 75:795, 1958.

181. Scadding JG: Sarcoidosis. London, Eyre & Spottiswoode, 1967, p 519.

182. Hilman BC, Aitken ML, Constantinescu M: Pregnancy in patients with cystic fibrosis. Clin Obstet Gynecol 39:70, 1996.

183. Kerem B, Rommens JM, Buchanan JA, et al: Identification of the cystic fibrosis gene: genetic analysis. Science 245:1073, 1989.

184. Riordan JR, Rommens JM, Kerem B, et al: Identification of the cystic fibrosis gene: cloning and characterization of complementary DNA. Science 245:1066, 1989.

185. Rommens JM, Iannuzzi MC, Kerem B, et al: Identification of the cystic fibrosis gene: chromosome walking and jumping. Science 245:1059, 1989.

186. Kotloff RM, FitzSimmons SC, Fiel SB: Fertility and pregnancy in patients with cystic fibrosis. Clin Chest Med 13:623, 1992.

187. Kopito LE, Kosasky HJ, Shwachman H: Water and electrolytes in cervical mucus from patients with cystic fibrosis. Fertil Steril 24:512, 1973.

188. Siegel B, Siegel S: Pregnancy and delivery in a patient with CF of the pancreas; report of a case. Obstet Gynecol 16:439, 1960.

189. Grand RJ, Talamo RC, di Sant' Agnese PA, et al: Pregnancy in cystic fibrosis of the pancreas. JAMA 195:993, 1966.

190. Cohen LF, di Sant' Agnese PA, Friedlander J: Cystic fibrosis and pregnancy: a national survey. Lancet 2:842, 1980.

191. Weinberger SE, Weiss ST, Cohen WR, et al: Pregnancy and the lung. Am Rev Respir Dis 121:559, 1980.

192. McAnulty JH, Metcalfe J, Ueland K: Cardiovascular disease. *In* Burrow GN, Ferris TF (eds): Medical Complications During Pregnancy, 3rd ed. Philadelphia, WB Saunders Company, 1988.

193. Gleicher N, Midwall J, Hochberger D, et al: Eisenmenger's syndrome and pregnancy. Obstet Gynecol Surv 34:721, 1979.

194. Rush D, Johnstone FD, King JC: Nutrition and pregnancy. *In* Burrows GN, Ferris TF (eds): Medical Complications During Pregnancy, 3rd ed. Philadelphia, WB Saunders Company, 1988.

195. Novy MJ, Tyler JM, Shwachman H, et al: Cystic fibrosis and pregnancy. Report of a case with a study of pulmonary function and arterial blood gases. Obstet Gynecol 30:530, 1967.

196. Palmer J, Dillon-Baker C, Tecklin JS, et al: Pregnancy in patients with cystic fibrosis. Ann Intern Med 99:596, 1983.

197. Corkey CWB, Newth CJL, Corey M, et al: Pregnancy in cystic fibrosis: a better prognosis in patients with pancreatic function. Am J Obstet Gynecol 140:737, 1981.

198. Canny GJ, Corey M, Livingstone RA, et al: Pregnancy and cystic fibrosis. Obstet Gynecol 77:850, 1991.

199. Kent NE, Farquharson DF: Cystic fibrosis in pregnancy. Can Med Assoc J 149:809, 1993.

200. Edenborough FP, Stableforth DE, Webb AK, et al: Outcome of pregnancy in women with cystic fibrosis. Thorax 50:170, 1995.

201. Olson GL: Cystic fibrosis in pregnancy. Semin Perinatol 21:307, 1997.

202. Heikkila A, Erkkola R: Review of β-lactam antibiotics in pregnancy: the need for adjustment of dosage schedules. Clin Pharmacokinet 27:49, 1994.

203. Jusko WJ, Mosovich LL, Gerbracht LM, et al: Enhanced renal excretion of dicloxacillin in patients with cystic fibrosis. Pediatrics 56:1038, 1975.

204. Yaffe SJ, Gerbracht LM, Mosovich LL, et al: Pharmacokinetics of methicillin in patients with cystic fibrosis. J Infect Dis 135:828, 1977.

205. Spino M, Chai RP, Isles AF, et al: Cloxacillin absorption and disposition in cystic fibrosis. J Pediatr 105:829, 1984.

206. De Groot R, Smith AL: Antibiotic pharmacokinetics in cystic fibrosis: differences and clinical significance. Clin Pharmacokinet 13:228, 1987.

207. MacDonald NE, Anas NG, Peterson RG, et al: Renal clearance of gentamicin in cystic fibrosis. J Pediatr 103:985, 1983.

208. Lemna WK, Feldman GL, Kerem B, et al: Mutation analysis for heterozygote detection and the prenatal diagnosis of cystic fibrosis. N Engl J Med 322:291, 1990.

209. Cole BN, Seltzer MH, Kassabian J, et al: Parenteral nutrition in a pregnant cystic fibrosis patient. JPEN J Parenter Enteral Nutr 11:205, 1987.

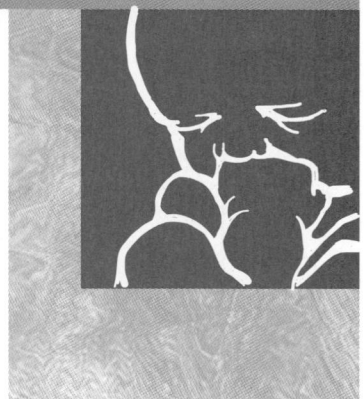

Chapter 31

Renal Disease

PHILIP SAMUELS AND DAVID F. COLOMBO

Of all the organ systems in the human body, one could argue that none are altered more in pregnancy than the kidney and urinary collecting system. Prior to the 1970s, patients with preexisting renal disease were strongly discouraged from even attempting pregnancy secondary to the expectation of increased perinatal morbidity and mortality and the likelihood of progression of renal disease. Currently, through our better understanding of renal disease in pregnancy, most of these women can look forward to a good outcome. This holds true even for women who have undergone a renal transplant.

This chapter discusses the normal changes in the kidney and urinary collecting system in pregnancy, the basic evaluation of renal status, acute and chronic renal disorders in pregnancy, and the treatment of the renal transplant patient.

ALTERED RENAL PHYSIOLOGY IN PREGNANCY

Pregnancy is associated with significant anatomic changes in the kidney and its collecting system (see Chapter 3). These changes begin to occur shortly after conception and may persist for several months postpartum.[1,2] The kidney itself is noted to increase in size and weight during the course of a pregnancy. Of more clinical significance is the marked dilatation of the collecting system including both the renal pelvis and ureters. This dilatation is most often greater on the right than on the left (Fig. 31–1). Etiologies for this change include hormonal changes (i.e., progesterone, endothelin, relaxin) and mechanical obstruction by the uterus itself.[3–5]

Renal plasma flow (RPF) increases greatly during pregnancy.[6] It peaks in the first trimester and, although it decreases near term, remains higher than in the nonpregnant patient. This change is due in part to increased cardiac output and decreased renal vascular resistance. The glomerular filtration rate (GFR) increases by 50 percent during a normal gestation.[7] It rises early in pregnancy and remains elevated through delivery. The percentage increase in GFR is greater than the percentage increase in RPF. This elevation of the filtration fraction leads to a fall in the blood urea nitrogen (BUN) and serum creatinine values.

Because GFR increases to such a great degree, electrolytes, glucose, and other filtered substances reach the renal tubules in greater amounts. The kidney handles sodium efficiently, reabsorbing most of the filtered load in the proximal convoluted tubule. Glucose reabsorption, however, does not increase proportionately during pregnancy. The average renal threshold for glucose is reduced to 155 mg/dl from 194 mg/dl in the nonpregnant individual.[8] Therefore, glycosuria can be seen in the normal gravida.

Urate is handled by filtration and secretion. Its clearance increases early in pregnancy, leading to lower serum levels of uric acid. In late pregnancy, urate clearance and serum urate levels return to their prepregnancy values. Serum urate levels are elevated in patients with preeclampsia. Whether this is due to decreased RPF, hemoconcentration, renal tubular dysfunction, or other renal circulatory changes remains uncertain. A summary of the renal changes in normal pregnancy is shown in Table 31–1.[9]

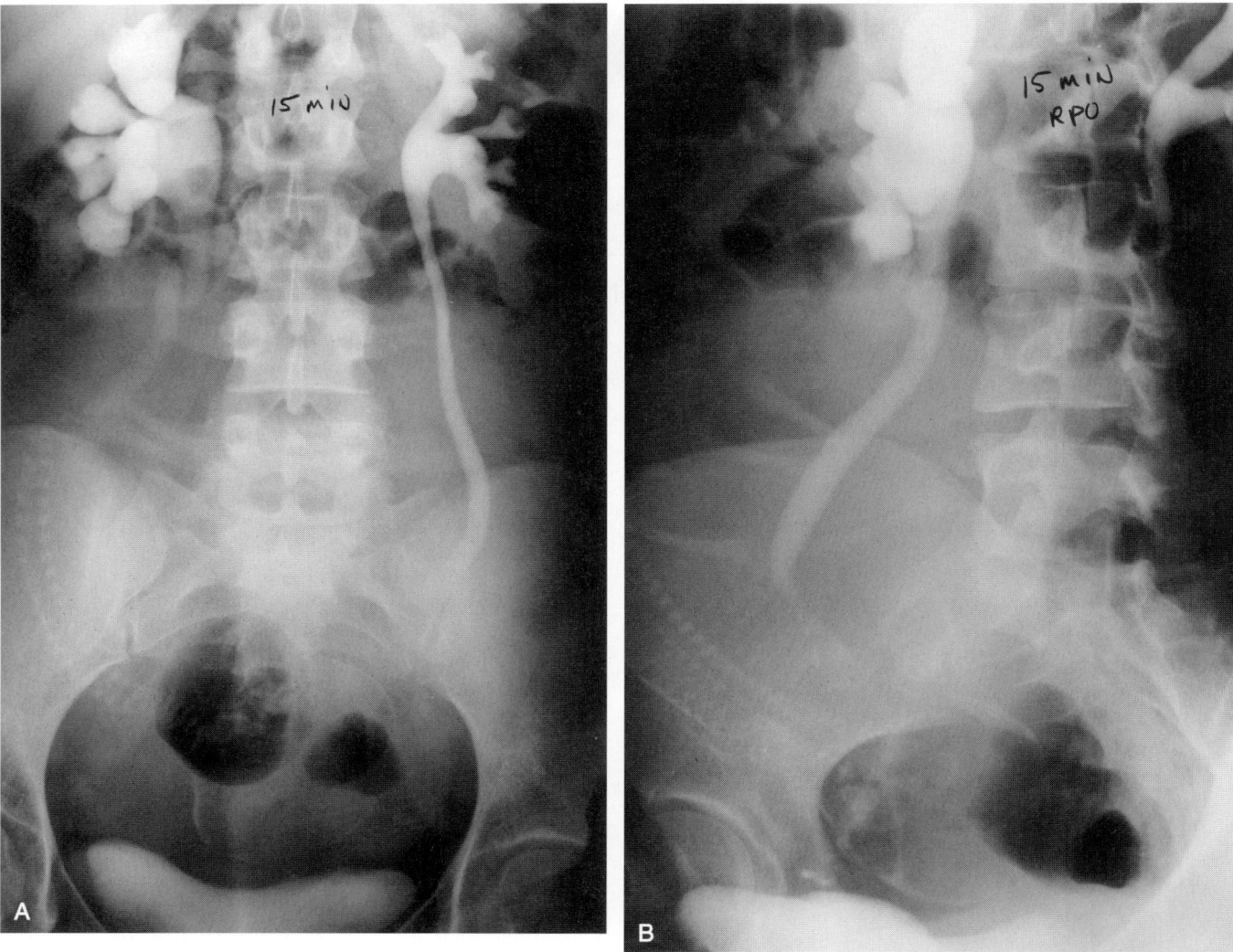

Figure 31–1. *A,* An intravenous pyelogram of a gravid patient presenting in late second trimester with flank pain. The image was taken in the anteroposterior view 15 minutes after the instillation of contrast dye. Note the dilatation of the renal pelves bilaterally, with the right side more dilated than the left. The fetus is seen in the vertex position. *B,* The same patient in the right lateral view.

Table 31–1. SUMMARY OF RENAL CHANGES IN NORMAL PREGNANCY

Alteration	Manifestation	Clinical Relevance
Increased renal size	Renal length about 1 cm greater on radiographs.	Postpartum decreases in size should not be mistaken for parenchymal loss.
Dilatation of pelves, calyces, and ureters	Resembles hydronephrosis on ultrasound or IVP (usually more prominent on the right).	Not to be mistaken for obstructive uropathy. Upper urinary tract infections are more virulent.
Changes in acid-base metabolism	Renal bicarbonate reabsorption threshold decreases.	Serum bicarbonate is 4–5 mM/L lower in pregnancy. PCO_2 is 10 mm Hg lower in normal pregnancy. PCO_2 of 40 mm Hg actually represents retention in pregnancy.
Renal water-handling	Osmoregulation altered as the osmotic thresholds for AVP release decreased.	Serum osmolarity decreased by approximately 10 mOsm/L.

IVP, intravenous pyelography; AVP, vasopressin; PCO_2, carbon dioxide tension. Adapted from Lindheimer M, Grünfeld JP, Davison JM: Renal disorders. *In* Barron WM, Lindheimer M (eds): Medical Disorders During Pregnancy. St. Louis, Mosby, 2000, p 39.

EVALUATION OF RENAL STATUS

As in the nonpregnant population, the evaluation of the urine can give critical insights as to the function of the kidney as well as the presence of urinary tract infection. The most frequently utilized method to evaluate the urine is the spot *urinalysis*. With the exception of the glucose, the study can be utilized as it would in the nonpregnant patient. It is, however, only a screening tool. If there is a concern that a patient has a change in her renal status or the possibility of bacteruria, further testing is needed.

One of the best methods to evaluate kidney function is collection of a *24-hour urine sample* for total protein analysis. The nonpregnant patient will usually spill less than 150 mg/day of protein. Most investigators consider up to 260 mg/day of total urinary protein and 29 mg/day of albumin normal in the gravid patient.[10] It should be noted that when one is using serial 24-hour urine samples to evaluate a change in renal status, it is crucial that the collection is standardized. The best method of comparing two urine collections is to evaluate the total amount of creatinine excreted in the 24-hour period. The amount a creatinine cleared in a day should remain constant during the course of a pregnancy for a given patient. If there is a large discrepancy in total creatinine between two samples, the difference in protein measured should be suspect. Another factor that must be considered is postural proteinuria. A patient may have an elevation in her urinary protein when ambulatory that resolves once the patient is recumbent.

Urinalysis has also been used to screen bacteruria. A recent study by McNair et al.[11] compared urinalysis to urine culture in the diagnosis of asymptomatic bacteriuria. They found that urinalysis has a sensitivity of 80.6 percent with a specificity of 71.5 percent. Given the false-negative rate of 19.4 percent in their population and the significant morbidity of undiagnosed bacteriuria, it was their recommendation that a urine culture be used as the primary method of screening all pregnant patients.

INFECTION OF THE URINARY TRACT
(SEE CHAPTER 40)

Asymptomatic Bacteriuria

Asymptomatic bacteriuria has been associated with multiple complications in pregnancy including low birth weight, preterm delivery, hypertension, preeclampsia, and maternal anemia.[12,13] The diagnosis of asymptomatic bacteriuria (ASB) is based on a clean-catch voided urine culture revealing greater than 100,000 colonies/ml of a single organism.[14] Some investigators have suggested that two consecutively voided specimens should contain the same organism before making the diagnosis of bacteriuria.[15,16] Between 1.2 and 5 percent of young girls will demonstrate ASB at some time before puberty.[17] After puberty, with the onset of sexual activity, the prevalence of ASB may increase to 10 percent.[17] Of women with ASB, approximately 35 percent have bacteria arising from the kidneys rather than from the lower urinary tract.

It is important to diagnose and treat ASB in pregnancy. Left untreated, a symptomatic urinary tract infection (UTI) will develop in up to 40 percent of these patients.[18,19] Recognition and therapy for ASB can eliminate 70 percent of acute UTIs in pregnancy. Nonetheless, 2 percent of pregnant women with negative urine cultures develop symptomatic cystitis or pyelonephritis. This group accounts for 30 percent of the cases of acute UTI that develop during gestation. We advocate screening of all women for ASB at their first prenatal visit.

Escherichia coli is the organism responsible for most cases of ASB. Patients can therefore be safely treated with nitrofurantoin, ampicillin, cephalosporins, and short-acting sulfa drugs (see the box "Antimicrobial Treatment for the Pregnant Patient with Bacteriuria.") Sulfa compounds should be avoided near term, as they compete for bilirubin-binding sites on albumin in the fetus and newborn and could cause kernicterus. Nitrofurantoin should not be used in patients with glucose-6-phosphate dehydrogenase deficiency, as there is a risk for hemolytic crisis. If the fetus has this enzyme deficiency, it may also experience hemolysis. Therapy for ASB should be continued for 3 to 7 days. The patient should have another culture performed 1 to 2 weeks after discontinuing therapy. Approximately 15 percent

---

Antimicrobial Treatment for the Pregnant Patient with Bacteriuria

- Amoxicillin 500 mg three times a day
- Ampicillin 250 mg four times a day
- Cephalosporin 250 mg four times a day
- Nitrofurantoin 100 mg four times a day
- Sustained release nitrofurantoin 100 mg two times a day
- Trimethoprim (160 mg)/sulfamethoxazole (800 mg) two times a day

The agent of choice should be given for a 3- to 7-day course. A repeat urine culture is recommended 2 weeks after the treatment has been completed.

of patients will experience a reinfection and/or will not respond to initial therapy. Therapy should be reinstituted after careful microbial sensitivity testing. Patients with recurrent UTI during pregnancy and those with a history of pyelonephritis should undergo radiographic evaluation of the upper urinary tract. This procedure should be delayed until the patient is 3 months postpartum so that the anatomic and physiologic changes of pregnancy can regress. Of women in the above categories, 20 percent will show a structural abnormality, but most will be insignificant.

Pyelonephritis

Occurring in approximately 1 to 2 percent of all pregnancies, pyelonephritis is an important source of maternal morbidity. Pyelonephritis is the most common nonobstetric cause of hospitalization during pregnancy.[20] Recurrent pyelonephritis has been implicated as a cause of fetal death and intrauterine growth restriction (IUGR). There appears to be an association between acute pyelonephritis and preterm labor.[21,22] Fan and co-workers,[23] however, have shown that if pyelonephritis is aggressively treated, it does not increase the likelihood of preterm labor, premature delivery, or low-birth-weight infants.

Occasionally, it is difficult to distinguish severe cystitis from pyelonephritis. Although the drugs used for treatment are similar, pyelonephritis requires intravenous antibiotics. Sandberg et al.[24] studied symptomatic UTI in 174 women. They found that C-reactive protein was elevated in 91 percent of pregnant women with acute pyelonephritis and only 5 percent of women with cystitis. They also noted that the urine-concentrating ability was lower in women with acute pyelonephritis. Because the erythrocyte sedimentation rate (ESR) is normally elevated in pregnancy, ESR was not a useful parameter for distinguishing pyelonephritis from cystitis. The most common symptoms of pyelonephritis include high fever, chills, acute tenderness over the kidneys in the costovertebral angle area (unilateral or bilateral), myalgias, nausea, and vomiting. During gestation, the right side is most often affected, as engorged blood vessels may inhibit ureteral drainage of the kidney. The fever curve noted in these patients will often have a "spiked" appearance, with periods of fever separated by periods of hypothermia. This pattern will usually persist even after treatment is initiated. The laboratory findings often include a urine sediment with numerous leukocytes and bacteria. In addition, patients will have a significantly elevated leukocyte count with a left shift.

Acute pyelonephritis should be initially treated on an inpatient basis, utilizing intravenous antibiotics. Empiric therapy should be begun as soon as the presumptive diagnosis is made. Therapy can be tailored to the specific organism after sensitivities have been obtained approximately 48 hours later. Because septicemia is present in approximately 15 percent of cases of pyelonephritis, blood cultures should be obtained if patients do not respond rapidly to initial antibiotic therapy. E. coli is the most common organism isolated in pyelonephritis. Generally, a broad-spectrum first-generation cephalosporin is the initial therapy of choice. Fan et al.[23] reviewed 107 cases of pyelonephritis in 103 pregnant women. They reported that 33 percent were resistant to ampicillin and 13 percent to first-generation cephalosporins. Since this study was published 9 years ago, the resistance to ampicillin and first-generation cephalosporins has increased. That is why it is so important to treat these women initially as inpatients. If resistance to more common therapies is encountered, a later generation cephalosporin or an aminoglycoside can safely be administered. During the febrile period, acetaminophen should be employed to keep the patient's temperature below 38°C. Small doses of acetaminophen will not mask the fever and symptoms of a patient who is unresponsive to treatment.

Intravenous antibiotic therapy should be continued for 24 to 48 hours after the patient becomes afebrile and costovertebral angle tenderness disappears. After the cessation of intravenous therapy, treatment with appropriate oral antibiotics should be continued for 1 to 2 weeks. Upon termination of therapy, urine cultures should be obtained on a regular basis for the remainder of gestation. After an episode of acute pyelonephritis, antibiotic suppression should be implemented and continued. Nitrofurantoin 100 mg once or twice daily is an acceptable regimen for suppression. In a study by Van Dorsten and colleagues,[25] the overall frequency of positive urine cultures following hospitalization for pyelonephritis was 38 percent. Nitrofurantoin suppression reduced the rate to 8 percent. Nitrofurantoin did not lower the rate of positive cultures if the inpatient antibiotic selection was inappropriate or if the culture was positive at the time of discharge.[25] Today, there is increased pressure to treat pregnant women with pyelonephritis as outpatients. Although not ideal, this approach is possible if daily nursing contact is maintained during the acute phase of the disease and appropriate laboratory parameters are followed.

Cunningham and co-workers[26] point out that pulmonary injury resembling adult respiratory distress syndrome (ARDS) can occur in patients with acute pyelonephritis. Clinical manifestations of this complication usually occur 24 to 48 hours after the patient is admitted for pyelonephritis.[26,27] Some of these patients will require endotracheal intubation, mechanical ventilation,[28] and positive end-expiratory pressure (PEEP). In Cunningham's series, there was no evidence that pulmonary edema was caused by intravenous fluid overload.[26] This ARDS-type picture probably results from endotoxin-induced alveolar capillary membrane injury. Towers et al. found pulmonary injury in 11 of 130 patients with pyelonephritis. A fever of greater than 103°F, a maternal heart rate above 110 bpm, and a gestation greater than 20 weeks placed the patient at increased risk for pulmonary injury. The most predictive factors for ARDS were fluid overload and tocolytic therapy.[29]

Austenfeld and Snow[30] studied 64 pregnancies in 30 women who had previously undergone ureteral reimplantation for vesicoureteral reflux. During pregnancy, 57 percent of these women had one or more UTIs, and 17 percent had more than one UTI or an episode of pyelonephritis.[30] More frequent urine cultures and aggressive therapy during pregnancy are recommended for this group of patients.

ACUTE RENAL DISEASE IN PREGNANCY

Urolithiasis

The prevalence of urolithiasis during pregnancy is 0.03 percent, with an incidence no higher than that of the general population.[31] Colicky abdominal pain, recurrent UTI, and hematuria suggest urolithiasis. If the diagnosis is suspected, intravenous pyelography should be undertaken, limiting this study to the minimum number of exposures necessary to make the diagnosis. Ultrasound can often be used to establish the diagnosis without radiation exposure. Newer ultrasound flow studies can actually follow flow from the ureter to the bladder and detect obstruction without the use of ionizing radiation. Urine microscopy can often detect crystals and help distinguish the type of stone before it is passed. For any patient suspected or proved to have renal stones, serum calcium and phosphorous levels should be measured to rule out hyperparathyroidism. Serum urate should also be determined.

Because of the physiologic hydroureter characteristic of pregnancy, most patients with symptomatic urolithiasis will spontaneously pass their stones. Treatment should be conservative, consisting of hydration and narcotic analgesia for pain relief.[32] Epidural anesthesia has been advocated to establish a segmental block from T11 to L2. While this approach may promote passage of the stone, it remains controversial. Lithotripsy is contraindicated during pregnancy.

Recurrent UTI with urease-containing organisms causes precipitation of calcium phosphate in the kidney that may lead to the development of staghorn calculi. Surgery is rarely indicated in these patients, especially during gestation. Patients with staghorn calculi should have frequent urine cultures, and bacteriuria should be treated aggressively. Recurrent infections can lead to chronic pyelonephritis with resultant loss of kidney function.

Glomerulonephritis

Acute glomerulonephritis is an uncommon complication of pregnancy, with an estimated incidence of 1 per 40,000 pregnancies.[33] Poststreptococcal glomerulonephritis rarely occurs in adults. In this disorder, renal function tends to deteriorate during the acute phase of the disease, but usually later recovers.[34] Acute glomerulonephritis can be difficult to distinguish from preeclampsia. Periorbital edema, a striking clinical feature of acute glomerulonephritis, is often seen in preeclampsia as well. Hematuria, red blood cell (RBC) casts in the urine sediment, and depressed serum complement levels indicate glomerular disease. In poststreptococcal acute glomerulonephritis, antistreptolysin O titers rise.

Treatment of acute glomerulonephritis in pregnancy is similar to that for the nonpregnant patient. Blood pressure control is essential, and careful attention to fluid balance is imperative. Sodium intake should be restricted to 500 mg/day during the acute disease. Serum potassium levels must also be carefully monitored.

Packham and co-workers[35] extensively reviewed 395 pregnancies in 238 women with primary glomerulonephritis. Only 51 percent of infants were born after 36 weeks' gestation. Excluding therapeutic abortion, 20 percent of fetuses were lost, 15 percent after 20 weeks' gestation. IUGR was noted in 15 percent of these cases. Maternal renal function deteriorated in 15 percent of pregnancies and failed to resolve postpartum in 5 percent.[35] Hypertension was recorded in 52 percent of the pregnancies and developed before 32 weeks' gestation in 26 percent. This blood pressure elevation was not an exacerbation of previously diagnosed hypertension, as in only 12 percent of pregnancies was there noted to be antecedent hypertension. Eighteen percent of the women who developed de novo hypertension in pregnancy remained hypertensive postpartum. Increased proteinuria was recorded in 59 percent of these pregnancies and was irreversible in 15 percent.[35] The highest incidence of fetal and maternal complications occurred in patients with primary focal and segmental hyalinosis and sclerosis. The lowest incidence of complications was observed in non–immunoglobulin A (IgA) diffuse mesangial proliferative glomerulonephritis.[35] The presence of severe vessel lesions on renal biopsy was associated with a significantly higher rate of fetal loss after 20 weeks' gestation.

Packham and co-workers[36] also studied 33 pregnancies in 24 patients with biopsy-proven membranous glomerulonephritis. Fetal loss occurred in 24 percent of pregnancies, preterm delivery in 43 percent, and a term liveborn in only 33 percent of patients. Hypertension was noted in 46 percent of these pregnant women. Thirty percent of patients had proteinuria in the nephrotic range in the first trimester.[36] The presence of heavy proteinuria during the first trimester correlated with a poor fetal and maternal outcome.[36] Jungers et al.[37] described 69 pregnancies in 34 patients with IgA glomerulonephritis. The fetal loss rate in this group was 15 percent. Preexisting hypertension was statistically associated with poor fetal outcome. Hypertension at the time of conception also correlated with a deterioration of maternal renal function during pregnancy. Hypertension in the first pregnancy was highly predictive of recurrence of hypertension in a subsequent pregnancy.[37]

Kincaid-Smith and Fairley[38] analyzed 102 pregnancies in 65 women with IgA glomerulonephritis. They noted that hypertension occurred in 63 percent of pregnancies, with 18 percent being severe. They also observed a decrease in renal function in 22 percent of these women.[38] Abe[39] retrospectively studied 240 pregnancies in 166 women with preexisting glomerular disease between 1976 and 1988. Eight percent of the pregnancies resulted in a spontaneous abortion, 6 percent resulted in stillbirth, and 86 percent were liveborn. Most losses occurred in women with a GFR less than 70 ml/min and preexisting hypertension. Even though the majority of women with renal insufficiency had good pregnancy outcomes, the long-term prognosis of the kidney disease was worse if the GFR was less than 50 ml/min and the serum creatinine was more than 1.5 mg/dl.[39] Renal complications were worse in patients with membranoproliferative glomerulonephritis, with 29 percent developing hypertension and 33 percent developing a long-term decrease in renal function.

Imbasciati and Ponticelli[40] summarized six studies containing a total of 906 pregnancies in 558 women with preexisting glomerular disease. This review, of course, has the limitations of including patients from a wide span of years and varying geographic locations. Nonetheless, broad generalizations can be made. The overall perinatal mortality was 13 percent. Hypertension, renal insufficiency, and nephrotic range proteinuria were the strongest prognostic factors for a poor pregnancy outcome. Having two of these factors was a particularly strong harbinger of fetal loss. The histologic type of glomerulonephritis had little correlation with pregnancy outcome. Hypertension persisted in 3 to 12 percent of patients who developed hypertension for the first time during pregnancy. In 25 percent of patients, hypertension worsened during pregnancy and corrected postpartum.[40] This presentation suggests superimposed preeclampsia, but that diagnosis is difficult to make in a patient who already has hypertension and proteinuria. In 3 percent of these 166 women, the course of their glomerular disease accelerated after pregnancy.

Acute Renal Failure in Pregnancy

Acute renal failure (ARF) is defined as a urine output of less than 400 ml in 24 hours. To make the diagnosis, ureteral and urethral obstruction must be excluded. The incidence of ARF during pregnancy is approximately 1 per 10,000. It is seen most frequently in septic first-trimester abortions and in cases of sudden severe volume depletion resulting from hemorrhage caused by placenta previa, placental abruption, or postpartum uterine atony.[41] It is also observed in the marked volume contraction associated with severe preeclampsia[42] and with acute fatty liver of pregnancy.[42,43]

The incidence of ARF in pregnancy has decreased over the years. Stratta and colleagues[44] reported 81 cases of pregnancy-related ARF between 1958 and 1987, accounting for 9 percent of the total number of ARF cases needing dialysis during that interval. In three successive 10-year periods (1958 to 1967, 1968 to 1977, and 1978 to 1987), the incidence of pregnancy-related ARF fell from 43 percent to 2.8 percent of the total number of cases of ARF. The incidence changed from 1 in 3,000 to 1 in 15,000 pregnancies over the study period.[44] In these 81 ARF cases, 11.6 percent experienced irreversible renal damage, the majority of which involved severe preeclampsia/eclampsia.[44]

Renal ischemia is the common denominator in all cases of ARF. With mild ischemia, quickly reversible prerenal failure results. With more prolonged ischemia, acute tubular necrosis occurs. This process is also reversible, as glomeruli are not affected. Severe ischemia, however, may produce acute cortical necrosis. This pathology is irreversible, although on occasion a small amount of renal function is preserved.[45] Stratta and colleagues[46] have reported 17 cases of ARF occurring over 15 years, and all were due to preeclampsia/eclampsia. Cortical necrosis occurred in 29.5 percent of the cases.[46] Whether or not ARF was associated with cortical necrosis did not appear to be related to chronologic age, parity, gestational age at which preeclampsia commenced, duration of preeclampsia prior to delivery, or eclamptic seizures. The only statistically significant factor associated with the appearance of cortical necrosis was placental abruption.[46] In another study, Turney and co-workers[47] demonstrated that acute cortical necrosis, which occurred in 12.7 percent of their patients with ARF, carried a 100 percent mortality within 6 years.

Sibai and colleagues[48] studied the remote prognosis in 31 consecutive cases of ARF in patients with hypertensive disorders of pregnancy. Eighteen of the 31 patients had "pure" preeclampsia, while 13 pregnancies had other hypertensive disorders and renal disease. Five percent of the 18 patients with pure preeclampsia required dialysis during hospitalization, and all had acute tubular necrosis. Of the other 13 women, 42 percent required dialysis and three patients had bilateral cortical necrosis. The majority of pregnancies in both groups were complicated by placental abruption and hemorrhage.[48] All 16 surviving patients in the pure preeclampsia group had normal renal function on long-term follow-up. Conversely, 9 of the 11 surviving patients in the other group required long-term dialysis, and four ultimately died of end-stage renal disease.[48] Turney and colleagues[47] also performed follow-up examinations of their patients. They found that maternal survival was adversely affected by increasing age. Their 1-year maternal survival rate was 78.6 percent. Follow-up of survivors showed normal renal function up to 31 years after ARF.[47]

Clinically, patients with reversible ARF first experience a period of oliguria of variable duration. Polyuria then occurs. It is important to recognize that BUN and serum creatinine levels continue to rise early in the polyuric phase. During the recovery phase, urine output approaches normal. In these patients, it is important to monitor electrolytes frequently and to treat any imbalance carefully. The urine/plasma osmolality ratio should be determined early in the course of the disease. If the ratio is 1.5 or greater, prerenal pathology is likely, and the disorder tends to be of shorter duration and less severity. A ratio near 1.0 suggests acute tubular necrosis.

The main goal of treatment is elimination of the underlying cause. Volume and electrolyte balance must receive constant scrutiny. To assess volume requirements, invasive hemodynamic monitoring is useful and lessens the need for clinical guesswork. This is especially true during the polyuric phase. Central hyperalimentation may also be required if renal failure is prolonged.

Acidosis frequently occurs in cases of ARF. Arterial blood gases therefore should be followed regularly. Acidosis must be treated promptly to prevent hyperkalemia, which may develop rapidly and can be fatal. Absolute restriction of potassium intake should be instituted immediately. Sodium bicarbonate, used to treat acidosis, may overload the patient with sodium and water. In this case, peritoneal or hemodialysis may be instituted. The main indications for dialysis in ARF of pregnancy are hypernatremia, hyperkalemia, severe acidosis, volume overload, and worsening uremia.

Hemolytic Uremic Syndrome

The postpartum hemolytic uremic syndrome is a rare idiopathic disorder that must be considered when a patient shows signs of hemolysis and decreasing renal function in the postpartum period. This idiopathic syndrome was first described in 1968 and may occur as early as the first trimester and up to 2 months postpartum.[49–52] In fact, it has even been reported following an ectopic pregnancy.[53] Most patients have no predisposing factors. Prodromal symptoms include vomiting, diarrhea, and a flu-like illness. Forty-nine cases have been reported, with a 61 percent mortality rate.[51] These cases date back to 1968; with improved intensive care monitoring and treatment, the prognosis has improved. Coratelli and co-workers[49] reported a case of hemolytic uremic syndrome that was diagnosed at 13 weeks' gestation and confirmed by renal biopsy. Circulating endotoxin was detected and was progressively reduced by hemodialysis performed daily from the third to the ninth days of the disease. Complete normalization of renal function occurred by day 34. These investigators propose that initiation of early dialysis may play an important role in supporting patients through the disease process. They also propose that endotoxins are key pathogenic factors in the disorder.[49] Conversely, Li and co-workers[54] discovered hemolytic uremic syndrome in a patient recovering from an uncomplicated cesarean delivery. No endotoxins were found in the patient's serum, stool, or renal biopsy material. The patient underwent dialysis and recovered.[54] Conte and co-workers[55] suggest that plasma exchange in cases of acute renal failure caused by the postpartum hemolytic uremic syndrome can play a vital role in supporting a patient through the illness. This does appear to be the key to therapy today.

Disseminated intravascular coagulation (DIC) with hemolysis usually accompanies the renal failure. However, DIC is not the cause of the syndrome. Microscopically, the kidney shows thrombotic microangiopathy. The glomerular capillary wall is thick, and biopsy specimens taken later in the course of the disease show severe nephrosclerosis and deposition of the third component of complement (C3).

Some researchers believe that this syndrome is due to decreased production of prostacyclin in the kidneys.[56,57] Prostacyclin infusions have been used to treat patients, but this therapy still remains experimental. One observer noted a decrease in antithrombin III in a patient with postpartum hemolytic uremic syndrome. This patient was successfully treated with an infusion of antithrombin III concentrate,[58] a preparation that is readily available today.

Polycystic Kidney Disease

Adult polycystic kidney disease is an autosomal dominant disorder that usually manifests itself in the fifth decade of life. Patients may occasionally display symptoms earlier. Hypertension is part of this disorder. If a patient with adult polycystic kidney disease becomes pregnant, hypertension may be exacerbated and not improve postpartum.[40] The overall prognosis for the disorder does not appear to worsen with an increasing number of pregnancies.

Vesicoureteral Reflux

Vesicoureteral reflux increases with pregnancy. It usually does not cause problems unless the reflux is severe. If it is severe enough to warrant surgery, this should be done before pregnancy. Even with surgical correction, patients with ureterovesical reflux are at increased risk for pyelonephritis and should have cultures performed frequently.[40] If an individual was receiving antibiotic prophylaxis prior to pregnancy, this should be continued. If the patient was not on prophylaxis, the obstetrician may wish to begin treatment with nitrofurantoin, depending on the clinical situation.

Brandes and Fritsche[59] report a case of acute renal failure due to obstruction of the ureters by a gravid uterus. Only 13 other cases have been reported prior to this case, a twin pregnancy complicated by polyhydramnios at 34 weeks' gestation. The serum creatinine level peaked at 12.2 mg/dl, but resolved immediately after amniotomy.[59] In cases remote from term, ureteral stenting or dialysis may be necessary.

Renal Artery Stenosis

Renal artery stenosis is an extremely rare complication of pregnancy.[60] This disorder may present as chronic hypertension with superimposed preeclampsia or as recurrent isolated preeclampsia. Although Doppler flow studies may be suggestive, renal angiography is the most specific and sensitive diagnostic procedure. Percutaneous transluminal angioplasty can be carried out at the time of angiography. Heyborne et al.[60] present a case in which this procedure was accomplished at $26\frac{1}{2}$ weeks' gestation.

Nephrotic Syndrome

The nephrotic syndrome was initially described as a 24-hour urine protein excretion of 3.5 g or more, reduced serum albumin, edema, and hyperlipidemia.[61] Currently, the syndrome is defined by massive proteinuria alone, which is often the result of damage to the glomeruli.[61] The most common etiology of nephrotic syndrome in pregnancy (especially the third trimester) is preeclampsia. Other etiologies include proliferative glomerulonephritis, minimal change disease, lupus nephropathy, hereditary nephritis, diabetic nephropathy, renal vein thrombosis, and amyloidosis.[62]

Patients with newly diagnosed or persistent nephrotic syndrome must be followed closely in pregnancy. Whenever possible, the etiology of the proteinuria should be determined. In many cases, steroid therapy may be employed; however, its use can in some cases aggravate the underlying disease process.[62] One common complication of nephrotic syndrome in pregnancy is profound edema secondary to massive protein excretion in addition to the normal decline in serum albumin associated with pregnancy.[62] A second area of concern is a possible hypercoagulable state precipitated by urinary losses of antithrombin III, reduced levels of protein C and S, hyperfibrinogenemia, and enhanced platelet aggregation.[63]

CHRONIC RENAL DISEASE IN PREGNANCY

Chronic renal disease can be silent until its advanced stages. Because obstetricians routinely examine the patient's urine for the presence of protein, glucose, and ketones, they may be the first to detect chronic renal disease.

Any gravida with more than trace proteinuria should collect a 24-hour urine specimen for creatinine clearance and total protein excretion. This test is safe, inexpensive, and of only minor inconvenience to the patient. Creatinine clearance is elevated in pregnancy and, during the first trimester, may exceed 140 ml/min. Before pregnancy, 24-hour urinary protein excretion should not exceed 0.2 g. During gestation, quantities up to 0.3 g/day may be normal. Moderate proteinuria (<2 g/day) is seen in glomerular disease, most commonly lipoid nephrosis, systemic lupus erythematosus, and glomerulonephritis.

Microscopic examination of the urine can reveal much about the patient's renal status. If renal disease is suspected, a catheterized specimen should be obtained. More RBCs than one to two per high-power field or RBC casts are indicative of renal disease. RBCs usually indicate glomerular disease or collagen vascular disease. Less frequently, they suggest trauma or malignant hypertension. Increased numbers of white blood cells (WBCs), more than one to two per high-power field, or the appearance of WBC casts is usually indicative of acute or chronic infection. Cellular casts are found in the presence of renal tubular dysfunction, and hyaline casts suggest significant proteinuria. A single bacterium seen in an unspun catheterized urine specimen is suggestive of significant bacteriuria, and a follow-up culture should be performed.

The obstetrician can easily be misled when relying solely on the BUN and serum creatinine to assess renal function. A 70 percent decline in creatinine clearance, an indirect measure of GFR, can be seen before a significant rise in the BUN or serum creatinine occurs. In fact, little change in the serum creatinine or the BUN is seen until the creatinine clearance falls to 50 ml/min. Below that level, small decrements in creatinine clearance can lead to large increases in the BUN and creatinine. A single creatinine clearance value less than 100 ml/min is not diagnostic of renal diseases. An incomplete 24-hour urine collection is the most frequent cause of this finding. An abnormal clearance rate should therefore be restudied.

Serum urate is an often overlooked but helpful parameter in detecting renal dysfunction. Excretion of uric acid is dependent not only on glomerular filtration but also on tubular secretion. An elevated serum urate in the presence of a normal BUN and serum creatinine may therefore implicate tubular disease. A solitary increase in uric acid may also signify impending or early preeclampsia.

Effect of Pregnancy on Renal Function

Although baseline creatinine clearance is decreased in patients with chronic renal insufficiency, it should still rise during gestation. A moderate fall in creatinine clearance is often observed during late gestation in patients with renal disease. This decrease is typically more severe in patients with diffuse glomerular disease. It usually reverses after delivery.

The long-term effect of pregnancy on renal disease remains controversial. If the patient's serum creatinine is less than 1.5 mg/dl, pregnancy should have little effect on the long-term prognosis of the patient's kidney disease. Pregnancy, however, is associated with an increased incidence of pyelonephritis in patients with chronic renal disease. There are few data concerning the long-term effect of pregnancy on renal disease in women with true renal insufficiency. Occasionally, some patients with a baseline serum creatinine of more than 1.5 mg/dl will experience a significant decrease in renal function during gestation that does not improve during the postpartum period.[40,64,65] This deterioration occurs more frequently in women with diffuse glomerulonephritis. It is not possible, however, to predict which patients with renal insufficiency will experience a permanent reduction in renal function. If renal function significantly worsens during gestation, termination of pregnancy may not reverse the process. Abortion therefore cannot be routinely recommended for patients who become pregnant and whose baseline serum creatinine level exceeds 1.5 mg/dl. Ideally, patients with chronic renal disease should be thoroughly counseled about the possible consequences of pregnancy before conception.

Severe hypertension is the greatest threat to the pregnant patient with chronic renal disease. Left uncontrolled, hypertension can lead to intracerebral hemorrhage as well as deteriorating renal function. In most pregnancies complicated by chronic renal dysfunction, some degree of hypertension is present.[64,66] Approximately 50 percent of these patients will have worsening hypertension as pregnancy progresses, and diastolic blood pressures of 110 mm Hg or greater will develop in about 20 percent of cases.[67] Those patients with diffuse proliferative glomerulonephritis and nephrosclerosis are at greatest risk for the development of severe hypertension. Blood pressure control is the cornerstone of successful treatment of chronic renal disease in pregnancy.

Worsening proteinuria is common during pregnancy complicated by chronic renal disease and often reaches the nephrotic range.[67] In general, massive proteinuria does not indicate an increased risk for mother or fetus.[68] Low serum albumin, however, has been correlated with low birth weight.[69] The development of massive proteinuria is not necessarily a harbinger of preeclampsia. Nevertheless, in late pregnancy it is often difficult to differentiate impending preeclampsia from worsening chronic renal disease.

Effect of Chronic Renal Disease on Pregnancy

More than 85 percent of women with chronic renal disease will have a surviving infant if renal function is well preserved. Earlier reports were more pessimistic, citing a 5.8 percent incidence of stillbirth, a 4.9 percent incidence of neonatal deaths, and an increase in second-trimester losses.[67] If hypertension is not controlled and if renal function is not well preserved, there is still a high likelihood of pregnancy loss.[35] Antepartum fetal surveillance and advances in neonatal care have made great strides in improving perinatal outcome in these patients. One study reported a total fetal loss rate of 13.8 percent, including miscarriage, stillbirths, and neonatal deaths,[66] not very different from the general population.

The outlook for women with severe renal insufficiency whose baseline serum creatinine level exceeds 1.5 mg/dl is less clear. This is due in part to the limited number of pregnancies in such patients as well as to the large number who undergo elective abortion. One study reported no surviving infants when the maternal BUN was greater than 60 mg/dl.[68] Other investigations, however, have found that about 80 percent of such pregnancies resulted in surviving infants.[66,70] Preterm births and IUGR remain important problems in these pregnancies. The reported incidence of preterm birth ranges from 20 to 50 percent.[67,71]

Imbasciati and Ponticelli[40] summarize three studies containing 81 pregnancies in 78 women with serum creatinine concentrations less than 1.4 mg/dl.[40] The perinatal loss rate was only 9 percent. However, 33 percent of the infants were growth restricted, and 50 percent were born preterm secondary to either maternal or fetal indications. Disturbingly, 33 percent of the women showed acceleration of their renal disease after delivery. Some researchers believe that growth restriction may be due to the lack of plasma volume increase as the pregnancy progresses. In one study, Cunningham et al.[72] showed that women with moderate renal dysfunction did have increased creatinine clearances and plasma volumes during gestation, whereas women with severe renal dysfunction did not.[72]

Hemodialysis in Pregnancy

Patients with chronic hemodialysis can have successful pregnancies.[73–79] Many women with chronic renal failure, however, experience oligomenorrhea, and their fertility is often impaired.[80] These women commonly fail to use a method of contraception. It is therefore important that a serum human chorionic gonadotropin (hCG) level be assessed whenever pregnancy is suspected.

As in all patients with impaired renal function, the most important aspect of care is meticulous control of blood pressure. During dialysis, wide fluctuations in blood pressure often occur. One case report describes fetal distress associated with hypotension during dialysis.[81] Sudden volume shifts, therefore, should be avoided.[79] In late pregnancy, continuous fetal heart rate monitoring should be carried out during dialysis. If possible, the patient should be positioned on her left side with the uterus displaced from the vena cava. During dialysis, one must pay particular attention to electrolyte balance. Pregnant patients are in a state of chronic compensated respiratory alkalosis, and large drops in serum bicarbonate should be prevented. Dialysates containing glucose and bicarbonate are preferred, and those containing citrates should be avoided.[79]

Patients should be counseled that a successful pregnancy will require longer and more frequent periods of dialysis.[74,79,81] Patients must also follow a careful diet, ingesting at least 70 g of protein and 1.5 g of calcium daily. Weight gain should be limited to 0.5 kg between dialysis sessions.

Chronic anemia is often a problem in hemodialysis patients. The hematocrit should be kept above 25 percent, and transfusion with packed RBCs or erythropoietin therapy may be necessary to accomplish this objective.[74] Polyhydramnios appears to be a frequent complication in pregnant patients undergoing hemodialysis.[79,82]

The point at which to initiate hemodialysis is controversial. Cohen and co-investigators[76] believe that the early initiation of regular hemodialysis in patients with moderate renal insufficiency may improve pregnancy outcome. In two cases, when regular hemodialysis was begun in the second trimester, both patients carried to term, although the infants were growth restricted.[76] Redrow and co-workers[77] report 14 pregnancies in 13

women undergoing dialysis. Ten of those pregnancies were successful.

Chronic ambulatory peritoneal dialysis or chronic cycling peritoneal dialysis has also been associated with successful outcomes in pregnancy. Redrow et al.[77] hypothesize several advantages for peritoneal dialysis. These include a more constant chemical and extracellular environment for the fetus, higher hematocrit levels, infrequent episodes of hypotension, and no heparin requirement. They also postulate that intraperitoneal insulin facilitates the management of blood glucose in diabetic patients and that intraperitoneal magnesium used in the dialysate reduces the likelihood of preterm labor.

Preterm birth does occur more frequently in patients undergoing dialysis.[83] Progesterone is removed during dialysis, and at least one group has advocated that parenteral progesterone therapy should be administered to the patient undergoing dialysis.[84] In their review, Yasin and Doun[79] report a 40.7 percent incidence of premature contractions. Although it is tempting to consider cesarean delivery when the patient approaches term, this method should not be routine for these patients. Its use should be based only on obstetric indications.

The Europeans have compiled a registry of pregnant women requiring dialysis. There has been a 23 percent pregnancy success rate in 70 women with end-stage renal disease requiring dialysis.[82] The mean gestational age was 33.2 weeks. Most preterm births were due to growth restriction, hypertension, preterm labor, and abruption. These findings suggest that more frequent dialysis results in more uniform control of uremia and less fluctuation in blood volume, which should result in better pregnancy outcomes.

MANAGEMENT OF CHRONIC RENAL DISEASE IN PREGNANCY

A 24-hour urine collection for creatinine clearance and total protein excretion should be obtained as soon as the pregnancy is confirmed. These parameters should be monitored monthly. The patient should be seen once every 2 weeks until 32 weeks' gestation and weekly thereafter. These are general guidelines, and more frequent visits may be necessary in individual cases.

Control of hypertension is critical in managing patients with chronic renal disease. β-Blockers, calcium channel blockers, and hydralazine can be used to treat blood pressure effectively as long as the dosages are monitored carefully. Clonidine is occasionally useful in refractory patients. Doxazosin and prazosin may be used if necessary. Angiotensin-converting enzyme (ACE) inhibitors should be avoided during pregnancy. These drugs have been associated with fetal and neonatal oliguria/anuria.[85,86] In one study, 1 of 19 infants had anuria and required dialysis.[85] In another study, an infant required peritoneal dialysis.[86] Furthermore, congenital anomalies, including microcephaly and encephalocele,[85] have been associated with the use of ACE inhibitors.

The use of diuretics in pregnancy is controversial.[87,88] For massive debilitating edema, a short course of diuretics can be helpful. Electrolytes must be monitored carefully. Salt restriction does not appear to be beneficial once edema has developed. Salt restriction, however, should be instituted without hesitation in pregnant women with true renal insufficiency.

Fetal growth should be assessed with serial ultrasonography, because growth restriction is common in women with chronic renal disease. Antepartum fetal heart rate testing should be started at 28 weeks' gestation.[89]

Obstetricians should have a low threshold for hospitalizing patients with chronic renal disease. Increasing hypertension and decreasing renal function warrant immediate hospitalization. A sudden deterioration of renal function may be due to infection, dehydration, electrolyte imbalance, or obstruction.

The timing of delivery must be individualized. Maternal indications for delivery include uncontrollable hypertension, the development of superimposed preeclampsia, and decreasing renal function after fetal viability has been reached. Fetal indications are dictated by the assessment of fetal growth and fetal well-being.

Renal biopsy is rarely indicated during pregnancy. It is never indicated after 34 weeks' gestation, when delivery of the fetus and subsequent biopsy would be a safer alternative. Excessive bleeding secondary to the greatly increased renal blood flow has been reported by some[90] but not all[91] observers. If coagulation indices are normal and blood pressure is well controlled, morbidity should be no greater than that observed in the nonpregnant patient.[92] Packham and Fairley[93] report a series of 111 renal biopsies performed in 104 pregnant women over 20 years. The complication rate was 4.5 percent. The most likely clinical dilemma necessitating renal biopsy in a pregnant woman would be the development of nephrotic syndrome and increasing hypertension between 22 and 32 weeks' gestation. In this case, renal biopsy may distinguish chronic renal disease from preeclampsia and impact significantly on the treatment plan.

RENAL TRANSPLANTATION

Pregnancy following renal transplantation has become increasingly common. Many previously anovulatory patients begin ovulating postoperatively and regain fertility as renal function normalizes.[94] As in the case of women on hemodialysis, many transplant recipients have failed to realize they are pregnant until well into the second trimester.

Upon learning they are pregnant, many women stop taking all medications. The importance of continuing immunosuppressive therapy cannot be emphasized strongly enough to renal allograft recipients. Glucocorticoids, especially prednisone, are metabolized in the placenta by 11 β-ol-dehydrogenase, with only limited amounts reaching the fetus. No studies have documented an increased rate of malformations. Adrenocortical insufficiency has been rarely reported in infants born to mothers taking glucocorticoids.[95] Nevertheless, a pediatrician should be present at the delivery and should be aware of this possibility.

Azathioprine cannot be activated in the fetus because of its lack of inosinate pyrophosphorylase.[96] Azathioprine has been shown to cause decreased levels of IgG and IgM as well as a smaller thymic shadow on chest x-ray in these neonates.[97] Chromosomal aberrations, which cleared within 20 to 32 months, have also been demonstrated in lymphocytes of infants exposed to azathioprine in utero.[98] The long-term implications of this treatment are not yet known. IUGR has been reported in infants born to mothers receiving azathioprine.[99] These risks are outweighed, however, by the disastrous consequences of allograft rejection that may occur if the patient stops her medication.

Cyclosporin A appears to be relatively safe for use during gestation, but does hold some risks. Patients may develop arterial hypertension secondary to its interference with the normal hemodynamic adaptation to pregnancy.[100] Cyclosporin A crosses the placenta, but there is no evidence of teratogenesis.[101,102] Intrauterine growth restriction, in the absence of maternal hypertension, has been reported in a patient taking cyclosporin A during pregnancy.[103] Most women taking cyclosporin A have had no complications attributable to the drug, and the risk of allograft rejection certainly outweighs the fetal risk of the medication. Therefore, the medication should be continued throughout gestation.

Davison[104] reviewed 1,569 renal transplants in 1,009 women. He found that 22 percent of the women elected to abort their pregnancies, 16 percent had a spontaneous abortion, and 8 percent experienced perinatal deaths. Furthermore, he observed that 45 percent of the surviving pregnancies were delivered preterm and 22 percent were complicated by intrauterine growth restriction.[104] Three percent of the infants were born with major malformations, a rate no different from expected in the background population. Preeclampsia complicated 30 percent of the pregnancies but, as previously noted, the diagnosis is difficult to make in a patient who may already have hypertension and proteinuria.

The allograft rejection rate in these women was 9 percent, no different from that expected in a nonpregnant population.[104] Also, the long-term rejection rate was the same as for women who had not experienced a pregnancy.

During pregnancy, renal allograft recipients must be carefully watched for signs of rejection. As previously mentioned, significant episodes of rejection may occur in as many as 9 percent of transplant recipients during gestation. This figure is no greater than that expected in the nonpregnant population. Unfortunately, the clinical hallmarks of rejection—fever, oliguria, tenderness, and decreasing renal function—are not always exhibited by the pregnant patient. Occasionally, rejection may mimic pyelonephritis or preeclampsia, which occurs in approximately one third of renal transplant patients. In these cases, renal biopsy is indicated to distinguish rejection from preeclampsia. Rejection has been known to occur during the puerperium, when maternal immune competence returns to its prepregnancy level.[105] Therefore, it may be advisable to increase the dose of immunosuppressive medications in the immediate postpartum period.

Infection can be disastrous for the renal allograft. Therefore, urine cultures should be obtained at least monthly during pregnancy, and any bacteriuria should be aggressively treated. It is crucial to remember that the allograft is denervated, and the patient may experience no pain with pyelonephritis. The only symptoms may be fever and nausea.

Renal function, as determined by 24-hour creatinine clearance and protein excretion, should be assessed monthly. Approximately 15 percent of transplant recipients will exhibit a significant decrease in renal function in late pregnancy.[106] This condition usually, but not always, reverses after pregnancy. Proteinuria develops in about 40 percent of patients near term, but most often disappears soon after delivery unless significant hypertension is present.

As for patients with chronic renal disease, serial ultrasonography should be used to assess fetal growth, and antepartum fetal heart rate testing should be started at 28 weeks' gestation. Approximately 50 percent of renal allograft recipients will deliver preterm. Preterm labor, preterm rupture of membranes, and IUGR are common. Vaginal delivery should be accomplished when possible, with cesarean delivery reserved for obstetric indications. Allograft recipients may have an increased frequency of cephalopelvic disproportion from pelvic osteodystrophy,[107] resulting from prolonged renal disease with hypercalcemia or extended steroid use. The transplanted kidney, however, rarely obstructs vaginal delivery despite its pelvic location.

Although there have been many successful pregnancies in renal allograft recipients, no group has devised

---

Guidelines for Renal Allograft Recipients Who Wish to Conceive

Absolute Criteria
- Wait 2 years after cadaver transplant or 1 year after graft from living donor
- Immunosuppression should be at maintenance levels

Relative Criteria
- Plasma creatinine <1.5 mg/dl
- Absent or easily controlled hypertension
- No or minimal proteinuria
- No evidence of active graft rejection
- No pelvicalyceal distention on a recent ultrasound or intravenous pyelogram
- Prednisone dose 15 mg/day
- Azathioprine dose 2 mg/kg/day
- Cyclosporin A dose 2–4 mg/kg (available data on the use of this drug in pregnancy includes <150 patients)

Adapted from Lindheimer M, Katz A: Pregnancy in the renal transplant patient. Am J Kidney Dis 19:173, 2000.

---

criteria to determine when it is safest to conceive after transplantation. In a recent editorial, Lindheimer and Katz,[108] leading authorities on renal disease in pregnancy, have suggested guidelines, which are summarized in the box "Guidelines for Renal Allograft Recipients Who Wish to Conceive."

Key Points

➤ Asymptomatic bacteriuria complicates 10 percent of pregnancies, and if left untreated will result in symptomatic urinary tract infections in 40 percent of patients.

➤ Pyelonephritis complicates 1 to 2 percent of pregnancies, making it the most frequent nonobstetric cause of hospitalization during pregnancy.

➤ Patients with glomerulonephritis can have successful pregnancies, but pregnancy loss rates increase greatly if the patient has preexisting hypertension.

➤ Creatinine clearance can decline 70 percent before significant increases are seen in the BUN or serum creatinine level. Therefore, a 24-hour urine specimen for creatinine clearance should be collected in any patient when renal disease is suspected.

➤ The chance of successful pregnancy is reduced if the creatinine clearance is less than 50 ml/min or if the serum creatinine level is more than 1.5 mg/dl.

➤ Severe hypertension is the greatest threat to the pregnant woman with chronic renal disease.

➤ Growth restriction and preeclampsia are common in women with chronic renal disease. These patients should have frequent sonograms and should start antepartum fetal surveillance at 28 weeks' gestation.

➤ Patients with chronic renal disease are often anovulatory. After transplantation, as renal function returns, they ovulate and may become pregnant unexpectedly.

➤ Patients should wait 2 years after receiving a cadaver renal allograft and 1 year after receiving a living allograft before contemplating pregnancy. Furthermore, there should be no signs of allograft rejection.

➤ Renal transplant patients should remain on their immunosuppressive medications throughout gestation.

REFERENCES

1. Citiak KA, Newton JR: Serial quantitative maternal nephrosonography in pregnancy. Br J Radiol 58:405, 1985.
2. Citiak KA, Newton JR: Serial qualitative maternal nephrosonography in pregnancy. Br J Radiol 58:399, 1985.
3. Rassmussen PE, Nielson FR: Hydronephrosis during pregnancy: a literature survey. Eur J Obstet Gynecol Reprod Biol 27:249, 1988.
4. Danielson LA, Sherwood OD, Conrad KP: Relaxin is a potent vasodilator in conscious rats. J Clin Invest 103:525, 1999.
5. Conrad KP, Gandley RE, Ogawa T, et al: Endothelin mediates renal vasodilatation and hyperfiltration during pregnancy in chronically instrumented conscious rats. Am J Physiol 276: 767, 1999.
6. DeAlvarez R: Renal glomerulotubular mechanisms during normal pregnancy: glomerular filtration rate, renal plasma flow, and creatinine clearence. Am J Obstet Gynecol 75:931, 1958.
7. Davidson J: Changes in renal function and other aspects of homeostasis in early pregnancy. J Obstet Gynaecol Br Commonw 81:1003, 1974.
8. Christensen P: Tubular reabsorbtion of glucose during pregnancy. Scand J Clin Lab Invest 10:364, 1958.
9. Lindheimer M, Grünfeld JP, Davison JM: Renal disorders. In Barron WM, Lindheimer M (eds): Medical Disorders During Pregnancy. St. Louis, CV Mosby, 2000, p 39.
10. Higby K, Suiter CR, Phelps JY, et al: Normal values of urinary albumin and total protein excretion during pregnancy. Am J Obstet Gynecol 171:984, 1994.
11. McNair RD, MacDonald SR, Dooley SL, Peterson LR: Evaluation of the centrifuged and Gram-stained smear, urinalysis, and reagnet strip testing to detect asymptomatic bacteriuria in obstetric patients. Am J Obstet Gynecol 182:1076, 2000.
12. Romero R, Oyarzum E, Mazor M, et al: Meta-analysis of relationship between asymptomatic bacteriuria and preterm delivery/low birth weight babies. Obstet Gynecol 73:576, 1989.
13. Davison JM, Sprott MS, Selkon JB: The effect of covert bacteriuria in schoolgirls on renal function at 18 years and during pregnancy. Lancet 2:651, 1984.
14. Kass E: Asymptomatic infections of the urinary tract. Trans Assoc Am Physicians 60:56, 1956.
15. Norden C, Kass E: Bacteriuria of pregnancy—a critical reappraisal. Annu Rev Med 19:431, 1968.
16. McFadyen I, Eykryn S, Gardner N: Bacteriuria of pregnancy. J Obstet Gynaecol Br Commonw 80:385, 1973.
17. Kunin C: The natural history of recurrent bacteriuria in schoolgirls. N Engl J Med 282:1443, 1970.
18. Savage W, Hajj S, Kass E: Demographic and prognostic characteristics of bacteriuria in pregnancy. Medicine (Baltimore) 46:385, 1967.
19. Whalley P: Bacteriuria of pregnancy. Am J Obstet Gynecol 97:723, 1967.
20. Plattner MS: Pylonephritis in pregnancy. J Perinatol Neonat Nurs 8:20, 1994.
21. Brumfitt W: The significance of symptomatic and asymptomatic infection in pregnancy. Contrib Nephrol 25:23, 1981.
22. Gilstrap L, Leveno K, Cunningham F, et al: Renal infections and pregnanacy outcome. Am J Obstet Gynecol 141:709, 1981.
23. Fan YD, Pastorek JG II, Miller JM, Mulvey J: Acute pylonephritis in pregnancy. Am J Perinatol 4:324, 1987.
24. Sandberg T, Likin-Janson G, Eden CS: Host response in women with symptomatic urinary tract infection. Scand J Infect Dis 21:67, 1989.
25. Van Dorsten JP, Lenke RR, Schifrin BS: Pylonephritis in pregnancy: the role of in-hospital management and nitrofurantoin suppression. J Reprod Med 32:895, 1987.
26. Cunningham FG, Lucas MJ, Hankins GD: Pulmonary injury complicating antepartum pyelonephritis. Am J Obstet Gynecol 156:797, 1987.
27. Pruett K, Faro S: Pylonephritis associated with respiratory distress. Obstet Gynecol 69:444, 1987.
28. Goorman G, Schlaeffer E, Kopernic G: Adult respiratory distress syndrome as a complication of acute pylonephritis during pregnancy. Eur J Obstet Gynecol Reprod Biol 36:75, 1990.
29. Towers CV, Kaminskas CM, Garite CM, et al: Pulmonary injury associated with antepartum pylonephritis: can at risk patients be identified? Am J Obstet Gynecol 164:974, 1991.
30. Austenfeld MS, Snow BW: Complications of pregnancy in women after reimplantation for vesicoureteral reflux. J Urol 140:1103, 1988.
31. Harris R, Dunnihoo D: The incidence and significance of urinary calculi in pregnancy. Am J Obstet Gynecol 99:237, 1967.
32. Strong D, Murchison R, Lynch D: The management of ureteral calculi during pregnancy. Obstet Gynecol Surv 146:604, 1978.

33. Nadler N, Salinas-Madrigal L, Charles A, Pollack V: Acute glomerulonephritis during late pregnancy. Obstet Gynecol 34: 277, 1969.

34. Wilson C: Changes in renal function. *In* Morris N, Browne J (eds): Nontoxemic Hypertension in Pregnancy. Boston, Little, Brown, 1958, p 177.

35. Packham DK, North RA, Fairly KF, et al: Primary glomerulonephritis and pregnancy. Q J Med 71:537, 1989.

36. Packham DK, North RA, Fairly KF, et al: Membranous glomerulonephritis and pregnancy. Clin Nephrol 30:487, 1988.

37. Jungers P, Forget D, Houillier P, et al: Pregnancy in IgA nephropathy, reflux nephropathy, and focal glomerular sclerosis. Am J Kidney Dis 9:334, 1987.

38. Kincaid-Smith P, Fairley KF: Renal disease in pregnancy: three controversial areas: mesangial IgA nephropathy, focal glomerular sclerosis (focal and segmental hyalinosis and sclerosis), and reflux nephropathy. Am J Kidney Dis 9:328, 1987.

39. Abe S: An overview of pregnancy in women with underlying renal disease. Am J Kidney Dis 17:112, 1991.

40. Imbasciati E, Ponticelli C: Pregnancy and renal disease: predictors for fetal and maternal outcome. Am J Nephrol 11: 353, 1991.

41. Davison J: Renal disease. *In* deSwiet M (ed): Medical Disorders in Obstetric Practice. Oxford, Blackwell, 1984, p 236.

42. Pertuiset N, Grunfeld JP: Acute renal failure in pregnancy. Baillieres Clin Obstet Gynaecol 1:873, 1987.

43. Grunfeld JP, Pertuiset N: Acute renal failure in pregnancy. Am J Kidney Dis 9:359, 1987.

44. Stratta P, Canavese C, Dogliani M, et al: Pregnancy related acute renal failure. Clin Nephrol 32:14, 1989.

45. Grunfeld JP, Ganeval D, Bournerias F: Acute renal failure in pregnancy. Kidney Int 18:179, 1980.

46. Stratta P, Canavese C, Colla L, et al: Acute renal failure in preeclampsia-eclampsia. Gynecol Obstet Invest 27:225, 1987.

47. Turney JH, Ellis CM, Parsons FM: Obstetric acute renal failure 1956–1987. Br J Obstet Gynaecol 96:679, 1989.

48. Sibai B, Villar MA, Mabie BC: Acute renal failure in hypertensive disorders of pregnancy: pregnancy outcome and remote prognosis in thirty-one consecutive cases. Am J Obstet Gynecol 162:777, 1990.

49. Coratelli P, Buongiorno E, Passavanti G: Endotoxemia in hemolytic uremic syndrome. Nephron 50:365, 1988.

50. Robson J, Martin A, Burkley V: Irreversible postpartum renal failure: a new syndrome. Q J Med 37:423, 1968.

51. Seconds A, Louradour N, Suc J, Orfila C: Postpartum hemolytic uremic syndrome: a study of three cases with a review of the literature. Clin Nephrol 12:229, 1979.

52. Wagoner R, Holley K, Johnson W: Accelerated nephrosclerosis and postpartum acute renal failure in normotensive patients. Ann Intern Med 69:237, 1968.

53. Creasey GW, Morgan J: Hemolytic uremic syndrome after ectopic pregnancy: postectopic nephrosclerosis. Obstet Gynecol 69:448, 1987.

54. Li PK, Lai FM, Tam JS, Lai KN: Acute renal failure due to postpartum haemolytic uremic syndrome. Aust N Z J Obstet Gynaecol 28:228, 1988.

55. Conte F, Mewroni M, Battini G, et al: Plasma exchange in acute renal failure due to postpartum hemolytic-uremic syndrome: report of a case. Nephron 50:167, 1988.

56. Remuzzi G, Misiani R, Marchesi D, et al: Treatment of hemolytic uremic syndrome with plasma. Clin Nephrol 12:279, 1979.

57. Webster J, Rees A, Lewis P, Hensby C: Prostacyclin deficiency in haemolytic uraemic syndrome. BMJ 281:271, 1980.

58. Brandt P, Jesperson J, Gregerson G: Post-partum haemolytic-uremic syndrome successfully treated with antithrombin III. BMJ 281:449, 1980.

59. Brandes JC, Fritsche C: Obstructive acute renal failure by a gravid uterus: a case report and review. Am J Kidney Dis 18: 398, 1991.

60. Hayborn KD, Schultz MF, Goodlin RC, Durham JD: Renal artery stenosis during pregnancy: a review. Obstet Gynecol Surv 46:509, 1991.

61. Coe FL, Brenner BM: Approach to the patient with diseases of the kidney and urinary tract. *In* Fauci AS, Braunwald E, Isselbacher KJ, et al (eds). New York, McGraw-Hill, 1998, p 1495.

62. Davison JM, Baylis C: Pregnancy in patients with underlying renal disease. *In* Davison AM, Cameron JC, Grünfeld JP, et al (eds): Oxford, Oxford University Press, 1998, p 2327.

63. Denker BM, Brenner BM: Cardinal manifestations of renal disease. *In* Fauci AS, Braunwald E, Isselbacher KJ, et al (eds): New York, McGraw-Hill, 1998, p 258.

64. Bear R: Pregnancy in patients with renal disease: a study of 44 cases. Obstet Gynecol 48:13, 1976.

65. Hou S: Pregnancy in women with chronic renal disease. N Engl J Med 312:839, 1985.

66. Hou S, Grossman S, Madias N: Pregnancy in women with renal disease and moderate renal insufficiency. Am J Med 78: 185, 1985.

67. Katz A, Davison J, Hayslett J, et al: Pregnancy in women with kidney disease. Kidney Int 18:192, 1980.

68. Mackay E: Pregnancy and renal disease: a ten-year study. Aust N Z J Obstet Gynaecol 3:21, 1963.

69. Studd J, Blainey J: Pregnancy and the nephrotic syndrome. BMJ 1:276, 1969.

70. Kincaid-Smith P, Fairley K, Bullen M: Kidney disease and pregnancy. Med J Aust 11:1155, 1967.

71. Surian M, Imbasciati E, Banfi G, et al: Glomerular disease and pregnancy. Nephron 36:101, 1984.

72. Cunningham FG, Cox SG, Harstad TW, et al: Chronic renal disease and pregnancy outcome. Am J Obstet Gynecol 163: 453, 1990.

73. Ackrill P, Goodwin F, Marsh F, et al: Successful pregnancy in patient on regular dialysis. BMJ 2:172, 1975.

74. Kobayashi H, Matsumoto Y, Otsubo O, et al: Successful pregnancy in a patient undergoing chronic hemodialysis. Obstet Gynecol 57:382, 1981.

75. Savdie E, Caterson R, Mahony J, Clifton-Bligh P: Successful pregnancies treated by haemodialysis. Med J Aust 2:9, 1982.

76. Cohen D, Frenkel Y, Maschiach S, Eliahou HE: Dialysis during pregnancy in advanced chronic renal failure patients: outcome and progression. Clin Nephrol 29:144, 1988.

77. Redrow M, Cherem L, Elliott J, et al: Dialysis in the management of pregnant patients with renal insufficiency. Medicine 67:199, 1988.

78. Hou S: Pregnancy in women requiring dialysis for renal failure. Am J Kidney Dis 9:368, 1987.

79. Yasin SY, Doun SWB: Hemodialysis in pregnancy. Obstet Gynecol Surv 43:655, 1988.

80. Lim V, Henriquez C, Sievertsen G, Prohman L: Ovarian function in chronic renal failure: evidence suggesting hypothalamic anovulation. Ann Intern Med 57:7, 1980.

81. Nageotte MP, Grundy HO: Pregnancy outcome in women requiring chronic hemodialysis. Obstet Gynecol 72:456, 1988.

82. EDTA Registration Committee: Successful pregnancies in women treated by dialysis and kidney tranplantation. Br J Obstet Gynaecol 87:839, 1980.

83. Fine L, Barnett E, Danovitch G, et al: Systemic lupus erythematosus in pregnancy. Ann Intern Med 94:667, 1981.

84. Johnson T, Lorenz R, Menon K, Nolan G: Successful outcome of a pregnancy requiring dialysis: effects on serum progesterone and estrogens. J Reprod Med 22:217, 1979.

85. Piper JM, Ray WA, Rosa FW: Pregnancy outcome following

exposure to angiotensin-converting enzyme inhibitors. Obstet Gynecol 80:429, 1992.

86. Hulton SA, Thompson PD, Cooper PA, Rothberg AD: Angiotensin-converting enzyme inhibitors in pregnancy may result in neonatal renal failure. S Afr Med J 78:673, 1990.

87. Sibai B, Grossman R, Grossman H: Effects of diuretics on plasma volume in pregnancy with long term hypertension. Am J Obstet Gynecol 150:831, 1984.

88. Rodriquez S, Leikin S, Hillar M: Neonatal thrombocytopenia associated with antepartum administration of thiazide drugs. N Engl J Med 270:881, 1964.

89. Sanchez-Casajuz A, Famos I, Santos M: Monitorization fetal en el transcurso de hemodialissi durante el embarazo. Rev Clin Esp 149:187, 1978.

90. Schewitz L, Friedman E, Pollak V: Bleeding after renal biopsy in pregnancy. Obstet Gynecol 26:1965, 1965.

91. Lindheimer M, Spargo B, Katz A: Renal biopsy in pregnancy-induced hypertension. J Reprod Med 15:189, 1975.

92. Lindheimer M, Fisher K, Spargo B, Katz A: Hypertension in pregnancy: a biopsy with long term follow-up. Contrib Nephrol 25:71, 1981.

93. Packham DK, Fairley K: Renal biopsy: indications and complications in pregnancy. Br J Obstet Gynaecol 94:935, 1987.

94. Merkatz I, Schwartz G, David D, et al: Resumption of female reproductive function following renal transplantation. JAMA 216:1749, 1971.

95. Penn I, Markowski E, Harris P: Parenthood following renal transplantation. Kidney Int 8:221, 1980.

96. Saarikoski S, Sappala M: Immunosuppression during pregnancy: transmission of azathioprine and its metabolites from mother to fetus. Am J Obstet Gynecol 115:1100, 1973.

97. Cote C, Meuwissen H, Picketing R: Effects on the neonate of prednisone and azathioprine administered to the mother during pregnancy. J Pediatr 85:324, 1974.

98. Price H, Salaman J, Laurence K, Langmaid H: Immunosuppressive drugs and the fetus. Transplantation 21:294, 1976.

99. Scott J: Fetal growth retardation associated with maternal administration of immunosuppressive drugs. Am J Obstet Gynecol 128:668, 1977.

100. Ponticelli C, Montagnino G: Causes of arterial hypertension in kidney transplantation. Contrib Nephrol 54:226, 1987.

101. Derfler K, Schuller A, Herold C, et al: Successful outcome of a complicated pregnancy in a renal transplant recipient taking cyclosporin A. Clin Nephrol 29:96, 1988.

102. Salamalekis EE, Mortakis AE, Phocas I, et al: Successful pregnancy in a renal transplant recipient taking cyclosporin A: hormonal and immunological studies. Int J Gynaecol Obstet 30:267, 1989.

103. Pickerell MD, Sawers R, Michael J: Pregnanacy after renal transplantation: severe intrauterine growth retardation during treatment with cyclosporin A. BMJ 1:825, 1988.

104. Davison J: Renal transplantation and pregnancy. Am J Kidney Dis 9:374, 1987.

105. Parsons V, Bewick M, Elias J, et al: Pregnancy following renal transplantation. J R Soc Med 72:815, 1979.

106. Davison J, Lindheimer M: Pregnancy in women with renal allografts. Semin Nephrol 4:240, 1984.

107. Huffer W, Kuzela D, Popovtzer M: Metabolic bone disease in chronic renal failure in renal transplant patients. Am J Pathol 78:385, 1975.

108. Lindheimer M, Katz A: Pregnancy in the renal transplant patient. Am J Kidney Dis 19:173, 2000.

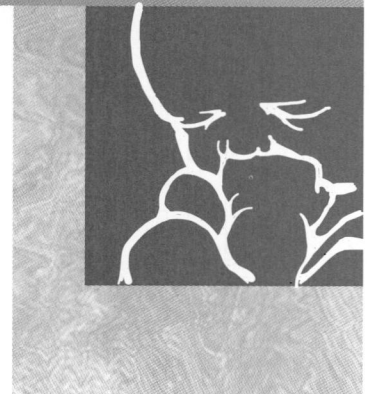

Chapter 32

Diabetes Mellitus

MARK B. LANDON, PATRICK M. CATALANO, AND STEVEN G. GABBE

The introduction of insulin therapy 80 years ago remains an important landmark in the care of pregnancy for the diabetic woman. Before insulin became available, pregnancy was uncommon and was likely to be accompanied by fetal mortality and a substantial risk for maternal death. Management techniques have been developed over the past 30 years to prevent complications based on an understanding of the pathophysiology of diabetic pregnancy. These advances have resulted in perinatal mortality rates in optimally managed cases that approach that of the normal population. This dramatic improvement in perinatal outcome has been largely attributed to clinical efforts to establish improved maternal glycemic control both prior to conception and during gestation (Fig. 32–1). Excluding major congenital malformations, which continue to plague pregnancies in the insulin-dependent woman, perinatal loss for the diabetic woman has fortunately become an uncommon event.

While the benefit of careful regulation of maternal glucose levels is well accepted, failure to establish optimal glycemic control as well as other factors continue to result in significant perinatal morbidity. For this reason, both clinical and basic laboratory research efforts continue to focus on the etiology of congenital malformations, fetal growth disorders, and intrauterine death. Clinical experience has also resulted in a more realistic appreciation of the impact that vascular complications can have on pregnancy and the manner in which pregnancy may impact these disease processes. With modern management techniques and an organized team approach, successful pregnancies have become the norm even for women with the most complicated diabetes. Before considering these clinical issues, it is important to understand the metabolic effects of pregnancy in relation to the pathophysiology of diabetes mellitus.

PATHOPHYSIOLOGY

Normal Glucose Tolerance

There are significant alterations in maternal metabolism during pregnancy, which provide for adequate nutritional stores in early gestation in order to meet the increased maternal and fetal demands of late gestation and lactation. Although we are apt to think of diabetes mellitus as a disorder exclusively of maternal glucose metabolism, in fact diabetes mellitus affects all aspects of maternal nutrient metabolism. In this section we consider maternal glucose metabolism as it relates to pancreatic β-cell production of insulin and insulin clearance, endogenous (i.e., primarily hepatic) glucose production and suppression with insulin, and peripheral insulin sensitivity. We also address maternal protein and lipid insulin metabolism. Lastly, the impact of these alternations on maternal metabolism is examined as they relate to maternal energy expenditure and fetal growth.

Glucose Metabolism

Normal pregnancy has been characterized as a "diabetogenic state" because of the progressive increase in postprandial glucose levels and insulin response in late gestation. However, early gestation can be viewed as an anabolic condition because of the increases in maternal fat stores and decrease in free fatty acid concentrations. Weiss et al.[1] have described significant decreases in maternal insulin requirements early in gestation in insulin-dependent women with optimal glucose control prior to conception. The mechanisms for this decrease in insulin requirements have been ascribed to various factors in-

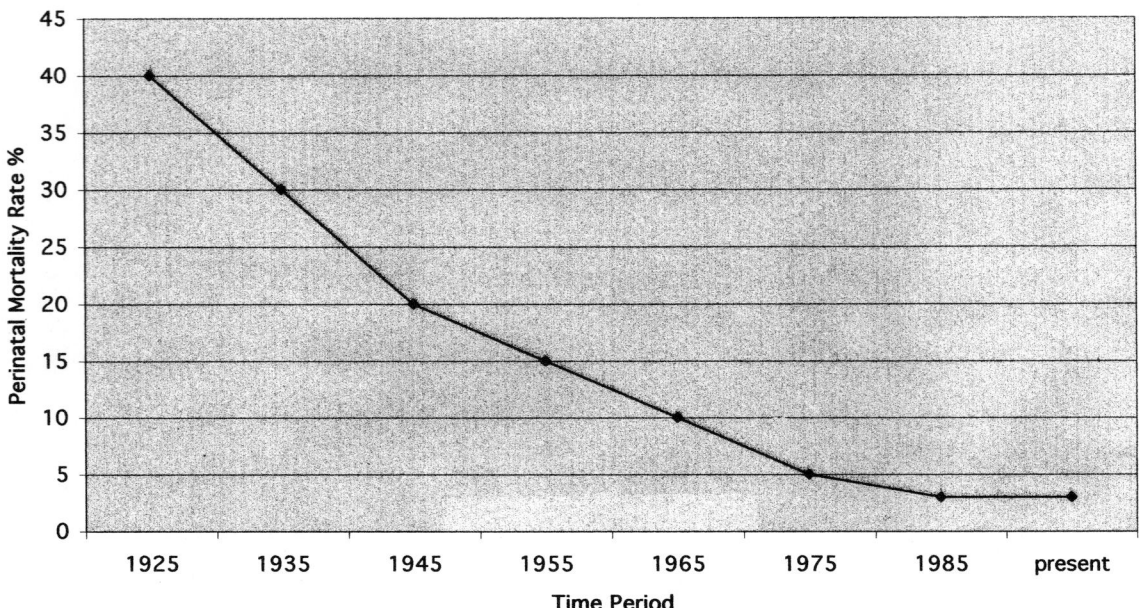

Figure 32–1. Perinatal mortality rates in pregnancy complicated by type 1 diabetes mellitus.

cluding insulin sensitivity, decreased substrate availability secondary to factors such as nausea, the fetus acting as a glucose sink, or enhanced maternal insulin secretion. Longitudinal studies in women with normal glucose tolerance have shown significant progressive alterations in all aspects of glucose metabolism as early as the end of the first trimester.[2]

There are progressive increases in insulin secretion in response to an intravenous glucose challenge with advancing gestation (Fig. 32–2). The increases in insulin concentration are more pronounced in lean as com-

pared to obese women, most probably as a response to the greater decreases in insulin sensitivity in lean women as will be described later. Data regarding insulin clearance in pregnancy are limited. In separate studies Bellman and Hartman,[3] Lind et al.,[4] and Burt and Davidson[5] reported no difference in insulin disappearance rate when insulin was infused intravenously in late gestation in comparison with nongravid subjects. In contrast, Goodner and Freinkel,[6] using a radiolabeled insulin, described a 25 percent increase in insulin turnover in a pregnant as compared with a nonpregnant rat

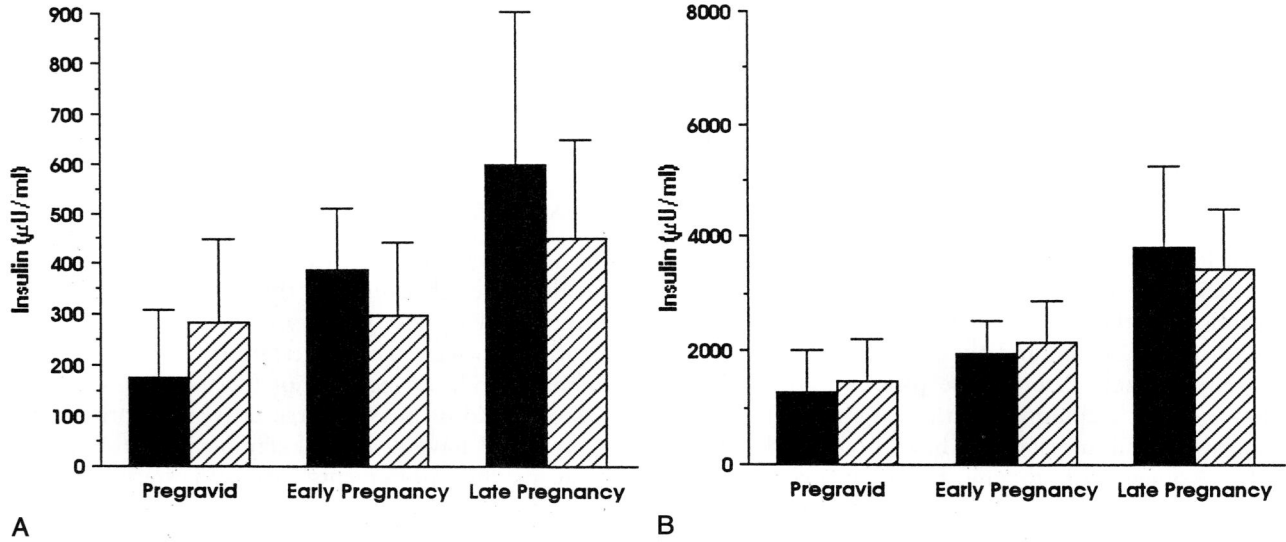

Figure 32–2. Longitudinal increase in insulin response to an intravenous glucose challenge in lean and obese women with normal glucose tolerance, pregravid, early and late pregnancy. *A*, First phase: area under the curve from 0 to 5 minutes. *B*, Second phase: area under the curve from 5 to 60 minutes.

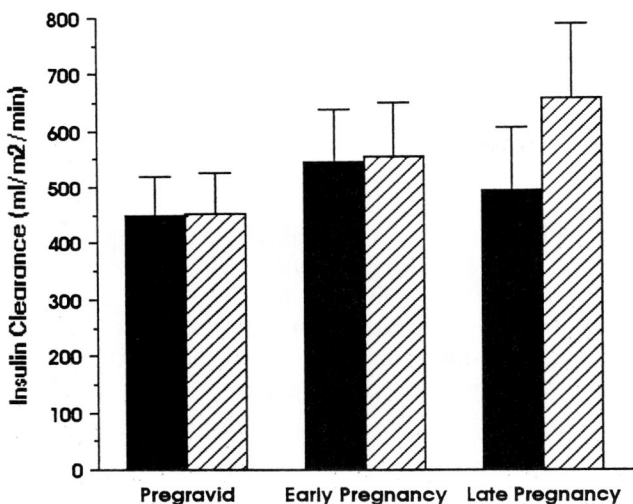

Figure 32–3. Longitudinal increases in metabolic clearance rate of insulin (ml/m²/min) in lean and obese women with normal glucose tolerance; pregravid, early, and late pregnancy.

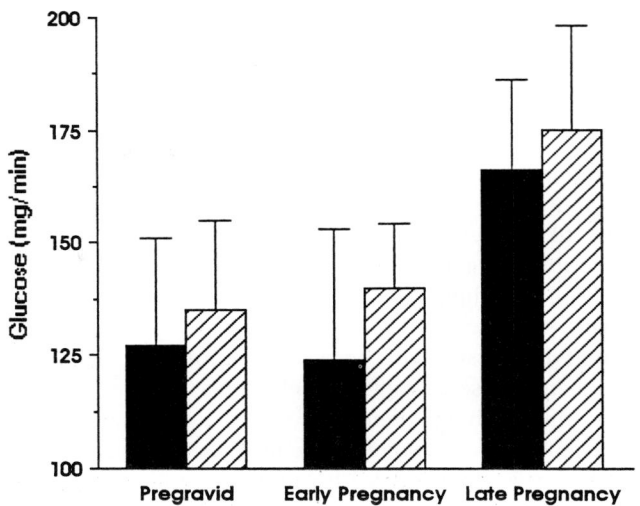

Figure 32–4. Longitudinal increase in basal endogenous (primarily hepatic) glucose production (mg/min) in lean and obese women with normal glucose tolerance; pregravid, early, and late pregnancy.

model. Catalano et al.[7] using the euglycemic-clamp model reported a 20 percent increase in insulin clearance in lean women and a 30 percent increase in insulin clearance in obese women by late pregnancy (Fig. 32–3). Although the placenta is rich in insulinase, the exact mechanism for the increased insulin clearance in pregnancy remains speculative.

Although there is a progressive decrease in fasting glucose with advancing gestation, the decrease is most probably a result of the increase in plasma volume in early gestation and increase in fetoplacental glucose utilization in late gestation. Kalhan and Cowett[9] using various stable isotope methodologies in cross-sectional study designs were the first to describe increased fasting hepatic glucose production in late pregnancy. Additionally, Catalano et al.[10] using a stable isotope of glucose in a prospective longitudinal study design reported a 30 percent increase in maternal fasting hepatic glucose production with advancing gestation (Fig. 32–4), which remained significant even when adjusted for maternal weight gain. Tissue sensitivity to insulin involves both liver and peripheral tissues, primarily skeletal muscle. The increase in fasting maternal hepatic glucose production occurred despite a significant increase in fasting insulin concentration, thereby indicating a decrease in maternal hepatic glucose sensitivity in women with normal glucose tolerance. Additionally, in obese women there was a decreased ability of infused insulin to suppress hepatic glucose production in late gestation as compared with pregravid and early pregnancy measurements, thereby indicating a further decrease in hepatic insulin sensitivity[11] in obese women.

Estimates of peripheral insulin sensitivity in pregnancy have included the measurement of insulin response to a fixed oral or intravenous glucose challenge

or the ratio of insulin to glucose under a variety of experimental conditions. In recent years, newer methodologies such as the Bergman minimal model[12] and the euglycemic-hyperinsulinemic[13] clamp have improved our ability to quantify peripheral insulin sensitivity. In lean women in early gestation, Catalano et al.[14] reported a 40 percent decrease in maternal peripheral insulin sensitivity using the euglycemic-hyperinsulinemic clamp. However, when adjusted for changes in insulin concentrations during the clamp and residual hepatic glucose production (i.e., the insulin sensitivity index), insulin sensitivity decreased only 10 percent (Fig. 32–5).

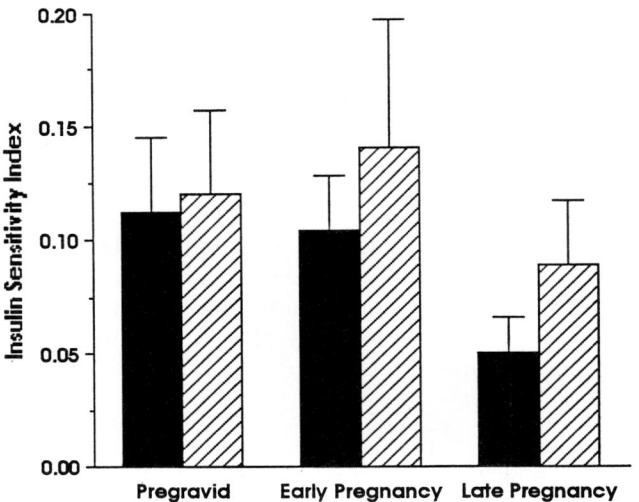

Figure 32–5. Longitudinal changes in the insulin sensitivity index (glucose infusion rate adjusted for residual endogenous glucose production and insulin concentrations achieved during the glucose clamp) in lean and obese women with normal glucose tolerance; pregravid, early, and late gestation.

In contrast, there was a 15 percent increase in the insulin sensitivity index in obese women in early pregnancy as compared with pregravid estimates.[15] Hence, the decrease in insulin requirements in early gestation observed in some women requiring insulin may be a consequence of a relative increase in insulin sensitivity, particularly in women with decreased insulin sensitivity prior to conception. As compared with the metabolic alterations in early pregnancy, there is a uniformity of opinion regarding the decrease in peripheral insulin sensitivity in late gestation. Spellacy and Goetz[16] were among the first investigators to report an increase in insulin response to a glucose challenge in late gestation. Additionally, Burt[17] demonstrated that pregnant women experienced less hypoglycemia in response to exogenous insulin in comparison with nonpregnant subjects. Later research by Fisher et al.[18] using a high-dose glucose infusion test, Buchanan et al.[19] using the Bergman minimal model, and Ryan et al.[20] and Catalano et al.[2] using the euglycemic-hyperinsulinemic clamp all have demonstrated a decrease in insulin sensitivity ranging from 33 to 78 percent. It should be noted, however, that all these quantitative estimates of insulin sensitivity are very likely overestimates due to non–insulin-mediated glucose disposal by the fetus and placenta. Hay et al.[21] reported that in the pregnant ewe model, approximately one third of maternal glucose utilization was accounted for by uterine, placental, and fetal tissue. Additionally, Marconi et al.[22] observed that based on human fetal blood sampling, fetal glucose concentration was a function of fetal size and gestational age in addition to maternal glucose concentration.

Placental glucose transport is a non–energy-requiring process and takes place through facilitated diffusion. Glucose transport is dependent on a family of glucose transporters referred to as the GLUT glucose transporter family. The principal glucose transporter in the placenta is GLUT 1, which is found in the syncytiotrophoblast.[23] GLUT 1 is located on both the microvillus and basal membranes. Basal membrane GLUT 1 may be the rate-limiting step in placental glucose transport. There is a two- to threefold increase in the expression of syncytiotrophoblast glucose transporters with advancing gestation.[24] Although GLUT 3 and GLUT 4 expression have been identified in placental endothelial cells and intervillous nontrophoblastic cells, respectively, the role they may play in placental glucose transport remains speculative.[25,26]

DIABETES MELLITUS

Diabetes mellitus is a chronic metabolic disorder characterized by either absolute or relative insulin deficiency, resulting in increased glucose concentrations. Although glucose intolerance is the common outcome of diabetes mellitus, the pathophysiology remains heterogeneous. The two major classifications of diabetes mellitus are type 1, formerly referred to as insulin-dependent diabetes or juvenile onset diabetes, and type 2, formerly referred to as non–insulin-dependent or adult-onset diabetes. During pregnancy, classification of women with diabetes has often relied on the White classification,[27] first proposed in the 1940s. This classification is based on factors such as the age of onset of diabetes and duration as well as end-organ involvement, primarily retinal and renal.

Type 1 Diabetes

Type 1 diabetes is usually characterized by an abrupt onset at a young age and absolute insulinopenia with lifelong requirements for insulin replacement. In some populations, the onset of type 1 diabetes may occur in individuals in the third or fourth decades of life. Patients with diabetes mellitus may have a genetic predisposition for antibodies directed against their pancreatic islet cells. The degree of concordance for the development of type 1 diabetes in monozygotic twins is 33 percent, suggesting that the events subsequent to the development of autoantibodies and appearance of glucose intolerance are also related to environmental factors. Because of the complete dependence on exogenous insulin, pregnant women with type 1 diabetes are at increased risk for the development of diabetic ketoacidosis. Additionally, because intensive insulin therapy is used in women with type 1 to decrease the risk for spontaneous abortion and congenital anomalies in early gestation, these women are at greater risk of hypoglycemic reactions. Studies by Diamond et al.[28] and Rosenn et al.[29] have shown that women with type 1 diabetes are at increased risk for hypoglycemic reactions during pregnancy because of diminished counterregulatory epinephrine and glucagon response to hypoglycemia. The deficiency in counterregulatory response may be in part due to an independent effect of pregnancy.

The alterations in glucose metabolism in women with type 1 diabetes are not well characterized. Because of maternal insulinopenia, insulin response during gestation can only be estimated relative to pregravid requirements. Estimates of the change in insulin requirements are complicated by the degree of preconceptional glucose control and frequent presence of insulin antibodies. Weiss and Hoffman[1] reported on the change in insulin requirements in women with type 1 diabetes and strict glucose control either prior to conception or before 10 weeks' gestation. There was a 12 percent decrease in insulin requirements from 10 to 17 weeks' gestation and a 50 percent increase in insulin requirement from 17 weeks' until delivery as compared with pregravid requirements. After 36 weeks' gestation there was a decrease in insulin requirements. A 5 percent decrease in insulin requirements after 36 weeks' gestation was also noted by McManus and Ryan.[30] The decrease in insulin requirements was associated with a longer duration of diabetes mellitus but not with adverse perinatal outcome. The fall in insulin requirements in early pregnancy in women with type 1 diabetes may be a reflection of decreased pregravid insulin sensitivity as will be described later.

Schmitz et al.[31] have evaluated the longitudinal changes in insulin sensitivity in women with type 1 diabetes in early and late pregnancy as well as postpartum in comparison with nonpregnant women with type 1 diabetes. In pregnant women with type 1 diabetes there was a 50 percent decrease in insulin sensitivity only in late gestation. There was no significant difference in insulin sensitivity in pregnant women with type 1 diabetes in early pregnancy or within 1 week of delivery as compared with the nonpregnant women with type 1 diabetes. Therefore, based on the available data, women with type 1 diabetes appear to have a similar decrease in insulin sensitivity when compared with women with normal glucose tolerance.

Relative to the issue of placental transporters (GLUT 1), there is a report by Jansson and Powell[32] describing an increase in both basal GLUT 1 expression and glucose transport activity from placental tissue in women with White Class D pregnancies.

Type 2 Diabetes/Gestational Diabetes

The pathophysiology of type 2 diabetes involves abnormalities of both insulin-sensitive tissues (i.e., a decrease in skeletal muscle and hepatic sensitivity to insulin) and β-cell response as manifested by an inadequate insulin response for a given degree of glycemia. Initially in the course of development of type 2 diabetes, the insulin response to a glucose challenge may be increased relative to that of individuals with normal glucose tolerance but is inadequate to maintain normoglycemia. Whether or not decreased insulin sensitivity (increased insulin resistance) precedes β-cell dysfunction in the development of type 2 diabetes continues to be debated. Arguments and experimental data support both hypotheses. As noted by Sims and Calles-Escadon,[33] heterogeneity of metabolic abnormalities exists in any classification of diabetes mellitus.

Despite the limitations of any classification system, certain generalizations can be made regarding women with type 2 or gestational diabetes mellitus (GDM). These individuals are typically older and more often heavier as compared with individuals with type 1 diabetes or normal glucose tolerance. The onset of the disorder is usually insidious with few patients complaining of the classic triad of polydipsia, polyphagia, and polyuria. Individuals with type 2 diabetes are often initially recommended to lose weight, increase their activity (i.e., exercise), and follow a diet that is low in fats and high in complex carbohydrates. Oral agents are often used to either increase insulin response or, with newer drugs, enhance insulin sensitivity. Individuals with type 2 diabetes may eventually require insulin therapy to maintain euglycemia but are not at risk for diabetic ketoacidosis. Data from monozygotic twin studies have reported a lifetime risk of both twins developing type 2 diabetes that ranges between 58 percent and almost 100 percent, suggesting that the disorder has a strong genetic component.

Women with type 2 diabetes are usually classified as Class B diabetes according to the White classification system. Women developing gestational diabetes (i.e., glucose intolerance first recognized during pregnancy) share many of the metabolic characteristics of women with type 2 diabetes. Although earlier studies reported a 10 to 35 percent incidence of islet cell antibodies in women with gestational diabetes as measured by immunofluorescence techniques,[34,35] more recent data using specific monoclonal antibodies have described a much lower incidence on the order of 1 to 2 percent,[36] suggesting a low risk of type 1 diabetes in women with gestational diabetes. Furthermore, postpartum studies of women with gestational diabetes have demonstrated defects in insulin secretory response[37] and decreased insulin sensitivity,[38] indicating that typical type 2 abnormalities in glucose metabolism are present in women with gestational diabetes. Of interest, the alterations in insulin secretory response and insulin resistance in women with a previous history of GDM as compared with a weight-matched control group may differ depending on whether or not the women with previous gestational diabetes are lean or obese.[39] Thus, in women with gestational diabetes, the hormonal events of pregnancy may represent an unmasking of a genetic susceptibility to type 2 diabetes.

There are significant alterations in glucose metabolism in women who develop gestational diabetes relative to the changes in glucose metabolism in women with normal glucose tolerance. Decreased insulin response to a glucose challenge has been demonstrated by Yen et al.,[40] Fisher et al.,[41] and Buchanan et al.[19] in women with gestational diabetes in late gestation. In prospective longitudinal studies of both lean and obese women with gestational diabetes, Catalano et al.[14] also showed a progressive decrease in first-phase insulin response in late gestation in lean women developing gestational diabetes as compared with a weight-matched control group (Fig. 32-6A). In contrast, in obese women developing gestational diabetes, there was no difference in first-phase insulin response but rather a significant increase in second-phase insulin response to an intravenous glucose challenge as compared with a

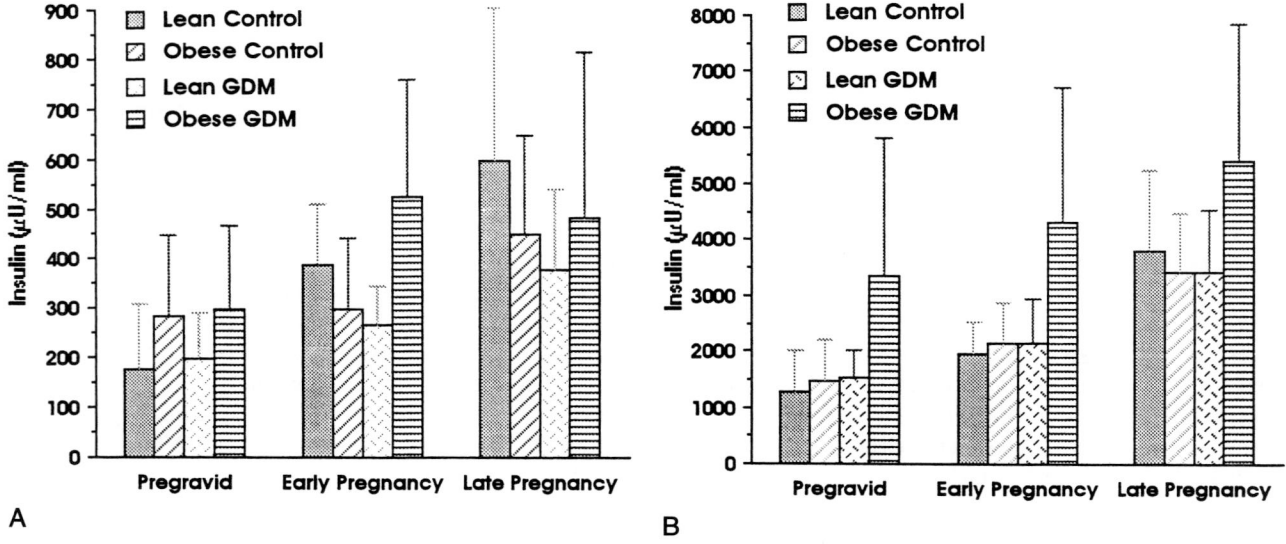

Figure 32–6. Longitudinal increase in insulin response to an intravenous glucose challenge in lean and obese women with normal glucose tolerance and gestational diabetes; pregravid, early, and late pregnancy. *A*, First phase: area under the curve from 0 to 5 minutes. *B*, Second phase: area under the curve from 5 to 60 minutes.

weight-matched control group (Fig. 32–6*B*). These differences in insulin response may be related to the ethnicity of the various study groups. Although there is an increase in the metabolic clearance rate of insulin with advancing gestation, there is no evidence that there is a significant difference between women with normal glucose tolerance and gestational diabetes.[15]

There is a significant decline in fasting glucose concentrations with advancing gestation in women developing gestational diabetes. In late fasting, glucose and hepatic glucose production pregnancy increases in women with gestational diabetes in comparison with a control group.[42] Whereas there was no significant difference in either fasting glucose concentration or hepatic glucose production in the longitudinal studies of Catalano et al.,[14,15] these differences may again be population specific. However, to date all reports indicate that in late gestation, women with gestational diabetes have increased fasting insulin concentrations (Fig. 32–7) and less suppression of hepatic glucose production during insulin infusion, thereby indicating decreased hepatic glucose insulin sensitivity in women with gestational diabetes as compared with a weight-matched control group.[14,15,42] In the studies of Xiang et al.,[42] there was significant correlation between fasting free fatty acid concentrations and hepatic glucose production, suggesting that insulin resistance in fat cells may contribute to hepatic insulin resistance.

Women with gestational diabetes have decreased insulin sensitivity in comparison with weight-matched control groups. Ryan et al.[20] was the first to report a 40 percent decrease in insulin sensitivity in women with gestational diabetes in comparison with a pregnant control group in late pregnancy using a hyperinsulinemic-

euglycemic clamp. Xiang et al.[42] found that women with gestational diabetes who had normal glucose tolerance within 6 months of delivery had significantly decreased insulin sensitivity as estimated by the glucose clearance rate during a hyperinsulinemic-euglycemic clamp, as compared with a matched control group with normal glucose tolerance during the third trimester. Catalano et al.[14,15] using similar techniques described the longitudinal changes in insulin sensitivity in both lean and obese women developing gestational diabetes in comparison with a matched control group. Women developing gestational diabetes had decreased insulin sensitivity as compared with the matched control group

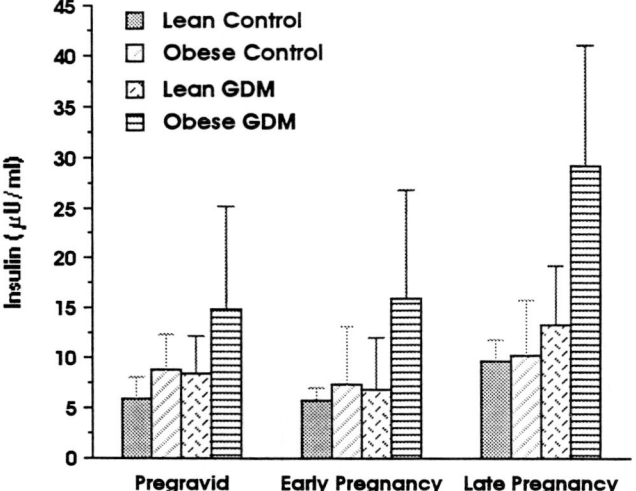

Figure 32–7. Longitudinal increase in basal or fasting insulin (μU/ml) in lean and obese women with normal glucose tolerance and gestational diabetes; pregravid, early, and later pregnancy.

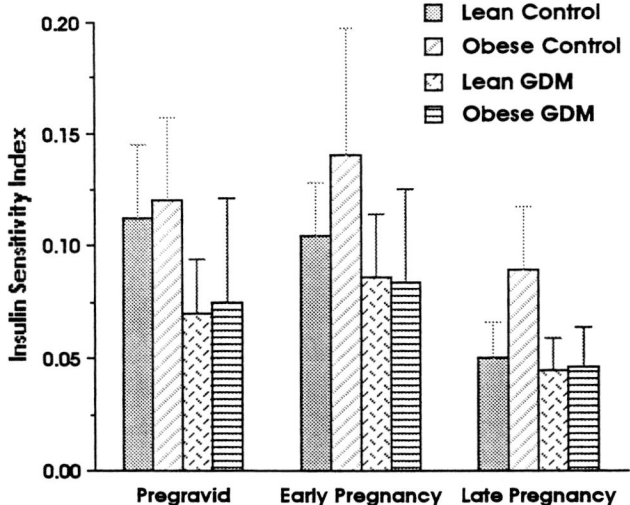

Figure 32–8. Longitudinal changes in the insulin sensitivity index (glucose infusion rate adjusted for residual endogenous glucose production and insulin concentrations achieved during the glucose clamp) in lean and obese women with normal glucose tolerance and gestational diabetes; pregravid, early, and late pregnancy.

(Fig. 32–8). The differences in insulin sensitivity were greatest before and during early gestation, and by late gestation the differences in insulin sensitivity between the groups were less pronounced but still significant. Of interest, there was an increase in insulin sensitivity from the time prior to conception through early pregnancy (12 to 14 weeks), particularly in those women with greatest decreases in insulin sensitivity prior to conception. The changes in insulin sensitivity from the time prior to conception through early pregnancy were significantly correlated with changes in maternal weight gain and energy expenditure.[43] The relationship between these alterations in maternal glucose insulin sensitivity and weight gain and energy expenditure may help explain the decrease in maternal weight gain and insulin requirements in women with diabetes in early gestation.[1]

Studies in human skeletal muscle and adipose tissue have demonstrated that postreceptor defects in the insulin signaling cascade are related to decreased insulin sensitivity in pregnancy. Garvey et al.[44] were the first to demonstrate that there were no significant differences in the glucose transporter (GLUT 4) responsible for insulin action and skeletal muscle in pregnant as compared with nonpregnant women. Based on the studies of Friedman et al.[45] in both pregnant women with normal glucose tolerance and gestational diabetes as well as weight-matched nonpregnant control subjects there appeared to be defects in the insulin signaling cascade in pregnancy as well as what may be additional abnormalities in women with gestational diabetes. All pregnant women appeared to have a decrease in insulin receptor substrate-1 (IRS-1) expression. The down-regulation of the IRS-1 protein closely parallels the decreased ability of insulin to induce additional steps in the insulin signaling cascade, resulting in movement of the GLUT 4 to the cell surface membrane and facilitating glucose transport into the cell. The down-regulation of IRS-1 protein closely parallels the ability of insulin to stimulate 2-deoxyglucose uptake in vitro. In addition to the above mechanisms, women with gestational diabetes mellitus demonstrate a distinct decrease in the ability of the insulin receptor β (that component of the insulin receptor not on the cell surface) to undergo tyrosine phosphorylation. The additional defect in the insulin signaling cascade results in a 25 percent lower glucose transport activity.

Amino Acid Metabolism

Although glucose is the primary source of energy for the fetus and placenta, there are not appreciable amounts of glucose stored as glycogen in the fetus or placenta. However, accretion of protein is essential for growth of fetoplacental tissue. There is increased nitrogen retention in pregnancy in both maternal and fetal compartments. There is an increase of approximately 0.9 kg of maternal fat-free mass by 27 weeks.[46] There is significant decrease in most fasting maternal amino acid concentrations in early pregnancy prior to the accretion of significant maternal or fetal tissue.[47] These anticipatory changes in fasting amnio acid metabolism occur after a shorter period of fasting in comparison with nonpregnant women, and may be another example of the accelerated starvation of pregnancy as described by Freinkel et al.[48] Furthermore, amino acid concentrations such as serine correlate significantly with fetal growth in both early and late gestation.[49] Maternal amino acid concentrations were significantly decreased in mothers of small-for-gestational-age neonates in comparison with maternal concentration in appropriately grown neonates.[50]

There is also a significant conservation of nitrogen/protein in late gestation. There is a decrease in maternal plasma urea nitrogen concentrations as well as a decrease in urea nitrogen synthesis and excretion.[51] In evaluating the balance between protein breakdown and resynthesis, estimates of amino acid turnover using stable isotopes of leucine are useful. Studies by Denne et al.[52] have shown that the rates of basal or fasting proteolysis or protein turnover are similar in pregnant and nonpregnant subjects, indicating that there may be no change in fasting amino acid insulin sensitivity in pregnancy. Additionally, there are no published studies evaluating the effect of infused insulin on amino acid turnover during pregnancy in either pregnant women with normal or abnormal glucose tolerance. Therefore, based on studies of whole-body protein turnover in late gestation, there may be a slight decrease in the rate of protein breakdown during fasting[53] and a small increase on protein turnover during the day.[54] Additional studies will be required to understand the alterations in amino acid metabolism during pregnancy in normal and abnormal maternal and fetoplacental growth and development.

Amino acids are actively transported across the placenta from mother to fetus via energy-requiring amino acid transporters. These transporters are highly stereospecific, but have low substrate specificity. Additionally, they may vary with location between the microvillus and basal membranes.[55] Decreased amino acid concentrations have been reported in growth-restricted neonates in comparison with appropriately grown neonates. Decreased amino acid transporter activity has been implicated as a possible mechanism. However, the potential role if any of placental amino acid transporters in the development of fetal macrosomia in women with diabetes is currently unknown.[56]

Lipid Metabolism

While there is ample literature regarding the changes in glucose metabolism during gestation, the data regarding the alterations in lipid metabolism are meager by comparison. Knopp et al.[57] have reported that there is a two- to fourfold increase in total triglyceride concentration and a 25 to 50 percent increase in total cholesterol concentration during gestation. Additionally, there is a 50 percent increase in low-density lipoprotein (LDL) cholesterol and a 30 percent increase in high-density lipoprotein (HDL) cholesterol by midgestation, which decreases slightly in the third trimester. Maternal triglyceride and very-low-density lipoprotein (VLDL) triglyceride levels in late gestation are positively correlated with maternal estriol and insulin concentrations.

The increase in maternal lipid concentration in late gestation, in particular free fatty acids, has been hypothesized as one mechanism responsible for the decrease in maternal insulin sensitivity.[58] Free fatty acids have been associated with fetal overgrowth, particularly of fetal adipose tissue. There is a significant difference in the arteriovenous free fatty acid concentration at birth much as there is with arteriovenous glucose concentration. Knopp et al.[59,60] reported that neonatal birth weight was positively correlated with triglyceride and free fatty acid concentrations in late pregnancy. Similar conclusions were reached by Ogburn et al.,[61] who showed that higher fetal insulin levels decrease free fatty acid concentrations, inhibit lipolysis, and result in increased fat deposition in the fetus. Lastly, Kleigman et al.[62] reported that infants of obese women had an increased birth weight and skinfold thickness and higher free fatty acid levels when compared with infants of lean women.

Lipid metabolism in women with diabetes mellitus is influenced by whether the woman has type 1 or type 2 diabetes. This also applies when these women become pregnant. In women with type 2 diabetes and gestational diabetes, Knopp et al.[63] reported an increase in triglyceride and decrease in HDL concentrations. However, Montelongo et al.[64] reported little change in free fatty acid concentrations through all three trimesters after a 12-hour fast. Recently, Koukkou et al.[65] reported an increase in total triglyceride but a lower LDL cholesterol in women with gestational diabetes. In women with type 1 diabetes, there was no change in total triglyceride, but a lower cholesterol concentration, secondary to a decrease in HDL. This is of interest because HDL acts as a plasma antioxidant and thus may be related to the increase in congenital malformations in women with type 1 diabetes. Oxidative stress has been implicated as a potential factor in the incidence of anomalies in women with type 1 diabetes.

Maternal Weight Gain and Energy Expenditure

Estimates of the energy requirements of pregnancy range from a cost of 80,000 kcal to a net saving of up to 10,000 kcal.[66] As a result, the recommendations for nutritional intake in pregnancy are diverse and depend on the population being evaluated. Furthermore, based on more recent data, recommendations for individuals within a population may be more diverse than previously believed, making general guidelines for nutritional intake difficult.[67]

The theoretical energy cost of pregnancy was originally estimated by Hytten[46] using a factorial method. The additional cost of pregnancy consisted of (1) the additional maternal and fetoplacental tissue accrued during pregnancy and (2) the additional "running cost" of pregnancy (e.g., the increased cardiac output). In Hytten's model, the greatest increases in maternal energy expenditure occur between 10 and 30 weeks' gestation, primarily because of maternal accretion of adipose tissue. However, the mean increases in maternal adipose tissue vary considerably among various ethnic groups. Forsum et al.[68] reported a mean increase of over 5 kg of adipose tissue in Swedish women, whereas Lawrence et al.[69] found no increase in adipose tissue stores in women from the Gambia.

Basal metabolic rate accounts for 60 to 70 percent of total energy expenditure in individuals not engaged in competitive physical activity and correlates well with total energy expenditure. As with the changes in maternal accretion of adipose tissue, there are wide variations in the change in maternal basal metabolic rate during gestation, not only in different populations but again within relatively homogeneous groups. The cumulative energy changes in basal metabolic rate range from a high of 52,000 kcal in Swedish women[70] to net savings of 10,700 kcal in women from the Gambia[69] without nutritional supplementation. The mean increase in basal metabolic rate in Western women relative to a nonpregnant, nonlactating control group averages approximately 20 percent.[71] However, the coefficient of variation of basal metabolic rate in these populations during gestation ranges from 93 percent in women in the United Kingdom[72] to over 200 percent in Swedish women.[70] When assessing energy intake in relation to energy expenditure, however, estimated energy intake remains significantly lower than the estimates of total energy expenditure. These discrepancies have usually been explained by factors such as (1) increased metabolic efficiency during gestation,[73] (2) decreased maternal activity,[74] and (3) unreliable assessment of food intake.[72]

Data in nonpregnant subjects may help us understand some of the wide variations in metabolic parameters during human gestation, even with homogeneous populations. Swinburn et al.[75] reported that in the Pima Indian population, subjects with decreased insulin sensitivity gained less weight when compared with more insulin sensitive subjects (3.1 vs. 7.6 kg) over a period of 4 years. Furthermore, the percentage weight change per year was highly correlated with glucose disposal as estimated from clamp studies. Catalano et al.[43] conducted a prospective longitudinal study in early pregnancy of the changes in maternal accretion of body fat and basal metabolic rate in women with normal glucose tolerance and gestational diabetes. Women with gestational diabetes had decreased glucose insulin sensitivity in early gestation as compared with the control group and had significantly smaller increases in body fat than women with normal glucose tolerance. There was a significant inverse correlation between the changes in fat accretion and insulin sensitivity (i.e., women with decreased pregravid insulin sensitivity had less accretion of body fat as compared with women with increased pregravid insulin sensitivity). These results are consistent with a previous report showing that total weight gain in women with gestational diabetes was 2.5 kg less as compared to a weight-matched control group.[76]

In these same subjects there was also a significant inverse correlation between changes in basal metabolic rate and basal hepatic glucose production.[43] In early gestation, there was a 7 percent increase in basal metabolic rate in women with normal glucose tolerance and only a 2 percent increase in women with gestational diabetes. As before, there was a significant negative correlation between the changes in basal metabolic rate and estimates of glucose metabolism, in this case basal hepatic glucose production. The results of these studies show that there is a relationship between the changes in maternal insulin sensitivity and changes in basal metabolic rate and accretion of adipose tissue in early gesta-

tion. The ability of women with decreased pregravid glucose insulin sensitivity to conserve energy, increase body fat, and make sufficient nutrients available to produce a healthy fetus supports the hypothesis that decreased maternal insulin sensitivity may have a reproductive metabolic advantage in women when food availability is marginal. In contrast, decreased maternal insulin sensitivity before conception in areas where food is plentiful and a sedentary lifestyle is more common may manifest itself as gestational diabetes and increase the long-term risk for both diabetes and obesity in the woman and her offspring.

PERINATAL MORBIDITY AND MORTALITY

Fetal Death

In the past, sudden and unexplained stillbirth occurred in 10 to 30 percent of pregnancies complicated by type 1 (insulin-dependant) diabetes mellitus.[77,78] Although relatively uncommon today, such losses still plague the pregnancies of patients who do not receive optimal care. Stillbirths have been observed most often after the 36th week of pregnancy in patients with vascular disease, poor glycemic control, hydramnios, fetal macrosomia, or preeclampsia. Women with vascular complications may develop fetal growth restriction and intrauterine demise as early as the second trimester. In the past, prevention of intrauterine death led to a strategy of scheduled preterm deliveries for type 1 diabetic women. This empiric approach reduced the number of stillbirths, but errors in estimation of fetal size and gestational age as well as the functional immaturity characteristic of the infant of the diabetic mother (IDM) contributed to many neonatal deaths from hyaline membrane disease (HMD).

The precise cause of the excessive stillbirth rate in pregnancies complicated by diabetes remains unknown. Because extramedullary hematopoiesis is frequently observed in stillborn IDMs, chronic intrauterine hypoxia has been cited as a likely cause of these intrauterine fetal deaths. Recent studies of fetal umbilical cord blood samples from pregnant women with type 1 diabetics have demonstrated "relative fetal erythremia and lactic acidemia."[79] Maternal diabetes may also produce alterations in red blood cell oxygen release and placental blood flow.[80]

Reduced uterine blood flow is thought to contribute to the increased incidence of intrauterine growth restriction (IUGR) observed in pregnancies complicated by diabetic vasculopathy. Investigations using radioactive tracers have also suggested a relationship between poor maternal metabolic control and reduced uteroplacental

Table 32–1. FREQUENCY OF CONGENITAL MALFORMATIONS IN INFANTS OF DIABETIC MOTHERS

Study	Frequency	%
Ylinen et al.[225]	11/142	7.7
Mills et al.[88]	25/279	9.0
Greene[226]	35/451	7.7
Steel and Duncan[237]	12/239	7.8
Fuhrmann et al.[222]	22/292	7.5
Simpson et al.[87]	9/106	8.5
Albert et al.[86]	29/289	10.0

blood flow.[81] Ketoacidosis and preeclampsia, two factors known to be associated with an increased incidence of intrauterine deaths, may further decrease uterine blood flow. In diabetic ketoacidosis, hypovolemia and hypotension caused by dehydration may reduce flow through the intervillous space, while in preeclampsia, narrowing and vasospasm of spiral arterioles may result.

Alterations in fetal carbohydrate metabolism also may contribute to intrauterine asphyxia.[82–84] There is considerable evidence linking hyperinsulinemia and fetal hypoxia. Hyperinsulinemia induced in fetal lambs by an infusion of exogenous insulin produces an increase in oxygen consumption and a decrease in arterial oxygen content.[85] Persistent maternal–fetal hyperglycemia occurs independent of maternal uterine blood flow, which may not be increased enough to allow for enhanced oxygen delivery in the face of increased metabolic demands. Thus, hyperinsulinemia in the fetus of the diabetic mother appears to increase fetal metabolic rate and oxygen requirement in the face of several factors such as hyperglycemia, ketoacidosis, preeclampsia, and maternal vasculopathy, which can reduce placental blood flow and fetal oxygenation.

Congenital Malformations

With the reduction in intrauterine deaths and a marked decrease in neonatal mortality related to HMD and traumatic delivery, congenital malformations have emerged as the most important cause of perinatal loss in pregnancies complicated by type 1 and type 2 diabetes mellitus. In the past, these anomalies were responsible for approximately 10 percent of all perinatal deaths. At present, however, malformations account for 30 to 50 percent of perinatal mortality.[78] Neonatal deaths now exceed stillbirths in pregnancies complicated by pregestational diabetes mellitus, and fatal congenital malformations account for this changing pattern.

Most studies have documented a two- to sixfold increase in major malformations in infants of type 1 and type 2 diabetic mothers. At The Ohio State University Diabetes in Pregnancy Program, we have observed 29 congenital anomalies in 289 (10 percent) women enrolled from 1987 through 1993.[86] In a prospective analysis, Simpson et al. observed an 8.5 percent incidence of major anomalies in the diabetic population, while the malformation rate in a small group of concurrently gathered control subjects was 2.4 percent.[87] Similar figures were obtained in the Diabetes in Early Pregnancy Study in the United States.[88] The incidence of major anomalies was 2.1 percent in 389 control patients and 9.0 percent in 279 diabetic women. In general, the incidence of major malformations in worldwide studies of offspring of diabetic mothers has ranged from 5 to 10 percent (Table 32–1).

The insult that causes malformations in IDM impacts on most organ systems and must act before the seventh week of gestation.[82] Central nervous system malformations, particularly anencephaly, open spina bifida and, possibly, holoprosencephaly, are increased 10-fold.[90] Cardiac anomalies, especially ventricular septal defects and complex lesions such as transposition of the great vessels, are increased fivefold. The congenital defect thought to be most characteristic of diabetic embryopathy is sacral agenesis or caudal dysplasia, an anomaly found 200 to 400 times more often in offspring of diabetic women (Fig. 32–9). However, this defect is not pathognomonic for diabetes, since it also occurs in nondiabetic pregnancies.

Impaired glycemic control and associated derangements in maternal metabolism appear to contribute to abnormal embryogenesis. The notion of excess glucose as the single teratogenic agent in diabetic pregnancy has thus been replaced with the view of a multifactorial etiology[89] (see the box "Proposed Factors Associated with Teratogenesis in Pregnancy Complicated by Diabetes Mellitus").

Maternal hyperglycemia has been proposed by most investigators as the primary teratogenic factor, but hyperketonemia, hypoglycemia, somatomedin inhibitor excess, and excess free oxygen radicals have also been

---

Proposed Factors Associated with Teratogenesis in Pregnancy Complicated By Diabetes Mellitus

- Hyperglycemia
- Ketone body excess
- Somatomedin inhibition
- Arachidonic acid deficiency
- Free oxygen radical excess

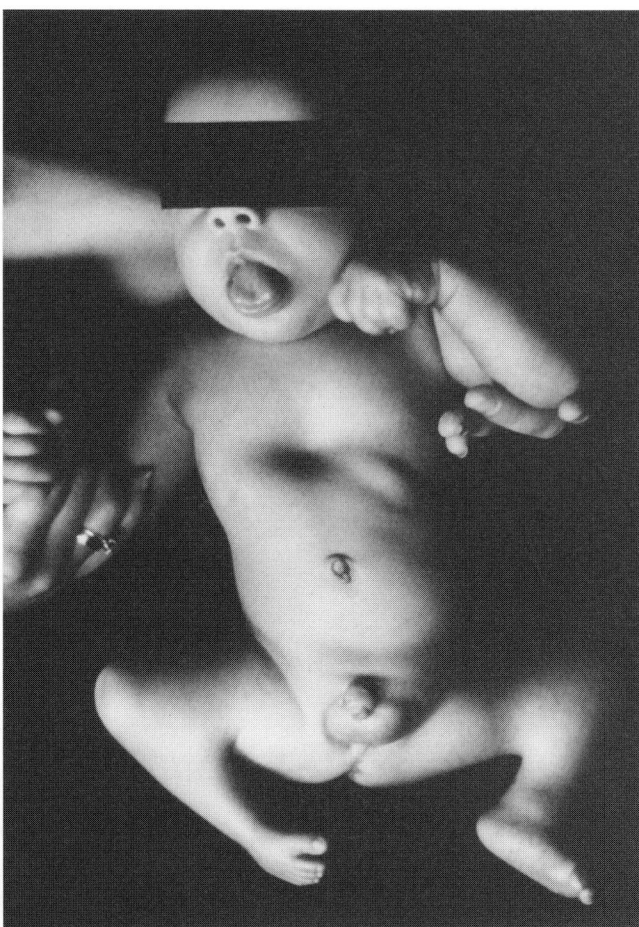

Figure 32–9. Infant of a diabetic mother with caudal regression syndrome. The mother of this infant presented with class F diabetes at 26 weeks, in poor glycemic control. Ultrasound examination revealed absent lower lumbar spine and sacrum and hypoplastic lower extremities.

suggested.[89] The profile of a woman most likely to produce an anomalous infant would include a patient with poor periconceptional control, long-standing diabetes, and vascular disease.[90] Genetic susceptibility to the teratogenic influence of diabetes may be a factor. Koppe and Smoremberg-School as well as Simpson and colleagues have suggested that certain maternal HLA types may be more often associated with anomalies.[91,92]

Several mechanisms have been proposed by which the above teratogenic factors produce malformations. Freinkel et al. suggested that anomalies might arise from inhibition of glycolysis, the key energy-producing process during embryogenesis. He found that D-mannose added to the culture medium of rat embryos inhibited glycolysis and produced growth restriction and derangement of neural tube closure.[93] Freinkel et al. stressed the sensitivity of normal embryogenesis to alterations in these key energy-producing pathways, a process he labeled "fuel-mediated" teratogenesis. Goldman and Baker have suggested that the mechanism responsible for the increased incidence of neural tube defects in embryos cultured in a hyperglycemic medium may involve a functional deficiency of arachidonic acid, because supplementation with arachidonic acid or my-oinositol will reduce the frequency of neural tube defects in this experimental model.[94] Pinter and Reece and Pinter et al. have confirmed these studies and demonstrated that hyperglycemia induced alterations in neural tube closure include disordered cells, decreased mitoses, and changes indicating premature maturation. These authors have further demonstrated that hyperglycemia during organogenesis has a primary deleterious effect on yolk sac function with resultant embryopathy.[95,96]

Altered oxidative metabolism from maternal diabetes may cause increased production of free oxygen radicals in the developing embryo, which are likely teratogenic. Supplementation of oxygen radical scavenging enzymes, such as superoxide dismutase to culture medium of rat embryos, protects against growth delay and excess malformations.[97] It has been suggested that excess free oxygen radicals may have a direct effect on embryonic prostaglandin biosynthesis. Free oxygen radical excess may enhance lipid peroxidation and, in turn, generated hydroperoxides might stimulate thromboxane biosynthesis and inhibit prostacyclin production, an imbalance that could have profound effects on embryonic development.[89]

Fetal Macrosomia

Macrosomia has been variously defined as birth weight greater than 4,000 to 4,500 g as well as large for gestational age where birth weight is above the 90th percentile for population and sex-specific growth curves. Fetal macrosomia complicates as many as 50 percent of pregnancies in women with gestational diabetes and 40 percent of pregnancies complicated by type 1 diabetes, including some women treated with intensive glycemic control (Fig. 32–10). Delivery of an infant weighing greater than 4,500 g occurs 10 times more often in women with diabetes as compared with a population of women with normal glucose tolerance.[98]

According to the Pedersen hypothesis, maternal hyperglycemia results in fetal hyperglycemia and hyperinsulinemia, resulting in excessive fetal growth. Increased fetal β-cell mass may be identified as early as the second trimester.[99] Evidence supporting the Pedersen hypothesis has come from the studies of amniotic fluid and cord blood insulin and C-peptide concentrations. Both are increased in the amniotic fluid of insulin-treated women with diabetes at term[100] and correlate with neonatal fat mass.[101] Lipids and amino acids, which are elevated in pregnancies complicated by gesta-

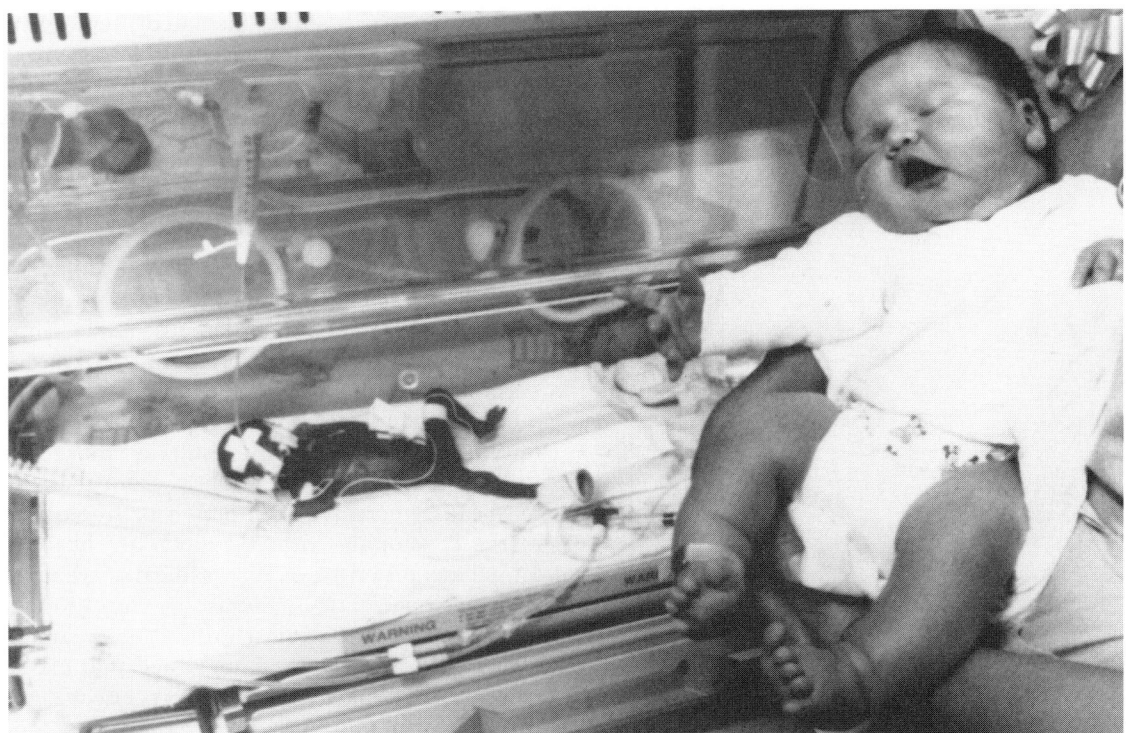

Figure 32–10. Two extremes of growth abnormalities in infants of diabetic mothers. The small growth-retarded infant on the left weighed 470 g and is the offspring of a woman with nephropathy and hypertension, delivered at 28 weeks' gestation. The neonate on the right is the 5,100-g baby of a woman with suboptimally controlled class C diabetes.

tional diabetes, may also play a role in excessive fetal growth by stimulating the release of insulin and other growth factors from the fetal pancreatic β-cells and placenta. Infants of mothers with gestational diabetes have an increase in fat mass as compared with fat-free mass.[102] Additionally, their growth is disproportionate, with chest/head and shoulder/head ratios larger than those of infants of women with normal glucose tolerance. This factor may contribute to the higher rate of shoulder dystocia and birth trauma observed in these infants.[103]

The results of several clinical series have validated the Pedersen hypothesis inasmuch as tight maternal glycemic control has been associated with a decline in the incidence of macrosomia. In a series of 260 insulin-dependent women achieving fasting plasma glucose concentrations between 109 and 140 mg/dl, Gabbe et al.[104] observed 58 (22 percent) macrosomic infants. Kitzmiller and Cloherty[105] reported that 11 percent of 134 women achieving fasting glucose concentrations between 105 and 121 mg/dl were delivered of an infant with a birth weight in excess of 4,000 g. A more dramatic reduction in the rate of macrosomia has been reported when more physiologic control has been achieved. Roversi and Gargiulo[106] instituted a program of "maximally tolerated" insulin administration and observed macrosomia in only 6 percent of cases. Jova-

novic and coworkers[107] eliminated macrosomia in 52 women who achieved mean glucose levels of 80 to 87 mg/dl throughout gestation. Landon and colleagues[108] using daily capillary glucose values obtained during the second and third trimesters in insulin-dependent women reported a 9 percent rate of macrosomia when mean values were below 110 mg/dl compared with 34 percent when less optimal control was achieved. Jovanovic et al.[109] have suggested that 1-hour postprandial glucose measurements correlate best with the frequency of macrosomia. After controlling for other factors, these authors noted that the strongest prediction for birth weight was third-trimester nonfasting glucose measurements.

In a series of metabolic studies, Catalano et al.[110] estimated body composition in 186 neonates using anthropometry. Fat-free mass that comprised 86 percent of mean birth weight accounted for 83 percent of the variance in birth weight, and fat mass, which comprised only 14 percent of birth weight, accounted for 46 percent of the variance in birth weight. There was also significantly greater fat-free mass in male as compared with female infants. Using independent variables such as maternal height, pregravid weight, weight gain during pregnancy, parity, paternal height and weight, neonatal sex, and gestational age, the authors accounted for 29 percent of the variance in birth weight,

30 percent of the variance in fat-free mass, and 17 percent of the variance in fat mass.[111] Including estimates of maternal insulin sensitivity in 16 additional subjects, they were able to explain 48 percent of the variance in birth weight, 53 percent in fat-free mass, and 46 percent in fat mass.[112] Studies by Caruso et al.[113] have corroborated these findings, reporting that women with unexplained fetal growth restriction had greater insulin sensitivity as compared with a control group of women whose infants were appropriate weight for gestational age. A positive correlation between birth weight and weight gain has been observed in women with normal glucose tolerance, but there is a negative correlation in women with gestational diabetes. In women with normal glucose tolerance, the correlation was strongest in women who were lean before conception and became progressively weaker as pregravid weight for height increased.[76] In women with gestational diabetes, there was no significant correlation between maternal weight gain and birth weight, irrespective of pregravid weight for height. These studies emphasize the role of the maternal metabolic environment and fetal growth.

In addition to an increased risk of birth trauma, fetal macrosomia in infants of women with abnormal glucose tolerance may be associated with significant long-term risks. The birth weight of these infants tends to normalize by 1 year of age but increases in early childhood.[114] These children are at greater risk for obesity at ages 1 to 9 and in adolescence. Silverman and colleagues[114] have reported a strong correlation between amniotic fluid insulin levels and increased body mass index (wt/ht^2) at ages 14 to 17 years, indicating an association between islet cell activation in utero and development of childhood obesity. Childhood obesity then predisposes to obesity in the adult. Pettitt and colleagues have shown that infants born to Pima Indian women with impaired glucose tolerance were more obese as children than infants of women with normal glucose tolerance, even when the later group developed diabetes later in life.[115] These data suggest that there are both in utero maternal metabolic factors as well as genetic factors leading to the later development of obesity and type 2 diabetes.

Hypoglycemia

Neonatal hypoglycemia, a blood glucose below 35 to 40 mg/dl during the first 12 hours of life, results from a rapid fall in plasma glucose concentrations following clamping of the umbilical cord. Hypoglycemia is particularly common in macrosomic newborns, with rates exceeding 50 percent. With near physiologic control of maternal glucose levels during pregnancy, overall rates of 5 to 15 percent have been reported.[106,107] The degree

of hypoglycemia may be influenced by at least two factors: (1) maternal glucose control during the latter half of pregnancy, and (2) maternal glucose control during labor and delivery. Maternal blood glucose levels greater than 90 mg/dl during delivery have been found to increase significantly the frequency of neonatal hypoglycemia.[116] Presumably, prior poor maternal glucose control can result in fetal β-cell hyperplasia, leading to exaggerated insulin release following delivery. IDMs exhibiting hypoglycemia have elevated cord C-peptide and free insulin levels at birth and an exaggerated pancreatic response to glucose loading.[117]

Respiratory Distress Syndrome

The precise mechanism by which maternal diabetes alters pulmonary development remains unknown. Experimental animal studies have focused primarily on the effects of hyperglycemia and hyperinsulinemia on pulmonary surfactant biosynthesis. An extensive review of the literature confirms that both of these factors are involved in delayed pulmonary maturation in the IDM.[118]

In vitro studies have documented that insulin can interfere with substrate availability for surfactant biosynthesis.[119,120] Smith has postulated that insulin interferes with the normal timing of glucocorticoid-induced pulmonary maturation in the fetus.[120] Cortisol apparently acts on pulmonary fibroblasts to induce synthesis of fibroblast-pneumocyte factor, which then acts on type II cells to stimulate phospholipid synthesis.[121] Carlson and coworkers have shown that insulin blocks cortisol action at the level of the fibroblast by reducing the production of fibroblast-pneumocyte factor.[122]

Clinical studies investigating the effect of maternal diabetes on fetal lung maturation have produced conflicting data. With the introduction of protocols that have emphasized glucose control and antepartum surveillance until lung maturity has been established, respiratory distress syndrome (RDS) has become a less common occurrence in the IDM. Several studies agree that in well-controlled diabetic women delivered at term, the risk of RDS is no higher than that observed in the general population.[123,124] Kjos et al. studied the outcome of 526 diabetic gestations delivered within 5 days of amniotic fluid fetal lung maturation testing and reported hyaline membrane disease in five neonates (0.95 percent), all of whom were delivered prior to 34 weeks' gestation.[124] Mimouni et al. compared outcomes of 127 IDMs with matched controls and concluded that diabetes in pregnancy as currently managed is not a direct risk factor for the development of RDS. Yet, cesarean delivery not preceded by labor and prematurity, both of which are increased in diabetic pregnancies, clearly increase the likelihood of neonatal respiratory disease.[125]

Calcium and Magnesium Metabolism

Neonatal hypocalcemia, serum levels below 7 mg/dl, occurs at an increased rate in the IDM when one controls for predisposing factors such as prematurity and birth asphyxia.[58] Hypocalcemia in the IDM has been associated with a failure to increase parathyroid hormone synthesis following birth.[126] Decreased serum magnesium levels have also been documented in pregnant diabetic women as well as their infants. Mimouni et al. described reduced amniotic fluid magnesium concentrations in women with diabetes.[127] These findings may be explained by reduced fetal urinary magnesium excretion, which would accompany a relative magnesium-deficient state. Magnesium deficiency may paradoxically inhibit fetal parathyroid hormone secretion.

Hyperbilirubinemia and Polycythemia

Hyperbilirubinemia is frequently observed in the IDM. Neonatal jaundice has been reported in as many as 53 percent of pregnancies complicated by diabetes and 38 percent of pregnancies with GDM.[128,129] Although several mechanisms have been proposed to explain these clinical findings, the pathogenesis of hyperbilirubinemia remains uncertain. In the past, the jaundice observed in the IDM was often attributed to prematurity. Studies that have analyzed morbidity carefully, according to gestational age, however, have rejected this concept.[130]

Although severe hyperbilirubinemia may be observed independent of polycythemia, a common pathway for these complications most likely involves increased red blood cell production, stimulated by increased erythropoietin in the IDM. Presumably, the major stimulus for red cell production is a state of relative hypoxia in utero, as described previously. Although cord erythropoietin levels generally are normal in IDMs whose mothers demonstrate good glycemic control during gestation, Shannon and Ylinen found that glycosylated hemoglobin values in late pregnancy were significantly elevated in mothers of hyperbilirubinemic infants.[129,131] Fetal hyperinsulinemia may also stimulate erythropoiesis.[79]

MATERNAL CLASSIFICATION AND RISK ASSESSMENT

Priscilla White[132] first noted that the patient's age at onset of diabetes, the duration of the disease, and the presence of vasculopathy significantly influenced perinatal outcome. Her pioneering work led to a classification system that has been widely applied to pregnant women with diabetes.[132] A modification of this scheme is presented in Table 32–2. Counseling a patient and

Table 32–2. MODIFIED WHITE CLASSIFICATION OF PREGNANT DIABETIC WOMEN

Class	Diabetes Onset Age (yr)	Duration (yr)	Vascular Disease	Insulin Need
Gestational diabetes				
A1	Any	Any	0	0
A2	Any	Any	0	+
Pregestational diabetes				
B	>20	<10	0	+
C	10–19 or	10–19	0	+
D	<10 or	>20	+	+
F	Any	Any	+	+
R	Any	Any	+	+
T	Any	Any	+	+
H	Any	Any	+	+

Modified from White P: Pregnancy complicating diabetes. Am J Med 7:609, 1949.

formulating a plan of management requires assessment of both maternal and fetal risk. The White classification facilitates this evaluation.

Class A_1 diabetes mellitus includes those patients who have demonstrated carbohydrate intolerance during a 100-g 3-hour oral glucose tolerance test (OGTT); however, their fasting and 2-hour postprandial glucose levels are less than 95 mg/dl and 120 mg/dl, respectively. These patients are generally managed by dietary regulation alone. If the fasting value of the OGTT is elevated (>95 mg/dl) and/or 2-hour postprandial glucose levels exceed 120 mg/dl, patients are designated Class A_2. Insulin is most often required for these women.

The Second and Third International Workshop-Conferences on Gestational Diabetes sponsored by the American Diabetes Association in cooperation with the American College of Obstetricians and Gynecologists (ACOG) recommended that the term gestational diabetes rather than Class A diabetes be used to describe women with carbohydrate intolerance of variable severity with onset or recognition during the present pregnancy.[133,134] The term gestational diabetes fails to specify whether the patient requires dietary adjustment alone or treatment with diet and insulin. This distinction is important because those patients who are normoglycemic while fasting appear to have a significantly lower perinatal mortality rate.[135] Women with gestational diabetes who require insulin are at greater risk for a poor perinatal outcome than those controlled by diet alone.

Patients requiring insulin are designated by the letters B, C, D, R, F, and T. Class B patients are those whose onset of disease occurs after age 20. They have had diabetes less than 10 years and have no vascular complications. Included in this subgroup of patients are those who have been previously treated with oral hypoglycemic agents.

Class C diabetes includes patients who have the onset of their disease between the ages of 10 and 19 or have had the disease for 10 to 19 years. Vascular disease is not present.

Class D represents women whose disease is of 20 years' duration or more, or whose onset occurred before age 10, or who have benign retinopathy. The latter includes microaneurysms, exudates, and venous dilation.

In summary, risk assessment may be simplified by evaluating the patient's blood glucose and blood vessels. Patients with excellent glucose control and no blood vessel disease should do well. Those in poor control and with vasculopathy are at increased risk for fetal death, IUGR, preeclampsia, and preterm delivery.

Nephropathy

Renal disease develops in 25 to 30 percent of women with type 1 diabetes mellitus, with a peak incidence after approximately 16 years of diabetes.[136] Women with diabetic nephropathy have a significantly reduced life expectancy. In women with overt nephropathy, end-stage renal disease occurs in 50 percent by 10 years and in greater than 75 percent of cases by 20 years. Class F describes the 5 to 10 percent of pregnant patients with underlying renal disease. This includes those with reduced creatinine clearance and/or proteinuria of at least 400 mg in 24 hours measured during the first 20 weeks of gestation. Two factors present prior to 20 weeks' gestation appear to be predictive of perinatal outcome in these women (e.g., preterm delivery, low birth weight, or preeclampsia): proteinuria greater than 3.0 g/24 h and serum creatinine greater than 1.5 mg/dl.

In our series of 45 Class F women, 12 women had such risk factors.[137] Preeclampsia developed in 92 percent, with a mean gestational age at delivery of 34 weeks compared to an incidence of preeclampsia of 36 percent in 33 women without these risk factors who reached an average gestational age of 36 weeks. Remarkably, perinatal survival was 100 percent in this series, and no deliveries occurred prior to 30 weeks' gestation. Comparable series detailing perinatal outcomes in Class F patients are presented in Table 32–3.

The management of the diabetic woman with nephropathy requires great expertise. Limitation of dietary protein, which may reduce protein excretion in nonpregnant patients, has not been adequately studied during pregnancy. Although controversial, some nephrologists recommend a modified reduction in protein intake for pregnant women with nephropathy. Control of hypertension in pregnant women with diabetic nephropathy is crucial to prevent further deterioration of kidney function and to optimize pregnancy outcome. Although debatable, some cautiously use diuretics when patients are extremely nephrotic, as this group may be prone to volume-dependent forms of hypertension. Angiotensin-converting enzyme (ACE) inhibitors, which reduce intraglomerular pressure and improve proteinuria in nonpregnant diabetic patients, should be avoided during pregnancy, as these agents can affect fetal urine production resulting in oligohydramnios.

Several studies have failed to demonstrate a permanent worsening of diabetic renal disease as a result of pregnancy.[137–139] Furthermore, it has been suggested that pregnancy itself does not increase the risk of devel-

Table 32–3. COMPARATIVE STUDIES IN OUTCOMES IN CLASS F DIABETES MELLITUS

	Kitzmiller et al.[138] (n = 26)	Grenfel et al.[244] (n = 20)	Reece et al.[139] (n = 31)	Gordon et al.[137] (n = 45)	Rosenn et al.[141] (n = 61)
Chronic HTN	31%	27%	22%	26%	47%
Initial Creatinine >1.9 mg/dl	38%	10%	22%	11%	—
Initial proteinuria >3.0 g/24 h	8.3%	—	22%	13%	—
Preeclampsia	15%	55%	35%	53%	51%
Cesarean delivery	—	72%	70%	80%	82%
Perinatal survival (%)	88.9	100	93.5	100	94%
Major anomalies	3 (11.1%)	1 (4.3%)	3 (9.7%)	2 (4%)	4 (6%)
IUGR (%)	20.8	NA	19.4	11.0	11%
Delivery					
<34 wk (%)	30.8	27	22.5	15.5	25%
34–36 wk (%)	40.7	23	32.3	35.5	28%
>36 wk (%)	28.5	50	45.2	49	47%

oping nephropathy, although development of proteinuria and poor glycemic control are markers for subsequent renal disease. Kitzmiller and colleagues reviewed 35 pregnancies complicated by diabetic nephropathy.[138] Proteinuria increased in 69 percent and hypertension developed in 73 percent. Following delivery, proteinuria declined in 65 percent of cases. In only two patients did protein excretion increase after gestation. In Gordon's series, 26 women (58 percent) had more than a 1-g increase in proteinuria, and by the third trimester, 25 (56 percent) excreted more than 3.0 g/24 h.[137] In the vast majority of cases, protein excretion returned to baseline levels following gestation. Changes in creatinine clearance during pregnancy are variable in Class F patients. Kitzmiller, in reviewing 44 patients from the literature, noted that about one third of women had an expected rise in creatinine clearance during gestation, compared to one third who had a decline of more than 15 percent by the third trimester.[140] In Gordon's series, 12 of 16 women whose clearance fell developed preeclampsia. Of interest, most patients with a severe reduction in creatinine clearance (<50 ml/min) do not demonstrate a further reduction in first-trimester clearance during pregnancy.[137] However, a decline in renal function can be anticipated in 20 to 30 percent of cases. Several authors have suggested that any deterioration of renal function after pregnancy is probably consistent with the natural course of diabetic nephropathy and is not related to pregnancy per se.[141] Thus, women with early stage nephropathy (<1 g/24 h of proteinuria and normal creatinine clearance) entering pregnancy are unlikely to manifest a decline in renal function in 1 to 2 years of follow-up.[137]

With improved survival of diabetic patients following renal transplantation, a small group of kidney recipients has now achieved pregnancy (Class T). Nine cases of pregnancy complicated by diabetes and prior renal transplantation have been described.[142] In this series, there were no episodes of renal allograft rejection. Prednisone and azathioprine were administered throughout gestation. A single maternal death and two fetal deaths did occur in patients with preexisting peripheral vascular disease. Superimposed preeclampsia occurred in six patients. All seven surviving infants were delivered prior to term, with fetal compromise evident in six of these cases.

Retinopathy

Class R diabetes designates patients with proliferative retinopathy. As with nephropathy, prevalence of retinal disease is highly related to the duration of diabetes. At 20 years, nearly 80 percent of diabetic individuals will have some element of retinopathy. Excellent glycemic control prevents retinopathy and may slow its progression. Parity is not associated with a risk for subsequent retinopathy.[143] However, pregnancy does convey a greater than twofold independent risk for progression of existing retinopathy.[144] Progression of diabetic retinopathy during pregnancy is associated with hypertensive disease.[145] Retinopathy may worsen significantly during pregnancy in spite of the major advances that have been made in diagnosis and treatment of existing retinopathy. Ideally, women planning a pregnancy should have a comprehensive eye examination and treatment prior to conception. For those discovered to have proliferative changes during pregnancy, laser photocoagulation therapy with careful follow-up has helped maintain many pregnancies to a gestational age at which neonatal survival is likely.

In a large series of 172 patients, including 40 cases with background retinopathy and 11 with proliferative changes, only one patient developed new-onset proliferative retinopathy during pregnancy.[146] A review of the literature by Kitzmiller confirms the observation that progression to proliferative retinopathy during pregnancy rarely occurs in women with background retinopathy or those without any eye ground changes.[147] Of the 561 women in these two categories, only 17 (3.0 percent) developed neovascularization during gestation.[147] In contrast, 23 of 26 (88.5 percent) with untreated proliferative disease experienced worsening retinopathy during pregnancy.

Pregnancy may increase the prevalence of some background retinal changes.[148] Characteristic streak-blob hemorrhages and soft exudates have been noted and retinopathy may progress despite strict metabolic control. At least two studies have related worsening retinal disease to plasma glucose at the first prenatal visit as well as the magnitude of improvement in glycemia during early pregnancy.[149,150] In a subset of 140 women without proliferative retinopathy at baseline followed in the Diabetes in Early Pregnancy Study, progression of retinopathy was seen in 10.3, 21.1, 18.8, and 54.8 percent of patients with no retinopathy, microaneurysms only, mild nonproliferative retinopathy, and moderate to severe nonproliferative retinopathy at baseline, respectively. Elevated glycosylated hemoglobin at baseline and the magnitude of improvement of glucose control through week 14 was associated with higher risk of progression of retinopathy.[150] Women with an initial glycohemoglobin greater than 6 SD above the control mean compared with those within 2 SD of the mean were nearly three times as likely to experience worsening retinopathy. Whether improving control or simply suboptimal control itself contributes to a deterioration of background retinopathy remains uncertain. Hypertension may also be a significant risk factor for the progression of retinopathy during pregnancy.[145] Rosenn and colleagues reported that worsening of retinopathy occurred in 55 percent of women with a hypertensive disorder of pregnancy compared to 25 percent of women without chronic hypertension or preeclampsia.

For women with proliferative changes, laser photocoagulation is indicated and most will respond to this therapy. However, those women who demonstrate severe florid disc neovascularization that is unresponsive to laser therapy during early pregnancy may be at great risk for deterioration of their vision. Termination of pregnancy should be considered in this group of patients.

In addition to background and proliferative eye disease, vaso-occlusive lesions associated with the development of macular edema have been described during pregnancy.[151] Cystic macular edema is most often found in patients with proteinuric nephropathy, anemia, and hypertensive disease leading to retinal edema. Macular capillary permeability is a feature of this process. The degree of macular edema is directly related to the fall in plasma oncotic pressure present in these women. In Sinclair's series, seven women with minimal or no retinopathy before becoming pregnant developed severe macular edema associated with preproliferative or proliferative retinopathy during the course of their pregnancies. Although proliferation was controlled with photocoagulation, the macular edema worsened until delivery in all cases and was often aggravated by photocoagulation.[151] While both macular edema and retinopathy regressed after delivery in some patients, in others these pathologic processes persisted, resulting in significant visual loss.

Coronary Artery Disease

Class H diabetes refers to the presence of diabetes of any duration associated with ischemic myocardial disease. There is evidence that the small number of women who have coronary artery disease are at an increased risk for mortality during gestation. This is particularly true for women who suffer an infarction during pregnancy.[152] For these cases, the maternal mortality rate is approximately 50 percent and fetal loss is common as well.[153] A high index of suspicion for ischemic heart disease should be maintained in women with long-standing diabetes, since anginal symptoms may be minimal and infarction may thus present as congestive heart failure.[153] While there are a few reports of successful pregnancies following myocardial infarction in diabetic women, cardiac status should be carefully assessed early in gestation or preferably prior to pregnancy. If electrocardiographic abnormalities are encountered, echocardiography may be used to assess ventricular function or modified stress testing may be performed. The decision to undertake a pregnancy in a woman with diabetes and coronary artery disease needs

to be made only after serious consideration. The potential for morbidity and mortality must be thoroughly reviewed with the patient and her family. The management of myocardial infarction during pregnancy is discussed in Chapter 29.

DETECTION OF DIABETES IN PREGNANCY

It has been estimated that 2 to 3 percent of pregnancies are complicated by diabetes mellitus and that 90 percent of the cases represent women with GDM.[154] An increased prevalence of GDM is found in women of Hispanic, African, Native American, South or East Asian, and Pacific Island ancestry.[155] Women with GDM represent a group with significant risk for developing glucose intolerance later in life. Whereas O'Sullivan projected that 50 percent of GDM would become diabetic in follow-up study of 22 to 28 years, more recent series by Dornhorst and Rossi suggest this level of risk may be manifest by 5 years after the index pregnancy.[156,157] The likelihood for subsequent diabetes apparently increases when GDM is diagnosed in early pregnancy, and is accompanied by impaired β-cell function and obesity.

As noted above, GDM is a state restricted to pregnant women whose impaired glucose tolerance is discovered during pregnancy. Because, in most cases, patients with GDM have normal fasting glucose levels, some challenge of glucose tolerance must be undertaken. Traditionally, obstetricians relied on historical and clinical risk factors to select those patients most likely to develop GDM. This group included patients with a family history of diabetes, or those whose past pregnancies were marked by an unexplained stillbirth, or the delivery of a malformed or macrosomic infant. Obesity, hypertension, glycosuria, and maternal age over 25 were other indications for screening. Interestingly, over half of all patients who exhibit an abnormal GTT lack the risk factors mentioned above. Coustan and colleagues have reported in a series of 6,214 women that using historical risk factors and an arbitrary age cut-off of 30 years for screening would miss 35 percent of cases of GDM.[158]

In the summary and recommendations of the Second and Third International Workshop-Conference on GDM, screening was recommended for all pregnant women. Following the Fourth International Workshop-Conference in 1997, universal screening was recommended for women in ethnic groups with relatively high rates of carbohydrate intolerance during pregnancy and diabetes later in life.[159] If was recognized

Screening Strategy for Detection of GDM

Risk assessment for GDM should be ascertained at the first prenatal visit.

Low risk

Blood glucose testing is not routinely required if all of the following characteristics are present:

Member of an ethnic group with a low prevalence of GDM

No known diabetes in first-degree relatives

Age <25 years

Weight normal before pregnancy

No history of abnormal glucose metabolism

No history of poor obstetric outcome

Average risk

Perform blood glucose screening at 24 to 28 weeks using one of the following:

Two-step procedure: 50-g GCT followed by a diagnostic OGTT in those meeting the threshold value in the GCT

One-step procedure: diagnostic OGTT performed on all subjects

High risk

Perform blood glucose testing as soon as feasible, using the procedures described above.

If GDM is not diagnosed, blood glucose testing should be repeated at 24 to 28 weeks or at any time a patient has symptoms or signs suggestive of hyperglycemia.

Adapted from Fourth International Workshop-Conference on Gestational Diabetes Mellitus. Diabetes Care 21(Suppl 2): B161, 1998.

that certain features place women at low risk for GDM (see the box "Screening Strategy for Detection of GDM"), and it may not be cost-effective to screen this subgroup of women. Those at low risk include women who are not members of ethnic groups at increased risk for developing type 2 diabetes, those who have no previous history of abnormal glucose tolerance or poor obstetric outcomes usually associated with GDM, and those who have all of the following characteristics: age less than 25 years, normal body weight, and no family history of diabetes. Similarly, the ACOG first suggested that whereas selective screening for GDM may be appropriate in some clinical settings such as teen clinics (low-risk populations), universal screening may be more appropriate in other settings (high-risk populations).[160] It should be noted that in some countries, experts have questioned the benefit of GDM screening programs.[161]

The criteria for the diagnosis of GDM originally des-

ignated a population at increased risk for the development of type 2 diabetes in later life. The fact that O'Sullivan's original work establishing the criteria used for the diagnosis of GDM failed to evaluate an association between mild carbohydrate tolerance and perinatal outcome has led many to question the overall significance of this diagnosis. It has been further suggested that the criteria for the diagnosis of GDM are conceptually flawed in that they represent a dichotomous definition of normal and abnormal gestational glucose tolerance, when the risk of adverse maternal–fetal outcomes and later diabetes should be logically graded upward with higher values on the OGTT and with the degree of fasting hyperglycemia.[162] Two studies have in fact addressed the relationship between mild degrees of carbohydrate tolerance and rates of neonatal macrosomia. In a study of 3,637 women without GDM, Sermer and colleagues demonstrated a graded increase in adverse outcomes (including large infants) with increasing maternal carbohydrate intolerance.[163] Similarly, Sacks identified fasting and 2-hour glucose values as independent risk factors for macrosomia in a multivariate analysis of over 3,500 pregnant women. However, as no clinically meaningful glucose threshold could be identified, Sacks concluded that the criteria for GDM will likely be established by consensus.[164] There remains a compelling need to develop diagnostic criteria for GDM that are based on specific relationships between hyperglycemia and risk of adverse outcome.[165]

The screening test for GDM, a 50-g oral glucose challenge, may be performed in the fasting or fed state. Sensitivity is improved if the test is performed in the fasting state.[166,167] A plasma value between 130 and 140 mg/dl is commonly used as a threshold for performing a 3-hour OGTT. Coustan et al. have demonstrated that 10 percent of GDM women will have screening test values between 130 and 139 mg/dl.[166] This study indicated that the sensitivity of screening would be increased from 90 percent to nearly 100 percent if universal screening were employed using a threshold of 130 mg/dl. The prevalence of positive screening tests requiring further diagnostic testing increases from 14 percent (140 mg/dl) to 23 percent (130 mg/dl), and is accompanied by an approximately 12 percent increase in the overall cost to diagnose each case of GDM.

Whereas most women can be screened for GDM at approximately 24 to 28 weeks' gestation, it is advisable to screen earlier in pregnancy those with strong risk factors such as morbid obesity, family history in first-degree relatives, or previous GDM.[168] If initial screening is negative, repeat testing is performed at 24 to 28 weeks. Utilizing the plasma cut-off of 140 mg/dl, one can expect approximately 15 percent of patients with an abnormal screening value to have an abnormal 3-hour OGTT. Patients whose 1-hour screening value

Table 32–4. DETECTION OF GESTATIONAL DIABETES—UPPER LIMITS OF NORMAL

Screening Test (50-g) 1-Hour	Plasma (mg/dl) (130–140)	
Oral GTT*	NDDG	Carpenter and Coustan[169]
Fasting	105	95
1-hour	190	180
2-hour	165	155
3-hour	145	140

* Diagnosis of gestational diabetes is made when any two values are met or exceeded.
NDDG, National Diabetes Data Group.
From the National Institutes of Health Diabetes Data Group: Classification and diagnosis of diabetes mellitus and other categories of glucose intolerance. Diabetes 28:1039, 1979.

exceeds 190 mg/dl (10.5 mmol/L) rarely exhibit a normal OGTT.[169] In these women, it is preferable to check a fasting blood glucose level before administering a 100-g carbohydrate load. If the fasting glucose is 95 mg/dl or greater, the patient is treated for GDM.

The criteria for establishing the diagnosis of gestational diabetes are listed in Table 32–4. The U.S. National Diabetes Data Group criteria represent a calculated conversion of O'Sullivan's thresholds in whole blood. Carpenter and Coustan prefer to use another modification of these data that is supported by a comparison of the older Somogyi-Nelson method and current plasma glucose oxidase assays.[170] These criteria have been modified by the Fourth International Workshop-Conference on GDM. Several studies have confirmed that patients diagnosed using the less stringent Carpenter criteria experience as much perinatal morbidity as subjects diagnosed by the National Diabetes Data Group Criteria.[171] Using either criteria, the patient must have a normal fasting value and two abnormal postprandial glucose determinations to be designated as Class A_1.

TREATMENT OF THE INSULIN-DEPENDENT PATIENT

As fetal glucose levels reflect those of the mother, it is not surprising that clinical efforts aimed at optimizing maternal control are considered paramount in the decline in perinatal death seen in pregnancies type 1 diabetics over the last few decades. Self-blood glucose monitoring combined with aggressive insulin therapy has made the maintenance of maternal normoglycemia (levels of 60 to 120 mg/dl) a therapeutic reality (Table 32–5). In most institutions, patients are taught to mon-

itor their glucose control using glucose-oxidase–impregnated reagent strips and a meter.[172]

To achieve the best glycemic control possible for each patient, conventional insulin therapy often needs to be abandoned during pregnancy in favor of intensive therapy. Insulin regimens have classically included multiple injections of insulin usually prior to breakfast, the evening meal, and often bedtime, complemented by self-blood glucose monitoring and adjustments of insulin dose according to glucose profiles. Patients are instructed on dietary composition, insulin action, recognition and treatment of hypoglycemia, adjusting insulin dosage for exercise and sick days, as well as monitoring for hyperglycemia and potential ketosis. These principles form the foundation for intensive insulin therapy in which an attempt is made to simulate physiologic insulin requirements. Insulin administration is provided for both basal needs and meals, and rapid adjustments are made in response to glucose measurements. The treatment regimen generally involves three to four daily injections or the use of a continuous subcutaneous insulin infusion (CSII) device, the insulin pump. With either approach, frequent self-blood glucose monitoring is fundamental to achieve the therapeutic objective of physiologic glucose control. Glucose determinations are made in the fasting state and before lunch, dinner, and bedtime. Postprandial and nocturnal values are also helpful. Patients are instructed on an insulin dose for each meal and at bedtime if necessary. Meal-time insulin needs are determined by the composition of the meal, the premeal glucose measurement, and the level of activity anticipated following the meal. Basal or intermediate-acting insulin requirements are determined by periodic 2 A.M. to 4 A.M. glucose measurements as well as late afternoon values, which reflect morning neutral protamine Hagedorn (NPH) or Lente action. During pregnancy, diabetic women should develop the self-management skills that are essential to an intensive insulin therapy regimen.

Glycosylated hemoglobin measurements in each trimester can be used to assess glucose control in the previous 6 to 8 weeks. A hemoglobin A_{1c} level of 5 to 6 percent is desirable. The mean glucose represented by the hemoglobin A_{1c} level can be calculated using the "rule of 8's." A value of 8 percent equals 180 mg/dl,

Table 32–5. TARGET PLASMA GLUCOSE LEVELS IN PREGNANCY

Time	mg/dl
Before breakfast	60–90
Before lunch, supper, bedtime snack	60–105
Two hours after meals	≤120
2 A.M. to 6 A.M.	>60

and each 1 percent increase or decrease represents ± 30 mg/dl.

In patients who are not well controlled, a brief period of hospitalization is often necessary for the initiation of therapy. Individual adjustments to the regimens implemented can then be made. It is gratifying for many patients to feel they can take charge of their own diabetic control. Women who have previously followed a prescribed dosage regimen for years gain confidence in making adjustments in their insulin dosage after a short period of time. Patients are encouraged to contact their physician at any time if questions should arise concerning the management of their diabetes. During early pregnancy, patients are instructed to report their glucose values by telephone at least weekly.

Insulin therapy must be individualized with dosage determinations tailored to diet and exercise. Beef and pork insulin have largely been replaced by semisynthetic human insulin preparations. Most recently, insulin lispro has been introduced. A rapid-acting insulin preparation, this insulin, which features reversal of proline and lysine at positions B28 and B29, remains in monomeric form, and is rapidly absorbed. Its action begins in 15 minutes and peaks in 2 to 3 hours. Because its duration of action is shorter than that of regular insulin, unexpected hypoglycemia hours after an injection is avoided. Insulin lispro is not yet approved for use in pregnancy, but it is a category B drug. While an early report raised some question regarding a possible association between insulin lispro and progression of retinopathy in pregnancy, recent experience suggests this is not the case.[173,174]

Insulin is generally administered in two to three injections. We prefer a three-injection regimen, although most patients present taking a combination of intermediate-acting and short-acting insulin before dinner and breakfast. As a general rule, the amount of intermediate-acting insulin will exceed the short-acting component by a 2:1 ratio. Patients usually receive two thirds their total dose with breakfast and the remaining third in the evening as a combined dose with dinner or split into components with short-acting insulin at dinner time and intermediate-acting insulin at bedtime in an effort to minimize periods of nocturnal hypoglycemia. These episodes frequently occur when the mother is in a relative fasting state while placental and fetal glucose consumption continue. Finally, some women may require a small dose of short-acting insulin before lunch, thus constituting a four-injection regimen.

There has now been considerable experience with open-loop CSII pump therapy during pregnancy. The pump is a battery-powered unit, which may be worn, like a pager, during most daily activities. These systems provide continuous short-acting insulin via a subcutaneous infusion. The basal infusion rate and bolus doses to cover meals are determined by frequent self-monitoring of blood glucose. The basal infusion rate is generally close to 1 unit/h.

Initiation of pump therapy requires a highly motivated patient and a knowledgeable health care team. Many pregnant patients will be able to start using a pump without hospitalization.[176] Women must be educated regarding the strategy of continuous infusion and bolus doses. This requires that multiple blood glucose determinations be made to prevent periods of hyper- and hypoglycemia. Glucose values will quickly become normalized with minimal amplitude of daily excursions in most patients.[176]

Episodes of severe hypoglycemia are generally reduced with pump therapy.[176] When they occur, these events are usually secondary to errors in dose selection or failure to adhere to the required diet. The risk of nocturnal hypoglycemia, which is increased in the pregnant state, is reduced by lowering the basal rate from late evening until early morning. The basal rate can be programed to increase in the early morning hours to counteract the "dawn phenomenon."

The mechanics of the pump system are relatively simple. A fine-gauge butterfly needle device is attached by connecting tubing to the pump. This cannula is reimplanted every 2 to 3 days at a different site, usually in the anterior abdominal wall. Short-acting insulin is stored in the pump syringe. Infusion occurs at a basal rate, which can be fixed or altered for a specific time of day and duration. As noted above, the basal rate can be programmed for a lower rate at night. The size of preprandial boluses is based on the composition of each meal or snack. Approximately 60 percent of the total daily insulin dose is usually given as the basal rate and the remainder as premeal boluses infused. The largest bolus (30 to 35 percent) is administered with breakfast, followed by 25 percent before lunch and dinner and 15 to 20 percent before snacks.

Patients without any pancreatic reserve may have rapid elevations of blood glucose if there is pump failure or intercurrent infection. For this reason, many clinicians recommend that patients using a pump check their glucose level at 2 to 3 A.M. to detect hyperglycemia resulting from pump failure. Since the advent of buffered insulin, insulin aggregation leading to occlusion of the Silastic infusion tubing is uncommon.

Increasing numbers of patients are using pumps, in large part because they provide greater flexibility in lifestyle. However, the benefits and risks associated with the use of the pump in pregnancy have not been well studied. In the largest prospective, randomized investigation, Coustan and colleagues randomized 22 pregnant patients to intensive conventional therapy with multiple injections versus pump therapy.[175] There were no differences between the two treatment groups with respect to outpatient mean glucose levels, glycosyl-ated hemoglobin levels, or glycemic excursions. Gabbe et al. recently reported a large retrospective cohort study of women who began pump therapy during ges-tation as compared to a group treated with multiple insulin injections. Patients using the pump, many with insulin lispro, had fewer hypoglycemic reactions and comparable glucose control and pregnancy outcomes. Most continued using the pump after delivery, and their control was significantly better than that of pa-tients on multiple injections.[176]

Diet therapy is critical to successful regulation of ma-ternal diabetes. A program consisting of three meals and several snacks is used for most patients. Dietary composition should be 50 to 60 percent carbohydrate, 20 percent protein, and 25 to 30 percent fat with less than 10 percent saturated fats, up to 10 percent poly-unsaturated fatty acids, and the remainder derived from monosaturated sources.[177] Caloric intake is established based on prepregnancy weight and weight gain during gestation. Weight reduction is not advised. Patients should consume approximately 35 kcal/kg ideal body weight. Obese women may be managed with an intake as low as 1,600 cal/day, although if ketonuria develops, this allowance may be increased.

The presence of maternal vasculopathy should be thoroughly assessed early in pregnancy. The patient should be evaluated by an ophthalmologist familiar with diabetic retinopathy. Ophthalmologic examina-tions are performed during each trimester and repeated more often if retinopathy is detected. Baseline renal function is established by assaying a 24-hour urine col-lection for creatinine clearance and protein. An electro-cardiogram, thyroid function studies, and a urine cul-ture are also obtained.

Most patients are followed with outpatient visits at 1- to 2-week intervals. At each visit, control is assessed and adjustments in insulin dosage and diet are made. However, patients should be instructed to call at any time if periods of hypoglycemia (<50 mg/dl) or hyper-glycemia (>200 mg/dl) occur. The increased risk of hy-poglycemia in pregnant individuals may be related to defective glucose counterregulatory hormone mecha-nisms.[108] Both epinephrine and glucagon appear to be suppressed in pregnant diabetic women during hypogly-cemia.[28,129] For these reasons, family members should be instructed on how and when to administer a gluca-gon injection for the treatment of severe reactions.

KETOACIDOSIS

With the implementation of antenatal care, programs stressing strict metabolic control of blood glucose levels

for type 1 and type 2 diabetic women, diabetic ketoaci-dosis (DKA) has fortunately become a less common occurrence. Kilvert and colleagues reported 11 cases of ketoacidosis in 635 insulin-treated pregnancies between 1971 and 1990. One fetal loss and one spontaneous miscarriage complicated the pregnancies affected by DKA.[178]

Diabetic ketoacidosis can occur in the newly diag-nosed diabetic patient, and the hormonal milieu of pregnancy may become the background for this phenomenon. As pregnancy is a state of relative insulin resistance marked by enhanced lipolysis and ketogenesis, diabetic ketoacidosis may develop in a pregnant woman with glucose levels barely exceeding 200 mg/dl (11.1 mmol/L). Thus, DKA may be diag-nosed during pregnancy with minimal hyperglycemia accompanied by a fall in plasma bicarbonate and a pH value less than 7.30. Serum acetone is positive at a 1:2 dilution.

Early recognition of signs and symptoms of DKA will improve both maternal and fetal outcome. As in the nonpregnant state, clinical signs of volume depletion follow the symptoms of hyperglycemia, which include polydipsia and polyuria. Malaise, headache, nausea, and vomiting are common complaints. Occasionally, di-abetic ketoacidosis may present in an undiagnosed dia-betic woman receiving β-mimetic agents to arrest pre-term labor. Because of the risk of hyperglycemia and diabetic ketoacidosis in diabetic women receiving intra-venous medications such as a terbutaline, magnesium sulfate has become the preferred tocolytic for cases of preterm labor in these cases. Administration of antena-tal corticosteroids to accelerate fetal lung maturation can cause significant maternal hyperglycemia and pre-cipitate DKA. These patients must be closely followed in an acute care setting for at least 48 to 72 hours after corticosteroids have been given. An intravenous insulin infusion will usually be required and is adjusted on the basis of frequent capillary glucose measure-ments.

Once the diagnosis of DKA is established and the patient is stabilized, she should be transported to a facility where tertiary care in both perinatology and neonatology is available. Therapy hinges on the meticu-lous correction of metabolic and fluid abnormalities. An attempt at treatment of any underlying cause for ketoacidosis, such as infection, should be instituted as well (see the box "Management of DKA during Preg-nancy"). Diabetic ketoacidosis does represent a substan-tial risk for fetal compromise. However, successful fetal resuscitation will often accompany correction of mater-nal acidosis. Every effort should therefore be made to correct maternal condition before intervening and deliv-ering a preterm infant.

Management of DKA during Pregnancy

1. Laboratory assessment:
   Obtain arterial blood gases to document degree of acidosis present; measure glucose, ketones, electrolytes, at 1- to 2-hour intervals.
2. Insulin:
   Low-dose, intravenous (IV)
   Loading dose: 0.2–0.4 units/kg
   Maintenance: 2.0–10.0 units/h
3. Fluids:
   Isotonic NaCl
   Total replacement in first 12 h = 4–6 L
   1 L in first hour
   500–1,000 ml/h for 2–4 h
   250 ml/h until 80% replaced
4. Glucose:
   Begin 5% D/NS* when plasma level reaches 250 mg/dl (14 mmol/L)
5. Potassium:
   If initially normal or reduced, an infusion rate up to 15 to 20 mEq/h may be required; if elevated, wait until levels decline into the normal range, then add to IV solution in a concentration of 20–30 mEq/L
6. Bicarbonate:
   Add one ampule (44 mEq) to 1 L of 0.45 NS if pH is <7.10

*D/NS, dextrose in normal saline.

ANTEPARTUM FETAL EVALUATION

Over the past 20 years, protocols for antepartum fetal assessment in pregnancies complicated by diabetes mellitus have been incorporated into a program of outpatient monitoring during the third trimester. During this time period, when the risk of sudden intrauterine death increases, a program of fetal surveillance is initiated. As improvement in maternal control has played a major role in reducing perinatal mortality in pregnancies complicated by diabetes, antepartum fetal monitoring tests are now used primarily to reassure the obstetrician and avoid unnecessary premature intervention. These techniques have few false-negative results, and in a patient who is well controlled and exhibits no vasculopathy or significant hypertension, reassuring antepartum testing allows the fetus to benefit from further maturation in utero.

Maternal assessment of fetal activity serves as a screening technique in a program of fetal surveillance. To date, few studies have applied this method to a large number of women with diabetes mellitus. Patients with a variety of high-risk antepartum conditions including diabetes appear to have an increased incidence of alarming fetal activity patterns.[179] While the false-negative rate with maternal monitoring of fetal activity is low (~1 percent), the false-positive rate may be as high as 60 percent. Maternal hypoglycemia, while generally believed to be associated with decreased fetal movement, may actually stimulate fetal activity.[180]

Sadovsky and coworkers[181] reported that fetal movement at 25 to 33 weeks' gestation in 67 diabetic pregnancies was lower than in controls, while in the final 2 months of pregnancy, activity levels were similar to the nondiabetic population. In this series, there were four cases of cessation of fetal movement. Two fetuses died in utero 10 and 11 hours after maternal perception that activity had stopped, an interval shorter than that seen in other complications of pregnancy.

The nonstress test (NST) remains the preferred method to assess antepartum fetal well-being in the patient with diabetes mellitus.[182] If the NST is nonreactive, a biophysical profile (BPP) or contraction stress test is then performed (Fig. 32–11). Heart rate monitoring is begun early in the third trimester, usually by 32 weeks' gestation. Barrett et al.[183] documented six antepartum deaths in 425 patients having weekly tests,

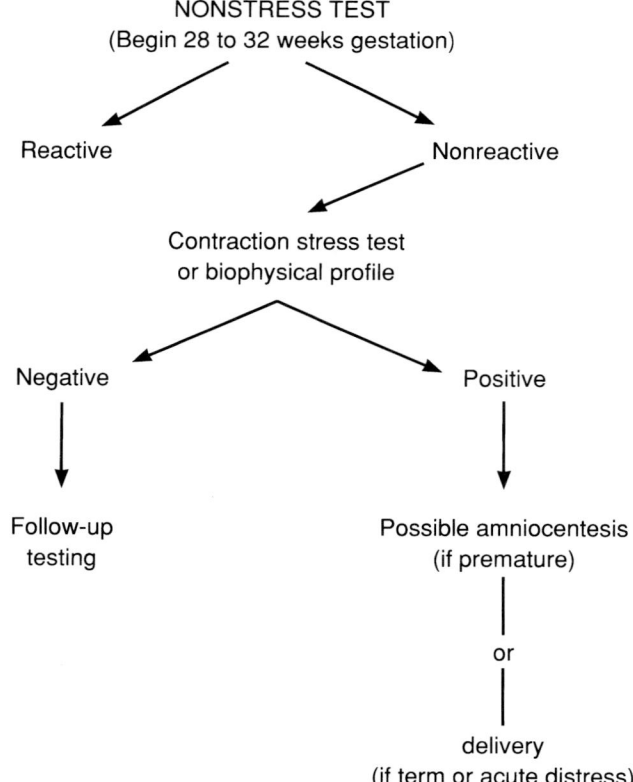

Figure 32–11. Scheme for antepartum fetal testing in pregnancy complicated by diabetes mellitus.

Table 32–6. ANTEPARTUM FETAL SURVEILLANCE IN LOW-RISK INSULIN-DEPENDENT DIABETES MELLITUS*

	Study
Ultrasonography at 4 to 6-week intervals	Yes
Maternal assessment of fetal activity, daily at 28 weeks	Yes
Nonstress test (NST) weekly at 28 weeks	Yes
	Twice weekly at 34 weeks
Contraction stress test or biophysical profile if NST nonreactive L/S, lung profile	Yes, if elective delivery planned prior to 39 weeks

* Low-risk pregestational diabetes mellitus: excellent control (60–120 mg/dl), no vasculopathy (classes B, C), no stillbirth.

a significantly greater fetal death rate than in other high-risk pregnancies. Other studies have also demonstrated an increased fetal death rate within 1 week of a reactive NST in pregnancies complicated by diabetes mellitus when compared with other high-risk gestations.[184] If the NST is to be used as the primary method of antepartum heart rate testing, we prefer that it be done at least twice weekly once the patient reaches 32 weeks' gestation. In patients with vascular disease or poor control, in whom the incidence of abnormal tests and intrauterine deaths is greater, testing is often performed earlier and more frequently.

Doppler umbilical artery velocimetry has been proposed as a clinical tool for antepartum fetal surveillance in pregnancies at risk for placental vascular disease. We have found that Doppler studies of the umbilical artery may be predictive of fetal outcome in diabetic pregnancies complicated by vascular disease.[185] Elevated placental resistance as evidenced by an increased systolic/diastolic ratio is associated with fetal growth restriction and preeclampsia in these high-risk patients.[185] In contrast, well-controlled patients without vascular disease rarely demonstrate abnormal fetal umbilical artery waveforms.

Johnstone and colleagues[186] have reported the largest experience with serial Doppler umbilical waveforms in pregnancies complicated by diabetes. In their study of 128 women, significant abnormal flow patterns were observed in 9 cases. Three of these women had nephropathy and three had preeclampsia. All of these pregnancies had normal outcomes. Importantly, several cases of fetal distress as defined by abnormal biophysical testing were accompanied by normal Doppler studies. Therefore, it appears that undue reliance should not be placed on normal waveform values in the diabetic pregnancy.[186]

It is important to include not only the results of antepartum fetal testing but to weigh all the clinical features involving mother and fetus before a decision is made to intervene for suspected fetal distress, especially if this decision may result in a preterm delivery (Tables 32–6 and 32–7). In reviewing nine series involving 993 diabetic patients, an abnormal test of fetal condition led to delivery 5 percent of the time.[187] It appears that outpatient testing protocols work well in type 1 and type 2 patients. Whether such testing is required for all women with diabetes mellitus remains controversial.[188] In a study of 114 well-controlled women, 10 patients were delivered for abnormal fetal testing. Eight of these 10 women had nephropathy or hypertension. Nephropathy or hypertension was associated with intervention for fetal well-being in 8 of 20 women with these risk factors in comparison with 2 of 94 without these complications. It thus appears that women whose diabetes is poorly controlled, who have hypertension, or who have significant vasculopathy that may be associated with fetal growth restriction are at increased risk for fetal compromise and probably benefit most from a program of antepartum fetal surveillance.

Ultrasound is a valuable tool in evaluating fetal growth, estimating fetal weight, and detecting hydramnios and malformations. A determination of maternal serum α-fetoprotein (MSAFP) at 16 weeks' gestation is often used in association with a detailed ultrasound study during the second trimester in an attempt to detect neural tube defects and other anomalies. Normal values of MSAFP for diabetic women are lower than in the nondiabetic population.[189] A lower threshold for the upper limit of normal may thus be preferable in pregnancies complicated by diabetes mellitus in order to help detect spina bifida and other major malformations that are increased in this population.

Fetal echocardiography is performed at 20 to 22 weeks' gestation for the investigation of possible cardiac anomalies. Using such an approach, Greene and Benacerraf detected 18 of 32 malformations in a series

Table 32–7. ANTEPARTUM FETAL SURVEILLANCE IN HIGH-RISK PREGESTATIONAL DIABETES MELLITUS*

	Study
Ultrasonography at 4 to 6-week intervals	Yes
Maternal assessment of fetal activity, daily at 28 weeks	Yes
Nonstress test (NST)	Minimum twice weekly
Contraction stress test or biophysical profile if NST nonreactive L/S, lung profile at 37–38 weeks	Yes

* High-risk pregestational diabetes mellitus: poor control (macrosomia, hydramnios), vasculopathy (classes D, F, R), prior stillbirth.

of 432 diabetic pregnancies.[190] The specificity was in excess of 99 percent and the negative predictive value was 97 percent. Spina bifida was identified in all cases; however, ventricular septal defects, limb abnormalities, and facial clefts were missed. A review of the prenatal diagnosis experience in 289 diabetic women in The Ohio State University Diabetes in Pregnancy Program revealed 29 anomalies in which 12 were cardiac, 14 were noncardiac, and 3 were combined.[86] Twelve of 15 (80 percent) cardiac and 10 of 17 (59 percent) noncardiac lesions were identified prenatally. When considering cardiac defects alone, we could not identify a glycosylated hemoglobin cut-off for these anomalies. Therefore, we believe detailed cardiac imaging should be offered to all women with pregestational diabetes mellitus to assist in the detection of cardiac lesions, especially those of the great vessels and cardiac septum.

Ultrasound examinations should be repeated at 4- to 6-week intervals to assess fetal growth. The detection of fetal macrosomia, the leading risk factor for shoulder dystocia, is important in the selection of patients who are best delivered by cesarean section. An increased rate of cephalopelvic disproportion and shoulder dystocia accompanied by significant risk of traumatic birth injury and asphyxia have been consistently associated with the vaginal delivery of large infants. The risk of such complications rises exponentially when birth weight exceeds 4 kg and is greater for the fetus of a diabetic mother when compared to a fetus with similar weight whose mother does not have diabetes.[191] Sonographic measurements of the fetal abdominal circumference have proved most helpful in predicting fetal macrosomia.[192] The abdomen is likely to be large because of increased glycogen deposition in the fetal liver and subcutaneous fat deposition. Using serial sonographic examinations, accelerated abdominal growth can be identified by 32 weeks' gestation.[193]

TIMING AND MODE OF DELIVERY

Delivery should be delayed until fetal maturation has taken place, provided that the patient's diabetes is well controlled and antepartum surveillance remains normal. In our practice, elective induction of labor is often planned at 38 to 40 weeks' gestation in well-controlled patients without vascular disease. Patients with vascular disease are delivered prior to term only if hypertension worsens or fetal growth restriction mandates early delivery. Before elective delivery prior to 39 weeks' gestation, an amniocentesis may be performed to document fetal pulmonary maturity. There is much evidence that tests of fetal lung maturity have the same predictive value in diabetic pregnancies as they do in the normal population.[124]

The presence of the acidic phospholipid phosphatidylglycerol (PG) is the final marker of fetal pulmonary maturation. Several authors have suggested that fetal hyperinsulinemia may be associated with delayed appearance of PG and an increased incidence of RDS. Landon et al.[108] have correlated the appearance of PG in amniotic fluid with maternal glycemic control during gestation. RDS may occur in the IDM with a mature lecithin/sphingomyelin ratio or fetal lung maturity index but absent PG. It follows that the clinician must be familiar with the laboratory analysis of amniotic fluid in his or her institution and the neonatal outcome associated with the results of fetal lung maturity testing.

When antepartum testing suggests fetal compromise, delivery must be considered. If amniotic fluid analysis yields a mature test result, delivery should be accomplished promptly. In the presence of presumed lung immaturity, the decision to proceed with delivery should be based on confirmation of deteriorating fetal condition by several abnormal tests. For example, if the NST as well as the BPP indicates fetal compromise, delivery is indicated. Finally, there remain several maternal indications for delivery including preeclampsia, worsening renal function, or deteriorating vision secondary to proliferative retinopathy.

The route of delivery for the diabetic patient remains controversial. Cousins,[194] in reviewing over 1,600 (White Class B, C, D, R) patients in the literature between 1965 and 1985, noted a cesarean section rate of approximately 45 percent. This figure is likely to represent the practice trends of most obstetricians and perinatologists in the United States.[182] Delivery by cesarean section usually is favored when fetal distress has been suggested by antepartum heart rate monitoring. If a patient reaches 38 weeks' gestation with a mature fetal lung profile and is at significant risk for intrauterine demise because of poor control or a history of a prior stillbirth, an elective delivery is planned.

The increased rate of shoulder dystocia and brachial plexus injury in the offspring of diabetic women has prompted adoption of early induction strategies as well as selection of patients for cesarean section based on ultrasound estimation of fetal size. Kjos and colleagues demonstrated that induction at 38 weeks in a population of GDM women was associated with a lower frequency of large-for-gestational age infants and shoulder dystocia without an increased cesarean rate.[195] This is in contrast to studies of nondiabetic women in which suspected macrosomia is apparently associated with an increased cesarean rate.[196] In a sophisticated decision tree analysis of cost effectiveness, Rouse and colleagues found that whereas elective cesarean delivery for macrosomia to prevent permanent brachial plexus injury

Table 32–8. RATE OF SHOULDER DYSTOCIA RELATED TO BIRTH WEIGHT AND DIABETIC STATUS

Birth Weight (g)	Without Diabetes (%)	With Diabetes (%)
<4,000	0.1–1.1	0.6–3.7
4,000–4,449	1.1–10.0	4.9–23.1
>4,500	4.1–22.6	20.0–50.0

Adapted from ACOG Practice Patterns No. 7, October 1997.

was prohibitively expensive in the nondiabetic woman at a cost of several million dollars per injury prevented, 489 cesarean sections at a cost per avoided birth injury of $880,000 per case for diabetic pregnancies with an estimated fetal size greater than 4,000 g seemed to be at least tenable.[197]

During labor, continuous fetal heart rate monitoring is mandatory. Labor is allowed to progress as long as normal rates of cervical dilatation and descent are documented. Acker et al.[198] have reported that the overall risk for shoulder dystocia in the macrosomic IDM is greater than for the large, normal infant. In their series of diabetic women, the risk for shoulder dystocia with a fetal weight greater than 4,000 g was approximately 30 percent. Somewhat less impressive yet significantly greater frequencies of shoulder dystocia for delivery of macrosomic IDMs versus non-IDMs have been reported by Nesbitt and colleagues[191] (Table 32–8). Despite attempts to select patients with obvious fetal macrosomia for elective cesarean delivery, arrest of dilatation or descent despite adequate labor should alert the physician to the possibility of cephalopelvic disproportion. About 25 percent of macrosomic infants (>4,000 g) delivered after a prolonged second stage will have shoulder dystocia.[199] It follows that cesarean delivery should be considered in a patient who demonstrates significant protracted labor or failure of descent.

GLUCOREGULATION DURING LABOR AND DELIVERY

As neonatal hypoglycemia is in part related to maternal glucose levels during labor, it is important to maintain maternal plasma glucose levels within the physiologic normal range. The patient is given nothing by mouth after midnight of the evening before induction or elective cesarean delivery. The usual bedtime dose of insulin is administered or, for women receiving pump therapy, the infusion is continued overnight. Upon arrival to labor and delivery early in the morning, the patient's capillary glucose level is assessed with a bedside meter. Continuous infusion of both insulin and glucose are then administered based on maternal glucose levels (see the box "Insulin Management during Labor and Delivery"). Ten units of regular insulin may be added to 1,000 ml of solution containing 5 percent dextrose. An infusion rate of 100 to 125 ml/h (1 unit/h) will, in most cases, result in good glucose control. Insulin may also be infused from a syringe pump at a dose of 0.25 to 2.0 units/h, and adjusted to maintain normal glucose values. Glucose levels are recorded hourly, and the infusion rate is adjusted accordingly. Jovanovic and Peterson have noted that well-controlled patients will often be euglycemic once active labor begins and will then require glucose at an infusion rate of 2.5 mg/kg/min.[200] It may be necessary to increase the insulin infusion during the second stage of labor with increased catecholamine secretion.

When cesarean delivery is to be performed, it should be scheduled for early morning. This simplifies intrapartum glucose control and allows the neonatal team to prepare for the care of the newborn. The patient is given nothing by mouth, and her usual morning insulin dose is withheld. If her surgery is not performed early in the day, one third to one half of the patient's intermediate-acting dose of insulin may be administered. Regional anesthesia is preferred because an awake patient permits earlier detection of hypoglycemia. Following surgery, glucose levels are monitored every 2 hours and an intravenous solution of 5 percent dextrose is administered.

Insulin Management during Labor and Delivery

- Usual dose of intermediate-acting insulin is given at bedtime.
- Morning dose of insulin is withheld.
- Intravenous infusion of normal saline is begun.
- Once active labor begins or glucose levels fall below 70 mg/dl, the infusion is changed from saline to 5% dextrose and delivered at a rate of 2.5 mg/kg/min.
- Glucose levels are checked hourly using a portable meter allowing for adjustment in the infusion rate.
- Regular (short-acting) insulin in administered by intravenous infusion if glucose levels exceed 140 mg/dl.

Adapted from Jovanovic L, Peterson CM: Management of the pregnant, insulin-dependent diabetic woman. Diabetes Care 3: 63, 1980.

After delivery, insulin requirements are usually significantly lower than were pregnancy or prepregnancy needs. The objective of "tight control" used in the antepartum period is relaxed for the first 24 to 48 hours. Patients delivered vaginally, who are able to eat a regular diet, are given one third to one half of their end-of-pregnancy dose of NPH insulin and short-acting insulin the morning of the first postpartum day. Frequent glucose determinations are used to guide insulin dosage. Most patients are stabilized on this regimen within a few days after delivery.

Women with diabetes are encouraged to breast-feed. The additional 500 kcal required daily are given as approximately 100 g of carbohydrate and 20 g of protein.[201] The insulin dose may be somewhat lower in lactating diabetic women. Hypoglycemia appears to be common in the first week following delivery and immediately after nursing.

MANAGEMENT OF THE PATIENT WITH GESTATIONAL DIABETES

The mainstay of treatment of GDM is nutritional counseling and dietary intervention. The optimal diet should provide caloric and nutrient needs to sustain pregnancy without resulting in significant postprandial hyperglycemia.[202] Women with GDM generally do not need hospitalization for dietary instruction and management. Once the diagnosis is established, patients are begun on a dietary program of 2,000 to 2,500 kcal daily.[202] This represents approximately 35 kcal/kg present pregnancy weight. Jovanovic-Peterson and Peterson have noted that such a diet composed of 50 to 60 percent carbohydrate will cause excessive weight gain and postprandial hyperglycemia, and will require insulin therapy in 50 percent of patients.[203] For this reason, several groups have studied the use of calorie-restricted diets. Algert and colleagues[204] have reported that obese women with GDM may be managed on as little as 1,700 to 1,800 kcal/day with less weight gain and no apparent reduction in fetal size. Magee et al.[205] designed a study to evaluate strict caloric restriction as a treatment for obese subjects with GDM. They randomized patients to a 2,400 kcal/day diet compared to a 1,200 kcal/day group. Average glucose levels and fasting insulin were reduced in the hypocaloric group. However, fasting glucose levels and postchallenge glucose levels were not significantly different. Significant ketonuria did develop in the restricted group, which may have a detrimental effect on fetal neurologic development.[206] The authors thus went on to study a 1,800-kcal diet, which improved glycemia and did not increase serum ketone levels.[207] Similar results have been reported by Peterson and Jovanovic-Peterson, who recommend 30 kcal/kg present pregnant weight for normal weight women, 24 kcal/kg for overweight women, and 12 kcal/kg for morbidly obese women.[208] These authors indicate that mild caloric restriction with modification of the carbohydrate component may be advised in obese GDM women.[209]

Once the patient with GDM is placed on an appropriate diet, surveillance of blood glucose levels is necessary to be certain that glycemic control has been established. At a minimum, practitioners have performed weekly assessment of fasting or postprandial glucose levels or both at clinic or office visits. Some clinicians prefer to have patients perform daily self-blood glucose monitoring, which in two retrospective studies has been associated with a decline in macrosomia at the expense of nearly half of all women requiring insulin therapy.[210,211] A practical approach may be to provide women with GDM with a glucose meter; however, if after a few weeks, both fasting and postprandial measurements are within the normal range, the frequency of testing can be reduced accordingly.

Whereas the ACOG has recommended that fasting plasma glucose levels be maintained below 105 mg/dl and 2-hour postprandial values be less than 120 mg/dl, therapeutic thresholds of fasting below 95 mg/dl and 1-hour postprandial below 140 mg/dl as well as 2-hour postprandial below 120 mg/dl have been suggested by the Fourth International Workshop-Conference.[212] If a patient repetitively exceeds these thresholds, then insulin therapy is suggested. The use of the above cutoffs for initiating insulin are based on data regarding increased perinatal morbidity when such values are exceeded in women with preexisting diabetes. Currently, there are no data from controlled trials to identify ideal glycemic targets for prevention of fetal risk for women with GDM.

Langer and colleagues[213] have critically evaluated thresholds for insulin therapy in GDM and concluded that to evaluate the effect of therapy, appropriate endpoints should include fetal macrosomia or large-for-gestational-age (LGA) infants, and neonatal metabolic complications. Langer and colleagues[213] evaluated insulin secretion patterns in women with GDM and non-GDM during an oral glucose tolerance test. Patients with fasting plasma glucose below 95 mg/dl had significantly greater insulin production than those with a glucose level greater than or equal to 95 mg/dl. To test whether the assignment to insulin therapy for a patient with a fasting value of 95 mg/dl or higher was appropriate, Langer et al.[213] compared rates of delivery of LGA infants among women with GDM grouped according to their fasting plasma glucose levels and whether diet or diet and insulin were used. He found that patients with a fasting glucose between 96 and 105 mg/dl had a greater incidence of LGA infants (28.6 percent) when receiving diet therapy alone versus obese women with GDM receiving both diet and insulin. Whereas Langer and co-workers[211] have documented a relationship between maternal glycemia and macrosomia in GDM, which would establish guidelines for insulin therapy, some authors have suggested that estimation of glycemia alone may be sufficient to optimally prescribe insulin therapy in these cases.

Buchanan and colleagues have reviewed the utility of fetal ultrasound measurements to guide insulin therapy in women with GDM.[214] In their study of diet-treated GDM, ultrasound performed at 29 to 33 weeks was used to identify pregnancies with fetuses having a large abdominal circumference (>75th percentile). These cases were then randomized to diet versus diet and insulin treatment. The insulin-treated group ultimately had a frequency of LGA infants of 13 percent, which was far below the 45 percent present in the diet-treated group. The cost-effectiveness of this approach needs to be compared to administration of insulin to women with fasting hyperglycemia on diet therapy, since approximately two thirds of women require insulin therapy for a large fetal abdominal circumference (on ultrasound examination) in this range of maternal glycemia.

In addition to aggressive insulin therapy and hypocaloric diet regimens, exercise has recently been studied as an alternative primary treatment for GDM. Such an approach is beneficial for nonpregnant type 2 diabetic patients in whom physical training increases insulin sensitivity. Fasting and postprandial insulin concentrations and glucose excursions are lowered in both obese and physically fit individuals who exercise. This effect apparently is sustained up to 5 to 7 days after the last training session. Three 20-minute aerobic exercise sessions weekly are recommended. Brisk walking is ideal.

Bung and colleagues[215] conducted a prospective study of the utility of exercise in the treatment of GDM. These authors randomized 41 women with GDM who manifested elevated fasting glucose levels, which would normally require insulin therapy. In the final analysis, 17 women completed a supervised bicycle ergometry training program compared with 17 women receiving insulin treatment. No statistical differences were observed in weekly blood glucose determinations between study groups. All fetal heart rate patterns were reactive before and after exercise. Thus, exercise programs for the treatment of GDM appear to be safe and may obviate the need for insulin therapy in some individuals.

Most recently, Langer and colleagues[216] have suggested that oral hypoglycemic therapy may be a suitable alternative to insulin treatment in women with GDM.[216] These investigators randomized 404 women to insulin versus glyburide and reported similar improvement in glycemia with both regimens. Most importantly, the frequency of macrosomia and neonatal hypoglycemia was similar in the two study groups. Fur-

ther studies will be necessary to establish the safety of this regimen.

Patients with GDM who are well controlled are at low risk for an intrauterine death. For this reason, we do not routinely institute antepartum fetal heart rate testing in uncomplicated diet-controlled GDM patients unless the patient has a hypertensive disorder, history of a prior stillbirth, or suspected macrosomia.[217] Women in these categories as well as those who require insulin treatment of GDM undergo twice-weekly heart rate testing at 32 weeks' gestation. Women with uncomplicated GDM do undergo fetal heart rate testing at 40 weeks' gestation. Using such a protocol at The Ohio State University Hospital Diabetes in Pregnancy Program, only two intrauterine deaths in over 1,500 cases of uncomplicated GDM have been observed in the last 12 years. Thus, it appears that the third-trimester stillbirth rate in these patients is no higher than that of the general obstetric population. A study of 389 women with GDM documented an antepartum stillbirth rate of 7.7 per 1,000, which was not significantly different from the rate of 4.8 per 1,000 observed in nondiabetic low-risk patients.[218] In this study, because 7 percent of fetuses were delivered for a low biophysical profile score, the benefit of testing all GDM pregnancies was raised. In the absence of a large prospective study comparing outcomes in monitored and nonmonitored GDM women without other risk factors, it is not possible to determine if any benefit exists to antepartum fetal surveillance in this apparently low-risk population.

Because many obstetricians have extrapolated the increased risk for stillbirth in pregestational diabetic women to those with GDM, a remarkable number of these pregnancies are subject to scheduled delivery at term. If glycemic control is suboptimal, or maternal hypertension or a previous stillbirth exists, such an approach seems warranted. As with antepartum fetal testing, should elective induction be the standard approach for uncomplicated GDM pregnancies? Lurie and co-workers[219] have in part addressed this issue by retrospectively comparing the outcomes of 124 GDM women delivered beyond 40 weeks' gestation compared with the same number of GDM women delivered before their expected date of confinement. Antepartum fetal surveillance was not routinely begun until 40 weeks' gestation. No significant differences in perinatal outcome, cesarean delivery rates, or shoulder dystocia were found between study groups. A vaginal delivery rate of 75.8 percent was achieved in GDM women delivering beyond 40 weeks' gestation. These authors concluded that elective induction before 40 weeks' gestation should be avoided and every attempt should be made to allow women with GDM, both diet- and insulin-treated, to proceed to spontaneous labor. In contrast, a follow-up prospective study from the same institution of 96 insulin-requiring women with GDM demonstrated that induction at 38 to 39 weeks was associated with a shoulder dystocia rate of 1.4 percent versus 10.2 percent in historic controls.[220]

Kjos and colleagues[195] have conducted a prospective randomized trial of active induction of labor at 38 weeks' gestation versus expectant management in a series which included 187 insulin-requiring women with GDM. The cesarean delivery rate was not significantly different in the expectant-management group (31 percent) from the active-induction group (25 percent). However, an increased prevalence of LGA infants (23 percent vs. 10 percent) was observed in the expectant management group. Moreover, the frequency of shoulder dystocia was 3 percent in this group, with no cases reported in those undergoing induction at 38 weeks' gestation. These data led the authors to conclude that elective delivery be considered in insulin-requiring patients with GDM because it does not increase the risk for macrosomia, shoulder dystocia, and cesarean delivery, and lowers the risk for fetal death. In patients managed expectantly, careful monitoring of fetal growth should be performed because of an apparent increasing risk for macrosomia with advancing gestational age in this population.

COUNSELING THE DIABETIC PATIENT

Anomalies of the cardiac, renal, and central nervous systems arise during the first 7 weeks of gestation, a time when it is most unusual for patients to seek prenatal care. Therefore, the management and counseling of women with diabetes in the reproductive age group should begin prior to conception. Unfortunately, it has been estimated that less than 20 percent of diabetic women in the United States obtain prepregnancy counseling.[182]

A reduced rate of major congenital malformation in patients optimally managed before conception is observed with special diabetes clinics (Table 32–9). In

Table 32–9. COMPARATIVE RATES OF MAJOR MALFORMATIONS IN OFFSPRING OF DIABETIC WOMEN RECEIVING PRECONCEPTIONAL COUNSELING

Study	With Preconceptional Counseling	Without Preconceptional Counseling
Fuhrmann et al.[222]	1/128 (0.8%)	22/292 (7.5%)
Steel and Duncan[237]	2/143 (1.4%)	10/96 (10.4%)
Kitzmiller et al.[224]	1/84 (1.2%)	12/110 (10.9%)
Whillhoite et al.[228]	1/62 (1.6%)	8/123 (6.5%)

Copenhagen, the rate of malformations fell from 19.4 percent to 8.5 percent in Class D and F patients who attended a prepregnancy clinic.[221] Fuhrmann et al.[222] found that intensive treatment begun prior to conception in 307 East German diabetic women reduced the malformation rate to 1 percent. Nearly 90 percent of women in this study maintained mean glucose levels less than 100 mg/dl (5.6 mmol/L). In contrast, the incidence of anomalies in the offspring of 593 diabetic women who registered for care after 8 weeks' gestation was 8.0 percent (47 of 593). Only 205 of those women had mean daily glucose levels of less than 100 mg/dl (5.6 mmol/L). Mills et al.[88] have reported that diabetic women registered prior to pregnancy had fewer infants with anomalies when compared to late registrants (4.9 percent vs. 9.0 percent). While the incidence of 4.9 percent is higher than that in a normal control population (2 percent), normalization of glycemia was not established in the early entry group.

Kitzmiller and colleagues studied 84 women with pregestational diabetes who were recruited for preconception education and management during a 7-year period.[224] A group of 110 pregnancy diabetic women presenting in the first trimester without preconceptional counseling served as controls in this study. One anomaly (1.2 percent) occurred in the preconception group versus 12 (10.9 percent) malformations in the control population.

Glycosylated hemoglobin levels obtained during the first trimester may be used to counsel diabetic women regarding the risk for an anomalous infant. In a retrospective study of 116 women at the Joslin Clinic, Miller and colleagues[223] observed that elevated hemoglobin A_{1c} concentrations early in pregnancy correlated with an increased incidence of malformations. In 58 patients with elevated glycosylated hemoglobin levels, 13 (22 percent) malformed infants were noted. This is in contrast to a 3.4 percent incidence of major malformations in 58 women whose glycosylated hemoglobin levels were in the normal range. Their findings were confirmed by Ylinen et al.,[225] who measured glycosylated hemoglobin before the 15th week of gestation in 142 pregnancies. In pregnancies complicated by fetal malformations, mean values were significantly higher than in pregnancies without malformations. In the subgroup of patients with glycosylated hemoglobin values greater than 10 percent (normal, <8 percent), fetal malformations were present in 6 of 17 cases. Overall, the risk of a major fetal anomaly may be as high as 1 in 4 or 1 in 5 when the glycosylated hemoglobin level is several percent above normal values. Greene[226] has reported that 14 of 35 pregnancies with a glycosylated hemoglobin exceeding 12.8 percent were complicated by major malformations. In his series from the Joslin Clinic, the risk for major anomalies did not become evident until glycosylated hemoglobin values exceed 6 SD above the mean. In contrast to the studies cited above is the Diabetes in Early Pregnancy (DIEP) study, in which malformation rates in IDMs were not correlated with first-trimester maternal glycosylated hemoglobin levels.[88] The authors suggested that more sensitive measures are needed to identify teratogenic mechanisms or that not all malformations can be prevented by good glycemic control. Further review of these data, which included glycosylated hemoglobin levels only in the early entry patients, demonstrates that these women were a relatively homogeneous group with respect to glycemic control; 93 percent had glycosylated hemoglobin levels less than 7 SD below the mean, a level of control that barely increases the risk for anomalies according to Greene's data.[226] Regardless of the glycosylated hemoglobin value obtained, all patients require a careful program of surveillance, as outlined earlier, to detect fetal malformations. The risk for spontaneous abortion also appears to be increased with marked elevations in glycosylated hemoglobin. However, for diabetic women in good control, there appears to be no greater likelihood of miscarriage.[227]

With the increasing evidence that poor control is responsible for the congenital malformations seen in pregnancies complicated by diabetes, it is apparent that preconception counseling involving the patient and her family should be instituted.[224,228] Physicians who care for young women with diabetes must be aware of the importance of such counseling. At this time, the nonpregnant patient may learn techniques for self-glucose monitoring as well as the need for proper dietary management. Folic acid dietary supplementation at a dose of at least 0.4 mg daily should be prescribed, as there is increasing evidence that this vitamin may reduce the frequency of neural tube defects, although it has not specifically been studied in the diabetic population.[229,230] During counseling, questions may be answered regarding risk factors for complications and the plan for general management of diabetes in pregnancy. Planning for pregnancy should optimally be accomplished over several months. Glycosylated hemoglobin measurements are performed to aid in the timing of conception. As a conservative recommendation, the patient should attempt to achieve a glycosylated hemoglobin level within 2 SD of the mean for the reference laboratory.[231]

CONTRACEPTION

There is no evidence that diabetes mellitus impairs fertility. Family planning is thus an important consideration for the diabetic woman. A careful history and complete gynecologic examination and counseling are required before selecting a method of contraception. Barrier methods continue to be a safe and inexpensive method of birth control. The diaphragm, used correctly with a spermicide, has a failure rate of less than 10 percent. Because there are no inherent risks to the diaphragm and other barrier methods, these have become the preferred interim method of contraception for women with diabetes. The intrauterine device may also be used by diabetic women without an increased risk of infection.[232]

Combined oral contraceptives (OCs) are the most effective reversible method of contraception, with failure rates generally less than 1 percent. There is, however, continued controversy regarding their use in the diabetic woman. The serious side effects of pill use, including thromboembolic disease and myocardial infarction, may be increased in diabetic women using combined OCs. In a retrospective study, Steel and Duncan[233] observed five cardiovascular complications in 136 diabetic women using primarily low-dose pills. Three patients had cerebrovascular accidents, one had a myocardial infarction, and one an axillary vein thrombosis. In a recent retrospective case-control study, despite diabetes increasing the risk for cerebral thromboembolism fivefold compared with controls, this risk was not enhanced by use of combined oral contraceptives.[234]

In Steel and Duncan's report, several women exhibited rapid progression of retinopathy. Klein and colleagues[235] studied OC use in a cross-sectional study of 384 type 1 diabetic women and reported no association between OCs and progression of vascular complications. For physicians who prescribe low-dose OCs to diabetic women, their use should probably be restricted to patients without serious vascular complications or additional risk factors such as a strong family history of myocardial disease. In these women, a monophasic preparation (progestin only) may be considered. In women receiving oral contraceptives, the lowest dose of estrogen and progesterone should be employed. Patients should have blood pressure monitoring after the first cycle and quarterly with baseline and follow-up lipid levels as well.

Women using the OCs may demonstrate increased resistance to insulin as a result of a diminished concentration of insulin receptors.[236] Despite the fact that carbohydrate metabolism may be affected by the progestin component of the pill, disturbances in diabetic control are actually uncommon with its use. In Steel and Duncan's study,[237] 81 percent of patients using the pill did not require a change in insulin dose. Triphasic OCs may also be used safely in former GDM women without other risk factors. Skouby et al.[238] have demonstrated that normal glucose tolerance and lipid levels can be expected in nonobese former GDM women followed after 6 months of therapy. Kjos and colleagues[239] performed a prospective randomized study of 230 women with recent GDM. OC users were randomized to low-dose norethindrone or levonorgestrel preparations in combination with ethinyl estradiol. The rate of subsequent diabetes in OC users was 15 to 20 percent, after 1-year follow-up. This rate was not significantly different from non-OC users (17 percent). Importantly, no adverse effects on total cholesterol, LDL, HDL, or triglycerides were found with OC use.

At present, there is little information available concerning long-acting progestins in women with diabetes or previous GDM. A statistically significant, yet clinically limited deterioration in carbohydrate tolerance has been reported in healthy depomedroxyprogesterone acetate (Depo-Provera; DMPA) users.[240] A decrease in serum triglyceride and HDL cholesterol levels, but not total cholesterol or LDL cholesterol has also been demonstrated with Depo-Provera.[241] Similarly, the subdermal implant, Norplant, which releases levonorgestrel, has been associated with elevated glucose and insulin levels in the nondiabetic population.[242] For these reasons, neither DMPA nor Norplant are recommended as first-line methods of contraception for women with diabetes. The progestin-only oral contraceptive would be preferred, as it does not produce significant metabolic effects in diabetic women. Kjos et al. have reported that progestin-only OCs administered to breast-feeding Hispanic women with prior gestational diabetes may accelerate the progression to type 2 diabetes.[243]

Key Points

➤ Pregnancy has been characterized as a diabetogenic state because of increased postprandial glucose levels in a late gestation.

➤ Both hepatic and peripheral (tissue) insulin sensitivity are reduced in normal pregnancy. As a result, a progressive increase in insulin secretion follows a glucose challenge.

➤ In women with gestational diabetes, the hormonal milieu of pregnancy may represent an unmasking of a susceptibility to the development of type 2 diabetes mellitus.

➤ According to the Pedersen hypothesis, maternal hyperglycemia results in fetal hyperglycemia and hyperinsulinemia, resulting in excessive fetal growth. Physiologic maternal glycemic control is associated with a reduced risk for fetal macrosomia.

➤ Congenital malformations occur with a two to sixfold increased rate in offspring of type 1 and type 2 diabetic women compared with the normal population. Impaired glycemic control and the associated derangement in maternal metabolism appear to contribute to abnormal embryogenesis.

➤ Women with Class F (nephropathy) diabetes have an increased risk for preeclampsia and preterm delivery which correlates with their degree of renal impairment.

➤ Diabetic retinopathy may worsen during pregnancy, yet for women optimally treated with laser photocoagulation *prior* to pregnancy, significant deterioration of vision is uncommon.

➤ Screening for GDM is generally performed between 24–28 weeks gestation. Screening strategies include universal screening or limiting screening to women over age 25 with risk factors for developing type 2 diabetes mellitus.

➤ Treatment of the insulin-dependent woman during pregnancy requires intensive therapy consisting of frequent self blood glucose monitoring and aggressive insulin dosing by multiple injections or continous subcutaneous infusion (insulin pump).

➤ The cornerstone of treatment for GDM is dietary therapy. Insulin or glyburide are reserved for individuals who manifest significant fasting hyperglycemia or postprandial glucose elevations despite dietary intervention.

➤ Antepartum fetal assessment for both pregestational and GDM pregnancies is based on the degree of risk believed to be present in each case. Glycemic control, prior obstetric history, and the presence of vascular disease or hypertension are important considerations.

➤ Delivery should be delayed until fetal maturation has occurred, provided that diabetes is well controlled and fetal surveillance remains normal. The mode of delivery for the suspected large fetus remains controversial. In cases of suspected macrosomia, a low threshold for cesarean section has been recommended to prevent traumatic delivery.

➤ Women with type 1 and type 2 diabetes mellitus should seek prepregnancy consultation. Efforts to improve glycemic control prior to conception have been associated with a significant reduction in the rate of congenital malformations in the offspring of such women.

REFERENCES

1. Weiss PAM, Hoffman H: Intensified conventional insulin therapy for the pregnant diabetic patient. Obstet Gynecol 64: 629, 1984.

2. Catalano PM, Tyzbir ED, Roman NM, et al: Longitudinal changes in insulin release and insulin resistance in non-obese pregnant women. Am J Obstet Gynecol 165:1667, 1991.

3. Bellman O, Hartman E: Influence of pregnancy on the kinetics of insulin. Am J Obstet Gynecol 122:829, 1975.

4. Lind T, Bell S, Gilmore E: Insulin disappearance rate in pregnant and non-pregnant women and in non-pregnant women given GHRH. Eur J Clin Invest 7:47, 1977.

5. Burt RL, Davidson IWF: Insulin half-life and utilization in normal pregnancy. Obstet Gynecol 43:161, 1974.

6. Goodner CJ, Freinkel N: Carbohydrate metabolism in pregnancy: the degradation of insulin by extracts of maternal and fetal structures in the pregnant rat. Endocrinology 65:957, 1959.

7. Catalano PM, Drago NM, Amini SB: Longitudinal changes in pancreatic b cell function and metabolic clearance rate of insulin in pregnant women with normal and abnormal glucose tolerance. Diabetes Care 21:403, 1998.

8. Kalhan SC, D'Angelo LJ, Savin SM, et al: Glucose production in pregnant women at term gestation: sources of glucose for human fetus. J Clin Invest 63:388, 1979.

9. Cowett RA, Susa JB, Kahn CB, et al: Glucose kinetics in nondiabetic and diabetic women during the third trimester of pregnancy. Am J Obstet Gynecol 146:773, 1983.

10. Catalano PM, Tyzbir ED, Wolfe RR, et al: Longitudinal changes in basal hepatic glucose production and suppression during insulin infusion in normal pregnant women. Am J Obstet Gynecol 167:913, 1992.

11. Sivan E, Chen X, Hombo CJ, et al: Longitudinal study of carbohydrate metabolism in healthy obese women. Diabetes Care 20:1470, 1997.

12. Pacini G, Bergman RN: MINMOD: a computer program to calculate insulin sensitivity and pancreatic responsitivity from the frequently sampled intravenous glucose tolerance test. Comput Methods Programs Biomed 23:113, 1986.

13. DeFronzo RA, Tobin JD, Andres R: Glucose clamp technique: a method for quantifying insulin secretion and resistance. Am J Physiol 237:E214, 1979.

14. Catalano PM, Tyzbir ED, Wolfe RR, et al: Carbohydrate metabolism during pregnancy in control subjects and women with gestational diabetes. Am J Physiol 264:E60, 1993.

15. Catalano PM, Huston L, Amini SB, Kalhan SC: Longitudinal changes in glucose metabolism during pregnancy in obese women with normal glucose tolerance and gestational diabetes. Am J Obstet Gynecol 180:903, 1999.

16. Spellacy WN, Goetz FC, Greenberg BZ, et al: Plasma insulin normal "early" pregnancy. Obstet Gynecol 25:862, 1965.

17. Burt RL: Peripheral utilization of glucose in pregnancy. III. Insulin intolerance. Obstet Gynecol 2:558, 1956.

18. Fisher PM, Sutherland HW, Bewsher PD: The insulin response to glucose infusion in normal human pregnancy. Diabetologia 19:15, 1980.

19. Buchanan TZ, Metzger BE, Freinkel N, et al: Insulin sensitivity and b-cell responsiveness to glucose during late pregnancy in lean and moderately obese women with normal glucose tolerance or mild gestational diabetes. Am J Obstet Gynecol 162:1008, 1990.

20. Ryan EA, O'Sullivan MJ, Skyler JS: Insulin action during pregnancy. Studies with the euglycemic clamp technique. Diabetes 34:380, 1985.

21. Hay WW, Sparks JW, Wilkening RB, et al: Partition of maternal glucose production between conceptus and maternal tissue in sheep. Am J Physiol 234:E347, 1983.

22. Marconi AM, Paolini C, Buscaglia M, et al: The impact of gestational age and fetal growth on the maternal-fetal glucose concentration difference. Obstet Gynecol 87:937, 1996.

23. Barros LF, Yudilevich DL, Jarvis SM, et al: Quantitation and immunolocalization of glucose transporters in the human placenta. Placenta 16:623, 1995.

24. Jansson T, Wennergren M, Illsley NP: Glucose transporter expression and distribution in the human placenta throughout gestation and in intrauterine growth retardation. J Clin Endocrinol Metab 77:1554, 1993.

25. Hauguel-de Mouzon S, Challier J, Kacemi A, et al: The GLUT3 glucose transporter isoform is differentially expressed with the human placental cell types. J Clin Endocrinol Metab 82:2689, 1997.

26. Xing A, Cauzac M, Challier J, et al: Unexpected expression of GLUT 4 glucose transporter in villous stromal cells of human placenta. J Clin Endocrinol Metab 83:4097, 1999.

27. White P: Pregnancy complicating diabetes. Am J Med 7:609, 1949.

28. Diamond MP, Reece EA, Caprios L, et al: Impairment of counter regulatory hormone responses to hypoglycemia in pregnant women with insulin-dependent diabetes mellitus. Am J Obstet Gynecol 166:70, 1992.

29. Rosenn BM, Miodovnik M, Khoury JC, et al: Counter regulatory hormonal responses to hypoglycemic during pregnancy. Obstet Gynecol 87:568, 1996.

30. McManus RM, Ryan EA: Insulin requirements in insulin-dependent and insulin-requiring GDM women during the final month of pregnancy. Diabetes Care 15:1323, 1992.

31. Schmitz O, Klebe J, Moller J, et al: In vivo insulin action in type 1 (insulin-dependent) diabetic pregnant women as assessed by the insulin clamp technique. J Clin Endocrinol Metab 61:877, 1985.

32. Jansson T, Powell TL: Glucose transport and GLUT1 expression are upregulated in placentas from pregnancies complicated by severe diabetes [abstract]. Placenta 18:A30, 1997.

33. Sims EAH, Calles-Escadon J: Classification of diabetes: a fresh look for the 1990s? Diabetes Care 13:1123, 1990.

34. Steel JM, Irvine WJ, Clark BJ: The significance of pancreatic islet cell antibody and abnormal glucose tolerance during pregnancy. J Clin Lab Immunol 4:83, 1980.

35. Ginsberg-Fellner F, Mark EM, Nechemias C, et al: Autoantibodies to islet cells: comparison of methods [letter]. Lancet 2:1218, 1982.

36. Catalano PM, Tyzbir ED, Sims EAH: Incidence and significance of islet cell antibodies in women with previous gestational diabetes mellitus. Diabetes Care 13:478, 1990.

37. Ward WK, Johnson CLW, Beard JC, et al: Abnormalities of islet b-cell function, insulin action and fat distribution in women with histories of gestational diabetes: relationship to obesity. J Clin Endocrinol Metab 61:1039, 1985.

38. Catalano PM, Bernstein IM, Wolfe RR, et al: Subclinical abnormalities of glucose metabolism in subjects with previous gestational diabetes. Am J Obstet Gynecol 166:1255, 1986.

39. Ryan EA, Imes S, Liu D, et al: Defects in insulin secretion and action in women with a history of gestational diabetes. Diabetes 44:506, 1995.

40. Yen SCC, Tsai CC, Vela P: Gestational diabetogenesis: quantitative analysis of glucose-insulin interrelationship between normal pregnancy and pregnancy with gestational diabetes. Am J Obstet Gynecol 111:792, 1971.

41. Fisher PM, Sutherland HW, Bewsher PD: The insulin response to glucose infusion in gestational diabetes. Diabetologia 19:14, 1980.

42. Xiang AH, Peters RH, Trigo E, et al: Multiple metabolic defects during late pregnancy in women at high risk for type 2 diabetes. Diabetes 48:848, 1999.

43. Catalano PM, Roman-Drago N, Amini SB, Sims EAH: Longitudinal changes in body composition and energy balance in lean women with normal and abnormal glucose tolerance during pregnancy. Am J Obstet Gynecol 179:156, 1998.

44. Garvey WT, Maianu L, Hancock JA, et al: Gene expression of GLUT4 in skeletal muscle from insulin-resistance patients with obesity, IGT, GDM, and NIDDM. Diabetes 41:465, 1992.

45. Friedman JE, Ishizuka T, Shao J, et al: Impaired glucose transport and insulin receptor tyrosine phosphorylation in skeletal muscle from obese women with gestational diabetes. Diabetes 48:1807, 1999.

46. Hytten FE, Leitch I: The gross composition of the components of weight gain. *In* The Physiology of Human Pregnancy. 2nd ed. London, Blackwell Scientific, 1971, p 371.

47. Metzger BD, Unger RH, Freinkel N: Carbohydrate metabolism in pregnancy. XIV. Relationships between circulation glucagon, insulin, glucose and amino acids in response to a "mixed meal" in late pregnancy. Metabolism 26:151, 1977.

48. Freinkel N, Metzger BE, Nitzan M, et al: "Accelerated starvation" and mechanisms for the conservation of maternal nitrogen during pregnancy. Israel J Med Sci 8:426, 1972.

49. Kalkhoff RK, Kandaraki E, Morrow PG, et al: Relationship between neonatal birth weight and maternal plasma amino acids profiles in lean and obese nondiabetic women with type 1 diabetic pregnant women. Metabolism 37:234, 1988.

50. McClain PE, Metcoff J, Crosby WM, Costiloe JP: Relationship of maternal amino acid profiles at 25 weeks of gestation to fetal growth. Am J Clin Nutr 31:401, 1978.

51. Kalhan SC, Tserng K, Gilfillan C, Dierker LJ: Metabolism of urea and glucose in normal and diabetic pregnancy. Metabolism 31:824, 1982.

52. Denne SC, Kalhan SC: Leucine metabolism in human newborns. Am J Physiol 253:E608, 1987.

53. Debenoist B, Jackson AA, Hall JSE, Persuad C: Whole body protein turnover in Jamaican women during pregnancy. Hum Nutr Clin Hutr 39:167, 1985.

54. Fitch WL, King JC: Protein turnover and 3-methylhistidien excretion in non-pregnant, pregnant and gestational diabetic women. Hum Nutr Clin Nutr 41C:327, 1987.

55. Ogata ES: The small for gestational age neonate. *In* Consell RM (ed): Principles of Perinatal-Neonatal Metabolism. 2nd ed. New York, Springer-Verlag, 1998, p 1097.

56. Liechty EA, Boyle DW: Protein metabolism in the fetal placental unit. *In* Consell RM (ed): Principles of Perinatal-Neonatal Metabolism. 2nd ed. New York, Springer-Verlag, 1998, p 369.

57. Knopp RH, Humphery J, Irvin S: Biphasic metabolic control of hypertriglyceridemia in pregnancy. Clin Res 25:161A, 1977.

58. Sivan E, Homoko CJ, Chen X, et al: Effect of insulin in fat metabolism during and after normal pregnancy. Diabetes 44:384, 1999.

59. Knopp RH, Magee MS, Walden CE, et al: Prediction of infant birth weight by GDM screening tests. Diabetes Care 15:1605, 1992.

60. Knopp RH, Bergelin RO, Wahl PW, Walden CE: Relationships of infant birth size to maternal lipoproteins, apoproteins, fuels, hormones, clinical chemistries, and body weight at 36 weeks gestation. Diabetes 34(Suppl 2):71, 1985.

61. Ogburn PL, Goldstein M, Walker J, Stonestreet BS: Prolonged hyperinsulinemia reduces plasma fatty acid levels in the major lipid groups in fetal sheep. Am J Obstet Gynecol 161:728, 1989.

62. Kliegman R, Gross T, Morton S, Dunnington R: Intrauterine growth and post natal fasting metabolism in infants of obese mothers. J Pediatr 104:601, 1984.

63. Knopp RH, Chapman M, Bergeline RO, et al: Relationship of lipoprotein lipids to mild fasting hyperglycemia and diabetes in pregnancy. Diabetes Care 3:416, 1980.

64. Montelongo A, Lasuncion MA, Pallardo LF, Herrera E: Longitudinal study of plasma lipoproteins and hormones during pregnancy in normal and diabetic women. Diabetes 41:1651, 1992.

65. Koukkou E, Watts GF, Lowy C: Serum lipid, lipoprotein and apolipoprotein changes in gestational diabetes mellitus: a cross-sectional and prospective study. J Clin Pathol 49:634, 1996.

66. Catalano PM, Hollenbeck C: Energy requirements in pregnancy: a review. Obstet Gynecol Surv 47:368, 1992.

67. Goldberg GR, Prentice AM, Coward WA, et al: Longitudinal assessment of energy expenditure in pregnancy by the doubly labeled water method. Am J Clin Nutr 57:494, 1993.

68. Forsum E, Sadurskis A, Wager J: Resting metabolic rate and body composition of healthy Swedish women during pregnancy. Am J Clin Nutr 47:942, 1988.

69. Lawrence M, Lawrence F, Coward WA, et al: Energy requirements of pregnancy in the Gambia. Lancet 2:1072, 1987.

70. Forsum E, Kabir N, Sadurskis A, Westerterp K: Total energy expenditure of healthy Swedish women during pregnancy and lactation. Am J Clin Nutr 56:334, 1992.

71. King JC, Butte NF, Bronstein MN, et al: Energy metabolism during pregnancy: influence of maternal energy status. Am J Clin Nutr 59:4395, 1994.

72. Prentice AM, Poppitt SD, Goldberg CR, et al: Energy balance in pregnancy and lactation. *In* Allen L, King J, Lonnerdal B (eds): Nutrient Regulation During Pregnancy, Lactation and Infant Growth. New York, Plenum Press, 1994, p 11.

73. Prentice AM, Goldberg GR, Davies HL, et al: Energy-sparing adaptation in human pregnancy assessed by wholebody calorimetry. Br J Nutr 62:5, 1989.

74. DeGroot LCPGM, Boekhot HA, Spaaij CJK, et al: Energy balance of healthy Dutch women before and during pregnancy: limited scope for metabolic adaptations. Am J Clin Nutr 59:827, 1994.

75. Swinburn BA, Myomba BC, Saad MF, et al: Insulin resistance associated with lower rates of weight gain in Pima Indians. J Clin Invest 88:168, 1991.

76. Catalano PM, Roma NM, Tyzbir ED, et al: Weight gain in women with gestational diabetes. Obstet Gynecol 81:523, 1993.

77. Landon MB, Gabbe SG: Fetal surveillance in the pregnancy complicated by diabetes mellitus. *In* Landon MB (ed): Clinics in Perinatology. Philadelphia, WB Saunders Company, 1993, pp 20, 549.

78. Centers for Disease Control and Prevention: Perinatal mortality and congenital malformations in infants born to women with insulin dependent diabetes. MMWR Morb Mortal Wkly Rep 39:363, 1990.

79. Salversen DR, Brudenell MJ, Nicholaides KH: Fetal polycythemia and thrombocytopenia in pregnancies complicated by maternal diabetes. Am J Obstet Gynecol 166:1987, 1992.

80. Madsen H: Fetal oxygenation in diabetic pregnancy. Dan Med Bull 33:64, 1986.

81. Nylund L, Lunell NO, Lewander R, et al: Uteroplacental blood flow in diabetic pregnancy: measurements with indium 113m and a computer linked gamma camera. Am J Obstet Gynecol 144:298, 1982.

82. Kitzmiller JL, Phillippe M: Hyperglycemia hypoxia, and fetal acidosis in Rhesus monkeys [abstract]. Presented at the 28th Annual Meeting of the Society for Gynecologic Investigation, St. Louis, MO, March, 1981.

83. Phillips AF, Dubin JW, Matty PJ, et al: Arterial hypoxemia and hyperinsulinemia in the chronically hyperglycemia fetal lamb. Pediatr Res 16:653, 1982.

84. Shelley HJ, Bassett JM, Milner RD: Control of carbohydrate metabolism in the fetus and newborn. Br Med Bull 31:37, 1975.

85. Carson BS, Philipps AF, Simmons MA, et al: Effects of a

sustained insulin infusion upon glucose uptake and oxygenation of the ovine fetus. Pediatr Res 14:147, 1980.

86. Albert TJ, Landon MB, Wheller JJ, et al: Prenatal detection of fetal anomalies in pregnancies complicated by insulin-dependent diabetes mellitus. Am J Obstet Gynecol 174:1424, 1996.

87. Simpson JL, Elias S, Martin AO, et al: Diabetes in pregnancy, Northwestern University Series (1977–1981). I. Prospective study of anomalies in offspring of mothers with diabetes mellitus. Am J Obstet Gynecol 146:263, 1983.

88. Mills JL, Knopp RH, Simpson JP, et al: Lack of relations of increased malformation rates in infants of diabetic mothers to glycemic control during organogenesis. N Engl J Med 318:671, 1988.

89. Eriksson U: The pathogenesis of congenital malformations in diabetic pregnancy. Diabetes Metab Rev 11:63, 1995.

90. Reece EA, Hobbins JC: Diabetic embryopathy: pathogenesis, prenatal diagnosis and prevention. Obstet Gynecol Surv 41:325, 1986.

91. Koppe J, Smoremberg-School M: Diabetes, congenital malformations and HLA types. *In* Listen E, Band H, Frus-Hansen B (eds): Intensive Care in the Newborn. Vol 4. Newark, Masson Publishing, 1983, p 15.

92. Simpson JL, Mills J, Ober C, et al: DR3+ and DR4+ diabetes women have increased risk for anomalies [abstract 3901]. Presented at the 37th Annual Meeting of the Society for Gynecologic Investigation. St. Louis, MO, 1990.

93. Freinkel N, Lewis NJ, Akazawa S, et al: The honeybee syndrome: implication of the teratogenicity of mannose in rat-embryo culture. N Engl J Med 310:223, 1984.

94. Goldman AS, Baker L, Piddington R, et al: Hyperglycemia-induced teratogenesis is mediated by a functional deficiency of arachidonic acid. Proc Natl Acad Sci U S A 82:8227, 1985.

95. Pinter E, Reece EA: Arachidonic acid prevents hyperglycemia-associated yolk sac damage and embryopathy. Am J Obstet Gynecol 166:691, 1986.

96. Pinter E, Reece EA, Leranth CZ, et al: Yolk sac failure in embryopathy due to hyperglycemia ultrastructural analysis of yolk sac differentiation associated with embryopathy in rat conceptuses under hyperglycemic conditions. Teratology 33:73, 1986.

97. Eriksson NJ: Protection by free oxygen radical scavenging enzymes against glucose-induced embryonic malformations in vitro. Diabetologia 34:325, 1991.

98. Spellacy WN, Miller S, Winegar A, et al: Macrosomia-maternal characteristics and infant complications. Obstet Gynecol 66:185, 1985.

99. Reiher H, Fuhrmann K, Noack S, et al: Age-dependent insulin secretion of the endocrine pancreas in vitro from fetuses of diabetic and nondiabetic patients. Diabetes Care 6:446, 1983.

100. Fallucca F, Gargiulo P, Troili F, et al: Amniotic fluid insulin, C-peptide concentrations and fetal morbidity in infants of diabetic mothers. Am J Obstet Gynecol 153:534, 1985.

101. Krew MA, Kehl RJ, Thomas A, Catalano PM: Relationship of amniotic fluid C-peptide levels to neonatal body composition. Obstet Gynecol 84:96, 1994.

102. Brans YW, Shannon DL, Hunter MA, et al: Maternal diabetes and neonatal macrosomia, III. Neonatal anthropometric measurements. Early Hum Dev 8:297, 1983.

103. Modanlou HD, Komatsu G, Dorchester W, et al: Large-for-gestational age neonates: anthropometric reasons for shoulder dystocia. Obstet Gynecol 60:417, 1982.

104. Gabbe SG, Mestman JH, Freeman RK, et al: Management and outcome of pregnancy in diabetes mellitus, class B-R. Am J Obstet Gyencol 129:723, 1977.

105. Kitzmiller JL, Gloherty JP: Diabetic pregnancy and perinatal morbidity. Am J Obstet Gynecol 131:560, 1978.

106. Roversi GD, Gargiulo M: A new approach to the treatment

107. Jovanovic L, Druzin M, Peterson CM: Effect of euglycemia on the outcome of pregnancy in insulin-dependent diabetic women as compared with normal control subjects. Am J Med 72:921, 1981.

108. Landon MB, Gabbe SG, Piana R, et al: Neonatal morbidity in pregnancy complicated by diabetes mellitus: predictive value of maternal glycemic profiles. Am J Obstet Gynecol 156:1089, 1987.

109. Jovanovic-Peterson L, Peterson CM, Reed CF, et al: Maternal postprandial glucose levels and infant birthweight: the Diabetes in Early Pregnancy Study. Am J Obstet Gynecol 164:103, 1991.

110. Catalano PM, Tyzbir ED, Allen SR, et al: Evaluation of fetal growth by estimation of body composition. Obstet Gynecol 79:46, 1992.

111. Catalano PM, Drago NM, Amini SB: Factors affecting fetal growth and body composition. Am J Obstet Gynecol 172:1459, 1995.

112. Catalano PM, Drago NM, Amini SB: Maternal carbohydrate metabolism and its relationship to fetal growth and body composition. Am J Obstet Gynecol 172:1464, 1995.

113. Caruso A, Paradisi G, Ferrazzani S, et al: Effect of maternal carbohydrate metabolism on fetal growth. Obstet Gynecol 92:8, 1998.

114. Silverman BL, Rizzo TA, Cho NH, Metzger BE: Long-term effects of the intrauterine environment. Diabetes 21(Suppl 2):142, 1998.

115. Pettitt DJ, Nelson RG, Saad MF, et al: Diabetes and obesity in the offspring of Pima Indian women with diabetes during pregnancy. Diabetes Care 16:310, 1993.

116. Soler NG, Soler SM, Malins JM: Neonatal morbidity among infants of diabetic mothers. Diabetes Care 1:340, 1978.

117. Kuhl C, Anderson GE, Brandt NJ, et al: Metabolic events in infants of diabetic mothers during first 24 hours after birth. Acta Paediatr Scand 71:19, 1982.

118. Bourbon JR, Farrell PM: Fetal lung development in the diabetic pregnancy. Pediatr Res 19:253, 1985.

119. Smith BT, Giroud CJP, Robert M: Insulin antagonism of cortisol action on lecithin synthesis by cultures of fetal lung cells. J Pediatr 87:953, 1975.

120. Smith BT: Pulmonary surfactant during fetal development and neonatal adaptation: Hormonal control. *In* Robertson B, Van Golde LMB, Batenburg JJ (eds): Pulmonary Surfactant. Amsterdam, Elsevier, 1985, p 357.

121. Post M, Barsoumian A, Smith BT: The cellular mechanisms of glucocorticoid acceleration of fetal lung maturation. J Biol Chem 261:2179, 1986.

122. Carlson KS, Smith BT, Post M: Insulin acts on the fibroblast to inhibit glucocorticoid stimulation of lung maturation. J Appl Physiol 57:1577, 1984.

123. Dudley DKL, Black DM: Reliability of lecithin/sphingomyelin ratios in diabetic pregnancy. Obstet Gynecol 66:521, 1985.

124. Kjos SL, Walther F: Prevalence and etiology of respiratory distress in infants of diabetic mothers: predictive value of lung maturation tests. Am J Obstet Gynecol 163:898, 1990.

125. Mimouni F, Miodovnik M, Whittset J, et al: Respiratory distress syndrome in infants of diabetic mothers in the 1980s: no direct adverse effect of maternal diabetes with modern management. Obstet Gynecol 69:191, 1987.

126. Tsang RC, Chen I-W, Friedman MA, et al: Parathyroid function in infants of diabetic mothers. J Pediatr 86:399, 1975.

127. Mimouni F, Miodovnik M, Tsang RC, et al: Decreased amniotic fluid magnesium concentration in diabetic pregnancy. Obstet Gynecol 69:12, 1987.

128. Widness JA, Cowett RM, Coustan DR, et al: Neonatal mor-

bidities in infants of mothers with glucose intolerance in pregnancy. Diabetes 34(Suppl 2):61, 1985.

129. Ylinen K, Raivio K, Teramo K: Haemoglobin AIc predicts the perinatal outcome in insulin-dependent diabetic pregnancies. Br J Obstet Gynaecol 88:961, 1981.

130. Stevenson DK, Bartoletti AL, Ostrander CR, et al: Pulmonary excretion of carbon monoxide in the human infants as an index of bilirubin production. II. Infants of diabetic mothers. J Pediatr 94:956, 1979.

131. Shannon K, Davis JC, Kitzmiller JL, et al: Erythropoiesis in infants of diabetic mothers. Pediatr Res 30:161, 1986.

132. White P: Pregnancy complicating diabetes. Am J Med 7:609, 1949.

133. Summary and Recommendations of the Second International Workshop-Conference on Gestational Diabetes. Diabetes 34 (Suppl 2):123, 1985.

134. Summary and Recommendations of the Third International Workshop Conference on Gestational Diabetes. Diabetes 40 (Suppl 2):197, 1991.

135. Gabbe SG, Mestman JH, Freeman RK, et al: Management and outcome of class A diabetes mellitus. Am J Obstet Gynecol 127:465, 1977.

136. Selby JV, Fitzsimmons SC, Newman JM, et al: The natural history and epidemiology of diabetic nephropathy. JAMA 263:1954, 1990.

137. Gordon M, Landon MB, Samuels P, et al: Perinatal outcome and long-term follow-up associated with modern management of diabetic nephropathy (class F). Obstet Gynecol 87:401, 1996.

138. Kitzmiller JL, Brown ER, Phillippe M, et al: Diabetic nephropathy and perinatal outcome. Am J Obstet Gynecol 141: 741, 1981.

139. Reece EA, Coustan DR, Hayslett JP, et al: Diabetic nephropathy: pregnancy performance and fetomaternal outcome. Am J Obstet Gynecol 159:56, 1988.

140. Kitzmiller JP: Diabetic nephropathy. In Reece EA, Coustan DR (eds): Diabetes Mellitus in Pregnancy. Principles and Practice. New York, Churchill Livingstone, 1988, p 489.

141. Rosenn BM, Miodovnik M, Khoury JC, et al: Outcome of pregnancy in women with diabetic nephropathy. Am J Obstet Gynecol 176:S631, 1997.

142. Ogburn PL Jr, Kitzmiller JL, Hare JW, et al: Pregnancy following renal transplantation in class T diabetes mellitus. JAMA 255:911, 1986.

143. Carstensen LL, Frost-Lansen K, Fulgeberg S, Nerup J: Does pregnancy influence the prognosis of uncomplicated insulin-dependent diabetes? Diabetes Care 5:1, 1982.

144. Klein BEK, Moss SE, Klein R: Effect of pregnancy on the progression of diabetic retinopathy. Diabetes Care 13:34, 1990.

145. Rosenn B, Miodovnik KM, Kranias G, et al: Progression of diabetic retinopathy in pregnancy: association with hypertension in pregnancy. Am J Obstet Gynecol 166:1214, 1992.

146. Horvat M, Maclear H, Goldberg L, Crock CW: Diabetic retinopathy in pregnancy: a 12 year prospective study. Br J Ophthalmol 64:398, 1980.

147. Kitzmiller JL, Gavin LA, Gin GD, et al: Managing diabetes and pregnancy. Curn Probl Obstet Gynecol Fertil 11:113, 1988.

148. Moloney JBM, Drury MI: The effect of pregnancy on the natural course of diabetic retinopathy. Am J Ophthalmol 93: 745, 1982.

149. Phelps RL, Sakol P, Metzger BE, et al: Changes in diabetic retinopathy during pregnancy, correlations with regulation of hyperglycemia. Arch Ophthalmol 104:1806, 1986.

150. Chew EY, Mills JL, Metzger BE, et al: Metabolic control and progression of retinopathy. The Diabetes in Early Pregnancy Study. Diabetes Care 18:631, 1995.

151. Sinclair SH, Nesler C, Foxman B, et al: Macular edema and pregnancy in insulin dependent diabetes. Am J Ophthalmol 97:154, 1984.

152. Gordon MC, Landon MB, Boyle J, et al: Myocardial infarction during pregnancy in a patient with class R/F diabetes mellitus: a case report and review of literature on class H IDDM. Obstet Gynecol Surv 51:437, 1996.

153. Hare JW: Maternal complications. In Hare JW (ed): Diabetes Complicating Pregnancy. The Joslin Clinic Method. New York, Alan R Liss, 1989, p 96.

154. Stephenson MJ: Screening for gestational diabetes mellitus: a critical review. J Fam Pract 37:277, 1993.

155. Solomon CG, Willett WC, Carey VJ, et al: A prospective study of pregravid determinants of gestational diabetes mellitus. JAMA 278:1078, 1997.

156. O'Sullivan JB: Body weight and subsequent diabetes mellitus. JAMA 248:949, 1982.

157. Dornhorst A, Rossi M: Risk and prevention of type 2 diabetes in women with gestational diabetes. Diabetes Care 21: B43, 1998.

158. Coustan DR, Nelson C, Carpenter NW, et al: Maternal age and screening for gestational diabetes: a population based study. Obstet Gynecol 73:557, 1989.

159. Summary and Recommendations of the Third International Workshop-Conference on Gestational Diabetes. Diabetes 40: 197, 1991.

160. ACOG Technical Bulletin Number 200. Diabetes and Pregnancy, December, 1994.

161. Periodic Health Examination, 1992 update: 1. Screening for gestational diabetes mellitus. Can Med Assoc J 147:435, 1992.

162. Naylor CD: Diagnosing gestational diabetes mellitus: is the gold standard valid? Diabetes Care 12:565, 1989.

163. Sermer M, Naylor CD, Gore DJ, et al: Impact of increasing carbohydrate intolerance on maternal-fetal outcomes in 3637 women without gestational diabetes. Am J Obstet Gynecol 173:146, 1995.

164. Sacks DA, Greenspoon JS, Abu-Fadil S, et al: Toward universal criteria for gestational diabetes: the 75-gram glucose tolerance test in pregnancy. Am J Obstet Gynecol 172:607, 1995.

165. Gabbe SG: The gestational diabetes mellitus conferences. Diabetes Care 21:B1, 1998.

166. Coustan DR, Widness JA, Carpenter NW, et al: Should the fifty-gram, one-hour plasma glucose screening test be administered in the fasting or fed state? Am J Obstet Gynecol 154: 1031, 1986.

167. Sermer M, Naylor CD, Gare DJ, et al: Impact of time since last meal on the gestational glucose challenge test. Am J Obstet Gynecol 171:607, 1994.

168. Landon MB: Gestational diabetes mellitus: screening and diagnosis. Lab Med 21:527, 1990.

169. Carpenter MW, Coustan DR: Criteria for screening tests of gestational diabetes. Am J Obstet Gynecol 144:768, 1982.

170. Sacks DA, Abu-Fadil S, Greenspoon J, et al: Do the current standards for glucose tolerance testing in pregnancy represent a valid conversion of O'Sullivan's original criteria? Am J Obstet Gynecol 161:638, 1989.

171. Magee MS, Walden CE, Benedetti TJ, et al: Influence of diagnostic criteria on the incidence of gestational diabetes and perinatal morbidity. JAMA 269:609, 1993.

172. Landon MB, Gabbe SG: Insulin treatment of the pregnant patient with diabetes mellitus. In Reece EA, Coustan DR (eds): Diabetes Mellitus and Pregnancy. New York, Churchill Livingstone, 1995, p 173.

173. Kitzmiller JL, Main EK, Ward B, et al: Insulin lispro and the development of proliferative retinopathy during pregnancy. Diabetes Care 22:873, 1999.

174. Buchbinder A, Miodovnik M, McElvy S, et al: Is insulin lispro a culprit in the progression of diabetic retinopathy during pregnancy? Am J Obstet Gynecol 182:1162, 2000.

175. Coustan DR, Reece EA, Sherwin RS, et al: A randomized clinical trial of the insulin pump versus intensive conventional therapy in diabetic pregnancy. JAMA 255:631, 1986.

176. Gabbe SG, Holing E, Temple P, et al: Benefits, risks, costs, and patient satisfaction associated with insulin pump therapy for the pregnancy complicated by type 1 diabetes mellitus. Am J Obstet Gynecol 182:1283, 2000.

177. The American Diabetes Association: Principles of Nutrition and Dietary Recommendations for Individuals with Diabetes Mellitus. Diabetes 28:1027, 1979.

178. Kilvert JA, Nicholson HO, Wright AD: Ketoacidosis in diabetic pregnancy. Diabet Med 10:278, 1993.

179. Rayburn WF, McKean HE: Maternal perception of fetal movement and perinatal outcome. Obstet Gynecol 56:161, 1980.

180. Holden KP, Jovanovic L, Druzin M, et al: Increased fetal activity with low maternal blood glucose levels in pregnancies complicated by diabetes. Am J Perinatol 1:161, 1984.

181. Sadovsky E, Brjejinski A, Mor-Yosef S, et al: Fetal activity in diabetic pregnancy. J Fetal Med 3:1, 1983.

182. Landon MB, Gabbe SG, Sachs L: Management of diabetes mellitus and pregnancy: a survey of obstetricians and maternal-fetal specialists. Obstet Gynecol 75:635, 1990.

183. Barret JM, Salyer SL, Boehm FH: The non-stress test: an evaluation of 1000 patients. Am J Obstet Gynecol 141:153, 1981.

184. Miller JM, Horger EO: Antepartum heart rate testing in diabetic pregnancy. J Reprod Med 30:515, 1985.

185. Landon MB, Gabbe SG, Bruner JP, Ludmir J: Doppler umbilical artery velocimetry in pregnancy complicated by insulin dependent diabetes mellitus. Obstet Gynecol 73:961, 1989.

186. Johnstone FD, Steel JM, Haddad NG, et al: Doppler umbilical artery flow velocity waveforms in diabetic pregnancy. Br J Obstet Gynecol 99:135, 1992.

187. Landon MB, Gabbe SG: Fetal surveillance in the pregnancy complicated by diabetes mellitus. Clin Perinatol 20:549, 1993.

188. Landon MB, Langer O, Gabbe SG, et al: Fetal surveillance in pregnancies complicated by insulin dependent diabetes mellitus. Am J Obstet Gynecol 167:617, 1992.

189. Milunsky A, Alpert E, Kitzmiller JL, et al: Prenatal diagnosis of neural tube defects VIII. The importance of serum alpha-fetoprotein screening in diabetic pregnant women. Am J Obstet Gynecol 142:1030, 1982.

190. Greene MF, Benacerraf B: Prenatal diagnosis in diabetic gravidas: utility of ultrasound and MSAFP screening. Obstet Gynecol 77:420, 1991.

191. Nesbitt TS, Gilbert WM, Herrchen B: Shoulder dystocia and associated risk factors with macrosomic infants born in California. Am J Obstet Gynecol 179:476, 1998.

192. Tamura RK, Shabbagha RE, Depp R, et al: Diabetic macrosomia: accuracy of third trimester ultrasound. Obstet Gynecol 67:828, 1986.

193. Landon MB, Mintz MG, Gabbe SG: Sonographic evaluation of fetal abdominal growth: predictor of the large-for-gestational age infant in pregnancies. Am J Obstet Gynecol 160:115, 1989.

194. Cousins L: Pregnancy complications among diabetic women: review 1965–1985. Obstet Gynecol Surv 42:140, 1987.

195. Kjos S, Henry O, Montoro M, et al: Insulin-requiring diabetes in pregnancy: a randomized trial of active induction of labor and expectant management. Am J Obstet Gynecol 169:611, 1993.

196. Levine AB, Lockwood CJ, Brown B, et al: Sonographic diagnosis of the large for gestational age fetus at term: does it make a difference? Obstet Gynecol 79:55, 1992.

197. Rouse DJ, Owen J, Goldenberg RL, et al: The effectiveness and costs of elective cesarean delivery for fetal macrosomia diagnosed by ultrasound. JAMA 276:1480, 1996.

198. Acker DB, Sachs BP, Friedman EA: Risk factors for shoulder dystocia. Obstet Gynecol 6:762, 1985.

199. Benedetti TJ, Gabbe SG: Shoulder dystocia: a complication of fetal macrosomia and prolonged second stage of labor with midpelvic delivery. Obstet Gynecol 52:526, 1978.

200. Jovanovic L, Peterson CM: Management of the pregnant, insulin-dependent diabetic woman. Diabetes Care 3:63, 1980.

201. Hollingsworth DR, Ney DM: Dietary management of diabetes during pregnancy. In Reece EA, Coustan DR (eds): Diabetes Mellitus in Pregnancy: Principles and Practice. New York, Churchill Livingstone, 1988, p 285.

202. Mumford MI, Jovanovic-Peterson L, Peterson CM: Alternative therapies for the management of gestational diabetes. Clin Perinatol 20:619, 1993.

203. Jovanovic-Peterson L, Peterson CM: Nutritional management of the obese gestational diabetic pregnant women. J Am Coll Nutr 11:246, 1992.

204. Algert S, Shragg P, Hollingsworth DR: Moderate caloric restriction in obese women with gestational diabetes. Obstet Gynecol 65:487, 1985.

205. Magee MS, Knopp RH, Benedetti TJ: Metabolic effects of 1200 kcal diet in obese pregnant women with gestational diabetes. Diabetes 39:324, 1990.

206. Rizzo T, Metzger BE, Burns WJ, et al: Correlations between antepartum maternal metabolism and intelligence of offspring. N Engl J Med 325:911, 1991.

207. Knopp RH, Magee MS, Raisys V, et al: Hypocaloric diets and ketogenesis in the management of obese gestational diabetic women. J Am Coll Nutr 10:649, 1991.

208. Peterson CM, Jovanovic-Peterson L: Percentage of carbohydrate and glycemia response to breakfast, lunch, and dinner in women with gestational diabetes. Diabetes 40(Suppl 2):172, 1991.

209. Jovanovic L: American Diabetes Association's Fourth International Workshop Conference on Gestational Diabetes Mellitus: Summary and Discussion. Therapeutic Interventions. Diabetes Care 2(Suppl 2):B131, 1998.

210. Goldberg J, Franklin B, Lasser L, et al: Gestational diabetes: impact of home glucose monitoring on neonatal birth weight. Am J Obstet Gynecol 154:546, 1986.

211. Langer O, Rodriguez DA, Xenakis EMJ, et al: Intensified versus conventional management of gestational diabetes. Am J Obstet Gynecol 170:1036, 1994.

212. Metzger BE, Coustan DR: Summary and Recommendations of the Fourth International Workshop Conference on Gestational Diabetes Mellitus. Diabetes Care 21:B161, 1998.

213. Langer O, Brustman L, Anyaegbunam A, et al: Glycemic control in gestational diabetes mellitus—how tight is tight enough; small for gestational age versus large for gestational age? Am J Obstet Gynecol 161:645, 1989.

214. Buchanan TA, Kjos S, Schafer U, et al: Utility of fetal measurements in the management of GDM. Diabetes Care 21(Suppl 2):B99, 1998.

215. Bung P, Artal R, Khodiguian N, Kjos S: Exercise in gestational diabetes: an optional therapeutic approach? Diabetes 40(Suppl 2):182, 1991.

216. Langer O, Conway D, Berkus M, et al: A comparison of glyburide and insulin in women with gestational diabetes mellitus. N Engl J Med 343:1134, 2000.

217. Landon MB, Gabbe SG: Antepartum fetal surveillance in gestational diabetes mellitus. Diabetes 34(Suppl 2):50, 1985.

218. Girz BA, Divon MY, Merkatz IR: Sudden fetal death in women with well controlled, intensively monitored gestational diabetes. J Perinatol 12:229, 1992.

219. Lurie S, Matzkel A, Weissman A, et al: Outcome of pregnancy in class A1 and A2 gestational diabetic patients delivered beyond 40 weeks gestation. Am J Perinatol 9:484, 1992.

220. Lurie S, Insler V, Hagay Z: Induction of labor at 38 to 39 weeks of gestation reduces the incidence of shoulder dystocia in gestational diabetic patient class A2. Am J Perinatol 13:293, 1996.

221. Molsted-Pedersen L: Pregnancy and diabetes, a survey. Acta Endocrinol 94(Suppl):13, 1980.

222. Fuhrmann K, Reiher H, Semmler K, et al: Prevention of congenital malformations in infants of insulin-dependent diabetic mothers. Diabetes Care 6:219, 1983.

223. Miller E, Hare JW, Cloherty JP, et al: Elevated maternal HbA1 in early pregnancy and major congenital anomalies in infants of diabetic mothers. N Engl J Med 304:1331, 1981.

224. Kitzmiller JL, Gavin LA, Gin GD, et al: Preconception management of diabetes continued through early pregnancy prevents the excess frequency of major congenital anomalies in infants of diabetic mothers. JAMA 265:731, 1991.

225. Ylinen K, Aula P, Stnman UH, et al: Risk of minor and major fetal malformations in diabetics with high haemoglobin A1c values in early pregnancy. BMJ 289:345, 1984.

226. Greene MF: Prevention and diagnosis of congenital anomalies in diabetic pregnancies. Clin Perinatol 20:533, 1993.

227. Mills J, Simpson JL, Drisoll SG, et al: Incidence of spontaneous abortion among normal and insulin-dependent diabetic women whose pregnancies were identified within 21 days of conception. N Engl J Med 319:1617, 1988.

228. Whillhoite MB, Bennert HW, Palomaki GE, et al: The impact of preconception counseling on pregnancy outcomes. The experience of the Maine Diabetes in Pregnancy Program. Diabetes Care 16:450, 1993.

229. Centers for Disease Control and Prevention: Recommendations for the use of folic acid to reduce the number of cases of spina bifida and other neural tube defects. MMWR Morb Mortal Wkly Rep 417:1, 1992.

230. MRC Vitamin Study Research Group: Prevention of neural tube defects; results of the medical research council vitamin study. Lancet 338:131, 1991.

231. Freinkel N: Diabetic embryopathy and fuel-mediated organ teratogenesis: lessons from animal models. Horm Metabol Res 20:463, 1988.

232. Kjos SL, Ballagh SA, LaCour M, et al: The copper T380A intrauterine device in women with type II diabetes mellitus. Obstet Gynecol 84:1006, 1994.

233. Steel JM, Duncan LJP: Serious complications of oral contraceptives in insulin-dependent diabetes. Contraception 17:291, 1978.

234. Lidegard O: Oral contraceptives, pregnancy, and the risk of cerebral thromboembolism: the influence of diabetes, hypertension, migraine and previous thrombotic disease. Br J Obstet Gynecol 102:153, 1995.

235. Klein BEK, Moss SE, Klein R: Oral contraceptives in women with diabetes. Diabetes Care 13:L895, 1990.

236. DePiaro R, Forte F, Bertoli A, et al: Changes in insulin receptors during oral contraception. J Clin Endocrinol Metab 52:29, 1981.

237. Steel JM, Duncan LJP: The effect of oral contraceptives on insulin requirements in diabetes. Br J Fam Plan 3:77, 1978.

238. Skouby S, Kuhl C, Molsted-Pederson L, et al: Triphasic oral contraception: metabolic effects in normal women and those with previous gestational diabetes. Am J Obstet Gynecol 163:495, 1985.

239. Kjos SL, Shoupe D, Dougan S, et al: Effect of low-dose oral contraceptives on carbohydrate and lipid metabolism in women with recent gestational diabetes: results of a controlled randomized prospective study. Am J Obstet Gynecol 163:1822, 1990.

240. Liew DFM, Ng CSA, Yong YM, et al: Long term effects of Depo-Provera on carbohydrate and lipid metabolism. Contraception 31:51, 1985.

241. DeSlypere JP, Thiery N, Vermeulen A: Effect of longterm hormonal contraception on plasma lipids. Contraception 31:633, 1985.

242. Konje JC, Otolorin EO, Ladipo AO: The effect of continuous subdermal levonorgestrel on carbohydrate metabolism. Am J Obstet Gynecol 166:15, 1992.

243. Kjos SL, Peters RK, Xiang A, et al: Contraception and the risk of type 2 diabetes mellitus in Latina women with prior gestational diabetes mellitus. JAMA 280:533, 1998.

244. Grenfel A, Brudnell JM, Doddridge MC, Watkins PJ: Pregnancy in diabetic women who have proteinuria. Q J Med 59:379, 1986.

Endocrine Diseases in Pregnancy

JORGE H. MESTMAN

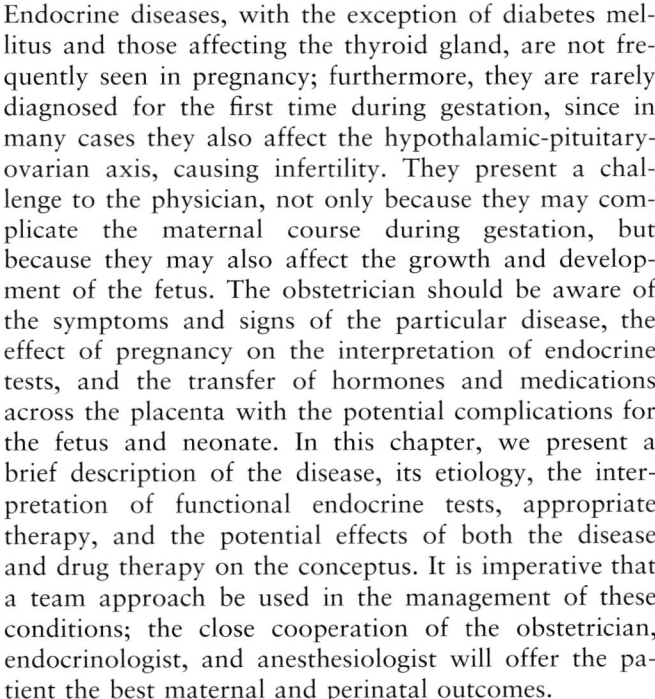

Endocrine diseases, with the exception of diabetes mellitus and those affecting the thyroid gland, are not frequently seen in pregnancy; furthermore, they are rarely diagnosed for the first time during gestation, since in many cases they also affect the hypothalamic-pituitary-ovarian axis, causing infertility. They present a challenge to the physician, not only because they may complicate the maternal course during gestation, but because they may also affect the growth and development of the fetus. The obstetrician should be aware of the symptoms and signs of the particular disease, the effect of pregnancy on the interpretation of endocrine tests, and the transfer of hormones and medications across the placenta with the potential complications for the fetus and neonate. In this chapter, we present a brief description of the disease, its etiology, the interpretation of functional endocrine tests, appropriate therapy, and the potential effects of both the disease and drug therapy on the conceptus. It is imperative that a team approach be used in the management of these conditions; the close cooperation of the obstetrician, endocrinologist, and anesthesiologist will offer the patient the best maternal and perinatal outcomes.

PITUITARY DISEASES

The pituitary gland enlarges during gestation, but the growth does not have clinical repercussions, unless a pathologic process is present. The enlargement is due to hyperplasia of the lactotroph cells, producers of prolactin (PRL).[1] Normal hormonal changes with progression of pregnancy will be discussed in relation to a specific disease.

Anterior Pituitary Insufficiency

Hypopituitarism is defined as a constellation of signs and symptoms resulting from a partial or total deficiency of hormones secreted by the pituitary gland. The pathologic lesion may be localized in the pituitary gland itself or in the hypothalamus: if the hypothalamus is involved, there will be a decrease in the secretion of hypothalamic releasing hormones. The most common etiologies of anterior pituitary insufficiency include destruction of the anterior pituitary gland by tumors, infarction (postpartum necrosis, or Sheehan's syndrome), an autoimmune process (lymphocytic hypophysitis), infiltrative lesions (tuberculosis, sarcoidosis), pituitary apoplexy,[2] idiopathic disease (Simmonds' disease), the empty sella syndrome, previous pituitary surgery, and radiotherapy to the pituitary gland. Recently, several reports of hypopituitarism as a result of mutations in the genes that encode the transcription factors for the differentiation of anterior pituitary cells have been published.[3,4] As a result of these mutations, both sporadic and familial congenital deficiencies of single or multiple hormones have been described. Mass lesions in the hypothalamus, history of radiation to the hypothalamic area, infiltrative lesions, head trauma, and infections account for some of the causes of partial or total hypopituitarism. Diabetes insipidus (DI) is usually present when the lesion is in the hypothalamic region. In a study of 172 adults with hypopituitarism, the disorder was due to a pituitary tumor or the consequence of the tumor in almost 80 percent, whereas 13 percent had extrapituitary disease, with sarcoidosis in 1 percent and Sheehan's syndrome in 0.5 percent.[5]

Sheehan's syndrome or postpartum pituitary necrosis due to severe blood loss during delivery has been considered the most common cause of panhypopituitarism in women of childbearing age. The pathogenesis is not clear, although Sheehan in his original description did associate it with severe postpartum hemorrhage.[6] The classic clinical presentation of Sheehan's syndrome is severe bleeding during delivery or immediately postpartum in about 90 percent of patients; in more than 10 percent of patients no catastrophic event is elicited. In some cases, acute adrenal insufficiency with hypotension and shock results; in most cases, however, a more insidious onset occurs with lack of lactation following delivery, amenorrhea, loss of pubic and axillary hair or failure of pubic hair to grow back following cesarean delivery, anorexia and nausea, lethargy, weakness, and weight loss. The disease may be recognized in the few days or weeks following delivery or many years after the original event.[7] On physical examination, the findings depend on the severity and duration of the disease. Commonly, the skin has a waxy character with fine wrinkles about the eyes and mouth. There is some periorbital edema, and a decrease in pigmentation is often seen. Axillary and pubic hair becomes increasingly sparse. Atrophy of the breast tissue may be present. Even in those patients losing weight, cachexia is not a feature of the disease. Postural hypotension is not uncommon, patients complaining of dizziness on arising in the morning or when getting up from a sitting position. Normocytic anemia is common. Serum electrolytes may be within normal limits, unless severe vomiting is present. Most of the gastrointestinal and postural hypotension symptoms are due to secondary adrenal insufficiency, although the serum potassium remains normal because aldosterone production by the adrenal gland is not affected. This constellation of symptoms does not occur in every patient, and it is not unusual for the full-blown picture to take 10 to 20 years to develop. Occasionally, the diagnosis is made when the patient develops acute adrenal insufficiency secondary to a stressful situation such as infection, trauma, or surgery.

The diagnosis is confirmed by the use of appropriate tests to investigate each of the pituitary hormones. Baseline or random determination of serum pituitary hormone concentrations is of little value, and dynamic tests to evaluate hypothalamic-pituitary hormonal reserve must be used. The most practical tests are presented in Table 33–1. However, their use in pregnancy is limited because, in most cases, the response is blunted.

Partial pituitary insufficiency is common. In a review of anterior pituitary function in patients with pituitary apoplexy due to different causes, growth hormone deficiency was common and occurred in almost 90 percent of patients; adrenocorticotropic hormone (ACTH) deficiency in about 66 percent, hypothyroidism caused by thyroid-stimulating hormone (TSH) deficiency in about 42 percent, and hypogonadism in 65 percent, whereas the incidence of diabetes insipidus was less than 5 percent.[8]

Several reports of successful pregnancies following the diagnosis of Sheehan's syndrome have been reported.[9–11] Placental function is not altered in patients with pituitary insufficiency. Although several patients conceived after treatment with gonadotropin, others have conceived spontaneously, an indication of partial pituitary failure. The outcome of pregnancy in women with Sheehan's syndrome is good in those receiving

Table 33–1. TESTS OF ANTERIOR PITUITARY HORMONE RESERVE

Hormone	Basal Levels	Test	Normal Response	Response In Pregnancy
GH	Suppressed	L-Dopa 500 mg, GH levels at 0, 1, 2 h	↑ by 10 ng/dl	Blunted
		Insulin hypoglycemia 0.1 U regular IV/kg GH at 0, 20, 60, 90 min	↑ by 10 ng/dl	Blunted
ACTH	Small rise	Insulin hypoglycemia (see above) Cortisol at 0, 20, 60, 90 min	↑ by 10 μg/dl	Blunted
		Metyrapone 750 mg every 4 h × 6	↑ urinary 17-KGS ↑ serum substance S	Blunted
TSH	First trimester: may be suppressed; second and third trimester normal	TRH 500 μg IV 0, 30, 50 min	↑ by 5 μl/ml	First may be blunted; second & third nl or increased
Prolactin	Increased	TRH (see above); prolactin 0, 30, 60 min	↑ × 2 baseline	Exaggerated
LH-FSH	Suppressed	LHRH IU 500 μg IV; LH + FSH 0, 30, 60 min	↑ × 2 baseline	Blunted

GH, growth hormone; ACTH, corticotropin; TSH, thyrotropin-stimulating hormone; TRH, thyrotropin-releasing hormone; LH, luteinizing hormone; FSH, follicle stimulating hormone; LHRH, luteinizing hormone-releasing hormone; 17-KGS, 17 ketogenic steroids; S, 11-desoxycortisol; IV, intravenous.
From Montoro MN, Mestman JH: Pituitary diseases during pregnancy. Infertil Reprod Med Clin North Am 5:732, 1994.

proper replacement therapy. In one review, 87 percent had live births and 13 percent had spontaneous abortions.[9]

When anterior pituitary insufficiency develops for the first time in pregnancy or early postpartum, the clinical manifestations may be related to local signs and symptoms due to acute expansion of the pituitary gland or by those related to specific hormone deficiencies. Acute enlargement of the pituitary gland could be the result of acute edema of a known or unknown pituitary lesion or bleeding into a preexisting pituitary tumor. Severe, deep, midline headaches and nausea, vomiting, and visual disturbances are common. Symptoms of an acute endocrine deficiency are mainly related to reduced cortisol secretion: protracted hypoglycemia responding to glucocorticoid therapy, nausea, vomiting, and hypotension.[12-14]

Lymphocytic hypophysitis, first described in 1962 by Goudie and Pinkerton,[15] is being recognized with increasing frequency as a cause of partial or total hypopituitarism.[16-18] It is considered to have an autoimmune pathogenesis and occurs mainly in women during pregnancy or in the postpartum period. Association with other autoimmune endocrine disorders (thyroiditis, gastritis, and adrenalitis) has been reported.[15,19] Sheehan[6] reported lymphocytic infiltration of the pituitary gland in some women with postpartum pituitary insufficiency. The clinical presentation is characterized by headaches and visual disturbances related to pressure from the expanding lesion mimicking a pituitary tumor or symptoms and signs of hypopituitarism such as hypoglycemia, hypotension, nausea, and vomiting. It may also present in the postpartum period as pituitary insufficiency, similar to Sheehan's syndrome without the history of profound bleeding.[20] Lymphocytic hypophysitis may be precipitated by acute infections and labor. Asa and associates[16] reported two patients with severe headache, nausea, vomiting, and impaired vision, one of whom required pituitary surgery at 6 months' gestation, because of an enlarging pituitary mass. Light and electron microscopic studies of the pituitary gland were consistent with lymphoid hypophysitis. The authors found another eight cases of proven lymphocytic hypophysitis, five seen on postmortem examination, and three on biopsy. In five patients, the diagnosis was made during the postpartum period, and in four patients there was evidence of other autoimmune endocrine disease. In some of the reported cases, endocrine manifestations related to pituitary insufficiency manifested for the first time in the postpartum period. Postpartum thyroiditis with reversible ACTH deficiency was described by Bevan et al.[19] Hyperprolactinemia, partial pituitary insufficiency, with or without a pituitary mass, has been reported in the postpartum period.[21,22] When available, the pathologic specimen showed significant lymphocytic infiltration. The differential diagnosis between pituitary tumor and lymphocytic hypophysitis can be made only by histologic examination; indeed, in some cases surgery was performed in pregnancy with the preoperative diagnosis of pituitary tumor.

Over 100 cases of lymphocytic hypophysitis have been described in the English literature and were recently reviewed by Gagneja et al.[18] In most cases, the diagnosis was made on clinical grounds with a few confirmed by histologic examination. Spontaneous regression of the pituitary mass with recovery of endocrine function has been reported.[23,24] Two patients became pregnant after the initial episode and had an uneventful delivery.[18,25] Based on the above information, in the presence of a clinical diagnosis of lymphocytic hypophysitis and absence of visual field defects, surgical therapy may be safely withheld, with periodic reassessment of endocrine function and the size of the lesion. In the majority of cases reported, gonadotropin function has been spared, suggesting a possibility of future spontaneous pregnancies. The most frequent associations are ACTH and prolactin defects and the presence of autoimmune thyroid disease.

Patients with partial or total hypopituitarism who become pregnant spontaneously or after treatment with gonadotropin may carry a normal pregnancy with successful neonatal outcome. In women on glucocorticoid replacement therapy, no increase in the dose is needed; the usual amount of hydrocortisone in patients with pituitary insufficiency is between 20 and 30 mg/day, two thirds of the total amount in the morning and one third in the evening. Occasionally, the dose of hydrocortisone may be decreased by one third of the total dose owing to the potentiation of hydrocortisone effect during pregnancy by estrogen.[26] This potentiation does not occur when synthetic corticosteroids such as prednisone and dexamethasone are used. The equivalent amount of prednisone is 5.0 to 7.5 mg daily and of dexamethasone 0.5 to 0.75 mg daily (Table 33-2). Aldosterone secretion is preserved, since its adrenal secretion is independent from ACTH. Therefore, in contrast to primary adrenal insufficiency, there is no need for mineralocorticoid replacement therapy. In the presence of thyroid deficiency, the amount of L-thyroxine may need to be increased from early pregnancy; the usual replacement dose is between 0.075 and 0.15 mg daily. The amount should be adjusted to keep the free thyroxine in the upper third of normal; in patients with secondary hypothyroidism, such as in women with hypopituitarism, serum TSH cannot be followed as a marker for proper thyroxine replacement as is the case in primary hypothyroidism.

Acute adrenal insufficiency is an emergency and should be managed with intravenous glucocorticoids, 200 to 300 mg of hydrocortisone in 24 hours or equiv-

Table 33-2. RELATIVE BIOLOGIC EFFECTS OF CORTICOSTEROIDS

Steroid	Preparations		
	Anti-inflammatory Effect	Carbohydrate Effect	Sodium Retention
Cortisone	1	1	1
Hydrocortisone or cortisol	1.25	1.25	1.25
Prednisone	5	5	0
Prednisolone	5	5	0
6α-Methylprednisolone (Medrol)	6	6	0
Dexamethasone (Decadron)	30	30	0
Betamethasone (Celestone)	30	30	0
Fludrocortisone (Florinef)	10	10	400
Deoxycorticosterone (Doca)	0	0.01	40

From Montoro MN, Mestman JH: Pituitary disease during pregnancy. Infertil Reprod Med Clin North Am 5:734, 1994.

alent doses of synthetic corticosteroids. Aggressive intravenous fluid therapy with 5 percent dextrose/normal saline should be started immediately (see section Addison's Disease below).

Pregnancy in cases of isolated growth hormone deficiency has been reported.[27] Lactation was unimpaired, placental function studies were normal, and intrauterine growth was also normal.

Prolactinomas

Serum prolactin normally increases early in pregnancy, reaching values close to 140 ng/ml by the end of pregnancy.[28] Prolactinoma is the most common pituitary tumor diagnosed in women of childbearing age. Pituitary tumors are divided according to their size, into microadenomas, less than 10 mm in diameter, and macroadenomas; the latter are further classified according to suprasellar extension and invasion of adjacent structures. Serum prolactin concentrations correlate fairly well with the size of the tumor. Hyperprolactinemia may be diagnosed in the absence of an enlargement of the pituitary gland, known as idiopathic hyperprolactinemia. Hyperprolactinemia decreases gonadotropin-releasing hormone (GnRH) secretion, accounting for the infertility seen in these patients. However, high levels of serum prolactin in the presence of normal menses, normal fertility, and absence of a pituitary lesion have been reported.[29,30] The syndrome is due to the presence of large amounts of "big-big prolactin," that normally accounts for less than 10 percent of the total serum prolactin. Pregnancy outcome is excellent for both mother and infant.

Once the diagnosis of prolactinoma is confirmed, several types of therapy are available, the choice depending on tumor size, radiologic classification, local symptoms, and the patient's age and desire for pregnancy.[31]

Radiation therapy as the initial and only therapy is seldom indicated.[32] Radiation therapy is employed following surgery in those patients with a residual lesion in order to prevent recurrences.

Surgical treatment, mainly transsphenoidal adenectomy, has been effective as the sole form of therapy in restoring ovulation in patients with small tumors. The cure rate, that is, normalization of serum prolactin, is in the range of 60 to 70 percent.[33] However, the recurrence rate is between 25 and 40 percent. The cure rate is significantly lower for macroadenomas. Feigenbaum et al.[34] followed over 400 patients for a mean of 9.2 years after surgery for prolactinoma. Hyperprolactinemia recurred in 47 percent of all patients. The best results were obtained in those patients with microadenomas and with serum prolactin levels 1 day after surgery of less than 5 ng/ml.

Medical therapy with bromocriptine, a dopamine-receptor agonist, has been effective in producing ovulation in 80 to 90 percent of hyperprolactinemic women.[35] Most patients respond to doses between 2.5 and 5 mg/day, although occasionally a dose of 7.5 mg/day or more is needed. Bromocriptine is effective not only in normalizing prolactin levels but also in reducing the size of the tumor.[36,37] In women desiring a pregnancy, it is advisable to use mechanical contraception in the first few months of bromocriptine therapy, until normal menses have been established. In patients who have side effects such as nausea and vomiting, an oral bromocriptine tablet may be administered vaginally with normalization of prolactin levels.[38]

In patients with large tumors on bromocriptine therapy, the drug should be given for at least 1 year, since recurrence of tumors of this size has been reported when the drug is stopped before the completion of the first year of treatment.[39,40]

Once conception takes place, bromocriptine should

be discontinued and the patient followed closely. For those women whose initial prolactin levels are over 200 ng/ml, or who have abnormal magnetic resonance imaging (MRI) scans with suprasellar extension, bromocriptine therapy during pregnancy should be continued.[39,40] Although the experience is limited to approximately 100 women who have used bromocriptine throughout gestation, no abnormalities have been noted in the infants, except for one with an undescended testicle and one with a talipes deformity.[31]

Cabergoline, a dopamine agonist with long duration of action, has been used in a few patients with a prolactinoma. It is as effective as bromocriptine in lowering prolactin levels, reducing the size of the tumor, and inducing ovulation. Its advantages include its long duration of action, with a dose taken every 3 or 4 days, and less side effects than bromocriptine.[41,42] The weekly dose is between 0.5 and 3 mg. The incidence of spontaneous abortion, preterm delivery, and congenital malformation is similar to that in the general population.[43] However, the number of pregnancies treated with cabergoline is much lower than with bromocriptine; therefore, bromocriptine should be the drug of choice for women seeking conception.

Complications during pregnancy are directly related to tumor size.[7,31,44–48] In patients with microadenomas, following induction of ovulation with bromocriptine, the reported incidence of headaches and visual field disturbances is between 1 and 4 percent. The incidence is close to 35 percent for patients with macroadenomas. However, if the pituitary macroadenoma is treated before pregnancy with either surgery or radiotherapy, the complication rate is about 4 percent. Complications may occur with equal frequency at any stage of pregnancy. Therefore, the management of patients with prolactinomas or any type of pituitary tumor in pregnancy depends on the size of the tumor and previous therapy. For patients with microadenomas, visual fields are indicated only if there are signs and symptoms of tumor enlargement; if the visual fields are abnormal, then an MRI scan of the pituitary gland is obtained. In the presence of any objective evidence of tumor enlargement, bromocriptine is resumed and continued throughout pregnancy at a dose of up to 20 mg/day. If after a few days there is no improvement, dexamethasone 4 mg every 6 hours is indicated. Surgery is performed in those complicated cases not responding to the above therapies.

The determination of serum prolactin during gestation is not helpful in evaluating tumor growth. With a few exceptions, serum prolactin levels in women with prepregnancy hyperprolactinemia remained unchanged during pregnancy. In one study, serum prolactin levels remained stable in the majority of patients with prepregnancy baseline prolactin levels of over 60 ng/ml.[40]

However, in those patients with prolactin levels of less than 60 ng/ml, the mean level doubled at the end of pregnancy and returned to pretreatment levels at the end of lactation.

Potential perinatal complications due to the use of bromocriptine have been reported[46]; abortion rates (11.1 percent), multiple pregnancy rates (1.2 percent), and prematurity rates (10.1 percent) are similar to those seen in the infertile population. Early reports of cervical incompetence have not been confirmed. The congenital malformation rate of 3.5 percent for major and minor lesions is comparable to the rate of 2.7 percent reported in a control group. Although bromocriptine crosses the placenta, no abnormalities in mental and physical development were detected in a group of 64 children, age 6 months to 9 years, whose mothers took bromocriptine at some time during gestation.[49]

Breast-feeding is not contraindicated in mothers with prolactinoma. There is no increase in prolactin secretion after suckling, and the mean value of prolactin is not increased compared with that of pregnancy.[50] A concern about seizures and strokes in the puerperium of women taking bromocriptine was not confirmed by a well-controlled study.[51]

Following delivery, women should be followed carefully for assessment of tumor growth. In patients with microadenomas, prolactin levels are measured a few months after delivery; drug therapy is reinstituted in the presence of persistent hyperprolactinemia. An MRI scan should be repeated in cases of macroadenomas soon after delivery, to detect any change in the size of the tumor.[52]

Management of patients who wish to conceive is summarized in Table 33–3.[31,47] Although a serum prolactin level of less than 100 ng/ml and a normal radiologic examination before pregnancy are predictors of low complication rates, exceptions have been reported. It is suggested that treatment with bromocriptine be

Table 33–3. MANAGEMENT OF WOMEN WITH HYPERPROLACTINEMIA BEFORE CONCEPTION

Tumor	Management	Pregnancy Follow-up
No tumor	Bromocriptine	Visual field (?)
Microadenoma	Bromocriptine* or surgery	Visual field every trimester
Macroadenoma	(A) Surgery + bromocriptine	Visual field monthly
	(B) Radiotherapy + bromocriptine	Visual field monthly

* Therapy for 1 year before conception.
From Mestman JH: Endocrine diseases in pregnancy. *In* Sciarra JJ (ed): Gynecology and Obstetrics. Philadelphia, Lippincott-Raven, 1997, p 6.

continued for at least 12 months before conception, as it seems to reduce the risk of tumor enlargement during pregnancy.[40,48]

Acromegaly

Acromegaly is a chronic disease caused in the vast majority of cases by hypersecretion of growth hormone by the adenohypophysis. It is almost always associated with a benign pituitary tumor and is characterized by slow and progressive enlargement of the extremities. Facial changes are typical, but they develop so gradually that neither the family nor the patient recognizes the changes. As in other endocrine disorders, comparison of the patient's photographs taken over many years may be the only clue to the presence and progression of the disease. Symptoms may be due to local expansion of the tumor, with headaches and visual field disturbances, or due to the somatic effect of chronic excess growth hormone secretion, such as hyperhidrosis, weight gain, arthralgias, and acroparesthesia (carpal tunnel syndrome). Most women with acromegaly suffer from menstrual irregularities. Galactorrhea with hyperprolactinemia is a common finding, and therefore infertility is common. The diagnosis is confirmed by an elevation in plasma growth hormone levels and/or elevations in insulin-like growth factor I (IGF-I). The latter is now considered the test of choice in nonpregnant women.

The diagnosis of acromegaly during pregnancy is difficult to confirm, since the conventional radioimmunoassay for growth hormone (GH) does not distinguish normal pituitary GH from the variant produced by the placenta,[53] unless a special radioimmunoassay (RIA) is used. The placental variant is secreted continuously rather than in a pulsatile pattern as is pituitary GH, binds to GH receptors, and functions as a GH agonist.[54] After the first trimester of pregnancy, the placental GH variant is the major component of circulating GH. Using specific RIAs for the placental GH variant, to separate both hormones, the highly pulsatile secretion of pituitary GH seen in acromegaly may help establish the diagnosis. GH release after thyrotropin-releasing hormone (TRH) injection is observed in most patients with acromegaly; however, the placental GH variant is unresponsive.[54] IGF-I values are less useful in the diagnosis, as they are elevated during normal pregnancy.

Patients with acromegaly rarely ovulate spontaneously. However, with the advent of new medical therapy, successful pregnancies have been reported with increased frequency. In 1954, Abelove and co-workers[55] reported 35 cases; they followed 2 acromegalic women and reviewed 33 reported cases with active disease. With few exceptions, infant outcome was normal. In one case, the infant was born with acromegalic features; during the neonatal period, growth was above average, but subsequently a normal growth pattern returned.[56] Unfortunately, no neonatal GH determinations were obtained. The lack of acromegalic features in newborns is in accord with the demonstration by King and colleagues that GH does not cross the placental barrier.[57] Herman-Bonert et al.[58] described 24 pregnancies in acromegalic women, and individual cases were reviewed by Neal in a recent report of one of his own cases.[59]

During pregnancy, women with active acromegaly are at potential risk for developing gestational diabetes, worsening of impaired glucose metabolism, and enlargement of the pituitary tumor. It is estimated that overt diabetes mellitus will develop in 10 to 20 percent, impaired glucose tolerance in 30 percent, and hypertension in 25 to 35 percent. Carpal tunnel syndrome symptoms may worsen during gestation. Patients with acromegaly usually have cardiomegaly shown on routine chest x-ray. Coronary artery disease and a specific cardiomyopathy have been reported.[60]

Therapy of acromegaly in nonpregnant patients includes surgery and/or radiation, or medical therapy using the somatostatin analogues.[61,62] Bromocriptine was used with relative success until new agents, octreotide and lanreotide, became available. These somatostatin analogues inhibit the production of GH, as well as glucagon and insulin. Because a complete cure is not always achieved with surgery and/or radiation, chronic therapy with somatostatin analogues has proven effective in normalizing serum GH and IGF-I levels. The dose of octreotide is 300 to 1,500 μg in three divided doses by subcutaneous injection. Long-acting somatostatin analogs, octreotide LAR (octreotide acetate for injectable suspension) and slow-release lanreotide (lanreotide SR), have been introduced.[63] Both preparations are administered intramuscularly at intervals of either 28 days (octreotide LAR) or 10 to 14 days (lanreotide SR). The goal of therapy is to achieve a serum GH level of less than 1.0 ng/ml with the new sensitive assays and normalization of IGF-I. The dose is adjusted according to the result of GH and IGF-I levels done every 3 months. Normalization of IGF-I has been achieved in about 70 percent of patients treated for periods over 6 months. The two preparations are well tolerated, although cholelithiasis may develop in 20 percent of patients.

Few cases of pregnancy in acromegalic women treated with bromocriptine have been reported.[64–67] In each case, pregnancy occurred in spite of persistent elevation in GH levels. Pregnancies occurred when prolactin levels returned to normal following drug therapy.

Eight cases have been reported of successful pregnancy in acromegalic women treated with octreotide.[58,59,68,69] Octreotide has been reported to cross the placenta by passive diffusion without producing adverse effects in the fetus.[70] In most cases, octreotide was discontinued at the time of pregnancy diagnosis. However, in two cases the drug was continued throughout pregnancy. As in cases of prolactinoma, it is advisable to perform visual field examinations each trimester or as clinically indicated with severe headache or visual disturbances. MRI is reserved for those cases developing abnormal visual fields. If an enlargement of the pituitary tumor is detected, reinstitution of medical therapy and close follow-up is recommended.

Diabetes Insipidus

Women with isolated DI antedating pregnancy, and with normal anterior pituitary function, carry their pregnancies uneventfully and infant outcome is normal.

Shortly after conception, plasma osmolality decreases by about 9 to 10 mOsm/kg and remains low throughout pregnancy. Despite this decrease in plasma osmolality, basal levels of serum arginine vasopressin (AVP), the antidiuretic hormone, are similar to those seen in nonpregnant women.[71] It has been suggested that in pregnancy there is a resetting of the "thirst osmostat" with a decrease in the osmotic threshold for antidiuretic hormone release by 8 to 10 mOsm/kg. The ability to concentrate the urine remains unchanged.[72] The placenta produces vasopressinase, a cysteine aminopeptidase enzyme that degrades AVP. As the result of the increased production of the enzyme vasopressinase in the last part of pregnancy, a 1,000-fold increase between the 4th and 38th weeks of gestation, there is a threefold increase in endogenous AVP during pregnancy.[73] This rapid degradation of AVP may uncover latent forms of DI, and could explain the lack of response to injectable vasopressin, but a normal response to desmopressin, a drug that is not metabolized by vasopressinase.[74]

Diabetes insipidus is characterized clinically by polyuria (over 3 L/24 h) and polydipsia due to a deficiency of antidiuretic hormone (central or neurogenic diabetes insipidus), or to peripheral resistance to the action of the hormone at the level of the renal tubules (nephrogenic diabetes insipidus). Lesions at the level of the hypothalamus or pituitary gland are usually the cause of central diabetes insipidus. These include invasion of the neurohypophysis by tumors, metastatic lesions, including breast cancer, granulomas, infections, skull trauma, and following hypophysectomy. In 50 percent of cases, however, DI is considered idiopathic, probably on an autoimmune basis. It has recently been shown that many of the idiopathic cases are due to lymphocytic inflammation of the posterior pituitary gland, sometimes with partial involvement of the anterior pituitary gland.[75] MRI study shows thickening of the pituitary stalk, enlargement of the neurohypophysis, and normal appearance of the adenohypophysis. The term

lymphocytic infundibulohypophysitis (LIH) has been suggested for this clinical entity.[76] Nephrogenic diabetes insipidus is a hereditary disorder affecting males; therefore, symptomatic women carriers are extremely rare. Psychogenic diabetes insipidus, rarely reported in pregnancy,[77] is differentiated from the other forms by the results of the water deprivation test.

The clinical presentation of idiopathic central DI is generally acute, with polyuria and polydipsia developing in a few days. Patients usually remember the day their symptoms began, they prefer to drink cold water, and their urinary output varies between 4 and 15 L in 24 hours.

The diagnosis of DI is confirmed by the results of the water deprivation test.[78] (see the box "Steps in the Water Deprivation Test"). The test separates patients into five groups: (1) normal, (2) complete central DI, (3) partial central DI, (4) nephrogenic DI, and (5) compulsive water drinking. The test is started early in the morning; the patient's weight, pulse, and blood pressure are obtained along with baseline determinations of serum and urine osmolality, and determination of plasma vasopressin levels. Thereafter, urine osmolality is obtained with each voided specimen. The test is terminated when the patient loses 3 percent of body weight or when urinary osmolality shows no increment in two successive specimens. At the end of the test, serum osmolality and vasopressin levels are measured. Patients with DI, regardless of the cause, show no in-

---

Steps in the Water Deprivation Test*

1. Nothing by mouth after 7:00 A.M.
2. Baseline serum and urine osmolality and serum vasopressin levels.
3. Hourly measurements of urine osmolality and body weight.
4. Water deprivation is continued until two subsequent urine osmolalities vary by less than 10 percent or when 3 to 5 percent body weight is lost.
5. At this time, serum osmolality, serum sodium, and vasopressin levels are obtained.
6. Five units of aqueous vasopressin (Pitressin) are injected subcutaneously.
7. Urine osmolality 1 hour after the injection.

*The test must be performed under careful supervision to avoid either severe dehydration in patients with significant antidiuretic hormone deficiency or water intoxication in patients with primary polydipsia due to continuous water ingestion after the administration of vasopressin (Pitressin).
From Mestman JH: Endocrine diseases in pregnancy. *In* Sciarra JJ (ed): Gynecology and Obstetrics. Philadelphia, Lippincott-Raven, 1997, p 7, with permission.

crement in urinary osmolality, but plasma osmolarity does increase due to dehydration. Plasma vasopressin levels are low in central DI; they are inappropriately high in the nephrogenic type. Injection of aqueous vasopressin 5 U subcutaneously at the end of the test separates central DI from nephrogenic DI in the vast majority of cases. L-Deamino-8-arginine vasopressin (desmopressin, [dDAVP], a synthetic analog of vasopressin resistant to vasopressinase) is preferable in pregnancy, a dose of 10 μg given intranasally. In central DI, there is a decrease in urinary output and an increase in urinary osmolality. No changes are seen in the nephrogenic type. Patients with primary polydipsia or psychogenic DI respond with some increase in urine osmolality to the administration of dDAVP, but the increase is not as great as with patients who have central DI. In emergency situations, with acute onset of symptoms, such as cases of acute fatty liver of pregnancy or preeclampsia, treatment cannot be delayed, and diagnostic tests to assess the etiology of DI are limited to the determination of serum vasopressin, urinary, and plasma osmolality, with the dynamic test of water deprivation postponed until recovery from the acute injury.

In patients with newly diagnosed central DI, a complete evaluation to define the cause of the disease is imperative. Radiologic examination of the hypothalamic-pituitary area and hormonal studies for assessment of anterior pituitary function should be obtained. Long-term follow-up is indicated, as hypothalamic dysfunction may appear with time.[79]

Labor and delivery proceed normally in patients with DI, although an occasional patient with uterine atony has been reported. Plasma oxytocin concentrations have been reported as normal, with normal pulsatile release during labor and lactation.

DI during pregnancy may occur in different clinical settings[80]: (1) pregestational DI; (2) presenting for the first time in pregnancy and persisting thereafter; (3) transient, occurring during gestation or in the immediate postpartum period, associated with preeclampsia, liver disease, or HELLP (*h*emolysis, *e*levated *l*iver enzymes, and *l*ow *p*latelet count) syndrome; (4) transient, recurrent in pregnancy, patients with latent DI, manifesting only in pregnancy because of the increase in the placental vasopressinase; (5) postpartum DI in patients with acute pituitary insufficiency such as Sheehan's syndrome or hypophysitis; and (6) an unusual transient form of DI resistant both to vasopressin and dDAVP administration.

Hime and Richardson[81] reviewed 67 cases of DI in pregnancy, 1 case per 66,000 deliveries. Worsening of the symptoms occurred in over 50 percent of cases, spontaneous improvement in 20 percent, and no changes in the remainder. Labor progressed normally in the majority of cases, with few patients requiring induction of labor or cesarean section.

A form of transient vasopressin-resistant DI has been reported in the last trimester of pregnancy.[74,82] It is associated with preeclampsia, acute fatty liver of pregnancy, or HELLP syndrome, and responds to desmopressin but not AVP. DI was reported in a group of women in the last weeks of pregnancy associated with acute fatty liver. The presentation was characterized by nausea, vomiting, polyuria, and preeclampsia.[83] Diabetes insipidus resolved in the first weeks after delivery.

In the transient recurrent form of DI, relative deficiency of antidiuretic hormone (ADH) is manifested in pregnancy, because of the inability to increase the secretion of ADH in the presence of high levels of placenta vasopressinase. It could represent the development of the full clinical picture of DI in patients with a latent form of the disease.[84-86]

DI may present for the first time in the postpartum period, usually associated with partial anterior pituitary deficiency; the etiologies include lymphocytic hypophysitis or Sheehan's syndrome.[87,88]

Desmopressin is the drug of choice in the treatment of DI. Pitressin tannate in oil or water has been the standard drug of choice for many years and is still used occasionally. The antidiuretic effects of dDAVP last from 8 to 24 hours. dDAVP is available in three forms, nasal insufflation, parenteral and, most recently, tablet form. The usual dose of the nasal spray is 10 to 25 μg once or twice daily as needed to control polyuria. In the presence of rhinitis or other conditions that would interfere with absorption, or in the postoperative period, the parenteral form is used. Two to 4 μg is injected subcutaneously or intravenously and repeated every 12 to 24 hours, according to the control of symptoms, particularly nocturia, urinary osmolality, and 24-hour urinary output. Occasionally, lower extremity edema may result from an excessive dosage. Plasma electrolytes, fluid intake, and urinary output should be followed closely to avoid water intoxication. In patients with long-standing DI, complications are rare, the dosage of drug is stable, and electrolyte abnormalities are infrequent. There has been considerable experience with dDAVP in pregnancy.[89] The prepregnancy dose does not need to be modified in most cases. There are no adverse fetal effects, and the drug is safe in lactating mothers. In the rare case of nephrogenic DI, thiazide diuretics[90] are the only drugs that may be used, since nonsteroidal anti-inflammatory drugs are not recommended in pregnancy.

PARATHYROID DISEASES

Parathyroid diseases, uncommon in pregnancy, may produce significant perinatal and maternal morbidity and mortality if not diagnosed and properly managed.

After a brief review of calcium homeostasis during pregnancy, primary hyperparathyroidism, hypoparathyroidism, and osteoporosis are discussed. Several reviews on these topics have recently been published.[91-93]

Calcium Homeostasis during Pregnancy

Two hormones, parathyroid hormone (PTH) and 1,25-dihydroxyvitamin D, (1,25[OH]$_2$D$_3$) are responsible for maintaining calcium homeostasis. Approximately 50 percent of serum calcium is protein bound (mostly to albumin), 10 percent is complexed to anions, and 40 percent circulates free as ionized calcium. During pregnancy, there is an active transfer of maternal calcium to the fetus. A full-term infant requires 25 to 30 g of calcium during the course of pregnancy for new bone mineralization.

Total serum calcium during gestation is 8 percent below postpartum levels.[94] The upper limit of normal is 9.5 mg/dl. This decrease in total serum calcium is due to the physiologic hypoalbuminemia secondary to the normal expansion of the intravascular volume observed early in pregnancy. Ionized calcium levels, however, remain unchanged throughout gestation. Serum phosphate and renal tubular reabsorption of phosphorus also remain normal throughout pregnancy. Maternal serum PTH levels, when measured by a sensitive assay that accurately measures the levels of intact PTH, are slightly decreased in the second half of pregnancy.

Blood levels of 1,25(OH)$_2$D$_3$ (calcitriol), increase early in gestation as a result of stimulation of renal 1α-hydroxylase activity by estrogen, placental lactogen, and PTH, as well as synthesis of calcitriol by the placenta.[95] Both free and total 1,25(OH)$_2$D$_3$ are increased in pregnancy, the total because of an increase in vitamin D–binding protein.[96] Twenty-four-hour urinary calcium excretion also increases with each trimester of gestation and falls in the postpartum period,[97,98] reflecting the increased intestinal calcium absorption induced by higher levels of 1,25-hydroxyvitamin D during gestation. Pregnancy-induced hypertension is characterized by decreased urinary calcium excretion probably explained by a decrease in serum 1,25-vitamin D serum levels.[99]

Parathyroid hormone-related protein (PTHrP), a peptide responsible for the hypercalcemia found in many malignant tumors, increases in early pregnancy. Hirota et al.[100] measured PTHrP in each trimester of human pregnancy, in umbilical venous blood and postpartum. A steady increase in plasma values was observed throughout pregnancy, with a peak in the third trimester and high values in cord blood. The plasma concentration in the postpartum period was directly related to the degree of breast-feeding. The source of maternal serum PTHrP is unknown, and both fetal and maternal sites have been postulated. PTHrP is secreted by breast tissue and may be involved in the transfer of calcium

into milk.[101] PTHrP plays a role in placental calcium transport in sheep,[102] but its importance in human maternal physiology is less clear.

Serum calcitonin levels are higher during pregnancy and in the postpartum period, when compared with nonpregnant controls. In 20 percent of patients, the values exceed the normal nonpregnant range.[103] The origin of calcitonin is thyroidal C cells, breast, and placenta. Its role in pregnancy has not been elucidated, although it may protect the maternal skeleton from excessive resorption of calcium.[91]

Osteocalcin is a bone-specific protein released by osteoblasts into the circulation proportional to the rate of new bone formation. It is slightly decreased during the second trimester of pregnancy, with an increase in the postpartum period.[95,104] Markers of bone resorption increase during pregnancy, reaching values in the last trimester of pregnancy up to twice normal. These changes are consistent with the increase in bone turnover at the time of maximal transfer of maternal calcium to the fetus.

Following delivery, urinary calcium excretion is reduced; ionized serum calcium remains within normal limits; and total calcium, 1,25-hydroxyvitamin D, and serum PTH return to prepregnancy levels. Early concern of calcium loss in lactating mothers, with the development of osteopenia, has not been confirmed; and calcium supplementation during breast-feeding appears to be unnecessary. The alteration in calcium and bone metabolism that accompanies human lactation represents a physiologic response that is independent of calcium intake.[92,105]

Hyperparathyroidism

Primary hyperparathyroidism (PHP) is an uncommon disease in women of childbearing age. The incidence of the disease in pregnancy is unknown, but it is definitely rare; and most of the reported cases have been single ones complemented with a review of the literature. Over 150 cases have been reported in the English literature and have been recently reviewed.[106] Since the introduction of routine automated techniques in clinical medicine, the majority of patients with PHP are asymptomatic and their serum calcium elevation are mild. There are few clinical indications for ordering a serum calcium level in pregnancy.

The first case of PHP during pregnancy was reported in 1931.[107] Shortly thereafter, the first case of neonatal hypocalcemia causing tetany in a mother with undiagnosed hypercalcemia due to hyperparathyroidism was described by Friderichsen.[108] The most common cause of PHP in pregnancy is a single parathyroid adenoma, present in about 80 percent of all cases. Primary hyperplasia of the four parathyroid glands accounts for about 15 percent of the cases reported, 3 percent are due to multiple adenomas, and only four cases due to parathyroid carcinoma have been reported in the English literature.[109] In 1962, Ludwig[110] reviewed the literature on the subject, describing 21 women with 40 pregnancies. The incidence of fetal wastage was 27.5 percent. Neonatal tetany due to hypocalcemia representing the first indication of maternal hyperparathyroidism occurred in 19 percent of these cases. In 1972, Johnstone and co-workers[111] confirmed a perinatal mortality of 25 percent with a high incidence of neonatal hypocalcemia. Most of the patients reported in early years had significant metabolic complications of hyperparathyroidism, the two most common being renal and bone disease. In contrast to the previous high neonatal morbidity and mortality Kelly,[112] reviewing the literature from 1976 to 1990, found only 2 perinatal deaths (5 percent) among 37 infants born of hyperparathyroid mothers. Two additional cases of perinatal deaths were reported in mothers with hypercalcemic crisis.[113,114]

Today, in the nonpregnant state, almost 70 percent of patients are asymptomatic, and the diagnosis is made through the routine use of biochemical screening.[115] In pregnancy, since routine calcium determinations are not performed, manifestations of the disease are present in almost 70 percent of the diagnosed patients. In a review of 70 pregnant women, gastrointestinal symptoms such as nausea, vomiting, and anorexia were present in 36 percent of patients, whereas 34 percent presented with weakness and fatigue. In 26 percent, mental symptoms including headaches, lethargy, agitation, emotional lability, confusion, and inappropriate behavior were reported. Nephrolithiasis was detected in 36 percent, bone disease in 19 percent, acute pancreatitis in 13 percent, and hypertension in 10 percent. Only 24 percent of these patients were asymptomatic.[116]

Parathyroid cancer is a rare cause of hyperparathyroidism, with four cases documented in pregnancy. Serum calcium levels are significantly higher than in other causes of PHP.[108,117–119] Perinatal mortality and morbidity were significant. Hypercalcemia with values above 13 mg/dl in the presence of a palpable neck mass should raise a strong suspicion of parathyroid carcinoma. On the contrary, in the presence of mild hypercalcemia and a neck mass, the most common cause of the neck lesion is a thyroid nodule. One other clinical feature of parathyroid carcinoma is poor response to the usual clinical therapeutic measures such as intensive hydration and loop diuretics. Surgery is the only effective therapy.

Hyperparathyroidism should be considered in the differential diagnosis of acute pancreatitis during pregnancy. Acute pancreatitis has been reported in 13 percent of women with primary hyperparathyroidism. The incidence in nonpregnant hyperparathyroid women is about 1.5 percent, and is less than 1 percent in normal pregnancy.[120] This complication is associated with significant neonatal and maternal morbidity. It is more common in the primipara than in women who have had multiple pregnancies. Acute pancreatitis with PHP is mostly likely to occur during the last trimester of pregnancy or the postpartum period, but has also been reported in the first trimester of pregnancy, mimicking hyperemesis gravidarum. Indeed, in two cases hyperthyroidism was also present, which most likely represents the syndrome of transient hyperthyroidsm of hyperemesis gravidarum (see section Thyroid Diseases, below). Serum calcium should be obtained in any pregnant woman with persistent significant nausea, vomiting, and abdominal pain.

Hyperparathyroid crisis, a serious complication of PHP, has been reported during gestation and the postpartum period, and is characterized by severe nausea and vomiting, generalized weakness, changes in mental status, and severe dehydration. Hypertension may be present and should be differentiated from preeclampsia. The serum calcium is frequently over 14 mg/dl; hypokalemia and elevation in serum creatinine are routinely seen. If not recognized and treated promptly, hyperparathyroid crisis may progress to uremia, coma, and death. Of the 12 cases reported in the literature, 4 occurred in the postpartum period. Patients presented with severe nausea, vomiting, and elevation in serum creatinine due to dehydration. Serum calcium levels over 20 mg/dl were reported in three cases,[106,121,122] and three patients died.[121,123,124] Six cases have been associated with pancreatitis. Four fetal deaths have also been reported.

Bone disease in patients with PHP is now unusual. However, in early series, it was a common complication.[111] Radiologic evaluation of the bones showed diffuse demineralization, subperiosteal resorption of the phalanges and, in severe cases, single or multiple cystic lesions and generalized osteoporosis. A 27-year-old woman was described with generalized musculoskeletal pain and radiographic evidence of advanced bone disease at 34 weeks' gestation.[125]

The two most common causes of neonatal morbidity are prematurity and neonatal hypocalcemia, the latter related to levels of maternal hypercalcemia. In early reports it was frequently the only clue of maternal hyperparathyroidism. It develops between the 2nd and 14th day of life and last for a few days.[108,111]

The diagnosis of PHP is based on persistent hypercalcemia in the presence of increased serum PTH levels.[126] A persistent serum calcium value over 9.5 mg/dl is suspicious of hypercalcemia. Serum phosphorus is decreased in about 50 percent of pregnant women with PHP. A determination of 24-hour urinary calcium excretion is helpful in the diagnosis, since most women with PHP have an increase in urinary calcium excretion, above the usual hypercalciuria of normal pregnancy. Urinary calcium excretion is low or low normal in the syndrome of familial hypocalciuric hypercalcemia (FHH), another cause of hypercalcemia that needs to be included in the differential diagnosis. The serum alka-

Causes of Hypercalcemia in Pregnancy and the Puerperium

Primary hyperparathyroidism (most common)
Rare causes related to pregnancy
    Familial hypocalciuric hypercalcemia*
    Postpartum hypercalcemia in
      hypoparathyroidism
    PTHrP-induced hypercalcemia
Other causes not related to pregnancy
    Malignancy
    Endocrine
        Thyrotoxicosis
        Adrenal insufficiency
    Vitamin overdose
        Vitamin D
        Vitamin A
    Drugs
        Thiazide diuretics
        Lithium
    Granulomatous disease
        Sarcoidosis
        Tuberculosis
        Histoplasmosis
        Coccidioidomycosis
Milk alkali syndrome
Acute and chronic renal failure
Total parenteral nutrition

*Different expression with significant neonatal manifestations. From Mestman JH: Endocrine diseases in pregnancy. *In* Sciarra JJ (ed): Gynecology and Obstetrics. Philadelphia, Lippincott-Raven, 1997, p 11, with permission.

line phosphatase level may be increased in PHP. However, it is also increased in normal pregnancy. High-resolution ultrasonography of the neck is not useful, since it seldom differentiates a parathyroid lesion from thyroid nodular disease. Parathyroid imaging studies are contraindicated in pregnancy.

Differential Diagnosis of Hypercalcemia

Although most young women with hypercalcemia have PHP, other unusual causes should be ruled out, mainly endocrine disorders, vitamin D or A overdose, the use of thiazide diuretics, or granulomatous diseases (see the box "Causes of Hypercalcemia in Pregnancy and the Puerperium"). A brief discussion of three uncommon syndromes associated with hypercalcemia during pregnancy follows.

1. Familial hypocalciuric hypercalcemia (FHH) is an autosomal dominant condition with a high penetrance for hypercalcemia. The disorder is associated with an inactivating mutation in the gene for the calcium-sensor receptor.[127] The main function of the receptor is in the regulation of calcium balance via changes in the parathyroid and kidneys. Mild hypercalcemia, slight elevation in serum PTH, mild hypermagnesimia, and low urinary calcium excretion are the typical findings. There is moderate hyperplasia of the four parathyroid glands. Total parathyroidectomy is seldom indicated due to the benign course of the disease.[128] Infants born to mothers with FHH may present with different clinical manifestations. First, asymptomatic hypercalcemia can develop in an affected offspring if the mother is a carrier for FHH. In a second situation, severe neonatal hypocalcemia can occur in a mother with FHH syndrome. Although neonatal hypocalcemia could be severe, neonatal parathyroid function returns to normal a few weeks after delivery. In the third situation, severe neonatal hypercalcemia, also called neonatal severe hyperparathyroidism,[129] occurs in infants homozygous for the FHH gene defect. Some infants require parathyroidectomy soon after birth.

2. Postpartum hypercalcemia may occur in women with treated hypoparathyroidism.[130,131] The mechanism for hypercalcemia is not well understood. Nausea and vomiting develop a few days after delivery, dehydration ensues, and other manifestations of hypercalcemia develop, mainly mental changes. Serum calcium may be significantly elevated. Patients with treated hypoparathyroidism should be followed postpartum with serum calcium determinations, and vitamin D should be discontinued if hypercalcemia occurs. In severe cases, intravenous fluids and glucocorticoid therapy are required[132] (Fig. 33–1).

3. A few cases of hypercalcemia, mediated by PTHrP, during pregnancy and in the postpartum period have been reported.[133,134] In one case, hypercalcemia developed in two successive pregnancies. In the second pregnancy, serum PTHrP levels were elevated three times normal and the infant was born with mild hypercalcemia that returned to normal within 24 hours after delivery.[133] In the other case,[134] a 25-year-old woman had massive bilateral breast enlargement at 24 weeks' gestation. Her serum calcium level was 14.3 mg/dl, but her serum PTH level was undetectable. She underwent bilateral mastectomy during pregnancy. The immunohistochemical studies demonstrated PTHrP antigenic activity in breast tissue.

Therapy

Surgery is the only effective treatment for PHP. A novel oral agent that acts directly on the calcium sensor is being investigated. It has not been approved for clinical use.[135] Surgery is a safe procedure when performed by a surgeon with extensive experience in neck surgery.

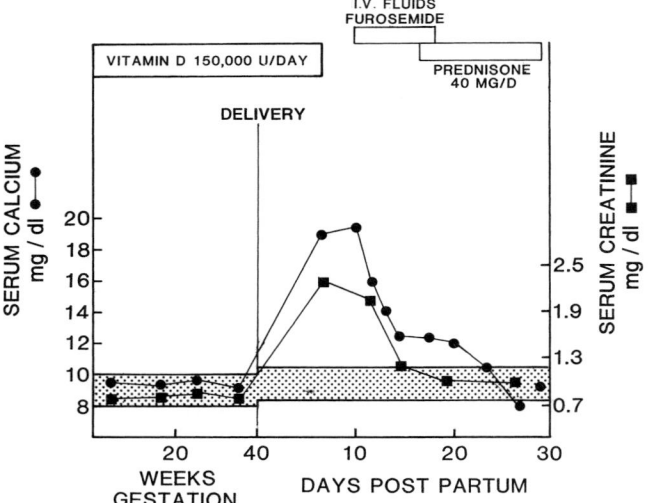

Figure 33–1. Serum calcium (*closed circles*) and creatinine (*closed squares*) levels during pregnancy and 1 month after delivery in a woman with hypoparathyroidism who was treated with vitamin D and calcium. IV, intravenously administered; stippled area, normal range.

Complications due to surgery, particularly in the presence of a single lesion, are low and the cure rate is excellent. In nonpregnant individuals without symptoms or complications and with a serum calcium below 12 mg/dl, the conservative approach is an alternative therapeutic choice.

Guidelines for the management of PHP in nonpregnant individuals have been suggested.[136] The proper management of PHP in pregnancy has not been uniformly agreed upon. For asymptomatic pregnant women in whom serum calcium is below 11 mg/dl, close follow-up with proper hydration and avoidance of medications that could elevate calcium such as thiazide diuretics is reasonable, although there are no studies in the literature supporting this or any other approach. Since most of the neonatal complications have been reported in patients with symptomatic disease, a surgical approach is indicated in these patients, as well as those with complications such as nephrolithiasis and bone disease and those with persistent hypercalcemia (>11 mg/dl). It is preferable to perform the surgery in the second trimester of pregnancy. In the series reported by Carella and Gossain,[116] 38 women underwent parathyroidectomy during pregnancy, 7 during the first trimester and the other 18 in the second trimester. In the total group of 25, there was only 1 fetal loss. In 12 women in whom surgery was performed during the third trimester of pregnancy, the incidence of perinatal complications was 58 percent.

For women with PHP first diagnosed after 28 weeks' gestation, the optimal treatment strategy is unclear, and the decision in such a situation should be based on general patient condition, severity of hypercalcemia, and other complicating circumstances.

Medical therapy is reserved for those patients with significant hypercalcemia that are not surgical candidates. Oral phosphate therapy of 1.5 to 2.5 g/day has been shown to be effective in controlling hypercalcemia.[137] Side effects of oral phosphate therapy include nausea, vomiting, and hypokalemia. These problems can be easily avoided by decreasing the dose of the medication. In patients in whom surgery is not advisable, it is important to prevent elevations in serum calcium. Good hydration, early treatment of urinary tract infections, and avoiding medications known to cause elevations in serum calcium such as vitamin D, vitamin A, aminophylline, and thiazide diuretics are all important. Serum calcium should be determined on a regular basis.

In patients undergoing surgical treatment, hypocalcemia, albeit transient, may occur after surgery in some cases. Serum calcium should be checked every 6 hours, and if the patient develops hypocalcemic symptoms, intravenous calcium in the form of calcium gluconate, 10 to 20 ml of a 10 percent solution, should be given over a period of 5 to 10 minutes. Intermittent infusions may be repeated or calcium gluconate can be diluted in 5 percent dextrose or isotonic saline and infused continuously at 1 mg/kg body weight per hour. In patients with bone disease, postsurgical hypocalcemia may be profound, and aggressive treatment is needed. These patients may benefit from vitamin D supplementation in the form of calcitriol 0.25 to 0.5 μg/day for a few days before operative intervention.[138]

Hypoparathyroidism

The most common etiology of hypoparathyroidism is damage to or removal of the parathyroid glands in the course of surgery for thyroid gland pathology. The incidence of permanent hypoparathyroidism following thyroid surgery has been estimated to be between 0.2 and 3.5 percent. In many cases, hypocalcemia in the immediate postoperative period is only transitory. Idiopathic hypoparathyroidism is a much less common cause of the disease, frequently associated with other autoimmune endocrinopathies, as part of the polyglandular autoimmune syndrome type 1. Antibodies directed against parathyroid calcium-sensing receptor have been detected in 56 percent of patients with idiopathic hypoparathyroidism.[139]

The requirement for calcium supplementation and vitamin D may decrease in some but not all women with hypoparathyroidism during the second half of pregnancy and lactation. In a few cases, hypocalcemic symptoms ameliorate with progression of pregnancy. The explanation for the above findings is not clear. It may be related to the increased intestinal absorption of calcium and/or the production of vitamin D by the placenta.

Clinical clues for the diagnosis of hypoparathyroidism include a previous history of thyroid surgery, and clinical, radiologic, and laboratory information. Typical symptoms of hypocalcemia are numbness and tingling of the fingers and toes and around the lips. Patients may complain of carpopedal spasm, laryngeal stridor, and dyspnea. Convulsions may be a manifestation of severe hypocalcemia. Symptoms of irritability, emotional lability, impairment of memory, and depression are common. On physical examination, patients with idiopathic hypoparathyroidism demonstrate changes in the teeth, skin, nails, and hair as well as papilledema and cataracts. Chvostek's sign, a twitch of the facial muscles, notably those of the upper lip, when a sharp tap is given over the facial nerve, is seen in many patients with hypocalcemia. Chvostek's sign has also been described in 10 percent of normal adults. Trousseau's sign is another sign of hypocalcemia. It is the induction of carpopedal spasm by reducing the circulation in the arm with a blood pressure cuff. The constriction should be maintained above the systolic blood pressure for 2 minutes before the test is considered negative.

The diagnosis of hypoparathyroidism is confirmed by the presence of persistent low serum calcium and high serum phosphate levels. Plasma alkaline phosphatase is usually normal. The differential diagnosis of hypocalcemia includes rickets, osteomalacia, and hypomagnesemia.

Marked hypocalcemia may occur in severely ill patients. The etiology is unclear, and a return to normal serum calcium is the rule following the recovery from the acute event.[140]

In 1942, Anderson and Musselman[141] published a review of the literature on hypoparathyroidism and tetany in pregnancy, collecting 240 cases. Twenty-six of the cases were due to postthyroid surgery, and 140 were the so-called idiopathic type. It is likely that in some of these cases tetany was not due to hypoparathyroidism. Therapeutic abortion was recommended because of the high fetal and maternal mortality. Other reports have confirmed that hypoparathyroidism, if not properly treated, may increase perinatal loss, including spontaneous abortions, stillbirths, and neonatal deaths.[142,143] Radiologic bone changes may be present in the newborn as a consequence of intrauterine hyperparathyroidism. They are characterized by generalized skeletal demineralization, subperiosteal bone resorption, bowing of the long bones, osteitis fibrosa cystica, and rib and limb deformities. Loughead et al.[144] described 16 infants of hypoparathyroid mothers. Secondary hyperparathyroidism in the infants resolved by 1 month of age.

Vitamin D deficiency in the mother has been associated with decreased fetal growth. Maternal serum calcium may be normal or slightly decreased. Brunvand et al.[145] followed 30 Pakistani women during pregnancy, 13 with elevated serum PTH levels at the time of delivery, and 29 with serum levels of 25-hydroxyvitamin D below normal. There was a positive correlation between serum maternal ionized calcium levels and the crown–heel length of the newborn. The authors suggested that vitamin D deficiency could interfere with fetal growth through an effect on maternal calcium homeostasis.

Treatment of hypoparathyroidism in pregnancy does not differ from the nonpregnant state, including a normal high-calcium diet and vitamin D supplementation. The normal calcium supplementation of pregnancy is about 1.2 g/day. Vitamin D requirements may decrease in some patients by the second half of gestation. Calcitriol 1 to 3 μg/day is used almost routinely in most patients affected with hypoparathyroidism.[132,146,147] Calcitriol must be given in single or divided doses, since its half-life is much shorter than vitamin D. If vitamin D is used, the dose is in the range of 50,000 to 150,000 IU/day. The importance of compliance with medications should be strongly emphasized, particularly when calcitriol is prescribed, in view of its short half-life. The major problem in the treatment of hypoparathyroidism is the recurrence of hypercalcemia and hypocalcemia. Therefore, serum calcium determinations should be performed at regular intervals. The most common symptoms of vitamin D intoxication are nausea, constipation, fatigue, headaches, and in more severe cases, vomiting and dehydration. It is important to assess serum calcium and phosphorous during pregnancy, particularly in the postpartum period, to detect the early onset of hypercalcemia (see above).[137,148]

Lactation in mothers taking vitamin D may be contraindicated, because a metabolite of vitamin D, 25-hydroxyvitamin D, has been detected in breast milk in high concentration in a mother taking 50,000 IU of vitamin D daily.[149] Regardless of the form of vitamin D prescribed, serum calcium determinations should be done in the postpartum period, particularly in breast-feeding mothers.

Pseudohypoparathyroidism

Pseudohypoparathyroidism encompasses several different disorders having as a common feature varying degrees of target organ resistance to PTH. Somatic changes are present in some forms of the syndrome, including short stature, obesity, round face, brachydactyly, and mental retardation, with brain calcifications. This variant is known as Albright's syndrome of type 1a. Most patients suffer from hypocalcemia, due to a derangement of renal 1α-hydroxylase and production of calcitriol. A few cases have been reported during pregnancy. Spontaneous normocalcemia occurred in two patients during four pregnancies. The authors provided evidence of placental synthesis of calcitriol to account for the normocalcemia. In both patients, serum PTH, which was significantly increased before pregnancy, was reduced by 50 percent during gestation. Serum cord calcium, phosphorus, and calcitriol concentrations were within normal limits.[150,151] These infants are at risk for intrauterine fetal hyperparathyroidism, perhaps because of the relative maternal hypocalcemia during pregnancy.[152]

Osteoporosis

The condition of idiopathic osteoporosis related to pregnancy was recognized in the 1950s.[153] In the last few years, there has been an increased interest in several clinical aspects of osteoporosis in pregnancy and lactation.[154-156] In general, osteoporosis is suspected in pregnancy when the patient presents with severe, persistent back or hip pain and radiologic examination shows signs of osteopenia. Studies measuring calcitrophic hormones and biochemical markers of bone reabsorption in each trimester in pregnancy and in the postpartum period showed a slight decrease in bone mass in the third trimester,[157] followed by recovery within the first 6 months postpartum. In a study of a group of white, upper middle class, postmenopausal women, there was no association between the number of pregnancies and lactation as predictors of decreased bone mineral density.[158]

Osteoporosis may be diagnosed during pregnancy or in the postpartum period. Whether these are two different syndromes or represent the same clinical entity is unclear, since the symptoms may begin during pregnancy, but the diagnosis is made for the first time after delivery. Osteoporosis diagnosed during pregnancy may be localized in the hip(s) or lumbar spine or both. Pain in one hip or back pain is the presenting symptom in most cases, usually in the second half of gestation. Spontaneous recovery is the usual course a few months postpartum.[159] A case has been reported of onset in the first trimester with recovery following abortion.[160]

Although osteoporosis has been diagnosed during pregnancy, pregnancy unmasks rather than causes low bone mass. As suggested by Rizzoli and Bonjour and others,[156,161,162] postural changes during pregnancy, including increased lordosis, when superimposed on a small and transient decrease in bone mass, may lead to pain and even fractures. In a study of 24 women with symptoms of bone pain for many years, 18 of them complained of back pain, 5 complained of hip pain, and 1 complained of ankle pain in late pregnancy or up to 8 months after delivery.[155] Radiologic examination of the spine showed vertebral deformities in 17. Bone mass was measured in 21, and 7 women had evidence of osteoporosis and 13 were osteopenic. The authors conclude that bone mass was probably low before pregnancy and that a transient and slight decrease in bone mass during pregnancy could have weakened the bone further. Radiologic examination of the localized painful

area and studies of bone density following delivery are indicated. In some cases, a short course of calcitonin or bisphosphonate therapy plus calcium supplementation may be needed.

The impact of lactation on the progression of osteoporosis is controversial. The study by Kritz-Silverstein et al. revealed that lactation by itself was not a determinant of bone mineral density.[158] Although one investigation reported that lactation for more than 8 months was associated with greater bone mineral at both the femoral neck and shaft,[163] another study found that nursing for longer than 9 months produced a greater decrease in bone mass than observed during the first 6- to 9-month period of nursing.[164] Given this controversy, the health care provider must decide if cessation of lactation is advisable in the management of osteoporosis.

Heparin-associated osteoporosis has been reported in several cases during pregnancy.[165] It may be related to the total dose of heparin. Treatment with calcium supplementation or calcitriol, although not proven, may be helpful in those patients receiving heparin therapy. Barbour et al.[166] followed 14 pregnant women requiring heparin therapy. Five of the 14 cases experienced a 10 percent decrease from baseline proximal femur bone density measurements as compared with none in a matched control group. They concluded that heparin adversely affected bone density in about one third of exposed patients.

ADRENAL DISEASES

Adrenal Gland Physiology

The adrenal gland secretes three main hormones: cortisol, aldosterone, and dehydroepiandrosterone (DHEA) and dehydroepiandrosterone-sulfate (DHEA-S) and some estrogen. Cortisol is present in the circulation bound to a specific binding protein, corticosteroid-binding globulin (CBG) or transcortin, bound to albumin, and in a free or biologically active form. In the nonpregnant woman, 70 to 80 percent is bound to CBG and only 10 to 15 percent remains in the free or unbound fraction. In pregnancy, there is an increase in plasma levels of CBG, and by the end of the third trimester the serum levels of CBG have doubled from prepregnancy levels. At the same time, there is an increase in free or unbound cortisol, its serum concentration increasing by the first trimester of gestation.[167,168]

Aldosterone is the most potent mineralocorticoid secreted by the adrenal cortex. The daily secretion rate in nonpregnant women is about 50 to 250 μg on a normal sodium intake. Its secretion is controlled by the renin-angiotensin system, by serum potassium levels, and to a lesser degree by ACTH. The aldosterone secretion rate and plasma concentration increase during pregnancy, with the first changes occurring as early as 2 weeks after conception.[169]

The adrenal cortex secretes hormones with weak androgenic properties: DHEA and DHEA-S. DHEA production rate is increased during pregnancy. It is aromatized to estradiol and estrone by the term placenta and contributes up to 9 percent of circulating estradiol.[170]

Cushing's Syndrome

Cushing's syndrome is a result of chronic tissue exposure to excessive amounts of glucocorticoids. Cushing's syndrome may be classified as ACTH dependent and ACTH nondependent (see the box "Classification of Cushing's Syndrome"). ACTH-dependent Cushing's syndrome is due to excessive or inappropriate secretion of ACTH by a pituitary tumor or hyperplasia, or by an ectopic tumor producing ACTH or ACTH-releasing hormone. ACTH-nondependent Cushing's syndrome is due to an intrinsic disorder of the adrenal gland, such as a benign or malignant tumor, or is iatrogenic, secondary to pharmacologic doses of glucocorticoids used in the treatment of systemic medical diseases. Women are nine times more likely than men to develop Cushing's syndrome, with a higher incidence between 20 and 40 years of age. In women of childbearing age, the most common cause of Cushing's syndrome is bilateral adrenal hyperplasia, accounting for 75 percent of all cases; 20 percent of cases are caused by an adrenal tumor, most commonly a single adenoma, whereas a few cases result from bilateral nodular adrenal hyperplasia and ectopic ACTH production. In pregnancy,

---

Classification of Cushing's Syndrome

ACTH dependent
    Chronic administration of ACTH
    Excessive production of pituitary ACTH
       (Cushing's disease) (Bilateral adrenal
       hyperplasia)
    Ectopic ACTH
Non-ACTH dependent
    Chronic administration of synthetic
       corticosteroids
    Adrenal adenoma
    Adrenal carcinoma

ACTH, adrenocorticotropic hormone.
From Mestman JH: Endocrine diseases in pregnancy. *In* Sciarra JJ (ed): Gynecology and Obstetrics. Philadelphia, Lippincott-Raven, 1997, p 15, with permission.

---

however, adrenal adenomas account for over 50 percent of Cushing's syndrome.[171-173] Adrenal carcinoma is rare, although it appears to be more common in pregnancy. Although ectopic ACTH syndrome is unusual in young women, an occasional case has been reported in pregnancy.[174]

Cushing's syndrome is characterized clinically by a protracted progression of symptoms, manifested by muscle weakness, personality changes, oligo- or amenorrhea, hirsutism, weight gain, and back pain due to osteoporosis. An increased incidence of thromboembolism also has been reported. One of the first common manifestations in women is oligomenorrhea, which progresses to amenorrhea; hence, pregnancy in women with Cushing's syndrome is unusual. Anovulation may be due to suppression of pituitary gonadotropin by high levels of glucocorticoids and/or high androgen levels.

On physical examination, hypertension, truncal obesity, fat deposition in the supraclavicular areas and upper dorsal spine areas (buffalo hump), moon face, atrophy of the skin that is easily bruised, and purple striae (over the abdomen, axillae, and hip areas) are common features. Weakness, due to muscular atrophy, can be marked, particularly in the quadriceps muscles, the patient being unable to rise from a deep knee bend without assistance. Headaches and visual field disturbances due to a large pituitary tumor are rare. Kidney stones due to hypercalciuria are reported to occur in 15 to 20 percent of patients. Hirsutism, sometimes of the lanugo type, is common. The severity of virilization depends on the amount of androgen produced by the adrenal lesion. In patients with an adrenal adenoma, the secretion of androgens is low, whereas it is moderately high in patients with bilateral adrenal hyperplasia. Masculinization is rare and when it occurs is due to an adrenal carcinoma producing large amounts of androgens.

An increase in hematocrit, leukocytosis with relative lymphopenia, and eosinopenia are usually seen. An abnormal glucose tolerance test has been reported in over 50 percent of patients, and frank diabetes in 20 to 30 percent. Mild hypokalemia with metabolic alkalosis is common. Radiologic examination of the chest may show an enlarged mediastinum secondary to fat deposition. Osteoporosis is also observed.

The clinical diagnosis may present difficulty during pregnancy because characteristically similar striae, weight gain, and hypertension are seen in both conditions.[175] Comparisons of close-up photographs from earlier years are helpful in detecting subtle changes. Some clinical features such as severe hypertension in the second trimester, significant hyperglycemia, mental changes, and muscle weakness may alert the physician to this rare disorder. Proper use and interpretation of tests assessing the hypothalamic-pituitary-adrenal axis function confirm the diagnosis.

A persistent elevation in urinary-free cortisol is the best indicator of excessive production by the adrenal gland(s). It should be kept in mind, however, that a slight elevation does occur in normal pregnancy. Mean urinary free cortisol levels of 127 μg/day (range, 68 to 252μg/day) as compared with nonpregnant levels of 37 μg/day (range, 11 to 83) have been reported in pregnancy.[176] Plasma cortisol increases three fold from the first to the third trimester of pregnancy, and random determinations of plasma cortisol are of little help in establishing this diagnosis, because values are normal in many patients with Cushing's syndrome. Furthermore, plasma cortisol is normally elevated due to an increase in CBG. The overnight dexamethasone suppression test, although an excellent screening test in nonpregnant patients, is of limited value during gestation. Lack of diurnal variation of serum cortisol is suggestive of the disease, but in order to properly assess the result of the test, specimens should be obtained between 7 A.M. and 9 A.M. in the morning and late in the evening, preferably at midnight.[177] In view of the normal elevation in serum cortisol, the criteria for evening levels is a decrease to less than 50 percent of morning levels.[178,179]

In pregnancy, the determination of free cortisol in a 24-hour urine specimen is the best screening test to rule out Cushing's syndrome. At least two collections of 24 hours are needed before proceeding to further diagnostic tests. Concomitant determination of urinary creatinine is necessary to ensure a complete urine collection. Once the diagnosis of Cushing's syndrome is confirmed, the etiology should be investigated. As noted above, the most common causes in pregnancy are adrenal hyperplasia and adrenal adenomas.

Plasma ACTH levels are helpful when interpreted in the light of urinary cortisol values. They are better if obtained in early morning (7 to 9 A.M.). A high-normal or elevated value in the presence of high urinary cortisol is suggestive of ACTH-dependent Cushing's syndrome (Cushing's disease). Low ACTH values are consistent with a unilateral adrenal tumor.

Further delineation of the pathologic cause is carried out with the use of the dexamethasone suppression test. Urinary cortisol is measured prior to and during 2 days, first with a small dose (0.5 mg every 6 hours) and then with a high dose of oral dexamethasone (2 mg every 6 hours). In normal pregnancy, urinary cortisol is suppressed to less than 55 nmol/24 h.[172] Patients with Cushing's syndrome, regardless of the cause, fail to suppress urinary cortisol excretion with the small doses (0.5 mg every 6 hours). On the high-dose dexamethasone regimen, patients with bilateral adrenal hyperplasia show a 50 percent or greater fall in urinary free cortisol, whereas there is no suppression in those patients with an adrenal tumor.

Intravenous administration of corticotropin-releasing hormone (CRH) with the determination of plasma ACTH and cortisol is used as an adjunctive test in establishing the etiology of Cushing's syndrome.[180,181] Plasma ACTH does not increase following the administration of CRH when the cause is an adrenal tumor or ectopic ACTH production. An increase in plasma ACTH of greater than 50 percent or serum cortisol of greater than 20 percent from baseline values has a 95 percent specificity and almost 90 percent sensitivity in the diagnosis of Cushing's disease.

In cases in which the diagnosis is not confirmed by the above tests, or when more specific localization of the pituitary lesion is desired in preparation for surgery, inferior petrosal sinus blood sampling is obtained for measuring both cortisol and ACTH. Venous blood is obtained by catheterization through the femoral vein. Comparison of central versus peripheral levels of ACTH allows for the separation between an ectopic source of ACTH from a pituitary lesion. In pregnancy, the jugular vein has been used instead of the femoral vein, in order to avoid excessive radiation exposure to the fetus. Although the procedure was successful in confirming the pituitary origin of Cushing's disease, it did not localize the site of the lesion.[182]

Once the diagnosis of Cushing's syndrome is confirmed by these hormonal tests, imaging of the pituitary or adrenal gland will demonstrate the presence of a lesion in the majority of cases. In pregnancy, MRI is the preferred method of imaging for both the adrenal and pituitary glands, because of the lack of radiation exposure for the fetus. In patients with Cushing's disease, MRI of the pituitary gland may identify a tumor or diffuse hyperplasia, diagnoses sometimes difficult to confirm because of the enlargement of the pituitary gland occurring during normal pregnancy. Imaging by itself without the validation of biochemical tests should be discouraged, since nonfunctional tumors or "incidentalomas" have been reported in at least 10 percent of a so-called normal population.[183,184]

Cushing's syndrome, itself an uncommon disorder, is rarely seen during pregnancy. Just over 100 cases have been reported in the English literature, most of them isolated reports. Several reviews have been published.[171–173] During pregnancy or in the postpartum period, spontaneous exacerbation[185–187] or amelioration[188–191] of symptoms have been described. Wallace et al.[192] presented a patient with recurrent Cushing's syndrome in three successive pregnancies. In this woman with "pregnancy induced Cushing's syndrome," hormonal and clinical features normalized postpartum. There was a lack of urinary cortisol suppression with the administration of dexamethasone. Although the authors were unable to detect any direct adrenal stimulation in vitro and in vivo from extracts of the placenta or maternal serum, the clinical course is suggestive of a stimulator originating in the fetoplacental unit. Estrogen-dependent nodular adrenal hyperplasia was the apparent cause in one woman. In another report with spontaneous resolution after delivery, the presence of gastric inhibitory polypeptide receptors was the cause of ACTH-independent Cushing's syndrome.[193]

Maternal and perinatal morbidity and mortality are significant in Cushing's syndrome. Arterial hypertension occurs in over 70 percent of cases,[171] overt diabetes in 30 percent, preeclampsia in 7 percent, and congestive heart failure in 7 percent. Maternal death has been reported in 4 percent of cases due to congestive heart failure in the postpartum period and sepsis.[174,194] Fetal wastage, including abortions, stillbirths, and neonatal deaths, approaches 30 percent. Prematurity has been reported in 52 percent of infants and intrauterine growth restriction in 25 percent.

The modality of treatment depends on the severity of the disease, the etiology, the gestational age at the time of diagnosis, and a frank discussion of potential benefits and risks of therapy with the patient and her family. There is some evidence that treatment during pregnancy improves fetal outcome. Buescher[173] reviewed 105 pregnancies in women with Cushing's disease and confirmed the high incidence of prematurity and a perinatal mortality of 12.4 percent, equally divided between neonatal and intrauterine deaths. Comparing a subgroup of 32 patients treated during pregnancy against 73 untreated women, the perinatal mortality was 6.3 percent in the former and 15.1 percent in the untreated group. However, there was no difference in the incidence of premature birth or intrauterine growth restriction. In another series, the outcome of pregnancy was significantly better in patients who underwent a bilateral adrenalectomy for hyperplasia or unilateral adrenalectomy for adenoma during pregnancy.[195]

Transsphenoidal pituitary surgery has been performed in several patients during pregnancy.[182,197–200] In one case, surgery was done at 22 weeks' gestation, and the patient was delivered at 30 weeks' gestation because of severe hypertension.[198] In two other patients, transsphenoidal surgery was performed in the second trimester, with a healthy infant delivered at 38 weeks' gestation in one case[197] and an intrauterine death at 33 weeks of pregnancy in another.[182]

Drugs such as metyrapone and particularly ketoconazole are used to treat Cushing's syndrome when surgery has failed, while awaiting the effect of radiation therapy to the pituitary gland, or in preparation for surgery. These medications have shown beneficial effects in some pregnant patients.[175,191,193,196,200,201,203–205] Metyrapone acts primarily to inhibit steroid 11β-hydroxylation, thereby decreasing the secretion of cortisol by the adrenal glands. Its main use is as a diagnostic tool to assess ACTH reserve. In one case,[200] metyrapone in doses between 250 and 1,000 mg daily was given from 29 weeks' gestation until the spontaneous onset of la-

bor at 36 weeks' gestation. The patient improved, and fetal growth and well-being were satisfactory. The newborn showed no signs of adrenal insufficiency.

Several cases of Nelson's syndrome (pituitary tumor with skin pigmentation following bilateral adrenalectomy for Cushing's disease) have been reported during pregnancy with good infant outcome.[206,207] Because ACTH does not cross the placenta, the fetal adrenal glands are not affected.

In summary, the etiology and gestational age may determine management of Cushing's syndrome in pregnancy. In the first two trimesters, adrenal surgery is indicated in the presence of an adrenal tumor; if MRI localizes the lesion in the pituitary gland, transsphenoidal surgery may be attempted in specialized centers. For patients in the third trimester, or those in whom the source of hypercorticolism cannot be localized, drug therapy with ketoconazole or metyrapone should be considered. Drug therapy during embryogenesis, however, should be used with great caution in view of the possible teratogenicity of these drugs, particularly ketoconazole.

Addison's Disease

Addison's disease, or primary adrenal insufficiency, results from the total destruction of the adrenal cortex, with deficiency of glucocorticoids (cortisol), mineralocorticoid (aldosterone), and the weak androgen dehydroepiandrosterone. When adrenal insufficiency is caused by a deficiency of pituitary ACTH (secondary adrenal insufficiency), aldosterone and adrenal androgen secretions are preserved. Autoimmune disease is the most common cause of primary adrenal insufficiency, accounting for about 70 percent of all cases. Other causes include granulomatous diseases, particularly tuberculosis, surgical bilateral adrenalectomy for systemic diseases, bilateral metastatic carcinoma, bilateral adrenal bleeding during anticoagulant therapy, as well as fungal infections and acquired immunodeficiency syndrome (AIDS). Severe systemic infections by meningococcus (Waterhouse-Friderichsen syndrome) may present as acute adrenal insufficiency characterized by vascular collapse and petechial hemorrhage in the skin and mucosa.

Secondary adrenal insufficiency occurs as a result of pituitary insufficiency, mainly through chronic suppression of pituitary ACTH in patients receiving corticosteroid therapy for various periods of time. In this situation, symptoms of adrenal insufficiency are manifested during periods of stress. It takes an average of 8 months for the hypothalamic-ACTH-adrenal axis to recover completely following the discontinuation of corticosteroid therapy.[208]

The most common symptoms of chronic primary adrenal insufficiency are weakness, fatigue, nausea and eventually vomiting early on awakening, and weight loss. Characteristically, these patients feel relatively well in the morning and experience increased fatigue and asthenia during the progression of the day. Blood pressure is low, and patients may complain of postural hypotension. Although pigmentation of the skin and mucosa is characteristically described in Addison's disease, it is not seen in all patients. The pigmentation is seen in body creases, such as palms of the hands, knuckles, knees, and elbows; in scars; and in the genital, gingival margin, and buccal mucosa. Vitiligo may be found in 10 to 15 percent of patients with Addison's disease. These lesions have been ascribed to autoimmune destruction of the melanocyte and occur in hyperpigmented areas. Gonadal function is disturbed, and in women, axillary and pubic hair may be reduced because of lack of adrenal androgens. Adrenal crisis, a medical emergency, is characterized by severe hypotension, nausea, vomiting, diarrhea, and severe dehydration. Patients may present with elevated body temperature, although infection is not always demonstrated.

Laboratory findings typically include mild anemia, hyponatremia, hyperkalemia, and increased serum blood urea nitrogen. However, in a significant number of patients, serum electrolytes remain within normal limits. Hypercalcemia may be seen during the acute phase of adrenal insufficiency. Hypoglycemia presents in the fasting state and during adrenal crisis.

Lack of cortisol response to ACTH administration or elevated plasma ACTH levels in the presence of a low serum cortisol concentration, or both,[209] confirm the diagnosis. Baseline or random serum cortisol levels are low in most patients with Addison's disease. However, normal cortisol levels do not rule out the disease, as cortisol levels are normally elevated due to the increased CBG. In nonpregnant patients, a serum cortisol value of less than 3 μg/dl provides presumptive evidence of adrenal insufficiency, whereas a value of less than 10 μg/dl suggests the diagnosis.[210] Basal values for diagnosing adrenal insufficiency in pregnancy have not been established. The diagnosis of adrenal insufficiency must be confirmed by dynamic tests, namely, the serum cortisol response to the administration of ACTH. There are several ways to perform ACTH stimulation tests:

Short ACTH Stimulation Test: This is the simplest available test to rule out the presence of Addison's disease. It can be performed at any time of the day. For the test, synthetic ACTH (1–24) (cosyntropin), 0.25 μg, is given as a rapid intravenous bolus and plasma cortisol is measured before and 30, 60, and 120 minutes after cosyntropin administration.[211] A peak cortisol response of 18 μg/dl over the baseline values rules out Addison's disease and almost all cases of secondary adrenal insufficiency, the exception being recent onset of secondary adrenal failure. In these cases, a low-dose, 1-μg

cosyntropin intravenous dose may detect patients with a mild form of secondary adrenal insufficiency.[212] However, a suboptimal or complete lack of response to ACTH administration does not confirm the diagnosis, and a more prolonged ACTH stimulation test is needed.[213]

Long ACTH Stimulation Test: There are several modifications of the original test; ACTH in the form of cosyntropin, 0.25 mg in 500 ml 5 percent dextrose in normal saline is given every 12 hours for 48 hours, and serum cortisol is measured before and every 12 hours. A serum plasma cortisol of over 30 μg/dl rules out the presence of primary adrenal insufficiency. To prevent acute adrenal crisis in symptomatic patients, dexamethasone, 0.5 mg, is added to the continuous ACTH infusion. In patients already on glucocorticoid replacement therapy, dexamethasone is substituted at least 24 hours before and during the test. This dose of corticosteroid does not interfere with the determination of serum cortisol and provides enough glucocorticoid activity to correct the patient's symptoms. The 48-hour continuous ACTH infusion can accurately distinguish between primary and secondary adrenal insufficiency. With the former, there is no increase in cortisol values; in the latter situation, serum cortisol levels increase after the first 24 hours of the test.

Plasma ACTH Determination: High serum ACTH and low cortisol levels are the hallmark of primary adrenal insufficiency. Normal ACTH values early in the morning are between 20 and 150 pg/ml. Baseline cortisol values less than 10 μg/dl and ACTH levels of greater than 250 pg/ml are diagnostic of primary adrenal insufficiency.

Patients with primary adrenal insufficiency require treatment for the remainder of their lives with occasional exceptions. Cortisone or hydrocortisone is the treatment of choice, in doses of 15 to 30 mg/day, with two thirds of the dose being given in the morning and one third in the evening. In most patients, a mineralocorticoid is added in the form of fluorohydrocortisone; the dosage varies from 0.05 to 0.2 mg daily. Although cortisol is the natural hormone produced by the adrenal gland and is the drug of choice, other synthetic glucocorticoids may be used. Prednisone and prednisolone are less expensive and more available than cortisone, and either may be used in doses of 3 to 5 mg in the morning and 1 to 3 mg in the evening. Dexamethasone (Decadron) is not recommended, because of its prolonged action (more than 24 hours).

Patient education is imperative to prevent medical catastrophes. Patients should wear visible identification with their diagnosis, therapy, and physician phone number. They should know that their dosage of corticosteroids should be doubled in cases of moderate stress, and they should have available an injectable form of glucocorticoid in case of vomiting. Available injectable preparations include dexamethasone 4 mg/ml, or hydrocortisone 100 mg/ml, for intramuscular injections.

Adrenal crisis is a medical emergency requiring immediate treatment. Dehydration is treated with intravenous fluids in the form of normal saline and glucose; 100 mg of hydrocortisone should be injected as a bolus intravenously. An additional 200 mg should be given during the first 24 hours. Appropriate therapy for hypotension should be instituted. In most cases, infection is responsible, and a careful search for the cause of the acute crisis should be made.

In patients with known adrenal insufficiency or on corticosteroid therapy undergoing elective surgery, cortisol should be given in total doses of 200 to 300 mg during the day of surgery. Many regimens have been proposed for the management of patients. However, we recommend cortisol, 100 mg intravenously every 8 hours, in continuous infusion for the first 24 hours and then decreased by 50 mg/day until the patient is able to take oral medications. The infusion should be started early on the morning of surgery. In most cases, by the fourth or fifth postoperative day the patient is able to return to her routine preoperative daily dosage. Because the amount of cortisol administered has adequate mineralocorticoid action, no mineralocorticoid supplementation is needed during this time. Daily determinations of serum electrolytes and glucose should be obtained to rule out hypokalemia and hyperglycemia resulting from the high dose of glucocorticoids. It has also been suggested that an injection of cortisone acetate, 50 to 100 mg intramuscularly, be given the day before surgery. The same regimen is applied to patients having received corticosteroid therapy in the past and having discontinued it within the last 12 months. An additional scheme is to use cortisone acetate, 50 mg intramuscularly, every 6 hours for the first day, every 8 hours during the second day, and every 12 hours for the fourth day after a surgical procedure. During surgery, 100 mg of hydrocortisone is added to the intravenous solution.

Women with Addison's disease have few complications during pregnancy. Early reports have indicated no increase in miscarriage rate, prematurity, or intrauterine death.[214–216] The amount of glucocorticoid needed does not increase during pregnancy. The dose may actually be reduced as a result of the potentiation of hydrocortisone's biological action by estrogen.[26] The requirement for glucocorticoid increases during the stress of labor. A booster dose of hydrocortisone 100 mg or equivalent amounts of synthetic preparations are given at the beginning of labor (see Table 33–2). Mineralocorticoid requirements remain the same throughout pregnancy.

Acute adrenal insufficiency developing in pregnancy or the puerperium is rare, and in most cases is secondary to an acute deficiency of pituitary ACTH such as in the reported cases of pituitary lymphocytic hypophysitis or bleeding into a pituitary tumor. The classic presentation is protracted hypoglycemia resistant to glucose administration but responding to glucocorticoid administration.[14]

Neonatal adrenal insufficiency is rare in infants of mothers receiving corticosteroid therapy. In a review of 260 pregnancies during which steroids were given to the mother for variable periods, only one infant was believed to have adrenal corticosteroid insufficiency.[217]

Congenital Adrenal Hyperplasia

Congenital adrenal hyperplasia (CAH)[218] is a hereditary disorder involving both adrenal glands. It is produced by a number of defects of corticosteroid biosynthesis that result in reduced production of cortisol, a secondary increase in ACTH secretion, which is then responsible for adrenal hyperplasia and accumulation of hormonal precursors. Defects of several enzymes related to the cytochrome P-450 group of oxidases can produce different clinical pictures (Fig. 33–2).

The 21-hydroxylation defect (CYP21A2) is most common, with impaired conversion of 17-hydroxyprogesterone to 11-deoxycortisol. This abnormality is found in more than 90 percent of patients with CAH. It is transmitted as an autosomal recessive disorder involving a gene on the short arm of chromosome 6 and affects approximately 1 of every 14,200 live births.[219,220] In the Caucasian population, the incidence of the mild nonclassic forms of the disorder have been estimated to be between 1 in 100 to 1 in 1,000.[221,222] In Caucasian women with clinical evidence of excessive androgen production, the incidence is about 2 percent, and is even slightly higher in Jewish women of European origin.[223]

The clinical manifestations depend on the severity of the abnormality in the 21-hydroxylase genes. The two classic presentations of CYP21A2 deficiency are a simple virilizing form presenting as genital ambiguity, and a sodium-wasting form, recognized at the time of delivery or soon thereafter. In the former, the 21-hydroxylase enzymatic activity is low but detectable; while in the salt-wasting form there is no enzymatic activity. The third form of the disease, nonclassic or late-onset CYP21A2 deficiency, is mild and is detected in childhood or adulthood, with manifestations of hirsutism and menstrual irregularities. These patients have 20 to 60 percent of normal enzymatic activity.[224]

Female infants affected by the disease have pseudohermaphroditism, while affected males have normal sexual development. Clitoral enlargement, labial fusion, and formation of a urogenital sinus are due to the

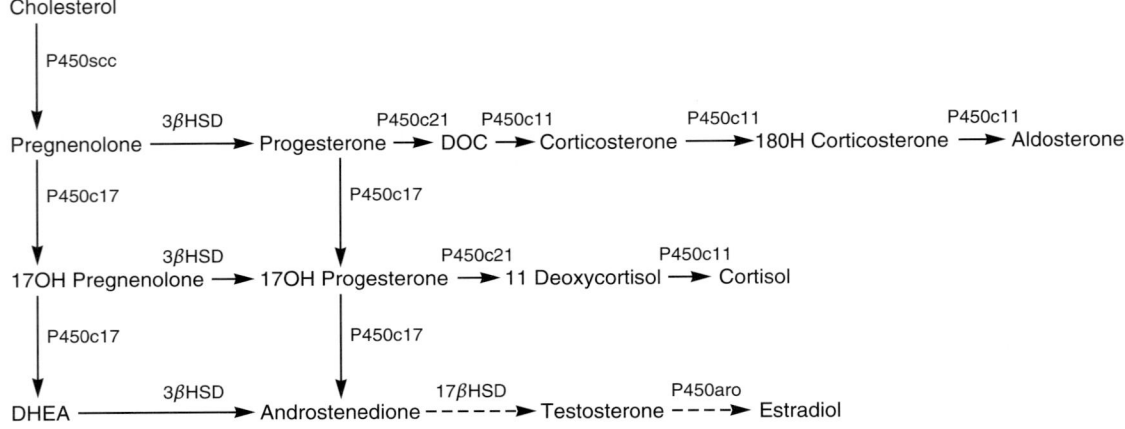

Figure 33–2. Adrenal steroid biosynthesis pathway.

effects of androgen excess in utero. Infants with the severe form of salt wasting, affecting more than two thirds of infants with this enzymatic defect, present with dehydration, hypovolemia, hypotension, hyponatremia, and hyperkalemia.

The diagnosis is based on the clinical picture and high serum 17-hydroxyprogesterone (17-OHP) levels. In addition, serum testosterone, progesterone, and DHEA-S levels are also elevated. In the salt-wasting type, low aldosterone and high renin levels are typically found. In patients with the nonclassic form or late-onset disease, serum 17-OHP levels are over 200 ng/dl in the basal state during the follicular phase of the menstrual cycle, and have an exaggerated response to the administration of ACTH, with values over 1,500 ng/dl.

Other types of defects include the 11β-hydroxylation (CYP11B1) deficiency and, more rarely, a defect of the 3β-hydroxysteroid-dehydrogenase enzyme.

The goal of treatment is to prevent adrenal insufficiency, to provide salt-retaining corticosteroids in cases of the salt-losing variety, to suppress androgen secretion to prevent virilization, and to normalize growth and later reproductive function. This is achieved with doses of hydrocortisone between 25 and 75 mg/day or 10 to 25 mg/m²/day, divided in two or three doses.[225] Dexamethasone with a longer half-life is preferred by some authors in doses of 0.25 to 0.75 mg/day.[226] Parameters of adequate glucocorticoid dosage are assessed by the determination of plasma 17-OHP, androstenedione (A), and testosterone (T); growth curve velocity; and the rate of skeletal maturation. Adult patients with the salt-losing variety also require mineralocorticoid therapy in the form of Florinef (fludrocortisone) 0.05 to 0.3 mg/day. The dose is adjusted to normalize plasma renin activity. The pediatric dose is 70 μg/m²/day. No adjustment is needed in pregnancy.[227] A free testosterone determination is the best test to assess glucocorticoid therapy during gestation.[227] However, the techniques for the determination of free

testosterone have not been universally refined at the present time. The fetal outcome may be normal. In spite of the lack of suppression of maternal androgens, placental aromatase activity has a protective effect not only on the fetal genitalia but also in preventing the effect of androgens on the fetal brain.[228]

Reproductive function may be impaired, particularly in those women with the salt-wasting form. The causes of a low rate of conception are multiple and have been discussed in a recent article.[229] In addition to anatomic vaginal problems, poor compliance with medications and other factors such as bisexuality or homosexuality, and decreased interest in sexual activity play an important role.

Klingensmith and co-workers[230] reported a group of 18 women, 10 years of age or older with CAH followed over many years. Initiation of menstruation was delayed in all of these patients when compared with the general population. Eight patients were treated for the first time after age 20 years, and none were able to conceive. Of 20 patients in whom treatment was started between ages 6 and 20 years, 64 percent who were sexually active had at least one pregnancy. For patients treated before age 6, the pregnancy rate was about 60 percent. The amount of cortisone needed was between 30 and 56 mg/m² in 24 hours, and the levels of urinary 17-ketosteroids were between 2.5 and 5.3 mg/day. All women were maintained during pregnancy on the prepregnancy dose of steroids. Of the 13 pregnancies, 9 were viable and only 1 resulted in an infant born with multiple congenital malformations. That mother had systemic lupus erythematosus and was treated with large doses of salicylate. All of the mothers underwent cesarean section, and there was only one case of a premature infant with mild residual cerebral palsy. No patient in this study had an infant with CAH. Overall, the fertility rate was low, and first-trimester abortions were common.[227,230–232]

Prenatal evaluation of the partner of a woman, who

has the disease or is a carrier, is needed to assess possible fetal risk. The partner has 1 to 6 percent chance of being a carrier of the disease. Determination of plasma 17-OHP at baseline and following the administration of ACTH allows the detection of the partner's heterozygous state in most cases.[218] Fetuses are considered "potentially affected" if (1) both parents are heterozygous, (2) both parents are homozygous, or (3) one parent is homozygous and the other heterozygous.

Prenatal diagnosis of CAH due to 21-hydroxylase deficiency is possible with detection of elevated amniotic fluid 17-OHP and adrenal androgen concentrations or with linkage analysis and HLA typing of cultured amniotic fluid cells. However, because these tests cannot be completed before 16 to 17 weeks' gestation, any preventive therapy should be given before the results of the tests become available, as masculinization of the female fetus occurs between 10 and 16 weeks' gestation.[233]

Chorionic villus biopsy at 8 to 10 weeks' gestation allows the earliest and most accurate prenatal diagnosis.[219] Early treatment, as soon as pregnancy is recognized, may prevent the development of masculinization of external genitalia in the affected female fetus. Dexamethasone is the drug of choice, since it crosses the placenta most readily and suppresses fetal adrenal androgen synthesis, reducing masculinization. Potentially affected mothers should be treated until fetal sex is known. Overall, this treatment is effective in about two thirds of patients.[234] The dose of dexamethasone is between 1.0 and 1.5 mg daily from early in pregnancy until delivery (20 μg/kg maternal weight). Maternal estriol levels are an accurate index of fetal adrenal function and genital development,[235] while amniotic fluid steroid levels have shown an inconsistent correlation with fetal masculinization. Pang et al.[236] reported maternal side effects of this therapy including cushingoid facial features; facial hirsutism; excessive weight gain; and permanent striae, hypertension, and gestational diabetes. The authors recommend that patients be made aware of potential side effects, that women receiving this treatment be closely monitored, and that the dose of dexamethasone be reduced during the second half of pregnancy, to reduce side effects.

Follow-up of 84 newborns whose mothers were treated with dexamethasone showed normal birth weight, birth length, and head circumference compared with untreated fetuses. In 43 neonates of mothers treated with dexamethasone,[237] 15 had congenital adrenal hyperplasia and 28 were unaffected. Five unaffected and three affected had postnatal failure to thrive and psychomotor developmental delay.

11 β-Hydroxylase (CYP11B1) deficiency is common in the Middle East, but rare in European populations, with a rate of only in 100,000 live births. It accounts for 8 percent of all cases of CAH.[238] The production of cortisol is reduced, with an excessive production of 11-deoxycortisol, 11-deoxycorticosterone, and adrenal androgens.[218] It is transmitted as an autosomal recessive disorder, caused by mutations of the CYP11B1 gene on the long arm of chromosome 8. The clinical manifestations may be present at birth, in children, or as a late-onset form.[239]

In the neonate, ambiguous genitalia in the female and penile enlargement are the clinical presentations.[240] In childhood, the disease may present as sexual precocity, early puberty in boys, or acne in men. Hirsutism, acne, and menstrual irregularities are the manifestations in puberty or young women. Hypertension and hypokalemia are the most common form of presentation along with virilization. The diagnosis may be made for the first time in adolescence or adulthood, when the patient presents with infertility, or oligomenorrhea, hirsutism, and short stature. Hypertension in the late-onset form is uncommon.

Laboratory findings include high serum levels of 11-deoxycortisol, 11-deoxycorticosterone, DHEA-S, androstenedione, and testosterone. In the late-onset form of the disease, ACTH stimulation is needed, since in most cases basal serum levels of 11-deoxycortisol are within normal limits.

Treatment with glucocorticoid normalizes infertility, and successful pregnancies have been reported.[241] Prenatal treatment may be effective in preventing the development of ambiguous genitalia. In one case, dexamethasone in doses of 20 μg/kg/day was started in the fifth week of gestation in a woman with two previous daughters affected by CYP11B1 deficiency. At 10 weeks' gestation, karyotyping by chorionic villus sampling showed the fetus to be female, and treatment was continued throughout pregnancy. The newborn female was normal without evidence of abnormal external genitalia.[242]

Primary Aldosteronism

Described by Conn in 1955, hypertension and hypokalemia due to excessive production of aldosterone by the adrenal gland(s) characterizes primary aldosteronism.[243] A single adrenal adenoma is the most common etiology, accounting for over 70 percent of cases: 20 to 30 percent of patients suffer from bilateral adrenal hyperplasia or multiple microadenomas.

Primary hyperaldosteronism is an uncommon cause of hypertension representing less than 0.5 percent of all etiologies. Serum potassium is decreased in more than 90 percent of the cases. Headaches and muscle weakness are frequently present. Severe hypokalemia may produce polyuria and nocturia resistant to the action of vasopressin.

Metabolic alkalosis with hypochloremia, an elevation in serum bicarbonate, and a serum sodium at the upper limits of normal are commonly seen. Urinary potassium excretion is elevated and inappropriate to the serum potassium levels. Renal function is within normal limits, and the pH of the urine is neutral or alkaline.

The diagnosis is suspected in those patients having hypertension and hypokalemia. All other causes of hypokalemia, particularly ingestion of diuretics, must be ruled out. High levels of urinary potassium in the presence of hypokalemia are very suggestive of primary hyperaldosteronism. The diagnosis is confirmed by (1) an elevation in serum or urinary aldosterone, (2) suppressed levels of plasma renin, (3) lack of plasma renin elevation with the administration of a potent diuretic such as furosemide or in the upright posture, and (4) failure of serum aldosterone level to be suppressed by the administration of 200 μg of 9α-fludrocortisone twice a day for 3 days.[244] It is important to normalize serum potassium levels before performing the above tests.

In pregnant patients with primary aldosteronism, the excretion of urinary potassium is lower than in nonpregnant patients with this disorder. The increased levels of progesterone in the pregnant patient blocks the action of aldosterone. In normal pregnancies, there is an increase in aldosterone secretion and plasma aldosterone levels, with a peak at 36 weeks' gestation at levels eightfold to tenfold higher than in nonpregnant women. This elevation in plasma aldosterone is normally suppressed in pregnancy by administration of 9α-fludrocortisone.[245] Plasma renin levels increase early in gestation, reaching a peak at 12 weeks and then remain elevated throughout pregnancy.

Few cases of primary hyperaldosteronism have been reported in pregnancy. Aldosterone levels were elevated, and plasma renin was suppressed.[246–252] Spontaneous remission occurred in one woman during pregnancy.[247] A case of unexplained virilization in the fetus has been reported.[248]

Treatment is based on the cause of aldosteronism. An MRI scan of the abdomen is effective in localizing the adrenal lesion. In most cases reported in pregnancy, a single adrenal tumor was the etiology, making adrenalectomy the treatment of choice. Several cases have been reported in which adrenalectomy was performed in the second trimester. In cases of bilateral adrenal hyperplasia, medical treatment with spironolactone is effective.[252] However, their use in pregnancy is not recommended, since this drug may cause feminization of a male fetus. Oral medications, with the exception of spirolactone, are not effective in controlling hypertension or reversing hypokalemia. Calcium channel blockers may have a place in these difficult cases.[253]

Pheochromocytoma

Pheochromocytoma is a rare syndrome accounting for about 0.5 percent of all cases of newly diagnosed hypertension. It occurs with equal frequency in both sexes and is more common in the third and fourth decades of life. A single adrenal adenoma is the cause in 80 percent of all cases. Approximately 15 percent are multiple adenomas, and 10 to 12 percent are malignant. In patients with a strong family history of pheochromocytoma, involvement of both adrenals is commonly seen, associated with the syndrome of multiple endocrine neoplasia type II (MEN types IIa and IIb), with Von Hippel-Lindau syndrome, in association with medullary carcinoma of the thyroid and in association with parathyroid adenoma (Sipple's syndrome). Five percent of patients with neurofibromatosis are also affected with pheochromocytoma.[254] In fewer than 10 percent of cases, the chromaffin tumors initiate from outside the adrenal gland in the organ of Zuckerkandl[255] and the bladder wall[256]; they are known as paragangliomas.

The classic symptoms of pheochromocytoma are episodic headaches, sweating, and tachycardia. Hypertension may be persistent or paroxysmal; in about half of patients, arterial hypertension is paroxysmal. Other common symptoms include nervousness, tremor, weakness, psychiatric disorders, anxiety, abdominal pain, and warm flashes. Weight loss is seen in some patients, with symptoms suggesting hyperthyroidism. Indeed, in the past, when basal metabolic rate (BMR) was determined as a diagnostic test for hyperthyroidism, it was frequently elevated in patients with a pheochromocytoma. In pregnancy, itself a normal hypermetabolic state, many of the symptoms of pheochromocytoma may be confused with those of a normal gestation. This disorder may present a real diagnostic challenge to the physician.[257] Induction of anesthesia, examination of the abdomen, or changes in the patient's position can precipitate paroxysmal attacks.

As with many other endocrine diseases, pheochromocytoma associated with pregnancy is uncommon. However, when present it poses a life-threatening situation for mother and fetus. In 1969, Fox and co-workers[258] described one case and reviewed 89 others published in the literature. In 1982, Schenker and Granat[259] reviewed 112 pregnancies in 89 patients with pheochromocytoma. In 22, the diagnosis was made for the first time during pregnancy. Both of these articles emphasized the poor prognosis for mother and fetus. The maternal mortality rate was 48 percent and the fetal mortality rate 54 percent when the disease remained undiagnosed during pregnancy. Most of the maternal mortality occurred within 72 hours after delivery. The causes of maternal death included cerebrovascular accidents, cardiac arrhythmia, shock, and acute pulmonary edema. Only 1 of 26 patients died when the diagnosis was made before delivery. In 17 cases, the symptoms remitted between pregnancies, and in two thirds of all cases it occurred in multiparous women. Hypertension, paroxysmal or sustained, was present in 82 percent of the patients, headaches in 66 percent, palpitations in 17

Table 33–4. SYMPTOMS OF PHEOCHROMOCYTOMA IN PREGNANCY

Symptom	Cases, (%)
Hypertension	90
Headaches	70
Palpitations	40
Sweating	35
Anxiety	30
Blurred vision	20
Convulsions	10
Dyspnea	10

From Mestman JH: Endocrine diseases in pregnancy. *In* Sciarra JJ (ed): Gynecology and Obstetrics. Philadelphia, Lippincott-Raven, 1997, p 24, with permission.

percent, anxiety in 15 percent, and convulsions in 10 percent. In several cases, sudden shock appeared spontaneously or was induced by anesthesia or vaginal delivery without previous symptoms (Table 33–4). Of 67 patients with pheochromocytoma in whom the disease remained undiagnosed during pregnancy, preeclampsia was diagnosed in 29 (43 percent) and essential hypertension in 11 (16.4 percent). Clues for the diagnosis are paroxysmal hypertension, diaphoresis, palpitations, a gestational age less than 20 weeks, significant blood pressure changes from supine to recumbent position, postural hypotension, and aggravation of the blood pressure in patients given β-blockers. The differential diagnosis from pregnancy-induced hypertension (PIH) could be difficult, particularly in the presence of proteinuria.

In 1989, fetal wastage was reviewed in 162 pregnancies.[260] Fetal loss was observed in 53 percent, spontaneous abortion in 12 percent, intrauterine death in 23 percent, and neonatal or intrapartum death in 18 percent. Both maternal and fetal morbidity and mortality have greatly improved in the last three decades, since therapy with α-adrenergic receptor blocking agents was routinely introduced in the management of the disease.

The demonstration of elevated levels of catecholamines or their metabolites norepinephrine and epinephrine, their methylated metabolites normetanephrine and metanephrine, and the methylated deaminated metabolite vanilly mandelic acid (VMA) confirms the diagnosis of pheochromocytoma. An elevation in VMA or metanephrines in a 24-hour urine specimen is suggestive of the diagnosis. Unfortunately, no one test is considered the best. Some authors prefer a determination of urinary metanephrine, since it is less likely to be altered by drugs or foods.[261] All abnormal values should be confirmed by a second 24-hour collection. The following recommendations have been suggested for the proper interpretation of urinary catecholamine and their metabolites:

1. Overnight or 24-hour urine collections are preferable to random ones. An overnight urine collection, however, has been reported to be as accurate as a 24-hour collection and is more convenient.[262] Urinary creatinine should be measured in each 24-hour collection to determine if the collection is complete.

2. It is preferable to collect the urine with the patient at rest, on no medications, and without recent exposure to radiographic contrast media. Among medications for hypertension, diuretics, adrenergic blocking agents, and hydralazine do not interfere with the assays appreciably.

3. Urine collection must be acidified (pH < 3.0) and kept cold during and after collection.

4. The diagnostic information is greater in patients with paroxysmal symptoms if a 24-hour collection is done when they experience the crisis.

Total urinary free catecholamines are elevated in most patients with pheochromocytoma. Normally, total catecholamine excretion is between 100 and 150 μg/day, similar to the nonpregnant state. However, it may be slightly elevated in preeclampsia[263] and also in stressed, working, normal, pregnant women.[264] Specific quantitation of epinephrine and norepinephrine may assist in the localization of a lesion. Increased epinephrine excretion in excess of 50 μg/day suggests an adrenal lesion. Excessive secretion of norepinephrine is suspicious, but not diagnostic of an extra-adrenal tumor. False-positive elevations may occur in patients taking methyldopa, labetalol, or aminophylline; undergoing strenuous exercise; or in the presence of increased intracranial pressure, hypoglycemia, or clonidine withdrawal.

Plasma levels of catecholamines may be measured, particularly during a paroxysmal episode. It is important to adhere strictly to the technique of blood collection. Values may fluctuate under routine stressful situations, such as exercise, venipuncture, or anxiety. It is recommended that the patient rest in the sitting position in a quiet environment for half an hour before blood is drawn. Blood is obtained through an indwelling catheter. The plasma should be centrifuged and the serum stored at −80°C until assayed.[265] A value above 2,000 pg/ml is diagnostic of pheochromocytoma.

In cases in which the diagnosis is in doubt, the clonidine suppression test may be used, with the caution that, in some cases, it may cause severe hypotension. For the test, 0.3 mg of oral clonidine is administered, with plasma catecholamine determinations before and 3 hours after. A normal response is a total catecholamine concentration of less than 500 pg/ml (3.0 nmol/L). Because of the risk of severe hypotension, the test should not be done in the presence of normal catecholamine concentrations, in patients taking other medications such as methyldopa, β-blockers, antidepressants, or diuretics, or in hypovolemic patients.[266]

As soon as the diagnosis is confirmed, α-adrenergic

blocking agents should be started.[267,268] The drug most frequently used is phenoxybenzamine (Dibenzyline). The starting dose is 10 mg daily, with increases of 10 mg every 2 to 3 days until blood pressure and symptoms are controlled. The usual blocking dose is 1.0 mg/kg body weight per day. The dose may require adjustment because the drug has a half-life of approximately 24 hours, and hence it is cumulative. The usual dose of phenoxybenzamine is 40 to 80 mg/day.[267] A 2-week course of an α-adrenergic receptor blocker is the cornerstone of preoperative management.[260]

β-Blockers are added to the regimen when tachycardia develops following administration of an α-adrenergic blocking agent.[254] Propranolol 10 mg 3 to 4 times a day is useful in maintaining the pulse rate between 80 and 100 beats/min.[269] Labetalol should not be used, since it has α and β-blocking properties in a ratio of 1:5. The danger of excess β-blockade with precipitation of a hypertensive crisis limits its usefulness.[269] Hypertensive crises are treated with intravenous phentolamine in doses of 1 to 5 mg. Intravenous therapy also may be used in cases of unstable hypertension in preparation for surgery.[270] A course of 10 and 14 days of α-blockade and β-adrenergic blockers is the usual therapy in preparation for surgery. Indicators of acceptable control include a blood pressure less than 165/90 mm Hg; orthostatic hypotension present, but with standing blood pressure greater than 90/45 mm Hg; no changes in the electrocardiogram (ECG) for the last 2 weeks (no ST-segment or T-wave abnormalities); and less than one premature ventricular contraction every 5 minutes.[271]

Surgical intervention is the treatment of choice. Tumor localization in 47 cases in pregnancy showed 25 percent of them in the right adrenal gland, 17 percent in the left, 17 percent bilateral, and 32 percent intraabdominal extra-adrenal.[260] Localization of the tumor is imperative and is achieved in most cases with modern radiologic techniques. In pregnancy, the use of the computed axial tomographic (CAT) scan, arteriography, and selected venous catheterization is contraindicated for obvious reasons. MRI is useful in localizing and diagnosing adrenal lesions and, in pregnancy, is the method of choice for localization of the tumor. The major advantages are lack of ionizing radiation, lack of contrast dye, and the ability to distinguish pheochromocytoma from other adrenal lesions with the high-intensity signal emitted in T2-weighted images. Ultrasonography is of little value; pressure exerted by the sonogram probe has been reported as the causative agent in a paroxysmal attack.[272]

When the diagnosis is made during the first trimester, elective termination of pregnancy followed by tumor excision is recommended by some, whereas others[264,273] recommend selective tumor resection without interruption of pregnancy. However, the incidence of spontaneous abortion occurring after surgery is high.

During the last two trimesters of pregnancy, medical treatment is preferred, with removal of the tumor at the time of delivery by cesarean section.[264,274] The best results are obtained when the pregnancy has advanced to viability, the fetus is delivered by cesarean section, and tumor exploration is done immediately after delivery. Cesarean section rather than vaginal delivery is strongly recommended as the safest procedure both for mother and for the fetus.[259] Fetal mortality has been reduced to 17 percent when the diagnosis was made in the first two trimesters of pregnancy. When the diagnosis is made in the third trimester, administration of an α-adrenergic blocking agent may eliminate fetal mortality, compared with fetal deaths of 42 percent in the group that did not receive α-adrenergic blocking agent. No maternal mortality has been reported in those patients treated with an α-adrenergic blocking agent.

Stenstrom and co-workers[275] reviewed 29 cases from the literature and added 3 of their own. In this series, the pheochromocytoma was diagnosed antepartum and treated with α-adrenergic receptor blockade. Fourteen patients underwent treatment of short duration, between 4 and 21 days, six underwent treatment from 46 to 91 days, and in nine cases the duration was unknown. The investigators recommended use of elective tumor resection in the first trimester, and medical treatment followed by cesarean section and tumor removal when the diagnosis was made after the first trimester. Fetal mortality in the treated cases was 19 percent compared with 50 percent in those without the benefit of α-adrenergic receptor blockade treatment. Laparoscopic adrenal surgery has been successful in pregnancy.[276,277] An anesthesiologist should be consulted and become closely involved in the management of patients with pheochromocytoma.[278,279]

Syndromes Due to Excessive Production of Androgens

Virilization in pregnancy is exceedingly rare (see the box "Causes of Fetal and Maternal Virilization in Pregnancy").[280,281] When signs of hyperandrogenism appear for the first time in pregnancy, a complete investigation is warranted because of the possibility, albeit low, of a malignant lesion as the cause of the excess androgen production. A medical history may reveal drugs responsible for hirsutism, the time of onset of the symptoms and signs, a similar history in previous pregnancies, the degree of virilization, and the presence of systemic symptoms. Virilization of the newborn does not always depend on the concentration of maternal androgens.

Drugs producing maternal hyperandrogenism, hirsutism, and even virilization in pregnancy, are those with the highest risk for fetal virilization. Progestins given before the 13th week of gestation for the treatment of habitual abortion has been responsible for labial fusion in a group of infants born to mothers treated with this drug[282] (see Chapter 9). Male fetuses are not affected.

Causes of Fetal and Maternal Virilization in Pregnancy

Drugs
  Dilantin
  Danazol*
  Progesterone
  Stilbestrol* (large doses)
Ovarian lesions
  Arrhenoblastomas*
  Luteoma of pregnancy*
  Krukenberg's tumor*
  Mucinous cystadenomas
  Leydig's cell tumor
  Lipoid cell tumor
  Granulosa–theca cell tumor
  Dermoid cysts
  Hyperreactio luteinalis
  Polycystic ovarian syndrome
Adrenal lesions
  Virilizing adenoma*
  Virilizing carcinoma*
  Aldosterone-producing tumor

*Lesions and drugs producing fetal virilization.
From Mestman JH: Endocrine diseases in pregnancy. *In* Sciarra JJ (ed): Gynecology and Obstetrics. Philadelphia, Lippincott-Raven, 1997, p 25, with permission.

Oral contraceptives or exposure to progestins after the completion of external genital development between 7 and 12 weeks of gestation do not produce virilization in the fetus.

The most common cause of hirsutism and virilization in pregnancy is a luteoma of pregnancy,[283–285] a benign human chorionic gonadotropin-dependent ovarian tumor that develops during pregnancy. It is a solid mass, consisting of hyperplastic lutein cells, is bilateral in 50 percent of cases, and is usually 6 to 10 cm in diameter. Luteomas disappear after delivery. Virilization occurs in about 25 to 40 percent of such patients due to high levels of testosterone and androstenedione. Patients develop hirsutism, acne, deepening of the voice, and clitoral enlargement, beginning early in the second trimester. Fetal virilization is seen in 65 percent of female newborns. Cord serum androgen concentrations have been measured in few infants.[285,286] Those born with virilization have higher concentrations of testosterone in cord blood. In the case reported by Thomas and co-workers, chorionic gonadotropin stimulation 8 months postpartum resulted in increased urinary excretion of 17-ketosteroids and ovarian enlargement in a patient with a history of virilization in prior pregnancies.[283]

The other common cause of hyperandrogenism in pregnancy is hyperractio luteinalis, an entity of benign hyperplastic luteinization of ovarian thecal cells believed to develop as the consequence of an abnormal ovarian response to human chorionic gonadotropin (hCG). The ovaries are involved bilaterally, with multiple amber-colored cysts. As in the case of luteomas, virilization regresses after delivery but may recur in future pregnancies.[287,288] Virilization has been reported in 25 percent of women. Serum testosterone and androstenedione concentrations are significantly elevated, but virilization has not been reported in the female fetus.[289]

Other causes of virilization are rare and are listed in the box "Causes of Fetal and Maternal Virilization in Pregnancy." A solid, unilateral lesion on ultrasound is suspicious of malignancy. The chances of malignancy in the presence of an ovarian tumor in a virilized woman are close to 50 percent. In such a case, laparotomy or laparoscopy should be considered.

An unusual case of maternal virilization due to placental aromatase deficiency has been reported.[290] The infant was virilized at birth.

THYROID DISEASES

Thyroid disorders in pregnancy present a unique opportunity for health care professionals to use a similar "team approach" that has successfully improved the care of diabetic women. Because of changes in thyroid economy occurring early in pregnancy, it is imperative to advise women with chronic thyroid diseases to plan their pregnancies and contact their health care professionals as soon as the diagnosis of pregnancy is made. Autoimmune thyroid disease occurs five to eight times more often in women than in men, and its course could be affected by the immunologic changes occurring in pregnancy and in the postpartum period.[291–293]

In early pregnancy, the maternal thyroid gland is challenged with an increased demand for thyroid hormone secretion, due mainly to three different factors: (1) the increase in thyroxine-binding globulin (TBG) due to the effect of estrogen on the liver, (2) the stimulatory effect of hCG on the TSH thyroid receptor, and (3) the supply of iodine available to the thyroid gland. This last factor is of importance in areas of iodine deficiency. In the United States, the iodine content in the diet, although decreased in the last decades, appears to be sufficient for pregnancy needs.[294] The normal thyroid gland is able to compensate for these demands by increasing the secretion of thyroid hormones and maintaining the serum levels of free hormones within normal limits. However, in those situations in which there is a subtle pathologic abnormality of the thyroid gland, such as chronic autoimmune thyroiditis, the normal increase in the production of thyroid hormones is not met. As a consequence, the pregnant woman could develop biochemical markers of hypothyroidism (i.e., an elevation in serum TSH, and an increase in the size of the thyroid gland).

Active secretion of thyroid hormones by the fetal thyroid gland commences at about 18 weeks' gestation, although iodine uptake occurs between 10 and 14 weeks.[297] Transfer of thyroxine from the mother to the embryo occurs from early pregnancy. Maternal thyroxine has been demonstrated in coelomic fluid at 6 weeks[298] and in the fetal brain at 9 weeks.[299] This maternal transfer continues until delivery, but only in significant amounts in the presence of fetal hypothyroidism.[300] Recently, thyroid hormone receptor gene expression has been shown in human fetal brain by 8 weeks' gestation, supporting the important role of maternal thyroid hormone during the first trimester of human pregnancy in fetal brain development.[301] Recent studies, that need to be confirmed, suggest that mild maternal thyroid deficiency in the first trimester could result in long-term neuropsychological damage to the offspring.[295,296]

The levels of maternal thyroid hormone concentrations, both total thyroxine (TT_4) and total triiodothyronine (TT_3) increase from early pregnancy as the result of an elevation in TBG and a reduced peripheral TBG degradation rate.[302] TBG reaches a plateau by 20 weeks' gestation and remains unchanged until delivery. In spite of these acute changes in total hormone concentration, the serum free fractions of both T_4 and T_3 remain within normal limits, unless there is a decreased supply of iodine to the mother or in the presence of abnormalities of the thyroid gland.[291]

Human chorionic gonadotropin is a weak thyroid stimulator, acting on the thyroid TSH receptor. It is estimated that a 10,000 IU/L increment in circulating hCG corresponds to a mean T_4 increment in serum of 0.1 ng/dl, and in turn to a lowering of TSH of 0.1 mU/L. In situations in which there is a high production of hCG, such as in cases of multiple pregnancies, hydatidiform mole, and hyperemesis gravidarum (HG), serum T_4 concentrations rise to levels seen in thyrotoxicosis with a transient suppression in serum TSH values. Low TSH values may be seen in 15 percent of uncomplicated pregnancies, returning to normal with progression of pregnancy.[303]

Thyroid Function Tests

In spite of the limitations in the interpretation of serum TSH in the first trimester, measurement of serum TSH is the most practical, simple, and economic screening test for thyroid dysfunction. A high TSH value is consistent with the diagnosis of primary hypothyroidism, whereas a suppressed one, with few exceptions, is suggestive of hyperthyroidism (Fig. 33–3). In the presence of an abnormal serum TSH value, the determination of FT_4 or its equivalent free thyroxine index (FT_4I), is obtained for the assessment of thyroid function. A low TSH value and high concentrations of FT_4 or FT_4I is diagnostic of hyperthyroidism. There are special situations in which hyperthyroidism may be present in the presence of normal concentrations of FT_4. In such cases, a serum FT_3 or FT_3I determination should be obtained. High values are diagnostic of hyperthyroid-

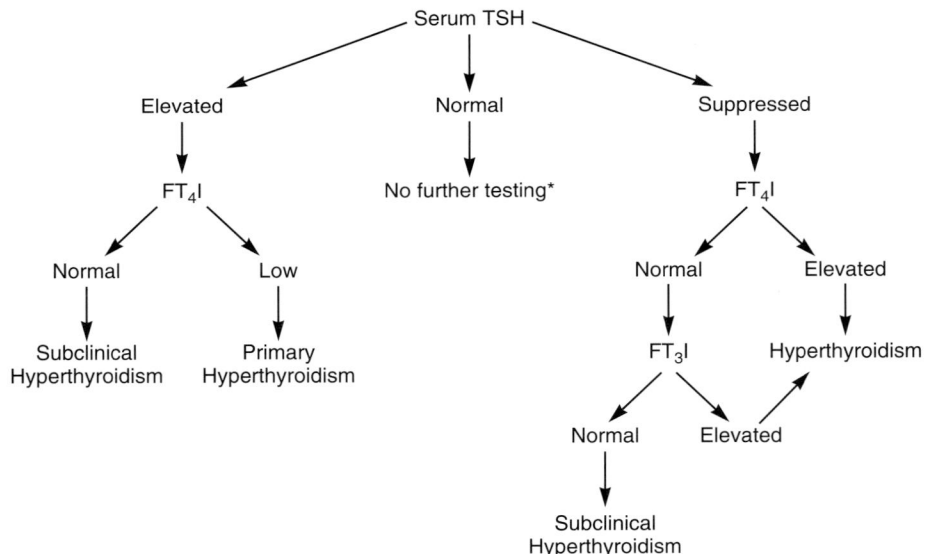

Figure 33–3. Algorithm for the diagnosis of thyroid disease. If there is clinical suspicion of secondary hypothyroidism, a determination of FT_4I is indicated. In this situation, the serum TSH is normal in the presence of low FT_4I. FT_4I, free thyroxine index or its equivalent, free thyroxine; FT_3I, free triiodothyronine index or its equivalent, free triiodothyronine; TSH, thyroid-stimulating hormone.

Indications for Maternal Determination of TSI or TRAb

Graves' disease (TSI)
  Fetal or neonatal hyperthyroidism in previous
    pregnancies
  Active disease, on treatment with antithyroid
    drugs
  Euthyroid, postablation, in the presence of:
    Fetal tachycardia
    Intrauterine growth restriction
    Incidental fetal goiter on ultrasound
Chronic thyroiditis without goiter (TRAb)
Incidental fetal goiter on ultrasound (TRAb)
Infant born with congenital hypothyroidism
  (TRAb)

TSI, TSH stimulating immunoglobulin; TRAb, TSH receptor antibodies.
From Mestman JH: Endocrine diseases in pregnancy. *In* Sciarra JJ (ed): Gynecology and Obstetrics. Philadelphia, Lippincott-Raven, 1997, p 27, with permission.

ism, the so-called T_3-toxicosis syndrome, sometimes seen in patients with an autonomous or "hot" thyroid nodule. Therefore, the use of a limited number of thyroid function tests (TFTs), properly ordered and interpreted, will allow the physician to assess thyroid function, and make the proper therapeutic decisions.[304]

The determination of TSH receptor antibodies (TSHRBAb or TRAb) is indicated in very special circumstances (see the box "Indications for Maternal Determination of TSI or TRAb"), in order to predict the possibility of fetal or neonatal thyroid dysfunction. These antibodies are immunoglobulins, usually of the IgG subclass, having different functional activity: stimulating (in most patients with Graves' disease) or blocking (in some patients with Hashimoto's thyroiditis, particularly in those without goiter) the TSH receptor of the thyroid gland. They do cross the placental barrier and may affect fetal thyroid function. The determination of TSHRAbs is commercially available using binding assays. These assays do not discriminate between stimulating or blocking antibodies. However, a specific bioassay is commercially available for the determination of stimulating antibodies (thyroid-stimulating immunoglobulins [TSIs]). Antibodies in the serum of patients with Graves' disease indicate a stimulating effect, and in the serum of patients with chronic or Hashimoto's thyroiditis suggest blocking or inhibitory effect. TSIs, formerly known as long-acting thyroid-stimulating antibody (LATS), when present in high concentrations in the maternal serum may cause fetal or neonatal hyperthyroidism.[305] Thyroid-blocking antibodies (TRBAb) in

high titers in the mother may produce neonatal hypothyroidism, a condition that is transient due to the short half-life of these antibodies.[306] Both antibodies may be present in patients with Graves' disease, and could explain the spontaneous improvement or aggravation of the disease with progression of pregnancy and in the postpartum period, respectively. The chances for the offspring to be affected by these maternal antibodies are very low (up to 2 percent of mothers with autoimmune thyroid disease). However, if mothers with high titers are not properly identified, the consequences for the infant could be irreversible neurologic and metabolic sequelae. Titers of these antibodies decrease with the progression of pregnancy. This could explain, in the case of Graves' disease, the tendency to spontaneous clinical improvement and the decrease in antithyroid drug requirement in the second half of pregnancy. A value of TSHRAb three to five times greater than normal is considered predictive of neonatal or fetal thyroid dysfunction.

Goiter is commonly seen in pregnancy in areas of iodine deficiency. However, in the United States and other areas of the world with sufficient iodine intake, the thyroid gland does not clinically increase in size during pregnancy. Therefore, the detection of a goiter in pregnancy is an abnormal finding that needs careful evaluation. The most common cause of diffuse goiter is chronic autoimmune thyroiditis or Hashimoto's thyroiditis. Most patients are euthyroid and the diagnosis is made by the determination of thyroid antibodies, mainly thyroid peroxidase (TPO). Antibody concentration decreases during pregnancy, and increases in the postpartum period. High values in the first trimester of pregnancy are predictors of the syndrome of postpartum thyroid dysfunction.[307]

The indications for requesting TFTs are represented

Indications for Thyroid Testing in Pregnancy

Family history of autoimmune thyroid disease
Women on thyroid therapy
Presence of goiter
Previous history of:
  High-dose neck radiation
  Therapy for hyperthyroidism
  Postpartum thyroid dysfunction
  Previous birth of an infant with thyroid disease
Type 1 diabetes mellitus

From Mestman JH: Thyroid diseases in pregnancy other than Graves' disease and postpartum thyroid dysfunction. Endocrinologist 9:924, 1999, with permission.

in the box "Indications for Thyroid Testing in Pregnancy." Whether routine thyroid screening in pregnant women is necessary remains a controversial issue, to be decided in the next few years, it is hoped, when more scientific information becomes available on the relationship of abnormal thyroid function early in pregnancy and neuropsychological and metabolic development of the offspring.

Prepregnancy Counseling

The physician may be faced with different clinical situations when counseling a woman contemplating pregnancy. With the advent of available information in the electronic media, it is important for the health care professional to offer the patient and her family objective and scientific data, supported by medical literature published in recognized peer-reviewed medical journals. The clinical situations may be summarized as follows:

1. *Hyperthyroidism under treatment:* A choice of the three classic therapeutic options for hyperthyroidism treatment should be given: (1) long-term antithyroid drug therapy, (2) radioactive ^{131}I ablation, and (3) near total thyroidectomy. Potential side effects of antithyroid drugs on the fetus should be discussed. If the patient opts for ablation therapy, there is no long-term effect of ^{131}I given to the future mother on the offspring. However, it its customary to wait 6 months after the therapeutic dose is administered before pregnancy is contemplated. Surgery is another option, selected by some physicians and patients concerned about the potential side effects of antithyroid drugs or radioactive treatment. Regardless of the form of therapy chosen, it is important for the patient to be euthyroid at the time of conception. In a large series of hyperthyroid pregnant women, a doubling in congenital malformations was reported when hyperthyroidism was not controlled in the first trimester of pregnancy as compared with women who were euthyroid early in gestation.[308]
2. *Previous ablation treatment for Graves' disease:* Two points are important: (1) the dose of thyroid replacement therapy needs to be increased in most women soon after conception[309,310]; and (2) in spite of euthyroidism, high maternal titers for TSI may be present, with the fetus being at risk of developing hyperthyroidism despite the mother being euthyroid.[311] Close follow-up during pregnancy and communication between the obstetrician and endocrinologist are essential.
3. *Previous treatment with ^{131}I for thyroid carcinoma:* Pregnancy does not affect the natural history of women previously treated for thyroid cancer. Spontaneous miscarriages have been reported to be as high as 40 percent in the first year after radiation treatment as compared with 18 percent in women who have received no radiation.[312] Therefore, it appears reasonable for patients with thyroid carcinoma to wait 1 year after completion of radioactive treatment before conception. Adjustment of the thyroid dose should be done early in pregnancy and in each trimester; serum TSH should be kept in the low normal range or undetectable.
4. *Treated hypothyroidism:* Women under treatment with thyroid hormone may require higher doses soon after conception.[309,310,313] As shown by Kaplan,[310] the amount of thyroid requirement increases according to the etiology of hypothyroidism. As soon as the diagnosis of pregnancy is made, thyroid tests should be performed, and thyroid doses adjusted accordingly. Following delivery, the dose should be reduced to prepregnancy levels. Common medications may affect the absorption of L-thyroxine, such as ferrous sulfate[314] and calcium,[315] among others. Patients should take L-thyroxine at least 2 hours apart from other medications.
5. *Euthyroid chronic thyroiditis:* Patients with Hashimoto's thyroiditis are at greater risk of spontaneous abortions and the development of postpartum thyroiditis.[316,317] Thyroid tests are indicated in early pregnancy to detect elevations in TSH and assess the need for treatment with thyroid hormones or to adjust the dose in patients already on thyroid therapy.

Maternal–Placental–Fetal Interactions

Studies in the last two decades have shown an important role of maternal thyroid hormones in embryogenesis.[318] It is accepted that maternal thyroxine crosses the placenta in the first half of pregnancy at the time when the fetal thyroid gland is not functional. Several studies have suggested an adverse effect on the intellectual development of children of mothers with mild thyroid deficiency in the first 20 weeks of gestation.[295,296]

Maternal TSH does not cross the placenta. TRH does cross the placental barrier, but its physiologic significance is unknown. TRH has been given to mothers to accelerate fetal lung maturation in premature infants.[319]

Methimazole (MM) and propylthiouracil (PTU), drugs used for the treatment of hyperthyroidism, cross the placenta, and if given in inappropriate doses may produce fetal goiter and hypothyroidism.[320] Preparations containing iodine given in large doses or for prolonged periods of time are contraindicated in pregnancy, since accumulation by the fetal thyroid may induce goiter and hypothyroidism.[321]

Hyperthyroidism

Hyperthyroidism is diagnosed in pregnancy in about 0.1 to 0.4 percent of patients.[322,323] Classically, it has been stated that Graves' disease is the most common

Etiologies of Hyperthyroidism in Pregnancy

Graves' disease
Nodular thyroid disease
Subacute thyroiditis
Iatrogenic
Hyperemesis gravidarum
Molar disease
Rare:
    Iodine induced
    TSH-producing pituitary tumor

cause of hyperthyroxinemia in pregnancy, with other etiologies being uncommon (see the box "Etiologies of Hyperthyroidism in Pregnancy"). As will be discussed subsequently, transient hyperthyroidism due to inappropriate secretion or action of hCG is becoming recognized as the most common cause of hyperthyroidism in pregnancy.[324,325] In our experience, single toxic adenoma and multinodular toxic goiter are found in less than 10 percent of cases. Subacute thyroiditis is rarely seen during gestation.

Transient Hyperthyroidism of Hyperemesis Gravidarum

This disorder is characterized by severe nausea and vomiting, with onset between 4 to 8 weeks' gestation, requiring frequent visits to the emergency room and sometimes repeated hospitalizations for intravenous hydration. Weight loss of at least 5 kg, ketonuria, abnormal liver function tests, and hypokalemia are common findings, depending on the severity of vomiting and dehydration. Free thyroxine levels are elevated, sometimes up to four to six times the normal values, whereas FT_3 is elevated in up to 40 percent of affected women, values not as high as serum FT_4. The T_3/T_4 ratio is less than 20, as compared with Graves hyperthyroidism, where the ratio is over 20. Serum TSH measured by a sensitive assay is consistently suppressed.[324-328] In spite of the significant biochemical hyperthyroidism, signs and symptoms of hypermetabolism are mild or absent. Patients may complain of mild palpitations and heat intolerance, but perspiration, proximal muscle weakness, and frequent bowel movements are rare. On physical examination, ophthalmopathy and goiter are absent, a mild tremor of the outstretched fingers is occasionally seen, and tachycardia may be present due in part to dehydration. Significant in the medical history is the lack of hyperthyroid symptoms before conception, since patients with Graves' disease diagnosed for the first time during gestation give the history of hypermetabolic symptoms several months be-

fore pregnancy. Spontaneous normalization of hyperthyroxinemia parallels the improvement in vomiting and weight gain, with most of the cases resolving spontaneously between 14 and 20 weeks' gestation, although persistence of hyperthyroidism beyond 20 weeks' gestation has been reported in 15 to 25 percent of cases.[326,327] Suppressed serum TSH may lag for a few more weeks after normalization of free thyroid hormone levels (Fig. 33–4). Antithyroid medications are not needed. In one series in which antithyroid medication was used, pregnancy outcome was not significantly different from a similar group of patients receiving no therapy.[326] Furthermore, a case has been reported in which normalization of serum thyroid levels with antithyroid medications did not resolve severe vomiting that was controlled only after first-trimester termination of pregnancy.[329] Occasionally, severe vomiting and hyperthyroidism may require parenteral nutrition.

The degree of thyroid abnormalities is directly related to the severity of vomiting and weight loss. In 67 patients studied by Goodwin et al.[324,330] liver and electrolyte abnormalities were routinely found in women with more symptomatology, including severe vomiting, weight loss of at least 5 kg, and significant dehydration. They also presented with more significant elevations in free thyroxine levels and suppression of serum TSH values. Those with a lesser degree of hyperemesis had a less severe disorder of thyroid function. Transient hyperthyroidism due to hyperemesis gravidarum should be suspected in women who present in the first few weeks after conception with the sudden onset of severe nausea and vomiting and thyroid tests in the hyperthyroid range. These patients do not complain of hypermetabolic symptoms antedating pregnancy, goiter is not detected by palpation, and symptoms or signs of tissue thyrotoxicosis are mild or absent. In addition, thyroid anti-TPO antibodies, markers of autoimmune thyroid disease, are negative. The differential diagnosis may also be difficult, as vomiting may also be a presenting symptom of hyperthyroidism of Graves' disease.[331]

The cause for the elevations of thyroid hormones in

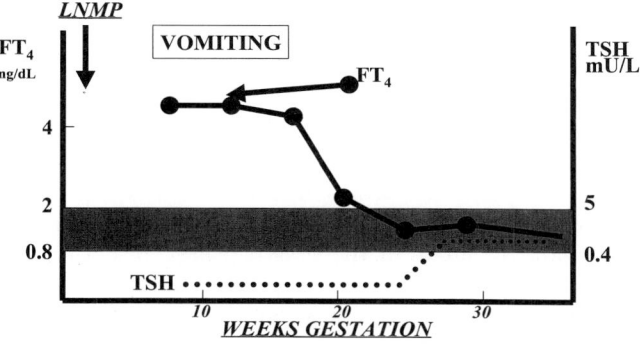

Figure 33–4. Clinical course of transient hyperthyroidism of hyperemesis gravidarum. LNMP, last normal menstrual period; FT_4, free thyroxine; TSH, thyroid-stimulating hormone.

patients with hyperemesis gravidarum remains controversial.[325,332] Most likely, high levels of hCG, a known stimulator of the TSH receptor, play an important role, as well as prolongation in its biologic activity as seen in twin pregnancies.[333] There is a significant, albeit weak correlation between the degree of thyroid stimulation and total hCG levels in normal women and those with hyperemesis.[330] It seems likely, however, that certain hCG fractions may be more important than the total hCG as thyroid simulators. The thyroid-stimulating activity of hCG in early pregnancy and in molar gestations correlates best with the percentage of basic, partially desialated hCG in serum.[325] A case has been reported in a mother and daughter with recurrent hyperemesis, in whom hCG levels were not elevated. Both were heterozygous for a missense mutation in the extracellular domain of the thyrotropin receptor. The mutant receptor was more sensitive than the wild-type receptor to hCG, thus accounting for the occurrence of hyperthyroidism despite the presence of normal hCG levels.[334]

The diagnosis of transient hyperthyroidism of hyperemesis gravidarum should be considered in women with severe vomiting, no clinical manifestations of Graves' disease, and biochemical evidence of hyperthyroidism in early pregnancy. Vomiting should be persistent and severe with a significant weight loss, since most women with morning sickness of pregnancy have normal thyroid function tests.[335] The syndrome may repeat in future pregnancies.

Gestational trophoblastic diseases, partial and complete hydatidiform moles, and choriocarcinoma are other causes of hyperthyroidism early in pregnancy.[334] Patients may present without symptoms in spite of chemical hyperthyroidism, or with various degrees of severity, including congestive heart failure. Evacuation of the mole eliminates the source of the excessive hCG and reverses the clinical and biochemical features of hyperthyroidism. Treatment with β-adrenergic blocking agents is effective in controlling the symptoms. Sodium iopanoate has been used to reduce the release of hormones by the thyroid gland and block peripheral conversion of T_4 to T_3.

Graves' Disease

The natural course of hyperthyroidism due to Graves' disease in pregnancy is characterized by an exacerbation of symptoms in the first trimester and during the postpartum period and an amelioration of symptoms in the second half of pregnancy. Stimulation of the thyroid gland by hCG in the first trimester has been suggested as the cause of exacerbation.[336] Immunologic responses caused by changes in lymphocyte subsets could explain spontaneous improvement in the second half of pregnancy and recurrences in the postpartum period.[337]

Table 33–5. POTENTIAL MATERNAL AND FETAL COMPLICATIONS IN UNCONTROLLED HYPERTHYROIDISM

Maternal	Fetal
Pregnancy-induced hypertension	Hyperthyroidism
Preterm delivery	Neonatal hyperthyroidism
Congestive heart failure	Intrauterine growth restriction
Thyroid storm	Small for gestational age
Miscarriage	Prematurity
Placental abruption	Stillbirth
Infection	

From Mestman JH: Hyperthyroidism in pregnancy. Endocrinol Metab Clin North Am 27:138, 1998, with permission.

Kung and Jones,[338] in a study comparing Graves' disease in pregnant and nonpregnant women, postulated that the amelioration of symptoms seen with progression of pregnancy was due to a decrease in the titers of TSHRAb with stimulating activity and an increase in TSHRBAb with thyroid-blocking activity. The reverse was true in the postpartum period, when aggravation of Graves' hyperthyroidism usually occurs.

When hyperthyroidism is properly managed throughout pregnancy, the outcome for mother and fetus is good; however, maternal and neonatal complications for untreated or poorly controlled mothers are significantly increased (Table 33–5).[339-342]

In the vast majority of patients in whom the diagnosis is made for the first time during pregnancy, hyperthyroid symptoms antedate conception. The clinical diagnosis of thyrotoxicosis may present difficulties during gestation, since many symptoms and signs are commonly seen in normal pregnancy, such as mild palpitations, heart rate between 90 and 100 beats/min, mild heat intolerance, shortness of breath on exercise, and warm skin. There are some clinical clues that increase the likelihood of the diagnosis of hyperthyroidism: presence of goiter, ophthalmopathy, proximal muscle weakness, tachycardia with a pulse rate over 100 beats/min, and weight loss or inability to gain weight in spite of a good appetite. Occasionally, the patient may be seen for the first time in congestive heart failure, and the etiologic diagnosis is difficult, since many of the physical findings are suggestive of cardiac valvular disease, particularly mitral insufficiency or stenosis. Hyperthyroidism under poor control is frequently complicated by preeclampsia. The physician should suspect hyperthyroidism in the presence of systolic hypertension with an inappropriately low diastolic blood pressure and a wide pulse pressure, also seen in other conditions such as aortic insufficiency.

Classic symptoms of hyperthyroidism include nervousness, increased sweating, increased appetite, heat intolerance, insomnia, proximal muscle weakness, irritability, changes in personality, frequent bowel movements, decreased tolerance to exercise (sometimes manifested as shortness of breath), eye irritation, frequent lacrimation, pruritus, and weight loss. Not all symptoms are present in a given patient. The physician should be aware of subtle complaints, particularly in the presence of weight loss or inability to gain weight. As mentioned above, in the first trimester of pregnancy the differential diagnosis from transient hyperthyroidism of hyperemesis gravidarum presents a real challenge for the health care professional.

On physical examination, the thyroid gland is enlarged in almost every patient with Graves' disease. Indeed, the absence of a goiter makes the diagnosis unlikely. The gland is diffusely enlarged, between two and six times the normal size, varies from soft to firm, sometimes being irregular to palpation, and with one lobe being more prominent than the other one. A thrill may be felt or a bruit may be heard, indications of a hyperdynamic circulation. Examination of the eyes may reveal obvious ophthalmopathy, but in the majority of cases exophthalmos is absent or mild, with one eye slightly more prominent than the other. Extraocular movements may be impaired on careful eye examination. Stare is common, as well as injection or edema of the conjunctiva. Pretibial myxedema is rare, seen in less than 10 percent of women. A hyperdynamic heart with a loud systolic murmur are common findings. Proximal muscle weakness, fine tremor of the outstretched fingers, and hyperkinetic symptoms are seen frequently. The skin is warm and moist, and palmar erythema is accentuated.

Free thyroxine determination or the calculation of the free thyroxine index (using total thyroxine levels and a test for assessment of TBG, such as resin T_3 uptake) are standard tests in most clinical laboratories, with the result available in 24 to 48 hours. Almost every patient with Graves' disease will have an elevated FT_4 concentration. A suppressed TSH value in the presence of a high FT_4 or FT_4 index confirms the diagnosis of hyperthyroidism.[304] It must be kept in mind, however, that a suppressed serum TSH is present in about 15 percent of normal pregnant women in the first trimester of pregnancy.[291] In some unusual situations, the serum FT_4 may be at the upper limit of normal or be slightly elevated, in which case the determination of FT_3 and the FT_3 index will confirm the diagnosis of hyperthyroidism. Thyroid peroxidase antibodies (anti-TPO) or thyroid antimicrosomal antibodies, markers of thyroid autoimmune disease, are elevated in most patients with Graves' disease; its determination is indicated in patients in whom the etiology of the hyperthyroidism is in doubt.

Significant maternal and perinatal morbidity and mortality were reported in early studies of pregnancies complicated by hyperthyroidism.[343,344] In the last 20 years, however, there has been a significant decrease in the incidence of maternal and fetal complications directly related to improved control of maternal hyperthyroidism.[340,342,345–348] The most common maternal complication is PIH. In women with uncontrolled hyperthyroidism, the risk of severe preeclampsia was five times greater than in those patients with controlled disease.[342] Other complications include preterm delivery, placental abruption, and miscarriage. Congestive heart failure may occur in women untreated or treated for a short period of time in the presence of PIH or operative delivery.[349,350] Left ventricular dysfunction is usually detected by echocardiography in women with cardiovascular manifestations. Although these changes are reversible, they may persist for several weeks after achieving a euthyroid state. In one study,[351] reduction in peripheral vascular resistance and higher cardiac output were still present in spite of normalization of thyroxine levels. This is an important finding with significant clinical implications. Left ventricular decompensation in hyperthyroid pregnant women may develop in the presence of superimposed preeclampsia, at the time of delivery or with intercurrent complications such as anemia or infection. We have seen congestive heart failure in the first half of pregnancy in women with longstanding hyperthyroidism. It is likely that the aggravation of hyperthyroidism seen in the first part of pregnancy played an important role in the development of this complication. Careful monitoring of fluid administration is imperative in these situations. Thyroid storm has been rarely reported in pregnancy.[352,353]

Fetal and neonatal complications are also related to maternal control of hyperthyroidism. Intrauterine growth restriction (IUGR), prematurity, stillbirth, and neonatal morbidity are the most common complications. Millar et al.[342] demonstrated that hyperthyroidism uncontrolled during the entire gestation was associated with a ninefold greater incidence of low-birth-weight infants as compared with the control population. It was almost 2.5 times greater in those whose hyperthyroidism was treated during pregnancy and became euthyroid at some time during gestation. In those mothers achieving a euthyroid state before or early in pregnancy, the incidence of low-birth-weight infants was no different from that in the control population. Mitzuda et al.[341] correlated the risk of delivering a small-for-gestational-age (SGA) infant with the presence of maternal thyrotoxicosis lasting more than 30 weeks of pregnancy, a duration of Graves' disease for most of 10 years, and onset of Graves' disease before age 20. Momotani and Ito[348] reported an incidence of spontaneous abortions (25.7 percent) and premature delivery (14.9 percent) in mothers hyperthyroid at the time of conception, as compared with 12.8 percent and 9.5 percent, respectively, in euthyroid mothers.

Treatment of hyperthyroidism is essential to prevent maternal, fetal, and neonatal complications (Table 33–5). The goal of treatment is normalization of thyroid tests as soon as possible and to maintain euthyroidism with the minimum amount of antithyroid medication. Excessive amounts of antithyroid drugs crossing the placenta may affect the fetal thyroid, with the development of hypothyroidism with or without goiter. Patients should be monitored at regular intervals and the dose of their medications adjusted to keep the FT_4 in the upper one third of the range of normal.[345] For this purpose, thyroid tests should be performed every 2 weeks at the beginning of treatment and every 2 to 4 weeks when euthyroidism is achieved. Patients with small goiters, a short duration of symptoms, and on minimal amounts of antithyroid medication will be able to discontinue antithyroid drugs by 34 weeks' gestation or beyond. It is not recommended to discontinue antithyroid therapy before 32 weeks' gestation, since in our experience relapses may occur in a significant number of patients.[354] In this country, the two antithyroid drugs available are PTU and methimazole (Tapazole). Both drugs are effective in controlling symptoms. To our knowledge, no studies have shown PTU to be superior to methimazole, both drugs having similar placental transfer kinetics.[355] Furthermore, when the efficacies of both drugs have been compared, euthyroidism was achieved with equivalent amounts of drugs and in the same period of time.[356,357] Neonatal outcomes were no different in both groups. Aplasia cutis, an unusual scalp lesion, occurred in a small group of patients taking methimazole,[358–360] but this is not a contraindication for its use in pregnancy. Isolated cases of esophageal atresia and choanal atresia were also reported with the use of methimazole, although the casual relationship was never proven.[361–363]

The initial recommended dose of PTU is 100 to 450 mg/day, and methimazole 10 to 40 mg/day divided in two daily doses.[364] Methimazole is preferable in the outpatient setting, since it is given once or twice daily, allowing for improvement in patient compliance. PTU, due to its shorter half-life, should be given every 8 hours. In our experience, 10 mg of methimazole twice a day or 100 to 150 mg of PTU three times a day is an effective initial dose in most patients. Those with large goiters and longer duration of the disease may need larger doses at initiation of therapy. In patients with minimum symptoms, an initial dose of 10 mg of Tapazole daily or PTU 50 mg two or three times a day may be initiated. In most patients, clinical improvement is seen in 2 to 6 weeks, and improvement in thyroid tests occurs within the first 2 weeks of therapy, with normalization to chemical euthyroidism in 3 to 7 weeks.[356] Resistance to drug therapy is unusual, most likely due to poor patient compliance.[365] Once clinical improvement occurs, mainly weight gain and reduction in tachycardia, the dose of antithyroid medication may be

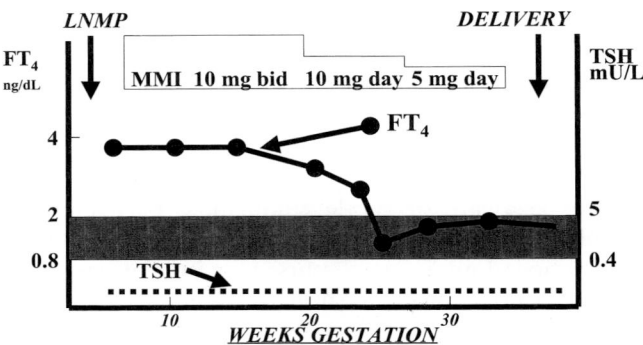

Figure 33–5. Management of hyperthyroidism. TSH, thyroid-stimulating hormone; FT_4, free thyroxine; LNMP, last normal menstrual period; MMI, methimazole.

reduced by half of the initial dose. The daily dose is adjusted every few weeks according to the clinical response and the results of thyroid tests. Serum TSH remains suppressed despite the normalization of thyroid hormone levels (Fig. 33–5). Normalization of serum TSH is an indicator to reduce the dose of medication. We do not recommend adding thyroxine to antithyroid drug therapy in the management of Graves' disease in pregnancy. If there is an exacerbation of symptoms or worsening of the thyroid tests, the amount of antithyroid medication is doubled. The main concern of maternal drug therapy is the potential side effect on the fetus; mainly, goiter and hypothyroidism. In most studies this has been prevented by using doses no greater than 200 mg PTU or 20 mg methimazole in the last few weeks of gestation.[366] However, small elevations in serum TSH in the neonate have been reported even with lower doses of antithyroid medication.[367] Furthermore, in one study, cord blood FT_4 values were not correlated to the antithyroid dose at term.[345]

Side effects of antithyroid drugs occur in 3 to 5 percent of treated patients.[368] The most common complications of both drugs are pruritus and skin rash. They usually resolve by switching to the other antithyroid medication. In general, the rash occurs 2 to 6 weeks after initiation of therapy. Since pruritus may be an initial symptom of hyperthyroidism, it is customary to ask the patient during the first visit if she is bothered by this. Other complications that are much less common are migratory polyarthritis, a lupus-like syndrome, and cholestatic jaundice. Agranulocytosis, a serious but unusual complication, has been reported in 1 in 300 patients receiving the drug.[369] It is manifested by fever, malaise, gingivitis, and sore throat. Agranulocytosis occurs in the first 12 weeks of therapy and appears to be related to the dose of medication.[370] Women should be made aware of the symptoms at the time the prescription is given, and advised to discontinue the drug and obtain a leukocyte count at once. Although some have recommended routine blood counts in patients on antithyroid therapy, it is not indicated, since granulocytopenia or agranulocytosis may appear without warning symptoms.

β-Adrenergic blocking agents (propranolol 20 to 40 mg every 6 hours or atenolol 25 to 50 mg/day) are very effective in controlling hyperdynamic symptoms and are indicated for the first few weeks in symptomatic patients.[322] One situation in which β-adrenergic blocking agents may be very effective is in the treatment of severe hyperthyroidsm during labor. In a case reported with both mother and fetus affected, labetalol was infused at a rate of 2 mg/min, controlling maternal and fetal tachycardia within 45 minutes.[371]

Subtotal thyroidectomy in pregnancy is effective in managing the disease; nowadays, indications for surgical treatment are few: allergy to antithyroid drugs,[372] very large goiters, patient preference, and the exceptional case of resistance to drug therapy.

[131]I therapy is contraindicated in pregnancy since, when given after 10 weeks' gestation, it produces fetal hypothyroidism.[373,374] A pregnancy test is mandatory in any woman of childbearing age before a therapeutic dose of ^{131}I is administered.

Iodine crosses the placenta. If given in large amounts and for prolonged periods, it may produce a fetal goiter and hypothyroidism.[321,375] Therefore, its use is not recommended in pregnancy. However, iodine has been used in small amounts, 6 to 40 mg/day in a group of pregnant Japanese women with mild hyperthyroidism.[376] Elevation in serum TSH was observed in 2 of 35 newborns, and the mothers were slightly hyperthyroid at the time of delivery. In spite of this observation, iodine therapy is not routinely indicated in the treatment of hyperthyroidism in pregnancy.

Excessive amounts of antithyroid drugs have induced fetal hypothyroidism and goiter. The diagnosis of goiter is made by ultrasonography, which shows hyperextension of the neck and a neck mass. Few cases of hypothyroidism have been confirmed by measuring serum thyroxine and TSH in fetal blood obtained by cordocentesis.[377] Treatment with intra-amniotic injection of L-thyroxine has resulted in resolution of the goiter.

Breast-feeding should be permitted if the daily dose of PTU or methimazole is less than 150 to 200 mg/day, respectively. It is prudent to give the total dose in divided doses after each feeding. The infant should be followed with thyroid function tests.[378] In a very provocative study, PTU was given to lactating hyperthyroid mothers whose infants were born with elevated serum TSH levels. Infant TSH levels normalized even with continuation of PTU therapy by the mothers.[379] In another study, thyroid tests were done at regular intervals in breast-fed infants of mothers taking up to 20 mg of methimazole daily, showing no evidence of hypothyroidism.[380]

Assessment of fetal well-being with the use of ultrasonography, the nonstress test, and a biophysical profile is indicated for cases in poor metabolic control, in the presence of fetal tachycardia and/or intrauterine growth restriction, in pregnancies complicated by PIH or any other obstetrical or medical complications.

Treatment of Thyroid Storm

Thyroid storm is a clinical diagnosis based on severe signs of thyrotoxicosis, with significant hyperpyrexia (>103°F), and neuropsychiatric symptoms that are essential for the clinical diagnosis. Tachycardia with a pulse rate exceeding 140 beats/min is not uncommon, and congestive heart failure is a frequent complication. Gastrointestinal symptoms such as nausea and vomiting, accompanied by liver compromise, have been reported. Laboratory tests show the classic hyperthyroid changes, although the actual elevation in FT_4 values does not help in the diagnosis.

Management includes the following:

1. Admission to the intensive care unit for supportive therapy such as fluids and correction of electrolyte abnormalities, oxygen therapy as needed, and control of hyperpyrexia. Acetaminophen is the drug of choice, since aspirin may increase free thyroid hormones.
2. Management of congestive heart failure, which may require large doses of digoxin.
3. Proper antibiotic therapy in case of infection.
4. β-Blocker therapy to control hyperadrenergic symptoms such as propranolol 60 to 80 mg every 4 hours orally or 1 mg/min intravenously. Esmolol, a short-acting β-acting antagonist given intravenously with a loading dose of 250 to 500 μg/kg of body weight followed by continuous infusion at 50 to 100 μg/kg/min may be used.
5. Methimazole 30 mg or PTU 300 mg every 6 hours (if unable to take oral medications a nasogastric tube may be needed); thionamides block the synthesis of thyroid hormones in a few hours.
6. One hour after the administration of thionamides, iodine is administered in the form of Lugol's solution, 10 drops three times a day or, if available, sodium iodide, given intravenously 1 g every 12 hours.
7. Glucocorticoids are also helpful, since they reduce the peripheral conversion of serum T_4 to T_3 in the form of hydrocortisone every 8 hours or equivalent amounts of other glucocorticoids.

In summary, thyroid storm is a life-threatening condition, requiring early recognition and aggressive therapy in an intensive unit care setting.

Neonatal Hyperthyroidism

Neonatal hyperthyroidism is infrequent, with an incidence of less than 1 percent of infants born to mothers with Graves' disease, therefore affecting 1 in 50,000 neonates. In the vast majority of cases, the disease is caused by the transfer of maternal immunoglobulin antibodies to the fetus. These stimulating thyroid antibodies to the TSH receptor (TSIs), when present in high concentrations in maternal serum, cross the placental barrier, stimulate the fetal thyroid gland, and may produce fetal or neonatal hyperthyroidism.[381] When the mother is treated with antithyroid medications, the fetus benefits from maternal therapy, remaining euthyroid during pregnancy. However, the protective effect of the antithyroid drug is lost after delivery, and neonatal hyperthyroidism may develop within a few days after birth. High titers of TSI receptor antibodies, a three- to fivefold increase over baseline, in the third trimester of pregnancy are predictors of neonatal hyperthyroidism.[341] If neonatal hyperthyroidism is not recognized and treated properly; neonatal mortality could be as high as 30 percent. Since the half-life of the antibodies is only a few weeks, complete resolution of neonatal hyperthyroidism is the rule.[382]

A few cases of familial neonatal Graves' disease[383] have been reported; the pathogenesis is not clearly understood. This condition may persist for several years.

Sporadic cases of neonatal hyperthyroidism without evidence of the presence of circulating TSI in mother or infant have recently been published.[384,385] Activation of mutations in the TSH receptor molecule are the cause of this entity. It is inherited as an autosomal dominant trait and, in contrast to Graves' neonatal hyperthyroidism, the condition persists indefinitely. Treatment with antithyroid medications followed by thyroid ablation therapy will eventually be needed.

Fetal Hyperthyroidism

In mothers with a history of Graves' disease previously treated with ablation therapy, either surgery or ^{131}I, concentrations of TSI may remain elevated, in spite of maternal euthyroidism. The concentration of these IgG immunoglobulins is low early in normal pregnancy, reaching a level in the fetus similar to that of the mother around 30 weeks' gestation. Therefore, the symptoms of fetal hyperthyroidism are not evident until 22 to 24 weeks of gestation. When TSI levels are present in high concentrations, fetal hyperthyroidism may result, characterized by fetal tachycardia, IUGR, oligohydramnios, and occasionally a goiter identified on ultrasonography by hyperextension of the fetal neck.[311,386-388] The diagnosis may be confirmed by measuring thyroid hormone levels in cord blood obtained by cordocentesis.[389,390] Heckel et al.[311] reviewed nine cases of fetal hyperthyroidism treated by maternal administration of antithyroid medications. Fetal tachycardia was the most frequent sign, whereas oligohydramnios and IUGR were reported in only two cases.

Fetal goiter was detected by ultrasonography in three cases. Treatment consisted of antithyroid medication given to the mother, PTU 100 to 400 mg/day or methimazole 10 to 20 mg/day. The dose is guided by the improvement and resolution of fetal tachycardia and normalization of fetal growth, both of which are indicators of good therapeutic response. Serial cordocentesis for the determination of thyroid hormone concentrations has also been used to monitor drug therapy.[391] The procedure should be reserved for centers with technical expertise in its use, since the complication rate is around 1 percent.[392]

In summary, the diagnosis of fetal hyperthyroidism should be suspected in the presence of fetal tachycardia with or without fetal goiter in mothers with a history of Graves' disease treated by ablation therapy and with high titers of serum TSI antibodies. The diagnosis can be confirmed by the determination of fetal thyroid hormones by cordocentesis.[392-394]

Hypothyroidism

Hypothyroidism in pregnancy is rarely diagnosed. Only a few series of patients have been reported.[395-397] However, subclinical hypothyroidism is more often encountered. Mild elevations in serum TSH are frequently detected in hypothyroid women on thyroid therapy soon after conception because of the increased demand for thyroid hormones in the first weeks of gestation.[309,310,398] The incidence of hypothyroidism, defined as any elevation in serum TSH above normal values, is between 0.19 and 2.5 percent.[399-403] In the above-mentioned studies, serum TSH was measured in the first half of pregnancy. The two most common etiologies of primary hypothyroidism are autoimmune thyroiditis (Hashimoto's thyroiditis) and postthyroid ablation therapy, surgical or ^{131}I treatment. Original studies reported a high incidence of congenital malformations, perinatal mortality, and impaired mental and somatic development in infants of hypothyroid women.[404] In contrast, recent reports showed no increase in the incidence of congenital malformations, and perinatal mortality is only slightly elevated.[395-397]

Regardless of the etiology, primary hypothyroidism is classified as subclinical hypothyroidism (normal FT_4 and elevated TSH) and overt hypothyroidism (low FT_4 and elevated TSH). The spectrum of women with hypothyroidism in pregnancy includes (1) women with subclinical and overt hypothyroidism diagnosed for the first time during pregnancy; (2) hypothyroid women who discontinue thyroid therapy at the time of conception because of poor medical advice or because of the misconception that thyroid medications affect the fetus; (3) those women on thyroid therapy requiring larger doses in pregnancy; (4) those women previously diagnosed but not compliant with their medication; (5) hyperthyroid patients on excessive amounts of antithyroid drug therapy; and (6) some patients on lithium or amiodarone therapy, as both drugs may impact thyroid function, particularly in women affected by chronic thyroiditis.[405,406]

The vast majority of patients with subclinical hypothyroidism are asymptomatic. Patients with overt hypothyroidism may complain of tiredness, cold intolerance, fatigue, muscle cramps, constipation, and deepening of the voice. On physical examination, the skin is dry and cold, deep tendon reflexes are delayed, and bradycardia may be detected as well as periorbital edema. A goiter is present in almost 80 percent of patients with chronic thyroiditis. The characteristic of the goiter is a diffuse enlargement, about two to three times the normal size, firm to palpation, painless, and with a rubbery consistency. In the other 20 percent, no goiter is found (atrophic thyroiditis, also known as primary myxedema or chronic thyroiditis without goiter).

The diagnosis of hypothyroidism is confirmed by the determination of serum TSH and FT_4 or FT_4I. The degree of severity of the clinical symptoms varies with the chemical thyroid abnormalities, although there is not always good correlation between clinical and chemical parameters. Serum thyroid antibodies (thyroid peroxidase antibodies [anti-TPO] formerly known as antimicrosomal antibodies [AMAs]), are elevated in patients with autoimmune thyroiditis. The titer of antibodies does not correlate with the size of the goiter or the clinical severity of hypothyroidism. In our series,[397] the mean TSH value at the time of diagnosis of overt hypothyroidism was 89.7 ± 86.2 mU/ml (normal, 0.4 to 5.0), with a mean FT_4I of 2.1 ± 1.5 (normal, 4.5 to 12). In the group with subclinical hypothyroidism, the mean serum TSH value was 28.4 ± 47.1 mU/mL with a mean FT_4I of 8.7 ± 3.6.

As in the case of hyperthyroidism, the most common complication in hypothyroid pregnant women is PIH, with an incidence of 21 percent in 60 patients with overt hypothyroidism (Table 33–6). Low birth weight was reported in 16.6 percent of infants. In one series,[397] 2 of 12 women with subclinical hypothyroidism developed postpartum hemorrhage. In our recent series of 23 women that conceived while being hypothyroid and completed their pregnancy in our institution, 10 presented with subclinical and 13 with overt hypothyroidism. In 13 of 23, the diagnosis of hypothyroidism was made for the first time during pregnancy, and the other 10 women had discontinued thyroid medication at least 3 months before conception. The incidence of complications was much less than in previous reports. No problems were seen in those women achieving euthyroidism before 24 weeks' gestation. The results of this study suggest that achieving euthyroidism early in pregnancy prevents late complications, even in women with severe hypothyroidism. The mean serum TSH in the overt hyperthyroid patients at presentation (16.1 weeks) was 90.4 IU/ml and the FT_4I was 1.4 (normal, 4.5–12).[407]

The impact of maternal hypothyroidism on the intellectual development of the offspring has been the subject of four studies, including two recent studies, one from this country and the other from Belgium.[295,296,408,409] In the study by Haddow et al.,[295] children born of mothers with mild elevations of serum TSH, measured between 16 and 18 weeks' gestation, were studied at age 7 to 9. They reported a 4-point decrease in IQ score on the Wechsler Intelligence Scale for Children. Pop et al.[296] detected a lower Baylor Psychomotor Developmental Index at 10 months of age in a small group of children the mothers of whom had low FT_4 but normal TSH at 12 weeks' gestation. In another study from Japan, Lui et al.[409] examined a group of eight children at age 4 and 10. IQs were compared in these children, whose mothers were hypothyroid in the first trimester, with their siblings. In the latter group, the mothers were euthyroid throughout gestation. There was no difference in the IQs of both groups of children. Mann et al.[408] had reported lower IQs in children from a group of mothers considered

Table 33–6. MATERNAL AND NEONATAL COMPLICATIONS OF HYPOTHYROIDISM IN PREGNANCY

	No. of Patients with Overt Hypothyroidism				No. of Patients with Subclinical Hypothyroidism		
	16	23	11	Total 50 (%)	12	45	Total 57 (%)
Pregnancy-induced hypertension	7	5	1	13 (26)	2	7	9 (15)
Placental abruption	3	0	0	3 (6)	0	0	0
Postpartum hemorrhage	3	1	0	4 (8)	2	0	2 (3.5)
Stillbirths	2	1	1	4 (8)	1	0	1 (1.7)
Congenital malformations	0	1	1	2 (3)	0	0	
Low birth weight	5	5	0	10 (20)	1	4	5 (8.7)
Anemia (HCT < 26%)	5	0	0	5 (10)	0	1	1 (1.7)

From Mestman JH: Endocrine diseases in pregnancy. *In* Sciarra JJ (ed): Gynecology and Obstetrics. Philadelphia, Lippincott-Raven, 1997, p 33, with permission.

hypothyroxinemic in pregnancy (serum TSH was not available at the time of the study). When they were studied at age 7, 5 of 21 (24 percent) had an IQ of less than 80, as compared with 10 percent of control children. These preliminary studies appear to support earlier animal research[410] showing the importance of maternal transfer of thyroxine in the first trimester of pregnancy, at a time when the fetal thyroid had not yet developed. From a practical point of view, these studies emphasize the importance of adjusting the dose of thyroxine in women under treatment for hypothyroidism soon after conception. Although we do not now support universal screening for hypothyroidism, we do recommend determination of thyroid tests early in pregnancy in those women at high risk for developing hypothyroidism (see the box "Indications for Thyroid Testing in Pregnancy").

Levothyroxine, or L-thyroxine, is the drug of choice for the treatment of hypothyroidism. In view of the complications mentioned above, it is important to normalize thyroid tests as soon as possible. An initial dose of 0.150 mg of levothyroxine is well tolerated by the majority of young hypothyroid patients. In those with severe hypothyroidism, there is a delay in the normalization of serum TSH, but normal serum FT_4 values are achieved in the first two weeks of therapy. The maintenance dose required for most patients is between 0.125 and 0.250 mg of levothyroxine per day. Higher doses may be required for patients after total thyroidectomy for thyroid carcinoma, since the goal in these cases is suppression of serum TSH.[313]

Patients on thyroid therapy before conception should have their TSH checked on their first visit and the amount of levothyroxine adjusted accordingly. The serum TSH should be repeated between 20 and 24 weeks and 28 and 32 weeks. Immediately after delivery, they should return to prepregnancy dosage. Interference in the absorption of thyroxine was discussed previously.[314,315]

Single Nodule of the Thyroid Gland

It is estimated that nodular thyroid disease is clinically detectable in 10 percent of pregnant women. In most cases, it is discovered during the first routine clinical examination or detected by the patient herself. The chances for a single or solitary thyroid nodule to be malignant are between 5 and 10 percent,[411] depending on risk factors such as previous radiation therapy to the upper body, rapid growth of a painless nodule, patient age, and family history of thyroid cancer. Papillary carcinoma accounts for almost 75 to 80 percent of malignant tumors, and follicular neoplasm for 15 to 20 percent; a few percent are represented by medullary thyroid carcinoma. Undifferentiated thyroid carcinoma is extremely rare in people under 50 years of age.

There is a paucity of information in the literature regarding the management and timing of the work-up in the presence of thyroid nodularity.[412–416] It is generally agreed that elective surgery should be avoided in the first trimester and after 24 weeks' gestation because of the potential risks of spontaneous abortion and premature delivery, respectively. In a selective group of patients operated on during or in the few months after delivery, the incidence of thyroid cancer was reported to be near 40 percent.[415,416] In both studies, fine-needle aspiration biopsy of the thyroid nodule was obtained before surgery, with findings consistent with papillary carcinoma or highly suspicious lesions.

Careful examination of the neck enables the physician to define and characterize the thyroid lesion. In addition to the size of the nodule, the consistency, tenderness, fixation to the skin, and presence of metastasis should be noted. A hard, painless nodule, measuring more than 2 cm in diameter, is suspicious of malignancy. High-resolution real-time ultrasound is very helpful in defining the size of the lesion, characterizing the dominant one, and identifying microcalcifications suspicious for either papillary or medullary thyroid carcinoma. Fine-needle aspiration biopsy is routinely used for diagnostic purposes.

In a recent retrospective study, a conservative approach to the management of a single thyroid nodule was recommended.[417] In this study, 61 women were pregnant at the time of the diagnosis of a differentiated thyroid carcinoma. The diagnosis was papillary cancer in 87 percent of them and follicular cancer in 13 percent. Fourteen women were operated on during pregnancy, whereas the other 47 women underwent surgical treatment 1 to 84 months after delivery. The outcome was compared with a group of 598 nonpregnant women matched for age. The median follow-up was 22.4 years as compared with 19.5 years in the nonpregnant group. Treatment and outcome were similar in both groups, those operated on during pregnancy and those in whom thyroidectomy was performed postpartum. The authors concluded that both diagnostic studies and initial therapy might be delayed until after delivery in most patients.

In the presence of a single thyroid nodule detected on physical examination, the following approach is recommended in our institution (Fig. 33–6)[416]:

1. *Serum TSH:* a suppressed serum TSH may indicate the presence of an autonomous nodule, which rarely is malignant.[418] In such cases, FT_4 and FT_3 are measured to rule out hyperthyroidism. It should be kept in mind that in normal first-trimester pregnancies, serum TSH level may be transiently low or undetected.[303]

2. If the serum TSH is within normal limits, the next step is *ultrasonography,* which will distinguish a

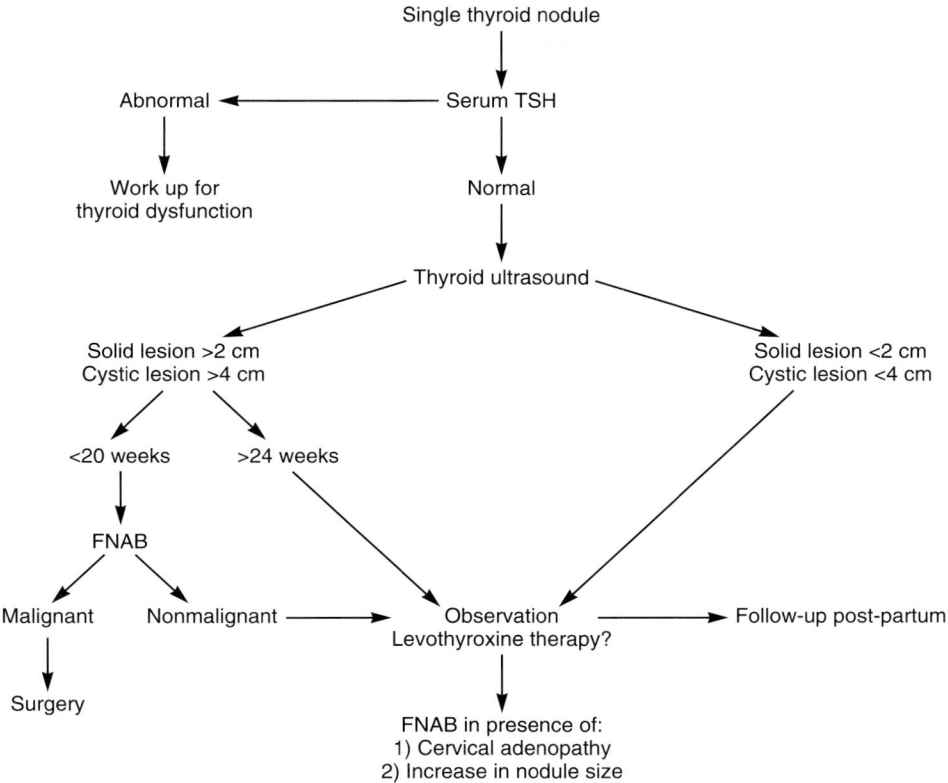

Figure 33–6. Evaluation of single thyroid nodules in pregnancy.

solid from a cystic lesion. In addition, it may show a multinodular gland not detected by palpation.

3. In the presence of a *solid lesion less than 2 cm or cystic lesion less than 4 cm* in diameter, observation with or without thyroxine suppression therapy is recommended. If clinically indicated, such as presence of cervical adenopathy or an increase in the size of the lesion with progression of pregnancy, fine-needle aspiration biopsy (FNAB) of the lesion is considered. It is important to point out the rarity of enlargement of these small nodules in the course of a few months of follow-up.

4. In patients with a *solid or mixed lesion on ultrasound greater than 2 cm or a cystic nodule greater than 4 cm*, the diagnostic approach differs according to gestational age: (a) *Before 20 weeks' gestation,* FNAB is done. The most important component of the FNAB is the cytopathologist's interpretation. A specific diagnosis is required: malignant, benign, follicular lesion, or inadequate specimen. In the latter, a repeat FNAB is recommended. (b) *For lesions diagnosed after 24 weeks' gestation,* FNAB may be postponed until after delivery, unless there is a strong suspicion of malignancy. Suppressive therapy with thyroxine to prevent further growth of the lesion, although considered controversial by some,[411] is the recommendation by our group. If there is

further growth of the lesion in spite of suppressive therapy, FNAB is recommended. (c) *For lesions diagnosed between 20 and 24 weeks' gestation,* the decision to wait until after delivery or to complete the work-up is made by the patient and her physician. The patient's anxiety and fear of having a potential malignant lesion should be considered when advice is given. Most malignant lesions of the thyroid gland are slow growing, and the long-term prognosis is good in the majority of patients.

5. *If the lesion is papillary carcinoma,* surgery is recommended before 24 weeks' gestation, although long-term follow-up of patients diagnosed in pregnancy indicates that postponement of surgery until after delivery does not affect morbidity or mortality.[417]

6. *For follicular lesions,* the decision about surgery is a personal one, since the chance for the lesion to be malignant is only between 15 and 20 percent. A similar approach is followed with Hürthle cell lesions.

The above protocol has been used in our institution for many years. In view of a recent publication discussed previously,[417] it is imperative for the physician to discuss the different therapeutic options with the patient and her family. If the lesion is diagnosed before

24 weeks' gestation, they should be informed of the recent data showing no deleterious effect in postponing therapy until after delivery. The anxiety of the patient and her family, and their wishes should be considered in making the final decision. The long-term prognosis of most thyroid cancers is exceptionally good, but patients should be followed for many years. General principles of care include the determination of serum thyroglobulin before surgery and at regular intervals thereafter; the decision to use radioactive iodine, which is indicated for completeness of thyroid ablation; and the importance of thyroid suppression therapy to keep the serum TSH suppressed in order to prevent possible recurrence of the lesion.[419]

Chronic Autoimmune Thyroiditis (Hashimoto's Thyroiditis)

Chronic or Hashimoto's thyroiditis[420] is an inflammatory disorder of the thyroid gland, the incidence depending on the definition of the entity. For example, in a long-term follow-up study in the Whickham survey,[421] there was an incidence in women of 3.5 cases per 1,000 per year, as contrasted with an incidence in men of 0.8 case per 1,000 per year. The prevalence increases with age. In most cases, there is a family history of thyroid disease, with 18 percent of relatives affected in one study[422] and 33 percent of siblings in another.[423] Chronic autoimmune thyroid disease is more common in women with other autoimmune diseases, particularly type 1 diabetes.[424] The classic clinic picture is characterized by the presence of a goiter, moderate in size, bilateral in most cases, with one lobe larger than the other, firm, rubbery consistency, and moving freely on swallowing. It is painless, although rapid growth of the gland may elicit some tenderness on palpation.

On presentation, most patients have no symptoms. The discovery of the goiter is made on routine physical examination, or detected by the patient or a family member. Occasionally, the patient may complain of mild to severe hypothyroid symptoms. The diagnosis may be suggested by a hyperechoic pattern on ultrasound of the thyroid.[425] The diagnosis is confirmed by the presence of thyroid autoantibodies (anti-TPO or antithyroglobulin autoantibodies). The actual antibody titer is not correlated with the size of the goiter, symptoms, or severity of the disease. From a practical point of view, there is no need to perform a determination of antithyroglobulin antibodies, since it does not add new information, increases the cost, and is not as sensitive as a determination of TPO autoantibodies. A serum TSH should be ordered to rule out thyroid dysfunction. If the serum TSH is elevated, a serum FT_4 will define if the patient suffers from subclinical or clinical hypothyroidism (see section Hypothyroidism, above). In some cases, goiter is not detected (atrophic thyroiditis or pri-

mary myxedema). Patients with euthyroid chronic thyroiditis may develop hypothyroidism over time. The odds ratio was 8 over 20 years in those women with a normal serum TSH and positive antibodies.[421]

The importance of diagnosing chronic thyroiditis in women of childbearing age relates to the potential consequences in pregnancy and the postpartum period. Women with chronic thyroiditis are at higher risk for spontaneous abortion, development of hypothyroidism for the first time in pregnancy, and postpartum thyroiditis.

Several investigators[426–428] have reported an association between thyroid autoantibodies and spontaneous miscarriages. Ongoing studies are evaluating the association of thyroid autoantibodies in women with recurrent spontaneous recurrent abortion.[429] Determination of serum TSH and anti-TPO antibodies should be performed in women with recurrent miscarriages. In the presence of normal TSH values, whether thyroid therapy is beneficial in preventing fetal loss in future pregnancies is not being systematically evaluated, although anecdotal information suggests a beneficial effect.

Women with chronic thyroiditis known to be euthyroid should be evaluated early in pregnancy, since some of them may develop hypothyroidism. Most euthyroid women will remain euthyroid throughout gestation, although there is a report suggesting an increased incidence of premature delivery in this group.[430]

In a subset of women with chronic thyroiditis, particularly those without a goiter (atrophic form), antibodies to the TSH receptor with blocking capabilities are present (TSHRBAb).[431] These antibodies cross the placenta, and in high titers may block the action of TSH in the fetal thyroid, causing transient congenital hypothyroidism.[432,433] The neonatal disease resolves spontaneously over 3 to 6 months as the maternal antibody is degraded.[434] In a population of 1,614,166 patients screened in New York, 9 mothers and their infants out of 788 infants with suspected congenital hypothyroidism had these antibodies.[435] Therefore, in mothers who have given birth to infants with congenital hypothyroidism, thyroid tests including TSHRBAb should be determined. In one study from Belgium, infants of euthyroid mothers with positive anti-TPO antibodies were evaluated for intellectual performance. A mild deficit was detected.[436] The significance of these findings needs to be confirmed by other long-term studies.

As will be discussed in the following section, the presence of thyroid antibodies, particularly high titers in the first trimester of pregnancy, predicts the development of the syndrome of postpartum thyroiditis.

Postpartum Thyroid Dysfunction

Thyroid dysfunction, hyper- and hypothyroidism, is recognized with increasing frequency in the 12 months following delivery, or following spontaneous or medi-

Postpartum Thyroid Dysfunction

Chronic thyroiditis
    Transient hyperthyroidism (low RAIU)
    Transient hypothyroidism
    Permanent hypothyroidism

Graves' disease
    Exacerbation of hyperthyroidism (high RAIU)
    Transient hyperthyroidism of chronic thyroiditis
    (low RAIU)

Hypothalamic pituitary disease
    Sheehan's syndrome
    Lymphocytic hypophysitis

RAIU, radioactive iodine uptake.
From Mestman JH: Endocrine diseases in pregnancy. *In* Sciarra JJ (ed): Gynecology and Obstetrics. Philadelphia, Lippincott-Raven, 1997, p 34, with permission.

cally induced abortions. Most of the cases are due to intrinsic thyroid disease, with a few due to hypothalamic or pituitary lesions (see the box "Postpartum Thyroid Dysfunction"). Patients with autoimmune thyroid disease, chronic thyroiditis, and Graves' disease are most frequently affected.

Postpartum thyroiditis (PPT), a variant of Hashimoto's or chronic thyroiditis, is the most common cause of thyroid dysfunction in the postpartum period. The prevalence is between 5 and 10 percent of all women,[430,437–440] with the exception of women with type 1 diabetes, where the incidence is close to 30 percent.[441] The clinical diagnosis is not always obvious and the clinician should be concerned about nonspecific symptoms such as tiredness, fatigue, depression, palpitations, and irritability in women following the birth of their child or a miscarriage or abortion. Fatigue is the most common complaint.[437] In some cases, the clinical symptoms resemble the syndrome of postpartum depression. Indeed, thyroid antibodies have been found more frequently in euthyroid women with postpartum depression, but this is still a controversial issue.[442] Since the clinical symptoms are mild, and many times are confused with the usual tiredness of women in the months following delivery, an argument can be made for routine screening in the postpartum period. This controversial issue has been recently reviewed.[443] It is the author's opinion that a careful history and physical examination will allow the physician to decide if thyroid tests are indicated in a given situation. Recognizing the mild degree of the symptoms, the presence of a goiter, history of similar symptoms in previous pregnancies, family history of thyroid disease, and type 1 diabetes mellitus, among other features, will prompt the health care professional to order serum TSH with anti-TPO antibodies. Those patients at risk should be evaluated in the first year postpartum because of the different manifestations of the disease.

Postpartum thyroiditis may also develop in women with negative antibodies. In a study from The Netherlands, the authors suggested two forms of PPT: an autoimmune form, which is most common and eventually will develop into chronic hypothyroidism, and a nonautoimmune form, without antibodies, that appears to be transient without progressing to permanent hypothyroidism.[444]

The clinical course is not uniform in the majority of patients. In about one third of the cases, mild symptoms of hyperthyroidism develop between 2 and 4 months postpartum. On physical examination, a goiter is felt in the majority of cases, firm and nontender to palpation. Tachycardia may be detected. The goiter may be discovered for the first time, or the patient may have noticed an increase in the size of a previously diagnosed goiter. Thyroid tests are in the hyperthyroid range and thyroid antibodies, anti-TPO antibody titers, are elevated in most cases. Spontaneously, without specific therapy, hypothyroidism develops in a few months, with spontaneous recovery and return to a euthyroid state by 7 to 12 months following delivery. Antibody titers have a tendency to increase during this process, and a change in the size of the goiter is usually noted. In a few patients, permanent hypothyroidism may develop. About 50 percent of patients, however, will develop permanent hypothyroidism within 5 years of the diagnosis of PPT.[445,446]

In one third of patients, the course of PPT is different, characterized by an initial episode of hypothyroidism between 3 and 7 months postpartum without the initial hyperthyroid phase. In the other one third of patients, the initial episode of hyperthyroidism is followed by a return to normal thyroid function. It has been suggested that some ultrasonographic changes of the thyroid gland, such as hypoechogenicity, are typical of PPT and may aid in the diagnosis of the syndrome.[447]

Postpartum thyroid dysfunction may also occur in patients with a known history of Graves' disease. It is common for women with Graves' disease to have an exacerbation of their symptoms in the first 2 months postpartum.[448] The symptoms of hyperthyroidism are more severe than those in patients with PPT. They may present with ophthalmopathy and the hypermetabolic findings. Therapy with antithyroid medications is needed in these cases. On the other hand, patients with Graves' disease may have a bout of hyperthyroidism secondary to a concomitant episode of PPT.[449,450] The differential diagnosis in this situation is important, since the treatment is different. If not contraindicated, as in breast-feeding mothers, a 4- or 24-hour thyroid radioactive iodine uptake (RAIU) is helpful. It will be very low in patients with PPT, whereas it is high normal or elevated in patients with recurrent hyperthyroid-

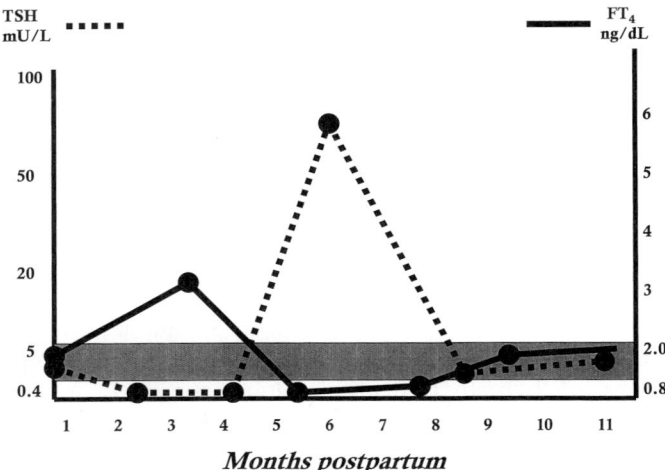

Figure 33–7. Clinical course of postpartum thyroiditis.

ism due to Graves' disease. When it is due to recurrent Graves' disease, treatment with antithyroid medications is indicated, or the physician may advise ablation therapy with ^{131}I.

Therefore, PPT is characterized by symptoms of thyroid dysfunction, that present in four different forms: (1) an episode of hyperthyroidism (2 to 4 months), followed by hypothyroidism (4 to 6 months) and reverting to euthyroidism (after the seventh month); (2) an episode of hyperthyroidism (3 to 4 months) reverting to euthyroidism; (3) an episode of hypothyroidism (4 to 6 months) reverting to a euthyroid state; and (4) permanent hypothyroidism after the hypothyroid phase (Fig. 33–7). However, there are exceptions to these chronologic phases. It is recommended that a diagnosis of PPT be considered for any thyroid abnormality occurring within 1 year after delivery or miscarriages.

Since most cases of postpartum thyroid dysfunction recover spontaneously, treatment is indicated for symptomatic patients. In the presence of hyperthyroid symptoms, β-adrenergic-blocking drugs (propranolol 20 to 40 mg every 6 hours or atenolol 25 to 50 mg every 24 hours) are effective in controlling the symptoms. Antithyroid medications are not effective, because the hyperthyroxinemia is secondary to the release of thyroid hormones due to the acute injury to the gland (destructive hyperthyroidism). There is no new hormone production, and therefore medications that work by blocking new thyroid hormone formation are ineffective. For hypothyroid symptoms, small amounts of levothyroxine 0.050 mg/day will control symptoms, allowing for a spontaneous recovery of thyroid function after discontinuation of the drug.

There are some features that may predict the development of PPT: presence of a goiter and high titers of thyroid antibodies in the first half of pregnancy, episodes of PPT in previous pregnancies, hypothyroidism

antedating pregnancy,[451] and a strong family history of autoimmune thyroid disease.[452] Women with type 1 diabetes mellitus are at high risk for developing PPT. PPT may recur in future pregnancies, with a recurrence rate between 30 and 70 percent.[453–455] PPT has been reported to be associated with other autoimmune endocrine disorders, such as adrenal insufficiency and lymphocytic hypophysitis.[19,456]

Key Points

➤ Hypopituitarism may present de novo in the second half of pregnancy, in the immediate postpartum period, or less commonly late postpartum. Severe hypoglycemia, responsive only to glucocorticoid therapy, is a characteristic feature. Lymphocytic hypophysitis with a normal or enlarged sella turcica on MRI appears to be the most common etiology.

➤ Idiopathic diabetes insipidus may manifest for the first time in pregnancy in patients with subclinical disease, or may occur as a complication of acute liver failure. An increase in polyuria and nocturia in a pregnant woman with normal serum glucose should alert the physician of such a diagnostic possibility.

➤ Cushing's disease is rare in pregnancy. The cause of Cushing's syndrome in pregnancy is the presence of an adrenal tumor in 50 percent of cases, versus 15 to 20 percent in nonpregnant patients.

➤ Hyperparathyroidism is almost always asymptomatic. Surgery is indicated in symptomatic patients and those with serum calcium levels over 11 mg/dl. The management of asymptomatic patients with levels of less than 11 mg/dl is unsettled.

➤ Hyperthyroidism due to Graves' disease needs to be differentiated in the first trimester of pregnancy from the syndrome of transient hyperthyroidism of hyperemesis gravidarum.

➤ Transient hyperthyroidism of hyperemesis gravidarum is the most common cause of hyperthyroxinemia in pregnancy; the cause is high or inappropriate levels of hCG.

➤ Both methimazole and PTU are used for the management of Graves' hyperthyroidism. The dosage should be adjusted frequently, aiming to use the minimum amount of drug that will keep the FT$_4$ at the upper limits of normal.

➤ Breast-feeding is not contraindicated in women on either methimazole or PTU, provided that the maximum daily dose is 200 mg of PTU and 20 mg of Tapazole.

➤ Hypothyroid women should have their thyroid tests checked early in pregnancy. An increase in dosage is needed in over 50 percent of patients.

➤ Postpartum thyroiditis affects between 5 and 10 percent of all women in the postpartum period. Women with chronic thyroiditis are at higher risk of developing the syndrome.

➤ When significant hirsutism with or without virilization occurs de novo in pregnancy, a complete endocrine evaluation should be carried out. The most common cause is a luteoma of pregnancy.

➤ Rare causes of hypertension in pregnancy include pheochromocytoma, Cushing's disease, and primary aldosteronism.

Acknowledgment

The author wishes to thank Elsa C. Ahumada for her secretarial assistance.

REFERENCES

1. Goluboff LG, Ezrin C: Effect of pregnancy on the somatotroph and the proclactin cell of the human adenohypophysis. J Clin Endocrinol Metab 29:1533, 1969.
2. Randeva HS, Schoebel J, Byrne J, et al: Classical pituitary apoplexy: clinical features, management and outcome. Clin Endocrinol (Oxf) 51:181, 1999.
3. Pellegrini-Bouiller I, Belicar P, Barlier A, et al: A new mutation of the gene encoding the transcription factor Pit-1 is responsible for combined pituitary hormone deficiency. J Clin Endocrinol Metab 81:2790, 1996.
4. Rosenbloom AL, Almonte AS, Brown MR, et al: Clinical and biochemical phenotype of familial anterior hypopituitarism from mutation of the PROP 1 gene. J Clin Endocrinol Metab 84:50, 1999.
5. Battes AS, Hoff W, Vant-Jones PJ, et al: The effect of hypopituitarism on life expectancy. J Clin Endocrinol Metab 81:1169, 1996.
6. Sheehan HL: Postpartum necrosis of the anterior pituitary. J Pathol Bacteriol 45:189, 1937.
7. Molitch ME: Pituitary disease in pregnancy. Semin Perinatol 22:457, 1998.
8. Veldhuis JD, Hammond JM: Endocrine function after spontaneous infarction of the human pituitary: report, review, and reappraisal. Endocr Rev 1:100, 1980.
9. Grimes HG, Brooks MH: Pregnancy in Sheehan's syndrome: report of a case and review. Obstet Gynecol Rev 35:481, 1980.
10. Singer PA, Mestman JH, Manning PR, et al: Hypothalamic hypothyroidism secondary to Sheehan's syndrome. West J Med 120:416, 1974.
11. Mestman JH: Endocrine disease in pregnancy. In Sciarra J (ed): Gynecology and Obstetrics. Philadelphia, Lippincott-Raven, 1997, p 1.
12. Smallridge RC, Corrigan DF, Thomason AM, et al: Hypoglycemia in pregnancy. Arch Intern Med 144:189, 1980.
13. Notterman RB, Jovanovic L, Peterson C, et al: Spontaneous hypoglycemia seizures in pregnancy: a manifestation of panhypopituitarism. Arch Intern Med 144:189, 1984.
14. Perlitz Y, Varkel J, Markovitz J, et al: Acute adrenal insufficiency during pregnancy and puerperium: case report and literature review. Obstet Gynecol Surv 54:717, 1999.
15. Goudie RB, Pinkerton PH: Anterior hypophysitis and Hashimoto's disease in a young woman. J Pathol Bacteriol 83:584, 1962.
16. Asa SL, Bilbao JM, Kovacks K, et al: Lymphocytic hypophysitis of pregnancy resulting in hypopituitarism: a distinct clinicopathologic entity. Ann Intern Med 95:166, 1981.
17. Thodou E, Asa SL, Kontogeorgos G, et al: Lymphocytic hypophysitis: clinicopathological findings. J Clin Endocrinol Metab 80:2302, 1995.
18. Gagneja H, Arafah B, Taylor HC: Histologically proven lymphocytic hypophysitis: spontaneous resolution and subsequent pregnancy. Mayo Clin Proc 74:150, 1999.
19. Bevan JS, Othman S, Lazarus JH, et al: Reversible adrenocorticotropin deficiency to probable autoimmune hypophysitis in a woman with postpartum thyroiditis. J Clin Endocrinol Metab 74:548, 1992.
20. Patel MC, Guneratne N, Haq N, et al: Peripartum hypopituitarism and lymphocytic hypophysitis. Q J Med 88:571, 1995.
21. Merker E, Futterweit W: Postpartum amenorrhea, diabetes insipidus and galactorrhea: report of five unusual cases with long-term follow up. Am J Med 56:554, 1974.
22. Stacpoole PW, Kandell TW, Fisher WR: Primary empty sella, hyperprolactinemia, and isolated ACTH deficiency after postpartum hemorrhage. Am J Med 74:905, 1983.
23. Zeller JR, Cerletty JM, Rabinovitch RA, et al: Spontaneous regression of a postpartum pituitary mass demonstrated by computed tomography. Arch Intern Med 142:373, 1982.
24. Leiba S, Schindel B, Weinstein R, et al: Spontaneous postpartum regression of pituitary mass with return of function. JAMA 255:230, 1986.
25. Ishihara T, Hino M, Kurahachi H, et al: Long term clinical course of two cases of lymphocytic adenohypophysitis. Endocr J 43:433, 1996.
26. Nelson DH, Tanney H, Mestman J, et al: Potentiation of the biologic effect administered hydrocortisone by estrogen treatment. J Clin Endocrinol Metab 23:261, 1963.
27. Tyson JE, Barnes AC, Merimee TJ, McKusick VA: Isolated growth hormone deficiency: studies in pregnancy. J Clin Endocrinol 31:147, 1970.
28. Rigg LA, Lein A, Yen SSC: Pattern of increase in circulating prolactin levels during human gestation. Am J Obstet Gynecol 129:454, 1997.
29. Jackson RD, Wortsman J, Malarkey WB: Persistence of large molecular weight prolactin secretion during pregnancy in women with macroprolactinaemia and its presence in fetal cord blood. J Clin Endocrinol Metab 68:1046, 1989.
30. Heaney AP, Laing I, Walton L, et al: Misleading hyperprolactinaemia in pregnancy. Lancet 353:720, 1999.
31. Molitch ME: Medical treatment of prolactinomas. Endocrinol Metab Clin North Am 28:143, 1999.
32. Grossman A, Cohen BL, Charlesworth M, et al: Treatment of

prolactinomas with megavoltage radiotherapy. BMJ 288: 1105, 1984.

33. Seri U, Rasio E, Beauregard H, et al: Recurrence of hyperprolactinemia after selective transsphenoidal adenomectomy in women with prolactinoma. N Engl J Med 309:280, 1983.

34. Feigenbaum SL, Downey DE, Wilson CB, Jaffe RB: Transsphenoidal pituitary resection for preoperative diagnosis of prolactin-secreting pituitary adenoma in women: long term follow up. J Clin Endocrinol Metab 81:1711, 1996.

35. Vance ML, Evans WS, Thorner MO: Bromocriptine. Ann Intern Med 100:78, 1984.

36. McGregor AM, Scanlon MF, Hall R, et al: Effects of bromocriptine on pituitary tumor size. BMJ 2:700, 1979.

37. Molitch ME, Elton RL, Blackwell RE, et al: Bromocriptine as a primary therapy for prolactin secreting macroadenomas: results of a prospective multicenter study. J Clin Endocrinol Metab 60:698, 1985.

38. Vermesh M, Fossum GT, Kletzky OA: Vaginal bromocriptine: pharmacology and effect on serum prolactin in normal women. Obstet Gynecol 73:693, 1988.

39. Konopka P, Raymond JP, Merceron RE, et al: Continuous administration of bromocriptine in the prevention of neurological complications in pregnant women with prolactinomas. Am J Obstet Gynecol 146:935, 1983.

40. Holmgren U, Bergstrand G, Hagenfeldt K, et al: Women with prolactinoma effect of pregnancy and lactation on serum prolactin and on tumor growth. Acta Endocrinol 111:452, 1986.

41. Webster J, Piscitelli G, Polli A, et al: A comparision of cabergoline and bromocriptine in the treatment of hyperprolactinemic amenorrhea. N Engl J Med 331:904, 1994.

42. Biller BMK, Molitch ME, Vance ML, et al: Treatment of prolactin secreting macroadenoma with the once weekly dopamine agonist cabergoline. J Clin Endocrinol Metab 81: 2338, 1996.

43. Robert E, Musatti L, Piscitelli G, et al: Pregnancy outcome after treatment with the ergot derivative, cabergoline. Reprod Toxicol 10:333, 1996.

44. Crosignani PG, Mattei AM, Severini V, et al: Long term effects of time, medical treatment and pregnancy in 176 hyperprolactinemic women. Eur J Obstet Gynecol Reprod Biol 44:175, 1992.

45. Cunnah D, Besser M: Management of prolactinomas. Clin Endocrinol 34:231, 1991.

46. Turkal JI, Braun P, Krupp P: Surveillance of bromocriptine in pregnancy. JAMA 247:1589, 1982.

47. Montoro MN, Mestman JH: Pituitary diseases during pregnancy. Infertil Reprod Med Clin North Am 24:41, 1994.

48. Kupersmith MJ, Rosenberg C, Kleinberg D: Visual loss in pregnant women with pituitary adenomas. Ann Intern Med 121:473, 1994.

49. Raymond JP, Goldstein E, Konopka P, et al: Follow up of children born of bromocriptine treated mothers. Horm Res 22:239, 1985.

50. Andersen AN, Tabor A, Hertz JB, et al: Abnormal prolactin levels and pituitary gonadal axis in the puerperium. Obstet Gynecol 57:725, 1981.

51. Rothman KJ, Funch DP, Dreyer NA: Bromocriptine and puerperal seizures. Epidemiology 1:232, 1990.

52. Rossi AM, Vilska S, Heinonen PK: Outcome of pregnancies in women with treated or untreated hyperprolactinemia. Eur J Obstet Gynecol Reprod Biol 63:143, 1995.

53. Frankenne F, Closset J, Gomez F, et al: The physiology of growth hormone (GHs) in pregnant women and partial characterization of the placental GH variant. J Clin Endocrinol Metab 66:1171, 1988.

54. Beckers A, Stevenaert A, Foidart JM, et al: Placental and pituitary growth hormone secretion during pregnancy in acromegalic women. J Clin Endocrinol Metab 71:725, 1990.

55. Abelove WA, Rupp JJ, Paschkis KE: Acromegaly and pregnancy. J Clin Endocrinol Metab 14:32, 1954.

56. Fisch RO, Prem KA, Feinberg SB, Gehrz PC: Acromegaly in a gravida and her infant. Obstet Gynecol 43:861, 1974.

57. King KC, Adam PAJ, Schwartz R, et al: Human placental transfer of human growth hormone 1125. Pediatrics 48:534, 1971.

58. Herman-Bonert V, Seliverstov M, Melmed S: Pregnancy in acromegaly: successful therapeutic outcome. J Clin Endocrinol Metab 83:727, 1998.

59. Neal JM: Successful pregnancy in a woman with acromegaly treated with octreotide. Endocr Pract 6:148, 2000.

60. Lopez-Velasco R, Escobar-Morreale HF, Vega B, et al: Cardiac involvement in acromegaly: specific myocardiopathy or consequence of systemic hypertension? J Clin Endocrinol Metab 82:1047, 1997.

61. Shimon I, Melmed S: Management of pituitary tumors. Ann Intern Med 129:472, 1998.

62. Newman CB: Medical therapy for acromegaly. Endocrinol Metab Clin North Am 28:171, 1999.

63. Stewart PM, Kane KF, Stewart SE, et al: Depot long acting somatostatin analog is an effective treatment for acromegaly. J Clin Endocrinol Metab 80:3267, 1995.

64. Bigazzi M, Ronga R, Lancranjan I, et al: A pregnancy in an acromegalic woman during bromocriptine treatment: effects on growth hormone and prolactin in the maternal, fetal and amniotic compartments. J Clin Endocrinol Metab 48:9, 1979.

65. Aono T, Shioji T, Kohno M, et al: Pregnancy following 2-bromo-a-ergocryptine (CB-154) induced ovulation in an acromegalic patient with galactorrhea and amenorrhea. Fertil Steril 27:341, 1976.

66. Luboshitzky R, Dickestein G, Barzalai D: Bromocriptine induced pregnancy in an acromegalic patients. JAMA 244:584, 1980.

67. Miyakawa I, Taniyama K, Koike H, et al: Successful pregnancy in an acromegalic patient during 2-Br-(alpha)-errocryptine (CB-154) therapy. Acta Endocrinol 101:333, 1982.

68. Landolt AS, Schmidt J, Wimpfheimer C, et al: Successful pregnancy in a previously infertile woman treated with octreotide for acromegaly. N Engl J Med 320:671, 1989.

69. Montani M, Pagani G, Gionola D, et al: Acromegaly and primary amenorrhea: ovulation and pregnancy induced by SMS 201-995 and bromocriptine. J Endocriol Invest 13:193, 1990.

70. Caron P, Gerbeau C, Pradayrol L: Maternal fetal transfer of octreotide. N Engl J Med 333:601, 1995.

71. Barron WM, Lindheimer MD: Renal sodium and water handling in pregnancy. Obstet Gynecol Annu 13:35, 1984.

72. Monson JP, Williams DJ: Osmoregulatory adaption in pregnancy and its disorders. J Endocrinol 132:7, 1992.

73. Davidson JM, Shiells EA, Barron WM, et al: Changes in the metabolic clearance of vasopressin and of plasma vasopressinase throughout human pregnancy. J Clin Invest 83:1313, 1989.

74. Durr JA: Diabetes insipidus in pregnancy. Am J Kidney Dis 9: 276, 1987.

75. Iglesias P, Diez JJ: Diabetes insipidus as a primary clinical manifestation of lymphocytic hypophysitis in a postmenopausal woman. Endocrinologist 10:127, 2000.

76. Miyagi K, Shingaki T, Ito K, et al: Lymphocytic infundibulo-hypophysitis with diabetes insipidus as a new clinical entity: a case report and review of the literature. No Shinkei Geka 25: 169, 1997.

77. Goodner DM, Arnas GM, Andros GJ, et al: Psychogenic

polydipsia causing acute water intoxication of pregnancy at term—a case report. Obstet Gynecol 37:873, 1971.

78. Robinson GA: Disorders of antidiuretic hormone secretion. Clin Endocrinol Metab 14:55, 1985.

79. Leger J, Velasquez A, Garel C, et al: Thickened pituitary stalk on magnetic resonance imaging in children with central diabetes insipidus. J Clin Endocrinol Metab 84:1954, 1999.

80. Durr JA, Lindheimer MD: Diabetes insipidus in pregnancy. Endocr Pract 2:353, 1996.

81. Hime MC, Richardson JA: Diabetes insipidus and pregnancy. Case report, incidence and review of the literature. Obstet Gynecol Surv 33:375, 1978.

82. Barron WM, Cohen LH, Ulland LA, et al: Transient vasopressin resistant diabetes insipidus of pregnancy. N Engl J Med 310:442, 1984.

83. Kennedy S, Hall PM, Seymour AE, et al: Transient diabetes insipidus and acute fatty liver of pregnancy. Br J Obstet Gynaecol 101:387, 1994.

84. Soule SG, Monson JP, Jacobs HS: Transient diabetes insipidus in pregnancy—a consequence of enhanced placental clearance of arginine vasopressin. Hum Reprod 10:3322, 1995.

85. William DJ, Metcalfe KA, Skingle L, et al: Pathophysiology of transient cranial diabetes insipidus during pregnancy. Clin Endocrinol 38:595, 1993.

86. Iwasaki Y, Oiso Y, Kondo K, et al: Aggravation of subclinical diabetes insipidus during pregnancy. N Engl J Med 324:522, 1991.

87. Raziel A, Rosenberg T, Schreyer P, et al: Transient postpartum diabetes insipidus. Am J Obstet Gynecol 164:616, 1991.

88. Ober KP, Elster A: Spontaneously resolving lymphocytic hypophysitis as a cause of postpartum diabetes insipidus. Endocrinologist 4:107, 1994.

89. Kallen BAJ, Carlsson SS, Bengtsson BKA: Diabetes inspidus and use of desmopressin (Minitrin) during pregnancy. Eur J Endocrinol 132:144, 1995.

90. Ford SM: Transient vasopressin-resistant diabetes insipidus of pregnancy. Obstet Gynecol 68:288, 1986.

91. Kovacs CS, Kronenberg HM: Maternal fetal calcium and bone metabolism during pregnancy, puerperium and lactation. Endocr Rev 18:832, 1997.

92. Mestman JH: Parathyroid disorders in pregnancy. Semin Perinatol 22:485, 1998.

93. Kohlmeirer L, Marcus R: Calcium disorders of pregnancy. Endocrine Metab Clin North Am 24:15, 1995.

94. Pitkin RM: Calcium metabolism in pregnancy and the perinatal period: a review. Am J Obstet Gynecol 151:99, 1985.

95. Seki K, Makimura N, Mitsui C, et al: Calcium regulating hormones and osteocalcin levels during pregnancy: a longitudinal study. Am J Obstet Gynecol 164:1248, 1991.

96. Seely EW, Brown EM, DeMaggio DM, et al: A prospective study of calciotrophic hormones in pregnancy and postpartum reciprocal changes in serum intact parathyroid hormone and 1,25 dihydroxyvitamin D. Am J Obstet Gynecol 176:214, 1997.

97. Gertner JM, Coustan DR, Kliger AS, et al: Pregnancy as a state of physiologic absorptive hypercalciuria. Am J Med 81:451, 1986.

98. Dahlman T, Sjoberg HE, Bucht E: Calcium homeostasis in normal pregnancy and puerperium: a longitudinal study. Acta Obstet Gynecol Scand 73:393, 1994.

99. Frenkl Y, Barkai G, Mashiach S, et al: Hypocalciuria of preeclampsia is independent of parathyroid hormone level. Obstet Gynecol 77:689, 1991.

100. Hirota Y, Anai T, Miyakawa I: Parathyroid hormone related protein levels in maternal and cord blood. Am J Obstet Gynecol 177:702, 1997.

101. Grill V, Hillary J, Ho PMW, et al: Parathyroid hormone related protein: a possible endocrine function in lactation. Clin Endocrinol 37:405, 1992.

102. Rodda CP, Kubota M, Heath JA, et al: Evidence for a novel parathyroid hormone related protein in fetal lamb parathyroid glands and sheep placenta: comparision with a similar protein implicated in humoral hypercalcemia of malignancy. J Endocrinol 117:261, 1988.

103. Samaan NA, Anderson GD, Adam-Mayne ME: Immunoreactive calcitonin in the mother, neonate, child and adult. Am J Obstet Gynecol 121:622, 1975.

104. Gallacher SJ, Fraser WD, Owens OJ, et al: Changes in calciotrophic hormones and biochemical markers of bone turnover in normal human pregnancy. Eur J Endocrinol 131:369, 1994.

105. Abrams SA: Bone turnover during lactation—can calcium supplementation make a difference? [Editorial]. J Clin Endocrinol Metab 83:1056, 1998.

106. Iqbal N, Aldasouqi S, Peacock M, et al: Life threatening hypercalcemia associated with primary hyperparathyroidism during pregnancy: case report and review of the literature. Endocr Pract 5:337, 1999.

107. Hunter D, Turnbull H: Hyperparathyroidism: generalized osteitis fibrosa with observations upon bones, parathyroid tumors and the normal parathyroid glands. Br J Surg 19:203, 1931.

108. Friderichsen D: Tetany in a suckling with latent osteitis fibrosis in the mother. Lancet 1:85, 1939.

109. Montoro MN, Paler RJ, Goodwin JM, et al: Parathyroid carcinoma during pregnancy. Obstet Gynecol 96:841, 2000.

110. Ludwing GD: Hyperparathyroidism in relation to pregnancy. N Engl J Med 267:637, 1962.

111. Johnstone RE II, Kreindler T, Johnstone RE: Hyperparathyroidism during pregnancy. Obstet Gynecol 40:580, 1972.

112. Kelly T: Primary hyperparathyroidism during pregnancy. Surgery 110:1028, 1991.

113. Croom RD III, Thomas CG Jr: Primary hyperparathyroidism during pregnancy. Am J Surg 131:328, 1976.

114. Clark D, Seeds JW, Cefalo R: Hyperparathyroid crisis in pregnancy. Am J Obstet Gynecol 140:841, 1981.

115. Silverberg SJ, Bilezikian JP: Evaluation and management of primary hyperparathyroidism. J Clin Endocrinol Metab 81:2036, 1996.

116. Carella M, Gossain V: Hyperparathyroidism and pregnancy: case report and review. J Gen Intern Med 7:448, 1992.

117. Hess HM, Dickson J, Fox HE: Hyperfunctioning parathyroid carcinoma presenting an acute pancreatitis in pregnancy. J Reprod Med 25:83, 1980.

118. Parham GP, Orr JW: Hyperparathyroidism secondary to parathyroid carcinoma in pregnancy: a case report. J Reprod Med 32:123, 1987.

119. Palmueri-Sevier A, Palmueri GMA, Baumgartner CJ, et al: Case report: long term remission of parathyroid cancer. Possible relation to Vitamin D and calcitriol therapy. Am J Med Sci 306:309, 1993.

120. Corlett RC, Mishell DR: Pancreatitis in pregnancy. Am J Obstet Gynecol 113:281, 1972.

121. Matthias GSH, Helliwell TR, Williams A: Postpartum hyperthyroid crisis: case report. Br J Obstet Gynaecol 94:807, 1987.

122. Stander JH, Ahern RE: The parathyroids in pregnancy. J Mt Sinai Hosp 14:629, 1947.

123. Schenker JG, Kallner B: Fatal postpartum hyperparathyroidism crisis due to primary chief cell hyperplasia of parathyroids: report of a case. Obstet Gynecol 25:705, 1965.

124. Soyannowo MA, McGeown MG, Bell M, et al: A case of

acute hyperparathyroidism with thyrotoxicosis and pancreatitis presenting as hyperemesis gravidarum. Postgrad Med J 44: 861, 1968.

125. Subrayen KT, Moodley SC, Jialal I, et al: Hyperparathyroidism in twin pregnancy: a case report. S Afr Med J 72:287, 1987.

126. Ficinski M, Mestman JH: Primary hyperparathyroidism during pregnancy. Endocr Pract 2:362, 1996.

127. Marx S: Familial hypocalciuric hypercalcemia. *In* Primer on the Metabolic Bone Diseases and Disorders of Mineral Metabolism. New York, Raven Press, 1993, p 166.

128. Pratt EI, Beren BB, et al: Hypercalcemia and idiopathic hyperplasia of the parathyroid glands in infant. J Pediatr 30:388, 1947.

129. Pollak M, Chou YH, Marx S, et al: Familial hypocalciuric hypercalcemia and neonatal severe hyperparathyroidism: the effect of mutant gene dosage on phenotype. J Clin Invest 93: 1108, 1994.

130. Wright AD, Joplin GF, Dixon HG: Postpartum hypercalcemia in treated hypoparathyroidism. BMJ 1:23, 1969.

131. Cundy T, Haining SA, Builland-Cumming DF: Remission of hypoparathyroidism during lactation: evidence for a physiological role for prolactin in the regulation of Vitamin D metabolism. Clin Endocrinol (Oxf) 26:667, 1987.

132. Caplan RH, Beguin EA: Hypercalcemia in a calcitriol treated hypoparathyroid woman during lactation. Obstet Gynecol 76: 485, 1990.

133. Lepre F, Grill V, Martin TJ: Hypercalcemia in pregnancy and lactation associated with parathyroid hormone-related protein. N Engl J Med 328:666, 1993.

134. Khosla S, VanHeerden JA, Gharib H, et al: Parathyroid hormone related protein and hypercalcemia secondary to massive mammary hyperplasia. N Engl J Med 322:1157, 1990.

135. Silverberg SJ, Bone HG, Marriott TB, et al: Short term inhibition of parathyroid hormone secretions by a calcium receptor agonist in patients with primary hyperparathyroidism. N Engl J Med 337:1506, 1997.

136. NIH Consensus Development Conference: Diagnosis and management of asymptomatic primary hyperparathyroidism. Ann Intern Med 114:593, 1991.

137. Montoro M, Collea JU, Mestman JH: Management of hyperparathyroidism in pregnancy with oral phosphate therapy. Obstet Gynecol 55:431, 1980.

138. Ledger GA: Hypocalcemia and hypoparathyroidism. *In* Bardin CW (ed): Current Therapy in Endocrinology and Metabolism, 4th ed. St. Louis, Mosby Yearbook, 1994, p 508.

139. Li Y, Song YH, Rais N, et al: Autoantibodies to the extracellular domain of the calcium sensing receptor in patients with acquired hypoparathyroidism. J Clin Invest 5:601, 1996.

140. Zaloga GP, Cerhnow B: The multifactorial basis for hypocalcemia during sepsis: studies of the PTH-vitamin D axis. Ann Intern Med 107:36, 1987.

141. Anderson GW, Musselman L: The treatment of tetany in pregnancy. Am J Obstet Gynecol 43:547, 1942.

142. Graham WP, Gordon GS, Loken HF, et al: Effect of pregnancy and of the menstrual cycle on hypoparathyroidism. J Clin Endocrinol Metab 24:512, 1964.

143. Bronsky D, Kiamko RT, Moncada R: Intrauterine hyperparathyroidism secondary to maternal hypoparathyroidism. Pediatrics 42:606, 1968.

144. Loughead JL, Mughal Z, Mimouni F, et al: Spectrum and natural history of congenital hyperparathyroidism secondary to maternal hypocalcemia. Am J Perinatol 7:350, 1990.

145. Brunvand L, Quistad E, Urdal P, et al: Vitamin D deficiency and fetal growth. Early Hum Dev 45:27, 1996.

146. Sadeghi-Nejad A, Wolfsdorf JI, Senior B: Hypoparathyroidism and pregnancy. Treatment with calcitrol. JAMA 243:254, 1980.

147. Salle BL, Berthezene F, Glorieux GH: Hypoparathyroidism during pregnancy: treatment with calcitriol. J Clin Endocrinol Metab 52:810, 1981.

148. Rude RK, Haussler MR, Singer FR: Postpartum resolution of hypocalcemia in a lactating hypoparathyroid patient. Endocr J 31:227, 1984.

149. Goldberg LD: Transmission of a vitamin D metabolite in breast milk. Lancet 2:1258, 1972.

150. Zerwekh JE, Breslau NA: Human placental production of 1a,25-dihydroxy-vitamin D: biochemical characterization and production in normal subjects and pateints with pseudohypoparathyroidism. J Clin Endocrinol Metab 62:192, 1986.

151. Breslau NA, Zerwekh JE: Relationship of estrogen and pregnancy to calcium homeostasis in pseudohypoparathyroidism. J Clin Endocrinol Metab 62:45, 1986.

152. Glass EJ, Barr DG: Transient neonatal hyperparathyroidism secondary to maternal pseudohypoparathyroidism. Arch Dis Child 56:565, 1981.

153. Nordin BEC, Roper A: Post pregnancy osteoporosis: a syndrome? Lancet 1:431, 1955.

154. Carbone LD, Palmieri GM, Graves SC, Smull K: Osteoporosis of pregnancy: Long term follow up of patients and their offspring. Obstet Gynecol 86:664, 1995.

155. Dunne F, Walters B, Marshall T, Heath DA: Pregnancy associated osteoporosis. Clin Endocrinol 39:487, 1993.

156. Rizzoli R, Bonjour JP: Pregnancy associated osteoporosis. Lancet 347:1274, 1996.

157. Drinkwater BL, Chesnut CH III: Bone density changes during pregnancy and lactation in active women: a longitudinal study. Bone Miner 14:153, 1991.

158. Kritz-Silverstein D, Barrett-Connor E, Hollenbach KA: Pregnancy and lactation as determinants of bone mineral density in postmenopausal women. Am J Epidemiol 136:1052, 1992.

159. Beaulieu J, Razzano C, Levine R: Transient osteoporosis of the hip in pregnancy. Clin Orthop 115:165, 1976.

160. Chigira M, Watanabe H, Udagawa E: Transient osteoporosis of the hip in the first trimester of pregnancy: a case report and review of the Japanese literature. Arch Orthop Trauma Surg 107:178, 1988.

161. Smith R, Athanasou NA, Ostlere SJ, Vipond SE: Pregnancy associated osteoporosis. Q J Med 88:865, 1995.

162. Goldman GA, Friedman S, Hod M, Ovadia J: Idiopathic transient osteoporosis of the hip in pregnancy. Int J Gynaecol Obstet 46:317, 1994.

163. Melton L, Bryant S, Wahner H, et al: Influence of breastfeeding and other reproductive factors on bone mass later in life. Osteoporos Int 3:76, 1993.

164. Sowers M, Crutchfield M, Jannausch M, et al: A prospective evaluation of bone mineral changes in pregnancy. Obstet Gynecol 77:841, 1991.

165. Dahlman T, Sjoberg H, Heligren M, et al: Calcium homeostasis in pregnancy during long term heparin treatment. Br J Obstet Gynaecol 99:412, 1992.

166. Barbour LA, Kick SD, Steiner JF, LoVerde ME: A prospective study of heparin induced osteoporosis in pregnancy using bone densitometry. Am J Obstet Gynecol 170:862, 1994.

167. Doe RP, Dickinson P, Zinneman HH, et al: Elevated nonprotein-bound cortisol (NPC) in pregnancy, during estrogen administration and in carcinoma of the prostate. J Clin Endocriol Metab 29:757, 1969.

168. Rosenthal HE, Slaunwhite WR Jr, Snadberh AA: Transcortin: a corticosteroid-binding protein of plasma. Cortisol and progesterone interplay and unbound levels of these steroids in pregnancy. J Clin Endocrinol Metab 29:352, 1969.

169. Nolten WE, Lindheimer MD, Oparil S, et al: Desoxycorticosterone in normal pregnancy. I. Sequential studies of the secre-

tory patterns desoxycorticosterone aldosterone and cortisol. Am J Obstet Gynecol 132:414, 1978.

170. Gant NF, Hutchinson HT, Siiteri PK, et al: Study of the metabolic clearance rate of dehydroisoandrosterone sulfate in pregnancy. Am J Obstet Gynecol 111:555, 1971.

171. Sheeler LR: Cushing's syndrome and pregnancy. Endocrinol Metab Clin North Am 23:619, 1994.

172. Hadden DR: Adrenal disorders of pregnancy: Endocrinol Metab Clin North Am 24:139, 1995.

173. Buescher MA: Cushing's syndrome in pregnancy. Endocrinologist 6:357, 1996.

174. Higgins T, Calabrese I, Sheeler LR: Opportunistic infections in patients with ectopic ACTH secreting tumors. Clev Clin Q 49:43, 1982.

175. Prebtani APH, Donat D, Ezzat S: Worrisome straie in pregnancy. Lancet 355:1692, 2000.

176. Lindholm J, Schultz-Moller N: Plasma and urinary cortisol in pregnancy and during estrogen-gestagen treatment. Scand J Clin Lab Invest 31:119, 1973.

177. Papanicolaou DA, Yanovski JA, Cutler GB, et al: A single midnight serum cortisol measurement distinguishes Cushing's syndrome from pseudo-Cushing states. J Clin Endocrinol Metab 83:1163, 1998.

178. Nolten WE, Lindheimer MD, Rveckert PA, et al: Diurnal patterns and regulations of cortisol secretion in pregnancy. J Clin Endocrinol Metab 51:466, 1980.

179. Anderson KJ, Walter WAW: Cushing's syndrome and pregnancy. Aust N Z J Obstet Gynaecol 43:861, 1974.

180. Kaye TB, Crapo L: The Cushing's syndrome: an update on diagnostic tests. Ann Intern Med 112:434, 1990.

181. Oldfield EH, Doppman JL, Nieman LK, et al: Petrosal sinus sampling with and without corticotropin-releasing hormones for the differential diagnosis of Cushing's syndrome. N Engl J Med 325:897, 1991.

182. Nieman LK, Oldfield EH, Wesley R, et al: A simplified morning ovine corticotropin-releasing hormone stimulation test for the differential diagnosis of adrenocorticotropin-dependent Cushing's syndrome. J Clin Endocrinol Metab 77:1308, 1993.

183. Molitch M, Russel E: The pituitary incidentaloma. Ann Intern Med 112:925, 1990.

184. Reincke M, Allolio B, Saeger W, et al: The incidentaloma of the pituitary gland: is neurosurgery required? JAMA 263:2772, 1990.

185. Liu L, Jaffe R, Borowski GD, et al: Exacerbation of Cushing's disease during pregnancy. Am J Obstet Gynceol 145:110, 1983.

186. Parra A, Cruz-Krohn J: Intercurrent Cushing's syndrome and pregnancy. Am J Med 40:961, 1966.

187. Calodney L, Eaton RP, Black W, et al: Exacerbation of Cushing's disease during pregnancy: report of a case. J Clin Endocrinol Metab 36:81, 1973.

188. Wieland RG, Shaffer MB Jr, Glove RP: Cushing's syndrome complicating pregnancy: case report. Am J Obstet Gynecol 38:841, 1971.

189. Bevan JS, Gough MH, Gillmer MDG, Burke CW: Cushing's syndrome in pregnancy: the timing of definite treatment. Clin Endocrinol 27:225, 1987.

190. Lee R, Rapoport A: Cushing's syndrome with amelioration during pregnacy. JAMA 221:392, 1972.

191. Reschini E, Giustina G, Crosignani P, et al: Spontaneous remission of Cushing's syndrome after termination of pregnancy. J Obstet Gynecol 51:598, 1978.

192. Wallace C, Toth E, Lewanczuk RZ, et al: Pregnancy induced Cushing's syndrome in multiple pregnancies. J Clin Endocrinol Metab 81:15, 1996.

193. Close CF, Mann MC, Watts JF, et al: ACTH independent Cushing's syndrome in pregnancy with spontaneous resolution after delivery: control of the hypercortisolism with metyrapone. Clin Endocrinol 39:375, 1993.

194. Koerten JM, Morales WJ, Washington SR, et al: Cushing's syndrome in pregnancy: a case report and literature review. Am J Obstet Gynecol 154:626, 1986.

195. Keely E: Endocrine causes of hypertension in pregnancy—when to start looking for zebras. Semin Perinatol 22:471, 1998.

196. Close CF, Mann MC, Watts JP, Taylor KG: ACTH independent Cushing's syndrome in pregnancy with spontaneous resolution after delivery: control of the hypercortisolism with metyrapone. Clin Endoc 39:375, 1993.

197. Ross RJM, Chew SL, Perry L, et al: Diagnosis and selective cure of Cushing's disease during pregnancy by transsphenoidal surgery. Eur J Endocrinol 132:722, 1995.

198. Pinetto MG, Pan Y, Oppenhiem D, et al: Bilateral inferior petrosal sinus corticotropin sampling in a pregnant patient with Cushing's syndrome. Am J Obstet Gynecol 171:563, 1994.

199. Mellor A, Harvey RD, Pobereskin LH, et al: Cushing's disease treated by transsphenoidal selective adenomectomy in mid-pregnancy. Br J Anaesth 80:850, 1998.

200. Gormley MJJ, Hadden DR, Kennedy TL, et al: Cushing's syndrome in pregnancy-treatment with metyrapone. Clin Endocrinol 16:283, 1982.

201. Connell JM, Cordiner J, Fraser R, et al: Pregnancy complicated by Cushing's syndrome: potential hazard of metyrapone therapy. Case report. Br J Obstet Gynaecol 92:1192, 1985.

202. Cabezon C, Bruno O, Cohen M, et al: Twin pregnancy in a patient with Cushing's disease. Fert Steril 72:371, 1999.

203. Amado JA, Pesquera C, Gonzalez EM, et al: Successful treatment with ketoconazole of Cushing's syndrome in pregnancy. Postgrad Med J 66:221, 1990.

204. Berwaerts J, Verhelst J, Mahler C, et al: Cushing's syndrome in pregnancy treated by ketoconazole: case report and review of the literature. Gynecol Endocrinol 13:175, 1999.

205. Kasperlik-Zaluska A, Migdalska B, Hartwick W, et al: Two pregnancies in women with Cushing's syndrome treated with cyproheptadine. Br J Obstet Gynaecol 87:1171, 1980.

206. Kasperlik-Kaluska AA, Nielubowicz J, Wislawski J, et al: Nelson's syndrome: incidence and prognosis. Clin Endocrinol 19:693, 1983.

207. Leiba S, Kaufman H, Winkelsberg G, Bahary CM: Pregnancy in a case of Nelson's syndrome. Acta Obstet Gynecol Scand 57:373, 1978.

208. Graber AL, Ney RL, Nicholson WE, et al: Natural history of pituitary-adrenal recovery following long term suppression with corticosteroids. J Clin Endocrinol Metab 25:11, 1965.

209. Grinspoon SK, Biller BM: Laboratory assessment of adrenal insufficiency. J Clin Endocrinol Metab 79:923, 1994.

210. Erturk E, Jaffe CA, Barkan AL: Evaluation of the integrity of the hypothalamic-pituitary-adrenal axis by insulin hypoglycemia test. J Clin Endocrinol Metab 83:2350, 1998.

211. Speckart PF, Nicoloff JT, Bethune JE: Screening for adrenocortical insufficiency with cosyntropin (synthetic ACTH). Arch Intern Med 128:761, 1971.

212. Tordjman K, Jaffe A, Grazas N, et al: The role of the low dose adrenocorticotropin test in the evaluation of patients with pituitary diseases. J Clin Endocrinol Metab 80:1301, 1995.

213. Rose LI, Williams GH, Jagger PI: The 48 hour adrenocorticotropin infusion test for adrenocortical insufficiency. Ann Intern Med 73:49, 1970.

214. Brent F: Addison's disease and pregnancy. Am J Surg 79:645, 1950.

215. Osler M: Addison's disease and pregnancy. Acta Endocrinol 41:67, 1962.

216. O'Shaughnessy RW, Hackett KJ: Maternal Addison's disease and fetal growth retardation. J Reprod Med 29:752, 1984.
217. Bongiovanni AM, McPadden AJ: Steroids during pregnancy and possible fetal consequences. Fertil Steril 11:181, 1960.
218. Garner PR: Congenital adrenal hyperplasia in pregnancy. Semin Perinatol 22:446, 1998.
219. Miller WL: Clinical review 54: genetics, diagnosis, and management of 21-hydroxylase deficiency. J Clin Endocrinol Metab 78:241, 1994.
220. Pang S, Murphey W, Levine LS, et al: A pilot newborn screening for congenital adrenal hyperplasia in Alaska. J Clin Endocrinol Metab 55:413, 1982.
221. Ferenczi A, Garami M, Kiss E, et al: Screening for mutations for 21-hydroxylase gene in Hungarian patients with congenital adrenal hyperplasia. J Clin Endocrinol Metab 84:2369, 1999.
222. Therrell BL, Berenbaum SA, Manter-Kapanke V, et al: Results of screening 1.9 million Texas newborns for 21-hydroxylase deficient congenital adrenal hyperplasia. Pediatrics 101:583, 1998.
223. Azziz R, Dewailly D, Owerbach D: Clinical review 56: nonclassic adrenal hyperplasia: current concepts. J Clin Endocrinol Metab 78:810, 1994.
224. Speiser PW, Dupont J, Zhu D, et al: Disease expression and molecular genotype in congenital adrenal hyperplasia due to 21-hydroxylase deficiency. J Clin Invest 90:584, 1992.
225. Pang S: Congenital adrenal hyperplasia. Curr Ther Endocrinol Metab 94:157, 1994.
226. Young MC, Hughes IA: Dexamethasone treatment for congenital adrenal hyperplasia. Arch Dis Child 65:312, 1990.
227. Garner PR: Managment of congenital adrenal hyperplasia in pregnancy. Endocr Pract 2:397, 1996.
228. Lo JC, Schwitzgebel VM, Tyrrell JB: Normal female infants born of mothers with classic congenital adrenal hyperplasia due to 21-hydroxylase deficiency. J Clin Endocrinol Metab 84:930, 1999.
229. Meyer-Bahlburg HF: What causes low rates of child bearing in congenital adrenal hyperplasia? J Clin Endocrinol Metab 84:1844, 1999.
230. Klingensmith GJ, Garcia SC, Jones HW Jr, et al: Glucocorticoid treatment of girls with congenital adrenal hyperplasia: effects on height, sexual maturation and fertility. Pediatrics 90:996, 1977.
231. Feldman S, Billaud L, Thalabard JC, et al: Fertility in women with late onset adrenal hyperplasia due to 21-hydroxylase deficiency. J Clin Endocrinol Metab 74:635, 1992.
232. Mulaikal RM, Migeon CJ, Rock JA: Fertility rates in female patients with congenital adrenal hyperlasia due to 21-hydroxylase deficiency. N Engl J Med 316:178, 1987.
233. Guerux B, Fiet J, Couillin P, et al: Prenatal diagnosis of 21-hydroxylase deficiency congenital hyperplasia by simultaneous radioimmunoassay of 21-deoxycortisol and 17-hydroxyprogesterone in amniotic fluid. J Clin Endocrinol Metab 66:534, 1988.
234. Mercado AB, Wilson RC, Cheng KC, et al: Prenatal treatment and diagnosis of congenital adrenal hyperplasia owing to steroid 21-hydroxylase deficiency. J Clin Endocrinol Metab 80:2014, 1995.
235. Evans MI, Chrousos GP, Mann DW, et al: Pharmacological suppression of the fetal adrenal gland in utero. Attempted prevention of abnormal external genital masculinization in suspected congenital adrenal hyperplasia. JAMA 253:1015, 1985.
236. Pang S, Clark AT, Freeman LC, et al: Maternal side effects of prenatal dexamethasone therapy for fetal congenital adrenal hyperplasia. J Clin Endocrinol Metab 75:249, 1992.
237. Lajic S, Wedell A, Bui TH, et al: Long term somatic follow up of prenatally treated children with congenital adrenal hyperplasia. J Clin Endocrinol Metab 83:3872, 1998.
238. Miller WL: Congenital adrenal hyperplasias. Endocrinol Metab Clin North Am 20:721, 1991.
239. White PC, Curnow KM, Pascoe L: Disorders of steroid 11-beta-hydroxylase isozymes. Endocr Rev 15:421, 1994.
240. Zachmann M, Tassinari D, Prader A: Clinical and biochemical variability of congenital adrenal hyperplasia due to 11-beta-hydroxylase deficiency. A study of 25 patients. J Clin Endocrinol Metab 56:222, 1983.
241. Rosler A, Weshler N, Leiberman E, et al: 11-hydroxylase deficiency congenital adrenal hyperplasia: update of prenatal diagnosis. J Clin Endocrinol Metab 66:830, 1988.
242. Cerame BL, Newfield RS, Pascoe L, et al: Prenatal diagnosis and treatment of 11-beta-hydroxylase deficiency congenital adrenal hyperplasia resulting in normal female genitalia. J Clin Endocrinol Metab 84:3129, 1999.
243. Conn JW: Primary aldosteronism: a new clinical syndrome. J Lab Clin Med 45:3, 1955.
244. Bravo EL: Primary aldosteronism: issues in diagnosis and treatment. Endocrinol Metab Clin North Am 23:271, 1994.
245. Ehrlich EH, Lindheimer MD: Effect of administered mineralocorticoid or ACTH in pregnant women: attenuation of kaliuretic influence of mineralocorticoids during pregnancy. J Clin Invest 51:1301, 1972.
246. Gordon RD, Tunny TJ: Aldosterone-producing-adenoma (A-P-A): effect of pregnancy. Clin Exp Hypertens 4:1685, 1982.
247. Biglieri EG, Slaton PE Jr: Pregnancy and primary aldosteronism. J Clin Endocrinol Metab 27:1628, 1967.
248. Elterman JJ, Hagen GA: Aldosteronism in pregnancy: association with virilization of female offspring. South Med J 76:514, 1983.
249. Solomon CG, Thiet MP, Moore F, et al: Primary hyperaldosteronism in pregnancy—a case report. J Reprod Med 41:255, 1996.
250. Webb JC, Bayliss P: Pregnancy complicated by primary aldosteronism. South Med J 90:243, 1997.
251. Baron F, Sprauve ME, Huddleston JF, et al: Diagnosis and surgical treatment of primary aldosteronism in pregnancy: a case report. Obstet Gynecol 86:644, 1995.
252. Brown JJ, Chinn RH, Ferris JB: Hypertension with hyperaldosteronism and low plasma renin concentration: the effect of prolonged treatment with spironolactone. Q J Med 39:631, 1970.
253. Laurel MT, Kabadi UM: Primary hyperaldosteronism. Endocr Pract 3:47, 1997.
254. Piouin PF, Chatellier G, Fofol I, et al: Tumor recurrence and hypertension persistence after successful pheochromocytoma operation. Hypertension 29:1133, 1997.
255. Greenberg M, Moawad AH, Wieties BM, et al: Extra-adrenal pheochromocytoma: detection during pregnancy using MRI. Radiology 161:475, 1986.
256. Bakri YN, Ingemansson SE, Ali A, et al: Pheochromocytoma in pregnancy. Acta Obstet Gynecol Scand 71:301, 1992.
257. Keely E: Endocrine causes of hypertension in pregnancy—when to start looking for zebras. Semin Perinatol 22:471, 1998.
258. Fox LP, Grandi J, Johnson AH, et al: Pheochromocytoma associated with pregnancy. Am J Obstet Gynecol 104:288, 1969.
259. Schenker JG, Granat M: Pheochromocytoma and pregnancy: an updated appraisal. Aust N Z J Obstet Gynaecol 22:1, 1982.
260. Harper MA, Murnaghan GA, Kennedy L, et al: Pheochromocytoma in pregnancy. Five cases and a review of the literature. Br J Obstet Gynaecol 96:594, 1989.
261. Bravo EL: Evolving concepts in the pathophysiology, diagno-

sis, and treatment of pheochromocytoma. Endocr Rev 15:356, 1994.

262. Peaston RT, Lennard TW, Lai LC: Overnight excretion of urinary catecholamines and metabolites in the detection of pheochromocytoma. J Clin Endocrinol Metab 4:1378, 1996.

263. Zuspan FP: Adrenal gland and sympathetic nervous system response in eclampsia. Am J Obstet Gynecol 114:304, 1972.

264. Katz VL, Jenkins T, Haley L, et al: Catecholamine levels in pregnant physicians and nurses. Obstet Gynecol 77:338, 1991.

265. Keely EJ: Pheochromocytoma in pregnancy. Curr Obstet Med 3:73, 1995.

266. Elliott WJ, Murphy MB: Reduced specificity of the clonidine suppression test in pregnancy with normal plasma catecholamine levels. Am J Med 84:419, 1988.

267. Griffith MMI, Felts JH, James FM, et al: Successful control of pheochromocytoma in pregnancy. JAMA 229:437, 1974.

268. Shapiro B: Imaging of catecholamine secreting tumours: uses of MIBG in diagnosis and treatment. Baillieres Clin Endocrinol Metab 7:741, 1993.

269. Sjoberg RJ, Simcic KJ, Kidd GS: The clonidine suppression test for pheochromocytoma: a review of its utility and pitfalls. Arch Intern Med 152:1193, 1992.

270. Burgess GE III, Cooper JR, Marino JR, et al: Anesthetic management of combined cesarean section and excision of pheochromocytoma. Anesth Analg 25:276, 1978.

271. Desmonds JM, Marty J: Anaesthetic management of patients with phaeochromocytoma. Br J Anaesth 56:781, 1984.

272. Velchik MG, Alavi A, Kressel HY, et al: Localization of pheochromocytoma MIBG, CT, and MRI correlation. J Nucl Med 30:328, 1989.

273. Burgess GE III: Alpha blockade and surgical intervention of pheochromocytoma in pregnancy. Obstet Gynecol 53:226, 1979.

274. Venuto R, Burstein P, Schneider R: Pheochromocytoma: antepartum diagnosis and management with tumor resection in the puerperium. Am J Obstet Gynecol 150:431, 1984.

275. Stenstrom G, Swolin K: Pheochromocytoma in pregnancy experience in treatment with phenoxybenzamine in three patients. Acta Obstet Gynecol Scand 64:367, 1985.

276. Finkenstedt G, Gasser RW, Hofle G, et al: Pheochromocytoma and subclinical Cushing's syndrome during pregnancy: diagnosis, medical pre-treatment and cure by laparoscopic unilateral adrenalectomy. J Endocrinol Invest 7:551, 1999.

277. Demeure MJ, Carlsen B, Traul D, et al: Laparoscopic removal of a right adrenal pheochromocytoma in a pregnant woman. J Laparoendosc Adv Surg Tech A 5:315, 1998.

278. Takahashi K, Sai Y, Nosaka S: Anaesthetic management for ceasarean section combined with removal of phaeochromocytoma. Eur J Anaesthesiol 15:364, 1998.

279. Desmonts JM, Marty J: Anaesthetic management of patients with pheochromocytoma. Br J Anaesthesiol 56:781, 1984.

280. McClamrock HD, Adashi EY: Gestational hyperandrogenism. Fertil Steril 57:257, 1992.

281. Manganiello PD, Adams LV, Harris RD, et al: Virilization during pregnancy with spontaneous resolution postpartum: a case report and review of the English literature. Obstet Gynecol Surv 50:404, 1995.

282. Grumbach MM, Ducharme JR, Moloshok RE: On the fetal masculinizing action of certain oral progestins. J Clin Endocrinol Metab 19:1369, 1959.

283. Thomas E, Mestman JH, Henneman C, et al: Bilateral luteomas of pregnancy with virilization: a case report. Obstet Gynecol 39:577, 1972.

284. Garcia-Bunuel R, Berek JS, Woodruff JD: Luteomas of pregnancy. Obstet Gynecol Surv 45:635, 1975.

285. Nagamani M, Gomes LG, Garza J: In vivo steorid studies in luteoma of pregnancy. Obstet Gynecol 59:105S, 1982.

286. Verkauf BS, Reiter EO, Hernandez L, et al: Virilization of mother and fetus associated with luteoma of pregnancy: a case report with endocrinologic studies. Am J Obstet Gynecol 129:274, 1977.

287. Hensleight PA, Carter RP, Grotjan HE: Fetal protection against masculinization with hyperreactio luteinalis and virilization. J Clin Endocrinol Metab 40:816, 1975.

288. Muechler EK, Fichter J, Zonogrone J: Human chorionic gonadotropin, estradiol, testosterone changes in two pregnancies with hyperreactio luteinalis. Am J Obstet Gynecol 157:1126, 1987.

289. Berger NG, Repke JT, Woodrull JD: Markedly elevated serum testosterone in pregnancy without fetal virilization. Obstet Gynecol 63:260, 1984.

290. Shozu M, Akasofu K, Harada T, et al: A new cause of female pseudohermaphroditism: placental aromatase deficiency. J Clin Endocrinol Metab 72:560, 1991.

291. Glinoer D: The regulation of thyroid function in pregnancy: pathways of endocrine adaptation from physiology to pathology. Endocr Rev 18:404, 1997.

292. Mestman JH: Thyroid diseases in pregnancy. Clin Obstet Gynecol 40:45, 1997.

293. Smallridge R: Symposium on thyroid disease in pregnancy and the postpartum period. Thyroid 9:629, 1999.

294. Hollowell JG, Staehling NW, Hannon WH, et al: Iodine nutrition in the United States. Trends and public health implications: iodine excretion data from National Health and Nutrition Examination Survey 1 and 3 (1971–1974 and 1988–1994). J Clin Endocrinol Metab 83:3401, 1998.

295. Haddow JE, Palomaki GE, Allan WC, et al: Maternal thyroid deficiency during pregnancy and subsequent neuropsychological development of the child. N Engl J Med 341:549, 1999.

296. Pop VJ, Kulipens JL, van Baar AL, et al: Low maternal free thyroxine concentrations during early pregnancy are associated with impaired pyschomotor development in infancy. Clin Endocrinol 50:149, 1999.

297. Thorpe-Beeston JG, Nicolaides KH, Felton CV, et al: Maturation of the secretion of thyroid hormone and thyroid stimulating hormone in the fetus. N Engl J Med 324:532, 1991.

298. Contempre B, Jauniaux E, Calvo R, et al: Detection of thyroid hormones in human embryonic cavities during the first trimester of pregnancy. J Clin Endocrinol Metab 77:1719, 1993.

299. Bernal J, Pekonen F: Ontogenesis of the nuclear 3,5,3′-triidothyronine receptor in the human fetal brain. Endocrinology 114:677, 1984.

300. Vulsma T, Gons MH, DeVijlder JJM: Maternal fetal transfer of thyroxine in congenital hypothyroidism due to a total organification defect or thyroid agenesis. N Engl J Med 321:13, 1989.

301. Iskaros J, Pickard M, Evans I, et al: Thyroid hormone receptor gene expression in first trimester human fetus brain. J Clin Endocrinol Metab 85:2620, 2000.

302. Ain KB, Mori Y, Refetoff S: Reduced clearance rate of thyroxine-binding globulin (TBG) with increased sialylation: a mechanism for estrogen-induced elevation of serum TBG concentration. J Clin Endocrinol Metab 65:686, 1987.

303. Glinoer D, DeNayer P, Bourdoux P, et al: Regulation of maternal thyroid during pregnancy. J Clin Endocrinol Metab 71:276, 1990.

304. Brent GA, Mestman JH: Physiology and tests of thyroid function. *In* Sciarra J (ed): Gynecology and Obstetrics, Vol 5. Philadelphia, Lippincott-Raven, 1999.

305. Zakarija M, McKenzie JM, Hoffman WH: Predications and

therapy of intrauterine and late onset neonatal hyperthyroidism. J Clin Endocriol Metab 62:368, 1986.

306. Iseki M, Shimizu M, Oikawa T, et al: Sequential serum measurements of thyrotropin binding inhibitor immunoglobulin G in transient familial neonatal hypothyroidism. J Clin Endocrinol Metab 57:384, 1983.

307. Stagnaro-Green A, Roman SH, Cobin RH, et al: A prospective study of lymphocyte-initiated immunosuppression in normal pregnancy: evidence of a T cell etiology for postpartum thyroid dysfunction. J Clin Endocrinol Metab 74:645, 1992.

308. Momotani N, Ito K, Hamada N, et al: Maternal hyperthyroidism and congential malformation of the offspring. Clin Endocrinol 20:695, 1984.

309. Mandel SL, Larsen PR, Seely EW, et al: Increased need for thyroxine during pregnancy in women with primary hypothyroidism. N Engl J Med 323:91, 1990.

310. Kaplan MM: Management of women on thyroxine therapy during pregnancy. Endocr Pract 2:281, 1996.

311. Heckel S, Favre R, Schlienger JL, et al: Diagnosis and successful in utero treatment of a fetal goitrous hyperthyroidism caused by maternal Graves' disease. Fetal Diagn Ther 12:54, 1997.

312. Schlumberger M, Vathaire F, Ceccarelli C, et al: Exposure to radioactive iodine 131 for scintigraphy or therapy does not preclude pregnancy in thyroid cancer patients. J Nucl Med 37:606, 1996.

313. Mestman JH: Thyroid hormone replacement during pregnancy. In Meikle AW (ed): Hormone Replacement Therapy. Philadelphia, Humana Press, 1997, p 119.

314. Campbell NRC, Hasinoff BB, Stalts H, et al: Ferrous sulfate reduces thyroxine efficacy in patients with hypothyroidism. Ann Intern Med 117:1010, 1992.

315. Singh N, Singh P, Hershman JM: Effect of calcium carbonate on the absorption of levothyroxine. JAMA 283:2822, 2000.

316. Amino N, Tada H, Hidaka Y: Postpartum autoimmune thyroid syndrome: a model of aggravation of autoimmune disease. Thyroid 9:705, 1999.

317. Caixas A, Albareda M, Garcia-Patterson A, et al: Postpartum thyroiditis in women with hypothyroidism antedating pregnancy? J Clin Endocrinol Metab 84:4000, 1999.

318. Porterfield SP, Hendrich CE: The role of thyroid hormones in prenatal and neonatal neurological development: current perspectives. Endocr Rev 14:94, 1993.

319. DeZegher F, Spitz B, Devlieger H: Prenatal treatment with thyrotropin releasing hormone to prevent neonatal respiratory distress. Arch Dis Child 67:450, 1992.

320. Burrow GN: Neonatal goiter after maternal propylithiouracil therapy. J Clin Endocrinol Metab 25:403, 1965.

321. Galina MP, Avnet NL, Einhorn A: Iodine during pregnancy: an apparent cause of neonatal death. N Engl J Med 267:1124, 1962.

322. Mestman JH: Hyperthyroidism in pregnancy. Endocrinol Metab Clin North Am 27:127, 1998.

323. Masiukiewicz U, Burrow GN: Hyperthyroidism in pregnancy. Diagnosis and treatment. Thyroid 9:647, 1999.

324. Goodwin TM, Montoro MN, Mestman JH: Transient hyperthyroidism and hyperemesis gravidarum: clinical aspects. Am J Obstet Gynecol 167:648, 1992.

325. Hershman JM: Human chorionic gonadotropin and the thyroid: hyperemesis gravidarum and trophoblastic tumors. Thyroid 9:653, 1999.

326. Bouillon R, Maesens M, Van Assche A, et al: Thyroid function in patients with hyperemesis gravidarum. Am J Obstet Gynecol 143:922, 1982.

327. Lao TT, Chin RKH, Chang AMZ: The outcome of hypermetic pregnancies complicated by transient hyperthyroidism. Aust N Z J Obstet Gynaecol 27:99, 1987.

328. Bober SA, McGill AC, Tunbridge WM: Thyroid function in hyperemesis gravidarum. Acta Endocrinol 111:404, 1986.

329. Kirshon B, Lee W, Cotton DB: Prompt resolution of hyperthyroidism and hyperemesis gravidarum after delivery. Obstet Gynecol 71:1032, 1988.

330. Goodwin TM, Montoro M, Mestman J, et al: The role of chorionic gonadotropin in transient hyperthyroidism of hyperemesis gravidarum. J Clin Endocrinol Metab 75:1333, 1992.

331. Rosenthal FD, Jones C, Lewis SI: Thyrotoxic vomiting. BMJ 2:209, 1976.

332. Goodwin TM, Hershman JM: Hyperthyroidism due to inappropriate production of human chorionic gonadotropin. Clin Obstet Gynceol 40:32, 1997.

333. Grun JP, Meuris S, De Nayer P, et al: The thyrotrophic role of human chorionic gonadotropin (hCG) in the early stages of twin (versus single) pregnancies. Clin Endocrinol 46:719, 1997.

334. Rodien P, Bremont C, Raffin-Sanson ML: Familial gestational hyperthyroidism caused by a mutant thyrotropin receptor hypersensitive to human chorionic gonadotropin. N Engl J Med 339:1823, 1998.

335. Mori M, Amino N, Tamaki H, et al: Morning sickness and thyroid function in normal pregnancy. Obstet Gynecol 72:355, 1988.

336. Tamaki H, Itoh E, Kaneda T, et al: Crucial role of serum human chorionic gonadotropin for the aggravation of thyrotoxicosis in early pregnancy in Graves' disease. Thyroid 3:189, 1993.

337. Weetman AP: The immunology of pregnancy. Thyroid 9:543, 1999.

338. Kung AWC, Jones BM: A change from stimulatory to blocking antibody activity in Graves' disease during pregnancy. J Clin Endocrinol Metab 83:514, 1998.

339. Mestman JH, Manning PR, Hodgman J: Hyperthyroidism and pregnancy. Arch Intern Med 134:434, 1974.

340. Davis LE, Lucas MJ, Hankins GDV, et al: Thyrotoxicosis complicating pregnancy. Am J Obstet Gynecol 160:63, 1988.

341. Mitsuda N, Tamaki H, Amino N, et al: Risk factors for developmental disorders in infants born to women with Graves' disease. Obstet Gynecol 80:359, 1992.

342. Millar LK, Wing DA, Leung AS, et al: Low birth weight and preeclampsia in pregnancies complicated by hyperthyroidism. Obstet Gynecol 84:946, 1994.

343. Bell GO, Hall J: Hyperthyroidism in pregnancy. Med Clin North Am 44:363, 1960.

344. Hawe P: The management of thyrotoxicosis during pregnancy. Br J Surg 52:731, 1965.

345. Momotani N, Noh J, Oyangi H, et al: Antithyroid drug therapy for Graves' disease during pregnancy: optimal regimen for fetal thyroid status. N Engl J Med 315:24, 1986.

346. Surgue D, Drury MI: Hyperthyroidism complicating pregnancy results of treatment by antithyroid drugs in 77 pregnancies. Br J Obstet Gynaecol 87:970, 1980.

347. Sherif IH, Dyan WT, Basairi S, et al: Treatment of hyperthyroidism in pregnancy. Acta Obstet Gynecol Scand 70:461, 1991.

348. Momatani N, Ito K: Treatment of pregnant patients with Basedow's disease. Exp Clin Endocrinol 97:268, 1991.

349. Clark SL, Phelan JP, Montoro MN, et al: Transient ventricular dysfunction associated with cesarean section in a patient with hyperthyroidism. Am J Obstet Gynecol 151:384, 1985.

350. Mestman JH: Severe hyperthyroidism in pregnancy. In Clark SL, Cotton DB, Hankins GDV, Phelan JP (eds): Critical Care Obstetrics, 2nd ed. London, Blackwell Scientific Publications, 1991, p 307.

351. Easterline TR, Schumacker BC, Carlson KL, et al: Maternal

hemodynamics in pregnancies complicated by hyperthyroidism. Obstet Gynecol 78:348, 1991.

352. Guenter KE, Friedland GA: Thyroid storm and placenta previa in a primigravida. Obstet Gynecol 44:403, 1965.

353. Mestman JH, Singer PA: Thyroid storm need not be lethal. Contemp Obstet Gynecol 22:135, 1983.

354. Mestman JH: Disorder of the thyroid gland. *In* Sciarra JJ (ed): Gynecology and Obstetrics. Philadelphia, Lippincott-Raven, 1996, p 1.

355. Mortimer RH, Cannell GR, Addison RS, et al: Methimazole and propylthiouracil equally cross the perfused human term placental lobule. J Clin Endocrinol Metab 82:3099, 1997.

356. Wing DA, Miller LK, Koonings PP: A comparision of propylthiouracil versus methimazole in the treatment of hyperroidism in pregnancy. Am J Obstet Gynecol 170:90, 1994.

357. Momotani N, Noh JY, Ishikawa N, et al: Effects of propylthiouracil and methimazole on fetal thyroid status in mothers with Graves' hyperthyroidism. J Clin Endocrinol Metab 82:3633, 1997.

358. Milham S: Scalp defects in infants of mothers treated for hyperthyroidism with methimazole or carbimazole during pregnancy. Teratology 32:321, 1985.

359. Van Dikje CP, Heydendael RJ, De Kleine MJ: Methimazole, carbimazole and congenital skin defects. Ann Intern Med 106:60, 1987.

360. Mandel SK, Brent GA, Larsen PR: Review of antithyroid drug use during pregnancy and report of a case of aplasia cutis. Thyroid 4:129, 1994.

361. Ramirez A, Espinoza de los Monteros A, Parra A, et al: Esophageal atresia and tracheoesophageal fistula in two infants born to hyperthyroid women receiving methimazole (Tapazole) during pregnancy. Am J Med Genet 44:200, 1992.

362. Johnsson E, Larsson G, Ljunggren M: Severe malformations in infants born to hyperthyroid mothers on methimazole. Lancet 350:1520, 1997.

363. Greenberg F: Choanal atresia and athelia: methimazole teratogenicity or a new syndrome? Am J Med Genet 28:931, 1987.

364. Cooper DS: Which antithyroid drug? Am J Med 80:1165, 1986.

365. Cooper DS: Propylthiouracil levels in hyperthyroid patients unresponsive to large doses. Ann Intern Med 192:328, 1985.

366. Burrow GN: Thyroid function and hyperfunction during gestation. Endocr Rev 14:194, 1993.

367. Cheron RG, Kaplan MM, Larsen PR, et al: Neonatal thyroid function after propylthiouracil therapy for maternal Graves' disease. N Engl J Med 304:525, 1981.

368. Franklyn JA: The management of hyperthyroidism. N Engl J Med 330:1731, 1994.

369. Rosove MH: Agranulocytosis and antithyroid drugs. West J Med 126:339, 1977.

370. Cooper DS, Golminz D, Levin AA, et al: Agranulocytosis associated with antithyroid drugs: effects of patient's age and drug dose. Ann Intern Med 98:26, 1983.

371. Bowman MI, Bergmann M, Smith JF: Intrapartum labetalol for the treatment of maternal and fetal thyrotoxicosis. Thyroid 8:795, 1988.

372. Bruner J, Landon MB, Gabbe SG: Diabetes mellitus and Graves' disease in pregnancy complicated by maternal allergies to antithyroid medication. Obstet Gynecol 72:443, 1988.

373. Stoffer SS, Hamburger JI: Inadvertent 131I therapy for hyperthyroidism in the first trimester of pregnancy. J Nucl Med 17:146, 1976.

374. Berg GE, Nystrom EH, Jacobson L, et al: Radioiodine treatment of hyperthyroidism in a pregnant woman. J Nucl Med 39:357, 1998.

375. Vicens-Calvet E, Potau N, Carreras E, et al: Diagnosis and treatment in utero of goiter with hypothyroidism caused by iodide overload. J Pediatr 133:147, 1998.

376. Momotani N, Hisaoka T, Noh J, et al: Effects of iodine on thyroid status of fetus versus mother in treatment of Graves' disease complicated by pregnancy. J Clin Endocrinol Metab 75:738, 1992.

377. Perelman AH, Johnson RL, Clemons RD, et al: Intrauterine diagnosis and treatment of fetal goitrous hypothyroidism. J Clin Endocinrol Metab 71:618, 1990.

378. Cooper DS: Antithyroid drugs: to breastfeed or not to breastfeed. Am J Obstet Gynecol 157:234, 1987.

379. Momotani N, Yamashita R, Yoshimoto M, et al: Recovery from fetal hypothyroidism: evidence for the safety of breastfeeding while taking propylthiouracil. Clin Endocrinol (Oxf) 31:591, 1989.

380. Azizi F: Effects of methimazole treatment of maternal thyrotoxicosis on thyroid function in breastfeeding infants. J Pediatr 128:855, 1996.

381. McKenzie JM, Zakarija M: Fetal and neonatal hyperthyroidism and hypothyroidism due to maternal TSH receptor antibodies. Thyroid 2:155, 1992.

382. Polak M: Hyperthyroidism in early infancy: pathogenesis, clinical features and diagnosis with a focus on neonatal hyperthyroidism. Thyroid 8:1171, 1998.

383. Hollingsworth DR, Mabry CC: Congential Graves' disase. Four familial cases with long term follow up and perspective. Am J Dis Child 130:148, 1976.

384. Kopp P, Van Sande J, Parma J, et al: Brief report: congenital hyperthyroidism caused by a mutation in the thyrotropin receptor gene. N Engl J Med 322:150, 1995.

385. De Roux N, Polak M, Coet J: A neomutation of thyroid stimulating hormone receptor in severe neonatal hyperthyroidism. J Clin Endocrinol Metab 81:2023, 1996.

386. Cove DH, Johnston P: Fetal hyperthyroidism: experience of treatment in four siblings. Lancet 1:430, 1985.

387. Perelman AH, Clemons RD: The fetus in maternal hyperthyroidism. Thyroid 2:225, 1992.

388. Wanstrom KD, Weiner CP, Williamson I, et al: Prenatal diagnosis of fetal hyperthyroidism using funipuncture. Obstet Gynecol 76:513, 1990.

389. Bruinse HW, Vermuelen-Weiner C, Wit JM: Fetal treatment for thyrotoxicosis in nonthyrotoxic pregnant women. Fetal Ther 3:152, 1988.

390. Porreco RP, Bloch CA: Fetal blood sampling in the management of intrauterine thyrotoxicosis. Obstet Gynecol 76:509, 1990.

391. Vali A, Wiles P, Thomas NB, et al: Relapse of maternal thyrotoxicosis presenting as a second trimester fetal goiter. Ultrasound Obstet Gynecol 3:429, 1993.

392. Pekonen F, Teramo K, Makinen T, et al: Prenatal diagnosis and treatment of fetal thyrotoxicosis. Am J Obstet Gynecol 1450:9893, 1984.

393. Skuza KA, Sills IN, Stene M, et al: Prediction of neonatal hyperthyroidism in infants born to mothers with Graves' disease. J Pediatr 128:264, 1996.

394. Zimmerman D: Fetal and neonatal hyperthyroidism. Thyroid 9:727, 1999.

395. Montoro MN, Collea JV, Frasier SD, et al: Successful outcome of pregnancy in women with hypothyroidism. Ann Intern Med 94:31, 1981.

396. Davis LE, Leveno KJ, Cunningham FG: Hypothyroidism complicating pregnancy. Obstet Gynecol 72:108, 1988.

397. Leung AS, Millar LK, Koonings PP, et al: Perinatal outcome in hypothyroid pregnancies. Obstet Gynecol 81:349, 1993.

398. Tamaki H, Amino N, Takeoka K, et al: Thyroxine requirements during pregnnacy for replacement therapy of hypothyroidism. Obstet Gynecol 76:230, 1990.

399. Klein RZ, Haddow JE, Faix JD, et al: Prevalence of thyroid deficiency in pregnant women. Clin Endocrinol (Oxf) 35:41, 1991.

400. Kamijo K, Saito T, Sato M, et al: Transient subclinical hypothyroidism in early pregnancy. Endocrinol J 37:397, 1990.

401. Lejeune B, Leomone M, Kinchac J, et al: The epidemiology of autoimmune and functional thyroid disorders in pregnancy [Abstract]. Endocrinol Invest 15(Suppl):77, 1992.

402. Dussault JH, Fisher DA: Thyroid function in mothers of hypothyroid newborns. Obstet Gynecol 93:15, 1999.

403. Fukushi M, Honma K, Fujita K: Maternal thyroid deficiency during pregnancy and subsequent neurophysiological development of the child (Letter). N Engl J Med 341:2016, 1999.

404. Man EB: Maternal hypothyroxinemia, development of 4 and 7 years old offspring. *In* Fisher DA, Burrows GN (eds): Perinatal Thyroid Physiology and Disease. New York, Raven Press, 1975, p 177.

405. Harjai KJ, Licata AA: Effects of amiodarone on thyroid function. Ann Intern Med 126:63, 1997.

406. Wilson R, McKillop KH, Crocket GT, et al: The effect of lithium therapy on parameters thought to be involved in the development of autoimmune thyroid disease. Clin Endocrinol (Oxf) 34:357, 1991.

407. Zograbyan A, Goodwin TM, Montoro MN, et al: What are the risk factors for perinatal complications in hypothyroidism. Abstract 142 presented at the 71st Annual Meeting of the American Thyroid Association, September 16, 1998, Portland, Oregon.

408. Man EB, Brown JF, Serunian SA: Maternal hypothyroxinemia: psychoneurological defects of progeny. Ann Clin Lab Sci 21:227, 1991.

409. Liu H, Momotani N, Yoshimura J, et al: Maternal hypothyroidism during early pregnancy and intellectual development of the progeny. Arch Intern Med 154:785, 1994.

410. de Escobar GM, Obregon JM, del Rey FE: Transfer of thyroid hormones from the mother to the fetus. *In* Delange F, Fisher DA, Glineor D (eds): Research in Congenital Hypothyroidism. New York, Plenum Press, 1988, p 15.

411. Singer PA, Cooper DS, Daniels G: Guidelines for the diagnosis and management of thyroid nodules and well differentiated thyroid cancer. Arch Intern Med 156:2165, 1996.

412. Hamberger JI: Thyroid nodules in pregnancy. Thyroid 2:165, 1992.

413. Hay ID: Nodular thyroid disease diagnosed during pregnancy: how and when to treat. Thyroid 9:667, 1999.

414. Tan GH, Gharib H, Goeliner JR, et al: Management of thyroid nodules in pregnancy. Arch Intern Med 156:2317, 1996.

415. Rosen JB, Walfish PG, Nikore V: Pregnancy and surgical thyroid disease. Surgery 98:1135, 1985.

416. Doherty CM, Shindo ML, Rice DH, et al: Management of thyroid nodules during pregnancy. Laryngoscope 105:251, 1995.

417. Moosa M, Mazzaferri EL: Outcome of differentiated thyroid cancer diagnosed in pregnant women. J Clin Endocrinol Metab 82:2862, 1997.

418. Cortelazzi D, Castagnone D, Tassis B, et al: Resolution of hyperthyroidism in a pregnant woman with toxic thyroid nodule by percutaneous ethanol injection. Thyroid 5:473, 1995.

419. Kamei N, Gullu S, Dagci Ilgin S, et al: Degree of thyrotropin suppression in differentiated thyroid cancer wihtout recurrence of metastases. Thyroid 9:1245, 1999.

420. Singer PA: Thyroiditis: acute, subacute, and chronic. Med Clin North Am 75:61, 1991.

421. Vanderpump MPJ, Tunbridge WMG, French JM, et al: The incidence of thyroid disorders in the community: a twenty year follow up of the Whickham Survey. Clin Endocrinol 43:55, 1995.

422. Doniach D, Roitt IM, Taylor KB: Autoimmunity in pernicious anemia and thyroiditis: a family study. Ann N Y Acad Sci 124:605, 1965.

423. Hall R, Stanbury JB: Familial studies of autoimmune thyroiditis. Clin Exp Immunol 2:719, 1967.

424. McCanlies E, O'Leary LA, Foley TP, et al: Hashimoto's thyroiditis and insulin dependent diabetes mellitus: differences among individuals with and without abnormal thyroid function. J Clin Endocrinol Metab 83:1548, 1998.

425. Gutekunst R, Hafermann W, Mansky T, et al: Ultrasonography related to clinical and laboratory findings in lymphocytic thyroiditis. Acta Endocrinol (Copenh) 121:129, 1989.

426. Stagnaro-Green A, Roman SH, Cobin RH, et al: Detection of at risk pregnancy by means of highly sensitive assays for thyroid autoantibodies. JAMA 264:1422, 1990.

427. Glineor D, Fernandez-Soto M, Bourdoux P, et al: Pregnancy in patients with mild thyroid abnormalities: maternal and fetal repercussions. J Clin Endocrinol Metab 73:421, 1991.

428. Singh A, Danta ZN, Stone S, et al: Presence of thyroid antibodies in early reproductive failure: biochemical versus clinical pregnancies. Fertil Steril 63:277, 1995.

429. Stagnaro-Green A: Recognizing, understanding and treating postpartum thyroiditis. Endocrinol Metab Clin North Am 29:417, 2000.

430. Glineor D, Riahi M, Grun JP, et al: Risk of subclinical hypothyroidism in pregnant women with asymptomatic autoimmune thyroid disorders. J Clin Endocrinol Metab 79:197, 1994.

431. Arikawa K, Ichikawa Y, Yoshida T, et al: Blocking type antithyrotropin receptor antibody in patients with nongoitrous hypothyroidism: its incidence and characteristics of action. J Clin Endocrinol Metab 60:953, 1985.

432. Matsuura N, Yamada Y, Nohara Y, et al: Familial neonatal transient hypothyroidism due to maternal TSH binding inhibitor immunoglobulins. N Engl J Med 303:738, 1980.

433. Ginsberg J, Walfish PG, Rafter DJ, et al: Thyrotropin blocking antibodies in the sera of mothers with congenitally hypothyroid infants. Clin Endocrinol 25:189, 1986.

434. LaFranchi S: Congenital hypothyroidism: etiologies, diagnosis, and management. Thyroid 9:735, 1999.

435. Brown RS, Bellasario RL, Botero D, et al: Incidence of transient congenital hypothyroidism due to maternal thyrotropin antibodies in over one million babies. J Clin Endocrinol Metab 81:1147, 1996.

436. Pop VJ, DeVries E, Van Baar AL, et al: Maternal thyroid peroxidase antibodies during pregnancy: a marker of impaired child development? J Clin Endocrinol Metab 80:3561, 1995.

437. Amino N, Mori H, Iwatani O, et al: High prevalence of transient postpartum thyrotoxicosis and hypothyroidism. N Engl J Med 306:849, 1982.

438. Roti E, Emerson SH: Postpartum thyroiditis. J Clin Endocrinol Metab 74:3, 1992.

439. Smallridge RC: Postpartum thyroid diseases through the ages: a historical view. Thyroid 9:671, 1999.

440. Gerstein HC: How common is postpartum thyroiditis? A methodologic overview of the literature. Arch Intern Med 150:1397, 1990.

441. Alvarez-Marfany M, Roman SH, Drexler AJ, et al: Long term prospective study of postpartum thyroid dysfunction in women with insulin dependent diabetes mellitus. J Clin Endocrinol Metab 79:10, 1994.

442. Kent GN, Stucky BG, Allen JR, et al: Postpartum thyroid dysfunction: clinical assessment and relationship to psychiatric affective morbidity. Clin Endocrinol (Oxf) 51:429, 1999.

443. Amino N, Tada H, Hidaka Y, et al: Therapeutic controversy: screening for postpartum thyroiditis. J Clin Endocrinol Metab 84:1813, 1999.

444. Kuijpens JL, Pop VJ, Vader HL, et al: Prediction of postpartum thyroid dysfunction: can it be improved? Eur J Endocrinol 139:36, 1998.

445. Othman S, Phillips DIW, Parkes AB, et al: A long term follow up of postpartum thyroiditis. Clin Endocrinol (Oxf) 32:559, 1990.

446. Tachi J, Amino N, Tamaki H, et al: Long term follow up and HLA association in patients with postpartum hypothyroidism. J Clin Endocrinol Metab 66:480, 1988.

447. Premawardhana LDKE, Parkes AB, Ammari F, et al: Postpartum thyroiditis and long term thyroid status prognostic influence of thyroid peroxidase antibodies and ultrasound echogenicity. J Clin Endocrinol Metab 85:71, 2000.

448. Amino N, Miyai K, Yamamoto T, et al: Transient recurrence of hyperthyroidism after delivery in Graves' disease. J Clin Endocrinol Metab 44:130, 1977.

449. Eckel RH, Green WL: Postpartum thyrotoxicosis in a patient with Graves' disease associated with low radioactive iodine uptake. JAMA 243:1545, 1980.

450. Momotani N, Noh J, Ishikawa N, et al: Relationship between silent thyroiditis and recurrent Graves' disease in the postpartum period. J Clin Endocrinol Metab 79:285, 1994.

451. Lazarus JH: Clinical manifestations of postpartum thyroid disease. Thyroid 9:685, 1999.

452. Jansson R, Bernander S, Karlsson A, et al: Autoimmune thyroid dysfunction in the postpartum period. J Clin Endocrinol Metab 58:681, 1984.

453. Amino N, Miyai K, Kuro P, et al: Transient postpartum hypothyroidism: fourteen cases with autoimmune thyroiditis. Ann Intern Med 87:155, 1977.

454. Dahlberg PA, Jansson R: Different aetiologies in postpartum thyroiditis. Acta Endocrinol 104:195, 1983.

455. Lazarus JH, Ammari F, Oretti R, et al: Clinical aspects of recurrent postpartum thyroiditis. J R Coll Gen Pract 47:305, 1996.

456. Mehta H, Badenhoop K, Walfish PG: Adrenal insufficiency after recurrent postpartum thyroiditis (postpartum Schmidt syndrome): a case report. Thyroid 8:269, 1998.

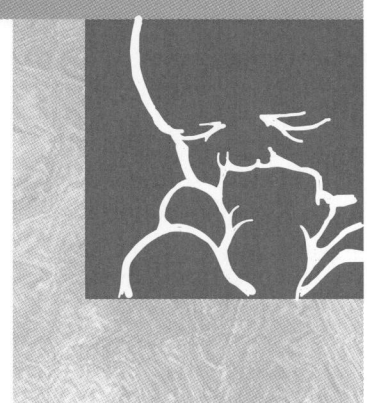

Hematologic Complications of Pregnancy

PHILIP SAMUELS

PREGNANCY-ASSOCIATED THROMBOCYTOPENIA

The widespread use of automated blood counts has led to the increased diagnosis of thrombocytopenia coexisting with pregnancy. Affecting approximately 4 percent of pregnancies, thrombocytopenia is the most frequent hematologic complication of pregnancy resulting in consultation. Hospital laboratories vary on their lower limit of a normal platelet count, but it is usually between 135,000 and 150,000/mm³. Platelet counts generally fall slightly, due to hemodilution and increased destruction, as gestation progresses. Platelet counts, however, should not fall below the normal range. In pregnancy, the vast majority of cases of mild to moderate thrombocytopenia are caused by gestational thrombocytopenia.[1] This form of thrombocytopenia has little chance of causing maternal or neonatal complications.[2] The obstetrician, however, is obliged to rule out other forms of thrombocytopenia that are associated with severe maternal or perinatal morbidity. The common and rare causes of thrombocytopenia in the gravida at term are shown in the box "Causes of Thrombocytopenia During Pregnancy." Until the late 1980s, it was assumed that all patients with an unexplained low platelet count carried a diagnosis of immune thrombocytopenic purpura (ITP), a recognized cause of neonatal thrombocytopenia. Unfortunately, traditional platelet antibody testing cannot distinguish among ITP, thrombocytopenia accompanying preeclampsia, and gestational thrombocytopenia.[3,4] Yet, the distinction between these disorders is important because each of these diagnoses carries distinct maternal and neonatal implications.

Gestational Thrombocytopenia

Patients with gestational thrombocytopenia usually present with mild (platelet count = 100,000 to 149,000/mm³) to moderate (platelet count = 50,000 to 99,000/mm³) thrombocytopenia.[5] These patients usually require no therapy, and the fetus appears to be at little, if any, risk of being born with profound thrombocytopenia (platelet count <50,000/mm³) or a bleeding diathesis. This distinct entity was first suggested but not specifically defined in a study published in 1986 by Hart et al.[6] In this study, 28 of 116 pregnant women (24 percent) who were evaluated prospectively during an 8-month period in 1983 had platelet counts less than 150,000/mm³ at least once during pregnancy. In all 17 patients who were followed after delivery, platelet counts returned to normal. Platelet-associated IgG (a positive direct test) was present in 79 percent of these 28 women, and 61 percent had serum antiplatelet IgG (a positive indirect test). None of these women had positive antibodies after delivery. Hart et al.[6] were actually describing gestational thrombocytopenia before the condition had been recognized as a distinct entity. They, furthermore, were the first to demonstrate that conventional platelet antibody testing cannot distinguish gestational thrombocytopenia from ITP.[6] Samuels et al.[3] also investigated 74 mothers with gestational thrombocytopenia. Forty-six (62 percent) of these patients had circulating antiplatelet IgG in their plasma (a positive indirect test); these women gave birth to two neonates with thrombocytopenia, both having platelet counts above 50,000/mm³. Burrows and Kelton[5,7,8] have further shown, in several large series, that there is little risk to the mother or neonate in cases of gestational thrombocytopenia. In one study no mother or

Causes of Thrombocytopenia During Pregnancy

Common causes
 Gestational thrombocytopenia
 Severe preeclampsia
 HELLP syndrome
 Immune thrombocytopenic purpura
 Disseminated intravascular coagulation
Rare causes
 Lupus anticoagulant/antiphospholipid antibody
  syndrome
 Systemic lupus erythematosus
 Thrombotic thrombocytopenic purpura
 Hemolytic uremic syndrome
 Type 2b von Willebrand's syndrome
 Folic acid deficiency
 Human immunodeficiency virus infection
 Hematologic malignancies
 May-Hegglin syndrome (congenital
  thrombocytopenia)

infant, in a group of 334 women with gestational thrombocytopenia, experienced bleeding complications.[8] In their earlier study of 1,357 healthy, pregnant women, 112 (8.3 percent) had platelet counts less than 150,000/mm³.[5] The lowest platelet count was 97,000/mm³. The incidence of thrombocytopenia (platelet count <150,000/mm³) in the infants of these 112 women was 4.3 percent, not statistically significantly different from infants born to healthy pregnant women without thrombocytopenia (1.5 percent). None of these infants had platelet counts less than 100,000/mm³. Indeed, the works by Samuels et al.[3] and Burrows and Kelton[5,7] have convincingly demonstrated that gestational thrombocytopenia is an entity distinct from ITP.

The decrease in platelet count, occurring in gestational thrombocytopenia, is not merely due to dilution of platelets with increasing blood volume. It appears to be due to an acceleration of the normal increase in platelet destruction that occurs during pregnancy.[1] This is demonstrated by the fact that the mean platelet volume (MPV) is increased in patients with gestational thrombocytopenia. The increase in platelet-associated IgG seen in these patients may merely reflect immune complexes adhering to the platelet surface rather than specific antiplatelet antibodies. Pregnant women who have gestational thrombocytopenia do not require any special therapy during the puerperium unless their platelet counts fall below 20,000/mm³ or if there is clinical bleeding. These complications, however, are rare, and it is difficult to determine whether these patients, with profound thrombocytopenia, have gesta-

tional thrombocytopenia or new onset of immune thrombocytopenic purpura.

Immune Thrombocytopenic Purpura

Although it only affects 1 to 3 per 1,000 pregnancies, ITP has received much attention in the obstetrics literature because of the potential for profound neonatal thrombocytopenia in infants born to mothers with this condition.

In 1954, Peterson and Larson[9] were the first to recognize that profound thrombocytopenia (platelet count <50,000/mm³) may develop in infants born to women with ITP. A subsequent report confirmed this observation.[10] In 1973, Territo et al.[11] made the first effort to predict which infants were at increased risk of being born with profound thrombocytopenia. They demonstrated, in a small number of patients, that fetuses born to mothers with platelet counts less than 100,000/mm³ were at highest risk. Many larger studies have since shown that this arbitrary cut-off, while generally true, is not useful in individual cases. Subsequently, a number of efforts have been made to use noninvasive parameters to assess the risk of severe neonatal thrombocytopenia, including the use of maternal glucocorticoids, whether or not the mother had undergone splenectomy, and the presence of maternal antiplatelet antibodies. None of these, however, has shown the desired positive or negative predictive values.[12-16]

In general, pregnancy has not been determined to cause ITP or to change its severity. Other studies, however, have demonstrated that in individual patients ITP exacerbations often occur during pregnancy and improve postpartum.[3,17,18] Harrington et al.[19] were the first to demonstrate that this disorder was humorally mediated. Shulman et al.[20] showed that the mediator of this disorder was IgG. These findings were confirmed when Cines and Schreiber[21] developed the first platelet antiglobulin test, a radioimmunoassay, in 1979. This test is now mostly performed by enzyme-linked immunosorbent assay (ELISA) or flow cytometry. New assays have shown that these autoantibodies may be directed against specific platelet surface glycoproteins, including the IIb/IIIa and Ib/IX complexes.[22] After the platelets are coated with antibody they are removed from circulation by binding to the Fc receptors of macrophages in the reticuloendothelial system, especially the spleen. Approximately 90 percent of women with ITP will have platelet-associated IgG.[21] Unfortunately, this is not specific for ITP, as studies have shown that these tests are also positive in women with gestational thrombocytopenia and preeclampsia.[3,4] Studies concerning the use of antibodies to specific epitopes on platelet surface glycoproteins are ongoing, and these tests eventually may be useful to distinguish among the various disorders.

To make the issue more confusing, the pathogenesis of ITP in children and adults usually differs. Childhood ITP usually follows a viral infection and clinically presents with petechiae and bleeding.[23] This form of ITP is generally self-limited and disappears over time. Adults, conversely, have milder bleeding and easy bruisability and are often diagnosed after a prolonged period of subtle symptoms. Adult ITP usually runs a chronic course, and long-term therapy is often eventually needed. Many pregnancies occur in women in their late teens and early twenties. In these women, with a history of ITP, it may be difficult to ascertain whether the patient has childhood ITP or adult ITP. Also, no study has shown whether the risk of neonatal thrombocytopenia is similar in both forms of ITP.

ITP is different from other causes of thrombocytopenia in pregnancy because of the aforementioned risk of profound neonatal thrombocytopenia. This has further been confounded by the fact that before 1990 it was assumed that all patients with unexplained thrombocytopenia during gestation had ITP. It was only after 1990 that gestational thrombocytopenia became recognized as a distinct entity.[2,3] This, therefore, has confounded studies because cases of gestational thrombocytopenia have diluted many studies, making it difficult to determine the true incidence of neonatal thrombocytopenia in women with ITP.

Table 34-1 lists several studies in which all patients had true ITP and delineates the rates of profound neonatal thrombocytopenia. Even these carefully performed studies show wide ranges in the rates of profound neonatal thrombocytopenia.

In 1980, Scott et al.[24] were the first to institute direct fetal platelet determination in a series of women with ITP by utilizing fetal scalp sampling. This procedure, however, requires operator skill, an engaged fetal vertex, a dilated cervix, ruptured membranes, and the ability to obtain a pure sample of fetal blood without any contamination with maternal blood or amniotic fluid. The procedure has proven to be technically difficult in the hands of many practicing obstetricians who do not perform fetal scalp sampling on a regular basis. In

many cases, amniotic fluid in the vagina contaminates the specimen. Amniotic fluid contains procoagulants, which cause fetal platelet clumping and spurious thrombocytopenia.

With the development and increased use of ultrasound-guided cordocentesis in the mid-1980s, accurate in utero sampling of fetal platelets has become feasible. Some authors advocate routine use of this technique in mothers with ITP.[25-27] Some maternal-fetal specialists believe that there is minimal risk involved with the cordocentesis. Ghidini and colleagues,[28] however, reviewed cordocentesis complications at medical centers where more than 100 procedures had been performed. They found a 1.4 percent risk of perinatal death in low-risk fetuses at more than 28 weeks' gestation undergoing the procedure. The complication rate may be appreciably higher when larger numbers of severely thrombocytopenic neonates have been studied. Bleeding may occur in up to 41 percent of cases, but most stop in less than 60 seconds. Complication rates will probably fall as experience increases and imaging, including color Doppler, improves. However, cordocentesis is expensive when including the price of the procedure, the physician consultation fee, the ultrasound guidance, and the fetal monitoring that must accompany the procedure. Indeed, the risks, associated costs, and low yield with which profoundly thrombocytopenic infants are identified do not justify the routine use of cordocentesis in all thrombocytopenic mothers.

The major reason why invasive testing has identified so few thrombocytopenic neonates is that many women with gestational thrombocytopenia were included in these series. Gestational thrombocytopenia, previously cited as the most common cause of thrombocytopenia in the third trimester, was not recognized until 1986. It was first alluded to by Hart et al.[6] In 1990, Burrows and Kelton,[8] as well as Samuels et al.[3] firmly established thrombocytopenia as an entity distinct from ITP. In the latter study, Samuels et al.[3] showed that roughly 50 percent of women referred to two major medical centers over 10 years with presumptive ITP actually had gestational thrombocytopenia. It is likely that the

Table 34-1. INCIDENCE OF PROFOUND NEONATAL THROMBOCYTOPENIA IN MOTHERS KNOWN TO HAVE IMMUNE THROMBOCYTOPENIC PURPURA

Reports	Total Patients with ITP	Infants with Platelet Count < 50,000/mm³	95% Confidence Interval
Karapatkin et al.[15]	19	6 (31.6%)	20.9%–52.5%
Burrows and Kelton[8]	60	3 (5%)	0%–10.5%
Noriega-Guerra et al.[13]	21	8 (38.1%)	17.3%–58.9%
Samuels et al.[3]	88	18 (20.5%)	12.0%–28.9%
Pooled (Crude)	*188*	*35 (18.6%)*	*13%–24%*

inclusion of large numbers of women with gestational thrombocytopenia in recent studies of maternal "ITP" has led to the spurious impression that the natural history of ITP has changed.

In a meta-analysis by Burrows and Kelton,[29] a 14.6 percent incidence of profound thrombocytopenia in infants born to mothers with ITP was reported. This meta-analysis did not, however, take into account that many of the studies included did not exclude patients with gestational thrombocytopenia. Therefore, the risks of profound thrombocytopenia may very well be greater than this reported incidence. These authors, also, reported a neonatal morbidity rate of 24 per 1,000 with few serious complications. This may only be low for the reasons mentioned above.

Samuels et al.[3] reported a neonatal morbidity rate of 278 per 1,000 infants born to mothers with true ITP. The sample size, however, was too small to determine if mode of delivery or degree of neonatal thrombocytopenia made an impact on this morbidity. This rate may be overly high, as these were patients referred to two large tertiary care centers. Nonetheless, this study does point out that ITP does not always carry a benign course for the neonate. The neonatal morbidities included intraventricular hemorrhage, hemopericardium, gastrointestinal bleeding, and extensive cutaneous manifestations of bleeding.[3] Regardless of the complication rates in profoundly thrombocytopenic fetuses, cordocentesis is rarely indicated in patients with ITP.

Thrombotic Thrombocytopenic Purpura and Hemolytic Uremic Syndrome

These two conditions are characterized by microangiopathic hemolytic anemia and severe thrombocytopenia. Pregnancy does not predispose a patient to these conditions, but these conditions should be considered when evaluating the gravida with severe thrombocytopenia. Thrombotic thrombocytopic purpura (TTP) is characterized by a pentad of findings, which are shown in the box "Pentad of Findings in TTP."[30,31] The complete pentad only occurs in approximately 40 percent of patients, but approximately 75 percent present with a triad of microangiopathic hemolytic anemia, thrombocytopenia, and neurologic changes.[32] Pathologically, these patients have thrombotic occlusion of arterioles and capillaries.[30] These occur in multiple organs, and there is no specific clinical manifestation for the disease. The clinical picture will reflect the organs that are involved. The pathophysiology of TTP remains elusive, but diffuse endothelial damage and impaired fibrinolytic activity are hallmarks of this disorder.[33] Weiner[34] has published the most extensive literature review concerning TTP. In this series of 45 patients, 40 developed the disease antepartum, with 58 percent occurring be-

---

Pentad of Findings in Thrombotic Thrombocytopenic Purpura (TTP)*

Microangiopathic hemolytic anemia†
Thrombocytopenia†
Neurologic abnormalities—confusion, headache, paresis, visual hallucinations, seizures
Fever
Renal dysfunction

---

*The classic pentad is only found in 40% of patients.
†These three findings are present in 74% of patients.[32]

---

fore 24 weeks' gestation. The mean gestational age at onset of symptoms was 23.5 weeks.

This finding may be helpful when trying to distinguish TTP from other causes of thrombocytopenia and microangiopathic hemolytic anemia occurring during gestation. In Weiner's review, the fetal and maternal mortality rates were 80 and 44 percent, respectively.[34] These mortality rates are overly pessimistic, as this series included many patients who contracted the disease before plasma infusion/exchange therapy was used for treating TTP. This disorder may be confused with rarely occurring early-onset severe preeclampsia. In preeclampsia, antithrombin III levels are frequently low, and this is not the case with TTP.[35] This test, therefore, may be a useful discriminator between these two disorders.

Although the hemolytic uremic syndrome (HUS) has many features in common with TTP, it usually has its onset in the postpartum period. Patients with HUS display a triad of microangiopathic hemolytic anemia, acute nephropathy, and thrombocytopenia. HUS is rare in adults, and the thrombocytopenia is usually milder than that seen in TTP, with only 50 percent of patients having a platelet count less than 100,000/mm³ at time of diagnosis. The thrombocytopenia worsens as the disease progresses.[36] A major difference between TTP and HUS is that 15 to 25 percent of patients with the latter develop chronic renal disease.[31] HUS often follows infections with verotoxin-producing enteric bacteria.[37] Cyclosporine therapy, cytoxic drugs, and oral contraceptives may predispose adults to develop HUS.[38–40] The majority of cases of HUS occurring in pregnancy develop at least 2 days after delivery.[31,33] In fact, in one series, only 9 of 62 cases (6.9 percent) of pregnancy-associated HUS occurred antepartum.[34] Four of those nine developed symptoms on the day of delivery. The mean time from delivery to development of HUS in patients in this series was 26.6 days. Maternal mortality may exceed 50 percent in postpartum HUS.

EVALUATION OF THROMBOCYTOPENIA DURING PREGNANCY AND THE PUERPERIUM

Before deciding on a course to follow in treating the patient with thrombocytopenia, the obstetrician must evaluate the patient and attempt to ascertain the etiology of her low platelet count. Important management decisions are dependent on arriving at an accurate diagnosis. A complete medical history, although time consuming, is critically important. It is essential to learn whether the patient has previously had a depressed platelet count or bleeding diathesis. It is also important to know whether these clinical conditions occur coincidentally with pregnancy. A complete medication history should be elicited, as certain medications, such as heparin, can result in profound maternal thrombocytopenia. The obstetric history should focus on whether there have been any maternal or neonatal bleeding problems in the past. Excessive bleeding from an episiotomy site or cesarean delivery incision site, a need for blood component therapy, easy bruising, or bleeding from intravenous sites during labor should alert the physician to the possibility of thrombocytopenia in the previous pregnancy. The obstetrician should also question whether the infant had any bleeding diathesis or if there was any problem following a circumcision. The obstetrician should also ask pertinent questions to determine whether severe preeclampsia or HELLP (Hemolysis, Elevated Liver Enzymes, Low Platelets) syndrome is the cause of her thrombocytopenia. The treatment of preeclampsia and HELLP is not discussed in this chapter, as they are covered elsewhere (see Chapter 28). Importantly, all thrombocytopenic pregnant women should be carefully evaluated for the presence of risk factors for human immunodeficiency virus (HIV) infection, as this infection can cause an ITP-like syndrome.

An accurate assessment of the gestational age should also be carried out. This is important, as some of the etiologies of thrombocytopenia in pregnancy are dependent on the gestational age. A thorough physical examination of the patient should also be performed. The physician should look for the presence of ecchymoses or petechiae. Blood pressure should be determined to ascertain whether the patient has impending preeclampsia. If the patient is developing HELLP syndrome, scleral icterus may be present. The eye grounds should be examined for evidence of arteriolar spasm or hemorrhage.

It is imperative that a peripheral blood smear be examined by an experienced hematologist or pathologist whenever a case of pregnancy-associated thrombocytopenia is diagnosed. This individual must determine if microangiopathic hemolysis is present. This will help in establishing a diagnosis. This specialist can also rule out platelet clumping, which will result in a factitious thrombocytopenia. Other laboratory evaluation should be performed as necessary to rule out preeclampsia and/or HELLP syndrome, as well as disseminated intravascular coagulopathy. If a diagnosis of ITP is entertained, appropriate platelet antibody testing should be performed.

After determining the etiology of thrombocytopenia, the physician can better determine whether imminent delivery is necessary, if the thrombocytopenia should be treated before initiating delivery, or if the low platelet count should be ignored.

THERAPY OF THROMBOCYTOPENIA DURING PREGNANCY

Gestational Thrombocytopenia

Gestational thrombocytopenia, the most common form encountered in the third trimester, requires no special therapy. The most important therapeutic issue is to refrain from therapies and testing that may lead to unnecessary intervention or iatrogenic preterm delivery. In patients with mild to moderate thrombocytopenia and no antenatal or antecedent history of thrombocytopenia, the patient should be treated like a normal pregnant patient. If the maternal platelet count drops below 50,000/mm³, the patient may still have gestational thrombocytopenia, but there are not enough data on mothers with counts this low to determine if there are any maternal or fetal risks. These patients, therefore, should be treated as if they have de novo ITP. Although approximately 4 percent of patients have gestational thrombocytopenia, less than 1 percent of uncomplicated pregnant women will have gestational thrombocytopenia with platelet counts less than 100,000/mm³.[8]

Immune Thrombocytopenic Purpura

Treatment of the gravida with ITP during pregnancy and the puerperium requires attention to both mother and fetus. As in other cases of thrombocytopenia, maternal therapy only needs to be instituted if there is evidence of a bleeding diathesis or to prevent a bleeding complication if surgery is anticipated. Again, there is usually no spontaneous bleeding unless the platelet count falls below 20,000/mm³. Surgical bleeding does not usually occur until the platelet count is less than 50,000/mm³. The conventional forms of raising a platelet count in the patient with ITP include glucocorticoid therapy, intravenous gammaglobulins, platelet transfusions, and splenectomy.

If the patient is having a bleeding diathesis or if the platelet count is below 20,000/mm³, there is usually a need to raise the platelet count in a relatively short period of time. Although oral glucocorticoids can be used, intravenous glucocorticoids may work more rapidly. Any steroid that has a glucocorticoid effect can be used. However, hematologists have the most experience with methylprednisolone. It can be given intravenously, and it has very little mineralocorticoid effect. It is important to avoid steroids with strong mineralocorticoid effects because these agents can disturb electrolyte balance, cause fluid retention, and result in hypertension. The usual dose of methylprednisolone is 1.0 to 1.5 mg/kg of *total body weight* intravenously daily in divided doses. It usually takes about 2 days to see a response, but it may take up to 10 days to see a maximum response. Even though it does have very little mineralocorticoid effect, there is some present. Because of the large dose that is being administered, it is important to follow the patient's electrolytes. There is little chance methylprednisolone will cause neonatal adrenal suppression because very little crosses the placenta. It is metabolized by placental 11-β-ol-dehydrogenase to an inactive 11-keto metabolite.

After the platelet count has risen satisfactorily using intravenous methylprednisolone, the patient can be switched to oral prednisone. The usual dose is 60 to 100 mg/day. It can be given in a single dose, but there is less gastrointestinal upset with divided doses. The physician can rapidly taper the dose to 30 or 40 mg/day, but slowly thereafter. Since the patient did have a very low platelet count before (or otherwise she would not be undergoing therapy), the physician should titrate the dose to keep the platelet count around 100,000/mm³. If the physician begins therapy with oral prednisone, the usual initial daily dose is 1 mg/kg total body weight. The response rate to glucocorticoids is about 70 percent. It is important to realize that if the patient has been taking glucocorticoids for a period of at least 2 to 3 weeks, she may have adrenal suppression and should undergo increased doses of steroids during labor and delivery in order to avoid an adrenal crisis. Tapering should be slowly thereafter. Also, if the patient has been on glucocorticoids for some time, she may experience significant side effects, including fluid retention, hirsutism, acne, striae, poor wound healing, and monilia vaginitis. In rare circumstances, patients on long-term steroids during gestation can develop osteoporosis or cataract formation. The chance of any fetal or neonatal side effects from the glucocorticoids, however, is remote.

Although glucocorticoids are the mainstays of treating maternal thrombocytopenia, up to 30 percent of patients will not respond to these medications. In this instance, the next medication to use is intravenous immunoglobulin. This agent probably works by binding to the Fc receptors on reticuloendothelial cells and preventing destruction of platelets. It may also adhere to receptors on platelets and prevent antiplatelet antibodies from binding to these sites. The usual dose is 0.4 g/kg/day for 3 to 5 days. However, it may be necessary to use as much as 1 g/kg/day. The response usually begins in 2 to 3 days and usually peaks in 5 days. An alternate regimen is to give 1 g/kg once and observe the patient. Often this single dose will result in an adequate increase in platelets. The length of this response is variable, and the timing of the dose is extremely important. If the obstetrician wants a peak platelet count for delivery, he or she should institute therapy about 5 to 8 days before the planned delivery.

Intravenous immunoglobulin is a blood product, but its method of preparation makes it safe for use. Plasma is thawed and pooled. After the cryoprecipitate is removed, it undergoes Cohn-Oncley cold ethanol fractionation.[41] This inactivates viruses.[42] Furthermore, the liquid form is incubated for 21 days at pH 4.25. This removes and inactivates both enveloped and nonenveloped model viruses,[43,44] including HIV, hepatitis C virus, hepatitis B virus, cytomegalovirus virus, Epstein-Barr virus, and herpes simplex virus. It has also been tested against RNA and DNA nonenveloped viruses.[45,46] A recent review of the literature uncovered no cases of viral transmission with the liquid formula of immunoglobulin that had been incubated at pH 4.25. Although intravenous immunoglobulin is very expensive, it should be used before contemplating splenectomy, as some patients with ITP will experience remission after delivery.[47]

In midtrimester, splenectomy can also be used to raise the maternal platelet count. This procedure is reserved for those who do not respond to medical management, with the platelet count remaining below 20,000/mm³. It can be performed postpartum if the patient does not respond to medical management. In extremely emergent cases of life-threatening bleeding or nonresponse, splenectomy can be safely performed at the time of cesarean section after extending a midline incision cephalad.

Platelet transfusions are indicated when there is clinically significant bleeding and while awaiting other therapies to become effective. Platelets can be given if the maternal platelet count is less than 50,000/mm³ during splenectomy, or during cesarean delivery if clinical bleeding is evident. They can be used before a vaginal delivery if the mother's platelet count is less than 20,000/mm³. Each "pack" of platelets will increase the platelet count by approximately 10,000/mm³. The half-life of these platelets is extremely short because the same antibodies and reticuloendothelial cell clearance rates that affect the mother's endogenous platelets will also affect the transfused platelets. However, if these platelets are transfused at the time the skin incision is made, it will allow enough hemostasis to carry out the surgical procedure.

If the patient with profound thrombocytopenia undergoes cesarean delivery, certain surgical precautions should be taken. The obstetrician should use electrocautery liberally. The bladder flap may be left open in order to avoid hematoma formation. If the parietal peritoneum is closed, subfascial drains are helpful if hemostasis is imperfect.

Although treating maternal thrombocytopenia is fairly straightforward, the need for evaluation of the fetal platelet count and how this information should alter patient management remain controversial. Although papers by Cooke[49] and Burrows and Kelton[29] have attempted to show that there is no risk in delivering a profoundly thrombocytopenic fetus vaginally, these meta-analyses are only generalizations. There is no one series large enough from which to draw adequate conclusions concerning mode of delivery of the profoundly thrombocytopenic fetus. There are no randomized studies concerning delivery of these patients. It is not our purpose to recommend a mode of delivery for the profoundly thrombocytopenic fetus, but to outline which fetuses are at risk of being born with thrombocytopenia and to allow the obstetrician to make decisions concerning delivery after discussion with the patient. As previously shown (Table 34–1), anywhere from 5 to 38 percent of infants born to mothers with ITP will have platelet counts less than 50,000/mm³. Several studies have tried to determine if administering glucocorticoids to the mother may have an effect on raising the fetal platelet count in utero.[12,13,15]

Although the study by Karapatkin et al.[15] was promising, other studies have not corroborated these findings. Furthermore, studies have shown that splenectomy has no bearing on neonatal platelet counts. The study by Samuels et al.[3] showed that 19.2 percent of ITP patients undergoing no therapy gave birth to profoundly thrombocytopenic infants compared with 22.7 percent of those receiving prednisone alone, 23 percent of those who had undergone a splenectomy and received prednisone, and 17.8 percent of those having undergone only splenectomy. The rate of profound neonatal thrombocytopenia was not significantly different among any of these groups. Even if there is not a difference in perinatal morbidity between vaginal and cesarean delivery, there are advantages of knowing whether a fetus is at risk of being born with a platelet count less than 50,000/mm³. The use of scalp electrodes and vacuum extractors are examples of interventions that may be avoided in the profoundly thrombocytopenic fetus. A prolonged second stage of labor in the nulliparous patient who is carrying a severely thrombocytopenic fetus should probably be avoided. Furthermore, because of the potential neonatal morbid-

ity, it might be safest if the profoundly thrombocytopenic infant were delivered in a tertiary care setting. In the study by Samuels et al.,[3] there were cases of severe gastrointestinal bleeding, hemopericardium, intraventricular hemorrhage, and severe cutaneous manifestations of bleeding in infants born to mothers with ITP.

The only method currently available to determine the fetal platelet count accurately before the onset of labor (cordocentesis) is both expensive and invasive. Furthermore, it carries an inherent risk of an adverse fetal outcome. Fear of an adverse outcome in the setting of a neonate with an unknown platelet count has led obstetricians to overutilize this invasive testing as well as surgical deliveries. There is almost no place for cordocentesis in the patient with ITP.

In summary, the treatment of thrombocytopenia during gestation is dependent on the etiology. The obstetrician need not act on the mother's platelet count unless it is below 20,000/mm³, or if it is below 50,000/mm³ with evidence of clinical bleeding or if surgery is anticipated. In these cases, the treatment will depend upon the diagnosis. Furthermore, whether delivery needs to be expedited or can be delayed is also dependent on the etiology of thrombocytopenia. The fetal/neonatal platelet count need only be considered if the mother carries a true diagnosis of ITP or, in the case of presumed gestational thrombocytopenia, when the platelet count is less than 75,000/mm³, as this may actually be de novo ITP. The key to managing these patients is to arrive at an accurate etiology for the thrombocytopenia and to approach the patient and her fetus rationally.

MANAGEMENT OF THROMBOTIC THROMBOCYTOPENIC PURPURA AND HEMOLYTIC UREMIC SYNDROME

Before the use of plasma exchange, maternal and fetal outcomes in cases complicated by TTP were uniformly poor.[34] The first cases treated with plasma exchange for TTP during pregnancy were reported in 1984.[50] One report described a patient who had previous fetal deaths from chronic TTP and experienced a successful pregnancy when treated with aspirin, dipyridamol, and plasma infusion.[51] There are no large series of patients with TTP in pregnancy. It does appear, however, through case reports, that the prognosis has improved greatly with plasma infusion and plasma exchange.

HUS has been much more difficult to treat. Only a few case reports have appeared. Supportive therapy remains the mainstay of these treatments.[34,50] Dialysis is often necessary with close attention to fluid management. Platelet function inhibitors have also been used in two cases during pregnancy.[52,53] Plasma infusion and plasma exchange can be attempted, but the results have not been as good as in cases of TTP.[54] Vincristine has been used with some success in nonpregnant patients but has not been tried with pregnancy, and prostacyclin infusion has been effective in children but has not been used during pregnancy.[53,55]

NEONATAL ALLOIMMUNE THROMBOCYTOPENIA

In neonatal alloimmune thrombocytopenia, a rare disorder, the mother lacks a specific platelet antigen and develops antibodies to this antigen. The disease is somewhat analogous to Rh isoimmunization, but involves platelets. If the fetus inherits this antigen from its father, maternal antibody can cross the placenta, resulting in severe neonatal thrombocytopenia. The mother, however, will have a normal platelet count. Deaver and co-investigators[56] reviewed 58 cases of neonatal alloimmune thrombocytopenia. The overall mortality rate was 9 percent, and the total incidence of suspected intracranial hemorrhage was 28 percent. The mortality rate was 24 percent for the firstborn infant and only 5 percent for subsequent offspring. The improved outcome in the latter group appeared to be related to more frequent utilization of cesarean delivery and to earlier use of corticosteroids in these children because obstetricians and pediatricians were expecting the disease.[56] The most common antibodies noted in these patients are anti-PLA 1 and BAK antibodies.[57] Transfusion of maternal platelets into the neonate also improved outcome in these cases. After birth or in utero the child can be transfused with the mother's platelets, since she lacks the antigen that would lead to platelet destruction by circulating antibodies. Bussel and colleagues[58] have demonstrated that the antenatal use of intravenous immunoglobulin may help to prevent thrombocytopenia in infants at risk for neonatal alloimmune thrombocytopenia. These investigators administered 1 g/kg per week to at-risk mothers and observed no toxicity. The concomitant use of glucocorticoids has not necessarily been shown to boost the effect of the intravenous immunoglobulin.[59] Because of the frequency with which very low platelet counts are encountered in these fetuses, there is a risk of fetal exsanguination with cordocentesis.[60] These patients should be cared for in a tertiary care center with experience caring for mothers and infants with this rare disorder.

IRON DEFICIENCY ANEMIA

During a singleton pregnancy, maternal plasma volume gradually expands by approximately 50 percent (1,000 ml). The total red blood cell (RBC) mass also increases, but only by approximately 300 ml (25 percent), and this starts later in pregnancy.[61] It is not surprising, therefore, that hemoglobin and hematocrit levels usually fall during gestation. These changes are not necessarily pathologic but usually represent a physiologic alteration of pregnancy. By 6 weeks postpartum, in the absence of excessive blood loss during the puerperium, hemoglobin and hematocrit levels have returned to normal.

Most researchers and clinicians diagnose anemia as a hemoglobin less than 11 g/dl or a hematocrit less than 32 percent. Using these criteria, 50 percent of pregnant woman are anemic. The incidence of anemia changes, depending on the population studied. It is unfortunate that this problem is often ignored, as most textbooks are published in industrialized nations, where anemia does not result in major morbidity and mortality. Yet, in the majority of the world, iron deficiency is an overwhelming problem. It does not receive the recognition it needs. It is not one of the "exciting subjects" that warrants significant federal funding in the United States. Yet, worldwide there are many maternal mortalities because of blood loss in women who are already anemic. The arbitrary cutoff for hemoglobin/hematocrit may need to be adjusted. Beaton suggests that these numbers should be adjusted downward and different targets should be established for different times in pregnancy.[62] Causes of anemia in pregnancy are shown in the box "Causes of Anemia During Pregnancy."

This is important because as pregnancy progresses, hemoglobin levels are often in the range of 10 to 10.5 g/dl in the late second and early third trimesters. These patients, if iron stores are present, do regain their normal hemoglobin/hematocrit postpartum. Approximately 75 percent of anemias that occur during pregnancy are secondary to iron deficiency.[61] Ho and co-investigators[63] performed elaborate hematologic evaluations of 221 term gravidas in Taiwan. None of the studied patients received an added iron preparation during gestation. Of the previously nonanemic patients, 10.4 percent developed clinical anemia after a full-term delivery. Of these 23 patients, 11 (47.8 percent) developed florid iron deficiency anemia, and another 11 developed moderate iron depletion.[63] The other anemic patients in the group had folate deficiency. Of the 198 nonanemic gravidas at term, 46.5 percent showed evidence of iron depletion even though they had a normal hematocrit.[63]

To distinguish the normal physiologic changes of pregnancy from those of pathologic iron deficiency, one

Causes of Anemia During Pregnancy

Common causes—85% of anemias
   Physiologic anemia
   Iron deficiency
Uncommon causes
   Folic acid deficiency
   Hemoglobinopathies
      Sickle cell disease
      Hemoglobin SC
      β-Thalassemia minor
Rare causes
   Hemoglobinopathies
      β-Thalassemia major
      α-Thalassemia
   Vitamin B_{12} deficiency
   Syndromes of chronic hemolysis
      Hereditary spherocytosis
      Paroxysmal nocturnal hemoglobinuria
   Hematologic malignancy
   Gastrointestinal bleeding

must understand the normal iron requirements of pregnancy (Table 34–2) and the proper use of hematologic laboratory parameters. In adult women, iron stores are located in the bone marrow, liver, and spleen in the form of ferritin. Ferritin constitutes approximately 25 percent (500 mg) of the 2 g of iron stores found in the normal woman. Approximately 65 percent of stored iron is in circulating RBCs.[61,64–66] If the dietary iron intake is poor, the interval between pregnancies is short, or the delivery is complicated by hemorrhage, iron deficiency anemia readily and rapidly develops.

The first pathologic change to occur in iron deficiency anemia is the depletion of bone marrow, liver, and spleen iron stores. The serum iron level falls, as does the percentage saturation of transferrin. The total iron-binding capacity rises, as this is a reflection of unbound transferrin. A falling hemoglobin and hematocrit follow. Microcytic hypochromic RBCs are released into the circulation. If iron deficiency is combined with folate deficiency, nomocytic and normochromic RBCs are observed on the peripheral blood smear.

Care must be taken when using laboratory parameters to establish the diagnosis of iron deficiency anemia during gestation. A serum iron concentration less than 60 mg/dl with less than 16 percent saturation of transferrin is suggestive of iron deficiency. An increase in iron-binding capacity, however, is not reliable, as 15 percent of pregnant women without iron deficiency will show an increase in this parameter.[67] Serum ferritin levels normally decrease mildly during pregnancy. A significantly reduced ferritin concentration is also indicative of iron deficiency anemia and is the best parameter with which to judge the degree of iron deficiency. Ferritin levels, however, can change 25 percent from one day to the next.[68] Harthoorn-Lasthuizen et al. examined erythrocyte zinc protoporphyrin testing in pregnancy.[69] They found that serum ferritin levels did not predict the development of iron deficient erythropoiesis. However, erythrocyte zinc protoporphyrin measurements did help determine which patients were developing iron deficiency before they developed frank anemia. These patients will benefit from iron therapy.[69] Van den Broek et al. felt that the erythrocyte zinc protoporphyrin level was not particularly helpful and that a serum ferritin of less than 30 μg/L is more than adequate to determine iron deficiency.[70] If a patient has been iron deficient for an extended period of time, her serum iron level can rise before she has depleted her iron stores. Also, if she takes a few iron pills before her prenatal visit, her serum iron level can rise to normal while her ferritin is still low. The ferritin level, at least, will indicate the total status of her iron stores.

Ahluwalia[71] feels that measuring serum transferrin receptors can give a better index of true iron status. Ferritin can be elevated in acute and chronic infections and transferrin receptors do not change in response to an infection. This is important in countries where chronic infection is common in pregnant women. Also, receptor concentrations are not confounded by the hemodynamic changes of pregnancy. This test is not yet readily available but may help us in the future to detect iron-deficient patients.[71] When hematologic parameters remain confusing, bone marrow aspiration usually provides the definitive diagnosis. The procedure, however, is rarely necessary.

Whether all women should receive prophylactic iron during pregnancy remains controversial. Long[72] believes that physiology is responsible for much of the decrease in hematocrit and, unless the patient is symptomatic or the hematocrit is very low, iron supplementation is unnecessary. Millman et al.[73] in reviewing the Cochrane database, found that 20 percent of fertile women have iron stores greater than 500 mg, which is the required minimum for pregnancy. They also noted that 40 percent of women have iron stores between 100 and 500 mg, and 40 percent have virtually no iron stores. This shows that the majority of individuals do need some iron supplementation.[73]

Table 34–2. IRON REQUIREMENTS FOR PREGNANCY AND THE PUERPERIUM

Increased red blood cell mass	450 mg
Fetus and placenta	360 mg
Vaginal delivery	190 mg
Lactation	1 mg/day

Table 34–3. ELEMENTAL IRON AVAILABLE FROM COMMON GENETIC IRON PREPARATIONS

Preparation	Elemental Iron (mg)
Ferrous gluconate, 325 mg	37–39
Ferrous sulfate, 325 mg	60–65
Ferrous fumarate, 325 mg	107

In pregnancy, iron absorption from the duodenum increases, providing 1.3 to 2.6 mg of elemental iron daily.[74,75] Iron is absorbed in the duodenum, and an acid environment helps this absorption. Therefore, the frequent use of antacid medications, commonly used by many patients, decreases the absorption of iron. Vitamin C, in addition to the iron, may increase the acid environment of the stomach and increase absorption. In patients who do not show clear signs of iron deficiency, it is uncertain whether prophylactic iron, in addition to what is in prenatal vitamins, leads to an increased hemoglobin concentration at term. Iron prophylaxis, however, is safe. With the exception of dyspepsia and constipation, side effects are few. One 325-mg tablet of ferrous sulfate daily provides adequate prophylaxis. It contains 60 mg of elemental iron, 10 percent of which is absorbed. If the iron is not needed, it will not be absorbed and will be excreted in the feces. The standard generic iron tablets and the amount of elemental iron they provide are listed in Table 34–3.

In iron-deficient patients, one iron tablet three times daily is recommended. I cannot ascertain the scientific source of this recommendation. Most individuals can absorb as much iron as they need taking iron twice daily. It should be taken 30 minutes before meals to allow maximum absorption. However, when taken in this manner, dyspepsia and nausea are more common. Therapy, therefore, must be individualized to maximize patient compliance.

Zavaleta et al. examined the use of zinc in addition to iron, since it is thought that zinc may help with hematopoiesis. They found that zinc, in addition to iron, did not increase the hemoglobin concentration in patients.[76] Young et al. studied the effectiveness of weekly iron supplementation as opposed to daily iron supplementation.[77] They found that weekly iron supplementation was almost as effective as daily supplementation in raising the hemoglobin concentration in iron-deficient patients. This approach can be used in patients with less than optimal compliance.

For those patients who are noncompliant or are unable to take oral iron and are severely anemic, intravenous iron can be given. Singh et al.[78] found that parenteral iron can be safely given and significantly raises the hematocrit in patients. It also raises the serum ferritin. There were no adverse effects in their study of patients.[78] Hallak et al.[79] looked at the safety and efficacy of parenteral iron administration. They administered parenteral iron to 26 patients. Only one patient developed signs of mild allergy during the test dose and was excluded from the study. The remaining 21 pregnant patients completed the course of therapy and received a mean of 1,000 mg of elemental iron. Their hemoglobin increased an average of 1.6 g/dl from the beginning to the end of therapy and rose another 0.8 g/dl during the following 2 weeks. Ferritin levels increased from 2.9 ng/ml at the beginning of therapy to 122.8 ng/ml by the end of therapy.[79] Ferritin levels only decreased to a mean of 109.4 ng/ml 2 weeks later. Only mild transient side effects were noted. The authors concluded that parenteral iron therapy is safe during pregnancy.[79]

Iron dextran comes in a concentration of 50 mg/ml. It can be given intramuscularly or intravenously. Intramuscular injection is very painful. Parenteral iron is indicated in those who cannot or will not take oral iron therapy and are not anemic enough to require transfusion. In fact, by building iron stores in the patients before delivery, we may be able to prevent a need for transfusion postpartum in the severely anemic patient. Unfortunately, iron dextran can cause anaphylaxis, which is caused by dissociation of the iron component and carbohydrate component. The reaction may be immediate or delayed. Therefore, a 0.5-ml test should be given and epinephrine should be readily available. This anaphylaxis usually occurs within several minutes but may take 2 days to develop. The dosage for iron dextran therapy is shown in the box "Iron Dextran Administration."

It is still not certain whether anemia results in an increased risk for poor pregnancy outcome. In a literature review, Scholl and Hediger[80] concluded that anemia diagnosed in early pregnancy is associated with preterm delivery and low birth weight. In this study, women with iron deficiency anemia had twice the risk of preterm delivery and thrice the risk of delivering a low-birth-weight infant.[80] Preterm labor, however, is a multifactorial problem, and there were many confounders in this study.

Iron Dextran Administration

$$\text{Dose(ml)} = 0.0442 \,(\text{Desired hgb-Observed hgb}) \times \text{LBW} + (0.26 \times \text{LBW})$$

---

hgb, hemoglobin; LBW, Lean body weight.

Yip[81] reviewed the literature concerning pregnancy outcome with anemia. He found through epidemiologic studies that there is an association between moderate anemia and poor perinatal outcome, yet he was unable to determine whether this relationship was causal.[81] Sifakis and Pharmakides[82] observed that hemoglobin concentrations less than 6 g/dl are associated with preterm birth, spontaneous abortion, low birth weight, and fetal deaths. Nevertheless, a mild to moderate anemia did not appear to have any significant effect on fetal outcome.[82] Hemminki and Starfield[83] reviewed controlled trials, concluding that routine iron administration did not decrease preterm labor or raise birth weight. Conversely, Stephansson et al. found an increased risk of stillbirth and growth-restricted infants in women with hemoglobin concentrations greater than 14.6 g/dl at their first prenatal visit.[84]

In summary, iron deficiency is very prevalent in the general pregnant population. In developing nations, it is alarmingly common and is a major cause of maternal morbidity and mortality. Routine iron administration should be used unless it is certain that the patient is iron replete. Iron prophylaxis can be taken as 1 iron tablet daily, or as one study showed, can be given on a weekly basis. There appears to be an association between poor pregnancy outcome and maternal anemia, especially severe anemia. It is uncertain, however, if this is a causal relationship.

FOLATE DEFICIENCY

Folic acid, a water-soluble vitamin, is found in green vegetables, peanuts, and liver. Folate stores are located primarily in the liver and are usually sufficient for 6 weeks. After 3 weeks of a diet deficient in folate, the serum folate level falls. Two weeks later, hypersegmentation of neutrophils occurs. After 17 weeks without folate ingestion, RBC folate levels drop. In the next week a megaloblastic bone marrow develops. During pregnancy, folate deficiency is the most common cause of megaloblastic anemia, as vitamin B_{12} deficiency is extremely rare. The daily folate requirement in the nonpregnant state is approximately 50 μg, but this rises three- to fourfold during gestation.[85] Fetal demands increase the requirement, as does the decrease in the gastrointestinal absorption of folate during pregnancy.[86]

Clinical megaloblastic anemia seldom occurs before the third trimester of pregnancy. If the patient is at risk for folate deficiency or has mild anemia, an attempt should be made to detect this disorder before megaloblastosis occurs. Serum folate and RBC folate levels are the best tests for folate deficiency.[87]

Folate deficiency rarely occurs in the fetus and is not a cause of significant perinatal morbidity. There is some evidence that fetuses that are homozygous for the C677T variant of the gene encoding for 5, 10-methylene tetrahydrofolate reductase have a 20 percent lower folate level and may be at risk for a neural tube defect.[88] Because infants born to pregestational diabetic mothers have an increased incidence of neural tube defects, Kaplan et al.[89] studied 31 pregnant diabetics and 54 controls to determine if there are aberrations in folate metabolism in patients with diabetes. They found that there were no differences in how ingested folate is processed in the diabetic pregnant patient.[89] Maternal morbidity, however, may result from the anemia, especially if the patient additionally suffers significant blood loss during the puerperium. Prenatal vitamins that require physician prescription contain 1 mg of folic acid. Most nonprescription prenatal vitamins contain 0.8 mg of folic acid. These amounts are more than adequate to prevent and treat folate deficiency. Women with significant hemoglobinopathies, patients ingesting anticonvulsant medications, women carrying a multiple gestation, and women with frequent conception may require more than 1 mg supplemental folate daily. If the patient is folic acid deficient, her reticulocyte count will be depressed. Within 3 days after the administration of sufficient folic acid, reticulocytosis usually occurs. In fact, folic acid deficiency should be considered when a patient has unexplained thrombocytopenia. (Leukopenia and thrombocytopenia, which accompany megaloblastosis, are rapidly reversed.) The hematocrit level may rise as much as 1 percent per day after 1 week of folate replacement.

Vollsett et al.[90] performed a retrospective analysis of 14,492 pregnancies in 5,883 women in Norway to determine if elevated homocysteine levels were associated with pregnancy complications. An elevated homocysteine level is often found with depressed folate levels. They compared those in the upper quartile homocysteine levels with those in the lower quartile. They noted a 32 percent (odds ratio: 1.32) higher risk for preeclampsia, 38 percent (odds ratio: 1.38) higher risk for prematurity, and a 10 percent (odds ratio: 2.01) higher risk for very low birth weight. All trends were statistically significant, but the limitations inherent in retrospective epidemiologic studies apply here.[90] Nelen et al.[91] found a relation between recurrent early pregnancy loss and genetic-related disturbances in folate and homocysteine metabolism.

Iron deficiency is frequently concomitant with folic acid deficiency. If a patient with folate deficiency does not develop a significant reticulocytosis within 1 week after administration of sufficient replacement therapy, appropriate tests for iron deficiency should be performed.

HEMOGLOBINOPATHIES

Since the last edition of this text, there has not been much change in the care of pregnant patients with sickle cell disease. The majority of research has focused on prenatal diagnosis of hemoglobinopathies.

Hemoglobin is a tetrameric protein composed of two pairs of polypeptide chains with a heme group attached to each chain.[92] The normal adult hemoglobin A_1 comprises 95 percent of hemoglobin. It consists of two α-chains and two β-chains. The remaining 5 percent of hemoglobin usually consists of hemoglobin A_2 (containing two α-chains and two δ-chains) and/or hemoglobin F (with two α-chains and two γ-chains). In the fetus, hemoglobin F (fetal hemoglobin) declines during the third trimester of pregnancy, reaching its permanent nadir several months after birth. Hemoglobinopathies arise when there is a change in the structure of a peptide chain or a defect in the ability to synthesize a specific polypeptide chain. The patterns of inheritance are often straightforward. The prevalences of the most common hemoglobinopathies are listed in Table 34–4.

Hemoglobin S

Hemoglobin S, an aberrant hemoglobin, is present in patients with sickle cell disease (hemoglobin SS) and sickle cell trait (hemoglobin AS). A single substitution of valine for glutamic acid at the sixth position in the β-polypeptide chain causes a significant change in the physical characteristics of this hemoglobin. At low oxygen tensions, RBCs containing hemoglobin S assume a sickle shape. Sludging in small vessels occurs, resulting in microinfarction of the affected organs. Sickle cells have a life span of 5 to 10 days, compared with 120 days for a normal RBC. Sickling is triggered by hypoxia, acidosis, or dehydration. Infants with sickle cell anemia show no signs of the disease until the concentration of hemoglobin F falls to adult levels. Some patients do not experience symptoms until adolescence.

Table 34–4. FREQUENCY OF COMMON HEMOGLOBINOPATHIES IN AFRICAN-AMERICAN ADULTS IN THE UNITED STATES

Hemoglobin Type	Frequency
Hemoglobin AS	1 in 12
Hemoglobin SS	1 in 708
Hemoglobin AC	1 in 41
Hemoglobin CC	1 in 4,790
Hemoglobin SC	1 in 757
Hemoglobin S/β-thalassemia	1 in 1,672

Approximately 1 of 12 African-American adults in the United States is heterozygous for hemoglobin S and, therefore, has sickle cell trait (hemoglobin AS) and carries the affected gene. These individuals generally have 35 to 45 percent hemoglobin S and are asymptomatic. The child of two individuals with sickle cell trait has a 50 percent probability of inheriting the trait and a 25 percent probability of actually having sickle cell disease. One of every 625 African-American children born in the United States is homozygous for hemoglobin S, and the frequency of sickle cell disease among adult African-Americans is 1 in 708.[93] I recommend that all at-risk patients undergo hemoglobin electrophoresis. Although it is more expensive, it will identify all patients with aberrant hemoglobin types. Chasen et al.[94] disagree with this protocol. By looking at RBC indices and sickle solubility testing, they saved $18 per patient. Using this testing, they missed only 4 of 36 carriers of a hemoglobinopathy.[94] I do not recommend this. In many practices, ancillary personnel often initially review and file laboratory test results. The interpretation of RBC indices is often confusing to the nonphysician.

The traditional teaching is that women with sickle cell trait are not at increased risk for maternal and perinatal morbidity. A study by Larrabee and Monga[95] question this. In their study, 162 women with hemoglobin AS had a 24.7 percent incidence of preeclampsia compared with 10.3 percent of controls. Furthermore, the mean birth weight of infants born to women with hemoglobin AS was 3,082 g compared with 3,369 g for controls ($p < 0.0001$). The rate of endometritis was 12.3 percent for sickle trait patients compared with 5.1 percent for controls ($p < 0.001$) despite similar rates for cesarean delivery.[95] This study indicates that our surveillance should be higher in patients with hemoglobin AS.

If a patient has hemoglobin AS, the spouse should be tested, and if both are carriers of a hemoglobinopathy, prenatal diagnosis should be offered. Prenatal diagnosis can be performed by DNA analysis with the polymerase chain reaction (PCR) and Southern blotting.[96,97] PCR amplification of DNA fragments can allow a more rapid laboratory diagnosis. Hemoglobin S can also be identified by hemoglobin electrophoresis and DNA analysis of fetal blood.[98] Wang et al.[99] reported on 500 prenatal diagnoses of sickle cell disease, 196 utilizing only Southern blotting and 304 utilizing PCR. PCR greatly shortened the time interval from sampling to diagnosis and resulted in an overall fourfold increase in diagnoses. They showed that a diagnosis made prior to 20 weeks' gestation increased the likelihood that the patient would elect pregnancy termination.[99] The odds ratio of termination in cases with earlier relative to later diagnosis was 4.7.

Painful vaso-occlusive episodes involving multiple organs are the clinical hallmark of sickle cell anemia. The most common sites for these episodes are the extremities, joints, and abdomen. Vaso-occlusive episodes can also occur in the lung, resulting in pulmonary infarction. Analgesia, oxygen, and hydration are the clinical foundations for treating these painful crises.

Sickle cell disease can affect virtually all organ systems. Osteomyelitis is common, and osteomyelitis caused by *Salmonella* is found almost exclusively in these patients. The risk of pyelonephritis is increased. Sickling may also occur in the renal medulla, where oxygen tension is reduced, resulting in papillary necrosis. These patients also exhibit renal tubular dysfunction and hyposthenuria. Because of chronic hemolysis and decreased RBC survival, patients with sickle cell anemia often demonstrate some degree of jaundice. Biliary stasis commonly occurs during crises, and cholelithiasis is seen in about 30 percent of cases.[100,101] Because of chronic anemia, high-output cardiac failure can occur. Left ventricular hypertrophy and cardiomegaly are not uncommon.

Many pregnancies complicated by sickle cell anemia are associated with poor perinatal outcomes. The rate of spontaneous abortion may be as high as 25 percent.[102–104] Perinatal mortality rates of up to 40 percent were reported in the past, but the current estimate is approximately 15 percent.[103–108] Powars and co-workers[109] studied 156 pregnancies in 79 women with sickle cell anemia. In this group, the perinatal mortality rate was 52.7 percent before 1972 and 22.7 percent after that time. In a report by Seoud and co-workers,[110] the perinatal mortality rate was 10.5 percent. Much of this poor perinatal outcome is related to preterm birth. Approximately 30 percent of infants born to mothers with sickle cell disease have birth weights below 2,500 g.[108] In the Seoud et al.[110] report, the mean birth weight was 2,443 g.[110] In a multicenter study, Smith et al.[111] reported that 21 percent of infants born to mothers with sickle cell disease were small for gestational age. It has been hypothesized that sickling in the uterine vessels may lead to decreased fetal oxygenation and intrauterine growth restriction.[112] Classic teaching is that increased levels of hemoglobin F in the mother spared her from increased painful crises during pregnancy and may also have a protective effect on the neonate. In a study by Anyaegbunam and colleagues,[113] hemoglobin F levels, however, were inversely correlated with birth weight percentile. In contrast, Morris et al.[114] studied 270 singleton pregnancies in 175 women with sickle cell disease. The overall fetal wastage rate was 32.2 percent. Mothers with high hemoglobin F levels had a significantly lower perinatal mortality rate. This finding may have real clinical significance for obstetricians in the future. Ohne-Frempong and Smith-Whitley[115] reviewed the use of hydroxyurea in children with sickle cell disease. This drug reduces the incidence of painful crises and increases hemoglobin F concentration.[115] The

safety of this drug in pregnancy has not been established. Further studies of its use in sickle cell disease are underway.

Stillbirth rates of 8 to 10 percent have been described in patients with sickle cell anemia.[103] These fetal deaths happen not only during crises but also unexpectedly. Careful antepartum fetal testing must therefore be utilized, including serial ultrasonography to assess fetal growth. In another study, Anyaegbunam and co-workers[116] studied Doppler flow velocimetry in patients with hemoglobinopathies. They showed abnormal systolic/diastolic ratios for the uterine or umbilical arteries in 88 percent of patients with hemoglobin SS compared with 7 percent with hemoglobin AS and 4 percent with hemoglobin AA. However, only 8 patients with hemoglobin SS were studied compared with 40 patients with hemoglobin AS and 48 women with hemoglobin AA.[116] Howard et al. showed that maternal exchange transfusions did not change uteroplacental Doppler blood flow velocimetry in these patients.[117] This demonstrates that although maternal well-being may be improved, there is no change in uteroplacental pathology.

Although maternal mortality is rare in patients with sickle cell anemia, maternal morbidity is great. Infections are common, occurring in 50 to 67 percent of women with hemoglobin SS. Most are urinary tract infections (UTIs), which can be detected by frequent urine cultures. Patients with hemoglobin AS are also at greater risk for a UTI and should be screened as well. Pulmonary infection and infarction are also common. Patients with sickle cell anemia should receive pneumococcal vaccine before pregnancy. Any infection demands prompt attention, because fever, dehydration, and acidosis will result in further sickling and painful crises. The incidence of pregnancy-induced hypertension is increased in patients with sickle cell anemia and may complicate almost one third of pregnancies in these patients.[106,111] Painful crises also appear to be more common during gestation.[118,119] This was not true, however, in one study.[111]

The care of the pregnant patient with sickle cell anemia must be individualized and meticulous. These patients will benefit from care in a medical center experienced in treating the multitude of problems that can complicate such pregnancies. From early gestation, good dietary habits should be promoted. A folate supplement of at least 1 mg/day should be administered as soon as pregnancy is confirmed. Although hemoglobin and hematocrit levels are decreased, iron supplements need not be routinely given. Serum iron and ferritin levels should be checked monthly and iron supplementation started only when these levels are diminished. Abudu and co-workers[120] found that serum ferritin values were significantly higher in pregnant women with hemoglobin SS disease than in those with hemoglobin AA. They concluded that the physiologic changes of pregnancy in patients with hemoglobin SS did not result in an iron deficiency state and that the use of prophylactic iron supplementations in these patients appears unjustified. Aken'Ova et al. found that ferritin and iron levels decreased in pregnant patients with sickle cell disease in Nigeria.[121] This points out that iron and ferritin levels should be checked during pregnancy. It must be emphasized that routine iron supplementation, even that in the prenatal vitamins, should not be given, as iron overload may lead to hemochromatosis.

The role of prophylactic transfusions in the gravida with sickle cell anemia is controversial. This therapy, which replaces the patient's sickle cells with normal RBCs, can both improve oxygen-carrying capacity and suppress the synthesis of sickle hemoglobin. A previous study showed a sevenfold reduction in perinatal mortality in patients receiving prophylactic transfusions.[122] In the same group of patients, there was a significant decrease in fetal growth restriction and preterm births. Morrison and co-workers[123] have also previously reported reduced perinatal wastage and maternal morbidity using a regimen of exchange transfusion. In contrast, workers at Johns Hopkins believe that meticulous prenatal care gives results as favorable as those obtained with prophylactic transfusion.[102] Many patients in that series, however, did require transfusion for painful crises and anemia. Koshy and co-investigators[124] followed 72 pregnant patients with sickle cell anemia, one half of whom received prophylactic transfusions and one half transfusions only for medical or obstetric emergencies. There was no significant difference in perinatal outcome between the offspring of mothers who received prophylactic transfusions and those who did not. Two risk factors were identified as harbingers of an unfavorable outcome: (1) the occurrence of a perinatal death in a previous pregnancy and (2) twins in the present pregnancy. Even though there was no difference in perinatal morbidity and mortality, prophylactic transfusion did appear to decrease significantly the incidence of painful crises. The investigators concluded that the omission of prophylactic RBC transfusion will not harm pregnant patients with sickle cell disease or their offspring.[124]

Tuck and co-workers[125] delineated the risks involved with exchange transfusion. In a study of 51 pregnancies transfused between 1978 and 1984, 22 percent developed atypical red cell antibodies and 14 percent had immediate minor transfusion reactions. These data showed no significant difference in maternal or fetal outcomes among patients who were transfused prophylactically and those who were not.[125] Mahomed[126] reviewed the Cochrane database and found there is not enough evidence to make any conclusions about the use of prophylactic RBC transfusion in patients with sickle cell disease. Many of the studies cited in this chapter did not show fetal benefits from exchange transfusion. They did not, however, attempt to quantify changes in maternal well-being. This needs to be carefully evaluated before stating that prophylactic transfusions should be eliminated from the care of the pregnant patient with sickle cell disease.

If one chooses to perform prophylactic transfusion, the goal is to maintain a percentage of hemoglobin A above 20 percent at all times and preferably above 40 percent, as well as to maintain the hematocrit above 25 percent. Morrison et al.[123] recommend that prophylactic transfusion begin at 28 weeks' gestation. Buffy-coat-poor washed RBCs are used to reduce the risk of isosensitization. Other risks of transfusion therapy include hepatitis, acquired immunodeficiency syndrome (AIDS), transfusion reactions, and hemochromatosis. HIV antibody testing and new tests for hepatitis C have made transfusions much safer.

Either booster or exchange transfusions can be used. Exchange transfusions are preferable because they result in less stress on the cardiovascular system, thus decreasing the possibility of congestive heart failure. Exchange transfusions also raise the percentage of hemoglobin A more efficiently. If only booster transfusions are utilized, diuretics should probably be administered to prevent fluid overload. Exchange transfusion can easily be performed by the pheresis unit of the hospital. This is faster and safer than older techniques. The patient should be positioned on her left side during the procedure to maximize uterine blood flow.

Vaginal delivery is preferred for patients with sickle cell disease. Cesarean delivery should be reserved for obstetric indications. Patients should labor in the left lateral recumbent position and receive supplemental oxygen. Although adequate hydration should be maintained, fluid overload must be avoided. Conduction anesthesia is recommended, as it provides excellent pain relief and can be used for cesarean delivery, if necessary. Figure 34–1 provides a schematic presentation for the care of patients with sickle cell anemia. It can be adapted to patients with other hemoglobinopathies.

Hemoglobin SC Disease

Hemoglobin C is another β-chain variant in which lysine is substituted for glutamic acid in the sixth position. Clinically significant hemoglobin SC disease occurs in 1 in 833 African-American adults in the United States.[93] Women with both S and C hemoglobin suffer less morbidity in pregnancy than do patients with only hemoglobin S.[99,102,104] As in sickle cell disease, however, there is an increased incidence of early spontaneous abortion and pregnancy-induced hypertension.[102–105]

Because patients with SC disease can have only mild symptoms, the hemoglobinopathy may remain undiagnosed until they suffer a crisis during pregnancy.

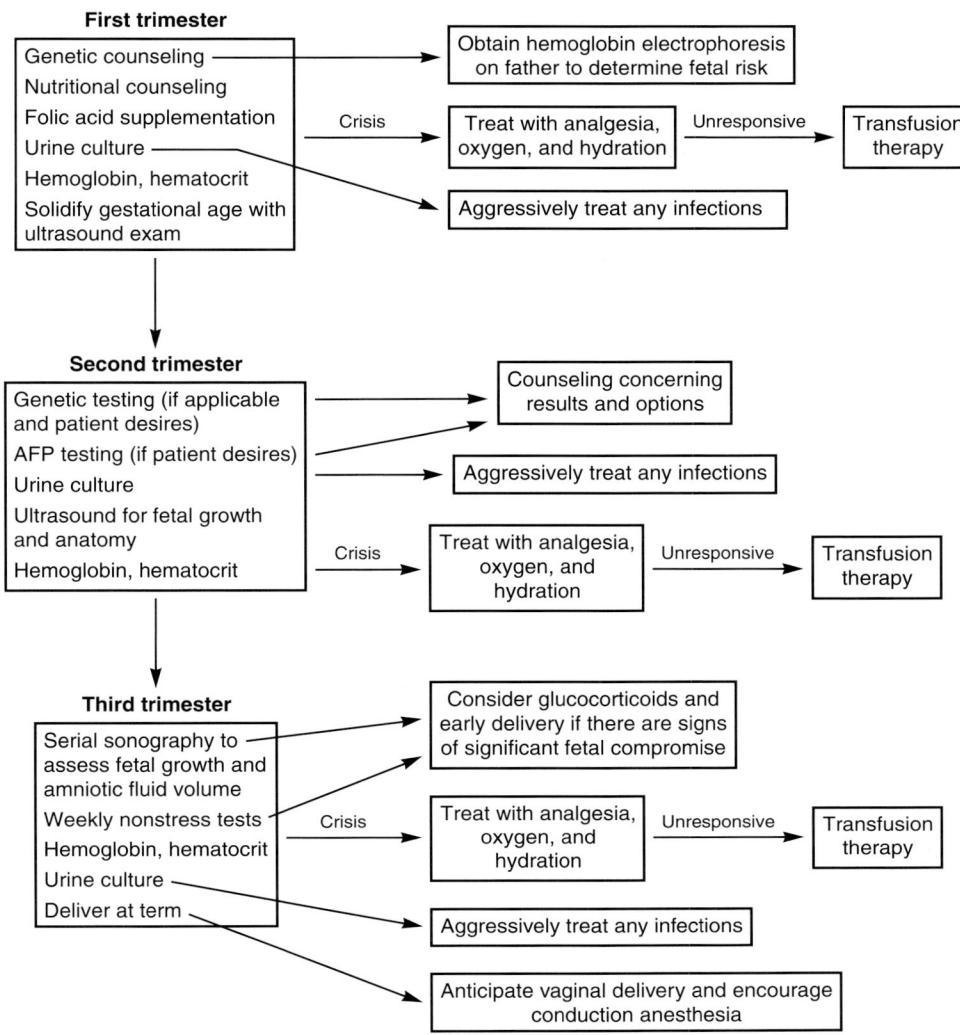

Figure 34–1. Schematic presentation of the care of patients with sickle cell anemia.

These crises may be marked by sequestration of a large volume of RBCs in the spleen accompanied by a dramatic fall in hematocrit.[127,128] Because these patients have increased splenic activity, they may be mildly thrombocytopenic throughout pregnancy. During gestation, patients with hemoglobin SC should receive the same program of prenatal care outlined for women with hemoglobin SS.

Thalassemia

Thalassemia results from a defect in the rate of globin chain synthesis. Any of the polypeptide chains can be affected. The disease may range from minimal suppression of synthesis of the affected chain to its complete absence. Either α- or β-thalassemia can occur. Heterozygous patients are often asymptomatic. Thalassemia can be detected by prenatal diagnosis. Wainscoat and co-workers[129] were able to offer prenatal diagnosis to

19 of 25 families with a potential for β-thalassemia using linkage analysis of restriction fragment length polymorphisms (RFLP). Cao and colleagues[130] reported their experience with prenatal diagnosis of β-thalassemia in 1,000 pregnancies followed at least 12 months after birth. Fetal blood sampling was carried out by placental aspiration, which yielded a sufficient amount of blood in 99 percent of cases. The fetal mortality rate associated with the fetal blood sampling, however, was 6.3 percent. With improvement in chorionic villous sampling and cordocentesis, prenatal diagnosis is now safe and the loss rate is much lower. Focharoen and co-workers[131] have been able to diagnose β-thalassemia in the second trimester by in vitro protein synthesis. They detect α-thalassemia by gene amplification in the first trimester.

Homozygous α-thalassemia results in the formation of tetramers of β-chains known as hemoglobin Bart. This hemoglobinopathy can result in hydrops fetalis.

Ghosh and co-investigators[132] reported their experience with 26 Chinese women who were at risk of giving birth to a fetus with homozygous α-thalassemia. Six of the 26 fetuses were affected. In two of the six cases, progressive fetal ascites appeared before 24 weeks' gestation. These pregnancies were terminated and the diagnoses confirmed. In the remaining four cases, there was evidence of intrauterine growth restriction by 28 weeks' gestation. At later gestational ages, an increase in the transverse cardiac diameter was seen in the affected fetuses.[132] Woo and colleagues[133] reported that umbilical artery velocimetry reveals a hyperdynamic circulatory state in fetuses that are hydropic because of α-thalassemia. In a study from Taiwan, Hsieh et al.[134] demonstrated that umbilical vein blood flow measurements can help to distinguish hydrops fetalis caused by hemoglobin Bart from hydrops fetalis having other causes. The umbilical vein diameter, blood velocity, and blood flow in fetuses with hemoglobin Bart were usually higher than those in fetuses with hydrops fetalis having other etiologies.

β-Thalassemia is the most common form of thalassemia. Patients with the heterozygous state are usually asymptomatic. They are detected by an increase in their level of hemoglobin A_2. In the homozygous state, synthesis of hemoglobin A_1 may be completely suppressed. This condition is characterized by an increase in both hemoglobin F and hemoglobin A_2. The homozygous state of β-thalassemia is known as thalassemia major, or Cooley's anemia. Patients with this disorder are transfusion dependent and have marked hepatosplenomegaly and bone changes secondary to increased hematopoiesis. These individuals usually die of infectious or cardiovascular complications before they reach childbearing age. Successful full-term pregnancies have been reported.[135] The few patients who do become pregnant generally exhibit severe anemia and congestive heart failure. Prenatal care is dependent on transfusion therapy similar to that used in the care of the patient with sickle cell disease.

Heterozygous β-thalassemia has different forms of expression. Patients with thalassemia minima have microcytosis but are asymptomatic. Those with thalassemia intermedia exhibit splenomegaly and significant anemia and may become transfusion dependent during pregnancy. Their anemia can be significant enough to produce high-output cardiac failure.[136] If these patients have not undergone splenectomy, they are at risk for a hypersplenic crisis.[137] Also, extramedullary hematopoiesis may impinge upon the spine, resulting in neurologic symptoms.[138]

These patients should be managed with a treatment program similar to that followed for patients with sickle cell disease. As in the case of sickle hemoglobinopathies, iron supplementation should only be given if necessary, as indiscriminate use of iron can lead to hemochromatosis. White and co-workers[139] have shown that patients with a β-thalassemia usually have a much higher ferritin concentration than normal patients and those who are α-thalassemia carriers. In β-thalassemia carriers, the incidence of iron deficiency anemia is four times less common than it is in α-thalassemia carriers and normal patients.[139] Van der Weyden and co-workers[140] have convincingly shown that red cell ferritin and plasma ferritin can be used in combination to determine if a patient has a potential for iron overload. Although iron is not necessary, folic acid supplementation appears important in β-thalassemia carriers. Leung and co-investigators[141] showed that the daily administration of folate significantly increased the predelivery hemoglobin concentration in both nulliparous and multiparous patients.

As in the case of sickle cell disease, antepartum fetal evaluation is essential in patients with thalassemia who are anemic. Asymptomatic thalassemia carriers need no special testing. However, patients with thalassemia should undergo frequent ultrasonography to assess fetal growth, as well as nonstress testing to evaluate fetal well-being.

Occasionally, individuals will inherit two hemoglobinopathies, such as sickle cell thalassemia (hemoglobin S thal). The prevalence of this disorder among adult blacks in the United States is 1 in 1,672.[142] The clinical course is variable. If minimal suppression of β-chains occurs, patients may be free of symptoms. However, with total suppression of β-chain synthesis, a clinical picture similar to that of sickle cell disease will develop. The course of these patients during pregnancy is quite variable, and their therapy must be individualized.

In summary, Figure 34–2 presents a stepwise approach to the work-up of anemia and the diagnosis of the conditions discussed in this chapter.

Von Willebrand's Disease

Von Willebrand's disease (vWD) is the most common congenital bleeding disorder in humans, and up to 1 percent of the population may have some form of the disorder.[143] Type 1 is an autosomal dominant disorder, whereas type 3 and occasionally type 2 are autosomal recessive.[144] Von Willebrand's disease is related to quantitative and/or qualitative abnormalities of von Willebrand's factor (vWF). This multimeric glycoprotein serves as carrier protein of factor VIII, an essential co-factor of coagulation in plasma, and promotes platelet adhesion to the damaged vessel and platelet aggregation. Distinct abnormalities of vWF are responsible for the three types of vWD. Types 1 and 3 are characterized by a quantitative defect of vWF, whereas type 2, comprising subtypes 2A, 2B, 2M, and 2N, refers to molecular variants with a qualitative defect of vWF. The knowledge of the structure of the vWF gene and

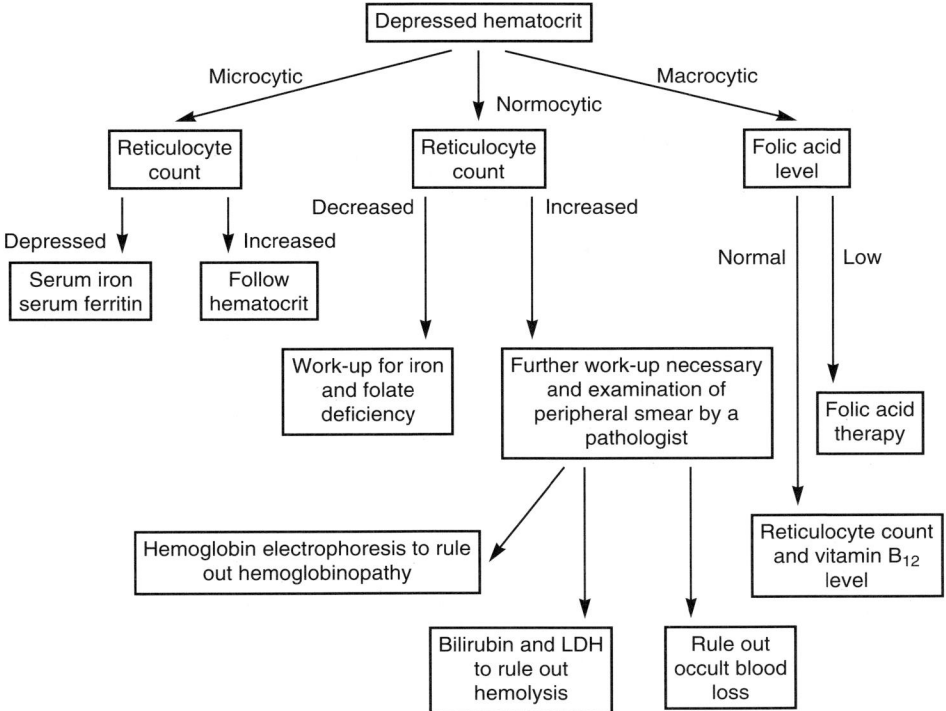

Figure 34–2. Evaluation of anemia.

the use of PCR have led to the identification of the molecular basis of vWD in a significant number of patients.[145] In type 2B, the only clinical symptom in pregnancy may be thrombocytopenia. This diagnosis, therefore, should be considered in the gravida presenting with isolated thrombocytopenia during pregnancy.[146,147]

The clinical severity of von Willebrand's disease is quite variable. Menorrhagia, easy bruising, gingival bleeding, and epistaxis are common. Menorrhagia is most severe in patients with type 2 and 3 vWD and most common in patients with type 1 disease.[148] In a compilation of two studies, 17 percent of women presenting with severe menorrhagia had a form of vWD.[148] Some patients may be entirely asymptomatic until they have severe bleeding after surgery or trauma.

Classically, the bleeding time is prolonged in patients with von Willebrand's disease as a result of diminished platelet aggregation. Occasionally, the activated partial thromboplastin time (APTT) will also be abnormal. In pregnancy, clotting factors including the factor VIII complex increase, and the patient's bleeding time may improve as gestation progresses.[148,149] This is especially true for type 1A von Willebrand's disease. In type 1B, the patient may not correct her bleeding time.[150] In type 2B, the platelet count will decrease. There will, however, be an improvement in the von Willebrand's factor multimeric pattern.[151] Heavy bleeding may be encountered in patients with von Willebrand's disease

undergoing elective or spontaneous first-trimester abortion because the levels of factor VIII have not yet risen.[152] Von Willebrand's disease does not appear to affect fetal growth or development. Postpartum hemorrhage may be a serious problem. The concentration of factor VIII C appears to determine the risk of hemorrhage. If the factor VIII C level is greater than 50 percent of normal and the patient has a normal bleeding time, she should not bleed excessively at vaginal delivery.[150,153–155] In a study by Kadir et al.,[152] 18.5 percent of patients with vWD experienced a significant postpartum hemorrhage, and 6 to 31 patients required transfusion. The clinical course during labor is quite variable. In a study by Chediak and co-workers,[156] bleeding complications were seen in six of eight (75 percent) pregnancies. Five of the newborns had von Willebrand's disease, one of whom was born with a scalp hematoma. Conti and associates,[157] conversely, reported no bleeding complications during the puerperium in five women with von Willebrand's disease. Ieko and colleagues[158] demonstrated that factor VIII concentrate could raise the platelet levels in patients with type 2B von Willebrand's disease. Ito et al. followed six women with type 1 vWD in 10 term pregnancies, 3 induced abortions, and 1 spontaneous abortion.[159] They found that bleeding complications occurred within 1 week after term delivery and immediately after both spontaneous and induced abortions.

Cryoprecipitate was, for many years, the treatment of

choice, as it contains all forms of both factor VIII C and the ristocetin cofactor. In those not responding to desmopressin, plasma-derived factor VIII/von Willebrand's factor concentrates should be used.[144] These concentrates can be treated with virucidal agents. The medium-purity and high-purity forms should be used, as they contain the most variety of multimers. Desmopressin (DDAVP) is the treatment of choice for type 1 von Willebrand's disease.[160] It elicits the release of von Willebrand's factor from endothelial cells. Intranasal preparations of 300 μg are usually used. In emergent or preoperative situations, 0.3 μg/kg can be given intravenously over 30 minutes.[144] It can rarely cause hyponatremia and fluid retention.

Bleeding during pregnancy is rare. Patients with classic type 1 von Willebrand's disease usually need no treatment with the increase in factor VIII levels during pregnancy. Those with a history of postpartum hemorrhage should be given an intravenous dose of desmopressin immediately after delivery, and the dose should be repeated 24 hours later. For those with type 2 and 3 disease, factor VIII/von Willebrand's factor concentrates are occasionally needed. Before a cesarean delivery, bleeding time should be measured. If it is prolonged, type 1 patients should be given desmopressin and type 2 or 3 patients should be given factor VIII/von Willebrand's factor concentrate.

HEREDITARY THROMBOPHILIAS

Venous thrombosis is the third most common vascular disease in the nation.[161] Pregnant women are particularly susceptible to this disorder. Virchow's triad, which is taught to most medical students, consists of vessel injury, venous stasis, and hypercoagulability. In pregnancy, we encounter venous stasis caused by hormonally related relaxation of vascular smooth muscle as well as mechanical compression of pelvic veins leading to decreased venous return to the vena cava. There are also changes in clotting factors, as all factors except V, XI, and XIII increase during pregnancy. Furthermore, there is a decrease in fibrinolytic activity. Therefore, deep vein thrombosis (DVT), occurring in 0.4 per 1,000 pregnancies, is six times more frequent during gestation as in nonpregnant individuals. In pregnancy, deep venous thrombosis usually involves the deep femoral and pelvic veins. If inadequately treated, these thromboses may lead to chronic venous insufficiency and leg ulcerations. These debilitating conditions are a major cause of disability in America.[162] If untreated, 24 percent of DVTs will result in pulmonary embolus, which occurs in 0.5 to 3.0 per 1,000 pregnancies. Without therapy, recurrent emboli will occur in 33.3 percent of patients.

The mortality rate from a pulmonary embolus is 15 percent in patients who are not treated for DVT, whereas the mortality rate is only 0.7 percent if prompt anticoagulation therapy is initiated. Therefore, prompt diagnosis and treatment are paramount. The diagnosis and treatment of pulmonary embolus is covered in Chapter 30. The purpose of this section is to address the causes, prevention, and treatment of DVT during pregnancy.

Before 1993, deficiencies or aberrations in protein S, C, antithrombin III, plasminogen, and fibrinogen were throught to be the only inheritable blood disorders that gave an individual a proclivity toward DVT and was responsible for 5 to 10 percent of all DVTs.[162] However, in 1993, activated protein C was added to the plasma of an individual with a pulmonary embolism, and the APTT was not prolonged.[163] This finding, activated protein C resistance, revolutionized the search for other etiologies of DVT. It has since been found that activated protein C resistance is responsible, at least in part, for about 40 percent of DVTs, fivefold more than any other single cause.[164]

How does activated protein C resistance lead to hypercoagulability? Figure 34–3 pictorially demonstrates what is discussed in this paragraph. Complexes of activated factors IX and VIII as well as activated factors V and X bind to the platelet surface and allow the amplification of thrombin (Fig. 34–3A), which catalyzes the conversion of fibrinogen to fibrin (the clot). When thrombin reaches a critical concentration, it stimulates thrombomodulin, which activates protein C. This in turn inactivates these factor complexes, thus turning off the production of thrombin (Fig. 34–3B). In the case of activated protein C resistance, protein C fails to turn off thrombin production by the activated factor V–X complex (Fig. 34–3C). Thrombin production, therefore, continues, leading to more conversion of fibrinogen to fibrin and thus a propensity toward clotting.

It has since been found that a single DNA point mutation at the activated protein C cleavage site on factor V, a substitution of arginine for glutamic acid at codon 506 (Arg506Gln), is responsible for 90 to 95 percent of activated protein C resistance.[165] This is known as the factor V_{Leiden} mutation. It is inheritable and fairly common. Homozygous and heterozygous forms exist. Heterozygous patients have a 5- to 10-fold clotting diathesis over the general population. Homozygotes, however, have a 50- to 100-fold increased risk.[166] It is unusual to find a homozygous patient that has not had thrombotic episodes prior to midlife. The frequency of this factor V_{Leiden} mutation varies with the population studied. The gene frequency in the United States is shown in the box "Population Frequency of Factor V_{Leiden} in the United States."

Higher plasma levels of homocysteine can lead to increased oxidation of homocysteine and the develop-

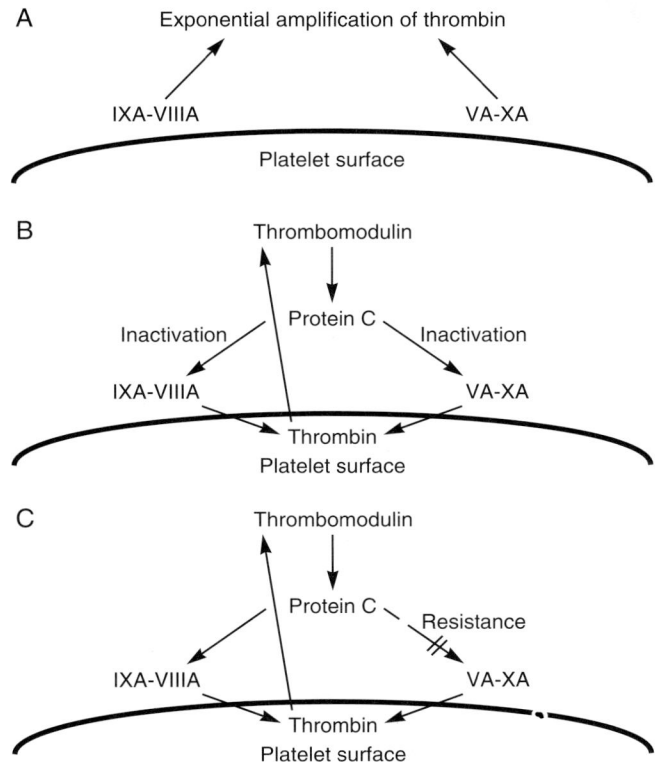

Figure 34–3. Activated protein C resistance and hypercoagulability. *A,* Binding of activated factors IX, VIII, V, and X to the platelet surface allows the amplification of thrombin, catalyzing the conversion of fibrinogen to fibrin. *B,* Stimulation of thrombomodulin leads to activation of protein C, which inactivates factor complexes and turns off the production of thrombin. *C,* In case of activated protein C resistance, protein C fails to turn off thrombin production by the activated factor V–X complex.

ment of superoxide radicals, which can damage endothelial cells, causing thrombus formation. Increased levels of homocysteine can occur when the compound is not converted to its natural metabolites methionine and cystathione. Figure 34–4 demonstrates the metabolism of homocysteine. As shown in these diagrams, folic acid, pyridoxine (vitamin B_6), and cyanocobalamin (vitamin B_{12}) are co-enzymes in the metabolism in homocysteine. Deficiencies of these B vitamins can, therefore, result in an excess of plasma homocysteine by limiting its conversion to cystathione and methionine. The most common cause of hyperhomocysteinemia, however, is caused by a mutation in the gene encoding for N^5,N^{10}-methylenetetrahydrofolate reductase, which is necessary for the metabolism of homocysteine to methionine (Fig. 34–4B). This mutation results in a thermolabile form of the enzyme that is less effective in the metabolism of homocysteine. The heterozygous state leads to a modest (if any) increase in homocysteine. The homozygous state, which is found in 9 percent of the general population, can cause significant increases in plasma homocysteine. Folic acid supplementation, even in individuals with normal serum folate levels, can lead to

Population Frequency of Factor V_{Leiden} in the United States

U.S. Caucasians 5.7%
African-Americans 1.2%
Hispanic-Americans 2.2%
Asian-Americans 0.45%
Native-Americans 1.25%

statistically significant reductions (up to 64.8 percent) in plasma homocysteine. Pyridoxine and vitamin B_{12} should also be used in an attempt to lower plasma homocysteine levels before prescribing anticoagulant therapy to the asymptomatic patient with elevated plasma homocysteine levels.

A mutation in the gene responsible for factor II (G20210A mutation) (prothrombin gene mutation) has also been identified. Individuals who are heterozygous for this gene mutation have an increased tendency toward thromboembolism, with an odds ratio of 2.8 to 3.8.[167]

Individuals with these thrombophilic conditions do not always develop thromboses. There are also exogenous factors that predispose individuals to thrombotic events. These are listed in the box "Nongenetic Synergistic Factors that May Predispose to Venous Thrombosis." If an individual has an inheritable tendency toward thrombosis, these exogenous factors may tip the scale in favor of thrombus development. These three relatively recently discovered gene mutations that predispose an individual toward thrombosis can be tested using DNA techniques. These are reliable tests, and results are not affected by anticoagulation or the physiologic changes of pregnancy.

The prevalence of the factor V_{Leiden} mutation in an obstetric population in Utah studied by Dizon-Towson

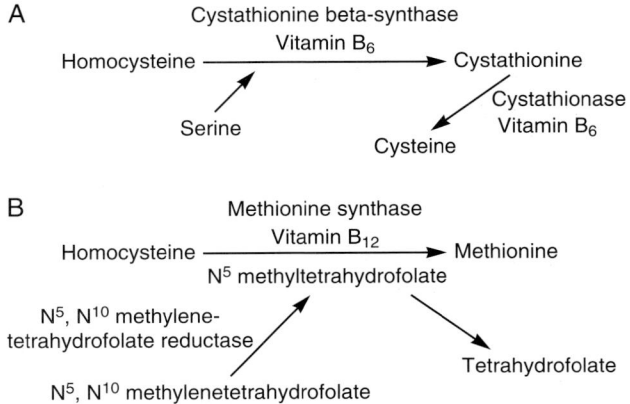

Figure 34–4. *A,* Metabolism of homocysteine to cystathionine. *B,* Metabolism of homocysteine to methionine.

Nongenetic Synergistic Factors that May Predispose to Venous Thrombosis

Pregnancy

Malignancy

Chronic infection

Diabetes mellitus

Trauma (including surgery)

Smoking

Obesity

Sedentary behavior (including bed rest for medical conditions)

Oral contraceptives (probable)

was 3.4 percent, which is similar to the published rate for nonobstetric populations.[168] Whereas less than 1 percent of patients without the mutation experienced a thromboembolic event during pregnancy, 28 percent of those with the factor V_{Leiden} mutation experienced such an event.[168] Indeed, the factor V_{Leiden} mutation appears to be a significant cause of deep vein thrombosis during gestation, especially when a patient has a predisposing factor such as those listed in the box "Nongenetic Synergistic Factors that May Predispose to Venous Thrombosis."

Hereditary thrombophilias may be associated with other pregnancy complications, especially those that may have a vascular component. It is not the purpose of this chapter to discuss these in detail. Briefly, several studies have demonstrated a relationship between the presence of factor V_{Leiden} mutation and preeclampsia.[169–171] These studies have not, however, demonstrated a causal role. Weiner-Megnagi and colleagues found that activated protein C resistance greatly increased the risk of placental abruption with an odds ratio of 8.16 ($p = 0.00125$).[172] Ridker and co-workers found that factor V_{Leiden} was present in 8 to 9 percent of patients with recurrent spontaneous pregnancy loss compared with 3.7 percent of controls.[173] Dizon-Towson reported that pregnancies with a fetus carrying the factor V_{Leiden} mutation were at increased risk for spontaneous abortion.[174]

The most dramatic data have been reported by Kupferminc and colleagues.[175] They determined the incidence of genetic thrombophilias in patients with severe preeclampsia, placental abruption, growth restriction, and stillbirth, pregnancy complications thought to have a strong vascular component. They found that 18 of 34 severe preeclamptic women had at least one of the three common gene mutations leading to thrombophilia. They also found at least one of these mutations in

12 of 20 abruptions, 22 of 44 pregnancies complicated by intrauterine growth restriction, and 5 of 12 stillbirths.[175]

The treatment of thrombosis during pregnancy consists of heparin therapy. If the patient has an active thrombosis, heparin can be dosed by a weight-based or non–weight-based regimen. The important component of this therapy is to check the APTT every 4 to 6 hours until the results are consistently about twice the control value. Obstetricians are increasingly using low-molecular-weight heparins. They are much more expensive, but may cause decreased heparin-induced thrombocytopenia and osteopenia. Monitoring the APTT is not necessary. Therefore, this therapy is more convenient for the patient. We have had the greatest experience using enoxaparin. The therapeutic dose is 1 mg/kg twice daily. Therapeutic levels can be ascertained by intermittent monitoring of activated factor X levels, as the pharmacokinetics of these drugs have not been reliably established in pregnancy.

Much research is needed concerning prophylactic anticoagulation in patients with factor V_{Leiden} mutation, patients with the thermolabile form of N^5,N^{10}-methylenetetrahydrofolate reductase, and patients with the prothrombin gene mutation. Because family members of patients with thrombotic events are being tested, we are identifying many patients who carry one of these genetic thrombophilias who have never experienced a sentinel event. We do not know if these individuals warrant prophylactic heparin during pregnancy, a time of hypercoagulability. It is our current practice to look for other risk factors such as those listed in the box "Nongenetic Synergistic Factors that May Predispose to Venous Thrombosis." We then have a long discussion concerning risks and benefits of prophylactic anticoagulation with the patient before a joint decision is made.

Key Points

> Four percent of pregnancies will be complicated by maternal platelet counts of less than 150,000/mm³. The vast majority of these patients will have gestational thrombocytopenia with a benign course and will need no intervention.

> Surgical bleeding occurs if the platelet count falls below 50,000/mm³ and spontaneous bleeding occurs if the platelet count falls below 20,000/mm³.

> Glucocorticoids are the first-line medication used to raise a low platelet count.

➤ Iron deficiency anemia is the most common cause of anemia in pregnancy and serum ferritin is the single best test to diagnose it.

➤ If a patient with presumed iron deficiency does increase her reticulocyte count with iron therapy, she may also have a concomitant folic acid deficiency.

➤ Patients pregnant with twins, those on anticonvulsant therapy, those with a hemoglobinopathy, and those who conceive frequently need supplemental folic acid during gestation.

➤ Most hereditary hemoglobinopathies can be detected in utero and prenatal diagnosis should be offered to the patient early in pregnancy.

➤ As in the nonpregnant patient, analgesia, hydration, and oxygen are the key factors in treating pregnant women with sickle cell crisis.

➤ Patients with sickle cell disease are at high risk of having a fetus with growth restriction and adverse fetal outcomes. Therefore, they warrant frequent sonography and antepartum fetal evaluation.

➤ Factor V_{Leiden} mutation occurs in up to 5 percent of the population and is responsible for a significant proportion of the thrombotic disease seen in pregnancy.

REFERENCES

1. McRae KR, Samuels P, Schreiber AD: Pregnancy-associated thrombocytopenia: pathogenesis and management. Blood 80: 2697, 1992.
2. Aster RH: Gestational thrombocytopenia. A plea for conservative management. N Engl J Med 323:264, 1990.
3. Samuels P, Bussel JB, Braitman LE, et al: Estimation of the risk of thrombocytopenia in the offspring of pregnant women with presumed immune thrombocytopenia purpura. N Engl J Med 323:229, 1990.
4. Samuels P, Main EK, Tomaski A, et al: Abnormalities in platelet antiglobulin tests in preeclamptic mothers and their neonates. Am J Obstet Gynecol 107:109, 1987.
5. Burrows RF, Kelton JG: Incidentally detected thrombocytopenia in healthy mothers and their infants. N Engl J Med 319: 142, 1988.
6. Hart D, Dunetz C, Nardi M, et al: An epidemic of maternal thrombocytopenia associated with elevated antiplatelet antibody in 116 consecutive pregnancies: relationship to neonatal platelet count. Am J Obstet Gynecol 154:878, 1986.
7. Burrows RF, Kelton JG: Fetal thrombocytopenia and its relation to maternal thrombocytopenia. N Engl J Med 329:1463, 1993.
8. Burrows RF, Kelton JG: Low fetal risks in pregnancies associated with idiopathic thrombocytopenia purpura. Am J Obstet Gynecol 163:1147, 1990.
9. Peterson OH Jr, Larson P: Thrombocytopenic purpura in pregnancy. Obstet Gynecol 4:454, 1954.
10. Tancer ML: Idiopathic thrombocytopenic purpura and pregnancy: report of 5 new cases and review of the literature. Am J Obstet Gynecol 79:148, 1960.
11. Territo J, Finkelstein J, Oh W, et al: Management of autoimmune thrombocytopenia in pregnancy and in the neonate. Obstet Gynecol 51:590, 1973.
12. Carloss HW, MacMillan R, Crosby WH: Management of pregnancy in women with immune thrombocytopenic purpura. JAMA 244:2756, 1980.
13. Noriega-Guerra L, Aviles-Miranda A, de la Cadena OA, et al: Pregnancy in patients with autoimmune thrombocytopenic purpura. Am J Obstet Gynecol 133:439, 1979.
14. Heys RFI: Child bearing and idiopathic thrombocytopenic purpura. J Obstet Gynaecol Br Commonw 73:205, 1966.
15. Karapatkin M, Porges RF, Karapatkin S: Platelet counts in infants of women with autoimmune thrombocytopenia: effects of steroid administration to the mother. N Engl J Med 305: 936, 1981.
16. Cines DB, Dusak B, Tomaski A, et al: Immune thrombocytopenic purpura and pregnancy. N Engl J Med 306:826, 1982.
17. Cines DB: Idiopathic thrombocytopenic purpura complicating pregnancy. Medical Grand Rounds 3:344, 1984.
18. Kelton JG, Inwood MJ, Narr RM, et al: The prenatal prediction of thrombocytopenia in infants of mothers with clinically diagnosed immune thrombocytopenia. Am J Obstet Gynecol 144:449, 1982.
19. Harrington WJ, Minnich V, Arimura G: The autoimmune thrombocytopenias. In Tascantins LM (ed): Progress in Hematology. New York, Grune Stratton, 1956, p 166.
20. Shulman NR, Marder VJ, Weinrach RS: Similarities between known antiplatelet antibodies and the factor responsible for thrombocytopenia in idiopathic purpura. Ann N Y Acad Sci 124:499, 1965.
21. Cines DB, Schreiber AD: Immune thrombocytopenia: use of a Coombs antiglobulin test to detect IgG and C3 on platelets. N Engl J Med 300:106, 1979.
22. He R, Reid DM, Jones CE, Shulman NR: Spectrum of Ig classes, specificities, and titers of serum antiglycoproteins in chronic idiopathic thrombocytopenic purpura. Blood 83:1024, 1994.
23. Yeager AM, Zinkham WH: Varicella-associated thrombocytopenia: clues to the etiology of childhood idiopathic thrombocytopenic purpura. Johns Hopkins Med J 146:270, 1980.
24. Scott JR, Cruikshank DR, Kochenour NK, et al: Fetal platelet counts in the obstetric management of immunologic thrombocytopenic purpura. Am J Obstet Gynecol 136:495, 1980.
25. Moise KJ, Carpenter RJ, Cotton DB, et al: Percutaneous umbilical cord blood sampling in the evaluation of fetal platelet counts in pregnant patients with autoimmune thrombocytopenic purpura. Obstet Gynecol 160:427, 1989.
26. Kaplan C, Daffos F, Forstier F, et al: Fetal platelet counts in thrombocytopenic pregnancy. Lancet 336:979, 1990.
27. Sciosia AL, Grannum PA, Copel JA, Hobbins JC: The use of percutaneous umbilical blood sampling in immune thrombocytopenic purpura. Am J Obstet Gynecol 159:1066, 1988.
28. Ghidini A, Sepulveda W, Lockwood CJ, Romero R: Complications of blood sampling. Am J Obstet Gynecol 168:1339, 1993.
29. Burrows RF, Kelton JG: Pregnancy in patients with idiopathic thrombocytopenic purpura: assessing the risks for the infant at delivery. Obstet Gynecol Surv 458:781, 1993.
30. Moschcowitz E: Hyaline thrombosis of the terminal arterioles

and capillaries: a hitherto undescribed disease. Proc N Y Pathol Soc 24:21, 1924.

31. Miller JM, Pastorek JG: Thrombotic thrombocytopenic purpura and the hemolytic uremic syndrome in pregnancy. Clin Obstet Gynecol 34:64, 1991.

32. Ridolfi RL, Bell WR: Thrombotic thrombocytopenic purpura: report of 25 cases and a review of the literature. Medicine 60:413, 1981.

33. Kwaan HC: Clinicopathologic features of thrombotic thrombocytopenic purpura. Semin Hematol 24:71, 1987.

34. Weiner CP: Thrombotic microangiopathy in pregnancy and the postpartum period. Semin Hematol 24:119, 1987.

35. Weiner CP, Kwaan HC, Xu C, et al: Antithrombin III activity in women with hypertension during pregnancy. Obstet Gynecol 65:301, 1985.

36. Nield GH: Haemolytic uraemic syndrome. Nephron 59:194, 1991.

37. Karmali MA, Petrie M, Lim C, et al: The association between idiopathic hemolytic uraemic syndrome and infection by verocytotoxin producing *Escherichia coli*. J Infect Dis 151:775, 1985.

38. Shulman H, Striker G, Deeg HJ, et al: Nephrotoxicity of cyclosporine A after allogeneic marrow transplantation: glomerular thromboses and tubular injury. N Engl J Med 305:1392, 1981.

39. Giroux L, Bettez P: Mitomycin C nephrotoxicity: a clinicopathologic study of 17 cases. Am J Kidney Dis 6:28, 1985.

40. Brown CG, Robson AP, Robson JG, et al: Haemolytic uraemic syndrome in a woman taking oral contraceptives. Lancet 1:1479, 1973.

41. Rousell RH: A new intravenous immunoglobulin in adult and childhood idiopathic thrombocytopenic purpura: a review. J Infect 15:59, 1987.

42. Mitra G, Wong MF, Mozen MM, et al: Elimination of infectious retroviruses during preparation of immunoglobulins. Transfusion 26:394, 1986.

43. Schwartz RS: Overview of the biochemistry and safety of a new native intravenous gammaglobulin, IGIV, pH 4.25. Am J Med 83:46, 1987.

44. Schwartz RS: Biochemistry and safety of native intravenous gammaglobulin (IGIV, pH 4.25). J Clin Apheresis 4:89, 1988.

45. Rousell RH, Budinger MD, Pirofsky B, Schiff RI: Prospective study on the hepatitis safety of intravenous immunoglobulin, pH 4.25. Vox Sang 60:65, 1991.

46. Rousell RH, Good RA, Pirofsky B, Schiff RI: Non-A non-B hepatitis and the safety of intravenous immunoglobulin pH 4.25: a retrospective survey. Vox Sang 54:6, 1988.

47. Kelton JG, Inwood MJ, Barr RM, et al: The prenatal prediction of thrombocytopenia in infants of mothers with clinically diagnosed immune thrombocytopenia. Am J Obstet Gynecol 144:449, 1982.

48. Moise KF Jr: Autoimmune thrombocytopenic purpura in pregnancy. Clin Obstet Gynecol 34:51, 1991.

49. Cooke RL, Miller RC, Katz VL, et al: Immune thrombocytopenic purpura in pregnancy: a reappraisal of management. Obstet Gynecol 78:578, 1991.

50. Lian ECY, Byrnes JJ, Harkness DR: Two successful pregnancies in a woman with chronic thrombotic thrombocytopenic purpura. Int J Obstet Gynecol 29:359, 1989.

51. Ezra Y, Mordel N, Sadovsky E, et al: Successful pregnancies of two patients with relapsing thrombotic thrombocytopenic purpura. Int J Obstet Gynecol 29:359, 1989.

52. Ponticelli C, Rivolta E, Imbasciatti E, et al: Hemolytic uremic syndrome in adults. Arch Int Med 140:353, 1980.

53. Beattie TJ, Murphy AV, Willoughby MLN, Belch JJF: Prostacyclin infusion in haemolytic-uraemic syndrome of children. BMJ 283:470, 1981.

54. Olah KS, Gee H: Postpartum haemolytic uraemic syndrome precipitated by antibiotics. Br J Obstet Gynaecol 97:83, 1990.

55. Gutterman LA, Levin DM, George BS, Sharma HM: The hemolytic-uremic syndrome: recovery after treatment with vincristine. Ann Intern Med 98:612, 1983.

56. Deaver JE, Leppert PC, Zaroulis CG: Neonatal alloimmune thrombocytopenic purpura. Am J Perinatol 3:127, 1986.

57. Okada N, Oda M, Sano T, et al: Intracranial hemorrhage in utero due to fetomaternal Bak(a) incompatibility. Nippon Ketsueki Gakkai Zasshi 51:1086, 1988.

58. Bussel JB, McFarland JG, Berkowitz R: Antenatal treatment of fetal alloimmune cytopenias. Blut 59:136, 1989.

59. Menell JS, Bussel JB: Antenatal management of thrombocytopenias. Clin Perinatol 21:591, 1994.

60. Paidas AH, Berkowitz RL, Lynch L, et al: Alloimmune thrombocytopenia: fetal and neonatal losses related to cordocentesis. Am J Obstet Gynecol 172:475, 1995.

61. Pitkin RM: Nutritional influences during pregnancy. Med Clin North Am 61:3, 1977.

62. Beaton GH: Iron needs during pregnancy: do we need to rethink our targets? Am J Clin Nutr, 72(Suppl):265S, 2000.

63. Ho CH, Yuan CC, Yeh SH: Serum ferritin, folate and cobalamin levels and their correlation with anemia in normal full-term pregnant women. Eur J Obstet Gynecol Reprod Biol 26:7, 1987.

64. DeLeeuw NKM, Lowenstein L, Hsieh YS: Iron deficiency and hydremia of normal pregnancy. Medicine 45:291, 1966.

65. Chopa J, Noe E, Matthew J, et al: Anemia in pregnancy. Am J Public Health 57:857, 1967.

66. Holly RG: Dynamics of iron metabolism in pregnancy. Am J Obstet Gynecol 93:370, 1965.

67. Carr MC: Serum iron/TIBC in the diagnosis of iron deficiency anemia during pregnancy. Obstet Gynecol 38:602, 1971.

68. Boued JL: Iron deficiency: assessment during pregnancy and its importance in pregnant adolescents. Am J Clin Nutr 59:5025, 1994.

69. Harthoorn-Lasthuizen EJ, Lindemans J, Langenhuijsen MM: Erythrocyte zinc protoporphyrin testing in pregnancy. Acta Obstet Gynecol Scand 79:660, 2000.

70. van den Broek NR, Letsky EA, White SA, Shenkin A: Iron status in pregnant women; which measurements are valid? Br J Haematol 103:817, 1998.

71. Ahluwalia N: Diagnostic utility of serum transferrin receptors measurement in assessing iron status. Nutr Rev 56:133, 1998.

72. Long PJ: Rethinking iron supplementation during pregnancy. J Nurse Midwifery 40:36, 1995.

73. Milman N, Bergholt T, Byg KE, et al: Iron status and iron balance during pregnancy. A critical reappraisal of iron supplementation. Acta Obstet Gynecol Scand 78:749, 1999.

74. Zuspan FP, Long WN, Russell JK, et al: Anemia in pregnancy. J Reprod Med 6:13, 1971.

75. Pritchard JA: Changes in the blood volume during pregnancy and delivery. Anesthesiology 26:393, 1965.

76. Zavaleta N, Caulfield LE, Garcia T: Changes in iron status during pregnancy in Peruvian women receiving prenatal iron and folic acid supplements with or without zinc. Am J Clin Nutr 71:956, 2000.

77. Young MW, Lupafya E, Kapenda E, Bobrow EA: The effectiveness of weekly iron supplementation in pregnant women of rural northern Malawi. Trop Doct 30:84, 2000.

78. Singh K, Fong YF, Kuperan P: A comparison between intravenous iron polymaltose complex (Ferrum Hausmann) and oral ferrous fumarate in the treatment of iron deficiency anaemia in pregnancy. Eur J Haematol 60:119, 1998.

79. Hallak M, Sharon AS, Diukman R, et al: Supplementing iron intravenously in pregnancy: a way to avoid blood transfusions. J Reprod Med 42:99, 1997.

80. Scholl TO, Hediger ML: Anemia and iron-deficiency anemia: compilation of data on pregnancy outcome. Am J Clin Nutr 59:492S, 1994.

81. Yip R: Significance of abnormally low or high hemoglobin concentration during pregnancy: special consideration of iron nutrition. Am J Clin Nutr 72:272S, 2000.

82. Sifakis S, Pharmakides G: Anemia in pregnancy. Ann N Y Acad Sci 900:125, 2000.

83. Hemminki E, Starfield B: Routine administration of iron and vitamins during pregnancy: review of controlled clinical trials. Br J Obstet Gynaecol 85:404, 1978.

84. Stephansson O, Dickman PW, Johansson A, Cnattingius S: Maternal hemoglobin concentration during pregnancy and risk of stillbirth. JAMA 284:2611, 2000.

85. Rothman D: Folic acid in pregnancy. Am J Obstet Gynecol 108:49, 1970.

86. Giles C, Ball EW: Iron and folic acid deficiency in pregnancy. BMJ 1:656, 1965.

87. Ek J: Plasma and red cell folate values in newborn infants and their mothers in relation to gestational age. J Pediatr 97:288, 1980.

88. Molloy AM, Mills JL, Kirke PN, et al: Folate status and neural tube defects. Biofactors 10:291, 1999.

89. Kaplan JS, Iqbal S, England BG, et al: Is pregnancy in diabetic women associated with folate deficiency? Diabetes Care 22:1017, 1999.

90. Vollsett SE, Refsum H, Irgens LM, et al: Plasma total homocysteine, pregnancy complications, and adverse pregnancy outcomes: the Hordaland homocysteine study. Am J Clin Nutr 71:962, 2000.

91. Nelen WL, van der Molen EF, Blom HJ, et al: Recurrent early pregnancy loss and genetic-related disturbances in folate and homocysteine metabolism. Br J Hosp Med 58:511, 1997.

92. Lambert EK, Bloom RN, Kosby M: Pregnancy in patients with hemoglobinopathies and thalassemias. J Reprod Med 19:193, 1977.

93. Motulsky AG: Frequency of sickling disorders in US blacks. N Engl J Med 288:31, 1973.

94. Chasen ST, Loeb-Zeitlin S, Landsberger EJ: Hemoglobinopathy screening in pregnancy: comparison of two protocols. Am J Perinatol 16:175, 1999.

95. Larrabee KD, Monga M: Women with sickle cell trait are at increased risk for preeclampsia. Am J Obstet Gynecol 177:425, 1997.

96. Lynch JR, Brown JM: The polymerase chain reaction: current and future clinical applications. J Med Genet 27:2, 1990.

97. Husain SM, Kalavathi P, Anandraj MP: Analysis of sickle cell gene using polymerase chain reaction and restriction enzyme Bsu 361. Ind J Med Res 101:273, 1995.

98. Posey YF, Shah D, Ulm JE, et al: Prenatal diagnosis of sickle cell anemia: hemoglobin electrophoresis versus DNA analysis. Am J Clin Pathol 92:347, 1989.

99. Wang X, Seeman C, Chen T, et al: Experience with 500 prenatal diagnoses of sickle cell disease. Prenat Diagn 14:851, 1994.

100. Barret-Connor E: Cholelithiasis in sickle cell anemia. Am J Med 45:889, 1968.

101. Cameron JL, Moddrey WC, Ziridema GD, et al: Biliary tract disease in sickle cell anemia: surgical considerations. Ann Surg 174:702, 1971.

102. Charache S, Scott J, Niebyl J, Bonds D: Management of sickle cell disease in pregnant patients. Obstet Gynecol 55:407, 1980.

103. Fort AT, Morrison JC, Berreras L, et al: Counseling the patient with sickle cell disease about reproduction: pregnancy outcome does not justify the maternal risk. Am J Obstet Gynecol 111:391, 1971.

104. Freeman MG, Ruth GJ: SS disease and SC disease—obstetric considerations and treatment. Clin Obstet Gynecol 12:134, 1969.

105. Curtis EM: Pregnancy in sickle cell anemia, sickle cell-hemoglobin C disease, and variants thereof. Am J Obstet Gynecol 77:1312, 1959.

106. Horger EO III: Sickle cell and sickle cell-hemoglobin disease during pregnancy. Obstet Gynecol 39:873, 1972.

107. Milner PF, Jones BR, Dobler J: Outcome of pregnancy in sickle cell anemia and sickle cell-hemoglobin C disease. Am J Obstet Gynecol 138:239, 1980.

108. Fessas P, Loukopoulos D: Beta thalassaemias. Clin Hematol 3:411, 1974.

109. Powars DR, Sandhu M, Niland-Weiss J, et al: Pregnancy in sickle cell disease. Obstet Gynecol 67:217, 1986.

110. Seoud MA, Cantwell C, Nobles G, Levy OL: Outcome of pregnancies complicated by sickle cell disease and sickle-c hemoglobinopathies. Am J Perinatol 11:187, 1994.

111. Smith JA, England M, Bellevue R, et al: Pregnancy in sickle cell disease: experience of the cooperative study of sickle cell disease. Obstet Gynecol 87:199, 1996.

112. Fiakpui EF, Moron EM: Pregnancy in sickle hemoglobins. J Reprod Med 11:28, 1973.

113. Anyaegbunam A, Billet HH, Langer O, et al: Maternal hemoglobin F levels may have an adverse effect on neonatal birth weight in pregnancies with sickle cell disease. Am J Obstet Gynecol 161:654, 1989.

114. Morris JS, Dunn DT, Poddorr D, Serjeant GR: Hematological risk factors for pregnancy outcome in Jamaican women with homozygous sickle cell disease. Br J Obstet Gynaecol 101:770, 1994.

115. Ohne-Frempong K, Smith-Whitley K: Use of hydroxyurea in children with sickle cell disease: what comes next? Semin Hematol 34:30, 1997.

116. Anyaegbunam A, Langer O, Brustman L, et al: The application of uterine and umbilical artery velocimetry to the antenatal supervision of pregnancies complicated by maternal sickle hemoglobinopathies. Am J Obstet Gynecol 159:544, 1988.

117. Howard RJ, Tuck SM, Pearson TC: Blood transfusion in pregnancy complicated by sickle cell disease: effects on blood rheology and uteroplacental Doppler velocimetry. Clin Lab Haematol 16:253, 1994.

118. Perkins RP: Inherited disorders of hemoglobin synthesis and pregnancy. Am J Obstet Gynecol 111:130, 1971.

119. Baum KF, Dunn DT, Maude GH, Serjeant GR: The painful crisis of homozygous sickle cell disease: a study of the risk factors. Arch Intern Med 147:1231, 1987.

120. Abudu OO, Macaulay K, Oluboyede OA: Serial evaluation of iron stores in pregnant Nigerians with hemoglobin SS or SC. J Natl Med Assoc 82:41, 1990.

121. Aken'Ova YA, Adeyefa I, Okunade M: Ferritin and serum iron levels in adult patients with sickle cell anaemia at Ibadan, Nigeria. Afr J Med Med Sci 26:39, 1997.

122. Cunningham FG, Pritchard JA, Mason R: Pregnancy and sickle cell hemoglobinopathies: results with and without prophylactic transfusions. Obstet Gynecol 62:419, 1983.

123. Morrison JC, Schneider JM, Whybrew WD, et al: Prophylactic transfusions in pregnant patients with sickle hemoglobinopathies: benefit versus risk. Obstet Gynecol 56:274, 1980.

124. Koshy M, Burd L, Wallace D, et al: Prophylactic red-cell transfusions in pregnant patients with sickle cell disease: a randomized cooperative study. N Engl J Med 319:1447, 1988.

125. Tuck SM, James CE, Brewster EM, et al: Prophylactic blood transfusion in maternal sickle cell syndromes. Br J Obstet Gynaecol 94:121, 1987.

126. Mahomed K: Prophylactic versus selective blood transfusion

for sickle cell anaemia during pregnancy. Cochrane Database Syst Rev 2: 2000.

127. Fullerton WT, Hendrickse J, Williams W, et al: Hemoglobin SC: clinical course. *In* Jonxis JHP (ed): Abnormal hemoglobins in Africa: A Symposium. Oxford, Blackwell Scientific Publications, 1965, p 215.

128. Solanki DL, Kletter GG, Castro O: Acute splenic sequestration crises in adults with sickle cell disease. Am J Med 80: 985, 1986.

129. Wainscoat JS, Work S, Sampietro M, et al: Feasibility of prenatal diagnosis of beta thalassaemia by DNA polymorphisms in an Italian population. Br J Haematol 62:495, 1986.

130. Cao A, Falchi AM, Tuveri T, et al: Prenatal diagnosis of thalassemia major by fetal blood analysis: experience with 1,000 cases. Prenat Diagn 6:159, 1986.

131. Focharoen S, Winichagoon P, Thonglairoam V: Prenatal diagnosis of thalassemia and hemoglobinopathies in Thailand: experience from 100 pregnancies. Southeast Asian J Trop Med Public Health 22:16, 1991.

132. Ghosh A, Tan MH, Liang ST, et al: Ultrasound evaluation of pregnancies at risk for homozygous alpha-thalassaemia-1. Prenat Diagn 7:307, 1987.

133. Woo JS, Liang ST, Lo RL, Chan FY: Doppler blood flow velocity waveforms in alpha-thalassemia hydrops fetalis. J Ultrasound Med 6:679, 1987.

134. Hsieh FJ, Chang FM, Huang HC, et al: Umbilical vein blood flow measurement in nonimmune hydrops fetalis. Obstet Gynecol 71:188, 1988.

135. Mordel N, Birkenfeld A, Goldfarb AN, Rachmilewitz EA: Successful full-term pregnancy in homozygous beta-thalassemia major: case report and review of the literature. Obstet Gynecol 73:837, 1989.

136. Necheles T: Obstetric complications associated with haemoglobinopathies. Clin Hematol 2:497, 1973.

137. Savona-Ventura C, Bonello F: Betathalassemia syndromes in pregnancy. Obstet Gynecol Survey 49:129, 1994.

138. Singounas EG, Sakas DE, Hadley OM: Paraplegia in a pregnant thalassemic woman due to extramedullary hematopoiesis: Successful management with transfusions. Surg Neurol 36: 210, 1991.

139. White JM, Richards R, Jelenski G, et al: Iron state in alpha and beta thalassaemia trait. J Clin Pathol 39:256, 1986.

140. Van der Weyden MB, Fong H, Hallam LJ, Harrison C: Red cell ferritin and iron overload in heterozygous beta-thalassemia. Am J Hematol 30:201, 1989.

141. Leung CF, Lao TT, Chang AM: Effect of folate supplement on pregnant women with beta-thalassaemia minor. Eur J Obstet Gynecol Reprod Biol 33:209, 1989.

142. Schmidt RM: Laboratory diagnosis of hemoglobinopathies. JAMA 224:1276, 1973.

143. Phillips MD, Santhouse A: von Willebrand disease: recent advances in pathophysiology and treatment. Am J Med Sci 316:77, 1998.

144. Castaman G, Rodeghiero F: Current management of von Willebrand's disease. Drugs 50:602, 1995.

145. Mazurier C, Ribba AS, Gaucher C, Meyer D: Molecular genetics of von Willebrand disease. Ann Genet 41:34, 1998.

146. Giles AR, Hoogendoorn H, Benford K: Type IIB von Willebrand's disease presenting as thrombocytopenia during pregnancy. Br J Haematol 67:349, 1987.

147. Rick ME, Williams SB, Sacher RA, McKeown LP: Thrombocytopenia associated with pregnancy in a patient with type IIB von Willebrand's disease. Blood 69:786, 1987.

148. Kouides PA: Females with von Willebrand disease: 72 years as the silent majority. Haemophilia 4:665, 1998.

149. Kasper CK, Hoags MS, Aggeler PM, Stone S: Blood clotting factors in pregnancy: factor VIII concentrations in normal and AHF-deficient women. Obstet Gynecol 24:242, 1984.

150. Takahashi H, Hayashi N, Shibata A: Type IB von Willebrand's disease and pregnancy: comparison of analytical methods of von Willebrand factor for classification of von Willebrand's disease subtypes. Thromb Res 50:409, 1988.

151. Casonato A, Sarrori MT, Bertomoro A, et al: Pregnancy-induced worsening of thrombocytopenia in a patient with type IIB von Willebrand's disease. Blood Coagul Fibrinolysis 2:33, 1991.

152. Kadir RA, Lee CA, Sabin CA, et al: Pregnancy in women with von Willebrand's disease or factor XI deficiency. Br J Obstet Gynaecol 105:314, 1998.

153. Noller KL, Bowie EJW, Kempers RD, Owen CA: von Willebrand's disease in pregnancy. Obstet Gynecol 41:865, 1973.

154. Evans P: Obstetric and gynecologic patients with von Willebrand's disease. Obstet Gynecol 38:37, 1971.

155. Lipton RA, Ayromlooi J, Coller BS: Severe von Willebrand's disease during labor and delivery. JAMA 248:1355, 1982.

156. Chediak JR, Alban GM, Maxey B: von Willebrand's disease and pregnancy: management during delivery and outcome of offspring. Am J Obstet Gynecol 155:618, 1986.

157. Conti M, Mari D, Conti E, et al: Pregnancy in women with different types of von Willebrand disease. Obstet Gynecol 68: 282, 1986.

158. Ieko M, Sakurama S, Sagan A, et al: Effect of factor VIII concentrate on type IIB von Willebrand's disease-associated thrombocytopenia presenting during pregnancy in identical twin mothers. Am J Hematol 35:26, 1990.

159. Ito M, Yoshimura K, Toyoda N, Wada H: Pregnancy and delivery in patient with von Willebrand's disease. J Obstet Gynaecol Res 23:37, 1997.

160. Mannucci PM: Treatment of von Willebrand's disease. J Intern Med Suppl 740:129, 1997.

161. Anderson FA, Wheeler HB, Goldberg RJ, et al: A population-based perspective of the hospital incidence and case-fatality rates of deep vein thrombosis and pulmonary embolism. Arch Intern Med 151:933, 1991.

162. Hooper WC, Evatt BL: The role of activated protein C resistance in the pathogenesis of venous thrombosis. Am J Med Sci 316:120, 1998.

163. Dahlback B, Carlsson M, Svensson PJ: Familial thrombophilia due to a previously unrecognized mechanism characterized by a poor anticoagulant response to activated protein C: prediction of a cofactor to activated protein C. Proc Natl Acad Sci U S A 90:1004, 1993.

164. Svensson PJ, Dahlback B: Resistance to activated protein C as a basis for venous thrombosis. N Engl J Med 330:517, 1994.

165. Bertina RM, Koeleman BPC, Koster T, et al: Mutation in blood coagulation factor V associated with resistance to activated protein C. Nature 369:64, 1994.

166. Rosendaal FR, Koster T, Vandenbroucke JP, Reitsma PH: High risk of thrombosis in patients homozygous for factor V Leiden (activated protein C resistance). Blood 85:1504, 1995.

167. Hillarp A, Zoller B, Svensson PJ, Dahlback B: The 20210 A allele of the prothrombin gene is a common risk factor among Swedish outpatients with verified deep venous thrombosis. Thromb Haemost 78:990, 1997.

168. Dizon-Towson DS, Nelson LM, Jang H, et al: The incidence of factor V Leiden mutation in an obstetric population and its relationship to deep vein thrombosis. Am J Obstet Gynecol 176:883, 1997.

169. Mimuro S, Lahous R, Beutler L, Trudinger B: Changes of resistance to activated protein C in the course of pregnancy and prevalence of factor V mutation. Aust N Z J Obstet Gynaecol 38:200, 1998.

170. Lindoff C, Ingemarsson I, Martinsson G, et al: Preeclampsia is associated with a reduced response to activated protein C. Am J Obstet Gynecol 176:457, 1997.
171. Kahn S: Severe preeclampsia associated with coinheritance of factor V Leiden mutation and protein S deficiency. Obstet Gynecol 91:812, 1998.
172. Wiener-Megnagi Z, Ben-Shlomo I, Goldberg Y, Shalev E: Resistance to activated protein C and the Leiden mutation: high prevalence in patients with abruptio placentae. Am J Obstet Gynecol 179:1565, 1998.
173. Ridker PM, Miletich JP, Buring JE, et al: Factor V Leiden mutation as a risk factor for recurrent pregnancy loss. Ann Intern Med 128:1000, 1998.
174. Dizon-Townson DS, Meline L, Nelson LM, et al: Fetal carriers of the factor V Leiden mutation are prone to miscarriage and placental infarction. Am J Obstet Gynecol 177:402, 1997.
175. Kuperminc MJ, Eldor A, Steinman N, et al: Increased frequency of genetic thrombophilia in women with complications of pregnancy. N Engl J Med 340:9, 1999.

Chapter 35

Collagen Vascular Diseases

PHILIP SAMUELS

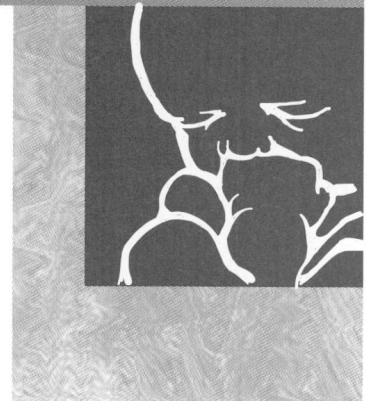

With the exception of rheumatoid arthritis, autoimmune diseases are associated with an increased risk of poor pregnancy outcome. Many of these diseases have a predisposition for women in their childbearing years. In fact, autoimmune diseases are occasionally first diagnosed during gestation. Often patients with recurrent pregnancy complications show evidence of autoimmunity but without significant criteria to allow a specific diagnosis.[1] These diseases are characterized by the production of autoantibodies—antibodies synthesized by an individual against a component of her own body. Increasingly sensitive and specific laboratory tests are being developed to aid in the diagnosis of these disorders (Tables 35–1 and 35–2).

SYSTEMIC LUPUS ERYTHEMATOSUS

Systemic lupus erythematosus (SLE) is a chronic disease with a great diversity of clinical and laboratory manifestations. Its onset is frequently insidious, and its diagnosis is often elusive and delayed. The course of SLE is characterized by chronic exacerbations and remissions. The prevalence of SLE is approximately 1 per 1,000 in the general population. The prevalence of the disease in women 15 to 64 years of age is estimated to be 1 per 700,[2] but in black women of the same age group the prevalence is 1 per 245.[3] The diagnosis of SLE is based on a patient meeting at least four of the diagnostic criteria accepted by the American Rheumatism Association (see the box "Revised Criteria for the Classification of Systemic Lupus Erythematosus [1982]").

Clinical Manifestations

Approximately 80 percent of patients with SLE demonstrate skin lesions. These may include the classic malar (butterfly) rash, alopecia, or discoid lesions that are often discolored. Photosensitivity is common. Arthralgias with some arthritis will be evident in 90 percent of patients. Nephritis and neurologic or psychiatric features are found in approximately 50 percent of cases. Because a patient can lose the majority of her renal function before she is symptomatic, renal pathology is often not diagnosed until other symptoms arise, which often delays the diagnosis of the disease.

The renal lesions of SLE include focal proliferative glomerulonephritis, membranous glomerulonephritis, mesangial nephritis, and diffuse proliferative glomerulonephritis. Patients with glomerulonephritis will excrete varying quantities of protein. The amount of proteinuria may range widely within the same individual, depending on disease activity. There are also diurnal variations; therefore, relying solely on a single voided specimen to determine the degree of proteinuria may be misleading. Those patients with focal and diffuse proliferative glomerulonephritis tend to have a worse long-term prognosis. Women with SLE may also present with seizures, peripheral neuropathy, or a psychotic episode. It is important to note that a recurrent fever of unknown etiology may also be the earliest manifestation of SLE.

Laboratory Diagnosis

More than 90 percent of patients with SLE will exhibit significant titers of antinuclear antibodies. In 80 to 90 percent of patients, an autoantibody directed against

Table 35–1. AUTOANTIBODIES OF DIAGNOSTIC SIGNIFICANCE

Autoantibody	Associated Disease
Antinuclear antibodies (ANA)	Most collagen vascular diseases
Antineutrophil cytoplasmic antibodies (ANCA)	70%–90% of patients with Wegner's granulomatosis, polyarteritis nodosa, crescentic glomerulonephritis
Anti-double-stranded DNA antibodies	80%–90% of SLE patients
High-affinity anti-DNA antibodies	Lupus nephritis
Antihistone antibodies	30%–60% of SLE patients, 95% of drug-induced lupus patients, 20% of rheumatoid arthritis patients
Antimitochondrial antibody	85%–95% of patients with primary biliary cirrhosis, 25%–30% of patients with chronic active hepatitis
Anti-Jo-1	Polymyositis, dermatomyositis
Anti-Ki	10% of SLE patients, especially with arthritis, pericarditis, and pulmonary hypertension
Anti-PM-1	Polymyositis
Antiscleroderma (SCL)-70 antibodies	20% of patients with scleroderma or progressive systemic sclerosis
Antiextractable nuclear antibodies (anti-Sm, anti-RNP, anti-SSA, anti-SSB)	SLE, Sjögren's syndrome, other collagen vascular diseases
Anti-RANA	Rheumatoid arthritis

double-stranded DNA will be detected. Anti-double-stranded DNA antibodies can be divided into subclasses. The high-affinity antibodies are seen more commonly in patients with renal involvement of their SLE, while the low-affinity antibodies are seen in milder forms of the disease. Extractable nuclear antibodies can be subdivided into antibodies against ribonuclear protein (anti-RNP, anti-SM), anti-SSA (Ro), and anti-SSB (La). The anti-SSA and -SSB antibodies are so named because they were initially identified in patients with Sjögren's syndrome. Anti-RNP antibodies are seen in 26 percent of patients with SLE; anti-SM antibodies are found in 28 percent of patients with SLE and can be correlated with renal involvement. Anti-SSA and anti-SSB antibodies, which are found in 25 and 12 percent of patients with SLE, respectively, have been associated with fetal and neonatal heart block. Anti-SSA antibodies are generally associated with manifestations of neonatal lupus. The extractable nuclear antibodies are usually seen in patients who have a speckled pattern of antinuclear antibodies.

Antihistone antibodies are seen in 30 to 60 percent of patients with SLE. They are seen in over 90 percent of patients with drug-induced lupus and are therefore useful in making this diagnosis. Anti-Ki antibodies are found in only 10 percent of patients with SLE, but correlate strongly with arthritis and with serious lupus systemic involvement such as pericarditis and pulmonary hypertension.

The Effects of Pregnancy on SLE

Pregnancy does not appear to affect or alter the long-term prognosis of patients with SLE.[4] Several studies, however, have documented increased flares of SLE dur-ing pregnancy and particularly during the puerperium.[4,5] It is difficult to compare and corroborate these studies, because there is no uniform definition of a lupus flare. Garsenstein et al.[4] predicted that the probability of a flare was three times greater during the first half of pregnancy, 1.5 times greater in the second half, and six times greater in the puerperium.[4] Meehan and Dorsey[6] examined the effects of pregnancy on the course of SLE in patients receiving glucocorticoids or azathioprine at conception. They found no statistically significant difference in the number of flares in pregnant women and nonpregnant controls when matched by disease duration and prior organ involvement. Lockshin[7] and Lockshin et al.[8] studied a variety of clinical markers of disease activity in 33 pregnancies in 28 women with SLE. They also demonstrated an absence of exacerbation during or after pregnancy. In a prospective study of 80 women, Lockshin[9] showed that exacerbation occurred in less than 13 percent of pregnant patients. He concluded, therefore, that there is no

Table 35–2. ANTINUCLEAR ANTIBODY PATTERNS IN RHEUMATOLOGIC DISEASE

Pattern	Disease State
Homogeneous	SLE, drug-induced lupus, chronic active hepatitis, many collagen vascular diseases
Speckled	SLE, Sjögren's syndrome, mixed connective tissue disease, rheumatoid arthritis
Nucleolar	Progressive systemic sclerosis, scleroderma, Sjögren's syndrome, subcutaneous SLE, SLE
Centromere	Scleroderma, CREST syndrome

Revised Criteria for the Classification of Systemic Lupus Erythematosus (1982)*

Malar rash

Discoid rash

Photosensitivity

Oral ulcers

Arthritis, nonerosive, involving two or more
peripheral joints

Serositis
  Pleuritis
  OR
  Pericarditis

Renal disorder
  Persistent proteinuria >0.5 g/day
  OR
  Cellular casts

Neurologic disorder
  Seizures
  OR
  Psychosis

Hematologic disorder
  Hemolytic anemia with reticulocytosis
  OR
  Leukopenia, <4,000/mm^3
  OR
  Lymphopenia, <1,500/mm^3
  OR
  Thrombocytopenia, <100,000/mm^3

Immunologic disorder
  Positive lupus erythematosus cell preparation
  Antibody to native DNA
  Anti-SM antibody
  False-positive serologic test for syphilis

Antinuclear antibodies in abnormal titers

---

*Four criteria necessary for diagnosis.
Adapted from Tan EM, Cohen AS, Fries JF, et al: The 1982 revised criteria for the classification of systemic lupus erythematosus. Arthritis Rheum 25:1274, 1982.

need for prophylactic glucocorticoids in the gravid patient with SLE. Derksen and co-workers[10] found that SLE patients who were in remission at the time of conception did not have any serious flares postpartum. In 82 percent of the 29 prospectively studied pregnancies, the disease remained quiescent throughout gestation.[10]

Conversely, Mintz and colleagues[11] showed an increase in SLE activity during pregnancy. This group studied 102 pregnancies in 75 women during a 10-year period. In this report, 59.7 percent of pregnancies that began with quiescent SLE experienced an exacerbation during pregnancy or the postpartum period. More than one half of these flares occurred in the first trimester and 20 percent during the puerperium. Most of the patients, however, readily responded to increased doses of glucocorticoids. Le Thi Huong and co-workers[12] in Paris found similar findings. Of 75 patients with inactive lupus at conception, 27 relapsed in pregnancy and 7 experienced postpartum flares.[12]

Although it remains debatable whether SLE is exacerbated by pregnancy, there is no dispute that there is a risk of major maternal morbidity and potentially of mortality in the gravida with SLE. Most maternal deaths occur during the puerperium as a result of pulmonary hemorrhage or lupus pneumonitis.[13,14] Rubin and colleagues[15] reported a case of pulmonary vasculitis resulting in pulmonary hypertension and death in a pregnant patient with SLE. Averbuch and co-workers[16] reported a case of cardiac tamponade occurring in the postpartum period caused by SLE. Marabani and co-workers[17] described a case of transverse myelitis during a pregnancy complicated by SLE. This complication responded quickly to steroids. In the study by Le Thi Huong et al.,[12] two women had nephrotic syndrome postpartum requiring high doses of steroids. They died of opportunistic infection secondary to immune suppression.[12] In our institution, we recently has a maternal death from SLE. The patient had a history of cocaine use and SLE. At the time of her admission, she had a negative toxicology screen but was experiencing lupus-related psychosis and had evidence of an old cerebral infarction on computed tomographic (CT) scan. Because of a low platelet count, general anesthesia was used for the ensuing cesarean delivery for fetal distress. She extended her cerebral infarction postoperatively and died. Gimovsky and associates[18] reviewed 108 pregnancies in 39 women affected with SLE and found that morbidity was rare in the immediate postpartum period. However, there was increased morbidity and mortality in the first few years after delivery.[18]

Most perinatologists advise their patients not to conceive during a time of increased lupus activity as this is associated with flares during pregnancy.[19] Although this seems logical, the volume of the literature to support this assertion is small.[20] The work by Mintz and colleagues[11] does, however, seem to favor this assumption. In general, a patient's disease should be quiescent for 5 to 7 months before conception. This recommendation is based on work by Hayslett and Lynn,[21] who observed that pregnancy outcome was good in 92 percent of women whose lupus had been in remission for at least 6 months prior to conception. This concept is also confirmed in the study of 35 pregnancies in 25 women observed by Derksen et al.[10] between 1987 and 1993. This is also confirmed in two review articles by Reichlin[22] and Julkunen.[19]

Women with lupus nephritis must be aware that there is a small but significant risk of permanent deterioration of renal function during pregnancy. Fine and co-workers[23] noted that in 9.6 percent of their patients renal function remained depressed for 3 to 12 months after delivery. Others have suggested that permanent renal deterioration during pregnancy is more frequent, perhaps as high as 50 percent.[24,25] In these studies, however, sample sizes were small. Conversely, Hayslett and Lynn[21] demonstrated no permanent change in renal function in pregnant patients with lupus nephritis. A summary of six studies reviewing 242 pregnancies in 156 patients revealed a 7.1 percent incidence of permanent renal dysfunction and a 30.2 percent incidence of transient renal dysfunction during gestation.[25] In this review, transient deterioration usually occurred in the third trimester. Poor pregnancy outcome is associated with active lupus nephropathy,[19] a serum creatinine level of at least 1.5 mg/dl, a BUN more than 50 mg/dl, and a creatinine clearance rate less than 50 ml/min.[19,21,26]

A lupus flare and preeclampsia present a difficult differential diagnosis, because they have similar signs and symptoms.[27] Both disorders often present with hypertension, edema, and proteinuria. To confound the issue, patients with lupus nephropathy are at an increased risk for developing superimposed preeclampsia during gestation. It is difficult, but very important, to make the distinction between these two phenomena. The treatment for preeclampsia is delivery, while the treatment for lupus nephritis is increased glucocorticoids and possibly azathioprine therapy. Buyon and co-workers[28] found that serum complement levels (C3 and C4) are valuable in differentiating between heightened lupus activity and preeclampsia. In normal pregnancy, complement levels tend to rise. They are, therefore, high or normal in the SLE patient with pure preeclampsia. Conversely, these levels fall with an exacerbation of lupus. If a patient develops hypertension and proteinuria in the second trimester, it is imperative to distinguish between preeclampsia and a lupus flare. If the diagnosis of preeclampsia is made, mandatory obstetric intervention could result in neonatal death or major morbidity from prematurity, depending on the gestational age. If serologic and chemical testing cannot make the distinction between the two conditions, a renal biopsy rarely may be indicated. Unfortunately, it is often impossible to distinguish between a lupus flare and severe preeclampsia necessitating an extremely preterm delivery.[27]

The Effects of SLE on Pregnancy

Although fertility is not impaired, SLE can have an adverse effect on pregnancy outcome in each trimester.[29] There is an increase in the spontaneous abortion rate, with the estimated incidence between 16 and 36 percent.[11,18,30–33] The risk of miscarriage is not necessarily related to disease activity. Mintz and co-workers[11]

reported a 16 percent spontaneous abortion rate regardless of disease activity.

In a study by Julkunen and colleagues,[34] patients with Sjögren's syndrome were compared with patients with SLE, and both were compared with controls. The relative risk of fetal loss was elevated in both patients with Sjögren's syndrome and SLE. Clinically significant intrauterine growth restriction was found more frequently in patients with SLE than in patients with Sjögren's syndrome.[34] Le Thi Huong et al.[12] examined 117 cases of SLE in pregnancy between 1987 and 1993. Twenty-eight infants were delivered full-term, while 48 were delivered prematurely. There were also 13 first-trimester losses, 2 second-trimester spontaneous abortions, and 3 third-trimester stillbirths, statistics above the expected rate of pregnancy loss. In this study, prematurity was related to a history of fetal loss, active SLE at onset of pregnancy, hypertension, and SLE requiring the patient to take at least 20 mg prednisone daily.[12] Growth restriction correlated with hypertension, low complement levels, and absence of anti-SSA antibodies.

In the study of Derksen et al.[10] of 35 pregnancies in 25 women, there were 8 first-trimester spontaneous abortions, no second-trimester losses, and 1 stillbirth. In a study by Ramsey-Goldman et al.,[35] a previous poor pregnancy outcome was the best predictor of a poor outcome in the present pregnancy.

In a large retrospective study, Petri and Albritton[36] reviewed 481 pregnancies in 203 women with SLE and used friends and family members without SLE as a control group. They found a 21 percent spontaneous abortion rate in women with SLE compared with 14 percent in friends and 8 percent in family members. Preterm delivery was found in 12 percent of lupus patients compared with 4 percent from each control group.[36] Hypertension requiring therapy, Raynaud's phenomenon, and not finishing high school were found to be significantly correlated with preterm delivery.[36]

In contrast to the study of Le Thi Huong et al.,[12] Leu and Lan[37] found anti-SSA antibodies were associated with growth restriction in pregnancies complicated by SLE. The presence of these antibodies, however, did not affect perinatal mortality. Kobayashi and co-workers studied 82 fetal outcomes in 55 women with SLE.[31] Live births occurred in 66 of 82 patients. They found a 50 percent incidence of growth restriction in infants born to mothers with low complement levels. This rate was significantly greater than infants born to women with normal complement levels.[31] Rahman and colleagues in Toronto[38] researched 141 pregnancies in 73 women with SLE between 1970 and 1995. They observed a 23.8 percent rate of spontaneous abortion, 2.2 percent rate of stillbirth, and a 7.9 percent rate of intrauterine growth restriction (IUGR).[38] They found that maternal renal disease was the only maternal predictor of fetal loss, and maternal hypertension was the only maternal predictor of pregnancy complications.[38] In studying 60 pregnancies in 46 patients in Spain, Carmona et al. found a mean duration of SLE of 6.25 years.[39] The rate of IUGR was 20.8 percent, had 18.9 percent of gravidas developed hypertension. Lupus flares occurred in 28.3 percent of patients postpartum.[39] Aggarwal et al. found IUGR in 40 percent of the offspring of the SLE patients in their study.[40]

Preterm birth is more frequent in women with SLE. Johnson et al.[41] attempted to determine the etiology of this preterm birth. In their study of 66 women in 58 pregnancies, they found that 39 percent of those delivering prematurely had experienced preterm premature rupture of the membranes.[41] This was not related to whether the patient was taking prednisone, the level of disease activity, or serologic studies. It appeared that rupture of the membranes was the single most frequent cause of preterm delivery in these patients. In Kleinman and colleagues review of 56 pregnancies spanning 19 years, the prematurity rate has 53 percent.[30] Analyzing 60 pregnancies in 46 SLE patients over 11 years, the prematurity rate was 20.8 percent.[39] This is increased, but not as dramatically as in the previously cited study.[30] Aggarwal et al. found a mean gestational age at delivery of 35.9 weeks, about 2 weeks earlier than their control group.[40]

Since the late 1980s, the lupus inhibitor and antiphospholipid antibodies have been the subject of concentrated research relating to recurrent miscarriage, infertility, and SLE. The diagnosis of the lupus inhibitor is often confusing. There is no single assay that is used to identify this phenomenon, and different assays have different sensitivities and specificities. Some clinicians and researchers rely solely on a prolongation of the activated partial thromboplastin time (aPTT) using platelet-poor plasma. A sensitive reagent must be used. Otherwise there will be many false-negative results. Other commonly used tests include the tissue thromboplastin inhibition test (TTI), kaolin clotting time (KCT), dilute Russell viper venom time, platelet neutralization procedure, and the hexagonal antibody. This variety of tests makes it difficult for the critical reader to compare different studies concerning the role of the lupus inhibitor in pregnancy outcome. One must also look at the years during which the study was performed when drawing conclusions about the results.

There is confusion concerning the difference between anticardiolipin antibodies and antiphospholipid antibodies. Antiphospholipid antibodies encompass many phospholipids, of which cardiolipin is only one. Antiphospholipid testing performed in different clinical laboratories may give discrepant results. The testing is not very specific due to the inherent wide spectrum for the antibodies which are tested. Harris, one of the pioneers in testing for antiphospholipid antibodies, feels that us-

ing β-2-glycoprotein 1 as an a alternative antigen may enhance the specificity of the test.[42] Ogasawara feels that β-2-glycoprotein 1–dependent antiphospholipid antibodies may be helpful in identifying autoimmune causes for habitual spontaneous abortion.[43]

The similarities and differences between the lupus inhibitor and anticardiolipin antibodies are also quite confusing. While many clinicians use the assays interchangeably, Rosove et al.[44] showed that the correlation between the two is not perfect, and both assays should be performed in order to maximize sensitivity. According to Field et al., antiphospholipid antibodies and lupus inhibitors favor different primary antigens.[45] The primary antigen for the lupus inhibitor appears to be prothrombin, while the primary antigen for antiphospholipid antibodies appears to be β-2-glycoprotein 1.[45] Munoz-Rodriguez and co-workers[46] have shown in a study of 177 patients with SLE and/or antiphospholipid syndrome that antibodies against antithrombin seems to be an independent risk factor for thrombosis, with an odds ratio of 3.7 ($p = 0.01$).[46]

Before concluding that the lupus inhibitor and anticardiolipin antibodies are a cause of poor pregnancy outcome, one must look at the prevalence of these phenomena in a normal pregnant population. Lockwood and co-workers,[47] in a study of 737 low-risk pregnancies, were the first to address this issue. Two of the 737 patients (0.27 percent) had a lupus inhibitor documented by a prolonged aPTT that did not correct after mixing with normal plasma. Both patients experienced a pregnancy loss. Elevated titers of IgM or IgG anticardiolipin antibodies were found in 16 patients (2.2 percent). Twelve of these 16 patients experienced an adverse pregnancy outcome. This study suggests that, while these phenomena are not widespread, the presence of the lupus inhibitor and anticardiolipin antibodies can be related to poor pregnancy outcome and placental infarction.[48,49] Ogishima and co-investigators recently examined the placentas of 150 patients with SLE, lupus inhibitor, and antiphospholipid antibodies.[50] They found the most extensive infarction and decidual vasculopathy in the placentas of patients who tested positive for both the lupus anticoagulant and antiphospholipid antibodies.[50] As shown by Lubbe et al.[51,52] in New Zealand, Branch et al.[53] in the United States, and Unander et al.[54] in Sweden, the lupus inhibitor and anticardiolipin antibodies are associated with recurrent spontaneous abortions even when there is no other evidence of collagen vascular disease. Also, in the absence of SLE, anticardiolipin antibodies can be associated with an increased risk for early preeclampsia, intrauterine growth restriction (IUGR), and fetal death.[53,54] Druzin et al.[56] and Lockshin and Druzin[57] have observed that patients with elevated anticardiolipin antibodies who have SLE are at significant risk to develop fetal distress in the second trimester with subsequent fetal death. Kutteh et al.[58] found that anticardiolipin antibodies were predictors of poor fetal outcome in patients with SLE. In their study, they found that the fetal loss rate was 39 percent in the patients with anticardiolipin antibodies and only 11 percent in those SLE patients without the antibodies.[58] Julkunen and colleagues[59] in Helsinki found that antiphospholipid antibodies were more sensitive in predicting fetal loss, but lupus inhibitor was more specific. Also, in this study, antiphospholipid antibodies did not correlate with prematurity or growth restriction.[59] Birdsall et al.[60] also found that antiphospholipid antibodies were present in 41 percent of women with recurrent miscarriage and 29 percent of women with a history of recent stillbirth. Their results were significant even in patients without signs suggestive of a collagen vascular disease.

Although treatment with heparin and aspirin has become the standard for treating lupus inhibitor and antiphospholipid antibodies, the precise population to be treated remains somewhat debatable. Furthermore, the type and dose of heparin has not been firmly established. Furthermore, the role of low-dose aspirin alone remains controversial.

Several studies report increased fetal survival and decreased morbidity and mortality in patients receiving prednisone in doses of 20 to 60 mg daily and low-dose aspirin.[53,60,61] It appears that this regimen will normalize a prolonged aPTT or other coagulation assay, but will have little effect on the level of circulating antiphospholipid antibody. These investigations, however, have not been controlled for the gestational age at which therapy was initiated. There have been no studies comparing prednisone alone to prednisone and aspirin.

Lockshin and co-workers[62] believe that prednisone may actually increase the incidence of fetal death in women with anticardiolipin antibodies. In their study of 21 women with a prior history of fetal death and a high titer of IgG anticardiolipin antibody, 11 were treated with prednisone. In the 11 treated women, 82 percent of the pregnancies ended in fetal death. In the untreated group, only 50 percent of pregnancies resulted in fetal death, a statistically significant difference. In patients treated with aspirin, there was no statistical difference in the outcomes of the groups. Based on these findings, Lockshin et al.[62] concluded that prednisone may actually worsen fetal outcome of the current pregnancy. Karp et al.[63] studied the outcomes of 27 pregnancies in 19 patients treated with prednisone and antiaggregants for the lupus inhibitor. There were only 13 successful outcomes, leading them to conclude that prednisone and antiaggregants may prevent second- and third-trimester losses but have only limited success in treating primary habitual abortion.[63] Nonetheless, there are other data that do support the use of prednisone and low-dose aspirin in treating patients with the

lupus inhibitor and the anticardiolipin antibody syndrome.[54,61,64] Landy and co-workers[65] followed 53 pregnancies complicated by lupus inhibitor or antiphospholipid antibodies. Thirty-three of these patients were treated with glucocorticoids and aspirin. They found that this therapy resulted in a 90.9 percent live-birth rate, higher than that achieved in patients only taking one medication. Geva et al. in Israel[66] treated 52 consecutive autoimmune patients with repeated failure of in vitro fertilization embryo transfer with prednisone and aspirin and observed a success rate in excess of 70 percent.[66]

Gatenby et al.[67] showed a dramatic improvement in patients receiving only aspirin therapy for elevated anticardiolipin antibodies. In patients with elevated antibodies and SLE, the pregnancy wastage rate dropped from 88 to 55 percent. In those with elevated antibodies alone, the rate of loss fell from 79 to 25 percent.[67] In their series, however, some of the patients were also receiving prednisone. Balasch and co-workers[68] studied 65 consecutive women with two or more spontaneous miscarriages. Seven (10.7 percent) were found to have anticardiolipin antibodies. Four of the seven women (57.1 percent) carried to term after being treated with low-dose aspirin alone. While the number of patients treated with aspirin alone is small, it does appear that this therapy might be beneficial in patients who have anticardiolipin antibodies.

Because infarctions are often found in the placentas of patients with anticardiolipin antibodies, researchers have begun using heparin therapy in this group. Rosove was one of the first to embark on anticoagulant therapy for antiphospholipid antibodies.[69] Rosove et al.[69] initiated heparin therapy at a mean gestational age of 10.3 weeks in 14 women with adverse pregnancy outcomes. The daily dosage ranged from 10,000 to 36,000 units. Live births occurred in 14 of 15 pregnancies (93.3 percent) with a mean gestational age of 36.1 weeks and a mean birth weight percentile of 57.[69] Heparin is now frequently used to treat patients with antiphospholipid antibodies. Low-dose heparin has less side effects than prednisone. Prednisone can be associated with increased striae, induction of gestational diabetes mellitus, poor wound healing, increased candidiasis, fluid retention, aseptic necrosis, cataracts, and other complications, especially when used in high doses. Branch et al.[70] found equivalent fetal survival when using heparin and aspirin; prednisone and aspirin; or heparin, prednisone, and aspirin. The maternal side effects were much less with a regimen that incorporated only heparin and low-dose aspirin. These authors advocate using 10,000 to 20,000 units of heparin daily. This study included 82 pregnancies in 54 women. It showed that the diagnosis of SLE, a history of preeclampsia, a history of thrombosis, a false-positive test for syphilis, and the titer of IgG anticardiolipin antibody made no difference regarding outcome of the current pregnancy.[70] The number of previous fetal deaths did correlate significantly with outcome in the current pregnancy. Heparin can result in heparin-induced thrombocytopenia, which can be life threatening. Danaparoid and r-hirudin (both heparinoids) have been used in such cases, as there is only a 10 to 20 percent cross-reactivity with heparin-associated antibodies.[71] There has been a great increase in the use of low-molecular-weight heparin in patients with antiphospholipid antibodies. The cost is greater than unfractionated heparin, but there is less heparin-induced thrombocytopenia and there may be less osteopenia associated with low-molecular-weight heparin. Granger and Farquharson showed excellent results using both low-molecular-weight heparin and low-dose aspirin.[72]

Intravenous immunoglobulin (IVIG) is currently being studied for use in treating patients with lupus inhibitor and/or antiphospholipid antibodies. Its mechanism of action is not entirely understood, but it may bind to receptors, preventing the binding of these deleterious antibodies. The correct dosage and dosage interval have not been elucidated. Clark et al. reviewed 19 pregnancies in 15 patients in whom IVIG was added to standard therapy.[73] There as a live birth rate of 84 percent, no growth restriction, and 75 percent delivered at or beyond 34 weeks' gestation. They felt that the cost was worthwhile if growth restriction and prematurity could be minimized.[73] Kaaja et al.[74] used high-dose immunoglobulin in conjunction with low-dose aspirin in four patients with good results. Somerset and co-workers[75] and Gordon and Kilby[76] also present evidence that IVIG is probably a useful adjuvant in the treatment of the antiphospholipid antibody syndrome in selected patients.

Anticardiolipin antibodies and the lupus inhibitor are associated with in vitro anticoagulation, but in vivo they are associated with thrombosis. These patients, therefore, are probably at some risk for thrombosis during gestation.[54,77–79] Mizoguchi et al.[78] described a 34-year-old woman with lupus inhibitor who had had six recurrent pregnancy losses without an intervening live birth. During her subsequent pregnancy, she developed multiple brain infarctions and hemiparesis. Rallings and co-workers[79] reported a 28-year-old primigravida who developed an acute anteroseptal myocardial infarction and died during gestation. She had a past history of thromboembolism. The only serologic abnormality noted was an elevated level of IgG anticardiolipin antibody.

We currently individualize our therapy of patients with lupus inhibitor and antiphospholipid antibodies. We take the patient's history and laboratory results into account when making decisions regarding therapy. Unfortunately, patients are occasionally tested for this syndrome after only having one spontaneous abortion. If this patient has equivocal or weakly positive testing,

we discourage therapy. For the patient whom we feel truly has this syndrome, we usually prescribe low-dose aspirin and heparin. Low-dose unfractionated heparin needs to be given twice daily. In these patients, low-molecular-weight heparin can probably be given once daily. The true key in treating these patients is to make certain they understand the potential side effects of the prescribed medication regimen and that they undergo the proper fetal and maternal surveillance throughout pregnancy.

Neonatal Manifestations of SLE

Complete congenital heart block, an infrequent complication of SLE, can be diagnosed prenatally. In the mid-trimester, a fetal heart rate of about 60 bpm with no baseline variability is indicative of congenital heart block. The patient should immediately undergo fetal echocardiography to rule out associated congenital cardiac malformations. Doppler studies can also locate the atrial ventricular disassociation. Fetal echocardiography can usually be carried out at 20 to 24 weeks' gestation and earlier in the asthenic patient. Affected fetuses usually show no evidence of congestive heart failure or hydrops, although occasionally this is observed. Therefore, fetuses with complete congenital heart block should be followed with serial ultrasonography every 1 to 2 weeks to ascertain if any evidence of anasarca has developed. Complete congenital heart block in the patient with SLE appears to be the result of immune complex deposition in fetal cardiac tissue as demonstrated by Litsey and co-workers.[80] This process leads to endocardiofibroelastosis and fibrosis of the conduction system.[81,82] Scott and colleagues[83] identified the anti-SSA (Ro) antibody in 83 percent of mothers delivering infants with complete congenital heart block. Anti-SSB (La) antibodies were found in a smaller but significant number of these mothers. Scheib and Waxman[84] have shown that these antibodies do bind to fetal cardiac tissue. They have described two successive pregnancies in a mother with anti-SSA antibody who gave birth to two antibody-positive children with complete congenital heart block. Derksen and Meilof[85] found that the level of anti-SSA antibody did not correlate with the development of complete congenital heart block. Le Thi Huong and co-workers[12] found manifestations of neonatal lupus in 3 of 22 infants whose mothers had anti-SSA antibody. Two had cutaneous manifestations and one had complete heart block. The titer of antibody did not appear to be related to the disease course. Conversely, Leu and Lan[37] found that patients with high titer anti-SSA antibody had a greater chance of having a neonate with manifestations of lupus. Three of 257 women with this antibody gave birth to an infant with complete congenital heart block.[37] All three had high antibody titers.

In most studies, mothers have had no symptoms of collagen vascular disease at the time of delivery. In the study of Vetter and Rashkad,[86] a large proportion of these women later developed SLE. According to Esscher and Scott,[87] the mother of a child born with complete congenital heart block has a 30 to 60 percent chance of developing a collagen vascular disease. Therefore, patients who deliver an infant with complete congenital heart block but who do not have SLE should have a careful clinical examination and undergo appropriate serologic tests on a routine basis. In future pregnancies, they should be treated as high-risk patients and undergo fetal echocardiography at the appropriate gestational age.

In the absence of structural cardiac anomalies, the neonatal mortality rate for infants born with complete congenital heart block is approximately 5 percent. In the studies of Vetter and Rashkad and Esscher and Scott[86,87] the mortality rate was 20 to 30 percent if a structural abnormality was also found. Falcini et al.[88] reported two cases of complete heart block and both mothers had anti-SSA/SSB antibodies. One child died of acute myocarditis at age 20 months. The other required cardiac surgery at age 10 years. Meng and Lockshin noted that childhood morbidity in children with anti-SSA/SSB heart block is high with 63 percent eventually requiring pacemakers.[89] They also found that the recurrence rate for complete congenital heart block is 12 to 16 percent.[86] Buyon and co-workers[90] aggressively treated a fetus with presumptive fetal myocarditis and heart block in a mother with SLE. They administered high doses of dexamethasone and performed plasmapheresis three times weekly. The patient responded well to therapy, showing a significant decrease in the titer of anti-SSB antibody. The infant was delivered at 31 weeks, and the heart block persisted. Others are attempting to treat early heart block in utero with steroids to decrease maternal antibody production and plasmapheresis to remove antibodies. Plasmapheresis is not without inherent risks and the utility of this therapy is yet to be determined.

Infants born to mothers with SLE may exhibit erythematous skin lesions of the face, scalp, and upper thorax.[12,91,92] These lesions usually disappear by 12 months of age. It appears that there is a higher incidence of anti-SSA antibodies in mothers giving birth to children with these skin lesions.[91] Anti-SSA antibody, furthermore, may be associated with an increased risk of miscarriage, even in the patient without SLE.[94]

Surveillance

Because of the increased risk of miscarriage, stillbirth, preterm delivery, and IUGR, the obstetrician caring for the patient with SLE should maintain close maternal and fetal surveillance. Any patient with a history of SLE should undergo preconceptual counseling and should have tests performed for the presence of the lupus inhibitor, anticardiolipin antibodies, anti-SSA (Ro) antibodies, anti-SSB (La) antibodies, and anti-double stranded DNA antibodies. As previously described, these findings are associated with a poorer pregnancy outcome. If indicated, therapy should be initiated after fully informing the patient of risks and benefits to both her and the fetus. If anti-SSA or anti-SSB antibodies are present, fetal echocardiography should be performed in the second trimester to rule out complete congenital heart block. Because of the risks of IUGR and preterm birth, accurate gestational dating is imperative in the patient with SLE. Patients should also have an examination of their urine sediment and a 24-hour urine collection for creatinine clearance and total protein excretion in early pregnancy to determine if there is any renal involvement of their SLE. Menstrual dating should be confirmed by ultrasonography at the first prenatal visit. At 18 to 20 weeks' gestation an additional ultrasound examination should be performed to confirm gestational age, ascertain appropriate fetal growth, and make certain that fetal anatomy is normal. IUGR in patients with SLE is usually asymmetric.[12] Fine et al.,[23] however, showed that symmetric IUGR can also occur. Because of the risk of IUGR and stillbirth, serial ultrasound examinations should be performed monthly after 20 weeks' gestation, with special attention to growth of the fetal abdomen, head, and femur.[93] The obstetrician should also be attentive to the volume of amniotic fluid, as decreased amniotic fluid can be the harbinger of fetal compromise and stillbirth.

At 28 weeks' gestation, weekly antepartum fetal heart rate testing should be initiated using the nonstress test. Antepartum fetal heart rate testing has been shown to improve fetal outcome in patients with systemic lupus erythematosus.[95] At 34 weeks, the frequency of testing should be increased to twice weekly. There are, however, no controlled studies showing that biweekly testing after 34 weeks improves perinatal outcome in the patient with SLE. Carroll[96] has shown that Doppler blood flow velocimetry is useful in following the gravida with the lupus inhibitor. In that study, abnormal umbilical artery systolic/diastolic ratios were found in five of six women with the lupus inhibitor who delivered growth-restricted fetuses. Only two of these patients demonstrated abnormally elevated uterine artery systolic/diastolic ratios. Ariyuki et al.[97] have demonstrated similar findings. Doppler may be a useful adjuvant in caring for the patient with SLE. Farine et al.[98] in Toronto found absent or reversed end-diastolic flow velocity in the umbilical artery of 11 percent of 56 patients with SLE. These patients had a high rate of preeclampsia, growth restriction, and fetal distress.[98]

Despite the sophisticated array of laboratory studies that are available to follow patients with SLE, the patient's clinical status remains of prime importance. There is no substitute for careful monitoring of maternal blood pressure and weight gain. These can be the earliest signs of superimposed preeclampsia, which is common in patients with SLE. They can also be the harbinger of a lupus flare.[27,99] Twenty-four-hour urine collections for creatinine clearance and total protein excretion should be carried out every 1 to 2 months. Serum creatinine, BUN, and uric acid levels should be determined whenever these urine collections are performed. A rise in serum uric acid can be a sign of impending preeclampsia. During a normal pregnancy, complement levels rise. A fall in the third or fourth components of complement (C3 or C4) or a fall in total hemolytic complement (CH50) has been associated with impending exacerbations of SLE.[100,101] Devoe and Aloy[102] found that a decrease in serum complement levels was also associated with a poor perinatal outcome. Because complement levels tend to rise during pregnancy, a single complement determination is of no value. A downward trend in complement levels, however, is significant, even though the level may fall within normal limits.

The timing of delivery is important and should be individualized. All too often, preterm delivery is performed merely to allay physician and patient anxiety. The obstetrician should strive for a vaginal delivery. If delivery is indicated near term and the patient's cervix is not favorable, cervical ripening agents may be employed. If the patient is taking glucocorticoids or if there is any evidence of lupus exacerbation, peripartum steroids should be administered parenterally. In the patient who undergoes cesarean delivery, intravenous steroids should be continued for 48 hours postoperatively, because adequate gastrointestinal absorption cannot be guaranteed until normal bowel function returns. Steroids should be tapered slowly and with great care in the postpartum period to prevent an exacerbation of SLE.[24,100]

Drug Therapy for SLE During Pregnancy

Patients with SLE are often hesitant to take their prescribed medications during pregnancy for fear of fetal effects. Many obstetricians are also reluctant to prescribe these medications for similar reasons. It is important for the obstetrician to be aware of the benefits and risks of medications used to treat SLE. Pregnancy is accompanied by a 40 to 50 percent increase in intravascular volume and an increase in interstitial fluid. Any steroid that has mineralocorticoid activity exacerbates interstitial fluid retention. This additive effect can cause maternal discomfort. The obstetrician should

therefore choose a steroid with minimal mineralocorticoid activity and maximum glucocorticoid activity. Steroids in combination with pregnancy may worsen acne and striae. Corticosteroid administration can also lead to gastrointestinal discomfort and ulceration. We therefore suggest that patients on chronic corticosteroid therapy use antacids after meals and at bedtime. Care should be taken, however, that antacid use does not interfere with the absorption of medications.

Chronic corticosteroid administration has been associated with bone demineralization and with an increased risk of hip fractures. For the gravida who is taking increased corticosteroids only during pregnancy, the actual risk is unknown. There is also a risk of cataract formation with long-term corticosteroid administration.

The induction of gestational diabetes from glucocorticoid administration is a distinct possibility. Approximately 3 percent of all pregnancies are complicated by gestational diabetes.[103] We perform 1-hour, 50-g oral glucose screening tests early and repeat them later in pregnancy in patients receiving long-term corticosteroids. We also test for diabetes later in gestation if there is any evidence of fetal macrosomia.

Pregnant women are often more concerned about the effects of the medication on their fetus than they are about the effects on themselves. The chronic ingestion of corticosteroids has not been associated with teratogenesis in humans.[104] An increase in the background incidence of cleft palate has been seen in rats and rabbits exposed to chronic corticosteroids but never in humans.[104-106] Neonatal adrenal suppression is a theoretical consideration in patients taking corticosteroids, but it has only rarely been reported. Nonetheless, the pediatrician should be informed when a mother has been taking corticosteroids antenatally.

Only a fraction of the steroids ingested by a pregnant woman reach the fetus. Prednisone, the most widely used glucocorticoid during gestation, is metabolized by the mother to its active form prednisolone. An 11-β-OH radical is responsible for prednisolone's physiologic activity. The placenta has an abundance of the metabolizing enzyme 11-β-ol dehydrogenase, which converts the active glucocorticoid to an inactive 11-keto metabolite. Depending on the study, only 10 to 50 percent of a dose of prednisone and only one sixth of a dose of hydrocortisone reach the fetus.[107-109] Levitz et al.[110] performed placental perfusion studies showing that steroids are rapidly cleared from the fetus. Beitins and coworkers[111] found that the maternal : fetal concentration gradient after intravenous administration of prednisolone was 10 : 1.

Dexamethasone and betamethasone cross the placenta more freely and for this reason are used to enhance fetal lung maturity. Blanford et al.[112] observed little conversion of dexamethasone or betamethasone to inactive forms. Work by Ballard et al.[107] and by Osathanondh et al.[109] demonstrate a maternal:fetal concentration gradient of 1:1 for dexamethasone and betamethasone.

To minimize potential fetal effects, prednisone should be the oral glucocorticoid of choice.[113] Both methylprednisolone and hydrocortisone are satisfactory for intravenous use when needed. Methylprednisolone has less mineralocorticoids effect and should create fewer maternal side effects.

Occasionally, azathioprine, a derivative of 6-mercaptopurine, will be required to control a patient's SLE. This medication readily crosses the placenta. In a study by Scott,[114] 64 to 93 percent of an administered dose appeared in fetal blood between 2.5 and 6 hours after intravenous administration. Azathioprine has not been shown to be teratogenic in humans, although congenital malformations have been observed in animal models.[115] Chronic azathioprine use during pregnancy has been associated with neonatal lymphopenia, lower serum IgG and IgM levels, and decreased thymic shadow on x-ray.[116] All of these changes have reversed with time. Scott[114,117] reports an increased incidence of IUGR in infants born to mothers who took azathioprine during pregnancy. As yet, no long-term information is available on immunologic development and later infection rates in children who were exposed to this medication in utero. Before administering azathioprine during pregnancy, however, the benefits and risks should be weighed carefully. Antimalarials occasionally are needed in women with SLE. These drugs bind to cells in the developing fetal eye, but no studies have identified any long-term effects. They should be used cautiously and only when clearly indicated in the patient with SLE.

RHEUMATOID ARTHRITIS

Rheumatoid arthritis is an autoimmune disease with a prevalence of approximately 2 percent. Its crippling chronic form occurs in about 0.35 percent of the population.[118] The onset of the disease is usually between the ages of 20 and 60 years, and women are two to three times more likely to be affected than are men.[119]

Diagnosis

The diagnosis of rheumatoid arthritis is based on guidelines set forth by the American Rheumatism Association (see the box "American Rheumatism Association Diagnostic Criteria for Rheumatoid Arthritis [RA]"). A list of exclusions has also been devised to make the

---

American Rheumatism Association Diagnostic Criteria for Rheumatoid Arthritis (RA)

Morning stiffness

Pain on motion or tenderness in at least one joint

Soft tissue swelling in at least one joint

Swelling in at least one other joint

Simultaneous symmetric joint swelling

Subcutaneous nodules

Radiologic changes typical of rheumatoid arthritis

Positive rheumatoid factor

Poor mucin precipitate from synovial fluid

Characteristic histologic changes in synovium

Characteristic histologic changes in subcutaneous nodules

A. Classic RA: 7 criteria

B. Definite RA: 5 criteria

C. Probable RA: 3 criteria

D. Signs and symptoms must persist for at least 6 weeks

E. No exclusions can be present

Adapted from Rodman GP, Schumacher HR: Appendix 2. *In* Primer on the Rheumatic Diseases, 9th ed. New York, Arthritis Foundation, 1988, p 207.

---

diagnosis more precise (see the box "Exclusions from Rheumatoid Arthritis").

Clinical Manifestations

Articular involvement is the hallmark of rheumatoid arthritis. The most common finding is an erythematous, warm, swollen metacarpophalangeal joint. The proximal interphalangeal and wrist joints may also be involved. Less frequently, metatarsophalangeal and shoulder joints are affected. Over time, cartilage destruction and pannus formation occur.[120] Carpal tunnel syndrome is often seen in patients with rheumatoid arthritis.[121]

Extra-articular features of rheumatoid arthritis are found in patients with the most joint involvement and the highest titers of rheumatoid factor.[122,123] Rheumatoid nodules, which occur in 20 percent of patients with rheumatoid arthritis, can appear in the heart and lungs and along any extremity.[124] Pericarditis, myocarditis, and endocarditis are occasionally seen in patients with rheumatoid arthritis. Vasculitis may result secondary to immune complex deposition and may affect the skin, peripheral nerves, and blood vessels.[125] Unlike

Exclusions From Rheumatoid Arthritis

Typical rash of systemic lupus erythematosus

Strongly positive lupus erythematosus cell preparation

Histologic evidence of periarteritis

Proximal muscle weakness consistent with dermatomyositis

Definite scleroderma

Clinical rheumatic fever

Clinical gouty arthritis

Tophi

Infectious arthritis

Tuberculous arthritis

Reiter syndrome

Clinical picture of shoulder-hand syndrome

Hypertrophic osteoarthropathy

Neuroarthropathy

Homogentisic aciduria

Sarcoidosis or positive Kveim test

Multiple myeloma

Erythema nodosum

Leukemia or lymphoma

Agammaglobulinemia

Adapted from Rodman GP, Schumacher HR: Appendix 2. *In* Primer on the Rheumatic Diseases, 9th ed. New York, Arthritis Foundation, 1988, p 207.

SLE, rheumatoid arthritis rarely involves the kidneys. It is important to note that after 10 years of disease more than 50 percent of patients are still able to work, and 15 percent will have a complete remission.[126]

Pathophysiology

Rheumatoid arthritis is characterized by proliferation and inflammation of synovial membranes. The membranes characteristically show a dense collection of lymphocytes in a diffuse nodular pattern.[127] T-cell function appears to be impaired, and there is an excessive number of T-suppressor cells.[128] Immune complexes, which activate the complement cascade, have been demonstrated in the blood, synovial fluid, and synovial membranes of patients with rheumatoid arthritis.[129,130] There appears to be a genetic predisposition to rheumatoid arthritis. A strong association between the histocompatibility antigen HLA-DR4 and rheumatoid arthritis has been shown.[131]

Laboratory Findings

Rheumatoid factors, IgM and IgG antibodies directed against the Fc fragment of IgG, are the hallmark laboratory finding of rheumatoid arthritis, but are not pathognomonic for this disorder. More severe disease is seen with higher titers of rheumatoid factor. Antinuclear antibodies are also found in approximately 20 percent of patients with rheumatoid arthritis.

Effects of Pregnancy on Rheumatoid Arthritis

Pope et al. determined that there is not an increase in infertility in women with rheumatoid arthritis.[132] In 1938, Hench[133] observed that many patients with rheumatoid arthritis experienced remissions during pregnancy. Persellin[134] noted that in pregnant women with rheumatoid arthritis 74 percent underwent remission during the first trimester, 20 percent in the second trimester, and 5 percent in the third trimester. In this series, however, 90 percent of patients experienced a postpartum exacerbation of their disease. Approximately 25 percent of these flares occurred in the first 4 weeks postpartum.[134] In a review, Klipple and Cecere[135] reported that approximately 70 percent of patients with rheumatoid arthritis experienced substantial improvements in disease activity during pregnancy including extra-articular symptoms. Most of these patients no longer required medications. This remission, however, was short lived, with more than 90 percent of women relapsing within 6 to 8 months postpartum. Klipple and Cecere[135] also found that in approximately 30 percent of patients with rheumatoid arthritis the course remained unchanged or worsened during gestation.

Quinn and colleagues[136] studied 24 pregnant women with rheumatoid arthritis, 21 of whom had quiescent disease activity during pregnancy. Nineteen of these 21 women had significant flares during the puerperium. These researchers noted that IgM rheumatoid factor levels increased during these flares while pregnancy-associated α_2-glycoprotein levels decreased. IgA rheumatoid factor was unaffected. These authors suggest that pregnancy-associated α_2-glycoprotein may be responsible for modulating the improvement in clinical symptoms in rheumatoid arthritis patients during gestation.[136] Nelson and colleagues[137] investigated HLA antigens in patients with rheumatoid arthritis and their offspring, as this autoimmune disorder has a known HLA class II antigen association. They found that amelioration of rheumatoid arthritis during gestation is associated with a disparity in HLA class II antigens between mother and fetus. They think that the maternal immune response to paternal HLA antigens may play a role in the remission in this disease that is often seen during pregnancy.[137] Lasink and co-workers[138] looked at the onset of rheumatoid arthritis in relation to pregnancy in 135 patients. They concluded that pregnancy may delay the clinical onset of disease in patients who will develop rheumatoid arthritis. Barrett et al. found an increase in relapse rate postpartum.[139] They compared disease activity in 38 first-time breast-feeding mothers, 50 repeat breast-feeding mothers, and 49 non-breast-feeding mothers.[140] They examined self-reported symptoms, joint counts (the number of involved joints), and C-reactive protein levels. They found that a postpartum flare may be induced by breast-feeding.[140] Iijima et al. checked for the presence of rheumatoid factors in 2,547 healthy women.[141] Only 2 (0.08 percent) of patients who could be followed developed rheumatoid arthritis within 12 months of delivery. One can conclude from this study that pregnancy does not trigger the onset of rheumatoid arthritis.[141]

Effect of Rheumatoid Arthritis on Pregnancy

Rheumatoid arthritis appears to have no adverse effects on pregnancy.[135,142,143] Spector and Silman[144] examined pregnancy outcomes in 195 women with rheumatoid arthritis and 462 controls. They found no increase in spontaneous abortions or stillbirths in patients with rheumatoid arthritis. They also concluded that a prior history of poor reproduction did not put the patient at risk for developing rheumatoid arthritis in the future.[144] A theoretical risk of uteroplacental insufficiency and IUGR does exist for patients with advanced extra-articular rheumatoid arthritis, and a case of IUGR attributed to vasculitis associated with severe disease has been described.[145]

To avoid pain and joint damage, care should be taken when positioning the patient with severe articular involvement on the delivery table. This is especially true if the patient has epidural or spinal anesthesia, because a joint can be damaged without the patient feeling pain. Obstetric anesthesiologists must also be cautious during rapid sequence induction of general anesthesia and intubation of patients with spinal involvement of rheumatoid arthritis. Subluxation of the atlanto-occipital joint is possible with devastating consequences. Popat et al.[146] describe these difficulties and the use of awake fiberoptic intubation in a patient with severe juvenile rheumatoid arthritis.

Effects of Medications Used to Treat Rheumatoid Arthritis

Nonsteroidal Anti-inflammatory Drugs

Acetylsalicylic acid (aspirin) was once the mainstay for the treatment of rheumatoid arthritis in pregnancy. The desired therapeutic blood level is 15 to 20 mg/dl. To achieve this the patient must take 3.6 to 4 g of acetyl-salicylic acid daily in three divided doses. Because salicylism, tinnitus, and deafness usually occur at levels of approximately 25 mg/dl, salicylate levels should be monitored regularly. Salicylate used throughout pregnancy may be associated with a prolonged gestation, long labor, increased blood loss at delivery, and postpartum hemorrhage.[147,148] These effects appear to be related to the inhibition of prostaglandin synthetase.[149] All nonsteroidals inhibit platelet aggregation. Inhibition by aspirin is irreversible while the effect on platelets by other nonsteroidals is reversible. The cyclooxygenase-2 inhibitors (cox-2) appear to have minimal, if any, effect on platelets.

There are many nonsteroidal anti-inflammatory agents currently available to treat rheumatoid arthritis. Physicians usually have their favorites, and the side-effect profiles differ somewhat, but not significantly. They have both analgesic and anti-inflammatory properties. There is considerable data available concerning indomethacin, as it is used as an adjuvant in the treatment of refractory preterm labor. Indomethacin, when used in late pregnancy, can cause premature closure of the fetal ductus arteriosus leading to pulmonary hypertension. Closure of the ductus arteriosus appears to be gestation-age dependent. These drugs, therefore, should be discontinued before 32 weeks' gestation if possible. Nonsteroidal anti-inflammatory agents can also cause changes in the fetal renal blood flow, resulting in oligohydramnios. It is unclear how long it takes these changes to occur. If at all possible, nonsteroidals should be avoided in the third trimester. Often, a short course of glucocorticoids can be used for symptoms in these patients. If, however, nonsteroidals must be used in late pregnancy, the amniotic fluid index must be carefully monitored.

Other Therapies

Penicillamine has been used successfully to treat rheumatoid arthritis in patients who are refractory to nonsteroidal agents. Penicillamine will reduce the titer of rheumatoid factor. Penicillamine freely crosses the placenta, and its use during pregnancy should be curtailed unless the benefits clearly outweigh the potential risks. Penicillamine has been successfully used in pregnancy without adverse effects.[150,151] Antimalarials are also used in refractory patients. A review by Koren showed no adverse fetal effects, even with first-trimester exposure.[152]

SCLERODERMA AND PROGRESSIVE SYSTEMIC SCLEROSIS

Progressive systemic sclerosis (PSS) and scleroderma are related collagen vascular diseases. They affect females four times more frequently than males, with onset usually between the ages of 30 and 50 years. The reported incidence is about 5 new cases per 1 million population per year. *Scleroderma,* the term used to describe the disorder when it is localized to the skin, is characterized by tight and bound down skin, sclerodactyly, and Raynaud's phenomenon. Clinical signs may precede development of the overt disease by several years.

In PSS, there is systemic involvement, including the gastrointestinal viscera as well as pulmonary vascular and parenchymal changes. Pulmonary hypertension with resultant right-sided heart failure is often the fatal consequence of PSS. With cardiac involvement, left-sided heart failure is occasionally seen.

It is now thought that a microchimeric state resulting from persistent fetal cells from prior pregnancies contributes to the development of scleroderma.[153] Class II HLA compatibility is common in patients with scleroderma.[154] In one study, 70.2 percent of women with scleroderma had this HLA-II compatibility compared to 21 percent of controls.[155] Scleroderma may, therefore, be a form of chronic graft-versus-host disease caused by fetal cells that have crossed the placenta during pregnancy and have remained unrecognized by the host due to class II HLA compatibility. Subsequent activation of these cells by as yet unknown stimuli results in the development of the disease.[155]

Laboratory Manifestations

Speckled-pattern antinuclear antibodies are observed in about 50 percent of patients, and 40 percent will demonstrate a rheumatoid factor. Anti-Scl-70, an extractable nuclear antibody, appears in the serum of 40 percent of patients with scleroderma and PSS. It appears to be fairly specific for this disease. Anti-Jo-1 antibodies are also occasionally seen in patients with scleroderma.

Effects of Pregnancy on Scleroderma and PSS

Johnson and co-workers[156] reported 18 cases of scleroderma and PSS complicating pregnancy. None of the women exhibited visceral involvement. In 39 percent of the patients, the disease showed no change or progressed at the same rate as prior to pregnancy. In an additional 39 percent the disease worsened, but no patient developed visceral involvement. In the remaining 22 percent some improvement was noted, but regression occurred after delivery. Several studies have described the onset of fatal renal involvement during pregnancy in patients with scleroderma and PSS.[157–160] In these reports, it is unclear whether visceral involvement antedated the pregnancy. Altieri and Cameron[161] reported a case of renal failure occurring in a pregnant woman with PSS. Partial recovery did follow the pregnancy. A successful pregnancy has been described in a patient with scleroderma complicated by renal disease and pulmonary hypertension who was treated with angiotensin-converting enzyme inhibitors.[162] The use of these agents during pregnancy is not recommended, but, because of the severity of the illness, they were used in this instance. Furthermore, Spiera et al.[163] reported a successful pregnancy in a patient with a previous hypertensive renal crisis caused by PSS. The patient was actually withdrawn from angiotensin-converting enzyme inhibitors when she became pregnant and had no renal complications during the pregnancy.[163] Jimenez[164] described a group of Spanish patients with scleroderma. Some improved, but several experienced worsening of skin thickening during pregnancy.[164] In a large review, Maymon and Fejgin[165] conducted a detailed literature search of scleroderma in pregnancy. Of 94 patients, 14 died during the course of pregnancy secondary to renal and cardiopulmonary involvement. It is important to note that this literature review covered many years. With more sophisticated maternal monitoring and therapy, the maternal mortality rate is probably much lower today.

Effects of Scleroderma on Pregnancy

Many theoretical complications exist, but few have been documented properly because of the rarity with which scleroderma and PSS coexist with pregnancy. Steen and Medsger[166] report no increase in infertility in patients with scleroderma. Also, the miscarriage rate was no different than their control population. This is in contrast to a previous study by Silman and Black.[167] Preterm birth, premature rupture of membranes, and stillbirth seem to be more common in patients with scleroderma and PSS.[168,169] Surviving infants show no evidence of scleroderma.[167,170] Steen et al.[171] examined pregnancy outcomes in 48 women with scleroderma and in two control groups matched for age and race. One control group contained normal patients and the other a group of women with rheumatoid arthritis. No difference was observed in the frequencies of miscarriage or perinatal death. Preterm births and infants with IUGR were found more frequently in patients with scleroderma and PSS. These data are favorable compared with those from the older literature reviewed by Maymon and Fejgin.[165] Steen and Medsger described pregnancy outcome between 1972 and 1986 in 214 women with scleroderma, 167 with rheumatoid arthritis, and 105 controls.[166] There were no significant differences in spontaneous abortion, preterm birth, growth restricted infants, or neonatal deaths amongst the three groups.[166]

Management During Pregnancy

If visceral involvement, especially pulmonary, cardiac, or renal, is documented, counseling should be undertaken before a patient attempts pregnancy. As previously mentioned, patients with renal involvement can carry to term, but gestation is often much more complicated. If scleroderma with only skin involvement exists, the patient may be followed expectantly. She should be aware that renal or cardiac involvement may be fatal. Steen suggests waiting until the disease stabilizes prior to conception.[172] A renal crisis with hypertension must be treated with angiotensin converting enzyme (ACE) inhibitors, even though these medications are usually contraindicated in pregnancy.[172] Anesthesia can be difficult in these patients, but several case reports have described how regional and general anesthesia can be safely employed in patients with scleroderma/progressive systemic sclerosis.[173–175]

MYASTHENIA GRAVIS

Although its prevalence is 1 per 25,000 in the general population, myasthenia gravis frequently coexists with pregnancy.[176] Women are twice as frequently affected as men and have an earlier onset of the disease, with a peak incidence occurring between the ages of 20 and 30 years. Even though 60 percent of patients with myasthenia gravis have enlargement of the thymus, only 8 percent have a malignant thymoma.[177] Thymectomy improves symptoms in up to two thirds of patients, but most still need additional medical therapy.[178] If the patient presents for prepregnancy counseling and is symptomatic despite large doses of medication, thymectomy should be undertaken before attempting pregnancy. Myasthenia gravis in pregnancy has been extensively studied by Plauché.[179] In a review of 314 pregnancies in 217 patients with myasthenia, he found no change in the myasthenic status throughout pregnancy, the puerperium, or the postpartum period in 31.5 percent of patients. In that review, exacerbations occurred in 40.8 percent of patients during pregnancy, including 30.6 percent during the puerperium. Another 28 percent showed a remission of their myasthenia during gestation.[179] Historically, there is a 25 to 60 percent preterm birth rate among patients with myasthenia gravis.[180,181] These are retrospective studies covering more than 40 years. With modern surveillance and therapy for preterm labor, this rate has probably decreased. Anti-acetylcholinesterase agents, which are used to treat myasthenia gravis, have an oxytocic action. It has been postulated that this could be the explanation for preterm labor observed in patients with myasthenia gravis.[182]

A team approach is necessary for proper treatment of the patient with myasthenia gravis. The neurologist and rheumatologist are not always familiar with the medications used by the obstetrician in treating complications of pregnancy. Conversely, because of the infrequency with which obstetricians see myasthenia gravis, they may be unfamiliar with the interactions between these medications and the disease.

Magnesium sulfate, for example, is absolutely contraindicated in the myasthenic patient. It further interferes with the neuromuscular blockade that is characteristic of the disease.[183] According to Castillo and Engbaek,[183] magnesium reduces the stimulating effect of acetylcholine on the muscle. It affects the amplitude of the endplate potential without affecting the muscle's resting potential. Cohen and co-workers[184] reported a near maternal death from administration of magnesium to a myasthenic patient. Catanzarite and co-investigators[182] described a respiratory arrest in a myasthenic patient with preterm labor who was treated with ritodrine and dexamethasone. They thought that the respiratory arrest was due to glucocorticoids. Although glucocorticoids generally ameliorate myasthenic symptoms, they may initially result in increased weakness in 25 to 80 percent of patients. Catanzarite and colleagues[182] proposed that this paradoxic effect, coupled with the hypokalemia caused by the ritodrine, led to the crisis.

Patient Management

Most patients with myasthenia gravis will be taking acetylcholinesterase inhibitors when they become pregnant. These medications are generally safe during gestation. The most commonly used medication, pyridostigmine, does not readily cross the placenta. Dosage adjustments, however, are frequently necessary because of the physiologic changes in vascular volume, renal blood flow, and hepatic function during pregnancy. Because myasthenia gravis is a disease of striated muscle, the smooth muscle of the uterus is generally not affected. The first stage of labor progresses at a normal pace. The second stage of labor involves voluntary pushing and the use of skeletal and pelvic girdle musculature.[185] These maternal expulsive efforts may be impaired because of the myasthenia gravis, and the obstetrician must be prepared to perform an operative vaginal delivery. Cesarean delivery should be reserved for obstetric indications. Patients are apt to undergo myasthenic crisis during labor, and the oral medications normally used have variable gastrointestinal absorption during this time. The obstetrician should therefore be prepared to use parenteral acetylcholinesterase inhibitors during labor and must be able to differentiate between an overdose of these medications and a myasthenic crisis.

Anesthesia and analgesia during labor present special challenges for the patient with myasthenia gravis. Although they are extremely sensitive to narcotics, patients with myasthenia gravis may be given these medications if carefully monitored.[186] Epidural anesthesia decreases the requirements for parenteral narcotics, prevents fatigue, and provides excellent anesthesia.[26] If, however, general anesthesia is elected for cesarean section, nondepolarizing muscle relaxants should be used with great care, if at all. Myasthenics are sensitive to these agents, and a prolonged response is usually seen.[186] It is also imperative to remember that certain inhalation agents may potentiate these agents. If general anesthesia is elected, the patient and her family should be warned that she may need ventilatory support for a period of time after the surgery.

If the patient develops a puerperal infection, aminoglycosides should be used with extreme caution. These agents can block the motor end-plate and cause a myasthenic crisis.[26]

Occasionally, myasthenia will be exacerbated during pregnancy. In such cases, therapy with extremely large doses of acetylcholinesterase inhibitors yields little response. These patients can be treated with plasmapheresis. The procedure may need to be repeated as needed, but dramatic results can be seen. After plasmapheresis, symptoms improve and the dose of acetylcholinesterase inhibitors can often be temporarily reduced. The procedure should be carried out with the patient in the left lateral position and with the uterus tilted off the inferior vena cava. It should be performed relatively slowly, with careful attention to maternal blood pressure. If plasmapheresis is being performed after 24 weeks' gestation, continuous fetal monitoring should be employed. Intravenous immunoglobulin (IVIG) is being used now in patients with myasthenia gravis. Dramatic results have been seen. The proposed mechanism, although oversimplistic, is that the infused antibody saturates muscle receptors so that the autoantibody has no sites to bind.

Neonatal Myasthenia Gravis

Neonatal myasthenia occurs in 10 to 25 percent of infants born to mothers with myasthenia gravis.[187–190] In his review series, Plauché[179] reported a 20.2 percent incidence of neonatal myasthenia, with a 2.1 percent stillbirth rate and a 3.8 percent neonatal mortality rate. Again, that study reviewed cases over a 40-year period. With modern neonatal care, the neonatal mortality rate is probably considerably lower. Neonatal myasthenia does not begin at birth but is usually evident within the first 2 days of life. For this reason, mothers with myasthenia gravis are not candidates for early discharge even if their disease is well controlled. It lasts an average of 3 weeks but can persist up to 15 weeks.[190] Symptoms usually include a weak cry, poor sucking effort, and, rarely, respiratory distress. Neonatal myasthenia is thought to be secondary to transplacental passage of IgG antibodies directed against acetylcholine receptors.

Key Points

- ➤ Systemic lupus erythematosus is associated with an increase in poor pregnancy outcome (i.e., from IUGR, stillbirth, and spontaneous abortion).

- ➤ The rate of pregnancy complications is decreased if patients with SLE have quiescent disease for 6 months prior to conception.

- ➤ Glucocorticoids are safe to use in pregnancy for the treatment of patients with SLE.

- ➤ The lupus inhibitor and anticardiolipin antibodies are found in 50 percent of patients with SLE. They are associated with an increased risk of pregnancy loss, including second- and third-trimester losses.

- ➤ Anti-SSA (Ro) and anti-SSB (La) antibodies are associated with complete congenital heart block and other manifestations of neonatal lupus.

- ➤ Low-dose heparin and low-dose aspirin are the therapies of choice for patients with lupus inhibitor/antiphospholipid antibodies who do not have active SLE.

- ➤ Rheumatoid arthritis tends to improve during pregnancy but may relapse in the postpartum period.

- ➤ Rheumatoid arthritis does not appear to have a major deleterious effect on pregnancy.

- ➤ Pyridostigmine can be safely used to treat patients with myasthenia gravis in pregnancy.

- ➤ Infants born to mothers with myasthenia gravis can have muscle weakness and even problems feeding. This usually manifests itself after the second day of life.

REFERENCES

1. Carbone J, Orera M, Rodriguez-Mahou M, et al: Immunological abnormalities in primary APS evolving into SLE: 6 years follow-up in women with repeated pregnancy loss. Lupus 8: 274, 1999.
2. Fessel WJ: Systemic lupus erythematosus in the community. Incidence, prevalence, outcome and first symptoms: the high

prevalence in black women. Arch Intern Med 134:1027, 1974.

3. Estes D, Christian CL: The natural history of systemic lupus erythematosus by prospective analysis. Medicine 50:85, 1971.

4. Garsenstein M, Pollak VE, Karik RM: Systemic lupus erythematosus and pregnancy. N Engl J Med 276:165, 1962.

5. Zurier RB: Systemic lupus erythematosus and pregnancy. Clin Rheum Dis 1:613, 1975.

6. Meehan RT, Dorsey JK: Pregnancy among patients with systemic lupus erythematosus receiving immuno-suppressive therapy. J Rheumatol 14:252, 1987.

7. Lockshin MD: Lupus erythematosus and allied disorders in pregnancy. Bull N Y Acad Med 63:797, 1987.

8. Lockshin MD, Reinitz E, Druzin ML, et al: Lupus pregnancy; case-control prospective study demonstrating absence of lupus exacerbation during or after pregnancy. Am J Med 77:893, 1984.

9. Lockshin MD: Pregnancy does not cause systemic lupus erythematosus to worsen. Arthritis Rheum 32:665, 1989.

10. Derksen FH, Bruinse HW, deGroot PG, Kater L: Pregnancy in systemic lupus erythematosus: a prospective study. Lupus 3:149, 1994.

11. Mintz G, Nitz J, Gutierrez G, et al: Prospective study of pregnancy in systemic lupus erythematosus: results of a multi-disciplinary approach. J Rheumatol 13:732, 1986.

12. Le Thi Huong D, Wechsler B, Piette JC, et al: Pregnancy and its outcome in systemic lupus erythematosus. Q J Med 87:721, 1994.

13. Ainslie WH, Britt K, Moshipur JA: Maternal death due to lupus pneumonitis in pregnancy. Mt Sinai J Med 46:494, 1979.

14. Leikin JB, Arof HM, Pearlman LM: Acute lupus pneumonitis in the postpartum period: a case history and review of the literature. Obstet Gynecol 68:295, 1986.

15. Rubin LA, Geran A, Rose TH, Cohen H: A fatal complication of lupus in pregnancy. Arthritis Rheum 38:710, 1995.

16. Averbuch M, Bojko A, Levo Y: Cardiac tamponade in the early postpartum period as the presenting and predominant manifestation of systemic lupus erythematosus. J Rheumatol 13:444, 1986.

17. Marabani M, Zoma A, Hadley D, Sturrock RD: Transverse myelitis occurring during pregnancy in a patient with systemic lupus erythematosus. Ann Rheum Dis 48:160, 1989.

18. Gimovsky ML, Montoro M, Paul RH: Pregnancy outcome in women with systemic lupus erythematosus. Obstet Gynecol 63:686, 1984.

19. Julkunen H: Renal lupus in pregnancy. Scand J Rheumatol Suppl 107:80, 1998.

20. Devoe L, Taylor RL: Systemic lupus erythematosus in pregnancy. Am J Obstet Gynecol 135:473, 1979.

21. Hayslett JP, Lynn RI: Effect of pregnancy in patients with lupus nephropathy. Kidney Int 18:207, 1980.

22. Reichlin M: Systemic lupus erythematosus and pregnancy. J Reprod Med 43:355, 1998.

23. Fine LG, Barnett EV, Danovitch GM, et al: Systemic lupus erythematosus in pregnancy. Ann Intern Med 94:667, 1981.

24. Mackey E: Pregnancy and renal disease: a ten-year study. Aust N Z J Obstet Gynaecol 3:21, 1963.

25. Ramsey-Goldman R: Pregnancy in systemic lupus erythematosus. Rheum Dis Clin North Am 14:119, 1988.

26. Foldes FF, McNall PG: Myasthenia gravis: a guide for anesthesiologists. Anesthesiology 23:837, 1962.

27. Repke JT: Hypertensive disorders of pregnancy. Differentiating preeclampsia from active systemic lupus erythematosus. J Reprod Med 43:350, 1998.

28. Buyon JP, Cronstein BN, Morris M, et al: Serum complement values (C_3 and C_4) to differentiate between systemic lupus activity and preeclampsia. Am J Med 81:194, 1986.

29. Fraga A, Mintz G, Orozco J, et al: Sterility and fertility rates, fetal wastage and maternal morbidity in systemic lupus erythematosus. J Rheumatol 1:1293, 1974.

30. Kleinman D, Katz VL, Kuller JA: Perinatal outcomes in women with systemic lupus erythematosus. J Perinatol 18:178, 1998.

31. Kobayashi N, Yamada H, Kishida T, et al: Hypocomplementemia correlates with intrauterine growth retardation in systemic lupus erythematosus. Am J Reprod Immunol 42:153, 1999.

32. Johns KR, Morand EF, Littlejohn GO: Pregnancy outcome in systemic lupus erythematosus (SLE): a review of 54 cases. Aust N Z J Med 28:18, 1998.

33. Zurier RG, Argyros T, Urman J, et al: Systemic lupus erythematosus: management during pregnancy. Obstet Gynecol 51:178, 1978.

34. Julkunen H, Kaaja R, Kurki P, et al: Fetal outcome in women with primary Sjögren's syndrome. A retrospective case-control study. Clin Exp Rheumatol 13:65, 1995.

35. Ramsey-Goldman R, Kutzer JE, Kuller LH, et al: Pregnancy outcome and anticardiolipin antibody in women with systemic lupus erythematosus. Am J Epidemiol 138:1057, 1993.

36. Petri M, Albritton J: Fetal outcome of lupus pregnancy: a retrospective case-control study of the Hopkins Lupus Cohort. J Rheumatol 20:650, 1993.

37. Leu LY, Lan JL: The influence on pregnancy of anti-SSA/Ro antibodies in systemic lupus erythematosus. Chi Mien I Hsueh Tsa Chih 25:12, 1992.

38. Rahman P, Gladman DD, Urowitz MB: Clinical predictors of fetal outcome in systemic lupus erythematosus. J Rheumatol 25:1526, 1998.

39. Carmona F, Font J, Cervera R, et al: Obstetrical outcome of pregnancy in patients with systemic lupus erythematosus. A study of 60 cases. Eur J Obstet Gynecol Reprod Biol 83:137, 1999.

40. Aggarwal N, Sawhney H, Vasishta K, et al: Pregnancy in patients with systemic lupus erythematosus. Aust N Z J Obstet Gynaecol 39:28, 1999.

41. Johnson MJ, Petri M, Witter FR, Repke JT: Evaluation of preterm delivery in a systemic lupus erythematosus pregnancy clinic. Obstet Gynecol 86:396, 1995.

42. Harris EN, Pierangeli SS, Gharavi AE: Diagnosis of the antiphospholipid syndrome: a proposal for use of laboratory tests. Lupus 7(Suppl):S144, 1998.

43. Ogasawara M, Aoki K, Katano K, et al: Prevalence of autoantibodies in patients with recurrent miscarriages. Am J Reprod Immunol 41:86, 1999.

44. Rosove MH, Brewer PM, Runge A, Hirji K: Simultaneous lupus anticoagulant and anticardiolipin assays and clinical detection of antiphospholipids. Am J Hematol 32:148, 1989.

45. Field SL, Brighton TA, McNeil HP, Chesterman CN: Recent insights into antiphospholipid antibody-mediated thrombosis. Baillieres Best Pract Res Clin Haematol 12:407, 1999.

46. Munoz-Rodriguez FJ, Reverter JC, Font J, et al: Prevalence and clinical significance of antiprothrombin antibodies in patients with systemic lupus erythematosus or with primary antiphospholipid syndrome. Haematologica 85:632, 2000.

47. Lockwood CJ, Romero R, Feinberg RF: The prevalence and biologic significance of lupus anticoagulant and anticardiolipin antibodies in a general obstetric population. Am J Obstet Gynecol 161:369, 1989.

48. Hanly JG, Gladman DD, Rose TH, et al: Lupus pregnancy, a

prospective study of placental changes. Arthritis Rheum 31:358, 1988.

49. Hedfors E, Lindahl G, Lindblad S: Anticardiolipin antibodies during pregnancy. J Rheumatol 14:160, 1987.

50. Ogishima D, Matsumoto T, Nakamura Y, et al: Placental pathology in systemic lupus erythematosus with antiphospholipid antibodies. Pathol Int 50:224, 2000.

51. Lubbe WF, Butler WS, Palmer SJ, et al: Lupus anticoagulant in pregnancy. Br J Obstet Gynaecol 97:357, 1984.

52. Lubbe WF, Butler WS, Liggins GC: The lupus-anticoagulant: clinical and obstetric implications. N Z Med J 97:398, 1984.

53. Branch DW, Scott JR, Kochenour NK, et al: Obstetric complications associated with the lupus anticoagulant. N Engl J Med 313:1322, 1985.

54. Unander AM, Norberg R, Hahn L, et al: Anticardiolipin antibodies and complement in ninety-nine women with habitual abortion. Am J Obstet Gynecol 156:114, 1987.

55. Lubbe WF, Walkom P, Alexander CJ: Hepatic and splenic haemorrhage as a complication of toxaemia of pregnancy in a patient with circulating lupus anticoagulant. N Z Med J 95:842, 1982.

56. Druzin ML, Lockshin M, Edersheim TG, et al: Second-trimester fetal monitoring and preterm delivery in pregnancies with systemic lupus erythematosus and/or circulating anticoagulant. Am J Obstet Gynecol 157:1503, 1987.

57. Lockshin MD, Druzin ML, Goei S, et al: Antibody to cardiolipin as a predictor of fetal distress or death in pregnant patients with systemic lupus erythematosus. N Engl J Med 313:152, 1985.

58. Kutteh WH, Lyda EC, Abraham SM, Wacholtz MC: Association of anticardiolipin antibodies and pregnancy loss in women with systemic lupus erythematosus. Fertil Steril 60:449, 1993.

59. Juikunen H, Jouhikainen T, Kaaja R, et al: Fetal outcome in lupus pregnancy: a retrospective case-control study of 242 pregnancies in 112 patients. Lupus 2:125, 1993.

60. Birdsall M, Pattison N, Chamley L: Antiphospholipid antibodies in pregnancy. Aust N Z J Obstet Gynaecol 32:328, 1992.

61. Lubbe WF, Palmer SJ, Butler WS, et al: Fetal survival after prednisone suppression of maternal lupus-anticoagulant. Lancet 1:1361, 1983.

62. Lockshin MD, Druzin ML, Qamar T: Prednisone does not prevent recurrent fetal death in women with antiphospholipid antibody. Am J Obstet Gynecol 160:439, 1989.

63. Karp HJ, Frenkel Y, Many A, et al: Fetal demise associated with lupus anticoagulant: clinical features and results of treatment. Gynecol Obstet Invest 28:178, 1989.

64. Ordi J, Barquinero J, Vilardell M, et al: Fetal loss treatment in patients with antiphospholipid antibodies. Ann Rheum Dis 48:798, 1989.

65. Landy HJ, Kessler C, Kelly WK, Weingold AB: Obstetric performance in patients with the lupus anticoagulant and/or anticardiolipin antibodies. Am J Perinatol 9:146, 1992.

66. Geva E, Amit A, Lerner-Geva L, et al: Prednisone and aspirin improve pregnancy rate in patients with reproductive failure and autoimmune antibodies: a prospective study. Am J Reprod Immunol 43:36, 2000.

67. Gatenby PA, Cameron K, Shearman RP: Pregnancy loss with phospholipid antibodies: improved outcome with aspirin containing treatment. Aust N Z J Obstet Gynaecol 29:294, 1989.

68. Balasch J, Font J, Lopez-Soto A, et al: Antiphospholipid antibodies in unselected patients with repeated abortion. Hum Reprod 5:43, 1990.

69. Rosove MH, Tabsh K, Wasserstrum N, et al: Heparin therapy for pregnant women with lupus anticoagulant or anticardiolipin antibodies. Obstet Gynecol 75:630, 1990.

70. Branch DW, Silver RM, Blackwell JL, et al: Outcome of treated pregnancies in women with antiphospholipid syndrome: an update of the Utah experience. Obstet Gynecol 80:614, 1992.

71. Huhle G, Geberth M, Hoffmann U, et al: Management of heparin-associated thrombocytopenia in pregnancy with subcutaneous r-hirudin. Gynecol Obstet Invest 49:67, 2000.

72. Granger KA, Farquharson RG: Obstetric outcome in antiphospholipid syndrome. Lupus 6:509, 1997.

73. Clark AL, Branch DW, Silver RM, et al: Pregnancy complicated by the antiphospholipid syndrome: outcomes with intravenous immunoglobulin therapy. Obstet Gynecol 93:437, 1999.

74. Kaaja R, Julkunen H, Ammala P, et al: Intravenous immunoglobulin treatment of pregnant patients with recurrent pregnancy losses associated with antiphospholipid antibodies. Acta Obstet Gynaecol Scand 72:63, 1993.

75. Somerset DA, Raine-Fenning N, Gordon C, et al: Intravenous immunoglobulin therapy in compromised pregnancies associated with antiphospholipid antibodies and systemic lupus erythematosus. Eur J Obstet Gynecol Reprod Biol 79:227, 1998.

76. Gordon C, Kilby MD: Use of intravenous immunoglobulin therapy in pregnancy in systemic lupus erythematosus an antiphospholipid antibody syndrome. Lupus 7:429, 1998.

77. Chamley LW, Pattison NS, McKay EJ: IgM lupus anticoagulants can be associated with recurrent fetal loss of thrombic episodes. Thromb Res 58:343, 1990.

78. Mizoguchi K, Kakisako S, Tanaka M, et al: Lupus anticoagulant as a risk factor for cerebral infarction and habitual abortions. Kurume Med J 36:113, 1989.

79. Rallings P, Exner T, Abraham R: Coronary artery vasculitis and myocardial infarction associated with antiphospholipid antibodies in a pregnant woman. Aust N Z J Med 19:347, 1989.

80. Litsey S, Noonan J, O'Connor W, et al: Maternal connective tissue disease and congenital heart block. N Engl J Med 312:98, 1985.

81. Draznin TH, Easterly NB, Fureu N, et al: Neonatal lupus erythematosus. J Am Acad Dermatol 1:437, 1979.

82. McCue C, Mantakas M, Tingelstad JB, et al: Congenital heart block in newborns of mothers with connective tissue disease. Circulation 56:82, 1977.

83. Scott JS, Maddison PJ, Tayler PV, et al: Connective-tissue disease, antibodies to ribonucleoprotein and congenital heart block. N Engl J Med 309:209, 1983.

84. Scheib JS, Waxman J: Congenital heart block in successive pregnancies: a case report and evaluation of risk with therapeutic consideration. Obstet Gynecol 73:481, 1989.

85. Derksen RH, Meilof JF: Anti-Ro/SS-A and anti La/SS-B autoantibody levels in relation to systemic lupus erythematosus disease activity and congenital heart block. A longitudinal study comprising two consecutive pregnancies in a patient with systemic lupus erythematosus. Arthritis Rheum 45:953, 1992.

86. Vetter VL, Rashkad WJ: Congenital complete heart block and connective tissue disease. N Engl J Med 309:236, 1983.

87. Esscher E, Scott JS: Congenital heart block and maternal systemic lupus erythematosus. BMJ 1:1235, 1979.

88. Falcini F, De Simone L, Donzelli G, Cerinic MM: Congenital conduction defects in children born to asymptomatic mothers with anti-SSA/SSB antibodies: report of two cases. Ann Ital Med Int 13:169, 1998.

89. Meng C, Lockshin M: Pregnancy in lupus. Curr Opin Rheumatol 11:348, 1999.

90. Buyon JP, Swersky SH, Fox HE, et al: Intrauterine therapy for presumptive fetal myocarditis with acquired heart block due to systemic lupus erythematosus. Arthritis Rheum 39:1, 1987.

91. Lockshin MD, Gibofsky A, Peebles CL, et al: Neonatal lupus erythematosus with heart block: family study of a patient with anti-SS-A and SS-B antibodies. Arthritis Rheum 26:210, 1983.

92. McCuiston CH, Schoch EP: Possible discoid lupus erythematosus in a newborn infant: report of case with subsequent development of acute systemic lupus erythematosus in mother. Arch Dermatol Syphilol 70:782, 1954.

93. McGee CD, Makowski EL: Systemic lupus erythematosus in pregnancy. Am J Obstet Gynecol 107:1008, 1970.

94. Mavragani CP, Dafni UG, Tzioufas AG, Moutsopoulos HM: Pregnancy outcome and anti-Ro/SSA in autoimmune diseases: a retrospective cohort study. Br J Rheumatol 37:740, 1998.

95. Adams D, Druzin MI, Edersheim T, et al: Condition specific antepartum testing: systemic lupus erythematosus and associated serologic abnormalities. Am J Reprod Immunol 28:159, 1992.

96. Carroll BA: Obstetric duplex sonography in patients with lupus anticoagulant syndrome. J Ultrasound Med 9:17, 1990.

97. Ariyuki Y, Hata T, Kitao M: Reverse end-diastolic umbilical artery velocity in a case of intrauterine fetal death at 14 weeks gestation. Am J Obstet Gynecol 169:1621, 1993.

98. Farine D, Granovsky-Grisaru S, Ryan G, et al: Umbilical artery blood flow velocity in pregnancies complicated by systemic lupus erythematosus. J Clin Ultrasound 26:379, 1998.

99. Buyon JP, Cronstein BN, Morris M, et al: Serum complement values (C_3 and C_4) to differentiate between systemic lupus activity and pre-eclampsia. Am J Med 81:194, 1986.

100. Tozman ECS, Urowitz MB, Gladman DD: Systemic lupus erythematosus and pregnancy. J Rheumatol 7:624, 1980.

101. Zulman MI, Talal N, Hoffman GS, et al: Problems associated with the management of pregnancies in patients with systemic lupus erythematosus. J Rheumatol 7:37, 1980.

102. Devoe LD, Aloy GL: Serum complement levels and perinatal outcome in pregnancies complicated by systemic lupus erythematosus. Obstet Gynecol 63:796, 1984.

103. Freinkel N: Gestational diabetes, 1979: philosophical and practical aspects of a major health problem. Diabetes Care 3:399, 1980

104. Bongiovanni AM, McPadden AJ: Steroids during pregnancy and possible fetal consequences. Fertil Steril 11:181, 1960.

105. Fainstat T: Cortisone-induced congenital cleft palate in rabbits. Endocrinology 55:502, 1954

106. Giannopoulos G, Tulchinsky D: The influence of hormones on fetal lung development. In Ryan KJ, Tulchinsky D (eds): Maternal-Fetal Endocrinology. Philadelphia, WB Saunders, 1988, p 310.

107. Ballard PL, Granberg P, Ballard RA: Glucocorticoid levels in maternal and cord serum after prenatal betamethasone therapy to prevent respiratory distress syndrome. J Clin Invest 56:15, 1975.

108. Blanford AT, Pearson-Murphy BE: In vitro metabolism of prednisolone, dexamethasone, betamethasone, and cortisol by the human placenta. Am J Obstet Gynecol 127:264, 1977.

109. Osathanondh R, Tulchinsky D, Kamali H, et al: Dexamethasone levels in treated pregnant women and newborn infants. J Pediatr 90:617, 1977.

110. Levitz M, Jansen V, Dancis J: The transfer and metabolism of corticosteroids in the perfused human placenta. Am J Obstet Gynecol 132:363, 1978.

111. Beitins IZ, Bayard F, Ances IG, et al: The transplacental passage of prednisone and prednisolone in pregnancy near term. J Pediatr 81:936, 1972.

112. Blanford AT, Pearson-Murphy BE: In vitro metabolism of prednisolone, dexamethasone, betamethasone, and cortisol by the human placenta. Am J Obstet Gynecol 127:264, 1977.

113. Gabbe SG: Drug therapy in autoimmune disease. Clin Obstet Gynecol 26:635, 1983.

114. Scott JR: Fetal growth retardation associated with maternal administration of immunosuppressive drugs. Am J Obstet Gynecol 128:668, 1977.

115. Davison JM, Lindheimer MD: Pregnancy in renal transplant recipients. J Reprod Med 27:613, 1982.

116. Cote CJ, Meuwissen HJ, Pickering RJ: Effects on the neonate of prednisone and azathioprine administered to the mother during pregnancy. J Pediatr 85:324, 1974.

117. Scott JR: Immunologic diseases in pregnancy. Prog Allergy 23:321, 1977.

118. Turnam GR: Rheumatoid arthritis. Clin Obstet Gynecol 26:560, 1983.

119. Masi AT, Maldonade-Cocco JA, Kaplan SB, et al: Prospective study of the early course of rheumatoid arthritis in young adults: comparison of patients with and without rheumatoid factor positivity at entry and identification of variables correlating with outcome. Semin Arthritis Rheum 5:299, 1976.

120. Baum J, Ziff M: Laboratory findings in rheumatoid arthritis. In McCary D (ed): Arthritis and Allied Conditions, 9th ed. Philadelphia, Lea & Febiger, 1979, p 491.

121. Harris ED Jr: The proliferative lesion in rheumatoid arthritis: manifestation and pathophysiology. In Harris ED Jr (ed): Rheumatoid Arthritis. New York, Medcom, 1974, p 374.

122. Gordon DA, Stein JL, Broder I: The extraarticular features of rheumatoid arthritis: a systemic analysis of 127 cases. Am J Med 54:445, 1973.

123. Hurd ER: Extraarticular manifestations of rheumatoid arthritis. Semin Arthritis Rheum 8:151, 1979.

124. Hollingsworth JW, Saykaly RJ: Systemic complications of rheumatoid arthritis. Med Clin North Am 61:217, 1977.

125. Williams RC: Adult and juvenile rheumatoid arthritis. In Parker GW (ed): Clinical Immunology. Philadelphia, WB Saunders, 1980, p 184.

126. Rodman GP (ed): Primer on the rheumatic diseases. JAMA 224(suppl):661, 1973.

127. Robbins SL, Cotran RS: The musculoskeletal system—joints and related structures. In Robbins SL, Cotran RS (eds): Pathologic Basis of Disease, 2nd ed. Philadelphia, WB Saunders, 1979, p 1452.

128. Yu DTY, Peter JB: Cellular immunological aspects of rheumatoid arthritis. Semin Arthritis Rheum 4:24, 1974.

129. McDuffie FC: Immune complexes in the rheumatic disease. J Allergy Clin Immunol 62:37, 1978.

130. Paget S, Gibofsky A: Immunopathogenesis of rheumatoid arthritis. Am J Med 67:961, 1979.

131. Stobo JD: Rheumatoid arthritis restriction maps. West J Med 137:109, 1982.

132. Pope JE, Bellamy N, Stevens A: The lack of associations between rheumatoid arthritis and both nulliparity and infertility. Semin Arthritis Rheum 28:342, 1999.

133. Hench PS: The ameliorating effect of pregnancy on chronic atrophic (infectious) rheumatoid arthritis, fibrositis and intermittent hydrarthrosis. Proc Mayo Clin 13:161, 1938.

134. Persellin RH: The effect of pregnancy on rheumatoid arthritis. Bull Rheum Dis 27:922, 1977.

135. Klipple GL, Cecere FA: Rheumatoid arthritis and pregnancy. Rheum Dis Clin North Am 15:213, 1989.

136. Quinn C, Mulpeter K, Casey EB, Feighery CF: Changes in levels of IgM RF and alpha 2 PAG correlate with increased

disease activity in rheumatoid arthritis during the puerperium. Scand J Rheumatol 22:273, 1993.

137. Nelson JL, Hughes KA, Smith AG, et al: Maternal-fetal disparity in HLA class II alloantigens and the pregnancy-induced amelioration of rheumatoid arthritis. N Engl J Med 329:466, 1993.

138. Lasink M, de Boer A, Kijkmans BA, et al: The onset of rheumatoid arthritis in relation to pregnancy and childbirth. Clin Exp Rheumatol 11:171, 1993.

139. Barrett JH, Brennan P, Fiddler M, Silman AJ: Does rheumatoid arthritis remit during pregnancy and relapse postpartum? Results from a nationwide study in the United Kingdom performed prospectively from late pregnancy. Arthritis Rheum 42:1219, 1999.

140. Barrett JH, Brennan P, Fiddler M, Silman A: Breast-feeding and postpartum relapse in women with rheumatoid and inflammatory arthritis. Arthritis Rheum 43:1010, 2000.

141. Iijima T, Tada H, Hidaka Y, et al: Prediction of postpartum onset of rheumatoid arthritis. Ann Rheum Dis 57:460, 1998.

142. Kaplan D, Diamond H: Rheumatoid arthritis and pregnancy. Clin Obstet Gynecol 8:286, 1965.

143. Betson JR, Dorn RV: Forty cases of arthritis and pregnancy. J Int Coll Surgeons 42:521, 1964.

144. Spector TD, Silman AJ: Is poor pregnancy outcome a risk factor in rheumatoid arthritis? Ann Rheum Dis 49:12, 1990.

145. Duhring JL: Pregnancy, rheumatoid arthritis, and intrauterine growth retardation. Am J Obstet Gynecol 108:325, 1970.

146. Popat MT, Chippa JH, Russell R: Awake fibreoptic intubation following failed regional anaesthesia for caesarean section in a parturient with Still's disease. Eur J Anaesthesiol 17:211, 2000.

147. Bulmash JM: Rheumatoid arthritis and pregnancy. Obstet Gynecol Annu 8:223, 1979.

148. Bulmash JM: Systemic lupus erythematosus and pregnancy. Obstet Gynecol Annu 7:153, 1978.

149. Lewis RB, Shulman JD: Influence of acetylsalicylic acid, an inhibitor of prostaglandin synthesis, on the duration of human gestation and labour. Lancet 2:1159, 1973.

150. Hlinst'ak K, Borovsky M, Hlinst'akova S: Pregnancy, labor, and early puerperium in a patient with Wilson's disease. Ceska Gynekol 64:198, 1999.

151. Messner U, Gunter HN, Niesert S: Wilson disease and pregnancy. Review of the literature and case report. Z Geburtshilfe Neonatal 202:77, 1998.

152. Koren G: Antimalarial drugs for rheumatoid disease during pregnancy. Can Fam Physician 45:2869, 1999.

153. Arlett CM, Smith JB, Jimenez SA: New perspectives on the etiology of systemic sclerosis. Mol Med Today 5:74, 1999.

154. Famularo G, DeSimone C: Systemic sclerosis from autoimmunity to alloimmunity. South Med J 92:472, 1999.

155. Arlett CM, Welsh KI, Black CM, Jimenez SA: Fetal-maternal HLA compatibility confers susceptibility to systemic sclerosis. Immunogenetics 47:17, 1997.

156. Johnson TR, Banner EA, Winkelmann RK: Scleroderma and pregnancy. Obstet Gynecol 23:467, 1964.

157. Fear RE: Eclampsia superimposed on renal scleroderma: a rare cause of maternal and fetal mortality. Obstet Gynecol 31:69, 1968.

158. Sood SV, Kohler HG: Maternal death from systemic sclerosis. J Obstet Gynaecol Br Commonw 77:1109, 1970.

159. Karlsen JR, Cook WA: Renal scleroderma and pregnancy. Obstet Gynecol 44:349, 1974.

160. Ehrenfeld M, Licht A, Stersman J, et al: Postpartum renal failure due to progressive systemic sclerosis treated with chronic hemodialysis. Nephron 18:175, 1977.

161. Altieri P, Cameron JS: Scleroderma renal crisis in a pregnant woman with late partial recovery of renal function. Nephrol Dial Transplant 3:677, 1988.

162. Baethge BA, Wolf RE: Successful pregnancy with scleroderma renal disease and pulmonary hypertension in a patient using angiotensin converting enzyme inhibitors. Ann Rheum Dis 48:776, 1989.

163. Spiera H, Krakoff L, Fishbane-Mayer J: Successful pregnancy after scleroderma hypertensive renal crisis. J Rheumatol 16:1597, 1989.

164. Jimenez FX, Simeon CP, Fonollosa V, et al: Scleroderma and pregnancy: obstetrical complications and impact of pregnancy on the course of the disease. Med Clin (Barc) 113:761, 1999.

165. Maymon R, Fejgin M: Scleroderma in pregnancy. Obstet Gynecol Surv 44:530, 1989.

166. Steen VD, Medsger TA Jr: Fertility and pregnancy outcome in women with systemic sclerosis. Arthritis Rheum 42:763, 1999.

167. Silman AJ, Black C: Increased incidence of spontaneous abortion and infertility in women with scleroderma before disease onset: a controlled study. Ann Rheum Dis 47:441, 1988

168. Spellacy WN: Scleroderma and pregnancy. Obstet Gynecol 23:297, 1964.

169. Slate WG, Graham AR: Scleroderma and pregnancy. Am J Gynecol 101:335, 1968.

170. Jones WR, Storey B: Perinatal aspects of maternal autoimmune disease. Aust Paediatr J 8:306, 1972.

171. Steen VD, Conte C, Day N, et al: Pregnancy in women with systemic sclerosis. Arthritis Rheum 32:151, 1989.

172. Steen VD: Scleroderma and pregnancy. Rheum Dis Clin North Am 23:133, 1997.

173. D'Angelo R, Miller R: Pregnancy complicated by severe preeclampsia and thrombocytopenia in a patient with scleroderma. Anesth Analg 85:839, 1997.

174. Hseu SS, Sung CS, Mao CC, et al: Anesthetic management in a porturient with progressive systemic sclerosis during cesarean section—a case report. Acta Anaesthesiol Sin 35:161, 1997.

175. Bailey AR, Wolmarans M, Rhodes S: Spinal anaesthesia for caesarean section in a patient with systemic sclerosis. Anaesthesia 54:355, 1999.

176. Kurtzke JF: Epidemiology of myasthenia gravis. Adv Neurol 19:545, 1978.

177. Hokkanen E: Myasthenia gravis. Ann Clin Res 1:94, 1969.

178. Havard CW, Fonseca V: New treatment approaches to myasthenia gravis. Drugs 39:66, 1990.

179. Plauché WC: Myasthenia gravis. Clin Obstet Gynecol 26:594, 1983.

180. Petri M, Golbus M, Anderson R, et al: Antinuclear antibody, lupus anticoagulant and anticardiolipin antibody in women with idiopathic habitual abortion. Arthritis Rheum 30:601, 1987.

181. Plauché WC: Myasthenia gravis in pregnancy: an update. Am J Obstet Gynecol 135:691, 1979.

182. Catanzarite VA, McHargue AM, Sandberg EC, et al: Respiratory arrest during therapy for premature labor in a patient with myasthenia gravis. Obstet Gynecol 64:819, 1984.

183. Castillo JD, Engbaek L: The nature of the neuromuscular block produced by magnesium. J Physiol 124:370, 1954.

184. Cohen BA, London RS, Goldstein PJ: Myasthenia gravis and pre-eclampsia. Obstet Gynecol 48:35, 1976.

185. McNall PG, Jafarnia MR: Management of myasthenia gravis in obstetrical patient. Am J Obstet Gynecol 92:518, 1965.

186. Rolbin SH, Levinson G, Shnider SM, et al: Anesthetic considerations for myasthenia gravis and pregnancy. Anesth Analog 57:441, 1978.

187. Barlow CF: Neonatal myasthenia gravis. Am J Dis Child 135: 209, 1981.
188. Donaldson JO, Penn AS, Lisak RP, et al: Antiacetylcholine receptor antibody in neonatal myasthenia gravis. Am J Dis Child 135:222, 1981.
189. Namba T, Brown SB, Grob D: Neonatal myasthenia gravis: report of two cases and review of the literature. Pediatrics 45: 488, 1970.
190. Scott JR: Immunologic diseases in pregnancy. Prog Allergy 23:321, 1977.

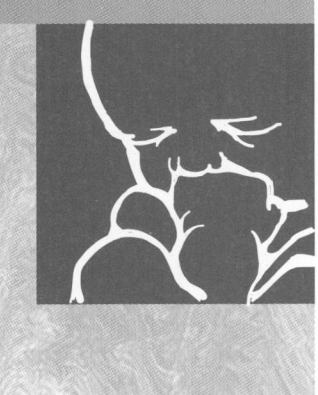

Chapter 36

Hepatic and Gastrointestinal Disease

Hepatic Disease

PHILIP SAMUELS

Liver dysfunction and disease occasionally complicate pregnancy. The most commonly seen problems include liver dysfunction associated with preeclampsia and hepatitis. These topics are covered in detail elsewhere in this text (see Chapters 28 and 40). This chapter focuses on acute fatty liver, intrahepatic cholestasis of pregnancy, and gallbladder disease associated with gestation (Table 36–1).

ACUTE FATTY LIVER

Acute fatty liver is a rare condition that has an incidence of between 1 in 6,692 and 1 in 15,900 pregnancies.[1-3] Since 1975, maternal survival has been reported as 72 percent, with neonatal survival slightly lower. The results are undoubtedly better now. These improved outcomes have been attributed to early recognition of the disorder followed by prompt delivery.[1,4-6] In a recent series, 28 cases of acute fatty liver of pregnancy were reviewed.[7] They occurred between 1982 and 1997, with an incidence of 1 in 6,659 births. There were no maternal mortalities and only two (7.6 percent) perinatal deaths.[7] Usually beginning late in the third trimester, acute fatty liver often presents with nausea and vomiting,[1,6,8] followed by severe abdominal pain and headache. The right upper quadrant is generally tender, but the liver is not enlarged to palpation. Within a few days, jaundice appears, and the patient becomes somnolent and eventually comatose. Hematemesis and spontaneous bleeding result when the patient develops hypoprothrombinemia and disseminated intravascular coagulation (DIC). Oliguria, metabolic acidosis, and eventually anuria occur in approximately 50 percent of patients with acute fatty liver of pregnancy.[8] Diabetes insipidus may also accompany the disease, but may not manifest itself until postpartum.[6,10] These patients may respond to desamino-cys-1-D-arginine-8-vasopressin (dDAVP) after delivery.[10] If the disease is allowed to progress, labor begins and the patient delivers a stillborn infant. The etiology of these fetal losses has not been convincingly demonstrated. Moise and Shah[2] suggest that uteroplacental insufficiency may be the cause of fetal distress and fetal death in these patients. During the immediate postpartum period, the mother becomes febrile, comatose and, without therapy, dies within a few days. DIC, renal failure, profound hypoglycemia, and occasionally pancreatitis are the most often cited immediate causes of death.[2,8,9] Two cases of liver rupture associated with acute fatty liver have also been reported.[11,12] In one case, a patient receiving intravenous heparin for thrombophlebitis suddenly expired as a result of rupture of a subcapsular hematoma of the liver.[12] The diagnosis of acute fatty liver in pregnancy was confirmed microscopically. It is important to note that although acute fatty liver is usually a disease of late pregnancy, it has been reported at 22 weeks' gestation.[13]

The primary differential diagnoses in cases of acute fatty liver include fulminant hepatitis and the liver dysfunction associated with the HELLP syndrome (*h*emolysis, *e*levated *l*iver enzymes, and *l*ow *p*latelet count) or preeclampsia (Table 36–1).[14-16] Several researchers have suggested a spectrum of diseases between acute fatty liver of pregnancy and preeclampsia.[14,16] Although it is often difficult, physicians are usually able to differentiate between these disorders based on physical and laboratory findings. An overdose of acetaminophen may mimic, to a certain extent, acute fatty liver of pregnancy; therefore, a careful drug history is imperative.

Etiology

The cause of acute fatty liver remains elusive. Brown et al.[17] have proposed a spectrum of diseases that includes the entire range from mild preeclampsia to acute fatty liver of pregnancy.

Treem and co-workers[18] note the similarities in clinical presentation and histologic appearance of the liver in pregnant women with acute fatty liver and in children with metabolic defects in the intramitochondrial β-oxidation pathway.[18] Sims et al.[19] found the same defect in affected children from three families, all of whose mothers had experienced acute fatty liver of

Table 36–1. DIFFERENTIAL DIAGNOSIS OF LIVER DISEASE IN PREGNANCY

	Serum Transaminase Levels (IU/L)	Bilirubin Level (mg/dl)	Coagulopathy	Histology	Other Features
Acute hepatitis B	>1,000	>5	–	Hepatocellular necrosis	Potential for perinatal transmission
Acute fatty liver	<500	<5	+	Fatty infiltration	Coma, renal failure, hypoglycemia
Intrahepatic cholestasis	<300	<5, mostly direct	–	Dilated bile canaliculi	Pruritus, increased bile acids
HELLP	>500	<5	+	Variable periportal necrosis	Hypertension, edema, thrombocytopenia

HELLP, *h*emolysis, *e*levated *l*iver enzymes, *l*ow *p*latelets; –, absent; +, present.

pregnancy. Schoeman et al.[20] discuss a similar case in which a mother had acute fatty liver in two successive pregnancies and delivered two healthy infants. Both infants died at approximately 6 months of age with fatty infiltration of the liver, with similar disorders of fatty acid oxidation. Ibdah et al. found that HELLP and acute fatty liver occur more frequently in women whose fetuses have a deficiency of long-chain 3-hydroxyacyl-CoA. This enzyme resides in the mitochondrial trifunctional protein, which also contains the active site of long-chain 2,3-enoyl CoA hydratase and long-chain 3-ketoacyl-CoA thiolase. While carrying fetuses with the homozygous mutation, 79 percent of mothers had acute fatty liver or HELLP.[21] Baldwin describes how this enzyme deficiency is similar to that found in pediatric Reye's syndrome and how the hepatic pathology of acute fatty liver and Reye's syndrome are similar.[22] Baldwin hypothesizes that the use of nonsteroidal anti-inflammatory agents in pregnancy may predispose the susceptible gravida to acute fatty liver. In Finland, Tyni et al.[23] examined 63 pregnancies in 18 mothers of 28 infants diagnosed with long-chain 3-hydroxyacyl-CoA dehydrogenase deficiency. Preeclampsia, HELLP, or acute fatty liver were found in 31 percent of pregnancies carrying an affected fetus, but in none of the pregnancies carrying a healthy fetus.[23]

Clinical Diagnosis

Malaise, nausea with vomiting, and epigastric and/or right upper quadrant pain are usually present. The duration of these prodromal symptoms and signs is variable. In a study of 14 cases over 8 years, Usta et al.[6] reported a mean gestational age of 34.5 weeks, with a range of 28 to 39 weeks. Four patients had hepatic encephalopathy, three had pulmonary edema, and three had ascites.[6] Reyes et al.[3] report lethargy and jaundice as the main presenting symptoms and signs in 11 patients with acute fatty liver of pregnancy in Chile. Unusual findings included seven patients with pruritus,

two of whom experienced itching weeks before the clinical onset of disease, and nine with polydypsia.[3] In his review, Bacq found that diabetes insipidus is a frequent finding.[24] Patients may also be febrile or present with hepatorenal syndrome.[25] By the time the diagnosis is made, patients often have a clinically manifested coagulopathy. Rarely, acute fatty liver may occur concomitantly with other diseases such as severe preclampsia,[25] chronic active hepatitis,[26] and pregnancy-induced cholestasis.[3,27] Pereira et al. found that 17 of 32 (53 percent) patients with acute fatty liver developed an infectious complication.[28]

Laboratory Diagnosis

In acute fatty liver of pregnancy, serum transaminase levels are elevated but usually remain below 500 IU/L.[5] In acute hepatitis, however, these levels are frequently above 1,000 IU/L. In liver dysfunction associated with preeclampsia or the HELLP syndrome, the transaminases are often in the same range as in acute fatty liver of pregnancy, but are occasionally higher. As a result of DIC, the prothrombin time and activated partial thromboplastin time (aPTT) are often prolonged. The prothrombin time is usually increased before the aPTT because it reflects the vitamin K–dependent clotting factors synthesized in the liver. A decreased fibrinogen level is accompanied by an elevation in fibrin degradation products, the D-dimer, and prothrombin.[1,2] Although the serum bilirubin level is elevated, it usually remains below 5 mg/dl and only rarely rises as high as 10 mg/dl, a level lower than one would expect in acute hepatitis. A liver biopsy specimen will reveal pericentral microvesicular fatty change. There is little inflammatory cell infiltration or hepatic necrosis. Periportal areas are usually preserved.[5,29] This picture is very different from fulminant hepatitis in which hepatocellular necrosis is significant. Special staining and electron microscopy yield no evidence of viral particles in acute fatty liver of pregnancy. The diagnosis can be made on frozen section of the liver biopsy material using oil red O stain. This staining is very sensitive but not specific for acute fatty liver of pregnancy. Similar staining is also seen in patients with severe preeclampsia and the HELLP syndrome. Barton and colleagues[30] believe that electron microscopy is more beneficial in establishing a definitive diagnosis. Reyes et al.[3] showed mega-mitochondria with paracrystalline inclusions in all patients who underwent liver biopsy. Because of the coagulopathy associated with acute fatty liver of pregnancy, liver biopsy is not advisable in most cases. If biopsy is essential to make the diagnosis and establish a plan of treatment, fresh frozen plasma can be administered to correct the coagulopathy before performing the procedure. Goodacre and colleagues[31] and Mabie and colleagues[32] believe that the diagnosis of acute fatty liver of pregnancy can occasionally be made using computed tomography (CT). The finding of decreased attenuation over the liver is consistent with fatty infiltration. Usta et al.[6] found that CT resulted in a large number of false-negative diagnoses. Thus, a negative scan does not rule out acute fatty liver of pregnancy. This finding was corroborated by Van Le and Podrasky.[33] In their study of five patients with acute fatty liver, none had an abnormal CT scan, and only one had an abnormal right upper quadrant ultrasound examination. Siegelman has demonstrated that fatty infiltration can be diagnosed with magnetic resonance imaging utilizing T2-weighted gradient-echo sequences.[34]

Management

Once the diagnosis has been established, delivery should be accomplished as quickly as is safely possible.[35] Important supportive measures must first be undertaken to ensure maternal well-being. The patient's coagulopathy must be corrected with fresh frozen plasma. If more concentrated fibrinogen is needed, cryoprecipitate can be administered. In a study by Castro et al.,[1] 28 patients with acute fatty liver were identified at the University of Southern California Medical Center. All 28 had evidence of persistent DIC, and 23 had a markedly depressed level of antithrombin III. Intravenous fluids containing adequate glucose should be given. This will prevent hypoglycemia, which can be fatal. If there is not a severe coagulopathy or the coagulopathy has been corrected, invasive hemodynamic monitoring may be instituted if necessary before delivery. This technique will allow the anesthesiologist and obstetrician to monitor the patient's fluid status.

Delivery soon after diagnosis is paramount. Vaginal delivery is preferable. If the patient's cervix is not ripe, cervical ripening agents may be employed to maximize the likelihood of a vaginal delivery. Cesarean delivery, however, is warranted if it appears that delivery cannot be effected in a timely fashion, and the patient is deteri-

orating. If the patient's coagulopathy has been corrected, epidural anesthesia is the best choice. Spinal anesthesia can also be used. Regional anesthesia is preferable, because it allows adequate assessment of the patient's level of consciousness. General anesthesia should be avoided if possible because of the hepatotoxicity of some anesthetic agents. Narcotic doses must be adjusted, as these drugs are metabolized by the liver.

Early diagnosis and delivery afford both mother and neonate an excellent chance for survival.[4,5] If delivery is effected before hepatic encephalopathy and renal failure develop, patients usually improve rather rapidly.[4–6,9,14] Davidson et al. report three cases of acute fatty liver occurring in triplet pregnancies.[36] All underwent cesarean delivery as soon as the diagnosis was suspected. All three had biopsy-proven disease and improved rapidly after delivery.[36] In Pereira's case review of extremely ill patients admitted to the Liver Failure Unit at Guy's Hospital in London, 4 of 32 women (12.5 percent) died, and the perinatal mortality was 9 percent.[28] Thus, even in the best tertiary care units, maternal mortality still occurs. Therefore, we must be vigilant and deliver these patients as soon as the diagnosis is seriously suspected. Ockner and colleagues[37] have reported a case in which the patient did not improve postpartum. After orthotopic liver transplantation, the multisystem failure rapidly reversed.[37] In that case, the diagnosis of acute fatty liver was documented histopathologically. Southern blot analysis for viral DNA was also negative, ruling out hepatitis. Amon et al.[25] also reported as successful postpartum liver transplant in a patient with acute fatty liver and severe preeclampsia.

The classic teaching is that there is little risk of recurrence of acute fatty liver in subsequent pregnancies. Barton and colleagues[30] described the first case of recurrent acute fatty liver in pregnancy confirmed by biopsy. Schoeman et al.[20] also reported a case of a mother who had acute fatty liver in two successive pregnancies. However, with the previously cited enzymatic defect found to be associated with acute fatty liver and with more pregnant women surviving the disease, we may encounter more recurrent cases in the future.

INTRAHEPATIC CHOLESTASIS OF PREGNANCY

Intrahepatic cholestasis is characterized by pruritus and mild jaundice usually occurring in the last trimester of pregnancy. It can, however, occur earlier in gestations. It has an uneven worldwide incidence of 1 in 1,000 to 1 in 10,000 deliveries.[39] The disease is reported to affect up to 14 percent of pregnancies in Chile.[39] Gonzalez et al.[40] determined the prevalence of intrahepatic cholestasis of pregnancy in Chile to be 4.7 percent in singleton pregnancies. In twin pregnancies, the incidence was 20.9 percent. The disease is also common in the Swedish population.[41] Berg et al.[41] reported the incidence in Sweden to be between 1 and 1.5 percent. In their study, the incidence of intrahepatic cholestasis of pregnancy had a distinct seasonal variation, peaking in November. This disorder is much less common in the United States, but appears to have a familial predisposition in Sweden.[42] In 1987, Wilson[43] reported the first case of intrahepatic cholestasis of pregnancy in an African-American patient. Abedin et al. found that cholestasis of pregnancy occurred in up to 1.5 percent of Asian women of Pakistani and Indian origin.[44] Intrahepatic cholestasis tends to recur in subsequent pregnancies, but the severity may vary from one pregnancy to the next. In their Chilean study, Gonzalez et al.[40] reported a recurrence rate of 70.5 percent in singleton pregnancies. Locatelli et al. found cholestasis of pregnancy in 15.9 percent of patients with hepatitis C compared with 0.8 percent of controls, suggesting that individuals with hepatitis C are more prone to cholestasis of preganacy.[45]

Clinical Manifestations

Patients with intrahepatic cholestasis usually begin having pruritus at night. It progresses, and the patient is soon experiencing bothersome pruritus continuously. Approximately 2 weeks later, clinical jaundice will develop in 50 percent of cases. The jaundice is usually mild, soon plateaus, and remains constant until delivery. The pruritus worsens with the onset of jaundice, and the patient's skin can become excoriated. The symptoms usually abate within 2 days after delivery. The differential diagnosis must include viral hepatitis and gallbladder disease. There is usually no fever or abdominal discomfort, as in hepatitis, or nausea or vomiting, as seen in hepatitis and gallbladder disease.

Laboratory Findings

Serum alkaline phosphatase levels are increased 5- to 10-fold in intrahepatic cholestasis of pregnancy. Alkaline phosphatase, however, is normally increased in pregnancy. This is due to placental production of this enzyme. Upon fractionation, most of the alkaline phosphatase is hepatic in origin rather than placental. Serum 5′-nucleotidase levels are also increased. Serum and urinary excretion of total sulfated progesterone metabolites are increased in cholestasis of pregnancy, whereas glucuronide metabolites are unchanged or low.[46] This shows that there is a primary change in the reductase metabolism of progesterone in cholestasis of pregnancy.[46] Bilirubin is elevated, but usually not above 5 mg/dl. Most is the direct, conjugated form. If intrahe-

patic cholestasis lasts for several weeks, liver dysfunction may result in decreased vitamin K reabsorption or decreased prothrombin production, leading to a prolongation of the prothrombin time. Serum transaminase levels are usually normal or moderately elevated, remaining well below the levels associated with viral hepatitis. Serum cholesterol and triglyceride levels may also be markedly elevated.

The serum bile acids (chenodeoxycholic acid, deoxycholic acid, and cholic acid) are increased. The levels are often more than 10 times the normal concentration. These acids are deposited in the skin and probably cause the extreme pruritus. The degree of pruritus, however, is not always related to the serum level of bile acids.[47] To make the diagnosis of intrahepatic cholestasis of pregnancy, the fasting levels of serum bile acids should be at least three times the upper limit of normal. Elevation of serum bile acids alone cannot be used to make the diagnosis. The patient must also have clinical symptoms. Serum transaminase levels may also be elevated 5 to 10 times normal. Reyes et al. found that serum copper is significantly higher and selenium levels are significantly lower in individuals with cholestasis of pregnancy.[48] Wojcicka-Jagodzinska and colleagues[49] reported that carbohydrate metabolism is disturbed in patients with intrahepatic cholestasis of pregnancy. These patients should therefore be screened for gestational diabetes when the diagnosis of cholestasis is made.

Histologically, the periportal areas show no change, and the hepatocellular architecture remains undisturbed. The centrilobular areas, however, reveal dilated bile canaliculi, many containing bile plugs. Ultrastructurally, there appears to be some destruction and atrophy of microvilli in the bile canaliculi.[50] These changes tend to regress after pregnancy.

Perinatal Outcome

The risk of preterm birth and fetal death may be increased in patients suffering from intrahepatic cholestasis of pregnancy.[51–54] Fisk and Storey[55] studied 83 pregnancies complicated by intrahepatic cholestasis over a 10-year period. Meconium staining occurred in 45 percent of the pregnancies, spontaneous preterm labor occurred in 44 percent, and intrapartum fetal distress complicated 22 percent. Of the 86 infants, 2 were stillborn and 1 died soon after birth. The overall perinatal mortality in this group of patients was 35 per 1,000.[55] Nonstress tests, serial ultrasonography to assess amniotic fluid volume, and estriol determinations failed to predict fetal compromise. Early intervention was indicated in 49 pregnancies, 12 because of suspected fetal distress. In light of this study, antepartum fetal heart rate testing and intense surveillance should be undertaken in gravidas with intrahepatic cholestasis of pregnancy. It may also be prudent to induce labor at term or when amniotic fluid studies indicate fetal lung maturity.[55] Heinonen and Kirkinen[52] reviewed 91 cases of cholestasis in pregnancy in Finland from 1990 to 1996. The cesarean section rate was 10 percent higher in the group of women with cholestasis. The risk of preterm delivery was higher (odds ratio, 2.73) and the need for neonatal intensive care was also higher (odds ratio, 2.15).[52] Matos et al.[54] report a full-term infant with unexplained intracerebral hemorrhage in a patient with cholestasis of pregnancy.

Management

Treatment is aimed at reducing the intense pruritus. Diphenhydramine, hydroxyzine, and other antihistamines help only slightly. Cholestyramine is an anion-binding resin that interrupts the enterohepatic circulation, reducing the reabsorption of bile acids. A total of 8 to 16 g/day in three to four divided doses is often helpful in relieving pruritus. It is most effective if started as soon as the pruritus is noted, before it becomes severe. It often takes up to 2 weeks to work. Because cholestyramine also interferes with vitamin K absorption, the prothrombin time should be checked at least weekly. If prolonged, parenteral vitamin K should be administered. When the prothrombin time returns to normal, the frequency of injections can be decreased. Cholestyramine causes a sensation of bloating and often results in constipation. Cholestyramine also can interfere with the absorption of other ingested medications, including prenatal vitamins. If the patient cannot tolerate cholestyramine, antacids containing aluminum may be used to bind bile acids. These medications are usually not as effective as cholestyramine. Phenobarbital, in a dose of up to 90 mg daily given at bedtime, can be helpful. Phenobarbital induces hepatic microsomal enzymes, increasing bile salt secretion and bile flow.[56-58] This medication usually takes more than 1 week to be effective. It has not been shown to change the serum concentration of bile acids.[59] It is important to remember that phenobarbital must not be given within 2 hours of cholestyramine, or the phenobarbital will be bound and excreted without being absorbed. The key to treating pregnancy-induced cholestasis is to begin therapy as soon as the diagnosis is made.

Dexamethasone has also been used with some success in treating pregnancy-induced cholestasis. Dexamethasone suppresses fetal–placental estrogen production, which is out of balance in the patient with cholestasis of pregnancy. Leslie et al., however, have shown that downstream placental production of estrogen is compromised in patients with cholestasis of pregnancy.[61] Two studies have investigated using guar gum, a gel-forming fiber that increases fecal elimination of bile acids, to treat the pruritus associated with pregnancy-induced cholestasis.[62,63] This dietary fiber was randomly assigned to 24 of 48 women with cholestasis of pregnancy in Finland.[62] In patients taking the guar gum, bile acids remained stable, whereas they increased in those taking the placebo. Pruritus improved in those taking guar gum and worsened in the placebo group.[62] Similar results were obtained in 48 patients in a more recent study in Finland.[63]

The two most recently studied medications for the treatment of intrahepatic cholestasis of pregnancy are S-adenyl-methionine (SAM-e) and ursodeoxycholic acid (UDCA). SAM-e may work by reversing estrogen-induced impairment of bile secretion. UDCA is a naturally occurring hydrophilic bile acid that replaces other more cytotoxic bile acids. Nicastri et al. studied 32 women with intrahepatic cholestasis.[64] There were four study groups: the first group received DCA; the second SAM-e; the third both drugs; and the fourth received placebo. A combination of both drugs was more effective than either drug alone.[64] Palma et al. compared 1 g daily of UDCA with a placebo over 3 weeks and found a significant decrease in pruritus and a significant decrease in liver function studies.[65] Other studies have shown similar results.[66,67] It appears that the proper dosage of UDCA is 14 to 16 mg/kg/day.[65,66] Because of intolerable pruritus and the possible impact on perinatal outcome, delivery may be undertaken at term or as soon as fetal lung maturity has been documented. Jaundice usually disappears within 2 days after delivery. The patient should be counseled that the condition may recur during subsequent pregnancies.[40] It is also important to note that some patients may manifest symptoms of intrahepatic cholestasis when taking oral contraceptives.[41,68]

PREGNANCY AND LIVER TRANSPLANTATION

At present, pregnancy in the liver transplant patient is a rare occurrence. As the procedure becomes more widespread, more liver transplant recipients will become pregnant. Laifer and colleagues[69] reported the results of eight pregnancies in women with liver transplants. Seven of the eight patients conceived between 3 weeks and 24 months after transplantation. Six had live births, and one electively terminated her pregnancy. Five patients developed pregnancy-induced hypertension, including three with severe preeclampsia. The six infants born to these women were delivered between 26 and 37 weeks.[69] Five of the six infants survived, and none had structural anomalies. One patient underwent orthotopic liver transplantation at 26 weeks' gestation after presenting in hepatic coma from fulminant hepatitis B. She was delivered on postoperative day 7 because of fetal distress. Laifer et al.[69] concluded that pregnancy does not appear to have a deleterious effect on hepatic graft function or survival. All eight of the patients in their series survived without permanent sequelae. As in the case of patients with a renal allograft, liver transplant recipients should continue their immunosuppressive medications throughout pregnancy. Furthermore, they should wait several years before conception to make certain that liver function is acceptable and there are no signs of rejection. As previously cited, liver transplantation has been used in acute fatty liver of pregnancy.[37,38]

GALLBLADDER DISEASE

Cholelithiasis is responsible for approximately 7 percent of cases of jaundice occurring during gestation.[70] Gallstones are present in 12 percent of all pregnancies.[71] Pregnancy appears to increase the likelihood of gallstone formation but not the risk of developing acute cholecystitis.[72–74]

Pregnancy markedly alters gallbladder function. Ultrasound studies performed after 14 weeks' gestation have shown that fasting gallbladder volume is twice normal, the rate of gallbladder emptying is decreased, and the percentage of emptying is lower, thus leaving a higher residual than in the nonpregnant patient.[73] Cholecystokinin is the major stimulus for gallbladder contraction. It appears that estrogen and/or progesterone may make these contractions less effective, leading to an increased residual volume.

Once the diagnosis is confirmed, attacks of biliary colic should be treated symptomatically during gestation. Ultrasound examination of the gallbladder will aid in the evaluation and diagnosis of these patients. Hiatt and colleagues[75] report that ultrasound successfully confirmed the presence of gallstones in 18 of 26 patients. Before resorting to surgery, attempts should be made to treat these patients medically. Attacks usually respond to intravenous hydration, analgesics, nasogastric suction, and antibiotics. Lockwood and associates[76] have also utilized total parenteral nutrition. Their patient did well with no fetal or maternal morbidity.

If possible, cholecystectomy should be postponed until after delivery. In their study of 26 patients, Hiatt and co-workers[75] found it necessary to perform cholecystectomy and cholangiography on 19 women, with 4 requiring common bile duct explorations. They noted that only two of seven patients who presented in the first trimester with cholecystitis carried their pregnancies to term. Daradkeh and colleagues studied 42 women suffering from gallstones during pregnancy.[77] In this study, 26 of 42 patients responded to conservative therapy and were able to postpone surgery until after delivery.

If ascending cholangitis develops, cholecystectomy should not be postponed. Cholecystectomy should also be performed if common bile duct obstruction occurs or severe pancreatitis develops. Certainly, surgery should not be delayed if an acute abdomen develops. In these instances, temporizing will only increase perinatal and maternal risk.[72] If cholecystectomy is performed in the second or third trimester, fetal mortality is less than 5 percent.[74] If pancreatitis secondary to biliary tract stones remains untreated, however, the fetal mortality approaches 60 percent.[74]

Dixon and colleagues,[78] reviewing their experience with 44 patients, found that conservative management of cholecystitis was followed by recurrent episodes of biliary tract symptoms requiring multiple hospitalizations. Cholecystectomy performed in the second trimester was associated with little maternal morbidity, no fetal loss, and a substantial reduction of total hospital days.

Laparoscopic cholecystectomy has been safely carried out in a number of pregnancies. In Austria, seven patients underwent laparoscopic cholecystectomy between 13 and 32 weeks with no complications and all deliveries occurring at term.[71] Insufflation pressures were 8 to 10 mm Hg. Mean operating time was 62 minutes. Cosenza et al. compared 12 laparoscopic cholecystectomies to 20 open cholecystectomies between 1993 and 1997.[78] There were no perinatal mortalities or major maternal morbidities in those undergoing laparoscopy.[78] Affleck and co-workers report 45 laparoscopic cholecystectomies and 22 laparoscopic appendectomies performed during pregnancy from 1990 to 1998.[79] Lemaire and van Erp report performing a laparoscopic cholecystectomy in a patient at 33 weeks gestation without incident.[80] Barone et al. compared 20 laparoscopic with 26 open cholecystectomies performed between 1992 and 1996.[81] Each group experienced one fetal death. Only one patient undergoing laparoscopic cholecystectomy developed preterm contractions compared with the open group. Indeed, there is a growing body of literature indicating that laparoscopic cholecystectomy is safe during pregnancy.

Finally, as obstetricians, it is our duty to help establish the proper diagnosis and, if therapy is out of our field, to encourage our colleagues to undertake appropriate therapy in a manner that is most beneficial to mother and fetus.

Key Points

➤ Acute fatty liver of pregnancy is a medical emergency requiring stabilization of the patient and timely delivery. Almost all cases will be complicated by disseminated intravascular coagulation.

➤ Liver transaminase levels in acute fatty liver of pregnancy are lower than what one would see in acute hepatitis.

➤ Profound hypoglycemia is a frequent concomitant of acute fatty liver and can cause death if untreated.

➤ Pregnancy-induced cholestasis usually occurs in the third trimester, causing intense pruritus and jaundice. Elevated serum bile acids are the best laboratory test for making the diagnosis in symptomatic patients.

REFERENCES

1. Castro MA, Goodwin TM, Shaw KJ, et al: Disseminated intravascular coagulation and antithrombin III depression in acute fatty liver of pregnancy. Am J Obstet Gynecol 174:211, 1996.
2. Moise KJ Jr, Shah DM: Acute fatty liver of pregnancy: etiology of fetal distress and fetal wastage. Obstet Gynecol 69:482, 1987.
3. Reyes H, Sandoval L, Wainstein A, et al: Acute fatty liver of pregnancy: a clinical study of 12 episodes in 11 patients. Gut 35:101, 1994.
4. Hou SH, Levin S, Ahola S, et al: Acute fatty liver of pregnancy: survival with early cesarean section. Dig Dis Sci 29:449, 1984.
5. Ebert EC, Sun EA, Wright SH, et al: Does early diagnosis and delivery in acute fatty liver of pregnancy lead to improvement in maternal and infant survival? Dig Dis Sci 29:453, 1984.
6. Usta IM, Barton JR, Amon EA, et al: Acute fatty liver of pregnancy: an experience in the diagnosis and management of fourteen cases. Am J Obstet Gynecol 171:1342, 1994.
7. Castro MA, Fassett MJ, Reynolds TB, et al: Reversible peripartum liver failure: a new perspective on the diagnosis, treatment, and cause of acute fatty liver of pregnancy, based on 28 consecutive cases. Am J Obstet Gynecol 181:389, 1999.
8. Purdie JM, Walters BN: Acute fatty liver of pregnancy: clinical features and diagnosis. Aust N Z J Obstet Gynaecol 28:62, 1988.
9. Shaffer EA: Liver disease in pregnancy. Curr Probl Obstet Gynecol 7:15, 1984.
10. Kennedy S, Hall PM, Seymour AE, Hague WM: Transient diabetes insipidus and acute fatty liver of pregnancy. Br J Obstet Gynaecol 101:387, 1994.
11. Minuk GY, Lui RC, Kelly JK: Rupture of the liver associated with acute fatty liver of pregnancy. Am J Gastroenterol 82:457, 1987.
12. Roh LS: Subcapsular hematoma in fatty liver of pregnancy. J Forensic Sci 31:1509, 1986.
13. Monga M, Katz AR: Acute fatty liver in the second trimester. Obstet Gynecol 93:811, 1999.
14. Riley CA, Romero R, Duffy TP: Hepatic dysfunction with disseminated intravascular coagulation in toxemia of pregnancy: a distinct clinical syndrome. Gastroenterology 80:1346, 1981.
15. Brown MS, Reddy KR, Hensley GT, et al: The initial presentation of fatty liver of pregnancy mimicking acute viral hepatitis. Am J Gastroenterol 82:554, 1987.
16. Riley CA, Latham PS, Romero R, Duffy TP: Acute fatty liver of pregnancy: a reassessment based on observations in nine patients. Ann Intern Med 106:703, 1987.
17. Brown MA, Pasaris G, Carlton MA: Pregnancy-induced hypertension and acute fatty liver of pregnancy: atypical presentations. Am J Obstet Gynecol 164:154, 1990.
18. Treem WR, Rinaldo P, Hale DE, et al: Acute fatty liver of pregnancy and long-chain 3-hydroxyacyl-coenzyme A dehydrogenase deficiency. Hepatology 19:339, 1994.
19. Sims HF, Brackett JC, Powell CK, et al: The molecular basis of pediatric long chain 3-hydroxyacyl-CoA dehydrogenase deficiency associated with maternal acute fatty liver of pregnancy. Proc Natl Acad Sci U S A 92:841, 1995.
20. Schoeman MN, Batey RG, Wilcken B: Recurrent acute fatty liver of pregnancy associated with a fatty-acid oxidation defect in the offspring. Gastroenterology 100:544, 1991.
21. Ibdah JA, Bennett MJ, Rinaldo P, et al: A fetal fatty-acid oxidation disorder as a cause of liver disease in pregnant women. N Engl J Med 340:1723, 1999.
22. Baldwin GS: Do NSAIDs contribute to acute fatty liver of pregnancy? Med Hypotheses 54:846, 2000.
23. Tyni T, Ekholm E, Pihko H: Pregnancy complications are frequent in long-chain 3-hydroxyacyl-coenzyme A dehydrogenase deficiency. Am J Obstet Gynecol 178:603, 1998.
24. Bacq Y: Acute fatty liver of pregnancy. Semin Perinatol 22:134, 1998.
25. Amon E, Allen SR, Petrie RH, Belew JE: Acute fatty liver of pregnancy associated with preeclampsia: management of hepatic failure with postpartum liver transplantation. Am J Perinatol 8:278, 1991.
26. Minton D, Yancey MK, Dolson DJ, Duff P: Acute fatty liver of pregnancy in a patient with chronic active hepatitis and associated hepatocyte alpha 1-antrypsin inclusions. Obstet Gynecol 81:819, 1993.
27. Vanjak D, Moreau R, Roche-Sicot J, et al: Intrahepatic cholestasis of pregnancy and acute fatty liver of pregnancy: an unusual, but favorable association? Gastroenterology 100:1123, 1991.
28. Pereira SP, O'Donohue J, Wendon J, Williams R: Maternal and perinatal outcome in severe pregnancy-related liver disease. Hepatology 26:1258, 1997.
29. Snyder RR, Hankins GD: Etiology and management of acute fatty liver of pregnancy. Clin Perinatol 13:813, 1986.
30. Barton JR, Sibai BM, Mabie WC, Shanklin DR: Recurrent acute fatty liver of pregnancy. Am J Obstet Gynecol 163:534, 1990.
31. Goodacre RL, Hunter DJ, Millward S, et al: The diagnosis of acute fatty liver of pregnancy by computed tomography. J Clin Gastroenterol 10:680, 1988.
32. Mabie WC, Dacus JV, Sibai BM, et al: Computed tomography in acute fatty liver of pregnancy. Am J Obstet Gynecol 158:142, 1988.
33. Van Le L, Podrasky A: Computed tomographic and ultrasonographic findings in women with acute fatty liver of pregnancy. J Reprod Med 35:815, 1990.
34. Siegelman ES: MR imaging of diffuse liver disease. Hepatic fat and iron. Magn Reson Imaging Clin N Am 5:347, 1997.

35. Bacq Y, Riely CA: Acute fatty liver of pregnancy: the hepatologist's view. Gastroenterologist 1:257, 1993.

36. Davidson KM, Simpson LL, Knox TA, D'Alton ME: Acute fatty liver of pregnancy in triplet gestation. Obstet Gynecol 91: 806, 1998.

37. Ockner SA, Brunt EM, Cohn SM, et al: Fulminant hepatic failure caused by acute fatty liver of pregnancy treated by orthotopic liver transplantation. Hepatology 11:59, 1990.

38. Franco J, Newcomer J, Adams M, Saeian K: Auxiliary liver transplant in acute fatty liver of pregnancy. Obstet Gynecol 95: 1042, 2000.

39. Reyes H: Intrahepatic cholestasis of pregnancy: an estrogen related disease. Semin Liver Dis 13:289, 1993.

40. Gonzalez MC, Reyes H, Arrese M, et al: Intrahepatic cholestasis of pregnancy in twin pregnancies. J Hepatol 9:84, 1989.

41. Berg B, Helm G, Petersohn L, Tryding N: Cholestasis of pregnancy: clinical and laboratory studies. Acta Obstet Gynecol Scand 65:107, 1986.

42. Dalen E, Westerholm B: Occurrence of hepatic impairment in women jaundiced by oral contraceptives and in their mothers and sisters. Acta Med Scand 195:459, 1994.

43. Wilson JA: Intrahepatic cholestasis of pregnancy with marked elevation of transaminases in a black American. Dig Dis Sci 32:665, 1987.

44. Abedin P, Weaver JB, Egginton E: Intrahepatic cholestasis of pregnancy: prevalence and ethnic distribution. Ethn Health 4: 35, 1997.

45. Locatelli A, Roncaglia N, Acreghini A, et al: Hepatitic C virus infection is associated with a higher incidence of cholestasis of pregnancy. Br J Obstet Gynaecol 106:498, 1999.

46. Meng LJ, Reyes H, Palma J, et al: Profiles of bile acids and progesterone metabolites in the urine and serum of women with intrahepatic cholestasis of pregnancy. J Hepatol 32:542, 2000.

47. Ghent CN, Bloomer JR, Koatska G: Elevations in skin tissue levels of bile acids in humans with cholestasis: relation to serum levels and to pruritus. Gastroenterology 73:125, 1977.

48. Reyes H, Baez ME, Gonzalez MC, et al: Selenium, zinc, and copper plasma levels in intrahepatic cholestasis of pregnancy, in normal pregnancy and in healthy individuals in Chile. J Hepatol 32:542, 2000.

49. Wojcicka-Jagodzinska J, Kuczynska-Sicinska J, Czajkowski K, Smolarczyk R: Carbohydrate metabolism in the course of intrahepatic cholestasis in pregnancy. Am J Obstet Gynecol 161: 959, 1989.

50. Adlercreutz H, Svanbor A, Anber A: Recurrent jaundice in pregnancy. I. A clinical and ultrastructural study. Am J Med 42:335, 1967.

51. Johnson WG, Baskett TF: Obstetric cholestasis: a 14 year review. Am J Obstet Gynecol 143:299, 1979.

52. Heinonen S, Kirkinen P: Pregnancy outcome with intrahepatic cholestasis. Obstet Gynecol 94:189, 1999.

53. Gaudet R, Merviel P, Berkane N, et al: Fetal input of cholestasis of pregnancy: experience at Tenon Hospital and literature review. Fetal Diagn Ther 15:191, 2000.

54. Matos A, Bernandes J, Ayres-de-Campos D, Patricio B: Antepartum fetal cerebral hemorrhage not predicted by current surveillance methods in cholestasis of pregnancy. Obstet Gynecol 89:803, 1997.

55. Fisk NM, Storey GN: Fetal outcome in obstetric cholestasis. Br J Obstet Gynaecol 95:1137, 1988.

56. Espinoza J, Barnaf L, Schnaidt E: The effect of phenobarbital on intrahepatic cholestasis of pregnancy. Am J Obstet Gynecol 119:234, 1974.

57. Bloomer JR, Bower JL: Phenobarbital effects in cholestasis liver disease. Ann Intern Med 82:310, 1975.

58. Laatikinen T: Effect of cholestyramine and phenobarbital on pruritus and serum bile acid levels in cholestasis of pregnancy. Am J Obstet Gynecol 132:501, 1978.

59. Heikkinen J, Maentausta O, Ylostal OP, et al: Serum bile acids in intrahepatic cholestasis of pregnancy during treatment with phenobarbital or cholestyramine. Eur J Obstet Gynecol Reprod Biol 14:153, 1982.

60. Hirvioja ML, Tuimala R: The treatment of intrahepatic cholestasis of pregnancy by dexamethasone. Br J Obstet Gynaecol 99:109, 1992.

61. Leslie KK, Reznikov L, Simon FR, et al: Estrogens in intrahepatic cholestasis of pregnancy. Obstet Gynecol 95:372, 2000.

62. Gylling H, Riikonen S, Nikkila K, et al: Oral guar gum treatment of intrahepatic cholestasis and pruritus in pregnant women: effects on serum cholestanol and other non-cholesterol sterols. Eur J Clin Invest 28:359, 1998.

63. Riikonen S, Savonius H, Gylling H, et al: Oral guar gum, a gel forming dietary fiber relieves pruritus in intrahepatic cholestasis of pregnancy. Acta Obstet Gynecol Scand 79:260, 2000.

64. Nicastri PL, Diaferio A, Tortagni M, et al: A randomised placebo-controlled trial of ursodeoxycholic acid and S-adenosyl methionine in the treatment of intrahepatic cholestasis of pregnancy. Br J Obstet Gynaecol 105:1205, 1998.

65. Palma J, Reyes H, Ribalta J, et al: Ursodeoxycholic acid in the treatment of cholestasis of pregnancy: a randomized, double blind study controlled with placebo. J Hepatol 27:1022, 1997.

66. Brites D, Rodriguez CM, Oliveira N, et al: Correction of maternal serum bile acid profile during ursodeoxycholic acid therapy in cholestasis of pregnancy. J Hepatol 28:91, 1998.

67. Meng LJ, Reyes H, Palma J, et al: Effects of ursodeoxycholic acid on conjugated bile acids and progesterone metabolites in serum and urine of patients with intrahepatic cholestasis of pregnancy. J Hepatol 27:1024, 1997.

68. Connolly TJ, Zuckerman AL: Contraception in the patient with liver disease. Semin Perinatol 22:178, 1998.

69. Laifer SA, Darby MJ, Scantlebury VP, et al: Pregnancy and liver transplantation. Obstet Gynecol 76:1083, 1990.

70. Riley CA, Romero R, Duffy TP: Hepatic dysfunction with disseminated intravascular coagulation in toxemia of pregnancy: a distinct clinical syndrome. Gastroenterology 80:1346, 1981.

71. Sung H-P, Heinerman PM, Steiner H, Waclowiczek HW: Laparoscopic cholecystectomy and interventional endoscopy for gall stone complications during pregnancy. Surg Endosc 14:267, 2000.

72. Kammerer WS: Nonobstetric surgery during pregnancy. Med Clin North Am 63:1157, 1979.

73. Bennion LJ, Grundy SM: Risk factors for the development of cholelithiasis in man. N Engl J Med 299:1221, 1978.

74. Printen KJ, Ott RA: Cholecystectomy during pregnancy. Am Surg 44:432, 1978.

75. Hiatt JR, Hiatt JC, Williams RA, Klein SR: Biliary disease in pregnancy: strategy for surgical management. Am J Surg 151: 263, 1986.

76. Lockwood C, Stiller RJ, Bolognese RJ: Maternal total parenteral nutrition in chronic cholecystitis: a case report. J Reprod Med 32:785, 1987.

77. Daradkeh S, Sumrein I, Paoud F, et al: Management of gallbladder stones during pregnancy: conservative treatment or cholecystectomy? Hepatogastroenterology 46:3074, 1999.

78. Dixon NP, Faddis DM, Silberman H: Aggressive management of cholecystitis during pregnancy. Am J Surg 154:292, 1987.

79. Affleck DG, Handrahan DL, Egger MJ, et al: The laparoscopic management of appendicitis and cholelithiasis during pregnancy. Am J Surg 178:523, 1999.

80. Lemaire BM, van Erp WF: Laparoscopic surgery during pregnancy. Surg Endosc 11:15, 1997.

81. Barone JE, Bears S, Chen S, et al: Outcome study of cholecystectomy during pregnancy. Am J Surg 177:232, 1999.

Gastrointestinal Disease

MARK B. LANDON

PEPTIC ULCER DISEASE

The symptoms and complications of peptic ulcer seem to decrease during pregnancy. This observation is supported by Clark, who interviewed pregnant women with a previous history of peptic ulcer disease and found that in 313 pregnancies, 44 percent became asymptomatic and 44 percent demonstrated a marked improvement in symptoms.[1] Only 12 percent remained the same or experienced worsening symptoms during gestation. There were no serious complications reported in this series. Of note, nearly half of the patients relapsed by 3 months postpartum and 75 percent of the patients questioned had experienced recurrent symptoms by 6 months after delivery. Vessey and colleagues have also reported a low rate of hospitalization for peptic ulcer disease in pregnant women and users of the contraceptive pill.[2] Of 175 women hospitalized for advanced symptoms of ulcer disease, none were pregnant.

Several factors that might improve the clinical course of patients with peptic ulcer disease during pregnancy have been investigated. It is well known that patients with duodenal ulcer have higher levels of basal and stimulated acid secretion. It has been suggested that the amelioration of symptoms during pregnancy may in part be secondary to progesterone-induced lower gastric acid output as well as increased mucus production. The latter may exert a protective effect on the intestinal mucosa. The placenta is also rich in histaminase, which may inactivate histamine or block its action at the level of the parietal cell. Plasma levels of histaminase increase dramatically during pregnancy and may be responsible for a decline in gastric acid output in patients who exhibit hyperacidity in the nonpregnant state.[3] Finally, pregnancy may favorably affect the gastric and duodenal mucosa's ability to regenerate as a result of increased levels of epidermal growth factor.[4]

The interplay of acid secretion and mucosal resistance is believed to be important in the pathogenesis of peptic ulceration. Infection of the stomach and duodenum with *Helicobacter pylori* has been implicated as a significant factor, as well. This organism is found in nearly all patients with duodenal ulceration. Its presence, however, is associated with ulcer formation in a minority of individuals.[5] Various physiologic alterations affecting acid secretion can result from *H. pylori* infection, which when combined with destruction of the hydrophobic phospholipid surface within the mucosa, predispose to ulcer formation. Host response, bacterial virulence, genetic predisposition, stress, and nonsteroidal anti-inflammatory drug use are other factors involved in the pathogenesis of ulcer disease.

Most physicians, when evaluating pregnant women with dyspepsia, attribute this complaint to gastric reflux in the lower esophagus. Heartburn is most often observed in the second and third trimesters. It usually responds to antacid therapy, and minimizing reflux by having the mother assume a semirecumbent position when she is supine. This regimen will often bring relief to patients with underlying peptic ulcer disease as well, and further diagnostic procedures are rarely needed. Duodenal ulcers produce either sharp or burning epigastric pain that is episodic following meals or it may awaken patients from sleep. Pain radiating to the back suggests posterior penetration. In patients with profound pain that is unresponsive to antacid regimens, panendoscopic examination of the stomach and upper duodenum may be performed. These procedures performed with appropriate analgesia are generally well tolerated during pregnancy.

The primary medical treatment for the symptomatic patient with peptic ulcer disease during pregnancy remains antacid therapy and diet. Administration of antacid 1 hour after meals and at bedtime usually provides relief of symptoms and promotes ulcer healing. In refractory cases, a dose may be added at 3 hours after meals. It is important to be aware that potential side effects of antacid therapy exist. Patients with peptic ulcer disease should be maintained on a normal diet, avoiding caffeine, salicylates, ethanol, or any gastric stimulant that aggravates their condition. Because basal acid output may normally rise during evening hours, it follows that patients should avoid bedtime snacks.

H_2 antagonists (cimetidine, ranitidine, famotidine)

continue to remain a second-line choice for therapy in pregnancy. If possible, these agents should be reserved for use during the second and third trimesters.[6] Cimetidine, ranitidine, and famotidine are category B medications.[7] The use of omeprazole, a powerful inhibitor of acid secretion, has been limited during pregnancy. This compound blocks hydrogen potassium ATPase in gastric parietal cells. Studies have suggested a potential for teratogenesis in animal studies, and this drug is category C.[8] Elective treatment of *H. pylori* with antibiotics and bismuth subsalicylate is generally recommended following delivery and breast-feeding.

Fewer than 100 cases of pregnant women who developed serious complications from peptic ulcer disease have been reported in the literature.[9] Bleeding, perforation, and obstruction should be treated as they would be in nonpregnant patients. Becker-Andersen and Husfelt, in reviewing 30 cases of hemorrhage from peptic ulcer during pregnancy, clearly demonstrated a decrease in maternal and fetal mortality rates with prompt surgical exploration.[9] The only two maternal deaths in their series occurred in patients who were in shock at the time of operation. However, a 44 percent fetal mortality rate was recorded in cases that were first managed conservatively. These authors stress that perforation and hemorrhage must be treated surgically using the same indications as in nonpregnant patients. If a partial gastrectomy is to be performed in the third trimester, it may be advisable to begin the procedure with a cesarean section. The fetus appears to be quite sensitive to maternal circulatory failure due to hypovolemia, and, in addition, gastric surgery may be facilitated after the gravid uterus has been evacuated.

ACUTE PANCREATITIS

The true incidence of pancreatitis complicating pregnancy is difficult to ascertain. In a review of 500 cases of acute pancreatitis, only 7 patients developed the disease while pregnant.[10] Reported incidences have ranged from 1 in 1,066 pregnancies to 1 in 2,888 deliveries.[11,12] Maternal death is uncommon compared with decades ago, especially if the diagnosis is established promptly.[11] There appears to be a greater association of gallstones with the development of pancreatitis during gestation. McKay et al. noted that 18 of 20 patients who developed pancreatitis while pregnant or within 5 months postpartum had cholelithiasis.[10] In a 22-year study, Block and Kelly reported that all 21 cases of pancreatitis during pregnancy in their institution were associated with gallstones.[13] In nonpregnant individuals, alcoholism is by far the most common etiologic factor. Other causes for pancreatitis include hyperlipidemia, idiopathic factors, infection, previous surgery, preeclampsia, hyperparathyroidism, thiazide ingestion, and penetrating duodenal ulcer. The normal hypertriglyceridemia of pregnancy may be exaggerated in patients with hyperlipidemia, thereby inducing acute pancreatitis.[14] These rare cases have been treated with either hyperalimentation or lipoprotein apheresis when dietary fat restriction failed to improve symptoms during pregnancy.[14,15]

The clinical presentation of pancreatitis is not significantly altered in pregnancy. The disease may occur at any stage of gestation, but is more common in the third trimester and the puerperium. Epigastric pain, which may radiate to the flanks or shoulders along with abdominal tenderness, should prompt appropriate laboratory investigation. Occasionally, a patient will present with nausea and vomiting as her only complaints. Mild fever and leukocytosis may be present. Radiographic examination of the abdomen may simply reveal an adynamic ileus. Ultrasound imaging of the pancreas can be difficult. Therefore, if significant pancreatic necrosis is suspected, CT imaging becomes preferable. Such images should be limited to reduce fetal exposure. In most cases, this radiologic study is unnecessary.

In evaluating the pregnant patient with suspected pancreatitis, the differential diagnosis includes most causes of abdominal pain in young women. These are principally peptic ulcer disease including perforation, acute cholecystitis, biliary colic, and intestinal obstruction. Specific tests employed to corroborate the diagnosis of pancreatitis rely on the measurement of pancreatic enzymes, principally amylase. Elevated values should suggest pancreatitis, although they may be present with other conditions such as cholecystitis, intestinal obstruction, peptic ulcer disease, hepatic trauma, and ruptured ectopic pregnancy. There is controversy as to whether serum amylase values are affected during gestation.[16] For this reason, serum lipase levels should be measured in suspected cases.

In most cases, acute pancreatitis resolves spontaneously within several days. However, in some 10 percent of cases, the illness is complicated and such patients are best managed in an intensive care environment. Pancreatic secretory activity should be reduced by keeping the patient NPO. Nasogastric suction is reserved for those with nausea and vomiting. Meperidine is the drug of choice for analgesia as, unlike morphine, it does not constrict the sphincter of Oddi. Fluid and electrolyte replacement, and serial laboratory assays of hemoglobin, white blood cell count, amylase, liver function enzymes, glucose, and calcium are essential. In advanced cases, hypocalcemia may be present, and calcium replacement is necessary. Patients who have been unable to eat for periods of greater than 1 week may benefit from intravenous alimentation.

Percutaneous aspiration of pancreatic exudate is important in refractory cases. This CT-guided procedure may be necessary to distinguish between sterile and infected pancreatic necrosis. For infected cases, surgical drainage of the pancreatic exudate is necessary. Jacobs et al. found that profoundly ill patients survived twice as often if they underwent surgical drainage.[17] Of course, laparotomy, carries with it the added risks of preterm labor and delivery. Patients who relapse may also develop a pseudocyst. This complication requires surgical intervention after a period of time in which an adequate drainage procedure can be accomplished. In spite of the high rate of preterm labor even in conservatively managed cases, the fetal salvage rate, in cases of maternal pancreatitis, has been reported to be as high as 89 percent.[12]

INFLAMMATORY BOWEL DISEASE

The inflammatory bowel diseases, ulcerative colitis (UC) and Crohn's disease (CD), or regional enteritis, are idiopathic disorders that have their peak incidence in the reproductive age group. UC is a disease of the colon or rectum, marked by acute attacks of bloody stools, diarrhea, cramping, abdominal pain, weight loss, and dehydration. The histologic findings include a decreased number of goblet cells, crypt abscesses, ulcerations, and an inflammatory infiltrate consisting of lymphocytes, plasma cells, and polymorphonuclear cells. The prevalence of UC in the female population under 40 years of age is 40 to 100 per 100,000.[18] CD is considerably less common than UC with an incidence of 2 to 4 per 100,000. The average age of onset is between 20 and 30 years. CD, in contrast to UC, tends to run a more subacute and chronic course, with symptoms including fever, diarrhea, and cramping abdominal pain.[19] CD may be found anywhere from mouth to anus including the perineum. However, the distal ileum, colon, and anorectal region are most frequently involved. Histologically, the inflammation is focal with fissuring, ulcerations and prominent lymphoid aggregates present. The hallmark of the histologic diagnosis is transmural involvement of the bowel coupled with the presence of multiple noncaseating granulomas. Because CD may involve only the colon, histologic differentiation from UC becomes important.

Ulcerative Colitis

The primary symptom in UC is bloody diarrhea. Frequent bowel movements with pus, intestinal cramping, fever, dehydration, and anemia are also observed with flaring of disease. Physical examination and laboratory data are nonspecific, with the diagnosis resting on endoscopic examination and biopsy.

Most studies have failed to provide adequate information on the specific effects of this disease on fertility. Early reports suggested a fertility rate of 15 to 31 percent, however, few data were provided about fertility assessment in these women as well as their partners.[20,21] Subsequently, Willoughby and Truelove provided data that suggested that UC had little if any effect on fertility.[22] Of 137 women desiring pregnancy, 119 (87 percent) conceived, a rate similar to most normal populations. This study, however, spanned 10 years and may not reflect periods of impaired fertility related to increased activity of the disease.

Data describing the influence of UC on pregnancy outcome is more conclusive. Abramson first described the pregnancy outcome of patients with UC according to their disease during gestation.[24] In this report, group I consisted of women with inactive disease at the start of pregnancy; group II, patients with active disease in early pregnancy; group III, patients with onset of disease during gestation; and group IV, patients in whom disease developed during the puerperium.[24] The data revealed that patients in group I had the best prognosis, as 18 of 20 had full-term pregnancies, with 7 experiencing exacerbation of disease during gestation or in the postpartum period. Of 12 patients in group II, all had term pregnancies marked by exacerbation of disease during pregnancy or the puerperium. Of five women in group III whose disease commenced during pregnancy, three fetal deaths occurred. It should be remembered, however, that this report antedated the use of steroids and other medications presently available to control active disease.

In 1956, Crohn et al. published their experience with UC in pregnancy.[25] They analyzed the perinatal outcomes in 110 women during 150 pregnancies using Abramson's classification. Group I contained 74 pregnancies in which 62 were successful. The disease was reactivated in 54 percent of cases including all six spontaneous abortions. Group II patients suffered reactivation of disease during pregnancy or postpartum in nearly 75 percent of cases. Pregnancy was successful in 84 percent (32 of 38) of women in this group. The Crohn et al. data suggested that patients with reactivation of quiescent disease during pregnancy had higher rates of abortion.[25] However, their 19 group III patients with new-onset disease experienced only one stillbirth and no spontaneous losses. In contrast, a Danish study demonstrated a higher probability of miscarriage in women with active disease at conception. Seven of 19 women in this category versus 9 of 133 with quiescent disease suffered a miscarriage.[26]

Willoughby and Truelove have confirmed that a good outcome can generally be expected in pregnancies complicated by UC.[22] Furthermore, their study described a group of 102 patients treated with modern therapies, including either steroids, sulfasalazine, or both. They recorded a spontaneous abortion rate of only 11 percent in 216 women followed over a 20-year period.[25] Women with quiescent disease at conception had a slightly greater chance of successfully reaching term when compared with patients whose disease was active during pregnancy. The proportion of low-birth-weight babies and the incidence of anomalies was similar to that of the general population. This study also examined the effect of pregnancy on UC. Of the 129 pregnancies in which colitis was quiescent at the time of conception, 90 (70 percent) of the patients remained free of symptoms throughout pregnancy and the puerperium.

Crohn's Disease

As Crohn's disease may affect any part of the gastrointestinal tract, its clinical presentation depends on the area of involvement. In most cases, abdominal pain with fever and nonbloody diarrhea are observed.

It has been difficult to determine the effect of CD on fertility. In studies that lacked full evaluation and follow-up, Crohn et al.[27] and Fielding and Cooke[28] reported infertility rates of 38 percent and 26 percent, respectively. Interestingly, Fielding and Cooke's study revealed a much higher infertility rate (67 percent) if CD involved the colon. DeDombal et al.[29] have confirmed that a high proportion of patients with large bowel disease are "subfertile." They suggest that temporary infertility may be related to the activity of the disease.[22] Khosla et al.[30] described infertility in 112 patients with CD and reported a 12 percent rate, similar to that seen in the general population. In a case-control study, the number of offspring of women with CD was 57 percent of that of paired controls. This study concluded that disease location had no influence on fertility.[31]

Studies describing the effect of CD on pregnancy suggest minimal if any increased risk to both mother and fetus. In Crohn's original report, 53 patients with regional ileitis had 84 pregnancies, and 75 (89 percent) infants survived. Seventy-one of these deliveries occurred at term.[27] However, the three patients who developed CD during pregnancy suffered two stillbirths and one preterm delivery. The only maternal death occurred in this group. Fielding and Cooke also reported favorable outcomes in a series of patients with both regional ileitis and Crohn's colitis. Their study described an 85 percent live-birth rate among 52 women in 98 pregnancies. Other studies confirm these excellent results, with full-term delivery rates of 73 to 83 percent.[32,33]

Three investigations suggest that active CD carries with it a greater risk of spontaneous miscarriage.[30,32,33] Khosla et al.[30] reported a spontaneous loss rate of 35 percent in patients with active disease at the time of conception and 50 percent in patients with severe disease. These data are supported by Danish and Canadian studies in which the risk of both preterm delivery and spontaneous abortion were found to be significantly higher in women with active disease at conception.[32,33]

A subgroup of patients deserves further mention, those who first develop disease during pregnancy. The caution about unfavorable outcomes in such patients has been supported by Martimbeau et al.[34] They reported 10 patients including one with twins in whom infant deaths occurred. Four of these neonatal deaths followed an operative procedure. However, tocolytics and neonatal intensive care were unavailable in most of these cases.

The effect of pregnancy on CD is similar to that reported for patients with UC. DeDombal et al.[29] reported that 73 percent of patients had no change in disease activity, 15 percent improved and 10 percent worsened during pregnancy. If a woman conceives while CD is in remission, she is just as likely to remain in remission as a nonpregnant patient. In Woolfson et al.'s study, 18 of 73 (25 percent) women with quiescent CD at conception relapsed during pregnancy.[33] Maintenance on medication did not affect the relapse rate. In a study by Khosla et al.,[30] postpartum flare-ups were virtually absent in contrast to DeDombal et al.'s[29] report of a 40 percent postpartum recurrence rate. Khosla et al.[30] also noted that patients with clinically active disease at the time of conception usually continue to have symptoms during pregnancy. Only 7 of 20 patients (35 percent) in this category went into remission or had slight improvement with pregnancy. Overall, the risk of exacerbation during pregnancy is not higher than that in the nonpregnant population.[31]

Treatment of Inflammatory Bowel Disease During Pregnancy

The medical treatment of inflammatory bowel disease is not altered greatly by pregnancy. All patients should be followed closely so that the activity of their disease may be assessed and psychological support can be provided. Since emotional tension may adversely affect both UC and CD, it is important that patients with inflammatory bowel disease have the opportunity to discuss the stress of pregnancy openly. Dietary counseling for patients with UC should emphasize proper nutritional intake. Patients with mild disease may respond to a low-roughage diet or the exclusion of milk products if they are lactose intolerant. In contrast, patients with CD often benefit from low-residue diets, presumably because the caliber of their small bowel may be limited by inflammation.

The initial therapy for inflammatory bowel disease during pregnancy is 5-aminosalicylic acid (5-ASA) products and corticosteroid therapy. The safety of both of these classes of medication has been well established in pregnancy. Sulfasalazine (Azulfidine) is most effective in maintaining remission and preventing further attacks. Patients who present early in pregnancy on sulfasalazine for a recent flare of their disease should probably be maintained on this therapy, as active colitis may develop if the drug is discontinued. The active metabolite of sulfasalazine, 5-ASA and its N-acetyl derivative, are also available for treatment.[35] These medications (Rowasa, Penta, Asocol) are all category B drugs. Concerns about the use of sulfasalazine in late pregnancy centered on its ability to cross the placenta, displace bilirubin, and cause kernicterus. However, the active fetal metabolite, sulfapyridine, has weak bilirubin displacing activity, and the actual risk is small. Jaundice was not increased in 209 neonates of women treated with Azulfidine. The safety of sulfasalazine in breastfeeding has raised some concern. The concentration of sulfapyridine in breast milk is approximately 45 percent that of maternal serum. Similarly, concentrations of 5-ASA are lower in fetal plasma and breast milk than in maternal serum.[35] Thus, sulfasalazine and 5-ASA can be given safely to nursing mothers.[36]

Steroids are indicated in patients who fail to respond to simple supportive measures. Steroid retention enemas may be effective for mild to moderate distal colitis or proctitis. Patients with severe disease are initially treated with high doses of intravenous hydrocortisone or its equivalent. Oral prednisone can then be substituted and tapered as the attack subsides. The safety of corticosteroids and sulfasalazine in pregnancy associated with inflammatory bowel disease was addressed in a national survey by Mogadam et al.[36] In examining 287 pregnancies in which either or both drugs were employed versus 244 untreated patients, no adverse effects could be found that were attributable to these drugs. The higher complication rates associated with severe CD in this study seemed to be more related to disease activity rather than the use of medication.

Occasionally, patients with inflammatory bowel disease may receive azathioprine for treatment. The safety of this medication during pregnancy remains controversial. Similarly, mercaptopurine (class D) or cyclosporine (class C) should be avoided in most cases during pregnancy. Alstead and colleagues[37] recently reported 16 pregnancies in 14 women receiving azathioprine for inflammatory bowel disease. There was one infectious complication of pregnancy (hepatitis B infection), but no congenital abnormalities or health problems in the offspring.[37] The decision to utilize this medication must be made after consultation with the patient including weighing the risk of exacerbation of disease upon discontinuation.

Patients with severe disease who become profoundly dehydrated require hospitalization and intravenous flu-

ids. The development of significant hypoalbuminemia coupled with inadequate caloric intake may require the institution of parenteral hyperalimentation. The benefits of such nutritional therapy include diminished gastrointestinal secretion and motility, potential relief of partial obstruction, closure of fistulas, and renewal of immunocompetence. Anemia should also be treated aggressively by transfusion, although mild anemias will generally respond to oral iron therapy.

Surgical Treatment

Although most acute episodes of inflammatory bowel disease respond to medical treatment, operative intervention will occasionally be necessary to treat perforation, obstruction, or patients unresponsive to standard therapies. While elective surgery for medically intractable disease or recurrent dysplastic lesions of the colon is best accomplished following pregnancy, patients who have undergone definitive surgical procedures for UC seem to fare well during pregnancy. Surgery during pregnancy does carry a significant risk of preterm delivery, probably due to the amount of uterine manipulation required during efforts to reach the distal colon. Surgery should not be delayed, however, in cases of perforation or complete obstruction. Anderson and colleagues[38] have reported three cases of emergency colectomy during pregnancy for toxic megacolon in women with fulminant UC. There were no maternal deaths; however, two stillbirths occurred as well as one preterm delivery.[38]

Ileostomy function during pregnancy is normal in most cases. Of 84 term pregnancies reported by Hudson, intestinal obstruction occurred in just 7 cases.[39] Of 17 cesarean sections performed in his series, all were done for obstetric indications. Similarly, Gopal and colleagues[40] described 82 pregnancies in 66 women following colostomy or ileostomy. Stomal dysfunction responded to conservative measures in all but three women who required surgery for intestinal obstruction. Complications from an episiotomy have been uncommon in patients previously operated on for UC. Data is not available for CD. However, the higher rate of perineal involvement in these patients should warrant a thorough evaluation before contemplating vaginal delivery.

Surgery for CD, unlike UC, in generally not curative. It is estimated that 40 percent of patients with ileitis will require surgery at some time for obstruction, perforation, extensive fistulas, or perirectal suppuration.[38] Most surgical procedures must limit the amount of bowel resection because of the diffuse nature of this disease. Prior bowel resection has been associated with increased risk of preterm delivery and spontaneous miscarriage.

Patients with Crohn's colitis who have undergone

proctocolectomy are at substantial risk for recurrent disease including persistent perineal wounds in up to 60 percent of cases.[41] Cesarean delivery should be considered for patients with perianal disease who have been diverted to promote healing. Those patients with CD who require surgery during pregnancy are usually operated on for obstruction.[42] As with UC, there may be a high incidence of fetal loss. The decision to perform a simultaneous cesarean delivery must be individualized according to the type of procedure involved, its indications and the gestational age of the pregnancy.

Key Points

➤ Women with peptic ulcer disease usually have improvement in symptoms during pregnancy. Primary medical treatment for symptomatic cases is antacid therapy and diet. Secondary therapy is H$_2$ blockers.

➤ Most cases of pancreatitis during pregnancy are associated with gallstones. Conservative supportive care aimed at decreasing pancreatic secretion is generally successful.

➤ Women with active ulcerative colitis in early pregnancy usually have recurrent flare-ups during gestation and postpartum.

➤ The onset of ulcerative colitis or Crohn's disease during pregnancy is associated with increased miscarriage and fetal loss rates.

➤ Sulfasalazine (Azulfidine) and 5-ASA metabolite drugs may be safely used to treat inflammatory bowel disease during pregnancy and in lactating women.

References

1. Clark DH: Peptic ulcer in women. BMJ 1:1259, 1953.
2. Vessey MP, Villard-Mackintoch L, Painter R: Oral contraceptives and pregnancy in relation to peptic ulcer. Contraception 46:349, 1992.
3. Clark DH, Tankel HI: Gastric acid and plasma histaminase during pregnancy. Lancet 2:886, 1954.
4. Warzech S, Spiro HM, Schwartz RD, Pilot ML: Peptic ulcer in pregnancy. A serial study of gastric secretion during pregnancy. Am J Dig Dis 4:289, 1959.
5. VanThiel DH, Gavaler JS, Joshi SN, et al: Heartburn of pregnancy. Gastroenterology 72:666, 1977.
6. Lewis JH, Weingold AB: The use of gastrointestinal drugs during pregnancy and lactation. Am J Gastroenterol 80:912, 1985.
7. Parker S, Schade R, Pohl C, et al: Prenatal and neonatal exposure of male rats to cimetidine but not ranitidine adversely affect subsequent sexual functioning. Gastroenterology 86:675, 1984.
8. Baron TH, Ramirez B, Richter JE: Gastrointestinal motility disorders during pregnancy. Ann Intern Med 118:306, 1993.
9. Becker-Anderson H, Husfelt V: Peptic ulcer in pregnancy. Acta Obstet Gynecol Scand 59:391, 1971.
10. McKay AJ, O'Neill J, Imrie CW: Pancreatitis, pregnancy, and gallstones. Br J Obstet Gynaecol 87:47, 1980.
11. Corlett RC, Mishell DR: Pancreatitis in pregnancy. Am J Obstet Gynecol 113:281, 1972.
12. Wilkinson EJ: Acute pancreatitis in pregnancy: a review of 98 cases and a report of 8 new cases. Obstet Gynecol Surv 28:281, 1973.
13. Block P, Kelly TR: Management of gallstone pancreatitis during pregnancy and the postpartum period. Surg Gynecol Obstet 168:426, 1989.
14. Achard JM, Westeel PF, Morniere P, et al: Pancreatitis related to severe acute hypertriglyceridemia during pregnancy: treatment with lipoprotein apheresis. Intensive Care Med 17:236, 1991.
15. Sanderson SL, Iverius PH, Wilson DE: Successful hyperlipemic pregnancy. JAMA 265:1858, 1991.
16. DeVore GR, Bracken M, Berkowitz RL: The amylase/creatinine clearance ratio in normal pregnancy and pregnancies complicated by pancreatitis, hyperemesis gravidarum, and toxemia. Am J Obstet Gynecol 136:747, 1980.
17. Jacobs ML, Daggett WM, Civetta JM: Acute pancreatitis: analysis of factors influencing survival. Ann Surg 185:43, 1977.
18. Kirsner JB, Shorter RG: Recent developments in non-specific inflammatory bowel disease. N Engl J Med 306:775, 1982.
19. Sorokin JJ, Levine SM: Pregnancy and inflammatory bowel disease: a review of the literature. Obstet Gynecol 62:247, 1983.
20. MacDougall I: Ulcerative colitis and pregnancy. Lancet 271:641, 1956.
21. Hudson M, Flett G, Sinclar TS, et al: Fertility and pregnancy in inflammatory bowel disease. Int J Gynaecol Obstet 58:229, 1997.
22. Willoughby CP, Truelove SC: Ulcerative colitis and pregnancy. Gut 21:469, 1980.
23. Felsen J, Wolarsky W: Chronic ulcerative colitis and pregnancy. Am J Obstet Gynecol 56:751, 1948.
24. Abramson D, Jankelson IR, Milner LR: Pregnancy in idiopathic ulcerative colitis. Am J Obstet Gynecol 6:121, 1951.
25. Crohn BB, Yarnis H, Cohen EB, et al: Ulcerative colitis and pregnancy. Gastroenterology 30:391, 1956.
26. Nielson OH, Andreasson B, Dondesen S, et al: Pregnancy in ulcerative colitis. Scand J Gastroenterol 18:735, 1986.
27. Crohn BB, Yarnis H, Korelitz BI: Regional ileitis complicating pregnancy. Gastroenterology 31:615, 1956.
28. Fielding JF, Cooke WT: Pregnancy and Crohn's disease. BMJ 2:76, 1970.
29. DeDombal FT, Burton IL, Goligher JC: Crohn's disease and pregnancy. BMJ 3:550, 1972.
30. Khosla R, Willoughby CP, Jewell DP: Crohn's disease and pregnancy. Gut 25:52, 1984.
31. Mayberry JF, Weterman IT: European survey of fertility and pregnancy in women with Crohn's disease: a case control study by European collaborative group. Gut 27:821, 1986.
32. Haagen Nielsen O, Andreasson B, Bondesen B, et al: Pregnancy in Crohn's disease. Scand J Gastroenterol 19:724, 1984.
33. Woolfson K, Cohen Z, McLeod RS: Crohn's disease and pregnancy. Dis Colon Rectum 33:869, 1990.
34. Martimbeau PW, Welch JS, Weiland LH: Crohn's disease and pregnancy. Am J Obstet Gynecol 122:746, 1975.
35. Christensen LA, Rasmussen SN, Hansen SH: Disposition of

5-aminosalicylic acid and N-acetyl-5-aminosalicylic acid in fetal and maternal body fluids during treatment with different 5-aminosalicylic acid preparation. Acta Obstet Scand 73:399, 1994.

36. Mogadam M, Dibbins MO, Korelitz BI, Ahmed SW: Pregnancy and inflammatory bowel disease: effect of sulfasalazine and corticosteroids on fetal outcome. Gastroenterology 80:72, 1981.

37. Alstead EM, Ritchie JK, Lennard-Jones JE, et al: Safety of azathioprine in pregnancy in inflammatory bowel disease. Gastroenterology 99:443, 1990.

38. Anderson JB, Turner GM, Williamson RCN: Fulminant ulcerative colitis in late pregnancy and the puerperium. Proc R Soc Med 80:492, 1987.

39. Hudson CN: Ileostomy in pregnancy. Proc R Soc Med 65:281, 1972.

40. Gopal KA, Amshel AL, Shonberg IL, et al: Ostomy and pregnancy. Dis Colon Rectum 28:912, 1985.

41. Block GE: Surgical management of Crohn's colitis. N Engl J Med 302:1068, 1980.

42. Davis MR, Bohon CJ: Intestinal obstruction in pregnancy. Clin Obstet Gynecol 26:832, 1983.

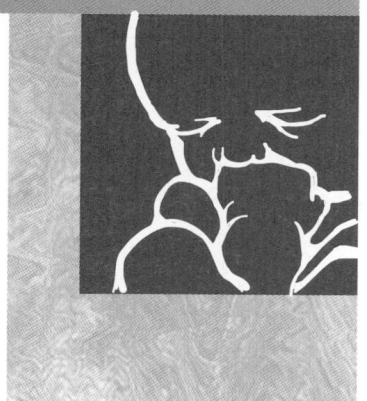

Chapter 37

Neurologic Disorders

PHILIP SAMUELS

SEIZURE DISORDERS

Affecting approximately 1 percent of the general population, seizure disorders are the most frequent major neurologic complication encountered in pregnancy. Seizure disorders may be divided into those that are acquired and those that are idiopathic. Acquired seizure disorders, which account for less than 15 percent of all seizures, may result from trauma, infection, space-occupying lesions, or metabolic disorders. Over 85 percent of seizure disorders are classified as idiopathic, meaning that no etiologic agent or inciting incident can be identified. Idiopathic seizures can be divided into types such as tonic-clonic, partial complex with or without generalization, myoclonic, focal, or absence.

In general, initial therapy is based on the type of seizure disorder experienced by the patient. There are, however, many crossovers, and patients may respond differently to each medication despite their seizure type. It is, therefore, not unusual to encounter a patient with any seizure type who may be taking any of the major antiepileptic medications. Furthermore, patients may be placed on a certain medication because they did not tolerate the side-effect profile of another anticonvulsant (Table 37–1). Because of the prevalence of this group of disorders in women of childbearing age, the stigmata surrounding epilepsy, and the misguided fears many patients and physicians have surrounding epilepsy in pregnancy, the treatment of the pregnant patient with a seizure disorder can create quite a challenge for the obstetrician. In addition, many patients with epilepsy have done very well on their medications so they have not been evaluated by a neurologist in many years. Some patients have been seizure free for many years and have stopped their medications, while others have been seizure free for many years but have continued to take their medication without being reevaluated. Still others have poorly controlled seizures, and it is unclear whether this is due to noncompliance with or ineffectiveness of their medication regimen. Other patients may be taking two medications when they may need only one. The obstetrician and neurologist must work closely together to guide the patient through her pregnancy and find the safest and most effective medical therapy for the patient. Through this cooperation, the vast majority of pregnant women with seizure disorders can have a successful pregnancy with minimal risk to mother and fetus.

Effects of Epilepsy on Reproductive Function

Women with seizure disorders should seek care from an obstetrician/gynecologist as soon as they become sexually active. Contraception may present a challenge to women with epilepsy, and the use of oral contraceptives may require special adjustments. Certain antiepileptic medications have been associated with contraceptive failure. Carbamazepine, phenobarbital, and phenytoin enhance the activities of hepatic microsomal oxidative enzymes.[1] The cytochrome P450 system is shared by these medications as well as by the steroid hormones. This increased enzymatic activity may lead to rapid clearance of these hormones, which may allow ovulation to occur. Therefore, medicated patients taking low-dose oral contraceptives, which are being prescribed with increasing frequency, may have more breakthrough bleeding[2] and may be at increased risk for unplanned pregnancy.[3,4] This rapid clearance does not appear to be induced by valproate or benzodiazepines.[1]

Fertility rates may be lower in patients with epilepsy.

Table 37–1. COMMON SIDE EFFECTS OF ANTICONVULSANTS

Drug	Maternal Effects	Fetal Effects
Phenytoin	Nystagmus, ataxia, hirsutism, gingival hyperplasia, megaloblastic anemia	Possible teratogenesis and carcinogenesis, coagulopathy, hypocalcemia
Phenobarbital	Drowsiness, ataxia	Possible teratogenesis, coagulopathy, neonatal depression, withdrawal
Primidone	Drowsiness, ataxia, nausea	Possible teratogenesis, coagulopathy, neonatal depression
Carbamazepine	Drowsiness, leukopenia, ataxia, mild hepatotoxicity	Possible craniofacial and neural tube defects
Valproic acid	Ataxia, drowsiness, alopecia, hepatotoxicity, thrombocytopenia	Neural tube defects and possible craniofacial and skeletal defects
Ethosuximide	Nausea, hepatotoxicity, leukopenia, thrombocytopenia	Possible teratogenesis

A retrospective study by Webber and colleagues[5] reviewed fertility rates in individuals with epilepsy over a 50-year period. They found that fertility rates were significantly lower in both men and women with epilepsy and that this could not be explained solely by the rate of marriage in these patients. Men appeared to be more adversely affected than women. Women with epilepsy had fertility rates 85 percent of the expected. Furthermore, in this retrospective review, women with partial seizures seemed to have lower fertility rates than those with generalized seizures. In a study by Dansky et al.,[6] fertility rates appeared to be lower in those women with early-onset epilepsy than those with late onset. Cramer and Jones[1] also reviewed a study published in Poland in 1979 that investigated the fertility rate in 263 unselected patients with epilepsy. They found that the fertility rate was half that of the general population, and 25 percent of married patients had no children.[1] All of these cited studies concerning lower fertility rates have many methodologic problems. Yet, even in these studies, the majority of patients with epilepsy were able to conceive without difficulty. Nonetheless, the practicing obstetrician/gynecologist should be prepared to undertake an infertility evaluation of these patients or to refer them to an infertility specialist should the need arise.

Effect of Pregnancy on Epilepsy

It has been taught that between 30 percent and 50 percent of patients will show an increase in seizure frequency during pregnancy. This was confirmed in the classic study of Knight and Rhind[7] of 153 pregnancies in 59 patients between 1953 and 1973. In that study, 45 percent of patients showed an increase in seizure frequency during pregnancy, while 50 percent had no change and 4.8 percent experienced a decrease. It is very important to note that anticonvulsant levels could not be readily measured until the mid 1970s. When the study of Knight and Rhind[7] was performed, anticonvul-

sant doses were usually only increased by physicians when patients had breakthrough seizures. An important finding from that study, however, was that patients with more frequent seizures tended to have exacerbations during pregnancy.[8] In fact, virtually all patients who had more than one seizure each month experienced worsening of their epilepsy during pregnancy, whereas only about 25 percent of patients who had not had a seizure in over 9 months experienced exacerbation of epilepsy during pregnancy. With the introduction of new medications and the ability to monitor anticonvulsant levels, these absolute numbers are no longer true. The relationship, however, does remain. Patients with more frequent seizures tend to have exacerbations of seizures during pregnancy. In a large study by Schmidt et al.,[8] 63 percent of patients had no change or a decrease in seizure frequency during pregnancy, while only 37 percent of patients had an increase of seizures during pregnancy. Importantly, in 34 of the 50 patients who showed an increase in seizure frequency during pregnancy, the increase was associated with noncompliance with their drug regimen or sleep deprivation. Conversely, in 7 of the 18 pregnancies in which improvement of seizure frequency was shown, this was related to improved compliance with the drug regimen or a correction of sleep deprivation for the 9 months preceding pregnancy. In a study by Tanganelli and Regesta,[9] seizure frequency did not change or improved in 82.6 percent of pregnancies. As has been shown in other studies, increases in seizure frequency were often due to noncompliance with medication regimens as well as frequent seizures in the preconception period. In contrast, Sabers et al. summarized 151 pregnancies in 124 women with epilepsy between 1978 and 1992.[10] They found 21 percent of patients has exacerbations of their seizures during pregnancy and 71 percent were only taking one medication.[10]

In summary, we now have the means to monitor anticonvulsant levels in patients frequently, and we have the medications to control seizures. We also understand that sleep deprivation can be a catalyst for seizures. With patient cooperation and close surveillance, seizure frequency should remain the same or even improve in most epileptic patients during pregnancy.

Effects of Pregnancy on the Disposition of Anticonvulsant Medications

It is well known that the levels of anticonvulsant medications can change dramatically during pregnancy. They usually decrease in total concentration as pregnancy progresses. Many factors including altered protein binding, delayed gastric emptying, nausea and vomiting, changes in plasma volume, and changes in the volume of distribution can affect the levels of anticonvulsant medications. It is beyond the scope of this chapter to elucidate these mechanisms. Without some understanding of this subject, however, it is difficult to manage the patient with epilepsy correctly. Therefore, some of the salient points of this topic are covered.

As phenytoin is one of the most widely prescribed anticonvulsant medications, its metabolism and elimination are discussed. Landon and Kirkley[11] and Kochenour et al.[12] showed that the serum concentration of phenytoin tends to fall during pregnancy and rise again during the puerperium and postpartum periods. Several factors can account for this. In early gestation, patients often have nausea and vomiting. Phenytoin is usually administered on a once-daily basis. If the patient vomits the medication, the drug levels will be highly variable. Furthermore, an increase in calcium intake during pregnancy, as well as the use of antacids, will lead to the formation of insoluble complexes with phenytoin, resulting in lower total drug levels. Also, with delayed gastric emptying in pregnancy, the time to peak drug level will be lengthened. Phenytoin is inactivated in the liver. Its rate of conversion may increase greatly during pregnancy, as the activity of oxidative enzymes increases. This is due to increased progesterone levels, which induce enzyme activity. This may also be enhanced by increased folic acid, which serves as a cofactor in these metabolic processes. Outside of pregnancy, approximately 90 percent of phenytoin is protein bound. Plasma albumin levels decrease during pregnancy while other protein levels may rise. This will cause changes in the total phenytoin level that do not necessarily reflect the free, active phenytoin concentrations. This effect is also enhanced by free fatty acids displacing phenytoin from albumin. In a recent study by Yerby et al.,[13] free levels of phenobarbital, carbamazepine, and phenytoin rose significantly throughout pregnancy while total levels fell. Therefore, the nonpregnant relationship between total drug and free (active) drug is not maintained. Free phenytoin levels, therefore, should be measured if possible. If free levels

are unavailable, drug doses should be adjusted according to the total serum level and the clinical picture. If the patient has increased seizure activity, medication doses should be increased as long as the patient is not showing signs of toxicity. Likewise, if the medication level is low but the patient is seizure free, no adjustment in dosing is necessary.

Similar pharmacokinetic changes occur in phenobarbital and carbamazepine, but to different degrees. Both of these drugs also show changes in protein binding and increased hepatic clearance during pregnancy. With phenobarbital, the protein binding is considerably less than phenytoin, and changes in plasma protein are less likely to be clinically significant. Primidone is an anticonvulsant medication that is metabolized to phenobarbital and another active metabolite, phenylethylmalonic acid diamide. When checking primidone levels, one must also check levels of phenobarbital. Infants born to mothers who have been taking barbiturates during pregnancy may exhibit some withdrawal symptoms that begin about 1 week after birth and usually last 1 to 2 weeks.[14] These symptoms usually involve minor irritability but may occasionally be more serious.

Carbamazepine also has an active metabolite, carbamazepine 10,11-epoxide. This metabolite can be measured and this measurement can be clinically useful in many instances. Carbamazepine is not as highly protein bound as phenytoin and is therefore not subject to as wide a fluctuation due to changes in protein levels. Carbamazepine also induces its own metabolic enzymes in the liver, so the half-life changes as the dose increases.[12]

All anticonvulsants interfere with folic acid metabolism. Patients on anticonvulsants may actually become folic acid deficient and develop macrocytic anemia. Folic acid deficiency has been associated with neural tube defects and other congenital malformations.[15,16] Because organogenesis occurs during the first weeks after conception, folic acid supplementation should be begun before pregnancy if possible. A dose of 4 mg daily is more than sufficient. As previously stated, increasing folic acid ingestion may increase the activity of hepatic microsomal enzymes and thus the clearance of anticonvulsant medications. Levels should be checked frequently, therefore, after folic acid therapy is implemented. Furthermore, therapy with phenytoin may result in increased metabolism of vitamin D, leading to decreased vitamin D levels. This has been shown to cause neonatal hypocalcemia in one case report.[17] The patient should be reminded to take her prenatal vitamins, which include an adequate amount of vitamin D to prevent problems.

Neonatal hemorrhage, due to decreased vitamin K–dependent clotting factors (II, VII, IX, X), has been seen in infants born to mothers taking phenobarbital, phenytoin, and primidone.[18] In one series,[18] 8 of 16 infants exposed to these medications had a cord blood coagulation pattern similar to that of a vitamin K deficiency. This occurred earlier than the customary hemorrhagic disease of the newborn. These infants responded to vitamin K infusion. Bleyer and Skinner[19] reviewed a case of their own and another 21 cases of hemorrhagic disease following anticonvulsant therapy that have appeared in the literature. They reached similar conclusions that these cases are vitamin K–dependent clotting factors deficiencies and that, at birth, infants should be given 1 mg of vitamin K intramuscularly.

Effect of Epilepsy on Pregnancy

The majority of women with seizure disorders who become pregnant will have an uneventful pregnancy with an excellent outcome. There appear, however, to be several pregnancy complications that are more prevalent in the mother with epilepsy than in the general population. In a review of all birth certificates for infants born in the state of Washington in 1980–81, Yerby and co-workers[20] identified 200 births to mothers with seizure disorders. Although birth certificate studies are often limited, these researchers controlled for many variables including previous adverse pregnancy outcome and socioeconomic status.[20] They found that mothers with seizure disorders were 2.66 times more likely to have had a previous fetal death after 20 weeks' gestation than the control population. Because of the retrospective nature of this study, the authors were unable to correlate this with growth restriction or other fetal problems. This increased incidence of stillbirth is confirmed in other studies.[7,21,22] It is unclear in any of these studies what type of fetal surveillance was utilized and if there were any predictors that these fetuses were at risk. Because of the long duration of many of these studies, many patients were pregnant during the 1970s and early 1980s. With the increased use of ultrasound to identify fetal growth restriction, malformations, and oligohydramnios, many of the stillborn fetuses may have been identified as being at risk and might have undergone antepartum fetal testing and intervention before the fetal demise occurred. These studies also were not stratified by medications taken, dosages, drug levels, or seizure activity during pregnancy.

Hiilesmaa et al.,[23] in a study of 150 pregnant women with seizure disorders, found no difference in perinatal mortality between patients and controls. There were, however, three third-trimester stillbirths in the epileptic group and two in the control group. Yerby and colleagues[19] also found an increased incidence of preeclampsia in women with seizure disorders. This has also been identified in other large retrospective studies.[7,21] Hiilesmaa et al.,[23] however, found no difference in the rate of preeclampsia between pregnant women with epilepsy and controls. Yerby et al.[20] also showed a 2.79-fold increase in low-birth-weight infants. In a

carefully performed study in Italy, Mastroiacovo and co-workers[24] found that the mean birth weight in neonates born to women with epilepsy was 107 g lower than controls. The mean birth weight in the epilepsy group, however, still fell within the normal range for gestational age. The clinical significance of this finding, therefore, is questionable. When considering all commonly used anticonvulsants, this decrease in neonatal weight appeared to be more common in infants exposed in utero to phenobarbital.

Mastroiacovo et al.[24] also found a decrease in head circumference in infants of mothers with epilepsy. This effect was seen both in untreated women with epilepsy and in those receiving medications.[24] Although this change was statistically significant, the mean head circumferences of both study and control infants still fell within the normal range. These authors found no difference in neonatal length comparing groups of mothers with epilepsy and control populations. Hiilesmaa et al.[25] also found a decrease in head circumference in neonates born to women with epilepsy. This decrease was most marked in women taking carbamazepine both alone or in combination with phenobarbital. Again, the mean head circumferences, however, were still within the expected normal range.[25] In the follow-up of this study, head circumferences were still smaller at 18 months of age.

Along similar lines, Hvas et al. compared pregnancy outcomes in 193 women with epilepsy to 24,094 women without epilepsy delivering between 1989 and 1997.[26] They found that birth weight of infants born to women with epilepsy was 208 g less than those born to women without a seizure disorder. The odds ratio that a woman treated with epilepsy would give birth to an infant with IUGR was 1.9.[26] Head circumference and body length were also diminished in the infants born to women taking antiepileptic drugs. When smokers with and without epilepsy were compared, there was an increased risk of preterm birth in those who smoked.[26] Battine et al. examined anthropometrics in children born to women with epilepsy in Canada, Japan, and Italy.[27] They found some distinct geographic differences in risk for decreased head circumference that may or may not be drug regimen related. The relative risk for small head circumference in infants exposed to more than one medication (polytherapy) was 2.7.[27] A dose-dependent response for both head circumference and body weight was seen with the use of phenobarbital and primidone.[27] The authors state that in addition to drug regimen, genetic, ethnic, and environmental effects should be taken into account when considering explanations for decreased head circumference and birthweight in infants born to women treated for epilepsy.[27]

Yerby and colleagues[20] found a sixfold increased rate of maternal herpes in women with epilepsy. There is no readily available explanation for this, and it has not been seen in other studies, although it is doubtful that anyone has looked for this as an endpoint. They further found a significant decrease in 1- and 5-minute Apgar scores. This may be attributed to fetal effect of maternal depressant medications such as phenobarbital. Conversely, Hiilesmaa et al.[23,25] found no increase in pregnancy complications in women with epilepsy. They found no increase in preterm labor, bleeding, pregnancy-induced hypertension, operative vaginal delivery, or cesarean delivery rates. These authors imply that the lack of increased operative deliveries in their study is due to the comfort of the obstetrician in caring for patients with seizure disorders. However, Yerby et al.[20] found an increased rate of cesarean deliveries in their review. For uncertain reasons, they also found an unexplained increase in third trimester amniocentesis and labor inductions. This may be construed as insecurity on the part of the obstetrician in caring for the patient with a seizure disorder and the desire to effect a delivery as soon as fetal pulmonary maturity could be documented.

In summary, there appears to be an increased risk of stillbirths in women with seizure disorders. The cause of this is not readily apparent but may be due to factors that are easily detectable today (such as intrauterine growth restriction) that were not detected when these studies were carried out. It also appears that infants born to mothers with seizure disorders, on average, are smaller than their control counterparts. It is uncertain whether the incidence of actual intrauterine growth restriction is higher. Furthermore, the incidence of preeclampsia may be higher in mothers with seizure disorders. The vast majority of pregnancies, however, will be uncomplicated with no increase in complications over the expected rate. Nonetheless, because of these few potential problems, the obstetrician should be more surveillant for pregnancy-related complications in pregnant women with seizure disorders.

Effects of Anticonvulsant Medications on the Fetus

There is little doubt that anticonvulsant medications are associated with an increase in congenital malformations, but the magnitude of this risk and the association of certain anomalies with specific drugs remain debatable. Although there was some evidence for teratogenicity related to phenytoin in the 1960s, Hanson and Smith[28] identified a specific fetal hydantoin syndrome in 1975. They noted growth and performance delays, craniofacial abnormalities (including clefting), and limb anomalies (including hypoplasia of nails and distal phalanges). They first reported this syndrome in five infants exposed to phenytoin in utero. Hanson et al.[29] later reported that 7 to 11 percent of infants exposed to phenytoin had this recognizable pattern of malforma-

tions. They furthermore found that 31 percent of exposed fetuses had some aspects of the syndrome. Yet in 1988 Gaily et al.[30] reported no evidence of the hydantoin syndrome in 82 women exposed in utero to phenytoin. Some of the patients had hypertelorism and hypoplasia of the distal phalanges, but none had the full hydantoin syndrome.

Since the original reports by Hanson and colleagues, many studies have reported congenital malformations in infants born to mothers taking anticonvulsant medications. These reports typify the discrepancies that fill the medical literature concerning this subject. There are studies that report each of the commonly used anticonvulsant medications (phenytoin, phenobarbital, carbamazepine, and valproate) is the worst teratogen, yet there are other studies that report each of these medications has a weak teratogenic potential. It remains of prime importance, therefore, to treat the patient with the medication that best controls her seizures. Another example of discrepancies and the need for more research involves the incidence of facial clefting among infants born to mothers with epilepsy. This is one of the most common anomalies found in these neonates. In a study by Friis et al.[31] untreated epileptics had an incidence of facial clefting 2.7 times the expected rate, whereas infants of mothers treated with anticonvulsants had 4.7 times the expected rate of clefting. All of the observed clefts in these groups were cleft lip with or without cleft palate. There was no increased incidence of isolated cleft palate. These authors concluded that epilepsy itself may increase the risk for cleft lip, with anticonvulsant medications increasing the risk even more.[31] A study by Kelly et al.[32] demonstrated that the association between epilepsy and facial clefting is in large part due to shared causal determinants that are probably both genetic and environmental in origin. They believe that the role of anticonvulsant medications in this association seems to be overestimated and probably represents only a modest additive influence. In contrast, however, Hecht et al.[33] in an epidemiologic study, found no evidence for familial association between epilepsy and clefting disorders.

It has now been two decades since Nakane and colleagues[34] published the first major, multi-institutional study investigating the teratogenecity of antiepileptic medications. This study, carried out between 1974 and 1977, examined 902 pregnancies in mothers with idiopathic epilepsy. The overall rate of congenital malformations was 7.2 percent. This included 8.7 percent in the mothers who received anticonvulsant medications during pregnancy and 1.9 percent in nonmedicated mothers. Looking only at liveborn infants, 9.9 percent had malformations (11.5 percent in the medicated group and 2.3 percent in the nonmedicated group). The incidence of malformations in mothers receiving anticonvulsant therapy was therefore about five times that of the nonmedicated group. Interestingly, Canger et al.[35] began collecting data in Italy at the time Nakane's group completed their data collection. Canger and co-workers studied 517 women with epilepsy throughout pregnancy. They found a 9.7 percent rate of malformations, a proportion strikingly similar to that of Nakane.[34]

In Nakane's study,[34] the predominant malformations were cleft lip/palate (3.14 percent) and cardiovascular malformations (2.95 percent). Nakane et al. also noted that as the number of anticonvulsant medications used in combination during pregnancy increased, the incidence of fetal malformations rose dramatically.[34] The malformation rate was less than 5 percent when one medication (monotherapy) was used and was greater than 20 percent when four medications were used. Of note, 537 patients were taking two or more medications while 93 patients were only taking one medication. This is fairly reflective of the prescribing patterns for anticonvulsant medications in the 1970s and shows why many of the studies and case reports from the 1970s are not relevant today, as many more patients are receiving monotherapy. In this study, only 15 percent of patients were treated with a single antiepileptic medication.[34] Congenital heart disease was significantly higher in infants born to mothers taking phenobarbital, and cleft lip/palate was more common in infants born to women taking primidone.

Kaneko and colleagues performed a prospective study to determine primary factors responsible for the increased incidence of malformations in infants born to mothers being treated with anticonvulsants.[36] They specifically looked at various drug combinations. The overall malformation rate was 14 percent. In the 16.1 percent of patients who were receiving a single medication, the malformation rate was 6.5 percent.[36] The malformation rate for those treated with multiple medications was 15.6 percent. There was no dose-dependent increase in the incidence of malformations associated with any individual medication. In this study there was also no relationship between the type of defect and the individual anticonvulsant. This contrasts with the study by Nakane et al.[34] In that study, polypharmacy had a significantly higher risk of causing congenital malformations than other medications.[29]

Kaneko et al.[37] published a follow-up study looking at malformations in infants exposed in utero to anticonvulsant medications. They compared these results with their previous study.[36] The first study looked at infants born between 1978 and 1984, while the later study looked at infants born between 1985 and 1989. Whereas 14 percent of infants had some malformation in the previous study, the malformation rate was only 6.3 percent in the second group.[37] Again, there was no relationship between the medication taken and the type of malformation found.[37] The lower rate of malforma-

tions may be attributable to the increase in patients receiving monotherapy. In the earlier study 16.1 percent of patients received a single medication, whereas 63.4 percent received a single medication in the later study.[37] Jick and Terris[38] matched 2 nonexposed pregnant women to each of 297 pregnant women exposed to antiepileptic medication. The rate of anomalies in infants born to women with epilepsy was 3.4 percent,[38] a rate even lower than that found by Kaneko et al. in their 1992 study.[37] In fact, 3.4 percent does not appear to be much higher than the background rate for congenital anomalies. Nonetheless, Jick and Terris found the relative risk for a woman on antiepileptic medications to give birth to an infant with an anomaly was 3.3.[38]

Most neurologists are treating patients with a single agent. Now that blood levels of anticonvulsant medications can be easily measured, single medications can be given at higher doses to make certain that therapeutic levels are achieved. This has lessened the need for multiple medications in the same patient. Prior to the ability to measure these levels, empiric doses of medication were given. If the patient continued to have seizures, another medication was often added rather than increasing the dose of the initial medication.

The same concept was verified in a study by Lindhout et al.[39] They compared the pattern of malformations in the offspring of two cohorts of women with seizure disorders, one from 1972 to 1979 and one from 1980 to 1985. In the earlier cohort, 15 of 151 (10 percent) of liveborn infants had at least one congenital anomaly. The most common anomalies were those most frequently reported for anticonvulsant medications: congenital heart defects, facial clefts, facial dysmorphism, and developmental retardation. In the later cohort, 13 of 172 infants (7.6 percent) exposed in utero to anticonvulsant medications had congenital malformations.[42] The most frequent anomalies in this group were spinal defects and hypospadias. All of these were associated with maternal therapy with valproate, carbamazepine, or both.[39] In the earlier cohort of patients, the mean number of drugs used during gestation was 2.2 compared with 1.7 in the later cohort. Whereas only 28 percent of women in the earlier cohort received only one medication, 47 percent of the women received monotherapy in the second group of patients. The lower overall rate of malformations in the latter cohort appeared to be due to the reduction in the number of pregnancies during which a combination of medications was used.[39] It is also apparent in this study that neither the duration of maternal epilepsy nor the maternal age was associated with malformations in the infants born to these mothers.

Dravet et al.[40] studied 227 women participating in a prospective study between 1984 and 1988. In that study there was a 7 percent malformation rate among infants born to mothers taking antiepileptic medications compared with 1.36 percent in the control group. Therefore, fetuses exposed in utero to anticonvulsants had a relative risk of 6.9 of being born with a congenital malformation. This is double the risk demonstrated by Jick and Terris.[38] In this study, the frequency of spina bifida was 17 times more than would be expected in the general population, and heart defects were 9.6 times greater than expected. Cleft lip with or without cleft palate was 8.4 times more frequent than expected in the general population. Using logistic regression, these authors concluded that valproate and phenytoin were the two most teratogenic medications.[40] Also in this study, there was a high correlation with congenital heart defects and maternal ingestion of phenobarbital.[40] This finding confirms that of Nakane et al.[34] The cases of neural tube defect and congenital heart defect were studied carefully and could not be related to a familial disposition to these defects. As other studies have shown, there was a higher incidence of malformations in infants born to mothers receiving polytherapy (16 percent) than in those receiving monotherapy (6 percent).

A study by Koch et al.[41] however, shows no difference between the rate of malformations in mothers receiving polytherapy and mothers receiving a single medication. Furthermore, they found that the infants born to mothers with epilepsy, regardless of therapy, had only twice as many major malformations as infants born to the control population. The number of minor anomalies, however, was approximately three times greater in infants born to mothers receiving anticonvulsant medication than in the control group. In the mothers receiving monotherapy, those taking valproate had the highest rate of minor malformations.[41] In this study, there appeared to be a link between the dose of valproate and the rate of malformations.

Gaily and Granstrom[42] also investigated minor anomalies in children of mothers with epilepsy. These authors point out that many of the supposedly specific syndromes resulting from intrauterine exposure to certain medications have many common features. They argue that specific syndromes and their association with specific drugs, as well as the frequencies of these syndromes, have not been confirmed in epidemiologic studies. They found that many of the minor anomalies that are thought to be specific features of a medication appear to be genetically linked with epilepsy.[42] Indeed, this is in contrast to many of the other published studies. In this study only distal digital hypoplasia appeared to be a specific marker for phenytoin teratogenicity. Again, this points out that there is no uniform consensus concerning the teratogenicity of anticonvulsant medications.

Yerby and colleagues[43] also looked prospectively at malformations in infants born to mothers with epilepsy. They further investigated whether pure folate deficiency might be responsible for the malformations. None of the women in their study had deficient folate levels. There was no difference in major malformations between patients and controls in this study.[43] The infants born to mothers taking anticonvulsant medications, however, had a higher mean number of minor anomalies. They found no difference in the number of minor anomalies whether the child was exposed in utero to one anticonvulsant medication or to several.[43] The only specific minor anomaly that was found statistically more frequently in infants born to mothers with epilepsy than in the control population was a prominent occiput. The authors also confirm the great overlap in minor anomalies and various medications, further casting doubt upon whether individual medications cause specific syndromes.[43]

Nulman and colleagues[44] examined 36 mother–child pairs exposed to carbamazepine, 34 pairs exposed to phenytoin, 9 pairs of nonmedicated epileptic women and matched each to 9 mother–child pairs exposed to nonteratogens. Minor anomalies were more common in offspring of mothers exposed to either carbamazepine or phenytoin (relative risk 2.1).[44] In a blended study of 43 children exposed to in utero antiepileptic medications and 47 controls, Fahnehjelm et al. found no difference in eye anomalies, nystagmus, or visual acuity between the two groups.[45]

Teenagers are often treated with valproate as the anticonvulsant of choice because of its low side-effect profile in this age group. It has, however, been reported to be associated with specific anomalies. DiLiberti et al.[46] in 1984, reported a specific fetal valproate syndrome. This was based on seven infants. They found a consistent facial phenotype in all seven children and other birth defects in four. This syndrome phenotype was confirmed by Ardinger and colleagues[47] in 1988. Jager-Roman et al.,[48] in 1986, reported fetal distress in 50 percent of 14 infants receiving valproate. Furthermore, 28 percent had low Apgar scores. They also found the same craniofacial defects as reported by DiLiberti et al.[46] Lindhout and Schmidt[49] confirmed the association between neural tube defects and valproate exposure in utero. They contend that there is a 1.5 percent risk of an infant being born with a neural tube defect if the mothers took valproate in the first trimester. Lindhout et al.[50] also studied 34 cases of neural tube defects in mothers taking anticonvulsant medications. In 33 of the 34 cases, mothers were exposed to either valproate or carbamazepine. Most of the cases of neural tube defects were lumbosacral. There was only one case of anencephaly. This implies that these medications have a predisposition to cause lumbosacral defects, since in the general population spina bifida and anencephaly are equally distributed. In only two cases were other major malformations found. The development of neural tube defects in these infants of mothers taking valproate also appeared to be a dose-dependent phenomenon. Wegner and Nau[51] have shown, in a mouse model, that valproate alters folic acid metabolism in embryos. This could account for the increased risk of neural tube defects in infants born to mothers who have taken valproate.

Carbamazepine, at one time, was thought to be safer than the other anticonvulsant medications for use in pregnancy. In 1989, Jones et al.[52] reported a pattern of minor craniofacial defects, fingernail hypoplasia, and developmental delay in infants exposed in utero to carbamazepine. Rosa[53] has also shown that there is a 1 percent risk of spina bifida in infants of mothers taking carbamazepine. Because this spectrum of defects (except spina bifida) is similar to that in the fetal hydantoin syndrome, Jones et al.[52] hypothesized that, as both drugs are metabolized through an arene oxide pathway, perhaps an epoxide intermediary is the teratogenic agent. Those fetuses with low levels of epoxide hydrolase are exposed to higher levels of epoxide intermediaries, and this may lead to an increase in malformations. Conversely, fetuses with high enzyme levels clear epoxides rapidly, minimizing exposure to the potential teratogens. Phenytoin, phenobarbital, and, to a lesser extent, carbamazepine are metabolized through this pathway.[54] Much work in this area is being performed by Finnell et al.,[54] who believe that low levels of epoxide hydrolase activity may be the common link explaining why only certain fetuses exposed to anticonvulsant medications in utero develop congenital malformations.

New antiepileptic drugs have been approved and rapidly clinically adopted since the last edition of this text. There is a need for these medications because 25 to 30 percent of epileptic patients are not adequately controlled by conventional therapies.[55] These newer medications work at the level of neurotransmitters such as γ aminobutyric acid (GABA) and also by blockade of sodium channels. Table 37-2 lists these drugs, with their dosages, and describes other considerations in their use. Gabapentin is probably the most frequently used of these medications. Many other applications have been found for this medication. It is used in chronic pain, mood stabilization, and neuropathies. The obstetrician, therefore, may encounter patients other than those with epilepsy on gabapentin. In epilepsy, it is only approved for use as an adjunct to other medications, but may soon have an indication for monotherapy. The usual maintenance dose is 900 to 2,400 mg daily in three divided doses, but doses up to 3,600 mg have been administered with only a minor increase in side effects. At present there are no studies of its use in pregnancy, although we have encountered 12 patients treated throughout pregnancy without incident. Nevertheless, patients should be warned that we do not know enough about the drug to appropriately counsel about its effects on the developing fetus. Nonetheless, if this medication is necessary to keep seizures under control, it should be used.

Lamotrigine is an adjunctive therapy for the treatment of simple and complex seizures with and without secondary generalization. It is important to note that approximately 10 percent of patients discontinue the medication because of a rash.[56] Severe rashes such as Stevens-Johnson syndrome and toxic epidermal necrolysis have been reported. It is important to note that the severe rashes have occurred with more frequency in pediatric patients. In a more recent study, rash necessitating discontinuation of therapy was found in only 2 percent of 11,316 treated patients.[57] The incidence was much higher in children aged 2 to 12. Ohman et al. report a successful pregnancy and note that the cord blood levels of lamotrigine were equal to those of maternal serum.[58] Also, the median milk/maternal plasma concentration ratio of 0.61 indicates that there are significant milk levels. We still do not have enough data to counsel patients concerning the use of this medication during pregnancy.

Topiramate and tiagabine are also used as adjunctive therapies for epilepsy. Both are effective, but there is little information on the use of these medications in pregnancy. The information will eventually be reported, as all four drugs are being administered more frequently.

I still believe that the neurologist and obstetrician should work together and use whichever medication(s)

Table 37-2. NEWER ANTIEPILEPTIC AGENTS

Medication	Usual Dose (mg/day)	Doses/Day	Special Notes
Gabapentin	1,200–3,600	3	Not enzyme inducer Antacids interfere
Lamotrigine	300–500	1 or 2	Rash in 11.2% Half-life affected by meds
Topiramate	100–400	2	May interfere with O.C.s
Tiagabine	8–56	2 to 4	Does not interfere with O.C.s

works best for the patient. It is bothersome, however, that after so many years of leading patients toward monotherapy, neurologists are swinging back toward using two drugs. As several studies that were previously reviewed in this chapter show, using multiple drugs in pregnancy increases the risk of a poorer pregnancy outcome.

There has been much debate over whether epilepsy itself and/or the use of antiepileptic medications is associated with psychomotor delays or mental retardation. In the landmark study by Nelson and Ellenberg,[21] an IQ below 70 was seen in 65.2 per 1,000 7-year-old children in the seizure group compared with 34 per 1,000 in the age-matched control group, a statistically significant difference. Before generalizations can be made, many confounding factors must be evaluated including other anomalies and social environment. In a review by Granstrom and Gaily,[59] none of the major antiepileptic medications appeared to carry special risk for mental retardation. They suggest, however, that polytherapy and inherited deviations in antiepileptic medication metabolism in the fetus increase the risk for mental retardation. This study is important because these researchers stress that other factors associated with maternal epilepsy such as seizures during pregnancy, inherited brain disorders, and a nonoptimal psychosocial environment can also affect a child's psychomotor development.[59] These factors are hard to control in any study. In a study by Gaily et al.,[60] 2 of 48 (4.1 percent) infants of mothers with epilepsy had mental retardation, and two additional infants had borderline intelligence. The mean IQ of the infants exposed in utero to anticonvulsant medications was statistically lower than the control group. When these four children were excluded from the analysis, the difference in mean IQ disappeared.[60] There was no increased risk of low intelligence attributable to fetal exposure either to antiepileptic medications below toxic levels or to brief maternal convulsions. No particular medication appeared to be associated with a lower IQ. Social class also appeared to play a role in the differences in IQs in these patients.[60] Moore et al.[61] reviewed 57 infants with fetal anticonvulsant syndromes. Eighty-one percent reported behavioral problems, with hyperactivity being the most common (34 percent). Two or more autistic features were found in 34 (60 percent) of the 57 children. Four were diagnosed with autism and two with Asberger's syndrome. Learning difficulties were found in 77 percent; and speech delay in 81 percent. Gross and fine motor delays were identified in 60 percent and 42 percent, respectively.[61] These percentages seem high, but it is important to remember that all of these children had already been identified as having an anticonvulsant syndrome.

In short, there appears to be a small, undefined risk of a slightly lower IQ and an increase in behavior problems in infants born to mothers with epilepsy. It does not appear that any particular medication results in a higher risk of this outcome.

Preconceptual Counseling for the Reproductive Age Woman with a Seizure Disorder

Although not always possible, it is preferable to counsel the patient with epilepsy before she becomes pregnant. A detailed history should be taken to see if there are any seizure disorders or congenital malformations in the family. This could provide a clue for fetal risks. The obstetrician must stress that the patient has greater than a 90 percent chance of having a successful pregnancy resulting in a normal newborn. A detailed history of medication use and seizure frequency should be obtained. The patient must be informed that if she has frequent seizures before conception, this pattern will probably continue. If she has frequent seizures, she should delay conception until control is better, even if this entails a change or addition of medication. The obstetrician must stress that controlling seizures is of primary importance and that the patient will need to take whatever medication(s) are necessary to achieve this goal throughout her pregnancy. If the patient has had no seizures during the past 2 to 5 years, an attempt may be made to withdraw her from anticonvulsant medications. This is usually done over a 1- to 3-month period, slowly reducing the medication. Up to 50 percent of patients will relapse and need to start their medications again. This withdrawal should be attempted only if the patient is completely seizure-free and only with the help of a neurologist. During the period of withdrawal from medications, patients should refrain from driving.

Furthermore, as previously shown, it is best to have the patient taking a single medication during pregnancy. If the patient is on multiple medications, the patient can be changed to monotherapy (over a several month period). The drug of choice for the specific type of epilepsy should be the one chosen for monotherapy. As the other medications are gradually withdrawn, levels of the remaining medication should be monitored frequently to make certain that the level remains therapeutic. When other medications are withdrawn, the level of the primary medication often increases without a dose increment. If it does not, however, the dose of the primary medication may need to be increased. The patient should refrain from conceiving until seizures have been well controlled for several months on the single medication. The patient must also be counseled that she should get adequate rest and sleep during pregnancy, as sleep deprivation is associated with increased seizure frequency.

The choice of antiepileptic medication depends on the seizure type. As the foregoing literature review has shown, there are studies claiming teratogenesis for each of the major anticonvulsant medications, yet there are also studies showing that each medication individually may not be particularly teratogenic. The most important point is to control maternal seizures. There may be some additional concern for using valproate in pregnancy due to the reported increased incidence of fetal distress.[48] It is important to note that this finding has not been corroborated in other studies. Therefore, if valproate is the anticonvulsant that works best for the patient, it should be used without hesitation. If valproate is used, the dose should be divided over three to four administrations daily to avoid high peak plasma levels.

In the past, it was thought that carbamazepine was the anticonvulsant of choice and had the least teratogenic effect. As has been shown in the foregoing literature review, there are studies that report malformations with the use of carbamazepine.[46,47] It is important to stress again that the anticonvulsant that does the best job of controlling seizures is the one that should be used for the patient. There is little information concerning the newer antiepileptic drugs and teratogenesis. If, however, they need to be used for good seizure control, they should be implemented as part of the patient's therapy.

Folic acid supplementation should be begun before or early in pregnancy. Folic acid supplementation may help to prevent neural tube defects, which are more common in treatment with carbamazepine and valproate but have been reported in women taking other anticonvulsants. Studies have shown that folic acid may decrease the incidence of neural tube defects in at-risk women.[16] It is important that this be implemented early in pregnancy, as open neural tube defects occur by the end of the fifth week of gestation. Furthermore, low folate levels have been associated with an increase in adverse pregnancy outcomes in women taking anticonvulsants.[62] Anticonvulsant levels should be checked frequently after implementing or increasing folic acid ad-

ministration, as it leads to lower anticonvulsant levels.[62] A daily dose of 4 mg/day should be more than ample. Patients should also be encouraged to take their prenatal vitamins, which contain vitamin D. This is because anticonvulsants may interfere with the conversion of 25-hydroxycholecalciferol to 1-25-dihydroxycholecalciferol, the active form of vitamin D.

Whether or not they ask, all mothers with idiopathic epilepsy wonder if their child will develop epilepsy. There is a surprising paucity of studies in this area. Children of parents without seizures have a 0.5 to 1 percent risk of developing epilepsy. It appears that the infant born to a mother with a seizure disorder of unknown etiology has a four times greater chance of developing idiopathic epilepsy than the general population.[63] Furthermore, it appears that epilepsy in the father does not increase a child's risk of developing a seizure disorder. Many of the rare seizure disorders have a stronger genetic component.[64]

Care of the Patient During Pregnancy

Once the patient becomes pregnant, it is of the utmost importance to establish accurate gestational dating. This will prevent any confusion over fetal growth in later gestation. The patient's anticonvulsant level should be followed as needed and dosages adjusted accordingly to keep the patient seizure free. It is a common pitfall to monitor levels too frequently and adjust dosages in a likewise frequent manner. It is important to remember that it takes several half-lives for a medication to reach a steady state (Table 37–3). Drugs like phenobarbital have extremely long half-lives, and the levels should not be checked too frequently. If levels are measured before the drug reaches a steady state and the dosage is increased, the patient will eventually become toxic from the medication. Drug levels should be drawn immediately before the next dose (trough levels) in order to assess if dosing is adequate. If the patient is showing signs of toxicity, a peak level may be obtained.

At approximately 16 weeks' gestation, the patient should undergo blood testing for maternal serum

Table 37–3. ANTICONVULSANTS COMMONLY USED DURING PREGNANCY

Drug	Therapeutic Level (mg/L)	Usual Nonpregnant Dosage	Half-Life
Carbamazepine	4–10	600–1,200 mg/day in three or divided doses (Two doses if extended-release forms are used)	Initially 36 h, chronic therapy 16 h
Phenobarbital	15–40	90–180 mg/day in two or three divided doses	100 h
Phenytoin	10–20, total; 1–2, free	300–500 mg/day in single or divided doses*	Avg 24 h
Primidone	5–15	750–1,500 mg/day in three divided doses	8 h
Valproic acid	50–100	550–2,000 mg/day in three or divided doses	Avg 13 h

* If a total dose of more than 300 mg is needed, dividing the dose will result in a more stable serum concentration.

marker screening in an attempt to detect neural tube defect. This, coupled with ultrasonography, gives a more than 90 percent detection rate for open neural tube defects. If the patient is difficult to scan or if she wants to be even more certain that there is no neural tube defect, amniocentesis can be undertaken. This should be considered if the patient is taking valproate or carbamazepine, as these medications appear to carry almost the same risk as if the patient had a family history of a neural tube defect.[49,50,53] At 18 to 22 weeks, the patient should undergo a comprehensive, targeted, ultrasound examination by an experienced obstetric sonographer to look for congenital malformations. A fetal echocardiogram can be obtained at 20 to 22 weeks to look for cardiac malformations, which are among the more common malformations of women taking any antiepileptic medications. If fetal echocardiography is not readily available, it is reassuring to remember that an adequate "four-chamber view" of the heart on ultrasound will identify 68 to 95 percent of major cardiac anomalies.[65,66]

As previously noted, there appears to be an increased risk for intrauterine growth restriction for fetuses exposed in utero to anticonvulsant medications. If the patient's weight gain and fundal growth appear appropriate, regular ultrasound examinations for fetal weight assessment are probably unnecessary. If, however, there is a question of fundal growth or if the patient's habitus precludes adequate assessment of this clinical parameter, serial ultrasonography for fetal weight assessment can be performed.

In older and retrospective studies, there appears to be an increased risk of stillbirth in mothers taking anticonvulsant medications.[7,20-22] In a prospective study, however, this complication was not seen.[23] As previously noted, in the studies that showed an increase in stillbirths, factors such as intrauterine growth restriction or oligohydramnios were not prenatally identified. With modern surveillance and the more common use of ultrasonography, many of these risk factors can be detected before the fetus faces imminent risk. Non-stress testing, therefore, is not necessary in all mothers with seizure disorders. It should be limited to those who have other medical or obstetric complications that place the patient at increased risk of stillbirth.

If at all possible, the patient should be maintained on a single medication, and drug levels should be drawn at appropriate intervals to make certain that the patient is receiving enough medication. If the patient is taking phenytoin, free levels should be obtained if possible. A drug dosage should not be increased only because the total level of drug is falling. The free level of drug may still be therapeutic. If, however, the patient develops any seizure activity, dosages should then be adjusted upward. A brief seizure during pregnancy does not appear to be deleterious to the fetus.[24] It is best to use the lowest dose of a single medication possible that will keep the patient seizure free. This, however, must be individualized. For instance, if the patient usually experiences seizures during the day and drives, it is important to make certain that the patient remains seizure free. For this type of patient, drug dosages should be increased if levels fall. If, on the other hand, the patient only has brief partial complex seizures that do not generalize and occur only during her sleep, it is optimal to keep the medications at the lowest serum concentration that will keep her seizure free. An occasional seizure of this type would not harm either patient or fetus. The key to managing anticonvulsants in pregnancy is individualization of therapy.

Early hemorrhagic disease of the newborn can occur in infants exposed to anticonvulsants in utero, and this appears to be a deficiency of the vitamin K–dependent clotting factors II, VII, IX, and X. The use of vitamin K in the third trimester to prevent hemorrhagic disease is somewhat controversial. Although some advocate administering 10 to 20 mg of vitamin K orally, daily, to mothers during the final few weeks of pregnancy, this is certainly not the standard of care. There appears to be no adverse effect of administering this vitamin, but, on the other hand, its utility has not been clearly demonstrated. Very little hemorrhagic disease of the newborn is seen today, and this is probably because most infants receive 1 mg of vitamin K intramuscularly at birth. This certainly should be given to all infants of mothers receiving anticonvulsants. Because of early discharges and the shortened time of neonatal observation, it might be prudent to check a prothrombin time on the cord blood at birth. This can be done by taking fresh cord blood and placing it in a citrated blood tube and having it sent immediately for prothrombin time. This might be especially prudent if the child is to undergo a very early circumcision.

Labor and Delivery

Vaginal delivery is the route of choice for the mother with a seizure disorder. If the mother has frequent seizures brought on by the stress of labor, she may undergo cesarean delivery after stabilization. Furthermore, seizures during labor may cause transient fetal bradycardia.[23] The fetal heart rate should be given time to recover. If it does not, then one must assume fetal distress and/or placental abruption and deliver by cesarean section. Because stress often exacerbates seizure disorders, an epidural anesthetic can benefit many laboring patients with epilepsy.

Management of anticonvulsant medications during a prolonged labor presents a challenge. During labor, oral absorption of medications is erratic and, if the patient vomits, almost negligible. If the patient is taking phenytoin or phenobarbital, these medications may be administered parenterally. An anticonvulsant level should be obtained first to help ascertain the appropriate dosage. Phenobarbital may be given intramuscularly, and phenytoin may be given intravenously. Fosphenytoin, although expensive, is available and makes the administration of intravenous phenytoin much easier. If the patient's phenytoin level is normal, the usual daily dose may be administered intravenously. The medication may only be mixed in normal saline and must be administered at a rate no faster than 50 mg/min. Fosphenytoin is easier to use. Because of the long half-life of phenobarbital, if the patient's serum level is therapeutic, a 60- to 90-mg intramuscular dose will probably be sufficient to maintain the patient throughout labor and delivery. The main problem arises if the patient is taking carbamazepine. This medication is not manufactured in a parenteral form, although extended-release forms now exist. Oral administration may be attempted, but, if the patient has seizures or a pre-seizure aura, she may be loaded with a therapeutic dose of phenytoin to carry her through labor. The usual loading dose is 10 to 15 mg/kg administered intravenously at a rate no faster than

50 mg/min. This should be effective in controlling seizures. Benzodiazepines may also be used for acute seizures, but one must remember that they can cause early neonatal depression as well as maternal apnea.[67] Prenatal diagnostic techniques are not perfect. Even if the infant appears to have no anomalies, an experienced pediatrician should be present at the delivery of the infant born to a mother taking anticonvulsant medications.

New Onset of Seizures in Pregnancy and the Puerperium

Occasionally, seizures will be diagnosed for the first time during pregnancy. This may present a diagnostic dilemma (Table 37–4). If the seizures occur in the third trimester, they are eclampsia until proven otherwise and should be treated as such until the attending physician can perform a proper evaluation. The treatment of eclampsia is delivery, but the patient must first be stabilized. It is often difficult, however, to distinguish eclampsia from an epileptic seizure. The patient may be hypertensive initially after an epileptic seizure and may

Table 37–4. DIFFERENTIAL DIAGNOSIS OF PERIPARTUM SEIZURES

	Blood Pressure	Proteinuria	Seizures	Timing	CSF	Other Features
Eclampsia	+++	+++	+++	Third trimester	Early: RBC, 0–1,000; protein, 50–150 mg/dl Late: grossly bloody	Platelets normal or ↓ RBC normal
Epilepsy	Normal	Normal to +	+++	Any trimester	Normal	Low anticonvulsant levels
Subarachnoid hemorrhage	+ to +++ (labile)	0 to +	+	Any trimester	Grossly bloody	
Thrombotic thrombocytopenic purpura	Normal to +++	++	++	Third trimester	RBC 0–100	Platelets ↓ ↓ RBC fragmented
Amniotic fluid embolus	Shock	−	+	Intrapartum	Normal	Hypoxia, cyanosis Platelets ↓ ↓ RBC normal
Cerebral vein thrombosis	+	−	++	Postpartum	Normal (early)	Headache Occasional pelvic phlebitis
Water intoxication	Normal	−	++	Intrapartum	Normal	Oxytocin infusion rate >45 mU/min Serum Na <124 mEq/L
Pheochromocytoma	+++ (labile)	+	+	Any trimester	Normal	Neurofibromatosis
Autonomic stress syndrome of high paraplegics	+++ with labor pains	−	−	Intrapartum	Normal	Cardiac arrhythmia
Toxicity of local anesthetics	Variable	−	++	Intrapartum	Normal	

Modified from Donaldson JO: Peripartum convulsions. *In* Donaldson JO (ed): Neurology of Pregnancy. Philadelphia, WB Saunders, 1989, p 312.

exhibit some myoglobinuria secondary to muscle breakdown. The diagnosis becomes clearer over time, but in either case, rapid, thoughtful action must be undertaken. The first physician to attend a patient after a seizure may not be an obstetrician/gynecologist, and magnesium sulfate may not be started acutely. This should be remedied as soon as possible.

If the patient at an earlier gestational age develops seizures for the first time, she should be evaluated and started on the proper medication. The physician must be alert to look for acquired causes of seizures including trauma, infection, metabolic disorders, space-occupying lesions, central nervous system bleeding, and ingestion of drugs such as cocaine and amphetamines. The patient must be stabilized, and the physician must make certain that an adequate airway is established for the protection of both mother and fetus. The physician should also look for focal signs that may be more suggestive of a space-occupying lesion, central nervous system bleeding, or abscess.

Blood should be obtained for electrolytes, glucose, calcium, magnesium, renal function studies, and toxicologic studies, while intravenous access is being established. If the patient had a tonic-clonic seizure, and the attending physician feels that this is probably new-onset epilepsy, she should be started on the appropriate anticonvulsant medication while awaiting results of laboratory studies. If she is not in status epilepticus, this medication may be given orally.

If the patient presents with recurrent generalized seizures, status epilepticus, immediate therapeutic action must be taken. The drug of choice is intravenous phenytoin, as it is highly effective, has a long duration of action, and a low incidence of serious side effects. This medication should be administered in a loading dose of 18 to 20 mg/kg at a rate not exceeding 50 mg/min. Rapid infusion may cause transient hypotension and heart block. If possible, the patient should be placed on a cardiac monitor while receiving a loading dose of phenytoin. Also, this medication must be given in a glucose-free solution to avoid precipitation.[68] Fosphenytoin, if available, can be given more rapidly with fewer side effects. If phenytoin is unavailable, a benzodiazepine may be used as a first-line drug for status epilepticus. These drugs, however, cause respiratory depression, and the physician must have the ability to intubate the patient if necessary when these medications are used. If these measures are ineffective, an anesthesiologist and neurologist should be immediately consulted if they are not already involved in the patient's care.

Any patient experiencing seizures for the first time during pregnancy without a known cause should undergo an EEG and some type of intracranial imaging. In looking only at eclamptic patients, Sibai et al.[69] found that EEGs were initially abnormal in 75 percent of patients but normalized within 6 months in all patients studied. While this group found no uniform computed tomography (CT) abnormalities in this set of eclamptics, they did find that 46 and 33 percent of eclamptics had some abnormalities in the magnetic resonance imaging (MRI) and CT, respectively. Most of the findings were nonspecific and were not helpful in diagnosis or treatment. If the physician is not certain that the patient has eclampsia, an imaging study should be part of the evaluation described above.

Postpartum Period

The levels of anticonvulsant medications must be monitored frequently during the first few weeks postpartum, as they can rapidly rise. If the patient's medication dosages were increased during pregnancy, they will need to be decreased rather rapidly after delivery to prepregnancy levels. All of the major anticonvulsant medications cross into breast milk. The levels vary in breast milk from 18 to 79 percent of the plasma levels.[67,70] The use of these medications, however, is not a contraindication to breast-feeding. Primidone, phenobarbital, and benzodiazepines may have a sedative effect on the fetus with later withdrawal symptoms. Should the infant exhibit these types of symptoms, breast-feeding should be discontinued.

All methods of contraception are available to women with idiopathic seizure disorders. The majority of women are able to take oral contraceptives without any adverse side effects.[71] Oral contraceptive failures are more common in women taking anticonvulsants. This is due to the fact that all of the major anticonvulsant medications induce hepatic enzymes, which metabolize estrogen faster.[71,72] These patients may, therefore, require oral contraceptives with higher dosages of estrogens. The amount of enzyme induction, however, varies and oral contraceptive doses must be individualized.

In conclusion, the majority of women with idiopathic epilepsy will have an uneventful pregnancy with an excellent outcome. To optimize neonatal outcome, the patient should take only one medication and, when possible, use the lowest dose effective in keeping her free of seizures. It is important, though, for the patient to realize that prevention of seizures is the most important goal during pregnancy. Simple interventions such as taking folic acid prior to conception, taking prenatal vitamins containing vitamin D, and giving the infant vitamin K at birth will help to optimize the outcome. There is an increase in congenital malformations in infants exposed to anticonvulsant medications in utero. The majority of infants exposed to these medications, however, will have no malformations. With modern techniques for prenatal diagnosis, including ultrasound and α-fetoprotein determination, many of these malformations can be detected early. The majority of women with epilepsy will labor normally and have spontaneous vaginal deliveries. In short, with close cooperation and excellent communication among the obstetrician, neurologist, and pediatrician, the vast majority of these patients will have a safe pregnancy with an excellent outcome.

MIGRAINE

Headaches are extremely common in women, and the majority of migraine headaches occur in women of childbearing age. Migraines can be classified as those with aura (other neurologic signs and symptoms) and those without aura. Maggioni and colleagues[73] surveyed 430 women 3 days postpartum about their headache histories and 126 (29.3 percent) were found to be primary headache sufferers. Of these patients, 81 suffered from migraine without aura, 12 suffered from migraine with aura, and 33 had tension type headaches.[73] The headaches, which are associated with vasodilation of the cerebral vasculature, last a variable amount of time. They are often accompanied by photosensitivity and nausea. Migraines with aura may be accompanied by sensations in the extremities and other lateralizing signs, sometimes making them difficult to distinguish from transient ischemic attacks.

Migraine symptoms tend to improve during pregnancy[73–75] Maggioni et al. found that 80 percent of patients experienced either complete remission or a 50 percent reduction in headaches during pregnancy. Improvement was more common after the first trimester. Granella and co-workers[75] found that migraines disappeared during pregnancy in 67 percent of cases. Granella et al.[75] also confirmed this. Aube found that 60 to 70 percent of women either go into remission or improve significantly, usually in the second and third trimesters.[76] The migraine type did not seem to be a prognostic factor. Those with menstrual migraines showed the most improvement.[76] In this study, however, 4 to 8 percent showed significant worsening during pregnancy.[76] Chen and co-workers[77] identified 508 women with a history of migraine from the Collaborative Perinatal Project of the National Institute of Neurological and Communicative Disease Disorders and Stroke. They found that patients with migraines smoke more heavily and had a longer smoking history than did their headache-free peers. They also found that in nonsmokers migraine was often associated with allergies.[77]

Chancellor and colleagues[78] followed nine patients whose migraines first occurred during pregnancy at various gestational ages. They were followed for more than 4 years after pregnancy, and the prognosis for headache was excellent. Four of the nine patients developed complications of pregnancy, including preeclampsia in two.[78] Maggioni found no increase in pregnancy complications in patients with migraine.[73] It is unknown if the headaches were caused by developing preeclampsia. It is important to rule out other severe complications of pregnancy before assigning a new diagnosis of migraine to a pregnant patient. Jacobson and Redman[79] reported a patient who actually lost consciousness during pregnancy because of a basilar migraine.

Supportive therapy is recommended for patients who experience migraine attacks during gestation. Both narcotic and nonnarcotic analgesics can be used as necessary. The use of nonsteroidal anti-inflammatory agents should be avoided if possible in late pregnancy, because when used over a long period they can cause premature closure of the ductus arteriosus and/or oligohydramnios. Nonetheless, they can be used for brief periods under physician supervision. When pain is severe, parenteral narcotics and appropriate anti-emetic therapy may be used. β-Blockers may be safely administered during pregnancy for prophylaxis. The calcium channel blockers used in the treatment of migraine can also be safely administered during gestation. Fluoxetine is occasionally successfully used for migraine prophylaxis. The same is true for the tricyclic antidepressants and is generally safe for use during pregnancy.

Ergotamine is best avoided during pregnancy. Previous reports have suggested it may cause birth defects that have a vascular disruptive etiology. Hughes and Goldstein[80] report a case in which an infant showed evidence of early arrested cerebral maturation and paraplegia. They hypothesize that ergotamine, acting either alone or in synergy with propranolol and caffeine, produced fetal vasoconstriction resulting in tissue ischemia and subsequent malformation.[80] It is important to note that this etiology is strictly theoretical. In addition, ergots are uterotonic and have an abortifacient potential. These drugs, however, should be avoided during pregnancy. Sumatriptan, a serotonin receptor agonist, is very successful in treating migraines. It has a potential for vasoconstriction in the fetal placental unit. In a review by O'Quinn and colleagues, there were no untoward effects in 76 first-trimester exposures to sumatriptan.[81] Using logistic regression, Olesen and colleagues[82] compared 34 sumatriptan exposures to 89 migraine controls and 15,995 healthy women. They found the risk of preterm birth was elevated (odds ratio 6.3). They also found the risk of IUGR was greater.[82] They do state that they did not control for disease severity. Sumatriptan, therefore, should only be used if the physician feels that the potential benefit clearly outweighs the potential risk. Table 37–5 lists some medications that can be used for treating migraines.

Dietary factors may precipitate migraine attacks. Careful history may uncover foods that should be

Table 37–5. DRUG THERAPY FOR MIGRAINE HEADACHES IN PREGNANCY

Medication	Class	Use	Dosage	Route of Administration	Safe for Pregnancy
Acetaminophen	Pain reliever	Acute pain	4 g/day maximum	PO or PR	Yes
Codeine	Narcotic	Acute pain	30–90 mg q3–4 h	PO	Yes
Meperidine	Narcotic	Acute pain	25–100 mg q3–6 h	PO, IM, or IV	Yes
Ibuprofen	Nonsteroidal	Acute pain	2,400 mg/day in divided doses	PO	Do not use in late pregnancy
Prochloroperazine	Phenothiazine	Nausea	5–25 mg q2–8 h depending on route	PO, PR, IM, IV	Yes
Promethazine	Phenothiazine	Nausea	12.5–50 mg q2–8 h depending on route	PO, PR, IM, IV	Yes
Butalbital (50 mg), acetaminophen 325 mg, caffeine 40 mg	Sedative, pain reliever, vasoconstrictor	Acute migraine	2 tablets q4 h, not to exceed 6 tablets daily	PO	Yes
Isometheptene mucate (65 mg), Dichloralphenazone (100 mg), Acetaminophen (325 mg)	Vasoconstrictor, sedative, pain reliever	Acute migraine	2 capsules immediately followed by 1 hourly for no more than 5 capsules in 12 hours	PO	Yes
Caffeine	Vasoconstrictor	Acute pain	500 mg in 50 ml IV solution—may repeat	PO or IV	Yes
Sumatriptan	Vasoconstrictor	Acute pain relief	300 mg/day PO max 6 mg SQ × 2/day max	PO or SQ	No
Ergotamine with caffeine	Vasoconstrictor	Acute pain relief	2 mg/200 mg (PO), then 1 mg/100 mg q½ h for 6 tab/day max **or** 2 mg/100 mg PR and repeat once in 1 h	PO or PR	No
Nortriptyline	TCA	Prophylaxis	25–100 mg qhs	PO	Yes
Amitriptyline	TCA	Prophylaxis	50–150 mg qhs	PO	Yes
Sertraline	SSRI	Prophylaxis	50–100 mg qhs	PO	Probably
Fluoxetine	SSRI	Prophylaxis	20–40 mg qhs	PO	Probably
Propranolol	β-blocker	Prophylaxis	80–120 mg bid	PO	Small risk for IUGR
Nadolol	β-blocker	Prophylaxis	20–80 mg qd	PO	Caution for IUGR
Atenolol	β-blocker	Prophylaxis	25–100 mg qd	PO	Caution for IUGR
Carbamazepine	Membrane stabilizer	Prophylaxis	Up to 1,200 mg/day in three divided doses	PO	Risk of NTD, other problems

IUGR, intrauterine growth restriction; NTD, neural tube defect; SSRI, serotonin-selective reuptake inhibitor; TCA, tricyclic antidepressant.

avoided, including foods containing monosodium glutamate, red wine, cured meats, and strong cheeses containing tyramine. Relative hypoglycemia and alcohol can also trigger migraine attacks.

CEREBROVASCULAR DISEASES

Arterial Occlusion

Twelve percent of arterial occlusions occur in women between the ages of 15 and 45 years, and approximately one third of these patients may be pregnant.[83] In a study from India, 37 percent of patients affected with cerebrovascular disease were under the age of 40 years, with a significant number of thromboses occurring during pregnancy and the puerperium.[84] Overall, the incidence of cerebral arterial occlusion in pregnancy is approximately 1 per 20,000 live births.[83,85] The mortality rate for pregnant women with cerebral arterial occlusion is twice that of men and three times that of non-pregnant women. According to Jennett and Cross,[83] middle cerebral artery occlusion is most common during pregnancy, whereas internal carotid artery occlusion is observed most often in the puerperium.

Hemiplegia and dysphasia are frequent findings.[85] Predisposing factors such as preeclampsia, chronic hypertension, or hypotensive episodes can be demonstrated in about one third of these patients. Brick and Riggs[86] have shown that oral contraceptives also raise the risk of ischemic cerebral vascular disease. Perhaps because of its relative frequency in the general population, the factor V Leiden mutation may be a predisposing factor in many of these patients. One half of the pregnancy-related cases occur during the immediate postpartum period and the remainder during the second and third trimesters. In a recent study, Lidegaard[87] concluded that pregnancy was associated with an elevated odds ratio of only 1.3 for cerebral thromboembolism. Brick[88] reported the case of a woman who had a documented partial obstruction of the left middle cerebral artery during the third trimester of pregnancy. Following delivery, her symptoms abated, and angiography 11 weeks later revealed complete resolution of the obstruction. Brick[88] therefore thought that this lesion was the result of reversible intimal hyperplasia from the increased estrogen and progesterone levels of pregnancy.

In cases of cerebral arterial occlusion, care must be taken to avoid increased intracranial pressure. If signs of increased intracranial pressure develop, parenteral dexamethasone should be administered. Osmotic diuresis can be used if needed. Supportive measures are also necessary, including close monitoring of electrolytes to detect inappropriate secretion of antidiuretic hormone. Physical and rehabilitative therapy should be started as soon as possible. These patients can progress normally through pregnancy and deliver vaginally.

A case of maternal death from carotid artery thrombosis associated with the HELLP syndrome (hemolysis, elevated liver enzymes, and low platelet count) has been reported by Katz and Cefalo.[89] They proposed that the infarction occurred because the patient experienced a rebound thrombocytosis leading to a hypercoagulable state. They stress the importance of closely following patients with HELLP syndrome so that those who develop a reactive thrombocytosis can be monitored for signs and symptoms of cerebral thrombosis.

Cortical Vein Thrombosis

The chief symptoms in patients with cortical vein thrombosis are headache, lethargy, and vomiting. Hemiplegia has a gradual onset, and seizure activity is common (Table 37–4).[90,91] This disorder occurs most frequently during the immediate postpartum period and may be attributed to a hypercoagulable state.[92] An incidence of 1 in 10,000 pregnancies was suggested in one study.[93] With the availability of CT and MRI, accurate diagnosis is possible. The actual incidence may be higher if patients are asymptomatic. Many patients with cortical vein thrombosis show signs of seizure

activity, and prophylactic anticonvulsants were once routinely given.[90] The drug of choice is phenytoin. The patient should be given a loading dose of 10 mg/kg followed by 300 to 500 mg orally each day. Phenytoin levels should be checked frequently to make certain that they are therapeutic and that the patient does not develop phenytoin toxicity. Some neurosurgeons are advocating expectant management and do not routinely give anticonvulsants.

Subarachnoid Hemorrhage

The rate of subarachnoid hemorrhage complicating pregnancy is approximately 1 per 10,400.[94] With cocaine abuse occurring across the country, the incidence may rise, as the associated increase in vasospasm associated with this drug is bleeding from preexisting berry aneurysms and arterial-venous (A-V) malformations.[95] Most subarachnoid hemorrhages occurring in pregnant patients are caused either by rupture of a berry aneurysm or bleeding from a congenital A-V malformation. Most berry aneurysms are thought to be due to a congenital defect in the elastic and smooth muscle layers of cerebral blood vessels. They are usually located in the vessels of the circle of Willis or those arising from it. Robinson and co-workers[96] evaluated 26 patients with spontaneous subarachnoid hemorrhage during pregnancy and found that approximately one half were caused by berry aneurysms and one half by A-V malformations. They observed that A-V malformations are more common in patients below the age of 25 years and usually bleed before 20 weeks' gestation. Conversely, berry aneurysms occur in patients over the age of 30 years and usually bleed in the third trimester.[96] Pregnancy appears to increase the risk of bleeding from an A-V malformation. The maternal mortality rate associated with an untreated A-V malformation is reported to be 33 percent. This figure, however, is based on old data, and the rate is significantly lower today. Most are treated rapidly and aggressively.

Diagnosis and Treatment

Any patient with localized signs of cerebral or meningeal irritation must be thoroughly evaluated. If the clinical examination dictates that further evaluation is necessary, MRI/MRA or a CT scan should be performed. If necessary, contrast dyes may be used. Cerebral angiography can be safely used to pinpoint the origin of cerebral bleeding. Subarachnoid hemorrhages, whether caused by A-V malformations or berry aneurysms, should be treated surgically when possible. Surgery under hypothermia or hypotension appears to cause no adverse fetal effects. The fetal heart rate should be monitored. If fetal bradycardia occurs, blood pressure should be raised sufficiently to normalize the fetal heart rate.[97] Kawasaki and colleagues[98] report a case of cerebellar hemorrhage in a 32-week primigravida. She was treated conservatively until term and was delivered by elective cesarean section. Her surgery, which was delayed until after delivery, was successful. D'Haese et al. have reported a case of combined cesarean delivery and aneurysm clipping.[99]

If the patient has undergone corrective surgery for an aneurysm or A-V malformation, she should be allowed to deliver vaginally. Because the Valsalva maneuver can increase intracranial pressure,[96] epidural anesthesia is recommended. Interestingly, Szabo and colleagues[100] have reported that moderate increases in blood pressure do not cause spontaneous hemorrhage in nonpregnant patients with intracranial A-V malformations. If the aneurysm or A-V malformation has not been surgically corrected, Robinson et al.[96] recommend elective cesarean delivery. However, there are no hard data on which to make this decision. Therefore, the mode of delivery should be determined by the obstetrician after discussion about the individual case with neurologists, neurosurgeons, and anesthesiologists. Laidler and colleagues[101] discussed the advantages of regional anesthesia in these patients. Buckley and co-workers[102] have described a case of simultaneous cesarean delivery and ablation of a cerebral A-V malformation. Levy and Jaspan discuss the anesthetic and obstetric management of an untreated vascular anomaly that had bled earlier in pregnancy in a patient who developed severe preeclampsia.[103]

As pregnancy has a deleterious effect on A-V malformations, those patients with inoperable lesions should be counseled about the dangers of future childbearing. With improved imaging techniques, the patient should be thoroughly evaluated before any recommendations are made for permanent sterilization.

Venous-venous (V-V) malformations are low-pressure phenomena. Patients should progress to term and deliver vaginally without any hemorrhagic event or complications.

MULTIPLE SCLEROSIS

Multiple sclerosis (MS) is a demyelinating disease that attacks men and women equally. The onset of symptoms usually occurs between the ages of 20 and 40 years. In the United States, the disease is more common in those residing above 40 degrees north latitude. The prevalence for those living in the southern United States is 10 per 100,000, while it is approximately 50 per 100,000 in those living in the northern states.[104] MS has no clear genetic predisposition.

The diagnosis of MS is often made years after the initial onset of sensory symptoms. The onset is usually subtle. Common presenting symptoms include weakness of one or both lower extremities, visual complaints, and loss of coordination. Because the disease primarily affects the white matter of the central nervous system, symptoms attributable to disruption of gray matter are uncommon. The disease is characterized by exacerbations and remissions. Less than one third of patients show steady progression of their disease after its onset.

It is impossible to predict the long-range prognosis of a patient with MS. About one half of patients are still able to work at their usual profession 10 years after the onset of the illness. After 20 years, however, only about one third remain employed. In a study of 185 women with MS, Weinshenker and colleagues[105] showed that there was no association between long-term disability and (1) total number of term pregnancies, (2) the timing of pregnancy relative to the onset of MS, or (3) the worsening of MS in relation to a pregnancy. The average life expectancy in patients with MS is also impossible to predict. Patients may live with the disease for more than 25 years. When death does occur, it is usually attributable to infection.

MS and pregnancy can coexist without unusual complications. Leibowitz and colleagues[106] found no decrease in fertility and no increase in perinatal mortality in patients with MS. Their study suggested that pregnancy does not predispose a patient to MS but that patients with "premorbid" disease are more likely to have the onset of early symptoms during pregnancy.

In fact, Runmarker and Andersen[107] demonstrated that the risk of onset of MS is reduced during gestation while the risk of onset during the postpartum period was no different than for the nonpregnant state. Furthermore, these investigators demonstrated a lower risk of onset of MS in parous than in nulliparous patients. Of 170 pregnant patients with MS studied by Millar and co-workers,[108] relapses occurred in only 45, the majority during the puerperium and postpartum periods. Birk and co-investigators[109] carefully followed pregnancies in eight women with MS. None of the women worsened during pregnancy. Six of the eight women, however, experienced relapses within the first 7 weeks after delivery. They also reported that there were differences in suppressor T cell levels during pregnancy, but these were not predictive of changes in clinical disease.[109] Frith and McLeod[110] studied 85 pregnancies and found no increased risk of relapse during pregnancy. They noted that most of the relapses that did occur during pregnancy took place in the third trimester. In another series, Frith and McLeod[111] reported that relapses occur most frequently in the last trimester and also in the first 3 months postpartum. In a large study, Nelson and colleagues[112] analyzed 191 pregnancies in women with nonprogressive MS. The exacerbation rate during the 9-month postpartum period was 34 percent, three times that of the 9 months during pregnancy. The rate was highest in the 3 months immediately following delivery and stabilized after postpartum month 6.[112] The exacerbation rates were the same in breast-feeding and non–breast-feeding women. The average time to flare was also similar in both groups. This study verifies that it is safe for women with MS to breast-feed their newborns.[112]

Bernardi and colleagues showed a decreased risk of relapse during the 9 months of pregnancy and the first 6 months postpartum.[113] In this study of 52 women, these researchers concluded that pregnancy, as a whole, is a protective event. Worthington et al.,[114] however, found more frequent relapses in the first 6 months postpartum, but not after that. Long-term prognosis was unaffected by pregnancy.[114] Vendru et al.[115] demonstrated that pregnancy delays the onset of long-term disability. As an index of progression, they used the length of time from onset of disease until wheel chair dependence. In patients with at least one pregnancy after onset, the mean time to wheel chair dependence was 18.6 years compared with 12.5 years for other women.[115] In a study encompassing 12 European countries, Confavreux and colleagues studied 269 pregnancies in 254 women with multiple sclerosis.[116] They determined the relapse rate in each trimester using the Kuntzke Expanded Disability Status Scale with 0 as good function and 10 as very disabled. They found the rate of relapse declined during pregnancy, especially in the third trimester. Relapses increased in the first 3 months postpartum before returning to prepregnancy rates.[116] The Kuntzke Disability Score worsened at the same rate for the year prior to pregnancy, during the pregnancy, and the years postpartum. Neither breast-feeding nor epidural analgesia had an adverse effect on the rate of relapse or on the progression of disability.[116]

Paraplegic patients are more susceptible to urinary tract infections during pregnancy but may feel no symptoms. Therefore, they should be screened routinely. If the patient has become paraplegic as a result of MS, there may be little pain associated with labor. It might be difficult therefore for the patient to discern when labor begins. Uterine contractions occur normally, but voluntary expulsive efforts may be hindered in the second stage of labor. Delivery by forceps or vacuum extraction therefore may be indicated. Bader and colleagues[117] report that women with MS who receive epidural anesthesia for vaginal delivery do not have a significantly higher incidence of exacerbation of their MS than those receiving only local anesthesia.

Corticosteroids and immunosuppressive agents are occasionally used to treat multiple sclerosis. In one case report, plasmapheresis was used with dramatic improvement in a woman with rapidly progressive MS.[118] Orvieto et al. report using intravenous immunoglobu-

lins to successfully prevent multiple sclerosis relapses for 6 months postpartum in 14 patients.[119] There are several new drugs and biopharmaceuticals available for treatment of multiple sclerosis. There is virtually no pregnancy experience with many of these agents. Therefore, they should be used if the neurologist and obstetrician feel that the benefits outweigh the potential risks.

CARPAL TUNNEL SYNDROME

The medial border of the carpal tunnel consists of the pisiform and hamate bones, and its lateral border consists of the scaphoid and trapezium bones. They are covered on the palmar surface by the flexor retinaculum. The median nerve and flexor tendons pass through this carpal tunnel, which has little room for expansion. If the wrist is extremely flexed or extended, the volume of the carpal tunnel is reduced. In pregnancy, weight gain and edema can produce the carpal tunnel syndrome that results from compression of the median nerve. Wallace and Cook[120] first reported the association between carpal tunnel syndrome and pregnancy in 1957. Although 20 percent of pregnant women complain of pain on the palmar surface of the hand, few actually have the true carpal tunnel syndrome.[121] In a 1998 study, Stolp-Smith et al. found 50 of 14,579 (0.34 percent) pregnant patients presenting between 1987 and 1992 actually met criteria for carpal tunnel syndrome.[122] Commonly, the syndrome consists of pain, numbness, and/or tingling in the distribution of the median nerve in the hand and wrist. This includes the thumb, index finger, long finger, and radial side of the ring finger on the palmar aspect. Compressing the median nerve and percussing the wrist and forearm with a reflex hammer, the Tinel maneuver, often exacerbates the pain. In severe cases, weakness and decreased motor function can occur. The definitive diagnosis is made by electromyography, but this test is often unnecessary.

McLennan and co-workers[123] studied 1,216 consecutive pregnancies. Of these patients, 427 (35 percent) reported hand symptoms. Fewer than 20 percent of these 427 affected women described the classic carpal tunnel syndrome. No patient required operative intervention. Most symptoms were bilateral and commenced in the third trimester of pregnancy. Ekman-Ordeberg et al.[124] found a 2.3 percent incidence of carpal tunnel syndrome in a prospective study of 2,358 pregnancies. The syndrome appeared to be more common in primigravidas with generalized edema. Conservative therapy with splinting of the wrist at night completely relieved symptoms in 46 of 56 patients. Of the remaining 10, three required surgery before delivery. In Stolp-Smith's study, symptoms began with equal frequency in all trimesters, but diagnosis was delayed until the third trimester in 50 percent of patients.[122] Only four patients required surgical intervention during gestation, and three additional patients required surgery postpartum. Wand[125] retrospectively studied 40 women with carpal tunnel syndrome developing in pregnancy and 18 women with carpal tunnel syndrome that developed in the puerperium. He confirmed that the syndrome occurs most frequently in primigravidas over the age of 30 years. All cases that developed before delivery occurred during the third trimester and resolved within 2 weeks after delivery. In those cases developing during the puerperium in women who breast-fed their infants, the symptoms lasted longer, a mean of 5.8 months.[125] In another series, Wand[126] studied 27 women who developed carpal tunnel syndrome during the puerperium. The condition was associated with breast-feeding in 24 of these women. Symptoms lasted an average of 6.5 months in the breast-feeding women. Only two of these patients required surgical decompression.[126]

Supportive and conservative therapies are usually adequate for the treatment of carpal tunnel syndrome. Symptoms usually subside in the postpartum period as total body water returns to normal.[127] Splints placed on the dorsum of the hand, which keep the wrist in a neutral position and maximize the capacity of the carpal tunnel, often provide dramatic relief. Local injections of glucocorticoids may also be used in severe cases. Although diuretics may help to control carpal tunnel syndrome symptoms over a short period of time, their use is not recommended because the symptoms return rather rapidly after the cessation of treatment. In an uncontrolled series, Ellis[128] reported that pyridoxine in a dose of 100 to 200 mg daily for 12 weeks can provide relief in a large percentage of patients with carpal tunnel syndrome. Before this can be recommended, controlled trials need to be undertaken.

Surgical correction of this syndrome should not be delayed in patients with deteriorating muscle tone and motor function. Decompression surgery for carpal tunnel syndrome is a simple procedure that can be safely carried out during pregnancy using local anesthesia, an axillary block, or a Bier block. With new endoscopic procedures, the procedure is even less invasive. Assmus and Hashemi report 314 hands surgically treated during pregnancy or the puerperium for carpal tunnel syndrome.[129] One hundred thirty-three cases were performed during pregnancy, most in the last trimester including four who had both hands treated simultaneously. Of the patients, 98 percent reported good or excellent results.[129] There were no complications and local anesthesia was used in all cases. These authors recommend surgery if sensory loss is present or if motor latency is more than 5 msec.[129] It is important to warn patients that carpal tunnel syndrome can recur in future pregnancies.[130]

PSEUDOTUMOR CEREBRI

Pseudotumor cerebri may complicate as many as 1 in 870 births.[131] It is seen more frequently in pregnant women, particularly those who are obese.[132–134] However, in a study by Ireland and colleagues[135] the incidences in pregnant women and in oral contraceptive users were no higher than in control groups. More than 95 percent of these patients present with headaches, and 15 percent have diplopia. Papilledema is found in virtually all patients.[132,134] To establish the diagnosis, one must demonstrate elevated cerebrospinal fluid (CSF) pressure, normal CSF composition, and the absence of an intracranial mass on MRI or CT scan.[137]

The pathogenesis of this disorder is unknown. Bates and colleagues[138] found CSF prolactin to be markedly elevated in cases of pseudotumor cerebri. Prolactin appears to have an affinity for receptors in the choroid plexus, where CSF is produced. Prolactin has osmoregulatory functions and therefore may have a role in the increased CSF production found in pseudotumor cerebri.[132] Some believe that reduced CSF reabsorption is the etiology of pseudotumor cerebri. Ahlskog and O'Neill[139] noted an association between the occurrence of pseudotumor cerebri and the following conditions: corticosteroid therapy and its withdrawal, nalidixic acid therapy, nitrofurantoin therapy, tetracycline therapy, hypoparathyroidism, deficiencies or excesses of vitamin A, and iron deficiency anemia.

Pregnancy outcome appears to be unaffected by the illness.[132,136] There is no increase in fetal wastage or congenital anomalies.[132] Koppel and colleagues[140] reported a case of pseudotumor cerebri that presented in a 15-year-old primigravida following eclampsia. It lasted for 3 weeks. Wheatley and colleagues[141] noted a case of pseudotumor cerebri occurring in a diabetic pregnancy. They caution that it is important to make the distinction between symptoms of pseudotumor cerebri and visual impairment caused by diabetic retinopathy, as the treatments are different.[141] Thomas[142] described a case of pseudotumor cerebri occurring in two consecutive pregnancies in a woman with hemoglobin SC. In both instances, symptoms resolved following delivery and both infants were born at term.

Most patients respond well to conservative management.[131] The main objectives of treatment are relief of pain and preservation of vision. The patient should be followed closely with visual acuity and visual field determinations at intervals indicated by the clinical condition. In patients with mild disease, analgesics may be adequate. If pain persists, diuretics may be used. Acetazolamide, a carbonic anhydrase inhibitor, will reduce CSF production in many patients.[143] The usual dose is 500 mg twice daily. In more difficult cases, prednisone in doses of 40 to 60 mg daily usually provides good results.[131] Patients may be treated for 2 weeks, with the dose being tapered over the next month.[132] Serial lumbar punctures to reduce CSF pressure are rarely necessary today. Surgical approaches are reserved for refractory patients in whom rapid visual deterioration occurs.

Pseudotumor cerebri is not an indication for cesarean delivery. A review of the literature reveals that 73 percent of the reported patients delivered vaginally.[132] Cesarean delivery should be undertaken only for obstetric indications. Both epidural and spinal anesthesia, when expertly administered, can be safely used in patients with pseudotumor cerebri.[144] Bearing down, which can increase CSF pressure, should be avoided when possible. The second stage of labor should therefore be shortened by outlet forceps or by vacuum extraction.

The recurrence rate for pseudotumor cerebri appears to be between 10 and 12.3 percent in nonpregnant patients.[133,134] Pregnancy does not appear to predispose to a recurrence.[132]

Key Points

➤ Idiopathic seizures affect approximately 1 percent of the general population and are the most frequent neurologic complication of pregnancy.

➤ Prepregnancy counseling is imperative in the patient with a seizure disorder, and preconceptual folic acid therapy should be implemented under the direction of an obstetrician and a neurologist.

➤ Those with seizures occurring less than once each month will have the best control during pregnancy.

➤ The anticonvulsant medication that best controls the patient's seizures should be used during pregnancy.

➤ Because of the changes in plasma volume, drug distribution, and metabolism that occur during pregnancy, anticonvulsant levels should be checked frequently and dosages adjusted accordingly.

➤ Patients taking anticonvulsants have an increased risk of giving birth to an infant with both major and minor anomalies, but this risk is probably less than 10 percent. Therefore, the majority of patients with epilepsy will give birth to healthy infants.

➤ Carbamazepine and valproate are associated with neural tube defects, and these patients should receive 4 mg folic acid daily before and during early pregnancy.

➤ The vasoconstrictor drugs used to treat migraines should be avoided during pregnancy and lactation.

➤ Pregnancy does not hasten the onset of multiple sclerosis, nor does it hasten the onset of disability from multiple sclerosis.

➤ Carpal tunnel syndrome is common in pregnancy and usually responds to conservative splinting and/or glucocorticoid injection. Surgery can be safely undertaken if indicated during pregnancy.

REFERENCES

1. Cramer JA, Jones EE: Reproductive function in epilepsy. Epilepsia 32(Suppl 6):S19, 1991.
2. Back DJ, Bates M, Bowden A, et al: The interaction of phenobarbital and other anticonvulsants with oral contraceptive steroid therapy. Contraception 22:495, 1980.
3. Coulam CB, Annegers JF: Do anticonvulsants reduce the efficacy of oral contraceptives? Epilepsia 20:519, 1979.
4. Janz D, Schmidt D: Anti-epileptic drugs and failure of oral contraceptives. Lancet 1:1113, 1974.
5. Webber MP, Hauser WA, Ottman R, Annegers JF: Fertility in persons with epilepsy: 1935–1974. Epilepsia 27:746, 1986.
6. Dansky LV, Anderman E, Anderman F: Marriage and fertility in epileptic patients. Epilepsia 21:261, 1980.
7. Knight AH, Rhind EG: Epilepsy and pregnancy: a study of 153 pregnancies in 59 patients. Epilepsia 16:99, 1975.
8. Schmidt D, Canger R, Avanzini G, et al: Change of seizure frequency in pregnant epileptic women. J Neurol Neurosurg Psychiatry 46:751, 1983.
9. Tanganelli P, Regesta G: Epilepsy, pregnancy, and major birth anomalies: an Italian prospective, controlled study. Neurology 42(Suppl 5):89, 1992.
10. Sabers A, Rogvi-Hansen B, Dam M, et al: Pregnancy and epilepsy: a retrospective study of 151 pregnancies. Acta Neurol Scand 97:164, 1998.
11. Landon MJ, Kirkley M: Metabolism of diphenylhydantoin (phenytoin) during pregnancy. Br J Obstet Gynaecol 86:125, 1979.
12. Kochenour NK, Emery MG, Sawohuck RJ: Phenytoin metabolism in pregnancy. Obstet Gynecol 56:577, 1980.
13. Yerby MS, Friel PN, McCormick K, et al: Pharmacokinetics of anticonvulsants in pregnancy: alterations in plasma protein binding. Epilepsy Res 5:223, 1990.

14. Desmond MM, Schwanecke RP, Wilson GS, et al: Maternal barbiturate utilization and neonatal withdrawal symptomatology. J Pediatr 80:190, 1972.
15. Ogawa Y, Kaneko S, Otani K, Fukushima Y: Serum folic acid in epileptic mothers and their relationship to congenital malformations. Epilepsy Res 8:75, 1991.
16. Milunsky A, Jick H, Jick SS, et al: Multivitamin/folic acid supplementation in early pregnancy reduces the prevalence of neural tube defects. JAMA 262:2847, 1989.
17. Friis B, Sardemann H: Short reports: neonatal hypocalcaemia after intrauterine exposure to anticonvulsant drugs. Arch Dis Child 52:239, 1977.
18. Mountain KR, Hirsh J, Gallus AS: Neonatal coagulation defect due to anticonvulsant drug treatment in pregnancy. Lancet 1:265, 1970.
19. Bleyer WA, Skinner AL: Fatal neonatal hemorrhage after maternal anticonvulsant therapy. JAMA 235:626, 1976.
20. Yerby M, Koepsell T, Daling J: Pregnancy complications and outcomes in a cohort of women with epilepsy. Epilepsia 26:631, 1985.
21. Nelson KB, Ellenberg JH: Maternal seizure disorder, outcome of pregnancy, and neurologic abnormalities in the children. Neurology 32:1247, 1982.
22. Kallen B: A register study of maternal epilepsy and delivery outcome with special reference to drug use. Acta Neurol Scand 73:253, 1986.
23. Hiilesmaa VK, Bardy A, Teramo K: Obstetric outcome in women with epilepsy. Am J Obstet Gynecol 152:499, 1985.
24. Mastroiacovo P, Bertollini R, Licata D: Fetal growth in the offspring of epileptic women: results of an Italian multicentric cohort study. Acta Neurol Scand 78:110, 1988.
25. Hiilesmaa VK, Teramo K, Granstrom ML: Fetal head growth retardation associated with maternal antiepileptic drugs. Lancet 1:165, 1981.
26. Hvas CL, Henriksen TB, Ostergaard JR, Dam M: Epilepsy and pregnancy: effect of antiepileptic drugs and lifestyle on birthweight. Br J Obstet Gynaecol 107:896, 2000.
27. Battine D, Keneko S, Andermann E, et al: Intrauterine growth in the offspring of epileptic women: a prospective multicenter study. Epilepsy Res 36:53, 1999.
28. Hanson JW, Smith DW: The fetal hydantoin syndrome. J Pediatr 87:285, 1975.
29. Hanson JW, Myrianthopoulos NC, Sedgwick Harvey MA, Smith DW: Risks to the offspring of women treated with hydantoin anticonvulsants, with emphasis on the fetal hydantoin syndrome. J Pediatr 89:662, 1976.
30. Gaily E, Granstrom ML, Hiilesmaa V, Bardy A: Minor anomalies in offspring of epileptic mothers. J Pediatr 112:520, 1988.
31. Friis ML, Holm NV, Sindrup EH, et al: Facial clefts in sibs and children of epileptic patients. Neurology 36:346, 1986.
32. Kelly TE, Rein M, Edwards P: Teratogenicity of anticonvulsant drugs. Am J Med Genet 19:451, 1984.
33. Hecht JT, Annegers JF, Kurland LT: Epilepsy and clefting disorders: lack of evidence of a familial association. Am J Med Genet 33:244, 1989.
34. Nakane Y, Okuma T, Takahashi R, et al: Multi-institutional study on the teratogenicity and fetal toxicity of antiepileptic drugs: a report of a collaborative study group in Japan. Epilepsia 21:663, 1980.
35. Canger R, Battine D, Canevini MP, et al: Malformations in offspring of women with epilepsy: a prospective study. Epilepsia 40:1231, 1999.
36. Kaneko S, Otani K, Fukushima Y, et al: Teratogenicity of antiepileptic drugs: analysis of possible risk factors. Epilepsia 29:459, 1988.
37. Kaneko S, Otani K, Kondo T, et al: Malformation in infants

38. Jick SS, Terris BZ: Anticonvulsants and congenital malformations. Pharmacotherapy 17:561, 1997.
39. Lindhout D, Meinardi H, Meijer JWA, Nau H: Antiepileptic drugs and teratogenesis in two consecutive cohorts: changes in prescription policy paralleled by changes in pattern of malformations. Neurology 42(Suppl 5):94, 1992.
40. Dravet C, Julian C, Legras C, et al: Epilepsy, antiepileptic drugs, and malformations in children of women with epilepsy: a French prospective cohort study. Neurology 42(Suppl 5):75, 1992.
41. Koch S, Losche G, Jager-Roman E, et al: Major and minor birth malformations and antiepileptic drugs. Neurology 42(Suppl 5):83, 1992.
42. Gaily E, Granstrom ML: Minor anomalies in children of mothers with epilepsy. Neurology 42(Suppl 5):128, 1992.
43. Yerby MS, Leavitt A, Erickson M, et al: Antiepileptics and the development of congenital anomalies. Neurology 42(Suppl 5):132, 1992.
44. Nulman I, Scolnik D, Chitayat D, et al: Findings in children exposed in utero to phenytoin and carbamazepine monotherapy: independent effects of epilepsy and medications. Am J Med Genet 68:18, 1997.
45. Fahnehjelm KT, Wide K, Ygge J, et al: Visual and ocular outcome in children after prenatal exposure to antiepileptic drugs. Acta Ophthalmol Scand 77:530, 1999.
46. DiLiberti JH, Farndon PA, Dennis NR, Curry CJR: The fetal valproate syndrome. Am J Med Genet 19:473, 1984.
47. Ardinger HH, Atkin JF, Blackston RD, et al: Verification of the fetal valproate syndrome phenotype. Am J Med Genet 29:171, 1988.
48. Jager-Roman E, Deichl A, Jakob S, et al: Fetal growth, major malformations, and minor anomalies in infants born to women receiving valproic acid. J Pediatr 108:997, 1986.
49. Lindhout D, Schmidt D: In-utero exposure to valproate and neural tube defects. Lancet 2:1392, 1986.
50. Lindhout D, Omtzigt JGC, Cornel MC: Spectrum of neural-tube defects in 34 infants prenatally exposed to antiepileptic drugs. Neurology 42(Suppl 5):111, 1992.
51. Wegner C, Nau H: Alteration of embryonic folate metabolism by valproic acid during organogenesis: implications for mechanism of teratogenesis. Neurology 42(Suppl 5):17, 1992.
52. Jones KL, Lacro RV, Johnson KA, Adams J: Pattern of malformations in the children of women treated with carbamazepine during pregnancy. N Engl J Med 320:1661, 1989.
53. Rosa FW: Spina bifida in infants of women treated with carbamazepine during pregnancy. N Engl J Med 324:674, 1991.
54. Finnell RH, Buehler BA, Kerr BM, et al: Clinical and experimental studies linking oxidative metabolism to phenytoin-induced teratogenesis. Neurology 42(Suppl 5):25, 1992.
55. Dichter MA, Brodie MJ: New antiepileptic drugs. N Engl J Med 334:1583, 1996.
56. Gilman JT: Lamotrigine: an antiepileptic agent for the treatment of partial seizures. Ann Pharmacother 29:144, 1995.
57. Mackay FJ, Wilton LV, Pearce GL, et al: Safety of long-term lamotrigine in epilepsy. Epilepsia 38:881, 1997.
58. Ohman I, Vitols S, Tomson T: Lamotrigine in pregnancy: pharmacokinetics during delivery, in the neonate, and during lactation. Epilepsia 41:709, 2000.
59. Granstrom ML, Gaily E: Psychomotor development in children of mothers with epilepsy. Neurology 42(Suppl 5):144, 1992.
60. Gaily E, Kantola-Sorsa E, Granstrom ML: Intelligence of children of epileptic mothers. J Pediatr 113:677, 1988.
61. Moore SJ, Turnpenny P, Quinn A, et al: A clinical study of

57 children with fetal anticonvulsant syndromes. J Med Genet 37:489, 2000.

62. Dansky LV, Andermann E, Rosenblatt D, et al: Anticonvulsants, folate levels, and pregnancy outcome: a prospective study. Ann Neurol 21:176, 1987.

63. Annegers JF, Hauser WA, Elveback LR, et al: Seizure disorders in offspring of patients with a history of seizures—a maternal—paternal difference? Epilepsia 17:1, 1976.

64. Blandfort M, Tsuboi T, Vogel F: Genetic counseling in the epileptics. Hum Genet 76:303, 1987.

65. Bronshtein M, Zimmer EZ, Gerlis LM, et al: Early ultrasound diagnosis of fetal congenital heart defects in high-risk and low-risk pregnancies. Obstet Gynecol 82:225, 1993.

66. Wigton TR, Sabbagha RE, Tamura RK, et al: Sonographic diagnosis of congenital heart disease: comparison between the four-chamber view and multiple cardiac views. Obstet Gynecol 82:219, 1993.

67. Yerby MS: Problems and management of the pregnant woman with epilepsy. Epilepsia 28(Suppl 3):S29, 1987.

68. Orland MJ, Saltman RJ: Seizures. Washington Manual of Medical Therapeutics, 25th ed. 1986.

69. Sibai BM, Spinnato JA, Watson DL, et al: Eclampsia IV. Neurological findings and future outcome. Am J Obstet Gynecol 152:184, 1985.

70. Kaneko S, Sato T, Suzuki K: The levels of anticonvulsants in breast milk. Br J Clin Pharmacol 7:624, 1974.

71. Mattson RH, Cramer JA, Darney PD, Naftolin F: Use of oral contraceptives by women with epilepsy. JAMA 256:238, 1986.

72. Orme MLE: The clinical pharmacology of oral contraceptive steroids. Br J Clin Pharmacol 14:31, 1982.

73. Maggioni F, Alessi C, Maggino T, Zanchin G: Headache during pregnancy. Cephalalgia 17:765, 1997.

74. Somerville B: A study of migraine in pregnancy. Neurology 22:824, 1972.

75. Granella F, Sances G, Zanferrar C, et al: Migraine without aura and reproductive life events: a clinical epidemiological study of 1300 women. Headache 33:385, 1993.

76. Aube M: Migraine in pregnancy. Neurology 53(Suppl):S26, 1999.

77. Chen TC, Leviton A, Edelstein S, Ellenberg JH: Migraine and other diseases in women of reproductive age: the influence of smoking on observed associations. Arch Neurol 44:1024, 1987.

78. Chancellor AM, Wroe SJ, Cull RE: Migraine occurring for the first time in pregnancy. Headache 30:224, 1990.

79. Jacobson SL, Redman CW: Basilar migraine with loss of consciousness in pregnancy: case report. Br J Obstet Gynaecol 96:494, 1989.

80. Hughes HE, Goldstein DA: Birth defects following maternal exposure to ergotamine, beta blocker, and caffeine. J Med Genet 25:396, 1988.

81. O'Quinn S, Ephross SA, Williams V, et al: Pregnancy and perinatal outcomes in migraineurs using sumatriptan: a prospective study. Arch Gynecol Obstet 263:7, 1999.

82. Olesen C, Steffensen FH, Sorensen HT, et al: Pregnancy outcome following prescription for sumatriptan. Headache 40:20, 2000.

83. Jennett WB, Cross JN: Influence of pregnancy and oral contraception on the incidence of strokes in women of childbearing age. Lancet 1:1019, 1967.

84. Banerjee AK, Varma M, Vasista RK, Chopra JS: Cerebrovascular disease in north-west India: a study of necropsy material. J Neurol Neurosurg Psychiatry 52:512, 1989.

85. Cross JN, Castro PO, Jennett WB: Cerebral strokes associated with pregnancy in the puerperium. BMJ 3:214, 1968.

86. Brick JF, Riggs JE: Ischemic cerebrovascular disease in the young adult: emergence of oral contraceptive use and pregnancy as the major risk factors in the 1980s. W V Med J 85:7, 1989.

87. Lidegaard O: Oral contraceptives, pregnancy and the risk of cerebral thromboembolism: the influence of diabetes, hypertension, migraine, and previous thrombotic disease. Br J Obstet Gynaecol 102:153, 1995.

88. Brick JF: Vanishing cerebrovascular disease of pregnancy. Neurology 38:804, 1988.

89. Katz VL, Cefalo RC: Maternal death from carotid artery thrombosis associated with the syndrome of hemolysis, elevated liver function, and low platelets. Am J Perinatol 6:360, 1989.

90. Estanol B, Rodriguez A, Counte G, et al: Intracranial venous thrombosis in young women. Stroke 10:680, 1979.

91. Krayenbuhl HA: Cerebral venous and sinus thrombosis. Clin Neurosurg 14:1, 1967.

92. Bansal BC, Prakash C, Gupta RR, Brahmanandam KRV: Study of serum lipid and blood fibrinolytic activity in cases of cerebral venous/venous sinus thrombosis during the puerperium. Am J Obstet Gynecol 119:1079, 1974.

93. Abraham J, Rios PS, Inbaraj SG, et al: An epidemiological study of hemiplegia due to stroke in south India. Stroke 1:477, 1970.

94. Miller HJ, Hinkley CM: Berry aneurysms in pregnancy: a ten year report. South Med J 63:279, 1970.

95. Henderson CE, Torbey M: Rupture of intracranial aneurysm associated with cocaine use during pregnancy. Am J Perinatol 5:142, 1988.

96. Robinson JL, Hall CJ, Sevzimer CB: Arterial venous malformations, aneurysms, and pregnancy. J Neurosurg 41:63, 1974.

97. Minielly R, Yuzpe AA, Drake CC: Subarachnoid hemorrhage secondary to ruptured cerebral aneurysm in pregnancy. Obstet Gynecol 53:64, 1979.

98. Kawasaki N, Uchida T, Yamada M, et al: Conservative management of cerebellar hemorrhage in pregnancy. Int J Gynaecol Obstet 31:365, 1990.

99. D'Haese J, Christiaens F, d'Haens J, Camu F: Combined cesarean section and clipping of a ruptured cerebral aneurysm: a case report. J Neurosurg Anesthesiol 9:341, 1997.

100. Szabo MD, Crosby C, Sundaram P, et al: Hypertension does not cause spontaneous hemorrhage of intracranial arteriovenous malformations. Anesthesiology 70:761, 1989.

101. Laidler JA, Jackson IJ, Redfern N: The management of caesarean section in a patient with an intracranial arteriovenous malformation. Anaesthesia 44:490, 1989.

102. Buckley TA, Yau GH, Poon WS, Oh T: Caesarean section and ablation of a cerebral arteriovenous malformation. Anaesth Intensive Care 18:248, 1990.

103. Levy DM, Jaspan T: Anaesthesia for caesarean section in a patient with recent subarachnoid haemorrhage and severe pre-eclampsia. Anaesthesia 54:994, 1999.

104. McAlpine D, Lunisden CE, Acheson ED: Multiple Sclerosis, a Reappraisal, 2nd ed. Baltimore, Williams & Wilkins, 1972.

105. Weinshenker BG, Hader W, Carriere W, et al: The influence of pregnancy on disability from multiple sclerosis: a population-based study in Middlesex County, Ontario. Neurology 39:1438, 1989.

106. Liebowitz U, Antonovosky A, Katz R, et al: Does pregnancy increase the risk of multiple sclerosis? J Neurol Neurosurg Psychiatry 30:354, 1967.

107. Runmanker B, Andersen O: Pregnancy is associated with a lower risk of onset and a better prognosis in multiple sclerosis. Brain 118:253, 1995.

108. Millar JHD, Allison RS, Cheeseman EA: Pregnancy as a factor influencing relapse in disseminated sclerosis. Brain 82:417, 1959.

109. Birk K, Ford C, Smeltzer S, et al: The clinical course of multiple sclerosis during pregnancy and the puerperium. Arch Neurol 47:738, 1990.

110. Frith JA, McLeod JC: Pregnancy and multiple sclerosis. J Neurol Neurosurg Psychiatry 51:495, 1988.

111. Frith JA, McLeod JG: Pregnancy and multiple sclerosis: an Australian perspective. Clin Exp Neurol 24:1, 1987.

112. Nelson LM, Franklin GM, Jones MC: Risk of multiple sclerosis exacerbation during pregnancy and breast-feeding. JAMA 259:3441, 1988.

113. Bernardi S, Grasso MG, Bertollini R, et al: The influences of pregnancy on relapses of multiple sclerosis: a cohort study. Acta Neurol Scand 84:403, 1991.

114. Worthington J, Jones R, Crawford M, Forti A: Pregnancy and multiple sclerosis—a 3-year prospective study. J Neurol 241: 228, 1994.

115. Verdru P, Theys P, D'Hooghe MB, Carton H: Pregnancy and multiple sclerosis: the influence on longterm disability. Clin Neurol Neurosurg 96:38, 1994.

116. Confavreux C, Hutchinson M, Hours MM, et al: Rate of pregnancy-related relapse in multiple sclerosis. Pregnancy in Multiple Sclerosis Group. N Engl J Med 339:285, 1998.

117. Bader AM, Hunt CO, Datta S, et al: Anesthesia for the obstetric patient with multiple sclerosis. J Clin Anesth 1:21, 1988.

118. Khatri BO, D'Cruz O, Preissler G, et al: Plasmaphoresis in a pregnant patient with multiple sclerosis. Arch Neurol 47:11, 1990.

119. Orvieto R, Achiron R, Rotstein Z, et al: Pregnancy and multiple sclerosis: a 2-year experience. Eur J Obstet Gynecol Reprod Biol 82:191, 1999.

120. Wallace JT, Cook AW: Carpal tunnel syndrome in pregnancy. Am J Obstet Gynecol 73:1333, 1957.

121. Nicholas CG, Noone RB, Graham WP: Carpal tunnel syndrome in pregnancy. Hand 3:80, 1971.

122. Stolp-Smith KA, Pascoe MK, Ogburn PL Jr: Carpal tunnel syndrome in pregnancy: frequency severity and prognosis. Arch Phys Med Rehabil 79:1285, 1998.

123. McLennan HG, Oats JN, Walstab JE: Survey of hand symptoms in pregnancy. Med J Aust 147:542, 1987.

124. Ekman-Ordeberg G, Salgeback S, Ordeberg G: Carpal tunnel syndrome in pregnancy: a prospective study. Acta Obstet Gynecol Scand 66:233, 1987.

125. Wand JS: Carpal tunnel syndrome in pregnancy and lactation. J Hand Surg 15:93, 1990.

126. Wand JS: The natural history of carpal tunnel syndrome in lactation. J R Soc Med 82:349, 1989.

127. Massey EW: Carpal tunnel syndrome in pregnancy. Obstet Gynecol Surv 33:145, 1978.

128. Ellis JM: Treatment of carpal tunnel syndrome with vitamin B6. South Med J 80:882, 1987.

129. Assmus H, Hashemi B: Surgical treatment of carpal tunnel syndrome in pregnancy: results from 314 cases. Nervenarzt 71:470, 2000.

130. Tobin SM: Carpal tunnel syndrome in pregnancy. Am J Obstet Gynecol 97:493, 1967.

131. Katz VL, Peterson R, Cefalo RC: Pseudotumor cerebri and pregnancy. Am J Perinatol 6:442, 1989.

132. Peterson CM, Kelly JV: Pseudotumor cerebri in pregnancy: case reports and literature reviewed. Obstet Gynecol Surv 40: 323, 1985.

133. Weisberg LA: Benign intracranial hypertension. Medicine (Baltimore) 54:197, 1975.

134. Johnston I, Paterson A: Benign intracranial hypertension. II. CSF pressures and the circulation. Brain 97:301, 1974.

135. Ireland B, Corbett JJ, Wallace RB: The search for causes of idiopathic intracranial hypertension: a preliminary case-control study. Arch Neurol 47:315, 1990.

136. Koontz WL, Herbert WNP, Cefalo R: Pseudotumor cerebri in pregnancy. Obstet Gynecol 62:325, 1983.

137. Donaldson JO: Neurology in Pregnancy. Philadelphia, WB Saunders, 1978.

138. Bates GW, Whiteworth NS, Parker JL, et al: Elevated cerebrospinal fluid prolactin concentration in women with pseudotumor cerebri. South Med J 75:807, 1982.

139. Ahlskog JE, O'Neill BP: Pseudotumor cerebri. Ann Intern Med 97:249, 1982.

140. Koppel BS, Kaunitz AM, Tuchman AJ: Pseudotumor cerebri following eclampsia. Eur Neurol 30:6, 1990.

141. Wheatley T, Clark JD, Edwards OM, Jordan K: Retinal haemorrhages and papilloedema due to benign intracranial hypertension in a pregnant diabetic. Diabetic Med 3:482, 1986.

142. Thomas E: Recurrent benign intracranial hypertension associated with hemoglobin SC disease in pregnancy. Obstet Gynecol 67:7S, 1986.

143. Rubin RC, Henderson ES, Ommaya AK, et al: The production of cerebrospinal fluid in man and its modification by acetazolamide. J Neurosurg 25:430, 1966.

144. Palop R, Choed-Amphai E, Miller R: Epidural anesthesia for delivery complicated by benign intracranial hypertension. Anesthesiology 50:159, 1979.

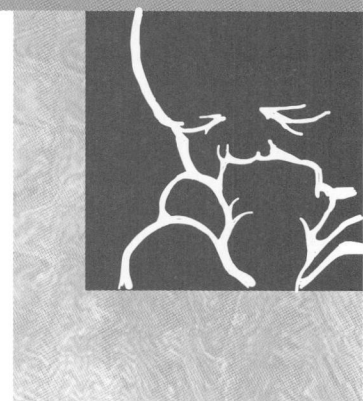

Chapter 38

Malignant Diseases and Pregnancy

LARRY J. COPELAND AND MARK B. LANDON

The juxtaposition of life and death presents numerous emotional and ethical conflicts to the patient, her family, and her physicians. The diagnosis of cancer for anyone is understandably frightening. To deal with cancer in the context of a pregnancy is particularly burdensome, since the patient may need to, or may perceive that she needs to, choose between her life or the life of her unborn. Cancer in pregnancy complicates the management of both the cancer and the pregnancy. Both diagnostic and therapeutic interventions must carefully address the associated risks to both the patient and the fetus. Informed decisions will require evaluation of a number of factors, and after careful counseling these considerations will be the foundation on which treatment decisions will be made. Over recent years there has been an evolution in the philosophy of care from one of total disregard of the pregnancy with frequent immediate termination to a more thoughtful approach in which management decisions attempt to balance the maternal and fetal interests ideally to limit risk of death or injury to both.

While cancer is the second most common cause of death for women in their reproductive years, only about 1 in 1,000 pregnancies[1] is complicated by cancer. Since there are no large prospective studies that address cancer treatment in pregnancy, physicians tend to base treatment strategies on small retrospective studies or anecdotal reports that occasionally present conflicting information.[2]

A successful outcome is dependent on a cooperative multidisciplinary approach. The management plan must be formulated within a medical, moral, ethical, legal, and religious framework acceptable to the patient and guided by and dependent on the communication and education resources of the health care team.

The malignancies most commonly encountered in the pregnant patient are, in descending order, breast cancer, cervical cancer, melanoma, ovarian cancer, thyroid cancer, leukemia, lymphoma, and colorectal cancer.[3] The frequencies of these diseases may increase secondary to the trend to delay childbearing. Before specific malignancies are discussed, some of the general issues are reviewed.

CHEMOTHERAPY DURING PREGNANCY

Pharmacology of Chemotherapy during Pregnancy

Since pregnancy alters physiology, there is the potential for altered pharmokinetics of the chemotherapy. Orally administered medications will be subjected to altered gastrointestinal motility. Peak drug concentrations will be decreased due to the 50 percent expansion in plasma volume, producing a longer drug half-life unless there is a concurrent increase in metabolism or excretion. The increase in plasma proteins and fall in albumin may alter drug availability, and amniotic fluid may act as a pharmacologic third space, potentially increasing toxicity due to delayed metabolism and excretion. Hepatic oxidation and renal blood flow are both elevated during pregnancy and may influence the metabolism and excretion of most drugs.[4] However, since pharmacologic studies in the pregnant woman are lacking, we currently assume that initial drug dosages are similar to the nonpregnant woman and adjustments to dose are based on toxicity on a course-by-course basis.

Since antineoplastic agents can be found in breast milk, breast-feeding is contraindicated.[5]

Drug Effects on the Fetus

Acute Effects

Because antineoplastic agents are targeted for the rapidly dividing malignant cell, one would expect the fetus with its accelerated growth pattern to be particularly subject to a high rate of serious toxicities. Clear documentation of such is not the case. Spontaneous abortions, fetal organ toxicity, premature birth, and low birth weight are potential risks in the pregnant patient receiving chemotherapy. Excluding the intentional use of abortifacients, it is difficult to demonstrate clearly that the use of chemotherapy results in an increase in the spontaneous abortion rate over the expected 15 to 20 percent. Fetal organ toxicity has not been reported as a major problem, although neonatal myelosuppression[6] and hearing loss in a 1-year-old[7] have been reported. Since early induction of labor or surgical delivery is often a component of the overall treatment plan, it is difficult to identify premature birth as a specific result of the chemotherapy. On the other hand, it appears that low birth weight is associated with the administration of chemotherapy in the second and third trimesters.[8]

Teratogenicity

All drugs undergo animal teratogenicity testing, and based on these results the drugs are assigned risk categories (Table 38–1) by the U.S. Food and Drug Administration (FDA).[9] Based on this system, most chemotherapeutic agents are rated as C, D, or X.[9] However, animal teratogenicity testing cannot always be reliably extrapolated to the human. For example, a drug (e.g., aspirin) may show teratogenic effects in animals and not affect humans. The opposite is also true and as such has serious potential to do harm; for example, a drug may show no animal teratogenicity (e.g., thalidomide) but cause serious human anomalies (see Chapters 7 and 9).

While the literature addressing chemotherapy administration during pregnancy is somewhat limited and dated, reviews by Nicholson[10] and Doll and colleagues[4] provide us with some information regarding the frequency of affected offspring. Nicholson reported that first-trimester exposure resulted in about a 10 percent frequency of major fetal malformations. For a similar situation, Doll and colleagues reported 17 and 25 percent frequencies for single-agent chemotherapy and combination chemotherapy, respectively. However, some of the patients from the later study also received irradiation, and exclusion of these cases drops the malformation rate to 6 percent. The risk of fetal malformation varies with the drug classification and specific drug. In general, antimetabolites and the alkylating agents appear to carry the highest risk.[11]

Table 38–1. FDA RISK CATEGORIES FOR DRUG USE DURING PREGNANCY

Category	Definition
A	Controlled studies have demonstrated no risk, and the possibility of fetal harm appears remote.
B	*Either* animal studies have failed to identify a risk but there are no controlled studies in women, *or* animal studies have shown an adverse effect that was not confirmed in controlled studies in women.
C	*Either* animal studies have revealed adverse effects and there are no controlled studies in women, *or* studies in women and animals are not available. Use drugs only if the potential benefit justifies the potential risk to the fetus.
D	There is evidence of fetal risk, but the benefits may be acceptable despite the risk in either a life-threatening situation or a serious disease for which safer drugs are ineffective.
X	Studies in animals or humans have demonstrated fetal abnormalities, and the risk of the drug in pregnant women clearly outweighs any possible benefit.

Adapted from Briggs GG, Freeman RK, Yaffe SJ: Instructions for use of the reference guide. *In* Briggs GG, Freeman RK, Yaffe SJ (eds): A Reference Guide to Fetal and Neonatal Risk: Drugs in Pregnancy and Lactation. 5th ed. Baltimore, Williams & Wilkins, 1998, p xxii.

ANTIMETABOLITES. Historically, aminopterin was used as an abortifacient, and in cases of failed abortion the risk of fetal malformation was about 50 percent. Methotrexate has replaced aminopterin for chemotherapeutic purposes, and, while similar types of anomalies occur, the 7 percent frequency is much reduced.[11] The use of low-dose methotrexate for systemic diseases (e.g., rheumatic disease and psoriasis) does not appear to produce teratogenicity.[12]

ALKYLATING AGENTS. The alkylating agents are a commonly used group of drugs for the management of malignancies. Unfortunately, most of the alkylating agents have demonstrated some teratogenic potential. Since these drugs are frequently given in combination with other nonalkylating agents, it is often difficult to identify the risk specific to the alkylating agent.

Because detailed ultrasonography may fail to identify subtle anatomic but serious functional abnormalities prior to 20 weeks' gestation, patients may want to consider the option of pregnancy termination if first-trimester chemotherapy is planned or administered. The risk of teratogenicity during the second and third trimesters is significantly reduced, possibly no different from that for pregnant woman who are not exposed to chemotherapy.[4]

ANTITUMOR ANTIBIOTICS. Even when administered in early pregnancy, antitumor antibodies appear to be associated with a low risk of teratogenicity. There is conflicting information in the literature as to whether the anthracyclines cross the placenta.[13–15] There is no evidence of bleomycin or dactinomycin teratogenicity.[16–18] Elit and colleagues report a fetus diagnosed with ventriculomegaly 1 week after one cycle of bleomycin, cisplatin, and etoposide for an ovarian germ cell malignancy. No baseline study was performed. The infant developed significant ventriculomegaly and cerebral atrophy. Causation between the chemotherapy and fetal complication seems unlikely but is unknown.[19]

VINCA ALKALOIDS. Vincristine and vinblastine, while potent teratogens in animals, do not appear to be as teratogenic in humans.[20]

MISCELLANEOUS. Cisplatin has been used in at least 10 pregnancies[7,16–26] without fetal malformation or toxicity, other than the possible abnormality reported by Elit and colleagues.[19] Henderson and colleagues[7] report bilateral sensorineural hearing loss at age 1 following in utero second-trimester exposure to carboplatinum. However, there were other potential causes of the hearing loss in this patient, including prematurity, prior cisplatin exposure, and neonatal gentamicin. Procarbazine and asparginase have both been associated with subsequent fetal malformations.[4,10,27]

COMBINATION CHEMOTHERAPY. There is no convincing evidence that there is a synergistic increase in malformations with the use of multiple-agent regimens when compared with single-agent therapy.[4,10]

NATIONAL REGISTRY. In 1984 the National Cancer Institute established a national registry for in utero exposure to chemotherapy.[28] The registry is currently located at the University of Oklahoma and is under the direction of Dr. John J. Mulvihill. Through August 2000, the registry had summaries of approximately 302 patients. Of the first 210 case studies there were 29 abnormal outcomes with a total of 52 defects. Only two abnormal outcomes were associated with exposure after the first trimester.

Delayed Effects

While second malignancies, impaired growth and development, intellectual impairment, and infertility have been reported after chemotherapy administration to children, the delayed effects of in utero exposure are less well documented.[6,29]

In summary, the risks of exposing a fetus to chemotherapy correlate highly with the gestational age at the time of the exposure. Most organogenesis occurs between 3 and 8 weeks of embryonic life, and it is during this time that major morphologic abnormalities are most likely to occur from exposure to any chemotherapeutic agent. Second- and third-trimester chemotherapy exposure does not appear to carry a significantly increased risk of major fetal anomalies.

RADIATION, DIAGNOSTIC AND THERAPEUTIC

The potential for fetal injury arises from exposure to ionizing radiation, both the low-dose diagnostic procedures and the more intense doses associated with radiation therapy. This subject is discussed in Chapter 7.

SURGERY AND ANESTHESIA, GENERAL FACTORS

While aspects of surgery are addressed below under the specific cancer sites, there are some general considerations worthy of review. Although complications of surgery can threaten the fetus, extraperitoneal surgery is not related to spontaneous abortion or preterm labor. Abdominal or pelvic surgery, if timing flexibility exists, is best performed in the second trimester to limit the risk of first-trimester spontaneous abortion or preterm labor. In the first trimester, progesterone therapy is indicated (weeks 7 to 12) following a bilateral oophorectomy. Perioperative cautions include attention to the relative safety of all drugs administered. Fever secondary to either infection or atelectasis should be treated promptly, since it may be associated with fetal abnormalities.

There is no evidence that there are significant risks of anesthesia independent of coexisting disease.[30] In the second and third trimesters, careful attention to positioning is required so as to avoid vena cava compression from the enlarged uterus.

PREGNANCY FOLLOWING CANCER TREATMENT

With improved survival rates for many childhood and adolescent malignancies, one must be prepared to offer prenatal counseling to the young woman who presents with a personal cancer history. Issues worthy of review and in need of clarification for the obstetrician and the patient are listed in the box "Counseling Issues for Pregnancy Following Cancer Treatment."

While previous abdominal irradiation for a Wilms' tumor appears to adversely affect the risk of pregnancy complications, including increased perinatal mortality, low birth weight, and abnormal pregnancy, a review of

Counseling Issues for Pregnancy Following Cancer Treatment

1. What is the risk of recurrence of the malignancy?
2. If a recurrence was diagnosed, depending on the most likely sites, what would be the nature of the probable treatment? How would such treatment compromise both the patient and the fetus?
3. Will prior treatments—pelvic surgery, radiation to pelvis or abdomen, or chemotherapy—affect fertility or reproductive outcome?
4. Will the hormonal milieu of pregnancy adversely affect an estrogen-receptor–positive tumor?

pregnancies following treatment for Hodgkin's lymphoma revealed no increased poor pregnancy outcome.[31] However, the rate of ovarian failure following the multiple drug combinations is over 50 percent in some reports.[32] Also, a combination of pelvic irradiation and chemotherapy for Hodgkin's disease results in an even higher rate of ovarian failure.

Will a pregnancy increase the risk of recurrence or accelerate recurrence? Even in women with estrogen receptor–positive breast cancer, there is no evidence that pregnancy adversely affects survival. In addition to the altered hormonal milieu, concern is also directed toward the potential for accelerated tumor activity associated with alterations in the pregnant patient's immune system. There are no data to support this concern. Long-term follow-up studies of children with in utero exposure to antineoplastic agents have not demonstrated any impairment in growth, despite an increased frequency of intrauterine growth restriction.[6,29] In those children who have been tested for intellectual development, no impairment has been identified.[33]

CANCER DURING PREGNANCY

General Considerations

The risk of having a coincident malignant tumor during pregnancy is approximately 0.1 percent. Approximately one third of recorded maternal deaths are secondary to a coexisting malignancy. Delays in diagnosis of the cancer during pregnancy are common for a number of reasons: (1) many of the presenting symptoms of cancer are often attributed to the pregnancy; (2) many of the physiologic and anatomic alterations of pregnancy can compromise the physical examination; (3) many serum tumor markers (β-human chorionic gonadotropin [hCGs], α-fetoprotein, CA 125, and others) are increased during pregnancy; and (4) our ability to perform either imaging studies or invasive diagnostic procedures is often altered during pregnancy.

Since the gestational age is significant when evaluating the risks of treatments, it is important to determine gestational age accurately. An early ultrasound evaluation may be useful in this regard.

BREAST CANCER

The predicted number of breast cancer cases in women in the United States for the year 2000 is 184,200, and the predicted number of related deaths is 41,200.[34] Approximately 2 to 3 percent of all breast cancers in women under age 40 occur concurrent with pregnancy or lactation, and approximately 1 in 1,360 to 3,330 pregnancies is complicated by breast cancer.[35] However, there may be an increase in the frequency of breast cancer complicating other forms of cancer due to delayed childbearing.[36]

In general, the risk of breast cancer is directly related to the duration of ovarian function. Therefore, both early menarche and late menopause appear to increase the likelihood of developing breast cancer. However, interruption of the normal cyclic ovarian function by pregnancy appears protective. This apparent protective effect may be secondary to the normal hormonal milieu of pregnancy that produces epithelial proliferation, followed by marked differentiation and mitotic rest. Multiparity and in particular multiparous patients who breast-feed have a lower risk of developing breast cancer than does the nulliparous woman. Based on one study of almost 90,000 women, breast-feeding may not be an independent protective factor.[37]

Paradoxically, carriers of BRCA1 and BRCA2 mutations may have an increased risk of developing breast cancer by having children.[38]

Diagnosis and Staging

Breast abnormalities should be evaluated in the same manner as if the patient were not pregnant. The most common presentation of breast cancer in pregnancy is a painless lump discovered by the patient. Despite the striking physiologic breast changes of pregnancy, including nipple enlargement and increases in glandular tissue resulting in engorgement and tenderness, breast cancer should be screened for during pregnancy. Since the breast changes become more pronounced in later pregnancy, it is important to perform a thorough breast examination at the initial visit. Diagnostic delays are often attributed to physician reluctance to evaluate breast complaints or abnormal findings in pregnancy. While bilateral serosanguinous discharge may be normal in late pregnancy, masses require prompt and definitive evaluation. The lengths of delays in diagnosis of breast cancer in pregnancy are commonly 3 to 7 months or longer.[39]

A case-control study from Princess Margaret Hospital suggested that pregnant patients are at higher risk of presenting with advanced disease because pregnancy impedes early detection.[40] Mammography in pregnancy is controversial. While the radiation exposure to the fetus is negligible,[41] the hyperplastic breast of pregnancy is characterized by increased tissue density, making interpretation more difficult.[42]

Fine-needle aspiration (FNA) of a mass for cytologic study is recommended. FNA is reliable for a diagnosis of carcinoma (false-positive results are rare), but if a solid mass is negative for tumor it should be evaluated by excisional biopsy. Similar to the nonpregnant patient, approximately 20 percent of breast biopsies performed in pregnancy reveal cancer. Tissue biopsies should be submitted for estrogen receptor (ER) and progesterone receptor (PR) analyses. Consistent with the fact that these patients are young, the majority are receptor negative.[43] There is concern that false-negative ER results performed by the ligand-binding method may occur in pregnancy because of either competitive inhibition by high levels of estrogens or by down-regulation. Immunologic assays that use monoclonal antibody recognize both occupied and unoccupied receptors and therefore may more accurately reflect the receptor status.

Prior to proceeding with treatment, the patient requires staging. All draining lymph nodes should be evaluated. The contralateral breast must be carefully assessed. Laboratory tests should include baseline liver function tests and serum tumor markers, carcinoembryonic antigen (CEA), and CA 15-3. CA 15-3 appears to be a useful tumor marker for monitoring breast cancer in pregnancy.[44] A chest x-ray is indicated and, if the liver function tests are abnormal, the liver can be evaluated by ultrasound. With precautions of good hydration and insertion of a urinary bladder catheter, a bone scan can be performed in pregnancy. However, in an asymptomatic patient with normal blood tests, the yield is low, and therefore it is not usually performed in those circumstances. In a symptomatic patient, radiographs of the specific symptomatic bones are advised.

While one report suggests an increased incidence of inflammatory breast cancer in pregnancy,[45] other reviews have not confirmed this observation, and it is generally thought that breast cancers in pregnancy are histologically identical to the nonpregnant patient of the same age. Because inflammatory breast cancer can be mistaken for mastitis, a biopsy of breast tissue should be performed when a breast suspected of being infected is incised and drained.

Treatment

The treatment of breast carcinoma at any time is often overshadowed by psychologic and emotional factors. Because of potential risks to the developing fetus, treatment decisions carry an additional burden. Patients with advanced disease and a poor prognosis may consider termination on this basis alone. Therapy, however, must be individualized in accordance with present knowledge and with the specific desires of the patient.

Local Therapy

The usual criteria for breast-preserving therapy versus modified radical mastectomy pertain to the patient with breast cancer, stages I to III.[46] However, the option of lumpectomy, axillary node dissection, and irradiation is complicated by the presence of the pregnancy. One publication presents a mathematical model suggesting the risk of axillary metastases due to treatment delay is minimal and may be acceptable to some third-trimester patients with early breast cancer who prefer lumpectomy with radiation postpartum.[47] Consideration should be given to the delay of irradiation until after delivery. Experimetal calculations suggest that a tumor dose of 5,000 cGy will expose the fetus to 10 to 15 cGy while the fetus is within the true pelvis. Later in pregnancy, parts of the fetus may receive as much as 200 cGy.[48] Brent[49] has suggested that 5 cGy is a relatively safe upper limit of fetal exposure. While the potential for teratogenesis is reduced later in pregnancy, radiation can affect fetal growth and may carry a risk for future carcinogenesis or secondary birth defects.

Pregnancy Termination

Since early studies suggested a poorer outcome in the pregnant patient, it was assumed that the hormonal changes of pregnancy contributed to rapid growth. Therefore, therapeutic abortion was frequently advised. At present, a harmful effect of continuing pregnancy has not been demonstrated in most published series (Table 38–2). However, it is difficult to evaluate the potential bias toward performing abortion in patients with advanced disease. Since young women tend to have hormone-receptor–negative tumors,[51] it is difficult to make an argument, based on hormonal concerns, for either termination of pregnancy or oophorectomy as an adjunct to therapy.[52–54]

Patients who present with either metastatic breast carcinoma or rapidly progressive inflammatory carci-

Table 38–2. SURVIVAL FROM BREAST CANCER IN PATIENTS UNDERGOING THERAPEUTIC ABORTION COMPARED TO THOSE NOT UNDERGOING ABORTION

Authors	Delivered		Therapeutic Abortion		Comments
	No. of Patients	5-Yr Survival	No. of Patients	5-Yr Survival	
Adair (1953)	36	44	23	70	25 pregnant at diagnosis, 34 pregnant after treatment for cancer. Only node-positive patients benefited from abortion
Holleb and Farrow (1962)	12	33	12	17	Surgery during first trimester
Rissanen (1968)	20	50	7	43	4 patients (1 aborted; 3 delivered) were stage IV
Clark and Reid (1978)	93	29	13	15	12% spontaneous abortion; 1 stillbirth. Abortion was not biased for more advanced disease
King et al. (1985)	35	67	18	53	For stage I patients: delivery vs. abortion: 18 vs. 4 patients; 5-yr survival is 88% vs. 33%

Modified from Holmes FA: Breast cancer during pregnancy. Cancer Bull 46:405, 1994.

noma frequently elect pregnancy termination. In general, delays of therapy should be avoided, especially for the patient with inflammatory breast cancer. Immediate initiation of chemotherapy is critical to providing the patient with inflammatory carcinoma with any chance for long-term survival. In the patient with a clinical indication for adjuvant chemotherapy, other than inflammatory carcinoma, the delay of instituting chemotherapy and awaiting fetal pulmonary maturity should be considered in select third-trimester situations. A recent French study reported 17 of 20 pregnancies, in patients treated with chemotherapy for breast carcinoma, resulted in live births.[55] Others concur with the use of chemotherapy in the second and third trimesters in the management of breast cancer.[56,57]

Prognosis

As with any malignant disease, the prognosis best correlates with the anatomic extent of disease at the time of diagnosis. The presence and extent of nodal involvement is especially predictive of prognosis in both nonpregnant and pregnant patients. Table 38–3 provides 5- and 10-year survival data by nodal status.[45,52,58–63] While nodal status is of prognostic significance, the number of positive nodes is also important. In the preg-

Table 38–3. 5- AND 10-YEAR SURVIVAL RATES, BY NODAL STATUS, OF PREGNANT OR LACTATING PATIENTS TREATED FOR BREAST CANCER

Investigators	No. of Patients	Overall		Node Negative		Node Positive	
		5-Yr (%)	10-Yr (%)	5-Yr (%)	10-Yr (%)	5-Yr (%)	10-Yr (%)
White and White[59]	806	13	9	21	13	7	6
Holleb and Farrow[52]	117	31	—	65	—	17	—
Byrd et al.[58]	29	55	—	100	80	28	6
Applewhite et al.[39]	48	25	15	56	22	18	13
Riberio and Palmer[61]	59	31	24	90	90	37	21
Clark and Reid[62]							
Pregnant	121	—	22	—	35	—	22
Lactating	80	—	32	—	69	—	18
King et al.[45]	63	53	49	82	71	36	36
Petrek et al.[63]	56	61	45	82	77	47	25

nant patient, the 5-year survival rate is 82 percent for patients with three or fewer positive nodes and 27 percent if greater than three nodes contain tumor.[45] Pregnancy, probably due to the associated delays in diagnosis, appears to increase the frequency of nodal disease, with 60 to 85 percent of patients exhibiting axillary nodal disease at diagnosis.[45,64]

When controlled for age and stage, pregnancy does not seem to affect prognosis adversely.[40,63,65,66] Some have suggested a worse prognosis if the cancer is diagnosed in the second trimester.[65]

Subsequent Pregnancy

While the consensus is that subsequent pregnancies do not adversely affect survival, there are recommendations regarding the timing of a subsequent pregnancy.[67,68] It is generally advised that women with node-negative disease wait for 2 to 3 years, and this interval should be extended to 5 years for patients with positive nodes. Others have advised that no delay is indicated for the patient with good prognostic disease who does not receive postoperative adjuvant chemotherapy.[69] It has been advised that patients should undergo a complete metastatic work-up prior to a subsequent pregnancy.

While no studies indicate that subsequent pregnancy adversely affects survival, the retrospective reports that suggest a potential favorable affect of subsequent pregnancy are too small to draw firm conclusions.[65,70] The trend to better survival is also noted in patients who received adjuvant chemotherapy and subsequently became pregnant.[71]

LACTATION AND BREAST RECONSTRUCTION

Lactation is possible in a small percentage of patients after breast-conserving therapy for early stage breast cancer.[72,73] Lumpectomy using a radial incision rather than the cosmetically preferred circumareolar incision is less likely to disrupt ductal anatomy. Disruption of the ductal system may increase the rate of mastitis. Breastfeeding is contraindicated in women receiving chemotherapy, since significant levels can be found in breast milk.

Breast reconstruction with the use of autologous tissue has increased secondary to questions about the use of silicone-filled implants. The transverse rectus myocutaneous flap (TRAM) is one popular method of breast reconstruction. Since the donor site is a portion of the anterior abdominal wall, there is potential concern when the patient develops abdominal distention from pregnancy. In one case report and review of the literature, nine cases of pregnancy following breast reconstruction experienced no problem with anterior abdominal wall integrity.[74]

HODGKIN'S DISEASE AND NON-HODGKIN'S LYMPHOMA

Hodgkin's Disease

Approximately 35,900 cases of lymphoma will be diagnosed in women in the United States in the year 2000, and only about 12 percent of these will be Hodgkin's disease.[34] Hodgkin's disease, commonly encountered in patients in their late teens and twenties, occurs at a mean age of 32 years. Non-Hodgkin's lymphomas occur at a mean age of 42 and therefore are reported less frequently in association with pregnancy. Lymphomas complicate approximately 1 in 6,000 pregnancies. Spontaneous abortion, stillbirth rates, and preterm births do not appear to be increased.[75,76] Pregnancy does not appear to affect adversely the course of the disease.[77,78] Routine termination of pregnancy should not be advised. While some advocate therapeutic abortion for the patient with a first-trimester pregnancy and Hodgkin's disease to allow complete staging, others, probably more appropriately, have limited the role of therapeutic abortion to those women requiring infradiaphragmatic irradiation or those with systemic symptoms or visceral disease, which are best managed with multiagent chemotherapy.

Hodgkin's disease frequently presents with enlarged cervical or axillary lymph nodes. The diagnosis is established by biopsy of the suspicious nodes. The presence of systemic symptoms such as night sweats, pruritis, or weight loss suggests more extensive disease. Two histologic variants, nodular sclerosis and lymphocyte-predominant, have a better prognosis than mixed cellularity and lymphocyte-depleted tumors.

Clinical staging for lymphoma necessitates the systemic evaluation by history, laboratory findings, bone marrow, and radiographic imaging. Clinical treatment and staging should be individualized. Pathologic staging for Hodgkin's disease may involve laparotomy and splenectomy; however, this is not usually necessary for non-Hodgkin's lymphoma, as disseminated disease can usually be documented without surgery. The minimal staging for Hodgkin's disease during pregnancy includes radiographic examination of the chest, liver function tests, bone marrow biopsy, complete blood count, and urinalysis. Chest tomography or computed tomographic (CT) scan of the mediastinum may be nec-

Table 38–4. STAGING CLASSIFICATION OF HODGKIN'S DISEASE*

Stage	Description
I	Involvement of a single lymph node region (I) or of a single extralymphatic organ site (I$_E$)
II	Involvement of two or more lymph node regions on the same side of the diaphragm (II) or localized involvement of an extralymphatic organ site and of one or more lymph node regions on the same side of the diaphragm (II$_E$)
III	Involvement of lymph node regions on both sides of the diaphragm (III), which also may be accompanied by localized involvement of an extralymphatic organ or site (III$_E$), of the spleen (III$_S$), or of both (III$_{SE}$)
IV	Diffuse or disseminated involvement of an extralymphatic organ with or without localized lymph node involvement (liver, bone marrow, lung, skin)

*Symptoms of unexplained fever, night sweats, and unexplained weight loss of 10 percent of normal body weight results in classification of patients as B; absence of these symptoms is denoted as A.

essary to evaluate nodal enlargement in the chest. Evaluation of the abdomen is compromised by the gravid uterus, and some consideration should be given to delaying abdominal imaging until after the first trimester. Magnetic resonance imaging (MRI) may be the safest technique for demonstrating intra-abdominal adenopathy. Isotope scans of the liver and bone are best avoided during pregnancy. A single-shot lymphangiogram results in an exposure of less than 1 rad to the fetus and is probably safe after the first trimester.[79] Ultrasonography is safe and may provide useful information.

Disease stage (Table 38–4) is the most important factor in treatment planning and prognosis. Survival for early-stage Hodgkin's disease exceeds 90 percent, whereas patients with disseminated nodal disease have a 5-year survival rate of about 50 percent. As expected, patients with stage IV disease have poor survival rates. While radiation therapy is the mainstay of treatment for early-stage Hodgkin's disease, combination chemotherapy is employed for the treatment of advanced-stage disease with organ involvement. The MOPP regimen (nitrogen mustard, vincristine, procarbazine, and prednisone) in combination with radiation is often used to treat patients with bulky, large mediastinal masses or disseminated nodal disease. Most investigators agree that treatment should not be withheld during pregnancy except in early-stage disease, particularly if the diagnosis is made in late gestation. Radiotherapy to the supradiaphragmatic regions may be performed with abdominal shielding after the first trimester. Thomas and Peckham[79] reported three cases of mantle field irradiation with abdominal shielding for supradiaphragmatic

disease. The estimated radiation exposures to the fetus for these patients at 10, 15, and 16 weeks were 2.5, 4.4, and 10.4 rad, respectively. While these pregnancies went to term with apparent normal outcomes, long-term follow-up on these infants was not presented. Spontaneous abortion has been reported with an estimated first-trimester fetal dose of 9 rad secondary to scatter from delivering 4,400 rad to the chest of a patient receiving treatment for a recurrence.[80] Another patient in the same report received 3,300 rad to a mantle field at 16 weeks' gestation, and no adverse affects were noted. In general, if the estimated exposure to a first-trimester fetus is expected to exceed 10 rad or if combination chemotherapy is planned for the first trimester, therapeutic abortion should be considered because of the risk of fetal malformation.[81] Asymptomatic early-stage disease presenting in the second half of pregnancy may be followed closely while preparations are made for early delivery.[80] The use of steroids and single-agent chemotherapy has been proposed for the patient with systemic symptoms.

Subdiaphragmatic or advanced disease requires chemotherapy. Since many of the most commonly used chemotherapeutic agents are known teratogens, such treatment is best avoided in the first trimester. Similar treatments should also be approached with caution later in pregnancy, although most case reports have documented only intrauterine growth restriction and neonatal neutropenia as complications. Long-term follow-up toxicity studies are lacking.

Following therapy for Hodgkin's disease, it has been suggested that pregnancy planning should take into consideration that about 80 percent of recurrences will manifest within 2 years. Treatments for Hodgkin's disease may compromise the reproductive potential of young patients.[32,82] As reflected in Figure 38–1, ovarian

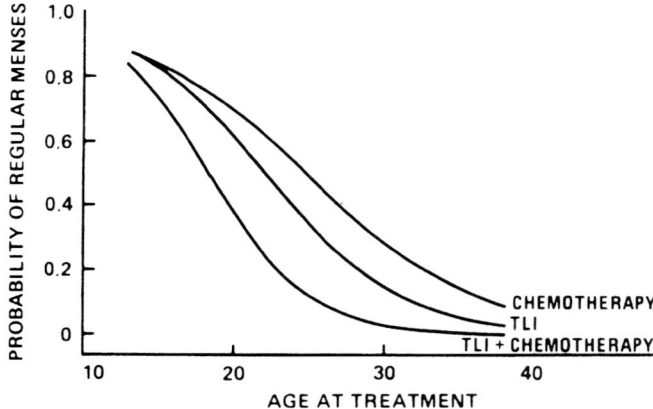

Figure 38–1. Probability of regular menses after chemotherapy, total lymphoid irradiation (TLI), and TLI and chemotherapy in patients with Hodgkin's disease. The synergistic effect is more apparent in younger women. (From Horning SJ, Hoppe RT, Kaplan HS: Female reproduction after treatment for Hodgkin's disease. N Engl J Med 304:1377, 1981, with permission.)

failure is more likely to occur in older patients, even if treated with fewer courses of chemotherapy.[83] Some studies have reported a rate of only 12 percent of normal ovarian function following therapy for Hodgkin's disease.[84] Combined treatment with irradiation and chemotherapy provides the highest risk of ovarian failure.

Bilateral midline oophoropexy at staging laparotomy has been advocated for the patient requiring pelvic node irradiation.[85] Even with this technique the ovaries may be exposed to a significant dose of irradiation, ranging from 600 to 3,500 rad.[79] Additionally, there are concerns of adhesions and ovum pick-up and transport. While combined oral contraceptives have been advocated to preserve ovarian function, there is no evidence that the gonads are protected.[85] Depending on their availability, new reproductive technologies, including oocyte donation and embryo cryopreservation, can be considered for select situations.[86]

Patients who become pregnant after treatment for Hodgkin's lymphoma do not demonstrate increased adverse perinatal outcomes such as fetal wastage, term birth, and birth defects when compared with sibling controls.[87,88] While fetal anomalies have occurred after treatment for Hodgkin's disease,[89] chromosomal abnormalities or a new gene mutation have not been diagnosed.[82] The absence of a repetitive pattern of malformations makes it difficult to imply a casual relationship between any birth defects observed and previous therapy for Hodgkin's disease.

Non-Hodgkin's Lymphoma

Non-Hodgkin's lymphoma occurs at a mean age of 42 years and therefore is reported less frequently than Hodgkin's disease in association with pregnancy. In general, non-Hodgkin's disease is more likely to affect a pregnancy adversely because patients usually have an aggressive histology and advanced-stage disease. Burkitt's lymphoma is usually rapidly progressive and may involve the breast and ovary. Lymphoma of the breast has a particularly poor prognosis, and it has been speculated that there may be a hormonal influence on this malignancy in pregnant patients.[90]

In a report by Ward and Weiss,[91] about 60 percent (12 of 21) of second- and third-trimester cases resulted in surviving infants. The perinatal mortality rate associated with patients who were either not treated or treated by surgery was almost 40 percent (5 of 13), while almost 90 percent (seven of eight) of infants of mothers treated by chemotherapy survived. Of the mothers treated with chemotherapy, 50 percent (four of eight) survived. Of the 13 patients who were not treated or who were treated with surgical resection, 5 (38 percent) survived. The nature of the presenting disease probably played a preselection role regarding the treatments. Including additional, more recent, reports, it is evident that about 60 to 70 percent of patients and about 75 percent of infants survive.

Adult T-cell leukemia/lymphoma, caused by the human T-cell lymphotropic virus type I, is found in Japan, the Caribbean, and the southern United States. The virus is present in familial clusters and is transmitted by sexual intercourse, blood transfusions, and breast milk. Infants seroconvert between 12 and 19 months of age at a rate of 20 to 25 percent.[92,93]

ACUTE LEUKEMIA

While the incidence of leukemia in pregnancy is not specifically known, it is estimated to occur in less than 1 in 75,000 pregnancies. Acute leukemia represents about 90 percent of leukemias coexisting with pregnancy. Acute myeloid leukemia accounts for about 60 percent and acute lymphoblastic leukemia (ALL) for about 30 percent of cases. Over three fourths of the cases are diagnosed after the first trimester.[6,94]

The prognosis for acute leukemia in pregnancy is guarded.[6,94–97] In adults, acute leukemia in the nonpregnant patient, if untreated, has a median survival of about 2 months.[98] In the treated patient, the median survival is between 1 and 2 years. Immediate and aggressive therapeutic intervention will yield complete remission rates of about 75 percent, and 40 percent of these are sustained. While there is no evidence that pregnancy adversely affects the prognosis of acute leukemia, a 1987 report identified a median survival of 16 months in the pregnant patient,[6] and another study in 1988 reported a median survival of 27.5 months in a nonpregnant population.[99] However, the differences in patient populations (the latter study was a report on the more favorable ALL) and the varied treatments precludes any reliable comparison.[98] Optimal care of the pregnant patient with acute leukemia necessitates a team effort and is best achieved in a cancer referral center.

The diagnosis of acute leukemia is rarely difficult. The signs and symptoms of anemia, granulocytopenia, and thrombocytopenia, including fatigue, fever, infection, and easy bleeding or petechiae, usually prompt a complete blood count. A normal or elevated white blood cell count is present in up to 90 percent of patients with ALL. Counts in excess of 50,000 are found in only one fourth of patients. In contrast, patients with acute nonlymphocytic leukemia (ANLL) may present with markedly elevated white blood cell counts, although one third will present with leukopenia.[100] The diagnosis of leukemia should be confirmed by bone marrow biopsy and aspirate. The biopsy material is usually hypercellular with leukemic cells. The smear of the aspirate reveals decreased erythocyte and granulocytic precursors as well as megakaryocytes. Leukemic cells comprise greater than one half of the marrow's cellular elements in most patients. The morphology of the marrow and the peripheral leukemic cells help to distinguish between lymphocytic and nonlymphocytic leukemias. This latter group includes acute myelocytic (granulocytic), promyelocytic, monocytic, and myelomonocytic leukemias, and erythroleukemia. Acute myelocytic leukemia is the most common form of ANLL. Patients who develop ANLL as a result of previous chemotherapy have a particularly poor response to treatment.

There are numerous reports of successful pregnancies in patients aggressively treated with combination chemotherapy for acute leukemia. Acute leukemia and its therapy are associated with an increase in stillbirths (approximately 15 percent), prematurity (approximately 50 percent), and growth restriction.[95,98] In 1988 and 1991, reports by Aviles and colleagues,[33,101] no serious long-term effects of in utero exposure to chemotherapy were reported. The first report included 17 children, aged 4 to 22, whose mothers received treatment for acute leukemia.[101] In the second report, 43 children who were born to mothers with a variety of hematologic malignancies were examined at 3 to 19 years of age.[33] In both studies, greater than 40 percent of the cases involved exposure during the first trimester.

If the mother is exposed to cytotoxic drugs within 1 month of delivery, the newborn should be monitored closely for evidence of granulocytopenia or thrombocytopenia.

CHRONIC LEUKEMIA

Chronic leukemia accounts for approximately 10 percent of cases of leukemia during pregnancy, with the majority of these being patients with chronic myelocytic leukemia (CML).[98] Chronic lymphocytic leukemia has a median age of onset of about 60 years, making cases during pregnancy rare. The median age of patients with CML is 35 years. CML is characterized by excessive production of mature myeloid cell elements, with granulocyte counts averaging 200,000/dl. Most patients have thrombocytosis and a mild normochromic normocytic anemia. Platelet function is often abnormal, although hemorrhage is usually limited to patients with marked thrombocytopenia. CML tends to be indolent, and normal hematopoiesis is only mildly affected in the early stages of disease. Therefore, delay of aggressive treatment is a more feasible option than with acute leukemia. Unless complications such as severe systemic

symptoms, autoimmune hemolytic anemia, recurrent infection, or symptomatic lymphatic enlargement occur, treatment for chronic leukemia should be withheld until after delivery. Therapy, when necessary, usually includes prednisone and an alkylating agent such as chlorambucil or cyclophosphamide. High dose steroids alone may be used to treat autoimmune hemolytic anemia. Currently, the median survival for CML is over 60 months, with survivals up to 10 years common.

Often, the diagnosis of CML antedates the pregnancy. While pregnancy does not appear to affect CML adversely, therapy does increase the frequency of preterm birth and low birth weight. Information about contemporary management and prognosis is scarce secondary to the fact that few recent cases of CML during pregnancy have been reported. There are reports of CML treatment with leukapheresis during pregnancy. This treatment appears to be both safe and effective. Leukapheresis results in improvement of blood counts, systemic symptoms, and splenomegaly. Also, this treatment, although costly and involved, offers less risk of teratogenesis than cytotoxic treatments.[94,102] Other treatment regimens reported include biologic modifiers, such as interferon-α[103,104] and hydroxyurea.[104–107]

Hairy cell leukemia during pregnancy is rare, with only six reported cases. A predilection for men and the older age groups is the reason for the infrequency. Interferon-α treatment has been used in two cases with no adverse fetal effects.[103]

MELANOMA

The incidence of malignant melanoma is increasing in the childbearing years, and it is estimated that 1 percent of the population will develop this disease.[108] Since the median age at onset is approximately 50 years, the disease is relatively uncommon. However, one study reported malignant melanoma in 2.8 per 1,000 deliveries.[109] The understanding of the natural history of melanoma has been advanced by the identification of prognostic variables.[110] Prognostic features of the primary tumor include tumor thickness, Clark's level of invasion, Breslow's modifications, and Chung's modifications (Fig. 38–2), ulceration, and body location.

A topic of continued debate is whether pregnancy exerts a negative effect on the course of malignant melanoma. Reports from the 1950s suggested that melanoma arising during pregnancy is associated with an aggressive clinical course.[112,113] Subsequent reports, some being controlled studies, suggest melanoma diagnosed during pregnancy is more likely to be diagnosed at an advanced stage.[114–116] Most of the more recent studies are limited to patients with stage I disease and

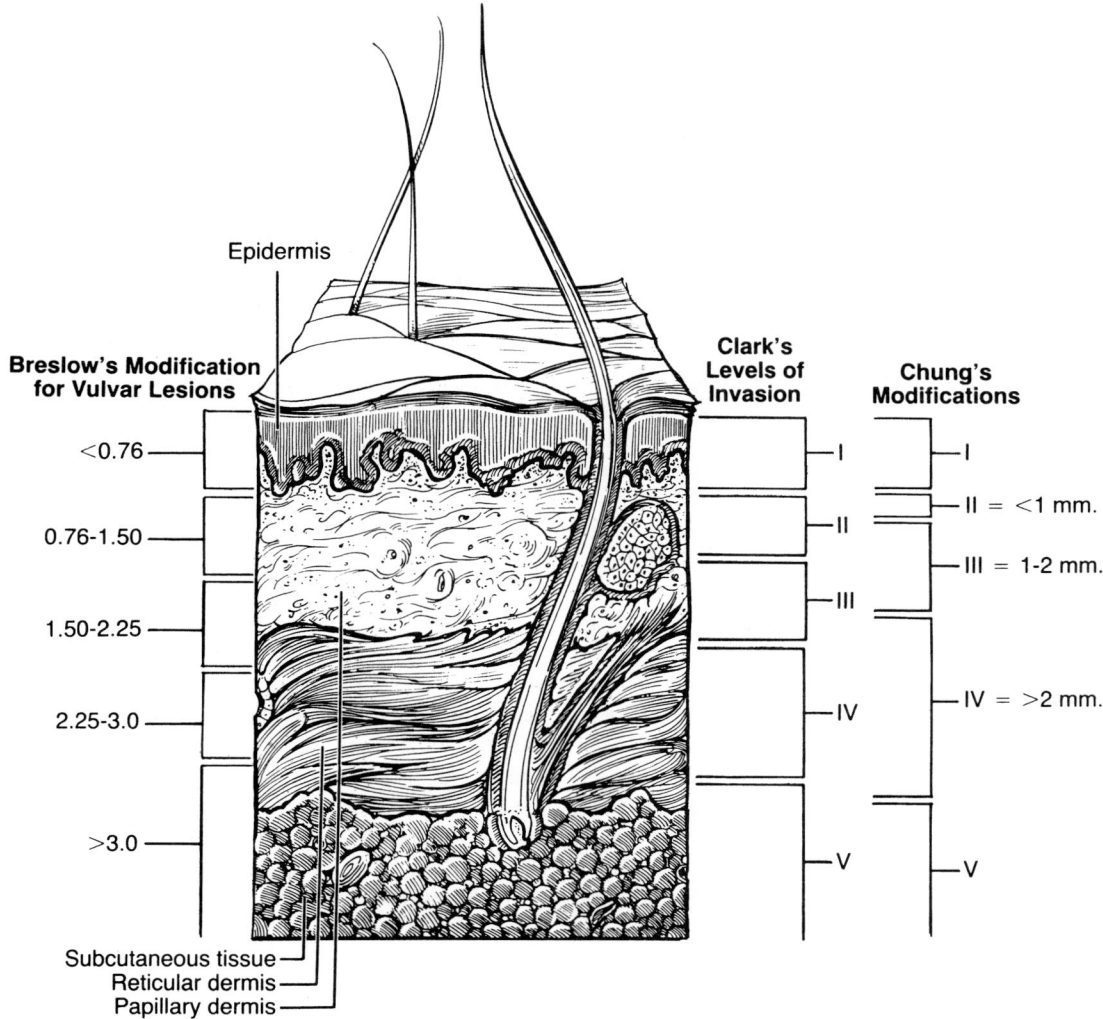

Figure 38–2. Schematic comparison of the different levels of invasion for melanoma. (From Gordon AN: Vulvar tumors. *In* Copeland LJ [ed]: Textbook of Gynecology. 2nd ed. Philadelphia, WB Saunders Company, 2000, p 1202, with permission.)

thus do not address this issue.[117,118] While many studies suggest that melanoma developing during pregnancy is more likely to appear in locations associated with a poor prognosis,[114–118] others show no increase in poor prognostic location of lesions in the pregnant patient.[119,120]

The World Health Organization (WHO) 1991 study examined the relevant prognostic features of melanoma in the childbearing years and in pregnancy.[118] This report suggested that patients who were diagnosed during pregnancy had tumors demonstrating significantly greater tumor thickness (Table 38–5). However, after correcting for tumor thickness, survival rates were similar. Additional studies from Massachusetts General Hospital and Duke University have supported the observation of greater tumor thickness in patients diagnosed during pregnancy (Table 38–6). Other investigators have found no difference in lesion thickness in pregnancy.[121] The issue remains unsettled, and explana-

tions for the increased tumor thickness include hormonal stimulation, growth factor stimulation, immunologic alterations of pregnancy, and delays in diagnosis. Delays in diagnosis are understandable, since it is not uncommon for pigmentation changes to take place during pregnancy. Therefore, tissue sampling is often delayed secondary to abnormalities being dismissed as a normal change of pregnancy.

Surgery remains the most effective modality for the treatment of melanoma. For patients with stage I or II tumors, the standard surgical excision with margins appropriate for tumor thickness should be performed. Regional lymph node dissection can be done in the patient with regional (stage III) disease. Since adjuvant chemotherapy is experimental and has not demonstrated improved survival, it is not recommended for the pregnant patient because of the potential risk to the fetus. Adjuvant interferon and vaccines for the nonpregnant patient are also under evaluation. These treatments hold more promise for the pregnant patient, based on fetal considerations. Advanced metastatic disease carries a poor prognosis. Since chemotherapy with dacarbazine results in a clinical response, usually of short duration, in no more than 30 percent of patients, it is usually most appropriate to plan for early delivery in cases of disseminated disease presenting late in pregnancy.

Is there a role for therapeutic abortion? Despite rare reports of regression after delivery, no studies support any therapeutic benefit associated with therapeutic abortion.[123,124] However, given the aggressive nature of the current therapies available for metastatic disease, it is not inappropriate to consider abortion when managing advanced disease presenting in the first trimester.[124]

The patient who has undergone apparent successful treatment for a malignant melanoma may express concern about the safety of a future pregnancy. No adverse impact on recurrence or survival has been identified in the majority of the literature on this issue.[115,118,119] However, the timing of the subsequent pregnancy deserves some consideration. The probability of survival of a specific cancer should be evaluated based on the known prognostic variables. The 5-year survival rate for the patient with a melanoma less than 1.5 mm thick is 90 percent. For a tumor of intermediate thickness (1.5 to 4 mm) the 5-year survival rate is 50 to 75 percent, and for a more deeply invasive tumor survival is less than 50 percent. While some report that approximately 60 to 70 percent of patients will develop their recurrence within 2 years and 80 to 90 percent within 5 years, the WHO study claimed that 83 percent of recurrences develop within the first 2 years.[124] Based on this information, it is generally recommended that patients wait 2 to 3 years before attempting another pregnancy, especially with nodal disease.[118] There are insufficient data on the select group of patients who develop their initial melanoma during pregnancy to make recommendations regarding the safety of a subsequent pregnancy.

Another issue of concern is which form of birth con-

Table 38–5. WHO STAGES I AND II STUDY OF MALIGNANT MELANOMA

Relationship to Time of Pregnancy	No. of Patients	Mean Tumor Thickness (mm)
Before	85	1.29
During	92	2.38*
After all	143	1.96
Between	68	1.78

* $p < 0.004$. When corrected for tumor thickness, survival rates were not different. Multivariate analysis identified tumor thickness as an independent prognostic variable, not pregnancy.
From MacKie RM, Bufalino R, Morabito A, et al: Lack of effect on pregnancy outcome of melanoma. Lancet 337:653, 1991, with permission.

Table 38–6. PRIMARY MELANOMA TUMOR THICKNESS IN PREGNANT AND NONPREGNANT PATIENTS

Study	Tumor Thickness (mm)		p Value
	Pregnant	Nonpregnant	
Singluff et al.[120]	2.7	1.5	0.052
Mackie et al.[118]	2.3	1.7	0.002
Travers et al.[122]	2.3	1.2	0.0001

trol should be used. The use of oral contraceptives has not been demonstrated to affect adversely the natural history of a previously treated melanoma.[125,126]

CERVICAL CANCER

Approximately 3 percent of all invasive cervical cancers occur during pregnancy. Cervical cancer is the most common gynecologic malignancy associated with pregnancy, occurring in approximately 1 per 2,200 pregnancies.[127–129]

However, the true incidence is difficult to ascertain due to the reporting biases associated with the reports originating from large referral centers. Also, various reports may include patients who have preinvasive lesions as well as patients who are diagnosed postpartum.

All pregnant patients should be evaluated on their initial obstetric visit with visualization of the cervix and cervical cytology, including an endocervical brush. The general principles of screening for cervical neoplasia apply to the pregnant patient. The Papanicolaou smear is used to screen the normal-appearing cervix. If the cervix appears friable, cervical cytology alone may not be sufficient to alert the physician to the presence of a malignant tumor. False-negative cervical cytology is at increased risk in pregnancy due to excess mucus and bleeding from cervical eversion. Therefore, it is necessary to obtain a biopsy to ensure that tissue friability is not secondary to tumor. Also, an ulcerative or exophytic lesion must have histologic sampling performed. While approximately one third of pregnant patients with cervical cancer are asymptomatic at the time of diagnosis, the most common symptoms are vaginal bleeding or discharge. Evaluation for the possibility of neoplastic disease of the lower genital tract is required in the evaluation of vaginal bleeding in the pregnant as well as the nonpregnant patient.

Considering the routine practice of performing cervical cytology in early pregnancy, one would expect there to be a preponderance of early-stage disease diagnosed in the first trimester. Surprisingly, this is not the situation. The diagnosis of cervical cancer is commonly made postpartum rather than during pregnancy and, while stage IB disease is the most commonly diagnosed stage, all stages are represented in significant numbers. Both patient and physician factors, including lack of prenatal care, failure to obtain cervical cytology or to biopsy gross cervical abnormalities, false-negative cytology, and failure to evaluate abnormal cytology or vaginal bleeding properly, contribute to the delays in diagnosis. Unfortunately, the complaint of spotting or bleeding during pregnancy is common and usually secondary to pregnancy-related conditions.

Cervical cytology suggestive of a squamous intraepithelial lesion or a report of atypical glandular cells during pregnancy requires appropriate clinical evaluation (Fig. 38–3). The colposcopic evaluation of the pregnant cervix is altered by the physiologic changes of pregnancy and, since most practicing physicians will diagnose invasive cervical cancer associated with pregnancy only once or twice in their careers, it may be prudent to consult a gynecologic oncologist. While colposcopy during pregnancy is usually enhanced by the physiologic eversion of the lower endocervical canal, vascular changes and redundant vagina may alter or obscure normal visualization. During pregnancy, failure to visualize the entire transformation zone and squamocolumnar junction is uncommon. While endocervical curettage is not generally recommended during pregnancy, lesions involving the lower endocervical canal can often be directly visualized and biopsied. While the pregnant cervix is hypervascular, serious hemorrhage from an outpatient biopsy is uncommon, and the risk of bleeding is offset by the risk of missing an early invasive cancer. Following a coloposcopic evaluation with appropriate tissue sampling, most patients with preinvasive lesions can be followed with repeat colposcopy at 6- to 8-week intervals to delivery.[130,131]

Patients then require a careful and complete colposcopic evaluation 6 weeks' postpartum. Cone biopsy during pregnancy, when necessary, should ideally be performed during the second trimester to reduce the risks of first-trimester abortion and rupture of membranes or premature labor in the third trimester.[132–134] Complications from conization of the pregnant cervix

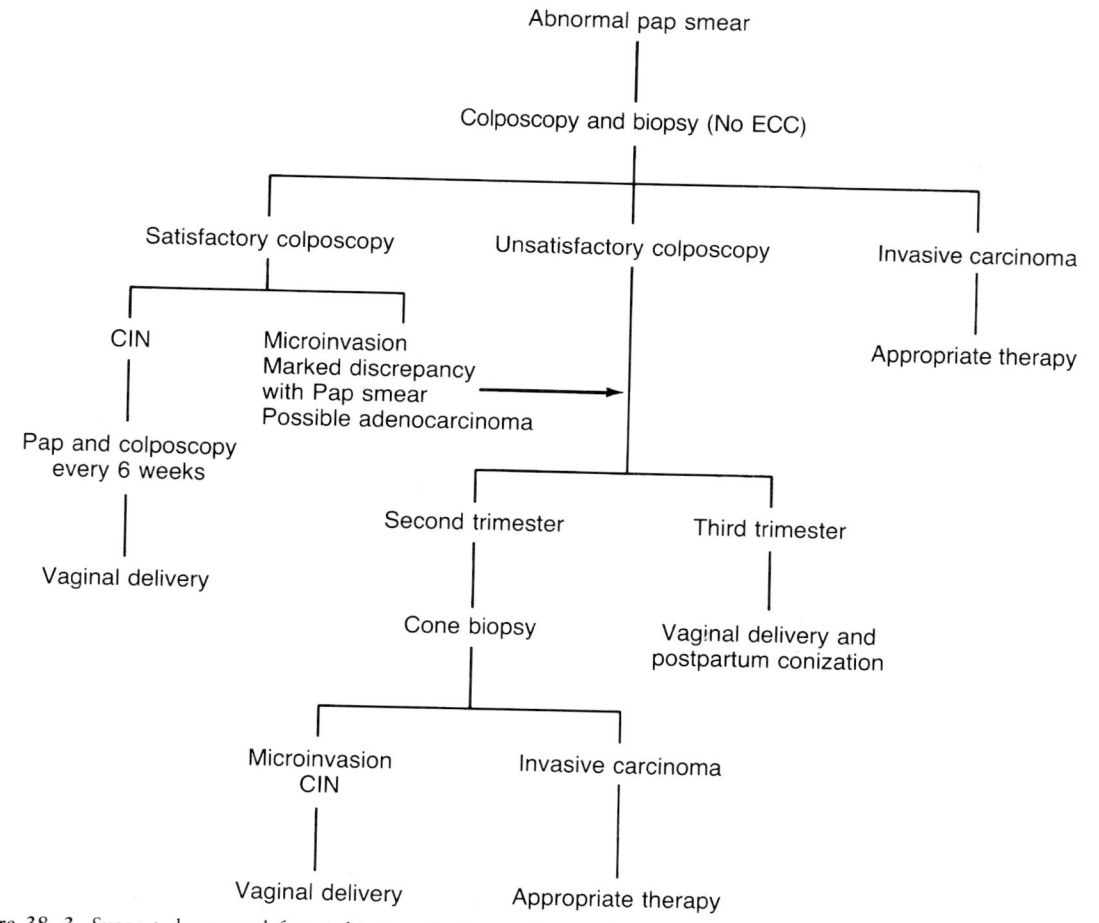

Figure 38–3. Suggested protocol for evaluation of abnormal cervical cytology in pregnancy. ECC, endocervical curettage; CIN, cervical intraepithelial neoplasia. (From Hacker NF, Berek JS, Lagasse LD, et al: Carcinoma of the cervix associated with pregnancy. Obstet Gynecol 59:735, 1982, with permission.)

are common. Therapeutic conization for intraepithelial squamous lesions is contraindicated during pregnancy. Diagnostic cone biopsy in pregnancy is reserved for patients whose colposcopic-directed biopsy has shown superficial invasion (suspect microinvasion) or in other situations where an invasive lesion is suspected but cannot be confirmed by biopsy. When a cone biopsy is necessary during pregnancy, one should keep in mind the anatomic alteration of the cervix secondary to pregnancy. A shallow disk-like cone is usually satisfactory to clarify the diagnosis with a minimum of morbidity. It should be kept in mind that patients who have had a conization during pregnancy are at higher risk for residual disease. Therefore, close follow-up is essential.

Following the diagnosis of invasive cervical cancer, a staging evaluation is indicated. The standard cervical staging is clinical and usually based on the results of physical examination, cystoscopy, proctoscopy, chest x-ray, and intravenous pyelogram. CT scan or, in some centers, lymphangiography is often performed to identify lymph node metastasis. In the pregnant patient, the standard staging evaluation is modified. The chest radiograph is performed with abdominal shielding. Sonography is used to detect hydronephrosis and, if additional retroperitoneal imaging is desired for the evaluation of lymphadenopathy, consideration should be given to using MRI. While the use of MRI during pregnancy is not approved, there have been no reported sequelae and the theoretical risks are less than the risks associated with ionizing radiation techniques.

Microinvasion

In patients with a microinvasive squamous carcinoma with negative margins on cone biopsy, consideration can be given to conservative management until delivery. The risk of occult metastatic disease is predominantly dependent on two pathologic features: (1) the depth of invasion and (2) the presence or absence of lymphovascular space involvement.[135] Whether the cone biopsy can be considered sufficient long-term therapy or whether a postpartum hysterectomy with or without lymphadenectomy should be performed is also based on the detailed analysis of the pathologic features of the cone biopsy. In these cases, consultation with a gynecologic oncologist is appropriate.

Invasive, Early-Stage Disease

Since the definitive treatment of invasive cervical cancer is not compatible with pregnancy continuation, the clinical question that must be addressed is when to conclude the pregnancy so that therapy can be completed. Considering this requirement, treatment options will be influenced by gestational age, tumor stage and metastatic evaluation, and maternal desires and expectations regarding the pregnancy. The management of early invasive cervical cancer (stages IB and IIA) in the young patient is usually by radical hysterectomy, pelvic lymphadenectomy, and aortic lymph node sampling.[136] The primary advantage over radiation therapy for these patients is preservation of ovarian function. For the patient with a high probability of having a poor prognostic lesion and therefore requiring postoperative irradiation, consideration can be given to performing a unilateral or bilateral oophoropexy at the time of the hysterectomy. The ovarian suspension should be intraperitoneal, as retroperitoneal placement seems to predispose to subsequent ovarian cyst formation. In the first trimester, this surgery is usually carried out with the fetus in utero. In the third trimester, the radical hysterectomy and pelvic lymphadenectomy are performed after completion of a high classic cesarean delivery. Delays in therapeutic intervention have not been reported to increase recurrence rates for patients with small-volume stage I disease.[138] While the pelvic vessels are large, the dissection is enhanced by more easily defined tissue planes.[139,140]

Second-trimester situations are more problematic. Serious consideration should be given to administering one to three cycles of platinum-based chemotherapy and thereby allowing an additional 7 to 15 weeks of fetal maturation. In one study, maturation from 26 to 27 weeks' gestation compared with 34 to 35 weeks increased fetal viability from 67 percent to 97 percent.[141] The neoadjuvant chemotherapy approach (chemotherapy prior to either surgery or irradiation) would unlikely compromise and may enhance the overall efficacy of treatment. Also, having passed the primary interval of organogenesis, it is unlikely that serious fetal sequelae will occur secondary to the chemotherapy. Certainly in terms of general fetal salvage and outcome, the risk of extreme prematurity would far outweigh the risk of the chemotherapy exposure. While this management of second-trimester cervical cancer presentations seems logical, there is scant information about this treatment approach. However, neoadjuvant chemotherapy with vincristine and platinum-based chemotherapy for ovarian cancers has been reported with no fetal sequelae identified.[20]

Invasive, Locally Advanced Disease

The management of the patient with more advanced local disease is based on treatment with chemotherapy and irradiation, both external beam to treat the regional nodes and shrink the central tumor and brachytherapy to complete the delivery of a tumoricidal dose to the cervix and adjacent tissues.[136] Coordinating a chemoradiation treatment plan for pregnant patients with stages IIB, stage III, and stage IVA is challenging. The patient with a first-trimester pregnancy can usually be treated in the standard fashion with initiation of chemotherapy and external therapy to the pelvis or extended field, as dictated by standard treatment guidelines. Most of these patients will proceed to abort spontaneously within 2 to 5 weeks of initialing the radiation. Patients in the late first trimester are least likely to abort spontaneously, and it may be necessary to perform a uterine evacuation on the completion of external therapy in some patients. Following either spontaneous abortion or uterine evacuation, the brachytherapy component of the radiation therapy can proceed in the standard fashion. Patients in either their second or third trimester should have a high classic cesarean delivery prior to starting standard chemotherapy and irradiation. Again, it would seem appropriate to strongly consider neoadjuvant chemotherapy for this group of patients, especially the patient with a second-trimester or early third-trimester presentation, when the opportunity for fetal maturation could be provided.

Invasive, Distant Metastasis

Metastatic disease to extrapelvic sites carries a poor prognosis. While a select few patients with aortic node metastasis may receive curative therapy, it is unlikely for the patient with pulmonary metastasis, bone metastasis, or supraclavicular lymph node metastasis to be cured. Personal patient choices and ethical considerations will be the major factors guiding treatment in these situations.

Small cell neuroendocrine tumors of the cervix associated with pregnancy are rare. Neoadjuvant or adjuvant chemotherapy with cisplatin, etoposide, and doxorubicin is recommended, and long-term survivors have been reported.[142,143]

Method of Delivery

Controversy continues to surround the issue of the method of delivery for the term patient with cervical cancer. It seems heroic and unjustifiably risky to encourage vaginal delivery of a patient with a large, firm, barrell-shaped tumor or a large friable and hemorrhagic exophytic tumor. However, many small-volume stage IB, IIA, and early IIB tumors are potential candidates for vaginal delivery. Whether vaginal delivery promotes systemic dissemination of tumor cells is unknown. While the general opinion is that survival rates are not influenced by the mode of delivery,[127,144] a recent multivariate analysis "showed a possible trend ($p = 0.08$) toward a negative outcome after vaginal delivery."[129]

Although systemic tumor dissemination secondary to vaginal delivery has not been documented, there are reports of episiotomy implants for both squamous carcinoma and adenocarcinoma following vaginal delivery.[145–147] Episiotomy implants are sufficiently rare that

the risk should not be a determining factor for a given patient. However, the episiotomy should be carefully followed in a cervical cancer patient who delivers vaginally. Episiotomy nodules in these patients must be promptly evaluated by biopsy, as an early diagnosis may permit curative therapy.[145] Diagnostic delays secondary to suspicion of the nodules representing stitch abscess should be avoided.

Survival

While some authors have suggested that the survival of patients with cervical cancer associated with pregnancy is compromised,[148] most reports indicate that the prognosis is not altered.[127–129,148,149]

OVARIAN CANCER

With the increased use of diagnostic ultrasound, ovarian cysts and masses are more frequently encountered in early pregnancy.[150] While adnexal masses are frequently encountered in pregnancy, only 2 to 5 percent are malignant ovarian tumors.[151,152] Ovarian cancer occurs in approximately 1 in 18,000 to 1 in 47,000 pregnancies.[153,154]

While the three major categories of ovarian tumors— epithelial, germ cell, and stromal—occur during pregnancy, there is a disproportionate number of patients with germ cell tumors compared with the nonpregnant patient. A review of the literature since 1984 reveals 40 patients having malignant primary ovarian tumors during pregnancy. Germ cell tumors account for 45 percent (Fig. 38–4); 37.5 percent are epithelial tumors, 10 percent are stromal tumors, and 7.5 percent are categorized as miscellaneous. This distribution is undoubtedly skewed by the reporting bias associated with rare tumors. Characteristic of epithelial tumors in young patients who are not pregnant, the majority of epithelial ovarian tumors complicating pregnancy are of low grade (grade 1 or low malignant potential) or early stage, not uncommonly both low grade and stage I.

Management of the adnexal mass in pregnancy is the subject of some controversy. The risks of surgical intervention may favor a conservative approach.[156] Serial sonograms may be of some value in determining the nature and biologic potential of the tumor. If the clinical presentation is consistent with torsion, rupture, or hemorrhage, immediate surgical intervention is indicated. Prompt surgical exploration is also performed for the mass associated with ascites or when there is evidence of metastatic disease. Since surgical exploration during pregnancy is associated with an increase in pregnancy loss and neonatal morbidity, it is ideal to

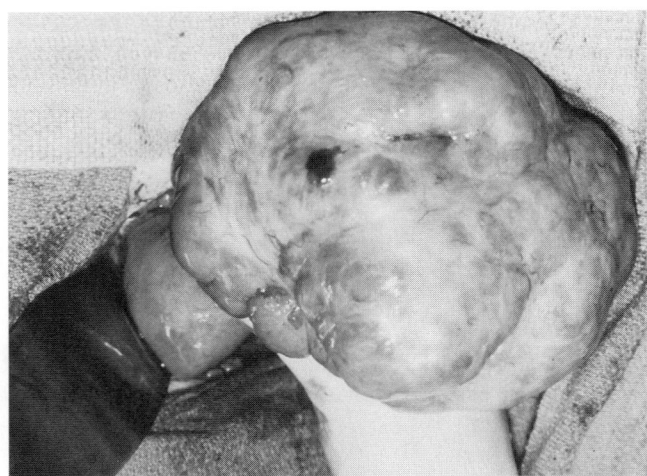

Figure 38–4. Dysgerminoma, the most common malignant ovarian neoplasm found in pregnancy, characterized by a lobulated solid gross appearance. (From Copeland LJ: Gestational trophoblastic neoplasia. *In* Copeland LJ [ed]: Textbook of Gynecology. 2nd ed. Philadelphia, WB Saunders Company, 2000, p 1391, with permission.)

delay surgical intervention until term or after delivery. A number of opposing risks require consideration prior to following a conservative approach. The risk of greatest concern is that a delay of surgical intervention could permit a malignant ovarian tumor to spread, resulting in a decreased opportunity for cure. However, considering the rarity of advanced-stage poorly differentiated epithelial tumors in this age group, this risk is relatively small. There does appear to be an increased probability that an adnexal mass during pregnancy will undergo torsion or rupture,[157,158] and surgical intervention for these events is associated with higher fetal loss than an elective procedure.[151,159] While ovarian tumors may be the cause of obstructed labor,[151] this is uncommon. Serial sonographic evaluations will identify the rare tumor that remains pelvic as the gestation progresses. Since most ovarian masses relocate to the abdomen as the pregnancy advances, other explanations should be considered for persistent pelvic masses, including pelvic kidney, uterine fibroids, and colorectal or bladder tumors.

When a malignant ovarian tumor is encountered at laparotomy, surgical intervention should be similar to that for the nonpregnant patient. If the patient is preterm and the tumor appears confined to one ovary, consideration should be given to limiting the staging to removal of the ovary, cytologic washings, and a thorough manual exploration of the abdomen and pelvis. The potential benefit of more extensive staging, including aortic node sampling, may be offset by higher pregnancy loss or neonatal morbidity. Prior to surgery, a comprehensive discussion with the patient should guide the extent of surgery if metastatic disease, especially a

high-grade epithelial lesion, is encountered. Depending on the gestational age and the patient's desires, limited surgery followed by chemotherapy and additional extirpative surgery following delivery must be offered in select cases.

Preoperative serum tumor markers are of limited value during pregnancy secondary to the physiologic increases in hCG, α-fetoprotein, and CA 125. Kobayashi and colleagues[160] have reported the mean CA 125 levels during pregnancy. CA 125 increases during the first trimester (mean, 72 U/ml) and then normalizes during the second trimester. CA 125 values tend to be significantly elevated following second-trimester abortion (mean, 447 U/ml) and term delivery (mean, 204 U/ml). Following diagnostic confirmation of a malignant ovarian tumor, the appropriate serum markers are useful to monitor the course of the disease.

Virilizing ovarian tumors during pregnancy are most commonly secondary to theca-lutein cysts, and their evaluation and management should be conservative. These benign exaggerated physiologic "tumors" may redevelop with subsequent pregnancies.[161]

Postoperative Adjuvant Therapy

Postoperative adjuvant therapy should follow the treatment guidelines for the nonpregnant patient. Following tumor debulking, patients with advanced epithelial tumors should receive combination chemotherapy. Until 1995, the standard therapy was a platinum and alkylating combination. However, with the recent demonstration of the superior effectiveness of the combination of cisplatinum and Taxol,[162] these agents may offer the patient a better survival. Unfortunately, there is no information available regarding the potential toxic effects of Taxol on a developing fetus. There are favorable case reports on the treatment of stage III serous ovarian carcinoma with postoperative platinum-based chemotherapy.[163–165] There are a number of favorable treatment outcomes reported in patients with malignant germ cell tumors and pregnancy.[166–176]

Young and colleagues[177] reviewed their collective experience with stromal ovarian tumors in pregnancy. One third of the patients presented with tumor rupture. Since the role of adjuvant chemotherapy for stromal tumors is complex and controversial, consultation with a gynecologic oncologist is recommended.

VULVAR AND VAGINAL CANCER

Since vulvar and vaginal cancers usually occur after age 40, the diagnosis of either disease concurrent with pregnancy is rare. Fewer than 20 cases of vulvar carcinoma diagnosed and treated during pregnancy have been reported.[178-180]

Vulvar carcinoma in pregnancy is usually stage I or II disease. The diagnosis is based on biopsy, and neither pregnancy nor the young age of a patient should discourage the biopsy of a vulvar mass. Since verrucous squamous carcinoma tends to be misdiagnosed as condyloma, it is important to inform the pathologist of the clinical characteristics of unusually large or aggressive condyloma-like lesions. Surgical management is similar to that used in the nonpregnant patient, with the preference being to perform surgery in the second trimester to avoid the fetal risks of anesthesia exposure in the first trimester and the maternal risks associated with operating on the hypervascular vulva in the third trimester. The surgical management of vulvar carcinoma is trending to more conservative procedures.[181] Vaginal delivery has been reported following surgical resection of vulvar cancers during pregnancy.[178,179]

Vaginal carcinoma is less common than vulvar carcinoma. The same limitations apply to vaginal cancer as apply to locally advanced cervical cancer in pregnancy. The cornerstone of treatment is irradiation therapy. Clear cell adenocarcinoma of the vagina has been reported in 16 pregnant patients, and 13 were long-term survivors.[182]

ENDOMETRIAL CANCER

Approximately 30 cases of endometrial cancer associated with pregnancy have been reported. While many of these cases are diagnosed in the first trimester, abnormal bleeding later in pregnancy or postpartum may be the presenting symptom of this tumor. Only about 30 percent of these cases are associated with a viable fetus.[183-186]

GASTROINTESTINAL CANCERS

Upper Gastrointestinal Cancers

The diagnostic delay in detecting an upper gastrointestinal cancer is often attributable to the frequency and duration of gastrointestinal symptoms in pregnancy. In the United States, stomach cancer is rarely diagnosed in women during the reproductive years. During pregnancy, persistent severe upper gastrointestinal symptoms are best evaluated by gastroduodenoscopy rather than radiologic studies. Since curative resection of lo-

calized stomach cancer is possible in only approximately 30 percent of patients, it is imperative that treatment not be delayed.

Malignant hepatic tumors are rare during the reproductive years. Hepatocellular tumors detected during pregnancy should be resected, since the maternal and fetal mortality associated with subcapsular hemorrhage and liver rupture during pregnancy is high. Elevated steroid levels may predispose the tumor to rupture during pregnancy. There is no increase in the vascularity of the liver during pregnancy. In patients with unresectable hepatomas, therapeutic abortion may be considered to decrease the risk of subsequent rupture and bleeding.

Colon and Rectal Cancer

The incidence of colon cancer during pregnancy is about 1 in 13,000 live-born deliveries.[187] Colorectal carcinoma is usually found in women beyond childbearing age, with only 8 percent of patients diagnosed before age 40. Over 200 cases of colorectal cancer in pregnancy have been reported.[188]

Since pregnancy is often accompanied by constipation and exacerbations of hemorrhoids and anal fissures, the symptoms of colorectal carcinoma, namely, rectal bleeding, constipation, pain, and backache, tend to be attributed to the pregnancy, and diagnostic delays occur. The majority of colorectal carcinomas during pregnancy are rectal and palpable on rectal examination, contrary to what is found in the nonpregnant patient (Table 38–7).[189] Patients with unexplained hypochromic microcytic anemia should be evaluated with stool guaiac testing. If a colorectal lesion is suspected, endoscopic methods of evaluation are preferred to radiologic imaging studies. Unfortunately, most cases of colorectal cancer are not diagnosed until late pregnancy or at the time of delivery. Delays in diagnosis are probably responsible for a higher likelihood of advanced stage colorectal cancer in pregnancy and an associated poor prognosis. The hormonal effect of pregnancy on tumor development is unknown.[188] A report by Woods

Table 38–7. DISTRIBUTION OF COLON AND RECTAL CARCINOMAS IN NONPREGNANT AND PREGNANT POPULATIONS

Patient Group	Total	Colon	Rectum
General population	1,704	1,244 (73%)	460 (27%)
Age under 40 years	186	127 (68%)	59 (32%)
Pregnant	244	41 (17%)	203 (83%)

From Medich DS, Fazio VW: Hemorrhoids, anal fissure, and carcinoma of the colon, rectum, and anus during pregnancy. Surg Clin North Am 75:77, 1995, with permission.

and colleagues[187] suggests that colorectal carcinoma in pregnancy adversely affects the pregnancy. Only 78 percent of their cases resulted in healthy live-born infants.[187]

Management of colon cancer is determined by gestational age at diagnosis and tumor stage. During the first half of pregnancy colon resection with anastomosis is indicated for colon cancers.[190] Abdominoperineal resection or low anterior resection has been accomplished up to 20 weeks' gestation without disturbing the gravid uterus. In some cases, access to the rectum may be impossible without a hysterectomy or uterine evacuation.

In late pregnancy, a diverting colostomy may be necessary to relieve a colonic obstruction and allow the development of fetal maturity before instituting definitive therapy. Some patients with a diagnosis after 20 weeks may opt to continue the pregnancy to fetal viability. Vaginal delivery is planned unless the tumor is obstructing the pelvis or is located on the anterior rectum. If cesarean delivery is performed, tumor resection can be accomplished immediately. Neoadjuvant chemotherapy or radiation therapy for colorectal carcinoma in the pregnant patient has not demonstrated sufficient response to risk fetal exposure.

In the most recent report, the stage-specific survival rates for pregnant patients with rectal cancer were 83, 27, and 0 percent for stages B, C, and D, respectively.[188] The corresponding survivals rates for the same stages of colon cancer were 75, 33, and 0 percent.[188] No Dukes' A classification rectal or colon cancer was reported, consistent with the frequency of diagnostic delays.[188]

URINARY TRACT CANCERS

Fewer than 50 cases of renal cell carcinoma and less than 10 cases of bladder cancer have been reported during pregnancy. Urethral carcinoma during pregnancy is also rare. The hallmark of urinary tract cancers is hematuria. The initial evaluation of hematuria in pregnancy should be urethrocystoscopy, urinary cytology, and renal ultrasonography. The primary therapy for renal cell carcinoma is surgery, and the survival rate for localized disease may exceed 50 percent. While preoperative arterial embolization may facilitate surgery on hypervascular tumors, improved survival rates have not been conclusively demonstrated. Adjuvant radiotherapy or chemotherapy tends to have minimal impact on long-term outcomes.

Transitional carcinoma of the bladder can be managed by local fulguration or resection if it is well differentiated and superficial. Less differentiated, deeply invasive, and recurrent tumors may require a partial or complete cystectomy. Urethral carcinoma treatment varies with the size and location. Distal urethral tumors are usually treated with excision and interstitial brachytherapy implants.

CENTRAL NERVOUS SYSTEM TUMORS

The spectrum of central nervous system tumors found in pregnant patients is similar to that of the nonpregnant patient.[191] In pregnancy, 32 percent of brain tumors are gliomas, 29 percent meningiomas, 15 percent acoustic neuromas, and the other 24 percent are divided among other more rare subtypes. Spinal tumors account for only about one eighth of the central nervous system tumors. Vertebral hemangiomas comprise 61 percent of the spinal tumors and meningiomas, 18 percent. Unfortunately, the presenting symptoms of headache and nausea and vomiting are often attributed to normal complaints of pregnancy, and delays in diagnosis result. Meningiomas, pituitary adenomas, acoustic neuromas, and vertebral hemangiomas may demonstrate rapid enlargement during pregnancy. This may be secondary to fluid retention, increase in blood volume, or hormonal stimulation.[192] MRI is the most common form of imaging used to diagnose intracranial neoplasms.

Since painful contractions and pushing increase intracranial pressure, it is recommended that labor be as pain free as possible, and the second stage of labor should be assisted with forceps to reduce the risk of herniation.[192] The anesthetic management of labor and delivery for patients with intracranial neoplasms has been reviewed by Finfer.[193]

While high-grade glial tumors should undergo prompt diagnosis and treatment, low-grade glial tumors such as astrocytomas and oligodendrogliomas do not usually require immediate intervention. Adjuvant cranial radiotherapy with abdominal shielding should be considered for patients with high-grade tumors. Adjuvant chemotherapy is not usually effective and therefore should probably be delayed until after delivery.

Successful surgical removal of a variety of central nervous system tumors has been reported.[192,194–198] Corticosteroids are recommended to reduce the surrounding edema of intracranial masses.

The use of bromocriptine in pregnancy is controversial. A report of no adverse fetal effects in over 1,400 pregnancies in which bromocriptine was taken in the first trimester supports the use of bromocriptine during pregnancy if expansion of a prolactinoma is detected.

MISCELLANEOUS TUMORS

Similar to the management for small cell neuroendocrine tumors of the cervix,[142] neuroendocrine tumors or neuroblastomas of other primary sites tend to demonstrate excellent response to chemotherapy.[199] Pheochromocytoma during pregnancy is rare and may mimic hypertensive disorders of pregnancy[200] (see Chapter 33).

FETAL–PLACENTAL METASTASIS

Metastatic spread of a maternal primary tumor to the placenta or fetus is rare. One review identified 45 cases of placental metastases and 7 cases of fetal metastases.[201] Malignant melanoma is the most frequently reported tumor metastatic to the placenta. Hematologic malignancies are the second most common tumor to spread to the placenta. Placental and fetal dissemination of lymphomas have been reported.[202–205] One case of vertical transmission of a mother's leukemia cell line was demonstrated through identification of a leukemia clone.[207] There is one case report of a central nervous system tumor metastatic to the placenta.[208] Choriocarcinoma metastatic to a fetus usually results in death within a few months of age.[209,210]

GESTATIONAL TROPHOBLASTIC DISEASE AND PREGNANCY-RELATED ISSUES

It is uncommon for a normal viable pregnancy to be complicated by gestational trophoblastic disease (GTD). A comprehensive summary of the evaluation and management of the complete spectrum of GTD is beyond the scope of this textbook. However, the aspects of GTD related to the general obstetric and postpartum care are reviewed.

Hydatidiform Mole (Complete Mole)

The incidence of hydatidiform mole has great geographic variability. In the United States it occurs in approximately 1 in 1,000 to 1 in 1,500 pregnancies. The two clinical risk factors that carry the highest risk of a molar pregnancy are (1) the extremes of the reproductive years (age 50 or older carries a relative risk of over 500)[211] and (2) the history of a prior hydatidiform mole (the risk for development of a second molar pregnancy is 1 to 2 percent,[212–214] and the risk of a third after two is approximately 25 percent).[215] Patients with these risk factors should have an ultrasound evaluation of uterine contents in the first trimester. While historically approximately 50 percent of patients were not diagnosed with a molar pregnancy prior to vaginal expulsion of molar tissue, currently in developed countries most patients are diagnosed either by ultrasound while asymptomatic or by ultrasound for the evaluation of vaginal spotting or cramping symptoms. Approximately 95 percent of complete hydatidiform moles have a 46,XX paternal homologous chromosomal pattern.

The safest technique of evacuating a hydatidiform mole is with the suction aspiration technique. Oxytocin should not be initiated until the patient is in the operating room and evacuation is imminent in order to minimize the risk of embolization of trophoblastic tissue. The alternative management for the elderly patient who requests concurrent sterilization is hysterectomy. Following either evacuation or hysterectomy, weekly β-hCG is drawn until the hCG titer is within normal limits for 3 weeks. The titers are then observed at monthly intervals for 6 to 12 months. Figure 38–5 illustrates an algorithm for molar pregnancy management.[216]

For the patient with a complete molar pregnancy, the risk of requiring chemotherapy for persistent GTD is approximately 20 percent. Clinical features that increase this risk include delayed hemorrhage, excessive uterine enlargement, theca-lutein cysts, serum hCG greater than 100,000 mIU/ml, and maternal age over 40. It is obviously particularly important not to misinterpret a rising β-hCG due to a new intervening pregnancy as persistent GTD, since intervention with chemotherapy would be a significant risk to a new gestation, inducing either abortion or possible teratogenic defects.

Invasive Mole (Chorioadenoma Destruens)

Since invasion of the myometrium by molar tissue is clinically occult, it is difficult to assess the true incidence, estimated to be between 5 and 10 percent. The clinical hallmark of invasive mole is hemorrhage, often severe, either vaginal or intraperitoneal.

Partial Hydatidiform Mole

Most partial moles have a triploid karyotype, and the next most common is a trisomy 16. A minority of partial moles exhibit normal diploidy. Karyotype analysis of the accompanying fetus is important in planning therapeutic intervention. A partial mole associated with a nonviable fetal chromosomal abnormality will require

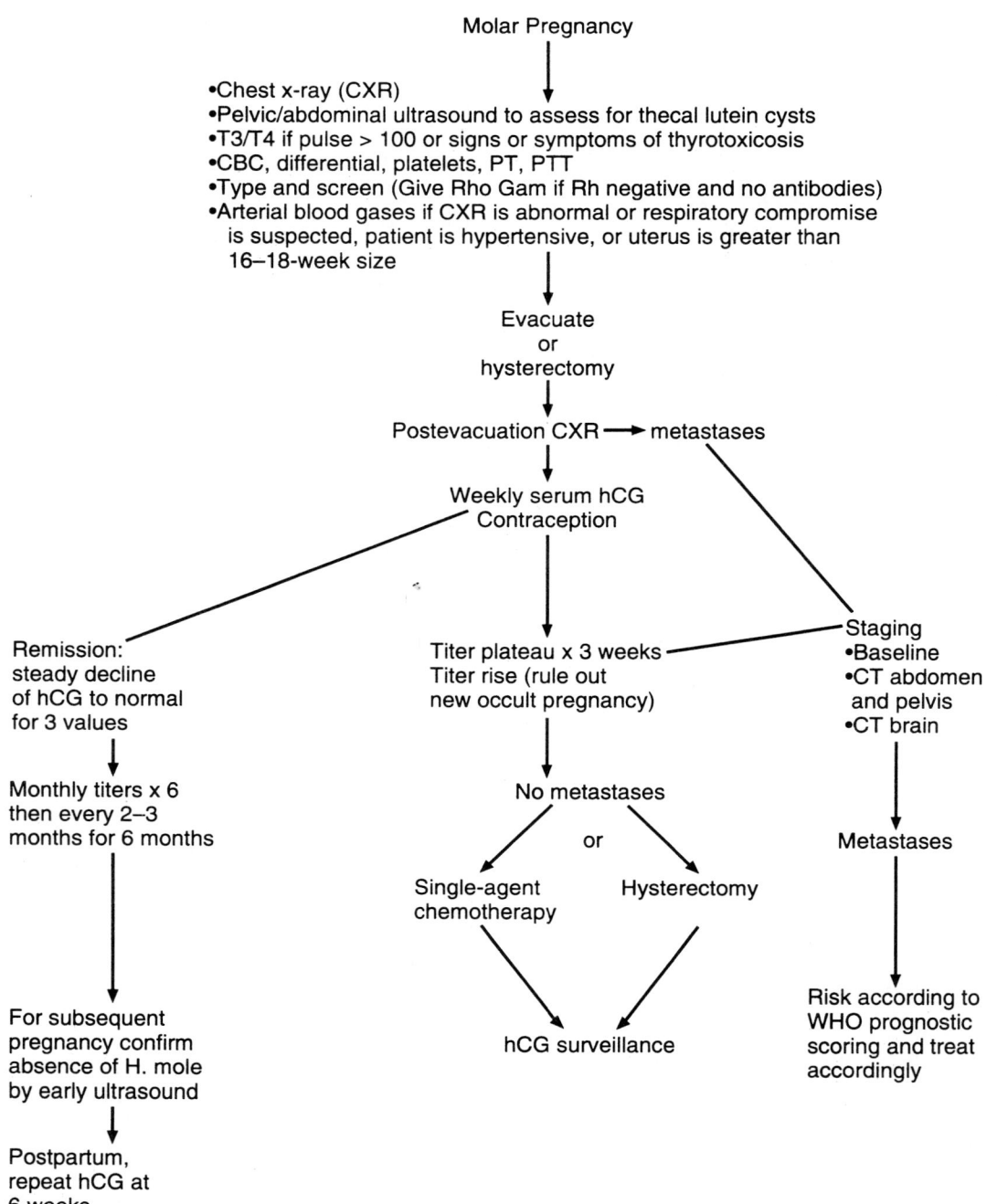

Figure 38–5. Algorithm for the management of molar pregnancy. (From Copeland LJ: Gestational trophoblastic neoplasia. *In* Copeland LJ [ed]: Textbook of Gynecology. 2nd ed. Philadelphia, WB Saunders Company, 2000, p 1414, with permission.)

either mechanical or medically induced uterine evacuation (Fig. 38–6). In the presence of an abundance of hydropic tissue, there is always the concern that trophoblastic tissue embolization may occur during uterine contractions induced to evacuate molar tissue. The management of a patient with sonographic findings suggestive of a diagnosis of a partial mole is particularly challenging if the karyotype analysis of the fetus is diploid, especially if the diagnosis is made in the second or third trimester. When a normal karyotype exists, it is appropriate to consider diagnostic possibilities other than partial mole, such as a twin gestation—one normal developing fetus and one molar pregnancy. Also, degenerative changes (hydropic villi), retroplacental hematomas, placental abnormalities (chorioangiomas), degenerative uterine myomas, and aborted tissue, sometimes referred to as a "transitional mole," may lead to imaging abnormalities that are difficult to interpret.

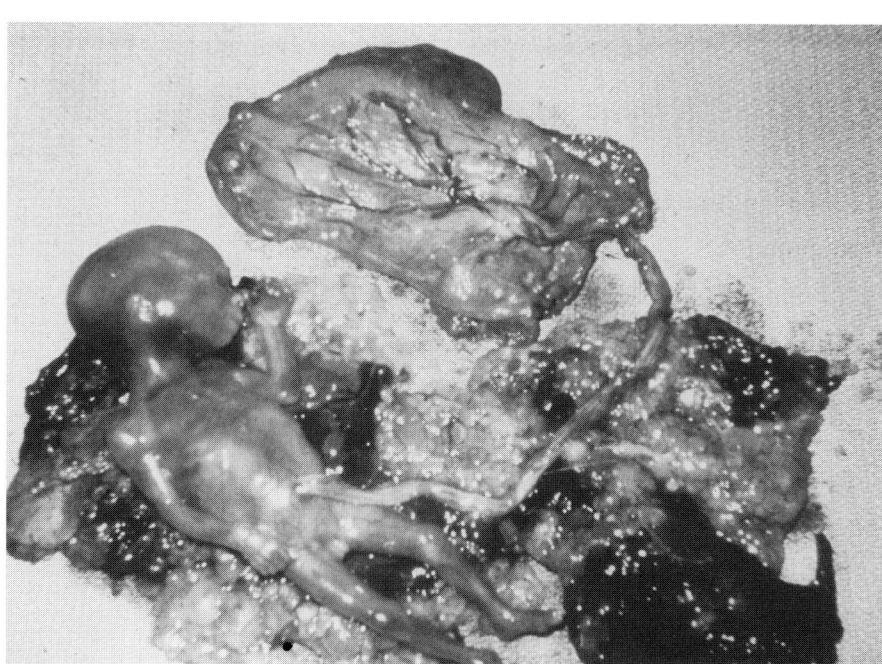

Figure 38–6. Partial mole with dead fetus of abnormal karyotype. (From Copeland LJ: Gestational trophoblastic neoplasia. *In* Copeland LJ [ed]: Textbook of Gynecology. 2nd ed. Philadelphia, WB Saunders Company, 2000, p 1416, with permission.)

Approximately 2 to 6 percent of patients develop persistent GTD after a partial molar pregnancy.[218,219] Therefore, these patients require the same postevacuation surveillance and management as the patient with a complete mole.

Placental Site Trophoblastic Tumor

Less than 1 percent of all patients with GTD have placental site trophoblastic tumor. While this tumor usually presents with abnormal vaginal bleeding following a term pregnancy, it can also be a sequela to a molar pregnancy or abortion. The postpartum presentation is characterized by a slightly enlarged uterus, per-

sistent bleeding or, occasionally, amenorrhea, and a slightly elevated β-hCG level. The hCG may not reliably reflect disease progression. The histologic diagnosis may be obtained by uterine curettage, possibly hysteroscopically directed. Since this disease tends to metastasize late and be somewhat resistant to chemotherapy, surgical excision (hysterectomy) should be considered.[220] If the patient is desirous of future childbearing, management considerations that have been reported with some success include systemic chemotherapy, regional infusion chemotherapy, uterine curettage, and local excision of tumor by hysterotomy and uterine reconstruction.[221]

Choriocarcinoma

Choriocarcinoma develops in approximately 1 in every 40,000 term pregnancies and this clinical presentation represents about one fourth of all cases of choriocarcinoma. The other cases follow molar disease or an abortion (spontaneous, therapeutic, or ectopic). GTD following a term pregnancy is always either choriocarcinoma or a placental site trophoblastic tumor, assuming a singleton pregnancy.

Choriocarcinoma is notorious for masquerading as other diseases. This is secondary to hemorrhagic metastases producing symptoms such as hematuria, hemoptysis, hematemesis, hematochezia, stroke, or vaginal bleeding. The common sites for metastatic disease are listed in Table 38–8. The diagnosis of choriocarcinoma is based on history, imaging studies, and a serum β-hCG level. Histologic confirmation is neither neces-

Table 38–8. COMMON SITES FOR METASTATIC CHORIOCARCINOMA*

Site	Percent
Lung	60–95
Vagina	40–50
Vulva/cervix	10–15
Brain	5–15
Liver	5–15
Kidney	0–5
Spleen	0–5
Gastrointestinal	0–5

* Frequencies vary, depending on whether data are based on autopsy studies or are obtained from pretreatment imaging.
From Copeland LJ: Gestational trophoblastic neoplasia. *In* Copeland LJ (ed): Textbook of Gynecology. 2nd ed. Philadelphia, WB Saunders Company, 2000, p 1391, with permission.

sary for the diagnosis nor a prerequisite to initiate therapy. Again, it is necessary to exclude the presence of a new gestation as the source of a rising β-hCG level prior to extensive diagnostic imaging or therapeutic intervention.

The complexities of the general treatment approach or treatment for special situations is beyond the scope of this textbook. It is recommended that the reader refer to a gynecology or gynecologic ontology resource for discussions of the therapeutic subtleties and pitfalls. Choriocarcinoma should be managed by a gynecologic oncologist, preferably one with a special interest in the disease.

Key Points

➤ Since many of the common complaints of pregnancy are also early symptoms of metastatic cancer, pregnant women with cancer are at risk for delays in diagnosis and therapeutic intervention.

➤ The safest interval for most cancer therapies in pregnancy is the second trimester, thereby avoiding induction of teratogenic risks or miscarriage in the first trimester and avoiding neonatal morbidity associated with preterm delivery in the third trimester.

➤ Antimetabolites and alkylating agents present the greatest hazard to the developing fetus.

➤ Diagnostic delays of breast cancer in pregnancy are often attributed to physician reluctance to properly evaluate breast complaints or abnormal findings in pregnancy.

➤ Treatment for Hodgkin's disease may compromise the reproductive potential, and combined treatment with irradiation and chemotherapy provides the highest risk of ovarian failure.

➤ If a mother is exposed to cytotoxic drugs within 1 month of delivery, the newborn should be monitored closely for evidence of granulocytopenia or thrombocytopenia.

➤ The effect of pregnancy on the clinical course of melanoma has been the subject of debate. When corrected for tumor thickness, pregnancy does not appear to be an independent prognostic variable for survival.

➤ After stratifying for stage and age, patients with pregnancy-associated cervical carcinoma have survival rates similar to the nonpregnant patient.

➤ Since most malignant ovarian tumors found in pregnancy are either germ cell tumors or low-grade, early-stage epithelial tumors, the therapeutic plan will usually permit continuation of the pregnancy and preservation of fertility.

➤ While rare, most colorectal carcinomas in pregnancy are detectable on rectal examination, underscoring the need for a rectal examination at the patient's first prenatal visit.

REFERENCES

1. Donnegan WL: Cancer and pregnancy. Cancer 33:194, 1983.
2. Koren G, Weiner L, Lishner M, et al: Cancer in pregnancy: identification of unanswered questions on maternal and fetal risks. Obstet Gynecol Surv 45:509, 1990.
3. Doll DC, Ringenberg QS, Yarbro JW: Management of cancer during pregnancy. Arch Intern Med 148:2058, 1988.
4. Doll DC, Ringenberg QS, Yarbro JW: Antineoplastic agents and pregnancy. Semin Oncol 16:337, 1989.
5. Ben-Baruch G, Menczer J, Goshen R, et al: Cisplatin excretion in human milk. J Natl Cancer Inst 84:451, 1992.
6. Reynoso EE, Shepherd FA, Messner HA, et al: Acute leukemia during pregnancy: the Toronto leukemia study group experience with long term follow-up in children exposed in utero to chemotherapeutic agents. J Clin Oncol 5:1098, 1987.
7. Henderson CE, Elia G, Garfinkel D, et al: Platinum chemotherapy during pregnancy for serous cystadenocarcinoma of the ovary. Gynecol Oncol 49:92, 1993.
8. Zemlickis D, Lishner M, Degendorfer P, et al: Fetal outcome after in utero exposure to cancer chemotherapy. Arch Intern Med 152:573, 1992.
9. Briggs GG, Freeman RK, Yaffe SJ: Instructions for use of the reference guide. In Briggs GG, Freeman RK, Yaffe SJ (eds): A Reference Guide to Fetal and Neonatal Risk: Drugs in Pregnancy and Lactation. 3rd ed. Baltimore, Williams & Wilkins, 1990, p xix.
10. Nicholson HO: Cytotoxic drugs in pregnancy. J Obstet Gynaecol Br Commonw 75:307, 1968.
11. Schardein JL: Cancer chemotherapeutic agents. In Schardein JL (ed): Chemically Induced Birth Defects, 2nd ed. New York, Marcel Dekker, 1993.
12. Kozlowski RD, Steinbrunner JV, Mackenzie AH, et al: Outcome of first-trimester exposure to low-dose methotrexate in eight patients with rheumatic disease. Am J Med 88:589, 1990.
13. Roboz J, Gleichner N, Wu K, et al: Does doxorubicin cross the placenta? Lancet 2:2691, 1979.
14. Barni S, Ardizzola A, Zanetta G, et al: Weekly doxorubicin chemotherapy for breast cancer in pregnancy: a case report. Tumori 78:349, 1992.
15. Karp GI, Von Oeyen P, Valone F, et al: Doxorubicin in pregnancy: possible transplacental passage. Cancer Treat Rep 67:773, 1983.
16. Malone JM, Gershenson DM, Creasy RK, et al: Endodermal sinus tumor of the ovary associated with pregnancy. Obstet Gynecol 68:86, 1986.

17. Kim DS, Park MI: Maternal and fetal survival following surgery and chemotherapy of endodermal sinus tumor of the ovary during pregnancy: a case report. Obstet Gynecol 73: 503, 1989.

18. Christman JE, Teng NNH, Lebovic GS, Sikic BI: Case report: delivery of a normal infant following cisplatin, vinblastine, and bleomycin chemotherapy for malignant teratoma of the ovary during pregnancy. Gynecol Oncol 37:292, 1990.

19. Elit L, Bocking A, Kenyon C, Natale R: An endodermal sinus tumor diagnosed in pregnancy: case report and review of the literature. Gynecol Oncol 72:123, 1999.

20. Tewari K, Cappuccini F, Gamkino A, et al: Neoadjuvant chemotherapy in the treatment of locally advanced cervical carcinoma in pregnancy. Cancer 82:1529, 1998.

21. Metz SA, Day TG, Pursell SH: Adjuvant chemotherapy in a pregnant patient with endodermal sinus tumor. Gynecol Oncol 32:371, 1989.

22. Malfetano JH, Goldkrand JW: Cisplatinum combination chemotherapy during pregnancy for advanced epithelial ovarian carcinoma. Obstet Gynecol 75:545, 1990.

23. King LA, Nevin PC, Williams PP, et al: Treatment of advanced epithelial ovarian carcinoma in pregnancy with cisplatin-based chemotherapy. Gynecol Oncol 41:78, 1991.

24. van der Zee AGJ, de Bruijn HWA, Bouma J, et al: Endodermal sinus tumor of the ovary during pregnancy: a case report. Am J Obstet Gynecol 164:504, 1991.

25. Farahmand SH, Marchetti DL, Asirwatham JE, Dewey MR: Case report: ovarian endodermal sinus tumor associated with pregnancy: review of the literature. Gynecol Oncol 41:156, 1991.

26. Horbelt D, Delmore J, Meisel R, et al: Mixed germ cell malignancy of the ovary concurrent with pregnancy. Obstet Gynecol 84:662, 1994.

27. Gilland J, Weinstein L: The effects of cancer chemotherapeutic agents on the developing fetus. Obstet Gynecol Surv 38:6, 1983.

28. Beidler N: Cancer treatment during pregnancy: there's strength in numbers for researchers. J Natl Cancer Inst 92: 372, 2000.

29. Garber JE: Long-term follow-up of children exposed in utero to antineoplastic agents. Semin Oncol 16:437, 1989.

30. Mazze RI, Kallen B: Reproductive outcome after anesthesia and operation during pregnancy: a registry study of 5405 cases. Am J Obstet Gynecol 161:1178, 1989.

31. Aisner J, Weirnik PH, Pearl P: Pregnancy outcome in patients treated for Hodgkin's disease. J Clin Oncol 11:507, 1993.

32. Clark ST, Radford JA, Crowther D, et al: Gonadal function following chemotherapy for Hodgkin disease: a comparative study of MVPP and a seven-drug hybrid regimen. J Clin Oncol 13:134, 1995.

33. Aviles A, Diaz-Maqueo JC, Talavera A, et al: Growth and development of children and mothers treated with chemotherapy during pregnancy; current status of 43 children. Am J Hematol 36:243, 1991.

34. Greenlee RT, Murray T, Bolden S, Wingo PA: Cancer statistics, 2000. CA Cancer J Clin 50:7, 2000.

35. Lewison EF: Breast cancer and pregnancy or lactation. Surg Gynecol Obstet 99:417, 1954.

36. White E: Projected changes in breast cancer incidence due to the trend toward delayed childbearing. Am J Public Health 77:495, 1987.

37. Michels KB, Willett WC, Rosner BA, et al: Prospective assessment of breastfeeding and breast cancer incidence among 89,877 women. Lancet 347:431, 1996.

38. Jernstrom H, Lerman C, Ghadirian P, et al: Pregnancy and risk of early breast cancer in carriers of BRCA1 and BRCA2. Lancet 354:1846, 1999.

39. Applewhite RR, Smith LR, DiVincenti F: Carcinoma of the breast associated with pregnancy and lactation. Ann Surg 39: 101, 1973.

40. Zemlickis D, Lishner M, Degendorfer P, et al: Maternal and fetal outcomes after breast cancer in pregnancy. Am J Obstet Gynecol 166:781, 1992.

41. Parente JT, Amsel M, Lerner R, Chinea F: Breast cancer associated with pregnancy. Obstet Gynecol 71:861, 1988.

42. Max MH, Lamer TW: Breast cancer in 120 women under 35 years old. Ann Surg 50:23, 1984.

43. Clark GM, Osborne CK, McGuire WL: Correlations between estrogen receptor, progesterone receptor, and patient characteristics in human breast cancer. J Clin Oncol 2:1102, 1984.

44. Botsis D, Sarandakou A, Kassanos D, et al: Breast cancer markers during normal pregnancy. Anticancer Res 19:3539, 1999.

45. King RM, Welch JS, Martin JK Jr, Coul CB: Carcinoma of the breast associated with pregnancy. Surg Gynecol Obstet 160:228, 1985.

46. Kinne DW: Primary treatment of breast cancer. *In* Harris JR, Hellman S, Henderson IC, Kinne DW (eds): Breast Diseases. 2nd ed. Philadelphia, JB Lippincott, 1991, p 356.

47. Nettleton J, Long J, Kuban D, et al: Breast cancer during pregnancy: quantifying the risk of treatment delay. Obstet Gynecol 87:414, 1996.

48. van der Vange N, van Donegan JA: Breast cancer and pregnancy. Eur J Surg Oncol 17:1, 1991.

49. Brent RL: The effect of embryonic and fetal exposure to x-ray, microwaves, and ultrasound: counseling the pregnant and nonpregnant patient about these risks. Semin Oncol 16: 347, 1989.

50. Holmes FA: Breast cancer during pregnancy. Cancer Bull 46: 405, 1994.

51. Elledge RM, Ciocca DR, Langione DR, et al: Estrogen receptor, progesterone receptor, and HER-2/neu protein in breast cancers from pregnant patients. Cancer 71:2499, 1993.

52. Holleb AI, Farrow JH: The relationship of carcinoma of the breast and pregnancy in 283 patients. Surg Gynecol Obstet 115:65, 1962.

53. Lee TN, Horz JM: Significance of ovarian metastases in therapeutic oophorectomy for advanced breast cancer. Cancer 27: 1374, 1971.

54. Ravdin RG, Lewison EF, Slack NH: The results of a clinical trial concerning the worth of prophylactic oophorectomy for breast cancer. Surg Gynecol Obstet 131:1055, 1970.

55. Giacolone PL, Laffargue F, Benos P: Chemotherapy for breast carcinoma during pregnancy: a French national survey. Cancer 86:2266, 1999.

56. Bernik SF, Bernik TR, Whooley BP, et al: Carcinoma of the breast during pregnancy: a review and update on treatment options. Surg Oncol 7:45, 1999.

57. Berry DL, Theriault RL, Holmes FA, et al: Management of breast cancer during pregnancy using a standardized protocol. J Clin Oncol 17:855, 1999.

58. Byrd BF Jr, Bayer DS, Robertson JC, Stephenson SE: Treatment of breast tumors associated with pregnancy and lactation. Ann Surg 155:940, 1962.

59. White TT, White WC: Breast cancer and pregnancy: report of 49 cases followed five years. Ann Surg 144:384, 1956.

60. Applewhite RR, Smith LR, DiVincenti F: Carcinoma of the breast associated with pregnancy and lactation. Ann Surg 39: 101, 1973.

61. Riberio GG, Palmer MK: Breast carcinoma associated with pregnancy: a clinician's dilemma. BMJ 2:1524, 1977.

62. Clark RM, Reid J: Carcinoma of the breast in pregnancy and lactation. Int Radiat Oncol Biol Phys 4:693, 1978.

63. Petrek JA, Dukoff R, Rogatko A: Prognosis of pregnancy-associated breast cancer. Cancer 67:869, 1991.

64. Donegan WL: Breast cancer and pregnancy. Obstet Gynecol 50:244, 1977.

65. Peters MV: The effect of pregnancy in breast cancer. *In* Forrest APM, Kunkler PB (eds): Prognostic Factors in Breast Cancer. Baltimore, Williams & Wilkins, 1968, p 120.

66. Nugent P, O'Connell TX: Breast cancer and pregnancy. Arch Surg 120:1221, 1985.

67. Danforth DN Jr: How subsequent pregnancy affects outcome in women with a prior breast cancer. Oncology 11:21, 1991.

68. Velentgas P, Daling JR, Malone KE, et al: Pregnancy after breast carcinoma: outcomes and influence on mortality. Cancer 85:2424, 1999.

69. Epstein RJ, Henderson IC: The Danforth article reviewed: the jury is in. Oncology 11:30, 1991.

70. Cooper DR, Butterfield J: Pregnancy subsequent to mastectomy for cancer of the breast. Ann Surg 171:429, 1970.

71. Sutton R, Buzdar AU, Hortobagyi GN: Pregnancy and offspring after adjuvant chemotherapy in breast cancer patients. Cancer 71:2499, 1990.

72. Higgins S, Haffty B: Pregnancy and lactation after breast-conserving therapy for early-stage breast cancer. Cancer 73:2175, 1994.

73. Tralins A: Is lactation possible after breast irradiation? Proc Am Soc Clin Oncol 12:77, 1993.

74. Miller MJ, Ross ME: Case report: pregnancy following breast reconstruction with autologous tissue. Cancer Bull 45:546, 1993.

75. Barry RM, Diamond HD, Craver LF: Influence of pregnancy on the course of Hodgkin's disease. Am J Obstet Gynecol 84:445, 1962.

76. Sweet DL Jr: Malignant lymphoma: implications during the reproductive years and pregnancy. J Reprod Med 17:198, 1976.

77. Lishner M, Zemlickis D, Degendorfer P, et al: Maternal and fetal outcome following Hodgkin's disease in pregnancy. Br J Cancer 65:114, 1992.

78. Gelb AB, van de Rijn M, Warnke RA: Pregnancy-associated lymphomas. A clinicopathologic study. Cancer 78:304, 1996.

79. Thomas PRM, Peckham MJ: The investigation and management of Hodgkin's disease in the pregnant patient. Cancer 38:1443, 1976.

80. Jacobs C, Donaldson SS, Rosenberg SA, Kaplan HS: Management of the pregnant patient with Hodgkin's disease. Ann Intern Med 95:649, 1981.

81. Friedman E, Jones GW: Fetal outcome after maternal radiation treatment of supradiaphragmatic Hodgkin's disease. Can Med Assoc J 149:1281, 1993.

82. Dein RA, Mennuti MT, Kovach P, Gabbe SG: The reproductive potential of young men and women with Hodgkin's disease. Obstet Gynecol Surv 39:474, 1984.

83. Horning SJ, Hoppe RT, Kaplan HS: Female reproduction after treatment for Hodgkin's disease. N Engl J Med 304:1377, 1981.

84. Chapman RM, Sutcliffe SB, Malpas JS: Cytotoxic induced ovarian failure in women with Hodgkin's disease. I. Hormone function. JAMA 242:1877, 1979.

85. Chapman RM, Sutcliffe SB, Lees LH: Cyclical combination chemotherapy and gonadal function. Lancet 1:285, 1979.

86. Jarrell JJ: Reproductive toxicology. *In* Copeland LJ (ed): Textbook of Gynecology. Philadelphia, WB Saunders Company, 2000, p 453.

87. Holmes GE, Holmes FF: Pregnancy outcome of patients treated for Hodgkin's disease. Cancer 41:1317, 1978.

88. Janov AJ, Anderson J, Cella DF, et al: Pregnancy outcome in survivors of advanced Hodgkin's disease. Cancer 70:688, 1992.

89. McKeen EA, Mulvill JJ, Rosner F, Zarrari MH: Pregnancy outcome in Hodgkin's disease. Lancet 2:590, 1979.

90. Selvais PL, Mazy G, Gosseye S, et al: Breast infiltration by acute lymphoblastic leukemia during pregnancy. Am J Obstet Gynecol 169:1619, 1993.

91. Ward FT, Weiss RB: Lymphoma and pregnancy. Semin Oncol 16:397, 1989.

92. Ohba T, Matusuo I, Katabuchi H, et al: Adult T-cell leukemia/lymphoma in pregnancy. Obstet Gynecol 72:445, 1988.

93. Manns A, Blattner WA: The epidemiology of the human T-cell lymphotropic virus type I and type II: etiologic role in human disease. Transfusion 31:67, 1991.

94. Caligiuri MA, Mayer RJ: Pregnancy and leukemia. Semin Oncol 16:338, 1989.

95. Catanzarite VA, Ferguson JE: Acute leukemia and pregnancy: a review of management and outcome, 1972–1982. Obstet Gynecol Surv 39:663, 1984.

96. Juarez S, Cuadrado JM, Feliu J, et al: Association of leukemia and pregnancy: clinical and obstetric aspects. Am J Clin Oncol 11:159, 1988.

97. Zuazu J, Julia A, Sierra J, et al: Pregnancy outcome in hematologic malignancies. Cancer 61:703, 1991.

98. Antonelli NM, Dotters DJ, Katz VL, Kuller JA: Cancer in pregnancy: a review of the literature. Part II. Obstet Gynecol Surv 51:135, 1996.

99. Hoelzer D, Thiel E, Loffler H, et al: Prognostic factors in a multicenter study for treatment of acute lymphoblastic leukemia in adults. Blood 71:123, 1988.

100. Wiernik PH: Acute leukemias of adults. *In* DeVita VT Jr, Hellman S, Rosenberg SA (eds): Cancer: Principles and Practice of Oncology. Philadelphia, JB Lippincott, 1982, p 302.

101. Aviles A, Niz J: Long term follow-up of children born to mothers with acute leukemia during pregnancy. Med Pediatr Oncol 16:3, 1988.

102. Bazarbashi MS, Smith MR, Karanes C, et al: Successful management of Ph chromosome chronic myelogenous leukemia with leukapheresis during pregnancy. Am J Hematol 38:235, 1991.

103. Baer MR, Ozer H, Foon KA: Interferon-alpha therapy during pregnancy in chronic myelogenous leukemia and hairy cell leukemia. Br J Haematol 81:167, 1992.

104. Delmer A, Rio B, Baudner F, et al: Pregnancy during myelosuppressive treatment for chronic myelogenous leukemia. Br J Haematol 82:783, 1992.

105. Jackson N, Shukri A, Ali K: Hydroxyurea treatment for chronic myeloid leukemia during pregnancy. Br J Haematol 85:203, 1993.

106. Patel M, Dukes IAF, Hill JC: Use of hydroxyurea in chronic myeloid leukemia during pregnancy: a case report. Am J Obstet Gynecol 165:565, 1991.

107. Tertian G, Tchernia G, Papiernik E, et al: Hydroxyurea and pregnancy. Am J Obstet Gynecol 166:1868, 1992.

108. Friedman RJ, Rigel DS, Kopf AW: Early detection of malignant melanoma: the role of the physician examination and self examination of the skin. CA Cancer J Clin 35:130, 1985.

109. Smith RS, Randall P: Melanoma during pregnancy. Obstet Gynecol 34:825, 1969.

110. Balch CM, Soong SJ, Milton GW, et al: A comparison of prognostic factors and surgical results in 1,786 patients with localized (stage I) melanoma treated in Alabama, USA, and New South Wales, Australia. Ann Surg 146:677, 1982.

111. Gordon AN: Vulvar tumors. *In* Copeland LJ (ed): Textbook of Gynecology. Philadelphia, WB Saunders Company, 2000, p 1202.

112. Pack GT, Scharnagel IM: The prognosis for malignant melanoma in the pregnant woman. Cancer 4:324, 1951.

113. Byrd BF, McGanty WJ: The effect of pregnancy on the normal course of malignant melanoma. South Med 47:324, 1951.

114. George PA, Fortner JG, Pack GT: Melanoma with pregnancy: a report of 115 cases. Cancer 13:854, 1960.

115. Shiu MH, Schottenfeld D, Maclean B, Fortner JG: Adverse effect of pregnancy on melanoma. Cancer 37:181, 1976.

116. Houghton AN, Flannery J, Viola MV: Malignant melanoma of the skin occurring during pregnancy. Cancer 48:407, 1981.

117. Wong DJ, Stassner HT: Melanoma in pregnancy. Clin Obstet Gynecol 33:782, 1990.

118. MacKie RM, Bufalino R, Morabito A, et al: Lack of effect on pregnancy outcome of melanoma. Lancet 337:653, 1991.

119. McManamny DS, Moss ALH, Pocock PV, et al: Melanoma and pregnancy: a long-term follow-up. Br J Obstet Gynaecol 96:1419, 1989.

120. Slingluff CL Jr, Reintgen D, Vollmer RT, et al: Malignant melanoma arising during pregnancy: a study of 100 patients. Ann Surg 211:552, 1990.

121. Lederman JS, Sober AJ: Effect of prior pregnancy on melanoma survival. Arch Dermatol 121:716, 1985.

122. Travers R, Sober A, Barnhill R, et al: Increased thickness of pregnancy-associated melanoma: a study of the MGH pigmented lesion clinic. Melanoma Res 3(Suppl):44, 1993.

123. Colburn DS, Nathanson L, Belilos E: Pregnancy and malignant melanoma. Semin Oncol 16:377, 1989.

124. Ross MI: Melanoma and pregnancy: prognostic and therapeutic considerations. Cancer Bull 46:412, 1994.

125. Ostelind A, Tucker MA, Stone BJ, et al: The Danish case control study of cutaneous malignant melanoma III: hormonal and reproductive factors in women. Int J Cancer 42:821, 1988.

126. Lederman JS, Lew RA, Koh HK, Sober AJ: Influence of estrogen administration on tumor characteristics and survival in women with cutaneous melanoma. J Natl Cancer Inst 74:981, 1985.

127. Hacker NF, Berek JS, Lagasse LD, et al: Carcinoma of the cervix associated with pregnancy. Obstet Gynecol 59:735, 1982.

128. Zemlickis D, Lishner M, Degendorfer P, et al: Maternal and fetal outcome after invasive cervical cancer in pregnancy. J Clin Oncol 9:1956, 1991.

129. Nevin D, Soeters R, Dehaeck K, et al: Cervical carcinoma associated with pregnancy. Obstet Gynecol Surv 50:228, 1995.

130. Benedet JL, Selke PA, Nickerson KG: Colposcopic evaluation of abnormal Papanicolaou smears in pregnancy. Am J Obstet Gynecol 157:932, 1987.

131. Economos K, Perez Veridiano N, Delke I, et al: Abnormal cervical cytology in pregnancy: a 17-year experience. Obstet Gynecol 81:915, 1993.

132. Averette HE, Nasser N, Yankow SL: Cervical conization in pregnancy. Am J Obstet Gynecol 106:543, 1970.

133. Hannigan EV, Whitehouse HH III, Atkinson WD, et al: Cone biopsy during pregnancy. Obstet Gynecol 60:450, 1982.

134. Hannigan EV: Cervical cancer in pregnancy. Clin Obstet Gynecol 33:837, 1990.

135. Copeland LJ, Silva EG, Gershenson DM, et al: Superficially invasive squamous cell carcinoma of the cervix. Gynecol Oncol 45:307, 1992.

136. Lewandowski GS, Copeland LJ, Vaccarello L: Surgical issues in the management of carcinoma of the cervix in pregnancy. Surg Clin North Am 75:89, 1995.

137. Duggan B, Muderspach LI, Roman LD, et al: Cervical cancer in pregnancy: reporting on planned delay in therapy. Obstet Gynecol 82:598, 1993.

138. Sood AK, Sorosky JL, Krogman S, et al: Surgical management of cervical cancer complicating pregnancy: a case-control study. Gynecol Oncol 63:294, 1996.

139. Monk BJ, Montz FJ: Invasive cervical cancer complicating intrauterine pregnancy. Treatment with hysterectomy. Obstet Gynecol 80:199, 1992.

140. Sivanesaratnam V, Javalakshmi P, Loo C: Surgical management of early invasive cancer of the uterine cervix associated with pregnancy. Gynecol Oncol 48:68, 1993.

141. Greer BE, Easterling TR, McLennan DA, et al: Fetal and maternal considerations in the management of stage IB cervical during pregnancy. Gynecol Oncol 34:61, 1989.

142. Lewandowski GS, Copeland LJ: A potential role for invasive chemotherapy in the treatment of small cell neuroendocrine tumors of the cervix. Gynecol Oncol 48:127, 1993.

143. Balderston KD, Tewari K, Gregory WT, et al: Neuroendocrine small cell cervix cancer in pregnancy: long-term survivor following combined therapy. Gynecol Oncol 71:128, 1998.

144. Shingleton HM, Orr JW: Cervical cancer complicating pregnancy. In Cancer of the Cervix. Edinburgh, Churchill Livingstone, 1983, p 284.

145. Copeland LJ, Saul PB, Sneige N: Cervical adenocarcinoma: tumor implantation in the episiotomy sites of two patients. Gynecol Oncol 28:230, 1987.

146. Gordon AN, Jensen R, Jones HW III: Squamous carcinoma of the cervix complicating pregnancy: recurrence in episiotomy after vaginal delivery. Obstet Gynecol 73:850, 1989.

147. Cliby WA, Dodson WA, Podratz KC: Cervical cancer complicated by pregnancy: episiotomy site recurrences following vaginal delivery. Obstet Gynecol 84:179, 1994.

148. Hopkins MP, Morley GW: The prognosis and management of cervical cancer associated with pregnancy. Obstet Gynecol 80: 9, 1992.

149. Jones WB, Shingleton HM, Russell A, et al: Cervical carcinoma and pregnancy. A national pattern of care study of the American College of Surgeons. Cancer 77:1479, 1996.

150. Fleischer AC, Shah DM, Entman SS: Sonographic evaluation of maternal disorders during pregnancy. Radiol Clin North Am 28:51, 1990.

151. Hess LW, Peaceman A, O'Brien W, et al: Adnexal mass occurring with intrauterine pregnancy: a report of 54 patients requiring laparotomy for definitive management. Am J Obstet Gynecol 158:1029, 1988.

152. El Yahia AR, Rahman J, Rahman MS, et al: Ovarian tumors in pregnancy. Aust N Z J Obstet Gynaecol 31:327, 1991.

153. Munnell EW: Primary ovarian cancer associated with pregnancy. Clin Obstet Gynecol 6:983, 1963.

154. Dgani R, Shoham Z, Atar E, et al: Ovarian carcinoma during pregnancy: a study of 23 cases in Israel between the years of 1960 and 1984. Gynecol Oncol 33:326, 1989.

155. Copeland LJ: Gestational trophoblastic neoplasia. In Copeland LJ (ed): Textbook of Gynecology. Philadelphia, WB Saunders Company, 2000, p 1391.

156. Platek DN, Henderson CE, Goldberg GL: The management of a persistent adnexal mass in pregnancy. Am J Obstet Gynecol 173:12236, 1995.

157. Jacob JH, Stringer CA: Diagnosis and management of cancer during pregnancy. Semin Perinatol 14:79, 1990.

158. Jolles CJ: Gynecologic cancer associated with pregnancy. Semin Oncol 16:417, 1989.

159. Katz VL, Watson WJ, Hansen WF, et al: Massive ovarian tumor complicating pregnancy: a case report. J Reprod Med 38:907, 1993.

160. Kobayashi F, Sagawa N, Nakamura K, et al: Mechanism and clinical significance of elevated CA 125 levels in the sera of pregnant women. Am J Obstet Gynecol 160:563, 1989.

161. VanSlooten AJ, Rechner SF, Dods WG: Recurrent maternal virilization during pregnancy caused by benign androgen-producing ovarian lesions. Am J Obstet Gynecol 167:1342, 1992.

162. McGuire WP, Hoskins WJ, Brady MF, et al: Cyclophosphamide and cisplatin compared with paclitaxel and cisplatin in patients with stage III and stage IV ovarian cancer. N Engl J Med 334:1, 1996.

163. Malfetano JH, Goldkrand JW: Cisplatinum combination chemotherapy during pregnancy for advanced epithelial ovarian carcinoma. Obstet Gynecol 75:545, 1990.

164. King LA, Nevin PC, Williams PP, Carson LF: Case report of treatment of advanced epithelial ovarian carcinoma in pregnancy with cisplatin-based chemotherapy. Gynecol Oncol 41:78, 1991.

165. Henderson CE, Giovanni E, Garfinkel D, et al: Case report: platinum chemotherapy during pregnancy for serous cystadenocarcinoma of the ovary. Gynecol Oncol 49:92, 1993.

166. Buller RE, Darrow V, Manetta A, et al: Conservative surgical management of dysgerminoma concomitant with pregnancy. Obstet Gynecol 79:887, 1992.

167. Weed JC, Roh RA, Mendenhall HW: Recurrent endodermal sinus tumor during pregnancy. Obstet Gynecol 54:653, 1979.

168. Petrucha RA, Ruffolo E, Messina AM, et al: Endodermal sinus tumor: report of a case associated with pregnancy. Obstet Gynecol 55(Suppl):90, 1980.

169. Schwartz RP, Chatwani AJ, Strimel W, Putong PB: Endodermal sinus tumors in pregnancy: report of a case and review of the literature. Gynecol Oncol 15:434, 1983.

170. Ito K, Teshima K, Suzuki H, Noda K: A case of ovarian endodermal sinus tumor associated with pregnancy. Tohoku J Exp Med 142:183, 1984.

171. Malone JM, Gershenson DM, Creasy RK, et al: Endodermal sinus tumor associated with pregnancy. Obstet Gynecol 68:86, 1984.

172. Kim DS, Park MI: Maternal and fetal survival following surgery and chemotherapy of endodermal sinus tumor of the ovary during pregnancy: a case report. Obstet Gynecol 73:503, 1989.

173. Metz SA, Day TG, Pursell SH: Adjuvant chemotherapy in a pregnant patient with endodermal sinus tumor. Gynecol Oncol 32:371, 1989.

174. van der Zee AGL, de Bruijn HWA, Bouma J, et al: Endodermal sinus tumor of the ovary during pregnancy: a case report. Am J Obstet Gynecol 164:504, 1991.

175. Farahmand SH, Marchetti DL, Asirwatham JE, Dewey MR: Case report: ovarian endodermal sinus tumor associated with pregnancy: review of the literature. Gynecol Oncol 41:156, 1991.

176. Horbelt D, Delmore J, Meisel R, et al: Mixed germ cell malignancy of the ovary concurrent with pregnancy. Obstet Gynecol 84:662, 1994.

177. Young RH, Dudley AG, Scully RE: Granulosa cell, Sertoli-Leydig cell and unclassified sex-cord stromal tumors associated with pregnancy: a clinical pathological analysis of 36 cases. Gynecol Oncol 18:181, 1984.

178. Collins CG, Barclay DL: Cancer of the vulva and cancer of the vagina in pregnancy. Clin Obstet Gynecol 6:927, 1973.

179. Lutz MH, Underwood PB, Rozier JC, et al: Genital malignancy in pregnancy. Am J Obstet Gynecol 129:536, 1977.

180. Moore DH, Fowler WC, Currie JL, Walton LA: Squamous cell carcinoma of the vulva in pregnancy. Gynecol Oncol 41:74, 1991.

181. Burke TW, Stringer CA, Gershenson DM, et al: Radical wide excision and selective inguinal node dissection for squamous cell carcinoma of the vulva. Gynecol Oncol 38:328, 1990.

182. Senekjian EK, Hubby M, Bell DA, et al: Clear cell adenocarcinoma of the vagina and cervix in association with pregnancy. Gynecol Oncol 24:207, 1986.

183. Schneller JG, Nicastri AD: Intrauterine pregnancy coincident with endometrial carcinoma: a case study and review of the literature. Gynecol Oncol 54:87, 1994.

184. Fine BA, Baker TR, Hempling RE, et al: Pregnancy coexisting with serous papillary adenocarcinoma involving both uterus and ovary. Gynecol Oncol 53:369, 1994.

185. Vaccarello L, Apte SM, Copeland LJ, et al: Endometrial carcinoma associated with pregnancy: a report of three cases and review of the literature. Gynecol Oncol 74:118, 1999.

186. Ayhan A, Gunalp S, Karaer C, et al: Endometrial adenocarcinoma in pregnancy. Gynecol Oncol 75:298, 1999.

187. Woods JB, Martin JN Jr, Ingram FH, et al: Pregnancy complicated by carcinoma of the colon above the rectum. Am J Perinatol 9:102, 1992.

188. Bernstein MA, Madoff RD, Caushaj PF: Colon and rectal cancer in pregnancy. Dis Colon Rectum 36:172, 1993.

189. Medich DS, Fazio VW: Hemorrhoids, anal fissure, and carcinoma of the colon, rectum, and anus during pregnancy. Surg Clin North Am 75:77, 1995.

190. Nesbitt JC, Moise KJ, Sawyers JL: Colorectal carcinoma in pregnancy. Arch Surg 120:636, 1985.

191. Roelvink NCA, Kamphorst W, van Alphen HAM, et al: Pregnancy-related primary brain and spinal tumors. Arch Neurol 44:209, 1987.

192. DeAngelis LM: Central nervous system neoplasms in pregnancy. Adv Neurol 64:139, 1994.

193. Finfer SR: Management of labor and delivery in patients with intracranial neoplasms. Br J Anaesth 67:784, 1991.

194. Lunardi P, Rizzo A, Missori P, et al: Pituitary apoplexy in an acromegalic woman operated on during pregnancy by transsphenoidal approach. Int J Gynecol Obstet 34:71, 1990.

195. Coyne TJ, Atkinson RL, Prins JB: Adrenocorticotropic hormone-secreting pituitary tumor associated with pregnancy. Case report. Neurosurgery 31:953, 1992.

196. Johnson RJ Jr, Voorhies RM, Witkin M, et al: Fertility following excision of a symptomatic craniopharyngioma during pregnancy: case report. Surg Neurol 39:257, 1993.

197. Tokuda Y, Hatayama T, Sakoda K: Metastasis of malignant struma ovarii to the cranial vault during pregnancy. Neurosurgery 33:515, 1993.

198. Doyle KJ, Luxford WM: Acoustic neuroma in pregnancy. Am J Otol 15:111, 1994.

199. Arango HA, Kalter CS, Decesare SL, et al: Management of chemotherapy in a pregnancy complicated by a large neuroblastoma. Obstet Gynecol 84:665, 1994.

200. Harper MA, Murnaghan GA, Kennedy L, et al: Pheochromocytoma in pregnancy. Five cases and a review of the literature. Br J Obstet Gynaecol 96:594, 1989.

201. Dildy GA III, Moise KJ Jr, Carpenter RJ Jr, et al: Maternal malignancy metastatic to the products of conception: a review. Obstet Gynecol Surv 44:535, 1989.

202. Rothman LA, Cohen CJ, Astarola J: Placental and fetal involvement by maternal malignancy: a report of rectal carcinoma and a review of the literature. Am J Obstet Gynecol 116:1023, 1973.

203. Kurtin PJ, Gaffney TA, Haberman TM: Peripheral T cell lymphoma involving the placenta. Cancer 70:2963, 1992.

204. Pollack RN, Sklarin NT, Rao S, et al: Metastatic placental lymphoma associated with maternal human immunodeficiency virus infection. Obstet Gynecol 81:856, 1993.

205. Tsujimura T, Matsumoto K, Aozasa K: Placental involvement by maternal non-Hodgkin's lymphoma. Arch Pathol Lab Med 117:325, 1993.

206. Catlin EA, Roberts JD Jr, Evana R, et al: Transplacental

transmission of natural-killer cell lymphoma. N Engl J Med 341:85, 1999.

207. Osada S, Horibe K, Oiwa K, et al: A case of infantile acute monocytic leukemia caused by vertical transmission of the mother's leukemic cells. Cancer 65:1146, 1990.

208. Pollack RN, Pollak M, Rochon L: Pregnancy complicated by medulloblastoma with metastases to the placenta. Obstet Gynecol 81:858, 1993.

209. Andreitchouk AE, Takahashi O, Kedama H, et al: Choriocarcinoma in infant and mother: a case report. J Obstet Gynaecol Res 22:585, 1996.

210. Kishkurno S, Ishida A, Takahashi Y, et al: A case of neonatal choriocarcinoma. Am J Perinatol 14:79, 1993.

211. Bandy LC, Clarke-Pearson DL, Hammond CB: Malignant potential of gestational trophoblastic disease at the extreme age of reproductive life. Obstet Gynecol 64:395, 1984.

212. Matalon M, Modan B: Epidemiologic aspects of hydatidiform mole in Israel. Am J Obstet Gynecol 112:107, 1972.

213. Lurain JR, Brewer JI, Turok EE, Halpern B: Gestational trophoblastic disease: treatment results at the Brewer Trophoblastic Disease Center. Obstet Gynecol 60:354, 1982.

214. Berkowitz RS, Goldstein DP, Bernstein MR, Sablinska B: Subsequent pregnancy outcomes in patients with molar pregnancies and gestational trophoblastic tumors. J Reprod Med 32:680, 1987.

215. Sand PK, Lurain JR, Brewer JI: Repeat gestational trophoblastic disease. Obstet Gynecol 63:140, 1984.

216. Copeland LJ: Gestational trophoblastic neoplasia. *In* Copeland LJ (ed): Textbook of Gynecology. 2nd ed. Philadelphia, WB Saunders Company, 2000, p 1414.

217. Copeland LJ: Gestational trophoblastic neoplasia. *In* Copeland LJ (ed): Textbook of Gynecology. 2nd ed. Philadelphia, WB Saunders Company, 2000, p 1416.

218. Rice LW, Berkowitz RS, Lage JM, Goldstein DP: Persistent gestational trophoblastic tumor after partial molar pregnancy. Gynecol Oncol 48:165, 1993.

219. Goto S, Yamada A, Ishizuka T, Tomoda Y: Development of post molar trophoblastic disease after partial molar pregnancy. Gynecol Oncol 48:165, 1993.

220. Chang YL, Chang TC, Hsueh S, et al: Prognostic factors and treatment for placental site trophoblastic tumor—report of 3 cases and analysis of 88 cases. Gynecol Oncol 73:216, 1999.

221. Leiserowitz GS, Webb MJ: Treatment of placental site trophoblastic tumor with hysterotomy and uterine reconstruction. Obstet Gynecol 88:696, 1996.

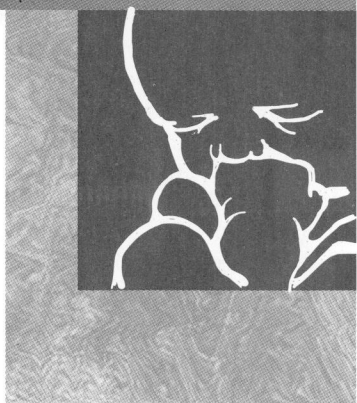

Dermatologic Disorders

ROXANNE STAMBUK AND ROY COLVEN

Most of the skin changes that occur during pregnancy are consequences of dramatic mechanical, hormonal, and blood volume changes. However, there are some specific dermatoses that only affect pregnant patients. This chapter first reviews the physiologic skin changes that occur during pregnancy and then discusses specific dermatoses associated with pregnancy. This chapter aims to enable the practitioner to distinguish between common skin changes with pregnancy and those that are more serious for the pregnant patient or her unborn child.

PHYSIOLOGIC SKIN CHANGES DURING PREGNANCY

Hypermelanosis

Hypermelanosis, or darker than constitutive skin color, occurs in 90 percent of pregnancies.[1,2] Darkly complected women are more likely to manifest hypermelanosis during pregnancy. The hypermelanosis may be generalized or localized to areas of increased melanocyte density. The areolae, umbilicus, vulva, and perianal skin may darken as early as the first trimester. The linea alba often becomes the hyperpigmented linea nigra. Pigmented nevi, freckles, and recent scars may also deepen in color.

Melasma, or chloasma, is an acquired facial hypermelanosis. It manifests with symmetric, well-defined hyperpigmented patches distributed on the cheeks, chin, eyebrows, nose and upper lip. Melasma affects at least 70 percent of pregnant women, with equal racial predilection.[3] Besides pregnancy, melasma can affect patients on oral contraceptive pills; with liver disease, hyperthyroidism, and nutritional deficiencies; and as a photo-

toxic reaction to certain cosmetics and medications. Melasma also uncommonly affects males, even in the absence of the above disorders or medications.

The pathogenesis of melasma is unknown. The role of hormonal factors such as melanocyte-stimulating hormone (MSH) is unclear. Levels of estrogen which, like MSH, can stimulate melanogenesis, are not consistently elevated in women with melasma.[4]

Ultraviolet (UV) radiation exposure, including sunlight, accentuates the hyperpigmentation. Patients with melasma should protect themselves from UV exposure by avoiding the most intense hours of sunlight, seeking shade, wearing shading clothing including a hat, and applying a broad-spectrum UV sunscreen of sun protection factor (SPF) 15 or greater. Melasma normally regresses or disappears in the majority of women. However, nearly 30 percent of patients will have persistent hyperpigmentation at 10 year follow-up.[1]

Women with persistent melasma may be treated with 2 to 4 percent hydroquinone cream combined with sunscreen applied in the morning. Hydroquinone cream combined with retinoic acid 0.05 to 0.1 percent cream,[5] and hydrocortisone 1 percent cream also appear to improve the condition, perhaps more rapidly.[6] Other options include chemical peels with trichloroacetic acid or glycolic acid performed postpartum by an experienced dermatologist.[7] Consistent sunscreen use must continue to avoid recurrence of melasma.

Melanocytic Nevi and Pregnancy

During pregnancy, some melanocytic nevi ("moles") may increase in size, and new nevi may develop.[8,9] If atypical clinical features are present, one may need to biopsy a suspicious pigmented lesion to rule out dysplasia or melanoma. A recent study of pregnant women without multiple nevi or a family history of melanoma showed no significant change in the sizes of their pigmented nevi.[10] However, a special subgroup of women with the "atypical mole syndrome" appear to be at increased risk for dysplastic changes during pregnancy.[11] These women have a family history of melanoma and multiple clinically atypical nevi.[11] The atypical mole syndrome itself in these pregnant women who were objectively studied more likely accounted for the dysplastic changes noted in the moles rather than the pregnancy.

Studies to date have not provided evidence that hormonal changes during pregnancy put the pregnant patient at increased risk of melanoma.[12-15] Although there are detectable estrogen-binding proteins on melanoma cells, there are no estrogen or progesterone receptors.[16]

When a pregnant woman is diagnosed with melanoma, the pregnancy does not adversely affect her prognosis.[12,17-20] Because melanoma incidence overall is increasing, all pregnant women with mole changes including asymmetry, increase in size or elevation, irregular border configuration, or variegation in color should be examined with the same care and scrutiny as all individuals with mole changes.

Hair Changes

Hirsutism

Hirsutism is excessive coarse, or terminal, body hair growth. Mild hirsutism commonly affects pregnant women. The face is frequently affected, though terminal hair growth may be pronounced on the extremities as well. Terminal hairs grow less commonly on the abdomen during pregnancy. Hirsutism is believed to be primarily an endocrinologic phenomenon. During normal pregnancy, the proportion of hair in the anagen (growing) phase is higher than that in the telogen (resting) phase. Hirsutism may result from placental androgen production during normal pregnancy. Mild hirsutism rarely requires therapy. It normally regresses following delivery, but does recur with subsequent pregnancies. Severe hirsutism with virilization should warrant investigation for an androgen-secreting tumor.

Telogen Effluvium

The normal hair cycle consists of three phases: anagen, the growing phase; telogen, or resting phase; and catagen, or the transitional phase in between anagen and telogen. Telogen hair normally sheds due to reactivation of the hair follicle with the beginning of anagen hair growth.[21] Eighty to ninety percent of hairs are in anagen, compared to 13 percent, on average, in telogen. *Telogen effluvium*, or hair loss after a proportional increase of anagen hairs becoming telogen, is often seen 4 to 6 months into the postpartum period, with average hair loss at two to three times the normal rate of 100 scalp hairs per day. The postpartum drop in estrogen levels precipitates telogen effluvium. Patients should be reassured that normal hair growth will occur 6 to 15 months postpartum, with reestablishment of normal hair cycle proportions. However, in rare circumstances, the hair may not return to its prepregnancy thickness. Persistent alopecia may indicate thyroid dysfunction or low iron stores.

Striae Distensae

Striae distensae, thin atrophic pink or purple linear bands that appear on the abdomen, breasts, and thighs, begin in the late second trimester in up to 90 percent of pregnant women.[4] Striae likely result from a combination of two factors. Stretching produces striae. Also, adrenocorticosteroids and estrogen promote tearing of the collagen matrix of the dermis and weakening of elastic fibers.[1] Electron microscopy demonstrates rearrangement and reduction of fibrillin fibers in biopsies of striae.[22] Most striae fade postpartum to thin flesh-colored atrophic bands.

Although treatment of early striae with topical retinoic acid improves stretch marks,[23] retinoids, even used topically, are contraindicated during pregnancy due to the potential risk of absorption and teratogenicity. Treatment of striae with a 585-nm pulsed dye laser increases dermal elastin and results in clinical improvement.[24] A trial of topical treatment of striae using glycolic acid and tretinoin versus glycolic acid and topical ascorbic acid demonstrated equal improvement and increased elastin after 12 weeks of daily application.[25] Despite these therapeutic advances, no evidence demonstrates complete resolution of striae with treatment.

Vascular Changes

Most pregnant women exhibit vascular changes within the skin. High levels of estrogen cause proliferation of cutaneous blood vessels. Vasomotor instability may also produce pallor, flushing, and mottling of the skin in response to temperature changes. Scattered petechiae may manifest on the lower extremities due to increased cutaneous capillary hydrostatic pressure and fragility common in late pregnancy. Mucous membranes may also manifest vascular changes; gingival swelling during gestation gives rise to pregnancy gingivitis.[26]

Spider angiomata occur in up to 70 percent of white women during pregnancy.[1] Blood quickly refills a compressed spider angioma from a central arteriole outward to tortuous radiating capillaries; the shape resembles a spider. One sees spider angiomata distributed sparsely on the face, trunk, and upper extremities, areas drained by the superior vena cava. Most lesions fade within 3 months during the postpartum period. Hepatic

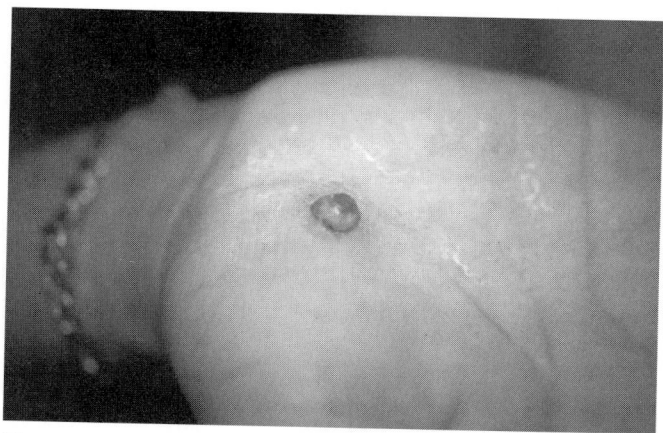

Figure 39–1. Pyogenic granuloma. This bright red papule appeared and grew to this size during 1 week. Due to its rapid appearance and friability, this pregnant patient in her second trimester sought medical attention promptly.

involute after delivery. Large hemangiomas may persist and rarely are associated with arteriovenous shunting and high-output cardiac failure.

Pyogenic granuloma (Fig. 39–1), also called granuloma gravidarum, occurs in 2 percent of pregnant women.[4] Usually solitary, a pyogenic granuloma develops rapidly as a brightly erythematous sessile or pedunculated friable papule with a collar of thickened epidermis at its base. They can be distributed anywhere on the skin or mucous membranes. Most women seek attention because of the granuloma's rapid growth and recurrent bleeding. This lesion consists of capillary proliferation and mixed inflammatory infiltrate, similar to granulation tissue. Pyogenic granuloma is thought to be an abnormal tissue response to trauma. However, most patients report no trauma history. Although these masses usually remit during the postpartum period, surgical excision may be required if the lesion fails to resolve.

cirrhosis also causes spider angiomata, likely due to higher circulating estrogen levels.

Similar to spider angiomata, *palmar erythema* affects two thirds of pregnant women. Erythema of the thenar and hypothenar eminences may occur as early as the first trimester as a result of a sixfold increase in blood flow to the hands.[27] Hepatic cirrhosis, systemic lupus erythematosus, and hyperthyroidism also cause palmar erythema. When a manifestation of pregnancy, palmar erythema typically resolves following delivery.

Small *capillary hemangiomas* may occur during the second and third trimesters in up to 5 percent of pregnant women.[1] Unlike spider angiomata, these lesions do not completely compress. Most small hemangiomas will

SPECIFIC DERMATOLOGIC CONDITIONS ASSOCIATED WITH PREGNANCY

Dermatologic disorders specific to pregnancy that present with pruritus as a common symptom include pemphigoid gestationis, polymorphic eruption of pregnancy, prurigo gestationis, and pruritic folliculitis of pregnancy (Table 39–1).[28-30] The difficulty in classifying and diagnosing these disorders stems from confusing nomenclature and lack of specific diagnostic crite-

Table 39–1. SPECIFIC INFLAMMATORY DERMATOSES OF PREGNANCY

Disease	Onset	Degree of Pruritus	Types of Lesions	Distribution	Increased Incidence of Fetal Morbidity or Mortality
Pemphigoid gestationis	First month to postpartum	Moderate to severe	Erythematous papules, vesicles, bullae	Abdomen, extremities, generalized	Unresolved
Prurigo gestationis	Fourth to ninth month	Moderate	Excoriated papules	Extensor surfaces of extremities	No
Impetigo herpetiformis	First to ninth month	Minimal	Pustules	Genitalia, medial thighs umbilicus, breasts, axillas	Yes
Polymorphic eruption of pregnancy	Third trimester	Severe	Erythematous urticarial papules and plaques	Abdomen, thighs, buttocks, occasionally arms and legs	No
Pruritic folliculitis of pregnancy	Third trimester	Moderate	Erythematous papules or pustules	Shoulder, back, arms, chest, abdomen	No
Cholestasis of pregnancy	Third trimester	Moderate to severe	None or excoriations	Generalized	Unresolved

ria, with the exception of pemphigoid gestationis. Newer classification schemes help to differentiate between these entities.[31-33] In general, it is most important to distinguish between pruritus without rash or with secondary excoriations versus pruritus with primary skin lesions.

Pruritus

Pruritus is a common symptom in pregnancy, occurring in 3 to 14 percent of all women.[34] In a prospective study of 3,192 pregnant women, 1.6 percent suffered from persistent pruritus severe enough to warrant treatment.[31] Pruritus is a common symptom in most pregnancy-specific inflammatory skin diseases. Atopic dermatitis, which may lead to considerable pruritus, is more prevalent than previously recognized in pregnant women.[35] Pruritus can also be caused by systemic entities such as liver disease, thyroid dysfunction, diabetes mellitus, drug eruptions, parasites, and malignancy.

Intrahepatic cholestasis, which occurs in 0.5 percent of pregnancies, is one of the most common causes of pregnancy-related pruritus. Intrahepatic cholestasis leads to increased levels of serum bile salts, and increased deposition of bile salts in the skin leads to itching.[32,34] Cholestatic pruritus occurs in the second or third trimester of pregnancy.[36] The pregnant patient experiences itch mainly on the palms and soles, although the itch can become generalized. There are no primary skin lesions. Changes on the skin are secondary from excoriations.[31] Liver function tests demonstrating increased serum levels of hepatic transaminases and bilirubin confirm the diagnosis of cholestasis.[37] Although the maternal prognosis is good, cholestasis has been associated with increased risks for the fetus, with risks of fetal prematurity and fetal death. Both estrogen and progesterone propagate cholestasis.[36]

Pemphigoid Gestationis

Pemphigoid gestationis is a rare, pruritic, autoimmune, bullous skin disease that occurs during the second and third trimesters of pregnancy and the puerperium.[38] The term *pemphigoid gestationis* supercedes the older term, *herpes gestationis*, because it does not involve the herpes viruses and because of its antigenic and clinical similarity to bullous pemphigoid. It affects only female patients and occurs only in the presence of placental tissue. Outside of pregnancy, choriocarcinoma and hydatidiform disease have also incited pemphigoid gestationis. The disease occurs in 1 per 1,700 to 50,000 pregnancies.[32,38,39] In a prospective study in which all pregnant women with pruritic skin lesions had skin biopsies, the incidence of pemphigoid gestationis was found to be 1 per 7,000.[40] The occurrence during the third trimester of pregnancy and the recurrence of pemphigoid gestationis with menstruation and with oral contraceptive use strongly implicates a hormonal influence. The increased frequency of certain histocompatibility locus antigens (HLA) in women with pemphigoid gestationis suggests a genetic predisposition. Up to 85 percent of women with pemphigoid gestationis have HLA-DR3, and 45 percent have the combination of HLA-DR3 and HLA-DR4.[38,41,42] An increased frequency of these HLA antigens also has been found with other autoimmune disorders. Graves' disease occurs in patients with pemphigoid gestationis with a higher than expected incidence.[43]

Clinically, pemphigoid gestationis typically presents with severely pruritic erythematous, urticarial, or hive-like, papules and plaques around the umbilicus (Fig. 39–2). Within days to weeks, the eruption spreads to involve the trunk, back, buttocks, forearms, palms, and soles, usually sparing the face, scalp, and mucosa. Within 2 to 4 weeks of the onset of the disease, vesicles and tense serum-filled bullae develop either at the margins of the edematous, erythematous plaques or de novo in clinically uninflamed skin. Sometimes vesicles and bullae do not develop, adding confusion to the diagnosis.[38] The lesions tend to heal without scarring if secondary infection does not ensue.

Pemphigoid gestationis usually presents during the second or third trimester, with a mean of 21 weeks' gestation, although patients may present with recurring crops of blisters at any time during pregnancy. It occurs for the first time during the early postpartum period in 20 percent of patients.[38] Many patients with pemphigoid gestationis transiently improve during the last 6 to 8 weeks of pregnancy only to experience an uncomfortable flare of their disease within 24 to 48 hours of delivery. The postpartum duration varies; the bullous lesions persist 5 to 24 weeks and urticarial lesions

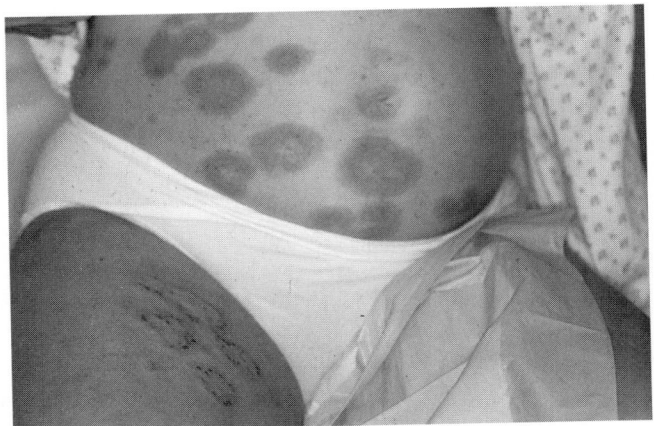

Figure 39–2. Pemphigoid gestationis during the third trimester. This patient developed erythematous urticarial superficial plaques on the thighs and abdomen that progressed to bullae formation. Biopsy revealed a heavy linear complement deposition at the basement membrane zone, consistent with pemphigoid gestationis.

longer.[38] Pemphigoid gestationis usually recurs and may be more severe with an earlier onset in subsequent pregnancies. A small proportion of women (8 percent) do not develop pemphigoid gestationis in subsequent pregnancies.[43]

One can easily make a presumptive diagnosis of pemphigoid gestationis in a pregnant woman with a typical distribution of vesicles and bullae. Skin biopsy, including a sample processed for direct immunofluorescence (DIF), confirms the diagnosis. This confirmation distinguishes pemphigoid gestationis from polymorphic eruption of pregnancy, which does not recur with subsequent pregnancies. Distinguishing these two diseases enables counseling of the patient about the recurrence risk in future pregnancies.

Skin sampling technique involves taking two 3-mm punch biopsies. One biopsy is taken from a new skin lesion and is placed in formalin for histologic evaluation. The second is taken from perilesional normal skin (within 1 to 2 cm of a lesion) and placed in transfer media for direct immunofluorescence studies. If the tissue sample for direct immunofluorescence is placed in formalin, the appropriate reactive antigens may be masked or destroyed.

Histology reveals intercellular epidermal edema, with basal keratinocyte necrosis, and occasionally eosinophils and lymphocytes along the dermal–epidermal junction. Subepidermal bullae containing eosinophils with edema of the papillary dermis are also seen. An inflammatory infiltrate of eosinophils and lymphocytes invades the dermis in a perivascular distribution. Immunopathology of these specimens demonstrates the third component of complement in a linear band of fluorescence along the basement membrane zone between the epidermis and dermis.[44] Immunoglobulin G (IgG) deposits in the basement membrane in a minority of cases.

A circulating IgG1 autoantibody with complement-fixing capability, previously referred to as the *herpes gestationis factor* (HG factor), incites the pathology of pemphigoid gestationis.[44,45] Like bullous pemphigoid, the autoantigen involved in pemphigoid gestationis is a 180-kDa transmembrane collagenous protein found in basal keratinocytes in the anchoring complex of the hemidesmosome.[46] This protein, called bullous pemphigoid antigen 180 (BP180), mediates the attachment of these keratinocytes to the underlying basement membrane.[45] Sera from patients with pemphigoid gestationis recognize a major epitope on the C-terminal domain of BP180.[47] Antibodies generated to this domain produce subepidermal blistering when injected into neonatal mice, implicating the importance of this domain in pathogenesis.[48] Circulating IgG1 autoantibodies have not been isolated from the sera of all affected women and, when found, rarely exceed a titer of 1:16.[38] Antibodies to BP180 are detectable with indirect immuno-

fluorescence on epithelial substrates for up to 5 months after the skin lesions have resolved.[49]

Investigators hypothesize that the expression of major histocompatibility complex (MHC) proteins in the placenta triggers an allogenic reaction between maternal lymphocytes and the paternal-derived MHC molecules. This results in the formation of an IgG1 autoantibody against a placental antigen that cross-reacts with maternal cutaneous basement membrane and causes the skin lesions.[50]

Pemphigoid gestationis does not increase the risk of maternal mortality. Therefore, treatment is aimed at controlling pruritus, suppressing formation of new vesicles and bullae, and preventing secondary infection of skin lesions. Topical steroids and antihistamines may be used initially if the symptoms are mild. Most patients, however, will require systemic corticosteroid therapy. Prednisone dosages start at 40 to 60 mg/day. With improvement of clinical symptoms and no new bullae formation, the dose can then be tapered to 10 to 20 mg/day if clinical improvement is noted. Azathioprine, dapsone and, rarely, plasmapheresis have been employed in cases that fail to respond to corticosteroids.[38] For postpartum patients who experience a flare of pemphigoid gestationis requiring continued steroids, prednisone doses of 20 mg/day still allow safe breast-feeding. McKenzie et al. suggest taking the steroid 4 hours prior to breast-feeding to minimize levels in breast milk.[51]

Prior to the development of immunologic techniques that permitted an accurate diagnosis, pemphigoid gestationis was believed to have minimal adverse effects on the fetus.[52] In 1969, Kolodny reported no increase in preterm births, stillbirths, or abortions.[39] However, Lawley et al. subsequently reviewed 40 immunologically proven cases of pemphigoid gestationis and documented serious fetal morbidity and mortality: preterm births occurred at a rate of 22 percent and three women suffered stillbirths.[53] These authors suggested that high levels of circulating antibasement membrane antibody and peripheral eosinophilia caused the increased fetal risk. Shornick and Black described 74 patients with pemphigoid gestationis confirmed by immunofluorescence studies.[54] They found an increased frequency of fetal growth restriction and prematurity, but not stillbirth or miscarriage.[54] The recent most comprehensive study of pemphigoid gestationis in 87 patients with a total of 278 pregnancies concludes that the rate of spontaneous abortion and ectopic pregnancy in women with pemphigoid gestationis is similar to the normal population.[43] Although there is evidence in the literature for prematurity with pemphigoid gestationis, all current studies indicate no increased risk of miscarriage or stillbirth. Not enough evidence currently exists to determine whether systemic therapy for pemphigoid gestationis reduces the risk of fetal prematurity.

The HG factor, which is now known to be IgG1

autoantibody, crosses the placenta, binds with the basement membrane of the amnion,[55] and deposits in fetal skin.[38] Transient newborn pemphigoid gestationis has been reported in up to 5 percent of newborns.[43,54] Neonatal pemphigoid gestationis is usually mild and presents with erythematous papules or frank bullae.[56] Passive transfer of antibody probably incites this process, which generally resolves within a short period of time.[56,57]

Polymorphic Eruption of Pregnancy

In 1979, Lawley et al. described seven patients with a severe pruritic eruption that first occurred during the third trimester of pregnancy.[58] The authors felt this eruption, termed *pruritic urticarial papules and plaques of pregnancy* (PUPPP), could be differentiated by clinical and histologic findings from any other previously described pregnancy-associated skin condition. In the United Kingdom, the term *polymorphic eruption of pregnancy* (PEP) was coined by Holmes and Black[29] to better describe the variable skin features of this disease. The incidence of PEP ranges from 1 in 240 to 1 in 200 pregnancies.[31,58]

The etiology and pathogenesis are unknown.[59] No hormonal or autoimmune abnormalities had been found previously in women with PEP.[60,61] A more recent study shows decreased cortisol levels in women with PEP.[35] Increased skin tension resulting in skin damage may play a role in the etiology of PEP. The majority of women affected by PEP are primigravidae with prominent striae or have uterine distention with twins or hydramnios.[32,35] Skin biopsies of lesions from affected women giving birth to male neonates demonstrate detectable fetal male DNA.[62] Seventy percent of pregnant women with PEP give birth to male fetuses.[35] A provocative new hypothesis proposes that fetal male DNA acting as a skin antigen precipitates PEP.[62]

The lesions of PEP typically begin in the abdominal striae distensae of primigravidas during the third trimester (Fig. 39–3). Lesions initially present as 1- to 2-mm erythematous papules, surrounded by a narrow pale halo of vasoconstriction, that coalesce into urticarial plaques.[63] Small vesicles also can develop on the plaques. Lesions usually spread to the thighs and may involve the buttocks and arms. In contrast to pemphigoid gestationis, the periumbilical area is often spared in PEP. The face is also spared. Most patients experience intense pruritus that improves rapidly following delivery and resolves 1 to 2 weeks postpartum. The mean onset of skin lesions is 36 weeks' gestation; PEP rarely commences postpartum.[63] In general, PEP does not recur with subsequent pregnancies.

Histologic findings in this disorder most often demonstrate a superficial perivascular dermal infiltrate of lymphocytes and histiocytes and edema of the papillary

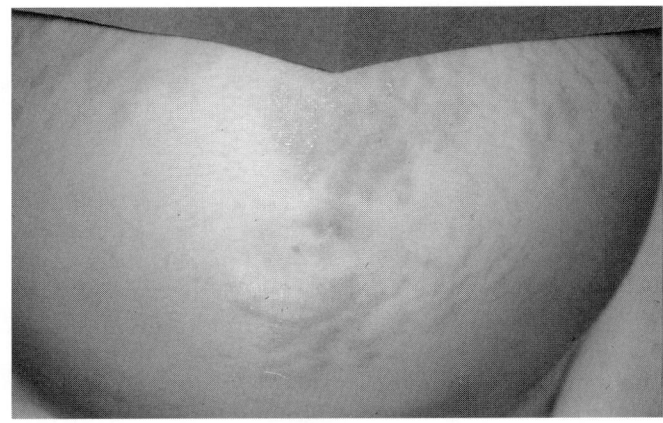

Figure 39–3. Polymorphic eruption of pregnancy (pruritic urticarial papules and plaques of pregnancy [PUPPP] syndrome). Erythematous urticarial plaques and small papules erupted on the abdomen of this patient pregnant with conjoined female twins during the third trimester.

dermis; the epidermis is normal.[58] Another histologic pattern shows spongiosis of the epidermis and marked dermal edema, with a dermal perivascular and interstitial infiltrate of lymphocytes and eosinophils.

In contrast to pemphigoid gestationis, PEP shows no specific immunofluorescence pattern from skin biopsies. Many patients' direct immunofluorescence demonstrate nonspecific immunoreactants and a small subset reveals granular deposits at the dermal–epidermal junction.[64,65] These histologic and immunofluorescence findings may be associated with many urticarial allergic responses and several viral exanthems.

As with pemphigoid gestationis, the main goal of therapy is symptomatic relief of the intense pruritus.[63] High-potency topical steroids generally effect a response in the vast majority of women, though some will require systemic steroids.[63] Antipruritic drugs such as hydroxyzine or diphenhydramine also may help. Fortunately, for these patients, delivery brings relief of both symptoms and lesions.[58] In some women, the severe pruritus will warrant induction of labor once fetal lung maturity is ensured.[66]

Prurigo Gestationis and Papular Dermatitis

Prurigo gestationis consists of pruritic excoriated papules usually limited to the extensor surfaces of the extremities. The disease occurs in 1 per 50 to 200 pregnancies.[67,68] Lesions generally appear during the second half of gestation as small, symmetrically distributed, 1- to 2-mm papules. Vesicle or bullae formation does not occur. The condition usually resolves following delivery. Maternal and fetal health is not impacted, and recurrence during subsequent gestations is uncommon.

Papular dermatitis likely represents a more severe and widespread form of prurigo gestationis. In the past, papular dermatitis was considered a separate skin disorder. Spangler et al. originally reported this disorder in association with increased urinary chorionic gonadotropin, decreased plasma hydrocortisone levels, and increased fetal risk.[69] However, because of inadequate assessment of fetal risk, absence of adequate controls of the biochemical findings, and lack of further reports substantiating this specific skin rash, most current authors do not recognize this as a separate entity with an impact on fetal health.[30–33]

The diagnosis of prurigo gestationis is made by the clinical appearance of a primary papular eruption in a woman without laboratory evidence of cholestasis of pregnancy. The histologic findings show a nonspecific dermal perivascular lymphohistiocytic infiltrate. The pruritus responds to mid- to high-strength topical steroids and oral antipruritics. Systemic corticosteroid therapy is rarely necessary for the treatment of prurigo gestationis.

Pruritic Folliculitis of Pregnancy

In 1981, Zoberman and Farmer first described *pruritic folliculitis of pregnancy* in six women who presented with a generalized erythematous, hair follicle–centered rash.[70] Roger et al. found the incidence of this skin disorder to be 1 per 3,000 pregnancies.[31] The eruption consists of numerous 2- to 4-mm follicular papules or pustules distributed on the shoulders, upper back, arms, chest, and abdomen, and clinically resembles acne. Most women present in the third trimester. Histopathologic findings show acute folliculitis with a neutrophilic infiltrate of the follicle and the surrounding dermis.[70] Cultures are usually sterile.

The exact etiology is unknown, but could be hormonally induced, since the lesions disappear within 2 to 3 weeks following delivery and look similar to corticosteroid-, androgen-, and progesterone-related acneiform eruptions.[32] A recent study of pregnant patients with pruritic neutrophilic folliculitis did not show any changes in androgen levels compared to controls.[71] No microorganism appears to cause the eruption.

The disorder does not cause significant maternal morbidity. In one study, however, fetal birth weight was significantly reduced compared to controls.[71] Treatment is similar to that of mild acne, using 10 percent benzoyl peroxide and oral antihistamines if severe pruritus exists.

Impetigo Herpetiformis

Though clinically similar to pustular psoriasis, *impetigo herpetiformis* typically occurs in women without a previous personal or family history of psoriasis. The condition is rare, with less than 100 pregnancies reported.[72] Authors disagree whether impetigo herpetiformis stands as a distinct entity caused by pregnancy or is a form of pustular psoriasis triggered by pregnancy.[73] A reported patient who developed impetigo herpetiformis 1 day postpartum[74] and a pregnant patient with both psoriatic pustules and typical psoriatic plaques[75] emphasize the relationship of this disorder to pustular psoriasis. Also, both pustular psoriasis and impetigo herpetiformis share the common feature of decreased levels of skin-derived antileukoproteinase.[77]

Impetigo herpetiformis begins in the second half of gestation, with groups of painful sterile pustules on an erythematous base distributed on the inner thighs and groin. The pustules coalesce and spread to the trunk and extremities. Lesions may become secondarily infected. Unlike many of the dermatoses of pregnancy, lesions do not itch. Mucous membranes are frequently affected. Histologically, impetigo herpetiformis demonstrates spongiform intraepidermal and subcorneal pustules. A dense lymphocytic infiltrate surrounds dermal blood vessels. The histopathologic features cannot be differentiated from pustular psoriasis.[73] Histologically, impetigo herpetiformis is distinguishable from impetigo, herpes, and pemphigoid gestationis.

Impetigo herpetiformis may incite systemic symptoms, including fever, chills, arthralgias, vomiting, diarrhea, and lymphadenopathy.[73] Prostration with septicemia, and cardiac and renal failure have rarely occurred in severe cases. Hypocalcemia and hyperphosphatemia are not uncommon in this setting and have led investigators to postulate that hypoparathyroidism is associated with this disorder.

Systemic corticosteroids are the first-line treatment for impetigo herpetiformis. Prednisone, or an equivalent steroid, in doses up to 60 mg/day, may be required. Once the disease responds, a slow taper is recommended, as too rapid a taper can cause disease rebound. Antibiotics are used for secondary infection when indicated. Some authors report only a moderate response to corticosteroid treatment.[73] However, other medications used for pustular psoriasis, including methotrexate, retinoids, and hydroxyurea, are contraindicated in pregnancy. Cyclosporin A has been used successfully and safely in one pregnant patient with psoriasis.[77]

The disease resolves following delivery, though it can recur in subsequent pregnancies. One reported patient had subsequent recurrences during each of eight pregnancies.[78] Increased fetal morbidity has been observed in a few cases. Authors have recommended close fetal surveillance and consideration of elective delivery after fetal lung maturity has been ensured.[78]

Key Points

➤ Pregnancy is associated with several physiologic changes of the skin that may concern the pregnant woman. These include hyperpigmentation, mild hirsutism, hair loss, striae distensae, and vascular changes.

➤ During pregnancy, some nevi may increase in size, and new nevi may develop. This may necessitate the need to perform a biopsy if one suspects melanoma.

➤ Pruritus is a common symptom in pregnancy and usually resolves postpartum; infrequently, it is due to a serious dermatologic disease. In addition to evaluating the pregnant woman for dermatologic diseases that occur unassociated with pregnancy, the health care provider must evaluate for pregnancy-specific dermatologic diseases.

➤ The most common pregnancy-specific causes of pruritic rashes are polymorphic eruption of pregnancy, prurigo gestationis, and cholestasis of pregnancy.

➤ Rare dermatologic conditions associated with pregnancy are pemphigoid gestationis, pruritic folliculitis of pregnancy, and impetigo herpetiformis.

➤ The only dermatologic diseases of pregnancy that have been shown to cause fetal morbidity are pemphigoid gestationis and impetigo herpetiformis. Antepartum testing for fetal well-being should be utilized in these women. Transient newborn pemphigoid gestationis has also been reported.

➤ Pemphigoid gestationis can be difficult to clinically distinguish from polymorphic eruption of pregnancy. Skin biopsies with immunofluorescence studies differentiates the two disorders.

➤ The treatment for pemphigoid gestationis is aimed at controlling symptoms. Most patients will require systemic corticosteroid therapy.

➤ Topical steroid therapy generally induces a response in the vast majority of women with polymorphic eruption of pregnancy, but some will require systemic steroids. The main goal of therapy is symptomatic relief of the intense pruritus. In some women, the pruritus will be significant enough to warrant induction of labor once fetal lung maturity is ensured.

REFERENCES

1. Wong RC, Ellis CN: Physiologic skin changes in pregnancy. J Am Acad Dermatol 10:929, 1984.
2. Muzaffar F, Hussain I, Haroon TS: Physiologic skin changes during pregnancy: a study of 140 cases. Int J Dermatol 37:429, 1998.
3. Sanchez NP, Pathak MA, Sato S, et al: Melasma: a clinical, light microscopic, ultrastructural, and immunofluorescence study. J Am Acad Dermatol 4:698, 1981.
4. Winston GB, Lewis CW: Dermatoses of pregnancy. J Am Acad Dermatol 6:977, 1982.
5. Griffiths CEM, Finkel LJ, Ditre CM, et al: Topical tretinoin (retinoic acid) improves melasma. A vehicle-controlled clinical trial. Br J Dermatol 129:415, 1993.
6. Murray JC: Pregnancy and the skin. Dermatol Clin 8:327, 1990.
7. Moy LS, Murad H, Moy RL: Glycolic acid peels for the treatment of wrinkles and photoaging. J Dermatol Surg Oncol 19:243, 1993.
8. Sanchez JL, Figueroa LD, Rodriguez E: Behavior of melanocytic nevi during pregnancy. Am J Dermatopathol 6:89, 1984.
9. Foucar E, Bentley TJ, Laube DW, et al: A histopathologic evaluation of nevocellular nevi in pregnancy. Arch Dermatol 121:350, 1985.
10. Pennoyer JW, Grin CM, Driscoll MS, et al: Changes in size of melanocytic nevi during pregnancy. J Am Acad Dermatol 36:378, 1999.
11. Ellis DL: Pregnancy and sex steroid hormone effects on nevi of patients with the dysplastic nevus syndrome. J Am Acad Dermatol 25:467, 1991.
12. Mackie RM, Bufalino R, Morabito A, et al: Lack of effect of pregnancy on outcome of melanoma. Lancet 337:653, 1991.
13. Driscoll MS, Grin-Jorgensen CM, Grant-Kels JM: Does pregnancy influence the prognosis of malignant melanoma? J Am Acad Dermatol 29:619, 1993.
14. Smith MA, Fine JA, Barnhill RL, et al: Hormonal and reproductive influences and risk of melanoma in women. Int J Epidemiol 27:751, 1998.
15. Squatrito RC, Harlow SP: Melanoma complicating pregnancy. Obstet Gynecol Clin North Am 25:407, 1998.
16. Duncan LM, Travers RL, Koerner FC, et al: Estrogen and progesterone receptor analysis in pregnancy-associated melanoma: absence of immunohistochemically detectable hormone receptors. Hum Pathol 25:36, 1994.
17. Reintgen DS, McCarty KS, Vollmer R, et al: Malignant melanoma and pregnancy. Cancer 55:1340, 1985.
18. McManamny DS, Moss ALH, Pocock PV, et al: Melanoma and pregnancy: a long-term follow-up. Br J Obstet Gynaecol 96:1419, 1989.
19. Wong JH, Sterns EE, Kopald KH, et al: Prognostic significance of pregnancy in stage I melanoma. Arch Surg 124:1227, 1989.
20. Slinguff CL Jr, Reintgen DS, Vollmer RT, et al: Malignant melanoma arising during pregnancy: a study of 100 patients. Ann Surg 211:552, 1990.
21. Headington JT: Telogen effluvium: new concepts and review. Arch Dermatol 129:556, 1993.
22. Watson RE, Parry EJ, Humphries JD, et al: Fibrillin microfibrils are reduced in skin exhibiting striae distensae. Br J Dermatol 138:931, 1998.
23. Kang S: Topical tretinoin therapy for management of early striae. J Am Acad Dermatol 38:S90, 1998.

24. Alster TS: Laser treatment of hypertrophic scars, keloids, and striae. Dermatol Clin 15:419, 1997.

25. Ash K, Lord J, Zukowski M, McDaniel DH: Comparison of topical therapy for striae alba (20 percent glycolic acid/0.05 percent tretinoin versus 20 percent glycolic acid/10 percent L-ascorbic acid). Dermatol Surg 24:849, 1998.

26. Parmley T, O'Brien TJ: Skin changes during pregnancy. Clin Obstet Gynecol 33:713, 1990.

27. Mattison MD: Transdermal drug absorption during pregnancy. Clin Obstet Gynecol 33:718, 1990.

28. Black MM, Stephens CJM: The specific dermatoses of pregnancy: the British perspective. Adv Dermatol 7:105, 1992.

29. Holmes RC, Black MM: The specific dermatoses of pregnancy: a reappraisal with specific emphasis on a proposed simplified clinical classification. Clin Exp Dermatol 7:65, 1982.

30. Vaughan Jones SA, Black MM: Pregnancy dermatoses. J Am Acad Dermatol 40:233, 1999.

31. Roger D, Vaillant L, Fignon A, et al: Specific pruritus diseases of pregnancy, a prospective study of 3,192 pregnant women. Arch Dermatol 130:734, 1994.

32. Holmes RC, Black MM: The specific dermatoses of pregnancy. J Am Acad Dermatol 8:405, 1983.

33. Borradori L, Saurat J: Specific dermatoses of pregnancy, toward a comprehensive view? Arch Dermatol 130:778, 1994.

34. Dacus JV: Pruritus in pregnancy. Clin Obstet Gynecol 33:738, 1990.

35. Vaughan Jones SA, Hern S, Nelson-Piercy C, et al: A prospective study of 200 women with dermatoses of pregnancy correlating clinical findings with hormonal and immunopathological profiles. Br J Dermatol 141:71, 1999.

36. Bacq Y: Intrahepatic cholestasis of pregnancy. Clin Liver Dis 3:1, 1999.

37. Heikkinen J: Serum bile acids in the early diagnosis of intrahepatic cholestasis of pregnancy. Obstet Gynecol 61:581, 1983.

38. Shornick JK: Herpes gestationis. J Am Acad Dermatol 17:539, 1987.

39. Kolodny R: Herpes gestationis: a new assessment of incidence, diagnosis, and fetal prognosis. Am J Obstet Gynecol 104:39, 1969.

40. Zurn A, Celebi CR, Bernard P, et al: A prospective immunofluorescence study of 111 cases of pruritic dermatosis of pregnancy: IgM anti-basement membrane zone antibodies as a novel finding. Br J Dermatol 126:474, 1992.

41. Holmes RC, Black MM: Herpes gestationis. Dermatol Clin 1:195, 1987.

42. Garcia-Gonzalez E, Castro-Llamas J, Karchmer S, et al: Class II major histocompatibility complex typing across the ethnic barrier in pemphigoid gestationis. A study in Mexicans. Int J Dermatol 38:46, 1999.

43. Jenkins RE, Hern S, Black MM: Clinical features and management of 87 patients with pemphigoid gestationis. Clin Exp Dermatol 124:255, 1999.

44. Jordon ER, Heine KG, Tappeiner G, et al: The immunopathology of herpes gestationis: immunofluorescence studies and characterization of "HG factor." J Clin Invest 57:1426, 1976.

45. Morrison LH, Labib RS, Zone JJ, et al: Herpes gestationis autoantibodies recognize a 180-kD human epidermal antigen. J Clin Invest 81:2023, 1988.

46. Mutasim DF, Takahashi Y, Labib RS, et al: A pool of bullous pemphigoid antigen(s) is intracellular and associated with the basal cell cytoskeleton-hemidesomosome complex. J Invest Dermatol 84:47, 1985.

47. Guidice GJ, Emery DJ, Zelickson BD, et al: Bullous pemphigoid and herpes gestationis autoantibodies recognize a common non-collagenous site on the BP 180 ectodomain. J Immunol 151:5742, 1993.

48. Liu Z, Diaz LA, Swartz SJ, et al: Molecular mapping of pathogenically relevant BP180 epitope associated with experimentally induced murine bullous pemphigoid. J Immunol 155:5449, 1995.

49. Satoh S, Seishima M, Sawada Y, et al: The time course of the change in antibody titres in herpes gestationis. Br J Dermatol 140:119, 1999.

50. Kelly SE, Black MM, Fleming S: Hypothesis: pemphigoid gestationis: a unique mechanism of initiation of an autoimmune response by MHC class II molecules? J Pathol 158:81, 1989.

51. McKenzie SA, Selley JA, Agnew JE: Secretion of prednisolone into breast milk. Arch Dis Child 50:894, 1975.

52. Carruthers JA: Herpes gestationis: clinical features of immunologically proven cases. Am J Obstet Gynecol 131:865, 1978.

53. Lawley TJ, Stingl G, Katz SI: Fetal and maternal risk factors in herpes gestationis. Arch Dermatol 114:552, 1978.

54. Shornick JK, Black MM: Fetal risks in herpes gestationis. J Am Acad Dermatol 26:63, 1992.

55. Ortonne JP, Hsi BL, Verrando P, et al: Herpes gestationis factor reacts with amniotic epithelial basement membrane. Br J Dermatol 117:147, 1987.

56. Chorzelski TP, Jablonska S, Beutner EH, et al: Herpes gestationis with identical lesions in the newborn: passive transfer of disease? Arch Dermatol 112:129, 1976.

57. Bonifazi E, Meneghini CL: Herpes gestationis with transient bullous lesions in the newborn. Pediatr Dermatol 34:715, 1984.

58. Lawley TJ, Hertz KC, Wade TR, et al: Pruritic urticarial papules and plaques of pregnancy. JAMA 241:1696, 1979.

59. Alcalay J, Wolf JE: Pruritic urticarial papules and plaques of pregnancy: the enigma and the confusion. J Am Acad of Dermatol 19:1115, 1988.

60. Alcalay J, Ingber A, Kafri B, et al: Hormonal evaluation and autoimmune background in pruritic urticarial papules and plaques of pregnancy. Am J Obstet Gynecol 158:417, 1988.

61. Spangler AS, Emerson K: Estrogen levels and estrogen therapy in papular dermatitis of pregnancy. Am J Obstet Gynecol 110:435, 1971.

62. Aractingi S, Berkane N, Bertheau PH, et al: Fetal DNA in skin of polymorphic eruptions of pregnancy. Lancet 352:1898, 1998.

63. Yancey KB, Hall RP, Lawley TJ: Pruritic urticarial papules and plaques of pregnancy. Clinical experience in 25 patients. J Am Acad Dermatol 10:473, 1984.

64. Goodall J: Immunofluorescence biopsy for pruritic urticarial papules and plaques of pregnancy. J Am Acad Dermatol 22:322, 1990.

65. Aronson I, Bond S, Fiedler VC, et al: Pruritic urticarial papules and plaques of pregnancy: clinical and immunopathologic observations in 57 patients. J Am Acad Dermatol 39:933, 1998.

66. Beltrani VP, Beltrani VS: Pruritic urticarial papules and plaques of pregnancy: a severe case requiring early delivery for relief of symptoms. J Am Acad Dermatol 26:266, 1992.

67. Ware M, Swinscow TDV, Thwaites JG: Pregnancy prurigo. BMJ 1:397, 1969.

68. Holmes RC, Black MM, Dann J, et al: A comparative study of toxic erythema of pregnancy and herpes gestationis. Br J Dermatol 106:499, 1982.

69. Spangler AS, Reddy W, Bardawil WA: Papular dermatitis of pregnancy: a new clinical entity? JAMA 181:577, 1962.

70. Zoberman E, Farmer ER: Pruritic folliculitis of pregnancy. Arch Dermatol 117:20, 1981.

71. Vaughan Jones SA, Hern S, Black MM: Neutrophil folliculitis and serum androgen levels. Clin Exp Dermatol 24:392, 1999.

72. Ott F, Krakowski A, Tur E, et al: Impetigo herpetiformis with lower serum level of vitamin D and its diminished intestinal absorption. Dermatologica 164:360, 1982.

73. Lotem M, Katzenelson V, Rotem A, et al: Impetigo herpetiformis: a variant of pustular psoriasis or a separate entity. J Am Acad Dermatol 20:338, 1989.

74. Katsambas A, Stavropoulos PG, Katsiboulas V, et al: Impetigo herpetiformis during the puerperium. Dermatology 198:400, 1998.

75. Breier-Maly J, Ortel B, Breier F, et al: Generalized pustular psoriasis of pregnancy (impetigo herpetiformis). Dermatology 198:61, 1999.

76. Kuijpers AL, Schalkwijk J, Rulo HF, et al: Extremely low levels of epidermal skin-derived antileucoproteinase/elafin in a patient with impetigo herpetiformis. Br J Dermatol 137:123, 1997.

77. Wright S, Glover M, Baker H: Psoriasis, cyclosporin, and pregnancy. Arch Dermatol 127:426, 1991.

78. Oumeish OY, Farraj SE, Bataineh A: Some aspects of impetigo herpetiformis. Arch Dermatol 118:103, 1982.

Chapter 40

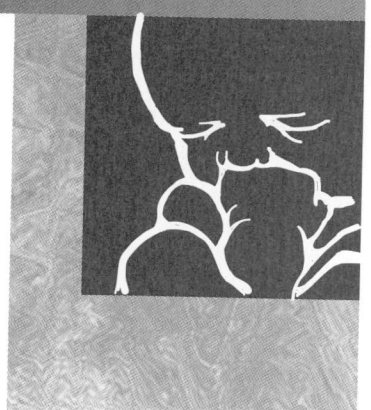

Maternal and Perinatal Infection

PATRICK DUFF

Infection is the single most common complication encountered by the obstetrician. Some infections such as puerperal endometritis, candidiasis, trichomoniasis, and lower urinary tract infection are of principal concern to the mother and pose little or no risk to the fetus or neonate. Others, such as rubella, cytomegalovirus infection, and parvovirus infection cause minimal maternal morbidity but devastating fetal injury. Still others, for example, chorioamnionitis, gonorrhea, syphilis, toxoplasmosis, pyelonephritis, group B streptococcal infection, rubeola, and human immunodeficiency virus (HIV) infection, may cause serious morbidity, and even mortality, for both the mother, fetus, and/or neonate.

The purpose of this chapter is to review in detail the major maternal and perinatal infections that the obstetrician confronts in clinical practice. The first portion of the chapter focuses primarily on bacterial infections of the lower and upper genital tract. The second portion considers the infections that pose special risks to the fetus. The principal features of these infections are summarized in Tables 40–1 and 40–2.

VAGINAL INFECTIONS

Bacterial Vaginosis

Epidemiology

Bacterial vaginosis (BV) is responsible for approximately 45 percent of cases of vaginitis. It is a polymicrobial infection, and the predominant pathogens are anaerobes, *Gardnerella vaginalis*, *Mobiluncus* species, and genital mycoplasmas.[1] BV usually results from disturbances in the normal vaginal ecosystem caused by hormonal changes, pregnancy, or antibiotic administra-

tion. The principal feature of this alteration in vaginal flora is a marked decrease in the lactobacilli species that produce lactic acid and a corresponding increase in anaerobic organisms. In some instances, BV can result from sexual contact with an infected partner. In contrast to trichomoniasis and candidiasis, symptomatic BV in pregnancy has been associated with several serious maternal complications, including preterm labor, preterm premature rupture of membranes, chorioamnionitis, and puerperal endometritis.[2–4]

Diagnosis

The most prominent clinical manifestation of BV is a thin, gray, homogeneous, malodorous vaginal discharge. The odor is often accentuated after intercourse. Vulvar or vaginal pruritus is uncommon, and the vaginal pH is characteristically greater than 4.5. When vaginal secretions are mixed with several drops of a 10 percent potassium hydroxide (KOH) solution, a pungent fishy odor is produced ("whiff test" or amine test). On microscopic examination of a saline preparation, the normal lactobacilli flora is largely replaced by multiple small bacilli and cocci. Motile, comma-shaped *Mobiluncus* species, and clue cells are present (Fig. 40–1). Culture of vaginal secretions is not indicated in routine clinical practice.[1]

Treatment

Symptomatic patients with BV should be treated.[5–7] In addition, asymptomatic patients who are at increased risk of preterm delivery (e.g., history of prior preterm birth) also should be screened for BV and treated if positive. Several investigations have demonstrated a decreased rate of preterm delivery and decreased frequency of maternal and neonatal infection when such

Table 40–1. ETIOLOGY, DIAGNOSIS, AND MANAGEMENT OF MAJOR OBSTETRIC INFECTIONS

Condition	Microbiology	Confirmatory Diagnostic Test	Treatment*
Vaginal infection			
Bacterial vaginosis	*Gardnerella vaginalis, Mobiluncus* species, anaerobes, mycoplasmas	Saline preparation Vaginal pH Amine test	Topical or oral clindamycin or metronidazole
Candidiasis	*Candida albicans, C. tropicalis, C. glabrata*	KOH preparation	Topical antifungal cream
Trichomoniasis	*Trichomonas vaginalis*	Saline preparation	Oral metronidazole
Endocervical infection			
Gonorrhea	*Neisseria gonorrhoeae*	Endocervical culture	Oral cefixime or intramuscular ceftriaxone
Chlamydia	*Chlamydia trachomatis*	Endocervical culture Antigen detection	Oral erythromycin, azithromycin, or amoxicillin
Urinary tract infection			
Urethritis	*N. gonorrhoeae*	Culture of urethral discharge	Oral cefixime or intramuscular ceftriaxone
	C. trachomatis	Culture of urethral discharge or antigen detection	Oral erythromycin, azithromycin, or amoxicillin
Asymptomatic bacteriuria or cystitis	*E. coli, Klebsiella pneumoniae, Proteus* species	Urinalysis Culture	Sulfisoxazole, nitrofurantoin monohydrate macrocrystals, trimethoprim-sulfamethoxazole DS
Pyelonephritis	As above	As above	Intravenous cefazolin and/or gentamicin or aztreonam
Chorioamnionitis	Group B streptococci, coliforms, anaerobes	Clinical examination Amniotic fluid leukocyte esterase, glucose, Gram's stain, and culture	Intravenous penicillin or ampicillin plus gentamicin; add clindamycin or metronidazole if cesarean delivery is required
Puerperal endometritis	Group B streptococci, coliforms, anaerobes	Clinical examination	Intravenous clindamycin plus gentamicin or extended spectrum cephalosporin or penicillin or carbapenem

* See text for detailed prescribing information.

patients received therapy.[8] However, the value of *routine* screening of asymptomatic, low-risk patients has *not* been confirmed.

The drug of choice for treating BV in pregnancy is oral metronidazole (250 mg three times daily for 7 days). For patients who are unable to tolerate metronidazole, clindamycin (300 mg orally [PO] twice daily for 7 days) can be used. Although the topical preparations of metronidazole and clindamycin are effective in eradicating BV from the vagina, they are not of proven value in preventing adverse pregnancy complications such as preterm delivery.[5–8]

Candidiasis

Epidemiology

Candidiasis is responsible for approximately 25 to 30 percent of all cases of vaginitis. The three principal candida species that cause symptomatic infection are, in descending order of frequency, *C. albicans, C. tropicalis,* and *C. glabrata.*[9] Candidiasis is not usually a sexually transmitted disease. Yeast are part of the nor-

mal vaginal flora in many women, and symptoms develop only when overgrowth of these organisms occurs. Several conditions predispose to symptomatic moniliasis, including recent antibiotic or corticosteroid therapy, diabetes, use of oral contraceptives, pregnancy, and immunodeficiency states. Although isolated cases of chorioamnionitis due to candida species have been reported, serious systemic infections are uncommon unless the patient is receiving hyperalimentation or is immunocompromised.

Diagnosis

Infected patients usually report vaginal and vulvar pruritus and a white, curd-like vaginal discharge. The vaginal pH is typically less than 4.5. The vaginal mucosa and vulva may be erythematous and edematous, and punctate, erythematous satellite lesions may be present on the lateral aspect of the vulva and medial aspect of the thighs.[9]

The simplest test for confirmation of this diagnosis is microscopic examination of a KOH preparation for hyphae, pseudohyphae, and budding yeast. Cultures are

Table 40-2. SUMMARY OF ETIOLOGY, DIAGNOSIS, AND MANAGEMENT OF MAJOR PERINATAL INFECTIONS

Condition	Complications Maternal	Complications Fetal/Neonatal	Diagnosis Maternal	Diagnosis Fetal/Neonatal	Management* Maternal	Management* Fetal/Neonatal
CMV	Chorioretinitis, pneumonia in immunocompromised patient	Congenital infection	Detection of antibody	Amniocentesis—culture amniotic fluid Ultrasound	Ganciclovir for severe infection	Consider pregnancy termination when mother has primary infection
Group B streptococci	UTI Chorioamnionitis Endometritis Wound infection Preterm labor PROM	Sepsis Pneumonia Meningitis	Culture	Culture	Intrapartum antibiotic prophylaxis	Treatment with ampicillin or penicillin
Hepatitis A	Rare	None	Detection of antibody	N/A	Prevention—hepatitis A vaccine	Administer immune globulin to neonate if mother acutely infected at delivery
B	Chronic liver disease	Neonatal infection	Detection of surface antigen	N/A	Supportive care Prevention—HBIG + HBV for susceptible household contacts	HBIG + HBV immediately after delivery
C	Chronic liver disease	Neonatal infection	Detection of antibody	N/A	Supportive care Interferon	Nonimmunoprophylaxis available
D	Chronic liver disease	Neonatal infection	Detection of antigen and antibody	N/A	Supportive care	HBIG + HBV immediately after delivery
E	Increased mortality	None	Detection of antibody	N/A	Supportive care	None
Herpes simplex	Disseminated infection in immunocompromised patient	Neonatal infection	Clinical examination, culture, PCR	Clinical examination, culture	Acyclovir, valacyclovir, or famciclovir for severe primary infection	Cesarean delivery when mother has overt infection
HIV infection	Opportunistic infection, malignancy	Congenital or perinatal infection	Detection of antibody or antigen	Same	Combination chemotherapy	Combination chemotherapy for prevention of vertical transmission
Parvovirus infection	Rare	Anemia hydrops	Detection of antibody	Ultrasound	Supportive care	Intrauterine transfusion for severe anemia
Rubella	Rare	Congenital infection	Detection of antibody	Ultrasound	Prevention—vaccination prior to pregnancy Supportive care	Pregnancy termination for affected fetus
Rubeola	Otitis media, pneumonia, encephalitis	Abortion, preterm delivery	Detection of antibody	N/A	Prevention—vaccination prior to pregnancy Supportive care	N/A
Syphilis	Aortitis Neurosyphilis	Congenital infection	Darkfield examination or serology	Ultrasound	Penicillin	Penicillin
Toxoplasmosis	Chorioretinitis, CNS infection	Congenital infection	Detection of antibody	Amniocentesis—detection of toxoplasma DNA by nucleic acid probe	Sulfadiazine Pyrimethamine Spiramycin	Treatment of mother prior to delivery reduces risk of fetal infection
Varicella	Pneumonia Encephalitis	Congenital infection	Clinical examination, detection of antibody	Ultrasound	VZIG, acyclovir for prophylaxis or treatment	VZIG, acyclovir for prophylaxis or treatment of neonate

UTI, urinary tract infection; CMV, cytomegalovirus; PROM, premature rupture of membranes; HBIG, hepatitis B immune globulin; HBV, hepatitis B vaccine; PCR, polymerase chain reaction; HIV, human immunodeficiency virus; CNS, central nervous system; DNA, deoxyribo-nucleic acid; VZIG, varicella zoster immune globulin.
* See text for detailed discussion of patient management.

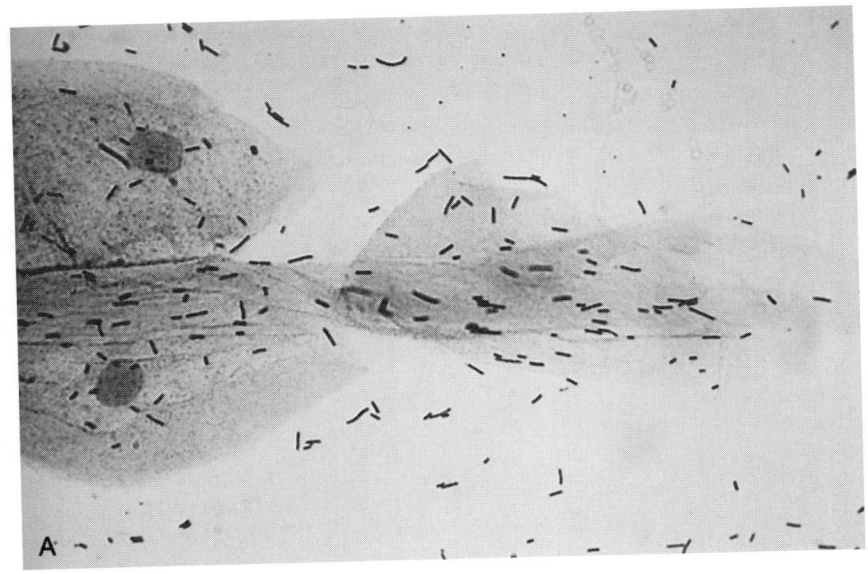

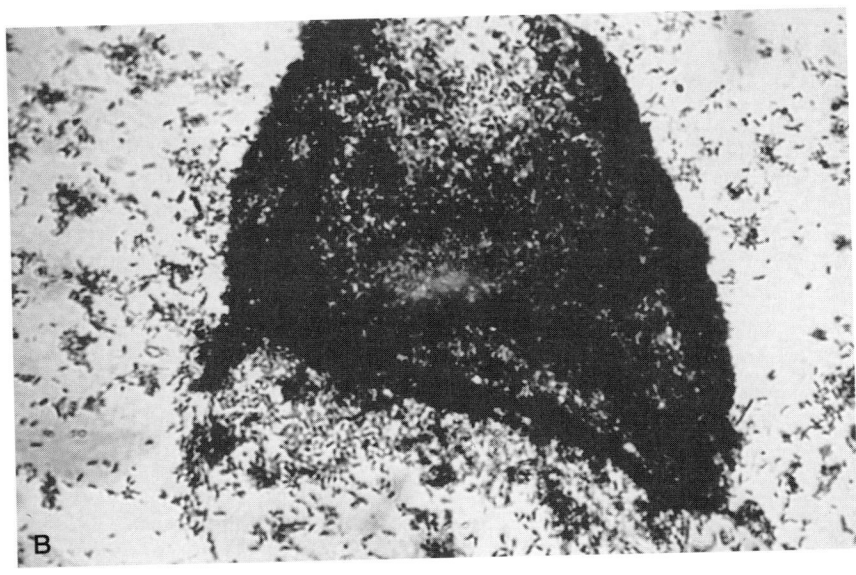

Figure 40–1. *A,* Gram's stain of normal vaginal secretions. Note the predominance of lactobacilli and the clear borders of the vaginal epithelial cells. *B,* Gram's stain of vaginal secretions in a patient with BV. Note the absence of lactobacilli, the abundance of other cocci and bacilli, and the epithelial cell studded with bacteria (clue cell). (Courtesy of Sharon L. Hillier, Ph.D., University of Washington.)

indicated only for patients who have persistent clinical findings and a negative microscopic examination and for those with recurrent infections who have had a poor response to treatment. Sabouraud's agar is the optimal medium for culture and may permit identification of a species of candida with an unusual pattern of sensitivity to antimicrobial compounds.

Treatment

For uncomplicated candida infections, topical therapy for 3 to 7 days with agents such as miconazole, terconazole, clotrimazole, and butoconazole is usually highly effective. Treatment of women with persistent or recurrent infection is more problematic. These patients should be counseled about preventive measures such as avoidance of bubble baths, use of cotton undergar-

ments, and close attention to perineal hygiene.[9,10] In particularly refractory cases, administration of systemic antimicrobials such as ketoconazole or fluconazole should be considered because of their greater activity against reservoirs of yeast in the gastrointestinal tract.[11–13] Neither drug has been studied extensively in pregnancy. However, fluconazole appears to have a more favorable toxicity profile. The appropriate oral dose of this compound for treatment of a refractory infection is 150 mg in a single dose.

Trichomoniasis

Epidemiology

Trichomoniasis is a sexually transmitted disease caused by the protozoan *Trichomonas vaginalis*. *Trichomonas* is responsible for approximately 25 percent of cases of vaginitis. It is an extremely contagious infection; virtually 100 percent of women who have sexual contact with an infected partner contract the disease.[1] Trichomoniasis is not commonly associated with serious maternal or neonatal complications.

Diagnosis

The usual symptoms of trichomoniasis are vaginal pruritus, superficial dyspareunia, frequency, dysuria, and a malodorous, yellow-green, frothy vaginal discharge. On physical examination, the vaginal mucosa is typically erythematous, and punctate hemorrhages may be present on the cervix ("strawberry cervix"). The pH of the vagina is usually in the range of 5 to 7.[1]

The most useful test for rapid confirmation of infection is direct visualization of the flagellated organisms in a saline preparation (wet mount). The sensitivity of this test is 60 to 80 percent, depending on the size of the inoculum and the thoroughness with which the slide is inspected. The Papanicolaou smear has similar sensitivity, but it is not as readily available to the office-based practitioner. T. vaginalis can be cultured on specialized media such as Hollander's medium or Feinberg-Whittington medium. However, culture is a more expensive and time consuming diagnostic test and, accordingly, it is rarely indicated in clinical practice.[1]

Treatment

Metronidazole is the only antibiotic with uniform activity against T. vaginalis. Treatment efficacy is 95 percent or higher if the patient is compliant and her sexual partner is treated concurrently. Absolute resistance of the organism to metronidazole is uncommon, and relative resistance can usually be overcome by administering the drug in higher doses for longer periods of time.[2,3]

Metronidazole can be given in three oral dosage regimens: a single dose of 2 g; 250 mg three times daily for 7 days, or 500 mg twice daily for 7 days. The former dosage schedule improves compliance and reduces expense.[8] In laboratory models, metronidazole has been associated with both mutagenicity and carcinogenicity. Although these effects have not been documented in humans (Food and Drug Administration [FDA] pregnancy category B), use of the drug in the first trimester of pregnancy raises theoretical concerns.[4,16] Accordingly, if the patient is relatively asymptomatic, treatment should be delayed until organogenesis is complete.

ENDOCERVICAL INFECTIONS

Chlamydia

Epidemiology

Chlamydia trachomatis is the most common sexually transmitted pathogen in Western nations. The organism can cause localized infection of the urethra, endocervix, and rectum. It also is the most common cause of perihepatitis (Fitz-Hugh–Curtis syndrome) and an occasional cause of pneumonia. In addition, in the developing nations of the world, C. trachomatis is responsible for inclusion conjunctivitis, a leading cause of blindness. Infants delivered to infected women may develop either conjunctivitis and/or pneumonia. The former complication occurs in up to 50 percent of infants delivered to infected mothers; the latter affects 3 to 18 percent of infants.[17,18]

Diagnosis and Clinical Management

C. trachomatis may be grown in tissue culture. However, this methodology is relatively expensive and time consuming. Fortunately, less expensive, rapid identification tests such as nucleic acid probes are sufficiently sensitive to justify their clinical use for identification of chlamydia infection. In high-risk populations, the sensitivity and specificity of the newest tests exceed 90 percent.[17,19]

Although tetracycline and doxycycline have the greatest activity against C. trachomatis, these drugs should not be used in pregnancy because of their harmful effects on fetal teeth. For several years, erythromycin had been considered the drug of choice for treatment of chlamydia infection in pregnancy. However, many pregnant patients fail to complete the full course of erythromycin because of gastrointestinal side effects.[20] Therefore, the preferred agent now is azithromycin, 1,000 mg (powder formulation) PO in a single dose.[21] Amoxicillin (500 mg PO three times a day for 7 days) also is an acceptable alternative.[22]

In view of the fact that 5 to 10 percent of patients do not respond to the initial course of treatment, a test of cure should be performed approximately 2 weeks after therapy is completed. In addition, infected patients should be screened for other sexually transmitted diseases such as gonorrhea, syphilis, hepatitis B, and human immunodeficiency virus infection. Neonates delivered to infected mothers should receive prophylaxis with tetracycline or erythromycin ophthalmic preparations and observed for evidence of an ensuing respiratory tract infection.

Gonorrhea

Epidemiology

Gonorrhea is caused by the gram-negative, intracellular diplococcus, *Neisseria gonorrhoeae*. The infection is transmitted primarily by sexual contact. Gonorrhea also may be transmitted perinatally from mother to infant and cause serious ophthalmic injury (*ophthalmia neonatorum*).

In pregnant women, gonorrhea may be manifested as an asymptomatic to mildly symptomatic localized infection of the urethra, endocervix, and/or rectum. Local infection may increase the risk of preterm labor and preterm premature rupture of membranes and predispose to intrapartum and postpartum infection. Gonorrhea also may present as a moderately severe pharyngitis or as a disseminated infection.[17] The most common manifestation of disseminated gonococcal infection is arthritis, typically affecting several small to medium size joints. The next most common manifestation is a diffuse violaceous, papular skin rash. Less common but potentially more serious sequelae of disseminated infection include meningitis, pericarditis, endocarditis, and perihepatitis (Fitz-Hugh–Curtis syndrome).[23]

Diagnosis and Management

The most reliable test for confirmation of gonococcal infection is culture of the organism on selective agar such as Thayer-Martin medium. Gram's stain and nucleic acid probes are helpful when positive, but their sensitivity varies widely.

The drugs of choice for treating *localized* gonococcal infection in pregnancy are ceftriaxone (125 intramuscularly [IM] in a single dose) and cefixime (400 mg PO once). The former drug is the preferred agent for treatment of *disseminated* infection and should be administered in a dose of 1 g intravenously (IV) or IM every 24 hours until a clinical response has been achieved.[8,17] Tetracyclines and quinolones should not be used in pregnancy because of their injurious effects on fetal teeth and cartilage. Patients who are allergic to β-lactam antibiotics may be treated with a single 2-g IM dose of spectinomycin.[8] Treatment of the neonate with either silver nitrate or tetracycline ophthalmic preparations is effective in preventing most cases of ophthalmia neonatorum.

Patients who test positive for gonorrhea should be screened for other sexually transmitted diseases. Because of the uniformly excellent activity of ceftriaxone and cefixime against *N. gonorrhoeae*, tests of cure are not *routinely* indicated when patients are treated with these agents. However, patients with persistent symptoms and/or signs of infection should be carefully reevaluated.

Acute Urethritis

Acute urethritis (acute urethral syndrome) is usually caused by one of three organisms: coliforms (principally *Escherichia coli*), *Neisseria gonorrhoeae*, or *Chlamydia trachomatis*. Coliform organisms are part of the normal vaginal and perineal flora and may be introduced into the urethra during intercourse or when wiping after defecation. *N. gonorrhoeae* and *C. trachomatis* are sexually transmitted pathogens.[24]

Affected patients typically experience frequency, urgency, and dysuria. Hesitancy, dribbling, and a mucopurulent urethral discharge also may be present. On microscopic examination, the urine usually has white blood cells (WBCs), but bacteria are not consistently present. Urine cultures may have low colony counts of coliform organisms, and cultures of the urethral discharge may be positive for gonorrhea and chlamydia. A rapid diagnostic test, such as a nucleic acid probe, may be used in lieu of culture for *C. trachomatis*.[24]

Most patients with acute urethritis warrant empiric treatment before the results of urine or urethral cultures are available. Infections caused by coliforms will usually respond to the antibiotics described below for treatment of asymptomatic bacteriuria and cystitis. If gonococcal infection is suspected, the patient should be treated with either oral cefixime (400 mg in a single dose) or intramuscular ceftriaxone (125 mg in a single dose).[8,17] The former is approximately one third the cost of the latter. If the patient is allergic to β-lactam antibiotics, an effective alternative is spectinomycin, administered intramuscularly in a single dose of 2 g. If chlamydial infection is suspected or confirmed, appropriate treatment regimens include: erythromycin base (500 mg PO four times daily for 7 days), amoxicillin (500 mg PO three times daily for 7 days), or azithromycin (1000 mg PO in a single dose).[8] The latter drug is a long-acting derivative of erythromycin and is presently the only antibiotic that is effective in a single dose against *C. trachomatis*. When administered in a powder formulation, it is relatively inexpensive and is a cost-effective alternative to multiday treatment regimens. Doxycycline or tetracycline should not be used in pregnancy because of their adverse effects on fetal bone and teeth.

Asymptomatic Bacteriuria and Acute Cystitis

The prevalence of asymptomatic bacteriuria in pregnancy is 5 to 10 percent, and the vast majority of cases antedate the onset of pregnancy. The frequency of acute cystitis in pregnancy is 1 to 3 percent. Some cases of cystitis arise de novo; others develop as a result of failure to identify and/or treat asymptomatic bacteriuria.[25]

E. coli is responsible for 80 to 90 percent of cases of *initial* infections and 70 to 80 percent of recurrent cases. *Klebsiella pneumoniae* and *Proteus* species also are important pathogens, particularly in patients who have a history of recurrent infection. Approximately 3 to 7 percent of infections will be caused by gram-positive organisms such as group B streptococci, enterococci, and staphylococci.[24,25]

All pregnant women should have a urine culture at their first prenatal appointment to detect preexisting asymptomatic bacteriuria. If the culture is negative, the likelihood of the patient subsequently developing an *asymptomatic* infection is 5 percent or less. If the culture is positive (defined as $\geq 10^5$ colonies/ml urine from a midstream clean-catch specimen), prompt treatment is necessary to prevent ascending infection.[25]

Patients with acute cystitis usually have symptoms of frequency, dysuria, urgency, suprapubic pain, hesitancy, and dribbling. Gross hematuria may be present, but high fever and systemic symptoms are uncommon. In symptomatic patients, the leukocyte esterase and nitrate tests will usually be positive. When a urine culture is obtained, a catheterized sample is preferred because it minimizes the probability that urine will be contaminated by vaginal flora. With a catheterized specimen, a colony count greater than or equal to 10^2/ml is considered indicative of infection.[26]

Asymptomatic bacteriuria and acute cystitis characteristically respond well to short courses of oral antibiotics. Single dose therapy is not as effective in pregnant women as in nonpregnant patients. However, a 3-day course of treatment appears to be comparable to a 7- to 10-day regimen for an initial infection.[24] The longer courses of therapy are most appropriate for patients with recurrent infections. Table 40–3 lists several antibiotics of value for treatment of asymptomatic bacteriuria and cystitis.

When sensitivity tests are available (e.g., in patients with asymptomatic bacteriuria), they may be used to guide antibiotic selection. When empiric treatment is indicated, the choice of antibiotics must be based on established patterns of susceptibility. In recent years, 20 to 30 percent of strains of *E. coli* have developed resistance to ampicillin. Thus, this drug should not be used when the results of sensitivity tests are unknown unless the suspected pathogen is enterococcus.[27]

When choosing among the drugs listed in Table 40–3, the clinician should consider the following factors. First, the sensitivity patterns of ampicillin, amoxicillin, and cephalexin will be the most variable.[27] Second, these drugs, along with amoxicillin-clavulanic acid, will also have the most pronounced effect on normal bowel and vaginal flora and thus be the most likely to cause diarrhea or monilial vulvovaginitis. Third, amoxicillin-clavulanic acid and trimethoprim-sulfamethoxazole will usually be the best empiric agents for treatment of patients with suspected drug-resistant pathogens.[28] In this situation, the latter drug offers a major cost advantage

---

Table 40–3. ANTIBIOTICS FOR TREATMENT OF ASYMPTOMATIC BACTERIURIA AND ACUTE CYSTITIS

Drug	Strength of Activity	Oral Dose × 3 Days	Relative Cost
Amoxicillin	Some *E. coli*, most *Proteus* species, group B streptococci, enterococci, some staphylococci	875 mg bid	Low
Amoxicillin-clavulanic acid (Augmentin)	Most gram-negative aerobic bacilli and gram-positive cocci	875 mg bid	High
Ampicillin	Some *E. coli*, most *Proteus* species, group B streptococci, enterococci, some staphylococci	250–500 mg qid	Low
Cephalexin (Keflex)	Most *E. coli*, most *Klebsiella* and *Proteus* species, group B streptococci, staphylococci	250 mg qid	Low
Nitrofurantoin monohydrate macrocrystals—sustained–release preparation (Macrobid)	Most gram-negative aerobic bacilli	100 mg bid	Moderate
Sulfisoxazole (Gantrisin)	Most gram-negative aerobic bacilli	2 g × 1 dose, then 1 g qid	Low
Trimethoprim-sulfamethoxazole–double strength (Bactrim-DS, or Septra-DS)	Most gram-negative aerobic bacilli	800 mg/160 mg bid	Low

bid, twice daily; qid, four times daily.
Modified from Duff P: Urinary tract infections. Prim Care Update Obstet Gynecol 1:12, 1994.

over the former. Finally, because of theoretical concerns about their effect on protein binding of bilirubin, sulfonamide drugs should probably be avoided near the time of delivery.

For patients who have an initial infection and experience a prompt response to treatment, a urine culture for test of cure is probably unnecessary.[29] Cultures during, or immediately after, treatment are indicated for patients who have a poor response to therapy or who have a history of recurrent infection. During subsequent clinic appointments, the patient's urine should be screened for nitrites and leukocyte esterase. If either of these tests is positive, repeat urine culture and retreatment are indicated.[30]

Acute Pyelonephritis

The incidence of pyelonephritis in pregnancy is 1 to 2 percent.[25] The vast majority of cases develop as a consequence of undiagnosed or inadequately treated lower urinary tract infection. Two major physiologic changes occur during pregnancy that predispose to ascending infection of the urinary tract. First, the high concentration of progesterone secreted by the placenta has an inhibitory effect on ureteral peristalsis. Second, the enlarging gravid uterus often compresses the ureters, particularly the right, at the pelvic brim, thus creating additional stasis. Stasis, in turn, facilitates migration of bacteria from the bladder into the ureters and renal parenchyma (Fig. 40–2).

Approximately 75 to 80 percent of cases of pyelonephritis occur on the right side. Ten to 15 percent are left sided, and a slightly smaller percentage are bilateral.[25] E. coli is again the principal pathogen.[25,27] Klebsiella pneumoniae and Proteus species also are important causes of infection, particularly in women with recurrent episodes of pyelonephritis.[27] Highly virulent gram-negative bacilli, such as Pseudomonas, Enterobacter, and Serratia are unusual isolates except in immunocompromised patients. Gram-positive cocci do not usually cause upper tract infection. Anaerobes also are unlikely pathogens unless the patient is chronically obstructed or instrumented.

The usual clinical manifestations of acute pyelonephritis in pregnancy are fever, chills, flank pain and tenderness, frequency, urgency, hematuria, and dysuria. Patients also may have signs of preterm labor, septic shock, and adult respiratory distress syndrome (ARDS). Urinalysis is usually positive for white cell casts, red blood cells, and bacteria. Urine colony counts greater than 10^2 colonies/ml, in samples collected by catheterization, confirm the diagnosis of infection.

Pregnant patients with pyelonephritis may be considered for outpatient therapy if their disease manifestations are mild, they are hemodynamically stable, and they have no evidence of preterm labor. If an outpa-

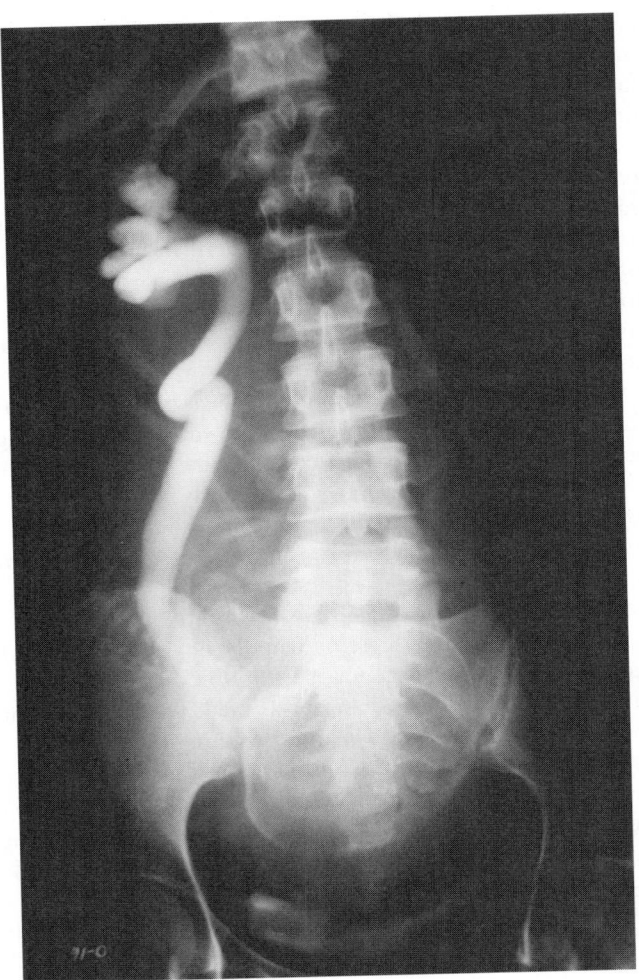

Figure 40–2. Intravenous pyelogram in a pregnant woman shows marked dilation of the right ureter and mild dilation of renal collecting system.

tient approach is adopted, the patient should be treated with agents that have a high level of activity against the common uropathogens. Acceptable oral agents include amoxicillin (875 mg)-clavulanic acid (125 mg), one tablet twice daily or trimethoprim-sulfamethoxazole-DS (one tablet twice daily for 7 to 10 days). Alternatively, a visiting home nurse may be contracted to administer a parenteral agent, such as ceftriaxone (2 g IM or IV once daily).

Pregnant patients who appear to be moderately to severely ill or who show any signs of preterm labor should be hospitalized for intravenous antibiotic therapy. They should receive appropriate supportive treatment and be monitored closely for complications such as sepsis, ARDS, and preterm labor. One of the best choices for empiric intravenous antibiotic therapy is cefazolin (1 to 2 g every 8 hours).[27] For hospitalized patients, this drug is less expensive to administer than the newer broader spectrum cephalosporins or penicillins and has an equivalent spectrum of activity against the coliform organisms most likely to be responsible for infection. If the patient is critically ill or is at high risk for a resistant organism, a second antibiotic, such as gentamicin (1.5 mg/kg every 8 hours) or aztreonam (500 mg to 1 g every 8 to 12 hours) should be administered, along with cefazolin, until the results of susceptibility tests are available.

Once antibiotic therapy is initiated, approximately 75 percent of patients defervesce within 48 hours. By the end of 72 hours, almost 95 percent of patients will be afebrile and asymptomatic.[31] The two most likely causes of treatment failure are a resistant microorganism or obstruction. The latter condition is best diagnosed with renal ultrasonography or intravenous pyelography and typically results from a stone or physical compression of the ureter by the gravid uterus.

Once the patient has begun to defervesce and her clinical examination has improved, she may be discharged from the hospital. Oral antibiotics should be prescribed to complete a total of 7 to 10 days of therapy. Selection of a specific oral agent should be based on considerations of efficacy, toxicity, and expense.

Approximately 20 to 30 percent of pregnant patients with acute pyelonephritis will develop a recurrent urinary tract infection later in pregnancy.[25] The most cost-effective way to reduce the frequency of recurrence is to administer a daily prophylactic dose of an antibiotic, such as sulfisoxazole (1 g) or nitrofurantoin monohydrate macrocrystals (100 mg). Patients receiving prophylaxis should have their urine screened for bacteria at each subsequent clinic appointment. They also should be questioned about recurrence of symptoms. If symptoms recur, or the dipstick test for nitrite or leukocyte esterase is positive, a urine culture should be obtained to determine if retreatment is necessary.

CHORIOAMNIONITIS

Epidemiology

Chorioamnionitis (amnionitis, intra-amniotic infection) occurs in approximately 1 to 5 percent of term pregnancies.[32] In patients with preterm delivery, the frequency of clinical or subclinical infection may approach 25 percent.[33] Although chorioamnionitis may result from hematogenous dissemination of microorganisms, it more commonly is an ascending infection caused by organisms that are part of the normal vaginal flora. The principal pathogens are *Bacteroides* and *Prevotella* species, *E. coli*, anaerobic streptococci, and group B streptococci.[34] Several clinical risk factors for chorioamnionitis have been identified. The most important are young age, low socioeconomic status, nulliparity, extended duration of labor and ruptured membranes, multiple vaginal examinations, and preexisting infections of the lower genital tract.[32]

Diagnosis

In most situations, the diagnosis of chorioamnionitis can be established on the basis of the clinical findings of maternal fever and maternal and fetal tachycardia, in the absence of other localizing signs of infection. In more severely ill patients, uterine tenderness and purulent amniotic fluid may be present.[32] The disorders that should be considered in the differential diagnosis of chorioamnionitis include upper respiratory infection, bronchitis, pneumonia, pyelonephritis, viral syndrome, and appendicitis.

Laboratory confirmation of the diagnosis of chorioamnionitis is not routinely necessary in term patients who are progressing to delivery. However, in preterm patients who are being evaluated for tocolysis or corticosteroids, laboratory assessment may be of value in excluding or establishing the diagnosis of intrauterine infection. In this clinical context, amniotic fluid should be obtained by transabdominal amniocentesis. Table 40–4 summarizes the abnormal laboratory findings that may be present in infected patients.[32,35–40]

Management

Both the mother and infant may experience serious complications when chorioamnionitis is present. Bacteremia occurs in 3 to 12 percent of infected women. When cesarean delivery is required, up to 8 percent of women develop a wound infection, and approximately 1 percent develop a pelvic abscess. Fortunately, maternal death due to infection is exceedingly rare.[32]

Five to 10 percent of neonates delivered to mothers with chorioamnionitis have pneumonia or bacteremia. The predominant organisms responsible for these infections are group B streptococci and *E. coli*. Meningitis occurs in 1 percent or less of term infants and in a slightly higher percentage of preterm infants. Mortality due to infection ranges from 1 to 4 percent in term neonates but may approach 15 percent in preterm infants because of the confounding effects of other complications such as hyaline membrane disease and intraventricular hemorrhage.[32]

In order to prevent maternal and neonatal complications, parenteral antibiotic therapy should be initiated as soon as the diagnosis of chorioamnionitis is made, unless delivery is imminent. Three separate investigations have demonstrated that mother–infant pairs who receive prompt intrapartum treatment have better outcomes than patients treated after delivery.[41–43] The principal benefits of early treatment include decreased frequency of neonatal bacteremia and pneumonia and

Table 40-4. DIAGNOSTIC TESTS FOR CHORIOAMNIONITIS

Test	Abnormal Finding	Comment
Maternal white blood cell (WBC) count[32]	≥ 15,000 cells/mm³ with preponderance of leukocytes	Labor and/or corticosteroids may result in elevation of WBC count.
Amniotic fluid glucose[35-37]	≤ 10 to 15 mg/dl	Excellent correlation with positive amniotic fluid culture and clinical infection.
Amniotic fluid interleukin-6[38]	≥ 7.9 ng/ml	Excellent correlation with positive amniotic fluid culture and clinical infection.
Amniotic fluid leukocyte esterase[39]	≥ 1 + reaction	Good correlation with positive amniotic fluid culture and clinical infection.
Amniotic fluid Gram's stain[32]	Any organism in an oil immersion field	Allows identification of particularly virulent organism such as group B streptococci; however, the test is very sensitive to inoculum effect. In addition, it cannot identify pathogens such as mycoplasmas.
Amniotic fluid culture[32]	Growth of aerobic or anaerobic microorganism	Results are not immediately available for clinical management.
Blood cultures[32,40]	Growth of aerobic or anaerobic microorganism	Will be positive in 5–10% of patients. However, will usually not be of value in making clinical decisions unless patient is at increased risk for bacterial endocarditis, is immunocompromised, or has a poor response to initial treatment.

decreased duration of maternal fever and hospitalization.

The most extensively tested intravenous antibiotic regimen for treatment of chorioamnionitis is the combination of ampicillin (2 g every 6 hours) or penicillin (5 million units every 6 hours) plus gentamicin (1.5 mg/kg every 8 hours).[15,32] These antibiotics specifically target the two organisms most likely to cause neonatal infection: group B streptococci and *E. coli*. With rare exceptions, gentamicin is preferred to tobramycin or amikacin because it is available in an inexpensive generic formulation. Amikacin should be reserved for immunocompromised patients who are particularly likely to be infected by highly virulent, drug-resistant, aerobic gram-negative bacilli. In patients who are allergic to β-lactam antibiotics, either vancomycin (500 mg every 6 hours or 1 g every 12 hours), erythromycin (1 g every 6 hours), or clindamycin (900 mg every 8 hours) can be substituted for ampicillin.

If a patient with chorioamnionitis requires cesarean delivery, a drug with activity against anaerobic organisms should be added to the antibiotic regimen. Either clindamycin (900 mg every 8 hours) or metronidazole (500 mg every 12 hours) is an excellent choice for this purpose. Failure to provide effective coverage of anaerobes may result in treatment failures in 20 to 30 percent of patients.

Extended spectrum cephalosporins, penicillins, and carbapenems also provide excellent coverage against the bacteria that cause chorioamnionitis. Dosages and dose intervals for several of these agents are listed in Table 40-5.[44] Less information is available concerning the effectiveness of these drugs compared to the ampicillin or penicillin plus gentamicin regimen. In addition, the toxicity profile for the fetus and neonate has not been as well delineated.

As a general rule, parenteral antibiotics should be continued until the patient has been afebrile and

Table 40-5. SINGLE AGENTS OF VALUE IN TREATMENT OF CHORIOAMNIONITIS

Drug	Dosage and Dose Interval	Relative Cost to the Pharmacy*
Extended spectrum cephalosporins		
Cefotaxime	2 g q8–12h	Intermediate
Cefotetan	2 g q12h	Low
Cefoxitin	2 g q6h	High
Ceftizoxime	2 g q12h	Intermediate
Extended spectrum penicillins		
Ampicillin-sulbactam	3 g q6h	Low
Mezlocillin	3–4 g q6h	Intermediate
Piperacillin	3–4 g q6h	Intermediate
Piperacillin-tazobactam	3.375 g q6h	Intermediate
Ticarcillin-clavulanic acid	3.1 g q6h	Low
Carbapenem		
Imipenem-cilastatin	500 mg q6h	High
Meropenem	1 g q12h	High

* Cost estimates do not include dose preparation fees and administration charges.

asymptomatic for approximately 24 hours. Once an adequate clinical response has been achieved, antibiotics may be discontinued and the patient discharged. A course of oral antibiotics administered as an outpatient is rarely indicated.[15,32,44]

There are two principal exceptions to the above rule. First, a patient with a documented staphylococcal bacteremia may require a longer period of intravenous therapy and, subsequently, an extended course of oral antibiotics. Second, the patient who has a vaginal delivery and then experiences a rapid defervescence may be a suitable candidate for a short course of oral antibiotics administered as an outpatient. In this situation, amoxicillin (875 mg)-clavulanic acid (125 mg), one tablet twice daily for 2–3 days, provides effective coverage against most of the organisms responsible for chorioamnionitis and is usually very well tolerated.

Patients with chorioamnionitis are at increased risk for dysfunctional labor. Approximately 75 percent require oxytocin for augmentation of labor, and up to 30 to 40 percent require cesarean delivery, usually for failure to progress in labor. While chorioamnionitis by itself should not be regarded as an indication for cesarean, affected patients need careful monitoring during labor to ensure that uterine contractility is optimized. In addition, the fetus also needs close surveillance. Fetal heart rate abnormalities such as tachycardia and decreased variability (Fig. 40–3) occur in over three fourths of cases, and additional tests such as vibroacoustic stimulation, scalp stimulation, or scalp pH assessment may be necessary to evaluate fetal wellbeing.[32,45]

PUERPERAL ENDOMETRITIS

Epidemiology

The frequency of puerperal endometritis in women having vaginal delivery is approximately 1 to 3 percent. In women having a scheduled cesarean prior to the onset of labor and rupture of membranes, the frequency of endometritis ranges from 5 to 15 percent. When cesarean delivery is performed after an extended period of labor and ruptured membranes, the incidence of infection is 30 to 35 percent without antibiotic prophylaxis and 15 to 20 percent with prophylaxis. In highly indigent patient populations, the frequency of infection may be almost double the figures cited above.[46]

Endometritis is a polymicrobial infection caused by microorganisms that are part of the normal vaginal flora. These bacteria gain access to the upper genital tract, peritoneal cavity and, occasionally, the bloodstream as a result of vaginal examinations during labor

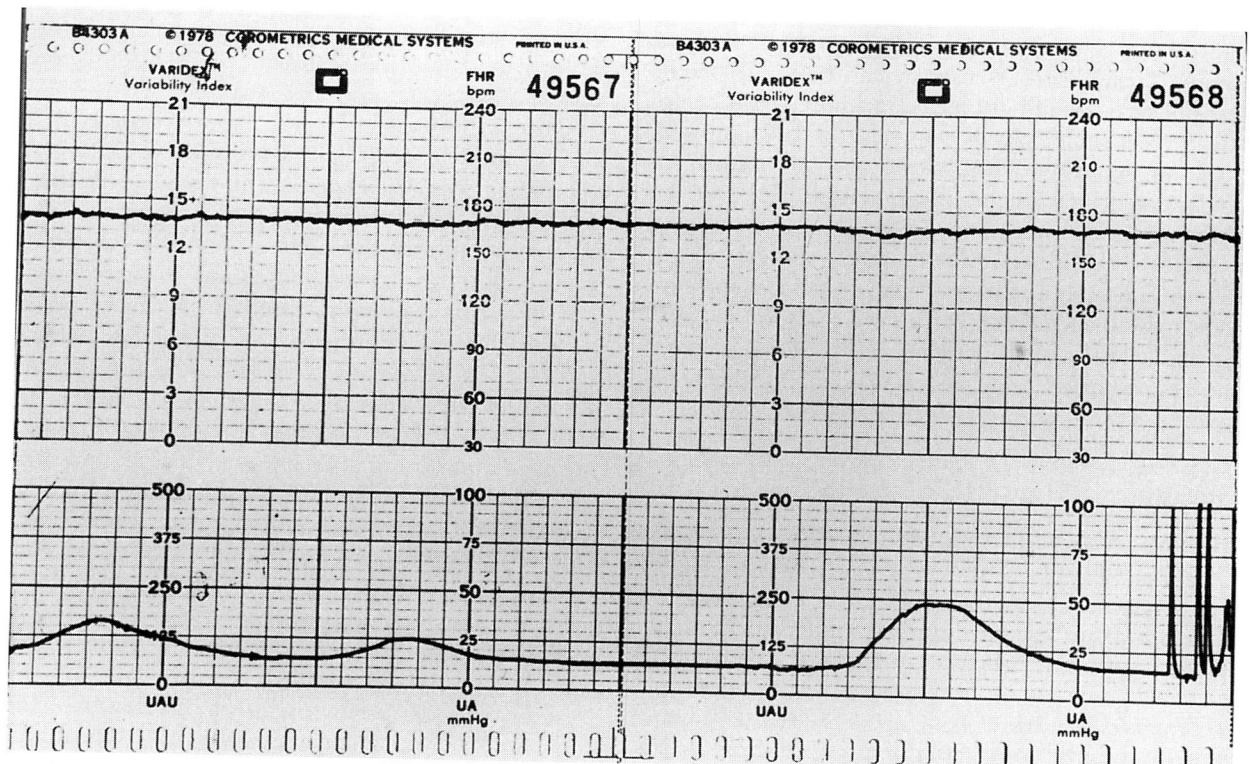

Figure 40–3. Fetal heart tracing from a patient with chorioamnionitis. Note the tachycardia of 170 beats/min and the decrease in both short- and long-term variability.

and manipulations during surgery. The most common pathogenic bacteria are group B streptococci, anaerobic streptococci, aerobic gram-negative bacilli (predominantly *E. coli, Klebsiella pneumoniae,* and *Proteus* species), and anaerobic gram-negative bacilli (principally *Bacteroides* and *Prevotella* species). *Chlamydia trachomatis* is not a common cause of early-onset puerperal endometritis but has been implicated in late-onset infection. The genital mycoplasmas may be pathogens in some patients, but they tend to be present in association with more highly virulent bacteria.[46]

The principal risk factors for endometritis are cesarean delivery, young age, low socioeconomic status, extended duration of labor and ruptured membranes, and multiple vaginal examinations. In addition, preexisting infection or colonization of the lower genital tract (gonorrhea, group B streptococci, bacterial vaginosis) also predisposes to ascending infection.[46]

Clinical Presentation and Diagnosis

Affected patients typically have a fever of 38°C or higher within 36 hours of delivery. Associated findings include malaise, tachycardia, lower abdominal pain and tenderness, uterine tenderness, and discolored, malodorous lochia. A small number of patients also may have a tender, indurated inflammatory mass in the broad ligament, posterior cul de sac, or retrovesical space.

The initial differential diagnosis of puerperal fever should include endometritis, atelectasis, pneumonia, viral syndrome, pyelonephritis, and appendicitis. Distinction among these disorders usually can be made on the basis of physical examination and a limited number of laboratory tests such as WBC count, urinalysis and culture and, in select patients, chest x-ray. Endometrial cultures are of primary value in evaluating patients who have a poor initial response to antibiotic treatment. When these cultures are obtained, they should be collected with a double-lumen instrument to prevent contamination by lower genital tract flora.[47] Blood cultures also are indicated in such patients and in those who are immunocompromised or at increased risk for bacterial endocarditis.[46]

Management

Patients who have mild to moderately severe infections, particularly after vaginal delivery, can be treated with short intravenous courses of single agents such as the extended spectrum cephalosporins and penicillins or carbapenem antibiotics such as imipenem-cilastatin and meropenem. Table 40–5 lists several antibiotics that have acceptable breadth of coverage against the polymicrobial genital tract flora. Combination antibiotic regimens should be considered for more severely ill patients, particularly those who are indigent and in poor general health and those who have had cesarean deliv-

Table 40–6. COMBINATION ANTIBIOTIC REGIMENS FOR TREATMENT OF PUERPERAL ENDOMETRITIS

Antibiotics	Intravenous Dose	Relative Cost to the Pharmacy*
Regimen 1		
Clindamycin	900 mg q8h	Intermediate
Gentamicin	1.5 mg/kg q8h	Low
	or	
	7 mg/kg ideal body weight q24h*†	
Regimen 2		
Clindamycin	900 mg q8h	Intermediate
Aztreonam	1–2 g q8h	High
Regimen 3		
Metronidazole	500 mg q12h	Low
Penicillin	5 million units q6h	Low
or		
Ampicillin	2 g q6h	Low
Gentamicin	1.5 mg/kg q8h	Low
	or	
	7 mg/kg ideal body weight q24h	

* Cost estimates do not include dose preparation fees and administration charges.
† Single daily dosing of aminoglycoside antibiotics is more effective and less expensive than multidose treatment. In addition, it is less likely to cause toxicity. At present, there is little information concerning the effects of single large doses of aminoglycosides on the developing fetus. Therefore, this regimen should be reserved for postpartum patients.

eries. Table 40–6 lists several antibiotic combinations of proven value in treatment of puerperal endometritis.[15,44]

Once antibiotics are begun, approximately 90 percent of patients will defervesce within 48 to 72 hours. When the patient has been afebrile and asymptomatic for approximately 24 hours, parenteral antibiotics should be discontinued, and the patient should be discharged. As a general rule, an extended course of oral antibiotics is not necessary following discharge.[48] There are at least two notable exceptions to this rule. First, patients who have had a vaginal delivery and who defervesce within 24 hours are candidates for early discharge. In these individuals, a short 2–3 day course of an oral antibiotic such as amoxicillin (875 mg)-clavulanic acid (125 mg), one tablet twice daily, may be substituted for continued parenteral therapy. Second, patients who have had a staphylococcal bacteremia require a more extended period of administration of parenteral and oral antibiotics with specific antistaphylococcal activity.[49]

Patients who fail to respond to the antibiotic therapy outlined above usually have one of two problems. The first is a drug-resistant organism. Table 40–7 lists possible weaknesses in coverage of selected antibiotics and indicates the appropriate change in treatment. The second major cause of treatment failure is a wound infection. Infected wounds should be opened completely to provide drainage. If extensive cellulitis at the margin of the incision is present, an antibiotic with specific coverage against staphylococci, such as nafcillin (2 g IV every 6 hours), should be added to the treatment regimen.

When changes in antibiotic therapy do not result in clinical improvement and no evidence of wound infection is present, several unusual disorders should be considered. The differential diagnosis of persistent puerperal fever is summarized in Table 40–8.[46]

Prevention of Puerperal Endometritis

Prophylactic antibiotics are clearly of value in reducing the frequency of postcesarean endometritis, particularly in women having surgery after an extended period of labor and ruptured membranes.[50] The most appropriate agent for prophylaxis is a limited spectrum (first-generation) cephalosporin, such as cefazolin. Cefazolin should be administered in an intravenous dose of 1 g immediately after the neonate's umbilical cord is clamped. A second dose is indicated approximately 8 hours after the first dose in high-risk patients, especially when operating time is prolonged beyond 1 hour. Although extended spectrum penicillins and cephalosporins are effective for prophylaxis, they offer no advantage over cefazolin and are severalfold more expensive. Moreover, widespread use of these drugs for prophylaxis may ultimately limit their usefulness for treatment of established infections.[50]

Patients who have an immediate hypersensitivity to β-lactam antibiotics pose a special problem. One alternative is to administer metronidazole, 500 mg IV. Another alternative is to administer a single dose of clindamycin (900 mg) plus gentamicin (1.5 mg/kg). Although these antibiotics are commonly used for treatment of overt infections, their administration is still warranted in penicillin-allergic patients who are at high risk for postoperative infection.

Table 40–8. DIFFERENTIAL DIAGNOSIS OF PERSISTENT PUERPERAL FEVER

Condition	Diagnostic Test(s)	Treatment
Resistant microorganism	Endometrial culture Blood culture	Modify antibiotic therapy
Wound infection	Physical examination Needle aspiration Ultrasound	Incision and drainage Antibiotics
Pelvic abscess	Physical examination Ultrasound CT MRI	Drainage Antibiotics
Septic pelvic vein thrombophlebitis	Ultrasound CT MRI	Heparin anticoagulation Antibiotics
Recrudescence of connective tissue disease	Serology	Corticosteroids
Drug fever	Inspection of temperature graph WBC— identify eosinophilia	Discontinue antibiotics
Mastitis	Physical examination	Modify antibiotic treatment to provide coverage of staphylococcal organisms

From Duff P: Antibiotic selection for infections in obstetric patients. Semin Perinatol 17:367, 1993, with permission.

Table 40–7. TREATMENT OF RESISTANT MICROORGANISMS IN PATIENTS WITH PUERPERAL ENDOMETRITIS

Initial Antibiotic(s)	Principal Weakness in Coverage	Modification of Therapy
Extended spectrum cephalosporins	Some aerobic and anaerobic gram-negative bacilli Enterococci	Change treatment to clindamycin or metronidazole plus penicillin or ampicillin plus gentamicin
Extended spectrum penicillins	Some aerobic and anaerobic gram-negative bacilli	As above
Clindamycin plus gentamicin or aztreonam	Enterococci Some anaerobic gram-negative bacilli	Add ampicillin or penicillin* Consider substitution of metronidazole for clindamycin

* Ampicillin alone is highly active against enterococci. Penicillin *plus* gentamicin work synergistically to provide excellent coverage against this organism.
From Duff P: Antibiotic selection for infections in obstetric patients. Semin Perinatol 17:367, 1993, with permission.

SERIOUS SEQUELAE OF PUERPERAL INFECTION

Wound Infection

Wound infection after cesarean delivery typically occurs in association with endometritis. Approximately 3 to 5 percent of patients with the latter disorder subsequently are found to have an incisional infection.[46] The major risk factors for wound infection are listed in the box "Principal Risk Factors for Postcesarean Wound Infection." The principal causative organisms are *Staphylo-*

Principal Risk Factors for Postcesarean Wound Infection

- Poor surgical technique
- Low socioeconomic status
- Extended duration of labor and ruptured membranes
- Preexisting infection such as chorioamnionitis
- Obesity
- Type 1 (insulin-dependent) diabetes
- Immunodeficiency disorder
- Corticosteroid therapy
- Immunosuppressive therapy

coccus aureus, aerobic streptococci, and aerobic and anaerobic bacilli.[51]

The diagnosis of wound infection always should be considered in patients who have a poor clinical response to antibiotic therapy for endometritis.[46] Clinical examination characteristically shows erythema, induration, and tenderness at the margins of the abdominal incision. When the wound is probed with either a cotton-tipped applicator or fine needle, pus usually exudes. Some patients, however, may have an extensive cellulitis without harboring frank pus in the incision. Clinical examination should be sufficient to establish the correct diagnosis. Gram's stain and culture of the wound exudate are not routinely needed, since the results of these tests rarely influence selection of antibiotics or duration of antibiotic treatment.

When pus is present in the incision, the wound must be opened and drained completely. Antibiotic therapy should be modified to provide coverage against staphylococci, since some regimens for endometritis may not specifically target this organism. Nafcillin (2 g IV every 6 hours) would be a suitable drug for this purpose. In a patient who is allergic to β-lactam antibiotics, vancomycin (1 g IV every 12 hours) is an acceptable alternative.[44]

Once the wound is opened, a careful inspection should be made to be certain that the fascial layer is intact. If it is disrupted, surgical intervention will be necessary to reapproximate the fascia. Otherwise, the wound should be irrigated two to three times daily with a solution such as warm saline, a clean dressing should be maintained, and the incision should be allowed to heal by secondary intention. Antibiotics should be continued until the base of the wound is clean and all signs of cellulitis have resolved. Patients usually can be treated at home once the acute signs of infection have subsided.

Necrotizing fasciitis is an uncommon but extremely serious complication of abdominal wound infection.[52] It also has been reported in association with infection of the episiotomy site.[53] This condition is most likely to occur in patients with type 1 (insulin-dependent) diabetes, cancer, or an immunosuppressive disorder. Multiple bacterial pathogens, particularly anaerobes, have been isolated from patients with necrotizing fasciitis.

Necrotizing fasciitis should be suspected when the margins of the wound become discolored, cyanotic, and devoid of sensation. When the wound is opened, the subcutaneous tissue is easily dissected free of the underlying fascia, but muscle tissue is not affected. If the diagnosis is uncertain, a tissue biopsy should be performed and examined by frozen section.

Necrotizing fasciitis is a life-threatening condition and requires aggressive medical and surgical management. Broad-spectrum antibiotics with activity against all potential aerobic and anaerobic pathogens should be administered. Intravascular volume should be maintained with infusions of crystalloid, and electrolyte abnormalities should be corrected. Finally, and most importantly, the wound must be debrided and all necrotic tissue removed. In many instances, the dissection must be quite extensive and may be best managed in conjunction with an experienced general or plastic surgeon.[52]

Pelvic Abscess

With the advent of modern antibiotics, pelvic abscesses after cesarean or vaginal delivery have become extremely rare. Less than 1 percent of patients with puerperal endometritis develop a pelvic abscess.[46] When present, abscess collections are typically located in the anterior or posterior cul de sac, most commonly the latter, or the broad ligament. The usual bacteria isolated from abscess cavities are coliforms and anaerobic gram-negative bacilli, particularly *Bacteroides* and *Prevotella* species.[54]

Patients with an abscess typically experience a persistent fever despite initial therapy for endometritis. In addition, they usually have malaise, tachycardia, lower abdominal pain and tenderness, and a palpable pelvic mass anterior, posterior, or lateral to the uterus. The peripheral WBC count is usually elevated, and there is a shift toward immature cell forms. Ultrasound, computed tomographic (CT) scan, and magnetic resonance imaging (MRI) may be used to confirm the diagnosis of pelvic abscess.[55] Although the latter two tests may be slightly more sensitive, the former offers the advantages of decreased expense and ready availability.

Patients with a pelvic abscess require surgical intervention to drain the purulent collection. When the abscess is in the posterior cul de sac, colpotomy drainage may be possible. For abscesses located anterior or lateral to the uterus, drainage may be accomplished by CT scan or ultrasound-guided placement of a catheter drain.[56] When access is limited or the abscess is extensive, open laparotomy is indicated.

Patients with a pelvic abscess must receive antibiotics

with excellent activity against coliform organisms and anaerobes.[54] One regimen that has been tested extensively in obstetric patients with serious infections is the combination of penicillin (5 million units IV every 6 hours) or ampicillin (2 g IV every 6 hours) plus gentamicin (1.5 mg/kg IV every 8 hours or 7 mg/kg of ideal body weight every 24 hours) plus clindamycin (900 mg IV every 8 hours) or metronidazole (500 mg IV every 12 hours). If a patient is allergic to β-lactam antibiotics, vancomycin (500 mg IV every 6 hours or 1 g IV every 12 hours) can be substituted for penicillin or ampicillin. Aztreonam (1 to 2 g IV every 8 hours) also can be used in lieu of gentamicin when the patient is at risk for nephrotoxicity. Alternatively, the single agents imipenem-cilastatin (500 mg IV every 6 hours) or meropenem (1 g every 8 hours) provide excellent coverage against the usual pathogens responsible for an abscess. Antibiotics should be continued until the patient has been afebrile and asymptomatic for a minimum of 24 to 48 hours.[46]

Septic Pelvic Vein Thrombophlebitis

Like pelvic abscess, septic pelvic vein thrombophlebitis is extremely rare, occurring in 1 in 2,000 pregnancies overall and in less than or equal to 1 percent of patients who have puerperal endometritis.[57] Intrauterine infection may cause seeding of pathogenic microorganisms into the venous circulation; in turn, these organisms may damage the vascular endothelium and initiate thrombosis.

Septic pelvic vein thrombophlebitis occurs in two distinct forms.[57] The most commonly described disorder is acute thrombosis of one (usually the right) or both ovarian veins (*ovarian vein syndrome*).[58] Affected patients typically develop a moderate temperature elevation in association with lower abdominal pain in the first 48 to 96 hours postpartum. Pain usually localizes to the side of the affected vein but may radiate into the groin, upper abdomen, or flank. Nausea, vomiting, and abdominal bloating may be present.

On physical examination, the patient's pulse is usually elevated. Tachypnea, stridor, and dyspnea may be evident if pulmonary embolization has occurred. The abdomen is tender, and bowel sounds are often decreased or absent. Most patients demonstrate voluntary and involuntary guarding, and 50 to 70 percent have a tender, rope-like mass originating near one cornua and extending laterally and cephalad toward the upper abdomen. The principal conditions that should be considered in the differential diagnosis of ovarian vein syndrome are pyelonephritis, nephrolithiasis, appendicitis, broad ligament hematoma, adnexal torsion, and pelvic abscess.

The second presentation of septic pelvic vein thrombophlebitis is termed *enigmatic fever*.[59] Initially, affected patients have clinical findings suggestive of endometritis and receive systemic antibiotics. Subsequently, they experience subjective improvement, with the exception of temperature instability. They do not appear to be seriously ill, and positive findings are limited to persistent fever and tachycardia. Disorders that should be considered in the differential diagnosis of enigmatic fever are drug fever, viral syndrome, collagen vascular disease, and pelvic abscess.

The diagnostic tests of greatest value in evaluating patients with suspected septic pelvic vein thrombophlebitis are CT scan and MRI (Fig. 40–4). These tests are most sensitive in detecting large thrombi in the major pelvic vessels. They are not as useful in identifying thrombi in smaller vessels. In such cases, the ultimate diagnosis may depend on the patient's response to an empiric trial of heparin.[60,61]

Patients with septic pelvic vein thrombophlebitis should be treated with therapeutic doses of intravenous heparin.[57,60] The dose of heparin should be adjusted to maintain the activated partial thromboplastin time (aPTT) at approximately 2 times normal or to achieve a serum heparin concentration of 0.2 to 0.7 IU/ml. Therapy should be continued for 7 to 10 days. Long-term anticoagulation with oral agents is probably unnecessary unless the patient has massive clotting throughout the pelvic venous plexus or has sustained a pulmonary embolism. Patients should be maintained on broad-spectrum antibiotics throughout the period of heparin administration.

Once medical therapy is initiated, the patient should have objective evidence of a response within 48 to 72 hours. If no improvement is noted, surgical intervention may be necessary.[57,60] The decision to perform surgery should be based on clinical assessment and the relative certainty of the diagnosis. The surgical approach, in turn, should be tailored to the specific intraoperative

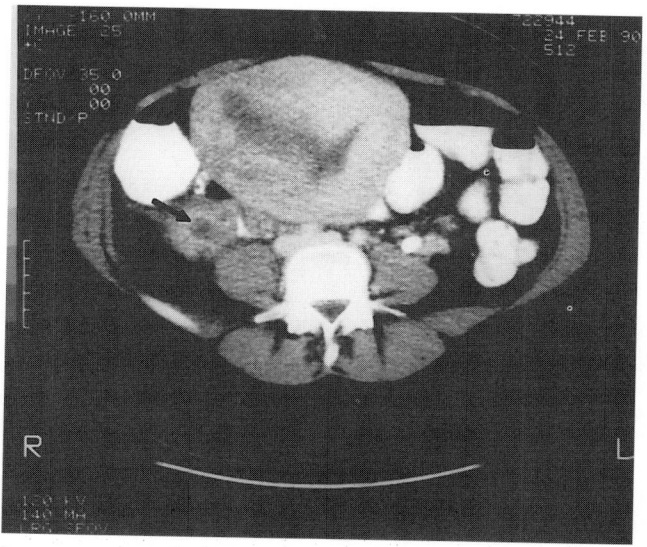

Figure 40–4. CT scan shows a thrombus (*arrow*) in right ovarian vein.

findings. In most instances, treatment requires only ligation of the affected vessel(s). Extension of the thrombosis along the vena cava to the point of origin of the renal veins may necessitate embolectomy. Excision of the infected vessel and removal of the ipsilateral adnexa and uterus are indicated only in the presence of a well-defined abscess. Whenever any of the above procedures are being considered, consultation with an experienced vascular surgeon is imperative.

SEPTIC SHOCK

Septic shock in obstetric patients is usually associated with four specific infections: septic abortion, acute pyelonephritis, and severe chorioamnionitis or endometritis.[13] Fortunately, fewer than 5 percent of patients with any of these infections develop septic shock. The most common organisms responsible for septic shock are the aerobic gram-negative bacilli, principally *E. coli, Kleb-*

siella pneumoniae, and *Proteus* species. Highly virulent, drug-resistant coliforms such as *Pseudomonas, Enterobacter,* and *Serratia* species are uncommon except in immunosuppressed patients.[62]

Aerobic gram-negative bacilli have a complex lipopolysaccharide in their cell wall that is termed *endotoxin.* When released into the systemic circulation, endotoxin is capable of causing a variety of immunologic, hematologic, neurohormonal, and hemodynamic derangements that ultimately result in multiorgan dysfunction. Figure 40–5 presents a simplified summary of the pathophysiology of endotoxic shock.[62]

In the early stages of septic shock, patients usually are restless, disoriented, tachycardic, and hypotensive. Although hypothermia is occasionally present, most patients have a relatively high fever (39° to 40°C). Their skin may be warm and flushed due to an initial phase of vasodilation (*warm shock*). Subsequently, as extensive vasoconstriction occurs, the skin becomes cool and clammy. Cardiac arrhythmias may be present, and signs of myocardial ischemia may occur. Jaundice, often due to hemolysis, may be evident. Urinary output typically

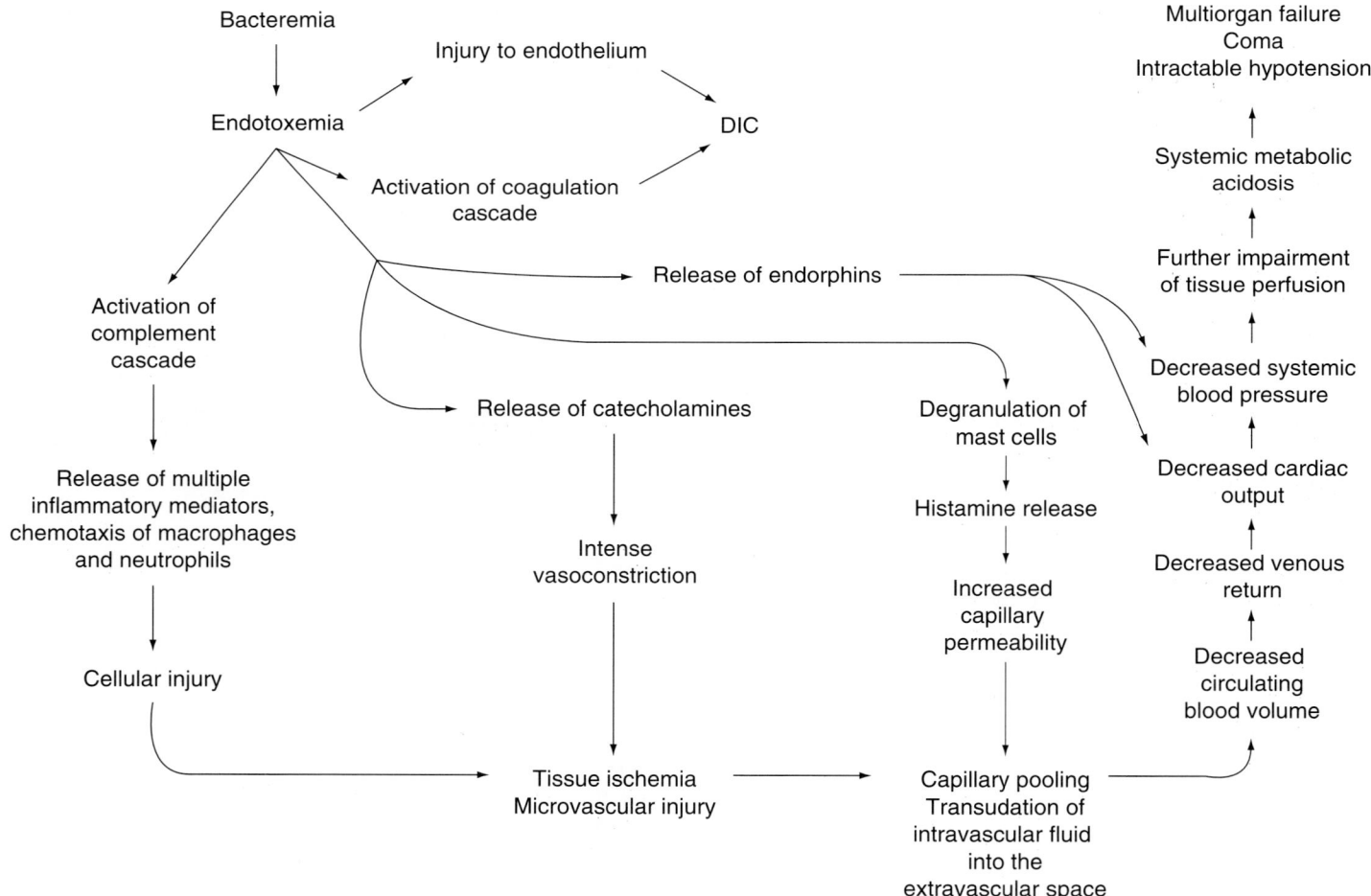

Figure 40–5. Pathophysiology of septic (endotoxic) shock.

decreases, and frank anuria may develop. Spontaneous bleeding from the genitourinary tract or venipuncture sites may occur as a result of disseminated intravascular coagulation (DIC). ARDS is a common complication of severe sepsis and is associated with manifestations such as dyspnea, stridor, cough, tachypnea, and bilateral rales and wheezing (Fig. 40–5).[63] In addition to these systemic signs and symptoms, affected patients also may have findings related to their primary site of infection such as purulent lochia, uterine tenderness, peritonitis, or flank tenderness.

The differential diagnosis of septic shock in obstetric patients includes hypovolemic and cardiogenic shock, diabetic ketoacidosis, anaphylactic reaction, anesthetic reaction, and amniotic fluid or venous embolism.[62] Distinction among these disorders usually can be made on the basis of a thorough history and physical examination and a limited number of laboratory studies. The WBC count initially may be decreased but, subsequently, is elevated in the majority of patients. A large percentage of bands is usually evident. The hematocrit may be decreased if blood loss has occurred. Tests of coagulation such as platelet count, serum fibrinogen concentration, serum concentration of fibrin degradation products, prothrombin time, and partial thromboplastin time are frequently abnormal. Serum concentrations of the transaminase enzymes and bilirubin are often increased. Similarly, increased concentrations of blood urea nitrogen (BUN) and creatinine reflect deterioration of renal function. Chest x-ray in patients with septic shock is indicated to determine if pneumonia or ARDS is present. In addition, CT scan, MRI, and ultrasound may be of value in localizing an abscess.[55] Affected patients also require electrocardiographic monitoring to detect arrhythmias or signs of ischemic injury.

The first goal of treatment of septic shock is to correct the hemodynamic derangements precipitated by endotoxin. Two large-bore intravenous catheters and a urinary catheter should be inserted. Isotonic crystalloid such as Ringer's lactate solution or normal saline should be administered and the infusion titrated in accordance with the patient's pulse, blood pressure, and urine output. Application of the military antishock garment also may be helpful in stabilizing the patient's blood pressure, especially when bleeding is occurring.

If the initial fluid infusion is not successful in restoring hemodynamic stability, a right heart catheter should be inserted to monitor pulmonary artery wedge pressure. In addition, dopamine should be administered.[64] In low doses, this vasopressor stimulates myocardial contractility and improves perfusion of central organs. In higher doses, the drug has primarily vasoconstrictive effects and may actually compromise tissue perfusion.

Corticosteroids no longer are recommended for treatment of septic shock. Although these drugs may initially improve hemodynamic instability, they ultimately promote superinfection with drug-resistant microorganisms and do not improve overall mortality.[65,66] In selected patients with refractory hypotension, intravenous administration of the narcotic antagonist naloxone has led to reversal of the shock state.[67] The dose and duration of administration of naloxone have not been standardized.

The second objective of treatment is to administer broad-spectrum antibiotics targeted against the most likely pathogens.[62] For genital tract infections, the combination of penicillin (5 million units IV every 6 hours) or ampicillin (2 g IV every 6 hours) plus clindamycin (900 mg IV every 8 hours) or metronidazole (500 mg IV every 12 hours) plus gentamicin (1.5 mg/kg IV every 8 hours or 7 mg/kg ideal body weight IV every 24 hours) or aztreonam (1 to 2 g IV every 8 hours) is an appropriate regimen. Alternatively, imipenem-cilastatin (500 mg IV every 6 hours) or meropenem (1 g every 8 hours) can be administered as single agents. Patients also may require surgery, for example, to evacuate infected products of conception, drain a pelvic abscess, or remove badly infected pelvic organs. Indicated surgery never should be delayed because a patient is unstable, because operative intervention may be precisely the step necessary to reverse the hemodynamic derangements of septic shock.

Other adjuncts in the treatment of infection include infusion of granulocytes and administration of antisera to the major antigens of coliform bacteria.[62,68] The former modality has its greatest application in treatment of neutropenic patients. The second intervention has appeared promising in some investigations but remains experimental.

Patients with septic shock require meticulous supportive care. Core temperature should be maintained as close to normal as possible by use of antipyretics and a cooling blanket. Coagulation abnormalities should be identified promptly and treated by infusion of platelets and coagulation factors, as indicated. Finally, patients should be given oxygen supplementation and observed closely for evidence of ARDS, one of the major causes of mortality in cases of severe sepsis.[14] Oxygenation should be monitored by means of a pulse oximeter or radial artery catheter. At the first sign of respiratory failure, the patient should be intubated and supported with mechanical ventilation.

The prognosis in patients with septic shock clearly depends on the severity of the patient's underlying illness. In patients with "rapidly fatal illnesses," such as hematopoietic malignancies, mortality approaches 80 percent. In patients with "ultimately fatal illnesses" (e.g., solid tumors), mortality decreases to 40 to 50 percent. However, in otherwise healthy patients, mortality rarely exceeds 15 percent.[69] Fortunately, most obstetric patients are in the latter category. Therefore, the prognosis for complete recovery is excellent provided that the patient receives competent, timely intervention.

CYTOMEGALOVIRUS INFECTION

Epidemiology

Cytomegalovirus (CMV) is a double-stranded DNA virus that replicates within the nucleus of an infected cell. Humans are its only known host. Like herpes simplex virus, CMV may remain latent in host cells after the initial infection. Recurrent infection is usually due to reactivation of endogenous latent virus rather than reinfection with a new strain of virus. Cell-mediated immunity is more important than humoral mechanisms in controlling infection.[70]

CMV is not highly contagious and, therefore, close personal contact is required for infection to occur. *Horizontal transmission* may result from receipt of an infected organ or blood, from sexual contact, or from contact with contaminated saliva or urine. *Vertical transmission* may occur as a result of transplacental infection, exposure to contaminated genital tract secretions during delivery, or breast-feeding. The incubation period of the virus ranges from 28 to 60 days, with a mean of 40 days.[70-72]

Among young children, the most important risk factor for infection is close contact with playmates, particularly in the setting of day-care. In an early report, Pass and co-workers[73] surveyed 70 children attending a day-care center in Birmingham, Alabama. Investigators obtained mouth swabs from 29 children and urine specimens from 68. Forty-five percent of mouth swabs and 53 percent of urine cultures were positive for CMV. Nine percent of infants less than 1 year of age shed virus in either saliva or urine; 83 percent of children 1 to 2 years of age shed virus.

Jones et al.[74] conducted a similar survey in a regular day-care center and a facility for developmentally delayed children. Twenty-two percent of children in both centers were viruric, and 11 percent shed virus in their saliva. Hutto and co-workers[75] surveyed 47 toddlers attending day-care. Fourteen (30 percent) shed virus in saliva. The highest rate of salivary excretion (80 percent) occurred in children 12 to 24 months of age. Forty percent of the children were viruric.

Infected children clearly pose a risk of transmitting virus to adult day-care workers. Adler[76] recently examined the rate of seroconversion to CMV among day-care employees. At the time of initial assessment, 202 workers were seronegative. Within 10 months, 19 (11 percent) had seroconverted. The rate of seroconversion

was greatest among employees who cared for children under 2 years of age.

Small children also pose a risk to members of their own family. Taber et al.[77] performed a serologic study and identified 68 families where both parents were seronegative for CMV. Over a 3-year period, seroconversion occurred in one or more members of 37 families (53 percent). Mean annual seroconversion rates were approximately 10 percent for fathers, mothers, and children. The index case was usually a child.

In addition to acquiring infection from young children, adolescents and adults may develop infection as a result of sexual contact. CMV infection is endemic among gay men and heterosexuals with multiple partners.[70,78] Additional risk factors for infection include lower socioeconomic status, history of abnormal cervical cytology, birth outside of North America, first pregnancy at less than 15 years, and co-infection with other sexually transmitted diseases (STDs) such as trichomoniasis.[79]

Clinical Manifestations in Children and Adults

Most children who acquire CMV infection are asymptomatic. When clinical manifestations are present, they usually are mild and include malaise, fever, lymphadenopathy, and hepatosplenomegaly. Similarly, most adults with either primary or recurrent CMV are asymptomatic. Symptomatic patients typically have findings suggestive of mononucleosis. Respiratory infection is uncommon in adults with normal immune function, but an increasing number of cases of serious CMV infection are likely to occur as a consequence of the rising prevalence of HIV infection in women.

Diagnosis of Infection in Adults and Children

The diagnosis of CMV infection can be confirmed by isolation of virus in tissue culture. The highest concentration of CMV is usually present in urine, seminal fluid, saliva, and breast milk. Several different cell lines have been used to support viral growth, and techniques such as the viral shell assay, immunofluorescent staining, monoclonal antibody, and polymerase chain reaction (PCR) permit identification of viral antigen within 24 hours.[80-83]

Serologic methods also are helpful in establishing the diagnosis of CMV infection, provided that the reference laboratory is skilled in performing such tests. In the acute phase of infection, virus-specific immunoglobulin M (IgM) antibody is present in serum. IgM titers usually decline rapidly over a period of 30 to 60 days, but they can remain elevated for several months. There is no absolute immunoglobulin G (IgG) titer that clearly will differentiate acute from recurrent infection. However, a fourfold or greater change in the IgG titer is consistent with recent acute infection.[70] Other laboratory tests suggestive of CMV infection include a differential WBC count showing atypical lymphocytes, low platelet count, and elevated serum transaminase concentrations.

Congenital and Perinatal Infection

As a result of exposure to either young children or an infected sexual partner, approximately 50 to 80 percent of adult women in the United States have serologic evidence of past CMV infection. Unfortunately, the presence of antibody is not perfectly protective against vertical transmission; thus, pregnant women with both recurrent and primary infection pose a special risk to their fetus. Fetal and neonatal CMV infection may occur at three distinct times: antepartum, intrapartum, and postpartum. Antepartum or congenital infection is the greatest risk to the fetus and is perhaps the most difficult to understand because of the often bewildering array of statistics reported in epidemiologic surveys.

Congenital (Antepartum) Infection

Congenital CMV infection results from hematogenous dissemination of virus across the placenta. Dissemination may occur with both primary and recurrent (reactivated) infection but is much more likely in the former setting. From 1 to 4 percent of uninfected women seroconvert during pregnancy.[84] In women who acquire primary infection, 40 to 50 percent of the fetuses will be infected. Based on work with a guinea pig model, Kumar and Prokay[85] have concluded that the overall risk of congenital infection is greatest when maternal infection occurs in the third trimester, but the probability of severe fetal injury is highest when maternal infection occurs in the first trimester.

Of fetuses with congenital infection, 5 to 18 percent will be overtly symptomatic at birth. The most common clinical manifestations are hepatosplenomegaly, intracranial calcifications, jaundice, growth restriction, microcephaly, chorioretinitis, and hearing loss. The most frequent laboratory abnormalities are thrombocytopenia, hyperbilirubinemia, and elevated serum transaminase concentrations. Approximately 30 percent of severely infected infants die. Eighty percent of the survivors have severe neurologic morbidity, ocular abnormalities, or sensorineural hearing loss.[86,87] Approximately 85 to 90 percent of infants delivered to mothers with primary infection will be asymptomatic at birth. Ten to 15 percent subsequently develop hearing loss, chorioretinitis, or dental defects within the first 2 years of life.

Pregnant women who experience recurrent CMV infection are much less likely to transmit infection to their fetus. Recurrent infection occurs predominantly as a result of reactivation of latent infection rather than reinfection with a new viral strain. The most recent, and probably clearest, delineation of fetal risk in this situation is the report by Fowler et al.[87] In an excellent epidemiologic investigation, these authors studied 125 women with serologic evidence of primary infection and 64 with recurrent infection. In the former group, 18 percent of infants were symptomatic at birth. An additional 7 percent developed at least one major sequela within 5 years of follow-up. Two percent died, 15 percent had sensorineural hearing loss, and 13 percent had IQs less than 70. In contrast, none of the infants delivered to mothers with recurrent infection were symptomatic at birth. During the period of surveillance, 8 percent had at least one sequela, but none had multiple defects. The most common sequela was hearing loss. The authors concluded that maternal antibody provided substantial, but not complete, protection against serious fetal infection.

Overall, approximately 1 percent of infants (40,000) born in the United States each year have congenital CMV infection. Approximately 3,000 to 4,000 infants are symptomatic at birth, and an additional 4,000 to 6,000 subsequently have neurologic or developmental problems in the first years of life. CMV infection is now the principal cause of hearing deficits in children. Public health officials estimate that the annual cost of caring for children with congenital CMV is $1.86 billion.[88]

Perinatal (Intrapartum and Postpartum) Infection

Perinatal infection may occur *during delivery* as a result of exposure to infected genital tract secretions. At the time of delivery, up to 10 percent of pregnant women may be shedding CMV in cervical secretions and/or urine. Twenty to 60 percent of exposed fetuses may subsequently shed virus in their pharynx and/or urine. The incubation period for this form of infection ranges from 7 to 12 weeks, with an average of 8 weeks. Fortunately, infected infants rarely have serious sequelae of infection acquired during delivery.[86,89]

Perinatal infection also may develop as a *result of breast-feeding*. Stagno et al.[90] surveyed 278 women who had recently delivered and who agreed to provide samples of breast milk. Thirty-eight (13 percent) had CMV isolated at least once from colostrum or milk. Twenty-eight of these women were shedding CMV only in breast milk. Nineteen of their neonates were breast-fed, and 11 (58 percent) acquired CMV infection, despite the presence of neutralizing antibody in breast milk. Fortunately, serious sequelae did not occur in infected infants.

Diagnosis of Fetal Infection

In recent years, much attention has focused on analysis of amniotic fluid and fetal serum as a means to diagnose congenital infection. Several authors have compared the relative value of the following diagnostic tests: viral culture of amniotic fluid and fetal serum, determination of total IgM concentration in fetal serum, identification of anti-CMV IgM in fetal serum, and assessment of fetal liver function tests. These reports uniformly have supported the superiority of amniotic fluid analysis (viral culture or nucleic acid probe for viral antigen) in confirming the diagnosis of congenital CMV infection.

Lange and co-workers[91] were the first to report successful diagnosis of congenital infection by sampling of fetal blood. They performed cordocentesis on a hydropic fetus at 25 weeks' gestation, and the fetal blood smear showed severe erythroblastosis. Total IgM concentration was normal, but virus-specific IgM antibody to CMV was detected by radioimmunoassay. Hohlfeld et al.[80] subsequently described their assessment of 15 women with documented primary CMV infection in pregnancy. Eight fetuses were infected, and all were correctly identified by detection of antigen in amniotic fluid by the shell vial assay. In each instance, the subsequent viral culture was positive. Only four fetuses (50 percent) had increased total IgM concentrations and abnormal liver function tests. Two fetuses had thrombocytopenia, and none had positive viral blood cultures. The finding of a negative amniotic fluid culture was 100 percent specific in predicting the absence of congenital infection.

Lynch and co-authors[82] recently described their experience with assessment of 12 patients, 7 of whom had serologically confirmed primary infection and 5 of whom were evaluated because of abnormal sonographic findings. Eleven of the patients had an amniocentesis and cordocentesis. Of the seven women with serologically confirmed primary CMV infection, only one fetus was infected. This fetus had a normal hematocrit and platelet count, negative IgM-specific antibody, elevated γ-glutamyltranspeptidase (GGTP) concentration, and positive amniotic fluid culture. In the group of five women with abnormal sonograms, all of the fetuses were infected. Four (80 percent) had positive amniotic fluid cultures, and none had a positive blood culture. One had thrombocytopenia, three had elevated GGTP, and four had elevated total IgM.

In the most recent and largest series of invasive diagnostic testing for congenital CMV infection, Donner et al.[83] assessed 52 fetuses at risk for congenital CMV.

Sixteen fetuses were infected, 13 of whom were diagnosed antenatally. Thirteen of 16 (81 percent) had at least one abnormal test. Detection of virus in amniotic fluid by culture or PCR methodology correctly identified 12 (75 percent) infected fetuses. Four patients required two amnioceteses to establish the diagnosis. Nine of 16 fetuses (56 percent) had virus-specific IgM antibody in cord blood. Six of 11 (55 percent) fetuses who had hematologic assays were thrombocytopenic. A negative amniotic fluid culture was 100 percent specific in identifying an uninfected fetus.

Although identification of virus in amniotic fluid appears to be the most sensitive and specific test for diagnosing congenital infection, it does not necessarily identify the *severity* of fetal injury. This issue is obviously of great importance in counseling parents about the prognosis for their infant. Fortunately, detailed sonography can be invaluable in providing information about severity of fetal impairment. The principal sonographic findings suggestive of serious fetal injury include microcephaly, ventriculomegaly, intracerebral calcifications, hydrops, growth restriction, and oligohydramnios.[92] Unusual findings that also may indicate a severely infected infant include fetal heart block,[93] intra-abdominal echodensities,[94] meconium peritonitis,[95] and isolated serous effusions.[92] Clinicians should be aware that the ultrasound examination may be normal early in the course of fetal infection. Therefore, fetuses at risk should have repeat examinations to determine if anomalies are apparent.

Treatment and Prevention

At the present time, a vaccine for CMV is not available. Antiviral agents such as ganciclovir and foscarnet have moderate activity against CMV, but their use is limited primarily to treatment of severe infections in immunocompromised patients. Accordingly, obstetrician–gynecologists should focus most of their attention on educating patients about preventive measures.

One of the most important interventions is helping patients understand that CMV infection can be a sexually transmitted disease and that sexual promiscuity significantly increases an individual's risk of acquiring the infection. Individuals who have multiple sexual partners should be counseled that latex condoms provide an effective barrier to transmission of CMV.[96] Another important intervention is educating health care workers, day-care workers, elementary school teachers, and mothers of young children about the importance of simple infection control measures such as handwashing and proper cleansing of environmental surfaces. Obstetricians and pediatricians must be consistently aware of the importance of transfusing only CMV-free blood products to fetuses, neonates, pregnant women, and immunocompromised patients, and screening potential donors of organs and semen for CMV infection.[71] Finally, health care workers must adhere to the principles of universal precautions when treating patients and handling potentially infected body fluids.[84]

For several reasons, routine prenatal screening for CMV infection is not recommended. First, laboratory resources could be overwhelmed if all pregnant women were screened. Second, if laboratories do not ensure a high level of quality control, the interpretation of serologic tests may be confusing and may lead to incorrect and irreversible interventions such as pregnancy termination. Third, neither antiviral chemotherapy nor immunoprophylaxis is available to protect the fetus or neonate. Accordingly, screening should be limited to women who have symptoms suggestive of acute CMV infection, who have had definite occupational exposure to CMV, or who are immunocompromised.

GROUP B STREPTOCOCCAL INFECTION

Epidemiology

Streptococcus agalactiae is a gram-positive encapsulated coccus that produces β-hemolysis when grown on blood agar. On average, approximately 20 to 25 percent of pregnant women harbor group B streptococci in their lower genital tract and/or rectum. The group B streptococcus is one of the most important causes of early-onset neonatal infection. The prevalence of neonatal group B streptococcal infection is 1 to 2 per 1,000 live births, and approximately 10,000 to 12,000 cases of neonatal streptococcal septicemia occur each year in the United States.[97,98]

Neonatal group B streptococcal infection can be divided into *early-onset* and *late-onset* infection. Approximately 80 to 85 percent of cases of neonatal group B streptococcal infection are early in onset and result almost exclusively from vertical transmission from a colonized mother. Early-onset infection presents primarily as a severe pneumonia and/or overwhelming septicemia. In preterm infants, the mortality from early-onset group B streptococcal infection approaches 25 percent. In term infants, the mortality is lower, averaging approximately 5 percent in recent investigations. Late-onset neonatal group B streptococcal infection occurs as a result of both vertical and horizontal transmission. It is typically manifested by bacteremia, meningitis, and pneumonia. The mortality from late onset infection is approximately 5 to 10 percent for both preterm and term infants.[97,98]

Unfortunately, obstetric interventions have proven ineffective in preventing late-onset neonatal infection. Therefore, the remainder of this discussion will focus on early-onset infection. Major risk factors for early-onset infection include preterm labor, especially when complicated by preterm premature rupture of membranes (PROM); intrapartum maternal fever (chorioamnionitis); prolonged rupture of membranes, defined as greater than 12–18 hours; and previous delivery of an infected infant.[97,99,100] Approximately 25 percent of pregnant women have at least one risk factor for group B streptococcal infection. The neonatal attack rate in colonized patients is 40 to 50 percent in the presence of a risk factor, and less than or equal to 5 percent in the absence of a risk factor. In infected infants, neonatal mortality approaches 30 to 35 percent when a maternal risk factor is present but is less than or equal to 5 percent when a risk factor is absent.[97–99]

Maternal Complications

Several obstetric complications occur with increased frequency in pregnant women who are colonized with group B streptococci.[97] The organism is a major cause of chorioamnionitis and postpartum endometritis. It also may cause postcesarean wound infection, usually in conjunction with other aerobic and anaerobic bacilli and staphylococci. Group B streptococci also are responsible for approximately 2 to 3 percent of lower urinary tract infections in pregnant women but usually do not cause pyelonephritis. Group B streptococcal urinary tract infection, in turn, is a risk factor for preterm labor. Thomsen et al.[101] recently reported a study of 69 women at 27 to 31 weeks' gestation who had streptococcal urinary tract infections. Patients were assigned to treatment with either penicillin or placebo. Treated patients had a significant reduction in the frequency of both preterm PROM and preterm labor. Other investigations have confirmed the association between group B streptococcal colonization and preterm labor and preterm PROM. Women with the latter complication who are colonized with group B streptococci tend to have a shorter latent period and higher frequency of chorioamnionitis and puerperal endometritis compared to noncolonized women.[102]

Diagnosis

The "gold standard" for the diagnosis of group B streptococcal infection is bacteriologic culture. Todd-Hewitt broth or selective blood agar is the preferred medium. Specimens for culture should be obtained from the lower vagina, perineum, and perianal area, using a simple cotton swab. In recent years, considerable research has been devoted to assessment of rapid diagnostic tests for the identification of colonized women. Table 40–9 summarizes the results of several investigations of rapid diagnostic tests. The information in this table is based on the review by Yancey et al.[103]

Table 40–9. RELIABILITY OF RAPID DIAGNOSTIC TESTS FOR GROUP B STREPTOCOCCI

Test	Test Performance			
	Sensitivity (%)	Specificity (%)	PV+ (%)	PV− (%)
Gram's stain	34–100	60–70	13–33	86–100
Growth in starch medium	93–98	98–99	65–98	89–99
Antigen detection (coagglutination, latex particle agglutination, enzyme immunoassay)	4–88*	92–100	15–100	76–99
DNA probe†	71	90	61	94

PV+, positive predictive value; PV−, negative predictive value.
* Sensitivities for identification of heavily colonized women ranged from 29–100%.
† Specimens were grown in culture for 3.5 hours before DNA probe was used.
Information in this table is from Yancey et al.[103]

These authors noted that, although the rapid diagnostic tests had reasonable sensitivity in identifying heavily colonized patients, they had poor sensitivity in identifying lightly and moderately colonized patients. This latter finding severely limits the usefulness of the rapid diagnostic tests in clinical practice.

Prevention of Group B Streptococcal Infection

In the past 20 years, several different strategies have been proposed for the prevention of neonatal group B streptococcal infection.[98–106] Each strategy has had major imperfections. In 1996, however, the Centers for Disease Control and Prevention (CDC) published a series of recommendations that incorporated the major advantages of previous protocols and minimized some of the more problematic aspects of selected strategies.[107] The CDC guidelines recommend universal culturing of all patients at 35 to 37 weeks. Samples should be obtained from the lower vagina, perineum, and perianal area and cultured in selective media such as Todd-Hewitt broth. Patients who are colonized should receive intrapartum prophylaxis with one of the antibiotic regimens listed in Table 40–10. If culture results are unavailable (e.g., a patient with preterm labor or a patient who failed to register for prenatal care), the patient should receive intrapartum prophylaxis if she has a recognized risk factor for early-onset neonatal group B streptococcal infection.

Ideally, antibiotics should be administered at least four hours prior to delivery. DeCueto et al.[109] recently demonstrated that the rate of neonatal group B streptococcal infection was significantly reduced when patients had been treated for at least this period of time. In a large population-based survey, Rosenstein and Schuchat[108] assessed the theoretical impact of the CDC recommendations and showed that a strategy of universal culturing and treatment of *all* colonized patients would prevent 78 percent of cases of neonatal infection. In contrast, only 41 percent of cases were prevented when patients were targeted for prophylaxis only on the basis of risk factors. In addition, Locksmith et al.[110] recently confirmed that the CDC strategy also was of value in decreasing the rate of maternal infection compared to a strategy of only treating on the basis of risk factors.

HEPATITIS

Hepatitis is one of the most common and most highly contagious viral infections. At present, six distinct types of hepatitis virus have been identified: A, B, C, D, E, and G. Each type of hepatitis has a slightly different clinical implication for the pregnant woman and her fetus.

Hepatitis A

Hepatitis A is responsible for approximately 30 to 35 percent of cases of hepatitis in the United States. It is caused by a 27-nm ribonucleic acid (RNA) virus that is a member of the picornavirus family. The virus is transmitted by person-to-person contact through fecal–oral contamination. Poor hygiene, poor sanitation, and intimate personal or sexual contact facilitate transmission. Epidemics frequently result from common exposure to

Table 40–10. ANTIBIOTICS WITH ACTIVITY AGAINST GROUP B STREPTOCOCCI

Drug	Dose for Intrapartum Prophylaxis
Ampicillin	2 g initially, then 1 g q4h
Penicillin	5 million units initially, then 2.5 million units q4h
Erythromycin	500 mg q6h
Clindamycin	900 mg q8h
Vancomycin	500 mg q6h

contaminated food and water. In the United States, individuals at particular risk for hepatitis A are those who have recently immigrated from, or traveled to, developing nations of the world where the disease is endemic.[111] Drug abusers, gay men, and children in day-care centers also are at increased risk of acquiring hepatitis A.[112,113]

The incubation period of hepatitis A ranges from 15 to 50 days, with a mean of 28 to 30 days. The highest concentration of viral particles is in fecal material. The virus is not normally excreted in urine or other body fluids.

Some patients with hepatitis A are relatively asymptomatic. When symptoms do occur, they usually include malaise, fatigue, anorexia, nausea and vomiting, and right upper quadrant pain. The characteristic physical findings of acute hepatitis A are jaundice, hepatic tenderness, darkened urine, and acholic stools.

The most useful diagnostic test for hepatitis A is detection of IgM-specific antibody. IgM antibody usually is detectable 25 to 30 days following the initial exposure and persists in the serum for up to 6 months. IgG antibody is detectable within 35 to 40 days of exposure and persists indefinitely, thus conferring lifelong immunity. In addition, the serum concentration of alanine aminotransferase (ALT), aspartate aminotransferase (AST), and bilirubin are usually moderately to markedly elevated. Liver biopsy is rarely indicated to confirm the diagnosis of viral hepatitis.[114] When performed, it characteristically shows extensive hepatocellular injury and a prominent inflammatory infiltrate (Fig. 40–6).

Fortunately, acute hepatitis A is usually a self-limited illness, and only supportive care is required for the vast majority of patients. Recovery is typically complete within 4 to 6 weeks. Fewer than 0.5 percent of affected patients develop fulminant hepatitis, coagulopathy, or encephalopathy. Such individuals clearly require hospitalization; others may be treated as outpatients. Infected patients should be advised of the need for sound nutrition. Physical activity should be limited to prevent upper abdominal trauma. Drugs with potential hepatotoxicity should be avoided. Sexual and household contacts should receive immunoprophylaxis with a single intramuscular dose of immune globulin, 0.02 ml/kg within 2 weeks of exposure. In addition, they also should receive the formalin-inactivated hepatitis A vaccine, in a single intramuscular dose of 0.06 ml. The vaccine is highly immunogenic and is safe for use in pregnancy.[115,116]

As a general rule, unless the pregnant mother becomes severely ill, hepatitis A does not pose a serious risk to the fetus. Perinatal transmission of infection rarely occurs, and a chronic carrier state does not exist. An infant delivered to an acutely infected mother should receive immune globulin to prevent horizontal transmission of infection after delivery.[114]

Hepatitis B

Approximately 40 to 45 percent of all cases of hepatitis in the United States are caused by hepatitis B virus. Over 300,000 new cases of hepatitis B occur annually,

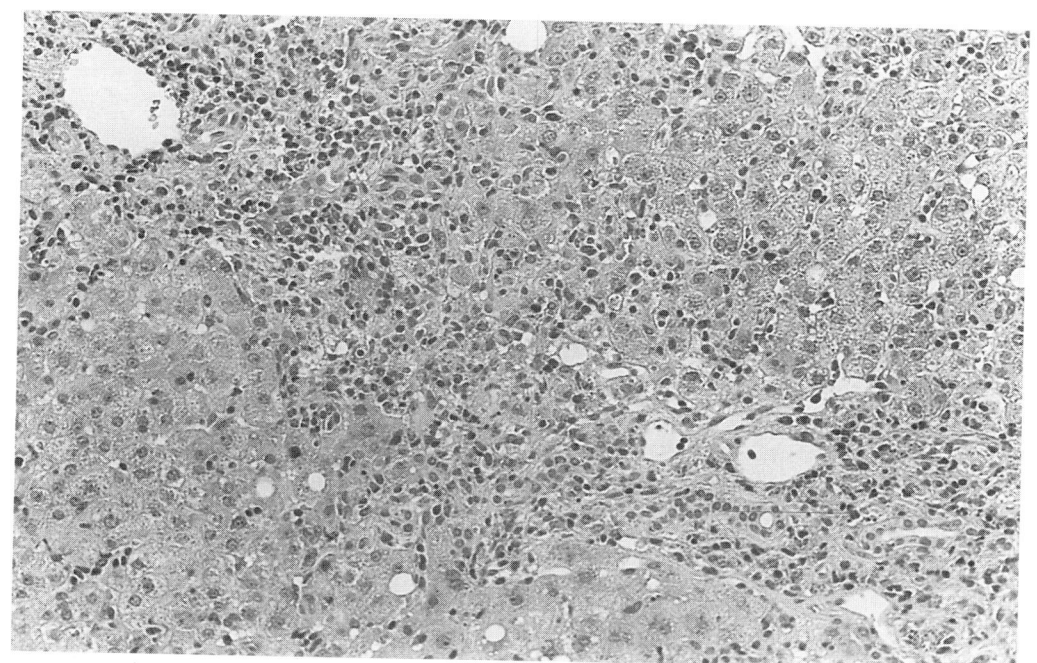

Figure 40–6. Photomicrograph of liver biopsy shows characteristic histologic changes of acute viral hepatitis. Note the intense inflammatory infiltrate.

and about 1 million Americans are chronic viral carriers. The frequencies of acute and chronic hepatitis B in pregnancy are 1 to 2 per 1,000 and 5 to 15 per 1,000, respectively.[117]

Hepatitis B is caused by a DNA virus, and the intact virus is termed the Dane particle. The virus has three major structural antigens: surface antigen (HBsAg), core antigen (HBcAg), and e antigen (HBeAg). Transmission of hepatitis B occurs primarily as a result of parenteral injection, sexual contact, and perinatal exposure.[114] Certain population groups have an increased prevalence of hepatitis B: Asians, Eskimos, drug addicts, transfusion recipients, dialysis patients, residents and employees of chronic care residencies, prisoners, and recipients of tattoos.

Following an acute infection caused by hepatitis B virus, less than 1 percent of patients develop fulminant hepatitis and die. Eighty-five to 90 percent experience complete resolution of their physical findings and develop protective levels of antibody. Ten to 15 percent of patients become chronically infected. Of these, 15 to 30 percent subsequently develop chronic active or persistent hepatitis or cirrhosis, and a small percentage develop hepatocellular carcinoma. Chronic liver disease is particularly likely to occur in patients who remain seropositive for HBeAg or who become superinfected with the hepatitis D virus.[114]

The diagnosis of *acute* hepatitis B is confirmed by detection of the surface antigen and IgM antibody to the core antigen. Identification of HBeAg is indicative of an exceptionally high viral inoculum and active viral replication. Patients who have *chronic* hepatitis B infection have persistence of the surface antigen in the serum and liver tissue. Some individuals, particularly Asians, also remain seropositive for HBeAg.[114,115,118]

Patients with acute and chronic hepatitis B infection pose a major threat of transmission to other household members, especially their sexual partner. In addition, infected women also may transmit infection to their fetus. Perinatal transmission occurs primarily as a result of the infant's exposure to infected blood and genital secretions during delivery. In the absence of immunoprophylaxis for the neonate, perinatal transmission occurs in 10 to 20 percent of women who are seropositive for HBsAg. The frequency of perinatal transmission increases to almost 90 percent in women who are seropositive for both HBsAg and HBeAg.[114,115,119]

Fortunately, a combination of passive and active immunization is highly effective in preventing both horizontal and vertical transmission of hepatitis B infection. All individuals who have had household or sexual exposure to another person with hepatitis B infection should be tested to determine if they have antibody to the virus. If they are seronegative, they should immediately receive immunoprophylaxis with hepatitis B immune globulin (HBIG), 0.06 ml/kg IM. They then should receive the hepatitis B vaccination series. Similarly, infants who are delivered to seropositive mothers should receive HBIG, 0.5 ml IM, immediately after birth. They then should begin the hepatitis B vaccination series within 12 hours of birth. At the present time, two recombinant hepatitis B vaccines are available, Recombivax-HB and Engerix-B.[114,115] Both products are composed of inactivated portions of the surface antigen and are prepared by recombinant DNA technology. Neither poses a risk of transmission of a bloodborne pathogen, and both are safe for administration during pregnancy to patients at risk.

Neonatal immunoprophylaxis is approximately 85 to 95 percent effective in preventing neonatal hepatitis B infection. In view of the extremely favorable results of immunoprophylaxis, the CDC recently recommended universal hepatitis B vaccination for all infants.[120] Dosage recommendations vary depending on the mother's serostatus. Infants born to seronegative mothers require only the vaccine. Infants born to seropositive mothers should receive both the vaccine and hepatitis B immune globulin. Therefore, obstetricians must continue to screen *all* of their patients for hepatitis B at some point during pregnancy. Selective screening on the basis of acknowledged risk factors will fail to identify 30 to 50 percent of seropositive women.[114]

Patients infected with hepatitis B virus also may transmit infection to medical and nursing personnel who care for them. Each year, approximately 12,000 American health care workers contract hepatitis B as a result of an occupational injury such as a needle stick or splash to a mucous membrane. Of these, approximately 200 develop fulminant hepatitis and subsequently die.[115,121] Health care workers can protect themselves from hepatitis in three principal ways. First, they should be vaccinated for hepatitis B. Second, they should encourage *all* young adults and other individuals who have a specific risk factor to receive the hepatitis B vaccine. Third, they should consistently follow universal precautions to prevent sharp injuries and splashes to exposed mucous membrane or skin surfaces.

Conversely, health care workers who are infected with hepatitis B also pose a risk to others. They, too, must observe safeguards to prevent horizontal transmission of infection to their patients. Infection is most likely to occur as a consequence of direct blood-to-blood exposure during invasive surgical procedures. Unless the patient has documented immunity to hepatitis B, the infected health care worker has an ethical obligation to inform her that some risk of transmission exists. The attendant should then perform the procedure only if the patient explicitly consents. During the actual procedure, the operator must take every precaution to ensure that a sharp injury and resultant blood-to-blood contact do not occur.

Non-A, Non-B Hepatitis

Non-A, non-B hepatitis accounts for 10 to 20 percent of cases of hepatitis in the United States. Non-A, non-B hepatitis occurs in two forms: parenterally transmitted hepatitis C and enterically transmitted hepatitis E.

Hepatitis C

Hepatitis C is a 30- to 38-nm, single-stranded RNA virus that is similar in structure to flaviviruses and pestiviruses. Its incubation period is 5 to 10 weeks. The principal risk factors for hepatitis C are intravenous drug abuse, transfusion, and sexual intercourse.[122] In a recent survey by Osmond and co-workers,[123] two thirds of a selected population of drug abusers were seropositive for hepatitis C. In a similar survey of patients attending an STD clinic in San Francisco, Weinstock et al.[124] found the prevalence of hepatitis C to be 7.7 percent. Approximately 90 percent of all cases of post-transfusion hepatitis are due to hepatitis C, and 2.5 to 15 percent of patients who receive multiple transfusions become infected with this virus. Hepatitis C is particularly likely to result in chronic liver disease. Approximately 50 percent of infected patients develop biochemical evidence of hepatic dysfunction. Of these, about 20 percent subsequently develop chronic active hepatitis or cirrhosis.[114]

Approximately 75 percent of patients with hepatitis C are asymptomatic. The diagnosis of hepatitis C infection is confirmed by identification of anti-C antibody. Initial screening for this antibody should be performed with an enzyme immunoassay (EIA). A positive EIA should be followed with a recombinant immunoblot assay (RIBA). The present RIBA is able to detect four specific viral antigens. If at least two antigens are identified, the test is considered positive. If only one antigen is identified, the test is considered indeterminant. The present generation of laboratory assays does not precisely discriminate between IgM and IgG antibody. Moreover, antibody may not be detectable until up to 22 weeks after the onset of clinical illness. Direct detection of antigen also is possible with PCR methodology, although this test is not yet widely available.[114]

In a general obstetric population, the prevalence of hepatitis C is 1 to 3 percent. The principal risk factors that identify an obstetric patient at high risk for hepatitis C include concurrent STDs such as hepatitis B and HIV infection, multiple sexual partners, history of recent multiple transfusions, and history of intravenous drug abuse.[125] The frequency of perinatal transmission is highly variable. In women who are co-infected with human immunodeficiency virus and/or who have high serum concentrations of hepatitis C RNA, the transmission rate may be as high as 40 percent. In other patients, the rate of transmission is less than or equal to 10 percent.[122,126]

At the present time, a vaccine for hepatitis C is not available. Passive immunization with immunoglobulin (0.06 ml/kg IM) should be administered following percutaneous exposure to a person with hepatitis C. The benefit of immunoprophylaxis for the neonate has not been proven in controlled clinical trials. Although interferon-α has shown some activity against the virus, relapses occur in 44 to 80 percent of patients within 6 to 12 months of discontinuation of therapy.[114]

Hepatitis E

The hepatitis E virus is an RNA virus that is closely related to the calicivirus family. It may present in both an icteric and anicteric form. The virus is transmitted by the fecal–oral route and, therefore, the epidemiology of hepatitis E is similar to that of hepatitis A. The incubation period ranges from 2 to 9 weeks, with a mean of 45 days.[127,128] Hepatitis E is rare in the United States but is endemic in developing countries.[129–131] In these countries, maternal mortality has been alarmingly high, ranging from 10 to 20 percent. Extreme poverty, coexisting medical illnesses, malnutrition, and poor prenatal care are at least partially responsible for the poor maternal prognosis. The only cases of hepatitis E in the United States have occurred in patients who traveled to countries where the disease was endemic.[132]

Three new diagnostic tests are available for confirmation of hepatitis E infection. Viral-like particles can be identified in the stool of infected patients by electron microscopy. These particles will agglutinate when combined with serum from the patient. In addition, a fluorescent antibody blocking assay and Western blot assay are now available for use.[114,132]

Women with hepatitis E require intensive supportive care. As a general rule, if the mother survives, fetal outcome is not adversely affected. A chronic carrier state does not occur, and perinatal transmission is distinctly uncommon. However, Khuroo et al.[133] recently described eight mothers who developed hepatitis E in the third trimester. Six of their infants had clinical and/or serologic evidence of hepatitis E. Two infants had hypothermia and hypoglycemia and died within 24 hours of birth.

Hepatitis D

Hepatitis D, or delta hepatitis, is caused by an RNA virus that is dependent on co-infection with the hepatitis B virus for replication. Hepatitis D has an external coat of hepatitis B surface antigen and an internal delta antigen that is encoded by its own genome. The epidemiology of hepatitis D is essentially identical to that of hepatitis B.[134]

Acute hepatitis D occurs in two forms: *co-infection* and *superinfection*. Co-infection represents the simultaneous occurrence of acute hepatitis B and D. It is usually a self-limited disorder and rarely leads to chronic liver disease. Superinfection occurs when *acute* hepatitis D develops in a patient who is a *chronic* hepatitis B carrier. Approximately 20 to 25 percent of patients with chronic hepatitis B ultimately become superinfected with the delta virus, and about 80 percent of these individuals subsequently develop chronic hepatitis. Of those who have chronic hepatitis, 70 to 80 percent develop cirrhosis and portal hypertension and, unfortunately, almost 25 percent ultimately die of hepatic failure.[134,135]

The clinical manifestations of acute hepatitis D are similar to those of any acute viral hepatitis. The diagnosis of *acute co-infection* can be confirmed by detection of delta antigen in hepatic tissue or serum and IgM-specific antibody in serum. In addition, the tests for HBsAg and HBcAb-IgM are positive. In patients with acute *superinfection,* serologic tests reflect acute hepatitis D (positive antigen, positive IgM antibody) and chronic hepatitis B infection (positive surface antigen, positive HBcAb-IgG). Patients with *chronic* hepatitis D usually have detectable serum levels of IgG-specific antibody for the delta virus and are seropositive for HBsAg. Unfortunately, IgG antibody does not eradicate the delta viremia, and the antigen still can be identified in serum and hepatic tissue.[114,134,135]

Patients with acute hepatitis D should receive the general supportive care outlined for hepatitis A. Patients with chronic infection should be monitored periodically for worsening hepatic function or coagulopathy. At present, there is no specific antiviral agent or immunotherapy that is curative for either acute or chronic delta infection. Perinatal transmission of hepatitis D virus has been reported. Fortunately, transmission is uncommon because the neonatal immunoprophylaxis for hepatitis B is almost uniformly effective against hepatitis D.[114]

Hepatitis G

Hepatitis G (HGV or GBV-C) is a recently discovered single-stranded RNA virus that is related to hepatitis C. It can cause acute and persistent infections in humans, but the disease is usually mild, and the clinical significance of infection is uncertain. Persistent infection is usually not associated with biochemical evidence of ongoing hepatic injury. Hepatitis G is more prevalent, but less virulent, than hepatitis C. Co-infection with hepatitis A, B, and C and HIV is common. A chronic carrier state has been described, and perinatal transmission has been documented. Hepatitis G nucleic acid can be detected by PCR, and an envelope protein can be identified by enzyme-linked immunosorbent assay (ELISA).

At present, no immunoprophylactic agent or antiviral chemotherapy for hepatitis G is available.[136]

HERPES SIMPLEX VIRUS INFECTION

Epidemiology

Herpes simplex virus (HSV), a double-stranded DNA virus, is transmitted by direct, intimate contact. Following the initial infection, the virus remains dormant in neuronal ganglia and may reactivate at later times. Two strains of the virus have been identified: HSV-1 and HSV-2. The former causes primarily oropharyngeal infection and the latter, genital tract infection. Approximately 0.5 to 1.0 percent of women have an overt herpetic infection during pregnancy. About 400 cases of neonatal herpes occur annually in the United States, and the estimated incidence of neonatal infection ranges from 1 in 7,500 to 1 in 30,000 live births.[137,138]

HSV infections are classified as *primary, nonprimary first episode,* and *recurrent* on the basis of historical and clinical findings and serologic testing.[137–140] Table 40–11 summarizes the criteria for each diagnosis. Approximately 20 to 40 percent of Americans are seropositive for HSV. Up to 80 percent of these individuals do not have a history of an overt primary infection.

Clinical Manifestations

The onset of HSV infection is usually heralded by a prodrome of neuralgias, paresthesias, and hypesthesias, followed by an eruption of painful vesicles in either the orolabial area or genitalia. The vesicles typically rupture, forming a shallow-based ulcer (Fig. 40–7), and then form a dry crust. Some vesicles become secondarily infected and evolve into frank pustules. Ultimately, the vesicles heal without scarring.[137,138]

In patients experiencing a primary HSV infection,

Table 40–11. CLASSIFICATION OF HERPES SIMPLEX VIRUS INFECTION

Classification	Criteria
Primary	First clinical infection
	No preexisting antibody
Nonprimary, first episode	No history of genital tract infection
	Positive antibody for the other strain of the virus (HSV1 or HSV2)
Recurrent	Prior history of clinical infection
	Positive antibody for the same strain of virus causing the present infection

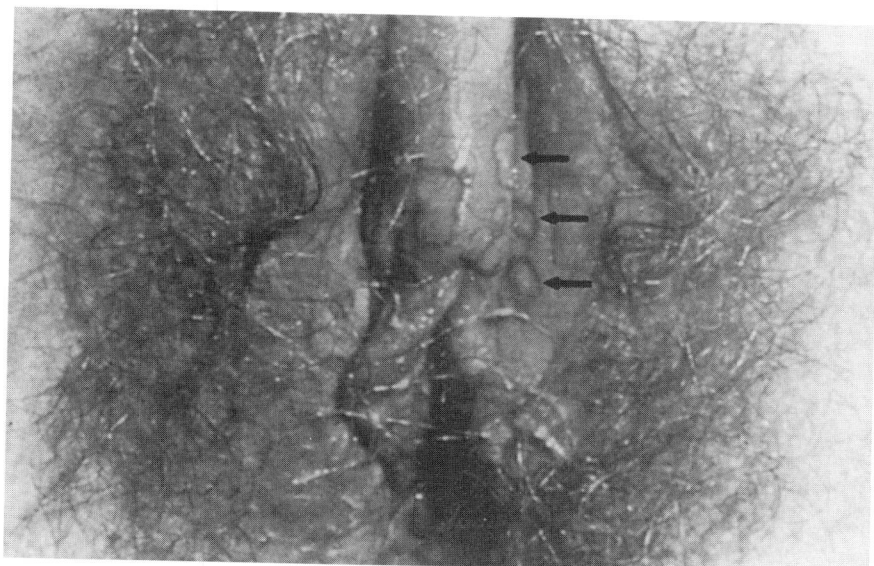

Figure 40–7. Ulcerated lesions (*arrows*) characteristic of herpes simplex infection. (From Duff P, Christian JS, Yancey MK: Infections associated with pregnancy. *In* Coulam CB, Faulk WP, McIntyre JA [eds]: Immunologic Obstetrics. New York, WW Norton & Co, 1992, p 578, with permission.)

vesicles may be present for up to 3 weeks. Systemic symptoms may be moderately severe, and local complications such as urinary retention may occur. In recurrent infections, overt vesicles are fewer in number and less painful and typically persist for less than or equal to 14 days. Table 40–12 compares the incubation period and clinical features of primary and recurrent HSV infection.[137]

In some patients, particularly those who are immunocompromised, HSV infection may be widely disseminated, affecting extensive areas of skin, mucosal membranes, and visceral organs. HSV also may cause a severe ocular infection, meningitis, encephalitis, and ascending myelitis.

Diagnosis

Several laboratory tests may be used to confirm the diagnosis of HSV infection. Cytologic preparations show characteristic multinucleated giant cells and intranuclear inclusions.[137,138] PCR assays are extremely sensitive in detecting low concentrations of viral DNA, but such assays are not yet widely available.[141] Serology is especially useful in classifying the initial herpetic episode as *primary* versus *nonprimary first episode*.[137,138] However, serologic testing is rarely indicated in patients who experience recurrent HSV infection.

Until the advent of PCR, viral isolation in tissue culture was considered the gold standard for confirmation of diagnosis. Viral isolation is usually possible within 72 to 96 hours of inoculation of the tissue culture. The highest rate of isolation is achieved when clinical specimens are obtained from fresh vesicles or pustules (Table 40–13). Vesicular fluid should be aspirated with a fine needle into a tuberculin syringe. Ulcers should be scraped vigorously with a wooden spatula or cotton-tipped applicator.[137,138]

Obstetric and Perinatal Complications

Severe primary HSV infection has been associated with spontaneous abortion, preterm delivery, and intrauterine growth restriction. Isolated case reports also have

Table 40–12. COMPARISON OF PRIMARY VERSUS RECURRENT HERPES SIMPLEX VIRUS INFECTION

	Type of Infection	
Stage of Illness	Primary	Recurrent
Incubation period and/or prodrome (days)	2–10	1–2
Vesicle, pustule (days)	6	2
Wet ulcer (days)	6	3
Dry crust (days)	8	7
Total	22–30	13–14

Table 40–13. FREQUENCY OF ISOLATION OF HERPES SIMPLEX VIRUS FROM SKIN LESIONS

Type of Lesion	Approximate Frequency of Viral Isolation
Vesicle	90%
Pustule	85%
Ulcer	70%
Crust	25%

been published documenting in utero infection even in the presence of intact membranes.[137,138,142] However, the greatest risk to the fetus occurs when overt HSV infection is present at the time of labor. In this situation, the principal mechanism of infection is direct contact with infected vesicles during the process of vaginal birth. The frequency of neonatal infection clearly is dependent on whether the mother has a primary or recurrent HSV infection. In the setting of a primary infection, the viral inoculum in the genital tract is high, and maternal antibody is not present. Approximately 40 percent of neonates delivered vaginally to such women will become infected. In the absence of antiviral chemotherapy, almost half of these infants die, and 35 to 40 percent experience severe neurologic morbidity such as chorioretinitis, microcephaly, mental retardation, seizures, and apnea. In women who have recurrent *symptomatic* HSV infection, the risk of neonatal infection following vaginal delivery is 5 percent or less. In women who have a history of recurrent HSV infection but no prodromal symptoms or overt lesions, the risk of neonatal infection with vaginal delivery is less than or equal to 1 in 1,000.[137,138,140,143–145]

Neonatal HSV infection may take many forms. In its simplest manifestation, it may appear as a localized abscess at the site of attachment of a scalp electrode or as isolated mucocutaneous lesions. In its more severe forms, neonatal HSV infection may present as widely disseminated mucocutaneous lesions, visceral infection, meningitis, and encephalitis. In such instances, mortality may approach 50 to 60 percent, and up to half of the survivors may have persistent morbidity.[137,138,140,142,143,146]

Management during Pregnancy

Clinical management of HSV infection has changed dramatically in recent years. For several reasons, surveillance cultures of the genital tract in patients with a history of HSV infection have been ineffective in preventing neonatal HSV infection.[147–149] First, cultures are not perfectly sensitive. In a recent report, Cone et al.[141] detected HSV DNA by PCR in 9 of 100 asymptomatic pregnant women who had negative viral cultures. Second, culture results are not always readily available at the time a patient is admitted for delivery. Third, most children with neonatal HSV infection are actually born to women who do not have a history of prior infection and who, hence, would not be targeted for surveillance cultures.[145,147–150]

Accordingly, the following simplified guidelines have now been recommended by the Infectious Diseases Society for Obstetrics and Gynecology and endorsed by the American College of Obstetricians and Gynecologists.[138,144] At the time of the patient's initial prenatal appointment, she should be questioned about a prior history of HSV infection. If her history is positive, she should be screened for other STDs such as gonorrhea, chlamydia, syphilis, hepatitis B and C, and HIV infection. When the patient ultimately is admitted for delivery, she should be asked about prodromal symptoms and examined thoroughly for cervical, vaginal, and vulvar lesions. If no prodromal symptoms or overt lesions are present, vaginal delivery should be anticipated. If symptoms or lesions are present, cesarean delivery should be performed. Cesarean secton is indicated even in the presence of ruptured membranes, since operative delivery significantly decreases the size of the viral inoculum to which the infant is exposed.

Mothers with symptomatic infection do not need to be isolated from their infants or other patients. They should wash their hands carefully before handling the infant and shield the baby from any contact with vesicular lesions. Breast-feeding is permissible as long as no skin lesions are present on the breast.

In addition to the guidelines outlined above, clinicians should be aware of possible indications for use of antiviral therapy during pregnancy. Immunocompromised patients with disseminated infections require hospitalization for treatment with intravenous acyclovir. Oral acyclovir (400 mg three times daily for 5 to 10 days) should be considered for immunocompetent patients who have *severe* herpetic infection (e.g., prominent systemic symptoms and urinary retention), especially near term.[151] Alternative regimens include valacyclovir (1,000 mg PO twice daily) or famciclovir (125 mg PO twice daily). Prophylactic treatment with oral acyclovir (400 mg twice daily) or valacyclovir (1,000 mg daily) may be appropriate in women with frequent recurrent infections in pregnancy, particularly near term.[151,152]

Acyclovir is classified by the FDA as a pregnancy category C drug. To date, the Acyclovir Registry has reported no increase in the frequency of adverse effects in infants exposed in utero to this antiviral agent.[153,154] Valaclovir and famciclovir are classified as pregnancy category B.

HUMAN IMMUNODEFICIENCY VIRUS INFECTION

Epidemiology

HIV infection is caused by a ribonucleic acid (RNA) retrovirus. The principal viral strain responsible for disease in the United States is HIV-1. HIV-2 is a related strain that is endemic in Africa, Portugal, and France. HIV-2 infection is uncommon in the United States except in individuals who have traveled to endemic areas or had sexual contact or shared needles with persons from endemic areas.[155,156]

HIV has a unique propensity to attack and infect CD4 lymphocytes. Upon entering the host cell, the virus uses its reverse transcriptase enzyme to synthesize DNA from RNA. It then integrates the DNA into the host genome. Subsequently, as the host cell replicates its nucleic acid, it also unwittingly replicates new viral nucleic acid. As viral replication continues, the CD4 lymphocyte is progressively weakened, and ultimately destroyed, thus rendering the host susceptible to an extensive variety of opportunistic infections and malignancies.[155]

HIV infection occurs in a continuum that can be divided arbitrarily into four stages. Stage 1 of the disease is the acute retroviral infection that develops several weeks after exposure to the virus. In this stage, the patient has symptoms similar to mononucleosis. Over a period of several weeks, the acute episode resolves, and the patient enters the latent phase of illness. During the latent phase, the patient is asymptomatic, but viral replication occurs, albeit slowly, in lymphatic tissue. The duration of the latent phase is approximately 5 to 10 years. Inexorably, the viral inoculum progressively increases, and the patient enters stage 3 of the disease. This stage is characterized by mild to moderately severe symptoms and debilitating, but usually not life-threatening, opportunistic infections. Ultimately, the patient develops acquired immunodeficiency syndrome (AIDS). Once symptomatic HIV infection develops, the patient's life expectancy is usually 3 to 5 years.[157]

At the present time, almost 500,000 Americans have AIDS, or have died from AIDS. An additional 1 million are infected with the virus but are not yet in the terminal stage of their illness. In the United States, approximately 15 to 20 percent of all cases of HIV infection occur in women. Almost 75 percent of infected women are black or Hispanic. In women, the two most important mechanisms of HIV infection are intravenous drug abuse and heterosexual contact with a high-risk male. In the general obstetric population in the United States, the frequency of HIV infection is approximately 1 per 1,000. However, in some inner city populations, the prevalence of infection is as high as 1 to 1.5 percent.[158–160]

Heterosexual transmission is increasing in importance as a mechanism of spread of HIV infection.[161] Several sexual practices have been shown to substantially increase the risk of transmission of infection. Of these, the most important is unprotected intercourse with multiple partners. Receptive anal intercourse is a particularly dangerous practice because the columnar epithelium of the anus and rectum is more susceptible to trauma than the stratified squamous epithelium of the vagina. The presence of other STDs that cause genital ulcers, such as herpes, syphilis, and chancroid, also is an important risk factor for HIV infection. Concurrent use of illicit intravenous drugs and crack cocaine and contact with a noncircumcised male also are independent risk factors for HIV infection.

Clinical Manifestations

Symptomatic patients with HIV infection typically have fever, malaise, fatigue, anorexia, nausea, vomiting, diarrhea, weight loss, and generalized lymphadenopathy. Neurologic manifestations may be quite prominent and debilitating, specifically peripheral neuropathy and dementia. These neurologic manifestations result both from direct injury of the central nervous system (CNS) by HIV and the effects of opportunistic infections such as toxoplasmosis.[155,157]

Opportunistic infections, of course, are the hallmark of HIV infection.[162] Among the most common are *Pneumocystis carinii* pneumonia, mycobacterium avium complex, pulmonary tuberculosis, toxoplasmosis, candidiasis, and cytomegalovirus infection. Genital herpes; hepatitis B, C, and D; and syphilis are common concurrent sexually transmitted diseases. Unusual malignancies occur with disturbing regularity in patients with HIV infection.[163] The two most common are Kaposi's sarcoma (rare in women, extremely common in homosexual men) and non-Hodgkin's lymphoma. The latter disorder has an alarming tendency for early invasion of the central nervous system.

Diagnosis

The diagnosis of HIV infection may be confirmed by direct culture of virus from peripheral blood lymphocytes and monocytes. The diagnosis also can be established by detection of viral antigen by PCR. Infected patients usually have a decreased number of CD4 cells and an inverted CD4:CD8 ratio. Serum immunoglobulin levels also are elevated.[164]

The principal diagnostic test at present is identification of virus-specific antibody.[164] The initial serologic screening test should be an enzyme immunoassay (EIA). This test is highly sensitive, inexpensive, and readily suited for screening large numbers of patients. If the initial EIA test is positive, the test should be repeated. If the second test is positive, a confirmatory Western blot assay or immunofluorescent antibody assay (IFA) should be performed. The Western blot test detects specific viral antigens and is considered positive when any two of the following three antigens are identified: p24 (viral core), gp-41 (envelope), and gp-120/160 (envelope). If a patient has two positive EIAs, followed by a confirmatory Western blot or IFA, the likelihood of a false-positive test is less than 1 in 10,000.[165,166]

As a general rule, patients in the United States should be routinely tested only for HIV-1 infection. Testing for HIV-2 infection is indicated if the patient has had sexual contact, or has shared needles, with a partner from an area of the world where HIV-2 infection is endemic. Testing also should be done if the patient has recently traveled to an endemic area or received a blood transfusion or nonsterile injection in such a locale. In addition, testing also should be performed in individuals who have clinical evidence of HIV infection, but in whom serologic tests for HIV-1 are nonconfirmatory. Screening for HIV-2 infection may be done with a specific EIA and Western blot. In addition, a commercial EIA is now available that simultaneously screens for HIV-1 and HIV-2.[156]

Perinatal Transmission

Approximately 90 percent of all cases of HIV infection in children are due to perinatal transmission. Perinatal transmission may occur as a result of hematogenous dissemination, but it is most likely to result from intrapartum exposure to infected maternal blood and genital tract secretions.[157,159] The frequency of vertical transmission of HIV infection varies from a low of 5 to 10 percent to a high of 50 to 60 percent. The average in most investigations has been 20 to 30 percent.[167,168] Factors that increase the likelihood of vertical transmission are summarized in Table 40–14.

Obstetric Complications

Studies of obstetric outcome in patients with HIV infection are difficult to interpret because affected patients have so many confounding conditions that may compli-

cate pregnancy. Such conditions include drug addiction, poor nutrition, limited access to prenatal care, poverty, and concurrent sexually transmitted diseases. When investigators have tried to control for these confounding variables, infected women appear to be at increased risk for several major complications: preterm delivery, preterm PROM, intrauterine growth restriction, increased perinatal mortality, and postpartum endometritis. Pregnancy per se probably does not significantly accelerate the progression of HIV infection.[157,159]

Management

All obstetric patients should be offered voluntary screening for HIV infection at the time of their first prenatal appointment. Selective screening only in patients presumed to be high risk will fail to identify approximately 50 percent of seropositive women.[169] Infected women should be counseled about the risk of perinatal transmission of infection and about potential obstetric complications. They should then be offered the option of pregnancy termination. In addition, arrangements should be made for patients to obtain assistance from appropriate support personnel such as social workers, nutritionists, and psychologists. Patients also should be advised to discontinue smoking, since this practice appears to accelerate the course of the disease.[157,159]

Infected patients should be screened for other sexually transmitted diseases such as gonorrhea, chlamydia, herpes, hepatitis B and C, and syphilis. They should be tested for antibody to cytomegalovirus and toxoplasmosis because both of these infections can cause severe chorioretinitis and central nervous system disease, and both are amenable to treatment with antimicrobial agents. Patients also should have a tuberculin skin test; if this test is positive, a chest x-ray should be per-

Table 40–14. FACTORS THAT INCREASE THE RISK OF VERTICAL TRANSMISSION OF HIV INFECTION

Risk Factor	Presumed Mechanism
HIV-1 vs. HIV-2	Risk is much greater with HIV-1, presumably as a result of greater virulence of HIV-1
History of previous child with HIV infection	Higher viral inoculum in mother
Mother with AIDS	Higher viral inoculum, decreased immunocompetence of the mother
Preterm delivery	Decreased neonatal immunocompetence
Decreased maternal CD4 count	Impaired maternal immunity
High maternal viral load	Higher viral inoculum
Firstborn twin	With vaginal delivery, firstborn twin has more prolonged exposure to infected blood and genital tract secretions
Chorioamnionitis	Placental vasculitis facilitates hematogenous dissemination of virus
Vaginal delivery, particularly in the setting of prolonged rupture of membranes	Greater fetal contact with infected blood and genital secretions
Intrapartum blood exposure (e.g., episiotomy, vaginal laceration, forceps delivery)	Greater fetal contact with infected blood and genital secretions

formed to identify active pulmonary disease. In addition, patients should receive vaccinations for hepatitis A and B, pneumococcal infection, and viral influenza. They should have a Papanicolaou smear to determine if cervical intraepithelial neoplasia is present. They also should have periodic assays for CD4 count and viral load (HIV RNA-PCR) to assess the state of their immune system and the progression or remission of their disease.

Patients also should receive treatment with antiviral chemotherapy. The rationale for treatment is twofold: prevention of perinatal transmission of HIV infection and improvement in the course of the mother's disease. Until recently, treatment guidelines in pregnancy focused primarily on the first objective and were based on the landmark study of the AIDS Clinical Trials Group (ACTG) Protocol 076.[170] This study was conducted in the United States and France and included a select group of obstetric patients: asymptomatic woman beyond the first trimester of pregnancy who had CD4 counts greater than $200/mm^3$ and who had not previously been treated with zidovudine. Women were randomized to receive placebo or zidovudine (100 mg PO five times daily) during the antepartum period. Patients then received intravenous zidovudine during labor, in a loading dose of 2 mg/kg over 1 hour, followed by 1 mg/kg/h throughout labor. Following delivery, infants in the treatment group received oral zidovudine (2 mg/kg every 6 hours) for six weeks postpartum. At the first interim data analysis, information was available for 363 infants. The independent safety monitor recommended that the study be discontinued because the frequency of perinatal transmission was 25.5 percent in the placebo arm versus 8.3 percent in the active treatment arm, representing a 67 percent reduction in the risk of vertical transmission ($p = 0.00006$).

Several other recent studies in developing nations have shown that shorter courses of inexpensive oral antiretroviral medications also are effective in decreasing the rate of perinatal transmission of HIV infection. One investigation was conducted in *non–breast-feeding* women in Thailand.[171] Patients received 300 mg of zidovudine twice daily, beginning at 36 weeks, and were treated with the same oral dose every 3 h during labor. The rate of perinatal transmission was reduced by 50 percent. In a similar trial in *breast-feeding* women in Cote d'Ivoire, perinatal transmission was reduced by 37 percent at 6 months postpartum.

In another investigation in sub-Saharan Africa (PE-TRA Trial),[172] patients received zidovudine (300 mg twice daily) plus lamivudine (150 mg twice daily) from 38 weeks until delivery. They also received zidovudine (200 mg) every 3 hours during labor, and the mother and baby were treated with combined therapy for 1 week postpartum. The rate of perinatal transmission was reduced by 51 percent in treated patients.

Finally, in the HIVNET 012 trial conducted in Kampala, Uganda,[173] patients were randomly assigned to treatment with nevirapine (200 mg PO at the onset of labor followed by oral treatment of the baby with a single dose of 2 mg/kg within 72 hours of birth) versus zidovudine (600 mg PO at the onset of labor and 300 mg every 3 hours until delivery followed by oral treatment of the baby with 4 mg/kg for 7 days after birth). Ninety-nine percent of the babies were breastfed. At 16 weeks after delivery, the rates of neonatal infection were 25 percent in the zidovudine group and 13 percent in the nevirapine group ($p = 0.0006$). Both regimens were well tolerated and very inexpensive compared to the treatment regimen used in the ACTG 076 trial.

In addition to these new findings related to intrapartum chemoprophylaxis, several treatment trials in nonpregnant patients have demonstrated a distinct advantage for multiagent regimens compared to monotherapy with respect to suppression of viral load, elevation of CD4 count, improvement in quality of life, and prolongation of disease-free interval. Accordingly, there is a growing consensus that these new treatment options should be offered to pregnant women as well.[174]

Table 40–15 lists the drugs most commonly used for treatment of HIV infection in pregnant women. Pending new information from ongoing trials, a reasonable approach is treatment with two nucleoside reverse transcriptase inhibitors and a protease inhibitor.[174] In view of the favorable results of the ACTG 076 study, one of the nucleosides should be zidovudine, administered in a dose of 300 mg orally, twice daily. Lamivudine (150 mg PO twice daily) also has an exceptionally good safety and efficacy profile. These two agents can be administered in a convenient combination formulation, Combivir, twice daily. Of the current protease inhibitors, the one with the best combination of safety, efficacy, and expense is nelfinavir (750 mg PO three times daily).

Other combinations of agents certainly have proved effective in studies in nonpregnant patients and should be considered if the regimen outlined above is ineffective or causes adverse effects.[174] In addition, pregnant women should be advised that the complete range of effects of these new drugs on the fetus has not been delineated.

In addition to specific antiviral chemotherapy, patients also should receive prophylaxis against the most common opportunistic infections. Table 40–16 summarizes selected guidelines for use of antibiotic prophylaxis in HIV-infected patients.[175]

When the physician is delivering the HIV-positive patient, every effort must be made to avoid instrumentation that would increase the neonate's exposure to infected maternal blood and secretions. Specifically, whenever feasible, the fetal membranes should be left

Table 40–15. AGENTS MOST COMMONLY USED FOR TREATMENT OF HIV INFECTION IN PREGNANT WOMEN

Agent	Usual Adult Dose	Remarks	Cost of 30-Day Treatment
Nucleoside analogs			
Lamivudine (3TC, Epivir)	150 mg bid	Adverse effects are similar to those of zidovudine, but are less frequent. Drug is eliminated by renal excretion.	$230.00
Zidovudine (Retrovir)	300 mg bid	Main adverse effect is marrow suppression.	$287.00
Nonnucleoside reverse transcriptase inhibitors			
Nevirapine (Viramure)	200 mg bid	Most common adverse effect is rash. If the rash is extensive, the drug should be permanently discontinued. Hepatitis is a rare side effect.	$248.00
Protease inhibitors			
Indinavir (Crixivan)	800 mg q8h	Well tolerated. Most serious adverse effect is nephrolithiasis. Most common side effect is GI upset. Less expensive than Ritonavir.	$450.00
Nelfinavir (Viracept)	750 mg tid or 1250 mg in am and 1000 mg in pm	Clinical efficacy data are limited. Most common adverse effects are diarrhea, fatigue, poor concentration.	$557.00

GI, gastrointestinal.

intact until delivery. In addition, application of the fetal scalp electrode and scalp pH sampling should be avoided.

Several recent reports have investigated the role of elective cesarean delivery as a method for reducing the rate of perinatal transmission of HIV infection. Perhaps the two of greatest interest are the reports from the French Perinatal Cohort[176] and the International Perinatal HIV Infection Group.[177] In the former investigation, in women receiving monotherapy with zidovudine, elective cesarean delivery before the onset of labor or rupture of membranes was associated with a lower rate of transmission than emergent cesarean section or vaginal delivery (0.8 percent vs. 11.4 percent vs. 6.6 percent, $p = 0.002$). The latter report was a meta-analysis of 15 prospective cohort studies from North America and Europe that included 8,533 mother–child pairs. The vast majority of women received monotherapy with zidovudine. Elective cesarean delivery was associated with approximately a 50 percent decrease in the rate of perinatal transmission of HIV infection (odds ratio [OR], 0.43; 95 percent confidence interval [CI], 0.33 to 0.56). When both elective cesarean delivery and antiretroviral therapy were used, the rate of transmission was re-

Table 40–16. PROPHYLACTIC ANTIBIOTIC REGIMENS FOR COMMON OPPORTUNISTIC INFECTIONS*

Condition	Indication for Prophylaxis	Antibiotic Regimen
Pneumocystis carinii pneumonia	Prior infection or CD4 < 200/mm³	TMP-SMX 1 DS tablet qd indefinitely
Toxoplasmic encephalitis	CD4 < 100/mm³ + serology	TMP-SMX 1 DS tablet qd indefinitely
Tuberculosis	+PPD > 5 mm No active disease on chest x-ray	INH; 300 mg qd, plus pyridoxine, 50 mg qd × 12 mo
Disseminated infection with mycobacterium avium complex (MAC)	CD4 < 50/mm³	Azithromycin 1200 mg weekly
Cryptococcosis	CD4 < 50/mm³	Routine prophylaxis not recommended Patients who have been treated for an acute cryptococcal infection should receive fluconazole, 200 mg qd, indefinitely

* Recommendations in this table are based on information presented in Centers for Disease Control and Prevention.[175]
TMP-SMX, trimethoprim-sulfamethoxazole; INH, isoniazid.

duced by 87 percent, and the actual frequency of transmission was 2 percent (95 percent CI, 0.0 to 4.0).

Although the results of these studies are impressive, they must be interpreted with caution. Neither study was prospective or randomized with respect to mode of delivery. Patients were not stratified according to viral load. Moreover, very few of the patients were treated with the highly active multiagent regimens currently recommended.

In light of the information presented above, elective cesarean appears to be indicated for the following patients: those receiving no antiviral treatment, those receiving monotherapy alone, and those receiving combination chemotherapy but who have detectable viral loads. Women receiving optimal combination chemotherapy who have undetectable viral loads should be advised that it is uncertain whether elective cesarean delivery offers an additional protective effect against perinatal transmission.[178]

In the postpartum period, the mother should be advised to avoid any contact between her body fluids and an open area on the skin or mucous membranes of the neonate. She also should be cautioned against breastfeeding. Initially, the risk of HIV transmission through breast milk was regarded as low. Recently, however, a report by Dunn et al.[179] called this original assumption into serious question. In this investigation of African women, the authors divided subjects into two groups, those who acquired HIV infection postnatally and those who were infected prenatally. In the former group, 29 percent of breast-fed infants became infected. In the latter group, the added risk of infection from breastfeeding (i.e., above the inherent risk associated with perinatal transmission) was 14 percent. Finally, infected patients should be urged to use secure contraception and adopt responsible sexual practices to prevent spread of infection to their partners.

PARVOVIRUS INFECTION

Epidemiology

Human parvovirus B19 is a member of the Parvoviridae family. It is a single-stranded DNA virus that codes for only a small number of proteins. Its reproductive capability is limited and, therefore, it can only replicate in cells that are dividing rapidly.[180,181] The virus is distributed worldwide, and infection may occur in both a sporadic and epidemic form. Humans are the only known host for the B19 virus. The organism is transmitted by respiratory droplets and infected blood components, and the incubation period is 4 to 20 days. Serum and respiratory secretions become positive for the virus several days before clinical symptoms develop. Once symptoms appear, respiratory secretions and serum are usually free of the virus.[180,181] Prevalence of antibody to parvovirus increases with age. In children age 1 to 5 years, approximately 2 to 15 percent are seropositive for antibody. In adolescents and adults, the seroprevalence increases to more than 60 percent.[180,181]

Clinical Manifestations

The most common clinical presentation of parvovirus infection is *erythema infectiosum* or *fifth disease*. This illness typically occurs in elementary school and daycare populations in the late winter and early spring. Patients usually have low-grade fever, malaise, adenopathy, and polyarthritis affecting the hands, wrists, and knees. In addition, they have a characteristic pruritic, erythematous "slapped cheek" rash on the face and a finely reticulated erythematous rash on the trunk and extremities (Fig. 40–8).The rash may wax and wane over a period of several months in response to stress, exercise, sunlight, or bathing. Erythema infectiosum is a

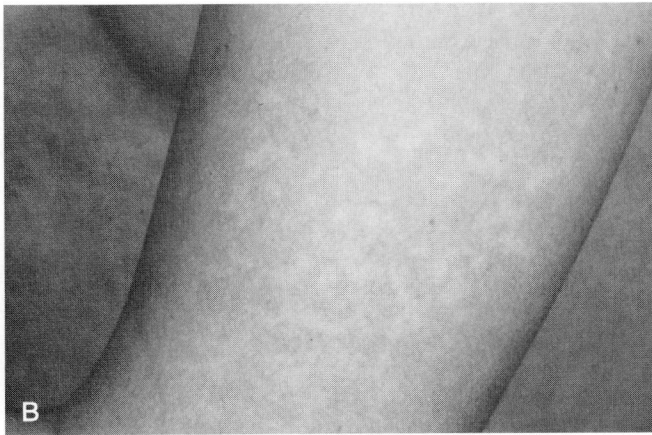

Figure 40–8. Characteristic "slapped cheek" rash of erythema infectiosum (*A*). Note lace-like rash on upper extremity (*B*).

self-limited illness. Complete recovery is the norm, and serious long-term sequelae rarely occur.[180,181]

The second major clinical presentation of parvovirus infection is *transient aplastic crisis*. This disorder occurs almost exclusively in individuals who have an underlying hemoglobinopathy and results from viral infection of the bone marrow, with resultant destruction of red blood cell precursors. Affected patients have prodromal symptoms similar to erythema infectiosum. One to 7 days after the onset of the prodrome, signs of anemia develop, such as pallor, weakness, and lethargy. Patients with transient aplastic crisis usually do not have a skin rash. Full recovery without sequelae is the usual outcome, provided the patient receives appropriate supportive care.[180,181]

Fetal Infection

The risk that a susceptible mother will acquire infection from an infected household member is 50 to 90 percent.[180–182] The risk of transmission in a day-care setting or classroom is lower, ranging from 20 to 30 percent.[182–184] Published information regarding subsequent risk of transmission to the fetus is based on one principal end point, namely, fetal hydrops. Hydrops appears to result primarily from viral infection of fetal erythroid stem cells, leading to an aplastic anemia and high-output congestive heart failure. Hydrops may also be due, at least in part, to direct infection of the myocardium by the virus.

The reported frequency of fetal hydrops or other adverse outcome following maternal infection has varied from 0 to 38 percent, with most authors citing frequencies in the range of 5 to 15 percent.[180–182,185–187] The risk of fetal infection is greatest when maternal illness occurs in the first trimester, as noted in Table 40–17.[182] Parvovirus does not typically cause a structural defect in the fetus.

Diagnosis of Maternal Infection

Parvovirus can be grown in tissue culture consisting of fresh bone marrow supplemented with erythropoietin.

Table 40–17. ASSOCIATION BETWEEN GESTATIONAL AGE AT TIME OF EXPOSURE AND RISK OF FETAL PARVOVIRUS INFECTION

Time of Exposure (Weeks' Gestation)	Frequency of Severely Affected Fetuses (%)
1–12	19
13–20	15
>20	6

Table 40–18. INTERPRETATION OF SEROLOGIC TESTS FOR MATERNAL PARVOVIRUS INFECTION

Condition	Maternal Antibody	
	IgM	IgG
Susceptible	–	–
Immune—infection > 120 days ago	–	+
Infection within 7 days	+	–
Infection within 7–120 days	+	+

The virus also can be detected by DNA hybridization assays using serum, leukocytes, respiratory secretions, urine, or tissue. In addition, infection can be documented by characteristic histologic changes in infected cells, such as eosinophilic inclusion bodies, marginated chromatin, and direct detection of viral particles by electron microscopy.[180–182] However, the mainstay of laboratory diagnosis is serologic testing. Antibody to parvovirus can be measured by ELISA, RIA, and Western blot. IgM-specific antibody is usually positive by the third day after symptoms develop. It typically disappears within 30 to 60 days, but may persist for up to 120 days. IgG antibody is detectable by the seventh day of illness and persists for life.[180–182] Table 40–18 summarizes the interpretation of serologic tests for parvovirus.

Diagnosis of Fetal Infection

The most valuable test for diagnosis of fetal parvovirus infection is ultrasound. Severely affected fetuses typically have evidence of hydrops. Since the incubation period of the virus may be longer in the fetus than in the child or adult, the patient should be followed with serial ultrasound examinations for 8 to 10 weeks after her acute illness. If the fetus shows no signs of hydrops during this observation period, additional diagnostic studies are unnecessary. If hydropic changes appear and the fetus is at an appropriate gestational age, cordocentesis is indicated (see below).[180–182,188]

Maternal Management

Following a documented exposure to parvovirus, the mother should immediately have a serologic test to determine if she is immune or susceptible to the virus. If preexisting IgG antibody is present, the patient can be reassured that second infections are extremely unlikely and that her fetus is not at risk. If the patient is susceptible, she should have a repeat serologic test in approximately 3 weeks to determine if she has seroconverted. If seroconversion is detected, serial ultrasound examinations should be performed over the ensuing 8 to 10 weeks to evaluate fetal well-being.

No antiviral agent or vaccine is presently available for treatment of parvovirus infection, but patients with erythema infectiosum rarely need more than simple supportive care. Patients with transient aplastic crisis may require red cell transfusion during the acute phase of their illness. As a general rule, isolation of patients with erythema infectiosum is not of value in reducing transmission of infection, since spread by respiratory droplets has already occurred by the time the patient has clear signs of clinical disease. Conversely, if patients with transient aplastic crisis are isolated early in the course of their illness, horizontal transmission to other susceptible individuals may be reduced.[180–182]

Fetal Management

If fetal hydrops is documented by ultrasound, cordocentesis should be performed if technically feasible. Fetal blood should be collected for determination of hematocrit and detection of IgM-specific antibody.[188] Although case reports have described spontaneous resolution of hydrops in infected fetuses, criteria predictive of such a good outcome are not well established.[189,190] Therefore, if severe anemia is present, intrauterine transfusion should be performed.[191,192] Fairley et al.[192] recently reported the outcome of 66 fetuses with hydrops due to congenital parvovirus infection. In 26 cases, the fetus was dead at the time of initial assessment, and in two cases, therapeutic abortion was performed. Twelve of the 38 fetuses who were alive at the time hydrops was diagnosed had intrauterine transfusions; 3 of the 12 died. Twenty-six fetuses did not undergo transfusion, and 13 died (OR, 0.14; 95 percent CI, 0.02 to 0.96).

In a similar analysis, Rodis et al.[193] surveyed members of the Society for Maternal-Fetal Medicine regarding management of patients with parvovirus infection. Members reported the outcome of 467 cases of fetal hydrops. Seven patients elected to have pregnancy terminations. One hundred sixty-four fetuses had intrauterine transfusions; 27 of these fetuses (16 percent) died. Of the 296 fetuses who *did not* undergo transfusion, 138 (47 percent) died ($p < 0.0001$).

Until recently, most authors had reported normal long-term development in surviving infants. However, in 1993, Conry and co-workers[194] described three children with persistent neurologic morbidity following parvovirus infection that occurred at 21 to 24 weeks' gestation. Neurologic abnormalities included hypotonia, arthrogryposis, motor developmental delay, infantile spasms, intracranial calcifications, and ventriculomegaly. One child died on the sixth day of life. In 1994, Brown et al.[195] described three infants with persistent

severe anemia following intrauterine transfusion for parvovirus infection. One of the children died, and autopsy demonstrated widespread viral infection. The other children required regular transfusions. In view of these recent unfavorable reports, clinicians should be cautious in counseling parents regarding the long-term prognosis in affected infants.

RUBELLA

Epidemiology

Rubella is an RNA virus that is a member of the togavirus family. Only a single serotype is known.[196] Rubella occurs primarily in young children and adolescents. The disease is most common in the springtime. Major epidemics of rubella occurred in the United States in 1935 and 1964; minor sporadic epidemics occurred approximately every 7 years until the late 1960s. With licensure of an effective rubella vaccine in 1969, the frequency of this infection has declined by almost 99 percent.[197] In 1992, a new low of 160 cases was reported to the CDC.[198] The persistence of this infection appears to be due to failure to vaccinate susceptible individuals rather than to lack of immunogenicity of the vaccine.

The rubella virus enters the host through the upper respiratory tract. From this site, the virus travels quickly to the cervical lymph nodes and then is disseminated hematogenously throughout the body. The incubation period is approximately 2 to 3 weeks. The virus is present in blood and nasopharyngeal secretions for several days before appearance of the characteristic rash; it also is shed from the nasopharynx for several days after appearance of the exanthem. Therefore, the patient can be contagious for an extended period of time.[196,199]

Antibody against rubella does not normally appear in the serum until after the rash has developed. Acquired immunity to rubella is usually lifelong. Second infections have occurred after both natural primary infections and vaccination. However, recurrent infections generally are not associated with serious illness, viremia, or congenital infection.

Clinical Manifestations

Most children and adults with rubella have mild constitutional symptoms such as malaise, headache, myalgias, and arthralgias. The principal clinical manifestation of this illness, of course, is a widely disseminated, nonpruritic, erythematous, maculopapular rash (Fig. 40–9).

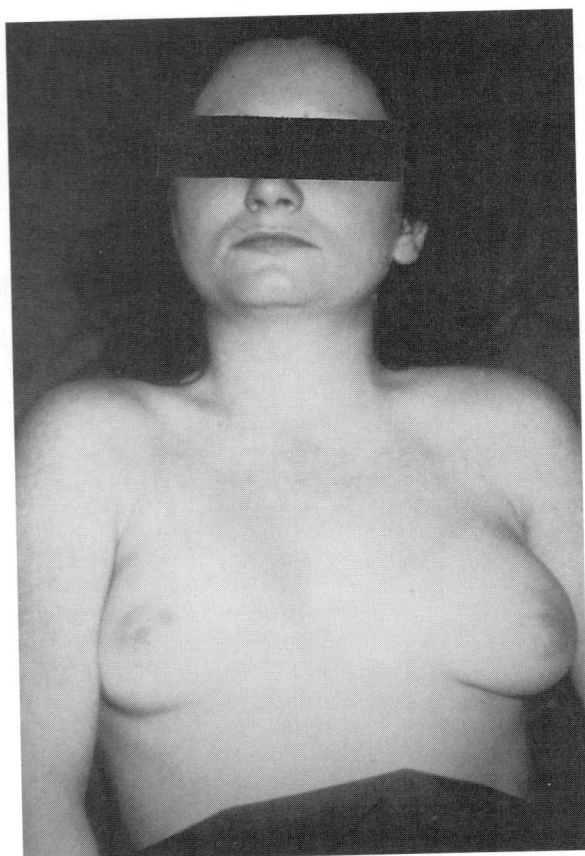

Figure 40–9. Photograph shows typical erythematous, maculopapular rash of rubella.

Postauricular adenopathy and mild conjunctivitis also are common. These clinical manifestations usually are short-lived and typically resolve within 3 to 5 days. The differential diagnosis of rubella includes rubeola, roseola, other viral exanthems, and drug reaction.[196]

Diagnosis

The diagnosis of rubella can usually be established on the basis of the patient's physical examination. If necessary, serologic tests can be used to confirm the diagnosis. IgM antibody usually reaches a peak 7 to 10 days after the onset of illness and then declines over a period of 4 weeks. The serum concentration of IgG antibody usually rises more slowly, but antibody levels persist throughout the lifetime of the individual. Several different types of antibody detection tests are available, including enzyme immunoassay, indirect immunofluorescence, and latex agglutination. In a recent comparative study, Sautter et al.[200] found that the enzyme immunoassay and latex agglutination tests were the most rapid and convenient methods for screening for antibody to rubella.

Congenital Rubella Syndrome

Because of the success of rubella vaccination campaigns, the incidence of congenital rubella syndrome in the United States has declined dramatically over the past 25 years.[196–198] In 1991, 31 cases of congenital rubella syndrome were reported to the CDC; in 1992, only five cases were reported.[198] Unfortunately, however, approximately 10 to 20 percent of women in the United States remain susceptible to rubella and, hence, their fetuses are at risk for serious injury should the mother become infected during pregnancy.

The rubella virus crosses the placenta by hematogenous dissemination, and the frequency of congenital infection is critically dependent on the time of exposure to the virus.[196,201,202] Approximately 50 percent of infants exposed to the virus within 4 weeks of conception will manifest signs of congenital infection. When maternal infection occurs in the second 4-week period after conception, approximately 25 percent of fetuses will be infected. When infection develops in the third month, approximately 10 percent of fetuses will be infected. When maternal infection occurs beyond this point in time, less than 1 percent of babies will be infected.

An entire spectrum of anomalies has been associated with congenital rubella syndrome. The four most common abnormalities are deafness (affecting 60 to 75 percent of fetuses), eye defects (10 to 30 percent), CNS anomalies (10 to 25 percent), and cardiac malformations (10 to 20 percent). The most common cardiac abnormality associated with congenital rubella is patent ductus arteriosus, although supravalvular pulmonic stenosis is perhaps the most pathognomonic. Other possible abnormalities include microcephaly, mental retardation, pneumonia, intrauterine growth restriction, hepatosplenomegaly, hemolytic anemia, and thrombocytopenia.[201,202]

A variety of tests have been proposed for the diagnosis of congenital rubella syndrome. Cordocentesis can be performed to determine the total serum IgM concentration in fetal blood and to detect virus-specific antibody. However, fetal immunoglobulin production usually cannot be detected prior to 19 to 22 weeks of gestation. Some authors have proposed chorionic villus sampling (CVS) as a diagnostic test because placental tissue infected with rubella virus produces a cytopathic effect when grown in tissue culture. Viral antigen also can be identified rapidly in tissue culture by RNA-DNA hybridization techniques, and amniotic fluid can be cultured for rubella virus. Unfortunately, although the tests outlined above can demonstrate that rubella virus is present in the fetal compartment, they do not indicate the degree of fetal injury. Accordingly, detailed ultrasound examination is the best test to determine if serious fetal injury has occurred. Abnormalities that can be identified accurately by ultrasound include intrauterine growth restriction, microcephaly, and cardiac malformations.

The prognosis for infants with congenital rubella syndrome is guarded. Approximately 50 percent of affected individuals have to attend schools for the hearing impaired. An additional 25 percent of infected children require at least some special schooling because of hearing impairment, and only 25 percent are able to attend mainstream regular schools. Some affected individuals develop insulin-dependent diabetes later in life, presumably secondary to in utero infection of the pancreas. The estimated lifetime cost of caring for a child with congenital rubella syndrome is approximately $200,000 to $300,000.[201–203]

Obstetric Management

Ideally, women of reproductive age should have a preconception appointment when they are contemplating pregnancy. At this time, they should be evaluated for immunity to rubella. If serologic testing demonstrates that they are susceptible, they should be vaccinated with rubella vaccine prior to conception.[196] When preconception counseling is not possible, all obstetric patients should have a test for rubella at the time of their first prenatal appointment. Women who are susceptible to rubella should be counseled to avoid exposure to other individuals who may have viral exanthems.

If a susceptible patient subsequently has exposure to rubella, serologic tests should be obtained to determine whether acute infection has occurred. If acute infection is documented, patients should be counseled about the risk of congenital rubella syndrome. Obviously, specific counseling should be based on the time in gestation when maternal infection occurred. The diagnostic tests for detection of in utero infection should be reviewed. Patients should be offered the option of pregnancy termination based on the assessed risk of serious fetal injury.[199]

Susceptible patients who are fortunate enough to escape infection during pregnancy should be vaccinated immediately postpartum. The present rubella vaccine is the RA 27/3 preparation.[197] It is much more immunogenic than the earlier HPV-77 and Cendehill vaccines and is available in a monovalent form, bivalent form (measles-rubella [MR]), and trivalent form (measles-mumps-rubella [MMR]). Approximately 95 percent of patients who receive rubella vaccine seroconvert. Antibody levels persist for at least 18 years in more than 90 percent of vaccinees.

There are few adverse effects of vaccination, even in adults. Less than 25 percent of patients experience mild constitutional symptoms such as low-grade fever and malaise. Less than 10 percent experience arthralgias, and less than 1 percent develop frank arthritis. Interestingly, when the vaccine is administered in the immediate postpartum period, these adverse effects are often delayed for up to 21 days. Women who have received the vaccine cannot transmit infection to susceptible contacts, such as younger children in the home. Breastfeeding is not a contraindication to vaccination. In addition, the vaccine can be administered in conjunction with other immune globulin preparations such as Rh-immune globulin.

Women who receive rubella vaccine should practice secure contraception for a minimum of 3 months after vaccination. For a number of years, the CDC maintained a registry of women who received the rubella vaccine within 3 months of conception. That registry included almost 400 patients, and fortunately there were no instances in which congenital rubella syndrome resulted from vaccination.[204] However, there were cases in which women elected to have abortions following vaccination and rubella virus was isolated from the products of the conception. The maximum theoretical risk of congenital rubella resulting from rubella vaccine in early pregnancy is 1 to 2 percent.

RUBEOLA (MEASLES)

Virology

The measles virus is a paramyxovirus that is closely related to the canine distemper virus. The organism was first successfully isolated by Enders and Peebles in 1954. The wild virus is pathogenic only for primates, and humans are the only natural host. The organism is a single-stranded RNA virus. It is quite labile and is extremely sensitive to acid, proteolytic enzymes, strong light, and drying.[205,206]

Epidemiology

Measles virus is highly contagious and is spread primarily by respiratory droplets. Seventy-five to 90 percent of susceptible contacts become infected after exposure. The incubation period is 10 to 14 days. Before a vaccine was available, virtually all children acquired measles. In 1963, however, inactivated and live attenuated vaccines were licensed. The inactivated vaccine was subsequently discontinued in 1967. The current vaccine used in the United States is an attenuated preparation that was licensed in 1968.[205–207]

Since licensure of the vaccine, the reported incidence of measles has decreased by almost 99 percent. As expected, children less than 10 years of age have shown the greatest decline in incidence of measles. During the mid 1980s, almost 60 percent of reported cases of measles affected children greater than 10 years of age, compared with only 10 percent during the period 1960 to 1964.[205-207] In recent years, two major types of measles outbreaks have been reported in the United States. One type has occurred among unvaccinated preschoolers, including children less than 15 months of age. Another has occurred among previously vaccinated school-age children and college students. Approximately one third of the cases in the latter type of outbreak have been in individuals who previously were vaccinated. Presumably, these cases result from either *primary failure* to respond to the first vaccine or *secondary failure,* a situation where an adequate serologic response initially develops but immunity wanes over time.[208,209]

Clinical Manifestations

The clinical manifestations of measles usually appear within 10 to 12 days of exposure. The most common are fever, malaise, coryza, sneezing, conjunctivitis, cough, and photophobia. All patients typically develop a generalized maculopapular rash, and the majority also have Koplik's spots, which are blue-gray specks on a red base that develop on the buccal mucosa opposite the second molars. The skin exanthem typically begins on the face and neck and then spreads to the trunk and extremities. It usually lasts for approximately 5 days and then recedes in the order in which it appeared. The duration of illness is approximately 7 to 10 days. Patients are contagious from 1 to 4 days before the onset of coryza. Immunity to measles should be lifelong following wild virus infection and is mediated by both humoral and cell-mediated mechanisms.

Although measles is typically a minor illness, some patients develop serious sequelae. Otitis media occurs in 7 to 9 percent of infected patients; bronchiolitis and pneumonia affect 1 to 6 percent. A severe form of hepatitis also may occur. In a recent report by Atmar and associates,[210] 7 of 13 (54 percent) pregnant women with measles developed hepatitis.

Encephalitis occurs in approximately 1 per 1,000 cases of measles. It results from both viral infection of the CNS and a hypersensitivity reaction to the systemic viral infection. Measles encephalitis may result in permanent neurologic impairment, including mental retardation; the mortality rate from this complication is approximately 15 to 33 percent.[205-207] Another unusual but extremely serious complication of measles is subacute sclerosing panencephalitis (SSPE). This complication occurs in 0.5 to 2 per 1,000 cases. The manifestations of SSPE typically develop approximately 7 years after the acute measles infection. SSPE is more common in children who had measles before the age of 2. The disorder is characterized by progressive neurologic debilitation and a virtually uniformly fatal outcome.

A final complication is an unusual condition, termed *atypical measles.* This disorder is a severe form of mea-

sles reinfection that affects young adults previously vaccinated with the formalin-inactivated killed measles vaccine that was distributed in the United States from 1963 to 1967. Affected patients have extremely high antibody titers to measles. They typically experience high fever; pneumonitis; pleural effusion; and a coarse, maculopapular, hemorrhagic, or urticarial rash. Although the disease is usually self-limited, atypical measles can lead to hepatic, cardiac, and renal failure. Interestingly, affected patients are not contagious to others. The risk of perinatal transmission with atypical measles has not been defined precisely.[206]

Diagnosis

Five clinical criteria should be present to establish the diagnosis of measles: fever greater than or equal to 38.3°C, a characteristic rash lasting longer than 3 days, cough, coryza, and conjunctivitis.[2] Although the virus can be cultured, the mainstay of diagnostic tests is detection of antibody to measles.[205-208] The simplest and most sensitive tests are the hemaglutination inhibition (HI) assay and the ELISA. The confirmation of acute measles virus infection is based on detection of IgM-specific antibody or a fourfold change in the IgG titer in convalescent, compared to acute, sera. The acute titer for IgG antibody should be obtained within 3 days of the onset of the rash and the convalescent titer should be obtained 10–20 days later.

The differential diagnosis of measles can be difficult. A variety of other infections must be considered, including rubella, scarlet fever, Rocky Mountain spotted fever, toxoplasmosis, enterovirus infection, mononucleosis, meningococcemia, and serum sickness.

Complications of Measles during Pregnancy

Several reports have described an increase in maternal mortality associated with measles infection during pregnancy. Most fatalities have been due to pulmonary complications. In one of the earliest reports, Christensen et al. described a serious epidemic of measles in Greenland in 1951.[211] Four of 83 pregnant women (4.8 percent) who developed measles died. An unspecified number of these women also had active tuberculosis. In the report by Atmar et al.,[210] 1 of 13 pregnant women (8 percent) with measles died because of severe respiratory infection. In another report, Eberhart-Phillips and co-workers[212] evaluated 58 pregnant women with measles. Thirty-five (60 percent) required hospitalization. Fifteen (26 percent) developed pneumonia, and two (3 percent) died.

Early reports described a slight increase in the frequency of preterm delivery and spontaneous abortion when women developed measles during pregnancy. In the recent report by Eberhart-Phillips et al.,[212] 13 of 50 (26 percent) women with continuing pregnancies delivered preterm. The frequency of congenital anomalies is not significantly increased in women who have measles during pregnancy, although Ekbom and associates[213] recently reported a possible association between perinatal measles infection and subsequent Crohn's disease.

Infants of mothers who are acutely infected at the time of delivery are at risk for neonatal measles. This infection typically develops within the first 10 days of life and results from transplacental viral dissemination. In some reports, the mortality in preterm and term infants with neonatal measles has been as high as 60 percent and 20 percent, respectively.[205,208,210,212,214] Of importance is the fact that these alarmingly high mortality figures were published prior to the era of skilled neonatal care and the availability of broad-spectrum antibiotics for treatment of secondary bacterial infections.

Management of Measles during Pregnancy

Pregnant women with measles should be observed carefully for evidence of serious complications such as otitis media, hepatitis, encephalitis, and pneumonia. Secondary bacterial infections should be treated promptly with antibiotics. Administration of aerosolized ribavirin may be of benefit in patients with severe viral pneumonitis.[210] The affected patient should be counseled that the risk of injury to her fetus is low. Probably the most effective method for evaluating the fetus for in utero infection is detailed ultrasound examination. Findings suggestive of in utero infection include microcephaly, growth restriction, and oligohydramnios. Neonates delivered to a mother who has developed measles within 7 to 10 days of delivery should receive intramuscular immune globulin in a dose of 0.25 mg/kg. These infants should subsequently receive the live measles vaccine when they are 15 months of age.[206,208]

Prevention of Infection

All children should receive measles vaccine when they are 15 months of age. The immunization should be administered as part of the trivalent MMR vaccine. The appropriate initial dose for young children is 0.5 ml subcutaneously. The original public health recommendations provided for only a single dose of measles vaccine. However, as noted previously, recent outbreaks of measles have occurred in individuals who received only one dose of the vaccine. Accordingly, the CDC now recommends that all individuals who have not been infected with the wild measles virus receive a second dose of vaccine. Children who receive their first dose at age 15 months should receive a second dose at 4 to 6

years of age. Children who are vaccinated with the live vaccine before their first birthday should be considered unvaccinated and should receive the full two-dose series. Individuals who received "further attenuated vaccine," accompanied by immune globulin or measles immune globulin, should be considered unvaccinated and receive two doses of the vaccine. Individuals who were given the inactivated vaccine during the period 1963 to 1967 are at risk for developing severe atypical measles syndrome if they are exposed to the natural virus. Accordingly, these individuals also should receive two doses of the live vaccine. Women of reproductive age who have only one documented measles vaccination also are candidates for a second immunization. The seroconversion rate with the new live virus vaccine is greater than or equal to 95 percent.[206,208]

There are three specific contraindications to vaccination: pregnancy, severe febrile illness, and history of anaphylactic reaction to egg protein or neomycin. The vaccine should not be given for 3 months after a person has received immune globulin, whole blood, or other antibody-containing blood products. However, the vaccine can be administered concurrently with Rh-immune globulin in the immediate postpartum period. Although no cases of congenital infection have been described as a result of the measles vaccine, patients receiving the vaccine should practice effective contraception for 3 months following inoculation.[206,208]

Few adverse effects are associated with measles vaccination. Approximately 5 to 15 percent of vaccinees develop a low-grade fever. Five percent or less develop a rash. Less than 1 percent have febrile seizures, and less than 1 per 1 million cases develop encephalitis.

When an outbreak of measles does occur, susceptible individuals should be targeted for post exposure prophylaxis. If they are not pregnant, they should receive the live measles vaccine within 72 hours of exposure. They also should receive immune globulin within 6 days of exposure. The appropriate dose of immune globulin is 0.25 ml/kg for immunocompetent patients and 0.5 ml/kg for immunocompromised individuals. The maximum dose of the immune globulin preparation is 15 ml. Pregnant patients should receive only immune globulin.[206,208]

SYPHILIS

Epidemiology

Syphilis is caused by the spirochete *Treponema pallidum*. Infection occurs primarily as a result of sexual contact. The organism penetrates mucosal barriers and is highly contagious. Infection develops in 10 percent of contacts after a single exposure and in 70 percent after multiple exposures.[215,216] Syphilis also may be transmitted perinatally, with devastating consequences for the fetus.

The prevalence of syphilis in the United States has increased dramatically in recent years, coincident with the upsurge in cases of HIV infection and the growing epidemic of drug abuse. The greatest increase has been in females, aged 15 to 24 years, and a disproportionate number of cases have occurred in blacks and Hispanics living in urban areas.[215,216]

Clinical Manifestations and Staging

Syphilis may be divided into four *clinical* categories: primary, secondary, tertiary, and neurosyphilis. In addition, syphilis may present as a latent infection. Latent syphilis is subdivided into early latent (<1 year duration) and late latent infection (>1 year).[215–217] The incubation period of syphilis ranges from 10 to 90 days. At the end of this period, the characteristic raised, painless chancre appears. In women, the chancre is usually on the cervix or vaginal wall and may not be apparent except on close inspection (Fig. 40–10). In some patients, the chancre may be present in extragenital sites such as the fingers, oropharynx, nipples, or anus. The chancre usually heals in 3 to 6 weeks even without specific antimicrobial treatment. The principal disorders that must be considered in the differential diagnosis of primary syphilis are herpes simplex virus infection, chancroid, trauma, scabies, Behçet's syndrome, Stevens-Johnson syndrome, and carcinoma.

Patients who receive either no treatment, or inadequate treatment, may develop secondary syphilis 2 to 6 months after their primary infection. The principal clinical manifestation of this stage of the infection is a generalized maculopapular rash that is most obvious on the palms of the hands and soles of the feet (Fig. 40–11). This rash may be confused with disseminated gonococcal infection, measles, rubella, scabies, psoriasis, and drug eruption. Other findings associated with secondary syphilis include mucous patches (Fig. 40–12), shallow, painless ulcerations in the oropharynx; and condylomata lata, grayish, raised papules that appear near the anus and vulva. In addition, bone tenderness, iritis, alopecia, and generalized lymphadenopathy also may be present. The lesions of secondary syphilis usually resolve spontaneously in 3 to 6 weeks, even without treatment. Untreated patients then enter a latent phase of their illness. In this phase, infected women pose only a small risk of horizontal transmission of infection to their sexual partner. However, vertical transmission to the fetus still may occur.[215–217]

Approximately one third of patients with untreated secondary disease ultimately develop tertiary syphilis after an interval of several years. Tertiary syphilis is distinguished by three principal findings: gumma formation, cardiac lesions, and central nervous system abnormalities (neurosyphilis). The characteristic cardiac lesions are aortic insufficiency and dissecting aortic aneurysm. Neurologic manifestations include meningovascular syphilis, cranial nerve palsies, generalized paresis, tabes dorsalis, optic atrophy, uveitis, and Argyll-Robertson pupils. Four to 9 percent of patients with untreated syphilis ultimately develop neurosyphilis. In some individuals, particularly those with concurrent HIV infection, neurologic manifestations may occur early in the course of syphilis and can be responsible for severe morbidity.[215–217]

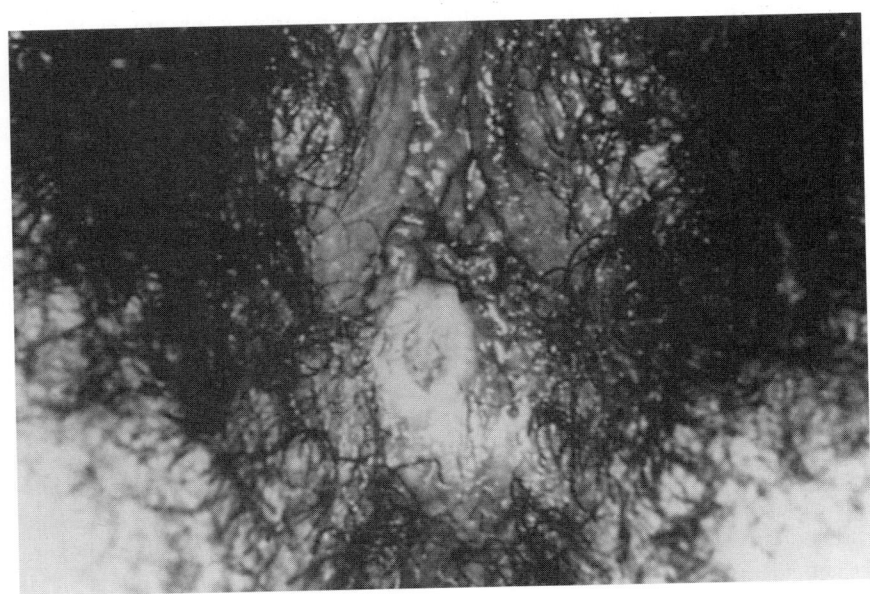

Figure 40–10. Painless chancre characteristic of primary syphilis. (From Duff P, Christian JS, Yancey MK: Infections associated with pregnancy. *In* Coulam CB, Faulk WP, McIntyre JA [eds]: Immunologic Obstetrics. New York, WW Norton & Co, 1992, p 578, with permission.)

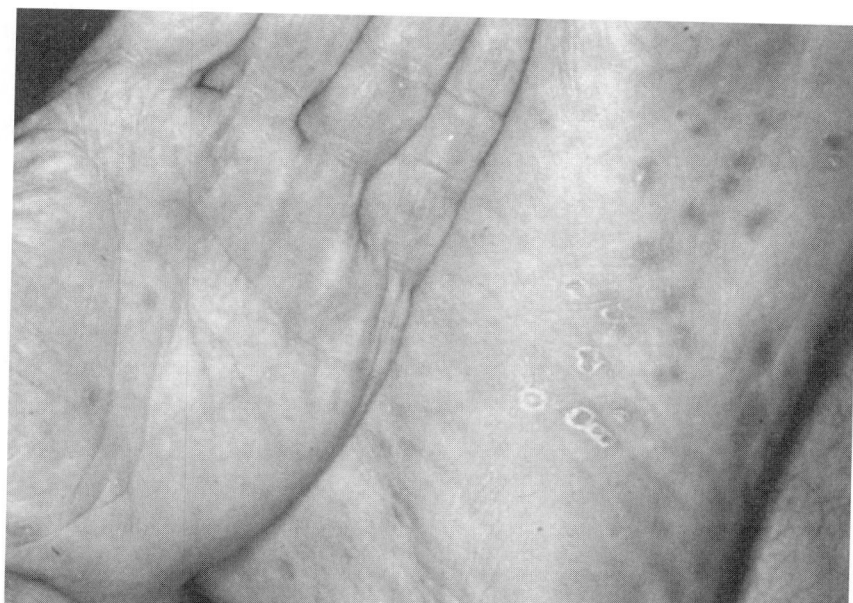

Figure 40–11. Maculopapular rash characteristic of secondary syphilis. (From Duff P, Christian JS, Yancey MK: Infections associated with pregnancy. *In* Coulam CB, Faulk WP, McIntyre JA [eds]: Immunologic Obstetrics. New York, WW Norton & Co, 1992, p 578, with permission.)

Diagnosis

T. pallidum cannot be cultured. It can be identified from overt lesions such as the chancre by darkfield microscopy and fluorescent antibody staining. However, most cases of infection, particularly those in the latent stage, are diagnosed by serology. The initial screening test for syphilis should be a nontreponemal assay such as the Venereal Disease Research Laboratories (VDRL) test or rapid plasma reagin (RPR) test. Several factors can cause biologically false-positive (BFP) test results such as collagen vascular disease, bacterial and viral infections, multiple myeloma, advanced cancer, chronic liver disease, IV drug use, multiple blood transfusions, and pregnancy. Accordingly, a positive screening test must be confirmed by a specific treponemal assay such as the fluorescent treponemal antibody absorption test (FTA-ABS) or microhemagglutination assay (MHATP). Biologic false-positive treponemal tests have been reported in patients with Lyme disease, leprosy, malaria, mononucleosis, and collagen vascular disease.

Lumbar puncture is indicated when neurosyphilis is suspected and in all patients who are co-infected with syphilis and HIV. Cerebrospinal fluid (CSF) abnormalities include a mononuclear pleocytosis (10 to 400 cells/mm^3), elevated protein (>45 mg/dl), and a positive VDRL test.[215–217]

Virtually 100 percent of patients will have a positive serologic test within 4 weeks of their primary infection. With appropriate antibiotic treatment, quantitative nontreponemal tests usually decrease fourfold within 3 months in patients with primary or secondary syphilis. When this decline does not occur, patients should be reevaluated and considered for a second course of treat-

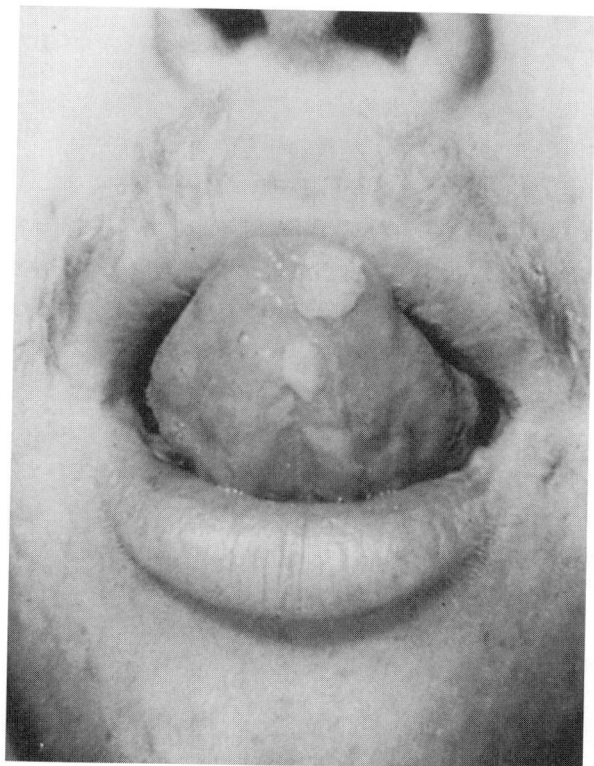

Figure 40–12. Mucous patch, characteristic of secondary syphilis. (From Duff P, Christian JS, Yancey MK: Infections associated with pregnancy. *In* Coulam CB, Faulk WP, McIntyre JA [eds]: Immunologic Obstetrics. New York, WW Norton & Co, 1992, p 578, with permission.)

Table 40–19. FREQUENCY OF VERTICAL TRANSMISSION OF SYPHILIS

Stage of Maternal Infection	Approximate Frequency of Congenital Syphilis
Primary	50%
Secondary	50%
Early latent	40%
Late latent	10%
Tertiary	10%

ment. Antibody titers may decline more slowly in patients with more advanced stages of disease. Specific treponemal tests typically remain positive for life even after adequate treatment, although 13 to 24 percent of patients may ultimately become seronegative.[215-217] Ideally, patients should be followed with quantitative titers for up to 12 to 18 months after their initial infection to determine if they become seronegative.

Perinatal Complications

Syphilis in pregnancy may be associated with an increased risk of fetal demise, intrauterine growth restriction, and preterm delivery.[218] It also may accelerate the course of HIV infection in pregnant women. However, the most frequent (and potentially ominous) complication of syphilis in pregnancy is congenital infection. *T. pallidum* can cross the placenta and infect the fetus *at any stage of gestation.* Up to one third of fetuses with congenital syphilis are stillborn.[4] The frequency of vertical transmission varies primarily with the stage of maternal disease, as noted in Table 40–19. The many possible clinical manifestations of congenital syphilis are summarized in Table 40–20 and illustrated in Figures 40–13 and 40–14.

Table 40–20. CLINICAL MANIFESTATIONS OF CONGENITAL SYPHILIS

Early	Late
Maculopapular rash	Hutchinson teeth
Snuffles (syphilitic rhinitis)	Mulberry molars
Mucous patches	Interstitial keratitis
Hepatosplenomegaly	Deafness
Jaundice	Saddle nose
Pneumonia	Rhagades
Lymphadenopathy	Saber shins
Osteochondritis	Mental retardation
Chorioretinitis	Hydrocephalus
Iritis	Generalized paresis
	Optic nerve atrophy
	Clutton joints (hydrarthosis)

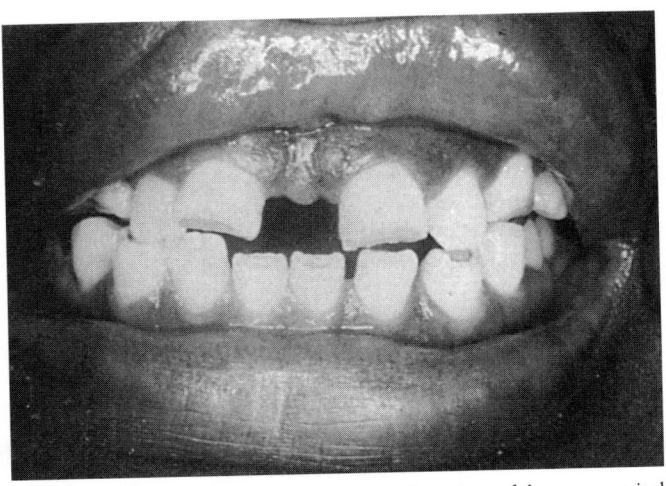

Figure 40–13. Hutchinson teeth, a manifestation of late congenital syphilis. (From Duff P, Christian JS, Yancey MK: Infections associated with pregnancy. *In* Coulam CB, Faulk WP, McIntyre JA [eds] Immunologic Obstetrics. New York, WW Norton & Co, 1992, p 578, with permission.)

T. pallidum has been recovered from fetal blood and amniotic fluid in cases of congenital infection.[219] However, the prenatal diagnostic test with the greatest potential for identifying the severely infected fetus is ultrasound. Ultrasound findings suggestive of in utero infection include placentomegaly, intrauterine growth restriction, microcephaly, hepatosplenomegaly, and hydrops.

Treatment

The treatment of syphilis in pregnancy is summarized in Table 40–21.[215-217] Clearly, penicillin is the drug of

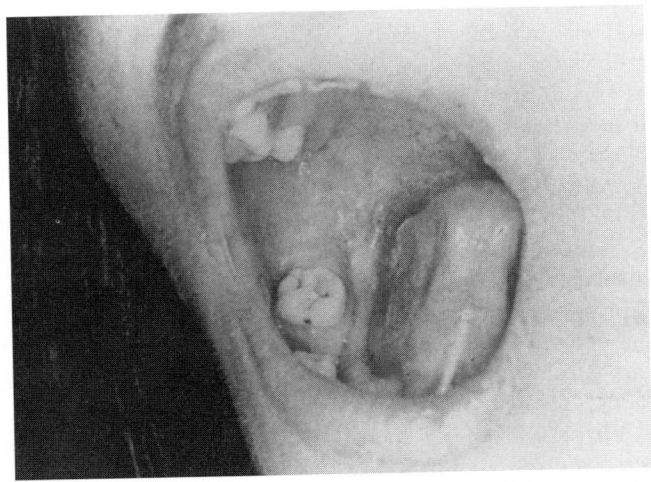

Figure 40–14. Mulberry molar, a manifestation of late congenital syphilis. (From Duff P, Christian JS, Yancey MK: Infections associated with pregnancy. *In* Coulam CB, Faulk WP, McIntyre JA [eds]: Immunologic Obstetrics. New York, WW Norton & Co, 1992, p 578, with permission.)

Table 40-21. RECOMMENDATIONS FOR TREATMENT OF SYPHILIS IN PREGNANCY

Stage of Disease	Principal Treatment	Alternate Treatment if Allergic To Penicillin*
Primary, secondary, or latent syphilis <1 year's duration	Benzathine penicillin G, 2.4 million units IM × 1†	Erythromycin 500 mg PO qid × 15 days Ceftriaxone 250 mg IM qd × 10 days
Latent syphilis >1 year's duration or cardiovascular syphilis	Benzathine penicillin G, 2.4 million units IM weekly × 3	Erythromycin 500 mg qid × 30 days
Neurosyphilis	Aqueous crystalline penicillin G, 3–4 million units q4h × 10–14 days, followed by benzathine penicillin G, 2.4 million units IM × 1 *or* Aqueous procaine penicillin G, 2.4 million units IM daily with probenecid, 500 mg PO qid, both for 10–14 days, followed by benzathine penicillin G, 2.4 million units IM × 1	No regimen of proven value other than penicillin

* These regimens should be administered only if desensitization to penicillin is unsuccessful.
† In patients who are concurrently infected with HIV, treat as outlined below for late latent or tertiary syphilis. Patients also should have a lumbar puncture to determine if neurosyphilis is present.

choice for this infection because of its proven ability to prevent congenital infection in most cases. Patients who have a previous history of an allergic reaction to penicillin should be skin tested to determine if their allergy persists.[215-217] In point of fact, approximately 10 percent of patients who report a history of severe allergy to penicillin remain allergic throughout life. They can be reliably identified by testing with major and minor penicillin determinants. If allergy is confirmed, patients should be desensitized with either oral or intravenous regimens.[215,217,220] Desensitization can usually be completed within 4 hours. It is best accomplished in consultation with an allergist and performed in an area of the hospital with immediate access to emergency resuscitative equipment. A simple regimen for desensitization is outlined by Ziaya et al.[220] Alternative antibiotic regimens are not of proven value for prevention of congenital syphilis or treatment of advanced stages of disease. Accordingly, they should be used only if desensitization is unsuccessful.

Pregnant women receiving penicillin for treatment of syphilis may develop uterine contractions and decreased fetal movement as a result of a Jarisch-Herxheimer reaction. In a recent report, Klein and co-workers[221] observed this reaction in 15 of 33 women (45 percent). The reaction was particularly likely in those patients who had primary and secondary syphilis, and the abnormalities typically appeared 2 to 8 hours after treatment and resolved within 24 hours. There are no reliable clinical or laboratory assessments that predict which patients will develop the Jarisch-Herxheimer reaction, and no specific treatment is available.

TOXOPLASMOSIS

Epidemiology

Toxoplasma gondii is a protozoan that has three distinct forms: trophozoite, cyst, and oocyst (Fig. 40–15). The life cycle of *T. gondii* is dependent on wild and domestic cats, which are the only host for the oocyst.

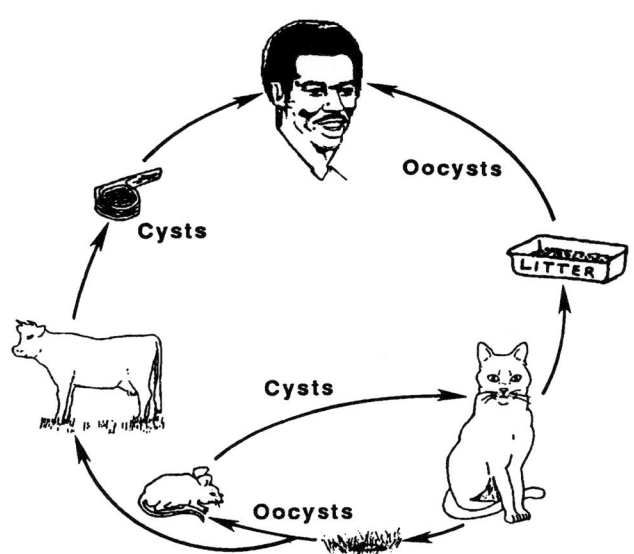

Figure 40–15. Life cycle of *Toxoplasma gondii*. (From Duff P, Christian JS, Yancey MK: Infections associated with pregnancy. *In* Coulam CB, Faulk WP, McIntyre JA [eds]: Immunologic Obstetrics. New York, WW Norton & Co, 1992, p 578, with permission.)

The oocyst is formed in the cat intestine and subsequently excreted in the feces. Mammals, such as cows, then ingest the oocyst, which is disrupted in the animal's intestine, releasing the invasive trophozoite. The trophozoite then is disseminated throughout the body, ultimately forming cysts in brain and muscle.

Human infection occurs when infected meat is ingested or when food is contaminated by cat feces (e.g., via flies, cockroaches, or fingers). Infection rates are highest in areas of poor sanitation and crowded living conditions. Stray cats and domestic cats that eat raw meat are most likely to carry the parasite. The cyst is destroyed by heat, and the practice of eating rare or raw meat in France may explain the high prevalence of infection in that country.[222]

Approximately 40 to 50 percent of adults in the United States have antibody to this organism, and the prevalence of antibody is highest in lower socioeconomic populations. The frequency of seroconversion during pregnancy is less than or equal to 5 percent, and approximately 3 in 1,000 infants show evidence of congenital infection. Clinically significant congenital toxoplasmosis occurs in approximately 1 in 8,000 pregnancies. Toxoplasmosis is more common in western Europe, particularly France. More than 80 percent of women of childbearing age in Paris have antibody to *T. gondii,* and congenital toxoplasmosis is about twice as frequent as in the United States.[222,223]

Clinical Manifestations

The ingested organism invades across the intestinal epithelium and spreads hematogenously throughout the body. Intracellular replication leads to cell destruction. Clinical manifestations of infection are the result of direct organ damage and the subsequent immunologic response to parasitemia and cell death. Host immunity is mediated primarily through T lymphocytes.

Most infections in humans are asymptomatic. Even in the absence of symptoms, however, patients may have evidence of multiorgan involvement, and clinical disease can follow a long period of asymptomatic infection. Symptomatic toxoplasmosis usually presents as an illness similar to mononucleosis.[222,223]

In contrast to infection in the immunocompetent host, toxoplasmosis can be a devastating infection in the immunosuppressed patient. Because immunity to *T. gondii* is cell-mediated, patients with HIV infection and those treated with chronic immunosuppressive therapy after organ transplantation are particularly susceptible to new or reactivated infection. In these patients, CNS dysfunction is the most common manifestation of infection. Findings typically include encephalitis, meningoencephalitis, and intracerebral mass lesions. Pneumonitis, myocarditis, and generalized lymphadenopathy also occur commonly.[222,223]

Diagnosis

The diagnosis of toxoplasmosis can be confirmed by serologic and histologic methods. Serologic tests that suggest an acute infection include detection of IgM-specific antibody, demonstration of an extremely high IgG antibody titer, and documentation of IgG seroconversion from negative to positive.[222,223] Clinicians should be aware that serologic assays for toxoplasmosis are not well standardized. When initial laboratory tests appear to indicate that an acute infection has occurred, repeat serology should be performed in a well-recognized reference laboratory.

The best tissue for identification of *T. gondii* is a lymph node or brain biopsy. Histologic preparations can be examined by light and electron microscopy. For light microscopy, specimens should be stained with either Giemsa or Wright stains.[222–224]

Congenital Toxoplasmosis

Congenital infection can occur if a woman develops *acute* toxoplasmosis during pregnancy. Chronic or latent infection is unlikely to cause fetal injury except perhaps in an immunosuppressed patient. Approximately 40 percent of neonates born to mothers with acute toxoplasmosis show evidence of infection. Congenital infection is most likely to occur when maternal infection develops in the third trimester. Less than half of affected infants are symptomatic at birth. The clinical manifestations of congenital toxoplasmosis are quite varied and are summarized in the box "Clinical Manifestations of Congenital Toxoplasmosis."[223–225]

The most valuable tests for antenatal diagnosis of congenital toxoplasmosis are ultrasound, cordocentesis, and amniocentesis. Ultrasound findings suggestive of infection include ventriculomegaly, intracranial calcifications, microcephaly, ascites, hepatosplenomegaly, and growth restriction. Fetal blood samples can be tested for IgM-specific antibody after 20 weeks of gestation. Fetal blood and amniotic fluid can be inoculated into

---

Clinical Manifestations of Congenital Toxoplasmosis

- Rash
- Hepatosplenomegaly
- Ascites
- Fever
- Chorioretinitis
- Periventricular calcifications
- Ventriculomegaly
- Seizures
- Mental retardation
- Uveitis

mice, and the organism can subsequently be recovered from the blood of infected animals. In addition, Hohlfeld et al.[226] have now identified a specific gene of *T. gondii* in amniotic fluid using a PCR test. In their investigation, 34 of 339 infants had congenital toxoplasmosis confirmed by serologic testing or autopsy. All amniotic fluid samples from affected pregnancies were positive by PCR. Test results were available within 1 day of specimen collection.

Management

Toxoplasmosis in the immunocompetent adult is usually an asymptomatic or self-limited illness and does not require treatment. Immunocompromised patients, however, should be treated, and the regimen of choice is a combination of oral sulfadiazine (4-g loading dose, then 1 g four times daily) plus pyrimethamine (50 to 100 mg initially, then 25 mg daily). In such patients, extended courses of treatment may be necessary to cure the infection.

Treatment also is indicated when acute toxoplasmosis occurs during pregnancy. Treatment of the mother clearly has been shown to reduce the risk of congenital infection and decrease the late sequelae of infection.[224,225] Pyrimethamine is not recommended for use during the first trimester of pregnancy because of possible teratogenicity. Sulfonamides can be used alone, but single-agent therapy appears to be less effective than combination therapy. In Europe, spiramycin has been used extensively in pregnancy with excellent success.[224,225] It is available for treatment in the United States through the CDC.

Aggressive early treatment of infants with congenital toxoplasmosis is indicated and consists of combination therapy with pyrimethamine, sulfadiazine, and leucovorin for 1 year.[227] Early treatment reduces, but does not eliminate, the late sequelae of toxoplasmosis such as chorioretinitis.

In the management of the pregnant patient, *prevention* of acute toxoplasmosis is of paramount importance. Pregnant women should be advised to avoid contact with stray cats or cat litter. They should always wash their hands after preparing meat for cooking and should never eat raw or rare meat. Fruits and vegetables also should be washed carefully to remove possible contamination by oocysts.

VARICELLA

Epidemiology

The varicella-zoster (VZ) virus is a DNA organism that is a member of the herpes virus family. Humans are the only known source of infection. Natural varicella infection occurs primarily during early childhood. Less than 10 percent of cases occur in individuals greater than 10 years of age; however, older patients account for more than 50 percent of all fatalities due to varicella. Varicella is transmitted by direct contact and respiratory droplets. The virus is highly infectious, and approximately 95 percent of susceptible household contacts become infected following exposure. The incubation period is 10 to 14 days. Patients are infectious from 1 day before the outbreak of the rash until all of the cutaneous lesions have dried and crusted over. Immunity to varicella is usually lifelong.[228]

Herpes zoster infection occurs as a result of reactivation of latent virus infection in a patient who already has had varicella. Because of the presence in the host of virus-specific antibody, herpes zoster is usually a much less serious disorder than varicella and rarely poses a major risk to either the mother or her baby unless the former is immunocompromised. However, susceptible patients may develop acute varicella when exposed to individuals with herpes zoster and, therefore, they must be counseled appropriately about this risk.[228]

Clinical Manifestations

The usual clinical manifestations of varicella are fever, malaise, and a skin rash. The characteristic skin lesions usually begin as pruritic macules that appear in crops. The macules progress to papules, then to vesicles, and finally to crusts. The lesions initially appear on the trunk and then spread centripetally to the extremities.

In immunocompetent children, serious complications of varicella are exceedingly rare. However, in adults, two life-threatening sequelae may develop: encephalitis and pneumonia. The former occurs in less than or equal to 1 percent of pregnant women; the latter may develop in up to 20 percent of patients. Prior to the development of acyclovir, the mortality associated with varicella pneumonia in pregnancy approached 40 percent.[228,229]

Diagnosis

The diagnosis of varicella is usually made by clinical examination alone. In problematic cases, the virus can be isolated in tissue culture and cytologic preparations may show multinucleated giant cells and eosinophilic intranuclear inclusions. Serologic assays are of primary value in assessing a patient's susceptibility to varicella immediately following exposure. The two most useful antibody assays are the fluorescent antimembrane antibody test (FAMA) and ELISA. Both assays show sustained elevations, usually lifelong, following natural infection.[228,230]

Management of Maternal Infection

The optimal approach to maternal varicella infection is *prevention*. All women of reproductive age should be assessed for immunity to varicella, ideally before they attempt pregnancy. Susceptible patients, particularly those who are likely to be exposed to varicella either at home or in the workplace, should be offered the new varicella vaccine. Varivax (Merck) is a live attenuated vaccine that is highly immunogenic and approximately 70 to 80 percent effective in protecting the patient against natural infection. Individuals greater than 12 years of age should receive two subcutaneous doses of the vaccine, 4 to 8 weeks apart. Vaccine recipients should use effective contraception for 3 months after immunization. The vaccine can be administered simultaneously with the MMR immunization, but it should not be given in conjunction with blood or blood products. In addition, the vaccine is contraindicated in patients who are pregnant, who have immunodeficiency disorders, or who have received high-dose systemic steroids within 30 days of vaccination.[231]

If the patient first presents for medical care when she is pregnant, she should be questioned about varicella immunity at the time of her first prenatal appointment. If she is uncertain about prior infection, an IgG varicella serology should be performed. If the serology is positive, the patient can be reassured that she is immune and that she and her fetus are not at risk should subsequent exposure occur. If the serology is negative, the patient should be counseled to avoid exposure to individuals who may have varicella or herpes zoster.

Unfortunately, however, the more common situation that the obstetrician encounters is a pregnant patient who has been exposed acutely to an individual who "may have had chickenpox." The clinician's first step in the approach to this situation is to verify that the index patient actually has varicella. If infection is confirmed, the pregnant woman should then be questioned about immunity to varicella. If immunity cannot be documented by history, an IgG varicella serology should be obtained, and the result should be reviewed within 24 to 48 hours of exposure. If the serology is positive, the patient can be reassured that her fetus is not at risk. If the serology is negative, the patient should receive varicella-zoster immune globulin (VZIG). This preparation is 60 to 80 percent effective in preventing infection if given within 72 to 96 hours of exposure. The dose of VZIG is one vial (125 units) per 10 kg of actual body weight, up to a maximum of 5 vials. In problematic cases, if waiting for the varicella serology will delay administration of VZIG for more than 96 hours after exposure, the immunization should be given without confirmatory serology.[228,232,233] Acyclovir also is effective in preventing varicella when given prophylactically. The appropriate dose is 800 mg PO five times daily for 5 to 7 days.[234]

Patients who receive VZIG, as well as those who present for care too late for passive immunoprophylaxis, should be counseled about the clinical signs and symptoms of varicella. In particular, they must be advised to report immediately if early manifestations of varicella encephalitis or pneumonia develop. If serious sequelae occur, the patient should be admitted to the hospital for intravenous therapy with acyclovir. The recommended dose of acyclovir is 500 mg/m^2 every 8 hours, and treatment should be continued until the patient's systemic symptoms have resolved and the cutaneous lesions have begun to crust. Immunocompromised patients should be treated with intravenous acyclovir immediately at the onset of clinical illness because they are at such increased risk for serious complications.[228,229] Otherwise, healthy patients also may be treated with oral acyclovir if they have moderate to severe systemic symptoms. The appropriate dose of acyclovir is 800 mg five times daily for 7 to 10 days.[228,229]

Congenital Infection

Congenital varicella results primarily from hematogenous dissemination of virus across the placenta. Ascending infection following rupture of membranes is possible but extremely unlikely. Congenital infection may lead to spontaneous abortion, intrauterine fetal demise, and varicella embryopathy. The latter disorder is manifested by multiple abnormalities such as cutaneous scars, limb hypoplasia, muscle atrophy, malformed digits, psychomotor retardation, microcephaly, cortical atrophy, cataracts, chorioretinitis, and microophthalmia.[228]

Fortunately, two recent investigations have demonstrated a relatively low frequency of anomalies even following exposure in the first half of pregnancy. Pastuszak et al.[235] reported a study of 106 women with varicella in the first 20 weeks of gestation. The frequency of varicella embryopathy was 1.2 percent, and the prevalence of preterm birth was 14 percent. Subsequently, Enders and co-workers[236] published the largest prospective study of varicella in pregnancy. They observed a 2 percent incidence of congenital infection when maternal varicella occurred at 13 to 20 weeks' gestation. The frequency of congenital infection was only 0.4 percent when maternal infection occurred before 13 weeks' gestation.

The presence of varicella virus in the fetal compartment can be identified by detection of virus-specific IgM antibody and elevated total IgM antibody in cord blood. Virus also can be cultured in amniotic fluid and identified by PCR in placental tissue. Unfortunately, identification of viral DNA, virus-specific antibody, or even the virus itself does not accurately predict the degree of fetal injury. For this purpose, ultrasonography is the preferred diagnostic modality. Sonographic findings suggestive of fetal varicella include polyhydramnios, hydrops, hyperechogenic foci in the abdominal organs (particularly the liver), cardiac malformations, limb deformities, microcephaly, and intrauterine growth restriction.[228]

Neonatal Infection

The final major complication of varicella infection in pregnancy is *neonatal varicella*. Infection of the neonate occurs in 10 to 20 percent of infants whose mothers have acute varicella within the period from 5 days before to 2 days after delivery.[228] Infection usually results from hematogenous dissemination of virus across the placenta at a time when no maternal antibody is present to provide passive immunity to the fetus. Less commonly, neonatal varicella results from postnatal exposure to the mother or another infected person.

The clinical course of neonatal varicella can be variable in progression and severity. The infant usually becomes symptomatic within 5 to 10 days of delivery. Some neonates have only scattered skin lesions and no systemic signs of illness. Others have a biphasic course, initially presenting with a cluster of skin lesions, followed by more widespread dissemination. Still others have a more severe acute illness associated with extensive cutaneous lesions and visceral infection. The most common life-threatening complication is pneumonia. In reports published before the widespread availability of acyclovir, the mortality associated with neonatal varicella was 20 to 30 percent.[228]

To prevent neonatal varicella, an effort should be made to delay delivery until 5 to 7 days after the onset of maternal illness. If delay is not possible, the neonate should receive VZIG (one vial, 125 units) immediately after birth. An important additional preventive measure is isolation of the infant from the mother until all vesicular lesions likely to come in contact with the infant have crusted over.[228,233]

Occasionally, herpes zoster is present in the newborn. This condition is usually a manifestation of intrauterine varicella that occurs in the second half of pregnancy. The clinical course is typically benign, but in rare instances, encephalitis has been documented.

▮ Key Points

➤ Vaginal infections occur commonly in pregnancy. Moniliasis is best treated with topical antifungal compounds such as miconazole, terconazole, or chlortrimazole. Metronidazole is the only antibiotic with uniform efficacy against trichomonas. Clindamycin and metronidazole,

administered either orally or topically, are effective for treatment of bacterial vaginosis.

➤ Urinary tract infections in pregnancy are caused primarily by *E. coli, Klebsiella pneumoniae,* and *Proteus* species. Pyelonephritis is a particularly serious infection in pregnancy because it may be complicated by preterm labor, bacteremia, and ARDS.

➤ Chorioamnionitis and puerperal endometritis are caused by multiple aerobic and anaerobic organisms. Antibiotic therapy should be directed against group B streptococci, aerobic gram-negative bacilli, and *Bacteroides* and *Prevotella* species.

➤ Primary maternal CMV infection during pregnancy is associated with a 40 percent risk of fetal infection. Ten to 15 percent of infected infants are severely affected at birth. Ultrasonography and amniotic fluid viral culture are the best methods for diagnosing fetal infection.

➤ All pregnant women should be screened for hepatitis B infections. Infants delivered to seropositive mothers should receive both hepatitis B immune globulin (HBIG) and hepatitis B vaccine shortly after birth.

➤ HSV infection may be classified as *primary, initial, nonprimary,* and *recurrent. Primary infection* poses the major risk of perinatal transmission. Women with prodromal symptoms or visible lesions should be delivered by cesarean section; asymptomatic women may deliver vaginally.

➤ All pregnant women should be screened for HIV infection. Prophylactic treatment of seropositive women with combination chemotherapy significantly reduces the risk of perinatal transmission of infection and prolongs maternal survival.

➤ Maternal parvovirus infection may result in fetal hydrops. Intrauterine transfusion may be a lifesaving intervention for the hydropic fetus.

➤ Primary maternal toxoplasmosis poses a serious risk of fetal infection. Fetal infection is best diagnosed by DNA analysis of amniotic fluid. Spiramycin is effective in treating both maternal and fetal infection.

➤ Varicella in pregnancy presents serious risk to both the mother and her infant. Susceptible women exposed to varicella should be treated with VZIG. Neonates delivered to mothers with acute varicella also should receive immunoprophylaxis with VZIG. Following delivery, susceptible women should be vaccinated with the new live virus vaccine, provided they are willing to use effective contraception for 3 months.

REFERENCES

1. Eschenbach DA, Hillier S, Critchlow C, et al: Diagnosis and clinical manifestations of bacterial vaginosis. Am J Obstet Gynecol 158:819, 1988.
2. Gravett MG, Hummel D, Eschenbach DA, Holmes KK: Preterm labor associated with subclinical amniotic fluid infection and with bacterial vaginosis. Obstet Gynecol 67:229, 1986.
3. Martius J, Krohn MA, Hillier SL, et al: Relationships of vaginal *Lactobacillus* species, cervical *Chlamydia trachomatis*, and bacterial vaginosis to preterm birth. Obstet Gynecol 71: 89, 1988.
4. Clark P, Kurtzer TA, Duff P: The role of bacterial vaginosis in peripartum infections. Infect Dis Obstet Gynecol 2:179, 1994.
5. Greaves WL, Chungafung J, Morris B, et al: Clindamycin versus metronidazole in the treatment of bacterial vaginosis. Obstet Gynecol 72:799, 1988.
6. Hillier S, Krohn MA, Watts H, et al: Microbiologic efficacy of intravaginal clindamycin cream for the treatment of bacterial vaginosis. Obstet Gynecol 76:407, 1990.
7. Hillier SL, Lipinski C, Briselden AM, Eschenbach DA: Efficacy of intravaginal 0.75% metronidazole gel for the treatment of bacterial vaginosis. Obstet Gynecol 81:963, 1993.
8. Centers for Disease Control and Prevention: 1998 guidelines for treatment of sexually transmitted diseases. MMWR Morb Mortal Wkly Rep 47 (Suppl):1, 1998.
9. Friedrich EG: Vaginitis. Am J Obstet Gynecol 152:247, 1985.
10. Vulvovaginitis. ACOG Technical Bulletin, No. 135, November 1989.
11. Sobel JD: Recurrent vulvovaginal candidiasis. N Engl J Med 315:1455, 1986.
12. Multicentre Study Group: Treatment of vaginal candidiasis with a single oral dose of fluconazole. Eur J Clin Microbiol Infect Dis 7:364, 1988.
13. Phillips RJM, Watson SA, McKay FF: An open multicentre study of the efficacy and safety of a single dose of fluconazole 150 mg in the treatment of vaginal candidiasis in general practice. Br J Clin Pharmacol 44:219, 1990.
14. Thomason JL, Gelbart SM: Trichomonas vaginalis. Obstet Gynecol 74:536, 1989.
15. Duff P: Antibiotic selection for infections in obstetric patients. Semin Perinatol 17:367, 1993.
16. Robbie M, Sweet RL: Metronidazole use in obstetrics and gynecology: a review. Am J Obstet Gynecol 145:865, 1983.
17. Duff P: Antibiotic selection in obstetric patients. Infect Dis Clin North Am 11:1, 1997.
18. Alexander ER, Harrison HR: Role of *Chlamydia trachomatis* in perinatal infection. Rev Infect Dis 5:713, 1983.
19. Baselski VS, McNeeley SG, Ryan G, Robison M: A comparison of nonculture-dependent methods for detection of *Chlamydia trachomatis* infections in pregnant women. Obstet Gynecol 70:47, 1987.
20. Schachter J, Sweet RL, Grossman M, et al: Experience with the routine use of erythromycin for chlamydial infections in pregnancy. N Engl J Med 314:276, 1986.
21. Martin DH, Mroczkowski TF, Dalu ZA, et al: A controlled trial of a single dose of azithromycin for the treatment of chlamydia urethritis and cervicitis. N Engl J Med 327:921, 1992.
22. Magat AH, Alger LS, Nagey DA, et al: Double-blind randomized study comparing amoxicillin and erythromycin for the treatment of *Chlamydia trachomatis* in pregnancy. Obstet Gynecol 81:745, 1993.
23. Al-Suleiman SA, Grimes EM, Jonas HS: Disseminated gonococcal infections. Obstet Gynecol 61:48, 1983.
24. Duff P: Urinary tract infections. Prim Care Update Obstet Gynecol 1:12, 1994.
25. Duff P: Pyelonephritis in pregnancy. Clin Obstet Gynecol 27: 17, 1984.
26. Stamm WE, Counts GW, Running KR, et al: Diagnosis of coliform infection in acutely dysuric women. N Engl J Med 307:463, 1982.
27. Dunlow S, Duff P: Prevalence of antibiotic-resistant uropathogens in obstetric patients with acute pyelonephritis. Obstet Gynecol 76:241, 1990.
28. Stamm WE, Hooton TM: Management of urinary tract infections in adults. N Engl J Med 329:1328, 1993.
29. MacMillan MC, Grimes DA: The limited usefulness of urine and blood cultures in treating pyelonephritis in pregnancy. Obstet Gynecol 78:745, 1991.
30. Robertson AW, Duff P: The nitrite and leukocyte esterase tests for the evaluation of asymptomatic bacteriuria in pregnant patients. Obstet Gynecol 71:878, 1988.
31. Cunningham FG, Morris GB, Mickal A: Acute pyelonephritis of pregnancy: a clinical review. Obstet Gynecol 43:112, 1973.
32. Gibbs RS, Duff P: Progress in pathogenesis and management of clinical intraamniotic infection. Am J Obstet Gynecol 164: 1317, 1991.
33. Armer TL, Duff P: Intraamniotic infection in patients with intact membranes and preterm labor. Obstet Gynecol Surv 46:589, 1991.
34. Gibbs RS, Blanco JD, St. Clair PJ, et al: Quantitative bacteriology of amniotic fluid from women with clinical intraamniotic infection at term. J Infect Dis 145:1, 1982.
35. Romero R, Jimenez C, Lohda AK, et al: Amniotic fluid glucose concentration: a rapid and simple method for the detection of intraamniotic infection in preterm labor. Am J Obstet Gynecol 163:968, 1990.
36. Kirshon B, Rosenfeld B, Mari G, Belfort M: Amniotic fluid glucose and intraamniotic infection. Am J Obstet Gynecol 164:818, 1991.
37. Gauthier DW, Meyer WJ, Bieniarz A: Correlation of amniotic fluid glucose concentration and intraamniotic infection in patients with preterm labor or premature rupture of membranes. Am J Obstet Gynecol 165:1105, 1991.
38. Romero R, Yoon BH, Mazor M, et al: The diagnostic and prognostic value of amniotic fluid white blood cell count, glucose, interleukin-6, and Gram stain in patients with preterm labor and intact membranes. Am J Obstet Gynecol 169: 805, 1993.
39. Hoskins IA, Johnson TRB, Winkel CA: Leukocyte esterase activity in human amniotic fluid for the rapid detection of chorioamnionitis. Am J Obstet Gynecol 157:730, 1987.
40. Locksmith G, Duff P: Assessment of the value of routine blood cultures in patients with chorioamnionitis: an outcome analysis. Infect Dis Obstet Gynecol 2:111, 1994.
41. Sperling RS, Ramamurthy RS, Gibbs RS: A comparison of intrapartum versus immediate postpartum treatment of intraamniotic infection. Obstet Gynecol 70:861, 1987.
42. Gilstrap LC, Leveno KJ, Cox SM, et al: Intrapartum treatment of acute chorioamnionitis: impact on neonatal sepsis. Am J Obstet Gynecol 159:579, 1988.

43. Gibbs RS, Dinsmoor MJ, Newton ER, et al: A randomized trial of intrapartum versus immediate postpartum treatment of women with intra-amniotic infection. Obstet Gynecol 72: 823, 1988.

44. Duff P: Antibiotics for pelvic infections. *In* Rayburn WF, Zuspan FP (eds): Drug Therapy in Obstetrics and Gynecology. 3rd ed. St. Louis, Mosby Year Book, 1992, p 577.

45. Duff P, Sanders R, Gibbs RS: The course of labor in term patients with chorioamnionitis. Am J Obstet Gynecol 147: 391, 1983.

46. Duff P: Pathophysiology and management of postcesarean endomyometritis. Obstet Gynecol 67:269, 1986.

47. Duff P, Gibbs RS, Blanco JD, et al: Endometrial culture techniques in puerperal patients. Obstet Gynecol 61:217, 1983.

48. Milligan DA, Brady K, Duff P: Short-term parenteral antibiotic therapy for puerperal endometritis. J Matern Fetal Med 1:60, 1992.

49. Duff P: Staphylococcal infections. *In* Gleicher N (ed): Principles and Practice of Medical Therapy in Pregnancy. 2nd ed. New York, Appleton & Lange, 1992, p 518.

50. Duff P: Prophylactic antibiotics for cesarean delivery: a simple cost-effective strategy for prevention of postoperative morbidity. Am J Obstet Gynecol 157:794, 1987.

51. Gibbs RS, Blanco JD, St. Clair PJ: A case-control study of wound abscess after cesarean delivery. Obstet Gynecol 62: 498, 1983.

52. Golde S, Ledger WJ: Necrotizing fasciitis in postpartum patients. Obstet Gynecol 50:670, 1977.

53. Shy KK, Eschenbach DA: Fatal perineal cellulitis from an episiotomy site. Obstet Gynecol 54:292, 1979.

54. Weinstein WM, Onderdonk AB, Bartlett JG, Gorbach SL: Experimental intra-abdominal abscesses in rats: development of an experimental model. Infect Immun 10:1250, 1974.

55. Knochel JQ, Koehler PR, Lee TG, Welch DM: Diagnosis of abdominal abscesses with computed tomography, ultrasound, and 111In leukocyte scans. Radiology 137:425, 1980.

56. Gerzof SG, Robbins AH, Johnson WC, et al: Percutaneous catheter drainage of abdominal abscesses. A five-year experience. N Engl J Med 305:653, 1981.

57. Duff P, Gibbs RS: Pelvic vein thrombophlebitis: diagnostic dilemma and therapeutic challenge. Obstet Gynecol Surv 38: 365, 1983.

58. Brown TK, Munsick RA: Puerperal ovarian vein thrombophlebitis: a syndrome. Am J Obstet Gynecol 109:263, 1971.

59. Dunn LJ, Van Voorhis LW: Enigmatic fever and pelvic thrombophlebitis. N Engl J Med 276:265, 1967.

60. Duff P: Septic pelvic vein thrombophlebitis. *In* Charles D (ed): Obstetric and Perinatal Infections. St. Louis, Mosby Year Book, 1993.

61. Brown CEL, Lowe TE, Cunningham FG, Weinreb JC: Puerperal pelvic vein thrombophlebitis: impact on diagnosis and treatment using x-ray computed tomography and magnetic resonance imaging. Obstet Gynecol 68:789, 1986.

62. Duff P, Gibbs RS: Maternal sepsis. *In* Berkowitz RL (ed): Critical Care of the Obstetric Patient. New York, Churchill Livingstone, 1983.

63. Kaplan RL, Sahn SA, Petty TL: Incidence and outcome of the respiratory distress syndrome in gram-negative sepsis. Arch Intern Med 139:867, 1979.

64. Goldberg LI: Dopamine—clinical uses of an endogenous catecholamine. N Engl J Med 291:707, 1974.

65. The Veterans Administration Systemic Sepsis Cooperative Study Group: Effect of high-dose glucocorticoid therapy on mortality in patients with clinical signs of systemic sepsis. N Engl J Med 317:659, 1987.

66. Sprung CL, Caralis PV, Marcial EH, et al: The effects of high dose corticosteroids in patients with septic shock. A prospective controlled study. N Engl J Med 311:1137, 1984.

67. Holaday JW, Faden AI: Nalaxone reversal of endotoxin hypotension suggests role of endorphins in shock. Nature 275: 450, 1979.

68. Ziegler EJ, McCutchan JA, Fierer J, et al: Treatment of gram-negative bacteremia and shock with human anti-serum to a mutant *Escherichia coli.* N Engl J Med 307:1225, 1982.

69. Freid MA, Vosti KL: The importance of underlying disease in patients with gram-negative bacteremia. Arch Intern Med 121:418, 1968.

70. Betts RF: Cytomegalovirus infection epidemiology and biology in adults. Semin Perinatol 7:22, 1983.

71. Wilhelm JA, Malter L, Schopfer K: The risk of transmitting cytomegalovirus to patients receiving blood transfusions. J Infect Dis 154:169, 1986.

72. Stagno S, Pass RF, Dworsky ME, Alford CA: Congenital and perinatal cytomegalovirus infections. Semin Perinatol 7:31, 1983.

73. Pass RF, August AM, Dworsky M, Reynolds DW: Cytomegalovirus infection in a day care center. N Engl J Med 307:477, 1982.

74. Jones LA, Duke-Duncan PM, Yeager AS: Cytomegaloviral infections in infant-toddler centers: centers for the developmentally delayed versus regular day care. J Infect Dis 151:953, 1985.

75. Hutto C, Little EA, Ricks R, et al: Isolation of cytomegalovirus from toys and hands in a day care center. J Infect Dis 154:527, 1986.

76. Adler SP: Cytomegalovirus and child day care. N Engl J Med 321:1290, 1989.

77. Taber LH, Frank AL, Yow MD, Bagley A: Acquisition of cytomegaloviral infections in families with young children: a serological study. J Infect Dis 151:948, 1985.

78. Demmler GJ, Schydlower M, Lampe RM: Texas, teenagers, and CMV. J Infect Dis 152:1350, 1985.

79. Chandler SH, Alexander ER, Holmes KK: Epidemiology of cytomegaloviral infection in a heterogeneous population of pregnant women. J Infect Dis 152:249, 1985.

80. Hohlfeld P, Vial Y, Maillard-Brignon C, et al: Cytomegalovirus fetal infection: prenatal diagnosis. Obstet Gynecol 78:615, 1991.

81. Lamy ME, Mulongo KN, Gadisseaux JF, et al: Prenatal diagnosis of fetal cytomegalovirus infection. Am J Obstet Gynecol 166:91, 1992.

82. Lynch L, Daffos F, Emanuel D, et al: Prenatal diagnosis of fetal cytomegalovirus infection. Am J Obstet Gynecol 165: 714, 1991.

83. Donner C, Liesnard C, Content J, et al: Prenatal diagnosis of 52 pregnancies at risk for congenital cytomegalovirus infection. Obstet Gynecol 82:481, 1993.

84. Adler SP: Cytomegalovirus and pregnancy. Curr Opin Obstet Gynecol 4:670, 1992.

85. Kumar ML, Prokay SL: Experimental primary cytomegalovirus infection in pregnancy: timing and fetal outcome. Am J Obstet Gynecol 145:56, 1983.

86. Stagno S, Pass RF, Dworsky ME, et al: Congenital cytomegalovirus infection. N Engl J Med 306:945, 1982.

87. Fowler KB, Stagno S, Pass RF, et al: The outcome of congenital cytomegalovirus infection in relation to maternal antibody status. N Engl J Med 326:663, 1992.

88. Dobbins JG, Stewart JA, Demmler GJ: Surveillance of congenital cytomegalovirus disease, 1990–1991. MMWR Morb Mortal Wkly Rep 41:35, 1992.

89. Reynolds DW, Stagno S, Hosty TS, et al: Maternal cytomegalovirus excretion and perinatal infection. N Engl J Med 289: 1, 1973.

90. Stagno S, Reynolds DW, Huang ES, et al: Congenital cytomegalovirus infection. N Engl J Med 296:1254, 1977.

91. Lange I, Rodeck CM, Morgan-Capner P, Simmons A: Prenatal serological diagnosis of intrauterine cytomegalovirus infection. BMJ 284:1673, 1982.

92. Grose C, Weiner CP: Prenatal diagnosis of congenital cytomegalovirus infection: two decades later. Am J Obstet Gynecol 163:447, 1990.

93. Lewis PE, Cefalo RC, Zaritsky AL: Fetal heart block caused by cytomegalovirus. Am J Obstet Gynecol 136:967, 1980.

94. Forouzan I: Fetal abdominal echogenic mass: an early sign of intrauterine cytomegalovirus infection. Obstet Gynecol 80: 535, 1992.

95. Pletcher BA, Williams MK, Mulivor RA, et al: Intrauterine cytomegalovirus infection presenting as fetal meconium peritonitis. Obstet Gynecol 78:903, 1991.

96. Katznelson S, Drew WL, Mintz L: Efficacy of the condom as a barrier to the transmission of cytomegalovirus. J Infect Dis 150:155, 1984.

97. Group B streptococcal infections in pregnancy. ACOG Technical Bulletin, No. 170, July 1992.

98. Yancey MK, Duff P: An analysis of the cost-effectiveness of selected protocols for the prevention of neonatal group B streptococcal infection. Obstet Gynecol 83:367, 1994.

99. Boyer KM, Gotoff SP: Prevention of early-onset neonatal group B streptococcal disease with selective intrapartum chemoprophylaxis. N Engl J Med 314:1665, 1986.

100. Committee on Infectious Diseases and Committee on Fetus and Newborn: Guidelines for prevention of group B streptococcal (GBS) infection by chemoprophylaxis. Pediatrics 90: 775, 1992.

101. Thomsen AC, Morup L, Hansen KB: Antibiotic elimination of group-B streptococci in urine in prevention of preterm labor. Lancet 1:591, 1987.

102. Newton ER, Clark M: Group B streptococcus and preterm rupture of membranes. Obstet Gynecol 71:198, 1988.

103. Yancey MK, Armer T, Clark P, Duff P: Assessment of rapid identification tests for genital carriage of group B streptococci. Obstet Gynecol 80:1038, 1992.

104. Siegel JD, McCracken GH, Threlkeld N, et al: Single-dose penicillin prophylaxis against neonatal group B streptococcal infections. N Engl J Med 303:769, 1980.

105. Yow MD, Mason EO, Leeds LJ, et al: Ampicillin prevents intrapartum transmission of group B streptococcus. JAMA 241:1245, 1979.

106. Boyer KM, Gadzala CA, Kelly PD, Gotoff SP: Selective intrapartum chemoprophylaxis of neonatal group B streptococcal early-onset disease. III. Interruption of mother-to-infant transmission. J Infect Dis 148:810, 1983.

107. Centers for Disease Control and Prevention: Prevention of perinatal group B streptococcal disease: a public health perspective. MMWR Morb Mortal Wkly Rep 45(Suppl): 1996.

108. Rosenstein NE, Schuchat A: Opportunities for prevention of perinatal group B streptococcal disease: a multistate surveillance analysis. Obstet Gynecol 90:901, 1997.

109. DeCueto M, Sanchez M-J, Sanpedro A, et al: Timing of intrapartum ampicillin and prevention of vertical transmission of group B streptococcus. Obstet Gynecol 91:112, 1998.

110. Locksmith GJ, Clark P, Duff P: Maternal and neonatal infection rates with three different protocols for prevention of group B streptococcal disease. Am J Obstet Gynecol 180:416, 1999.

111. Shapiro CN, Coleman PJ, McQuillan GM, et al: Epidemiology of hepatitis A: seroepidemiology and risk groups in the USA. Vaccine 10(Suppl 1):S59, 1992.

112. Centers for Disease Control: Hepatitis A among drug abusers. MMWR Morb Mortal Wkly Rep 37:297, 1988.

113. Centers for Disease Control: Hepatitis A among homosexual men—United States, Canada, and Australia. MMWR Morb Mortal Wkly Rep 41:155, 1992.

114. Hepatitis in pregnancy. ACOG Technical Bulletin 174:1, 1992.

115. Centers for Disease Control: Protection against viral hepatitis. Recommendations of the Immunization Practices Advisory Committee. MMWR Morb Mortal Wkly Rep 39(RR-2):1, 1990.

116. Duff B, Duff P: Hepatitis A vaccine: ready for prime time. Obstet Gynecol 91:468, 1998.

117. Syndman DR: Hepatitis in pregnancy. N Engl J Med 313: 1398, 1985.

118. Hoofnagle JH: Chronic hepatitis B. N Engl J Med 323:337, 1990.

119. Sweet RL: Hepatitis B infection in pregnancy. Obstet Gynecol Report 2:128, 1990.

120. Centers for Disease Control: Hepatitis B virus: A comprehensive strategy for eliminating transmission in the United States through universal vaccination: recommendations of the immunization practices advisory committee (ACIP). MMWR Morb Mortal Wkly Rep 40(RR-13):1, 1991.

121. Jagger J, Hunt EH, Brand-Elnaggar J, et al: Rates of needlestick injury caused by various devices in a university hospital. N Engl J Med 319:284, 1988.

122. Lynch-Salomon DI, Combs CA: Hepatitis C in obstetrics and gynecology. Obstet Gynecol 79:621, 1992.

123. Osmond DH, Padian NS, Sheppard HW, et al: Risk factors for hepatitis C virus positivity in heterosexual couples. JAMA 269:361, 1993.

124. Weinstock HS, Bolan G, Reingold AL, et al: Hepatitis C virus infection among patients attending a clinic for sexually transmitted diseases. JAMA 269:392, 1993.

125. Bohman VR, Stettler RW, Little BB, et al: Seroprevalence and risk factors for hepatitis C virus antibody in pregnant women. Obstet Gynecol 80:609, 1992.

126. Lau JY, Davis GL, Kniffen J, et al: Significance of serum hepatitis C virus RNA levels in chronic hepatitis C. Lancet 341:1501, 1993.

127. Chauhan A, Jameel S, Chawla YK, et al: Common aetiological agent for epidemic and sporadic non-A, non-B hepatitis. Lancet 339:1509, 1992.

128. Bradley DW, Maynard JE: Etiology and natural history of post-transfusion and enterically transmitted non-A, non-B hepatitis. Semin Liver Dis 6:56, 1986.

129. Velazquez O, Stetler HC, Avila C, et al: Epidemic transmission of enterically transmitted non-A, non-B hepatitis in Mexico, 1986–1987. JAMA 263:3281, 1990.

130. Wong DC, Purcell RH, Sreenivasan MA, et al: Epidemic and endemic hepatitis in India: evidence for a non-A, non-B hepatitis virus aetiology. Lancet 2:876, 1980.

131. Thomas DL, Mahley RW, Badur S, et al: Epidemiology of hepatitis E virus infection in Turkey. Lancet 341:1561, 1993.

132. Centers for Disease Control: Hepatitis E among U.S. travelers, 1989–1992. MMWR Morb Mortal Wkly Rep 42:1, 1993.

133. Khuroo MS, Kamili S, Jameel S: Vertical transmission of hepatitis E virus. Lancet 345:1025, 1995.

134. Rizzetto M: The delta agent. Hepatology 3:729, 1983.

135. Jacobson IM, Dienstag JL, Werner BG, et al: Epidemiology and clinical impact of hepatitis D virus (delta) infection. Hepatology 5:188, 1985.

136. Alter MJ, Gallagher M, Morris TT, et al: Acute non-A-E hepatitis in the United States and the role of hepatitis G virus infection. N Engl J Med 336:741, 1997.

137. Cook CR, Gall SA: Herpes in pregnancy. Infect Dis Obstet Gynecol 1:298, 1994.

138. Herpes simplex virus infection. ACOG Technical Bulletin No. 102, March 1987.

139. Brown ZA, Vontver LA, Benedetti J, et al: Effects on infants of a first episode of genital herpes during pregnancy. N Engl J Med 317:1246, 1987.

140. Brown ZA, Benedetti J, Ashley R, et al: Neonatal herpes simplex virus infection in relation to asymptomatic maternal infection at the time of labor. N Engl J Med 324:1247, 1991.

141. Cone RW, Hobson AC, Brown Z, et al: Frequent detection of genital herpes simplex virus DNA by polymerase chain reaction among pregnant women. JAMA 272:792, 1994.

142. Stone KM, Brooks CA, Guinan ME, Alexander ER: National surveillance for neonatal herpes simplex virus infections. Sex Transm Dis 16:152, 1989.

143. Prober CG, Sullender WM, Yasukawa LL, et al: Low risk of herpes simplex virus infections in neonates exposed to the virus at the time of vaginal delivery to mothers with recurrent genital herpes simplex virus infections. N Engl J Med 316:240, 1987.

144. Gibbs RS, Amstey MS, Sweet RL, et al: Management of genital herpes infection in pregnancy. Obstet Gynecol 71:779, 1988.

145. Gibbs RS, Mead PB: Preventing neonatal herpes—current strategies. N Engl J Med 326:946, 1992.

146. Whitley R, Arvin A, Prober C, et al: Predictors of morbidity and mortality in neonates with herpes simplex virus infections. N Engl J Med 324:450, 1991.

147. Kulhanjian JA, Soroush V, Au DS, et al: Identification of women at unsuspected risk of primary infection with herpes simplex virus type 2 during pregnancy. N Engl J Med 326:916, 1992.

148. Prober CG, Hensleigh PA, Boucher FD, et al: Use of routine viral cultures at delivery to identify neonates exposed to herpes simplex virus. N Engl J Med 318:887, 1988.

149. Arvin AM, Hensleigh PA, Prober CG, et al: Failure of antepartum maternal cultures to predict the infant's risk of exposure to herpes simplex virus at delivery. N Engl J Med 315:796, 1986.

150. Randolph AG, Washington AE, Prober CG: Cesarean delivery for women presenting with genital herpes lesions. Efficacy, risks, and costs. JAMA 270:77, 1993.

151. Brown ZA, Baker DA: Acyclovir therapy during pregnancy. Obstet Gynecol 73:526, 1989.

152. Goldberg LH, Kaufman R, Kurtz TO, et al: Long-term suppression of recurrent genital herpes with acyclovir. Arch Dermatol 129:582, 1993.

153. Centers for Disease Control: Pregnancy outcomes following systemic prenatal acyclovir exposure—June 1, 1984–June 30, 1993. MMWR Morb Mortal Wkly Rep 42:806, 1993.

154. Whitley RJ, Gramm JW: Acyclovir: a decade later. N Engl J Med 327:782, 1992.

155. Pantaleo G, Graziosi C, Fauci AS: The immunopathogenesis of human immunodeficiency virus infection. N Engl J Med 328:327, 1993.

156. O'Brien TR, George JR, Holmberg SD: Human immunodeficiency virus type 2 infection in the United States. JAMA 267:2775, 1992.

157. Human immunodeficiency virus infections. ACOG Technical Bulletin, No. 165, March 1992.

158. Curran JW, Morgan WM, Hardy AM, et al: The epidemiology of AIDS: current status and future prospects. Science 229:1352, 1985.

159. Minkoff HL, DeHovitz JA: Care of women infected with the human immunodeficiency virus. JAMA 266:2253, 1991.

160. Guinan ME, Hardy A: Epidemiology of AIDS in women in the United States. JAMA 257:2039, 1987.

161. Padian NS: Heterosexual transmission of acquired immunodeficiency syndrome: international perspectives and national projections. Rev Infect Dis 9:947, 1987.

162. Glatt AE, Chirgwin K, Landesman SH: Treatment of infections associated with human immunodeficiency virus. N Engl J Med 318:1439, 1988.

163. MacMahon EME, Glass JD, Hayward SD, et al: Epstein-Barr virus in AIDS-related primary central nervous system lymphoma. Lancet 338:969, 1991.

164. Sloand EM, Pitt E, Chiarello RJ, et al: HIV testing. State of the art. JAMA 266:2861, 1991.

165. Centers for Disease Control: Interpretation and use of the western blot assay for serodiagnosis of human immunodeficiency virus type 1 infections. MMWR Morb Mortal Wkly Rep 38:1, 1989.

166. McNeil JG, Brundage JF, Wann ZF, et al: Direct measurement of human immunodeficiency virus seroconversions in a serially tested population of young adults in the United States Army, October 1985 to October 1987. N Engl J Med 320:1581, 1989.

167. Italian Multicenter Study: Epidemiology, clinical features, and prognostic factors of paediatric HIV infection. Lancet 2:1043, 1988.

168. European Collaborative Study: Mother-to-child transmission of HIV infection. Lancet 2:1039, 1988.

169. Duff P: Prenatal screening for human immunodeficiency virus infection: purpose, priorities, protocol, and pitfalls. Obstet Gynecol 74:403, 1989.

170. Connor EM, Sperling RS, Gelber R, et al: Reduction of maternal-infant transmission of human immunodeficiency virus type 1 with zidovudine treatment. N Engl J Med 331:1173, 1994.

171. Shaffer N, Chuachoowong R, Mock PA, et al: Short-course zidovudine for perinatal HIV-1 transmission in Bangkok, Thailand: a randomized controlled trial. Lancet 353:773, 1999.

172. Dabis F, Msellati P, Meda N, et al: 6-month efficacy, tolerance, and acceptability of a short regimen of oral zidovudine to reduce vertical transmission of HIV in breastfed children in Cote d'Ivoire and Burkina Faso: a double-blind placebo-controlled multicentre trial. Lancet 353:786, 1999.

173. Guay LA, Musoke P, Fleming T, et al: Intrapartum and neonatal single-dose nevirapine compared with zidovudine for prevention of mother-to-child transmission of HIV-1 in Kampala, Uganda: HIVNET 012 randomised trial. Lancet 354:795, 1999.

174. Carpenter CCJ, Fischl MA, Hammer SM, et al: Antiretroviral therapy for HIV infection in 1998. JAMA 280:78, 1998.

175. Centers for Disease Control and Prevention: 1997 USPHS/IDSA guidelines for the prevention of opportunistic infections in persons infected with human immunodeficiency virus. MMWR Morb Mortal Wkly Rep 46(Suppl):1, 1997.

176. Mandelbrot L, LeChanadec J, Berrebi A, et al: Perinatal HIV-1 transmission. Interaction between zidovudine prophylaxis and mode of delivery in the French perinatal cohort. JAMA 280:55, 1998.

177. The International Perinatal HIV Group: The mode of delivery and the risk of vertical transmission of human immunodeficiency virus type I. N Engl J Med 340:977, 1999.

178. Scheduled cesarean delivery and the prevention of vertical transmission of HIV infection. ACOG Committee Opinion, No. 219, August 1999.

179. Dunn DT, Newell ML, Ades AE, et al: Risk of human immunodeficiency virus type 1 transmission through breastfeeding. Lancet 340:585, 1992.

180. Kumar ML: Human parvovirus B19 and its associated diseases. Clin Perinatol 18:209, 1991.

181. Thurn J: Human parvovirus B19: historical and clinical review. Rev Infect Dis 10:1005, 1988.

182. Centers for Disease Control: Risks associated with human parvovirus B19 infection. MMWR Morb Mortal Wkly Rep 38:81, 1989.

183. Cartter ML, Farley TA, Rosengren S, et al: Occupational risk factors for infection with parvovirus B19 among pregnant women. J Infect Dis 163:282, 1991.

184. Gillespie SM, Cartter ML, Asch S, et al: Occupation risk of human parvovirus B19 infection for school and day-care personnel during an outbreak of erythema infectiosum. JAMA 263:2061, 1990.

185. Rodis JF, Hovick TJ, Quinn DL, et al: Human parvovirus infection in pregnancy. Obstet Gynecol 72:733, 1988.

186. Rodis JF, Quinn DL, Gary W, et al: Management and outcomes of pregnancies complicated by human B19 parvovirus infection: a prospective study. Am J Obstet Gynecol 163:1168, 1990.

187. Public Health Laboratory Service Working Party on Fifth Disease: Prospective study of human parvovirus (B19) infection in pregnancy. BMJ 300:1166, 1990.

188. Peters MT, Nicolaides KH: Cordocentesis for the diagnosis and treatment of human fetal parvovirus infection. Obstet Gynecol 75:501, 1990.

189. Pryde PG, Nugent CE, Pridjian G, et al: Spontaneous resolution of nonimmune hydrops fetalis secondary to human parvovirus B19 infection. Obstet Gynecol 79:859, 1992.

190. Humphrey W, Magoon M, O'Shaughnessy R: Severe nonimmune hydrops secondary to parvovirus B19 infection: spontaneous reversal in utero and survival of a term infant. Obstet Gynecol 78:900, 1991.

191. Sahakian V, Weiner CP, Naides SJ, et al: Intrauterine transfusion treatment of nonimmune hydrops fetalis secondary to human parvovirus B19 infection. Am J Obstet Gynecol 164:1090, 1991.

192. Fairly CK, Smoleniec JS, Caul OE, Miller E: Observational study of effect of intrauterine transfusions on outcome after parvovirus B19 infection. Lancet 346:1335, 1995.

193. Rodis JF, Borgida AF, Wilson M, et al: Management of parvovirus infection in pregnancy and outcomes of hydrops: a survey of members of the Society of Perinatal Obstetricians. Am J Obstet Gynecol 179:985, 1998.

194. Conry JA, Torok T, Andrews I: Perinatal encephalopathy secondary to in utero human parvovirus B-19 (HPV) infection [Abstract] Neurology 43:A346, 1993.

195. Brown KE, Green SW, deMayolo JA, et al: Congenital anaemia after transplacental B19 parvovirus infection. Lancet 343:895, 1994.

196. Rubella and pregnancy. ACOG Technical Bulletin No. 171, August 1992.

197. Centers for Disease Control: Rubella prevention: Recommendations of the immunization practices advisory committee (ACIP). MMWR Morb Mortal Wkly Rep 39:1, 1990.

198. Centers for Disease Control: Rubella and congenital rubella syndrome—United States, January 1, 1991–May 7, 1994. MMWR Morb Mortal Wkly Rep 43:391, 1994.

199. Mann JM, Preblud SR, Hoffman RE, et al: Assessing risks of rubella infection during pregnancy. JAMA 245:1647, 1981.

200. Sautter RL, Crist AE, Johnson LM, LeBar WD: Comparison of five methods for the determination of rubella immunity. Infect Dis Obstet Gynecol 1:188, 1994.

201. Miller E, Cradock-Watson JE, Pollock TM: Consequences of confirmed maternal rubella at successive stages of pregnancy. Lancet 2:781, 1982.

202. Munro ND, Smithells RW, Sheppard S, et al: Temporal relations between maternal rubella and congenital defects. Lancet 2:201, 1987.

203. McIntosh EDG, Menser MA: A fifty-year follow-up of congenital rubella. Lancet 340:414, 1992.

204. Bart SW, Stetler HC, Preblud SR, et al: Fetal risk associated with rubella vaccine: an update. Rev Infect Dis 7:S95, 1985.

205. National Vaccine Advisory Committee: The measles epidemic. The problems, barriers, and recommendations. JAMA 266:1547, 1991.

206. Centers for Disease Control: Measles prevention: recommendations of the Immunization Practices Advisory Committee (ACIP). MMWR Morb Mortal Wkly Rep 38:1, 1989.

207. Hersh BS, Markowitz LE, Maes EF, et al: The geographic distribution of measles in the United States, 1980 through 1989. JAMA 267:1936, 1992.

208. Centers for Disease Control: Measles prevention: Supplementary statement. MMWR Morb Mortal Wkly Rep 38:11, 1992.

209. Atkinson WL, Hadler SC, Redd SB, Orenstein WA: Measles surveillance—United States, 1991. MMWR Morb Mortal Wkly Rep 41:1, 1992.

210. Atmar RL, Englund JA, Hammill H: Complications of measles during pregnancy. Clin Infect Dis 14:217, 1992.

211. Christensen PE, Schmidt H, Bang HO, et al: An epidemic of measles in Southern Greenland, 1951. Acta Med Scand 144:430, 1953.

212. Eberhart-Phillips JE, Frederick PD, Baron RC, Mascola L: Measles in pregnancy: a descriptive study of 58 cases. Obstet Gynecol 82:797, 1993.

213. Ekbom A, Wakefield AJ, Zack M, Adami HO: Perinatal measles infection and subsequent Crohn's disease. Lancet 344:508, 1994.

214. Stein SJ, Greenspoon JS: Rubeola during pregnancy. Obstet Gynecol 78:925, 1991.

215. Hook EW, Marra CM: Acquired syphilis in adults. N Engl J Med 326:1060, 1992.

216. Rolfs RT, Nakashima AK: Epidemiology of primary and secondary syphilis in the United States, 1981 through 1989. JAMA 264:1432, 1990.

217. Centers for Disease Control: 1993 Sexually transmitted diseases treatment guidelines. MMWR Morb Mortal Wkly Rep 42:1, 1993.

218. Ricci JM, Fojaco RM, O'Sullivan MJ: Congenital syphilis: the University of Miami/Jackson Memorial Medical Center experience, 1986–1988. Obstet Gynecol 74:687, 1989.

219. Wendel GD, Sanchez PJ, Peters MT, et al: Identification of *Treponema pallidum* in amniotic fluid and fetal blood from pregnancies complicated by congenital syphilis. Obstet Gynecol 78:890, 1991.

220. Ziaya PR, Hankins GDV, Gilstrap LC, Halsey AB: Intravenous penicillin desensitization and treatment during pregnancy. JAMA 256:2561, 1986.

221. Klein VR, Cox SM, Mitchell MD, Wendel GD: The Jarisch-Herxheimer reaction complicating syphilotherapy in pregnancy. Obstet Gynecol 75:375, 1990.

222. Krick JA, Remington JS: Toxoplasmosis in the adult—an overview. N Engl J Med 298:550, 1978.

223. Sever J: The dangers of toxoplasmosis in pregnancy. Contemp Obstet Gynecol 10:29, 1977.

224. Daffos F: Prenatal management of 746 pregnancies at risk for congenital toxoplasmosis. N Engl J Med 318:271, 1988.

225. Desmonts G, Couvreur J: Congenital toxoplasmosis. A prospective study of 378 pregnancies. N Engl J Med 290:1110, 1974.

226. Hohlfeld P, Daffos F, Costa JM, et al: Prenatal diagnosis of congenital toxoplasmosis with a polymerase-chain reaction test on amniotic fluid. N Engl J Med 331:695, 1994.

227. Guerina NG, Hsu HW, Meissner HC, et al: Neonatal sero-

logic screening and early treatment for congenital *Toxoplasma gondii* infection. N Engl J Med 330:1858, 1994.

228. Chapman S, Duff P: Varicella in pregnancy. Semin Perinatol 17:403, 1993.

229. Smego R, Asperilla MO: Use of acyclovir for varicella pneumonia during pregnancy. Obstet Gynecol 78:1112, 1991.

230. McGregor JA, Mark S, Crawford GP, Levin MJ: Varicella zoster antibody testing in the care of pregnant women exposed to varicella. Am J Obstet Gynecol 157:281, 1987.

231. Varicella vaccine. Med Lett Drugs Ther 37:55, 1995.

232. Duff P: Varicella in pregnancy: five priorities for clinicians. Infect Dis Obstet Gynecol 1:163, 1994.

233. Centers for Disease Control: Varicella-zoster immune globulin for the prevention of chickenpox. MMWR Morb Mortal Wkly Rep 33:83, 1984.

234. Asano Y, Yoshikawa T, Suga S, et al: Postexposure prophylaxis of varicella in family contact by oral acyclovir. Pediatrics 92:219, 1993.

235. Pastuszak AL, Levy M, Schick B, et al: Outcome after maternal varicella infection in the first 20 weeks of pregnancy. N Engl J Med 330:901, 1994.

236. Enders G, Miller E, Cradock-Watson J, et al: Consequences of varicella and herpes zoster in pregnancy: prospective study of 1739 cases. Lancet 343:1547, 1994.

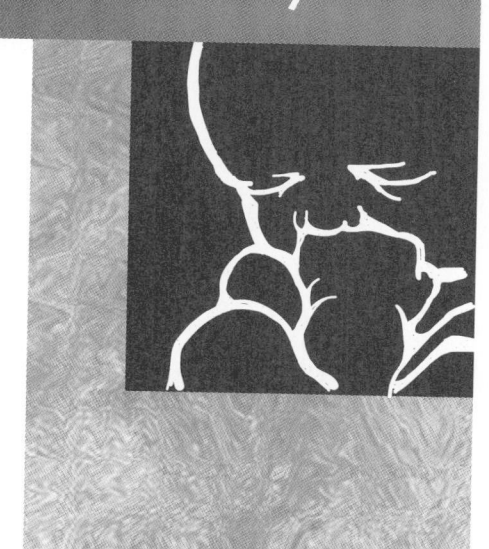

Legal and
Ethical Issues in
Perinatology

Legal and Ethical Issues in Obstetric Practice

GEORGE J. ANNAS AND SHERMAN ELIAS

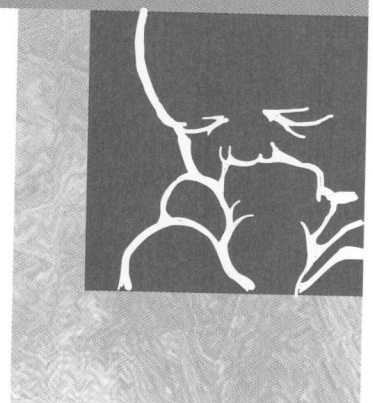

Society has great expectations that modern medical technologies will improve longevity and quality of human life, and nowhere are these expectations higher than in the practice of obstetrics and the desire and expectation of having a healthy child. Along with the rapidly expanding capabilities in diagnosis and treatment, physicians find themselves facing numerous ethical dilemmas while practicing in a medicolegal climate in which malpractice suits can threaten even the most competent and conscientious practitioner.

We cannot address in a single chapter the seemingly infinite ethical and legal controversies facing contemporary obstetric practice and research. Instead, we focus on several topics of particular relevance to the practicing obstetrician.

ABORTION*

The political debate over abortion during the past three decades has shifted among various dichotomous views of the world life: life versus choice, fetus versus woman, fetus versus baby, constitutional right versus states' rights, government versus physician, physician and patient versus state legislature. Hundreds of statutes and almost two dozen Supreme Court decisions on abortion later, the core aspects of *Roe v. Wade,*[2] the most controversial health-related decision by the Court ever, remain substantially the same as they were in 1973. Attempts to overturn *Roe* in both the courtroom and the legislature have failed. Pregnant women still have a constitutional right to abortion. The fetus is still not a person under the Constitution. States still cannot

*This section is adapted from Annas,[1] with permission.

make abortion a crime (either for the woman or the physician) before the fetus becomes viable. States still can outlaw abortion after the fetus becomes viable only if there is an exception that permits abortion to protect the life or health of the pregnant woman. And states still can impose restrictions on abortion before fetal viability only if those restrictions do not actually create a substantial obstacle to a pregnant woman's obtaining an abortion.

Political tactics have shifted from the use of antiabortion rhetoric to change the law concerning abortion to the use of legislative and judicial forums to change the rhetoric of abortion. The hope seems to be that more heated rhetoric will help turn the public and physicians against abortion itself, regardless of its constitutionally protected status.

Roe and Casey

More than 25 years ago, in *Roe v. Wade,* the Supreme Court held that women have a constitutional right of privacy that is "fundamental" and "broad enough to encompass a woman's decision . . . to terminate her pregnancy."[1] If a right is fundamental, the state must demonstrate a "compelling state interest" to restrict it. The Court determined that the state's interest in the life of the fetus becomes compelling only at the point of "viability," defined as the point at which the fetus can survive independent of its mother. Even after viability, the state cannot favor the life of the fetus over the life or health of the pregnant woman: physicians must be able to use their "medical judgement for the preservation of the life or health of the mother." *Roe*'s companion case, *Doe v. Bolton,* specifically included mental health in this determination, saying, "The medical judgment may be exercised in the light of all factors—physical, emotional, psychological, familial, and the woman's age—relevant to the well-being of the patient. All these factors may relate to health. This allows the attending physician the room he needs to make his best medical judgment."

When the Court heard *Planned Parenthood v. Casey*[3] in 1992, most commentators assumed that there were more than enough votes to overturn *Roe*. Instead, three seemingly anti-*Roe* Justices together wrote a joint opinion that while describing the abortion right as a liberty right (instead of a privacy right) and prohibiting the state from unduly burdening it prior to viability (instead of requiring the state to demonstrate a "compelling interest" in regulating abortion) nonetheless confirmed the "core holding" of *Roe*: that states could not outlaw abortion before the fetus becomes viable and could do so thereafter only when the life or health of the woman was not threatened by continuing the pregnancy.[4] Twenty-four-hour waiting periods were approved; spousal notification was ruled unconstitutional. With the loss of all hope that the Court would ever overturn *Roe*, antiabortion advocates needed a new approach to keep the abortion debate alive. They found it in so-called partial-birth abortions.

Partial-Birth Abortion in Congress

In June 1995, the first Partial-Birth Abortion Ban Bill was introduced in Congress to make it a federal crime to perform "an abortion in which the person performing the abortion partially vaginally delivers a living fetus before killing the fetus and completing the delivery." In March 1996, the House passed a revised Senate version, which provided in part:

> (a) Whoever, in or affecting interstate or foreign commerce, knowingly performs a partial-birth abortion and thereby kills a human fetus shall be fined under this title or imprisoned not more than two years or both.
> (b) . . . the term partial-birth abortion means an abortion in which the person performing the abortion partially vaginally delivers a living fetus before killing the fetus and completing the delivery . . . it is an affirmative defense . . . that the partial-birth abortion was performed by a physician who reasonably believed (1) the partial-birth abortion was necessary to save the life of the mother; and (2) no other procedure would suffice for that purpose.[5]

In April 1996, President Bill Clinton vetoed the bill at a White House press conference at which five women described how they made the decision to terminate their pregnancies with what could be considered a partial-birth abortion under the proposed law. He said that the debate was "not about the prochoice/prolife debate" but about the tragic circumstances of "a few hundred Americans every year who desperately want their children." The President said that he would sign a bill that was consistent with *Roe v. Wade*. In the President's words, "I will accept language that says serious,

adverse health consequences to the mother. Those three words."[6]

When the Senate voted in September 1996 to sustain the President's veto, the leader of the fight to override it was Senator Rick Santorum (R-Pa.), who was challenged as having no personal experience or expertise in this area. A week after the vote, Santorum had his own story to tell.[7] The senator's wife had been pregnant with their fourth child when they were informed that ultrasonography showed that their child had a "fatal defect," which turned out to be complete urinary tract obstruction. They were given three options: have an abortion, do nothing, or choose in utero surgery to insert a shunt. They chose the shunt procedure, which was successfully performed at 20 weeks' gestation. The procedure resulted in infection that put Karen Santorum in serious danger. An abortion would have removed the source of her infection, but she refused. Instead, she went into labor and gave birth to an extremely premature infant, Gabriel. Two hours later he died in his parents' arms.

This seemed to give Santorum the personal expertise to make him a more credible antiabortion advocate. But his experience also illustrates at least two major problems with the legislation he supports. First, his wife's actions can be considered praiseworthy only because she had a choice that is protected by current law. Second, the distinction between premature delivery and abortion on the edges of viability has always been problematic. Santorum, for example, has been quoted as having said, in relation to this experience, that even when the life of the mother is at stake, and "you have to end a pregnancy early . . . that does not necessarily mean having an abortion. You can induce labor, using a drug like Pitocin [oxytocin]."[8] If one accepts the standard medical definition of abortion (termination of a pregnancy when the fetus is not viable), this is a distinction without a difference. Whether a planned abortion is performed or labor is induced, both are intended to terminate a nonviable pregnancy. The real issue is not the method used to terminate the pregnancy, but the justification for terminating it. It is also reasonable to argue that after a fetus is viable, abortion is simply no longer possible by definition; the only option is premature delivery.

What makes the term "partial-birth abortion" so politically powerful is its inaccurate conflation of two polar-opposite results of pregnancy, birth and abortion. Senator Daniel Patrick Moynihan (D-N.Y.) has, for example, described it as "as close to infanticide as anything I have ever come upon."[9] But close is not identical. When Virginia attorney general Mark Earley describes the procedure as a "disturbing form of infanticide,"[10] he is making a legally inaccurate political statement. An almost born child is not yet born, and this is not a person under the Constitution. And, as the

Supreme Court has repeatedly held, if the viable fetus is killed for the sake of the woman's life or health, the act is not infanticide by definition.

Medical Practice and Medical Politics

In January 1997, Santorum reintroduced the Partial-Birth Abortion Ban Act in the Senate. Approximately 1 month later, the executive director of the National Coalition of Abortion Providers told reporters that he had lied in 1995 when he claimed that partial-birth abortions were rare and were performed only in extreme situations; instead, he said that "thousands" were performed annually, and most "on healthy fetuses and healthy mothers."[11] The total number of abortions performed in the United States has been steadily declining, although there are no accurate statistics on the frequency of partial-birth abortions. There were two important differences in Congress this time around: medical organizations took conflicting positions, and substantial compromises were attempted in the Senate. The first time around, the American Medical Association (AMA) had taken no position, and the American College of Obstetricians and Gynecologists (ACOG) had urged the President to veto the bill.

In January 1997, ACOG's executive board issued its first and only statement on "intact dilatation and extraction." The board wrote that it understood that the bill attempted to outlaw a procedure containing all of the following elements:

1. deliberated dilatation of the cervix, usually over a sequence of days;
2. instrumental conversion of the fetus to a footing breech;
3. breech extraction of the body excepting the head; and
4. partial evacuation of the intracranial contents of the living fetus to effect vaginal delivery of a dead but otherwise intact fetus.[12]

The board described this as "one method of terminating a pregnancy" after 16 weeks. The board noted that it was sometimes used to save the life or health of the mother, but that its "select panel . . . could identify no circumstances under which this procedure . . . would be the only option to save the life or preserve the health of the woman . . . [although it] may be the best or most appropriate procedure." The board's primary point was that only the woman's physician should make the decision about what particular procedure to use in individual circumstances, and that therefore "the intervention of legislative bodies into medical decision making is inappropriate, ill advised, and dangerous."

The AMA took a different position. On the eve of the Senate vote in May 1997, the AMA's board of trustees agreed to support the legislation if Santorum would add two physician-friendly procedural amendments.[13] These were a requirement that the physician's action be "deliberate and intentional," and a procedure to involve the state medical board in the trial of an accused physician. State bans on partial-birth abortion are based on the inherent police power that states have to protect the health and safety of the public. The federal government has no such power; the federal bill is instead based on the power of Congress to regulate interstate commerce. Because the AMA endorsed the federal bill, it implicitly agreed that what physicians do with individual patients in their offices is a matter of interstate commerce, and therefore subject to regulation by the federal government. This is a stunning concession.

Attempts to reach a real compromise that could have resulted in a bill that President Clinton could sign, and that would probably have been upheld by the courts as constitutional, were made primarily by Senator Dianne Feinstein (D-Calif.), Senator Barbara Boxer (D-Calif.), and Senator Thomas Daschle (D-S.D.). The Feinstein-Boxer amendment would have dealt specifically with the problem the President had with the original bill by adding "serious adverse health consequences to the woman" as an additional exception to the prohibition. Daschle offered to ban all abortions, by any technique, after viability. The only exception would be to save the life of the pregnant woman or to protect her from "grievous injury" to her physical health, defined as "a severely debilitating disease or impairment specifically caused by the pregnancy, or an inability to provide necessary treatment for a life-threatening condition."[14]

Daschle's bill defined the realm of the debate as the period after viability (roughly the third trimester) but nonetheless attempted to limit the reach of *Roe v. Wade* by restricting the exception regarding the health of the pregnant woman to physical (not mental) health and to the risk of "grievous" harm, at that. ACOG endorsed the Daschle compromise, but in doing so seemed to put politics over loyalty to patients, since the Daschle proposal limited the ability of a physician to act to protect the health of a patient after the fetus becomes viable.

In May 1997, the Senate adopted the Santorum bill by a vote of 64 to 36, and in October 1997, it was passed by the House and sent to the President. Two days later, President Clinton again vetoed the bill. He issued a three-paragraph message to the House of Representatives, in which he said he was vetoing the bill "for exactly the same reasons I returned an earlier substantially identical version . . . last year"—that is, because of its failure to include an exception for abortion to prevent "serious harm" to a woman's health.

In 2000, in *Stenberg v. Carhart,* the U.S. Supreme

Court ruled, 5 to 4, that state laws outlawing "partial birth abortions," that were worded substantially identical to the laws passed by Congress and vetoed by President Clinton, are unconstitutional.[15] The reasons are twofold. The first is that the law is unconstitutionally vague because the procedure it purports to outlaw is described in words that could be read to outlaw other abortion procedures that everyone agrees are constitutional. This places physicians in fear of prosecution, and may thus cause them not to perform abortions they otherwise would, putting an "undue burden" on pregnant women wishing to terminate their pregnancies. Secondly, the act makes no exception for the "health of the woman," and *Roe v. Wade* requires that this exception exist throughout the pregnancy. Ultimately, the central question regarding abortion remains who should make the decision: the state or women and their physicians together. The answer of the Supreme Court, as articulated in *Roe v. Wade,* and reinforced in *Stenberg,* is that the decision belongs to the woman and her physician together.[16]

Government Regulation of Medical Procedures

Both sides admit that even if the technique of intact dilatation and extraction is outlawed, it is unlikely that even one abortion will be prevented. Thus, perhaps the primary lesson of the past 25 years is that the controversy over abortion in America is not susceptible to political solution. Moreover, since neither Congress nor the states can alter the constitutional law of abortion as set forth in *Roe v. Wade* and *Casey,* if the debate about partial-birth abortion were only a debate about abortion itself, it would be of little practical consequence. The debate, however, exposes other important issues.

The chief issue is the proper role of the government in regulating medical care. Historically, prochoice forces have favored this framing of the abortion debate. When the debate about abortion is argued as a choice between having a woman and her physician make the decision and having the state legislature or Congress make it, the woman and her physician are the overwhelming choice of Americans. The government-versus-physician framework is also uncomfortable for Republicans, who tend to argue against government interference with private decision making. And even when government regulation seems appropriate, most Republicans prefer regulation by the individual states to regulation by the federal government.

A more focused way to frame the debate is to ask whether decisions about specific medical procedures should be made by physicians or legislators. The AMA's support of the ban on partial-birth abortion seems to be a repudiation of its historic position against

government interference in this realm. If the AMA believes that the federal government can outlaw a constitutionally protected procedure performed in the privacy of a physician's office on the basis of the federal government's power to regulate interstate commerce, then the AMA has conceded that the federal government can regulate all medical procedures. On the other hand, the AMA has never had a consistent position on abortion.[17]

The issue of who (the medical profession or the state—or health plans, for that matter) has the authority to determine what is and what is not a legitimate medical procedure has implications for everything done by physicians, not just for abortions.[18] *Roe v. Wade* and *Casey* both teach that government restrictions on legitimate medical procedures that are used to perform abortions before the fetus is viable are unconstitutional (at least if the use of such procedures does not increase the risks to the woman's health). These cases also teach that the failure to make exceptions to outlawed procedures (so that they can be used to protect the life and health of the pregnant woman) also makes the bills regulating partial-birth abortion unconstitutional as passed.

It has been primarily because of the failure to allow physicians to protect the woman's health after the fetus becomes viable, the vagueness of the definition of partial-birth abortion, and the application of the ban before fetal viability that courts have found that some of the similar laws regulating partial-birth abortion that have been passed in more than two dozen states are unconstitutional.[19-24] One U.S. Circuit court, however, did approve the law if it was very narrowly interpreted, although the reasoning of the majority in this 5 to 4 opinion is deeply flawed.[25]

In the only case to reach the Supreme Court before the President's veto, in March 1998, the Court refused to hear an appeal of a lower-court decision that the Ohio ban on partial-birth abortion was unconstitutional. Three Justices (Clarence Thomas, Antonin Scalia, and William Rehnquist), however, voted to hear the appeal so that the Court could reopen what has become the central issue in the debate: whether the Constitution requires an exception to a ban on abortion after viability that includes the pregnant woman's mental health.[26] Although we can only guess at why none of the other six Justices voted to hear this case (it takes four Justices to agree to hear an appeal to the Court), it would appear that all of them think that a woman's mental health is as protected under the Constitution as her physical health.

President Clinton was thus on strong constitutional grounds when he based his vetoes on the failure of these bills to allow for a physician's action to preserve a pregnant woman's health. He was also on strong grounds in insisting, like ACOG, that the proper person to make a judgment about the health of the woman is the physician (acting, of course, in partnership with the woman). As the Court put it in *Roe v. Wade,* this "decision vindicates the right of the physician to administer medical treatment according to his professional judgment." This means that if intact dilatation and extraction is a legitimate medical procedure, it is constitutionally protected under *Roe v. Wade.* If, however, it is not such a procedure, but rather in the category of nonmedical interventions, like female genital mutilation[27] and execution by lethal injection, it has (and deserves) no such protection. Therefore, another way to frame the debate about abortion is to ask who should have the authority to determine which procedures are legitimate medical procedures.

Efforts to reframe the abortion debate have always involved a dichotomy that allows us to ignore or marginalize either women or fetuses by asking us to avert our attention from abortion itself and concentrate on something else. Often, this something else is the physician and the relation of medicine to government. At other times, it is (appropriately, we think) the pregnant woman and her life and health. Pregnancy is a unique human condition; there is nothing else like it in medicine or life, and we must therefore deal with it on its own terms, and not by analogy. To do so is simply impossible in the political arena. Because abortion foes have never seemed to care whether or not the laws they propose are unconstitutional, they have promised to continue to try to pass such laws.

Professional organizations should set and follow the terms of their own specialties, and in this area ACOG is the proper body to make this determination. But when professional organizations determine the content and scope of reasonable medical practice not on the basis of their professional skills and the health interests of their patients, but rather on the basis of their reading of the prevailing political winds, they undermine their own credibility and explicitly agree that standards for medical practice should be set by politicians rather than by the medical profession.

GENETIC COUNSELING, SCREENING, AND PRENATAL DIAGNOSIS

Any woman who employs a physician for prenatal care should have the right to have the physician fully inform her of any reason the physician has to believe that her fetus might be handicapped and to inform her further of the existence of diagnostic tests that might identify the precise genetic condition. The physician incurs this duty to disclose because it is this type of information

that the pregnant woman seeks prenatal care to discover (i.e., to learn all she can to help her have a healthy child). It is therefore entirely reasonable for the pregnant woman to expect her physician to apprise her of any relevant information regarding her fetus and options she might have so that she and the child's father can determine what action to take.[28]

A wrongful birth suit must allege and prove not only that the physician was negligent in the care of the pregnant woman, but also that had the negligent act not been done the child would not have been born (e.g., had the woman been properly informed that she was at risk to have a child with Down syndrome, she could have sought amniocentesis or chorionic villus sampling and had an abortion if her fetus were so affected). A related but far more controversial lawsuit is brought by the child (through its parents or guardian) against the physician because it was born, a so-called wrongful life suit. Until recently, most courts rejected lawsuits by the child because they thought it was impossible to put a monetary value on life in an impaired condition compared with nonexistence. The choice for these children is *never* to be born healthy, but only to be born with a handicap (such as Down syndrome or Tay-Sachs disease) or not to be born at all. We think that future courts are likely to limit such actions to *serious* handicaps, those in which fetuses, if they could speak to us (which, of course, they can only do through their parents), would agree with an "objective societal consensus" that their own best interest would be served if they were aborted. Put another way, they would be better off *from their own perspective* if they never existed. Conditions like deafness and Down syndrome would not qualify, whereas conditions like Tay-Sachs would. Measuring damages *is* problematic, but courts are likely to award at least the added medical costs caused by the handicap itself. However, because medical costs can be recovered in a wrongful birth case directly, wrongful life cases are only likely to be brought in those rare instances in which for some reason (e.g., the child has been given up for adoption) the parents have lost the right to sue on their own behalf.[29]

Genetic Counseling and Prenatal Diagnosis

The following conclusions may be drawn regarding the legal and ethical obligations of the obstetrician in relationship to genetic counseling and prenatal diagnosis.

First, the law requires physicians to give accurate information to the parents and forbids the withholding of vital information from them. These principles are consistent with the doctrine of informed consent and the reasonable expectations of pregnant women under a physician's care. The physician does not guarantee a healthy child, but the reasonable expectation of the patient is that she will be apprised of any information the physician has that the child might be handicapped and of the alternative ways to proceed so that the patient can determine what action to take.[30]

Second, no obstetrician can be required to perform chorionic villus sampling or genetic amniocentesis. Indeed, many are not qualified to perform these procedures and for them to do so may itself be malpractice. As stated in an opinion of the Judicial Council of the American Medical Association[31]:

> Physicians who consider the legal and ethical requirements applicable to genetic counseling to be in conflict with their moral values and conscience may choose to limit such services to preconception diagnosis and advice or not provide any genetic services. However, there are circumstances in which the physician who is so disposed is nevertheless obligated to alert prospective parents that a potential genetic problem does exist, that the physician does not offer genetic services, and that the patient should seek medical genetic counseling from another qualified specialist.

Third, genetic counseling should be morally nondirective, that is, the counselor should remain impartial and objective in providing information that will allow competent counselees to make their own informed decision. The Judicial Council of the American Medical Association[31] has given the following opinion:

> Physicians, whether they oppose or do not oppose contraception, sterilization, or abortion, may decide that they can engage in genetic counseling and screening, but should avoid the imposition of their personal moral values and the substitution of their own moral judgment for that of the prospective parents. The ethical and moral decisions have to be made by the family and should not be imposed by the physician.

Fourth, to ensure the patient's interest in both autonomy and privacy, no information obtained in genetic counseling or screening should be disclosed to any third party, including insurers and employers, without the patient's informed consent.[32,33] Such strict nondisclosure policies should be maintained unless and until specific legislation is enacted that would clearly delineate the circumstance in which confidentiality must be breached, analogous to certain contagious diseases, gunshot wounds, and child abuse. On the other hand, counselors should be permitted to attempt to persuade patients to make disclosures of important information to potentially affected relatives if there is a high probability of serious harm and if the disclosure is limited to pertinent genetic information. We recommend that the genetic counselor make clear, both verbally and in writing, the policy that he or she follows so that the patient can refuse to be screened or counseled if he or she is not in agreement with the disclosure policy. Such agreements will serve to heighten the public's confidence in genetic counseling and will encourage people to participate voluntarily in both screening and counseling.

Genetic Screening[†]

Our ability to translate our expanding genetic knowledge into usable information for individual patients is at best uncertain. Taking a family history and, when indicated, recommending certain tests to identify carriers of genetic diseases are standard in obstetric care. Today's screening tests usually focus on conditions that occur either in the family or in the racial or ethnic group of one or both prospective parents. As our ability to identify genes associated with particular diseases increases, a panel of screening tests to identify carriers of numerous genes will be offered more routinely. It will then become increasingly difficult—if not impossible—to inform those offered screening or testing for reproductive purposes about all the genetic information that can be obtained and the implications of that information.

Consent for Screening

Our current model for screening and testing requires pretest counseling.[35] Such counseling is a method of obtaining informed consent, and the obligation to counsel can be seen as inherent in the fiduciary nature of the doctor–patient relationship.[36,37] For ordinary medical procedures, the physical risks and treatment alternatives are the chief items of information that must be disclosed. There are few physical risks in genetic screening. What must be conveyed in counseling regarding genetic screening is that the tests may yield new information that may ultimately force some unwelcome choices (such as whether to marry, abort, or adopt). Self-determination and rational decision making are the central values protected by informed consent.[36,37] In the setting of reproductive genetics, what is at stake is the right to decide whether or not to have a genetic test, with emphasis on the right to refuse if the potential harm (in terms of stigma or unacceptable choices) outweighs, for the individual person or family, the potential benefit.

Generic Consent for Genetic Screening

As the Human Genome Project nears conclusion, tens if not hundreds of new genetic screening tests will compete for introduction into routine clinical practice. Already some researchers have suggested population-based screening to identify carriers of the genes for such conditions as the fragile X syndrome and myo-

---

[†]This section has been adapted from Elias and Annas,[34] with permission.

tonic dystrophy. Each new screening test presents the same questions: What information should be given to which patients, when should it be presented, who should present it, and how and by whom should the results be conveyed? It will soon be impossible to do meaningful prescreening counseling about all available carrier tests. Giving too much information ("information overload") can amount to misinformation and make the entire counseling process either misleading or meaningless.[38] To prevent disclosure from being pointless or counterproductive, we believe that strategies based on general or "generic" consent should be developed for genetic screening. Their aim would be to provide sufficient information to permit patients to make informed decisions about carrier screening, yet avoid the information overload that could lead to "misinformed" consent.[39]

Traditionally, goals of reproductive genetic counseling, including counseling about screening carrier status, involve helping the person or family to

(1) comprehend the medical fact, including the diagnosis, the probable course of the disorder, and the available management; (2) appreciate the way heredity contributes to the disorder, and the risk of recurrence in specified relatives; (3) understand the options for dealing with the risk of recurrence; (4) choose the course of action which seems appropriate to them in view of their risk and their family goals and act in accordance with that decision; and (5) make the best possible adjustment to the disorder in an affected family member and/or to the risk of recurrence of that disorder.[40]

For example, in the current context of counseling a couple at least one of whom is of Italian ancestry, each of these issues would be discussed as it relates specifically to α-thalassemia, with explanation of the use of hemoglobin electrophoresis as a screening test to determine carrier status. If consideration of another prenatal test were appropriate—as in the case of screening of maternal serum for α-fetoprotein, human chorionic gonadotropin, and unconjugated estriol to detect fetal aneuploidy, open neural tube defects, and other abnormalities—a separate discussion about these tests, including information on their sensitivity and specificity, and of each of the possible associated fetal disorders would also be required. Even knowledgeable couples could become confused, frustrated, and anxious if faced with scores of such options for genetic screening.

By contrast, an approach based on generic consent would emphasize broader concepts and common-denominator issues in genetic screening. We envision a situation in which patients would be told of the availability of a panel of screening tests that can be performed on a single blood sample. They would be told that these tests could determine whether they carry genes that put them at increased risk of having a child with a birth defect that could involve serious physical

abnormalities, mental disabilities, or both. Several common examples could be given to indicate the frequency and spectrum of severity of each type or category of condition for which screening was being offered. For example, prenatal screening could include tests for fetal conditions such as neural tube defects and chromosome abnormalities such as cystic fibrosis and fragile X syndrome. In the future, a sample of fetal blood cells may be retrievable from maternal blood to be used not only for estimation of risks but also perhaps for definitive diagnosis.[41]

In the course of such counseling, important factors common to all genetic screening tests would be highlighted. Among these are the limitations of screening tests, especially the fact that negative results cannot guarantee a healthy infant; the possible need for additional, invasive tests, such as chorionic villus sampling or amniocentesis, to establish a definitive diagnosis; the reproductive options that might have to be considered, such as prenatal diagnosis, adoption, gamete donation, abortion, or acceptance of risks; the costs of screening; issues of confidentiality, including potential disclosure to other family members; and the possibility of social stigmatization, including discrimination in health insurance and employment. If carrier status is detected in the woman, it must be emphasized that the partner should also be screened. Before prenatal testing was agreed to in such cases, the woman would need to be told that she would be advised to consider abortion if the fetus was found to be affected with a nontreatable condition.[37]

This type of generic consent to genetic screening can be compared with obtaining consent to perform a physical examination. Patients know that the purpose of the examination is to locate potential problems that are likely to require additional follow-up and that could present them with choices they would rather not have to make. The patient is not generally told, however, about all the possible abnormalities that can be detected by a routine physical examination or routine blood work, but only the general purpose of each. On the other hand, tests that may produce especially sensitive and stigmatizing information, such as screening of blood for the human immunodeficiency virus, should not be performed without specific consent. Similarly, because of its reproductive implications, genetic testing has not traditionally been carried out without specific consent. Even in a generic model, tests for untreatable fatal diseases such as Huntington's disease should not be combined with other tests or performed without specific consent.[37]

What is central in the concept of generic consent for genetic screening is not a waiver of the individual patient's right to information. Rather, it would reflect a decision by the genetics community that the most reasonable way to conduct a panel of screening tests to identify carriers of serious conditions is to provide basic, general information to obtain consent for the screening and much more detailed information on specific conditions only after they have been detected. Since, in the vast majority of cases, no such conditions will in fact be found, this method is also the most efficient and cost effective.

Limits to Generic Consent

Some people require more specific and in-depth information on which to base their decision regarding screening. It is therefore essential to build into the screening program ample opportunity for patients to obtain all the additional information they need to help them make decisions. Clinicians, of course, must be open and responsive to the concerns and questions of patients. Counseling could be provided in person by a physician or other health professional. Alternatively, audiovisual aids could be used, which would help ensure consistency in the information provided, be more efficient, and respond to the shortage of genetic counselors.

Generic consent for genetic screening should help prevent information overload and wasting time on useless information. It would not, however, solve what is likely to be an even more central problem in genetic screening: are there genetic conditions for which screening should not be offered to prospective parents? Examples might include genes that predispose a person to a particular disease late in life (such as Alzheimer's disease, Parkinson's disease, or breast cancer).[37,42] From the perspective of the fetus, life with the possibility—or even the high probability—of developing these diseases in late adulthood is much to be preferred to no life at all. Thus, in this case, unlike that of the fetus with anencephaly, for example, no reasonable argument could be made that precluding abortion by denying this information could amount to forcing a "wrongful life" on the child.[35] Because of a personal experience with a friend or family member who suffered from one of these diseases, however, the couple might see abortion as a reasonable choice under such circumstances.

We must address this question directly and publicly. Are there genetic diseases and predispositions for which screening of prospective parents and testing of fetuses should not be offered as a matter of good medical practice and public policy, regardless of the technical ability to screen and the wishes of the couple? Offering carrier screening to assist couples in making reproductive decisions is not a neutral activity but, rather, implies that some action should be taken on the basis of the results of the test. Thus, for example, merely offering screening for a breast cancer or colon cancer gene suggests to couples that artificial insemination, adoption, and abortion are all reasonable choices if they are found to be carriers of such a gene. We do not believe that pregnancies in women who want to have a child should be terminated for this reason, and thus we believe carrier screening for the breast cancer gene should not be offered in the context of reproductive planning. In the absence of an effective way to set the standard of care for carrier screening, however, prenatal screening tests for these and similar genes will inevitably be offered by at least some commercial companies and private physicians.

A standard of care for genetic screening and consent in the face of hundreds of available genetic tests will inevitably be set. We believe the medical profession should take the lead in setting such standards and that, with public input, the model of generic consent for genetic screening will ultimately be accepted.

FORCED CESAREAN DELIVERY

In 1979, a group of Israeli obstetricians published a controversial article entitled "The fetal right to live," suggesting that when women in labor refuse cesarean delivery "It is probably that the patient hopes to be freed in this way of an undesired pregnancy . . . because it is an unplanned pregnancy, the woman is divorced or widowed, the pregnancy is an extramarital one, there are inheritance problems, etc."[43] The view that women who refuse cesarean delivery are in some way willfully abusing their fetuses seems prevalent and deeply held, at least by some male obstetricians and judges. This opinion is reflected in several cases in which judges have ordered women who were refusing cesarean delivery during labor to undergo the procedure "for the welfare of the unborn child."

In 1987, Kolder et al.[44] reported a U.S. national survey revealing that court orders have been obtained for cesarean deliveries in 11 states, for hospital detentions in 2 states, and for intrauterine transfusions in 1 state. Among 21 cases in which court orders were sought, the orders were obtained in 86 percent; in 88 percent of those cases, the orders were received within 6 hours. The majority of the women involved were black, Asian, or Hispanic, and all were poor. Nearly one half were unmarried and one fourth did not speak English as their primary language. In the survey, they also found that 46 percent of the heads of fellowship programs in fetomaternal medicine thought that women who refused medical advice and thereby endangered the life of the fetus should be detained. Forty-seven percent supported court orders for procedures such as intrauterine transfusions. Until 1990, with the exception of one case in the Georgia State Supreme Court, all cases had been decided by lower courts and therefore had little precedential importance.[45] In the vast majority of cases, judges were called on an emergency basis and ordered interventions within hours. The judge usually went to the hospital. Physicians should know what most lawyers and almost all judges know: when a judge arrives at the hospital in response to an emergency call, he or she is acting much more like a lay person than a jurist. Without time to analyze the issues, without representation for the pregnant woman, without briefing or thoughtful reflection on the situation, in almost total ignorance of the relevant law, and in an unfamiliar setting faced by a relatively calm physician and a woman who can easily be labeled "hysterical," the judge will almost always order whatever the doctor advises. There is nothing in *Roe v. Wade*[2] or any other appellate decision that gives either physicians or judges the right to favor the life or well-being of the fetus over that of the pregnant woman. Nor is there legal precedent for a mother being ordered to undergo surgery (e.g., kidney or partial liver transplant) to save the life of her dying child. It would be ironic and inconsistent if a woman could be forced to submit to more invasive surgical procedures for the sake of a fetus than a child. Forcing pregnant women to follow medical advice also places unwarranted faith in that advice. Physicians often disagree about the appropriateness of obstetric interventions, and they can be mistaken.[46] In three of the first five cases in which court-ordered cesarean delivery were sought, the women ultimately delivered vaginally and uneventfully. In the face of such uncertainty—uncertainty compounded by decades of changing and conflicting expert opinion on the management of pregnancy and childbirth—the moral and legal primacy of the competent, informed pregnant woman in decision making is overwhelming.[47]

Physicians may feel better after being "blessed" by the judge, but they should not. First, the appearance of legitimacy is deceptive; the judge has acted injudiciously, and there is no opportunity for meaningful appeal. Second, the medical situation has not changed, except that more time has been lost that should have been used to continue discussion with the woman directly. And, finally, the physician has now helped to transform himself or herself into an agent of the state's authority.[47]

The question of how to help a woman who continues to refuse intervention in the face of a court order remains. Do we really want to attempt to restrain and forcibly medicate and operate on a competent, refusing adult? Although such a procedure may be "legal," it is hardly humane. It is not what one generally associates with modern obstetric care and may cause harm. It also encourages an adversarial relationship between the obstetrician and the patient. Moreover, even from a strictly utilitarian perspective, this marriage of the state and medicine is likely to harm more fetuses than it

helps, because many women will quite reasonably avoid physicians altogether during pregnancy if failure to follow medical advice can result in forced treatment, involuntary confinement, or criminal charges.

Extending notions of child abuse to "fetal abuse" simply brings government into pregnancy with few, if any, benefits and with great potential for invasions of privacy and deprivations of liberty. It is not helpful to use the law to convert a woman's and society's moral responsibility to her fetus into the woman's legal responsibility alone.[35] After birth, the fetus becomes a child and can and should thereafter be treated in its own right. Before birth, however, we can obtain access to the fetus only through its mother and, in the absence of her informed consent, can do so only by treating her as a fetal container, a nonperson without rights to bodily integrity.

The American College of Obstetricians and Gynecologists has issued an opinion from its Committee on Ethics entitled "Patient Choice: Maternal Fetal Conflict"[48] that we believe provides thoughtful and useful guidance for the medical practitioner. The conclusions of this statement are as follows:

1. With advances in medical technology, the fetus has become more accessible to diagnostic and treatment modalities. The fetomaternal relationship remains a unique one, requiring a balance of maternal health, autonomy, and fetal needs. Every reasonable effort should be made to protect the fetus, but the pregnant woman's autonomy should be respected.
2. The vast majority of pregnant women are willing to assume significant risk for the welfare of the fetus. Problems arise only when this potentially beneficial advice is rejected. The role of the obstetrician should be one of an informed educator and counselor, weighing the risks and benefits to both patients as well as realizing that tests, judgments, and decisions are fallible. Consultation with others, including an institutional ethics committee, should be sought when appropriate to aid the pregnant woman and obstetrician in making decisions. The use of the courts to resolve these conflicts is almost never warranted.
3. Obstetricians should refrain from performing procedures that are unwanted by a pregnant woman. The use of judicial authority to implement treatment regimens in order to protect the fetus violates the pregnant woman's autonomy. Furthermore, inappropriate reliance on judicial authority may lead to undesirable societal consequences, such as the criminalization of noncompliance with medical recommendations.

In 1990, the District of Columbia Court of Appeals, in a strongly worded opinion, essentially adopted the

American College of Obstetricians and Gynecologists statement as law, holding that the decision of the pregnant woman must be honored in all but "extremely rare and truly exceptional" cases.[50]

FETAL RESEARCH

Federal Regulations

Society has a critical stake in both the treatment of fetal disorders and the maintenance of respect for the human dignity of the fetus. Fetal research and its regulation is one of the most controversial and complex areas in the entire field of human experimentation. The National Commission for the Protection of Human Subjects of Biomedical and Behavioral Research, for example, spent the first year of its existence working on the subject of fetal experimentation under a congressional mandate to make recommendations regarding fetal research before working on any other topic. This mandate itself was most influenced by the 1973 *Roe* decision discussed above. The consequence of this decision was an increase in the number of fetuses aborted; hence the amount of fetal material available for research also increased.

Before experimentation involving human fetuses begins, current U.S. Department of Health and Human Services (HHS) regulations require that appropriate animal studies be performed and that investigators play no role in any decision to terminate a pregnancy. The purpose of any in utero experiment must be to meet the health needs of the particular fetus, and the fetus must be placed at risk only to the minimum extent necessary to meet such needs. In the case of nontherapeutic research, the risk to the fetus must be "minimal" and the knowledge must be "important" and not obtainable by other means. The consent of both the mother and father is required, unless the father's identity is not known, he is not reasonably available, or the pregnancy resulted from rape. Fetal research protocols must be approved by an institutional review board (IRB), taking special care to review the subject selection process and the method of obtaining informed consent.

Technically, these federal regulations apply only to investigators who receive federal research funds or who are affiliated with institutions that have signed an agreement with HHS that all research performed in their institution and by their staff will be approved by an IRB under these regulations. We believe, however, the principles set forth by these regulations to be so fundamentally important to the protection of the integrity of the fetus, the potential parents, and the research enterprise itself that they provide the minimum guidelines that should be adhered to voluntarily in all institutions undertaking fetal research projects.

State Statutes

More state legislation has been enacted regarding fetal research than any other type of research, and the poor quality of the legislation has added to the complicated nature of this issue. About one half of the states currently have statutes regulating fetal research; 15 were passed soon after the *Roe* decision and in direct response to it. Most state statutes restrict both in utero and ex utero research, and the restrictions are generally more stringent than the federal regulations with the exception of New Mexico's statute, which is modeled after federal regulations. In Massachusetts, for example, it is a crime to study the fetus in utero unless the research does not "substantially jeopardize" the life or health of the fetus and the fetus is not the subject of an elected abortion. Because the law includes the embryo in its definition of a fetus, it could also inhibit stem cell research that involves the destruction of a human embryo.[51] Thus, therapeutic research, such as shunting procedures to treat fetal urinary tract obstruction, is permissible even in this restrictive state. Utah, the only state to deal exclusively with in utero fetuses, prohibits all research on "live unborn children." Some states limit their prohibition to the living abortus and thus do not apply to fetal surgery. California restricts experimentation only on ex utero fetuses, outlawing "any type of scientific or laboratory research or any other kind of experimentation or study, except to protect or preserve the life and health of the fetus." Thus there is little consistency or rationale among jurisdictions regarding regulations directly pertaining to fetal research. Nonetheless, one is bound by the laws of the state in which one performs fetal research, and knowledge of its provisions is obviously necessary in states that have such statutes.[52–54]

Consent

A fundamental premise of Anglo-American law is that no one can touch or treat a competent adult without the adult's informed consent. This doctrine is based primarily on the value we place on autonomy, or self-determination, and secondarily on rational decision-making. The first requires that individuals have the ultimate say concerning whether their bodies will be "invaded"; the latter requires disclosure of certain material information, including a description of the proposed procedure, risks of death and serious disability, alternatives, success rates, and problems of recuperation before one is asked to consent to an "invasion."[55]

These issues are relatively straightforward when dealing with an adult, but how do they apply when experimentation or therapy is directed toward a fetus? Unfortunately, the distinction between experimentation and therapy is often unclear. In general, therapy involves procedures performed primarily for the benefit of the patient that are considered "good and accepted practice," whereas experimentation involves new or innovative procedures not yet considered standard practice performed for the primary purpose of testing a hypothesis or gaining new knowledge.[56]

In the therapeutic setting, the consent of either one of the parents is usually sufficient for beneficial procedures to be performed on children. In the case of the fetus, however, if the proposed investigative therapeutic procedure will place the mother at any risk of death or serious disability, she alone has the right to consent and the corresponding right to withhold consent. Even after fetal viability, *Roe* and *Casey* give the woman and her physician the right to terminate the pregnancy if her life or health is endangered. This is consistent with the Court's ruling that where conflict exists between a potential father and the pregnant woman over the issue of an abortion, the woman's position should prevail because she has more at stake (e.g., her body, health risks) than the potential father.[57] The same logic applies here. Consent of the pregnant woman is a mandatory prerequisite for both investigative procedures and therapy. Her consent must be informed, and she should be told as clearly as possible about the proposed experimental procedure or therapy and its risks to herself and her fetus, as well as alternatives, success rates, and the likely problems of recuperation.[58,59]

Key Points

▶ So-called partial-birth abortion bans are unconstitutional unless they provide an exception for the pregnant woman's life and health.

▶ In *Roe v. Wade* (1973), the United States Supreme Court determined that a fundamental "right to privacy existed in the Fourteenth Amendment's concept of personal liberty" that is "broad enough to encompass a woman's decision whether or not to terminate a pregnancy" prior to fetal viability without state interference.

▶ In *Planned Parenthood of Southeastern Pennsylvania v. Casey* (1992) the United States Supreme Court reaffirmed the "core" of *Roe v. Wade* and ruled that prior to fetal viability states cannot "unduly burden" a woman's decision to terminate a pregnancy (i.e., although consent and waiting periods may be constitutionally acceptable, states cannot regulate abortion in ways that will prevent a significant number of women from obtaining them.)

▶ *Roe* and *Casey* are critical to understanding the rights of obstetricians (which are derived from the rights of their patients) because they are the major sources of law regarding how far states can go to regulate decisions made in the obstetrician–patient relationship.

▶ The legal and ethical obligations of an obstetrician in relationship to genetic counseling and prenatal diagnosis can be summarized as follows: (1) the physician must give accurate information to the parents and cannot withhold vital information from them; (2) no obstetrician can be required to perform prenatal diagnostic procedures; (3) prenatal genetic counseling should be morally nondirective; and (4) to protect patient privacy and autonomy, no information obtained in genetic counseling or screening should be disclosed to any third party without patient's authorization.

▶ "Generic" consent for genetic *screening* that emphasizes broad concepts and common-denominator issues should help maximize rational decision making by preventing information overload and wasting time on useless information.

▶ Fetal research protocols must be approved by an institutional review board, which must review the scientific protocol, the subject selection process, the consent form, and the method of obtaining informed consent from both the recipient and donor.

▶ Self-determination and rational decision making are the central purposes of informed consent, and information on recommended procedures, risks, benefits, and alternatives should be presented in a way that furthers these purposes.

▶ Consent of the pregnant woman is a mandatory prerequisite for both investigative procedures and therapy. Her consent must be informed, and she should be told as clearly as possible about the proposed experimental procedures or therapy, its risks to herself and her fetus, as well as alternatives, success rates, and the likely problems of recuperation.

▶ The fetomaternal relationship is a unique one that requires physicians to promote a balance of maternal health and fetal welfare while respecting maternal autonomy. Obstetricians should refrain from performing procedures that are refused by pregnant women: the decision of the competent pregnant woman must be honored in all but "extremely rare and truly exceptional" cases, although reasonable steps to persuade a woman to change her mind are appropriate.

REFERENCES

1. Annas GJ: Partial birth abortion, Congress and the Constitution. N Engl J Med 339:279, 1998.
2. *Roe v. Wade,* 410 U.S. 113 (1973).
3. *Planned Parenthood of Southeastern Pennsylvania v. Casey,* 502 U.S. 1056 (1992).
4. Annas GJ: The Supreme Court, liberty, and abortion. N Engl J Med 327:651, 1992.
5. H.R. 1833, 104th Cong.
6. Remarks on returning without approval to the House of Representatives partial birth abortion legislation Weekly Compilation of Presidential Documents. April 10, 1996;643.
7. Santorum R: A brief life that changed our lives forever. National Right to Life News. May 23, 1997;6.
8. Klein J: The senator's dilemma. New Yorker. January 5, 1998;30.
9. Vobejda B, Brown D: Harsh details shift tenor of abortion fight: both sides bend facts on late-term procedure. Washington Post. September 17, 1996;A1.
10. Hsu S: Virginia ban on certain abortions is blocked, law too vague U.S. judge says. Washington Post. June 26, 1998;C1.
11. Gianelli DM: Abortion rights leader urges end to 'half truths.' American Medical News. March 3, 1997;3, 28.
12. American College of Obstetrics and Gynecology: Statement on intact dilatation and extraction, January 12, 1997.
13. Gianelli DM: House affirms AMA stance on abortion. American Medical News. July 7, 1997;3, 30.
14. Seelye KQ: Democratic leader proposes measure to limit abortions. New York Times. May 9, 1997;A32.
15. *Stenberg v. Carhart,* 530 U.S. 914 (2000).
16. Annas GJ: "Partial-Birth Abortion" and the Supreme Court. N Engl J Med 344:152, 2001.
17. Wolinksy H, Brune T: The Serpent on the Staff: The Unhealthy Politics of the American Medical Association. New York, GP Putnam's Sons, 1994.
18. Kassirer JP: Practicing medicine without a license—the new intrusions by Congress. N Engl J Med 336:1747, 1997.
19. *Women's Medical Professional Corp. v. Voinovich,* 130 F.3d 187 (6th Cir. 1997).
20. *Planned Parenthood of So. Arizona v. Woods,* 982 F. Supp. 1369 (D. Arizona 1997).
21. *Carhart v. Stenberg,* 972 F. Supp. 507 (D. Nebraska 1997).
22. *Summit Medical Associates v. James,* 984 F. Supp. 1404 (M.D. Alabama 1998).
23. *Evans v. Kelley,* 977 F. Supp. 1283 (E.D. Michigan 1997).
24. Massie AM: So-called "partial-birth abortion" bans: bad medicine? Maybe. Bad Law? Definitely! U P H L Rev 59:301, 1998.
25. *Hope Clinic v. Ryan,* 1999 U.S. App. LEXIS 26925.
26. *Voinovich v. Women's Medical Professional Corp.,* 523 U.S. 1036 (1998).
27. Annas CL: Irreversible error: the power and prejudice of female genital mutilation. J Contemp Health Law Policy 12:325, 1996.
28. Annas GJ, Coyne B: "Fitness" for birth and reproduction: legal implication of genetic screening. Family Law Q 9:463, 1975.
29. Annas GJ, Elias S: Legal and ethical implications of fetal diagnosis and gene therapy. Am J Med Genet 35:215, 1990.
30. Annas GJ: Medical paternity and "wrongful life." Hastings Center Rep 11:8, 1981.
31. Recent opinions of the Judicial Council of the American Medical Association. JAMA 251:278, 1984.
32. Annas GJ: Problems of informed consent and confidentiality in genetic counseling. *In* Milunsky A, Annas GJ (eds): Genetics and the Law. New York, Plenum Press, 1975.
33. President's Commissions for the Study of Ethical Problems in Medicine and Biomedical and Behavioral Research: Screening and Counseling for Genetic Conditions, February 1983. Library of Congress No. 83-600502. Washington, DC, U.S. Government Printing Office, 1983.
34. Elias S, Annas GJ: Generic consent for genetic screening. N Engl J Med 330:1611, 1994.
35. Elias S, Annas GJ: Reproductive Genetics and the Law. Chicago, Yearbook, 1987.
36. Annas GJ: The Rights of Patients. 2nd ed. Carbondale, IL, Southern Illinois University Press, 1989.
37. Andrews LB, Fullarton JE, Holtsman NA, Motulsky AG (eds): Assessing genetic risks: implications for health and social policy. Washington, DC, National Academy Press, 1994.
38. Rodwin M: Medicine, Money and Morals. New York, Oxford University Press, 1993.
39. Social Policy Research Priorities for the Human Genome Project. *In* Annas GJ, Elias S (eds): Mapping Our Genes: Using Law and Ethics as Guides. New York, Oxford University Press, 1992, p 269.
40. Fraser FC: Genetic counseling. Am J Hum Genet 26:636, 1974.
41. Simpson JL, Elias S: Isolating fetal cells from maternal blood: advances in prenatal diagnosis through molecular technology. JAMA 270:2357, 1993.
42. Biesecker BB, Boehnke M, Calzone K, et al: Genetic counseling for families with inherited susceptibility to breast and ovarian cancer. JAMA 269:1970, 1993.
43. Lieberman JR, Mazor M, Chain W, et al: The fetal right to live. Obstet Gynecol 53:515, 1979.
44. Kolder VEB, Gallagher J, Parsons MT: Court-ordered obstetrical interventions. N Engl J Med 316:1192, 1987.
45. Nelson LJ, Milliken N: Compelled medical treatment of pregnant women. JAMA 259:1060, 1988.
46. Notzon FC, Placek PJ, Taffel SM: Comparisons of national cesarean-section rates. N Engl J Med 316:386, 1987.
47. Annas GJ: Protecting the liberty of pregnant patients. N Engl J Med 316:1213, 1987.
48. ACOG Committee Opinion: Patient Choice: Maternal-Fetal Conflict. Number 55. Washington DC, American College of Obstetricians and Gynecologist, October 1987.
49. *In Re A.C.,* 573 A 2d 1235 (DC App 1990).
50. Annas GJ: Standard of Care: The Law of American Bioethics. New York, Oxford University Press, 1993.
51. Annas GJ, Caplan A, Elias S: Stem cell politics, ethics and medical progress. Nat Med 5:13, 1999.
52. Annas GJ, Glantz LH, Katz BH: Informed Consent to Human Experimentation. Cambridge, MA, Ballinger, 1977.
53. Friedman JM: The federal fetal experimentation regulations: an establishment clause analysis. Minn Law Rev 61:961, 1977.
54. Brock EA: Fetal research: what price progress? Detroit Coll Law Rev 3:403, 1979.
55. Annas GJ, Densberger JE: Competence to refuse medical treatment: autonomy vs. paternalism. Toledo Law Rev 15:561, 1984.
56. Annas GJ, Glantz LH, Katz BF: The Rights of Doctors, Nurses and Allied Health Professionals. Cambridge, MA, Ballinger, 1981.
57. *Danforth v. Planned Parenthood,* 428 U.S. 52 (1976).
58. Elias S, Annas GJ: Perspectives on fetal surgery. Am J Obstet Gynecol 145:807, 1983.
59. Annas GJ: Waste and longing: the legal status of placental-blood banking. N Engl J Med 340:1521, 1999.

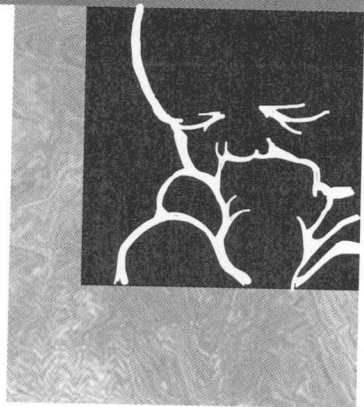

Anatomy of the Pelvis

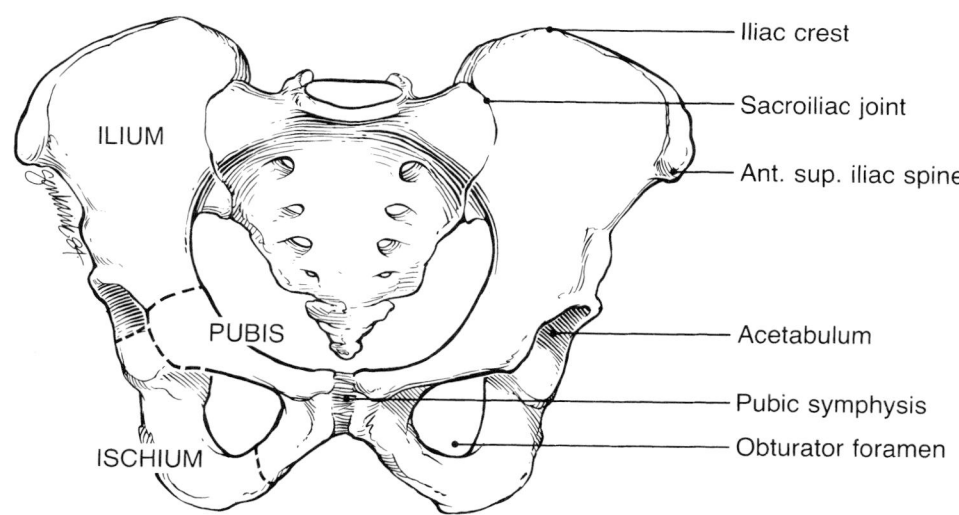

- Iliac crest
- Sacroiliac joint
- Ant. sup. iliac spine
- Acetabulum
- Pubic symphysis
- Obturator foramen

ILIUM

PUBIS

ISCHIUM

Figure A–1. Major components of the bony pelvis shown in a frontal superior view of the female pelvis. The plane of the pelvic brim faces forward and forms an angle of about 60 degrees to the horizontal. Features that most clearly distinguish the female from the male pelvis include a wider subpubic angle, wider sciatic notch, and greater distance from pubic symphysis and anterior edge of the acetabulum.

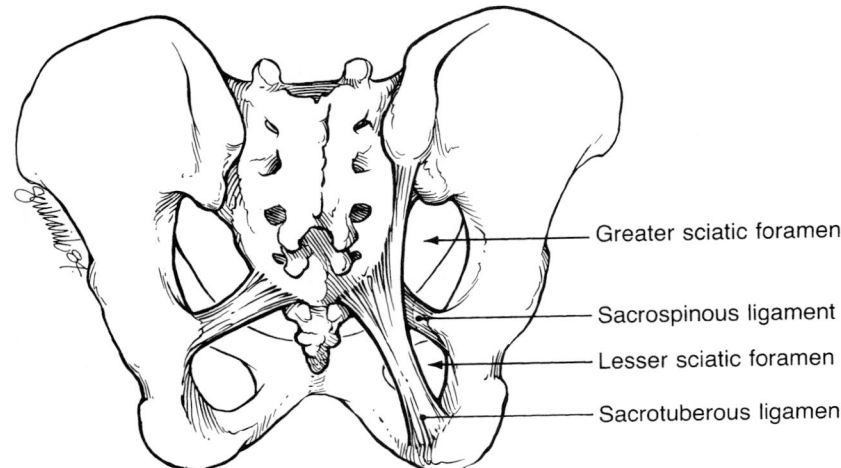

Figure A–2. Major ligaments and notches of the female pelvis, posterior view. During pregnancy, temporary changes take place in the ligaments that permit both movement of the joints and enlargement of the pelvic cavity. This becomes important during parturition.

Greater sciatic foramen

Sacrospinous ligament

Lesser sciatic foramen

Sacrotuberous ligament

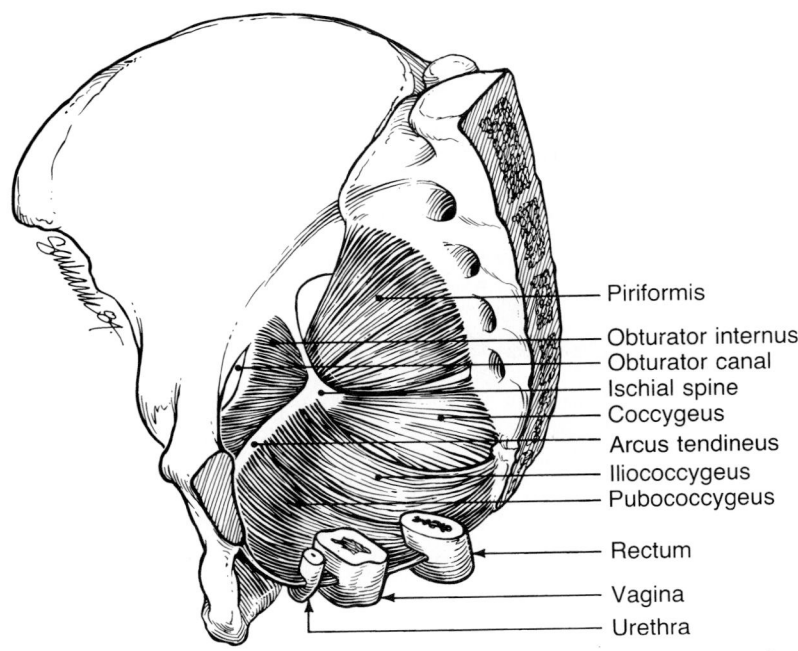

Piriformis

Obturator internus

Obturator canal

Ischial spine

Coccygeus

Arcus tendineus

Iliococcygeus

Pubococcygeus

Rectum

Vagina

Urethra

Figure A–3. Muscles of the pelvic diaphragm, oblique view. The pelvic diaphragm forms a muscular floor for the support of the pelvic organs. Note the location of the urethra, uterus, and rectum as they pierce the floor of the pelvic diaphragm.

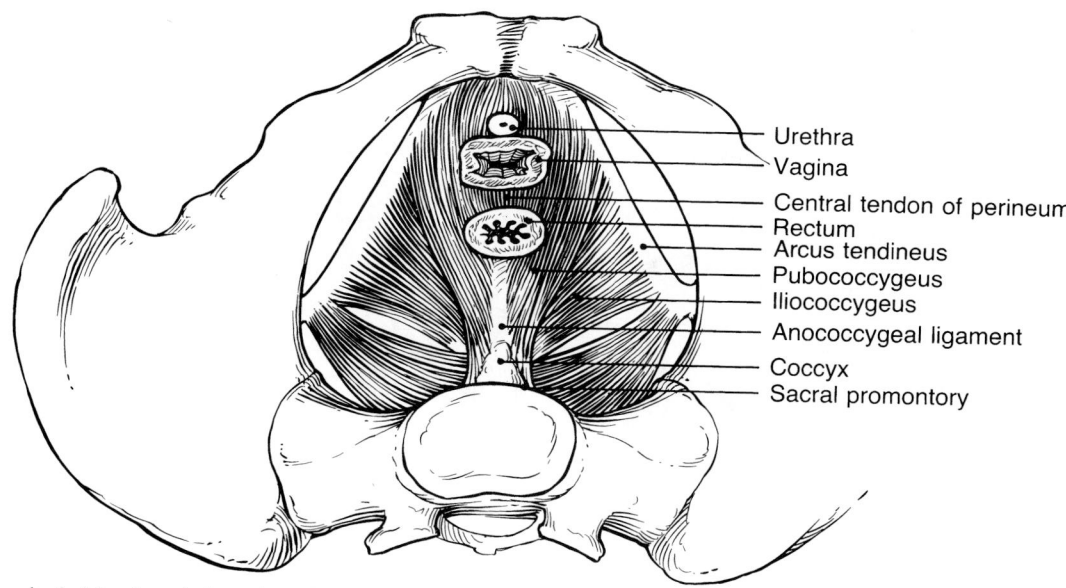

Figure A–4. Muscles of the pelvic diaphragm, superior view. As seen from above, the pelvic diaphragm consists of a number of different muscles and ligaments. The spaces between these muscles transmit a number of vessels and nerves as they leave the pelvis. Note the relationship of the central tendon of the perineum to the rectum and uterus.

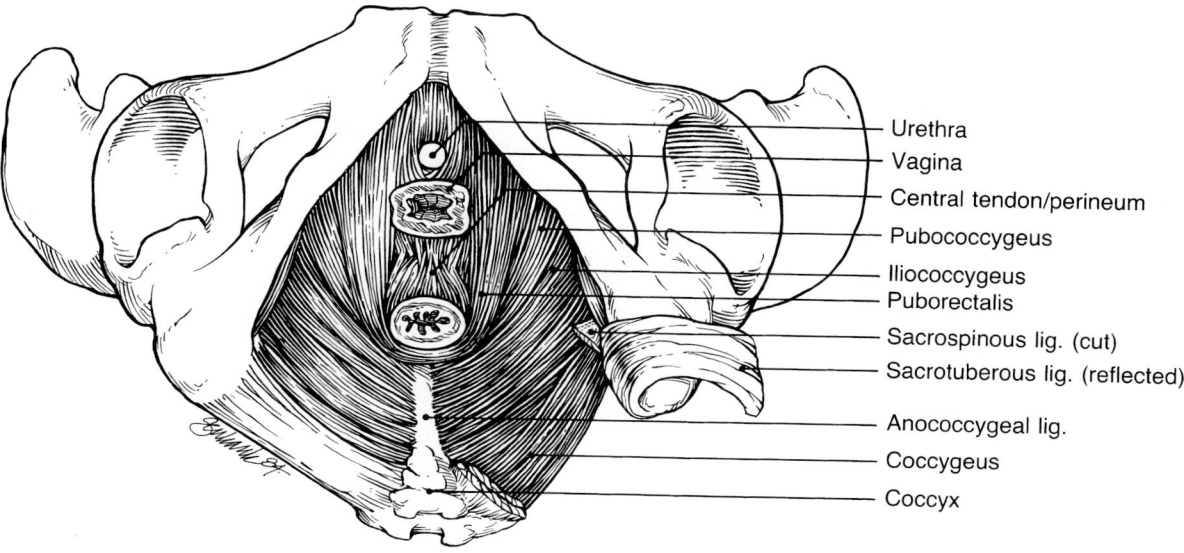

Figure A–5. Inferior view of muscles of the pelvic diaphragm. The pelvic diaphragm is bilaterally symmetric, with the perineal body (central tendon) and the anococcygeal ligament forming a strong median raphe. lig., ligament.

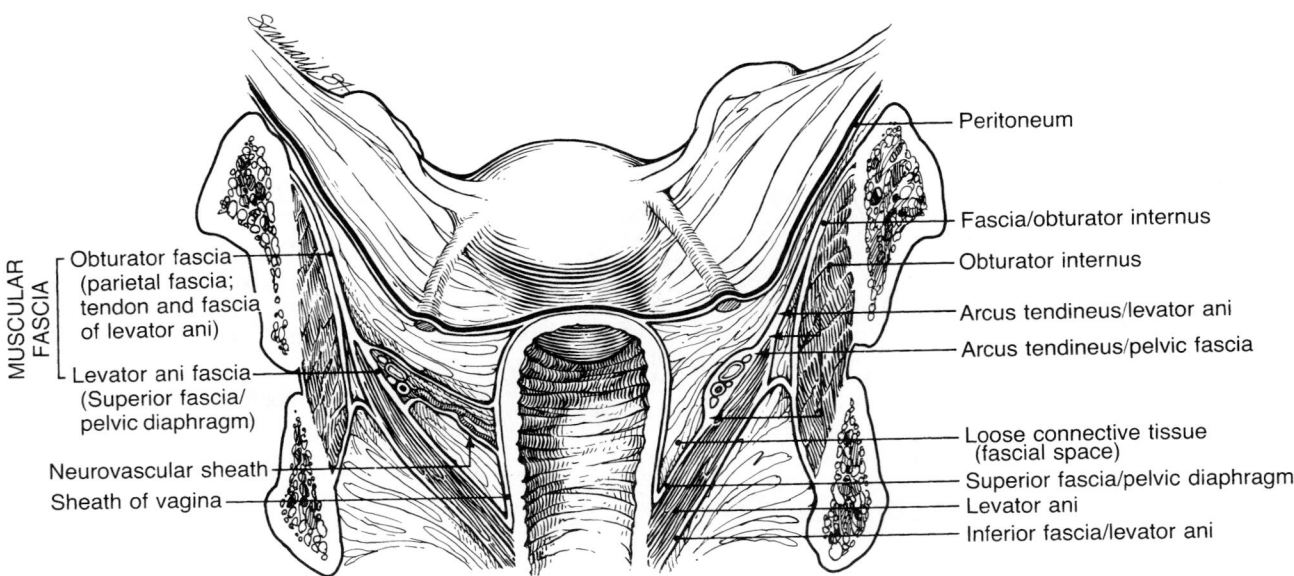

MUSCULAR FASCIA

Obturator fascia (parietal fascia; tendon and fascia of levator ani)

Levator ani fascia (Superior fascia/pelvic diaphragm)

Neurovascular sheath

Sheath of vagina

Peritoneum

Fascia/obturator internus

Obturator internus

Arcus tendineus/levator ani

Arcus tendineus/pelvic fascia

Loose connective tissue (fascial space)

Superior fascia/pelvic diaphragm

Levator ani

Inferior fascia/levator ani

Figure A–6. Fascial and peritoneal relationships of the pelvic diaphragm. In this frontal view of the pelvis, the levator ani can be seen to slope downward and medially, surrounding the vagina. The loose connective tissue beneath the pelvic peritoneum is variable in thickness, depending on the general adiposity of the individual. Note also the continuity of the different fascias as they merge to form the neurovascular sheaths.

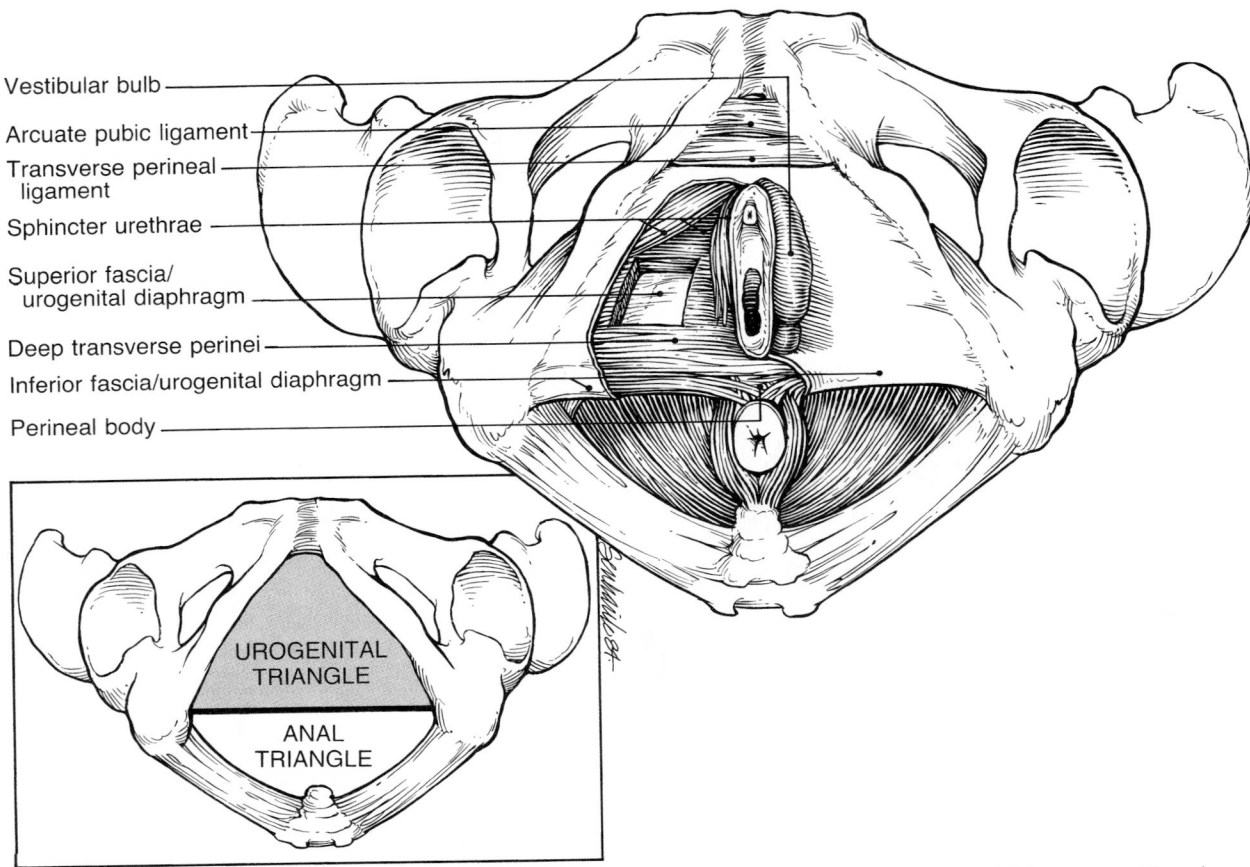

Vestibular bulb

Arcuate pubic ligament

Transverse perineal ligament

Sphincter urethrae

Superior fascia/urogenital diaphragm

Deep transverse perinei

Inferior fascia/urogenital diaphragm

Perineal body

UROGENITAL TRIANGLE

ANAL TRIANGLE

Figure A–7. Muscles of the deep perineal space, inferior view. As viewed with the patient in dorsal lithotomy position, the deep perineal space consists of smaller muscles than the superficial perineal space. Note that the vestibular bulb lies within the superficial perineal space. *Inset:* Division of the perineum into a urogenital (anterior) triangle and an anal (posterior) triangle.

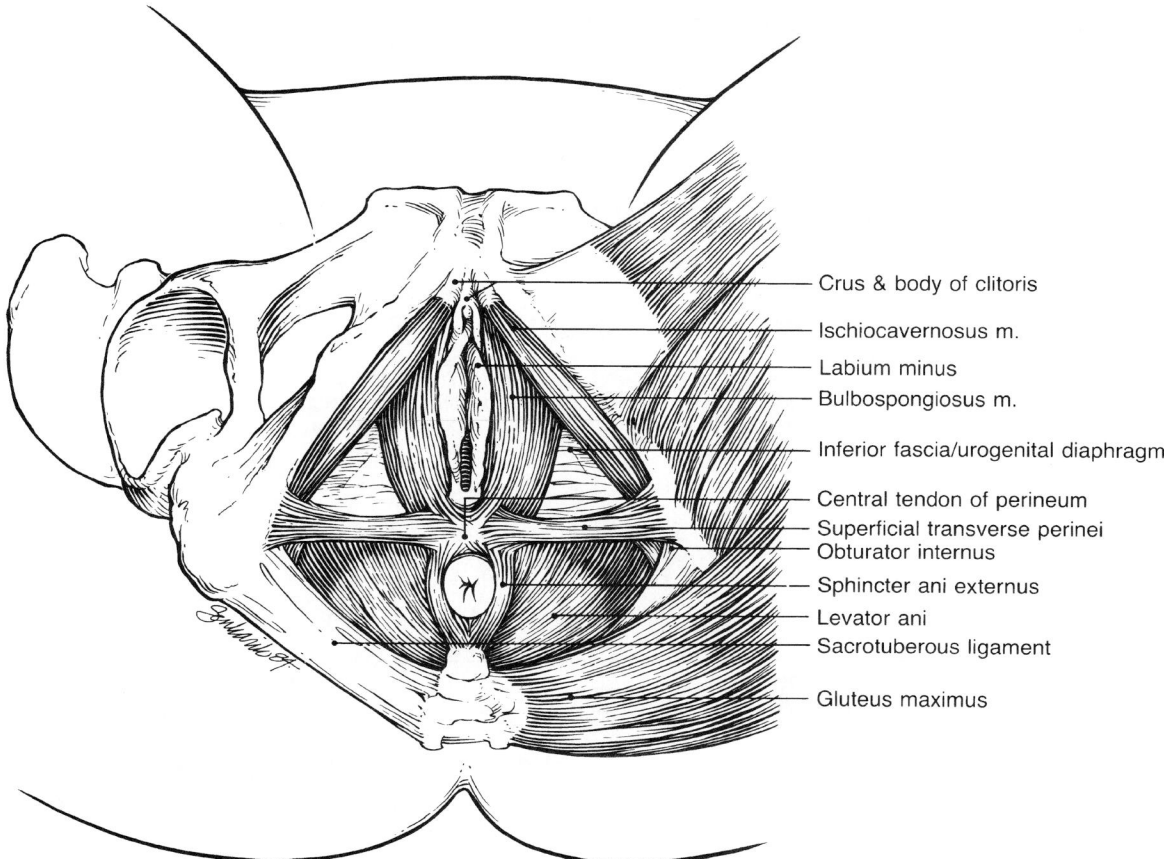

Crus & body of clitoris

Ischiocavernosus m.

Labium minus

Bulbospongiosus m.

Inferior fascia/urogenital diaphragm

Central tendon of perineum

Superficial transverse perinei

Obturator internus

Sphincter ani externus

Levator ani

Sacrotuberous ligament

Gluteus maximus

Figure A–8. Muscles of the superficial perineal space, from below. As viewed with the patient in dorsal lithotomy position, the muscles of the superficial perineal space of the urogenital triangle and the muscles of the anal triangle all converge in the midline. m., muscle.

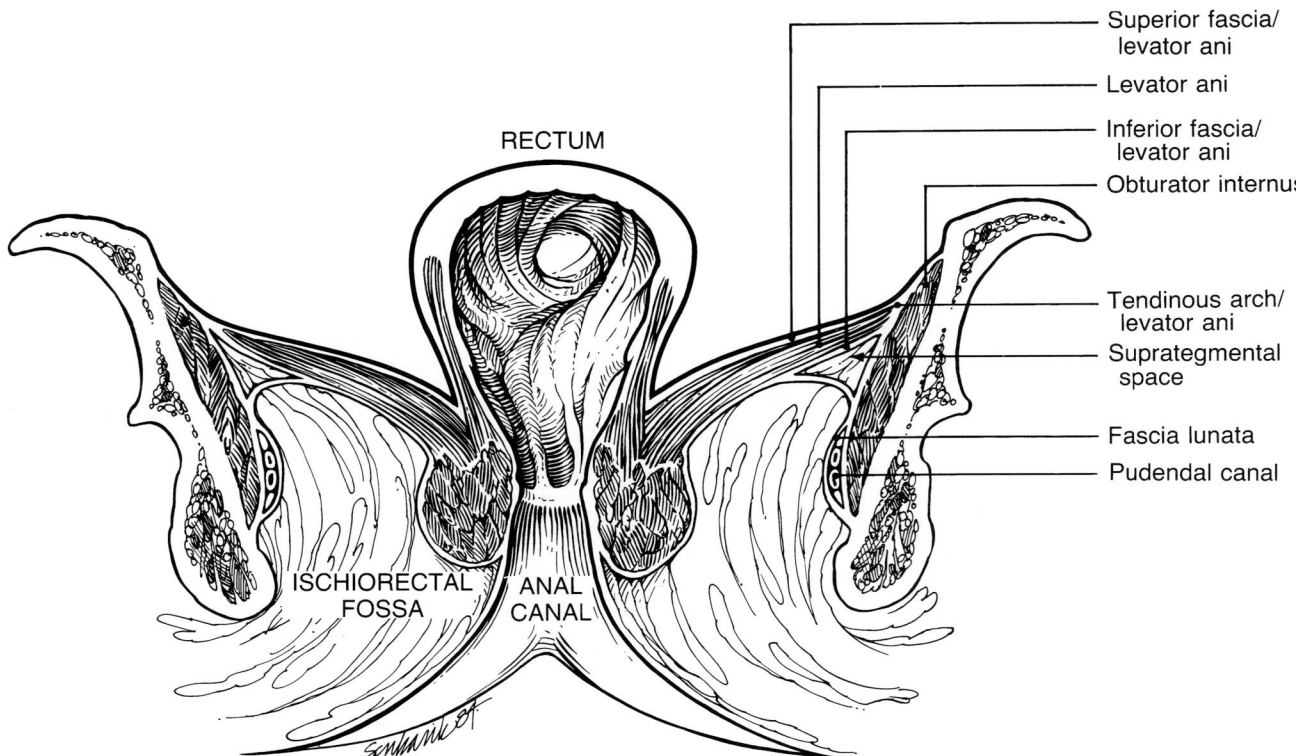

Figure A–9. Ischiorectal fossa, frontal section. The ischiorectal fossa surrounds the rectum and vagina and forms most of the potential space within the posterior triangle of the perineum. The fascia of the levator ani merges with the visceral sheath of the rectum and vagina to lend support.

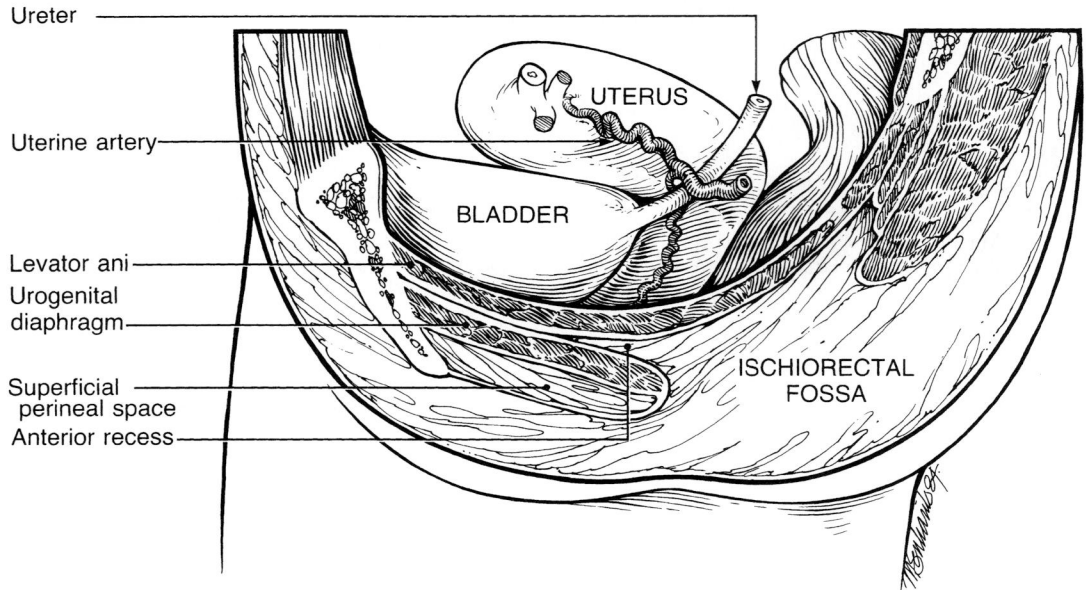

Figure A–10. Ischiorectal fossa and urogenital diaphragm, sagittal section. The ischiorectal fossa extends both forward and backward from the anal triangle. The urogenital diaphragm subdivides the urogenital triangle, with the anterior recess of the ischiorectal fossa superior to it. The subcutaneous fat between the inferior aspect of the superficial perineal space and the skin varies among individuals.

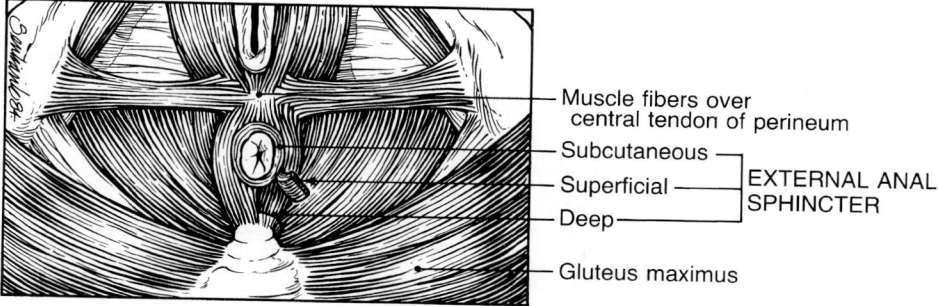

Figure A–11. External anal sphincter as viewed in dorsal lithotomy position. The external anal sphincter is composed of three muscles that arise from the coccyx and converge into the central tendon of the perineum. Midline or mediolateral episiotomy may damage this sphincter; proper reapproximation is essential for fecal continence.

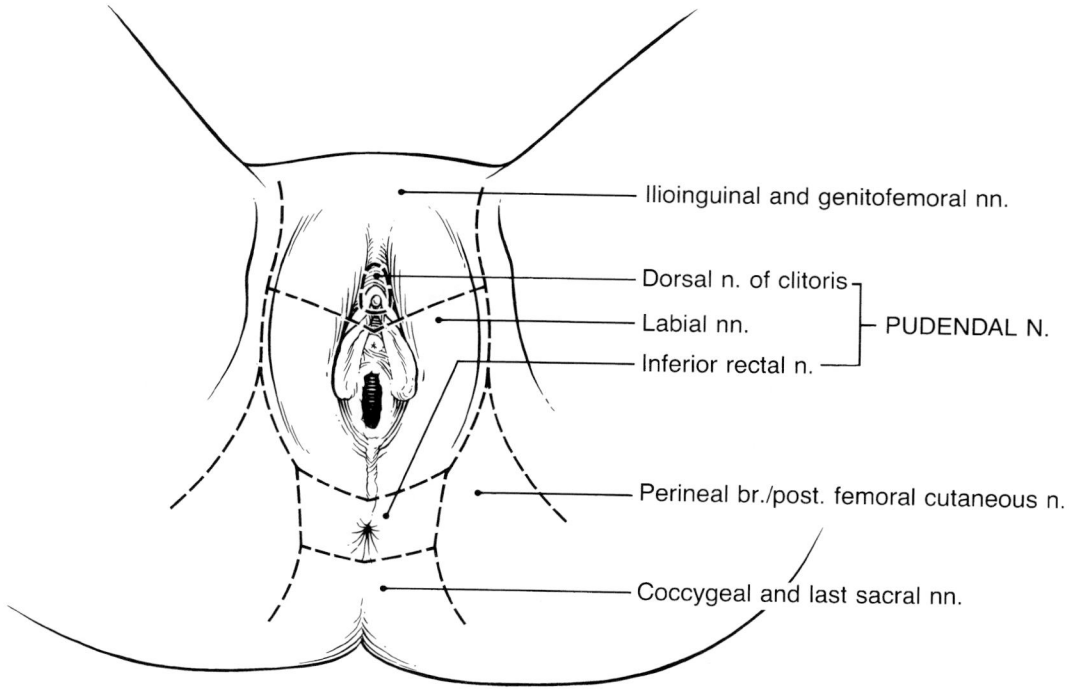

Figure A–12. Cutaneous nerve supply to the perineum. Most cutaneous innervation to the perineum comes from the pudendal nerve, but important regions are supplied by other sources. Pudendal block thus only anesthetizes a portion of the perineal surface. The exact limits of each specific nerve supply are variable. N., nerve; nn., nerves.

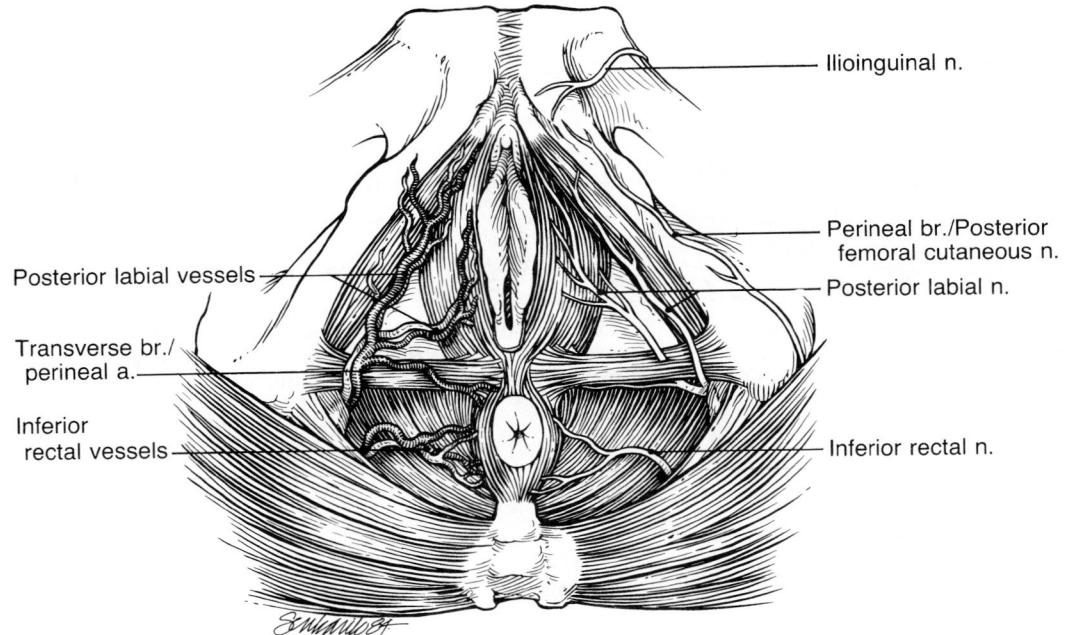

Figure A–13. Superficial perineal blood supply and nerves, as viewed with the patient in dorsal lithotomy position. The vessels and nerves to the superficial perineal space follow each other. The vasculature is markedly engorged during pregnancy, and there may be significant bleeding from these vessels because of laceration, trauma, or episiotomy. Note the transverse branch of the perineal artery, a vessel often encountered during routine midline or mediolateral episiotomy. br., branch; a., artery; n., nerve.

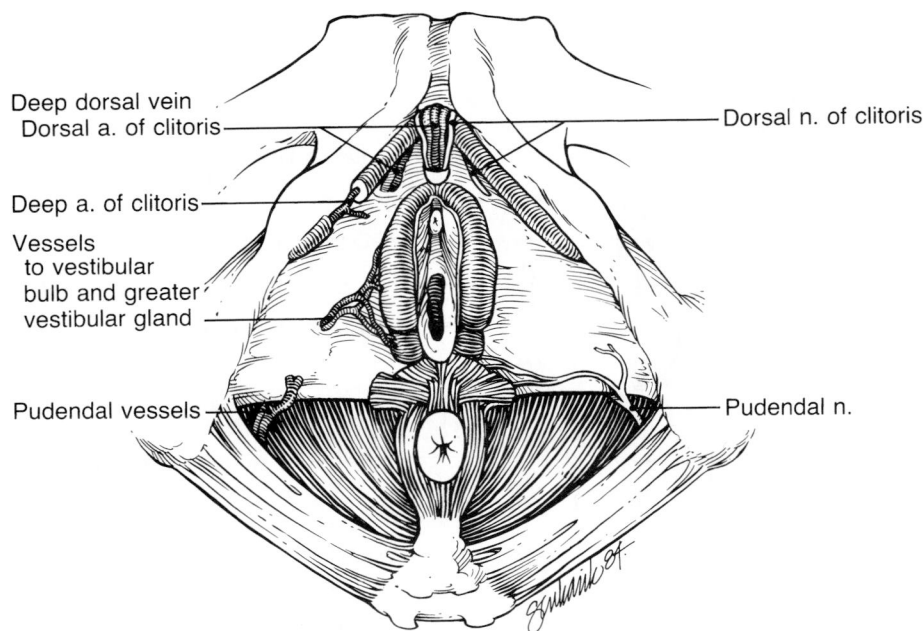

Figure A–14. Vessels and nerves of the deep perineal space. The vasculature and innervation to the deep perineal space enters the anterior triangle from superior to inferior, in contrast to the superficial perineal space vessels and nerves. Note that the blood supply and innervation to the vestibular bulb and greater vestibular gland (Bartholin's gland) are derived from the deep perineal vessels and nerves. a., artery; n., nerve.

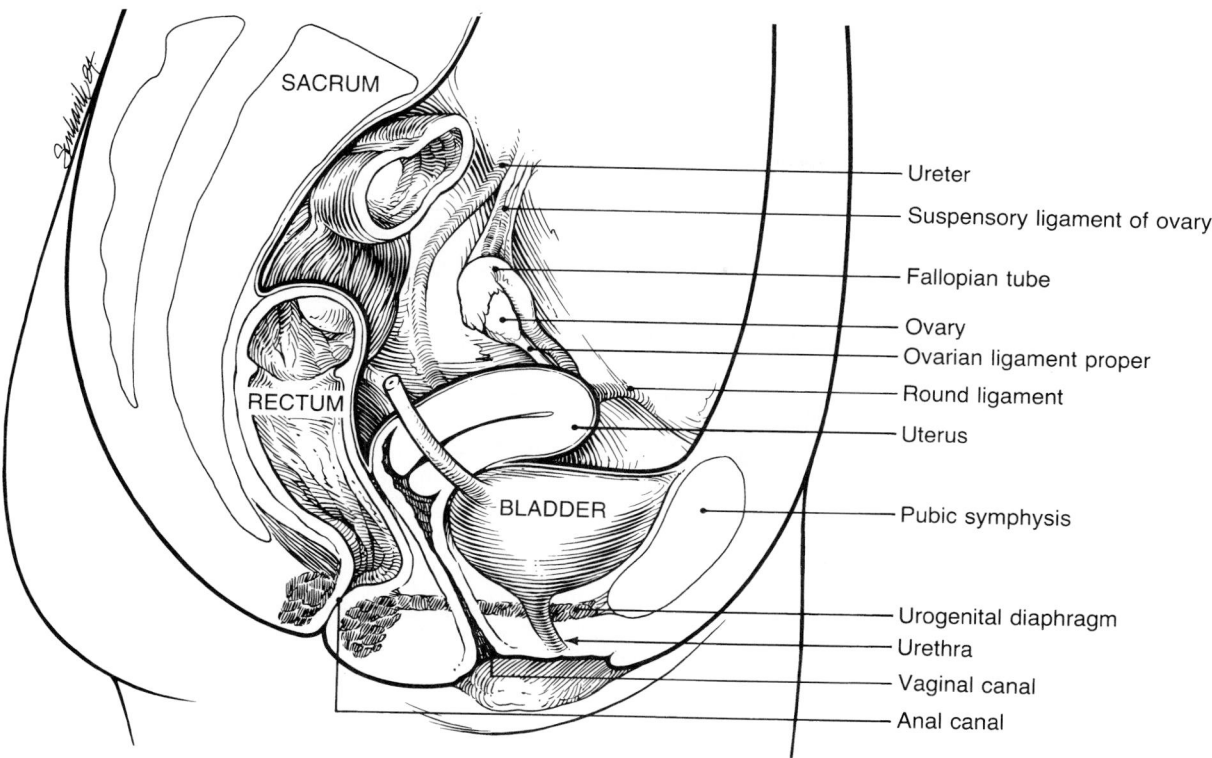

Figure A–15. Major organs of the pelvis, sagittal section. The internal organs of the pelvis are supported by the levator ani. Note how the anteverted, anteflexed uterus gains further support from both the urinary bladder and rectum. The ureter crosses the lateral aspect of the uterus at the level of the internal os on its way to the bladder. The actual position of the ovary and fimbriated end of the tube is quite variable.

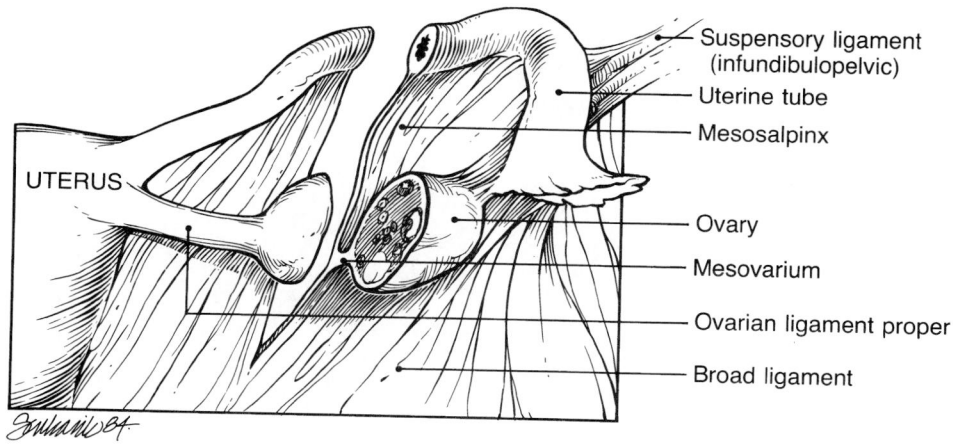

Figure A–16. Anatomy of the fallopian tube and ovary, posterior view. The ovary and tube are suspended by mesenteries derived as specialized portions of the broad ligament. The vasculature and nerves enter through the mesovarium and mesosalpinx.

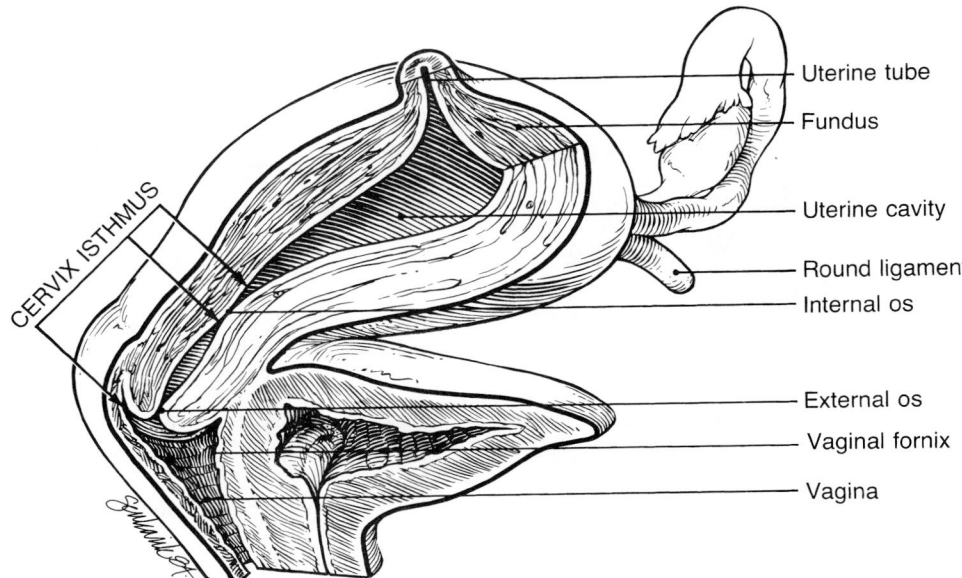

Figure A–17. Anatomic regions of the uterus, lateral view. The uterus is composed of cervix, isthmus, corpus, and fundus. Because the regions of the uterus grow at different rates during pregnancy, the distance between cornual fallopian tube and fundus increases markedly with increasing gestation. Note that the peritoneal reflection of the bladder occurs at the level of the uterine isthmus.

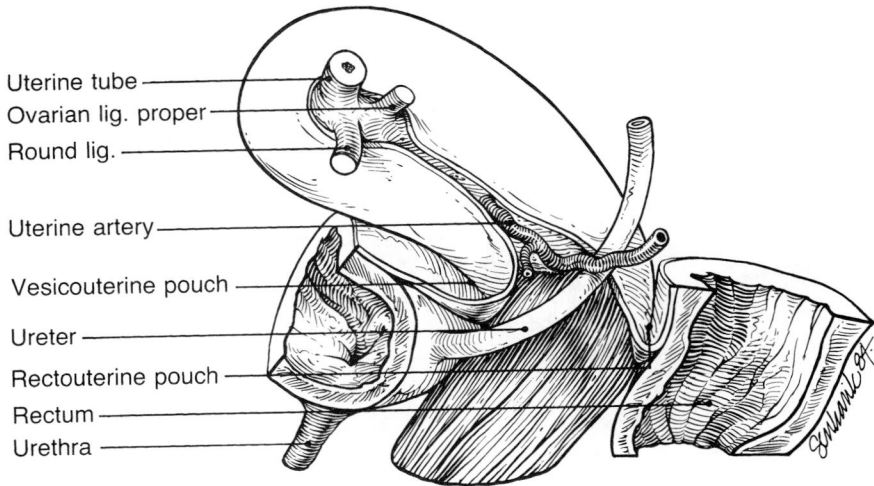

Figure A–18. Anatomic relationships of the uterus, lateral view. The broad ligament contains the uterus and forms an anterior and posterior covering. The triangular space along the lateral uterine wall lies between the leaves of the broad ligament. Note the relationship of the ureter to the uterine artery. lig., ligament.

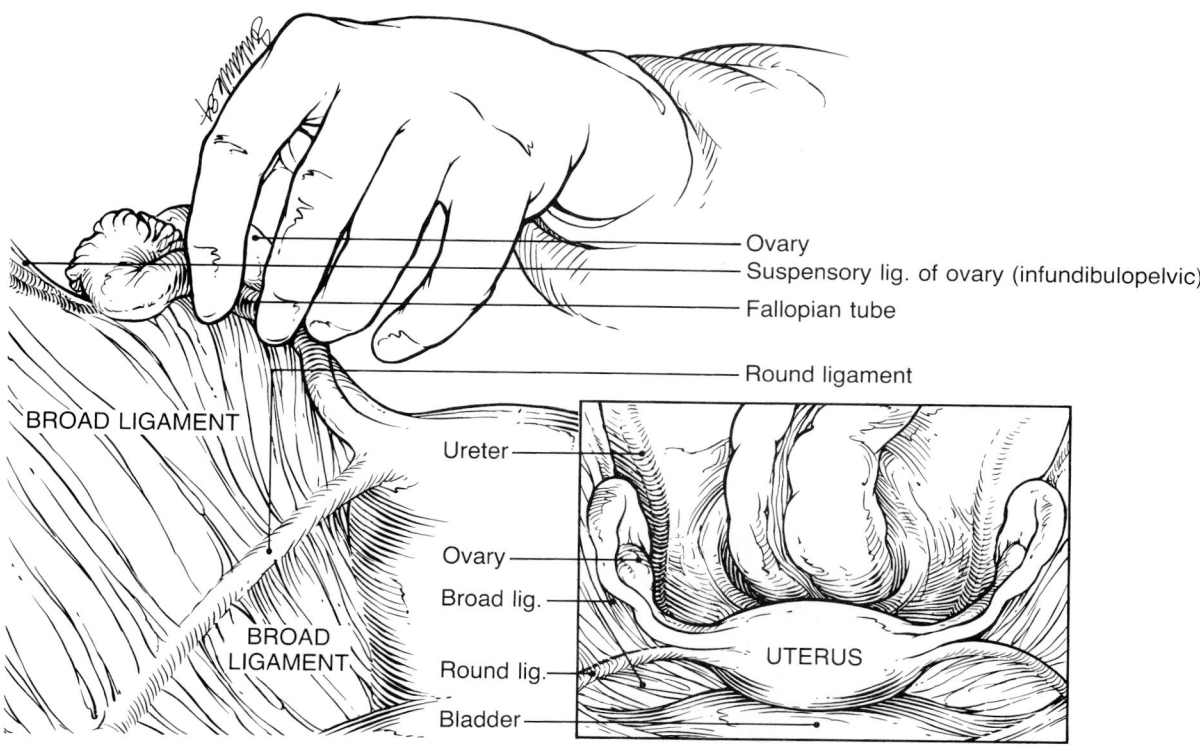

Figure A–19. Broad ligament and contained organs, frontal view. The round ligament runs within the anterior leaf of the broad ligament and inserts through the inguinal canal to the labium majus. *Inset:* The relationships as seen from an anterosuperior perspective. Note the rectovaginal pouch as seen from above and anteriorly. lig., ligament.

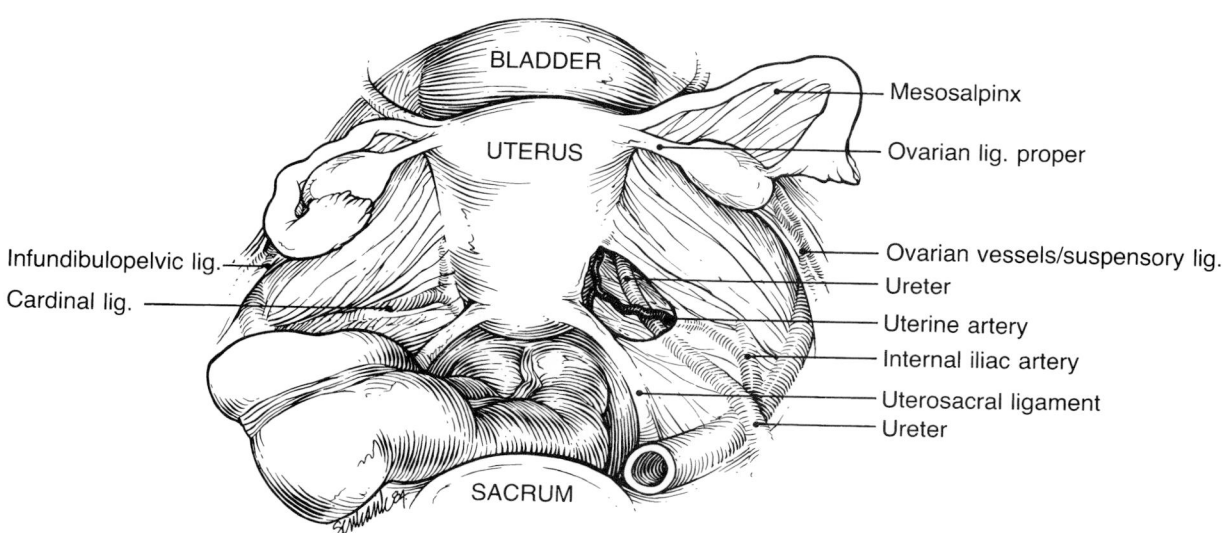

Figure A–20. Organs of the pelvis, posterior view. The rectouterine pouch is demarcated by the uterosacral ligaments. This pouch is often termed the *posterior cul-de-sac*. In this diagram, a section of the posterior leaf of the broad ligament has been removed to show the relationship of the uterine artery to the ureter. Intraligamentous tumors, infection, endometriosis, or previous surgery can often alter this relationship. lig., ligament.

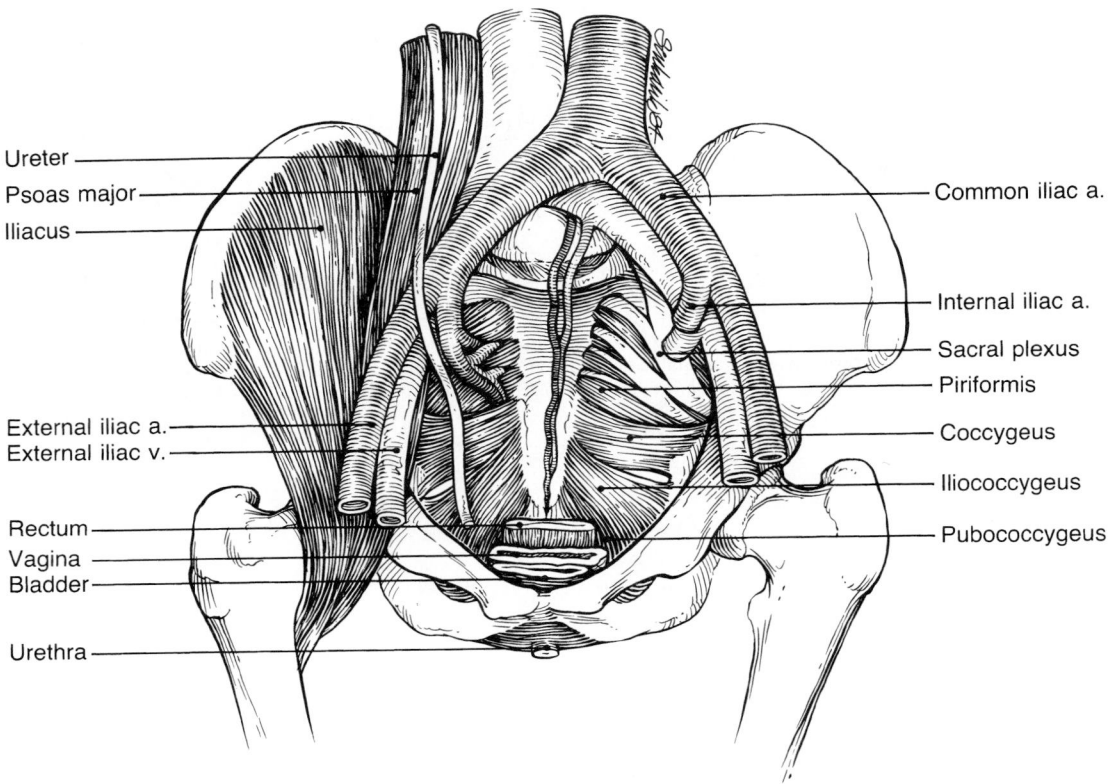

Ureter

Psoas major

Iliacus

External iliac a.

External iliac v.

Rectum

Vagina

Bladder

Urethra

Common iliac a.

Internal iliac a.

Sacral plexus

Piriformis

Coccygeus

Iliococcygeus

Pubococcygeus

Figure A–21. Major vessels of the pelvis, frontal view. The major vasculature of the pelvis is shown in relationship to the pelvic diaphragm. The proximity of the ureter to the internal iliac (hypogastric) artery is noteworthy. Ligation of the hypogastric artery may thus jeopardize the ureter unless care is taken. Note the anterior and posterior trunks of the internal iliac artery. a., artery; v., vein.

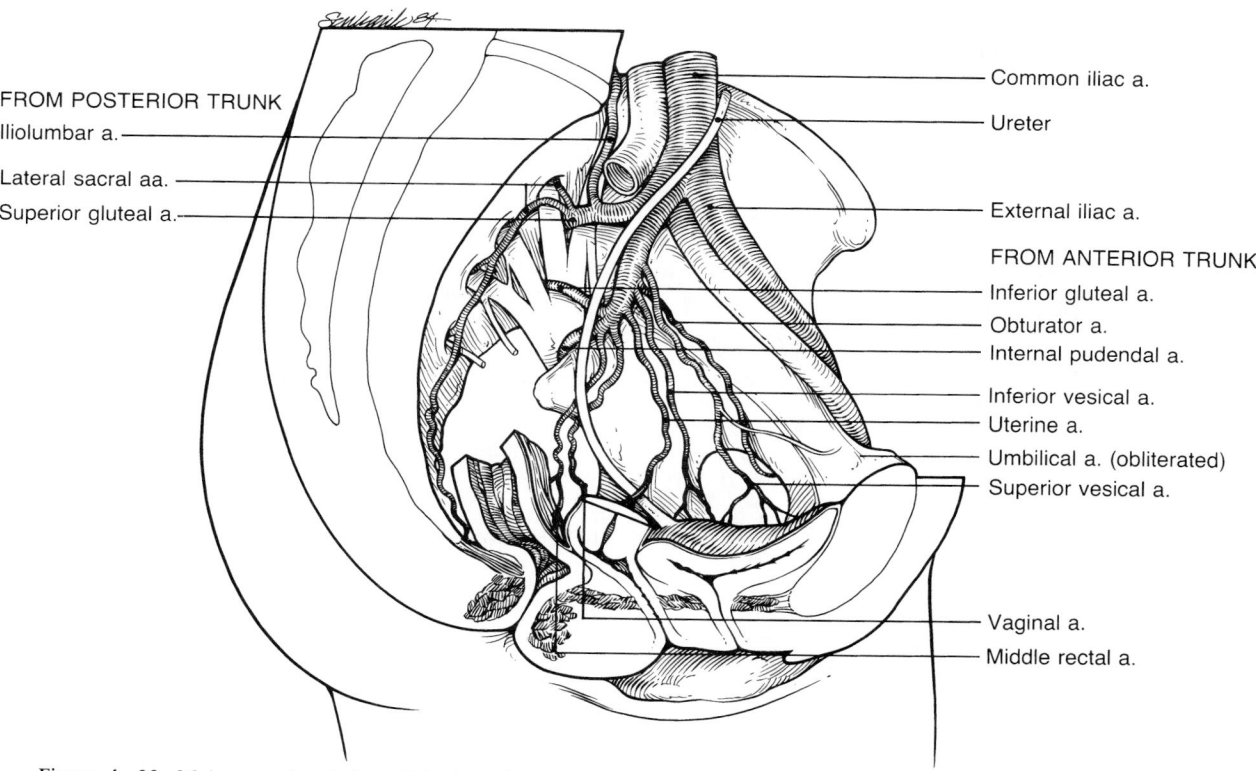

Figure A–22. Major vessels of the pelvis, lateral view. The major subdivisions of the anterior and posterior trunks are highly variable, and no singular branching pattern accounts for most patients. Note the relationship of the vessels to the sacral plexus. The uterus has been amputated at the level of the isthmus to permit a better view of the branching patterns of the anterior trunk. a., artery; aa., arteries.

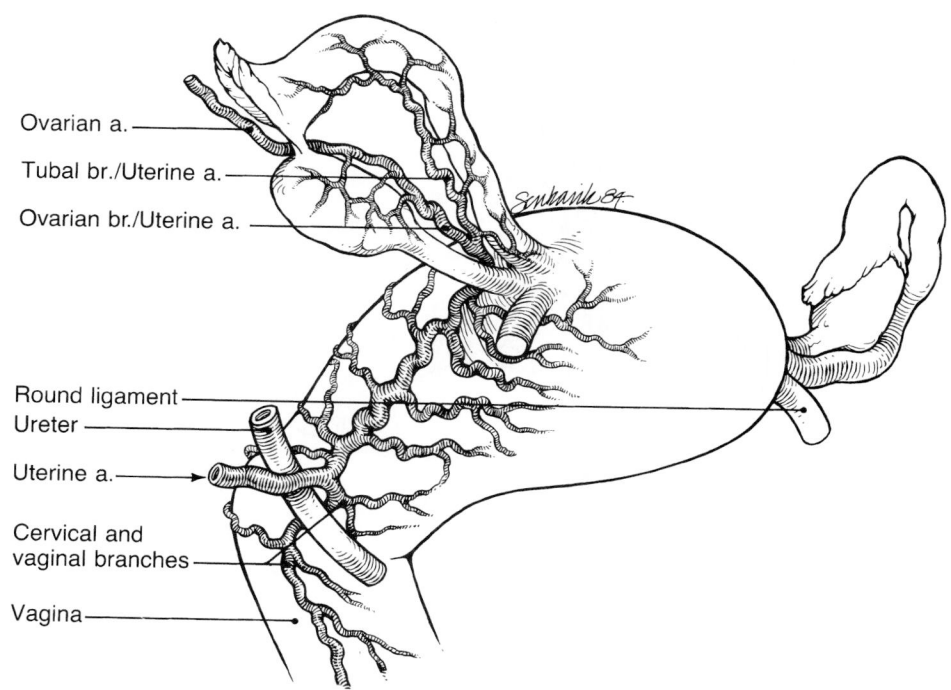

Figure A–23. Blood supply to the uterus, tube, and ovary. The vasculature supply to the major pelvic organs is derived from the internal iliac (uterine) artery and the ovarian artery. Note the anastomotic plexuses of vessels along the lateral aspect of the uterus at the region of the cornu. Descending branches from the uterine artery supply the cervix and vagina. a., artery; br., branch.

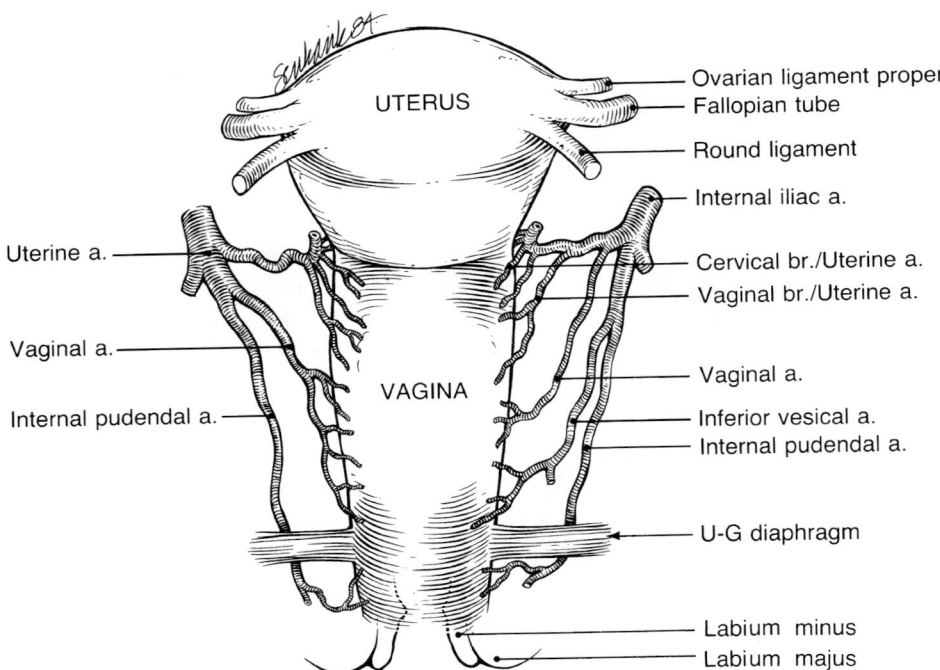

Ovarian ligament proper
Fallopian tube
Round ligament
Internal iliac a.
Cervical br./Uterine a.
Vaginal br./Uterine a.
Vaginal a.
Inferior vesical a.
Internal pudendal a.
U-G diaphragm
Labium minus
Labium majus

UTERUS
VAGINA
Uterine a.
Vaginal a.
Internal pudendal a.

Figure A–24. Blood supply to the vagina. Like the uterus, the vagina derives its blood supply from two major sources: the uterine and pudendal arteries. The internal pudendal artery supplies the vagina from inferior to superior. The vaginal artery, often a branch from the uterine artery, and the uterine artery itself supply the superior position of the vagina. a., artery; U-G, urogenital; br., branch.

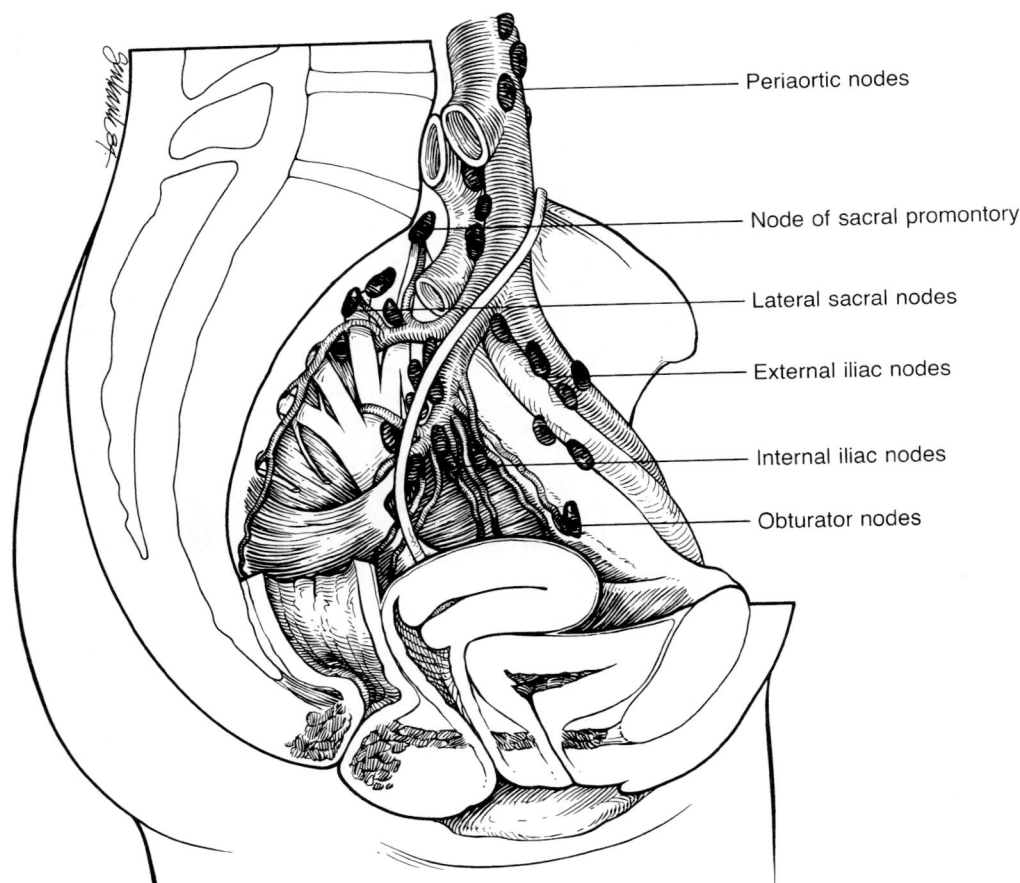

Periaortic nodes
Node of sacral promontory
Lateral sacral nodes
External iliac nodes
Internal iliac nodes
Obturator nodes

Figure A–25. Major lymphatics of the pelvis. The major lymph nodes of the pelvis follow the major vessels. Each group of nodes receives contributions from multiple organs. The groupings are somewhat arbitrary, for no distinct separation of individual node groups exists.

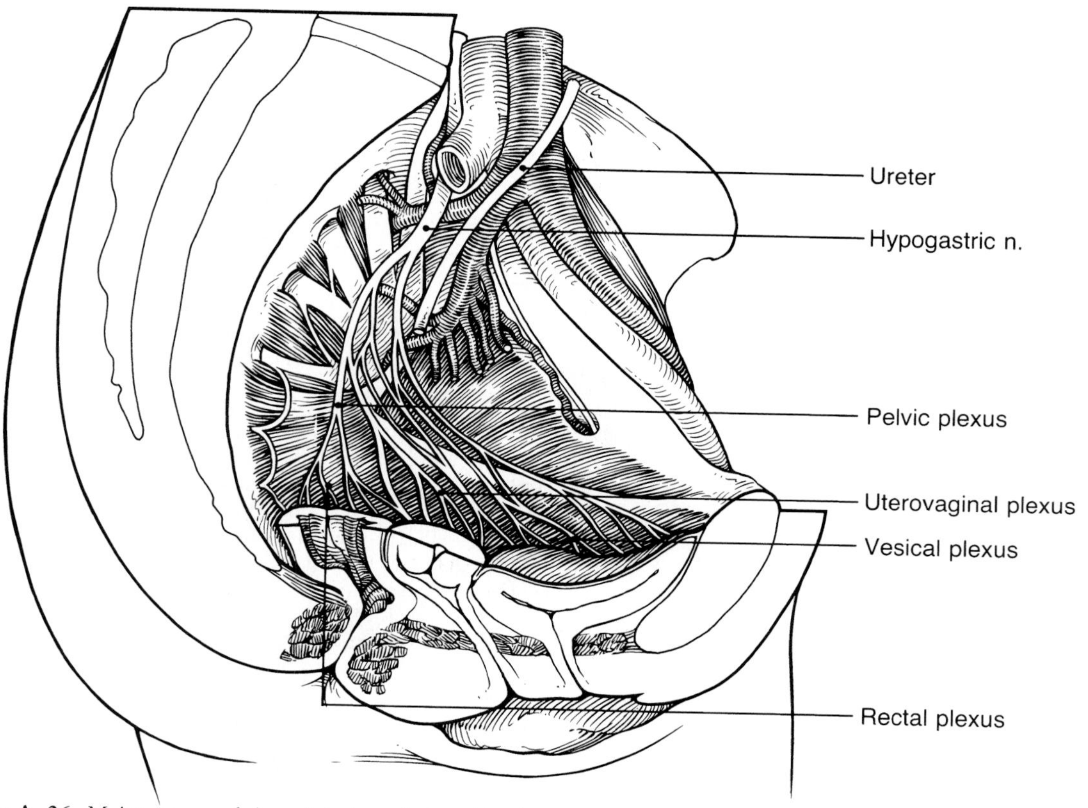

Ureter

Hypogastric n.

Pelvic plexus

Uterovaginal plexus

Vesical plexus

Rectal plexus

Figure A–26. Major nerves of the pelvis, lateral view. Few branches of the sacral plexus are evident, as these nerves leave the pelvis even as the branches are forming. Most of the pelvic plexus lies medial to the vasculature. n., nerve.

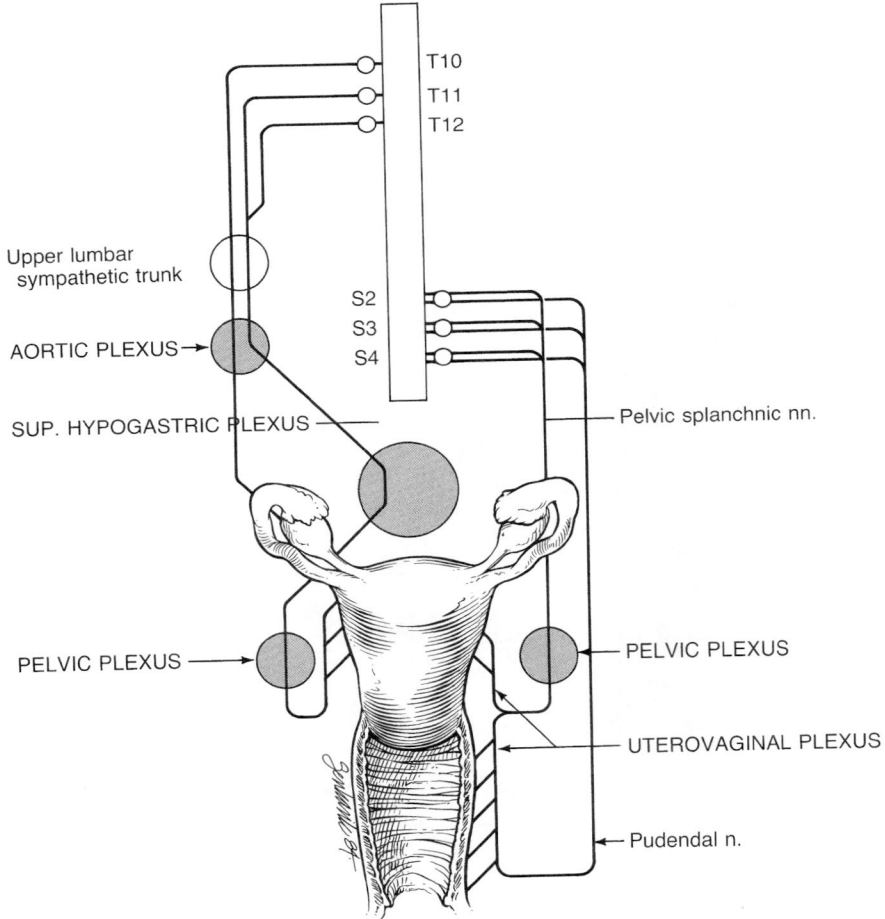

Figure A–27. Afferent innervation of the female genital tract. The left side of this diagram demonstrates the sympathetic nervous system. Fibers entering the spinal cord are illustrated on the right. The major afferent pain fibers for the uterus, tubes, and ovaries enter the cord at T10, T11, and T12. The afferent innervation of the vagina and external genitalia enter at S2, S3, and S4. sup., superior; n., nerve; nn., nerves.

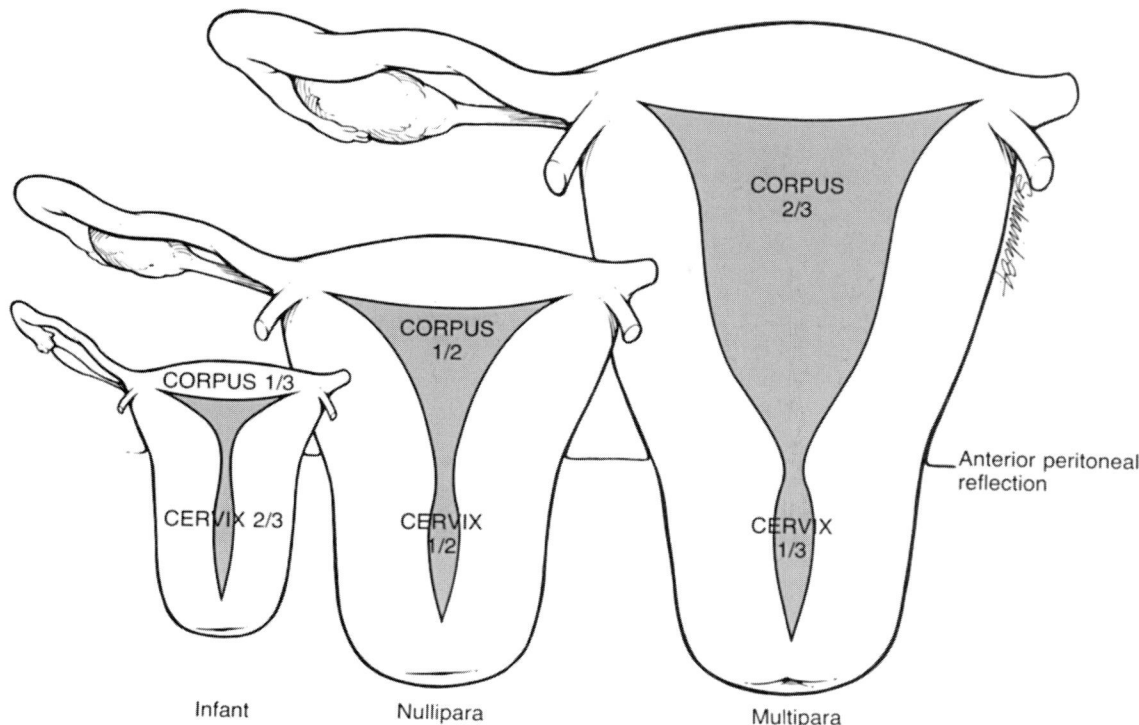

Figure A–28. Changes in the uterus with age and parity. At puberty, growth occurs primarily in the corpus and the fundus, although the cervix continues to grow as well. After menopause, the uterus regresses to a state more closely allied to that of the premenarcheal anatomy. During pregnancy, the cervical portion is relatively greater than in the nonpregnant state.

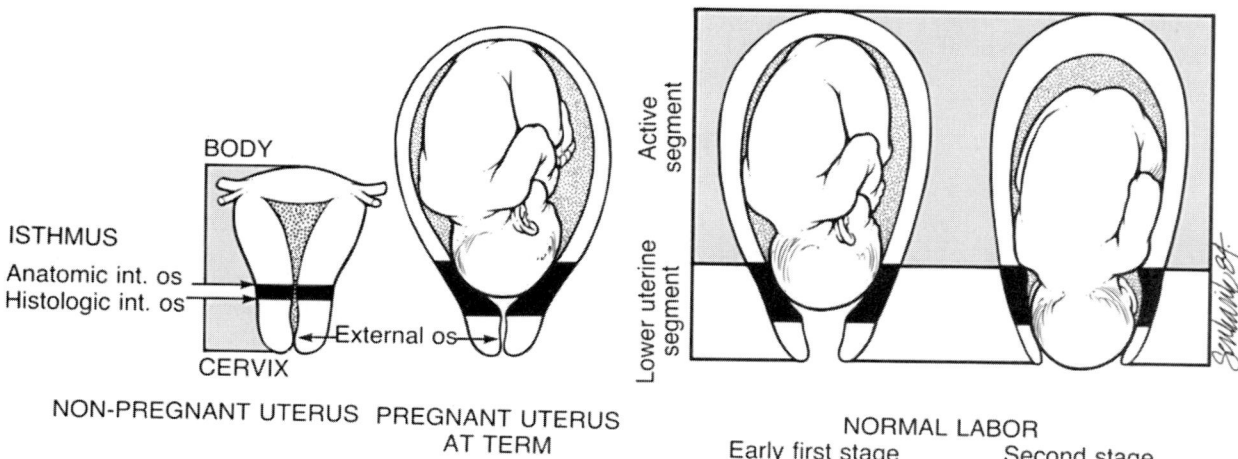

Figure A–29. Changes in the uterus caused by pregnancy and parturition. The hormonal changes of pregnancy as well as dynamic forces of labor cause the development of the lower uterine segment from the vestigial uterine isthmus. After parturition, these changes regress dramatically. Low transverse cesarean delivery inclusions are performed through this thinned isthmic region, known as the *lower uterine segment*.

Key Points

➤ To facilitate childbearing, the female pelvis—as opposed to the male pelvis—is characterized by a wider subpubic angle, increased width of the sciatic notch, and greater distance from the symphysis pubis to the anterior edge of the acetabulum.

➤ The levator ani, the major supporting structure for the pelvic viscera, is a tripartite muscle mass composed of the iliococcygeus, pubococcygeus, and puborectalis; the iliococcygeus is the broadest and most posterior portion.

➤ Innervation of the levator ani is through the third and fourth sacral nerves.

➤ The major nerve supply of the perineum is derived from the pudendal. However, the ilioinguinal, genitofemoral, perineal branch of the posterior femoral cutaneous, coccygeal, and last sacral nerve also contribute; thus, a pudendal nerve block anesthetizes only a portion of the perineum.

➤ The internal iliac (hypogastric) artery arises at the level of lumbosacral articulation. It can be distinguished from the external iliac by its smaller size and by its more medial and more posterior position.

➤ The ureter lies more superficially and is either medial or slightly anterior to the internal iliac artery.

➤ The cardinal ligaments are located at the base of the broad ligament, are continuous with the connective tissue of the parametrium, and are attached to the pelvic diaphragm through continuity with the superficial superior fascia of the levator ani.

➤ Since the origin of the uterine artery is quite variable, its isolation and ligation for control of postpartum bleeding are often fruitless. The uterine artery usually arises as an independent vessel from the internal iliac artery, but it may also arise from the inferior gluteal, internal pudendal, umbilical, or obturator arteries.

➤ Afferent pain fibers for the uterus, tubes, and ovary enter the cord at T10, T11, T12; thus, spinal or epidural anesthesia must extend to these levels. Fortunately, efferent fibers to the uterus enter above these levels, thus not interfering with contractions.

➤ The body of the nonpregnant uterus weighs approximately 70 g, whereas at term it weighs approximately 1,100 g.

SUGGESTED READINGS

Embryology

Sadler TW: Langman's Medical Embryology. 6th ed. Baltimore, Williams & Wilkins, 1990.

Gross Anatomy

Agur AMR: Grant's Atlas of Anatomy. 9th ed. Baltimore, Williams & Wilkins, 1991.

Gardner ED: Gardner-Gray-O'Rahilly Anatomy: A Regional Study of Human Structure. 5th ed. Philadelphia, WB Saunders, 1986.

Hamilton WJ: Textbook of Human Anatomy. St. Louis, CV Mosby, 1976.

Hollinshead WH: Anatomy for Surgeons. 3rd ed, Vol 3. New York, Harper & Row, 1982.

Moore K: Clinically Oriented Anatomy. 3rd ed. Baltimore, Williams & Wilkins, 1992.

Snell RS: Clinical Anatomy for Medical Students. 5th ed. Boston, Little, Brown, 1995.

Williams PL, Bannister LL, Berry M, et al: Gray's Anatomy. 38th ed. Edinburgh, Churchill Livingstone, 1995.

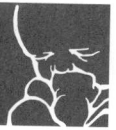
Note: Page numbers followed by the letter b refer to boxed material; those followed by the letter f refer to figures, and those followed by t refer to tables.

ISBN 0-443-06572-1

90071